FOURTH EDITION

LEWIS'S CHILD AND ADOLESCENT PSYCHIATRY

A COMPREHENSIVE TEXTBOOK

FOURTH EDITION

LEWIS'S CHILD AND ADOLESCENT PSYCHIATRY

A COMPREHENSIVE TEXTBOOK

Editors

Andrés Martin, MD, MPH
Associate Professor of Child Psychiatry and Psychiatry
Child Study Center
Yale University School of Medicine
New Haven, Connecticut

Fred R. Volkmar, MD
Irving Harris Professor of Child Psychiatry,
Psychology and Pediatrics; and Director,
Child Study Center
Yale University School of Medicine
New Haven, Connecticut

Wolters Kluwer Health | Lippincott Williams & Wilkins
Philadelphia • Baltimore • New York • London
Buenos Aires • Hong Kong • Sydney • Tokyo

Acquisitions Editor: Charley Mitchell
Managing Editor: Michelle LaPlante
Project Manager: Nicole Walz
Manufacturing Coordinator: Kathy Brown
Associate Director of Marketing: Adam Glazer
Design Coordinator: Terry Mallon
Cover Designer: Joseph DePinho
Production Services: Pine Tree Composition, Inc./Laserwords Private Limited
Printer: Quebecor Inc.

530 Walnut Street
Philadelphia, PA 19106 USA
LWW.com

Printed in the USA

Library of Congress Cataloging-in-Publication Data

Lewis's child and adolescent psychiatry : a comprehensive textbook / editors, Andrés Martin, Fred R. Volkmar ; editor emeritus, Melvin Lewis.–4th ed.
p. ; cm.
Rev. ed of: Child and adolescent psychiatry / edited by Melvin Lewis. 3rd ed. c2002.
Includes bibliographical references and index.
ISBN-13: 978-0-7817-6214-4
ISBN-10: 0-7817-6214-6
1. Child development. 2. Sick children–Psychology. 3. Child psychiatry. I. Martin, Andrés. II. Volkmar, Fred R. III. Lewis, Melvin, 1926- IV. Child and adolescent psychiatry. V. Title: Child and adolescent psychiatry.
[DNLM: 1. Mental Disorders. 2. Adolescent. 3. Child. 4. Infant. WS 350 L6755 2007]
RJ131.L42 2007
618.92′89—dc22

2007006352

Care has been taken to confirm the accuracy of the information presented and to describe generally accepted practices. However, the authors, editors, and publisher are not responsible for errors or omissions or for any consequences from application of the information in this book and make no warranty, expressed or implied, with respect to the currency, completeness, or accuracy of the contents of the publication. Application of this information in a particular situation remains the professional responsibility of the practitioner.

The authors, editors, and publisher have exerted every effort to ensure that drug selection and dosage set forth in this text are in accordance with current recommendations and practice at the time of publication. However, in view of ongoing research, changes in government regulations, and the constant flow of information relating to drug therapy and drug reactions, the reader is urged to check the package insert for each drug for any change in indications and dosage and for added warnings and precautions. This is particularly important when the recommended agent is a new or infrequently employed drug.

Some drugs and medical devices presented in this publication have Food and Drug Administration (FDA) clearance for limited use in restricted research settings. It is the responsibility of the health care provider to ascertain the FDA status of each drug or device planned for use in their clinical practice.

To purchase additional copies of this book, call our customer service department at (800) 638-3030 or fax orders to (301) 223-2320. International customers should call (301) 223-2300.

Visit Lippincott Williams & Wilkins on the Internet: at LWW.com. Lippincott Williams & Wilkins customer service representatives are available from 8:30 am to 6 pm, EST.

10 9 8 7 6 5 4 3 2 1

We dedicate this book

To our wives, Rebecca and Lisa;
To our children, Max, Ariela, Gabriela, and Jacob Donald; Lucy and Emily;
To the teachers and mentors from whom we have received so much;
To the patients, families, students, and colleagues
to whom we hope in some measure to have given back;
To all those dedicated to child and adolescent mental health,
working each day to make a difference.

■ FOREWORD

A WORD is dead
When it is said,
Some say.
I say it just
Begins to live
That day.

Emily Dickinson

The Belle of Amherst hit the nail on the head. Words are living things. And Emily Dickinson gave them meaning, with a new style, well ahead of its time. Words give meaning to our work, too. They form our knowledge base, which is itself a life in words that is always evolving. Yet basic developmental principles beneath that changing knowledge base offer continuity as well. Change mixed with continuity. That's what a textbook should offer.

The original *Child and Adolescent Psychiatry: A Comprehensive Textbook* was the first one published in our field since Leo Kanner's classic *Child Psychiatry* half a century before. Since then a number of other texts have been published, forming the excellent selection available today. But the latest edition of this volume continues to be the cornerstone of my library, and the first choice of many other child and adolescent psychiatrists. Its encyclopedic scope offers a broad reference that serves as a foundation for our field, as well as offering answers to the questions of everyday clinical practice and posing new ones that have yet to be answered.

A word about its development. Melvin Lewis, the pioneering editor of the first three editions of the *Textbook*, has given over responsibility for its fourth edition to the next generation—to a pair of valued colleagues with whom he has worked for years. The first, Andrés Martin, also follows in Lewis's footsteps as the new editor of the *Journal of the American Academy of Child and Adolescent Psychiatry*, a periodical that contains the cutting edge of research in our field. He is joined by co-editor Fred Volkmar, a distinguished scholar and world-renowned researcher in the area of autism. Together, they have assembled an impressive list of experts as contributors to this fourth edition.

A published book is a finished product, but it doesn't begin to live until its words are read and discussed, its inaccuracies debated and corrected, its truths corroborated and its hypotheses tested. *Lewis's Child and Adolescent Psychiatry: A Comprehensive Textbook, fourth edition* illustrates so well the changes in child and adolescent psychiatry, but it also insists upon the continuity of our field, teaching us how to listen to the young voices who are just setting on their course. Its words are alive; in them are both the continuity and the changes that are our field.

John F. McDermott, MD
Professor of Psychiatry Emeritus
University of Hawaii School of Medicine
Editor Emeritus
Journal of the American Academy of Child and Adolescent Psychiatry

PREFACE

LEWIS'S FOURTH

[T]he mission ... is not to pass on an unchanged truth through a succession of the learned but to host the endless labor, carried on from generation to generation, needed to come closer to the truth: the work of challenging the adequacy of what currently passes for the truth, attempting to seize it more fully, and making that understanding available to others so they can move beyond it to a yet fuller realization.

Richard Broadhead
Free Speech and its Discontents (2004)

Readers acquainted with the three earlier editions of this volume are as likely to be reassured as they are to be disoriented on seeing this latest version. The reassurances will come from the textbook's signature heft and color, a similar breadth in scope and depth in coverage, and the welcome resurfacing of many familiar names within. The disorientation should be slight but significant, perhaps beginning with the very name of the book, subtly but most certainly different from its predecessors'. The landmark *Child and Adolescent Psychiatry: A Comprehensive Textbook* that first appeared in 1991 had reached second and third editions within just eleven years (in 1996 and 2002, respectively). Today, 16 years after it first appeared onstage to set a new standard in the field, its latest edition comes forth, under the slightly altered title of *Lewis's Child and Adolescent Psychiatry: A Comprehensive Textbook.* The one-word change is at once subtle and momentous.

In this fourth edition, Melvin Lewis, for whom this landmark text has been a labor of love, makes way for two of his colleagues and students (not to mention admirers and friends) to continue his editorial vision and commitment. The book's new title reflects more than a semantic detail: in a fundamental way, *Lewis* embodies Mel's legacy and the values he has held dear for decades. His has been a model of professional and scholarly comportment that the two of us emulate each day. We are grateful for the opportunity granted us, and aware of the responsibility implicit in the stewardship we have been entrusted. We have strived for a new edition that includes the best of our science; that translates and makes it accessible and applicable; that provides cohesion for a rapidly evolving discipline; that welcomes and guides the novice as much as reminds the veteran of the richness of our work. An edition, in brief, that by becoming a vehicle to improve the mental health of children and adolescents will make Melvin Lewis proud.

This fourth edition's title and cover art are the first and most apparent differences, but not the only ones. Indeed, it is in its substantially revised, updated and reorganized inner structures that the book is very much a new edition. The better testament to *Lewis's* ability to advance Mel's legacy may be in how different, rather than in how similar, it is from earlier versions. An evolving discipline is reflected in organically changing books that refuse to become definitive: gauging from the changes to this tome from a mere five years ago, our field is a lively and thriving one.

An Approach to the Discipline, the first of seven sections, sets the tone for the volume as a whole. If there has been a guiding principle in assembling this textbook, it has been our effort to trace the links between multiple components of our field. We sought to identify continuities across the domains of clinical practice, research, training, and policy—a mutually enriching interplay at times more aspired to than real. We have opted for a reorganized structure in which aspects as varied as economics, diversity, or evidence-based practice are not treated as afterthoughts. On the contrary, we see such topics as a necessary foundation upon which to build. We have been deliberate in our choice of a first chapter that begins with the clinical care of a single child and ripples outward toward familial and societal dimensions: The care of children and families remains not only our foremost concern, but the place from where our major insights have almost invariably come.

The second section, *Scientific Foundations*, synthesizes three major domains of critical relevance to advance our knowledge base in childhood psychiatric disorders: epidemiology and prevention, genetics, and neuroscience. While this section could never be all-inclusive, it does aim to provide a basic level of scientific literacy required to be an informed consumer of the literature; one aware that today's arcane and seemingly esoteric finding may hold the key to tomorrow's breakthrough intervention. To provide a framework for understanding these or any other pertinent scientific approaches, the section includes an overarching chapter on research methodology and statistics.

We pause here to note with sadness the untimely passing of our colleague Robert Harmon during the making of this book. The very first chapter that we received came from Bob and his colleagues in Colorado. *Methodology and Statistics: A Relevant Primer and Overview* arrived with a characteristically encouraging and upbeat message from Bob. Of note, it appeared in our inboxes a full two days before the very first deadline, one so fashionably ignored by the other authors—ourselves included. We remember Bob with affection, and thank him not only for teaching and writing skills we all admire, but for punctuality that is an editor's dream.

The third section, *A Developmental Framework*, chronologically follows normal development from the prenatal period through late adolescence. While incorporating the more relevant theories of human development, its chapters have a stronger emphasis on clinical applicability than encyclopedic coverage of specific milestones or schools of thought. The section is very much in line with our experience of Mel's teaching and is capped with a review of developmental psychopathology, addressing the ways in which genetic endowment and environmental conditions can interact along the dimension of time to increase the likelihood of resilient or pathologic outcomes.

A fourth section on *Nosology, Classification, and Diagnostic Assessment* starts with an overview of the different ways in which child psychopathology has been historically classified. This chapter identifies differences across, and within, the major nosological schemes: the European ICD vs. the American DSM, and the various iterations of the latter. Although this discussion will eventually be eclipsed by the arrival of the forthcoming DSM-V, the more relevant point to make here is that this volume is not beholden to any given system: we have not imposed editorial consistency at this level, realizing that such classification schemes are fluid and perfectible products. Thus, some chapters stay within well-demarcated diagnostic lines, others see the limitations in existing criteria, while yet others take whatever is useful from different classifications. The longer part of this section is dedicated to the diagnostic and clinical assessment process, and includes chapters that range from specific forms of assessment to the integration of the rich complexity inherent in child psychiatric practice.

Specific Disorders and Syndromes is the fifth and longest section. We should note here that for many conditions we have followed groupings that made good clinical sense to us, even if our organization scheme was not necessarily the most traditional. The same can be said of the part on treatment in the sixth section, where we created a *Continuum of Care and Location-Specific Interventions* category that, while wordily titled, brings together aspects that are often as poorly interconnected in textbooks as they are out in the community.

The seventh and final section encompasses the very broadly ambassadorial *Interface Areas of Child and Adolescent Psychiatry*. Specifically, it includes our discipline's work on the borders—and often well within the territories—of pediatrics, schools, and the law.

Lewis comes up to 87 chapters, 155 contributing authors and over 1000 pages of text. What if anything can we make of these summary and impressive statistics? And what can we make of the fact that it has 46 *fewer* chapters and a significantly different line-up and content than its previous edition? More importantly, how does a discipline know that its knowledge base is moving in the right direction? When its truths become pickled into canonical and unchanging texts, or when they squirm out of our grasp and refuse to be fixed? When their tomes become thicker? When they become leaner? Perhaps it is when the tomes disappear altogether?

These questions are not rhetorical, nor are they simply meant to provoke. The fact is that books today are not what they used to be just a decade ago, and the place and function of the academic textbook needs to be reconsidered in light of today's hegemony of the internet as a source of living and constantly shifting knowledge. Knowledge that in turn brings up a whole new set of questions about the information available to clinicians, practitioners and patients: What is the least disorienting and most reassuring source of information after all? Do not get us wrong: neither one of us is a pessimist. We are proud of this book and confident that it will teach and, we hope, inspire the readers it reaches, that it can provide a sense of overarching coherence one would be hard pressed to find elsewhere. But we are realists and aware that some of the information contained in these pages will be out of date even before the book sees the light of day and that some more will gradually decay like so much radioactive material. The problem we now face is finding some sort of effective rapprochement between nimble cybernetics, with its propensity to conflate the constructive and responsible with the misleading and reckless through a simple mouse-click, and the solid consensus of the textbook, where rigorous methodology and transparent use of science and sources also risk reifying what is incorrect as authoritative.

Lewis's previous edition was already available as an e-book that included hypertext links. This new edition follows suit with updated technology, and a shorter, pocket companion version with self-assessment questions is planned. In these ways, this traditional textbook will continue to advance into electronic territory. As we look at the first three editions sitting on our shelves, we think back to the shelf of Professor Victor McCusick, father of modern human genetics and editor of the classic *Mendelian Inheritance in Man* first published in 1966. During the years under his watch, genetic information exploded, such that his svelte single tome evolved into a massive three-volume 12th edition by 1998. Paper stock and wet forests shuddered at the thought of what the next edition might entail. As it turns out, it entailed very little, at least by ways of paper: By then the resource had all but ceased to be a book, having migrated almost entirely to the web as OMIM (http://www.ncbi.nlm.nih.gov/omim).

Even as this and other textbooks are likely to continue merging, blending, and otherwise becoming complementary with electronic resources, we do not hold our breath for a complete migration to the web. But even if there is one, we wager that there are abiding values and clinical wisdom in these pages that will continue to hold true and guide our practice for years to come. The very first and the very last contributions to this communal effort reassure us of as much: we are indebted to Jack McDermott for his foreword, to Leon Eisenberg for his postscript, and to both for standing as beacons who direct us toward values and principles worth holding dear.

We are grateful to the superb lineup of contributing authors for their engagement, responsiveness and excellent work. We thank our advisory board members for their input and sage advice at critical junctures en route to the palpable reality of this book. We express special thanks to a Lippincott Williams and Wilkins team superbly orchestrated by Charley Mitchell. And to end as we began, our gratitude and deep appreciation to Melvin Lewis, whose passion and vision were the original ingredients for this textbook's secret recipe. Grateful though we are, we humbly recognize that the success of this edition should be measured by how much it helps move our field toward the fuller realization of helping children and families everywhere.

Andrés Martin
Fred R. Volkmar
Child Study Center
Yale University School of Medicine
New Haven, Connecticut

■ CONTENTS

SECTION III ■ A DEVELOPMENT FRAMEWORK

SECTION IV ■ NOSOLOGY, CLASSIFICATION, AND DIAGNOSTIC ASSESSMENT

SECTION V ■ SPECIFIC DISORDERS AND SYNDROMES

■ CONTRIBUTING AUTHORS

Jean Adnopoz, MPH
Clinical Professor
Child Study Center
Yale University School of Medicine
New Haven, Connecticut

Thomas F. Anders, MD
Distinguished Professor (Emeritus)
Department of Psychiatry and Behavioral Sciences
University of California, Davis
Davis, California

George M. Anderson, PhD
Research Scientist
Child Study Center
Yale University School of Medicine
New Haven, Connecticut

Adrian Angold, MRCPsych
Associate Professor
Department of Psychiatry and Behavioral Sciences
Duke University Medical Center
Durham, North Carolina

Eugene L. Arnold, MD
Professor Emeritus, Psychiatry
Department of Psychiatry
Ohio State University
Columbus, Ohio

Peter Ash, MD
Associate Professor, Psychiatry
Department of Psychiatry and Behavioral Sciences
Emory University
Atlanta, Georgia

Andrea Gottsegen Asnes, MD, MSW
Associate Research Scientist
Department of Pediatrics
Yale University School of Medicine
New Haven, Connecticut

David Axelson, MD
Assistant Professor, Psychiatry
Department of Psychiatry
University of Pittsburgh Medical Center
Pittsburgh, Pennsylvania

Steven J. Barreto, PhD
Clinical Assistant Professor
Department of Psychiatry and Human Behavior
Brown University Medical School
Providence, Rhode Island

Myron L. Belfer, MD, MPA
Professor, Psychiatry
Department of Social Medicine
Harvard Medical School
Boston, Massachusetts

Eugene V. Beresin, MA, MD
Associate Professor
Department of Psychiatry
Harvard Medical School
Boston, Massachusetts

Steven Berkowitz, MD
Assistant Professor
Child Study Center
Yale University School of Medicine
New Haven, Connecticut

Boris Birmaher, MD
Professor, Psychiatry
Department of Psychiatry
University of Pittsburgh Medical Center
Pittsburgh, Pennsylvania

Joseph C. Blader, PhD
Assistant Professor
Department of Psychiatry and Behavioral Science
State University of New York
Stony Brook, New York

Efrain Bleiberg, MD
Alicia Townsend Freidmen Professor of Psychiatry
Director, Division of Child and Adolescent Psychiatry
Menninger Department of Psychiatry and Behavioral Sciences
Baylor College of Medicine
Houston, Texas

Michael H. Bloch, MD
Resident, Integrated Child, Adolescent, and Adult Psychiatry Research Training Program
Child Study Center
Yale University School of Medicine
New Haven, Connecticut

John R. Boekamp, PhD
Clinical Assistant Professor, Psychiatry/Human Behavior
Department of Psychiatry and Human Behavior
Brown University Medical School
Providence, Rhode Island

Mendy A. Boettcher, PhD
Clinical Instructor
Division of Child and Adolescent Psychiatry
Stanford University Medical Center
Stanford, California

Jeff Q. Bostic, MD, EdD
Assistant Clinical Professor
Department of Psychiatry
Harvard Medical School
Boston, Massachusetts

David A. Brent, MD
Professor of Psychiatry, Pediatrics, and Epidemiology
Department of Psychiatry
University of Pittsburgh Medical Center
Pittsburgh, Pennsylvania

Rachel Margaret Ann Brown, MBBS
Associate Dean for Student Programs
Professor, Clinical Psychiatry
Department of Psychiatry
University of Missouri-Columbia School of Medicine
Columbia, Missouri

Jonathan M. Campbell, PhD
Associate Professor
Department of Educational Psychology
University of Georgia
Athens, Georgia

John V. Campo, MD
Professor
Department of Psychiatry
The Ohio State University
Columbus, Ohio

Laurie Cardona, PsyD
Chief, Psychology
Child Study Center
Yale University School of Medicine
New Haven, Connecticut

Lee Combrinck-Graham, MD
Associate Clinical Professor
Child Study Center
Yale University School of Medicine
New Haven, Connecticut

Edwin H. Cook, Jr., MD
Associate Professor, Psychiatry and Pediatrics
Department of Psychiatry
University of Illinois at Chicago
Chicago, Illinois

Elizabeth Jane Costello, PhD
Professor, Psychology
Department of Psychiatry and Behavioral Sciences
Duke University Medical Center
Durham, North Carolina

Peter T. Daniolos, MD
Assistant Professor
Department of Psychiatry
The George Washington University Medical Center
Washington, D.C.

Sujith Dhanasiri, BDS, MPhil
Research Officer
Health Services Research Department
King's College London, Institute of Psychiatry
London, United Kingdom

Melanie A. Dirks, MPhil
Graduate Student
Department of Psychology
Yale University School of Medicine
New Haven, Connecticut

Elisabeth M. Dykens, PhD
Professor
Psychology and Human Development
Vanderbilt University
Nashville, Tennessee

Helen Egger, MD
Assistant Professor
Department of Psychiatry and Behavioral Sciences
Duke University Medical Center
Durham, North Carolina

Leon Eisenberg, MD
Professor Emeritus, Social Medicine and Child Psychiatry
Department of Social Medicine
Harvard Medical School
Boston, Massachusetts

Maurice Eisenbruch, MD
Director, Institute for Health and Diversity
Vice Chancellor's Adviser on Diversity
Professor, Culture and Health
Institute for Health and Diversity
Victoria University
Melbourne, Australia

Thomas Fernandez, MD
Fellow
Child Study Center
Yale University School of Medicine
New Haven, Connecticut

Matia Finn-Stevenson, PhD
Research Scientist
Associate Director
Child Study Center
Yale University School of Medicine
New Haven, Connecticut

Michael First, MD
Professor, Clinical Psychiatry
Department of Psychiatry
Columbia College of Physicians and Surgeons
New York, New York

Carmel A. Foley, MD
Assistant Professor
Department of Psychiatry
Albert Einstein College of Medicine
Bronx, New York

Eric Fombonne, MD
Canada Research Chair/Professor of Child Psychiatry
Department of Psychiatry
McGill University
Montreal, Canada

Brian W.C. Forsyth, MB, ChB
Professor, Pediatrics
Department of Pediatrics
Yale University School of Medicine
New Haven, Connecticut

Geraldine S. Fox, MD, MHPE
Professor
Department of Psychiatry
University of Illinois at Chicago
Chicago, Illinois

Jennifer Freeman, PhD
Assistant Professor of Research
Department of Psychiatry and Human Behavior
Brown University Medical School
Providence, Rhode Island

Gregory K. Fritz, MD
Professor/Director, Child and Adolescent Psychiatry
Department of Psychiatry and Human Behavior
Brown University Medical School
Providence, Rhode Island

Abbe Garcia, PhD
Assistant Professor of Research
Department of Psychiatry and Human Behavior
Brown University Medical School
Providence, Rhode Island

Manely Ghaffari, MD
Fellow, Child and Adolescent Psychiatry
Child Study Center
New York University School of Medicine
New York, New York

Walter S. Gilliam, PhD
Assistant Professor, Child Psychiatry and Psychology
Child Study Center
Yale University School of Medicine
New Haven, Connecticut

John P. Glazer, MD
Head, Section of Child and Adolescent Psychiatry
Department of Psychiatry and Psychology
The Cleveland Clinic
Cleveland, Ohio

Mary Margaret Gleason, MD
Clinical Assistant Professor
Department of Psychiatry and Human Behavior
Brown University Medical School
Providence, Rhode Island

Jeffrey A. Gliner, PhD
Professor Emeritus
Department of Occupational Therapy
Colorado State University
Fort Collins, Colorado

Nitin Gogtay, MD
Staff Clinician
Child Psychiatry Branch
National Institute of Mental Health
Bethesda, Maryland

Joseph González-Heydrich, MD
Assistant Professor
Department of Psychiatry
Harvard Medical School
Boston, Massachusetts

Elena L. Grigorenko, PhD
Associate Professor
Child Study Center
Yale University School of Medicine
New Haven, Connecticut

Katherine A. Halmi, MD
Professor
Department of Psychiatry
Weill Medical College of Cornell University
White Plains, New York

John Hamilton, MD, MSc
Senior Physician
The Permanente Medical Group of California
Sacramento, California

Robert J. Harmon, MD (*Deceased*)
Department of Psychiatry
University of Colorado at Denver and Health Sciences Center
Denver, Colorado

Sharon M. Hasbani, MD
Fellow, Child and Adolescent Psychiatry
Child Study Center
Yale University School of Medicine
New Haven, Connecticut

David A. Hay, PhD
Professor
School of Psychology
Curtin University of Technology
Perth, Western Australia

Johannes Hebebrand, MD
Professor
Department of Child and Adolescent Psychiatry
University of Duisburg-Essen
Essen, Germany

Schuyler W. Henderson, MD
Department of Psychiatry
Columbia College of Physicians and Surgeons
New York, New York

Peter Hindley, MBBS, BSc
Consultant/Lead Psychiatrist, Child and Adolescent Psychiatrist
Children's Psychological Medicine
St. Thomas' Hospital
London, England

Robert M. Hodapp, PhD
Professor
Director, Center for the Advancement of Children's Mental Health
Department of Special Education
Vanderbilt University
Nashville, Tennessee

Christian Hopfer, MD
Associate Professor
Department of Psychiatry
University of Colorado at Denver and Health Sciences Center
Denver, Colorado

Peter S. Jensen, MD
Ruane Professor of Child Psychiatry
Director, Center for the Advancement of Children's Mental Health
Department of Psychiatry
Columbia College of Physicians and Surgeons
New York, New York

Joan Kaufman, PhD
Associate Professor
Harris Associate Professor of Child Psychology and Psychiatry
Department of Psychiatry
Yale University School of Medicine
New Haven, Connecticut

Robert A. King, MD
Professor of Child Psychiatry
Child Study Center
Yale University School of Medicine
New Haven, Connecticut

Ami Klin, PhD
Director, Autism Program
Harris Associate Professor of Child Psychology and Psychiatry
Child Study Center
Yale University School of Medicine
New Haven, Connecticut

Martin Knapp, PhD
Professor
Department of Social Policy
London School of Economics and Political Science
London, England

Amy L. Krain, PhD
Assistant Professor, Psychiatry
Child Study Center
New York University School of Medicine
New York, New York

Anlee D. Kuo, MD, JD
Assistant Clinical Professor
Department of Psychiatry
University of California, San Francisco
San Francisco, California

Nathaniel Laor, MD, PhD
Professor, Psychiatry and Behavioral Services
Department of Psychiatry and Behavioral Services
Sackler School of Medicine
Tel-Aviv University
Tel-Aviv, Israel

James F. Leckman, MD
Professor
Child Study Center
Yale University School of Medicine
New Haven, Connecticut

Henrietta Leonard, MD
Professor
Department of Psychiatry and Human Behavior
Brown University Medical School
Providence, Rhode Island

Robert J. Levine, MD
Professor, Medicine and Lecturer in Pharmacology
Co-Director, Interdisciplinary Center for Bioethics
Department of Internal Medicine
Yale University School of Medicine
New Haven, Connecticut

Moira Lewis, MS, CCC-SLP
Speech-Language Pathologist
Child Study Center
Yale University School of Medicine
New Haven, Connecticut

Paul J. Lombroso, MD
Professor
Child Study Center
Yale University School of Medicine
New Haven, Connecticut

Catherine Lord, PhD
Professor
Department of Psychology
University of Michigan
Ann Arbor, Michigan

Suniya S. Luthar, PhD
Professor, Clinical and Developmental Psychology
Department of Counseling and Clinical Psychology
Teachers College, Columbia University
New York, New York

Steven Marans, PhD
Professor, Child Psychiatry and Psychiatry
Child Study Center
Yale University School of Medicine
New Haven, Connecticut

Andrés Martin, MD, MPH
Associate Professor, Child Psychiatry and Psychiatry
Child Study Center
Yale University School of Medicine
New Haven, Connecticut

Linda C. Mayes, MD
Arnold Gessell Professor of Child Psychiatry, Pediatrics, and Psychology
Child Study Center
Yale University School of Medicine
New Haven, Connecticut

David P.A. McDaid, MSc, BSc
Research Fellow
Personal Social Services Research Unit
London School of Economics and Political Science
London, England

Edwin J. Mikkelsen, MD
Associate Professor
Department of Psychiatry
Harvard Medical School
Boston, Massachusetts

George A. Morgan, PhD
Professor Emeritus, Education and Human Development
Department of Education and Human Development
Colorado State University
Fort Collins, Colorado

Nancy E. Moss, PhD
Clinical Assistant Professor
Child Study Center
Yale University School of Medicine
New Haven, Connecticut

Corinne Moss-Racusin, BA
Doctoral Student
Department of Psychology
Rutgers, The State University of New Jersey
Piscataway, New Jersey

David A. Mrazek, MD
Professor, Psychiatry and Pediatrics
Department of Psychiatry
Mayo Clinic College of Medicine
Rochester, Minnesota

Patricia J. Mrazek, MSW, PhD
Mental Health Policy Consultant
Rochester, Minnesota

Laura Mufson, PhD
Associate Professor, Clinical Psychology
Department of Psychiatry
Columbia University College of Physicians and Surgeons
New York, New York

Robert A. Murphy, PhD
Associate Professor
Department of Psychiatry and Behavioral Sciences
Duke University Medical Center
Durham, North Carolina

David F. Musto, MD
Professor
Child Study Center
Yale University School of Medicine
New Haven, Connecticut

Barry Nurcombe, MD
Professor Emeritus
Department of Child and Adolescent Psychiatry
The University of Queensland
Brisbane, Australia

Karen J. O'Donnell, PhD
Associate Clinical Professor
Department of Psychiatry and Behavioral Sciences
Duke University Medical Center
Durham, NC

Jessica R. Oesterheld, MD
Lecturer
Department of Psychiatry
Tufts University School of Medicine
Boston, Massachusetts

Margaret Paccione-Dyszlewski, PhD
Clinical Assistant Professor
Division of Biology and Medicine
Brown University School of Medicine
Providence, Rhode Island

Rhea Paul, PhD
Professor
Child Study Center
Yale University School of Medicine
New Haven, Connecticut

Mani Pavuluri, MD, PhD
Associate Professor
Department of Psychiatry
University of Illinois at Chicago
Chicago, Illinois

Bradley S. Peterson, MD
Suzanne Crosby Murphy Professor
Department of Psychiatry
Columbia University College of Physicians and Surgeons
New York, New York

Cynthia R. Pfeffer, MD
Professor
Department of Psychiatry
Weill Medical College of Cornell University
White Plains, New York

John Piacentini, PhD, ABPP
Professor, Psychiatry and Biobehavorial Sciences
Department of Psychiatry and Biobehavorial Sciences
David Geffen School of Medicine
at the University of California, Los Angeles
Los Angeles, California

Daniel S. Pine, MD
Chief, Developmental Studies/Emotion and Development Branch
Emotion and Development Branch
National Institute of Mental Health
Bethesda, Maryland

Yann B. Poncin, MD
Associate Research Scientist
Child Study Center
Yale University School of Medicine
New Haven, Connecticut

Laura Prager, MD
Assistant Professor
Department of Psychiatry
Harvard University Medical School
Boston, Massachusetts

Rebecca P. Prince, BA
Graduate Student
Department of Counseling and Clinical Psychology
Teachers College, Columbia University
New York, New York

Kyle D. Pruett, MD
Clinical Professor, Psychiatry and Nursing
Child Study Center
Yale University School of Medicine
New Haven, Connecticut

Andres J. Pumariega, MD
Professor
Department of Psychiatry
Temple University School of Medicine
Philadelphia, Pennsylvania

Gary R. Racusin, PhD
Assistant Clinical Professor
Child Study Center
Yale University School of Medicine
New Haven, Connecticut

Guatami Rao, MD
Clinical Instructor
Department of Neurology
Yale University School of Medicine
New Haven, Connecticut

Judith Rapoport, MD
Chief
Child Psychiatry Branch
National Institute of Mental Health
Bethesda, Maryland

Joseph M. Rey, MBBS, PhD
Honorary Professor
Department of Psychological Medicine
University of Sydney
Sydney, Australia

Mark A. Riddle, MD
Professor
Department of Psychiatry and Behavioral Sciences
Johns Hopkins School of Medicine
Baltimore, Maryland

Paula Riggs, MD
Associate Professor, Psychiatry
Department of Psychiatry
University of Colorado at Denver and Health Sciences Center
Denver, Colorado

Rachel Z. Ritvo, MD
Assistant Clinical Professor, Psychiatry and Behavioral Sciences
Department of Psychiatry
The George Washington University Medical Center
Washington, D.C.

Samuel Ritvo, MD
Clinical Professor, Psychiatry
Child Study Center
Yale University School of Medicine
New Haven, Connecticut

Melisa D. Rowland, MD
Associate Professor
Department of Psychiatry and Behavioral Sciences
Medical University of South Carolina
Charleston, South Carolina

Alison Salt, MBBS, MSc
Honorary Senior Lecturer
Department of Neuroscience
Institude of Child Health
London, England

Lawrence Scahill, MSN, PhD
Professor
Child Study Center
Yale University School of Medicine
New Haven, Connecticut

Diane H. Schetky, MD
Clinical Professor
Department of Psychiatry
University of Vermont College of Medicine
Portland, Maine

Steven C. Schlozman, MD
Assistant Professor
Department of Psychiatry
Harvard Medical School
Boston, Massachusetts

David J. Schonfeld, MD
Thelma and Jack Rubinstein Professor of Pediactrics
Department of Pediactrics
University of Cincinnati College of Medicine
Cincinnati, Ohio

Robert Schultz, PhD
Associate Professor
Child Study Center
Yale University School of Medicine
New Haven, Connecticut

Mary Schwab-Stone, MD
Associate Professor, Child Psychiatry
Child Study Center
Yale University School of Medicine
New Haven, Connecticut

Richard I. Shader, MD
Professor, Psychiatry and Pharmacology
Department of Psychiatry
Tufts University School of Medicine
Boston, Massachussetts

Sarghi Sharma, MD
Assistant Professor, Psychiatry
Department of Psychiatry and Behavioral Sciences
University of Texas Medical Branch
Galveston, Texas

Carla Sharp, PhD
Assistant Professor
Menninger Department of Psychiatry and Behavioral Sciences
Baylor College of Medicine
Houston, Texas

G. Pirooz Sholevar, MD
Clinical Professor, Child Psychiatry
Department of Psychiatry
Jefferson Medical College
Philadelphia, Pennsylvania

John B. Sikorski, MD
Clinical Professor
Department of Psychiatry
University of California San Francisco
San Francisco, California

Laura Stout Sosinsky, PhD
Postdoctoral Associate
Child Study Center
Yale University School of Medicine
New Haven, Connecticut

Cesar A. Soutullo, MD, PhD
Assistant Professor
Department of Psychiatry
University of Navarra College of Medicine
Pamplona, Spain

Lacramioara Spetie, MD
Assistant Professor
Department of Psychiatry
The Ohio State University
Columbus, Ohio

Matthew W. State, MD, PhD
Harris Associate Professor
Child Study Center
Yale University School of Medicine
New Haven, Connecticut

Bradley Stein, MD, MPH
Associate Professor
Department of Psychiatry
University of Pittsburgh School of Medicine
Pittsburgh, Pennsylvania

Carla Smith Stover, PhD
Associate Research Scientist
Child Study Center
Yale University School of Medicine
New Haven, Connecticut

Dorothy E. Stubbe, MD
Associate Professor
Child Study Center
Yale University School of Medicine
New Haven, Connecticut

Cynthia J. Telingator, MD
Assistant Professor
Department of Psychiatry
Harvard Medical School
Boston, Massachusetts

Christopher R. Thomas, MD
Professor
Department of Psychiatry and Behavioral Sciences
University of Texas Medical Branch
Galveston, Texas

Lynelle E. Thomas, MD
Assistant Professor, Child Psychiatry
Child Study Center
Yale University School of Medicine
New Haven, Connecticut

Kenneth E. Towbin, MD
Professor
Department of Psychiatry
The George Washington University Medical Center
Washington, D.C.

Kathleen D. Tsatsanis, PhD
Associate Research Scientist
Child Study Center
Yale University School of Medicine
New Haven, Connecticut

Flora M. Vaccarino, MD
Associate Professor
Child Study Center
Yale University School of Medicine
New Haven, Connecticut

Fred R. Volkmar, MD
Professor, Director
Child Study Center
Yale University School of Medicine
New Haven, Connecticut

Garry Walter, MBBS, PhD
Professor
Department of Psychological Medicine
University of Sydney
Sydney, Australia

V. Robin Weersing, PhD
Assistant Professor
Joint Doctoral Program in Clinical Psychology
San Diego State University
University of California at San Diego
San Diego, California

Kathryn Whetten, PhD
Associate Professor of Public Policy, Nursing, and Community and Family Medicine
Center for Health Policy
Duke University School of Medicine
Durham, North Carolina

Daniel T. Williams, MD
Special Lecturer
Department of Psychiatry
Columbia College of Physicians and Surgeons
New York, New York

Nancy C. Winters, MD
Associate Professor
Residency Training Director
Department of Psychiatry
Oregon Health and Science University
Portland, Oregon

Leo Wolmer, PhD
Director of School Interventions
Department of Psychiatry and Behavioral Services
Sackler School of Medicine
Tel-Aviv University
Tel-Aviv, Israel

Joseph L. Woolston, MD
Vice Chair for Clinical Affairs
Child Study Center
Yale University School of Medicine
New Haven, Connecticut

Jami F. Young, PhD
Assistant Professor, Clinical Psychology
Department of Psychiatry
Columbia College of Physicians and Surgeons
New York, New York

Charles H. Zeanah, MD
Sellars Polchow Professor of Psychiatry
Department of Psychiatry
Tulane University Health Sciences Center
New Orleans, Louisiana

Bradley J. Zebrack, PhD, MSW
Assistant Professor
School of Social Work
University of Southern California
Los Angeles, California

Karen R. Zeff, PhD
Postdoctoral Fellow
Department of Psychiatry and Human Behavior
Brown University Medical School
Providence, Rhode Island

Edward F. Zigler, PhD
Sterling Professor of Psychology, Emeritus
The Edward Zigler Center in Child Development and Social Policy
Yale University School of Medicine
New Haven, Connecticut

Kenneth J. Zucker, PhD
Professor
Department of Psychiatry and Psychology
University of Toronto
Toronto, Canada

SECTION I
AN APPROACH TO THE DISCIPLINE

CHAPTER 1.1 ■ THE ART OF THE SCIENCE: A CHILD, FAMILY, AND SYSTEMS-CENTERED APPROACH

KYLE D. PRUETT

I keep picturing all these little kids playing some game in this big field of rye . . .
Thousands of little kids and nobody's around—nobody big, I mean—except me . . .
What I have to do, I have to catch everybody if they start over the cliff.

J.D. Salinger, *The Catcher in the Rye*

INVITATION TO THE PRACTICE OF CHILD AND ADOLESCENT PSYCHIATRY?

Like many medical students before me, I had been deeply moved and troubled by my first encounters with the life-shattering onset of schizophrenia in young adulthood: such pain and disorientation in the mind, at such a promising era of life. There simply had to be better ways to reduce the morbidity of these illnesses for these young people and their families, or at least to catch them before they crested Holden Caulfield's cliff.

Such thinking drew me away from pediatrics and adult psychiatry, and into working with ever younger children, looking earlier and earlier for when to help and how to comprehend their distress. I eventually found myself standing at NICU bassinettes with anyone I could find who could help me fathom how things could go so wrong, so fast, and so often for children. Luckily, I found smart, humane mentors in people like Al Solnit and Sally Provence who discouraged simplistic formulations and helped me embrace the complexity of early experience with all the intellectual rigor I could muster.

It struck me from the beginning that child and adolescent psychiatry had it right. It was onto something vitally important; the earlier the better—for diagnosis, treatment, parent guidance, and whatever we could do to help families grow with their vulnerable children. It also struck me as extremely shortsighted to dissect out the child—even intellectually—from the family for diagnostic studies, economies of time, convenience of intervention, or cost containment. Such myopia was like a celestial navigator trying to identify a constellation by fixing on but one star with his sextant; then as now, a really good way to get good and lost.

So how could one stay on course in this odyssey to effective intervention and prevention? Is it better to consult the gene map (nature) or the family tree (nurture) as primary navigational aids? From the beginning of developmental mental health explorations in the 1920s and 30s, child psychiatry seemed destined to distrust the facile nature vs. nurture dichotomy offered up as dogma by so many behavioral scientists. Careful clinical investigations and longitudinal inquiry fell short again and again of affirming it as the best way to formulate helpful interventions.

Contemporary science has further relieved us of this distraction, helping us to conceptualize the dichotomy less as competition, and more as dialogue or transaction. It has proven more illuminating to investigate how we nurture nature than to officiate at a face-off between the two. Tierney et al. highlight clearly the interaction between environment and genome as accounting for more of the variance in clinical outcomes of illness than either genetics or environment alone (1). The compelling studies by Caspi of G(ene) × E(xperience) (2), and Kaufman (3) of gene interactions and environmental modifiers of depression in children provide elegant empirical grounding to that effect. Taken together, their work addressing G × E interactions between severity of child abuse, 5HT transporter polymorphisms, and outcomes of depression and conduct disorder have profound implications for future societal and mental health intervention.

The outcomes of well designed longitudinal studies of young children and families at risk also encourage us to focus on this discourse between gene and environment so that we can design more effective and relevant service, policy, and research agendas. Sroufe concludes from his Minnesota Study of Risk and Adaptation from Birth to Adulthood that "early history is not destiny, important as it is . . . [D]ata suggest a renewed focus on the lived experience of the child and [less] preoccupation with inherent biological variations (4)."

This perspective protects us from too narrow a focus on the behavior of the child as we struggle to understand how to decrease the morbidity of psychopathology and increase resilience around vulnerabilities. Hechtman's discussion of the research into long-term outcomes of childhood disorders encourages us to cast a broad net as we hunt for salient factors affecting outcome that extend well beyond behavior (5). She reminds us to look beyond age, gender, IQ, comorbid conditions, physical, and emotional health to include socioeconomic status, family function, and composition, and child rearing practices.

It is the need to capture this complexity—not to avoid or oversimplify it—that defines child psychiatric clinical competence. We have tried to conceptualize this visually in textbook after textbook by drawing concentric circles outward from the child to include all the factors that shape development, per se; particularly when we adhere to classical definitions of development as the melding of genetic predisposition, or maturation, with experience. But such visuals typically fall short, because as Spitz so efficiently summarized, "Maturation is a useful concept, but in reality there is only development (6)." In the end, it is the environment that processes any given child's genetic blueprint, through maturation, into lived experience.

Herein lies the core purpose in diagnostic and intervention strategies: encompass and embrace the complexity of the child's experience to understand and treat, while fully incorporating age and circumstance. This is precisely what obligates the researching and treating physician to employ the child-, family-, and systems-centered approach embraced in this textbook.

Families render humans human. Era-specific developmental forces within the family and the child define the salient relationships and intimacies that draw the infant into the human race, one human transaction at a time. The family in all its permutations ultimately embraces that child's maturational promise and, through powerful reciprocal forces, converts tissue, synapse and instinct into human development. Although family processes seem linear (from birth and growth to decline and death, repeated through each generation), family process itself appears more helical. Each generation must accommodate to its own unique life cycle agenda simultaneously. Consequently, it may be more helpful to visualize family processes as intertwined developmental courses, not unlike Watson and Crick's double helix. Running parallel, the generations develop together, intimately connected to, but nevertheless distinct from, other generations in the family.

Another way to imagine the development of the family maintains this helical image, but consists of different conceptual strands. One axis is the trail of generational myths, expectations, attributes, memories, and secrets—the family's "givens." This is the family's narrative about itself, so eloquently described by Pincus and Dare (7) and Vangelisti (8). The narrative evolves much like folk songs in the oral tradition, passed on at home, as children are taught who and what their family is now, has been, and is hoped to be.

The other axis is the family's forward progression through time in its own life cycle. This encompasses the usual stresses and opportunities of the family's children's developmental requirements and the intrusion of "fateful events." How the family copes with the course of development, accidents, and intrusions from outside and within is determined in part by whether these two axes intersect at strong or weak points. Real trouble seems most likely when a vulnerable stretch on the transgenerational axis intersects with an equally vulnerable stretch on the developmental axis. For example: A family narrative axis carries the myth/expectation that "Jones boys always marry wild women" at a time when, on the developmental axis, the Jones' first born son is starting his adolescence by easing up on his academic discipline and testing behavioral boundaries. He tells his parents progressively less about his life and whereabouts (appropriately), especially where girls are concerned and voilà—his and his family's fantasies about "wild women" fuse and sparks fly.

Family development as a dynamic phenomenon is particularly hard to embrace because clinicians tend to encounter families at just one nodal point in time, depriving them of critical longitudinal perspective. Research suggests strong links between early loss, trauma, and disturbance in the family and later interpersonal dysfunction (9–11). At any given time in our interaction with a family, we may be uncertain about which direction the causal links may be moving (such as whether a vulnerable child destabilizes the family, or vice versa) (12). Nevertheless, we are wise to keep in mind that most mental illnesses are not the result of a sole inborn factor, or some single extraneous perturbation, but rather the multiply determined end result of human development gone awry, which has become apparent at some seemingly discrete moment.

THE CHANGING FAMILY SYSTEM

Sociologists have suggested that current cycles of family life are undergoing accelerating change. Lower birth rates, substantial (though declining) divorce rates, increasing remarriage rates, and longer life expectancies have reduced childbearing from being the major occupation of parents to what is now less than 50% of parents' lifelong commitment.

Typically, historians urge caution whenever referring to "unprecedented change." Demos (13), and Laslette and Wall (14), have dispelled the myth of the ideal three-generational family holding sway in pre-industrial family life. Nevertheless, a social process has occurred over the past several hundred years, and in particular over the past few decades, that has effected major changes in family functioning. Hareven summarizes: "Through a process of differentiation, the family gradually surrendered functions previously concentrated within it to other social institutions. During the pre-Industrial period, the family not only reared children, but also served as a workshop, a school, a church, and an asylum" (15) (p. 460). The difficulties faced by contemporary families are rooted in this diminished capacity to adapt and cope (partly because of smaller size) and the further narrowing in the range of the family's socioeconomic functions and independence.

The declining maternal and child death rates of the 1950s, combined with a higher marriage rate and longer life span created a higher percentage of children growing up in stable, two-parent families than had ever occurred in America's history. Beginning with the next decade, however, multiple determined trends began to reshape the ideal and real traditional nuclear family. The sexual revolution uncoupled the societal association of sexual and reproductive behavior, particularly for women. From 1971 to 2002, the percentage of unmarried American girls 15 to 19 years of age who engaged in sexual intercourse rose from 28% to 60%. Second, married women with children moved into the paid workforce: There was an increase from the 1960 level of 19% of married women with children younger than 6 years of age in the labor force to a real figure of 66% in 2001. Historian Robert Griswold noted that these forces, combined with attitudinal changes toward coparenting, have brought increasing numbers of fathers into the nurturing domain (16).

Fertility and fecundity also declined in the United States beginning in the 1960s. We are now at levels lower than those necessary for the replacement of the population, having moved from an average of 3.7 children per woman in 1960 to 1.79. Increased child survival over the last century, combined with women having their first children later, may also be contributing to families having fewer children.

The divorce rate in America, though currently slowing, brought us past a landmark in 1974, when for the first time in our history, more marriages concluded in divorce than in the death of a spouse. The percentages of unmarried couples, same-sex couples, serial and stepfamilies, and single-parent families (single by choice or not) have all increased, whereas nuclear unit percentages continue to decrease.

Finally, it is the opinion of many clinicians and researchers that the quality of life for children in the past 30 years has not improved at the same rate as it has for adults. Also, rates of distress seem to be on the rise. Achenbach and Howell studied the changes over 13 years in the prevalence of children in the general population with behavioral/emotional problems (17). They found more untreated children who needed psychological intervention in the 1989 sample than in the 1976 sample. The 2005 Kids Count Report by the Annie E. Casey Foundation documented a downturn in child well-being trends with increasing child poverty, infant low birthweight and mortality, and a teen death rate increase over the previous five-year report. This suggests that the trend noted by Achenbach has yet to reverse itself.

Though family structure continues to evolve to include different constellations, the majority of children continue to long for meaningful relationships with both biological parents in, his or her life (18). The family structure that is most influential in the child's development, however, is the one perceived by the child as his or her family, not the one perceived by the Census Bureau.

Many contemporary statistics illustrate an important, irreducible fact about change in the American family: Mothers are in the labor force to stay. The 2003 Bureau of Labor Statistics report documented that 16% of all married couple families have a wage-earning father and a stay-at-home mother; the number was 67% in 1940 (19). Child rearing families also tend to receive more societal and economic support when both parents are committed to the job in all its complexity. Families have changed, yet the institutions the families rely on most heavily, schools and the workplace, have been slow in responding to these changes in the family system.

MOTHERHOOD AND FATHERHOOD

Each child who enters the family changes it permanently and irreversibly, rendering the child's perception of the family unique to his or her own experience. Sameroff and Fiese have helped us move away from the restrictions of the linear, interactional model of child development, and toward one that better encompasses the progressive, dynamic, reciprocal forces that have helped children change families and vice versa (20). Their "transactional model" emphasizes the need for incorporating social and economic as well as biological forces. Proposing a "continuum of caretaking causality," such increased emphasis on the qualitative aspects of the nurturing domain, has encouraged clinicians and researchers to think anew about who in the family is doing what with the children, and not simply how long they are doing it.

The Berkeley Adult Attachment Interview (21) in its application to family development (22) serves as an example of growing skill in our capacity to assess the adult's state of mind (and not simply his or her behavior) with regard to attachment to his or her children, and vice versa. The interview for the Adult Attachment Classification System is done separately with mother and father. This is an example of how we are returning to the exploration of the overriding significance of the quality, sensitivity, and intent of the nurturing interaction, and not merely the biological predispositions of the interactors. Mothers, fathers, grandparents, aunts, uncles, and siblings—all form unique attachments to children that, in formative settings, are welcomed and easily integrated by the child into a mosaic of consistent, predictable, comforting internalizations of the nurturing experience. Therefore, internalization of the nurturing experience, be it positive or negative, is not merely the result of a single adult attachment.

Optimal child development is fostered by optimal family development, whatever shape that family takes. This occurs by translating the recognizable maturational stages of child development into the transactional modalities and developmental dynamics of the family. Optimal family development, as perceived by the child, begins with a secure individual relationship, which the infant typically makes with its primary caregiver, typically the mother. Fathers as primary caregivers, however, certainly have the capacity to rear their children without placing them at developmental risk (24–26). Radin and Harold-Goldsmith cite the advantages to young children of paternal involvement, independent of the reasons for the father's presence (27). The other optimal phenomenon for promoting development in the family network consists of the capacity of mothers and fathers to form reciprocal, empathic relationships with the child, aided by a broad and complete range of affective expression. Both parents must be ready to accept developmental progression and change, because it comes rapidly, particularly in the first year, aided by appreciation for the child's idiosyncratic traits, temperament, skills, and vulnerabilities.

Much clinical literature, however, falls short in its attempts to clarify distinct maternal and paternal antecedents to psychological syndromes. For example, although Bezirganian et al. found that maternal overinvolvement, paired with maternal inappropriateness, combined to form pathogenic predispositions toward borderline personality disorder in children (23), paternal measures, which were included, were not commented on in their discussion.

Despite the dramatic increase in the number of publications on fathering since the mid-1980s (28), fathers continue to be vastly underrepresented in the literature, though fathers are now more engaged with their young children than in any era since the Industrial Revolution; the father's share of childcare more than doubled between 1965 and 1998 (29). A typical example of how this remains neglected in the literature: A major prospective, longitudinal study on parental psychopathology, and parenting styles as related to the risk of social phobia in children failed to include any data on fathers (30).

Phares and Compas reviewed research papers in the major journals dealing with clinical child development published from 1984 to 1991 and found that nearly half of all studies involved mothers only (31). Nearly one-fourth of the remaining studies did include father-related material, but did not differentiate its effects. The final one-fourth did measure father–child effects and found them consistently present. So when researchers do bother to look for father effects, they typically find them. The authors suggested that the over-reliance on mothers as research participants has fostered not only an incomplete data set with regard to child development, but also one that is heavily gender biased because "relations cannot be found among variables that are not investigated (31)." (p. 406)

EVALUATING THE FAMILY

As the child psychiatrist works to understand the child's experience, despite such lacunae in the literature, he or she is best served by viewing the family as a system, in which change in one segment of the family resonates throughout the system; negative or positive change in one segment promotes or discourages development in others. Families must "raise the children" while socializing their young, balancing risk and protective factors (32), and simultaneously meeting the demands of rapidly evolving maturational forces in the child. It is crucial, then, to appropriately evaluate the family system's potential for preparing its children for adulthood.

Skinner et al. created the Family Assessment Measure, consisting of a general and dyadic scale to distinguish reliably between normal and problem families (33). Mrazek et al. developed the Parenting Risk Scale, which uses a semistructured interview to rate difficulties and concerns regarding parental commitment, knowledge base, control, psychiatric disturbance, and emotional availability (34). Fleck described an efficient, five-factor method for assessing the system's capacity to support the development of its children, consisting of a) leadership, b) boundaries, c) emotional climate, d) communication, and e) the establishment and accomplishment of goals and tasks throughout the life cycle (35). As we begin to examine the family's development across the life cycle, it is critical to remain conscious of these five factors.

Leadership is the decisionmaking, facilitating source of power and discipline used by the parents who lead the family unit. It is shaped by the presence or absence of mutual support and esteem, and by the effectiveness of the communication between the leaders of the family unit. Leadership itself is quite complex, as seen in the work of Minuchin, who has tracked its migration between family members and generations depending on the particular mix of strengths, vulnerabilities, or developmental demands that are preoccupying the family at any given moment.

Family boundaries refer to boundaries a) within the individual that define the self, b) between generations, and c) between the family and the community. It is important that these boundaries be semipermeable, permitting contact and discourse with others outside the family boundary. Self- and generational boundaries remain relatively stable throughout the life cycle, whereas family/community boundaries must become increasingly permeable as children cross them with increasing frequency to participate in the community around them.

The emotional climate or affectivity of the family unit is the connective tissue that binds the family together as a functioning entity. It sustains—or erodes—the family's capacity to care for and support one another, especially since the family has ceased to be such a self-contained economic unit. Chronic scapegoating of a family member, child abuse, and neglect are classic signs of failure in the family's emotional climate.

Communication within families is verbal and nonverbal. Communicative language and its uses for deepening relationships are learned best within the family, assuming a healthy emotional climate. Experiences and affect are shared through the medium of language, whereas values and culture are differentiated and reinforced by the consistency, tone, and content of communication within the family.

Finally, the expectation that families will nurture and socialize their young so that they develop into contributing members of society is the moral obligation placed on these functions. The success or failure of this expectation is determined by the way the family achieves its goals for individual members and sets the members' tasks toward reaching those goals. Goals and tasks throughout the life cycle change and evolve in complex ways and, unlike communication or boundaries, seem not to diminish in significance over time.

Cultural influences powerfully shape the tasks of the family across the life span. As child-rearing domains become increasingly complex, it is essential that clinicians and researchers remain vigilant for the health-promoting cultural and functional forces that frame a particular family's expectations, strengths, and vulnerabilities in their context (26, 36–37). Values about dependability, family loyalty, intimacy, privacy, autonomy, and extended family access vary widely and normatively across the whole range of families created by adoption and assisted reproductive technologies (38–39).

Appreciating particular values in context is critical for the growing number of children raised in families with multiple cultural influences. Social and cultural isolation of such children and their parents can frustrate the resilience and strength so common in the families that cross-race adopt, or take a chance on a multiple fostered child, making their task unnecessarily more complex. Same-sex parenting partners and their children can experience conflict in certain communities stemming from the failure to appreciate such a family's contextual needs and competencies (40), rendering the children at greater risk in certain developmental stages, especially the transition to adolescence (41).

THE ARTS OF CHILD PSYCHIATRY

Now that we have defined the parameters of our task, we can look in greater detail at the skills that child psychiatrists rely on to help them accomplish their goals, and what if anything is contributed by an artful or humanistic approach to their work. Child psychiatry as a field has had a historical influence on the country's general attitudes toward the need of its children that is well out of proportion to its number of practitioners. Child psychiatrists figure so prominently in the creation of the fields of mental health consultation and crisis intervention that one is compelled to ask "Why them?" Why have they consistently held such seminal leadership positions in public policy, from the landmark Joint Commission on the Mental Health of Children in 1965 right up to the Neurons to Neighborhoods Report of the National Institutes of Medicine in 2002? Why did the nation's media turn to them so frequently for consultation and guidance following the events of 9/11/01? Why this trusted provenance in the wellbeing of all children, and not simply the mentally ill, from this medical subspecialty at the local and national level?

The OED's attempts at defining "art" are instructive in understanding this penchant for hard-headed soft-heartedness among child and adolescent psychiatrists. A "skill in doing anything as a result of knowledge or practice" suggests that medical training in and of itself prepares and predisposes these practitioners and researchers to embrace interdisciplinary thinking automatically. Such thinking is essential to understanding child development, as one is constantly juggling competing theories to understand a particular child and family's vulnerability, be it behavioral, psychodynamic, cognitive, or all of the above. So, when it comes to working with a team on an inpatient unit, a military base or in school consultation, it is already second nature to be informed by other "systems" of understanding. It is likewise second nature to be thinking differentially about case-based diagnostic and symptomatic material the moment it is reported, heard, read, or encountered.

Another OED definition of "art" reads "human workmanship as opposed to natural [ability]." The ability to listen with nonjudgmental patience, discriminating care and open mindedness to children's verbal and nonverbal communication is one of the hallmarks of this specialty's competence. So many of our young patients trust us because they feel heard by us. This skill at listening to behavior, symptoms, play, artwork, or rationalizations develops over time in the clinic, supervision, team meetings, emergency departments, the movie theater or the waiting room, and can eventually start to resemble a "knack." However, as a teacher and supervisor of hundreds of practitioners in this field for over three decades, I am more persuaded by the "work(wo)manship" argument for developing the "knack" than the "nature" one.

This very skill or "intellectual instrument" undergirds the child psychiatrists' reputation for being among the best interviewers in medicine, whether the subject be child or adult. The daily experience with children and their families shapes one's judgment over time about what to ask and when, in investigating and fathoming the child's distress. The clinician knows that questions are never simply queries, but rather conveyances of judgment, concern, comprehension, or indifference, depending on how and when they are asked, and how carefully they attend to the answers. It is in the art of the interview itself that the potentially caring/healing relationship is introduced and shaped, and the empathic apprehension of the skilled listener/observer is established, whether with an individual child/infant, parent, couple, or entire family system.

Outside the interviewing domain, however, child psychiatrists also respect and embrace the complexity of the context in which the child of concern lives his or her daily life. It is this appreciation for contextual symptom expression that makes them so useful to the institutions that serve the needs of children in the community, and such effective advocates for policies that increase care and wellbeing of society's most vulnerable; hence, their historical role in establishing mental health consultation in community agencies and schools (42, 43), and crisis intervention in the first place.

This contextual predilection for information also renders typical child psychiatrists slower than the average general practitioner to prescribe medications with the potential to change behavior, understanding as they do the power of context to influence behavior. The longer amount of time with the child and family utilized by the child psychiatrist may predispose toward this difference, but it remains more a perceptual than a time management issue.

Another perceptual distinction that defines the child psychiatrist's unique approach to understanding and studying mental health and illness is the enduring respect for the power of development to predispose to health. Child psychiatrists, therefore, habitually embed a child's clinical presentation into the proper era/context of child and family development.

Family development itself is usually arbitrarily divided into stages for better understanding of the predictable developmental phenomena typical of a certain era. This approach risks oversimplifying the complexity of the relationship system which expands or contracts to support the entrance, development, and exit of family members emotionally, culturally, and historically. I review these stages with an eye to the contributions made by the nurturers and the "nurturants," examining the unique and differing roles of mothers and fathers as participants and facilitators of normal development across the life cycle.

A DEVELOPMENTAL APPROACH

Coupling and Family Formation

The human pair responsible for nurturing the newborn brings conscious and unconscious motivations, both libidinal and aggressive, to their coalition. The choice of mate is governed by a web of intrinsic and experiential factors, tempered by the degree of separation from the family of origin.

Making a deliberate, conscious decision about family formation predisposes toward health, just as an unconscious, nonjoint decision predisposes to risk. One of the strongest unconscious motivations toward coupling is the wish to acquire in one's mate a longed-for or unfinished aspect of oneself. This can strongly predispose toward stability in a marriage. There is evidence to suggest that this may have an ameliorating effect on eventual family formation despite previous negative experiences, particularly on the part of the mother in her own childhood nurturing interactions. Eichberg has found in her research using the Adult Attachment Inventory that the father's role is positively ameliorative (44) of a mother's negative experience with her own parents (45).

When the coupling results in marriage, it is a joining of two complex historical, interpersonal, emotional, and economic systems. Couples are marrying later and postponing birthing their children: The average age of marriage for women in 2004 was 23.1 and for men 24.9 years, and the birth of their first child came on average 1 year and 11 months later. This implies there is a relatively short time given to adjusting to this phase in the life cycle. Sociologists show us there does seem to be a relatively narrow window for the timing of this phase. Women are twice as likely to divorce if they marry before the age of 20 years than if they marry during their 20s. They are half again as likely to divorce if they marry after 30 years of age than if they marry during their 20s (46). A variety of other factors also can contribute to difficulty at this life cycle transition: a) the couple resides at either great distance or close proximity to either family of origin; b) the couple meets or marries in close proximity to a significant loss; c) the couple marries after knowing each other for fewer than six months or an engagement lasting over three years; d) the wedding is performed without family or friends; and e) the wife becomes pregnant before or within the first year of marriage (47, 48). It does seem that the rise in women's socioeconomic and political status is correlated (though not necessarily causally) with some degree of marital destabilization and with the increasing, although not absolute, marital dissatisfaction of their husbands. We are clearly in a transition toward more egalitarian relationships, and the educational and occupational equity of the sexes can be a creative catalyst (49, 50).

How people are choosing partners and who they are choosing has also changed, as trends in miscegenation and same-sex partnerships show, which brings new challenges, strengths and stressors to the new family.

First Conception, Birth, and Nurturance

This era begins with conception and ends at the end of the child's first year. There is much psychological work to be done by both parents in preparing for and dealing with conception. There also is enormous variability in the amount of conscious deliberation devoted to the decision to conceive a child. Once conception does take place, planned or unplanned, complex psychological responses follow in both wife and husband. The mother struggles with profound changes occurring in her body during pregnancy and after delivery.

Meanwhile, much of the psychological work is fueled by a conscious reassessment of the couple's own family experience. A new identity begins to come to fruition, that of being a parent, not just having one (50). What makes this riveting is that both maternal and paternal identifications are deeply rooted in each individual. The mother prepares herself psychologically for the coming attachment to her infant by drawing her attention to her own inner experience and her growing fetus, as her preoccupation with the outside world decreases.

Fathers are involved in psychological work of a different sort, albeit active and equally important in terms of preparation. Food cravings, somatic preoccupations such as vague gastrointestinal disorders, and nutritional changes are widely reported. Concern about his adequacy as a provider and protector may erode an expectant father's self-esteem. Mood changes, frequently expected in mothers, also occur in fathers: "Even before the birth of his child, the father's life, his body, and his mind are busy making ready in ways of which he may only have a passing awareness (25)." Birth preparation classes may be helpful and supportive to both mothers and fathers in promoting a sense of mutual commitment and in explaining the universal pleasures and fears during the pregnancy and birth phase. Both mothers and fathers have complex mental images of their children long before the child sees the light of day.

But nothing is more powerful than the parental experience of the birth in terms of its long-term impact. First impressions are enormously powerful for both mothers and fathers. Attachment and bonding research has clearly articulated for us the importance of the mother–infant haptic and tactile involvement in the hours after birth. Fathers who are present at the birth are more verbal about their babies, more accurate in describing them, and more intimately attached to them at followup (26).

The newborn's job is no less important—though more complex neurobiologically—than that of the parents (51). The neonate must first stabilize and regulate his or her internal life to the point where he or she is able to perceive and respond to events in the external world by processing sensory, vestibular, and human interactional input (52). Next, the newborn must use his or her repertoire of skills and intrinsic reflexes to elicit sensitive nurturing experiences from the human world, which will make it possible for newborns to enter into the dynamic, reciprocating intimacies of relating pleasurably to their caregivers (53).

Finally, infants must make use of pleasurable experiences to communicate with the important objects in the world in a meaningful and intimate way so that they will be entertained, stimulated, fed, and have attendance to their bodily functions. Both mothers and fathers, whether or not they have prior experience, learn by on-the-job training to read, as well as anticipate, their infant's signals. Empathic connections and the capacity to comfort, soothe, woo, and entertain are tasks common to both mothering and fathering. Qualitative differences are present, however, in the idiosyncratic ways in which mothers and fathers respond (26). Mothers tend to respond to their babies on a more intimate scale, facilitating fine motor development and affective differentiation. Fathers tend to be more active and gross-motor involved. Nevertheless, as shown by Parke and Sawin, fathers were able to feed their babies as effectively and efficiently, although somewhat differently stylistically, as their spouses (all couples in the study were married) (54).

Infants appear quite interested in and responsive to the differences between paternal and maternal interactive styles (55). Yogman noted that by the time infants were eight weeks old, they were responding differently to their fathers and mothers (56). At six weeks, infants hunched their shoulders and lifted their eyebrows when their fathers appeared in their visual field. The same infants, when they saw or heard their mothers, seemed to expect more routine functional handling, such as feeding or diapering and became settled rather than animated.

The involvement in the first year of life of two caring and competent adults appears to have a positive effect on overall cognitive development. Pedersen et al. found that the more actively involved a six-month-old had been with his or her father, the higher the infant's scores on the Bailey test of mental and motor development (57). Also, Parke, in examining children over the first eight weeks of life, found that the more fathers were involved in everyday, repetitive, boring aspects of care, such as bathing, feeding, dressing, and diapering, the more socially responsive the infants were (54). It is in the mutual pleasures of this early experience that the adults, who have now moved up a generation and become caretakers to the younger generation, feel their own personal development frequently propelled forward to new levels of empathic—even altruistic—connections, not only with their children but also with other important objects in their lives.

Given these important health-promoting interactions in the first year of life, we are wise to take seriously the potential effects on the infant of time-sensitive adult vulnerabilities during this era, such as post-partum depression. Well known research documents the prevalence of maternal post-partum depression and its potentially negative effects, if untreated, on the infant. Critically important newer research draws our attention to the unexpectedly high incidence of paternal post-partum depression in fathers, once researchers began to investigate it. Untreated, this can further complicate comorbidity in the mother and potentially further threaten the infant's wellbeing in the first year (58).

Toddlerhood and Individuation within the Family

The child's astounding increase in mental and physical resources propels him or her out of the omnipotence of the first year of life into a much more social context, in which new skills permit more active shaping of the need-satisfying environment. The development of language, increasing sophistication in cognitive structures, mastery over motility and sphincters, and the incorporation of gender identity and gender role expectations all prepare the child for the complex sequences of the vital separation-individuation process (59). Parents are alternately challenged through intense clinging and contentious interchange, giving this era ambivalence as its marquee. Aggression, caretaking, love, anger, and sensuous intimacy are now part of the toddler's repertoire (37). This makes limit setting a vital companion to the toddler's adventurous experimentation with challenging, aggressive, and seductive behaviors. At the same time, the parent is wise to be led by the toddler, rather than attempt to lead the toddler (60). By now, fathering styles are quite differentiated from mothering styles of interaction, with fathers initiating more rough-and-tumble, unusual, unpredictable, physical, and stimulating forms of play. Biller and Meredith noted that mothers tended to engage in more conventional, toy-mediated play, picking up their children to engage in caretaking and nurturing activities more than fathers (61).

The child's increased level of mastery over the internal environment makes more energy available to explore the boundaries of the external environment, giving separation tasks a much higher valence during waking life. Adjustments to the toddler's new, if clumsy, drive for autonomy are necessary to avoid prolonging the child's functional dependency. Because separation from the mother sometimes is the fuel for the sleep disturbances that are common during the second year of life, the father can help decrease the virulence of nighttime disruption by being the one who goes in to soothe and settle the child, sparing the child from another separation from the mother, while helping the child feel safe and secure.

Clearly, the child's unique temperament and style interact with parental values and experience with regard to personal autonomy, separateness from family of origin, and impulse and bodily control. The unique contributions of the father during these years have been increasingly recognized as vital to the success of this developmental era (62).

The Preschooler

The preschool child's appropriate use of personal pronouns, ability to say "no," and increasingly adaptive capacities all draw the family as a whole further into a new domain that will be characterized by the time the stage is complete, by three-party rather than two-party relationships. Curiosity, assertiveness, and the capacity to begin to delay gratification help the child regulate and moderate intense instinctual feelings and affects. Cognitive growth, meanwhile, assists the child in learning and remembering what the important objects in his or her life will or will not tolerate. By the beginning of this phase, parents should have largely discarded baby talk because both the child and the parents can have a more satisfactory communicative interaction. Reasonably adept parents are able to respond with affection, empathy, and a minimum of rejection to the preschool child's bid for intimate, controlling attention from the parent of the opposite sex. Appropriate, predictable limit setting and humor play important roles in helping the child and parent withstand the heavy weather of strong rivalrous feelings. By now, parents are able to yield most control over bodily functions to the child, relinquishing him or her as a physical possession, and admiring and encouraging his or her attributes as a separate, gender-specific human being who is beginning to understand the joys of the delay of gratification. During these preschool years, fathers interact with their children mainly through play and productivity. Through role modeling, the father provides opportunities for children of both sexes to build increasingly positive self-esteem (63).

The press of developmental needs during this period, highlighted in research, shows us a critical relationship between marital satisfaction and parental involvement. There is much research that indicates marital satisfaction to be at its lowest ebb during the childbearing years (64). Waldron and Routh note that marital satisfaction follows a U-shaped graph, with high levels of marital comfort before children are born and again after they leave home (65). Frequently, children place such significant demands on the couple that there is little energy left to fuel the marital relationship, although it is not suggested that children destroy marriages (even though in some instances they may be permitted or even encouraged to do so). Rapoport et al. report that marriage often is experienced by fathers as better than by mothers during this nadir of marital satisfaction because it is mothers who usually have more negative experiences with their children, feel more isolated, and are more vulnerable to psychosomatic stress ailments, including fatigue (66).

Although the discrepancies between maternal and paternal experience during this phase of the life cycle can be problematic, including occasional envy and jealousy on the part of the parent who is having the more difficult and challenging time with the preschool child, the long-term effects of having both parents involved intimately during this phase are strongly positive. One of the most dramatic findings in the father-infant care research is the relationship between early involvement and subsequent sexual abuse. If a man is involved in the physical care of his child before the age of three years, there is a dramatic drop in the probability that man will be involved later on in life with sexual abuse of his own or anyone else's children (67).

School Age and Family Unity

The timely differentiation of the child–parent relationship from interdependent dyad to more intergenerational autonomy allows the child to make powerful psychological investments in nonparental adults other than his or her own parents, initiating the first disillusionment in one's parents. Just as the child's body is relinquished from parental control, so is the child's mind. The family now helps the child separate for most of his or her waking hours to attend school and confront social and cognitive challenges. Interest seems to grow exponentially in relating to other children and adults, as well as for learning and problem solving. License must be granted for further exploration; at the same time, limits are placed in a reasonable, comfortable manner. The integration of family and tradition, as guided by societal mythology, serves as the hallmark of this period of development. Themes of internal control begin to compete with the pursuit of pleasure as the integrated seven- or eight-year-old strives for balance. During this period, it often is easier for a family to spend prolonged, uninterrupted segments of time with one another for travel, leisure activities, and neighborhood projects. Interestingly, girls may have only one or two friends they would call "best," whereas boys may name six or seven friends, who usually turn out to be somewhat more casual acquaintances. But during the school-age period, a father may serve as a confidant, a pal, even a friend or teacher (68). The opportunity for shared activities and mastery experiences with adults of the same sex is extremely important in terms of the solidification of gender role behavior and gender identity itself. Father absence, however (69), leads teachers to rate both boys and girls as more aggressive relative to mother–father families. Especially poignant was the finding that the protective factors for mother–father families were not as apparent among low-income families.

Adolescence and Generational Redefinition

Families of adolescents must use boundaries that are qualitatively different from those in families with younger children. The boundaries must now assist the children in managing their own impulses because parents no longer have as much authority as they once enjoyed. The boundaries between the family and the outside world must become more permeable without being destroyed. There is a normal careening between independence and dependence. A sense of self is beginning to be consolidated and shaped by values, the search for pleasure, and particular goals and tasks that sometimes stretch far out into the future and other times are immediate and impulsively sought.

The primary object relationship between the parents and the teenager now must be retooled for the transition from childhood to adulthood. The teenager is involved in a regular, normative struggle between independence and dependence. The adolescent also is becoming intensely interested in his or her constantly changing body. Previously accepted family values and "do unto others as they would have them do unto you" beliefs more typical of middle childhood are now subjected to greater scrutiny.

Developmental stress does not necessarily doom the family to turmoil during this phase, but profound physical and psychological changes threaten the previous level of homeostasis in the family. Adolescents notice weaknesses and vulnerabilities in their family, as well as in their own psychological functioning, but these may also be seen as possible points of departure for new adaptive functioning; this uncertainty as to where strengths and weaknesses lie, and intergenerational disagreement about the relevance of the strength or weakness, can lead to significant disputes. But adolescent observations are notoriously selective. Bulimic teenagers and young adults rated their fathers as showing less affection and more control toward them than their nonbulimic siblings, suggesting that the paternal relationship may be a source of nonshared environmental experience associated with bulimia nervosa (70).

Adolescence often is a period of significant stress in the family because both the adolescents and their parents are often experiencing physiologic and mental changes at the same time. Both generations may be scrutinizing their primary attachments anew and questioning their value and trustworthiness. Just as the adolescent is beginning to make choices regarding values and career goals at the beginning of his or her work life, the parents are needing to accept that certain cherished goals may never be achieved, and they may become quite preoccupied by the limited time left in their lives.

As the adolescent begins to pull further away from the nurturing domain through going to college or taking a full-time job, the parental response can be one of either pride in their child's capacity to cope with life's new challenges or sadness over what appears to be the permanent loss of one's own progeny. The family as a whole can have its homeostatic behavior deeply challenged by an adolescent's need to extract his or her autonomy from the parental nurturing domain.

Young adulthood and emancipation, the marriage of offspring (the middle family), and, finally, aging and senescence are the last three phases of normal family development. The kind of influence parents now have on their children is largely encompassed by their availability for discussion and advice and by bearing witness to their children's integrity, while being careful to plan and sustain their own autonomy. Grandchildren may come next, providing a rejuvenation of spirit and body, not to mention occasions of joy. The relaxations of retirement, the consolidation of the family around oneself as a patriarch or matriarch, and finally, the privileges and honor of the emeritus round out the pleasurable tableau of the senior family era.

The developmental tasks faced by the child and the child's caregivers are the same whether the structure of the family is nuclear or reconstituted. The energy and resources, both emotional and physical, to attend to those tasks are ["energy and resources ... are"] strongly influenced, however, by a particular family's structural limits and flexibility. Adoptive, single-parent, foster, and recombined family groupings are all subject to the same leadership, boundary, affectivity, communicative, and task and goal requirements. The issues of attachment, separation, emancipation, loss, and response to change are largely the same. Each exerts its own particular spin on normal development, but none is doomed to trouble by dint of family structure alone.

Adoptive families do not have the same biological preparation time, although given hard work, supportive professionals to encourage and nurture them, and some measure of good fortune, they can follow a similar psychological preparation sequence. The separate biological parents' narrative must be integrated into the family's mental history of itself in some fashion. Single-parent families, whether male- or female-headed, face depletion and isolation early and often and work best when social and medical support systems are available early and are flexible enough to supplement parental needs and childcare.

Recombined and reconstituted families—when a divorced, widowed, or never-married single parent forms a household with a new partner who may or may not be a parent—are also increasing exponentially. Depending on the mechanism of parental singleness (death, divorce, abandonment), the new parent may be seen as a threat or solution to intimacy between parent and child. Rivalry and jealousy frequently stimulate guilt and anxiety, especially when the same-sex parent has been displaced or replaced. Interestingly, Black and Pedro-Carroll have shown that the effects of interparental conflict on the psychological wellbeing of children were mediated more by the overall quality of parent–child relationships than by interadult conflict itself (71). Stepparents frequently are in risk situations, being tested by their "new children" while simultaneously feeling special loyalty to their "old children" and trying to sustain a new spousal relationship. Time (measured in years), patience, and liberal, frequent communication (sometimes new to everyone as a process) plus permission to parent are all essential. Society's myths do not help, either. *Stepmother* in English conjures up Cinderella's stepmother, and stepfather in Spanish is *padrastro*, which also means hangnail. On a smaller scale, all families face some of the same issues because families are always reconstituting, biologically and psychologically. Because of the relentless push of developmental and maturational forces in the individuals of our species, like the river, one can never step into one family in the same place twice.

AN INVITATION ACCEPTED

As we review these developmental trajectories for families, we are reminded of the parallel processes at work in the developmental trajectory of the career of the child psychiatrist. How is the art of the practice itself woven over time into the child psychiatrist's personal growth and development? Their own personal context shapes their practice, and their personal attitude toward it, in countless ways. For example, they do or do not become parents themselves, struggling with the same universal doubts, joys, slings and arrows of either path. I have heard my students wish aloud that they could revise some old piece of advice given or judgment made through the lens of their own personal experience of parenting or not. On the other hand, those who do have children may at times carry special burdens of self-doubt as the useless "expert" when they have no clue about how to help their own distressed offspring or despairing spouse manage some interpersonal or intrapsychic skirmish.

Child psychiatrists struggle with their own health issues, emotional and physical, suffer personal losses, and experience their own 15 minutes of fame, all the while trying to listen with great patience, when they are occasionally feeling unheard themselves. This is one of the compelling reasons that supervision and collegial support throughout one's professional life should be the rule, not the exception.

This is especially germane if the clinician holds to the standard "do unto others as you would have them do unto you." Highly desirable as this standard may be, it occasions personal depletion at a rapid clip. A lifelong trajectory of repletion through reflective supervision, continuing education, restorative play (mental and physical), and diversion will protect and preserve that knack for listening for meaning in what matters to our patients and their families.

For myself, I have grown less judgmental, softer, and I hope more effective and efficient with age. I am freer with my humor and compassion, and more grateful for what I have learned from my patients' shared experiences in our work together. I assume from the beginning that my patients—child and family—are doing the best they can, regardless of how troubled the results may at first appear.

At the same time, I somehow feel more demanding of myself and my patients, trusting our skills and creativities more than I did at the beginning of my career, when I thought life would somehow be more perfectible. Innovations seem to arise in more and more cases, partly as a function of the extraordinary pace of science's advance in this field. In fact, as I reflect on the beginning of my career, I wonder if we as a medical specialty got so good at asking questions because there were so few answers; this may be less the case today with the arrival of each new issue of our journals. In fact, it is hard to imagine a medical specialty with a broader intellectual horizon (a strong recruitment talking point whenever I get the chance).

That is precisely why I am simultaneously enthusiastic about and concerned for the current preoccupation with evidence-based medicine. On one hand, it will upgrade the quality of evidence that we use and generate, and upon which we rely to make diagnoses and develop treatment plans. On the other, "evidence" in isolation falls short of helping the clinician "do the right thing" because the patient's needs are embedded in the complex context of their culture-specific, value-laden, intergenerational "system" of beliefs and hopes [as are the clinicians!]. Few have said it better than Jeree Pawl (72):

> We learn over time that everything we think we know is a hypothesis; that we have ideas, but that we don't have truth. We learn that those [patients] with whom we work have all of the information we need, and that this is what we will work with. When we know this, our attitude conveys it; and the child and family sense themselves as sources, not objects. In this context, they become aware of a mutual effort. They do not feel weighed, measured or judged. They do feel listened to, seen and appreciated.

References

1. Tiernari P, Wynne LC, Sorri A, et al.: Genotype-environment interaction in schizophrenia-spectrum disorder: Long-term follow-up of Finnish adoptees. *Brit J Psychia* 184:216–222, 2004.
2. Caspi A, Sugden K, Moffitt TE, et al.: Influence of life stress on depression: moderation by a polymorphism in the 5_HTT gene. *Science* 301: 386–389, 2003.
3. Kaufman J, Yang BZ, Douglas-Palumberi H, et al.: Brain-derived neurotrophic factor-5-HTTLPR gene interaction and environmental modifiers of depression in children. *Biol Psychiatry* 59:958–965, 2006.
4. Sroufe LA, Egeland B, Carlson E, et al.: *The Development of the Person: Minnesota Study of Risk and Adaptation from Birth to Adulthood.* New York, Guilford Press, 2005.
5. Hechtman L, ed.: *Do They Grow Out of It? Long-term Outcomes of Childhood Disorders.* Washington DC, American Psychiatric Press, 1996.
6. Spitz RA: *The First Year of Life: A Psychoanalytic Study of Normal and Deviant Development of Object Relations.* New York, International Universities Press, 1965.
7. Pincus L, Dare C: *Secrets in the Family.* New York, Pantheon, 1978.
8. Vangelisti AL: Family secrets: forms, functions, and correlates. *J Social Pers Relationships* 11:113–135, 1994.
9. Ainsworth M, Eichberg C: Effects on infant–mother attachment of mother's unresolved loss of an attachment figure or other traumatic experience. In: Morris P, Parks C, Hinde R (eds): *Attachment Across the Life Cycle.* New York: Routledge Press, 1991, pp. 160–186.
10. Borkowski J, Ramey S: *Parenting and the Child's World: Influences on Academic, Intellectual and Socioeconomic Development.* New York, Erlbaum Press, 2001.
11. Bowen M: *Family Therapy in Clinical Practice.* New York, Aronson, 1978.
12. Wamboldt M, Wamboldt F: Role of the family in the onset and outcome of childhood disorders: selected research findings. *J Am Acad Child Adolesc Psychiatry* 39:1212–1219, 2000.
13. Demos J: *A Little Commonwealth: Family Life in Plymouth Colony.* New York, Oxford University Press, 1970.
14. Laslette P, Wall R, eds: *Household and Family in Past Time.* Cambridge, Cambridge University Press, 1972.
15. Hareven T: American families in transition: historical perspectives on change. In: Walsh F. (ed): *Normal Family Processes.* New York: Guilford, 1982, pp. 446–466.
16. Griswold R: *Fatherhood in America: A History.* New York, Basic Books, 1993.
17. Achenbach T, Howell C: Are American children's problems getting worse? A 13-year comparison. *J Am Acad Child Adolesc Psychiatry* 32:1145–1154, 1993.
18. Galinsky E: Family life and corporate policies. In: Yogman M, Brazelton B, (eds): *In Support of Families.* Cambridge, MA: Harvard University Press, 1986.
19. U.S. Bureau of Labor Statistics report, National Survey of Parents as Wage-Earners, 2003.
20. Sameroff A, Fiese B: The developmental ecology of early intervention. In: Shonkoff J, Meisels S (eds): *Handbook of Early Childhood Intervention.* 2nd ed. New York: Cambridge University Press, 2000, pp. 135–159.
21. George C, Kaplan N, Main M: *The Berkeley Adult Attachment Interview.* Berkeley, CA: University of California, Department of Psychology, 1985.
22. Main M, Kaplan N, Cassidy J: Security in infancy, childhood and adulthood: a move to the level of representation. *Monogr Soc Res Child Dev* 50:66–104, 1985.
23. Bezirganian S, Cohen P, Brook J: The impact of mother–child interaction on the development of borderline personality disorder. *Am J Psychiatry* 150:1836–1842, 1993.
24. Pruett K: Infants of primary nurturing fathers. *Psychoanal Study Child* 40:257–277, 1983.
25. Pruett K: *The Nurturing Father.* New York, Warner, 1987.
26. Pruett K: *Fatherneed: Why Father Care Is as Essential as Mother Care for Your Child.* New York, Free Press, 2000.
27. Radin N, Harold-Goldsmith R: The involvement of selected unemployed and employed men with their children. *Child Dev* 60;454–459, 1989.
28. Lamb M: *The Role of the Father in Child Development*, 3rd ed. New York, John Wiley & Sons, 1997.
29. Yeung W, Sandberg J, Davis-Kean P, Hofferth S: Children's time with fathers in intact families. *J Marriage and Family* 63:136–154, 2000.
30. Lieb R, Wittchen H, Hofler M, et al.: Parental psychopathology, parenting styles, and the risk of social phobia in offspring. *Arch Gen Psychiatry* 57:859–865, 2000.
31. Phares V, Compas BE: The role of fathers in child and adolescent psychopathology: make room for daddy. *Psychol Bull* 111:387–412, 1992.
32. Werner E: Protective factors and individual resilience. In: Shonkoff J, Meisels S, (eds).: *Handbook of Early Childhood Intervention*, 2nd ed. New York: Cambridge University Press, 2000.
33. Skinner HA, Steinhauer PD, Santa-Barbara J: The Family Assessment Measure. *Can J Ment Health* 2:91–105, 1983.
34. Mrazek D, Mrazek P, Klinnert M: Clinical assessment of parenting. *J Am Acad Child Adolesc Psychiatry* 34:272–282, 1995.
35. Fleck S, ed: *Psychiatric Prevention and the Family Life Cycle.* New York, Brunner/Mazel, 1989.
36. Johnson-Powell G, Yamamoto J, eds: *Transcultural Child Development.* New York, John Wiley & Sons, 1997.
37. Pruett K: *Me, Myself and I; How Children Build Their Sense of Self.* New York, Goddard, 1999.
38. Coll C, Magnuson K: Cultural differences as sources of developmental vulnerabilities and resources. In: Shonkoff J, Meisels J (eds).: *Handbook of Early Childhood Intervention*, 2nd ed. New York: Cambridge, 2000.
39. Rey J, Peng R, Morales-Blanquez C, et al.: Rating the quality of family environment in different cultures. *J Am Acad Child Adolesc Psychiatry* 39:1168–1174, 2000.
40. D'Augelli A, Patterson C: *Lesbian, Gay, and Bisexual Identities over the Lifespan: Psychological Perspectives.* New York, Oxford University Press, 1995.
41. Lock J, Steiner H: Gay and lesbian, and bisexual youth risks for emotional, physical, and social problems: results from a community-based survey. *J Am Acad Child Adolesc Psychiatry* 38:297–304, 1999.
42. Pruett K and Cotton P: The affective experience of residency training in community psychiatry. *Am J Psychiatry* 132(3);57–63, 1975.
43. Pruett K: Home treatment of two infants who witnessed their mother's murder. *J Amer Acad Child Psychiatry* 18:647–658, 1979.
44. Eichberg C: Quality of infant–parent attachment: related to mother's representation of her own relationship history. Presented at the meeting of the Society for Research in Child Development; 1987 Apr 19–22; Baltimore, MD.
45. Main M, Goldwyn R: Adult attachment classification system. In: Main M, (ed).: *A Typology of Human Attachment Organization: Assessed in Discourse, Drawings and Interviews.* New York, Cambridge University Press, 1992.
46. Glick P, Norton A: Marrying, divorcing, and living together in the US today. *Pop Bull* 38:3–38, 1978.
47. Bacon L: Early motherhood, accelerated role transition and social pathologies. *Soc Forces* 52:333–341, 1974.
48. Becker G: Economics of marital instability. *J Polit Econ* 85:1141–1187, 1987.
49. Burke R, Weir T: The relationships of wives' employment status to husband, wife and peer satisfaction. *J Marriage Fam* 2:279–287, 1976.
50. Cowan C, Cowan P: *When Partners Become Parents.* Mahwah, New Jersey, Earlbaum Associates Publishers, 2000.
51. Shonkoff J: Neurons to Neighborhoods, *National Institutes of Medicine* 2002.
52. Ramey C, Ramey S: *Right from Birth.* New York, Goddard Press, 1999.
53. Leckman J, Mayes L: Primary parental preoccupation: circuits, genes, and the crucial role of the environment, *J Neural Trans* 111:753–771, 2004.

54. Parke R, Sawin D: Infant characteristics and behavior as elicitors of maternal and paternal responsiveness in the newborn period. Presented at the meeting of the Society for Research in Child Development; 1975 Apr 17–20; Denver, CO.
55. Feldman R: Infant–mother and infant–father synchrony: the co-regulation of positive arousal. *Infant Mental Health J* 24:1–23, 2003.
56. Yogman M: Development of the father–infant relationship. In: Fitzgerald G, Lester F, Yogman M, (eds.): *Theory and Research in Behavioral Pediatrics* New York, Plenum, 1:221–297, 1982.
57. Pedersen F, Rubinstein J, Yarrow L: Infant development in father-absent families. *J Genet Psychol* 135:51–61, 1979.
58. Ramchandani P, Stein A, Evans J, O'Connor T: Paternal depression in the postnatal period and child development: a prospective longitudinal study. *Lancet* 365:2158–2159, 2005.
59. Zeanah C, Larrieu J, Heller S: Developmental assessment of infants and toddlers. In: Zeanah C, (ed.): *Handbook of Infant Mental Health*, 2nd ed. New York, Guilford Press, 2000.
60. Lieberman A: *The Emotional Life of the Toddler*. New York, Free Press, 1993.
61. Biller H, Meredith D: *Father Power*. New York, David McKay, 1974.
62. Greenspan S: The second other: the role of the father in early personality formation and the dyadic-phallic phase of development. In: Cath S, Gurwitt A, Ross JM, (eds.): *Father and Child: Developmental and Clinical Perspectives*. Boston, Little, Brown, 1982.
63. Sarnoff C: The father's role in latency. In: Cath S, Gurwitt A, Ross J, (eds.): *Father and Child: Developmental and Clinical Perspectives*. Boston, Little, Brown, 1982.
64. Glenn G, McLanahan S: Children and marital happiness: a further specification of the relationship. *J Marriage Fam* 44:63–72, 1982.
65. Waldron H, Routh D: The effect of the first child on the marital relationship. *J Marriage Fam* 43:785–788, 1981.
66. Rapoport R, Rapoport R, Strelitz Z: *Fathers, Mothers and Society*. New York, Basic Books, 1977.
67. Parker H, Parker S: Cultural roles, rituals and behavior regulation. *Am Anthropol* 86:584–600, 1984.
68. Benson L: *Fatherhood: A Sociological Perspective*. New York, Random House, 1968.
69. Pearson JL, Ialongo NS, Hunter AG, et al.: Family structure and aggressive behavior in a population of urban elementary school children. *J Am Acad Child Adolesc Psychiatry* 33:540–548, 1994.
70. Wonderlich S, Ukestad L, Perzacki R: Perceptions of nonshared childhood environment in bulimia nervosa. *J Am Acad Child Adolesc Psychiatry* 33:140–141, 1994.
71. Black A, Pedro-Carroll J: Role of parent–child relationship in mediating the effects of marital disruption. *J Am Acad Child Adolesc Psychiatry* 32:1019–1027, 1993.
72. Pawl J: The interpersonal center of the work that we do. *Zero to Three* 20(4):5–7, 2000.

CHAPTER 1.2 ■ PREVAILING AND SHIFTING PARADIGMS: A HISTORICAL PERSPECTIVE

DAVID F. MUSTO

INTRODUCTION

Child psychiatry is itself in its youth as a profession. During the first decades of the twentieth century, it emerged as a subspecialty of adult psychiatry even as that field was becoming established. Essential to the growth of child psychiatry was the acceptance by both the medical professions and society at large of the concept of childhood as a distinct period of human life, with characteristic stages from infancy through adolescence into young adulthood. Although there is some debate on the exact nature of concepts of childhood before the seventeenth century (1), by the nineteenth century, parents, educators, and legislators as well as the medical profession began to view children as in need of special protections and considerations in order to become healthy adults. The separation of childhood years as a focus of study and treatment accelerated near the end of the nineteenth century. Childhood (including adolescence) became an attractive subject of investigation, and many disciplines enlisted in the study of childhood's special characteristics, needs, disabilities, and therapies. As in the case of general psychiatry, psychologists, pediatricians, educators, and social workers all contributed to the intellectual and scientific foundations of child psychiatry.

Whether the techniques and discoveries of the new field could be expected to mold the child as he or she developed, or if behavior and personality were largely fixed by heredity, has been a source of constant controversy for centuries. In the eighteenth century, John Locke argued that, at birth, the human mind was a blank slate. This idea, supposing as it did that there was no such thing as hereditary privilege, subverted aristocratic claims of divine right and had far-reaching political and social consequences—not the least of which was our own Declaration of Independence, based on the notion that "all men are created equal." Belief in the power of environmental forces on individual development continued into the nineteenth century, though not without criticism. Severe mental illness, for example, was increasingly seen as hereditary and pretty much hopeless. Gregor Mendel's discoveries lent experimental evidence to the idea that traits were heritable and to some degree predictable. How to affect heredity in order to improve society (eugenics) was a puzzle, but in time the political, social, and scientific ramifications of hereditarian ideas were as significant as Locke's contrary faith in the malleability of the mind's tabula rasa. The debate between proponents of biological determinism (nature) and supporters of environmental explanations (nurture) for normative as well as deviant behavior among children has been with us in one form or another since the beginning of the psychiatric profession.

GS HALL AND NORMATIVE DEVELOPMENT

Two broad channels of research have merged into the creation of child psychiatry: first, the investigation of normative child development, as in education and psychological maturation; and second, the investigation of emotional disturbance and forms of disability. In the area of normative development, the leading figure in the United States at the end of the nineteenth century was G. Stanley Hall, a pioneer psychologist and educator (2). Hall engaged in a wide variety of investigations on behavior and psychological stages as part of what has been called the "child study movement." One technique he adopted was to send out questionnaires to see what children at various ages had learned and what they appeared capable of learning. He was interested in activities of children and in the attitudes of their parents and teachers. The questionnaire method was not an accurate device but for the time represented progress toward a scientific basis of child development. The range of Hall's topical syllabi, as he termed them in the journals Pedagogical Seminary and the American Journal of Psychology (which Hall founded), was extensive. Topics included "Anger," "Some Common Traits and Habits," "Thoughts and Feelings about Old Age," "The Teaching Instinct," and "Educational Ideals." The syllabi were one to four pages each and distributed to appropriate target groups such as teachers or children. Those returned were tabulated and the statistics reported. Other educators also employed the questionnaire method; one was Margaret E. Schallenberger, who in 1894 published results of an interesting inquiry into moral judgment. Schallenberger suggested that at about nine years of age children shift from a morality of consequences to a morality of intentions, an anticipation of more recent work on the moral and mental development of children (3).

An important feature of the child study movement is the simple fact of affirming sequential development from infancy to adulthood. When normal development could be described, the stage was set for more accurate accounts of deviation from the normal, lags in development, and finding lacunae in the broad front of development. Hall believed that the stages of development recapitulated the evolution of mankind (that, for example, adolescence is the "heroic age" of chivalry and derring-do), and that the inevitable unfolding of this developmental sequence is the foundation of all child study (4).

Several developments in American society, especially the perceived need for lengthier education in a work world characterized by growing bureaucracy and the requirement for business literacy, indirectly stimulated this emphasis on childhood and adolescence. Thus, not surprisingly, the child study movement had its greatest impact among educators, not academic psychologists. Some have suggested this appeal to educators was due to the improved status accorded the teacher when attention was focused on the schoolchild. The rising enrollment and actual attendance at high schools and the significance attached to teaching the majority of children through mid-adolescence made understanding the norms of youth fundamental to education policy and practice. Hence, child study and other approaches to the rules of development were of direct value to educators. Meanwhile these studies were not only of practical value to society but also touched on the more abstract understanding of human nature.

A series of professionals who have offered advice on child rearing, including Hall's student, Arnold Gesell, and Benjamin Spock, a student although not an adherent of Gesell's, trace the beginnings of their careers to Hall. In addition, new youth groups were modeled after the kind of analysis Hall had made in his massive, two-volume study Adolescence, published in 1904 (5). The Boy and Girl Scout movement in the period around World War I were intended to harmonize with the child's specific stages of development. Thus a stream of child development arose directed not at the disturbed or abnormal individual but toward the improvement and understanding of the average child growing up in American society. Again, the readers of this literature were commonly parents and teachers, rather than physicians or academicians.

ENVIRONMENT, HEREDITY AND PARENTAL BEHAVIOR

In the late nineteenth century, child development study began to focus on deviancy, coinciding with a trend in both popular and scientific thought that had its origins in darwinian concepts of evolutionary "progress"—the idea that both healthy development and pathology were based on genetics, and that reproduction among individuals thought to be the most fit would contribute to the betterment of mankind. Of course, Hall and similar researchers were interested in both normality and pathology, so a sharp demarcation cannot be drawn between the two areas of research, but centers increasingly established themselves as primarily concerned with juvenile delinquency, with the retarded, or with a study of emotional stresses or hereditary "defects" that might account for mental disorder.

A cluster of beginnings important to the history of child psychiatry started in 1896 and continued until 1924. In 1896, at the University of Pennsylvania, Lightner Witmer instituted a clinic chiefly devoted to the mentally retarded child; in 1909, William Healy established the Juvenile Psychopathic Institute in Chicago, which advised the juvenile court on the diagnoses of offenders; and in 1924 the American Orthopsychiatric Association (AOA) was established, which brought together the disciplines comprising psychiatric diagnosis and treatment of children with the professionals involved in child guidance: psychiatrists, psychologists, social workers, and the judiciary (6, 7). These three events symbolize the broad advance in the understanding and treatment of psychiatrically ill and mentally retarded children, which has continued to the present.

This was the period during which ideas now known as eugenics became prevalent in both scientific inquiries and popular culture, and powerful forces promoted reform of all sorts of social ills that were supposed to have deleterious effects on future generations of Americans. The drive to suppress alcohol consumption was just one aspect of this reformist atmosphere, but perhaps the one with the most profound effect on attitudes toward children and the consequences of parental behavior. Whether or not alcohol consumption affected the health of the developing fetus—or even its genetic structure—and thus the mental development of the child was a subject of heated controversy. Intense fear of the personal and social effects of alcohol pervaded society, and the belief in a safe threshold of alcohol use faded under an onslaught of real and pseudoscience, emotional public campaigns and single-issue politics. Even the smallest amount of alcohol was thought dangerous, for it did at least a little damage and could lead to further drinking and start the experimenter down the road to alcoholism.

Ordinary science, the kind found in peer-reviewed journals, supported the concern over alcohol, especially when a fetus or young children were involved. Researchers studied animals and found that alcohol had a deleterious effect on offspring of mice, rats, and guinea pigs. These studies indicated that alcohol could damage not only the fetus, especially in its early stages of development, but could permanently change the individual's genetics, so that damage in one generation would be transmitted to later generations. One scientist who provided this worrisome information was Dr. Charles Stockard, Professor of Anatomy at Cornell Medical School. In 1916 he reported his conclusion, after a study of guinea pigs, that:

> ...the experiments show the hereditary transmission through several generations of conditions resulting from an artificially induced change in the germ cells of one generation by treating them with alcohol (8).

Stockard's research was taken up by persons dealing with humans and quickly applied. A New York pediatrician wrote the next year on "Disease conditions in older babies that can be attributed to prenatal influences." Stockard's work and that of other laboratory workers and the observations quoted from clinicians would suggest that "cases of retarded development in older children, nervous and irritable conditions, epilepsy, and the various forms of infantilism and idiocy, are in many cases the result of alcoholism in one or both of the parents before conception or possibly of alcoholism in the grandparents or great-grandparents" (9).

A 1905 survey of school children in New York City showed that 53% of children of drinking parents were "dullards," while only 10% of 13,523 children of abstainers were "dullards" (10). A 1916 study of families showed that alcoholism in a given generation was followed "in the next two to three generations by epilepsy, imbecility, stillbirth, infant death, chorea and tremor" (11).

A contrary position was presented, most notably by the biometrician Karl Pearson, who studied schoolchildren and their parents, among other subjects, and concluded that parental alcohol use was not linked to defects in their offspring (12). Needless to say, the vast majority of writers on the subject attacked him, and even John Maynard Keynes wrote a refutation of Pearson's methods in the Journal of the Royal Statistical Society (13).

A second doubter was Henry H. Goddard, the renowned Director of Research at the Vineland Training School in New Jersey. Strongly disagreeing that alcoholism was a cause of feeblemindedness, he was surprised "that anyone could have reasoned so falsely" (14). Goddard found that the retardation observed in the families he studied could be accounted for by heredity and accidents, including disease in the child and mother. Goddard had made a famous study of the Kallikak family, a large group of related persons who were marked by retardation, antisocial behavior and poverty (15). He concluded that here too the cause was heredity that perpetuated feeblemindedness over several generations. His research bolstered the Supreme Court decision in 1927 that permitted sterilization of the mentally defective because, as Supreme Court Justice Oliver Wendell Holmes remarked, "Three generations of imbeciles are enough" (16).

The general attitude of writers on alcohol in the era just before national prohibition was summed up by Dr. Alfred Gordon, Professor of Physiology at Jefferson Medical School, when, in 1911, he warned that alcoholism "leads to a degeneration not only of the individual, but also of the species, to depopulation; it is dangerous to society as it produces a slow and progressive deterioration of the individual and an intellectual and physical sterility of the race (17)..."

This is echoed in a social scientist's warning from 1913:

> To sociologists it is evident that the question of maternal inebriety is one of national importance, for many women fail to realize that alcohol taken in small amounts, if taken every day, may have serious results (18).

Coincidentally with Goddard's work at Vineland, Witmer, at the University of Pennsylvania, and Walter Fernald, in Boston, concentrated on the problems of the mentally deficient. One of the earliest goals of these pioneers was to be able to measure degrees of mental deficiency. Through them, the intelligence tests that have become such a familiar aspect of life in America for the school-aged child were introduced. The mental tests of Binet and Simon were translated from the French, and variations were introduced in the transition to indigenous American tests for intelligence, of which the Scholastic Aptitude Tests and the Weschler Adult Intelligence Scale are contemporary examples (19).

WILLIAM HEALY AND "ENVIRONMENTALISM"

Dr. William Healy's leadership in the treatment of wayward children illustrates the commitment of a different group of professionals to understanding child development in the context of social environment. Several distinguished individuals in Chicago were interested in the problems of disadvantaged children who were referred to the justice system because of criminal acts. Prominent among those persons who brought Dr. Healy out of a neurology practice to a much more psychologically informed investigation of juvenile delinquents were Ethel S. Dummer, a philanthropist, Julia Lathrop, later the first head of the U.S. Children's Bureau (1912), and Jane Addams, social worker and founder of Hull House in Chicago, where the planning meetings were held for what would become the first juvenile court clinic. These individuals persuaded Healy to inform himself, through travel and study, on the best techniques for understanding and treating youthful offenders.

With the strong concurrence of Juvenile Court Judge Pinckney, who acknowledged the need for more information on the psychology of the offenders who stood before him, the Juvenile Psychopathic Institute was founded in April 1909. Dr. Healy eventually thought the title, which implied that "serious antisocial behavior betokened something pathological in the offender" was in error and reflected the attitude of organic causation, which he was to fight for the remainder of his life. Like Ethel Dummer, who had long believed in the importance of external events on mental life (20), Dr. Healy came to espouse a strong environmentalist approach to childhood emotional disturbance. He was deeply antagonistic to the prevalent views of such criminologists as Lombroso, who found criminal tendencies and degeneracy to be based on the heredity and constitutional elements in a person's body. To Healy, Lathrop, Addams, and Dummer, the misery of the slums was a more likely—and correctable—cause of crime than an inevitable biological makeup.

Dummer's five-year grant to maintain the Juvenile Psychopathic Institute came to an end in 1914, but the Cook County government, impressed with the value of a diagnostic facility for young offenders, assumed the financial burden with a slightly modified title, The Psychopathic Clinic of the Juvenile Court. Still, a lack of treatment facilities limited the usefulness of diagnosis. When Healy and his colleague Augusta F. Bronner were invited to Boston in 1916 to the Judge Baker Foundation, they were promised increased treatment resources and ten years' financial support. They accepted and opened the Boston Clinic in April 1917. Before his death in 1915, Judge Harvey H. Baker had expressed the hope that a full-time clinic would be established in Boston "for the intensive study of baffling cases" (21). Thus the association between the new psychology and the quandaries of the legal system grew closer. The basic research into behavior and treatment of children that was essential to the establishment of a distinct profession of child psychiatry was also furthered.

ARNOLD GESELL AND BIOLOGICAL BASES OF NORMAL DEVELOPMENT

During the same period, Arnold Gesell undertook a different approach to child development and behavior. Gesell, who received his doctorate in psychology from Clark University under Hall in 1906 and his medical degree from Yale University in 1915, started a juvenile "psycho-clinic" at the New Haven Dispensary in 1911. The clinic became the Yale Clinic of

Child Development and later the site of the Yale Child Study Center. Gesell, who had been a high school teacher, involved himself with schools in much the way Healy was associated with juvenile courts. He served as school psychologist for the Connecticut State Board of Education prior to World War I and was one of the earliest persons, if not the first, to hold such a post. He traveled around the state, at times by horse and buggy, to examine children in the schools, make diagnoses, and recommend appropriate treatment or placement (22). Gesell viewed child development as proceeding chiefly from a biological timetable, a more sophisticated form of Hall's approach to human development. His books on child development, based on a pioneer use of motion pictures for the study of infancy and childhood, were guides to child development in the United States for many parents in the second quarter of the twentieth century.

Gesell and Healy well represent the competing biological and environmental schools of thought that, as noted, have alternated in this country as the dominant view of behavior and therapy. Just before his career began at Yale, Gesell had decided that he wished to "make a thoroughgoing study of the developmental stages of childhood," and Healy recalled that what prompted his life of study was the desire to know why a particular person was a delinquent and how to modify or prevent antisocial behavior. One naturally looked to the discovery of a set order and progression of development, the other to origins of disturbed development and powerful therapies to interrupt it.

CHILD GUIDANCE CLINICS

What Healy established to acclaim in Chicago and then more firmly expanded in Boston became a model for the creation of child guidance clinics throughout the nation. The impetus for this expansion came from the Commonwealth Fund in 1921, whose funding permitted establishment of clinics in several cities to demonstrate the value of such services for children and their families. In 1923, Dr. Karl H. Menninger invited a group of psychiatrists to meet to consider the formation of a new group with its own journal that would be linked to corrective and preventative efforts directed at youthful offenders. As mentioned, the American Orthopsychiatric Association (AOA) was established the next year, and Dr. Healy was elected the first president. The strong support given to guidance clinics is reflected in the increasingly stringent requirements for membership, which by 1930 was limited to those who worked in a clinic that regularly used the coordinated services of a psychiatrist, clinical psychologist, and a psychiatric social worker. These specific requirements have more recently been liberalized, but the purpose of the rules earlier in AOA's history was to foster development of professions focused on childhood emotional disorders and to affirm the faith of many experts that a team approach was not only feasible but preferable (23).

WATSON AND FREUD

While professional interests in childhood were intensifying in the 1920s, the popular theories of the behaviorist John B. Watson were directing parents to establish rigid feeding schedules and to "condition" their children to proper behavior and attitudes. Watson influenced the Children's Bureau and the Bureau's child-care pamphlets to a marked degree. Whether parents followed Watson's ideas faithfully in large numbers (or followed any expert's opinions faithfully) is doubtful, but it is an irony that while guidance clinics were, in general, trying to create a more flexible approach to behavior problems, Watson's behaviorism was more likely to be the recommendation of government and some lay publications (24).

Watson denied the existence of the unconscious as well as the dominant influence of biological constitution. Understandably, his behaviorism was attacked on two fronts—by those who were sensitive to dynamic psychological factors in human behavior, such as William Healy, who stoutly defended the unconscious, and by hereditarians, such as Gesell, who held that biological patterns at birth substantially guided later development. The major theoretical concepts that supported the psychological outlook were psychoanalytic. Sigmund Freud, like Hall, had sought to discover the normative pattern of human development. In 1909 he published his pioneering attempt to analyze a child's phobic reaction in the case history of "Little Hans" (25). In his exploration of emotional and biological maturation, he eventually viewed the early years of life as crucial in establishing later patterns of behavior. His analysis also presented, through free association, a means for therapy and investigation and, to a further extent, particularly as perceived in the United States, practical insights into antisocial behavior and suggestions concerning the prevention and treatment of criminals and disturbed youth (26). In Europe, August Aichhorn influenced treatment of antisocial juveniles with the publication in 1925 of Verwahrloste Jugend, later translated into English as Wayward Youth (1935), which emphasized the need to deal with underlying determinants of latent delinquency.

The decision by Anna Freud to devote her life's studies to childhood and the treatment of children's difficulties represented a major evolution of the psychoanalytic movement to encompass detailed investigation of child development and pathology. Others, notably Erik Erikson, came under the influence of psychoanalytic thought in the 1930s and helped to roll back the dominance of behaviorism and replace a simplistic approach to child rearing with a more sensitive attuning of parents to the emotional needs and plasticity of infants and children.

PEDIATRICS AND CHILD PSYCHIATRY

The impact of psychoanalytic thinking on the child guidance movement, clinical psychology, and social work was large, but there was little appreciation for it among pediatricians in the 1920s and 1930s. Pediatrics was making great progress in the treatment of childhood disease, but the area of child development was more influenced by Watson and Gesell than by those advocating theories of dynamic mental and emotional development. A division can still be noted because pediatricians have, in general, taken a greater lead in the care of the retarded, while psychiatrists have been more prominent in the treatment of the emotionally disturbed child. Nevertheless, there is no arbitrary divide between physical and emotional health and development, and the ties between pediatrics and psychiatry have gradually improved. Milton Senn, in his historical studies of the growth of child development, places great emphasis on the appointment of Leo Kanner, in 1930, to be the liaison between pediatrics and psychiatry at Johns Hopkins University (27). Both Adolph Meyer, head of the Phipps Psychiatric Clinic, and Edwards Park, the eminent professor of pediatrics at Johns Hopkins University, held Kanner in great respect, which had much to do with his influence. The authority and esteem with which Park was held by pediatricians in turn enabled Kanner to reach many pediatricians who had found little of value in psychiatric evaluation of children. Meyer had long been associated with the treatment of children, and it was he, for example, who had recommended Healy to Julia Lathrop as the best person to investigate the psychological aspects of juvenile delinquency in 1908.

Kanner was the author of the first text on child psychiatry in the United States (1935), and is noted for, among other advances in child psychiatry, pioneer recognition and description of childhood autism (28, 29). The number of pediatricians who have subsequently been leaders in psychiatric aspects of childhood has been large and include Milton Senn and Benjamin Spock. In 1937, the Commonwealth Fund, expanding support for the training of psychiatrists and others in the mental health field, began to provide fellowships for pediatricians to spend two years studying child psychiatry as fellows at one of the major training centers, such as the Philadelphia Child Guidance Clinic or the New York Hospital/Cornell Medical College (30). Today, hospitals commonly have a consultation-liaison psychiatrist for pediatric services as well as pediatricians active on the psychiatric service.

DETERMINISM DISCREDITED—THE EXAMPLE OF ALCOHOL RESEARCH

During the late 1920s, public acceptance of national alcohol prohibition declined. Repeal of the eighteenth Amendment finally came in 1933 and with it, both science and popular culture came to scorn the arguments advanced by those in favor of alcohol control. Extreme claims about the dangers of alcohol were laughed into silence. Most telling from the point of view of attitudes toward child development, scientific research began to support the new, less deterministic view of alcohol. Even Dr. Stockard's conclusions began to change. In 1932, as repeal was imminent, he wrote:

> . . . what do we know of the nature of alcohol action on embryonic development? . . . In sufficient concentrations we have found that it is effective, but such alcohol concentrations as are necessary to directly effect [*sic*] the development of lower animals are far in excess of the possible alcohol content of human blood compatible with human survival. . . . Results from these experiments on the embryos of lower animals justify only the conclusion that if comparisons with human embryos are possible they indicate that the content of alcohol in human blood is fortunately never sufficiently high to present a danger to the developing embryo (31).

This was just the beginning of a new authoritative view of alcohol and the fetus that would dominate teaching and advice regarding alcohol for the next 40 years. Perhaps the leading American authority on alcohol during this period was E.M. Jellinek. In 1940, Jellinek commented on the danger of alcohol intake during pregnancy by declaring that "the idea of germ poisoning by alcohol in humans" was now "safely dismissed" by "practically unanimous opinion (32)." Two years later, Jellinek and Howard Haggard wrote in their book for the public, Alcohol Explored, that "no acceptable evidence has ever been offered to show that acute alcoholic intoxication has any effect whatsoever on the human germ, or has any influence in altering heredity, or is the cause of any abnormality in the child" (33).

In their 1975 review of research on alcohol and offspring, Warner and Rosset suggested that such a rejection of biological explanations for the apparent effects of alcohol was due to a broader shift toward understanding development in terms of external influences (34). This approach is more optimistic and more favorable to psychotherapy than is biological determinism, as it holds out the possibility of mental health and normal development for even disturbed individuals through psychiatric intervention—as well as, perhaps, improvement in living conditions, reorganization of communities, and education. The idea that the central fact of someone's life is the inexorable unfolding of innate biological patterns, the view championed by Arnold Gesell, now seemed discouraging and subversive of a belief in equal opportunity.

TRAINING, PROFESSIONALIZATION, AND ORGANIZATION

Training programs supported by the Commonwealth Fund and the Rockefeller Foundation (beginning in 1922 and 1924, respectively) provided training for 138 psychiatrists by 1940 (35). What the training should be was under constant debate, but it generally consisted of supervision in the activities of a major guidance clinic with the possible addition of neurologic and pediatric experience at a medical center. Psychoanalytic training also became a major element in this process because it appeared to deal directly with the child's mental development and, for many students, had abiding explanatory value for childhood behavior, as well as its relationship to adult altitudes and development (36).

World War II brought psychiatrists into the military and into armed services induction centers. A degree of leadership was accorded psychiatrists with experience in child psychiatry and child guidance clinics and, on their recommendation, hundreds of thousands of draftees were excluded from service. In retrospect, their sensitivity to possible abnormality may have been excessive, but one long-range effect of their efforts and those of psychiatrists near the battle fronts was to raise the prestige of psychiatry. Some leaders in the psychiatric profession and in the American political scene sought ways of applying to the home front the effective therapies applied or learned during the war. Shortly after the war ended, the National Mental Health Act (1946) permitted the federal government to provide training grants and, within two decades, thousands of psychiatrists were trained (37). As general psychiatry grew, so did the number of those specializing in child psychiatry. Child guidance clinics experienced a new growth in numbers and activity after having declined while many of their staffs participated in the war effort. A conviction developed that neither the field nor the clinics were any longer experimental, and that they would grow and would benefit from specific standards.

The organization of clinics, the American Association of Psychiatric Clinics for Children (AAPCC), grew out of needs recognized by the Division of Community Clinics of the National Committee for Mental Hygiene. It began with informal meetings of clinic directors during the annual meetings of the AOA. The first meeting was held in 1940 and gradually expanded to include the chief mental health professions from each clinic. Finally, in 1945, the AAPCC was established with Frederick H. Allen of Philadelphia as its first president, and two years later, the association promulgated formal guidelines for training in child psychiatry. These standards did not accredit an individual but did set the standard for a clinic that wished to be an approved training center (38). Still, no professional accreditation existed for child psychiatrists.

The first group to limit its membership only to child psychiatrists was the American Academy of Child Psychiatry, founded in 1953. Originally limited to a small fraction of all child psychiatrists, the academy has expanded to encompass the majority of those who describe themselves as child psychiatrists and almost all who have been accredited by the American Board of Psychiatry and Neurology. In the latter board, child psychiatry has also advanced as a specialty, because in 1957 the board recognized the field as a subspecialty and established standards for the training of child psychiatrists (39). Thus, child psychiatry moved from an occasional interest of a random psychiatrist earlier in the twentieth century to a well-defined specialty by midcentury.

THE RETURN TO GENETIC RESEARCH AND HEREDITARIAN THINKING

Today American science and society are once more considering the question of the roles of heredity, environment and parental (particularly maternal) behavior on child development. One study published in 1990 looked at women whose drinking habits were judged to be moderate but whose children at the age of seven years had an IQ estimated to be seven points lower than the control group. This suggested to the authors that even moderate drinking could cause measurable and persistent deficits (40). From studies like this The New York Times framed a headline that read "Lasting Costs for Child Are Found from a Few Early Drinks" (41).

Another study from the Journal of the American Medical Association in 1991 reported on fetal alcohol syndrome (FAS) among adolescents and older persons. Their mothers were often chronic alcoholics, so this was not a question of social drinking. The cost to society of caring for these affected persons was estimated to be $1.2 million in a lifetime. The incidence of FAS ranged from 1 in 700 in Seattle to as high as 1 in 8 in a British Columbia Indian village. The authors concluded: "Gestational exposure to alcohol can cause a wide spectrum of disabilities that have lifelong physical, mental, and behavioral implications (42)".

We can find numerous studies that implicate alcohol, even in moderation, for causing enduring intellectual and social deficits, sometimes so catastrophic that an individual is fated to become a ward of society.

A final historical irony is that the story of the Kallikaks, whose damaged lives Goddard attributed to heredity, not alcohol, reemerged in a study published in 1995 in the Archives of Pediatric and Adolescent Medicine. The article argues that after all it was alcohol that caused the Kallikaks' terrible outcome. Armed with the knowledge of FAS, the authors examined records, photographic and other evidence Goddard had collected and came to the conclusion that it "confirms the associations of parental alcoholism with mental retardation in childhood and with infant mortality" (43). Even the exceptions of 80 years ago, then, are being, so to speak, posthumously converted into support of alcohol's effects on the fetus.

The first two decades of the twentieth century and the present share other characteristics, one of the most important being a confidence in the biological basis of human behavior. The goal of eugenics was to devise ways in which the better, more productive physiologies could be promoted and the less desirable reduced. The quality individuals would be increased through, say, fertile marriages of good stock, while the undesirable stock would be curbed through sterilization.

These three eras—biological, then environmental and once again biological—prompt the question: Are we about to repeat the folly of eugenics, or will we put the power of new discoveries in genetics to work in the service of a more nuanced and sensitive understanding of the complex relationship between heredity and environment? Developments in psychiatry and related sciences, some of which are discussed throughout the present volume, allow us to be optimistic that the latter answer will prove true. Unlike earlier frustrating experiences of studying Mendelian inheritance without understanding how genes interact with the environment, a growing body of research is pinpointing segments of genetic material that can be closely studied in the laboratory as well as in the clinic. For example, Caspi et al. identified specific genes implicated in protecting some maltreated children from developing psychopathology in adulthood (44). Changed circumstances open remarkable opportunities. As outlined by Plomin and Rutter, new studies include twin and adoptee investigations of resilience, identification of genetic markers that confer protection or vulnerability, and sibling studies that would clarify the contributions of shared and nonshared environments on outcomes (45).

Researchers today have a greater appreciation of the new opportunities and the limitations of their methods. The public should also become informed about the new genetics so that the seductiveness of genetic explanations does not lead to the oversimplifications found in the eugenics movement earlier in the twentieth century.

CREDITS

This article is a revised and expanded version of one first published as:

Musto DF. Child psychiatry: An historical perspective. In: Michels R, Cavenar JO, Brodie HKH, Cooper AM, Guze SB, Judd LL, Klerman GL, Solnit AJ, eds..Psychiatry; Vol 2, Child Psychiatry. Philadelphia: JB Lippincott; 1985: 1–6.

The text also contains material edited and extracted from:

Musto DF. The impact of public attitudes on drug abuse research in the twentieth century. In: Glanz MD, Hartel CR, eds. Drug Abuse, Origins and Interventions. Washington, DC: American Psychological Association; 1999: 63–78.

References

1. Hendrick, H: Children and childhood. *Refresh—Recent Findings of Research in Economic & Social History* 1992; 15 <http://www.ehs.org.uk/society/pdfs/Hendrick%2015a.pdf>.
2. Ross D: *G. Stanley Hall: The Psychologist as Prophet*. Chicago, University of Chicago Press, 1972.
3. Siegel AW, White SH: The child study movement: Early growth and development of the symbolized child. *Adv Child Dev Bull* 17:256–262, 1982.
4. Kett JF: *Rites of Passage: Adolescence in America, 1790 to the Present*. New York, Basic Books, 1977.
5. Hall GS: *Adolescence, Its Psychology and Its Relations to Physiology, Anthropology, Sociology, Sex, Crime, Religion and Education*. New York, D Appleton, 1904.
6. Sears RR: *Your Ancients Revisited: A History of Child Development*. Chicago, University of Chicago Press, 1975.
7. Lowrey LG: The birth of orthopsychiatry. In: Lowrey LG, (ed.): *Orthopsychiatry, 1923–1948, Retrospect and Prospect*. New York, American Orthopsychiatric Association, pp. 190–208, 1948.
8. Stockard CR: The hereditary transmission of degeneracy and deformities by the descendants of alcoholized mammals. *Interstate Medical Journal* 23:385–403, 1916.
9. Freeman RG: Disease conditions in older babies that can be attributed to prenatal influences. *American Journal of Obstetrics* 77:459–462, 1917.
10. MacNicholl TA: Alcohol and the disabilities of children. *JAMA* 48:396–398, 1907.
11. Gordon A: The influence of alcohol on the progeniture. *Interstate Medical Journal* 23:431–436, 1916.
12. Elderton EM, Pearson K: A first study of the influence of parental alcoholism on the physique and ability of the offspring. *Eugenics Laboratory Memoirs* X, 1910.
13. Keynes JM: Influence of parental alcoholism (letter to the editors). *Journal of the Royal Statistical Society* 74:114–121, 1910.
14. Goddard HH: Alcoholism and feeble-mindedness. *Interstate Medical Journal* 23:442–445, 1916.
15. Goddard HH: *The Kallikak Family: A Study in the Heredity of Feeble-mindedness*. New York, MacMillan, 1912.
16. Buck v. Bell, 274 US 200, 207.

17. Gordon A: Parental alcoholism as a factor in the mental deficiency of children: A statistical study of 117 families. *Journal of Inebriation* 33:90–99, 1911.
18. Irwell L: Influence of parental alcoholism upon the human family. *The Medical Times* April:114–115, 1913.
19. Davies SP: *The Mentally Retarded in Society*. New York, Columbia University Press, pp. 26–32, 1959.
20. Dummer ES: Life in relation to time. In: Lowrey LG (ed.): *Orthopsychiatry 1923–1948, Retrospect and Prospect*. New York, American Orthopsychiatric Association, pp. 3–13, 1948.
21. Healy W, Bronner AF: The child guidance clinic. In: Lowrey LG (ed.): *Orthopsychiatry, 1923–1948, Retrospect and Prospect*. New York, American Orthopsychiatric Association, pp. 14–49, 1948.
22. Gesell A: Arnold Gesell. In: Boring EG, Langfeld HS, Werner H, et al. (eds.): *History of Psychology in Autobiography*. Vol 4. Worcester, MA, Clark University Press, pp. 123–142, 1952.
23. Musto DF: A short history of orthopsychiatry. In: Shore MF, Mannino FV (eds.): *Mental Health and Social Change: Fifty Years of Orthopsychiatry*. New York, AMS Press, pp. 5–15, 1975.
24. Kessen W: *The Child*. New York, John Wiley & Sons, pp. 230–231, 1965.
25. Freud S: Analysis of a phobia in a five-year-old boy. In: Strachey J (ed.): *The Standard Edition of the Complete Works of Sigmund Freud*. Vol 10. London, Hogarth Press, pp. 3–152, 1966–1972.
26. Hale NG: *Freud and the Americans: The Beginning of Psychoanalysis in the United States, 1876–1917*. New York, Oxford University Press, 1971.
27. Senn MJE: Pediatrics in orthopsychiatry. In: Lowrey LG, (ed.): *Orthopsychiatry, 1923–1948, Retrospect and Prospect*. New York, American Orthopsychiatric Association, pp. 300–309, 1948.
28. Kanner L: *Child Psychiatry*. Springfield, IL, Charles C Thomas, 1935.
29. Kanner L: Autistic disturbances of affective contact. *Nerv Child* 2:217–250, 1943.
30. Senn MJE: Pediatrics in orthopsychiatry. In: Lowrey LG (ed.): *Orthopsychiatry, 1923–1948, Retrospect and Prospect*. New York, American Orthopsychiatric Association, pp. 300–309, 1948.
31. Stockard CR: The effects of alcohol in development and heredity. In: Emerson H (ed.): *Alcohol and Man*. New York, Macmillan, pp. 102–119, 1932.
32. Jellinek EM, and Jolliffe N: Effect of alcohol on the individual: Review of the literature of 1939. *Quarterly Journal of Studies on Alcohol* 1:110–181, 1940.
33. Haggard HW, and Jellinek EM: *Alcohol Explored*. Garden City, NY, Doubleday, Doran, 1942.
34. Warner RH, and Rosset HL: The effects of drinking on offspring: An historical survey of the American and British literature. *Journal of Studies on Alcohol* 36:1395–1420, 1975.
35. Kirkpatrick ME: Fellowship training in orthopsychiatry. In: Lowrey LG (ed.): *Orthopsychiatry, 1923–1948, Retrospect and Prospect*. New York, American Orthopsychiatric Association, pp. 83–99, 1948.
36. Senn MJE: Insights into the child development movement in the United States. *Monogr Soc Res Child Dev* 40:38–47, 1975.
37. Musto DF: Whatever happened to "community mental health"? *Public Interest* Spring 53–79, 1975.
38. Curran F: *The American Association of Psychiatric Clinics for Children—History, Purpose, and Organization*. New York, American Association of Psychiatric Clinics for Children, 1957.
39. The history of the American Academy of Child Psychiatry. *J Am Acad Child Psychiatry* 1:196–202, 1962.
40. Streissguth AP, Barr HM, Sampson PD: Moderate prenatal alcohol exposure: Effects on child IQ and learning problems at age $7\frac{1}{2}$ years. *Alcoholism: Clinical and Experimental Research* 14:662–669, 1990.
41. *New York Times* 16 February 1989:B-16.
42. Streissguth AP, Ase JM, Clarren SK, Randels SP, LaDue RA, Smith DF: Fetal Alcohol Syndrome in adolescents and adults. *JAMA* 265:1961–1967, 1991.
43. Karp RJ, Qazi QH, Nikker JA, Angelo WA, Davis JM: Fetal Alcohol Syndrome at the turn of the 20th century. *Archives of Pediatrics and Adolescent Medicine* 149:45–47, 1995.
44. Caspi A, McClay J, Moffitt TE, et al.: Role of genotype in the cycle of violence in maltreated children. *Science* 297:851–854, 2002.
45. Plomin R, Rutter, M: Child development, molecular genetics, and what to do with genes once they are found. *Child Development* 69:1223–1242, 1998; see also, Rutter M: Nature, nurture, and development: from evangelism through science toward policy and practice. *Child Development* 73:1–21, 2002.

CHAPTER 1.3 ■ ETHICS

DIANE H. SCHETKY

OVERVIEW

Ethical codes in medicine date back to the fifth century BC, yet they received little attention in our medical literature until the 1990s. Greater awareness and interest in ethics can be attributed to a) an increasingly consumer-centered approach to medicine, with its attendant emphasis on patient rights; b) high-technology medical developments that offer choices unheard of in the past and, in turn, introduce the need for health care rationing and decisions about prolonging life; and c) changes in the delivery of health care that alter the physician's autonomy, impose the role of gatekeeper, and challenge our traditional ethical codes.

Ethical codes are not laws but standards of conduct expected from a professional. They exist to help professionals to reconcile providing service while also earning a living from that service. In medicine, these codes define the norms, duties, and virtues expected in our professional work. As noted by Reiser et al. (1), "Self-conscious reflection on standards of conduct is one of the defining characteristics of a profession." Ethical codes serve to protect the profession and benefit the patient and society as well. In maintaining the image and standard of conduct of the profession, they enable the patient to establish trust in the physician.

The Hippocratic oath originated in the fifth century BC, but it was not widely applied until the tenth century. It stresses the physician's power to heal and the need to divest this power from killing. In doing so, as noted by Margaret Mead (2), the code clearly separates the physician from the sorcerer or shaman, who has the power both to harm and to cure. The Hippocratic oath stresses the physician's obligation to the patient and the duty to keep confidences. It prohibits abortion, euthanasia, and sexual relationships with patients. Dyer (3) notes that the Hippocratic tradition has come under scrutiny by critics who contend that it is anachronistic. Critics argue that it does not deal with the technologic advances in medicine or with problems of cost containment. Many contend that it is too paternalistic and does not adequately address the rights of patients. Dyer (3) recommends that we accept the oath "symbolically in terms of the intent and the concept of the profession it outlines."

Psychiatrists today generally follow the Principles of Medical Ethics with Annotations Especially Applicable to Psychiatry (4). These guidelines provide us with a way of thinking about ethical dilemmas, but they do not necessarily solve them. Often competing ethical principles come in conflict, such as a woman's right to autonomy and to refuse a Cesarean section versus her physician's concern for the welfare of her fetus. To understand these ethical guidelines, it is helpful to appreciate the ethical principles that underlie them. The four basic moral principles that guide us in medical research and health care are analyzed in great detail by Beauchamp and Childress (5) and are briefly summarized here. Autonomy comes from the Greek words for "self" and "rule" and in medicine refers to the ability to make decisions for oneself without being controlled by others. Autonomy becomes the basis for informed consent and therapeutic privilege. Nonmaleficence is a concept derived from the Latin *Primum non nocere* (First do no harm), and originally stems from the Hippocratic oath, which states "I will use treatment to help the sick according to my ability and judgment, but I will never use it to injure or wrong them." The principle of beneficence refers to the obligation to help others to further their legitimate interests and, more specifically, to promote the welfare of the patient. The principle of justice refers to offering fair treatment to all.

NATURE OF THE DOCTOR–PATIENT RELATIONSHIP

A fiduciary relationship is one in which one person receives the trust or confidence of another and is under a duty to act for the benefit of that person. Examples include an attorney–client or broker–client relationship. Trust is the cornerstone of the fiduciary relationship that exists between physician and patient. The physician as fiduciary is expected to act for the benefit of the patient and not exploit that relationship for personal gain. Simon (6) reminds us that the psychiatrist's main source of gratification should arise from the psychotherapeutic process, and his or her only material reward is payment for service.

Trust is essential to both evaluation and treatment. Without trust, patients would be reluctant to divulge the intimate details about their lives that are often necessary to arrive at diagnoses and embark on treatment. The fiduciary relationship is less clearcut in regard to children. Issues of trust and confidentiality are more complex in child and adolescent psychiatry because we must deal with parents as well as the child. Parents' rights to know certain information about their child need to be balanced with the child's interests. Further, the age and cognitive maturity of the child have a bearing on the child's ability to participate in decisions about treatment or medication, as well as disclosures to others.

Doctor–patient relationships are also defined by boundaries that keep us in our professional role and prevent us from exploiting patients. Boundaries provide a sense of security to both physician and patient. They help us to maintain objectivity and allow us to focus on the patient's best interest. Boundaries discourage acting out by both patient and physician and foster respect for the patient's autonomy and dignity. The forces of both transference and countertransference threaten the therapist's neutrality and, if not recognized and resolved, may erode boundaries and undermine therapy. Straying from one's usual practices may be a warning sign of boundary violations. Psychiatrists who begin to see patients at unusual locales or times, who waive usual billing procedures, or who start socializing with patients and their families may be on a slippery slope. They need to reflect on that behavior and to consider the consequences, because seemingly benign boundary violations may lead to more serious ethical violations.

CONFIDENTIALITY

The terms confidentiality and privilege are often confused. Privilege, the narrower of the two terms, refers only to the patient's right to bar disclosure of information obtained during treatment in judicial or quasijudicial proceedings. Confidentiality, in contrast, refers to the disclosure of information learned in treatment to third parties. The physician's duty to maintain confidentiality is both a legal and an ethical one that derives from the right to privacy under common law and our ethical codes. Appelbaum and Gutheil (7) note that the ethical foundations for confidentiality are twofold. First is the concern that without assurance of confidentiality patients would be reluctant to seek treatment. Second is the argument that, having implied that communications are confidential, mental health professionals must keep their implicit or explicit promise.

Privilege and confidentiality can be waived only by the patient, with certain exceptions. Generally, these exceptions include when the patient is in danger of harming him or herself or others, such as a sexually active patient who is positive for human immunodeficiency virus and who refuses to take precautions or to inform sexual partners, and state laws mandating reporting of child abuse or impaired physicians. However, exceptions continue to grow and now include insurance company audits, which usually call for blanket rather than informed consent to release records, insurance fraud investigations involving either the psychiatrist or the patient (8), and limits to confidentiality under HIPAA regulations.

The psychiatrist may be faced with a moral dilemma when a subpoena demands patient records and their release is not in the best interest of that patient. The psychiatrist's conscience must guide him or her whether to defy the law or seek to quash the subpoena. For a discussion of the legal ramifications of breach of confidentiality and consent issues, see Chapter 7.3.

CONSENT

Minors, with some exceptions, are not competent to give consent to treatment, to medical research, or for release of medical information, but they may be asked to give their assent in accord with their developmental age. Consent must be obtained from parents or guardians unless state law allows adolescents to consent to treatment or unless they are emancipated. For consent to be informed, parties must know the nature of the condition treated, the risks and benefits of the proposed treatment and their choices, and the risks of no treatment. Further, they should be free to agree or disagree without undue influence. It is advisable to obtain consent in writing for high-risk treatments and for release of records. If parents are separated or divorced, consent must be obtained from the custodial parent. If the child is in a shared custody arrangement, the psychiatrist should attempt to contact the other parent regarding treatment decisions, because joint decision making on medical matters is usually part of shared custody arrangements. If one is in doubt about the terms of parental rights, one can always ask a parent to bring in the divorce decree.

The child and adolescent psychiatrist, perhaps more than the adult psychiatrist, faces many pressures to violate confidentiality owing to all the collateral contacts that arise during work with children. These include parents, teachers, guidance counselors, other therapists involved with the family, daycare providers, the child's physician, and sometimes personnel from protective services or other agencies. Even when there is consent for release of information, the psychiatrist must delicately balance how much information a school needs to know about a child's turbulent family life to help a child while respecting the family's wish for privacy. The child and adolescent psychiatrist may need to decide when it is necessary to override a child's plea not to disclose certain information, such as speaking to a teacher, when parents have authorized such communication. The following case illustrates the many levels at which we must weigh decisions about confidentiality.

Case Illustration

Sally Barnes, age 8 years, has been in treatment for an anxiety disorder that waxes and wanes. She lives with her recently widowed mother and younger sister. One day, she is brought to her weekly appointment by her grandmother and tells her therapist, Dr. Coles, that her mother is home, sick with the flu. Sally then reveals that her mother was drinking excessively the night before at a friend's house and drove Sally and her sister home while under the influence of alcohol. Sally heard her mother vomiting during the night, and in the morning her mother was so sick that she asked Sally to stay home to care for her little sister.

In this clinical scenario, Dr. Coles is confronted with the decisions regarding a) using Sally's disclosures to confront Mrs. Barnes; b) sharing concerns with Sally's grandmother; c) contacting Mrs. Barnes' therapist; and d) involving protective services.

Dr. Coles chooses to say nothing to the grandmother because she does not have the mother's permission to speak with her. Sally is eager for her therapist to talk to her mother. Dr. Coles calls Mrs. Barnes, who initially denies the allegations made by Sally but who then backs down and agrees to allow Dr. Coles to contact her own therapist. Later, she admits that things are very out of control in her life, agrees to an inpatient admission, and approaches her mother (Sally's grandmother) to help care for the children. Dr. Coles does not feel the need to involve protective services at this juncture. The question of how much to tell the school and daycare is discussed with Mrs. Barnes and is left to her discretion. Sally may have been afraid that Dr. Coles would speak to her mother about her drinking problem. In that case, she would have had to deal with Sally's fear around disclosing this secret and her rationale for overriding Sally's objections in taking the steps she did to insure her welfare.

LIMITS OF CONFIDENTIALITY

Child psychiatrists need to define to both patient and parents the limits of confidentiality at the onset of evaluation and treatment. The extent to which communications from parent to therapist will be shared with the child should be discussed. If the psychiatrist needs to share the child's confidences with the parents, there are several options. The first is to urge the child to do so or to meet jointly and discuss the issues. If this fails, the psychiatrist may then tell the child why he or she needs to share the information with the parents and what will be told.

In small, underserved communities, the psychiatrist may, like it or not, have to medicate and sometimes treat more than one family member or friends of patients. This poses a challenge to the psychiatrist in terms of double bookkeeping, that is, remembering what information was heard from whom and storing away what may have been heard but cannot be used because it was shared in confidence. Additional problems may arise around advocacy and issues of countertransference. In general, dual agency such as this is best avoided. If no alternatives exist, the psychiatrist should at least make each patient from the same family aware that he or she is seeing the other.

DOUBLE AGENTRY

Double agentry is a term that refers to serving two masters simultaneously. This is a problem that may arise from consultants when they are not clear about their roles. For instance, an adolescent may reveal to a psychiatrist performing a consult for a school that he or she is dealing drugs in school. If the psychiatrist shares this information with the school, the student is likely to be expelled and if not, other students are at risk. The psychiatrist needs to be clear that as a consultant his or her duty is to the school that hired him or her, not the student. The dilemma could be minimized by informing the student at the onset of the consultation about the limits of confidentiality. As illustrated below, double agentry may also arise when a therapist pursues the parents' agenda without regard to the child's best interests.

Case Illustration

Mr. and Mrs. Jones seek help from Dr. Smith in regard to their 14-year-old son, Tom. They complain that he is defiant, questions his father, talks back, and refuses to attend services at their church. They hope that Dr. Smith will render Tom more compliant and will bring back their "good little boy." If Dr. Smith colludes with their agenda, he risks becoming their agent. Tom, conversely, does not see that he needs help other than using Dr. Smith's authority to get his parents off his back so he can gain more freedom. An overidentified therapist could be tempted to collude with Tom's agenda. Dr. Smith empathizes with Tom's plight but views his role as helping Tom to separate and individuate from his family and to develop responsible autonomy. Unless he spells out where he stands with the family, therapy is not likely to succeed.

CONFIDENTIALITY AND THE MEDIA

Child and adolescent psychiatrists need to be on guard against violating confidences when giving press interviews. It is usually prudent to be circumspect and to limit comments to what is already public knowledge and to comment on overarching issues rather than on the specifics of a case. Parents may give consent for a therapist to talk with the media about their children, as in high-profile custody or abuse cases. However, parents who are caught up in the heat of litigation are not always the best judges about whether media attention will be harmful to their children.

The psychiatrist needs to guard against exploiting high-profile cases for his or her own personal gain. Similarly, they should avoid offering their services pro bono in such cases, as this raises questions regarding their motives for involvement. Occasionally, psychiatrists may be tempted to go above the law and try to justify rash actions such as releasing confidential reports to the media as being in the child's best interests. Rarely can such actions be justified, and when closely examined they usually represent grandiosity, narcissism, and unchecked countertransference on the part of the psychiatrist.

CONFIDENTIALITY IN PROFESSIONAL PRESENTATIONS AND PUBLICATIONS

Confidentiality must be preserved when psychiatrists write about patients or present them or their artwork at conferences. One has the choice of disguising material sufficiently to preserve the patient's identity or seeking permission from the child and his or her parents to use the material. Therapists may be tempted to write books about their patients. It is difficult to reconcile this with keeping the patient's interests foremost, and such an agenda is likely to derail therapy. Literary exploitation of therapy in the mass media is unsettling to the public and does not promote trust in the profession. Even if this occurs with the patient's consent, questions may be raised about how informed the consent was, as in the case of author Anne Sexton, whose psychiatrist released therapy tapes to her biographer after Sexton's death.

The advent of new technologies, and particularly the ease and affordability in access to digital videotaping and desktop editing, has introduced additional ethical considerations. Provisions regarding confidentiality and the limits of what may or may not be shared vary for the different purposes of clinical care or training and education, and according to the size and nature of the viewing group in question. For example, a video clip used by a multidisciplinary team treating a child has ethical and confidentiality implications quite different from those of a report aired on primetime television. A full discussion on the ethical implications of these new technologies is beyond the scope of this chapter. The interested reader is referred to recent publications on the topic, especially the volume on child psychiatry and the media edited by Beresin and Olson (9) (2005).

DUAL RELATIONSHIPS

Dual relationships pose a challenge to maintaining confidentiality. Anyone practicing near where they live or whose children attend the same school as their patients do is bound to encounter awkward situations. The child psychiatrist's children are unaware of who is or is not a patient of their parent. They may wish to invite patients to birthday parties, play at their homes, or share car pools. As the child psychiatrist's children grow older, attend larger schools, and engage in more extracurricular activities, it becomes increasingly difficult to screen patients for their potential ties to one's children. In small towns, one may end up evaluating or treating children of one's colleagues or one's children's teachers or future teachers. If there are no other resources, turning down requests for help in times of crises may be viewed as inhumane and does not help one's image. How well these dual relationships work often depends on the nature of the patient's disorder, the extent of family psychopathology, and the therapist's ability to maintain boundaries. Each new adult patient or parent of a child patient should be viewed as one less potential friend. The two-way give and take of friendships cannot exist in therapy, because the therapist may not use the relationship for his or her own personal needs. It may be necessary to explain this to certain families at the onset of one's professional involvement with them.

The longer one is in practice, the more likely one is to run into patients all over town. The psychiatrist may need to patronize parents of patients, be they shop owners, pharmacists, plumbers, or restaurant owners. Adult patients and patients' parents may be appointed to boards one sits on or may join one's organizations. The child and adolescent psychiatrist either learns to deal with these encounters or retreats to the high ground and becomes a recluse. There is much to be said for patients' seeing their psychiatrists as real persons, whether at the dump on a Saturday morning or at the local high school basketball game. Successfully negotiating these encounters requires that the psychiatrist be comfortable with his or her public persona, be able effectively to process these encounters, and maintain boundaries and confidentiality. In assessing how to address patients in public, one learns to take cues from them. Children may be unabashed about seeing their therapist in the supermarket, whereas their parents may be less comfortable. Teenagers may shirk from public contact or may surprise their therapists by wanting to introduce their friends.

The Psychiatrist's Family. One learns to train family members (and friends) not to ask "How do you know so and so?" Some psychiatrists develop nonverbal cues with spouses for handling awkward social situations. Should the psychiatrist's child learn the identity of a patient, he or she must appreciate that it is the patient's choice whether to disclose the psychiatrist–patient relationship. In some communities, children may be quite comfortable telling another child that they are patients of their parent. Conversely, I have had to curb my son's one-time enthusiasm for trying to refer classmates whom he perceived to be in need of help. Adult patients may deliberately attempt to become friends with their therapist's spouse, and this may become awkward if the spouse is unaware of the existing professional relationship. The therapist may have to intervene with the patient in such situations.

FORENSIC ISSUES

Forensic evaluations differ from regular diagnostic evaluations in that their intent is not therapeutic. Forensic evaluations are intended to help the court to find the truth and address the legal question at hand. To do so, the forensic psychiatrist must strive for impartiality and must avoid cases in which prior ties, be they social or professional, could tinge objectivity or neutrality. Whenever possible, forensic examinations should be separated from treatment (10–12). Therapists inevitably become advocates for their patients, and, in doing so, they may be less than objective. Furthermore, they rely on narrative rather than on historical truth and usually do not seek out the type of corroborative material relied on by the forensic psychiatrist. Another reason to avoid such a dual relationship is that confidentiality is compromised once the therapist has to testify in court. Some attorneys may try to draw therapists into child custody battles or may try to persuade them to change their opinions.

The forensic psychiatrist needs to clarify the nature of the examination and explicitly establish the terms of confidentiality at the onset of an exam with retaining families or third parties. It is not an unusual ploy for a parent to attempt to suppress an unfavorable custody report by stating that she went to the psychiatrist for therapy and that the therapist is therefore violating her confidences. From a practical standpoint, the forensic psychiatrist should request payment up front in the form of a retainer. This approach ensures payment, makes clear that one is being paid for one's time rather than for one's opinion, and lessens the possibility of bias. It is customary to charge more for forensic evaluations, because they require more expertise and can be very disruptive to one's practice. It is always unethical to accept a case on a contingency fee because this creates too much vested interest in the outcome of the case.

When court-appointed, the child psychiatrist may operate with quasi-judicial immunity, which protects the psychiatrist from liability. Practicing forensic psychiatry may increase the risk of being sued and it is important to be well trained and grounded in potential ethical problems that may arise before venturing into this arena. Anyone practicing in this area should be aware of the ethical guidelines of the American Academy of Psychiatry and Law, which are more specific to forensics than are the ethical guidelines of the American Psychiatric Association (APA) or the American Academy of Child and Adolescent Psychiatry (AACAP). In addition, the AACAP has useful practice guidelines pertaining to child custody (13) and to assessment of children who may have been abused (14). Psychiatrists who practice forensic psychiatry need to accept the limits of their experience, not inflate credentials, and avoid making unsubstantiated statements. For further discussion of the pitfalls in these cases, see Schetky (10, 15).

Forensic psychiatrists who perform assessments out of their own state should be aware that many states now require licensure for this activity. This is a result of the decision by the American Medical Association (AMA) that forensic psychiatry constitutes the practice of medicine. Failure to address local licensure requirements may result in not being allowed to testify, as well as possible civil or criminal liability (16). For a full discussion of forensic issues, the reader is referred to Forensics section of this volume.

DEALING WITH THIRD-PARTY PAYERS

An unwelcome downside of the current practice of medicine is having to deal with third-party payers and paperwork. With the advent of managed care, telephone trees and voice mail, and with the need for prior authorizations and written treatment plans, the task has become even more time consuming and unsavory. Ethical dilemmas arise when the patient's best interests and the psychiatrist's wish to be paid conflict with insurance companies' interest in minimizing cash outflow. This creates temptations on all sides to engage in unethical behaviors.

Insurance companies may deliberately lose or destroy claims, may reject claims for spurious reasons, or may endlessly "research" disputed claims as a delaying tactic. Noncustodial parents may pocket insurance payments. Patients or parents may request that diagnoses or codes be altered out of concerns about confidentiality so they can receive better reimbursement. The psychiatrist may be tempted to exaggerate the patient's condition in order to get necessary services approved or to obtain higher reimbursement rates. There may be the temptation to alter dates of service, as when Medicaid will not pay for a parent visit on the same day the child is seen, regardless of how far they have traveled. A similar problem arises when only one psychiatric visit is allowed per day, even if the patient needs admission and an intake assessment after an outpatient visit. Physicians may be tempted to exaggerate duration of visits to compensate for low rates of reimbursement. There clearly are perverse incentives to common practices such as "diagnostic upgrading." And yet, regardless of one's motives, these practices are fraudulent and, as such, subject to criminal prosecution. The psychiatrist who engages in fraud may also be subject to ethical investigations and sanctions. (For a complete discussion, refer to Chapter 7.3 and to the Annotations to the AACAP Ethical Code, with Special Reference to Evolving Health Care Delivery and Reimbursement Systems (17).

With the advent of healthcare rationing and a profit motive for managed-care companies, serious concerns arise around who is responsible for the patient once an insurance carrier decides that it will no longer pay for hospitalization or authorize further outpatient visits (18). Little regard is given to the impact on patients of forcing them to change therapists because their managed-care company changes as a result of a job change or a takeover of a managed-care organization. What are the ethics of managed-care companies that direct children of their subscribers to providers who lack adequate training in child therapy? Managed care further disrupts a practitioner's referral patterns if he or she is restricted to obtaining consultations from a list of providers in a particular company. Additional concerns arise over confidentiality as it becomes necessary to share more and more information about patients to justify ongoing treatment. Of particular concern are the blanket consent forms authorizing release of medical information that subscribers are expected to sign when they become insured by private health care companies, Medicaid, or Medicare. This sort of consent is not informed because the subscriber does not know or cannot anticipate what may be in the records being released. Physicians who refuse to release requested information may be penalized by the withholding of reimbursement or even recoupment notices regarding prior payments.

Managed care pressures physicians to become gatekeepers and to consider not only the patient's needs but society's needs when it comes to allocation of health resources. Levinsky (19) reminds us that this is an untenable position, as "physicians are required to do everything that they believe may benefit each patient without regard to costs or other societal considerations."

REPORTING ETHICAL VIOLATIONS

The APA Principles of Medical Ethics (4) states in Section 2, "A physician shall deal honestly with patients and colleagues and strive to expose those physicians deficient in character or competence, or who engage in fraud or deception." Reporting a colleague is a most unpleasant experience, yet necessary to maintain the welfare of patients and the credibility of the profession. Ethical complaints may be filed with the district branch of the APA, with local medical societies, or with state licensing boards. Complaints are handled confidentially. Where appropriate, the psychiatrist should urge patients to file a complaint. If an ethical violation is confirmed by the APA, there are four possible sanctions, ranging from admonishment or reprimand to suspension or expulsion from the association. The defendant psychiatrist is entitled to appeal. Because of the cost of conducting hearings regarding ethical complaints, the APA has urged district branches to take a more educational role in regard to complaints, i.e., stress prevention and early intervention through education, and refer the more egregious cases to state licensing boards. The AACAP Ethics Committee is available for consultation with members but lacks the financial and workforce resources to investigate complaints.

Reports of possible ethical violations may be based on our own observations, disclosures from patients, or external evidence. The psychiatrist may be reluctant to believe allegations by a patient, particularly if they involve sexual misconduct by a colleague known to the psychiatrist. The patient may feel protective of the abusing therapist or fearful of the investigation process and may not wish to disclose. The treating psychiatrist may be reluctant to act contrary to his patient's wishes. Anonymous complaints by a therapist or physician usually cannot be investigated. The APA Council on Ethical and Judicial Affairs (20) believes that physicians must report sexual misconduct to the appropriate authorities. One should also be aware of state laws regarding the reporting of an impaired physician or one involved in abusive behavior.

Reports based on extrinsic evidence pertain to information a psychiatrist may have read in a newspaper or an event based on a legal fact, such as when a psychiatrist adopts a patient.

Filing a complaint allows the ethics committee to look further into the matter. Extrinsic evidence may also be used to bypass an ethics hearing if the facts speak for themselves.

SUMMARY

Child and adolescent psychiatrists need to familiarize themselves with the ethical codes that govern their practices. They should not be pressured by patients or insurance companies into acting in ways contrary to the patient's interests or the profession's code of ethics, nor should they exploit insurance companies for their own financial gain. If in doubt as to whether a certain behavior is ethical, child and adolescent psychiatrists may refer to AACAP: Annotations to AACAP Ethics Code (17) or consult with the Ethics Committee of the AACAP or their APA district branch ethics committee.

APPENDIX: PRINCIPLES OF PRACTICE OF CHILD PSYCHIATRY

A child or adolescent and his or her family may expect the child psychiatrist to:

- Have as primary concerns the welfare and the optimal development of the individual child or adolescent assessed in the context of the family, school, and community based on scientific knowledge and collective and personal experience;
- Foster the unique and nurturing relationship among the child or adolescent and the parents or caretakers and the family;
- Recognize the child's or adolescent's need for the support of adults;
- Avoid all actions that may have a detrimental effect on the optimal development of the child;
- Use his or her unique relationship with the child or adolescent and family to foster their wellbeing and optimal development;
- Promote, by all appropriate means, the uniqueness of the individual;
- Seek to develop with the child or adolescent as thorough an understanding as possible of the child psychiatrist's role, opinions, conclusions, and recommendations;
- Protect specific confidences of the child or adolescent and the parents or guardians and others involved, unless this course would involve untenable risks or jeopardize caretaking responsibility;
- Seek to develop with those involved in the care or treatment of the child or adolescent (parents or guardians, and, when appropriate, the family, teacher and school, court or correctional agency, physician, and others) as thorough an understanding as possible of the child psychiatrist's role, opinions, conclusions, and recommendations;
- Help the child or adolescent to recognize the influence of his or her own relationship with family members and the consequences of his or her decisions;
- Help family members to resolve differences in their views of professional judgments or recommendations;
- Avoid acting solely as an agent of the parents, guardians, or agencies;
- Maintain the integrity of professional judgments and behaviors independent of influence of the source of compensation.

Adapted from the American Academy of Child Psychiatry Code of Ethics, May 16, 1982, with permission.

References

1. Reiser S, Dyck A, Curran W (eds.): *Historical Perspectives and Contemporary Concerns.* Cambridge, MA, MIT Press, p. 1, 1977.
2. Mead M: Cited in Levine M: *Psychiatry and Ethics.* New York, George Brasilier, pp. 324–325, 1972.
3. Dyer AR: *Ethics and Psychiatry.* Washington DC, American Psychiatric Press, 1988.
4. APA: *Principles of Medical Ethics.* Washington, DC, American Psychiatric Association, 1993.
5. Beauchamp T, Childress J: *Principles of Biomedical Ethics*, 3rd ed. New York, Oxford University Press, 1989.
6. Simon R: *Clinical Psychiatry and the Law.* Washington, DC, APPI Press, 1987.
7. Appelbaum P and Gutheil T: *Clinical Handbook of Psychiatry and the Law*, 2nd ed. Baltimore, Williams and Wilkins, 1991.
8. Schetky DH: Exceptions to confidentiality in criminal investigations. *AACAP News* 31:2, 2000.
9. Beresin EV and Olson CK: Child Psychiatry and the Media. *Child and Adolescent Psychiatric Clinics of North America* 14(3), 2005.
10. Schetky DH: Forensic Ethics. In: Schetky DH and Benedek EP (eds.): *Principles and Practice of Child and Adolescent Forensic Psychiatry.* Washington, DC, APPI Press, 2002.
11. Strasburger L, Gutheil T, Brodsky A: On wearing two hats: Role conflict in serving both as psychotherapist and expert witness. *Am J Psychiatry* 154:448–456, 1997.
12. Greenberg A and Shuman D: Irreconcilable Conflict Between Therapeutic and Forensic Roles. *Professional Psychology: Research and Practice* 28:50–57, 1997.
13. American Academy of Child and Adolescent Psychiatry: Practice Parameters for Child Custody Evaluations: <www.aacap.org/clinical/parameters/summaries/CUSTODY~1.HTM>.
14. American Academy of Child and Adolescent Psychiatry: Practice Parameters for Forensic Evaluation of Children and Adolescents Who May Have Been Physically or Sexually Abused. *Journal of the American Academy of Child and Adolescent Psychiatry* 36:10 G=Suppl, 37s–55s, 1997.
15. Schetky DH: Ethics and the clinician in custody disputes. *Child Psychiatr Clin North Am* 7:455–465, 1998.
16. Simon R and Shuman D: Conducting forensic examinations on the road: Are you practicing your profession without a license?. *J Am Acad Psychiatry Law* 27:75–82, 1999.
17. American Academy of Child and Adolescent Psychiatry: *Annotations to AACAP Ethics Code with Special Reference to Evolving Health Care Delivery and Reimbursement Systems.* Washington, DC, American Academy of Child and Adolescent Psychiatry, 1995.
18. Appelbaum P: Who is responsible when a patient's insurance runs out? *Psychiatr Serv* 47:361–362, 1997.
19. Levinsky N: The doctor's master. *N Engl J Med* 311:1573–169, 1994.
20. American Psychiatric Association Council on Ethical and Judicial Affairs, 1991.

CHAPTER 1.4 ■ EDUCATION AND TRAINING

DOROTHY E. STUBBE AND EUGENE V. BERESIN

If you treat an individual as he is, he will remain as he is. But if you treat him as if he were what he ought to be and could be, he will become what he ought to be and could be.

Johann Wolfgang von Goethe: Wilhelm Meister's Apprenticeship VIII-4

BACKGROUND AND CONTEXT

There is a dearth of child and adolescent psychiatrists to treat the nation's children and their families with serious mental health needs (1, 2). Epidemiological studies suggest that 5% to 9% of children suffer from "extreme functional impairments" from psychiatric disorders, and up to 10% to 20% have a diagnosable disorder (3). There are approximately 7,000 child and adolescent psychiatrists in the United States, considerably below the estimated 20,000 needed to provide the psychiatric care of seriously psychiatrically ill children and youth within a multidisciplinary system of care. Child and adolescent psychiatry researchers are similarly insufficient to meet the need to advance our knowledge on the etiology and treatment of these disorders (4–8).

Recruiting, training, and mentoring the next generation of child and adolescent psychiatrists is one of the major challenges, as well as one of the major opportunities, of the field. Graduates face a plethora of career opportunities in clinical practice, academics, and research. Lifestyle and improving remuneration also draw medical graduates to the field (9). Yet there are many challenges facing training programs and obstacles to recruitment. Enhanced training requirements, a paucity of funding for graduate medical education of subspecialties, and depleted faculty time to provide the required mentorship and teaching are ongoing challenges. The vigor, rejuvenation, and satisfaction of training the next generation of superior physician clinicians and scientists are the enduring rewards (10).

CHILD AND ADOLESCENT PSYCHIATRY RESIDENCY TRAINING IN THE UNITED STATES

Historical Note

Child psychiatry in this country began with the establishment of the child guidance clinics, the first of which was the Juvenile Psychopathic Institute in Chicago, established by Dr. William Healy in 1909. As child guidance clinics grew in number and in size, it became clear that psychiatrists who worked with children must have training that was more extensive and specific than that obtained in their general psychiatry residency. A major conference held in 1944 under the auspices of the Commonwealth Fund provided a standard set of skill areas that should be mastered by psychiatrists who treat children and their families (11). These skill areas included growth and development, psychodynamics, working with parents, administration, and community organizations.

In 1946, World War II was over and there was a renewed vigor to provide for the children of the new baby boom. The Mental Health Act of 1946 provided monies for the training of child psychiatrists. Additionally, the American Association of Psychiatric Clinics for Children (AAPCC) was formed. The training committee provided an approval process for potential training sites, including an application and survey. About half of the child guidance clinics were approved as training sites in this way.

The American Academy of Child Psychiatry (AACP) was founded in 1953. Initially a by-invitation-only organization, the AACP was committed to ensure training accreditation within the medical specialty, not only through child guidance clinics. After a debate of whether child psychiatry was more appropriately a pediatric or psychiatric subspecialty, the choice was made for psychiatry. The American Board of Medical Specialties approved the subspecialty and examined its first candidates in child psychiatry in 1959.

Inextricably linked to subspecialty certification are standardized training criteria formulated through the Accreditation Council of Graduate Medical Education (ACGME). The ACGME Residency Review Committee (RRC) in Psychiatry oversees periodic surveys and decides upon accreditation status of each program for training (12). This approach was much more medically oriented than the earlier AAPCC reviews. The ACGME demanded that child psychiatry training programs be linked to accredited general psychiatry residency programs and to medical centers approved by the Joint Commission on the Accreditation of Hospitals. These requirements forced the child guidance clinics interested in training to abscond from their exclusive community roots and to become attached to medical schools. It also stimulated the development of new child psychiatry training programs that were situated in medical centers, rather than freestanding in the community.

In 1969, the Academy opened its doors to all child psychiatrists who graduated from, or who were in training in, ACGME-approved programs. The AACP expanded to capture the treatment of adolescents into its purview in 1989, becoming the American Academy of Child and Adolescent Psychiatry (AACAP) of today. The American Association of directors of Psychiatric Residency Training (AADPRT) and the Association for Academic Psychiatry (AAP) are more recently formed organizations specifically devoted to education and training.

As with all of medicine, training and education is both an art and a science. A good training director serves as the conductor for the symphony—transmitting a serious and passionate commitment to the highest standards of comprehensive care for children, adolescents, and families, a dedication to residents and their personal and professional growth and excellence as physicians, and a vision of the field—where it is now and where it needs to go. In each institution, the instrumentation and symphonic music will vary, but the basic principles apply. Excellence in training requires coordinated and well constructed training experiences that adhere to all training requirements, within multiple systems (medical school, hospital, clinics), synchronized with the goals and structure of the broader administration (Dean, hospital administration, Chair of Department of Psychiatry, Division Chair, Directors of Residency Training) and harmonized with the resources and needs of the Division and Department.

Recruitment, Portals of Entry, and Training Program Types (Traditional and Novel) Recruitment and Workforce Issues

There is a nationwide shortage of child and adolescent psychiatrists. A survey by Beresin and Borus of accredited child psychiatry fellowships identified a shortage of recruits for residency and faculty positions in child and adolescent psychiatry in the late 1980s (13). This shortage has continued (1). Lack of exposure to child and adolescent psychiatry during medical school education, increasing levels of educational debt burden, long years of residency training, and relatively smaller income potential in general psychiatry, as well as in child and adolescent psychiatry, are factors that influence a medical student's career decision (14, 15). Other obstacles to recruitment include inadequate support in academic institutions, decreasing graduate medical education (GME) funding, and decreasing clinical revenues in the managed care environment (16).

In spite of the shortages, child and adolescent psychiatry has made impressive progress in its scientific knowledge base through research, especially in neuroscience, developmental science and genetics (17). Additionally, there is a growing recognition of the need for child and adolescent psychiatry by policymakers and the public at large. The Surgeon General's Conference on Children's Mental Health in 2000, and the President's New Freedom Commission on Mental Health in 2003, have both acknowledged the shortage as a national crisis. Pending legislation proposes loan forgiveness programs for child and adolescent psychiatry trainees and full GME funding for shortage specialties such as child and adolescent psychiatry. There is increasing media coverage on mental health problems of children and adolescents, as the public becomes more aware and concerned about these vital issues facing our youth. The public has become increasingly interested in issues of mental health and effective interventions, as the aftermaths of such disasters as the September 11th, 2001 attack on the World Trade Center and Hurricane Katrina in the Gulf Coast in August 2005 have left not only physical, but more permanently, mental health scars on the population.

Recruitment efforts in child and adolescent psychiatry focus on three salient areas: 1) ensuring that talented, interested physicians have positive exposure and engagement early in training to the field of child and adolescent psychiatry; 2) providing training opportunities that are appealing and ensure ongoing engagement of the resident in work with children and families; and 3) the positive aspects of lifestyle, remuneration, and the plethora of job opportunities for individuals seeking a career in the field.

The Transition from General Psychiatry Residency to Child and Adolescent Psychiatry

Developing a professional identity as a child and adolescent psychiatrist is a core aspect of residency education and training. While many residents have had a longstanding interest in children and families, and look forward with great enthusiasm finally to working in the field, assuming the role of a child and adolescent psychiatrist is fraught with challenges. Many stressors inherent in the transition from general psychiatry residency to child and adolescent residency may interfere with the educational process (18).

By the time a resident enters child and adolescent residency training he/she has had at least three initiations into new territory: medical school, internship, and general psychiatry residency. The entry into child and adolescent residency training is yet another "beginning," with the attendant narcissistic challenge of starting over and having to master new skills, having just achieved competence and confidence with adults. The loss of working with adults threatens losing skills acquired over three to four years.

Child and adolescent residents working clinically with children use nonverbal skills, deal with primitive defenses, and manage behavior in individuals who are far less able to use advanced cognitive skills and concepts than the adults with whom they previously were quite comfortable. They also have to manage new and complex countertransference problems, such as "adopting" their patients, undoing the actions of "incompetent" parents, and overidentifying with their child patients. They are mandated reporters, and must "turn in" parents to authorities. And they now must serve as authorities for schools, courts, and social service agencies in making decisions that have a profound effect on the child and family, including decisions about custody, placement, incarceration—all at a time when they have relatively limited knowledge and skill in the field. They must shoulder the responsibility of working with dying children and grieving parents. At a less intense level, they have to answer complex developmental and behavioral questions from parents, pediatricians, and allied professionals when they are themselves novices. The new residents have to face all this in the context of increased time demands for calls, emails, paperwork and meetings. They need to help deeply troubled children and families at a time when there are limited resources for outpatient and inpatient care, and far too few clinicians in all child-related healthcare disciplines to take on referrals for the comprehensive care of the children and families they serve. Finally, child and adolescent psychiatry is more demanding than general psychiatry, in that residents need to embrace a developmental model that requires greater integration of the many factors that impact child development, such as genetics, family, culture, educational systems, and social forces.

This stress is heightened by the loss of the previous peer group from general psychiatry residency. Colleagues from general residency are graduating and beginning their careers. Many child and adolescent psychiatry residents are shouldering high educational debt and have to put off their loan repayments for another two years. This training also occurs at a time when many residents are feeling pressure to establish new love relationships, or have started having families and struggle to make a living and spend precious time with their families, all while managing a rigorous and stressful residency program.

Training programs need to appreciate the difficulty of the transition, and promote means for residents to cope with these stresses. The effective collaboration between the residency training coordinator and the training director is crucial to this task. At the admissions level, screening for the most mature, adaptive, and resilient candidates is helpful. Trying to assemble a residency class that is cohesive and supportive is also useful. The program should provide time for residents to meet with faculty and discuss the issues and problems involved in the transition. Alerting the faculty to these transition issues is vital, so they may be addressed in individual supervision. Finding many opportunities to have residents observe faculty treating children and families and serving as consultants provides the means for them to learn skills and have working role models for identification. It may be valuable for some residents to continue treating adult patients, either in the program or through moonlighting, to help preserve previously acquired skills.

Traditional and Innovative Child and Adolescent Psychiatry Training Models

There has been an ongoing debate about the most effective, efficient, and appealing methods to train competent child and adolescent psychiatrists. There were early proposals that child and adolescent psychiatry should split from general psychiatry, as did pediatrics from internal medicine. There have been numerous other proposals, as well. The primary impetus for new and more innovative training portals are twofold: 1) a philosophy of training that endorses innovative training tracks to more fully ensure quality education of competent graduates by optimizing training methods; and 2) enhancing recruitment into the field by providing a variety of attractive and novel training portals.

Existing Portals

Traditional Child and Adolescent Psychiatry Training

Training in child and adolescent psychiatry generally occurs after medical school, and after a first post graduate (PG-1) year that includes at least four months of general medicine or pediatrics, two months of neurology, and two years of general psychiatry training. However, with recent revisions of the RRC training requirements, child and adolescent psychiatry training may commence any time following graduation from medical school. Training in child and adolescent psychiatry is for two years, and the first year of training may count for the PG-4 year of general psychiatry training. Thus, traditional training in child and adolescent psychiatry may be completed in either five or six years after completing medical school. Most residents enter at the PG-4 year. They experience pressures to finish training; to address family, finances, and career development issues, and for some, to plan ahead toward further training such as forensics, addictions, or research fellowships. Many residents are eager to work with children and families more quickly. Other residents prefer to complete the full four years of general psychiatry training prior to starting child and adolescent psychiatry residency. They wish to take advantage of the opportunity for elective experiences, chief residency, and/or to consolidate skills in their work with adults.

Integrated Training

Triple Board

An innovative five-year training sequence in pediatrics, general psychiatry, and child and adolescent psychiatry, better known as the "Triple Board," began as a pilot training experiment in 1985 and was approved nationwide as a combined residency in 1992 (19). The "Triple Board" concept was to create an alternative pathway of training to become a child and adolescent psychiatrist that would combine pediatric, general psychiatry and child and adolescent psychiatry training and would allow a path shorter than would be required in the conventional (additive) training sequence of seven or eight years. One of the goals of the combined training program was to create a nucleus of academically based child and adolescent psychiatrists who were trained and socialized as pediatricians, and who could bridge a gap between the pediatric and the child and adolescent psychiatry communities. Additionally, it was hoped that this core of "Triple Boarders" could serve as a magnet in the academic environment to attract medical students to the specialty field of child and adolescent psychiatry. This track is sponsored by the ABPN, the ABPN Committee on Certification in Child and Adolescent Psychiatry, and the American Board of Pediatrics. Followup suggests that this training track has trained competent and successful clinicians and scientists, most of whom practice predominantly child and adolescent psychiatry, although often in a setting with medically compromised children (20). Although the rotations and integration of the three specialties varies from program to program, all programs provide 24 months of pediatrics, and 18 months each of general and child and adolescent psychiatry. Upon completion of training, residents may sit for board examinations in all three disciplines. There are presently ten approved Triple Board training programs.

Integrated Training Tracks

Integrated training specifies a residency that combines training in two or more disciplines in a contiguous, rather than consecutive, training model. This approach, initially developed and implemented in the 1970s at the University of Pittsburgh by Peter Henderson, M.D., combined child and general psychiatry training from the onset of training. Since that time, a few more institutions have adopted similar models of integrated training. Other programs have the flexibility to initiate a variety of child and adolescent psychiatry clinical experiences within the general psychiatry residency for individuals with a declared interest. Although programs vary in the specific manner in which they configure training requirements, all share in common the principle of exposing residents early and continuously to children and childhood pathology (21).

Training programs with an integrated track meet all existing program requirements for residency education in both general psychiatry and child and adolescent psychiatry. Programs with integration seek to allow knowledge, skills and attitude-building in a developmental context of patient care, and to solidify the trainee's identity as a child psychiatrist early on. Most integrated training occurs within the context of a five-year clinical training program.

Academic Integrated Training Track

In the United States, there is a dearth of academic child and adolescent psychiatrists, and physicians adding to the research base on the etiologies and effective treatments of childhood psychiatric disorders (5, 22). Integrated training in general psychiatry, child and adolescent psychiatry, and research allows medical students to move directly into an integrated child-adult psychiatric residency and research training program that is constructed to do justice to the basic developmental sciences and efficacious interventions while not neglecting the fundamentals of psychiatry. The major goal of this alternative training route is to provide a national model to increase the number and quality of child and adolescent psychiatrists in research careers.

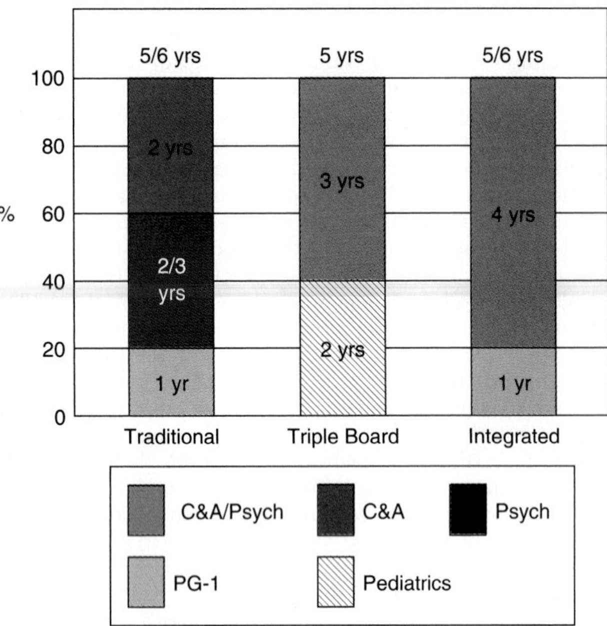

FIGURE 1.4.1. Current training options.

In response to the Institute of Medicine's report on the shortage of psychiatrist researchers, the National Institute of Mental Health established the National Psychiatry Training Council (NPTC) (23). With the support of the NPTC, of which he was co-chair, James Leckman, M.D. and others proposed a six-year integrated child and adolescent psychiatry academic track (24) that has become a reality at the Yale Child Study Center and the University of Colorado and is being considered in other institutions. This program highlights three basic principles: 1) early identity formation as a child and adolescent psychiatric researcher; 2) the developmental continuity of training; and 3) individualization of training and "tooling" opportunities to prepare the trainee for a research career. The program has a predominantly pediatric internship year, followed by a Basic Skills year that allows for the identification of a research team and mentor, appropriate coursework, as well as clinical experiences in evidence-based and long-term insight-oriented treatments. Martin and colleagues have provided a detailed program description of an academic track program (25). Research and clinical experiences with adults, children, adolescents and families are integrated throughout the residency. Figure 1.4.1 summarizes the current training options in child and adolescent psychiatry residency training.

Proposed Portals: Not Presently Approved

Post-Pediatric Training

A newly proposed portal utilizes the Triple Board model for training individuals who have fully completed three years of pediatric training. This model includes 18 months each of general psychiatry and child and adolescent psychiatry, and proposes to incur board eligibility in both general and child and adolescent psychiatry.

This model would allow newly graduated pediatricians or pediatricians who have been in practice for a number of years and wish to retool in child and adolescent psychiatry to do so in three years, rather than the usual four. Table 1.4.1 contrasts the potential advantages and disadvantages of post-pediatric training and triple board (TB) training.

TABLE 1.4.1

POST-PEDIATRIC TRAINING: COMPARISON WITH TRIPLE BOARD (TB) TRAINING

Advantages	Disadvantages
■ Extension of current TB concept	■ Six years vs. five years for TB
■ Can be organized in one department	■ Less integration than TB
■ Less stressful: Master one discipline first	■ Peer group less specified
■ A new way to bring good physicians into child psychiatry	■ Shift in cultures
■ Program includes 54 months of working with children and families	■ School loans and loss of income for experienced pediatricians
■ Child psychiatry with unfilled positions could use this portal to attract applicants	■ Complicated financing for programs

Fast Tracking

A more controversial discussion regards the creation of a four-year training pilot in child and adolescent psychiatry and general psychiatry. This would essentially include an internship year with four months of primary care and two months of neurology, followed by 30 months of general and child and adolescent psychiatry. This portal may have appeal to entering students for whom length of training and student debt are salient, and has the advantage of increasing the number of practitioners in the field more quickly. However, it does not have broad support as an option that provides sufficient training.

Another controversial portal is one in which child and adolescent psychiatry may be pursued directly, without training in general psychiatry. In many European and other developed countries, the major pathway to a career in child psychiatry is via a program that trains specifically in child psychiatry, including basic training in general psychiatry, pediatrics, and neurology. In most of these nations, child psychiatrists are not fully trained in adult psychiatry. The model would provide a direct pathway to child and adolescent psychiatry after pediatric internship and other pediatric experiences. The training may be four or five years. Again, this model has not received broad support of the training community or accrediting bodies.

Competency-Based Assessment in Child and Adolescent Psychiatry Training

Didactic and Clinical Components: The Core Competencies

The training of competent physicians is the goal of all residency training. However, until recently the exact definition of "competent" and the specific areas in which the practitioner was to have attained competency had been only vaguely defined. Thus, the Accreditation Council for Graduate Medical Education (26) identified six core areas in which a resident is required to obtain competence. Programs must define the specific knowledge, skills, and attitudes required for competence in each of the six Core Competencies, and provide educational

TABLE 1.4.2

CORE COMPETENCIES IN RESIDENCY TRAINING

Competency	Definition
Patient care	Compassionate, appropriate, and effective treatment of patients, which serves to promote health and recovery
Medical knowledge	Established and evolving biomedical, clinical, and cognate sciences, as well as the application of this knowledge to patient care
Practice-based learning and improvement	Investigation and evaluation of care for patients, the appraisal and assimilation of scientific evidence, and accessing of the evidence base for treatments to improve patient care
Interpersonal and Communication Skills	Effective exchange of information and collaboration with patients, their families, and other allied health professionals
Professionalism	Commitment to carrying out professional responsibilities, adherence to ethical principles, and sensitivity to patients of diverse backgrounds
Systems-Based Practice	Actions that demonstrate an awareness of and responsiveness to the larger context and system of health care, as well as the ability to call effectively on other resources in the system to provide optimal health care for patients

experiences as needed in order for residents to demonstrate competence (27, 28). Table 1.4.2 gives a summary of the Core Competencies in graduate medical education.

In medical practice, levels of expertise range from novice to master. The residency training requirements of "competence" is that level of expertise which may be expected of a new practitioner in the field. This vague definition is transformed into appropriate and identifiable benchmarks for competency. "Is this person safe to practice independently?" is the critical question to answer in the affirmative in the assessment of attainment of competency prior to graduation.

Competency-based training requires that programs:

- Specify training outcomes in competency terms
- Provide provisional predictors of competent professional performance
- Clarify educational goals for trainees before training is initiated
- Ensure that the curriculum is directly related to the ultimate goal of training the individual for the specialized professional role
- Clearly identify instructional learning objectives for each rotation
- Ensure that educational outcomes are related to identified objectives that are both observable and measurable

Evaluation: Formative and Summative Assessments

Broadly defined, professional competence includes a range of dimensions that must be integrated in the care of patients. Epstein and Hundert have defined this as "the habitual and judicious use of communication, knowledge, technical skills, clinical reasoning, emotions, values, and reflection in daily practice for the benefit of the individual and the community being served" (29). They see competence as more than simply a demonstration of specific knowledge, skills and attitudes, but rather as the integration of ways of thinking, feeling and behaving that are synthetic, ongoing, context dependent, mindful, and in continuous development. The assessment of competency is thus an extraordinarily complex task.

Before considering the means of assessment, it is useful to conceptualize evaluation as formative or summative. Formative assessment is done in order to further the learning process, whereas summative assessment is geared to evaluating the attainment of skills, usually at the completion of an educational experience such as a rotation, didactic seminar or at the end of a training year. Formative assessment is usually done early and often so residents may identify areas of strength or deficiency, allow for awareness of the weaknesses by residents and faculty, provide ongoing means for constructive change, and evaluate how targeted interventions have helped. The cornerstone of formative assessment is feedback. Summative assessments include examinations at the end of each year, such as the Child Psychiatric In-Training Examination (Child PRITE), a 200 multiple choice question examination modeled after Part I of the ABPN Board Examination, with nationally normed scores, and with all questions with referenced answers being returned to the residents following the examination. Another example of a summative examination is the annual oral examination of clinical skill, the "mock Boards," also modeled after Part II of the ABPN Child and Adolescent Psychiatry Examination.

Feedback is defined as an information exchange between resident and faculty describing performance in a particular activity. It is intended to assist in the acquisition of knowledge, skills, and attitudes. If executed properly, feedback should be done once specific goals and objective have been defined. It should be ongoing, face-to-face, based on first-hand data, objective, nonjudgmental, and allow a discussion of the process (30). An example of feedback would be the observation of a clinical evaluation of a child and family, with the faculty member present. Far too often in our medical schools and residency training programs, feedback is neglected, and residents receive either subjective superlative reviews (e.g., "good job!") or hear about their daily performance only if something goes wrong.

There are a number of considerations in evaluating the six ACGME competencies. Faculty must determine if the assessment measure should be formative or summative, if it is practical and do-able, what the constraints of time and cost entail, and the need for training of raters. The ACGME is committed to requiring increasing reliability and validity of outcomes in future years. Measures may be global or specific. Global ratings are typically performed by a wide range of evaluators. The best example of a global rating measure, and one that is currently required of all residency training programs regardless of specialty, is the "360 degree evaluation." Although training programs vary in the instrument used, the 360 degree evaluation is a scale that is completed by a diverse group of individuals involved with the resident in the care of patients. The evaluators may include attending physicians (either psychiatrists or pediatricians who have asked for consultation), nurses, social workers, other coworkers, support staff, teachers, patients, families and peers. It is best suited to measuring professionalism, interpersonal and communication skills, and systems-based practice. Specific assessment tools include chart-stimulated reviews, reviews of oral presentations or clinical interviews, standardized written examinations, or structured examination of simulated patients.

There are considerable challenges to effective assessment. The distinction must be made between evaluating knowing (and knowing how), showing (and showing how) and actually doing competent behaviors in routine practice when not observed (31). While the first area (knowing) is rather easy to measure, the second (showing) and third (doing) are more difficult, particularly in a reliable and valid manner. We need better tools and methods to ensure that faculty are seeing the same behaviors, and share the same benchmarks for competent performance. Furthermore, if we take competence as a developmental process, we need to define the benchmarks differently for residents just out of medical school compared to senior residents and practitioners working in the field.

One of the important consequences of a highly successful evaluation methodology is that it may provide an alternative model to the one used currently in residency training. Many of the ACGME requirements for residency training are timed: They require a certain period of time on a service or rotation for successful completion. This allows for a relatively stable and predictable process for training programs, but decreases flexibility for an individual resident. In a purely competency-based training model, if a resident can demonstrate competency at a relatively early stage of training in a given area, more time could be devoted to other, more advanced or elective experiences. This could open up the training process to facilitate specialty training in a wide range of clinical, academic or research endeavors.

Remediation

The enormous personal investment, as well as institutional and national investment in each physician, provides a crucial impetus to ensure that each resident competently completes training and enters the workforce to care for the large number of underserved children and families in need.

Surprisingly little has been written about the remediation of competency in medical education. In each of the six core competencies, a failure to meet the core competency criteria in knowledge or skills can be described as a "deficiency" that must be made up, for example, through access to a missed learning opportunity or repetition of previously offered material (32–35). In contrast, the "remediation" of attitudes is a more difficult definition, which suggests that a change is required in a resident's outlook (36). Health impairments, due to physical, psychiatric or substance abuse problems, are special challenges to remediation, and have federal and state guidelines that must be followed regarding the impaired physician and the safety of the public.

Remediation of competence is embedded within the overall philosophy of lifelong learning and improvement. At the start of any educational or training endeavor, the novice does not yet possess the knowledge, skills and attitudes required for competence. Remediation is the act of identifying areas that are not yet performed competently and addressing them. Learners who are not making the progress expected of a resident at their level of training require remediation to ensure that the skill level is consistent with the expertise needed to perform the tasks with competence. The steps in the competency process include:

- Defining competent practice
- Engaging faculty and trainees in the process of competency- based training, assessment, optimal feedback, and remediation if needed
- Use of assessment measures of competency that are fair, use multiple evaluators, and may include a variety of formats
- If competence is not attained, a plan for remediation is made, implemented, and monitored.

Competency-based training, assessment, and remediation utilize a skills-attainment model rather than an apprentice model of training. For many faculty and supervisors, this method of teaching and supervision may be new or foreign, and faculty require a great deal of education to ensure that supervision is optimally interactive, with ongoing constructive feedback, monitoring, and engagement in the difficult task of gaining the skills needed for superior practice. Except for the very rare circumstance in which a trainee has such an egregious violation of ethics and practice that termination is required, residents should receive constructive feedback on strengths and relative weaknesses in their skill set, and be engaged and motivated for self-improvement on an ongoing basis. From this theoretical stance, training and supervision may be conceptualized as ongoing remediation—or remediation may be conceptualized as ongoing improvement of medical practice. Remediation is not discipline. It is only when a resident does not meet required expectations for improvement of practice that the process may move forward into a more disciplinary procedure.

If a trainee displays deficiencies in competence that are severe, pose a danger to the public, or have not been modified by a concerted and comprehensive remediation plan, the remediation process may need to enter into a disciplinary phase. Each institution has a due process procedure in place for trainees, and the program director should be familiar with the process and ensure that all residents are informed, as well.

Steps in a remediation process include:

- Performance evaluations
- Written warnings
- Prescriptive/remedial procedures

Types of disciplinary action include:

- Probation—Strictly written expectations for which the trainee is closely monitored, with the explicit plan for termination if the expectations are not met
- Retention—Extending the training time to remediate areas of deficiency
- Non-renewal of appointment—Advanced warning and a planned nonrenewal of the training appointment prior to graduation
- Termination—Dismissal from the program—usually for egregious or ongoing professional violations
- Not certifying for Board qualification—Not recommended. This is when a resident completes the training period, but a letter certifying competency is not sent to the Board for specialty certification.

Directors of residency training are charged with the task of ensuring competent graduating physicians. The courts have strongly supported the academic judgment of professional faculty unless evidence of discrimination or other wrongdoing by the faculty exists. The courts view residents as clinician/faculty rather than students as far as disciplinary actions are concerned. As a matter of public policy regarding patient safety in medical care, less stringent due process is required for residents than for medical students. The courts support disciplinary actions, including dismissal of the resident, in the interest of public safety in the course of patient care.

Faculty Development in the Age of Competencies

The incorporation of a competency-based curriculum in medical education requires new challenges to the faculty. First, they need to understand the conceptual basis for looking at outcomes in the educational process, assimilate the new language of the competencies into their lexicon, and embrace the process as not simply additional bureaucratic burdens, but rather a different way of approaching the educational mission. There is no doubt that building an ongoing assessment into the daily process of working with residents will be more time consuming.

The faculty needs to learn how to provide ongoing objective feedback and the means of doing so. This will involve increased direct observation of resident–patient interactions, as well as codifying ways of observing them. Interrater reliability studies will need to be conducted among faculty members to ensure that assessments are internally consistent. Other standardized techniques, such as chart reviews and checklists for resident presentations, are needed. The faculty will increasingly be involved in 360-degree evaluations, and help implement these by engaging staff from other disciplines, and inviting patients and families to contribute. The faculty and residents will need to be more comfortable and familiar with the use of videotaped sessions, an excellent means of observing their interactions with patients. In-service programs are needed to help faculty learn new ways of teaching the core competencies. Examples include innovative collaborative rounds with pediatricians and schools in the care of patients with complex disorders as an effective method to teach systems-based practice. The Kalamazoo Consensus Statement on Communication Skills may be an effective means of learning to teach and assess Interpersonal and Communication Skills (37). Engaging faculty and residents in the creative endeavor of training keeps faculty up to date and fresh, as well as provides an optimal training environment for residents.

The competency movement and need for increased faculty training and participation comes at a time when the faculty is stretched more than ever. The increasing demand for productivity due to managed care has taken precious time away from teaching and academics. The child and adolescent faculty is already in high demand for teaching in multiple arenas: medical school, adult residency, child residency, and pediatrics. The rewards for the faculty include the enthusiasm and rejuvenation that comes with training the next generation of superior child and adolescent psychiatrists (10).

Program and Institutional Accreditation

Training in all of the medical specialties is well regulated for quality, to ensure that the training program is providing the full scope of experiences, didactics, and supervision in a suitable environment. The Accreditation Council for Graduate Medical Education (ACGME) is responsible for setting training requirements for all specialties and subspecialties approved by the American Board of Medical Specialties, and consists of representatives from the American Medical Association (AMA), the American Board of Medical Specialties (ABMS), the Association of American Medical Colleges (AAMC), the American Hospital Association, and the Council of Medical Specialty Societies.

The General or Institutional Requirements are the same regardless of the specialty being reviewed. They are concerned less with the particular training area than with the overall support and surveillance provided by the medical center in which the training program is embedded. These issues include requirements for the selection of trainees and assurance that there are procedures for evaluation, feedback, grievance reporting, duty hours, and due process. There also must be adequate compensation, an emphasis on education rather than on service, and acculturation help for those trainees who need it (12). The General Requirements necessitate that the institution provide adequate facilities and support to residency training programs. This has provided needed resources during fiscally conservative times and ensures the ongoing viability of residency training.

The Special Requirements are the essential training components that are specific to a particular specialty or subspecialty. They are revised every 5 to 10 years, although discrete changes or "minor revisions" may be made between revisions. The revisions of the Special Requirements and the evaluation of the ACGME surveys are the responsibility of the Residency Review Committee (RRC). There are RRCs for all accredited specialties, and the RRCs report to the ACGME. RRC members for psychiatry are nominated by three organizations: the American Medical Association (AMA), the American Board of Psychiatry and Neurology (ABPN), and the American Psychiatric Association (APA). At least every five years, accredited child and adolescent psychiatry residency training programs receive a reaccreditation site review—a full review of the program to determine if all of the Institutional and Special Requirements for training are being met. The Program Information Form (PIF) is well known to directors of the residency training program and training coordinators (the administrative personnel that coordinate the smooth functioning of the training program) as the document submitted to the RRC to denote the specifics of didactic and clinical training, competency evaluations, and program structure. It is upon this document, as well as the site visitor's review of the program and meeting with residents, faculty and administrators, that recommendations for accreditation are made. Accreditation may be full (5 years) or with citations (for areas of concern to be remedied), with ongoing accreditation for less than 5 years. Additionally, probationary status or nonaccreditation may occur for egregious lapses in the required training components.

In 1959, the first training programs for child psychiatry were accredited—a total of 11. As of 2005, there were 114 approved child and adolescent psychiatry residency programs in the United States, and 741 filled residency positions in child and adolescent psychiatry (38).

Board Certification in Child and Adolescent Psychiatry

ABPN Certification

It is the RRC's responsibility to accredit training programs, but it is the American Board of Psychiatry and Neurology (ABPN) that certifies individuals as competent to practice as specialists. The ABPN determines the accuracy of the applicant's credentials in regard to schooling and residency. To be a candidate for certification in child and adolescent psychiatry, one must have completed at least three postgraduate years of ACGME-approved residency in general psychiatry and a two-year approved residency in child and adolescent psychiatry. One also must have passed the written and oral ABPN examinations in general psychiatry.

In the past there was a clear distinction between the ACGME that accredited programs, and the ABPN that certified individuals. With the advent of the competency movement, the ACGME and ABPN have grown closer in their mission to ensure the competency of graduates. Plans are in place to initiate a new Part I of the ABPN certification examination of communication skills, which will be assessed during the second year of general psychiatry residency to ensure that each resident demonstrates an ability to conduct a psychiatric interview and develop rapport between doctor and patient. The current written examination for general psychiatry is planned to move into the last year of general (or first year of child and adolescent) residency training. The increased collaboration between these regulatory agencies may alter the manner in which residents are certified in the future.

Maintenance of Certification

In 1994 the ABPN moved from an unlimited certification to a time-limited certificate that requires recertification every ten years. As posited by the American Board of Medical Specialties (ABMS), of which the ABPN is a member, each physician must engage in the process of maintenance of certification that includes strategies that ensure a continuum of learning, self-assessment, professionalism, and cognitive growth through the maintenance of certification program. For psychiatry, this program requires participating in an annual self-assessment continuing education program that earns 30 Category I Continuing Medical Education (CME) credits from approved sources, maintenance of a full license to practice medicine, taking a multiple choice examination administered by the ABPN every ten years, and completing a "performance in practice module," although the latter requirement is planned but not yet implemented.

CHILD AND ADOLESCENT PSYCHIATRY TRAINING WITHIN BROADER MEDICAL EDUCATION

Medical Student Education in Child Psychiatry and Human Development

Lack of exposure to child and adolescent psychiatry has been identified as one of the major obstacles to recruitment into the field (1, 16). Medical schools vary considerably in their curricula and in the utilization of their child and adolescent psychiatry faculty. Some schools have faculty contributing to required courses in human development. Often, key elements of human development are "embedded" throughout the curriculum, and therefore potentially do not receive the same attention that human development enjoys when it exists as an independent course. In general, child psychiatry didactics are rare throughout medical school curricula, and often faculty teaching in the relatively short core clerkships are left to mention child psychiatry in the context of a more general psychiatric education experience. Most clerkships are heavily geared to teaching psychiatry in adult settings, largely inpatient units, and medical students rarely have an opportunity to see children and families. Some may see children and families when on call in emergency settings. The didactics that are involved in the core psychiatry clerkships often involve some child and adolescent psychiatry, though this is generally minimal—certainly not enough exposure in most schools to stimulate interest in the field. Medical students who have an interest in development and in the psychosocial issues of children and families often must choose elective rotations that provide educational experiences with these patients, or devise their own electives. Interested students may choose to work in community settings, schools, child and adolescent inpatient or residential programs, or in clinical settings around the United States and abroad. There are many opportunities, but much has been relegated to the creativity of students and their mentors.

One important and innovative program is the Donald Cohen/Klingenstein Third Generation Foundation Fellowship in Child and Adolescent Psychiatry. Begun at Yale Medical School, the Klingenstein Fellowship serves to mentor interested medical students in child and adolescent psychiatry from their first year through graduation. The program has been replicated to currently include six programs nationally: Harvard, Johns Hopkins, Mt. Sinai, Stanford, University of California at Davis, and the Yale Child Study Center. Students accepted into the program are assigned a mentor, based on their particular interests in the field. Most programs have the student follow a patient and family longitudinally for the duration of their medical school career. This may involve sitting in therapy sessions, going to the pediatrician for medical visits, making home visits, going to the child's school, attending births of siblings, etc. In short, the student is deeply involved with the child and family, including as many activities as possible to fully appreciate the many psychological, medical, social, and cultural forces that impact a child and family during the course of development. Other students may "shadow" faculty members in their clinical work in a variety of clinical service areas. On a monthly basis, the students at each medical school spend an evening with faculty that may involve clinical discussions, movies, or didactic presentations. Additional opportunities for mentoring, observing clinical work, or doing elective academic projects, including engaging in research are encouraged. While the Klingenstein project is in its early phases, it is an innovative and highly effective national effort to increase interest in child and adolescent psychiatry through the combination of clinical experience, mentoring, and academic experiences. This program, together with other initiatives to increase exposure and involvement of medical students to child psychiatry, has been recently reviewed (25).

The Continuum from Medical School through Residency Training

Unfortunately for residents who choose a traditional portal of entry into child and adolescent psychiatry and who did not have the good fortune of a Klingenstein or comparable fellowship experience, there is limited continuity in education and training from medical school through general psychiatry residency into child and adolescent psychiatry training. Medical schools are required to provide a course in human development, but do not have a requirement for clinical child and adolescent psychiatry. Elective opportunities are available, though not in all medical schools. Most medical students interested in child and adolescent psychiatry have an interest in pediatrics. In fact, many struggle with the career decision between child psychiatry and pediatrics. Such students will take many pediatric electives, though there may be few training opportunities in child psychiatry or the psychosocial aspects of pediatrics.

The general psychiatry residency requirement for child and adolescent psychiatry is for 2 months of clinical work with children and families. This may be done in inpatient, partial hospital, or outpatient settings. General psychiatry residents may take one of their two months of consultation psychiatry in child psychiatry and may take one of their two required months of neurology in pediatric neurology. In addition, the requirements for forensic and addictions may be completed with child and adolescent patients. For residents interested in child and adolescent psychiatry early on, if their program offers the opportunity, they may be able to have considerable child psychiatry training before their child psychiatry residency. For others, particularly the ones who discover child and adolescent psychiatry later in their generally psychiatry residency, there may be limited continuity between child and adolescent and general psychiatric residency training.

The Relationship Between Child Psychiatry and Pediatrics

Pediatric residencies are required to teach two months of Developmental Behavioral Pediatrics within their three years of training. This is taught largely within pediatric programs themselves, although some may use affiliated child and adolescent psychiatry faculty to train their residents. Child and adolescent psychiatry residency programs have a requirement for a rotation in consultation to pediatrics. All child and adolescent programs have a formal consultation service to pediatrics in which the residents rotate for this educational experience.

It is very important for child and adolescent and pediatric programs to develop and foster a close collaborative relationship. The high prevalence of psychiatric and psychosocial problems in children and families results in a tremendous burden on pediatricians. Given the shortage of child and adolescent psychiatrists nationally, our field can help pediatricians by providing consultation, education, and assistance in situations of psychiatric emergencies presenting to pediatrics and hospitalized children and families, and arranging an appropriate disposition for their patients. Consultation services at this time are largely devoted to inpatient pediatrics. Increasingly, however, we need to be able to provide pediatricians consultation for their outpatient services. Since the primary locus of pediatric care is in the outpatient setting, there is an acute and ongoing need for ambulatory consultation. How pediatrics will manage the rising need for psychiatric, psychological, and social services remains to be seen. What we can provide our colleagues at this time is education in the assessment and treatment of psychiatric disorders, so they will better be able to identify problems, discuss them in an informed manner with parents, and determine what treatments they may provide themselves, and what services must be triaged to allied professionals in mental health.

SPECIAL ISSUES IN EDUCATION AND TRAINING: MENTORSHIP, MORALE, LEADERSHIP LIFESTYLE, AND COMMUNITY

Professional Identity Formation: The Role of Mentors

Mentoring is frequently cited by trainees and early career psychiatrists as one of the most powerful influences in career development (39, 40). Williams and colleagues (40), in a focus group study of mentor–mentee relationships, identified qualities that mentors and mentees should possess that facilitate good mentoring relationships. "Specifically, mentors must be compatible on a personal level, active listeners, able to identify potential strengths in their mentees, and able to assist mentees in defining and reaching goals. Mentees must be proactive, willing to learn, and be selective in accepting advice from their mentors" (40).

Mentorship is an active process, which, when the key elements are present, may be a life-changing experience for both the mentor and the mentee. It is the power of the relationship that promotes development—the mentor's ability to envision in the mentee strengths, weaknesses and growth potential—not just what he/she is at the time, but what he/she has the potential to become (41). Idealization of the mentee by the mentor and vice versa makes for a powerful bond. However, there is much more than idealization. Realistic appraisal, insight, motivation, and career expertise are other qualities of mentorship that are required to effectively assist the mentee in genuine growth.

Mentorship has been acknowledged as a crucial element of research careers, as demonstrated by the National Institutes of Health (NIH) Mentored Career Development Awards. However, mentorship may help launch clinical, administrative, teaching, and other career paths as well. Mentors may be assigned or may be developed on the basis of mutual identification in a less formal process. A study by Ragins and Cotton (42) suggests that informal mentored relationships, developed on the basis of mutual identification, led to greater benefits for protégés than formal arrangements. Formally arranged mentorship arrangements typically last between six months and one year (43); informal ones between three and six years (44). Martin (41) has noted that "it is less physical proximity than meaningful intellectual, personal, and emotional connections that count most" (p. 1226) in the mentor–mentee relationship. "More than duration, internalization can be seen as providing a useful metric for the success of the experience. Those individuals capable of invoking and making use of the other (whether spontaneously or through active effort) have been effectively mentored" (p. 1228).

The risks inherent in the mentorship relationship are those that come with a power differential in a personal and intimate relationship. There is the potential for the mentor to use the relationship for his/her own aggrandizement or narcissistic gratification; the potential for romantic interests interwoven with professional ones; the potential to exploit the talents of the mentee or to plagiarize ideas; and the potential for the mentor to promise more than he/she can deliver and to lose interest or neglect commitments to the mentee. The mentee, as well, may idolize the mentor, and the potential for intense transference feelings is ever present. To be optimally successful, early and clear articulation of expectations of the work together in the mentorship relationship may provide the template and the scaffolding to build a relationship that launches a successful career. Frequent reassessment of the working relationship to ensure alignment of goals and expectations reinvigorates the work, and ensures the optimal effectiveness of the mentor–protégé bond. It is the sign of a successful mentorship relationship when the protégé becomes a mentor to others, thus rejuvenating and promulgating the transmission of values from generation to generation (41, 43).

Maintaining Morale and Values in Our Students, Residents, and Faculty

While departments may differ in their healthcare delivery system, the size and nature of the faculty, and in the population served, the core values and philosophy of all training programs remain the same. We share a profound and passionate commitment to the highest standard of care for children, adolescents, and families. From the standpoint of an academic program, the mission is to transmit the core knowledge, skills and attitudes necessary for this task. All departments must provide a culture in which students, residents, and faculty are treasured, where teaching is cherished, where deficiencies in individuals and in the program are sensitively remediated, and where deep trust and honest, open communication are shared and encouraged between all members of the community (16).

Yet there are innumerable obstacles to achieving these ideals. It may be difficult to provide comprehensive, longitudinal care for patients and their families due to insurance caps on numbers of outpatient visits, and shortened lengths of stay. Many departments have had to increase faculty demands for direct clinical service, resulting in the inevitable choice between meeting productivity demands and spending precious time with students and residents. Faculty are increasingly torn between making a living and doing what brought them to academic institutions—teaching and research. These pressures on the clinical faculty are compounded for the research faculty, given shrinking funds for investigation. All of these forces can breed demoralization among faculty and disappointment among the residents, who in many institutions have had to shoulder increased caseloads and less direct supervision and mentoring. Decreased federal funding of graduate medical education in combination with the impact of managed care has forced many hospitals and medical schools to downsize their training programs, and cap residency and fellowship positions (45). For the residents, these economic forces, coupled with the already mentioned difficulties in transitioning from general to child and adolescent residency training, are potential wellsprings of unhappiness.

How then can morale and the esteemed values of residency training and education be maintained? The training director is in a unique position to tackle these potential problems, though there are no quick fixes to such complex and systemic issues. The training director must help facilitate a "holding environment" for faculty and residents. First and foremost, the training director must have a key administrative position in the psychiatry department and academic medical center where he/she has an awareness of the flow of patients, service needs, and demands for academic leadership. He/she needs to have a close working relationship with the director of graduate medical education. Now that the ACGME has strengthened its mandates on the institution to provide support for the missions of the training programs, and with the institution held liable for citation if found deficient, there are new means to request needed resources for the department from the medical school and/or hospital. This may be of invaluable assistance to the department. The training director must have a very close relationship with the chief of the department and the chief of child and adolescent psychiatry in order to make the problems in the residency known and viewed as a priority. While the training director has no hiring or firing power over the faculty, he/she has significant authority, especially if his/her word is viewed by all as one with that of the Chair.

Obviously, engagement of the faculty is far different than providing marching orders. All faculty have chosen to work in the academic setting because of their love of teaching, mentoring, and advancing science. They are crucial to the establishment of the holding environment and are in the most direct contact with residents. The key to morale is finding any means possible to help the faculty feel honored and respected. The training director must have a close relationship with them, and be present in as many venues as possible—clinical, administrative, and academic. The training director must promote each faculty member's sense of connection to the mission of the department and the program. Frequent group and individual meetings are essential, as is being a direct conduit to the chief and chair. The training director may not be able to increase reimbursement for services or salaries, but can help the faculty in being recognized as key members of the academic program through committee appointments, promotion, having opportunities to give grand rounds and other presentations, and joining research teams. Every effort must be made to acknowledge faculty achievements, such as teaching awards, notices of local and national presentations, and publications. Faculty retreats and social gatherings are valuable ways to help foster a sense of group cohesion, even in times of increasing fragmentation. Group emails that help faculty make clinical referrals, distribute useful articles, or send other messages to each other may add to this sense of cohesion. Finally, faculty may be able to have forums for communication and updating in the residency program through a common program Webpage or training site on the Web. Most programs now have software for a common portal that allows for schedules, evaluations, and posting articles. These sites may serve multiple purposes for faculty as well as residents.

Morale in a residency class is critical for the functioning of a training program. A class that is tight, supportive, smooth functioning, and just plain fun is instrumental to the personal and professional development of the residents. The faculty and training director should see this as an important part of recruitment. The fit between each resident and between the residents and the program should not be underestimated. Group cohesion may also be fostered by keeping the residents together for seminars and meetings with the training director. Each resident should feel that he/she has an important contribution to make to the program, in clinical and academic contributions and in decisionmaking about the structure of the program. When the residents feel valued, that their feedback is heard and matters, and when they feel that their interests are advocated by the training director and faculty, they are much more likely to go the extra mile for each other and their clinical services. There is no substitute for the training director's nurturing a warm, personal relationship with each resident. This required face time provides humor, candid conversation, admission of personal and systemic faults, and a time for needed expression of gratitude as well as complaint. The relationship with each resident and with the residency class is no less than role modeling the kind of professional relationships we expect to foster through the competencies. Needless to say, the residents need the proper balance of supervision, mentoring, guidance, autonomy, time with each other, and time with friends and family. Morale is high when residents and faculty can truly say that they work hard, and play hard, and that they feel like family—and as in most families, there will be struggles and differences, but above all, unconditional love and support.

Teaching How to Teach: Leadership Development, Professional, and Public Education

The goal of child and adolescent psychiatry residency training is to train competent physicians and the next generation of leaders in the field. Integration of components of leadership training into the curriculum enhances this mission.

Graduates have identified lack of training in administrative, supervisory, and financial/managed care issues to be the areas of most deficiency in their training (39). Many child and adolescent psychiatrists are hired as team leaders and medical directors upon graduation. Thus, development of a high skill level in leadership, management, and teaching is needed in training.

Leaders may be defined as individuals who inspire others to go beyond what they think they are capable of doing, making it possible for a group to attain a goal that was previously thought unattainable by 1) inspiring trust, 2) acting consistently, and 3) motivating with words and deeds.

Components of training in leadership skills and enhancing leadership potential may be categorized into six primary arenas: 1) values transmission and formation of an identity as a leader; 2) competency in core knowledge and skills; 3) effective listening, learning, and integrating skills; 4) promoting creativity; 5) effective communication and collaboration skills; and 6) promoting by words and actions sacrifice for the greater goal (46, 47).

Programs have embedded components of leadership and management training to varying degrees. However, a more focused curriculum in leadership is needed. Teaching to teach (public speaking skills, how to put together a presentation, making presentations more interactive, mentored teaching experiences), a high level of collaborative skills, team building, and a deep and abiding vision are required for truly effective leadership. Providing team leadership experiences, seminars on teaching, effective supervision and mentorship—all of these are curricular aspects of promoting leadership skills in trainees. Other components of a training curriculum to promote leadership development includes interactive and experiential seminars on effective listening, learning and integrating, with constructive feedback on these skills by supervisors and others. A professional development seminar, working in and learning about systems, meeting creative leaders in the field to learn about their lives, career trajectories, motivations and advice, and ample elective time to explore areas of interest and promote creative projects are other options for promoting leadership within the residency training program. The options are numerous, and call on the creativity and resources of each program to individualize the professional development curriculum to the training mission of the institution.

Public education is a core professional responsibility of all physicians. Education begins in the office and hospital units with our patients, parents, and families. A parent and child need to understand principles of normal development and psychopathology and its treatment for a sound therapeutic alliance and effective collaboration with the physician. Child and adolescent psychiatrists are also frequently asked to speak at schools, religious organizations, and other community groups. Many of these talks help educate the public about normal development and its variations, as well as psychiatric problems and their treatment. Residencies are required to instruct residents in these patient-care-centered and public educational venues.

Research shows that Americans get much, if not most, of their mental health information from media news, including the Internet, and from public entertainment. Some programs perpetuate myths and misinformation. Others present controversial information that scares parents away from certain treatments. For example, the Federal Drug Administration's black box warnings on certain antidepressants and stimulants frightens parents, is often misrepresented by certain groups in the media, and casts doubt on some treatments frequently used by child and adolescent psychiatrists. Our residents and future practitioners need to be prepared to discuss these issues with patients and with the media. When used well, the many forms of mass and targeted media—including newspapers, radio, television, and the Internet—can counter inaccurate reports and destructive stereotypes. They can also provide information, reassurance, and perspective that can transform the lives of our patients and their families.

The expansion of mass media offers child and adolescent psychiatrists a new opportunity to influence public opinion and policy, and educate parents, teachers, and allied professionals who work with children and families. However, few residency programs prepare residents on how to interact with media (48, 49). Residents benefit from seminars that help them appreciate the complex interests and motivations of journalists and how different forms of the mass media operate; learn ways of ordering priorities for public presentations as opposed to professional lectures and seminars; acquire specific skills needed for managing different forms of media and using mass media as an extension of their clinical practice; and have ample opportunity to practice these skills with teachers who have experience in interactions with the media (48–50).

Community in Education: The Role of Local, Regional and National Organizations

Parker J. Palmer noted that "To teach is to create a space in which the community of truth is practiced" (51). Our community of truth is established by the close ties child and adolescent psychiatrists, pediatricians, and allied health professionals develop. Teaching requires a personal, inner commitment and devotion to our students, but cannot be separated from our community of practicing clinicians, researchers, educators, and administrators. How we establish "truth" is complex and communal. How we transmit, assess, and regulate the material of our field requires community. Sharing our research, empirical findings, clinical perspectives, standards of care or educational models requires a community of professionals who are in continual dialogue. In this way we advance child and adolescent psychiatry.

As our field moves more toward outcomes-based curricula, predicated on the acquisition of competencies, and as the attainment of knowledge, skills, and attitudes are viewed and assessed in a developmental context, we need ongoing collaboration between the national organizations that oversee educational programs. The Liaison Committee on Medical Education (LCME) and the Association of American Medical Colleges (AAMC), which oversee medical school education; the Accreditation Council for Continuing Medical Education (ACGME) and the American Board of Medical Specialties (ABMS), which oversee graduate medical education and certification; and the ABMS and the ACCME, which oversee continuing education and recertification, should actively work together to ensure that there is a real continuum between all levels of medical education. At this time the writers of the United States Medical Licensing Examination (USMLE) have no connection with writers of the ABMS certifying examinations, or any maintenance of certification examinations. Beyond examination writing, the accrediting bodies for undergraduate and graduate medical education ought to adopt the same categories of competencies, and have an organized method of viewing benchmarks for each level of professional advancement. This need not be a rigid system of control or oversight, but an open dialogue between regulatory agencies that have an impact on the training and education of our nation's physicians. Currently conversations are taking place between these organizations, and among the specialty organizations, such as the American Academy of Child and Adolescent Psychiatry (AACAP), the American Psychiatric Association (APA), and the American Association of Directors of Psychiatric Residency Training (AADPRT) to facilitate greater understanding of the benchmarks of competence throughout a professional's life cycle.

At local and regional levels, medical schools and residencies should share precious educational resources. Beyond exchanging teachers, examinations such as "mock oral Boards" could be shared between programs. Regional associations of our national organizations often have special events for medical students, residents, and faculty, and these enterprises should continue. It is not hard to offer mentors in a region for an interested medical student or resident. There are endless possibilities for developing and nurturing our educational community in child and adolescent psychiatry—for students, residents, faculty, and practicing clinicians. We must also not forget that our community has largely been confined to our medical schools and residencies. However, there are many allied professional schools, such as nursing, dental, public health, education, business, and law among others, that can prove invaluable by our facilitating crossfertilization of students and faculty. Beyond this, an untapped resource in our local community is the university, with its undergraduate college and graduate schools of arts and sciences. Medicine has remained rather distant from these campuses. However, our faculty could provide excellent teaching for undergraduates, as is occurring in many colleges that have majors combining neuroscience, psychology, and behavior. Further we are greatly underutilizing the many excellent faculty in sociology, anthropology, and related social sciences that may make a new and important contribution to the training and education of our students and residents, while expanding and enriching our community of scholars.

Lifestyle Issues

Child and adolescent psychiatry, as one of the most underserved medical specialties, provides for a plethora of job opportunities for graduates. According to a survey of all graduating residents and fellows in two states in 2001, child and adolescent psychiatry ranked first of 27 medical specialties in California, and second of 28 specialties in New York, in the average number of job offers per resident upon graduation (52, 53). Child and adolescent psychiatry also fared extremely well in graduates' ratings of diversity of practice options, work–life balance, and flexibility.

Child and adolescent psychiatrists have widely diverse and varied practice options, including academics, research, clinical practice in a variety of settings (private practice, group practice, clinics, and within a continuum of care from outpatient, day treatment programs, residential treatment programs and inpatient hospitalization). Consultations to schools, courts, hospitals, pediatric settings, and other agencies are common. Additionally, advocacy and public policy initiatives may be a formal or informal aspect of many child and adolescent psychiatry careers.

Child and adolescent psychiatry offers a unique opportunity to spend time with your patients and to watch them grow and develop over time and to their best potential. In a recent survey of early career child and adolescent psychiatrists, job satisfaction was rated very high overall—with a median overall career satisfaction rating of 5 on a 6-point Likert scale (9).

Lifestyle issues are being considered seriously by medical graduates when choosing a specialty. A carefully crafted career in child and adolescent psychiatry provides flexibility in work hours to allow a balance between career and family or other interests. Salaries are highly competitive. There are jobs in all parts of the country, allowing for geographic flexibility. Most institutions and agencies pay a higher salary to psychiatrists who have completed child and adolescent psychiatry training. According to 2000 and 2001 combined survey data, the median starting income for child and adolescent psychiatrists was $141,600, compared to $109,100 for adult psychiatrists (52).

Child and adolescent psychiatry remains a medical specialty with a serious shortage of physicians. However, the training and mentorship enterprise is thriving, with recruitment efforts starting from early in training. The superior training of the next generation of effective leaders in the field is the mission of residency training directors in child and adolescent psychiatry training programs. However, it "takes a village" to train a superior child and adolescent psychiatrist. Physicians, allied professionals, residency training coordinators, and patients and their families are all part of that village.

References

1. Kim WJ: Child and adolescent psychiatry workforce: a critical shortage and national challenge. *Acad Psychiatry* 27:277–282, 2003.
2. Sierles FS, Yager J, Weissman SH: Recruitment of U.S. medical graduates into psychiatry: reasons for optimism, sources of concern. *Acad Psychiatry* 27:252–259, 2003.
3. U.S. Department of Health and Human Services 1998: *Mental Health*. Rockville, MD, U.S. Department of Health and Human Services, 1998.
4. Fenton W, James R, Insel T: Psychiatry residency training, the physician-scientist, and the future of psychiatry. *Acad Psychiatry* 28:263–266, 2004.
5. Kupfer DJ, Hyman SE, Schatzberg AF, Pincus HA, Reynolds CF: Recruiting and retaining future generations of physician scientists in mental health. *Arch Gen Psychiatry* 59:657–660, 2002.
6. New Freedom Commission on Mental Health: *Achieving the Promise: Transforming Mental Health Care in America*. Final Report. DHHS Pub. No. SMA-03-3832. Rockville, MD, 2003.
7. U.S. Department of Health and Human Services: *Mental Health: A Report of the Surgeon General*. Rockville, MD, U.S. Department of Health and Human Services, 1999.
8. U.S. Public Health Service: *Report of the Surgeon General's Conference on Children's Mental Health: A National Action Agenda*. Washington, DC, Department of Health and Human Services, 2000.
9. Stubbe DE, Thomas WJ: A survey of early-career child and adolescent psychiatrists: Professional activities and perceptions. *J Am Acad Child Adolesc Psychiatry* 41(2):123–130, 2002.
10. Beresin EV: The administration of residency training programs. *Child and adolescent psychiatric clinics of North America* 11:67–89, 2002
11. Cohen RL: The history of training in child and adolescent psychiatry. In: Cohen RL, Dulcan MK (eds.): *Basic Handbook of Training in Child and Adolescent Psychiatry*. Springfield, IL, Charles C Thomas, 1987, pp. 10–23.
12. Schowalter JE: Program accreditation. In: Cohen RI, Dulcan MK (eds.): *Basic Handbook of Training in Child and Adolescent Psychiatry*. Springfield, IL, Charles C Thomas, 1987, pp. 391–401.
13. Beresin EV, Borus JF: Child psychiatry fellowship training: a crisis in recruitment and manpower. *Am J Psychiatry* 146:759–763, 1989.
14. Martin VL, Bennet DS, Pitale M: Medical students' perceptions of child psychiatry: pre- and post-psychiatry clerkship. *Acad Psychiatry* 29:362–367, 2005.
15. Szajnberg NM, Beck A: Medical student attitudes toward child psychiatry. [Letter] *J Am Acad Child Adolesc Psychiatry* 33(1):145, 1994.
16. Beresin EV: Child and adolescent psychiatry residency training: current issues and controversies. *J Am Acad Child Adolesc Psychiatry* 36:1339–1348, 1997.
17. Eisenberg L: The past 50 years of child and adolescent psychiatry: a personal memoir. *J Am Acad Child Adolesc Psychiatry* 40:743–748, 2001.
18. Beresin EV. Training in child and adolescent psychiatry. In: Noshpitz J (ed). *Handbook of Child and Adolescent Psychiatry: Volume 7: Advances and New Directions*. New York, John Wiley and Sons, 1998, pp. 509–532.
19. Schowalter, J. E.: Tinker to Evers to Chance: Triple Board Update. *J Am Acad Child Adolesc Psychiatry* 32:243, 1993.
20. Schowalter JE, Friedman CP, Scheiber SC, Juul D: An experiment in graduate medical education: combined residency training in pediatrics, psychiatry, and child and adolescent psychiatry. *Acad Psychiatry* 26:237–244, 2002.
21. Moran M: Residency program combines child, general psychiatry. *Psychiatr News* 41:9, 2006.
22. Institute of Medicine: *Research Training in Psychiatry Residency: Strategies for Reform*. Washington, DC, The National Academies Press, 2003.
23. Yager J, Greden J, Abrams M, Riba M: The Institute of Medicine's report on research training in psychiatry residency: strategies for reform—background, results and follow up. *Acad Psychiatry* 28:267–274, 2004.
24. Abrams MT, Patchan KM, Boat TF: *Research Training in Psychiatry Residency: Strategies for Reform*. Washington, DC, The National Academies Press, 2003.
25. Martin A, Bloch M, Stubbe D, Pruett K, Belitsky R, Ebert M, Leckman JF: From too little too late to early and often: child psychiatry education in medical school (and before and after). Child and adolescent psychiatric clinics of North America, in press.
26. Accreditation Council for Graduate Medical Education (ACGME) Outcome Project: *ACGME General Competencies Version 1.3*. Chicago, IL, ACGME, 2000.
27. Sargent J, Sexson S, Cuffe S, Drell M, Dugan T, Ferren P, Kim WJ, Stubbe D, Zima B, Brown T: Assessment of competency in child and adolescent psychiatry training. *Acad Psychiatry* 28:18–26, 2004.
28. Sexson S, Sargent J, Zima B, Beresin E, Cuffe S, Drell M, Dugan T, Fox G, Kim WJ, Matthews K, Sylvester C, Pope K: Sample core competencies in child and adolescent psychiatry training: a starting point. *Acad Psychiatry* 25:201–213, 2001.
29. Epstein R, Hundert EM: Defining and assessing professional competence. *JAMA* 287:226–235, 2002.
30. Ende J: Feedback in clinical medical education. *JAMA* 250:777–781, 1983.
31. Miller GE: Assessment of clinical skills/competence/performance. *Acad Medicine* 65 (Suppl):S63–S67, 1990.
32. Boiselle PM: A remedy for resident evaluation and remediation. *Acad Radiol* 12:894–900, 2005.
33. Doty CI, Lucchesi M: The value of a web-based testing system to identify residents who need early remediation: what are we waiting for? *Acad Emerg Med* 11:324, 2004.
34. Schwind CJ, Williams RG, Boehler ML, Dunnington GL: Do individual attendings' post-rotation performance ratings detect residents' clinical performance deficiencies? *Acad Med* 79:453–457, 2004.
35. Turnbull J, Carbotte R, Hanna E, Norman G, Cunnington J, Ferguson B, Kaigas T: Cognitive difficulties in physicians. *Acad Med* 75:177–181, 2000.
36. Hays RB, Jolly BC, Caldon LJ, McCrorie P, McAvoy PA, McManus IC, Rethans JJ: Is insight important? Measuring capacity to change performance. *Med Educ* 36:965–971, 2002.
37. Bayer-Fetzer Conference on Physician-Patient Communication in Medical Education: Essential elements of communication in medical encounters: the Kalamazoo Consensus Statement. *Academic Medicine* 76:390–393, 2001.
38. Accreditation Council for Graduate Medical Education: *ACGME Annual Survey*. Chicago, IL, ACGME, 2006.
39. Stubbe DE: Preparation for practice: Child and adolescent psychiatry graduates' assessment of training experiences. *J Am Acad Child Adolesc Psychiatry* 41(2):131–139, 2002.

40. Williams LL, Levine JB, Malhotra S, Holtzheimer P: The good-enough mentoring relationship. *Acad Psychiatry* 28:111–115, 2004.
41. Martin A: Ignition sequence: on mentorship. *J Am Acad Child Adolesc Psychiatry* 44:1225–1229, 2005.
42. Ragins BR, Cotton JL: Mentor functions and outcomes: a comparison of men and women in formal and informal mentoring relationships. *J Appl Psychol* 84:529–550, 1999.
43. Kram KE: *Mentoring at work: Developmental relationships in organizational life*. Glenview, IL, Scott Foresman, 1985.
44. Murray M: *Beyond the myths and magic of mentoring: How to facilitate an effective mentoring program*. San Francisco, Jossey-Bass, 1991.
45. Beresin EV: The changing economics of child and adolescent psychiatry training. *Harvard Rev Psychiatry* 4:218–220, 1996.
46. Goleman D: Leadership that gets results. *Harvard Business Review* 78:78–90, 2000.
47. Heifetz, R:. *Leadership without easy answers*. Cambridge, MA, Harvard University Press, 1994.
48. Kutner L, Beresin EV: Media training for psychiatry residents. *Academic Psychiatry* 23:227–232, 1997.
49. Kutner L, Beresin EV: Reaching out: mass media techniques for child and adolescent psychiatrists. *JAACAP* 39:1452–1454, 2000.
50. Olson CK, Kutner LA: Media outreach for child psychiatrists. In: Beresin EV, Olson CK (eds.), *Child and adolescent psychiatric clinics of North America*. Philadelphia, Saunders, 14:613–623, 2005.
51. Palmer PJ: *The Courage to Teach: Exploring the Inner Landscape of a Teacher's Life*. San Francisco, Jossey-Bass, 1998, p. 90.
52. Fox G: Choosing child and adolescent psychiatry as a career: the top ten questions. *DevelopMentor* fall 2005.
53. Nolan JA, Forte GJ, and Salsberg ES: *Physician Supply and Demand Indicators in New York and California: A Summary of Trends in Starting Income, Relative Demand, and GME Graduates in 35 Medical Specialties*. Rensselaer, NY, Center for Health Workforce Studies, School of Public Health, SUNY Albany, February 2003.

CHAPTER 1.5 ■ CHILD AND FAMILY POLICY: A ROLE FOR CHILD PSYCHIATRY AND ALLIED DISCIPLINES

WALTER S. GILLIAM, EDWARD F. ZIGLER, AND MATIA FINN-STEVENSON

Child and adolescent psychiatrists, as well as their allied discipline colleagues, have long understood many of the family and societal factors that impact children's development and functioning (e.g., poverty, community violence, substance abuse, substandard education, family discord). Many of these predictors and contributors to psychiatric impairment have been the focus of public concern, debate, and often policy development. Although child and adolescent psychiatrists and other mental health professionals have much to contribute to thinking about population-wide efforts to address these problems, few receive any training on how to understand effective policy development or their role in it.

In this chapter, we discuss some of the social changes we experience in our society, their impact on children and families, and policy responses to address these. We will also discuss the role of mental health professionals in the policy arena. It will become apparent in the course of the chapter that there are benefits as well as problems inherent in the utilization of mental health research in policy settings. A number of opportunities exist for mental health professionals to contribute to the development of policies for children and families. However, their effectiveness in this regard is dependent not only on their knowledge of scientific principles and findings from mental health research but also on their familiarity with the social policy process and their ability to work with policy makers.

WHAT IS POLICY?

Policy is any agreed-upon set of principles used to guide decisions or procedures. Policies often are codified in written forms, such as laws, governmental regulations, or organizational procedures. In many cases, however, policies are not explicated formally and exist simply as implicit assumptions about "the way things are done." The most formal type of policy is legislation—the laws enacted by state and federal government that create and fund service programs (public-funded prevention services, entitlement services for persons with disabilities), establish or alter rules for government services (procedures for arbitrating disputes regarding special education), and regulate the way individuals and private businesses may interact (mental health parity laws regarding insurance providers, laws regarding domestic violence and protection). Some policies are sets of governmental procedures and definitions that are developed by agency staff to guide the provision of their services, but do not rise to the formalized level of legislation. Even the rules and position statements of professional organizations, such as the American Academy of Child and Adolescent Psychiatry, are policies. What differentiates policies is the degree to which they have been formalized, who they regulate, the consequences that can be imposed for breaking them, and how difficult it is to change them. What all policies have in common is that in all cases someone first envisioned the need for a policy, someone decided what the policy should be, and some individuals or group of people actively or implicitly agreed to it. In many cases the persons writing and deciding policies understand the policy process very well, but may have little or no knowledge of the systems they are regulating or the implications of their policies.

THE NEED FOR EFFECTIVE CHILD AND FAMILY SOCIAL POLICY DEVELOPMENT

Over recent decades, researchers and clinicians in psychiatry, developmental psychology, and other disciplines related to mental health have become increasingly involved in the shaping of policies and legislation designed to address the mental health problems of children and youth. While the focus of legislative action on behalf of children is not new, the presence of researchers and clinicians in the debate has added a different dimension, offering new opportunities for interaction between research and policy. Mental health professionals are directing their work toward the understanding of how contemporary social problems contribute to mental dysfunction in children, not only reporting their research but also underscoring the policy implications inherent in their findings and suggesting a course of action. By participating in the policy process and conducting studies relevant to social issues, they are contributing to the accumulation of knowledge, thus enhancing their understanding of development as well as improving the nation's capacity to address the needs of children.

The interest in social policy among mental health professionals was precipitated by a number of developments. One of these was the implementation during the 1960s and 1970s of federally sponsored social programs such as Project Head Start (1–3). The proliferation of such programs, and the funds made available for them, enabled researchers and clinicians to apply their knowledge and training to such areas as program development and evaluation, which had not previously received their attention (4–6). A related development is that in order to secure funding for research, it is often necessary to demonstrate the practical application of findings and their potential to address societal needs (7).

Another development that fueled the interest in social policy was the recognition that children develop within the social context; they are influenced by various aspects of their immediate environment as well as by the more remote social institutions such as the school, the workplace, government, and the mass media, areas over which children and parents have little, if any, control (8). This realization gave impetus to a number of ecological studies and the compilation of information on children's behavior, achievement, and physical and mental health (9). On the basis of data generated by these efforts, it has become apparent that an ever-growing number of children and adolescents in the United States face serious problems that often result in mental dysfunction (10).

CHILD MENTAL HEALTH NEEDS: SCOPE OF THE PROBLEM

The problem of unmet psychiatric needs in children has been acknowledged for decades, as well as the contributory societal forces needed for proactive policy remedies. A committee of the Institute of Medicine (11), convened at the request of the National Institute of Mental Health (NIMH), studied the mental health status of children and adolescents. It found that at least 12% of children under age 18 (7.5 million children) have a diagnosable mental illness and that many other children exhibit broader indicators of dysfunction, including substance abuse, teen pregnancy, and school dropout, which the committee defined as consequences of or risk factors for developing mental disorders. These findings are echoed in more recent studies. One of these studies estimates that 20% of youths aged 9–17 years have a diagnosable emotional or behavioral disorder and that 9–13% of them suffer from serious emotional disturbances that interfere with their daily functioning (12). Another study focuses on even younger children, indicating that 10% of 3- to 17-year-olds in the United States receive treatment for emotional and behavioral disorders (13).

That so many children are affected by mental disorders suggests that the problem is of national concern. The costs involved in treating mental health disorders are difficult to estimate, in part because of comorbidity with other problems such as substance abuse, making it difficult to separate the costs of care associated with each disorder. Additionally, the information needed to calculate the personal, social, and other costs of childhood mental disorders has not been systematically collected, thus rendering any cost analyses conservative estimates at best. Nevertheless, the studies that are available suggest that the costs of childhood mental disorders are staggering. Rice and colleagues (14) found that treatment services for mentally ill children aged 14 and under exceed $1.5 billion a year. Others suggest that the costs of mental illness in children are much higher since, besides treatment costs, there are indirect costs and costs for nonhealth services, which are borne by families, the schools, the juvenile justice system, and other social institutions (15). As an indication of the costs involved, the estimated direct and indirect cost of mental illness for the total population of the United States was $150 billion in 1996, the latest year for which data are available (16). Clearly, more definitive analyses are needed to establish the actual costs of childhood mental disorders, and such information is important if we are to have a context within which to make decisions about the care of mentally ill children and the allocation of funds to address their needs.

This is a critical issue, given the widely held belief that many children do not have access to mental health services. Two major points are noted in this regard. First, only a small proportion of the overall health budget is directed at children (17). Second, the recent health care reforms that have replaced fee-for-service care with managed care have had both a positive and negative impact on mental health care for children and adolescents. According to the National Health Care Reform Tracking Project (HCRTP), a 5-year study of the impact of managed behavioral health care, access to health services in general has increased for young people (18). However, with the emphasis on brief, problem-oriented approaches, it has become more difficult for children with serious emotional disorders (the "high-utilizers") and the uninsured to obtain the care needed. Additionally, 90% of health care expenditures for children are consumed by the 15% of children who have chronic illness and disability, leaving little for mental health care. In budget allocation decisions that are made when Medicaid funds are decreased, for example, mental health services are often eliminated.

CONTRIBUTING FACTORS AT THE COMMUNITY AND FAMILY LEVELS

Perhaps even more significant than the findings on the prevalence and potential costs associated with childhood mental disorders are the findings on the factors that contribute to the development of such disorders. More research is needed to unravel the causes and determinants of childhood mental illness. However, much progress has been made in the past several decades, producing multiple lines of evidence that suggest that a variety of biological, psychological, social, and environmental factors are involved as causal agents, and that in some cases, an interaction between these factors exacerbates vulnerability to mental disorders. Of significance is the fact that in increasing numbers of children, social and environmental risk factors are implicated in the onset of mental dysfunction (19, 20). Included among these risk factors are prolonged separations between the parent and child (21), physical or sexual abuse (22, 23), poverty (24–26), marital discord (27, 28), parental psychopathology (29), instability in the family environment (30), and a variety of other stressors related to family life (11, 20, 31). Rutter (32) points out that children who experience one of these risk factors may not be any more likely to suffer serious consequences than children with no risk factors. However, the more risks or stressors that are present in children's lives, the greater the probability of damaging outcomes.

It is also noted that some risk factors compound other problems, such as low birth weight and central nervous system difficulties, which, when they occur in isolation, may have no negative effects. Infant central nervous system difficulties, for example, may be overcome if the child is reared in a stable and supportive environment, but are exacerbated if the child is raised in an unstable, poorly educated, low-income, or otherwise stressful family environment (33, 34). Likewise, premature low birth weight babies, who are more vulnerable to environmental insufficiencies than are full-term babies, may experience developmental problems if they are reared by unresponsive adults but may suffer no negative consequences if they receive appropriate care (35).

Poverty

Poverty remains a grave concern, with increasing numbers of families with young children experiencing serious economic problems. This is in part due to the growth in the number of single-parent households, which are the largest and fastest growing family type (36). According to the Current Population Survey in 1998 (37), children under 6 living with a single mother were five times more likely to be poor than those living with both parents. Other contributing factors are cuts in public assistance and the decline in the real value of family income (36, 38). The United States provides far less public income assistance to single-parent families than many other industrialized nations (36). Instead, welfare reform initiatives emphasize labor force participation as the route out of poverty. However, whereas in the past, economic prosperity and employment were effective means of reducing the poverty rate, they are no longer sufficient as an antipoverty strategy for single-parent families because of the decline in wage rates, particularly for less skilled workers (36). For example, in the 1980s, each 1% expansion in the aggregate economy correlated with a $.32 decline in weekly wages. Comparing two strong economic years, high school dropouts earned 22% less in 1993 than 1979, while high school graduates earned 12% less. This compares to a rise in income of 10% for college-educated men and 22% for men with post-college degrees (36). For two-parent families, the wage decline has been partly offset by the entry of increasing numbers of women into the labor force, but for single-parent families the escape from poverty is more difficult.

Poverty's Effects on Children

The decline in real income affects adults and children. However, for children the consequences are particularly serious since, as noted earlier, a significant percentage of families in poverty are those with young children. Indeed, even though the overall poverty rate has declined in recent years, poverty among children under 18 remains high at 18.9%. Children under 6 are particularly vulnerable, with a poverty rate of 20.6% (37).

The ramifications of living in poverty are numerous and include assaults on children's physical and mental health (39). Klerman (40) found that poor families have no access to health care and that other conditions associated with poverty, such as lack of money to spend on health-promoting activities, hunger, and lack of transportation and adequate housing further exacerbate the problem. As a result, poor children experience more health problems and have a higher mortality rate. In several other studies, it is indicated that there is a powerful, albeit indirect, link between poverty and mental health disorders, leading mental health professionals to the conclusion that poverty is one of the major risk factors in such disorders (26, 41, 42). Although at one time mental dysfunction, low achievement, and other problems associated with poverty were discussed in terms of assumed negative traits of poor children, researchers now realize that the major sources of psychopathology associated with poverty stem from environmental stresses and feelings of powerlessness and frustration (41, 43). Also, it is noted that, among poor families, there is a high incidence of poor prenatal care, low birth weight, and malnutrition (44, 45), which are known to contribute to children's vulnerabilities to environmental stress (11). Parental depression and substance misuse are also heightened among poor families, increasing the risk of child neglect and abuse and contributing to mental health disorders (16, 23, 46).

Welfare Reform: Effects and Side Effects

The most dramatic piece of legislation for children and families in recent years is the Personal Responsibility and Work Opportunity Reconciliation Act of 1996. By replacing Aid to Families with Dependent Children (AFDC) with Temporary Assistance to Needy Families (TANF), the government effectively reduced public entitlement to cash benefits. States are now granted greater flexibility in the use of welfare funds while obliged to impose work requirements and a 5-year lifetime limit on receipt of federal assistance.

What has been the impact on children and families? The plethora of research studies on the impact of welfare reform reveals success in achieving a 40% reduction in the numbers of dependent families, along with a substantial increase in labor force participation by mothers (47). However, these positive indicators may mask unmet needs. First, a primary implication of increased employment is the need for child care. Research indicates that many parents lack access to high quality care for their children, either through poor provision or because it is too expensive. These findings were highlighted in the first wave of results from a study of the impact of welfare reform in California, Florida, and Connecticut (48). The study noted that the majority of children were in home-based care, and only 13% of this care was deemed to be of good or excellent quality. A second implication of the welfare reform emphasis on employment is that some parents who have difficulty maintaining employment may be rendered ineligible for financial assistance, thus increasing the poverty of their family. For example, the long-term unemployed are likely to require support to maintain their jobs; some poor people, through depression, domestic violence, addictions or mild mental retardation, may be unable to sustain employment. The figures indicating reduction in welfare dependency do not account for those who have been diverted from welfare assistance without entering employment (47). Thirdly, welfare and immigration legislation has reduced access to noncash services such as Medicaid and food stamps, affecting 20% of the children living in the United States (47). Aber and colleagues (49) further indicate that overall welfare reform does not appear to have reduced child poverty, despite the increased levels of parental employment. However, the researchers note that some specific groups, such as children of teen parents, may fare well as long as they are provided with sufficient support services to mediate any negative impact associated with welfare reform.

Parental Psychopathology

A substantial body of literature supports the observation that children of psychiatrically impaired or substance-abusing parents have an increased risk of developing mental health problems compared to children of normal parents (29). It has long been recognized that maternal depression is widespread, particularly among families in receipt of welfare (50). Kagan and Fuller (48) observed in their sample of 948 single mothers with young children, that the incidence of depression was three times higher than the national average, resulting in disengaged parenting practices likely to result in poor development.

Another area of increasing concern is parental substance misuse. There are an estimated 11 million children under the age of 18 with alcohol-dependent parents, and an unknown number of children whose parents abuse drugs (46). Negative influences are transmitted to children through a variety of mechanisms. One leading area of research addresses the consequences of prenatal exposure to cocaine, identifying disruptions to development, such as impaired arousal regulation, which lowers the threshold for coping with stressful conditions (51). Other scholars have documented the relationship between parental substance abuse and subsequent psychopathology in children, emphasizing the role of mediating factors such as family conflict, lack of family rituals, poor home management, ineffective parenting strategies, physical violence, abuse, isolation, stress and frequent family moves (23, 46). With rates of drug misuse increasing, it is important to provide medical and social support to families to ensure healthy child development.

Domestic and Community Violence

Another area of particular concern for researchers and policymakers alike is the "epidemic of youth violence (52)." Although exact numbers are hard to quantify, there is little doubt that a large and growing number of children are exposed to violence in their homes, schools, and communities as victims, observers, or perpetrators. For example, a study in New Haven, Connecticut, revealed that 41% of sixth, eighth, and tenth grade students in public schools reported having witnessed at least one violent crime in the past year, and almost all of the eighth graders knew someone who had been killed through violence (53). The findings of such studies are troubling not only because of the threat to children's safety, but because of the short- and long-term impact on their healthy development. It is not unusual for children exposed to violence to experience disruptions in sleeping, eating, and toileting, and to display generalized fear and flashbacks. Repeated exposure increases the likelihood of depression, anxiety, post-traumatic stress disorder, low school attainment and high alcohol use (52).

There are important policy implications arising from research into the prevalence and effects of exposure to violence among children and youth. Studies of resilience indicate that a key protective factor is a relationship with a caring, responsible adult, usually a parent (54). However, in some instances, parents may be emotionally or practically unavailable to their children, either because they themselves are the victims or perpetrators of violence or because they are numbed by the exposure to violence in their communities. Therefore, the resources of other adults in the community need to be tapped. Research reveals great potential for school-based programs to lead the way in reducing violence among young people and to promote resilience. Other agencies are also well placed to intervene. One example is the Child Development and Community Policing program (CDCP), which fosters collaboration among schools, mental health services, and the police department, and includes training professionals to work within a developmental perspective (52). An evaluation of the program is currently underway, but anecdotal evidence suggests that the CDCP program has resulted in reduced fear of crime, improved relationships between the police and community, increased referrals of children to mental health agencies, reduced rates of violence, and improved adjustment among children (52).

Domestic Violence

Many children also experience violence in their home. While the issue of domestic violence has been on the policy and research agenda for several decades, the impact on children has received less attention. It is estimated that between 3.3 million and 10 million children in the United States are exposed to domestic violence each year (55). While such violence cuts across social strata, it is more prevalent among families living in poverty and is associated with multiple stressors, including substance abuse and other forms of violence. According to recent research, in 30–60% of families experiencing domestic violence, child maltreatment is also present (56). Possible consequences for these children include behavioral problems and depression, and in adulthood they may develop low self-esteem, and resort to violence and criminal behavior (55). Programs do exist in health care, child welfare, mental health, and law enforcement agencies, but rigorous evaluations have not yet measured their effectiveness.

School Violence

Recent media attention has focused on violence in schools (57, 58). Although the high-profile incidents of schools shootings are relatively rare, a large number of young people are exposed to violence of varying levels (59). Statistics from the National Crime Victimization Survey (NCVS) and the Youth Risk Behavior Survey (YRBS) indicate a decline in rates of violence, which may be due in part to the proliferation of prevention programs, but rates of violent crime among youth remain high (58, 60). The results from a recent study indicated no decrease in feeling too unsafe to go to school, being threatened or injured with a weapon on school property, or having property stolen or deliberately damaged at school (58). In addition to the immediate consequences of exposure to violence, the longer term mental health of young people may be affected. In a survey of 1,100 youth in an urban school, there was a strong correlation between exposure to violence and the development of internalizing and externalizing disorders (59). Children in middle school were found to be particularly vulnerable.

However, while the picture looks bleak, recent violence prevention strategies have yielded promising results. One of the largest and longest running school-based violence prevention programs in the United States—the Resolving Conflict Creatively Program (RCCP)—is currently implemented in over 60 New York City schools and in 12 other school systems across the country (57). The skills taught in the classroom include communicating clearly and listening carefully, expressing feelings and dealing with anger, resolving conflicts, fostering cooperation, appreciating diversity, and countering bias. A recent 3-year evaluation of the program indicated positive outcomes, where an average of 25 lessons were taught in a year, according to child and teacher reports and objective measures.

Family Fragmentation and Mobility

Many children today experience potentially damaging experiences that stem from difficult conditions in family life. During the past 30 years, our society has undergone vast economic and social changes that have transformed the structure of the family and the roles and responsibilities of men and women. These changes have created stressful conditions for children and adults.

Consider, for example, the increased fragmentation and isolation of the family. Currently, one of every four children in the United States lives in a single-parent family, and among African Americans the numbers are one of every two children (61). The growth in the number of single-parent families is particularly disturbing since it is often associated with multiple stressors for both parents and children. The presence of a female head of household and young children, poverty, and maternal depression, are characteristic traits (although not ubiquitous ones) of single-parent families (48, 62). The rise in single-parent households is attributable largely to the increasing number of births to unmarried mothers (36, 63). While the birth rate for married women has declined since 1980, the birth rate for unmarried women increased 49% between 1980 and 1990 and remained constant through to 1995, reflecting the growing preference for nonmarriage (64). The percentage of nonmarital births to African American women is particularly high at 69.7% (36).

Family Mobility and Isolation

American families are increasingly diverse. Currently, 20% of children under 18 living in the United States are immigrants, and this percentage is likely to increase (47). The profile of immigrants in America is changing; they are arriving from increasingly diverse countries of origin and experiencing more limited economic opportunities upon arrival in the United States than was the case with previous generations of immigrants. Research indicates that, despite the great diversity between and within immigrant groups, many share particular needs arising from the experience of stress, depression and isolation in the years following their arrival in the United States (65). Furthermore, because many immigrants lack full access to education, health, and social services, the healthy development of children is jeopardized. There has also been a significant rise in racial and ethnic diversity within the United States population, and this development too raises concerns regarding the availability, access to, and nature of social services. It is projected that by 2030, 50% of children living in the United States will be nonwhite (63). It is thus increasingly important that services for children are tailored to the cultural diversity of the population. The increased diversity also poses a challenge for policymakers to design effective antipoverty strategies, since the poverty rate is higher among some racial and ethnic groups than in the general population.

A related change in family life is the relative isolation and lack of social support that have occurred because of the increasing mobility of people in search of employment and other opportunities (66). As a result, many families no longer live near or have access to the support and assistance of friends and relatives. Referred to by some as a decrease in "social capital (67)," the lack of social support is notable, since having access to a support system often mediates the negative consequences of stress (25, 50, 68).

Divorce

Another reality for many families is divorce. The rate of divorce, particularly among families with children, rose dramatically between 1965 and 1979. Since 1979, the rate of divorce has declined and seems to have leveled off (69). Nevertheless, it is estimated that half of all first marriages will end in divorce (70). The presence of children is not a deterrent for divorce: Roughly 60% of all current divorces involve children (71). Most children will experience the remarriage of one or both of their parents and live in reconstituted families (72). This is illustrated by the following data. Although 71.8% of American children lived with a mother and father figure, the percentage of children living with their biological parents is much lower—64.9% of white children, 23.6% of African-American children, and 53.4% of Hispanic children (70). While the rate of divorce has remained constant after a significant rise in the 1960s and '70s, roughly 40% of children will nevertheless experience the divorce of their parents (73). The rate of divorce is higher among African Americans (70). While divorce is not necessarily a disaster for children, stresses arising from the disruption and subsequent remarriage of parents often lead to psychological difficulties among children (72, 74).

A great deal of controversy surrounds the impact of divorce and remarriage on children. Emery (72) draws four salient points in his review of the research. First, divorce is a source of great stress for children, whether through loss of contact with a parent or due to economic hardship. Second, divorce makes psychological problems as much as twice as likely for children: Even though children may appear to adapt well initially, there may be delayed negative effects (27, 28, 75). Third, despite the risks, most children from divorced families function as well as those from married families, demonstrating resilience (74). Fourth, resilience does not preclude vulnerability: Children experience difficult feelings despite coping well. The outcomes of divorce for children depend on many factors, including age, gender, ethnicity, and socioeconomic status. Tschara and colleagues (76), for example, found that children have difficulty adjusting to the divorce if they were older, had prior psychological problems, and had parents with more marital conflict. Hetherington and colleagues (77) found that the long-term effects of divorce and remarriage appear to be related to a number of factors, including the child's developmental status, sex, and temperament; the quality of the home environment; and availability of support systems both to the parents and the child.

The number of stressors the child experiences is also a factor, since, as noted earlier, a single stress typically does not carry with it appreciable psychiatric risk, but multiple stressors increase the risk for mental dysfunction (32). Particular concern is noted for children whose custodial parent experiences extreme economic difficulties for an extended period of time and/or whose noncustodial parent fails to pay for child support (72, 78). In 1991, only 54% of single parents with children had awards for child support, and only half of these awards were paid in full (72, 79). Even where awards were paid, the average amount was small, at $3,011. Part of the problem is that the noncustodial parent also has a low income, but often, noncustodial parents simply refuse to acknowledge financial responsibility for their children.

Children whose parents suffer emotional and psychological difficulties as a result of divorce are also likely to experience multiple stressors. Researchers have found that when parents' distress is acute, the parents fail to attend to the needs of their children, they do not recognize the children's painful experience with the divorce, or they burden the children with their own adjustment difficulties (80).

Also at substantial risk are children who are involved in prolonged custody fights. These children are the most vulnerable of children of divorce, since custody battles can continue indefinitely. Judges attempt to make custody decisions on the basis of the best interests of the child. However, neither judges nor lawyers are prepared for the arduous task of determining the best interests of the child. Nor are they trained to interview the child, consider his or her needs and concerns, or weigh the urgency of the child's condition and circumstances (81). Recognizing the child as the hidden client in divorce proceedings, Goldstein, Freud, and Solnit (82, 83) have attempted to provide guidance to lawyers and judges by incorporating legal considerations within the framework of principles drawn from developmental psychology and psychiatry. They recommend that decisions regarding child custody be made quickly, that an effort be made to avoid prolonged proceedings, and that whatever decision is made have final effect that is not reversible. They further recommend that judges award full custody of the child to one "psychological parent." There is controversy surrounding this latter recommendation. Some psychiatrists emphasize the psychological value for some children of maintaining a close relationship with both parents, even those involved in a bitter dispute over custody issues (84). Although some of their recommendations are controversial, Goldstein and colleagues paved the way for other psychiatrists to think about the use of knowledge and theoretical principles in establishing criteria for practical decisions that involve children.

The need for mental health professionals to consider the policy implications of their work is underscored by Wallerstein (27, 81). Wallerstein further notes that although an increasing number of policymakers and legal professionals are seeking guidance from the mental health professions, the accumulation of psychological knowledge has not kept up with rapid changes that have occurred in family law. Hetherington and Camara (85) make a similar point, indicating that the knowledge about the effects of divorce on children and postdivorce parent–child relationships is still fragmentary, with several important questions remaining to be addressed.

Although more research is needed, sufficient information currently exists for us to appreciate the widespread implications of the research and the opportunities that exist to mediate the consequences of divorce. In this regard, the knowledge of how divorce affects children and parents should be disseminated not only among mental health professionals but also among other professionals who work with children. Teachers, for example, need to be alerted to these findings so they can be sensitive to any changes in children's behavior and offer them and their parents support and counsel about ways they can cope with the changes in their lives (86, 87). Additionally, as noted earlier, the legal profession needs to be made aware of the research and its implications. Ideally, psychological support for parents and children should be made available immediately when the divorce proceedings begin. One important policy development has been the use of mediation services in divorce cases. These services are staffed by mental health professionals who have access to legal advice. Although initially begun as a way to curtail the high costs of divorce, families who have used mediation services note that one of the major benefits of the services is the availability of psychological support (88).

The importance of psychological support for children of divorce should be made known to policymakers, who can make it a national priority to ensure that these children have access to support services. Several successful support programs for children of divorce have been developed in schools across the United States (89). However, they are few in number and meet the needs of only a small percentage of the children who stand to benefit from such programs. Given the number of children who need such support, these programs should be made available in all schools, or at least in some schools in every community. The federal government can take a leadership role by making available funds that would finance the development of such programs.

MATERNAL EMPLOYMENT

Another complex societal change affecting all children, regardless of family income, has been the entry of a large number of women into the labor force. This phenomenon is especially apparent among women who have children. For women with school-age children, full-time employment has been relatively common for about three decades, with upwards of 70% of such mothers now working out of the home. Among women with infants and preschool children, more dramatic changes have taken place. In 1973, 30% of mothers with children under 6, and 50% of mothers with school-age children were working. By 1997, these figures had risen to 65% and 77%, respectively (61). Among mothers with infants, the rise has been even more dramatic. In 1987, less than 30% of women with infants 1 year old and under were working. By 1998, 55% of mothers returned to full-time work within a few weeks of the baby's birth (61, 90).

The research on the effects of maternal employment on children has found that in and of itself maternal employment is not necessarily associated with either negative or positive effects (91–93). Rather, parental attitudes to the mother's employment are more significant in their effects on children than is employment itself (93, 94). But researchers point out that although maternal employment appears to be benign in its effects on children, in many dual-worker families both the parents and the children experience an inordinate amount of stress. In general, women have assumed new roles in the workplace, but they have not abdicated their traditional responsibilities to family life and childrearing. This has resulted in role conflict and guilt (93, 95), as well as changes in lifestyle and difficulties that permeate the whole family system. Studies have found that close to 40% of employed parents, women and men, indicate that they experience severe conflict, guilt, and stress (96). For children, this state of affairs means that not only do they have less time with their parents, but they are affected by the fact that their parents are under stress from trying to do too much.

Other institutions besides the family are affected by the increase in women's participation in the out-of-home labor force. Employers, concerned about worker productivity, are raising questions about women's juggling work and family responsibilities, and some of them are also beginning to realize that they may be losing valued female employees when childrearing conflicts with full-time work. There are also pressures on such institutions as the school, which have to implement changes in order to accommodate the needs of children not only during school hours but before and after school (97, 98). Additionally, changes have occurred in some professions that were previously associated with flexible work schedules that enabled mothers to work and at the same time rear their children. Teachers, for example, are finding that they have to extend their workday and thus disrupt their own family life because many of their students' parents are working and unavailable for parent conferences and other school events during the day (99).

Increased Demand for Child Care

Although numerous societal changes and problems are associated with women's participation in the labor force, none are as significant as the unprecedented demand for child care services. Today, child care is one of the most widely recognized social problems. Virtually everyone, from working parents to chief executives of major corporations, is discussing the lack of good-quality, affordable child care services. Child care is also the subject of debate at state and local level governments, where the need for child care services is noted. The attention to the child care issue is not surprising, given the increase in the number of infants and children who need it. However, it belies the fact that it has been a major social problem for over three decades. At the 1970 White House Conference on Children, the need for child care services was noted as the number one priority for the nation to address. However, two obstacles—ideological arguments against the use of child care, as well as the lack of public awareness of the need for child care services—stood in the way of policy action on the issue (100). As a result, the problem worsened, reaching crisis proportions before finally attracting national recognition.

Notwithstanding the attention that the issue now receives, child care continues to be regarded as an individual family problem to be addressed by parents. This is evident in that the majority of businesses do not make provisions to ease the stresses associated with balancing work and family life, and that despite the enactment of the Family Support Act and the Child Care and Development Block Grant, which provide needy families with financial assistance for child care, we are still far short of having a comprehensive solution to the problem (98, 101).

There are numerous facets to the child care problem, one of these being the high cost of services. This is a major concern for parents, some of whom choose a child care facility solely on the basis of cost. This point is made by Hofferth and Wissoker (102), who found that parents not only choose child care on the basis of cost, but also that they switch facilities if the price increases. Precise data on what families spend on child care are not available, but it is known that child care costs are anywhere between $1,500 and $10,000 a year, depending on the quality of care and the age of the children involved. It is estimated that full-time child care for preschoolers costs an average of $3,000 a year, and that for infants the costs can exceed $9,600 a year. With the cost of care being so prohibitive, it is not surprising that it is one of the major factors in choosing child care.

From a policy perspective, the high cost of care is significant for at least two other reasons. First, child care costs are a major expenditure for families, and the amount of money families spend on child care is directly related to their income (103). Low-income families spend less on child care in absolute terms than do higher income families, but the proportion of the family budget that is taken up by child care costs is greater among low-income families, who have to allocate as much as 27% of their earnings to child care (104). Even for middle-income families, the burden of child care costs are great, as they do not qualify for state subsidies and pay higher taxes on their earnings (105). Second, there is a relationship between the cost and quality of care, with good-quality care costing substantially more than poor quality, custodial care. This being the case, there are inequalities in the quality of child care children experience depending on their family's income. The fact that good-quality care is a privilege that only some children are enjoying is of concern, because child care is an environment where children spend a large portion of every day. As such, it has significant effects on children's development and wellbeing. For example, recent research highlights the link between educational child care programs and reduced rates of violence and crime (106).

In an attempt to define good-quality care, mental health professionals make a distinction between developmentally appropriate care that is responsive to the needs of children and care that is merely custodial in nature (4). The determinants of good-quality care have been found to be an age-appropriate staff–child ratio and group size, as well as the presence of providers who have knowledge of and training in child development (107, 108). Training in child development—rather than years of experience working with children—sets apart nurturing providers who respond to the varied and individual needs of young children from providers who are unable to provide children with appropriate experiences (107).

Researchers have used this information in important ways to address the needs of children and to promote national awareness of the lack of quality child care and its impact on children. For example, in the Cost, Quality, and Outcomes study (109), researchers examined child care centers in four states, looking at the relationships between the cost of child care, the actual experiences of the children in the centers, and the effects of these experiences on children's development. The study noted several disturbing findings, the major one being that although child care centers vary widely, most centers are mediocre in quality and "sufficiently poor to interfere with children's emotional and intellectual development (109)." Forty percent of the infants and toddlers in center-based care were found to be at risk as a result of poor health and safety standards. In the recent followup to this study, it was confirmed that children in poor quality care do indeed experience developmental problems that persist when the children are of school age (110). Another study focused on the quality of care in family day care homes and the homes of relatives, which are popular child care choices among parents, especially low-income parents and parents of infants and toddlers. The study found that only 1 in nine family day care homes offered good quality care and that the quality of care by relatives was even worse (111).

Researchers used child care quality indicators in other ways as well, for example, the development of training programs and accreditation for child care providers and child care facilities (112, 113), and in the establishment of guidelines for the operation of child care programs (114) and evaluative tools to assess the quality of child care facilities (115). Young and colleagues (116) used quality indicators to determine if the standards governing states' child care licensing requirements are adequate. They found that although state regulations represent a basic minimum in terms of ensuring the health and safety of children, the regulations in most states fall below even that minimum. In other words, a child care facility may be licensed by a state, but that does not mean that it provides good quality care. The researchers not only analyzed states' regulatory standards, but also recommended changes that states can make to upgrade the quality of child care.

These and other similar efforts underscore two important points about the link between research and policy: a) that research findings can be brought to bear on social problems and serve as the impetus for appropriate action (117), and b), that a thorough understanding of the problem—in this case, the factors that influence quality care—is essential if mental health researchers are to be able to make recommendations for appropriate action.

The research on child care discussed only briefly in this chapter has also focused on the effects of child care on infants as well as other issues such as supply and demand, and the availability of child care services. The research has been important, providing indications that although the supply of child care facilities for preschoolers has increased since 1977, there are still regions in the country where demand exceeds supply (118). Studies also suggest that the demand for child care is going to increase, given the growing presence of women in the labor force as well as other demographic factors and employment trends (69, 119). Additionally, it has been found that in two segments of child care, child care for infants and toddlers (120) and child care for school-age children, the demand far exceeds the supply (121). On this latter point, the research has led to policy action, with the federal government allocating substantial amounts of funds for the establishment of supervised programs for children during time when they are out of school. This is important since for adolescents, the peak time for violence, crime and sexual activity is after school hours, between 3 PM and 6 PM, when many are unsupervised by an adult (122).

Workplace Changes to Support Families

The high cost of child care and lack of good quality care is an issue not only due to the possible harm to children, but also because it is a source of stress for parents. This has prompted discussions of the need to make changes in the workplace to create conditions that are supportive of family life. Several suggestions have been made, including corporate support of child care services. Although a few companies have developed on-site child care centers for their employees, and others partially offset the cost of child care for their employees or provide other supportive services, such as information and referral, the need for child care is too large for corporations to address alone. Corporate involvement can thus be conceived, at best, as only one part of a comprehensive solution to the child care problem.

However, there are other ways for corporations to support family life. For example, some corporations may be able to implement flexible schedules to allow employees time for childrearing responsibilities (123). Some corporations provide this option to their employees, but the majority do not (96, 124). In some businesses, flexible work schedules may prove to be counterproductive and therefore unworkable as a means to enhance family life. However, among some corporations, such changes can be effectively implemented if steps are taken to alert the corporate world to the need and importance of such changes in the workplace. It has been suggested that mental health researchers can help by engaging in relevant studies. Among the questions that need to be addressed, Stipek and McCroskey (125) note that there is little research currently available on the different work schedules that support employees in their role as parents; the increased productivity, if any, associated with different work schedules; and other important questions, such as how different work schedules for parents affect the frequency with which children are sent to school ill or are examined by a doctor. This latter research question is important in part because even in cases where parents have good child care arrangements, they need to be at home with their children when the children are ill. Parents' inability to take time off from work, however, has resulted not in any workplace policy changes but rather in the development of child care facilities that specialize in the care of sick children. This is disturbing, since children who are ill need to be with their parents. No studies are needed to establish this fact, but the American Academy of Pediatrics indicates that studies substantiate the fact that children's ability to overcome illness and benefit from medical treatment is directly related to their being with their parents during the illness. However, due to lack of advocacy on the issue, society's response to the care of sick children has been child care for sick children rather than the institution of flexible work schedules for parents.

Family Leave Policies

Related to flexible work schedules is the need for parental leave policies that would enable parents to spend time with their infants during the first several months after birth. The first few months of life represent a critical period for the development of attachment between parents and the infant and that within the context of a secure parent–infant relationship, the growing child thrives and is encouraged to become more autonomous (126, 127). The first few months of life also represent a very stressful period that necessitate the adjustment of all family members to the newborn (128).

A Blue Ribbon Committee on Infant Care Leave studied the issue and found that an increasing number of women return to work very shortly after the birth of their babies. The committee recommended that in the interests of infant mental health as well as parents' wellbeing, one of the parents should be given the option of a paid leave of absence from work for the first 6 months after birth (129). Although the importance of such leave is noted on the basis of medical and social science research (129, 130), adequate parental leave is not available to most parents in the United States.

This is despite the passage of the Family and Medical Leave Act (FMLA) in 1993, which granted 12 weeks unpaid leave in any 12-month period to employees in companies of 50 or more workers. The impact of the federal legislation was limited for three major reasons: First, 34 states had already passed laws prior to the FMLA (131, 132). Second, as much as 40% of the workforce were ineligible for leave because of the size of their companies, since the majority of workers are in small businesses (133, 134). The business community is adamantly against any interference with their policies and has thus lobbied to exclude small companies from eligibility. Third, the leave granted was unpaid, and research shows that many have been discouraged from taking leave for financial reasons (135). However, the FMLA is significant as the first national move toward parental leave, and has prompted discussions about paid leave at the federal level, and in some states such as Connecticut. Again, the issue of parental leave is instructive, revealing how findings from research can lead to policy.

THE NEED FOR INTERACTION BETWEEN SCIENCE, CLINICAL KNOWLEDGE, AND POLICY DEVELOPMENT

Although many American families are affected by the societal factors described earlier, social policies in the United States have not kept pace with societal changes. Our society is, as a result, in a state of disequilibrium wherein social policies are not in synchrony with the realities of family life. It is this disequilibrium that is creating difficulties for families. Not all mental health disorders in children stem from such difficulties. However, the stressful conditions under which many children live place a burden on children's ability to cope with the demands of school, the family, and relationships with peers. The problems that emanate from the changing conditions of family life touch on economic realities, traditions, and institutional structures, so solutions may be slow to evolve (99). Nevertheless, mental health professionals can have a positive effect on family life in several ways. For example, they can alert policymakers and the general public to how stress in families negatively affects the very core of society. They can also call for further studies of the conditions under which children live and children's responses to these realities. This focus on research is important. It can deepen our understanding of how children are affected by different conditions and of why some children are able to cope with difficulties in their lives, whereas other children succumb (25, 54). The research can also enhance our understanding of the ways children cope with problems so that we can devise useful strategies for intervention and prevention.

Policies and Programs to Support Children and Their Families

In response to the widespread need for such programs, a host of family support services has been developed and implemented in recent years. The programs range from informal, grass-roots, self-help services such as Parents Anonymous and Parents without Partners (136) to more formal types of services that include professional assistance (137). These programs have been referred to as a "new breed" of programs in that they are rooted in the premise that the most effective way to create and sustain benefits for children is to improve their families and communities. However, this premise is hardly new and can be traced to Project Head Start (138). Project Head Start, along with other social programs, was initiated over three decades ago in an effort to enhance the lives of young children. It was, and continues to be, an innovative program that includes a cycle of experimentation and revision that helps ascertain which types of services are best suited for and have the most impact on children. As a result of this cycle of experimentation and revision, and of recent research interest in the ecological study of children, the conventional wisdom about how to address the needs of children has shifted from child-centered programs to programs that focus not only on the child but also on the family as a whole (139, 140).

Although the development of family support programs is conceptually traced to previously developed social programs, they differ in a number of ways. Most important, many family support programs are nongovernmental initiatives. Rather, they began as grass-roots efforts, initiated and sustained by individuals in response to stressful situations in their lives, and in the absence of any other form of social support. Although several states have initiated family support programs (89, 141), such programs are still characterized by the lack of government support. Another characteristic of family support programs is that although they are varied in the type of services rendered and the population served, they share a commitment to provide emotional, informational, and instrumental assistance to family members, enabling individuals to cope with whatever problems they may have (142, 143).

Primary Prevention

In helping individuals in these ways, family support programs exemplify a primary prevention strategy that focuses on the prevention of mental health disorders (43, 144). As noted earlier in this chapter, there is a clear and consistent relation in research findings between adaptive difficulties and heightened levels of stress (145–147). Other studies have established that both personal and situational variables may mediate this reaction and enable individuals who are vulnerable to become better able to cope. One such variable is social support. Social support has been found to improve an individual's ability to withstand stress (43, 148), to mediate the consequences of life crises (68), and to enhance general adjustment and wellbeing. Social support systems should not be conceived of as the propping up of someone who is in danger of falling (144). Rather, they refer to efforts to augment an individual's strengths in order to facilitate mastery of the environment. Social support as a means of primary prevention in mental health should not be perceived as a one-time intervention but rather as an enduring pattern of continuous or intermittent ties that help maintain the psychological and physical integrity of the individual (144).

Families, like individuals, have a certain life course in which, at particular points, stresses and crises are a natural state of affairs. At those times, support programs can be invaluable in helping family members to utilize their strengths and rally to cope with the problem, thus warding off severe family dysfunction and mental health disorders (149). Although family support programs have this primary prevention potential, the degree to which they are effective in preventing mental disorders is not yet known. This is due to the fact that the growth and proliferation of family support programs has not been matched by evaluations of their efficacy (150). The reason for this may be that the programs are grass-roots efforts that were not known to or recognized by many researchers in the field of mental health until recently (136, 151). An additional reason is that many such programs are difficult to evaluate. For example, it is often difficult, if not impossible, to randomly select individuals for participation in a program—a basic requirement needed to meet scientific standards.

However, the lack of evaluation data is a characteristic not only of family support programs but of other types of primary prevention programs as well. Cowen (152) notes that evaluation studies are needed to separate some of the good and effective prevention programs now being tried from others that are simply "maintained by inertia or falsely placed conviction." Addressing the problem caused by the lack of evaluation data, Zigler and Freedman (153) observe that although family support programs have proliferated, they have done so without any clear indication as to the direction their course of growth should take. Moreover, those evaluation studies that do exist are varied in quality of design, appropriateness of data collection measures, and validity of conclusions (154). On a more practical level, Cowen (152) notes that the future of prevention programs in general and family support programs in particular depends on evaluations of their effectiveness, since the funding and therefore the continued existence of many programs is often dependent on the answer to a single question: Are these programs beneficial and cost effective?

The evaluation of family support programs, although important, is not a simple task. In many cases, the programs have no explicitly stated goals, thus rendering an evaluation difficult (155). Additionally, many of these programs are in the formative stage, too early to evaluate results accurately (156); these and other problems associated with the evaluation of programs are not insurmountable. Indeed, they are being addressed by many researchers in mental health, who are finding that by participating in program evaluation, they not only contribute to the development of more valid evaluation methodologies (157); they are also contributing to a theoretical understanding of children's development, thereby opening up new vistas for research and practice. For example, on the basis of a review of existing evaluations of family support programs, researchers have found that those that are successful in addressing the multiple needs of families have four common features: They are comprehensive; they are flexible; they are located in the community; and they are results oriented, their ultimate goal being to strengthen families (158). These findings about family support services are useful, for they provide directions for implementation and the replication of the services on a wider scale (150, 159).

Program Development and Evaluation

The importance of support services is noted for a wide variety of families who encounter different types of stressful life events. Many families—for example, those who have premature or medically fragile babies (160–162) or who experience the illness or death of family members—have difficulty coping and are in need of some kind of support. Likewise, there are many people who need assistance with childrearing: Many parents need help gaining the ability to simultaneously nurture and discipline children, or need assistance coping with transitional problems encountered during different stages of their children's development (43).

Support services are also needed to prevent chronic juvenile delinquency. Yoshikawa (163) notes that there has been an increase in juvenile crime in the United States. There has been a 60.1% increase over a 10-year period in arrests of youths under age 18 for murder and manslaughter (164). Juvenile crime is linked to the violence that has become part of the daily lives of families, especially those who are poor; it is experienced by increasingly younger children (165). Yoshikawa (163) documents several factors that are predictive of chronic delinquency: low socioeconomic status, convicted parents, low intelligence, poor parental childrearing, troublesomeness, and conduct disorders. His review of the research further suggests that programs that combine early family support and education and which include, among several aspects, a parent-focused informational and emotional support component, represent a promising direction for the primary prevention of early-onset, chronic delinquency. Other studies (166, 167) suggest that early childhood intervention and support programs are linked to the prevention of juvenile delinquency.

EFFECTING POLICY CHANGE

In order to effect positive policy change on behalf of children and families, it is important to note both the promise and problems inherent in research-informed policy decisions, as well as the need for a cadre of professionals well trained to work at the intersect of clinical knowledge, research, and policy development.

Promise and Problems in Research-Informed Policy Decisions

There are numerous contributions that mental health professionals have made. For example, school-based programs have been developed by psychiatrists such as James Comer in an effort to prevent affective disorders in children and ensure responsivity to children's mental health needs. The authors of this chapter have also developed a school-based early care and family support program which has been implemented in over 1,300 schools across the country (98). Indeed, as a result of their involvement in program development and evaluation, mental health researchers have accumulated a vast amount of knowledge that "totally transforms the nation's capacity to improve outcomes for vulnerable children (159, 168)." This knowledge, derived from over three decades of program development and evaluation, includes evidence of the effectiveness of a number of programs that reduce the burdens of risk factors in childhood, thereby reducing the probability of later damage (159, 169).

Mental health professionals further note that there is evidence that it is not necessary to change everything—the structure of opportunity, the neighborhood environment, and other aspects of the child's life—to make a crucial difference for children at risk (159). However, this knowledge is not being utilized to alter the life path of many of the children who are growing up under stressful conditions (159, 170).

The failure to utilize knowledge from the research stems from several problems. One such problem is that the information on effective programs is generally not shared with the public or with policymakers (171, 172). Thus, these programs, many of them at the demonstration stage, fail to be replicated on a larger scale. Even in cases where programs' potential benefits are known, there is skepticism that such programs, once they are replicated, will continue to be effective. Although this is a valid concern, Schorr (159) notes that successful programs can be built upon if we can attract and train enough skilled and motivated individuals, if we devise a variety of replication strategies, and if we resist the lure of replication through dilution. This latter point is noted given the fact that in efforts to serve as many children as possible or due to lack of sufficient funds, programs are diluted, thus diminishing their quality and potential benefits. Zigler and Berman (139) note that the inclusion of more children at the expense of program quality has occurred even in such well known programs as Project Head Start. They suggest continued monitoring of programs as a means of ensuring their effectiveness.

This point needs to be conveyed to policymakers and others who are in charge of the allocation of funds for program development and replication. However, although an increasing number of mental health researchers are working in the policy arena, there is still a rather uneasy relationship between them and policymakers (7). Maccoby and colleagues (173) note that policymakers often regard researchers as impractical. From their perspective, they may be skeptical of policy recommendations coming from researchers who do not seem to understand the complexities of achieving a consensus among rival constituencies. Researchers, on the other hand, seem to regard policymakers as disingenuous and too willing to compromise even when the research evidence does not justify such action. Meltsner (174) also observes that part of the tension and mistrust between policymakers and mental health researchers emanates from the assumption that knowledge from research is value free, whereas policies are made in a value-laden context. However, this characterization of research and policy is misleading. Often, scientific research takes on the values of the investigators, as is evident in the questions asked, methodologies employed, and the interpretation and presentation of the findings.

Problems such as these serve to impede the utilization of research in policy settings. The problems are further exacerbated by the fact that researchers are often perceived as unable to provide clear answers to policy questions, or, looked at from another perspective, that policymakers are unable to ask questions in a way that would lead to valid and reliable research (173). In part, this problem stems from the unrealistic expectations among policymakers and the inability of many of them to appreciate that single studies cannot, in and of themselves, provide definitive answers to questions. But researchers also contribute to the problem. Sheldon White (171) notes that often researchers are unfamiliar with the policy process or are unable to "read" political issues. They hold to long, slow standards of proof and refutation that are, in the policy arena, "obstructive and nihilistic." Thompson (175) makes a similar point, noting that, often, policy issues do not lend themselves easily to research and that research findings are often limited in their applicability to policy because of sampling and measurement issues. Although it is imperative that researchers uphold their professional standards and credibility as scientists (117), there are times when findings from the research, even if they are not entirely conclusive, can nonetheless provide a direction for policy. For example, the research on the effects of child care on children's development was controversial, yielding conflicting findings that served to confuse the public and policymakers (176). Although research on the topic continues, researchers were able to convene and come to a consensus that indicated that as long as young children are in a good-quality child care settings, they will not be adversely affected by their experiences in child care.

This led to a policy recommendation for efforts to monitor the quality of care children receive and ensure that all children receive care that is conducive to optimal development (120). It is apparent that there are circumstances, such as the increasing number of children in child care, when awaiting definitive conclusions from the research is counterproductive, especially when action can be taken at the same time that research on a particular issue is continuing.

A different problem occurs when research findings are misused by academics or the media to support a vested policy interest. An example is the controversial issue of the importance of the early years in child development. The research on brain development is a case in point. Magnetic resonance imaging and other techniques that were once confined to medical diagnoses have been used to examine the development of the brain. The findings on brain research have been illuminating, although in many cases preliminary, and have shown the developmental importance of the first three years of life. Such studies have captured media and policy attention. Some researchers, excited by the window of opportunity for action on behalf of children, made exaggerated and distorted claims not substantiated by the research. These were refuted by Bruer (177), who noted that some researchers, in emphasizing the potential for brain development in the 0 to 3 years period, ignored other critical periods through to adulthood. However, Bruer himself went to the other extreme, denouncing the importance of the first 3 years of life and ignoring findings from social science that have shown that prevention and intervention in the early years are critical. The debate has been taken up by the national media, with viewpoints expressed through sound bites, undermining the complex scientific findings of decades of research. In the process, there is danger that the polarization of the issue could result in a policy retreat from children's services and continued misunderstanding of the research on brain development (178).

Training the Next Generation of Policy Shapers

Understanding what impedes the use of research in policy is important if mental health researchers are to have an impact in the policy arena. Lindblom (179) identified four general guidelines for researchers to follow in order to encourage the use of research in carving out policy directions: a) that researchers be concerned in a nonpartisan way with the values and interests of society in general and children in particular, b) that they take a practical approach and suggest policies that are feasible and have a chance of attracting widespread political and public support, c) that they respond to the needs of policymakers and provide them with recommendations for action on the basis of research findings, and d) that they become cognizant of and responsive to the policy process.

It is also suggested that researchers make serious attempts to disseminate the findings from the research, not only to policymakers but to the general public. No society acts until it has a sense of the immediacy of the problem (180). The Great Society programs of the 1960s illustrate this point. During that time, social issues were covered in major newspapers and were in the forefront of national attention. There were daily stories on welfare mothers, reports on poverty, and expositions on hunger in the United States. Hence there was sympathy for the poor and support for the War on Poverty (3).

Although for a time thereafter there was appreciably less interest in issues pertaining to children and families, there are indications that this is changing. First, developmental psychologists, psychiatrists, and other mental health professionals are becoming aware of the need for public education on the needs of children (181). And, in a departure from their past practices, many mental health professionals are no longer satisfied with simply sharing information with one another. Rather, they disseminate their knowledge not only by presenting their findings directly to policymakers but by taking steps to ensure that the information is covered in the popular media. Indeed, the dissemination of research in the context of the popular media has come to be accepted as an important aspect of the training received by some professionals in the field of mental health (7).

Many mental health professionals are also receiving training in the integration of child development research and social policy, learning not only about the policy process but also about some of the ways to merge their knowledge with that of policymakers in the formation of programs and policies for children. For example, with support from the Bush Foundation in Minnesota, several training centers were established, one of which was the Bush Center in Child Development and Social Policy at Yale University, renamed the Edward Zigler Center in 2005. The Zigler Center has prepared doctoral students and postdoctoral fellows in a variety of disciplines related to mental health to apply their knowledge in the policy arena. Many graduates of the Bush Center have gone on to work in the policy arena or in other universities where they have established courses and programs on the integration of child development research and social policy. The success of the training centers is evident not only in the increased number of researchers who apply their work to the policy arena, but also in the numerous issues, such as child care, parental leave, and the need for family support services, that only a few years ago were not discussed but that now command national attention. The success of these efforts is further evident in the fact that an increasing number of policymakers are now acknowledging the importance of knowledge from the research in the formulation of policies and are actively seeking the collaboration of professionals in the field of mental health. If mental health professionals and policymakers continue to work together in this spirit of collaboration, we will be able to bring about much-needed changes that will assist family life.

References

1. Zigler E, Styfco S: *Head Start and Beyond: A National Plan for Extended Childhood Intervention.* New Haven, CT, Yale University Press, 1993.
2. Zigler E, Muenchow S: *Head Start: The Inside Story of America's Most Successful Educational Experiment.* New York, Basic Books, 1992.
3. Zigler E, Valentine J (eds): *Project Head Start: A Legacy of the War on Poverty.* New York, Free Press, 1979.
4. Phillips D. *Quality child care: What does the research tell us?* Washington, DC, National Association for the Education of Young Children; 1987.
5. Salkind NJ: The effectiveness of early intervention. In: Goets EM, Allen KE (eds): *Early Childhood Education: Special Environmental, Policy, and Legal Considerations.* Gaithersburg, MD, Aspen, 1983.
6. Takanishi R, DeLeon P, Pallack MS: Psychology and public policy affecting children, youth, and families. *American Psychologist* 38:67–69, 1983.
7. Zigler E: A place of value for applied and policy studies. *Child Development* 69(2):532–542, 1998.
8. Bronfenbrenner U: *The Ecology of Human Development.* Cambridge, MA, Harvard University Press, 1979.
9. Garbarino J, Kostelny K: Parenting and Social Policy. In: Bornstein M (ed): *Handbook of Parenting. Vol 3: Status and Social Conditions of Parenting.* Mahwah, NJ, Lawrence Erlbaum Associates, 1995.
10. Miringoff M: *The Index of Social Health.* New York, United Nations Children's Fund, 1993.
11. Institute of Medicine: *Research on Children and Adolescents with Mental, Behavioral and Developmental Disorders.* Washington, DC, National Academy Press, 1989.
12. Manderscheid R, Sonnenschein MA (eds): *Mental Health, United States, 1996.* Washington, DC, U.S. Government Printing Office, 1996.
13. Kazdin AE: *Psychotherapy for Children and Adolescents: Directions for Research and Practice.* New York, OUP, 2000.
14. Rice DP, Kelman S, Dunmeyer S: *The Economic Costs of Alcohol and Drug Abuse and Mental Illness: 1985 (Report to the Office of Financing and*

Coverage Policy, Alcohol, Drug Abuse and Mental Health Administration, U.S. Department of Health and Human Services). San Francisco: Institutes for Health and Aging, University of California, 1990.
15. Office of Technology Assessment: *Children's Mental Health: Problems and Services—A Background Paper.* Washington, DC, U.S. Government Printing Office, 1986, publication no. OTA-BP-H33.
16. U.S. Department of Health and Human Services: *Healthy People 2010: Understanding and Improving Health.* Washington, DC: U.S. Department of Health and Human Services, 2000.
17. Deal LW, Shiono PH, Behrman RE: Children and managed health care: Analysis and recommendations. *The Future of Children* 8(2):4–24, 1998.
18. Stroul BA, Pires SA, Armstrong MI, Meyers JC: The impact of managed care on mental health services for children and their families. *The Future of Children* 8(2):119–133, 1998.
19. Galston W: *Causes of Declining Well Being among U.S. Children.* New York, 1993.
20. Tuma JM: Mental health services for children. *American Psychologist* 44:188–199, 1989.
21. Tennant C: Parental loss in childhood. *Archives of General Psychiatry* 45:1045–1050, 1988.
22. Rutter M, Smith D (eds): *Psychosocial Disorders in Young People: Time Trends and Their Causes.* Chichester: John Wiley; 1995.
23. Widom CS: Childhood victimization: Early adversity and subsequent psychopathology. In: Dohrenwend BP (ed): *Adversity, Stress, and Psychopathology*, OUP, 1998.
24. Brooks-Gunn J, Duncan GJ: The effects of poverty on children. *The Future of Children* 7(2):55–71, 1997.
25. Garmezy M: Stress-resistant children: The search for protective factors. In: Stevenson JE (ed): *Recent Research in Developmental Psychopathology.* Oxford, Pergamon, pp. 213–233, 1985.
26. Rutter M: Institute of psychiatry department of child and adolescent psychiatry. *Psychological Medicine* 6:505–516, 1976.
27. Wallerstein JS: *Surviving the Breakup.* New York: Basic Books; 1988.
28. Wallerstein JS, Corbin S: The child and the vicissitudes of divorce. In: Lewis M (ed): *Child and adolescent psychiatry: A comprehensive textbook*, 2nd ed. Baltimore, MD, Williams and Wilkins, pp. 1118–1126, 1996.
29. Beardslee WR, Versage EM, Gladstone TRG: Children of affectively ill parents: A review of the past 10 years. *Journal of the American Academy of Child and Adolescent Psychiatry* 37:1134–1141, 1998.
30. Rutter M: Parental mental disorder as a psychiatric risk factor. In: Hales R, Frances A, eds. *APA annual review* (vol 6). Washington, DC, American Psychiatric Press, 647–663, 1987.
31. American Psychiatric Association. *Diagnostic and Statistical Manual of Mental Disorders.* 4th (ed): Washington, DC, American Psychiatric Association Press, 1994.
32. Rutter M: *Changing youth in a changing society.* Cambridge, MA: Harvard University Press, 1980.
33. Hughes D, Simpson L: The role of social change in preventing low birthweight. *The Future of Children* 5(1):87–102, 1995.
34. Sameroff AJ, Seifer R, Zax M, et al.: Early indicators of developmental risk: The Rochester longitudinal study. *Schizophrenia Bulletin* 13:383–394, 1987.
35. Hack M, Klein N, Taylor HG: Long-term developmental outcomes of low birth-weight infants. *The Future of Children* 5(1):176–196, 1995.
36. Blank RM: *It Takes a Nation: A New Agenda for Fighting Poverty*: Russell Sage Foundation, 1997.
37. U.S. Bureau of the Census. *Poverty in the United States 1998.* Washington, DC, U.S. Bureau of the Census, 1999.
38. Children's Defense Fund. *State of America's Children.* Washington, DC, Children's Defense Fund, 1993.
39. Wolfe B: Economic issues of healthcare. In: Chase-Lansdale PL, Brooks-Gunn J (eds): *Escape from Poverty: What Makes a Difference to Children?* New York, Cambridge, 1995; pp.170–188.
40. Klerman L: *Alive and well? Health care for children in America.* New York: National Center for Children in Poverty, 1991.
41. Albee GW: Toward a just society: Lessons from observations on the primary prevention of psychopathology. *American Psychologist* 41:891–898, 1986.
42. Webster-Stratton C: Preventing conduct problems in Head Start children: Strengthening parenting competencies. *Journal of Consulting and Clinical Psychology* 66(5):715–730, 1998.
43. Albee GW, Gullotta TP: *Primary prevention works.* Thousand Oaks, CA, Sage Publications, 1997.
44. Brown JL: *The link between nutrition and cognition.* Medford, MA, Tufts University, 1998.
45. Chomitz V, Cheung L, Lieberman E: The role of lifestyle in preventing low birth weight. *The Future of Children* 5(1):121–138, 1995.
46. Johnson JL, Leff M: Children of substance abusers: Overview of research findings. *Pediatrics* 103(5):1085–1099, 1999.
47. Blum BB, Berrey EC: *Welfare Research Perspectives: Past, Present and Future.* New York, National Center for Children in Poverty, 1999.
48. Kagan SL, Fuller B: *Executive Summary: Remember the Children: Mothers Balance Work and Child Care under Welfare Reform—The Connecticut perspective.* The Bush Center in Child Development and Social Policy, Yale University, February 2000.
49. Aber L, Brooks-Gunn J, Maynard R: The effects of welfare reform on teenage parents and their children. *The Future of Children* 5(2):53–71, 1995.
50. Brown GW, Harris TO. *Social Origins of Depression: A Study of Psychiatric Disorder in Women.* New York, Free Press, 1978.
51. Mayes LC, Grillon C, Granger R, Schottenfeld R: Regulation of arousal and attention in preschool children exposed to cocaine prenatally. *Annals of the New York Academy of Sciences* 846:126–143, 1998.
52. Marans S, Schaefer MC: Community policing, schools and mental health: The challenge of collaboration. In: Elliott DE, Hamburg BA, Williams KR (eds): *Violence in American Schools: A New Perspective.* New York, Cambridge University Press, 1998.
53. Schwab-Stone M, Ayers T, Kasprow W, et al.: No safe haven: A study of violence exposure in an urban community. *Journal of the American Academy of Child and Adolescent Psychiatry* 34(10):1343–1352, 1995.
54. Gunnar M: *Quality Care and the Buffering of Stress Physiology: Its Potential in Protecting the Developing Human Brain.* Minneapolis: University of Minnesota, Institute of Child Development, 1996.
55. *The Future of Children: Domestic Violence and Children* 9(3) [entire issue], 1999.
56. Edelson JL: The overlap between child maltreatment and woman battering. *Violence Against Women* 5:134–154, 1999.
57. Aber JL, Brown JL, Henrich CC. *Teaching Conflict Resolution: An Effective Approach to Violence Prevention.* New York, National Center for Children in Poverty, 1999.
58. Brener ND, Simon TR, Krug EG, Lowry R. Recent trends in violence-related behaviors among high school students in the United States. *Journal of the American Medical Association* 282(5):440–446, 1999.
59. Schwab-Stone M, Chen C, Greenberger E, Silver D, Lichtman J, Voyce C. No safe haven II: The effects of violence exposure on urban youth. *Journal of the American Academy of Child and Adolescent Psychiatry* 38(2):359–367, 1999.
60. Federal Interagency Forum on Child and Family Statistics. *1999.* Washington, DC, National Center for Health Statistics; America's Children 1999: Indicators of youth violent crime and victimization show continuing declines.
61. Children's Defense Fund. *The State of America's Children Yearbook 1998.* Washington, DC, Children's Defense Fund, 1998.
62. U. S. Bureau of the Census: Money, income, and poverty status of families and persons in the United States. In: *Current Population Reports.* Washington, DC, Government Printing Office, 1988, p. 60.
63. Hernandez DJ. Economic and social disadvantages of young children: Alternative policy responses. In: Barnett WS, Boocock SS (eds): *Early care and education for children in poverty: Promises, programs, and long-term results.* New York: State University of New York Press; 1998.
64. U.S. National Center for Health Statistics: *Vital and Health Statistics: Trends in Pregnancies and Pregnancy Rates by Outcome: Estimates for the U.S. 1976–1996.* Washington, DC, Centers for Disease Control and Prevention, January 2000.
65. Board on Children and Families: Immigrant children and their families: Issues for research and policy. *The Future of Children* 5(2):72–89, 1995.
66. McCullough S: Testimony presented to the U.S. House Select Committee on Children, Youth and Families, 1987.
67. Coleman JS. Families and schools. *Education Researcher* 1987;16:32.
68. Gore S: Stress-buffering functions of social supports: An appraisal and clarification of research models. In: Dohrenwend BS, Dohrenwend BP (eds): *Stressful Life Events: Their Nature and Effects*, New York, Wiley, 1980.
69. Hernandez DJ: Demographic trends and the living arrangements of children. In: Hetherington EM, Arsteh ID, (eds): *Impact of Divorce, Single-Parenting, and Step-parenting on Children*, Hillsdale, NJ, Erlbaum, 1988.
70. U.S. Bureau of the Census: *Marriage, Divorce and Remarriage in the 1990s. Current population reports.* Washington, DC, Government Printing Office, 1992.
71. National Center for Health Statistics. 1995.
72. Emery RE: *Marriage, Divorce, and Children's adjustment*, 2nd ed. Thousand Oaks, CA, Sage Publications, 1999.
73. Behrman R, Quinn L. Children and divorce: Overview and analysis. *The Future of Children* 4(1):4–14, 1994.
74. Twaite JA, Silitsky D, Luchow AK: *Children of Divorce: Adjustment, Parental Conflict, Custody, Remarriage, and Recommendations for Clinician*, Jason Aronson, Inc., 1998.
75. Wallerstein JS: Tailoring the intervention to the child in the separating and divorced family. *Family and Conciliation Courts Review* 29:448–459, 1991.
76. Tschara JM, Johnson JR, Kline M, et al.: Conflict, loss, change and parent-child relationships: Predicting children's adjustment during divorce. *Journal of Divorce* 13:1–22, 1990.
77. Hetherington EM, Hagan MS, Anderson ER: Marital transition: A child's perspective. *American Psychologist* 44:303–312, 1989.
78. Haskins R, Schwartz JB, Akin JS, et al.: How much support can absent fathers pay? *Policy Studies* 14:201, 1985.
79. U.S. Bureau of the Census: Child support for custodial mothers and fathers: 1991. In: *Current Population Reports.* Washington, DC, Government Printing Office, 1995.
80. Kurdek LA, Blisk D: Dimensions and correlates of mothers' divorce experiences. *Journal of Divorce* 6:1–24, 1983.

81. Wallerstein J: Child of divorce: An overview. *Behav Sci Law* 4:105–118, 1986.
82. Goldstein J, Freud A, Solnit A: *Beyond the Best Interests of the Child.* New York: Free Press, 1973.
83. Goldstein J, Freud A, Solnit A: *Before the Best Interests of the Child*, 2nd ed. New York, Free Press, 1979.
84. Guidibaldi J, Cleminshaw HK, Perry JD, et al.: The effects of divorce on child development. *School Psychology Review* 13:300–323, 1983.
85. Hetherington EM, Camara KA: Families in transition: The process of dissolution and reconstitution. In: Parke RD (ed): *Review of Child Development Research.* Vol 7: The Family. Chicago: University of Chicago Press; 1984.
86. Kurdek LA: An integrative perspective on children's divorce adjustment. *American Psychologist* 36:856–866, 1981.
87. Miller PA, Ryan P, Morrison W: Practical strategies for helping children of divorce in today's classroom. *Childhood Education: Infancy Through Early Adolescence* 75(5), 1999.
88. Bahr SJ: Divorce mediation: An evaluation of an alternative divorce policy. 2:1, 1981.
89. Weiss HB: *State Leadership in Family Support Programs.* Cambridge, MA: Harvard Family Research Project, Harvard University, 1989.
90. U.S. Department of Labor: *Labor-Force Participation of Women with Children under Age 6.* Washington, DC, U.S. Bureau of Labor Statistics, 1997.
91. Zaslow MJ, Emig CA: When low-income mothers go to work: Implications for children. *The Future of Children* 7(1):110–115, 1997.
92. Greenberger E. Bronfenbrenner et al.: revisited: Maternal employment and the perception of young children. Paper presented at the 97th Annual Convention of the American Psychological Association, August 11, 1989, New Orleans.
93. Hoffman LW: Effects of maternal employment in the two-parent family. *American Psychologist* 44:283–292, 1989.
94. Hoffman LW: Work, family and the child. In: Pallak MS, Perloff RO (eds): *Psychology and Work: Productivity, Change and Employment.* Washington, DC, American Psychological Association Press, 1986.
95. Moen P, Dempster MC: Employed parents: Role strain, work time and preferences for working less. *Journal of Marriage and Family* 49:579, 1987.
96. Friedman D: *Family Supportive Policies: The Corporate Decision Making Process.* New York: The Conference Board, 1987.
97. Zigler E: The school of the 21st century. *American Journal of Orthopsychiatry* 36:31–32,55-59, 1989.
98. Finn-Stevenson M, Zigler E: *Schools of the 21st Century: Linking Child Care and Education.* Westview Press, 1999.
99. Zeitlin J: *Work and Family Responsibilities: Achieving a Balance.* New York, Ford Foundation, 1989.
100. Nelson JR, Jr.: The politics of federal day care regulation. In: Zigler E, Gordon E (eds): *Day Care: Scientific and Social Policy Issues.* Boston, Auburn House, 1982.
101. Zigler E, Lang M: *Child Care Choices: Balancing the Needs of Children, Families, and Society.* New York, Free Press, 1991.
102. Hofferth SL, Wissoker DA: Price, quality, and income in child care choice. *Journal of Human Resources* 27:70–111, 1992.
103. *The Future of Children: Financing Child Care* 6(2) [entire issue]; 1996.
104. Kagan SL, Cohen N: *Funding and Financing Early Care and Education.* New Haven, CT, Bush Center on Child Development and Social Policy, Yale University, 1997.
105. Betson DM, Michael RT: Why so many children are poor. *The Future of Children* 7(2):25–39, 1997.
106. Newman S, Brazelton TB, Zigler E, et al.: *America's Child Care Crisis: A Crime Prevention Tragedy.* Washington, DC, Fight Crime: Invest in Kids, 2000.
107. Arnett J: Caregivers in day care centers: Does training matter? *Journal of Applied Developmental Psychology* 10:541–552, 1989.
108. Roupp R, Travers J, Glantz F, et al.: *Children at the center: Final report of the National Day Care Study* Vol 1. Cambridge, MA: Abt Associates, 1979.
109. Helburn S (ed): *Cost, Quality, and Child Outcomes in Child Care Centers: Technical Report.* Denver, Center for Research in Economic and Social Policy, University of Colorado, 1995.
110. Peisner-Feinberg ES, Burchinal MR, Clifford RM, et al.: *The Children of the Cost, Quality, and Outcomes Study Go to School: Technical Report.* Chapel Hill, University of North Carolina at Chapel Hill, Frank Porter Graham Child Development Center, 1999.
111. Galinsky E, Howes C, Kontos S, Shinn MB: *The Study of Children in Family Child Care and Relative Care.* New York, Families and Work Institute, 1994.
112. Ward EH: Credentializing for day care. *Voice for Children* 9:15, 1976.
113. Bredenkamp S, Copple C: *Developmentally Appropriate Practice in Early Childhood Programs*, revised ed. Washington, DC, National Association for the Education of Young Children, 1997.
114. Provence S: Infant day care. The relationship between theory and practice. In: Zigler E, Gordon E (eds): *Day care: Scientific and Social Policy Issues.* Boston, Auburn House, 1982.
115. Harms T, Clifford RM, Cryer D: *Early Childhood Environment Rating Scale (rev. ed.).* New York, Teachers College Press, 1998.
116. Young KT, Marsland KW, Zigler E: Regulatory status of center-based infant and toddler child care. *American Journal of Orthopsychiatry* 67:535–544, 1997.
117. Zigler E, Finn-Stevenson M: Applied developmental psychology. In: Lamb M, Bornstein M (eds): *Developmental Psychology: An Advanced Textbook.* Hillsdale, NJ, Erlbaum, 1987.
118. Kisker EE, Hofferth SL, Phillips DA, et al.: *A Profile of Child Care Settings: Early Education and Care in 1990.* Washington, DC, U.S. Department of Education, 1991.
119. Child Care Action Campaign: *Child Care: The Bottom Line.* New York, Child Care Action Campaign, 1988.
120. National Center for Clinical Infant Programs: *Who Will Mind the Babies?* Washington, DC, National Center for Clinical Infant Programs, 1988.
121. Seligson M: *School-Age Child Care: Developmental and Programmatic Issues.* New Haven, CT, The Bush Center in Child Development and Social Policy, Yale University, 1989.
122. Besharov DJ: *America's Disconnected Youth: Toward a Preventive Strategy*: CWLA Press, 1999.
123. Bureau of National Affairs: *Special Report. Work and Family: A Changing Dynamic.* Rockville, MD, Bureau of National Affairs, 1986.
124. Kamerman SB: Child care services: A national picture. *Monthly Labor Review* 448–464, 1983.
125. Stipek D, McCroskey J: Investing in children: Government and workplace policies for parents. *American Psychologist* 44:416–432, 1989.
126. Ainsworth MDS, Blehar MC, Waters E, et al.: *Patterns of Attachment: A Psychological Study of the Strange Situation.* Hillsdale, NJ, Erlbaum, 1978.
127. Cicchetti D, Cummings M, Greenberg M, et al.: An organizational perspective on attachment beyond infancy: Implications for theory, measurement, and research. In: Greenberg M, Cicchetti D, Cummings M (eds): *Attachment in the Preschool Years: Theory, Research, and Intervention.* Chicago, University of Chicago Press, 1990.
128. Brazelton TB: Issues for working parents. *American Journal of Orthopsychiatry* 56:14–25, 1985.
129. Zigler E, Frank M (eds): *The Parental Leave Crisis: Toward a National Policy.* New Haven, CT, Yale University Press, 1988.
130. Hopper P, Zigler E: The medical and social science basis for a national infant care leave policy. *American Journal of Orthopsychiatry* 58:324–338, 1988.
131. Finn-Stevenson M, Trzcinski E: Mandated leave: An analysis of federal and state legislation. *American Journal of Orthopsychiatry* 61:567–575, 1991.
132. Trzcinski E, Finn-Stevenson M: A response to arguments against mandated parental leave: Findings from the Connecticut survey of parental leave policies. *Journal of Marriage and Family* 53:445–460, 1991.
133. Wisensale SK: Family leave policy: An assessment of the past, a look toward the future. Paper presented at: Bush Center Social Policy Luncheon Series, Yale University, New Haven, CT, February 18, 2000.
134. U. S. Department of Labor, Commission on Family and Medical Leave. *A Workable Balance: Report to the Congress on Family and Medical Leave Policies.* Washington, DC, U.S. Department of Labor, Women's Bureau, 1996.
135. Waldfogel J: The impact of the family and medical leave act. *Journal of Policy Analysis and Management* 18(2):281–302, 1999.
136. Whittaker J, Garbarino J: *Social Support Networks: Informal Helping in the Human Services.* New York, Aldine, 1983.
137. Gullotta TP: Operationalizing Albee's incidence formula. In: Albee GW, Gullotta TP (eds): *Primary Prevention Works.* Thousand Oaks, CA, Sage Publications, 1997, pp. 3–22.
138. Zigler E, Freedman J: Head Start: A pioneer of family support. In: Kagan S, Powell D, Weissbourd B, et al. (eds): *Family Support Programs: The State of the Art.* New Haven, CT, Yale University Press, 1987.
139. Zigler E, Berman W: Discerning the future of early childhood intervention. *American Psychologist* 38:894–906, 1983.
140. Bronfenbrenner U, Weiss H: Beyond policies without people: An ecological perspective on child and family policy. In: Zigler E, Kagan SL, Klugman E (eds): *Children, Families, and Government: Perspectives on American Policy.* Cambridge, MA, Harvard University Press, 1983.
141. Powell DR: How schools support families: Critical policy tensions. *Elementary School Journal* 91:307–319, 1991.
142. Weiss CH: Nothing as practical as good theory: Exploring theory-based evaluation for comprehensive community initiatives for children and families. In: Connell JP, Kubisch AC, Schorr LB, Weiss CH (eds): *New Approaches to Evaluating Community Initiatives: Concepts, Methods, and Contexts.* Washington, DC, Aspen Institute, 1995.
143. Zigler E, Weiss H: Family support systems: An ecological approach to child development. In: Rapoport N (ed): *Children, Youth, and Families: The Action Research Relationship.* New York, Cambridge University Press, 1985.
144. Caplan G: *Support Systems and Community Mental Health.* New York, Behavioral Publications, 1974.
145. Bloom BL: Prevention of mental disorders: Recent advances in theory and practice. *Community Mental Health Journal* 15:179–191, 1979.
146. Cowen EL: The wooing of primary prevention. *American Journal of Community Psychology* 5:258–284, 1980.
147. Hamburg D: An outlook on stress research and health. In: Elliot G, Eisdorfer C (eds): *Stress and Human Health.* New York, Springer, 1982.

148. Cassell J: The contributions of the social environment to host resistance. *American Journal of Epidemiology* 104:107–123, 1976.
149. Riessman F: Support groups as preventive intervention. In: Kessler M, Goldston SE (eds): *A* Decade of Progress in Primary Prevention. Hanover, NH: University Press of New England, 1986.
150. Elias MJ: Reinterpreting dissemination of prevention program as widespread implementation with effectiveness and fidelity. In: Weissberg R, Gullotta T, Hampton R, Ryan B, Adams G (eds): *Establishing Preventive Services*. Thousand Oaks, CA, Sage Publications, 1997, pp. 282–289.
151. Weiss HB: Introduction. In: Payne C (ed): *Programs to Strengthen Families: A Resource Guide*. Chicago: Yale University and The Family Resource Coalition, 1984.
152. Cowen EL: Expanding horizons in prevention research. *Contemporary Psychology* 31:260–261, 1986.
153. Zigler E, Freedman J: Evaluating family support programs. In: Kagan S, Powell D, Weissbourd B, et al. (eds): *Family Support Programs: The State of the Art*. New Haven, CT, Yale University Press, 1987.
154. Roth J, Murray LF, Brooks-Gunn J, Foster WH: Youth development programs. In: Besharov DJ (ed): *America's Disconnected Youth: Toward a Prevention Strategy*. CWLA Press, 1999.
155. Weiss HB, Jacobs FH: *Evaluating Family Programs*. New York, Aldine De Gruyter, 1988.
156. Rossi PH: Evaluating community development programs: Prospects and problems. In: Ferguson R, Dickens W (eds): *Community Development Programs*. Washington, DC, Brookings, 1998.
157. Green BL, MacAllister C: Theory-based participatory evaluation: A powerful tool for evaluating family support programs. *Zero to Three* 18(4):30–36, 1998.
158. Carnegie Corporation of New York: *Starting Points: Meeting the Needs of Our Youngest Children*. New York, Carnegie Corporation of New York, 1994.
159. Schorr LB: *Common Purpose: Strengthening Families and Neighborhoods to Rebuild America*. New York, Anchor Books, 1997.
160. Field TM, Goldberg S, Stern S, et al. (eds): *High-risk Infants and Children: Adult and Peer Interaction*. New York, Academic, 1980.
161. Goldberg S, DiVitto BA: *Born Too Soon: Pre-Term Birth and Early Development*. New York, Freeman, 1983.
162. Shiono P, Behrman R: Low birth-weight: Analysis and recommendations. *The Future of Children* 5(1):4–18, 1995.
163. Yoshikawa H: Prevention as cumulative protection: Effects of early family support and education on chronic delinquency and its risks. *Psychol Bull* 115:28–54, 1994.
164. Federal Bureau of Investigation: *Uniform Crime Reports for the United States, 1990*. Washington, DC, U.S. Government Printing Office, 1991.
165. Osofsky J, Fenichel E (eds): *Caring for Infants and Toddlers in Violent Environments: Hurt, Healing and Hope*. Washington, DC, Zero to Three/National Center for Clinical Infant Programs, 1994.
166. Zigler E, Taussig C, Black K: Early childhood intervention: A promising preventative for juvenile delinquency. *American Psychologist* 47:997–1006, 1992.
167. Berrueta-Clemant JR, Schweinhart JJ, Barnett WS, Epstein AS, Weikert DP: *Changed Lives: The Effects of the Perry Preschool Program on Youths Through Age 19*. Ypsilanti, MI, High/Scope Press, 1984.
168. Schorr LB, Schorr D: *Within Our Reach: Breaking the Cycle of Disadvantage*. New York, Doubleday, 1988.
169. Price RH, Cowen EL, Lorion RP, et al. (eds): *Fourteen Ounces of Prevention: A Casebook for Practitioners*. Washington, DC, American Psychological Association Press, 1988.
170. Hamburg D: Testimony before the U.S. House Select Committee on Children, Youth and Families, 1987.
171. White S: Review of "Within Our Reach." *Young Children* 66–70, September 1988.
172. Zervigon-Hakes A: Culture clash: Translating research findings into public policy. In: Barnett WS, Boocock SS (eds): *Early Care and Education for Children in Poverty: Promises, Programs, and Long-Term Results*. New York, State University of New York Press, 1998.
173. Maccoby EE, Kahn A, Everett BA: The role of psychology research in the formation of policies affecting children. *American Psychologist* 38:80–84, 1983.
174. Meltsner AI: The seven deadly sins of policy analysis. *Knowledge: Creation, Diffusion, Utilization* 7:367–382, 1986.
175. Thompson R: Developmental research and legal policy: Toward a two-way street. In: Cicchetti D, Toth S (eds): *Child Abuse, Child Development and Social Policy*. Norwood, NJ, Ablex, 1993.
176. Clarke-Stewart KA: Infant day care: Maligned or malignant? *American Psychologist* 44:266–273, 1989.
177. Bruer JT: *Myth of the First Three Years: A New Understanding of Early Brain Development and Lifelong Learning*. New York, Free Press, 1999.
178. Zigler E, Finn-Stevenson M, Hall N: *Brain Development and Social Policy: The Controversy*. In press.
179. Lindblom CE: Who needs what social research for policy making? *Knowledge: Creation, Diffusion, Utilization* 7:345–366, 1986.
180. Zigler E, Finn M: From problem to solution: Changing public policy as it affects children and families. *Young Children* 36:31–32, 55–59, 1981.
181. McCall RB, Gregory TG, Murray JP: Community developmental research results to the general public through television. *Developmental Psychology* 20:45–54, 1984.

CHAPTER 1.6 ■ MONEY MATTERS: FUNDING CARE

MARTIN KNAPP, DAVID P.A. McDAID, AND SUJITH DHANASIRI

INTRODUCTION

The primary concerns of anyone working with children and adolescents with mental health problems are alleviation of symptoms, promotion of quality of life, support of families, and improvement of broad life chances. These should also be the primary concerns of those with responsibility for resource allocation, whether it is deciding how much funding can be made available, how it is shared between competing uses, or how to improve efficiency in its use. These latter can be seen as economic questions, but they cannot be answered without a clear understanding of child and family needs and the outcomes of interventions.

Interventions for children and adolescents include primary prevention of behavioral and emotional problems, services that respond to the emergence of such problems, treatments that directly address symptoms and their immediate consequences, and actions targeted on longer term, broader implications for individuals and communities. For almost any such intervention to be successful—indeed, for it to be initiated—skilled staff are needed, supported by appropriate physical and other resources. In turn, because little in life is free, this requires commitment of the necessary finances.

The purpose of this chapter is to explore these links between finances, resources, and achievements. We first introduce a conceptual framework that summarizes the main connections linking resources to individual and family outcomes. One source of complexity that runs throughout the arguments in this chapter is that many children and adolescents have multiple needs, often prompting multiple responses—from health care, education, social work, criminal justice, and other services. Each of these service sectors has its own funding streams and associated arrangements for allocating resources; we consider this mixed economy in the third section. We then turn to a discussion of financing arrangements: How are child and adolescent mental health services funded? In judging whether financing arrangements are delivering the services and outcomes needed and wanted, we refer to two widely discussed performance criteria: efficiency (the balance between outcomes and what it costs to achieve them) and equity (whether outcomes, access, and burdens are fairly distributed). Achieving better performance by those criteria is often hampered: We therefore next discuss the resource barriers in the way of progress. The concluding section summarizes the key messages.

THE PRODUCTION OF WELFARE

- As a starting point, it is helpful to explicate the links between budgets, staff, and other resources hired or purchased, treatments and other services thereby delivered, and health and quality of life improvements hopefully experienced by individuals, families, and communities. A simple representation of a treatment and care systems helps to identify the probable connections between key entities (Figure 1.6.1): Revenue collection is the process by which health, education, social services, and other systems receive money from individuals, households, employers, and other organizations.
- The funds thereby available to those systems are the purchasing budgets, to be allocated between competing needs and demands.
- Commissioning is the process by which purchasers (e.g., insurance funds and government departments) transfer funds to service providers in return for (usually) contractually agreed-upon services.
- Providing budgets are the funds available to the bodies that actually deliver services.
- For those services to be delivered (whether health promotion, assessment, treatment, or supervision), resource inputs are employed: staff, buildings, equipment, medications, and other consumables.
- Some resources are not bought and sold in markets, such as family care, volunteer inputs, and support from faith and community groups. But these inputs are not really "free": using them in one activity (in supporting children with behavioral problems, say) means they are unavailable for other uses (such as a volunteer or parent getting a paid job). In other words, there are opportunity costs.
- Services produced from combinations of the resource inputs can be labeled intermediate outputs. They indicate success: Deploying funds to hire staff to deliver services is an achievement in its own right. But they are not the ultimate goals of mental health systems (which are usually expressed in terms of health and quality of life improvement). Relevant questions about these intermediate outputs concern volume (How many therapy sessions are delivered? How many children are supported in a school-based program?), quality of care, and the characteristics of service users (case-mix, in healthcare parlance).
- Final outcomes are the focal point of the whole system: symptom alleviation, fewer behavioral problems, improved functioning, educational attainment, and quality of life enhancement. Potentially, there are also outcomes for communities. Some final outcomes take years to reveal themselves fully.
- In between services (the intermediate outputs) and outcomes are a number of mediating factors, such as the care-setting social milieu, young people's care histories, individual and family resilience, and staff attitudes. Although potentially very influential in determining the success of an intervention, they do not have a readily identified cost (since they are not usually marketed) and so they might get overlooked when attention focuses on how services are financed and what they achieve. These can be called nonresource inputs.

This representation was originally called the production of welfare framework (1) and developed to underpin discussion of the economics of care systems because (loose) analogies could be drawn between production processes as studied in mainstream economics and care and support approaches used in health, social services, and education to promote individual and family welfare. There is no suggestion here of mechanistic processes of treatment or care. The stylized framework in Figure 1.6.1 has the signal virtues of highlighting the core connections between what goes in (finances, the resource inputs they purchase, and the unfunded contributions of family members and volunteers) and what comes out (services delivered, and improved outcomes for children, adolescents, and families). And although it looks highly simplified to anyone familiar with psychiatric, education, social services, or justice systems, in fact it is more complicated than often appears to be assumed by strategic decision makers looking for quick fixes. Pumping more money into a system will only generate better outcomes for children, adolescents, and families if all the necessary links are in place and are functioning properly. Thus, revenue generation or collection needs to be planned carefully to avoid creating perverse incentives, and skilled staff need to be supported by other resources if they are to deliver services that families need. Equally, the organization of those services and the therapeutic approaches they employ need to be chosen carefully to maximize the chances of successful resolution. This means looking not only at whether there is evidence of therapeutic effectiveness but also whether it is cost effective.

Succinctly expressed, the success of a child and adolescent mental health system in improving health and quality of life will depend on the mix, volume, and deployment of resource inputs and the services they deliver, which in turn are dependent on available finances.

A MIXED ECONOMY

Child and adolescent mental health services as narrowly defined and conventionally viewed sit in the middle of a complex, multiservice, multibudget world. The reason is simple: Children and adolescents with behavioral or emotional problems and their families often have multiple needs. In well developed, well resourced systems, these needs could be identified, assessed, and addressed by numerous agencies (including pediatrics, child psychiatry, education, social work, and youth justice).

Many examples could be given. Farmer et al. (2) documented the various entry points to, and movement within, part of the U.S. mental health service system: Sixty percent of all youths entered through education, 27% through specialty mental health, and 13% through the general medical sector. Glied and Evans Cuellar (3) describe how 92% of children with serious emotional disturbances in another study received services from more than two systems, and 19% from more than four. In Scotland, 10% of new referrals to child and adolescent psychiatry outpatient services were already under social work supervision (4). Two studies, one in the United States (5) and one in the U.K. (6), illustrate the multiple needs

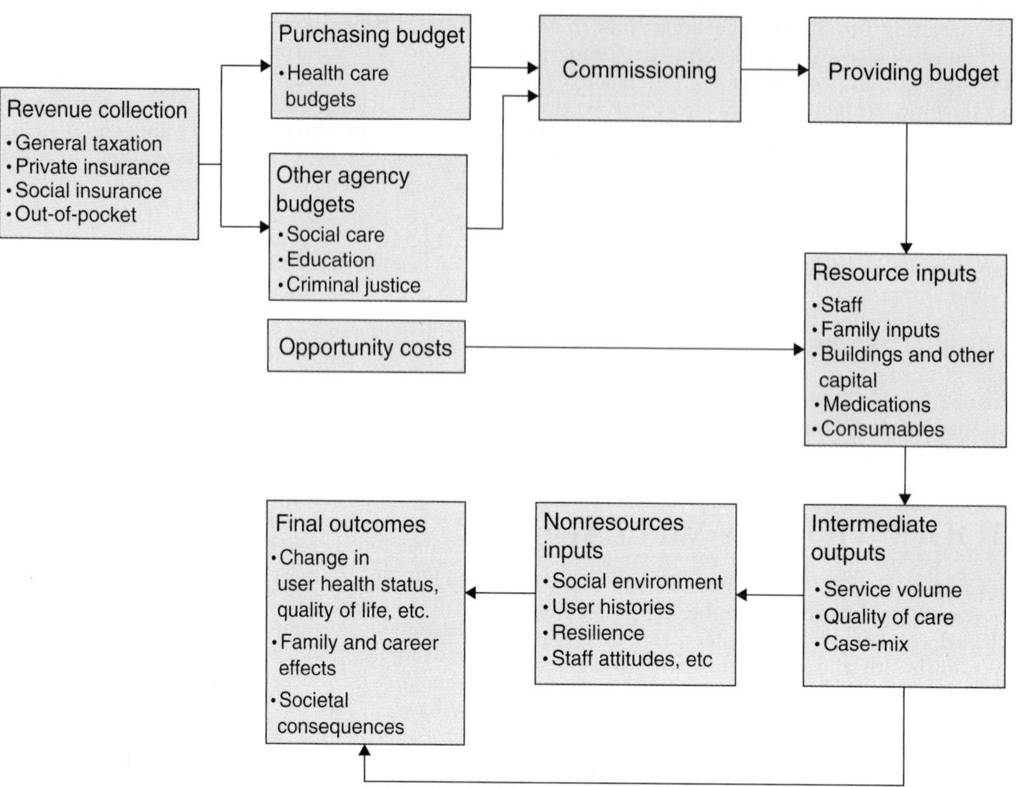

FIGURE 1.6.1. The production of welfare framework, revenue collection, and commissioning.

of children with conduct disorder and the multiple budgets that contribute to meeting them.

Multiple Provider Sectors

The resources described in Figure 1.6.1 might therefore come from social work, education, housing, employment, criminal justice, or other systems. These services could be delivered by government (public sector), for-profit, or nonprofit organizations. Indeed, most countries have a thriving mixed economy of provision. There are additionally the multifarious contributions of parents, other family caregivers, and volunteers. Even health promotion strategies, which tend to be coordinated by national and local government bodies, still need inputs from others, such as local communities (the social capital effect).

Do these provider distinctions matter? Entities with different legal forms often behave differently in response to incentives, and can be motivated by slightly different goals. For instance, a government hospital may have different objectives and constraints from a for-profit hospital or a charitable hospital linked to a faith community. This may affect their modus operandi, patterns of resource dependency, and styles of governance. Distinctive motivations could influence how they respond to changes in funding levels and routes, market prices for staff or medications, and competition, with implications for costs, case-mix, quality of care, and outcomes (7).

Multiple Funding Sources

Another reason for distinguishing between provider types and the sectors in which they are located is because they are likely to have different funding bases. A treatment facility in the public sector—where most are located in the U.K., for example—is likely to be heavily reliant on tax revenues, whereas a for-profit provider will probably receive more of its funding from insurance plans or user fees. School-based social work services in some countries may be funded through the general education budget, which itself is usually funded through some form of taxation. Services run by nonprofit organizations might be funded under contract or grant from government and by insurance payments, but could also receive charitable donations. Family caregivers, although ostensibly unpaid, might actually receive social security support or disability allowances tied to children's needs. Matching the diversity in provision, therefore, is a mixed economy of funding.

Interconnections: Transaction Types

Crossclassifying the main funding and provider types generates a large number of possible interconnections. The matrix in Figure 1.6.2 describes just the broadest categorization of provider sectors and funding sources, but it is already immediately clear that the mixed economy of child mental health care is a highly pluralist system. And each combination of funding arrangement and provider sector could apply to the health, education, social services, criminal justice, and other systems.

There are many transaction types. For example, tax revenues that support for-profit providers could be linked through performance-related contracts, tax breaks, or lump-sum cash subsidies. Insurance payments to providers could be made through fee-for-service, capitation, or other mechanisms. Each transaction type has accompanying needs for regulatory frameworks to control, auditing, and monitoring.

Charting the broad contours of the mixed economy in this way helps to identify the range and volume of services offered to and used by children, adolescents, and families, and the means by which they are funded. It also emphasizes the inherent financial interdependence of different services and

Revenue Collection (Funding)	Mode or Sector of Provision			
	Public/Government Sector	Nonprofit/NGO Sector	For-Profit Sector	Informal Sector
General taxation				
Social insurance				
Voluntary (private) insurance				
Charitable				
Foreign governments				
Out-of-pocket				
No exchange				

Source: Adapted from (Knapp 1984).

FIGURE 1.6.2. The mixed economy of child mental health.

agencies. One recent U.S. study demonstrated how improved community mental health services for young people affected public expenditures in other sectors, "including inpatient hospitalization, the juvenile justice system, the child welfare system, and the special education system. . . . The full fiscal impact of improved mental health services can be assessed only in the context of their impact on other sectors" (5) (p. 50). Child and adolescent mental health services in England's national health service allocated as much as 15% of their core budgets to school programs (8). The "expanded school mental health framework" initiated by the U.S. government encourages education services to liaise with community mental health centers, health departments, hospitals, and others to broaden mental health promotion and intervention, although funding is "patchy and tenuous" (9).

Coordination

Good interagency coordination is imperative if individual and family needs are to be met, which requires collaborative approaches to financing. Without effective coordination, yawning gaps could open up in the spectrum of support: Even in well resourced care systems there are large numbers of young people whose needs go unrecognized or undertreated. Wasteful duplication of effort is another possibility. Countries, states, and municipalities differ in their service and agency definitions, responsibilities and arrangements, and therefore in their interagency boundaries and the kinds of connected action that spans them. One of the major organizational resource challenges, therefore, is to coordinate the funding of services in ways that are effective, cost-effective, and fair. Cost shifting and problem dumping between agencies will not help children and families, but recognition of economic symbiosis could help decisionmakers fashion improved responses to needs through pooled budgets, jointly commissioned programs, and other whole system initiatives (3, 8, 10).

FINANCING ARRANGEMENTS

Accessing health care services is not like buying groceries, which is why most high- and middle-income countries rely on prepayment systems of revenue collection. Prepayment is organized through tax contributions, social insurance, or private insurance (more accurately labeled voluntary insurance). Prepayment is widely held to be preferable to out-of-pocket payments as the main way to finance health care. An individual's risk of needing health care is very uncertain, but when the need arises, the attendant costs (of treatment) and losses (of earnings) could be catastrophic. Prepayment contributions pool risks, and have the potential to redistribute benefits toward people with greater health needs. They can also be made progressive, so that poorer individuals pay less for equivalent health care than richer people. Out-of-pocket-payment systems cannot achieve such targeting unless accompanied by well informed systems of payment exemptions that are closely monitored to ensure implementation and prevent abuse.

Prepayment systems have their problems. If there is no charge at the point at which a service is used there may be excessive utilization—the so-called moral hazard problem that might be addressed by introducing copayments at point of use. Another potential difficulty is adverse selection: High-risk individuals are denied coverage or face unaffordable premiums. Additionally, in attempts to cap expenditures, some insurance or managed care arrangements exclude mental health coverage, with predictable consequences for access, knock-on costs, societal inefficiencies, and inequity. Legal intervention, regulation, or subsidy may be needed as countermeasures, or universal coverage guaranteed by public financing (taxation or social insurance) to provide a safety net. Whatever the merits of prepayment systems, there are obstacles to their wider use in low-income countries, including the state of the economy, unstable governance structures, and the informality of much employment. Consequently, out-of-pocket payments dominate in many low-income countries, where foreign donors may provide significant additional resources, generally in-kind rather than funds.

Financing can be public or private. Public systems are normally tax based, while private systems include voluntary health insurance (sometimes called private insurance, taken up and paid for at the discretion of individuals) and out-of-pocket payments. Social health insurance systems—common in parts of continental Europe—are quasi-public, as the funding is managed by agencies established by government.

Globally, and looking at health systems as a whole, the most common method of financing is tax based (60%), followed by social insurance (19%), out-of-pocket payments (16%), external grants (3%) and voluntary insurance (2%) (11). As far as mental health systems are concerned, almost every country has a mix of public and private funding.

Two particular questions need to be addressed: What do these various revenue collection arrangements mean for child and adolescent mental health services? And what are the consequences of different commissioning processes (fee-for-service, capitation, and so on) to which they give rise?

Tax-Based Financing

Many health, education, and other systems are funded from national, regional, or local taxes. Income tax is usually described as progressive because it can be structured to capture progressively larger income shares from wealthier individuals. Indirect taxes such as sales tax tend to be regressive, as poorer individuals often contribute larger proportions of their incomes. Tax-based systems of health financing are seen as the most progressive and equitable (12). Payments are mandatory, and scale economies can be achieved in administration, risk management and purchasing power (13). For those who advocate health as a right, taxation-based health systems fit the bill, while those with conservative leanings view such arrangements as an erosion of personal responsibilities and freedom.

Tax-based systems have limitations. Health care funding levels often fluctuate with the state of the national economy: When an economy is not doing well, there is a tendency to cut back on publicly funded programs (10, 14). Competing political and economic objectives also make a tax-based system less transparent, and bureaucracy can add to the inefficiency, reflected perhaps in long waiting lists (although these are also symptomatic of underfunding). Patients tend to view tax-based systems as offering them less choice, but uninsured individuals in an alternative financing system might argue that they face no choice whatsoever.

The U.S. health system is obviously a mixture of public and private finance, with the tax-based part organized at state level but delivered primarily through nongovernment providers. Medicaid is one such approach, supporting low-income individuals, financed jointly by the federal government and the states, and covering a substantial proportion of all child and adolescent mental health expenditure across the country (3). The U.S. Congress enacted the State Children's Health Insurance Program (SCHIP) in 1997 to expand health insurance coverage among children: It provided states with federal matching funds to insure low-income children who were not eligible for Medicaid. In 2003, 26% of children with a diagnosed mental health problem in the United States were publicly insured, but another 10% did not have any health insurance coverage (15). Even to access state-funded school mental health programs, students were required to have active insurance and a clinical diagnosis (9). Another grim reality is the custody for care, where middle class families that do not qualify for Medicaid transfer custody of their children to child welfare or juvenile justice services simply in order to access mental health care (10). However, there have been improvements. The proportion of adolescents in poor and near-poor families without insurance decreased between 1995 and 2002 (16). Another reason for improved access to care has been suggested: "The expanded evidence base and armamentarium of drugs have led to tremendous growth in the number of children who receive treatment for mental health problems" (3) (p. 41).

Publicly funded mental health care in the United States is delivered mostly through privately owned/managed health maintenance organizations (HMOs), preferred provider organizations (PPOs), or physicians in private practice. In contrast, the tax-funded Swedish health system, with its predominantly regionally organized financing and administration, relies on provision through public rather than private institutions. So too do the child and adolescent mental health systems in countries such as the U.K. and Malaysia, although nationally collected taxes are the mainstay of the resource base there.

Social Health Insurance

Health and other systems based on social health insurance (SHI) generate their revenues from salary-based contributions administered and managed by quasi-public bodies (sometimes called sickness funds). Employers also make contributions, and transfers are made from general taxation to sickness funds to provide cover for unemployed, retired, and other disadvantaged or vulnerable people—clearly pertinent for people with mental problems. This is common in South and Central America. In Belgium, France, and the Netherlands, tax revenues are used to cover SHI deficits or fund services like hospitalization. In Albania, Latvia, Poland, Romania, and Russia, despite having established systems of social health insurance, taxation continues to dominate health care financing because the formal working population is too small to generate sufficient revenue to cover the population eligible to receive benefits (17).

Enrollment is usually mandatory, and although premiums are not risk adjusted, they tend to be linked to income so that pooling allows for redistribution according to need and income. Entitlement to health care services through taxation or social insurance is commonplace in most European countries, and in fact accounts for over 70% of total health spending in most western European states. In low- and middle-income countries, where tax compliance and collection are difficult, SHI has been seen as a viable alternative for health care funding (18). However, the link between health financing and employment constrains job mobility and hence economic competitiveness. Both tax-based and social insurance-dominated systems take account of ability to pay and cover vulnerable and low-income groups (12).

Even where universal entitlement under tax or SHI predominates, entitlement to mental health services may be limited, and arguably inequitable. In Austria, social health insurance excludes most mental health disorders on the grounds that they are chronic rather than curable, and as much as one-third of social care expenditure for mental health is realized through private out-of-pocket payments (19). Similarly, in Germany only medical aspects of psychosocial care are covered under health insurance: Long-term care needs for people with chronic mental health problems are classed as social rehabilitation or social reintegration and are the responsibility instead of social welfare agencies, which are tax financed and operate means-testing to decide what payments must be made by service users or their families. In fact, many European countries are shifting mental health services out of the health sector, opening up greater possibilities for copayments that could inhibit access (20).

Voluntary (Private) Health Insurance

Voluntary health insurance (VHI) is taken up and paid for at the discretion of individuals (or employers on behalf of individuals) and offered by public, quasi-public, for-profit, or nonprofit organizations. Generally speaking, VHI plays only a marginal role in Europe (21). Countries like Germany, the Netherlands, and Spain allow VHI as a substitute for a statutory protection. In the Netherlands, people can take up exclusive VHI packages that cover expensive services like mental health, a practice that is growing (20).

In contrast, VHI accounts for half of health care expenditure in the United States, and 63% of children below 18 years access healthcare through private (employer-sponsored) insurance (15). However, chronic conditions such as many mental health problems have found themselves squeezed out, which stimulated the Mental Health Parity Act of 1996. In response, employers substituted utilization limits for dollar limits (22). Around 80% of individuals with private, employer-sponsored health insurance had inpatient or outpatient visit limits on their coverage; 23% did not meet the benchmark level of 30 inpatient days, 20 outpatient visits, and prescription drug coverage, while another 3% had no mental health benefits at all (23). Children's services have been particularly affected (3). An assessment of children's mental health care coverage in 98 of the most common plans in the United States found that prescription drug benefits were excluded in 20%, another 20% excluded drug coverage to those with ADHD or behavioral disorders in general, and a higher proportion excluded coverage for residential treatment and partial hospitalizations (10). The trend to carve out managed care plans for mental health raises the danger of undertreatment (24).

People individually purchasing insurance have lower bargaining power, which affects the benefits that are covered. As we have just seen, inherent also in this financing system are disadvantages like adverse selection and cream skimming: Higher risk groups (such as those with mental health problems) may find insurance unaffordable, especially as mental health problems are more prevalent among lower income groups, and lower risk groups may feel that their own premiums are too high. Most insurance plans also exempt existing conditions from the benefit packages. Only 11 U.S. states require every insurer in the individual market to accept all applicants regardless of health status (23).

Out-of-Pocket Payments

In prepayment systems, out-of-pocket payments may be co-payments (specific amount to be paid), coinsurance (agreed percentage of expenses) or deductibles (agreed amount to be paid before insurance kicks in). Though the objectives for introducing out-of-pocket payments differ, the impact remains common everywhere in adversely affecting access and equity. Out-of-pocket payments are justified by the economic rationale that they discourage unnecessary service use (moral hazard) and create price sensitivity that might help direct patients to more cost-effective and appropriate treatments. However, in the long run they might defeat the very purpose of cost efficiency, as delayed treatments might substantially increase costs. About half of all western European countries levy some out-of-pocket charges for specialist mental health services within their publicly funded health systems (20), while they are even more prevalent in parts of central and eastern Europe (25), and are often the only means of health finance in low-income countries (26).

The share of total funding coming from out-of-pocket payments for the typical child with a mental health problem in the United States fell by 45% between 1987 and 1998. This was partly because of the growth of Medicaid and SCHIP funds for these children, but also because VHI plans substituted utilization management for cost sharing, primary care assumed a greater share of treatment responsibility (and is not usually treated as a mental health benefit), and prescription drug coverage grew (3). But the burden of out-of-pocket payments remains for many families, a regressive practice that discourages the use of essential as well as nonessential services. Given the stigma associated with mental health problems, their chronicity, and the damage they can reap, heavy reliance on out-of-pocket funds is inadvisable.

Commissioning

In order to move revenues collected from taxes or insurance premiums to service providers, a variety of commissioning or purchasing mechanisms can be used. Provider reimbursements can be retrospective (fee-for-service) or prospective (capitation and budgets). Historically, fee-for-service arrangements dominated health care commissioning, and although they encourage productivity, they also perversely encourage resource consumption through unnecessary visits, diagnostic investigations, and hospitalizations, and so push up overall costs. Consequently, prospective payments have increasingly been substituted, particularly as part of managed care developments, to encourage cost consciousness among providers. Capitation is one such method: A fixed payment is made for a defined set of benefits (in input and/or outcome terms). It encourages efficiency, but risks selection and cream skimming. Providers might narrow their practice and undermine the objectives of managed care to provide primary and preventive interventions (27). Such behavior shifts costs onto other providers. Some prospective payment methods use diagnosis-related groups (DRGs), a case-mix classification system that groups patients with a similar clinical diagnosis and treatment process to calculate the funds to be allocated. One early calculation suggested that 20% of Medicare hospital costs were saved through the introduction of DRG-based pricing (28). DRG based pricing can help save costs but to get around this providers might resort to up-coding or "DRG creep," which is the practice of billing using a DRG code that provides a higher payment rate than the DRG code that accurately reflects the service furnished to or needed by the patient.

Public financing systems have increasingly adopted commissioning methods from the private insurance market, with emphasis on managed plans. Within Medicaid, for example, enrollment in some form of managed care increased from 10% of the covered population in 1991 to 58% in 2002 (29). One consequence was to shift the balance of care away from inpatient treatment (30), but perhaps there is now a higher risk that seriously ill children will be undertreated (3).

A study comparing three different arrangements—fee-for-service (FFS), health maintenance organization, and carved-out managed care plans—found no significant differences in access rates, but the FFS plan was favorable for children with an increased risk profile (31). Another study found that satisfaction ratings were much higher in Medicaid for FFS than for managed plans (32).

TARGETING, EFFICIENCY, AND EQUITY

There are never likely to be enough resources to meet all mental health needs. Choices must be made. For example, to what extent should child psychiatric services be delivered from a hospital base or from a community clinic? If there are more children and adolescents needing to see specialist staff than there are treatment sessions available, who should get priority? What proportion of a mental budget should be diverted away from treating identified needs in order instead to uncover previously unrecognized needs? What investment should be made to support a broader health promotion strategy? When does it make sense to stop treating or supporting one particular child or family and to use the time to initiate a treatment program for a newly referred child?

Decisionmakers—from those who control the budgets to those who actually deliver the services—need to be clear about the basis upon which they choose one option over another. In a world that is increasingly seeking evidence-based approaches to policy and practice while recognizing resource scarcity, a number of resource-related criteria are likely to be invoked to guide such decisions. These might include maximizing the therapeutic impact from available resources, integrating more children with behavioral problems into mainstream education, broadening access to effective pharmacotherapies or parenting programs, improving fairness in the amount families have to pay for treatment, and improving targeting of services on needs. Many of these resource-related criteria fall into two groups: efficiency and equity.

Efficiency

Efficiency means achieving the maximum effects in terms of services delivered or outcomes achieved (such as needs met or quality of life improved) from a specified volume of resources (such as an available budget).

Many factors might prevent a mental health system from being fully efficient. It may be that too many resources are used up in the administration of the system itself: Are there, for example, too many managers supervising the frontline staff who actually deliver treatment? Another source of inefficiency could be that resources are used in inappropriate combinations: A child psychiatrist is likely to be more effective, for example, if they have access to a range of therapies supported by a multidisciplinary team. Or there may be poor target efficiency in that available services are not provided to the people who need them most, because insufficient efforts are made to identify and prioritize needs or to encourage families to come forward for treatment. Another reason for inefficiency could simply be that little is known about the relationship between resources expended and outcomes achieved. This is where cost-effectiveness analyses can contribute.

Cost-Effectiveness Evidence

When considering whether to use or recommend a particular treatment for a specified problem, decisionmakers must first get an answer to the clinical question Is the treatment effective in improving health and quality of life? They will then usually want an answer to the second question: Is it cost effective? That is, does the treatment achieve the outcomes at a cost that is worth paying? Not surprisingly, the second question—the economic question—can generate howls of concern that it encourages rationing or in some other way denies people access to services or a better quality of life.

These two questions lie at the heart of cost-effectiveness analysis. They compare the two parts of the chain in Figure 1.6.1 that link what gets spent to what gets achieved. While it is always likely to be necessary to reformulate the clinical and economic questions in ways that make them answerable with empirical research, we should not forget their inherently straightforward intent.

Given what we have already discussed in relation to the broad mixed economies of provision and financing, it is obvious that we need to view both costs and outcomes in quite broad terms:

- There are many inputs to a child and adolescent mental health system—health, social services, education, criminal justice, and so on—plus economic impacts in terms of lost productivity, premature mortality and family burden. Each of these has associated costs (6, 33).
- Good mental health care is not just about tackling clinical symptoms, but about improving someone's ability to function in ways that are valued by them and about promoting quality of life. There are also likely to be impacts on parents, siblings, classmates, and communities.

There have been relatively few studies of cost effectiveness of interventions for children and adolescents with mental health problems. Most have been undertaken in North America, western Europe, or Australia. This geographical unevenness needs emphasis because the results of economic evaluations may not transfer readily from one country to another: Differences in health systems, financing arrangements, incentive structures, and relative prices hamper generalization.

A recent systematic review identified 14 English-language studies assessing both costs and outcomes (34). There is insufficient space to give details here, but completed cost-effectiveness studies ranged widely in focus, looking at the roles of hospital and community-based service delivery, medications, parent training, early intervention, psychological treatment, skills development, educational programs, support system models, and care management. Taken together, these studies demonstrate the potential for devising targeted, problem-specific treatments and coordinated services, but they still cover only a fragment of the full mental health system. Moreover, and regrettably, the cost-effectiveness evidence is also patchy in quality: A number of the studies harbor methodological weaknesses. Today there are numerous studies underway that will eventually offer a better evidence platform for pursuing the efficiency improvements that promote health, education, and quality of life improvements from available budgets.

Equity

Equity relates to the distribution of outcomes, access and payment. One very relevant equity question is whether individual financial contributions are linked to ability to pay, indeed whether there needs to be a redistributive effort so that families with lower incomes contribute proportionately lower amounts. We touched on this question in discussing financing, and arrangements can be made to improve distribution. Equity in relation to the outcomes is another matter. Certainly, equity in final outcomes is a laudable but probably very ambitious goal, primarily because those outcomes are influenced by many factors over and above the resources devoted to mental health care, including income and its distribution, housing, family dynamics, lifestyle, and personality traits. Consequently, equity in access—perhaps expressed as equal access to treatment for equal need—is a more frequently discussed criterion, but still one that is hard to achieve.

It is clear that rates of service utilization by children and adolescents with mental health problems remain low across many countries, and that patterns of access are unevenly distributed (35–38). From an egalitarian standpoint it could be argued that utilization should not be influenced by "extraneous" factors such as ability to pay or geographical location.

Why do children, adolescents, and families not utilize services? One enduring reason is the stigma widely associated with mental illness. Another is the low rate of identification of needs. A third, obviously, is inability to pay for treatments. Many factors therefore contribute to inequality and numerous solutions have been propounded, including actions to improve public awareness and reduce discrimination, redistributive financing arrangements that are less disadvantageous to poor families, and so on.

BARRIERS AND OPPORTUNITIES

Even when there is an evidence base—i.e., even when there is a good appreciation of how to enhance child and family health and quality of life, or improve system efficiency, or improve the distribution of payments or access—there could be resource barriers in the way (39). These barriers challenge child and adolescent mental health systems across the world.

One of the most insidious and seemingly insurmountable barriers is resource insufficiency: Child and adolescent mental health services are underfunded, sometimes grossly so. This is clearly a major issue for countries where the proportion of national income devoted to healthcare is low, as in most of the poorer countries of the world, or where the proportion of the health budget allocated to child and adolescent mental health is minimal. Without funds it is difficult to build any kind of service system. Resource insufficiency leads inevitably to shortages of skilled staff (3, 36), and difficulties in recruiting and training appropriate personnel. Such shortages might energize the search for treatment modalities that make more cost-effective use of what is actually available, but there are limits to what can be achieved.

Increasing the resources available for child and adolescent mental health care would help overcome these challenges, but even when resources are committed, available services might be poorly distributed, available at the wrong place or time relative to the distribution of needs. They may be available only if delivered by specialist clinics or particular schools, or concentrated in urban areas, or available only to certain population groups (usually those with higher incomes). This resource distribution barrier is often related to the fundamental precepts of how a health or education system is financed or structured. In centrally coordinated systems, resources could perhaps be allocated according to need, but systems built on voluntary health insurance financing have few such opportunities.

A more general difficulty is resource inappropriateness: Available services do not match what is needed or preferred. Treatment or support arrangements may be too rigidly organized, leaving service systems unable to respond to differences in individual needs or preferences, or to community circumstances. Such inflexibility is common when there is scant information on population or individual needs, or when families have few opportunities to participate in treatment decisions, or when there is deep-rooted reluctance to move away from hospital-based services.

A linked challenge is resource dislocation: Services may potentially be available to meet individual and family needs, but they are poorly coordinated. Such a situation can be compounded by professional rivalry, performance assessment regimes, stultifying bureaucracy or "silo budgeting" (resources held in one agency's "silo" cannot be allocated to other uses), and some forms of managed care. Improved coordination might be achieved by reducing budgetary conflicts between agencies, rewarding efficiency and equity improvements, and encouraging individual and family participation in decision-making. These arrangements have their own (transaction) costs, of course, and a careful spending balance must be struck between using resources to deliver services using them simply to coordinate. The Fort Bragg demonstration program illustrates that service content is as important as coordination itself (3, 40, 41).

The timing problem can be quite insidious. For a start, most intended improvements to practice take a long time to work their way through to improved health outcomes, cost-effectiveness gains, or fairer access. Moreover, evidence for improved practice may have been gathered under experimental circumstances and the advantages suggested by research may not actually get realized in real-world settings. There could be transitional or longer term difficulties recruiting suitable professionals, or opening new facilities. Decisionmakers must also be encouraged to think long, for the immediate consequences of many interventions could be modest, but the long-term benefits immense (42,43).

Attitudes can put up other barriers. A population survey in Germany offers cogent evidence: The general public was clearly less willing to safeguard spending on mental health compared with other health conditions (44). The low priority accorded mental health was attributed to ignorance that conditions could be treated, beliefs that they were self-inflicted, and underestimation of individual susceptibility to psychiatric illness. Of course, people naturally want to give priority to treating life-threatening conditions, and most mental health problems are not seen in that light, but deep-rooted ignorance and stigma were probably largely influential in shaping these attitudes.

CONCLUSION

Child and adolescent mental health systems—interpreting this term broadly to include health, education, social work, and criminal justice components—are often in a state of flux. It may be a shift of emphasis from inpatient to community-based services, or the broadening of treatment eligibility criteria, or the expansion of insurance coverage. It could be the reconfiguration of multiprofessional staff teams, or new school-based proposals for identifying need. Changes of this kind usually raise economic questions. How are these initiatives to be financed? What cost implications will these changes have? Can they be afforded? Will they prove cost effective? What will they imply for the distribution of payment, access, and outcome?

There are many ways to raise and distribute the funds for child and adolescent mental health services, but there is no agreement on the best form of prepayment system—whether it should be via tax financing or social insurance or voluntary insurance—or about whether some level of out-of-pocket payment creates appropriate incentives, or about whether fee-for-service, capitation, or some other approach is the best way to commission services from providers. But there is growing experience of using each of these approaches, and growing evidence about what they might imply in particular for children and families affected by emotional or behavioral problems.

Given the comparatively high prevalence of these problems among poorer groups in the population and the often high costs of accessing effective treatments, governments need to make commitments to redistributive policies. They need to set in place the structures that encourage efficient and equitable links between the fundamental aims of improving the lives of children, adolescents, and families; the services and interventions that can deliver those improvements; and the financing mechanisms and purchasing systems that get the funds to providers. And they need to do so across many service sectors—certainly looking at specialist mental health, general medical care, education, social work, supported housing, social security, and criminal justice.

References

1. Knapp M: *The Economics of Social Care*. Macmillan, London, 1984.
2. Farmer EMZ, Burns BJ, Phillips SD, Angold A, Costello EJ: Pathways into and through mental health services for children and adolescents. *Psychiatric Services* 54:60–6, 2003.
3. Glied S, Evans Cuellar A: Trends and issues in child and adolescent mental health. *Health Affairs* 22:39–50, 2003.
4. Hoare P, Norton B, Chisholm D, Parry-Jones W: An audit of 7000 successive child and adolescent psychiatry referrals in Scotland. *Clinical Child Psychology and Psychiatry* 1:229–49, 1996.
5. Foster EM, Connor MS: Public costs of better mental health services for children and adolescents. *Psychiatric Services* 56:50–5, 2005.
6. Romeo R, Knapp M, Scott S: Children with antisocial behaviour: what do they cost and who pays? *British Journal of Psychiatry* 188:547–53, 2006.
7. Frank RG, McGuire T: Economics and mental health. In: Culyer AJ, Newhouse JP, (eds.): *Handbook of health economics*. Elsevier, Amsterdam, 2000.
8. Pettitt B: *Effective joint working between child and adolescent mental health services and schools*. Department for Education and Skills, London, 2003.
9. Weist MD, Goldstein J, Evans SW, Lever NA, Axlerod J, Schereters R, Pruitt D: Funding a full continuum of mental health promotion and intervention programs in the schools. *Journal of Adolescent Health* 32:S70–8, 2003.
10. Koppelman J: Children with mental disorders: making sense of their needs and the systems that help them. *National Health Policy Forum Issue Brief* 799:1–24, 2004.
11. Saxena S, Sharan P, Saracen B: Budget and financing of mental health services: baseline information on 89 countries from WHO's project atlas. *Journal of Mental Health Policy and Economics* 6:135–43, 2003.
12. Mossialos E, Dixon A, Figueras J, Kutzin J, (eds.): *Funding health care: options for Europe*. Open University Press, Buckingham, 2002.
13. Savedoff W: *Tax-based financing for health systems: options and experiences*. World Health Organization, Geneva, 2004.
14. Kavanagh S, Knapp M: Market rationales, rationing and rationality? Mental health care reform in England. *Health Affairs* 14:260–68, 1995.
15. Center for Disease Control and Prevention: *Health insurance coverage—National Center for Health Statistics*, 2003. <http://www.cdc.gov/nchs/fastats/hinsure.htm>.
16. Newacheck PW, Kim SE: A national profile of healthcare utilization and expenditure for children with special healthcare needs. *Archives of Pediatrics and Adolescent Medicine* 159:10–7, 2005.
17. Preker A, Jakab M et al.: Health financing reforms in Eastern Europe and Central Asia. In: Mossialos E et al. (eds.): *Funding health care: options for Europe*. Buckingham Open University Press, 2001.
18. Carrin G: Social health insurance in developing countries: a continuing challenge. *International Social Security Review* 55:57–69, 2002.
19. Zechmeister I, Osterle A, Denk P, Katschnig H: Incentives in financing mental health care in Austria. *Journal of Mental Health Economics and Policy* 5:121–29, 2002.
20. Knapp M, McDaid D: Economic realities: financing, resourcing, challenging, resolving. In: Knapp M, McDaid D, Mossialos E, Thornicroft G (eds.): *Mental health policy and practice across Europe*. Open University Press, Buckingham, forthcoming.
21. Mossialos E, Thomson S: *Voluntary health insurance in the European Union*. European Observatory on Health Systems and Policies, 2003.
22. Mark TL, Coffey RM: What drove private health insurance spending on mental health and substance abuse care between 1992–1999? *Health Affairs* 22:165–72, 2003.
23. Substance Abuse and Mental Health Service Administration: *National estimates of mental health insurance benefits*. National Mental Health Information Center, Center for Mental Health Services, 2006.
24. Libby AM, Cueller A, Snowden LR, Orton HD: Substitution in a Medicaid mental health carve-out: services and costs. *Journal of Healthcare Financing* 28:11–23, 2006.
25. Zaluska M, Suchecka D, Traczewska J, Paszko J: Implementation of social services for the chronically mentally ill in a Polish health district: consequences for service use and costs. *Journal of Mental Health Policy and Economics* 8:37–44, 2005.
26. Dixon A, McDaid D, Knapp M, Curran C: Financing mental health: equity and efficiency concerns for low and middle income countries. *Health Policy and Planning* 21:171–82, 2006.
27. Robinson CJ: Theory and practice in the design of physician payment incentives. *Milbank Quarterly* 79:2, 2001.
28. Russell LB, Manning CL: The effect of prospective payment on Medicare expenditures. *New England Journal of Medicine* 16:439–44, 1989.
29. Buck JB: Medicaid, health care financing trends, and the future of state-based public mental health services. *Psychiatric Services* 54:969–75, 2003.
30. Simpson L, Zodet MW, Chevarley FM, Owens PL, Dougherty D, McCormick M: Health care for children and youth in the United States: 2002 report on trends in access, utilization, quality and expenditures. *Ambulatory Pediatrics* 4:131–53, 2004.
31. Mandell DS, Boothroyd RA, Stiles PG: Children's use of mental health services in different Medicaid insurance plans. *Journal of Behavioral Health Services Research* 30:230–40, 2003.
32. Heflinger CA, Simpkins CG, Scholle SH, Kelleher KJ: Parent/caregiver satisfaction with their child's Medicaid plan and behavioral health providers. *Mental Health Services Research* 6, 23–31 2004.
33. Foster EM, Jones DE and the Conduct Problems Prevention Research Group: The high costs of aggression: public expenditures resulting from conduct disorders. *American Journal of Public Health* 95:1767–72, 2005.
34. Romeo R, Byford S, Knapp M: Economic evaluations of child and adolescent mental health interventions: a systematic review. *Journal of Child Psychology and Psychiatry* 46:919–30, 2005.
35. Leaf PJ, Algeria M, Cohen P, Goodman SH, Horwitz S, Hoven CW, Narrow WE, Vaden-Kiernan M, Regier DA: Mental health service use in the community and schools: results from the four-community MECA study. *Journal of the American Academy of Child and Adolescent Psychiatry* 35:889–97, 1996.
36. Levav I, Jacobsson L, Tsiantis J, Kolaitis G, Ponizovsky A: Psychiatric services and training for children and adolescents in Europe: results from a country survey. *European Child and Adolescent Psychiatry* 13:395–401, 2004.
37. Offord DR, Boyle MH, Szatmari P, Rae-Grant NI, Links PS, Cadman DT, Byles JA, Crawford JW, Blum HM, Byrne C, Thomas H, Woodward CA: Ontario child health study. Six-month prevalence of disorder and rates of service utilization. *Archives of General Psychiatry* 44:832–38, 1987.
38. Sourander A, Helstela L, Ristkari T, Ikaheimo K, Helenius H, Piha J: Child and adolescent mental health service use in Finland. *Social Psychiatry and Psychiatric Epidemiology* 36:294–98, 2001.
39. Knapp M, Funk M, Curran C, Prince M, Gibbs M, McDaid D: Mental health in low- and middle-income countries: economic barriers to better practice and policy. *Health Policy and Planning* 21:157–70, 2006.
40. Bickman L: A continuum of care: more is not always better. *American Psychologist* 51:921–33, 1996.
41. Foster EM, Bickman L: Refining the costs analyses of the Fort Bragg evaluation: the impact of cost offset and cost shifting. *Mental Health Services Research* 2:13–25, 2000.
42. Fergusson DM, Horwood LJ, Ridder EM: Show me the child at seven: the consequences of conduct problems in childhood for psychosocial functioning in adulthood. *Journal of Child Psychology and Psychiatry* 46:837–49, 2005.
43. Scott S, Knapp M, Henderson J, Maughan B: Financial cost of social exclusion: follow-up study of antisocial children into adulthood. *British Medical Journal* 323:191–94, 2001.
44. Matschinger H, Angemeyer M: The public's preference concerning the allocation of financial resources to health care: results from a representative population survey in Germany. *European Psychiatry* 19:478–82, 2004.

1.7 ■ DIVERSE POPULATIONS

CHAPTER 1.7.1 ■ CULTURAL CHILD AND ADOLESCENT PSYCHIATRY

G. PIROOZ SHOLEVAR

INTRODUCTION

Cultural child and adolescent psychiatry consists of a body of theoretical and technical knowledge that informs high quality psychiatric evaluation, treatment and assessment of developmental process across cultural and language barriers to children, adolescents, and families. Clinicians are increasingly called upon to evaluate or treat patients from multiple cultural and linguistic groups. In our multicultural American society, treating a patient who speaks a different language or holds beliefs at variance with the majority culture requires the knowledge and skills that constitute cultural psychiatry (1). Cultural psychiatry defines the impact of culture on psychiatric evaluation and diagnosis and provides guidelines for culturally competent and sensitive psychiatric treatment and systems of care (1–3). It is characterized by introducing the vast diversity of human experience into an understanding of the complexities of mental health and illness.

Cultural psychiatry has evolved consistently throughout the past century. Initially and at the beginning of the twentieth century it was primarily concerned with comparison of manifestations of mental disorders in different cultures and countries. It described the exotic and special features of different syndromes and disorders discovered in Africa, the Far East, and other non-Western countries. The descriptions were based on a universalist (and Western) viewpoint of psychiatry and mental disorders. In the mid-twentieth century prominent anthropologists such as Ruth Benedict, Margaret Mead, and Bronislaw Malinowski incorporated psychoanalytic constructs into their cultural investigations of the impact of culture on personality development and disorders (4). This highly productive collaboration between psychiatry and anthropology also included Emile Durkhiem's landmark study on suicide and George Herbert Mead's Symbolic Interactionalist Theory.

The interest in sound methodological measures in the mid-twentieth century resulted in the construction of a number of crossculturally validated epidemiological and diagnostic instruments. Recent findings based partially on such methodology have resulted in a gradual shift from a universalist viewpoint to a more culturally specific perspective (1, 2, 5).

The value orientation theory was originally proposed by Kluckhohn (6). It is based on variations in generalized cultural values. According to Kluckhohn, there are three possible variations in solution to the problems of time (past, present, future); activity (doing, being, being-in-becoming); relationship in groups (individual, collateral, linear); man–nature relationship (harmony-with-nature, mastery-over-nature, subjugated-to-nature); and basic nature of man (neutral/mixed, good, evil).

Cultures vary widely in these dimensions. For example, American culture emphasizes a future time orientation, a "doing" mode of activity, an "individualistic" relational orientation focusing on autonomy; mastery over nature; and the nature of man as neutral or mixed. Using this now-dated typology, Spiegel (7) pointed how Southern Italians in contrast are oriented toward present, being, collateral relational view, subjugation by nature and a mixed view of human nature, while Southern Irish are oriented toward present, being, lineal relationships, subjugation by nature and the evil nature of man. In their views, the contrast between variable value orientations can create interpersonal tension and conflicts, such as in a crosscultural marriage.

The *cultural relativist* perspective of current cultural psychiatry is in contrast to the *universalist* one, and asserts that cultural values and meanings are relative to and embedded in their cultural context and cannot be measured against a universal system. It uses locally meaningful categories to describe indigenous syndromes, their phenomenology, and native explanatory models based on an ethnographic perspective (8). They make strong attempts to avoid the categorical fallacy.

Category fallacy refers to application of a category that is valid within one cultural context to a culture where the category has no diagnostic validity or relevance. It stems from a universalist approach to assigning meaning to behaviors transculturally. In contrast, cultural relativists propose that cultural meanings and values are relative and fundamentally embedded in their cultural context. The latter perspective is referred to as *emic*, in contract to the former approach, known as ethic, which applies Western diagnostic categories to another cultural context (8).

Definitions

Culture consists of those patterns of behavior, acquired and transferred over time, which prescribe the norms, customs, roles, and values inherent in political, economic, religious, and social aspects of family life. Culture provides the set of rules and standards that guide people's actions, makes their behavior understandable to one another, and helps to explain individuals' relationships to their sociobiological context.

Ethnicity refers to the sense of belonging and having a rootedness in history that reaches beyond religion, race, or national or geographic origin. Ethnicity is our basic identity—who we are in relation to other human groups. It frames our manner of dress, style, and communication through language and rituals, as well as how we feel about life, death, and illness (9, 10). The concept is derived from the Greek work *ethnos*, or people of a nation. We are born with an ethnic identity. Throughout life we experience and adopt different cultures, thereby living with expectations and values from both a majority culture (i.e., the American culture) and minority culture—our culture of origin. We carry with us both the values, assumptions, traditions, and worldviews transmitted over generations within our ethnic group and the concurrent—sometimes competing—view of the cultural context in which we live. As noted by McGoldrick et al. (10) and Herr (11), ethnic traditions still affect third and fourth generations in subtle ways and are often experienced as cultural conflicts between members of the younger generation.

Cultural context refers to the sociocultural environment in which people live and interact. The combination of ethnic origin and cultural context, together with the pressures imposed by cultural transitions and/or migration, inevitably creates difficulties that family groups must resolve. Landau (12) discusses the challenge minorities face in balancing the demands of living within two cultures—the culture of origin and the majority culture. She notes that if the stresses and differences are too great, the family network is too remote or too weak to help, the family must either adapt to the culture or turn inward on itself, becoming isolated and enmeshed as a family group. As a consequence of the ethnocentric defense, very often the family resists accepting help from outsiders unless their problems become too great to handle alone.

Cultural identity refers to the patient's cultural or ethnic reference group and the degree of involvement with both host culture and culture of origin. This internalized self-definition selectively incorporates values, beliefs and historical elements from those available in the person's environmental values and contains self-experiences related to ethnicity, gender, values, and a wide range of beliefs.

Ethnic identity describes a sense of commonality transmitted over generations by the family and reinforced by the surrounding community (10). An ethnic group is defined as "those who conceive themselves as alike by virtue of their common ancestry, real or fictitious, and who are so regarded by others" (13). It is perceived as "we" in contrast to "they." Ethnic identity develops as the product of ethnic socialization by children acquiring the values, attitudes, behaviors, and perceptions of an ethnic group, and perception of themselves and others as members of the group (14).

Cultural mask, Montalvo and Gutierrez (15), refers to the family's use of real elements in their culture to conceal their problematic behavior and interactions. For example, the family can use the rationale: "We are Latin, we are expected to have hot tempers." The family thus uses culturally sanctioned behavior in a defensive fashion in order to protect crucial underlying issues. The family presents to the therapist a view of who they are based on what they think is expected of them instead of showing how they actually behave when trying to resolve problems or even interact with one another. Montalvo and Gutierrez caution the therapist to search for the problemsolving approach of the family and not get caught up in exotic or unusual behavior patterns unique to the family's culture.

Acculturation

Acculturation refers to the process of behavioral and attitudinal changes in a cultural subgroup as a result of exposure to the practices of a different dominant group (16). Initially it was hypothesized that a high level of acculturation decreases stress and the risk of psychological disorder in members of cultural subgroups. Subsequent studies have further recognized the complexity of the process; the concurrent relationship between a high level of acculturation and increased psychological distress probably due to social role conflicts and the partial loss of traditional support received from the original culture (1, 17, 18).

The culturally sensitive clinician can be well served by paying close attention to the unique experiences of each individual in the acculturation process as it is manifested by intense rejection or blind acceptance of cultural elements of the host or original cultures, or a defensive resistance to assimilation into the broader culture. The complexity of the acculturation process in child/adolescent and family psychiatry can be significant because of different levels of acculturation achieved by children and their parents. Children born in the host country can achieve a very high level of acculturation, while parents may adhere strongly to the practices of their original culture and reject the values of the host culture. Fathers may develop a much higher level of linguistic and cultural competence due to their workplace experiences in contrast to the mothers, who may not learn the new language and cultural practices if primarily functioning in the household. The level of acculturation of younger children may also differ significantly from that of older children, particularly if born and initially raised in the previous culture and exhibiting sharp differences from their younger and Americanized siblings.

The degree and nature of the acculturation process can be determined by inquiry into age at immigration, number of years in the United States, language proficiency, and participation in the host culture's social activities and social networks (1, 16).

Culture-Bound Syndromes

Culture-bound syndromes consist of disturbances in mood, behavior or belief systems that appear restricted to a particular cultural context. They are frequently viewed as exotic or covert illness phenomena occurring in the context of a local culture. Many culture-bound syndromes have been described worldwide. For example, some syndromes can exhibit acute episodes of anxiety, such as *ataques de nervios* in Latin America or Koro in Malaysia. The former syndrome manifests by trembling, shouting, crying, fainting, seizure-like activity or suicidal gestures. The person may return to normal functioning rapidly. As with many similar syndromes, it is a pattern of behavior that is understood locally as a meaningful manifestation of distress, acceptable within the cultural context. Such symptoms signal distress and activate a culturally specific response to the situation. The symptoms are recognized and interpreted through the appropriate attribution, which is part of the common socialization process for the cultural subgroup (8).

Effect of Culture and Ethnicity on Child Development

Recent trends have brought the cultural context of child and personality development into bold relief. Among these are the global demographic trend toward cultural heterogeneity, and contributions from crosscultural psychiatry and psychology. It is generally established now that culture influences the development of children and shapes personality from infancy through adulthood. The childrearing practices of parents and family provide the infant with the basic nurturance needed for development. Equally important is the role of parents and family in transmitting cultural rules, standards, and values to the child through the process of socialization. Cultures vary widely and differ from each other in the way the tasks of socialization are carried out, the specific rules and values transmitted, and the behavioral and conceptual outcome of socialization process in terms of beliefs and world views adopted by the children (19–21).

It is also firmly established that much of our information on child development is based on norms that are almost exclusively Western, middle class and male oriented. Most of the observations and studies have been conducted in Western settings and are nonrepresentative of the world's population. These studies perpetuate a given view of the universe and tell us little about how children develop in so-called "minority cultures" in Western societies (22, 23). Child rearing practices vary widely in different cultures. In many cultures, particularly Western ones, the main parenting person is the mother, with the father assuming an important but secondary parental role. In African societies, older siblings assume a significant role in raising infants and young children. Other family members and grandparents assume important childrearing roles in Asian and some other countries. Other caretakers offer the children a different or expanded view of the world (24, 25). Socialization occurs not only through explicit teaching but also through day-to-day experience of childhood and through the structure of the settings where the children live and play.

Cultural Impact on Developmental Stages

Examination of influence of different cultures on different developmental stages is gaining intense interest among investigators. We briefly review the investigations of several developmental stages.

Crosscultural Research on Infancy

A strong theme in literature is the "precocity" of babies from traditional, nonindustrialized societies. They may stand or sit two to four or more weeks earlier than American and European norms. At times the precocity in Africa has been linked with reports of precocity at birth. The clusters of advanced behaviors are to a large degree correlated with environmental factors (26, 27).

Putting aside the multiple and complex methodological shortcomings in many studies, it is generally established that African babies reared in relatively traditional ways achieve many motor functions, particularly in the first year of life, before their European and American counterparts. The findings from studies in Uganda have been subsequently supported by multiple studies in other African Countries (26, 27). The advanced skills frequently coincide with deliberate teachings of the infants by the mothers and other caretakers of how to walk, sit, and help the babies practice those skills. They may use props to facilitate those tasks. The encouragement of sitting and carrying the baby on the caretaker's back is more helpful in the development of trunk, buttocks, and thigh muscles in comparison to having the child sit on an infant seat (26, 27, 29). Similar findings have been reported in Asian countries, including India (28, 30).

Lester and Brazelton (31) propose that African childrearing practices are built on the infant's responsiveness to being handled in the neonatal period and facilitate motor precocity. Motor excitement of infants may elicit intense interpersonal handling from the caregiver, thus enhancing developmental progression. Normal infants in different traditional cultures appear to exhibit critical cognitive developmental levels at about the same time throughout the world (26, 31).

Temperament

In studying temperament, cultural affiliation is a strong predictor of infant temperament in the first year of life and is exquisitely sensitive to environmental influences. McDermott (25) has proposed that temperament should be viewed as a constellation of traits with a threshold of expression that varies from culture to culture. Considering two broad clusters of temperament, namely rhythmicity and activity, significant cultural variations are evident. Chinese American, Japanese American, and Navajo Indians are temperamentally less excitable than other groups who exhibit lower levels of arousal and are easily consoled. Mexican Indians and Kenyan infants have smoother transitions from one state to another and maintain quiet, alert states for longer periods and are higher on motor maturity (25, 32, 33).

Examining the investigations of Jerome Kagan (34, 35) on shyness and social/behavioral inhibition, McDermott (25) proposed that cultures impart meanings to the behavior but also determine how others perceive and react to the behavior. Inhibited and shy children are more readily accepted by mothers in the Chinese culture, as opposed to the North American. Shy-anxious children in China are valued and accepted by society and peers and adjust well to their social environment (34–36). In the West, shyness and social withdrawal are associated with peer rejection and isolation, reflecting strong emphasis of the West on the need for self-expression and self-confidence (34–36). In contrast, the ready acceptance of this biologically determined behavior by parents, teachers, and peers in Asian culture reflect a low level of apprehension about this trait. McDermott proposes that Chess and Thomas's model of goodness-of-fit be applied at the cultural as well as the individual level.

The first large-scale investigation of children living in multiple cultures was undertaken by the anthropological team of Beatrice and John Whiting (37, 38). They compared the behavior of children and the adults' expectation of them in six different cultures: India, Kenya, Mexico, Okinawa, Philippines, and the United States. Children in nonindustrialized cultures were given tasks important to the well being of the families, such as caring for younger siblings and tending to a goat so the family did not go without milk. Children showed nurturing and responsible behavior. Children in industrialized cultures were not expected to contribute to their family's survival, were more self-centered and dependent, and their self-centered orientation was tolerated by their families. The self-centeredness may be actually an asset in Western cultures and enhance the desire for personal profit (19). Whiting and Whiting found the influence of peers on young children to be very powerful and occur early. Additionally, parental efforts to control and redirect the aggression of their children emerged more strongly than their nurturance in all of the above cultures (25, 37, 38).

Being part of a group, rather than individual assertiveness, is highly valued in many cultures. Being agreeable, respectful, emotionally mature, courteous, and self-controlled are considered major assets as they promote interdependence. Traditional Japanese culture views newborns as independent and making them dependent, bound to and part of the group, is considered a fundamental task of the family. The Japanese traditional practice of keeping young children close to the mother all the time fosters a high level of social and personal closeness and interdependence characteristics that are very different from American culture (19, 39).

Preschoolers

Preschool Chinese children are expected to pay close attention during lessons, unlike American preschoolers. Chinese nursery school teachers initiate and organize most of the daily activities, while the children listen, follow directions, take turns, and share. The activity structure teaches the children the value of self-control, obedience, and cooperation with other children. In contrast, the American nursery school provides a wide range of toys that can be used by children in their own way in free play, transmitting the importance of self-expression and individuality in the American culture (19, 39).

Children's inclination to compete or cooperate emerges as a signification differential point among Anglo-American and many non-Western or nonindustrialized cultures. Madsen used a cooperation game for two players, where only one child could partially win if s/he cooperated with the other person but both children lost if they competed. Madsen (35, 41) found dramatic behavioral differences between urban

Anglo-American and rural Mexican children. The Anglo-American children, particularly the older ones, were far more competitive even when it did not benefit them. The rural Mexican children were far more cooperative, even when they did not directly benefit. The strategies of both groups of children were adaptive within their culture (19).

Culture and School Achievement

Daily experiences of Japanese and many Asian children conveys the high level of cultural value placed on formal education, which explains the much higher score of Japanese students on math and science in comparison to American students. Starting in elementary school, Japanese students spend many more hours in the classroom and doing homework than American students. They also receive extensive tutoring after hours for exams, and enrichment courses (19, 39, 41). The emphasis of Japanese parents on education reflects their cultural belief that achievement depends on effort; parents are rarely satisfied with their children's academic achievement and urge them to work harder. In contrast, American parents believe that academic success depends primarily on innate ability and assume their children are doing their best (19).

Transition to school is frequently difficult for children from a cultural subgroup attending a school representing the radically different social interactional pattern of the majority culture. Middle-class American children enter school already feeling very familiar and at ease with being asked many questions, particularly *test-type questions* with the answers already known by the adults. African-American children from a lower socioeconomic class were usually unfamiliar with this type of questions and more accustomed to *story-starter* or *accusation* or *analogy type questions* and acted unresponsively to the test-type questions (19, 43). The same cultural mismatch between children's usual style of interacting with adults and the expected social style in school has been described with other minority groups, including Native American children and East Indian children in England. This cultural mismatch makes the transition to school more difficult for children from cultural subgroups. It interferes with the shift to decontextualized thought, learning to solve problems that are abstract and removed from the immediate context by applying their informal problemsolving skills learned at home in everyday life (19, 43). It can affect how much children can learn from their school experience and explain the lower average achievement test scores for African-American and Latino children and their higher rate of school dropout and school failure in comparison to Anglo-Americans (44).

Cultural Bias in Testing Intelligence

Any test to measure intelligence (IQ test) is a product of a certain culture and the level of knowledge of that culture affects how well one performs on that test. There are subtle ways in which cultural background can influence test scores. Cultures vary in their definition of intelligence and the preferred way of performing a cognitive task (45). The interpersonal setting and the racial or ethnic identity of the tester can reduce the accuracy of test results; children feel more comfortable being tested by members of their own ethnic group. Some children from cultural subgroups feel confused by an adult asking a series of questions when he already knows the answers to them.

To reduce the problem of cultural bias, *culture-free tests* (no culture-based content) and *culture-fair tests* have been developed. In one such test, the problems are presented visually to eliminate the use of language. However, the difference in performance scores on these tests for some cultural groups were unreliably high (45, 46). Culture-fair IQ tests uses items that are appropriate to all cultures, but the problem of accurate assessment has remained unsolved. Therefore, intelligence tests remain an effective tool for comparison of intellectual ability within the same culture, but not for comparison across cultures (19).

Cross-Cultural Studies of Adolescence

Adolescence marks the transition from childhood to adult roles in different cultures and has been studied by multiple investigators since the initial observations of Margaret Mead in Samoa in the 1920s. The complexities of adult roles in Western industrialized societies require a very protracted period of learning to acquire the social and technical skills necessary to assume adult roles and gain privileges such as driving (in most states at age 16), voting (19), and drinking (usually at 21). Adolescents have to be dependent on their parents financially for a protracted period of time and feel as "marginal" people in a no-man's-land (47), denied full adult social and sexual roles (19). The inner feeling of frustration can lead to a period of conflictual relationship with parents.

In contrast to the experience of adolescents in industrialized societies, anthropologist Margaret Mead found the adolescent transition to adult roles in Samoan culture to be nonstressful and gradual; the adolescent's interests and activities matured progressively and without significant stress or conflicts (4). Her basic conclusions in this area has been supported by subsequent investigations (19).

In some cultures, such as certain tribes in Kenya, transition to adulthood is somewhat abrupt as the growing children's duties expand over a short period of time (19, 36, 47). Such societies have special ceremonies called "rites of passage" to mark entry into adult roles, which are anticipated by the children for years in advance (19).

The universally accepted dual developmental tasks of adolescence, namely preparation for adulthood and identity formation, follows differential patterns in different cultures. Western cultures tend to encourage achievement through academic endeavors and physical sports. In Confucian-influenced Asian cultures, emphasis is on self-discipline, subjugation of desires and self-refinement as the preferred methods of accomplishment of inner peace (47). Canino and Canino (48) point out that assertiveness, competitiveness and independence, which are highly valued in Western culture, can be contradictory to core Puerto Rican values and create conflict in Puerto Rican families who live in the mainland United States.

Puberty has been studied extensively crossculturally. The major noticeable changes of puberty occur over a time span of four years and in girls between the ages nine to 16. Girls in industrialized countries tend to reach menarche earlier than girls in nonindustrialized and developing countries because malnutrition and chronic illnesses are more common. The median age for menarche in North America, Japan and Western Europe is 12.5 to 13.5, in contrast to Africa, where it is 14 to 17 years. Across a wide range of cultures and countries, girls from higher income families with adequate nutrition reach menarche sooner than girls from lower income families. There is no crosscultural difference in the age of onset of menarche between girls in groups from comparable income families (19, 49).

Cross-Cultural Psychiatric Evaluation and Treatment

Cross-cultural psychiatric evaluation and treatment describe the skills required to provide care across cultural and linguistic barriers when a clinician consults with a patient from a different cultural/ethnic group who holds a different system of belief values and may speak a different language. In addition to the goal of conducting a comprehensive clinical evaluation, the clinician should assess the contributions of culturally derived forces and stressors to the patient's symptomatology and the adequacy of protective factors in the patient's social environment to mediate stress and promote healthy adjustment.

Religion, faith, and healing are often so intertwined that in certain cultures, when a psychiatric condition occurs, diagnosis and remedy may be more influenced by spiritual rather than medical interpretation. For example, in Hispanic cultures there is a condition called *susto*, which describes a type of terror or fright that occurs consequent to some trauma. The victim of *susto* or trauma suffers a "soul loss" through fright. As in posttraumatic stress disorder (PTSD), the trauma can manifest clinically as anxiety, panic, fear, or depression. The cure consists of the intervention of a person skilled in healing—a *curandero*, or healer, who allows the patient to release fears and hostilities (17, 50). Treatment consists of medicine, some ritual or ceremony with friends and relatives, and the support of a network of friends. Ultimately the person is "reassured" through a type of transferential cure—a combined systemic approach that includes a spiritual orientation, the support of friends and family, and faith in the healer.

The evaluator should have an adequate understanding of the patient's culture of origin and the impact of the cultural—or immigration—issues on the child's developmental process. He should inquire about the expectations of parents from the psychiatric treatment, based on their culture of origin. Many patients, particularly Asian, have initially tried folk healers, exorcists, and herbal medicine, prior to evaluation. Such efforts should be explored respectfully and with an accepting attitude. Many Asian families only come for psychiatric evaluation under pressure from school, social agencies, or family court, and their ambivalence about treatment should be respected (17, 47, 48). Frequently, there is a profound feeling of failure and alienation in the family because they have attempted unsuccessfully to solve the problem on their own for a prolonged period of time. The pain of the family should be acknowledged empathically, while countering their feelings of being a failure as a family; one should also disavow the family's view of themselves as a "mental illness family" rather than a family with a problem who are actively attempting to find a solution (47, 48). The impact of the child's emotional disorder on the internal family environment, interpersonal dynamics, and weakening of the parental authority should be explored.

The initial evaluative session serves the multiple tasks of forging a relationship with all family members, collecting data, and enlisting their active partnership in the treatment process. It requires continuous respect and empathy, particularly around inquiries into the parents' explanation for the child's behavior, and addressing their questions and fears. Clinicians can often perform these tasks more comfortably in separate sessions with parents and children. However, clinicians who are proficient in family and individual therapy can effectively accomplish these goals in child-centered conjoint family sessions.

Contrary to the initial view of many clinicians, the contemporary field of cultural psychiatry considers that comprehensive and meaningful evaluations across cultural boundaries can be performed by clinicians who are from a background radically different from a patient's culture as far as the principles and guideline outlined in this chapter are applied.

Clinical Interview

Interview across the cultural barrier requires a high level of attention and sensitivity to the establishment of rapport and empathy with the patient and the family. Respect and deference to the elders and head of households can facilitate acceptance by the patients. Comments on positive assets of family members, such as children's good looks and manners, can enhance the sense of pride in all family members. Clinician should adopt the preferred communication style of the family; the patient may feel more comfortable with a formal conversational method of inquiry rather than an informal one, or with asking rapid-fire questions from a checklist. Some Latino patients, particularly in inner city populations, should be allowed extra time initially to describe the symptoms in great detail; every daily call from the school about the child's disruptiveness; the child's poor eating habits; irregular sleeping routine; disrespect for the parents. This communication style should only be redirected in a way that avoids alienating the person. Certain content carries stigma, such as discussion of overt aggression, suicidality, or sexuality with certain Asian groups. The patient's preference should be respected and handled with special tact, as if one were conducting a complex defense/resistance analysis.

Language proficiency as a barrier to health care is a formidable obstacle to the care of several cultural groups, particularly with the increasing number of Latino and Asian immigrants. It is estimated that 50% of these groups are monolingual and the level of language proficiency and language independence of many patients in the remaining half may fall short of what is needed for an accurate and comprehensive psychiatric assessment. Therefore, a variety of translators, interpreters, specially trained translators, and cultural/linguistic consultants are engaged to facilitate the communication process between the clinician and the patient. The highest level of assistance can be rendered by cultural/linguistic consultants, who work closely with members of the clinical team, and are especially trained and sensitized to recognize rich affective and cognitive context accompanying the patient's verbal communication in order to arrive at the *connotative meaning* of their expressions, rather than just the literal ones. There are guidelines for the use of translators, using the necessary translation time to make additional observations about the patient's behavior, resistance, and to recognize errors in translation based on patient's response. Frequently, patients can recognize intuitively the translation errors of the interpreter and they should be empowered to point them out. The evaluator should have the necessary skills to recognize the patient/translator "transference," translator-patient "countertransference," and ways of avoiding splitting the authority (transference) between the translator and the clinician. Many fully bilingual patients—particularly Latinos—may choose to use an interpreter in the sessions in order to focus their efforts on describing their situation. They frequently correct the interpreter during translation errors. This phenomenon should not be misunderstood as a power-struggle maneuver, but as a preferred communication style. Furthermore, the language proficiency of a fully bilingual person can fall short during the description of traumatic events from the past that are laden with intense affect (51–54).

Cultural Formulation

Cultural formulation is a key concept in the biopsychosocial assessment and diagnosis of mental disorders, similar to psychodynamic or biological formulations. The DSM IV recommends inclusion of a number of components into such a formulation to make it serve as a sensitive instrument to address the requirements of a comprehensive assessment in culturally diverse or multicultural groups (1, 54). The formulation should include: a) the cultural identity of the patient; b) cultural explanations of the patient's illness; c) cultural factors related to the psychosocial environment; and d) overall cultural assessment for diagnosis and treatment.

For immigrants, cultural formulations should include pre-immigration history, including major conflicts, losses, or traumas that may have contributed to the immigration. For example, a 13-year-old girl who lived with her grandmother in Puerto Rico for most of her life was sent to the United States abruptly after she was sexually abused by a relative. The trauma of the sexual abuse, the abrupt loss of the relationship with her primary psychological caregiver, and the unpreparedness of the mother to care for the daughter after many years of separation were not included in the formulation.

Mental Health and Psychiatric Care: Effect of Culture in Help-Seeking

Need assessment surveys of the general population have consistently shown that most people with serious emotional problems do not seek professional help, particularly from mental health professionals. With a culturally diverse population, special powerful barriers are operative, which explains the low level of utilization of mental health services by minorities and culturally diverse groups, as emphasized in the 2000 Surgeon General's report (55). Chief among them is fear of stigmatization and discrimination, which combines with attitudinal, demographic and system-dependent factors.

The fear of discrimination particularly due to linguistic barrier is a formidable deterrent for many members of certain cultural groups. Equally significant is the fear of disregard, disrespect, or misunderstanding the patient's culture and customs. Fear of disregard for the status of parents and elders, and the importance of the children's respect for parents, parental values, and loyalty to the family keeps many families from seeking help. Essential clinician variables are: empathy, skillful perceptiveness, effective communication, straightforwardness, honesty, flexibility, intellectual curiosity, openmindedness, and tolerance for psychological challenges of adolescents and children (56, 57). Adequate inquiry into parental views of the problems, their explanation for the behavior, their expectations of treatment outcome, keeping them informed of the treatment progress, and addressing crisis situations by involving the family can help forge a strong therapeutic alliance with the family. Rogler and Colleagues (16) recommend the following requirements for providing mental health services to culturally diverse populations: 1) locating mental health services in minority neighborhoods and close to public transportation, as minority groups such as Asians and Latinos tend to congregate closely to each other; 2) employing mental health workers and clinicians who share the linguistic and cultural backgrounds of the patients; and 3) creating an ambiance that reflects the cultural heritage of the patient population in outpatient and hospital settings.

Culturally specific therapies are increasingly emerging in the clinical research literature and incorporate specific elements from the patient's native culture into therapeutic interventions (1). Such approaches modify conventional psychiatric treatments by incorporating folk rituals, herbs, and the patient's own cultural conception of the illness into therapeutic interventions.

A large number of patients in the majority culture tend to seek treatment for their emotional disorders from a primary care physician. In a seemingly parallel phenomenon, many members of minority groups tend to seek treatment relief and support from outside the mental health system from people such as a *curandero* and folk healers in Latino cultures. Mental health programs can penetrate the lay referral structure by assembling some credible members of the ethnic network into their professional structure (47, 48). Informal and immediate registration of the patient for the initial contact with treatment can reduce the barrier to care (47, 48, 58).

Psychopharmacology

Many cultural groups, particularly the Latino, hold a culturally shared belief that emotional disorders are somatically based and best treated with medication; they expect a rapid rate of recovery from target symptoms and are alarmed by side effects that they relate to "toxicity." The Chinese, Korean, and Japanese tend to require much lower medication doses, at times one-half or one-third of the conventional doses, to achieve therapeutic response (1, 47). Therefore crossethnic variations in drug responses are becoming a focus of increased attention.

Cytochrome P450 isoenzymes are key in the metabolism of psychotropic and nonpsychotropic drugs (Chapter 6.1.2). The genetic defects in poor metabolizers are unequally distributed among ethnic populations. The percentage of CYP2D6 poor metabolizers is lower in Asians and higher in Caucasians. Similar interethnic variance exists in frequency of poor metabolizers of CYP2Cmp; low among whites (3 percent), intermediate for African Americans (18 percent), and higher in Asians and Japanese (up to 20 percent). Immigrants and members of many subcultural groups commonly use herbal medicines. Inquiry into the use of the traditional herbal medicines of Asians, Latinos, and other immigrants to the United States is essential because many of these herbs possess high levels of psychoactive activities. Others such as ginseng may stimulate or inhibit cytochrome P450 enzymes (1, 47).

The American Multicultural Society

Since the start of the twenty-first century, American society and the global community have become increasingly heterogeneous with respect to racial, ethnic, and cultural composition. The Latino population is growing at a particularly high rate in the United States. They have become more numerous than African Americans, to constitute the largest American minority group at 14.2% of the population (in comparison to African Americans at 12.2%, Asians at 4.2%, and Native Americans at 0.8%) (*Source*: United States 2004 American Community profile.). The number of children in Latino and African-American families is proportionally higher than in Caucasian families, which has significant implications for child and adolescent psychiatric and mental health services. In many urban areas, particularly ones with low economic resources, people of color constitute the majority population (59). It has been estimated that by the year 2050, 50% of the American population will be composed of people of color, and Latinos will comprise 25% of the American population (59).

Global demographic trends reveal a world in which the majority is characterized by cultural heterogeneity rather than "ethnic purity." A recent report has revealed that for the first time, the majority of the parents are living in cultural settings other than those where they themselves were brought up (58). The multicultural profile of American and global families has given rise to the theoretical orientation of multiculturalism. Multiculturalism is based on the assumption that there is no one way to conceptualize human behavior, explain the realities and experiences of diverse cultural groups, and that no particular set of competencies have proven effective with every form of diversity (58, 59, 62).

The following section describes characteristics of three major cultural subgroups in American Society.

CHARACTERISTICS OF FAMILIES FROM THREE CULTURES

African-American Families

African Americans compose 12.2% of the population in the United States of America (U.S. Census Bureau 2004) (58). A majority of African Americans have migrated from the American south to northern and western states. Issues of parity and equality with other cultural groups are most evident in the job market, where African Americans made 80% of what whites earned (63). Presently, there has been a strong upsurge of African psychology sensibility that seeks to expose the richness and strengths of African-American culture, for a more balanced perspective.

Although slavery and its aftermath disrupted the structure and support of the tribal experience for those Africans who were torn from their homeland, the tribal kin "network" remained a vital part of their heritage (64, 65). This focus on kin and the kinship network is relived in many parts of African-American life through religion, childcare, and foster family care, and constitutes a significant aspect of African-American life. Kinship bonds are a central residual part of the African culture, as in the rich delineations created by the extended family. Other arrangements include households where the children are not related to the head of the household, and arrangement that Billingsley (65) refers to as "augmented families."

Mothering and informal adoption are crucial concepts in African-American culture. It is common within the African culture for women to nurse other women's children as needed. In the United States, informal adoption is quite common and part of a very old slave tradition, whereby friends or relatives "took in" children who could not be cared for by their own parents. "Child keeping," as it is referred to by Stack (67), is indicative of the strong network operating within this culture.

Upward Mobility

Upward mobility is highly valued in the "American Dream" of individualism and ownership of material goods (65). However, as described by Pinderhughes (64), the American dream is always in conflict with the "victim value system." The victim value system is a name given to the struggle to overcome obstacles that threaten self-esteem. Often this struggle leads to the paradoxical erection of barriers to opportunity through inadequate education that limits employment opportunities.

Children and Responsibility

In many African-American families the role of the parent is often delegated to a child who takes on responsibility for other children while the parent(s) works. Parentification denotes how the child assumes a parental role both emotionally and physically. From an early age, children take the task of "mothering" very seriously. Reasonability also extends to aging grandparents and is characterized by respect and recognition for what the grandparents have done for the family as children. Elderly people are respected and cared for within the family network rather than institutions or agencies. A corresponding social myth depicts the black father as peripheral, a myth that has been overemphasized in psychiatric literature and further reifies deficit perspectives (63–65).

The Role of the Church and Spirituality

The role of the church and spirituality are crucial to African-American culture and can be traced throughout African history: "Spirituality is deeply embedded in the Black psyche" Knox (66). The church is seen as the one institution that remains a refuge against the painful experiences of life, including racism and discrimination.

Latino-American Families

Latino is the more contemporary term used to refer to a cultural group that shares a language, values, and customs. There are several regional subcultures that are referred to collectively as the "Latino culture." (Note that *Latino* is used to describe the general culture, but *Latina* and *Latino* are used to describe female and male members of the culture, respectively.) Gonzalez (67) correctly notes that for many in this very diverse population, the word Hispanic projects a politically conservative perspective, whereas Latino is considered a much less political demarcation and more in keeping with a sense of vitality and ethnocultural progressiveness. Chicano denotes people of American birth but of Mexican descent who do not align themselves with either culture. Latinos are a heterogeneous group. Mexicans are the largest subgroup (64%), followed by Puerto Ricans (9.6%) and Cubans (3.6%). Latinos from other Latin American countries comprise 22.9% of the total Latino populations in the United States. Relatively recent changes to Latino culture include large numbers of immigrants from Central and South America countries, each bringing another nuance to the Latino population (68).

This diversity requires very careful use of cultural context, since race is no longer a biological concept. For example, when treating an individual who is of Hispanic origin, yet physically looks African American, which cultural lens do we apply?

Spiritism

Spiritism pervades Latino culture and is the belief that the visible work is influenced by powerful good and evil personages that inhabit a larger invisible world. Rituals help maintain this belief. Emotional problems are often attributed to spiritual problems; therefore, the sufferer is likely to consult a *spiritist*. Rituals to remove or cleanse individuals are frequently performed by *espiritistas* and *curanderos* in these rituals, or *limpias* (17).

Integrity and Respeto

Personalismo, or individualism, emphasizes inner virtues and enables an individual to respect him- or herself regardless of the level of material success achieved. Respect for authority and self is the basis for dignity in the Puerto Rican culture. It is maintained in the family and community through the enforcement of a system of rules. Respect for men and for the elderly is emphasized. Children learn to respect adults through a system of *compadrazgo*, which is a kinshiplike tradition or copaternity of children by *compadres* (godparents) and biological parents. In the *compadrezgo* tradition, there are expectations of mutual aid among family members and the practice of the rules of respect (17, 68).

The often-used term *machismo*, or the cult of manliness, is well established in the social sciences lore and has iconic symbolism. However, the notion of being a gentleman, or *caballero*, is also essential and more accurate. Corresponding to this is the cult of the Virgin Mary and *Marianismo*, or living according to the traits Mary exemplified. Comas-Diaz (69) observed that at home Latinas are expected to adhere to their *marianista* side and at work they are expected to show their determination, or *hembrismo* side.

Kinship Bonds and the Extended Family

Kinship bonds in Latino culture are strong, and the family pledges to support all of its members as long as they remain within the family system (17, 68, 69). The unity and dignity of the family are highly valued. The extended family, rather than the nuclear family, is emphasized and includes the godparents (*compadres*) and adopted children, as well as relatives by blood or marriage. During times of crisis, children are often moved from one nuclear family to another within the family system.

The Role of Migration

Migration (e.g., in search of work) can affect family structure and behavior in a variety of ways because it often involves shifts in the male dominance of the marital dyad. The reversal of sex roles (e.g., the wife may earn more money than the husband) may create marital conflict and cultural dissonance (17, 68).

Children and Childrearing

Children provide a source of closeness for the mother. The Hispanic mother characteristically demonstrates this during the first three years of a child's life by doing everything for the child and being very permissive. Dependence on the mother is fostered and maintained, especially for the male child. The male adolescent is given more social freedom than the female, while having his everyday needs met by his mother or sister. The female adolescent more typically is encouraged to begin caring for the younger children. She remains at home with her parents and thinks less about her own independence (17, 68).

Asian-American Families

In Asian cultures, the tenets of Confucianism and Buddhism, symbolism within the language, the cultural view of health and wellness, migration trends, kinship bonds, and sex roles are instrumental in defining behavior. The value orientations of Asian-American communities in America are very different from the values of mainstream America.

The diversity within Asian-American families makes it essential to become familiar with Asian experiences of migration and immigration. Lee (70) describes three types of Asian families within the United States: 1) immigrant families who have recently arrived and are in need of basic survival skills; 2) immigrant-American families (usually foreign-born parents with American-born children), who often experience parent–child value conflicts; and 3) immigrant-descended families of American-born parents with children. This third group usually speaks English at home and lives according to Western cultural values, thus experiencing far less value conflict. The variety of Asian-American groups include Chinese, Filipino, Korean, Japanese, Samoan, and Southeast Asian families. They all have different family values and characteristics.

The Roles of Confucianism and Buddhism

In Asian culture there is an emphasis, reinforced by religion, on the primacy of the group over the individual. Confucianism and Buddhism assign hierarchical roles for all members and dictate highly formalized rules of behavior and conduct. Autonomy and independence are not encouraged; relationships among and between family members are strictly prescribed. Since forces outside the individual dictate behavior, the feeling of control from within is diminished. In the East Asian family the concept of family encompasses many generations. This unlimited familial timeframe is reinforced by such customs as ancestor worship, family record books, and marriage arrangements that are designed to mark the continuation of the family line, not necessarily the start of a new family. It is believed that through marriage, the woman leaves her family of origin and becomes absorbed into her husband's family—past and present (17, 47).

Sex Roles and Family Roles

Within the East Asian family unit, the father assumes the role of leader, decisionmaker, authority figure, and primary disciplinarian. East Asian fathers can appear stern, distant, and generally less approachable that East Asian mothers (71). The community views the family's successes and failures as the father's responsibility. Mothers, by contrast, are the nurturers of husband and children and are emotionally devoted caregivers. The children's strongest emotional ties are with the mother. Generally, sons are more highly valued than daughters, since the family name and linkage are passed through the male side. The most important child is the oldest son, since he becomes the head of the family when his father dies. He is also devoted to his mother and is heavily influence by her. In this way, the mother indirectly controls the family upon the death of her husband.

Obligation and Shame

Obligation and shame are strong determinants of interpersonal relationships within the context of East Asian culture. Obligation is incurred through assigned roles or stature and through acts of kindness or helpfulness for which obligation is due (70, 71). A family member's greatest obligation is to his or her parents.

Communication among family members and with society is shaped by age, sex, education, occupation, social status, and family background. There is an ever-present fear that social error will be committed, resulting in *tiu lien*, or shame (literally, "loss of face"). This can occur through the public exposure of misconduct and can result in the withdrawal of support for an individual from family, community, and society. The loss of support produces tremendous feelings of anxiety and abandonment; therefore, there is a silence and watchfulness for the correct cues to follow in social situations (70–72).

The Role of Migration and Transition

There are tremendous cultural conflicts imposed on the Asian American in trying to live within two cultures. The experience of migration and the process of transition and acculturation can produce interpersonal and intrapsychic conflict for recently immigrated Asian families. Adaptation to a new culture is a complex process and is determined by several factors: 1) the extent to which the original expectations of migration coincide with reality, 2) the availability of support systems, 3) the degree to which the immigrant family structure is similar to the family structure of the newly adopted culture, and 4) how the cultures fit together within the larger society (12).

View of Psychiatric Symptoms and Psychiatry in Asian Culture

In Asian culture, somatization is the usual manner in which psychological problems and complaints are presented. Rather than using the word depressed, the person will talk about his stomach hurting or her head being empty. If a person is angry, he or she may present symptoms related to the gallbladder or liver but not present a psychological complaint. Furthermore, the words for psychiatry—*fing sheng bin shue*—have nothing to do with psychiatry, the term referring to a kidney-heart specialty. Therefore, the person of the psychiatrist is viewed as a kidney-heart doctor who is going to treat the emotions. When Asian Americans come for treatment they are probably expecting some form of physical intervention, not talk therapy. The father in an Asian-American family may resist bringing the children for family therapy because it may be stressful or shameful and the child would be seen as a type of "mental patient." As Uzee (72) has noted, in Asian culture "there is no concept of being a little bit sick. If you are sick and you go to a psychiatrist or counselor that means you are very, very sick—you are psychotic, suicidal, homicidal, or something is severely wrong. That reflects not only upon you, but your whole family." The customary way to avoid this shame is to hide the person from the community to save face.

CONCLUSIONS

Cultural child and adolescent psychiatry describes the body of theoretical and technical knowledge necessary for clinicians to provide competent psychiatric care across cultural and language barriers to children, adolescents, and families. It is based on the theoretical orientation of multiculturalism, which assumes that there is no one way to conceptualize human behavior, explain the realities and experience of various forms of cultural diversity, and no particular set of competencies that have proven effective in all cultural settings. The cultural relativist perspective asserts that cultural values and meanings are relative to and embedded in their cultural context and cannot be measured against a universal system. It uses locally meaningful observations to examine the impact of cultural context on the developmental processes in children and their ultimate personality characteristics.

The increasingly multicultural American and global communities have acted as a compelling force for the growth of the field of cultural psychiatry and psychology. The incorporation of a vast body of cultural knowledge into descriptions of developmental processes, psychiatric diagnosis, clinical formulation, and culturally sensitive treatments will soon require the expansion of our fundamental biopsychosocial model as described by Engel 50 years ago. That model can be expanded into a *biopsychosociocultural model* to address the complexities of the clinical and developmental processes in a heterogeneous group in respect to their racial, ethnic, and cultural composition. It would allow evaluation and description of the experience of individuals from one cultural group with another dominant culture, their acculturations process and tensions, as well as the opportunities created by their unique differences.

References

1. Trujillo M: Cultural Psychiatry. In: Saddock B and Sadock V., eds.: *Comprehensive Textbook of Psychiatry*, Seventh Edition. Baltimore, Williams and Wilkins, ch. 44, pp. 492–499, 2000.
2. Kleinman A: *Rethinking Psychiatry: From Cultural Category to Personal Experience*. New York, The Free Press, 1988.
3. Mezzich JE, Kleinman A, Fabrega H, Parron DL, (ed.): *Culture and Psychiatric Diagnosis: A DSM-IV Perspective*. Washington, DC, American Psychiatric Press, 1996.
4. Mead M: *Coming of Age in Samoa*. New York: William Morrow, 1925/1939.
5. Alarcon R (ed.): Cultural psychiatry. *Psychiatry Clin North Am* 18:3, 1995.
6. Kluckhohn FR, Strodtbeck, FL: *Variations in Value Orientations*. New York, Harper & Row, 1961.
7. Spiegel J: Ethnicity and Family Therapy: An overview. In: Mc Goldrick M, Pearce J, Giordano J., eds.: *Ethnicity and Family Therapy*, 2nd edition, New York, Guilford Press, ch 1, pp. 3–30, 1996.
8. Becker A, Kleinman A: Anthropology and psychiatry. In: Saddock and Saddock V, (eds.): *Comprehensive Textbook of Psychiatry*, 7th edition, Philadelphia, Lippincott, Williams and Wilkins, Ch. 4.1, pp. 463–475, 2000.
9. Giordano J, Giordano GP: *The Ethno-Cultural Factor in Mental Health: A Literature Review and Bibliography*. New York, Institute on Pluralism and Group Identity, 1977.
10. Mc Goldrick et al.: *Ethnicity and Family Therapy*. 2nd edition, New York, Guilford Press, 1996.
11. Herr DM: Intermarriage. In: Thernstrom S, Orlov A, Handlin O, (eds.): *Harvard Encyclopedia of American Ethnic Groups*. Cambridge, Harvard University Press, 1980.
12. Landau J: Therapy with families in cultural transition. In: McGoldrick M, Pearce JK, Giordano J (eds.): *Ethnicity and Family Therapy*. New York, Grune & Stratton, 1982, pp. 552–571.
13. Shibutani T, Kwan, KM: *Ethnic Stratification*. New York, Macmillan, 1965.
14. Rothernram MJ, Phinney JS: Introduction: definitions and perspectives in the study of children's ethnic socialization. In: Phinney JS, Rotheram MJ (eds.): *Children's Ethnic Socialization: Pluralism and Development*. Newbury Park, CA, Sage, 1986, pp. 10–28.
15. Montalvo B, Gutierrez M: A perspective for the use of the cultural dimension in family therapy. In: Hansen IJ, Falicov CJ (ed.): *Cultural Perspectives in Family Therapy*. Rockville, MD, Aspen Systems, 1983, pp. 15–31.
16. Rogler LH, Gurak DT, Cooney RS: The migration experience and mental health: Formulation relevant to Hispanics and other immigrants. In: M Gaviria, JD Arana (eds.): *Health and Behavior: Research Agenda for Hispanics*, Simon Bolivar Research Agenda for Hispanics I, University of Illinois, Chicago, 1987.
17. Schwoeri L, Sholevar P, Combs, M: Impact of culture and ethnicity on Family Interventions. In: Sholevar P (ed.), *Textbook* Washington DC, Appi Press, ch 34, pp. 725–745.
18. Escobar JI: Immigration and mental health: Why are immigrants better off. *Arch Gen Psychiatry* 55:781,1998.
19. De Hart GB, Sroufe LA and Cooper RG.: *Child Development: Its Nature and Course*, 4th edition, Boston, McGraw Hill Co., 2000.
20. Bronfenbrenner U: *The Ecology of Human Development*. Cambridge, MA, Harvard University Press, 1979.
21. Bronfenbrenner U: Ecological systems theory. *Annals of Child Development* 6:187–249, 1989.
22. Nugent JK, Greene S, Wieczoreck-Deering D, Mazor K, Hendler J, Bombardier C: The cultural context of mother–infant play in the newborn period. In: Macdonald K, (ed.): *Parent–child Play*. Albany, NY, State University of New York Press, 1993, pp. 367–389.
23. Nugent JJ, Lester BM, Brazelton TB: *The Cultural Context of Infancy*, Vol. 3. Norwood, NJ, Ablex, 1995.
24. Earls F: Cultural and national differences in the epidemiology of behavior problems of preschool children. *Cult Med Psychiatry* 6:45–56, 1982.
25. Mc Dermott J: Effects of Culture and Ethnicity on Child and Adolescent Development. In: Melvin Lewis, (ed.): *Child and Adolescent Psychiatry: A Comprehensive Textbook*, 3rd edition, Philadelphia, Lippincott Williams and Wilkins, ch. 38, pp. 494–498, 2002.
26. Super CM: Environmental effects on motor development: The case of African infant precocity. *Developmental Medicine and Child Neurology* 18:561–567, 1976.
27. Super CM: Behavioral development in infancy. In: Munroe RL, Munroe RH, Whiting BB, (eds.): *Handbook of Cross-cultural Human Development*. New York, Garland Press, 1980.
28. Lucknow children: A longitudinal study. *Indian Journal of Pediatrics* 40:1–7.
29. Gerber M, Dean RFA: The state of development of newborn African children. *Lancet* 272 (1):1216–1219, 1957.
30. Das VK Sharma NL: Developmental milestones in a selective sample of Lucknow children: A longitudinal study. *Indian Journal of Pediatrics* 40:1–7, 1973.
31. Lester BM, Brazelton TB: Cross-cultural assessment of neonatal behavior. In: Stevenson HW, Wagner DA (eds.): *Cultural perspectives on child development*.
32. Scarr-Salapatck S: An evolutionary perspective on infant intelligence: Species patterns and individual variations. In: Lewis M (ed.): *Origins of Intelligence*. New York: Plenum, 1976.
33. De Vries M, Samaroff A. Culture and temperament: Influences of infant temperament in three East African Societies. *Am J Orthopsychiatry* 54:83–96, 1984.
34. LeVine RA (1998). Human parental care: Universal goals, cultural strategies, individual behavior. In RA LeVine, PM Miller, and MM West, eds., New Directions for Child Development: No. 40. *Parental behavior in diverse societies* (pp. 3–12). San Francisco: Jossey-Bass.
35. Kagan S, Madsen M: Experimental analyses of cooperation and competition of Anglo-American and Mexican Children. *Developmental Psychology* 6:49–59, 1972.
36. Chen X, Rubin K, Cen G, et al.: Child rearing attitudes and behavioral inhibition in Chinese and Canadian toddler: A cross cultural study. *Dev Psychol* 34:677–686, 1998.
37. Whiting BB, Edwards CP: *Children of Different Worlds*. Cambridge, MA, Harvard University Press, 1988.
38. Whiting B, and Whiting J: *Children of Six Cultures: A Psycho-cultural Analysis*. Cambridge, MA, Harvard University Press, 1975.
39. Stevenson HW, Azuma H, Hakuta K: *Child Development and Education in Japan*. New York, Freeman, 1986.
40. LeVine RA: Parental goals: A cross-cultural view. *Teachers College Record* 76:226–239, 1974.
41. Madsen M: Development and cross-cultural differences in cooperative and competitive behavior of young children. *Journal of Cross-Cultural Psychology* 2:365–371, 1971.
42. Stevenson HC: Missed, dissed, and pissed: Making meaning of neighborhood risk, fear and anger management in urban Black youth. *Cultural Diversity and Mental Health* 3:37–52, 1997.

43. Tharp R: Psychocultural variables and constants: Effects on teaching and learning. *American Psychologist* 44:349–359, 1989.
44. Goodnow JJ: The nature of intelligent behavior: Questions raised by cross-culture studies. In: Resnick L (ed): *The nature of intelligence*. Hillsdale, NJ, Erlbaum. 169–1880, 1976.
45. Sternberg RJ: Beyond IQ: *A Triarchic Theory of Human Intelligence*. New York, Cambridge University Press, 1985.
46. Levine ES Padilla AM: *Crossing Cultures in Therapy: Pluralistic Counseling for the Hispanic*. Monterey, CA, Brooks/Cole, 1980.
47. Kim P: Culture and child and adolescent psychiatry. In: Tseng, Wen-Shing, Streltzer, Jon (eds): *Cultural competence in clinical psychiatry*. Washington, DC, American Psychiatric Publishing, Inc., 2004, pp. 125–145.
48. Canino IA, Canino G: Impact of stress on the Puerto Rican family: treatment considerations. *Am J Orthopsychiatry* 50:535–541,1980.
49. Tseng W-S, McDermott J: *Culture, Mind and Therapy: An Introduction to Cultural Psychiatry*. New York, Brunner/Mazel, 1981.
50. Sholevar P: "My child does not respect me," presented at the Annual meeting of the American Academy of Child/Adolescent Psychiatry, Honolulu, Hawaii, October, 2000.
51. Sholevar P: Mental Health Treatment of Latino patients, Annual Scientific meeting, Philadelphia Psychiatric Society, October 2005.
52. Marcos LR, Trujillo M: Culture, language and communicative behavior: The psychiatric examination of Spanish-Americans. In: RP Duran (ed.) *Latino Language and Communicative Behavior*, Norwood, NJ, Ablex Publishing, 1981.
53. Marcos LR: Linguistic dimensions in the bilingual patient. *AM J Psychoanal* 36:347, 1976.
54. Lu, Russel, Mezzich, JE: Issues in the assessment and diagnosis of culturally diverse individuals. In: Oldham J, Riba M, (ed.) *Annual Review of Psychiatry, vol. 14*, Washington, DC, American Psychiatric Press, 1995.
55. U.S. Public Health Service: *Report of the Surgeon General's Conference on Children's Mental Health: A National Action Agenda*. Washington, DC, Department of Health and Human Services, 2000.
56. Canino IA, Spurlock J: *Culturally Diverse Children and Adolescents: Assessment, Diagnosis and Treatment*. New York, Guilford, 1994.
57. Flores JL: The utilization of a community mental health service by Mexican Americans. *Int. J Soc. Psychiatry* 24:271–275, 1978.
58. McLoyd VC: Changing demographics in the American population: Implications for research on minority children and adolescents. In: McLoyd VC, Steinberg L (eds.): *Studying minority adolescents: Conceptual, methodological, and theoretical issues* Mahwah, NJ, Lawrence Erlbaum Associates, 1998, pp. 3–28.
59. Day, JC: *Population projections of the United States by age, sex, race, and Hispanic origin: 1995 to 2050, U.S. Bureau of the Census, Current Population Reports, P25-1130*. Washington, DC, US Government Printing Office, 1996.
60. Nugent JK, Lester BM, Brazelton TB: *The cultural context of infancy*, vol. 3. Norwood, NJ, Ablex, 1995.
61. Bingham R, Porche-Burke L, James S, Sue D, Vazquez, M: Report on the National Multicultural Conference and Summit II, in *Cultural Diversity and Ethnic Minority Psychology* vol. 8, no. 2, 75–87, 2002.
62. O'Hare W, Pollard K, Mann T, et al. African Americans in the 1990s. *Popul Bull* 46:8–10, 1991.
63. Boyd-Franklin N: *Black Families in Therapy: A Multisystems Approach*. New York, Guilford, 1989.
64. Pinderhughes E: Afro-American families and the victim system. In: McGoldrick M, Pearce J (eds.), *Ethnicity and Family Therapy*. New York, Guilford, 1982, pp. 108–122.
65. Billingsley A: *Black Families in White America*. Englewood Cliffs, NJ, Prentice-Hall, 1968.
66. Knox D: Spirituality: A tool in the assessment and treatment of black alcoholics and their families. *Alcoholism Treatment Quarterly* 2[3/4]:31–44, 1985.
67. Gonzalez D: What is the problem with Hispanic? Just ask a Latino. *New York Times* 1992.
68. Garcia-Preto N: *Latino families: An overview. In Ethnicity and Family Therapy*, 2nd edition. McGoldrick M, Giordano J, Pearce JK (eds.). New York, Guilford, 1996, pp. 141–154; Latino families and overview, p. 846.
69. Comas-Diaz L: Lati Negra. *Journal of Feminist Family Therapy* 5[3/4]:35–74, 1994.
70. Lee E: A social system approach to assessment and treatment for Chinese-American families. In: McGoldrick M, Pearce JK, Giordano J. (eds.), *Ethnicity and Family Therapy*. New York, Grune & Stratton, 1982, pp. 552–571.
71. Shon SP, Ja DY: Asian families. In: McGoldrick M, Pearce JK, Giordano J (eds.) *Ethnicity and Family Therapy*. New York, Guilford, 1982, pp. 208–228.
72. Uzee E: Videotaped discussion of working with Asian-American families [Working With Minority Families]. Symposium conducted at the 142nd annual meeting of the American Psychiatric Association, San Francisco, CA, May 6–11, 1989.

CHAPTER 1.7.2 ■ THE HEARING OR VISUALLY IMPAIRED CHILD

PETER HINDLEY AND ALISON SALT

MODELS OF DEAFNESS, VISUAL IMPAIRMENT, AND DEAF-BLINDNESS: CULTURE AND DISABILITY

Deafness and severe visual impairment (SVI) are low-incidence conditions which, alone and in combination, can have a significant effect on a child's development and mental wellbeing. Less severe degrees of hearing and visual impairment are more common but have a less significant impact on child development. This chapter provides an overview of hearing and visual impairment and a more detailed account of deaf, SVI, and deaf-blind children's development and mental health. Two Web sites (www.raisingdeafkids.org and www.boystownhospital.org) provide an overview of deafness and an online research facility. The American Federation for the Blind website (www.afb.org) is a useful source of information as well.

The sensory impairments can be defined in a variety of ways. Two key models are used, medical and cultural. Medical definitions of sensory impairments focus on the severity of impairment, the site and type of impairment, the age of onset of the impairment and the presence or absence of additional disabilities. The cultural model of sensory impairment challenges the notion that a deaf or visually impaired person is disabled. Cultural models focus on the social experience of deafness or blindness and the strengths of deaf and blind communities and individuals (Table 1.7.2.1).

Being a deaf, SVI, or deaf-blind young person does not necessarily increase the risk of developing mental health problems. Three sets of factors, which are linked to sensory impairments, do. First are the consequences of being deaf,

TABLE 1.7.2.1

DEFINITIONS OF SENSORY IMPAIRMENT

Hearing Impairment	Visual Impairment	Deaf-Blindness
Severity: mild <40dB in better ear; moderate <70dB; severe <95dB; profound 96dB<(BSA 1988) **Age of onset:** congenital, early onset, acquired and progressive **Site:** conductive or sensorineural	**Severity:** Partially sighted; low vision; legally blind (<20/200 Snellen or 20° visual field); totally blind (AFB 1995) **Age of onset:** congenital, early onset and acquired **Site:** peripheral or central	**Severity:** either deafness and any visual impairment or legally blind and any hearing impairment **Age of onset:** congenital, early onset and acquired **Site:** conductive or sensorineural HI and peripheral or central VI
Descriptors: Children with profound deafness in the better ear are commonly called **deaf.** Children with moderate to severe deafness are commonly called **hard of hearing.**		Children with combinations of visual impairment and deafness are called **deaf-blind.**
Cultural: use of sign language, experiencing the world visually, identification with other deaf people, attitude of majority community—"assimilating" or "oppositional" (4)	**Cultural:** constructing the world as a narrative, not as a gestalt (67)	**Cultural:** use of hand-on signing or hands on finger-spelling. Identification with other deaf-blind people and experience of oppression

SVI, or deaf-blind in a world which is oriented to the needs of hearing and sighted people. The goodness or poorness of fit between the needs of sensorially impaired children and their environment has an impact from early in the child's life—in particular, since the vast majority of deaf and SVI children are born into hearing and sighted families, how the family adjusts to the needs of their deaf or SVI child. Second, brain insults and other physical illnesses linked to the cause of deafness or blindness may confer additional neuropsychological vulnerabilities. Third, children with sensory impairments are more vulnerable to all forms of abuse and neglect.

DEAF, HARD OF HEARING AND HEARING-IMPAIRED CHILDREN

Epidemiology and Etiology of Hearing Impairment

Hearing impairment affects approximately 17/1,000 children under the age of 18 in the United States (1). The most common forms of hearing loss are those resulting from middle ear effusions, although these are often time limited. It is not always possible to establish the age of onset of hearing impairment, but among children with permanent hearing impairment just under 60% have congenital hearing loss and approximately 25% acquired hearing loss (2). Genetic causes are the most common causes of permanent sensorineural hearing loss, followed by the complications of severe prematurity and intrauterine and postnatal infections (Table 1.7.2.2).

Otitis Media with Effusion, Unilateral Deafness, and Hard of Hearing Children

Acute otitis media (AOM) affects about 2/3 of children in the age range 6–24 months. AOM is very uncommon after 6 years of age. About 45% of children with AOM have a middle ear effusion (MEE) one month after an episode of AOM and approximately 10% have one three months after an episode of AOM. MEE can cause hearing loss, and where this is greater than 20 dB loss, surgical insertion of PEC tubes is indicated. Chronic MEE with hearing impairment can cause language delay in children (www.e-medicine.com). Unilateral deafness affects approximately 1/1,000 live births (3), of which approximately 35% have profound unilateral hearing impairment. Hearing impairment as a result of MEE and as a result of unilateral sensorineural deafness can cause significant difficulties for the child in the classroom and in conversational settings. Common effects of these forms of hearing impairment include: localization of sound; understanding what people say when there is other noise at the same time; paying attention in class; following directions in class; and learning new concepts. The possibility of an undetected hearing impairment should always be considered in children referred for attention problems.

Children with moderate to severe hearing impairment need an initial multidisciplinary assessment by audiologists, pediatricians, speech and language therapists, teachers of the deaf, and where appropriate, geneticists. The main intervention for these children will be the provision of hearing aids with support from teachers of the deaf to ensure that classroom provision and teaching practice meet the individual child's needs. Hearing aids amplify the sound being transmitted to the middle ear. Digital hearing aids allow specific adjustments to be made to improve comfort and amplify specific frequencies, but they need careful fitting (4).

Despite their advantages, digital hearing aid users still face a variety of problems. Children can still experience excessive amplification of background noise, which makes noisy environments particularly difficult. Recruitment, perceiving greater increases in sound loudness than would be expected (e.g., a sound at 70 dB is tolerable but intolerable at 110 dB), can cause pain and distress. Finally, acoustic feedback, leading to high-pitched whistling, can occur if hearing aids are not fitting properly. This is a particular problem for young children who are growing rapidly.

The majority of hard of hearing children who have received appropriate audiological and educational intervention will develop effective spoken language. They are likely to experience a degree of language delay and may have pragmatic and syntactic deficits. This is also true of many, but not all, deaf children who receive early (i.e., before two years) cochlear implantation (see below).

TABLE 1.7.2.2

PREVALENCE AND ETIOLOGY OF SENSORY IMPAIRMENT

Hard of Hearing and Deafness	SVI and Blindness
Prevalence:	*Prevalence:*
Early onset: 101/100,000	Early onset: 4/10,000
Acquired: 21/100,000[1]	Acquired: 2/10,000[2]
Additional impairments:	*Additional impairments:*
Total: 20–40%[3]	Total: 77%[2]
Visual: 4%	
Mental retardation: 8%	n.b.: mortality of 10% in SVI/blind with additional or SVI/Blind+[2]
Emotional and behavioral: 4%	
Learning: 9%	
Etiology and timing (%s)[1]:	*Etiology and timing (%s)*[2]:
Early onset Acquired	SVI/Blind SVI/Blind+
	Prenatal 83.3 54.5
Genetic 44.7 24.7	Neonatal+ 2.9 21.7
Prenatal 4.0 1.0	Perinatal
Perinatal 17.6 11.3	Childhood 7.8 20.8
Postnatal 0.0 41.2	All
CFA* 2.9 0.0	Hereditary 33
Other 1.0 3.0	Hypoxia/ischaemia 18
Missing 25.7 18.6	Tumour 4
	Infection 3
	Hydrocephalus 3
	Injury (AI and NAI) 3
	Systemic 2
	Other 5
	Unknown 25
	Cause and timing unknown 9
	n.b. % > because some children have multiple aetiology
Site (%s):	*Site (%s):*
Sensorineural 91.5	SVI/Blind SVI/Blind+
Conductive 8.5	Cerebral/visual 5.9 60.1
	Pathway
	Optic nerve 16.7 31.3
	Retina 60.8 19.1
	Whole globe 9.8 5.7
	Other anterior** 22.6 8.9
	Other 2.9 1.5
	n.b. % >100 because some children have multiple sites

*Cranio-facial abnormalities
**Uvea, lens, cornea, and glaucoma
[1]Data from Davis A & Mencher G. Epidemiology of permanent hearing impairment. In: Newton VE, editor. *Paediatric Audiological Medicine.* London and Philadelphia: Whurr Publishers; 2002. pp. 65–90.
[2]Data from Rahi JS & Cable N on behalf of the British Childhood Visual Impairment Study Group. *Severe visual impairment and blindness in children in the UK.* The Lancet. 2003; 362: 1359–65.
[3]Data from Knoors H & Vervloed PJ. *Educational Programming for Deaf Children with Multiple Disabilities.* In: Marschark M & Spencer PE, editors. *The Oxford Handbook of Deaf Studies, Language and Education.* Oxford and New York: Oxford University Press; 2003. pp. 82–96.

Cultural Aspects of Deafness

There are historical references to deaf people and the use of sign language dating back to the classical period (5), but the modern study of the cultural aspects of deafness began in the 1960s with Bob Stokoe's (6) studies of American Sign Language (ASL). The Deaf community came to be defined by a series of key experiences. Central among these were the use of sign language, experiencing the world visually and the experience of oppression by the majority culture (7). More recent studies have suggested that the types of community that emerge, e.g., distinct and separate deaf communities, merged communities of deaf and hearing people, or single deaf people within hearing communities, depend in part on the attitude of the majority hearing community toward deafness (4). Majority communities can be seen on a continuum. At one end are those that make no distinction between the role and function of deaf and hearing people, so-called *assimilating communities.* These tend to occur in rural communities and lead to merged communities of deaf and hearing people, such as the community described in nineteenth century Martha's Vineyard (8). At the other end of the continuum are communities in which the role and function of deaf people is significantly restricted and their cultural practices, such as the use of sign language, are suppressed. These are so called *oppositional communities.* Most industrial communities of the nineteenth and twentieth century shared these characteristics and lead to the distinct deaf communities described by Meadow-Orlans and Erting.

A key feature of oppositional deaf communities is cultural discontinuity; 90–95% of deaf children are born into hearing families (deaf children of hearing parents [DOH]), the vast majority with no previous experience of deafness (9). Approximately 90% of deaf parents have hearing children (10). Historically DOH children joined the deaf community through key experiences such as attending residential schools and joining deaf clubs. Changes in education legislation and practice have lead to the vast majority of American deaf children being educated in mainstream classes or special education classes in mainstream schools. Early intervention and cochlear implants are changing the experiences of deaf children and their hearing families. At the same time, fewer deaf people seem to be active in formal social organizations such as deaf clubs and changes in communication technology (email, close captioning and video-telephony) are making communication much easier.

Sign Languages

Sign languages are naturally occurring languages that develop whenever significant numbers of deaf people come together (11). In the Western world, prior to formal education, this occurred in areas with high rates of congenital deafness, such as Martha's Vineyard. This continues to happen in parts of the developing world, such as Yucatan (4). Formal education of deaf children began in Europe in the sixteenth and seventeenth centuries and was first established in the United States in 1817.

The American founders of deaf education brought French teachers of the deaf from Paris. American Sign Language (ASL) origins appear to be in *Langue des Signes Française*, the native sign language of Martha's Vineyard and the sign language of North American Indians (Sherman and Wilcox 2003). There are strong linguistic and neurological arguments to support the contention that language originally emerged from early gesture and that sign language antedates spoken language (11).

ASL, like other natural sign languages, differs both syntactically and lexically from spoken English. Fischer and Huslt (12) provide a comprehensive overview of the structure of ASL. ASL uses movements and shapes of both hands, facial expression, eye gaze, and upper body movements to convey both lexical and syntactic features. Spoken languages, except for tonal languages, tend to rely on sequences of sounds to convey meaning. In contrast, sign languages can present information simultaneously, e.g., two hands, facial expression, body movement, and eye gaze can all change simultaneously. ASL has been adapted to accommodate syntactic and lexical aspects of spoken English as Manually Coded English (MCE). These artificial pidgins tend to be both less efficient and less flexible than either spoken English or ASL.

The evidence from lesion studies and functional scanning studies suggest that native signers (deaf and hearing), in the main, use the same areas of the brain that hearing people do when they use spoken language (13). Deaf children of deaf parents (DOD) who are exposed to ASL from birth develop ASL at the same rate that hearing children develop spoken language (14). Features of early language similar to those seen in spoken language, such as manual babbling, have all been observed in DOD infants (14). Hearing infants are able to divide their auditory and visual attention so that they can listen to their caregivers and attend to play activities. This is not possible for deaf infants, who have to divide their attention within the visual channel. Deaf parents use a variety of approaches to manage this task, such as signing onto the infant's body and bringing objects into the infant's visual field (15). In broad terms, DOD children's social and emotional development follows milestones similar to hearing children (16), and their academic and vocational outcomes tend to be better than DOH children.

Development of DOH Children

The causes of the differences in development between DOD and DOH children can be understood in a number of ways—first, the effect of the diagnosis of deafness on family relationships. Prior to the introduction of universal neonatal screening, most deaf children would not have been diagnosed until at least six months of age, although for some it was considerably later. This period of time gave parents the opportunity to adapt intuitively to their deaf child's needs. For the vast majority, the diagnosis of deafness came as a shock with accompanying feelings of loss and anger (17). The majority of hearing parents appear to make a good adjustment, but for those who have difficulty in accepting their child's deafness there appears to be an increased risk of an insecure attachment relationship developing. Second, the "goodness of fit" between the child and their parents (18) can be considered in terms of the transaction between the child's temperamental style, the parenting style, and their external resource. These factors are important for deaf children, but in addition we need to consider goodness of fit of communication. The majority of deaf children will need some form of signed communication, but not all parents will wish to use and may be advised not to use sign language. Lack of access to early language is probably the single most important developmental risk factor for DOH children.

However, this picture has been significantly affected by three recent changes in the management of deafness: the introduction of universal neonatal hearing screening or UNHS (19); the development of early intervention programs linked to UNHS programs (20); and the increasing use of cochlear implants with deaf infants (4, 21).

Neonatal Screening and Early Intervention

UNHS programs generally use a two-stage approach to screening for hearing loss. Evoked otoacoustic emissions (EOAE) or automated ABR (see below) is used in newborn infants to ascertain those as risk of hearing loss. EOAE detects the signal generated by the hair cells in response to sound. Both EOAE and automated ABR have false positive rates of approximately 20% (19). All infants screened positive by EOAE or automated ABR are tested using a diagnostic auditory brainstem response. ABR tests the auditory systems response up to the nuclei and neural pathways of the brainstem to confirm bilateral deafness of moderate or greater severity (>40 dB in the better ear). UNHS will not ascertain all children with early onset deafness. Children with auditory neuropathy, cortical deafness, and children with progressive deafness may not be detected and so ongoing surveillance is needed.

UNHS programs have been advocated because research has found that deaf children receiving intervention before six months show significant gains in language development, both spoken and signed, when compared with children receiving intervention after six months (20). One of the problems in the United States has been that these post-diagnosis interventions have not been provided consistently (19). The programs with the best outcomes, such as the Colorado Hearing Impaired Program or CHIPS, provide a range of interventions. Parents are provided with early psychological support to adjust to the diagnosis and to make decisions about which language, signed or spoken, they plan to use with their child. Language interventions are provided in parents' homes and parents also have access to parent groups and deaf mentors.

Cochlear implants (4, 21) are sophisticated hearing aids which allow an electronic signal to be delivered directly to the cochlea, thereby avoiding all of the problems of amplification associated with conventional aids. Implantation involves neurosurgery, which is generally safe but has rare, serious, and extremely infrequently fatal side effects. They are generally most effective in the earliest years of life and can lead to profoundly deaf children functioning as a severely deaf child. They are not universally effective. There was considerable controversy within the deaf community when cochlear implants were first used with deaf children, as they were seen as a potential threat to the community. This controversy has lessened with time and ongoing debate.

Social and Emotional Development

Most hearing parents adapt successfully to the needs of their deaf infant (18). However, for many the presence of a deaf infant leads to higher levels of stress, both in terms of daily hassles, additional financial burdens, and reduced social networks. In families where parents have difficulties in accepting their deaf infant, insecure attachment relationships are more likely to emerge. When there is poor matching of communication needs between the deaf infant and their hearing parents, less mutually satisfying interaction will occur and more directive parental styles can develop.

Most deaf children in the United States are educated in some form of integrated setting (22). Studies of peer interactions of deaf children tend to focus on the early years (23). The findings from these studies are not wholly consistent but suggest that deaf children tend to interact less than hearing children. They tend to interact more with other deaf children, but interactions with hearing peers occurs more often if the peer is familiar to them. Deaf children show more social interaction and more cooperative play the more well developed language they have. Generally deaf children tend to show less symbolic play and less sophisticated interaction skills than hearing peers. These difficulties in interaction, both in the family setting and in early education, have an impact on deaf children's social and emotional development. They are more likely to show delays in development of theory of mind (24), and to have a more limited emotional vocabulary and social understanding (25). It is important to point out that this does not affect all DOH children. Those that have developed early language and experienced positive peer relationships may show none of these delays. However, all deaf children experience difficulty in accessing incidental learning (the everyday learning that naturally occurs when children interact spontaneously with their social environments) and many deaf adolescents in integrated settings describe significant difficulties in peer relationships (26). School-based interventions aimed at promoting deaf children's social and emotional functioning are crucial to preventing mental health problems (25).

Deaf children who have been raised in standard early intervention and educational settings are at higher risk of significant reading and writing delays. These delays, linked in turn to difficulties in accessing incidental learning, may account for the significant academic underachievement still seen in many deaf children (27). Finally deaf children, like many children with disabilities, are at greater risk of all forms of abuse. In some residential deaf schools this abuse has become transgenerational (28).

Deaf-Blind Children

Best (29) estimated that 0.01/1,000 children are deaf-blind, but this is likely to be an underestimate. In the past, congenital rubella has accounted for a third to a half of cases (30) but this has fallen as a result of universal rubella immunization in many countries. Genetic conditions such as Usher syndrome and brain abnormalities associated with severe prematurity are now likely to account for the majority. Approximately 3–6% of deaf and hard of hearing children have Usher's syndrome (1). Additional impairments are very common, with intellectual impairment in a third to a half, and brain abnormalities in a quarter (30).

Deaf-blindness is one of the most devastating (31) and least understood (32) of handicapping conditions. Its impact on children and their families is influenced by the severity of the sensory impairments and the nature and severity of associated impairments (33). Responses to sensory losses may include feelings of anxiety, isolation, denial, resentment, or distortion of body image. The parents of deaf-blind children have to make major adaptations. In the case of Usher syndrome, many parents appear devastated and unable to imagine their child's future when they are informed that their already deaf child may well go progressively blind (34).

Cultural Aspects

In areas where there is high incidence of Usher syndrome, such as in the Cajun community of LA, deaf-blind communities have formed. A similar community has formed in Seattle, WA, primarily through migration. Miner (35) provides guidance on therapeutic techniques when working with deaf-blind people [see also the deaf-blind Website (36)]. Differential diagnostic problems for deaf-blind children are similar to those of deaf and SVI children. It can be particularly difficult to differentiate between complex neuropsychiatric conditions such as autism and the social and emotional consequences of dual sensory impairments.

Psychiatric Aspects of Deafness

Most studies have shown that the rate of psychopathology is increased in deaf and HOH children (hereon called deaf children) compared with the general population, although the majority do not have a mental disorder (37). However, comparisons across studies are difficult because of differences in methodology. Only four studies have used information from teachers and parents, including parental interviews (38–41). Of these, only the last two included interviews with young people. These studies showed increased rates of emotional and behavioral disorders (Table 1.7.2.3).

TABLE 1.7.2.3

PREVALENCE AND ETIOLOGY OF MENTAL HEALTH PROBLEMS IN DEAF, VI, AND DEAF-BLIND CHILDREN

Hard of Hearing and Deaf	SVI and Blind
Prevalence: Deaf: 22–42% HoH: 16–60% (37) Increase in both emotional and behavioral disorder Autistic spectrum disorder 5% Psychotic disorder increased in congenital rubella and CMV	*Prevalence*: 21% emotional and behavioral deficit—insecurity or withdrawal, attachment problem, inattentiveness, impulsive or hyperactive oppositional-defiant behavior, temper tantrums, and toileting problems. Autistic spectrum disorder—30% of PVI
Etiological factors: Genetic and chromosomal anomalies Intrauterine and perinatal/neonatal insults linked to pervasive brain damage Early language and experiential deprivation Sexual, physical and emotional abuse and neglect Bullying at school Identity problems, especially for hard of hearing children	*Etiological factors*: Associated pervasive brain damage Early mother-child interaction Early sleep difficulties Separation anxiety Relationships with peers Associated learning disability (MR) Overprotection in adolescence, making the development of personal and sexual relationships more difficult

The range of psychiatric disorders is, in the main, the same as in hearing children (40) but deaf children are exposed to a range of additional risk factors (37, 40). Pervasive developmental disorders are more common among deaf children (see below). It is not clear whether or not children in mainstream or special schools are at higher risk of mental health problems. Smith and Sharp (42) found that deaf children in mainstream schools were particularly likely to be bullied. On the other hand, deaf children in residential schools appear to be more vulnerable to abuse (28).

Psychiatric Assessment

Deaf children rely on visual communication. When interviewing them, the room needs to be uncluttered and well lit but without a bright light, such as a window behind the interviewer. Lipreading requires a clear view of the lips, and bushy beards and mustaches can cause problems. No more than 25% of spoken language is seen through lip patterns alone (43). Deaf people have to make educated guesses when lipreading (44), and a strong foreign accent can make that more difficult.

When clinicians have limited signing skills, their efforts to engage signing deaf children can blunt their capacity to detect subtle emotional signals, thereby missing emotional disorders (45). In these circumstances it is better to engage a professional sign language interpreter, preferably with experience in child mental health and with an opportunity to meet the child prior to the interview and for debriefing afterward. This is particularly important because the interpreter will have the child's eye contact and may have picked up subtle emotional cues (46). The coexistence of deafness and psychiatric disorder can lead clinicians to an unwarranted assumption that deafness explains all—the phenomenon of "diagnostic shadowing" (47).

Psychological Assessments

Caution is needed in interpreting psychological test findings in deaf children, because most tests have been validated exclusively in hearing populations. A knowledge of developmental and cultural aspects of deafness is essential (48).

Disruptive Behavior

The overrepresentation of deaf children with disruptive behavior among those referred to clinics may partially reflect referral patterns. However, there may be associations with brain pathology that occur with some types of deafness (49). In a longitudinal study of children affected by congenital rubella, Chess and Fernandez (50, 51) found that early impulsiveness in those with deafness alone disappeared as the children acquired language and self-control skills. By contrast, impulsiveness persisted in deaf children with additional impairments. Oppositional behavior can be an expression of underlying feelings of impotence, anxiety, or sadness, or an expression of frustration with difficulties of communication (49). Symptoms of distractibility and overactivity may reflect a distracting visual environment or poor language matching in the classroom, leading to boredom or to undetected intellectual or language impairments, or seizure disorders or the side effects of drugs (49).

Emotional Disorders

The underrepresentation of emotional disorders in deaf children seen in the specialist services runs counter to the epidemiological evidence. Using the CBCL, van Eldik (52) found significantly higher scores on the anxious/depressive scale among deaf teenagers than among hearing peers. Emotional problems may be missed because poor signing skills prevent parents and teachers from recognizing mood disturbance.

Schizophrenia and Other Psychoses

Psychotic disorders are not more common in most deaf young people (47). However, one study has found increased rates in deaf young people, with deafness arising from congenital rubella or CMV (53). Because the syntax of sign language is very different from spoken language, disorders of thinking can be misattributed (33). Equally, accurate assessments of thought disorder and abnormal experiences can be difficult (47). Nevertheless, phenomena such as clang associations and flight of ideas have been clearly identified in deaf adults with psychotic disorders (47).

Autism and Related Disorders

Two studies of deaf children attending audiology clinics found autism and related disorders to be more common than in hearing children. Juré, Rapin, and Tuchman (54) estimated a prevalence of 5.3% and Rosenhall et al. (55) 3.5%. In the latter study, intellectual impairment did not account for the higher rate. One of the assumed causes of an increased prevalence of autism in deaf children is a common underlying cause arising from brain damage caused by agents such a intrauterine rubella (50) and cytomegalovirus (56). However, deaf children with autism and genetic causes of deafness, such as Connexin 26, have been reported (57).

The age of diagnosis is frequently later in deaf children (54), in part reflecting diagnostic shadowing. This is despite the fact that the basic impairments associated with autism are qualitatively different from what is seen in other deaf children. Nevertheless, poor language skills stemming from deafness may be associated with delayed but not impaired imaginative play. Unusual communication patterns and passivity are more common in deaf children with intellectual impairment who do not have autism, and even clinicians with good signing skills can have difficulty in detecting language disorder in sign. Some deaf children with autism show significant improvements in social functioning when educated in signing environments (54, 58).

Intervention

The majority of deaf children who are referred to mental health services come from hearing families. Many of these children will have experienced difficulties in everyday communication within their families and with their peers (26). Their personal narratives and personal coping skills are often patchy and fragmented (26). These experiences of difficulties in communication are frequently repeated in their interaction with mental health services. Although many programs claim to be accessible to deaf children, frequently this is through provision of ASL interpreters or by single practitioners with varying ASL skills (59).

There appears to be no specialized inpatient psychiatric program for deaf children and adolescents in the United States (59). There are a limited number of culturally affirmative programs run from Residential Treatment Centers. These are programs with deaf and hearing staff with ASL skills and understanding of the cultural and psychosocial consequences of deafness (60). The programs strongly associated with residential schools for the deaf are more likely to provide a spectrum of provision and have stronger links to the local deaf community (e.g., Pressley Ridge and West Philadelphia School for the Deaf). Deaf children admitted to RTCs are likely to have complex needs, given the high rates of sexual abuse and multiple disabilities seen in this population (61).

Elliott et al. (62) describe specific pitfalls in the psychotherapy of deaf children, as well as the value of deaf therapists. Interpreters in family and group therapy may become incorporated into transference relationships (63). Medication may involve effects that impede communication because they influence the skills needed for signing, lip reading, speaking, and writing (47). Deaf children are sometimes unable to describe the effects and side effects of the medication prescribed.

Hearing Children of Deaf Parents (HOD)

Knowledge on the development of hearing children of deaf parents is relatively limited (10, 64). The most comprehensive report is an anthropological study of 150 grownup children of signing deaf parents (65).

Most deaf parents are competent and caring, but they experience stresses as a result of being deaf in a hearing world (10). Hearing children of deaf parents are at the center of interaction between deaf and hearing cultures. Although use of sign language is a central component of being deaf and often a source of pride, some deaf people see their sign language as less valued than spoken language and may experience shame when using sign outside their deaf community. This may lead some to choose not to use sign with their hearing child and to rely on inadequate spoken language. In other circumstances hearing children are drawn into the role of communicator/interpreter for their parents. These experiences can be seen as adverse, "parentifying" the child at an early age, but to others these experiences lead to "greater adaptiveness, resourcefulness, curiosity and "worldliness" (10).

Deaf parents may have difficulty in accessing information about parenting, and their own childhood within a hearing family may not have provided them with good models of parenting. This may lead to their feeling unconfident or incompetent as parents (10).

In some respects, the experience of deaf parents of hearing children can be compared to that of parents raising children from different ethnic backgrounds to their own (10). Most of the grownup hearing children of deaf parents studied by Preston (65) acknowledged some difficulties in their childhood but attributed these as much to the hearing society's response to their parents as to their parent's failings. Their roles as interpreters and advocates were linked to experiences that were both fulfilling and hurtful. In a similar vein, many described loyalties that were divided between their deaf parents and their hearing grandparents.

Little is known about the psychological wellbeing of hearing children of deaf parents. There is a small number of studies (66) of parents or children referred to clinical services that suggest that these children are at risk of social and emotional difficulties, language delay, and mild learning disabilities. Charlson (66) studied deaf parents referred to child protection services in California. She describes a number of parental risk factors: maternal substance abuse, deaf mother's married to hearing partner, parental childhood abuse, and lack of contact with the deaf community. She emphasizes the difficulty that these parents have in accessing suitable community resources.

Children with Visual Impairment and Blindness

The Epidemiology and Etiology of Visual Impairment. The cumulative incidence of severe visual impairment (SVI) was reported as 5.9/10,000 (95% CI 5.33, 6.45/10,000) in children aged 0–16 in a recent comprehensive survey in the U.K. (4) (Table 1.7.2.2). The most common cause was hereditary (33%), followed by hypoxia/ischemia. Seventy-seven percent of the group had additional impairments (SVI/Blind+). There were differences between children with only visual impairment (VI) and the SVI/Blind+ group. In the SVI/Blind group, the onset of the VI was more likely to be prenatal and the site of impairment was more likely to be peripheral. In the SVI/Blind+ group there were more children with postnatal onset and the site of impairment was more likely to be central or visual pathways. These kinds of lesions are also more strongly associated with pervasive brain abnormalities.

Cultural Aspects of Visual Impairment. Investigation of the sociocultural perspectives on blindness has been relatively limited compared to that of deaf culture. Fogel (67) suggested that the central experience of blindness involves construction of the world as a narrative rather than a gestalt, and that this constitutes the essential strength of the blind person.

Family Response to VI. Parents may often react with shock and disbelief to the diagnosis of VI (68, 69). Some parents experience considerable distress, and it has been suggested that parental depression and lack of understanding of their baby's apparent lack of response can lead to decreased interaction between child and parent (70–72). Eventual positive adaptation to these reactions is usual but may need appropriate support (73).

The quality of language used by parents is also affected by the presence of visual impairment. Parents have been found to be more directive and less contingent on their children's communicative cues (71). Moore and McConachie (74) found that mothers of blind children, when playing with their child, talked less about objects that their child was actually attending to at the time. The findings suggested that it is very difficult for parents to "think themselves into" what their child finds salient (75) and to ascertain what a blind child is actually focusing attention on and hence what to talk about.

Blind parents of blind babies appear to have fewer obstacles to natural effective communication and have greater reliance on close proximity and touch (76). Given the child's dependence on gaining information through language, maintaining a "stream" of language (77), which is responsive to the child's activities and interests (78, 79), appears important.

Although there is a lack of systematic research, longitudinal studies of early development in children with VI suggest that attachment formation may be significantly affected (71).

Screening for Visual Impairment and Early Intervention. Universal screening for visual impairment requires a broader approach than for deafness because of the large number of eye conditions that lead to visual impairment and their diverse presentations. Early universal screening is recommended in the U.K. soon after birth and at six weeks (80) and the American Academy of Pediatrics (AAP) recommends vision screening be performed at all well-child visits for children starting in the newborn period to three years (81) by ocular history, vision assessment, external inspection of the eyes and lids, ocular motility assessment, pupil examination, and red reflex examination. These screening efforts have generally been ineffective in early identification of visual impairment and have had an impact on the timely introduction of early intervention and support for families (82).

Sonksen designed and applied a systematic visual and developmental program for babies and preschoolers (83) that continues to be delivered by the multidisciplinary team at the Wolfson Centre, Great Ormond Street Hospital for Children, London and has been promoted through the published booklet "Show me what my friends can see" (84). More recently, the Department for Education in the U.K. has supported the development of a monitoring protocol and guide for parents and the professionals working with them to support and promote early development (85). Similar support services are available in the United States (http://www.afb.org/).

The first two years of life appear to be a particularly critical time for development of the blind child and specific intervention to support the development of "form" vision (86) and to support early social interaction, especially precursors of joint attention and joint object–related communication and play, are especially important (87). (Table 1.7.2.4)

Development of Children with Visual Impairment. Visual impairment has a significant and farreaching effect on all areas

TABLE 1.7.2.4

EARLY INTERVENTION APPROACHES

Hard of Hearing and Deaf	SVI and Blind
Early intervention has best outcomes	Promotion of visual development
Long term planning of resources	Promotion of development in all areas, including:
Access to early language—signed or spoken	Mobility and spatial awareness
Psychological support to parents	Perceptual understanding
Parental peer group support	Language
Access to deaf mentors for parents and children	Social interaction especially—joint attention
Cochlear implants most effective under two years	

of development. Delay in all milestones is most evident in the preschool period, although obvious challenges remain in making progress at school. These delays are inevitable when consideration is given to the increased cognitive demand of tasks achieved without the benefit of the information provided by vision (e.g., the concept of object permanence and joint attention) (88). Children with vision limited to only awareness of light or light-reflecting objects (classified as profound visual impairment [PVI]) show the greatest delay (89), between one to two years' delay compared to sighted peers. Children with SVI will also show a lesser degree of delay (90).

It has been argued that many aspects of delayed development are the result not of the visual impairment itself but of environmental or condition-specific variables that tend to accompany VI (71). Approximately 77% of children with VI have additional impairments (91), especially those with damage to the visual cortex or posterior visual pathways, seen in up to 30% of children with visual impairments. Understanding the etiology of "delayed" development requires acknowledgment of the complex issues involved, including factors relevant to the child's own learning potential, which may be genetic or related to the etiology of the condition leading to VI, the physical and social–emotional environment, and the level of or timing of onset of the VI itself.

These factors are evident in considering individual differences seen in developmental achievements of children with visual impairment and emphasize the need to ensure maximum support through early intervention, to ensure children have the optimum support for visual promotion and optimal environment for learning. The child who has only awareness of light or light-reflecting objects and whose visual loss is congenital and affecting only the eyes or visual pathways with no additional potential neurological or brain involvement (referred to by Sonksen and Dale as congenital disorders of the primary visual system [CDPVS] (89)) provide the purest model for considering the impact of visual impairment on development.

The constraints of lack of vision on learning are complex and the impact of delay in one area of development is likely to have secondary effects on other areas of development, so that the effects are cumulative (92). The routes to learning are therefore likely to be different to fully sighted peers.

Sonksen argues that visual impairment itself could theoretically have an impact on functional organization and reorganization of the cerebral cortex, e.g., through cortical template formation and networking and on the cortical visual system during crucial early brain development, and hence the impact is likely to be far reaching (89).

Dale et al. in a cohort of CDPVS children between the ages of 2.5 to 3 years showed a much higher prevalence of mental retardation (19 to 33%) than in a sighted population (10–15%) (89). Severe mental retardation (DQ <55) ranged from 10 to 13% compared to 1–2% in the sighted population (93).

Areas of Development

Motor and Perceptual Development. Learning to move requires understanding of the physical world, including the concept of the continuity of the physical world around the baby—the floor as a permanent base that can be moved across or reached for to balance when learning to sit. Vision also provides the motivation to move or reach out to explore (94). The environment may interact in limiting acquisition of skills when parents are more protective and cautious about giving their blind child the opportunities to explore. Temperamental factors in young children will also play a role; for example, a timid child, having learned to walk, may be more reluctant to "launch" herself into the world than a more adventurous one.

Developing reach and interest in play depend on developing concepts of sound localization and object permanence. Babies without vision require the support of their parents and caregivers to learn these concepts (86, 95).

Language Development. Language development relies on an understanding of joint reference and developing the concept of symbolic understanding. The early opportunities that sighted children have to see objects and to establish joint reference to objects named by parents repeatedly in the first year of life before language develops is lost to the blind infant. Limited experience in general, and not only visual, may play a role in delaying language acquisition, as may parenting style.

Early acquisition of babble is not affected significantly by visual impairment (96, 97). The rate of word acquisition varies between studies, with some reporting delays and others no difference. McConachie and Moore (98), looking at a group of children with no additional developmental problems, did find a delay in the acquisition of first words, although they found that subsequent development of words was often more rapid than in children with full sight. Variations in the pattern of acquisition of subsequent words have been reported, e.g., the use of specific or general nominals, and an increase in use of action words mainly describing the child's own actions (98, 99). Differences in the style of language development have also been described, e.g., the use of multiword phrases, linked to familiar social routines, before the use of noun labels. This has been referred to as a more expressive rather than referential style of language use (100). Children with VI also have a tendency to continue with immediate echolalia longer than sighted peers (101). Delays are also seen in the appropriate use of personal and other pronouns and the use of spatial–relational words (e.g., here–there) (102).

Cognitive Development. Cognition is a complex construct and Warren (71) provides an excellent review of the subject in children with VI. Delays have been reported in areas such as the development of classification, abstract concepts, and conservation of weight and volume in children with VI. However, results are often conflicting due to sample variability and the complex interactions of "innate IQ," experience, and other factors that are difficult to disentangle.

The role of visual imagery in language learning in children with VI also shows considerable individual variation, enhancing learning for some and interfering with learning for others (71). The presence of VI has been thought by some to influence cognitive style, leading to a more global (diffuse and unstructured) rather than articulated (structured) style (71), although this is refuted by other research. Short-term or long-term memory does not appear to be influenced by VI. Finally, research into processing of phonological and tactile information in children with VI suggests that the two are separate but interdependent (71). This is particularly important with respect to the reading of Braille.

Academic Achievement. Accessing literacy through Braille or through suitable adaptation of written material through enlargement and appropriate use of low-vision aids is a major challenge for children with VI. Learning to read through the use of Braille is potentially a more complex process than learning to read using vision, because it entails linguistic, motor, and spatial skills (71, 103). Children with VI may therefore make slower progress in the early stages of acquiring literacy, and this may also delay the recognition of other specific learning difficulties. The long-term followup study of children with VI by Freeman et al. (104) found better than expected academic outcomes, with 76% having completed secondary education and 19% having attended or attending university.

Social and Emotional Development. Children with VI face considerable challenges in social and emotional development (70, 105, 106). Attainment of social skills, such as learning to read nonverbal communication cues, initiating and maintaining interactions, and using eye gaze to regulate interactions (107) are highly visually dependent. Despite this limited feedback from their environment, Mulford (108) found that most blind children (aged 5–6 years) had established a range of verbal and nonverbal communication strategies for establishing referential communication. However, Preisler (109) found that blind children rarely initiated and had difficulty maintaining social interactions and related much more to adults. Interaction with peers was more extended in structured play but they had more difficulty in free play settings. A long-term followup of children with VI into adult life (104) found that half had a romantic relationship and 20% were in partnerships, all with sighted people.

Mental Health Problems in Children with Visual Impairment

Visual impairment is associated with an increased rate of psychopathology. As with deafness, psychiatric disorder in children with VI is more likely when there are additional impairments. As described above, congenital blindness has a more pervasive effect on psychological development, but acquired VI may lead to a greater sense of loss for both parents and children (69) (Table 1.7.2.5).

Jan et al. (69) studied 86 children and young people (0–20 years) who were blind and partially sighted compared to neighborhood controls and found that 57% showed psychiatric or cognitive disorder. A third of this population had mental retardation or a developmental disorder. The psychiatric diagnoses included adjustment reaction, personality disorder, and behavior disorder. More children with VI were prescribed more psychotropic medication, and more had sleep and nutritional problems. In a study of preschool children with severe VI and mental retardation, a third of the group showed social withdrawal, lack of relationships with other children, self-injurious behavior and/or poor compliance at bedtime (110). A more recent study of young children (n = 74) with "isolated" SVI (0–5 years) found a lower rate of problems; 21% of children had a significant emotional and behavioral deficit, including insecurity or withdrawal, attachment problem, inattentiveness, impulsive or hyperactive oppositional-defiant behavior, temper tantrums, and toileting problems (111).

Emotional and behavioral difficulties in adolescents with VI have been reported in a number of studies: higher mean scores than sighted controls on the parent, teacher, and self-report versions of the CBCL (112), with higher scores in those at residential compared to public school (113), an increased rate of loneliness and difficulties making friends, but not of depression, compared with controls (114). Ollendick et al. (115) noted increased fears in a pattern that reflected the dangers that children with VI faced in their everyday world. The particular challenges faced by adolescents with VI in making friends and the benefits of these friendships is discussed by Rosenblum and emphasizes the need for families and professionals to provide sensitive support in this area (116, 117).

Dale (118), using a specially designed questionnaire for parents of children with VI, found that social communication skills are particularly prone to disruption in the second year of life, children with PVI having particular difficulty in sharing of interests and attention to objects with an interacting adult, compared to sighted children and children with SVI. Other cohort studies and case series have reported similar difficulty (71).

These findings are of theoretical interest when considering the underlying etiology of the high incidence of autism or autistic-like features noted in children with PVI. Cass et al. (119) postulated that the stage of attention control and behavioral independence in the second and third years of life are periods of increased vulnerability to setback and regression (the first signs of which are increasingly negative behavior, failure of social communication and social relating, and increased self-stimulation and stereotypies). This study of 32 children with a range of visual disorders found 10 with "developmental setback," which has features similar to autistic regression, compared with 1/72 children with SVI. Compare this to the prevalence in sighted children 0.05 to

TABLE 1.7.2.5

COMMON DEVELOPMENTAL DELAYS IN SENSORIALLY IMPAIRED CHILDREN

Hard of Hearing and Deaf	SVI and Blind
Motor/perceptual: Generally no significant effect; occasional motor delay linked to balance problems	*Motor/perceptual*: Gross motor milestones delayed in some children Acquisition of all perceptual motor concepts requires higher cognitive demands and therefore delayed, e.g., sound localization, object permanence, object relationships Delay most significant in PVI
Language: Significant language delay if not provided with appropriate intervention Significant problems with literacy common in deaf children	*Language*: Delay in acquisition of first words Variations in use of specific nominals and general nominals More action words describing the child's own actions More use of multiword phrases linked to familiar social routines More immediate echolalia Delays in the appropriate use of personal pronouns Delay in the use spatial–relational words Delay most significant in PVI
Social/emotional: Delays in metacognitive development Delays in developing emotional understanding and vocabulary	*Social/emotional*: Limitations in - Developing joint attention - Developing joint reference to objects - Learning to read nonverbal communication cues - Initiating and maintaining interactions - Using eye gaze to regulate interactions Delay most significant in PVI
Cognitive/academic: Literacy problems linked to academic underachievement	*Cognitive/academic*: Need for suitable appropriate reference ranges Increased demands of learning Braille or adaptation for large print

2 per 10,000 (120). In a subsequent study of children with CDPVS a similar prevalence (33%) was found in 27 children with PVI in contrast to 3% in the 37 children with SVI, suggesting that PVI is the main risk factor. Others have found similar prevalence of autistic-like features (70, 121, 122)

Specific abnormalities in the behavior and psychological functioning of children with visual impairment show resemblance to those seen in sighted autistic children (122), including impairment in social communicative competence, emotional recognition, creative symbolic play, and language, including echolalia and confusion in use of personal pronouns, stereotypies, mannerisms and ritualistic behavior, and uneven profiles of cognitive abilities including difficulty with abstract thinking and problems of "theory of mind" (123).

Some of these behaviors have been described as *blindisms*. However, a systematic approach considering the pattern of behaviors, their intensity, duration, and how difficult it is to redirect the behavior advocated by Gense and Gense (124) can distinguish between those children with VI and autism and those with visual impairment alone.

Hobson (125) has suggested that there may be overlap in the functional developmental psychopathology of congenitally blind and autistic children. He suggests that deprivation of social-emotional experience, e.g., understanding and identifying with other people's attitudes and emotions, may contribute to a range of blind children's social, cognitive and linguistic delays and abnormalities.

Young adults with VI have also been reported to have an excess of emotional disorders (126). Increased depression and anxiety has been reported among adults who become blind at a later age (127).

Psychiatric Assessment. The assessment of children with VI and their families is comparable to that of deaf children. However, the clinician needs to be familiar with the diversity of developmental patterns in young visually impaired children and be aware of their own reactions to the child with VI; one study showed that there was a tendency to make a more favorable assessment of cognitive and social capacities when the blind child used gaze direction (128).

Specific areas of potential difficulty need emphasis in history taking, including the impact of early mother–child interaction, early sleep difficulties relating to circadian cycle disturbances (129) or perception of social cues relating to sleep (130) and separation anxiety (70, 131). In adolescence, overprotection may make the development of personal and sexual relationships more difficult (132).

The environment for the psychiatric interview needs to be adapted to the child with VI; obstacles should be minimized, lighting should be optimum for a partially sighted child (note that some children with VI are photophobic), and children need to be given time to explore and adapt to the new environment (133). The clinician must take the time to describe and respond to questions about the contents of the room and the toys, and about the purpose and procedures of the assessment and be prepared to have more physical contact with the child than with fully sighted children (33). The clinical appraisal should also include an adequate physical assessment given the frequency of additional impairments.

Psychological Assessment. As has been argued earlier, cognitive development will be influenced by the level of vision which will influence not only the rate of learning but also the child's experiences; therefore assessment must take account of the level of VI. Few assessments are available with suitably appropriate reference ranges (see psychological assessment). It is also important to ensure that the test materials themselves are within the child's experience (71). In addition to the specific impact of visual impairment on cognition, other physical and sensory impairments and associated conditions may be associated with learning disability.

Assessment of young children will often require more time than their sighted peers, as they may need more time to adjust to introduction of many new materials and will often use touch and oral manipulation to become familiar with toys and test objects.

As described above, visual impairment has a potential profound impact on all areas of development and experience. Therefore the results of tests standardized for sighted children even if sight is apparently not required to complete the test (e.g., the verbal subscales of the WISC IV) or the tests have been translated into Braille or large print (134) must be interpreted with caution (71). Ideally, tests designed specifically for children with VI with appropriate reference ranges should be used (e.g., the Reynell-Zinkin-Reynell (90), ITVIC (135), and Blindness Aptitude test (136)). In the preschool age group there is a need for updated norms (89). Care is also needed in relation to the implications regarding comparisons with standardization data (137).

Interventions

Standard therapeutic interventions and styles of therapist–child interaction may need some modification for children and young people with VI. Fewer specific specialized psychiatric in- and outpatient services for children and adolescents with VI are available, compared to deaf children.

Modifications include the need for therapists to translate their nonverbal communication, conveyed through posture and facial expressions, into words and to appreciate the limitations of the child's use of directed gaze, facial expression, and posture to convey their feelings. As with deaf children, careful monitoring of the effects and side effects of medication is very important in relation to possible influences on sensory functioning. The American Federation of the Blind has recently published a comprehensive guide for intervening with blind children with autism (Table 1.7.2.6).

Adult Outcomes. There have been few longitudinal studies of children with VI into adult life. The most detailed (104) followed a heterogeneous sample of children with VI previously studied by Jan et al. (69). Those with mental retardation and those whose vision deteriorated showed the worst psychiatric outcome. Mannerisms were most likely to continue in those with multiple handicaps.

Adverse experiences in childhood were reported in a high proportion; a third of the women and one in nine of the men reported that they had been sexually molested or abused and nearly three-quarters said they had been cruelly teased at school. There was a strong tendency for the partially sighted to want to pass as normal and misunderstandings tended to be worse for these students, as their visual abilities were more difficult for others to recognize. Only 40% were employed.

CONCLUSIONS

Hearing and visual impairments have contrasting impacts on children's development and wellbeing. Both groups of children are more vulnerable to mental health problems but with differing patterns of problems. SVI/blind children appear particularly vulnerable to autistic spectrum disorders. This increased vulnerability appears to be the consequence of the combined effects of visual impairment on social relatedness and the impact of pervasive brain damage. Although deaf children are more vulnerable to autistic spectrum disorders than hearing children, it is not to the same extent as SVI/blind children. Deaf children appear vulnerable to both emotional and behavioral disorders. Although the etiology is not completely clear, early language and experiential deprivation appear key factors.

TABLE 1.7.2.6

PLANNING AND INTERPRETING ASSESSMENTS AND INTERVENTIONS

Hard of Hearing and Deaf	SVI and Blind
Setting: Avoid bright background lighting behind clinician Bushy moustaches and beards make lipreading difficult	*Setting*: Diversity of developmental patterns Obstacles minimized Lighting optimum Children given time to explore and adapt to the new environment
Language and communication: Ensure good access to communication Sign language interpreter if necessary Simplify written communication Written sign language can be misinterpreted as thought disordered English	*Language and communication*: Describe contents of the room, toys, and purposes and procedures of assessment
Activities: Visual activities, role play and nonlanguage activities play to deaf children's strengths	*Activities*: More physical contact with the child than with fully sighted children Physical assessment required to exclude additional impairments
Assessor's emotional response: Common feeling of disempowerment when faced by deaf child, especially if sign language user, tendency to use exaggerated positive affect to engage child	*Assessor's emotional response*: Tendency to make a more favorable assessment of cognitive and social capacities when the blind child uses gaze direction

Sadly, service development and provision does not appear to reflect the specific needs of blind and deaf children. There are relatively few specialized services for them, and current commissioning structures do not seem to reflect adequately the specific needs of these groups of children.

References

1. <http://www.nidcd.nih.gov/health/statistics/hearing.asp>. Accessed on 21 Jan 2006.
2. Parving A, Hauch A-M: <http://www.int-pediatrics.org/PDF/Volume% 2016/16-1/parving.pdf>. Accessed 21 Jan 2006.
3. Vartainen E & Karjalainen S: Prevalence and etiology of unilateral sensorineural hearing impairment in a Finnish childhood population. *International Journal of Pediatric Otorhinolaryngology* 43: 253–259, 1998.
4. Harkins JE, Bakke M: Technologies for Communication: Status and Trends. In: Marschark M & Spencer PE (eds.): *The Oxford Handbook of Deaf Studies, Language and Education*. Oxford and New York: Oxford University Press; 2003, pp. 406–419.
5. Woll B, Ladd P: Deaf Communities. In: Marschark M & Spencer PE, (eds.): *The Oxford Handbook of Deaf Studies, Language and Education*. Oxford and New York: Oxford University Press; 2003, pp. 151–163.
6. Stokoe B: *Sign language structure: An outline of the visual communication systems of the American deaf (Occasional papers 8)*. Buffalo, University of Buffalo Department of Anthropology.and Linguistics, 1960. (Reprinted Burtonsville, MD: Linstock Press; 1993).
7. Meadow-Orlans KP, Erting C: Deaf People in Society. In: Hindley P, Kitson N, (eds.): *Mental Health and Deafness*. London and Philadelphia: Whurr Publishers, 2000, pp. 3–24.
8. Groce N: *Everyone here spoke sign language*. Cambridge, MA, Harvard University Press, 1985.
9. Rawlings BW, Jensema CJ: *Two Studies of the Families of Hearing Impaired Children*. Washington, DC, Gallaudet University Office of Demographic Studies, 1977.
10. Singleton JL, Tittle MD: Deaf parents and their hearing children. *Journal of Deaf Studies and Deaf Education* 5: 221–236, 2000.
11. Armstrong DF, Wilcox S: Origins of Sign Language. In: Marschark M, Spencer PE, (eds.): *The Oxford Handbook of Deaf Studies, Language and Education*. Oxford and New York: Oxford University Press; 2003, pp. 305–318.
12. Fischer SD, van der Hulst H: Sign Language Structures. In: Marschark M & Spencer PE, (eds.): *The Oxford Handbook of Deaf Studies, Language and Education*. Oxford and New York: Oxford University Press; 2003, pp. 319–331.
13. Emmorey K: The Neural Systems Underlying Sign Language. In: Marschark M & Spencer PE (eds.): *The Oxford Handbook of Deaf Studies, Language and Education*. Oxford and New York; Oxford University Press; 2003, pp. 361–378.
14. Schick B: The Development of American Sign Language and Manually Coded English Systems. In: Marschark M, Spencer PE, (eds.): *The Oxford Handbook of Deaf Studies, Language and Education*. Oxford and New York: Oxford University Press; 2003, pp. 219–231.
15. Harris M: *Language Experience and Early Language Development: From Input to Uptake*. Hove (U.K.) and Hillsdale, NJ, Essays in Developmental Psychology Series, Lawrence Erlbaum, 1992.
16. Meadow-Orlans KP, Spencer PE, Koester LS: *The World of Deaf Infants: A Longitudinal Study*. Oxford and New York, Oxford University Press, 2004.
17. Luterman D, Kurtzer-White E, Seewald R: *The Young Deaf Child*. Austen, Texas, Pro-Ed, 2001.
18. Traci M, Koester LS: Parent-Infant Interactions: A Transactional Approach to Understanding the Development of Deaf Infants. In: Marschark M, Spencer PE, (eds.): *The Oxford Handbook of Deaf Studies, Language and Education*. Oxford and New York, Oxford University Press, 2003, pp. 190–202.
19. Cone-Wesson B: Screening and Assessment of Hearing Loss in Infants. In: Marschark M, Spencer PE (eds.): *The Oxford Handbook of Deaf Studies, Language and Education*. Oxford and New York, Oxford University Press, 2003, pp. 420–433.
20. Sass-Lehrer M, Bodner-Johnson M: Early Intervention: Current Approaches to Family Centred Programming. In: Marschark M, Spencer PE (eds.): *The Oxford Handbook of Deaf Studies, Language and Education*. Oxford and New York, Oxford University Press, 2003, pp. 65–81.
21. Spencer PE, Marschark M: Cochlear Implants: Issues and Implications. In: Marschark M, Spencer PE (eds.): *The Oxford Handbook of Deaf Studies, Language and Education*. Oxford and New York, Oxford University Press, 2003, pp. 434–451.
22. Holden-Pitt L, Diaz JA: Thirty years of the Annual Survey of Deaf and Hard of Hearing Children and Youth: A glance over the decades. *American Annals of the Deaf*. 143: 72–76, 1998.
23. Antia SD, Kreimeyer KH: Peer Interactions in Deaf and Hard of Hearing Children. In: Marschark M, Spencer PE (eds.): *The Oxford Handbook of Deaf Studies, Language and Education*. Oxford and New York, Oxford University Press, 2003, pp. 164–176.
24. Remmel E, Bettger JG, Weinberg AM: Theory of Mind Development in Deaf Children. In: Clark MD, Marschark M, Karchmer M (eds.): *Context, Cognition and Deafness*. Washington DC, Gallaudet University Press, 2001.
25. Calderon R, Greenberg M: Social and Emotional Development in Deaf Children: Family, School and Program Effects. In: Marschark M, Spencer PE (eds.): *The Oxford Handbook of Deaf Studies, Language and Education*. Oxford and New York, Oxford University Press, 2003, pp 177–189.
26. Steinberg A: Autobiographical Narrative on Growing Up Deaf. In: Spencer PE, Erting CJ, Marschark M (eds.): *The Deaf Child in the Family and School: Essays in Honor of Kathryn P. Meadow-Orlans*. Mahwah, NJ, Lawrence Erlbaum Associates, 2000.
27. Karchmer MA, Mitchell RE: Demographic and Achievement Characteristics of Deaf and Hard-of-Hearing Students. In: Marschark M, Spencer PE (eds.): *The Oxford Handbook of Deaf Studies, Language and Education*. Oxford and New York, Oxford University Press, 2003, pp. 21–37.
28. Sullivan P, Brookhouser P, Scanlan M: Maltreatment of Deaf and Hard of Hearing Children. In: Hindley P, Kitson N (eds.): *Mental Health and Deafness*. London and Philadelphia, Whurr Publishers, 2000. pp. 149–184.
29. Best C: The "new" deaf-blind? Results of a national survey of deaf-blind children in ESN (S) and hospital schools. *British Journal of Visual Impairment* 1: 11–13, 1983.
30. Trybus RJ: Demographics and population character research in deaf-blindness. In: Stahlecker JE, Glass LE, Machalow S (eds.): *State of the Art:*

Research Priorities in Deaf-Blindness. UCSF, CA, Center on Deafness, 1985.

31. Adler MA: Psychosocial interventions with deaf-blind youths and adults. In: Heller BW, Flohr LM, Zegans LS (eds.): *Psychosocial Interventions with Sensorially Disabled Persons.* London, Grune & Stratton, 1987.
32. McInnes JM, Treffry JA: *Deaf-Blind Infants and Children: A Developmental Guide.* Milton Keynes, Open University Press; 1982.
33. Jenkins IR, Chess S: Psychiatric evaluation of perceptually impaired children: Hearing and visual impairments. In: Lewis M (ed.): *Child and Adolescent Psychiatry: A Comprehensive Textbook*, 2nd ed. Baltimore, Williams & Wilkins; 1996, pp. 526–534.
34. Miner ID: Psychosocial implications of Usher syndrome, type I, throughout the life cycle. *Journal of Visual Impairment & Blindness* 89: 287–296. 1995.
35. Miner ID: Psychotherapy for People with Usher Syndrome. In: Leigh IW (ed.): *Psychotherapy with Deaf Clients from Diverse Client Groups.* Washington DC, Gallaudet University Press, 1999, pp. 302–327.
36. www.deafblind.com (accessed Jan 19 2006).
37. Hindley PA: Psychiatric aspects of hearing impairments. *Journal of Child Psychology and Psychiatry* 38: 101–117 1997.
38. Rutter M, Graham P, Yule W: A neuropsychiatric study in in childhood. *Clinics in Developmental Medicine Nos. 35/36.* London, Spastics International Medical Publications, 1970.
39. Freeman RD, Malkin SF, Hastings JO: Psychological problems of deaf children and their families: A comparative study. *American Annals of the Deaf* 120: 275–304 1975.
40. Hindley PA, Hill PD, McGuigan S, Kitson N: Psychiatric disorder in deaf and hearing impaired children and young people: A prevalence study. *Journal of Child Psychology and Psychiatry* 35: 917–934, 1994.
41. Van Gent T, Goedhart AW, Hindley PA, Treffers PDA: Prevalence of psychopathology in a population of deaf adolescents, assessed by a multi-method, multi-informant approach. Submitted to *Journal of the American Academy of Child and Adolescent Psychiatry*, 2005.
42. Smith PK, Sharp S: *School Bullying: Insights and Perspectives.* London, Routledge, 1994.
43. Conrad R: *The Deaf Schoolchild.* London, Harper & Row Ltd, 1979.
44. Beck G, de Jong E: *Opgroaien in een Horende vereld.* Twello, NL, van Tricht, 1990.
45. Hindley PA, Hill PD, Bond D: Interviewing deaf children, the interviewer effect: A research note. *Journal of Child Psychology and Psychiatry* 34: 1461–1467, 1993.
46. Turner J, Klein H, Kitson N: Interpreters in mental health settings. In: Hindley P & Kitson N (eds): *Mental Health and Deafness.* London and Philadelphia, Whurr Publishers, 2000, pp. 297–310.
47. Kitson N, Thacker, A: Adult psychiatry. In: Hindley P, Kitson N (eds): *Mental Health and Deafness.* London and Philadelphia: Whurr Publishers, 2000, pp. 75–98.
48. Maller SJ: Intellectual assessment of deaf people: A critical review of core concepts and issues. In: Marschark M, Spencer PE (eds.): *The Oxford Handbook of Deaf Studies, Language and Education.* Oxford and New York, Oxford University Press, 2003, pp. 451–463.
49. Kelly D, Forney J, Parker-Fischer S, Jones M: The challenge of attention deficit disorder in children who are deaf or hard of hearing. *American Annals of the Deaf* 138: 343–348, 1993.
50. Chess S, Korn SJ, Fernandez PB: *Psychiatric Disorders of Children with Congenital Rubella.* New York, Brunner & Mazel, 1971.
51. Chess S, Fernandez P: Do deaf children have a typical personality? *Journal of the American Academy of Child Psychiatry* 19: 654–664, 1980.
52. Van Eldik T: *Mental health problems, family stress, family functioning and stressful life events of deaf children.* PhD thesis, Erasmus Universiteit Rotterdam, 1998.
53. Brown AS, Cohen P, Greenwald S, Susser E: Nonaffective Psychosis after Prenatal Exposure to Rubella. *American Journal of Psychiatry* 157: 438–443, 2000.
54. Juré R, Rapin I, Tuchman RF: Hearing impaired autistic children. *Developmental Medicine and Child Neurology* 33: 1062–1072, 1991.
55. Rosenhall U, Nordin V, Sandström M, Ahlsen G, Gillberg C: Autism and hearing loss. *Journal of Autism and Developmental Disorders* 29: 349–357, 1999.
56. Van Gent T, Heijnen CJ, Treffers PhDA: Autism and the immune system. *Journal of Child Psychology and Psychiatry* 38: 337–349, 1997.
57. Hindley PA: Recent advances in autism and sensory impairments. *Social Brain 2, Glasgow*, March 2006.
58. Roberts C, Hindley P: Practitioner review: The assessment and treatment of deaf children with psychiatric disorders. *Journal of Child Psychology and Psychiatry* 40: 151–167, 1999.
59. Hamerdinger S, Hill E: Serving Severely Emotionally Disturbed Deaf Youth: A Statewide Program Model, (submitted for publication). 2005.
60. Vreeland J, Tourangeau J: Culturally affirmative residential treatment services for deaf children with emotional and behavioral disorders. In: Glickman NS, Gulati S (eds.): *Mental Health Care of Deaf People: A Culturally Affirmative Approach.* Mahwah, NJ, Erlbaum, 2003, pp. 239–260.
61. Willis WG, Vernon M: Residential psychiatric treatment of emotionally disturbed deaf youth. *American Annals of the Deaf* 147: 31–38, 2002.
62. Elliot H, Glass L, Evans JW: *Mental Health Assessment of Deaf Clients: A Practical Manual.* Boston, College Hill Press, 1987.
63. Hoyt MF, Siegelman EY, Schlesinger HS: Special Issues Regarding Psychotherapy with the Deaf. *American Journal of Psychiatry* 138: 807–811, 1981.
64. Meadow-Orlans K: Parenting with a sensory or physical disability. In: Borstein M (ed.): *Handbook of Parenting*, Vol 4: *Applied and Practical Considerations.* Hillsdale, NJ, Erlbaum, 1995, pp. 57–84.
65. Preston P: *Mother–Father Deaf.* Cambridge, MA, Harvard University Press, 1994.
66. Charlson E.S: At-risk deaf parents and their children. In: Austen S & Crocker S (eds.): *Deafness in Mind: Working Psychologically with Deaf People across the Lifespan.* London and Philadelphia, Whurr Publishers, 2004, pp. 222–234.
67. Fogel A: Seeing and being seen. In: Lewis V, Collis GM (eds.): *Blindness and Psychological Development.* Leicester, BPS Books, 1997, pp. 86–98.
68. Sonksen PM: Constraints on parenting: Experience of a paediatrician. *Child: care, health and development* 15: 29–36, 1989.
69. Jan, JE, Freeman RD, Scott EP: *Visual Impairment in Children and Adolescents.* New York, Grune & Stratton, 1977.
70. Fraiberg S: *Insights from the Blind: Comparative Studies of Blind and Sighted Children.* New York, Basic Books, 1977.
71. Warren DH: *Blindness and Children: An Individual Differences Approach.* Cambridge, Cambridge University Press, 1994.
72. Sandler AM, Hobson RP: On engaging with people in early childhood: The case of congenital blindness. *Clinical Child Psychology and Psychiatry* 6: 205–222, 2001.
73. Als H, Troninck E, Brazelton TB: Affective reciprocity and the development of autonomy: The study of a blind infant. *Journal of the American Academy of Child Psychiatry* 19: 22–40, 1980.
74. Moore V, McConachie H: Communication between blind and severely visually impaired children and their parents. *British Journal of Developmental Psychology* 12; 491–502, 1994.
75. Preisler G: Early patterns of interaction between blind parents and their sighted infants. *Child: Care, health and development* 17: 65–90, 1991.
76. Rowbury C: *Referential communication between a blind mother and a blind child.* Paper presented at Developmental Section Conference, British Psychological Society, Cambridge, September, 1991.
77. Recchia SL: Play and concept development in infants and young children with severe visual impairments: A constructivist's view. *Journal of Visual Impairment* 91: 401–406, 1997.
78. Rowland C: Patterns of interaction between three blind infants and their mothers. In: Mills AE (ed.): *Language Acquisition in the Blind Child.* Beckenham, Croom Helm, 1983, pp. 114–132.
79. Peters AM: The interdependence of social, cognitive and linguistic development: Evidence from a visually impaired child. In: Tager-Flusberg H (ed.): *Constraints on Language Acquisition: Studies of Atypical Children.* Hillsdale, NJ, Lawrence Erlbaum, 1994, pp. 195–219.
80. Hall DM, Elliman D: *Health for all children*, 4th ed. Oxford, Oxford University Press, 2003.
81. <http://www.ahrq.gov/clinic/uspstf/uspsvsch.htm>. Accessed 21/01/2006.
82. Blaikie AJ, Ravenscroft J, Dutton GD, MacEwen C, Visual Impairment Scotland Team: *A New System of Notification of Childhood Visual Impairment and the Information It Has Provided on the Services for Scottish Children.* Edinburgh, Visual Impairment Scotland, 2003.
83. Sonksen PM, Petrie A, Drew KJ: Promotion of visual development of severely visually impaired babies: Evaluation of a developmentally based programme. *Developmental Medicine and Child Neurology* 33; 320–335, 1991.
84. Sonksen PM, Stiff B: Show me what my friends can see. London, Wolfson Centre, 1991.
85. <http://www.earlysupport.org.uk/Materials/Materialsindevelopment/visuallyimpairedchildren/tabid/344/Default.aspx>. Accessed 21/01/2006.
86. Sonksen PM: The assessment of "vision for development" in severely visually handicapped babies. *Acta Ophthalmologica* Supplement 157: 82–90, 1983.
87. Dale N: Early signs of developmental setback and autism in infants with severe visual impairment. In: Pring L (ed.): *Autism and Blindness.* London and Philadelphia, Whurr Publishers, 2004.
88. Bigelow AE: The development of joint attention in blind infants. *Development and Psychopathology* 15: 259–275, 2003.
89. Sonksen PM, Dale N: Visual impairment in infancy: Impact on neurodevelopmental and neurobiological processes. *Developmental Medicine and Child Neurology* 44: 782–791, 2002.
90. Reynell J: *Manual for the Reynell-Zinkin Developmental Scales for Young Visually-Handicapped Children. Part I.* Windsor, NFER, 1979.
91. Rahi JS, Cable N, on behalf of the British Childhood Visual Impairment Study Group: Severe visual impairment and blindness in children in the UK. *The Lancet* 362: 1359–1365, 2003.
92. Sonksen PM: Vision and early development. In: Wybar R, Taylor D (eds.): *Paediatric Ophthalmology: Current Aspects.* New York, Marcel Dekker, 1983, pp 85–95.
93. Dale N, Sonksen P: Developmental outcome, including setback, in young children with severe visual impairment. *Developmental Medicine and Child Neurology* 44:613–622, 2002.

94. Sonksen PM, Levitt SL, Kitzinger M: Identification of constraints acting on motor development in young visually disabled children and principles of remediation. *Child: Care, health and development* 10:273–286, 1984.
95. Bigelow AE: Locomotion and search behavior in blind infants. *Infant behavior and development* 15:179–189, 1992.
96. Andersen ES, Dunlea A, Kekelis LS: Blind children's language: Resolving some differences. *Journal of Child Language* 11:645–664, 1984.
97. Bigelow AE: Early words of blind children. *Journal of Child Language* 14:47–56, 1987.
98. McConachie H, Moore V: Early expressive language of severely visually impaired children. *Developmental Medicine and Child Neurology* 36: 230–240, 1994.
99. Mulford RC: First words of the blind child. In: Smith MD, Locke JL (eds.): *The emergent lexicon: The child's development of a linguistic vocabulary.* New York, Academic Press, 1988, pp. 293–338.
100. Nelson K: Individual differences in language development: Implications for development and language. *Developmental Psychology* 17: 170–187, 1981.
101. Prizant BM: Toward an understanding of language symptomatology of visually impaired children. In: Sykanda AM, Buchanan BK, Jan JE, Groenveld M, Blockberger SJ (eds.): *Insight in sight: Proceedings of the fifth Canadian interdisciplinary conference on the visually impaired child.* Vancouver, CNIB, 1984, pp. 70–87.
102. Fraiberg S, Andelson E: Self representation in young blind children. In: Jastrzembska JS (ed.): *The effects of blindness and other impairments on early development.* New York: American Foundation for the Blind, 1976, pp. 136–159.
103. Millar S: Reading without vision. In: Lewis V, Collis GM (eds.): *Blindness and Psychological Development.* Leicester: BPS Books, 1997, pp. 86–98.
104. Freeman RD, Goetz E, Richards DP et al.: Defiers of negative prediction: a 14-year follow-up study of legally blind children. *Journal of Visual Impairment and Blindness*, 85: 365–370, 1991.
105. McGurk H: Affective motivation and development of communication competence in blind and sighted children. In: Mills AE (ed.): *Language Acquisition in the Blind Child: Normal and Deficient.* London: Croom Helm, 1983, pp. 108–113.
106. Hobson R, Brown R, Minter EM, Lee A: Autism "revisited": The case of congenital blindness. In: Lewis V, Collis GM (eds.): *Blindness and Psychological Development.* Leicester: BPS Books, 1997, pp. 99–115.
107. Kekelis LS: Peer interactions in childhood: The impact of visual impairment. In: Sacks SZ, Kekelis LS, Gaylord-Ross RJ (eds.): *The Development of Social Skills by Blind and Visually Impaired Students.* New York: American Foundation for the Blind, 1992, pp. 13–35.
108. Mulford RC: Referential development in blind children. In: Mills AE (ed.): *Language Acquisition in the Blind Child.* Beckenham: Croom Helm, 1983, pp. 89–107.
109. Preisler G: Social and emotional development of blind children: A longitudinal study. In: Lewis V, Collis GM (eds.): *Blindness and Psychological Development.* Leicester: BPS Books, 1997, pp. 69–85.
110. Kitzinger M, Hunt H: The effect of residential setting on sleep and behaviour patterns of young visually-handicapped children. In: Stevenson JE (ed.): *Recent Research in Developmental Psychopathology.* Oxford: Pergamon Press, 1985, pp. 73–80.
111. Ophir-Cohen M, Ashkenazy E, Cohen A, Tirosh E: Emotional Status and Development in Children Who Are Visually Impaired. *Journal of Visual Impairment and Blindness.* 99:478–485, 2005.
112. Achenbach TM, Edelbrock CS: *Manual for the Child Behavior Checklist and Revised Behavior Profile.* Burlington VT, University of Vermont Department of Psychiatry, 1983.
113. Van Hasselt VB, Kazdin AE, Hersen M: Assessment of problem behavior in visually handicapped adolescents. *Journal of Clinical Child Psychology* 15: 134–141, 1986.
114. Huure TM, Aro HM: Psychosocial development among adolescents with visual impairment. *European Child and Adolescent Psychiatry* 7:73–78, 1998.
115. Ollendick TH, Matson JL, Helsel WJ: Fears in visually impaired and normally-sighted youths. *Behavior Research and Therapy* 3: 375–378, 1985.
116. Rosenblum LP: Perceptions of the impact of visual impairment on the lives of adolescents. *Journal of Visual Impairment and Blindness* 94: 434–445, 2000.
117. Peavey KO, Leff D: Social acceptance of adolescent mainstreamed students with visual impairments. *Journal of Visual Impairment & Blindness* 96: 808–811, 2002.
118. Dale N: Personal communication, 2006.
119. Cass H, Sonksen PM, McConachie HR: Developmental setback in severe visual impairment. *Archives of Disease in Childhood* 70: 192–196, 1994.
120. Gillberg C, Steffenburg S, Schaumann H: Is autism more common now than ten years ago? *British Journal of Psychiatry* 158: 403–409, 1991.
121. Norris M, Spalding PJ, Brodie FH: *Blindness in Children.* Chicago, University of Chicago Press, 1957.
122. Brown R, Hobson RP, Lee A, Stevenson J: Are there 'autistic-like' features in congenitally blind children? *Journal of Child Psychology & Psychiatry* 38: 693–703, 1997.
123. McAlpine LM, Moore C: The development of social understanding in children with visual impairments. *Journal of Visual Impairment and Blindness* 89: 349–358, 1995.
124. Gense MH, Gense DJ: Identifying autism in children with blindness and visual impairments. *Re:view* 26: 55–62, 1994.
125. Hobson RP: *Autism and the Development of the Mind.* Hove, UK, Erlbaum, 1993.
126. Yoshida T, Ichikawa T, Ishikawa T, Hori M: Mental health of visually and hearing impaired students from the viewpoint of the University Personality Inventory. *Psychiatry and Clinical Neurosciences* 52: 413–418, 1998.
127. De Leo D, Hickey PA, Meneghel G, Cantor CH: Blindness, fear of sight loss, and suicide. *Psychosomatics* 40: 339–344, 1999.
128. Raver-Lampman SA: Effect of gaze direction on evaluation of visually impaired children by informed respondents. *Journal of Visual Impairment & Blindness.* 84: 67–70, 1990.
129. Sasaki H, Nakata H, Murakami S, Uesugi R, Harada S, Teranishi M: Circadian sleep–wake rhythm disturbance in blind adolescence. *Japanese Journal of Psychiatry and Neurology* 46: 209, 1992.
130. Sadeh A, Klitzke M, Anders TF, Acebo C: Case study: sleep and aggressive behavior in a blind, retarded adolescent. A concomitant schedule disorder? *Journal of the American Academy of Child and Adolescent Psychiatry* 34: 820–824, 1995.
131. Burlingham D: *Psychoanalytic Studies of the Sighted and the Blind.* New York International University Press, 1972.
132. Scholl GT: The psychosocial effects of blindness: Implications for program planning in sex education. *New Outlook for the Blind* 68: 210–215, 1974.
133. Hansen R, Young J, Ulrey G: Assessment considerations with the visually handicapped child. In: Ulrey G, Rogers S (eds.): *Psychological Assessment of Handicapped Infants and Young Children.* New York: Thieme-Stratton, 1982.
134. Van Hasselt VB, Sisson LA: Visual impairment. In: van Hasselt VB, Hersen M (eds.): *Psychological Evaluation of the Developmentally and Physically Disabled.* New York: Grune & Stratton, 1987.
135. Dekker R, & Koole FD: Visually impaired children's visual characteristics and intelligence. *Developmental Medicine and Child Neurology* 34: 123–133, 1992.
136. Newland TE: The blind aptitude test. *Journal of Visual Impairment & Blindness* 73: 134–139, 1979.
137. Serjeant J, Taylor E: Psychological Testing and Observation. In: Rutter M, Taylor E, (eds.): *Child and Adolescent Psychiatry*, 4th Ed. Oxford: Blackwell Scientific, 2002, pp. 87–102.

CHAPTER 1.7.3 ■ SEXUAL MINORITY YOUTH

CYNTHIA J. TELINGATOR AND PETER T. DANIOLOS

IDENTITY, ROLE, AND ORIENTATION

It is challenging to write a chapter on sexual minority youth and avoid the trap of further entrenching a dichotomous discussion about sexuality, rather than advance a discussion about the multidimensionality of an individual. Sexual minority youth is a term used to describe adolescents who are not exclusively heterosexual. In this chapter we will use this term to refer to youth with same sex attractions, relationships, or behaviors, regardless of their self-identification as lesbian, gay, or bisexual (1).

The youth of today are resisting the categorization of their emotional attachments as well as their intimate relations. Although the categorization of gay, lesbian, and bisexual has been helpful in the past to find community, in many parts of the world it no longer is necessary to segregate oneself with others who label themselves in a similar way in order to find acceptance. Schools and the media have played an important role in redefining community for youth who are sexual minorities. They have created role models that have supported the idea that it is possible to understand one's sexual identity in a more complex manner. There is increasing visibility of adults who partner, have children, and create a home and a life outside of a heterosexual construct.

The variation in adolescent sexual identity development is as complicated as any aspect of identity development. It is not known what aspects of biological, environmental, psychological, and sociocultural influences are critical to a sexual minority identity, but relevant current research will be presented in this chapter, along with stressors adolescents may experience that might lead an adolescent and/or a family to seek psychiatric consultation. While the problems these adolescents face require the full empathy and support of a trained professional, it is important to acknowledge that not all sexual minority adolescents face these challenges with the same degree of severity. There are many recognized cases of individuals whom, for whatever reason, whether it is a solid support system, a loving environment, or their own abilities to maneuver the many complex challenges most adolescents in these stages of development face, are able to enter adulthood fully self-accepting and secure in their feelings regarding their sexual identity.

As child and adolescent clinicians we often see the most vulnerable youth. This vulnerability occurs secondary to complex interactions of the child within a family, culture, and society. Although research findings often find higher rates of mental health risk in adolescent sexual minority populations, it is difficult to isolate what is due to internalized homophobia and external stressors that sexual minority youth experience, versus other biological and psychosocial factors. The defenses used to cope with both internal and external stressors can lead to compartmentalization to protect this aspect of one's identity from being known. Youth may consciously and unconsciously do this as a shelter from rejection, as well as from emotional and physical harm by family members, peers, communities, and religious affiliations.

DEFINITIONS

Although in the literature and in clinical discussion definitions may vary, some core concepts are defined here and used within the chapter. *Gender identity* refers to the youngster's internally perceived gender, regardless of chromosomal constitution, gonadal/hormonal secretions, or genitalia. Most children develop a stable gender identity that is concordant with their biology around the age of three. This process is likely driven by biologic determinants, but environmental psychosocial factors may also play a role. This chapter will not explore the experience of transsexual youth, as this is a distinct population and thus beyond the scope of this chapter.

Gender role refers to culturally underwritten masculine and feminine behaviors, attitudes, and personality traits, partly biologically driven, and partly shaped by environment. "Aspects of sex-typed behavior in childhood and adulthood are affected by hormones that were present very early in development, confirming findings in other mammalian species (2)." This is often noticeable as early as age two or three, although in some children there can be flexibility until age five or later. In younger children, gender role can be observed by stereotypic "feminine" affiliative, nurturant play involving dolls and feminine dressup and also in "masculine" rough and tumble play, with a greater interest in automotives and action toys. It includes play and work preferences, friendships, extracurricular interests, and courting patterns, and can variably shift over the course of one's life. Children's books and the media play a role in reinforcing stereotypes.

Gender roles are enforced by peers. Anxiety about atypical gender behavior may lead to peers teasing and ostracizing gender atypical youth, and to parents bringing their child for a mental health evaluation. For some, gender-variant roles in childhood may coincide with a later homosexual identity. The association between sexual orientation in adults and retrospective reports of gender nonconformity in children is substantially higher among men than among women (3).

Sexual orientation is the predominance of erotic feelings, thoughts, and fantasies one has for members of one sex, or both sexes. Some consider it to be biologically driven, immutable, stable over time, and resistant to conscious control (4). Diamond states that these beliefs are derived primarily from gay male populations and posits that women differ. She states, "In contrast to this premise, female same-sex orientations often exhibit late and abrupt development, and inconsistencies among women's prior and current behavior, ideation and attractions have been extensively documented (5)." Freud stated in Analysis Terminable and Interminable, "We have come to learn, however, that every human being is bisexual in this sense and that his libido is distributed, either in a manifest or a latent fashion, over objects of both sexes (6)." Savin Williams believes that sexual identity—which refers to one's identity as a sexual being, and is distinct from gender identity—and behavior—not orientation—are most subject to conscious choice and thus fluid over time (4). Both Savin Williams and Diamond posit that sexual orientation exists along a continuum, with the possibility of a multitude of expressions over the lifespan of an individual. Sexual orientation may not be within conscious control but may shift along a bisexual continuum for some, and for others remain in a fixed position.

Sexual behavior and one's identity as heterosexual, gay, lesbian, or bisexual can be malleable over time. "The fluidity of sexual desire, behavior and identity may be a fundamental characteristic of sexuality during the teenage years (7)." Complicated cultural and social identities will influence sexual identity as well. Savin Williams and Diamond compared the genders and looked at sexual identity trajectories among sexual minority youth. This research led them to conclude that differences among youths can not be explained by gender alone. "No singular sexual identity model is capable of representing the diverse trajectories of male and female sexual identity development." They found that the context for sexual identity development was more likely to be emotionally oriented for female adolescents and sexually oriented for male adolescents (8).

HISTORICAL OVERVIEW AND EPIDEMIOLOGY

Although the existence of divergent attractions and sexual behaviors is not a new phenomenon, public and professional discourse have changed over time. It was only in 1973 that homosexuality was deleted from the Diagnostic and Statistical Manual (DSM II) of the American Psychiatric Association, following the work of Evelyn Hooker that did not find increased rates of psychopathology among homosexuals (9). The Stonewall Rebellion in 1969, when the visibility of the gay, lesbian, bisexual, and transgendered community was increased in the media, had an influence as well. The social movement that began at that time has accelerated with the help of popular culture in the United States in recent years. Youth today are rejecting the labels that have served to help identify community in the past, and those who need or want to affix a label to themselves are sometimes choosing broader categories such as queer, polysexual, heteroflexible, and polyamorous.

In 1992, Gary Remefedi et al. conducted a survey of Minnesota junior and senior high school students. In this early study Remefedi found that 1.6% of males and 0.9% of females identified themselves as either bisexual or predominantly homosexual, and more than 10% were "not sure (10)." Of the 36,706 students, 52% reported having some heterosexual experience and 1% as having had a homosexual experience. Interestingly only 27.1% of the students with homosexual experience self-identified as homosexual or bisexual. He also found that even though a larger number of adolescent boys reported a homosexual identification, more adolescent girls reported same-sex attractions and fantasies (10).

This does not necessarily correlate with assuming a gay, lesbian, or bisexual identity. In a study sample of Massachusetts students, which asked about same-sex experiences rather than self-labels, 6.4% of sexually experienced students reported same-sex sexual contact. In addition, they found that an equal number of male and female adolescents had same-sex experiences (11).

More adolescents are self-identifying as lesbian, gay, and bisexual. D'Augelli collected data in the late '80s and again in the late '90s in social and recreational programs for gay, lesbian, and bisexual youth in America and Canada. His final sample included 542 youths, 62% male and 38% female. He found that 74% identified as gay or lesbian, and 20% reported being bisexual, but mostly gay or lesbian; and 6% said they were bisexual, but equally gay or lesbian and heterosexual. The bisexual group was significantly more represented by females. They also reported being aware of same-sex feelings around age ten for male youth and 11 for female youths. Self-labeling occurred on average five years after initial awareness. This is a significant decrease in the age that sexual minority youth are self-identifying from the literature of only a decade age. More sexual minority youth are self-identifying while they are still of high school age and living at home even if they are not sexually active (7).

Recent studies have shown that same-sex contact occurs a year or two prior to a boy's gay identification, while a girl is more likely to have her first same-sex contact after identifying as lesbian. The context for first same-sex sexual contact and self-labeling were found to be more emotionally or relationship oriented for young women and sexually oriented for young men (8). Although the data on this has varied, it probably represents diverse trajectories that sexual minority youth take in their development (12–14). Many adolescence begin to explore their sexuality during this developmental period. While this is normative for heterosexual youth, sexual minority youth may not have this experience, due to stigma and internalized homophobia, which may delay the exploration of their sexuality (1).

Sexual minority youth face similar and different developmental tasks than their heterosexual peers as they try to assimilate this aspect of their identity into their lives and their social and emotional relationships. Adolescents who are raised in families and communities where heterosexuality is considered normative often hide or deny their same-sex feelings and interests. The implications of this for identity development are unknown. Since many of these teens are being raised in families where the parents have a different sexual orientation, it is difficult to make use of parental identifications to help with the process of self-exploration (15).

Increased homosexual and bisexual role models are a result of a shifting culture, with greater tolerance for homosexuality. A virtual community now exists where youth can explore the notion that distinct and rigidly defined categories of sexual arousal, attractions, fantasies, and behaviors are not necessarily concordant with individual feelings and experiences. Teens have more access to discourse about sexuality through TV, books, magazines, school and community support groups, and the Internet. The deconstruction of the heterosexual paradigm as uniquely normative has allowed the possibility for more youths to begin to experience both the social and emotional incorporation of a sexual minority identity. D'Augelli found that even though society has become more accepting, "youths spent one-third of their lives aware of same-sex feelings but not revealing this to others (7)." But simultaneously, increasing numbers of high school students today personally know someone who is in a sexual minority. A recent *Washington Post*/Henry J. Kaiser Family Foundation/Harvard University sponsored survey noted that 57% of Washington, DC–area teens had a friend who is gay or lesbian (16).

In his study, D'Augelli found that half of the sexual minority males and three-quarters of the females had had heterosexual experiences, with more females having had heterosexual sex prior to having a same-sex experience. More males (84%) than females (60%) in this study were aware of their same-sex feelings prior to engaging in heterosexual sex (7). Sexual identity, sexual behavior, and sexual orientation are not stable or necessarily congruent for many adolescents during this period of development. This is particularly relevant for the mental health clinician who relies on the description of sexual behavior to define a patient's sexual orientation or sexual identity.

ADOLESCENT SEXUAL DEVELOPMENT

Kinsey first described a nonbinary understanding of sexual orientation as a spectrum with exclusive homosexuality (0) on one end of a continuum and exclusive heterosexuality (6) on the other. He found that for both men and women sexual behavior could be very fluid over time (17, 18). Sexual behavior in adolescence does not necessarily predict future patterns of sexual arousal, emotional and romantic feelings, or fantasies.

Contributions made by Troiden, Cass, and others helped to begin a dialogue in the field about "normal" development for sexual minorities. The literature on heterosexual identity development is sparse as it is has been considered "normative development" and little research has been done to understand it. Troiden, Cass, and others described a linear stage model of sexual identity development that depicts a pathway to a full integration of one's sexual identity. Troiden used retrospective data from predominantly openly identified gay men with same-sex attractions. Troiden's model begins with a stage of Sensitization. It is described in the literature as a sense of being different from peers (21), with this sense of difference often stemming from nonconforming gender roles. The correlation of early feelings of "being different," and later same-sex orientations, correlates more strongly for men than for women (5, 22, 23).

The second Troiden stage is called Identity Confusion. Beginning in adolescence the youngster wonders if he is homosexual, based on his same-sex sexual interests, and feels threatened by the social mandate for heterosexual identity. This is qualitatively distinct from heterosexual youth who may have transient same-gender sexual interests and experimentation. Such youngsters cope by trying to pass as heterosexual, and may immerse themselves in heterosexual sex to prove to self and others that they are heterosexual.

Troiden's third stage is called Identity Assumption. There is gradual acceptance of one's homosexual identity through contact with gay and lesbian individuals and a supportive homosexual culture, if that is available in the community. Selective self-disclosure occurs first to other openly homosexual youth and adults and then to selected heterosexual peers and adults. Rural and minority youth have a much harder time, the former due to lack of available role models and the latter due to double discrimination or stronger cultural bias against homosexuality within their minority community.

Troiden and Cass expanded on the work of Goffman (24) to describe the impact of stigma on gay and lesbian youth who are consolidating their identities. Such youth tend to use "impression management" skills, as described in the work of Goffman in reference to members of other stigmatized groups who use "covering" defenses, in order to minimize the impact of stigma and the risk of rejection. They do this by selectively disclosing to those most likely to be accepting, while minimizing to others aspects of their identity which they fear might lead to rejection. Goffman also described the process of "spoiled identities," as identity becomes reduced to the stigmatized aspects, denying membership in other aspects of the self, such as ethnicity and religious affiliation. This concept has been extended to sexual minority youth by authors such as Martin in his article *Learning to Hide: The Socialization of the Gay Adolescent*, and has been revisited by many others, including Yoshino's recent book on "covering (25–27)."

Troiden's fourth stage is called Commitment. Homosexual identity is internalized with more acceptance "with the fusion of sexuality and emotionality into a significant whole." There is increasing disclosure to peers and family. Management of stigma shifts from the personal to political and educational efforts in the broader community. Cass adds two additional stages. Stage five is called Identity Pride. This represents a stage where the individual is self-accepting and more involved with the community. Stage six is Synthesis. In this stage identity is fully incorporated into their lives, both socially and professionally (28).

Diamond, Garnets, Savin Williams, Klein, and others have challenged these models of linear progression, and have introduced a concept of a multidimensional approach to sexual identity development (8, 29, 30). Fritz Klein developed an alternative multidimensional model of sexuality, which includes a grid of seven variables: sexual attraction, sexual behavior, sexual fantasies, emotional preference, social preference, self identification, and hetero/homosexual lifestyle, all plotted along a time course (8, 17–20).

Galatzer-Levy addressing clinical aspects of treatment stated, "In non-linear systems models, like epigenetic models, the fact that processes share initial and end points does not indicate that the paths joining these points are the same. Instead it leaves us free, in each case to explore the path taken by the individual and suggests that there will often be multiple paths between various developmental points (31)." Other critiques of earlier linear models include using male retrospective experiences as the norm, and not taking cultural factors into account (30, 32). At the time the linear models were constructed there was little data on the development of sexual identity in women.

Diamond has written extensively on the development of female same-sex orientation. "Women appear more likely to exhibit situational and environmental plasticity in sexual attractions, behavior, and identifications (33)." She argues that thinking about sexual identity development in women as an evolving process may be more helpful in understanding their development with regard to both emotional and sexual attractions. In this study some women maintain a stable same-sex attraction and behaviors over their lifespan and others are more fluid. In another study Lisa Diamond conducted, women with same-sex attractions did not have the same childhood profiles as men. Men were found to have an early age of same-sex attractions, gender atypicality, and an early age of first same-sex contact (5). The sexual minority women she studied were more likely to have had a late and abrupt development of same-sex attractions.

Rosario et al. looked at ethnic and racial differences in the coming-out process. They looked at a sample of black, Latino, and white youths and found that there were no significant differences in the sexual developmental milestones, sexual orientation, sexual behavior, or sexual identity between groups. They found that cultural factors did not impede the formation of identity but might cause a delay in identity integration due to familial and cultural factors. Cultural factors (which include religious beliefs) may delay integration of a gay identity, as manifested by limiting involvement in gay-related social activities, due to the impact of stigma. They reported that black sexual minority youth were involved in fewer gay-related social activities, and also reported less comfort with others knowing about their sexual orientation, and disclosed less frequently to others, than did white youth. Latino youths also disclosed to fewer people than white youth. Black youth reported greater increases in positive attitudes regarding their sexual identity than did white youths over time. Negotiating multiple identities impacted in sexual minority identity formation in males and females of varied ethnic backgrounds (34–37).

Denizet-Lewis writes about the phenomenon of DL, or Down Low, among African-American young men. "Rejecting a gay culture they perceive as white and effeminate, many black men have settled on a new identity, with its own vocabulary and customs and its own name: Down Low." These young men often lead outwardly "straight" lives, and secretly engage in sex with other men. They identify not as gay but as black.

Many are young, urban men who live in a hypermasculine "thug" culture. To be gay is to shame and let down the black community (38).

Joseph Carrier wrote about the youth in Guadalajara, Mexico, where sexual orientation is defined both by gender behavior and sexual practices. "Feminine males are especially denigrated because it is unthinkable that a masculine male could be a 'real homosexual.' Generally speaking, only male receivers in homosexual intercourse are considered 'homosexual'." He also notes that "all people exhibiting traits of the opposite sex are considered to be homosexual (13)." Some racial and ethnic groups present barriers to the expression of one's sexual identity, while others permit it within a defined construct.

A number of authors have also looked at resiliency and coping skills in sexual minority youth. A study by Lewis et al. (39) found that lesbian adults who had lower levels of "stigma consciousness" had fewer negative psychological and physical outcomes. Laseer and Tharinger (40), extending the work of Bandura on social learning theory, noted that gay, lesbian, and bisexual youth utilized a strategy termed "visibility management" to negotiate their environment. This refers to how these youth make decisions about to whom to disclose what, and how to go about disclosing their sexual orientation. This is similar to the work of Goffman regarding "impression management" skills often found among stigmatized groups (24).

Developmental Challenges

All adolescents face unique developmental challenges. There has been debate in the literature about whether sexual minority youth are more at risk. Concerns remain about the sampling bias involved on both sides of the debate. Most of the studies in the past decade have not been longitudinal, but cross sectional, with the preponderance focusing on male gay-identified youth. Many studies inadvertently exclude youth who may engage in same-sex behaviors, but do not self-identify as a sexual minority. In 1994, prior to the societal changes taking place that have supported a sexual minority identity, Savin-Williams wrote "In actuality, the vast majority of gay male, bisexual and lesbian youths cope with their daily, chronic stressors to become healthy individuals who make significant contributions to their culture (41)."

Some sexual minority youth face stress and distress related to their sexual minority status that may lead them to consult a child psychiatrist. Studies conducted in the last decade have found that lesbian, gay, and bisexual youth face increased health risk factors, both physical and emotional, as well as increased health risk behaviors (42), although "the causal link between these stressors and outcomes has not been scientifically established (41)." Increased risk is related to both external and internal stressors. External stress has been defined in the literature as experiences of violence, verbal abuse, rejection, and other acts that are perpetrated against sexual minority youth or those who are assumed to be sexual minority youth (43, 44). The internal stresses that sexual minority youth often face may shift, reflecting developmental factors at different life stages as well as different stages of "coming out," and tend to represent the internalization of society's negative attitudes toward homosexuality (45).

Erik Erikson (46) stated, "the sad truth is that in any system based on suppression, exclusion, and exploitation, the suppressed, excluded, and exploited unconsciously accept the evil image they are made to represent by those who are dominant." As is the case for many minority populations, stigma and shame play powerful roles in the lives and mental wellbeing of lesbian, gay, bisexual, and questioning youth. Stress results from chronic rejection, scapegoating, social isolation, bullying, and physical and verbal assaults (42, 47). Family, peer, and community support for these youngsters can be protective, as noted in the work of Remafedi (48). Gay youth often learn to hide their homosexual orientation by attempting to present themselves as heterosexual. This facade can become a process of deception at all levels, living a lie in order to obtain acceptance in their larger peer group, and keeping a protective distance from peers and parents from whom they hide their homosexuality (25).

Adolescents who disclose a sexual minority identity to their parents may experience increased family conflict, as well as family rejection. Social service agencies have reported that approximately one-third of homeless youth in large urban centers are gay or lesbian (49). A study done by D'Augelli (7) looked at gay, lesbian, and bisexual self-identified youth during two periods: 1987–1989 and 1995–1997 at community centers. There was some geographic as well as cultural diversity in the sampling. He found that 81% of the 542 youth sampled reported verbal abuse related to being a sexual minority youth; "38% had been threatened with physical attacks, 22% had objects thrown at them, 15% had been physically assaulted, 6% had been assaulted with a weapon, and 16% had been sexually assaulted." All of these incidents were reported by the youth as being related to their sexual minority status. Some of this abuse occurred at school, some at home, and some in the community. Fear of being victimized was prevalent. Youths who were aware of their minority sexual orientation at earlier ages, self-identified earlier and self-disclosed earlier, reported more lifetime victimization. Some have reported that highly effeminate boys are targeted more than others as many have had atypical gender roles since childhood and have experienced social ostracism since an early age (50).

In 1989, the United States government's report of the Secretary's Task Force on Youth Suicide showed that suicide was the leading cause of death among sexual minority youth. In this report "up to" 30% was quoted as the percentage of sexual minority youth who commit suicide annually. The author of this report went on to say that "gay youth are 2-3 times more likely to suicide than other youth (51)."

In 1995 the Center for Disease Control and Prevention conducted a school-based survey which was known as the YRBS, or the Youth Risk Behavior Survey. Garafalo et al. used the data from the YRBS and discovered that gay, lesbian, and bisexual youth were more likely than their peers to have been victimized or threatened, and engaged in risk behaviors that included suicide attempts, substance abuse, and sexual risk behaviors. He reviewed the data from male adolescents with multiple same-sex partners and compared them to male adolescents with multiple other sex partners and found the former to have an increased risk of victimization, violent behavior, and substance use. He also looked at suicide risk in sexual minority youth and those who reported "not sure" when asked about sexual orientation. He found a significantly increased frequency of suicide attempts. "Sexual orientation has an independent association with suicide attempts for males, while for females the association of sexual orientation with suicidality may be mediated by drug use and violence/victimization (43, 52)."

Lock and Steiner, using a community sample of approximately 1,800 students in an upper middle class area of high school students ages 12–18, found that gay, lesbian, and bisexual (GLB) youth had higher general health, mental health, and sexual risks, compared to their heterosexual peers (53). This data is consistent with other studies. The increased risk of homelessness for sexual minority youth is due in part to family rejection; with a number of these youth resorting to prostitution and sexually risky behaviors, which leave them vulnerable to STDs, hepatitis, HIV, and pregnancy.

Fergusson et al. studied a birth cohort from Christchurch, New Zealand to age 21 years and found that sexual minority youth are at increased risk of psychiatric disorder and suicidal behavior. In this study they found this to be true for both males and females. Their analysis of their data showed that there were few differences in the social, family, and childhood backgrounds of these youth compared to other cohort members, which lessened the likelihood of a sampling bias (54).

At this time, the National Longitudinal Study of Adolescent Health (Add Health Study) is the most comprehensive study of adolescents in the United States. Of the approximately 12,000 youth who responded, 7% reported having same-sex attraction or relationships. This was found to be slightly more common among males than females. Youth were not asked specifically about sexual identity, but rather experiences and attractions. This broadened the sample from previous studies. Russell and Joyner looked at the data to attempt to better understand previously reported risk of suicidality in sexual minority youth. They found that "regardless of age and family background, males and females who reported same-sex romantic attraction or relationships were more likely than their peers to report suicidal thoughts." Their results were consistent with those reported in a 1989 U.S. government report showing that youth with same-sex orientation were two times more likely than their same-sex peers to attempt suicide, and were more likely than their peers to report suicidal thoughts (55). They looked at risk factors associated with increased suicidal ideation and attempts, and found that these youth were more likely to feel hopeless, depressed, victimized, to abuse alcohol, and to have a close relative or peer attempt suicide. They went further to say that even though these risk factors are similar to suicide risk factors for all adolescents, "there is a strong link between same-sex sexual orientation and adolescent suicidal thoughts and attempts." These convenience samples support that sexual minority youth have a high rate of suicide attempts, although currently no empirical evidence has shown that they are overrepresented among those adolescents who have completed suicide (47, 56, 57).

Others have contested the theory that gay youth are more likely to attempt suicide. Savin Williams feels that many of the studies finding gay youth at higher risk are flawed due to convenience samples, with higher risk groups studied rather than truly normative samples. David Shaffer found that other risk factors such as depression and substance abuse increase the risk of suicide, rather then whether a child is homosexual or bisexual (59). Galatzer-Levy, emphasizing that the vast majority of sexual minority youth emerge as healthy young adults, similar to their heterosexual peers, writes, "It is important that society as a whole come to terms with this new generation of well-adjusted, competent young men and women, who differ from their peers in terms of sexual orientation but little else (58)."

PSYCHO-BIOLOGICAL THEORIES

Charlotte Patterson writes, "Is sexual orientation best thought of as an inborn characteristic determined by genetic factors? Or should it be regarded as socially constructed and malleable across the lifespan?" (60). The answer to this question is unknown. The development of a homosexual identity may be a complex and nonuniform interplay among genetics, in utero exposure to hormones, and neurodevelopmental, dynamic and experiential factors. Given the breadth and fluidity of sexuality, one can theorize that there will never be a simple explanation for the development of sexual orientation (61–63).

Elevated concordance of homosexuality has been identified in several studies of identical male twins separated early in life and raised apart. Concordance for lesbian women has been shown as well, but at a lower rate than for homosexual men. Dean Hamer identified a sequence of markers at the tip of the X chromosome (xq28) in 33 of 40 pairs of homosexual brothers. This finding has not been replicated nor has a similar study been done with lesbian sisters (3, 44, 64–66). Several studies have shown monozygotic male twins to have concordance rates between 52% and 66%, and lower for women at 48%.For dizygotic twins male concordance has been shown to be 22–30% while for women it was 16% (64, 67–69).

The role of prenatal sex hormones in humans in the development of structural differences in the brain and sex-linked behaviors is being explored. Exposure of the fetus to testosterone at six to 12 weeks' gestation alters the neuronal migration in the hypothalamus, preoptic area, corpus callosum, planum temporale, cerebellum, and amygdala. Gorski described an area in the hypothalamus of rats, which he labeled the "sexually dimorphic nucleus" that is eight times larger in males than in females, leading to studies on the hypothalamic nuclei of humans. Allen et al. found that two out of the four anterior hypothalamic interstitial nuclei have been found to be larger in men than in women, with one nucleus larger in heterosexual than in homosexual men.

A study done by LeVay found that this hypothalamic nucleus (INAH3) was two to three times larger in heterosexual men than in women and homosexual men, who had similarly sized nuclei, and postulated that this was linked to prenatal testosterone levels. This study was based on autopsies which included heterosexual and homosexual men who had died of AIDS, and one woman who had died of AIDS. If homosexuality was not listed in the medical record, then the presumption of a heterosexual orientation was made. This study has not been replicated (70).

In 2005 Swedish researchers using pheromones to access sexual arousal in gay and heterosexual men found a connection between sexual orientation and the hypothalamus. Later that year scientists in Vienna announced they had found a master switch for sexual orientation in the fruit fly. Research into this question will continue as scientists pursue the question of the role of genetics in sexual orientation (71).

EVALUATION AND INTERVENTION

In his seminal article from 1982 A. Damien Martin states, "It is my contention that homosexuality is a normal variation in both sexual orientation and sexual behavior (25)." He speaks about the prejudice sexual minority youth face, which he states is similar to other minority groups, but is dissimilar in a significant way. Sexual minority youth often have a different sexual orientation than their parents, and therefore are not able to use positive identification along this dimension to help them navigate this aspect of their identity development. It can be a challenge to access a group supportive of their personal and social identity, especially during adolescence. Due to the necessity to "hide" in order to avoid ostracism and victimization, the "socialization of the gay adolescent becomes a process of deception at all levels, with the ability to play a role assuming primary significance (25)."

Secondary to the need to maintain "normative" sexuality, many sexual minority youth engage in sexual intimacy with opposite-gendered peers secondary to conscious and subconscious fears of being gay. This may also occur secondary to attractions to the opposite sex, peer group pressures, parental pressures, religious and community pressures, and fear of physical and emotional abuse. The impact of such psychosocial forces on development varies individually.

Russell and Consolacion reviewed the Add Health study and found that although the numbers of sexual minority youth were small in this study, they have potential clinical relevance. The data showed that "adolescents engaged in a diverse range of relationships, regardless of their romantic attractions. Most of the 12,000 adolescents responding (93%) reported heterosexual attractions. Of those, 26% were single, 73% were other-sex daters, and 1% were same-sex daters. Among the 7% self-identified sexual minority adolescents, 27% were single, 64% were other-sex daters, and only 9% were same sex daters," highlighting the impact of socially sanctioned dating norms. They found that sexual minority youth who were single were at greatest risk for anxiety and depression, and sexual minority other-sex daters may be at greater risk as well. Sexual minority same-sex daters were most likely to be suicidal (1).

The clinician should be aware of both the internal and external negotiations and compromises that sexual minority youth need to face, and explore the adolescents' identity across the dimensions of emotional and physical attractions, intimate relationships, and behavior. The initial responsiveness and openness of the clinician will set the tone for the therapeutic encounter. Closed-ended questions will often foreclose on the possibility of developing trust and openness on the part of the sexual minority youth, as will a premature resolution of sexual identity. The patient is less likely to speak about same-sex attractions if the clinician assumes a cross-sex attraction. Alternatively, identifying an adolescent with same-sex desires as gay or lesbian, without the adolescent labeling themselves as such, may prohibit exploration of other sex attractions or behaviors.

The exploration of the adolescent's sexuality and positive and negative feelings about their sexual orientation should take place in a therapeutic relationship in which the therapist can remain neutral. The adolescent is vulnerable to the internalization of the stigma associated with being a sexual minority youth. The therapist is similarly vulnerable. If he or she is unaware of this, it may impede both exploration and assimilation of this aspect of the patient's identity. Adolescents may not have conscious access to aspects of their sexual identity that are causing stress and emotional pain, but awareness may emerge through the creation of a safe therapeutic space. Dr. Hanley-Hackenbruck stated in her paper on *Coming Out and Psychotherapy* how "Given that doctor and patient have society's attitudes in common, homophobia will be both a transference and counter transference issue (72)."

Gay youth are emotionally vulnerable due to questions and concerns about disclosing their sexual minority status and the possible consequences on their lives from family, peers, institutions, and themselves (73). Because of their fear of rejection, discrimination, and violence, they often hide it from their parents, teachers, and other important adults. These youth often lack positive role models to support them in the development of their sexual identity. Margolies, Becker and Jackson-Brewer state in their paper *Internalized Homophobia: Identifying and Treating the Oppressor Within* that "Internalized homophobia functions as a defense mechanism resulting from the ego's struggle between rules and desires. Rather than a single entity, internalized homophobia is comprised of a constellation of defense methods. Allowing for individual variations, the cluster usually includes rationalization, denial, projection, and identification with the aggressor (74)."

The therapist is faced with tolerating anxiety about knowing a core part of their patient's identity, which may still be a secret from the parents. Many gay youth are conflicted as they discover that their sexual orientation does not coincide with their families' hopes and dreams for their future. The fear of causing psychic pain to themselves, as well as their parents, often contributes to the adolescent's decision to maintain this core aspect of their identity as a secret. To many parents, their child's homosexual identity is experienced as a fundamental betrayal. Parents' values are often part of the teenagers internalized value system. The parental fantasy about their adolescent's sexuality and sexual orientation is often infused with fantasies about their child's future relationships and creation of a family (78). This fantasy usually assumes heterosexuality. "Sexual orientation for gay men and lesbians is not recognized or acknowledged from birth, but is an achieved status rather than an ascribed status (77)."

Hanley-Hackenbruck writes, "Incorporated into the superego of each potentially gay and lesbian child are proscriptions against homosexual identity. The form, content, and intensity of these internalized attitudes vary and account for much of the variation in both the coming out process and psychotherapy process (72)." Cultural factors linked to stigmatization can impact the decision to disclose to parents as well (75).

The sexual minority identity of an adolescent may be a secret which binds the therapist and the patient together, but complicates work with the family. Bok speaks to the "conflicted ambivalent experience of secrecy" (76), in which one must remain mindful of both the protective and harmful aspects of secrets in a family. The therapist must respect the boundaries of confidentiality. When the adolescent wants to disclose his or her sexual identity to peers, siblings, and parents, the therapist may have a role in helping prepare for the multitude of reactions he or she may face.

As with any patient, the therapist should assess the adolescent's safety with the awareness of the risk factors involved. This should include a mental status exam, substance use history, and a history of violence and victimization in the home, as well as in school and the community. The potential for violence directed toward the patient should be reviewed. The possibility of self-harm should be addressed and includes cutting, eating disorders, substance abuse, unsafe sexual practices, and suicidal ideation. The use of Internet pornography and chat rooms should be assessed along with discussion and education about Internet predators.

Hershberger and D'Augelli looked at resiliency in the face of victimization and found that the primary predictor for mental health was self-acceptance (57). "A general sense of personal worth, coupled with a positive view of their sexual orientation, appears to be critical for the youths' mental health." They found that family support was an important variable that helped the sexual minority youth withstand (low level) emotional and physical attacks in the community. Family support was found to be associated with a greater sense of self-acceptance.

For some families, the discovery of the adolescent's nonheterosexual orientation can lead them to seek a "cure." Reparative Therapy claims to "cure" homosexuality, and is endorsed by groups who view homosexuality as pathology or sinful. Health and mental health professional organizations have rejected this "treatment." They do not support the idea that homosexuality is a mental disorder, or that the emergence of same-gender sexual desires among some adolescents is in any way abnormal or mentally unhealthy. The organizations which have issued public statements denouncing reparative therapy include the American Academy of Pediatrics, the American Psychiatric Association, the American Psychological Association, the National Association of Social Workers, and the American Counseling Association (79). The American Psychiatric Association stated in their 2000 position statement, "APA recommends that ethical practitioners refrain from attempts to change individuals' sexual orientation, keeping in mind the medical dictum to first, do no harm (80)." Such forms of psychotherapy ally with societal homophobia, and seek to increase the distress of gay, lesbian, and bisexual youth in order to effect a "shift" to heterosexuality.

Sexual minority adolescents are developmentally heterogeneous. Many may negotiate this aspect of their identity development without difficulty. Family and community support as well as healthy coping mechanisms will likely impact their psychological wellbeing. Eccles and others have advocated for schools providing environments that do not tolerate harassment. Support networks for parents of sexual minority youth have also been found to be helpful in the renegotiation of the parent's assumptions and expectations they hold for their children (81).

Gay-Straight Alliances (GSA) now exist in over 2,000 schools across the country, with the first started by Virginia Uribe in 1984 as Project 10, in California. Schools have played an important role in the positive changes that have occurred in peer groups with sexual minority youth. GSAs serve as sources of support for youth, even those too fearful to attend, and raise school awareness of the needs of sexual minority youth. In 1989 Project 10 East, located in Cambridge, MA was founded. This GSA was among the most popular school clubs, and was largely attended by "straight allies" of gay peers. In 1992 a Governor's Commission on Gay and Lesbian Youth was formed in Massachusetts, in part due to lobbying efforts of members of Project 10 East. This led to the Massachusetts "Safe Schools Act," which explicitly bans discrimination against sexual minority youth. As a result of this act there are close to 200 schools participating in the program in that state alone. A primary focus was to educate teachers and staff, and to support sexual minority youth in creating safe school environments where they could learn.

The Gay, Lesbian and Straight Education Network (GLSEN) is a valuable resource to access support in schools, although this is limited in parts of the country. The fall 2004 GLSEN newsletter *Respect* highlighted the need for national protection in schools for GBLT youth, finding that two-thirds of all elementary and secondary students in this country have no explicit school protections from harassment and discrimination based on their sexual orientation and gender identity/expression. Parents, Families and Friends of Lesbian and Gays (PFLAG) is another national organization that has chapters and support groups in all 50 states, offering support to parents.

CONCLUSION

Sexual minority youth have much in common with their heterosexual peers, and face similar developmental tasks. However, their path is complicated by the powerful forces of stigma, which deeply impacts their mental health, their core identity, and their sense of being a competent, "normal" sexual being able to connect with others on an intimate level. Mental health professionals can offer a safe space in which such youth can find acknowledgment, support, and fortification, allowing them to continue navigating their life course. Self-acceptance and family support play an important role in the psychological wellbeing of these adolescents (57).

Sexuality is a core aspect of identity. Sexual identity emerges over time, impacted by biological, familial, and environmental forces. For those whose identity outcome is not acceptable in their communities and families, development can be strained. In addition, the overwhelming psychic burden contributes to the development of symptoms of emotional illness, and for some serious psychopathology. For others, greater resilience may alter the outcome, due to the capacity to respond to internal and external conflicts without the same psychological cost. As culture shifts and transforms, formerly ostracized minorities are sometimes finding themselves to be accepted members of society. This has allowed some sexual minority youth to exist without the same pressures to develop "covering" defenses, or to "pass" as heterosexual. However, many others do not have this freedom due to cultural, familial, or intrapsychic factors.

The role of the child and adolescent psychiatrist is to understand the child regardless of what self-labels are used, and to help facilitate the integration of their sexuality with other aspects of their identity. The hoped for outcome is the emergence of a child less "spoiled" by stigma, and less "reduced" to any one aspect of their identity, a person well equipped for the emotional growth needed to emerge as a complex and multidimensional individual.

References

1. Russell ST, Consolacion TB: Adolescent romance and emotional health in the United States: beyond binaries. *J Clin Child Adolesc Psychol* 32(4):499–508, 2003.
2. Pescovitz OH Eugster EA: *Pediatric Endocrinology: Mechanisms, Manifestations, and Management.* Philadelphia, Lippincott Williams & Wilkins. xii, 839, 2004.
3. Bailey JM, Zucker KJ: Childhood Sex-Typed Behavior and Sexual Orientation: A Conceptual Analysis and Quantitative Review, *Developmental Psychology* 31(1):43–55, 1995.
4. Savin-Williams RC: The new gay teenager. *Adolescent lives; 3.* Cambridge, MA, Harvard University Press 2005, xi, 272.
5. Diamond L: Development of Sexual Orientation Among Adolescent and Young Adult Women, *Developmental Psychology* 34(5):1085–1095, 1998.
6. Freud S: Analysis Terminable and Interminable (1937). *The Complete Psychological Works of Sigmond Freud.* Vol. 23, London: Hogarth Press, 211–253, 1964.
7. Omoto AM, HS Kurtzman: Sexual Orientation and Mental Health: Examining Identity and Development in Lesbian, Gay, and Bisexual People, 1st ed. Contemporary Perspectives on Lesbian, Gay, and Bisexual Psychology. Washington, DC, *American Psychological Association* xi, 323, 2006.
8. Savin-Williams RC, LM, Diamond: Sexual Identity Trajectories among Sexual-Minority Youths: Gender Comparisons. *Arch Sex Behav* 29(6):607–627, 2000.
9. Hooker E: The Adjustment of the Male Overt Homosexual. *J Proj Tech* 21(1), 18–31, 1957.
10. Remafedi G, et al.: Demography of Sexual Orientation in Adolescents. *Pediatrics* 89(4 Pt 2): 714–721, 1992.
11. Faulkner AH, Cranston K: Correlates of Same-Sex Sexual Behavior in a Random Sample of Massachusetts High School Students. *Am J Public Health*, 88(2):262–266, 1998.
12. D'Augelli AR, Hershberger SL: Lesbian, Gay, and Bisexual Youth in Community Settings: Personal Challenges and Mental Health Problems. *Am J Community Psychol* 21(4):421–48, 1993.
13. Herdt GH, Boxer A: *Children of Horizons: How Gay and Lesbian Teens are Leading a New Way Out of the Closet*, Boston, Beacon Press, xxi, 290, 1993.
14. Rosario M, Rotheram-Borus MJ, Reid H: Gay-related Stress and its Correlates Among Gay and Bisexual Male Adolescents of Predominantly Black and Hispanic Background. *Journal of Community Psychiatry* 24:136–159, 1996.
15. Rotheram-Borus MJ Fernandez MI: Sexual orientation and Developmental challenges Experienced by Gay and Lesbian Youths. *Suicide Life Threat Behav*, 25 Suppl: 26–34; 1995 discussion 35–39.
16. Morin R: What Teens Really Think, In: the *Washington Post.* Washington, D.C. 14–19, 2005.
17. Kinsey AC, Pomeroy WB, Martin CE: Sexual Behavior in the Human Male. Philadelphia, WB Saunders Co, 1948 xv, 804.
18. Kinsey AC, Institute for Sex Research: *Sexual Behavior in the Human Female*, Philadelphia, Saunders, 1953, xxx, 842.
19. Fausto-Sterling A: *Sexing the Body: Gender Politics and the Construction of Sexuality*, 1st ed. New York,: Basic Books, 2000 xii, 473.
20. Klein F ed: The Need to View Sexual Orientation as a Multivariable Dynamic Process: A Theoretical Perspective In: McWhirter D Sanders SA Reinisch JM (eds): *Homosexuality/Heterosexuality: Concepts of Sexual Orientation*, Oxford University Press, New York, 1990, 277–82.
21. Troiden RR: The Formation of Homosexual Identities. *J Homosex* 17(1-2):43–73, 1989.
22. Green R: *The "Sissy Boy Syndrome" and the Development of Homosexuality.* New Haven, CT, Yale University Press, 1987.
23. Zugar B: Early Effeminate Behavior in Boys: Outcome and Significance for Homosexuality. *Journal of Nervous and Mental Disease* 172:90–97, 1984.
24. Goffman E: *Stigma; Notes on the Management of Spoiled Identity.* Englewood Cliffs, Prentice Hall. p. 147, 1963.
25. Martin AD: Learning to Hide: the socialization of the gay adolescent. *Adolesc Psychiatry* 10:52–65, 1982.

26. Yoshino K: *Covering: The Hidden Assault on our Civil Rights*. 1st ed. New York, Random House, p. 282, xiv, 2006.
27. Eliason MJ: Identity Formation for Lesbian, Bisexual, and Gay Persons: Beyond a "Minoritizing" View. *J Homosex* 30(3): p. 31–58, 1996.
28. Cass VC: Homosexual identity formation: A theoretical model. *Journal of Homosexuality* 4:219–235, 1979.
29. Garnets LD: Sexual orientations in perspective. *Cultur Divers Ethnic Minor Psychol* 8(2):115–129, 2002.
30. Peplau LA et al.: The Development of Sexual Orientation in Women. *Annu Rev Sex Res* 10: p. 70–99, 1999.
31. Galatzer-Levy: Chaotic Possibilities: Toward a new model of development. *International Journal of Psychoanalysis* 85:419–442, 2004.
32. Chung YB, K., M, Assessment of sexual orientation in lesbian/gay/bisexual studies. *Journal of Homosexuality* 30:49–62, 1996.
33. Diamond L: A new view of lesbian subtypes: stable versus fluid identity trajectories over an 8-year period. *Psychology of Women* 29:119–128, 2005.
34. Rosario M, Schrimshaw EW, Hunter J: Ethnic/racial differences in the coming-out process of lesbian, gay, and bisexual youths: a comparison of sexual identity development over time. *Cultur Divers Ethnic Minor Psychol* 10(3):215–228, 2004.
35. Dube EM, Savin-Williams RC: Sexual identity development among ethnic sexual-minority male youths. *Dev Psychol* 35(6):1389–1398, 1999.
36. Parks CA, Hughes TL, Matthews AK: Race/ethnicity and sexual orientation: intersecting identities. *Cultur Divers Ethnic Minor Psychol* 10(3):241–254, 2004.
37. Consolacion TB, Russell ST, Sue S: Sex, race/ethnicity, and romantic attractions: multiple minority status adolescents and mental health. *Cultur Divers Ethnic Minor Psychol* 10(3):200–214, 2004.
38. Denizet-Lewis B: *Living (and dying) on the down low*. New York, *New York Times*. 30, 2003.
39. Lewis R, et al.: Stigma Consciousness, Social Constraints, and Lesbian Well-Being. *Journal of Counseling Psychology* 53:48–56, 2006.
40. Lasser J, Tharinger D: Visibility management in school and beyond: a qualitative study of gay, lesbian, bisexual youth. *J Adolesc* 26(2):233–44, 2003.
41. Savin-Williams RC: Verbal and physical abuse as stressors in the lives of lesbian, gay male, and bisexual youths: associations with school problems, running away, substance abuse, prostitution, and suicide. *J Consult Clin Psychol* 62(2):261–269, 1994.
42. Bontempo DE D'Augelli AR: Effects of at-school victimization and sexual orientation on lesbian, gay, or bisexual youths' health risk behavior. *J Adolesc Health* 30(5):364–374, 2002.
43. Garofalo R, et al.: The association between health risk behaviors and sexual orientation among a school-based sample of adolescents. *Pediatrics* 101(5):895–902, 1998.
44. Bailey JM, et al.: A family history study of male sexual orientation using three independent samples. *Behav Genet* 29(2):79–86, 1999.
45. Friedman RC, Downey JI: Homosexuality. *N Engl J Med* 331(14):923–930, 1994.
46. Erikson EH: *Childhood and Society*. New York, Norton, 445, 1993.
47. DuRant RH, Krowchuk DP Sinal SH: Victimization, use of violence, and drug use at school among male adolescents who engage in same-sex sexual behavior. *J Pediatr* 133(1):113–118, 1998.
48. Remafedi G, Farrow JA, Deisher RW: Risk factors for attempted suicide in gay and bisexual youth. *Pediatrics* 87(6):869–875, 1991.
49. Kruks G: Gay and lesbian homeless/street youth: special issues and concerns. *J Adolesc Health* 12(7):515–518, 1991.
50. Remafedi G: *Death by denial: studies of suicide in gay and lesbian teenagers*. 1st ed. Boston, Alyson Publications, 205, 1994.
51. Gibson P: U.S. Department of Health and Human Services. Report of the Secretary's Task Force on Youth Suicide: Prevention and Interventions in Youth Suicide. In: *U.S. Department of Health and Human Services*. 1989.
52. Garofalo R, et al.: Sexual orientation and risk of suicide attempts among a representative sample of youth. *Arch Pediatr Adolesc Med* 153(5):487–493, 1999.
53. Lock J, Steiner H: Gay, lesbian, and bisexual youth risks for emotional, physical, and social problems: results from a community-based survey. *J Am Acad Child Adolesc Psychiatry* 38(3):297–304, 1999.
54. Fergusson DM, Horwood LJ, Beautrais AL: Is sexual orientation related to mental health problems and suicidality in young people? *Arch Gen Psychiatry* 56(10):876–880, 1999.
55. Russell ST Joyner K: Adolescent sexual orientation and suicide risk: evidence from a national study. *Am J Public Health* 91(8):1276–1281, 2001.
56. Rosario M, et al.: Gay-related stress and emotional distress among gay, lesbian, and bisexual youths: a longitudinal examination. *J Consult Clin Psychol* 70(4):967–975, 2002.
57. Hersberger S, D'Augelli AR: The Impact of Victimization on the Mental Health and Suicidality of Lesbian, Gay and Bisexual Youth. *Developmental Psychology* 31(1):65–74, 1995.
58. Cohler BJ, Galatzer-Levy RM: *The Course of Gay and Lesbian Lives: Social and Psychoanalytic Perspectives*. Chicago, University of Chicago Press, xviii, 537, 2000.
59. Schaffer D, et al.: Sexual orientation in adolescents who commit suicide. *Suicide and Life Threat Behavior* 25:64–71, 1995.
60. Patterson C: Sexual Orientation and Human Development: An Overview. *Developmental Psychology* 31(1): 3–11, 1995.
61. Meyer-Bahlburg H, et al.: *Prenatal Estrogens and the Development of Homosexual Orientation. Developmental Psychology* 31(1):12–21, 1995.
62. Byne W, Parsons B: Human sexual orientation. The biologic theories reappraised. *Arch Gen Psychiatry* 50(3):228–239, 1993.
63. Berenbaum S, Snyder E: Early hormonal influences on childhood sex-typed activity and playmate preferences: implications for the development of sexual orientation. *Developmental Psychology* 31(1):31–42, 1995.
64. Bailey JM, et al.: Heritable factors influence sexual orientation in women. *Arch Gen Psychiatry* 50(3):217–223, 1993.
65. Hamer DH, et al.: A linkage between DNA markers on the X chromosome and male sexual orientation. *Science* 261(5119):321–327, 1993.
66. Turner WJ: Homosexuality, type 1: an Xq28 phenomenon. *Arch Sex Behav* 24(2):109–134, 1995.
67. Bailey JM, Pillard RC: A genetic study of male sexual orientation. *Arch Gen Psychiatry* 48(12):1089–1096, 1991.
68. Perrin EC, ebrary Inc: *Sexual orientation in child and adolescent health care*. 2002 [cited; 199].
69. Whitam FL, Diamond M, Martin J: Homosexual orientation in twins: a report on 61 pairs and three triplet sets. *Arch Sex Behav* 22(3):187–206, 1993.
70. LeVay S: A difference in hypothalamic structure between heterosexual and homosexual men. *Science* 253(5023): 1034–1037, 1991.
71. Swidey, N: *What Makes People Gay?*, in *Boston Globe*. 2005: Boston. p. 33–37.
72. Hanley-Hackenbruck P: "Coming Out" and Psychotherapy. *Psychiatric Annals* 18(1):29–32, 1988.
73. Rotheram-Borus MJ, Marelich WD, Srinivasan S: HIV risk among homosexual, bisexual, and heterosexual male and female youths. *Arch Sex Behav* 28(2):159–177, 1999.
74. Margolies L, Becker M, Jackson-Brewer K: *Internalized homophobia: identifying and treating the oppressor within*. In: BLP Collectives (ed): *Lesbian Psychologies: explorations and challenges*, Chicago: University of Illinois Press, 229–242, 1987.
75. Meyer IH: Prejudice, social stress, and mental health in lesbian, gay, and bisexual populations: conceptual issues and research evidence. *Psychol Bull* 129(5):674–697, 2003.
76. Bok S: *Secrets: on the Ethics of Secrets and Relevation*. New York, Vintage, 1983.
77. Weinberg MS, Williams CJ, Pryor DW: Dual attraction: understanding bisexuality. New York, Oxford University Press, x, 437 1994.
78. Savin-Williams RC, Ream GL: Sex variations in the disclosure to parents of same-sex attractions. *J Fam Psychol* 17(3):429–438, 2003.
79. NARTH: *American Counseling Association Passes Resolution to Oppose Reparative Therapy*. 1999 [cited; available from: <http://www.narth.com/docs/acaresolution.html>].
80. APA: *COPP Position Statement on Therapies Focused on Attempts to Change Sexual Orientation Reparative or Conversion Therapies*. 2000.
81. Eccles TA, et al.: More normal than not: a qualitative assessment of the developmental experiences of gay male youth. *J Adolesc Health* 35(5):425 e11–8, 2004.

CHAPTER 1.8 ■ INTERNATIONAL CHILD AND ADOLESCENT MENTAL HEALTH

MYRON L. BELFER AND MAURICE EISENBRUCH

GOAL

This chapter delineates areas of concern in international child and adolescent mental health and focuses on issues of particular clinical import to child and adolescent psychiatrists and other child mental health clinicians. Many of the topics that are addressed are now relevant to domestic practice given widespread global immigration patterns.

OVERVIEW

International child and adolescent mental health embraces the world view on the place of children in society, the appreciation of diverse behavioral styles, the identification of psychopathology, and the setting of priorities for the use of scarce resources. As noted in the seminal articles on child psychiatry in developing countries (1–3), child and adolescent mental health is influenced by the economics of countries and societies within countries, by the internal and external displacement of children and adolescents through war and catastrophe, by the role of the child in the family, and by the place of women in society. New knowledge and greater recognition of the impact on children of exposure to trauma, sexual and physical abuse, inhumane living and working situations, inadequate health care, and drug abuse have heightened interest in approaches to ameliorating the impact on child and adolescent health and mental health of these potentially pathogenic influences. It is a challenge to child and adolescent psychiatrists and allied professionals to be active participants in understanding the nature of the problems faced and in being a part of the solution (4).

The overall health and wellbeing of children are international concerns. All countries with the exception of the United States of America have ratified the 1989 United Nations Convention on the Rights of the Child (5, 6). It commits countries to "ensure that all children have the right to develop physically and mentally to their full potential, to express their opinions freely, and to be protected against all forms of abuse and exploitation." The concern among some countries was the perception that ratification of the treaty would intrude on sovereign rights and/or traditional views of the child in a dependent position in society. In the end these concerns did not impede ratification but do impact implementation. In some countries that are party to the treaty, the affirmation of the rights of children has not resulted in benign policies toward the protection of children from harm or the fostering of positive development.

In the international arena, and increasingly in multicultural societies, child mental health and child psychopathology cannot be gauged solely from a Western perspective. It is simplistic to state, but meaningful to understand, that what may appear pathologic in one country or society, or to one cultural or subcultural group within a country, may be deemed normative or adaptive in another. This does not imply that it may not be helpful to have a consensus about a frame of reference regarding psychopathologic conditions, but the interested party must keep an open mind in attributing cause to behaviors, interpreting responses to events, or judging parental or familial interactions with children. The complexity of understanding children and adolescents embraces anthropologic, social, psychological, political, and rights dimensions. For the domestic practitioner, understanding the culture of the individual is important. For example, Murthy (7) reports that studies have found that suicide rates among immigrants are more closely aligned to the rates in the country of origin than to the rates in the country of adoption. Generally, suicide rates of immigrant populations are higher than in the country of origin. The methods of suicide are those used traditionally in the culture of origin. Canino et al. (8) also documented the persistence of the importance of culture-bound syndromes.

In many resource-poor countries, educational institutions represent the most coherent system embracing children and adolescents. As never before, the value placed on education in societies is being emphasized as agrarian pursuits have become commercialized or made nonviable. In resource-poor countries, the impact of technology is differentially affecting parts of society. On the one hand, technologic advance offers an unprecedented opportunity to the educated, but on the other, it accelerates inequality with the less educated. Urbanization combines with the technology revolution further to challenge accustomed ways that may stress individuals and families (9). Children and adolescents, as students or as part of a family, experience new stresses that convey either advantage or disadvantage, depending on access, intelligence, and resources. In response to these changes in society, resilience-building programs in schools, along with primary care health programs in communities, have evolved. While the emphasis on education may be profound in urban settings in resource-poor countries, the role of traditional healing for child mental health disorders, especially in rural settings, remains powerful (10–15). For instance, in Cambodia, the taxonomies and explanatory models of childhood illnesses are embedded in powerful beliefs about the role of ancestral spirits and the preceding mother from the child's previous incarnation (16).

The role and responsibilities of child and adolescent psychiatrists and other child mental health professionals vary in resource-poor countries. The competencies of the child and adolescent psychiatrist must fit the needs of the society in which they exist. For example, epilepsy and mental retardation clearly fall within the expected clinical competencies of child and adolescent psychiatrists in resource-poor countries but not in resource-rich countries. The infrastructure in some countries post conflict may have decimated the child mental health workforce. In Cambodia, for example, where the country's entire infrastructure, including the health system, was destroyed during the Khmer Rouge regime none of 43 surviving medical doctors in Cambodia were psychiatrists (17). When child psychiatry is a very scarce resource, there may be the opportunity for only a consultative role, limited diagnostics, and an inability to be part of or to stimulate discussion of national policy. Child and adolescent psychiatrists coming to resource-poor countries may play a vital role in educating others but must be willing to increase their cultural competence, self-reflection and in this way to increase their mindfulness of the local cultural context, inherent capacity of the existing systems, and ways to ensure the provision of appropriate education.

In understanding the impact of child and adolescent psychiatric disorders, it is not sufficient to understand diagnosis alone. Significant gains have been made in raising the consciousness about the mental health of children and adolescents, as well as adults, by bringing attention to the "burden" of mental illness (18) The global burden of disease is now most often measured in disability-adjusted life-years (DALYs). This approach makes possible a more standardized assessment of the burden of disease as measured by lost opportunity, diminished function, and the cost of treatment and rehabilitation, and it has gained a supportive response from policymakers. From the child mental health perspective, DALYs have limitations in that they do not quantify negative or positive effects of behaviors but only address outcomes. As a result, the importance of behaviors that start during childhood and adolescence but result in disease and death only later in life may be underestimated by this approach.

CONTEXTUAL CONCERNS ASSOCIATED WITH MENTAL DYSFUNCTION

Displacement

The global problem of displacement from family, home, community, and country are of enormous importance to the mental health of populations. Displacement by war resulted in approximately 21.5 million refugees in 1999. An additional 30 million, 80% of whom are children and women, were displaced internally. Fullilove (19) emphasizes the importance of "place" in the healthy development of individuals. Sampson et al. (20) specifically address the importance of the community as a mediator and contributor to the impact of violence on children and adolescents. The delineation of the importance of "collective efficacy" in communities is an important concept when one considers the impact of imposed poverty, housing disruption, and displacement in ethnic conflicts affecting previously closely aligned groups. In resource-poor countries, the notion of "place" and community are of equal or greater importance. The disruption of traditional communities by war, famine, and natural disaster leave children and adolescents in vulnerable situations that affect mental health. Internal displacement by war and famine leads to the breakup of families, months and years of uncertainty, disruption of education, and physical illness. Forced emigration and the loss of parents and relatives in war often mean abandonment or orphaning of children and adolescents. Although these stressors may serve to demonstrate the enormous resiliency of youth, they often lead to depression, suicide, and a range of stress responses.

The problems of displacement from homes, families, communities, and countries affect children in a host of ways. Zivic (21), in a study of Croatian children during war, found significantly higher depressive and phobic symptoms in displaced refugee children than in local children in stable social conditions. Laor et al. (22), in a developmental study of Israeli children exposed to Scud missile attacks, found higher externalizing and stress symptoms in displaced children as opposed to those able to maintain family and community connections. Children in these circumstances may find themselves without the protection and support of parents at critical junctures in their lives. Children are forced to act in more mature ways far earlier than normal development would dictate or allow. Displaced children are faced with exposure to war and violence that may have included seeing family members murdered. Less often, but even more horrific, some children have been forced into being the murderers of their family or conscripted to serve as child soldiers. Others find themselves either displaced to other countries or internally displaced and left to fend for themselves. Street children engage in survival tactics that include criminal activity and prostitution. In an effort to find a context for survival, the formation of youth gangs is increasingly evident, especially in societies where there is a lapse in government organization and control. More often than not, the children are the victims rather than the perpetrators.

Eisenbruch et al. note that one out of every 275 persons on Earth is "of concern" to the United Nations High Commissioner for Refugees (23). More than 21 million are displaced within their own country, a 25 percent increase from the year before. Eighty per cent of refugees are women and children (24). Families face the added stress of high infant mortality rates, and resort where possible to culturally familiar coping strategies (15). War brings in its wake many unaccompanied minors who face life without their parents (25).

Many refugees live in camps that have become "total institutions" with the attendant "process of mortification" (26). Dependency is a feature in many camps and especially in those that reproduce the authoritarian regimes from which the refugees escaped (27). Others are suffering from the multiple traumatic effects of torture. An outbreak of peace may mean fewer violent deaths, but entering the repatriation and resettlement phase of the cycle is yet another challenge for the disempowered (28, 29).

Children Exposed to Conflict

The priority concern of international child and adolescent mental health is often the acute and continuing tragedies that involve youth in armed conflict or its aftermath. Eighty percent of the victims of war are reported to be children and women (30). The result of armed conflict is often displacement externally as refugees or asylum seekers or internally within settings of civil war. Thabet and Vostanis (31) investigated anxiety symptoms and disorders in children living in the Gaza strip and their relation to social adversities. Children completed the revised manifest anxiety scale (a questionnaire with yes/no answers for 28 anxiety items and nine lie items), and teachers completed the Rutter scale (a questionnaire of 26 items of child mental health problems rated on a scale of 0–2: "certainly applies," "applies somewhat," "doesn't apply"). Children reported high rates of significant anxiety problems and teachers reported high rates of mental health problems that would justify clinical assessment. Anxiety problems, particularly negative cognitions, increased with age and were significantly higher among girls. Low socioeconomic status (father unemployed or unskilled worker) was the strongest predictor of general mental health problems. Living in inner city areas or camps, both common among refugees, was strongly associated with anxiety problems.

Thabet et al. (32) examined the mental health profile among 322 Arab children living in the Gaza strip. Western categories of mental health problems did not clearly emerge from the factor analysis, the main difference appearing to operate in parents' perceptions of emotional problems in preschool children. The authors warn of the need to establish indigenously meaningful constructs within this population and culture, and subsequently revise measures of child mental health problems

More attention is needed to culturally appropriate trauma therapy for children. Culture mediates the possible range of child responses (33). More than half of children exposed to war meet the criteria of PTSD (34), levels of stress were related to war exposure (35), the Impact of Event Scale (IES) persists after the war (36), and those who do are at higher risk of comorbid psychiatric diagnosis (37).

"Child Soldiers" and Exploitation of Children

In the turmoil of some resource-poor countries, children are now being forced to become child soldiers, and others are drawn into the conflict as sexual slaves. Child soldiers reportedly suffer posttraumatic stress disorder (38–43). Somasundaram states that to prevent children becoming soldiers we need first to understand why children choose to fight due to push factors (traumatization, brutalization, deprivation, institutionalized violence, and sociocultural factors) and pull factors (military drill from early childhood), as well as society's complicity (44).

These horrific experiences place an as yet undefined burden on the psychological development of the victim. Understanding these experiences may shed additional light on the extremes to which resiliency may allow future healthy development, but perhaps more likely it will demonstrate the more permanent scarring evidenced in disturbed interpersonal relationships, distorted defenses, heightened aggression, reduced empathy, and self-destructive behavior. The data are not yet available to ascertain whether these young people evidence posttraumatic stress disorder (PTSD) in the classic sense or whether, because of the early age of induction into the culture of war, they develop in a different way as a survival response. Huge challenges face child mental health clinicians in helping to reclaim the lives of former child soldiers (45, 46).

As for trafficking in children, worldwide, an estimated 1 million children are forced into prostitution every year and the total number of prostituted children could be as high as 10 million (47). Children are trafficked worldwide (48–56). The most urgent attention is paid to combating the trafficking (57), but the management of the psychological sequelae for the children will need to be given further attention. Nongovernmental organizations have been taking a lead in developing programs for children and adolescents freed from trafficking. Another issue of concern is the trafficking of children for child labor and other forms of exploitation. The International Labor Organization has taken this up as a major concern (58). The psychological consequences of child labor are complex, involving distorted relationships of children to their families and the assumption of adult roles prematurely.

HIV/AIDS

In sub-Saharan Africa, Russia, and parts of Asia, acquired immunodeficiency syndrome (AIDS) is now a pandemic. Special attention needs to be given to the consequences of AIDS on children and youth. The direct impact on children and adolescents is evident in India, other parts of Asia, and Africa, where sexual exploitation has led to a high incidence of youth infected, with the inevitable outcome of death as a result of lack of available treatment. An estimated 1.5 million children under 15 years old are living with human immunodeficiency virus (HIV) infection or AIDS (59). More than one-fourth of the young population in sub-Saharan Africa is infected. Among the ten most affected countries all in sub-Saharan Africa, approximately 6 million children younger than 15 lost their mother or both parents to AIDS.

As documented by Carlson and Earls (61), whether through social policy as evidenced in the Leagane children of Romania, or as the consequence of the pandemic of AIDS, the rearing of children in orphanages or in other situations that deprive children of appropriate stimulation and nurturance has potentially long-lasting consequences for societies. Those infected but struggling with the illness face the prospect of having to adjust to declining physical and mental functioning and often living isolated lives. Thus, the mental health consequences of AIDS as a chronic and pervasive illness must be considered. There is the obvious concern with the direct effect of AIDS on the youth with manifestations of neuropsychological dysfunction including dementia, depression, and other disorders, which go largely untreated. These children and adolescents living as orphans or in stigmatized environments are vulnerable because of the loss of parent figures, malnutrition, and disenfranchisement from societies that have a stigmatized view of AIDS-affected and HIV-infected persons.

The mental health consequences are similar in the international arena and are well documented in U.S. studies (60). The caution in developing countries is that recognition of the neuropsychological consequences will be overshadowed by the totality of the devastation. This lack of recognition of depression, dementing illness, and other consequences of HIV infection may contribute to the continuing spread of the epidemic.

Substance Abuse

Substance abuse in children and adolescents is a worldwide problem (62). In resource-poor countries, the problem is of no less importance than in Western countries and exacts a tremendous toll in terms of morbidity and mortality. Illicit drugs and psychoactive substances not defined as drugs of abuse (such as khat, inhalants, and alcohol) are used by youth regardless of economic circumstance or religious prohibition. Remarkably, in some Muslim countries, alcohol use and abuse are significant contributors to psychological morbidity. Khat or miraa (*Catha edulis*) is used extensively in East Africa and the Middle East. In Somalia, Ethiopia, and Kenya, the leaves of khat are chewed at all levels of society from about the age of ten (63). Khat may induce a mild euphoria and excitement that can progress to hypomania. In youth, khat use, especially if it is combined with the use of other psychoactive substances, may lead to psychosis.

Homeless street children are now found worldwide and appear particularly vulnerable to substance abuse and other high-risk behavior (64). Senayayake et al. (65) studied the background, life styles, health, and prevalence of abuse of street children in Colombo. Family disintegration was mentioned as the cause for life on the streets by 36%; child labor was reported in 38%; 16% admitted to being sexually abused; 20% were tobacco smokers. Homeless children also are prominent among those groups using inhalants and who are caught in cycles of physical and sexual abuse, often under the influence of drugs. Road accidents among those using drugs are also high.

Solvent and inhalant use is associated with poor economies. In South America, inhalant use is a dominant factor in the presentation of youth affected by psychoactive substances. In São Paolo, Brazil it is reported that up to 25% of children age 9 to 18 years abuse solvents (66). In the Sudan, gasoline is the inhalant of choice, whereas in Mexico, Brazil, and elsewhere in Latin America, paint thinner, plastic cement, shoe dye, and industrial glue are often used. Solvent use is also found among the aboriginal groups in Australia and on Native Canadian reservations (67). In Mexico, three of every 1,000 people between the ages of 14 and 24 years use inhalants on a regular basis (68). These figures do not include two high-risk groups, the homeless population and those less than 14 years old, whose rates of inhalant abuse are much greater. Several community studies carried out in different parts of Mexico show that starting ages are as young as five or six years (68). Data suggest that the percentage of young people using inhalants decreases with age, as other substances such as alcohol and marijuana are substituted. Inhalant use decreases as educational level increases (69).

Wittig et al. (70) examine the hypothesis that drug use among Honduran street children is a function of developmental social isolation from cultural and structural influences. Data from 1,244 children working and/or living on the streets of Tegucigalpa are described, separating "market" from "street" children. The latter group is then divided into those who sniff glue and those who do not to identify salient distinguishing factors. Family relations, length of time on the street, and delinquency are the most important factors.

Forster et al. (71) studied the self-reported activities engaged in by children found wandering on the streets of Porto Alegre, Brazil, aiming to describe their drug abuse habits and practice of thefts or mendicancy. Regular abuse of inhalants was reported much more frequently by the street subgroup of children, reaching a prevalence of 40%. The practice of theft was self-reported mainly by the children from the street group and only by the ones who used illicit drugs. These results show that very poor children might spend many hours of the day by themselves in the streets of a big city accompanied by children who are never under adult supervision. In spite of being alone for some hours a day and making friends with others who might use drugs, having a family and regularly attending school decreases the risk of delinquent acts and drug use.

Violence and Abuse

Violence to and by children and adolescents now appears to be all too prevalent worldwide (72). Bullying, corporal punishment, victimization of parents by children and adolescents has now been reported worldwide. It is beyond the scope of this chapter to address all forms of violence; it will focus on specifics related to child abuse. Understanding child abuse requires understanding the vast cultural diversity in which children and adolescents live, and there is a need for greater attention to be given to possible country-specific interventions (73). What is termed abuse varies between cultures.

There are differences in cross-cultural definitions, incidence in developed and developing countries across continents, and measures that have been instituted to prevent and manage child maltreatment (74). The literature suggests that child maltreatment is less likely in countries in which children are highly valued for their economic utility, for perpetuating family lines, and as sources of emotional pleasure and satisfaction. However, even in societies that value children, some children are valued more than others (75). Ethnicity has been found to play a role in the epidemiology of pediatric injury (76). There is a diverse culture-specific literature on abuse (77–79).

There are reports of structural models of the determinants of harsh parenting, for example, among Mexican mothers, where cultural beliefs play a major role in parenting within the framework of Mexican family relations (80). Changing cultural norms and attitudes in a given setting (e.g., Korea) can lead to children being at risk of abuse in the name of discipline or other seemingly appropriate parental or authority responses (81–83). Child abuse might increase in certain cultural groups as a result of cultural change rather than emerging from their traditions (84). Child psychiatrists with insufficient awareness about normative practices by parents, for example, dermabrasion or *cao gao* in Vietnam (85), may jump to the conclusion that hematomas around the child's head, neck, or chest signals that the parents may have been wrongdoers who abused their child. A culturally competent child psychiatrist, while not dismissing abuse out of hand, would also evaluate the alternative possibility, that the parents, with the best interests of the child in mind, submitted him/her to ritual treatment, for which the bruising acts as a public signal to the community that the child has been unwell.

Shalhoub-Kevorkian (86) reported a survey of victims of sexual abuse among Palestinian Israeli girls aged 14 to 16 years. Data revealed that the girls' attitudes not only conformed to general findings on disclosure of sexual abuse but also reflected sociopolitical fears and stressors. Helpers struggled between their beliefs that they should abide by the state's formal legal policies and their consideration of the victim's context. The study reveals how decontextualizing child protection laws and policies can keep sexually abused girls from seeking help.

The legal implications of child abuse are affected by practices which may be normative in certain cultural settings, for example, female genital mutilation (87). Some ethnic groups may carry out procedures on their children as a sign of caring rather than as a punitive measure. For instance in Cambodian and Vietnam there are cases with facial burns associated with what was termed "innocent cultural belief" (88). Thus, factors that lead to underreporting by physicians have included ethnic and cultural issues (89). Ethnographic data point to the importance of the social fabric in accounting for differences in child maltreatment report rates by predominant neighborhood ethnicity (90). There can be mismatches between the definition of child abuse between the culture of the professional and the culture of the families (91). There is much to be learned about the use of cultural evidence in child maltreatment law (92).

Case Illustration

Child abuse is subject to the definitions of various audiences rather than being intrinsic to the act. There are a few studies concerning the effect of culture and context of the *professionals* (as opposed to the families)—as in a study of Palestinian health/social workers where people agreed on what was child abuse but disagreed on when it should be reported. The results indicated a high level of agreement among students in viewing situations of abuse as well as neglect as maltreatment. Differences were found in their willingness to report situations of maltreatment. An inclination was found among students to minimize social and cultural factors as risk factors and to disregard signs that did not contain explicit signals of danger as characteristics of maltreated children (93). Baker and Dwairy (94) examined intervention in sexual abuse cases among the Palestinian community in Israel. They suggest that in many collective societies people live in interdependence with their families. Enforcing the laws against sexual perpetrators typically threatens the unity and reputation of the family, and therefore this option is rejected and the family turns against the victim. Instead of punishing the perpetrator, families often protect him and blame the victim. The punishment of the abuser results in the revictimization of the abused since the family possesses authority. Baker and Dwairy (94) suggest a culturally sensitive model of intervention that includes a condemning, apologizing, and punishing ceremony. In this way, exploiting the power of the family for the benefit of the victim of abuse before enforcing the law may achieve the same legal objectives as state intervention, without threatening the reputation and the unity of the family, and therefore save the victim from harm.

TAXONOMY AND CLASSIFICATION

Munir and Beardslee (95) are critical of DSM approaches and propose a developmental and psychobiologic framework for understanding the role of culture in child and adolescent psychiatry. Beauchaine (96) notes that developmental psychopathologists have criticized categorical classification systems for their inability to account for within-group heterogeneity in cultural influences on behavior. Appendix I of DSM-IV includes an Outline for Cultural Formulation to assist in evaluating cultural context on diagnosis and treatment, but this has not been crafted for cultural formulations of child and adolescent psychopathology. Novins et al. (97) attempted cultural case formulations for four American Indian children and identified several gaps concerning cultural identity and cultural elements of the therapeutic relationship.

Culture and Assessment

There has been a growing recognition in child psychiatry in Western settings to consider cultural context in the assessment of psychopathology (8). A culturally competent framework for assessment in resource-poor countries, while sorely needed, has not been developed. A simplistic attribution to culture of seemingly bizarre symptoms that in fact represent treatable mental illness would deflect energy from the development of effective treatment and prevention efforts. At the same time, an understanding of the cultural construction of major psychiatric disorders (including culture-bound disorders affecting young people) would minimize inaccurate diagnoses. This view has to be balanced with the understanding of less severe psychopathology, in which the observation of Neki (98) holds true, that ethnodynamics determine psychodynamics. In India, where the cultural ideal of an independent adult is not an autonomous adult, dependency is inculcated from childhood through a prolonged dependency relationship between mother and child. Dependency has a negative, pejorative connotation in Western thought, which is not so in the Indian context. The fostering of dependency is coupled with a high degree of control, low autonomy, and strict discipline, enforced within the broad framework of the family system. When this is identified by clinicians as representing a degree of pathology, decreased emphasis on the expression of thoughts and emotions in children could explain the greater preponderance of neurotic, psychosomatic, and somatization disorders (99). Thus, cultural context influences the definition of normalcy or disorder. It proscribes the values and ideals for the behavior of individuals, it determines the threshold of acceptance of pathology, and it provides guidelines for the handling of pathology and its correction (100).

Cultural issues also affect assessment because of problems with cultural validation of instruments. A German study showed problems in applying the United States factor structure of the Conners Parent Rating Scale (CPRS), with lack of correspondence of the impulsiveness/hyperactivity scale (101). A Greek study of the Conners-28 teacher questionnaire in a Greek community sample of primary schoolchildren found that the factor structure was similar to that originally reported by the United States, with a high level of discrimination between the referred and nonreferred sample, especially for the inattentive-passive scale (102).

Rey et al. (103) noted the lack of simple, reliable measures of the quality of the environment in which a child was reared which could be used in clinical research and practice. They developed a global scale to appraise retrospectively the quality of that environment and found good interrater reliability with clinicians from Australia, Hong Kong, and the People's Republic of China. Goodman et al. (104) developed a computerized algorithm to predict child psychiatric diagnoses on the basis of the symptom and impact scores derived from Strengths and Difficulties Questionnaires (SDQs) completed by parents, teachers, and young people. The predictive algorithm generates ratings for conduct disorders, emotional disorders, hyperactivity disorders, and any psychiatric disorder. The algorithm was applied to patients attending child mental health clinics in Britain and Bangladesh. SDQ prediction for any given disorder correctly identified 81–91% of the children who had that diagnosis.

Epidemiology

Determining the epidemiology of childhood mental disorders in Western society is a challenge. On the international scene, the ability to determine the precise magnitude of mental disorders is even more complex. Reporting systems are inadequate, the definition or recognition of disorders varies or has variable interpretations, and the cultural component of what constitutes a disorder is only now being more fully appreciated by epidemiologists and researchers. Of significance in resource-poor countries is that any measure of mental disorder takes place against a background of child and adolescent mortality and morbidity that makes the epidemiology of psychiatric disorder not only inaccurate, but often of a lower priority. Thus, in studying the epidemiology of psychiatric disorder in children and adolescents in resource-poor countries, it is important to define not only the prevalence and incidence of the disorders, but also the degree of impairment and burden of disease. No single study or consistent set of independent studies on the epidemiology of child and adolescent disorders since 1980 can be identified as definitive or relevant across societies. Those studies carried out in the 1980s reflect the deficiencies noted earlier and certainly do not reflect the current realities of the countries from which the data were reported (105, 106). Weiss has defined a new epidemiological approach combining qualitative study with classic epidemiologic methods (107–109). This new "cultural epidemiologic" approach has not yet been applied to child and adolescent mental disorders but holds the promise of gaining a more satisfactory understanding of the nature and extent of child and adolescent mental disorders worldwide.

Until now, when one has been faced with the realities of resource-poor countries, as noted, there is the danger of becoming a diagnostic nihilist in attempting to understand mental disorders in youth. However, for example, responsible investigators in Western Ethiopia clearly identified disordered mental functioning that meets a set of defined criteria (110). There is clear evidence that depression, psychosis, and mania can be defined and treated. The problem arises when one considers the context for the presentation of child and adolescent mental disorders. Is a hallucination during a ritual a disturbance in need of treatment? If the hallucination persists, should it be treated? What diagnostic label is appropriate? Giel and Van Lujik (111) found, in the pre-HIV/AIDS era, and counter to prevailing belief, that mental disorders were diagnosed more frequently than infectious diseases in the health centers in Africa that they studied. Until reporting is adequate and accurate, it cannot be assumed that the current state of mental health in the developing world actually supports the too prevalent minimalist and optimistic view. This sense is supported by the finding from WHO studies of primary care clinicians that showed that many patients seeking care had mental disorders, and their communities were aware of the problem (112). In the current era, Omigbodun (113) documented the psychosocial problems in a child and adolescent psychiatric clinic population in Nigeria: 62.2% of new referrals to the clinic had significant psychosocial stressors in the year preceding presentation. Problems with primary support, such as separation from parents to live with relatives, disruption of the family, abandonment by the mother, psychiatric illness in a parent, and sexual/physical abuse occurred in 39.4%. Significantly more children and adolescents with disruptive behavior disorders and disorders like enuresis, separation anxiety, and suicidal behavior had psychosocial stressors when compared to children with psychotic conditions, autistic disorder, and epilepsy.

Prevalence

Although it is interesting to consider epidemiological reports of more esoteric disorders, these are a distraction from the significant burden of disease that needs to be addressed in the mainstream of care. In most studies, the methodological inadequacies and other constraints do not permit these studies to be of use for program planning or needs assessment. However, most countries today have access to appropriate epidemiologic study guidelines, and it is a matter of setting a national priority and allocating resources to ascertain the data. For example, a study in India by Malhotra (114) used a sophisticated three-stage assessment of the epidemiology of disorders in school children aged 4 to 12 years. In this study, assessments by teachers, parents, and clinicians were compared. The teacher assessment on the Rutter B scale, a generally accepted measurement instrument, had a low concordance rate with the clinical assessment. When children tested positive on both the teacher and parent assessment, there was a diagnostic rate of 92.3% on the clinical assessment. The evidence pointed to a prevalence rate of psychiatric disorder ranging between 7% and 20%. The diagnostic possibilities included enuresis, mental retardation, and epilepsy, among others. Overall, the most conservative estimate of severe psychiatric disorder in India is 10% of the population younger than age 14 years, representing 35 million children (100).

Giel et al. (115) demonstrated in four countries (Sudan, Philippines, Colombia, and India) that between 12% and 29% of children aged 5 to 15 years showed mental health problems. The types of disorder identified in these resource-poor countries were reported as being no different from those encountered in industrialized countries. However, recognizable diagnoses were not given in the article. Thabet and Vostanis (116) report a pattern of anxiety symptoms and disorders among children living in the Gaza Strip comparable to previous epidemiologic research in Western societies. There were high rates of anxiety disorders and school-related mental health problems. Thabet and Vostanis find the same prevalence rate (21%) of anxiety-related disorders as do Kashani and Orvaschel (117). Thabet and Vostanis (116) state that their findings do not support the commonly held belief that in non-Western societies anxiety and other mental health symptoms are predominantly expressed through somatizing symptoms. Citing Nikapota, they state that child mental health symptoms do not differ significantly across cultures, and culture-specific mental health disorders are rare.

Most recently, Tadesse et al. (118) report a prevalence in Western Ethiopia of childhood behavioral disorder of 17.7%. The behavioral disorders are more frequent in boys than in girls. These latter data were gathered with a version of the Reporting Questionnaire for Children developed by WHO. Studies of Hackett et al. (119) and Bird et al. (120) find an excess of male patients with externalizing disorders.

What of the disorders that now occupy considerable attention in developed countries such as attention deficit hyperactivity disorder, autism, and anorexia nervosa? The diagnosis and treatment of these disorders highlight both a weakness and a strength of having an international perspective. The recognition and labeling of disorders come as a result of improved international communication. However, the process of assessment must take into account a host of cultural as well as formal diagnostic criteria, and this is too often ignored. Cultural concepts of what is normal or abnormal and how parents perceive the presence or absence of a diagnosable disorder (106) are essential to consider. In the case of eating disorders, there is clear evidence that the incidence may be affected by Western influences (121). In the diagnosis of attention deficit hyperactivity disorder (ADHD) pharmaceutical companies are now a primary source of both public and professional education and they often focus on the use of the diagnosis for the purpose of implementing a pharmacological intervention. This trend may provide an indirect incentive for the overdiagnosis of disorders such as ADHD and bipolar disorder. The understanding of the influence of increased public education on diagnosis requires further study.

Fayyad et al. (122), discussing the development of systems of care in resource-poor countries, focuses on ADHD and the development of a comprehensive system of care around it in Lebanon. In a study of adolescents in Bahrain diagnosed with adjustment disorder, al-Ansari and Matar (123) examined the type of life stressors that initiated their referrals to a child psychiatry unit. Disappointment in relationships with a family member or with a friend of the opposite sex was found to be the main stressor. Eating disorders classically are rare in resource-poor countries such as India (124), but anecdotal evidence suggests that with globalization and migration the rates are increasing (125–128). Autism is reported around the world, including in resource-poor countries (129–131), and with a cross-national consistency (132, 133). However, high rates of autism, almost 200 times higher than in the general population of children, have been reported among boys born in Sweden to mothers born in Uganda (134, 135).

Specific Mental Disorders

Posttraumatic Stress Disorder

It is a challenge that as mental health professionals we know so little about the consequences of exposure to natural disaster and armed conflict on long-term healthy mental development. In relation to adults it is clear that armed conflict leads to persistent negative functional consequences from exposure to trauma. As for children and adolescents, there are conflicting views on the impact of the traumas noted earlier (136–139). The resiliency of children over the long term seems to be a consistent dominant finding, but individual investigators identify specific consequences, with depression, externalizing behaviors, and PTSD as evident consequences (22). Diagnostic status does not relate to functional status according to Sack et al. (140). Sack et al. (139) not only show persistence of PTSD but also demonstrate a sometimes delayed onset of symptoms. Even in those youth demonstrating delayed PTSD, symptoms of depression diminished over time. Terr (141) demonstrated persistent effects on children from trauma, with lasting functional deficits. Studies related to children from Kuwait (142) and Iran (143) show the persistence of PTSD. Nader et al. (144) report moderate to severe PTSD in 70% of Kuwaiti children after the Gulf War. Thabet and Vostanis (116) found in the Gaza Strip that the prevalence among children ages 6 to 11 years of at least mild PTSD is 73%, and 39% presented with moderate to severe symptoms. Ahmad (145) reports that 25% of displaced

Kurdish children had evidence of PTSD, and Weine et al. (138) found similar rates in Bosnian adolescents who moved to the United States during the war. Hussain et al. (146), reporting on the impact of the siege of Sarajevo, noted that it is not the exposure to sniper fire, but the loss of a family member and deprivation of food, water, and shelter that have a severe adverse impact on children. The clinical manifestations of the trauma are avoidance and reexperiencing symptoms. Of concern is the implementation of clinical interventions that may inadvertently lead to an exacerbation or prolongation of symptoms: For example, the use of "ventilation" and retelling of the trauma through various means has been shown to have negative effects (147), whereas reestablishing families and returning to normal routines, including school attendance, has a salutary impact.

Conduct Disorder and Delinquency

A study of the adjustment of children in Sri Lanka using the Strengths and Difficulties Questionnaire (Goodman) with parent, teacher, and child informants, found problems consistent with other international studies of child mental health. Compared with Muslim and Singhalese children, Tamil children were rated as more hyperactive, with more emotional symptoms, conduct problems, and total behavioral difficulties. Relationships between behavioral adjustment and Tamil ethnicity and Hindu religion could be associated with longstanding ethnic conflict in Sri Lanka and confirms the need for development of child and adolescent health services in civil war–torn countries such as Sri Lanka (148).

A descriptive survey of Flemish delinquent adolescents found significant difference between ethnic groups on self-report scores (149). Tramontina et al. (118) evaluated the association between DSM-IV conduct disorder (CD) and school dropout in a sample of students from the state schools in the capital of the southernmost state of Brazil. The prevalence of DSM-IV CD was higher in the school-dropout group than in controls. The odds ratio for school dropout was higher in the presence of DSM-IV CD, even after controlling for potential confounding factors such as family structure and income. A crosscultural study of delinquency among West Indian boys (151) had comparable findings.

Depression

Childhood depression is gaining prominence worldwide (152). A crosscultural evaluation of depression in children in Egypt, Kuwait, and the United States (121) showed similar clinical patterns. Depressive and anxiety disorders should not be overshadowed by the attention currently being given to PTSD in developing countries in the aftermath of natural disasters and post-conflict situations.

The obverse side of childhood depression—and pertinent in resource-poor countries—is the depression that results in the death of a child. Few losses hurt as much as the death of a child, no less so in countries with high infant mortality rates. The constant threat that a child may die will influence the climate of parenting and family life. The Chagga regard childhood malnutrition, or *kuvimba*, as a sign of displeasure by the ancestral spirits (154). Howard and Millard (155) point out that as perceptions of young children have changed, there has been a diminution in the rituals to do with birth practices, ancestral spirits, and the child. Serious childhood illnesses continue to raise suspicions, however, of sorcery as a sign of community disharmony. Spells can be cast on children by hiding or swallowing some of their body substances such as hair or feces, or by introducing some foreign substance into the child's body. The threat of infant mortality [which tends to be consecutive (156)] may even change the cultural concepts of infancy, as among Canadian aboriginal children, where high infant mortality rates contributed to a delay in conferring personhood on the child (157). Scheper-Hughes (158) argued that maternal detachment and indifference toward their infants judged too weak to survive may lead to sick babies being left without attention.

Suicide

Suicide in youth is a pervasive world mental health problem. In Western cultures, suicide is overwhelmingly associated with defined mental illness. Suicide is the second leading cause of death for American Indian and Alaska Native youth (159). Elsewhere in the world, it may be very difficult to identify the mental illness associated with the suicidal act—and in the face of overwhelming helplessness, suicide may appear from the perspective of the protagonists as the only way out, with no clearly labeled mental illness. Studies of suicide in the West have focused on risk factors associated with cognitive distortions, substance use, and familial factors (160). In trying to assess the high rates of suicide in some resource-poor countries, it appears that the balance in determining suicidal risk may rest with environmental stressors and the perception of no way out. Expectations may often be more determinant of suicidal angst than reality (161). According to one view expressed by Murthy (162), the traditional protective effect of religion in certain cultures seems not to operate among the younger generation.

Chan et al. (163) consider suicide in China as a response to change due to globalization, in which Chinese values are more closely identified with the global culture. The high suicide rate is thus not seen as a reflection of psychiatric disorder but of sociocultural factors. It seems more apparent that suicide is viewed by those without demonstrable mental illness as a solution to social and personal dilemmas that bring with them thwarted expectations for a happy or successful life. For example, from this perspective, in India and in other resource-poor countries, the focus of the suicidal individual is not on achieving some exalted goal, but on being able to have enough of a dowry to be married, to not be isolated because of rape, or to be successful in passing a school advancement examination. This relative alteration in emphasis is important in the consideration of intervention strategies and in the training of workers to perform triage and to treat suicidal children and adolescents. A survey of adolescent health in nine Caribbean countries identified risk and protective factors predisposing to suicide attempts (164). In Hong Kong, amid the impressive high-rise buildings and fancy stores, reside families barely able to subsist. In this context of economic hardship, the result in part of massive economic adjustment in the Far East, the phenomenon of family suicide exists. Chan reports that families come together and, in a well planned manner, seal themselves in their small apartments and light a charcoal heater (165). In a relatively brief time, the members of the family are asphyxiated. This has become an acceptable form of suicide in that the bodies remain intact and have an attractive appearance because of the monoxide poisoning. To the extent that it has been possible to determine the psychological state of the family before the suicides, major psychiatric disturbance has not been reported.

Case Illustration

In India, four sisters aged 16 to 24 years committed suicide by hanging after an evening during which they bought sweet cakes and samosas and played word games. The context was that they were part of a once prosperous family in which the father died of tuberculosis for lack of medical treatment. Now they were periodically without sufficient food, but with a mother too proud to ask for help. This family was socially isolated because of parental marriage across religious lines, and they had suffered an unexpected financial downturn as a result of a road-widening project that took their once-fertile land. Suicide rates in India, although lower than the international average of 16 per 100,000, have been steadily rising. Psychiatrists believe this is in part a result of the accelerating pace of social and economic change. Whereas the biggest risk factor in the West is mental illness, studies in India have consistently found that the dominant risk factor is a combination of social and economic strain. Farmers in debt may take pesticide, and ostracized women who are victims of the dowry system in economically stretched circumstances might immolate themselves (166).

Disabilities, Mental Retardation, and Epilepsy

Disability—whether physical or mental—is all too common in resource-poor countries, especially those post conflict. In Cambodia, for example, between 2 to 3 percent of the population, or about one out of every 40 Cambodians, have physical disabilities (including 50,000 landmine survivors, many of them young people; 60,000 with paralysis from polio; 100,000 who are blind; 120,000 who are deaf; 102,000 to 178,500 with mental retardation; 20,400 to 40,800 people with severe mental disorders; and 154,000 to 408,000 people with epilepsy) (167).

Mental retardation and epilepsy are major disorders that often dominate the services of child mental health and pediatric professionals in resource-poor countries. In the 1980s, prevalence rates in resource-poor countries were estimated to be in the range of eight to 12 per 1,000 for children aged three to 10 years (168–170). Mental retardation and epilepsy are the most common mental disorders in India (171, 172). The rate of serious mental retardation in some resource-poor countries ranges from 5 to 16.2 per 1,000 population (173), significantly higher than the rate in the West. Cerebral palsy and postnatal causes of mental retardation are much more common in transitional societies than in developed countries. Untreated epilepsy limits a person's potential to participate in society. Unfortunately, although the cost of medication is relatively low, access to care is often limited. The care of the mentally retarded varies widely in resource-poor countries. In some countries, special effort is made to provide for productive lives with meaningful vocational education, especially in agrarian economies. All too often, the moderately and severely retarded are housed in minimal care institutions where premature death and illness are common.

Kim and Kumar (174) describe *Dousa-hou* as a Japanese psychological rehabilitation method widely used in Japan for children with mental retardation, cerebral palsy, and autism. The focus is to improve bodily movements and posture as well as to introduce social support to patients and their first-degree relatives. Analysis showed mothers got more social support interacting with their child's trainer and supervisor during *Dousa-hou*. Trainers were more interactive than mothers in the Indian group, followed by the Japanese and Korean cultural groups.

Children with disability such as epilepsy are among the most marginalized in many resource-poor countries. In Cambodia, for example, they have limited access to education, vocational training, employment, and income-generating opportunities and other services. Childhood epilepsy is viewed traditionally as caused by the attack of the preceding mother from the previous incarnation of the infant, and treatment may be sought by parents from *kruu*, or traditional healers, to ward off her attacks. The children may be cared for in the Buddhist temple, or kept indoors out of the sight of neighbors.

SERVICES

The World Health Organization, through the Atlas project, has developed the first objective profile of resources for services related to child and adolescent mental health (175). The findings confirm the worldwide gap in services to address child and adolescent mental health (176); the gaps exist in both resource poor and resource rich countries. The lack of services is tied to insufficient and unstable financing, lack of trained professionals, and lack of policy to support the development of child and adolescent mental health services.

Resource-poor countries lack the child mental health personnel to mount large-scale programs of treatment with fully trained staff members. The prospect of training large numbers of child mental health workers remains a continuing goal, whereas the training of child and adolescent psychiatrists to meet the potential need is beyond the realm of possibility. In the interim, what can be done to provide a way to intervene for the promotion of child mental health? Obviously, one focus is on developing prevention programs in general health and education systems. Second, training primary care practitioners from numerous disciplines is needed to provide basic child mental health services. Basic assessment and treatment are possible, with triage of the most severely disturbed.

McKelvey et al. (177) illustrate the differing priorities for child psychiatric services in Vietnam, where there is a focus on infectious diseases and malnutrition. Treatment is reserved for the most severely afflicted, especially patients with epilepsy and mental retardation. Specialized care is available in only a few urban centers. In rural areas treatment is provided by allied health personnel, paraprofessionals and community organizations.

In some countries, the lack of child mental health personnel has stimulated some remarkable efforts to train persons from diverse backgrounds to be effective in identifying and intervening to ameliorate child mental health problems. In Alexandria, Egypt, child counselors have been trained to develop sophisticated interventions in schools (178).

Program Illustration

In Alexandria, the Department of Community Medicine has supported the development of a cadre of school counselors. These counselors come from the ranks of volunteers, social workers, and psychologists. Without prior child mental health training, the workers are provided with coursework on common child mental health problems and then are supervised in field placements. The counselors work with parents around children identified by both the school and parents as having some type of behavioral problem. They also serve as contact points for the school, parents, or pediatricians to bring children with more severe behavioral disturbance to the attention of the few fully trained mental health professionals.

Leaders in child mental health programming in resource-poor countries are emphatic when faced with the reality of program implementation that Western models of care by specialists are neither feasible nor desirable. Indigenous methods and models of care need to be developed that are not dependent on specialists. Conversely, the development of these models that use parents, teachers, pediatricians, and others can be informed by the best thinking of child psychiatrists and other specialists. This has led to an emphasis on the training of primary care practitioners. Furthermore, short-term, focused training in specific areas related to diagnosis or intervention can be provided by specialists or through specialized child psychiatric centers that have a broad regional or national area of responsibility.

The development of child mental health training for primary care practitioners is well established in many sites, but the WHO Atlas documents that the utilization of primary care providers falls far short of the goal in both developing and developed countries. Murthy (7) describes the use of primary health care providers in resource-poor countries. In India, with 1.5 billion people, there are only 5,000 mental health providers—of whom only a fraction are psychiatrists—35,000 psychiatric beds, and a dearth of emergency services. The primary care provider, when adequately trained, is a valuable and essential point of contact and treatment for the mentally ill. In India, it has been demonstrated that primary care providers can provide a level of professional care that reduces morbidity and mortality. However, without appropriate training, primary practitioners have been shown to have a poor record of recognizing mental disorders. Giel et al. (179) report in their study in resource-poor countries that primary care practitioners identified only 10% to 20% of the disorders that the researchers were able to diagnose. WHO has devoted considerable efforts to the development and distribution of training manuals to aid primary care practitioners in the recognition of mental disorders (180, 181).

Moreover, India has developed the *anganwadi* system to provide basic nutrition and educational support in villages. This is both an appropriate preventive intervention and a way to assess youngsters presenting with disorders (182). The *anganwadi* system focuses on providing essential services to very young children. Like Head Start, the program provides nutrition, basic education, socialization, and a venue for more specialized intervention for children perceived to be at risk or in need of additional services (183). There must be a concern in the development of these indigenous systems of care that not too much dependence be placed on family structure and support at a time when urbanization and industrialization are eroding the traditional family structure. With the absence of security, and often living at a subsistence level, the new nuclear family faces previously unknown challenges and may be particularly vulnerable over this and the next generation.

Some programs are international in scope. For instance, WHO, as part of its Program on Mental Health, has fostered the use of life skills education (184). The goal of the Life Skills Program is to foster psychosocial competence. For children and adolescents, the Life Skills Program is taught in schools. The program itself as promulgated by WHO is based on the social learning theory of Bandura (185). Many similar models are operative throughout the world. A "training the trainer" component affects the overall resource of a community to provide for the mental health needs of some children and adolescents who are at risk. Among the obvious limitations in the developing world are the absence of universal education and the capacities of the teachers to go beyond essential educational tasks. Kapur et al. (186) demonstrate that the training of teachers as counselors was effective in India.

The prospect for the future of child mental health practice in resource-poor countries is tied to economic growth, health literacy, and reduction of stigma. The creative efforts to develop programs to reach children and adolescents in resource-poor countries need to be supported. Child and adolescent psychiatry will remain a scarce resource to be used in ways that will have a duplicative impact. This means that the training of volunteers, the training of peers, the support of family intervention programming, and the use of community-based early intervention need to be the focus of attention. Kim (187) proposed a curriculum guideline of cultural competence for child and adolescent psychiatric residencies. These guidelines stress ethnogeneric and developmental perspectives, which can be expanded further to include ethnospecific issues depending on the needs of each training program.

The notion of a continuum of care as advocated as a goal in developed countries is but a fantasy in the developing world, where there remains a reliance on inpatient care for the most seriously disturbed, and where outpatient care is often sparse. In some developing countries the Western model of managed care and the institution of various insurance schemes are underway. Unfortunately, the negative consequences of these aspects of care systems are too often unrecognized. In some countries the introduction of insurance has had the unintended consequence of reducing access for uncovered populations and has led to flight of health professionals into the private sector.

RESEARCH

Earls and Eisenberg (188) highlight three areas for enhanced research activity in relation to child and adolescent mental health. First is research to understand how the changes in contemporary society are reflected in the prevalence and incidence of mental disorders. Second is research to enhance the understanding of how different childrearing methods affect normal and deviant behavioral and emotional development. Third involves research on the design and delivery of mental health services. Mohler (189) describes and discusses the major challenges in crosscultural research on child mental health. Nelson and Quintana (190) present strategies for designing and conducting qualitative investigations, and address ethical issues involved in conducting qualitative research with minors. International child development and mental health studies often call for a mixed-methods approach (191).

Eisenbruch (192) has defined a template for the steps needed to ensure cultural competence in research, namely cultural competence in community engagement; communicating with research subjects; design; crosscultural validation of research instruments; sampling; calibrating diversity variables; demographic variables measured in datasets; research ethics; data collection techniques; data processing and analysis; and dissemination and action. Culturally competent community engagement by the researcher, for example, depends on a) building community partnerships; b) developing interventions that are acceptable and relevant; c) promoting successful recruitment, participation, and retention of participants; and d) developing a diverse, cohesive, and committed research team and effective managerial information support systems. International child psychiatry research program should pay attention to participation from the perspective of community members (193–195). International child psychiatric research should avoid sampling barriers among culturally diverse communities to do, for example, with lack of tolerance of diverse groups, social stigma, concern for issues of confidentiality, and fear of exposure because of possible threats to security (196). The research should avoid the use of instruments developed in one culture transferred to another given the cultural differences in the interpretation of certain items. The research should avoid definition of diversity with only a single variable. Cultural, racial, religious, and immigrant groups are not homogeneous. For example, any one population includes native-born, migrant, and immigrant peoples with distinctive national origins and regional settlement patterns, and varied and complex demographic structures. Data collection should be clear about descriptions of ethnic or racial measurement and reasons for including or excluding clearly defined populations. The research should be open to innovative recipes for data collection, for example, as proposed by Roszak (197) with clarity about (1) who provides information; (2) when data are collected; (3) which racial and ethnic categories are used—all hospitals should use standard racial and ethnic categories; (4) how data are stored; and (5) responses to patients' concerns. Nikapota (1) underscores the importance of determining "culture-appropriate" criteria to permit consistency in diagnosis. In doing research, it is important to consider the characteristics of the interviewer as well as the informant.

Fontes (198), drawing on his experiences conducting research on sexual abuse in a shantytown in Chile and with Puerto Ricans, examined ethical issues in crosscultural research on family violence. It was emphasized that special attention needs to be given to informed consent, definition of the sample, composition of the research team, research methods, and potential harm and benefit. Munir and Earls (199) articulate a set of ethical parameters for research that must be considered in doing research among children and adolescents of resource-poor countries. To apply a different standard justified by the difficulty of implementing protocols would violate the very support of a rights framework so essential for progress to be made on behalf of children in resource-poor countries.

An area of great interest is the development of assessment tools that incorporate the diversity of cultural parameters. Increasing numbers of instruments have been translated and back-translated for use in crosscultural studies. Instruments exist for the assessment of depression, anxiety, PTSD, quality of life, and other conditions. It remains for there to be a sufficient body of crosscultural research with modern standards for the conduct of the research that yields information on the reliability and validity of the instruments in their revised versions. Few instruments meet an agreed standard for use across all cultures in their current form.

As described by Earls (200), compulsory schooling leads to the need to understand the impact of learning disorders better. The appropriate diagnosis and remediation of these disorders are first-order priorities in countries where technologic advance places a premium on knowledge acquisition and use. As yet, research in this area has not been implemented in resource-poor countries, but the pressure to implement such studies is mounting.

Research into the understanding of the differential impact of childrearing methods should be an area of collaborative inquiry between those interested in mental health and those concerned with the role of women and the family in evolving societies. It is not evident that any one method of childrearing is superior to another. Perhaps developing and developed societies can learn from one another about the optimal methods for childrearing in the presence of the evolution of individual societies. The experience with the effects of urbanization, industrialization, changing roles of women, and increased survivorship of children in developed countries may form the basis for translation into the programs for resource-poor countries. Conversely, the healthy development of youngsters growing up in adversity in resource-poor countries may provide information on how to enhance understanding and to develop new interventions for children at risk in developed countries.

Attention needs to be focused on the important developments in global and international child mental health that are published in peer reviewed journals in languages other than English. A mechanism is needed to ensure that these key findings are not lost to the English-speaking world (201).

PREVENTION

It appears that prevention of mental disorders is the way to approach the problem of reducing the toll of mental illness in resource-poor countries. Many of the mental health issues that need to addressed are inextricably related to contextual issues, as noted earlier. One area too often overlooked in considering a way in which mental health problems can be prevented is through the overall reduction in malnutrition. The effect of malnutrition in societies impacts both the child directly and the parent who cares for the child. Both lead to significant mental health consequences that are preventable. The consequences from malnutrition can be delayed cognitive development, but also more subtle behavioral manifestations with attentional problems and learning disabilities (183, 202, 203). Some studies suggest that the behavior disorders associated with malnutrition are secondary to impaired maternal capacities and not to the malnutrition itself, because malnutrition does not appear to contribute to behavioral disturbance later in life (204, 205). Thus, mental health professionals working in the international arena must be mindful of this issue and consider it in their assessment of mental functioning, as well as advocating for proper nutrition as a preventive measure (206). There is an opportunity to reduce some behavioral and cognitive problems through a reduction in malnutrition.

Maternal depression associated with malnutrition, poor health, social deprivation, abuse, or other stressors affects the child and adolescent as well as the mother. This too is a preventable cause of childhood mental disorder, as demonstrated by Beardslee et al. (207). Using a family-based approach, Beardslee and colleagues sought to reduce risk factors and enhance protective factors for early adolescents. They demonstrated that providing parents with information about their affective state, equipping them with enhanced communication skills, and fostering parent–child dialogue led to an improvement in children's self-understanding and children's depressive symptomatology. This program is now being replicated in Finland, Costa Rica, and elsewhere (208).

Life skills education promoted by the WHO is the backbone of prevention programming in many resource-poor countries (209). Life skills' training is provided in the context of the school curriculum as a program to enhance psychosocial competencies. The training focuses on basic, generic skills such as decisionmaking and problemsolving, creative and critical thinking, communication and other interpersonal skills, self-awareness and empathic skills, and coping with stress and with emotions. The aims are to promote mental wellbeing and to enable children to take more responsibility for their lives and feel more effective (210).

The WPA Presidential Global Program for Child Mental Health identified school dropout as a major issue in both developing and developed countries. Intervention to prevent dropout was considered to be an important preventive strategy related to child mental health. The program conducted research on school dropout and prepared materials for use by clinicians and educators (211). The Global Program has produced other materials to support preventive intervention in resource poor countries (212).

SYSTEMIC ISSUES

Throughout the world, it is rare to see child mental health being incorporated into national health policy (213). In many countries, developed or developing, no coherent health policy exists that would provide a framework for program development. In countries with a health policy, child mental health rarely rises to a prominent position. Until child mental health becomes integrated into health policy, stable budgetary support for child and adolescent mental health programs will not be realized.

Advocacy for child and adolescent mental health is evident throughout the world, but competition with other interests often forces the issue off the policy agenda. When crises involve children, such as child soldiers in the Sudan or female genital mutilation, the issue of child mental health, for a time, gains the spotlight. Unfortunately, the advocacy and concern diminish with time and rarely find a sustaining constituency.

Nongovernmental organizations play an important role in promoting child mental health, in disseminating information, in providing a forum for professional exchange, and in advocating for specific causes. The constituent base of these organizations differs, but they generally have broad representation and provide an opportunity for interested persons to learn more about specific topics or develop ideas in a context of knowledgeable individuals. Many of the nongovernmental organizations have affiliated regional organizations that permit ongoing local involvement. National organizations have often taken leadership roles in advocacy efforts and crisis response. The following are some of the more established international nongovernmental organizations focused on child and adolescent mental health: the International Association for Child and Adolescent Psychiatry and Allied Professions, the World Association for Infant Mental Health, the International Association for Adolescent Psychiatry and Psychology, and the World Federation for Mental Health.

The lack of trained individuals in resource-poor countries and the maldistribution of professionals in developed countries is a significant impediment to the development of child and adolescent mental health services. The limitation for program implementation is the availability of trained persons for leadership and "training of the trainer." The lack of individuals within non-Western societies leads to the too-facile adoption of interventions and strategies that do not fully appreciate local culture and the appropriate utilization of available resources. Further, there is the need for these programs to be able to access tertiary diagnostic and treatment services for those with manifest psychiatric disorder. Efforts to support training are now ongoing through many nongovernmental and governmental efforts. The training of a sufficient number of individuals to implement appropriate, accessible care will be an ongoing challenge.

LESSONS TO BE LEARNED

It would be wrong to focus only on the areas where it appears that more could be done to enhance child and adolescent mental health services. Western mental health professionals and program developers can learn from the programmatic necessities and innate capacities of individuals and families in resource-poor countries.

Family participation in the care of the mentally ill or retarded children in resource-poor countries is impressive by any standard. The acceptance by communities of the special needs of affected families is often dramatic. Likewise, the willingness and ability of families to care for children, including the appropriate use of medication, for children with epilepsy and other disorders challenge Western concepts of continuity of care and the role of providers.

While the West has flirted with the enhanced use of primary care providers in the delivery of mental health services, but in resource-poor countries, necessity has led to impressive models for the training of primary care practitioners, as noted earlier. This is true in many countries, notably India and Thailand. Primary care training for specific mental health interventions is also part of a WHO strategy.

Conversely, there is a global trend toward the imposition of managed care on mental health services. This is occurring in countries, such as China and Eastern Europe, which have hardly met their child and adolescent mental health needs. The need is felt to control the cost of mental health services. Perhaps uncritically, economies throughout the world are adopting managed mental health care. From a Western perspective, it is obvious that although all mental health services suffer in a managed-care environment, child and adolescent mental health services are often most vulnerable to reductions and the use of the lowest-common-denominator service. Research into managed care and health services has not had the beneficial impact of stimulating the development of innovative systems of care. Unfortunately the investment needed to foster these systems of care and the social network needed to provide "wraparound" services do not exist in resource-poor countries. It remains to be seen whether traditional systems of care can be integrated into a meaningful continuum.

EMERGING ISSUES

The impact of globalization and political change underpins much of this chapter. Globalization and modernization bring new challenges to the attention of child and adolescent mental health professionals. In Japan, changes in society associated with rapid economic development are affecting the mental health of children and families, with concern about levels of school refusal, bullying, suicidal behavior, and delinquency (214). Lewis et al. (215) note the impact of the transition of the Eastern European countries from communist to democratic societies on children's mental health, both positively and negatively. On the positive side for child mental health is growing support for a democratic process within the family, the depoliticization of mental illness, the passage of laws assuring basic children's rights, services for and public awareness about child abuse, reforms in education, the proliferation of mental health clinics and support centers, and the resumption of training of mental health professionals in many countries. International adoption, the use of telepsychiatry in the developing and developed world, the role of industry and the for-profit sector in program development and education, and the increased recognition of the need to address the mental health consequences of conflict and natural disaster will be an ongoing challenge to professionals and those impacted by mental illness.

CONCLUSION

International child and adolescent mental health is no longer an exotic topic for theoretical discussion. With our global village, knowledge of child and adolescent mental health problems throughout the world is an important part of the education of all child and adolescent psychiatrists and allied professionals. The perspective gained from appreciating the stressors of children and adolescents in parts of the world embroiled in conflict and the nature of the responses offers the opportunity to learn more about the resilience of children and adolescents and about what we must do to develop more effective intervention programs.

The dearth of trained child and adolescent psychiatrists and allied professionals in developing countries challenges us to find the most effective means for inculcating knowledge and providing meaningful services. It is unrealistic to assume that any effort will meet the needs of child and adolescent psychiatry as determined by conventional planning assumptions. As services evolve in developed countries, there is probably much that can be learned from the way in which less developed countries have found the means to support families and individual persons to be relatively self-sufficient even when they are affected by mental disorders.

Given the enormity of the challenge to extend child mental health in a meaningful manner globally, the establishment of regional centers of excellence should be considered. These centers would incorporate resource libraries, have access to consultants, support training, and in some instances provide clinical diagnostic functions. Ultimately, the goal is to establish a sufficient cadre of child mental health professionals trained to an acceptable standard, with the capacity to relate in a culturally appropriate manner to the mental disorders of children and adolescents, and to be able to support the healthy development of children and adolescents worldwide.

References

1. Nikapota AD: Child psychiatry in developing countries. [Review] [70 refs]. *British Journal of Psychiatry* June; 158:743–51, 1991.
2. Velasco D: [Child psychiatry in developing countries] [French]. *Annales Medico-Psychologiques* June, 139(6):626–628, 1981.
3. Minde K: Child psychiatry in developing countries. *Journal of Child Psychology and Psychiatry and Allied Disciplines* January, 17(1):79–83, 1976.
4. Sugar JA, Kleinman A, Eisenberg L: Psychiatric morbidity in developing countries and American psychiatry's role in international health. *Hospital and Community Psychiatry* April, 43(4):355–60, 1992.
5. United Nations, Centre for Human Rights, UNICEF: *The Convention on the Rights of the Child*, adopted by the General Assembly of the United Nations 20 November 1989. London, UNICEF, 1990.
6. United States, Congress, Senate, Committee on Foreign Relations: The Optional Protocol to the Convention on the Rights of the Child on the Sale of Children, Child Prostitution and Child Pornography and the Optional Protocol to the Convention on the Rights of the Child on the Involvement of Children in Armed Conflict—Report (to accompany Treaty doc. 106-37). Washington, D.C: U.S. GPO; 2002.
7. Murthy RS: Rural psychiatry in developing countries. *Psychiatr Serv* July, 49(7):967–9, 1998.
8. Canino I, Chou JC, Christmas JJ, Chu P, Fabrega H, Jr., Fernandez-Pol B et al.: Cross-cultural issues and treatments of psychiatric disorders. *American Journal of Psychiatry* April, 148(4):543–4, 1991.
9. Rahim SI, Cederblad M: Effects of rapid urbanization on child behaviour and health in a part of Khartoum, Sudan: II. Psycho-social influences on behaviour. *Social Science and Medicine* 22(7):723–30, 1986.
10. Adelekan ML, Makanjuola AB, Ndom RJ: Traditional mental health practitioners in Kwara State, Nigeria. *East African Medical Journal* April, 78(4):190–6, 2001.
11. Reynolds P: *Traditional healers and childhood in Zimbabwe*. Athens, Ohio University Press, 1996.
12. Manci M: Clinical experience of treating STD's with traditional medicines, leading to treatment and prevention of HIV/AIDS. Int Conf AIDS, 1994 August 7, 10:215.
13. Robertson BA, Kottler A: Cultural issues in the psychiatric assessment of Xhosa children and adolescents. *S Afr Med J* March, 83(3):207–8, 1993.
14. Somasundaram DJ, van de Put WA, Eisenbruch M, de Jong JT: Starting mental health services in Cambodia. *Social Science & Medicine* April, 48(8):1029–46, 1999.
15. Suryani LK, Jensen GD: Psychiatrist, traditional healer and culture integrated in clinical practice in Bali. *Med Anthropol* January, 13(4):301–14, 1992.
16. Eisenbruch M: The ritual space of patients and traditional healers in Cambodia. *Bulletin de l'École Française d'Extrême-Orient* 79[2], 283–316, 1992.
17. Savin D: Developing psychiatric training and services in Cambodia. *Psychiatric services: A journal of the American Psychiatric Association* July, 51(7):935, 2000.
18. Desjarlais R, Eisenberg L, Good B, Kleinman A: *World mental health: Problems and priorities in low-income countries*. 10th ed. New York, Oxford University Press, 1995.
19. Fullilove MT: Psychiatric implications of displacement: Contributions from the psychology of place. *American Journal of Psychiatry* 153:1516–23, 1996.
20. Sampson RJ, Raudenbush SW, Earls F: Neighborhoods and violent crime: A multilevel study of collective efficacy. *Science* August 15, 277(5328):918–24, 1997.
21. Zivciç I: Emotional reactions of children to war stress in Croatia. *Journal of the American Academy of Child and Adolescent Psychiatry* July, 32(4):709–13, 1993.
22. Laor N, Wolmer L, Mayes LC, Golomb A, Silverberg DS, Weizman R et al.: Israeli preschoolers under SCUD missile attacks. A developmental perspective on risk-modifying factors. *Archives of General Psychiatry* May, 53(5):416–23, 1996.
23. UNHCR: *Refugees by Numbers*, 2001 Edition. <http://www unhcr ch/cgi-bin/texis/vtx/home/opendoc htm?tbl=STATISTICS&id=3d075d374&page=statistics>, 2002.
24. Forbes M: *Refugee Women*. London, Zed Press, 1992.
25. Williamson J, Moser A, Ford Foundation, International Committee of the Red Cross, Redd b, Office of the United Nations High Commissioner for Refugees et al.: *Unaccompanied children in emergencies—A field guide for their care and protection*. Geneva, International Social Service, 1987.
26. Goffman I: *Asylums*. Garden City, Anchor of Doubleday, 1961.
27. Marsella AJE, Bornemann TE, Ekblad SE, Orley JE: *Amidst peril and pain: The mental health and well-being of the world's refugees*. 20th ed. Washington, DC, American Psychological Association, 1994.
28. Eisenbruch M: The cry for the lost placenta: Cultural bereavement and cultural survival among Cambodians who resettled, were repatriated, or who stayed at home. In: van Tilburg M, Vingerhoets A (eds.): *Home is where the heart is: The psychological aspects of permanent and temporary geographical moves*. Tilburg, Tilburg University Press, 1997. pp. 119–142.
29. Tseng WS, Cheng TA, Chen YS, Hwang PL, Hsu J: Psychiatric complications of family reunion after four decades of separation. *American Journal of Psychiatry* April, 150(4):614–9, 1993.
30. Lee I: Second International Conference on Wartime Medical Services. *Medicine and War* April, 7(2):120–8, 1991.
31. Thabet AA, Vostanis P: Social adversities and anxiety disorders in the Gaza Strip. *Arch Dis Child* May, 78(5):439–42, 1998.
32. Thabet AA, Stretch D, Vostanis P: Child mental health problems in Arab children: Application of the strengths and difficulties questionnaire. *International Journal of Social Psychiatry* 46(4):266–80, 2000.
33. Aptekar L, Stocklin D: Children in particularly difficult circumstances. In: nd e, editor. *Handbook of cross-cultural psychology*, Vol. Inc., Boston, Allyn & Bacon, 1997, pp. 377–412.
34. Allwood MA, Bell-Dolan D, Husain SA: Children's trauma and adjustment reactions to violent and nonviolent war experiences. *Journal of the American Academy of Child and Adolescent Psychiatry* 41(4):450–7, 2002 April.
35. Smith P, Perrin S, Yule W, Hacam B, Stuvland R: War exposure among children from Bosnia-Hercegovina: Psychological adjustment in a community sample. *Journal of Traumatic Stress* April, 15(2):147–56, 2002.
36. Dyregrov A, Gjestad R, Raundalen M: Children exposed to warfare: A longitudinal study. *Journal of Traumatic Stress* 15(1):59–68, 2002 February.
37. Donnelly CL, Amaya-Jackson L: Post-traumatic stress disorder in children and adolescents: Epidemiology, diagnosis and treatment options. *Paediatric Drugs* 4(3):159–70, 2002.
38. Singh S: Post-traumatic stress in former Ugandan child soldiers.[comment]. *Lancet* May 15, 363(9421):1648, 2004.
39. Kuruppuarachchi K, Wijeratne LT: Post-traumatic stress in former Ugandan child soldiers.[comment]. *Lancet* May 15, 363(9421):1648, 2004.
40. Magambo C, Lett R: Post-traumatic stress in former Ugandan child soldiers.[comment]. *Lancet* May 15, 363(9421):1647–8, 2004.
41. McKay S, Wessells MG: Post-traumatic stress in former Ugandan child soldiers.[comment]. *Lancet* May 15, 363(9421):1646–7, 2004.
42. Derluyn I, Broekaert E, Schuyten G, De TE: Post-traumatic stress in former Ugandan child soldiers.[see comment]. *Lancet* March 13, 363(9412):861–3, 2004.
43. Moszynski P: Child soldiers forgotten in Angola. *BMJ* May 10, 326(7397):1003, 2003.
44. Somasundaram D: Child soldiers: Understanding the context. [Review] [11 refs]. *BMJ* May 25, 324(7348):1268–71, 2002.
45. Lamberg L: Reclaiming child soldiers' lost lives. *JAMA* August 4, 292(5):553–4, 2004.
46. Bracken PJ, Giller JE, Ssekiwanuka JK: The rehabilitation of child soldiers: Defining needs and appropriate responses. *Medicine, Conflict and Survival* April, 12(2):114–25, 1996.
47. Willis BM, Levy BS: Child prostitution: Global health burden, research needs, and interventions. *The Lancet* April 20, 359(9315):1417–22, 2002.
48. UNICEF, Innocenti Research Centre: *Trafficking in human beings, especially women and children, in Africa*. Florence, Italy, UNICEF Innocenti Research Center, 2003.
49. International Organization for Migration: *Trafficking in women and children from the Republic of Armenia: A study*. Yerevan, International Organization for Migration, 2001.
50. Jalalza'i MK: *Children trafficking in Pakistan*. Karachi, Royal Book Co, 2003.
51. Subedi G, Trafficking iC, International Labour Org: *Trafficking and Sexual Abuse among Street Children in Kathmandu*, 1st ed. Kathmandu International Labour Organization, 2002.
52. Sorajjakool S: *Child Prostitution in Thailand: Listening to Rahab*. New York, Haworth Press, 2003. 0
53. Rozario MR, Kesari P, Rasool J: *Trafficking in Women and Children in India: Sexual Exploitation and Sale*. New Delhi, Uppal Public House, 1988.
54. International Office for Migration: *Victims Trafficking in the Balkans: A study of Trafficking in Women and Children for Sexual Exploitation to,*

through, and from the Balkan Region. Vienna, Geneva, IOM International Organization for Migration, 2001.
55. Commission of the European Communities: *Combating Trafficking in Human Beings and Combating the Sexual Exploitation of Children and Child Pornography*. Brussels, Commission of the European Communities, 2001.
56. Inter-American Commission of Women: Trafficking of women and children for sexual exploitation in the Americas—An introduction to trafficking in the Americas; 2001.
57. Asian DB: *Combating Trafficking of Women and Children in South Asia—Regional Synthesis Paper for Bangladesh, India, and Nepal*. Manila, Asian Development Bank, 2003.
58. International Labour Organisation, International Programme on the Elimination of Child Labour: Combating trafficking in children for labour exploitation in the Mekong sub-region : A proposed framework for ILO-IPEC action and proceedings of a Mekong sub-regional consultation. ILO/IPEC, 1998.
59. UNICEF: *The State of the World's Children*. New York, UNICEF, 2000.
60. Munir K, Belfer ML: HIV and AIDS: Global and United States Perspectives. In: Wiener JM, Dulcan MK (eds.): *Textbook of child and adolescent psychiatry*. 3rd edition. Washington, DC, American Psychiatric Publishing, Inc, 2004, pp. 869–889.
61. Carlson M, Earls F: Psychological and neuroendocrinological sequelae of early social deprivation in institutionalized children in Romania. In: Carter CS, Lederhendler II, Kirkpatrick B (eds.): *The integrative neurobiology of affiliation*. New York Academy of Sciences, 1997. pp. 419–28.
62. Belfer M, Heggenhougen K: Substance abuse. In: Desjarlais R, Eisenberg L, Good B, Kleinman A (eds): *World Mental Health: Problems and Priorities in Low-income Countries*. New York, Oxford University Press, 1995. pp. 87–115.
63. Alem A, Kebede D, Kullgren G: The prevalence and socio-demographic correlates of khat chewing in Butajira, Ethiopia. *Acta psychiatrica Scandinavica Supplementum* 397:84–91, 1999.
64. Raffaelli M, Larson RW: *Homeless and Working Youth Around the World—Exploring Developmental Issues*. San Francisco, Jossey-Bass, 1999.
65. Senanayake MP, Ranasinghe A, Balasuriya C: Street children—A preliminary study. *Ceylon Medical Journal* December, 43(4):191–3, 1998.
66. Carlini-Cotrim B, Carlini EA: The use of solvents and other drugs among children and adolescents from a low socioeconomic background: a study in São Paulo, Brazil. *The International journal of the addictions* November, 23(11):1145–56, 1988.
67. Cameron FJ, Debelle GD: No more Pacific island paradises. *Lancet* June 2, 1(8388):1238, 1984.
68. Belasso G: The international challenge of drug abuse: The Mexican experience. In: Petersen RC, National Institute on Drug Abuse (eds.): *The International Challenge of Drug Abuse*, 19th ed. Rockville, MD, Dept. of Health, Education, and Welfare, Public Health Service, Alcohol, Drug Abuse, and Mental Health Administration, National Institute on Drug Abuse, Division of Research, 1978.
69. Cravioto P, Anchondo R-L, de la Rosa B: Risk factors associated with inhalant use among Mexican juvenile delinquents. In: National Institute on Drug Abuse, Community Epidemiology Work Group, Johnson B&S, (eds.): *Epidemiologic Trends in Drug Abuse*. Rockville, MD: U.S. Dept. of Health and Human Services, Public Health Service, Alcohol, Drug Abuse, and Mental Health Administration, Division of Epidemiology and Prevention Research, National Institute on Drug Abuse, 1992. pp. 472–477.
70. Wittig MC, Wright JD, Kaminsky DC: Substance use among street children in Honduras. *Substance Use & Misuse* June 1997: 32(7–8):805–827.
71. Forster LM, Tannhauser M, Barros HM: Drug use among street children in southern Brazil. *Drug & Alcohol Dependence* December 2 1996: 43(1–2):57–62.
72. World Health Organization: *World Report on Violence and Health*. Geneva, Switzerland, 2002.
73. Djeddah C, Facchin P, Ranzato C, Romer C: Child abuse: Current problems and key public health challenges. *Social Science and Medicine* September 15 2000: 51(6):905–15.
74. Ohtsuji M, Ohshima T, Kondo T, Godoy MR, Oehmichen M: [Fatal child abuse in Japan and Germany. Comparative retrospective study] [German]. *Archiv für Kriminologie* July 1998: 202(1–2):8–16.
75. D'Antonio IJ, Darwish AM, McLean M: Child maltreatment: International perspectives. *Maternal Child Nursing Journal* April 1993: 21(2):39–52.
76. Mazurek AJ: Epidemiology of paediatric injury. *J Accid Emerg Med* March 1994: 11(1):9–16.
77. Marzouki M, Hadh Fredj A, Chelli M: Child abuse and cultural attitudes: The example of Tunisia. *Child Abuse and Neglect* 11(1):137–41, 1987.
78. Agathonos H, Stathacopoulou N, Adam H, Nakou S: Child abuse and neglect in Greece: Sociomedical aspects. *Child Abuse Negl* 6(3):307–11, 1982.
79. Santana-Tavira R, Sanchez-Ahedo R, Herrera-Basto E: [Child abuse: a world problem]. *Salud Publica Mex* January 1998: 40(1):58–65.
80. Frias-Armenta M, McCloskey LA: Determinants of harsh parenting in Mexico. *Journal of Abnormal Child Psychology* April 1998: 26(2):129–139.
81. Doe SS: Cultural Factors in Child Maltreatment and Domestic Violence in Korea. *Children and Youth Services Review* 22(3–4):231–236, 2000.
82. Qureshi B: Cultural aspects of child abuse in Britain. *Midwife, Health Visitor & Community Nurse* October 1988: 24(10):412–413.
83. Reid S: Cultural difference and child abuse intervention with undocumented Spanish-speaking families in Los Angeles. *Child Abuse Negl* 8(1):109–112 1984.
84. Loening W-EK: Child abuse among the Zulus: A people in cultural transition. *Child Abuse and Neglect* 5(1):3–7, 1981.
85. Davis RE: Cultural health care or child abuse? The Southeast Asian practice of *cao gio*. *Journal of the American Academy of Nurse Practitioners* March 2000: 12(3):89–95.
86. Shalhoub-Kevorkian N: Disclosure of child abuse in conflict areas. *Violence Against Women* October 2005: 11(10):1263–91.
87. Hopkins SRMRDOCC: A discussion of the legal aspects of female genital mutilation. *A Adv Nurs* October 1999: 30(4):926–933.
88. Ho WS, Ying SY, Wong TW: Bizarre paediatric facial burns. *Burns* August 1 2000: 26(5):504–506.
89. Warner JE, Hansen DJ: The identification and reporting of physical abuse by physicians: A review and implications for research. *Child Abuse Negl* January 1994: 18(1):11–25.
90. Korbin JE, Coulton CJ, Chard S, Platt-Houston C, Su M: Impoverishment and child maltreatment in African American and European American neighborhoods. *Dev Psychopathol* 10(2):215–33, 1998.
91. Maitra B: Child abuse: a universal "diagnostic" category? The implication of culture in definition and assessment. *The International Journal of Social Psychiatry* 42(4):287–304, 1996.
92. Levesque RJ: Cultural evidence, child maltreatment, and the law. *Child Maltreat* May 2000: 5(2):146–160.
93. Haj YM, Shor R: Child maltreatment as perceived by Arab students of social science in the West Bank. *Child Abuse Negl* October 1995: 19(10):1209–1219.
94. Baker KA, Dwairy M: Cultural norms versus state law in treating incest: A suggested model for Arab families.[see comment]. *Child Abuse and Neglect* January 2003: 27(1):109–123.
95. Munir KM, Beardslee WR: A developmental and psychobiologic framework for understanding the role of culture in child and adolescent psychiatry. *Child and Adolescent Psychiatric Clinics of North America* October 2001: 10(4):667–677.
96. Beauchaine TP: Taxometrics and developmental psychopathology. [Review] [198 refs]. *Development & Psychopathology* 15(3):501–527, 2003.
97. Novins DK, Bechtold DW, Sack WH, Thompson J, Carter DR, Manson SM: The DSM-IV Outline for Cultural Formulation: a Critical demonstration with American Indian children.*Journal of the American Academy of Child and Adolescent Psychiatry* September 1997: 36(9):1244–1251.
98. Neki JS: An examination of the cultural relativism of dependence as a dynamic of social and therapeutic relationships. I. Socio-developmental. *British Journal of Medical Psychology* March 1976: 49(1):1–10.
99. Malhotra S, Malhotra A, Varma VK: *Child mental Health in India*. Delhi, Macmillan India Limited, 1992.
100. Malhotra S: Challenges in providing mental health services for children and adolescents in India. In: Young JG, Ferrari P (eds): *Designing Mental Health Services and Systems for Children and Adolescents—A Shrewd Investment*. Philadelphia, PA, Brunner/Mazel, 1998. pp. 321–334.
101. Huss M, Iseler A, Lehmkuhl U. [Cross-cultural comparison of Conners Scales: Can the US-American factorial structure be replicated on German clinical sample?] [German]. *Zeitschrift fur Kinder-und Jugendpsychiatrie und Psychotherapie* February 2001: 29(1):16–24.
102. Roussos A, Richardson C, Politikou K, Marketos S, Kyprianos S, Karajianni S et al.: The Conners–28 teacher questionnaire in clinical and nonclinical samples of Greek children 6–12 years old. *European Child and Adolescent Psychiatry* December 1999: 8(4):260–267.
103. Rey JM, Singh M, Hung SF, Dossetor DR, Newman L, Plapp JM et al.: A global scale to measure the quality of the family environment.[see comment]. *Archives of General Psychiatry* September 1997: 54(9):817–822.
104. Goodman R, Renfrew D, Mullick M: Predicting type of psychiatric disorder from Strengths and Difficulties Questionnaire (SDQ) scores in child mental health clinics in London and Dhaka. *European Child & Adolescent Psychiatry* June 2000: 9(2):129–134.
105. Odejide AO, Oyewunmi LK, Ohaeri JU: Psychiatry in Africa: An overview. *American Journal of Psychiatry* June 1989: 146(6):708–716.
106. Hackett R, Hackett L: Child psychiatry across cultures. *International Review of Psychiatry* May 1999: 11(2):225–235.
107. Taeb O, Heidenreich F, Baubet T, Moro MR: [Finding a meaning for illness: from medical anthropology to cultural epidemiology]. *Meddecine et maladies infectieuses* April 2005: 35(4):173–185.
108. Raguram R, Raghu TM, Vounatsou P, Weiss MG: Schizophrenia and the cultural epidemiology of stigma in Bangalore, India.*Journal of Nervous and Mental Disease* November 2004: 192(11):734–734.
109. DiGiacomo SM: Can there be a "cultural epidemiology"? *Med Anthropol Q* December 1999: 13(4):436–457.
110. Tadesse B, Kebede D, Tegegne T, Alem A: Childhood behavioural disorders in Ambo district, western Ethiopia. I. Prevalence estimates. *Acta Psychiatrica Scandinavica Supplementum* 397:92–97, 1999.

111. Giel R, Van LN: Psychiatric morbidity in a small Ethiopian town. *Rev Med Psychosom Psychol Med* October 1969: 11(4):435–456.
112. Harding TW, De Arango MV, Baltazar J, Climent CE, Ibrahim HH, Ladrido-Ignacio L et al.: Mental disorders in primary health care: A study of their frequency and diagnosis in four developing countries. *Psychol Med* May 1980: 10(2):231–241.
113. Omigbodun OO: Psychosocial issues in a child and adolescent psychiatric clinic population in Nigeria. *Social Psychiatry and Psychiatric Epidemiology* August 2004: 39(8):667–672.
114. Malhotra, S: Study of Psychosocial Correlates of Developmental Psychopathology in School Children: Report to Indian Council for Medical Research. New Delhi, Indian Council for Medical Research, 1995.
115. Giel R, de Arango MV, Clement, CE, et al.: Childhood mental disorders in primary health care: Results of observations in four developing countries. *Pediatrics* 68: 677–683, 1981.
116. Thabet AA, Vostanis P: Social adversities and anxiety disorders in the Gaza Strip. *Arch Dis Child* May 1998: 78(5):439–442.
117. Kashani JH, Orvaschel H: A community study of anxiety in children and adolescents. *American Journal of Psychiatry* March 1990: 147(3):313–318.
118. Tadesse B, Kebede D, Tegegne T, Alem A: Childhood behavioural disorders in Ambo district, western Ethiopia. II.Validation of the RQC. *Acta Psychiatrica Scandinavica Supplementum* 397:98–101, 1999.
119. Hackett RJ, Hackett L, Bhakta P, Gowers S: The prevalence and associations of psychiatric disorder in children in Kerala, South India. *Journal of Child Psychology and Psychiatry* July 1999: 40(5):801–807.
120. Bird HR, Gould MS, Yager T, Staghezza B, Canino G: Risk factors for maladjustment in Puerto Rican children. *Journal of the American Academy of Child and Adolescent Psychiatry* November 1989: 28(6):847–850.
121. Becker AE: *Body, Self and Society—The View from Fiji*. Philadelphia, University of Pennsylvania Press, 1995.
122. Fayyad JA, Jahshan CS, Karam EG: Systems development of child mental health services in developing countries. *Child and Adolescent Psychiatric Clinics of North America* 10(4):745–762, 2001.
123. al-Ansari A, Matar AM: Recent stressful life events among Bahraini adolescents with adjustment disorder. *Adolescence* 28(110):339–346, 1993.
124. Khandelwal SK, Sharan P, Saxena S: Eating disorders: An Indian perspective. *International Journal of Social Psychiatry* 41(2):132–146, 1995.
125. Littlewood R: Psychopathology and personal agency: Modernity, culture change and eating disorders in South Asian societies. *British Journal of Medical Psychology* March 1995: 68(1):45–63.
126. Hill AJ, Bhatti R: Body shape perception and dieting in preadolescent British Asian girls: links with eating disorders. *Int J Eat Disord* March 1995: 17(2):175–183.
127. Bryant WR, Lask B: Anorexia nervosa in a group of Asian children living in Britain [see comments]. *Br J Psychiatry* February 1991: 158:229–233.
128. le Grange D, Telch CF, Tibbs J: Eating attitudes and behaviors in 1,435 South African Caucasian and non-Caucasian college students.[see comment]. *American Journal of Psychiatry* February 1998: 155(2):250–254.
129. Gupta N: Autism: Some conceptual issues.[comment]. *Indian Pediatrics* September 2001: 38(9):1065–1067.
130. Yeargin-Allsopp M, Boyle C: Overview: The epidemiology of neurodevelopmental disorders. *Mental Retardation & Developmental Disabilities Research Reviews* 8(3):113–116, 2002.
131. Lotter V: Childhood autism in africa. *Journal of Child Psychology and Psychiatry and Allied Disciplines* July 1978: 19(3):231–244.
132. Chung SY, Luk SL, Lee PW: A follow-up study of infantile autism in Hong Kong. *Journal of Autism and Developmental Disorders* June 1990: 20(2):221–232.
133. Takei N: Childhood autism in Japan.[comment]. *British Journal of Psychiatry* November 1996: 169(5):671–672.
134. Gillberg C, Schaumann H, Gillberg IC: Autism in immigrants: Children born in Sweden to mothers born in Uganda. *Journal of Intellectual Disability Research* April 1995: 39(Pt. 2):141–144.
135. Gillberg IC, Gillberg C: Autism in immigrants: A population-based study from Swedish rural and urban areas. *Journal of Intellectual Disability Research* February 1996: 40(Pt. 1):24–31.
136. Mollica RF, Poole C, Son L, Murray CC, Tor S: Effects of war trauma on Cambodian refugee adolescents' functional health and mental health status. *Journal of the American Academy of Child and Adolescent Psychiatry* August 1997: 36(8):1098–1106.
137. Pynoos RS, Frederick C, Nader K, Arroyo W, Steinberg A, Eth S et al.: Life threat and posttraumatic stress in school-age children. *Arch Gen Psychiatry* December 1987: 44(12):1057–1063.
138. Weine SM, Vojvoda D, Becker DF, McGlashan TH, Hodzic E, Laub D et al.: PTSD symptoms in Bosnian refugees 1 year after resettlement in the United States. *Am J Psychiatry* April 1998: 155(4):562–564.
139. Sack WH, Him C, Dickason D: Twelve-year follow-up study of Khmer youths who suffered massive war trauma as children. *Journal of the American Academy of Child and Adolescent Psychiatry* September 1999: 38(9):1173–1179.
140. Sack WH, Clarke GN, Kinney R, Belestos G, Him C, Seeley J: The Khmer Adolescent Project. II: Functional capacities in two generations of Cambodian refugees. *J Nerv Ment Dis* March 1995: 183(3):177–181.
141. Terr LC: Chowchilla revisited: The effects of psychic trauma four years after a school-bus kidnapping. *American Journal of Psychiatry* December 1983: 140(12):1543–1560.
142. Abdel-Mawgoud M: A survey of fears associated with Iraqi aggression among Kuwaiti children and adolescents: A factorial study 5.7 years after the Gulf War. *Psychological Reports* August 1997: 81(1):247–255.
143. Almqvist K, Brandell-Forsberg M: Refugee children in Sweden: Post-traumatic stress disorder in Iranian preschool children exposed to organized violence. *Child Abuse Negl* April 1997: 21(4):351–366.
144. Nader KO, Pynoos RS, Fairbanks LA, al-Ajeel M, al-Asfour A: A preliminary study of PTSD and grief among the children of Kuwait following the Gulf crisis. *British Journal of Clinical Psychology* November 1993: 32(Pt. 4):407–416.
145. Ahmad A: Symptoms of posttraumatic stress disorder among displaced Kurdish children in Iraq: Victims of a man-made disaster after the Gulf war. *Nordic Journal of Psychiatry* 46(5):315–9, 1992.
146. Hussain SA, Nair J, Holcomb W, Reid JC, Vargas V, Nair SS: Stress reactions of children and adolescents in war and siege conditions. *American J Psychiatry* December 1998: 155(12):1718–1719.
147. Responding to Emergency Situations, World Health Organization, Department of Mental Health and Substance Abuse, 2005.
148. Prior M, Virasinghe S, Smart D: Behavioural problems in Sri Lankan schoolchildren: Associations with socio-economic status, age, gender, academic progress, ethnicity and religion. *Social Psychiatry and Psychiatric Epidemiology* August 2005: 40(8):654–662.
149. Vermeiren R, De CA, Deboutte D: A descriptive survey of Flemish delinquent adolescents. *Journal of Adolescence* June 2000: 23(3):277–285.
150. Tramontina S, Martins S, Michalowski MB, Ketzer CR, Eizirik M, Biederman J et al.: School dropout and conduct disorder in Brazilian elementary school students. *Canadian Journal of Psychiatry—Revue Canadienne de Psychiatrie* December 2001: 46(10):941–947.
151. Burke AW: A cross-cultural study of delinquency among West Indian boys. *International Journal of Social Psychiatry* 26(2):81–87, 1980.
152. World Health Organization: *WHO Guide to Mental and Neurological Health in Primary Care—A Guide to Mental and Neurological Ill Health in Adults, Adolescents and Children*. 2nd ed. London, Royal Society of Medicine Press, 2004.
153. Abdel-Khalek AM, Soliman HH: A cross-cultural evaluation of depression in children in Egypt, Kuwait, and the United States. *Psychological Reports* December 1999: 85(3 Pt. 1):973–980.
154. Gutmann, Bruno: *Das Recht der Dschagga. Munich*. New Haven, Human Relations Area Files, 1926.
155. Howard M, Millard AV: *Hunger and Shame: Poverty and Child Malnutrition on Mount Kilimanjaro*. New York and London, Routledge, 1997.
156. Gubhaju BB: The Effect of Previous Child Death on Infant and Child Mortality in Rural Nepal. *Studies in Family Planning* 16(4):231–236, 1985.
157. Moffat T: Infant mortality and cultural concepts of infancy: A case study from an early twentieth century aboriginal community. Special issue: The anthropology of infancy. *Pre and Peri Natal Psychology Journal* 8(4):259–273, 1994.
158. Scheper-Hughes N. Infant Mortality and Infant Care: Cultural and Economic Constraints on Nurturing in Northeast Brazil. *Social Science and Medicine* 19(5):535–546, 1984.
159. Borowsky IW, Resnick MD, Ireland M, Blum RW: Suicide attempts among American Indian and Alaska Native youth: Risk and protective factors. *Archives of Pediatrics & Adolescent Medicine* June 1999: 153(6):573–580.
160. Shaffer D: The epidemiology of teen suicide: An examination of risk factors. *Journal of Clinical Psychiatry* September 1988: 49 Suppl:36–41.
161. Bertolote J: Department of Mental Health and Substance Abuse, World Health Organization, Geneva, Switzerland. Personal communication, 2003.
162. Murthy RS: Approaches to suicide prevention in Asia and the Far East. In: Hawton K, Van Heeringen K (eds.): *International Handbook of Suicide and Attempted Suicide*. London, Wiley, 2000. pp. 625–637.
163. Chan KP, Hung SF, Yip PS: Suicide in response to changing societies. *Child and Adolescent Psychiatric Clinics of North America* October 2001: 10(4):777–795.
164. Blum RW, Halcon L, Beuhring T, Pate E, Campell-Forrester S, Venema A: Adolescent health in the Caribbean: Risk and protective factors. *American Journal of Public Health* March 2003: 93(3):456–460.
165. Chan K: Hong Kong, China. Personal communication. 2003.
166. Dugge C: A mirror for India: Suicide of 4 sisters. *International Herald Tribune* 2000.
167. United Nations, Economic and Social Commission for Asia and the Pacific: Focus on ability, celebrate diversity—Highlights of the Asian and Pacific decade of disabled persons, 1993–2003. New York, United Nations, 2003.
168. Belmont, L: The international pilot study of severe childhood disability—Final report—*Screening for Severe Mental Retardation in Developing Countries*. Utrecht, Bishop Bekkers Institute; 1984.
169. Narayanan H: A study of the prevalence of mental retardation in Southern India. *International Journal of Mental Health* 10:128–136, 1981.
170. Tao K: Mentally retarded persons in the People's Republic of China: A review of epidemiological studies and services. *American Journal on Mental Retardation* 93:193–199, 1988.

171. Lal N, Sethi B: Estimate of mental ill-health in children in an urban community. *Indian Journal of Pediatrics* 44(55):64, 1977.
172. Malhotra S, Chaturvedi S: Patterns of childhood psychiatric disorders in India. *Indian Pediatric Journal* 51:235–240, 1984.
173. Stein Z, Durkin M, Belmont L: "Serious" mental retardation in developing countries: An epidemiologic approach. *Annals of the New York Academy of Sciences* 477:8–21, 1986.
174. Kim YS, Kumar S: Cross-cultural examination of social interactions during a one-week *dousa-hou* (Japanese psychorehabilitation) camp. *Psychological Reports* December, 2004: 95(3 Pt. 1):1050–1054.
175. Atlas on child and adolescent mental health resources—Global concerns: Implications for the future. World Health Organization, Geneva, Switzerland, 2005.
176. Belfer ML, Saxena S: WHO Child Atlas Project. *Lancet* 367:551–552, 2006.
177. McKelvey RS, Sang DL, Tu HC: Is there a role for child psychiatry in Vietnam? *Australian and New Zealand Journal of Psychiatry* February, 1997: 31(1):114–119.
178. El-Din A, Moustafa A, Mohit A: A multisectoral approach to school mental health, Alexandria, Egypt. II. *Health Serv J East Medit Reg* 7(34):40, 1993.
179. Giel R, De Arango MV, Climent CE, Harding TW, Ibrahim HH, Ladrido-Ignacio L et al.: Childhood mental disorders in primary health care: Results of observations in four developing countries. A report from the WHO Collaborative Study on Strategies for Extending Mental Health Care. *Pediatrics* November: 1981 68(5):677–683.
180. Graham P, Orley J: WHO and the mental health of children. *World Health Forum* 19(3):268–272, 1998.
181. Nikapota, AD: *Recognition and Management of Children with Functional Complaints—A Training Package for the Primary Care Physician.* New Delhi, WHO Regional Office for South-East Asia, 1993.
182. Mathur G, Mathur S, Singh Y: Detection and prevention of childhood disability with the help of *anganwadi* workers. *Indian Pediatric Journal* 32:773–777, 1995.
183. Jazaïry I, International Fund for Agricultural Development: *The State of World Rural Poverty—An Inquiry into Its Causes and Consequences.* New York, Published for the International Fund for Agricultural Development by New York University Press, 1992.
184. World Health Organization Division of Mental Health: Life skills education in schools. WHO, 1994.
185. Bandura A: *Social Learning Theory.* Englewood Cliffs, NJ, Prentice Hall, 1977.
186. Kapur M, Cariapa I, Parthasarathy R: Evaluation of an orientation course for teachers on emotional problems amongst school children. *Indian Journal of Clinical Psychology* September, 1980: 7(2):103–107.
187. Kim WJ: A training guideline of cultural competence for child and adolescent psychiatric residencies. *Child Psychiatry and Human Development* 6(2):125–136, 1995.
188. Earls F, Eisenberg L: International perspective in child psychiatry. In: Lewis M (ed.): *Child and Adolescent Psychiatry—A Comprehensive Textbook.* Baltimore: Williams & Wilkins, 1991, p. 1189–1196.
189. Mohler B: Cross-cultural issues in research on child mental health. *Child and Adolescent Psychiatric Clinics of North America* 10(4):763–776 2001.
190. Nelson ML, Quintana SM: Qualitative clinical research with children and adolescents. [Review] [60 refs]. *Journal of Clinical Child & Adolescent Psychology* June 2005: 34(2):344–356.
191. Weisner TS: *Discovering Successful Pathways in Children's Development—Mixed Methods in the Study of Childhood and Family Life.* Chicago, University of Chicago Press, 2005.
192. Eisenbruch M: The lens of culture, the lens of health: Toward a framework and toolkit for cultural competence. Resource document, for UNESCO Asia-Pacific Regional Training Workshop on Cultural Mapping and Cultural Diversity Programming Lens to Safeguard Tangible and Intangible Cultural Expressions and Protect Cultural Diversity, Bangkok, 15–19 December 2004; 2004, pp. 1–248.
193. Lindenberg CS, Solorzano RM, Vilaro FM, Westbrook LO: Challenges and strategies for conducting intervention research with culturally diverse populations. [Review] [30 refs]. *J Transcult Nurs* April 2001: 12(2):132–139.
194. Lindgren T, Lipson JG: Finding a way: Afghan women's experience in community participation. *J Transcult Nurs* April 2004: 15(2):122–130.
195. Penrod J, Preston DB, Cain RE, Starks MT: A discussion of chain referral as a method of sampling hard-to-reach populations. *J Transcult Nurs* April 2003: 14(2):100–107.
196. Portillo CJ, Villarruel A, de Leon Siantz ML, Peragallo N, Calvillo ER, Eribes CM: Research agenda for Hispanics in the United States: A nursing perspective. [Review] [70 refs]. *Nurs Outlook* 2001 November: 49(6):263–269.
197. Roszak DJ: To eliminate racial/ethic disparities, hospitals must standardize data collection. *Hospitals & Health Networks* 78(6):78, 2004.
198. Fontes LA: Ethics in family violence research: Cross-cultural issues. *Family Relations: Journal of Applied Family & Child Studies* January 1998: 47(1):53–61.
199. Munir K, Earls F: Ethical principles governing research in child and adolescent psychiatry. *Journal of the American Academy of Child and Adolescent Psychiatry* May 1992: 31(3):408–414.
200. Earls F: Child psychiatry in an international context: With remarks on the current status of child psychiatry in China. In: Super CM (ed.): *The Role of Culture in Developmental Disorder.* San Diego, Academic Press, 1987, pp. 235–248.
201. Patel V, Sumathipala A: International representation in psychiatric literature: Survey of six leading journals. *Brit J Psychiatry.* 178:406–409, 2001.
202. Galler JR, Ramsey F, Solimano G, Lowell WE, Mason E: The influence of early malnutrition on subsequent behavioral development. I. Degree of impairment in intellectual performance. *Journal of the American Academy of Child Psychiatry* January 1983: 22(1):8–15.
203. Agarwal DK, Upadhyay SK, Agarwal KN, Singh RD, Tripathi AM: Anaemia and mental functions in rural primary school children. *Annals of Tropical Paediatrics* December 1989: 9(4):194–198.
204. Galler JR, Ramsey F: A follow-up study of the influence of early malnutrition on development: Behavior at home and at school. *Journal of the American Academy of Child and Adolescent Psychiatry* March 1989: 28(2):254–261.
205. Miranda CT, Paula CS, Santos L, Nobrega FJ, Hundeide K, Orley J: Association between mother–child interaction and mental health among mothers of malnourished children. *Journal of Tropical Pediatrics* October 2000: 46(5):314.
206. Gillespie S, Mclachlan M, Shrimpton R, World B, Human DN, UNICEF: *Combating Malnutrition—Time to Act.* Washington, DC, World Bank, 2003.
207. Beardslee WR, Gladstone TR, Wright EJ, Cooper AB: A family-based approach to the prevention of depressive symptoms in children at risk: evidence of parental and child change. *Pediatrics* 112(2):119–313 2003.
208. Beardslee: Personal communication, 2005.
209. Graham P, Orley J: WHO's activities related to psychosocial aspects of health (including child and adolescent health and development). In: de Girolamo G, Sartorius N (eds.): *Promoting Mental Health Internationally.* London, Gaskell, 1999, pp. 117–131.
210. Focusing Resources on Effective School Health: A FRESH Start to Enhancing the Quality and Equity of Education. <www.unesco.org/education?index.shtml>; <www.unicef.org/programme/lifeskills/mainmenu.html>; <www.who.int/hpr.fshi/index.htm>; <www.schoolsandhealth.org>.
211. Remschmidt, H, Belfer, ML: Mental health care for children and adolescents worldwide: A review. *World Psychiatry* 4(3):147–153, 2005.
212. International Association for Child and Adolescent Psychiatry and Allied Professions Webpage <www.iacapap.org>.
213. Shatkin JP Belfer, ML: The global absence of child and adolescent mental health policy. *Child and Adolescent Mental Health* 9:104–108, 2004.
214. McClure M, Shirataki S: Child psychiatry in Japan. *Journal of the American Academy of Child and Adolescent Psychiatry* July 1989: 28(4):488–492.
215. Lewis O, Sargent J, Friedrich W, Chaffin M, Cunningham N, Cantor PS: The impact of social change on child mental health in Eastern Europe. *Child and Adolescent Psychiatric Clinics of North America* October 2001: 10(4):815–824.

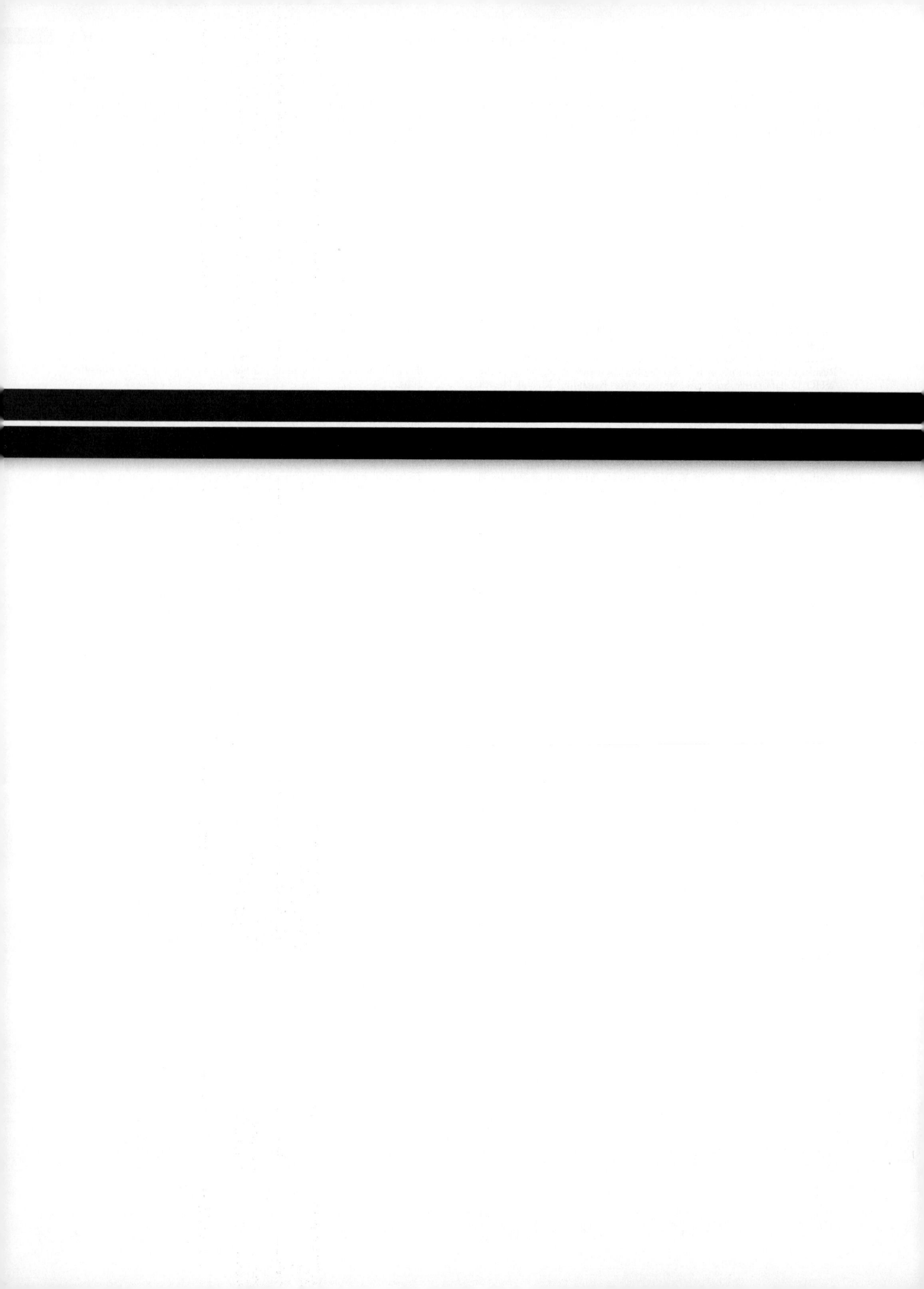

SECTION II
SCIENTIFIC FOUNDATIONS

2.1 ■ RESEARCH METHODOLOGY

CHAPTER 2.1.1 ■ UNDERSTANDING RESEARCH METHODS AND STATISTICS: A PRIMER FOR CLINICIANS

GEORGE A. MORGAN, JEFFREY A. GLINER, AND ROBERT J. HARMON

INTRODUCTION

Purposes of Research

Research has two general purposes: a) increasing knowledge within the discipline and b) increasing knowledge as a professional consumer of research in order to understand and evaluate research developments within the discipline. For many clinicians, the ability to understand research in one's discipline may be even more important than making research contributions. Dissemination occurs through an exceptionally large number of professional journals, workshops, and continuing education courses, as well as popular literature. Today's professional cannot simply rely on the statements of a workshop instructor to determine what should be included in an intervention. Even journal articles need to be scrutinized for weak designs, inappropriate data analyses, or incorrect interpretation of these analyses. Current professionals must have the research and reasoning skills to be able to make sound decisions and support them.

Research Dimensions and Dichotomies

Self-Report versus Researcher Observation

In some studies the participants report to the researcher about their attitudes, intentions, or behavior. In other studies the researcher directly observes and records the behavior of the participant. Sometimes instruments such as heart rate monitors are used by researchers to "observe" the participants' physiological functioning. Self-reports may be influenced by biases such as the halo effect, or participants may have forgotten or not thought about the topic. Many researchers prefer observed behavioral data. However, sensitive, well trained interviewers may be able to alleviate some of the biases inherent in self-reports.

Quantitative versus Qualitative Research

We believe that this topic is more appropriately thought of as two related dimensions. The first dimension deals with philosophical or paradigm differences between the quantitative (positivist) approach and the qualitative (constructivist) approach to research (1). The second dimension, which is often what people mean when referring to this dichotomy, deals with the type of data, data collection, and data analysis. We think that, in distinguishing between qualitative and quantitative research, the first dimension is the most important.

Positivist Versus Constructivist Paradigms. Although there is disagreement about the appropriateness of these labels, they help us separate the philosophical or paradigm distinction from the data collection and analysis issues. A study could be theoretically positivistic, but the data could be subjective or qualitative. In fact, this combination is quite common. However, qualitative data, methods, and analyses often go with the constructivist paradigm, and quantitative data, methods, and analyses are usually used with the positivist paradigm. This chapter is within the framework of the positivist paradigm, but the constructivist paradigm provides us with useful reminders that human participants are complex and different from other animals and inanimate objects.

Quantitative Versus Qualitative Data, Data Collection, and Analysis. Quantitative data are said to be "objective," which indicates that the behaviors are easily and reliably classified or quantified by the researcher. Qualitative data are more difficult to describe. They are said to be "subjective," which indicates that they are hard to classify or score. Some examples are perceptions of pain and attitudes toward therapy. Usually these data are gathered from interviews, observations, or documents. Quantitative/positivist researchers also gather these types of data but usually translate such perceptions and attitudes into numbers. Qualitative/constructivist researchers, on the other hand, usually do not try to quantify such perceptions; instead, they categorize them.

Data analysis for quantitative researchers usually involves well defined statistical methods, most often providing a test of the null hypothesis. Qualitative researchers are more interested in examining their data for similarities or themes which might occur among all of the participants on a particular topic.

VARIABLES AND THEIR MEASUREMENT

Research Problems and Variables

Research Problems

The research process begins with a problem. A research problem is an interrogative sentence about the relationship between two or more variables. Prior to the problem statement, the scientist usually perceives an obstacle to understanding.

Variables

A variable must be able to vary or have different values. For example, gender is a variable because it has two values, female or male. Age is a variable that has a large number of potential values. Type of treatment/intervention is a variable if there is more than one treatment or a treatment and a control group. However, if one studies only girls or only 12-month-olds, gender and age are not variables; they are constants. Thus, we can define *variable* as a characteristic of the participants or situation that has different values *in the study*.

Operational Definitions of Variables

An operational definition describes or defines a variable in terms of the operations used to produce it or techniques used to measure it. Demographic variables like age or ethnic group are usually measured by checking official records or simply by asking the participant to choose the appropriate category from among those listed. Treatments are described in some detail. Likewise, abstract concepts like mastery motivation need to be defined operationally by spelling out how they were measured.

Independent Variables

We do not restrict the term *independent variable* to interventions or treatments. We define an independent variable broadly to include any predictors, antecedents, or *presumed* causes or influences under investigation in the study.

Active Independent Variables. An active independent variable such as an intervention or treatment is *given* to a group of participants (experimental) but not to another (control group), within a specified period of time during the study. Thus, a pretest and posttest should be possible.

Attribute Independent Variables. A variable that could not be manipulated is called an *attribute independent variable* because it is an attribute of the person (e.g., gender, age, and ethnic group) or the person's usual environment (e.g., child abuse). For ethical and practical reasons, many aspects of the environment (child abuse) cannot be manipulated or given and are thus attribute variables. This distinction between active and attribute independent variables is important for determining what can be said about cause and effect. Research where an apparent intervention is studied after the fact is sometimes called *ex post facto*. We consider the independent variables in such studies to be attributes.

Dependent Variables

The dependent variable is the outcome or criterion. It is assumed to measure or assess the effect of the independent variable. Dependent variables are scores from a test, ratings on questionnaires, or readings from instruments (electrocardiogram). It is common for a study to have several dependent variables (performance and satisfaction).

Extraneous Variables

These are variables that are not of interest in a particular study but could influence the dependent variable and need to be controlled. Environmental factors, other attributes of the participants, and characteristics of the investigator are possible extraneous variables.

Levels of a Variable

The word *level* is commonly used to describe the values of an independent variable. This does not necessarily imply that the values are ordered. If an investigator was interested in comparing two different treatments and a no-treatment control group, the study has one independent variable, treatment type, with three levels, the two treatment conditions and the control condition.

We have tried to be consistent and clear about the terms we use; unfortunately, there is not one agreed-upon term for many research and statistical concepts. At the end of most sections, we have included a table similar to Table 2.1.1.1 that lists a number of key terms used in this chapter alongside other terms for essentially the same concept used by some other researchers. In addition to these tables of different terms for the same concept, we have appended a list of partially similar terms or phrases (such as independent variable vs. independent samples) which do not have the same meaning and should be differentiated.

Measurement and Descriptive Statistics

Measurement

Measurement is introduced when variables are translated into labels (categories) or numbers. For statistical purposes, we

TABLE 2.1.1.1

SIMILAR RELATED TERMS ABOUT VARIABLES

- Active independent variable ≈ manipulated variable ≈ intervention ≈ treatment
- Attribute independent variable ≈ measured variable ≈ individual difference variable
- Dependent variable (DV) ≈ outcome ≈ criterion
- Independent variable (IV) ≈ antecedent ≈ predictor ≈ presumed cause ≈ factor
- Levels (of a variable) ≈ categories ≈ values ≈ groups ≈ samples

Note. The term we use most often is listed on the left. Similar terms (indicated by ≈) used by other researchers and/or us are listed to the right.

and many statisticians (2) do not find the traditional scales of measurement (nominal, ordinal, interval, or ratio) useful. We prefer the following: a) *dichotomous* or binary (a variable having only two values or levels), b) *nominal* (a categorical variable with three or more values that are not ordered), c) *ordinal* (a variable with three or more values that are ordered, but not normally distributed), and d) *normally distributed* (an ordered variable with a distribution that is approximately normal [bell-shaped] in the population sampled). This measurement classification is similar to one proposed by Helena Chmura Kraemer (personal communication, March 16, 1999).

Descriptive Statistics and Plots

Researchers use descriptive statistics to summarize the data from their samples in terms of frequency, central tendency, and variability. Inferential statistics, on the other hand, are used to make inferences from the sample to the population.

Central Tendency. The three main measures of the center of a distribution are mean, median, and mode (the most frequent score). The *mean* or arithmetic average takes into account all of the available information in computing the central tendency of a frequency distribution; thus, it is the statistic of choice if the data are normally distributed. The *median* or middle score is the appropriate measure of central tendency for ordinal-level data.

Variability. Measures of variability tell us about the spread of the scores. If all of the scores in a distribution are the same, there is no variability. If they are all different and widely spaced apart, the variability is high. The *standard deviation* is the most common measure of variability, but it is appropriate only when one has normally distributed data. For nominal/categorical data, the measure of spread is the number of possible response categories.

Normal Curve

The normal curve is important because many of the variables that we examine in research are distributed in the form of the normal curve. Examples of variables that in the population fit a normal curve are height, weight, IQ, and many personality measures. For each of these examples, most participants would fall toward the middle of the curve, with fewer people at each extreme.

As shown in Figure 2.1.1.1, if a variable is normally distributed, about 68% of the participants lie within one standard deviation from either side of the mean, and 95% are within two standard deviations from the mean. For example, assume that 100 is the average IQ and the standard deviation is 15. The probability that a person will have an IQ between 85 and 115 is .68. Furthermore, only 5% (.05) would be expected to have an IQ less than 70 or more than 130. It is important to be able to conceptualize area under the normal curve in the form of probabilities because statistical convention sets acceptable probability levels for rejecting the null hypothesis at .05 or .01.

Conclusions about Measurement and the Use of Statistics

Table 2.1.1.2 summarizes information about the appropriate use of various kinds of plots and descriptive statistics, given nominal, dichotomous, ordinal, or normal data. Statistics based on means and standard deviation are valid for normally distributed (normal) data. Typically, these data are used in the most powerful (analysis of variance) statistical tests, called parametric statistics. However, if the data are ordered but grossly nonnormal (ordinal), means and standard deviations may not give meaningful answers. Then the median and a nonparametric test based on rank order would be preferred. Nonparametric tests have less power than parametric tests (they are less able to reject the null hypothesis when it should be rejected), but the sacrifice in power for nonparametric tests based on ranks usually is relatively minor. If the data are nominal (unordered), one would have to use the mode or frequency counts. In this case, there would be a major sacrifice in power. It would be misleading to use tests that assume the dependent variable is ordinal or normally distributed when the dependent variable is, in fact, nominal/not ordered. Table 2.1.1.3 provides examples of potentially confusing, essentially equivalent terms about measurement and descriptive statistics.

Measurement Reliability

Measurement reliability and measurement validity are two parts of overall research validity, the quality of the whole study. Reliability refers to consistency of scores on a particular instrument. It is incorrect to state that a test is reliable because reliability takes into account the sample that took the test. For example, there may be strong evidence for reliability for adults, but scores of depressed adolescents on this test

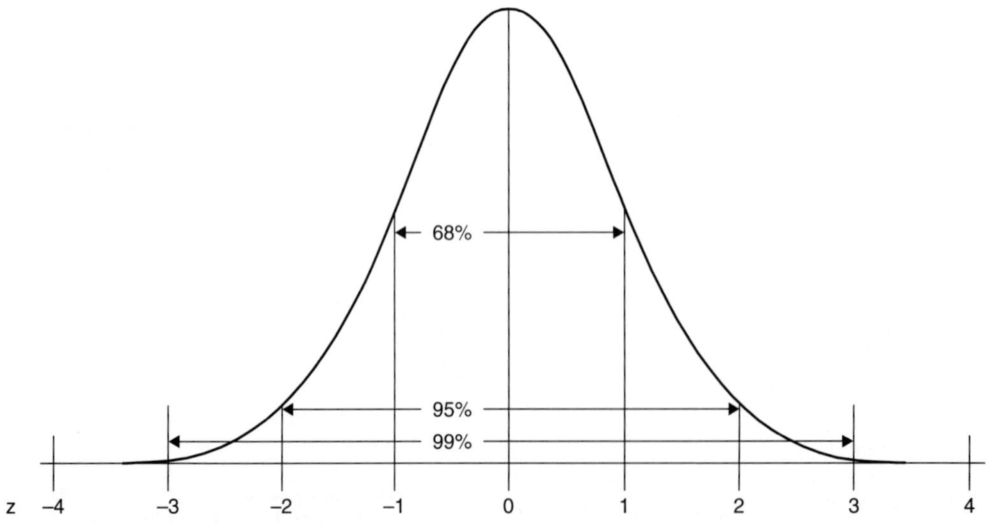

FIGURE 2.1.1.1. Frequency distribution and areas under the normal and standardized curve.

TABLE 2.1.1.2

SELECTION OF APPROPRIATE DESCRIPTIVE STATISTICS AND PLOTS

	Nominal	Dichotomous	Ordinal	Normal
Graphic Depiction (Plot)				
Frequency Distribution	Yes[a]	Yes	Yes	OK[b]
Bar chart	Yes	Yes	Yes	OK
Histogram	No[c]	No	OK	Yes
Frequency polygon	No	No	OK	Yes
Box and whiskers plot	No	No	Yes	Yes
Central Tendency				
Mean	No	OK	Of ranks, OK	Yes
Median	No	OK = mode	Yes	OK
Mode	Yes	Yes	OK	OK
Variability				
Range	No	Always 1	Yes	Yes
Standard deviation	No	No	Of ranks, OK	Yes
Interquartile range	No	No	OK	OK
How many categories	Yes	Always 2	OK	Not if truly continuous
Shape				
Skewness	No	No	Yes	Yes

[a]Yes means a good choice with this level of measurement.
[b]OK means OK to use, but not the best choice at this level of measurement.
[c]No means not appropriate at this level of measurement.

may be highly inconsistent. When researchers use tests or other instruments to measure outcomes, they need to make sure that the tests provide consistent data. If the outcome measure is not reliable, then one cannot accurately assess the results.

Conceptually, reliability is consistency. When evaluating instruments it is important to be able to express reliability numerically. The correlation coefficient, often used to evaluate reliability, is usually expressed as the letter r, which indicates the strength of a relationship. The values of r range between −1 and +1. A value of 0 indicates no relationship between two variables or scores, whereas values close to −1 or +1 indicate very strong relationships between two variables. A strong positive relationship indicates that people who score high on one test also score high on a second test. To say that a measurement is reliable, one would expect a coefficient between +.7 and +1.0. Others have suggested even stricter criteria. For example, reliability coefficients of .8 are acceptable for research, but .9 is necessary for measures that will be used to make clinical decisions about individuals. However, it is common to see published journal articles in which one or a few reliability coefficients are below .7, usually .6 or greater. Although correlations of −.7 to −1.0 indicate a strong (negative) correlation, they are totally unacceptable as evidence for reliability.

There are four different types of evidence for reliability, such as test-retest reliability, that are listed in Table 2.1.1.4, along with synonyms that you may see in the literature. In addition, there are many different methods to compute these different types of reliability. See Morgan, Gliner and Harmon (3) for specifics about these approaches to assessing reliability.

TABLE 2.1.1.3

SIMILAR TERMS ABOUT MEASUREMENT

- Categorical variable ≈ usually nominal, but variables may have discrete ordered *categories*
- Dichotomous ≈ binary ≈ dummy variable ≈ nominal with two categories
- Interval scale ≈ numeric ≈ continuous variable ≈ quantitative ≈ scale data
- Mean ≈ average ≈ arithmetic average
- Median ≈ midpoint
- Normal ≈ (approximately) normally distributed variable ≈ interval and ratio data ≈ quantitative ≈ continuous
- Nominal scale ≈ unordered categorical variable ≈ qualitative ≈ discrete
- Ordered variable ≈ ordinal or interval scale
- Ordinal scale ≈ unequal-interval scale ≈ discrete ordered categorical variable
- Range ≈ spread

Note. The term we use most often is listed on the left. Similar terms (indicated by ≈) used by other researchers and/or us are listed to the right.

TABLE 2.1.1.4

SIMILAR TERMS ABOUT MEASUREMENT RELIABILITY

- Alternate forms reliability ≈ equivalent forms ≈ parallel forms ≈ coefficient of equivalence
- Internal consistency reliability ≈ interitem reliability ≈ Cronbach's alpha
- Interrater reliability ≈ interobserver reliability
- Measurement reliability ≈ reliability ≈ test, instrument, or score reliability
- Test-retest reliability ≈ coefficient of stability

Note. The term we use most often is listed on the left. Similar terms (indicated by ≈) used by other researchers and/or us are listed to the right.

Measurement Validity

Validity is concerned with establishing evidence for the use of a particular measure or instrument in a particular setting with a particular population for a specific purpose. Here we will discuss what we call measurement validity; others might use terms such as *test validity, score validity*, or just *validity*. We use the modifier *measurement* to distinguish it from internal, external, and overall research validity and to point out that it is the measures or scores that provide evidence for validity. It is inappropriate to say that a test is "valid" or "invalid." Note also that an instrument may produce consistent data (provide evidence for reliability), but the data may not be a valid index of the intended construct.

In research articles, there is usually more evidence for the reliability of the instrument than for the validity of the instrument because evidence for validity is more difficult to obtain. To establish validity, one ideally needs a "gold standard" or "criterion" related to the particular purpose of the measure. To obtain such a criterion is often not an easy matter, so other types of evidence to support the validity of a measure are necessary.

There are five broad types of evidence to support the validity of a test or measure: a) content, b) responses, c) internal structure, d) relations to other variables, and e) the consequences of testing (4). Note that the five types of evidence are *not* separate types of validity and that any one type of evidence is insufficient. Validation should integrate all the pertinent evidence from as many of the five types of evidence as possible. Preferably validation should include some evidence in addition to content evidence, which is probably the most common and easiest to obtain. Table 2.1.1.5 shows the traditional names for the types of validity evidence and how they line up with the types of evidence from the current standards (4).

Evaluation of evidence for validity is often based on correlations with other variables, but there are no well established guidelines. Our suggestion is to use Cohen's (5) guidelines for interpreting effect sizes, which are measures of the strength of a relationship. We describe several measures of effect size and how to interpret them. Cohen suggested that generally, in the applied behavioral sciences, a correlation of $r = .5$ could be considered a large effect, and in this context we would consider $r = .5$ or greater to be strong support for measurement validity. In general, an acceptable level of support would be provided by $r \geq .3$, and some weak support might result from $r \geq .1$, assuming that such an r was statistically significant. However, for concurrent, criterion evidence, if the criterion and test being validated are two similar measures of the same concept (e.g., IQ), the correlation would be expected to be very high, perhaps .8 or .9. On the other hand, for convergent evidence, the measures should not be that highly correlated because they should be measures of different concepts. If the measures were very highly related, one might ask whether they were instead really measuring the same concept.

The strength of the evidence for the measurement of validity is extremely important for research in applied settings because without measures that have strong evidence for validity the results of the study can be misleading. Validation is an ongoing, never fully achieved, process based on integration of all the evidence from as many sources as possible.

TABLE 2.1.1.5

SIMILAR TERMS ABOUT VALIDITY

Concurrent validity ≈ now part of "evidence based on relations to other variables"
Construct validity ≈ now part of "evidence based on relations to other variables"
Content validity ≈ now part of "content evidence for validity"
Convergent validity ≈ now part of "evidence based on relations to other variables"
Criterion validity ≈ now part of "evidence based on relations to other variables"
Discriminant validity ≈ now part of "evidence based on relations to other variables"
Face validity ≈ (no longer used)
Factorial validity ≈ now part of "evidence based on internal structure"
Predictive validity ≈ now part of "evidence based on relations to other variables"
Validity (of a specific measure) ≈ measurement validity ≈ test, instrument, or score validity
Validity (of the design of a study) ≈ research validity ≈ internal or external validity

Note. In this table the traditional term is provided on the left. Similar terms, used in the current standards (4) are on the right. (See also Figure 2.1.1.7.)

RESEARCH APPROACHES, QUESTIONS, AND DESIGNS

Quantitative Research Approaches

Our conceptual framework includes five quantitative research approaches (randomized experimental, quasiexperimental, comparative, associational, and descriptive). This framework is helpful because it provides appropriate guidance about inferring cause and effect.

Figure 2.1.1.2 indicates that the general purpose of four of the five approaches is to explore relationships between or among variables. This is consistent with the notion that all common parametric statistics are relational and with the typical phrasing of research questions and hypotheses as investigating the relationship between two or more variables. Figure 2.1.1.2 also indicates the specific purpose, type of research question, and general type of statistic used in each of the five approaches.

Research Approaches with an Active Independent Variable

Randomized Experimental Research Approach. This approach provides the best evidence about cause and effect. For a research approach to be called randomized experimental, two criteria must be met. First, the independent variable must be active (be a variable that is *given* to the participant, such as a treatment). Second, the researcher must randomly assign participants to groups or conditions prior to the intervention; this is what differentiates experiments from quasiexperiments. More discussion of specific quasiexperimental and randomized designs is provided below.

Quasiexperimental Research Approach. Researchers do not agree on the definition of a quasiexperiment. Our definition is that there must be an active/manipulated independent variable, but the participants are not randomly assigned to the groups. In much applied research participants are already in groups such as clinics, and it is not possible to change those assignments and divide the participants randomly into experimental and control groups.

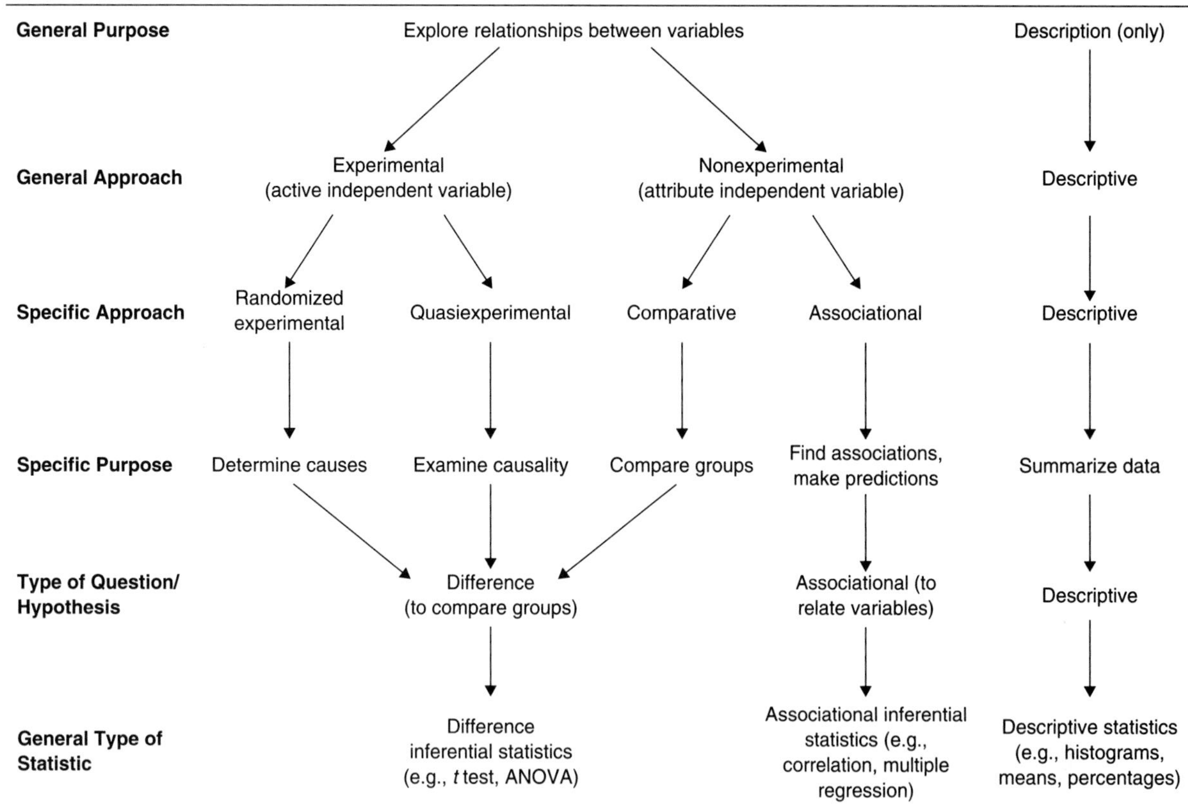

FIGURE 2.1.1.2. Schematic diagram showing how the general type of statistic and hypothesis or question used in a study corresponds to the purposes and the approach.

Research Approaches That Have Attribute Independent Variables

In most ways the associational and comparative approaches are similar. We call both nonexperimental approaches, as shown in Figure 2.1.1.2. The distinction between them, which is implied but not stated in most research textbooks, is in terms of the number of levels of the independent variable.

It is common for *survey research* to include both comparative and associational as well as descriptive research questions, and therefore to use all three approaches. It is also common for experimental studies to include attribute independent variables, such as gender, as well as an active independent variable and thus to use both experimental and comparative approaches. The approaches are tied to types of independent variables and research questions, not necessarily to whole studies.

Comparative Research Approach. Like randomized experiments and quasiexperiments, the comparative approach, which is sometimes called *causal-comparative*, or *ex post facto*, usually has a few levels (typically two to four) or categories for the independent variable and makes comparisons between groups.

Associational Research Approach. This approach is similar to the comparative approach because the independent variable is an attribute. In this approach, the independent variable is often continuous or has a number of ordered categories, usually five or more. We prefer to label this approach *associational* rather *correlational,* used by some researchers, because the approach is more than, and should not be confused with, a specific statistic.

Descriptive Research Approach

The term *descriptive research* refers to questions and studies that use only descriptive statistics, such as averages, percentages, histograms, and frequency distributions, which are not tested for statistical significance. This approach is different from the other four in that only one variable is considered at a time so that no comparisons or associations are determined. Although most research studies include some descriptive questions (at least to describe the sample), few stop there.

Research Questions and Hypotheses

Three Types of Basic Hypotheses or Research Questions

A *hypothesis* is a predictive statement about the relationship between two or more variables. *Research questions* are similar to hypotheses, but they are in question format. Research questions can be further divided into three types: *difference questions, associational questions*, and *descriptive questions* (see Figure 2.1.1.2).

For difference questions, one compares groups or levels derived from the independent variable in terms of their scores on the dependent variable. This type of question typically is used with the randomized experimental, quasiexperimental, and comparative approaches. For an associational question, one associates or relates the independent and dependent variables. Our descriptive questions are not answered with inferential statistics; they merely describe or summarize data.

As implied by Figure 2.1.1.2, it is appropriate to phrase any difference or associational research question as simply a *relationship* between the independent variable(s) and the dependent variable. However, we think that phrasing the research questions/hypotheses as a difference between groups or as a relationship between variables helps match the question

TABLE 2.1.1.6

SIMILAR TERMS ABOUT RESEARCH APPROACHES AND QUESTIONS

- Associational approach ≈ correlational ≈ survey ≈ descriptive
- Associational questions ≈ correlational questions
- Comparative approach ≈ causal-comparative ≈ ex post facto
- Descriptive approach ≈ exploratory research
- Difference questions ≈ group comparisons
- Nonexperimental research (comparative, associational, and descriptive approaches) ≈ some writers call all three descriptive

Note. The term we use most often is listed on the left. Similar terms (indicated by ≈) used by other researchers and/or us are listed to the right.

to the appropriate statistical analysis. Table 2.1.1.6 shows the terms other researchers sometimes use that correspond to those for our research approaches and questions.

EXPERIMENTAL DESIGNS

We describe here specific designs for both quasiexperiments and randomized experiments. This should help the reader visualize the independent variables, levels of these variables, and whether the participants are assessed on the dependent variable more than once.

Quasiexperimental Designs

The randomized experimental and quasiexperimental approaches have an active independent variable, which has two or more values, called levels. The dependent variable is the outcome measure or criterion of the study.

In both randomized and quasiexperimental approaches, the active independent variable has at least one level that is some type of intervention given to participants in the experimental group during the study. Usually there is also a comparison or control group, which is the other level of the independent variable. There can be more than two levels or groups (e.g., two or more different interventions plus one or more comparison groups).

The key difference between quasiexperiments and randomized experiments is whether the participants are assigned randomly to the groups or levels of the independent variable. In quasiexperiments random assignment of the participants is not done; thus, the groups are always considered to be nonequivalent, and there are alternative interpretations of the results that make definitive conclusions about cause and effect difficult. For example, if some children diagnosed with attention-deficit/hyperactivity disorder were treated with stimulants and others were not, later differences between the groups could be due to many factors. Families who volunteer (or agree) to have their children medicated may be different, in important ways, from those who do not. Or perhaps the more disruptive children were given stimulants. Thus, later problem behaviors (or positive outcomes) could be due to initial differences between the groups.

Poor Quasiexperimental Designs

Results from these designs (sometimes called *preexperimental*) are hard to interpret and should not be used. These designs lack a comparison (control) group, a pretest, or both.

Better Quasiexperimental Designs

Pretest-Posttest Nonequivalent-Groups Design. As with all quasiexperiments, there is no random assignment of the participants to the groups in this design. First, measurements (O_1) are taken on the groups prior to an intervention. Then one group (E) receives a new treatment (X), which the other (comparison) group (C) does not receive (~X); often the comparison group receives the usual or traditional treatment. At the end of the intervention period, both groups are measured again (O_2) to determine whether there are differences between the two groups. The design is considered to be nonequivalent because the participants are not randomly assigned (NR) to one or the other group. Even if the two groups have the same mean score on the pretest, there may be characteristics that have not been measured that may interact with the treatment to cause differences between the two groups that are not due strictly to the intervention. The following diagram illustrates the procedures for the pretest-posttest nonequivalent groups design:

NR	E	O_1	X	O_2
NR	C	O_1	~X	O_2

Table 2.1.1.7 summarizes two issues that determine the strength (from weak to strong) of the pretest-posttest nonequivalent groups design. These designs vary, as shown, on whether the *treatments* are randomly assigned to the groups or not and on the likelihood that the groups are similar in terms of attributes or characteristics of the participants. In none of the quasiexperimental designs are the *individual participants* randomly assigned to the groups, so the groups are always considered nonequivalent, but the participant characteristics may be similar if there was no bias in how the participants were assigned (got into) the groups.

Time-Series Designs. Time-series designs are different from the more traditional designs discussed above because they have multiple measurement (time) periods rather than just the pre- and post-periods. These designs often are referred to as *interrupted* time series because the treatment interrupts the baseline from posttreatment measures. The two most common types are single-group time-series designs and multiple-group time-series designs (6). Within each type, the treatment can be temporary or continuous. The logic behind any time-series

TABLE 2.1.1.7

ISSUES THAT DETERMINE THE STRENGTH OF QUASIEXPERIMENTAL DESIGNS

Strength of Design	Random Assignment of *Treatments* to Intact Groups	Participant Characteristics Likely to Be Similar
Poor (or pre)	No	No, because no comparison group or no pretest
Weak	No	Not likely, because participants decide which group to join (self-assign to groups)
Moderate	No	Maybe, because participants did not self-assign to groups and no known assignment bias
Strong	Yes	Maybe, because participants did not self-assign to groups and no known assignment bias

design involves convincing others that a baseline (several pretests) is stable prior to an intervention so that one can conclude that the change in the dependent variable is due to the intervention and not other environmental events or maturation. It is common in time-series designs to have multiple measures before and after the intervention, but there must be multiple (at least three) pretests to establish a baseline. One of the hallmarks of time-series designs is the visual display of the data, which are often quite convincing. However, these visual displays also can be misleading due to the lack of independence of the data points, and therefore always must be statistically analyzed.

Randomized Experimental Designs

In randomized designs the participants are randomly assigned to the experimental and control groups. Random assignment of participants to groups should eliminate bias on all characteristics before the independent variable is introduced. This elimination of bias is one necessary condition for the results to provide convincing evidence that the independent variable caused differences between the groups on the dependent variable. For cause to be demonstrated, other biases in environmental and experience variables occurring during the study also must be eliminated.

Three types of randomized experimental designs are discussed. For each we describe and diagram the design and present some of the advantages and disadvantages. The diagrams and discussion are limited to two groups, but more than two groups may be used with any of these designs. The experimental group receives the intervention, and the "control" group(s) receives the standard (traditional) treatment, a placebo, and/or another (comparison) treatment. For ethical reasons, it is unusual and not desirable for the control group to receive no treatment at all, but it is difficult to decide which type of control group is appropriate. Here we label all such options the *control treatment*.

Posttest-Only Control Group Design

The posttest-only control group design can be shown as follows:

R	E:	X	O
R	C:	~X	O

The sequential operations of the design are to randomly (R) assign participants to either an experimental (E) or control (C) group. Then the experimental group receives the intended intervention (X) and the control group (~X) does not. At the end of the intervention period, both groups are measured (O), using some form of instrumentation related to the study (dependent variable).

The key point for the posttest-only control group design is the random assignment of participants to groups. If participants are assigned randomly to one or the other group, the two groups should not be biased on *any* variable prior to the intervention. Therefore, if there are differences on the dependent measure following the intervention, it can be assumed that the differences are due to the intervention and not due to differences in participant characteristics.

Pretest-Posttest Control Group Design

The pretest-posttest control group design can be shown as follows:

R	E:	O_1	X	O_2
R	C:	O_1	~X	O_2

Reasons for using this design compared with the posttest-only control group design are to check for equivalence of groups before the intervention and to describe the population from which both groups are drawn. Another advantage of this design is that posttest scores could be adjusted statistically through analysis of covariance based on pretest score differences between the treatment and control groups. On the other hand, a problem could be created if a pretest is used. The pretest could bias the participants as to what to expect in the study, and practice on the pretest could influence the posttest (there could be carryover effects). Also, if the dependent variable is invasive (spinal tap), one would not want to use it as a pretest. Random assignment does mean that the groups will not differ substantially on the average, but this assurance is adequate only if the sample is large. In small-sample clinical research, it is not uncommon to find some large differences in important characteristics even when the participants were randomly assigned to groups.

Within-Subjects Randomized Experimental (or Crossover) Design

In the simplest case, this design has two levels and can be shown as follows:

		Condition 1	Test	Condition 2	Test
R	Order 1	X	O_1	~X	O_2
R	Order 2	~X	O_1	X	O_2

The participants are randomly assigned to order 1, which receives the experimental condition first and then the control condition, or to order 2, which receives the control condition and then the experimental. This type of design is frequently used in studies in which participants are asked to evaluate diets, exercise, and similar events assumed from previous research not to have carryover effects. The strength of this design is that participants act as their own control, which reduces error variance. This design can have problems if there are carryover effects from the experimental condition. Furthermore, one must be extremely cautious with this design when comparing a new treatment with a traditional treatment. The problem, often referred to as *asymmetrical transfer effects*, occurs when the impact of one order (perhaps the traditional treatment before the new treatment) is greater than the impact of the other order (new treatment before the traditional treatment).

Many possible variants of the above quasiexperimental and experimental designs are discussed in Shadish, Cook, and Campbell (7).

GENERAL DESIGN CLASSIFICATIONS

General design classifications are important for determining appropriate statistical methods to be used in data analysis. Within the randomized experimental, quasiexperimental, and comparative approaches, all designs must fit into one of three categories or labels (between, within, or mixed). These design classifications do not apply to the associational or descriptive approaches.

Between-Groups Designs

Between-groups designs are defined as designs in which each participant in the research study is in one and only one condition or group. For example, in a study investigating the effects of medication on the dependent variable, number of symptoms in hyperactive children, there might be two groups (or conditions or levels) of the independent variable: the current medication and a new medication. In a between-groups design, each participant receives only one of the two conditions or levels: either the current medication or the new one.

Within-Subjects or Repeated-Measures Designs

Within-subjects designs, the second type of general design classification, are conceptually the opposite of between-groups designs. In these designs, each participant in the research receives or experiences all of the conditions or levels of the independent variable. If we use the hyperactive children example just given, there still would be two conditions or levels to the independent variable. In a within-subjects design, each participant would be given first one medication, then the second medication and would be measured for the number of symptoms on both conditions. Because each participant is assessed more than once (for each condition), these designs are also referred to as repeated-measures designs.

Within-subjects designs have appeal due to the reduction in participants needed and to reduction in error variance because each participant is his or her own control. However, often these designs are less appropriate than between-groups designs because of the possibility of *carryover effects*. If the purpose of the study is to investigate conditions that may result in a long-term or permanent change, such as learning, it is not possible for a participant to be in one condition and then "unlearn" that condition to be in the same previous state to start the next condition. Within-subjects designs may be appropriate if the effects of order of presentation are negligible, as when participants are asked to evaluate several topics or when a medication effect would not be long lasting.

Matching is a second situation where a design is judged to be within subjects. When pairs of subjects in a comparison group and an experimental group are matched on key characteristics, the design is treated statistically as within subjects.

Mixed Designs

A mixed design has at least one between-groups independent variable and at least one within-subjects independent variable; thus there are a minimum of two independent variables. A between-groups independent variable is any independent variable that sets up between-groups conditions. A within-subjects independent variable is any independent variable that sets up within-subjects conditions.

Change Over Time (or Trials) as an Independent Variable

In within-subjects designs, there can be a third type (neither active nor attribute) of independent variable, called change over time or trials. This third type of independent variable is extremely important in randomized experimental and quasiexperimental designs because pretest and posttest are two levels of this type of independent variable. Longitudinal studies, in which the same participants are assessed at several time periods or ages, are another important case in which change over time is the independent variable.

Table 2.1.1.8 provides examples of terms for research designs sometimes used by other researchers that have meanings similar to ours.

TABLE 2.1.1.8

SIMILAR TERMS ABOUT RESEARCH DESIGNS

- Between groups ≈ independent samples
- Comparison group ≈ control group ≈ placebo group
- Factorial design ≈ two or more independent variables ≈ complex design
- Poor quasi-experimental designs ≈ preexperiments
- Random assignment to groups ≈ randomized design
- Randomized experiment ≈ true experiment ≈ randomized clinical trial ≈ randomized control trials ≈ RCT
- Single factor design ≈ one independent variable ≈ basic design
- Within subjects ≈ repeated measures ≈ related samples ≈ paired samples ≈ matched groups ≈ correlated samples ≈ within groups ≈ dependent samples

Note. The term we use most often is listed on the left. Similar terms (indicated by ≈) used by other researchers and/or us are listed to the right.

DIMENSIONS OF RESEARCH VALIDITY

Research validity refers to the merit of the design of a whole study, as distinguished from validity of the measurement of a variable. Based on the work of Cook and Campbell (6), we (3) divide research validity into four key components:

1. *Measurement reliability and statistics* We discussed the former above and will discuss the appropriate use and interpretation of statistics below.
2. *Internal validity* to be discussed below.
3. *Overall measurement validity of the constructs* which was discussed briefly above.
4. *External validity* which is how well the results of the study generalize to other populations, settings, treatments, and measures.

The next section describes briefly the issue of cause and effect, which is key to understanding internal validity.

Inferring Cause

A major goal of scientific research is to be able to identify a causal relationship between variables. However, there is disagreement among scholars as to what is necessary to prove that a causal relationship exists. Researchers note that even if they cannot identify all the causes or the most important causal factor of an outcome, they can identify a variable as one (or a partial) cause, under certain circumstances. Three criteria that must occur to infer a causal relationship: a) the independent variable must precede in time the dependent variable; b) there must be a relationship between the independent variable and the dependent variable (in the behavioral sciences this is usually determined statistically); and c) there must be no plausible third (extraneous) variable that also could account for a relationship between the independent and dependent variables.

Four of the five specific research approaches (except the descriptive) attempt to satisfy the three prerequisites. All four can, but do not always, meet the first two criteria, the independent variable preceding the dependent variable and establishing a relationship between variables. The randomized experimental and, to a much lesser extent, the quasiexperimental approaches can be successful in meeting the third condition, elimination of extraneous variables. The comparative and associational approaches are not well suited to establishing causes, but things can be done to control for some extraneous variables. Although the comparative and associational approaches are limited in what can be said about causation, they can lead to strong conclusions about the differences between groups and about associations between variables, respectively. Strong associations (correlations) between variables can generate equations where knowing a score on one variable allows one to predict, with some degree of accuracy, the score on the other variable (linear regression). The descriptive approach, as we define it, does not attempt to identify causal relationships or, in fact, any relationships. It focuses on describing variables.

Internal Validity

Cook and Campbell (6) defined internal validity as "the approximate validity with which we can infer that a relationship is causal." Internal validity depends on the strength or soundness of the design and influences whether one can conclude that the independent variable or intervention caused the dependent variable to change. Although internal validity is often discussed only with respect to randomized and quasiexperiments, we believe the concept also applies to research with attribute independent variables (and nonexperimental studies).

We group the Shadish et al. (7) threats to internal validity into two main types: *equivalence of the groups on participant characteristics* (equivalence of the intervention and control groups prior to the intervention) and *control of extraneous experience and environmental variables.*

Equivalence of Groups on Participant Characteristics

In research that compares differences among groups, a key question is whether the *groups* that are compared are *equivalent in all respects* prior to the introduction of the independent variable or variables. Using the randomized experimental approach, equivalence is approximately achieved through random assignment of participants to groups, especially if the sample size in each group is large. Random assignment of participants to the groups, which is characteristic of randomized experiments but not quasiexperiments, is the best way to ensure equivalent, or at least unbiased, groups. However, in quasiexperimental, comparative, or associational research, random assignment of participants to groups has not been or cannot be done.

Control of Extraneous Experience and Environment Variables

We have grouped several other "threats" to internal validity under a category that deals with the effects of extraneous (variables other than the independent variables) experiences or environmental conditions during the study. Thus, we have called this internal validity dimension *control of extraneous experience and environment variables.* Many of these threats occur because participants gain information about the purpose of the study while the study is taking place. An important aspect of this dimension has to do with whether extraneous variables or events *affect one group more* than the other. For example, if participants learn that they are in a control group, they may give up or not try as hard, exaggerating differences between the intervention and control groups. Or the opposite may occur and peers in the control group overcompensate, eliminating differences between the two groups.

Control of extraneous experiences and the environment depends on the specific study, but it is generally better for randomized experiments and for studies done in controlled environments such as laboratories.

Threats to Internal Validity

Table 2.1.1.9 provides a current list of threats to interval validity as described by Shadish et al. (7). Some of the names for the various threats are confusing, but the concepts are important. We have added a column for our suggested names.

TABLE 2.1.1.9

THREATS TO INTERNAL VALIDITY

Shadish, Cook, and Campbell (7)	Morgan, Gliner, and Harmon (3)
	Equivalence of groups
Regression	Use of extreme groups
Attrition/mortality	Participant dropouts/attrition during the study
Selection	Bias in assignment to groups
	Control of extraneous variables
Maturation	Changes due to time or growth/development
History	Extraneous events
Testing	Repeated testing, carryover effects
Instrumentation	Measurement inconsistency
Additive and interactive threats	Combinations of two or more threats
Ambiguous temporal precedence	Did the independent variable occur before the dependent variable?

Sampling and Population External Validity

Sampling is the process of selecting part of a larger group with the intent of generalizing from the smaller group, called the *sample*, to the *population*, the larger group. If we are to make valid inferences about the population, we must select the sample so that it is *representative* of the population. With a few notable exceptions, modern survey techniques have proven to be quite accurate in predicting or reporting information about the attitudes of the American public.

Steps in Selecting a Sample and Generalizing Results

There are many ways to select a sample from a population. The goal is to have an *actual sample* in which each participant represents a known fraction of the *theoretical* or *target population* so that characteristics of the population can be recreated from the sample. Obtaining a *representative sample* is not easy because things can go wrong at three stages of the research process. Figure 2.1.1.3 shows the key sampling concepts and the three steps (shown with arrows).

Types of Sampling

There are two major types of sampling designs that are used in obtaining the selected sample: probability (often considered unbiased sampling) and nonprobability (often considered biased sampling).

Probability Sampling. In probability sampling, every participant has a known, nonzero chance of being selected. The participants or elements of the population are usually people, but could be groups, animals, or events. With probability samples, researchers are able to make an estimate of the extent to which results based on the sample are likely to differ from what would have been found by studying the entire population. There are several types of probability sampling. The most basic is the *simple random sample*, which occurs when all participants have an equal and independent chance of being included in the sample. This technique can be implemented using a random number table to select participants from a list, the sampling frame, of the accessible population.

If some important characteristics of the accessible population such as gender or race are known ahead of time, one can reduce the sampling variation and increase the likelihood that

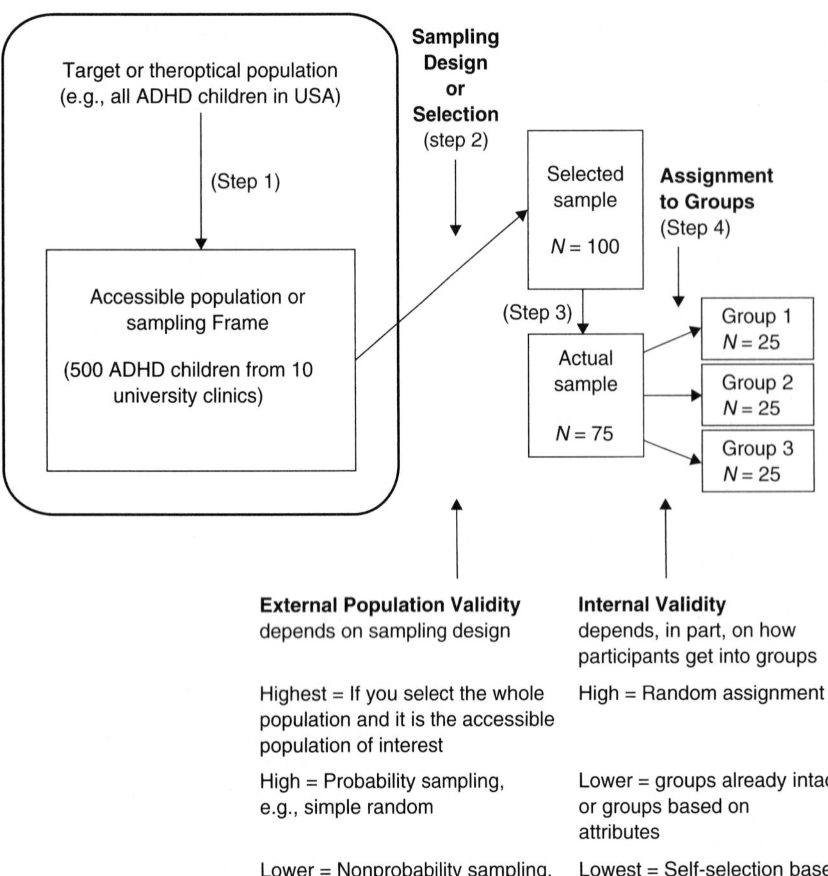

FIGURE 2.1.1.3. Schematic diagram of the sampling process and the distinction between random sampling and random assignment.

the sample will be representative of the population by using *stratified random sampling.*

Nonprobability Sampling. These samples are ones in which the probability of being selected is unknown. Time and cost constraints lead many researchers to use nonprobability samples. The most common type of nonprobability sample is called a *convenience sample.* A sample is considered a convenience sample if the researcher selected either the accessible population or some participants from the accessible population based on convenience. An extended discussion of the types of sampling and the advantages and disadvantages of each can be found in Fowler (8).

How Many Participants?

The question, "How many participants are needed for this study?" is asked often. One part of the answer depends on whom you ask and their discipline (9). The size of the sample should be large enough so one does not fail to detect important findings, but a large sample will not necessarily help one distinguish the merely statistically significant from societally important findings. *Statistical power analysis* can help one compute the sample size needed to find a statistically significant result given certain assumptions.

Sampling and the Internal and External Validity of a Study

We have discussed the internal and external validity of a study and noted that external validity is influenced by the representativeness of the sample. Note, as indicated in Figure 2.1.1.3, that the internal validity of a study is not directly affected by the sampling design or the type of sampling. Figure 2.1.1.3 also shows how the two uses of the word *random* have quite different meanings and different effects on internal and external validity. *Random selection,* or some other probability sampling method, of who is asked to participate in the study is important for high external validity. On the other hand, *random assignment,* or placement of persons who agree to participate into groups (Step 4), is important for high internal validity.

Table 2.1.1.10 provides alternate terms used by researchers for various aspects of the sampling process.

TABLE 2.1.1.10

SIMILAR TERMS ABOUT SAMPLING

- Accessible population ≈ sampling frame
- Actual sample ≈ sample ≈ final sample
- Convenience sampling ≈ nonprobability sampling ≈ biased sampling
- Random selection ≈ random sampling ≈ probability sampling
- Response rate ≈ return rate ≈ percent of selected sample participating
- Selected sample ≈ participants sampled
- Theoretical population ≈ target population ≈ population of interest

Note: The term we use most often is listed on the left. Similar terms (indicated by ≈) used by other researchers and/or us are listed to the right.

INFERENTIAL STATISTICS AND THEIR INTERPRETATION

Introduction to Inferential Statistics and Hypothesis Testing

When performing research, rarely are we able to work with an entire population of individuals. Instead, we usually conduct the study on a sample of individuals from a population. It is hoped that if the sample is representative we can infer that the results from our sample apply to the population of interest. Inferential statistics involves making inferences from sample statistics, such as the sample mean and the sample standard deviation, to population parameters such as the population mean and the population standard deviation.

The Hypothesis Testing Process

The goal of null hypothesis significance testing (NHST) is to reject the null hypothesis in favor of an alternative hypothesis. The *null hypothesis* states that the mean of the population of those who receive the intervention is equal to the mean of the population of those who do not. In other words, the intervention is not successful. An alternative hypothesis (our hypothesis of interest) states that the mean of the population of those who receive the intervention will be greater than the mean of the population of those who do not. If the null hypothesis is false, or rejected, the intervention is considered to be successful. Note that the null hypothesis was stated as a "no difference" null hypothesis, that is, that there is no difference between the population means of the treatment and control groups. However, especially in practical applications, the null hypothesis could be stated, but isn't often, as some specific functionally important difference between the means of the two populations. In that case, to reject the null hypothesis, the treatment group would have to exceed the control group by an amount necessary to make a *functional* difference. This is referred to as a *non nil null hypothesis.*

The hypothesis testing process can be summarized as a series of steps that the researcher takes to conduct the study. From the accessible population, a sample is selected. Participants in this sample are then assigned, randomly under the best circumstances, to one of two groups, an intervention group and a comparison group. (More than two groups could be used, such as two treatment groups and a comparison group.) Next, the participants in the intervention group undergo the new treatment and the participants in the comparison group receive the standard or traditional treatment. At the end of the treatment period, both groups are measured on the dependent variable and a comparison is made, usually between the means of the two groups.

How much of a difference between the two means is needed before one can conclude that there is a statistically significant difference? Inferential statistics provide an outcome (a statistic) that helps make the decision about how much of a difference is needed. However, even after performing inferential statistics, one is still making a decision with some degree of uncertainty.

An outcome that is highly unlikely (i.e., one that results in a low probability value) if the null hypothesis were true leads one to reject the null hypothesis. Most researchers set this probability value (alpha) as five times in 100, or .05. An outcome that is more likely (> .05) will result in a failure to reject the null hypothesis.

Type I and Type II Errors

Although inferential statistics help one make a decision (e.g., reject or not reject the null hypothesis), there is still a possibility that the decision made may be incorrect because the decision is based on the *probability* of a given outcome. Figure 2.1.1.4 shows that four outcomes are possible; two of the outcomes are correct decisions and two are errors. The correct outcomes are a) to not reject the null hypothesis when it is true (there is, in fact, no difference) and b) to reject the null hypothesis when it is false (a correct decision that there is a difference). The error of commission is c) to reject the null hypothesis when, in fact, it is true—type I error (saying that there is a difference when there really was no difference). The error of omission is d) to not reject the null hypothesis when it is false—type II error (saying that there was no difference when there really was a difference).

Statistical Power

Statistical power is the probability of a correct decision to *reject the null hypothesis when it is false.* Conventionally, the desired statistical power of a study is .80. Because statistical power is inversely related to a type II error, that error would be .20 if power is .80.

Although there are numerous methods to increase statistical power, the most common is to increase the size of the sample. In order to determine how many participants to include in a study, one must know the significance level (usually established at .05), type of hypothesis (directional or nondirectional), desired power (.8 if possible), and an estimate of the effect size (the strength of the relationship between the independent variable and the dependent variable, often stated in standard deviation units). Effect size information comes from a review of the literature on the topic. Most current research syntheses contain a metaanalysis that results in an effect size estimate.

Once the information (significance level, type of hypothesis, amount of power, and effect size) has been obtained, a power table or computer program can be used to determine the needed number of participants. Although increasing the number of participants in a study is a good way to increase statistical power, often this option is not possible. In program evaluation, frequently the number of participants is fixed, often below that desired for adequate power. There are other methods to increase power, such as using homogeneous groups, making sure the measure has strong evidence for reliability, and sometimes choosing a within-subjects design to reduce variability. Lipsey (10) and Cohen (5) provided valuable information on this topic.

		True in the population	
		Null is true (No real difference)	Null is false (Really is a difference)
Decision based on data from sample	Reject null	(c) Type I error (alpha)	(b) Correction decision (power)
	Do not reject null	(a) Correction decision	(d) Type II error (beta)

FIGURE 2.1.1.4. Correct decisions and type I and type II errors when testing a null hypothesis.

More Points about Hypothesis Testing

Three more points about inferential statistics and hypothesis testing need to be considered. First, when the null hypothesis is not rejected, it is never actually accepted. There could be many reasons why the study did not result in a rejection of the null hypothesis. Perhaps another more powerful or better designed study might result in a rejection of the null hypothesis.

Second, testing the null hypothesis is a key part of all types of inferential statistical procedures used with all of our research approaches except the descriptive approach.

Last, in order to provide a fair test of the null hypothesis, there must be adequate statistical power. A power analysis should be planned prior to the study.

Interpreting Inferential Statistics

Practical Significance versus Statistical Significance

A common misinterpretation is to assume that statistically significant results are practically or clinically important, but statistical significance is not the same as practical significance or importance. With large samples, statistical significance can be obtained even when the differences or associations are very small/weak. Thus, in addition to statistical significance, it is important to examine confidence intervals and/or the effect size.

Confidence Intervals

One alternative to null hypothesis significance testing (NHST) is to create confidence intervals. These intervals provide more information than NHST and may provide more practical information. For example, suppose one knew that an increase in scores of more than five points, on a particular instrument, would lead to a functional increase in performance. Two different methods of therapy were compared. The result showed that clients who used the new method scored statistically significantly higher than those who used the other method. According to NHST, we would reject the null hypothesis of no difference between methods and conclude that our new method is better. If we apply confidence intervals to this same study, we can determine an interval that we are quite confident contains the *population mean difference*. Using the preceding example, if the lower boundary of the confidence interval is greater than five points, we can conclude that using this method would lead to a practical or functional increase in performance. If, however, the confidence interval ranged from one to 11, the result would be statistically significant, but the mean difference in the population might be as small as one point, or as large as 11 points. Given those results, we could not be confident that there would be a *practical* or functional increase using the new method.

Confidence intervals (CI) use the same information that is needed to perform NHST. Whereas NHST is stated as an alpha level, alpha, usually .05, confidence intervals are stated as a lower and upper boundary and a percentage, usually 95%. When one uses a more conservative p value, say .01, then the probability of making a type I error decreases; the corresponding CI increases from 95% to 99%, and confidence that the true population mean is in the interval also increases. However, other things being equal, the range (breadth) of the confidence interval also increases.

Effect Size

A statistically significant outcome does not give information about the strength or size of the outcome or the effect. Effect size is the strength of the relationship between the independent variable and the dependent variable and/or the magnitude of the difference between levels of the independent variable with respect to the dependent variable. Statisticians have proposed effect size measures that fall mainly into three types or families: the r family, the d family, and measures of risk potency. We discuss these effect sizes and clinical significance in more detail below.

Steps in Interpreting Inferential Statistics

To fully interpret the results of an inferential statistic, the author should consider four issues. First, decide whether to reject the null hypothesis, as discussed earlier.

Second, the direction of the effect should be stated. Difference inferential statistics compare groups, so which group performed better should be noted. For associational inferential statistics (e.g., correlation), the sign is very important, so whether the association or relationship is positive or negative should be clear.

Third, the effect size should be included in the description of the results or, at the least, the information to compute it should be presented. The interpretation of the effect size is subjective.

Fourth, the researcher or the consumer of the research (clinician and patient/client) should make a judgment about whether the result has practical or clinical significance or importance. To do so the effect size, the costs of implementing change, and the probability and severity of any side effects or unintended consequences need to be taken into account.

Examples of the Use and Interpretation of Statistics

In Figure 2.1.1.2 we divided research questions into difference questions and associational questions. *Difference questions* compare groups and utilize the statistics, which we call *difference inferential statistics* (t test and analysis of variance). *Associational questions* examine the association or relationship between two or more variables. They utilize *associational inferential statistics* (correlation and regression). Figure 2.1.1.5 is a decision tree that shows how researchers might make a decision about what type of inferential statistic to use. A clinician/reader might work backward from a reported statistic to understand a rationale for the choice of a statistic.

The following examples are from articles published in the *Journal of the American Academy of Child and Adolescent Psychiatry*. Readers can find the original study in the reference list or they can see an expanded version of our description of the study and how the cited statistic was interpreted in Morgan et al. (3).

Basic (2 Variable) Difference Questions and Statistics. For the *independent samples t test* and *one-way ANOVA*, the article we selected was by Herpertz et al. (11), who compared three groups of boys on psychophysiological and other measures (e.g., IQ). They had three levels of the independent variable, (ADHD, ADHD + CD, and a comparison group without ADHD), a between or independent groups design (unrelated children in each group), and a normally distributed dependent variable (IQ), so an appropriate statistic was one-way ANOVA to compare the three levels or groups. A nonparametric statistic could have been used to compare the three groups of boys if the ANOVA assumptions had been markedly violated. If Herpertz et al. had just compared two of the groups (e.g., ADHD and ADHD+CD) they could have used an independent samples t test.

To illustrate the *paired samples t test* and *repeated-measures ANOVA*, we chose an article by Compton et al. (12), who assessed the benefits of sertraline in adolescents with social anxiety disorder in an open 8-week trial. They applied the paired t test to assess whether there was a change from the baseline to the end of the trial on the behavior avoidance test. They used repeated-measures ANOVA to determine whether

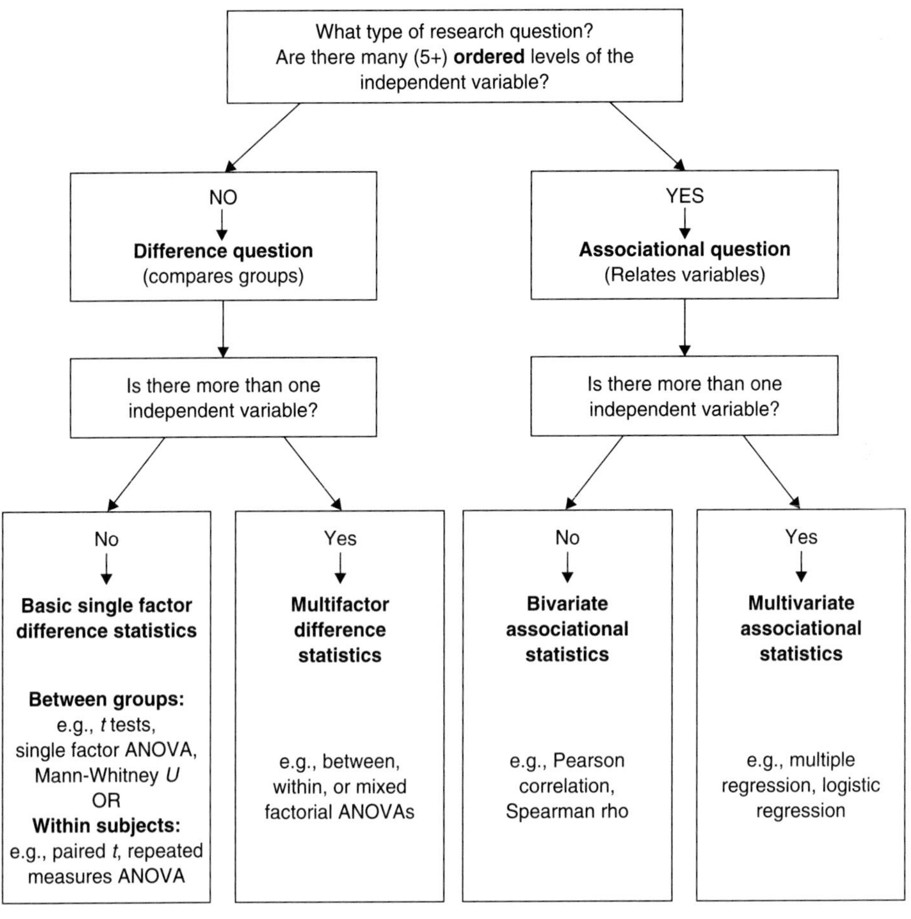

FIGURE 2.1.1.5. A decision tree for the selection of an appropriate inferential statistic.

there was clinical improvement at 2, 4, 6, and 8 weeks compared to the baseline. These statistics were used because there was one group of adolescents assessed repeatedly (within subjects design).

Basic (2 Variable) Associational Questions and Statistics. Dierker et al. (13) chose *Pearson correlations* to study the association or relationship between depression (CES-D scale) and anxiety (RCMAS). Note that both variables had many levels ranging from low to high, and these variables were at least approximately normally distributed.

A study by Wolfe et al. (14) was selected to illustrate the applicability of *chi-square.* They examined the relationship between family intactness (yes or no) and maltreatment classification (maltreated in the past or not). Note that both variables were dichotomous and produce a 2 × 2 contingency table. We will discuss risk potency effect size measures such as odds ratio and risk ratio, which are commonly used to help researchers and clinicians interpret data from 2 × 2 tables.

Complex (Three or more Variable) Questions and Statistics. When there are three or more variables, we call the statistics complex rather than multivariate, because there is not unanimity about the definition of multivariate, and several such complex statistics (factorial ANOVA) are not usually classified as multivariate. It is possible to break down a complex research problem or question into a series of basic (bivariate) questions and analyses as above. However, there are advantages to combining several bivariate questions into one complex analysis: Additional information is provided and a more accurate overall picture is obtained.

Conners et al. (15) selected *factorial ANOVA* to study the effects of four types of treatment and six treatment sites (a 4 × 6 factorial design) on a composite change or improvement scores in children with ADHD. Note that there are two between-groups independent variables (treatment type and site) and one dependent variable (improvement in ADHD symptoms).

Multiple regression was chosen by Logan and King (16) to study the extent of parents' ability to identify signs of depression in their adolescents (the dependent variable). They examined whether a combination of several independent variables would predict the degree to which parents could identify depression. Some of those independent variables were continuous and some were dichotomous.

Mick et al. (17) selected *logistic regression* to study whether children who had been diagnosed with ADHD or not (the dependent variable) seemed to be influenced by prenatal exposure to smoking, alcohol and/or drug use. These and several of the "control" independent variables were dichotomous (parent smoked or did not smoke).

When there is a design similar to that appropriate for a *t* test or ANOVA but there are *two or more* normally distributed dependent variables that are moderately interrelated, it is desirable to consider treating the variables simultaneously with a *multivariate analysis of variance* (MANOVA). Marmorstein and Iacono (18) chose MANOVA to study differences between depression (yes or no) and conduct disorder (yes or no) on a linear combination of several dependent variables (grade point average, number of school suspensions, number of substance abuse symptoms) considered together.

The General Linear Model

Exploring the *relationship between variables can be addressed in two ways* as shown in Figure 2.1.1.6. Researchers choose to use either difference or associational statistics, but statisticians

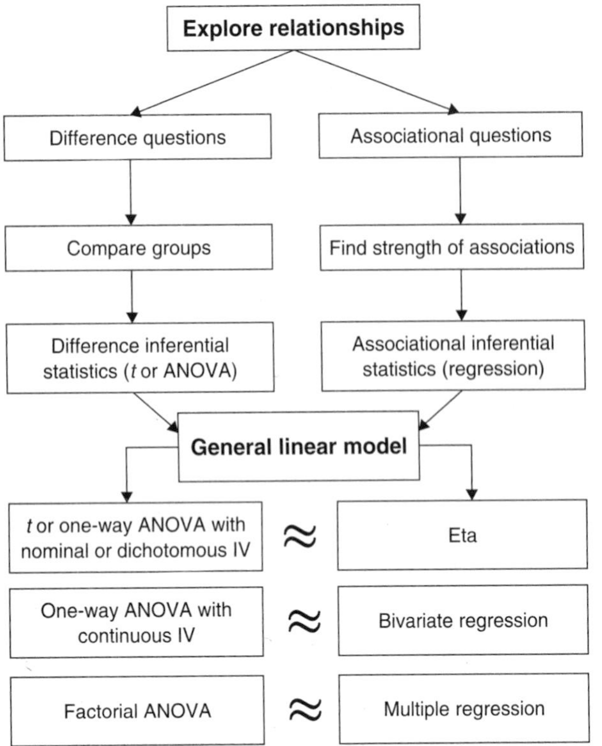

FIGURE 2.1.1.6. Schematic diagram showing how the general linear model is related to the purposes for and types of inferential statistics.

TABLE 2.1.1.11

SIMILAR TERMS ABOUT STATISTICS

- Alternative hypothesis ≈ research hypothesis ≈ H_1
- ANOVA ≈ F ≈ analysis of variance ≈ overall or omnibus F
- Associate variables ≈ relate ≈ predict → correlation or regression
- AUC ≈ probability of a superior (better) outcome
- Basic inferential statistics ≈ univariate statistics (one IV and one DV) ≈ also called bivariate statistics
- Compare groups ≈ test differences → t or ANOVA
- Complex inferential statistics ≈ multifactor statistics (more than one IV) ≈ multivariate statistics (usually more than one DV)
- Data mining ≈ fishing ≈ snooping ≈ multiple significance tests (without clear hypotheses)
- Multiple regression ≈ multiple linear regression
- Null hypothesis ≈ H_0
- Post hoc test ≈ follow-up tests ≈ multiple comparisons
- Repeated-measures ANOVA ≈ within-subject ANOVA
- Risk difference ≈ absolute risk reduction
- Significance level ≈ alpha level ≈ α
- Significance test ≈ null hypothesis significance test ≈ NHST
- Single-factor ANOVA ≈ one-way ANOVA

Note: The term we use most often is listed on the left. Similar terms (indicated by ≈) used by other researchers and/or us are listed to the right, and → means "leads to."

point out that the distinction between difference and associational statistics is artificial, as both serve the purpose of exploring and describing relationships (top box) and both are subsumed by the *general linear model* (middle box); that is, all common parametric statistics are relational. Thus, all of the methods used to analyze one continuous dependent variable and one or more independent variables, either continuous or categorical, are mathematically equivalent.

The bottom part of Figure 2.1.1.6 indicates that a t test or one-way ANOVA with a nominal or dichotomous independent variable is analogous to eta, which is a correlation coefficient for a nominal independent variable and a continuous dependent variable. Likewise, a one-way ANOVA with a continuous independent variable is analogous to bivariate regression. Thus, if there is a continuous, normally distributed dependent/outcome variable and there are five or more levels of a normally distributed independent variable, it would be appropriate to analyze it with either regression or a one-way ANOVA. Finally, as shown in the lowest boxes in Figure 2.1.1.6, factorial ANOVA and multiple regression are analogous mathematically.

Although our distinction between difference and associational parametric statistics is a simplification, we think it is useful educationally. Table 2.1.1.11 provides a list of sometimes confusing statistical terms and alternative names for them. The appendix provides a list of some research terms which are partially similar (or overlapping), but need to be distinguished.

SUMMARIZING STATISTICAL OUTCOMES

Metaanalysis: Formulation and Interpretation

Metaanalysis is a research synthesis of a set of studies that uses a quantitative measure, effect size, to indicate the strength of relationship between the treatment or other independent variable and the dependent variables. Not all research syntheses are metaanalyses. Often, the purpose of a research synthesis is to provide a description of a subject area, illustrating the studies that have been undertaken. In other cases, the studies are too varied in nature to provide a meaningful effect size index. The focus of this section, however, is on research syntheses that result in a metaanalysis. (For a more detailed discussion see Lipsey and Wilson, 19.)

One advantage of performing a metaanalysis includes the computation of a summary statistic for a large number of studies. This summary statistic provides an overall estimate of the strength of relationship between independent and dependent variables. A second advantage of metaanalysis is that it provides evidence of the reliability of a research finding. Researchers have more confidence in the findings of multiple studies than in the results of a single study. A third advantage is that it takes into account studies that failed to find statistical significance and may not have been published, perhaps because of a lack of statistical power (reduced sample size). A fourth advantage of metaanalysis is increased external validity. Many studies, strong in internal validity (design characteristics), do not use a representative sample of subjects. This limits the generalization of results. However, including many studies increases the variation of the sample and strengthens external validity.

Although there are many advantages to metaanalysis, there also has been considerable criticism. The most frequent criticism of metaanalysis is that it may combine "apples and oranges." Synthesizing studies that might differ on both independent and dependent variables brings into question the usefulness of the end product. Furthermore, many studies have similar independent and dependent variables, but differ in the strength of design. Should these studies be combined? Another criticism concerns small sample size. Introducing a large proportion of studies with inadequate statistical power into a metaanalysis could introduce bias into the overall effect size. Last, even though the statistics used in metaanalysis are quite sophisticated, the end product will never be better than the individual studies that make up the metaanalysis.

Criteria for Review

Although much of the focus of metaanalysis is on statistical procedures, perhaps the most important part of a metaanalysis is the planning of inclusion and exclusion criteria for selecting a study into the metaanalysis. These inclusion and exclusion criteria are often related to internal validity and external validity. Most researchers feel that metaanalyses composed of randomized control trials (RCT) represent the gold standard for clinical research.

Statistical Computations for Individual Studies

Type of Effect Size. There are numerous types of effect size indices. Briefly, the *d* effect size indicates the strength of a relationship between an independent and dependent variable in standard deviation units. The most common effect size indices used in meta-analyses are *d*, *r*, and odds ratio (OR), although risk ratio (RR) and number needed to treat (NNT) also have been used.

Number of Effect Sizes. Each study in the metaanalysis should yield at least one effect size. It is not uncommon, however, to observe studies that compare a treatment group with a control group on many measures. An effect size could be computed for each measure of the study. However, when studies have more than one measure, the measures are usually related or correlated. Thus, computing more than one effect size yields redundant information and gives too much weight to that particular study. Therefore, the researcher should select one representative measure from the study or use a statistical method to determine a representative measure.

Weights. For the most part, each study included in the meta-analysis is based on a different sample size. Studies with larger sample sizes are likely to be better estimates than studies with small sample sizes. Therefore, in order to take sample size into consideration when the effect sizes are averaged, a weight is computed for each effect size. Effect sizes also can be weighted by other important indices, such as quality of the study.

Computation of Combined Effect Size for Studies and Related Statistics

When all studies that meet the criteria for inclusion in the metaanalysis have been coded and effect size data entered, a *combined effect size* can be computed. Frequently there is an effect size computed for each construct. In addition to a mean effect size index computed for each construct, a confidence interval, usually 95%, also is obtained. Analyses also are performed to test for statistical significance, computing a z statistic, and to test for homogeneity, computing a Q statistic. If Q is statistically significant, the null hypothesis of homogeneity is rejected and the researcher assumes a heterogeneous distribution.

The most common followup procedure when a test for homogeneity of effect size distribution is statistically significant is to attempt to identify the variability that is contributing to the heterogeneity. Most often, the researcher has in mind, prior to the metaanalysis, certain hypotheses about which variables might contribute to variability in the mean effect size. These variables (such as strength of research design, sample subgroups, gender) are usually referred to as *moderator* variables.

Moderator variables are variables that interact with the independent variable to *cause* the change in the dependent variable. For example, gender might be a moderator variable that interacts with treatment such that there is only a success in women and not men. Moderator variables are often confused with *mediator* variables. Mediator variables are intervening variables between the independent and dependent variables that help explain the change in the dependent variable. For example, a metaanalysis might find class size (independent variable) is inversely related to student achievement (dependent variable). The mediator variable might be teacher attention, which intervenes between the independent and dependent variables.

Metaanalysis is a valuable tool for both the researcher and the clinician. Summarizing the results of many studies as an effect size index provides important strength of relationship information. Caution always should be used concerning the types of studies that went into the metaanalysis; especially, one should be aware of design issues.

Effect Sizes and Clinical Significance

Behavioral scientists are interested in answering three basic questions when examining the relationships between variables (20). First, should an observed result be attributed to chance or is it real (statistical significance)? Second, if the result is real, how large is it (effect size)? Third, is the result large enough to be meaningful and useful (clinical or practical significance)? In this chapter, we treat clinical significance as equivalent to practical significance.

Clinical Significance

The clinical significance of a treatment is based on external standards provided by clinicians, patients, and/or researchers. Judgments by the researcher and the consumers (clinicians and patients) regarding clinical significance should consider factors such as clinical benefit, cost, and side effects. Although there is no formal statistical test of clinical significance, we suggest using an effect size measure to assist in interpreting clinical significance. Each of these measures, however, has limitations that require the clinician to be cautious about interpretation.

Effect Size Measures

Statisticians have proposed many effect size measures. They fall mainly into three types or families: the *r* family, the *d* family, and measures of risk potency.

The *r* Family. One method of expressing effect sizes is in terms of strength of association, with statistics such as the Pearson product moment correlation coefficient, *r*, used when both the independent and the dependent measures are normally distributed. Such effect sizes vary between −1.0 and +1.0, with 0 representing no effect. This family of effect sizes also includes associational statistics such as the Spearman or Kendall rank correlation coefficients, and the multiple correlation coefficient (*R*).

The *d* Family. These effect sizes are used when the independent variable is binary (dichotomous) and the dependent variable is normally distributed. The *d* family effect sizes use different formulas, but they all express the mean difference in standard deviation units. Effect sizes for *d* range from minus to plus infinity, with zero indicating no effect; however, it is unusual to find *d* values in the applied behavioral sciences much greater than 1.

Measures of Risk Potency. These effect sizes are used when both the independent and the dependent variable are binary. There are many such effect sizes, but in this section we discuss five common ones: odds ratio, risk ratio, relative risk reduction, risk difference, and number needed to treat (NNT). Odds ratios and risk ratios vary from 0 to infinity, with 1 indicating no effect. Relative risk reduction and risk difference range from −1 to 1, with zero indicating no effect. NNT ranges from 1 to plus infinity, with very *large values* indicating no treatment effect.

AUC or Probability of a Superior Outcome. Finally we discuss an index that can be used when the independent variable is binary, but the dependent variable can be either binary or ordered. AUC stands for *area under the curve* but could be called the probability of a superior (better) outcome of one treatment over another. AUC integrates many of the other effect size indices and is directly related to clinical significance. Kraemer et al. (21) and Grissom and Kim (22) provide more information on this relatively new effect size.

Unfortunately, there is little agreement about which effect size to use for each situation. The most commonly discussed effect size in the behavioral sciences, especially for experiments, is *d*, but the correlation coefficient, *r*, and other measures of the strength of association are common in survey research. In medical journals, an odds ratio is most common.

In the remainder of this section, we discuss the use and interpretation of each of the above measures and discuss the advantages and disadvantages of each as indicators of clinical significance. In this discussion, we focus on positive association only—that is, effect sizes ranging from the value that indicates no effect to the value indicating maximal effect.

Interpreting *d* and *r* Effect Sizes

Table 2.1.1.12 provides general guidelines for interpreting the size of the effect for five measures discussed in this section. Cohen (5) provided research examples of what he labeled small, medium, and large effects suggested by *d* and *r* values. Most researchers would not consider a correlation (*r*) of .5 to be very strong because only 25% of the variance in the dependent variable is predicted. However, Cohen argued that when the two variables measure different constructs, an *r* of .3 is typical and .5 is about as large as correlations in applied behavioral sciences get. When, as in test-retest reliability measures, the two variables measure the same construct, typical correlations are much higher, for example, .7 or more.

Cohen (5) also pointed out that effects with a *d* of .8 are "grossly perceptible and therefore large differences...". Cohen's medium size effect is "visible to the naked eye. That is, in the course of normal experiences, one would become aware of an average difference." Kazdin and Bass (23), based on a review of psychotherapy research, found that *d* was approximately .8 when comparing a new active treatment against an inactive (treatment withheld) placebo. Comparing a new effective treatment with a usual or comparison treatment would produce a *d* of about .5.

The *d* and *r* guidelines in Table 2.1.1.12 are based on the effect sizes commonly found in studies in the applied behavioral sciences. They do not have absolute meaning; Cohen's "large," "medium," and "small" were meant to be relative to typical findings in behavioral research in general. For that reason, we suggest using "larger than typical" instead of "large," "typical" instead of "medium," and "smaller than typical" instead of "small." However, as suggested by the Kazdin and Bass (23) results, it is advisable to examine the research literature to see if there is information about typical effect sizes for those variables, in that context. The standards expressed in Table 2.1.1.12 then would need to be adjusted accordingly.

There are disadvantages of the *d* and *r* effect sizes as measures of clinical significance. First, they are relatively abstract, and consequently may not be meaningful to patients and clinicians, or even to researchers. They were not originally intended to be indices of clinical significance and are not readily interpretable in terms of how much *individuals* are affected by treatment.

Interpreting Measures of Risk Potency

Clinicians must make categorical decisions about whether or not to use a treatment (medication, therapy, hospitalization), and the outcomes also are often binary. For example, a child is classified as having ADHD or not, or being at risk for some negative outcome or not. In comparing two treatments, a positive outcome might indicate that the patient is sufficiently improved (or not) to meet the criteria for a clinically significant change. These binary decisions and outcomes provide data in a 2 × 2 contingency table. In some cases, a 2 × 2 table results when initially continuous outcome data are dichotomized (when responses on an ordered outcome measure in a clinical trial are reclassified as "success" and "failure"). Such dichotomization not only results in a loss of information, but, dichotomizing can result in inconsistent and arbitrary effect size indices due to different choices of the cut point or threshold for failure.

Odds Ratio. OR is the most commonly reported of these measures. However, a major limitation of the odds ratio as an effect size index is that the magnitude of the odds ratio may approach infinity if the outcome is rare or very common, even when the association is near random or no effect. The magnitude of the OR varies strongly with the choice of cut point.

Risk Ratio. Again, the choice of cut point and which risk ratio (failure or success) is chosen change the magnitude of the risk ratio, making it hard to interpret. Because the RR may approach infinity when the risk in the denominator approaches zero, there can be no agreed-on standards for assessing the magnitude or clinical significance of RR.

TABLE 2.1.1.12

INTERPRETATION OF THE STRENGTH (EFFECT SIZE) OF A POSITIVE RELATIONSHIP

	The *d* family:	The *r* family	2 x 2 Associations		
General Interpretation of the Strength of a Relationship	*d*	*r*	*AUC*	*RD*	NNT
Much larger than typical	≥1.00	≥.70	≥76%	≥52%	≤1.9
Large or larger than typical	.80	.50	71%	43%	2.3
Medium or typical	.50	.30	64%	28%	3.6
Small or smaller than typical	.20	.10	56%	11%	8.9

Note: We interpret the numbers in this table as a range of values. For example, a *d* greater than .90 (or less than −.90) would be described as much "larger than typical," in the applied behavioral sciences, a *d* between say .70 and .90 would be called "larger than typical," and *d* between say .60 and .70 would be "typical to larger than typical." We interpret the other columns similarly. AUC = Area under the curve, or probability of a superior outcome; RD = Risk difference; NNT = Number needed to treat.

Relative Risk Reduction. RRR can vary between 0 and 1.0. Because the "failure" RRR may be very small when the "success" RRR is large, RRR is difficult to interpret in terms of clinical significance, and there are no agreed-upon standards for judging its magnitude.

Risk Difference. RD, also called absolute risk reduction (ARR), can vary from 0% to 100%. When the RD is near zero, it indicates near random association. If the success or failure rates are extreme, the RD is likely to be near 0%. It is troublesome in terms of interpreting clinical significance that the RD is often very near zero when the odds ratio and one of the risk ratios are very large.

Number Needed to Treat. NNT is a relatively new measure that has been recommended for improving the reporting of effect sizes, but it has not yet been widely used. NNT is the number of patients who must be treated to generate one more success or one less failure than would have resulted had all persons been given the comparison treatment. Mathematically, NNT is the reciprocal of the risk difference. A result of 1.0 means the treatment is perfect, that every treatment subject succeeds and every comparison subject fails. An NNT greater than 1.0 means that the treatment is less than ideally effective, and the larger the NNT, the relatively less effective the treatment.

AUC or the Probability of a Superior/Better Outcome. This relatively new effect size might substitute for either *d* family measures or measures of risk potency. It represents the probability that a randomly selected participant in the treatment group has a better result than a randomly selected one in the comparison group. As shown in Table 2.1.1.12, one can define guidelines for interpreting AUC that correspond to those for *d*. For example, a medium or typical effect size of $d = .5$ corresponds to AUC = 64%. Thus, when comparing a treatment subject against a comparison subject, 64% of the time the treatment subject would have a better response.

AUC is of special interest because it can be computed based on clinical judgments alone. One could randomly select pairs of subjects, one of each pair in the treatment and one in the comparison group, and submit their clinical records to experts with group membership masked. The experts would then be asked which of the two had a better outcome. The proportion of the pairs for which the experts selected the treatment group subject as better off is an estimate of AUC.

Conclusion

Nuovo et al. (24) pointed out that the Consolidated Standards on Reporting Trials (CONSORT) recommends reporting the number needed to treat (NNT) or the risk difference (RD). However, often RD can seem unimpressively small, and NNT may seem very large, suggesting very little effect of treatment. In many such cases with small RD or large NNT, one of the risk ratios and one of the relative risk reduction measures and, most of all, the odds ratio can give an inflated impression of the size of the effect, thus exaggerating apparent clinical significance. For this reason, our preferred effect size for understanding clinical significance would tend to be AUC (the probability of a superior outcome), but remember that *d*, NNT, and RD are all mathematically equivalent and can be converted to AUC.

We have provided some general guidelines for interpreting measures of clinical significance. It is not possible, however, to provide any fixed standards that a clinician could use to conclude that an effect size was clinically significant. It makes a difference whether the treatment is for a deadly disease or for the common cold, and whether the treatment is risky and costly or safe and free. The context in which an effect size is used matters in interpreting the size of the effect; the effect size only facilitates consideration of clinical significance.

EVALUATING THE DESIGN AND METHODS OF A RESEARCH STUDY

This concluding section provides an overview of the evaluation of *research validity*, the validity of the design and methods of a study as a whole.

Research Validity versus Measurement Reliability and Measurement Validity

It is important to distinguish between evidence for the merit or worth of the whole study (*research validity*) as opposed to evidence in support of the quality of a specific instrument or test used in a study (*measurement validity*). Figure 2.1.1.7 shows that measurement reliability and validity (the upper two boxes) are different from, but related to, research reliability and validity (lower boxes), and the figure shows how all four fit into an overall conception of reliability and validity. The horizontal arrow indicates that measurement reliability is a necessary prerequisite for measurement validity (a measure cannot provide evidence for validity if it is not consistent/reliable). The vertical arrow indicates that the validity of a whole study depends to some extent on the reliability and validity of the specific measures or instruments used in the study.

Rating Scales to Evaluate Research Validity

A good study should have moderate to high internal *and* external validity. However, it is hard, in any given study, to achieve this goal. Using our research validity framework, a reader would evaluate a study from low to high on each of the four scales or dimensions shown in Figures 2.1.1.8 and 2.1.1.9. In Morgan, et al (3), we provide a comprehensive framework for evaluating the research validity of an article, including four additional rating scales.

Internal Validity

The top part of Figure 2.1.1.8 indicates the key features we use to rate the dimension of *equivalence of the groups on participant characteristics*. The bottom of Figure 2.1.1.8 shows the five issues that we use to rate the *control of experiences and the environment during the study*, i.e., contamination.

External Validity

External validity broadly defined asks about generalizability to other populations, settings, treatment variables, and measurement variables. If a study is not rated high on external validity, the author should at least be cautious about generalizing the findings. We use the three issues in the top of Figure 2.1.1.9 to evaluate *population external validity* and the five issues listed in the bottom part of Figure 2.1.1.9 to evaluate *ecological external validity*, whether the setting, testers, procedures and timing of the study are natural and, thus, whether the result of the specific study can be generalized.

ACKNOWLEDGMENTS

This chapter draws heavily on our book, *Understanding and Evaluating Research in Applied and Clinical Settings* (3) published recently by Lawrence Erlbaum Associates. We appreciate their permission to reprint or adapt from that book all the tables and figures used in this chapter.

RELIABILITY Stability or Consistency	**VALIDITY** Accuracy and Representativeness
Measurement (or test) reliability The participant gets the same or a very similar score from a specific *test*, *observation*, or *rating* when it is used for a similar purpose with a similar population. →	**Measurement (or test) validity** The score accurately reflects/measures what it was designed or intended to measure when used for a similar purpose with a similar population. ↓
Research (or study) reliability If repeated, the *study* would produce similar results. This is called *replication.* Meta analysis examines several similar studies in part to examine the consistency of their results.	**Research (or study) validity** The results of the study are accurate and generalizable. Two major dimensions of the *validity of a study* are: ▪ **Internal validity**—Strength of design. If high, one can make valid interferences about causes. • Equivalence of groups on participant characteristics. • Control of extraneous experience and environmental variables ▪ **External validity**—If high, the results may generalize to other populations, settings, and variables. • Population validity • Ecological validity

FIGURE 2.1.1.7. Relationships and differences between measurement reliability and validity and research reliability and validity.

INTERNAL VALIDITY

Equivalence of Groups on Participant Characteristics

Based rating on:

a) Were the participants randomly assigned to the groups?
b) If not, were there adequate attempts to make groups similar (e.g., ANCOVA) or *check* similarity on a *pretest?*
c) If no randomization, were there adequate attempts to make groups similar or check similarity on *other key variables*?
d) Was retention during the study high and similar across groups?

LOW	MEDIUM	HIGH
Groups very different, marked differential attrition	Some attempts to equate groups or groups found to be similar	Random assignment to groups and low attrition

Control of Experiences and Environment Variables (Contamination)

Based rating on:

a) Was the study conducted in a controlled environment (e.g., a lab)?
b) Were extraneous variables that could affect one group more than the others controlled? Did the groups have the same type of environment?
c) Was there a no treatment group (placebo) or usual treatment group?
d) Were extraneous variables that could affect all groups and obscure the true effect controlled?
e) Were attempts to reduce other extraneous influences adequate?

LOW	MEDIUM	HIGH
Extraneous variables not controlled, no comparison group (field setting)	Attempts to control experiences and environment	All extraneous variables controlled, eliminated or balanced (controlled lab)

FIGURE 2.1.1.8. Rating scales to evaluate the internal validity of the findings of a study.

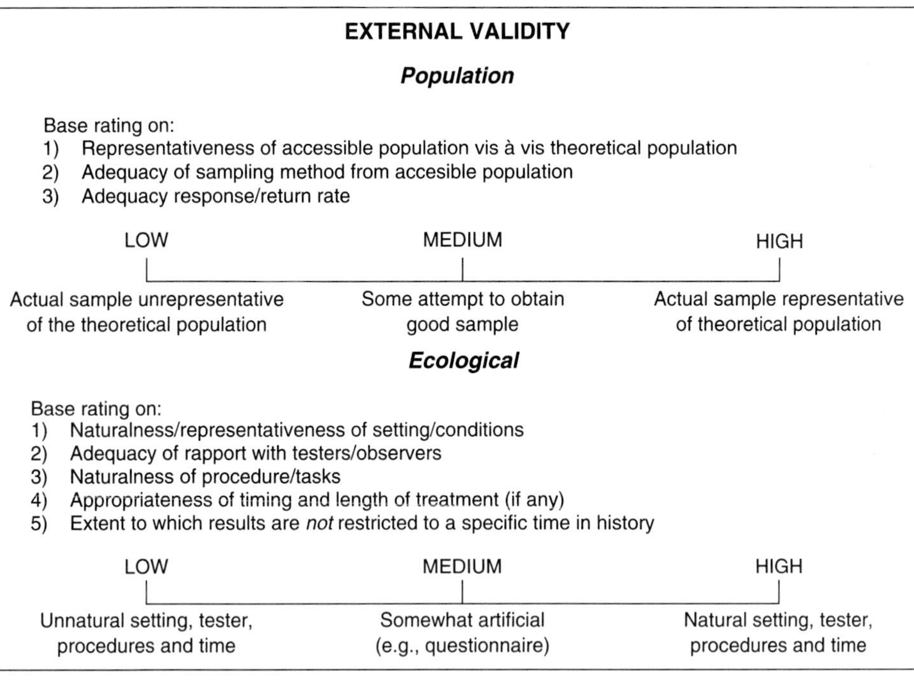

FIGURE 2.1.1.9. Rating scales to evaluate the external validity of the findings of a study.

Earlier versions of the tables, figures and text were published as a series of articles, "Clinicians' Guide to Research Methods and Statistics," published between 1999 and 2003 in the *Journal of the American Academy of Child and Adolescent Psychiatry* (JAACAP) by Lippincott, Williams, and Wilkins. We especially appreciate the critiques and statistical advice on the JAACAP series from Helena Chmura Kramer, professor of biostatistics at the Stanford University Medical School.

We also acknowledge the advice and encouragement of Andrés Martin, editor of this book, and we thank the Developmental Psychobiology Research Group (DPRG), Department of Psychiatry, University of Colorado School of Medicine, for support over many years. Dr. Harmon whose unexpected death was a loss to us personally, was supported by a Grant from the Irving B. Harris Foundation. We could not have completed the chapter without the word processing skills of Catherine Lamana and Alana Stewart.

APPENDIX: PARTIALLY SIMILAR TERMS FOR DIFFERENT CONCEPTS[1]

- Cronbach's *alpha* ≠ *alpha* (significance) level
- *Dependent* variable ≠ *dependent* samples design or statistic
- *Discriminant* analysis ≠ *discriminant* evidence for measurement validity
- *Factor* (i.e., independent variable) ≠ *factor* analysis
- Factorial *design* ≠ *factorial evidence* for measurement validity
- *Independent* variable ≠ *independent* samples
- *Levels* (of a variable) ≠ *level* of measurement
- *Odds* ratio ≠ *odds*
- *Outcome* (dependent) variable ≠ *outcome* (results) of the study
- Research *question* ≠ questionnaire *question* or item
- *Random* assignment of participants to groups ≠ *random* assignment of treatments to groups
- *Random* assignment (of participants to groups) ≠ *random* selection (or sampling of participants to be included in the study) ≠ *random* order
- Odds *ratio* ≠ risk *ratio*
- *Related* samples design ≠ variables that are *related*
- Random *samples* ≠ paired/related *samples* ≠ independent *samples*
- Measurement *scale* ≠ a rating *scale* ≠ summated/composite *scale*
- *Theoretical* research ≠ *theoretical* population
- Measurement *validity* ≠ research *validity*

[1]Italicized terms are listed alphabetically; ≠ means "not equal to."

References

1. Patton MQ: *Qualitative research and evaluation methods*, 3rd ed. Thousand Oaks, Sage, 2002.
2. Velleman PF, Wilkinson L: Nominal, ordinal, interval, and ratio typologies are misleading. *Am Statistician* 47:65–72, 1993.
3. Morgan GA, Gliner JA, Harmon RJ: *Understanding and evaluating research in applied and clinical settings*, Mahwah, Lawrence Erlbaum Associates, 2006.
4. American Educational Research Association, American Psychological Association, and National Council on Measurement in Education: *Standards for Educational and Psychological Testing*, Washington, DC: American Educational Research Association, 1999.
5. Cohen J: *Statistical Power Analysis for the Behavioral Sciences*. 2nd ed. Hillsdale, Lawrence Erlbaum Associates, 1988.
6. Cook TD, Campbell DT: *Quasi-experimentation: Design and Analysis Issues for Field Settings*. Boston, Houghton Mifflin, 1979.
7. Shadish WR, Cook TD, Campbell DT: *Experimental and Quasi-experimental Designs for Generalized Casual Influence*. Boston, Houghton Mifflin, 2002.
8. Fowler FJ Jr.: *Survey Research Methods*. 3rd ed. Thousand Oaks, Sage, 2001.
9. Kraemer HC, Thiemann S: *How Many Subjects? Statistical Power Analysis in Research*. Newbury Park, Sage, 1987.
10. Lipsey MW: *Design Sensitivity: Statistical Power for Experimental Research*. Newbury Park, Sage, 1990.
11. Herpertz SC, Wenning B, Mueller B, et al.: Psychophysiological responses in ADHD boys with and without conduct disorder: Implications for adult antisocial behavior. *J Am Acad Child Adolesc Psychiatry* 40:1222–1230, 2001.
12. Compton SN, Grant PJ, Chrisman AK, et al.: Sertraline in children and adolescents with social anxiety disorder: An open trial. *J Am Acad Child Adolesc Psychiatry* 40:564–571, 2001.
13. Dierker LC, Albano AM, Clarke GN, et al.: Screening for anxiety and depression in early adolescence. *J Am Acad Child Adolesc Psychiatry* 40:929–936, 2001.

14. Wolfe DA, Scott K, Wekerle C, et al.: Child maltreatment: Risk of adjustment problems and dating violence in adolescence. *J Am Acad Child Adolesc Psychiatry* 40:282–289, 2001.
15. Conners CK, Epstein JN, March JS, et al.: Multimodal treatment of ADHD in the MTA: An alternative outcome analysis. *J Am Acad Child Adolesc Psychiatry* 40:159–167, 2001.
16. Logan DE, King CA: Parental identification of depression and mental health service use among depressed adolescents. *J Am Acad Child Adolesc Psychiatry* 41:296–304, 2002.
17. Mick E, Biederman J, Faraone SV, et al.: Case-control study of attention-deficit hyperactivity disorder and maternal smoking, alcohol use, and drug use during pregnancy. *J Am Acad Child Adolesc Psychiatry* 41:378–385, 2002.
18. Marmorstein NR, Iacono WG: Major depression and conduct disorder in a twin sample: Gender, functioning, and risk for future psychopathology. *J Am Acad Child Adolesc Psychiatry* 42:225–233, 2003.
19. Lipsey MW, Wilson DB: *Practical meta-analysis*, Thousand Oaks, Sage, 2000.
20. Kirk RE: Promoting good statistical practices: Some suggestions. *Educ Psychol Meas* 61:213–218, 2001.
21. Kraemer HC, Morgan GA, Leech NL, et al.: Measures of clinical significance. *J Am Acad Child Adolesc Psychiatry* 42:1524–1529, 2003.
22. Grissom RJ, Kim JJ: *Effect sizes for research: A broad practical approach*. Mahwah, Lawrence Erlbaum Associates, 2005.
23. Kazdin AE, Bass D: Power to detect differences between alternative treatments in comparative psychotherapy outcome research. *J Consult Clin Psychol* 57:138–147, 1989.
24. Nuovo J, Melnikov J, Chang D: Reporting number needed to treat and risk difference in randomized controlled trials. *JAMA* 287:2813–2814, 2002.

CHAPTER 2.1.2 ■ EVIDENCE-BASED PRACTICE AS A CONCEPTUAL FRAMEWORK

JOHN HAMILTON

INTRODUCTION

David Sackett, an internist and epidemiologist, historically defined an evidence-based medicine approach as consisting of five steps:

1. Converting the need for information (about prevention, diagnosis, prognosis, therapy, causation) into an answerable question;
2. Searching for the best evidence to answer that question;
3. Critically appraising the discovered evidence for its validity, the size of the demonstrated effect, and its relevance to the clinical population at hand;
4. Integrating these conclusions with clinical expertise, patient preference, and a patient's unique circumstances, values, and biology; and
5. Evaluating the efficiency and effectiveness of these efforts with the goal of improvement in the next cycle (1).

Although Sackett's classic definition of an evidence-based approach is invaluable, this chapter focuses on the unique context of doing pediatric mental health. Child psychiatry is not internal medicine. It is typically practiced in outpatient multiprofessional teams where psychosocial interventions have a much greater role than in internal medicine. Readers seeking textbooks on basic principles of EBP might consult multiple guidebooks, journal articles, and the Internet (1–5).

This chapter begins with how various professional groups use the phrase "evidence-based." It then proceeds to make a case for how processes based on evidence-based practice (EBP) are useful and significantly different than usual practice. It continues with common objections to EBP, but offers a rebuttal for each and the evidence supporting EBP. The second part of this chapter presents selected elements of EBP within the context of pediatric mental health: tips on searching the most relevant databases, diagnostic approaches consistent with EBP, choosing a treatment, developing local data, and ideas about developing evidence-based systems.

THREE STREAMS OF EMPIRICISM: EBM, EBS, EBT

Varied authors and groups have used "evidence-based" (EB) as a modifying phrase. Evidence-based practice, or EBP (6, 7), is the term used here, but there is also evidence-based medicine, or EBM (5), evidence-based services, or EBS (8), and evidence-based treatments, or EBTs (9). The phrase "empirically supported treatments," or ESTs, is often used interchangeably with EBT (10). To oversimplify, there are three groups. The first group, using the term EBM, is often associated with medication issues and child psychiatrists. The second group, using the term EBT, is associated with psychologists, psychosocial treatments and the American Psychological Association (APA). The third group, EBS, is associated with systems striving to better use empirical results to improve outcomes. In this chapter, when we refer to EBP, we're including all three groups. These multiple terms share a common interest in the evidence of empirical data, both about our patients and our own functioning as well as off the shelf in the literature; combined, these three terms contain a powerful flood of ideas.

There is considerable overlap between EBM, EBT, and EBS, but each retains its distinct flavor. EBM authors often focus on changing individual practitioner behavior. For example, EBM tries to interest practitioners in researching "answerable questions" regarding individual patients. Often examples used involve medications. Many well known EBM leaders like David Sackett are epidemiologists or internists. On the other hand, EBT authors tend to focus more on studying specific manualized psychosocial treatments. EBT authors are often university-affiliated psychologists who study the effectiveness of a psychosocial intervention for a specific disorder. They also study how a psychosocial intervention "travels" when it is "exported" to sites other than where it was developed. Finally, evidence-based services (EBS) is a term used by clinicians in delivery systems trying to improve outcomes by better

TABLE 2.1.2.1

EVIDENCE-BASED MEDICINE (EBM), EMPIRICALLY SUPPORTED TREATMENTS (EST), AND EVIDENCE-BASED SYSTEMS (EBS)

	EBM	EST*	EBS
Origins	Many ideas developed at McMaster University in Ontario, Canada	American Psychological Association Task Force 12	State of Hawaii Child and Adolescent Mental Health Division (CAMHD)
Central Ideas	PICO (Population/Intervention/ Control or Comparison/Outcome) based on epidemiological thinking is core idea; "Bringing the literature to the bedside"	Focus on efficacy and effectiveness of well defined psychosocial interventions; lab–clinic gap a major hurdle	Feasible but proven treatments; extensive use of locally generated data; systemwide consensus on effective interventions
Frequent Members	University-based physicians	University-based psychologists	Large systems wanting improved results

*Also called Evidence-Based Treatments.

use of empirical evidence (11). In EBS a consensus-building group of providers, administrators, and consumers agrees on a menu of effective interventions including both EBTs and medications. These three empirical approaches are summarized in Table 2.1.2.1. The term evidence-based practices, or EBPs, used here is an umbrella term for processes based on all three groups while valuing patient preference and clinical expertise as well. EBP welcomes the use of clinical expertise, for example, in formulating the context of symptoms (12). And, while including both medication and psychosocial interventions, EBP is neutral in choosing between them, an advantage on a multidisciplinary team.

Significant boundaries between child psychology and child psychiatry have shaped these three streams of empiricism. Child psychologists and child psychiatrists typically belong to different professional organizations, attend different conventions, publish in different journals, and occupy different niches in clinical organizations such as state clinics or hospitals. These different worlds naturally evolve different ways of thinking, sometimes referred to as cognitive boundaries (13). In fact, the prevailing paradigm in each discipline may be so different that each discipline has distinct cognitive assumptions and may advance different claims to knowledge. At their worst, boundaries can be sufficiently extreme that there is no common ground for productive dialogue (14).

EBP is a helpful antidote to the tendency of practitioners to identify with a particular discipline or treatment. For example, a practitioner may think of himself as primarily a psychopharmacologist, or as a family therapist, a play therapist, a behavior therapist, or as an expert in delivering a specific manualized therapy. EBP as conceived here, on the other hand, is not attached to a specific treatment modality or profession. Instead, EBP chooses those feasible treatments proven in the most valid studies to deliver the most rapid, complete, and long lasting improvement in functioning and symptoms with the least harm. A commitment to EBP therefore significantly changes the identity of practitioners: A commitment to finding and using both published and "local" evidence becomes a central value.

In a multidisciplinary team, the processes of making a diagnosis, choosing a treatment, and assessing its results are all significantly different in a team committed to EBP than in a team proceeding "as usual." Table 2.1.2.2 lists a chain of clinical processes fundamental to EBP, and highlights differences between the EBP approach and usual practice in defining the clinical population, in choosing an intervention, and in evaluating its effects relative to a comparison or control group. This order is the familiar PICO format derived from epidemiology: Population, Intervention (or Exposure), Control (or Comparison), and Outcome. Of course, a solo practitioner can also use many of these processes. For example, both the well known PubMed site as well as the Internet site for the Journal of the American Academy of Child and Adolescent Psychiatry offer extensive resources for searching answerable questions. A major issue for practitioners, however, is how to offer ESTs that often require extensive training. Parent Management Training for Oppositional Defiant Disorder, for example (15), or Cognitive-Behavioral Treatment or Interpersonal Therapy for depression (16) all require training. Yet a practitioner may choose to obtain training in those ESTs which will be most useful in the practice she has developed. Informal subspecialization among community therapists is also an option.

WHY BOTHER? COMMON OBJECTIONS TO EBP, WITH REBUTTALS

At EBP lectures and informally in conversations with colleagues, certain objections to EBP seem inevitable. Here are some common ones; each is followed by a rebuttal.

There isn't much evidence in child psychiatry anyway.

A variant of this complaint is *There aren't RCTs for everything*. This objection fails to note that the EBP practitioner is committed to the judicious use of the most valid and relevant evidence available, not just RCTs. EBP does use a hierarchy of evidence based on validity of research design, and RCTs are high up in that hierarchy. But if only case reports exist, then the EBP approach is to use them as evidence. However, the rapid growth of information about the treatment of child psychiatric disorders in the past decade makes this increasingly unnecessary.

EBP misses the point, because treatment is all about the therapeutic relationship.

How closely are therapeutic relationship variables and outcomes associated in youth psychotherapy? How is that association moderated by age, presenting problem (emotional or behavioral), treatment type, and structure (behavioral or not, manualized or not), and whether the treatment was received from an ongoing clinical service or a "one-time" research team? And do therapeutic relationship variables function as the change mechanism itself? Or are they "merely" a necessary factor to promote attendance at sessions? Understanding these

TABLE 2.1.2.2

FUNCTIONS AND PROCESSES: TREATMENT AS USUAL VERSUS EBP

Function or Process	Treatment as Usual	Team Committed to EBP
Defining characteristics of clinical population at intake	Highly variable, narrative intake note DSM-IV as guide	Functioning and psychopathology measured with defined instruments while clinical interview establishes alliance and context of symptoms
Defining primary outcome variable(s)	Usually not done	Preference for choosing primary outcome variable(s) at time of evaluation [or assessment]
Choosing an intervention	Chosen on basis of familiarity, ease of use, often clinician specific	Pyramid of evidence has central role, evidence updated regularly
Evaluating local effect of interventions proven elsewhere	Often ignored	Always an issue, addressed via collecting local data
Collecting and making use of composite local diagnostic and outcome data	Rarely done	Always done, including benchmarking results to compare with natural history and published outcomes
Use of outcome data to inform provider, consumer, and administrator	Case outcome often not tracked with reliable measure; minimal aggregate outcome data	Provider, administration, consumer all interested in outcome data, individual and aggregate
Teaching staff EBP	Minimally structured case conferences or traditional supervision	Staff learns EBP in programwide projects and has access to EBP instruction
Linking providers to the literature	Conferences and reading	Conferences and reading; high-speed Internet connections to most useful databases; answerable questions searched often
Overall team culture	Multiple general practices; each clinician on her own	Clinicians specialize often; empirical results direct teamwide consensus

issues is made more difficult because effective therapy improves clients' perceptions of the relationship. The client's perception of progress in the therapy therefore inflates ratings of the alliance if the alliance is measured late in the course of therapy. Furthermore, understanding the impact of variables measuring the therapeutic relationship in youth psychotherapy is made more complex by the variety of psychotherapies, varying developmental levels, varying presenting problems, and no unifying agreement about how to measure relationship variables (17). In the adult psychotherapy literature, two meta-analytic reviews of the relationship between alliance and outcome have demonstrated a significant albeit modest effect (18).

In the youth literature, a meta-analysis of 23 studies with a median length of treatment of 19 sessions using numerous scales to measure the alliance/therapeutic relationship showed a small effect (estimated weighted effect size of .21) (17). There was no significant moderator effect for children vs. adolescents, behavioral vs. nonbehavioral, manualized vs. nonmanualized treatments, but the relationship was more important in youth with externalizing problems than those with internalizing problems.

And finally, because some of the studies measured the alliance late in treatment, high relationship ratings may reflect at least in part positive perceptions of the relationship based on a positive treatment response achieved by means other than the relationship. Other studies have shown that behaviorally oriented psychotherapists may be more inclined to see a positive relationship as essential to ensure attendance, whereas psychodynamic ones may see a positive relationship as a change mechanism in its own right (19).

In community-based child therapy, a strong therapeutic relationship supported continuing to attend sessions (20). In addition, the parent–therapist alliance was associated with reductions in internalizing psychopathology, while a close child–therapist alliance assessed during treatment was associated with a reduction in anxiety symptoms (21, 22). In summary, the therapeutic alliance matters in promoting attendance, in dealing with externalizing, and internalizing disorders, as well in community based child therapy. Nevertheless, these results suggest that the alliance by itself is inadequate to produce the larger effects clinicians and patients seek.

> The therapist is an artist, and psychotherapy is a subjective human encounter with a unique youth that can never be captured in an RCT.

At least some therapists object to EBP because they note it examines outcomes for groups of youths and thereby loses the individuality of each youth. According to this argument, EBP conclusions based on groups of youth fail to respond to each youth's uniqueness since no two youth share exactly the same genetic makeup, cultural heritage, social circumstances, developmental history, and family background. Yet it is a caricature of EBP interventions that they are applied indiscriminately without any interest in the individual. Consider an EBP psychosocial intervention as having a hard core but a soft exterior (23): Whereas the outside can be modified and individualized to make it easy to swallow, the hard inner core contains the essential components which create change.

In addition, newer generations of ESTs are sensitive to the criticism that a manualized treatment needs to be individualized as well as lively and engaging. Consider a recent study of collaborative problem solving in moody children with ODD (24). The design of this study allows for therapists providing the intervention to determine session content on the basis of their assessment of the clinical needs of the child and family. Other authors have also called for blending creativity and flexibility into a manualized treatment to allow individual variation within a defined intervention (25).

Finally, the first paradigm of the therapist as artist, working with the unique patient to create a unique solution, and the second paradigm of the therapist as adherent to the results of the best science, may be growing toward each other in recent years. For example, some recent EBM articles have softened their position towards the value of experience and clinical judgement (26), while the American Psychological Association has hardened its position about the importance of randomized trials (27). Both perspectives can be valued by a practitioner sensitive to multiple inputs: patient preference, his own experience, the nuances of each child, and the most valid available evidence.

THE CASE FOR EBP

Community care of clinically referred youth too often shows unimpressive results.

Two studies have shown that, in real-world practice settings, it is difficult for child mental health interventions to show an effect compared to a control group (28, 29). In the first, a randomized study by Bickman and colleagues (1999), one arm of the study received an increase in resources. Interviews were conducted for two years following collection of baseline data. Results in measures of symptoms and functioning showed that, while the arm with a considerable increase in resources did have improved access to care and in fact actually received more care, these access differences did not translate into improved clinical outcomes. In addition, children who did not receive any services improved at the same rate as treated children. This sobering conclusion is supported by Weisz and Jensen's review of the effectiveness of both medication and psychosocial intervention in the context of the real world of caring for clinically referred youth. The authors note that evidence, where available, on the effectiveness of such treatment is minimal when compared to the large body of evidence on efficacy. It seems reasonable to conclude that such null results suggest the need for change.

The evidence-based system in Hawaii's clinics appears to have improved outcome results.

In contrast to the sobering conclusions of these null results, committed efforts to build an evidence-based system of care in Hawaii's Child and Adolescent Mental Health Division (CAMHD) appear to have improved outcomes. This story begins in 1994 when federal courts charged the state with establishing a system of care to provide effective mental health and special education services for children and youth as required by federal law (11). The initial system responses to the court's decree included planning efforts and increases in service capacity, allowing more youth to access a wider variety of services, as well as increased quality monitoring and more interagency coordination. The statewide quality monitoring included basic quantitative feedback; this feedback demonstrated more youth being served by more services at a higher cost. Since stakeholders wanted assurances of efficiency, the focus turned to asking whether the increase in resources had led to improved symptomatic and functional outcomes with empirical results as the arbiter. In addition, CAMHD's leaders wanted the system to develop in a way that frontline decisions about patient care were based on the best available evidence. They focused, therefore, on linking the best and most relevant evidence to clinical decisions (11).

To accomplish this linking, the Hawaii Department of Health organized a task force on empirical services in October, 1999 (10); the only requirement for membership was, and remains today, regular attendance and willingness to read and review studies. Its membership has included clinicians from several disciplines, university faculty, parents, administrators, and CAMHD employees. This task force is charged with conducting ongoing multidisciplinary evaluation of psychosocial interventions for common disorders using methodology developed in the Clinical Division of the American Psychological Association. Additional topics can be reviewed as well, such as the efficacy of seclusion procedures. Each search uses a structured methodology; results are evaluated with a five-level system ranking the efficacy and effectiveness of each intervention. (Effectiveness is based on the performance of the intervention under naturalistic, or real-world, conditions.) The task force begins with a literature-based approach but its diverse constituency tempers the results to fit local conditions.

The result of the task force's work has been a "menu" of recommended treatments distributed to clinicians on a single sheet of blue paper, creating the nickname "blue menu," summarizing recommended psychosocial treatments. It is also posted on the Internet. A one-page review of the task force's conclusions regarding psychotropic medications' efficacy and effectiveness for the children of Hawaii is also distributed and posted on the Internet. Both are updated biennially.

CAMHD also tracks its own results at case, clinic, and system levels wide as well with the Child and Adolescent Functional Assessment Scale, or CAFAS (30), the Child Behavior Check List, Teacher Report Form, and Youth Self-Report (31). Following individual cases allows clinical staff to identify whether or not a youth is improving. Documented ongoing progress leads to the recommendation of continuing the present treatment. If a youth is not improving, the clinicians can reexamine whether there is a problem in treatment selection; if so, a more favorable intervention is sought (11).

Quarterly outcomes based on parent, teacher, and clinician reports for Hawaiian youths treated improved significantly during the years 2001 through 2004, years when the system was actively moving toward evidence-based practice (32). The slope of mean improvement in functioning as rated by the CAFAS showed a 146% increase; the slope of mean improvement in CBCL showed a 271% increase, and the TRF a 50% increase over the course of the three-year period (32). The proportion of youth showing a pattern of improvement during the service episode based on CBCL data rose from 54.7% to 68.2%, based on TRF data from 50.7 to 58.6, and based on the CAFAS from 66.5 to 69.0%.

These results are consistent with the hypothesis that implementing evidence-based services significantly impacts both functional outcome and symptomatic outcome. Furthermore, the results are large and clinically significant. Whether the changes in functioning improvement and symptom reduction stabilize here or continue to improve requires continued study. Although this study did not control for such potentially confounding variables as diagnostic mix, gender, or ethnicity impacting the results, it nevertheless shows consistent and large results across three separate informant groups—parent, teacher, and clinician. If EBP seems, therefore, well worth the effort, let's turn now to its core ideas.

CENTRAL CONCEPTS IN EBP

Number needed to treat, number needed to harm

The number needed to treat, or NNT, for any given intervention in a defined population, is the number of patients we need to treat with the intervention in order to prevent one additional bad outcome (1). This is calculated as follows:

NNT = 1/(Proportion of subjects in control group with bad outcome minus proportion of subjects in intervention group with bad outcome)

The denominator in the NNT equation is called the absolute risk reduction (ARR). Hence, a brief version of the formula is:

$$\text{NNT} = 1/\text{ARR}$$

As an example of NNTs, consider the Treatment for Adolescents with Depression Study (TADS). The "bad outcome" chosen was a failure to score either much improved or very much improved when assessed by an independent rater using the Clinical Global Impression (CGI) scale. Using this definition of bad outcome, 39.4% of subjects in the fluoxetine cell had a bad outcome versus 65.2% of subjects in the placebo cell. Thus:

$$NNT = 1(.652\text{–}.394) = 1/.258 = 3.87$$

Therefore the NNT reported for fluoxetine alone was 4, with 95% CI 3 to 8 when response is defined as a Clinical Global Impression score of much improved or very much improved at the end of treatment. The calculated NNT for combined treatment with CBT and fluoxetine using the identical definition of response was 3, with 95% CI 2 to 4 (33). The value of adding CBT to fluoxetine is evident not only in the improved NNT but also in the much narrower confidence intervals. Table 2.1.2.3 calculates NNTs in child and adolescent psychiatry for a variety of other disorders as well. Note that, in general, these NNTs hold up well in comparison with many standard interventions in medicine: Sackett (2000) notes that the NNT for preventing diabetic neuropathy with 6.5 years of intensive insulin treatment is 15, and that the risk of preventing a death over five weeks using streptokinase infusion in patients with acute myocardial infarction is 19. The NNTs in this table are a reflection of the progress made in recent decades in child and adolescent psychiatry.

By convention, NNT is always a whole number, rounded off to an integer. Note that NNT is impacted by several factors in addition to the effect of the intervention itself. First, how recovery is defined affects NNT; choosing a cutoff that makes it "easy" to achieve recovery produces a lower NNT. Second, how many in the control group spontaneously recover affects NNT; the more spontaneous recoveries in the control group, the more difficult it is to achieve a low NNT. Third, when the data are "sliced" to compare the intervention and comparison group may affect the NNT; time periods when the control and intervention groups diverge the most, such as longer followup times, produce lower NNTs. Ideally, NNTs are presented with 95% confidence intervals.

Note that classically, the NNT is calculated relative to a placebo group. However, some studies are purposefully designed without a placebo group for ethical or other reasons. Studies in Table 2.1.2.3 without a placebo arm are the MTA study, the Brent 1997 study, and the Kazdin 1992 study. Consider, for example, the MTA study, and the calculated NNT of 3 in the medication arm. This means it would be necessary to treat about 3 children with the carefully crafted medication management strategy in order to get 1 to reach the defined threshold for improvement who would not have reached that threshold if he had been treated in the community treatment arm. These studies, therefore, set an upper bound on the true NNT: the NNT relative to a true placebo, the formal definition of NNT. Therefore this column is indicated NNT $\leq$. The only exception to the upper bound rule is the study of PMT and PSST where no change is assumed as a control in the calculation, based on the natural history of the disorder.

The number needed to harm (NNH) is a useful measure of the frequency of undesired consequences from a treatment, and is calculated the same as the NNT, but based on the proportion of patients with the undesired consequence in the intervention group compared to the comparison group. For example, in the TADS study, 3.7% of the fluoxetine alone group had either an elevated mood, mania, or hypomania during the study, versus 1.78% of the placebo group (33). To put this number in context, however, it is important to note that adolescents with known bipolar disorder were excluded, and so were adolescents hospitalized for dangerousness to self or others within three months of consent or were deemed "high risk" for suicide. (The NNH regards a mood "switch" for fluoxetine in this sample is therefore 53.) In the same study, the adverse events of irritable or depressed mood including a worsening of depression or irritability or hypersensitivity or anger occurred in 4.6% of the fluoxetine group and. 9% of the placebo group, generating an NNH of 22 . One or more adverse events occurred in 18.3% of youth in the fluoxetine arm and 8.0% in the placebo group, for an NNH of ten for at least one adverse event.

Both NNT and NNH are ideally stated with 95% confidence intervals. In practice, few parents wish to hear technical discussions of sample size and confidence intervals. Nevertheless, the issue of confidence intervals can be included with verbal statements like "this has been studied so well we are quite certain about this" if the confidence intervals are narrow. Alternatively, for large confidence intervals, the clinician may state something like "the studies so far have not been definitive, so there's a big range of possible answers once this gets studied in more detail."

Hierarchies of Evidence

If potential "evidence" in EBP is defined as "any empirical observation about the apparent relation between events," (34) then it is useful to have a system for rating such empirical observations about the relation between events, with the least biased studies at the top. In EBP, this is done by creating a vertical hierarchy: Each step of the hierarchy represents a certain level of bias within the research design. With each step downward on the hierarchy, more bias is introduced.

The hierarchy of evidence from EBM in Table 2.1.2.4 shows the weight given randomized controlled trials and the even higher weight given systematic reviews of such trials. The N of 1 randomized controlled trial is at the very top position, but it is useful only for certain kinds of interventions, such as a stimulant medication dose which can be randomized to "on" or "off" in the same patient during subsequent time periods. For stimulant dose trials, N of 1 trial data are very good evidence indeed, since they come directly from the patient of interest and concern the treatments under consideration. Unfortunately, however, most other treatments cannot be so easily studied in an N of 1 trial.

Guyatt's "classical EBM" hierarchy of evidence is only a beginning, however, in choosing a treatment. The American Psychological Association's clinical division (Division 12) has established a hierarchy of evidence for rating psychosocial treatments with several levels. "Well established" requires two independent randomized trials with active controls. "Probably efficacious" requires one randomized trial with an active control or two trials with wait-list controls (10). Yet many questions remain in either of these approaches to creating a hierarchy. Even if a treatment is proven to have efficacy in two independent research studies, for example, the question of its effectiveness in a real-world setting remains.

Furthermore, treatment decisions depend not only on the strength of the methods used to establish efficacy or effectiveness, but also on a weighing of benefits against the risks and costs of treatment (35). Table 2.1.2.5 shows an approach to creating a hierarchy of recommendations about treatments based on combining the methodologic strength of the supporting evidence and the clarity of the balance between risk and benefit for that treatment. At the top of this hierarchy are treatments with excellent evidence for efficacy and/or effectiveness as well as clearly defined benefits outweighing clearly defined risks and costs. The number summarizes the clarity of the risk/benefit balance and the letter summarizes the

TABLE 2.1.2.3

ABSOLUTE RISK REDUCTION (ARR) AND NUMBER NEEDED TO TREAT (NNT)[a] FOR SELECTED COMMON DISORDERS IN CHILD AND ADOLESCENT PSYCHIATRY

Disorder/Population	Intervention	Metric	Respond (%) Treatment	Respond (%) Control[1]	ARR	NNT ≤
ADHD (MTA) (70)	Medication	SNAP-IV^{PT} <1.0[b]	56		31	3
	Behavioral R_x		34		9	11
	Both		68		43	2–3
	Community			25		
MDD/Age 12–17	Fluoxetine	CGI[c]	60.6		25.8	4
	CBT		43.2		8.4	12
Outpatient TADS Team (33)	Fluox + CBT		71.0		36.2	3
	Placebo			34.8		
MDD (71)	CBT	BDI <9[d] 3 weeks in a row	64.7		25.3	4
	Supportive R_x			39.4		
POTS (72)	CBT alone	CY-BOCS ≤10	39.3		35.7	3
	Sertraline alone		21.4		17.8	6
	CBT+sertraline		53.6		50	2
	Placebo			3.6		
ODD, Conduct Disorder (73)	PMT alone	CBCL Total Behavior Problems ≤90	38.9	Assume 0.0[e]	38.9	3
	PSST alone		33.3		33.0	3
	Combined		64.0		64.0	2
Mania (74)	Divalproex + quetiapine	YMRS	87		34	3
	Divalproex + placebo			53		
Recurrent MDD (75)	Fluoxetine	Relapse over 32 weeks	CDRS-R >40 + 2 weeks doing poorly[f]	34	16	7
	Placebo			60		

ADHD = Attention deficit hyperactivity disorder
BPR = Brief psychiatric rating—children
CBT = Cognitive behavioral therapy
CD = Conduct disorder
CDRS-R = Children's depression rating scale—revised
CY-BOCS = Children's Yale-Brown obsessive-compulsive scale
MDD = Major depressive disorder
MTA = Multimodal treatment of ADHD
ODD = Oppositional defiant disorder
PMT = Parent management training
POTS = Pediatric Obsessive-Compulsive Disorder Treatment Study
PSST = Problemsolving skills training
TADS = Treatment of Adolescent Depression Study
YMRS = Young Mania Rating Scale

[a] How the NNT is calculated varies from study to study, and this needs to be considered when understanding what NNT means for that study (see below).
[b] SNAP-IV = Swanson, Nolan, Pelham, Version IV, parent and teacher rating scale, mean of parent and teacher score.
[c] CGI- Clinical Global Impression score, evaluator-rated, improved or very much improved.
[d] Control received nondirective supportive therapy.
[e] No control used; since the natural history of conduct disorder is that symptoms tend to persist over time, the assumption of no change in symptoms was assumed as the best estimate for a control (76).
[f] Or physician rater's impression of relapse.

TABLE 2.1.2.4

A HIERARCHY OF STRENGTH OF EVIDENCE FOR TREATMENT DECISIONS

N of 1 randomized controlled trials
Systematic reviews of randomized trials
Single randomized trial
Systematic review of observational studies addressing patient-important outcomes
Single observational study addressing patient-important outcomes
Physiological studies
Unsystematic clinical observations

(From Guyatt, G., et al., *Introduction: The Philosophy of Evidence-Based Medicine, in Users' Guides to the Medical Literature: A Manual for Evidence-Based Clinical Practice,* G. Guyatt and D. Rennie, Editors. 2002, AMA Press: Chicago, IL. pp. 3–12, with permission.)

likelihood that the supporting evidence is free from bias (or methodologic strength).

SEARCHING THE LITERATURE

General Tips on Searching

The most relevant databases for clinicians are Medline, PsycINFO, the Cochrane Library's Central Register of Controlled Trials (CENTRAL), and the Website for the Journal of the American Academy of Child and Adolescent Psychiatry. A clinician familiar with these four databases and how they work is able to quickly answer many useful questions. Table 2.1.2.6 demonstrates results from searching three of these sites for answers to varied answerable questions. Results are shown as the number of retrieved publications, or "hits." The first search in the table arose treating a 14-year-old boy with Tourette's Syndrome and ADHD. He was taking desipramine (DMI) after stimulants had greatly worsened his tics and atomoxetine had made him nauseous. When he started DMI his grades improved markedly, and he reported being able to focus. Four years later, he was continuing to do well, but his physician wondered whether there was new information regarding desipramine and sudden death in youth. He quickly found an article raising further concerns (36) and spoke with the family about retrying atomoxetine. The second search regards information on parent management training began because a multidisciplinary team was looking for an EST to use with oppositional and defiant youth. The quotation marks around the phrase "parent management training" (PMT) greatly improve the specificity of the search, reducing hits from 299 to only ten highly relevant ones. The quotation marks specify that these three words must be found as a phrase, rather than appearing individually throughout the title or abstract. The clinician in this case quickly found support for learning it (37).

TABLE 2.1.2.5

GRADING TREATMENTS BASED ON RISK/BENEFIT CLARITY AND STRENGTH OF EVIDENCE

Grade	Clarity of Risks + Costs vs. Benefits	Strength of Evidence
1A	Clear	Multiple RCTs with no important flaws
1B	Clear	One or more RCTs with significant flaws and/or inconsistent results
1C+	Clear	No RCTs for this population, but RCT results can be extrapolated to the present patient *or* Overwhelming evidence from observational studies
1C	Clear	Observational studies
2A	Unclear	RCTs without significant limitations
2B	Unclear	RCTs with methodologic flaws and/or inconsistent results
2C	Unclear	Observational studies

Adapted from Guyatt et al. [35].

Several Tips About Using These Four Databases are Helpful in Searching.

1. *Especially if your time is limited, start with searches yielding information high in the pyramid of evidence such as those available at the Clinical Queries site.* The idea is to discover the best evidence immediately. In PubMed, take advantage of the Clinical Queries site, which offers filters if your question is primarily about the efficacy of a therapy (38). Using the filters for a narrow, specific search is a good starting point in evaluating a therapy since the site will now retrieve only RCTs. If the result is negative, then move on to the "sensitive" search filter that will include nonrandomized studies as well; your search is moving down the pyramid of evidence. On the other hand, if time is not an issue, consider starting with a sensitive search and being as inclusive (sensitive) as possible; only later narrow the search by becoming increasingly narrow (specific).

2. *Consider starting with preappraised evidence such as a Systematic Review.* Not all review articles are systematic. To constitute a systematic review, the authors need to 1) explicitly state inclusion and exclusion criteria regarding studies; 2) perform a comprehensive search with a transparent search strategy; 3) summarize the results according to explicit rules, including noting varied effects in different subgroups (39).

Unfortunately, the Cochrane Library has very few systematic reviews regarding current issues in child psychiatry. The journal Evidence-Based Mental Health contains some cogent summaries. The biannually updated Clinical Evidence is a book and compact disk with hyperlinked references; it uses exemplary methodology to answer clinically relevant questions, but its coverage of topics in child psychiatry is limited.

If such preappraised evidence is unavailable, often a good search strategy is to look for a meta-analysis around the issue in question. Searching in PubMed "ADHD AND meta-analysis[Ti]" (the Ti in brackets means the article will be retrieved only if the word "meta-analysis" is in the title, not just the abstract) is a successful search strategy for revealing 25 meta-analyses on ADHD; these references cover such subjects as the comparative efficacy of methylphenidate and Adderall (40).

3. *Be familiar with Medical Subject Headings (MeSH) and how to "explode" or restrict MeSH subheadings, as well as how to use search tools such as Boolean operators and "wildcards."* Asking the search to explode a MeSH term means the program will now look for all subheadings of that

TABLE 2.1.2.6

"HITS" (RETRIEVED REFERENCES) IN SELECTED DATABASES ACCESSED VIA OVID[a]

Database	Search Terms	Limits	Hits	Comments
PubMed	Desipramine *and* death	Age 0 to 18 Last 5 years	4	PubMed is a good place to begin for search terms like desipramine or atomoxetine, i.e., for information regarding medications.
	Desipramine *and* "Death, sudden" [77]	Age 0 to 18 No time limits	15	
	Parent Management Training	Age 0 to 18 Last 5 years	299	
	"Parent Management Training"	None	20	
Clinical Queries at PubMed ("therapy" box)	"Parent Management Training"	Specific search	4	Clinical Queries' specific searches retrieve only randomized trials.
		Sensitive search	8	
Cochrane Library's CCRCT via Ovid	Parent management training	None	7	The Cochrane Library databases are more difficult to use than these other Websites; they lack the "limits" options, for example, of other sites
	"Parent management training"	None	7	
PsycINFO (1985–2004) via Ovid)	"Parent management training"	None	79	PsycINFO is a good place to begin for search terms like "bullying" or "stepfamily problems."
	"Parent management training"	None	79	
Evidence Based Mental Health Online	Desipramine	None	16	Many references to child/adolescent literature.
	Desipramine *and* death		1	
	"Parent management training"		9	Requires subscription to search beyond first 150 words of article.
	"Parent management training"		2	

[a] Ovid accessed at www.ovid.com via The Permanente Medical Group portal, September 9, 2005 (except desipramine search done February 6, 2006).

MeSH term in addition to the term itself. At times this is useful; at other times, it is more useful to search only one or more specific subheadings of a MeSH term.

Become familiar with how to use the MeSH "tree" of terms and subheadings, and note that PsycINFO does not use MeSH, but uses its own thesaurus. Become familiar as well with Boolean operators like "and," "or," and "not," which can quickly either expand or limit a search. Wildcards are useful in allowing searching with multiple terms in a single search. "Adolesc*" in MedLine will retrieve, for example, articles on adolescence, adolescents, and adolescent. All databases have a tutorial function that explains its wildcards and its thesaurus; these are database-specific.

4. *Understand the strengths and weaknesses of each database related to the journals it does and does not contain.* PubMed retrieves many references for medications but omits many significant journals in psychology. PsycINFO includes an extensive array of psychology journal articles of variable quality; this database has its own thesaurus of index terms as well. The JAACAP Website offers AACAP members full text access to articles published since 1995, but only from a single, albeit highly relevant, journal. The Cochrane Library's Central Register of Controlled Trials is helpful as a complete source for RCT data; its Systematic Reviews library rarely has completed reviews in child psychiatry. Table 2.1.2.6 summarizes characteristics of these databases.

5. *Understand which databases are available and whether each produces an abstract alone or a full text article.* Both Medline via Entrez PubMed at the National Center for Biotechnology Information (NCBI) and the Website of the Journal of the American Academy of Child and Adolescent Psychiatry are available to most child psychiatrists. The former is in the public domain and generates abstracts, while the latter is included in membership in the American Academy of Child and Adolescent Psychiatry. Three other databases often available via an institutional affiliation are the Cochrane Library's Central Register of Controlled Trials (CENTRAL), its database of Systematic Reviews, and the database PsycINFO from the American Psychological Association. Most clinical "answerable questions" can be usefully searched using a combination of JAACAP, PubMed, CENTRAL, and PsycINFO. But in most organizational affiliations with Ovid, only some journals will supply full text access to the retrieved articles and abstracts. Hence, an advantage in searching the JAACAP site first is its access to full text articles; this avoids the frustration of finding excellent sources but being unable to obtain a full text copy immediately.

6. *Use branching out from a good specific reference whenever possible.* Look in the bibliography and expand from there. Look for other articles by the same author or by authors cited in the bibliography. Also note the MeSH subject term for a reference you find very helpful and use it for a MeSH search. This approach often quickly creates an expanding web of relevant references. One of the best examples of the "one good reference leads to another" strategy is Greenhalgh's review article

on disseminating an innovation (23). Note also that databases like PubMed offer searching of "Relevant Articles" as a link.

7. *Search a single aspect of a multiitem search at a time, then combine sets of references using Boolean operators.* For example, in searching Medline for outbreaks of suicide attempts in adolescents, search the MeSH term for suicide attempts separately initially. Search the MeSH term for outbreaks separately as well. Only then combine the sets of references using the Boolean operator "and" to find references in both sets. Finally, add limits such as age, year of publication, language of publication, and publication type serially one at a time. The advantage of this approach is transparency. How many hits were achieved at each stage and the effect of combining sets, as well as the effect of each limit, is clear. This transparency is useful because, if necessary, you can immediately revise your search based on the results. Dropping references should also be done using a transparent methodology. Justifying each step of winnowing is worthwhile, since each such narrowing step means lost information. "Hand searching" simply means scanning the abstracts or even whole articles and deciding their relevance and quality for the purpose at hand. Hand searching is the final step after winnowing through limits.

8. *Know what to do when the search retrieves far too many references to examine.* In Medline, consider using the subheadings under MeSH terms to refine the search. For example, adding "Major" (abbreviated [MAJR]) after the term restricts the search to only those articles where the subject is a major topic heading in that journal article. Similarly, subheadings to MeSH terms like "prevention and control" or "statistics" can be helpful in limiting large searches if those are areas of primary concern. Using the "Limits" feature in databases also narrows the number of references. Common limits are either specifying a specific publication type, such as only meta-analyses or only RCTs, or only a specific age group such as adolescents, or only the most recent references from perhaps the last five or ten years. Suppose, for example, a reader is interested in doing a comprehensive search on psychodynamic psychotherapy in children. He might start by searching the term "Psychotherapy [MeSH]" which uses the MeSH category psychotherapy, generating over 97,000 references. Limiting to age six to 12 reduces the number to about 14,000. Searching Medline with the term "psychodynamic" as a keyword and the limit of age six to 12 generates a more manageable 257. Combining these two sets generates a manageable list of 116 references to sort through. This list is a good start.

Tips on PubMed

To use PubMed well, it pays to understand MeSH terms, the National Library of Medicine's controlled vocabulary for medical subject headings. MeSH index words provides a consistent way to retrieve information even though articles may use varied terminology for the same concept. In other words, the MeSH term is the "official" term used by the database to organize all references relevant to a single subject that may be referred to using multiple words. Using MeSH terms in a search ensures that all references relevant to that subject are included. Furthermore, MeSH terms are organized as nested sets, becoming more and more specific; each term higher in the tree contains all the terms below it. Medline allows the searcher to visualize these nested sets of terms and choose the most specific term he can find for the subject of interest. This allows only highly specific articles to be retrieved. MeSH searches also allow the searcher to specify whether he wants articles retrieved if the MeSH term is found anywhere in the article, or whether he wants articles retrieved only if the MeSH term is a major heading in the article.

A therapist interested in alternatives to Dialectical Behavior Therapy (DBT), for example, searched "parasuicidal"—meaning frequent cutting or comparable low lethality self-harm attempts— in the MeSH tree of index terms. MeSH recognizes the term parasuicide, and suggests the term "Self-Injurious Behavior." This official MeSH term is defined as "behavior in which persons hurt or harm themselves without the motive of suicide or of sexual deviation " (41). The MeSH tree then looks like this:

Self-Injurious Behavior (SIB)
- Self-Mutilation
- Suicide
  - Suicide, Assisted
  - Suicide, Attempted

The therapist might want to search "self-injurious behavior" as a MeSH term (simply put [MeSH] after the term). The therapist might choose not to explode the term (meaning the search also would include all four items nested underneath Self-Injurious Behavior) if the goal is to find alternatives to DBT. The unexploded term will be more specific because it will find articles based on the above definition of SIB only and not include the lower terms. The search Psychotherapy[MeSH] AND "Self-Injurious Behavior [MeSH:NoExp]" limited to the age group of adolescence generates 75 references which can be used as a base to answer the therapist's question. By contrast, a less specific search that allows the search to explode the SIB term and include subheadings retrieves over 792 references—far too many to hand search. In summary, exploding a MeSH term—meaning that all the MeSH terms underneath this item will also be searched—is only desirable if all the subheadings are of potential interest.

Tips on PsycINFO

PsycINFO is a database that includes nearly 2,000 journals as well as some books, book chapters, and dissertations. Operated by the American Psychological Association, it is especially strong in searching questions related to psychosocial interventions.

A search generates abstracts and not full text articles. PsycINFO uses a thesaurus of index terms, providing a controlled vocabulary to structure the subject matter (23). The thesaurus includes more psychological terms than MeSH. "Pretend play," "Bullying," and "Parental involvement," for example, are legitimate thesaurus terms in PsycINFO. Yet in MeSH, "Bullying" has no suggested search strategy, and "Pretend play" in the MeSH tree returns "Play therapy" and "Play and playthings," a subset of Recreation. The PsycINFO thesaurus is available online.

However, not all searches do best with a thesaurus term. For example, searching the term "parent management training" in Ovid's PsycINFO thesaurus shows Parent Training as an index term which includes PMT. But because this index term also includes many forms of parent training, it retrieves 2,756 hits. A more successful strategy for a clinician seeking information about Patterson's well known Parent Management Training is the keyword search for the phrase in quotes, "parent management training" (see Table 2.1.2.6). Options regards "limits" are also different than those in PubMed. PsycINFO, rather than offering a premade filter to choose only randomized trials, offers the filter "clinical trial" instead.

The searcher can search by index terms from the thesaurus or by keyword. PsycINFO also lists classification codes—large categories with an accompanying number such as "cognitive therapy" (3311) or "group and family therapy" (3313).

Searching by keywords is uncontrolled in that any search term can be tried. PsycINFO then searches for those words in the title or abstract. When building combined searches using more than one combination of keywords, classifications, or index terms, build the search one step at a time to maximize transparency of the process. For example, typing in "psychodynamic child psychotherapy" into the thesaurus, the index term is "child psychotherapy." The term itself generates 3,433 hits. Searching this index term exploded generates 4,732 hits. "Psychodynamic" searched in the Thesaurus returns "psychodynamics" as a thesaurus index term. Exploded, this term generates 8,049 hits.

Now combining this set with the results from exploding "child psychotherapy" with the Boolean "AND" creates a manageable set of 41 references. Another approach is to search "psychodynamic$" with "$ " being a wildcard—it can represent any letter or combination of letters—and combine it with the results of exploding the index term "child psychotherapy": The result is 205 references.

The Cochrane Library

The Cochrane Central Register of Controlled Trials (CCRCT) is an efficient way to begin a search for those with access, because CCRCT strives to be complete, with over 350,000 registered controlled trials; importantly, it includes only controlled trials. Its advantage over a search for RCTs using the Clinical Queries PubMed site is that CCRCT attempts a search for any randomized trial published anywhere in the world (not just RCTs published in a journal indexed by PubMed). A parent seeking help regarding the usefulness of the Feingold diet could find a quick answer in CCRCT. A quick look for Feingold diet at the PubMed Clinical Query site, set for narrow searches, works equally well, and quickly reveals the same negative 1981 trial found in CCRCT. Moreover, the search options at the Clinical Queries PubMed site are easier to use, including the capacity to limit articles retrieved to only adolescents, for example. For this reason the Clinical Queries site may be more relevant for most clinicians unless no trials have been reported, in which case checking CCRCT may be worthwhile.

Historical Perspective: Archie Cochrane and the Virtual Library Named after Him

In 1972, the British epidemiologist Archie Cochrane wrote an influential book, Effectiveness and Efficiency: Random Reflections on Health Services, in which he pointed out that resources for health care would always be limited. Therefore, he concluded, using evidence from randomized controlled trials is critical, because the information they provide is more reliable than other sources of evidence. In 1979, he continued to advocate for the usefulness not only of RCTs, but also for efforts to summarize such trials in one place. "It is surely a great criticism of our profession," he wrote, "that we have not organized a critical summary, by specialty or subspecialty, adapted periodically, of all relevant randomized controlled trials." His remarks and influence were such that an international collaboration, the Oxford Database of Perinatal Trials (ODPT), developed around his way of thinking. The systematic review of randomized trials resulting from this collaboration became a centerpiece of what came to be called "the Cochrane approach": the structured method of presenting overview data summarizing multiple trials. This approach became a hallmark of the Cochrane Database of Systematic Reviews (CDSR), an online "library" that began in the 1980s with the ODPT. The Cochrane Collaboration was subsequently founded in 1993, five years after his death.

The symbol for the Cochrane Collaboration is two Cs facing each other and containing a closed circle with a central vertical line. The vertical line represents the null result, that is an odds ratio of 1.0. Each horizontal line represents the results of a single randomized controlled trial. The length of the line represents the 95% confidence intervals for the primary outcome variable studied in that trial; the shorter the line, the more certain the results. Some horizontal lines cross the central vertical line, meaning that the null hypothesis was not refuted within 95% confidence intervals. The horizontal lines that do not cross the central vertical line represent a study inconsistent with the null hypothesis as regards the primary outcome variable at the 95% confidence level. This makes it easy to scan the figure visually to see which studies reached significance and which did not. Furthermore, at the bottom there is a small diamond just to the left of the central vertical line. The diamond summarizes the pooled effect estimate from summing over the results of all the trials within the circle.

The specific horizontal lines and diamond used in the Cochrane Collaboration logo (Figure 2.1.2.1) represent a metaanalysis of randomized trials as regards administering a short, inexpensive course of a corticosteroid to women about to give birth prematurely. The first of these RCTs was reported in 1972. The logo summarizes the evidence that would have been revealed had the available RCTs been reviewed systematically in about 1982; the position of the diamond demonstrates that corticosteroids reduce the risk of babies dying from the complications of immaturity. In fact, more modern estimates are that this treatment reduces the odds of premature infants dying from the complications of immaturity by 30 to 50% (42). But because no systematic review of these

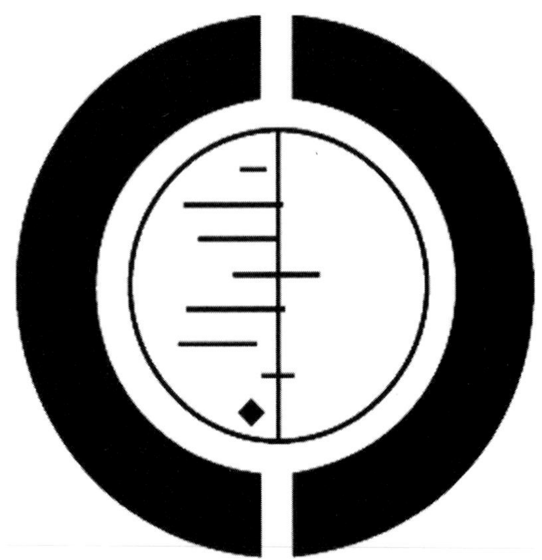

FIGURE 2.1.2.1. The Cochrane Collaboration logo. (Used with permission, courtesy of the Cochrane Colloquium.)

TABLE 2.1.2.7

USEFUL DATABASES: URLS AND AVAILABILITY

Site/URL	Sources/Abstracts(A) Full Text (FT)	Classification System Used	Strengths	Weaknesses
PubMed http://www.ncbi.nlm.nih.gov/entrez/query.fcgi	Extensive medical journal base A, Some FT	MeSH terms	MeSH allows specific searching.	DSM disorders not always MESH terms
PubMedClinical Queries http://www.ncbi.nlm.nih.gov/entrez/query/static/clinical.shtml	Same as PubMed	Same	Filters allow either searching for RCTs only or more sensitive search.	Systematic review less well defined than in CDSR
MeSH Database http://www.ncbi.nlm.nih.gov/entrez/query.fcgi?db=mesh	MeSH "tree" of terms	Branching "tree" of terms	Allows searching with controlled vocabulary.	Excludes many less medical terms (e.g., bullying).
PsycINFO, PsycARTICLES http://www.psycinfo.com/psycarticles/	Extensive psychology journal base A, Fee-based FT	Index terms Classification Keywords	Allows very specific searching (e.g., bullying).	No RCT filter Variable quality "Publication type" filter not crisp
CRCT http://www.nelh.nhs.uk/cochrane.asp	All RCTs No A or FT unless U.K., Australia	Keyword	Immediate discovery of RCTs on subject; uniform data presentation	Mostly via institutions in United States No charge in U.K., Australia, Latin America
CDSR http://www.cochrane.org/reviews/index.htm	Only if SR completed A but no FT	Keyword	Uniform data presentation Updated	Limited regarding child psychiatry
JAACAP www.jaacap.com	JAACAP to 1995 A. FT also if AACAP member	Keyword	Full text option Highly specific Included in AACAP membership	Limited to one journal No filters
EBMH Online http://ebmh.bmjjournals.com/	EB Mental Health. First 150 words available; FT requires subscription	Keyword	Preappraised evidence only	Requires subscription for full access; mixed with adult literature

trials had been published until 1989, this evidence was not widely disseminated and many premature babies presumably died unnecessarily. Hence, the logo is a rather grim reminder of the high stakes in performing systematic, timely reviews of relevant randomized controlled trials.

Abstracts of Cochrane systemic reviews are available for no charge (see Table 2.1.2.7) but access to the full text of the review usually occurs through affiliation with an institution that subscribes. The systematic reviews are updated regularly as more information becomes available, and in response to comments. The methodology is transparent. The "Library" exists only virtually in cyberspace. This system allows updates to include more recent studies and any criticism and comments (43). Comparisons with reviews in traditional journals have given the edge to the Cochrane Library versions (44). Cochrane systematic reviews are exclusively electronic and frequent review and openness to comments have been designed to take advantage of the electronic form (43).

The Cochrane Library thus developed a way of summarizing healthcare information that was systematic, completely electronic, up to date, open to criticism, and clearly distinguishing between trials based on their quality. The "system" used does not vary from review to review. Therefore once the consumer becomes accustomed to the format, he can quickly understand the results of any systematic review. Furthermore, the results are transparent, since each study's individual results are also summarized, as is the methodology. Finally, since the entire library is electronic, updating by teams working around the globe becomes feasible in a regular way through sharing the work in cyberspace. The Cochrane library has thus raised the bar for how medical knowledge is organized and disseminated, and been closely associated with the development of EBM.

For answerable questions in child psychiatry, the CCRCT is often useful as a good place to start searching an answerable question. Paradoxically, the Cochrane Library of Systematic Reviews is often not useful to child psychiatrists, because a systematic review has most often not been done on the child psychiatric topic of interest. Searching for reviews on ADHD, for example, retrieves 13 reviews but none specifically devoted to ADHD. Searching for reviews on major depression in adolescents is similarly unfruitful. By contrast, searching the Clinical Query site of NCBI in the Find Systematic Reviews box retrieves 229 references with many devoted exclusively to ADHD and many highly relevant to a practitioner (see Table 2.1.2.7). Nevertheless, the Cochrane Library's emphasis on the importance to practitioners of systematic reviews, published in cyberspace and updated frequently, remains at the heart of EBM.

DIAGNOSTIC PATHS CONSISTENT WITH EBP PRINCIPLES

EBP differs significantly from conventional clinical practice in how it approaches differential diagnosis. Whereas clinicians often use an unstructured interview and their familiarity with the categories of DSM-IV TM, EBP encourages feasible routes to more definitive diagnoses compatible with research studies for that disorder. In other words, EBP supports the importance of test/retest and interrater reliability and the multiple forms of validity (45) in the diagnostic process, while also recognizing the process must be feasible. An EBP approach to diagnosis is not new at all; it is merely trying to make feasible the more rigorous diagnostic approaches used in research for some time. In this way EBP is a useful bridge between the culture of research and the culture of clinical care, striving to help clinicians find rigorous yet practical diagnostic methods. EBP also encourages a thorough yet feasible search in symptom domains other than the presenting problem, since comorbid disorders are common and easily missed (46). Let's begin with how EBM approaches arriving at a clear conclusion in the domain of a primary diagnostic concern and return to the issue of assessing comorbid disorders.

In diagnostic work, the EBM practitioner should try to create a link between his patient's disorders and the research base on effective treatments. It is important, therefore, that the diagnostic procedures are not idiosyncratic to that practitioner or clinic. The diagnostic system used must also generate data capable of becoming useful information when compiled. The EBS youth mental health clinics in Hawaii, for example, establish an initial baseline of functioning using the Child and Adolescent Functional Assessment Scale, or CAFAS (30). When the CAFAS is repeated 3 months later, its mean and median slope are useful measures of changes in functioning in the population served by these clinics (11).

The clinician may at times elect to use a component of a research-level instrument, especially in the domain of primary concern. For example, the K-SADS-P/L modules for selected diagnoses such as MDD, bipolar, bulimia nervosa, alcohol abuse and multiple other disorders can be given as "stand-alone" modules within the context of a clinical interview as a compromise. Of course administration of the complete K-SADS provides a more thorough evaluation. This semistructured approach with clear anchor points to determine the presence or absence of symptoms is markedly less ambiguous than simply working from an open copy of DSM-IV. Furthermore, K-SADS modules are available free on the Internet (47). Another feasible research-level instrument is the computerized Diagnostic Schedule Interview for Children (DISC), which can be administered only for the domain of interest or in multiple domains in a wide search for psychopathology (48).

Another approach is to use an instrument which has been studied as a proxy for a research-level instrument, and been shown to be a feasible substitute. For example, in pediatric bipolar disorder (PBD), the parent version of the Young Mania Rating Scale (P-YMRS) has been studied as a proxy for a semistructured interview (49). Higher scores on the P-YMRS predict increasing likelihood of PBD on semistructured interviews. In order to use these likelihood ratios, it is necessary to estimate the base rate of BPD among patients presenting to the clinic (50). Such a base rate can either be estimated using published data or from local data generated at the clinic itself. The latter process is recommended only if the diagnostic process used locally has been adequate. Using data from the literature to calculate a base rate for common disorders like ADHD, MDD, bipolar disorder, and substance abuse disorders has advantages: The sample sizes are larger, and use peer-reviewed data typically generated with well defined diagnostic processes.

Bayes' theorem can be used to combine the information from an estimated base rate, family history, and parent-completed instrument assessing bipolar symptoms. Consider the example of a 9 year-old patient with episodes of extreme aggression, problems concentrating, and high levels of motor activity (50). To begin, the base rate for bipolar disorder in children entering community mental health center clinics is roughly 6%; this figure, therefore, becomes the initial estimated probability of bipolar disorder. Since this boy had a biological father with Bipolar I and a meta-analysis showed that children with a biological parent with bipolar disorder are five times as likely to have a bipolar diagnosis themselves, Bayes' theorem allows the clinician to combine these two independent sources of information as follows (2):

$$\text{Initial estimate of odds of bipolar disorder} = \text{Odds of having bipolar disorder in clinic} \times \text{likelihood ratio from family history}$$

Note that Bayes' theorem uses the odds, rather than the probability, of the boy having bipolar disorder. The information given as regards a base rate of 6% is actually a probability, which would need to be converted to odds for use in Bayes' theorem. A nomogram uses probabilities and avoids the clumsiness of converting probabilities to odds for use in Bayes theorem and then back again to probability, the more familiar concept (see Figure 2.1.2.2). The nomogram shows that this boy's probability rises to 24% from 6% on the basis of his positive family history.

Bayes' theorem allows the clinician to further refine the probability of this boy's meeting diagnostic criteria for bipolar disorder by using his mother's reports of his symptoms as reported on the externalizing score on the Child Behavior Check List. This process is especially helpful in ruling out bipolar disorder, i.e., showing that the probability of the boy's having bipolar disorder is sufficiently low and that no further testing is required. On the other hand, a high externalizing score on the CBCL should trigger use of a specific parent report regarding bipolar symptoms, such as the Parent Young Mania Rating Scale (P-YMRS). In such a case, continue to use Bayes' theorem with the boy in the example (51):

$$\text{Refined odds of bipolar disorder} = (\text{Odds for probability of } 24) \times (\text{likelihood ratio from that patient's score on P} - \text{YMRS})$$

Again, using a nomogram that translates probability into odds and back again to probability after the calculation makes things easier. With a likelihood ratio of 6 from his P-YMRS score, this boy's probability of having bipolar disorder jumps to 68.

This is not a diagnosis, but it is an easily arrived-at probability which should trigger a full-scale evaluation for bipolar disorder (see Youngstrom's discussion [51]). This methodology can be used to estimate the probability for other disorders such as ADHD as well (50).

In addition to feasible but empirically supported approaches to a primary diagnosis, data support using a broad assessment of psychopathology and functioning. There are many possible instruments. Achenbach's multiple-informant System of Empirically Based Assessment (ASEBA) is one feasible approach, as is a computerized structured interview such as the parent and child versions of the Diagnostic Interview Schedule for Children (48). Broadbased structured systems like ASEBA and the DISC are more likely to note comorbid anxiety disorders, substance abuse disorders, and the presence of multiple disorders than an unstructured clinical interview (52).

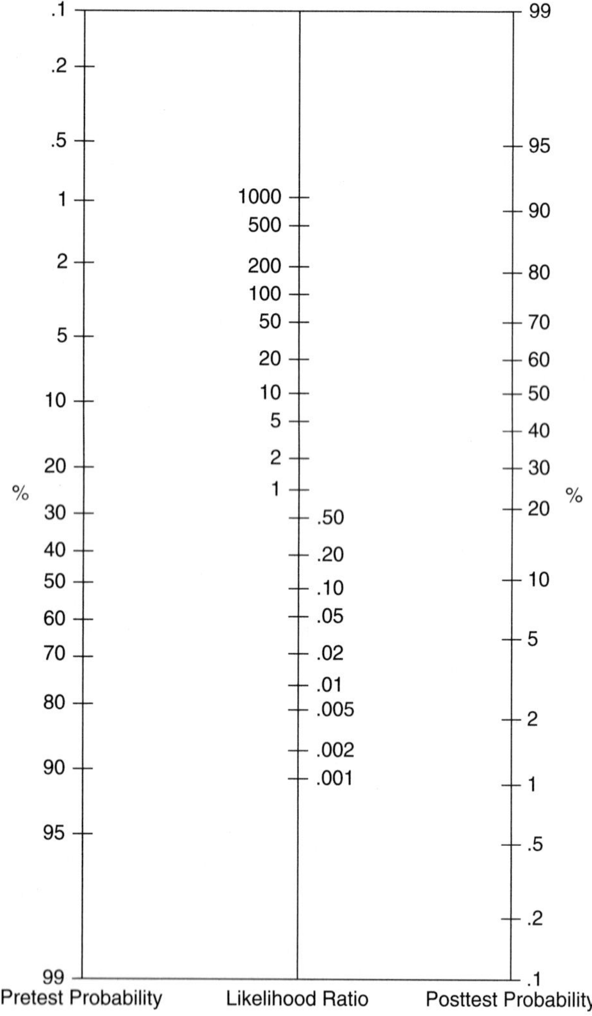

FIGURE 2.1.2.2. Nomogram for combining probability and likelihood ratio. (From Youngstrom EA, Youngstrom JK. Evidence-Based Assessment of Pediatric Bipolar Disorder, Part II: Incorporating Information from Behavior Checklists, *JAACP* 44:823–828, 2005, with permission.)

In comparing DISC diagnoses to diagnoses generated by clinicians in unstructured interviews, for example, agreement was higher for externalizing than for internalizing disorders, and clinicians were more likely than the DISC to assign a single diagnosis and less likely to assign no diagnosis. Systems like the ASEBA and DISC avoid the heuristic biases present in an unstructured diagnostic interview and their results are useful in building a local database. Such systems allow the interviewer more time and energy to pursue individual aspects of that child's psychosocial functioning and the context of his symptoms—favorite Internet sites and bands, friendships with peers, relationships with parents and teachers, idealized heroes and heroines, and cell phone ring tone (53). In other words, broadbased, structured assessments can complement a clinical interview. The goal is to provide both a technically sound measure of psychopathology and function as well as a youth-friendly, youth-relevant experience.

In summary, there is no single diagnostic process consistent with EBP; there are many. The goals include a complete, wide-ranging assessment of functioning, impairment, and psychopathology that is unlikely to miss disorders with significant morbidity. The approach also ideally uses feasible methods to provide a solid empirical link to major studies in the field, as well as a baseline for tracking outcome and generating local data. Sound yet practical diagnostic and/or tracking tools useful in everyday practice are noted in Table 2.1.2.8; each is either in the public domain or reasonably priced.

ENACTING EVIDENCE-INFORMED CARE IN CLINICAL ORGANIZATIONS

The task of moving an organization from its current practices toward functioning with processes more consistent with EBP has been called implementation. But projects designed to do this have taken much longer than originally intended (14), creating an implementation gap. More recently, some have suggested the term enactment of evidence-informed health care as a replacement for the term implementation (14). The term enactment comes from enactment theory, which focuses on subjective issues in how organizations function rather than on formal organizational charts. A clinical team is, therefore, enacted by individuals based on their own social perceptions of a negotiated order based on repeated interpersonal processes (54).

Leading a multiprofessional organization towards EBP is complex, with many disputes about the meaning of the change. Furthermore, the available evidence in favor of any particular innovation is often ambiguous; it is inevitably open to at least some interpretation and will be contested. Varied professional groups each have their own way of thinking about what constitutes evidence and its meaning, leading inevitably to competing claims on the truth. Each professional group has its own paradigms and cognitive assumptions, leading to each advancing different claims to knowledge (55). As a result, it is often difficult to find common ground for productive dialogue. Instead, each discipline proceeds almost on its own path, resulting in a complex situation which actually allows the end-user clinician increased choice among the competing claims (14). In addition, managerial control over elite professional groups is limited, since autonomy over working practices is a core value for elite professionals (14).

Creating change in a multiprofessional health care organization is complex for several other reasons as well. First, the context of change efforts to enact EBP varies enormously from one organization to another, and varies over time even within the same organization (56). What external pressure is there on the organization to survive in a competitive market? How do union–management issues and interprofessional "turf" issues shape the organization? How does its history shape its culture? This series of questions is only a start. In other words, no context is discrete; complex connections and interactions are the rule. Assessing outcome is also complex. Basic issues as when change is assessed and what is measured can change results markedly. Also, large healthcare organizations respond not only to multiple professional groups inside the organization, but to accrediting bodies and government agencies outside its boundaries. Consider, for example, the complexity of disputes about the safety and benefits of selective serotonin reuptake inhibitors in depressed youth. Government agencies, the press, national professional organizations, and research evidence were all involved.

Tips on Enacting Evidence-Informed Health Care in Organizations

A review of six studies designed to implement EBP for varied medical conditions came to several conclusions. First,

TABLE 2.1.2.8

FEASIBLE EVERYDAY INSTRUMENTS

Tracks or Aids Dx	Instrument	Reference	Informant
ADHD	SWAN	[66]	Teacher or Parent
Anxiety disorders	SCARED	[78]	Parent
Depressive disorders	Center for Epidemiological Studies—Depression CES-D	[79]	Youth
Depressive disorders	Johns Hopkins Depression Scale	[80]	Parent
Functioning	Columbia Impairment Scale (CIS)	[81]	Parent or youth
Multiple categorical diagnoses	Diagnostic Interview Schedule for Children (DISC)	[48]	Parent or youth
Multiple scales of psychopathology	Achenbach System of Empirically Based Assessment (ASEBA)	[31]	Parent (CBCL) Youth (YSR) Teacher (TRF)
Pediatric bipolar disorders	Young Mania Rating Scale—Parent (YMRS-P)	[82]	Parent
Acute stress and posttraumatic symptoms	Child Stress Disorders Checklist	[83]*	Parent

*Actual instrument in ArticlePlus feature on JAACAP Website.

implementing change is facilitated by open access to membership in key groups that filter the literature and create guidelines and educational initiatives (11, 56). In Hawaii's successful efforts to develop an EBS for youth mental health, groups of clinicians, administrators, and community members involved in the project had open membership; anyone willing to do the reading and attend regularly was allowed to join (8). Second, the hierarchical structure of the local team or hospital staff influences adoption of EBP; a more "flat" hierarchy offers less resistance to adoption. In a vertical hierarchy, junior staff members defer to more senior members regardless of the evidence, slowing adoption of EBP. Third, networks of social/professional relationships, rather than individuals, are central in whatever actions result from implementation efforts. Individuals live within and are a part of these networks.

From these studies, several useful guidelines appear for those interested in implementing EBP within the context of their own organization:

1. *An evidence-based perspective becomes reality only when it is enacted in local clinical settings by frontline clinicians.* Adopting a formal policy of adopting evidence-based practices is insufficient by itself to create enactment by frontline clinical groups over which senior management has limited control (14).

2. *Think of context not as a stage for the action of change, but rather as an active element in the change process.* A shift toward EBP—like other organizational change processes—is highly context dependent (14), where context is defined as multidimensional, multifaceted configurations of forces, often developing historically as negotiated interpersonal patterns. Because these forces interact in complex ways, unexpected outcomes from a planned change are common. (13). Individuals are influenced by the context of a network of social relationships beyond their immediate circle. Hence no context is discrete or separate.

3. *Key leaders are able to influence innovation towards EBP.* Although it is clear that the process is often complex, a senior, powerful, and skillful leader can stimulate innovation. (13)

4. *Take into account the distinctive nature of the multiprofessional organization.* Boundaries—educational, cognitive and social—between different professional groups inhibit the spread of EB ideas. Child psychiatrists may read only child psychiatry journals and not child psychology journals and vice versa, or attend only their own professional organizational meetings and vice versa. Knowledge can be powerful and threaten specific interest groups, which are then motivated to reject it (13).

5. *Use the extensive literature on "exporting" psychosocial interventions from development sites to practice sites and distilling components of effective treatments.* How to train practitioners to use manualized therapies developed at other sites is a topic that has been widely discussed elsewhere (57, 58). Another approach is to use a process of distilling the common elements in evidence-based interventions and then match these with profiles of target symptoms from individual clients (59). This latter approach is novel and has great potential.

6. *Use multiple means to motivate practitioners to adopt EB processes.* A project to disseminate synthesized evidence to pediatric clinicians concluded that multiple routes of evidence are necessary to convince practitioners to apply evidence in daily patient care (60). An organization is more able to tip toward applying evidence to direct patient care when the organization recognizes a local problem in how it uses research results, and differentiates among classes of evidence. Data showing results from the state of Hawaii's efforts to implement EBP makes a compelling case for the value research can add to practice; it also illustrates how Hawaii's clinicians differentiate among classes of evidence (32). Established means of influencing practitioners' behaviors, such as "best practice" groups, are also useful means to convey EBP ideas (60). Building on such natural social groups is more likely to result in behavioral change in practitioners than efforts to impose major changes in a top-down approach (54).

7. *Because context is complex and multiple routes are necessary to persuade practitioners to change, enacting evidence-based approaches in child mental health needs to be uniquely tailored for each organization and each desired change.* Summaries of how organizations change to include new practitioner behavior more grounded in evidence suggest multiple processes or activities are necessary to create change (23, 61). In brief, activities known to promote change successfully include skill-based training, evaluation of therapist fidelity and of programs, practice-based coaching, a facilitative administration, a well defined implementation team, a high level of facilitator involvement, clarity in defining the core components being implemented, hiring practices, and organizational readiness. The latter is defined by a clear need for change, funding, the confidence of the implementation team, and the involvement of stakeholders (23).

Enacting Evidence-Informed Health Care: An Outpatient Team, an Individual Practitioner

Despite the conclusions that certain drivers of change within health care organizations are effective, there is no single way to implement EBP because context is all-important. For example, an opinion leader physician at an outpatient child psychiatry team chose to initiate and support context-sensitive efforts to improve the functioning and quality of life in a larger proportion of the youth served, to make these improvements more substantial, and to make them occur more quickly. Aware that organizational change processes like a shift to evidence-based practice are highly context dependent, she first made an effort to understand the team's context (62). One key aspect, she realized, was the multidisciplinary nature of the team—psychologists, physicians, and social workers. Such diverse professional groups do not share a universal, communal and disinterested approach to knowledge; rather, each discipline displays distinct cognitive assumptions, often with clear boundaries around the discipline's knowledge, making knowledge often difficult to transfer from one discipline to another (63). Not only may the paradigms for generating knowledge in each profession be different, they may be so different that they lack common ground for productive dialogue. Each professional group may therefore produce bodies of knowledge that are not seen as authoritative within other groups (14).

She solved this by creating a work group open to anyone on the team willing to attend meetings and do the work required to complete the project. The group's first task would be to create a plan for how the team would approach youth with anxiety disorders. She led the group towards reviewing the work of the principal leaders in this field but also reviewing all published RCTs studying youth with panic disorder, generalized anxiety disorder, social anxiety disorder, separation anxiety disorder, or a phobia. Using the PubMed Clinical Queries site and limiting the search to recent publications focused on children or adolescents, she found a workable number of references for each disorder, and the group began its work. The work group's goal was to put together a short list of those core components appearing frequently in the most effective treatments. The group then chose those core components that both appeared frequently in effective treatments and were also feasible to use in the context of their setting, characterized by high volume and limited therapist availability. The work group stayed in touch via email and at team meetings with those staff members not participating in the literature review and feasibility discussions. The core components chosen as feasible within that context and supported by more than 1 RCT were exposure, relaxation training, cognitive restructuring, and fluoxetine. The approach she used—distillation of the literature into core components, and subsequently matching those components to a specific client in treatment—was well accepted by therapists. It helped that the process used was inclusive, open, and transparent; it may also have helped that the process respected therapists' autonomy and expertise in matching components and specific patients (64). The work group is currently developing ways to monitor fidelity to these core components.

Just as in organizations, there is no single path to implementing EBP among practitioners. Studies have shown that EBP is best learned in small group teaching experiences. Yet some practitioners may be able to improve their practice simply by being inquisitive, searching for evidence regards the answerable question as originally developed by EBM teachers (5). Resolving to improve his method of tracking response to treatment, for example, one practitioner began tracking symptoms in adolescents with anxiety disorders using an available instrument he uncovered through a Medline search (65). Similarly, he found that tracking responses of attention deficit/hyperactivity youth to stimulant treatment was inexpensive and feasible using an available brief report instrument (66) similar to the instrument used in the MTA study (67). This allowed him to build an alliance with parents by discussing likely outcomes. Parents appreciated the more thoughtful followup and their appreciation reinforced his change in behavior.

Solo practitioners can also benefit from joining the organization that uses their combined results to answer research questions, the Child and Adolescent Psychiatry Trials Network (67), allowing them to participate in research studies and inevitably piquing curiosity. In general, changing even an individual's practice begins with an action—a commitment to do something differently, be it a diagnostic process, a treatment decision, or choosing a followup methodology. Published summaries of EBP processes in child and adolescent psychiatry may be useful in reflecting on a starting point that is a good fit for a specific practitioner (68).

CONCLUSION

Contemporary child psychiatry requires a practice model realistic enough to recognize the vast array of contexts in which evaluations and treatments are delivered, yet rigorous enough to insist that each youth receive the most proven diagnostic process and treatment feasible in that setting. Clearly this is vastly different from each clinician's relying on personal preference—it is more time-consuming and more difficult than practice as usual. Results from the Hawaii group suggest it can make a substantial change in the bottom line of youth outcome, however, making the effort well worthwhile.

Readers are referred to the Clinicians' Guide to Evidence-Based Practice available on the Internet for further examples and discussion (69).

References

1. Sackett D et al.: *Evidence-Based Medicine: How to Practice and Teach EBM*. London, Churchill Livingstone, 2000, p. 261.
2. Friedland DJ (ed.): *Evidence-Based Medicine: A Framework for Clinical Practice*. Stamford, CT, Appleton & Lange, 1998, p. 263.
3. Guyatt GH, Rennie D: *Users' Guides to the Medical Literature: A Manual for Evidence-Based Clinical Practice*. Chicago, AMA Press, 2002, p. 705.
4. Hamilton J: Clinicians' guide to evidence-based practice: The answerable question and a hierarchy of evidence. *J Am Acad Child Adolesc Psychiatry* 44(6):596–600, 2005.
5. March JS et al.: Using and teaching evidence-based medicine: The Duke University child and adolescent psychiatry model. *Child Adolesc Psychiatric Clin N Am* 14:273–296, 2005.
6. Guyatt GH, Rennie D (eds.): *Users' Guides to the Medical Literature*. Chicago, IL, AMA Press, 2002, p. 706.
7. Burns B, Hoagwood KE: Preface. *Child & Adolescent Psychiatric Clinics of North America*, 13:717–728, 2005.
8. Chorpita BF et al.: Toward large-scale implementation of empirically supported treatments for children: A review and observations by the Hawaii empirical basis to services task force. *Clinical Psychology: Science and Practice*, 9(2):166–190, 2002.
9. Kazdin A: Evidence-based treatments: Challenges and priorities for practice and research. *Child & Adolescent Psychiatric Clinics of North America* 13(4):923–940, 2005.
10. Chorpita BF: The Frontier of Evidence-Based Practice, in Evidence-Based Psychotherapies for Children and Adolescents, A. Kazdin and J. Weisz Editors. New York, NY, Guilford Press, 2003, pp. 42–59.
11. Daleiden EL, Chorpita BF: From data to wisdom: Quality improvement strategies supporting large-scale implementation of evidence-based services. *Child & Adolescent Psychiatric Clinics of North America* 14(2):329–350, 2005.
12. Jellinek M, McDermott J: Formulation: Putting the diagnosis into a therapeutic context and treatment plan. *J Am Acad Child Adolesc Psychiatry* 43(7):913–916, 2004.
13. Ferlie E: Conclusion: From Evidence to Actionable Knowledge?. In: Dopson S, Fitzgerald L (eds.): *Knowledge to Action? Evidence-Based Health Care in Context*. Oxford University Press, Oxford, 2005, p. 182–197.

14. Ferlie E, Dopson S: Studying Complex Organizations in Health Care. In: Dopson S, Fitzgerald L (eds.): *Knowledge to Action? Evidence-based Health Care in Context.* Oxford University Press, Oxford, 2005, p. 8–26.
15. Kazdin AE: *Parent Management Training Treatment for Oppositional, Aggressive, and Antisocial Behavior in Children and Adolescents.* Oxford, Oxford University Press, 2005.
16. Mufson L et al.: *Interpersonal Psychotherapy for Depressed Adolescents*, 2nd ed. New York, Guilford, 2004.
17. Shirk SR, Karver M: Prediction of treatment outcome from relationship variables in child and adolescent therapy: A meta-analytic review. *Journal of Clinical and Consulting Psychology* 71(3):452–464, 2003.
18. Martin D, Graske J, Davis M: Relation of the therapeutic alliance with outcome and other variables: A meta-analytic review. *Journal of Consulting and Clinical Psychology* 68:438–450, 2000.
19. Shirk S, Russell R: *Change Processes in Child Psychotherapy: Revitalizing Treatment and Research.* New York, Guilford Press, 1996.
20. Garcia JA, Weisz JR: When youth mental health care stops: Therapeutic relationship problems and other reasons for ending youth outpatient treatment. *J Consulting and Clinical Psychology* 70(2):439–443, 2002.
21. Hawley K, Weisz J: Youth versus parent working alliance in usual clinical care: distinctive association with retention, satisfaction, and treatment outcome. *Journal of Clinical Child and Adolescent Psychology* 34(1):117–128, 2005.
22. McLeod BD, Weisz JR: The therapy process observational coding system–alliance scale: Measure characteristics and prediction of outcome in usual clinical practice. *Journal of Consulting and Clinical Psychology* 73(2): 323–333, 2005.
23. Greenhalgh T et al.: Spreading and sustaining innovations in health service delivery and organization. <http://www.sdo.lshtm.ac.uk/publications.htm>, 2004.
24. Greene RW et al.: Effectiveness of collaborative problem solving in affectively dysregulated children with oppositional-defiant disorder: Initial findings. *Journal of Consulting and Clinical Psychology* 72(6):1157–1164, 2004.
25. Kendall PC et al.: Breathing life into a manual: Flexibility and creativity with manual-based treatments. *Cognitive and Behavioral Practice* 5:177–198, 1998.
26. Haynes B, Devereaux P, Guyatt G: Clinical expertise in the era of evidence-based medicine and patient choice. *ACP J Club* 136:A11, 2002.
27. Levant RF: Evidence-Based Practice in Psychology. American Psychological Association, 2005.
28. Bickman L, Noser K, Summerfelt W: Long-term effects of a system of care on children and adolescents. *J Behav Health Services & Research* 26(2):185–202, 1999.
29. Weisz J, Jensen P: Efficacy and effectiveness of child and adolescent psychotherapy and pharmacotherapy. *Mental Health Services Research* 1:125–157, 1999.
30. Hodges K: *Child and Adolescent Functional Assessment Scale (CAFAS).* Ann Arbor, Michigan, Functional Assessment Systems, 1998.
31. Achenbach TM, McConaughy SH: *Empirically-Based Assessment of Child and Adolescent Psychopathology: Practical Applications.* Thousands Oaks, CA, Sage Publications, 1997.
32. Daleiden EL: Child Status Measurement: System Performance Improvements During Fiscal Years 2002–2004. State of Hawaii Department of Health, Child and Adolescent Mental Health Division, 2004.
33. March J et al.: Fluoxetine, cognitive-behavioral therapy, and their combination for adolescents with depression: Treatment for adolescents with depression study. *JAMA* 292(7):807–820, 2004.
34. Guyatt G et al.: Introduction: The philosophy of evidence-based medicine. In: Guyatt G, Rennie D (eds.): *Users' Guides to the Medical Literature: A Manual for Evidence-Based Clinical Practice.* Chicago, IL. AMA Press, 2002, p. 3–12.
35. Guyatt G et al.: Moving from evidence to action: Grading recommendations—a qualitative approach. In: Guyatt G, Rennie D (eds.): *Users' Guides to the Medical Literature: A Manual for Evidence-Based Clinical Practice.* Chicago, IL, AMA Press, 2002 p. 567–658.
36. Amitai Y, Frischer H: Excess fatality from desipramine in children and adolescents. *J Am Acad Child Adolesc Psychiatry* 45(1): 54–60, 2006.
37. Mabe P, Turner M, Josephson A: Parent management training. *Child Adolesc Psychiatr Clin N Am* 10(3): 451–464, 2001.
38. Medicine NLo, NCBI PubMed Clinical Queries. 2005.
39. Guyatt GH et al.: Moving from Evidence to Action. In: Rennie D (ed.): *Users' Guide to the Medical Literature: A Manual for Evidence-Based Clinical Practice*, Chicago, JAMA, 2002, pp. 175–199.
40. Faraone S, Biederman J, Roe C: Comparative efficacy of Adderall and methylphenidate in attention-deficit/hyperactivity disorder: A meta-analysis. *J Clin Psychopharmacol* 6(2): 43, 2002.
41. Medicine NLo, MeSH. 2005.
42. Collaboration TC, The Cochrane Collaboration Logo. 1993.
43. Starr M, Chalmers I: *The Evolution of the Cochrane Library: 1988 to 1993.* 2003.
44. Jadad A et al.: Methodology and reports of systematic reviews and meta-analyses: a comparison of Cochrane reviews with articles published in paper-based journals. *JAMA* 280: 278–280, 1998.
45. Streiner DL, Norman GR: *Health Measurement Scales: A Practical Guide to Their Development and Use.* 2nd ed. Oxford, Oxford University Press, 1995 p. 231.
46. Jensen AL: Evidence-based diagnosis: Incorporating diagnostic instruments into clinical practice. *J Am Acad Child Adolesc Psychiatry* 44:947–952, 2005.
47. Kaufman J et al.: Kiddie-Sads-Present and Lifetime Version (K-SADS-PL). Department of Psychiatry, University of Pittsburgh School of Medicine, 1997.
48. Shaffer D et al.: NIMH diagnostic interview schedule for children version IV (NIMH DISC-IV): Description, differences from previous versions, and reliability of some common diagnoses. *J Am Acad Child Adolesc Psychiatry* 39(1):28–38, 2000.
49. Youngstrom E et al.: Comparing the diagnostic accuracy of six potential screening instruments for bipolar disorder in youths aged 5 to 17 years. *J Am Acad Child Adolesc Psychiatry* 43:847–858, 2004.
50. Youngstrom EA, Duax J: Evidence-based assessment of pediatric bipolar disorder, Part I: Base rate and family history. *J Am Acad Child Adolesc Psychiatry* 44(7):712–717, 2005.
51. Youngstrom EA, Youngstrom JK: Evidence-based assessment of pediatric bipolar disorder, Part II: Incorporating information from behavior checklists. *J Am Acad Child Adolesc Psychiatry* 44(8):823–828, 2005.
52. Jensen AL, Weisz JR: Assessing match and mismatch between practitioner-generated and standardized interview-generated diagnoses for clinic-referred children and adolescents. *J Consult Clinc Psychol* 7(1):158–168, 2002.
53. Rosenblum DS et al.: Adolescents and popular culture: A psychodynamic overview. In: Solnit AJ, et al. (eds): *Psychoanalytic Study of the Child*, Volume, New Haven, CT. Yale University Press, 1999 pp. 319–338.
54. Weick KE: *Making Sense of the Organization.* Malden, MA: Blackwell, 2001.
55. Burrell G, Morgan G: *Sociological Paradigms and Organizational Analysis.* London, Heinemann Educational Books, 1979.
56. Dopson S, Fitzgerald L: *The Active Role of Context, in Knowledge to Action? Evidence-Based Health Care in Context.* Fitzgerald L. (ed.) Oxford. Oxford University Press, 2004, pp. 79–103.
57. Hoagwood KE: Making the translation from research to its application. *Clinical Psychology: Science and Practice* 9(2): 210–213, 2002.
58. Schoenwald SK, Hoagwood K: Effectiveness, transportability, and dissemination of interventions: What matters when? *Psychiatric Services* 52(9): 1190–1197, 2001.
59. Chorpita BF, Daleiden EL, Weisz JR: Identifying and selecting the common elements of evidence based interventions: A distillation and marching model. *Mental Health Services Research* 7(1): 5–20, 2005.
60. Lomas J: Retailing research: Increasing the role of evidence in clinical services for childbirth. *The Millbank Quarterly* 71(3): 439–474, 1993.
61. Fixsen D et al.: Implementation Research: A Synthesis of the Literature. University of South Florida, Louis de la Parte Florida Mental Health Institute, The National Implementation Research Network (FMHI Publication #231), 2005.
62. Dopson S, Fitzgerald L: The Active Role of Context. In: Dopson S, Fitzgerald L, (eds.): *Knowledge to Action? Evidence-Based Health Care in Context.* Oxford, Oxford University Press: 2005, pp. 79–103.
63. Fitzgerald L, Dopson S: Professional Boundaries and the Diffusion of Innovation. In: Dopson S., Fitzgerald L., (eds.): *Knowledge to Action? Evidence-Based Health Care in Context.* Oxford. Oxford University Press: 2005, pp. 104–131.
64. Chorpita BF, Daleiden EL, Weisz JR: Identifying and selecting the common elements of evidence based interventions: A distillation and matching model. *Mental Health Services Research* 7(1): 5–20, 2005.
65. Birmaher B et al.: The screen for child anxiety related emotional disorders (SCARED): Scale construction and psychometric characteristics. *Journal of the American Academy of Child and Adolescent Psychiatry* 36(4): 545–553, 1997.
66. Swanson J: SWAN Rating Scale. James Swanson, 2004.
67. Group TMC: A 14-month randomized clinical trial of treatment strategies for attention-deficit/hyperactivity disorder. *Archives General Psychiatry* 56: 1073–1086, 1999.
68. Hamilton JD: Evidence-Based Practice for Outpatient Clinical Teams. *J Am Acad Child Adolesc Psychiatry*, 2006. In press.
69. Group E: Clinicians' Guide to Evidence-Based Practice. *Journal of the American Academy of Child and Adolescent Psychiatry*, 2006.
70. Swanson J et al.: Clinical relevance of the primary findings of the MTA: Success rates based on severity of ADHD and ODD symptoms at the end of treatment. *J Am Acad Child Psychiatry* 40(2): 168–179, 2001.
71. Brent DA et al.: A clinical psychotherapy trial for adolescent depression comparing cognitive, family, and supportive therapy. *Archives of General Psychiatry* 54(9): 877–1885, 1997.
72. POTS Team: Cognitive-behavior therapy, sertraline, and their combination for children and adolescents with obsessive-compulsive disorder: The pediatric OCD treatment study (POTS) randomized controlled trial. *JAMA* 292(16): 1969–1976, 2004.
73. Kazdin A, Siegel T, Bass D: Cognitive problem-solving skills training and parent management training in the treatment of antisocial behavior in children. *J Consult Clinc Psychol* 60:733–747, 1992.

74. Delbello M, et al.: A double-blind, randomized, placebo-controlled study of quetiapine as adjunctive treatment for adolescent mania. *J Am Acad Child Adolesc Psychiatry* 41(10):1216–1223, 2002.
75. Emslie GJ, et al.: Fluoxetine treatment for prevention of relapse of depression in children and adolescents: A double-blind, placebo-controlled study. *J Am Acad Child Adolesc Psychiatry* 43(11):1397–1405, 2004.
76. Robins L, Rutter M (eds.): *Straight and Devious Pathways from Childhood to Adulthood*. London, Oxford University Press, 1990.
77. CASP, C.S.A.P., MeSH terms transcription to closest equivalent. 2004.
78. Birmaher B, et al.: Psychometric properties of the Screen for Child Anxiety Related Emotional Disorders (SCARED): A replication study. *J Am Acad Child Adolesc Psychiatry* 38(10):1230–1236, 1999.
79. Radloff L: A CES-D Scale: A self-report depression scale for research in the general population. *Applied Psychological Measurement* 1:385–401, 1977.
80. Joshi PT, Capozzoli JA, Coyle JT: The Johns Hopkins Depression Scale: Normative data and validation in child psychiatry patients. *J Am Acad Child Adolesc Psychiatry* 29(2):283–288, 1990.
81. Bird HR, et al.: The Columbia Impairment Scale (CIS): Piliot findings on a measure of global impairment for children and adolescents. *International Journal of Methods in Psychiatric Research* 3:167–176, 1993.
82. Gracious BL, et al.: Discriminative validity of a parent version of the young mania rating scale. *J Am Acad Child Adolesc Psychiatry* 41(11):1350–1359, 2002.
83. Saxe G, et al.: Child stress disorders checklist: A measure of ASD and PTSD in children. *J Am Acad Child Adolesc Psychiatry* 42(8):972–978, 2003.

CHAPTER 2.1.3 ■ RESPECT FOR CHILDREN AS RESEARCH SUBJECTS

ROBERT J. LEVINE

"So act as to treat humanity, whether in thine own person or in that of any other, in every case as an end withal, never as a means only." The German philosopher Immanuel Kant, writing late in the eighteenth century, provided this formal statement of the ethical principle of respect for persons. Persons are to be regarded as ultimate values in and of themselves; they are not to be used merely as means to another's goals.

Those who conduct research involving human subjects first define their goals and then identify persons whom they use as means to accomplish these goals. This is not unethical. What is proscribed is the use of persons merely as means—"as means only." To avoid this, researchers are required both ethically and legally to secure the approval of persons to be used as research subjects through a process called informed consent. If this approval entails acceptance of the researcher's goals, then the subject is not used merely as a means. Rather, the subject freely chooses to embrace the goals as his or her own and thus remains an end.

This chapter is concerned with informed consent and other issues related to the principle of respect for persons (e.g., privacy and confidentiality) as they relate to the involvement as research subjects of adolescents and children of various ages.

ETHICAL PRINCIPLES

The basic ethical principles identified by the National Commission for the Protection of Human Subjects of Biomedical and Behavioral Research (1) as those that should underlie the conduct of research involving human subjects are "respect for persons," "beneficence," and "justice." These principles were endorsed subsequently by the President's Commission for the Study of Ethical Problems in Medicine and Biomedical and Behavioral Research (2) as "basic values" for medical practice as well as for biomedical and behavioral research, calling them by somewhat different names: "respect," "well being," and "equity." According to these authoritative commissions, research involving human subjects should be conducted in accord with norms or rules designed to uphold and embody these basic principles or values. These rules are assembled in federal regulations for the "protection of human research subjects"; most relevant to the present concerns are those of the Department of Health and Human Services (Code of Federal Regulations, Title 45, Part 46; hereafter abbreviated as 45 CFR 46)[1] and the Food and Drug Administration (Code of Federal Regulations, Title 21, Parts 50 and 56; hereafter abbreviated as 21 CFR 50 and 21 CFR 56).

In this chapter there are frequent references to federal regulations. This is not intended to suggest that all ethical considerations are reflected adequately in the law. Rather, the regulations in this field generally represent a broad social consensus about what ought and ought not to be done. Even for research not covered by the regulations, they have come to be regarded as establishing a community standard, departures from which require justification (3). The regulations include both substantive and procedural rules (norms). A substantive rule specifies behaviors that are required (or forbidden) because they are morally right (or wrong). Some procedural rules specify procedures that should be performed to determine the most appropriate behavior when the behavior has not been specified by a substantive rule. Other procedural rules are designed either to assist in the adherence to the requirements of a substantive rule or to provide documentary evidence that

[1]SubPart A of 45 CFR 46, the basic DHHS regulations for the protection of human subjects are customarily referred to as the Common Rule because, with minor variations, they have been endorsed and adopted by almost all of the federal departments that conduct or support research involving human subjects. The other parts of the regulations providing special protections for fetuses and pregnant women (SubPart B), prisoners (SubPart C), and children (SubPart D) have not been adopted as part of the Common Rule. To avoid confusion in this chapter all DHHS regulations are referred to as 45 CFR 46. At the time of this writing, the DHHS Secretary's Advisory Committee on Human Research Protections is reviewing SubPart D with the aim of clarifying their definitions and the concepts. Their Website is revised from time to time to show the current state of their deliberations. (www.hhs.gov/ohrp/sachrp/index.html)

research has been conducted in accord with the relevant substantive rules (3).

AN ILLUSTRATION

The principle of respect for persons requires that human persons must be treated as autonomous agents. The substantive norm that requires informed consent is a specification of one way in which this principle is to be made operational in the conduct of research involving human subjects. The procedural norm that requires review and approval by an institutional review board affords a method for determining what specific bits of information must be divulged to prospective subjects in a particular research protocol. Another procedural norm that requires the signing of a consent form provides documentary evidence that the behavior required by the substantive norm has been accomplished. The form itself assists the investigator's efforts to comply with the substantive rule.

According to the National Commission:

> Respect for persons incorporates at least two basic ethical convictions: First, that individuals should be treated as autonomous agents, and second, that persons with diminished autonomy and thus in need of protection are entitled to such protections. An autonomous person is . . . an individual capable of deliberation about personal goals and of acting under the direction of such deliberation (1).

To show respect for autonomous persons requires that we leave them alone, even to the point of allowing them to choose activities that might be harmful (e.g., hang gliding), unless they agree or consent that we may do otherwise. We are not to touch them or encroach on their private spaces unless such touching or encroachment is in accord with their wishes. Our actions should be designed to affirm their authority and enhance their capacity to be self-determining; we are not to obstruct their actions unless they are clearly detrimental to others. We show disrespect for autonomous persons when we either repudiate their considered judgments or deny them the freedom to act on those judgments in the absence of compelling reasons to do so.

Clearly, not every human being is capable of self-determination. The capacity for self-determination matures during a person's life; some lose this capacity partially or completely, owing to illness or mental disability or in situations that severely restrict liberty, such as prisons. Respect for the immature or incapacitated may require one to offer protection to them as they mature or while they are incapacitated.

Because the central focus of this chapter is on respect for persons, it is necessary to emphasize that the other two principles are of equal importance in the sense that they have equal moral force. Research involving human subjects can be considered ethically justified if, and only if, it is adequately responsive to each of the three basic ethical principles (3). As we shall see, considerations of justice and beneficence place constraints on, for example, whom we can ask to serve as research subjects and how much risk we may ask them to accept in the interests of research.

INFORMED CONSENT

Principle I of the Nuremberg Code (4) provides the definition of consent from which definitions supplied in all subsequent codes and regulations are derived:

> The *voluntary* consent of the human subject is absolutely essential.
>
> This means that the person involved should have *legal capacity* to give consent; should be so situated as to be able to exercise *free power of choice,* without the intervention of any element of force, fraud, deceit, duress, over-reaching or other ulterior form of constraint or coercion; and should have sufficient *knowledge* and *comprehension* of the elements of the subject matter involved as to enable him to make an understanding and enlightened decision [emphasis added].

Thus, consent is recognized as valid if it has each of these four essential attributes: It must be competent (legally), voluntary, informed, and comprehending (or understanding).

It is through informed consent that the investigator and subject enter into a relationship, defining mutual expectations and their limits. This relationship differs from ordinary commercial transactions in which each party is responsible for informing himself or herself of the terms and implications of any of their agreements. Professionals who intervene in the lives of others are held to higher standards. They are obligated to inform the layperson of the consequences of their mutual agreements.

It is worth noticing that the Nuremberg Code defines and requires "voluntary consent." Since 1957 this term has been replaced by "informed consent," a term that reflects an idealized vision of the person as a rational, self-determining agent (5).

Federal regulations identify "elements" of information that must be transmitted during the negotiations for informed consent (45 CFR 46.116a); these are:

1. A statement that the study involves research, an explanation of the purposes of the research, and the expected duration of the subject's participation, a description of the procedures to be followed, and identification of any procedures that are experimental
2. A description of any reasonably foreseeable risks or discomforts to the subject
3. A description of any benefits to the subject or others that may reasonably be expected from the research
4. A disclosure of appropriate alternative procedures or courses of treatment, if any, which might be advantageous to the subject
5. A statement describing the extent, if any, to which confidentiality of records identifying the subject will be maintained
6. For research involving more than minimal risk, an explanation as to whether any compensation and an explanation as to whether any medical treatments are available if injury occurs and, if so, what they may consist of or where further information may be obtained
7. An explanation of whom to contact for answers to pertinent questions about the research and research subjects' rights, and whom to contact in the event of a research-related injury to the subject
8. A statement that participation is voluntary, refusal to participate will involve no penalty or loss of benefits to which the subject is otherwise entitled, and the subject may discontinue participation at any time without penalty or loss of benefits to which the subject is otherwise entitled

In addition, according to the regulations, the following elements must be provided "when appropriate" (45 CFR 46.116b):

1. A statement that the particular treatment or procedure may involve risks to the subject (or to the embryo or fetus, if the subject is or may become pregnant) that are currently unforeseeable
2. Anticipated circumstances under which the subject's participation may be terminated by the investigator without regard to the subject's consent
3. Any additional costs to the subject that may result from participation in research
4. The consequences of a subject's decision to withdraw from the research and procedures for orderly termination of participation by the subject

5. A statement that significant new findings developed during the course of the research that may relate to the subject's willingness to continue participation will be provided to the subject
6. The approximate number of subjects involved in the study

The regulations define only minimum standards for informed consent. In most cases it seems appropriate to supplement these basic requirements with additional elements of information (3). For example, prospective subjects should be told why they have been selected as invitees to participate in the research; ordinarily, this consists of a statement of the major inclusion and exclusion criteria for the protocol. In addition to the statement of "additional costs to the subject" required by the regulations, there should also be accurate statements of any cash payments or other economic advantages associated with participation in the research as a subject.

How does one determine whether any particular fact (e.g., any particular risk of injury) must be disclosed? The legal criterion for disclosure in the context of medical practice is "material risk," that is, any fact that is material to the patient's decision must be disclosed (3, 6). The determination of which risks are material in that they must be disclosed may be accomplished according to three different standards or tests (3, 7). Until recently, the prevailing standard was that of the "reasonable physician"; the determination of whether any particular risk or other fact should be disclosed was made on the basis of whether it was customary to do so in the community of practicing physicians.

The standard that is now applied most commonly is the "reasonable person" or "prudent patient" test. In the case of *Canterbury* v. *Spence* (8), the court held that the disclosure required was determined by the patient's right of self-decision, a right that can be effectively exercised only if the patient possesses enough information to enable an intelligent choice. A risk is thus material when a reasonable person, in what the physician knows or should know to be the patient's position, would be likely to attach significance to the risks or cluster of risks in deciding whether or not to forego the proposed therapy.

Some courts have adopted the rule that a risk is material if the particular patient making the choice or decision considers it material. Of the three standards, this rule, which some call the idiosyncratic person standard, is most responsive to the requirements of the ethical principle of respect for persons. It is, however, a highly impractical standard.

In the author's view, the reasonable person standard should determine the minimum amount of information that should be imparted by the researcher to each and every prospective subject. Then, in the course of the consent discussions, the researcher should attempt to learn from each prospective subject what more he or she would like to know.

Federal regulations permit "a consent procedure which does not include, or which alters, some or all of the elements of informed consent" or, in some cases, waiver of the entire requirement for informed consent, if:

> [a] The research involves no more than minimal risk to the subjects, [b] The waiver or alteration will not adversely affect the rights and welfare of the subjects, [c] The research could not practicably be carried out without the waiver or alteration, and [d] Whenever appropriate, the subjects will be provided with additional pertinent information after participation (45 CFR 46.116d).

Implicit in these conditions—particularly the second condition—is recognition of the standard of materiality. One may not withhold any material information without adversely affecting the rights of subjects. Waivers and alterations are commonly used in research involving medical records, "left-over" specimens of tissues and body fluids from which personal identifying information has been removed, survey research, and so on. It is more problematic when researchers propose to alter information for purposes of deceiving prospective research subjects (3).

The Department of Health and Human Services (DHHS) makes it clear that, "Nothing in these regulations is intended to limit the authority of a physician to provide emergency medical care, to the extent the physician is permitted to do so under applicable federal, state, or local law" (45 CFR 46.116f). Implicit in this rule is a recognition of two exceptions to the legal requirement for informed consent: the emergency exception and therapeutic privilege.[2]

The Food and Drug Administration (FDA) permits waiver of the consent requirement for the use of investigational new drugs (or other regulated test articles) in the treatment of individuals in "life-threatening situations" in which "informed consent cannot be obtained ... because of an inability to communicate with, or obtain legally effective consent from, the subject" (21 CFR 50.23). There is also a provision in FDA regulations for an exception from informed consent requirements for emergency research; this exception is designed for research activities in which most or all of the prospective subject population will be unable to consent and it will not be feasible (usually owing to lack of time) to get consent from a legally authorized representative (21 CFR 50.24).[3]

CONSENT FORMS

Thus far we have been considering informed consent, a process designed to show respect for subjects, fostering their interests by empowering them to pursue and protect their own interests. The consent form, by contrast, is an instrument designed to protect the interests of researchers and their institutions by defending them against civil or criminal liability. I believe that one of the reasons there has been so little successful litigation against investigators, as compared with practicing physicians, is the very formal and thorough documentation of informed consent on consent forms. Consent forms may be detrimental to the subject's interests not only in adversarial proceedings; signed consent forms in institutional records may lead to violations of privacy and confidentiality (3).

> DHHS regulations require:
> A written consent document that embodies the elements of informed consent.... This form may be read to the subject or the subject's legally authorized representative, but, in any event, the investigator shall give either the subject or the representative adequate opportunity to read it before it is signed (45 CFR 46.117).[4]

Although the primary purpose of the consent form is to protect the interests of researchers and their institutions, it is forbidden by federal regulations to:

> include any exculpatory language through which the subject or the representative is made to waive or appear to waive any of the subject's legal rights, or releases or appears to release the

[2]For an authoritative commentary on these two exceptions, see Appendix 1 of the President's Commission's Report, Making Health Care Decisions (2). For a more concise discussion see Levine (3).

[3]There are further conditions specified by FDA in its regulations. For further discussion of 21 CFR 50.23, see Levine (3). For 21 CFR 50.24 see Brody (42).

[4]The Department of Health and Human Services regulations also permit use of a "short" form. Use of this form of documentation seems even more complicated and cumbersome than use of the standard consent form. Moreover, its use requires a witness to the consent discussion (3).

investigator, the sponsor, the institution or its agents from liability for negligence.[5]

DHHS requires that "[a] copy shall be given to the person signing the form" (45 CFR 46.117). The primary purpose of the form notwithstanding, it can and should be designed to be helpful to the subjects. Having a copy of the form will afford them an opportunity to continue to get more information as additional questions occur to them. It can also serve as a reminder of the plans they must follow in order to accomplish the purposes of research, of the symptoms they should watch for to protect their own safety, of the perils of omitting doses of drugs, and so on. It can serve as a guide to conversations they might choose to have with family, friends, personal doctors, and other trusted advisors about whether they should consent; in some cases such conversations should be recommended during the consent negotiations. In the use of these forms, however, the researcher should heed the words of the President's Commission (9): "Ethically valid consent is a process of shared decision-making based upon mutual respect and participation, not a ritual to be equated with reciting the contents of a form that details the risks of particular treatments."

No consent form can be designed so as to anticipate all of any particular prospective subject's wishes to be informed. The consent form is most effective when it is viewed by the researcher as a guide to the negotiations with the prospective subject. The consent form should contain at least the minimum amount of information and advice that should be presented during the negotiations. If any substantive new understandings are developed in the process of negotiations that have any bearing on the prospective subject's willingness to participate, these should be added to the consent form signed by that individual.

DHHS regulations (45 CFR 46.117) permit waiver of the requirement for documentation of informed consent if:

1. The only record linking the subject and the research would be the consent document and the principal risk would be potential harm resulting from a breach of confidentiality.
2. The research presents no more than minimal risk of harm to subjects and involves no procedures for which written consent is normally required outside of the research context.

In some cases in which the regulations permit waiver of the requirements for documentation, it may be advisable to provide subjects with information sheets. These documents provide a written account of all information that could serve subjects' interests in ways suggested earlier. They differ from consent forms primarily in that they are not signed by subjects and retained by researchers. Thus, they afford limited protection to the researcher and the institution.

JUSTIFICATION OF RESEARCH INVOLVING CHILDREN

Children, as a class of persons, lack the legal capacity to consent. Moreover, many of them, particularly the younger ones, are not only incapable of sufficient comprehension to meet the Nuremberg Code's standard but are also not "so situated as to be able to exercise free power of choice." It is necessary to rely on other devices to show respect for children because they cannot consent. Two of these devices are permission and assent.

[5]Such language is also forbidden in the consent discussion (45 CFR 46.116).

Permission of one or both parents or of the legal guardian is closely related to what was formerly called proxy consent. With few exceptions, federal regulators regard permission as a necessary condition for authorizing the involvement of a child as a research subject; for children who cannot assent, it is usually a sufficient condition as well. The transactions involved in negotiating a valid permission are in all respects identical to those of informed consent.

Assent by the child should be as close an approximation of consent as the child's capabilities permit.

Before proceeding with our discussion of permission and assent, it is necessary to return to a consideration of the basic ethical principles.

Respect for persons requires that we treat individuals as autonomous agents only to the extent that they are autonomous. As noted earlier, "[p]ersons with diminished autonomy and thus in need of protection are entitled to such protections (1)." In response to this ethical conviction, there is established in federal regulations a standard called "minimal risk," which "means that the probability and magnitude of harm or discomfort anticipated in the research are not greater in and of themselves than those ordinarily encountered in daily life or during the performance of routine physical or psychological examinations or tests" (45 CFR 46).[6] Minimal risk serves as a threshold standard in that plans to involve children in research that presents more than minimal risk require special justification and procedural protections.

But many therapeutic procedures present far more than minimal risk, and it is not customary to obstruct children's access to them by calling for special procedural protections. The regulations make it clear that the minimal risk standard is applicable only to procedures that do not "hold out the prospect of direct benefit for the individual subjects" (45 CFR 46.405). Therapeutic procedures, by contrast, are to be authorized and justified precisely as they are in the practice of medicine. That is to say, the risk of any procedure is justified in terms of the benefit expected for the individual child-subject who will bear that risk. Also, as in medical practice, the relationship of anticipated benefit to the risk presented by the procedure must be at least as advantageous to the subject as that presented by any available alternative, unless, of course, the subject (or his or her parents) has considered and refused to accept a superior alternative. These rules are responsive to the ethical principle of beneficence, which as articulated by the National Commission (1) is expressed in the form of two general rules: " (1) Do no harm; and (2) maximize possible benefits and minimize possible harms."

Justice, as envisioned by the National Commission, requires a fair sharing of the burdens and benefits of society (1, 3). In the distribution of these burdens and benefits, special consideration is to be given to those who are vulnerable or disadvantaged. Children are considered vulnerable and are to be protected from exploitation because they lack the capacity to consent. They are not to be involved in research that is irrelevant to the class of person of which they are representative. When appropriate, research should be done first on adults and then on older children before involving younger children and infants (3).

In summary, children and their parents are not completely free to do their own thing. There are constraints grounded in ethical considerations and enforced by regulations regarding whom researchers may invite to serve as subjects and how

[6]The term minimal risk presents many problems. As it is defined, it may be interpreted in several different ways. For a discussion of its deficiencies, see Levine (3) and Kopelman (43). For an excellent discussion relating the concept of risk to the child's level of development, see Thompson (39).

much risk they may be asked to assume for research purposes. With these constraints in mind, we now turn to further consideration of assent and permission.

ASSENT

Respect for children does not require that we leave them alone even to the point of allowing them to choose dangerous activities unless they agree that we may do otherwise. Young children have no such liberty rights. What they have instead is a right to custody (10). We show respect for them by fostering their well being, protecting them from harm, and guiding them to become "the right kind of people."

As we have already noticed, federal regulations reflect the obligation to protect children from harm and to secure their well being. Let us now consider the obligation to guide their moral and social development—an obligation not recognized explicitly in the regulations.

In the 1970s there was a spirited debate over the legitimacy of using persons who are incapable of consent ("unconsenting subjects") as research subjects. Paul Ramsey (11) argued that it is always morally wrong. Richard McCormick (12), arguing the opposing viewpoint, pointed out that members of a moral community have certain obligations. One of these is to contribute to the general welfare when to do so requires little or no sacrifice. In the case of children, one may presume that they would consent if they could; he calls this a "correctly construed consent." In his view, when supplemented with parental permission, correctly construed consent authorized the use of children as subjects in research that fulfilled an important social need and involved "no discernible risk."

At this point, Terrence Ackerman (13) entered the debate, arguing that we tend to fool ourselves with procedures designed to show respect for the child's very limited autonomy. He claims that the child tends to follow "the course of action that is recommended overtly or covertly by the adults who are responsible for the child's well-being." He further contends that, in general, this is as it ought to be. "Once we recognize our duty to guide the child and his inclination to be guided the task becomes that of guiding him in ways which will involve his well-being and contribute to his becoming the right kind of person."

Willard Gaylin (14) tells the story of a man who acted in accord with Ackerman's position. After directing his 10-year-old son to cooperate with a venipuncture for research purposes, he explained that his direction arose from his perceived moral obligation to teach his child that there are certain things one does to serve the interests of others even if it does cause a bit of pain:

> This is my child. I was less concerned with the research involved than with the kind of boy I was raising. I'll be damned if I was going to allow my child, because of some idiotic concept of children's rights, to assume that he was entitled to be a selfish, narcissistic little bastard.

Parenthetically, while it is appropriate to guide and persuade a 10-year-old boy to submit to a venipuncture for research purposes, it is not ethically defensible to command him to do so against his will; it is also contrary to the requirements of federal regulations. Guiding children to become the "right kind of persons" entails teaching them about and encouraging them to embrace the sense of obligation to the moral community discussed before. It further entails showing respect for their maturing capacities for self-determination; one hopes the child will learn to choose to do unto others as the child would wish them to do unto her or him.

At what age does a child become capable of assent? Federal regulations specify no age, leaving it to the discretion of the Institutional Review Board (IRB), taking into account not only the age but also the maturity and psychological state of the children involved.

As the assent regulation is written, it seems to reflect a presumption that the capability to assent is an all-or-none phenomenon; the child is either capable or incapable of assent. This presumption is incorrect (15, 16) and, the author believes, unintended by the regulation writers. In the author's view the regulations are intended to be interpreted to permit a determination that prospective child-subjects may be capable of understanding some but not all of the elements of informed consent. Thus, for example, it may be appropriate to provide some children with "a description of any reasonably foreseeable risks or discomforts," without providing "an explanation as to whether any compensation [is] available if injury occurs."

It is possible to make some general comments on the capabilities to assent of children having normal cognitive development in various age groups. According to Lois Weithorn (15), who relates her empirical findings to Piaget's concepts of cognitive development:

> ... in general, developmental research suggests that most school-aged children are capable of meaningful assent for participation in most types of research studies. This means that the children probably are capable of comprehending the nature of the proposed procedures, the general purpose of the research, and of expressing a preference regarding participation. Research suggests that normal children ages 6 and older are quite capable of thoughtful and reasoned consideration of the types of information that investigators may provide.

Typically, at about age 11, children's cognitive development enters the "stage of formal operations," during which they become increasingly sophisticated in their capacities to reason about "possibility" and other abstract concepts. From ages seven to 11, in the "stage of concrete operations," the child is more or less limited to thinking about matters that are not too far removed from concrete reality. Thus, there are those who argue that the "age of assent" should be around six or seven, and others who say it should be around 11 or 12.[7]

Weithorn (15) continues:

> Early empirical findings also suggest that, although they may not be legally authorized to provide independent consent for treatment or research in most jurisdictions, normal adolescents age 14 and older may be as capable as adults of making competent decisions about such participation, according to the more stringent legal standards of competency.

The authority of mature and emancipated minors to consent is discussed subsequently in this chapter.

PERMISSION

Parental permission is envisioned by the National Commission as a reflection of the collective judgment of the family that an infant or child may participate in research (3, 17). In most cases the permission of one parent is sufficient; one may assume that he or she will represent the family's wishes satisfactorily.

---

[7] According to the National Commission (17), a child with normal cognitive development becomes capable of meaningful assent at about the age of 7 years, although some may be younger and some older. The Department of Health and Human Services (DHHS) did not accept this recommendation. Rather, at the time the proposed regulations were published, DHHS solicited public comment on which of three options it should adopt for nontherapeutic procedures: either age 7, age 12, or leaving the age to the discretion of the IRB. The final regulations reflect the third of these options.

When more than minimal risk is presented by a nontherapeutic procedure, the permission of both parents is required unless one is "deceased, unknown, incompetent, or not reasonably available, or when only one person has legal responsibility for the care or custody of the child" (45 CFR 46.408).

There are three additional criteria for justification of nontherapeutic procedures that present more than minimal risk (45 CFR 46.406): First, the degree of risk is limited to "a minor increase over minimal risk." Second, the procedure or intervention must be "likely to yield generalizable knowledge which is of vital importance for the understanding or amelioration of the subject's disorder or condition."[8] Third, the procedure or intervention must present "experiences to subjects that are reasonably commensurate with those inherent in their actual or expected medical, dental, psychological, social or educational situations." This means that the procedures must be ones that they or others with the specific disorder or condition under study will ordinarily experience by virtue of their having or being treated for that disorder or condition. Thus, it might be appropriate to invite a child with leukemia who has had several bone marrow examinations to consider having another for research purposes.

The requirement of commensurability reflects the National Commission's judgment that children who have had a procedure performed on them might be more capable than are those who are not so experienced of basing their assent on some familiarity with the procedure and its attendant discomforts; thus their decision to participate will be more knowledgeable.

Even though the parent gives permission, the child's refusal to assent to nontherapeutic interventions should be respected. Those who are incapable of assent may have some capacity to make their wishes known. The term *deliberate objection* is used to recognize that some children who are incapable of meaningful assent are able to communicate their disapproval or refusal of a proposed procedure. A four-year-old may protest, "No, I don't want to be stuck with a needle." However, an infant who might in certain circumstances cry or withdraw in response to almost any stimulus is not regarded as capable of deliberate objection. A child's deliberate objection usually should be regarded as a veto to his or her involvement in research (3, 17).

In the case of therapeutic interventions or procedures, the situation is much different. Federal regulations state simply, the assent of children is not a necessary condition (45 CFR 46.408). Parents have both the right and responsibility to override the objection of school-age children to necessary therapy. With regard to teenagers, decisions regarding authorization of investigational therapies are about as complicated as they are in the practice of medicine. The law recognizes the authority of emancipated and some mature minors to consent to or refuse standard or accepted therapy; these rules are not recognized explicitly in federal regulations regarding investigational therapies.

In the practical world of decisionmaking about who can authorize a therapeutic procedure, whether it is investigational or accepted, it rarely suffices to point to the law and thereby identify the person who has the legal right to make the decision. Many factors must be taken into account in reaching judgments about the capability of various persons to participate in and, in the event of irreconcilable disputes, prevail in such choices. In general, these judgments become more complicated as the child gets older or the stakes get higher (14, 18).

[8]What constitutes "minor increase" and "vital importance" is not defined in the regulations. Responsibility for deciding such matters in relation to particular research proposals is assigned to the IRB. If the IRB cannot decide or if it does decide that the degree of risk is more than a minor increase over minimal risk, it must refer the judgment to the Secretary of The Department of Health and Human Services (3).

IRBs have the authority to waive the requirement for permission when "it is not a reasonable requirement ... provided an appropriate mechanism for protecting the children is substituted" (45 CFR 46.408). The regulations suggest as an example of research in which a requirement for parental permission might not be reasonable is that on "neglected or abused children." The National Commission (17) specified several other examples:

> Research designed to identify factors related to the incidence or treatment of certain conditions in adolescents for which, in certain jurisdictions, they may legally receive treatment without parental consent; research in which the subjects are "mature minors" and the procedures involved entail essentially no more than minimal risk that such individuals might reasonably assume on their own; research designed to meet the needs of children designated by their parents as "in need of supervision," and research involving children whose parents are legally or functionally incompetent.

THE NATIONAL COMMISSION (17) FURTHER ELABORATES:

> There is no single mechanism that can be substituted for parental permission in every instance. In some cases the consent of mature minors should be sufficient. In other cases court approval may be required. The mechanism involved will vary with the research and the age, status and condition of the prospective subject....
>
> Assent of ... mature minors should be considered sufficient with respect to research about conditions for which they have the legal authority to consent on their own to treatment. An appropriate mechanism for protecting such subjects might be to require that a clinic nurse or physician, unrelated to the research, explain the nature and the purpose of the research ... emphasizing that participation is unrelated to provision of care. Another alternative might be to appoint a social worker, pediatric nurse, or physician to act as surrogate parent when the research is designed, for example, to study neglected or battered children. Such surrogate parents would be expected to participate not only in the process of soliciting the children's cooperation but also in the conduct of the research, in order to provide reassurance for the subject and to intervene or support their desires to withdraw if participation becomes too stressful.

The recommendations of the National Commission reflected their assumption that the "normal" family is one in which the members stand in a loving relationship to one another and that the parents in such a family will strive to protect the interests and welfare of their children. This point notwithstanding, they were aware of the fact that there are exceptions. In obvious cases (e.g., neglected or abused children) they recommended that the IRB should have the authority to waive the requirement for parental permission. In the less obvious cases, of which there may be many, decisions as to whether the parents are loyal to their children and welfare require sophisticated professional judgment. The National Commission wisely refrained from recommending that IRBs engage in micromanagement of such cases. Implicitly, the responsibility for such judgments is assigned to the investigator. The National Commission provided a margin of safety by recommending special substantive and procedural protections in cases in which more than minimal risk is presented by interventions that do not hold out the prospect of direct benefit for the individual child-subject.

In recent years there has been increasing interest in giving mature minors independent authority to authorize their own participation in certain types of research without requiring permission of their parents or guardians. To some extent this interest reflects a general trend in public policy toward facilitating inclusion as research subjects members of groups who were previously excluded (19). This interest also represents a pragmatic response to problems presented by the AIDS pandemic; specifically, many, and perhaps most, adolescents will not enroll as research subjects if this necessarily entails allowing their parents or guardians to learn or even suspect certain details of their sexual or drug-taking experience (20).

Most of the current federal regulations for the protection of human subjects reflect the attitude that prevailed in the 1960s and 1970s when they were written, that investigational drugs and participation in research were dangerous and researchers were likely to exploit subjects. Since the mid-1980s, primarily as a consequence of the efforts of AIDS activists, this vision has been largely replaced by one that research participation and access to investigational drugs are both more beneficial than burdensome. As a result of this shift in perception, public policies that were designed to protect persons from harm and exploitation, particularly those persons who are considered vulnerable by reason of limitation in their capacity to give informed consent, are being reinterpreted or rewritten to assure the same classes of persons equitable access to the benefits of investigational drugs as well as to the benefits of participation in research (19).

It has long been known that restrictive policies on involvement of children in research have resulted in a class injustice. Children as a class have been deprived of the benefits of the new knowledge that could result from carrying out research involving children as subjects. This deprivation is exemplified by the fact that approximately 80% of the drugs approved by the FDA for commercial distribution are not labeled for use in children, usually because sufficient studies have not been conducted in children (21, 22). In recent years agencies of the federal government have begun to respond to this class injustice. The National Institutes of Health now require that applications for grants or contracts to conduct research involving human subjects must include plans to enroll children unless the applicant can justify their exclusion (23). Similarly, the Food and Drug Administration requires inclusion of children in research done to support an application for a marketing permit unless the sponsor can justify their exclusion (24, 25, Public Law 105–115; Center for Drug Evaluation and Research).

At the time of this writing, federal policies have not been revised to permit involvement of mature minors as research subjects on their own authority except as discussed earlier in this chapter. However, it seems reasonable to predict that in the near future there could be such changes in the relevant policies or their interpretation. Santelli and associates (26) and Levine (27) have published examples of specific proposals. Inclusion of children who are wards (e.g., of the state) in research in which more than minimal risk is presented by nontherapeutic interventions requires special procedural protections that are beyond the scope of this discussion (45 CFR 46.409) (3). Many states and cities have regulations designed to protect the interests of foster children.

Concern has been expressed recently that such regulations often create formidable bureaucratic barriers to involving such children in randomized clinical trials or gaining them access to investigational drugs. For two reasons this presents a special problem to children with AIDS: a) A large percentage of such children are foster children; and b) many apparently effective therapies for AIDS and its complications are investigational drugs (28).

DOCUMENTATION

The regulatory requirement for documentation of permission is exactly the same as it is for informed consent. In circumstances in which there is no requirement for permission because the minor is authorized to assent for himself or herself the same requirements for documentation obtain. Apart from this, when children are asked to sign forms, as they often and quite properly are, the principal purpose, in the author's view, is to enhance their sense of participation in the process.

PRIVACY AND CONFIDENTIALITY

Privacy is "the freedom of the individual to pick and choose for himself the time and circumstances under which, and most importantly, the extent to which, his attitudes, beliefs, behavior and opinions are to be shared with or withheld from others (29)." Because this is the definition used in this chapter, some matters considered by the law to fall under the rubric of privacy are excluded (the right to abortion and contraception). In general, in clinical research, intrusions into individuals' privacy are permitted only with their informed consent. There is no invasion when an informed person allows a researcher into his or her private space.

Confidentiality is a term that is all too often used interchangeably with *privacy*. Confidentiality refers to a mode of management of private information; if a subject shares private information with (confides in) a researcher, the researcher is expected to refrain from sharing this information with others without either the subject's authorization or some other justification.

The ethical grounding for the requirement to respect the privacy of persons may be found in the principle of respect for persons. The ethical justification for confidentiality, according to Sissela Bok (30), is grounded in four premises, three of which support confidentiality in general; the fourth supports professional confidentiality in particular.

First and foremost, we must respect the individual's autonomy regarding personal information. To the extent they wish, and to the extent they are capable of doing so, they are entitled to have secrets. This facilitates their ability to live according to their own life plans.

Closely related is the second premise, which recognizes the legitimacy not only of having personal secrets but also of sharing them with whomever one chooses. This premise, which embodies an obligation to show respect for relationships among human beings and respect for intimacy, is exemplified by the marital privilege upheld in American law, according to which one spouse cannot be forced to testify against the other.

The third premise draws on the general requirement to keep promises. A pledge of confidentiality creates an obligation beyond the respect owing to persons and existing relationships. Once we are bound by a promise, we may no longer be fully impartial in our dealings with the promisee.

These three premises, taken together, provide strong prima facie reasons to support confidentiality. That is to say, they are binding on those who have accepted information in confidence unless there are sufficiently powerful reasons to do otherwise—as, for example, when maintaining confidentiality would cause serious harm to innocent third parties.

Bok's fourth premise adds strength to the pledge of silence given by professionals. The professional's duty to maintain confidentiality goes beyond ordinary loyalty, "because of its utility to persons and to society ... Individuals benefit from such confidentiality because it allows them to seek help they might otherwise fear to ask for" from doctors or others who can provide it.

Investigators, of course, are not necessarily professionals to whom individuals turn for professional help. Thus, only part of the fourth premise applies to investigators, the part that grounds the justification and requirement for confidentiality in its social utility. If researchers violated the confidence of their subjects, subjects would refuse to cooperate with them. This, in turn, would make it difficult, if not impossible, for researchers to contribute to the development of generalizable knowledge.

Over the millennia, the professions have viewed the obligation to maintain confidentiality as very important. The Hippocratic Oath requires, "What I may see or hear in the course of the treatment or even outside the treatment in regard to the life of men, which on no account one must spread abroad, I will keep to myself holding such things shameful to be spoken about."

Thomas Percival's *Code of Medical Ethics* (31), on which was based the first code of ethics of the American Medical Association, incorporated the following exhortation: "Patients should be interrogated concerning their complaints in a tone of voice which cannot be overheard."

In all states, the law not only recognizes the obligation of physicians and many other professionals to maintain confidentiality, it requires it. In many states, there are statutes granting testimonial privilege to information secured by physicians from patients in the course of medical practice (32). Testimonial privilege means that physicians cannot be compelled to disclose such information even under subpoena. Although the United States Supreme Court refused to extend the constitutional protections of privacy to physician–patient communications, the *Federal Rules of Evidence,* promulgated by the Judicial Conference, defer to state law on physician–patient privilege (32).

Most state laws on physician–patient privilege contain various exceptions, including mandatory reporting of information regarding battered and abused children, various communicable diseases, gunshot wounds, and certain proceedings concerned with health issues, including workers' compensation and insurance claims (32).

In 1974, in the case of *Tarasoff* v. *Board of Regents,* the supreme court of California ruled that a psychiatrist has a duty to protect the intended victim of a patient's threat of violence, if it is likely that such a threat would be carried out (33); this often but not always entails a duty to warn the intended victim. Subsequently, this duty has been recognized in many other states. The same principle is often invoked in debates over whether state laws should be changed to either permit or require doctors to warn sexual partners of persons infected with the HIV virus if they are unwilling to do so themselves (34).

It must be recognized that the right to confidentiality or privilege belongs to the patient. The patient may authorize sharing of private information for whatever purposes he or she chooses. In civil or criminal litigation where the patient makes the information in his or her medical record material to the support of his or her position, as so often happens in child custody cases or malpractice litigation, the court usually requires that the contents of the record be disclosed (33).

CONFIDENTIALITY IN RESEARCH

Most direct social injuries to research subjects result from breaches of confidentiality. An investigator may identify a subject as a drug or alcohol abuser, as a participant in various deviant sexual practices, as having any of a variety of diseases that may be deemed unacceptable by his or her family or social or political group, as having a higher or lower income than acquaintances might have predicted, as a felon, and so on. If certain individuals know such information, it might cost the subject his or her reputation, job, social standing, credit, or citizenship.

In recognition of these threats of social injury, federal regulations require the IRB to determine that "Where appropriate, there are adequate provisions to protect the privacy of subjects and to maintain the confidentiality of data" (45 CFR 46.111a).

How does one determine that provisions to maintain confidentiality are "adequate"? The first step is to become aware of the variety of factors that may pose threats to confidentiality in the research context. The second is to become aware of the various devices that are available to secure the confidentiality of research data.

The National Commission (35) offered some suggestions for safeguards of confidentiality: Depending on the degree of sensitivity of the data, appropriate methods may include coding or removal of individual identifiers as soon as possible, limitation of access to data, or the use of locked file cabinets. Researchers occasionally collect data that, if disclosed, would put subjects in legal jeopardy. Because research records are subject to subpoena, the National Commission suggests that when the identity of subjects who have committed crimes is to be recorded, the study should be conducted under assurances of confidentiality that are available from DHHS as well as the Department of Justice. For detailed information on these assurances of confidentiality, which provide immunity from subpoena, see (36).

CONSENT

As mentioned in the preceding, informed consent regulations require "a statement describing the extent, if any, to which confidentiality of records identifying the subject will be maintained." Statements about confidentiality of research records should not promise more than the researchers can guarantee. For most studies in which the private information to be collected is not especially sensitive, it suffices to state that the researchers intend to maintain confidentiality, that they will take precautions against violations, and that all reports of the research will be in the form of aggregated data and devoid of identifiers. When dealing with more sensitive information, it may be useful to specify some of the precautions; for example, videotapes will be destroyed within 60 days or, if the subject so requests, earlier; data will be kept in locked files; individuals will be identified by a code and only a small number of researchers will have access to the key that links code numbers to identifiers.

Plans to incorporate data in the subject's medical record should be made explicit. In general, when these data are relevant to patient management, they should be incorporated unless the subject objects. Incorporation of the results of nonvalidated diagnostic tests may lead to false diagnostic inferences, with adverse consequences to the patient's medical care or insurability. Most people do not understand the full implications of signing forms that release their medical records to insurance companies (37).

It is essential to disclose all serious threats of confidentiality breaches that can be anticipated. One such disclosure was used in a study of devices designed to encourage young children who are thought to have been abused sexually to speak freely of their experiences. A portion of the permission form for the normal control subjects reads as follows (3):

> Because this study is not intended to be related to either diagnosis or therapy for you or your child, you are entitled to decide whether the information obtained during this study should be entered into the medical record. If, however, during your child's interview, his or her behavior raises a concern of sexual abuse, a clinical evaluation of your child will be performed.... If after that evaluation the suspicion of sexual abuse persists, the case will be reported as mandated by law.

FDA regulations require (21 CFR 50.25a) "a statement describing the extent, if any, to which confidentiality of records identifying the subject will be maintained and notes the possibility that the [FDA] may inspect the records."

As noted earlier, federal regulations permit waiver of the informed consent requirement under certain conditions. These conditions are usually but not invariably met in studies of medical records (given adequate safeguards of confidentiality) or of "leftover" specimens obtained at autopsy, surgery, or collection for diagnostic purposes of body fluids such as blood or urine. In general, use of tissues or fluids without consent is justified if two conditions are satisfied (3): a) No more tissue or fluid is removed than the amount needed to accomplish the medically indicated purpose of removal; and b) the specimens are obtained by the researcher under conditions of anonymity (the diagnostic laboratory removes all personal identifiers before giving the specimens to the researcher).[9]

The practices just described are invasions of privacy. In such cases, patients are said to have a right of notice, that is, a right to be notified that such practices occur in the institution. These notices, which partially mitigate the invasion, are commonly printed in patient information brochures and on permission forms for surgery or autopsy. Although they are designed to afford patients opportunities to object, objections are rare. For examples of such notices, see Levine (3).

In some cases, with suitable justification, even the right of notice may be waived. Examples of such activities include collections of cord blood from neonates under conditions of anonymity in a nationwide study to determine the prevalence of HIV antibodies (3); monitoring for compliance in some randomized clinical trials (3); and covert observation or recording of public behavior (3). Further discussion of these activities and their justification is beyond the scope of this chapter. It must be noted that covert observation is a mild form of deception. In some cases even stronger forms of deception may be justified (3, 38).

Researchers commonly use medical or laboratory records to identify patients who might be suitable subjects for their studies. Having identified them, they then contact them by telephone or mail with invitations to participate in research. Those who are contacted usually do not recall having read notices describing such activities in hospital brochures. Some will wonder why a stranger who knows his or her diagnosis is calling. Careful plans must be made to avoid offending patients in such activities (3).

CHILDREN AND PRIVACY

The concerns of young children about privacy are different from those of older children and adolescents (39). Young children first develop territorial privacy ("This is my room") and possessional privacy ("This is my tricycle") and only later begin to develop informational privacy (concerns about others' knowledge of one's activities, associations, and interests). Thus young children may not know that what they say to others may be detrimental to the privacy interests of their families.

DHHS regulations are responsive to this concern. There are several classes of research that are generally considered so free of complicated ethical problems that they are exempted from coverage by the regulations (45 CFR 46.101b). Two of these exemptions do not apply to research involving children: a) research involving survey or interview procedures; and b) research involving observation of public behavior in which the researcher is a participant. These activities are not exempt in cases in which they "could reasonably place the subject at risk of criminal or civil liability or be damaging to the subject's financial standing or employability."

Researchers often must secure the approval of various custodians of children to involve them in research. Such custodians may be teachers, daycare workers, camp counselors, and the like. At times it is important to withhold or disguise some of the purposes of the research in order to protect the family's privacy or to avoid prejudicial treatment of children. For example, one would generally avoid telling teachers that the children are selected because they are offspring of parents with emotional disturbances.

As mentioned, informed consent requires "an explanation of the purpose of research." Does this mean that parents must always receive a full disclosure of purposes? Suppose the purpose is—as it was in one study—to determine whether little boys with XYY chromosome patterns are more likely than those with XY patterns to develop violent behavior. Disclosure of such a purpose could become a self-fulfilling prophecy. For further discussion of withholding the purpose of research and its justification, see Levine (3).

As mentioned earlier, the requirement for parental permission may be waived in "research designed to identify factors related to the incidence or treatment of certain conditions in adolescents for which ... they may legally receive treatment without parental consent." In general, the types of activities contemplated by this rule are treatment of sexually transmitted diseases, provision of contraceptive advice, and other matters that teenagers consider highly sensitive. We recognize the teenager's right to privacy, but how far should we go to protect it? Some of the factors that require consideration are illustrated in the following exchange.

Herceg-Baron (40) published a case study in which she detailed some of the special problems involved in research in the field of family planning involving minors as subjects. Many adolescents wish to seek advice about such matters as contraception without the awareness of such others as their parents. She details her institution's policy for protecting the minors' confidentiality. For instance, with regard to followup, investigators are required to offer various options, for example, telephone calls during certain hours when the minor knows she will be at home alone; contacts through school personnel such as nurses, teachers, or counselors; contacts by mail containing no agency letterhead or other identifying information; or leaving messages with friends.

In commenting on this case study, Carol Levine (41) raises several concerns. First, she suggests that many adolescents are ambivalent about clandestine sex and would, with some encouragement, welcome open discussion with their parents. The great concern with privacy seems to undermine the possibility for what could be valuable communication within the family. Levine is further concerned about the fact that the institution not only approves deception, it collaborates with the adolescent in deceiving her parents. This, she argues, sets a very poor example for the adolescent.

This brings us back to a point discussed in the preceding. Parents are not the only adults having responsibility for guiding the child to become the "right kind of person." Professionals must be aware of the fact that children see them as models of proper behavior. Consciously or otherwise, they provide examples that children will emulate. Accordingly, they should be especially careful not to suggest by example that promises (e.g., of confidentiality), truthfulness, and other ethical matters discussed in this chapter are to be taken lightly. In short, they should help children understand the importance of showing respect for persons.

ACKNOWLEDGMENTS

This work was funded in part by grant 1 P30 MH 62294 01A1 from the National Institute of Mental Health and a grant

[9] In some cases it may be impossible to remove identifiers, as when the patient's physician is also the researcher. In such cases the requirement for consent may be waived if the research will not yield any information having diagnostic significance. For further discussion of this point, see Levine (3).

from the Patrick and Catherine Weldon Donaghue Medical Research Foundation.

Portions of this chapter are excerpted or adapted from Levine RJ: *Ethics and Regulation of Clinical Research*, 2nd ed. New Haven, CT, Yale University Press, 1988.

References

1. National Commission for the Protection of Human Subjects of Biomedical and Behavioral Research: *The Belmont Report: Ethical Principles and Guidelines for the Protection of Human Subjects of Research*. (DHEW publication no. [OS] 78-0012). Washington, DC, U.S. Department of Health, Education, and Welfare, 1978.
2. President's Commission for the Study of Ethical Problems in Medicine and Biomedical and Behavioral Research. *Summing Up* (stock no. 040-000-00475-1). Washington, DC, U.S. Government Printing Office, 1983.
3. Levine RJ: *Ethics and Regulation of Clinical Research*, 2nd ed. New Haven, Yale University Press, 1988.
4. Nuremberg Code (in) Trials of War Criminals before the Nuremberg Military Tribunals: Control Council Law no. 10 (vol. 2). Washington, DC, U.S. Government Printing Office, 1949, pp. 181–182.
5. Katz J: *The Silent World of Doctor and Patient*. New York, Free Press, 1984.
6. Holder AR: *Medical Malpractice Law*, 2nd ed. New York, Wiley, 1978.
7. Curran WJ: Ethical issues in short term and long term psychiatric research. In: Ayd FJ (ed): *Medical, Moral, and Legal Issues in Mental Health Care*. Baltimore, Williams & Wilkins, 1974.
8. *Canterbury* v. *Spence*, 464 F 2d 72, CA DC 1972.
9. President's Commission for the Study of Ethical Problems in Medicine and Biomedical and Behavioral Research: *Making Health Care Decisions: The Ethical and Legal Implications of Informed Consent in the Patient–Practitioner Relationship* (stock no. 040-000-00459-9). Washington, DC, U.S. Government Printing Office, 1982.
10. Freedman B: A moral theory of informed consent. *Hastings Ctr Rep* 5(4):32–39, 1975.
11. Ramsey P: The enforcement of morals: Nontherapeutic research on children. *Hastings Ctr Rep* 6(4):21–30, 1976.
12. McCormick RA: Proxy consent in the experimentation situation. *Perspect Biol Med* 18(2):2–20, 1974.
13. Ackerman TF: Fooling ourselves with child autonomy and assent in nontherapeutic clinical research. *Clin Res* 27:345–348, 1979.
14. Gaylin W: Competence: No longer all or none. In: Gaylin W, Macklin R (eds): *Who Speaks for the Child?* New York, Plenum, 1982, pp. 27–54.
15. Weithorn LA: Children's capacities to decide about participation in research. *IRB: Rev Hum Subjects Res* 5(2):1–5, 1983.
16. Weithorn LA: Involving children in decisions involving their own welfare. In: Melton GB, Koocher GP, Saks MI (eds): *Children's Competence to Consent*. New York, Plenum, 1983, pp. 235–260.
17. National Commission for the Protection of Human Subjects of Biomedical and Behavioral Research: *Research Involving Children: Report and Recommendations* (DHEW publication no. [OS] 77-0004). Washington, DC, U.S. Department of Health, Education, and Welfare, 1977.
18. Thomasma DC, Mauer AM: Ethical complications of clinical therapeutic research on children. *Soc Sci Med* 16:913–919, 1982.
19. Levine RJ: The impact of HIV infection on society's perception of clinical trials. *Kennedy Inst Ethics J* 4:93–98, 1994.
20. Rogers AS, D'Angelo L, Futterman D: Guidelines for adolescent participation in research: Current realities and possible resolutions. *IRB: Rev Hum Subjects Res* 16(4):1–6, 1994.
21. American Academy of Pediatrics, Committee on Drugs: Guidelines for the ethical conduct of studies to evaluate drugs in pediatric populations. *Pediatrics* 95:286–294, 1995.
22. Groopman, J: The pediatric gap. *New Yorker*. January 10, 2005, 32–37.
23. National Institutes of Health: NIH policy and guidelines on the inclusion of children as participants in research involving human subjects. March 6, 1998. http://grants.nih.govgrantsguidenotice-filesnot 98-024.html.
24. Public Law 105–115: Food and Drug Administration Modernization Act of 1997. Subtitle B. Section 111. Pediatric Studies of Drugs.
25. Center for Drug Evaluation and Research: Frequently asked questions on pediatric exclusivity (505A), the pediatric "rule," and their interaction. http://www.fda.govcderpediatricfaqs.htm.
26. Santelli, JS, Rogers, AS, Rosenfeld, WD et al.: Guidelines for adolescent health Research: A position paper of the Society for Adolescent Medicine. *Journal of Adolescent Health* 33:396–409, 2003.
27. Levine RJ: Adolescents as research subjects without permission of their parents or guardians: Ethical considerations. *J Adolesc Health* 17:287–297, 1995.
28. Secretary's Work Group on Pediatric HIV Infection and Disease: *Final Report* (NIH Publication no. 89-3063). Washington, DC, Department of Health and Human Services, 1988.
29. Kelman HC: Privacy and research with human beings. *J Soc Issues* 33:169–195, 1977.
30. Bok S: *Secrets: On the Ethics of Concealment and Revelation*. New York, Pantheon, 1982.
31. Percival T: *Medical Ethics*. London, Russell, 1803. Reprint edited by Leake CD, Baltimore, Williams & Wilkins, 1927.
32. Brennan TA: Research records. Litigation and confidentiality: The case of research on toxic substances. *IRB: Rev Hum Subjects Res* 5(5):6–9, 1983.
33. Holder AR: *Legal Issues in Pediatrics and Adolescent Medicine*, 2nd ed. New Haven, CT, Yale University Press, 1985.
34. Gostin LD: Public health strategies for confronting AIDS: Legislative and regulatory policy in the United States. *JAMA* 261:1621–1630, 1989.
35. National Commission for the Protection of Human Subjects of Biomedical and Behavioral Research: *Institutional Review Boards: Report and Recommendations* (DHEW publication no; [OS] 78-0010). Washington, DC, U.S. Department of Health, Education, and Welfare, 1978.
36. Office for Human Research Protections (OHRP): Guidance on Certificates of Confidentiality. February 25, 2003 http://www.hhs.gov/ohrp/humansubjects/guidance/certconf.htm.
37. Siegler M: Confidentiality in medicine—A decrepit concept. *N Engl J Med* 307:1518–1521, 1982.
38. American Psychological Association: *Ethical Principles of Psychologists and Code of Conduct 2002*, http://www.apa.org/ethics/.
39. Thompson RA: Behavioral research involving children: A developmental perspective on research risk. *IRB: Rev Hum Subjects Res* 12(2):1–6, 1990.
40. Herceg-Baron R: Parental consent and family planning research involving minors. *IRB: Rev Hum Subjects Res* 3(9):5–8, 1981.
41. Levine C: Commentary: Teenagers, research and family involvement. *IRB: Rev Hum Subjects Res* 3: (9):8, 1981.
42. Brody B: Human subjects research, law, FDA rules. In: Murray TH, Mehlman MJ (eds): *Encyclopedia of Ethical, Legal and Policy Issues in Biotechnology*. New York, Wiley Interscience, 2000, pp. 675–683.
43. Kopelman L: Children as research subjects: A dilemma. *Journal of Medicine and Philosophy* Millennium Issue 25(6):745–764, 2000.

2.2 ■ EPIDEMIOLOGY AND PUBLIC HEALTH

CHAPTER 2.2.1 ■ EPIDEMIOLOGY

ERIC FOMBONNE

This chapter introduces the reader to basic concepts and terminology used in epidemiological research. In the first part, we illustrate how epidemiologists measure disease occurrence, design studies, and select samples to identify risk factors, and evaluate data to establish the causal nature of statistical relationships. In the second part, some achievements of 40 years of epidemiological research in child psychiatry are reviewed briefly. We first review issues specific to psychiatric epidemiology as they apply to the definition and assessment of child psychopathology in relation to the differentiation between normal and abnormal development, the use of dimensional or categorical approaches to case definition, the need to use impairment measures and to combine data from multiple informants, the need to take into account high rates of comorbidity between disorders, and the implications of pervasiveness or situational specificity of behaviors in estimating rates and risk associations for psychiatric disorders. Basic principles of measurement (reliability and validity) are defined as well as techniques used to screen and evaluate the performance of instruments. We then summarize findings on global psychiatric morbidity in children and adolescents as estimated from recent major population surveys and discuss issues relevant to special groups or new methodologies.

GENERAL EPIDEMIOLOGY

Definition and Historical Background

Epidemiology is the study of the distribution of diseases in human populations and of the factors that influence that distribution. The focus of epidemiology is to study patterns of disease occurrence in order to identify factors that are causally associated with the *onset* of disease in some individuals. Epidemiology relies essentially on *observational* (nonexperimental) methods. *Descriptive* epidemiology is mostly concerned with estimating rates of the disease for public health, or for administrative or monitoring purposes. *Analytical* or causative epidemiology concentrates on the identification of causes of disease occurrence in humans. *Clinical* epidemiology encompasses activities that use epidemiological methods to study other aspects of a disease, such as its natural history, factors that facilitate offset or persistence of the disorder, or relapse or other outcomes (i.e., mortality). One part of clinical epidemiology employs *experimental* methods (randomized clinical trials), where investigators can manipulate (through randomization) variables (treatments to which patients will be exposed) in designs that facilitate the derivation of causal inferences. Other types of epidemiology (genetic, occupational, psychiatric, ...) are defined both by the substantive area of research and by appropriate modifications of epidemiological techniques and tools, although epidemiological concepts and theories remain essentially the same across domains of application. The rest of the chapter is concerned with observational studies.

Epidemiology started in the nineteenth century with studies of infectious diseases, such as with the discovery of the infectious nature and mode of transmission of cholera in a London epidemic. In psychiatry, early efforts at the turn of the twentieth century helped to uncover the carential nature of the pellagra encephalopathy; or ecological studies of suicide led to hypotheses linking suicide rates and social change. After World War II, major epidemiological studies contributed to the understanding of the risk for cardiovascular disease or demonstrated the causal association between smoking and lung cancer. Explaining this relatively recent development, epidemiological studies require the collection of large amount of data that may be difficult and costly to acquire. In the last 30 years, epidemiology has developed as an independent discipline, with its own set of concepts and approaches. Medical and biological knowledge and statistical techniques are used by epidemiologists but epidemiology goes much beyond the statistical analysis of medical data.

Measures of Disease Occurrence

Several measures of disease occurrence are used by epidemiologists. We define here the three most commonly used: incidence rate, cumulative incidence or incidence proportion, and prevalence.

Incidence Rate and Cumulative Incidence

To calculate incidence, individuals initially free of the disease must be observed over a period of time. The example in Figure 2.2.1.1 illustrate new onsets of disease (or death, or relapse, or any other health event) among six individuals observed during a period of ten units of time (i.e., months or years). Some individuals (subject 1) are observed for the whole observation period, whereas others (individuals 4 to 6) have reduced observation times as they join or leave the sample during the observation period. Three disease onsets (individuals 2, 3, and 5) are observed; for these individuals, the period of observation ceases when the event has occurred, as subsequently they are no longer at risk of developing the disease and the observation time following the event becomes uninformative. The length of the line for each individual in Figure 2.2.1.1 represents the *person-time* experience of this individual and its own contribution to the denominator of the incidence rate. Only events occurring in individuals who are contributing to the person-time denominator are counted.

The incidence rate (IR) is calculated as follows:

$$\text{IR} = \frac{\text{N of new onsets of disease}}{\text{Sum of observation time across individuals}}$$

In the Figure 2.2.1.1 example, the incidence is $\text{IR} = 3/36 = 0.083$ time units^{-1}. IR can vary from 0 to infinite. It has the inverse of time as a unit (i.e., 0.083 per year) which, under some circumstances, can be interpreted as an average waiting

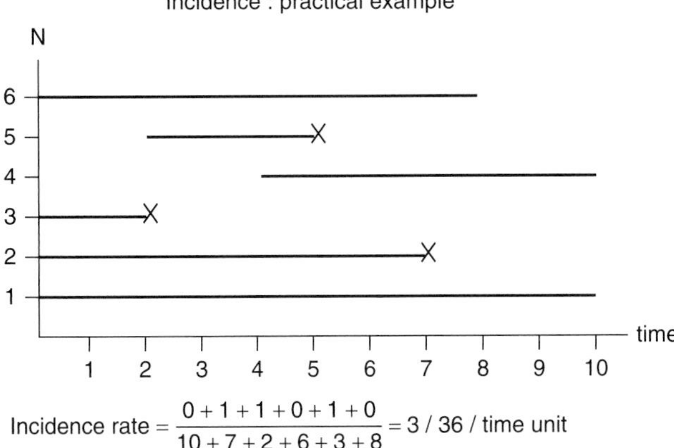

FIGURE 2.2.1.1. Calculating incidence.

time before disease onset. With a fixed number of events, the incidence increases if the person-time denominator decreases, as when the onset of new cases of disease occurs more rapidly, reflecting a faster penetration of the disease in the population. Calculation of incidence rates are more complex in real circumstances, depending on particular assumptions that hold true for the observed population (open [in steady state] or closed population, migration in or out, consideration of competing risks). Common examples of incidence rates are mortality rates, which have an easy intuitive meaning. For example, a young male suicide rate of 20/100,000/ year or 0.0002 year^{-1} means that, if one were to follow up 100,000 young males for a duration of one year each, 20 suicidal events would have been occurring during that observation period. However, the same incidence rate could be obtained with four suicidal deaths observed in following 2,000 subjects over a ten-year period. The numerical value of an incidence rate can therefore have different meanings depending on the study methodology.

Because incidence rates are not always that easy to interpret, epidemiologists use other measures of disease occurrence such as cumulative incidence (or incidence proportion). This measure is generally used for a closed population observed over a fixed period of time, all subjects being free of the disease at the beginning of the observation period. For example, if nine of 100 siblings of autistic probands develop autism from birth (the beginning of the observation period) to age three, the cumulative incidence of autism in this high-risk sample would be reported as 0.09 or 9% *over the first three years* of life. Unlike incidence rate, this figure is a proportion, dimensionless, and varying from 0 to 1. To be interpreted correctly, this cumulative incidence *must* be reported in conjunction to the length of the observation period, as the cumulative incidence will vary as a function of the followup time. In the previous example, if the sample is followed further from age three to five, another six cases might be newly diagnosed with autism, leading to a cumulative incidence of 0.15 *over five years* of observation. The intuitive interpretation of cumulative incidence is that it represents the average risk of developing the disease in the population under study (i.e., the summation of individual risks across individuals from the study population). One variant of incidence proportion is survival proportion, which is the complement of incidence proportion (survival versus death, no recurrence versus recurrence) and is often used in clinical epidemiological studies.

Prevalence

Prevalence focuses on disease *status* of individuals within a population rather than on the pattern of *onset* of new cases in that population. Prevalence is not a dynamic measure and, contrary to incidence rate or proportion, no passage of time is required for its calculation. Prevalence is calculated as the proportion of individuals in a population who, at a given point in time, have the disease. Prevalence (P) is a proportion[1] that is dimensionless and varies from 0 to 1. It is calculated as:

$$P = \frac{\text{N of subjects with the disease}}{\text{Population/sample size}}$$

Prevalence incorporates in its numerator recent and past onsets of the disease, and therefore the duration of the disease will influence the prevalence. If the disease is rapidly lethal or if it can be cured rapidly, the number of diseased individuals at any time point will drop and so will the prevalence. Thus, a prevalence rate reflects not only the incidence of the disease but factors that are associated with other aspects of the disease process (availability of treatments, natural history, lethality, . . .). The relationship of prevalence to incidence can be estimated, under some circumstances, as:

$$\frac{N_c}{N - N_c} \approx P \approx I \times D$$

where D is the average duration of the disease, I the incidence, N_c the number of cases in the population, N the population size and P the prevalence proportion. If the prevalence is small enough (i.e. <0.10), the formula simplifies to: $P = I \times D$. As I and D have respectively time^{-1} and time as units, P is dimensionless; it is a proportion that varies from 0 to 1. Prevalence rates can be useful as descriptors of the morbidity due to specific causes. They are useful for planning health and educational services. In some circumstances, they may also help generate hypotheses about causal factors associated with disease onset.

In psychiatry, prevalence rates are often referred to specific time periods. For example, a subject who has experienced a major depressive episode during the last 12 months but has now remitted might still contribute to the numerator of a prevalence rate if prevalence in that study is defined as 12-months *period prevalence*. In this example, any individual who met criteria for depression at any time point during the 12 months preceding the survey date would be defined as a case that would contribute to the prevalence pool (the numerator). The most commonly used period prevalence rates are 3-, 6-, and 12-months prevalence rates. Prevalence rates for longer periods of time can be useful to capture events that are either rare or episodic. Because the onset of symptoms of psychiatric disorder are often difficult to determine, psychiatric epidemiologists have often used the concept of *lifetime* prevalence. Thus, any individual who would have experienced a major depressive episode at any point during his lifespan would be counted at the numerator of a lifetime prevalence rate estimate, irrespective of his current disease status, of the age of first onset and of the total number of depressive episodes experienced by this individual over his life span.

Study Designs

The goal of epidemiologic studies is to examine whether or not particular variables are associated with a variation in disease occurrence. These variables are commonly referred to as exposures, as in the example of prenatal exposure to alcohol increasing the risk of neurodevelopmental and behavioral

[1]Technically, prevalence is a true proportion and not a rate (that implies different units of measurement for the numerator and denominator) although it is commonly referred to as a "rate," as we do later in the text.

abnormalities in children. Exposures can be susceptibility genes, prenatal or later life exposure to biological factors, a positive family history, psychosocial stressors, cognitive style or capacity, specific life events, and so on. When exposure to a variable of interest is associated with a demonstrated variation in the risk of the disorder, this variable is referred to as a risk factor for that disorder. A risk factor is statistically predicting of the disorder, but this relationship may or not be causal. The design and analysis of epidemiological studies aims at identifying risk factors and at evaluating the causal nature of their association with the disorder of interest.

Cohort Study

In cohort (or incidence) studies, the starting point consists of selecting two cohorts of subjects initially all free of the disease (Figure 2.2.1.2A). One cohort has experienced the exposure (exposed cohort) whereas the other (reference) cohort has not experienced it (unexposed cohort). Then, the person-time experience is measured in each cohort and the incidence of the disease can be estimated in each. The incidence in the exposed and unexposed cohorts is then compared by calculating an *incidence rate ratio* (Figure 2.2.1.2B) that is not different from 1 if there is no association between the exposure and the incidence. Conversely, if the exposure is associated with an increased risk of the disease, the IRR will be higher than 1. When the measure of disease occurrence available is the cumulative incidence, the relative effect of exposure on the disease is estimated by the *risk ratio*, obtained by dividing the cumulative incidence in the exposed cohort by that from the unexposed cohort.

Cohorts are defined by the exposure status of their members. Sometimes, one single cohort will be available, but measurement of the exposure for each subject will allow the construction of two or several cohorts according to exposure levels (unexposed vs. exposed; or nil, medium or high exposure). Cohort studies are difficult and costly to perform as they involve sometimes long periods of observation and therefore attrition can occur. One advantage of cohort studies is that several outcomes can be studied in relation to the initial exposure. Cohort studies are impractical if the disease incidence is low (rare disease), as the sample size required would be prohibitive. In some but not all studies, the investigator would be present at t_0 and wait for the cohort to mature (t_1) and live through the period at risk of developing the disease (*prospective cohort study*). In other studies (*retrospective cohort study*), the cohort study can be designed historically from data already collected. An example of this is the study showing a twofold increase in the risk of adult schizophrenia among subjects exposed to prenatal nutritional deficiency during the Dutch hunger winter in 1944–45 (1), a finding recently replicated for the Chinese famine in 1959–61 (2). Thus, the temporal position of the investigator regarding the data collection in a cohort study varies from study to study and is not what defines a cohort design. Knowledge of the biological mechanisms that might underlie an association and of the disease model under investigation are critical in designing cohort studies. Some exposures might have a long induction period (e.g., parental loss in childhood in relation to adult female risk of depression), which must inform the definition of the observational period and the data collection process.

Case-Control Study

In a case-control study, two groups are selected according to their present health status (with or without the disease of interest) and contrasted with respect to their past experiences of exposure to potential risk experiences (Fig. 2.2.1.3A). Case ascertainment must be as complete as possible in order to represent the full spectrum of the disease and to avoid selection biases, particularly when case sampling is not independent of the exposure. Cases can be selected from

A. Cohort study: design

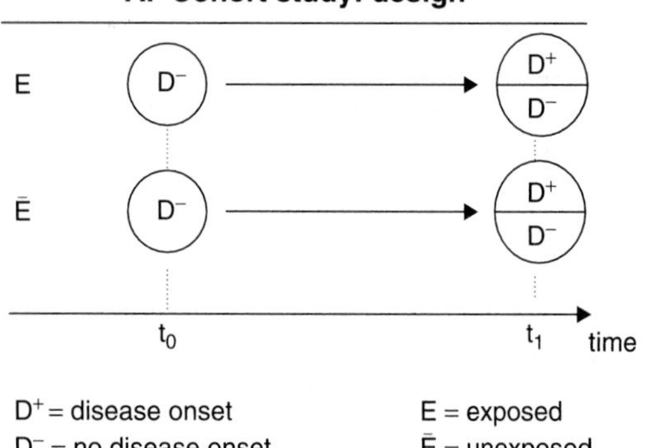

B. Presentation of data

	Exposed	Unexposed
Events	a	b
Person – years denominator	N_e	$N_{\bar{e}}$

a/N_e = incidence amongst exposed subjects

$b/N_{\bar{e}}$ = incidence amongst unexposed subjects

IRR = incidence rate ratio $= \dfrac{a/N_e}{b/N_{\bar{e}}}$

FIGURE 2.2.1.2. Design and presentation of data in cohort studies.

A. Case-control study: design

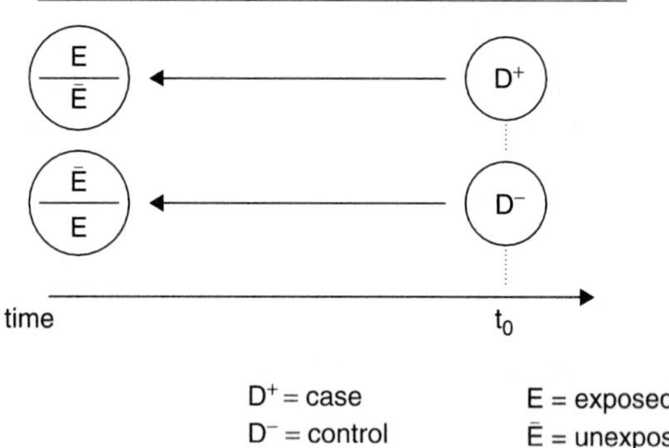

B. Case-control study: presentation of data

	Exposed	Unexposed
Cases	a	b
Controls	c	d

$$\text{OR} = \text{Odds–ratio} = \frac{a/b}{c/d} = \frac{a/c}{b/d} = \frac{a \times d}{b \times c}$$

FIGURE 2.2.1.3. Design and presentation of data in case-control studies.

the general population, but complete ascertainment may be difficult under these circumstances (i.e., identifying all cases of illness through hospitals, private clinics, and practices). Alternatively, cases may be selected in a cohort where more complete ascertainment can be achieved. Control selection is one of the most difficult design challenge in case-control studies. It is useful to conceptualize that the cases originated from a source population from which the controls should be selected, independently from knowledge of their exposure status. Controls should therefore represent adequately the distribution of the exposure in the source population from which cases originated. Only when this is achieved can the case-control analysis evaluate if the exposure experience differs meaningfully between the cases and the controls. An implication for this conceptualization is that it is usually wrong to select controls among healthy volunteers who are likely to underrepresent the frequency of exposure (supernormal controls or healthy worker effect in occupational studies) in the source population and bias upward the estimates of association. Approaches to the selection of controls that rely on friends, neighborhood, or classroom controls are appealing due to their convenience but may also pose threats to the validity. Numerous examples of such problems are found in the psychiatric or psychological literature, when patient data are compared to healthy volunteer data (i.e., referred depressed adolescents compared to high school students) or other convenient series of controls (classmates, friends, ...) leading to spurious "positive" findings.

To address the difficulty of control selection, two or more control groups may be selected that differ for their selection procedure and thus for the possible sampling biases that they each introduce. While intellectually appealing, this approach may be practically very labor intensive. Furthermore, there is no guarantee of the absence of bias when similar estimates are obtained when comparing the case series to each control group; conversely, if diverging estimates are obtained with each control group, the investigator is left with the difficult (and often impossible) task of determining where from and in which group the source of bias operates.

Exposure data are often (but not necessarily) collected retrospectively, making the study vulnerable to measurement biases due to differential recall (or recall bias) or missing data. For example, when interviewed and compared to nondepressed controls, currently depressed individuals might overreport past negative life experiences simply because their threshold for remembering and evaluating as negative particular events might be affected by their current mood state. Incidence rates are not available in a case-control study; estimates of the association between the candidate risk factor and the disease are calculated by comparing the odds of exposure among the cases and the controls (Figure 2.2.1.3B). One sometimes calculates the case/control ratio among exposed (a/c) and unexposed subjects (b/d), which leads mathematically to the same computation of the odds ratio. This calculation also illustrates how case-control studies converge toward cohort studies provided that the controls provide an adequate representation of the exposure distribution in the source population (i.e., when c and d converge towards N_e and $N_{\bar{e}}$, (see Figures 2.2.1.2B and 2.2.1.3B). The resulting odds ratio (OR) is an estimate of the incidence rate ratio obtained in cohort studies. Case-control studies can be performed more rapidly and are efficient. They are particularly required for rare diseases. Case-control studies also allow for the evaluation of several exposures in relation to a given disease.

Cross-Sectional Study

Cross-sectional studies are studies of large and representative samples of populations at a given point in time. Usually, disease status and exposure status are measured at the same time, and these data can then be used to calculate prevalence rates and prevalence rate ratios. Prevalence rates can be informative for planning and services purposes. Prevalence rates can also be compared in various subgroups of the population (males vs. females, high or low SES, rural vs. urban, ...) in order to identify characteristics or risk factors associated with disease status. Limitations of cross-sectional studies are that duration of the disease and other factors (earlier diagnosis, efficacious treatments ...) unrelated to disease onset influence the size of the prevalence pool (see above).

Ecological Study

In ecologic (or aggregate) studies, the unit of observation is the group rather than the individual. The level of analysis could be classrooms, schools, neighborhoods, municipalities, states, or countries. If both exposure and health outcome data are available at that level of analysis, their relationships can then be examined. For example, county suicide rates could be positively correlated with county unemployment rates, suggesting that unemployment leads to suicide. However, the joint distribution of exposure and disease is generally not known at the individual level, and it is possible that those individuals who commit suicide are not those who are unemployed (e.g., suicide might be occurring among young people, whereas unemployment would affect those over age 50). This interpretation problem has been identified as the *ecological fallacy* or ecological bias. In these studies, information about confounding factors (age, in the previous example) is usually very limited; in addition, the temporal sequence between disease events and exposure (that must precede the health outcome) can be difficult to determine. Ecological studies have the advantage of being simple and cheap to perform considering the wide availability of vital statistics and sociodemographic indicators in many countries. Time trend analyses and crossnational comparisons are also forms of ecological studies that may yield useful information not readily available otherwise. Ecological analyses can also be informative in circumstances where levels of individual exposure lack variability (i.e., all individuals in a population are unexposed or all are exposed). For example, studies examining risk of autism in relation to exposure to vaccination might be uninformative if every child in the study population has been vaccinated. Comparing rates of autism in areas or time periods that *differ* for their rates of vaccine uptake (an ecological comparison) might be the most informative approach. For example, rates of pervasive developmental disorders (PDD) increased in Quebec from 1987 to 1998 but, as levels of exposure to thimerosal through vaccines varied from medium to high and then nil during the same period, investigators used this natural experiment to show that trends in PDD rates were unrelated to exposure to varying thimerosal levels (3). In some investigations, ecological effects are also the focus of interest even when individual-level data are available. For example, one might want to examine the respective contribution to the individual risk of engaging in antisocial behavior from both child and familial characteristics (individual level) and of community characteristics (group level). Multilevel analyses of that kind have often been conducted in the social sciences.

Other Designs

Other study designs or mixed designs can be used in epidemiology. For example, a case-control study can be *nested* in a cohort study, which provides opportunities to ascertain a representative sample of cases and of controls and to rely on prospective (less biased) measurements of risk factors. In that instance, the case-control study would be referred to as a *prospective* case-control study owing to the fact that the measurement of risk factors *precedes* that of the onset of disease. Other study designs are discussed extensively elsewhere (4).

Issues of Sampling and Data Analysis

Sampling

In large population-based cross-sectional surveys that have been typical of psychiatric epidemiology in the last 40 years, sampling techniques vary from simple random sampling (SRS) to more complex stratified or cluster sampling strategies that aim to increase the precision of estimates, while optimizing survey resources and reducing costs. A typical example of a complex survey design would be a survey where two strata defined by the type of classrooms (special education versus mainstream) are selected and children from special education classrooms are sampled with a higher sampling fraction than their counterparts. In addition, if all the subjects within each classroom are selected, the natural occurrence of these clusters must be taken into account, as observations are no longer independent (the same would apply to household surveys). For example, the same teachers would be providing data on several children who also happen to share common experiences that may be determinants of behavioral disorders (teaching quality, physical characteristics of the classroom).

In selecting children for inclusion in the study sample, it is crucial to note the probability of each child being selected, so that subsequently these probabilities can be used to weight back the observations (usually with weights that are the inverse of the sampling fraction) for extrapolation to the target population. This allows oversampling of some subgroups without distortion of the final estimates, provided that proper weights are devised and applied. Taking into account the clusters and strata used initially as sampling frames is also required in order to derive unbiased variance estimators. The analysis of two-phase or more complex survey designs is discussed further by Dunn et al. (5).

Registers or Population-Based Electronic Databases

Registers are data collection systems maintained by administrative or public health authorities over time to monitor health indicators. Several psychiatric case registers exist that have been used in epidemiological investigations. When well maintained, they can provide an easy way to access and an efficient sampling source, from which various case-control or cohort studies can be derived in no time. Thus, national health and psychiatric registers available in Denmark or the General Practitioner Database in the U.K. have been invaluable tools for epidemiologists to allow them to test rapidly emerging hypotheses, such as on the risk of autism in relation to exposure to measles-mumps-rubella vaccine, or to the thimerosal content of children's immunizations. Different research designs were used from those sources, and including cohort (6, 7), case-control (8) or ecological (9) studies, all of which failed to detect any association.

Sample Size and Precision

In each study, the goal is to estimate rates or measures of association with as much precision as possible. Precision is decreased by various sources of random error, including imperfect measurements of exposure or disease status (see below), or sampling errors. In order to limit the loss of precision due to sampling error, increasing the sample size is a common technique that involves detailed calculations at the designing stage of the study that consider cost of sampling, sample availability, and preliminary estimation (based on past studies or conceptual considerations) of the likely range of values for the rates differences or risk ratios to be estimated. A tradeoff between gaining more precision by increasing sample size and the expanding costs of the study is often a consideration. In some case-control studies, the study efficiency can be tremendously improved by selecting several controls for each case. This would apply to circumstances where the number of available cases is limited, more statistical power is required, and controls are ubiquitous and cheap to obtain. Matching up to four or five controls to each case would maximize the power of the study. Beyond that number, the gains of matching extra controls become rapidly smaller and not worth pursuing.

Missing Data

Methods for dealing with missing data are crucial and have been addressed more efficiently in recent surveys. Participation rates in child psychiatry surveys have generally been high, often well over 80%. Bias in the estimates of prevalence and risk associations might result, nevertheless, if those who do not participate have higher rates of disorders, more severe disorders or disorders arising through different mechanisms. Empirical findings indicate that nonrespondents often differ systematically from respondents. For example, in a survey of school-age children, behavioral disturbances reported by teachers were 60% higher among nonparticipants than participants, but survey weights could be used to correct for this bias in the final prevalence estimation (10). Similarly, attrition bias in longitudinal studies may attenuate predictions regarding the persistence of disorders over time (11).

Missing data can also occur at the item level, with respondents omitting items on a checklist or failing to answer all questions in an interview. This may jeopardize data collection (if incomplete screens are deemed ineligible for further interview) or analysis (if incomplete interviews are not dealt with separately). Sophisticated statistical and imputation techniques are available to take account of missing data, different according to the reasons that they are missing (12, 13).

Statistical Testing

Point estimates of disease occurrence (incidence, prevalence) and of measures of association (relative risks, such as rate, risk and odds ratios) derive from the particular samples studied by investigators. The values obtained in one study are meant to be robust and unbiased estimators of the true population value, also called population parameters. In any one study, there is imprecision attached to each point estimate and epidemiologists communicate findings with 95% confidence intervals calculated around point estimates. For example, the odds ratio in a case control study could be expressed as: OR = 2.2 [95% confidence interval: 1.5—3.4]. A 95% confidence interval can be construed around all measures of disease occurrence and of association reviewed earlier. Confidence intervals provide a range of values that are consistent with the true population parameter under the present study circumstances. For measures of association, a relative risk of 1 is the expected value under the null hypothesis of no association between the exposure and the disease. If a 95% confidence interval around a point estimate for the relative risk includes 1, the null hypothesis is not rejected. If 1 is not included in the 95% confidence interval (as in the above example), the null hypothesis is rejected at the 0.05 significance level. Too much emphasis is sometimes placed on statistical testing. Statistical testing is necessary in circumstances where decisions must be made (treat this patient or not). In most studies, epidemiologists are interested in evaluating causal relationships, and a probabilistic rather than a black and white (significant or not) approach to this problem is warranted. Suffice it to remember that a very small effect (OR = 1.2; 95% CI: 1.05–1.45) of unlikely biological or clinical relevance could reach statistical significance only because the study has huge statistical power due to a very large sample size. Conversely, a larger, but statistically not significant, effect (OR = 2.9; 95% CI: 0.9–5.4) could point toward true associations of moderate magnitude. In those circumstances, epidemiologists who pursue causality will pay more attention to the strength of the association (the point estimate) and its interpretability in the larger context of the study design and findings. Causality assessment is better viewed as an ongoing, continuous, interpretative process that might be jeopardized with premature decision making rules embodied by classical statistical rules.

Bias and Confounding

Whereas sample size can influence the precision of a study, sample selection can limit the validity of the estimates obtained by introducing systematic (as opposed to random) error in the rate or risk ratio estimates. Various other sources of bias are well recognized in epidemiology, which are also briefly described here.

Selection Bias. Selection bias occurs when subjects who participate in the study differ systematically from the population that they represent for characteristics associated to the disease or exposure under study. Several examples have been discussed above. One other example of selection bias is selective attrition when, in a cohort study, subjects who are lost to follow-up differ from the cohort subjects with respect to the incidence of the disease. Migration in or out of a population or differential mortality are similarly potential sources of bias. When selection biases of that kind are suspected, it is critical for investigators to use baseline data to empirically test whether or not subjects lost to followup are systematically different from those who are not. Selection biases are a particular concern in case-control studies, especially with respect to the selection of controls.

Information Bias and Misclassification. A valid measure of the association between the exposure and the disease depends on the accuracy of measurement of both variables. Due to measurement error, a diseased subject could be classified as control, or an unexposed subject as exposed. Measurement errors on dichotomous classifications of exposure and disease status are described with concepts of sensitivity and specificity (see below). Classification errors are referred to as *misclassification* and a more general discussion of measurement principles and errors as it applies particularly to psychiatric research is provided below.

In an epidemiological study where the goal is to estimate without bias an association, a critical feature of misclassification is whether or not it occurs independently of other variables. *Differential misclassification* occurs when the measurement error affects cases or controls, or exposed versus unexposed subjects, with different patterns. A typical example of differential misclassification is recall bias. For example, in a case-control study of a severe birth neurodevelopmental abnormality of unknown origin at the time, mothers of cases reported significantly more psychosocial stressors during pregnancy (financial difficulties, marital difficulties) than mothers of controls (14). This suggested that psychosocial stress could be a cause of the negative birth outcome. It turned out that the abnormality was Down syndrome, the chromosomal etiology of which was only discovered in the months that followed. The only explanation for the spurious association between Down syndrome and psychosocial stressors during pregnancy in Stott's study lies in the differential reporting by mothers of cases (in search of a cause for their child's anomaly) of their past psychosocial experiences. It is important to consider that measurement error itself is not the problem if it affects subjects across groups equally. The bias arises from the fact that cases and controls do not report their exposure experience in a comparable fashion. Recall bias is a well recognized problem of retrospective case-control studies that can be addressed and prevented. For example, obtaining evidence from other sources of information, preferably collected before the onset of the disease (past medical or educational records), or through informants who are blind to the case status of study subjects, would limit the possibility of differential misclassification. Differential misclassification can inflate measures of association as in the previous example, or they may also attenuate them.

Nondifferential misclassification occurs when classification errors on exposure or on disease occur independently of each other. This type of misclassification almost always attenuates measures of association and biases the study results toward the null hypothesis of no association between the exposure and the disease. For example, in a case-control study free of measurement error of 200 depressed adolescents compared to 200 nondepressed controls, the presence of two or more negative life events (LE+) compared to one or less events (LE−) in the 12 months preceding the onset of depression is a risk factor for adolescent depression, with the ratio of exposure (LE + /LE−) being 80/120 in the cases and 40/160 in the controls, which translates into an odds-ratio of 2.7 (see Figure 2.2.1.3B). If one assumes now that life events are measured with an imperfect questionnaire method that misclassifies 20% of subjects truly LE+ as LE− and 20% of truly LE− subjects as LE+, and that this occurs equally among cases and controls (the misclassification is nondifferential, as it is independent of disease status), the ratio of exposure (LE + /LE−) is now 88/112 in the cases and 64/136 in the controls, which translates into an odds ratio of 1.7. In this example, the odds ratio is biased towards the null value of no association due to an unwelcome mixture of exposed and unexposed subjects in both cases and controls that blurs the true contrast of exposure distribution that exists between cases and controls in the absence of measurement error. Similar biases would occur if nondifferential misclassification applied to disease status. In general, therefore, nondifferential errors must be discussed in relation to negative studies or studies with associations of small magnitude. Differences in the error rate of measurement across studies may explain inconsistent or discrepant findings. In psychiatry, reliance on questionnaires and interviews, on lifetime measures of risk or disease experience, and on broad diagnostic groupings, are potential sources of considerable misclassification.

Confounding. Confounding factors are variables that may be responsible for a distortion of the relationship between the exposure and the disease. As such, confounding factors might over- or underestimate an association, and sometimes may even change the direction of the association. Confounding variables operate in all aspects of research, including in experiments. However, methods exist in experimental research (e.g., randomization) to limit the distorting effects of confounding factors. In nonexperimental designs, the control of confounding factors may be more difficult to achieve. To be a confounding factor, a variable must be shown (or known) to be associated with both the exposure and the disease independently. Furthermore, a confounding factor cannot merely be an intermediate variable in the causal chain linking exposure to disease. In a study where smoking during pregnancy is associated with later behavioral problems in the child, maternal antisocial behavior is a likely confounding factor. Maternal antisocial behavior is associated to smoking during pregnancy, and quite separately, it is associated with increased risk of child behavioral problems independently of its association to maternal prenatal smoking. Thus, the association between prenatal maternal smoking and later child behavioral problems could be entirely accounted by the confounding effects of maternal antisocial behavior. In other words, the cooccurrence of smoking and behavioral problems could be artefactual and entirely driven by their background association to maternal antisocial behavior.

Confounding factors must therefore be dealt with both at the planning and analysis stages of a study. When designing a study, it is important to include in the data collection careful and valid measurements of potential confounders. Confounders can be identified a priori by investigators based on past studies or on theoretical and biological knowledge about the disease and risk mechanisms under scrutiny. Another strategy is to restrict the study to particular sub-groups using exclusion criteria. For example, gender would be recognized as a potential confounding factor in a study examining the relationship between plasma levels of sex hormones and adolescent depressive symptomatology, since gender is associated with sex hormones levels and with the risk of depression. Restricting the study to females only is an effective solution but it has the disadvantage to limit the degree to which the findings can be generalized (nothing can be said about males). Another approach used by epidemiologists consists in stratifying the data at the analysis stage to obtain unconfounded stratum-specific estimates of the association that can be subsequently pooled together. Other techniques rely on statistical modeling, and techniques such as multiple logistic regression are often used to adjust the measures of association and remove the effects of confounders on the estimates. Detection, measurement and adjustment on confounding factors is an important task of investigators that is never ending. Thus, it always remains possible in every study that an observed association is explained by residual confounding effects or by unobserved and unmeasured confounding variables. Thus, replication of associations across studies is important to offer additional evidence for the validity of an association.

Causality Assessment

Risk Association and Causality Assessment. Measures of association in epidemiological studies (risk and odds ratios) are tested for statistical significance. When the risk or odds ratio departs sufficiently away from the value 1 that is expected under the null hypothesis, the null hypothesis of no association between the exposure and the disease under study can then be rejected. Two important features of this conclusion are to be noted. First, a significant association between exposure and disease reflects a statistical association between two variables. Demonstrating that this association is also causal is the ultimate goal of the epidemiologist, but requires several other types of evidence than a "statistically significant" result. Second, like statistical tests, the conclusion of epidemiological studies is asymmetrical. When the study fails to detect an association (the null hypothesis is not rejected), it cannot be regarded as proof that no association exists in the nature. Rather, the lack of association could reflect poor research design, sampling bias, or nondifferential misclassification. Conversely, when a significant association is reported, epidemiologists reject the null hypothesis of no association but causality cannot generally be definitely inferred from that conclusion.

Hill's Criteria. Stronger evidence for a causal association can nevertheless be evaluated using different sets of criteria. Hill (15) laid out nine criteria that he proposed as guides for evaluating the causal nature of an association. There are: 1) strength of the association, where higher odds or risk ratios are more likely to indicate a causal relationship; 2) consistency, where an association is replicated in different samples studied with different methods; 3) specificity, where causality is more likely if the association between the exposure is confined to that disease, as opposed to leading to multiple, unrelated, negative outcomes; 4) dose–response, where the risk of the disease increases with increasing levels of exposure; 5) temporality, where the exposure must precede the onset of disease in order to be causal; 6) plausibility, whereby the association could be referred to a biologically plausible mechanism; 7) coherence, where the causal nature of the association must be consistent with other aspects of the biological knowledge available about the disease; 8) experimental evidence, where the association is supported by the results of experimental manipulations of the exposure (in laboratory or human experiments, or field studies); and 9) analogy, when comparable associations can be identified in other domains of inquiry. Perhaps with the exception of the criterion of temporality, none of Hill's criteria is sufficient or necessary to establish causality. Thus, they should not be used as a mechanical checklist to "add" to the causal evidence, but simply as a set of arguments that may (or not) guide the interpretation of a given result.

Replication. An important argumentation for evaluating causality lies in the replication of findings across studies, preferably performed by different investigators, in different populations, and with different instrumentation. If findings converge (either for or against association) in studies that are otherwise likely to differ drastically in their potential sources of bias and imprecision, then the confidence in the interpretation increases substantially (although there remains no definite proof). For example, the recent hypothesis linking autism to exposure to the measles component of the measles-mumps-rubella (MMR) vaccine given to children in their second year of life was extensively tested by different epidemiological approaches that included cohort (6), case-control (8, 16) and ecological (3) designs that failed to reject the null hypothesis of no association. The consistent failure across studies to estimate a positive association should be taken as stronger evidence of the lack of association than that deriving from each study taken in isolation. Conversely, consistent positive associations between an exposure and a disease across studies strengthen the argument for causality. Metaanalysis is a technique that provides a quantitative route toward evaluating jointly the evidence arising from separate studies.

Public Health Relevance of Epidemiology

Epidemiology is the fundamental discipline of public health insofar as both the research methodology and the substantive findings of epidemiological studies are necessary to inform public health activities. Surveillance by public health agencies such as the Centers for Disease Control (CDC) is critical to the monitoring of the health of a population and for identifying variations in time and place in rates of disorders. Surveillance systems are also critical to respond to the emergence of new diseases (as in the AIDS example) or to changes in the incidence or prevalence of known illness (as suggested recently for autism). Vital statistics, including morbidity and mortality reports, have been traditional ways to monitor population health. They are often supplemented by specific and repeated surveys of disorders or events of importance for public health. Public health agencies have also the task to implement and evaluate universal or targeted preventive programs. Evaluation of models of service delivery, factors influencing access to health care, and more generally health services research, are public health activities that require the knowledge bases and contribution of epidemiological methods and studies.

Examples of the contribution of child psychiatric epidemiological studies to public health and surveillance programs are found easily. Several surveillance systems are in place in the United States to capture trends in child psychiatric disorders or problem behaviors. For example, as part of the Monitoring the

Future Study, annual surveys of large samples of high school students have been conducted since the 1970s to monitor rates of marijuana and other drug use. From the early 1990s onward, the CDC Youth Risk Behavior Surveillance System (YRBSS) have performed national, state, and local school-based surveys conducted by education and health agencies to monitor several categories of health-risk behaviors, including unintentional injuries and violence, tobacco, alcohol and other drug use, risky sexual behaviors, and suicidal behaviors. These surveys have been instrumental in showing that annual rates of suicide attempts are around 8%, affecting a substantial minority of teenagers. Monitoring time trends in the incidence of disorders has also been possible with epidemiological studies that relied on registers to identify cases over several decades. Thus, the Mayo Clinic register in Rochester, MN, has allowed investigators to detect changes in the incidence of disorders such as anorexia nervosa (17) or autism (18). Recently, the CDC has started a surveillance program of autism and related disorders in response to worldwide concerns about a possible increase in the incidence of pervasive developmental disorders.

CHILD PSYCHIATRY EPIDEMIOLOGY

Brief History and Landmark Studies

Child psychiatric epidemiology started in the mid-'60s with the British Isle of Wight surveys (19, 20). Prior to this landmark study, there had been few investigations of rates of behavioral problems in general population samples of children. One such survey emphasized the high prevalence of fears and worries and the discrepancies in rates of problems according to the informant (21). Most knowledge at the time relied on observations drawn from clinical case series. Behaviors were interpreted and theoretical inferences were made without having a proper calibration system of those behaviors that discriminated best between children seen in clinics and nonreferred children. Epidemiology, with its focus on general population samples and on comparisons between individuals with or without disorders, provided an obvious tool for the empirical investigation of child psychopathology.

The Isle of Wight surveys had key design characteristics that provided a model for surveys in the years after (22). A two-phase design was used with a systematic questionnaire screening of a large sample, followed by indepth assessments administered only to a subsample selected according to their positive and negative results at screening. Multiple informants were used at both phases, involving parents, teachers and children. The value of asking direct questions to children was established and interviews subsequently replaced the old indirect techniques (projective tests and free play) as investigation tools. Questionnaires and diagnostic interviews of known reliability and validity were employed for the first time to gather data. *Caseness* was defined according to both a recognizable behavioral pattern *and* evidence of impairment in the child's functioning. The surveys also adopted longitudinal approaches to measure prospectively risk factors and chart the natural history of disorders, and behavioral outcomes were related to neurological and educational risk factors (20). These methodological advances have been developed further in surveys conducted since. Two-phase designs are cost-effective ways to conduct cross-sectional surveys of large population-based samples and they have been employed in numerous child psychiatry epidemiological investigations (see Table 2.2.1.1 surveys). However, the value of longitudinal studies has been increasingly recognized by developmental psychopathologists and, wherever feasible, cohort or longitudinal approaches are preferred to study causal mechanisms underlying the onset of psychiatric disorders.

Measurement in Psychiatry

The planning of epidemiological studies requires precise methods to ascertain "cases" of the disorder under study (23). A definition of "caseness" must be adopted at the outset. Its nature should be shaped by the goals of the survey. A survey of autism to identify representative cases for inclusion in genetic studies will require detailed phenotypic assessments, precise diagnostic subtyping and exclusion of autistic syndromes associated with known medical disorders. If, on the other hand, the goal of the autism survey is to generate estimates of special educational needs for service planning, then a less restrictive and broader approach to caseness may be sufficient. Following the adoption of the most appropriate concept of the disorder, decisions must be made about the choice of various assessment procedures and instruments to evaluate caseness in study participants.

Definitions of Caseness

All epidemiological surveys have shown the high frequency of individual emotional or behavioral difficulties (19, 24). However, whereas some have a strong association with psychiatric disorder, others do not. Thus, in the Isle of Wight survey, thumb-sucking, nail-biting and bilious attacks all had very weak associations with psychiatric disorder (19). Similarly, item scores for *Asthma* and *Allergy* have been removed from the computation of the total score of the Child Behavior Checklist after consistent evidence that these were not associated with psychiatric referral. By contrast, the symptom of *Depressed mood* has been shown to account for much of the variance in comparisons of matched samples of nonreferred and referred children (24, 25).

However, continuities and discontinuities between individual symptoms and disorder may involve crucial transitions. Thus, depressed mood is experienced by about a third of adolescents in the general population (26) but the rate of depressive disorder is only about 5%. Similarly, some half of female adolescents diet, but anorexia nervosa occurs in less than 1% (27). The situation with substance use and abuse and with disruptive behavior is directly comparable. Many problem behaviors have a continuous distribution in the population and quantitative, rather than qualitative, deviance often defines psychopathology.

Dimensions and Categories

Because of this, most epidemiological studies use a mixture of dimensional and categorical approaches. The former are needed both to assess symptom severity and to allow the adoption of different cutoffs for different purposes. The latter is required for clinical decision making with respect to individual diagnosis and service planning. The issues are not specific to psychopathology; rather, they apply throughout most of medicine (as exemplified by asthma, hypertension, diabetes—all of which have dimensional parallels). Sometimes it is assumed that dimensional measures are synonymous with questionnaires and categorical ones with interview assessments, but that is not so. All standardized interviews provide for various forms of quantification of severity or numbers of symptoms. Conversely, most questionnaires provide the means for deriving categories from dimensional scores with appropriate cutoff points.

The most appropriate choice of measure constitutes a crucial step in any epidemiological study (Table 2.2.1.2).

TABLE 2.2.1.1

PREVALENCE FINDINGS FROM RECENT EPIDEMIOLOGICAL SURVEYS

Authors/year	Site	Age	N	Instruments/Diagnosis	Prevalence			
					Period	Any Emotional Disorder	Any Behavioral Disorder	Any Disorder
Anderson et al. 1987 (101)	Dunedin, New-Zealand	11	925	DISC-C/DSM-III	1 year	7.3	11.6	17.6
Offord et al. 1987 (95)	Ontario, Canada	4–16	2,679	Structured interview/ DSM-III like	6 months	—	—	18.1
Bird et al. 1988 (70)	Puerto-Rico	4–16	777	DISC/DSM-III	6 months	—	—	17.9
Esser et al. 1990 (102)	Mannheim, Germany	8	1,444	Clinical interview/ ICD-9	6 months	6.0	6.0	16.2
Morita et al. 1990 (103)	Gunma prefecture, Japan	12–15	1,999	Isle of Wight interview/ICD-9	3 months	—	—	15.0
Jeffers and Fitzgerald 1991 (104)	Dublin, Ireland	9–12	2,029	Isle of Wight interview/ICD-9	3 months	—	—	25.4
Fergusson et al. 1993 (105)	Christchurch, New-Zealand	15	986	DISC/DSM-III-R	—	—	—	22.1^{C} 13.0^{P}
Lewinsohn et al. 1993 (106)	Oregon, USA	16–18	1,710	K-SADS/DSM-III-R	Current	—	1.8	9.6
Fombonne 1994 (10)	Chartres, France	6–11	2,441	ICD-9/Isle of Wight module	3 months	5.9^{P}	6.5^{P}	12.4^{P}
Costello et al. 1996 (107)	Great Smoky Mountains, North Carolina, USA	9,11,13	4,500	CAPA/DSM-III-R	3 months	6.8	6.6	20.3
Verhulst et al. 1997 (30)	Nationwide, Netherlands	13–18	780	DISC C & P/DSM-III-R	6 months	—	7.9$^{C\ or\ P}$ 0.9$^{C\ \&\ P}$	35.5$^{C\ or\ P}$ 4.0$^{C\ \&\ P}$
Simonoff et al. 1997 (72)	Virginia, USA	8–16	2,762	CAPA/DSM-III-R	3 months	8.9	7.1	14.2
Steinhausen et al. 1998 (108)	Zurich, Switzerland	7–16	1,964	DISC-P/DSM-III-R	6 months	—	6.5	22.5
Breton et al. 1999 (109)	Quebec, Canada	6–14	2,400	Dominic-DISC2/ DSM-III-R	6 months	—	—	19.9^{P} 15.8^{C}
Ford et al. 2003 (88)	Nationwide, England and Wales	5–15	10,438	DAWBA/ICD-10	3 months	4.3 0.9^{b} 3.8^{c}	5.9	9.5
Costello et al. 2003 (73)	Great Smoky Mountains, North Carolina, USA	9–16	6,674	CAPA, DSM-IV	3 months	6.8$^{a,\ C\ or\ P}$	7.0$^{C\ or\ P}$	13.3$^{C\ or\ P}$
Canino et al. 2004 (74)	Puerto Rico	4–17	1,897	DISC-IV/DSM-IV	12 months	3.4$^{b,\ C\ or\ P}$ 6.9$^{c,\ C\ or\ P}$	11.1$^{C\ or\ P}$	16.4$^{C\ or\ P}$

^{C}: based on child as informant; ^{P}: based on parent as informant;
^{a}: any serious emotional disturbance;
^{b}:any depressive disorder;
^{c}: any anxiety disorder

Obviously, that choice should be driven by the main purposes of the study. Questionnaires have all the advantages of economy and simplicity and may be the first preference if the goal involves only group differences and trends. They will almost always be used in the first screening phase of multistage studies. On the other hand, they are less suitable for individual diagnosis or for the assessment of uncommon disorders involving qualitative departures from normality. Standardized interviews have the opposite set of strengths and weaknesses. The chief decision issue with interviews is whether to use an investigator-based (semistructured) interview that obtains descriptions of behavior that are rated using a standardized research-driven concept or a respondent-based (structured) interview that obtains yes/no answers to carefully structured questions. Each has its own merits and researchers will need to consider carefully which is most likely to meet the needs for the particular investigation to be undertaken. A further decision is needed on whether to choose a broad-based measure designed to tap all the common varieties of psychopathology or rather to use one or more focused instruments. The former will meet most needs but are less suitable for uncommon or unusual disorders such as autism, schizophrenia, or Tourette syndrome. Whatever the particular choice of instrument, investigators will usually need to test their chosen set of measures and data collection procedures in pilot studies of adequately sized samples to determine the procedural feasibility and its acceptability by respondents. Pilot studies should be analyzed carefully using quantitative methods whenever appropriate.

TABLE 2.2.1.2

CRITERIA FOR SELECTING AN INSTRUMENT

	Interview	Questionnaire
Purpose	Screening/Diagnosis	Screening/Assessment
Main use	Epidemiological/clinical	Epidemiological/clinical
Reliability	Test-retest	Test-retest
	Inter-rater	Split-half, internal consistency
Validity	Content, discriminant, concurrent, predictive	Content, discriminant, concurrent, predictive
	Cross-cultural	Factorial/construct validity
		Cross-cultural
Coverage/content	Diagnostic categories	Psychopathological constructs
	Number of disorders	Number of items
Method	Face-to-face interview	Self-report (usually) or other informant (parent, teacher, clinician)
Response format	Yes/No (highly structured)	Interval
	All informants' descriptions (semi-structured)	Likert scaling
		Visual analogue
Completion time	Long (hours)	Brief (minutes)
Informant	Subject	Subject (over 10 years)
	Parent	Parent, teacher
	Other	Clinician, interviewer, other
Time frame	Current (last 3 or 6 months)	Current, last week
	Last year	Last 3 to 12 months
	Lifetime	
Age assessed	Depends on informant and content	Depends on informant and content
Training	Required clinical for semi-structured, basic for highly structured	None (self-administered) or minimal (interviewer-assisted)
	Availability of training packages	Literacy requirement
	Availability of manual	Availability of manual
Version	Paper & pencil	Paper & pencil
	Computer-assisted	Computer administered
	Computer administered	
Data entry	Laborious (unless computerized)	Easy (optical forms. . .)
Scoring	Diagnostic algorithms	Norms, centiles, cut-offs
Costs	High	Low
Repeat assessments	Modularity of the interview	Easy, demonstrated sensitivity to change
	Scale scores available	
Extra features:		
- other domains	i.e., personal and family details, impairment, burden, etc.	i.e., personal and family details, scholastic achievement, etc.
- suitability for longitudinal studies	Adult diagnostic interviews	Parallel adult forms
- observational assessments	Companion observational schedule	Parallel observational scale
- cultural context	Availability in other languages	Availability in other languages
	Validity in different populations	Validity in different populations

Situation Specificity, Multiple Informants

From the Isle of Wight studies onward, it has been evident that the agreement on childhood psychopathology between different informants is typically low, and is only moderate at best. Thus, in an epidemiological survey of six to 11 year olds, only a quarter of children scoring above the cutoff on at least one screening measure were scoring above threshold on both parent *and* teacher questionnaires (28). In a metaanalysis of 119 studies, Achenbach et al. (29) found that the agreement was best (circa 60) when the pairs of informants had similar roles in relation to the child (such as with mother–father or teacher–teacher), whereas the mean correlation fell to the. 20s for other types of pairs (such as parent–child or parent–teacher).

There are many possible reasons for this low agreement between informants. These include random error in measurement; different perceptions of behavior according to the perspective of the observer; different frames of reference and variations in the child's behavior according to both setting and interpersonal features. The relative importance of these different possibilities is not known. However, it is clear that multiple informants are essential for any adequate epidemiological study. That is partly because each informant contributes uniquely to the measurement of psychopathology (as well as contributing to shared variance); because when studying the correlates of disorder it is necessary to go across informants (or use composite ratings) in order to avoid halo effect artifacts; and because of the importance of differentiating between situation-specific and pervasive disorders.

That leaves open the crucially important (but largely unresolved) question of how to combine the data from different informants and from different settings. Although there is some evidence that different informants have different strengths, only rarely will it be desirable to adopt a hierarchical approach in which the report of one informant is automatically given precedence over those of others. Nevertheless, child self-reports are particularly important for the assessment of mood and other emotional disturbances. Conversely, they are of very limited use for the assessment of hyperactivity. Similarly, teachers are generally better at the assessment of disruptive behavior than they are of depressed mood. As the findings from Verhulst et al. (30) show dramatically (see Table 2.2.1.1), prevalence findings are often hugely affected by how multiple ratings are dealt with.

Clinical interviewers usually use their "best" judgment in order to weigh the symptoms endorsed by each informant, resolving discrepancies by personal rules derived from a combination of experience and theoretical predictions. That is likely to result in different clinicians combining data in different ways. Another approach is trying to seek to resolve discrepancies between informants through a conjoint interview involving different informants (such as parent and child). This might be helpful in eliminating some errors due to miscomprehension and in "reconciling" the informants (31); however, the method is far from free of problems, most especially in giving rise to delicate situations that threaten to breach confidentiality. Nevertheless, this judgment method is recommended for some diagnostic interviews, such as the K-SADS (32), in order to allow the generation of a single unique score for each symptom rating. A third commonly used approach uses computer generation of diagnoses based on predefined algorithms. The method has the advantage of accuracy and speed. The algorithms must, however, deal with differences in reporting by informants according to specified rules. Usually, a symptom is counted as positive when it is reported by at least one informant—the so-called "or" rule (33). This technique typically leads to high numbers of generated diagnoses.

For dimensional assessments, Achenbach (34) has revised the data collected through his set of questionnaires in order to solve this cross-informant problem. Based on systematic analyses of the CBCL, the TRF and the YSR, he identified common syndromes on each of these questionnaires, and core syndromes that appeared consistent across sex and age subgroups. Then, a set of cross-informant core syndromes that spanned at least two instruments was selected. These were subsequently scaled with the relevant normative sample. This approach does not resolve the problem of how to combine data from discrepant informants, but it helps in increasing the interpretability of a profile of scores for a given child (35, 36). More sophisticated statistical techniques are available to researchers to deal with the measurement problems associated with multiple data sources and discrepancies between informants (see below), or are being developed (37).

Reliability and Validity Principles

At the core of medicine, and of any scientific inquiry, is measurement theory. In essence, this specifies the relationship between a conceptual construct and empirical measures. With respect to psychopathology, the construct cannot be directly observed (such as self-esteem, for example). There is a good deal of evidence for some of the key psychiatric diagnostic concepts such as autism or schizophrenia. Nevertheless, there has to be an empirical means of going from observables (whether those be signs or symptoms) to the postulated diagnostic entity. Child psychiatry research has progressed tremendously in that direction over the last two decades. Far from being a question mattering uniquely to researchers, the same measurement considerations and needs apply to everyday clinical practice. In that sense, the choice is not between measuring or not (or between research and clinical practice), but rather between measuring with known and replicable procedures or with unspecified idiosyncratic approaches.

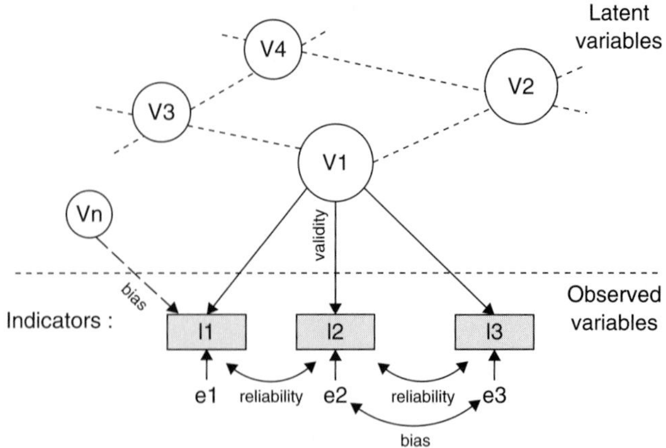

FIGURE 2.2.1.4. Measurement model.

Two major properties, validity and reliability, are examined in the evaluation of assessment procedures (clinical or research instruments, but also the simple clinical judgment) for which Figure 2.2.1.4 provides a convenient representation. Data collected as part of clinical or research assessments can be seen as empirical indicators of the underlying (unobserved) constructs of interest.

Reliability is the tendency of measures to yield consistent results over repeated trials. Reliability concerns the replicability of measures and the extent to which each measurement is affected by random error. Reliability can therefore be examined empirically (see bottom level on Figure 2.2.1.4). Typical procedures to estimate reliability are the test-retest paradigm, interrater agreement, and techniques based on correlations between subsets of instruments (split-half reliability), or among items composing a questionnaire (internal consistency). The reliability of the measurement is assessed within each procedure by specific statistics such as the kappa coefficient for categorical measurements (38), the intraclass correlation coefficient for quantitative scores (39), and other statistics [e.g., Cronbach's (40) alpha coefficient]. Reliability is a necessary condition, but not a sufficient one, for validity. If empirical indicators are unduly contaminated by random error (so that measurements cannot be replicated), then the question of their relationship to the constructs (the validity question) that they are purported to tap cannot be assessed meaningfully. On the other hand, high replicability does not necessarily mean good validity.

Validity concerns the crucially important relationship between the empirical observables and the postulated latent construct (a diagnosis, a psychological concept, etc.) as represented by the connections between the bottom and top levels on Figure 2.2.1.4. Several types of validity have been described. *Content* validity is concerned with the extent to which an instrument is representative of the universe of empirical indicators that are related to the concept measured. It is usually assessed by reliance on experts or on agreement with established instruments tapping the same concept. *Criterion-related* validity is the most empirical form of validity. It allows an index to be compared to an independent external criterion thought to assess the same concept. This can be either *concurrent* (high stress predicts cortisol levels) or *predictive* (IQ predicts later academic achievement). *Construct* validity is the most elusive and theoretical type of validity. Basically, it concerns the extent to which individual items or measures intercorrelate or group together to produce derived higher order constructs. Factor analysis has often been used for this purpose in the field of psychopathology. Thus, numerous factor analyses of questionnaires have consistently identified separate dimensions (or constructs) of psychopathology (such as attention problems, conduct symptoms, or emotional disturbances). These tend to map onto a broad bipartite division into internalizing/emotional problems and externalizing/disruptive behaviors (41, 42). Consistency of these factor analyses results has been taken as evidence of the construct validity of these psychopathology dimensions.

Diagnostic Reliability and Validity

In psychiatry, multiple efforts have been made to evaluate and improve the properties of psychiatric diagnosis. Since the first collaborative efforts sponsored by the World Health Organization to improve diagnosis in psychiatry, reliability studies have been undertaken to examine interrater agreement and to improve the definition, and thereby the diagnostic reproducibility, of disorders (43). In the late 1970s, with the development of research diagnostic criteria (44) and of standardized diagnostic interviews, emphasis was placed on the development of operational diagnostic criteria. This was embodied in the DSM-III (45) and its successors, and in the clinical and research versions of ICD-10 (46, 47). Studies of the reliability of child psychiatric diagnoses have been conducted with various schemes and instruments, giving rise to broadly similar overall conclusions (43).

Diagnostic reliability involves three rather different potential sources of error or variability: *information* variation (how data are collected); *interpretation* variance (how data are weighted and put together); and *criterion* variance (how algorithms are used to produce diagnoses). The first may be examined through test-retest studies to examine the extent to which the same answers are obtained on two consecutive occasions. On the whole, the findings have been of moderate to good reliability that is higher for symptom dimensions than for categorical diagnoses (48). This is affected, however, by the tendency for informants to report less psychopathology on the second occasion (48, 49). This is more pronounced with highly structured interviews but can be reduced somewhat by attention to both details of wording of questions and interview organization (50).

Interpretation variance can be assessed by determining the extent to which two informants agree (see above), or two investigators agreeing on their ratings of behavioral descriptions (51, 52), or two different diagnostic instruments giving the same answer. Typically this form of variance is greater—particularly across informant and across instruments. *Criterion* variance needs to be evaluated by comparing different ways of putting the data together. Standardization aims to keep this to a minimum but it is clear that different systems often give different answers (see, for example, the findings with respect to age of onset in ADHD (53), number of symptoms in antisocial diagnoses (54) or diagnostic algorithms in autism (55)).

Diagnostic validity concerns the extent to which a diagnostic construct truly reflects a syndrome that is different from others. The testing of validity, therefore, requires research that examines correlates of diagnosis with respect to basic features that are external to the behaviors that define the hypothesized diagnostic construct (56). Such correlates might include genetic influences, neuropathology, biological indices, course, and response to specific treatments. From a measurement perspective, validity concerns the extent to which empirical measures tap the crucial features that provide the basis of the diagnostic construct—that is the vertical connections between the top level (latent construct) and the bottom level (empirical measures) in Figure 2.2.1.4. The main measurement issue concerns the possible operation of biases in those vertical connections, expressed as Vn in Figure 2.2.1.4.

The main, possibly biasing, factor considered up to now has been the mental state of the informant (e.g., a depressed mother might overreport psychopathology in her child). To test that possibility it is necessary to determine whether maternal depression alters the pattern of associations between maternal reports of child psychopathology and teacher or child reports (57). The key statistic here relates to pattern differences and not to correlations as such. Thus, with respect to maternal depression the issue is whether a difference in child psychopathology is found on maternal reports that is not evident on reports from others. If there is, a bias is suggested. The weight of evidence from a range of studies indicates that there is some biasing effect, although not a great one. Recently, attention has broadened to consider whether depression in one parent alters the rating of the *other* parent by virtue of its influence on the overall family context (58). A comparable rating bias concern was raised with respect to possible *contrast* effects in parental ratings of twins. Thus, it was hypothesized that parents, in their ratings, might exaggerate differences between dizygotic (nonidentical) twins. Again, the test involves pattern effects in relation to the others. Such contrast effect biases have been found with respect to parental ratings of hyperactivity but, interestingly, not of other forms of disruptive behavior (59). Other examples of such possible rating biases concern the effects of a person's current social situation and mental state on their retrospective rating of negative childhood experiences (60). Findings suggest that there is a slight tendency for people who are doing well to *under* report past adversities but no tendency for people who are not doing well to *over*report (an illustration of recall bias). Obviously, to test this possibility, it is necessary to have longitudinal data involving contemporaneous measurement of the adverse experiences. Yet another example concerns the possibility that people with a mental disorder may overreport comparable disorders in relatives (61, 62). In all these examples the tests have involved some form of pattern difference that involves comparisons among different informants. Usually, the biases found have been small, but equally they have not been zero. The implication is that investigators need to use multiple informants and need to test for such possible biases, statistically correcting for them when required.

Latent Measurement Models

Historically, researchers tended to deal with these measurement problems either by choosing what seemed to be the "best" informant or alternatively by combining the ratings in some way (such as by adding them together or counting a report of a behavior if it comes from just one of a number of informants). Such composite strategies have the advantage of simplicity and, for this reason, they continue to have a worthwhile place in research. However, they fail to make use of all the data, they do not deal quantitatively with possible biases, and they do not remove random measurement error. Latent variable models were developed to deal with these issues [see Fergusson (63, 64) for clear descriptions of the rationale and the assumptions involved]. In brief, multivariate statistics are used to *infer* the latent construct (which can be either dimensional or categorical) that underlies the associations among a variety of behavioral measures. The focus is on the variance that is *shared* across measures—in effect putting to one side that which is unique to just one measure on the ground that, whatever its intrinsic importance, it is not measuring that which is common across measures. This "special" component is not thrown away but it can be isolated and examined in its own right. Latent variable methods also take into account prior probabilities and assessments in evaluating measurement error. Applications of latent construct measures in child psychiatry include studies of the impact of maternal depression on ratings of child psychopathology (65, 66), the crossinformant correlations of behavioral reports (67, 68), or the adult outcomes of antisocial behavior (69).

Impairment

The importance of including impaired functioning in case definition was well shown in Bird et al.'s (70) general population epidemiological study. The prevalence of psychiatric disorder was 50% if assessed on the basis of symptoms alone, without taking account of impairment, but 18% if the latter was required for case definition (70). Similar results have been found in other studies (71–74).

The need to assess functional impairment is now generally accepted but it has proved difficult to define and measure in a valid fashion. Impairment is related to concepts of role performance that reflect the adaptation of individual's adaptation into his social environment (75). This must be related to developmental level and sociocultural context. Typically, impairment resulting from psychopathology is assessed in four domains: interpersonal relationships, academic/work performance, social and leisure activities, and ability to enjoy and obtain satisfaction from life. These need to be evaluated with respect to functioning at home, school and in the community.

In earlier epidemiological surveys (76) and in most classification schemes (46, 77), the assessment of impairment was left largely to a global clinical judgment by the interviewer. In the early 1980s, instruments were developed to address this issue with the development of the Children's Global Assessment Scale (78). This instrument was shown to have adequate psychometric properties but it still relied on an experienced clinician, and did not specify how impairment data should be obtained. Further developments of this scale led to a simplified nonclinician version (75, 79). Another instrument, the Columbia Impairment Scale (80), was devised to be completed by both parent and adolescent respondents; it has the advantage of being brief and providing scores for specific domains. Preliminary data suggest that it is a useful measure, with the parent CIS having consistently better validity than the children's version. Other instruments exist, such as the Social Adjustment Inventory for Children and Adolescents (81) and the Child and Adolescent Functional Assessment Scale (75).

The issues to be addressed still include: 1) the differentiation between impairment and psychiatric symptoms (for example, aggression to peers is both a symptom of conduct disorder and a reflection of impaired functioning with respect of peer relationships); 2) how to determine causal connections between symptoms and impairment [preliminary findings suggest that informants found this difficult (75) and interrater agreement was low (82)]; 3) the difference between impairment and symptom severity; and 4) how to partition and attribute impairment in the case of comorbid presentations. Pickles et al. (83) found that depressive symptoms predicted later depression equally well with and without the presence of impairment; by contrast, the predictive power of conduct symptoms was increased in the presence of impairment. Angold et al. (84) found, in a community study, that over a fifth of children showed impairment even though their number of symptoms fell below specified cutoffs for diagnosis. These impaired children with subthreshold disorders were likely later to be referred to services, especially to school services in one study (74). Conversely, disorders without impairment tended to have a good outcome (85). The findings from the Ontario study tell much the same story (82).

Diagnostic interviews now include separate measures of impairment associated with disorders and symptoms (86, 87). However, research is still needed on the origins of impairment; it cannot be presupposed that they will necessarily be the same as for symptoms.

Case Identification and Screening

Case Identification

Once a case definition has been established, case identification methods are selected. Adequate sampling techniques are required to provide unbiased estimates of rates and risk factors associated with disorders. Drawing of a sample requires the availability of a sampling frame and of sampling units covering the population of interest. In child psychiatry, surveys have often relied upon school rosters [e.g., Fombonne (10)] because, with compulsory education, they provide comprehensive sampling frames. Alternatively, households may be used as sampling units [e.g., Bird et al. (70); Ford et al. (88)]. These approaches will still miss some children, such as homeless or street children (see Bird (70)) or those from families who migrate seasonally for employment reasons. Children in long-term residential facilities may also be overlooked. These losses will bias the findings if psychosocial factors associated with these unusual living circumstances are also risk factors for psychiatric disorders. Other sampling issues were discussed earlier.

Samples used in psychiatric surveys are often large, and direct interviewing of all study participants is not always convenient or possible. The two-phase design used in the Isle of Wight survey (76) has been frequently employed to deal with this difficulty. It requires a first phase of screening of all subjects with questionnaires easy to administer, followed by a diagnostic confirmation phase, more labor intensive, on a subsample of participants selected according to their results at the screening phase. The importance of understanding how screening instruments operate and how to measure their properties cannot therefore be overlooked.

Screening: Sensitivity, Specificity, Predictive Values

Dimensional measurements (whether by questionnaire or interview) lead to total scores ranging from a minimum (usually implying normality) to a maximum (mostly implying psychopathology). For both clinical and research reasons, investigators may want to transform these scores into categories (e.g., inferred normality versus inferred disorder). Figure 2.2.1.5 depicts a fairly common situation in which scores among normal (noncases) are plotted next to those with a disorder (cases) and show a degree of overlap. Any cutoff will partition these two distributions into four groups, designated false and true positives and false and true negatives. All cutoffs (obtained by moving the vertical line C to the right or to the left in Figure 2.2.1.5) would of course result in some degree of misclassification. The measurement question concerns the determination of what score provides the best discrimination between cases and

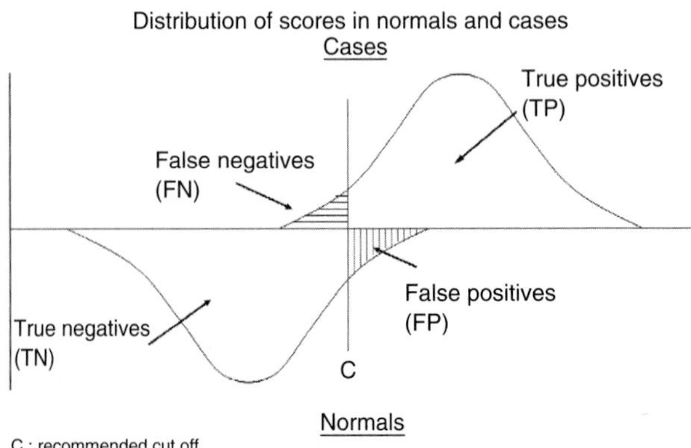

FIGURE 2.2.1.5. Distribution of scores in normals and cases.

TABLE 2.2.1.3

TYPICAL RESULTS OF A SCREENING EXERCISE

	Cases D	Normal $\bar{D}$	
Test positive : T+	a	b	a+b
Test negative : T−	c	d	c+d
	a + c	b + d	a + b + c + d = N

True positives : TP = a False negatives : FN = c D = diseased
False positives : FP = b True negatives : TN = d $\bar{D}$ = non-diseased
Sensitivity (or rate of true positives : RTP) : Se = a/a + c = p(T + /D)
Specificity (or rate of true negatives : RTN) : Sp = d/b + d = p(T − /$\bar{D}$)
Rate of false negatives : RFN = c/a + c = p(T − /D)
Rate of false positives : RFP = b/b + d = p(T + /$\bar{D}$)
Prevalence : P = a + c/N = p(D)
Positive predictive value : PPV = a/a + b = p(D/T+)
Negative predictive value : NPV = d/c + d = p($\bar{D}$/T−)

noncases and how the screening instrument performs in general. In practice, a cutoff has often been chosen before going to the field, and the results of the screening phase of an epidemiological survey would lead to a tabular presentation as illustrated in Table 2.2.1.3. Various important indices can be used to summarize the data in this situation, including specificity, sensitivity, and positive predictive value. Sensitivity and specificity are two important proportions that are often quoted to summarize the properties of an instrument. Investigators wish both of them to be high, but as is obvious from Table 2.2.1.3 and Figure 2.2.1.5, they vary in opposite directions.

Estimating Prevalence from Screening Data

One consequence of the imperfection of our screening instruments is that the prevalence of a disorder cannot be directly estimated from the screening data of a survey. Unfortunately, some authors sometimes report the "prevalence" of a condition to be equivalent to the proportion of subjects who scored above the cutoff during the screening phase (the prevalence of eating disorders or that of depression has often been reported as the proportion of subjects scoring high on eating or depression inventories). This approach is wrong as the proportion of screened positives in a survey is made of the sum of true positives and false positives (a+b/N in Table 2.2.1.3), which is very different from the prevalence rate that corresponds to the sum of true positives and false negatives (a+c/N in Table 2.2.1.3). To take a practical example, assuming that a near-perfect screening instrument is available with a sensitivity and specificity of 90%, the results of the hypothetical screening of 1,000 individuals are shown in Table 2.2.1.4 under two separate hypotheses regarding the true population prevalence rate. In both examples, the prevalence rate is different than the proportion of screened positives and, in the case of a low prevalence rate of 0.01 (Table 2.2.1.4A), the proportion of screen positives (10.8%) overestimates the prevalence by a factor greater than 10. Thus, the results of any screening test administered in a population cannot be directly interpreted in terms of prevalence, unless sensitivity and specificity are known for this survey and taken into account in a more complex estimating function.

Screening At-Risk Individuals

Another implication of the lack of perfect measurements has to do with screening particular individuals for the disorder of interest. If screening was perfect, we could infer in an individual with a positive screening score that he has the disorder; furthermore, we would expect that all individuals with the disorder would be picked up by the screening instrument. This ideal (but unrealistic) situation would correspond to a sensitivity and specificity of the screening tool of 100% (b and c would be equal to 0 in Table 2.2.1.3). As shown in the practical example of Table 2.2.1.4, the probability of detecting a disorder in a screened positive individual is in fact variable, and disappointing in the case of a low prevalence rate (Table 2.2.1.4A). This is despite using an instrument with excellent performance in terms of its sensitivity and specificity (both fixed at 90%). When the prevalence is low, cases in the screen positive group remain too few in comparison to false positives, making inferences about the presence of the disorder in a screen-positive individual child too hazardous to draw. The situation is much different when the prevalence is higher (Table 2.2.1.4B). Examples of this problem are widespread in child psychiatry, where detection and prevention programs have been evaluated, a case in point being the disappointing results in detecting individuals at risk for suicide with otherwise well devised screening measures of suicidal ideation (89). A corollary message is that properties of an instrument are context-specific and *not* inherent qualities of the instrument. Sensitivity, specificity, and positive predictive value are empirical, tangible indices of the validity of a measuring instrument. The example shows that some of these properties can be affected by the context of their application (the prevalence) and that validity is not an intrinsic, absolute, instrument property. Rather, validity must be (re)evaluated according to the goals and context of a study and validity assessment is best viewed as an ongoing process.

Receiving Operating Characteristics (ROC) Analysis

A scale or questionnaire is generally presented with one suggested cutoff point apparently associated with optimal

TABLE 2.2.1.4

TWO SCREENING EXAMPLES

A: Prevalence of 0.01				B: Prevalence of 0.30			
	Cases	Noncases			Cases	Noncases	
Screen +	9	99	108	Screen +	270	70	340
Screen −	1	891	892	Screen −	30	630	660
	10	990	1,000		300	700	1,000
P = 0.01	Sp = 0.90			P = 0.30	Sp = 0.90		
Se = 0.90	PPV = 9/108 = 0.083			Se = 0.90	PPV = 270/340 = 0.794		

P = prevalence; Sp = specificity; Se = sensitivity; PPV = positive predictive value.

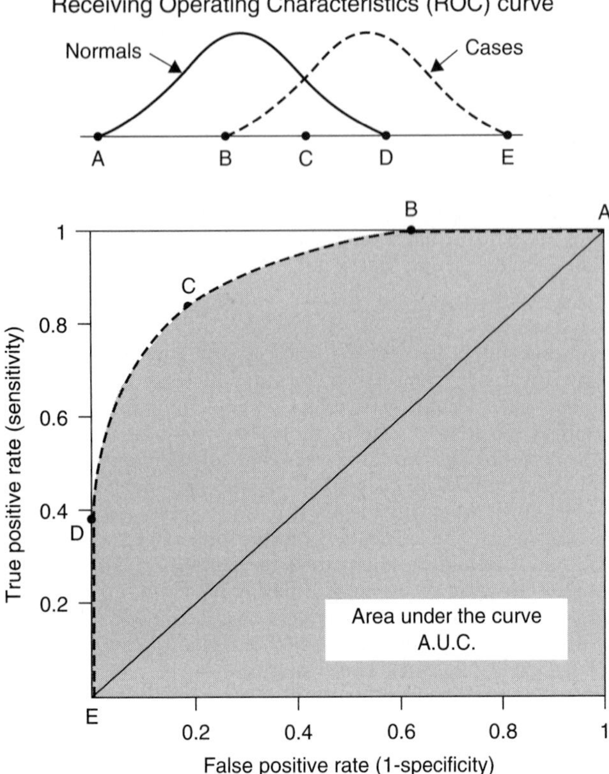

FIGURE 2.2.1.6. Receiving Operating Characteristics (ROC) curve.

performances (sensitivity and specificity). It is obvious that, as we move the cutoff point along the scale values, we would obtain different pairs of values for sensitivity and specificity. The investigator may want to vary the cutoff of an instrument to maximize sensitivity or specificity, depending on their study goals, the consequences of misclassification (sometimes, it is highly desirable to limit the false positive rate [increase the specificity] even at the expense of sensitivity, as in some biological or genetic studies), or on the prevalence of the disorder. The ROC curve simply plots sensitivity on one axis of a graph and the false positive rate (1-specificity) on the other for all possible cut points on a scale (see Figure 2.2.1.6). An ROC curve close to the diagonal corresponds to a poorly discriminant instrument, whereas the discriminant power of the instrument increases the farther on the upper left the ROC curve deviates. The area under the curve (AUC) is used as an overall summary index of the discriminant power of the scale. AUCs can be statistically compared to gauge the screening properties of different instruments, or to evaluate the gains or losses of discriminant power of a given tool when scoring instructions are changed, or items added or subtracted from the questionnaire. ROC analyses can also take into account the effect of the prevalence of the disorder on determining a best cutoff and evaluating the overall performance of an instrument, of the severity of cases under detection, and of the consequences of all types of misclassification errors (90, 91). ROC analyses have been helpful in promoting a flexible use of instruments that can suit better investigators' needs in their research contexts.

Major Psychiatric Surveys

It is outside the scope of this chapter to review the substantive findings of child psychiatry epidemiological surveys. Data on the incidence or prevalence of individual psychiatric disorders can be found in other chapters. In this section, we concentrate on current figures for overall psychiatric morbidity attributable to the most common internalizing and externalizing disorders.

Psychiatric Morbidity Among Children and Adolescents. Epidemiological surveys to assess prevalence usually rely on cross-sectional methods. Numerous prevalence surveys have now been conducted across the world [see Verhulst and Koot (23), Canino et al. (92), Bird, (71), Roberts et al. (93)]. Table 2.2.1.1 presents the main results of recent surveys. The overall rates of psychiatric disorders underscore the most important finding. Psychopathology in young people is common, most studies estimating the prevalence to be between 10% and 20%. Verhulst and Koot (23) reviewed 49 surveys and computed an average rate of 12.9%. Emotional disturbances and disorders of disruptive behavior are equally common (with rates of 6 to 8%). It should be noted that many of these surveys will not have included neurodevelopmental disorders such as autism and may not have picked up psychotic, bipolar, or eating disorders with an onset in late adolescence.

Community samples have also shown that only a small proportion (typically between 10 and 30%) of children with a disorder have had contact with specialist mental health services (88, 94–97). Disorders involving disruptive behavior (88, 98), and those that are severe or of long duration (99) are more likely to get referred. However, contextual factors (such as parental psychopathology) and family features also influence referral (100). The findings therefore indicate the need for caution in extrapolating from clinical samples or experience. Children seen in clinics often differ in systematic ways from nonreferred children with comparable levels of psychopathology. Epidemiological findings are needed for the development of psychopathological models.

Age of Onset. Age of onset is a definitional feature of several disorders. Enuresis cannot be diagnosed before the age of five, ADHD symptoms must be present before age seven and Asperger syndrome is differentiated from high-functioning autism by the absence of a significant language delay by age three. Age of onset is usually assessed retrospectively. However, the interrater and retest reliabilities of age of onset have been found to be poor outside the last three months for disorders with a recent onset and outside one year for those with a longer duration (110). Imperfect measurement of onset and offset of disorder can therefore influence prevalence estimates that are contingent upon specific time periods.

Age of onset also indexes differential outcomes. Moffitt (111) found that conduct disorders with an adolescent onset differed from early-onset conduct problems, with the latter more likely to be associated with neuropsychological impairments and with a worse long-term outlook. Similarly, adolescent-onset depression is associated with a particularly strong risk of recurrence in adult life (112, 113), whereas the course and correlates of depression beginning before puberty is rather different (114–116). The timing of onset is also crucial in order to explore the direction of causal effects in patterns of comorbidity. The demonstration that ADHD is a risk factor for later conduct disorder (but that the reverse does not apply) (117, 118) and that dysthymic disorder is a gateway to major depressive disorders (119) provide examples of this issue. Retrospective assessment of age of onset is also an issue in adult studies (120), particularly as accurate assessment of this variable can influence results from familial studies (121) and from studies of secular trends (122). One way to avoid the problem of unreliability in the timing of onsets is to use lifetime prevalence estimates [e.g., Lewinsohn et al. (106)]. These have the advantage of avoiding the problem of unreliability in the timing of onset and are probably the best approach for disorders present at the time of assessments. However, doubts arise over the reliability and validity of reports of past disorders that are no longer present. Such doubts probably apply less to disorders in childhood than in adult life because time spans are shorter and because multiple instruments are available.

Risk Factors. A detailed review of risk factors for child psychiatric disorders identified in epidemiological studies is out of the scope of this chapter (see chapters on individual disorders). Nevertheless, multiple risk mechanisms are now solidly established for specific disorders that have led to the development and systematic testing of treatments targeting these risk factors and to the consolidation of evidence-based practices. For example, the relationship between parenting problems, lack of maternal warmth, harsh discipline, marital discord, and the onset of antisocial symptoms in children has subsequently led to effective parent–child interventions (123). For many disorders, risk factors have been identified within the child (prenatal exposures, low birth weight, developmental delays, medical and especially brain disorders, IQ, cognitive style), in the family (parental psychopathology, marital discord, maternal sensitivity and warmth), in the school (classroom size, peer relationships, discipline practices, teaching styles), in the community (poverty, crime rates, access to drugs) and in broader societal factors (media viewing, body ideals).

There have been recent exciting developments in the systematic testing of causal mechanisms in child psychiatry epidemiology. Two are worth mentioning. First, the need is not only to identify a long collection of individual risk factors associated with psychiatric disorders but to develop models of psychopathology by examining the joint contribution of several risk factors operating in different domains (biological *and* psychological *and* social) and in the course of individual development. Thus, the first examples of the importance of gene and environmental interactions were found in a cohort study where young adults homozygous for the short allele of the serotonin transporter gene were found to be at much increase risk of depression when (and only when) exposed to negative life events as compared to those individuals homozygous for the long allele (124). The findings clearly indicated that psychosocial risk factors operate differently in individuals according to their genetic background. The simultaneous study of risk factors is necessary to refine our understanding of child psychopathology and move beyond the frequent oversimplified explanations that are in use in clinical settings (the patient *is* depressed because something bad happened to her). The key point, though, is that carefully selected epidemiological samples and measures, adequate sample sizes and longitudinal designs are necessary to fully evaluate these complex explanatory models. Second, new techniques of analyses of complex longitudinal data (trajectory methods) have shifted the focus from classical group-based predictor–outcome relationships to the identification of patterns of individual trajectories. Predictors of trajectory membership can then be identified, such as in the studies by Tremblay et al. (125) on the persistence or desistance of aggression over time. These methods are particularly suitable to the life span study of psychopathology and to a focus on individual differences in the onset and offset of psychopathological conditions.

Comorbidity. The high frequency of cooccurrence of two supposedly separate forms of psychopathology was noted in the Isle of Wight studies over 30 years ago (76). However, it is only in the last 15 years that it has received much conceptual attention and empirical study (31, 35, 126–129). In their thorough review of the topic, Angold et al. (31) concluded that artifacts cannot account entirely for the frequency and patterns of comorbidity and that mechanisms underlying comorbid presentations should be studied more systematically, preferably with epidemiological samples. Several research findings show how comorbidity may carry meaning. For example, the results of a family study of depression changed once comorbidity in the probands was properly taken into account (130) and a trend emerged for a positive drug response to tricyclic antidepressants in noncomorbid depressed subjects when results from a clinical trial were stratified according to the presence or absence of comorbid conduct disorder (131).

However, in order to undertake research using comorbidity it is necessary that the epidemiological studies' methods of measurement are adequate for dealing with the assessment of psychopathology that involves comorbid patterns.

Special Topics

Preschool Studies. Epidemiological investigations of preschool samples have been surprisingly few (132–138). Nevertheless, studies have shown that psychiatric disorders starting in the preschool years show a high degree of persistence over time and that their course is systematically associated with identifiable risk and protective factors. For example, a difficult temperament in the child interacts with characteristics of family dysfunction to increase the risk of psychopathology five years later (139); and a shy, inhibited style of interaction predicts later onset of anxiety disorders in childhood (140). Furthermore, evidence has accumulated that developmental disorders usually identified in the early years have short (141) and long-term consequences (142) with respect to psychosocial disturbances and functioning. Long-term followup of birth cohorts have also shown continuities between preschool behavior and adult psychopathology (143). Thus, identification of preschool problems is important, especially since early intervention might be more effective in the case of some disorders (144).

There are, however, particular challenges in the assessment of preschoolers (145). Infants and toddlers present with disturbances that tend to be closely associated with somatic development. Thus, feeding and sleeping difficulties are common in this age group. It is also an age when the effects of prenatal/perinatal risk factors may be particularly marked. Second, infants' behavior is closely intertwined with interactions with their caregivers. Accordingly, it is necessary to consider the extent to which any disturbance reflects psychopathology in the child rather than difficulties in a dyadic relationship. Third, specific developmental delays such as language or social relationships are first evident in the preschool years and call for a multifaceted developmental assessment. Fourth, very few dimensional measures assessing behavioral/emotional deviance have been properly validated for children below the age of four. Finally, current diagnostic schemes have acknowledged limitations for use with very young children (146). Scales such as the Temperament and Atypical Behavior Scale (147) and classifications such as the Zero-to-Three diagnostic classification (148) have been developed for infants and toddlers but they are based on particular conceptual frameworks and are closely linked to intervention strategies. However, downward extensions of psychiatric interviews have been recently developed and tested in preschoolers and have shown good psychometric properties (149). The use of this new generation of instruments in population-based samples of preschool children indicates that both rates and patterns of disorders and comorbidity in preschool samples are comparable to those of older children (150).

Norm-Referenced Instruments. Reference to normative data is implicit in the assessment of psychopathology. However, it was only in the late 1950s that systematic surveys of children's behaviors and emotions were undertaken on large samples of nonreferred children (21). The epidemiological surveys of child psychiatric disorders that followed helped to promote knowledge of normative behavior at different ages with the useful development of standardized questionnaires for use with multiple informants (23, 24, 76, 151). Increasingly, data from large representative samples of nonreferred children have been used to calibrate measures in order to provide the best identification of probable psychopathology. However, not all standardizations have used fully representative general population samples. There must be reservations about generalizability when convenience samples have been used. Second, norms are derived from particular regional or national samples and the query is whether it is justifiable to extrapolate to other regions or countries. For example, a 10- to 15-point difference in mean CBCL total scores has been reported among American, Australian (152), French (153) and Puerto Rican children (154). The question is whether these differences reflect true regional differences in psychopathology or rating tendencies that have been influenced by cultural contextual features. Both possibilities have to be considered seriously, but their differentiation requires the use of external validators of some kind. The Isle of Wight–Inner London comparison indicated that a true difference in rate of psychopathology was likely (155), whereas the U.K.–Hong Kong comparison with respect to hyperactivity suggested a rating difference effect (156). Investigators are well advised to be cautious about assumptions that one set of norms can be generalized to different populations.

Similar issues concern extrapolations from one large representative population to subgroups within. For example, are associations between social class and behavioral disturbance (24, 25) a true reflection of valid differences or a contextual rating bias effect? The same applies to age and gender differences. An automatic assumption that subgroup norms should be used or that any differences from total population norms are necessarily valid should be resisted. As ever, external validation is essential.

Third, norms apply to one particular point in time. Evidence has accumulated that there have been secular changes in the incidence of various psychosocial disorders (157–159) and of individual behavioral problems. Thus, Achenbach and Howell (160) compared two large representative samples of American youth surveyed 13 years apart and found increased scores on 46 of 118 behavioral problems and on all scale scores (the mean total score increasing from 18 to 24.2) in the most recent birth cohorts. Periodic recalibration of instruments is necessary in child psychopathology, just as it is for other measures such as psychometric tests (161, 162) or physical indices such as height, weight, head circumference and pubertal maturation (163).

Cultural Issues. Most industrialized societies today are multicultural, multiethnic, and multilingual, a fact that has important implications for clinical practice. In addition, it has implications for the assessment of psychopathology by means of standardized interviews or questionnaires. It would be a mistake to exaggerate the methodological difficulties. Rating scales have usually been found to function in much the same way across cultures (164–167) with, for example, comparable gender differences (152, 153, 167, 168).

Nevertheless, three issues require attention. First, there is a concern to ensure linguistic equivalence. This is usually accomplished by a series of back-translations from one language to the other by independent bilingual translators who are familiar with the psychopathological concepts. The last specification is important to ensure that the appropriate words are selected to tap the intended meaning. That is relevant, too, in relation to the need to ensure equivalence between American and British versions of instruments. The problems of going across languages are even greater and it is crucial that the translators appreciate the intended meaning in relation to psychopathology. Issues in relation to the translation of diagnostic interviews for Hispanics were described by Canino and Bravo (169) and examples of translation inaccuracies and of their effects on deviance scores were noted by Woodward et al. (170).

Second, there is the question of conceptual and perceptual equivalence. Thus, Weisz et al. (171) reported differences between Thai and American adults in their concern over particular behaviors; Lee (172) queried whether a morbid fear of fatness had the same implications for anorexia nervosa in Hong Kong as it does in Western societies; and King and Bhugra (173) posed the same question with respect to questions on dieting when used in cultures where this is part of religious practice. It cannot be claimed that there is an adequate database to show either the importance of these concerns or how they are best dealt with, but investigators need to be alert to their possible effects on measurement. They are likely to have effects because most ratings involve an explicit or implicit comparison with some norms, the behaviors being normal at a low level but abnormal at some higher level.

Third, there is diagnostic equivalence. Some cultures have syndromes that appear to have no obvious equivalent in other cultures, although systematic evidence on this is largely lacking. From a measurement perspective, perhaps the key point is that when different cultures express the same disorder through differently expressed manifestations, there needs to be caution in the application of diagnostic algorithms. For example, there is evidence that cultures vary in the extent to which they express depression in reports of feelings of misery; some are more likely to report these in terms of somatic complaints (174). Similar issues arise with respect to age variations, as reflected in the different role given to irritability in the diagnosis of depression in childhood and in adult life (77). Once more, there is at least as much of a danger of wrongly assuming an age (or cultural) difference as of overlooking a real difference. The arbitration has to lie in empirical studies. Recent systematic comparisons of children's emotional and behavioral problems assessed in over 30 cultures with the same instruments indicate that cultural differences are relatively small across countries, with mean scores for most samples falling close to the omnicultural mean (168, 175, 176).

Language of Assessment. Practically, as population samples in most countries reflect a mixture of cultures and languages, it has become essential for epidemiologists but also for clinicians to have access to instruments adequately translated and validated in different languages. The common instruments used to evaluate general psychopathology in children and adolescents are available in multiple languages. For example, access to non-English versions is obtained through specific Websites associated to the corresponding instruments, e.g., http://www.aseba.org/ordering/translations.html for the 74 international versions of the Child Behavior Checklist and http://www.sdqinfo.com/b3.html for the 61 translations of the Strengths and Difficulties Questionnaire. Translated versions of various instruments tapping specific dimensions of child psychopathology also exist and are available either from their authors or commercial distributors. Non-English versions of various diagnostic interviews also exist in different languages, although the work is less advanced than that for general psychopathological rating scales. It is prudent to check with the original authors of an instrument whether or not an available translation has been approved by them and properly established.

Studying Transitions to Adulthood. With a growing emphasis on life span perspectives on developmental psychopathology and an increasing focus on the study of continuities and discontinuities between child and adult disorders, psychiatric epidemiologists have now developed adult versions of child instruments that are suitable for longitudinal research and provide investigators with measurements that are highly consistent across age groups. For example, adolescent samples evaluated with a combination of the Child Behavior Checklist and Youth Self-Report Form can be followed as young adults with parallel adult versions of these instruments such as the Adult Self-Report and the Adult Behavior Checklist that can be used up to age 59. Versions for subjects aged 60 or older are also available (http://www.aseba.org). Similarly, adult extensions of child psychiatric interviews such as the CAPA or the DISC are being developed.

Interviewing and Computer Technology. Modern technology has allowed many assessment procedures to be computerized. For example, Berg et al. (177) compared the reliability, concurrent and criterion validity of two standard and computer-assisted procedures to collect data using two common psychopathology scales, the Rutter A2 scale and the CBCL. Psychometric properties were similar with the two procedures, suggesting that computer-assisted technologies might be used more extensively in routine practice.

There are numerous advantages to computerization: It eliminates observer bias; it ensures that all respondents receive precisely the same instructions and questions; by having a voice read the questions aloud it avoids illiteracy problems; it allows more complex and flexible skip and branching patterns than possible with paper and pencil procedures; it makes immediate checking of the consistency and range of responses possible; and it provides error-free computation of scores with or without reference to existing norms. Data are stored readily in a format that allows for further analysis; computer storage also makes the data collection procedure less vulnerable to errors such as accidental loss of data, theft, or inadvertent disclosure of confidential materials.

Several structured diagnostic interviews already have computerized versions. The role of the computer does, however, vary considerably. Computers are sometimes used to assist interviewers in their task of conducting the interview. In this instance, the interviewer still performs a face-to-face interview and records the answers of the respondent on a laptop computer as the interview proceeds. This procedure has both the advantage and disadvantage of allowing some degree of interviewer judgment. Fully computerized diagnostic interviews tend to be highly structured, with restricted response options. Computer-aided administration is particularly useful in helping the interviewer to follow complex skip rules and to track respondent's answers that require followup questions in the course of the interview. The NIMH DISC-IV (86) is typical of such interviews devised for large-scale epidemiological surveys. The DAWBA (178), used in the U.K. National Survey of Child Mental Health (88), provides another example, with the additional feature that space is allocated to record respondents' descriptions verbatim as well, so allowing a subsequent overarching clinical interpretation of all structured data and the addition of open-ended commentaries. This procedure, however, detracts somewhat from the greater efficiency of the computerized interviews—a major selling point. In other developments, computers are used to replace interviewers fully. Some sound versions of diagnostic interviews have now been developed for full self-administration, using headphones or speakers. The Voice DISC (86) and a substance abuse module of the CAPA (87) are examples of such developments, which totally eliminate interviewer costs.

Investigator-based interviews have been, for obvious reasons, less amenable to computerization, although some attempts have been made, such as with the DICA (179). One diagnostic interview relying on displays of pictures or cartoons to elicit symptomatic data has been released in computerized form [Interactive Dominic Questionnaire (180)], but more data are still needed on its basic properties.

Computerized interviewing does not usually decrease the time needed to administer the interview, but it can lead to substantial savings in terms of interviewer time (and costs) by eliminating that used for coding and interpretation. Successful use has been achieved in recent epidemiological surveys (88, 181).

It is possible, too, that computerized interviews may be better at eliciting potentially embarrassing personal information, because it eliminates the interpersonal context. Reich et al. (182) found that children enjoyed the computerized DICA-R interview, preferred it over a person interview, and said that they would tell things to the computer that they would not tell to a person. Survey research has shown that rates of at-risk behaviors involving sexual contacts and use of addictive substances were three times higher when questions were asked via audio-computerized methods than when asked face to face (183). Similar results have been found regarding suicidal behaviors [e.g., Reich et al. (182)].

It is too early to draw firm conclusions on the merits and demerits of computerized interviews. Clearly, they have very important advantages for some purposes and there is no doubt that they will be used more in the future. However, for some purposes, their chief advantage of eliminating the need to interviewers may be a disadvantage just because it eliminates personal contact. The structural format, too, will be limiting in relation to the eliciting of important unexpected information.

Computerized Clinical Databases. The progress made in the measurement of child psychopathology in epidemiological research has been paralleled by similar advances in the systematic evaluation of patients referred to mental health teams. Multiaxial diagnostic formulations and use of norm-referenced general psychopathology questionnaires are now standards in most clinical centers. Yet, despite the easy access to computers and databases, the data collected are usually not made readily available for research applications to clinical researchers (be they epidemiologists or clinicians). A good example of the usefulness of such clinical data recording systems is the Item Sheet that has been in place at the Maudsley Hospital for over half a century and which records diagnoses, symptoms, demographic details, psychosocial features, test findings, details of referral, and rating of clinical outcome. This large computerized database has allowed for the study of specific problem behaviors, sampling for long-term followup studies, patient comparisons between centers in different countries, the investigation of trends over time in specific behavioral problems and of their causes, and the study of comorbid patterns, e.g., Fombonne (112, 158, 159, 184). More streamlined data recording systems could easily achieve the same goals if a core set of variables were defined. Also, centers could decide to add on, for specific groups of patients of interest, or for defined periods of time, more exhaustive data recording procedures, because databases can easily be managed on modularity principles. Progress in information technology has made it easy and cheap to set up such databases and to exchange data when appropriate. Indeed, the need to audit services and to be accountable with regard to services activity for the health service will make such systems increasingly mandatory in most countries. Timely recognition of these needs and of the usefulness of these databases will help mental health professionals to influence these information systems in a way that might be more clinically relevant and useful for their own research and practice.

CONCLUSION

Progresses in child psychiatric epidemiology have been impressive in the last 30 years and have been made possible by the development of empirical and replicable measurement approaches to children's maladaptive behaviors and psychiatric disorders. The impact of epidemiology has been on several areas. For clinical practice, epidemiology has provided normative data on child behavior that are necessary to evaluate problems seen in clinical settings. As physiology is needed in medicine to understand disease pathology, knowledge of typically developing children acquired through epidemiological inquiries is needed for understanding child psychopathology.

Knowledge of the clinical significance of individual symptoms, of the risk factors associated with psychiatric disorders, of their population prevalence and incidence, is required for developing appropriate models of child psychopathology. For public health, surveys have drawn the attention on the importance of global morbidity in children due to mental health problems. In addition, disorders with an onset in childhood or adolescence have strong continuities with adult disorders, thus contributing to the burden of mental illness across the life span. Unfortunately, and despite increasing availability of evidence-based practices with demonstrated efficacy in controlled studies, access to services is insufficient in most countries. At a time where several indicators have shown upward trends in rates of behavioral disturbances in young people, service planners and policymakers should be made aware of this discrepancy. Progress in understanding causal mechanisms underlying some disorders has been substantial. Several risk factors are now well established that could be targeted by treatment and prevention programs. More refined understanding of child psychopathology is emerging, with new studies that now incorporate a joint assessment of genetic, biological and psychosocial factors, and combine longitudinal and developmental approaches in genetically informative designs to test competing hypotheses on psychopathological mechanisms.

References

1. Susser E, Neugebauer R, Hoek HW, Brown AS, Lin S, Labovitz D, Gorman JM: Schizophrenia after prenatal famine. Further evidence [see comments]. *Archives of General Psychiatry* 53(1):25–31, 1996.
2. St Clair D, Xu M, Wang P, Yu Y, Fang Y, Zhang F, Zheng X, Gu N, Feng G, Sham P, He L: Rates of adult schizophrenia following prenatal exposure to the Chinese famine of 1959–1961. *Jama* 294(5):557–62, 2005.
3. Fombonne E, Zakarian R, Bennett A, Meng L, McLean-Heywood D: Pervasive developmental disorders in Montreal, Quebec, Canada: prevalence and links with immunizations. *Pediatrics* 118(1):e139–50, 2006.
4. Rothman K G S: *Modern epidemiology*, Philadelphia, Lippincott-Raven, 1998.
5. Dunn G, Pickles A, Tansella M, Vazquez-Barquero JL: Two-phase epidemiological surveys in psychiatric research. *Br J Psychiatry* 174:95–100, 1999.
6. Madsen KM, Hviid A, Vestergaard M, Schendel D, Wohlfahrt J, Thorsen P, Olsen J, Melbye M: A population-based study of measles, mumps, and rubella vaccination and autism. *N Engl J Med* 347(19):1477–82, 2002.
7. Hviid A, Stellfeld M, Wohlfahrt J, Melbye M: Association between thimerosal-containing vaccine and autism. *Jama* 290(13):1763–6, 2003.
8. Smeeth L, Cook C, Fombonne E, Heavey L, Rodrigues LC, Smith PG, Hall AJ: MMR vaccination and pervasive developmental disorders: a case-control study. *Lancet* 364(9438):963–9, 2004.
9. Madsen KM, Lauritsen MB, Pedersen CB, Thorsen P, Plesner AM, Andersen PH, Mortensen PB: Thimerosal and the occurrence of autism: negative ecological evidence from Danish population-based data. *Pediatrics* 112(3 Pt. 1):604–6, 2003.
10. Fombonne E: The Chartres study: I. Prevalence of psychiatric disorders among French school-aged children. *British Journal of Psychiatry* 164:69–79, 1994.
11. Boyle MH, Offord DR, Racine YA, Catlin G: Ontario Child Health Study follow-up: evaluation of sample loss. *Journal of the American Academy of Child & Adolescent Psychiatry* 30(3):449–56, 1991.
12. Kalton G: *Compensating for Missing Data.* Ann Arbor, Institute for Social Research, 1983.
13. Little DRaR: *Statistical Analysis with Missing Data.* New York, Wiley, 1987.
14. Stott DH: Some psychosomatic aspects of casualty in reproduction. *J Psychosom Res* 3(1):42–55, 1958.
15. Hill AB: The environment and disease: association or causation? *Proc R Soc Med* 58:295–300, 1965.
16. Fombonne E, Chakrabarti S: No evidence for a new variant of measles-mumps-rubella–induced autism. *Pediatrics* 108(4):E58, 2001.
17. Lucas AR, Beard CM, O'Fallon WM, Kurland LT: 50-year trends in the incidence of anorexia nervosa in Rochester, Minn.: a population-based study. *Am J Psychiatry* 148(7):917–22, 1991.
18. Barbaresi WJ, Katusic SK, Colligan RC, Weaver AL, Jacobsen SJ: The incidence of autism in Olmsted County, Minnesota, 1976–1997: results from a population-based study. *Arch Pediatr Adolesc Med* 159(1):37–44, 2005.
19. Rutter M, Tizard J, Whitmore K: *Education, Health and Behavior.* New York, Robert E. Krieber Publishing, 1970.
20. Rutter M, Tizard J, Yule W, Graham P, Whitmore K: Research report: Isle of Wight studies, 1964–1974. *Psychological Medicine* 6:313–32, 1976.
21. Lapouse R, Monk M: An epidemiologic study of behaviour characteristics in children. *American Journal of Public Health* 48:1134–44, 1958.
22. Rutter M: Isle of Wight revisited: twenty-five years of child psychiatric epidemiology. *Journal of the American Academy of Child and Adolescent Psychiatry* 28:633–53, 1989.
23. Verhulst F, Koot H: *The Epidemiology of Child and Adolescent Psychopathology*, Oxford, U.K., Oxford University Press, 1995.
24. Achenbach TM, Edelbrock CS: Behavioral problems and competencies reported by parents of normal and disturbed children aged four through sixteen. *Monographs of the Society for Research in Child Development* 46(1):82, 1981.
25. Fombonne E: Parent reports on behaviour and competencies among 6–21-year-old French children. *European Child & Adolescent Psychiatry* 1 (4):233–43, 1992.
26. Petersen A, Compas B, Brooks-Gunn J, Stemmler M, Ey S, Grant K: Depression in adolescence. *American Psychologist* 48:155–68, 1993.
27. Fombonne E: Eating disorders: time trends and explanatory mechanisms, In: *Psychosocial disorders in young people: time trends and their causes.* Rutter M, Smith D (eds): Chichester, Wiley, 1995, pp 616–85.
28. Fombonne E: The Chartres Study: I. Prevalence of psychiatric disorders among French school-age children. *British Journal of Psychiatry* 164(1):69–79, 1994.
29. Achenbach TM, McConaughy SH, Howell CT: Child/adolescent behavioral and emotional problems: implications of cross-informant correlations for situational specificity. *Psychological Bulletin* 101(2):213–32, 1987.
30. Verhulst F, van der Ende J, Ferdinand R, Kasius M: The prevalence of DSM-111-R diagnoses in a national sample of Dutch adolescents. *Archives of General Psychiatry* 54(April):329–36, 1997.
31. Angold A, Costello E, Erkanli A: Comorbidity. *Journal of Child Psychology and Psychiatry* 40(1):57–87, 1999.
32. Ambrosini PJ: Historical development and present status of the schedule for affective disorders and schizophrenia for school-age children (K-SADS). *J Am Acad Child Adolesc Psychiatry* 39(1):49–58, 2000.
33. Bird HR, Gould MS, Staghezza B: Aggregating data from multiple informants in child psychiatry epidemiological research. *J Am Acad Child Adolesc Psychiatry* 31(1):78–85, 1992.
34. Achenbach TM: *Integrative guide for the 1991 CBCL/4-18, YSR and TRF profiles.* Burlington, VT, University of Vermont, Department of Psychiatry, 1991.
35. Achenbach T: "Comorbidity" in child and adolescent psychiatry: categorical and quantitative perspectives. *Journal of Child and Adolescent Psychopharmacology* 1:271–78, 1991.
36. Achenbach TM: Diagnosis, assessment, and comorbidity in psychosocial treatment research. *Journal of Abnormal Child Psychology* 23(1):45–65, 1995.
37. Kraemer HC, Measelle JR, Ablow JC, Essex MJ, Boyce WT, Kupfer DJ: A new approach to integrating data from multiple informants in psychiatric assessment and research: mixing and matching contexts and perspectives. *Am J Psychiatry* 160(9):1566–77, 2003.
38. Spitzer RL, Endicott J, Cohen J, Fleiss JL: Constraints on the validity of computer diagnosis. *Archives of General Psychiatry* 31(2):197–203, 1974.
39. Bartko JJ: On various intraclass correlation reliability coefficients. *Psychological Bulletin* 83(5):762–65, 1976.
40. Cronbach L: Coefficient alpha and the internal structure of tests. *Psychometrika* 16:297–334, 1951.
41. Elander J, Rutter M: Use and development of the Rutter Parents' and Teachers' Scales. *International Journal of Methods in Psychiatric Research* 5(151):1–16, 1995.
42. Achenbach TM, Edelbrock CS: The classification of child psychopathology: a review and analysis of empirical efforts. *Psychological Bulletin* 85(6):1275–1301, 1978.
43. Rutter M TA, Lann I (eds): *Assessment and Diagnosis in Child Psychopathology.* London, David Fulton, 1988.
44. Spitzer R, Endicott J, Robins E: Research diagnostic criteria: rationale and reliability. *Archives of General Psychiatry* 35:773–82, 1978.
45. American PA: *Diagnostic and Statistical Manual of Mental Disorders—DSM III*, Washington, DC, American Psychiatric Association, 1980.
46. World Health Organization: *The ICD-10 classification of mental and behavioural disorders: clinical descriptions and diagnostic guidelines.* Geneva, Switzerland, World Health Organization, 1992.
47. World Health Organisation: *The ICD-10 Classification of Mental and Behavioural Disorders—Diagnostic criteria for research.* Geneva, World Health Organisation, 1993.
48. Shaffer D, Lucas C, Richters J: *Diagnostic Assessment in Child and Adolescent Psychopathology*, New York, Guilford, 1999.

49. Piacentini J, Roper M, Jensen P, Lucas C, Fisher P, Bird H, Bourdon K, Schwab-Stone M, Rubio-Stipec M, Davies M, Dulcan M: Informant-based determinants of symptom attenuation in structured child psychiatric interviews. *Journal of Abnormal Child Psychology* 27(6):417–28, 1999.
50. Lucas CP, Fisher P, Piacentini J, Zhang H, Jensen PS, Shaffer D, Dulcan M, Schwab-Stone M, Regier D, Canino G: Features of interviews questions associated with attenuation of symptom reports. *Journal of Abnormal Child Psychology* 27(6):429–37, 1999.
51. Gould M, Rutter M, Shaffer D, Sturge C: UK/WHO study of ICD 9, in *Assessment and diagnosis in child psychopathology*. Edited by Rutter M, Tuma A, Lann I. David Fulton, London, 1988.
52. Prendergast M, Taylor E, Rapoport JL, Bartko J, Donnelly M, Zametkin A, Ahearn MB, Dunn G, Wieselberg HM: The diagnosis of childhood hyperactivity: a U.S.–U.K. cross-national study of DSM-III and ICD-9. *Journal of Child Psychology & Psychiatry & Allied Disciplines* 29(3):289–300, 1988.
53. Applegate B, Lahey BB, Hart EL, Biederman J, Hynd GW, et al.: Validity of the age-of-onset criterion for ADHD: a report from the DSM-IV field trials. *Journal of the American Academy of Child & Adolescent Psychiatry* 36(9):1211–21, 1997.
54. Lahey BB, Applegate B, Barkley RA, Garfinkel B, McBurnett K, Kerdyk L, Greenhill L, Hynd GW, Frick PJ, Newcorn J, et al.: DSM-IV field trials for oppositional defiant disorder and conduct disorder in children and adolescents. *American Journal of Psychiatry* 151(8):1163–71, 1994.
55. Volkmar FR, Klin A, Siegel B, Szatmari P, Lord C, Campbell M, Freeman BJ, Cicchetti DV, Rutter M, Kline W, et al.: Field trial for autistic disorder in DSM-IV. *American Journal of Psychiatry* 151(9):1361–7, 1994.
56. Rutter M: Diagnostic validity in child psychiatry. *Advances in Biological Psychiatry* 2:2–22, 1978.
57. Chilcoat HD, Breslau N: Does psychiatric history bias mothers' reports? An application of a new analytic approach. *J Am Acad Child Adolesc Psychiatry* 36(7):971–9, 1997.
58. Borge A, Samuelsen, S., Rutter, M.: Observer variance within families: Confluence among maternal, paternal and child ratings. *International Journal of Methods in Psychiatric Research* 10:11–21, 2001.
59. Simonoff E, Pickles A, Hervas A, Silberg JL, Rutter M, Eaves L: Genetic influences on childhood hyperactivity: contrast effects imply parental rating bias, not sibling interaction. *Psychological Medicine* 28(4):825–37, 1998.
60. Maughan B, Rutter M: Retrospective reporting of childhood adversity: issues in assessing long-term recall. *Journal of Personality Disorders* 11(1):19–33, 1997.
61. Kendler K, Silberg J, Neale M, Kessler R, Heath A, Eaves L: The family history method: whose psychiatric history is measured? *American Journal of Psychiatry* 148:1501–04, 1991.
62. Rende R, Weissman M: Assessment of family history of psychiatric disorder, in *Diagnostic assessment in child and adolescent psychopathology*. Shaffer D, Lucas C, Richters J (eds): New York, Guilford, 1999, pp. 230–55.
63. Fergusson D: A brief introduction to structural equation models, Verhulst F, Koot H (eds): In: *The Epidemiology of Child and Adolescent Psychopathology*. Oxford, U.K., Oxford University Press, 1995, pp. 122–45.
64. Fergusson DM: Structural equation models in developmental research. *Journal of Child Psychology & Psychiatry & Allied Disciplines* 38(8):877–87, 1997.
65. Boyle MH, Pickles AR: Influence of maternal depressive symptoms on ratings of childhood behavior. *Journal of Abnormal Child Psychology* 25(5):399–412, 1997.
66. Boyle MH, Pickles A: Maternal depressive symptoms and ratings of emotional disorder symptoms in children and adolescents. *Journal of Child Psychology & Psychiatry & Allied Disciplines* 38(8):981–92, 1997.
67. Fergusson D, Horwod L: The trait and method components of ratings of conduct disorder. Part 1: Maternal and teacher evaluations of conduct disorder in young children. *Journal of Child Psychology and Psychiatry* 28:249–60, 1987.
68. Fergusson DM, Horwood LJ: The trait and method components of ratings of conduct disorder—Part II. Factors related to the trait component of conduct disorder scores. *J Child Psychol Psychiatry* 28(2):261–72, 1987.
69. Zoccolillo M, Pickles A, Quinton D, Rutter M: The outcome of childhood conduct disorder: implications for defining adult personality disorder and conduct disorder. *Psychological Medicine* 22(4):971–86, 1992.
70. Bird HR, Canino G, Rubio-Stipec M, Gould MS, Ribera J, Sesman M, Woodbury M, Huertas-Goldman S, Pagan A, Sanchez-Lacay A, et al.: Estimates of the prevalence of childhood maladjustment in a community survey in Puerto Rico. The use of combined measures [published erratum appears in Arch Gen Psychiatry 1994 May;51 (5):429]. *Archives of General Psychiatry* 45(12):1120–6, 1988.
71. Bird HR: Epidemiology of childhood disorders in a cross-cultural context. *Journal of Child Psychology and Psychiatry* 37(1):35–49, 1996.
72. Simonoff E, Pickles A, Meyer JM, Silberg JL, Maes HH, Loeber R, Rutter M, Hewitt JK, Eaves LJ: The Virginia Twin Study of Adolescent Behavioral Development. Influences of age, sex, and impairment on rates of disorder [see comments]. *Archives of General Psychiatry* 54(9):801–8, 1997.
73. Costello EJ, Mustillo S, Erkanli A, Keeler G, Angold A: Prevalence and development of psychiatric disorders in childhood and adolescence. *Arch Gen Psychiatry* 60(8):837–44, 2003.
74. Canino G, Shrout PE, Rubio-Stipec M, Bird HR, Bravo M, etal.: The DSM-IV rates of child and adolescent disorders in Puerto Rico: prevalence, correlates, service use, and the effects of impairment. *Arch Gen Psychiatry* 61(1):85–93, 2004.
75. Bird H: The assessment of functional impairment, In: Shaffer D, Lucas C, Richters J (eds): *Diagnostic Assessment in Child and Adolescent Psychopathology*. Edited by New York, Guilford Press, 1999.
76. Rutter M, Tizard J, Whitmore K: *Education, Health and Behaviour*, New York, Robert E Krieber Publishing Co, 1970.
77. American Psychiatric Association: *Diagnostic and statistical manual of mental disorders—DSM IV*. Washington, DC, American Psychiatric Association, 1994.
78. Shaffer D, Gould MS, Brasic J, Ambrosini P, Fisher P, Bird H, Aluwahlia S: A children's global assessment scale (CGAS). *Archives of General Psychiatry* 40(11):1228–31, 1983.
79. Bird H, Andrews H, Schwab-Stone M, Goodman S, Dulcan M, et al.: Global measures of impairment for epidemiologic and clinical use with children and adolescents. *Internal Journal of Methods in Psychiatric Research* 6:1–13, 1996.
80. Bird H, Shaffer D, Fisher P, Gould M, Staghezza B, Chen J, Hoven C: The Columbia Impairment Scale (CIS): Pilot findings on a measure of global impairment for children and adolescents. *International Journal of Methods in Psychiatric Research* 3:167–76, 1993.
81. John K, Gammon GD, Prusoff BA, Warner V: The Social Adjustment Inventory for Children and Adolescents (SAICA): testing of a new semistructured interview. *Journal of the American Academy of Child & Adolescent Psychiatry* 26(6):898–911, 1987.
82. Sanford MN, Offord DR, Boyle MH, Peace A, Racine YA: Ontario child health study: social and school impairments in children aged 6 to 16 years. *J Am Acad Child Adolesc Psychiatry* 31(1):60–7, 1992.
83. Pickles A, Rowe R, Simonoff E, Foley D, Rutter M, Silberg J: Child psychiatric symptoms and psychosocial impairment: relationship and prognostic significance. *Br J Psychiatry* 179:230–5, 2001.
84. Angold A, Costello E, Farmer E, Burners B, Erkanli A: Impaired but undiagnosed. *Journal of the American Academy of Child and Adolescent Psychiatry* 38(2):129–137, 1999.
85. Costello E, Angold A, Keeler G: Adolescent outcomes of childhood disorders: the consequences of severity and impairment. *Journal of the American Academy of Child and Adolescent Psychiatry* 38(2):121–8, 1999.
86. Shaffer D, Fisher P, Lucas CP, Dulcan MK, Schwab-Stone ME: NIMH Diagnostic Interview Schedule for Children Version IV (NIMH DISC-IV): description, differences from previous versions, and reliability of some common diagnoses. *Journal of the American Academy of Child & Adolescent Psychiatry* Jan 39(1):28–38, 2000.
87. Angold A, Costello EJ: The Child and Adolescent Psychiatric Assessment (CAPA). *Journal of the American Academy of Child & Adolescent Psychiatry* 39(1):39–48, 2000.
88. Ford T, Goodman R, Meltzer H: The British Child and Adolescent Mental Health Survey 1999: the prevalence of DSM-IV disorders. *J Am Acad Child Adolesc Psychiatry* 42(10):1203–11, 2003.
89. Shaffer D, Scott M, Wilcox H, Maslow C, Hicks R, Lucas CP, Garfinkel R, Greenwald S: The Columbia Suicide Screen: validity and reliability of a screen for youth suicide and depression. *J Am Acad Child Adolesc Psychiatry* 43(1):71–9, 2004.
90. Fombonne E: The use of questionnaires in child psychiatry research: Measuring their performance and choosing an optimal cut-off. *Journal of Child Psychology & Psychiatry & Allied Disciplines* 32(4):677–93, 1991.
91. Hsiao J, Bartko J, Potter W: Diagnosing diagnoses. *Archives of General Psychiatry* 46:664–7, 1989.
92. Canino G, Bird H, Rubio Smaritza, Bravo M: Child psychiatric epidemiology: what we have learned and what we need to learn. *International Journal of Methods in Psychiatric Research* (special issue):79–92, 1995.
93. Roberts RE, Attkisson CC, Rosenblatt A: Prevalence of psychopathology among children and adolescents. *American Journal of Psychiatry* 155(6):715–25, 1998.
94. Leaf PJ, Alegria M, Cohen P, Goodman SH, Horwitz SM, et al.: Mental health service use in the community and schools: results from the four-community MECA Study. Methods for the Epidemiology of Child and Adolescent Mental Disorders Study. *Journal of the American Academy of Child & Adolescent Psychiatry* 35(7):889–97, 1996.
95. Offord DR, Boyle MH, Szatmari P, Rae-Grant NI, Links PS, Cadman DT, Byles JA, Crawford JW, Blum HM, Byrne C, et al.: Ontario Child Health Study. II: Six-month prevalence of disorder and rates of service utilization. *Archives of General Psychiatry* 44(9):832–6, 1987.
96. Costello EJ, Janiszewski S: Who gets treated? Factors associated with referral in children with psychiatric disorders. *Acta Psychiatrica Scandinavica* 81(6):523–9, 1990.
97. Zahner GE, Pawelkiewicz W, DeFrancesco JJ, Adnopoz J: Children's mental health service needs and utilization patterns in an urban community: an epidemiological assessment. *Journal of the American Academy of Child & Adolescent Psychiatry* 31(5):951–60, 1992.
98. Verhulst F, Koot H: *Child Psychiatric Epidemiology: Concepts, Methods and Findings*. Newbury Park, Sage Publications, 1992.
99. Whitaker A, Johnson J, Rapoport J, Kalikow K, Walsh B, Davies M, Braiman S, Dolinsky A: Uncommon troubles in young people: prevalance

estimates of selected psychiatric disorders in a nonreferred adolescent population. *Archives of General Psychiatry* 47(May):487–96, 1990.

100. Jensen P, Bloedau L, Davis H: Children at risk. L II: Risk factors and clinic utilization. *Journal of the American Academy of Child and Adolescent Psychiatry* 29:804–12, 1990.
101. Anderson JC, Franz CP, Williams S, McGee R, Silva PA: DSM-III disorders in preadolescent children. *Archives of General Psychiatry* 44:69–76, 1987.
102. Esser G, Schmidt MH, Woerner W: Epidemiology and course of psychiatric disorders in school-age children—results of a longitudinal study. *Journal of Child Psychology and Psychiatry* 31:243–63, 1990.
103. Morita H, Suzuki M, Kamoshita S: Screening measures for detecting psychiatric disorders in Japanese secondary school children. *Journal of Child Psychology & Psychiatry & Allied Disciplines* 31(4):603–17, 1990.
104. Jeffers A, Fitzgerald M: *Irish Families Under Stress. Vol. 2*. Dublin, Eastern Health Board, 1991.
105. Fergusson DM, Horwood LJ, Lynskey MT: Prevalence and comorbidity of DSM-III-R diagnoses in a birth cohort of 15 year olds. *Journal of the American Academy of Child & Adolescent Psychiatry* 32(6):1127–34, 1993.
106. Lewinsohn PM, Hops H, Roberts RE, Seeley JR, Andrews JA: Age cohort changes in the lifetime occurrence of depression and other mental disorders. *Journal of Abnormal Psychology* 102(1):110–120, 1993.
107. Costello E, Angold A, Burns B, Erkanli A, Stangl D, Tweed D: The Great Smoky Mountains Study of Youth: Functional impairment and serious emotional disturbance. *Archives of General Psychiatry* 53:1137–43, 1996.
108. Steinhausen H, Meier M, Angst J: The Zurich long-term outcome study of child and adolescent psychiatric disorders in males. *Psychological Medicine* 28:375–83, 1998.
109. Breton JJ, Bergeron L, Valla JP, Berthiaume C, Gaudet N, Lambert J, St-Georges M, Houde L, Lepine S: Quebec child mental health survey: prevalence of DSM-III-R mental health disorders. *Journal of Child Psychology & Psychiatry & Allied Disciplines* 40(3):375–84, 1999.
110. Angold A, Erkanli A, Costello EJ, Rutter M: Precision, reliability and accuracy in the dating of symptom onsets in child and adolescent psychopathology. *Journal of Child Psychology & Psychiatry & Allied Disciplines* 37(6):657–64, 1996.
111. Moffitt TE: Adolescence-limited and life-course-persistent antisocial behavior: a developmental taxonomy. *Psychological Review* 100(4):674–701, 1993.
112. Fombonne E, Wostear G, Cooper V, Harrington R, Rutter M: The Maudsley long-term follow-up study of adolescent depression: I. Adult rates of psychiatric disorders. *British Journal of Psychiatry* 179:210–217, 2004.
113. Weissman MM, Wolk S, Goldstein RB, Moreau D, Adams P, Greenwald S, Klier CM, Ryan ND, Dahl RE, Wickramaratne P: Depressed adolescents grown up. *Jama* 281(18):1707–13, 1999.
114. Weissman M, Wolk S, Wickramaratne P, Goldstein R, Adams P, Greenwald S, Ryan N, Dahl R, Steinberg D: Children with prepubertal-onset major depressive disorder and anxiety grown up. *Archives of General Psychiatry* 56:794–801, 1999.
115. Harrington R, Rutter M, Weissman M, Fudge H, Groothues C, Bredenkamp D, Pickles A, Rende R, Wickramaratne P: Psychiatric disorders in the relatives of depressed probands. I. Comparison of prepubertal, adolescent and early adult onset cases. *Journal of Affective Disorders* 42(1):9–22, 1997.
116. Rende R, Weissman M, Rutter M, Wickramaratne P, Harrington R, Pickles A: Psychiatric disorders in the relatives of depressed probands. II. Familial loading for comorbid nondepressive disorders based upon proband age of onset. *Journal of Affective Disorders* 42(1):23–8, 1997.
117. Taylor E, Chadwick O, Heptinstall E, Danckaerts M: Hyperactivity and conduct problems as risk factors for adolescent development. *Journal of the American Academy of Child & Adolescent Psychiatry* 35(9):1213–26, 1996.
118. Taylor E: Developmental neuropsychopathology of attention deficit and impulsiveness. *Development & Psychopathology* 11(3):607–28, 1999.
119. Kovacs M, Akiskal H, Gatsonis C, Parrone P: Childhood onset dysthymic disorder. Clinical features and prospective naturalistic outcome. *Archives of General Psychiatry* 51:365–74, 1994.
120. Kessler R, Mroczek D, Belli R: Retrospective adult assessment of childhood psychopathology, In: Shaffer D, Lucas C, Richters J (eds): *Diagnostic assessment in child and adolescent psychopathology*. New York, Guilford, 1999, pp. 256–84.
121. Schurhoff F, Bellivier F, Jouvent R, Mouren-Simeoni M-C, Bouvard M, Alilaire J-F, Leboyer M: Early and late onset bipolar disorders: two different forms of manic depressive illness? *Journal of Affective Disorders* 58:215–21, 2000.
122. Simon G, Von Korff M: Re-evaluation of secular trends in depression rates. *American Journal of Epidemiology* 135:1411–22, 1992.
123. Webster-Stratton C, Reid MJ, Hammond M: Treating children with early-onset conduct problems: intervention outcomes for parent, child, and teacher training. *J Clin Child Adolesc Psychol* 33(1):105–24, 2004.
124. Caspi A, Sugden K, Moffitt TE, Taylor A, Craig IW, Harrington H, McClay J, Mill J, Martin J, Braithwaite A, Poulton R: Influence of life stress on depression: moderation by a polymorphism in the 5-HTT gene. *Science* 301(5631):386–9, 2003.
125. Tremblay RE, Nagin DS, Seguin JR, Zoccolillo M, Zelazo PD, Boivin M, Perusse D, Japel C: Physical aggression during early childhood: trajectories and predictors. *Pediatrics* 114(1):43–50, 2004.
126. Rutter M: Comorbidity: concepts, claims and choices. *Criminal Behaviour and Mental Health* 7:265–85, 1997.
127. Caron C, Rutter M: Comorbidity in child psychopathology: concepts, issues and research strategies. *Journal of Child Psychology & Psychiatry & Allied Disciplines* 32(7):1063–80, 1991.
128. Hinshaw S, Lahey B, Hart E: Issues of taxonomy and comorbidity in the development of conduct disorder. *Development and Psychophatology Special Issue: Toward a development perspective on conduct disorder* 5:310–49, 1993.
129. Nottelmann E, Jensen P: Comorbidity of disorders in children and adolescents: developmental perspectives, In: Ollendick T, Prinz R. (eds): *Advances in Clinical Child Psychology*, vol 17. New York, Plenum Press, pp 109–55, 1995.
130. Merikangas KR, Mehta RL, Molnar BE, Walters EE, Swendsen JD, Aguilar-Gaziola S, Bijl R, Borges G, Caraveo-Anduaga JJ, DeWit DJ, Kolody B, Vega WA, Wittchen HU, Kessler RC: Comorbidity of substance use disorders with mood and anxiety disorders: results of the International Consortium in Psychiatric Epidemiology. *Addictive Behaviors* 23(6):893–907, 1998.
131. Hughes C, Sheldon H, Preskorn S, Weller E, Weller R, Hassanein R, Tucker S: The effect of concomitant disorder in childhood depression on predicting treatment response. *Psychopharmacological Bulletin* 26:235–38, 1990.
132. Richman N, Stevenson J, Graham P: *Pre-school to school: a behavioural study*, London, Academic Press, 1982.
133. Earls F: Prevalence of behavior problems in 3-year-old children. *Archives of General Psychiatry* 37:1153–57, 1980.
134. van den Oord E, Koot H, Boomsma D, Verhulst F, Orlebeke J: A twin-singleton comparison of problem behaviour in 2–3-year-olds. *Journal of Child Psychology & Psychiatry* 36:449–58, 1995.
135. Lavigne JV, Gibbons RD, Christoffel KK, Arend R, Rosenbaum D, Binns H, Dawson N, Sobel H, Isaacs C: Prevalence rates and correlates of psychiatric disorders among preschool children. *Journal of the American Academy of Child & Adolescent Psychiatry* 35(2):204–14, 1996.
136. Pianta R, Castaldi J: Stability of internalizing symptoms from kindergarten to first grade and factors related to instability. *Developmental Psychopathology* 1:305–16, 1989.
137. Pianta R, Caldwell C: Stability of externalizing symptoms from kindergarten to first grade and factors related to instability. *Developmental Psychopathology* 2:246–58, 1990.
138. Cohen S, Bromet E: Maternal predictors of behavioral disturbance in preschool children: a research note. *Journal of Child Psychology & Psychiatry & Allied Disciplines* 33(5):941–6, 1992.
139. Maziade M, Cote R, Boutin P, Bernier H, Thivierge J: Temperament and intellectual development: a longitudinal study from infancy to four years. *American Journal of Psychiatry* 144(2):144–50, 1987.
140. Kagan J, Snidman N, Arcus D: Childhood derivatives of high and low reactivity in infancy. *Child Development* 69(6):1483–93, 1998.
141. Stevenson J, Richman N, Graham P: Behaviour problems and language abilities at three years and behavioural deviance at eight years. *Journal of Child Psychology & Psychiatry & Allied Disciplines* 26(2):215–30, 1985.
142. Mawhood L, Howlin P, Rutter M: Autism and developmental receptive language disorder—a comparative follow-up in early adult life. I: Cognitive and language outcomes. *Journal of Child Psychology & Psychiatry & Allied Disciplines* 41(5):547–59, 2001.
143. Caspi A, Moffitt TE, Newman DL, Silva PA: Behavioral observations at age 3 years predict adult psychiatric disorders: Longitudinal evidence from a birth cohort. *Archives of General Psychiatry* 53:1033–39, 1996.
144. Rogers S: Empirically supported comprehensive treatments for young children with autism. *Journal of Clinical Child Psychology* 27(2):168–79, 1998.
145. Mayes LC: Addressing mental health needs of infants and young children. *Child & Adolescent Psychiatric Clinics of North America* 8(2):209–24, 1999.
146. Emde R, Bingham R, Harmon R: Classification and the diagnostic process in infancy, In: Zeanah C (ed): *Handbook of Infant Mental Health*. New York, Guilford, 1993.
147. Bagnato S, Neisworth J, Salvia J: *Early childhood indicators of developmental dysfunction*, Baltimore, Paul H Brookes, 1999.
148. Zero to Three: Diagnostic Classification—DC:0–3: *Diagnostic classification of mental health and developmental disorders of infancy and early childhood*. Washington, DC, National Center for Clinical Infant Programs, 1994.
149. Egger HL, Erkanli A, Keeler G, Potts E, Walter BK, Angold A: Test-Retest Reliability of the Preschool Age Psychiatric Assessment (PAPA). *J Am Acad Child Adolesc Psychiatry* 45(5):538–49, 2006.
150. Egger HL, Angold A: Common emotional and behavioral disorders in preschool children: presentation, nosology, and epidemiology. *J Child Psychol Psychiatry* 47(3–4):313–37, 2006.
151. Bourdon KH, Goodman R, Rae DS, Simpson G, Koretz DS: The Strengths and Difficulties Questionnaire: U.S. normative data and psychometric properties. *J Am Acad Child Adolesc Psychiatry* 44(6):557–64, 2005.

152. Achenbach TM, Hensley VR, Phares V, Grayson D: Problems and competencies reported by parents of Australian and American children. *Journal of Child Psychology & Psychiatry & Allied Disciplines* 31(2):265–86, 1990.
153. Stanger C, Fombonne E, Achenbach TM: Epidemiological comparisons of American and French children: Parent reports of problems and competencies for ages 6–21. *European Child & Adolescent Psychiatry* 3(1):16–28, 1994.
154. Achenbach TM, Bird HR, Canino G, Phares V, Gould MS, Rubio-Stipec M: Epidemiological comparisons of Puerto Rican and U.S. mainland children: parent, teacher, and self-reports. *Journal of the American Academy of Child & Adolescent Psychiatry* 29(1):84–93, 1990.
155. Rutter M QD: Psychiatric disorder: Ecological factors and concepts of causation, In: McGurk H (ed): *Ecological factors in human development.* Amsterdam, North Holland, 1977, pp 173–87.
156. Leung PW, Luk SL, Ho TP, Taylor E, Mak FL, Bacon-Shone J: The diagnosis and prevalence of hyperactivity in Chinese schoolboys. *British Journal of Psychiatry* 168(4):486–96, 1996.
157. M Rutter DS (ed): *Psychosocial Disorders in Young People: Time trends and their causes*, Chichester, Wiley, 1995.
158. Fombonne E: Increased rates of psychosocial disorders in youth. *European Archives of Psychiatry & Clinical Neuroscience* 248(1):14–21, 1998.
159. Fombonne E: Suicidal behaviours in vulnerable adolescents. Time trends and their correlates. *British Journal of Psychiatry* 173:154–9, 1998.
160. Achenbach TM, Howell CT: Are American children's problems getting worse? A 13-year comparison. *Journal of the American Academy of Child & Adolescent Psychiatry* 32(6):1145–54, 1993.
161. Flynn J: Massive IQ gains in 14 nations: What IQ tests really measure. *Psychological Bulletin* 101:171–91, 1987.
162. Fuggle PW, Tokar S, Grant DB, Smith I: Rising IQ scores in British children: recent evidence. *Journal of Child Psychology & Psychiatry & Allied Disciplines* 33(7):1241–7, 1992.
163. Fredriks AM, van Buuren S, Burgmeijer RJ, Meulmeester JF, Beuker RJ, Brugman E, Roede MJ, Verloove-Vanhorick SP, Wit JM: Continuing positive secular growth change in The Netherlands 1955–1997. *Pediatric Research* 47(3):316–23, 2000.
164. Verhulst FC, Achenbach TM: Empirically based assessment and taxonomy of psychopathology: Cross-cultural applications. A review. *European Child and Adolescent Psychiatry* 4(2):61–76, 1995.
165. Weisz J, Eastman, K: Cross-national research on child and adolescent psychopathology, In: Koot FVaH (ed): *The Epidemiology of Child and Adolescent Psychopathology*. Oxford, Oxford University Press, 1995, pp 42–65.
166. Ivanova M AT, Dumenci L, Rescorla L, Almqvist F, Bilenberg N, Bird H, Chen W, Domuta A, Dopfner M, Erol N, Fombonne E: Testing the configural invariance of the Child Behavior Checklist Syndromes in 30 cultures. *Journal of Clinical Child and Adolescent Psychology* (in press).
167. Crijnen AAM, Achenbach TM, Verhulst FC: Problems reported by parents of children in multiple cultures: The Child Behavior Checklist syndrome constructs. *American Journal of Psychiatry* 156(4):569–74, 1999.
168. Ivanova M, Achenbach T, Dumenci L, Rescorla L, Almqvist F, Bilenberg N, Bird H, Chen W, Domuta A, Dopfner M, Erol N, Fombonne E: Testing the configural invariance of the Child Behavior Checklist Syndromes in 30 cultures. *Journal of Child Psychology and Psychiatry.*
169. Canino G, Bravo M: The translation and adaptation of diagnostic instruments for cross-cultural use, In: Shaffer D, Lucas C, Richters J (eds): *Diagnostic assessment in child and adolescent psychopathology.* New York, Guilford Press, 1999.
170. Woodward CA, Thomas HB, Boyle MH, Links PS, et al.: Methodologic note for child epidemiological surveys: The effects of instructions on estimates of behavior prevalence. *Journal of Child Psychology & Psychiatry & Allied Disciplines* 30(6):919–24, 1989.
171. Weisz JR, Suwanlert S, Chaiyasit W, Weiss B, Walter BR, Anderson WW: Thai and American perspectives on over- and undercontrolled child behavior problems: exploring the threshold model among parents, teachers, and psychologists. *Journal of Consulting & Clinical Psychology* 56(4):601–9, 1988.
172. Lee S: Anorexia nervosa in Hong Kong: a Chinese perspective. *Psychological Medicine* 21:703–11, 1991.
173. King M, Bhugra D: Eating disorders: lessons from a cross-cultural study. *Psychological Medicine* 19:955–58, 1989.
174. Kleinman A, Good B: *Culture and Depression: Studies in the Anthopology and Cross-cultural Psychiatry of Affect and Disorder*, Berkeley, University of California, 1985.
175. Rescorla L, Achenbach M, Bilenberg N, Domuta A, Dopfner M, Erol N, Fombonne E, Fonseca A, Frigerio A, Hannesdottir H, et al.: Problems reported by parents of children ages 6 to 16 in 30 cultures. (submitted).
176. Rescorla L, Achenbach TM, Ginzburg S, Ivanova M, Dumenci L, Amlmqvist F, Bathiche M, Bilenberg N, Bird H, Domuta A, Erol N, Fombonne E, et al.: Problems reported by teachers of children ages 6 to 15 in 20 cultures. *School Psychology Review* (in press).
177. Berg I, Lucas C, McGuire R: Measurement of behaviour difficulties in children using standard scales administered to mothers by computer: reliability and validity. *European Child and Adolescent Psychiatry* 1 (1):14–23, 1992.
178. Goodman R, Ford T, Richards H, Gatward R, Meltzer H: The development and well-being assessment: description and initial validation of an integrated assessment of child and adolescent psychopathology. *Journal of Child Psychology and Psychiatry* 41:645–56, 2000.
179. Reich W: Diagnostic interview for children and adolescents (DICA). *Journal of the American Academy of Child & Adolescent Psychiatry* 39(1):59–66, 2000.
180. Valla J, Bergeron L, Smolla N: The Dominiv-R: a pictorial interview for 6- to 11-year old children. *Journal of the American Academy of Child and Adolescent Psychiatry* 39(1):85–93, 2000.
181. Patton GC, Coffey C, Posterino M, Carlin JB, Wolfe R, Bowes G: A computerised screening instrument for adolescent depression: population-based validation and application to a two-phase case-control study. *Social Psychiatry & Psychiatric Epidemiology* 34(3):166–72, 1999.
182. Reich W, Cottler L, McCallum K, Corwin D, Eerdewegh V: Computerized interviews as a method of assessing psychopathology in children. *Comprehensive Psychiatry* 36:40–45, 1995.
183. Turner C, Ku L, Rogers S, Lindberg L, Pleck J, Sonenstein F: Adolescent sexual behavior, drug use, and violence: increased reporting with computer survey technology. *Science* 280:867–73, 1998.
184. Simic M, Fombonne E: Depressive conduct disorder: symptom patterns and correlates in referred children and adolescents. *Journal of Affective Disorders* 62:175–85, 2001.

CHAPTER 2.2.2 ■ PREVENTION OF PSYCHIATRIC DISORDERS

DAVID A. MRAZEK AND PATRICIA J. MRAZEK

INTRODUCTION

The research evidence that supports preventive interventions has developed to a point that it is reasonable to establish public health goals that are designed to decrease the incidence of risk factors associated with the onset of mental illness. A number of malleable influences on child and adolescent development have been identified, and well validated preventive intervention programs are now being implemented.

However, preventive interventions have not been widely adopted, and even when psychiatrically ill children are identified, many do not receive treatment. Given this context, it has been difficult to initiate preventive interventions for children who are only beginning to develop early symptoms that are associated with the onset of a psychiatric disorder. Furthermore, there is still insufficient political conviction that a public health investment in preventive interventions would result in a decrease in the prevalence and ultimately the cost of psychiatric illnesses.

Randomized controlled trials have demonstrated that it is possible to reduce the risk factors that are associated with mental illness. The majority of preventive trials have focused on the prenatal period, early infancy, childhood, and adolescence rather than on adulthood. Early studies have demonstrated that some positive outcomes have persisted for twenty years. More recently, the prevention of the initial onset of depression, anxiety, and psychosis has been demonstrated. The implementation of these interventions on a wider scale will hopefully provide convincing evidence that further validates that these interventions are effective.

Child and adolescent psychiatrists play critical roles in the initiation of clinical preventive interventions. This can occur as a consequence of their direct clinical care of children or their consultations to the community systems regarding the creation and improvement of prevention activities (1).

Research has begun to demonstrate that the prevention of mental disorders can be accomplished. This is an important development beyond earlier demonstrations of the prevention of behaviors that were linked with these disorders. Child and adolescent psychiatrists are in an ideal position to become more involved in these prevention research efforts given that they are the most intensively trained clinicians who routinely evaluate and treat severe mental illness in young patients. Importantly, psychiatric clinicians regularly work with psychiatrically ill children on a daily basis. Therefore, they are in key positions to identify and intervene with those children who are at highest risk. Preventive intervention research has benefited from interactions between academicians who are experts in research methodology and psychiatric practitioners who have extensive experience with children who are symptomatic and at risk for developing severe psychiatric illnesses.

HISTORY

In 1957, a series of definitions were put forward to organize the field of prevention of physical and emotional illnesses. Primary prevention was defined as an intervention designed to decrease the number of new cases of a disorder or illness. Secondary prevention was defined as an intervention designed to lower the rate of established cases of the disorder or illness. Tertiary prevention was defined as an intervention designed to decrease the amount of disability associated with existing illnesses. While all three of these "preventive" interventions are designed to have positive outcomes, only primary preventive interventions result in a decrease in the incidence of an illness in a given population at risk. In contrast, secondary and tertiary preventive interventions are initiated after the onset of the disorder and are better described as treatments designed to minimize the morbidity of already expressed diseases.

This older terminology was defined in *Principles of Preventive Psychiatry*, which was written in 1964 immediately following the mental health initiative that was advanced by the Kennedy administration (2). Ironically, despite this early recognition of the importance of prevention, child and adolescent psychiatrists have not played a central role in many of the more recently developed preventive intervention initiatives.

DEVELOPMENT OF CONTEMPORARY DEFINITIONS OF PREVENTIVE INTERVENTIONS

In the late 1980s a review of prevention research efforts at the National Institute of Mental Health suggested that more prevention research was needed. As a direct consequence of this recognition, an Institute of Medicine (IOM) committee on the prevention of mental disorders was created through a Congressional mandate. An important action of this IOM committee was to recommend the adoption of an alternative taxonomy for mental health interventions that more effectively differentiated prevention, treatment, and maintenance. The use of the term prevention in this classification system was restricted to interventions provided prior to a patient receiving a psychiatric diagnosis. The term treatment was reserved for therapeutic interventions provided to individuals who met diagnostic criteria. The term maintenance referred to long-term care provided to patients with chronic mental illness that reduced relapse and recurrence of symptoms and decreased the disability associated with the disorder (3). This classification system created a "spectrum of interventions" (Figure 2.2.2.1).

The IOM Committee recommended that three new sub-categories of preventive interventions be formed in order to

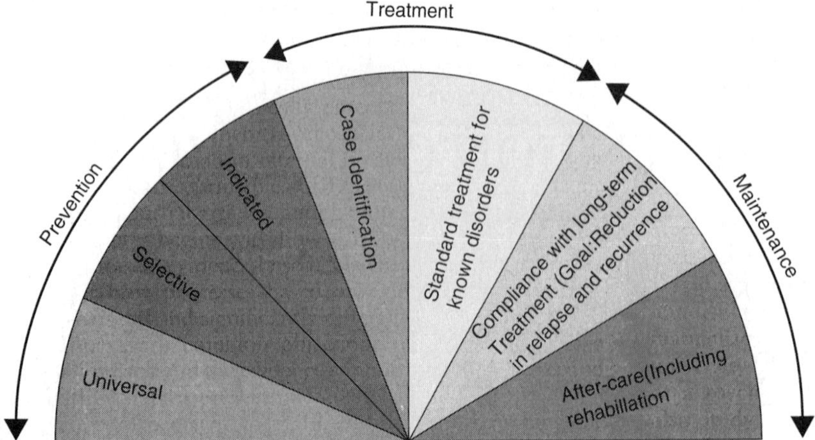

FIGURE 2.2.2.1. The Mental Health Intervention Spectrum for Mental Disorders.

TABLE 2.2.2.1

CLASSIFICATION OF PREVENTIVE INTERVENTIONS FOR MENTAL DISORDERS

Indicated preventive interventions for mental disorders are targeted to high-risk individuals who are identified as having minimal but detectable signs or symptoms foreshadowing mental disorder, but who do not meet standard diagnostic criteria that define a mental disorder.

Selective preventive interventions for mental disorders are targeted to individuals or a subgroup of the population whose risk of developing mental disorders is significantly higher than average. The risk may be imminent or it may be a lifetime risk. Risk groups may be identified on the basis of biological, psychological or social risk factors that are known to be associated with the onset of a mental disorder.

Universal preventive interventions are targeted to the general public or a whole population group that has not been identified on the basis of individual risk. The intervention is desirable for everyone in that group.

better differentiate the wide variety of interventions that had previously been referred to as primary preventions. All three subcategories shared the defining characteristic that they were designed to be administered to populations prior to the initial onset of a psychiatric diagnosis. These categories were referred to as *indicated*, *selective*, and *universal preventive interventions* and were differentiated from each other based on their targeted populations. This nomenclature has become the standard method of describing preventive interventions (see Table 2.2.2.1).

RISK AND PROTECTIVE FACTORS

The term risk factor is used in both prevention and treatment, but the implications of risk within these two types of intervention are different. In prevention, a risk factor must predate the onset of the illness and can be a silent characteristic that is used to identify a target population. The reduction of risk factors that are both causal and malleable is a goal of preventive interventions. Once the diagnosis of an illness has been made, risk factors that are subsequently identified should be used to guide treatment decisions and influence the assessment of prognosis.

The concept of protective factors is parallel to risk factors. An individual who is characterized as having one or more protective factors is determined to be less at risk for the development of a specific form of psychopathology than an individual without the protective factor. The majority of protective factors are nonspecific and perceived to be universally beneficial. Common examples of protective factors include a supportive family environment or superior general intelligence.

While there is essentially a balance of positive protective factors and negative risk factors for every individual, there has not been a universally accepted methodology for the creation of an overall quantification of risk for a particular child. What may prove to be useful in the individual analysis of risk is to consider the relative weight of each identified risk and protective factor for a given individual. An analytic method with variably weighted coefficients recognizes that risk factors vary in their pathogenic effect. It also recognizes that biological and psychosocial risk factors as well as biological and psychosocial protective factors must be analyzed within the context of the developmental capacities of an individual child.

PREVENTION-MINDED TREATMENT

In a very practical sense, child and adolescent psychiatrists have begun to expand their practices to include a modified form of treatment referred to as prevention-minded treatment (1). Prevention-minded treatment has been subdivided into two types. The first subtype of prevention-minded treatment involves the provision of traditional individual treatment, but includes strategies that are designed to indirectly benefit other family members. With this approach to prevention-minded treatment, the practitioner provides the direct treatment for the patient but considers the effects of his interventions on other family members who do not participate in the episode of care. The goal of this type of intervention is to provide indirect preventive interventions through the patient for another family member and it requires an appreciation of symptoms or exposure to risk factors of the other family member. An example of this approach is illustrated by the treatment of a mother with a major depressive disorder who has young children. If the clinician who is treating the mother becomes aware that her preschool child is developing behavioral symptoms such as an exaggerated concern for the safety of his mother, the clinician could bring these problems to the attention of her patient as well as providing her patient some guidance on how to handle these behaviors. Providing the mother a better understanding of the possible origins of the anxiety that her child is experiencing and providing the mother specific guidance in how to effectively reassure her child can be effective interventions. These interventions are designed to help both the mother and her child, but they would be a targeted preventive intervention for the child. Empirical evidence that effective treatment of major depressive disorders in women who have young children has a positive outcome not only on the women, but also on their children represents another example of indirect prevention-minded treatment (4).

The second type of prevention-minded treatment is a direct intervention involving other family members as a part of the treatment for the primary patient. This form of intervention often involves the invitation of other family members, including the children of a patient, to actively participate in therapy sessions. The therapist is open to the possibility of providing preventive interventions directly to other family members. Many forms of family therapy are designed to consider the adaptation of all members of the family system. An example could be an identified patient who is an adolescent with early prodromal symptoms of bipolar disorder whose family actively participates in family therapy. The ability of the teenager to monitor his own behavior may be severely compromised during hypomanic intervals. By recruiting family members to help the adolescent regulate his behavior, the anticipated escalation of these hypomanic symptoms may be averted. At the same time, this strategy can minimize the probability that the parents and siblings might develop symptoms. It does so by providing them with an intellectual context for dealing with the symptoms of bipolar illness and by preserving the quality of their interpersonal relationships.

PREVENTIVE INTERVENTION RESEARCH

Preventive intervention research is a maturing scientific endeavor. The Society for Prevention Research is an interdisciplinary professional organization that is dedicated to promoting evidence-based programs and for increasing the quality of research projects in the field. The standards of evidence of the Society for Prevention Research for efficacy, effectiveness, and dissemination of prevention programs and policies are now quite sophisticated (5). Specific issues related to the analysis of the outcomes of preventive intervention programs have been increasingly well addressed (6).

Many earlier preventive intervention research efforts did not designate presence or absence of psychiatric diagnosis as a primary outcome measure. However, preventive interventions focused on minimizing exposure to risk factors may well have an indirect positive benefit of preventing or delaying the onset of psychiatric disorders. The Prevention Research Program at the University of Arizona has demonstrated that preventive interventions can have multiple effects that improve function as well as reduce rates of psychiatric symptoms and psychiatric disorders (7). Their *New Beginnings Program,* a selective preventive intervention, targeted children whose parents had divorced. Approximately a third of the children of parents who divorce develop a psychiatric illness. Given this level of risk, these children are a very appropriate population for an early intervention. Using a randomized controlled clinical trial design, two well described preventive interventions were tested. The first intervention involved the mothers of the children and consisted of 11 group sessions and two individual sessions. The second intervention provided this same program for the mothers but also included 11 sessions for the children. The results of the six-year followup of both the program for the mothers and the program that involved both the mothers and children demonstrated that the children who received either of the interventions did better than the comparison group. The adolescents who had received these interventions were shown to have reduced symptoms of psychiatric disorder, lower rates of psychiatric diagnoses, less use of marijuana and alcohol, and fewer sexual partners. This program also resulted in parents having a greater sense of empowerment in their ability to be able to help their children. The consistency of these positive findings over multiple and varied outcome measures provides evidence to support the hypothesis that targeted preventive intervention efforts can simultaneously have broad beneficial effects and prevent psychiatric disorders. This program has addressed other important at-risk populations, including children who have experienced the death of a parent (8).

PREVENTION OF BEHAVIORAL DISORDERS

Webster-Stratton originally developed a treatment intervention for young conduct-disordered children and their families. This intervention included a therapist-led group discussion that emphasized parent training. The program involved the viewing of standardized videotapes that presented parents and their children engaging in both desirable and problematic interactions. This treatment was later modified to become an indicated preventive intervention for children with early symptoms of conduct disorder who did not meet diagnostic criteria. The intervention was modified again to allow it to be used as a selective intervention for children who were at high risk for behavior problems and enrolled in Head Start programs. These children were not symptomatic at the time of the intervention. The intervention program, known as "The Incredible Years," is now used widely (9, 10).

A decrease in the development of antisocial disorder in adulthood has been demonstrated through the implementation of a universal classroom-based preventive intervention for children in the first and second grades (11). The intervention has been named the "Good Behavior Game" and it is directed at improving the classroom management skills of teachers to allow them to support the social development of students and reduce the frequency of aggressive and disruptive behaviors. A randomized controlled trial was carried out in 40 first-grade classrooms in 18 elementary schools in Baltimore, Maryland. Positive outcomes were demonstrated, which varied by gender, baseline level of risk, and cohort. Generally, children judged to be at the highest level of risk benefited more from the intervention than children who were assessed to be at a lower level of risk. The most aggressive boys in first grade were the children who demonstrated the greatest reduction in aggressive behavior over the course of the first through seventh grades. These boys were less likely to develop an antisocial personality disorder as adults. They also had a 50 percent reduction in lifetime illicit drug use.

Another classic study designed to minimize behavioral problems was the Prenatal/Early Infancy Project (12–14). This home visitation project was a selective preventive intervention that was eventually renamed the Nurse–Family Partnership. The intervention began before the children were born and continued until they were 24 months of age. The risk factors that were used focused on psychosocial disadvantage and included the mothers being eighteen or younger, being a single parent, or having low socioeconomic status. This very early intervention involved parent education and the reinforcement of the mother's social support network. The intervention was shown to have a wide number of positive outcomes, including fewer behavioral disturbances in the target children many years after the initial home visits.

PREVENTION OF DEPRESSION AND SUICIDE

Two independent randomized controlled trials demonstrated that the prevention of unipolar depressive disorder in adolescents is possible with an indicated preventive intervention. In the first study, ninth and tenth graders were evaluated for depressive symptoms using a standard screening instrument and then subsequently interviewed (15). Students who met the criteria for current major depressive disorder or dysthymic disorder were referred for treatment. Other students who had a high level of subthreshold symptoms were offered a cognitive group intervention consisting of 15 after-school sessions led by mental health clinicians. At one-year follow-up, the students who were treated had fewer new cases of major depressive disorder and dysthymic disorder than did students in the control group.

The second study was based in a health maintenance organization (16). Adolescent children of depressed parents were identified by screening HMO pharmacy records of their parents to identify those parents who had been prescribed antidepressant medication within the previous 12 months. Parental diagnosis was confirmed through an assessment using the F-SADS. The adolescents were between the ages of 13 to 18 and were assessed using the K-SADS-E to obtain DSM-III-R diagnoses. Subjects were then assigned to one of three groups based on the severity of their depression. The middle-severity group reported subdiagnostic levels of depressive symptoms, which did not meet criteria for a DSM-III-R diagnosis. These youth were randomized to usual care provided by the HMO or to usual care and 15 sessions of a group cognitive therapy prevention program led by a therapist with a master's degree. The adolescents were taught cognitive restructuring techniques to identify and challenge irrational, unrealistic, or overly negative thoughts. This cognitive intervention specifically focused on their beliefs about depression and their thoughts of being the child of a depressed parent. When these subjects were evaluated 15 months after the intervention, the intervention group had a 9.3 percent cumulative incidence of major depression, as compared to the usual-care control group, which had a 28.8 percent cumulative incidence. A review of the cost-effectiveness of the program found its cost was comparable to the cost of standard treatments for depression and other mental health interventions (17).

The *Preventive Intervention Project (PIP)* is another example of a preventive intervention targeted at children who are at an increased risk for the development of depression (18–20). This intervention was designed for children between the ages of eight and 15 who were living with a biological parent with a mood disorder. Two manual-based programs were tested. The first intervention targeted the depressed parents and used a lecture format as well as two separate group sessions. This intervention did not involve the at-risk children. The second intervention used a clinician-facilitated format consisting of six to 11 sessions. This intervention included separate meetings with the parents and children as well as family meetings. In both formats, psychoeducational information about mood disorders was provided and parents were helped to better support the initiatives of their children. In the clinician-facilitated format, efforts were made to link information about mood disorders to the depressive illness experiences of the parent in the intervention. Two and a half years after the completion of the interventions, the parents who had received either the lecture format or the clinician-facilitated intervention reported improvements in the behaviors and attitudes of their children. There was a significant relationship between the number of positive changes that the parents reported in the behavior of their children and their improved understanding of the course and treatment of mood disorders. Furthermore, the internalizing symptom scores of the children who had received either of the interventions improved when they were assessed at followup. This family-based approach is particularly applicable to implementation in a clinical setting. Implementation could be accomplished by adding a relatively small number of additional sessions to the standard treatment of those adult patients with mood disorder who have children in the therapeutic age range. A particularly attractive aspect of this method of implementing a selective intervention is that billing for these additional sessions could be accomplished by using traditionally recognized family therapy codes that are linked to the diagnostic code of the parent.

A related issue in dealing with prevention efforts that are targeted to deal with depression is the prevention of suicide. A systematic review of a wide range of approaches designed to prevent suicide has recently been completed (21). The conclusion of this analysis suggested that the primary interventions that were demonstrated to be most effective were relatively nonspecific. Both physician education in the recognition of depression and its treatment and the absolute restriction of lethal methods of suicide were associated with a decrease in suicide.

An alternative strategy to consider in the prevention of suicide is to identify high risk individuals based on genetic testing. The genes that are most highly associated with suicide were recently reviewed (22). The strongest association was to the tryptophan hydroxylase gene (TPH). However, there was also an association with the promoter region polymorphism of the serotonin transporter gene (SLC 6A4) in patients with violent suicidal behavior. Interestingly, the association with the monoamine oxidase gene (MAO) appears to be nonspecific, and variations in this gene appear to be related to more aggressive or violent behavior rather than to the increased likelihood of suicide. Identification of adolescents or young adults at risk for depression who were demonstrated to have one or more polymorphisms of these susceptibility genes would be a particularly high risk group for a selective preventive intervention.

PREVENTION OF PSYCHOSIS

Adolescents and young adults who are at high risk for the development of schizophrenia have been the focus of many preventive intervention research initiatives. The goal of this work includes the identification of risk factors and biological markers to allow for interventions for subjects who are at very high risk. Many of these studies have been designed to prevent the onset of an initial episode of psychosis. While all of these intervention strategies have involved multidimensional components, the most controversial aspect of these interventions has been the use of antipsychotic medications prior to subjects meeting the formal diagnostic criteria of a psychotic illness.

The work of the Edinburgh High Risk Study has focused on the early identification of a range of characteristics that identify individuals who are at an increased risk for the development of schizophrenia (23). These characteristics have included cognitive, anatomical, and other physical markers. A range of atypical emotional and behavioral problems have been described, including situational anxiety, depression, and changes in cognitive perceptions such as isolated hallucinations. In addition to social anxiety, a higher frequency of social withdrawal and schizotypal features has been reported in those adolescents who subsequently develop schizophrenia (24). Formalized psychological testing further demonstrated that the at-risk individuals who developed schizophrenia were found to have lower verbal IQ scores than those who did not go on to develop schizophrenia (25). In considering neuroanatomic structural variations using structural MRI scans, decreased volumes in the temporal lobes were associated with development of schizophrenia (26). Using a voxel-based morphology technique, a decrease in grey matter was also demonstrated bilaterally in the anterior cingulate (27). Finally, dermatoglyphs, or fingerprints, were evaluated, and those subjects who developed schizophrenia were demonstrated to have the least complex fingerprints (28). This well conducted research effort clearly provides an increasingly coherent pattern of variation which will ultimately provide guidance on the identification of those patients who are most at risk for developing schizophrenia and those who would be most likely to benefit from selective preventive interventions.

The Early Psychosis Prevention and Intervention Center in South Australia has similarly conducted studies designed to identify individuals at high risk for the development of schizophrenia and have systematically assessed their responses to treatment (29). A combination of cognitive behavioral therapy and low dose risperidone treatment was associated with a delay in the progression of the development of psychotic symptoms (30). An early intervention using a specific suicide prevention therapy was also shown to decrease some of the symptoms associated with depression, but did not result in a decrease in the frequency of suicidal ideation (31). Neuroanatomical changes were examined, and decreased volumes of grey matter demonstrated in the right medial temporal, lateral temporal, and inferior frontal cortex were found to occur more frequently in those patients who developed psychotic illness. Less grey matter was also demonstrated bilaterally in the cingulate cortex in those patients who developed schizophrenia (32). These researchers have been strong advocates for initiating early interventions for these patients who have been shown to be at high risk for the development of schizophrenia (33). They support judicious pharmacotherapy for high-risk patients who are seeking treatment for their symptoms based on the modest improvements that have been demonstrated by empirical research. However, the benefit has not been sufficiently established to recommend the implementation of a screening procedure to identify potential patients with prodromal symptoms of schizophrenia who are not seeking treatment (34).

An experienced team of prevention investigators at Yale University are currently supporting the conduct of more research to better define how to prevent psychotic symptoms prior to moving forward with intervention initiatives. This group completed an initial preventive intervention to determine whether olanzapine at low doses (e.g., 5 to 15 mgm) could decrease symptoms in patients experiencing the prodromal symptoms of schizophrenia. Preliminary reports from this research did identify both a delay in the onset of symptoms, as well as modest weight gain (35). More recent findings confirm that there was some delay in the initiation of symptoms, but this finding did not reach statistical significance as a consequence of considerable subject attrition (36). However, the intervention group who received olanzapine did continue to have a significant weight gain in comparison to the comparison group (37). The risk–benefit ratio in this study has generally been assessed to be equivocal. Further research has been recommended to evaluate an alternative antipsychotic medication that was not associated with weight gain but would be successful in delaying the onset of psychotic symptoms.

The effectiveness of selective and indicated preventive interventions for schizophrenia could be greatly enhanced by screening children who are at risk for schizophrenia based on having an affected parent and then subsequently screening these at-risk children for a panel of susceptibility genes associated with the onset of schizophrenia. Eight genes have been repeatedly associated with having an increased risk for the onset of schizophrenia and are listed in Table 2.2.2.2 (38). Given that genotyping can be done reliably and prior to birth, the development of very early selective preventive interventions are now possible.

Given that schizophrenia is a highly heritable condition, it is possible to design either selective or indicated preventive interventions for children of parents with schizophrenia using genotyping to identify those adolescents at greatest risk. The most efficient strategy would be to target those individuals who have extensive family pedigrees with multiple affected family members as well as having multiple polymorphisms of susceptibility genes that put them at very high risk. Schizophrenia does not result from a problem with a single gene, but rather is the consequence of the interacting influences of a number of pathological genetic variations that influence many neural pathways (39–41). If the design of the intervention was modified to include children who were already showing some of the symptoms of schizophrenia, but did not meet clinical diagnostic criteria for the disorder, the correct term to describe the intervention would be an "indicated" preventive intervention.

TABLE 2.2.2.2

SCHIZOPHRENIA SUSCEPTIBILITY GENES

Gene (Abbreviated Full Name)	Chromosome Locus
COMT (catechol-O-methyltransferase)	22q11
DTNBP1 (dystrobrevin-binding protein 1)	6p22
NRG1 (neuregulin 1)	8p12–21
RGS4 (regulator of G-protein signaling 4)	1q21–22
GRM3 (glutamate receptor, metabotropic 3)	7q21–22
DISC1 (disrupted in schizophrenia 1)	1q42
G72 (G72)	13q32–34
DAAO (D-animo acid oxidase)	12q24

SOCIAL POLICY AND THE PREVENTION OF MENTAL ILLNESS

The demonstration of the positive cost benefit ratio for the implementation of universal interventions in psychiatry has not yet been clearly achieved. Generally, universal prevention studies have shown that the most positive results occur in those children who are at highest risk. In contrast, many children who are at minimal or no risk do not benefit at all from these interventions. This pattern of response supports the view that early screening and the development of interventions targeted to populations who are clearly at high risk or have early symptoms is a more practical approach.

It is now possible to implement currently demonstrated evidence-based selective and indicated preventive interventions to minimize risk factors and early symptoms associated with the onset of mental disorders. However, the implementation of these preventive interventions for children at risk for depression or conduct disorder will require political commitment. Given that these programs are predicted to decrease overall public health expenditures, there is reason to be optimistic about the future implementation of these programs.

The next generation of interventions designed to prevent serious psychiatric disorders will hopefully have an even more dramatic impact on the incidence and prevalence of serious mental illnesses. The combination of being able to determine genetic risk on a highly quantitative basis as a result of low cost and rapid genotyping throughput and the implementation of evidence-based preventive interventions designed to minimize psychosocial risk factors should make selective and indicated preventive interventions highly cost effective.

References

1. Mrazek, PJ and Ritchie, GF: *Becoming a Preventionist: A Guide to Expand Your Mental Health Practice*. Rockville, MD, U.S. Department of Health and Human Services, Substance Abuse and Mental Health Services Administration, Center for Mental Health Services (in press).
2. Caplan, G: *Principles of Preventive Psychiatry*. New York, Basic Books, Inc., 1964.
3. Mrazek, PJ and Haggerty, RJ (eds.): *Institute of Medicine: Reducing Risks for Mental Disorders: Frontiers for Preventive Intervention Research*. Washington, DC, National Academy Press, 1994.
4. Weissman, MM, Pilowsky, DJ, Wickramaratne, PJ, et al.: STAR*D-Child Team: Remissions in maternal depression and child psychopathology, a Star D-child report. *JAMA* 295(12):1389–1398, 2006.
5. Flay, BR, Biglan, A, Boruch, RF, et al.: Standards of evidence: Criteria for efficacy, effectiveness and dissemination. *Prev Sci* 6 (3):151–175, 2005.
6. Cuijper, P: Examining the effects of prevention programs on the incidence of new cases of mental disorders: The lack of statistical power. *Amer J Psych* 160 (8):1385–1391, 2003.
7. Wolchik, SA, Sandler, IN, Millsap, RE, et al.: Six-year follow-up of preventive interventions for children of divorce: A randomized controlled trial. *JAMA* 288(15):1874–1881, 2002.
8. Sandler, IN, Ayers, TS, Wolchik, SA, et al.: The family bereavement program: Efficacy evaluation of a theory-based prevention program for parentally bereaved children and adolescents. *J Consult Clin Psych* 71(3):587–600, 2003.
9. Webster-Stratton, C, Reid, MJ, Hammond, M: Preventing conduct problems, promoting social competence: A parent and teacher training partnership in Head Start. *J Clin Child Psych* 30(3):283–302, 2001.
10. Webster-Stratton, C, Taylor, T: Nipping early risk factors in the bud: Preventing substance abuse, delinquency, and violence in adolescence through interventions targeted at young children (0–8 years). *Prev Sci* 2(3):165–192, 2001.
11. Kellam, SG, Anthony, JC: Targeting early antecedents to prevent tobacco smoking: Findings from an epidemiologically based randomized field trial. *Amer J Pub Health* 88(10):1490–1495, 1998.
12. Olds, DL, Eckenrode, J, Henderson, CR, Jr., et al.: Long-term effects of home visitation on maternal life course and child abuse and neglect. Fifteen-year follow-up of a randomized trial. *JAMA* 278:637–643, 1997.

13. Olds, D, Henderson, CR, Jr., Cole, R, et al.: Long-term effect of nurse home visitation on children's criminal and antisocial behavior: Fifteen-year follow-up of a randomized controlled trial. *JAMA* 280(14):1238–1244, 1998.
14. Izzo, CV, Eckenrode, JJ, Smith, EG, et al.: Reducing the impact of uncontrollable stressful life events through a program of nurse home visitation for new parents. *Prev Sci* 6 (4):259–267, 2005.
15. Clarke, GN, Hornbrook, M, Lynch, F, et al.: A randomized trial of a group cognitive intervention for preventing depression in adolescent offspring of depressed parents. *Arch Gen Psych* 58:1127–1134, 2001.
16. Clarke, GN, Hornbrook, M, Lynch, F, et al.: Group cognitive-behavioral treatment for depressed adolescent offspring of depressed parents in a health maintenance organization. *J Am Acad Child Adolesc Psych* 41(3):305–313, 2002.
17. Lynch, FL, Hornbrook M, Clarke, GN, et al.: Cost-effectiveness of an intervention to prevent depression in at-risk teens. *Arch Gen Psych* 62:1241–1248, 2005.
18. Beardslee, WR: Outreach supported antidepressant treatment and cognitive behavioural therapy are effective for depression in low income minority women. *Evid Based Ment Health* 7:21, 2004.
19. Beardslee, WR, Gladstone, TRG: Prevention of childhood depression: Recent findings and future prospects. *Biol Psych* 49:1101–1110, 2001.
20. Beardslee, WR, Gladstone, TRG, Wright, EJ, Cooper, AB: A family-based approach to the prevention of depressive symptoms in children at risk: Evidence of parental and child change. *Ped* 112(2):e119–e131, 2003.
21. Mann, JJ, Apter, A, Bertolote, J, et al.: Suicide prevention strategies: A systematic review. *JAMA* 294(16):2064–2074, 2005.
22. Bondy, B, Buettner, A, Zill, P: Genetics of suicide. *Molec Psych* (11) pp 336–351, 2006.
23. Cunningham Owens, DG, Miller, P, Lawrie, SM, Johnstone, EC: Pathogenesis of schizophrenia: A psychopathological perspective. *Br J Psych* 186:386–393, 2005.
24. Johnstone, EC, Ebmeier, KP, Miller, P, Owens, DGC, Lawrie, SM: Predicting schizophrenia: Findings from the Edinburgh High-Risk Study. *Br J Psych* 186:18–25, 2005.
25. Byrne, M, Clafferty, BA, Cosway, R, et al.: Neuropsychology, genetic liability, and psychotic symptoms in those at high risk of schizophrenia. *J Abnorm Psych* 112(1):38–48, 2003.
26. Lawrie, SM, Whalley, HC, Abukmeil, SS, et al.: Temporal lobe volume changes in people at high risk of schizophrenia with psychotic symptoms. *Br J Psych* 181:138–143, 2002.
27. Job, DE, Whalley, HC, McConnell, S, Glabus, M, Johnstone, EC, Lawrie, SM: Voxel-based morphometry of grey matter densities in subjects at high risk of schizophrenia. *Schizoph Res* 64:1–13, 2003.
28. Langsley, N, Miller, P, Byrne, M, et al.: Dermatoglyphics and schizophrenia: findings from the Edinburgh high risk study. *Schizoph Res* 74:122–124, 2005.
29. Yung, AR, Phillips, LJ, Yuen, HP, McGorry, PD: Risk factors for psychosis in an ultra high-risk group: psychopathology and clinical features. *Schizophr Res* 67:131–142, 2004.
30. McGorry, PD, Yung, AR, Phillips, LJ, et al.: Randomized controlled trial of interventions designed to reduce the risk of progression to first-episode psychosis in a clinical sample with subthreshold symptoms. *Arch Gen Psych* 59:921–928, 2002.
31. Power, PJR, Bell, RJ, Mills, R, et al.: Suicide prevention in first episode psychosis: The development of a randomized controlled trial of cognitive therapy for acutely suicidal patient with early psychosis. *Aust NZ J Psych* 37:414–420, 2003.
32. Pantelis, C, Velakoulis, D, McGorry, PD, et al.: Neuroanatomical abnormalities before and after onset of psychosis: A cross-sectional and longitudinal MRI comparison. *The Lancet* 361:281–288, 2003.
33. McGorry, PD, Yung, AR: Early intervention psychosis: An overdue reform. *Aust NZ J Psych* 37:393–398, 2003.
34. McGorry, PD: Early intervention in psychotic disorders: Beyond debate to solving problems. *Br J Psych* 187(Suppl.48):s108-s110, 2005.
35. Woods, SW, Breier, A, Zipursky, RB, et al.: Randomized trial of olanzapine versus placebo in the symptomatic acute treatment of the schizophrenic prodome. *Biol Psych* 54:453–464, 2003.
36. Melle, I, Johannesen, JO, Friis, S, et al.: Early detection of the first episode of schizophrenia and suicidal behavior. *Amer J Psych* 163(5):800–804, 2006.
37. McGlashan, TH, Zipursky, RB, Perkins, D, et al.: Randomized, double-blind trial of olanzapine versus placebo in patients prodromally symptomatic for psychosis. *Amer J Psych* 163(5):790–799, 2006.
38. Harrison, PJ, Weinberger, DR: Schizophrenia genes, gene expression, and neuropathology: On the matter of their convergence. *Molec Psych* 10(1):40–68, image 5, 2005.
39. Weinberger, DR (2005). Genetic mechanisms of psychosis: *In vivo* and postmortem genomics. National Institutes of Health, Clinical Brain Disorders Branch, Genes, Cognition and Psychosis Program, Bethesda, Maryland. *Clin Ther* 27: Supplement A, S8–15, 2005.
40. Weinberger, DR (2006). New directions in psychiatric therapeutics. *J Amer Soc Exp Neurother* 3(1):1–2, 2006.
41. Prathikanti, S, Weinberger, DR: Psychiatric genetics—the new era: genetic research and some clinical implications. *Br Med Bull* December 19:73–74:107–122, 2005.

2.3 ■ GENETICS

CHAPTER 2.3.1 ■ FROM GENES TO BRAIN: DEVELOPMENTAL NEUROBIOLOGY

JAMES F. LECKMAN, FLORA M. VACCARINO, AND PAUL J. LOMBROSO

Human beings are complex living organisms that can be characterized by their appearance and behavior at each point in their life cycle. Many of these characteristics are uniquely human, such as the array of languages that facilitate interpersonal communication and permit a meaningful interplay of ideas and emotions. Other characteristics, such as affection and aggression, are less distinctive and place our species as one among many that populate the earth. Scientific advances over the past 150 years clearly indicate that hereditary factors that are transmitted from generation to generation account for much of the observed variation among and within species. Although the complexities of human existence cannot be reduced simply to the effects of genes, it is inescapable that genetic factors provide the biological basis for many of our potentialities and vulnerabilities as human beings (1).

Our genetic endowment, as a species, is a unique collection of discrete units of heredity (genes) that for the most part are linearly arranged on 46 chromosomes (22 pairs of homologous chromosomes and two sex chromosomes) (Figure 2.3.1.1). It is apparent from the completion of the human genome sequencing project that there are approximately 35,000 genes on our chromosomes. This collection of genes makes us both alike and different from other organisms. Although the precise genetic determinants of our interspecies similarities and differences are largely obscure, it is probable that many of the responsible genetic factors will be identified. For example, investigators are in the midst of discovering the cascade of genes that have contributed to the remarkable neuroanatomical and functional evolution of the cerebral neocortices across different mammalian species over the past 50 million years (2).

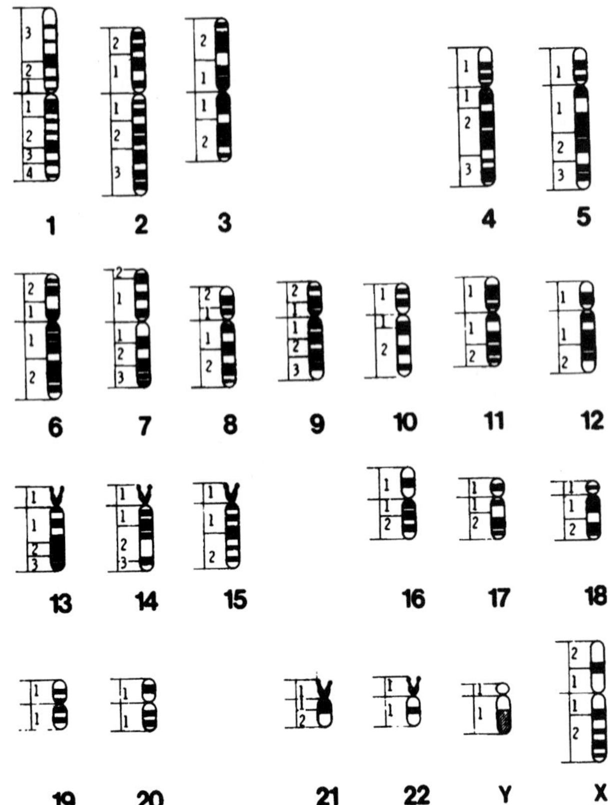

FIGURE 2.3.1.1. Depiction of high-resolution banded human chromosomes. (Adapted from *Yale-HHMI Human Gene Mapping Library Chromosome Plots*, Number 5. New Haven, CT, Howard Hughes Medical Institute, 1989.)

Genetic factors also contribute to variations within species. A large number of physical and psychological traits, including gender, height, and intelligence, have been shown to be under at least partial genetic control. One need only examine the striking physical and psychological similarities between monozygotic (genetically identical) twins reared apart to recognize the powerful influence of genes in determining who we are. (3, 4) Some of these intraspecies differences, such as gender, are due to actual differences in the number and type of genes present in the individual. For example, genes on the Y chromosome are present in males and are transmitted from father to son. Other intraspecies differences are due to multiple forms (polymorphic alleles) of specific genes that are distributed within the population. The polymorphisms are due to differences in the basic elements of genes, namely the linear sequence of nucleotides that form our chromosomes. For the most part, these polymorphisms are silent in the sense that they do not change the proteins that are encoded. However, some of the changes lead to differences in the structure, activity or level of expression of proteins, which may then contribute to traits such as blood type, height, or eye color. In others, the changes within the genes are subtler, and make the individual more susceptible to additional factors, be they genetic or environmental, that may lead to phenotypic expression of clinical significance.

Some allelic variations are so significant that we use the term mutation to signify that the changes will usually lead to disease states such as Rett syndrome, Huntington's disease, Marfan syndrome, or sickle cell anemia, disorders in which other ameliorating factors will have little effect. Finally, some intraspecies differences may depend on which parent passed on a particular piece of genetic material, a process termed genetic *imprinting*. (5) Briefly, imprinting affects the structure of the deoxyribonucleic acid (DNA) molecule but not the nucleotide sequence itself. Mechanisms that modify the DNA structure without changing the nucleotide sequence are termed *epigenetic phenomena*. For example, proteins that regulate gene expression are not able to gain access to imprinted genes, and genes within an imprinted chromosomal region are effectively silenced. The most dramatic example of imprinting concerns two distinctively different developmental disorders, Prader-Willi and Angelman's syndrome, that are due to alterations of DNA in the same general chromosomal region on chromosome 15 (6).

Apart from interspecies and intraspecies variations, it is also important to recognize that differences over the life span of an individual member of a species can also be due to genetic factors. Simply put, this means that not all genes are active at the same time. For example, the hemoglobin genes active during fetal life are different from those that are active in adulthood. Differences in the pattern of expression of genes over the life span are largely responsible for the physical and cognitive functioning of individual organisms, from *Drosophila* to humans. These differences are also responsible for the allocation of specific characteristics and functions to specific cells of the body, e.g., for making muscle cells different from brain cells, and are orchestrated by master developmental genes in a precise manner. As the temporal patterns of gene expression during human development become known, we may come to be able to better predict each individual's genetic potential.

The next two sections, Genes and Regulation of Gene Function, present a condensed summary of some of the fundamental aspects of the structure and function of genes and gene products. Several excellent general references cover this material in greater depth (7, 8).

GENES

Mendel first postulated the existence of discrete hereditary factors or genes in 1865 (9) but their importance was not appreciated until the early 1900s. As indicated above, genes are arranged linearly on chromosomes that are found in the nuclei of most cells (Figure 2.3.1.2). They are composed of DNA. DNA consists of a string of nucleotides (complex molecules that contain a sugar moiety, a phosphate group, and either a purine or a pyrimidine base) that are linked together. These linkages involve connecting the carbon atom of one sugar moiety to the carbon atom of the next nucleotide through a phosphate group. Four separate nucleotides are found in DNA. Two contain purine bases (adenine and guanine) and two contain pyrimidine bases (thymine and cytosine).

Genetic information is conveyed by the nucleotide sequence of a particular DNA molecule. Most DNA molecules exist in a double helical structure composed of two polynucleotide chains held together by a series of hydrogen bonds between complementary base pairs (adenine is bonded to thymine and guanine to cytosine) (Figure 2.3.1.3). This structure confers stability of the molecule and provides the basis for replication. Since each strand of DNA in the double helix is exactly complementary to the other, knowing the sequence of one strand provides precise knowledge of the sequence of the other.

The sequence of nucleotides on a DNA molecule determines the order of the 20 different amino acids in proteins. As a consequence, the information contained in DNA provides the instructions for cells to grow and divide, set in motion developmental sequences that lead to orderly differentiation

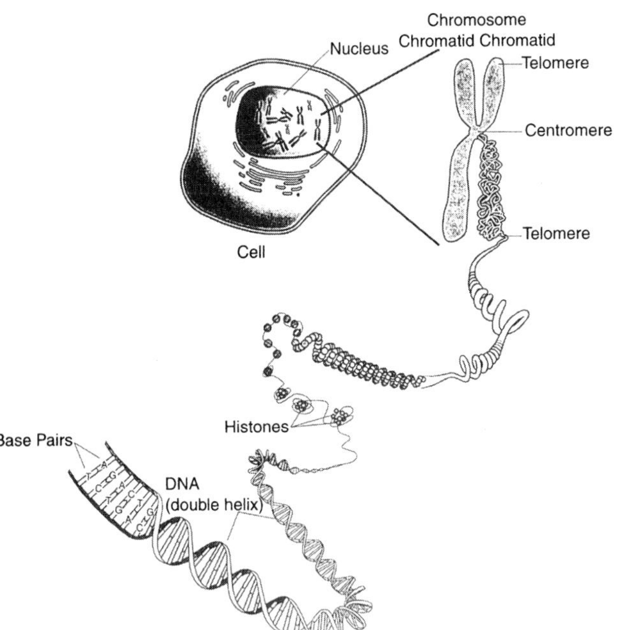

FIGURE 2.3.1.2. The structure of chromosomes. Chromosomes are thread-like packages of DNA in the nucleus of a cell. This drawing also depicts a diagram of the DNA double helix in its common form showing the antiparallel orientation of the complementary strands and the wrapping of DNA around histone cores. (Adapted from the *Glossary of Genetic Terms* and associated illustrations found on the Website of the National Genome Research Institute, 2000.)

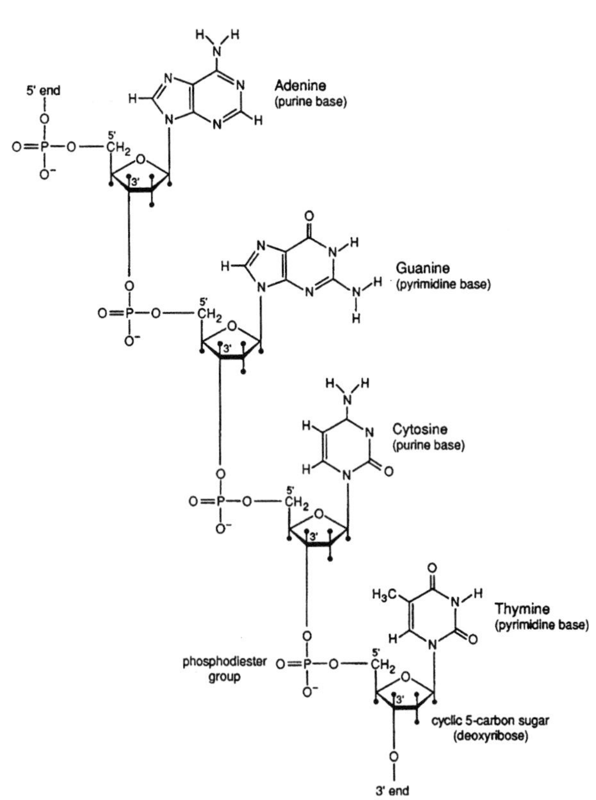

FIGURE 2.3.1.3. Chemical structure of DNA, showing the phosphodiester 3′-5′ linkages that connect the nucleotides. (Adapted from Watson JD, Hopkins NH, Roberts JW, et al.: *Molecular Biology of the Cell.* Menlo Park, CA, Benjamin/Cummings, 1987.)

of cell types, and provide for the maintenance of a diversified population of cells that are necessary for the successful functioning of complex organisms.

The nucleotide sequence, however, does not provide a direct template for protein synthesis. Instead, there are a series of intervening steps that require the DNA to be transcribed into messenger ribonucleic acid (mRNA). Messenger RNA molecules are very similar in composition to DNA and can hybridize with complementary DNA sequences. Mature mRNA molecules are rapidly transported out of the nucleus, where they serve as the template for protein synthesis.

The translation of a message into a specific amino acid sequence occurs at ribosomes located in either the cytoplasm or attached to the endoplasmic reticulum. The amino acid sequence is determined by the sequence of bases, with sets of three bases constituting a codon that stands for an amino acid. At the ribosome, codons of an mRNA molecule bind to complementary anticodons of transfer RNAs (tRNAs), which then transfer specific amino acids to the growing protein chain. The basic elements of this "central dogma" of protein production were first proposed by Crick (10).

Genes are normally extremely stable and are precisely copied during the chromosomal duplications that precede cell divisions (mitosis). Obviously, any mistakes that occur have the potential of disturbing the normal sequence of amino acids in a protein. There are a number of proteins within the nucleus whose function it is to recognize and repair errors within the DNA sequence. Very rarely, however, mistakes go uncorrected and will result in changes in the original nucleotide sequence. The majority of such changes have no effects as they occur in regions on the DNA molecule that do not encode for protein. However, mutations that occur within the sequence that encodes for protein or within regulatory portions of genes may have functional consequences. First, they may slightly change the enzymatic function of the protein, leading to the allelic variations discussed above. Second, when a critical amino acid is mutated, there may be dramatic changes in the function of the encoded protein and, ultimately, to the organism. Finally, this capacity for change can, in rare instances, lead to positive consequences that serve as the basis for evolution.

REGULATION OF GENE FUNCTION

According to some estimates, only about 1 percent of the genome is being expressed at a given time in higher eukaryotic cells (8). Different sets of genes are active during development compared to the mature organism, and different genes are required in the various tissues. Some genes are expressed continuously, while others are required during specific periods, and others are only expressed in response to hormonal or environmentally triggered changes. Regulation of gene function can occur at any of the many steps required for gene expression (Figure 2.3.1.4).

Transcriptional Factors

The basic flow of biological information is from DNA to RNA (transcription) and from RNA to protein (translation). Transcription of mRNA is initiated by the binding of a protein complex containing RNA polymerase II to the regulatory region of a gene, termed the promoter. These regions are usually found immediately upstream of the transcriptional start site. Sequences of highly conserved nucleotides within the

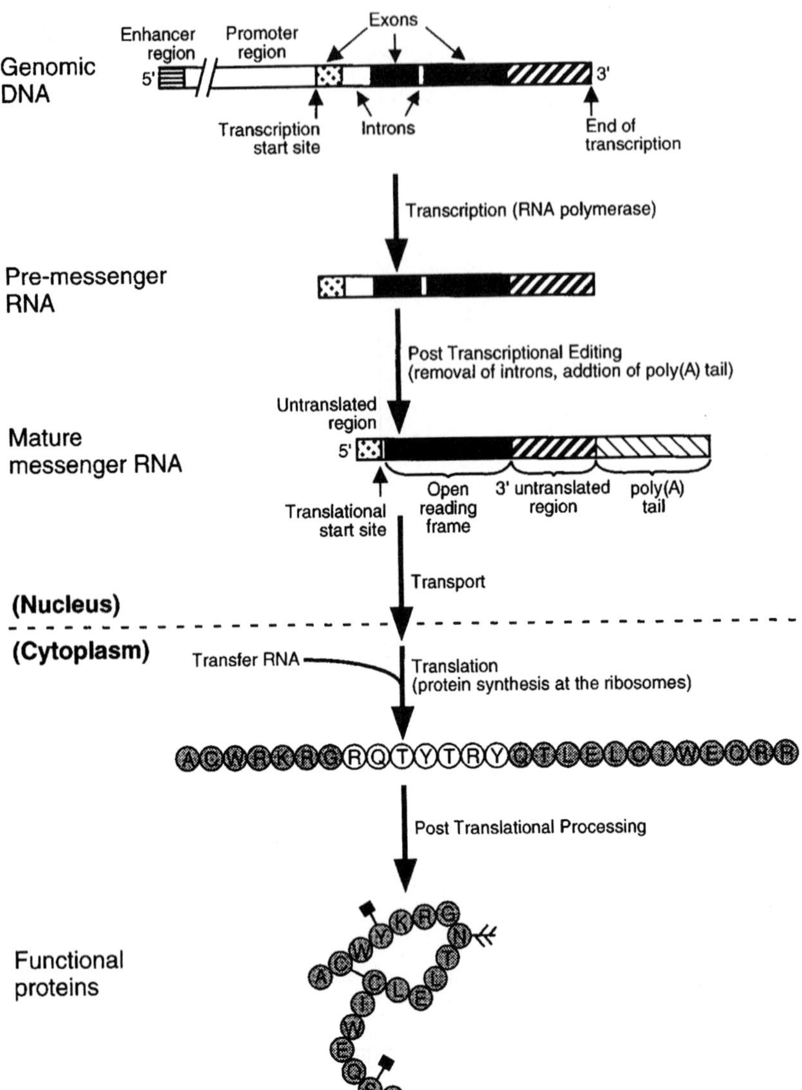

FIGURE 2.3.1.4. Sequence of events leading to gene expression. A protein-coding gene comprises a stretch of genomic DNA that contains an open reading frame. This region contains instructions for making the protein, as well as adjacent control regions—promoters and enhancers—where the gene's transcriptional mechanism is switched on or off. The promoter region is the site at which RNA polymerase binds and starts transcribing. The enhancer regions may be thousands of base pairs distant from the promoter. Transcription of the gene into mRNA may be either stimulated or inhibited by transcription factors that bind to promoter and enhancer regions. The mRNA formed by transcription is spliced to remove introns and processed within the cell nucleus to produce mRNAs that are exported to the cytoplasm for translation into protein at the ribosomes. Some proteins go through posttranslational modification to become biologically active. The four examples depicted include: cleavage of precursor proteins, conformational change through covalent cysteine–cysteine (C–C) bonds, phosphorylation of serine (S) or tyrosine (Y) *(black squares)*, and glycosylation of asparagines (N, branching motif).

promoter serve as binding sites for the regulatory proteins required to initiate transcription. After binding, the two DNA strands unravel and the sense strand is accessible to the polymerase enzyme. In addition, other highly conserved DNA sequences have been identified that either enhance or repress the transcription of target genes. These sequences are usually found near the regulatory promoter region or in further upstream regions of DNA. Enhancer or repressor sequences bind regulatory proteins called transcription factors to form complexes that allow the RNA polymerase II complex to bind more or less efficiently to the underlying gene. In this way, specific sets of genes are expressed while others are repressed, depending on the precise mixture of enhancers, repressors, and transcription factors present in the cell. It should be pointed out that mutations that occur within the promoter regions of genes can have a dramatic effect on the expression of the encoded protein by disrupting the binding sites of the basal transcriptional machinery, repressors, or enhancer proteins.

Some of these highly conserved repetitive DNA sequences in the promoter regions of genes serve as phylogenetic "footprints," which are reliable guides to regulatory regions of genes (11). As such, their presence is being used as one element of algorithms to identify putative novel genes within the vast sequence data bases generated by the human genome project and related commercial efforts (12).

Several classes of DNA-binding proteins exist and regulate the transcription of most genes. The best characterized of these transcription factors contain conserved amino acid regions that bind to specific DNA sequences. For example, homeodomain transcription factors have a highly conserved 60-amino acid region with a helix-turn-helix structure. This structure contains two helices that bind a specific DNA sequence in the major groove of the double helix of DNA (13). Other transcriptional factors have different tertiary structures known as *zinc fingers* and *leucine zippers* that also bind to DNA regulatory sequences within the promoter and regulate the initiation of transcription (14, 15).

Another major issue concerns the mechanisms by which genes remain quiescent in some cell lineages or are repressed after a period of activity (16). This is a critical issue during the complex cascade in time and space of the genes necessary for the formation of the brain. During specific points in development, different genes are sequestered within heritable forms of chromatin complex that preclude transcription. Developmental repression of adult gene expression is remarkably efficient. Ratios of 1:10,000,000 or more have been estimated for the level of globin or growth hormone transcripts in cells not expressing these genes compared with those that are (17, 18).

One way to achieve gene repression is for transcription factors to modify the structure of the DNA molecule itself.

One such process is through the acetylation of histones. In normal transcription, histone acetylation causes an unwinding of the DNA that permits the transcriptional machinery to bind to the promoter region. Consequently, factors that activate histone acetylases promote gene transcription.

Another important mechanism of gene regulation is achieved through CpG islands that are present within the regulatory regions of most genes. "CpG islands" refer to the presence of nucleotide sequences rich in C + G nucleotides. The protein methyl-CpG binding protein (Mecp2) is thought to bind to methylated CpG dinucleotides in the mammalian genome and to recruit the repressor Sin3A and histone deacetylase (Hdac) (19–21). In addition, Mecp2 associates with both histone H2 Lys9 methyltransferase and with the DNA methyltransferase Dnmt1 (22, 23), which are potent inhibitors of transcription. Intriguingly, mutations in Mecp2 have been identified in most individuals with Rett syndrome (24). Repression of transcription via Mecp2 and associated proteins has emerged as being an important factor in two neurodevelopmental disorders, Rett and fragile X syndrome (25) (see Chapter 2.3.3, Lombroso, for a more detailed examination of these two syndromes), as well as the molecular events leading to various cancers.

DNA in somatic tissue is characterized by a bimodal pattern of methylation, which is established through a series of developmental events (26). Very early in development, most DNA is unmethylated, but after implantation, a wave of *de novo* methylation modifies most of the genome, excluding the majority of CpG islands, which are mainly associated with housekeeping genes. These genomic methylation patterns are broadly maintained during the life of the organism by maintenance methylation and generally correlate with gene expression.

"Gene dosage" is another crucial issue in the regulation of genes. Under normal circumstances in adults there are classes of genes where only one of the two inherited copies is active. Two prominent examples include genes that are not expressed due to the early coordinated inactivation of one copy of the two X chromosomes in women, and those genes that are not expressed due to genomic imprinting. Imprinting involves the coordinated silencing of contiguous genes coming either from the father or mother. Although the mechanisms that underlie such events are poorly understood, significant progress is being made to understand these processes at the molecular level (27–29).

It is evident from this description that gene transcription depends on a complex combination of regulatory mechanisms. A different pattern of gene expression will emerge depending on which nucleotide sequences are present within a promoter region as well as which transcription factors, enhancers, or repressor proteins are present within the cell. Moreover, this interplay of regulatory factors will determine whether and how much of a specific protein is transcribed. We will return to these concepts below when we describe exactly how certain growth factors as well as environmental factors interplay with transcription factors to either initiate or repress expression of genes within the brain.

A species' genetic program unfolds in a largely predictable fashion despite its formidable complexity from the earliest gene expression in the zygote through the entire morphogenesis of the organism. This uniformity may depend, in part, on the presence of redundant pathways and in part from the fact that development proceeds largely in the direction of increasing complexity, but lesser potential.

Posttranscriptional Events

Transcribed RNA typically goes through a number of modifications before it is ready for export from the nucleus. An early step includes the excision of intervening regions of the RNA, termed introns that do not encode for protein; the remaining expressed sequences, or exons, are joined together. This processing of immature RNA molecules occurs through a mechanism called splicing, in which nucleotide splice sites are recognized by proteins whose function it is to bind to these sites, remove the introns, and splice together the exons. The end result is a mature message containing the sequence of nucleotides that encode the amino acids that form the protein.

Several splice sites are often present within a gene and allow for different exons of the gene to be brought together, while excluding other exons. This flexibility in mRNA formation has several important functions. A single gene may produce several nearly identical proteins that differ in certain critical amino acid regions, or domains. The resulting proteins may have different enzymatic functions or binding affinities for target proteins. Alternatively spliced messages are particularly enriched within the central nervous system (CNS), where they are often expressed at different developmental periods. For example, one version of a protein may only be expressed during embryonic development, while an alternatively spliced variant is only expressed during adulthood. The former protein may be required for early neuronal development or may be targeted to the nucleus. An alternatively spliced adult form may have a novel domain that targets it to the synapse, where it participates in specific signaling pathways. Alternative splicing of genes is a regulatory mechanism that permits proteins to be expressed in different forms, within differing tissues, or at varying developmental periods.

Another gene regulatory mechanism involves the addition of long stretches of adenine nucleotides, the poly(A) tail, to the mRNA message prior to its being shuttled out of the nucleus and into the cytoplasm. The function of the poly(A) tail is to regulate the timing of translation of the mRNA into functional protein, and provide stability to the mRNA molecule.

Translational Factors

The process of translating mRNA molecules into proteins occurs outside of the nucleus. A number of RNA-binding proteins as well as the ribosomes themselves bind to the messages and initiate a complex series of events, many of which are themselves under regulatory control. Although regulatory mechanisms at this level may seem unnecessary, they do provide a means of rapidly controlling synthesis of gene products by cells. Mutations in proteins that regulate the translation of messages can lead to a number of developmental disorders, including fragile X syndrome.

The stability of a mature mRNA that has entered the cytosol is a critical determinant of how many copies of a protein will be synthesized by the ribosomal apparatus. Certain base sequences in the message as well as the poly(A) tail are thought to influence the stability of many mRNA molecules and their rate of degradation.

Posttranslational Processing

Once a protein has been formed, it often undergoes further modification. For example, sulfhydryl groups in two cysteine residues may form a covalent bond with each other and this provides stability for the protein as it folds into a final tertiary structure. Several other chemical modifications also occur, such as the phosphorylation of serine, tyrosine, and threonine residues, the glycosylation of the amino acid asparagine, the acetylation of the NH2 terminal amino acids, or the hydroxylation of proline and lysine residues. Glycoproteins are formed by the addition of various sugar moieties to the free hydroxyl group of serine or threonine (30).

The removal of certain amino acid stretches from a protein is another posttranslational modification that occurs. One example is the formation of neuropeptides that often involves the cleavage of precursor proteins at specific sites. For example, the processing of prodynorphin molecules leads to a variety of dynorphin moieties and leuenkephalin. Intriguingly, differential processing of prodynorphin, as well as other precursor proteins, in different tissues is commonplace, so that the form of dynorphin found in the anterior lobe of the pituitary is different from the form of dynorphin found in the neurointermediate lobe (31).

ENVIRONMENTAL EFFECTS ON GENE TRANSCRIPTION

Growth Factors

Growth factors have been implicated in a broad range of developmental processes in which cell specification, growth, migration, and survival have to be coordinated across tissues or germ layers. For example, in early embryonic development, interactions between the ectoderm and the underlaying mesoderm are critical for the formation of neural tissue; in particular, factors are synthesized and secreted as a result of these cell movements that repress epidermal cell fate and promote neural fate via an antagonism of Wnt and transforming growth factor signaling (32). Subsequently, fibroblast growth factors (FGF) and sonic hedgehog (Shh), which are synthesized within the neural tube itself or are diffusing in it from the mesoderm, regulate early brain growth and patterning along the antero–posterior and dorso–ventral axes. Different factors are critical for the growth of specific portions of the brain; for example, basic fibroblast growth factor (FGF2) is necessary for cell proliferation and neurogenesis in the developing cerebral cortex (33, 34) while still unidentified FGF family members, acting primarily through the FGF receptor 1, are required for the growth of the hippocampus (35). Interestingly, the same factors are used later in brain development to promote the growth of neuronal connections, the initial formation of synaptic connections, and the migration and maturation of glial cells (36–39) (Smith et al., in press). Finally, in postnatal development, different growth factor families, particularly neurotrophins which include brain-derived neurotrophic factor (BDNF), are thought to participate in the activity-dependent retraction and pruning of connections and synapses (40, 41). These processes are thought to mediate learning and memory formation (42). Thus, growth factors are required for multiple steps during both development and mature CNS functioning (43).

While many different growth factors are produced within the CNS, often only minute amounts of these molecules are secreted. The end result is that neurons compete for the small amounts of trophic factors present. The receptors for the various growth factors lie on the outer membrane and bind their specific growth factor. Once bound, a cascade of signals is initiated that promotes the growth, differentiation, and long-term survival of cells, as well as the development of the synaptic connections that are required for synaptic plasticity during learning and memory.

Most receptors have two functional domains: an extracellular portion that binds to the signaling molecule and an intracellular domain that passes along the signal. The binding of a growth factor to its receptor often results in two ligand–receptor complexes coming together on the membrane to form dimers (Figure 2.3.1.5). The intracellular catalytic domains of the receptors are protein kinases (proteins that add phosphate groups to substrate molecules), and dimerization positions the activated receptors in close proximity to each other to permit the cross phosphorylation of each receptor molecule.

Several events then occur in rapid succession. A number of proteins are recruited from the cytoplasm to form complexes of signaling proteins at the plasma membrane. These newly recruited proteins are often themselves phosphorylated by the activated receptors and a cascade of signals is initiated that ultimately leads to the activation of transcription factors and the transcription of specific sets of genes. For example, one of the best studied signaling pathways necessary for learning and memory leads through a series of successive phosphorylations to the activation of a protein called "mitogen activated protein kinase" (MAPK). One of the functions of MAPK follows from its rapid transportation into the nucleus where it phosphorylates specific transcription factors and initiates the transcription of genes required for synaptic plasticity. Other intracellular signaling molecules include protein kinase C and phosphatidylinositol kinases.

In summary, the binding of growth factors to their receptors on the cell surface leads to the rapid transmission of the signal into the neuron. It is not surprising that mutations in some of these receptor proteins disrupt the normal transmission of intracellular signaling, leading to a number of developmental disorders affecting the structure and function of the CNS (44–46).

Hormones

Hormones use a related mechanism to transmit signals into cells (47). There are many different types of hormones within our bodies. We review one of these that has an important role within the CNS. Hydrocortisone is a glucocorticoid hormone secreted in response to stressful events. Although stress responses are critical for our survival as a species, too much stress has adverse effects on our physiology and may damage neuronal structure and function (48, 49).

Hydrocortisone is synthesized in the cortex of the adrenal gland, where it is released into the blood stream. Similar to most steroid hormones, hydrocortisone is a lipid-soluble molecule. This fact leads to several important differences between this family of signaling proteins and the growth factors.

Growth factor receptors lie on the plasma membrane, where they are able to directly bind their ligand. In contrast, the receptors for most hormones are concentrated in the cytosol or nucleus. Lipid soluble hormones pass directly across the membrane and bind to their receptors within the cells to initiate specific cascades of signals.

A second difference between receptors on the surface of membranes and hormone receptors is the fact that hormone receptors act directly as transcription factors. Prior to binding their respective hormones, hormone receptors are in an inactive state, as they are tightly associated with an inhibitory protein. The inhibitory protein is released when the hormone binds to the receptor and a DNA-binding domain on the receptor–hormone complex becomes unmasked. The complex is now able to interact with specific DNA sequences within the promoter region of genes. In this way, hormone receptors initiate the transcription of genes required by the cell at that moment.

Most hormones exert their effects in two stages. Initially, the hormone receptor induces the transcription of a small number of genes. This effect usually occurs within 30 minutes and is known as the primary hormonal response. Because many of these genes are themselves transcription factors, a cascade of transcription is begun. Steroid hormones thus are able to exert much longer lasting responses than growth factors. Typically, the immediate effects of growth factors disappear within seconds or milliseconds, although their action can be prolonged

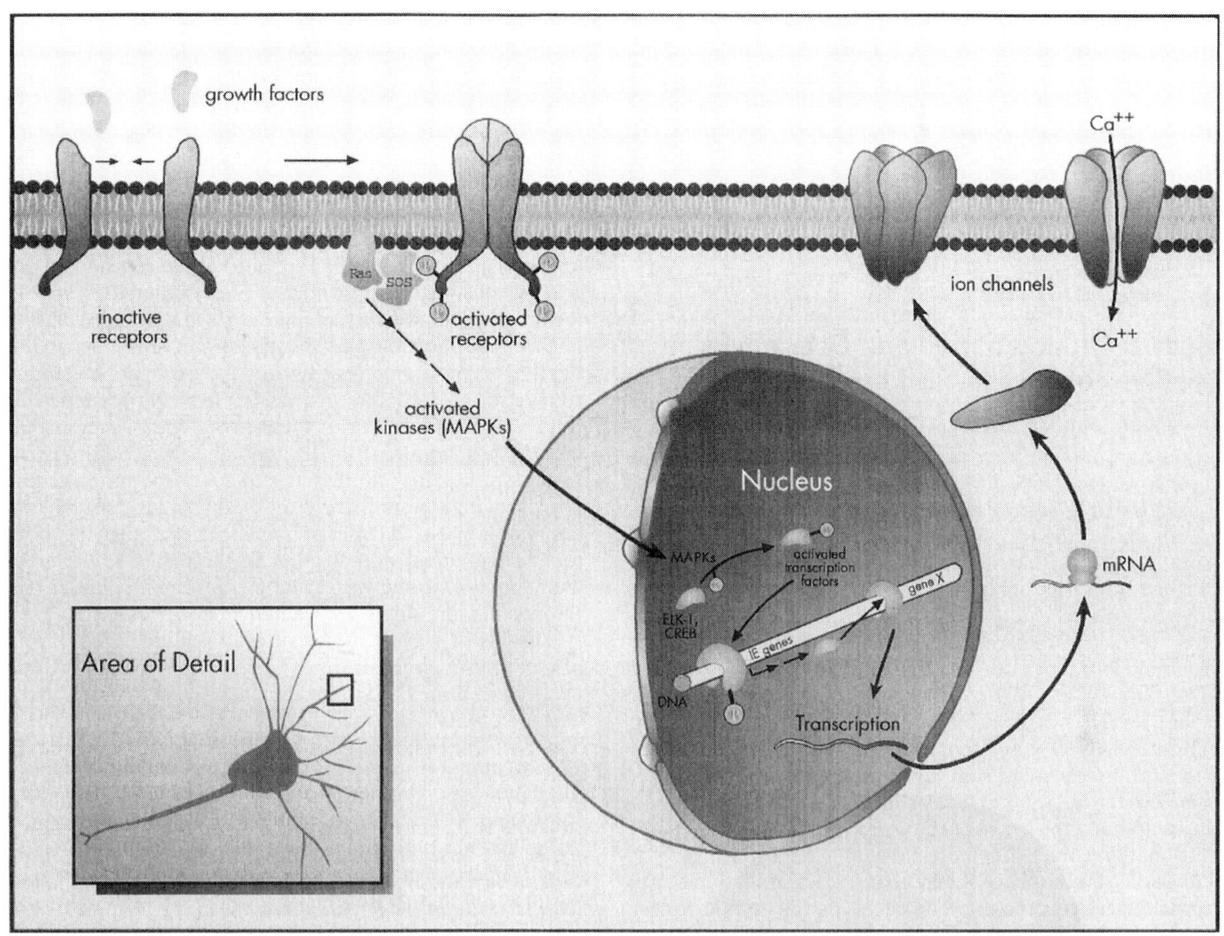

FIGURE 2.3.1.5. Signal transduction and the action of growth factors. Growth factors generate signals in a cell by binding to specific receptors on the plasma surface and initiating transcription of needed proteins. Two molecules of a growth factor are shown binding to their receptor. The receptors are transmembrane tyrosine kinases receptors that associate with each other after ligand binding and become phosphorylated. In their phosphorylated state, the receptors attract other signaling proteins, including the adapter protein SOS and the enzyme, Ras. The newly formed complex of proteins activates several kinase pathways, one of which is shown here (MAPKs). In this pathway, transcription factors (Elk-1, Jun) are activated by phosphorylation within the nucleus and initiate the transcription of genes, some of which are themselves transcription factors (immediate early, or IE, genes). The IE transcription factors initiate transcription of additional genes, and their mRNA messages are transported back into the cytoplasm and translated into proteins, such as the ion channels shown. In this example, an ion channel is being synthesized and leads to an increased level of the second messenger, Ca^{2+}. (Adapted from Vaccarino FM, Lombroso PJ. Growth factors. *J Am Acad Child Adol Psychiatry* 37:789–790, 1998.) (See color plate.)

by the activation of downstream signaling pathways. In contrast, hormones such as hydrocortisone persist in the blood for hours, whereas the thyroid hormones last even longer and their actions persist for days. The newly synthesized transcription factors activate additional genes in a delayed or secondary hormonal response. A single hormone, therefore, can initiate a persistent and complex pattern of gene expression.

GENES AND THE CREATION AND MAINTENANCE OF THE NERVOUS SYSTEM

Although the precise number of genes that regulate the growth and development of the CNS is unknown, some investigators have estimated that at least one-third of the mammalian genome is devoted exclusively to this task (50). Recent estimates from the human genome sequencing project suggest that over 35,000 genes exist in the human genome. Thus, approximately 10,000 of these are specifically expressed within the human CNS. This figure does not include constitutively expressed genes that maintain the basic functions of cellular life, including the regulation of the cell cycle, production of subcellular organelles, and maintenance of the cellular structure.

The process of development is a heritable feature of all organisms. The unfolding of gene expression must provide virtually all of the information necessary to guide the orderly succession of events that will transform portions of the fertilized egg into a fully developed CNS. The morphogenesis of the nervous system involves at least five major genetically regulated processes: the birth of specific cell types, their migration to their final destination, their growth, the development of neural connections, and cell death (51, 52). A fundamental understanding of these processes would require precise knowledge of: a) the developmental information relevant to the CNS that is encoded in the human genome, b) how this information is regulated and utilized in "morphogenetic" time and space, and c) how the products of these genes endow the differentiating and differentiated cells of the embryonic CNS with their functional characteristics (16). Although we remain largely ignorant of the critical determinants of these processes, remarkable progress toward understanding them has been made during the past decade (53). Genetic studies of the development of the CNS in flies, worms, and other model systems have led the way to many of our most fundamental discoveries.

Spatial Differentiation and Determination of Specific Cell Lineages

Interestingly, mRNAs synthesized by the mother during oogenesis are present after fertilization and provide the basis for most of the biosynthetic capacity of early embryos. Thousands of mRNAs are formed during oogenesis and remain dormant within the egg until fertilization occurs. One of the reasons for this is that much of the machinery required for the proper transcription, translation, and processing of mature proteins is not yet available in the very early embryo. In some species, the set of maternal genes constitutes the majority of all genomic loci active during ontogeny (16).

The maternal mRNAs persist until the blastula stage, when they are replaced by transcripts produced by the developing organism. Many of these transcripts are homologous with the maternal transcripts, but some are novel genes not included in the maternal set. An instructive example of this transition from maternal to zygotic transcription concerns several evolutionarily conserved proteins that act as a trigger for cell divisions. Studies have shown that the accumulation of the maternally derived protein cyclin serves as the mitotic trigger for early cellular divisions, whereas later cell divisions depend on the production of a different trigger protein produced by the developing zygote (54).

Two other important classes of genes active at this point in development are segmentation and homeotic genes. These genes have been best characterized in *Drosophila,* where they determine the number and polarity of body segments and the identity and sequence of body segments (55). Most of these genes are evolutionarily conserved and present in the human genome.

Although the precise functions of homeotic genes in mammalian development have not been fully established, they are known to be differentially expressed in the central and peripheral nervous systems, as well as in mesodermal derivatives (56). Intriguingly, some of these genes exist in multigene clusters related by duplication and divergence. In some instances, the relative chromosomal position of the gene in a cluster corresponds to the domain of expression in the developing embryo (Figure 2.3.1.6). Many of these genes code for transcription factors. As a consequence, attention has focused on their roles in organizing the differential expression of other genes that are ultimately responsible for establishing distinctive cellular phenotypes. Their expression patterns provide evidence for the segmental organization of the rostral CNS, although their function in the vertebrate CNS is more complex than in *Drosophila* and often not well understood (57).

Dozens of regulator genes have been identified during the past decade that appear to play crucial roles in the development of the vertebrate CNS. These include the vertebrate homologs of *Drosophila* segment polarity genes *engrailed* and *wingless* (58). The first forebrain-specific homeodomain-containing genes including the *distaless, gastrulation- and brain-specific gene, orthodenticle,* and *empty-spiracle* gene families were isolated and characterized by the early 1990s (59–62). Subsequently, vertebrate genes encoding for secreted morphogens such as Shh and FGFs were found to be expressed in longitudinal and transverse domains along the entire neural axis (63). In many cases growth factors induce homeodomain gene expression, although the converse is also true. The intricate cascade of genetic and molecular events that lead to the development

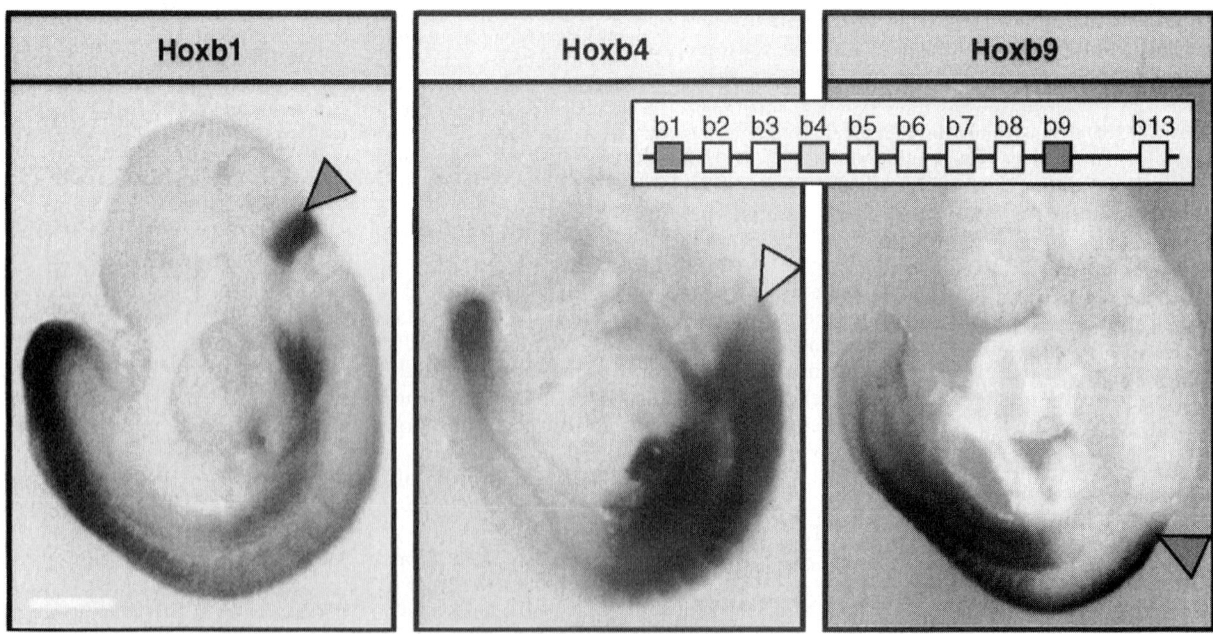

FIGURE 2.3.1.6. Homeodomain-containing genes and their expression in the neural axis. Hox gene expression in the mouse embryo. The three panels show lateral views of 9.5-day-old mouse embryos stained with antibodies specific for the protein products of *Hoxb1, Hoxb4,* and *Hoxb9* genes. (Adapted from Wolpert L, Beddington J, Brockes J, et al.: *Principles of Development.* Oxford: Oxford University Press, 1998, p. 103.) (See color plate.)

of the mammalian CNS is one of the most exciting stories in developmental neuroscience.

Not surprisingly, defects in the human homologues of homodomain transcription factors and growth factor genes are being recognized with increasing frequency as a cause of cortical malformations due to aberrant neuronal proliferation and differentiation (64). Examples of this phenomenon are dystonia (65) mental retardation associated with schizencephaly or with other disorders of cortical migration (66–69).

Finally, it has also become clear that neurogenesis occurs in adults as well as in the prenatal period. New neurons have been identified that originate in the subventricular zone and then migrate through the white matter to the neocortex, where they extend axons, and become functionally active (70).

Migration of Neurons

The early embryonic development of the nervous system is characterized in part by the migration of populations of neurons. Examples of this phenomenon include the migration of neural crest cells to form elements of the peripheral nervous system (autonomic and sensory ganglia, glial cells, and adrenomedullary cells) and the migration of neurons born within the ventricular zone to their final destination within the cortical laminae. A range of factors mediate these events, and some have been identified, including proteins that contribute to inherent directional preferences, chemotaxis, and differential adhesion of cells as they migrate (71).

In the case of corticogenesis, it has been established that the newly formed glutamatergic projection neurons migrate along radial glial guides that stretch between the ventricular surface and outer cortical surface (72). It is likely that cytoskeletal proteins, molecular motors and adhesion molecules are necessary for this migratory process to occur (73–75). One example is the extracellular glycoprotein reelin, which is secreted by interneurons in the cortical and hippocampal marginal zone, and whose deficiency results in aberrant migratory patterns and layering of glutamate projection neurons in cerebral cortex and hippocampus (as is seen in the "reeler" mouse mutant) (76, 77). Another example is the microtubule-binding protein doublecortin, which is selectively expressed by newly generated, migrating neurons. Cortical neurons are unable to complete their migration when doublecortin expression is decreased in mouse models (78). Inborn mutations in the doublecortin gene and other genes that govern neuronal migration have been implicated in a number of human disorders, including X-linked lissenencephaly, focal pachypolymicrogyria, and the "double-cortex" syndrome (79, 80) (next chapter). In many instances, however, the genes responsible for the abnormal migration have not yet been identified (81).

A second type of migration has recently been described, which is independent from radial glial cell guides, and involves the rapid "tangential" movement of GABAergic neurons from their site of origin in the medial, lateral, and caudal ganglionic eminences to the cerebral cortex, hippocampus, basal ganglia, and olfactory bulb (82–84). An abnormal number and location of GABAergic cells in prefrontal regions of the cortex is considered the most replicated biological abnormality in schizophrenia (85), and an abnormal distribution of GABAergic neurons has been also found in severe cases of Tourette syndrome and possibly other hyperactivity disorders (86, 87). Hence, the regulation of tangential migration, which is the focus of considerable attention in current neuroscience research, may turn out to be of fundamental importance for the pathogenesis of common neuropsychiatric disorders.

Neural Connectivity and Survival

Developing nerve cells have the remarkable characteristic of being able to maintain contact with literally thousands of other nerve cells by extending cellular processes over substantial distances. These contacts are of crucial importance in establishing and maintaining the functional integrity of the nervous system. These processes initially develop by way of local extension and retraction of specialized areas on the surface of the neurons called growth cones. A variety of external signals regulate the formation, maintenance, and/or degradation of these neuronal connections, including mechanical guides, differential adhesiveness, the influence of electrical fields, and interaction with gradients of trophic substances (71, 88, 89).

Once neuronal processes reach their target field, the neurons acquire obligatory trophic dependencies. Target fields contain growth factors such as nerve growth factor that bind to the axons projecting to that field and are retrogradely transported to the afferent cell body. A given target field, however, is able to support only a limited number of neurons, and the "extra" neurons are lost. For example, although nerve growth factor (NGF) does not attract sensory nerve fibers to their target fields, it is intimately involved in the target-mediated survival of neurons. Indeed, from the first appearance of the neuronal processes in the target field, there is a marked increase in the rate of transcription of the NGF gene and the amount of NGF in the target field. There is also a rapid appearance of cell surface receptors for NGF on the sensory neurons (mediated by the transcription of the NGF receptor gene) (90).

Genetic factors are likely to play an important facilitatory role in neurite outgrowth and synaptogenesis throughout life. The dynamic equilibrium between neurite outgrowth and the formation of synapses versus neurite pruning and synapse withdrawal may well be a crucial mechanism that allows organisms to modify their behavior or "learn" as a result of experience. Although the precise genetic mechanisms that underlie these complex processes are not well understood, one mechanism may involve those genes that regulate the expression of molecules involved in neuronal communication. For example, *in vitro* and *in vivo* studies have indicated that many neurotransmitters and neuromodulators, in addition to their communicative function in mature neural systems, play important roles in the development and maintenance of these systems by promoting or inhibiting the growth of neural processes (91).

Recently, a carboxypeptidase A inhibitor, latexin, has been identified that appears to play a role in cortical projection neurons that are fated to establish links between the primary sensory and motor cortex and secondary association areas (92). A number of mouse mutants are also providing valuable insights into the genes, molecules, and mechanisms that mediate the connection of cortical neurons to cortical and subcortical targets (93).

The Role of Early Life Experience

The development of the nervous system depends on environmental as well as genetic factors. At each level and stage of development, the microenvironments and macroenvironments of the organism play a crucial role. The unfolding of the genetic program, with its complex sequences and patterns of gene expression, depends in large measure on the presence of transcriptional factors in the microenvironment of the nucleus. This means that our ability to separate out the relative contributions of genetic and epigenetic influences is difficult because the genes influence the environment through the production of various proteins and the environment, in turn, alters the expression of genes (Figure 2.3.1.7).

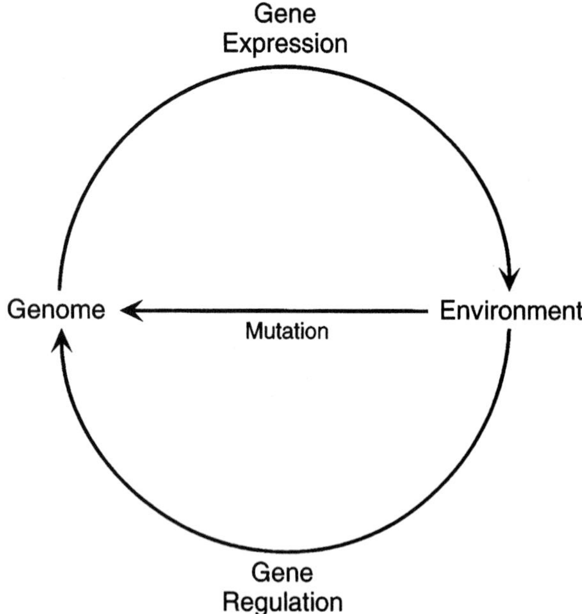

FIGURE 2.3.1.7. Gene–environment interactions. (Adapted from Purves D, Lichtrnan JW. *Principles of Neural Development.* Sunderland, MA: Sinauer, 1985.)

This reciprocal relationship between genes and the environment is played out over the entire course of development. Developmental biologists have long been interested in characterizing the sequence of microenvironmental changes occurring within the CNS that allow for the normal unfolding of early brain development. In fact, a great deal has been learned regarding the orderly turning on of various transcription factors that organize the body plan, including the brain (Figure 2.3.1.5). A growing list of growth factors and cell surface molecules present in the microenvironment influence these events by altering the synthesis or the posttranslational processing of transcription factors by activating signaling pathways that were discussed in the preceding sections.

This is not to say that external environmental factors cannot influence some of these early developmental events. It is well established that drugs, alcohol, altered nutrition (including a lack of oxygen, or hypoxia), and infectious illnesses disrupt the orderly progression of neuronal growth during critical periods of brain development. However, the brain of a healthy fetus in a "normal" environment will develop because of the instructions contained in its genetic code.

The situation changes significantly during the latter part of gestation onward as the CNS becomes functionally active. In humans as well as other mammals, there is a tremendous growth in the number of synaptic connections (94). Moreover, as neuronal connections form, the proper ones are strengthened throughout early infancy by the expansion of functioning synaptic contacts. Although neuronal connections can be made throughout life, it is during the early childhood years and again during puberty that the greatest amount of change occurs in synapses throughout the nervous system.

A great deal of experimental evidence has indicated that neuronal activity is required for the proliferation of these connections, as well as their later refinement (95, 96). Neuronal activity is triggered by interactions of the developing organism with its intrauterine and postnatal environments. Ultimately, genes within the brain must be activated, while others must be repressed to permit the normal development of axonal growth cones and the elaboration of synapses, as well as the pruning back of unwanted or unnecessary connections. Much of what developmental neurobiologists have learned regarding these processes began with the seminal work of Hubel and Wiesel over 30 years ago. These investigators were interested in determining how the visual cortex develops and organizes itself. The visual cortex is a region of the brain that encompasses approximately 30% of the cortex when its associated regions are included. Their work clearly established that the connectivity of the adult visual cortex is critically dependent on early synaptic input (97, 98). Visual experience is required for the development in the primary visual cortex of what are termed ocular dominance columns. In order to function properly, visual input from the right or left eye must be separated into alternating columns in the visual cortex. Prior to and immediately following birth, inputs from the eyes are not separated but, rather, make overlapping synaptic contacts. Once visual activity is initiated after birth, there is a progressive segregation of the visual inputs into adjacent columns. This reshaping of the axonal connections within the cortex by visual experience is referred to as activity-dependent plasticy (99).

What was unexpected from the work of Hubel and Wiesel was the discovery that the orderly segregation requires visual experience during a critical period of time. Normal ocular dominance columns will not develop if an animal, such as a kitten, is raised for the first six weeks with vision permitted only through one eye. The columns receiving input from the occluded eye shrink, while those receiving from the open eye expand, and the occluded eye becomes disconnected from the cortex. Consequently, if vision is then restored to the deprived eye, a "catch-up" does not occur, and the failure to develop properly segregated columns becomes permanent. The visual cortex remains abnormally organized throughout the animal's life (100).

Similar deficits are seen in humans who do not experience normal visual inputs during their first years of life. The clinical examples most commonly described are the abnormalities that occur in an infant born with either unilateral or bilateral cataracts. If the cataract is not diagnosed and surgically removed early in life, the child will never develop vision in the affected eye(s). There is a critical period in human infants when proper synaptic connections within the visual cortex must be formed. This is in contrast to the situation in adulthood, where cataracts may be present for years; however, once removed, the individual regains visual acuity.

More recent research has revised this concept and revealed that ocular dominance columns develop before any activity is detectable in the cortex (101, 102). Hence, it appears that experience modifies rather than establishes cortical architecture. This activity-dependent refinement occurs in many regions of the cortex involved in sensory perception (100). One example comes from the work of investigators interested in what happens to cortical regions after amputation of a finger (103). The earlier this occurs, the more plastic is the cortex in remodeling. Regions that used to subserve the amputated finger regress and nearby digits expand their representations into the region. An extreme example of neural plasticity and the capacity for the brain to reorganize connections involves the rewiring of visual projections to the auditory cortex early in life that allows the animal to "see" using its auditory cortex (104).

Another example relates to how much easier it is to learn a second language early in life. Functional magnetic resonance imaging studies were used to determine the areas of the brain that are metabolically activated during language acquisition in individuals who learn both native and second languages. When a child learns two languages, both languages are represented in a single language center; however, when an adult attempts to learn a second language, a new language center is established that is clearly distinguishable from the primary language center (105).

The sphere of influences acting on the nervous system continually enlarges during development (71). The cytoplasm of the egg, with its maternally derived biosynthetic apparatus, provides the initial milieu, a "good enough" environment to support development. Later, local cellular interactions between the mesoderm and the nervous tissue, between neurons and glia, and the reciprocal activity networks of neurons influence the microenvironment of the discrete cell lineages and regulate morphogenesis. Finally, the nervous system is also shaped by hormones and other substances carried by the vasculature and by wholly external events in the prenatal and postnatal world.

Consistent with this view, evidence for a critical period in which maternal stimuli and pup–mother interactions shape the future behavior of the progeny has recently been presented (106). In these animal studies, the level of maternal care as measured by licking and grooming by the mothers profoundly influenced the quality of maternal care offered by the female adult offspring. It also established an enduring pattern of stress response in the pups as they matured. The pups raised by the attentive dams were more likely to show less stress in response to novel environments (107). These findings are also consistent with other studies that have documented the enduring impact of maternal stress in the perinatal period (108, 109). Importantly, many of these effects appear to result from environmental effects on gene expression in limbic regions of the brain. For example, the level of licking and grooming by the mother regulates the DNA methylation and histone acetylation of the glucorticoid receptor gene promoter, and the subsequent transcription of this gene in the hippocampus in the offspring (110, 111). It is also likely that alterations in these neurobiological systems may alter an individual's vulnerability to later psychopathology, including mood and affective disorders (112).

Finally, it is likely that events in early family life, interactions with peers, and educational opportunities shape the course of development just as surely as the developing individual profoundly influences his or her environment. The developmental perspectives of child psychiatry echo in the study of developmental neurobiology.

FUTURE PROSPECTS

Genetics and the developmental neurosciences are on the threshold of a new era in which the sequence of the human genome is widely available, and the intricate cascade of molecular events that govern brain development are being elucidated. DNA "chips" containing fragments of virtually all the mRNAs coded for by the human genome are now available to investigators in commercial, as well as academic, settings. Using these tools, the genetic underpinning of neuropsychiatric syndromes can be explored (113–117) and animal models of these diseases are likely to be successfully developed.

Although the scientific, information management, and logistical challenges to understanding the complexity of the human genome vis à vis brain development are daunting, they are likely to pale in comparison to the ethical dilemmas to be faced as information about our vulnerability genes becomes accessible. The ethical problems will multiply as commercial firms develop even more potent pharmacological tools to influence these developing neurobiological systems. We also predict that this new knowledge will emphasize the importance of early life events in shaping the CNS and will point the way to the profound and enduring importance of selective early interventions for families at high risk (118–120).

References

1. Leckman JF, Mayes LC: Understanding developmental psychopathology: how useful are evolutionary accounts? *J Am Acad Child Adolesc Psychiatry* 37(10):1011–1021, 1998.
2. Northcutt RG, Kaas JH: The emergence and evolution of mammalian neocortex. *Trends Neurosci* Sep 1995:18(9):373–379.
3. Shields J: *Monozygotic Twins, Brought Up Apart and Brought Up Together*. London, New York, Oxford University Press, 1962.
4. Juel-Nielsen N: *Individual and Environment: Monozygotic Twins Reared Apart*. Rev. ed. New York, International Universities Press, 1980.
5. Moore T, Haig D: Genomic imprinting in mammalian development: a parental tug-of-war. *Trends Genet* Feb 1991:7(2):45–49.
6. Knoll JH, Wagstaff J, Lalande M: Cytogenetic and molecular studies in the Prader-Willi and Angelman syndromes: an overview. *Am J Med Genet* Apr 1 1993:46(1):2–6.
7. Alberts B, Johnson A, Lewis J, Raff M, Roberts K, Walter P: *Molecular Biology of the Cell*. Garland Science, 2002.
8. Watson JD: *Molecular Biology of the Gene*. 5th ed. San Francisco, Pearson/Benjamin Cummings, 2004.
9. Mendel G, Tschermak E: *Versuche èuber Pflanzenhybriden. Zwei abhandlungen (1865 und 1869)*. Leipzig, W. Engelmann, 1901.
10. Crick FH, Barnett L, Brenner S, Watts-Tobin RJ: General nature of the genetic code for proteins. *Nature* Dec 30 1961:192:1227–1232.
11. Gumucio DL, Shelton DA, Zhu W, et al.: Evolutionary strategies for the elucidation of cis and trans factors that regulate the developmental switching programs of the beta-like globin genes. *Mol Phylogenet Evol* Feb 1996:5(1):18–32.
12. Hardison R, Slightom JL, Gumucio DL, Goodman M, Stojanovic N, Miller W: Locus control regions of mammalian beta-globin gene clusters: combining phylogenetic analyses and experimental results to gain functional insights. *Gene* Dec 31 1997:205(1–2):73–94.
13. McGinnis W, Levine MS, Hafen E, Kuroiwa A, Gehring WJ: A conserved DNA sequence in homoeotic genes of the Drosophila Antennapedia and bithorax complexes. *Nature* Mar 29–Apr 4 1984:308(5958):428–433.
14. Landschulz WH, Johnson PF, McKnight SL: The leucine zipper: a hypothetical structure common to a new class of DNA binding proteins. *Science* Jun 24 1988:240(4860):1759–1764.
15. Miller J, McLachlan AD, Klug A: Repetitive zinc-binding domains in the protein transcription factor IIIA from Xenopus oocytes. *Embo J* Jun 1985:4(6):1609–1614.
16. Davidson EH: *Gene Activity in Early Development*. Orlando, FL, Academic Press, 1986.
17. Groudine M, Weintraub H: Rous sarcoma virus activates embryonic globin genes in chicken fibroblasts. *Proc Natl Acad Sci USA* Nov 1975:72(11):4464–4468.
18. Ivarie RD, Schacter BS, O'Farrell PH: The level of expression of the rat growth hormone gene in liver tumor cells is at least eight orders of magnitude less than that in anterior pituitary cells. *Mol Cell Biol* Aug 1983:3(8):1460–1467.
19. Nan X, Ng HH, Johnson CA, et al.: Transcriptional repression by the methyl-CpG-binding protein MeCP2 involves a histone deacetylase complex. *Nature* May 28 1998:393(6683):386–389.
20. Jones PL, Veenstra GJ, Wade PA, et al.: Methylated DNA and MeCP2 recruit histone deacetylase to repress transcription. *Nat Genet* Jun 1998:19(2):187–191.
21. Klose RJ, Bird AP: MeCP2 behaves as an elongated monomer that does not stably associate with the Sin3a chromatin remodeling complex. *J Biol Chem* Nov 5 2004:279(45):46490–46496.
22. Fuks F, Hurd PJ, Wolf D, Nan X, Bird AP, Kouzarides T: The methyl-CpG-binding protein MeCP2 links DNA methylation to histone methylation. *J Biol Chem* Feb 7 2003:278(6):4035–4040.
23. Kimura H, Shiota K: Methyl-CpG-binding protein, MeCP2, is a target molecule for maintenance DNA methyltransferase, Dnmt1. *J Biol Chem* Feb 14 2003:278(7):4806–4812.
24. Amir RE, Van den Veyver IB, Wan M, Tran CQ, Francke U, Zoghbi HY: Rett syndrome is caused by mutations in X-linked MECP2, encoding methyl-CpG-binding protein 2. *Nat Genet* Oct 1999:23(2):185–188.
25. Horike S, Cai S, Miyano M, Cheng JF, Kohwi-Shigematsu T: Loss of silent-chromatin looping and impaired imprinting of DLX5 in Rett syndrome. *Nat Genet* Jan 2005:37(1):31–40.
26. Greally JM, State MW: Genetics of childhood disorders: XIII. Genomic imprinting: the indelible mark of the gamete. *J Am Acad Child Adolesc Psychiatry* Apr 2000:39(4):532–535.
27. Marahrens Y: X-inactivation by chromosomal pairing events. *Genes Dev* Oct 15 1999:13(20):2624–2632.
28. Sleutels F, Barlow DP: The origins of genomic imprinting in mammals. *Adv Genet* 46:119–163, 2002.
29. Sleutels F, Barlow DP, Lyle R: The uniqueness of the imprinting mechanism. *Curr Opin Genet Dev* Apr 2000:10(2):229–233.
30. Freifelder D: *Molecular Biology*. Boston, Jones & Bartlett, 1987.
31. Molineaux CJ, Hassen AH, Rosenberger JG, Cox BM: Response of rat pituitary anterior lobe prodynorphin products to changes in gonadal steroid environment. *Endocrinology* Nov 1986:119(5):2297–2305.
32. Wilson SW, Rubenstein JL: Induction and dorsoventral patterning of the telencephalon. *Neuron* 28(3):641–651, 2000.
33. Raballo R, Rhee J, Lyn-Cook R, Leckman JF, Schwartz ML, Vaccarino FM: Basic fibroblast growth factor (Fgf2) is necessary for cell proliferation and neurogenesis in the developing cerebral cortex. *J Neurosci* 20(13):5012–5023, 2000.

34. Vaccarino FM, Schwartz ML, Raballo R, et al.: Changes in cerebral cortex size are governed by Fibroblast Growth Factor during embryogenesis. *Nature Neuroscience* 2:246–253, 1999.
35. Ohkubo Y, Uchida AO, Shin D, Partanen J, Vaccarino FM: Fibroblast growth factor receptor 1 is required for the proliferation of hippocampal progenitor cells and for hippocampal growth in mouse. *J Neurosci* Jul 7 2004:24(27):6057–6069.
36. Oh LY, Denninger A, Colvin JS, et al.: Fibroblast growth factor receptor 3 signaling regulates the onset of oligodendrocyte terminal differentiation. *J Neurosci* Feb 1 2003:23(3):883–894.
37. Umemori H, Linhoff MW, Ornitz DM, Sanes JR: FGF22 and its close relatives are presynaptic organizing molecules in the mammalian brain. *Cell* Jul 23 2004:118(2):257–270.
38. Salinas PC: The morphogen sonic hedgehog collaborates with netrin-1 to guide axons in the spinal cord. *Trends Neurosci* Dec 2003:26(12):641–643.
39. Charron F, Stein E, Jeong J, McMahon AP, Tessier-Lavigne M: The morphogen sonic hedgehog is an axonal chemoattractant that collaborates with netrin-1 in midline axon guidance. *Cell* Apr 4 2003:113(1):11–23.
40. Cabelli RJ, Shelton DL, Segal RA, Shatz CJ: Blockade of endogenous ligands of trkB inhibits formation of ocular dominance columns. *Neuron* Jul 1997:19(1):63–76.
41. Gianfranceschi L, Siciliano R, Walls J, et al.: Visual cortex is rescued from the effects of dark rearing by overexpression of BDNF. *Proc Natl Acad Sci USA* Oct 14 2003:100(21):12486–12491.
42. Klintsova AY, Greenough WT: Synaptic plasticity in cortical systems. *Curr Opin Neurobiol* Apr 1999:9(2):203–208.
43. Vaccarino FM, Schwartz ML, Raballo R, Rhee J, Lyn-Cook R: Fibroblast growth factor signaling regulates growth and morphogenesis at multiple steps during brain development. In: Pedersen RA, Shatten G (eds): *Current Topics in Developmental Biology*. Vol. 46. San Diego, CA, Academic Press, 1999, pp. 179–200.
44. Sweatt JD: Mitogen-activated protein kinases in synaptic plasticity and memory. *Curr Opin Neurobiol* Jun 2004:14(3):311–317.
45. Sweatt JD, Weeber EJ, Lombroso PJ: Genetics of childhood disorders: LI. Learning and memory, Part 4: Human cognitive disorders and the ras/ERK/CREB pathway. *J Am Acad Child Adolesc Psychiatry* Jun 2003:42(6):741–744.
46. Passos-Bueno MR, Wilcox WR, Jabs EW, Sertie AL, Alonso LG, Kitoh H: Clinical spectrum of fibroblast growth factor receptor mutations. *Hum Mutat* 14(2):115–125, 1999.
47. Evans RM: The steroid and thyroid receptor superfamily. *Science* 240:889–895, 1988.
48. Post RM, Weiss SR, Li H, et al.: Neural plasticity and emotional memory. *Dev Psychopathol* Fall 1998:10(4):829–855.
49. Sapolsky RM: Depression, antidepressants, and the shrinking hippocampus. *Proc Natl Acad Sci USA* Oct 23 2001:98(22):12320–12322.
50. Hahn WE, Van Ness J, Chaudhar N: Overview of the molecular genetics of mouse brain. In: Schmitt FO, Bloom FE (eds.): *Molecular Genetic Neuroscience*. New York: Raven Press, 1982, p. 332.
51. Jacobson M, Rao MS: *Developmental neurobiology*. 4th ed. New York, Kluwer Academic/Plenum, 2005.
52. Vaccarino FM, Leckman JF: Overview of brain development. In: Martin A, Scahill L, Charney D, Leckman JL (eds.): *Textbook of Child and Adolescent Psychopharmacology*. Oxford University Press, 2002.
53. Rubenstein JLR, Rakic P: Genetic control of cortical development. *Cereb Cortex* 9:521–523, 1999.
54. O'Farrell PH, Edgar BA, Lakich D, Lehner CF: Directing cell division during development. *Science* Nov 3 1989:246(4930):635–640.
55. Gehring WJ: Homeo boxes in the study of development. *Science* Jun 5 1987:236(4806):1245–1252.
56. Graham A, Papalopulu N, Krumlauf R: The murine and Drosophila homeobox gene complexes have common features of organization and expression. *Cell* May 5 1989:57(3):367–378.
57. Puelles L, Rubenstein JL: Forebrain gene expression domains and the evolving prosomeric model. *Trends Neurosci* Sep 2003:26(9):469–476.
58. Joyner AL: Engrailed, Wnt and Pax genes regulate midbrain–hindbrain development. *Trends in Genetics* 12(1):15–20, 1996.
59. Boncinelli E, Gulisano M, Broccoli V: Emx and Otx homeobox genes in the developing mouse brain. *J Neurobiol* 24:1356–1366, 1993.
60. Murtha MT, Leckman JF, Ruddle FH: Detection of homeobox genes in development and evolution. *Proc Natl Acad Sci USA* 88:10711–10715, 1991.
61. Rubenstein JL, Puelles L: Homeobox gene expression during development of the vertebrate brain. *Curr Top Dev Biol* 29:1–63, 1994.
62. Simeone A, Acampora D, Gulisano M, Stornaiuolo A, Boncinelli E: Nested expression domains of four homeobox genes in developing rostral brain. *Nature* 358:687–690, 1992.
63. Tanabe Y, Jessel TM: Diversity and pattern in the spinal cord. *Science* 274:1115–1123, 1997.
64. Raymond AA, Fish DR, Sisodiya SM, Alsanjari N, Stevens JM, Shorvon SD: Abnormalities of gyration, heterotopias, tuberous sclerosis, focal cortical dysplasia, microdysgenesis, dysembryoplastic neuroepithelial tumour and dysgenesis of the archicortex in epilepsy. Clinical, EEG and neuroimaging features in 100 adult patients. *Brain* Jun 1995:118(Pt. 3):629–660.
65. Pohlenz J, Dumitrescu A, Zundel D, et al.: Partial deficiency of thyroid transcription factor 1 produces predominantly neurological defects in humans and mice. *J Clin Invest* Feb 2002:109(4):469–473.
66. Kato M, Dobyns WB: X-linked lissencephaly with abnormal genitalia as a tangential migration disorder causing intractable epilepsy: proposal for a new term, "interneuronopathy." *J Child Neurol* Apr 2005:20(4):392–397.
67. Stepp ML, Cason AL, Finnis M, et al.: XLMR in MRX families 29, 32, 33 and 38 results from the dup24 mutation in the ARX (Aristaless related homeobox) gene. *BMC Med Genet* Apr 25 2005:6:16.
68. Brunelli S, Faiella A, Capra V, et al.: Germline mutations in the homeobox gene *EMX2* in patients with severe schizencephaly. *Nature Gen* 12:94–96, 1996.
69. Friocourt G, Poirier K, Rakic S, Parnavelas JG, Chelly J: The role of ARX in cortical development. *Eur J Neurosci* Feb 2006:23(4):869–876.
70. Gage FH: Neurogenesis in the adult brain. *J Neurosci* Feb 1 2002:22(3):612–613.
71. Purves D, Lichtman JW: *Principles of neural development*. Sunderland, MA, Sinauer Associates, 1985.
72. Rakic P: Specification of cerebral cortical areas. *Science* 241:170–176, 1988.
73. Hatten ME, Mason CA: Neuron-astroglia interactions *in vitro* and *in vivo*. *Trends Neurosci* 9:168–174, 1986.
74. Rakic P: Neuronal-glial interactions during brain development. *Trends Neurosci* 4:184–187, 1981.
75. Rakic P: Defects of neuronal migration and the pathogenesis of cortical malformations. *Prog Brain Res* 73:15–37, 1988.
76. Rakic P, Sidman RL: Organization of cerebellar cortex secondary to deficit of granule cells in weaver mutant mice. *J Comp Neurol* Nov 15 1973:152(2):133–161.
77. Rakic P, Sidman RL: Sequence of developmental abnormalities leading to granule cell deficit in cerebellar cortex of weaver mutant mice. *J Comp Neurol* Nov 15 1973:152(2):103–132.
78. Bai J, Ramos RL, Ackman JB, Thomas AM, Lee RV, LoTurco JJ: RNAi reveals doublecortin is required for radial migration in rat neocortex. *Nat Neurosci* Dec 2003:6(12):1277–1283.
79. Walsh CA, Goffinet AM: Potential mechanisms of mutations that affect neuronal migration in man and mouse. *Current Opinion in Genetics & Development* 10(3):270–274, 2000.
80. Gleeson JG, Walsh CA: Neuronal migration disorders: from genetic diseases to developmental mechanisms. *TINS* 23:352–359, 2000.
81. Yoshimura K, Hamada F, Tomoda T, Wakiguchi H, Kurashige T: Focal pachypolymicrogyria in three siblings. *Pediatr Neurol* May 1998:18(5):435–438.
82. Lavdas AA, Grigoriou M, Pachnis V, Parnavelas JG: The medial ganglionic eminence gives rise to a population of early neurons in the developing cerebral cortex. *Journal of Neuroscience* 19(18):7881–7888, 1999.
83. Nadarajah B, Parnavelas JG: Modes of neuronal migration in the developing cerebral cortex. *Nat Rev Neurosci* Jun 2002:3(6):423–432.
84. Anderson SA, Eisenstat DD, Shi L, Rubenstein JL: Interneuron migration from basal forebrain to neocortex: dependence on Dlx genes. *Science* 278:474–476, 1997.
85. Lewis DA, Volk DW, Hashimoto T: Selective alterations in prefrontal cortical GABA neurotransmission in schizophrenia: a novel target for the treatment of working memory dysfunction. *Psychopharmacology (Berl)* Jun 2004:174(1):143–150.
86. Kleiner-Fisman G, Calingasan NY, Putt M, Chen J, Beal MF, Lang AE: Alterations of striatal neurons in benign hereditary chorea. *Mov Disord* Jun 28 2005.
87. Kalanithi PS, Zheng W, Kataoka Y, et al.: Altered parvalbumin-positive neuron distribution in basal ganglia of individuals with Tourette syndrome. *Proc Natl Acad Sci USA* Sep 13 2005:102(37):13307–13312.
88. Guan KL, Rao Y: Signalling mechanisms mediating neuronal responses to guidance cues. *Nat Rev Neurosci* Dec 2003:4(12):941–956.
89. Kalil RE, Dubin MW, Scott G, Stark LA: Elimination of action potentials blocks the structural development of retinogeniculate synapses. *Nature* Sep 11–17 1986:323(6084):156–158.
90. Davies AM, Bandtlow C, Heumann R, Korsching S, Rohrer H, Thoenen H: Timing and site of nerve growth factor synthesis in developing skin in relation to innervation and expression of the receptor. *Nature* Mar 26–Apr 1 1987:326(6111):353–358.
91. Lipton SA, Kater SB: Neurotransmitter regulation of neuronal outgrowth, plasticity and survival. *Trends Neurosci* Jul 1989:12(7):265–270.
92. Arimatsu Y, Ishida M, Sato M, Kojima M: Corticocortical associative neurons expressing latexin: specific cortical connectivity formed *in vivo* and *in vitro*. *Cereb Cortex* Sep 1999:9(6):569–576.
93. O'Leary DD, Yates PA, McLaughlin T: Molecular development of sensory maps: representing sights and smells in the brain. *Cell* Jan 22 1999:96(2):255–269.
94. Bourgeois JP, Rakic P: Changes of synaptic density in the primary visual cortex of the macaque monkey from fetal to adult stage. *J Neurosci* Jul 1993:13(7):2801–2820.
95. Edelman G: *Neural Darwinism: The Theory of Neuronal Group Selection*. New York, Basic Books, 1987.
96. Shatz CJ: Impulse activity and the patterning of connections during CNS development. *Neuron* Dec 1990:5(6):745–756.
97. Hubel DH: *Eye, Brain, and Vision*. New York, Scientific American Library, distributed by W.H. Freeman, 1988.
98. Wiesel TN: Postnatal development of the visual cortex and the influence of environment. *Nature* Oct 14 1982:299(5884):583–591.

99. Purves D: *Neural Activity and the Growth of the Brain*. Cambridge [England], New York, Cambridge University Press, 1994.
100. Katz LC, Shatz CJ: Synaptic activity and the construction of cortical circuits. *Science* 274:1133–1138, 1996.
101. Crowley JC, Katz LC: Ocular dominance development revisited. *Curr Opin Neurobiol* Feb 2002:12(1):104–109.
102. Crowley JC, Katz LC: Early development of ocular dominance columns. *Science* Nov 17 2000:290(5495):1321–1324.
103. Merzenich MM, Kaas JH, Wall JT, Sur M, Nelson RJ, Felleman DJ: Progression of change following median nerve section in the cortical representation of the hand in areas 3b and 1 in adult owl and squirrel monkeys. *Neuroscience* Nov 1983:10(3):639–665.
104. Von Melchner L, Pallas SL, Sur M: Visual behaviour mediated by retinal projections directed to the auditory pathway. *Nature* Apr 20 2000:404(6780):871–876.
105. Kim KH, Relkin NR, Lee KM, Hirsch J: Distinct cortical areas associated with native and second languages. *Nature* Jul 10 1997:388(6638):171–174.
106. Francis D, Diorio J, Liu D, Meaney MJ: Nongenomic transmission across generations of maternal behavior and stress responses in the rat. *Science* 286(5442):1155–1158, 1999.
107. Meaney MJ: Maternal care, gene expression, and the transmission of individual differences in stress reactivity across generations. *Annual Review of Neuroscience* 24:1161–1192, 2001.
108. Ladd CO, Huot RL, Thrivikraman KV, Nemeroff CB, Meaney MJ, Plotsky PM: Long-term behavioral and neuroendocrine adaptations to adverse early experience. *Prog Brain Res* 122:81–103, 2000.
109. Vallee M, MacCari S, Dellu F, Simon H, Le Moal M, Mayo W: Long-term effects of prenatal stress and postnatal handling on age-related glucocorticoid secretion and cognitive performance: a longitudinal study in the rat. *Eur J Neurosci* Aug 1999:11(8):2906–2916.
110. Weaver IC, Cervoni N, Champagne FA, et al.: Epigenetic programming by maternal behavior. *Nat Neurosci* Aug 2004:7(8):847–854.
111. Fish EW, Shahrokh D, Bagot R, et al.: Epigenetic programming of stress responses through variations in maternal care. *Ann NY Acad Sci* Dec 2004:1036:167–180.
112. Heim C, Nemeroff CB: The impact of early adverse experiences on brain systems involved in the pathophysiology of anxiety and affective disorders. *Biol Psychiatry* Dec 1 1999:46(11):1509–1522.
113. Evans SJ, Choudary PV, Neal CR, et al.: Dysregulation of the fibroblast growth factor system in major depression. *Proc Natl Acad Sci USA* Oct 26 2004:101(43):15506–15511.
114. Mirnics K, Middleton FA, Lewis DA, Levitt P: Delineating novel signature patterns of altered gene expression in schizophrenia using gene microarrays. *Scientific World Journal* Apr 4 2001:1:114–116.
115. Mirnics K, Levitt P, Lewis DA: Critical appraisal of DNA microarrays in psychiatric genomics. *Biol Psychiatry* Apr 14 2006.
116. Vawter MP, Atz ME, Rollins BL, Cooper-Casey KM, Shao L, Byerley WF: Genome scans and gene expression microarrays converge to identify gene regulatory loci relevant in schizophrenia. *Hum Genet* Jun 2006:119(5):558–570.
117. Altar CA, Jurata LW, Charles V, et al.: Deficient hippocampal neuron expression of proteasome, ubiquitin, and mitochondrial genes in multiple schizophrenia cohorts. *Biol Psychiatry* Jul 15 2005:58(2):85–96.
118. Olds DL, Kitzman H, Cole R, et al.: Effects of nurse home-visiting on maternal life course and child development: age 6 follow-up results of a randomized trial. *Pediatrics* Dec 2004:114(6):1550–1559.
119. Olds D, Henderson CR, Jr., Cole R, et al.: Long-term effects of nurse home visitation on children's criminal and antisocial behavior: 15-year follow-up of a randomized controlled trial. *JAMA* Oct 14 1998:280(14):1238–1244.
120. Harris IB: *Children in Jeopardy: Can We Break the Cycle of Poverty?* New Haven, Yale University Press, 1996.

CHAPTER 2.3.2 ■ ASSESSING RISK: GENE DISCOVERY

THOMAS FERNANDEZ AND MATTHEW W. STATE

INTRODUCTION

There is indisputable evidence for the heritability of most early-onset psychiatric illnesses. However, the specific genes conveying risk for these disorders remain largely unknown. Given the strength of the data regarding genetic contributions to childhood disorders, the process of gene discovery has been surprisingly slow and frustrating. This, of course, has not been for lack of effort, ingenuity, or determination on the part of patients, families, and researchers. The obstacles that have impeded progress in child psychiatry have presented similar formidable challenges to other medical disciplines that contend with common, multifactorial illnesses. Fortunately, as in these other cases, the fruits of decades of labor in gene hunting are now beginning to be harvested.

Converging forces have resulted in widespread and well justified optimism about the prospects for major discoveries in the genetics of developmental neuropsychiatric disorders: the combination of hard-won insights into the genetic mechanisms underlying neuropsychiatric disorders of childhood, revolutionary advances in genomic technologies, an extraordinary level of involvement among parent and advocacy groups, and broad interdisciplinary research efforts involving clinicians, geneticists, and neuroscientists is transforming the field. Indeed, over the past several years, the first strong evidence for specific genetic contributions to child psychiatric and developmental disorders has been identified. Over the next decade, numerous genetic risks for childhood disorders will be identified, dramatically altering our understanding of the basic mechanisms of child psychiatric disease and fundamentally influencing clinical practice.

In this chapter we will address the challenges to gene identification that have confounded investigations of child psychiatric disorders and outline the major research strategies aimed at overcoming these obstacles. This discussion is intended to lay the groundwork for subsequent chapters, which will review genetic findings relevant to specific disorders, describe the interplay of environment and genetics in conferring both risk and resilience, and highlight the potential contribution of genetics to research in the areas of psychopharmacology and neuroimaging.

OBSTACLES TO GENE DISCOVERY IN CHILDHOOD DISORDERS

Multiple Interacting Genes

Over the last three decades, the identification of disease-causing genes has become commonplace (1). These successes have largely been in the area of single gene disorders exhibiting Mendelian patterns of inheritance: that is, dominant, recessive, or X-linked (Table 2.3.2.1). As a general proposition, the inheritance of psychiatric disorders, such as schizophrenia, bipolar disorder, autism, and Tourette syndrome do not appear to fall into this category, in the sense that they cannot be accounted for by the transmission of a single gene. Rather, the commonly accepted view is that, for the most part, these disorders will be found to be the result of multiple interacting alleles, each with relatively small contributions, compared to the genetic effects observed in Mendelian disorders. For instance, in the case of autism spectrum disorders, analysis of linkage data and family studies has led to widespread acceptance of the hypothesis that at least 15 genes are likely to be involved (2).

Many psychiatric conditions are also strongly influenced by nongenetic factors. For instance, in the case of schizophrenia, the monozygotic concordance rate (see Table 2.3.2.1) is approximately 50 percent (3, 4). The observation that twins sharing all their genetic material share a diagnosis only half the time strongly suggests that influences apart from the sequence of their DNA is contributing to disease risk. These influences may be environmental in the classic sense, or may involve heritable genetic mechanisms that are not coded for in the sequence of DNA (so-called epigenetic factors). The elaboration of the extent and nature of gene–environment interactions in developmental neuropsychiatric disorders is a vibrant area of research that has resulted in important recent insights into the etiopathology of mood and attentional disorders, among others. These findings are reviewed in more detail subsequently in the text.

An Uncertain Genetic Architecture

The combination of multigene inheritance, environmental, and epigenetic influences present significant challenges to researchers interested in gene identification. In addition, fundamental questions remain regarding the genetic architecture of nearly every childhood neuropsychiatric disorder. For instance, it is not known whether genetic variation that is common or rare in the population is likely to carry the lion's share of risk for common childhood psychiatric conditions. As will be discussed subsequently, this issue is critically important in selecting appropriate research strategies to identify contributing genes as well as in interpreting the resulting findings.

As a general proposition, two alternatives are most commonly investigated: One is the so-called "common disease-common variant" hypothesis, which holds that most of the risk for complex neuropsychiatric disorders will be accounted for by variations, or alleles, that are common in the population. By definition, these are genetic polymorphisms that are present in more than 1 percent of individuals. An often-cited example is Alzheimer's disease and the increased risk conferred by the e4 allele at the apoliporotein E (APOE) gene locus, a variance that occurs with relatively high frequency in the general population (5, 6).

It is widely accepted that in the case of common disorders that begin late in life, common alleles are likely to play a major role. This is because natural selection is likely to favor variations whose effects occur after the age at which individuals typically reproduce. Hence, deleterious alleles contributing to late-onset conditions may attain a substantial frequency in the general population.

This same logic, with minor modifications, can be applied to early-onset disorders: if one presumes that such conditions result from the conspiracy of multiple genes and that each contributing genetic variation has a relatively small effect, selection against any individual allele may be weak, allowing disease-related variations to become common in the population (7–9). In addition, it is possible that certain ancient alleles may have historically conferred some selective advantage, and only more recently contributed to disease. This is thought to be the case with respect to the recent identification of a common genetic variant associated with both childhood and adult-onset obesity (10). One can imagine that a gene allele predisposing to higher body mass index could have previously been advantageous during times of scarcity, and that relatively recent environmental changes would have transformed this into a genetic risk.

The common disease-common variant hypothesis is also consistent with what is known about the overall structure of the normal human genome (11). The majority of overall variation within a population is accounted for by common alleles. It would follow then that if selective pressure were not acting to limit the frequency of incrementally contributing loci, common diseases would reflect this underlying structure, i.e., common variation would account for common disease.

An alternate possibility is that a significant proportion of early-onset child psychiatric disorders may be the result of rare genetic variation. This could occur via several scenarios: either through the accumulation of many different rare mutations within one or a small number of genes (so-called allelic heterogeneity), or rare mutations in any of a large number of genes resulting in a similar or overlapping phenotype (locus heterogeneity). Moreover, these two mechanisms, locus and allelic heterogeneity, could combine within what is now considered a single psychiatric syndrome, a scenario which would present significant challenges to progress in genetic research.

The rare variant hypothesis is intuitively attractive, particularly in the case of severe early-onset illnesses. One could imagine that a genetic variation contributing to fundamental impairments in social functioning arising early in life could be subject to selective pressures, as affected individuals might be less likely to have offspring than those who are unaffected.

If one looks to other areas of medicine for clues, it is most likely that a combination of rare and common variants will be found to play a role in child psychiatric illness. For instance, in the case of diseases such as hypertension and breast cancer, rare alleles carrying significant disease risks have been identified. However, these mutations do not appear to account for the majority of population risk. Nonetheless, the discovery of rare alleles has provided vitally important insights into the pathophysiology of these disorders (12, 13).

As noted, the question of whether child psychiatric disorders involve common or rare genetic variation is highly relevant because those methods and study designs that may be most appropriate to identify the contribution of one type of risk may have little ability to identify the other. This issue will be addressed as the various approaches to gene hunting are presented below.

Phenotypic Heterogeneity

In addition to the obstacles presented by complex inheritance and an uncertain mode of inheritance, diagnostic issues in child psychiatric disorders present major challenges to geneticists. Ultimately, irrespective of the specific methodology employed, disease-gene hunting involves identifying observable clinical phenomena that bring together individuals with some degree of shared genetic risk and then uncovering the responsible or contributing variation(s) within the genome. If one has difficulty identifying a group of affected individuals who share a proportion of their risk in common, gene identification can be quite difficult.

The absence of reliable and specific physiological markers for childhood psychiatric illnesses presents a significant challenge. Of course, one problem is that our current diagnostic

TABLE 2.3.2.1

GLOSSARY OF SELECTED TERMS. (COURTESY OF NATIONAL HUMAN GENOME RESEARCH INSTITUTE)

Term	Definition
Allele	One of the variant forms of a gene at a particular locus (gene location), on a particular chromosome. Different alleles may have functional significance or may be normal variants.
Association study	These studies examine the relative allele frequencies among populations with and without a phenotype of interest.
Candidate gene	A gene suspected of being involved in a disease, based on prior suggestive evidence. For example, the gene may be located within a region of a chromosome detected by linkage analysis, the gene's protein product may suggest that it could be associated with a disease, or the gene may be located near a chromosomal abnormality.
Chromosome	One of the threadlike "packages" of DNA in the nucleus of a cell. Humans normally have 23 pairs of chromosomes, with 22 pairs of autosomes and 1 pair of sex chromosomes. Each parent contributes one chromosome to each pair.
Concordance	The presence of a given trait or phenotype in both members of a twin pair.
Deletion	A particular kind of mutation: Loss of a piece of DNA from a chromosome. Deletion of a gene or part of a gene can lead to a disease or abnormality, but can also be benign.
Dominant	A Mendelian pattern of inheritance in which a single transmitted gene variant results in a specific phenotypic characteristic, including, for example, a disease. Typically there is a strong relationship between carrying the genetic variant and having the disease. With a dominant gene, the chance of passing on the gene (and therefore the disease) to children is 50 percent in each pregnancy.
Duplication	An extra copy or copies of a chromosome segment.
Exon	The region of a gene that contains the code for producing the gene's protein. Each exon codes for a specific portion of the complete protein.
FISH	Fluorescence *in situ* hybridization. A technique that uses fluorescent probes that attach to unique known regions of chromosomes. It is useful for determining the location and extent of chromosomal abnormalities and for gene mapping.
Gene	The basic functional and physical unit of heredity passed from parent to offspring. Genes are pieces of DNA, and most genes contain the information for making a specific protein.
Genome	The complete sequence of DNA contained in an organism or a cell, which includes all chromosomes within the nucleus and the DNA in mitochondria.
Insertion	A type of chromosomal abnormality in which a DNA sequence is inserted into a gene, likely disrupting the normal structure and function of that gene.
Intron	The region of a gene containing a sequence of DNA that does not code for the gene's protein product.
Linkage	The relationship between genes and/or markers that lie near each other on a chromosome. Linked genes and markers tend to be inherited together. A marker and a phenotype are linked when they are inherited together.
Linkage analysis	Statistical examination of the likelihood that markers are linked to a particular phenotype by tracing inheritance through families. A high likelihood of linkage (expressed as a LOD score) at a locus suggests that the variation causing or contributing to disease is near the marker(s) being investigated.
Locus	The location on a chromosome where a specific gene is located.
LOD score	Logarithm of the odds. A likelihood ratio that expresses the statistical evidence in favor of linkage.
Marker	A variable segment of DNA with an identifiable physical location on a chromosome and whose inheritance can be followed. Because DNA segments that lie near each other on a chromosome tend to be inherited together, markers are often used as an indirect means of tracking the inheritance pattern of a gene that has not yet been identified.
Mutation	A permanent structural alteration in DNA. DNA changes may have no effect, may cause harm, or may improve an organism's chance of surviving and passing this alteration on to descendants.
Phenotype	The observable traits or characteristics of an organism (hair color, weight, or the presence or absence of a disease). Phenotypic traits are not necessarily genetic.
Polymorphism	A common variation in the sequence of DNA among individuals, typically defined as frequency of 1 percent or greater.
Recessive	A Mendelian pattern of inheritance in which two copies of a mutant gene, one from each parent, are necessary to cause a genetic disorder.
Sequencing	Determining the exact order of the base pairs in a segment of DNA.
SNPs	Single nucleotide polymorphisms. Variations at a single nucleotide that occur in human DNA at a frequency of approximately one every 1,000 bases. These variations can be used as markers to track inheritance in families and to analyze linkage with a phenotype. By definition a SNP with a population frequency of greater than 1 percent is defined as "common"
Translocation	Breakage and removal of a large segment of DNA from one chromosome, followed by the segment's attachment to a different chromosome. May be unbalanced (loss of DNA) or balanced (no loss of DNA)
X-linked	A Mendelian pattern of inheritance in which a disease gene variant is located on the X chromosome, often causing X-linked diseases to be seen preferentially in males or to have a more severe manifestation in males (due to the presence of one normal copy of the gene in females carrying two X chromosomes).

approaches may have weak correlations with underlying biological mechanisms. It is not yet possible to determine, for instance, whether similar genetic liabilities may underlie several diagnostic categories that are considered as quite separate within the boundaries imposed by current systems of classification (14). The high frequency of comorbidities and wide-ranging clinical presentations seen in child psychiatric syndromes certainly suggests that this may be the case. In addition, while severe forms of any disorder may be quite easily recognized, more subtle manifestations may be difficult to assess and verify. The unambiguous delineation of affected versus unaffected individuals, even within an extended family, can also be complicated by clinical phenomena that change through the course of development, either through an age-dependent onset, a waxing and waning course, or symptoms that decrease markedly in adulthood.

The issue of diagnostic uncertainty in child psychiatry can also pose significant logistical problems in that it can be quite difficult to ascertain comparable samples across sites that are geographically remote. For example, in the case of hypertension, large-scale studies of individuals may be undertaken in which the diagnostic measures may involve little more than multiple readings from a blood pressure cuff. Contrast this with what is typically required for a state-of-the-art psychiatric diagnosis in almost any disorder. One can imagine that the effort and expense required to collect useful data on large numbers of patients in child psychiatry is considerably more challenging than in many other fields of medicine.

Alternatives to categorical approaches to phenotypic assignment aimed at addressing these challenges are discussed in some detail below.

APPROACHES TO GENE DISCOVERY AND CHARACTERIZATION

Assessing Heritability and Patterns of Transmission

Most often, gene discovery efforts are preceded by epidemiology investigations aimed at determining the general nature and extent of the genetic risk. Such studies typically seek to identify whether a particular disorder aggregates within families and, if so, whether there is an identifiable pattern of transmission. Such investigations may, for example, evaluate the risk to a relative of an affected individual as compared to the overall incidence of a disorder. The resulting quantity is referred to as λ with a subscript denoting the degree of relatedness. For example a λ_{sib} would refer to the relative risk to a sibling of an affected individual. This calculation can be quite useful, first in identifying whether genes might be involved. Moreover, a comparison of this risk among different degrees of relatedness may provide a clue as to the nature of the genetic transmission (15, 16).

However, such investigations typically cannot determine whether the observed familial aggregation or increased risk is the direct result of genetic influences. In this regard, both twin and adoption studies play a critical role in teasing apart the relative contribution of genetic factors versus environmental factors in disease etiology. For twin studies, the rates at which monozygotic twins (MZ) share a diagnosis are compared to the rates for dizygotic twins (DZ). An assumption is made that both types of same-sex twins will have a similar degree of shared environmental influences. Consequently, if genes "trump" environment in the etiology of a disorder, those siblings that share all of their DNA (MZ) should be more likely to share a diagnosis than twins who share the same amount of DNA as any sibling pair (DZ). Conversely, if environment predominates as a contributing factor, rates of concordance should not fundamentally differ based on the amount of shared genetic material. Adoption studies accomplish a similar goal by comparing monozygotic twins who are raised together versus those in which twins are "adopted away." These types of investigations are quite powerful, but are less common in the literature than twin studies.

For autism spectrum disorders (ASDs), MZ concordance has been found to be in the neighborhood of 60 percent for the full syndrome and 90 percent for the broad spectrum. In contrast, DZ concordance has been found to be relatively low, about 3–15 percent, depending on the diagnostic criteria employed. These data support the conclusion that the observed familial clustering is largely the result of genetic factors and translate into an estimate of heritability that places ASDs among the most strongly genetic of all neuropsychiatric conditions (for reviews, see (17, 18)).

Once family, twin, and adoption studies have demonstrated that genetic factors are likely to play a role in the pathogenesis of a disorder, there are several different means to identify the specific genes involved. Direct approaches include three overlapping methodologies: linkage analysis, including whole genome screens in affected sibling pairs; gene association studies, including candidate gene studies and family-based studies of association; and cytogenetic methods, including karyotyping, fluorescence *in situ* hybridization (FISH), and microarray comparative genomic hybridization (CGH). We will next examine the basic principles behind these methods, as well as advantages and pitfalls of each as they relate to the search for disease susceptibility genes in child psychiatry.

Linkage Analysis

Linkage analysis assesses the probability that a given phenotype and a particular genetic marker (or series of markers) are transmitted together from one generation to another (Figure 2.3.2.1A). To appreciate how the investigation of evenly spaced "anonymous" markers, which are typically known bits of "nonfunctional" DNA, may lead to the identification of a disease gene, one needs to refer to basic genetic principles. When egg and sperm are formed, homologous chromosomes from each of the 22 pairs of autosomes have a tendency to exchange information through a process known as crossing over. Thus, each of the chromosomes in the haploid gamete is, on average, a mixture of its two parental chromosomes. During this process of gamete formation, the likelihood that any two points on a parental chromosome will have a crossover between them is a function of how far apart they are: Loci at opposite ends of a chromosome will be likely to be separated by a crossover. Loci close to each other will be less likely to have a crossover between them and will tend to pass together through multiple generations.

Thus, if one were to investigate a simple dominant disorder due to a gene of major effect using random markers spaced throughout the genome, the closer a particular marker was to the gene mutation causing the disorder, the more likely it would be that that marker would reliably appear in each affected individual (and would not appear in unaffected individuals). Through the investigation of many markers in many affected persons, one can begin to close in on a region of a chromosome containing a disease-related gene. This process is known as positional cloning, given that one is initially narrowing in on a location within the genome without knowing in advance anything about the genes present in that chromosomal segment.

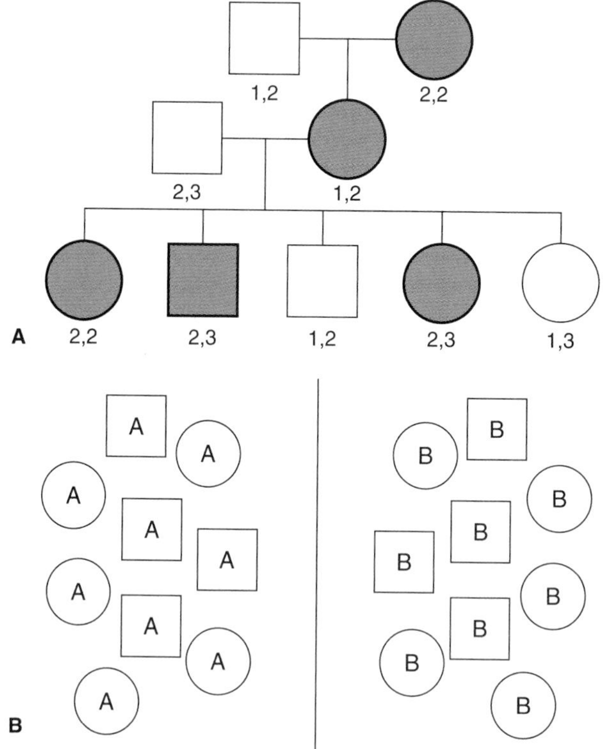

FIGURE 2.3.2.1. **Schematic illustrations of linkage and association principles. A.** Linkage analysis. A pedigree showing disease (solid shade) among males (squares) and females (circles) in multiple generations. The pair of numbers under each member of the pedigree represents the alleles of a DNA marker which was used to genotype the family. By analyzing the pattern of affected status within pedigrees, one may hypothesize the pattern of disease inheritance (dominant in this case) and then use a parametric linkage approach. By analyzing the frequency with which a particular genotype occurs along with disease in one or multiple families, it may be possible to conclude that a gene involved in disease phenotype is likely to lie in close proximity to a DNA marker. In this case, grandmaternal marker allele 2 appears to be linked to disease. **B.** Association studies. Individuals with a particular disorder or phenotype (labeled A) are compared with control subjects without the disease or phenotype (labeled B) to determine whether one group is more likely to carry particular allele(s) of the gene(s) being studied.

As a general matter, two basic approaches to linkage analysis predominate in the hunt for human disease genes. The first is known as parametric linkage analysis. In this case, one specifies a hypothesis about the nature of the proposed genetic transmission (for instance, that a disorder is the result of a dominantly acting mutation that is rare in the population) and then calculates the odds of seeing the observed pattern of transmission given the proposed model versus the odds of observing the same pattern of transmission if there were no linkage (free recombination). Results are expressed as a logarithm of the odds (LOD) score, such that, for example, an LOD score of 3 indicates the odds in favor of linkage between a marker and the disease are 10^3:1. Indeed, this particular score is taken as the threshold for statistical significance in an investigation of the whole genome, due to the fact that multiple comparisons are conducted (one simultaneously investigates multiple markers). Roughly, 1000:1 odds in favor of linkage at a marker (LOD score of 3) corresponds to a genome-wide p value of 0.05.

Parametric linkage analysis is a tremendously powerful approach to investigate Mendelian disorders as demonstrated by a host of dramatic discoveries, including the identification of genes for Huntington's disease, hypertension, mental retardation, and various cancers (1, 12, 19). These successes are directly attributable to the presence of genes of major effect exhibiting simple transmission in the families under study. In those instances in which this approach to linkage has been used successfully in complex disorders, it is typically the result of the identification of a rare family demonstrating inheritance that is simpler than what is presumed to be the norm.

As has been discussed, common child psychiatric disorders are unlikely to be exclusively inherited in a Mendelian fashion. Moreover, while it is presumed that many genes will conspire in any affected individual, the way in which any gene carries such risks or interacts with other genes is not yet know. As a result, some researchers have come to favor an alternative approach known as nonparametric linkage. These investigations do not require the specification of a hypothesis regarding the mode or character of inheritance. Instead, one seeks to identify any region of the genome that is shared among affected related individuals (or not shared in affected–unaffected relative pairs) more often than would be expected by chance. Presently, the most commonly used strategy in this regard relies on affected sibling pairs. Although generally less powerful than parametric linkage, nonparametric analyses are more robust in that they are not sensitive to misspecifications of the mode inheritance. As is the case with parametric studies, results are often presented as LOD scores and there are widely accepted statistical thresholds: LOD scores of greater than 2.2 but less than 3.6 are denoted "suggestive" linkage, scores greater than or equal to 3.6 but less than 5.4 are considered statistically significant, and LOD scores of 5.4 or greater are thought to be highly significant (20). These thresholds can be translated into a more practical metric: A suggestive LOD score of 2.2 is likely to be found by chance (erroneously) once per each genome wide scan; an LOD score of 3.6 will be identified by chance once per every 20 scans (20).

While there was initially considerable optimism about the power of nonparametric approaches, early returns in several areas of child psychiatry were not as rewarding as anticipated. For instance, with respect to Tourette syndrome (TS), when early parametric linkage studies did not identify TS-related loci, an international genetics consortium turned to nonparametric approaches. However, the first scan conducted using this approach did not detect statistically significant linkage either (21). With respect to autism, nine independent nonparametric genome-wide studies have been performed in the last decade. While several regions of suggestive or significant linkage have been found in individual studies, until very recently, no scan was able to replicate any other at precisely the same marker or markers (22, 23).

The reasons for these difficulties may be due in part to contrasting inclusion criteria, the choice of analytical methods, the specific genetic markers used in the various studies, and very likely the combination of locus and allelic heterogeneity. In addition, in all likelihood there was an initial tendency to underestimate the number of patients needed to detect the contribution of individual genes with quite small effects. As a consequence, increasing the number of well characterized samples through collaborative efforts and metaanalyses is now seen as imperative across the range of childhood psychiatric disorders.

In addition, several alternative approaches are simultaneously being employed to increase the power of linkage studies, through the stratification of patients and/or the identification of so-called endophenotypes, which are measurable phenomena that exist in the causal chain between genetic variation and categorical diagnoses. These approaches, discussed below, have the potential to increase the gene-finding power of linkage studies by identifying a more genetically homogenous group of subjects for study.

Endophenotypes and Sample Stratification

As noted, genome scans in the area of autism spectrum disorders have shown relatively limited evidence for significant linkage and, with few exceptions, the results have not converged at the same genetic locus (defined as the same marker or set of markers; for review see (22)). As noted, one explanation for these divergent results may be issues of phenotypic classification. It is possible that current methods of psychiatric disease classification, which are typically reflected in inclusion criteria for genetic studies, have little correlation with biological mechanisms. This scenario would increase genetic heterogeneity in research samples, weakening the statistical power of linkage analyses. In light of this possibility, many investigators have experimented with alternative approaches to phenotypic assignment, with the hope that this will lead to more genetically homogeneous subgroups and thus more consistency in the genetic findings.

Much work has focused on defining intermediate phenotypes, or endophenotypes, with the assumption that these are heritable traits that are more closely related to the biology of the disorder than is the categorical diagnosis (24). Endophenotypes may include anatomical, neurophysiological, biochemical, or other measurable traits of a syndrome, which may be measured and specified with more reliability and validity than is possible for the overall disorder diagnosis. If child psychiatric disorders are not a single entity but a collection of overlapping traits resulting from the combined action of multiple risk alleles, one can imagine that the expression of one such trait may involve fewer genes than the overall disorder, thereby decreasing the genetic heterogeneity of study samples if they are defined by these endophenotypes as opposed to broader diagnostic categories (23, 25).

For instance, in the case of autism, Buxbaum et al. (2001) chose to evaluate a sample based on language characteristics, one of the three symptom clusters that define the diagnosis. A genome screen for susceptibility genes in 95 families with two or more individuals affected with ASDs showed an LOD score of 2.39 at 2q31.3. By restricting the sample to a subset of 49 families showing phrase speech delay (PSD), defined as the absence of phrased speech until >36 months, the evidence in favor of linkage improved to an LOD of 3.32, approaching statistical significance (26). A similar finding was reported by a second group, using an independent sample and a similar method of restricting analysis by endophenotype. A genomic-screen linkage analysis of 99 families with autistic disorder found an LOD score of 1.12 at 2q33. After restricting analysis to 45 families that exhibited PSD, evidence for linkage increased, with an LOD score of 2.86 at this same locus (27).

A similar strategy involves sample stratification in an effort to increase the power of linkage studies. This approach differs from endophenotyping only in the sense that the criteria for creating a subset does not necessary reflect a hypothesis regarding an intermediate state between diagnosis and gene. For instance, one may stratify a sample based on age, sex, or various categorical diagnostic formulations. The power of this approach to increase the homogeneity of a sample has recently also been demonstrated in the autism literature. The largest genome-wide scan, which resulted in a maximum LOD score in the suggestive range on chromosome 17 (28), was reevaluated based on whether males only (MO) or both males and females were in an affected sibling pair (29). Using the MO families, the LOD score at chromosome 17 increased to a statistically significant level. A subsequent full-genome linkage scan in an independent sample of MO families also reached statistical significance at chromosome 17 and showed the first formal replication in the autism linkage literature at a single marker (30).

These studies are one example among many in which the identification of endophenotypes and sample stratification appear to increase genetic homogeneity and the power of linkage studies. One must be cautious, however, about the number of endophenotypes or stratified subsets examined. The statistical thresholds presented previously with respect to linkage were established for the case of genome-wide scans examining a unitary diagnostic entity. As one multiplies the number of subsets evaluated in a study, it will be essential to be attentive to correcting for multiple comparisons, if the number of false-positive findings is not to be inflated. In this regard, the ultimate test of any linkage study is not the resulting statistic, but finally the identification of a risk allele in the linkage interval. The increased power of the aforementioned approaches will be clearly demonstrated when studies are able to go beyond the initial identification of a significant LOD score, to replication and risk allele confirmation.

Genetic Association

In contrast to linkage studies, which examine transmission within families, association studies assess gene frequencies within populations. Until recently, these types of studies typically investigated one or a number of known, common genetic polymorphisms (markers) in or near predetermined "candidate genes" of interest. In essence, the methodology is a variation on the classic case-control design. In general, in the field of human genetics, one seeks to determine if individuals with a particular disorder or phenotype are significantly more (or less) likely than controls to carry particular allele(s) of the gene or genes being studied (Figure 2.3.2.1B).

Association methods have been shown to be more powerful than linkage methods under a number of conditions that typically prevail in complex disease. In particular, they are considered to be more powerful in detecting common susceptibility variants of relatively small effect, unlike linkage analysis, which requires relatively strong genetic effects given feasible sample sizes (14, 24, 31, 32).

Association studies are also popular for practical reasons. The most commonly used designs study either affected individuals versus unrelated controls, or as is often the case in pediatric disorders, affected probands and their parents (where the nontransmitted parental alleles are used as the control). This contrasts with parametric linkage analyses, in which extended families must be identified and characterized, or nonparametric linkage studies that often require the identification of two affected siblings, thus excluding a significant number of patients who present to clinic. As a result, association studies make the study of large numbers of subjects reasonably practical and allow this type of investigation to dovetail often with other case-control studies being conducted simultaneously (such as pharmacological studies).

While both the ability to detect genes of small effect and the logistical advantages of association studies make them popular across all fields of medicine, they are not without limitations. For example, association strategies may have difficulty identifying a relevant gene, even when it is under direct investigation. This may be a consequence of the common polymorphism(s) chosen as markers for a particular study. The power of a study to detect association is influenced by a number of factors. For instance, studies are most powerful if one is fortunate enough to be investigating the genetic variation within a gene that is actually causing the problem. If this is not the case, then the power to detect association rests in part on how similar the marker frequency is to the frequency of the unknown disease allele being sought within the population under study.

A second important limitation of association studies is their vulnerability to false-positive results. In a recent review, only a small fraction of published positive associations in the literature were able to be replicated in more than one additional study (33). One source of this error may be population stratification. This results from variations in the frequencies of certain genetic markers among different ethnic groups. If one compares individuals with a particular phenotype to controls, and the two groups are not ethnically similar, a genetic marker that is found more frequently in the affected group will erroneously appear to be associated with the identified phenotype. An approach commonly used to avoid population stratification bias is that of family-based association testing, which takes advantage of internal controls. In this strategy, an affected individual and their parents are genotyped at one or several loci. The alleles at these loci that are transmitted to the affected individual are compared to remaining alleles that have not been transmitted (control alleles). In fact these studies are a hybrid of a linkage and association strategy. They are linkage studies in the sense that they investigate transmission from one generation to the next within families, and association studies in the sense that they are investigating the allele frequency among an unrelated group of probands compared to a control.

An alternative approach to protect against population stratification called genomic control can be used in traditional case-control studies. This strategy involves the genotyping of a number of polymorphic markers in the study population that are not hypothesized to be related to disease at the same time that candidate genes are evaluated. The former markers should then indicate whether there is marked stratification within a cohort.

It is important to note that an association can only be detected if the genetic marker studied is very close to or within the susceptibility gene. For this reason, this strategy has often been used to narrow a region believed to contain a susceptibility gene after linkage analysis, or to test for association between a phenotype and a candidate gene (for instance, a gene hypothesized to underlie susceptibility to the phenotype based on what is known about its biology or its proximity to chromosomal abnormalities seen in those with the phenotype). However, with recent dramatic expansions in the number of characterized polymorphic markers providing dense coverage across most of the entire human genome, it is becoming possible to systematically screen large sections of the genome for genes of small effect, without requiring prior hypotheses about pathophysiology or location.

Recent advances in microarray technologies, in which many thousands of spots of DNA can be arranged on a single microscope slide, are now allowing researchers to query hundreds of thousands of single nucleotide polymorphism (SNP) gene markers, evenly spaced throughout the genome, in a single reaction and at relatively low cost. This is allowing even small laboratories to conduct whole-genome association studies without having to choose candidate genes in advance. The power and potential of this approach was recently highlighted by the identification an association between the complement factor H gene and age-related macular degeneration (34) and more recently in the identification of a risk allele for childhood as well as adult-onset obesity (10). We will very likely soon see advances toward understanding genetic susceptibility in child psychiatric disorders using genome-wide association methodologies.

An example of a recent gene discovery that draws from a combination of linkage, association, and endophenotyping is that of DCDC2 as a susceptibility gene for reading disability (RD) or developmental dyslexia, a common complex neurobehavioral disorder in children. Over the last two decades, independent linkage studies have produced several overlapping findings suggesting an RD locus at 6p21.3–22 (35–42). An association study using 29 markers spanning the region with the most consistent evidence for linkage identified a strong association between one of these markers (JA04) and performance on an orthographic choice reading task in patients with RD (41). In a followup association study by this same group, 147 SNP markers surrounding JA04 were examined in a larger sample of families with RD (43). By using such a high-density marker panel in a region of the genome implicated by linkage and an earlier association study employing endophenotypes, this group identified significant association between markers within DCDC2 and a quantitative phenotype reflecting RD (a composite score including reading recognition, reading comprehension, and spelling subtests of a standardized achievement test). In addition, a large polymorphic deletion within an intron of DCDC2 was identified, which disrupts a regulatory region important for function of this gene. RT-PCR data showed that DCDC2 localizes to areas of the brain important for reading, and RNAi studies showed that down-regulating DCDC2 leads to abnormal neuronal migration in these same brain regions (43). This evidence supports DCDC2 as a susceptibility gene for RD, and illustrates the importance of using multiple methodologies for disease gene discovery in complex disorders.

Molecular Cytogenetics

Molecular cytogenetics refers to the use of molecular probes to study chromosomes. Techniques such as fluorescence *in situ* hybridization (FISH) may be used in the identification of susceptibility genes by identifying patients with chromosomal abnormalities (translocations, deletions, duplications) and then identifying genes in this region that may be disrupted as a result (Figures 2.3.2.2 and 2.3.2.3). This approach has been used successfully in helping to identify the genes for multiple medical disorders (1) as well as a host of mental retardation syndromes (19). For complex child psychiatric disorders, it is assumed that genes affected by such rare gross chromosomal abnormalities are unlikely to account for any significant portion of susceptibility risk in most of the overall affected population. However, identifying genes involved in these rearrangements may identify loci that are mutated in affected but cytogenetically normal individuals or identify genetic pathways providing insights into the pathogenesis of more common forms of these disorders.

Recent findings with respect to Tourette syndrome (TS) point to the potential value of this approach in common complex psychiatric disorders. As noted previously, neither parametric nor nonparametric studies had been able to identify a disease-related gene in TS. Abelson et al. (2005) studied a de novo chromosomal inversion in the only member of a family affected with TS (Fig. 2.3.2.3). One of the two breakpoints identified in this child mapped near a gene known as SLIT and Trk-Like family member 1 (SLITRK1). The other three genes mapping closest to the two breakpoints were thought to be less likely candidates, in part because SLITRK1 was known to be expressed in brain regions thought relevant to TS and related disorders.

Given a starting hypothesis that mutations in SLITRK1 would likely be rare among individuals with TS, the authors directly queried the entire coding and regulatory regions of SLITRK1 among unrelated affected individuals. They identified a mutation in a second family with TS and related disorders that was predicted to lead to a truncation of the resulting protein, and which was not present in several thousand control individuals. Additional screening also demonstrated a rare variation in a regulatory region of SLITRK1 that was present in two unrelated affected persons and absent in several thousand unrelated controls (44).

The work by Abelson and colleagues demonstrated both the important strengths as well as the potential weaknesses of

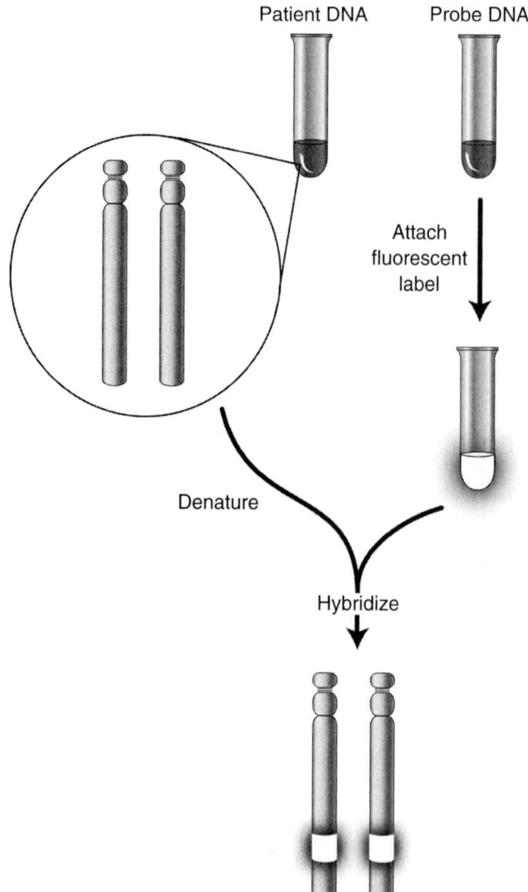

FIGURE 2.3.2.2. Fluorescence *in situ* hybridization (FISH). A technique that uses fluorescent-labeled probes that attach to unique known regions of chromosomes. Probe DNA is labeled with a fluorescent dye and hybridized to denatured genomic patient DNA on a microscope slide. Under normal circumstances (no chromosomal abnormalities), when viewing metaphase chromosomes after hybridization, two fluorescent signals per probe will be seen (one for each homologous chromosome). However, chromosomal abnormalities (deletions, duplications, translocations) may alter the number and locations of these signals if the probes localize to the affected regions (see Figure 2.3.2.3). In this way, FISH is useful for determining the location and extent of chromosomal abnormalities and for gene mapping.

the molecular cytogenetic approach. On the positive side, the work was able to identify both a specific candidate disease gene as well as specific functional genetic changes for further investigation. Moreover, the initial studies implicated *SLITRK1* in the regulation of dendritic growth in cortical pyramidal cells, offering potentially important opportunities to study this biological pathway in relation to TS.

The study also demonstrated the liabilities of searching for rare genetic variants in a common disease. By definition, the results are likely to affect only a small number of individuals and no single piece of evidence may be a "smoking gun." These authors chose to pursue multiple lines of investigation, including mutation screening, case-control analysis, and *in vitro* neurobiological studies to support a role for SLITRK1 in TS. However, the ultimate implications of the work will likely only be clear in retrospect, through the identification of additional rare families with clear mutations in this gene, the elaboration of a biological pathway including other genes that may carry risk for TS, and through the study of animal models, which may offer more clues as to the relationship of SLITRK1 to TS and related phenomena.

In the same way that a chromosomal abnormality led to the discovery of SLTIRK1 as a strong candidate gene in TS, cytogenetic abnormalities have provided leads toward the identification of susceptibility genes in schizophrenia and autism as well. The observation of a balanced translocation involving chromosomes 1 and 11 that segregated with schizophrenia and affective disorders in a multigenerational Scottish family (45, 46) led to the identification of DISC1 at one of the breakpoints (1q42) (47), and evidence for linkage of schizophrenia to this region has since been reported in several independent samples (48–50). Furthermore, several association studies found evidence relating different allelic variations at DISC1 to schizophrenia (51–54), while several DISC1 polymorphisms appear to be associated with altered hippocampal structure, activation on fMRI, and cognitive function (55–58). Taken together, the evidence so far suggests that *DISC1* is a susceptibility gene in schizophrenia, and may contribute to this disorder through an effect on hippocampal development and function.

With respect to autism and pervasive developmental disorders (PDD), this approach has recently led to the identification of Neuroligin 4 (NLGN4) as one of the first confirmed transcripts in which clearly functional mutations are associated with idiopathic or nonsyndromic autism and ASDs. In this case, cytogenetic studies found X-chromosome deletions in three autistic patients (59). This led to screening of the candidate interval, resulting in the demonstration of a functional mutation that segregated with ASDs in a European family (60). A second group has provided independent confirmation of these initial findings for NLGN4 using parametric linkage analysis (61), and others have demonstrated the functional relevance of the identified NLGN4 mutations (62) as well as the importance of neuroligin-family gene expression in normal synaptic development (63–65).

Subsequent studies indicate that the overall frequency of NLGN4 mutations in patients with ASD is likely to be very low (66–68). While the contribution of neuroligins to ASD risk in the overall patient population appears to be small, these findings are important in that they provide a critical starting point for investigations of the molecular and cellular mechanisms underlying ASD biology. In similar ways, using cytogenetic techniques to characterize rare chromosomal abnormalities for other child psychiatric disorders, while unlikely to lead to the identification of a common risk allele, may provide first clues to disease pathways and novel therapeutic insights.

THE IMPACT OF GENOMIC TECHNOLOGIES ON GENE DISCOVERY

The foregoing discussion has focused on the complex nature of genetic transmission in childhood psychiatric disorders and the methodologies used to identify genes under these circumstances. The recent genetic findings presented above and those discussed throughout the text are a cause for considerable optimism. What is equally remarkable, however, is the ongoing revolution in genomic technologies that has allowed for these breakthroughs and that continues to transform our understanding of the genome.

The sequencing of the human genome has and will continue to have a profound impact on the process of gene discovery. Prior to this landmark accomplishment, undertaking each of the aforementioned approaches to gene discovery represented a Herculean task. For instance, efforts at linkage analysis had to contend with a relatively small number of available polymorphic markers and, very often, uncertainty regarding their precise location within the genome. Only within the

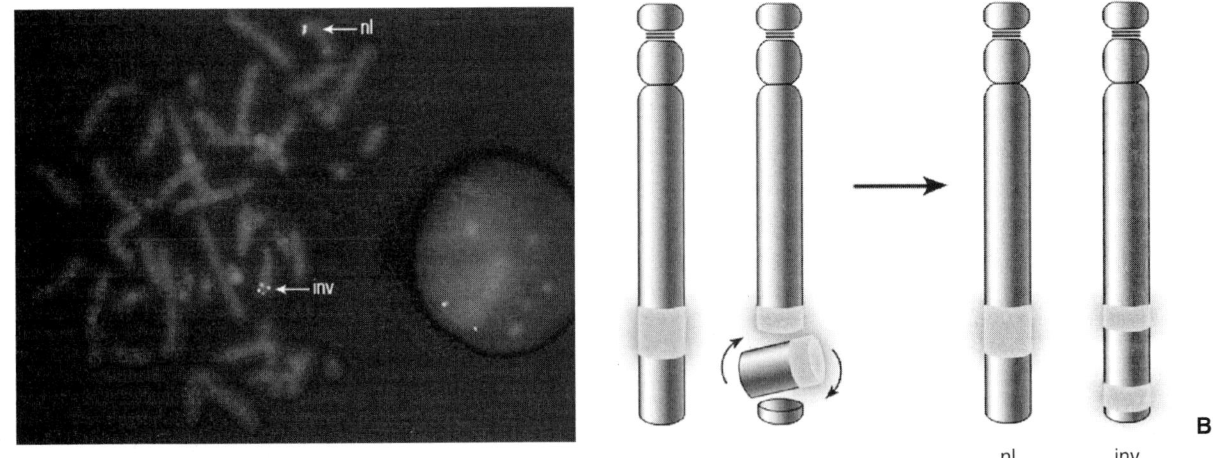

FIGURE 2.3.2.3. **Using FISH to map a chromosome 13 inversion in a patient with TS. A.** Photograph of metaphase chromosomes under 100× objective lens after hybridization with a fluorescent-labeled probe specific for a DNA sequence at 13q31.1. The experimental probe is visualized at the expected position on the normal (nl) chromosome 13. Two fluorescence signals are visible on the inverted (inv) chromosome 13, indicating that this probe spans the breakpoint. **B.** Illustration of how the chromosome 13 inversion results in two fluorescence signals when the DNA probe spans one of the inversion breakpoints. In this case, the breakpoint at 13q31.1 mapped near the gene SLITRK1 and further investigation of its sequence revealed rare mutations in three unrelated individuals affected with TS. (See color insert.)

preceding decade had a sufficient number of polymorphic markers become available to reliably investigate the entire genome. Moreover, once a candidate interval was defined, it would very often take years of work to determine what the sequence of the DNA was within that interval, what known and potential genes were present, and, finally, where a causal mutation might be located.

In the wake of the creation of public databases containing the human genome sequence, this type of information is now only a mouse-click away. Accordingly, the rate of genetic investigation has accelerated dramatically. For example, at present, when a candidate interval is characterized, the identity of every known gene in that interval is immediately available with links to information on all known polymorphisms and mutations in that gene, what is understood about the function of its protein product, often its precise expression pattern determined both by microarray and in-situ hybridizations, and its degree of conservation across species, among many other attributes (for instance, see http://genome.ucsc.edu).

Another consequence of the human genome project has been the rapid development of genomic microarray technologies. These advances have helped transform the initial phases of linkage and association studies. For example, as the basic sequence of the human genome has been revealed, so too has the precise location and nature of genetic polymorphisms, including SNPs that are found on average one every 1,000 nucleotides in the human genome. As noted previously, assays for these polymorphisms may be arrayed on glass slides allowing researchers, in a single reaction, to investigate hundreds of thousands of genetic markers simultaneously in a single individual. This is in contrast to previous approaches to genotyping that required a separate experimental reaction for each of several hundred polymorphic markers. In short, the efficiency of genotyping has increased substantially and, simultaneously, the cost of doing so has fallen precipitously. This combination now permits nearly every laboratory with an interest to pursue genome-wide investigations of patients at a scale that would have been unthinkable just a half-dozen years ago.

In addition, the combination of genome sequencing and the development of microarrays has also transformed the process of identifying chromosomal deletions or duplications. There are several approaches at present, with one of the most widely employed being array-based comparative genomic hybridization (array-CGH, Figure 2.3.2.4). In array-CGH, equal quantities of patient DNA, labeled with one fluorescent dye, are mixed with control DNA, labeled with a different fluorescent dye. This mixture is then hybridized to a slide containing hundreds of thousands (and soon millions) of small bits of known DNA sequences (probes) spotted in a grid, with each probe corresponding to a unique position in the genome. The ratio of fluorescence signals at each spot is then queried. At any one of these, excess signal from the fluorescent marker linked to the patient DNA is evidence for duplication of the patient's DNA in the region of the genome represented by that probe. Conversely, excess signal from the fluorescent marker linked to the control DNA suggests that there is a loss of patient DNA (a deletion) at that point in the genome. Already, this approach has resulted in investigations that are 100–1,000 times more sensitive than conventional cytogenetics.

As this technology has developed, it has become increasingly clear that there is much more structural variation in the normal human genome than previously expected. It appears that duplications and deletions are quite frequent in normal individuals, even in regions known to contain genes with important biological functions (69–71). The nature of these variations, now referred to as copy number polymorphisms, is a new and intriguing area of genomic investigation.

One immediate result of the ability to detect the many deletions and duplications in the normal genome is that it is no longer possible to draw simple conclusions regarding cytogenetic abnormalities. The discovery of the loss of genetic material in affected individuals was often previously accepted as the cause of their phenotype. Now it is necessary to investigate whether such a loss (or gain) might simply represent a benign variation in the genome. Moreover, as in the case of other types of common variation, it is certainly possible that copy number variations might contribute to disease risk in an incremental (dose-related) and interactive manner.

Finally, a critically important advance over the last several years has been the increased availability of DNA repositories consisting of samples from well characterized patients with

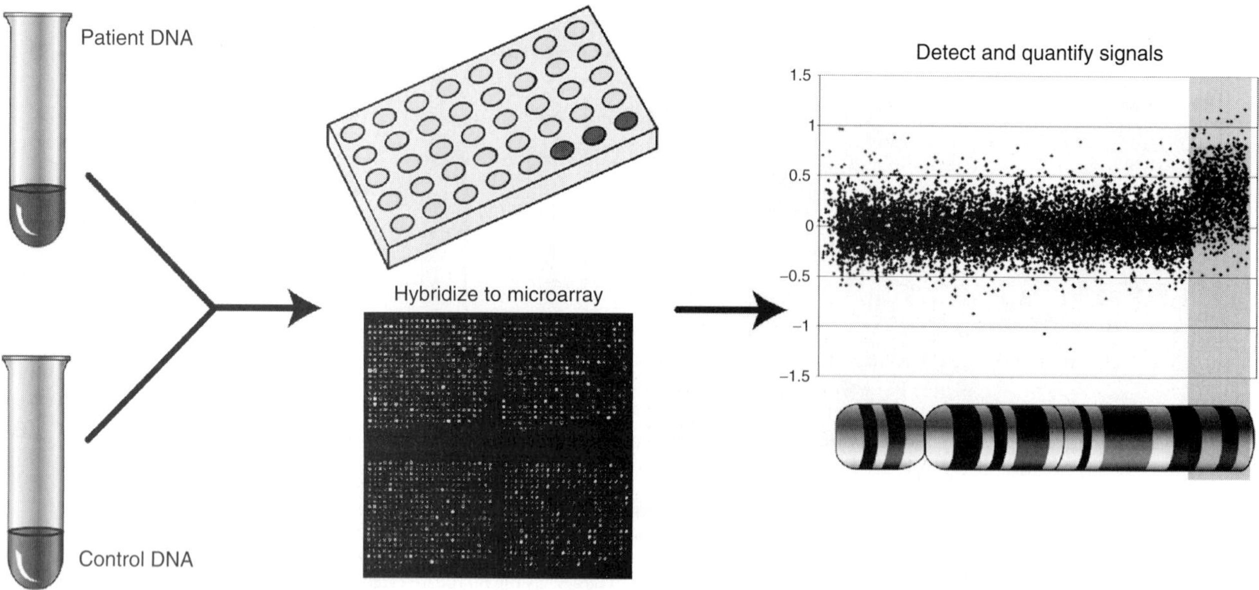

FIGURE 2.3.2.4. **Array-based comparative genome hybridization (array-CGH).** Equal quantities of patient and control DNA, each labeled with a different fluorescent dye, is hybridized to a slide containing many known DNA sequence probes spotted in a grid (array), with each probe corresponding to a unique position in the genome. After hybridization, the ratio of fluorescence signals at each probe on the array is detected and quantified. Excess signal from the fluorescent dye linked to the patient DNA (red) at each array probe is evidence for duplication of patient DNA in the region of the genome represented by the probe(s). Conversely, excess green signal would represent deletion of patient DNA. In this example, the signal ratios detected on the array are plotted onto a graph which reveals a duplication of the distal aspect of the long arm of chromosome 9 (red shade). (See color insert.)

child psychiatric disorders. The development of these resources has had a substantial impact. For instance, researchers from outside a field who might have been reluctant to make a substantial investment to study a child psychiatric disorder are now able to test novel hypotheses with relatively low risk and at low cost. In addition, established laboratories have been able to markedly increase their samples sizes and/or use available DNA resources as a confirmation group. As new genomic technologies and information have become widely distributed, the issue of the availability of samples for study promises to play an increasingly large role. Consequently, the hard work of parent groups, patient advocates, researchers, and, in the United States, the National Institutes of Health to develop these large sample repositories, promises to be as important to the field of gene discovery as the extraordinary advances in genomic technologies witnessed over the past decade.

CONCLUSION

Developmental neuropsychiatric disorders are, as a general proposition, complex genetic disorders. The interaction of multiple genes with environmental factors and, likely, epigenetic influences has made the process of identifying disease-related genes problematic. As has been the case in other complex disorders, a variety of gene-hunting strategies, including linkage, association, and molecular cytogenetic approaches, targeting both common and rare variation, are likely to be most successful in unraveling the genetics of these conditions. Over the past several years, significant progress has been made in the identification of specific risk alleles. The combination of advances in genomic technologies, as well as the increased availability of large samples of well characterized patients, promises a period of rapid and dramatic discovery in the near future.

ACKNOWLEDGMENTS

The authors would like to thank Thomas Morgan, M.D., of the Yale Child Study Center and Department of Genetics for his review and helpful suggestions during the preparation of this manuscript.

References

1. Collins FS: Positional cloning: Let's not call it reverse anymore. *Nat Genet* 1:3–6, 1992.
2. Risch N, Spiker D, Lotspeich L, et al.: A genomic screen of autism: Evidence for a multilocus etiology. *Am J Hum Genet* 65:493–507, 1999.
3. Kendler KS: Overview: A current perspective on twin studies of schizophrenia. *Am J Psychiatry* 140:1413–1425, 1983.
4. Cardno AG, Marshall EJ, Coid B, et al.: Heritability estimates for psychotic disorders: The Maudsley twin psychosis series. *Arch Gen Psychiatry* 56:162–168, 1999.
5. Corder EH, Saunders AM, Strittmatter WJ, et al.: Gene dose of apolipoprotein E type 4 allele and the risk of Alzheimer's disease in late onset families. *Science* 261:921–923, 1993.
6. Fullerton SM, Clark AG, Weiss KM, et al.: Apolipoprotein E variation at the sequence haplotype level: Implications for the origin and maintenance of a major human polymorphism. *Am J Hum Genet* 67:881–900, 2000.
7. Reich DE, Lander ES: On the allelic spectrum of human disease. *Trends Genet* 17:502–510, 2001.
8. Pritchard JK, Cox NJ: The allelic architecture of human disease genes: Common disease-common variant ... or not? *Hum Mol Genet* 11:2417–2423, 2002.
9. Pritchard JK: Are rare variants responsible for susceptibility to complex diseases? *Am J Hum Genet* 69:124–137, 2001.
10. Herbert A, Gerry NP, McQueen MB, et al.: A common genetic variant is associated with adult and childhood obesity. *Science* 312:279–283, 2006.
11. Altshuler D, Brooks LD, Chakravarti A, et al.: A haplotype map of the human genome. *Nature* 437:1299–1320, 2005.
12. Lifton RP, Gharavi AG, Geller DS: Molecular mechanisms of human hypertension. *Cell* 104:545–556, 2001.
13. Welcsh PL, King MC: BRCA1 and BRCA2 and the genetics of breast and ovarian cancer. *Hum Mol Genet* 10:705–713, 2001.

14. Rutter M, Silberg J, O'Connor T, Simonoff E: Genetics and child psychiatry: I. Advances in quantitative and molecular genetics. *J Child Psychol Psychiatry* 40:3–18, 1999.
15. Risch N: Linkage strategies for genetically complex traits. II. The power of affected relative pairs. *Am J Hum Genet* 46:229–241, 1990.
16. Risch N: Linkage strategies for genetically complex traits. I. Multilocus models. *Am J Hum Genet* 46:222–228, 1990.
17. Rutter M: Genetic studies of autism: From the 1970s into the millennium. *J Abnorm Child Psychol* 28:3–14, 2000.
18. Folstein SE, Rosen-Sheidley B: Genetics of autism: Complex aetiology for a heterogeneous disorder. *Nat Rev Genet* 2:943–955, 2001.
19. Ropers HH, Hamel BC: X-linked mental retardation. *Nat Rev Genet* 6:46–57, 2005.
20. Lander E, Kruglyak L: Genetic dissection of complex traits: Guidelines for interpreting and reporting linkage results. *Nat Genet* 11:241–247, 1995.
21. A complete genome screen in sib pairs affected by Gilles de la Tourette syndrome. The Tourette syndrome association international consortium for genetics. *Am J Hum Genet* 65:1428–1436, 1999.
22. Bacchelli E, Maestrini E: Autism spectrum disorders: Molecular genetic advances. *Am J Med Genet C Semin Med Genet* 142:13–23, 2006.
23. Veenstra-VanderWeele J, Christiann SL, Cook EHJ: Autism as a paradigmatic complex genetic disorder. *Annu Rev Genomics Hum Genetics* 5:379–405, 2004.
24. Sanders AR, Duan J, Gejman PV: Complexities in psychiatric genetics. *Int Rev Psychiatry* 16:284–293, 2004.
25. Gottesman II, Gould TD: The endophenotype concept in psychiatry: Etymology and strategic intentions. *Am J Psychiatry* 160:636–645, 2003.
26. Buxbaum JD, Silverman JM, Smith CJ, et al.: Evidence for a susceptibility gene for autism on chromosome 2 and for genetic heterogeneity. *Am J Hum Genet* 68:1514–1520, 2001.
27. Shao Y, Raiford KL, Wolpert CM, et al.: Phenotypic homogeneity provides increased support for linkage on chromosome 2 in autistic disorder. *Am J Hum Genet* 70:1058–1061, 2002.
28. Yonan AL, Alarcon M, Cheng R, et al.: A genomewide screen of 345 families for autism-susceptibility loci. *Am J Hum Genet* 73:886–897, 2003.
29. Stone JL, Merriman B, Cantor RM, et al.: Evidence for sex-specific risk alleles in autism spectrum disorder. *Am J Hum Genet* 75:1117–1123, 2004.
30. Cantor RM, Kono N, Duvall JA, et al.: Replication of autism linkage: Fine-mapping peak at 17q21. *Am J Hum Genet* 76:1050–1056, 2005.
31. Risch N, Merikangas K: The future of genetic studies of complex human diseases. *Science* 273:1516–1517, 1996.
32. Risch NJ: Searching for genetic determinants in the new millennium. *Nature* 405:847–856, 2000.
33. Hirschhorn JN, Lohmueller K, Byrne E, Hirschhorn K: A comprehensive review of genetic association studies. *Genet Med* 4:45–61, 2002.
34. Klein RJ, Zeiss C, Chew EY, et al.: Complement factor H polymorphism in age-related macular degeneration. *Science* 308:385–389, 2005.
35. Cardon LR, Smith SD, Fulker DW, Kimberling WJ, Pennington BF, DeFries JC: Quantitative trait locus for reading disability: Correction. *Science* 268:1553, 1995.
36. Cardon LR, Smith SD, Fulker DW, Kimberling WJ, Pennington BF, DeFries JC: Quantitative trait locus for reading disability on chromosome 6. *Science* 266:276–279, 1994.
37. Fisher SE, Marlow AJ, Lamb J, et al.: A quantitative-trait locus on chromosome 6p influences different aspects of developmental dyslexia. *Am J Hum Genet* 64:146–156, 1999.
38. Gayan J, Smith SD, Cherny SS, et al.: Quantitative-trait locus for specific language and reading deficits on chromosome 6p. *Am J Hum Genet* 64:157–164, 1999.
39. Grigorenko EL, Wood FB, Meyer MS, et al.: Susceptibility loci for distinct components of developmental dyslexia on chromosomes 6 and 15. *Am J Hum Genet* 60:27–39, 1997.
40. Grigorenko EL, Wood FB, Meyer MS, Pauls DL: Chromosome 6p influences on different dyslexia-related cognitive processes: Further confirmation. *Am J Hum Genet* 66:715–723, 2000.
41. Kaplan DE, Gayan J, Ahn J, et al.: Evidence for linkage and association with reading disability on 6p21.3-22. *Am J Hum Genet* 70:1287–1298, 2002.
42. Turic D, Robinson L, Duke M, et al.: Linkage disequilibrium mapping provides further evidence of a gene for reading disability on chromosome 6p21.3-22. *Mol Psychiatry* 8:176–185, 2003.
43. Meng H, Smith SD, Hager K, et al.: DCDC2 is associated with reading disability and modulates neuronal development in the brain. *Proc Natl Acad Sci USA* 102:17053–17058, 2005.
44. Abelson JF, Kwan KY, O'Roak BJ, et al.: Sequence variants in SLITRK1 are associated with Tourette's syndrome. *Science* 310:317–320, 2005.
45. St Clair D, Blackwood D, Muir W, et al.: Association within a family of a balanced autosomal translocation with major mental illness. *Lancet* 336:13–16, 1990.
46. Blackwood DH, Fordyce A, Walker MT, St Clair DM, Porteous DJ, Muir WJ: Schizophrenia and affective disorders—cosegregation with a translocation at chromosome 1q42 that directly disrupts brain-expressed genes: Clinical and P300 findings in a family. *Am J Hum Genet* 69:428–433, 2001.
47. Millar JK, Wilson-Annan JC, Anderson S, et al.: Disruption of two novel genes by a translocation co-segregating with schizophrenia. *Hum Mol Genet* 9:1415–1423, 2000.
48. Ekelund J, Hennah W, Hiekkalinna T, et al.: Replication of 1q42 linkage in Finnish schizophrenia pedigrees. *Mol Psychiatry* 9:1037–1041, 2004.
49. Ekelund J, Hovatta I, Parker A, et al.: Chromosome 1 loci in Finnish schizophrenia families. *Hum Mol Genet* 10:1611–1617, 2001.
50. Hwu HG, Liu CM, Fann CS, Ou-Yang WC, Lee SF: Linkage of schizophrenia with chromosome 1q loci in Taiwanese families. *Mol Psychiatry* 8:445–452, 2003.
51. Callicott JH, Straub RE, Pezawas L, et al.: Variation in DISC1 affects hippocampal structure and function and increases risk for schizophrenia. *Proc Natl Acad Sci USA* 102:8627–8632, 2005.
52. Hennah W, Varilo T, Kestila M, et al.: Haplotype transmission analysis provides evidence of association for DISC1 to schizophrenia and suggests sex-dependent effects. *Hum Mol Genet* 12:3151–3159, 2003.
53. Zhang X, Tochigi M, Ohashi J, et al.: Association study of the DISC1/TRAX locus with schizophrenia in a Japanese population. *Schizophr Res* 79:175–180, 2005.
54. Hodgkinson CA, Goldman D, Jaeger J, et al.: Disrupted in schizophrenia 1 (DISC1): Association with schizophrenia, schizoaffective disorder, and bipolar disorder. *Am J Hum Genet* 75:862–872, 2004.
55. Cannon TD, Hennah W, van Erp TG, et al.: Association of DISC1/TRAX haplotypes with schizophrenia, reduced prefrontal gray matter, and impaired short- and long-term memory. *Arch Gen Psychiatry* 62:1205–1213, 2005.
56. Burdick KE, Hodgkinson CA, Szeszko PR, et al.: DISC1 and neurocognitive function in schizophrenia. *Neuroreport* 16:1399–1402, 2005.
57. Hennah W, Tuulio-Henriksson A, Paunio T, et al.: A haplotype within the DISC1 gene is associated with visual memory functions in families with a high density of schizophrenia. *Mol Psychiatry* 10:1097–1103, 2005.
58. Thomson PA, Wray NR, Millar JK, et al.: Association between the TRAX/DISC locus and both bipolar disorder and schizophrenia in the Scottish population. *Mol Psychiatry* 10:657–68, 616, 2005.
59. Thomas NS, Sharp AJ, Browne CE, Skuse D, Hardie C, Dennis NR: Xp deletions associated with autism in three females. *Hum Genet* 104:43–48, 1999.
60. Jamain S, Quach H, Betancur C, et al.: Mutations of the X-linked genes encoding neuroligins NLGN3 and NLGN4 are associated with autism. *Nat Genet* 34:27–29, 2003.
61. Laumonnier F, Bonnet-Brilhault F, Gomot M, et al.: X-linked mental retardation and autism are associated with a mutation in the NLGN4 gene, a member of the neuroligin family. *Am J Hum Genet* 74:552–557, 2004.
62. Chih B, Afridi SK, Clark L, Scheiffele P: Disorder-associated mutations lead to functional inactivation of neuroligins. *Hum Mol Genet* 13:1471–1477, 2004.
63. Chih B, Engelman H, Scheiffele P: Control of excitatory and inhibitory synapse formation by neuroligins. *Science* 307:1324–1328, 2005.
64. Chubykin AA, Liu X, Comoletti D, Tsigelny I, Taylor P, Sudhof TC: Dissection of synapse induction by neuroligins: Effect of a neuroligin mutation associated with autism. *J Biol Chem* 280:22365–22374, 2005.
65. Comoletti D, De Jaco A, Jennings LL, et al.: The Arg451Cys-neuroligin-3 mutation associated with autism reveals a defect in protein processing. *J Neurosci* 24:4889–4893, 2004.
66. Blasi F, Bacchelli E, Pesaresi G, Carone S, Bailey AJ, Maestrini E: Absence of coding mutations in the X-linked genes neuroligin 3 and neuroligin 4 in individuals with autism from the IMGSAC collection. Am J Med Genet B *Neuropsychiatr Genet* 141B:220–221, 2006.
67. Gauthier J, Bonnel A, St-Onge J, et al.: NLGN3/NLGN4 gene mutations are not responsible for autism in the Quebec population. *Am J Med Genet B Neuropsychiatr Genet* 132:74–75, 2005.
68. Vincent JB, Kolozsvari D, Roberts WS, Bolton PF, Gurling HM, Scherer SW: Mutation screening of X-chromosomal neuroligin genes: No mutations in 196 autism probands. *Am J Med Genet B Neuropsychiatr Genet* 129:82–84, 2004.
69. Sebat J, Lakshmi B, Troge J, et al.: Large-scale copy number polymorphism in the human genome. *Science* 305:525–528, 2004.
70. Iafrate AJ, Feuk L, Rivera MN, et al.: Detection of large-scale variation in the human genome. *Nat Genet* 36:949–951, 2004.
71. Eichler EE: Widening the spectrum of human genetic variation. *Nat Genet* 38:9–11, 2006.

CHAPTER 2.3.3 ■ MOLECULAR BASIS OF SELECT CHILDHOOD PSYCHIATRIC DISORDERS

PAUL J. LOMBROSO AND JAMES F. LECKMAN

The past decade has seen remarkable progress in the application of molecular genetic strategies to the study of neurologic and neuropsychiatric disorders (1, 2). The chromosomal location for a number of autosomal-dominant, autosomal-recessive, and X-linked disorders has been accomplished (Table 2.3.3.1). The genes that are mutated in many of these illnesses have been mapped or identified. Determining the function of both the normal and mutated proteins has begun. This chapter reviews some of the important accomplishments in this area. It begins with a discussion of the molecular bases for normal learning and memory and how mutations of key signaling proteins lead to developmental disorders, and concludes with a brief consideration of the molecular basis of additional child psychiatric disorders.

LEARNING AND MEMORY

The ability to learn something new and then consolidate that information into long-term memories is part of normal development. As clinicians, we are often asked to evaluate whether a child is developing appropriately. Are specific skills emerging at the appropriate time points or are they delayed? Landmarks include the ability of a child to speak, to read, or to interact appropriately with peers. The mechanisms by which children learn to sit and crawl, walk and talk, and develop social skills have been the intensive focus of psychologists and psychiatrists over the years.

It is only in the past few decades that investigators have begun to study these questions at a molecular level (3, 4). What has emerged is a fascinating story of how cells within the central nervous system communicate with each other during learning and initiate a series of events that lead to the formation of long-term memories. Equally interesting is the finding that disruptions to these normal processes contribute to several developmental disorders. We will first review some of the mechanisms by which normal learning develops before discussing disorders that occur when these processes are disrupted.

A central concept to emerge from research on learning and memory is that the formation of long-term memories requires both biochemical and structural modifications within neurons. The transformation of short-term, labile memories into more stable, long-term memories requires growth at specialized points of neuronal contact termed synapses. Synapses change shape as learning proceeds—new synapses are formed or old ones are strengthened. This phenomenon, termed synaptic plasticity, is found in all parts of the brain where memories are formed.

When an action potential arrives at the end of the axon, synaptic vesicles fuse with the presynaptic terminal membrane and release one or more of a variety of neurotransmitters. The transmitters diffuse across the narrow synaptic cleft and bind to receptors on the postsynaptic terminal. Neurons communicate in this way, and the subsequent processing of the incoming signal at the postsynaptic terminal results in long-lasting changes in both the shape and biochemical composition of synapses.

A tremendous amount of research has been devoted to understanding this process over the last decade (5). To summarize, a signal arrives at the surface of a neuron and induces the production of proteins required for the morphological and biochemical changes at the synapse. This experience-induced synaptic plasticity underlies how memories are formed, and the molecular mechanisms by which this occurs will be reviewed next.

A key player in these events is a member of the mitogen-activated protein kinase (MAPK) family of proteins, the extracellular-signal regulated kinase (ERK) (6–8). The arrival of a signal at the postsynaptic terminal activates a cascade of signaling proteins that leads to the activation of ERK (Figure 2.3.3.1). The ERK pathway is activated in all brain regions where synaptic plasticity occurs and is necessary for the formation of new long-term memories (5). This has been demonstrated by blocking the activity of ERK by injecting inhibitors of this enzyme into specific brain regions, such as the amygdala. The formation of memories that are normally consolidated within that structure does not occur (e.g., fear conditioning) (9, 10). Similarly, if ERK activity is blocked within the hippocampus, the formation of memories that require the hippocampus is prevented (visual-spatial learning) (11).

ERKs are members of a family of enzymes termed kinases that add phosphate groups to substrate proteins. The addition of bulky, negatively charged phosphate groups often results in a change in the three-dimensional shape of the phosphorylated protein. The conformational change in turn often exposes a previously hidden amino acid domain buried deep within the structure of the protein. The exposure of the domain now permits interactions of the protein with other polypeptides or molecules further downstream in a cascade. For example, phosphorylation and activation of ERK leads in turn to the phosphorylation of a set of transcription factors. The transcription factors are now capable of initiating gene transcription (12).

In this way, a signal originating at the surface of a postsynaptic neuron is communicated to the interior of the cell, and a group of genes are transcribed. The proteins produced are necessary for the modifications at the spine that accompany synaptic plasticity. As a consequence, the neuron becomes more sensitive to future synaptic input: It responds with higher excitatory potentials than before. Moreover, the increase in responsiveness may last for prolonged periods of time, months or longer. This phenomenon, termed long-term potentiation, is thought to underlie the molecular changes that occur during the formation of stable, long-term memories (5, 13).

A key point in the present discussion is that a series of proteins are "upstream" of ERK and necessary for its

TABLE 2.3.3.1

CHROMOSOMAL LOCALIZATION AND GENE ABNORMALITIES IN SELECTED PSYCHIATRIC AND NEUROLOGIC DISORDERS

Genetic Disorder	Chromosomal Location	Genetic Mutation (Protein)
Autosomal dominant		
Amyotrophic lateral sclerosis	21q22.1	Point mutations (superoxide dismutase)
Benign familial neonatal convulsions 1	20q13.2	Point mutations (voltage-gated potassium channel)
Benign familial neonatal convulsions 2	8q24	Point mutations (a second voltage-gated potassium channel)
Charcot-Marie-Tooth disease		
Type 1A	17p11.2	Gene duplication, deletions, point mutations (peripheral myelin protein-22, PMP22)
Type 1B	1q22	Point mutations (myelin protein zero protein)
Alzheimer disease		
AD1	21q21	Point mutations (amyloid precursor protein)
AD2	19q13.2	Increased frequency of apoE4 allele
AD3	14q24.3	Point mutations (presenilin-1)
AD4	1q31-q42	Point mutations (presenilin-2)
Huntington disease	4p16.3	Triplet repeat (huntintin)
Myotonic dystrophy	19q13.2	Triplet repeat (myotonin protein kinase)
Neurofibromatosis		
Von Recklinhausen	17q11.2	Deletions, insertions, translocations, and point mutations (neurofibromin)
Acoustic neuroma	22q.12.2	Translocations, deletions, point mutations (merlin)
Parkinson disease	4q21	Point mutations (α-synuclein)
Spinocerebral ataxia	6p23	Triplet repeat (SCA1)
Imprinting disorders		
Angelman syndrome	15q11-12	Deletion, uniparental disomy, point mutations, imprinting center mutation (UBE3A)
Prader-Willi syndrome	15q11-12	Deletion, uniparental disomy, imprinting center mutation (candidate protein: SNRNP)
Autosomal recessive		
Ataxia telangiectasia	11q23	Translocation, deletions, point mutations (ATM)
Gaucher disease	1q21	Point mutations (glucocerebrosidase)
Lissencephaly		
Miller-Dieker	17q13.3	Deletions (lissencephaly 1)
Milder lissencephaly	17q13.3	Point mutations (lissencephaly 1)
Phenylketonuria	12q24	Deletions, point mutations (phenylalanine hydroxylase)
Parkinson disease	6q25.2-q27	Point mutations, deletions (parkin)
Retinoblastoma	13q14	Deletions, point mutation (retinoblastoma)
Rubinstein-Taybi syndrome	16p13.3	Translocation, deletions, point mutations (CREB-binding protein)
Schizencephaly	3q25-q26	Candidate gene (homoeobox gene emx2)
Waardenburg syndrome	2q35	Deletions, point mutation (Pax-3)
Williams syndrome	7q11.23	Deletions (multiple candidate genes)
Wilson disease	13q14.21	Point mutations, deletions (copper-transporting ATPase)
Velocardiofacial syndrome	22q11	Candidate gene (UFDIL)
X-linked recessive		
Muscular dystrophy		
Duchenne dystrophy	Xp21.21	Large deletion (dystrophin)
Becker dystrophy	Xp21.21	Small deletion (dystrophin)
Fragile X syndrome	Xq27.3	Triplet repeat (FMR-1)
Lesch-Nyhan syndrome	Xq27	Deletions, point mutations (HGPRT)
Lissencephaly (double-cortex)	Xq22.3	Translocation, point mutations (doublecortin)
Rett syndrome	Xq28	Point mutations (MeCP2)
Spinobulbar muscular atrophy	Xp21.3	Triplet repeat (androgen receptor)
Mitochondrial diseases with maternal transmission		
Leber hereditary optic atrophy	Mitochondria	Point mutations (NADH dehydrogenase)
Mitochondrial myopathy	Mitochondria	Deletion (candidate genes: Cox II and cytochrome b)

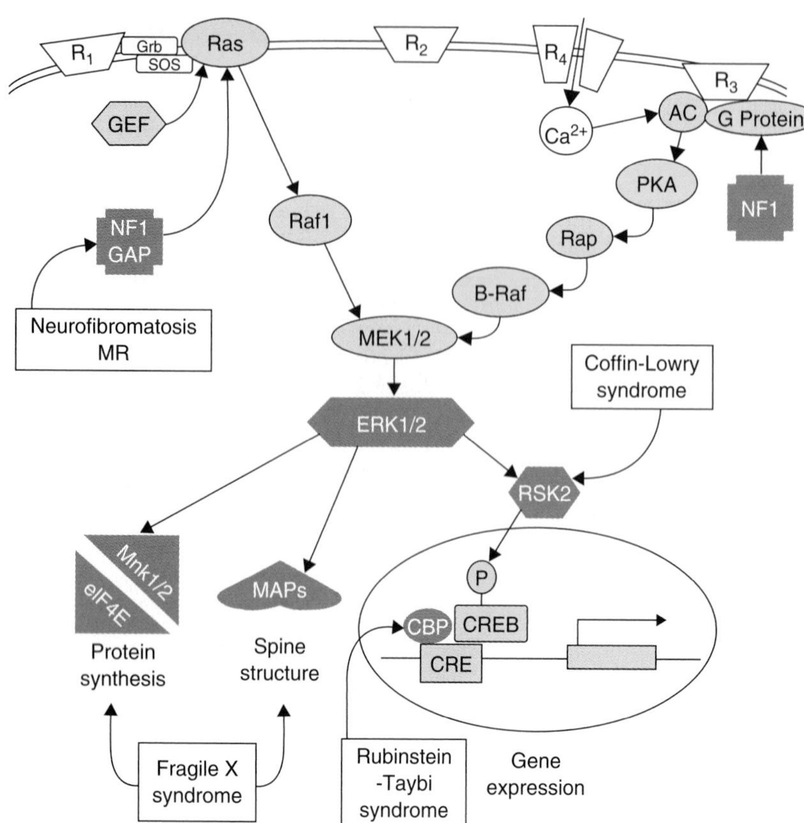

FIGURE 2.3.3.1. The ERK MAPK cascade is affected in human mental retardation syndromes. The mitogen-activated protein kinase (MAPK) family includes two important members that are involved in many different forms of learning and memory. These proteins are termed extracellular-signal–regulated kinases (ERKs) to reflect the fact that they were initially characterized as kinases that became activated after growth factors bound to specific receptors at the outer surface of a cell's membrane. Upstream regulators and selected potential downstream targets of the ERK MAP kinase cascade are shown, along with known sites of derangement in human mental retardation syndromes. One current model is that MAPK plays multiple roles in memory formation: Modulating the induction of lasting synaptic changes through regulating voltage-dependent potassium channels and triggering long-lasting changes through regulating gene expression via CREB phosphorylation. Other possible sites of action are regulating local protein synthesis, regulating cytoskeletal proteins, and regulating other ion channels such as the AMPA subtype of glutamate receptor. (Adapted with permission from Sweatt JD, Weeber EJ, Lombroso PJ: Cognitive disorders and the ras/ERK/CREB pathway. *J Am Acad Child Adol Psychiatry* 42:741–744, 2003.)

activation, while a series of proteins are "downstream" of activated ERK and are required for transcriptional activation. It follows that disruption of components of this multistep pathway might in turn disrupt the development of synaptic plasticity. Mutations have recently been discovered in several genes involved in this pathway and these mutations lead to the three developmental disorders that are discussed next (Figure 2.3.3.1).

Neurofibromatosis is an autosomal dominant disease with clinical features that include neural-derived tumors, and café-au-lait spots throughout the body. Approximately half of the affected individuals are also mentally retarded (14). The gene that causes neurofibromatosis (NF1) was recently characterized and several different mutations were identified in affected patients (15). Variability in the types of mutations (point mutations, insertions, or deletions) reflects the high level of phenotypic heterogeneity seen in affected individuals.

The region of the gene that is mutated determines whether or not the child develops cognitive deficits, in addition to the characteristic benign tumors. In other words, the normal neurofibromin protein has several amino acid domains with distinct cellular functions. One of the domains regulates cellular proliferation, and mutations within this region of the gene lead to the formation of tumors. Another portion of the protein regulates the ERK pathway, and mutations within this region interfere with the ability of neurofibromin to regulate the ERK pathway. As a consequence, the ERK pathway is overactive and does not respond appropriately to incoming neuronal signals. Normal synaptic plasticity does not occur and individuals with this type of mutation are mentally retarded (16).

A mutation in a second protein in the classical ERK pathway leads to Coffin-Lowry mental retardation syndrome (17). One of the downstream targets of the ERK pathway is a kinase called ribosomal S6 kinase (RSK2). RSK2 is a protein kinase that rapidly enters the nucleus upon activation and phosphorylates the important transcription factor, CREB. This transcription factor targets specific genes and induces their expression; in the absence of phosphorylation, CREB remains less active. Mutations in the RSK2 gene disrupt the normal cascade from the neuronal surface to the nucleus, interfere with gene transcription, and proteins that are required for synaptic modifications are not expressed (18).

A third disorder associated with mutations in the ERK pathway is Rubinstein-Taybi syndrome (RTS) (19). RTS individuals have characteristic clinical signs that include facial abnormalities, broad digits, and mental retardation. Recently, a mutation to the CREB binding protein gene (CBP) was discovered in patients with the RTS phenotype. The CBP protein is required for the normal unwinding of DNA that precedes the binding of transcription factors to promoter regions. As a result of the mutation, the transcription factor CREB cannot bind properly to the targeted DNA sequences and gene transcription does not occur. Once again, synaptic plasticity is disrupted and normal learning does not develop.

FRAGILE X SYNDROME

The molecular biology of fragile X syndrome has advanced dramatically over the past decade (20). This disorder is the second most common cause of mental retardation after Down syndrome and affects as many as 1 in 750 to 1,000 males, and 1 in 500 to 750 females (21) (Chapter 5.1.2).

Children with fragile X syndrome are born with mild to severe mental retardation. Additional clinical symptoms include facial, testicular, and connective tissue abnormalities (22, 23). Abnormal speech patterns are present in the majority of cases and include echolalia and high-pitched speech, as well as poor articulation, dysfluency, and dyspraxia. There is often gaze aversion among these children, as well as stereotypic behaviors, hyperactivity, and attentional difficulties. Aggressive and self-injurious behaviors are prominent features in some cases (24). Although there has been some interest in identifying specific linguistic, cognitive, or behavioral deficits among affected individuals, these have not been found (21, 25–27). This is of some interest given the recent molecular discoveries discussed below indicating a general disruption to synaptic plasticity throughout the brain.

Fragile X syndrome is transmitted from one generation to the next as an X-linked disorder. It has been known for many years that the phenotype of fragile X syndrome often cosegregates with what appears to be a "fragile" site on the X chromosome. In a certain proportion of cells grown in the absence of the nutrient, folic acid, a break point becomes visible on one of the X chromosomes (Figure 2.3.3.2) (28). The chromosomal region is not in fact separated but rather does not stain normally on karyotype analyses. These findings suggested that the gene or gene(s) involved in the disorder might lie near the disrupted site.

Several unusual aspects of the disorder were noted before the gene was actually cloned. Approximately 20 percent of the males who carry the abnormal gene are not mentally impaired. If the gene lay on the X chromosome, why were these individuals not affected, as they have no normal copy of the gene to compensate for the mutated gene? These men were called "normal transmitting males," and pass the abnormal gene to their daughters, who may also be unaffected. However, their grandsons are at high risk for the full syndrome. This progression in severity over several generations is known as *anticipation.*

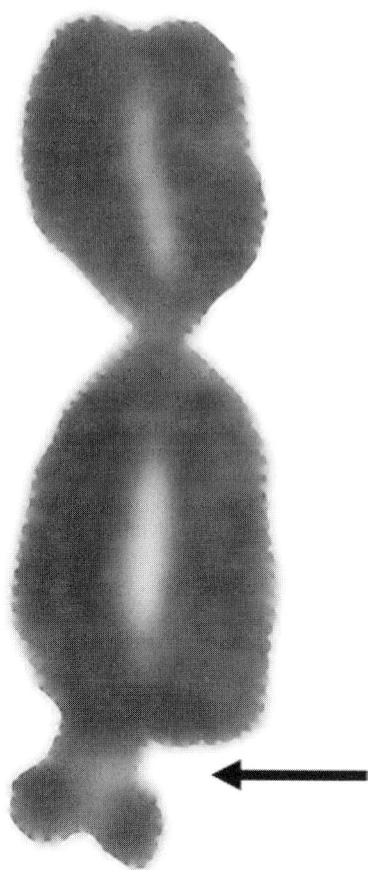

FIGURE 2.3.3.2. Fragile X site. The fragile site is shown on an affected chromosome of an individual with fragile X syndrome. (Adapted with permission from Lubs H: A marker X chromosome. *Am J Hum Gen* 21:231–244, 1969.)

The molecular basis for anticipation is now understood, and relates to the molecular defect found in the affected FMR-1 gene (29). A novel type of mutation was identified, termed a triplet repeat expansion. Triplet repeats refer to any three bases in the nucleotide sequence that are repeated as a unit several times. In the case of fragile X syndrome, the three repeated nucleotides are cytosine-guanine-guanine (CGG). Normal individuals have between six and 50 repeats of these bases in their FMR-1 gene, with 29 repeats being the most frequent number seen (29). Affected individuals, however, have a dramatic increase in the number of repeated sequences, with 200 to 1,000 repeats typically. Mothers of affected probands often have numbers of CGG repeats that fall in between those seen in normal individuals and those affected with the full fragile X syndrome. Carriers thus typically have between 50 and 200 CGG repeats (29); repeats in this range are called *premutations.*

Some individuals who carry the premutation of the *FMR-1* gene have mild cognitive and behavioral symptoms (30). Heterozygotic fragile X females perform poorly on visuospatial and/or memory subtests (31, 32). Moreover, magnetic resonance imaging (MRI) and positron emission tomography (PET) analysis have shown premutation female carriers to have significant decreases in total brain volumes, as well as metabolic increases in the hippocampus and cerebellum (33). Mothers who have the premutation are at a much higher risk of expanding the triplet repeat in the next generation to produce affected children with the full mutation. Although why it happens remains unclear, the expansion change from premutation to the full mutation is the molecular basis for the phenomenon of anticipation.

Two separate phenotypes recently have been described in premutation carriers. Premature ovarian failure is reported to affect 16 percent to 24 percent of female carriers (34). One-third of male premutation carriers over the age of 50 develop fragile X–associated tremor and ataxia syndrome (35, 36). The molecular biology of these two distinct disorders remains unclear and does not appear directly related either to the CGG triplet repeat size or to the extent of FMRP deficit.

In addition to the 200 to 1,000 CGG repeats in affected individuals, other abnormalities in the DNA have been noted. CpG islands were discussed in the previous chapter, and are regions often found within promoter regions with high content of the two bases, cytosine and guanosine. Cytosines may be chemically modified by the addition of a methyl group, and large regions of methylated nucleotides regulate whether a gene is expressed or not. The relatively small triplet repeat found in unaffected individuals is present immediately downstream of the promoter region, in a region of the FMR message that does not encode protein (37).

The triplet repeat expansion in fragile X produces a large increase in the number of methylated CpG islands (38). The extent of methylation over the region correlates directly with the loss of functional protein (39). The methylated region also explains the "fragile site" that is observed, as this region of DNA does not stain well on karyotype analyses and appears as a broken chromosomal region. To summarize, the abnormal methylation pattern is adjacent to the promoter region, interferes with normal transcription of the gene, and ultimately leads to the absence of functional protein in most affected individuals.

What is the normal function of the FMR-1 protein and how does its absence lead to clinical symptoms? Soon after the gene was isolated in 1991, researchers noticed that the protein contained three domains with highly conserved amino acid patterns. These domains are homologous to a motif found in proteins that bind to ribonucleic acid (RNA) molecules. These proteins are called RNA-binding proteins and are involved at multiple steps during the processing, trafficking, or translating of transcripts within cells (40–42). A mutation in an RNA-binding protein might seriously impair the ability of cells to produce mature messages or translate those messages into protein.

This was in fact described in a fragile X patient who did not have the expected triplet repeat expansion, but instead had a point mutation that changed a single highly conserved amino acid normally present within one of the RNA-binding motifs (42–44). The domain thus appeared to be critical for the proper function of FMR-1 protein, and mutations in this domain interfere with its ability to bind RNA molecules and to process them correctly. In addition, this case indicated that although the majority of cases are caused by a triplet repeat expansion fragile X syndrome, any mutation that disrupts the functional activity of the FMR-1 protein could reasonably lead to a similar clinical syndrome. It is a good example of allelic heterogeneity, where mutations in different parts of a single gene lead to the identical phenotype.

Knowledge of the intracellular location of the FMR-1 protein has extended our understanding of its function. The fragile X protein binds to ribosomes, the organelles within cells that are made from ribosomal RNA and various RNA-binding proteins and function as factories that translate mRNA transcripts into proteins (45).

Studies of the expression pattern of the FMR-1 gene during development show the areas of the brain that normally have the highest level of expression. These include the basal forebrain and hippocampus (46). Both are involved in short-term memory and sequential processing of information, and are affected in some neurodegenerative disorders, such as Alzheimer's disease. In addition, clinical neuroimaging studies have detected age-related volumetric changes in fragile X individuals in the cerebellar vermis, fourth ventricle, and hippocampus (47–49). Finally, the production of animal models, such as knockout mice, has been helpful in studying the underlying processes that are disrupted. Many of the clinical features seen in fragile X syndrome are present in these knockout mice (51).

A major advance in our understanding of the normal role of FMR-1 has come from two lines of investigation. The first has to do with the question of where proteins are translated within neurons. The older dogma was that messages produced within the nucleus were rapidly transported into the cytoplasm where they attached to ribosomes and deposited the translated proteins into the endoplasmic reticulum for further processing. This is the case for the vast majority of messages. However, within neurons, recent work has suggested that a population of messages is actually transported throughout the dendrites and into the spines themselves. They remain there until an incoming signal arrives and initiates local protein synthesis at the very spines where the proteins are needed.

This new model has been helpful in solving a major difficulty with the earlier dogma. A typical neuron has up to 10,000 spines. Incoming synaptic activity arrives at perhaps several hundred of these spines. The previous model would have had the incoming signal travel to the nucleus, to initiate gene transcription and protein translation in the perinuclear region. The problem that arose was how proteins were then transported to the minority of spines where synaptic modifications were required.

The new model posits that messages themselves are transported throughout the dendrites to the spines, ready for an incoming signal. Evidence for this model has been extensive over the past several years, as various components of the translational machinery have been detected throughout dendrites and within the spines (51). These include the messages themselves as well as ribosomes and various proteins required for local protein synthesis (52).

It should be added that local proteins synthesis does not preclude a signal from being sent from the activated spines back to the nucleus to initiate gene transcription. In fact, these signals must occur for long-term potentiation to be maintained and long-term memories consolidated. There is an initial burst of local protein synthesis that *induces* long-term potentiation, and a later phase during which mRNA messages must be transcribed to *maintain* the long-term potentiation. An interesting consequence of this can be demonstrated by injecting transcriptional inhibitors into specific brain regions. If these inhibitors are injected into the amygdala, for example, *short-term* fear conditioning memories are formed, but this learning is not consolidated into *long-term* memories, as the maintenance of LTP requires protein synthesis.

Having solved one problem, researchers were left with another. Obviously, the messages that are transported down the neurites must not be translated until the proper synaptic input arrives. Recent work from several laboratories has suggested that inhibition of translation is an important function of FRMP (20). FMRP attaches to newly synthesized mRNAs in the nucleus, accompanies these messages throughout the neuronal network and into spines, all along inhibiting translation of the messages into proteins. When a signal arrives that normally would induce synaptic plasticity, the inhibitory actions of FMRP end and the message is translated into proteins.

Exactly how this happens is not yet understood (53). One interesting possibility is that the kinase ERK is involved. It is now known that one of the functions of activated ERK, besides its ability to transduce signals into the nucleus as described above, is to participate in the regulation of local protein synthesis at the spine itself (54, 55). Presumably, these functions of ERK work in parallel: one to initiate rapid local protein synthesis and the second to translocate into the nucleus and activate gene transcription.

The messages that are transported to the spines are a subset of messages found in neurons: messages that encode for proteins necessary for the biochemical and structural modifications occurring at the synapse (56, 57). It should be pointed out that FMRP is probably only one of a number of proteins required for this process. Many proteins are needed to support the transport of messages, their inhibition or activation at the spine, as well as providing the scaffolding support for local translation of proteins. Although this is more speculative, it is likely that mutations that disrupt these proteins will be found to also disrupt synaptic plasticity to varying degrees and produce cognitive deficits in affected individuals.

The model presented in the previous paragraphs leads to certain predictions. If FMRP is necessary for synaptic plasticity to develop, then the absence of this key player might result in detectable disruptions in spine morphology. William Greenough and his colleagues have looked at this question and have found evidence supporting the hypothesis. They used anatomical techniques to examine spines from patients with fragile X syndrome as well as a mouse model of the syndrome (58, 59). Compared to the controls, they found larger numbers of long, spindly, and immature-looking spines in the fragile X cases, and fewer numbers of short, mushroom-shaped, and mature-looking spines. Taken together, these studies suggest that FMRP is involved in development of spines through regulation of the shape, number, and maturity of spines, and that this occurs through FMRP's regulation of local protein synthesis.

Expansion of the FMR-1 gene through triplet repeats was originally thought to be a genetic anomaly unique to fragile X syndrome. More than a dozen other triplet repeat disorders have now been identified (Figure 2.3.3.3), including Huntington's chorea, Friedreich's ataxia, and myotonic dystrophy (60–62). The phenomenon of anticipation had been apparent in most of these disorders but early investigators dismissed it as the result of ascertainment bias. The discovery of triplet repeat expansions, however, provided the molecular

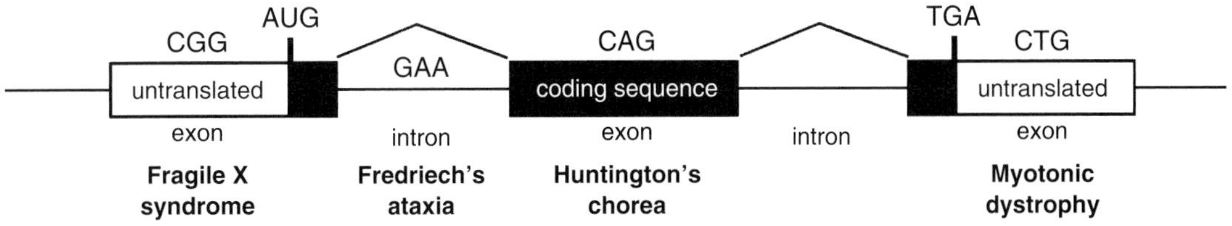

CGG AUG GAA CAG TGA CTG
untranslated exon | intron | coding sequence exon | intron | untranslated exon
Fragile X syndrome | **Fredriech's ataxia** | **Huntington's chorea** | **Myotonic dystrophy**

FIGURE 2.3.3.3. **Triplet repeat disorders.** A hypothetical gene is shown prior to the splicing together of exons and the removal of introns to produce a mature RNA message. Triplet repeat expansions have been discovered in all regions of a gene. In fragile X syndrome, the cytosine-guanine-guanine (CGG) repeat lies in the 5′ untranslated region immediately adjacent to the promoter region. The expansion to 1,000 to 2,000 repeats leads to abnormal methylation patterns and disrupts normal transcription of the gene. In myotonic dystrophy, the cytosine-adenine-guanine (CAG) repeat is found at the other end of the gene within the 3′ untranslated region. It is believed that the expansion there results in an unstable mRNA prone to degradation, as well as perhaps affecting the transcription of a second nearby homeobox gene. In Huntington's chorea, the triplet repeat expansion occurs in the open reading frame of the gene and leads to the inappropriate incorporation of an amino acid, in this case glutamine, within the protein sequence. Triplet repeat expansions have also been found in introns, where they presumably interfere with the proper splicing of the message. Friedreich's ataxia is an example of this type of expansion.

explanation for this phenomenon. The degree of anticipation can be quite remarkable (Figure 2.3.3.4). In myotonic dystrophy, for example, expansions that are just above the threshold for disease may only result in individuals developing cataracts late in life. Several generations later, descendants have the full expansion with long repeats and fatal congenital illness (63). Interestingly, anticipation has been described in families with schizophrenia and bipolar disorder, and some investigators believe triplet repeat expansions may account for a subset of these affected patients (64–68).

PRADER-WILLI AND ANGELMAN SYNDROMES

Half of our 46 chromosomes derive from our mothers and the other half from our fathers. For years, it had been assumed that genes that lay on either chromosomal pair were equivalent and that each produced the same amount of functional protein. Mutations present in one gene could often be overcome through the actions of the normal protein derived from the homologous gene.

This is an accurate description of the molecular events for the majority of genes; however, recent studies over the past decade have demonstrated that some gene pairs are not functionally equivalent. Instead, only one of the two genes is active and the other is repressed. The production of functional proteins depends on whether the gene that encodes it lies on the chromosome derived from the mother or the one from the father. In some cases, the maternal gene is the only one expressed; in others cases, the paternal gene. This phenomenon is termed *genomic imprinting*.

For the majority of disorders, mutations change the specific nucleotide sequence of a gene and thereby change the amino acid sequence of the encoded protein. For a smaller group of disorders, mutations of nucleotide sequences are not involved. Rather, factors other than the underlying nucleotide sequence determine whether the DNA produces useful patterns of gene expression. These factors are known as *epigenetic* phenomena to distinguish them from events that have an effect on the actual nucleotide sequences. We have discussed some epigenetic factors earlier in our discussion of methylation in fragile X syndrome and will do so again below when we discuss Rett syndrome. In these disorders, the actual packaging of chromatin and DNA influences gene expression, rather than a mutation to the nucleotide sequence.

Approximately 30 genes have been discovered to date that are imprinted. Many of them play a key role in the growth and differentiation of various tissues. Disruption of these genes is implicated in a number of cancers and developmental disorders. These advances are reviewed in the following with an emphasis on two developmental disorders caused by imprinting defects—Prader-Willi and Angelman syndromes.

Prader-Willi syndrome (PWS) is a rare disorder with a prevalence of 1 in 10,000 births. A constellation of symptoms arises shortly after birth (69). Infants are often hypotonic and fail to thrive; however, their dietary habits change within the first year or two of life, and these individuals typically become hyperphagic and obese (70). They are often mildly to moderately mentally retarded and have a number of additional behavioral problems that include temper tantrums, aggressive behaviors, and obsessive-compulsive symptoms outside of the compulsive food-related behaviors (71–73).

Angelman syndrome is also a relatively rare disorder with a prevalence of 1 in 10,000 births. Individuals with the disorder

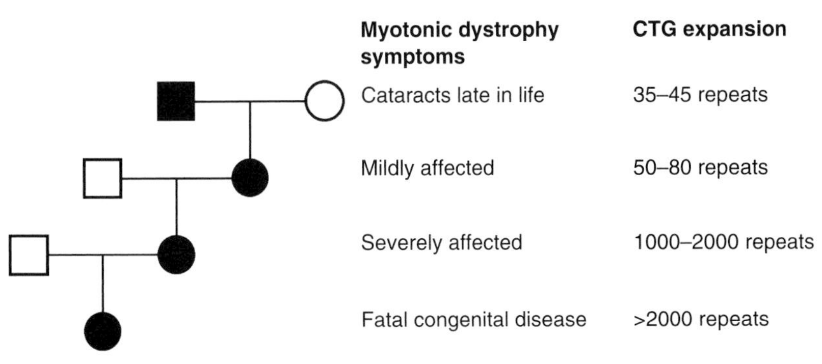

FIGURE 2.3.3.4. **Anticipation.** Anticipation refers to the increase in severity for a disorder over several generations. In myotonic dystrophy, for example, the increase in symptoms ranges from cataracts late in life in a great-grandfather, to milder symptoms in a grandfather, and then more severe muscle disorder in the father, to fatal congenital illness in the proband. A corresponding increase is found in the triplet repeat expansion for cytosine-thymidine-guanine (CTG).

are also hypotonic as infants and develop motor delays and moderate to severe mental retardation. They have a characteristic facies with a large mandible with an open-mouth expression, abnormal gait, and puppet-like limb movements; they rarely develop speech. Affected individuals often have an abnormal electroencephalogram and develop epilepsy early in life (74).

By the mid-1980s, it was known that both disorders are caused by a deletion on chromosome 15 (15q11–q13). Cytogenetic and molecular techniques showed that the same region is deleted in individuals with either syndrome. This result was somewhat puzzling because the disorders are very different, yet the identical deletion seemed to cause PWS in some cases and Angelman syndrome in others (75, 76).

It was then discovered that the clinical symptoms depend on which parent donates the deleted chromosome (77). The deletion derives from the father in most cases of PWS. In contrast, most individuals with Angelman syndrome have a deletion on the chromosome that derives from the mother.

A further clarification of the underlying mechanism came when the region for each disorder was pinpointed to a small region on chromosome 15. The section of DNA responsible for PWS is distinct but very close to the area responsible for Angelman syndrome. Part of the puzzle was thus clarified. A large deletion often occurs that spans both regions. The child will develop PWS if the deletion occurs on the paternal chromosome and Angelman syndrome if the deletion occurs on the maternal copy.

These two nearby regions on chromosome 15 are differentially imprinted. Normally, genes within the PWS region are expressed on chromosomes that derive from the father. Immediately downstream a second set of genes lie within the Angelman-critical region. These paternal-derived genes are imprinted and not expressed. The opposite expression pattern is found on the maternal chromosome. Genes within the Angelman region are expressed, whereas genes within the PWS region are silenced (Figure 2.3.3.5) (78, 79).

Deletions are responsible for approximately 70 percent of cases of both PWS and Angelman syndrome. A second mechanism, however, exists. The illnesses may be caused when children receive two copies of chromosome 15 from one of their parents (80). This unusual mechanism is called uniparental disomy (UPD). It occurs after an initial trisomy event in which two chromosomes from one parent are inappropriately passed along with one copy of the chromosome from the other parent, resulting in a total of three (rather than two) chromosomes. One chromosome is lost during gamete formation. If the initial trisomy involves two maternal and one paternal chromosomes, then loss of the extra paternal copy would result in two maternal chromosomes, or maternal UPD. If the initial trisomy involves two paternal and one maternal chromosome, then loss of the extra maternal copy would result in paternal UPD.

Maternal UPD results to PWS (81). In this situation, the genes that lie within the PWS region are present but on two maternal chromosomes. All the genes within the critical region are imprinted and no functional proteins are produced. Paternal UPD represents the opposite situation. PWS genes are present on both paternal chromosomes and both sets are expressed. However, the genes that lie adjacent within the Angelman region are imprinted; therefore, even though there

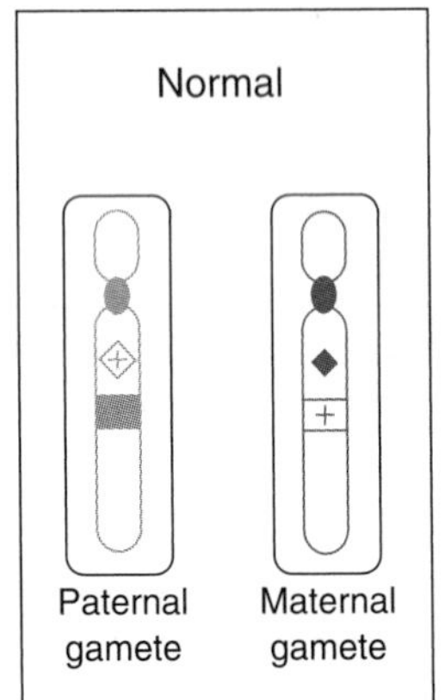

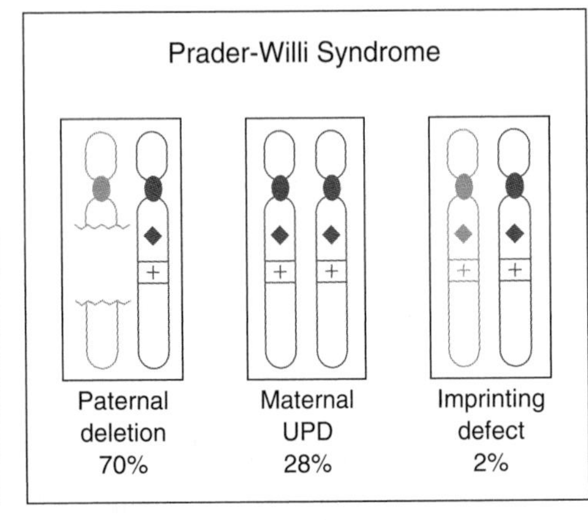

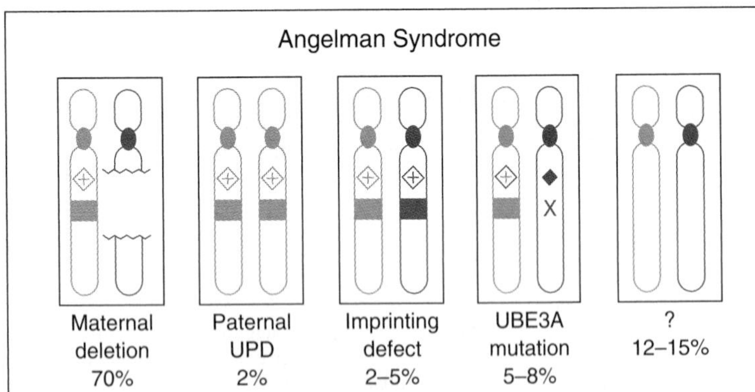

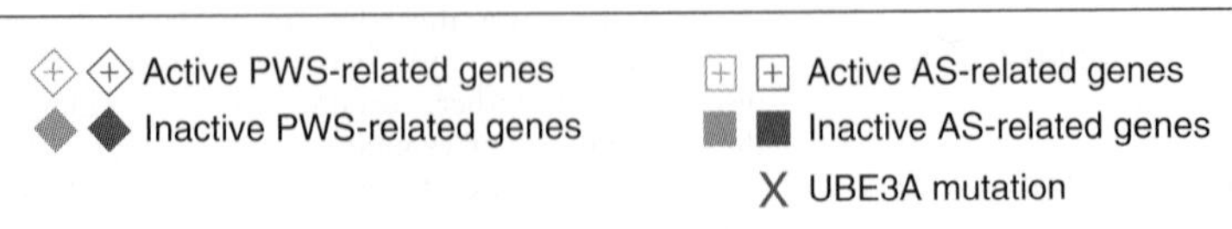

FIGURE 2.3.3.5. Imprinting in Prader-Willi and Angelman syndromes. Imprinting refers to the silencing of certain genes. It is a stable and reversible event that depends on the parental origin of the chromosome on which the gene lies and results in repression of a gene. For some genes, the paternal gene is silenced, whereas for other genes, it is the maternal gene. On chromosome 15, two adjacent regions are imprinted. In the normal situation (shown in the left, top panel), genes in the Prader-Willi syndrome (PWS) region are expressed on the paternal chromosome, whereas genes in the Angelman region are imprinted. The opposite situation exists on the maternal chromosome: genes in the PWS region are repressed, whereas genes in the Angelman region are expressed. Three mechanisms for developing PWS are shown, whereas four mechanisms have been discovered for Angelman syndrome (AS). The key at the bottom indicates genes, imprinting patterns, and mutations in both disorders. The relative proportion of each type of genetic abnormality in each syndrome is also shown. UPD, uniparental disomy. (Adapted with permission from Everman D, Cassidy S: Genomic imprinting: breaking the rules. *J Am Acad Child Adol Psychiatry* 39:386–389, 1999.) (See color insert.)

are two copies of all the genes, both sets are repressed and no protein is expressed.

A third mechanism that leads to these disorders involves a region of DNA called the imprinting center. This center controls imprinting by regulating the extent of methylation and chromatin compaction for hundreds of kilobases of DNA on either side. It appears that one center determines the state of imprinting within both the PWS- and Angelman-critical regions. Mutations within the imprinting center have been discovered that lead to inappropriate imprinting or a lack of imprinting where it should normally occur. These types of mutations cause PWS or Angelman syndrome in about 2 percent to 3 percent of affected individuals (82).

Finally, a fourth mechanism exists that causes Angelman syndrome in approximately 10 percent of the cases. This is a mutation within a single gene lying within the Angelman-critical region called UBE3A (83–85). The protein encoded by this gene normally regulates the life span of other proteins within the cell by regulating their proteolysis (Figure 2.3.3.6).

Many proteins must be quickly degraded and removed from the intracellular environment to ensure proper cell function. These include signaling proteins in which rapid turnover permits repeated signaling. It is also critical to remove certain enzymes that have become damaged before they interfere with normal intracellular signaling pathways. Several copies of a small molecule are added to proteins destined for degradation. This molecule, ubiquitin, acts as a flag to target the protein for degradation. The UBE3A gene is required in this process. It is one of several proteins that act in sequential order to attach ubiquitin molecules to targeted proteins. Intracellular organelles called proteosomes recognize ubiquitinated proteins, bind to them, and activate proteases that cut the protein into its constitutive amino acids. When this protein is mutated and unable to function properly, it is thought that an inappropriate accumulation of proteins occurs within CNS neurons and disrupts their normal function.

Several enzymes in addition to UBE3A are required in the series of enzymatic reactions that ends with the addition of ubiquitin molecules to proteins targeted for destruction. It is possible that mutations in these other genes will be found and lead to similar clinical problems. These mutations would represent examples of locus heterogeneity in which mutations in distinctly different genes produce the same phenotype. A number

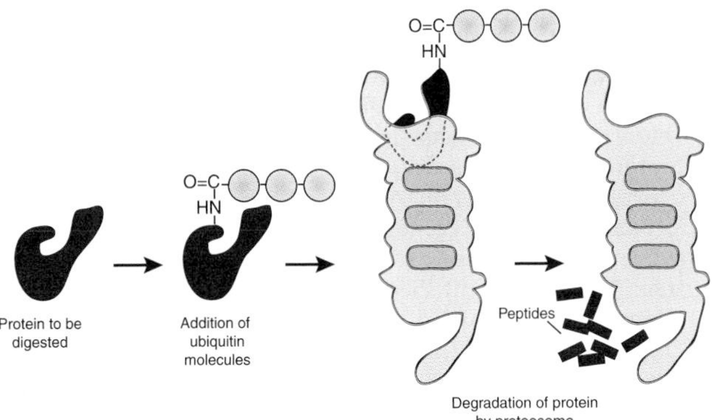

FIGURE 2.3.3.6. Angelman syndrome. It is critical to remove unwanted proteins from within cells before they disrupt cellular metabolism. Several steps are involved in this process and lead to the addition of one or more ubiquitin molecules to proteins targeted for degradation. The addition of ubiquitin to the protein serves as a signal to the proteosome, an organelle that breaks down proteins and serves as the cellular equivalent of a garbage disposal for a cell's unwanted proteins. (Adapted with permission from Lombroso PJ: Genetics of childhood disorders: XVI Angelman syndrome. *J Am Acad Child Adol Psychiatry*, 2000.)

of laboratories are actively investigating this possibility. On the other hand, no single gene mutation has yet been found in patients with PWS, and it remains unclear at present whether the absence of a single gene or the deletion of several genes within the critical PWS region are necessary for the disorder.

Two final notes should be made regarding Angelman syndrome. Recent work suggests that the maternally imprinted genes are differentially imprinted depending on the brain region where they are expressed (86). In addition, one of the genes within the Angelman region encodes for a subunit of the $GABA_A$ receptor (87). The absence of this gene and a related disturbance in GABA transmission is believed to be responsible for the seizure disorders present in individuals with the full deletion syndrome. As expected, individuals with a point mutation within only the UBE3A gene do not have epilepsy.

WILLIAMS SYNDROME

Deletions that span a number of genes and cause a constellation of symptoms are called *contiguous gene syndromes.* Williams syndrome is one such disorder, caused by a deletion on chromosome 7. This developmental disorder is characterized by distinct facial features, a variable degree of mental retardation, cardiovascular disease, and a very distinctive cognitive profile (88). The cognitive problems consist of visual–spatial deficits. Affected children are unable to integrate the parts of a picture into a whole pattern (89). Interestingly, these children frequently exhibit strengths in other cognitive areas, such as verbal skills. Indeed, some elements of their speech are normal, such as the quality of their vocabulary, auditory memory, and social use of language. Moreover, many patients sing or play musical instruments with considerable talent. The disorder, first described by Williams (90) in 1961, has a rather low prevalence of 1 per 20,000 live births, but remains a topic of considerable interest because of the striking disparity in cognitive strengths and weaknesses (91–93).

This disparity raises the possibility that the gene(s) responsible for Williams syndrome influence(s) the development of specific cortical regions and related cognitive abilities. This is in contrast to other forms of mental retardation, such as fragile X syndrome, where a more uniform depression is seen across many cognitive skills. As such, Williams syndrome has the potential to help identify factors that are important for acquisition of cognitive abilities during normal development.

Functional imaging studies have helped clarify some of the underlying neuropathologic mechanisms in Williams syndrome (94). In a rigorous study, the investigators examined regions that might be responsible for the visuospatial difficulties that are so prevalent among affected individuals. They identified a localized region within the dorsal pathway of the visual system around the intraparietal sulcus that appears to be responsible for the deficits in visuospatial processing. Jernigan and Bellugi (95) conducted MRIs on IQ- and age-matched subjects with Williams and Down syndromes. The cerebral cortices of both groups showed an overall decrease in volume. Cerebellar size, on the other hand, differentiated the two conditions. It was normal among the Williams syndrome subjects but significantly hypoplastic among the Down subjects.

Jernigan and coworkers extended this study by focusing in greater detail on the morphologic abnormalities in the cortices of Williams subjects (96). The overall volume of the cerebral cortex was reduced compared to normal subjects, but there was a relative sparing of the frontal areas and limbic structures, as well as a greater degree of hypoplasia in more posterior cortical structures. Different cortical regions are apparently affected to different degrees in Williams subjects.

Additional morphologic data comes from the autopsy of a Williams subject. Galaburda and colleagues found abnormal organization among the neurons in posterior cortical regions (area 17), an increase in cell packing density throughout cortical regions, and abnormal neuronal clustering (97). It is a single autopsy case, however, and additional work is necessary to clarify the underlying pathologic process.

Taken together, these findings suggest that abnormal, nonuniform development of the cerebral cortex may be responsible for the nonuniform cognitive findings that characterize these patients. The relatively intact cognitive skills related to affective recognition, face processing, and linguistic skills may be a consequence of the relatively normal development of limbic and frontal cortices and perhaps the relatively normal cerebellar structures. Poor functioning in visuospatial skills may be owing, at least in part, to the abnormalities in the posterior cortical structures, such as the parietal and occipital cortices known to be involved in visual processing. It is reasonable to suggest that the gene or genes affected in Williams syndrome may have their greatest impact on the development or normal functioning of more posterior regions of the cerebral cortex.

Nearly all patients with Williams syndrome have a large deletion of a segment of chromosome 7 (98, 99). A number of researchers note that the cardiovascular symptoms seen in many patients cosegregate with a gene in the deleted region, elastin. Elastin is a major component of skin, blood vessels, and lung tissues. The haplodeficiency caused by the deletion of elastin is likely to cause the vascular abnormalities and characteristic facies in these patients (98). Elastin, however, is not detectable in fetal or adult nervous tissue and probably does not contribute to the cognitive abnormalities (100).

Tassabehji and colleagues (101) (1996) were the first to report the deletion of a second gene in 20 out of 20 Williams syndrome patients. The sequence of this gene is nearly identical to a previously characterized gene called LIM kinase 1. Because it is expressed in high concentrations in the brain (102, 103), mutations in this gene are being searched for and are possible candidates responsible for the cognitive deficits seen in Williams syndrome patients (104). In fact, LIM kinase knockout mice have disrupted LTP, abnormalities in synaptic morphology, and deficits in learning (105). The specific cognitive deficits were intriguing: These mice have difficulties "unlearning." For example, once they have learned the position of a hidden platform in the Water Maze test, they are unable to learn the new location for the platform when it is relocated, something that normal mice can adapt to (105).

For a brief period, it was thought that elastin and LIM kinase 1 were the only genes within the deleted region. It is now known, however, that approximately 20 genes are present within the Williams syndrome critical region (Figure 2.3.3.7). In addition to elastin (89, 99) and the LIM kinase 1 (100, 101), other genes include syntaxin 1A (106), CLIP-115 (107), and Frizzled 9, a receptor for Wnt signaling (108), the replication factor C subunit (109), and the general transcription factor 2I (110). Several laboratories are currently investigating the function of these genes (111).

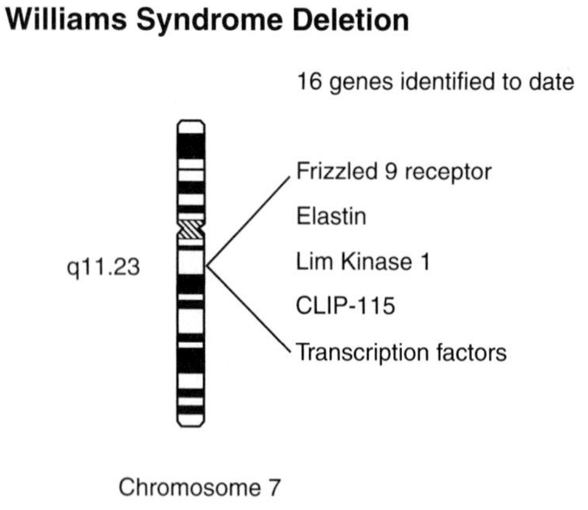

Williams Syndrome Deletion

FIGURE 2.3.3.7. Williams syndrome. The deletion at 7q11.23 in patients with Williams syndrome contains at least 16 genes. Several of these genes are expressed within the central nervous system. Shown are candidate genes for the neuropsychiatric symptoms observed in subjects with Williams syndrome. When several genes contribute to the expression of a disorder through their deletion, the illness is termed a contiguous gene syndrome.

RETT SYNDROME

Rett syndrome is a disorder within the autism spectrum (112). It has a prevalence of 1 in 10,000. Affected children develop normally and reach developmental milestones within the first year of life; parents are unaware of any abnormalities. One of the first clinical symptoms is the loss of purposeful hand movements. Other clinical findings soon emerge, including loss of speech, growth retardation with microcephaly, ataxia, and a severe disruption of normal cognitive functioning. Clinical symptoms stabilize for the next several decades of life after this initial rapid regression (113).

One unusual feature of the disorder is that females are almost exclusively affected. An early explanation for the preponderance of affected females is that the mutated gene is located on the X chromosome. There are many examples of X-linked disorders in which males die *in utero* because males only have one X chromosome and only a single copy of the gene in question. Females have a second copy of the gene on their other X chromosome, and it appears that transcription of this gene in a significant subset of cells provides some degree of protection during fetal development and early postnatal life. However, symptoms may eventually emerge because haploinsufficiency, a single functional copy of a gene, is unable to confer lasting protection.

The chromosomal location for the gene was facilitated by analysis of affected sisters, and its approximate position was identified at Xq28 (114). Candidate genes known to be present in this region were carefully studied. A number were systematically excluded as analyses of their nucleotide sequences revealed no mutations compared to the identical sequences from normal individuals; however, a gene was recently discovered that is mutated in several affected individuals (115). The protein encoded by this gene is methyl CpG-binding protein 2 (MeCP2), and mutations in two of its functional domains have now been characterized (Figure 2.3.3.8).

How are mutations in this gene related to clinical symptoms? As discussed in the previous chapter, many genes are expressed in certain tissues and not in others. Of the approximately 35,000 genes on the human genome, only about one-third are expressed exclusively within the central nervous system (CNS). Some of these genes and their protein products are important for normal development during critical periods of brain development. Others are needed only after birth, whereas others must be expressed at all times because they are involved in normal housekeeping functions required of the cell. This illustrates how carefully gene expression must be regulated for normal development and maintenance of tissues to proceed.

The previous chapter reviewed how transcription factors and other regulatory proteins such as enhancers and repressors bind to promoter regions of genes and either initiate transcription of specific subsets of genes or maintain their stable repression. The proteins involved in these regulatory events bind to specific deoxyribonucleic acid (DNA) sequences within the promoter regions that control gene expression.

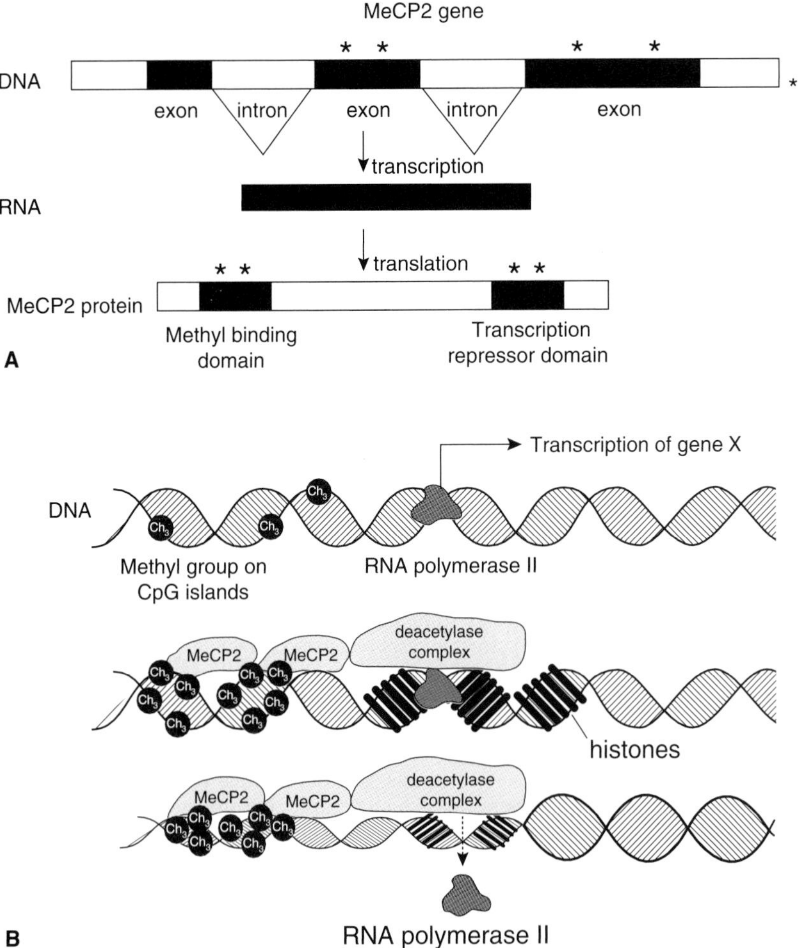

FIGURE 2.3.3.8. Rett syndrome. *A.* The *MeCP2* gene consists of three exons separated by two introns. The exons are spliced together to produce a mature RNA message that is translated into MeCP2 protein. The gene has been implicated in Rett syndrome after several mutations were found within the coding regions in a number of patients. These are indicated by asterisks (*) in the nucleotide sequence and protein. Mutations to date have been found to change the amino acid sequence within two functional domains of the protein. *B.* MeCP2 protein, through one of its functional domains, binds to methylated cytosine nucleotides present in CpG islands that are enriched within regulatory regions of many genes. After binding to DNA, the second functional domain is activated and recruits a deacetylase complex that chemically modifies nearby histone molecules. The chemical modification of histones leads to a further compacting of the DNA into chromatin. The transcriptional machinery, including DNA polymerase II, no longer has easy access to the underlying DNA and is unable to initiate transcription. (Adapted with permission from Lombroso PJ: Rett syndrome. *J Am Acad Child Adol Psychiatry,* 2000.)

The protein that is mutated in Rett syndrome plays a critical role in regulating gene expression. The accessibility of DNA sequences depends to a large extent on the degree of methylation present within the regulatory regions (116). Methylation is a chemical modification to DNA that occurs when methyl groups are added to cytosine nucleotides. It is particularly prevalent in regions of DNA that contain a high content of cytosine and guanine pairs, so-called CpG islands. Although CpG islands are present throughout the genome, they are most enriched within the promoter regions of genes. In fact, one approach to identifying transcriptional start sites is to look for CpG islands because they are often found immediately upstream of the transcriptional start site.

It was thought that DNA methylation alone was capable of repressing gene expression. RNA polymerase II is the enzyme that transcribes most DNA into RNA. Methylation of CpG islands within promoter regions was initially believed to be sufficient to prevent the enzyme from gaining access to these regions and initiating transcription; however, what actually occurs is somewhat more complicated.

The protein implicated in Rett syndrome, MeCP2, has two functional domains. One end of the protein recognizes methylated cytosines and binds tightly to them. The second domain is then activated and functions by recruiting another set of proteins, the histone deacetylase complex, to the immediate vicinity. Histones are a family of proteins present within the nuclei of all cells. Their role in modifying the secondary structure of DNA has been recognized for some time because they provide a core of protein around which the chromosomal DNA is wrapped (117). The histone deacetylase complex that has been recruited by MeCP2 chemically modifies histones. The result is a compaction of the DNA surrounding the promoter region such that the transcriptional machinery of the nucleus is no longer able to gain efficient access to the gene. This effectively silences it.

The initial report on Rett syndrome found six distinct mutations among the patients who had a mutation of their MeCP2 gene (115). Several of these are missense mutations that replace critical amino acids within the protein. Mutations of this type are located within the methyl-binding domain and disrupt its ability to recognize and interact with methyl groups. The remaining mutations are found in the second functional region, the domain that recruits the deacetylation complex. Two types of mutations are present in this second domain. One is the insertion of a single nucleotide that leads to a shift in the downstream codons. A shift such as this results in the translation of a new amino acid sequence downstream of the point of mutation. The second mutation results in a novel stop codon. This type of mutation leads to the production of a shortened or truncated protein. Each of the mutations results in an impaired or nonfunctional protein (115).

Only certain regions of the MeCP2 gene were actually sequenced in this initial study. The regions sequenced were those that contain the open reading frame or that portion of the DNA that encodes for protein. These regions are often analyzed first because they require far fewer nucleotides to be sequenced compared to an analysis of the entire gene with its multiple introns and regulatory regions. Mutations in open reading frame, therefore, are the first to be detected, although regulatory regions of a gene also may be disrupted by mutations. For example, mutations at a promoter area may interfere with the proper initiation of transcription, whereas mutations in introns may interfere with the proper splicing together of exons by disrupting a splice site regulatory sequence. In fact, as additional regions of the gene were analyzed, over 80 percent of individuals with Rett syndrome have mutations in the MeCP2 gene.

Allelic heterogeneity refers to the presence of different mutations within a single gene. In the majority of disease-causing mutations studied so far, the same or a very similar clinical phenotype is seen when different functional domains of a single gene are mutated. This type of allelic heterogeneity was demonstrated in the initial study on Rett syndrome (115). Six distinct mutations were found in different regions of the same gene, and all the patients had the same disorder. It is likely that additional mutations will be found within regulatory sequences of MeCP2 that result in a similar phenotype. On the other hand, mutations to a single gene occasionally cause very different clinical presentations. For example, several mutations within the receptor for the fibroblast growth factor are responsible for a number of distinctly different skeletal and growth abnormalities (118).

By way of contrast, *locus heterogeneity* refers to mutations in different genes that result in a similar clinical presentation among affected individuals. This can happen, for example, when several proteins are involved in a series of related enzymatic reactions. For example, MeCP2 encodes for one member of a larger family of proteins. At least two other members have been discovered that also bind to DNA and are involved in the recruitment of the histone deacetylation complex. Each of these proteins is now being examined to determine whether mutations in their genes also cause Rett syndrome. Moreover, as discussed, a number of proteins besides MeCP2 are required to properly repress target genes. Mutations of any of these other genes may result in a related clinical phenotype. In fact, mutations have now been documented in a second gene that results in a clinical phenotype very similar to Rett syndrome (119, 120).

The recent findings with Rett syndrome raise a number of interesting questions. One relates to the predominance of neurologic symptoms in the clinical examination. MeCP2 is not uniquely expressed in the brain but is found in many other tissues. Nevertheless, symptoms outside of the brain are not a predominant part of the disorder. It appears that the CNS is particularly vulnerable to disruptions of this gene. A similar situation occurs in Huntington's chorea, where neurologic symptoms are also the central part of an illness, although the mutated gene is expressed in many tissues.

A second related question concerns the normal developmental trajectory early in life that precedes the development of symptoms. Much longer delays are seen with a number of neurodegenerative disorders where symptoms are not detected until the fourth or fifth decade of life. One explanation put forward is that toxic compounds are slowly produced over time and must accumulate before neuronal damage occurs. Free radicals are examples of toxic compounds implicated in a number of neurodegenerative disorders, including Huntington's chorea. Normally, enzymes are present that detoxify free radicals within cells. If these enzymes lose their full functional activity through a mutation or are expressed in smaller amounts, then the toxins will accumulate over time and eventually interfere with normal neuronal function.

This may be what happens in the brains of Rett syndrome patients. As discussed, the normal function of the MeCP2 protein is to repress transcription of several additional genes. These downstream target genes are not yet known, but it is reasonable to assume that mutations to MeCP2 lead to the inappropriate expression of these genes. It is possible that the products of these genes are themselves toxic, or interfere with the normal signaling pathways that function during this developmental period. Neuroanatomic studies might clarify this hypothesis. The literature contains a single autopsy report (121), and abnormalities were detected in pyramidal neurons in layers II–III of the cerebral cortex. They had fewer dendrites than normal and many fewer dendritic arborizations.

LISSENCEPHALY

The cerebral cortex is formed of billions of cells that are born during just a few months of embryonic life from a small population of progenitor cells. The cells that are born must differentiate and migrate to reach their final resting place in the appropriate layer of the cortex.

However, a number of disorders are caused by mutations in genes whose proteins are required for the orderly progression from neuronal birth, differentiation into appropriate neuronal subtypes, migration, and eventual elaboration of synaptic connections.

Neurogenesis occurs in a region called the ventricular zone, which lies adjacent to the lumen of the neural tube. Although neurogenesis primarily occurs during the development of the brain *in utero*, some degree of neurogenesis occurs throughout life (122). In the cerebral cortex, neurons must migrate past layers of earlier born cells to reach their final destinations. Those born at later periods have more complex migratory routes. Many employ a guidance system composed of radial glial cells (123). The radial glial cells are thought to send a process that spans the developing cortex and serves as scaffolding along which certain neurons migrate. Chemotaxic signals are produced that keep the neuron moving along the radial glial process. When it reaches its final destination, other signaling molecules are produced that instruct the neuron to stop migrating, enter the proper lamina, and begin to elaborate processes (124).

Disruption of the normal migration of neurons causes several human disorders. The most common of these are the lissencephalies that consist of several syndromes: isolated lissencephaly (ILS), Miller-Dieker syndrome (MDS), and X-linked lissencephaly (125). In each, disruption of the normal neuronal migration is reflected in a smooth cortical surface that lacks the normal pattern of gyri and sulci. In addition, although the cerebral cortex normally has six layers, cortices of affected individuals have only four (Figure 2.3.3.9).

In 1993, a large deletion on chromosome 17 was found in two patients with MDS. The search then began to clone the gene responsible for the disorder, and it was soon isolated and termed LIS-1 (126). The deletion spans this gene and genes on either side of it and is another example of a contiguous gene syndrome. The absence of several genes is believed to be responsible for the more severe MDS phenotype, which also has numerous congenital abnormalities. Point mutations in the same LIS-1 gene were soon found in other affected individuals. These individuals had the milder form of lissencephaly (ILS).

How does a mutation in LIS-1 cause the observed cortical abnormalities? LIS-1 encodes for a regulatory protein that controls the activity of a second protein, termed platelet activating factor (PAF)-acetyl hydrolase (127, 128). PAF acts as a signaling protein that binds to the surface of neurons. The ensuing cascade of signals is required for the normal migration of neurons (129). LIS-1 is expressed at its highest levels in the developing cortex, consistent with the protein's putative role in signaling. Exactly how mutations in LIS-1 interfere with normal migration is not well understood, although one model suggests that a disruption occurs to cytoskeletal proteins that need to rearrange themselves at the growing tip of the migrating neuron (130).

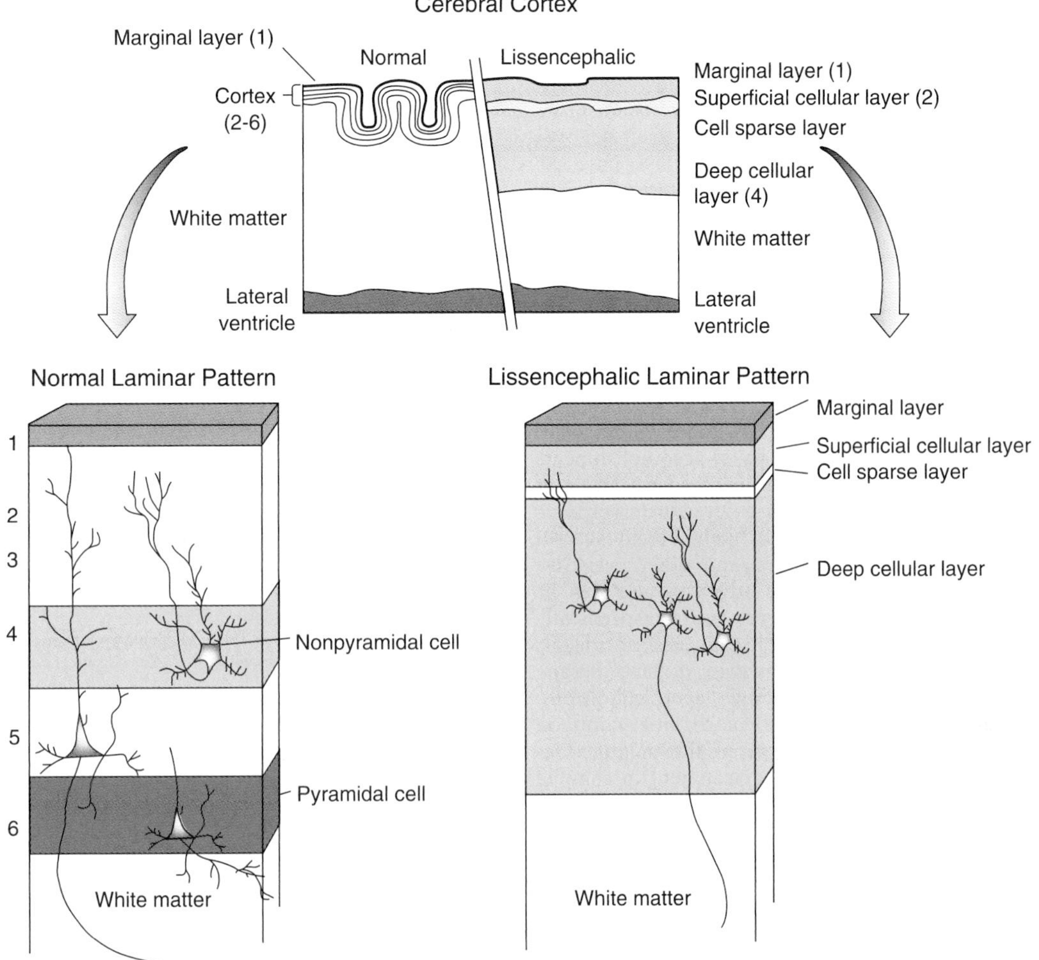

FIGURE 2.3.3.9. Lissencephaly. The normal cerebral cortex is a highly organized structure, and its six layers are shown on the left (1–6). In contrast, the lissencephalic brain lacks the normal pattern of sulci and gyri, and there are only four layers. (Adapted with permission from Reiner O, Lombroso PJ: Lissencephaly. *J Am Acad Child Adol Psychiatry* 37:231–232, 1998.)

A second disorder that affects neuronal migration is termed subcortical band heterotopia (131). This disorder, also known as X-linked lissencephaly or double cortex, is associated with mental retardation and epilepsy. The histological findings are made of bilateral bands of gray matter consisting of disorganized neurons present in the central white matter between the cortex and ventricular wall. The degree of mental retardation is directly related to the thickness of the extra neuronal tissue.

The gene that causes double cortex was recently cloned (132, 133). The gene encodes for the protein double cortin (DCX). Structurally, this protein is highly homologous to a family of kinases, called calcium calmodulin–dependent kinases. Although its exact role in neuronal migration remains to be clarified, recent studies indicate that it binds to and appears to stabilize cytoskeletal proteins required for the normal movement of neurons (134, 135).

It is interesting to note that 20 percent of individuals with lissencephaly have no detectable mutation in LIS-1, whereas a similar number of individuals with subcortical band heterotopia have no detectable mutation of DCX. It is possible that additional studies will detect novel mutations within these genes; however, it is likely that different genes are mutated and lead to similar cortical abnormalities—another example of locus heterogeneity.

COMMON CHILD PSYCHIATRIC DISORDERS

Child psychiatry has yet to establish the molecular basis for most of its more common disorders. The reasons for this failure lie beyond the scope of this chapter, but genetic complexity is one culprit. Many of the disorders described in the preceding sections exhibit Mendelian patterns of inheritance, such as the X-linked transmission of Rett and fragile X syndromes; however, pedigree studies of most common child and adolescent mental disorders fail to show such a pattern of vertical transmission across generations. The presence of non–Mendelian patterns of transmission does not necessarily imply that genetic factors are unimportant, only that their role in the transmission and expression of disease phenotypes is complex. Examples include polygenetic transmission, in which a multiplicity of genetic and environmental factors is causative. Height and intelligence are good examples of polygenetic traits and it may be that some forms of childhood-onset anxiety disorders and attention deficit hyperactivity disorder will also fall into this category. Interestingly, the alleles that contribute to the vulnerability to develop these disorders may be common in the population and be seen as normal variants. However, when they act in concert with other vulnerability alleles or with adverse environments, they may lead to the syndrome in question.

Understanding the genetics of complex disorders is relevant to other fields of medicine and significant progress has been made in areas such as breast cancer and hypertension (136, 137). Our field is posed to take advantage of their success. If child psychiatric disorders follow in a similar course, we can expect that in rare instances single gene mutations will be responsible for common disease phenotype. Such observations will then set the stage for animal studies that will serve a valuable heuristic role in elucidating additional genes and relevant neurobiological pathways.

CONCLUSION

Advances in genomics, molecular genetics, and developmental neuroscience provide an impressive array of accomplishments that are laying the foundation for a deeper understanding of the biological bases of some childhood-onset neuropsychiatric disorders. Success in these areas will likely herald success in other rare diseases, such as autism and other pervasive developmental disorders. Therapeutic advances also can be anticipated as therapeutic agents are developed that specifically target the molecular and cellular consequences of specific genetic mutations. Perhaps even the promise of gene therapy can be realized for some of the single gene conditions. Nevertheless, the road ahead, particularly for common disorders, will not be an easy one given the complexities involved and the crucial role of the environment in shaping and reshaping the CNS within the constraints of our genetic endowment.

ACKNOWLEDGMENTS

This work was supported by the National Association of Research on Schizophrenia and Depression (NARSAD, PJL), and the National Institute of Health grant MH01527. Portions of this work have appeared in: Lombroso P: Learning and memory. *Rev Bras Psiquiatr* 26:207–210, 2004.

References

1. Kandel ER: A new intellectual framework for psychiatry. *Am J Psychiatry* 155:457–469, 1998.
2. Nestler EJ, Barrot M, DiLeone RJ, Eisch AJ, Gold SJ, Monteggia LM: Neurobiology of depression. *Neuron* 34:13–25, 2002.
3. Weeber EJ, Levenson JM, Sweatt JD: Molecular genetics of human cognition. *Mol Interv* 2:376–379, 2002.
4. Squire LR, Kandel ER: *Memory: From Mind to Molecule*, New York: Scientific American Library, 1999.
5. Sweatt JD: *Mechanisms of Memory*, New York: Elsevier Press, 2003.
6. Roberson ED, English JD, Adams JP, Selcher JC, Kondratick C, Sweatt JD: The mitogen-activated protein kinase cascade couples PKA and PKC to CREB phosphorylation in area CA1 of hippocampus. *J Neuroscience* 19:4337–4348, 1999.
7. Orban PC, Chapman PF, Brambilla R: Is the Ras-MAPK signalling pathway necessary for long-term memory formation? *Trends Neurosci* 22:38–44, 1999.
8. Atkins CM, Selcher JC, Petraitis JJ, Trzaskos JM, Sweatt JD: The MAP kinase cascade is required for mammalian associative learning. *Nature Neuroscience* 1:602–609, 1998.
9. Rodrigues SM, Schafe GE, LeDoux JE: Molecular mechanisms underlying emotional learning and memory in the lateral amygdala. *Neuron* 44:75–91, 2004.
10. Schafe GE, Atkins CM, Swank MW, Bauer EP, Sweatt JD, LeDoux JE: Activation of ERK/MAP kinase in the amygdala is required for memory consolidation of Pavlovian fear conditioning. *J Neurosci* 20:8177–8187, 2000.
11. Blum S, Moore AN, Adams F, Dash PK: A mitogen-activated protein kinase cascade in the CA1/CA2 subfield of the dorsal hippocampus is essential for long-term spatial memory. *J Neurosci* 19:3535–3544, 1999.
12. Impey S, Obrietan K, Wong ST, et al.: Cross talk between ERK and PKA is required for Ca2+ stimulation of CREB-dependent transcription and ERK nuclear translocation. *Neuron* 21:869–883, 1998.
13. English JD, Sweatt JD: A requirement for the mitogen-activated protein kinase cascade in hippocampal long-term potentiation. *J Biol Chem* 272:19103–19106. 1997.
14. Silva AJ, Elgersma Y, Costa RM: Molecular and cellular mechanisms of cognitive function: implications for psychiatric disorders. *Biol Psychiatry* 47:200–209, 2000.
15. Costa RM, Federov NB, Kogan JH, et al.: Mechanism for the learning deficits in a mouse model of neurofibromatosis type 1. *Nature* 415:526–530, 2002.
16. Weeber EJ, Sweatt JD: Molecular neurobiology of human cognition. *Neuron* 33:845–848, 2002.
17. Jacquot S, Merienne K, De Cesare D, et al.: Mutation analysis of the RSK2 gene in Coffin-Lowry patients: extensive allelic heterogeneity and a high rate of de novo mutations. *Am J Hum Genet* 63:1631–1640, 1998.
18. Johnston MV: Clinical disorders of brain plasticity. *Brain Dev* 26:73–80, 2004.
19. Petrij F, Giles RH, Dauwerse HG, et al.: Rubinstein-Taybi syndrome caused by mutations in the transcriptional co-activator CBP. *Nature* 376:348–351, 1995.
20. Bagni C, Greenough WT: From mRNP trafficking to spine dysmorphogenesis: the roots of fragile X syndrome. *Nat Rev Neurosci* 6:376–387, 2005.
21. Dykens EM, Hodapp RM, Ort SI, et al.: Trajectory of adaptive behavior in males with fragile X syndrome. *J Autism Dev Disord* 23:135–145, 1993.
22. Martin JP, Bell J: A pedigree of mental defect showing sex-linkage. *J Neurol Psychiatry* 6:154–157, 1943.
23. Baumgardner T, Reiss A, Freund L, et al.: Specification of the neurobehavioral phenotype in males with fragile X syndrome. *J Pediatrics* 95:744–752, 1995.
24. Bregman J, Dykens E, Watson M, et al.: Fragile X syndrome: variability of phenotypic expression. *J Amer Acad Child Adoles Psychiatry* 4:463–471, 1987.
25. Freund LS, Reiss AL, Hagerman Rm, et al.: Chromosome fragility and psychopathology in obligate female carriers of the fragile X chromosome. *Arch Gen Psychiatry* 49:54–60, 1992.
26. Fryns JP: The female and the fragile X. A study of 144 obligate female carriers. *Am J Med Gen* 23:157–169, 1986.
27. Hodapp RM, Leckman JF, Dykens EM, et al.: ABC profiles in children with fragile X syndrome, Down syndrome, and nonspecific mental retardation. *Am J Men Retardation* 97:39–46, 1992.
28. Lubs H: A marker X chromosome. *Am J Hum Gen* 21:231–244, 1969.
29. Fu Y-H, Kuhl DP, Pizzuti A, et al.: Variation of the CGG repeat at the fragile site results in genetic instability: resolution of the Sherman paradox. *Cell* 67:1047–1058, 1991.
30. Hagerman RJ, Staley LW, O'Conner R, et al.: Learning-disabled males with a fragile X CGG expansion in the upper premutation size range. *Pediatrics* 97:122–126, 1996.
31. de von Flindt R, Bybel B, Chudley AE, et al.: Short-term memory and cognitive variability in adult fragile X females. *Am J Med Genet* 38:488–492, 1991.
32. Kemper M, Hagerman R, Ahmad R, et al.: Cognitive profiles and the spectrum of clinical manifestations in heterozygous fra(X) females. *Am J Med Gen* 23:139–156, 1986.
33. Murphy DG, Mentis MJ, Pietrini P, et al.: Premutation female carriers of fragile X syndrome: A pilot study on brain anatomy and metabolism. *J Am Acad Child Adolesc Psychiatry* 38:1294–1301, 1999.
34. Allingham-Hawkins DJ, Babul-Hirji R, et al.: Fragile X premutation is a significant risk factor for premature ovarian failure: The international collaborative POF in fragile X study—preliminary data. *Am J Med Genet* 83:322–325, 1999.
35. Jacquemont S, Hagerman RJ, Leehey MA, et al.: Penetrance of the fragile X-associated tremor/ataxia syndrome in a premutation carrier population. *J Am Med Asso* 291:460–469, 2004.
36. Hagerman PJ, Hagerman RJ: Fragile X-associated tremor/ataxia syndrome (FXTAS). *Ment Retard Dev Disabil Res Rev* 10:25–30, 2004.
37. Nelson D: The fragile X syndromes. *Semin Cell Biol* 6:5–11, 1995.
38. Oberle I, Rousseau F, Heitz D, et al.: Instability of a 550-base pair DNA segment and abnormal methylation in fragile X syndrome. *Science* 252:1097–1110, 1991.
39. Pieretti M, Zhang F, Fu Y-H, et al.: Absence of expression of the FMR-1 gene in fragile X syndrome. *Cell* 66:817–822, 1991.
40. Eichler EE, Richards S, Gibbs RA, et al.: Fine structure of the human FMR1 gene. *Hum Mol Genet* 2:1147–1153, 1993.
41. Siomi H, Siomi M, Nussbaum R, et al.: The protein product of the fragile X gene, FMR1, has characteristics of an RNA-binding protein. *Cell* 74:291–298, 1993.
42. Siomi H, Choi M, Siomi M, et al.: Essential role for KH domains in RNA binding: Impaired RNA binding mutation in the KH domain of FMR1 that causes fragile X syndrome. *Cell* 77:33–39, 1994.
43. De Boulle K, Verkerk AJ, Reymers E, et al.: A point mutation in the FMR-1 gene associated with fragile X mental retardation. *Nat Genet* 3:31–35, 1993.

44. Musco G, Stier G, Joseph C, et al.: Three dimensional structure and stability of the KH domain: molecular insights into the fragile X syndrome. *Cell* 85:237–245, 1996.
45. Khandijan E, Corbin F, Woerly S, et al.: The fragile X mental retardation protein is associated with ribosomes. *Nat Genet* 12:91–93, 1996.
46. Abitbol M, Menim C, Delezoide A-L, et al.: Nucleus basalis magno cellularis and hippocampus are the major sites of FMR-1 expression in human fetal brain. *Nat Genet* 4:147–152, 1993.
47. Mostofsky SH, Mazzocco MM, Aakalu G, et al.: Decreased cerebellar posterior vermis size in fragile X syndrome: correlation with neurocognitive performance. *Neurology* 50:121–130, 1998.
48. Mostofsky SH, Reiss AL, Lockhart P, et al.: Evaluation of cerebellar size in attention-deficit hyperactivity disorder. *J Child Neurol* 13:434–439, 1998.
49. Reiss AL, Lee J, Freund L: Neuroanatomy of fragile X syndrome: the temporal lobe. *Neurology* 44:1317–1324, 1994.
50. Dutch-Belgian Fragile X Consortium: FMR-1 knockout mice: a model to study fragile X mental retardation. *Cell* 78:23–33, 1994.
51. Steward O, Schuman EM: Protein synthesis at synaptic sites on dendrites. *Annu Rev Neurosci* 24:299–325, 2001.
52. Ostroff LE, Fiala JC, Allwardt B, et al.: Polyribosomes redistribute from dendritic shafts into spines with enlarged synapses during LTP in developing rat hippocampal slices. *Neuron* 35:535–545, 2002.
53. Zalfa F, Giorgi M, Primerano B, et al.: The fragile X syndrome protein FMRP associates with BC1 RNA and regulates the translation of specific mRNAs at synapses. *Cell* 112:317–327, 2003.
54. Kelleher, RJ, Govindarajan A, Tonegawa S: Translational regulatory mechanisms in persistent forms of synaptic plasticity. *Neuron* 44:59–73, 2004.
55. Kelleher RJ 3rd, Govindarajan A, Jung HY, Kang H, Tonegawa S: Translational control by MAPK signaling in long-term synaptic plasticity and memory. *Cell* 116:467–479, 2004.
56. Brown V, Jin P, Ceman S, Darnell JC, et al.: Microarray identification of FMRP-associated brain mRNAs and altered mRNA translational profiles in fragile X syndrome. *Cell* 107:477–487, 2001.
57. Darnell JC, Jensen KB, Jin P, Brown V, Warren ST, Darnell RB: Fragile X mental retardation protein targets G quartet mRNAs important for neuronal function. *Cell* 107:489–499, 2001.
58. Irwin SA, Patel B, Idupulapati M, Harris JB, et al.: Abnormal dendritic spine characteristics in the temporal and visual cortices of patients with fragile-X syndrome: a quantitative examination. *Am J Med Genet* 98:161–167, 2001.
59. Comery TA, Harris JB, Willems PJ, et al.: Abnormal dendritic spines in fragile X knockout mice: Maturation and pruning deficits. *Proc Natl Acad Sci USA* 94:5401–5404, 1997.
60. Caskey CT, Pizzuti A, Fu Y-H, et al.: Triplet repeat mutations in human disease. *Science* 256:784–789, 1992.
61. Nelson D, Warren S: Trinucleotide repeat instability: When and where? *Nat Genet* 4:107–108, 1993.
62. Warren S: The expanding world of trinucleotide repeats. *Science* 271:1374–1375, 1996.
63. Fu Y-H, Pizzuti A, Fenwick RG Jr, et al.: An unstable triplet repeat in a gene related to myotonic dystrophy. *Science* 255:1256–1258, 1992.
64. Fortune MT, Kennedy JL, Vincent JB: Anticipation and CAG*CTG repeat expansion in schizophrenia and bipolar affective disorder. *Curr Psychiatry Rep* 5:145–154, 2003.
65. Margolis RL, McInnis MG, Rosenblatt A, Ross CA: Trinucleotide repeat expansion and neuropsychiatric disease. *Arch Gen Psychiatry* 56:1019–1031, 1999.
66. McInnis MG, McMahon FJ, Chase GA, et al.: Anticipation in bipolar affective disorder. *Am J Hum Genet* 53:385–390, 1993.
67. Morris AG, Gaitonde E, McKenna PJ, et al.: CAG repeat expansions and schizophrenia association with disease in females and with early age-at-onset. *Hum Mol Gen* 4:1957–1961, 1995.
68. O'Donovan MC, Guy C, Craddock N, et al.: Expanded CAG repeats in schizophrenia and bipolar disorder. *Nat Genet* 10:380–381, 1995.
69. Prader A, Labhart A, Willi H: Ein Syndrom von Adipositas, Kleinwuchs, Kryptorchismus und Oligophrenie nach Myatonieartigem Zustand im Neugeborenenalter. *Schweiz Med Wschr* 86:1260–1261, 1956.
70. Holm VA, Cassidy SB, Butler MG, et al.: Prader-Willi syndrome: consensus diagnostic criteria. *Pediatrics* 91:398–402, 1993.
71. Dykens EM, Cassidy SB: Correlates of maladaptive behavior in children and adults with Prader-Willi syndrome. *Am J Med Genet* 60:546–549, 1995.
72. Dykens EM, Leckman JF, Cassidy SB: Obsessions and compulsions in Prader-Willi syndrome. *J Child Psychol Psychia Allied Disc* 37:995–1002, 1996.
73. State MW, Dykens EM, Rosner B, et al.: Obsessive-compulsive symptoms in Prader-Willi and "Prader-Willi-like" patients. *J Am Acad Child Adoles Psychiatry* 38:329–334, 1999.
74. Angelman H: "Puppet children": A report of three cases. *Dev Med Child Neurol* 7:681–688, 1965.
75. Ledbetter DH, Riccardi VM, Airhart SD, et al.: Deletions of chromosome 15 as a cause of the Prader-Willi syndrome. *N Engl J Med* 304:325–329, 1981.
76. Magenis RE, Brown MG, Lacy DA, et al.: Is Angelman syndrome an alternate result of del(15) (q11q13)? *Am J Med Genet* 28:829–838, 1987.
77. Cassidy SB, Schwartz S: Prader-Willi and Angelman syndromes: Disorders of genomic imprinting. *Medicine* 77:140–151, 1998.
78. Cassidy SB: Prader-Willi syndrome. *J Med Genet* 34:917–923, 1997.
79. Nicholls RD, Saitoh S, Horsthemke B: Imprinting in Prader-Willi and Angelman syndromes. *Trends Genet* 14:194–200, 1998.
80. Ledbetter D, Engel E: Uniparental disomy in humans: Development of an imprinting map and its implications for prenatal diagnosis. *Hum Mol Genet* 4:1757–1764, 1995.
81. Nicholls RD, Knoll JHM, Butler MG, et al.: Genetic imprinting suggested by maternal heterodisomy in non-deletion Prader-Willi syndrome. *Nature* 342:281–285, 1989.
82. Ohta T, Gray TA, Rogan PK, et al.: Imprinting-mutation mechanisms in Prader-Willi syndrome. *Am J Hum Genet* 64:397–413, 1999.
83. Kishino T, Lalande M, Wagstaff J: UBE3A/E6-AP mutations cause Angelman syndrome. *Nat Genet* 15:70–73, 1997.
84. Matsuura T, Sutcliffe JS, Fang P, et al.: De novo truncating mutations in E6-AP ubiquitin-protein ligase gene (UBE3A) in Angelman syndrome. *Nat Genet* 15:74–77, 1997.
85. Nicholls RD: Strange bedfellows? Protein degradation and neurological dysfunction. *Neuron* 21:647–649, 1998.
86. Albrecht U, Sutcliffe JS, Cattanach BM, et al.: Imprinted expression of the murine Angelman syndrome gene, Ube3a, in hippocampal and Purkinje neurons. *Nat Genet* 17:75–78, 1997.
87. DeLorey TM, Handforth A, Anagnostaras SG, et al.: Mice lacking the beta3 subunit of the $GABA_A$ receptor have the epilepsy phenotype and many of the behavioral characteristics of Angelman syndrome. *J Neurosci* 18:8505–8514, 1998.
88. Pober BR, Dykens EM: Williams syndrome: An overview of medical, cognitive, and behavioral features. *Child Adolesc Psychiatr Clin North Am* 5:929–943, 1996.
89. Ewart A, Morris C, Atkinson D, et al.: Hemizygosity at the elastin locus in a developmental disorder, Williams syndrome. *Nat Genet* 5:11–16, 1993.
90. Williams J, Barratt-Boyes B, Lowe J: Supravalvular aortic stenosis. *Circulation* 24:1311–1318, 1961.
91. Bellugi U, Bihrle A, Jernigan T, et al.: Neuropsychological, neurological, and neuroanatomical profile of Williams syndrome. *Am J Med Genet* 6:115–125, 1990.
92. Bellugi U, Lichtenberger L, Jones W, Lai Z, St George M: I. The neurocognitive profile of Williams Syndrome: a complex pattern of strengths and weaknesses. *J Cogn Neurosci* 12 Suppl 1:7–29, 2000.
93. Wang P, Doherty S, Rourke SB, et al.: Unique profile of visuo-perceptual skills in a genetic syndrome. *Brain Cogn* 29:54–65, 1995.
94. Meyer-Lindenberg A, Hariri AR, et al.: Neural correlates of genetically abnormal social cognition in Williams syndrome. *Nat Neurosci* 2005.
95. Jernigan TL, Bellugi U: Anomalous brain morphology on magnetic resonance images in Williams syndrome and Down syndrome. *Arch Neurol* 47:529–533, 1990.
96. Jernigan TL, Bellugi U, Sowell E, et al.: Cerebral morphologic distinctions between Williams and Down syndromes. *Arch Neurol* 50:186–191, 1993.
97. Galaburda A, Wang P, Bellugi U, et al.: Cytoarchitectonic anomalies in a genetically based disorder: Williams syndrome. *Neuroreports* 5:753–757, 1994.
98. Lowery M, Morris C, Ewart A, et al.: Strong correlation of elastin deletions, detected by FISH, with Williams syndrome: Evaluation of 235 patients. *Am J Hum Gen* 57:49–53, 1995.
99. Nickerson E, Greenberg F, Keating M, et al.: Deletions of the elastin gene at 7q.11.23 occur in approximately 90 percent of patients with Williams syndrome. *Am J Hum Gen* 56:1156–1161, 1995.
100. Frangiskakis J, Ewart A, Morris C, et al.: LIM-kinase 1 hemizygosity implicated in impaired visuospatial constructive cognition. *Cell* 86:59–69, 1996.
101. Tassabehji M, Metcalfe K, Fergusson W, et al.: LIM-kinase deleted in Williams syndrome. *Nat Genet* 13:272–273, 1996.
102. Mizuno K, Okano I, Ohashi K, et al.: Identification of a human cDNA encoding a novel protein kinase with two repeats of the LIM/double zinc finger motif. *Oncogene* 9:1605–1612, 1994.
103. Proschel C, Blouin MJ, Gutowski NJ, et al.: Limk1 is predominantly expressed in neural tissues and phosphorylates, threonine and tyrosine residues *in vitro*. *Oncogene* 11:1271–1281, 1995.
104. Hoogenraad CC, Akhmanova A, Galjart N, De Zeeuw CI: LIMK1 and CLIP-115: linking cytoskeletal defects to Williams syndrome. *Bioessays* 26:141–150, 2004.
105. Meng Y, Zhang Y, Tregoubov V, et al.: Abnormal spine morphology and enhanced LTP in LIMK-1 knockout mice. *Neuron* 35:121–133, 2002.
106. Osborne LR, Soder S, Xiao-Mei S, et al.: Hemizygous deletion of the syntaxin 1A gene in individuals with Williams syndrome. *Am J Hum Genet* 61:449–452, 1997.
107. Osborne LR, Martindale D, Scherer SW, et al.: Identification of genes from a 500 kb region at 7q11.23 that is commonly deleted in Williams syndrome. *Genomics* 36:328–336, 1996.
108. Wang Y, Samos C, Peoples R, et al.: A novel human homologue of the *Drosophila* frizzled wnt receptor gene binds wingless proteins and is in

the Williams syndrome deletion at 7q11.23. *Hum Mol Genet* 6:465–472, 1997.
109. Peoples R, Perez-Jurado L, Wang Y, et al.: The gene for replication factor C subunit 2 (RFC2) is within the 7q11.23 Williams syndrome deletion. *Am J Hum Genet* 58:1370–1373, 1996.
110. Perez Jurado LA, Wang YK, et al.: A duplicated gene in the breakpoint regions of the 7q11.23 Williams-Beuren syndrome deletion encodes the initiator binding protein TFII-I and BAP-135, a phosphorylation target of BTK. *Hum Mol Genet* 7:325–334, 1998.
111. Zhao C, Aviles C, Abel RA, et al.: Hippocampal and visuospatial learning defects in mice with a deletion of frizzled 9, a gene in the Williams syndrome deletion interval. *Development* 132:2917–2927, 2005.
112. Rett A: *Über ein zerebral-atrophisches syndrome bei Hypesammonemie*. Vienna, Bruder Hollinek, 1966.
113. Naidu S: Rett syndrome: Natural history and underlying disease mechanisms. *Eur Child Adol Psychiatry* 6:14–17, 1997.
114. Webb T, Clarke A, Hanefeld F, et al.: Linkage analysis in Rett syndrome families suggests that there may be a critical region at Xq28. *J Med Genet* 35:997–1003, 1998.
115. Amir RE, Van den Veyver IB, Wan M, et al.: Rett syndrome is caused by mutations in X-linked MECP2, encoding methyl-CpG-binding protein 2. *Nat Genet* 23:185–188, 1999.
116. Kass SU, Pruss D, Wolffe AP: How does DNA methylation repress transcription? *Trends Genet* 13:444–440, 1997.
117. Nan X, Campoy J, Bird A: MeCP2 is a transcriptional repressor with abundant binding sites in genomic chromatin. *Cell* 88:471–481, 1997.
118. Park WJ, Meyers GA, Li X, et al.: Novel FGFR2 mutations in Crouzon and Jackson-Weiss syndromes show allelic heterogeneity and phenotypic variability. *Hum Mol Genet* 4:1229–1233, 1995.
119. Weaving LS, Christodoulou J, Williamson SL et al.: Mutations of CDKL5 cause a severe neurodevelopmental disorder with infantile spasms and mental retardation. *Am J Hum Genet* 75:1079–1093, 2004.
120. Evans JC, Archer HL, Colley JP, et al.: Early onset seizures and Rett-like features associated with mutations in CDKL5. *Eur J Hum Genet* 2005.
121. Belichenko PV, Oldfors A, Hagberg B, et al.: Rett syndrome: 3-D confocal microscopy of cortical pyramidal dendrites and afferents. *Neuroreport* 5:1509–1513, 1994.
122. Gould E, Tanapat P: Stress and hippocampal neurogenesis. *Biol Psychiatry* 46:1472–1479, 1999.
123. Rakic P: Mode of cell migration to the superficial layers of monkey neocortex. *J Comp Neurol* 145:61–84, 1972.
124. Rakic P, Cameron RS, Komuro H: Recognition, adhesion, transmembrane signaling and cell motility in guided neuronal migration. *Curr Opin Neurobiol* 4:63–69, 1994.
125. Dobyns WB, Truwit CL: Lissencephaly and other malformations of cortical development: 1995 update. *Neuropediatrics* 26:132–147, 1995.
126. Reiner O, Carrozzo R, Shen Y, et al.: Isolation of a Miller-Dieker lissencephaly gene containing G protein beta-subunit–like repeats. *Nature* 364:717–721, 1993.
127. Hattori M, Adachi H, Aoki J, et al.: Cloning and expression of a cDNA encoding the beta-subunit (30-kDa subunit) of bovine brain platelet-activating factor acetyl hydrolase. *JBC* 270:31345–31352, 1995.
128. Hattori M, Adachi H, Tsujimoto M, et al.: Miller-Dieker lissencephaly gene encodes a subunit of brain platelet-activating factor. *Nature* 370:216–218, 1994.
129. Reiner O, Albrecht U, Gordon M, et al.: Lissencephaly gene expression in the CNS suggests a role in neuronal migration. *J Neurosci* 15:3730–3738, 1995.
130. Sapir T, Cahana A, Seger R, et al.: LIS1 is a microtubule-associated phosphoprotein. *Eur J Biochem* 265:181–188, 1999.
131. Walsh CA: Genetic malformations of the human cerebral cortex. *Neuron* 23:19–29, 1999.
132. Des Portes V, Francis F, Pinard JM, et al.: Doublecortin is the major gene causing X-linked subcortical laminar heterotopia (SCLH). *Hum Mol Genet* 7:1063–1070, 1998.
133. Gleeson JG, Allen KM, Fox JW, et al.: Doublecortin, a brain-specific gene mutated in human X-linked lissencephaly and double cortex syndrome, encodes a putative signaling protein. *Cell* 92:63–72, 1998.
134. Francis F, Koulakoff A, Boucher D, et al.: Doublecortin is a developmentally regulated, microtubule-associated protein expressed in migrating and differentiating neurons. *Neuron* 23:247–256, 1999.
135. Gleeson JG, Lin PT, Flanagan LA, et al.: Doublecortin is a microtubule-associated protein and is expressed widely by migrating neurons. *Neuron* 23:257–271, 1999.
136. Lifton RP: Molecular genetics of human blood pressure variation. *Science* 272:676–680, 1996.
137. Miki Y, Swensen J, Shattuck-Eidens D, et al.: A strong candidate for the breast and ovarian cancer susceptibility gene BRCA1. *Science* 266:66–71, 1994.

2.4 ■ NEUROSCIENCES

CHAPTER 2.4.1 ■ NEUROIMAGING METHODS IN THE STUDY OF CHILDHOOD PSYCHIATRIC DISORDERS

THE MRI UNIT AT COLUMBIA UNIVERSITY AND NEW YORK STATE PSYCHIATRIC INSTITUTE

ABBREVIATIONS

AC	Anterior Commissure
ADHD	Attention-Deficit/Hyperactivity Disorder
BOLD	Blood Oxygen Level Dependent
CSF	Cerebrospinal Fluid
CT	Computed Tomography
DTI	Diffusion Tensor Imaging
DW	Diffusion-Weighted
EEG	Electroencephalography
fMRI	Functional Magnetic Resonance Imaging
GABA	γ aminobutyric acid
FOV	Field of view
ICA	Independent component analysis
Ins	Myo-inositol
ISI	Inter-Stimulus interval
MEG	Magnetoencephalography
MRI	Magnetic Resonance Imaging
MRS	Magnetic Resonance Spectroscopy
NAA	N-acetyl aspartate
PC	Posterior Commissure
PET	Positron Emission Tomography
PPM	Parts per Million
ROI	Region of Interest

SNR	Signal-to-Noise Ratio
SPECT	Single Photon Emission Computer Tomography
T	Tesla
tCh	Total Choline
tCr	Total Creatine
TS	Tourette Syndrome

OVERVIEW

The direct observation of the structural and functional organization of the brain using neuroimaging methodologies is playing an increasingly important role in the study of childhood psychiatric disorders. Ultimately, this improved understanding of the causes of psychiatric disturbances in children will suggest new and more specific treatments for these conditions, including the means for planning individualized treatments and for monitoring therapeutic response.

We aim to provide herein a comprehensive introduction to neuroimaging methods that will help readers to become informed consumers of such research. In particular, our goal is to describe the advantages and limitations of each technology that must be appreciated when gauging the merits of an imaging study. We will also provide brief examples of the implementation of these techniques to the study of childhood psychopathologies and the kinds of insight into pathophysiology that they can provide.

We will review a range of existing and emerging technologies that are useful in neuroimaging studies of normal and abnormal brain development, focusing in particular on magnetic resonance imaging (MRI) because of its relative safety and widespread use compared with other imaging methods. We will discuss only briefly the principles of positron emission tomography (PET) and single photon emission computer tomography (SPECT) because these require the administration of radioactive tracers. Although some investigators have argued persuasively that the degree of radiation exposure (often less than the equivalent of a chest x-ray) poses no significant risk to children (1, 2), these methods are unlikely to find widespread acceptance in research protocols, particularly in those that include healthy control children. MRI will therefore almost certainly continue to be the most widely used imaging modality for the study of children. We will also briefly review electroencephalography (EEG) and magnetoencephalography (MEG), given their increasing use in the study of brain function in children.

What Is an Image?

The basic unit of a two-dimensional digital image is a picture element or "pixel." A pixel is a two-dimensional square that has a single level of grayness ranging from black to white. Each pixel represents a corresponding three-dimensional cube of tissue in the brain called a volume element or "voxel." Many pixels assembled into a larger square or rectangular array constitute an image that represents a corresponding three-dimensional "slice" of brain tissue. Each pixel of the image has associated with it a number that represents some feature of the corresponding voxel in the brain. This feature may be, for example, the degree of x-ray attenuation or tissue density (in x-ray and computed tomography, CT), the magnitude of reflected sound waves from soft tissue interfaces within the body (by ultrasound, US), the concentration of photons emitted by the radioisotopes delivered to a specific tissue or chemical receptor within the patient's body (PET and SPECT), the number of protons in the tissue (in anatomical MRI), the relative concentration of deoxyhemoglobin (in functional MRI or fMRI), or the concentration of a chemical compound (in magnetic resonance spectroscopy or MRS). This physical characteristic of the tissue is encoded within a signal coming from the brain. In a gray-scale image, the number associated with a pixel, and therefore the physical feature of the brain that it represents, is assigned a level of grayness ranging from black to white. The strength of the signal coming from a single voxel, and therefore the level of grayness of its corresponding pixel, will differ between neighboring voxels if the average physical or chemical features of those voxels differ. The differing levels of grayness across an image thus represent differences in the physical property (e.g., density, water content, protons, deoxyhemoglobin, or chemical compounds) of the brain as measured by a particular imaging modality.

The quality of an image depends on the characteristics of the signal within and across pixels, which include resolution, signal-to-noise ratio, and contrast. *Resolution* refers to the size of the voxels from which a radio signal is being measured. The smaller the voxels, the better the resolution. Higher resolution allows for greater discrimination of neighboring structures within the brain (Figure 2.4.1.2). At a lower resolution, two differing structures may be included within the same voxel; the signal that originates within each of the two structures will be averaged into a single signal (called a *partial volume* effect). The pixel representing this averaged signal will be assigned a single level of grayness.

As with any measurement process, repeated measures of the physical properties of a voxel in the brain will have some degree of error that centers around an average value. Random error, or *noise*, in the measurement of signal within each voxel degrades the quality of the image. The ratio of the strength of the signal to the noise of the signal within each pixel provides a useful index of image quality. Whenever signal strength decreases, or when noise increases, the signal-to-noise ratio (SNR) decreases and image quality degrades (Figure 2.4.1.1). For example, in MRI, the strength of the magnetic field, a primary determinant of SNR, is measured in Tesla (T), a unit of measurement that represents the number of magnetized water molecules within a specific volume of tissue. With a magnetic field of a higher strength, the number of hydrogen protons excited within magnetized water molecules is greater. This in turn increases the strength of the signal coming from any given voxel, thus improving the quality of the image.

On any MRI scanner, a common way to improve SNR is to increase the size of voxels, thereby increasing the volume of brain tissue that provides the radio signal for each pixel. Voxel size can be increased by increasing slice thickness or by increasing the dimensions of the voxels in the imaging plane, which in turn is achieved by decreasing the number of voxels into which an image is divided (termed the "matrix" of the image). The field of view (FOV) of the image (the height and width of the two-dimensional slice of brain tissue being imaged), is approximately 25 cm × 25 cm in a human. In a typical image from MRI, this FOV is broken into 256 segments, or matrixes, in each direction. Therefore, the matrix size for the 2D slice is said to be 256 × 256, making each voxel slightly smaller than 1 mm × 1 mm in size within the slice of the brain being imaged (250 mm broken into 256 segments yields individual segments of 250/256 = 0.98 mm in length for each of the two dimensions of the FOV). Thus, in order to increase the voxel size and subsequently the SNR, one must either increase the FOV or decrease the matrix size,

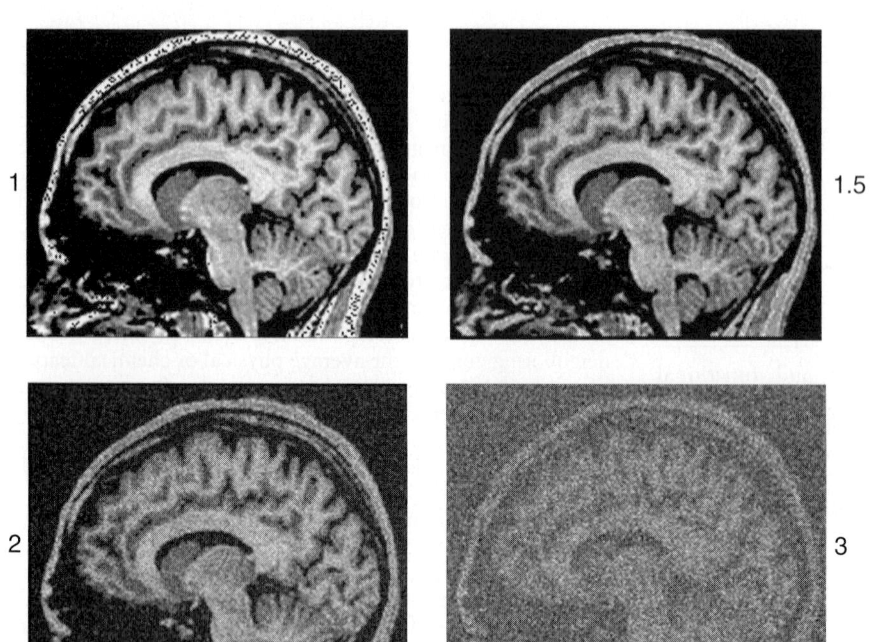

FIGURE 2.4.1.1. **Signal-to-noise ratio.** The noise of a single cross-sectional sagittal view of the brain is varied from the original image (upper left) to a value that is: 1.5 times larger (upper right), 2 times larger (lower left), or 3 times larger (lower right). Increasing the noise three-fold makes this particular image barely discernible.

both of which will decrease the spatial resolution of the image. Conversely, increasing the resolution in an MR image will typically decrease the SNR.

Finally, image *contrast* refers to the difference in the strength of signal acquired from adjacent tissues. The level of contrast reflects how well signals that originate in voxels of differing tissue types in the brain are discriminated, as reflected by the differing levels of grayness across the pixels of the image. Recall that the range of biological information acquired during the scanning process is recast in terms of gray scale in order to generate a 2D black and white image. By convention, most such MR images are assigned gray-scale values ranging from 0 (pure black) to 255 (pure white). Pixels with no relative contrast would all be assigned a single value and therefore would appear as uniformly black, white, or gray in an image. Pixels with maximum contrast would receive a gray-scale value of either 0 (black) or 255 (white), with no intervening values (Figure 2.4.1.2). An image with optimal contrast would assign the most widely differing gray-scale values to voxels whose signal strengths may differ only slightly, but in a way crucial for the investigative purposes of the scan. For example, to distinguish gray from white matter optimally, gray-scale values would discriminate portions of the white matter that are more "white" (i.e., that have a higher myelin content or some other actual tissue characteristic that differs across the brain) from other portions that are less "white" (i.e., that have a lower myelin content). The exquisite contrast of MR images makes this imaging modality superior to its historical predecessors for clinical and research applications, particularly CT (Figure 2.4.1.3), although contrast in CT images has improved considerably in recent years.

BRAIN IMAGING MODALITIES

Computed Tomography (CT)

Computed tomography (CT or CAT scanning) uses x-ray beams to penetrate through body parts and provide views of internal body structures. The images in CT are generated by quantifying the degree of absorption of the x-ray beam by the

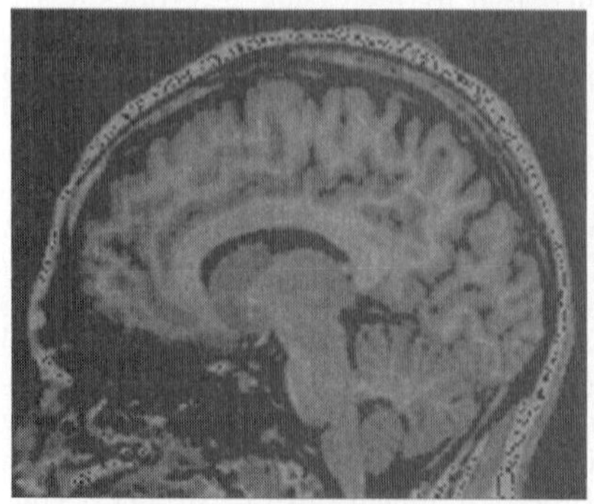

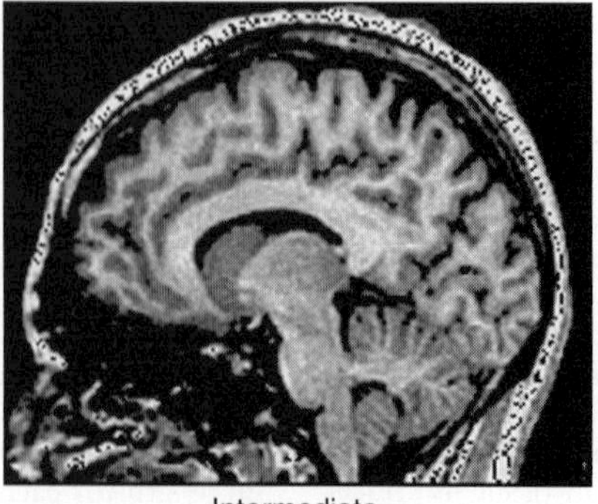

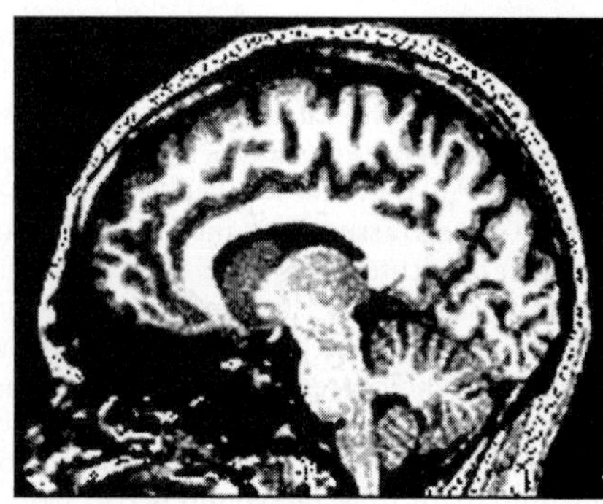

FIGURE 2.4.1.2. **Contrast.** The effects of varying levels of contrast are shown for a single cross-sectional sagittal view of the brain. Contrast varies from lowest on the left and intermediate in the middle to highest on the right.

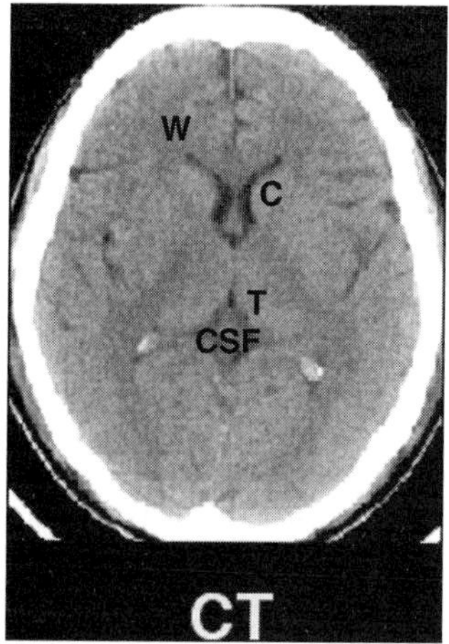

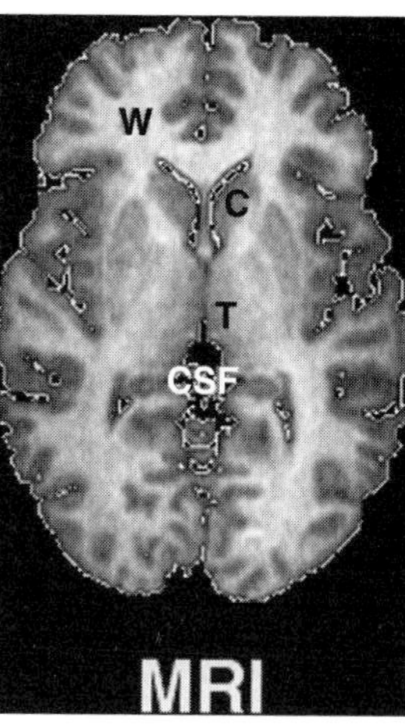

FIGURE 2.4.1.3. MRI vs. CT contrast. The contrast obtainable by MRI and CT is compared in axial images acquired at the level of the basal ganglia. Contrast characteristics are vastly superior in MRI. Letters are shown overlaying various tissue types and anatomical structures: C = caudate nucleus (subcortical gray matter); T = thalamus; CSF = cerebral spinal fluid; W = white matter of the frontal lobes. (See color insert.)

various body parts through which it passes. In a conventional x-ray, such as that of the chest or abdomen made for clinical diagnosis, all the organs through which the x-rays pass are collapsed onto the single, two-dimensional x-ray film, so that distinguishing the features of differing organs is difficult. CT imaging, however, uses an array of detectors placed around the subject to measure the reduction in strength, or attenuation, of *multiple* x-ray beams passing through the same body region from many different angles. Reconstruction of an image using attenuation measures from all of these beams gives an accurate representation of the tissues located at differing depths within the body through which the beam passes. CT has excellent depth penetration and sensitivity, although it provides low contrast to discriminate among various soft tissues. The spatial resolution of CT images is approximately 1 mm, and the imaging plane is limited to axial sections.

In a so-called "spiral," multidetector CT scanner, each detector records the transmitted x-ray beam as the source of the beam spirals around the body. Measurement of attenuation in beam intensity enters into a large set of equations used to calculate the densities of the tissues through which the beam has passed. These densities are mapped to each voxel of a set of thin 2D slices in the brain. When stacked one on top of another, many such 2D slices constitute a 3D imaging volume of the brain. Because the number of detectors and their packing density determines the resolution of the scanner, increasing the number of detector elements has become a major focus of the development of CT scanners. A higher number of detectors also enables a more rapid acquisition of individual slices. State-of-the-art CT scanners have tightly packed detectors that enable acquisition of up to 64 slices, thereby increasing brain coverage and the ability of CT to image smaller structures. Recently, hybrid PET/CT scanners have been constructed that combine the ability of PET to image blood flow and neurotransmitter systems with the ability of CT to provide high-resolution anatomical images of the brain. In addition, CT is being used to monitor the targeted delivery of medications and to individualize therapy for patients with cancer. Use of high-speed CT scanners in conjunction with administration of a contrast agent makes possible the measurement of blood flow in brain tissues, permitting the rapid assessment of possible stroke patients and evaluating the need for thrombolytic medications.

Positron Emission Tomography (PET)

PET uses radiotracers to track and then produce images of various in vivo biochemical and neurophysiological processes. Radiotracers are compounds of simple molecules, such as glucose, that are labeled with radioactive nuclei, such as ^{11}C and ^{18}F, ^{13}N, or ^{15}O, that emit positrons after they are injected into the subject being imaged. Within a short distance (<3 mm) from the site where the positron is emitted, the positron collides with electrons that present naturally within molecules of the surrounding tissue. The colliding positrons and electrons annihilate one another, producing two gamma rays that are emitted at 180° trajectories from one another. These two gamma rays then pass out of the tissue and are recorded by detectors positioned in the axial plane surrounding the head. The precise localization of the origination of the gamma rays can be determined by noting which detections occur simultaneously at 180° orientations.

The locations where positrons (and the subsequent gamma rays) originate, and the information they provide about brain physiology, will vary depending upon the pharmacological properties of the particular radiotracer used. Some tracers, for instance, are located primarily to the intravascular space and are used to measure blood flow. Other tracers, like 2-deoxyglucose, are treated as energy substrates and thus are taken up by neurons and phosphorylated; because phosphorylated deoxyglucose cannot be metabolized, however, the radioactive tracer accumulates and can be measured as an index of the metabolic activity of the neurons containing them. Still other tracers act as ligands for specific neurotransmitter receptors, including various receptor subtypes for the dopamine, serotonin, and GABA receptors. The resolution of the images constructed using various tracers is determined in part by the tissue compartment in which the tracer is located, because this determines the distance between the site of positron emission and annihilation from each of the isotopes. In-plane resolution for typical PET scanners is 6 mm, while the newest high-resolution scanners have an improved in-plane resolution of 2 to 3 mm.

The radioactive isotopes used in the synthesis of various PET tracers have relatively short half-lives. The half life for ^{15}O, which is incorporated into water molecules in studies of cerebral blood flow, is two minutes. That for ^{11}C, which is incorporated into various molecules that bind to neurotransmitter receptors, is 20 minutes; and that for ^{18}F, which is incorporated into deoxyglucose for studies of brain metabolism, is 110 minutes. Because of these short half-lives, the radionuclides must be produced in a cyclotron located at or near the site of the PET scanner. The cost of constructing and maintaining this cyclotron contributes to the great expense of PET imaging relative to other imaging modalities.

Single Photon Emission Computed Tomography (SPECT)

SPECT is similar to PET in that it measures gamma ray emissions from minute amounts of radioactively labeled molecules that have been injected, ingested, or inhaled. Whereas PET tracers emit positrons that produce two gamma rays oriented at 180° trajectories from each other, SPECT tracers emit photons whose spatial orientations and times of emission, are independent of those for any other photon released—hence the "single photon emission" in the SPECT moniker. These photons pass through brain tissue and are subjected to scattering before they are detected and measured using collimators. The density and spatial organization of these collimators will determine the precision with which the trajectories and sites of origin of the emitted photons can be determined. More collimators therefore improve the spatial resolution of a SPECT scanner. Increasing the number of collimators, however, also proportionately reduces the number of photons that enter each of the detectors and thus reduces sensitivity, or the SNR, of the scanner. Desires for improved resolution and SNR therefore must be weighed against one another with SPECT imaging, just as they are with other imaging modalities. The resolution of typical SPECT images is 6 to 10 mm, while newer scanners yield resolutions of 5 to 6 mm.

SPECT ligands typically incorporate isotopes of technetium and iodine, which have long half-lives and that therefore, unlike PET ligands, do not need to be synthesized on site in a large and expensive cyclotron. This is a major cost-saving advantage of SPECT compared with PET. In addition, the development of pharmacologically specific tracers is often easier with SPECT than with PET. Compared with PET, SPECT can detect slower kinetic processes because of the longer half-life of its tracers. The most common use of SPECT in the study of psychiatric diseases has been the measurement of regional cerebral blood flow, although it has also been used commonly to study neurotransmitter systems.

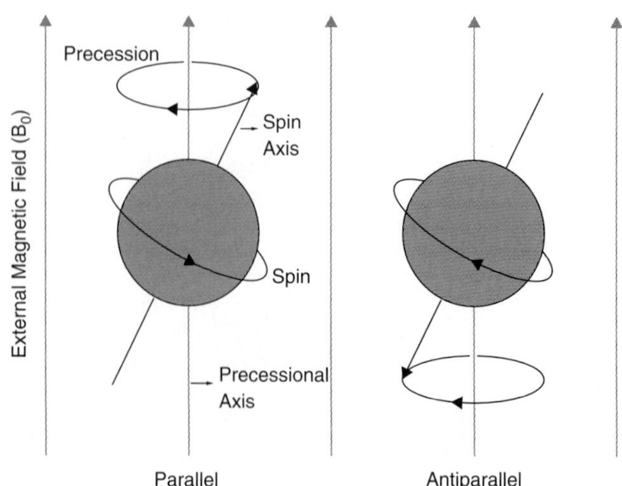

FIGURE 2.4.1.4. Schematic representation of the alignment of spin magnetic dipole moment (m) with a strong external magnetic field (B_0). Only two spin states are allowed: one with m parallel to B_0 and one with m opposing or antiparallel to B_0.

Magnetic Resonance Imaging (MRI)

In general use since the early 1980s, MRI is perhaps still most commonly regarded as a clinical tool that provides exquisite images of brain anatomy. MRI, however, has seen extraordinary growth in its use for studying brain activity associated with specific cognitive tasks, and more recently, it has also been used to study the concentration of certain metabolites and neurotransmitters in the brain, as well as to assess the integrity and orientation of nerve fiber tracts. To understand what these modalities can and cannot tell us about brain structure and function, one must become familiar with the basic processes by which MRI captures and represents within an image the features of brain structure and function.

Biological tissues are as much as 70 percent water by weight. Each water molecule contains two hydrogen atoms whose nuclei comprise a single proton each. MRI uses these single-proton nuclei to generate a radio signal from the brain that carries information about the microscopic environment in which the hydrogen nucleus finds itself. This information and the anatomical location from which it originated is decoded by computer software in the MRI scanner and then assigned an intensity (a level of grayness) within the corresponding pixel of the image. This intensity represents that quantity of the particular biological information encoded by the radio signal coming from the brain, which is selected and tuned by the scanner. The biological information being probed by the scanner determines the modality of the MRI study being conducted—i.e., whether it is studying the density of tissue in anatomical MRI, the oxygen content of the tissue in functional MRI, the diffusion of water in diffusion tensor imaging, or the concentration of certain neurometabolites in MRI spectroscopy. The brain is turned into a radiotransmitter through a combination of the powerful magnetic field within the MRI scanner and the transmission by the scanner of a series of pulses of radio waves that the brain tissue absorbs and then returns as another series of radio waves, now encoding the desired information about the tissue being imaged. We will now describe in greater detail precisely how this combination of magnetic field and radio waves from the MRI scanner turn the brain into a radio transmitter.

The nuclei of hydrogen atoms within biological tissues normally and inherently spin on an axis, like a spinning top or the earth. In the absence of a strong magnetic field, the axis of a spinning proton is oriented randomly in space. However, when biological tissues are placed within the powerful magnetic field of an MRI scanner, the spinning protons align in one of two directions, either parallel or antiparallel with the direction of the magnetic field (Figure 2.4.1.4). The number of protons aligned in parallel with the magnetic field is always slightly higher than the number of protons aligned antiparallel to the magnetic field. Because the magnetic fields produced by spinning protons aligned in opposite directions cancel each other, only the "excess" protons aligned parallel to the magnetic field contribute to the measurable radio signal used to generate an MR image. Nevertheless, because the numbers of molecules present in each cubic centimeter of tissue are enormous, the numbers of excess protons are still sufficient to produce a detectable and measurable signal. Thus, MRI has inherently low sensitivity in measuring the physical characteristics of brain tissue compared with other imaging modalities, because an MRI signal cannot be acquired from every molecule within a given voxel. On average, a few molecules per million participate in the process of image formation using MRI. At higher magnetic fields, the number of participating protons increases, hence providing the constant drive toward building scanners that operate at higher field strengths.

In addition to spinning on an axis that is parallel to the magnetic field, these hydrogen nuclei also gyrate, or "precess," when exposed to the magnetic field of the scanner, much like a spinning top or gyroscope in the presence of the earth's gravitational field (Figure 2.4.1.4). Similar to the orientation of the spin of the proton, precession also occurs on an axis that is parallel to the magnetic field and at a particular frequency. The scanner then emits pulses of radiofrequency (RF) energy whose frequencies match precisely the frequency at which the protons are precessing. The coincidence of the two frequencies, that of proton precession and that of the RF pulses, creates the *resonance* effect of MRI through which the precessing protons absorb the energy within the RF pulses (the resonance frequency of precession happens to equal precisely the spin frequency of the protons). This absorption of energy excites the precessing protons, causing the axis of their spins to tilt toward the plane perpendicular to both the axis of precession and the static magnetic field. Following application of the RF pulse, the excited protons will slowly "relax," tending to realign their spin axes with the main magnetic field. Because the spin itself of each proton creates a radio signal, the rate of energy relaxation can be measured, a rate that differs from proton to proton depending on the nature of the surrounding tissue. Differences in the rate of relaxation between the protons of differing tissue types translate into contrast between those differing tissues types within an MR image. Application of additional magnetic field *gradients* in precise patterns too complicated to review here encodes the location of the proton emitting the signal. All MRI modalities use these same basic techniques to encode information about various physiological features and location of brain tissue.

MRI MODALITIES

Anatomical MRI

This imaging modality most often provides clinical information concerning the presence of localized lesions or anatomical defects within the brain. Most neuropsychiatric disorders, however, are not reliably associated with anatomical lesions that can be identified by gross inspection of the image. The utility of anatomical MRI in studying neuropsychiatric disorders therefore lies in its ability to provide more subtle information about brain structure—most commonly, information concerning the volumes and occasionally the shapes of particular brain regions. Although image resolution in most current anatomical imaging studies is approximately a cubic millimeter, in practice, the reliability of measures of regional brain volume is poor for structures smaller than a few cubic centimeters.

Image Analysis

The volumetric measurement of anatomical images depends critically on the methods used to analyze the images. Image analysis typically involves initial preprocessing steps, which tend to vary considerably from lab to lab. Preprocessing, however, usually involves some attempt to reduce the noise and improve the contrast of the images. One important step that is usually required, especially when a goal of analysis is the differentiation of tissue types across spatially distant portions of the brain, is correction of a systematic drift in intensity of the pixels that is caused by systematic and artifactual variation in the intensity within the image. Systematic and artifactual variation is produced by variations either in the magnetic field or in the radiofrequency pulse from the scanner that is used to turn the brain itself into a radio transmitter (3, 4). This systematic drift in intensity will make some pixels that represent cortical gray matter, for instance, look more like higher intensity white-matter pixels.

The next steps in image analysis after preprocessing usually involve some way to differentiate one kind of tissue in the brain from another, termed tissue *segmentation*, and then subdivision of individual tissue types into subregions, a process termed tissue *parcellation*. Both of these steps may be performed using manual definition, computerized automation, or some combination of both. Segmentation may be used to help isolate brain from nonbrain tissues (i.e., in differentiating cortical gray matter from cerebrospinal fluid [CSF] in the sulci), in differentiating gray matter from white matter, or in differentiating CSF in the ventricles from surrounding white matter. Although the methods used to segment tissue types are many and varied (5–12), they all rely considerably on differences in pixel intensity across gray matter, white matter, and CSF. The simplest automated method of segmenting tissues is simply to define the tissue types based on a range of gray-level values, which typically is based on features of the histogram across the entire image or in some portion of it. Even the most sophisticated techniques for tissue segmentation rely to some extent on these image histograms.

Once tissues are segmented one from another, they often are subdivided to provide more anatomically relevant subregions. Cortical gray matter, for example, may be divided according to prefrontal, motor, sensory, or parietal cortices. Ventricular CSF may be divided into the lateral bodies, temporal horns, or the 3rd and 4th ventricles (Figure 2.4.1.5), subcortical gray matter might be divided into caudate, putamen, globus pallidus, and nucleus accumbens (Figure 2.4.1.6), and the cerebral hemispheres can be divided into a variable number of sections (Figure 2.4.1.7). Like segmentation, parcellation may be performed either manually or with the aid of computer automation. Parcellation may involve definition of borders and contours using primarily differences in the gray-scale intensity of the pixels across regions of interest. More automated methods of tissue parcellation include the use of natural boundaries between tissue types, such as the boundaries of cortical sulci and gray matter, to help subdivide gray matter of the cerebral cortex (13). The assumption, however, that divisions based on the cortical sulci follow boundaries between cytoarchitectonically unique subregions, such as those described in the classifications of Brodmann (14) or others (15, 16) is true only to a first approximation (17, 18). Another common method of tissue parcellation is the use of anatomical landmarks within the brain to divide tissues around those landmarks into subregions. These kinds of landmarks, such as the anterior and posterior commissures, are generally considered relatively invariant across individuals in their spatial relationship to other structures within the brain, although this assumption is largely untested (19–21). A

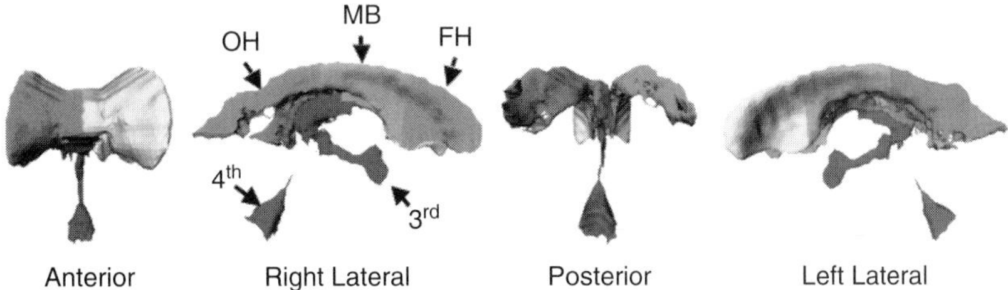

FIGURE 2.4.1.5. Parcellation of the cerebral ventricles. After segmentation, the cerebral ventricles are parcellated. The lateral bodies of the ventricles are divided into three subregions using two coronal planes, one through the anterior commissure (AC) and one through the posterior commissure (PC). The temporal horns are separated from the lateral bodies using an axial plane containing both the AC and PC. The third ventricle is separated from the lateral ventricles at the foramen of Monroe, and the fourth ventricle is separated from the third at the top of the cerebral aqueduct. Subdivisions are shown in four views: anterior, right lateral, posterior, and left lateral. FH = frontal horn; MB = midbody; OH = occipital horn; TH = temporal horn; 3rd = third ventricle; 4th = fourth ventricle. (See color insert.)

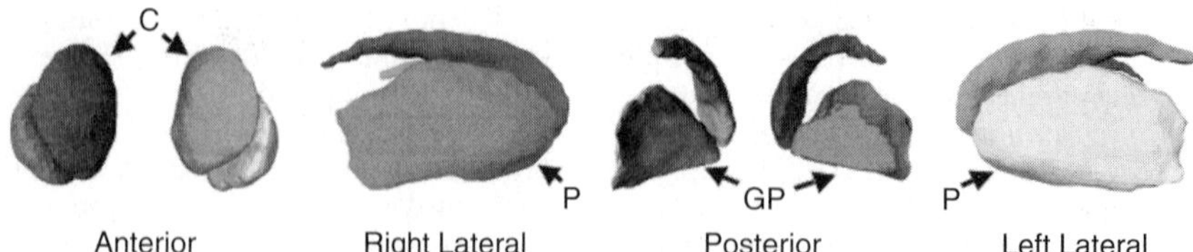

FIGURE 2.4.1.6. **Hand-tracing the basal ganglia.** To delineate basal ganglia, the anatomical MR image was first cropped to the cortices surrounding the basal ganglia, and then the contrast between structures in the cropped image was enhanced by histogram equalization. Finally, we hand-traced the caudate, putamen, and globus pallidus nuclei in the transaxial plane. The head of the caudate nucleus was delineated from the accumbens nucleus by drawing a straight line in the coronal plane from the inferior tip of the internal capsule to the inferior tip of the lateral ventricles. C = caudate; P = putamen; GP = globus pallidus. (See color insert.)

number of computerized methods using statistical models of shape have also been proposed for the more precise delineation of anatomical subregions in the brain; however, these methods require expert knowledge at various levels (22–32). These methods first learn shape (i.e., by computing various statistics of the shape) for a specific brain region from an example set of 20 or more regions that were previously delineated by an expert and then use these computed statistics to delineate the region in a new subject image. Most studies use some combination of these various parcellation schemes to define anatomical subregions within tissue types (33).

A number of laboratories have introduced more novel, largely automated methods of image analysis that segment and parcellate much of the brain (34–37). These methods offer the promise of establishing large, normative databases in which the data from individuals and groups can be compared. Although the details of these methods of course vary considerably across laboratories, they tend to have in common with one another the warping of individual brains into a standardized brain space, so that a voxel in one brain is superimposed to the greatest extent possible on the corresponding voxel in another brain, called image *coregistration*. The simplest way to coregister images involves manual reformatting (rotation, translation, and scaling, and then reslicing) of one image (called the *float*) until the reformatted image superimposes on the other image (called the *target*) to the greatest extent possible. More advanced computerized methods use information (such as externally placed markers, pixel intensities, or other image features, including edges) from the images to be registered, and therefore are fast, consistent, precise, and do not require human interaction (38–53). Once images from differing subjects are coregistered, the methods then either find some way to measure the deviation of each voxel in one individual or group from the mean of the sample or from the mean of another group. Any number of characteristics can be compared across groups, but common features include estimates of relative volume, shape, thickness of the cortical mantel, or correlations of these local brain-based measures with the clinical measures of subjects at particular points of the cerebral surface (Figure 2.4.1.8), local white matter intensities, and volumes of the subcortical nuclei.

Applications

Anatomical MR images have been extensively used to define brain structures and to study correlates of brain measures, including volumes of entire structures and local changes in volumes, with various clinical and genetic measures within and across groups of subjects (54, 55). Additionally, because anatomical MR images have high spatial resolution, SNR, and tissue contrast, these images are used for anatomical localization of brain activations and deactivations in functional MR studies, white matter fiber pathways in diffusion tensor studies, and concentration of brain metabolites in MR spectroscopy studies. Furthermore, anatomical MR images play the key role in coregistering unique information from various MR modalities within a multimodal framework that will greatly help an investigator to constrain interpretations regarding the neural bases of developmental psychopathologies.

Limitations

Measurements of regional brain volumes tell us little or nothing about the brain's ultrastructural features, such as the number, anatomical integrity, or connectivity of the cellular elements that constitute the volume of the tissue being measured. The

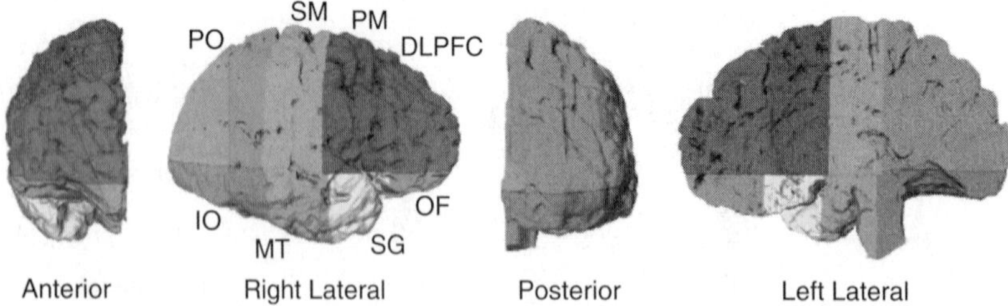

FIGURE 2.4.1.7. **Parcellating right hemisphere into eight anatomical sectors.** Here the brain is isolated by using an isointensity contour function in conjunction with manual editing. We then used a curvilinear plane positioned through standard midline landmarks to divide the brain into hemispheres. We used one axial plane containing the anterior-commissure (AC) and posterior-commissure (PC), and three coronal planes (one tangential to the anterior border of the AC, one through the PC, and one tangential to the genu of the corpus callosum) to divide the right hemisphere into eight anatomical sectors. DLPF = dorsal prefrontal; PM = premotor; SM = sensorimotor; PO = parietooccipital; IO = inferior occipital; MT = midtemporal; SG = subgenual; OF = orbitofrontal. (See color insert.)

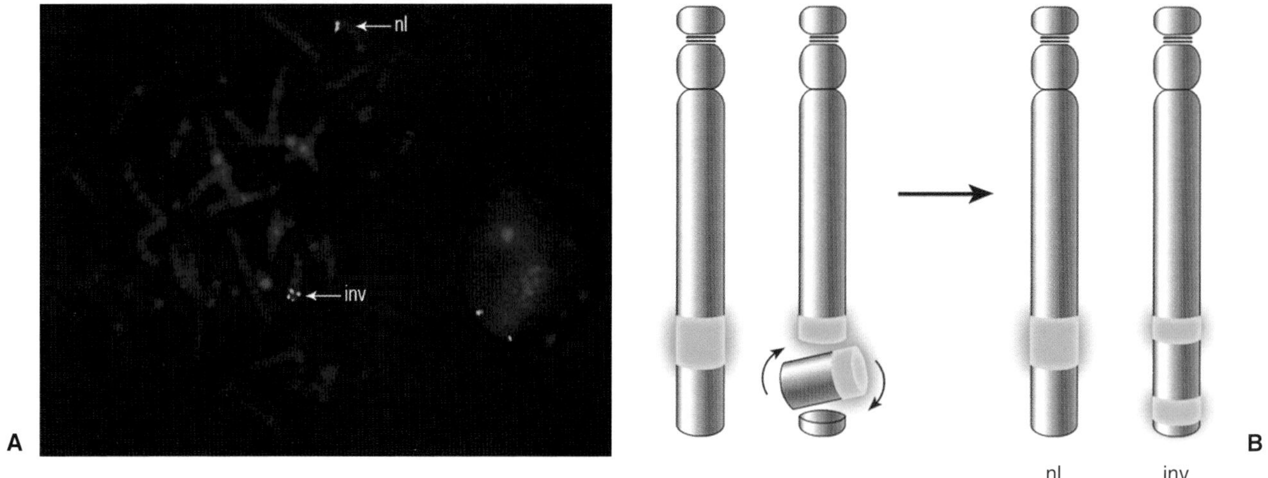

FIGURE 2.3.2.3.

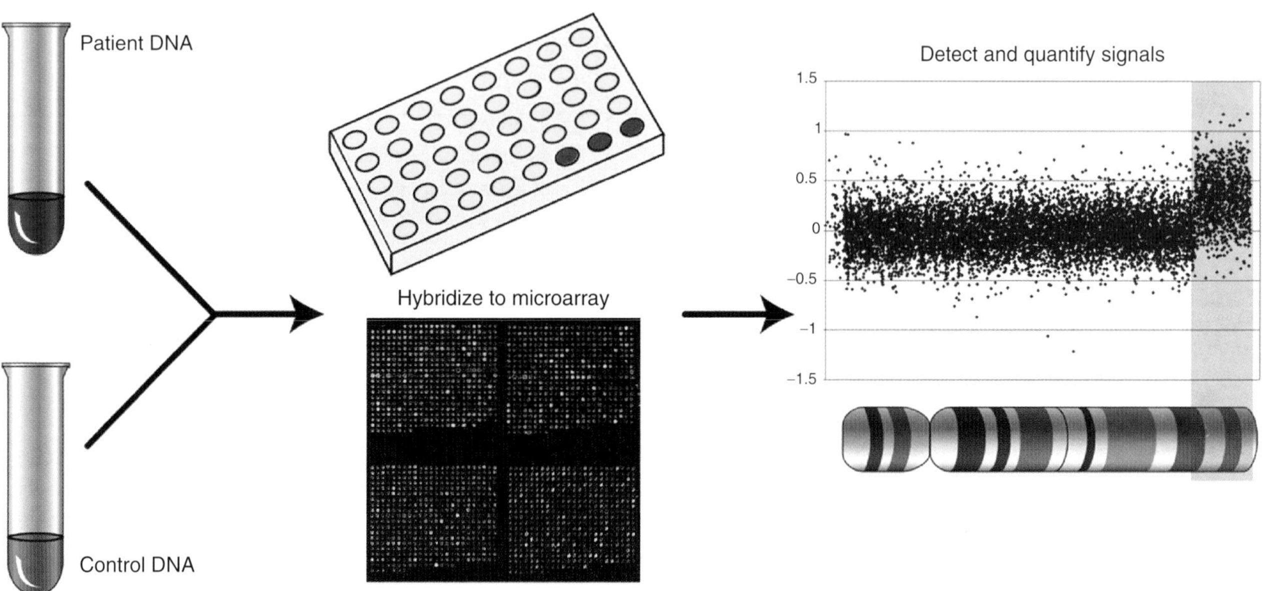

FIGURE 2.3.2.4.

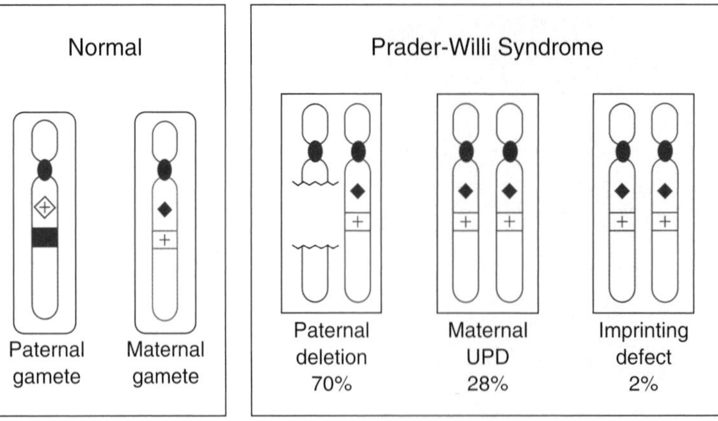

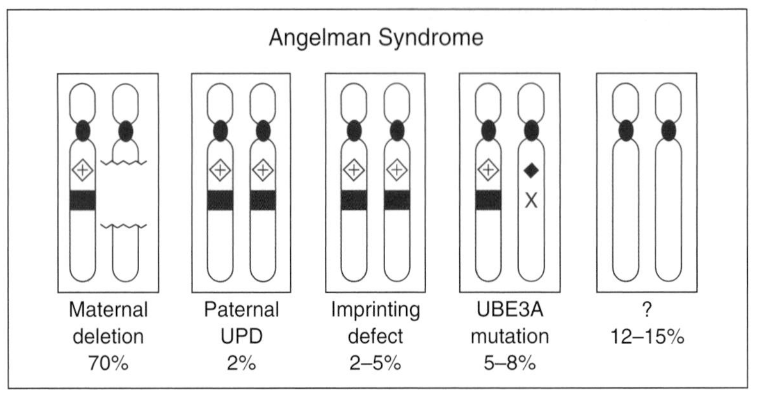

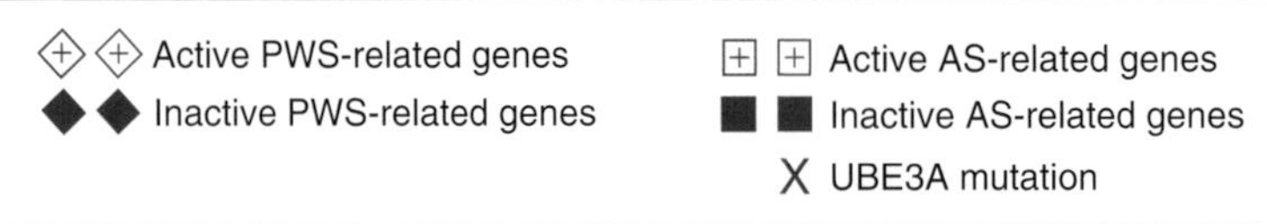

FIGURE 2.3.3.5.

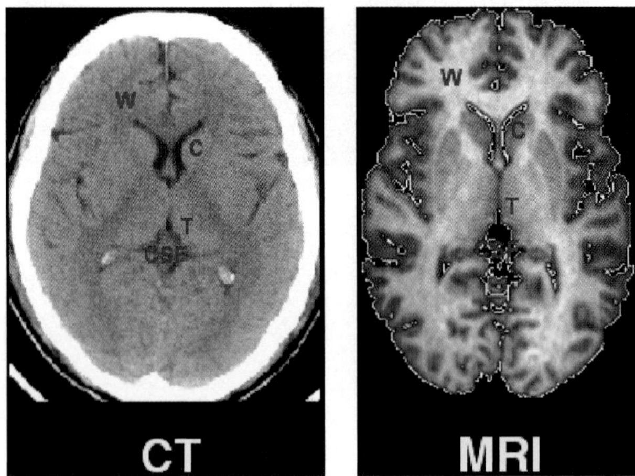

FIGURE 2.4.1.3.

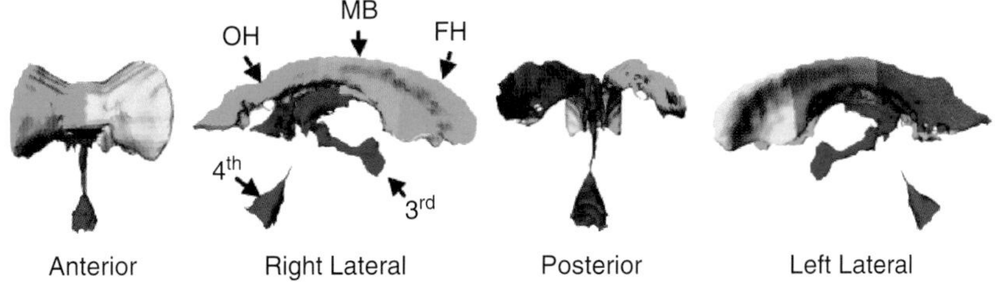

FIGURE 2.4.1.5.

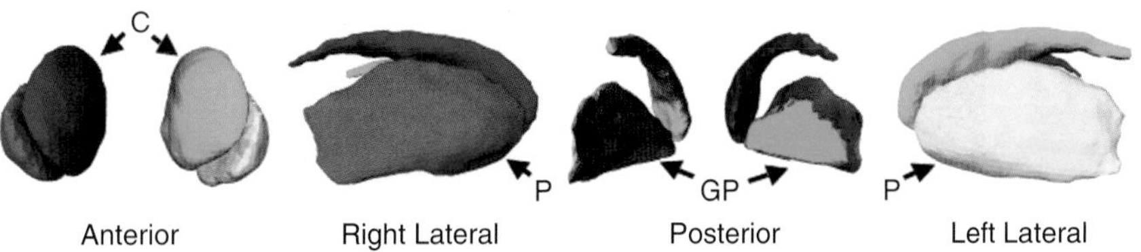

FIGURE 2.4.1.6.

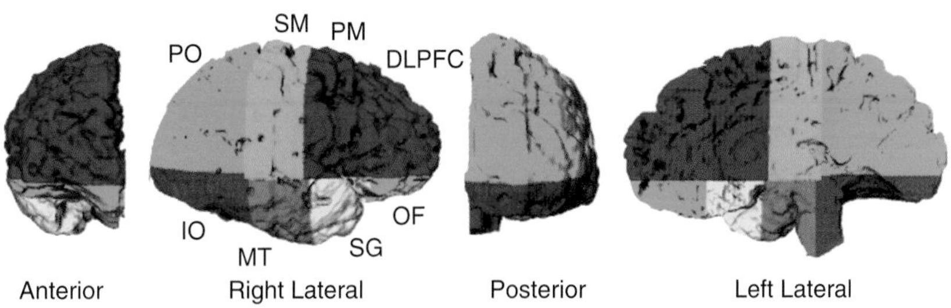

FIGURE 2.4.1.7.

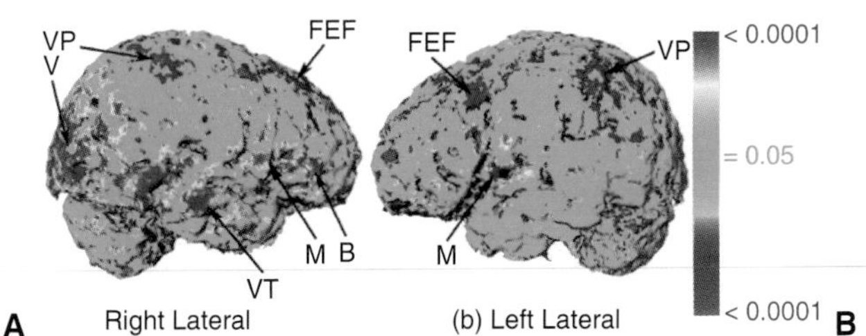

FIGURE 2.4.1.8.

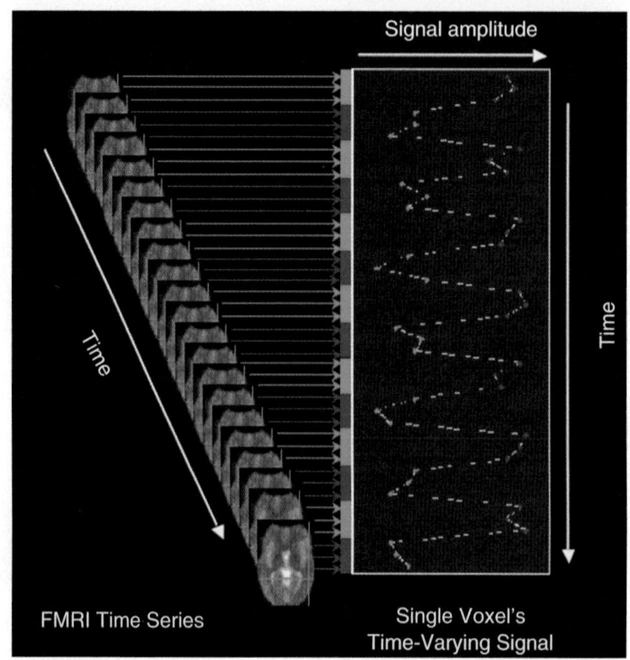

FIGURE 2.4.1.9.

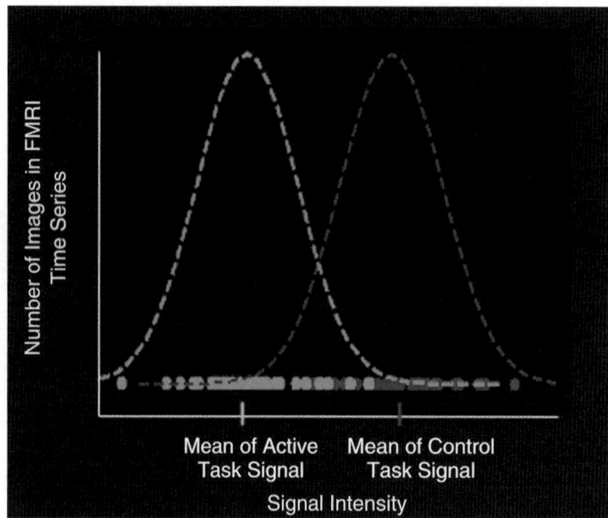

FIGURE 2.4.1.10.

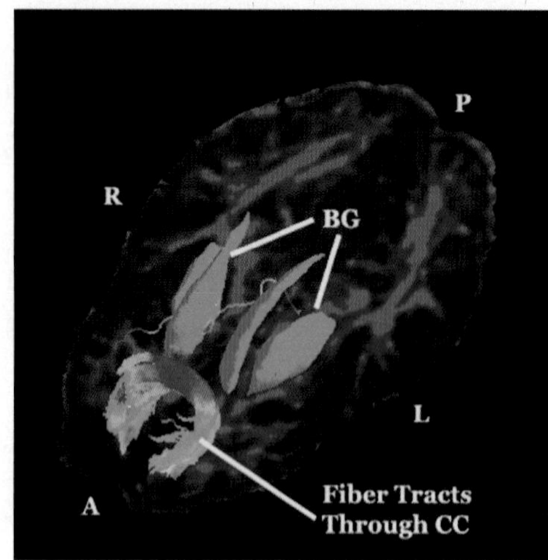

FIGURE 2.4.1.11.

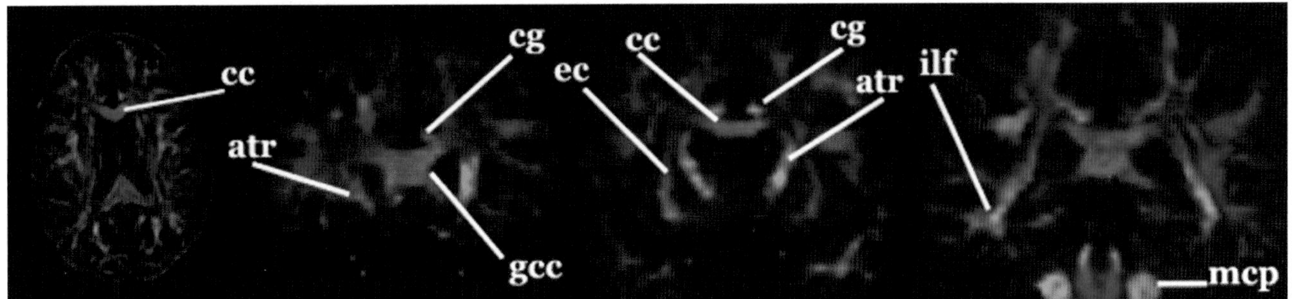

FIGURE 2.4.1.12.

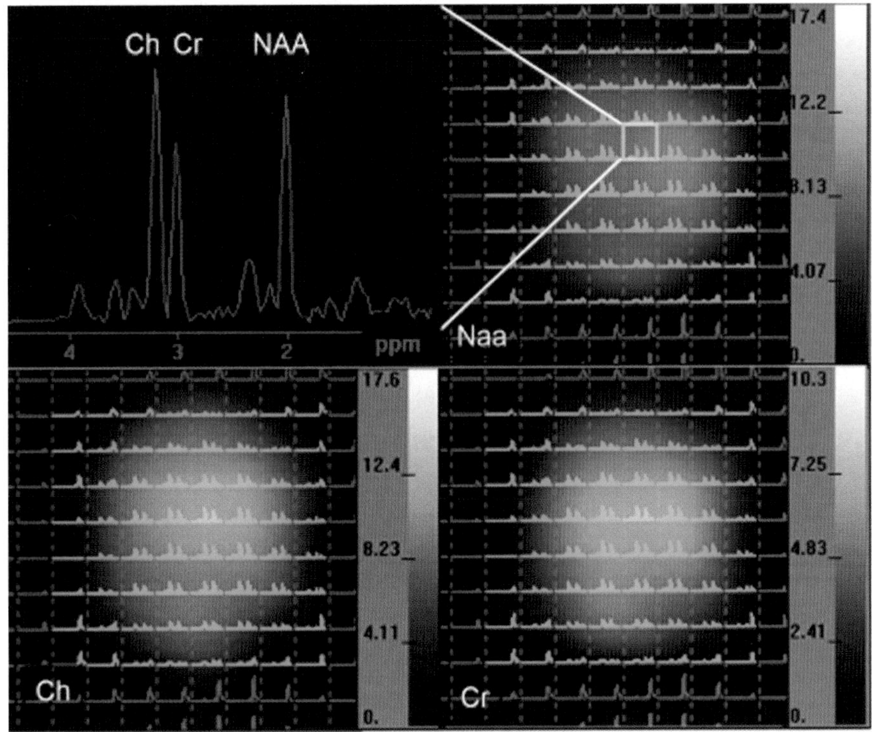

FIGURE 2.4.1.13.

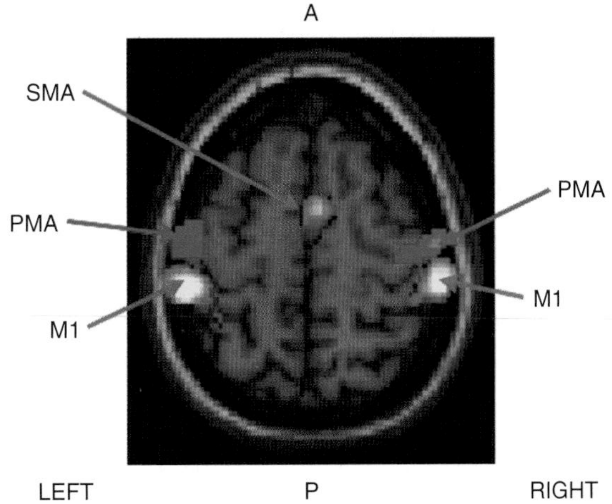

FIGURE 2.4.1.14.

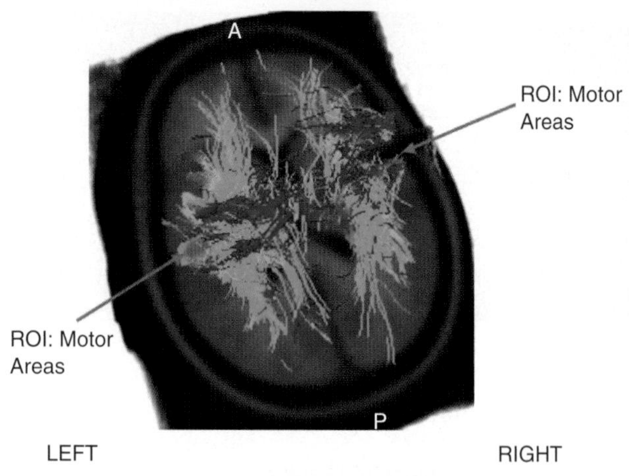

FIGURE 2.4.1.15.

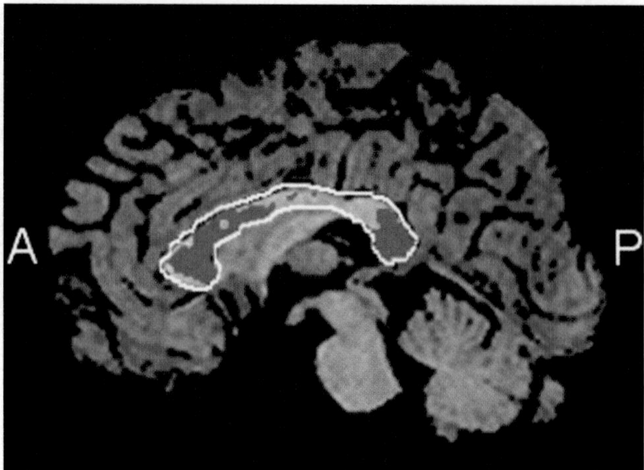

FIGURE 2.4.1.16.

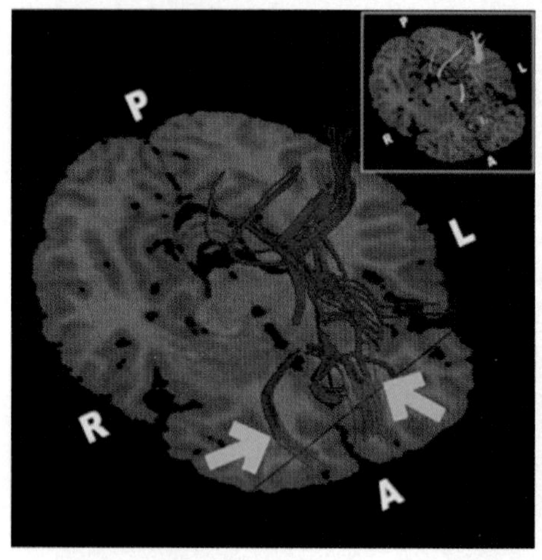

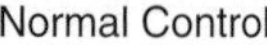

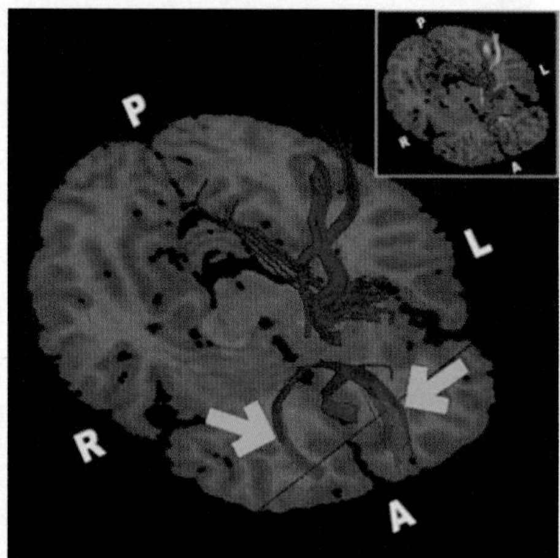

TS

FIGURE 2.4.1.17.

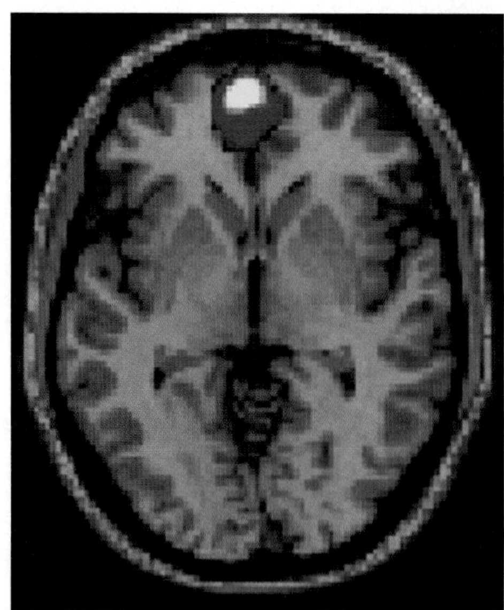

FIGURE 2.4.1.18.

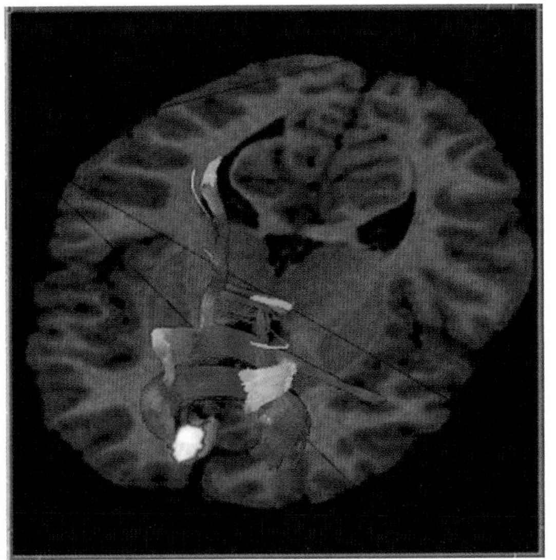

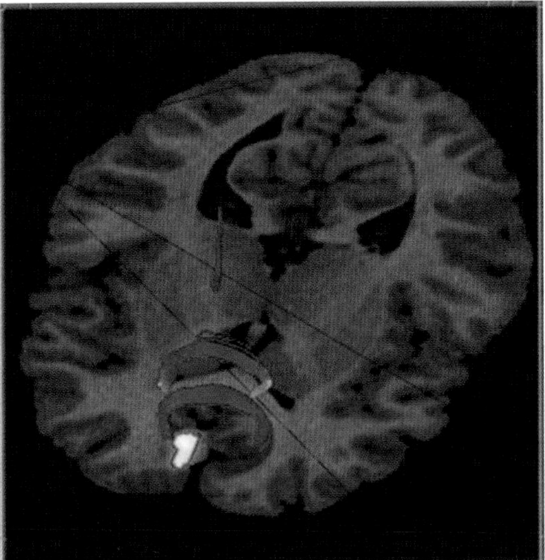

FIGURE 2.4.1.19.

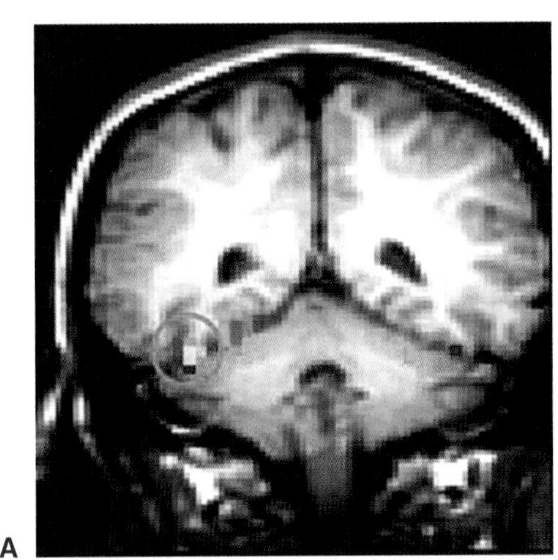

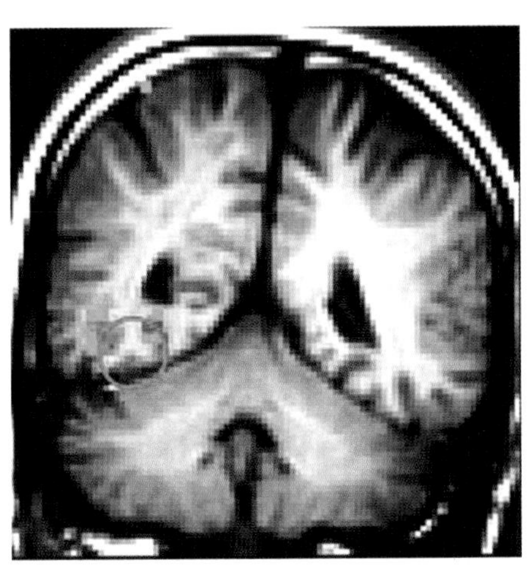

FIGURE 5.1.1.1a.

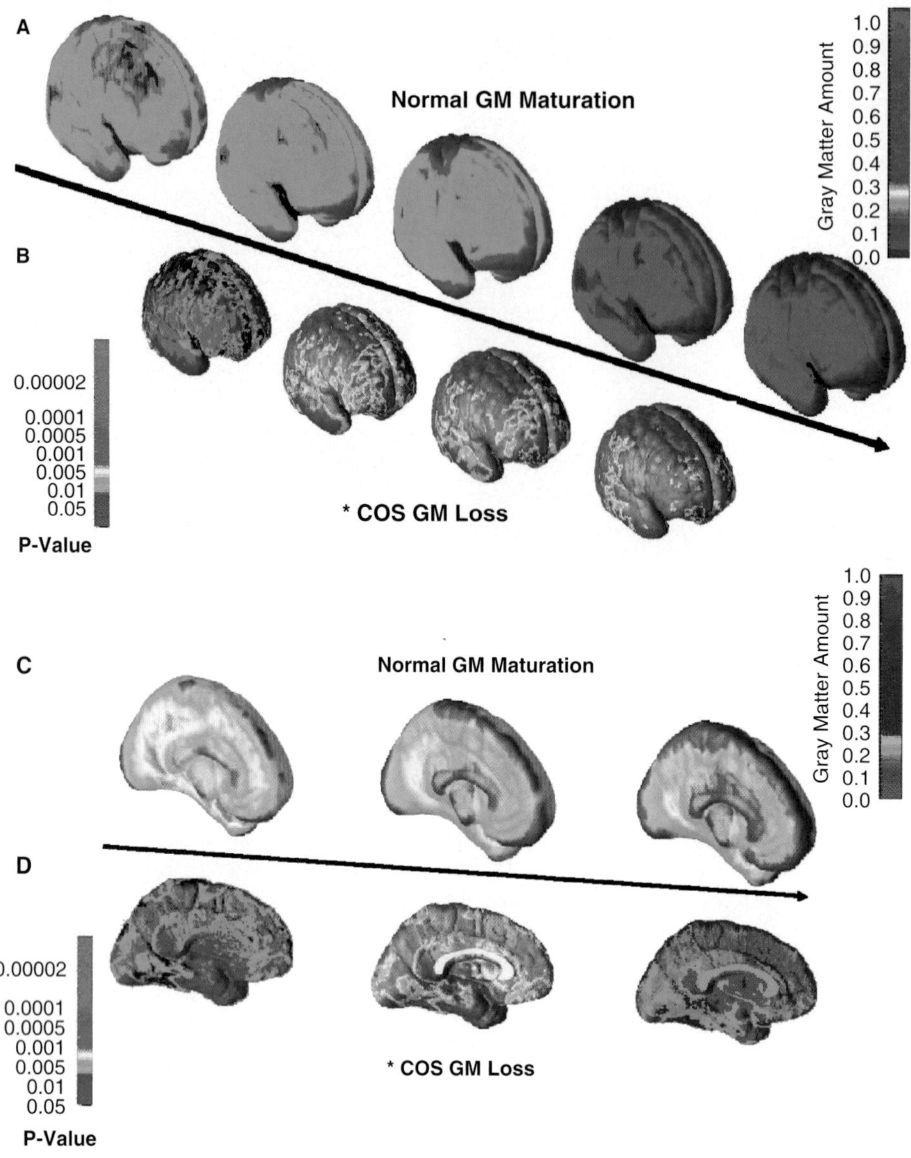

FIGURE 5.3.3.

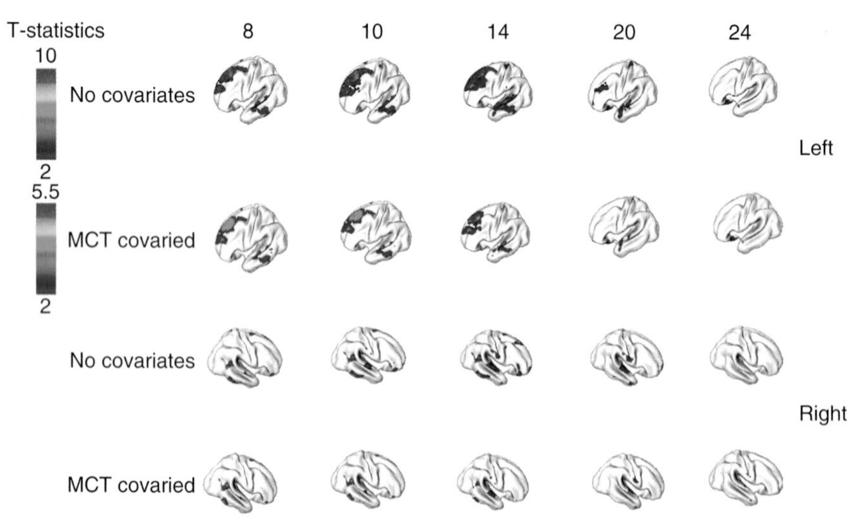

FIGURE 5.3.4.

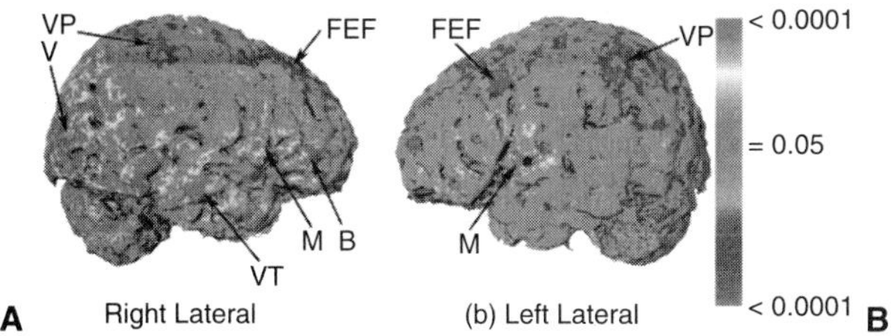

FIGURE 2.4.1.8. Correlating IQ and shape. Statistical analyses of the correlations between intelligence quotient (IQ) and the shape of the cortex for a group of 32 healthy subjects. The color-encoded *p-values* of the correlations (violet denotes negative and red denotes positive) between IQ and cortical surface are plotted across the entire surface of the cortex of a subject selected as reference. B = Broca's region; FEF = frontal eye fields; M = motor; V = vision; VP = visual parietal; VT = visual temporal. (See color insert.)

ultimate significance of individual or group differences in regional volumes that can be detected by imaging studies is therefore still an open question. Nevertheless, recent clinical and preclinical studies suggest that individual variance in the macroscopic volumes that we measure on MR images may arise from genetic differences (56) as well as from experience-dependent effects (57) that influence the addition, subtraction, or reorganization of cellular elements within that volume. These effects of neural plasticity are known to influence brain structure at all levels, from the remodeling of synaptic architecture to the organization of cortical maps (57–59). Volumetric data may therefore carry information about the effects of genetic liabilities and past experiences on the macroscopic structure of the brain.

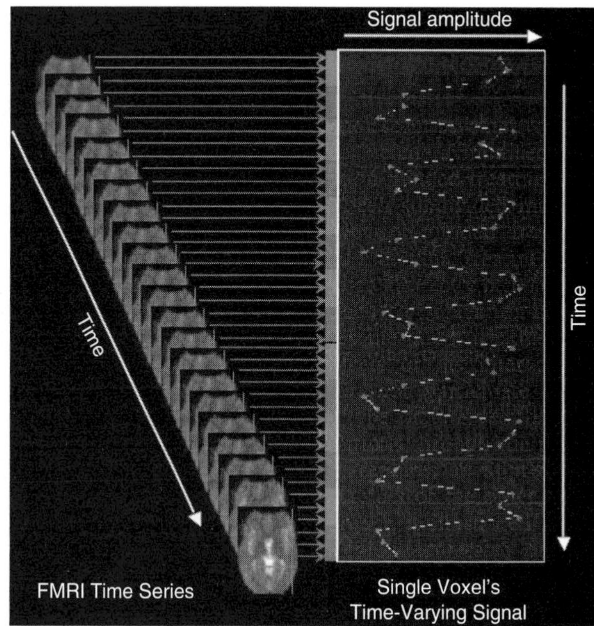

FIGURE 2.4.1.9. FMRI time series. Left: Functional MR images were acquired sequentially as a subject performed an active task (in green) and a control task (in red) during successive blocks of time. **Right:** A corresponding hypothetical time course for the fMRI signal in a single voxel is shown, with green representing fMRI signal acquired during the active task and red representing fMRI signal acquired during the control condition. Increasing signal amplitude is toward the right and advancing time is toward the bottom in this time series. (See color insert.)

Functional MRI

The discovery that the MRI signal represented in the gray-scale values of an MR image can, when tuned to encode certain features of the volume being imaged, vary during performance of a cognitive or behavioral task was first reported in 1991 (60). This time-varying signal has been found to reflect primarily changes in deoxyhemoglobin concentration within the corresponding voxel of the brain. Deoxyhemoglobin concentration is a complex function of the temporal variation in oxygen use and blood supply (termed the blood oxygen level dependent or BOLD response), which ultimately depends on the corresponding temporal variation in the activity of neurons within that voxel. The change in MRI signal during a task is therefore an indirect measure of the change in neuronal activity associated with the performance of that task.

FMRI Time Series

The variation in fMRI signal associated with performance of a task is monitored and tested statistically by acquiring many images in rapid succession while subjects perform in alteration at least two tasks, one of which is the baseline (or control) task and the other of which is the primary task of interest. A typical fMRI experiment might acquire an image in each slice every 1–2 seconds, for a total of several hundred to several thousand images per experiment in that slice per subject. The signal within any single pixel at the times of acquisition of those images will therefore constitute a time-ordered series of signal values, or an *fMRI time series*. If the neuronal activity within a voxel of brain tissue varies systematically through time with the change in performance of one task to the other, the signal in the corresponding pixel's time series will also vary systematically through time with the change in task (Figure 2.4.1.9). The time-dependent variation in the fMRI signal or, equivalently, in the pixel's gray scale, can then be tested statistically to determine whether it varies with the change in task at a level that is beyond chance. Although this task-dependence of the time-varying fMRI signal can be tested using many more or less sophisticated statistical procedures, the simplest is to sort the signal values of the time series into two populations—those acquired during the baseline task and those acquired during performance of the primary task of interest. The means of these populations of signal values are then tested using any number of parametric or nonparametric statistics, the most common of which is a t-statistic (Figure 2.4.1.10). The magnitude of the t-statistic or its corresponding probability value is typically color-coded and then painted on the pixel of the image that represents a voxel in the corresponding slice of brain. Pixels in which the t- or p-value surpasses a predefined threshold are then considered "active" during the primary task of interest relative to the baseline task. FMRI methodologies depend critically upon comparing signal intensities within each pixel across two or more tasks to determine where in the brain neural activity varies systematically with the change in performance of one task to another.

Subtraction Paradigms

If this task-dependent variation in fMRI signal is to have any discernible physiological meaning, the tasks for which the fMRI signals (and, by extension, the local neural activities) are being compared must be most carefully and appropriately selected. This is because activity in any given brain region may well differ between any two tasks, for innumerable reasons. Differential brain activity associated with the tasks, for example, could be caused by differences in the physical properties (hue, saturation, brightness of color, shape, contour, texture) of the visual stimuli across tasks. Differential brain

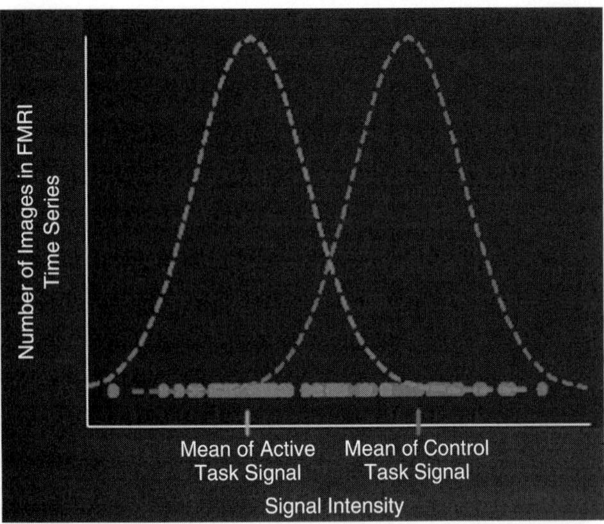

FIGURE 2.4.1.10. Statistical testing of fMRI signal changes. Shown here are the hypothetical distributions of signal intensity within a single pixel during the active (green) and control (red) task conditions in an fMRI time series. Because many images are acquired as the task varies, the signal intensity is sampled many times over the course of an experiment (once for each time point at which an image is acquired). These measurements of signal intensity will have a mean value and a distribution around that mean for each of the two task conditions. The two populations of signal intensities, one for each task condition, can then be compared statistically to assess whether the fMRI signal in that voxel and, presumably, the underlying neuronal activity in the corresponding voxel of the brain, varies significantly with the change in performance of one task to the other. In this example, the mean signal acquired during the active task is lower than the mean signal during the control task. (See color insert.)

activity could also be caused by differences in the comparative difficulties of the two tasks (which might produce systematic differences in orienting, alerting, vigilance, effort, confusion, uncertainty, search strategies, or motor response times). It could also be caused by differences in the cognitive strategy used to perform the tasks, in the thoughts and affects uniquely associated with each of the tasks, or in any number of other differences in brain and mental functioning associated with the tasks. Therefore, if the differential brain activity detected in an fMRI experiment is to be understood at all, the "baseline" task must differ from the primary task of interest by a single or more realistically a few features that range from basic physical features of the stimulus to higher order physiological, affective, and cognitive components. When these features of the tasks are tightly controlled, the brain activity associated with the control task is said, in colloquial terms, to "subtract out" from brain activity associated with the primary task of interest. In the maps that represent the comparison of brain activity in the two tasks, this subtraction leaves only the brain activity associated with the cognitive processing components that are *unique* to the primary task of interest. This general strategy of comparing brain activity associated with two or more tasks is therefore typically termed a "subtraction paradigm."

Assumptions and Examples of Subtraction Paradigms

Implicit in the majority of these subtraction methodologies used in functional imaging studies (including many PET and SPECT, as well as fMRI studies) is the assumption that the brain processes information in a serial and additive fashion. This assumption is perhaps most classically exemplified in imaging studies of language processing, in which each level of a hierarchy of tasks serves as the control for the task above it (61). For example, gaze fixation may serve as the control task for the passive viewing of written symbols that resemble letters. This subtraction might represent differential brain activity associated with, say, orthographic processing. Viewing of the same written symbols might then be compared with the passive viewing of strings of letters from the alphabet (but arranged so as not to spell real words) to represent cognitive processes associated uniquely with letter recognition or phonological processing. Viewing of these pseudoword letter strings, compared with viewing of letter strings that represent real words, might represent brain activity associated with semantic processing (i.e., with the processing of word meanings). Viewing of real words that are nouns, compared with viewing of the same words while subjects generate verbs associated with those nouns, might represent brain activity associated with word generation, or more expressive language functions. Each of these subtractions in a functional imaging experiment represents brain activity associated with one task when compared with another. When interpreting task-related signal changes, this differential brain activity is conceptualized as one step or one stage of information processing within a larger, hierarchically ordered series of stages of information processing.

Subtraction paradigms such as these are not unique to functional imaging studies—indeed, subtraction paradigms have long been used in cognitive neuroscience, particularly in the study of the differential effects of a hierarchy of tasks on reaction times. The strong assumptions of these paradigms—that the brain is a serial processor, that cognitive functions are linearly additive (and can therefore be "subtracted" one from another), and that cognitive processing is highly modular (and therefore serially ordered modules can be spatially localized within functional brain imaging studies)—have been roundly and convincingly criticized numerous times throughout the history of cognitive neuroscience (62–66). Nevertheless, the experimental results of these subtraction paradigms in imaging studies have proved to be reasonably robust and reproducible, at least in well-designed experiments. Furthermore, they have arguably, in some instances at least, produced results that support some of these strong assumptions.

The dependence on subtraction methodologies is both a strength and a weakness of using fMRI for the study of neuropsychiatric disorders. It is a strength because the method permits probing very specific mental processes in healthy and ill individuals. It is a weakness because it confines investigation to a very narrow domain of brain functioning. FMRI currently is not able to measure and compare resting brain activity across individuals in the way that PET and SPECT can. The utility of fMRI in studying any particular neuropsychiatric illness will therefore depend critically on the appropriateness of the selection of the mental process that is being probed with the subtraction paradigm and on the success in designing and implementing the corresponding subtraction paradigm. The problem is that our knowledge of the pathophysiology of any illness is currently too limited to provide an adequate guide for the selection of a probe for a particular cognitive process that will prove to illuminate the features of pathophysiology that are central to that illness, rather than being simply correlated with or peripheral to epiphenomena of the disorder.

Experimental Design

The early experimental paradigms used in fMRI study are mostly the "blocked design," in which a series of trials in one condition is presented for an extended period of time (67, 68). The signal acquired during one blocked condition is first temporally integrated, then compared with that acquired under another blocked condition. In a typical blocked experimental design, the functional responses evoked by an individual stimulus presented within blocks are not resolved; instead, only the average differences in brain activity across the two conditions can be discerned. In addition, understanding of the differences in functional responses across these two conditions may be compromised by a number of factors, including the differing expectancies, motivation, strategies, and attentional states of the subjects as they prepare for and process stimuli within and between blocks of each task condition.

"Event-related designs" have been developed in the attempt to overcome some of the problems associated with blocked stimulus designs (69, 70). This type of design uses a series of single trials at a relatively slow rate of stimulus presentation to reduce the overlap of the hemodynamic responses evoked by consecutive individual trials. Event-related designs isolate individual trial events and therefore allow images to be formed of the transient neuronal changes associated with individual cognitive and sensory processes. However, this method often limits the number of trials that can be collected in individual experiments because of their long interstimuli intervals (ISI).

Rapid event-related fMRI paradigms have been developed to overcome problems associated with block stimulus designs and the long interstimulus intervals of many conventional event-related designs. The introduction of "jitter" (i.e., a variable temporal delay between successive trials) significantly reduces the duration of the interstimulus interval in an experiment, while providing enough information for the estimation of the BOLD response. In rapid event-related designs, the trial ordering and temporal jittering between trials is critical for minimizing the dependence of the BOLD response on the previous trial. Very often, the presentations of differing stimuli conditions are randomized and counterbalanced across time.

Group Comparisons

Comparing the differential fMRI signal change associated with a task across diagnostic groups, an intuitively obvious goal for fMRI studies of neuropsychiatric disorders, is a nontrivial matter. A group difference in the pattern or intensity of brain activation may be attributable to some intrinsic qualifier, such as diagnostic group. However, apparent group differences may be introduced by the presence of other confounding features that differ across groups, such as age, sex, or intelligence. Therefore, in order to minimize the effects of these experimental confounds, either groups should be matched on these kinds of features, or these features should be controlled in the statistical analyses that compare brain activation across groups.

Group comparisons typically are performed in one of two ways: voxel-based or region-of-interest (ROI)-based analyses. Voxel-based analyses usually provide information about which parts of the brain are activated during a specific task, whereas ROI-based solutions provide information about how a specific brain region changes its hemodynamic activity when the subject performs a task. These two approaches differ considerably in many respects, but in essence their differences arise from the ways in which they identify the pixels of the image whose mean signal intensities will be compared across the diagnostic groups. The voxel-based approach compares individuals on a single voxel-by-voxel basis, after individual brains are warped into a standard volume, shape, and spatial orientation and then superimposed one on top of the other. Corresponding voxels in the images from each person are then assumed to represent these same voxels of tissue across the brains of individual subjects. Therefore, after this warping procedure, the location of a voxel in the prefrontal cortex of one person is assumed to be in precisely the same location as the voxel identified in the prefrontal cortex of another person. The warping of the brains is usually performed with reference to a set of standard anatomical landmarks—the anterior commissure (AC), the posterior commissure (PC), and an imaginary box that bounds all sides of the brain. Voxels are most commonly identified using a coordinate system along the x, y, and z axes that are oriented with respect to these landmarks. This particular "Talairach" coordinate system derives its name from one of its developers (71). Mean signal changes across the task are calculated for each individual in the study, and at each voxel. Every voxel therefore has associated with it two populations of signal changes, one for each diagnostic group, which are then compared with one another using any number of standard statistical techniques. These statistical tests are performed individually for each pixel in the image.

ROI-based comparisons of group activations, in contrast, define in some way an ROI on the unwarped images of each individual—it may be defined, for example, by manually circumscribing the boundary of the structure on the anatomical images, upon which are plotted the functional images or their mean signal changes at each voxel. The mean signal changes at each voxel within the larger ROI are then either summed or averaged to provide a descriptive statistic that represents the overall task-dependent change in fMRI signal within the entire ROI. That measure of ROI-based signal change for each individual is then used to compare activation in that ROI across diagnostic groups.

Limitations

The greatest limitation of voxel-based approaches for fMRI analyses is the assumption that, except for differences in scaling (i.e., in overall volume) and head orientation, the anatomy and corresponding localization of function is the same across individuals and across diagnostic groups—an assumption that is demonstrably false. Because of known differences in the anatomy of brains of patients who have neuropsychiatric illnesses compared with normal subjects, the brains of neuropsychiatric patients on average would not be expected to superimpose well when warped into the Talairach coordinate system. It is therefore possible, for instance, that corresponding pixels in the images of these individuals might represent prefrontal gray matter in one group and prefrontal white matter in the other group. Because task-related signal change should occur in cortical gray matter rather than in the underlying white matter, the voxel-based comparison across groups at this point will appear to show more activation in the first group compared with the second. This group difference, however, would simply be an artifact. The ROI-based approach is not vulnerable to this artifact because it defines boundaries of the ROI based on the relevant anatomy or anatomical landmarks of each individual in the study. The ROI approach, in contrast, assumes that anatomically and functionally relevant regions can actually be defined with some precision, in a valid and reliable manner. In some regions, such as the cerebral cortex, this assumption is highly questionable, given the improbability of defining cytoarchitectonically valid regions using the gray-scale values of MR images. This difficulty is only compounded when ROIs are superimposed on functional MR images that typically have resolutions on the order of 70–100 mm^3, because the cytoarchitectonic regions and their boundaries will be averaged into these large pixels of the image.

Diffusion Tensor Imaging

Developed relatively recently, diffusion tensor imaging (DTI) is a modality of MRI that can provide information about the direction and integrity of neural fiber tracks in the brain in vivo. DTI operates by mathematically describing the directional diffusion of water in brain tissues. At locations in the brain where the diffusion of water molecules is not constrained in a particular direction by the structure of a tissue having a directional orientation (e.g., the unconstrained cerebrospinal fluid in the ventricles), the probability of locating a water molecule that has been "tagged" with MRI-based excitation is statistically equal in all directions (a probabilistic sphere). However, at locations where tissues do have structures with clear directional orientation, water molecules tend to diffuse parallel to that direction. Under these conditions, the probability of locating a tagged water molecule appears more elliptical than spherical. Myelinated axons within the white matter of the brain, as well as in muscles and tendons in the body, are primary examples of biological tissues with well organized, directional orientation. Thus by measuring the diffusion of water molecules along the directional orientation of myelinated axons, investigators can track the pathways of the axons themselves.

DTI pulse sequences are used to measure the diffusion of water in many spatial directions at each voxel, thereby generating a diffusion-weighted (DW) image for every direction of measurement. The spatial direction for measurement is determined by applying a *directional magnetic gradient*, such that only the MRI signal that is sensitive to the spatial direction of that magnetic gradient can be detected. More precisely, the image intensities in a DW image are attenuated according to the direction and strength of the gradient, as well as the characteristics of the local microstructure. Lesser intensities indicate greater diffusion. DW images are in turn used to construct *diffusion tensors*, ellipsoid geometrical representations of the diffusional properties of water at a given voxel. A tensor can be expressed mathematically by a 3×3 numerical matrix containing 6 unknown variables (3 of which represent components of the vector along the 3 spatial dimensions, and 3 that represent the corresponding magnitudes of those spatial components). Because 6 variables are required to define a tensor at each voxel, DW images must be acquired along at least 6 gradient directions, in addition to acquisition of one or more DW images without a directional gradient (i.e., a baseline image). In general, the more DW images used in constructing a tensor, the greater the accuracy of the estimated tensor's mathematical profile and its corresponding 3D geometrical representation.

Many useful measurements can be derived from diffusion tensors. Measures of *diffusion anisotropy* (i.e., the degree of directional dependence of diffusion), including fractional anisotropy and relative anisotropy, are indices that describe the local anisotropy of water diffusion and that range from 0.0 (isotropic, diffusing equally in every direction) to 1.0 (non-isotropic, diffusing strongly in one direction). In brain tissues, the *principal direction* of a tensor (i.e., the orientation of an ellipsoid's longest axis) usually represents the local orientation of the underlying fibers. Using *DTI tractography*, investigators can study the connectivity of white matter in the brain by reconstructing the pathways of nerve fiber bundles based on the principal direction of diffusion and other information inferred from diffusion tensors (Figure 2.4.1.11). In addition, color-coded maps generated with DTI and based on the principal directions of tensors can be used to parcellate more easily some tissues that are difficult to segment using conventional anatomical images (Figure 2.4.1.12).

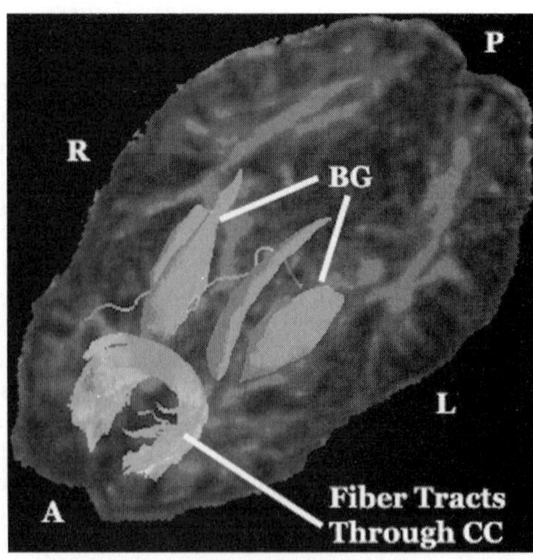

FIGURE 2.4.1.11. An example of fiber bundles tracked in the brain passing through the corpus callosum (CC). A = anterior; P = posterior; L = left; R = right. The fibers are painted in colors according to their running direction. Left–right are depicted in red, anterior–posterior in green and inferior–superior in blue. The basal ganglia are painted in green for reference. The image slice is translucent and some of the fibers are actually underneath the axial brain slice. (See color insert.)

Applications

Clinical applications of DTI have focused on determining the integrity of white matter tracts, as measured by the local anisotropy of diffusion (the more highly organized an axon bundle, the less isotropic will be the diffusion). The first major clinical application of DTI was in the diagnosis of stroke. DTI demonstrated changes in contrast between tissues within minutes following an ischemic insult, whereas conventional imaging showed changes only after many hours (72). Moreover, DTI has been used to demonstrate the loss of white matter in multiple sclerosis (73), schizophrenia (74–76), dyslexia (77), and preterm birth (78). Because this imaging method provides an entirely new perspective on brain structure, its application in neuroimaging studies is sure to increase in coming years.

Limitations

Although MRI technology itself has advanced significantly in recent years, DTI remains relatively immature in its applied uses in the study of childhood psychopathologies. Because the spatial resolution of DTI is low compared with the diameter of a single nerve fiber, partial volume effects (e.g., the value of a voxel in the images could represent signals from more than one tissue type) are unavoidable. Consequently, only major fiber bundles can be reconstructed and examined reliably. Because the diffusion tensor is a relatively simple model of the diffusivity of water, DTI has difficulty depicting regions near boundaries between differing types of tissue (such as cortical gray and white matter) as well as in regions where fiber pathways cross. Recently, however, more advanced models of water diffusivity have been proposed that attempt to overcome the weaknesses of the diffusion tensor model, including q-space imaging and generalized diffusion tensor imaging.

In addition, processing DTI data is computationally more difficult compared with other MRI modalities, for several reasons. First, DTI data demand enormous amounts of storage space: one DT image is usually 24 times the size of a conventional anatomical MR image. Second, while other MRI modalities use images that encode a single number with a gray-scale intensity at each voxel, diffusion tensors contain high-dimensional spatial and geometrical information at each voxel; because this information in tensors is biologically meaningful, maintaining integrity of this information during image processing is vitally important. Thus, developing standardized procedures for the processing and analysis of DTI data is challenging. Processing DTI data is further complicated by the presence of noise, imaging artifact, and distortion in DT images that are caused by the sensitivity of the data to inherent imperfections in scanner performance.

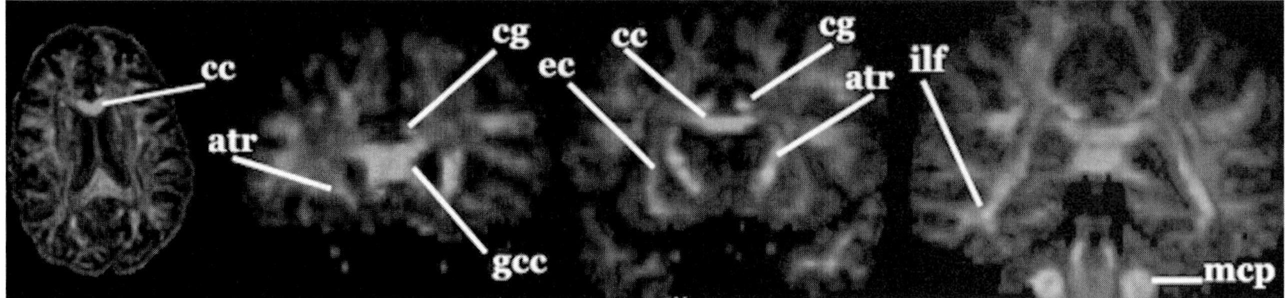

FIGURE 2.4.1.12. Examples of DTI color maps showing the principal direction of prominent white matter tracts. (left) Axial slice; (right) coronal slices. cg = cingulum, ec = external capsule, atr = anterior thalamic radiation; cc = corpus callosum; gcc = genu of the corpus callosum; ilf = inferior longitudinal fasciculus; mcp = middle cerebellar peduncle. Color schema: red = left–right; green = inferior–superior; blue = anterior–posterior. (See color insert.)

Furthermore, when fiber pathways have been constructed from DTI data, the statistical analysis of nerve fibers remains mathematically challenging because of the large number of fibers, as well as their great variability in length, orientation, and shape. Therefore, no mathematical models can yet convincingly and reliably measure and compare the similarity of two fibers across individuals or groups of subjects. In group analyses currently, we are generally limited to voxel-wise comparisons of invariant measures, such as fractional anisotropy or deviations in principal directions of the tensors. Nevertheless, despite these limitations, DTI is gaining importance in both research and clinical applications.

Magnetic Resonance Spectroscopy

Magnetic resonance spectroscopy (MRS) is an akin but quite complementary technique to MRI. Whereas MRI provides anatomical information of the subject in the form of images based on the signals from protons in tissue water, MRS provides biochemical information of the subject in the form of a *spectrum*, a series of spectral peaks of differing intensities at differing radiofrequencies in the MRI signal originating from various nuclei in the metabolites. The commonly used nuclei in in vivo MRS are proton (^{1}H), phosphorus (^{31}P) and carbon 13 (^{13}C), and the corresponding MRS imaging technique is denoted by ^{1}H MRS, ^{31}P MRS and ^{13}C MRS, respectively. ^{1}H MRS is the most widely used technique because it provides the greatest sensitivity for detecting a signal from biologically significant metabolites. Over two decades of development, MRS has improved greatly in the techniques used for data acquisition, providing greatly improved spatial and spectral resolution and higher SNR, as well as in techniques for processing of the imaging data, including the accuracy of metabolite quantification and the number of metabolites that can be quantified. The increasing availability and application of MRS have led to valuable findings concerning the roles of metabolite concentrations in the pathophysiologies of neuropsychiatric disorders.

The important parameters of the MR spectra are "frequency" and "intensity" of the resonance signal. The resonant frequency depends on the species of the nucleus, the strength of the magnetic field (B_0) of the scanner and, most importantly, on the internal magnetic field generated by the local distribution of electrons around the nucleus. In practice, the frequency, or the position of an MR spectral peak, termed its chemical shift, is recorded relative to the position of a reference signal in units of ppm (parts per million), defined as $\delta = (\gamma - \gamma_{Ref}) \times 10^6/\gamma_{Ref}$, where γ and γ_{Ref} are the respective frequencies of the nucleus and the reference. In this case, the positions of the MR spectral peaks are determined only by the internal chemical environment that the nuclei experience, not by B_0. Therefore, the nuclei are regarded as tiny probes within the molecules themselves, and their spectra are regarded as the fingerprints that reflect the structural information of the sample. The intensity, or the area under a spectral peak, is proportional to the number of the nuclei that contribute to the peak, and it can be used to deduce the concentration of the corresponding metabolite. The upper left panel of Figure 2.4.1.13 shows an example of ^{1}H MR spectrum of a healthy newborn. The chemical shifts of three prominent single peaks (termed *singlets*) are assigned to three major metabolites: N-acetyl aspartate (NAA) at 2.01 ppm, total creatine (tCr) at 3.04 ppm, and choline-containing compounds (tCh) at 3.24 ppm.

By employing methods of spatial encoding and localization that are used in all MRI modalities, in vivo MRS technique allows the acquisition not only of a spectrum from a single voxel in the body (a technique often referred to as single voxel MR spectroscopy), but also of i) a 2D matrix of spectra from a matrix of voxels in a slice, ii) multiple 2D matrices of spectra from several slices, and iii) a 3D matrix of spectra from a 3D volume. These techniques of 2D or 3D multiple-voxel MRS not only present the data as a matrix of resonance spectra (as shown in Figure 2.4.1.13), but also can depict the data in the form of images, similar to those of conventional MRI; 2D and 3D MRSs are therefore referred to as *MR spectroscopic imaging*, or MRSI.

The purposes of MRS and MRSI are to measure the concentrations and the distributions of metabolites within the brain. This can be achieved by comparing the signals of metabolites and the signal of a reference with a known concentration. The reference can be internal, such as tissue water or, more commonly, it can be the concentrations of other metabolites that are assumed to be normal, such as creatine; the reference can also be external to the brain, such as water in a vial attached close to the head of the subject. The concentration is often expressed in units of millimoles per liter (mM).

The most frequently measured brain metabolites in ^{1}H MRS are NAA, tCr, and tCh, mainly because of their high concentrations and prominent singlets (i.e., their peaks are discrete and not contaminated strongly by their overlap with other metabolites), and because of the simplicity of their quantification during image processing. In addition, several other metabolites can be quantified that are significant in studies of psychiatric illnesses, such as glutamate/glutamine, γ-amino (GABA), and myo-inositol (Ins). Measuring these metabolites has been challenging because of their lower concentrations, weak signals, and complex spectral structures. However, with the proliferation of advanced MR spectroscopy techniques and high magnetic field strengths that improve SNR, measurements

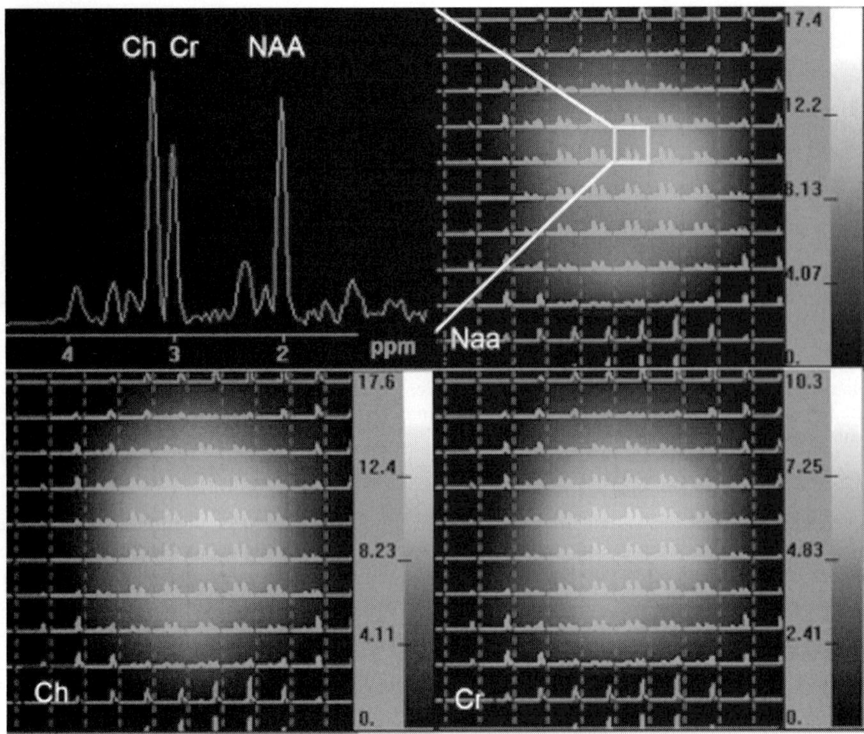

FIGURE 2.4.1.13. Proton MR spectra and MRS images of the newborn brain. The upper left panel is a spectrum from the voxel marked in the upper right panel. The other three panels show spectra matrices. The spectra in the regions of interest (ROIs) depicted in green exhibit spectral structures that are similar to the voxel spectrum shown in the upper left panel. However, the individual peak areas differ from voxel to voxel because of the differing spatial distributions of the metabolite concentrations. The background in the upper right and the lower panels are the spectroscopic images (SI) of NAA, tCh, and tCr, respectively, obtained by integrating the corresponding peak areas in each voxel and interpolating to an apparent higher resolution. These SIs depict the distributions of the metabolites. The scales on the right-hand sides of the panels are in arbitrary units and represent the relative concentrations of the metabolites. (See color insert.)

of these metabolites is becoming increasingly common and more reliable.

Applications

Several groups have reported alterations in levels of NAA, tCh, Ins, glutamate/glutamine, and GABA in patients with major depression, bipolar disorder, panic disorder, or attention-deficit/hyperactivity disorder (ADHD). A recent study of adolescent bipolar disorder, for example, showed reductions of NAA and tCh concentrations in gray matter of the frontal lobe (79). Similarly, higher mean concentrations of NAA were detected in the left centrum semiovale of children with ADHD than in children with autism and healthy controls (80). Other studies suggested increased glutamate/glutamine concentrations in the frontal cortex (81) and anterior cingulate cortex (82) of children with ADHD. Reduced or abnormal GABA concentrations have been reported in anxiety disorders, major depression, and drug addiction (83). Abnormal levels of inositol, an important second messenger in brain metabolism, have been reported in many psychiatric disorders, including bipolar disorder, depression, panic disorder, and schizophrenia (84).

Limitations

Although MRS techniques have been improving rapidly, intrinsic limitations should be considered when designing MRS studies and when interpreting their results. Compared with anatomical and functional MRI, for example, the spatial and temporal resolutions of MRS, as well its SNR, are relatively low. Currently, a typical voxel size in ^{1}H MRS is 1 cc. The typical scanning time required for single-voxel ^{1}H MRS is several minutes and more than 20 minutes for 2D MRSI having a matrix of 32 × 32. The spatial and temporal resolutions and SNR of MRS of other nuclei are even lower. Moreover, the low spatial resolution and low SNR of MRS impairs the accuracy and reproducibility of measurement compared with other MRI modalities. Finally, absolute quantification of metabolite concentrations, rather than quantification relative to another metabolite, is highly desirable. Absolute quantification requires correction for various imperfections in the imaging data, such as the contributions of multiple tissue types within voxels, imperfections in the magnetic field or radiofrequency signals of the scanner, and difficulties finding and implementing reliable references to standardize the measurements. Addressing these difficulties is far from trivial, so that thus far only NAA, total creatine, and total choline-containing compounds that have prominent singlets can be quantified with reasonably good accuracy in human studies. With concerted efforts across the MRS community, however, these challenges will be addressed in the years to come.

Methods for Studying Functional and Anatomical Connectivity

Distributed neural networks govern human behavior (85, 86), and in recent years, investigating these networks noninvasively has become increasingly possible using functional brain imaging (86). A common objective in functional brain imaging is to characterize the activity in a particular brain region in terms of the interactions among inputs from other regions. The analysis of fMRI time-series data recorded from the human brain therefore can provide information not only about task-related activity, but also about the connectivity among brain regions.

Recent fMRI studies have shown that low-frequency physiological fluctuations ($<$0.08 Hz, or $<$4.8 cycles per minute) are temporally correlated between functionally related areas (such as motor, auditory, and visual regions) and are therefore deemed to reflect underlying connectivity, possibly through numerous synaptic connections (87–89). Detecting and quantifying these low-frequency correlations in functional imaging data, however, is challenging. Several new mathematical algorithms, such as clustering analyses based on self-organized maps (SOMs), artificial neural networks (ANNs), principal component analysis (PCA), and independent component analysis (ICA), have been proposed for exploring the interregional connectivity of brain functioning either at rest or during

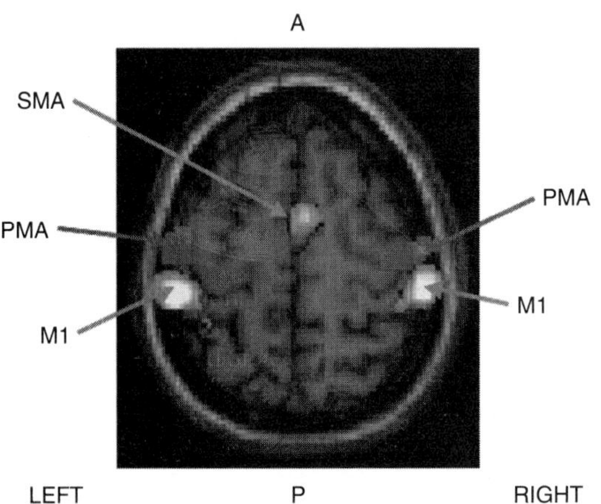

FIGURE 2.4.1.14. Functional connectivity map from a simple finger tapping task. Primary motor area (M1) and supplementary motor area (SMA) are depicted in red, the premotor area (PMA) in blue. (See color insert.)

performance of a cognitive task. Using the map of regions that are functionally connected, DTI fiber tacking can then be used to study the extent to which these regions are also anatomically connected (Figures 2.4.1.14 and 2.4.1.15).

Applications

Methods for measuring functional connectivity have been used increasingly in psychiatry to study disturbances in underlying brain circuitry that are associated with psychiatric disorders. Patients with schizophrenia and their siblings, for example, have been shown to have significantly reduced functional connectivity between frontal and temporal regions as assessed using the coherence of EEG recordings (90). Using fMRI and PET, others have found abnormal connectivity of the amygdala across hemispheres in depressed subjects, suggesting the presence of dysfunctional interactions of frontal cortices with the amygdala (91).

Data-driven methods for the analysis of fMRI signal, such as ICA, can identify functional connectivity in subjects at rest, therefore obviating the usual need to perform a cognitive task in studies of brain function (89, 92). These methods offer the promise of studying functional brain connectivity in studies even of very young children, who have difficulty performing a cognitive task in the scanner.

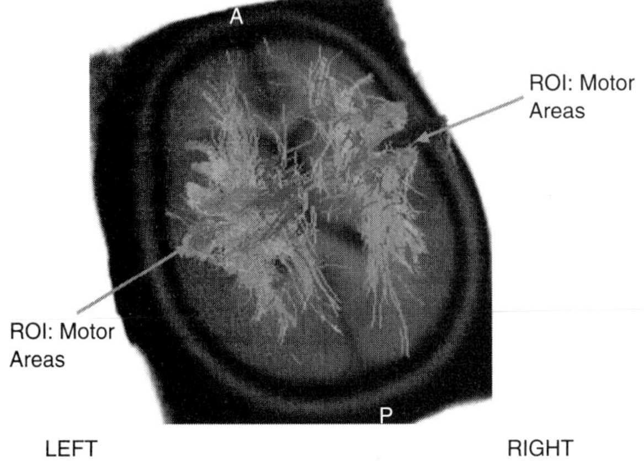

FIGURE 2.4.1.15. Fiber tracks based on the functional connectivity map shown in Figure 2.4.1.14 (ROI = regions of interest). (See color insert.)

Multimodal MRI

Multimodal MRI incorporates data for individual subjects from two or more MRI modalities. Because each imaging modality provides unique information concerning brain structure and function, data from differing modalities are complementary and mutually informative. In combination, these data help to constrain interpretations regarding the neural basis of developmental psychopathologies, thereby improving the neurobiological validity of those interpretations (7, 93–96). Anatomical MRI, for example, provides high-resolution images of brain structure, which can then serve as the basis for anatomical mapping of the neuronal activations detected by fMRI, the white matter fiber pathways studied with DTI, or the concentrations of neurochemicals measured with MRS. The processing of multimodal imaging data, however, involves three major challenges: coregistration, identification of the regions to be studied, and the valid and efficient display of information in this multidimensional variable space.

Coregistration

The combination of multiple imaging modalities requires that data from differing modalities be coregistered, i.e., aligned within a common "template space," such that corresponding points between images from different modalities lie in the same, or nearly the same, spatial position. However, coregistering images from various modalities can be difficult because images from those modalities differ significantly in many respects, including, but not limited to, their contrast, resolution, and SNR. For example, T1-weighted and T2-weighted images (two types of anatomical images) show the same brain tissues in very different levels of brightness and contrast. Moreover, anatomical images consist solely of scalar values at each voxel, whereas DT images contain a three-dimensional mathematical matrix at each voxel. And unlike data from other modalities, fMRI data are four-dimensional, containing both spatial and temporal information.

Coregistration typically entails the acquisition of a high-resolution, T1-weighted MR image that corresponds in alignment with an image acquired in another modality. This T1-weighted image is then normalized (i.e., a combination of coregistration plus a manipulation or "warping" of the image "matches up" corresponding points between images of each modality) to a predesignated (usually a T1-weighted) template image. This normalization process generates a "deformation field" that defines mathematically how the T1-weighted image was warped to fit the template brain. Because the T1-weighted image aligns with the corresponding image from another modality (e.g., a DT image), the deformation field obtained by normalizing the T1-weighted image to the template image can then be applied to the image from that other modality as well, thereby coregistering it to the template. Coregistration methods usually operate on the basis of matching, on a voxel-by-voxel basis, the gray-scale intensities of the images from each of the modalities (7).

Exploring Specific Regions of Interest (ROIs)

Used in tandem, images from one modality can be useful in defining ROIs required for study in another modality. For example, fMRI can be used to identify the functional fields of activation associated with a particular behavioral task, and the corresponding anatomical MRI images can then be used to identify the neuroanatomical location of those activations. Those activations can then serve as ROIs for "seed points" (starting points) in DTI-based tracking of the anatomical connectivity of those activations. DTI can similarly help to determine whether anatomical disturbances in multiple brain regions (detected using anatomical MRI) are associated with underlying disturbances in anatomical connectivity between those regions, and thus whether abnormalities in differing brain regions are anatomically related (94). In addition, MRS can help to determine whether differences in regional volumes and their associated disturbances in anatomical connectivity are likely associated with disturbances in the health or number of neurons, or with disturbances in levels of neurotransmitters, such as glutamate or GABA, in those regions.

Information Display

Graphical representation, or "visualization," of coregistered, multimodal imaging data is one of the most effective ways to explore the massive amount of information contained in these datasets. Visualization provides great insight into the nature of the correlations between information from the various MRI modalities. However, because the brain contains many functionally independent and dependent subregions, as well as a vast number of nerve fibers and metabolites, visualizing the massive amount of data that can be gleaned from multimodal imaging requires a strategic approach to selecting what will and will not be displayed. If all information from a multimodal dataset were displayed without discrimination, the resulting visualization would be unwieldy, with features of interest buried among details of less significance. Moreover, differences in resolution between modalities must be considered during the process of visualization. For example, voxel sizes vary widely between modalities (approximately 1 mm^3 in anatomical MRI, 2–5 mm^3 in DTI[6], 50-100 mm^3 in fMRI, and 1000–2000 mm^3 in MRS). These differences in resolution pose challenges for the interpretation and visualization of data across modalities because data from a larger voxel of one modality, if displayed together with higher resolution data from multiple, smaller voxels in another modality, may give the false impression that such data are of high resolution and that its measures are thus of a constant value across those multiple, smaller voxels.

Visualization can be effected using basic two-dimensional (2D) slice displays or more advanced three-dimensional (3D) graphic renderings. Displays of overlaid 2D slices can reveal correlations between data from differing modalities by showing merged data on a slice-by-slice basis. Graphic displays in 3D can show the spatial relationship between data across modalities using either surface or volume rendering techniques. Measures of brain structure, function, and chemical concentrations can be mapped onto anatomical data and displayed together using a surface definition of key brain components. On an even more sophisticated level, volume rendering can display the coregistered multimodal data as a semitransparent gel. To extract and display the information that is most relevant to investigators, a carefully designed schema should be used to determine at each region which modalities provide data that are potentially more correlated with other data and that are thus most likely to be responsible for the abnormality or neural function under investigation. Modalities thus selected can be modified during interactive navigation. Using visual inspection to identify ROIs that contain global associations of data between modalities, one can initiate more localized analyses of the intercorrelations of interest.

Illustration

We first identified disturbances in the anatomical MRIs of a group of 22 patients with Tourette syndrome (TS) compared with 25 normal control subjects, aged 10 to 17 years. These regional abnormalities were then used as ROI seed points for fiber tracking with DTI and a subsequent analysis of connectivity (94). An automated procedure first identified morphological differences between groups in spatially normalized, T1-weighted anatomical images, and those regions

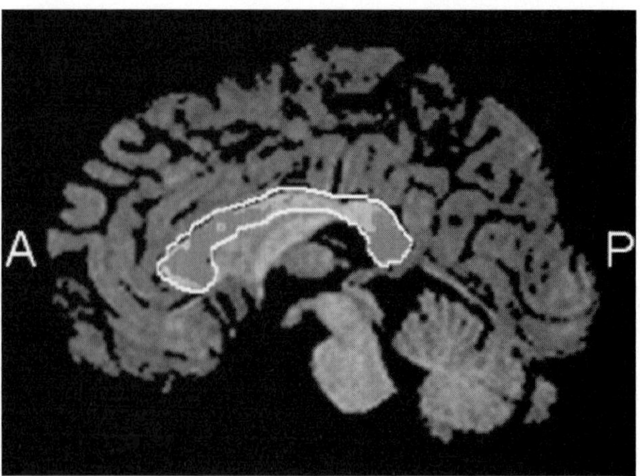

FIGURE 2.4.1.16. Volume difference identified statistically on midsagittal slices. The ROIs (shown in pink) in the corpus callosum (CC) are the regions where the CC in the TS group is smaller than in the control group. These ROIs are used for fiber tracking in DTI data (A = anterior; P = posterior). (See color insert.)

within the corpus callosum served as the a priori seed points for the tracking of a subset of all fibers within the brain. Approximately 362 fibers in the TS group and 292 in the control groups were tracked (Figures 2.4.1.16 and 2.4.1.17), and several regions of differing trajectories of fiber tracts were identified across groups, suggesting that not only are the brains of the children with TS anatomically abnormal, but also the fiber connections arising from those regions (Figures 2.4.1.18 and 2.4.1.19).

NON–MRI-BASED TECHNIQUES FOR FUNCTIONAL IMAGING

Electroencephalography

Recent advances in the technology of applied electroencephalography (EEG) have moved this imaging modality from being a largely clinical tool to one that is useful for research. The attraction of EEG has always been its ability to measure brain electrical activity directly, and therefore neuronal activity directly, rather than some more distant proxy for neuronal activity, such as the regional relative metabolic rate (in PET), blood flow (PET and SPECT), or deoxyhemoglobin (fMRI). Moreover, the millisecond temporal resolution of EEG, which is far superior to that of other imaging modalities, is on the time scale of the firing of individual neurons. The greatest limitation of EEG has always been its poor spatial resolution, which is caused by the blurring of the EEG signal across electrodes by differences in conductivity of the highly resistive skull, as well as CSF and other tissues. The spatial resolution that can be obtained with EEG has been improved considerably by the use of more than 100 scalp electrodes (spaced less than 2.5 cm apart), compared with the more standard clinical 16 or 32 electrode array (spaced 6 cm apart). This higher density of electrode recordings has been combined with other imaging modalities, such as anatomical and functional MRI, improving the mathematical modeling of tissue conductivity to "deblur" the EEG signal measured at the scalp (97) and to constrain the mathematical solution of the "inverse problem" required for the localization of the source of EEG activity (98, 99).

In principle, EEG is a relatively inexpensive imaging modality, although it is much more expensive if MRI is used to improve source localization. In contrast to other

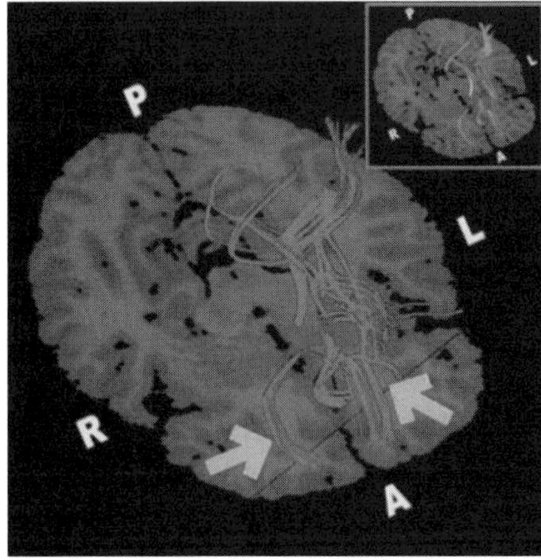

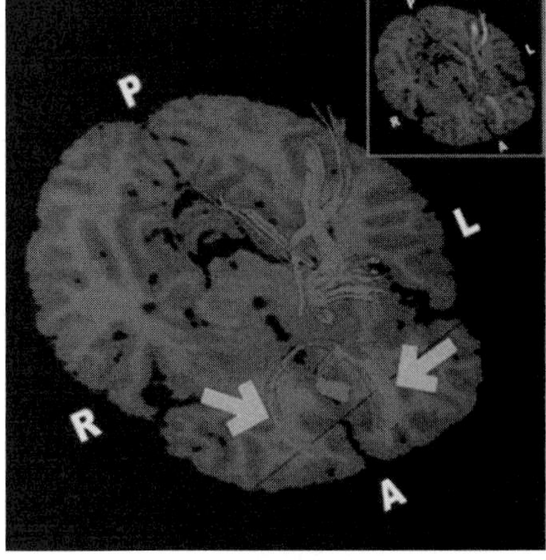

FIGURE 2.4.1.17. Fiber tracts based on the ROIs from Figure 2.4.1.16, viewed from above and superimposed on one axial slice of the template brain. The normal control group is shown on the left and the TS group on the right. At the tips of the light blue arrows, fibers grow downward from superior to inferior (i.e., below the translucent axial slice). In the insets, fibers are colored in accordance with their running directions: red for anterior–posterior; green for superior–inferior; blue for left–right. A = anterior; P = posterior; L = left; R = right. (See color insert.)

imaging modalities, EEG avoids the expense and problems associated with special shielding, cyclotrons, or radioisotopes needed for other imaging modalities. The major disadvantage of EEG—the blurring of EEG signal by the skull, CSF, and connective tissues—is not overcome entirely yet by the methodologies of high-resolution EEG, so that its current limit in resolution (several centimeters) is still inferior to that of most other imaging modalities. Moreover, the localization of EEG signal is seriously constrained by the assumption of a single source of brain activity associated with a cognitive task at any one point in time. This assumption seems implausible at its face value in that it requires the brain to be a purely serial processor, even for higher cognitive tasks. This assumption would appear to be more valid for the early components of the EEG signal, compared with its longer latency features. Furthermore, the underlying sources identified for any given surface EEG recording are not unique, so that identification of the most probable source is something of an art, one that requires the invocation of numerous assumptions and constraints. The resistance of the skull and other intervening tissues also interferes with hemispheric localization of the EEG signal. Moreover, the EEG signal is sensitive to motion artifact, which is always a problem with ill children. Finally, application of the many electrodes required for high-resolution EEG can be difficult, although newer electrode caps have reduced this difficulty considerably.

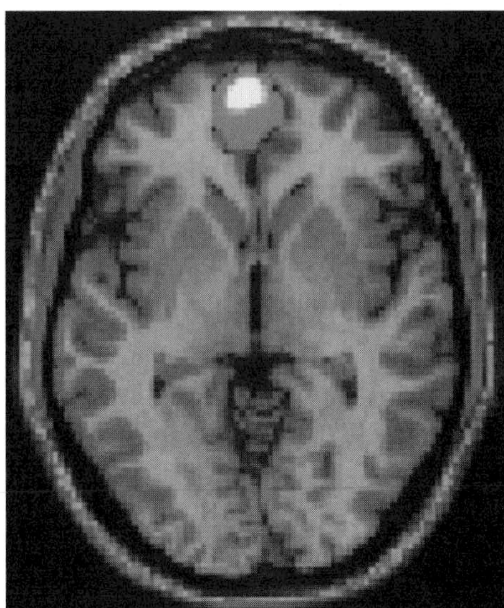

FIGURE 2.4.1.18. Activation of the cingulum identified using independent component analysis (ICA) as ROIs (shown in red and yellow) from fMRI data, superimposed on a coregistered DTI template, and used as seeds for fiber tracking in DTI data. (See color insert.)

Magnetoencephalography

Every electrical current has associated with it a magnetic field, and therefore the electrical currents in the brain produce magnetic fields that can be measured. Magnetoencephalography (MEG) measures extracranial magnetic fields produced by the intraneuronal ionic current flow within appropriately oriented cortical pyramidal cells. MEG is therefore the only imaging modality available that provides a quantitative index of intraneuronal current flow (as opposed to the extraneuronal current flow measured using EEG). MEG can record up to several hundred channels simultaneously without the nuisance of using scalp electrodes. MEG is less vulnerable than EEG to the conductance effects of intervening media such as skull, CSF, air, and other tissues; it therefore provides less blurring and better hemispheric localization than does EEG. With an accuracy of localization of 2–5 mm, MEG also provides better spatial resolution than does EEG, and it has a similarly excellent temporal resolution (<1 msec). As MEG does not require the use of scalp electrodes, it is less prone than EEG to motion artifact from the scalp.

MEG shares several disadvantages with EEG, including the inability to measure activity in subcortical structures, the constraint of assuming a single source of brain activity at any instant in time, and the nonuniqueness of the solutions for localizing sources of MEG activity. As with high-resolution EEG, coregistered MRIs can help to constrain the solutions for source localization. The unique disadvantage of MEG compared with EEG is that MEG hardware is extremely expensive, and it requires a magnetically shielded room, adding to the expense and hindering the feasibility of this imaging modality. Despite these limitations, the advantages of MEG make it a rapidly growing and increasingly popular functional imaging modality.

STATISTICAL ISSUES

Statistical methods for the analysis of MRI data remain largely underdeveloped because of practical constraints and associated

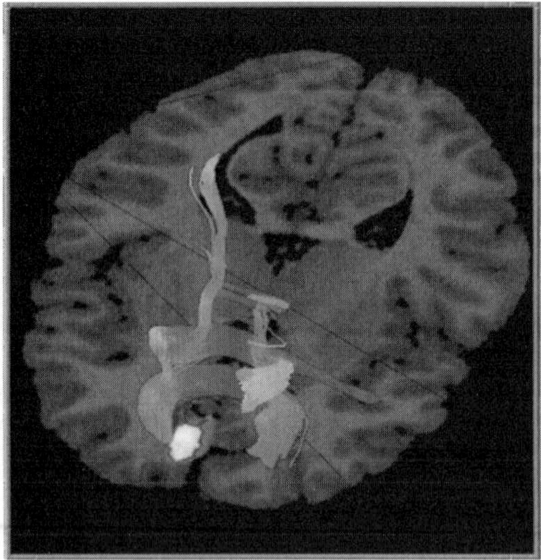

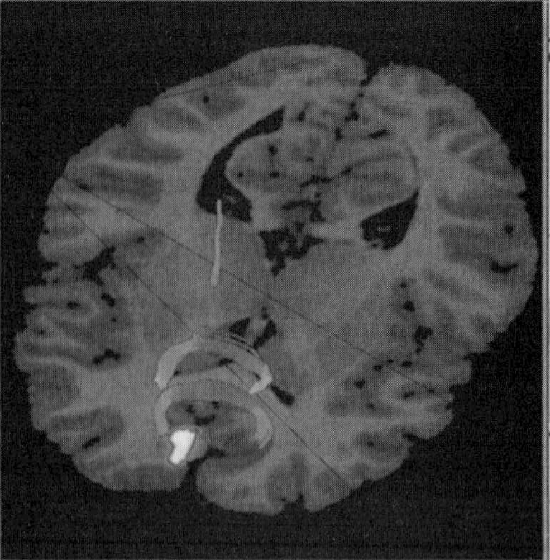

FIGURE 2.4.1.19. Fibers in ROIs from two groups: L = normal control; R = TS. For the normal control group, 3,612 fiber tracts were longer than 50 mm. In contrast, for the TS group, only 48 fiber tracts were longer than 50 mm, 342 tracts longer than 30 mm, and 498 tracts longer than 20 mm. (See color insert.)

theoretical difficulties. The first practical constraint is the small sample size (less than 20 subjects) used for many imaging studies. A small sample size not only eliminates many statistical tools (test statistics) that presuppose a large sample size (greater than 100), but it also produces poor reproducibility of findings, particularly because of the high intersubject variability of imaging data. A second practical constraint is the sheer quantity of data generated in imaging datasets. For instance, a typical fMRI experiment with 30 subjects will acquire several hundred to several thousand images for each subject, and each image contains approximately 100,000 voxels and a corresponding number of data points—thus totaling billions of data points in an entire study. Analyzing a vast amount of imaging data eliminates the possibility of applying more sophisticated statistical methods that detect, for example, complex spatial and temporal correlations, because of the sheer computational intensity that this would involve. A third practical constraint is the complexity of imaging data itself—for example, the high-dimensional information encoded in DT images greatly complicates its statistical analysis. Although comparing diffusion tensors across groups (e.g., healthy controls and patients) can be accomplished by treating each diffusion tensor as a single point in an abstract space, called a *manifold*, this requires a highly advanced knowledge of statistics and mathematics. Moreover, special care must be taken in the statistical analyses to account for imaging data that generally are highly intercorrelated across space and time.

Anatomical MRI Data

Two important considerations in the statistical analysis of anatomical MRI data are accounting for morphological scaling and the intercorrelation among regional brain volumes. "Scaling" refers to the ubiquitous correlation of brain size with body size, and the ubiquitous correlations of the sizes of subregions in the brain with overall brain size (100). Compared with women, for instance, men on average have larger brains, and this difference in brain size is primarily attributable to larger body size. Thus, any statistical analysis of volumetric data should take into account scaling effects, although how best to account for scaling effects remains controversial (101, 102). Moreover, because regional volumes within the same brains are intercorrelated, any statistical analysis of multiple regions should account for these intercorrelations using such procedures as linear mixed models with repeated measures over a spatial domain.

fMRI Data

Statistical methods for fMRI data must take into account two important noise characteristics, the spatial and temporal autocorrelation of the fMRI time series. "Spatial correlation" refers to the intercorrelation of the signal intensities of the fMRI time series across neighboring voxels, which may derive from the presence of multiple voxels within a single biological field of activation (e.g., the multiple voxels within Brodmann's area) (103) or simply derive from the inherent physical limitations of the scanning process and the construction of the image itself. Regardless of its cause, the presence of intercorrelation across voxels violates common statistical assumptions concerning the independence of observations in the dataset. Specific statistical methods, including Markov random fields, can be used to account for spatial autocorrelation, but the computations involved are enormous (104). To complicate matters further, fMRI data are also correlated across time within voxels, the degree of which may differ across the brain. Autoregressive modeling is the most popular statistical tool for handling autocorrelation in fMRI data (105). Properly accounting for spatial and temporal correlation improves the detection of neuronal activation associated with experimental tasks.

Multiple Comparisons

A central goal of imaging brain structure and function is to identify brain regions that are differentially associated with a response or covariate of interest, such as diagnosis, behavioral task, severity of disease, age, or IQ. Testing these associations across multiple brain regions or across the many voxels of the imaging volume involves multiple statistical comparisons. For instance, in an fMRI study, 100,000 statistical tests are usually performed simultaneously. However, when conducting these numerous tests, one must control for false positive, or Type I, errors as well as for false negative, or Type II, errors. When 100,000 tests are performed simultaneously at a significance level of 5 percent, 5,000 (= 100,000 × 0.05) false positive findings would be expected on the basis of chance alone. Procedures for controlling Type I error rate when performing multiple comparisons include use of single-step procedures, step-up and step-down procedures, random field theory, false discovery rates, and resampling methods (106–109).

PRACTICAL, METHODOLOGICAL, AND CONCEPTUAL CHALLENGES IN PEDIATRIC IMAGING STUDIES

Despite the major technological advances in the ability to measure brain structure, function, metabolites and fiber tracts, the successful scanning of children requires addressing adequately a wide variety of practical problems. Even healthy children, for example, find it difficult to remain still during a scanning session, and this difficulty is only compounded by the presence of hyperactivity, fidgetiness, anxiety, and impaired impulse control in children who have psychiatric illnesses. These difficulties can be addressed by (1) adequately preparing children for the procedures prior to and during the scan, (2) providing a calm setting with familiar faces at the scanning session, and (3) use of techniques for relaxing and desensitizing the children to the scanning environment, including the use of a mock scanner. In younger children, scanning during sleep is frequently advantageous and can be facilitated by scanning children at night. Because of the difficulty in acquiring data that are free of motion artifact and the possibility that such artifact may systematically affect data quality in ill, compared with healthier children, raw data should be evaluated blindly for quality, across diagnostic groups to rule out the presence of these systematic group differences.

In addition to the practical challenges of scanning children, many methodological and conceptual issues make difficult the valid interpretation of imaging data. For example, measurements obtained with MRI tell us more about macroscopic features of brain structure and activity than about its ultrastructural features (the number of neurons or axons, their anatomical connectivity, or connectivity of the cellular elements in a tissue). FMRI signals, for example, are averaged together from the change in blood oxygenation that is associated with the activity of all synapses within a voxel. Projections to and from neurons in other brain regions, however, also contribute to the averaged signal that supposedly represents the activity in that particular voxel.

Another interpretive challenge inherent to imaging data is determining the exact location of a given measurement in the brain. To overcome this problem of localization, gray-scale information is often used to identify cortical sulci and to define ROIs (110). These sulci are assumed to represent the borders of specific cytoarchitectural units (14); however, the spatial extent of these units does not always follow sulcal boundaries (17, 18). Another method of localization, planar stereotaxy, uses anatomical landmarks to define ROIs, yet this method is a crude approximation of underlying cytoarchitecture. Moreover, the assumption that these landmarks conform in an invariant spatial relationship to other brain areas has not been tested formally (111).

In all imaging studies, a major challenge is distinguishing the cause of an illness from possible compensatory effects. The presence of debilitating symptoms from chronic illness likely causes adaptive changes to neural systems throughout the brain, and these changes are often difficult to distinguish from the events that may cause the symptoms in the first place (112). This issue is particularly relevant in cross-sectional designs, the most common type of study reported in the imaging literature. Group differences between affected and unaffected individuals are often interpreted as representing an abnormality in the patient group that is causally linked to the disease. Cross-sectional findings, however, preclude us from distinguishing cause from effect: Is the group difference a precipitating factor or a consequence of the disorder? Larger volumes of a particular brain structure in a patient group, for example, could represent a compensatory effect of illness, such as the need to rely on that structure to suppress symptoms. In clinical groups, correlations of deviations in brain morphology with symptom severity can help to disentangle causes from compensatory effects (113–115).

A challenge particular to pediatric imaging is interpreting cross-sectional imaging studies from a developmental perspective. These interpretations are often made under the false assumption that members of younger age cohorts will eventually resemble their older counterparts who have the same biological illness. Most childhood illnesses, however, differ from their adult counterparts in clinical phenotype, associated comorbidities, and natural history. Thus cross-sectional studies can lead us to misunderstand the developmental correlates of an illness (116, 117). Longitudinal brain imaging studies of affected individuals are often favored for tracking changes in brain structure and function over time. Interpretations of findings from longitudinal studies, however, are similarly limited by the difficulty of distinguishing cause from consequence, although compensatory effects may be detected more easily in this kind of design. Assessing associations of imaging measures with the exacerbation or remission of symptoms over time, for example, cannot prove whether the brain changes caused the changes in symptoms, or whether the changes in symptoms caused the changes in the brain properties being measured (117–119).

The high frequency of comorbid conditions in children with neuropsychiatric disorders raises another challenge to studying these disorders. Comorbidity can be accounted for by including covariates for comorbid conditions and by testing their influence on the outcome measures. An alternative approach is to build a pure group of the experimental condition and distinct samples of patients with coexisting conditions and then compare the individuals in these groups with their healthy control counterparts.

Potential Solutions to These Challenges

Possible solutions to these conceptual challenges do exist; however, undertaking them can be both costly and time consuming. Extending imaging studies to progressively younger or high-risk cohorts would be an ideal approach for disentangling causes from compensatory effects. Studies of young children who are at risk for certain illnesses would permit identification of trait markers for disease vulnerability that, in the absence of symptoms, are independent of the compensatory effects of having a given illness. Prospective longitudinal studies that involve scanning high-risk samples at multiple time points would enable us to identify the switches from trait vulnerabilities to state disturbances while, at the same time, allowing the study of these disturbances early in their course. By comparing these early disturbances with those that occur during illness onset and progression, we could determine how compensatory mechanisms may exert their effects on brain structure and function, and ultimately distinguish these effects from the neurobiological causes of the illness.

Another possible, albeit difficult, solution involves studying gene–brain–behavior correlations in both healthy and ill children. Determining the morphological and functional correlates in the human brain of genetic variants would allow us to assess whether genotypes correlate with measures of brain morphology and brain function as measured by both imaging and neuropsychological testing (120). Combining these measures could, in turn, account more powerfully for individual and group differences in behavior both within and across clinical diagnostic groups than do either measure alone. Both genetic and environmentally based disturbances likely contribute to the pathophysiology of many childhood neuropsychiatric illnesses. Thus studying gene–brain–behavior correlations would allow us to identify better the pathophysiologic mechanisms that determine the presence of childhood disorders and, eventually, distinguish their causes from the neuroplastic and compensatory responses that contribute to either the attenuation or remission of symptoms. However, despite the virtually universal recognition of the importance of studying the roles of genes, environment, and their interactions in determining brain structure and function, very few in vivo human studies have assessed these associations formally.

A third possible solution is to yoke imaging studies to clinical trials while experimentally controlling and manipulating a potentially causal variable. The use of appropriately designed experiments with appropriate contrast groups and a sufficiently large sample would allow any treatment-specific neurobiological effects to be distinguished from the effects that are associated with the mere presence of an illness. The brain-based effects of a given medication, when assessed in a clinical trial that includes a placebo control group of children, for example, would be discernible from the compensatory neurobiological effects of the spontaneous remission of symptoms that arises with development.

The growing number of brain imaging modalities that can be applied safely in children offers the exciting promise of rapidly improving our knowledge of pediatric brain structure and function in health and illness in the years and decades to come. Technological advances that allow the acquisition of multiple imaging modalities within the same children will enable us to begin identifying the correlates of brain structure, function, behavior, and ultimately clinical phenotype within and across individuals. Although practical, methodological, and conceptual challenges to pediatric neuroimaging exist, we have enumerated some experimental approaches as possible solutions that will likely allow further progress in understanding normative developmental processes and in understanding the etiologies and pathophysiologies of developmental disorders.

ACKNOWLEDGMENTS

This work was supported in part by NIMH grants MH36197, MH068318, K02-74677, 1T32MH16434, and 5T32MH18264, and NIDA grant DA017820, as well as by the Suzanne Crosby Murphy Endowment at Columbia University Medical Center and the Thomas D. Klingenstein and Nancy D. Perlman Family Fund.

References

1. Ernst M, Freed ME, Zametkin AJ: Health hazards of radiation exposure in the context of brain imaging research: Special consideration for children. *J Nucl Med* Apr 1998: 39(4):689–98.
2. Zametkin A, Liotta W: The future of brain imaging in child psychiatry. *Child and Adolescent Psychiatric Clinics of North America* 6:447–460, 1997.
3. Arnold JB, Liow J-S, Schaper KA, Stern JJ, Sled JG, Shattuck DW, et al.: Qualitative and quantitative evaluation of six algorithms for correcting intensity nonuniformity effects. *Neuroimage* 13:931–943, 2001.
4. Sled JG, Zijdenbos AP, Evans AC: A nonparametric method for automatic correction of intensity nonuniformity in MRI data. *IEEE Trans Med Imaging* Feb 1998: 17(1):87–97.
5. Clarke LP, Velthuizen RP, Camacho MA, Heine JJ, Vaidyanathan M, Hall LO, et al.: MRI segmentation: Methods and applications. *Magn Reson Imaging* 13:343–368, 1995.
6. Pham DL, Xu C, Prince JL: Current methods in medical image segmentation. *Annual Review of Biomedical Engineering* 2:315–337, 2000.
7. Viergever MA, Maintz JB, Niessen WJ, Noordmans HJ, Pluim JP, Stokking R, et al. Registration, segmentation, and visualization of multimodal brain images. *Comput Med Imaging Graph* Mar–Apr 2001: 25(2):147–151.
8. Bezdek J, Hall L, Clarke L: Review of MR image segmentation techniques using pattern recognition. *Med Phys* 20(4):1033–1048, 1993.
9. Lim KO, Pfferbaum A: Segmentation of MR brain images into cerebrospinal fluid spaces, white and gray matter. *J Computer Assisted Tomography* 13(4):588–593, 1989.
10. Rigau J, Feixas M, Sbert M, Bardera A, Boada I: Medical image segmentation based on mutual information maximization. In: Barillot C, Haynor DR, Hellier P (eds).: *Med Image Computing and Computer Assisted Interventions*; Berlin, Springer-Verlag, 2004, pp. 135–142.
11. Sethi IK, Sarvarayudu GPR: Hierarchical classifier design using mutual information. *IEEE Transactions on Pattern Analysis and Machine Intelligence* 4(4):441–445, 1982.
12. Wells WM, Grimson WEL, Kikinis R, Jolesz FA: Adaptive Segmentation of MRI Data. *IEEE Trans on Medical Imaging* 15(4):429–442, 1996.
13. Caviness VSJ, Meyer J, Makris N, Kennedy DN: MRI-based topographic parcellation of human neocortex: An anatomically specified method with estimate of reliability. *J Cogn Neurosci* 8:566–587, 1996.
14. Brodmann K: *Vergleichende Lokalisationslehre der Grosshirnrinde*. Leipzig, Barth, 1909.
15. Braak H: *Architectonics of the Human Telencephalic Cortex*. Berlin, Springer-Verlag, 1980.
16. Flechsig P: *Anatomie des menschlichen Gehirns und Rückenmarks auf myelogenetischer Grundlage*. Leipzig, G. Thieme, 1920.
17. Dabringhaus A, Schormann T, Steinmetz H, Schlaug G, Zilles K, Roland PE: What is a standard brain? Intersubject variability of the shape of the human forebrain. *Human Brain Mapping* 1:64, 1995.
18. Zilles K, Schleicher A, Langemann C, et al.: Quantitative analysis of sulci in the human cerebral cortex: Development, regional heterogeneity, gender difference, asymmetry, intersubject variability, and cortical architecture. *Human Brain Mapping* 5:218–221, 1997.
19. Andreasen NC, Flashman L, Flaum M, Arndt S, Swayze Vn, O'Leary DS, et al.: Regional brain abnormalities in schizophrenia measured with magnetic resonance imaging. *JAMA* 272(22):1763–1769, 1994.
20. Kates WR, Warsofsky IS, Patwardhan A, Abrams MT, Liu AM, Naidu S, et al.: Automated Talairach atlas-based parcellation and measurement of cerebral lobes in children. *Psychiatry Research* 91(1):11–30, 1999.
21. Peterson BS, Staib L, Scahill L, Zhang H, Anderson C, Leckman JF, et al.: Regional brain and ventricular volumes in Tourette syndrome. *Arch Gen Psychiatry* 58(5):427–440, 2001.
22. Collins D, Zijdenbos A, Barre W, Evans A: Animal + insect: Improved cortical structure segmentation. *Information Processing in Medical Imaging* 1999; 1613.
23. Cootes TF, Hill A, Taylor CJ, Haslam J: The use of active shape models for locating structures in medical imaging. Information Processing in Medical Imaging; 1993; Flagstaff, USA: 1993. p. 33–47.
24. Cootes TF, Taylor CJ, Cooper DH, Graham J: Training models of shape from sets of examples. *Proceedings of British Machine Vision Conference* 1992:9–18.
25. Fischl B, Kouwe Avd, Destrieux C, Halgren E, Sgonne F, Salat D, et al.: Automatically parcellating the human cerebral cortex. *Cerebral Cortex* 14:11–22, 2004.
26. Kass M, Witkin A, Terzopoulos D: Snakes: Active contour models. *Int J Comp Vision* 1:321–331, 1988.
27. Leventon M, Grimson W, Faugeras O: Statistical shape influence in geodesic active contours. *Computer Vision and Pattern Recognition* 2000:1316–1323.
28. Staib LH, Duncan JS: Boundary finding with parametrically deformable models. *IEEE Trans Pattern Anal Machine Intell* 14:1061–1075, 1992.
29. Staib LH, Duncan JS: Boundary finding with parametrically deformable models. *IEEE Trans Pattern Anal Machine Intell* 14:1061–1075, 1992.
30. Terzopoulos D, Metaxas D: Dynamic 3-D models with local and global deformations: Deformable superquadrics. *IEEE Pattern Analysis and Machine Analysis* 13:703–14, 1991.
31. Vemuri BC, Radisavljevic A: Multiresolution stochastic hybrid shape models with fractal priors. *ACM Trans Graphics* 13:177–200, 1994.
32. Wen SW, Smith G, Yang Q, Walker M: Epidemiology of preterm birth and neonatal outcome. *Semin Fetal Neonatal Med* 9(6):429–435, Dec: 2004.
33. Caviness VSJ, Meyer J, Makris N, Kennedy DN: MRI-based topographic parcellation of human neocortex: An anatomically specified method with estimate of reliability. *J Cogn Neurosci* 8:566–587, 1996.
34. Le Goualher G, Procyk E, Collins DL, Venugopal R, Barillot C, Evans AC: Automated extraction and variability analysis of sulcal neuroanatomy. *IEEE Transactions on Medical Imaging* 18(3):206–217, 1999.
35. MacDonald D, Kabani N, Avis D, Evans AC: Automated 3-D extraction of inner and outer surfaces of cerebral cortex from MRI. *Neuroimage* 12(3):340–356, 2000.
36. Toga AW, Thompson PM: New approaches in brain morphometry. *American Journal of Geriatric Psychiatry* 10(1):13–23, 2002.
37. Zilles K, Kawashima R, Dabringhaus A, Fukuda H, Schormann T: Hemispheric shape of European and Japanese brains: 3-D MRI analysis of intersubject variability, ethnical and gender differences. *Neuroimage* 13:262–271, 2001.

38. Anderson JLR, Sundin A, Valind S: A method for coregistration of PET and MR brain images. *J of Nuclear Medicine* 36:1307–1315, 1995.
39. Arun KS, Huang TS, Blostein SD: Least-squares fitting of two 3-D point sets. *IEEE Trans on Pattern Analysis and Machine Intelligence* 5:698–700, 1987.
40. Ayache N, Gueziec A, Thirion J, Gourdon A, Knoplioch J: Evaluating 3D registration of CT-scan images using crest lines. In: Wilson DC, Wilson JN (eds.): *Mathematical Methods in Medical Imaging*. Bellingham, WA: SPIE Press, 1993, pp. 60–71.
41. Bajcsy R, Lieberson R, Reivich M: A computerized system for the elastic matching of deformed radiographic images to idealized atlas images. *J of Computer Assisted Tomography* 7(4):618–625, 1983.
42. Barillot C, Lemoine D, le Bricquer L, Lachmann F, Gibaud B: Data fusion in medical imaging: Merging multimodal and multipatient images, identification of structures, and 3D display aspects. *European Journal of Radiology* 17:22–27, 1993.
43. Besl PJ, McKay ND: A method for registration of 3D shapes. *IEEE Trans on Pattern Analysis and Machine Intelligence* 14(2):239–256, 1992.
44. Christensen GE, Miller MI, Marsh JL, Vannier MW: Automatic Analysis of Medical Images Using a Deformable Textbook. Computer Assisted Radiology: Berlin, Springer-Verlag, 1995, pp. 146–151.
45. Collignon A, Maes F, Delaere D, Vandermeulen P, Seutens P, Mar G: Automated multimodality image registration using information theory. *Proceedings of the 14th International Conference* 1995:263–274.
46. Davatzikos C, Prince JL: Brain Image Registration Based on Curve Mapping. *IEEE Workshop on Biomedical Image Analysis*. Los Alamitos, CA, IEEE Computer Society Press; 1994, pp. 245–254.
47. Feldmar J, Ayache N: Rigid, affine and locally affine registration of free-form surfaces. *Int J Comp Vision* 18(2):99–119, 1996.
48. Gilhuijs KGA, van den Ven PJH, van Herk M: Automatic three-dimensional inspection of patient setup in radiation therapy using portal images, simulator images, and computed tomography data. *Medical Physics* 23(3):389–399, 1996.
49. Wells WM, Grimson WEL, Kikinis R, Jolesz FA: Adaptive segmentation of MRI data. *IEEE Trans Med Img* 15:429–442, 1996.
50. Lavallee S, Szeliski R, Brunie L: Anatomy-based registration of three-dimensional models using octree-splines. In: Taylor R, Lavallee S, Burdea GC, Mosges R (eds.): *Computer-Integrated Surgery, Technology and Clinical Applications*. Cambridge, MA: MIT Press, 1996. pp. 115–143.
51. Maes F, Collignon A, Vandermeulen D, Marchal G, Suetens P: Multimodal Image Registration by Maximizing Mutual Information. *Mathematical Methods in Biomedical Image Analysis*. Los Alamitos, CA, IEEE Computer Society Press, 1996. pp. 14–22.
52. Viola P, Wells WM: *Alignment by maximization of mutual information*. Int Conf on Computer Vision, 1995. Los Alamitos, CA, IEEE Computer Society Press, 1995 pp. 16–23.
53. Woods RP, Maziotta JC, Cherry SR: MRI-PET registration with automated algorithm. *J of Computer Assisted Tomography* 17(4):536–546, 1993.
54. Peterson BS: Neuroimaging studies of Tourette syndrome: A decade of progress. *Adv Neurol* 85:179–196, 2001.
55. Peterson BS, Staib L, Scahill L, Zhang H, Anderson C, Leckman JF, et al.: Regional brain and ventricular volumes in Tourette syndrome. *Arch Gen Psychiatry* May 2001: 58(5):427–440.
56. Thompson PM, Cannon TD, Narr KL, van Erp T, Poutanen VP, Huttunen M, et al.: Genetic influences on brain structure. *Nature Neuroscience* 4(12):1253–1258, 2001.
57. Hann DM, Huffman LC, Lederhendler II, Meinecke D (eds.): *Advancing Research on Developmental Plasticity: Integrating the Behavioral Science and Neuroscience of Mental Health*. Washington, DC, National Institute of Mental Health, 1998.
58. Buonomano DV, Merzenich MM: Cortical plasticity: From synapses to maps. *Annual Review of Neuroscience* 21:149–186, 1998.
59. Elbert T, Pantev C, Wienbruch C, Rockstroh B, Taub E: Increased cortical representation of the fingers of the left hand in string players. *Science* 270:305–307, 1995.
60. Belliveau JW, Kennedy DNJ, McKinstry RC, Buchbinder BR, Weisskoff RM, Cohen MS, et al.: Functional mapping of the human visual cortex by magnetic resonance imaging. *Science* 254:716–719, 1991.
61. Frackowiak RS: Functional mapping of verbal memory and language. *Trends Neurosci* Mar 1994: 17(3):109–115.
62. Nemeroff CB, Kilts CD, Berns GS: Functional brain imaging: Twenty-first century phrenology of psychological advance for the millennium? *Am J Psychiatry* 156:671–673, 1999.
63. Poeppel D: A critical review of PET studies of phonological processing. *Brain Lang* Dec 1996: 55(3):317–351, discussion 52–85.
64. Wexler BE: A model of brain function: Its implications for psychiatric research. *Br J Psychiatry* Apr 1986 148:357–362.
65. Sternberg S: The discovery of processing stages: Extensions of Donder's method. In: Koster W (ed): *Attention and Performance II*. Amsterdam: North-Holland Publishing Co, 1969.
66. Donders FC: On the speed of mental processes. *Acta Psychol (Amst)* 30:412–431, 1969.
67. Bandettini PA, Wong EC, Hinks RS, Tikofsky RS, Hyde JS: Time course EPI of human brain function during task activation. *Magn Reson Med* Jun 1992: 25(2):390–397.
68. Puce A, Allison T, Asgari M, Gore JC, McCarthy G: Differential sensitivity of human visual cortex to faces, letterstrings, and textures: A functional magnetic resonance imaging study. *J Neurosci* Aug 15 1996: 16(16):5205–5215.
69. Zarahn E, Aguirre G, D'Esposito M: A trial-based experimental design for fMRI. *Neuroimage* Aug 1997: 6(2):122–138.
70. McCarthy G, Luby M, Gore J, Goldman-Rakic P: Infrequent events transiently activate human prefrontal and parietal cortex as measured by functional MRI. *J Neurophysiol* Mar 1997: 77(3):1630–1634.
71. Talairach J, Tournoux P: *Co-planar Stereotaxic Atlas of the Human Brain*. New York, Thieme Medical Publishers, 1988.
72. Moseley ME, Cohen Y, Mintorovitch J, Chileuitt L, Shimizu H, Kucharczyk J, et al.: Early detection of regional cerebral ischemia in cats: Comparison of diffusion- and T2-weighted MRI and spectroscopy. *Magn Reson Med* May 1990: 14(2):330–346.
73. Werring DJ, Clark CA, Barker GJ, Thompson AJ, Miller DH: Diffusion tensor imaging of lesions and normal-appearing white matter in multiple sclerosis. *Neurology* May 12 1999: 52(8):1626–1632.
74. Buchsbaum MS, Tang CY, Peled S, Gudbjartsson H, Lu D, Hazlett EA, et al.: MRI white matter diffusion anisotropy and PET metabolic rate in schizophrenia. *Neuroreport* Feb 16 1998:9(3):425–430.
75. Foong J, Maier M, Clark CA, Barker GJ, Miller DH, Ron MA: Neuropathological abnormalities of the corpus callosum in schizophrenia: A diffusion tensor imaging study. *J Neurol Neurosurg Psychiatry* Feb: 2000 68(2):242–244.
76. Lim KO, Hedehus M, Moseley M, de Crespigny A, Sullivan EV, Pfefferbaum A: Compromised white matter tract integrity in schizophrenia inferred from diffusion tensor imaging. *Arch Gen Psychiatry* Apr 1999: 56(4):367–374.
77. Klingberg T, Hedehus M, Temple E, Salz T, Gabrieli JD, Moseley ME, et al.: Microstructure of temporo-parietal white matter as a basis for reading ability: Evidence from diffusion tensor magnetic resonance imaging. *Neuron* Feb 2000: 25(2):493–500.
78. Huppi PS, Maier SE, Peled S, Zientara GP, Barnes PD, Jolesz FA, et al.: Microstructural development of human newborn cerebral white matter assessed in vivo by diffusion tensor magnetic resonance imaging. *Pediatr Res* Oct 1998: 44(4):584–590.
79. Cecil KM, DelBello MP, Morey R, Strakowski SM: Frontal lobe differences in bipolar disorder as determined by proton MR spectroscopy. *Bipolar Disord* Dec 2002: 4(6):357–365.
80. Fayed N, Modrego PJ: Comparative study of cerebral white matter in autism and attention-deficit/hyperactivity disorder by means of magnetic resonance spectroscopy. *Acad Radiol* May 2005: 12(5):566–569.
81. Courvoisie H, Hooper SR, Fine C, Kwock L, Castillo M: Neurometabolic functioning and neuropsychological correlates in children with ADHD-H: Preliminary findings. *J Neuropsychiatry Clin Neurosci* Winter 2004: 16(1):63–69.
82. Moore CM, Biederman J, Wozniak J, Mick E, Aleardi M, Wardrop M, et al.: Differences in brain chemistry in children and adolescents with attention deficit hyperactivity disorder with and without comorbid bipolar disorder: A proton magnetic resonance spectroscopy study. *Am J Psychiatry* Feb 2006: 163(2):316–318.
83. Chang L, Cloak CC, Ernst T: Magnetic resonance spectroscopy studies of GABA in neuropsychiatric disorders. *J Clin Psychiatry* 64 Suppl 3:7–14, 2003.
84. Kim H, McGrath BM, Silverstone PH: A review of the possible relevance of inositol and the phosphatidylinositol second messenger system (PI-cycle) to psychiatric disorders—focus on magnetic resonance spectroscopy (MRS) studies. *Hum Psychopharmacol* Jul 2005: 20(5):309–326.
85. Friston K: Functional integration and inference in the brain. *Progress in Neurobiology* 68:113–143, 2002.
86. Huettel SA, Song, AW, McCarthy, G: *Magnetic Resonance Imaging*. Sinauer Associates Press, 2004.
87. Biswal B, Yetkin FZ, Haughton VM, Hyde JS: Functional connectivity in the motor cortex of resting human brain using echo-planar MRI. *Magn Reson Med* 34:537–541, 1995.
88. Lowe MJ, Mock, BJ, Sorenson, JA: Functional connectivity in single and multislice echo-planar imaging using resting-state fluctuations. *Neuroimage* 7:119–132, 1998.
89. Van de Ven VG, Formisano E, Prvulovic D, Christian HR, Linden DEJ: Functional connectivity as revealed by spatial independent component analysis of fMRI measurements during rest. *Human Brain Mapping* 22:165–178, 2004.
90. Winterer G CR, Egan MF, Goldberg TE, Weinberger DR: Functional and effective frontotemporal connectivity and genetic risk for schizophrenia. *Biol Psychiatry* 54(11):1181–1192, 2003.
91. Irwin W AM, Abercrombie HC, Schaefer SM, Kalin NH, Davidson RJ: Amygdalar interhemispheric functional connectivity differs between the non-depressed and depressed human brain. *Neuroimage* 21(2):674–686, 2004.
92. Greicius MD KB, Reiss AL, Menon V: Functional connectivity in the resting brain: A network analysis of the default mode hypothesis. *Proc Natl Acad Sci USA* 100(1):253–258, 2002.
93. Xu D, Wang Z, Bansal R, Plessen KJ, Peterson BS: An automated DTI study using fMRI data. *Human Brain Mapping*, In press.

94. Xu D, Hao Z, Bansal R, Plessen KJ, Geng WD, Peterson BS: Bridging anatomical MRI and DTI studies using volume preserved warping. *Journal of Magnetic Resonance Imaging*, submitted.
95. Krakow K, Wieshmann UC, Woermann FG, Symms MR, McLean MA, Lemieux L, et al.: Multimodal MR imaging: Functional, diffusion tensor, and chemical shift imaging in a patient with localization-related epilepsy. *Epilepsia* Oct 1999: 40(10):1459–1462.
96. Kidwell CS, Alger JR, Saver JL: Beyond mismatch: Evolving paradigms in imaging the ischemic penumbra with multimodal magnetic resonance imaging. *Stroke* Nov 2003: 34(11):2729–2735.
97. Gevins A, Le J, Leong H, McEvoy LK, Smith ME: Deblurring. *J Clin Neurophysiol* May 1999: 16(3):204–213.
98. Dale AM, Halgren E: Spatiotemporal mapping of brain activity by integration of multiple imaging modalities. *Curr Opin Neurobiol* Apr 2001: 11(2):202–208.
99. Gevins A, Le J, Brickett P, Reutter B, Desmond J: Seeing through the skull: Advanced EEGs use MRIs to accurately measure cortical activity from the scalp. *Brain Topogr* Winter 1991: 4(2):125–131.
100. Gould SJ: *The Mismeasure of Man*. New York, W.W.Norton, 1981.
101. Andreasen NC, Arndt S, Cohen G, Alliger R, Swayze VW: Correction for head size. *Psychiatry Research* 50:121–139, 1993.
102. Mathalon DH, Sullivan EV, Rawles JM, Pfefferbaum A: Correction for head size in brain imaging measurements. *Psychiatry Research: Neuroimaging* 50:121–139, 1993.
103. Roland PE: *Brain Activation*. New York, Wiley-Liss, 1993.
104. Gossl C, Auer DP, Fahrmeir L: Bayesian spatial-temporal inference in functional magnetic resonance imaging. *Biometrics* 57:554–562, 2001.
105. Worsley KJ, Liao C, Grabove M, Petre V, Ha B, Evans AC: A general statistical analysis for fMRI data. *NeuroImage* 15:1–15, 2002.
106. Shaffer JP: Multiple hypothesis testing: A review. *Annual Review of Psychology* 46:561–584, 1995.
107. Westfall PH, Young SS: *Resampling-Based Multiple Testing: Examples and Methods for p-Value Adjustment*. New York, Wiley, 1993.
108. Dudoit S, Shaffer JP, Boldrick JC: Multiple hypothesis testing in microarray experiments. *Statistical Science* 18:71–103, 2003.
109. Nichols T, Hayasaka S: Controlling the family-wise error rate in functional neuroimaging: A comparative review. *Stat Meth Med Res* 12:419–446, 2003.
110. Caviness VSJ, Meyer J, Makris N, Kennedy DN: MRI-based topographic parcellation of human neocortex: An anatomically specified method with estimate of reliability. *J Cogn Neurosci* 8:566–587, 1996.
111. Peterson BS, Staib L, Scahill L, Zhang H, Anderson C, Leckman JF, et al.: Regional brain and ventricular volumes in Tourette syndrome. *Arch Gen Psychiatry* 58:427–440, 2001.
112. Peterson BS: Conceptual, methodological, and statistical challenges in brain imaging studies of developmentally based psychopathologies. *Develop Psychopath* 15:811–832, 2003.
113. Peterson BS, Staib L, Scahill L, Zhang H, Anderson C, Leckman JF, et al.: Regional brain and ventricular volumes in Tourette syndrome. *Arch Gen Psychiatry* 58:427–440, 2001.
114. Peterson BS: Conceptual, methodological, and statistical challenges in brain imaging studies of developmentally based psychopathologies. *Develop Psychopath* 15:811–832, 2003.
115. Plessen KJ, Wentzel-Larsen T, Hugdahl K, Feineigle P, Klein J, Staib LH, et al.: Altered interhemispheric connectivity in individuals with Tourette's disorder. *Am J Psychiatry* Nov 2004: 161(11):2028–2037.
116. Kraemer HC, Yesavage JA, Taylor JL, Kupfer D: How can we learn about developmental processes from cross-sectional studies, or can we? *Am J Psychiatry* 157:163–171, 2000.
117. Gerard E, Peterson BS: Developmental processes and brain imaging studies in Tourette syndrome. *J Psychosom Res* Jul 2003: 55(1):13–22.
118. Peterson BS: Conceptual, methodological, and statistical challenges in brain imaging studies of developmentally based psychopathologies. *Develop Psychopath* 15:811–832, 2003.
119. Peterson BS, Thomas P: Functional brain imaging in Tourette's syndrome: What are we really imaging? In: Ernst M, Rumsey J (eds.): *Functional Neuroimaging in Child Psychiatry*. Cambridge, Cambridge University Press, 2000. pp. 242–265.
120. Gottesman, II, Gould TD: The endophenotype concept in psychiatry: Etymology and strategic intentions. *Am J Psychiatry* Apr 2003: 160(4): 636–645.

CHAPTER 2.4.2 ■ NEUROCHEMISTRY, PHARMACODYNAMICS, AND BIOLOGICAL PSYCHIATRY

GEORGE M. ANDERSON AND ANDRÉS MARTIN

INTRODUCTION

Continuing advances in basic neurobiology and psychopharmacology have led to a greatly expanded knowledge of brain functioning and hold the promise of better treatment and fuller understanding of childhood psychiatric disorders (1, 2). The recent elucidation of the genetic bases of a number of single-gene childhood psychiatric disorders provides additional hope, and to some extent directions, for tackling the more complex molecular and biological influences in autism, attention deficit/hyperactivity disorder (ADHD), Tourette syndrome, anxiety, posttraumatic stress disorder (PTSD), depression, and suicide. Identification of causative factors in Parkinson's disease, Huntington's disease and Alzheimer's disease further encourages the notion that the pharmacology of childhood psychiatric disorders can be made more rational and effective, and the biological bases of the relevant behaviors ascertained.

The three entwined areas of neurobiology, pharmacodynamics, and biological psychiatry can be introduced by first considering basic concepts in the separate realms of inquiry. Relevant neurobiology includes findings in the areas of neuronal circuitry, neural transmission and intracellular signaling. Phamacodynamics concerns the short- and long-term effects of drugs on neuronal function and structure. Insights and serendipitous findings from psychopharmacology reciprocally inform basic neuroscience and also have often been central to the hypotheses pursued in biological psychiatry. Recognition of the importance of genetics and complexity of psychiatric disorders is changing in fundamental ways how biological psychiatry is approached. Whether the field is termed molecular psychiatry, biological psychiatry, or clinical neuroscience, an increased focus on genetic influences and on behavioral components or endophenotypes has been prompted by a better appreciation of the scope and complexity of the endeavor.

GENERAL CONSIDERATIONS OF CNS FUNCTIONING

Overview

Neuronal circuitry, synaptic neurotransmission, and intracellular information processing constitute three major levels of central nervous system (CNS) functioning critical to understanding mechanisms of psychotropic drug action and the biological basis of cognitive and behavioral processes.

Neuronal circuitry to a large extent defines and reflects the functional activity and organization of the CNS. Neuronal communication via neurotransmitter release is a fundamental mechanism of brain function. The release of neurotransmitters and neuromodulators, their mechanisms of action, and their effect on target neurons are complex and still not fully understood; however, despite the diversity of neurotransmitters and receptors in the human brain, all forms of neural communication have the common goal of modulating neuronal activity. This is achieved by changing either the electrical or biochemical properties of the cell. The balance of intracellular and extracellular ions characterizes the electrical properties of the neuron. At rest, there are more negatively charged ions inside than outside the cell, thereby creating a negative resting membrane potential. Decreasing the resting potential leads to excitation, increasing it, to inhibition. The more enduring properties of the neuron are determined by longer term processes regulating the expression of specific genes, the production of proteins, and the creation of a distinct metabolism.

Neuronal Circuitry

The adult human cerebral cortex has about 100 billion neurons; each neuron establishes about a thousand to ten thousand connections to other neurons. Neurons are arranged in distributed networks that play critical roles in the expression of human behavior (3). This involves the collection of sensory information through perceptual modules, the creation of a representation, and the production of a response. Here we focus on four major anatomic systems that are crucial for these three steps of information processing: the cortex, thalamus, basal ganglia, and medial temporal lobe (Figure 2.4.2.1).

1. The thalamus is the gateway to cortical processing of all incoming sensory information, here represented by the three major systems: somatosensory, auditory, and visual (Figure 2.4.2.1). Primary sensory cortices receive information from the appropriate input modules (sensory organ + thalamus).
2. The association cortex integrates information from primary cortices, subcortical structures, and brain areas affiliated with memory to create an internal representation of the sensory information.
3. The medial temporal lobe (including the hippocampus and amygdala) serves two major functions in the brain: to integrate multimodal sensory information for storage into and retrieval from memory, and to attach limbic valence to sensory information (e.g., pleasant or unpleasant, fight or flight).
4. The basal ganglia are primarily involved in the integration of input from cortical areas. The basal ganglia modulate cortical activity via a cortico-striato-pallido-thalamo-cortical (CSPTC) loop. The most prominent projections to the striatum arise from the motor cortex.

All major projections (solid lines) in this basic circuitry (Figure 2.4.2.1) are glutamatergic (using the amino acid neurotransmitter glutamate), except for the projections from the

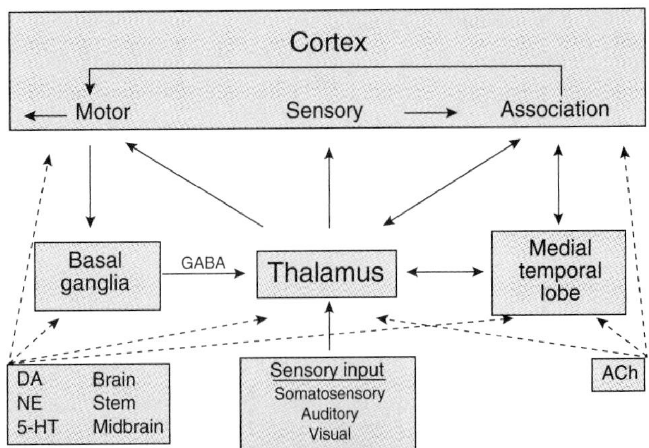

FIGURE 2.4.2.1. Neuronal circuitry. Basic scheme of information processing in the human brain. Straight arrows indicate glutamatergic pathways. The BG–thalamus projection is GABAergic. The broken arrows indicate the widespread, neurotransmitter-specific projections arising from the basal forebrain (ACh) and brain stem (DA, NE, 5-HT). A1, primary auditory cortex; ACh, acetylcholine; BG, basal ganglia; DA, dopamine; 5-HT, serotonin; see text for further details.

basal ganglia toward the thalamus, which are GABAergic (employing γ-aminobutyric acid). The glutamatergic neurons within each of the major components or regions of the circuit are under inhibitory control by GABAergic interneurons. In addition, four groups of densely packed neurons provide diffuse projections to all areas of the brain to modulate their functions: cholinergic neurons in the basal forebrain and brain stem, dopaminergic neurons in the substantia nigra and ventral tegmental area, noradrenergic neurons in the locus ceruleus, and serotonergic neurons in the raphe nuclei. The broken arrows in Figure 2.4.2.1 indicate the four neurotransmitter-specific projection systems. The relay of information from one neuron to another in these various circuits is usually effected by synaptic neurotransmission.

General Aspects of Synaptic Neurotransmission

Dendrites create a network of fibers providing the cell body of the neuron with input from other cells (Figure 2.4.2.2). The cell integrates these different inputs through modulation of the membrane potential, changes in second messenger systems and at the level of the nucleus (regulation of gene expression). The cell body is also the site of synthesis of nearly all cell-specific proteins, including transporters, receptors, and the enzymes needed for neurotransmitter production.

The axon is the output station of the neuron. The axon can be short (local circuit neuron) or long (projection neuron). If a deviation from the resting membrane potential is above a certain threshold, an action potential is created and travels downstream rapidly. The nerve terminal is the widened terminal part of the axon. It provides a small area of close contact with dendrites of communicating neurons: the synapse. Variations of this typical scheme include synapses between two terminals, two dendrites, and neurotransmitter release in medial parts of the axon.

As seen in Figure 2.4.2.2, the presynaptic neuron releases the vesicular stored neurotransmitter into the synapse and can express two types of proteins that affect synaptic communication: Presynaptic membrane-bound receptors can bind the intrinsic neurotransmitter (at autoreceptors) or transmitters of neighboring neurons (at heteroreceptors) and

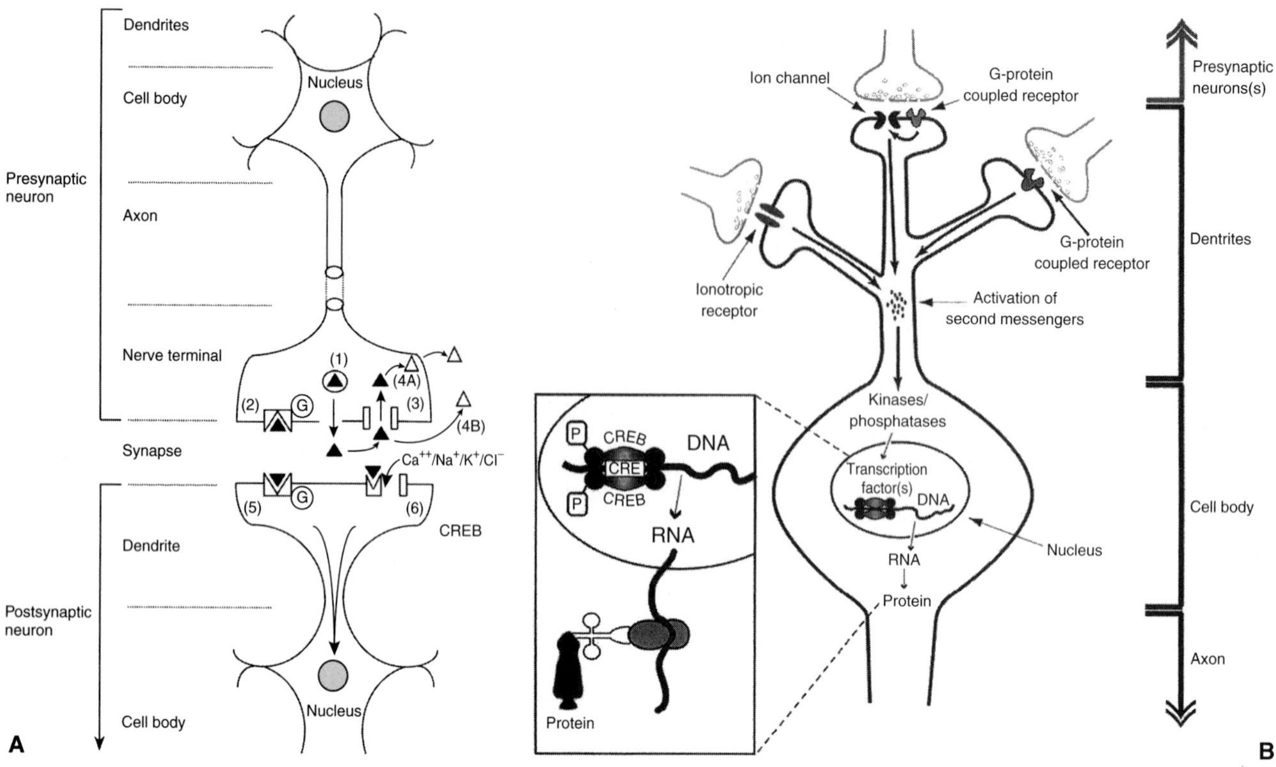

FIGURE 2.4.2.2. A. Anatomy of the neuron with major aspects of typical pre- and postsynaptic neurons labeled. Also depicted are six major mechanisms of synaptic neurotransmission: 1) release of neurotransmitter stored in vesicles; 2) binding of transmitter to presynaptic autoreceptor; 3) clearance of transmitter by reuptake; 4) A-intracellular metabolism of transmitter, B-extracellular metabolism of transmitter; 5) binding of transmitter to G-protein coupled receptor; 6) binding of transmitter to ion channel coupled receptor; see text for details. **B.** Intracellular information processing. Neurotransmitters released from the presynaptic neuron activate receptors at the postsynaptic neuron. Second messengers either enter the neuron (e.g., Ca^{2+} through ligand-gated ion channels) or are newly synthesized inside the neuron (e.g., G-protein–coupled receptors stimulate adenylate cyclase and the synthesis of cyclic AMP). Neurons usually have multiple receptor types and are able to integrate information from a variety of synaptic inputs. Second messengers stimulate protein kinases and protein phosphatases to control the state of phosphorylation of various proteins inside the neuron. Transcription factors such as CREB are regulated by kinases and phosphatases. A high level of discrimination is observed, although some transcription factors integrate information from different second messenger pathways. Thus, kinases and phosphatases regulate groups of genes under the control of specific transcription factors. **Inset:** Phosphorylation of CREB stimulates the transcription from DNA into RNA, which is transported out of the nucleus and translated (with ribosomes and tRNA) into protein.

affect the cell via intracellular messengers. One response, for example, is the modulation of neurotransmitter release (4). Presynaptic membrane-bound reuptake transporters pump the released neurotransmitter back into the cell (5). The released transmitter can undergo intracellular, extracellular metabolism (*4B*), or be repackaged in vesicules for rerelease.

The neuron receiving the input (postsynaptic cell) can be modulated via two different types of receptors (Figure 2.4.2.2). In the case of fast-acting, class I (ionotropic) receptors, the neurotransmitter binds to the receptor protein and within milliseconds this leads to a change in the permeability of the associated ion channel, allowing the influx of ions such as Ca^{2+}, Na^{+}, K^{+}, or Cl^{-}. In contrast, with slow-acting, class II (G-protein-coupled) receptors, the binding of the neurotransmitter to the receptor protein leads to a change in the protein conformation. This change is relayed to an associated G-protein, so called because it binds guanidine triphosphate (GTP) in order to be activated. G-proteins regulate two major classes of effector molecules: ion channels and second messenger generating enzymes. This general pattern and form of synaptic neurotransmission is repeated across the six major neurotransmitters. However, the differences seen across the glutamatergic, GABAergic, dopaminergic, noradrenergic, serotonergic and cholinergic systems are intriguing, form the bases of specific psychopharmacological effects, and underlie still prevailing neurobiological theories of biological psychiatry.

INTRACELLULAR INFORMATION PROCESSING

Our understanding of how neurons relay information between each other has moved beyond the role of synaptic transmission and into that of processes that take place within cells. Each neuron is the target of many projections from local and distant neurons. These influences are integrated at the level of the cell membrane and cell nucleus. The neurotransmitter-mediated activation of ion channels in the cell membrane can lead to an increase or decrease of the resting membrane potential. This may lead to the creation of an action potential. At the level of the cell nucleus, the various receptors and ion channels expressed on the cell membrane may influence gene and protein expression.

Gene expression is regulated by transcription factors that bind to specific sequences of the DNA in the nucleus (Figure 2.4.2.2B); therefore, membrane-bound receptors or ion channels in distal parts of the neuron must be able to activate intraneuronal signal transduction pathways that can span long distances and translocate to the nucleus. Because proteins assemble the neuron and determine neuronal properties, gene expression regulates neuronal function and may cause malfunction. Many psychopharmacologic agents with delayed therapeutic effects are thought to produce their therapeutic benefits through modulation of gene expression (6, 7).

Release of neurotransmitters from the presynaptic neuron into the synapse activates receptors on the postsynaptic neuron (see Figure 2.4.2.2B). Ions such as calcium enter the cell and act as second messengers on activation of inotropic receptors. Activation of G-protein–coupled receptors facilitates the opening of neighboring ion channels or the synthesis of second messengers such as cyclic AMP. Second messengers (calcium, cyclic AMP) regulate the activity of protein kinases (proteins that transfer phosphate groups to a substrate protein) and phosphatases (proteins that remove phosphate groups from a substrate protein). In all cases investigated to date, the activation of neurotransmitter receptors changes the state of phosphorylation of neuronal proteins.

The transcription factors are one group of proteins regulated by phosphorylation. Transcription factors operate by recruiting the transcription initiation complex and RNA polymerase to particular genes. The RNA polymerase then transcribes the DNA template into an RNA molecule, which is translated into protein outside the nucleus.

Among the best-studied transcription factors in the brain is the Ca^{2+}- and cyclic AMP-responsive element binding protein (CREB). The study of CREB has provided us with an insight into the complex consequences of transcription factor activation and gene expression on higher brain function. A variety of signal transduction pathways are integrated into CREB-mediated gene expression, such as those activated by G_s-proteins, inotropic receptors, or growth factors. Cyclic AMP-responsive element binding protein is activated by phosphorylation and regulates the expression of several target genes (e.g., genes for peptide neurotransmitters, enzymes involved in neurotransmitter synthesis, and growth factors). The discovery that CREB plays a vital role in processes such as learning and memory provided a link between gene regulation and cognitive function.

Small but persistent abnormalities in neurotransmission can have far-reaching consequences because neurotransmitters and receptors influence gene and protein expression in the brain. An understanding of signal transduction pathways and transcription factors such as CREB may be instrumental in providing new therapeutic avenues in psychopharmacology.

Pharmacodynamics Overview

Pharmacodynamic principles are concerned with the biochemical and physiologic effects of drugs at their active sites, that is, with their specific mechanisms of action. Stated succinctly, "pharmacokinetics describes what the body does to a drug; pharmacodynamics what a drug does to the body" (see Chapter 6.1.1 {Oesterheld, Shader & Martin}). The effects of a medication may change during development, as brain regions or neurotransmitter systems develop and mature. Most psychopharmacological agents exert their effects by interacting with specific protein targets—receptors, ion channels, transporters, or enzymes. Each of the major neurotransmitter systems have, therefore, a number of routes by which they can be manipulated (as are delineated in subsequent sections). The nature of the drug effect depends upon the site targeted while the selectivity of action is often a function of the relative affinity of the agent for the target site versus its other, often multiple, sites of interaction. Adverse drug effects are often the result of relatively nonselective agents and can severely limit their clinical utility.

Biological Psychiatry Overview

Research in biological psychiatry has made it increasingly clear that the genetics and biology of the common disorders are complex, in that multiple genes appear to contribute to the syndromes (Chapters 2.3.2 {Fernandez & State} and 2.3.1 {Leckman, Lombroso & Vaccarino}). This is not surprising given the complex and diffuse nature of the neural systems that subserve the relevant brain processes (8). The genetic complexity is further multiplied by the wealth of variation arising from gene–environment interactions: Illuminating the complexity will require the application of new and appropriate genetic methods (9–11).

An emerging overarching theme is that all biological, neuropharmacologic, and behavioral investigation needs to be performed in a genetic context. There is also a greater focus on components or domains of behavior and a greater interest in quantifying the traits or variables of interest. The rationale for examining what have been referred to as elementary units of psychological dysfunction (12), core or candidate symptoms, quantitative phenotypes (13), endophenotypes (14), or core psychopathological processes (15, 16) is becoming more and more compelling.

One formulation of the interrelated aspects of biological psychiatry is presented in Figure 2.4.2.3. The mutual interacting influences of genetic and environmental factors

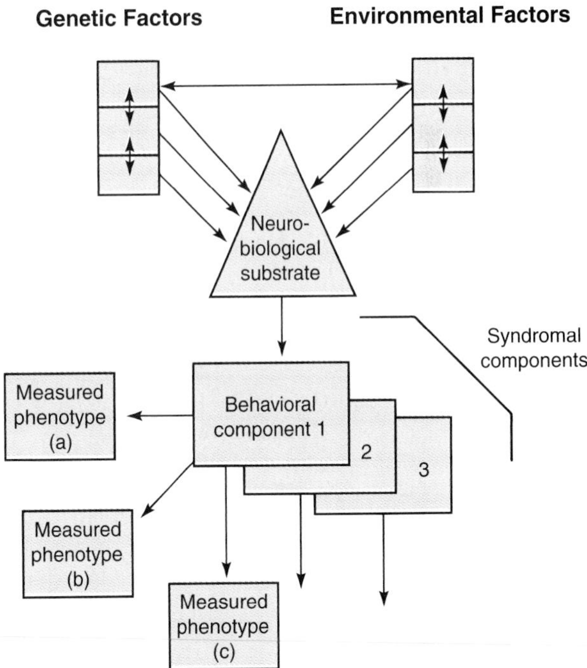

FIGURE 2.4.2.3. Schematic of the interrelated factors underlying biological psychiatry. The mutual interacting influences of genetic and environmental factors are shown determining the neurobiological systems that combine to form the substrate of relevant behaviors. The behaviors can be assessed through a range of measured phenotypes (*a–c*). The multiple behavioral components of most syndromes and disorders are depicted by the receding additional behavioral components (1–3).

are shown determining the neurobiological systems that, in combination, form the substrate of relevant behaviors. The field of biological psychiatry has traditionally emphasized neurochemical and neuroendocrinologic approaches. Other fields that are now proving critical to advancing an understanding of brain neural transmission in psychiatry include neurophysiology, neuropsychology, neuroimaging (17) and pharmacogenetics (18). Elucidation of the bases of the childhood disorders can be expected to proceed through an iterative process involving mutually beneficial relationships among all of the perspectives (19, 20). It is clear that one should be ever mindful of the developmental context when studying childhood psychiatric disorders (21, 22).

NEUROTRANSMITTER SYSTEMS

Overview

The major neurotransmitter systems can be divided into two groups based on their anatomic distribution. The first group comprises the serotonergic, dopaminergic, noradrenergic and cholinergic neurons. These four systems originate from small groups of neurons, densely packed in circumscribed areas of the forebrain or brain stem, and project to their target areas typically by long-ranging projection fibers. The second group includes the glutamatergic and GABAergic systems. Their neurons are by far the most prevalent and widely distributed types in the human brain. As mentioned, a number of similarities and parallels are apparent across the neurotransmitter system. Each system will be considered from the standpoint of its anatomy and neural transmission mechanisms, its pharmacodynamics or psychopharmacology, and the relevant biological psychiatry investigation.

SEROTONERGIC SYSTEM

Serotoninergic Neural Transmission/Neuroanatomy

Most serotonergic cells overlap with the distribution of the raphe nuclei in the brainstem. A rostral group (B6–8 neurons) projects to the thalamus, hypothalamus, amygdala, striatum, and cortex (23). The remaining two groups (B1–5 neurons) project to other brainstem neurons, the cerebellum, and the spinal cord. A schematic diagram of a serotonergic neuron and the metabolism of serotonin (5-HT) are depicted in Figure 2.4.2.4. Serotonin is produced after hydroxylation and decarboxylation of the essential amino acid tryptophan. Serotonin produced can be taken up by the vesicular monoamine transporter (VMAT2) and stored in vesicles for subsequent release or metabolized by the mitochondrial enzyme monoamine oxidase (MAO). Once released, 5-HT can interact with presynaptic or postsynaptic receptors, diffuse to extrasynaptic sites, or be taken up by neuronal or glial membrane 5-HT transporters (5-HTTs).

Serotonin acts at two different classes of receptors: at an inotropic receptor (5-HT_3 receptor) or at slower acting

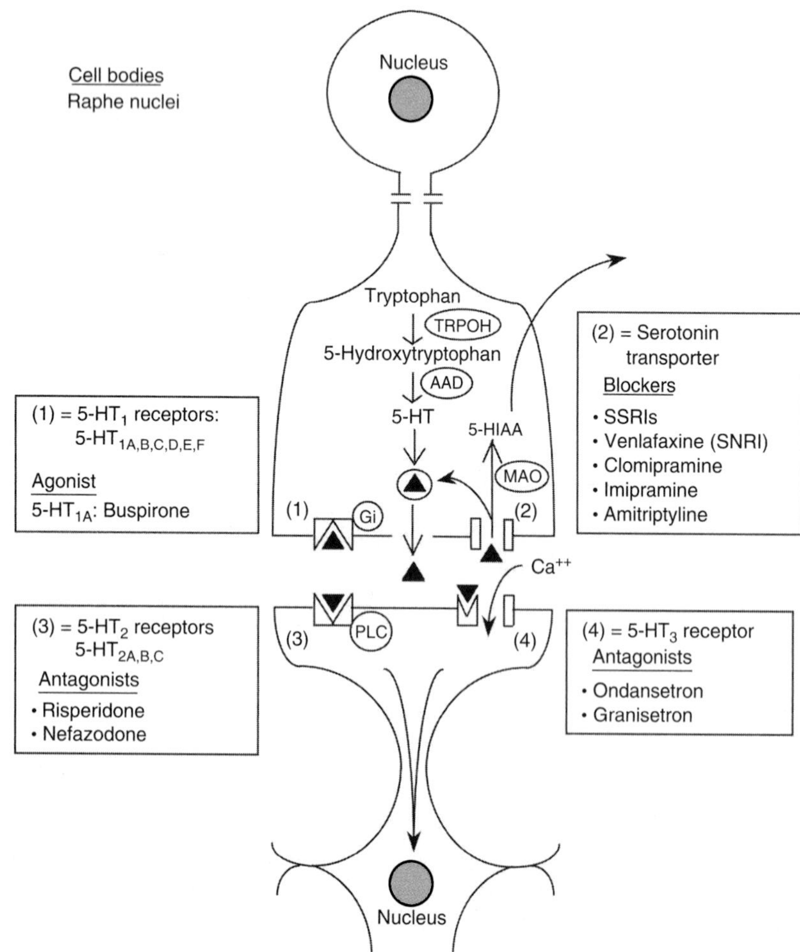

FIGURE 2.4.2.4. Serotonergic neurotransmission. Diagrammatic illustration of a serotonergic neuron. Serotonin (5-HT) synthesized from tryptophan (TRP) by the rate-limiting enzyme tryptophan hydroxylase (TRPOH) can be taken up by the vesicular monoamine transporter (VMAT2) and stored in vesicles for subsequent release or metabolized by the mitochondrial enzyme monoamine oxidase (MAO). Released 5-HT can interact with presynaptic or postsynaptic receptors, diffuse to extrasynaptic sites, or be taken up by neuronal or glial membrane 5-HT transporters (5-HTTs). Inhibition of the 5-HTT by selective serotonin reuptake inhibitors (SSRIs) results in higher levels of synaptic and extracellular fluid 5-HT, leading to greater 5-HT receptor stimulation.

receptors, coupled either to phospholipase C (5-HT_2 receptors) or to G-proteins (5-H $T_{1,4-7}$ receptors) (24). The 5-HT_1 receptors (5-$HT_{1A,B,C,D,E,F}$) (Figure 2.4.2.4) are coupled to G_i and lead to a decrease of cyclic AMP. The 5-HT_{1A} receptor is also directly coupled to a K^+ channel leading to increased opening of the channel. The 5-HT_1 receptors are the predominant serotonergic autoreceptors. 5-HT_2 receptors (5-$_{HT2A-C}$) are coupled to phospholipase C and lead to a variety of intracellular effects (mainly depolarization). Three receptors (5-$HT_{4,\ 6\ \&\ 7}$) are coupled to G_s and activate adenylate cyclase. The 5-HT_3 receptor is the only monoamine receptor coupled to an ion channel, and is found in the cortex, hippocampus, and in the area postrema, where it mediates nausea and emesis. It is typically localized presynaptically and regulates neurotransmitter release.

Serotonergic Pharmacodynamics

Serotonin is linked to many brain functions because of the widespread serotonergic projections and heterogeneity of the serotonergic receptors (23, 25). For example, modulation of serotonergic receptors and the reuptake site is beneficial (among others) in the treatment of anxiety, depression, obsessive-compulsive disorder, and schizophrenia (26). Interest in central 5-HT functioning derives from 5-HT's important role in processes as diverse and important as sleep, mood, appetite, perception, and hormone secretion (25), as well as its critical role in neurodevelopment (27).

Blockade of the serotonin transporter by selective serotonin reuptake inhibitors (SSRIs), such as fluoxetine (Prozac), results in higher levels of synaptic and extracellular fluid 5-HT and leads to greater pre- and postsynaptic 5-HT receptor stimulation. The serotonin transporter is the primary target site for several antidepressants, including the selective serotonin reuptake inhibitors (SSRIs), venlafaxine, and tricyclic antidepressants such as clomipramine and, to a lesser extent, imipramine and amitriptyline (Figure 2.4.2.4). Recent work in nonhuman primates has indicated that the increase in functionally active 5-HT occur within hours and is relatively constant over the course of treatment.

The atypical neuroleptics, such as risperidone, ziprasidone, and olanzapine all act as antagonists at 5-HT_2 receptors, as well as having blocking properties at dopamine receptors. The beneficial antipsychotic effects of the drugs appear to be at least partly mediated through their effects at cortical 5-HT_{2A} receptors. In particular, it appears that 5-HT_{2A} receptors on apical dendrites of cortical pyramidal cells may be especially important in gating sensory input. The critical role of the 5-HT_{2A} receptor in perception is underscored by a consideration of the effects of the 5-HT_{2A} agonist lysergic acid diethylamide (LSD). Adverse effects of the atypical neuroleptics on appetite and the associated weight gain appear to be at least partly due to effects at the 5-HT_{2C} receptor, while the substantial and enduring hyperprolactinemia frequently observed is a consequence of the dopamine D_2 receptor blockade in the pituitary.

Other serotonergic agents include the atypical anxiolytic buspirone, which acts as an agonist at the 5-HT_{1A} receptor. Newer antimigraine drugs such as sumatriptan have agonist effects at arterial 5-$HT_{1B/D}$ receptors, while the antiemetic odansetron acts to antagonize 5-HT_3 receptor sites in the intestine and perhaps in the brain.

Biological Psychiatry of Serotonin

Autism. Initial interest in a role for 5-HT in autism stemmed in part from the powerful effects of serotonergic agents, such as LSD, on perception. Research in the area was further stimulated by early reports of elevated 5-HT in blood of autistic children (28, 29). Beneficial effects of treatment with serotonin reuptake inhibitors (30) and exacerbation observed after tryptophan depletion (31) have also heightened interest in the role of 5-HT in autism. Although most of the 5-HT-related research has focused on the hyperserotonemia of autism, a number of studies of CSF 5-HIAA and several neuroendocrinologic studies of central 5-HT functioning have been reported (32). CSF studies are in general agreement that few or no differences exist between autistic and control groups' mean levels of 5-HIAA (33). A series of studies has provided converging evidence that 5-HT_{2A} receptor function and expression may be altered in autism. In 1989, McBride and colleagues reported that central and peripheral 5-HT_{2A} receptor functioning appeared reduced in autism (34). Thus, a diminished 5-HT_{2A} -mediated neuroendocrine response was paralleled by a reduced 5-HT_{2A} -mediated platelet aggregation response and lower platelet 5-HT_{2A} receptor binding in autism. Alterations in platelet 5-HT_{2A} binding indices were also reported by Cook et al. (35), with 5-HT_{2A} receptor measures inversely related to platelet 5-HT levels. These reports are paralleled by two neuroimaging studies reporting reduced 5-HT_{2A} receptor density in cortical regions (36).

TS/OCD. A role for 5-HT has been hypothesized because of the close connection between TS and obsessive-compulsive disorder (37). Effective treatment of obsessive-compulsive symptoms in patients with TS with the serotonergic uptake inhibitors fluvoxamine and fluoxetine has further stimulated research on the connection. The largest study of the 5-HT metabolite, 5-hydroxyindoleacetice acid (5-HIAA), found similar levels in patients with TS, OCD, or TS plus OCD, and the normal control group (38). No studies of 5-HT receptor functioning have been carried out in patients with TS, and early reports of benefit from the immediate 5-HT precursor, 5-hydroxytryptophan, have not been replicated. Research examining postmortem brain tissue has found decreases in 5-HT, 5-HIAA, and tryptophan across nearly all cortical and subcortical areas in TS (39, 40). Further post-mortem research is necessary in order to replicate the findings; however, the results tend to increase the possibility that 5-HT may be a factor in the symptomatology of TS.

ADHD. Interest in a role for 5-HT in ADHD was stimulated by early reports of decreased platelet 5-HT in affected children. Subsequent studies have not replicated this finding and have found normal levels of platelet and urine 5-HIAA, as well as normal numbers and affinities of platelet imipramine-binding sites in subjects with ADHD. In addition, studies of CSF 5-HIAA have not found differences between ADHD and control subjects. On the whole, the neurochemical research and the minimal treatment response to serotonergic agents have made it seem less likely that a 5-HT alteration is etiologic. Even so, it appears that the role of 5-HT in disruptive behaviors, particularly with respect to impulse control, deserves further consideration.

DOPAMINERGIC SYSTEM

Dopaminergic Neural Transmission/Neuroanatomy

Dopaminergic neurons can be divided into three major groups based on the length of their efferent fibers: a) ultrashort systems in the retina and olfactory bulb; b) intermediate-length systems originating in the hypothalamus and projecting to the pituitary gland; and c) wide-ranging systems originating from two areas, the substantia nigra (SN) and the ventral tegmental area (VTA). The SN neurons (also called A9 neurons) project to caudate and putamen, whereas the VTA neurons (also called A10 neurons) project to limbic areas such as nucleus accumbens and amygdala (i.e., mesolimbic projections) and several cortical areas such as frontal, cingulate, and entorhinal cortex (i.e., mesocortical projections).

The metabolism of the catecholamine dopamine (DA) is shown in Figure 2.4.2.5. DA is synthesized from tyrosine, after hydroxylation to dihydroxyphenylalanine (DOPA) and decarboxylation by aromatic acid decarboxylase (AAAD), and is found in highest concentration in the midbrain, although extensive cortical projections also occur. Dopamine has been shown to be critical in reward, modulating movement, and cognition. Dopamine is released into the synapse from vesicles (Figure 2.4.2.5) and subsequently removed from the synapse by two mechanisms. First, catechol-O-methyl-transferase (COMT) degrades intrasynaptic DA. Second, the dopamine transporter (DAT), a Na^+/Cl^- dependent neurotransmitter transporter, transports DA out of the synaptic cleft (Figure 2.4.2.5). Parenthetically, and of relevance to the action of stimulants, the transporter can actually function in either direction, depending on the concentration gradient. Free intracellular DA can either be taken back up into vesicles or metabolized by mitochondrial monoamine oxidase (MOA).

Dopamine acts at two different classes of dopamine receptors in the CNS, the D_1 and D_2 receptor families (Figure 2.4.2.5) (41). The D_1 receptor family includes the D_1 and D_5 receptors. Both are coupled to G_s (G-stimulating) and lead to an increase of cyclic AMP. The D_2 receptor family includes the D_2, D_3, and D_4 receptors. All are coupled to G_i (G-inhibitory) and lead to a decrease of cyclic AMP. There is a predilection of the different dopamine receptors for expression in specific brain areas (e.g., D_1 receptors are found in the striatum and cortex, D_2 receptors in the striatum and pituitary gland, and D_3 receptors in the nucleus accumbens). Presynaptic dopaminergic receptors are typically of the D_2 type and found on most portions of the dopaminergic neuron (as autoreceptors). They regulate DA synthesis and release, as well as the firing rate of DA neurons. Autoreceptors are 5 to 10 times more sensitive to DA agonists than postsynaptic receptors.

Dopamine affects several brain functions primarily by modulation of other neurotransmitter systems (42). Dopaminergic neurons of the SN project to the striatum and modulate the function of striatal GABAergic interneurons. Dopaminergic projections of the VTA to limbic structures such as the nucleus accumbens are known to be involved in reward behavior and the development of addiction to drugs such as ethanol, cocaine, nicotine, and opiates (43, 44). Dopaminergic projections from the VTA to the cortex play a role in the fine-tuning of cortical neurons (i.e., modulation of signal-to-noise ratio) (45).

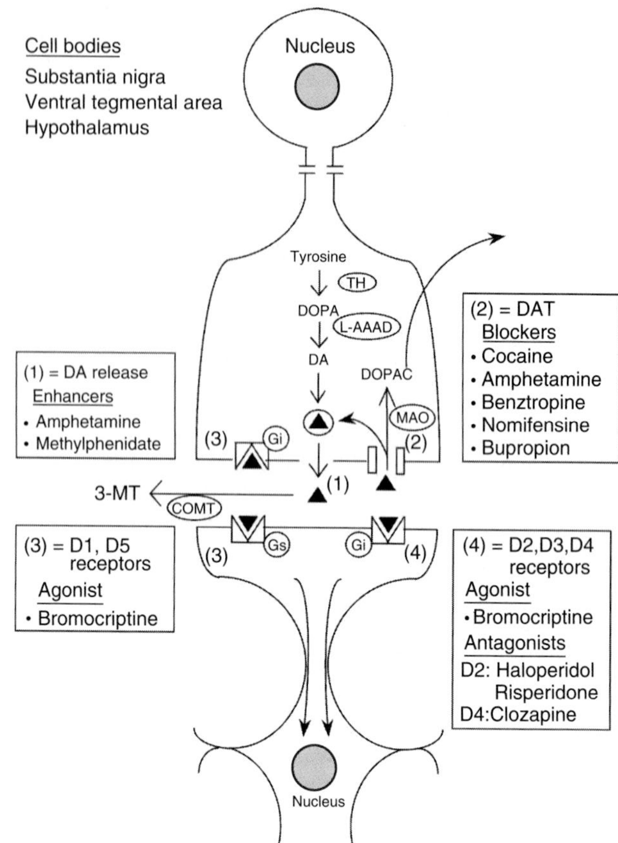

FIGURE 2.4.2.5. Dopaminergic neurotransmission. Diagrammatic illustration of a dopaminergic neuron. Dopamine (DA) synthesized from tyrosine by the rate limiting enzyme tyrosine hydroxylase (TH) can be taken up by the vesicular monoamine transporter (VMAT2) and stored in vesicles for subsequent release, or metabolized by the mitochondrial enzyme monoamine oxidase. Released DA can interact with presynaptic or postsynaptic receptors. Inhibition of the DA transporter (DAT) by DA reuptake inhibitors (DAT blockers) results in higher levels of synaptic and extracellular fluid of DA and leads to greater DA receptor stimulation.

Dopaminergic Pharmacodynamics

Dopamine receptor blockade, particularly at D_2 sites in the frontal cortex, is a major mechanism of action of most antipsychotic drugs (Figure 2.4.2.5). Both the older typical neuroleptics like the phenothaizines (e.g., chlorpromazine) and butyrophenones (e.g., haloperidol), as well as newer atypical neuroleptics including risperidone, ziprasidone and olanzapine, have anatogonist effects at D_2 receptors. The most recently introduced atypical antipsychotic drug, aripiprazole, appears to work by serving as a partial agonist at both pre- and post-synaptic dopamine receptors. By so doing, aripiprazole may moderate dopaminergic function, reducing presynaptic dopamine release while modestly stimulating postsynaptic receptors.

Dopamine is released into the synapse from vesicles (Figure 2.4.2.5) and this process is facilitated by the stimulants methylphenidate and amphetamine. Stimulant drugs such as amphetamine and cocaine also potently block the dopamine transporter (DAT). The euphoriant properties of the stimulants appear to be principally mediated through their enhancement of dopaminegic transmission in the striatum (specifically, the nucleus accumbens).

Biological Psychiatry of Dopamine

ADHD. The symptomatology of attention deficit hyperactivity disorder (ADHD) includes inattention, distractibility, and impulsivity, with or without hyperactivity (46). The remarkable effects of stimulants on children with ADHD have led to a longstanding and continuing interest in the role of DA. Family and twin studies have strongly supported the idea that there are inherited components to the disorder (47).

A large number of neurobiological studies have been carried out; the majority involves the measurement of neurotransmitter metabolites in blood and urine, either at baseline or after pharmacological perturbation. An increasing number of brain-imaging studies have been reported (48). These studies have tended to focus attention on the frontal cortex and midbrain DA nuclei and their projection areas. The well replicated genetic findings of an association between ADHD symptomatology and alleles of the dopamine transporter and D4 DA receptor genes (18) have further increased interest in DA. Although the neurochemical investigation has been extensive and includes studies of dopamine and its principal metabolite, homovanillic acid (HVA), in CSF, plasma and urine, it has failed to establish definitive alterations in ADHD. Neuroendocrine studies in ADHD are limited and also provide no definite information regarding possible group differences.

Tourette Syndrome (TS). Neuroanatomic and neuropharmacologic considerations have prompted a number of neurochemical studies with a focus on the monoamines DA, 5-HT, and NE in TS (49, 50). A role for DA is suggested by the amelioration of tics by neuroleptics, exacerbation of symptomatology after administration of stimulants, and importance of DA pathways in modulating basal ganglia output (51). The measurement of the DA metabolite HVA in CSF has not revealed consistent differences between mean levels in TS and control groups (38). Studies of post-mortem brain from a small number of patients with TS have yielded conflicting results. Singer and colleagues (50, 52) have found increased densities of the DA transporter in basal ganglia regions and suggested that the increased densities are a reflection of increased DA innervation within the striatum; however, observations of the normal striatal levels of DA, homovanillic acid, and tyrosine hydroxylase do not support this idea (39, 40). Although an initial imaging study reported higher striatal DA transporter binding in Tourette patients, subsequent studies have not confirmed this elevation (50). Interest in possible alterations in relative densities of brain D2 and D1 DA receptors has increased following a report of a relationship between density and tic severity in twins (53).

Autism. A case for altered DA functioning in autism can be made, based on its clear role in mediating motoric disturbances (e.g., stereotypies) and the observation that DA blockers are effective in treating some aspects of autism. The majority of relevant neurochemical studies have examined levels of HVA (32). The concentration of HVA in CSF does not appear to be altered (54). Measurements of HVA in urine have been inconsistent and the only study of plasma HVA reported similar levels in autistic and control subjects (55). Other relevant measures include urinary DA, reportedly normal in autism, and plasma prolactin, which also has been reported to be normal in autistic subjects (55). Taken together, the studies suggest that central dopaminergic functioning, to the extent it can be assessed by the measures employed, is normal in autism.

NORADRENERGIC SYSTEM

Noradrenergic Neural Transmission/Neuroanatomy

About half of all noradrenergic neurons (i.e., 12,000 on each side of the brain stem) are located in the locus ceruleus. They provide the extensive noradrenergic innervation of the cortex, hippocampus, thalamus, cerebellum, and spinal cord. The remaining neurons are distributed in the tegmental region. They innervate predominantly the hypothalamus, basal forebrain, and spinal cord. Norepinephrine (NE) is released into the synapse from vesicles; amphetamine facilitates this release (Figure 2.4.2.6). Norepinephrine acts in the CNS at two different types of noradrenergic receptors, α and β.

Adrenergic α receptors can be subdivided into $\alpha 1$ receptors, which are coupled to phospholipase and located postsynaptically, and $\alpha 2$ receptors, which are coupled to G_i and located primarily presynaptically (Figure 2.4.2.6). Adrenergic β receptors in the CNS are predominantly of the $\beta 1$ subtype. Beta-1 receptors are coupled to G_s and lead to an increase of cyclic AMP. Norepinephrine is removed from the synapse by catabolism by catechol-O-methyltransferase (COMT) and through uptake by the norepinephrine transporter (NET), a Na^+/Cl^- dependent neurotransmitter transporter. Once internalized, NE can be degraded by the intracellular enzyme monoamine oxidase (MAO); metabolic end-products include 3-methoxy-4-hydroxyphenylethleneglycol (MHPG) and vanillylmandelic acid (VMA).

Noradrenergic projections modulate sleep cycles, appetite, mood, and cognition by targeting the thalamus, limbic structures, and cortex. Also, the locus ceruleus (LC) receives afferents from the sensory systems that monitor the internal and external environments. The widespread LC efferents lead to an inhibition of spontaneous discharge in the target neurons. Stress responses, central and peripheral arousal, and learning and memory are all critically modulated by noradrenergic neurons (56, 57). The critical role of the noradrenergic system in the stress response is shown in Figure 2.4.2.7. The extensive interaction of the central/peripheral NE system with the hypothalamic-pituitary-adrenal (HPA) axis is evident and is summarized in the review of Chrousos and Gold (58).

Noradrenergic Pharmacodynamics

Noradenergic agents function through a variety of mechanisms. Monoamine oxidase inhibitors (MAOIs) act to increase intra- and extracellular NE by inhibiting enzymatic catabolism by MAO. A number of antidepressant drugs, including desipramine, nortriptyline, atomoxetine, and venlafaxine increase extracellular NE via blockade of the norepinephrine transporter (Figure 2.4.2.6) (59). Clonidine and guanfacine are potent $\alpha 2$ receptor agonists and tend to decrease noradrenergic tone by stimulating presynaptic $\alpha 2$ autoreceptors in the locus coeruleus. This can lead to sedating and hypotensive effects. However, their actions at post-synaptic $\alpha 2$ receptors in the cortex may be important to their apparent beneficial effects on attention and impulse control (57). The other major class of adrenergic receptors consists of the $\beta 1$ and $\beta 2$ adrenergic receptors. The $\beta 1$ subtype are found in the cerebral cortex, while both types are found in peripheral vasculature. While the more lipophilic β-blockers (e.g., propranolol) can antagonize both central and peripheral β-receptors, peripheral blockade effected by less lipophilic agents (e.g., nadolol) may be sufficient to have behavioral effects.

Biological Psychiatry of Norepinephrine

Given the apparent importance of stress and trauma in affecting the onset, expression, and severity of various forms of psychopathology, it is not surprising that NE has been extensively investigated in biological psychiatry. Certainly, central NE and the noradrenergic sympathetic nervous system play a central role in arousal and the stress response.

Tourette Syndrome (TS). The importance of noradrenergic projections from the locus ceruleus in controlling states of arousal, as well as reports of symptom amelioration after treatment with the α_2-agonist clonidine (60), are suggestive evidence for altered noradrenergic functioning in Tourette syndrome (TS). There are several reports of lowered urinary excretion of MHPG in TS; however, this finding has not been consistently replicated. Assessment of the sympathetic

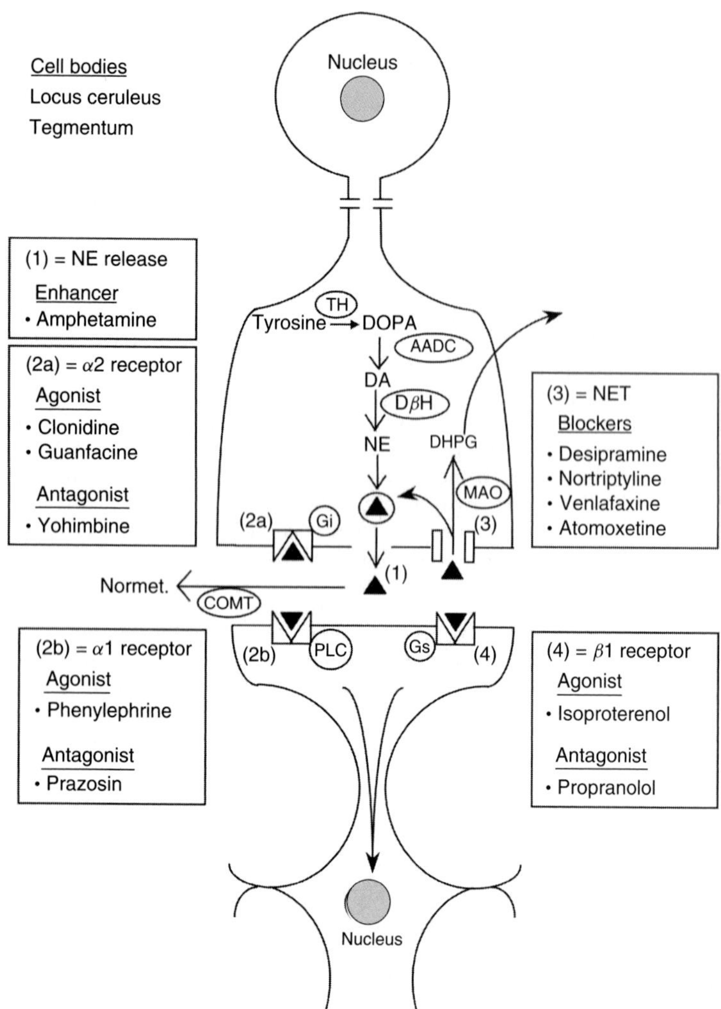

FIGURE 2.4.2.6. Noradrenergic neurotransmission. Diagrammatic illustration of a noradrenergic neuron. Norepinephrine (NE) synthesized from dopamine by the enzyme dopamine-beta-hydroxylase (DBH) can be taken up by the vesicular monoamine transporter (VMAT2) and stored in vesicles for subsequent release or metabolized by the mitochondrial enzyme monoamine oxidase. Released NE can interact with presynaptic or postsynaptic receptors. Inhibition of the norepinephrine transporter (NET) by NE reuptake blockers results in higher levels of synaptic and extracellular fluid of NE and leads to greater NE receptor stimulation.

nervous system by measurement of autonomic cardiovascular measures has not revealed any substantial differences in the TS group (61). However, studies of plasma, urinary, and CSF stress hormones before and after a lumbar puncture clearly suggest that at least some patients with TS have an increased stress response (62, 63). This conclusion is consistent with the results of the largest study of NE and MHPG in CSF, which found that, although MHPG levels were normal, concentrations of NE were elevated nearly twofold (38). Given the much shorter half-life of NE compared to MHPG, the results are indicative of normal basal stress response functioning and increased acute stress responsivity.

ADHD. Arousal mechanisms almost certainly play an important part in ADHD-associated symptoms of hyperactivity, impulsivity, distractibility, and inattention (64, 65). The crucial role of the central noradrenergic system and sympathetic nervous system (SNS) in regulating arousal, together with noradrenergic effects of stimulant medication, has led to hypotheses of noradrenergic involvement in ADHD (66, 67). Treatment studies employing the noradrenergic-specific agents clonidine and guanfacine, as well as an increasing appreciation of the role of central NE in attention and cognition (56, 57, 68), have served to maintain interest in the role of NE in the symptoms of ADHD.

Baseline measurements of NE in serum and MHPG in plasma have not revealed differences between ADHD and control subjects. The data with respect to MHPG and NE in urine are less consistent, with MHPG excretion, for instance, decreased, unchanged, or increased in ADHD (69). Research establishing a positive association between classroom performance and epinephrine (EPI) excretion (70), along with reports of stimulant-induced EPI release and longstanding observations of cognitive enhancing effects of systemically administered EPI, suggest a possible role for EPI in attention. Several reviews have discussed how altered interaction of the adrenergic and noradrenergic systems might contribute to symptoms of ADHD (66, 67, 71). Although studies of baseline EPI excretion have not found differences between ADHD and control groups, three studies (72–74) have found substantially lower rates of EPI excretion during cognitive testing in ADHD patients compared to normal controls. In studies examining the effects of amphetamine or methylphenidate in patients with ADHD, both drugs increased EPI excretion, but relatively smaller adrenomedullary responses were seen in patients compared to controls following acute (75) or chronic (76) dosing. A similar reduced adrenomedullary response was observed in children with ADHD during hypoglycemic challenge when plasma levels of epinephrine were measured. Thus, the finding of a blunted epinephrine response in ADHD has been seen consistently across a number of situations. In the most recent study (72), the blunted response appeared to be specific to the inattention component or domain of ADHD. Further work in this area appears warranted: It would not be surprising if genetically determined variations in the functioning of each of the catecholamines contributed some part to one or more of the component behaviors of ADHD.

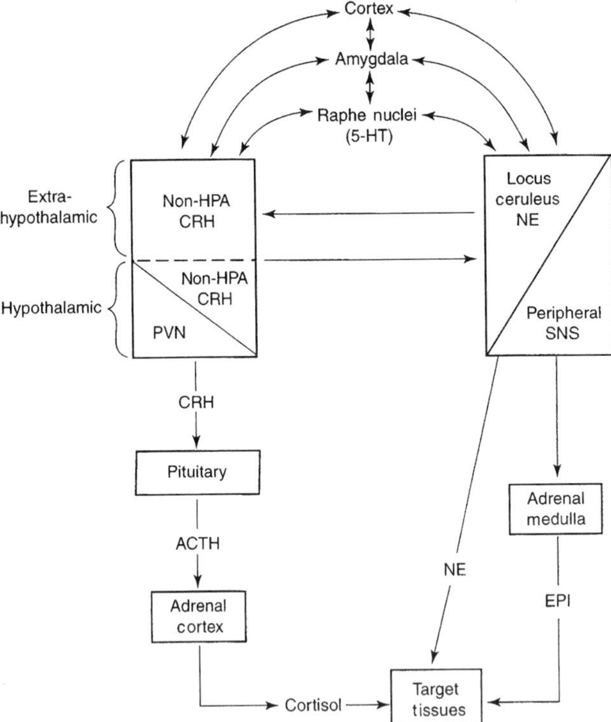

FIGURE 2.4.2.7. Stress response system. Diagram of the two major components of the stress response system: the central noradrenergic/sympathoadrenomedullary system and the hypothalamic-pituitary-adrenal (HPA) axis. The extensive interaction of the central/peripheral norepinephrine systems with the HPA axis is evident. Not shown are the extensive hormonal and neuronal inputs and feedback occurring from the periphery to the central nervous system.

Autism. As one of the two major components of the stress response system (58), the sympathetic/adrenomedullary system has been of interest in autism owing to the hyperarousal, hyperactivity, and overreaction to novel situations often seen in autism. It should be mentioned that the HPA axis, the other major component of the stress response (Figure 2.4.2.7), has also been well studied in autism. The functioning of the sympathetic/adrenomedullary system has been assessed through measurements of norepinephrine (NE) and epinephrine (EPI) in plasma or urine. In addition, plasma and urine levels of the major NE metabolites, 3-methoxy-4-hydroxyphenylethylglycol (MHPG) and vanillylmandelic acid (VMA) have been determined. Serum levels of dopamine-β-hydroxylase—the synthetic enzyme secreted along with NE from sympathetic neurons—also have been studied (77). In nearly all cases, indices that reflect basal functioning of the sympathetic/adrenomedullary system were found to be normal in patients with autism. On the other hand, most of the studies measuring indices of acute stress response have found elevations in patients with autism when they are exposed to the stress of a venipuncture or neuropsychological test. Taken together, the data support the idea that stress response systems are hyperresponsive when individuals with autism are stressed, but that autistic patients are not in a chronic state of hyperarousal. Findings from studies of HPA axis function are consistent with the sympathetic/adrenomedullary results, and support the same conclusions.

The apparent increased response to stressors could result from a difference in the level of perceived stress, an overelicitation of the physiologic response, or an abnormality in the stress response systems themselves. It will be difficult to determine whether the individual with autism experiences a greater threat, if the response to the threat is less well regulated, or both. Despite the difficulties encountered in stress response research in autism, further research in this area is warranted, given the clinical relevance and possible etiologic nature of alterations in this area.

GLUTAMATERGIC SYSTEM

Glutamatergic Neural Transmission/Neuroanatomy

Glutamatergic neurons are widely distributed throughout the brain (see Figure 2.4.2.1). Prominent glutamatergic pathways are the cortico-cortical projections, connections between thalamus and cortex, and projections from cortex to striatum (extrapyramidal pathway) and to brain stem/spinal cord (pyramidal pathway) (78).

Glutamate acts at three different types of inotropic receptors (Figure 2.4.2.8) and at a family of G-protein–coupled (metabotropic) receptors (79, 80). Binding of glutamate to the inotropic receptor opens an ion channel allowing the influx of Na^+ and Ca^{2+} into the cell. NMDA receptors bind glutamate and *N*-methyl-D-aspartate. The receptor is comprised of two different subunits: NMDAR1 (seven variants) and NMDAR2 (four variants). The NMDA receptor is highly regulated at several sites. For example, the receptor is virtually ineffective unless a ligand binds to the glycine site and it is blocked by binding of ligands (e.g., ketamine and phencyclidine = PCP) to the PCP site inside the channel. AMPA receptors bind glutamate, AMPA, and quisqualic acid, whereas kainate receptors bind glutamate and kainic acid.

The metabotropic glutamate receptor family includes at least seven different types of G-protein–coupled receptors (mGluR1-7). They are linked to different second messenger systems and lead to the increase of intracellular Ca^{2+} or the decrease of cyclic AMP. The increase of intracellular Ca^{2+} leads to the phosphorylation of target proteins in the cell. Glutamate is removed from the synapse by high-affinity reuptake; two transporter proteins are expressed in glial cells and one in neurons (Figure 2.4.2.8). After uptake into glia, glutamate is converted to glutamine by glutamine synthetase. Glutamine can then diffuse back into the neuron to replenish neuronal glutamate after hydrolysis by mitochondrial glutaminase completing this cycle, termed the glutamine–glutamate shunt.

Glutamate has an effect on many brain functions. For example, glutamatergic neurons and NMDA receptors in the hippocampus are important in the creation of long-term potentiation, a crucial component in the formation of memory (81). Excess stimulation of glutamatergic receptors, as seen in seizures or stroke, can lead to unregulated Ca^{2+} influx and neuronal damage (82–84). Decreased glutamatergic function is thought to be involved in the creation of psychotic symptoms.

GLUTAMATERGIC PHARMACODYNAMICS

Glutamate appears ineffective at the NMDA receptor unless glycine or serine is bound at the strychnine-insensitive glycine modulatory site. Phencyclidine (PCP) and ketamine can block activity of the NMDA receptor by binding to the PCP site within the NMDA-associated ion channel. Ketamine and PCP can induce psychotic symptoms, though ketamine may prove to be useful therapeutically in certain circumstances. Conversely, serine, *d*-cycloserine, glycine or inhibitors of glycine uptake

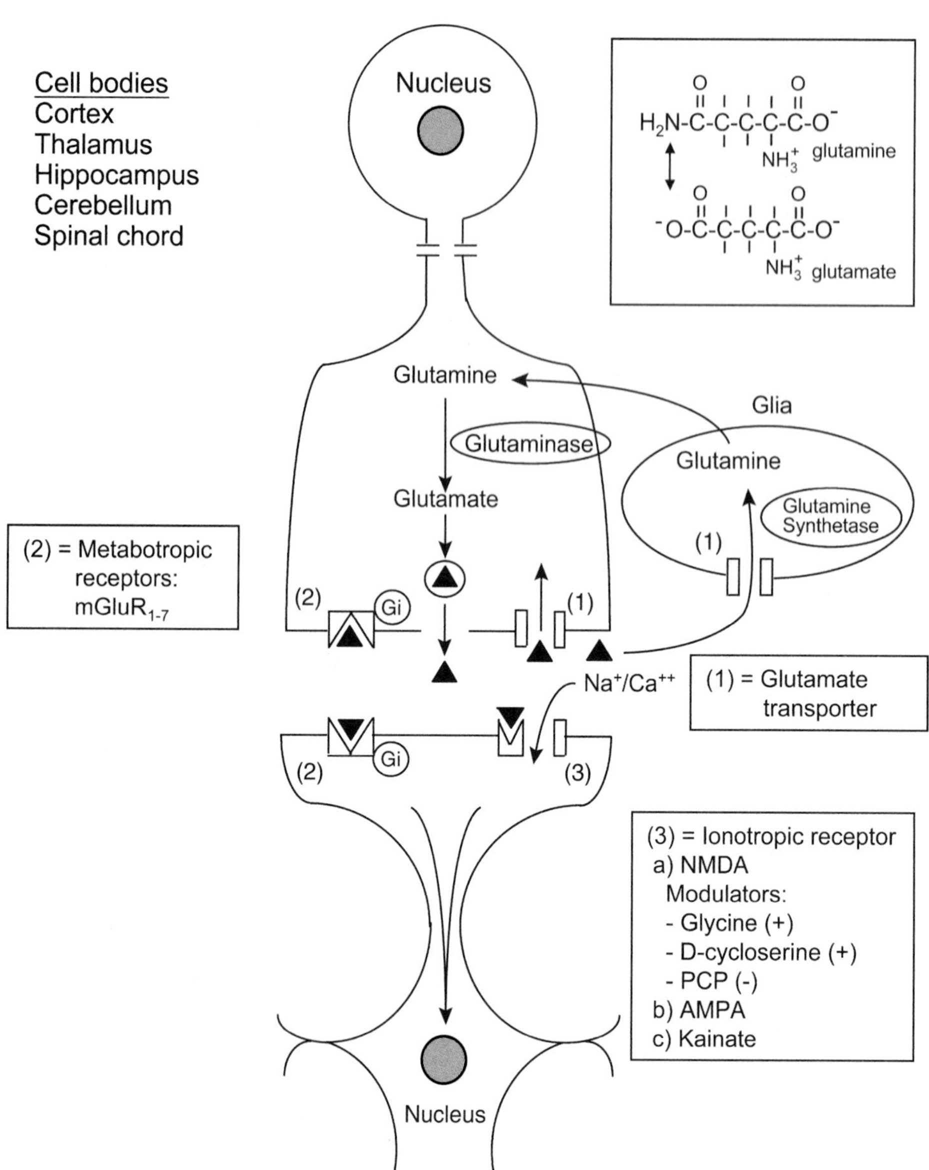

FIGURE 2.4.2.8. Glutamatergic neurotransmission. Diagram of the glutamatergic neuron with the pertinent processes of neural transmission and metabolism depicted. Intraneuronal glutamate is taken up into vesicles by the vesicular glutamate transporter. Released glutamate can stimulate pre- and postsynaptic receptors and be taken up by the membrane glutamate transporter (*1*). The glutamate-glutamine shunt through glial cells is an importance source of releasable glutamate. An inset depicts the interconversion of glutamate (glutamic acid) and glutamine.

have been reported to be useful in decreasing psychotic and/or negative symptoms in schizophrenia (85–87); however, more recent trials have not been impressive in this regard (88).

Antagonists at the AMPA receptor are being studied as possible therapeutic agents in infantile seizures, while ampakines or positive modulators of the receptor complex may offer a fruitful approach in schizophrenia. Investigation of various ways to manipulate glutamatergic functioning in schizophrenia will remain an active area of research (89)and advances may have relevance to autism and early-onset psychosis.

Biological Psychiatry of Glutamate

Schizophrenia. Although a hypoglutamatergic theory of schizophrenia has been widely touted, the theory is based mainly on consideration of the opposing interrelationships between the dopaminergic and glutamatergic systems and on the psychotomimetic effects of glutamatergic agents, including PCP and ketamine. Postmortem brain research has yet to yield consistent findings with respect to glutamatergic markers in schizophrenia.

TS. In the one study of central excitatory amino acids in Tourette's syndrome (TS), postmortem brain levels of glutamate were lowered in the three projection areas of the subthalamic nucleus; (40) it was hypothesized that this might lead to disinhibition of the thalamocortical circuit. This would tend to place TS in the group of hyperkinetic movement disorders, including Huntington's disorder and hemiballismus. As reviewed by Swerdlow and Young (90), further research is needed to clarify basal ganglia functioning in TS. Imaging studies (91) and postmortem research have provided interesting leads to consider with respect to the functioning of cortico-striato-pallido-thalamocortical pathways.

GABAERGIC SYSTEM

Gabaergic Neural Transmision/Neuroanatomy

GABAergic neurons can be divided into two groups (Figure 2.4.2.1): a) Short-ranging neurons (also called interneurons or local circuit neurons) in the cortex, thalamus, striatum, cerebellum, and spinal cord; and b) medium- and long-ranging neurons in the basal ganglia, septum, and substantia nigra.

GABA acts at two types of receptors, the $GABA_A$ and $GABA_B$ receptors. The $GABA_A$ receptor is a receptor-channel complex comprised of five subunits (92). Activation leads to the opening of the channel, allowing chloride ions to enter the cell, resulting in decreased excitability. Five distinct classes of subunits and multiple variations in the composition of the $GABA_A$ receptor are known. The receptor can be modulated by benzodiazepines at the benzodiazepine (BZ) subunit and by barbiturates and ethanol near the chloride channel (Figure 2.4.2.9). The BZ site is further subclassified into $\alpha 1$, $\alpha 2$, and $\alpha 3$ and 4 types.

The $GABA_B$ receptor is a G-protein–coupled receptor with similarity to the metabotropic glutamate receptor (93, 94). The $GABA_B$ receptor is linked to G_i (decreasing cyclic AMP and opening of K^+ channels) and G_o (closing Ca^{2+} channels). GABA is removed from the synapse by a sodium-dependent GABA uptake transporter (Figure 2.4.2.9). Cortical and thalamic GABAergic neurons are crucial for the inhibition of excitatory neurons.

GABAergic Pharmacodynamics

Positive modulation of $GABA_A$ receptors is beneficial in the treatment of anxiety disorders, insomnia, and agitation—most likely because of a general inhibition of neuronal activity. The benzodiazepines, including lorazepam, clonazepam, and midazolam, are widely used to treat anxiety despite problems with tolerance and dependence. Somewhat more $\alpha 1$-specific agents such as zolpidem (Ambien) and related compounds are useful in reducing sleep latency and increasing overall time asleep, and appear to do so without tolerance or rebound effects even after long-term treatment. Furthermore, GABAergic agonists such as benzodiazepines or barbiturates are efficacious in the treatment and prevention of seizures (95). The wide and age-old use of alcohol for self-medication of a number of life's problems is an enduring testament to the importance of the GABAergic system.

GABAergic Biological Psychiatry

The importance of GABA in basal ganglia neural transmission has led to treatment studies of GABAergic agents (96) in

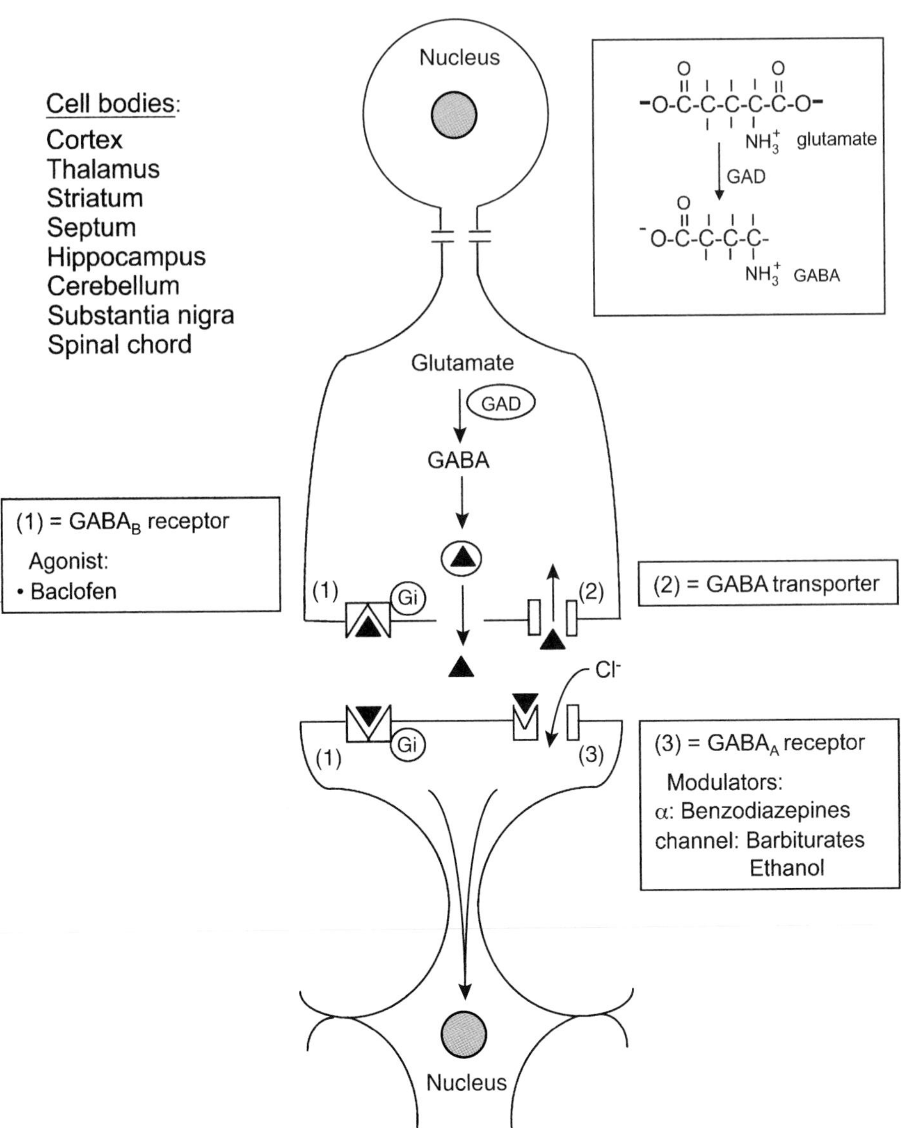

FIGURE 2.4.2.9. GABAergic neurotransmission. Diagram of the GABAergic neuron with the pertinent processes of neural transmission and metabolism depicted. Glutamate serves as the major precursor for GABA, with conversion to GABA occurring through the action of glutamic acid decarboxyalse (GAD). An inset depicts the conversion of glutamate (glutamic acid) to GABA. Released GABA can stimulate pre- and postsynaptic receptors and be taken up by the membrane GABA transporter (2).

TS. However, studies of CSF GABA have not found group differences in patients with TS and studies of postmortem tissue have not revealed alterations in GABA concentrations. A series of recent studies have indicated that cortical GABA may be reduced in depression and that levels may normalize during treatment with antidepressants (97, 98).

CHOLINERGIC SYSTEM

Cholinergic Neural Transmission/Neuroanatomy

Cholinergic neurons in the central nervous system are either wide-ranging projection neurons or short-ranging interneurons. Projection neurons in the basal forebrain (septum, diagonal band, nucleus basalis of Meynert) project to the entire cortex, hippocampus, and amygdala, and projection neurons located in the brain stem project predominantly to the thalamus. Cholinergic interneurons in the striatum modulate the activity of GABAergic striatal neurons.

Acetylcholine (Ach) acts at two different types of cholinergic receptors. Muscarinic receptors bind ACh as well as other agonists (muscarine, pilocarpine, bethanechol) and antagonists (atropine, scopolamine). There are at least five different types of muscarinic receptors (M1 to M5). All have slow response times and can be coupled to G-proteins and a variety of second messenger systems. When activated, the final effect can be to open or close channels for K^+, Ca^{2+}, or Cl^- (99).

Nicotinic receptors are less abundant than the muscarinic type in the CNS. They bind ACh as well as agonists such as nicotine (Figure 2.4.2.10) or antagonists such as *d*-tubocurarine. The fast-acting, ionotropic nicotinic receptor allows influx of $Na^+ > K^+ > Ca^{2+}$ into the cell. Acetylcholine is removed from the synapse through hydrolysis into acetyl CoA and choline by the enzyme acetyl cholinesterase (AChE).

Acetylcholine modulates attention, novelty seeking, and memory via the basal forebrain projections to the cortex and limbic structures. Anticholinergic delirium and Alzheimer's disease are examples of a cholinergic deficit state (100, 101). Furthermore, cholinergic interneurons modulate striatal neurons by opposing the effects of dopamine.

Cholinegic Pharmacodynamics

Stimulation of the fast-acting, ionotropic nicotinic receptor with nicotine leads to improvements in attention; however, the addictive properties of nicotine have greatly restricted its use in attentional problems. The acetylcholinesterase inhibitors (AChEIs) are widely used to increase cholinergic function in

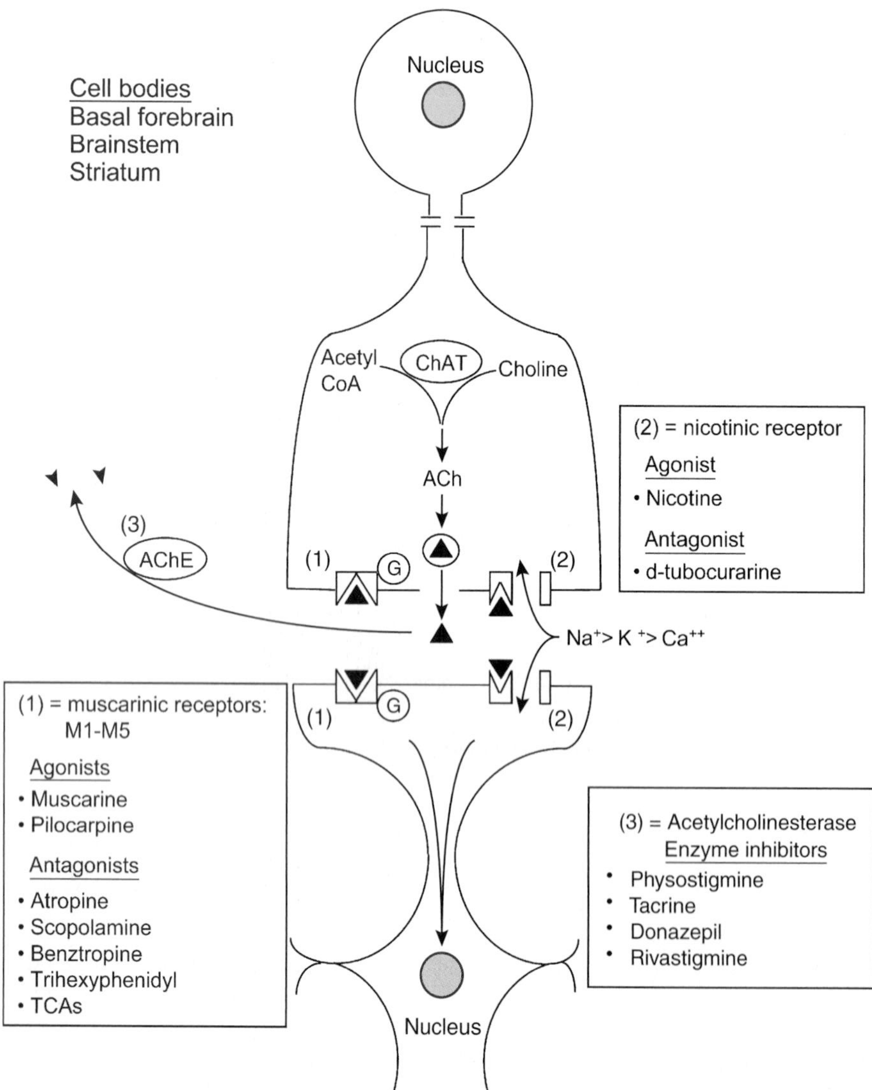

FIGURE 2.4.2.10. Cholinergic neurotransmission. Diagram of the cholinergic neuron with the pertinent processes of neural transmission and metabolism depicted. Acetylcholine (Ach) is formed by the action of choline acetyltransferase (ChAT), and is metabolized after release by the enzyme acetylcholine esterase (AChE) (3).

a more general manner. The AChEIs are most often used to treat the dementia of Alzheimer's; benefits have also been reported in Parkinson and Down syndromes. Like Alzheimer's, the latter disorder appears to have an associated cholinergic deficit. It remains to be seen whether AChEIs like rivastigmine and donepezil will prove of use in treating attention deficits in ADHD and autism.

Cholinergic Biological Psychiatry

Autism. Studies of peripheral cholinergic markers in autism are limited. However, several studies have reported decreased nicotinic receptor binding in postmortem brain tissue despite relatively normal levels of the presynaptic markers choline acetyltransferase (ChAT) and AChE, and normal muscarinic receptor binding (102). Thus, epibatidine binding to the $\alpha 4\beta 2$ nicotinic receptor was reported to be markedly lower throughout the cortex in brain of subjects with autism. Replication of the finding is necessary, but the results to date raise intriguing issues about the possible etiological role of altered cholinergic functioning during development and the possible therapeutic effects of early manipulation of the cholinergic system.

ADHD. The cholinergic system has been hypothesized to be involved in ADHD, based on its important role in attention and cognition, the high rate of smoking in ADHD (possible self-medication phenomenon), high rates of gestational exposure to maternal smoking, the enhancing effects of nicotine on catecholaminergic systems, and the limited data available on therapeutic effects of nicotinic agents in ADHD. It is not clear whether cholinergic agents, including the AChEIs, will prove to be useful in treating ADHD-related problems.

TS. The importance of ACh in basal ganglia neural transmission has led to treatment studies using choline and other cholinergic agents (103, 104). However, studies of CSF acetylcholinesterase have not found group differences. Though reports of increased red blood cell choline have appeared (105) and muscarinic receptor binding in white blood cells has been reported to be drastically lowered in TS (106), neither observation can be considered definitive.

ACKNOWLEDGMENT

The authors thank Dr. Stephan Heckers of Vanderbilt University for his contributions to an earlier version of this manuscript, and for allowing them to modify and use some of the figures presented.

References

1. Andreasen NC: Linking mind and brain in the study of mental illnesses: a project for a scientific psychopathology. *Science* 275(5306):1586–1593, 1997.
2. Kandel ER, Squire LR: Neuroscience: breaking down scientific barriers to the study of brain and mind. *Science* 290(5494):1113–1120, 2000.
3. Mesulam MM: *Principles of Behavioral Neurology*. New York, Oxford University Press, 2000.
4. Langer SZ: 25 years since the discovery of presynaptic receptors: present knowledge and future perspectives. *Trends Pharmacol Sci* 18(3):95–99, 1997.
5. Lester HA, Cao Y, Mager S: Listening to neurotransmitter transporters. *Neuron* 17(5):807–810, 1996.
6. Duman RS, Heninger GR, Nestler EJ: A molecular and cellular theory of depression [see comments]. *Arch Gen Psychiatry* 54(7):597–606, 1997.
7. Hyman S: Mental illness: genetically complex disorders of neural circuitry and neural communication. *Neuron* 28(2):321–323, 2000.
8. Heninger GR: Special challenges in the investigation of the neurobiology of mental illness. In: Charney DS, Nestler EJ, Bunney BS (eds.): *Neurobiology of Mental Illness*. New York, Oxford University Press, 1999, pp. 89–99.
9. Burmeister M: Basic concepts in the study of diseases with complex genetics. *Biol Psychiatry* 45(5):522–532, 1999.
10. Collier DA, Curran S, Asherson P: Mission: not impossible? Candidate gene studies in child psychiatric disorders. *Mol Psychiatry* 5(5):457–460, 2000.
11. Petronis A, Gottesman, II, Crow TJ, et al.: Psychiatric epigenetics: a new focus for the new century. *Mol Psychiatry* 5(4):342–346, 2000.
12. Van Praag HM: Over the mainstream: diagnostic requirements for biological psychiatric research. *Psychiatry Res* 72(3):201–212, 1997.
13. Leckman JF, Zhang H, Alsobrook JP, Pauls DL: Symptom dimensions in obsessive-compulsive disorder: toward quantitative phenotypes. *Am J Med Genet* 105(1):28–30, 2001.
14. Almasy L, Blangero J: Endophenotypes as quantitative risk factors for psychiatric disease: rationale and study design. *Am J Med Genet* 105(1):42–44, 2001.
15. Krueger RF: The structure of common mental disorders. *Arch Gen Psychiatry* 56(10):921–926, 1999.
16. Wittchen HU, Hofler M, Merikangas K: Toward the identification of core psychopathological processes? *Arch Gen Psychiatry* 56(10):929–931, 1999.
17. Hendren RL, De Backer I, Pandina GJ: Review of neuroimaging studies of child and adolescent psychiatric disorders from the past 10 years. *J Am Acad Child Adolesc Psychiatry* 39(7):815–828, 2000.
18. Anderson GM, Cook EH: Pharmacogenetics. Promise and potential in child and adolescent psychiatry. *Child Adolesc Psychiatr Clin N Am* 9(1): 23–42, viii, 2000.
19. Bailey A, Phillips W, Rutter M: Autism: toward an integration of clinical, genetic, neuropsychological, and neurobiological perspectives. *J Child Psychol Psychiatry* 37(1):89–126, 1996.
20. McBride PA, Anderson GM, Shapiro T: Autism research: bringing together approaches to pull apart the disorder. *Arch Gen Psychiatry* 53(11):980–983, 1996.
21. Dawson G, Ashman SB, Carver LJ: The role of early experience in shaping behavioral and brain development and its implications for social policy. *Dev Psychopathol* 12(4):695–712, 2000.
22. Skuse DH: Behavioural neuroscience and child psychopathology: insights from model systems. *J Child Psychol Psychiatry* 41(1):3–31, 2000.
23. Jacobs BL, Azmitia EC: Structure and function of the brain serotonin system. *Physiol Rev* 72(1):165–229, 1992.
24. Julius D: Molecular biology of serotonin receptors. *Annu Rev Neurosci* 14:335–60, 1991.
25. Lucki I: The spectrum of behaviors influenced by serotonin. *Biol Psychiatry* 44(3):151–162, 1998.
26. Murphy DL, Andrews AM, Wichems CH, Li Q, Tohda M, Greenberg B: Brain serotonin neurotransmission: an overview and update with an emphasis on serotonin subsystem heterogeneity, multiple receptors, interactions with other neurotransmitter systems, and consequent implications for understanding the actions of serotonergic drugs. *J Clin Psychiatry* 59(Suppl 15):4–12, 1998.
27. Rubenstein JLR: Development of serotonergic neurons and their projections. *Biol Psychiatry* 44:145–150, 1998.
28. Hanley HG, Stahl SM, Freedman DX: Hyperserotonemia and amine metabolites in autistic and retarded children. *Arch Gen Psychiatry* 34(5): 521–531, 1977.
29. Schain RJ, Freedman DX: Studies on 5-hydroxyindole metabolism in autistic and other mentally retarded children. *J Pediatr* 58:315–320, 1961.
30. McDougle CJ, Naylor ST, Cohen DJ, Volkmar FR, Heninger GR, Price LH: A double-blind, placebo-controlled study of fluvoxamine in adults with autistic disorder. *Arch Gen Psychiatry* 53(11):1001–1008, 1996.
31. McDougle CJ, Naylor ST, Cohen DJ, Aghajanian GK, Heninger GR, Price LH: Effects of tryptophan depletion in drug-free adults with autistic disorder. *Arch Gen Psychiatry* 53(11):993–1000, 1996.
32. Anderson GM, Hoshino Y: Neurochemical studies of autism. In: Cohen DJ, Donnellan AM (eds.): *Handbook of Autism and Pervasive Developmental Disorders*, 2nd ed. New York, Wiley, 1997, pp. 166–191.
33. Anderson GM: Studies on the neurochemistry of autism. In: Bauman ML, Kemper TL (eds.): *The Neurobiology of Autism*. Baltimore, Johns Hopkins University Press, 1994, pp. 227–242.
34. McBride PA, Anderson GM, Hertzig ME, et al.: Serotonergic responsivity in male young adults with autistic disorder. Results of a pilot study. *Arch Gen Psychiatry* 46(3):213–221, 1989.
35. Cook EH, Jr., Arora RC, Anderson GM, et al.: Platelet serotonin studies in hyperserotonemic relatives of children with autistic disorder. *Life Sci* 52(25):2005–2015, 1993.
36. Murphy DG, Daly E, Schmitz N, et al.: Cortical serotonin 5-HT2A receptor binding and social communication in adults with Asperger's syndrome: an in vivo SPECT study. *Am J Psychiatry* 163(5):934–936, 2006.
37. Grad LR, Pelcovitz D, Olson M, Matthews M, Grad GJ: Obsessive-compulsive symptomatology in children with Tourette's syndrome. *J Am Acad Child Adolesc Psychiatry* 26(1):69–73, 1987.
38. Leckman JF, Goodman WK, Anderson GM, et al.: Cerebrospinal fluid biogenic amines in obsessive compulsive disorder, Tourette's syndrome, and healthy controls. *Neuropsychopharmacology* 12(1):73–86, 1995.
39. Anderson GM, Pollak ES, Chatterjee D, Leckman JF, Riddle MA, Cohen DJ: Brain monoamines and amino acids in Gilles de la Tourette's

syndrome: a preliminary study of subcortical regions. *Arch Gen Psychiatry* 49(7):584–586, 1992.
40. Anderson GM, Pollak ES, Chatterjee D, Leckman JF, Riddle MA, Cohen DJ: Postmortem analysis of subcortical monoamines and amino acids in Tourette syndrome. *Adv Neurol* 58:123–133, 1992.
41. Baldessarini RJ, Tarazi FI: Brain dopamine receptors: a primer on their current status, basic and clinical. *Harv Rev Psychiatry* 3(6):301–325, 1996.
42. Missale C, Nash SR, Robinson SW, Jaber M, Caron MG: Dopamine receptors: from structure to function. *Physiol Rev* 78(1):189–225, 1998.
43. Diana M: Drugs of abuse and dopamine cell activity. *Adv Pharmacol* 42:998–1001, 1998.
44. Koob GF: Circuits, drugs, and drug addiction. *Adv Pharmacol* 42:978–982, 1998.
45. Goldman-Rakic PS: The cortical dopamine system: role in memory and cognition. *Adv Pharmacol* 42:707–711, 1998.
46. Carey WB: A suggested solution to the confusion in attention deficit diagnoses. *Clin Pediatr (Phila)* 27(7):348–349, 1988.
47. Faraone SV, Doyle AE: The nature and heritability of attention-deficit/hyperactivity disorder. *Child & Adolescent Psychiatric Clinics of North America* 10:299–316, 2001.
48. Castellanos FX, Giedd JN, Marsh WL, et al.: Quantitative brain magnetic resonance imaging in attention-deficit hyperactivity disorder. *Arch Gen Psychiatry* 53(7):607–616, 1996.
49. Cohen DJ, Leckman JF: Developmental psychopathology and neurobiology of Tourette's syndrome. *J Am Acad Child Adolesc Psychiatry* 33(1):2–15, 1994.
50. Singer HS, Wendlandt JT: Neurochemistry and synaptic neurotransmission in Tourette syndrome. *Adv Neurol* 85:163–178, 2001.
51. Leckman JF, Riddle MA: Tourette's syndrome: when habit-forming systems form habits of their own? *Neuron* 28(2):349–354, 2000.
52. Singer HS, Hahn IH, Moran TH: Abnormal dopamine uptake sites in postmortem striatum from patients with Tourette's syndrome. *Ann Neurol* 30(4):558–562, 1991.
53. Wolf SS, Jones DW, Knable MB, et al.: Tourette syndrome: prediction of phenotypic variation in monozygotic twins by caudate nucleus D2 receptor binding. *Science* 273(5279):1225–1227, 1996.
54. Narayan M, Srinath S, Anderson GM, Meundi DB: Cerebrospinal fluid levels of homovanillic acid and 5-hydroxyindoleacetic acid in autism. *Biol Psychiatry* 33(8–9):630–635, 1993.
55. Minderaa RB, Anderson GM, Volkmar FR, Akkerhuis GW, Cohen DJ: Neurochemical study of dopamine functioning in autistic and normal subjects. *J Am Acad Child Adolesc Psychiatry* 28(2):190–194, 1989.
56. Aston-Jones G, Chiang C, Alexinsky T: Discharge of noradrenergic locus coeruleus neurons in behaving rats and monkeys suggests a role in vigilance. *Prog Brain Res* 88:501–520, 1991.
57. Arnsten AF: Catecholamine regulation of the prefrontal cortex. *J Psychopharmacol* 11(2):151–162, 1997.
58. Chrousos GP, Gold PW: The concepts of stress and stress system disorders. Overview of physical and behavioral homeostasis. *JAMA* 267(9):1244–1252, 1992.
59. Charney DS: Monoamine dysfunction and the pathophysiology and treatment of depression. *J Clin Psychiatry* 59(Suppl 14):11–14, 1998.
60. Leckman JF, Hardin MT, Riddle MA, Stevenson J, Ort SI, Cohen DJ: Clonidine treatment of Gilles de la Tourette's syndrome. *Arch Gen Psychiatry* 48(4):324–328, 1991.
61. Van Dijk JG, Koenderink M, Kramer CG, den Heijer JC, Roos RA: Non-invasive assessment of autonomic nervous function in Gilles de la Tourette syndrome. *Clin Neurol Neurosurg* 94(2):157–159, 1992.
62. Chappell PB, Leckman JF, Scahill LD, Hardin MT, Anderson G, Cohen DJ: Neuroendocrine and behavioral effects of the selective kappa agonist spiradoline in Tourette's syndrome: a pilot study. *Psychiatry Res* 47(3):267–280, 1993.
63. Chappell PB, McSwiggan-Hardin MT, Scahill L, et al.: Videotape tic counts in the assessment of Tourette's syndrome: stability, reliability, and validity. *J Am Acad Child Adolesc Psychiatry* 33(3):386–393, 1994.
64. Halperin JM, Newcorn JH, Koda VH, Pick L, McKay KE, Knott P: Noradrenergic mechanisms in ADHD children with and without reading disabilities: a replication and extension. *J Am Acad Child Adolesc Psychiatry* 36(12):1688–1697, 1997.
65. Ornitz EM, Gabikian P, Russell AT, Guthrie D, Hirano C, Gehricke JG: Affective valence and arousal in ADHD and normal boys during a startle habituation experiment. *J Am Acad Child Adolesc Psychiatry* 36(12):1698–1705, 1997.
66. Mefford IN, Potter WZ: A neuroanatomical and biochemical basis for attention deficit disorder with hyperactivity in children: a defect in tonic adrenaline mediated inhibition of locus coeruleus stimulation. *Med Hypotheses* 29(1):33–42, 1989.
67. Pliszka SR, McCracken JT, Maas JW: Catecholamines in attention-deficit hyperactivity disorder: current perspectives. *J Am Acad Child Adolesc Psychiatry* 35(3):264–272, 1996.
68. Arnsten AF, Steere JC, Hunt RD: The contribution of alpha 2-noradrenergic mechanisms of prefrontal cortical cognitive function. Potential significance for attention-deficit hyperactivity disorder. *Arch Gen Psychiatry* 53(5):448–455, 1996.
69. Baker GB, Bornstein RA, Douglass AB, Van Muyden JC, Ashton S, Bazylewich TL: Urinary excretion of MHPG and normetanephrine in attention deficit hyperactivity disorder. *Mol Chem Neuropathol* 18 (1-2):173–178, 1993.
70. Frankenhaeuser M: Behavior and circulating catecholamines. *Brain Res* 31(2):241–262, 1971.
71. McCracken JT: A two-part model of stimulant action on attention-deficit hyperactivity disorder in children. *J Neuropsychiatry Clin Neurosci* 3(2):201–209, 1991.
72. Anderson GM, Dover MA, Yang BP, et al.: Adrenomedullary function during cognitive testing in attention-deficit/hyperactivity disorder. *J Am Acad Child Adolesc Psychiatry* 39(5):635–643, 2000.
73. Hanna GL, Ornitz EM, Hariharan M: Urinary epinephrine excretion during intelligence testing in attention-deficit hyperactivity disorder and normal boys. *Biol Psychiatry* 40(6):553–555, 1996.
74. Pliszka SR, Maas JW, Javors MA, Rogeness GA, Baker J: Urinary catecholamines in attention-deficit hyperactivity disorder with and without comorbid anxiety. *J Am Acad Child Adolesc Psychiatry* 33(8):1165–1173, 1994.
75. Rapoport JL, Mikkelsen EJ, Ebert MH, Brown GL, Weise VK, Kopin IJ: Urinary catecholamines and amphetamine excretion in hyperactive and normal boys. *J Nerv Ment Dis* 166(10):731–737, 1978.
76. Elia J, Borcherding BG, Potter WZ, Mefford IN, Rapoport JL, Keysor CS: Stimulant drug treatment of hyperactivity: biochemical correlates. *Clin Pharmacol Ther* 48(1):57–66, 1990.
77. Minderaa RB, Anderson GM, Volkmar FR, Akkerhuis GW, Cohen DJ: Noradrenergic and adrenergic functioning in autism. *Biol Psychiatry* 36(4):237–241, 1994.
78. Ozawa S, Kamiya H, Tsuzuki K: Glutamate receptors in the mammalian central nervous system. *Prog Neurobiol* 54(5):581–618, 1998.
79. Nakanishi S: Molecular diversity of glutamate receptors and implications for brain function. *Science* 258(5082):597–603, 1992.
80. Nakanishi S, Nakajima Y, Masu M, et al.: Glutamate receptors: brain function and signal transduction. *Brain Res Brain Res Rev* 26(2–3):230–235, 1998.
81. Wilson MA, Tonegawa S: Synaptic plasticity, place cells and spatial memory: study with second generation knockouts. *Trends Neurosci* 20(3):102–106, 1997.
82. Coyle JT, Puttfarcken P: Oxidative stress, glutamate, and neurodegenerative disorders. *Science* 262(5134):689–695, 1993.
83. Loscher W: Pharmacology of glutamate receptor antagonists in the kindling model of epilepsy. *Prog Neurobiol* 54(6):721–741, 1998.
84. Dingledine R, McBain CJ, McNamara JO: Excitatory amino acid receptors in epilepsy. *Trends Pharmacol Sci* 11(8):334–338, 1990.
85. Farber NB, Newcomer JW, Olney JW: Glycine agonists: what can they teach us about schizophrenia? *Arch Gen Psychiatry* 56(1):13–17, 1999.
86. Goff DC, Tsai G, Levitt J, et al.: A placebo-controlled trial of D-cycloserine added to conventional neuroleptics in patients with schizophrenia. *Arch Gen Psychiatry* 56(1):21–27, 1999.
87. Heresco-Levy U, Ermilov M, Lichtenberg P, Bar G, Javitt DC: High-dose glycine added to olanzapine and risperidone for the treatment of schizophrenia. *Biol Psychiatry* 55(2):165–171, 2004.
88. Lane HY, Chang YC, Liu YC, Chiu CC, Tsai GE: Sarcosine or D-serine add-on treatment for acute exacerbation of schizophrenia: a randomized, double-blind, placebo-controlled study. *Arch Gen Psychiatry* 62(11):1196–1204, 2005.
89. Moghaddam B: Targeting metabotropic glutamate receptors for treatment of the cognitive symptoms of schizophrenia. *Psychopharmacology (Berl)* 174(1):39–44, 2004.
90. Swerdlow NR, Young AB: Neuropathology in Tourette syndrome: an update. *Adv Neurol* 85:151–161, 2001.
91. Peterson BS: Neuroimaging studies of Tourette syndrome: a decade of progress. *Adv Neurol* 85:179–196, 2001.
92. Lüddens H, Korpi E: GABAa receptors: Pharmacology, behavioral roles, and motor disorders. *Neuroscientist* 2:15–23, 1996.
93. Bettler B, Kaupmann K, Bowery N: GABAB receptors: drugs meet clones. *Curr Opin Neurobiol* 8(3):345–350, 1998.
94. Kaupmann K, Huggel K, Heid J, et al.: Expression cloning of GABA(B) receptors uncovers similarity to metabotropic glutamate receptors. *Nature* 386(6622):239–246, 1997.
95. Bazil CW, Pedley TA: Advances in the medical treatment of epilepsy. *Annu Rev Med* 49:135–162, 1998.
96. Mondrup K, Dupont E, Braendgaard H: Progabide in the treatment of hyperkinetic extrapyramidal movement disorders. *Acta Neurol Scand* 72(3):341–343, 1985.
97. Sanacora G, Mason GF, Krystal JH: Impairment of GABAergic transmission in depression: new insights from neuroimaging studies. *Crit Rev Neurobiol* 14(1):23–45, 2000.
98. Sanacora G, Mason GF, Rothman DL, Krystal JH: Increased occipital cortex GABA concentrations in depressed patients after therapy with selective serotonin reuptake inhibitors. *Am J Psychiatry* 159(4):663–665, 2002.
99. Bonner TI: The molecular basis of muscarinic receptor diversity. *Trends Neurosci* 12(4):148–151, 1989.
100. Geula C: Abnormalities of neural circuitry in Alzheimer's disease: hippocampus and cortical cholinergic innervation. *Neurology* 51(1 Suppl 1):S18–29; discussion S65–17, 1998.

101. Giacobini E: Cholinergic foundations of Alzheimer's disease therapy. *J Physiol Paris* 92(3–4):283–287, 1998.
102. Perry EK, Lee ML, Martin-Ruiz CM, et al.: Cholinergic activity in autism: abnormalities in the cerebral cortex and basal forebrain. *Am J Psychiatry* 158(7):1058–1066, 2001.
103. Dursun SM, Hewitt S, King AL, Reveley MA: Treatment of blepharospasm with nicotine nasal spray. *Lancet* 348(9019):60, 1996.
104. Stahl SM, Berger PA: Physostigmine in Tourette syndrome: evidence for cholinergic underactivity. *Am J Psychiatry* 138(2):240–242, 1981.
105. Sallee FR, Kopp U, Hanin I: Controlled study of erythrocyte choline in Tourette syndrome. *Biol Psychiatry* 31(12):1204–1212, 1992.
106. Rabey JM, Lewis A, Graff E, Korczyn AD: Decreased (3H) quinuclidinyl benzilate binding to lymphocytes in Gilles de la Tourette syndrome. *Biol Psychiatry* 31(9):889–895, 1992.

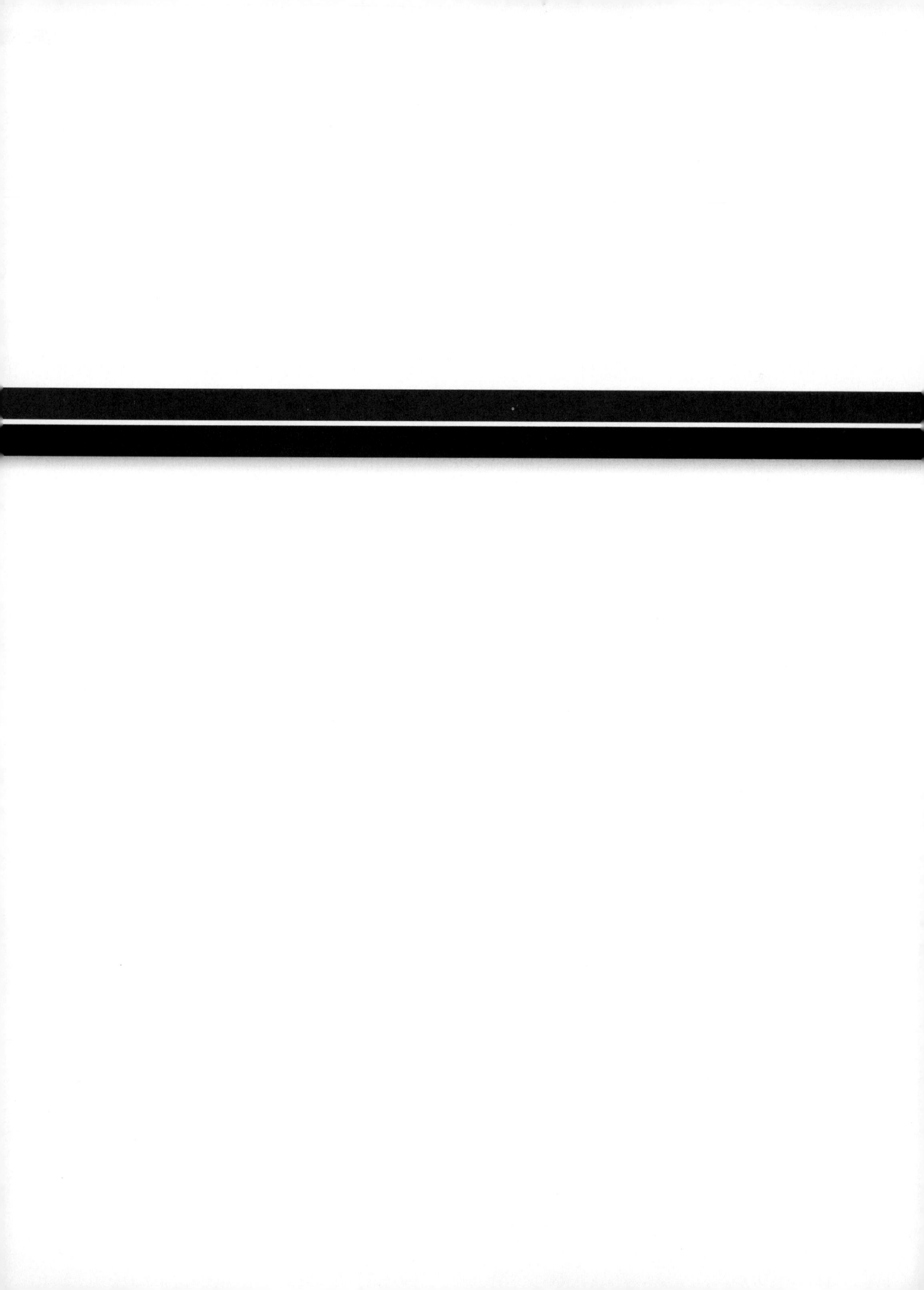

SECTION III
A DEVELOPMENT FRAMEWORK

3.1 ■ NORMAL DEVELOPMENT

CHAPTER 3.1.1 ■ THE INFANT AND TODDLER

LINDA C. MAYES, WALTER S. GILLIAM, AND LAURA STOUT SOSINSKY

The role of child psychiatry in care of infants and toddlers is expanding especially as the diagnostic nosology for serious early development disorders such as autism or attachment disorders becomes increasingly refined. Further, as child psychiatrists collaborate actively with pediatricians (1), they often are called upon to assess infants and toddlers for apparent developmental delays, behavioral difficulties, or parent–child problems. The interface between child psychiatry and pediatrics also means child psychiatrists may consult with parents during their pregnancy or as they anticipate their older child's response to the birth of a new sibling. As child psychiatrists also provide consultation to a range of child care and early education settings, they are more often consulting with parents about child care decisions and settings. Each of these consultative settings requires that child psychiatrists have a solid understanding of normative early development. In this chapter, we provide guidelines for thinking about normal early development and the basic phases of infant and toddler development especially as these are relevant to the clinical practice of child psychiatry. We also provide an overview of salient issues regarding the environments of infants and toddlers again as these are relevant to clinically salient issues in the development of young children.

Most scientists and clinicians define the periods of infancy and toddlerhood as being the first three years of postpartum life. More specifically, infancy refers to the time before the beginning of expressive verbal communication that occurs at about 18 months. The developmental shift that occurs at this time has a dramatic transformational impact on the child's ability to reason cognitively, deepen elaborate social relationships, and mediate emotional experiences linguistically. Toddlerhood is a period of increasing autonomy in which the child uses his or her new skills to explore their world, physically, cognitively, and socially. Regardless of the exact chronological time frame, infancy and toddlerhood encompass the most rapid and contextually transactional period of neurodevelopmental change throughout the postpartum life span. Therefore, all clinical work in child psychiatry with infants and toddlers is framed by the context of rapidly changing, growing systems that may be in or out of synchrony with one another.

NORMATIVE DEVELOPMENTAL FORCES

Development is characterized by processes by which each individual uniquely adapts and integrates his or her own nature with the opportunities and limitations of his or her experience across time. The developmental transactional ecological framework posits a child's behavior at any point in time as a product of reciprocal transactions among the child's characteristics (genetic/biological/physical, cognitive/linguistic, and social/emotional competencies) and the caregiving environment (dynamic interrelationships among child behavior, caregiver responses to such behavior, and the dyadic relationship) and the broader ecological context (multiple levels of social organization, including family, neighborhood, and child care) (2–7).

Developmental psychopathology is similarly characterized by patterns of behavioral adaptation over time and in context, rather than by static, isolated, or domain-specific problems (7–9). The average environment often can sufficiently compensate for problems when they occur. But when a child's unique needs or difficulties are present in an environment lacking adequate nurturance and support, they combine to produce "initial patterns of maladjustment which then spin their way into diagnosable pathology (7)."

Interacting Factors in Development

There are several interacting factors that drive or moderate developmental processes. Indeed, clinical assessment of infants and their families represents a process of gaining a better understanding of these interacting forces. Five specific areas are discussed: a) the interaction of innate and experiential factors, b) maturational processes, c) the essential role of relationships with others for healthy development; d) the broader context of relationships and the environment; and e) developmental stages and critical or sensitive periods. While each of these areas is interrelated, there are points that are unique to each.

The Interaction of Innate and Experiential Factors

The interactive balance between innate and experiential factors is a well worn controversy in developmental science, and even now it is possible to find proponents emphasizing the singular importance of one over the other. Rarely are these issues clearly distinguishable in a clinical evaluation. At the least, infants bring a set of innate capacities that influence how they respond to the environment and how it responds to them. The clinician is always faced with considering how intrinsic and extrinsic factors have interacted to contribute to an infant's developmental difficulties or strengths. Infants are more vulnerable to developmental dysfunction, even with a supportive environment, if there is biological dysfunction, as in genetic disorders or severe prematurity. Conversely, even "well endowed" infants are at risk for developmental dysfunction if their environment provides inadequate or inconsistent nurturing. A combination of an impoverished or dangerous environment combined with biological or genetic risks is a significant predictor of developmental dysfunction, and as the number of risk factors increase so increases the likelihood for poor outcomes (10, 11). Indeed, in an extensive review of genetic research conducted by a special task force of the American Psychological Association, it was concluded that genes, the environment, and the interaction of these two forces each play a large role in cognitive development (12). This transactional model of child development, which stresses the dynamic interplay between individual- (genes, experience) and contextual-level (aspects of environment, culture) factors, is the prevailing paradigm (13) and there are now several compelling examples of apparent gene–environment interaction including, for example, older children's risk for depression in the face of early trauma with social support being the contextual or mediating factor (14).

Maturational Processes

Depending on the clinician's frame of mind, maturation, or the progressive unfolding and differentiation of intrinsic capacities, presents either a complication or a challenge in the process of developmental assessment. Infants change rapidly, and the appearance of behaviors and responses can be highly variable despite certain expected sequences. Also, although very young infants begin life in a relatively undifferentiated state, within the first months, perceptual and motor systems differentiate rapidly. Implicitly, a stage-based model of infant development guides much of clinical perspectives by acknowledging that sequences of development *generally* are based upon orderly maturational steps that have been well described and defined. This sequence and the knowledge of when children typically achieve certain skills can be used to establish norms, against which an individual infant's developmental skills can be contrasted. As Provence (15) has stated, "Maturation ... is a necessary construct, an invisible process represented by observable behaviors."

As described above, environment, genetic predisposition, and the interaction of both can alter maturational forces significantly. For example, we expect grasping patterns to follow an expectable, regular sequence of neurological maturation but know that the timetable for infants' use of a particular grasp to hold a toy or explore a box is individually variable and can be highly related to the infant's exposure. Or, although the infant may have the neurological capacity for a responsive smile and the perceptual–motor integration to extend his or her arms toward an adult, experience in interaction with the environment is a necessary factor for such observable behaviors to emerge. Also, it is true that variants of typical maturational processes exist that are not necessarily associated with later problems. For example, it is typical for infants to learn to crawl on hands and knees at eight to nine months old and then walk at 12 months. However, various alternative pathways of infant locomotion are fairly common and are not necessarily related to underlying problems, and researchers have long known that age of walking alone is not a good predictor of developmental outcomes (16).

It is important to draw a distinction between developmental processes that are primarily delayed versus those that represent a qualitative deviation from the typical progression of skills. For example, some infants and young children present a pattern of development that approximates the typical orderly progression of developmental skills, but are nonetheless developing along that track at a pace significantly behind their same-age peers. Others, however, may evidence patterns of development that are substantially different from the normal progression or show signs of qualitative differences in neuromuscular development (localized or diffuse hypotonia, abnormal reflex patterns). Significantly deviant patterns of development appear to be more common in children whose overall development is very delayed relative to chronological age expectations.

Relationships

It is impossible to overstate the role of human relationships in development. The essential role of stable and nurturing human relationships is well established and universally acknowledged among researchers (17). However, most formal infant assessment techniques were developed to focus exclusively on the measurement of maturational forces, as if assuming that development proceeds relatively independent of environmental input. Thus, it is important to emphasize *that every infant assessment* must consider the other individuals in that infant's life. Understanding normal, delayed, or deviant development requires some understanding of the infant's experiences with adults. The younger the child, the more central are such individuals to the child's safety and total well-being. Such serious events as traumatic separation, physical abuse, witnessing violence, deprivation, loss, and neglect often have devastating effects on a child's development (18). Moreover, less extreme variations in children's environments have profound effects on every aspect of early development, with relationships and interactions with primary caregivers being of acute importance in the very early years.

Understanding the early environment in which infants and toddlers develop is a vast topic that encompasses individual differences in parenting style, the impact of parental psychopathology such as depression, family disruption such as divorce, and how parents adapt their behaviors to the emerging developmental skills of the infant, each areas of extensive clinical scholarship and research. In this section is highlighted the areas most relevant for child psychiatrists beginning to evaluate a young child or work with the parents of an infant or toddler.

Relationships and interactions with primary caregivers, most often the mother and/or father, directly affect and dynamically interact with multiple domains of child development. These domains include attachment and social-emotional development; behavior, cooperation, and development of morality; early learning, exploration, and cognitive and language development; and health and physical development. Parents also indirectly transmit to their children, through their impact on caregiving behaviors, the effects of more distal environmental factors such as poverty (19–21), parental life circumstances (21, 22), and parental beliefs and attitudes (23). Parents can also shape their child's environment indirectly through provision of stimulating and supportive social and material resources in the home environment, through choice of neighborhood, and, most crucially in early childhood, through their decisions regarding nonparental child care (21, 24–26). Furthermore, the same distal environmental factors, like poverty, that affect parenting also limit parents' ability to choose and shape their child's home, neighborhood, and child care environments (17, 20, 21, 25, 26).

Infants are strongly motivated and primed to develop attachments with adult caregivers to ensure close, protective, and nurturing contact. When parenting (or primary caregiving) is reliably sensitive and contingently responsive to a child's cues and needs, the child is more likely to develop a secure attachment. Secure attachment behaviors include using the parent as a secure base from which to comfortably explore, monitoring and seeking proximity with the parent, seeking contact eagerly after separation or if frightened, and evidence of trust and delight in the parent. When parenting is detached, intrusive, erratic, inconsistent, or rejecting, children are more likely to develop an insecure attachment, characterized by disrupted play, preoccupation with the parent's presence, avoidance or resistance to contact and distress or anger at reunion after separation, or difficulty being comforted. Secure attachment has been associated longitudinally with development of social and emotional competence, a child's confidence and sense of efficacy in novel or challenging situations and ability to manage stress, and greater self-efficacy, and is shown to set the stage for future positive relationships with others (16, 28).

Adequate care and nurturing for an infant involves a balance among gratification, comfort, and support and the frustration inevitable in all developmental phases. Adequacy in caregiving, difficult as it is to define, generally includes attempts to mediate painful, tension-producing situations and to adjust the balance between comfort and frustration. The appropriate balance varies depending on the child's age. For example, the infant's frustration at not being fed immediately is different from the toddler's frustration at being unable to reach a favorite toy, and each requires a different response from the parents. In one instance, frustration may produce a painful, tense state; in another, it may lead to an adaptive solution that enhances further learning and appropriate individuation and independence.

Parenting is associated powerfully with other domains of child development beyond attachment, although the lines between various parenting behaviors and areas of child development are blurred by dynamic transactions and integration over time. Sensitivity, contingent, appropriate responsiveness, and consistency are associated with all areas of social-emotional development (including competencies such as sustained attention, compliance, empathy, prosocial peer interactions, and emotion regulation) and also support children's early learning. Parents promote their child's language and cognitive abilities when they understand their child's current abilities and structure learning opportunities accordingly, provide a rich verbal environment, and adjust their support and stimulation as the child's capacities emerge (16, 29).

Furthermore, while encouragement rather than restriction of exploration is helpful, limit setting and consistent and firm standards are also important especially for a toddler's development of cooperation, behavioral control, and sense of conscience. Authoritative (rather than harsh or permissive) setting and enforcement of limits, incentives, and punishments, modeling of desired behaviors, and consistent routines all positively affect child's behavioral development. Rather than a static "parenting style," these behaviors are dynamic, adjust for changing child characteristics, and involve give and take. Toddlers' developing cognitive capacities integrate parental expectations and standards, in turn affecting development of self-regulation, conflict management, empathy, cooperation, and awareness of the feelings and perspectives of others (16, 29).

Often clinicians are not always dealing with gross parenting deficits or failures, such as in serious abuse and neglect (30). For many infants and young children, there are crucial experiences that may have adverse effects that are much harder to identify. For example, we are only beginning to understand the critical effect of maternal depression in the first month to one year, when the mother is psychologically and sometimes physically unavailable to her infant (22, 31, 32). A growing body of research on the issue of caregiver mental illness, however, suggests that serious psychopathology in caregivers can significantly alter dyadic and familial interaction patterns, which in turn lead to altered developmental courses for infants. Caregiver psychopathology is a forceful example of how parental life circumstances might alter parenting and, thereby, infant and toddler development. Other factors internal to the parent—such as parenting stress (negative perceptions of child behavior, the parent–child relationship, and the self as parent) and child rearing beliefs (nonauthoritarian or progressive child-centered child rearing beliefs; such as belief that children learn actively, versus traditional or adult-centered child rearing beliefs; such as approval of uniform treatment and encouragement of obedience to authority)—also shape parenting behaviors. Life circumstances, such as single parenthood, low parental education, substance abuse, and, most pervasively, poverty, can strain the parent's ability to respond sensitively and contingently to their infant's cues and needs (17, 20, 21). Caregivers, however articulate and enlightened, may be unaware of their own difficulties in responding to their infants, or of how their mood states, worries, and frustrations affect their parental responsiveness. It is at this level that the importance of establishing a working relationship between parents and evaluator is clearest.

Broader Context and Environment

The early environment in which infants and toddlers develop is influenced by the broader ecological context. The broader ecological context includes the home environment, other caregiving environments such as nonparental child care, broader family circumstances and risks, and the neighborhood. These contextual influences on child development may be direct, as in the case of a nonparental caregiver's interactions with the child, indirect, as in the effect of poverty on parenting behaviors and available resources, or both direct and indirect, as when poverty limits a parent's child care choices, thus exposing the child to poorer quality child care.

The Home Environment. Within the family setting, the materials, activities, and transactions that are supportive of early learning have been shown to be associated with children's IQ, cognitive and language development, and later school performance (24). The supportiveness and stimulation of home environments vary greatly by family socioeconomic and ethnic status, and such variations, even in the very early years, demonstrate differential effects on child outcomes. Parents' provision of social resources, such as opportunities to interact with peers, also influence child development (17, 20, 21).

Understanding a young child's typical "environment" is a crucial part of any thorough child psychiatric assessment. Who cares for the infant during the day? Is there a live-in nanny or do the parents take their baby to grandparents, older aunt or uncle, or a family childcare program neighbor? Often these individuals may actually spend more direct care time with a young infant than parents themselves and in addition to being able to provide extensive history about the infant's daily routines and emerging skills, are also important attachment figures for the infant. Furthermore, infants and toddlers adapt differently to different caregivers and not uncommonly, may behave differently with different adults or show fewer or more symptoms depending on the adult caring for them at the time. Hence, it is very important to have multiple informants regarding an infant or young child's development and behavior when she or he is being evaluated.

Nonparental Child Care. A very young child's relationship and interactions with his or her parent (or primary caregiver) may be most salient and central to early development, but other caregiving experiences also impact child well-being. For the vast majority of young children today in the United States, nonparental child care is "second only to the immediate family" as a developmental context (17). The impact of relationships and interactions with nonparental child care providers on child development is similar in many ways to the influence of parental relationships. Children can form attachment bonds with nonparental caregivers and receive supports for early learning and language development. In addition, in many settings, young children experience peer interactions and a school-like environment.

To put the scope of child care environments in context, about 10.7 million young children are regularly in care by someone other than their parents, largely due to the vast increase in employment of mothers of young children in recent decades. The largest increase in the last decade and a half has been in child care use by infants and toddlers, with 41% of infants and 53% of toddlers in child care (17). Child care settings, which vary widely, fall into four broad categories, listed from the least to the most formal: relative care, in-home nonrelative care (nannies, au pairs), family day care, and center-based care. Parents more often utilize home-based care for infants and toddlers, in part due to greater preference, flexibility, and availability, and sometimes to lower cost. Almost one-third of infants and toddlers in care are in family day care homes.

The quality, as well as the quantity and type, of child care experienced by young children contributes to child development. High quality child care is characterized by warm, responsive, and stimulating interactions between children and caregivers. For example, high-quality interactions are characterized by caregivers who express positive feelings in interactions with children, are emotionally involved, engaged, and aware of the child's needs and sensitive and responsive to their initiations, speak directly with children in a manner that is elaborative and stimulating while being age-appropriate, and ask questions and encourage children's ideas and verbalizations. Structural quality features of the setting, including ratio of children to adults, group size, and caregiver education and training, act indirectly on child outcomes by facilitating high-quality child–caregiver interactions. To illustrate, it would be difficult for even the most sensitive and stimulating provider to provide high-quality interactions with each child if she was the sole caregiver of 10 toddlers (33).

Disentangling the effects of nonparental caregiving on child development is complex, as the type, quantity, and quality of child care to which children are exposed is not random but selected by parents. Recent research programs, especially that of the NICHD Study of Early Child Care and Youth Development, have made strides in this direction (33). Furthermore, as parents choose child care, it can be considered indirect parenting (even by many parents (34), and is another important avenue by which parents impact their young children's early development. The magnitude of the effects of parenting and family factors on child development is about twice that of child care factors (35). However, after adjusting for family characteristics, child care retains unique influence on child development, to about half the magnitude of the effect of parenting. The greater strength of effect of parenting is to be expected, as biological parents share genetic characteristics with their children, which most nonparental child caregivers do not (or share less genetic similarity, in the case of grandparents or other relatives). Plus, parents (whether biological parents or not) are typically stable, consistent, central presences in their children's early years, whereas most nonparental caregivers come in and out of the children's lives, and many times children have multiple caregivers (and even multiple arrangements) simultaneously. Changes in nonparental care can be disruptive for young children, and are important factors for clinicians to consider in assessment and treatment. The effects of child care characteristics on child development are highlighted next.

A child's experience of child care per se is not related to better or worse outcomes for children compared to child's experience of exclusive maternal care (35). Earlier research suggested that child care exposure in the first year of life may interfere with the mother–child attachment bond (36). However, subsequent research demonstrated that child care use by itself did not affect attachment. Only when combined with low maternal sensitivity and responsiveness did poor-quality child care, larger quantities of child care, or multiple child care arrangements predict greater likelihood of insecure attachment (37). Beyond the question of attachment, the longitudinal effects of child care quality, quantity, and type on child outcomes have been examined extensively, demonstrating that child care quality is a consistent and modest predictor of child outcomes across most domains of development, child care quantity is a consistent, modest predictor of social behavior, and child care type is an inconsistent, modest predictor of cognitive and social outcomes, adjusting for family factors (parental income, education, and race/ethnicity, family structure, parental sensitivity) (35).

Children who experienced higher quality child care performed better than other children on cognitive, language, and academic skill tests and, at some points in early childhood, were rated as showing more prosocial skills and fewer behavior problems and negative peer interactions. Compared to these effects, which were relatively consistent and modest in magnitude, the effects of parenting quality on the same outcomes are consistent and strong, being about twice as strong as the effects of child care quality (35).

Quantity of child care is related only to social outcomes. Children who spend more time in any kind of child care are rated or observed at some points in the preschool period to display more problem behaviors, more teacher–child conflict, and more negative behaviors in interactions with friends. The magnitude of these effects of child care hours on social outcomes are modest (35).

Finally, type of care shows mixed associations with child outcomes. Although findings vary across age, children who experience more center care have stronger cognitive, language, and memory skills and display more positive behaviors in interactions with a friend, but also show fewer prosocial skills and more behavior problems. These effects of center-based care on child outcomes were less consistent and modest compared to other reported effects (35).

The disturbing fact is that, despite the importance of high-quality child care for child development, several large studies have found that most child care is of "poor to mediocre" quality (33, 38, 39). In one study, only 14% of centers (8% of center-based infant care) were found to provide developmentally appropriate care, while 12% scored at minimal levels that compromised health and safety (40% for infant care) (38). Similarly, in another study, 58% of family day care homes provided adequate or custodial care, and only 8% provided good care (39). Unfortunately, children with the greatest amount of family risk may be the most likely to receive child care that is substandard in quality. However, many children from lower risk families also receive lower quality care, and despite their advantages at home, these children may not be protected from the negative effects of poor-quality care (40).

For most parents, finding child care that they can afford, access, manage, and accept as a good environment for their child is a very difficult process, and one many parents find distressing (25, 41). Not only is affordable and accessible child care hard to find, many parents are worried about how their child will fare in child care. Many parents worry that their child will feel distressed by group settings, will suffer from separation from the parents, or will even be subjected to neglect or abuse. This worry is especially likely among low-income parents with fewer family and community resources to draw upon (41). A smaller proportion of parents may think of child care only as babysitting, and may not consider consequences for their child's development so long as the child is safe and warm. These parents may be less likely to select a high-quality child care arrangement, which is especially problematic if the family is facing socioeconomic challenges that already place them at risk of receiving lower quality care for their children (42). Complicating the problem, many parents feel that little organized, helpful professional guidance in choosing child care is available (25). Furthermore, parents are the purchasers but not the recipients of care, and are not in the best position to judge its quality. In addition, many parents are first-time consumers of child care with little experience and very immediate needs, selecting care in a market that does little to provide them with useful information about child care arrangements (43).

Child professionals may be many parents' only source of professional consultation regarding their child. Child psychiatrists can emphasize the importance of high quality care for an infant's or toddler's development, describe how it looks and provide referrals and information on how to find and select high-quality child care. Furthermore, child psychiatrists can help parents determine how to adjust child care arrangements to best meet their child's specific needs (eating and sleeping habits, enhanced language classrooms). Parents may also request a child psychiatrist's assistance in evaluating a program for their child. Child psychiatrists may find it important to see an infant or toddler in their child care setting and to meet the teachers and staff. Increasingly child psychiatrists are called upon to serve as consultants to such settings, both to evaluate individual children and also to consult to the teachers and staff about program development and continued staff education.

Developmental Stages and Critical Periods

Historically, theories of development have conceptualized the phenomena as primarily either quantitative or qualitative. A quantitative conceptualization portrays development primarily as a continuous orderly accumulation of skills, dependent on the mastering of prerequisite skills. Qualitative conceptualizations, in contrast, stress the importance of various developmental stages that are each qualitatively different and represent a marked shift in the manner in which the person perceives, understands, and interacts with the environment. In short, the quantitative conceptions represent development as a continuous process, whereas qualitative theories propose that development is a process marked by periodic discontinuities or reorganizations. The concept of developmental stages involves such theories as Freud's theory of psychosexual stages, Erikson's theory of psychosocial stages, and Piaget's theories of cognitive stages. Clinically, the concept is a valuable one in that it provides schemata for understanding development. Extant research provides some support for both conceptualizations, and the developmental continuity versus discontinuity debate continues.

Research suggesting the existence of certain *critical periods* in human development has provided some support for conceptualizing development as occurring in qualitative different stages. The concept of critical periods for the optimal development of different functions suggests that certain capabilities are optimally mastered at certain times, and difficulties arise when this optimal period is disrupted. Although the concept of critical periods was first clearly established in animal models, it has been demonstrated in humans, especially in the areas of social competence and language acquisition. Indeed, it appears clinically true that when the critical period passes without optimal organization of a given function, mastery is fully achieved with far more difficulty, if ever. It is also a clinical truism that when a function is newly emerging, it is most vulnerable to environmental stresses. This statement is supported by the common observation that an infant may stop talking if hospitalized just as the first words appear. Similarly, for an infant, chronic environmental stressors may result in a delay of appearance of age-appropriate skills. For example, a parent's anxiety over a toddler's growing motoric independence may slow the development of motor skills and the elaboration of exploration. An infant's particular stage of development may influence which issues are most salient and most vulnerable to stress. During an *evaluation* session, stage-specific developmental characteristics also may influence not only the child's ability to demonstrate mastery of certain developmental skills, but also how the infant approaches challenges, including challenges elicited during a developmental assessment. For example, toddlers struggling with emerging independence may react differently to an evaluator's *assessment* tasks than would the younger infant who is focused more establishing social reciprocity and engaging his or her surrounding environment.

Reviewing research over the past decade, Zeanah and colleagues (44) concluded that there exist four distinct stages of qualitative reorganization during the first three years of life. [See also Greenspan (45).] Although their perspective is primarily focused on social-emotional aspects of development and draws from recent research and theory, the stages correspond rather closely to those of earlier developmentalists, especially Piaget (46). Indeed, many of the qualitative changes in cognitive development first proposed by Piaget seem to provide the prerequisites for qualitative changes in social and emotional functioning now being proposed. The following description of different stages during infancy and toddlerhood illustrate these qualitative changes, as well as the dynamic interaction between maturational processes and social relationships and the interactive nature of development across cognitive, sensorial, social, linguistic, and motoric domains.

Five Qualitative Stages of Infancy and Toddlerhood

The Stage 1 Prenatal Development

Although infants with birth defects or malformations are not routinely brought to child psychiatry as the first referral, child psychiatrists working with young children and their families necessarily consider the child's pregnancy. In instances of developmental delays, careful histories regarding exposures to illness or toxins during pregnancy, rate of maternal weight gain, ease or difficulty of delivery, or immediate postnatal complications are important landmarks for charting the health of the pregnancy. Additionally, and especially relevant to child psychiatry, are parental expectations and wishes for the unborn infant. Does the pregnancy come at an optimal or a stressful time for the parent or parents? Have there been major life events during the pregnancy that the parents now associate with their child's development such as the illness of an elderly parent, a job loss, a sudden move? How do the parents imagine their infant to be (a process sometimes referred to as developing a mental portrait of the baby)? This may include imagined personality or physical characteristics, attributions to the fetal patterns of movement during the day ("This is going to be a very active baby—kicks all the time"), or perceptions of how the fetus is apparently responding to the parents' likes and dislikes such as to favorite foods or music. Does the parent perceive the pregnancy as a burden and the fetus as complicating unnecessarily the parent's life, or is the pregnancy viewed as a positively life-changing event, transforming the parent's views of self and of life in general? The "psychological background" of a pregnancy is critical information for understanding how that infant fits into the family and the parents' perceptions and expectations for that child, especially when young children are referred for behavioral or early regulatory difficulties. These mental portraits are equally important information in instances when infants are severely compromised medically (47).

The Stage 2 Infant (0–2 Months)

During the first couple of months postpartum, infants work primarily toward achieving homeostasis, or the capacity for maintaining physiological equilibrium, in the face of internal and external stimulation. However, they are also surprisingly active and sophisticated learners, capable of crossmodally exploring and perceiving his or her environment, visually tracking objects as they move through space, habituating to invariant stimuli, discriminating novelty, and even anticipating caregiver actions (48).

The Stage 3 Infant (2–7 Months)

The second stage (2 to 7 months) is marked primarily by increased social reciprocity between the infant and caregiver(s). This qualitative change follows increased awareness of the external world (made possibly by greatly enhanced visual abilities) and improved coordination of sensory input and nonreflexive (voluntary) motor output occurring at about 1 month of age. During the second stage, the infant's responsive cooing, repertoire of increasingly differentiated emotional responses, and a proclivity toward direct imitation of others' behaviors starting at about 4 months serve to facilitate reciprocal or contingent social interactions. During the latter half of the second stage (beginning as early as about 4 1/2 months), infants start to show an understanding of *object permanence* (the understanding that objects and people continue to exist even when they are no longer within sight or sound) and a rudimentary understanding of the principles of *cause and effect*. These two epiphanies transform the infant's perception of the world and provide the requisite abilities for all future social-cognitive development. The concept of object permanence allows the infant to create mental representations of objects and others. It is therefore a prerequisite skill for imagining and for visual differentiation between caregivers and strangers. Cause-and-effect reasoning leads to increased intentionality of actions. Both of these newfound cognitive abilities make possible simple interactive games between infants and caregivers, such as peek-a-boo.

The Stage 4 Infant (7–18 Months)

At about 7 to 9 months another qualitative shift occurs with profound impacts on reciprocal communication and social preference or familial belonging. At this time infants develop a sense of *intersubjectivity*, the understanding that their thought, feelings, gestures, and sounds can be understood by others. Also, at about this age, most infants begin to demonstrate means–end reasoning leading to goal-directed behavior. They can string together several behaviors (more than one) in order to achieve a final outcome, often the attainment of some desired object. Through intersubjectivity and means–ends reasoning, the infant is able to consider caregivers as objects that can be used to get their needs and wants met. (And the Stage 3 infant's now solid grasp of object permanence gives him or her a large inventory of these wants and needs.) Together, intersubjectivity and means–end reasoning lead to the beginning of *communicative gesturing* (e.g., the moment when stretching for an object just out of reach becomes pointing to that object while looking at the caregiver in order to request assistance). In the context of all of these qualitative changes in the way in which the infant interacts with others, social preferences are established and become increasingly salient. At about 6 to 8 months of age, *separation anxiety* is first observable with most infants, peaking at about 14 to 18 months and declining thereafter (49). Relatedly, *stranger anxiety* appears to begin at about 8 months, peaks at about 24 months, and steadily declines thereafter.

By the second half of Stage 3 (starting at about 12 months), several new skills in the cognitive, language and motor domains create profound changes. At about 12 months infants typically first learn to walk, and this new form of independent locomotion, more so than crawling, heralds increased independence and a broadening world. Cognitively, the infant's reasoning becomes strikingly less rigid and more open to alternative solutions. For example, prior to about 12 months, infants who learn that an object is hidden in a particular place will persist in looking for that object at that same location even after watching someone relocate that object to a different location. This is commonly referred to as the AB error. However, after about 12 months the infant's ability to hold increasingly larger amounts of information and to discard outdated information allows for a fluidity of reasoning such that the AB error diminishes or disappears. Given this increased cognitive capacity and fluidity of reasoning, *trial-and-error problem solving* begins to replace conditioned response learning. Also, from about 12 to 18 months infants develop rudimentary communicative speech. By 12 months most infants understand the meaning of several words and may have an expressive vocabulary of about five or six words. By the time they reach 18 months of age, infants typically understand the meaning of an amazing number of words, can communicate in one-word sentences, and have doubled their expressive vocabulary to about 10 words. Their melodic, jargoned speech patterns now closely resemble the inflections and turn-taking pauses observed in conversation.

The Stage 5 Infant (18–36 Months)

At about 18 months an increased ability to use *symbolic representation* transforms the infant's cognitive and social world. About 12 months earlier, object permanence marked the beginning of the infant's ability to hold in the mind mental representations of objects. The Stage 4 infant is now well able to allow symbols to stand for objects, heralding greatly increased language proficiency. The use of words marks a qualitative change in the way infants think about the world and interact with others, and, likely, the reverse is true as well (50). The beginning of this transformation appears to be marked by a move from direct imitation of others to *deferred imitation*, where the behaviors of others are remembered and then practiced later. *Symbolic play* appears as the infant uses a doll to symbolize a baby, and the infant begins to combine words and gestures in order to label objects in his or her world or make needs and wants known to caregivers. By 18 months these skills are becoming solidified, and the infant's interactions

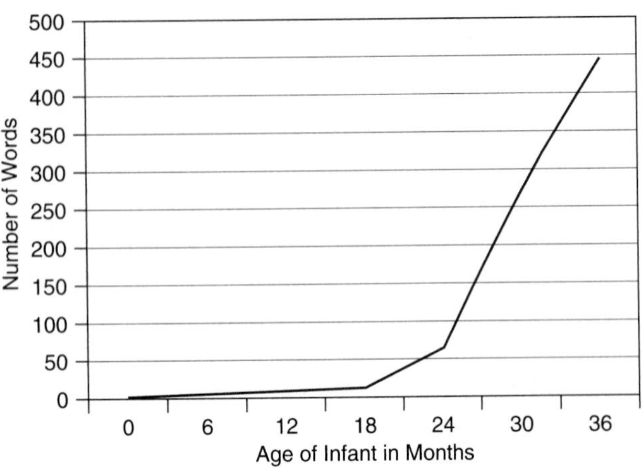

FIGURE 3.1.1.1. Typical rate of increase in expressive vocabulary of infants.

with others change dramatically. Additionally, at about 18 to 24 months, *internal problem solving* begins to replace trial-and-error problem solving, as the infant's ability to mentally hold and manipulate internal representations increases. From 18 to 24 months, toddlers' expressive vocabularies typically increase from about 10 words to about 50 to 75 words. By 30 months, the toddler's expressive vocabulary has increased to nearly 300 words, and by 36 months many toddlers have an expressive vocabulary of 500 to 1,000 words and typically speak in three- to four-word sentences (51) (Figures 3.1.1.1 and 3.1.1.2).

FORCES THAT MAY COMPROMISE NORMATIVE DEVELOPMENT

A variety of both endogenous and exogenous forces may compromise normal infant and toddler development. These are described briefly below and listed in Table 3.1.1.1.

Regulatory Disturbances

These include disturbances in self-regulatory capacities, such as sleep or eating disturbances, including food refusal, night terrors, repeated waking, or problems in impulse control such as excessively aggressive behavior. Low frustration tolerance is another mark of regulatory difficulties. Self-stimulatory behaviors, such as rocking or head banging, may indicate a variety of social or regulatory difficulties, may be a manifestation of environmental stress, or may signify more profound difficulties in relatedness, as in pervasive developmental disorder.

TABLE 3.1.1.1

FORCES THAT MAY COMPROMISE NORMATIVE DEVELOPMENTAL PROCESSES

1. **Regulatory Disturbances**
   - A. Sleep disturbances (frequent waking)
   - B. Excessive crying or irritability
   - C. Eating difficulties (finicky eating or food refusal)
   - D. Low frustration tolerance
   - E. Self-stimulatory/unusual movements (rocking, head banging, excessive finger sucking)
2. **Social/environmental Disturbances**
   - A. Failure to discriminate caregiver
   - B. Apathetic, withdrawn, no expression of affect or interest in social interaction
   - C. Excessive negativism
   - D. No interest in objects or play
   - E. Abuse, neglect, or multiple placements or caregivers
   - F. Repeated or prolonged separations from caregivers
3. **Psychophysiological Disturbances**
   - A. Nonorganic failure to thrive
   - B. Recurrent vomiting or chronic diarrhea
   - C. Recurrent dermatitis
   - D. Recurrent wheezing
4. **Developmental Delays**
   - A. Specific delays (gross motor, language)
   - B. General delays or arrested development
5. **Genetic and Metabolic Disorders with Known Neurodevelopmental Sequelae**
   - A. Down syndrome
   - B. Fragile X syndrome
   - C. Inborn errors of metabolism
6. **Exposure to Toxins**
   - A. Fetal alcohol syndrome
   - B. Lead poisoning
7. **Central Nervous System Damage**
   - A. Traumatic brain injuries
   - B. Intraventricular hemorrhages
8. **Prematurity and Serious Illnesses Early in Life**

Social/Environmental Disturbances

Disturbances in social development and/or the caregiving environment, including serious and profound problems in differentiating mother or caregiver, such as might be seen in pervasive developmental disorder or infantile autism, and disturbances in predominant mood. Infants who are predominantly withdrawn and apathetic are at great risk for developmental difficulties. In this category are also included environmental conditions such as repeated or prolonged separations or neglect, abuse, and exposure to violence, all of which place infants at risk for social and affective disturbances (30).

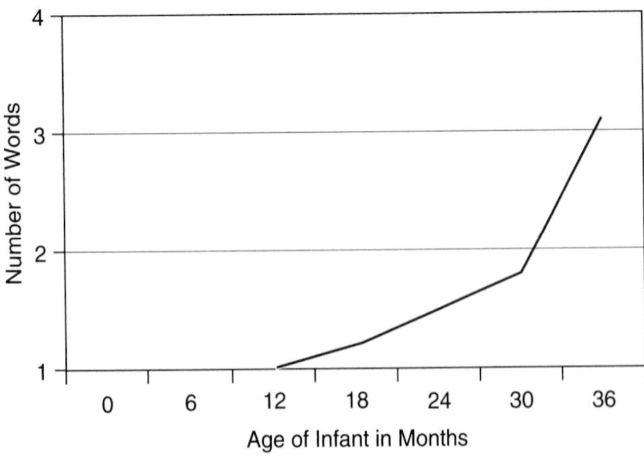

FIGURE 3.1.1.2. Typical rate of increase in number of words per sentence in infants.

Psychophysiological Disturbances

These include, among others, failure to thrive, recurrent vomiting, wheezing, or chronic skin rashes. The younger the child, the more likely the response to an environmental stress will be a global one involving several organ systems (e.g., failure to thrive). Clearly, any one of these problems may have physical causes, but clinicians should be alert to the close connection between physiological and psychological adjustment in young children.

Developmental Delays

Delays in specific areas of development, including motor development and activity, language and communication, awareness of others and degree of relatedness to others (seen often together with language delay), or delays in more than one of these areas. Such delays may be more common among infants with complicated perinatal courses such as those born severely premature or following parental substance abuse and prenatal exposure to alcohol, cocaine, or other drugs. Thus, infants with such histories will more often be referred for assessments early in order to plan for appropriate interventions.

Genetic and Metabolic Disorders with Known Neurodevelopmental Sequelae

Various genetic and metabolic disorders have known neurodevelopmental sequelae. These include, but are not limited to, Down syndrome, fragile X, Prader-Willi, certain sex chromosome anomalies (e.g., Klinefelter's syndrome), and poorly managed phenylketonuria (PKU) (52). Although certain developmental and behavioral sequelae are associated with these conditions, the extent can often vary considerably, and developmental assessment can be useful to document its course and better target psychosocial interventions.

Exposure to Toxins

Exposure to environmental toxins, such as the case with fetal alcohol syndrome and lead poisoning, has been associated with both developmental delays and behavioral disregulation. Though useful in treatment planning, assessments are not able to determine the proportion of the developmental presentation attributable to these potential causal factors.

Central Nervous System Damage

Central nervous system damage (e.g., traumatic brain injuries and intraventricular hemorrhages) can, of course, lead to developmental sequealae, and followup with a developmentalist can be invaluable in understanding the level of functional impairment and tracking recovery.

Prematurity and Early Illnesses

Prematurity and other serious medical conditions that may result in hospitalization or other restriction of appropriate stimulation early in a child's life, may lead to altered parent–child interaction and adversely affect development (53).

Extant research suggests that the specific disturbances and conditions listed above are highly interrelated and mediated by the social context of the child (44). For example, failure to thrive may also indicate social (the family and caregiver–child dyadic relationships) and/or environmental disturbances, or general developmental delay may occur with repeated separations or in a withdrawn, apathetic child. A particular developmental profile, such as delayed language skills but age-appropriate motor and problem-solving skills, may occur with different presenting difficulties, and thus it is not possible to specify a characteristic diagnostic developmental pattern for failure to thrive, sleep disturbances, or the other problems listed in the table.

In addition to the above caveats, three general points are important to remember. First, language and communication skills are particularly vulnerable to biological and environmental stresses. Moreover, problems in communication also affect personal-social development. For most of the problems listed under social/environmental disturbances, the infant will likely show minimally delayed language and personal-social development. Also, any adaptive or motor items that require interaction with the examiner will be affected by disturbances in relatedness, and the child's skills in these areas will appear scattered not necessarily because of motor impairment but because of the necessity for social interaction for administering the item. Second, it is possible for an infant presenting with some of the difficulties outlined in the table to have an age-appropriate developmental profile in terms of what things the child can and cannot do. In this case, the qualitative observations of how the infant approaches the setting are crucial. The qualitative aspects of the child's interactions with the caregiver and the evaluator, motivations, problemsolving processes, and mood state are infinitely more important than a simple inventory of the infant's skills. Third, an infant's or toddler's level of developmental functioning may vary considerably between domains. Infants with psychophysiological disturbances often show such a "scattered" developmental profile. Qualitative observations are again important with this kind of profile, as well as repeated assessments over time in order to gain a better sense of the child's developmental trajectory.

Generally, a comprehensive assessment of a young child provides a description of the child's functional capacities, the relationships among the various domains such as language and socialization, the child's ability to adapt, and the range of coping strategies. For the very young infant, developmental assessments describe neurodevelopmental functioning and individual regulatory capacities. For caregivers, the evaluation provides information about both their child and the potential therapeutic value of the alliance established with the clinician. For the referring clinician, the assessment may provide a more integrated view of the infant's psychological as well as physical status. Finally, infant assessments often serve the purpose of facilitating referrals to appropriate educational or rehabilitative services. In such cases, the useful question is not whether or not the infant is delayed or has problems, but what are the most appropriate services to ameliorate these problems or to compensate for these conditions. In cases such as these, the evaluating clinicians will need to be collaborators themselves with individuals directing intervention and educational services for infants. (Several excellent reviews of the effectiveness of early intervention services for infants are available (54–56).)

SUMMARY

Infant psychiatry is a developing field that brings child psychiatrists into closer work with very young children and their parents. Disorders such as autism have long been recognized as specific developmental disorders requiring intensive child psychiatric care but more recently, early regulatory disturbances, disruptions in attachments, prematurity, and other biological disruptions have come into the purview of child psychiatrists. Working with infants and toddlers brings child psychiatrists into close contact with rapidly developing systems and infant psychiatry requires a detailed appreciation of the range of normative as well as abnormal development and an understanding of how different caregiving environments may dramatically alter developmental trajectories, especially in the first years of life. The child psychiatrist with a special interest in infancy and early childhood by virtue of his or her medical training has a special appreciation of the biological aspects of early development. The contemporary infant psychiatrist has available the wealth of data from many infant observational studies, from genetic and neurobiological perspectives, and from a rich multidisciplinary environment of professionals working with infants, toddlers, and their families that includes developmental psychologists, social workers, pediatricians, geneticists, and developmental neurobiologists. Further, the infant psychiatrist is constantly integrating biology with an understanding of the infant's adult caring environment and assessing the relationship between infant and family as much as the developmental integrity of the infant.

References

1. Mayes LC: Collaboration between child psychiatrists and pediatricians. In: Cavenar JO (ed.): *Psychiatry (Revised Edition)*. Philadelphia: J.B. Lippincott; 1992, Chap. 73.
2. Bronfenbrenner U: Contexts of child rearing: Problems and prospects. *American Psychologist* 34(10):844–850, 1979.
3. Bronfenbrenner U: Ecology of the family as a context for human development: Research perspectives. *Developmental Psychology* 22(6):723–742, 1986.
4. Bronfenbrenner U: Environments in developmental perspective: Theoretical and operational models. In: Friedman SL, Wachs TD (eds): *Measuring environment across the life span: Emerging methods and concepts*. Washington, DC: American Psychological Association, 1999, pp. 3–28.
5. Sameroff AJ: Transactional models in early social relations. *Human Development* 18(1–2):65–79, 1975.
6. Sameroff AJ: The social context of development. In: Eisenberg N (ed): *Contemporary topics in development*. New York: Wiley, 1987.
7. Sameroff AJ: Developmental systems and psychopathology. *Development & Psychopathology*. Sum 2000;12(3):297–312.
8. Sroufe L, Rutter M: The domain of developmental psychopathology. *Child Development*. Vol 55(1), Feb 1984, 17–29.
9. Cicchetti D: Developmental psychopathology: Reactions, reflections, projections. *Developmental Review*. Dec 1993;13(4):471–502.
10. Sameroff AJ, Chandler MJ: Reproductive risk and the continuum of caretaking causality. In: Horowitz FD, Hetherington M, Scarr-Salapatek S, et al. (eds): *Review of child development research*. Vol 4. Chicago: University of Chicago Press, 1975, pp. 187–244.
11. Peck S, Sameroff A, Ramey S, Ramey C: Transition into school: Ecological risks for adaptation and achievement in a national sample. Paper presented at: Biennial Meeting of the Society for Research in Child Development; April, 1999; Albuquerque, NM.
12. Neisser U, Boodoo G, Bouchard TJ, et al: Intelligence: Knowns and unknowns. *American Psychologist* 51:77–101, 1996.
13. Sameroff AJ, Fiese BH: Models of development and developmental risk. In: Zeanah CH (ed): *Handbook of infant mental health*. 2nd ed. New York: Guilford Press, 2000, pp. 3–19.
14. Kaufman J, Yang BZ, Douglas-Palumberi H, et al: Brain-derived neurotrophic factor-5-HHTLPR gene interactions and environmental modifiers of depression in children. *Biological Psychiatry* 59(8):673–680, 2006.
15. Provence S: Developmental assessment: Principles and process. In: Brennemann (ed): *Practice of pediatrics*. Vol 1. Hagerstown, MD: Harper & Row, 1972, Chap 5.
16. McGraw MB: From reflex to muscular control in the assumption of an erect posture and ambulation of the human foot. *Child Development* 3:291–297, 1932.
17. Shonkoff JP, Phillips DA (eds): *From neurons to neighborhoods: The science of early childhood development*. Washington, DC, National Academy Press, 2000.
18. Rogeness GA, Suchakorn A, Amrung SA, et al.: Psychopathology in abused children. *Journal of the American Academy of Child and Adolescent Psychiatry* 25:659–665, 1986.
19. Brooks-Gunn J, Duncan GJ. The effects of poverty on children. *Future of Children*. Sum–Fal 1997;7(2):55–71.
20. Bornstein MH, Bradley RH. *Socioeconomic status, parenting, and child development*. Mahwah, NJ, Lawrence Erlbaum Associates, 2003.
21. Aber JL, Jones SM, Cohen J. The impact of poverty on the mental health and development of very young children. In: Zeanah CH, ed. *Handbook of Infant Mental Health*. New York: Guilford Press; 2000.
22. Cicchetti D, Rogosch FA, Toth SL: Maternal depressive disorder and contextual risk: Contributions to the development of attachment insecurity and behavior problems in toddlerhood. *Development and Psychopathology*. Spr 1998;10(2):283–300.
23. Kochanska G: Maternal beliefs as long-term predictors of mother–child interaction and report. *Child Development*. Dec 1990;61(6):1934–1943.
24. Bradley RH, Caldwell BM: Home observation for measurement of the environment: A revision of the preschool scale. *American Journal of Mental Deficiency* 84(3):235–244, 1979.
25. Pungello EP, Kurtz-Costes B: Why and how working women choose child care: A review with a focus on infancy. *Developmental Review* 19(1):31–96, 1999.
26. Gable S, Cole K: Parents' child care arrangements and their ecological correlates. *Early Education & Development* 11(5):549–572, 2000.
27. Oates J, Lewis C, Lamb ME: Parenting and attachment. In: Ding S, Littleton K (eds.): *Children's personal and social development*. 2005, pp. 12–51.
28. Baumwell L, Tamis-LeMonda CS, Bornstein MH: Maternal verbal sensitivity and child language comprehension. *Infant Behavior & Development* 20(2):247–258, 1997.
29. Kochanska G, Thompson RA: The emergence and development of conscience in toddlerhood and early childhood. In: Grusec JE, Kuczynski L (eds.): *Parenting and children's internalization of values: A handbook of contemporary theory*. New York: John Wiley & Sons, Inc, 1997, pp. 53–77.
30. Kaufman J, Henrich C: *Exposure to Violence and Early Childhood Trauma*. Zeanah, Charles H Jr, 2000.
31. Garrison WT, Earls FT: Epidemiology and perspectives on maternal depression and the young child. In: Tronick E, Field T (eds.): *Maternal depression and infant disturbance*. San Francisco: Jossey-Bass New Divisions for Child Development, 1986, pp. 13–30.
32. Murray L, Cooper PJ: *Postpartum Depression and Child Development*. New York, NY. Guilford Press, 1997.
33. NICHD Early Child Care Research Network. *Child care and child development: Results from the NICHD study of early child care and youth development*. New York: Guilford Press, 2005.
34. Uttal L: Custodial care, surrogate care, and coordinated care: Employed mothers and the meaning of child care. *Gender & Society* 10(3):291–311, 1996.
35. NICHD Early Child Care Research Network. Child-care effect sizes for the NICHD study of early child care and youth development. *American Psychologist*. Feb–Mar 2006;61(2):99–116.
36. Belsky J, Rovine MJ. Nonmaternal care in the first year of life and the security of infant–parent attachment. *Child Development*. Vol 59(1), Feb 1988, 157–167.
37. NICHD Early Child Care Research Network. The effects of infant child care on infant–mother attachment security: Results of the NICHD study of early child care. *Child Development* 68(5):860–879, 1997.
38. Helburn SW (ed.): *Cost, quality, and child outcomes in child care centers: Public report*. 2nd ed. Denver, CO, Department of Economics, Center for Research in Economic and Social Policy, University of Colorado, 1995.
39. Kontos S, Howes C, Shinn M, Galinsky E: *Quality in family child care and relative care*. New York, Teachers College Press, 1995.
40. Peisner-Feinberg ES, Burchinal MR: Relations between preschool children's child-care experiences and concurrent development: The cost, quality, and outcomes study. *Merrill-Palmer Quarterly* 43(3):451–477, Jul 1997.
41. Farkas S, Duffet A, Johnson J: *Necessary compromises: How parents, employers, and children's advocates view child care today*. Washington, DC, Public Agenda, 2000.
42. Sosinsky LS: *Parental selection of child care quality: Income, demographic risk, and beliefs about harm of maternal employment to children* [Dissertation]. New Haven, CT, Department of Psychology, Yale University, 2005.
43. Helburn SW: Preface. *The Annals of the American Academy of Political and Social Science* 563(1):8–19, 1999.
44. Zeanah CH, Boris NW, Larrieu JA: Infant development and developmental risk: A review of the past 10 years. *Journal of the American Academy of Child and Adolescent Psychiatry* 36(2):165–178, 1997.
45. Greenspan S: *Psychopathology and adaptation in infancy and early childhood*. New York, International Universities Press, 1981.
46. Piaget J, Inhelder B: *La psychologie de l'enfant [The psychology of the child]*. Paris, Presses Universitaires de France, 1966.
47. Mayes LC: The assessment and treatment of the psychiatric needs of medically compromised infants: Consultation with preterm infants and their families. *Child and Adolescent Psychiatric Clinics of North America* 4(3):555–569, 1995.
48. Bremner G, Fogel A: *The Blackwell Handbook of Infant Development*. Oxford, Blackwell Publishing, 2004.
49. Kagan J. Emergent themes in human development. *American Scientist* 64:190, 1976.
50. Hollich GJ, Hirsh-Pasek K, Golinkoff RM: Breaking the language barrier: An emergentist coalition model for the origins of word learning. *Monographs of the Society for Research in Child Development* 65(3), 2000.
51. Ulrey G: Assessment considerations with language impaired children. In: Ulrey G, Rogers SJ (eds): *Psychological assessment of handicapped infants and young children*. New York, Thieme-Stratton, 1982.
52. Madrid A, Marachi JP: Medical assessment: Its role in comprehensive psychiatric evaluation. *Child and Adolescent Psychiatric Clinics of North America* 8:257–270, 1999.
53. Minde K: Prematurity and serious medical conditions in infancy: Implications for development, behavior, and intervention. In: C. H. Zeanah J (ed.):

Handbook of infant mental health. 2nd ed. New York: Guilford Press, 2000, pp. 176–194.
54. Clarke-Stewart K, Fein GG: Early childhood programs. In: Haith MM, Campos JJ (eds): *Handbook of child psychology*. Vol 2. New York: Wiley, 1983, pp. 917–999.
55. Guralnick MJ (ed): *The effectiveness of early intervention*. Baltimore, Brookes, 1997.
56. Shonkoff JP, Meisels SJ: Early childhood intervention: The evolution of a concept. In: Meisels SJ, Shonkoff J (eds): *Handbook of early childhood intervention*. New York: Cambridge University Press, 1990, pp. 3–31.

CHAPTER 3.1.2 ■ THE PRESCHOOL CHILD

LAURA STOUT SOSINSKY, WALTER S. GILLIAM, AND LINDA C. MAYES

Between the ages of two to five years and under average conditions, children's cognitive, social, and emotional worlds are rapidly expanding and changing (1). Their language abilities expand their capacity for imagination and symbolic thinking and for enlarging social relationships. Their changing cognitive capacities expand their ability for problemsolving and learning about the world. They develop the ability to name their own and others' feelings and to relate behavior to emotional states and expressions. During the preschool period of development, children are even more commonly in broader social worlds, such as child care and early childhood education programs, and may also experience the birth of a new sibling. While pediatricians remain the most likely professional to be consulted by parents when they are concerned about their two- to five-year-old child's health and development, a number of other professionals are very likely to be involved in a preschooler's life, including child care and educational professionals. (Throughout this chapter, the use of the word "parent" is inclusive of all adults that assume an important and regular role in providing care to the child.) Also, this developmental period marks the beginning of more common referrals to child psychiatrists. These referrals come from teachers, parents, and pediatricians most commonly for behavioral problems, especially excessive aggression with peers or other adults, separation difficulties when faced with school and child care programs, developmental delays, especially of speech and language, and concerns about social delays, especially as these relate to social disabilities such as autism.

Development of behavior and competencies is a process of change over time as a child's characteristics reciprocally transact with the immediate caregiving environment and the broader ecological context, as discussed in the previous chapter on infant and toddler development (2–6; see Chapter 3.1.1). In the preschool years, specific features of these elements that differ from the earlier infancy and toddlerhood period include, for most preschoolers, increasing sophistication and capacity of cognitive, communicative, and social-emotional skills, a longer history of more varied experiences with parents and primary caregivers, and the high likelihood of exposure, often extensive, to nonparental early care and education contexts, perhaps for the first time.

As with infancy and toddlerhood, the diagnostic nosology for specific disorders among preschool children is only beginning to emerge and only a few diagnostic labels, such as autism and the related social disabilities, are commonly used. Furthermore, social-emotional well-being has received lesser emphasis relative to the impact of cognitive and linguistic competencies on later child outcomes. In addition, developmental change in early childhood is rapid, and assessment of normal and problematic behaviors can be challenging. However, there is a growing body of research evidence that social-emotional and behavioral problems in early childhood are real, not transient, and that occurrence and persistence are associated both with cooccurrence of other problems and with family and parenting difficulties (7). From this and other work, there is general consensus that the understanding of a child's development requires an appreciation of the caregiving contexts which support, protect, and nurture the child during this period of dependence on adults (8).

In this chapter we review several areas relevant to preschool children's development and those issues about which child psychiatrists may be most often called upon to consult with families and teachers. The basic developmental areas of normative preschool development include a) robust language learning, including the word-learning explosion and use of language to express emotions and convey more complex or hypothetical information; b) emerging thinking and learning capacities, including executive functioning skills as well as the young child's emerging ability to reflect on his own and others' mental activities—feelings, dreams, beliefs, and thoughts; c) emerging peer relationships and the capacity for imaginary play (and imaginary friends); and d) normative issues regarding separation and individuation. Consideration is given to each of these areas' transactions over time with each other, with caregiving, and with the broader environmental context. Understanding these basic developmental areas is key to a child psychiatrist's ability to consult effectively when parents and teachers bring developmental concerns about a young child.

In terms of specific consultative questions, we cover three areas in brief—fears and apparent anxiety, aggressive behavior, and child psychiatric consultation to preschool settings as examples of the more common reasons for child psychiatric involvement with preschool children. Specific diagnoses including autism, conduct or oppositional difficulties, attentional problems, and assessment for developmental delay are covered elsewhere in this volume.

LANGUAGE

A word-learning language explosion begins at about 18 months and continues through the preschool years, during which children learn on average about nine words per day. Language acquisition is robust, with children learning vocabulary and the fundamentals of linguistic semantics by age 4 or 5, even with very little environmental support (as exemplified by deaf children's early communication even without language input). However, there appears to be a sensitive period for language proficiency. The specific language a child learns and linguistic qualities such as morphology, grammar, phonology, verbal expression of emotions, and conveyance of information about past, present, or hypothetical events are best learned by the preschool period. The difference among children of differing language proficiency levels on these linguistic qualities is not as much whether or not they can use these linguistic skills, but in the frequency and effectiveness with which they use them in their daily lives. The ease at which these skills can be learned begins to decline at about 6 or 7 years of age (9).

As language proficiency is pivotal for subsequent cognitive and social development, especially school readiness and success, the contributors to development of language proficiency are of great interest. There is evidence that the amount of talk caregivers (usually mothers) direct toward their young children is associated with vocabulary growth and preliteracy skills. The amount and richness of the vocabulary children are exposed to, both child- and other-directed, is also related to language development (10). The genetic contribution of parents is of course important, but so is the family's socioeconomic status, with children of lower income, less educated parents receiving less quantity and quality of linguistic exposure and demonstrating lower levels of language proficiency (9).

EMERGING MINDS

Beginning around two years of age, young children start to form more stable concepts of the world around them. They begin to think symbolically—to use one object to stand for others. For example, young children use scribbled drawings to represent houses, people, animals—and to tell stories using these scribbled bits.

Moreover, in the preschool period, there begin to be vast individual differences in children's executive functioning—a child's capabilities to self-regulate, sequence, plan, and organize. The development of these executive controls has a global and lasting effect on later competencies, and problems in executive functioning can lead to later school problems. In contrast, there is little individual variation in normally developing preschoolers' disposition towards a positive motivation. Young children are intrinsically motivated to explore, try, and learn. In the preschool period, this intrinsic motivation is related to self-attributions about their abilities that are indiscriminately positive. Typically developing preschoolers often perceive themselves as being the best at everything, and to be getting better and better everyday. This disposition often declines on school entry, which may be related to improved cognitive abilities of self-appraisal and social comparison, but is also likely associated with a greater exposure to peers and the increased judgment and potential for criticism in formal school environments. Early education, whether formal or informal by parents and caregivers, should have as a goal encouragement of a child's natural inclination to explore and learn, not only to foster cognitive skills but also a positive motivation toward learning (9).

The preschool period is also marked by the beginnings of concerted attention to a child's skills and abilities considered basic to school readiness, as well as basic self-care skills. Children acquire skills best when caregivers present them with tasks that are just a bit too difficult to accomplish independently, but are possible with appropriate assistance. This highly effective approach to teaching young children requires a certain degree of sensitivity to the child's developmental level, often referred to as the child's "zone of proximal development (11)." In addition to this type of parent–child interaction, parents encourage their child's preliteracy and premath skills with activities such as reading, quantitative games, and provision of opportunities such as trips to the library. These activities are most influential when undertaken in warm and nurturing routines. Being read to has the most impact when the child is comfortably and regularly cuddled in a parent's lap for a bedtime story (9).

By the time children are four to five years old, they have acquired the ability to understand that their thoughts, beliefs, and feelings are their own and that others may feel differently, even believe differently from them. Interpreting the behaviors and words of others as being a part of their feelings and thoughts is a major part of being human and getting along in a social world. This capacity is a remarkable developmental achievement covered broadly under the term *developing theory of mind*—the notion that a part of social development is seeing the world in both physical and nonphysical terms, with the latter being invisible or imagined states of thoughts, feelings, and beliefs. There is a large literature on the emerging theory of mind in young children, especially as a capacity that does not develop fully in autistic children, and several have proposed distinct stages in this developmental progression—from a physical stance (the world is as we see it, and we predict the world based on the laws of nature) to an intentional stance in which we understand and predict the world at the level of mental states—beliefs, feelings, fears, worries. The boy is crying because he misses his grandmother, or the girl is happy because she got the present she was hoping to receive.

Once children begin to see the world through the lens of mental states, their understanding of their own self and others greatly expands. They are capable then, for example, of playful deceit—hiding something in a way that sends another person down the wrong path because they understand that by providing deceptive clues, the other person develops a false belief as to the whereabouts of an object. They become capable of subtle sarcasm, understanding that just by a change in a tone of voice, someone else reads their intent and not just the meaning of their words. However, during the preschool years, these capacities are just emerging and tend to disappear at moments of fatigue or stress. Thus, a clinician working with a four-year-old who has been remarkably clear about his feelings and the feelings of others may be very surprised when a usually competent boy melts in disappointment or anger because he was sure his mother knew exactly what he was thinking about for his birthday. Further, under stress or unusually severe trauma and neglect, it is very difficult for children to fully develop or allow themselves to imagine the intentions of others who may have been hurtful or neglectful and thus, clinicians working with severely disadvantaged populations may see a delay in the appearance of these very important social perspective-taking capacities. Thus, in addition to understanding where their patients are in basic developmental domains such as cognition, language, fine and gross motor, child psychiatrists working with young children need also to evaluate where their preschool patient is in his/her capacity to think about his own feelings and beliefs as well as those of others. This is most evident in their play (see next section) and less often through direct questions of "How do you feel?" or "What do you think?" though they may answer such questions indirectly about characters in a story or in a play sequence of their own.

PLAY

Play, broadly defined, covers many activities. One is the rough and tumble play of children running, jumping, chasing, and wrestling with one another. This form is universal across most cultures, and even across different species. Play also includes verbal forms that are uniquely human, in which children play with sounds and words, even inventing their own language and rhymes—and it is this capacity that is most central to a child psychiatrist's ability to communicate with younger children through the special language of play. Manipulating and exploring toys and other objects is a form of play that gives young children a chance to learn by looking, feeling, tasting, listening—a form of trial and error, hands-on learning.

Pretend Play

Children's pretend play varies remarkably in quality, content, intensity, and engagement with other children and adults. In part, their developmental maturity defines the type of play they are capable of creating. Pretend play begins around age two, or just before children are able to let a real object stand for another or for something imaginary. When a toddler begins to brush a doll's hair, this is the very beginning of her ability to pretend. She is using a toy (a doll) with a real object (a brush) to represent a real action. When she starts to feed the doll with a spoon, making lip-smacking noises and blowing on the spoon to cool the soup, she has gone one step further. She is "representing" imaginary food. And when she offers that food to another doll or an adult, the full ability to pretend—to represent her mental world through play—is in evidence.

The ability to pretend requires the ability to symbolize—to let one thing stand for another, just as a picture of a car stands for a real car. The ability to create symbols or representations is part of entering a more complex and layered world of social communication. There are several different levels or stages in learning to use symbols. In the earliest, a baby picks up a spoon and touches it to the edge of a bowl. She thus shows she understands this object's use—what actions a spoon is associated with, even when she is not using it for that action. A variant on this later stage is when a child "eats" from an empty spoon and looks with a smile to her father as she nibbles. Similarly, a toddler can act out sleep, closing his eyes for a few seconds before looking to see if a parent is watching. When a preschooler pretends to feed a doll and read it a story, he shows he is capable of a more complicated level of pretense. And when children begin turning one representation into another, such as having a cup be a hat, their pretend abilities are at an even more sophisticated level. That opens up more avenues for expression.

Peer Play

Play with peers and establishing relationships with other children is "one of the major developmental tasks of early childhood (9)." Both the type and the complexity of play has been studied, specifically in regard to prosocial play, engaged behavior, and emotional expression during play. A child's acceptance among peers also begins to vary in the preschool years, although peer like- or dislike-nominations are very unstable at this time. A striking increase in social skills occurs in the preschool years, and peer play increasingly involves pretense (described further below) and expanded numbers of children.

Very young children under three years of age often play alone with a toy or other object. They may roll a truck around and make authentic truck sounds. But they make no special effort to invite others to join their play. In "parallel play," also characteristic of children three years of age and younger, two or more children play by themselves but close to each other. They may even use similar toys, such as a bucket and sand, but they are not playing with one another. They are simply in close proximity.

Children three to four years old begin to engage one another. They share toys, pass them back and forth, even talk about the same activity and follow one another. Their play is still not completely cooperative, however. If preschoolers have no real companion nearby, they may engage an imaginary friend as a playmate. When children are around four years and older, they begin to engage one another in games in which they must share a goal and a story. They assign roles, direct action, even carry stories and games from day to day.

Peer play is influenced by caregivers. Secure attachment relationships have been associated with higher levels of social competence, greater preschool popularity, and more positive friendships (12, 13). In addition, parents' role in helping children play well with others and provision of peer play opportunities, monitoring of peer interactions, modeling and coaching acceptable behaviors, and discouraging unacceptable behaviors are all associated with more positive peer relationships (9).

A child's temperament is also related to his or her peer interactions. Inhibition hinders children's peer interactions, although excessive exuberance can also cause difficulties. More importantly, the child's ability to regulate his or her individual temperament is associated with peer-interaction skills. A child's competencies at sustained attention, controlled expression of negative emotion, and ability to inhibit certain actions is more related to positive peer interactions and relationships than is underlying temperament as such (9).

Clinical Use of Play

One of the important skills for a child psychiatrist working with younger children is learning how to use play therapeutically and as a means of communicating with young children about what is uppermost in their minds. Often children who have been neglected or otherwise stressed and traumatized are unable to use play adaptively and unable to engage in imaginative fantasy play. If we consider play as a special language for communication with younger children, it is appropriate to work with a young child to enhance their ability to play as a means of expression of anxieties and worries (though play should never be taken as a veridical account of children's past experiences). To use play therapeutically requires different techniques from simply joining in with children's play. For one, the child psychiatrist is always trying to understand what a child may be conveying through his or her play—why this burst of anger in the animals surrounding the house, why the lonely child whose cries are never heard? At the same time, direct interpretation of play, that is, taking the imaginary action and translating it into questions about the child's own experiences, is not always effective inasmuch as young children are not always able or aware of using play characters and themes to tell stories directly reflective of their own experiences. Their play may reflect what is concerning to them—how to handle being angry or feeling lonely—but this is not the same as interpreting, for example, the lonely crying child in the play as being a direct statement of an experience the patient must have had. Thus, while there is a considerable literature on this issue, child psychiatrists using play as a therapeutic technique may be more effective by staying "within the play" and, for example, introducing another character who also feels very lonely and lost and does not know what to do or a character who comes along to help. Either way, the therapist is working within the child's story to try to help the child expand his expression of his feelings and his beliefs in a way that helps the therapist better understand the patient.

Many preschool children—up to half, according to some surveys—create imaginary companions and insist on their reality. For children under five, the boundary between fact and fantasy is often more fluid. But if pressed, most preschoolers will agree that their friends are not really visible, not really hungry, not really sleeping beside them. Imaginary friends seem to serve a number of normative purposes including companionship. Indeed, the forms that imaginary friends take often reflect children's concerns and anxieties, just as their games do. An imaginary friend can offer a child psychological protection from her worries by taking on magical powers, or even by succumbing to dangers in the child's place. Child psychiatrists are often faced with distinguishing between the normative use of an imaginary friend and a young child's more than expected difficulty in distinguishing real from pretend. With younger children, this distinction may be especially difficult and require seeing the child in more than one setting and over time.

SEPARATION

Typically developing preschool-aged children are struggling between independence and dependence, to be both "grown up" and at the same time able to turn to their parents. Especially around separations and transitions, preschoolers are often unpredictable and emotionally labile. They can effortlessly separate for child care one day and the next tearfully cling to their parents. An outside stress, such as the birth of a new baby, may make separation more difficult. Many preschoolers have had some successful experiences with separations, such as going to child care or staying at home with a babysitter. Each separation successfully weathered enhances the preschooler's ability to withstand the next.

Preschoolers often struggle to deal with separations because their repertoire of coping abilities is still developing. Older children can call on their increased cognitive abilities and a repertoire of past experiences, but preschool children do not always have the cognitive abilities to reassure themselves that each separation will work out. This is why it is very common for a preschool child to question her parents repeatedly, even about daily experiences like child care, and ask to be reassured about when parents will return, where they will be during the day, and who will pick them up. Parents often feel confused, frustrated, and guilty hearing these questions repeated, but preschool children ask because they are using their newfound language skills to deal with uncertainty.

Preschool children's emerging symbolic capacities also help them cope with separations—a stuffed animal or other favorite toy, a picture, or even something belonging to their parent can stand for a person they miss. Preschoolers' use of symbolic possessions also shows their newfound capacity for "object constancy," the knowledge that something can be out of sight but nonetheless continue to exist. Preschool children are just beginning to grasp this idea as it pertains to people. They are starting to create mental images of their absent parents and to wonder what people are doing when they are not with them. Nearly every young child worries about being left alone or separated from his parents. This is true no matter how thoughtful or careful parents have been or even if they have not been separated from their preschoolers. Children especially need their parents close when they are afraid, feeling sick, or going through important changes, such as moving or starting a new school.

Parents are often surprised at how hard it is for a preschooler to say goodbye to a favorite teacher at the end of the year, or accept a new teacher the following year. Children this age also mourn the loss of a regular babysitter or nanny, and do not easily replace that person with someone new. Preschoolers need help in mastering the experience of parting with people outside the family. They need to be reassured that their caregiver did not leave because of them. Visits with an old nanny or teacher after the farewell are helpful, as are pictures, letters, and phone calls. Sometimes parents think continued contact will make it harder for their children to get used to a new teacher or nanny, and feel that it is best for the child to experience a "clean break" with their previous teacher or nanny. This approach, however, rarely helps preschoolers. Even years later, children may mention an early teacher or babysitter parents had long forgotten. They return time and time again to rework the separation and think about what that person meant in their lives.

An especially difficult separation for young children may be during parental separation and divorce (14). How does the nearly inevitable conflict between parents that accompanies divorce affect a young child still concerned about consistency and object constancy? What is the impact of parental loss versus shared custody? Goldstein, Freud, and Solnit (15) emphasized the critical roles of clinical expertise and opinion in serving the best interests of young children in custody disputes, and it is an increasingly common consultation for child psychiatrists to be asked either by a court or by parents to consult about how best to help a young child in the instance of parental conflict and divorce.

The principle of continuity of care, so often stressed for young children as essential for their ability to deal with separation, comes into practical application in two major decisions during divorce—custody and visitation. By and large, for preschool children, single parent—rather than two-parent—custody remains the most common decision of courts but joint custody is increasing as fathers want to be more involved in their childrens' lives and more mothers face the difficulties of working full time and raising a family. While there is no firm empirical evidence to support either alternative, experiential case reports do suggest that younger children do better when parents are able to minimize the degree of discord and conflict and/or avoid catching the child in the middle of their disputes. Similarly there are few to no systematic data about appropriate visitation models but it is clear that consistency, structure, and predictability are key, especially as preschoolers are highly dependent on routines and dependable structure. Child psychiatrists specializing in work with younger children may be involved not only in consultation to the court but in ongoing consultation to one or both parents for how best to care for their child and how both parents, if they so desire or if appropriate, may have a role in their child's life.

FEARS AND ANXIETY

Fears, worries, and anxiety are often more evident in children's second and third years, even as separation and stranger anxiety wane. This fearfulness and caution is normative. It keeps a very young, very small child from straying too far. While it may sound paradoxical, children who are well cared for are more able to experience normal fear and worry and thus to run back to their parents for comfort and reassurance. Children who have been neglected and abused are more often heedless of danger. They cannot easily recognize normal feelings of fear and worry as protective signals (16).

Despite their energy and enormous interest in the world, two- and three-year-old children are still quite dependent on adults and are still often preoccupied, even in the most optimal of situations, with the constancy of the important people in their lives. They feel apprehensive not just about new things they encounter but also about what appears in their thoughts and fantasies. They may feel particularly uneasy at bedtime when they are about to be left alone. Preschool children soothe their worries through constancy and routines. Indeed, such rituals are the essence of this age. If a child can keep things around her unchanging and predictable, the world seems a little less uncertain and daunting. For the child psychiatrist asked to evaluate a young child who becomes inconsolable with the slightest change in routine, the question is how normative versus how rigid such routines are, what purpose they serve, and how they fit in the child's daily routine.

Fears and worries also become more evident in the preschool years because, as discussed earlier, this is when the capacities for imagination greatly expand—and usually what young children imagine is far more frightening than their actual experiences. Their bad dreams seem real, and for them there is only a thin line between scary thoughts and actual events. Playing about monsters, they may suddenly become quite scared when they hear a door open elsewhere in the house. Two- and three-year-olds are certain that just by thinking about scary things, they can sometimes make them happen. They are sure that everyone knows about their occasionally angry thoughts, and that such anger can actually harm others. Young children thus feel simultaneously powerful and helpless, at the center of their world and insignificant. They have the power to make things happen and, at the same time, are so small in the face of the bad things they can imagine in the world. All this is cause for normal anxieties but once again, often poses a diagnostic challenge for a child psychiatrist who must distinguish between what is usual for age and what has gone beyond the bounds of normative to be constrictive and maladaptive.

Unlike older children and adults, preschoolers cannot always talk explicitly about their worries or try to avoid the thoughts or situations that frighten them. Often, therefore, they show their fears in paradoxical ways. Afraid of the vacuum cleaner, they may actively avoid it, or they may constantly try to explore and master it. Fearing the dark, they may play with turning the lights on and off or be frantic whenever they are left alone in their beds at night. They may become ever more insistent on certain rituals. Some preschoolers meet any change in their routine with irritability. Young children going through a particularly worrisome time may have routines about food, clothing, bathing, and going to school. These routines are soothingly predictable whenever the child feels uncertain and confused. At the same time, insistence on sameness is a characteristic of a number of early developmental disorders and the consulting child psychiatrist faces, as with other issues raised in this chapter, the dilemma of sorting normative from maladaptive.

Often young children show their worry and fear in ways that seem unexpected, such that the more anxious they are, the more active and uncontrollable they become. Often they are so excited that they cannot heed their parents' or teachers' efforts to help them. Some adults might interpret this behavior as willful or oppositional, but it often reflects a state of such internal overstimulation and anxiety that the child simply cannot control himself. For some children, worries and fears are not simply responses to developmental pressures or the stresses of ordinary living. Rather, their strong, often overwhelming feelings grow out of proportion to their experiences. Anxieties interfere with their lives at school and home, with their friendships, and with their pleasure in play. This increase in worry can be a part of a stressful life event, such as the birth of a new sibling, an illness, or a death in the family.

AGGRESSION

Aggression is a complex set of behaviors, especially in preschool children that reflects a balance between response to frustration versus assertiveness and individuation. Aggressive behavior is one of the more common reasons for child psychiatry consultation, especially in the context of a young child's placement in a child care or educational setting. Furthermore, out of control, aggressive behavior may be one of the most common difficulties between young children and their parents that prompt families to seek mental health consultation. Thus, understanding aggression as both a normative developmental requirement and a possible symptom is key to effective child psychiatric consultation.

Aggressive behavior in young children has many roots and serves some important social roles. Furthermore, adults have considerable influence over how children view and express their aggressive thoughts. While some variables in a child's aggression, such as her basic tolerance for frustration, may depend in part on genetic endowment and/or early experience, many others are shaped by what he or she learns from her experiences with parents and teachers.

At the very least, aggressive behaviors always express some needs and feelings of the child. Also, children who enter their second year of life with few words sometimes may exhibit greater levels of physical aggression than their more verbose peers because they have no other means to express their needs and frustrations. Some children rarely, if ever, express themselves through aggressive behaviors, while others find aggressive behaviors a ready and comfortable way of communicating. Reliance on aggressive behaviors to meet needs can be modeled by parents, other adults, peers, and siblings, and screen media (television, videos, movies, computer games).

For very young children, aggressive behavior is also a way of expressing independence, as in "Mine!" "Me do!" and "Go away!" These firm statements may be unpleasant, even hurtful, to another person or anger an adult. Toddlers' temper tantrums, while surely tempestuous and irritating for parents, are statements of frustration. These young children often feel small, dependent, and powerless, but as they grow their need for independence grows, too. Thus, developmentally, temper tantrums begin as children start to experiment with separation from their parents. The more they move away from the emotionally secure base of the parent, the more dependent and little they may feel, and the more vulnerable to frustration and tantrums they may become.

Aggressive feelings and thoughts, not necessarily expressed in behavior, are also a central part of young children's fantasy lives. They are small and dependent upon a much larger, stronger adult world. They struggle for independence—to be "grown up." Pretending to be very powerful, even scary and aggressive, is one way to play with getting bigger. In preschool children, aggressive behaviors have different intents, causes, and outcomes.

In trying to figure out why a child is biting or hitting, it is important for the child psychiatrist to ask where she directs her violence: toward other people or only toward inanimate objects? In other words, does she kick and break toys or kick and hurt her classmates, siblings, and parents? What typically starts the aggressive behavior? Is she frustrated by wanting a toy she cannot have, or by wishing to be hugged by a very busy parent or teacher? Is she very tired or very excited—at the end of the day or just after a puppeteer has visited the child care center? Is she reacting to another child's teasing about her hair, how she fell on the playground, or how she cried when her father left? Did another child hit or push her? It is also wise to consider the apparent intent of a child's aggressive behavior. Is it a means to an end—to get the desired toy or make a place on the teacher's lap? Is it to create a personal space—a kind of "don't tread on me" signal? Does the goal seem to injure or destroy, or is it really to gain another's attention, to win in a game, or get the best seat in circle time? No child acts aggressively in the same way for the same reasons in every situation. By identifying what a child really wants, her caregivers can tell her not to push or hit while also showing her a better way to achieve her aim, thus reducing her frustration and need to act out.

When evaluating a child's aggression, it is also important to consider how it might be linked to his fears and worries. Such behavior may be a way for him to express how he is really worried deep down without acting fearful. Not all aggressive feelings in children reflect deeper fears and anxiety, but when they do, it is very important for parents and teachers to be made aware of these fears and worries. For most young children, physically aggressive behavior—hitting, biting, pushing, kicking—begins to subside by their third, or at the latest their fourth, birthdays. On the other hand, verbal aggression—shouting, yelling, name-calling—increases between the ages of two and four years as children gain more language skills. Most often, all kinds of hostile behaviors, verbal and physical, diminish in frequency by five or six years of age when children enter first and second grade. Younger children are most aggressive around asserting their physical needs and wants. Older children, in contrast, focus their aggression on social situations and needs. Indeed, as children get older, their aggression is more often related to a perceived hurt or slight; they want to pay back an insult to their self-esteem which they perceive from a particular person. Thus, paradoxically, as children get older, they are far less aggressive, but when they are, their actions may be more often intended to harm another person.

Although significant behavior problems during the early years are often stable and predictive of later behavioral difficulties (7), it is not guaranteed that an aggressive preschooler will grow into an aggressive school-age child. Despite parents' and teachers' concerns, the hitting, kicking, biting three-year-old is not guaranteed to become an aggressive school-age child. What matters most is how adults understand and meet aggressive behavior in younger children. By finding methods for young children to strive for mastery, self-assertion, and self-protection, adults support these important developmental tasks without encouraging hostile or violent behavior. Aggression met with aggression is far more likely to convey the message that people can express frustration and anger only through shouting, name-calling, or physical action. Aggression met with an effort to understand what a young child is trying to communicate shows that when people feel frustrated and angry, they can think about how to express those feelings in ways other people understand.

CHILD PSYCHIATRIC CONSULTATION IN PRESCHOOL SETTINGS

There are more preschoolers enrolled in early education and child care programs than ever before (17, 18). The recent increase in the number of preschoolers enrolled in formal care outside means that a greater number of young children are coming into contact with potential referral agents (preschool teachers, child care providers), which translates into more psychiatric referrals at lower ages than ever. Rather than simply waiting for these young children and their families to present at the child psychiatrist's office, many child psychiatrists and clinicians of other disciplines have sought to address the referral issues in the child care or preschool setting (19, 20).

There are many advantages to providing child psychiatric services as part of a consultative service to early care and education programs (21). Consultative delivery models afford the clinician an opportunity to observe the patient in a natural setting (e.g., the child care program), observe interactions with often several peers, obtain information about the child's functioning from other adults in addition to the parents, and enlist the assistance of many adults in supporting treatment recommendations. Additionally, children often behave very differently at home versus in their child care programs, where the degree of structure and behavioral expectations may vary considerably. The opportunity to observe the child across these different settings is often invaluable as a way of better understanding potential environmental triggers for the behavioral concerns and understanding the child's capacity to modulate her behavior to match different environmental contexts.

Mental health consultation in early education programs can take many forms. Consultation can be focused solely on classroom specific reduction of particular behaviors that the teacher finds difficult to manage (peer aggression, tantrumming, running out of the classroom), or it can be more global in focus, such as using the classroom experiences to create opportunities for the child to develop competencies that can lead to increased self-efficacy. Sometimes the consultation is focused specifically on the child, but often the consultation may include systemic assistance to the teaching staff regarding how to improve the overall mental health climate in the classroom, facilitating teachers' understanding of children's behaviors and teacher behavior management skills, creating a more efficient and effective system of screening and identifying children in need of assistance, and sometimes even addressing mental health needs in the teaching staff.

Attention paid to the overall functioning of preschool and child care classroom (from the physical setting to interactions between teachers and children) can provide clues to understanding the child's behavior and how best to intervene. When a child and family presents in a psychiatric office, it is essential to understand the effect of familial psychopathology on the young child (22). Similarly, the metal health of preschool teachers, who sometimes spend as many or more waking hours with a preschooler than do his parents, can impact child–adult interactions and contribute to emotional and behavioral difficulties. For example, child care provider depression has been associated with child care that is less sensitive, more detached from the children, and (when not detached) more intrusive or negative (23). Also, child care teachers who report elevated levels of depression or job stress, or depressed levels of job satisfaction, are more likely to report having expelled a preschooler from their classroom in the past year (24). Of course, low wages and relatively high levels of job turnover in the child care workforce (25) may contribute significantly to teacher burnout. Unfortunately, mental health consultation in child care settings may often ignore adult functioning.

SUMMARY

Between two and five years of age is a time of very rapid development, especially in social and cognitive skills that expand the world for preschool children. They gradually acquire the ability to think in terms of mental states such as feelings and beliefs, to understand others' intentionality, and to play symbolically and imaginatively. Increasingly, they are venturing further from the home, forming relationships with peers and nonfamilial adults in child care and early education settings. Child psychiatrists working with children of this age are often faced with distinguishing normative heightened anxiety, preference for routines, and aggression from presentations in which these same characteristics are maladaptive and in need of intervention. Hence, this developmental period especially calls for a thorough understanding of normal as well as abnormal development. Further, as with infancy, this period of development also brings child psychiatrists in close collaboration and consultation with pediatricians and early childhood education settings.

References

1. Goswami U: *Blackwell Handbook of Childhood Cognitive Development*. Oxford, Blackwell Publishing, 2004.
2. Bronfenbrenner U: Contexts of child rearing: Problems and prospects. *American Psychologist* 34:844–850, 1979.
3. Bronfenbrenner U: Ecology of the family as a context for human development: Research perspectives. *Developmental Psychology* 22:723–742, 1986.
4. Bronfenbrenner U: Environments in developmental perspective: Theoretical and operational models. In: Friedman SL, Wachs TD (eds.): *Measuring environment across the life span: Emerging methods and concepts*. Washington, DC: American Psychological Association, 1999 pp. 3–28.
5. Sameroff AJ: Transactional models in early social relations. *Human Development* 18:65–79, 1975.
6. Sameroff AJ: The social context of development. In: Eisenberg N (ed.): *Contemporary topics in development*. New York, Wiley, 1987.
7. Briggs-Gowan MJ, Carter AS, Bosson-Heenan J, Guyer AE, Horwitz SM: Are infant-toddler social-emotional and behavioral problems transient? *Journal of the American Academy of Child and Adolescent Psychiatry* 45:849–858, 2006.
8. Carter AS, Briggs-Gowan MJ, Davis NO: Assessment of young children's social-emotional development and psychopathology: Recent advances and recommendations for practice. *Journal of Child Psychology and Psychiatry and Allied Disciplines* 45:109–134, 2004.
9. Shonkoff JP, Phillips DA: *From neurons to neighborhoods: The science of early childhood development*. Washington, DC, National Academy Press, 2000.
10. Hart B, Risley TR: *Meaningful differences in the everyday experience of young American children*. Baltimore, Paul H Brookes Publishing, 1995.
11. Vygotsky L: Tool and symbol in child development and internalization of higher psychological functions. In: Cole M, John-Steiner V, Scribner S, Souberman E (eds.): *L. Vygotsky, Mind in society*. Cambridge, MA: Harvard University Press, 1978.
12. Howes C: The earliest friendships. In: Bukowski WM, Newcomb AF, Hartup WW (eds.): *The Company They Keep: Friendship in Childhood and Adolescence*. New York: Cambridge University Press, 1996 pp. 66–86.
13. Park KA, Waters E: Security of attachment and preschool friendships. *Child Development* 60:1076–1081, 1989.
14. Mayes LC, Siegl AM: In: Galatzer-Levy R, Kraus L (eds.): *The Scientific Basis of Child Custody Decisions*. New York: John Wiley and Sons; 1999 pp. 188–204.
15. Goldstein J, Freud A, Solnit AJ: Beyond the Best Interest of the Child. New York: Free Press, 1973.
16. Crittenden PM, Ainsworth MDS: Child maltreatment and attachment theory. In: Cicchetti D, Carlson V (eds.): *Child Maltreatment: Theory and Research on the Causes and Consequences of Child Abuse and Neglect*. New York: Cambridge University Press, 1989 pp. 432–463.
17. Barnett WS, Hustedt JT, Robin KB, Schulman KL: *The State of Preschool: 2005 State Preschool Yearbook*. New Brunswick, NJ, Rutgers University, National Institute for Early Education Research, 2005.
18. Gilliam WS, Zigler EF: A critical meta-analysis of all evaluations of state-funded preschool from 1977 to 1998: Implications for policy, service delivery and program evaluation. *Early Childhood Research Quarterly* 15:441–473, 2000.
19. Kaplan M: In: Mayes LC, Gilliam W (eds.): *Child and Adolescent Psychiatric Clinics: Comprehensive Psychiatric Assessment of Young children*. Philadelphia: Saunders, 1999 pp. 379–394.
20. Sosinsky LS, Gilliam WS: Child care: How pediatricians can support children and families. In: Kliegman RM, Behrman RE, Jenson HB, Stanton BF (eds.): *Nelson Textbook of Pediatrics*. 18th ed. Philadelphia: Elsevier; in press.
21. Donohue PJ, Falk B, Provet AG: *Mental Health Consultation in Early Childhood*. Baltimore, Paul H. Brookes, 2000.
22. Cicchetti D, Rogosch FA, Toth SL: Maternal depressive disorder and contextual risk: Contributions to the development of attachment insecurity and behavior problems in toddlerhood. *Development and Psychopathology* 10:283–300, 1998.
23. Hamre BK, Pianta RC: Self-reported depression in nonfamilial caregivers: Prevalence and associations with caregiver behavior in child-care settings. *Early Childhood Research Quarterly* 19:297–318, 2004.
24. Gilliam WS, Shahar G: Preschool and child care expulsion and suspension: Rates and predictors in one state. *Infants and Young Children* 19:228–245, 2006.
25. Whitebook M, Sakai L: Turnover begets turnover: An examination of job and occupational instability among child care center staff. *Early Childhood Research Quarterly* 18:273–293, 2003.

CHAPTER 3.1.3 ■ DEVELOPMENT OF SCHOOL-AGE CHILDREN

LEE COMBRINCK-GRAHAM AND GERALDINE S. FOX

INTRODUCTION

The middle years of childhood, spanning the age from when a child enters primary school through the onset of adolescence, are also referred to as "the school-age period" because of the critical importance of school in development in our society. Many classical theorists have classified this time as the period when a child enters society and begins to establish the basis for becoming a contributing member of his/her community.

Sigmund Freud, and other drive theorists, described middle childhood as a sexually dormant interlude between the mastery of Oedipal strivings with establishment of the superego, and the pubertal reawakening of sexual desire in a true genital phase. It has since been established that latency is a myth. Erik Erikson lent a more enduring characterization of this period when he described the critical psychological issue: "Industry versus Inferiority (1)." In formal schooling a child is attempting to master the basics of the industry of our society, to build on academic abilities. Failure to progress in school and in the peer context can establish a sense of inferiority rather than support the momentum of a drive for competence. Neofreudians (Sullivan, Horney, Thompson) added an emphasis on social context as the critical shaping force on how this developmental period is negotiated. Harry Stack Sullivan, for example, observed that this "juvenile era" provides the first opportunity for society to "correct" the influence of the family.

Freud, Erickson, and Sullivan defined the important work of this period. Research into the details of cognitive, emotional, and social development confirm that civilization and being-in-society are the essentials of development in the school-age period. Thus, thinking about the child's psychological well-being must extend beyond the child to include not only the family but also the social, economic, and political contexts that define its functioning. Vygotsky's concept of "mind in society" and Bateson's "ecology of mind" point to the dynamic exchange of experience, accomplishment, and social response and effectiveness.

The best way to emphasize the remarkable growth that occurs during middle childhood is to contrast the skills of children when they enter and exit grade school (Table 3.1.3.1).

Table 3.1.3.1 describes what can be seen in normal average children in the United States, whether they come from poor, inner city neighborhoods, rural settings, or more privileged and educated family backgrounds. Children may be more advanced if they have been provided with educationally stimulating experiences. Children who do not perform at the levels indicated in the table require closer examination to determine whether "delays" are due to disabilities, emotional factors, or contextual factors.

Abundant information supports a rich understanding of how the innate physical, cognitive, psychosexual, and moral maturation of children between the ages of 6 and 10 is meshed with the children's increasing presence in societies outside of the family: the school, the neighborhood, and the extended "family" of the family's community. This evidence bears out that without the interaction of children in these societies in such a way that the child's presence and role is identified, confirmed, and appreciated, it is likely that the child will experience the catastrophe of the developmental failure of this period, inferiority, and all of its consequences.

In this chapter we will review current information about how children advance from preschool to preadolescence, examining the areas of central nervous system maturation, emotion, gender differences, moral development, social development, and cognition. These areas must be understood in the contexts of the child's internal life, and in relation to family, peers, and school. We will focus greater attention on issues of schooling because, since school-aged children spend most of their waking lives in school, the school environment is vital to every aspect of the child's development, including how the child views the family, how the family views itself in relation to the child, and ultimately how the child views himself.

MATURATION OF THE CENTRAL NERVOUS SYSTEM

The brain undergoes a period of rapid growth through age 2, then develops at a much slower rate until puberty. At birth the brain is estimated to be about 10% of adult volume. It grows to 90% of adult volume by age 5 and completes its growth slowly over the next 9 years. What is more significant than actual volume, however, is the modification of anatomical structures and myelinization, which is almost completed around the age of 7 (2). Synaptic pruning in the prefrontal cortex (the area affecting social judgment) continues as an ongoing process through adolescence.

MRI studies of school-aged children's brains have confirmed these observations. By the age of 7 the child's brain is about the size of the adult brain. Boys' brains are about 10% larger than girls' and this total volume difference persists into adulthood (3, 4). Differences, too, are found in the basal ganglia, where the globus pallidus is larger in boys, while the caudate is larger in girls. Boys show a relatively greater increase in size of the amygdala, while girls have more growth of the hippocampus. These relative differences are consistent with findings of androgen receptors in the amygdala and of estrogen receptors in the hippocampus. There are also findings of greater lateral ventricular expansion in boys (2). Caveness, et al. (5) found that subcortical gray structures are at adult volume in girls and are greater than their adult volumes in males, while the volume of central white matter is smaller in the female brain. As the frontal lobes develop, children become increasingly able to cognitively inhibit—that is, to focus their attention and refrain from being distracted by irrelevant stimuli (6).

Some data on neurotransmitter development may further sharpen our view of the intrinsic maturational schedule of the child and elucidate the emergence of the abilities of school-age children. Noradrenergic systems develop early and exert early influence on the formation of the cortex. In contrast, dopaminergic systems (associated with attention regulation) and serotoninergic systems (associated with mood and aggression) have a more gradual effect on crucial connections between brainstem nuclei and cortical structures. Cholinergic systems, associated with memory and higher cortical functions, develop relatively late (7).

These refinements in brain structure and function result in the maturation of higher cortical functions, correlating with improved abilities in motor coordination, increased attention and focus, increased self-regulation, and expanded consideration for others. The speed of information processing increases significantly between 6 and 12 years of age, which parallels synaptic pruning and myelination (8). For example, tasks of writing, organizing work on a page, coordinating sounds with visual cues (e.g., deciphering words and spelling phonetically) require control in ear and eye–hand coordination. First-graders who write letters or words backwards, or who write their names with the correct letters but in a different order, are not necessarily showing signs of learning disability. Rather, they have not yet developed mastery of the conventions involving direction and order that are necessary to read and write and perform arithmetic functions. It is normal and expectable to not fully master these conventions until second grade.

GENDER DIFFERENCES IN DEVELOPMENT

Psychosexual Development

According to psychoanalytic theory, sexual development is biphasic, with a "latent" period during the school-age years. Freud believed that latency was a distinguishing feature of humans over animals, and hoped to discover anatomical evidence of this through then-promising studies of changes in the interstitial portions of the "sex glands" (9). However, contemporary studies of sex hormones do not support the biphasic theory. Infants have relatively high but varying proportions of sex hormones in cord blood. The levels of sex hormones fall after birth and begin to rise, due to endogenous production, during the school-age period (ages 7–8 in girls, and about 2 years later in boys). Sex hormones begin a gradual upsurge around age 8, continuing through the pubertal peak. Children engage in some sexual play with self and others. Retrospective interviews with homosexual adults generally pinpoint middle childhood as the time when sexual preference was established. Some have postulated that school-age children's greater sexual awareness may be reflected in their expressed feelings of disgust and shame and the strong sense of modesty that develops during the school years. Others have reported that sex play among school children is a natural extension of that of preschoolers (10). Infants and toddlers masturbate; preschoolers also engage in mutual exploration. Psychoanalytic theory posits that sexual strivings in the Oedipal child are overcome with the development of defense mechanisms. Children often enter middle childhood with a few good friends of the opposite sex. Around, age 8, however, the same-sex groupings become polarized, with the opposite gender having developing "cooties" and being generally avoided or teased. Moving toward preadolescence, however, the "yuckiness" of the opposite sex gradually gives way to admiring certain individuals from a distance. Older school-age girls' budding attraction to movie stars and rock

TABLE 3.1.3.1

CHARACTERISTICS OF THE SCHOOL-AGED CHILD

	Child Entering First Grade (5–6 Years Old)	Completing Fifth Grade (10–11 Years Old)
Motor	Hop, skip, jump, throw, catch, kick a ball Reasonable balance, able to stand still and hold arms steady; stands on one foot, left and right General sense of left and right, not always consistent Able to do rapid alternating movements Mild synkinesis on fine finger movements	Hop, skip, jump, throw, catch, and kick a ball with ease. Elaborates: e.g., dance steps; throw behind back or trick the receiver Balance is good; tandem walking with ease. Accurate distinction of left and right. No synkinesis
Writing and drawing	Able to name and copy circle, square, triangle, and cross easily; some copy diamond and asterisk Five pointed star is possible, if child has been exposed to this in kindergarten Draws person with body, arms, and legs Can put detailed features, but often leaves them out; can draw house and tree, as well	Circle, square, triangle, diamond, asterisk, five-pointed star. Cube can be accomplished, but often only after shown how to draw it Draws more detailed person with hands, feet, action figures. Girls with more decorative detail. Boys with more action detail
Stories	About drawings, persons are largely self-referential. Even if a figure has a different name, the life circumstances are usually identical to the child's	May draw someone who is not self and can have a story about another, even made-up family. Creates complex plots, using well developed descriptive language
Fund of knowledge (depends on exposure)	Recites alphabet; counts beyond 20, writes name, first and last. Recognizes printed letters and numbers (not cursive). Writes most letters and numbers. May have some reversals.	Reads aloud and to self with comprehension; performs double-digit addition and subtraction in head; multiplies, divides, and does fractions on paper; knows details about historical figures, geography, natural phenomena, body systems
Cognitive	Egocentric; idiosyncratic definitions of "scientific" observations; centration, defining by only one dimension; beginning concrete operations: conservation and classification	Conservation of number, weight and volume; flexibility of operational skills, including reversibility
Moral	Defines right and wrong in terms of punishment and pain, or other personal and idiosyncratic rationales. Interested in how the world works, including life and death, religion; uses magical thinking	Defines right and wrong through internal principles Has empathy and can weigh issues from another's position
Social	Enjoys the company of other children Names several friends Interactional play with rules, often externally determined Creative play is imitative Peers judged by whether they are nice to child Games of individual prowess. May play on team, but cooperates based on rules rather than complex strategizing.	Likely to have a best friend and a close circle of friends Activities with peers are increasingly independent of parental supervision Able to create games and make up rules; consideration for others, particularly with girls Increasing self-reliance and responsibility Peers judged by their qualities Teamwork
Self-view	Dependent on others' descriptions	Dependent on view of success, competence, and evaluation by internal standards, as well as comparison with peers and social pressures. Selects from multiple available models to define standard for "cool" for self and select friends
Sex	Interested in sexual differences; pleasure from touching oneself; generally play with same-sex friends but comfortable with organized co-ed activities	Secondary sexual changes from Tanner stages II-V, girls usually 2 years ahead of boys. Prefers same sex friends. Some awkwardness about growth (slouching, embarrassment about breast development and foot size). Wide range of pubertal onset in peer group may create challenges to individual self-esteem. Some admiration of individual members of the opposite sex versus thinking others are "yucky." Interest expressed through teasing, messages sent through others.
Family	Identification with parents or siblings, primarily same-sex Participates in family rituals and routines around meals and bedtimes	Compare parents with other adults, including teachers and other children's parents More independent of family rituals and routines More responsibility for household tasks, own self-care, and homework

idols serves a group interactional function, as well as helping to define identity. As with preschoolers, if school-age children are preoccupied with sexual themes, it is wise to look for the possibility of sexually stimulating experiences, such as sexual abuse or witnessing of sex acts.

There is a wide range of both timing and tempo of pubertal onset, and it begins for many girls near the end of what is traditionally termed middle childhood. The onset of puberty at age 9–11, as measured through breast growth, correlates with a positive body image, positive peer relationships, and superior adjustment in girls (11). Conversely, a slower maturational pace may wreak havoc on social relationships, as peers realign themselves with children who are perceived to possess more attractive or desirable traits.

It is well established that children adopt a firm gender identity by age 3. This expression of their maleness or femaleness is manifested early by choices of role models and friends. With gender differences, as with so many of the other issues discussed in this chapter, the question of what is innate and what is the outcome of socialization remains intriguing.

John Money's (12, 13) studies of infants with ambiguous genitalia established that gender identity was primarily determined through socialization. But explorations of differences in sexual preference and transsexual behaviors have raised questions about the roles of sex hormones in determining gendered behaviors. Carol Jacklin (14) reviewed a number of purported relationships of hormones to behavior. There were no consistent findings and many weaknesses with the studies. Jacklin proposed that the internal representation of one's gender, which she refers to as schemata (changing and evolving networks of associations to filter and organize information about oneself, one's gender, and its meaning) evolve out of diverse information, including modes of behavior, properties of objects, attitudes, and feeling states. Information is both presented and processed differently for boys and girls. For example, Jacklin notes how rare it is to see someone compliment a girl on how strong she is getting, or a boy on how nurturing he is. Although observational research documents little difference in parental treatment of boys versus girls (15), children's sex-stereotyped views of parental roles in society nevertheless become ingrained and persist through the school years into adolescence (16).

A number of characteristics are associated with being male or female in the school-age period. Carol Gilligan (17) cites Janet Lever's studies of 181 fifth-grade children at play. She observed that boys play outdoors in large and heterogeneous groups, and they play competitive games that last longer than those of girls. The games played by boys are full of disputes that seem to add interest to the interaction and do not derail the game. Similar observations of children playing led Jean Piaget to conclude that boys were more advanced in moral development because of their fascination with legal procedures and experience at generating fair arbitration of disputes. Many others concluded similarly that in the area of moral development and the development of the capacity to exert effective leadership in complex groups, boys preceded girls; few girls ever caught up.

In proposing that women listen to the demands of socialization and morality "in a different voice," Gilligan added new value to this "instrumental versus expressive" gender dichotomy. Gilligan's descriptions of different lines of moral development for boys and girls will be discussed later in the review of moral development during school age.

Recognizing that boys generally develop instrumental functions and girls expressive ones has provided explanations for other observed differences between boys and girls. In academic achievement, for example, girls traditionally have tended to do better in verbal areas, while boys have done better in math and science. Even as the causes of these differences are being explored, they are also being denied and recharacterized. Feminism apparently has had its effects on gender identity and gender role behaviors in both girls and their mothers. For example, the widely held view that boys are more mathematically capable than girls has been demonstrated to be more an effect of socialization than innate capability. Math anxiety was related to gender-stereotyped beliefs of parents, the mothers being most influential (18). Furthermore, gender differences in academic skills that had been previously noted are now not found on many tests of academic competence (14). It is likely that other so-called innate gender differences will be similarly reevaluated in the future. Still, Gilligan et al. (19), in a Harvard research study, describe "hitting the cultural wall"; when preadolescent girls realize that society values appearance more than accomplishment, they become more self-critical and worry about their weight. A negative body image was found to be associated with high IQ. In the American Association of University Women's *Shortchanging Girls, Shortchanging America*, a study of 3,000 girls and boys in fourth through tenth grade concluded that girls lose their positive self-esteem and switch to appearance as the primary way to measure themselves (20). Other studies (21, 22) support that preadolescent girls are more likely to get depressed, have their IQ scores drop, and decline in math and science.

Cognitive Development

The standard by which school-age children's cognitive competence has been evaluated is the achievement of what Jean Piaget termed "concrete operations." The preschooler's preoperational thought is a creative effort to grasp causality and make meaning of experience using idiosyncratic and egocentric logic. In contrast, school-age children master important operations that increase their objectivity and their ability to be conventional.

Classification and conservation are the two crucial achievements of concrete operational thinking. Classification is the ability to group objects or concepts; conservation is the ability to recognize constant qualities/quantities of material even when the material undergoes changes in morphology. The concrete logical operations enable the child to deal systematically with hierarchies and categories, series and sequences, alternative and equivalent ways of getting to the same place, and reciprocal relationships. They include:

1. Composition—Combining elements leads to another class (e.g., red and blue leads to purple);
2. Associativity—Combinations may be made in different orders with the same result;
3. Reversibility—being able to return mentally to an earlier point in the process;
4. Seriation—the ability to create an orderly sequence along a quantitative dimension such as height, and
5. Decentration—simultaneously relating several aspects of a problem. This includes the ability to picture mentally another's frame of reference, which affects not only spatial reasoning, but the potential for increasingly empathic understanding of another's point of view. (23)

Logical operations are crucial to mastering basic reading and mathematics skills, and they are also necessary for conducting social interaction, with its increasing complexity of groups, games, and rules. Acquisition of the ability to do conventional and objective mental operations is associated with an interest in the scientific workings of the birth process, and a grasp of the finality, universality, and inevitability of death.

Successful school-age children have not just the ability to perform the specific concrete operations themselves but also the ability to communicate about them in conventional ways. They understand that there are conventions of conversation, response to questions on tests, and social comportment. With cognition, as with almost every other aspect of the school-age youngster's development, joining society and sharing conventions is the key to success. This interest in conventions and rules is frequently accompanied by a fascination with ordering and ritual. For example, school-age children often develop favorite numbers, magical rituals ("Step on a crack, break your grandmother's back"), or the need to do things in even pairs. They may also become collectors of coins, stamps, insects, baseball cards, comic books, and such and may spend a great deal of time reviewing and ordering their collections.

During middle childhood, attention becomes increasingly selective. The ability to plan before taking action also develops (24). The school-age child's theory of mind (metacognition) is increasingly sophisticated, viewing the mind as an active and reflective information processor (25). Children become aware of their own mental processes, private speech, and choice of memory strategies. However, school-age children are just beginning to develop cognitive self-regulation. One predictor of academic success is the ability to effectively self-regulate (26).

Morality

Along with the development of concrete operations, a child's sense of morality, that is, the appreciation of consequences and justice, evolves from an egocentric, idiosyncratic, and often harsh system of evaluations of behavior by punishment, to adopting internalized rules for evaluating behavior.

Piaget (27) posited that school-age children's morality is in the "interpretation of rules" stage. This accomplishment permits the child to understand the spirit of a rule and to make subjective moral judgments.

Kohlberg (28) described the moral development that most school-age children reach as the level of "conventional morality." Conventional morality contains two stages: "interpersonal concordance" and "orientation toward authority." In the stage of "interpersonal concordance" a child measures behavior and judges it on the basis of whether it pleases those he looks up to. These mutual interpersonal expectations are those of a "good girl" or "good boy," who wants to please her or his parents and teachers, and obeys the Golden Rule ("Do unto others as you would have them do unto you"). The next stage in conventional morality, "orientation toward authority," reflects the societal values of duty, respect, and law and order. This differs from the stage of interpersonal concordance in that the child's moral compass is now set by the social system instead of the immediate social context of family, school, or neighborhood. The child supports the rules of society, believes that it is essential not to break these rules in order for society to function, and makes moral judgments based on how well an individual situation conforms to the rules of the social system.

Gilligan's (14) studies of girls' and women's moral development led her to emphasize the importance of relationships. In contrast to the traditionally masculine, seemingly quasimathematical system for evaluating moral choices, Gilligan finds that girls use a form of narrative that evolves solutions within conversations and interpersonal action. Thus, Gilligan interprets the fifth-grade girls' play observed by Lever (described earlier) not as poorly developed or socially immature but as valuing different aspects of the social experience. Gilligan describes the different response of an 11-year-old boy and girl, both of whom were at the top of their sixth grade class in a private elementary school in an academic community. The moral test question was that of the man whose wife is gravely ill and whose survival depends on receiving a specific medicine. The medicine is too expensive and the pharmacist will not reduce the price. The man breaks into the pharmacy and steals the medicine for his wife. In responding to the question of what should happen to the man, the boy thoughtfully weighed the problem of laws against stealing and a higher law valuing life. The girl, on the other hand, felt that the various parties needed talk to each other, and could not render an opinion about what should happen to him. She was aware of the rules, but felt that the conflict was such that mediation was needed to reach a resolution.

There has been significant critical reanalysis of Gilligan's data and conceptualization of the gender differences in moral reasoning. For both girls and boys, the development of morality reflects conventional thinking and measuring their evaluations with the rules of their society, as they understand them. Although moral reasoning continues to evolve through and beyond adolescence, many of the standards that are developed for our own behavior during middle childhood are likely to remain internalized and used as self-evaluation measures into adulthood.

Stilwell, et al., in a study of 132 students aged 5–17 years, describes moral development as a natural outgrowth of attachment, evolving through five stages (29). First, the child's sense of security and experience of empathic responsiveness become paired with a sense of moral obligation. Next, the caretaker's rules are incorporated. Then, an understanding develops of how empathy can modify strict rule following. Next, ideals and role models are selected that reflect earlier learning in attachment relationships. Finally, the self is visualized as a keeper of moral standards. These stages roughly correlate with Kohlberg's stages of morality, but emphasize the grounding of morality and conscience in the early and fundamental experience of attachment and secure base, out of which empathy develops.

EMOTIONAL ISSUES

The most significant emotional issues in the lives of school-aged children concern personal worth that is determined by a sense of competence and place (in family, peer group, and communities). Competence is reflected in all of the places a child may live, at home by accomplishing tasks of caring for self (completing dressing, including tying shoes) and at school by accomplishing the academic material presented. Robert White (30, 31) postulated a "drive" to competence that he felt to be as important as libidinal drives. In the school-age period, competence is not just experienced by the child succeeding at a task, but by others' evaluation of his or her performance.

As Erickson warned, the emotional risk for the school-aged child is the possibility of feeling inferior if the child evaluates him- or herself as not being able to accomplish tasks. This evaluation comes first from outside, from a teacher expressing disappointment or frustration, from other children laughing, from parents' disappointment with grades, or a teacher's report. Increasingly through the school-aged period, children can evaluate their own performance and measure it against that of others. Failures in one area may be compensated by accomplishments in another, eventually, but the early school-aged child who has not yet learned about compensation, may just feel dejected. By the end of middle childhood, each child has constructed a composite evaluation of his or her own relative areas of competence and weakness, and has come up with his own answer to the questions, "What am I good at? Can I get the job done?" Again, these characterizations tend to persist into adulthood.

The fears of a school-aged child are quite different from those of a preschooler. Because school-aged children are out and about in society, they are much more likely to witness or hear about catastrophic events that could happen to them. Their vulnerability to catastrophic fears is increased by the development, during the school-aged period, of understanding of the irreversibility and inevitability of death. Many school-aged children's dreams reflect efforts to master these fears by setting themselves up as heroes who save whole families or communities from robbers, murderers, fires, storms, or other disasters. Children who don't feel competent may be overwhelmed by these fears and have repeated dreams in which they are attacked and victimized and helpless.

Harry Stack Sullivan (32) was one of the first to emphasize the social influence on development. He described a series of internal processes by which the child gradually substitutes his or her own standards of evaluation for those of family members. Stimulated by models outside the family, these processes unfold throughout the early school period.

- *Social subordination* reflects a change in the child's acceptance of authority from the specifics of personal caretakers to general categories such as the principal, police, crossing guards, and teachers. The child first evaluates peers in terms of how they are regarded by these authority figures.
- *Social accommodation* is a process of acknowledging that there are differences between people. Early school-age children are intolerant of differences and can be cruel, but (with socialization and education) gradually differences may come to be respected.
- *Differentiation of authority figures* is the child's emerging ability to compare adults (comparing parents to school-based authorities).
- *Control of focal awareness* refers to the child's response to social pressure to abandon some of his or her egocentric ideas and adopt a more conventional stance.
- *Sublimatory reformation* refers to the reorientation of focal awareness to the group-approved satisfactory behavior.
- *Supervisory patterns* reflect an awareness of one's behavior in groups. The supervisory patterns are almost like imaginary characters that develop in order to monitor oneself and eventually become internalized.

Self in Society

By the time they enter the school-age period, children have developed four basic areas of self-esteem: academic competence, social competence, physical/athletic competence, and physical appearance (33). As they progress through middle childhood, children continue to develop and refine their self-concept and sense of self-esteem, measuring and rating themselves within the context of their families, peers, and culture. The most salient achievement of the school-age period is a sense of oneself as a member of society. To accomplish this, maturation is required, as has been described. But the most significant arenas for advancing and refining the sense of self both in the present and in anticipating the future are the interpersonal arenas of family, peers, and school.

Home and Family

According to Heinz Kohut, the development of self occurs through a process of mirroring and idealization. In order to develop healthy narcissism, the child needs grownups to admire him and demonstrate attunement to his feelings ("mirroring"). The child also needs to be able to look up to his parents and other role models, and aspire to be like them without being unduly distracted by their faults and shortcomings ("idealization").

Similarly, parenting styles have been classified by Diana Baumrind (34) according to "responsivity" (accurately assessing and responding to children's needs) and "demandingness" (setting high expectations). Parents with high responsivity and high demandingness ("authoritative" style) tend to have the best outcome, with children who do well academically and socially. Low responsivity/low demandingness describes the neglectful or uninvolved parent; and high responsivity/low demandingness describes the permissive parent. Low responsivity/high demandingness is characteristic of an authoritarian style, which may be predictive of a positive outcome in some minority families. Inadequate parental monitoring correlates strongly with a risk of delinquent behaviors, while parental involvement positively contributes to the child's cognitive and social competence (35).

The parent's optimal role in middle childhood may be that of a consultant or facilitator, coaching the child's development of his own skills and opinions, assisting as needed when help is requested, but allowing mistakes to be made and independent striving to occur in a supportive environment whenever feasible. This approach is congruent with an authoritative style, in that high responsivity and high expectations can coexist with allowing self-exploration on the part of the child.

The "goodness of fit (36)" between parenting style and child temperament is a moving target, constantly in flux. As the child encounters new challenges and develops new competencies, the parallel parental challenge is to be sensitive to the child's ever-changing needs, providing progressive responsibility and supervised autonomy as appropriate (37). Recent research on genotypes and family relationships suggests that parent–child interactions are genetically influenced. Children's genotypes evoke specific parental responses; similarly, parental response patterns evoked by their children's particular behaviors show evidence of heritability (38). Targeted interventions can favorably alter these parental responses to difficult behaviors (39), hopefully changing their expression. The familiar social context of the family and neighborhood (that also includes extended family and religious communities with which the family may be involved) are altered in the school-age period through several processes. The first is a practical one: When children spend more time in school, parents may spend more time doing things other than caring for their children. For parents who were already working, or who remain at home caring for younger children, or who choose to home-school their children, this may not be a significant change. In general, however, this creates a significant shift from the family organized for care of itself and its young children, drawn inward by primarily centripetal forces, to the more outwardly oriented family of adolescent children, where forces seem to be centrifugal, drawing family members out into interactions with the society at large. Combrinck-Graham (40) described the decreasing centripetal forces of the school-aged child's family as "a house in the summertime; it is sturdy but has doors and windows open for circulation. Everyone comes in to share the family meal, to take shelter from the rain, and to sleep."

A second process that changes the family environment is the evaluation that comes about from children bringing home their experiences with other children, other children's parents, and other adults whom they meet independently of their own families. Children make statements: John's mother lets him do this; Martha's mother doesn't do that; Sandy's father doesn't live with them. Or they ask questions: Why doesn't Daddy stay home with us the way George's father does? How come you don't pick me up at school?—Randy's mother does. Are we rich or poor? Are we Republican or Democrat? Why don't we celebrate Christmas? And so on. Or children reflect frank criticism: You don't know as much as my teacher. Smoking is bad for you; you shouldn't smoke.

A third process of family change is through children's relatively greater involvement in activities outside the home. Visits to friends, after-school activities, membership in clubs, or participation on teams takes time out from family routines after school and on weekends. Adolescents are far more involved in activities outside the home, but most school-aged children's families have the opportunity to assemble for dinner and an evening routine that allows for completing homework and some form of age-appropriate bedtime routine. Exceptions are largely due to complicated work schedules of caregivers, who may work second shift or overtime.

A fourth process of family change is the possible social enrichment of all family life through involvement with the school as a community. This can be through socializing with families of other children, involvement in school and after-school activities, and through advocacy about school issues (PTA or participation on the school board). All family members, not just the children, usually become more involved in social experiences outside the family during the school-age period.

Family/community relationships that have been stable prior to the school-age period are subject to change in similar ways. In the early school-age period children are developing skills that facilitate interaction with peers in the neighborhood (mastering a two-wheel bike; accomplishments in the pick-up sport of the neighborhood, such as soccer or basketball). Children may have different experiences with other children in the home area and in school. At home, in the neighborhood, a child may be included in a group of different-aged children and accepted because of familiarity or the relationships between the families. For example, children may be a part of a Sunday school group that is also part of the social context of the congregation. This peer group reflects the child's place in a family's place in a community. As the child grows older through school age in such a community, the child becomes more identified by distinct contributions to the community (such as participating in the music program, mastery of religious lessons, contributions to recreational activities) rather than just by membership in a family.

Children may assume more distinct roles in their neighborhood society or Sunday school group as they develop in school, or they may be less involved, as they become more interested in other things. Hobbies and collections are characteristic passions of school-aged children and often become the basis for formation of new social groupings. Social contacts may be conducted on line as children come together around a particular interest.

The roles of television, video games, and personal music players, access to the Internet, and instant messaging are only beginning to be evaluated (41). While these forms of occupation or entertainment, and even communication, now have an established place in the lives of American school children, such activities tend to isolate children from the daily commerce with their families and peers, and may stimulate an increasingly unrealistic view of life, one's role in it, and one's abilities. These activities may be comforting to children who are otherwise struggling either with learning, attention, or socialization, though this comfort may further cut them off from activities that involve them in their society. Some concerns about the role of TV watching in interfering with the "function of brains . . . to interact with each other to form families and societies," are explored by Kramer (42) when he writes about the biology of family culture. Finally, these activities are sedentary and often accompanied by eating, and there is increasing concern about obesity, diabetes, and other health problems associated with this lifestyle.

Peers

The peer group can be one of the most facilitating influences in school-aged children's development, or it can be disastrously inhibiting. As with other developmental tasks, each child brings a particular pattern of prior experience to the task of developing a social self. There is considerable evidence that peers themselves have their own attractions and that a substantial if not primary influence over a child's social self-development comes from the outside, predominantly through peer culture and its particular draw on the child's drives for mastery and competence. Robert White's (31, 32) description of the growth of competence drives in the school-age period includes how to get along with others in the sense of competing, compromising, learning the rules of the game, and protecting oneself from injury. White points out that other children afford an opportunity to do something interesting with the environment and that gradually the world of contemporaries competes with the family circle. Bemporad (43) describes the juvenile era as a period between separation and procreation in which peers are the intermediaries. Erickson's focus on how children master industry overemphasizes individual achievement at the expense of cooperation. In a crosscultural comparison, Kagan (44) credits the society of peers for advancing the development of children in San Marcos. He describes rural Guatemalan Indian infants and preschoolers who by all culturally relevant measures are "retarded" but who at 11 perform at the same level as American children in tests of cognitive functioning. The Guatemalan infant is unstimulated and left alone; only basic physical needs are attended to. Thus, Guatemalan infants do not have the assertive interaction with environment that is so prized in American infants and preschoolers. Kagan suggests that in the school-age period, where the relative neglect of these children by adults leaves them to form their own social groupings, Guatemalan youngsters begin to practice and learn assertiveness through jockeying for social position. Grunebaum and Solomon (45) refer to Harry Harlow's studies, concluding that young rhesus monkeys leave their mothers because peer relationships are interesting, not because their mothers reject them. There has been some recent debate about the relative influence of peer group versus parents on development, with some taking the view that the peer effect is significant, while the parent effect is negligible (46).

Regardless of the relative weight placed on each of these factors, it seems that the drive for inclusion and acceptance, and the judgments of the other children that the child selects as his peer group, impact heavily on the school-age child's development of his own self-image and values. At the same time, the child's ongoing internal self-definition in turn influences his selection of peers to identify with and measure himself against. By around age 8, there has been a significant shift in a child's ability to compare and assess his own skills in comparison to others, combined with feedback from parents, teachers, and peers. He begins to rank himself in various arenas, and to combine these multiple assessments into his own ongoing "report card." This constant evaluation of self in social context becomes internalized into his own kinetic sense of identity. For better or worse, the opinions and descriptions we form of ourselves in middle childhood tend to continue throughout life. Personal "style," preferences, values, and self-assessment in comparison with others all have their foundation during the school-age period. How do children's attributions (explanations for why we act as we do) affect their self-esteem? Was their performance due to luck, ability, or effort? Children who make "mastery-oriented attributions" (47) give credit to their ability when they succeed ("I'm great at math"), and attribute failure to factors that are controllable ("I need to study harder") or not fundamental ("This was an especially tough exam"). By contrast, children who attribute their failure to an innate lack of ability ("learned helplessness") may develop a downward spiral in which they stop trying to succeed (48). Attribution retraining and help with self-regulation can be helpful, especially when started early (49).

Stages of peer development have been identified and described by Grunebaum and Solomon (50):

- Unilateral partners and one-way assistance—the preschool child,
- Bilateral partners and fair-weather cooperation—middle childhood, and
- Chumship and consensual exchange—preadolescence

The first school-age phase is characterized by membership in peer groups and is based on playmates' willingness and ability to play the way the child wishes. The second school-age stage (from about age 9) advances friendship to a closeness that Sullivan referred to as "chumship" with a peer of the same sex with whom an intimacy is formed, which paves the way for heterosexual intimacy and caring beginning in adolescence. A study that examined second, fifth, and eighth graders' attitudes and choices for companionship and intimacy found that family members were the most important sources for companionship for both second and fifth graders. Same-sex peers were important throughout school age, but were increasingly important as the subjects grew older. Girls tended to report intimate disclosure to peers earlier than boys, probably reflecting that girls may value intimacy more than boys (51).

As peer interaction and the view of self in relation to others is vital to cognitive and intellectual development, so cognitive operations are vital to a child's emerging social self in the school-age period. Minuchin (52) points out that children move from games such as "Simon Says," "Mother May I," and "Follow the Leader," in which the children in groups follow the directions of a leader, to games in which the rules are set and governed by the players themselves, to games that involve contributions to the efforts of a team. This evolution involves shifts in the ways in which others are evaluated. Children begin the period by deeming others good if they give them things and bad if they take things away, and move to recognizing skills and personal attributes, to finally acknowledging and valuing social attributes, such as fairness. This shift, in turn, requires the expansion of perspective, which permits a child to see a situation from another's point of view. This decentering may be seen as a cognitive component to empathy and the development of more sophisticated morality.

With social development, as with intellectual development, preparation and prior experience are substantial influences. Patterns of behavior involving aggression are established early, and generalized aggressive disposition and the tendency to exhibit aggression in the context of specific relationships are quite stable (53). Aggressiveness is also associated with social rejection in the school-age period (54, 55). One view of the stability of aggression is that it is constitutionally determined. Another view is that aggression develops and is maintained in interpersonal sequences. For example, one researcher reported that "early-timing" mothers, those whose first children are born when they are in their 20s, have more difficulty setting limits on their children than "late-timing" mothers do (56). Children of early-timing mothers are more likely to be aggressive, and in the absence of good limit setting within the family, the aggression becomes less amenable to social intervention. It is most likely that aggression levels are determined by an ongoing interaction of biological tendency with psychosocial context.

Sociometric studies of school-age children yield up to five groups: popular, average, rejected, neglected, and controversial (57). There are two subgroups of rejected children, those who undervalue themselves and have low self-esteem, even in comparison to their teachers' evaluations of them; and those who have a positive view of themselves but are seen as defensive and aggressive (54). When children in different sociometric groups were asked to evaluate themselves and one another, it was expected that aggressive children would show attributional biases not shown by nonaggressive children. But in fact, these children's evaluations of others were not out of line, even though other children clearly identified the reputation of rejected children. Additionally, negative reputation increasingly separates the rejected group at older ages (55). Aggression and consequent rejection and social isolation during middle childhood is a primary predictor of maladjustment in later years. Rejected children often form social groups with other unpopular peers, which unfortunately may compound the problem by reinforcing poor social skills (58).

Contemporary reviews of peer relationships in the middle years point to the difficulties in researching this ever-changing set of connections. For example, peer relationships occur in a context. The grouping of children in a classroom may not be the same as how these children seek each other's company and friendship out of school. Furthermore, how children relate to one another in the classroom is very much affected by whether the educational style facilitates interaction between the students or not.

How children group, the size of their network, how popularity is related to friendship—all of these conditions of peer relationships seem to evolve through the school-age period, but researchers are still not clear about identifying the best tools for assessing and therefore understanding the processes of peer interaction (59–61).

SCHOOLING

Schooling refers to the ecological setting in which children learn. It refers to the environment, the size, the philosophy, the characteristic transactions between teachers and students, and the culture of the school. How the child *can* function, what he or she can do, how the child perceives him- or herself, especially in terms of competence and the accompanying confidence to be able to accomplish, and finally, how the child is a part of communities/societies—all of these are substantially forged and reshaped in the school environment.

We will discuss four aspects of schooling:

1. Preparation: the effects of prior experience;
2. Attunement to children's learning styles and needs;
3. Concordance or discordance with the patient's family/community ethos; and
4. How the school serves as a model for a community in which a child finds a role.

The Effect of Experience and Preparation on Children's School Functioning

Children arrive at school with diverse experiences. Most dramatically different are the experiences of children from middle-class, educated families and those from poor, minority, inner city families. The former are more likely to have attended educationally oriented preschools, have traveled at least in their own communities, have visited libraries and museums, and have been read to by their parents and teachers; the latter have more likely been involved with complex family and "adoptive" family relationships ("play" mamas and many "aunts" and "uncles"), have experienced comings and goings of people in their daily worlds, and have been exposed to situations of danger and hardship with little sense of control over these situations. Children from immigrant families may not speak English, or, alternatively, may be the only members of their family who do speak English. Some minority youngsters may never have seen a book, a piece of paper, or a crayon by the time they enter school. But many of them may have been assuming responsibilities in the household, such as caring for younger children, getting meals, caring for themselves while adults are away, and translating for their parents. The former group has been prepared to enter school since toddlerhood, while the latter group is prepared to manage an entirely different set of experiences, which may not be compatible with what is expected in school (62–64).

There is abundant evidence that the parents' education is related to children's achievement. Davis-Kean (65) researched this premise and found that this relationship is true of both white and African American families. Regardless of race, parental education relates indirectly to children's achievement through reading and providing a warm and supportive environment.

There has been considerable exploration of the relationship between attachment style and adjustment to school in recent years (66). Granot and Mayseless (67) examined the relationship between attachment styles and adjustment in school, as measured by teacher ratings and student sociograms. Their sample of nineteen 10–12-year-olds in Israel found that 66% were secure, 15% avoidant, 6% ambivalent, and 13% disorganized. As expected, the secure children had the highest adjustment scores and the fewest negative nominations on the sociogram. The ambivalently attached children were intermediate in scholastic and emotional adjustment and had the highest number of negative nominations in the sociogram, corresponding with significantly lower levels of social adjustment than the secure children. Importantly, there was no relationship between attachment style and cognitive achievements.

Studies of the effects of model preschool programs and general application of Head Start programs for poor and minority children demonstrate that there is some advantage to having had a preschool experience, and this advantage is more dramatic and more lasting if the experience was in a model preschool program (68). In followup throughout the remainder of their school lives, children from model preschools were significantly less likely to be placed in special education programs than controls, but most often effects disappeared in 3–6 years, after the children entered formal public school (69). This suggests that preparation, alone, does not suffice to ensure a positive school experience. It is important to note that the most effective early education programs involved the parents in the school effort, so that the fit between home culture and school culture was enhanced.

Reading comprehension is largely thought to be text-based (content oriented) and interactional (develops within a relationship). It is increasingly evident that reading success is heavily influenced by the preparation of the reader, who brings to the task his or her expectations, prior knowledge of the content and structure of the material, and cultural background (70). Studies support this observation. One study reported that a group of 4-year-olds given simple instructions in segmenting and blending words of two and three syllables 10 minutes a day for 13 weeks resulted in dramatically higher reading scores than those of children involved in nonspecific reading-related activities (71). Coles reported a study of the families of children with reading disabilities found that there is a significant lack of preparation of these children for reading. Other studies found that in some families, messages about expectations of failure were transmitted, while in others there were failures to provide exposure to preparatory material; in still others there was obvious evidence of "communication deviance" whereby the explanatory frameworks of language were so odd or idiosyncratic to the family that the child had unusual difficulty mastering conventional rules needed to learn to read (72). In addition to insufficient preparation, other etiologies of reading difficulty must be considered. These include learning disability (due to underlying processing deficits, auditory discrimination problems, decoding difficulties), mental retardation, and knowledge deficits in oral language or vocabulary. Basic prereading skills include the ability to bring background knowledge to bear on a new situation, self-questioning behavior, and predictive skills.

Attunement to Children's Learning Styles and Needs

The second aspect of schooling involves the interaction around learning. Many use Vygotsky's ideas about the evolving mind in society to better understand how children learn successfully. In this framework, learning represents the transfer of responsibility for reaching a particular goal (73). This transfer takes place in the "zone of proximal development (ZPD)," which is defined as "the distance between the actual developmental level as determined by independent problem solving and the level of potential development as determined through problem solving under adult guidance or in collaboration with more capable peers" [Vygotsky, cited in Slavin (74)]. The ZPD is a useful measure of learning potential because it includes the instructional context (or, in the case of psychometrics, the relationship between child and examiner) as indispensable to the measured achievement. When children are tested to see whether or not they can adopt strategies presented at various ZPD levels and apply them to other, similar situations without further instruction, those presented in the lower area of the ZPD are readily generalized, those in the midrange are adopted and gradually generalized, and those toward the higher end of the zone may not be adopted at all (68). The child's readiness, and the instructor's attunement to presenting material at a level that stretches already established abilities but is not so novel as to be overwhelming, are crucial to the "transfer of responsibility" that defines successful learning.

Fellow students as well as teachers provide assistance with developing more sophisticated problem solving, as is stated in Vygotsky's definition of the ZPD. There are specific methods of peer involvement in learning that have come to be known as "cooperative learning." Cooperative learning refers to any number of types of student groupings for learning but differs from peer tutoring in that the material is presented by the teacher rather than by the peers. Students are given problems to solve or projects to complete, and the incentive to work together is encouraged either by rewarding the group's efforts, rewarding each individual child on the basis of the group's efforts, or rewarding the group on the basis of each child's achievement. Children can and will positively influence one another's progress. This is particularly true when some children in the group are more advanced than others, but it is also true when all children are struggling to master a new challenge. For example, using the Piagetian description of accomplishment of conservation, nonconserving children learn from peers who have mastered conservation, but they also progress in conservation skills when struggling with conservation problems with other nonconserving children (74). The process of working together must be specifically supervised and rewarded, because otherwise the more competent children take most of the responsibility for accomplishing the objectives or completing the project, while the less competent children do not contribute. But properly conceived, the value of cooperative teaching extends beyond the opportunities it creates for learning. It also provides a framework for learning about others, valuing differences, observing and utilizing the strengths of others, helping one another, and making a contribution to a community goal.

Regardless of the rate children learn and the specific strengths and weaknesses they may have in mastering certain materials, attunement to each child's zone of proximal development and pitching the new material to the appropriate level will inevitably enhance not only the child's success but enthusiasm for learning.

Howard Gardner's theory of multiple intelligences suggests eight areas of aptitude with different processing operations and skill sets (75). These areas include linguistic, logical-mathematical, musical, spatial, bodily-kinesthetic, naturalist, interpersonal, and intrapersonal. By expanding the traditional narrow definition of intelligence, this view challenges families and schools to help realize each child's unique potential.

Gardner's theory of multiple intelligences is echoed in Mel Levine's neurodevelopmental profiling (76). In these and other approaches being utilized in innovative educational strategies, the principle is that different children have specific learning styles. According to these theories, it is incumbent upon the teacher to ask, "How does this particular child learn best?" and to design an educational strategy that utilizes the appropriate mode.

Concordance or Discordance with the Patient's Family/Community Ethos

Two facets of congruence between the style of school and family as interfacing systems have been studied. The first involves expectations in the areas of educational goals, what is expected of the child, rules, and areas of permissiveness. Since the education system has been established by the majority culture, generally goals are congruent between school and majority families. Parents expect their children to attend school regularly, to be respectful, to be motivated, and to achieve. Problems come up when children can't or don't fulfill these expectations, which are ordinarily shared by family and school systems. They also come up, however, when these expectations are not shared by family and school systems. Then the all-too-common complaint that the child misbehaves at school but is fine at home, or, less commonly, the reverse, is brought to the attention of a counselor or mental health professional. This type of problem is most likely to be found in children from ethnic and cultural minority families and can be ameliorated when parents are intimately involved in school life (77). The second facet concerns the congruence of the way school and family systems are organized. In general systems terms, interpersonal systems can be open and relatively closed, referring to characteristics of freedom of exchange with other systems, definition of system boundaries, and amount of variety that is encouraged or tolerated within the system. Some schools that have been founded around specific religions are examples of closed systems, and these often serve a specific population with shared rules and values, constituting a good fit. Rules about conduct, limits, and privacy are consistent across school and family and may differentiate each from the rest of society. Some schools have a more closed system than many of the families of children attending. That is, the schools have clear rules and expectations about everything from dress to punctuality, while the families' own are more loosely organized. The school personnel tend to see these families as irresponsible and incompetent, and themselves as more capable caretakers. Open families sending their children to closed schools feel criticized and defensive, and a child is caught between the two systems, as he may want to conform to the school's expectations but depends upon the family to provide appropriate support. Open school systems allow for variability and have the potential of being flexible. But in many instances, open school systems interfacing with open family systems may have such a lack of definition that the children have no clear framework within which to define themselves. This kind of congruence between open family and open school systems often results in the involvement of the child with more systems, such as welfare, juvenile justice, or mental health (78).

Other aspects of the child and family's community relationships also support commitment to and investment in schooling. One study examining African American students in different socioeconomic circumstances found that more important than poverty or prevalence of crime in a neighborhood was the effect of "collective socialization." (79) Collective socialization occurs in a community where adults recognize the children, speak to them, comment on their behavior, and will report to their parents or other authorities, if indicated. The study was primarily exploring the effect of collective socialization on conduct problems, and did note that in communities with collective socialization, there was a reduced risk for conduct problems. Schooling was a much more successful and valued part of the children's lives in these communities, as well.

How the School Serves as a Model for a Community in Which a Child Finds a Role

A list of characteristics of effective schools includes strong leadership, an atmosphere that is orderly and not oppressive, teachers who participate in decision making, school staff that has high expectations of students, and frequent monitoring of student progress (80). A specific aspect of school environment that has been studied is school size. It has been shown that large schools are often overmanned, meaning that there are more students than role opportunities. This means that there are not enough opportunities in student government, arts, sports programs, or for individual distinction to recognize more than a very few children. In undermanned schools there are opportunities for students to be involved in activities and to take more initiative. The environmental role demands on the students in undermanned schools increase the levels of student participation so that they can contribute to the school community, develop identified roles in this community, and become known to themselves and each other as distinctive individuals. In large schools there is the danger of anonymity and ultimately a high rate of dropping out and involvement in antisocial behavior and substance abuse. The movement to consolidate schools thus increases the chances that students will not have a positive experience in school, unless the student population is broken down into smaller units within which students experience a manageable-size community (80).

Summary of Salient Features of Schooling

For school to be most effective at supporting the crucial development in school-aged children, there has to be attention to the preparation children have had prior to entering school, and assistance to those whose experience has not primed them to take advantage of the school experience. Second, each child's learning style and readiness needs to be understood sufficiently that educational material is presented that stimulates a child's drive to competence, without being so overwhelming that the child gives up. Most curricula are established to meet the levels of most children in the grade. But there are always children who are either more advanced or slower to whom learning tasks need to be thoughtfully and individually offered. Third, attention needs to be placed on the congruence between expectations of school personnel and those of parents. Involving parents in school activities is the most effective way to collaborate and close any gaps that could cause confusion and loyalty conflicts for the children. Finally, schools need to form manageable-sized communities in which children can distinguish themselves. Even if the total school size is very large, there are ways to subdivide into smaller communities.

We have increasingly come to think of the school as a learning community in which the students' membership and identity must be nurtured and respected. The desired emphasis on students learning together in optimally sized schools and classrooms that allow for the recognition of each student's unique place and contributions to the learning community, as described above, is unfortunately not a conscious part of many children's educational experience. Particularly with the No Child Left Behind legislation (81), school curriculum and teacher concentration has been refocused on individual children's performance, as both the schools' and teachers' evaluations and federal funding are based on this. This refocus puts this very important community function of schooling at great risk, in our view.

There are cultures where children learn the "industry" of their society other than in school, primarily through various forms of apprenticeship. Schools in our society offer both the opportunity for learning the industry and for learning one's place in society. We would be remiss if we did not point out that children in our Western society are privileged to have time set aside in their development for schooling. Although child labor is almost nonexistent in the United States and Europe, there are currently 250 million child laborers in the world between the ages of 5 and 14 (90% in Asia and Africa), living in extreme poverty, engaged in repetitive and physically demanding tasks, who do not have the opportunity to go to school at all, and have limited opportunity to play and learn (82).

FAILURES OF DEVELOPMENT IN THE SCHOOL-AGE PERIOD

From this discussion of normal developmental processes and influences on developmental outcome, understanding many failures of development is straightforward. Maturational deviations or delays (such as developmental disabilities, mental retardation, or pervasive developmental disorders) limit a child's developmental progress in all the spheres we have discussed. The child is able to master neither the learning nor social tasks. In addition, the family does not develop the independence and social integration characterized by the school-age family, often because these families are tied into attending the needs of their special children. Similar limitations of development often occur in families with children with chronic medical illnesses, as well. The challenge for mental health professionals who use a developmental approach in their work is to find arenas where handicapped children can be competent and interact socially. Lowering expectations of performance, providing ability-appropriate responsibilities for children to meet, and encouraging reciprocal social interaction are interventions that can maximize developmental accomplishments of these special youngsters.

Interference with learning may be on the basis of immaturity, or, as is more commonly diagnosed, due to disorders of focus, attention, impulse management, or specific learning dysfunction. Understanding the crucial developmental issues of establishing a view of oneself as a functioning person in a community can focus mental health consultants' attention on helping child, family, and teachers find strategies for managing areas of difficulty. Medication is often used to support such efforts, but is most effective when the child and the people closest to him or her are concentrating on competence and strategies for becoming competent.

Inferiority and defeat are the principal emotional pitfalls of school-aged children, because of the importance of mastery and recognition within the communities in which children participate. Depression is both a cause and an outcome of failure to progress in the manner that the child believes others expect. Assessment and treatment of depression in school-aged children must always include assessment of the developmental issues of competence and how a child is viewed by his or her peers so that in addition to psychotherapy and medication assistance with social functioning and academic mastery will be included. Disabling anxiety may occur as a result of either separation fears or performance worries. Both of these scenarios require that the school-aged child learn how to reassure himself. The developmental challenge is to find a secure sense of self, moving comfortably between his nuclear family and his peer group, and setting reasonable internal standards for success in the face of external expectations. Externalizing behavior disorders drastically interfere with children's developmental progress in this era by disrupting learning and social accomplishment. Many such behaviors may be viewed as a defense against a sense of failure and inferiority (better to be seen as bad than dumb). Developmental approaches to treatment must include attention to academic progress along with several approaches to helping such children be accountable for their behavior. Behavioral management with consequences may be helpful, but will be more so in this age group if there are exercises in putting oneself in another's place and developing empathy, so that these children can function in society.

ACKNOWLEDGMENTS

The assistance of Margo McClelland in the preparation of this chapter is gratefully acknowledged.

References

1. Erikson E: *Childhood in Society.* New York, Norton, 1950.
2. Shapiro T, Perry R: Latency revisited: The age of 7 plus or minus 1. *Psychoanal Study Child* 31:79–105, 1976.
3. Giedd JN, Castellanos FX, Jagath CR, et al.: Sexual dimorphism of the developing human brain. *Prog Neuropsychopharmacol Biol* 21:1185–1201, 1997.
4. Reiss AL, Abrams MT, Singer HS, et al.: Brain development, gender and IQ in children: A volumetric imaging study. *Brain* 119:1763–1774, 1996.
5. Caveness VS Jr, Kennedy DN, Richelme C, et al.: The human brain age 7–11 years: A volumetric analysis based on magnetic resonance images. *Cereb Cortex* 6:726–736, 1996.
6. Dempster FN, Corkill, AJ: Interference and inhibition in cognition and behavior: Unifying themes for educational psychology. *Educational Psychology Review* 11:1–88, 1999.
7. Coyle JT, Harris JC: The development of neurotransmitters and neuropeptides. In: Noshpitz J (ed.): *Textbook of Child Psychiatry*, vol 7. New York: Basic Books, 1987 pp. 14–25.
8. Kail R: Speed of information processing: Developmental change and links to intelligence. *Journal of School Psychology* 38:51–61, 2000.
9. Buxbaum E: Between the Oedipus complex and adolescence: The "quiet" time. In: Greenspan SI, Pollock GH (eds.): *Psychoanalytic Contributions Toward Understanding Personality Development*, vol 2: Latency, Adolescence, and Youth. Rockville, MD: National Institute of Mental Health, 1980 pp. 121–136.
10. Rutter M: Normal psychosexual development. *J Child Psychol Psychiatry* 11:259–283, 1971.
11. Brooks-Gunn J: Antecedents and consequences of variation in girls' maturational timing. *J of Adol Health Care* 9:365–373, 1988.
12. Money J, Hampson JG, and Hampson JL: An examination of some basic sexual concepts: The evidence of human hermaphroditism. *Bulletin of the Johns Hopkins Hospital* 97:301–319, 1955.
13. Money J, Hampson JG, and Hampson JL: Hermaphroditism: Recommendations concerning assignment of sex, change of sex and psychological management. *Bulletin of the Johns Hopkins Hospital* 97:284–300, 1955.
14. Jacklin CN: Female and male: Issues of gender. *Am Psychol* 44:127–133, 1989.
15. Lytton H, Romney DM: Parents' differential socialization of boys and girls: A meta-analysis. *Psychological Bulletin* 109:267–296, 1991.
16. Goldman JDC, Goldman RJ: Children's Performance of parents and their roles: A cross-national study on Australia, England, North America, and Sweden. *Sex Roles* 9:791–812, 1983.
17. Gilligan C: *In a Different Voice: Psychological Theory and Women Development.* Cambridge, MA, Harvard University Press, 1982.

18. Eccles JS, Jacobs JE: Social forces shape math attitudes and performance. *Signs* 11:367–389, 1986.
19. Gilligan C, Lyons N, Hanmer T (eds.): *Making Connections: The Relational Worlds of Adolescent Girls at Emma Willard School*. Cambridge, MA, Harvard University Press, 1990.
20. Greenberg-Lake Analysis Group: *Shortchanging girls, shortchanging America: A nationwide poll of students ages 9–15*. Research commissioned by American Association of University Women. American Association of University Women, Washington, DC, 1991.
21. Debold E, Wilson M, Malave I. *Mother–daughter revolution: From betrayal to power*. New York: Addison-Wesley, 1993.
22. Sadker D. *Failing at fairness: How our schools cheat girls*. New York: Simon & Schuster, 1995.
23. Piaget J, Inhelder B. *The psychology of the child*. New York: Basic Books, 1969.
24. Scholnick EK. Knowing and constructing plans. SRCD Newsletter, Fall issue, 1995; 17:1–2.
25. Kuhn D. Metacognitive development. Current Directions in Psychological Science. 2000; 9, 5:178–181.
26. Joyner MH, Kurtz-Costes B. Metamemory development. In W Schneider and FE Weinert, eds. *Memory performance and competencies: Issues in growth and development*. Hillsdale, NJ: Erlbaum, 1997: 275–300.
27. Piaget J. *The moral judgement of the child*. New York, Free Press, 1948.
28. Kohlberg L. Stage and sequence: The cognitive-development approach to socialization. In: Goslin DA, ed. *Handbook of socialization theory and research*. Chicago: Rand-McNally, 1969.
29. Stilwell B, Galvin M, Kopta SM, et al.: Moralization of attachment: A fourth domain of conscience functioning. *J Am Acad Child Adolesc Psychiatry* 36:1140–1147, 1997.
30. White RW: Motivation reconsidered: The concept of competence. *Psychol Rev* 66:297–333, 1959.
31. White RW: Competence and the psychosexual stages of development. Nebraska Symposium on Motivation, 1960 pp. 97–141.
32. Sullivan HS: *The Interpersonal Theory of Psychiatry*. New York, Norton, 1953.
33. Marsh HW: The structure of academic self-concept: The Marsh/Shavelson mode. *Journal of Educational Psychology* 82:623–636, 1990.
34. Baumrind D: The discipline controversy revisited. *Fam Relat* 45:405–414, 1996.
35. Andrews DW, Dishion TJ: The microsocial structure underpinnings of adolescent problem behavior. In: Ketterlinus L RD, Lamb ME (eds.): *Theories of theories of mind*. Cambridge, England: Cambridge University, 1994: 184–199.
36. Thomas A, Chess S: Genesis and evolution of behavioral disorders: From infancy to early adult life. *Am. J. Psychiatry* 141(1):1–9, 1984.
37. Goodnow JJ: From household practices to parents' ideas about work and interpersonal relationships. In: Harkness S, Super C (eds.): *Parents' cultural belief systems*. New York: Guilford, 1996 pp. 313–344.
38. Reiss D: The interplay between genotypes and family relationships. Current Directions in Psychological Science. *American Psychological Society* 14(3):139–143, 2005.
39. Bakermans-Kranenburg MJ, van Ijzendoorn MH, Juffer F: Less is more: Meta-analyses of sensitivity and attachment interventions in early childhood. *Psychological Bulletin* 129:195–215, 2003.
40. Combrinck-Graham L: A developmental model for family systems. *Fam Proc* 24:139–150, 1985.
41. Villani VS, Olson CK, Jellinek MS: Media literacy for clinicians and parents. *Child and Adol Psychiat Clinics of North America* 14(3):523–553, 2005.
42. Kramer DA: The biology of family culture. In: Combrinck-Graham, (ed.): *Children in family contexts*, 2nd ed. New York: Guilford, 2006.
43. Bemporad JR: From attachment to affiliation. *Am J Psychoanal* 44:792–799, 1984.
44. Kagan J, Klein RE: Cross-cultural perspectives on early development. *Am Psychol* 28:947–961, 1973.
45. Grunebaum H, Solomon L: Toward a peer theory of group psychotherapy: I. On the developmental significance of peers and play. *Int J Group Psychother* 30:23–49, 1980.
46. Harris JR: *The Nurture Assumption: Why Children Turn Out the Way They Do*. New York, Free Press, 1998.
47. Heyman GD, Dweck CS: Children's thinking about traits: Implications for judgments of the self and others. *Child Development* 69:391–403, 1998.
48. Pomerantz EM, Saxon JL: Conceptions of ability as stable and self-evaluative processes: A longitudinal examination. *Child Development* 72:152–173, 2001.
49. Eccles JS, Wigfield A, Schiefele U: Motivation to succeed. In: N Eisenberg (ed.): *Handbook of child psychology:* Vol. 3. *Social, emotional, and personality development*, 5th ed. New York: Wiley, 1998: 1017–1095.
50. Grunebaum H, Solomon L: Toward a theory of peer relationships: II. On the stages of social development and their relationship to group psychotherapy. *Int J Group Psychother* 32:283–307, 1982.
51. Buhrmester D, Furman W: The development of companionship and intimacy. *Child Dev* 58:1101–1113, 1987.
52. Minuchin P: *The middle years of childhood*. Belmont, CA, Brooks-Cole, 1977.
53. Cummings EM, Iannotti RJ, Zahn-Waxler C: Aggression between peers in early childhood: Individual continuity and developmental change. *Child Dev* 60:887–895, 1989.
54. Boivin M, Begin G: Peer status and self-perception among early elementary school children: The case of the rejected children. *Child Dev* 60:591–596, 1989.
55. Rogosch FA, Newcomb AF: Children's perceptions of peer reputations and their social reputations among peers. *Child Dev* 60:597–610, 1989.
56. Hartup WW: Social relationships and their developmental significance. *Am Psychol* 44:120–126, 1989.
57. Coie JD, Dodge K A, and Coppotelli H: Dimensions and types of social status: A cross-age perspective. *Developmental Psychology* 18:557–570, 1982.
58. Bagwell CL, Schmidt ME, Newcomb AF, Bukowski WM: Friendship and peer rejection as predictors of adult adjustment. In: Nangle DW, and Erdley CA (eds.): *The Role of Friendship in Psychological Adjustment*. San Francisco: Jossey-Bass, 2001 pp. 25–49.
59. Gifford-Smith MD, Brownell CA: Childhood peer relationships: Social acceptance, friendships, and peer networks. *J School Psychol* 41:235–284, 2003.
60. Sheridan SM, Buhs ES, Warnes ED: Childhood peer relationships in context. *J School Psychol* 41:285–292, 2003.
61. Brownell CA, Gifford-Smith ME: Context and development in children's school-based peer relations: Implications for research and practice. *J School Psychol* 41:305–310, 2003.
62. Heath SB: Oral and literate traditions among black Americans living in poverty. *Am Psychol* 44:367–373, 1989.
63. Miller-Jones D: Culture and testing. *Am Psychol* 44:360–366, 1989.
64. Wilson MN: Child development in the context of the black extended family. *Am Psychol* 44:380–385, 1989.
65. Davis-Kean PE: The influence of parent education and family income on child achievement: The indirect role of parental expectations and the home environment. *J Family Psychol* 19(2):294–304, 2005.
66. Humber N, Moss E: The relationship of preschool and early school age attachment to mother–child interaction. *Am J Orthopsychiatry* 75(1):128–141, 2005.
67. Granot D, Mayseless O: Attachment security and adjustment to school in middle childhood. *International J of Behavioral Development* 25(6):530–541, 2001.
68. Haskins R: Beyond metaphor: The efficacy of early childhood education. *Am Psychol* 44:274–282, 1989.
69. Bradley RH, Caldwell BM, Rock SL: Home environment and school performance: A ten-year follow-up and examination of three models of environmental action. *Child Dev* 69:852–867, 1988.
70. Hall WS: Reading comprehension. *Am Psychol* 44:157–161, 1989.
71. Coles G: *The Learning Mystique*. New York, Pantheon, 1987.
72. Ditton P, Green RJ, Singer MT: Communication deviances: A comparison between parents of learning-disabled and normally achieving students. *Fam Process* 26:75–87, 1987.
73. Belmont JM: Cognitive strategies and strategic learning: The socio-instructional approach. *Am Psychol* 44:142–148, 1989.
74. Slavin R: Developmental and motivational perspectives on cooperative learnings: A reconciliation. *Child Dev* 58:1161–1167, 1987.
75. Gardner H: *Intelligence Reframed: Multiple Intelligences for the 21st Century*. New York, Basic Books, 1999.
76. Levine M, et al.: Learning disabilities: An interactive developmental paradigm. In: Lyon GR, Gray DB (eds.): *Better Understanding Learning Disabilities: New Voices from Research and Their Implications for Education and Public Policies*. Baltimore: Paul H. Brookes, 1993 pp. 229–250.
77. Phinney J, Rotheram MJ: *Children's ethnic socialization: Pluralism and development*. New York, Sage, 1986.
78. Rotheram MJ: The family and the school. In: Combrinck-Graham L (ed): *Children in Family Contexts*. New York: Guilford, 1989 pp. 347–368.
79. Simons LG, Simons RL, Conger RD, Brody GH: Collective socialization and child conduct problems: A multilevel analysis with an African American sample. *Youth and Society* 35(3):267–292, 2004.
80. Linney JA, Siedman E: The future of schooling. *Am Psychol* 44:336–340, 1989.
81. No Child Left Behind Act. PL 107–110. 2001.
82. Jones PM: From Childhood, A Life of Hard Labor [Statistical sources: U.S. Department of Labor, International Labor Organization]. *Chicago Tribune*, p. 1, June 25, 2000.

CHAPTER 3.1.4 ■ ADOLESCENCE

ROBERT A. KING

We are born, so to speak, twice over. Born in existence and born into life; born a human being and born a man.

—Rousseau, *Emile*

Adolescence in contemporary Western industrial society is shaped and defined by the interplay of complex biological, cultural, economic, and historical forces. This lengthy transitional state, which may last a decade or more, is a distinctive period in which a youngster is no longer a child nor yet fully adult, but partakes of some of the challenges, privileges, and expectations of both epochs.

Adolescence is a period of paradoxes, as youngsters reach physical and sexual maturity well before they are fully cognitively and emotionally mature. On one hand, a secular trend toward earlier puberty over the past century and half means that defining maturational changes often begin by age 9–12, and that by 13 years of age many youngsters are potentially fertile and sexually attuned, if not yet fully active. On the other hand, the educational demands of a complex modern economy have prolonged formal education and raised the age of mandatory school attendance to approximately 16 years, whereas social welfare concerns have abolished child labor and legally restricted adolescent employment, thus postponing entry into the world of work. [Some measure of this shift may be seen in the contrast between 1900, when many Americans still lived on family farms, and only 10% of 14- to 17-year-olds attended high school, and the present 95% high school attendance rate (1).]

As a result, full economic emancipation usually is not possible until the later teens, at the earliest, and in the case of young people pursuing college or postgraduate education, often not until the middle to late 20s.

In the United States, the legal status of adolescents is a confusing mixture of privileges and strictures that attempts to balance the need for control and protection with the incremental granting of autonomy (2). For example, a 14-year-old may fly a plane, but not legally drive a car, whereas a 17-year-old may serve in the army, but not vote until 18 years of age, when he or she still is not legally allowed to drink. In many jurisdictions, a 14-year-old may legally obtain an abortion without her parents' knowledge or consent but needs her parents' permission to be absent from school to do so.

Despite the restrictions on their full-time employment, young adolescent consumers are a potent economic force, controlling billions of dollars in disposable income annually. Teenagers, hence, comprise an eagerly sought-after demographic target for marketers, advertisers, and the broadcast, print, and electronic media. In turn, to attract and hold these young viewers and readers, media programming directed to them increasingly emphasizes sex and violence as prominent themes; sexual themes are estimated to make up approximately one-third of the content of prime time shows popular with teens (3).

Winnicott once remarked aphoristically, "There is no such thing as a baby," meaning that the baby could not be considered apart from its relationship with its mother. Although adolescence is the epoch *par excellence* of individuation and autonomy striving, it is similarly impossible to have a full understanding of adolescent development apart from its specific biological, family, community, cultural, and historical contexts (4). Thus, while recent theoretical perspectives on adolescence acknowledge the development of *independence* and autonomy from parents, there is now an increased awareness of the complementary dynamic of the adolescent's developing capacity for *interdependence* and the ability to form and sustain mutually supportive relationships outside the family. Paralleling this relational perspective is an increased emphasis on the *ecological* perspective, which sees individual adolescents and their relationships as embedded in the interconnected contexts of family, school, neighborhood, and culture (5).

The interactions among these factors are complex and multidirectional. Not only are adolescents influenced by their families, but they reshape their families' dynamics as they grow. Although important aspects of adolescents' development are genetically and biologically determined, the effects of these determinants may be mediated or influenced by psychosocial factors. For example, family factors influence not only the impact of the timing of puberty but may actually affect the timing of puberty itself, with earlier and more rapid maturation in adolescents raised in more conflictual, less supportive homes (6–8). Behavioral genetics studies that have revealed the importance of nonshared environmental factors suggest that adolescent siblings evoke different interactional and social environments even within the same family (9).

It is important to bear in mind the great diversity of social and family contexts in which today's adolescents grow up (10, 11). In the United States, despite some commonalities, the experiences of adolescent who are immigrants, gay or lesbian, or growing up in poverty, foster care, single-parent, or other nontraditional family structures differ in important ways from the general patterns presented later in this chapter. Even greater differences exist between the majority culture of the West and more traditional societies, with less emphasis on individual autonomy and fewer expectations that adolescence should be a period of vocational choice or attaining full independence from families (12). Some anthropologic studies have concluded that in such preindustrial societies, there may be less adolescent turmoil and conflict with parents (13, 14).

One important research question concerns the impact on adolescence as the processes of modernization (demographic shift to longer life span, smaller families, urbanization, shift from agrarian to manufacturing and service economies,) and globalization (with development of an "information society") expose more and more teenagers in such societies to the same media and cultural influences as in the West (11–13). As 85% of the world's adolescents, age 10 to 19 years old, live in developing countries, where they comprise one-third of the national populations, these influences will play a fateful role in shaping the coming century's culture, politics, and economy (15).

One facet of globalization transforming important aspects of adolescence is the near-ubiquitous availability, at least in the industrialized world, of various electronic media, such

TABLE 3.1.4.1

TIME SPENT BY YOUTH 8–18 Y.O. WITH MEDIA AND SELECTED NONMEDIA ACTIVITIES IN A TYPICAL DAY

	Activity Time in Hours (Nonexclusive Categories)
Watching TV	3:04
Hanging out with parents	2:17
Hanging out with friends*	2:16
Listening to music	1:44
Exercising, sports, etc.	1:25
Watching movies/videos	1:11
Using a computer	1:02
Pursuing hobbies, clubs, etc.	1:00
Talking on the telephone*	0:53
Doing homework*	0:50
Playing video games	0:49
Reading	0:43
Working at a job*	0:35
Doing chores*	0:32

*Asked only of seventh- to twelfth-graders.
From Roberts et al., 2005 (18).

as TV, video games, cellular telephones, and the Internet (including instant messaging, e-mail, downloading music and videos, and social networking sites, such as Facebook and MySpace). At least 3/4 of American teens instant message and as many as 1/3 maintain blogs (16). The Youth Risk Behavior Survey (17) found that one-fifth of high school students reported 3 or more hours a day spent on an average school day playing video or computer games or using a computer for something other than schoolwork. A recent Kaiser Family Foundation Study (18) documented the relative amounts of time youngsters, age 8–18 years old, spent daily on these activities, compared with nonmedia activities (see Table 3.1.4.1; note that the times are not mutually exclusive; for example a youngster may talk on the phone while watching TV. Indeed, about 25% of youngsters reported multitasking (using more than one medium at the same time)). Over and above the sheer number of hours spent on these various media and their impact on youngsters' attention and cognitive style, youngsters are now exposed, for good or ill, and often without much adult supervision, to a plethora of global influences and virtual subcommunities, ranging from pornography to fellow aficionados of various cultural, athletic, or intellectual interests. Many adolescents now live much of their lives in an on-line social context; how this will influence their emotional and social development remains a vast experiment in progress (16).

PHYSICAL CHANGES AT ADOLESCENCE

The term *puberty* (from the Latin *pubertas*, meaning age of manhood) is used to refer to the physiologic and morphologic changes that mark the transition from childhood to adulthood.

Hormonally Mediated Changes

The most visibly dramatic aspects of adolescence relate to the hormonally mediated changes of puberty: the development of primary and secondary sexual characteristics; marked growth in stature, muscle mass, and strength; and increased sebaceous gland activity. These changes are the result of three different sets of hormonal changes: 1) adrenarche, 2) gonadarche, and 3) increased growth hormone secretion.

Adrenarche, the steady increase in adrenally produced androgens, begins as early as 6 to 8 years of age, leading to increased skeletal growth and the beginning appearance of body hair even before the surge of gonadal hormones associated with puberty proper.

Puberty proper is marked by *gonadarche,* in which the pulsatile release of gonadotropin-releasing hormone produces increased pituitary release of follicle-stimulating hormone and luteinizing hormone that in turn drive the production of gonadal hormones (primarily testosterone in boys, estrogen in girls). Together with these gonadal hormones, increased release of growth hormone stimulates the pubertal growth spurt.

The triggers for this activation of the pituitary–gonadal axis are unclear, but have been speculated to include leptin (serving as a metabolic signal of adequate body weight/composition), neurotransmitter-mediated attenuation of inhibitory tone or increased excitatory tone at the level of the hypothalamic gonadostat, and altered hypothalamus–amygdala interactions (19, 20).

The process of puberty takes approximately 4 to 5 years from start to finish, with girls (in the industrialized world) beginning the process on average at 9 to 11 years of age, approximately 2 years earlier than the average onset for boys. The various stages of this process, as indicated by pubic hair, breast development, height spurt, and menarche in girls, and pubic hair, penile and testicular growth, and height spurt in boys, have been classified by Tanner (21) into stages I through V. Although Tanner staging of a child's pubertal development is done most accurately by direct physical examination, alternative methods include the self-report Pubertal Development Questionnaire, or asking youngsters to identify their stage of development using a set of standard, gender-specific photographs (7).

The first harbinger of impending puberty usually is acceleration in linear growth, as much as 10 cm per year, which usually precedes increases in muscle mass and strength, thereby producing the gangly appearance of many early adolescents.

For girls, the initial stages of puberty are the beginnings of breast development [mean age 8.9 years (Standard deviation [SD], 1.9) for African-American girls and 10.0 years (SD, 1.8) for white girls] and the appearance of pubic hair [mean age 8.8 years (SD, 2.0) and 10.5 years (SD 1.7), respectively] (22).

The clearest marker of puberty in girls is the onset of menses, or *menarche*. Girls' periods initially remain irregular for some time, and despite the high rates of early teen pregnancy, ovulation and full fertility may require 2 years to develop. Most modern girls have been well prepared for menarche by health classes, peers, and mothers, and news of who has (or has not) yet begun her periods is the topic of excited exchanges of confidences among middle school girls.

A critical body weight and fat/muscle ratio appears to be a necessary condition for menarche; hence, girls who train intensively for athletics or dance or who are anorectic may have delayed menarche. Probably related to the permissive role of adequate nutrition and body weight, there has been a steady secular decrease in the age of menarche since the Industrial Revolution, at the rate of approximately 2.3 months per decade. Currently, the average age of menarche is 12.9 years (SD, 1.2) in white girls and 12.2 years (SD, 1.2) in African American girls (22). (As in preindustrial Europe, the age of menarche remains approximately 17 years in many developing countries). In recent years, there has been controversy about the appropriate norms for deciding at what age female pubertal development should be considered premature, because one large study found that by 7 to 8 years of age, 5% of white girls and 15.4% of African-American girls were at Tanner stage II or greater for breast development and 2.8% and 17.7%, respectively, were at Tanner II stage or greater for pubic hair. Further study is needed as to whether this represents an increased prevalence of very early puberty in girls, and if so, what its implications are regarding potential causes and indications for suppressive treatment (23, 24).

In boys, growth of the penis and testes and beginning spermatogenesis occur in early and middle adolescence. In contrast to menarche, however, "semenarche" or the beginning of ejaculation, whether by masturbation or spontaneous nocturnal emissions, usually remains a very private matter among Western boys (25).

Detailed longitudinal studies reveal considerable variation in the onset and progress of the various stages of puberty, both within and between genders. Thus, peak growth velocity in girls occurs approximately 2 years earlier than in boys, whereas pubic hair appearance often is only approximately 9 months earlier.

Much research has examined the question of the developmental impact on adjustment of early versus late maturation in boys and girls (19, 26, 27). In general, these studies show that, for boys, early maturation is advantageous in terms of popularity, self-esteem, and intellectual abilities, but does confer some increased risk for delinquent or problem behaviors, perhaps because of friendships with older peers (8). For girls, the picture is more complex, with early maturing girls tending to have more adjustment difficulties (including lower self-image and greater vulnerability to depression, anxiety, and eating disorders), to engage in more risky behaviors, and to experience early sexual intercourse. The impact of early versus late maturation in girls, however, also depends on social context variables such as social class, pubertal status of peers, cultural norms, and timing of concomitant changes (e.g., school transition), as well as prepubertal adjustment (8, 19, 28).

For many decades, an emphasis on the psychological effects of pubertal hormonal changes dominated discussions of the psychobiology of adolescence—what might be termed the "raging hormones" theory of adolescent psychology. However, only limited and equivocal associations have been found between various forms of adolescent psychopathology and gonadal hormonal levels (29, 30), with hormonal levels accounting for only a very small proportion of the variance in negative affects, compared with the influence of social factors.

Neurobiological Changes in Adolescence

Recent research has underlined the magnitude of neurobiological changes in the adolescent brain, especially in the forebrain and mesocortical and limbic regions (31, 32). To what extent these are influenced by or dependent on prenatal or pubertal hormonal factors is not clear.

One of the most dramatic changes in adolescent brain reorganization is a massive elimination or "pruning" of cortical synapses, with an estimated loss of up to 30,000 synapses per second during adolescence (33, 34). The resulting loss of approximately half of the cortical synaptic connections present before puberty is believed to affect preferentially excitatory synapses and is accompanied by declines in brain glucose metabolism, oxygen utilization, and blood flow; decreased overall electroencephalographic amplitude; and more complex and focal patterns of brain activation. The neuropsychological and neurochemical consequences of this synaptic remodeling are especially prominent in the prefrontal cortex, with loss of excitatory glutamatergic inputs, but also marked changes in dopaminergic input.

Longitudinal magnetic resonance imaging studies find a rostrocaudal wave of growth in the corpus callosum during childhood, with growth rates in the fibers connecting the temporoparietal cortical association and language areas peaking in early adolescence and then declining (perhaps paralleling the ending of the critical period for second-language acquisition). Cortical volume changes varied by region, with enlargement in the temporoparietal regions, but up to 50% loss in the subcortical gray matter of the head of the caudate (35). A longitudinal MRI study of youngsters 7–19 years of age found that intelligence was associated with the trajectory of cortical development, especially in the frontal regions. More intelligent children had a "particularly plastic cortex, with an initial acceleration and prolonged phase of cortical increase [peaking at about age 11 years], which yields to an equally vigorous cortical thinning by early adolescence" (32).

The full extent and significance of these changes in brain architecture and functioning are not yet clear (20, 32, 35). It seems likely, however, that they are reflected in the adolescent's burgeoning intellectual capacities, as well as a shift in various motivational, attentional, and emotional realms. For example, various neuropsychological tasks of executive functioning and inhibition that are believed to involve prefrontal cortical functioning continue to improve through adolescence (36).

Studies of schizophrenia, mood disorders, and other conditions have shed light on the pathogenic potential of these adolescent brain developments (see extensive review by Spear (20)). For example, the neurodevelopmental theory of schizophrenia (37) draws on the observation that although the infectious, neuromigratory, and nutritional insults predisposing to the disorder occur prenatally (usually in the second trimester), overt schizophrenic symptoms typically do not appear until late adolescence. Drawing on various animal models, Weinberger (37) and colleagues suggest that the behavioral effects of early lesions remain largely silent until unmasked by abnormalities in the usual late-adolescent maturational changes in the prefrontal cortex, hippocampus, or other limbic regions; these maturational changes are hypothesized to lead to the overt symptoms of schizophrenia, perhaps because of increased sensitivity to normative adolescent stressors. The normal adolescent maturation of the dorsolateral prefrontal cortex and working memory capacity is in part related to developmental changes in GABAergic neurons and their synapses, which are essential for the fine tuning of inhibitory control. Evidence from a variety of sources suggests that these developmental changes in GABAergic neurons are disrupted in schizophrenia (38).

The normative pubertal maturational changes in neuronal connectivity and functioning may interact with specific genetic vulnerabilities to influence the development of psychopathology. For example, Gothelf et al. (39) showed that over the course of adolescence in velo-cardio-facial syndrome (22q11.2 deletion syndrome), youngsters with the low-activity allelic form of catechol-O-methyltransferase (COMT) were at increased risk of decline in prefrontal cortical volume and cognitive functioning, as well as development of psychosis, compared to subjects with the high-activity allelic form. (It is of interest that the propensity of adolescent marijuana use to produce psychosis is also moderated by these same COMT polymorphisms (40)).

Other Biological Changes

Along with puberty come changes in appetite and sleep patterns.

Across species, the adolescence-associated growth spurt results in more time spent feeding and foraging for food. Most families with teenagers can attest to their youngsters' elevated metabolic rate and what has been termed *developmental hyperphagia* (20, 41).

Adolescence also sees a shift in sleep patterns, with a sleep phase delay or tendency to fall asleep later and wake up later (42). On average, 10- to 12-year-old children sleep approximately 9.3 hours a night and awaken spontaneously. In contrast, the mean length of sleep for high school students is 7.5 hours per night, with one-fourth of students sleeping 6.5 hours or less per night. Laboratory studies, however, suggest that the actual average sleep need for high school students is closer to 10 hours per night (43).

Part of this phase shift appears to be biological; later night-onset and later morning-termination of melatonin secretion make it difficult for the adolescent to go to sleep earlier or to wake up alert in time for school, which, deleteriously for many teenagers, may begin as early as 7:20 AM. This shift in sleep patterns also has a psychosocial component. Adolescents are given greater autonomy by their parents in controlling their own bedtimes, whereas the expansion of social contacts outside the home and increased social stimulation (in the form of phone, instant messaging, and e-mail) keep the teenager up later.

As a result of both these environmental and neurobiological factors, many adolescents suffer from "too little sleep at the wrong circadian phase," (43) especially on school days, with consequent difficulty getting up, frequent daytime drowsiness, and impaired alertness and cognitive functioning. Such adolescents are also at increased risk of learning difficulties, impaired academic performance, depressed mood, and accident-proneness.

COGNITIVE CHANGES IN ADOLESCENCE

Adolescence is marked by dramatic quantitative and qualitative growth in cognitive abilities (44). Although not a universal achievement, adolescence marks the attainment for many youngsters of what Piaget termed the stage of formal operations, with the ability to construct "contrary-to-fact" propositions and a growth in hypothetico-deductive problem-solving ability and understanding of propositional logic and probability (45). Along with a greater capacity for abstraction, adolescence often sees the flowering of passionate intellectual and aesthetic interests, with impressive achievements in areas such as music, mathematics, computer science, or physics. Interestingly, adolescent works of genius are more commonly in these abstract areas than in those involving the empirical sciences or the humanities.

Although the validity of Piaget's views have been debated, there is a general consensus that adolescents' cognitive abilities are characterized by growing complexity, the ability to think about possibilities, and increased speed and efficiency of information processing.

These cognitive changes also have their counterpart in the adolescent's social cognition and moral development (46). The development of formal operational thinking permits a growth in social perspective-taking and a decline in childhood egocentrism; it enables the adolescent to contemplate better what a social situation might look like from another person's point of view. As described by Kohlberg (47), moral reasoning becomes more complex and expands to include orientation to interpersonal relationships, maintenance of social order, notions of social contract and general rights, and, finally, reference to universal ethical principles. (Gilligan (48) has criticized Kohlberg's purportedly universal hierarchy of stages of moral reasoning as male-oriented in its emphasis on rules and universal principles and "moral logic of justice," in contrast to what she sees as the more interpersonal and nurturant bases of women's values in the "moral logic of care.")

Despite greater cognitive abilities, however, adolescents do not always use these capacities for sound decisionmaking, in part, perhaps, because their cognitive performance in real-life situations (as opposed to optimal test conditions) is more vulnerable to disruption by strong affects, everyday stresses, and peer influences (46, 49–52).

On a practical level, the adolescent develops a more mature time sense, a greater awareness of the finality of death, and, along with wider knowledge of the outside world, a keener sense of the diversity and relativity of moral codes. This moral awakening may be accompanied by an intensified interest in and sophistication about politics, ideology, or religion. This wider vision, as most eloquently described in the work of Erik Erikson (53), provides both opportunities and hazards. Along with a penchant for philosophical musings, the adolescent may experience a sense of moral confusion and at least transient feelings of anomie. The anxieties of what Seltzer (54) has termed *frameworklessness* may lead some adolescents to a fanatical embrace of some ideology or religion on one hand or a posture of nihilism on the other.

PSYCHOLOGICAL TASKS OF ADOLESCENCE

The physical, neurobiological, and cognitive changes described previously herald dramatic shifts in the adolescent's relationship to his or her own body, appetites, parents, peers, and self-image. In this next section, we turn to the psychological tasks of adaptation these shifts impose on the developing teenager (Table 3.1.4.2).

Coping with a Changing Body Image

Save for pregnancy or devastating illness, no other epoch sees such dramatic changes in the body and its self-representation as does adolescence. Although often welcome, these changes also are unsettling. Body and facial hair begins to grow. Menstrual discharges, erections, or ejaculation can occur at unexpected and embarrassing times. Acne and body odors make their appearance and are a source of anxiety. Boys' voices may break unexpectedly as they deepen. Changes in the distribution of fat and muscle alter body outlines. Not only must girls deal with breast development, but, to their embarrassment, many boys develop gynecomastia.

Adolescents compare their development carefully with that of their peers and are acutely aware of their self-perceived imperfections. Much time is spent brooding in front of the mirror, examining every potential blemish and trying to catch

TABLE 3.1.4.2

GROWTH TASKS BY DEVELOPMENTAL PHASE

The normative psychological tasks of adolescence are:

- Developing a satisfactory and realistic body image
- Developing increased independence from parents and adequate capacities for self-care and regulation
- Developing satisfying relationships outside the family
- Developing appropriate control and expression of increased sexual and aggressive drives
- Identity consolidation, including a personal moral code and at least provisional plans for a vocation and economic self-sufficiency

a glimpse of the self. A single pimple may seem to loom as large as the Matterhorn, its stigma increased by the sense that it is as glaringly obvious to everyone else as it is to the adolescent.

In Western society, girls in particular are very preoccupied with the body image ideal of thinness held up to them by the media (55). Girls' levels of satisfaction with their bodies and physical appearance decline as they pass through adolescence. This is especially problematic for girls who are earlier maturing. The National Health Examination Survey (56) found that most adolescent boys with body weights less than the top 10th percentile were satisfied with their weight; in contrast, even among girls whose weight was in the 50th percentile, 25% of lower socioeconomic group girls and over 40% of high socioeconomic group girls wanted to be thinner. The Youth Risk Behavior Survey (17) found that although 32% of high school boys and 25% of girls were overweight or at risk of being overweight (defined as having a body mass index equal to or greater than the 85th percentile for age and sex), only 25% of boys thought they were overweight, compared with 38% of girls; furthermore, only 30% of boys were trying to lose weight during the preceding 30 days, compared with 62% of girls. Compared with black girls, a higher proportion of white and Hispanic girls considered themselves overweight or were trying to lose weight.

Pathologic eating behaviors are common in adolescent girls. For example, a survey of two private girls' secondary schools found that 18% of the girls reported at least one major symptom of an eating disorder: 8% to 15% thought about food all the time, 6% to 12% induced vomiting to control their weight, over 2% used laxatives for weight control, and 7% often fasted or starved to lose weight (57). The most recent Youth Risk Behavior Survey (17) found that 4.5% of high school students report vomiting or taking laxatives within the past month to lose or control weight; the prevalence was higher among girls (6.2%) than boys (2.8%), with white and Hispanic girls reporting a higher prevalence (6.7 and 6.8% respectively) than black females (4.0%). These endemically high levels of body dissatisfaction and pathologic eating attitudes and behaviors provide a large reservoir of vulnerable adolescent girls from whose ranks those with frank bulimia and anorexia are recruited.

More research is needed, however, to understand better the cultural factors that influence the wide variations in the prevalence of disordered eating attitudes and behaviors across different communities and ethnic groups and over time.

The adolescent's body is also a representation of the adolescent's self. Hence, not surprisingly, teenagers spend great amounts of time, energy, and money trying to make their appearance conform to some perceived ideal. Boys in middle adolescence may try to bulk up their gangling habitus or firm up a pudgy physique by weight lifting, bodybuilding, nutritional supplements, and even anabolic steroids in an effort to transform their self-image from weak, dependent, or vulnerable to that of a "hard body"—tough, masculine, and strong. Girls endlessly experiment with makeup and consult friends and teen magazines regarding "makeovers." Both sexes may go through a dizzying panoply of clothing and hairstyles, trying on in rapid succession a kaleidoscope of fashions and styles that also represent possible social selves: slut, punk, home-boy, preppie, grunge, jock, Goth, and so forth. Multiple body piercings and tattoos convey more permanent, but potentially disfiguring personal statements. (By tattooing on a lover's name, the bearer seeks self-reassuringly to reinforce the permanence of a relationship (58).)

Beyond its role as a source of anxiety or pleasure, the body also may be the vehicle for painful or self-destructive means of reducing psychic tension (e.g., through delicate cutting) or dealing with conflicts over dependency or instinctual longings (bulimia, anorexia nervosa) (59).

Changing Relations with Parents

Surveys such as those of Offer and Schonert-Reichl (60) have emphasized that most adolescents regard their relations with their parents as stable, trusting, and sustaining and continue to turn toward parents as important, primary sources of advice, comfort, and assistance. Although this appears to be objectively true for most adolescents, on a subjective level, for both the parents and youngster, there are important shifts in the emotional terms of the relationship (8, 61).

LOOSENING TIES TO PARENTS

Time spent with family decreases during adolescence, from 25% of waking hours for high school freshmen to only 15% for seniors (62). Furthermore, there is a shift in the affective tone of time spent with parents and in the adolescent's view of the parents.

The teenager's own parents often are de-idealized. This is a painful process for parents as their previously admiring child develops a keen (sometimes distorted, sometimes all-too-accurate) sense of their shortcomings. Even those many teens who retain warm and supportive relations with their parents experience an increased sense of loneliness because the youngster feels no longer able or willing to share many intimate concerns or longings as of old. The adolescent may alternate between wishes for autonomy and wishes to be taken care of. Feelings of dependency may have to be warded off with disparagement, indifference, or oppositionality (63). As a result, well meaning parents often are bewildered as to which side of the child's ambivalence they are dealing with at any given moment (hence, the titles to various guides for the parents of teens, such as *Get Out of My Life, but First Could You Drive Me and Cheryl to the Mall?* (64)).

CONFLICT WITH PARENTS

Csikszentmihalyi and Larson (62) remark that "friction appears to be an endemic feature of family life" in families with adolescents, noting that "adults and adolescents live in separate, if overlapping, realities," often viewing the same events quite differently. This is true not only of specific events, but of family life in general, with adolescents tending to underestimate parental influence on them, and parents tending to overestimate their influence. Similarly, parents usually perceive the family's cohesion and adaptability as more satisfactory than do their teenagers who, in turn, report more conflicts with their parents than do the parents themselves (45, 61, 65).

Conflicts between parents and children increase with the beginning of adolescence. In early adolescence, these clashes concern household rules, chores, room cleaning, bedtime, diet, friends, dress, and hygiene; later in adolescence, issues such as dating and curfews become more prominent. Montemayor and Hanson's (66) naturalistic study of early adolescents found that conflicts with parents and siblings occurred at the rate of approximately 20 per month, or one every three days. Metaanalytic studies find that although the frequency of parent–child conflicts declines from early adolescence through late adolescence, the negative affective intensity of conflicts peaks in midadolescence (65).

Mothers appear to bear the brunt of most of these clashes, especially with early adolescent daughters (67); father–son clashes in particular take on greater affective intensity in mid-adolescence (65). Early maturation in girls and problems such as adolescent depression or substance abuse increase the likelihood of conflict (12).

This squabbling and bickering take a toll on the psychological well-being of the parents, as well as the adolescent, with many parents reporting difficulty adjusting to their teenager's strivings for autonomy (8).

The quality of daily family life, thus, becomes more turbulent in families with adolescents, with minor, but frequent "daily hassles"; for example, as boys approach puberty, there is a deterioration in family communication as both parents and child interrupt each other more frequently and explain themselves less (62) (Steinberg, 1981, cited in Csikszentmihalyi and Larson, 1984). Time sampling studies find that when with their families, adolescents' negative thoughts outnumber positive ones by ten to one (62).

The apparent decrease in parent–child conflict in middle adolescence coincides with decreased time spent with parents and a turn toward greater involvement and reliance on peers, leading Laursen et al. (65) to speculate that "it is likely that parents and children disagree less simply because they are together less. Increases in conflict affective intensity coincide with increases in autonomy and emotional dysphoria that occur as adolescents spend more time alone and with peers."

Despite the mutual stresses of increased conflict, most parent–child relationships remain solid. As Arnett (12) notes, "Even amidst relatively high conflict, parents and adolescents tend to report that overall their relationships are good, that they share a wide range of core values, and that they retain a considerable amount of mutual affection and attachment."

Seen from one perspective, the immediate *causa belli* of many typical parent–adolescent clashes appear seemingly trivial: hairstyle, clothes, chores, curfew, or volume and taste in music. The intensity of conflict, however, usually reflects the parents' or child's perception (accurate or not) that vital issues are at stake: for the parents, issues of loyalty, respect, responsibility, and the dangers of sex, substance abuse, or other risky behavior; for the adolescents, issues of autonomy, control of their own body, and connections to friends.

Adolescents whose parents are able to hold firm and maintain balance in the face of these upheavals, without being overly permissive, harshly authoritarian, or indifferent, appear to do best. Numerous studies conclude that what has been termed *authoritative parenting*—combining warmth and responsiveness on one hand with firmness and demandingness—is associated with a wide range of adolescent competencies, academic achievement, and positive outcomes (61).

By later adolescence, in most cases, volatility and strife decrease and some degree of equilibrium is restored to the parent–adolescent relationship, albeit on a newer and more egalitarian basis, with the youngster having more autonomy and involvement in family decision making.

TRANSITION TO SELF-CARE

As adolescence progresses, youngsters gradually claim or are ceded greater control over their diet, hygiene, sleep schedule, and dress, as well as responsibility for their school work. Nonetheless, these remain topics of frequent minor skirmishes, at least in early adolescence, with much parental nagging about junk food, skipped meals, slovenly or inappropriate dress, time spent on the phone (or Internet), and the like.

Although adolescence is a time of general good physical health, it also is the period during which many attitudes and habits are established with respect to diet, exercise, substance use, smoking, driving, and sexual behaviors that will constitute long-term risk (or protective) factors for health in later life (68).

Ironically, for many youngsters with serious chronic illnesses, such as type 1 diabetes mellitus or cystic fibrosis, despite their greater cognitive understanding of the exigencies of their condition, the quality of their care frequently deteriorates as they take over the responsibility for adherence to their treatment regimen (26, 69). Thus, many adolescent diabetic patients fail to adhere to their diet, blood glucose testing, and insulin regimen. Adolescent diabetic girls may even deliberately permit themselves to spill sugar in their urine as an ill-advised form of weight control. Some chronically ill youngsters may stop their medication, including chemotherapy or immunosuppressant therapy, with potentially fatal consequences.

Unlike health-conscious adults, many adolescents perceive the need to pay extra attention to their physical condition as anxiety provoking, stigmatizing, or frighteningly threatening to their wish for autonomy and invulnerability; hence, rather than responding to their medical condition with heightened attentiveness, they may try to avoid thinking about or dealing with their illness altogether.

Developing Satisfying Relationships Outside the Family

As dependence on parents becomes less acceptable to adolescents, they turn increasingly to peers for companionship, advice, support, and intimacy (70). Csikszentmihalyi et al. (71) found that during the school year, adolescents spend one-third of their waking time talking with peers, but less than 8% of waking time talking with adults. Talking with friends was the activity that teens reported made them the happiest.

Parents may be bemused or annoyed by their adolescent's intense need to hang out with and be with peers, regardless of any family plans. As Seltzer (54) points out, this is not merely for the immediate pleasures of the event. Rather, the need for continuing access to peers is driven by an intense need to relate, to compare, and to try out aspects of the developing self. It is this developmental need that explains "why adolescents never seem to tire of being with one another.... [I]t is not the overt social activity or the content of the event (e.g., a rock concert, a football game, a dance) that feeds the drive. It is *being with one another*—looking, listening, and resultant comparing. Adolescents report details of who was there, what they did or said, and what they wore in far greater detail than they describe the content of the event."

With adolescence, the communicative, supportive, and intimate aspects of friendship take on increased importance. Although nonromantic opposite-sex friendships occur in later adolescence, close friendships in early adolescence tend to be with the same sex. Among girls, intimate conversations are most often the cement of friendships, whereas for boys, it tends to be shared activities. With age, the need for control and conformity decreases, and there is greater tolerance for differences between friends (8).

The choice of friends is a complex matter. Although the range of possibilities is defined by the given community and school population, the adolescent's specific choices of friends reflect an important and often fateful aspect of self-definition. Adolescents most often choose friends who share their behaviors, attitudes, interests, and identities (8). Friends, however, also may be chosen on many other grounds, including perceived virtues or aspects of the self that the adolescent consciously repudiates or feels he or she lacks. Friends may serve as sources of support or admiration, as collusive companions for regression or delinquency, objects of sexual or aggressive exploitation, targets for projection—the list is endless. The choice of friend may be used to try on or borrow self-attributes; for example, a girl who perceives herself as unattractive or unpopular may hang out with a girl whom she sees as beautiful or popular. A boy who feels himself to be overly compliant, timid, or passive may chose to hang out for a while with a more venturesome or delinquent peer. Friendships pursued out of such interests may be transient or unstable as the youngster comes to feel in greater possession of the desired attribute himself or herself, or repudiates the wish for it.

Empirical studies have examined what personal attributes of peers are most salient to adolescents. For example, Midwestern high school students were asked to rate a list of attributes as to the frequency with which they were noticed in age mates. The top 10 attributes most frequently rated as "always of interest" were (in decreasing order): cleanliness, loyalty to friends, clothes, dependability, trustworthiness, general physical appearance, maturity, popularity with opposite sex, figure/build/physique, and honesty. Despite some gender and age differences, appearance and dependability were widely viewed as very important, whereas specific skills and abilities were of little interest (54).

Over the course of high school, adolescents shift in the gender and group size with whom they associate (70). Thus, freshmen hang out predominantly in same-sex groups, sophomores in same-sex dyads, juniors in mixed-sex groups, and seniors predominantly in small groups of heterosexual couples (62). In early adolescence, the adolescent's crowd consists of a large group of peers with similar reputations and role stereotypes (preppies, goths, brains, jocks, nerds). Younger adolescents value crowd affiliation as fostering friendships, providing support, facilitating interactions, and providing a source of identity and status (according to where the adolescent's particular crowd fits in the school or community hierarchy). Attitudes toward being "part of a crowd" do, however, change over the course of adolescence (70). Older adolescents are more likely to be dissatisfied with the perceived conformity demands of crowds and prefer smaller, more intimate groups. By the later high school years, the salient peer group may be the clique, a smaller group of peers similar in terms of activities, attitudes, status, age, and race.

Ironically, many adolescents, while resisting parental advice in the name of autonomy, are slavishly compliant with the perceived tastes and values of peers, especially regarding fashions and preferences in dress, slang, music, television, and movies.

As Steinberg and Morris (8) point out, however, peers influence each other in positive ways, including prosocial behaviors and academic achievement, as well as in negative ways, such as delinquency or substance use. These influences are not necessarily coercive or conformist, but also stem from emulatory admiration and a community of attitudes and interests that form the basis for the friendship in the first place.

Adolescents' relationships with their parents are an important influence on peer relationships. Authoritative parenting styles appear to lessen the negative effects of peer influences; conversely, teenagers from less cohesive families are more likely to be influenced by peers than by parents (8). A tendency to look to peers rather than to parents for guidance and values, especially when combined with a choice of peers with delinquent behavior, low academic aspirations, or with values markedly divergent from the adolescent's parents, is an important risk factor for a wide range of problem behaviors (72).

Sexual and Aggressive Drives

Adolescence sees the epochal development of experiencing sexual attraction toward others and perceiving oneself as the object of others' sexual desire. How these subjectivities unfold and are given individual and social meanings is a complex process with physiologic, cultural, and individual dimensions (73). The interplay of these factors has been the focus of much anthropologic, psychoanalytic, and developmental study (26, 74, 75).

After a period of fairly open genital interests and play during the preschool years, overt sexual behavior and interests diminish markedly during the school years (76). Although even in these years before adolescence, sexual interests are never completely latent, masturbation, if it continues, is more furtive, and the child becomes more modest and inhibited about discussing sexual and romantic matters.

Beginning at approximately 10 years of age, feelings of sexual awareness and attraction make their conscious appearance. This development, which appears to be linked to rising adrenal androgens, occurs even before the onset of gonadal puberty proper. The reticence of children at this age makes the phenomenon difficult to study in Western culture, but in many preliterate cultures, such as Melanesia, sexual rites of passage, at least for boys, occur as early as 10 years of age (74). It is also around the age of 10 to 11 years that some children become aware of same-sex attractions and homoerotic fantasy.

In early adolescence, genital excitement and sexual interests often occur independently of liking, intimacy, or wish for emotional closeness. For young adolescent boys, the objects of sexual fantasy and masturbatory excitement frequently are magazine models or television and movie figures, rather than actual acquaintances. In keeping with their burgeoning attunement to social relationships, early adolescent girls are usually intensely interested in the romantic relationships, real and fantasied, of their peers, with endless discussions of who is "going out" or has broken up with whom. However, the early teen boys who are their age-peers often are unpromising candidates as romantic partners, hence many girls' crushes and eroticized longings focus on media figures, such as the various "boy bands" marketed to this audience. Although movies and television have long provided the raw materials for adolescent sexual fantasy, it is not yet clear what the recent increases in the ubiquity, sexual explicitness, and violence of mass media (including now the Internet) will be on the sexual socialization of teens (3).

With adolescence, there also is a resurgence of overt sexual activity (76, 77). The rate of explicit masturbation increases from approximately 10% at age 7 to approximately 80% at age 13 years, whereas that of heterosexual play rises to approximately 65% at age 13 years; homosexual play also is not uncommon in early adolescence, with 25% to 30% of 13-year-old boys reporting at least one episode of same-sex play.

The transition from childhood masturbation to that of adolescence involves more than an increased physiologic capacity for arousal and orgasm. Most teens report consciously fantasizing when masturbating to orgasm, and even those who do not seem aware of some sort of sexual imagery (75). Sexual fantasies (which also occur without overt masturbation) become an intense and important part of the adolescent's psychological inner life. Beyond serving as a source of pleasure and compensatory wish fulfillment in lieu of other sexual outlets, these fantasies provide the occasion for the adolescent to elaborate or explicate his or her idiosyncratic and personal erotic scripts: who, doing what, with whom, with what body parts, with what implicit and explicit emotional tone and interpersonal interactions, and with what admixture of dominance or submission, control or abandonment, sadism or masochism, and admiration or degradation. (Laufer (78) has coined the term *central masturbatory fantasy* to describe the organizing aspects of these not always fully conscious fantasies in relationship to arousal and orgasm.) These fantasies are more than just a form of rehearsal or anticipatory coping; they help the adolescent explore and become aware of what is pleasurable, anxiety provoking, transgressive, or deeply compelling in his or her longings and to become familiar with individual preconditions for erotic excitement and fulfillment.

A key task of adolescence is to bring these erotic longings adaptively into the interpersonal arena as a vehicle for intimacy, emotional closeness, and ultimately the formation of a stable partnership for the conception and rearing of the next generation.

Although early adolescence sees the transition from largely autoerotic sexual activity to sexual interactions with peers, this takes place at different rates in different social and ethnic groups and with different interpersonal meanings (26, 75, 79). The prevalence of ever having had sexual intercourse is about 34% in the ninth grade and 63% by the twelfth grade, with higher rates among males than females; the respective rates among black high school students are 68%, Hispanic students 51%, and white students 43% (17).

For girls, the relational aspect of sexual involvement usually is paramount, and girls may engage in petting, oral sex, or intercourse as an attempted means of winning or retaining a boy's perceived interest, affection, or commitment. For young adolescent boys, sexual activity often has a more exploitative nature, with less interest in the relational aspect of the activity. However, these gender distinctions are not universal, with some research suggesting that "girls are more sexually oriented and boys more romantically oriented" (73) (p. 221) than previously believed (80).

(For a detailed account of the epidemiology and other aspects of adolescent sexuality, as well the implications for prevention of pregnancy and acquired immunodeficiency syndrome (AIDS), see Chapter 7.1.3.3.

Falling in love is an important part of adolescence, even when not accompanied by sexual intimacy (5, 79). Adolescence's most intense longings, keenest pleasures, painful frustrations, and bitterest disappointments center on the quest for a reciprocated love that helps to define the still inchoate self and assuage the loneliness of individuation.

Adolescent sexuality stirs in adults a variable reactive mixture of envy, apprehension, or repressiveness. Parents who may be facing their own midlife crises must contend with their sons' or daughters' burgeoning sexuality. Many of the parent–child conflicts in midadolescence, such as those around clothes, friends, dating, curfews, and driving, although seemingly trivial, have the subtext of the parents' attempts to control the pace, scope, and direction of their adolescent's sexual activity. (A few parents who are overidentified with their adolescent's sexuality or take too much vicarious excitement in it collusively encourage their teen's transition to sexual activity.)

Despite much forgetfulness about the travails of their adolescence, most adults retain evocative, bittersweet memories of their own adolescent romantic longings. It is not surprising then, that from *Romeo and Juliet* on, the pangs and passions of adolescent love, whether thwarted or fulfilled, have remained an enduring theme of plays, novels, poetry, movies, and songs.

Identity

In his seminal work *Childhood and society*, Erik Erikson (53) describes the challenge of identity formation as follows:

> [I]n puberty and adolescence all samenesses and continuities relied on earlier are more or less questioned again.... The growing and developing youths, faced with [the] physiological revolution within them, and with tangible adult tasks ahead of them are now primarily concerned with what they appear to be in the eyes of others as compared with what they feel they are, and with the question of how to connect the roles and skills cultivated earlier with the occupational prototypes of the day.... [It is the ability] to integrate all identifications with the vicissitudes of the libido, with the aptitudes developed out of endowment, and with the opportunities offered in social roles. [The desired outcome] is the accrued confidence that the inner sameness and continuity prepared in the past are matched by the sameness and continuity of one's meaning for others.

One of the most influential empirical extensions of Erikson's work was Marcia's taxonomy for classifying adolescents into four identity statuses: the *identity-confused* subject who has not yet experienced an identity crisis or made a role commitment; the *foreclosed* subject, who has made unexamined commitments, usually as received from parents and others; the *moratorium* subject, who is actively struggling to define values and commitments; and the *identity-achieved* subject, who has resolved these crises (81).

In contemporary society, many of these identity issues are not fully engaged until the college years or beyond (1).

Empirical research has shifted away from global notions of identity to focus more on the development of specific self-concepts (8, 82). With their growing cognitive sophistication, adolescents' views of themselves become more differentiated and better organized. Harter (83) and others have examined the distinct dimensions of adolescents' self-concept across several realms, such as social relations, appearance, academics, athletics, and morality, and their relationship to global self-worth. Adolescents weigh these dimensions differently depending on whether they are interacting with peers, parents, or teachers, and it is only over time that these discrepancies decline to produce a more consonant, better integrated self-image. [Behavioral genetic studies of siblings suggest that heritable factors may exert more of an influence than do shared environmental factors on perceived scholastic and athletic competence, physical appearance, and general self-worth; perceived social competence appears to be primarily determined by nonshared environmental factors reflecting each sibling's unique family and social experiences (9, 84).]

In addition to the ubiquitous categories of adolescent self-concept described by Harter, ethnic and sexual minority adolescents also must consolidate a sense of identity vis-à-vis both their minority group and the mainstream culture (8).

CLINICAL ASPECTS OF ADOLESCENCE

On the basis of many epidemiologic studies, it now appears that only approximately 20% of adolescents have diagnosable clinical disorders. However, it is equally clear that during adolescence, a substantial proportion of youngsters experience increased conflicts with parents and mood difficulties and engage in risk behaviors.

The Storm and Stress Debate Revisited

For many years, debate has continued over the frequency and severity with which adolescent turmoil occurs and the extent to which it should be considered normative in American culture or universal across epochs and cultures (for a review of this issue, see Arnett (12)).

Classical writers, such as Aristotle and Plato, saw the period we now call adolescence as a time of changeability and vulnerability that required careful character education and social constraints. Aristotle noted in his *Rhetorica*:

> Young men have strong passions, and tend to gratify them indiscriminately. Of the bodily desires, it is the sexual by which they are most swayed and in which they show absence of self-control.... They are changeable and fickle in their desires, which are violent while they last, but quickly over: their impulses are keen but not deep-rooted.... They cannot bear being slighted, and are indignant if they imagine themselves being unfairly treated" (quoted in Muus (81)).

Although, over the centuries, adolescents have at times been idealized for their beauty and grace or as bearing the hope of the future, they also have been regarded by their elders with deep misgivings and dismay as potentially disruptive and subversive, not only difficult to handle, but threatening to undermine society's strictures regarding sex, aggression, and respect for elders. Hence, the old shepherd laments in *The Winter's Tale:*

> I would that there were no age between ten and three-and-twenty, or that youth would sleep out the rest, for there is nothing in between but getting wenches with child, wronging the ancientry, stealing, fighting ... (Act III, scene iii).

In his seminal 1904 work, G. Stanley Hall (85) noted "a period of semicriminality is normal for all healthy [adolescent] boys" (quoted in Arnett (12)). Speaking of the internal upheavals of adolescence, rather than overt deviant behavior, Anna Freud (63) noted, "the upholding of a steady equilibrium during the adolescent process is in itself abnormal." She observed that:

> it is normal for an adolescent to behave for a considerable length of time in an inconsistent and unpredictable manner; to fight his impulses and to accept them; to ward them off successfully and to be overrun by them; to love his parents and to hate them; to revolt against them and to be dependent on them ... to thrive on imitation of and identification with others while searching unceasingly for his own identity; to be more idealistic, artistic, generous and unselfish than he will ever be again, but also the opposite—self-centered, egoistic, and calculating.

In more recent years, this view of adolescence as inherently tumultuous has come under attack as an overgeneralization from mental health professionals' clinical samples, from a romantic notion of youthful struggle (86), or from popular authors' vivid portrayals of their own idiosyncratic adolescent experiences. For example, in an article polemically entitled *Debunking the myths of adolescence: Findings from recent research*, Offer and Schonert-Reichl (60) characterize the "myth" that normative adolescence is tumultuous as assuming that "[t]he 'typical' adolescent is ... out of control, in constant conflict with his or her family, and incapable of rational thought." In contrast, they observe, on the basis of nonclinical samples, that "adolescence is not a time of severe disturbance for all adolescents. Moreover, ... a significant percentage of adolescents (80%) do not experience adolescent turmoil, relate well to their families and peers, and are comfortable with their social and cultural values.... [T]eenagers who exhibit little disequilibrium are normal ... [and] ... adolescence is a period of development that can be traversed without turmoil and that the transition to adulthood is accomplished gradually and without undue upheaval."

As with many debates, the truth lies somewhere in the middle of these dichotomies and depends on the terms of the argument and matters of degree (e.g., what type and severity of turmoil). In a review of the topic, Arnett (12) concluded:

> [T]here is support for Hall's (1904) view that a tendency toward some aspects of storm and stress exists in adolescence. In their conflicts with parents, in their mood disruptions, and in their heightened rates of a variety of types of risk behavior, many adolescents exhibit a heightened degree of storm and stress compared with other periods of life. Their parents, too, often experience difficulty—from increased conflict when their children are in early adolescence, from mood disruptions during mid-adolescence, and from anxiety over the increased possibilities of risk behavior when children are in late adolescence. However ... there are cultural differences in storm and stress, and within cultures there are individual differences in the extent to which adolescents exhibit the different aspects of it. [However], [e]ven amidst the storm and stress of adolescence, most adolescents take pleasure in many aspects of their lives, are satisfied with most of their relationships most of the time, and are hopeful about the future.

Having examined conflicts with parents, we turn to a more detailed consideration of mood problems and risk behaviors.

Mood Difficulties and Perceived Stress

Adolescence is a time of rising incidence for major depression, with the risk of depression and the preponderance of affected girls versus boys increasing not only with age, but more specifically with advancing pubertal status.

Only a minority of adolescents develop a full-blown affective disorder. Nonetheless, adolescence sees a marked increase in emotional lability, depressed mood, and negative emotions (anxiety and self-consciousness), with over one-third of adolescents in nonclinical samples reporting high levels of depressed mood (12, 29, 87, 88). For example, the national Youth Risk Behavior Survey (17) of high school students found that, during the preceding year, 37% of girls and 20% of boys felt sad or hopeless almost every day for at least 2 weeks in a row and 22% and 12%, respectively, seriously considered attempting suicide. Mood disruptions are associated with higher levels of negative life events (89). Comparing fifth graders and ninth graders, Larson and Richards (87) describe the dramatic decline in the proportion of time youngsters feel "very happy," "proud," or "in control" as an emotional fall from grace.

Girls appear especially prone to negative moods. For example, Offer and colleagues (82) (1988) found marked gender differences in emotional vulnerability across adolescence. Compared with boys, girls described themselves as moodier, sadder, lonelier, more prone to uncontrollable crying, more easily hurt, less autonomous and more other-directed, and more ashamed of their bodies.

Adolescents also report a substantial increase in the number of negative life events. It is difficult to determine to what extent this reflects a more stressful environment, greater sensitivity to events, or shifts in the types of situations that precipitate negative emotions (90, 91).

The nature and sources of perceived stress change over the course of adolescence, with early adolescents experiencing stress in relationship to peers and older adolescents with respect to academic issues. Especially in early adolescence, girls appear to experience more stress than at other ages and to perceive more stressful events than do boys (91–93).

Although significant life events, such as parental separations or unemployment, moves, or deaths, have a serious impact on adolescents, many of the fluctuations in adolescent mood reflect the less dramatic daily hassles—homework, tests, disagreements with friends—and the minor disappointments, stresses, and embarrassments that form the fabric of adolescent life. It may be deceptive, however, to try to conceptualize and quantify these hassles as completely independent external variables because unlike many major life events, the intensity, valence, and even the occurrence of such episodes often lie largely in the eye of the adolescent beholder (62).

Time sampling studies of adolescent mood in community samples find that, compared with adults, adolescents have greater mood variability as measured by both the width of their mood swings (between extreme highs and lows) and the evanescence of these extremes (62). In the nonclinical high school population studied, greater subjectively experienced mood lability was not associated with poorer adjustment or other pathologic processes.

Neurobiological factors also may influence the impaired mood regulation and increased stress reactivity observed in adolescence (52). A longitudinal study by Angold and colleagues (94) found that reaching Tanner stage III was associated with increased levels of depression in girls; however, hormonal levels of testosterone and estradiol were more closely associated with levels of depression than age or Tanner stage per se. Although this suggests that it is not morphologic body changes themselves that render pubertal girls more prone to depression, it is unclear whether these findings reflect direct depressogenic endocrine influences on the central nervous system or hormonally mediated changes in responsivity to life events and stress.

Spear (20) proposed that age-related changes in the balance of dopamine regulation in the prefrontal cortex relative to mesolimbic brain regions lead to shifts in the incentive value and motivational power of different reinforcers. Drawing on both human and animal data, Spear proposes a transient relative "reward deficiency syndrome" or "adolescent anhedonia" that results in previously pleasurable activities being experienced as less rewarding and leads to a compensatory search for new and more intense forms of stimulation (greater novelty seeking, risk taking, and increases in consummatory behaviors, such as food and drugs). Arnsten and Shansky (52) note that even mild stress impairs prefrontal cortical cognitive functioning and that several aspects of adolescent brain development may amplify these stress-induced deficits.

Risk-Taking Behaviors

Adolescent risk-taking behavior is a significant source of morbidity and mortality in this otherwise vigorous age group. In contrast to persons 25 years of age or older, for whom two-thirds of all deaths are due to cardiovascular disease and cancer, three-fourths of all deaths for youths 10 to 24 years of age are due to motor vehicle crashes, other unintentional injuries, homicide, and suicide, with AIDS also becoming a rapidly rising cause of death for young adults. Behaviors that increase the risk of these adverse outcomes are common among teenagers. The Centers for Disease Control and Prevention (17) national Youth Risk Behavior Survey found that for the 30 days preceding the survey, 10% of high school students reported rarely or never wearing a seat belt, 28% had ridden with a driver who had been drinking and 10% had driven a vehicle when they had been drinking, 19% had carried a weapon, 43% had drunk alcohol, 23% had smoked tobacco, 20% had used marijuana, and 8.4% had attempted suicide in the prior 12 months. Other health-impairing behaviors also were common. About half of the students had had sexual intercourse; of these, 37% had not used a condom at last intercourse.

These risk behaviors are not uniformly distributed across the adolescent population. For example, among ninth graders, 22% are estimated to be at low risk, with no involvement with any risk behaviors such as substance use, sex, depression/suicide, antisocial behavior, school problems, unsafe vehicle use, or bulimia (95). Another 29% report only one such risk indicator, 18% report two, and 31% report three or more. High-risk youth (those reporting multiple risk behaviors) are characterized by early onset of high-risk behaviors, absence of nurturing parenting, child abuse, lack of involvement with school, susceptibility to peer influence, depression, disadvantaged neighborhoods, and lack of gainfully employed role models.

Certain patterns of autonomic reactivity may also predispose to increased risk-taking under certain circumstances (96), and data from nonhuman primates suggest important interactions between genetically determined variations in neurotransmitter regulation and early rearing environment (see below).

It is important to distinguish between occasional experimentation and persistent patterns of dangerous behavior (8). Although most adolescents will experiment with alcohol or minor delinquent behaviors, in most cases these behaviors do not persist into adulthood. Studies in both human and nonhuman adolescents suggest that certain aspects of the neurobiology of the adolescent brain may make adolescents more vulnerable to substance abuse (97, 98). (In turn, chronic alcohol or nicotine use during adolescence may have long-lasting deleterious effects on cognitive functioning (99). Animal research also suggests that certain genotypes may predispose adolescents to alcohol or nicotine abuse (100).

The prevalence of problem behaviors does increase in adolescence and early adulthood, but persistence in problem behaviors, such as substance use or antisocial behavior, usually is associated with difficulties in earlier childhood (101). The work of Jessor (72) and others (102) suggests that risk-taking behaviors such as sexual activity, substance use, reckless driving, and delinquency not only increase over adolescence but frequently are associated with each other and share common psychosocial antecedents. These behaviors are not simply arbitrary, perverse, or motivated only by sensation-seeking or exploratory motives, but are in part purposeful, meaningful, goal-oriented, and functional. For example, Jessor (72) observes that such behaviors also can serve the instrumental ends of gaining peer acceptance, establishing autonomy from parents, defying conventional authority, relieving anxiety or frustration, or affirming the transition to a more adult status.

Although the propensity to impulsivity, risk-taking, and sensation seeking has important family and social determinants, it also appears to reflect developmental immaturities in the neural mechanisms underlying inhibitory control, emotional processing, and executive functioning (103). Shifts in reward sensitivity occur early in adolescence and "drive adolescents to seek higher levels of novelty and stimulation than they did as children (49)," while the more slow maturing regulatory competencies that might check this novelty and stimulation-seeking do not come online until later in adolescence (104). (Psychiatric and medical testimony regarding this relative immaturity played a role in the important U.S. Supreme Court decision (*Roper* vs. *Simmons*) banning the death penalty for crimes committed prior to age 18 (103, 105).

ETHOLOGIC PERSPECTIVES

Examination of the transition from youth to adulthood in other mammalian (especially nonhuman primate) species suggests animal models for the counterpart of human adolescence. Like human adolescents, the young of other species exhibit increases in peer-directed social interactions and greater novelty-seeking and risk-taking behaviors (20, 106, 107). Spear has suggested that these shared behavioral features represent ontogenetic adaptations that help individuals in this transitional period in "acquiring the necessary skills to permit survival away from parental caretakers. Increased affiliation with peers and the taking of risks via exploring novel areas, behaviors, and reenforcers may also help facilitate the dispersal of adolescents away from the natal family unit" (20), with the adaptive goal of avoiding inbreeding. Similarly, human adolescents and many pubertal nonhuman primates spend increased time in social interactions with peers, including aggressive fighting, but also in reconciliatory and affiliative behaviors; paralleling this shift in social orientation from adults to peers is an increase in conflicts between the adolescent and parents, which also may help to encourage separation from the natal family unit (108, 109). Increased risk taking also is seen across species, with increased exploratory behavior and novelty seeking, but also increased mortality. From an evolutionary perspective, such risks "may be—or at least once were—means of securing physical resources, attracting mates, and denying mating opportunities to competitors" (109).

Research on nonhuman primates also provides clues about the complex interplay of heritable and environmental factors that shape risky behaviors during adolescence. Juvenile rhesus males with low CSF 5-HIAA are at increased risk of being expelled early from their natal troop and have very high mortality rates (46%) over a 4-year period compared to their peers with higher 5-CSF HIAA (0%) (110). Their high mortality rates (and unpopularity) reflect their excessively aggressive and impulsive behaviors, including inappropriate attacks on peers and higher ranking adults and other risky behaviors, such as excessively dangerous leaps from tree to tree. Although 5-HIAA is a highly heritable trait in rhesus monkeys, it is also strongly influenced by early social experiences, especially attachment relationships, with peer-reared monkeys exhibiting lower CSF 5-HIAA levels throughout their life span than mother-reared counterparts. Gene × environment interaction is apparent in the finding that the impact of serotonin transporter (5-HTT) genotype is strongly influenced by early rearing conditions (peer- vs. mother-rearing). Among monkeys heterozygous for the "short" allelic variant of the 5-HTT gene, peer-reared monkeys had much lower CSF 5-HIAA levels and poor attention and motor maturity than did their mother-reared counterparts. However, for monkeys homozygous for the "long" 5-HTT allele, peer- vs. mother-rearing did not substantially diminish CSF 5-HIAA levels, suggesting that mother rearing may "buffer" the potential vulnerability conferred by the heterozygous genotype (100, 111). Similarly, allelic variations of the monoamine oxidase A (MAOA) gene influence aggressive behavior in rhesus monkeys, but the behavioral expression of MAOA genotype is influenced by early rearing (112).

THE CLOSE OF ADOLESCENCE

The pubertal changes that are the hallmark of adolescence provide a relatively clear marker for the beginning of adolescence. In contrast, the close of adolescence in contemporary society is less clearly defined. At one time in the United States and even today in traditional societies, the end of adolescence and assumption of adult status was usually marked by a discrete event, such as marriage, beginning of full-time employment, or military service. Currently, however, the same forces that have helped to create adolescence as a distinctive period of life in industrial and postindustrial society also have blurred the end of adolescence (1). College and postgraduate education has become increasingly important, and the proportion of youth pursuing post–high school education has risen from 14% in 1940 to over 60% in the 1990s. Correspondingly, the median age of marriage in the United States rose from 21 years for women and 23 years for men in 1970 to 25 years for women and 27 years for men in 1996. Thus, for many young people, entry into adult roles regarding work, marriage, and parenthood is delayed until the late 20s or even early 30s.

Arnett (1) has proposed that the period from the late teens through the 20s be considered a distinctive period he terms *emerging adulthood*. In contrast to adolescents, 95% of whom live in a parental home, most young people age 18 years or older in the United States leave home, approximately one-third to live in a college setting and approximately 40% to live independently and work full time. Approximately two-thirds cohabit for a time with a romantic partner. However, despite high rates of residential mobility in the 20s, many young people retain some degree of dependence on their parents.

Hence, adolescence gives way to a prolonged period of quasi-autonomy and continued identity and vocational exploration that only gradually draws to a close in the third decade of life with the consolidation of an adult work identity, the capacity for adult friendships and a lasting intimate relationship, the emergence of a more mutual and equal relationship with parents, the integration of new attitudes toward time, and the beginning contemplation of parenthood (113).

References

1. Arnett JJ: Emerging adulthood: A theory of development from the late teens through the twenties. *Am Psychol* 55:469–480, 2000.
2. Scott E, Woolard J: The legal regulation of adolescence. In: Lerner R, Steinberg L (eds.): *Handbook of adolescent psychology*. 2nd ed. Hoboken, NJ: Wiley, 2004, pp. 523–550.
3. Chapin JR: Adolescent sex and mass media: A developmental approach. *Adolescence* 35:799–811, 2000.
4. Lerner RM, Galambos NL: Adolescent development: Challenges and opportunities for research, programs, and policies. *Annu Rev Psychol* 49:413–446, 1998.
5. Collins WA, Steinberg L: Adolescent development in interpersonal context. In: Damon W, Lerner RM (eds.): *Handbook of Child Psychology*. Vol 3. 6th ed. Hoboken, NJ: John Wiley & Sons, 2006, pp. 1003–1067.
6. Graber JA, Brooks-Gunn J, Warren MP: The antecedents of menarcheal age: Heredity, family environment, and stressful life events. *Child Dev* 66:346–359, 1995.
7. Graber JA, Petersen AC, Brooks-Gunn J: Pubertal processes: Methods, measures, and models. In: Graber JA B-GJ, Petersen AC (eds.): *Transitions through adolescence: Interpersonal domains and context*. Mahwah, NJ: Lawrence Erlbaum Associates, 1996, pp. 23–53.
8. Steinberg L, Morris AS: Adolescent development. *Annu Rev Psychol*. 2001: 52.
9. Reiss D: *The Relationship Code: Deciphering Genetic and Social Influences on Adolescent Development*. Cambridge, MA, Harvard University Press, 2000.
10. Way N, Chu JY (eds.): *Adolescent Boys: Exploring diverse cultures of boyhood*. New York: New York University Press, 2004.
11. Larson R, Wilson S: Adolescence across place and time: Globalization and the changing pathways to adulthood. In: Lerner R, Steinberg L (eds.): *Handbook of Adolescent Psychology*. 2nd ed. Hoboken, NJ: Wiley, 2004, pp. 299–330.
12. Arnett J: Adolescent storm and stress, reconsidered. *Am Psychol* 54:317–326, 1999.
13. Schlegel A: The global spread of adolescent culture. In: Crockett LJ, Silbereisen RK (eds.): *Negotiating Adolescence in a Time of Social Change*. Cambridge, UK: Cambridge University Press, 2000, pp. 71–81.
14. Schlegel A, Barry HI: *Adolescence: An Anthropological inquiry*. New York, Free Press; 1991.
15. Richter LM: Studying adolescence *Science* June 30, 2006 312:1902–1905.
16. Bradley K: Internet lives: Social context and moral domain in adolescent development. *New Directions for Youth Development* 108:57–76, 2005.
17. Centers for Disease Control and Prevention: Youth risk behavior surveillance—United States, 2005. *Morb Mortal Wkly Rep* 55(SS-5): 1–108, 2006.
18. Roberts DF, Foehr UG, Rideout V: Generation M: Media in the lives of 8–18 year-olds. A Kaiser Family Foundation Study. March 2005. <http://www.kff.org/entmedia/7251.cfm.> Accessed June 17, 2006.
19. Susman EJ, Rogol A: Puberty and psychological development. In: Lerner R, Steinberg L (eds.): *Handbook of adolescent psychology*. 2nd ed. Hoboken, NJ: Wiley, 2004, pp. 15–44.
20. Spear LP: The adolescent brain and age-related behavioral manifestations. *Neurosci Biobehav Rev* 24:417–463, 2000.
21. Tanner JM: Sequence and tempo in the somatic changes in puberty. In: Grumbach MM GG, Mayer FE (eds.): *Control of the onset of puberty*. New York: John Wiley & Sons, 1974.
22. Herman-Giddens ME, Slora EJ, Wasserman RC, et al.: Secondary sexual characteristics and menses in young girls seen in office practice: A study from the Pediatric Research in Office Settings network. *Pediatrics* 99:505–512, 1997.
23. Kaplowitz PB, Oberfield SE: Drug and Therapeutics and Executive Committees of the Lawson Wilkins Pediatric Endocrine Society. Reexamination of the age limit for defining when puberty is precocious in girls in the United States: Implications for evaluation and treatment. *Pediatrics* 104:936–941, 1999.
24. Endocrine Society and Lawson Wilkins Pediatric Endocrine Society: Press release. March 1, 2001; <www.endo-society.org.>
25. Stein JH, Reiser LW: A study of white middle-class adolescent boys' responses to "semenarche" (the first ejaculation). *J Youth Adolesc* 23:373–384, 1994.
26. Brooks-Gunn J, Paikoff R: Sexuality and developmental transitions during adolescence. In: Schulenberg J, Maggs J, Hurrelmann K (eds.): *Health risks and developmental transitions during adolescence*. Cambridge, UK: Cambridge University Press, 1997, pp. 190–219.
27. Graber JA, Lewinsohn PM, Seeley JR, et al.: Is psychopathology associated with the timing of pubertal development? *J Am Acad Child Adolesc Psychiatry* 36:1768–1776, 1997.
28. Ge X, Kim IJ, Brody GH, Conger RD, Simons RL, Gibbons FX: It's about timing and change: Pubertal transition effects on symptoms of major depression among African American youths. *Developmental Psychology* 39:430–439, 2003.
29. Buchanan CM, Eccles JS, Becker JB: Are adolescents the victims of raging hormones? Evidence for activational effects of hormones on moods and behavior at adolescence. *Psychol Bull* 111:62–107, 1992.

30. Cameron JL: Interrelationships between hormones, behavior, and affect during adolescence: Understanding hormonal, physical, and brain changes occurring in association with pubertal activation of the reproductive axis. *Annals of the New York Academy of Sciences* 1021:110–123, 2004.
31. White T, Nelson CA: Neurobiological development during childhood and adolescence. In: Findling FL, Schultz SC (eds.): *Schizophrenia in Adolescents and Children: Assessment, Neurobiology, and Treatment.* Baltimore: Johns Hopkins University Press, 2004.
32. Shaw P, Greenstein D, Lerch J, et al.: Intellectual ability and cortical development in children and adolescents. *Nature* Mar 30, 2006:440(7084): 676–679.
33. Bourgeois J-P, Rakic P: Changes of synaptic density in the primary visual cortex of the macaque monkey from fetal to adult stage. *J Neurosci* 13:2801–2820, 1993.
34. Rakic P, Bourgeois J-P, Goldman-Rakic PS: Synaptic development of the cerebral cortex: Implications for learning, memory, and mental illness. *Prog Brain Res* 102:227–243, 1994.
35. Thompson PM, Giedd JN, R.P. W, et al.: Growth patterns in the developing brain detected by using continuum mechanical tensor maps. *Nature* 404: 190–193, 2000.
36. Luna B, Sweeney JA: The emergence of collaborative brain function: fMRI Studies of the development of response inhibition. *Ann NY Acad Sci* 1021: 296–309, 2004.
37. Weinberger DR: Schizophrenia as a neurodevelopmental disorder. In: Hirsch SR, Weinberger DR (eds.): *Schizophrenia.* Oxford: Blackwell Science, 1995, pp. 293–323.
38. Lewis DA, Cruz D, Eggan S, Erickson S: Postnatal development of prefrontal inhibitory circuits and the pathophysiology of cognitive dysfunction in schizophrenia. *Ann NY Acad Sci* 1021:64–76, 2004.
39. Gothelf D, Eliez S, Thompson T, et al.: COMT genotype predicts longitudinal cognitive decline and psychosis in 22q11.2 deletion syndrome. *Nature Neuroscience* 8(11):1500–1502, 2005.
40. Caspi A, Moffitt TE, Cannon M, et al.: Moderation of the effect of adolescent-onset cannabis use on adult psychosis by a functional polymorphism in the catechol-O-methyltransferase gene: Longitudinal evidence of a gene X environment interaction. *Biological Psychiatry* 57(10):1117–1127, 2005.
41. Post GB, Kemper HCG: Nutrient intake and biological maturation during adolescence: The Amsterdam Growth and Health Longitudinal Study. *Eur J Clin Nutr* 47:400–408, 1993.
42. National Research Council and Institute of Medicine: *Sleep Needs, Patterns, and Difficulties of Adolescents.* Washington, DC, National Academy Press, 2000.
43. Carskadon MA, Acebo M, Jenni OG: Regulation of adolescent sleep: Implications for behavior. *Ann NY Acad Sci* 1021:276–291, 2004.
44. Keating DP: Cognitive and brain development. In: Lerner R, Steinberg L (eds.): *Handbook of Adolescent Psychology.* 2nd ed. Hoboken, NJ: Wiley, 2004, pp. 45–84.
45. Coleman JC, Hendry L: *The Nature of Adolescence.* 2nd ed. London, Routledge, 1990.
46. Eisenberg N, Morris AS: Moral cognitions and prosocial responding in adolescence. In: Lerner R, Steinberg L (eds.): *Handbook of Adolescent Psychology.* 2nd ed. Hoboken, NJ: Wiley, 2004, pp. 155–188.
47. Kohlberg L: *Stages in the Development of Moral Thought and Action.* Holt, Rinehart & Winston, 1969.
48. Gilligan C: *In a Different voice: Psychological theory and women's development.* Cambridge, MA, Harvard University Press, 1982.
49. Steinberg L: Risk taking in adolescence: What changes, and why? *Ann NY Acad Sci* 1021:51–58, 2004.
50. Beyth-Marom R, Fischhoff B: Adolescents' decisions about risks: A cognitive perspective. In: Schulenberg J, Maggs J, Hurrelmann K (eds.): *Health Risks and Developmental Transitions During Adolescence.* Cambridge, UK: Cambridge University Press, 1997 pp. 110–135.
51. Dahl RE: The development of affect regulation: Bringing together basic and clinical perspectives. *Ann NY Acad Sci* 1008:183–188, 2003.
52. Arnsten AFT, Shansky RM: Adolescence: Vulnerable period for stress-induced prefrontal cortical function? *Ann NY Acad Sci* 1021: 143–147, 2004.
53. Erikson EH: *Childhood and Society.* 2nd (revised) ed. New York, Norton, 1963.
54. Seltzer VC: *Psychosocial Worlds of the Adolescent: Public and Private.* New York, John Wiley & Sons, 1989.
55. Roberts DF, L H, Foehr UG: Adolescents and media. In: Lerner R, Steinberg L (eds.): *Handbook of Adolescent Psychology.* 2nd ed. Hoboken, NJ: Wiley; 2004 pp. 487–521.
56. Gross RT, Duke PM: Effects of early vs. late physical maturation on adolescent behavior. In: Levine MD CW, Crocker AC et al. (ed.): *Developmental-Behavioral Pediatrics.* Philadelphia: WB Saunders, 1983, pp. 149–156.
57. Hendren RL, Barber JK, Sigafoos A: Eating-disordered symptoms in a nonclinical population: A study of female adolescents in two private schools. *J Am Acad Child Psychiatry* 25:836–840, 1986.
58. Martin A: On teenagers and tattoos. *J Am Acad Child Adolesc Psychiatry* 860–861, 1997.
59. Ritvo S: The image and uses of the body in psychic conflict: With special reference to eating disorders in adolescence. *Psychoanal Study Child* 39:449–469, 1984.
60. Offer D, Schonert-Reichl KA: Debunking the myths of adolescence: Findings from recent research. *J Am Acad Child Adolesc Psychiatry* 31:1003–1014, 1992.
61. Collins WA, Laursen B: Parent-adolescent relationships and influences. In: Lerner R, Steinberg L (eds.): *Handbook of adolescent psychology.* 2nd ed. Hoboken, NJ: Wiley, 2004, pp. 331–361.
62. Csikszentmihalyi M, Larson R: *Being Adolescent: Conflict and Growth in the Teenage Years.* New York, Basic Books, 1984.
63. Freud A: Adolescence. *The writings of Anna Freud,* Vol V (1956–1965). New York, International Universities Press, 1958/1969 pp. 136–166.
64. Wolf AE: *Get Out of My Life, but First Could You Drive Me and Cheryl to the Mall?: A Parent's Guide to the New Teenager.* New York, Noonday Press, 1991.
65. Laursen B, Coy KC, Collins WA: Reconsidering changes in parent–child conflict across adolescence: A meta-analysis. *Child Dev* 69:817–832, 1998.
66. Montemayor R, Hanson E: A naturalistic view of conflict between adolescents and their parents and siblings. *J Early Adolesc* 5:23–30, 1985.
67. Graber JA, Brooks-Gunn J: "Sometimes I think that you don't like me": How mothers and daughters negotiate the transition into adolescence. In: Cox MJ, Brooks-Gunn J, et al. (eds.): *Conflict and Cohesion in Families: Causes and Consequences.* Mahwah, NJ:207–242, 1999.
68. DiClemente RJ, Hansen WB, Ponton LE (eds.): *Handbook of Adolescent Health Risk Behavior.* New York, Plenum, 1996.
69. King RA, Lewis M: The difficult child. *Child Adolesc Psychiatr Clin North Am* 3:531–541, 1994.
70. Brown BB: Adolescents' relationships with peers. In: Lerner R, Steinberg L (eds.): *Handbook of Adolescent Psychology,* 2nd ed. Hoboken, NJ: Wiley, 2004, pp. 363–394.
71. Csikszentmihalyi M, Larson R, Prescott S: The ecology of adolescent activity and experience. *J Youth Adolesc* 6:281–294, 1977.
72. Jessor R: Risk behavior in adolescence: A psychosocial framework for understanding and action. *J Adolesc Health Care* 12:597–605, 1991.
73. Savin-Williams RC, Diamond LM: Sex. In: Lerner R, Steinberg L (eds.): *Handbook of Adolescent Psychology,* 2nd ed. Hoboken, NJ: Wiley, 2004, pp. 189–231.
74. Herdt G, McClintock M: The magical age of 10. *Arch Sex Behav* 29:587–606, 2000.
75. Katchadourian H: Sexuality. *At the Threshold: The Developing Adolescent.* Cambridge, MA, Harvard University Press, 1990, pp. 330–351.
76. Friedrich WN, Grambsch P, Broughton D, et al.: Normative sexual behavior in children. *Pediatrics* 88:456–464, 1991.
77. Rutter M: Normal psychosexual development. *J Child Psychol Psychiatry* 11:259–283, 1971.
78. Laufer M: The central masturbation fantasy, the final sexual organization, and adolescence. *Psychoanal Study Child* 31:297–316, 1976.
79. Furman W, Brown BB, Feiring C (eds.): *The Development of Romantic Relationships in Adolescence.* New York, Cambridge University Press, 1999.
80. Kuczynski A: She's got to be a macho girl. *New York Times.* November 3, 2002, 9:1,12.
81. Muus RE. *Theories of Adolescence,* 5th ed. New York, Random House, 1988.
82. Offer D, Ostrov E, Howard KI, et al.: *The Teenage World: Adolescents' Self-Image in Ten Countries.* New York, Plenum Medical, 1988.
83. Harter S: *The Construction of the Self: A Developmental Perspective.* New York, Guilford Press, 1999.
84. McGuire S, Manke B, Saudino KJ, et al.: Perceived competence and self-worth during adolescence: A longitudinal behavioral genetic study. *Child Dev* 70:1283–1296, 1999.
85. Hall GS: *Adolescence: Its Psychology and Its Relation to Physiology, Anthropology, Sociology, Sex, Crime, Religion and Education* Vols 1 and 2. Englewood Cliffs, NJ, Prentice Hall, 1904.
86. Rakoff VM: Nietzsche and the romantic construction of adolescence. *Adolescent psychiatry: Developmental and clinical studies* 22:39–56, 1998.
87. Larson R, Richards MH: *Divergent Realities: The Emotional Lives of Mothers, Fathers, and Adolescents.* New York, Basic Books, 1994.
88. Petersen AC, Compas BE, J B-G, et al.: Depression in adolescence. *Am Psychol* 48:155–168, 1993.
89. Brooks-Gunn J, Warren M: Biological and social contributions to negative affect in young adolescent girls. *Child Dev* 60:40–55, 1989.
90. Larson R, Asmussen L: Anger, worry, and hurt in early adolescence: An enlarging world of negative emotions. In: Colten ME, Gore S (eds.): *Adolescent Stress: Causes and Consequences.* New York: Aldine de Gruyter, 1991, pp. 21–41.
91. Wagner BM, Compas BE: Gender, instrumentality, and expressivity: Moderators of the relation between stress and psychological symptoms during adolescence. *Am J Commun Psychol* 18:383–406, 1990.
92. Ge X, Lorenz FO, Conger RD, et al.: Trajectories of stressful life events and depressive symptoms during adolescence. *Dev Psychol* 30:467–483, 1994.
93. Vik P, Brown SA: Life events and substance abuse during adolescence. In: Miller TW (ed.): *Children of Trauma.* Madison, CT: International Universities Press, 1999, pp. 179–204.

94. Angold A, Costello EJ, Erkanli A, Worthman CM: Pubertal changes in hormone levels and depression in girls. *Psychol Med* 29:1043–1053, 1999.
95. Dryfoos JG: *Safe Passage: Making It Through Adolescence in a Risky Society*. Oxford, U.K., Oxford University Press, 1998.
96. Liang SW, Jemerin JM, Tschann JM, et al.: Life events, cardiovascular reactivity, and risk behavior in adolescent boys. *Pediatrics* 96:1101–1105, 1995.
97. Spear LP, Varlinskaya EI: Adolescence: Alcohol sensitivity, tolerance, and intake. *Recent Developments in Alcoholism* 17:143–159, 2005.
98. Merikangas KR: The importance of adolescence in the development of nicotine dependence. *Annals of the New York Academy of Sciences* 1021: 198–201, 2004.
99. Jacobsen LK, Krystal JH, Mencl WE, Westerveld M, Frost SJ, Pugh KR: Effects of smoking and smoking abstinence on cognition in adolescent tobacco smokers. *Biological Psychiatry* 57:56–66, 2005.
100. Suomi SJ: Gene–environment interactions and the neurobiology of social conflict. *Annals of the New York Academy of Sciences* 1008:132–139, 2003.
101. Arnett J: Reckless behavior in adolescence: A developmental perspective. *Dev Rev* 12:339–373, 1992.
102. Igra V, Irwin CE, Jr.: Theories of adolescent risk-taking behavior. In: DiClemente RJ HW, Ponton LE (ed.): *Handbook of Adolescent Health Risk Behavior*. New York: Plenum, 1996, pp. 35–51.
103. Beckman M: Crime, culpability, and the adolescent brain. *Science* 305(5684):596–599, 2004.
104. Steinberg L, Dahl R, Keating D, Kupfer DJ, Masten AS, Pine DS: The study of developmental psychopathology in adolescence: Integrating affective neruoscience with the study of context. In: Cicchetti D, Cohen DJ (eds.): *Developmental Psychopathology*, Vol 2. 2nd ed. Hoboken, NJ: John Wiley & Sons, 2006, pp., 710–741.
105. Kaplan A: When is it "cruel and unusual punishment"? Supreme Court bans juvenile death penalty. *Psychiatric Times* May 1, 2005: 1.
106. Kelley AE, Schochet T, Landry CF: Risk taking and novelty seeking in adolescence. *Ann NY Acad Sci* 1021:27–32, 2004.
107. Spear LP: Adolescent brain development and animal models. *Ann NY Acad Sci* 1021:23–26, 2004.
108. Steinberg L: Pubertal maturation and parent–adolescent distance: An evolutionary perspective. In: Adams GR, Montemayor R, Gullotta TP (eds.): *Advances in Adolescent Behavior and Development*. Newbury Park, CA: Sage Publications, 1989, pp. 71–97.
109. Steinberg L, Belsky J: An evolutionary perspective on psychopathology in adolescence. *Rochester Symposium on Developmental Psychopathology. Adolescence: Opportunities and Challenges*, Vol 7. Rochester, NY, University of Rochester Press, 1996, pp. 93–124.
110. Higley JD, Mehlman PT, Higley SB, et al.: Excessive mortality in young free-ranging male nonhuman primates with low cerebrospinal fluid 5-hydroxyindoleacetic acid concentrations. *Archives of General Psychiatry* 53:537–543, 1996.
111. Barr CS, Newman TK, Becker ML, et al.: The utility of the non-human primate model for studying gene by environment interactions in behavioral research. *Genes, Brain & Behavior* 2(6):336–340, 2003.
112. Newman TK, Syagailo YV, Barr CS, et al.: Monoamine oxidase: A gene promoter variation and rearing experience influences aggressive behavior in rhesus monkeys. *Biological Psychiatry* 57:167–172, 2005.
113. Colarusso CA: Adulthood. In: Kaplan HI, Kaplan VA (eds.): *Kaplan and Sadock's Comprehensive Textbook of Psychiatry*, Vol 2, 8th ed. Baltimore: Williams and Wilkins, 2005, pp. 3565–3586.

CHAPTER 3.2 ■ DEVELOPMENTAL PSYCHOPATHOLOGY

SUNIYA S. LUTHAR AND REBECCA P. PRINCE

DEVELOPMENTAL PSYCHOPATHOLOGY DEFINED: MAJOR FEATURES

Developmental psychopathology is an integrative discipline, wherein principles from classical developmental theory are applied to investigate clinical and psychiatric phenomena (1–4). This integration of perspectives is invaluable because it promotes our understanding of atypical development and also illuminates understanding of normative developmental processes. To illustrate, applications of developmental theories such as those of Werner, Piaget, and Erikson provide critical insights into the organization and causes of different forms of maladjustment. Conversely, studies of pathology enhance our knowledge of normal development, particularly in terms of individual differences in development as well as risk and protective processes associated with different types of outcomes.

Whereas developmental and clinical psychology are integral elements in the field of developmental psychopathology, the scope of this integrative discipline extends beyond these areas. Theory and methods from these domains are integrated with those from various others, including epidemiology, biology, neuroscience, sociology, and anthropology. Such multidomain, multicontextual approaches to inquiry are essential in moving toward the long-term goal of a more comprehensive understanding of the development of psychopathology.

A final feature of developmental psychopathology is that it bridges the often wide span between empirical research and the application of knowledge, to benefit at-risk populations. Investigators in this tradition design and implement interventions that are based in developmental theory and research on risk and protective processes, such that they inform both preventive interventions and social policy.

To summarize, the four central characteristics that define the field of developmental psychopathology are 1) the use of classical developmental theory and research to inform issues of psychopathology, 2) the use of insights from at-risk or atypical populations to increase our understanding of normal developmental processes, 3) integration of developmental and clinical perspectives with those from other disciplines, and 4) the derivation of implications for preventive and therapeutic interventions, and for social policy.

RISK

In developmental psychopathology research, risk is defined in terms of statistical probabilities: A high-risk condition is one that carries high odds for measured maladjustment in critical domains (5). Exposure to community violence, for example, constitutes high risk given that children experiencing it reflect significantly greater maladjustment than those who do not (6). Similarly, maternal depression is a risk factor in that children of mothers with depressive diagnoses can be as much as eight times as likely as others to develop depressive disorders themselves by the adolescent years (7).

In addition to establishing discrete risk dimensions such as community violence, poverty, or parent mental illness, researchers have also examined composites of multiple risk indices such as parents' low income and education, their histories of mental illness, and disorganization in their neighborhoods. Seminal research by Rutter (8) demonstrated that when risks such as these coexist (as they often do, in the real world), effects tend to be synergistic, with children's outcomes being far poorer than when any of these risks existed in isolation. Use of this cumulative risk approach is well exemplified in work by Sameroff and his colleagues (9, 10). These authors computed a total risk score across 10 different dimensions, assigning for each one, a score of 1 (versus 0) if the child fell in the highest quartile of continuous risk dimensions, and for dichotomous dimensions such as single parent family status, if they were present in that child's life. An alternative approach, exemplified in work by Masten and her colleagues (11), involves standardizing values on different risk scales and adding them to obtain a composite.

Decisions regarding the use of single- or multiple-risk indices in resilience research depend on the substantive research questions. The former is used, obviously, when applied researchers seek to identify factors that might modify the effects of particular environmental risks known to have strong adverse effects, so as to eventually derive specific directions for interventions. Examples are parental divorce or bereavement; knowledge of what ameliorates the ill effects of these particular adversities has been valuable in designing appropriate interventions (12, 13). Additive approaches are more constrained in this respect, precluding identification, for example, of which of the indices subsumed in the composite are more influential than others. On the other hand, composite risk indices generally explain more variance in adjustment than do any of them considered alone, and as noted earlier, they may be more realistic in that many of these risks do cooccur in actuality (5, 14).

Risk is rarely absolute; the potential for deleterious outcomes varies according to age as well as other child characteristics. Prolonged separation from the primary caregiver, for example, is more harmful for infants and toddlers than for older children, whereas community violence is less likely to affect preschoolers than older youth who are more able to move about the neighborhood independently. By the same token, there are some risks relatively unique to particular groups. An example is racial discrimination, which affects ethnic minority groups but not children of Caucasian heritage.

The same construct can connote risk in one setting but be relatively benign or even beneficial in others. An example is stringency of parent discipline. Whereas high levels of control and strictness are often seen as deleterious for children, a series of studies have shown that they are actually beneficial for youngsters living in dangerous inner city neighborhoods (15–18).

DISORDER

In developmental psychopathology as in child psychiatry, the notion of disorder often represents psychiatric diagnoses. Researchers typically assess diagnoses via structured interviews such as the Schedule for Affective Disorders and Schizophrenia for School-Aged Children (K-SADS-PL) (19) or the Diagnostic Interview Schedule for Children (NIMH DISC-IV) (20), which are usually administered to the child aged 5 and older as well as the primary caregiver. For each diagnostic category, these interviews have a series of initial probes to determine the existence of a disorder, and if responses are in the affirmative, then additional probes are asked to determine if diagnostic criteria are met.

The other approach, also commonly used, is to assess overall children's symptom levels on different maladjustment domains, via instruments such as the Behavior Assessment System for Children, (BASC) (21) or the Child Behavior Checklist (CBCL) (22) [and its variants, the Teacher Rating Form (TRF) and the Youth Self Report (YSR) (23)]. These measures include a list of symptoms from diverse maladjustment domains which collectively yield scores on discrete subscales (such as attention, conduct, or depressive problems); in turn, composite scores across related subscales indicate overall maladjustment, such as internalizing and externalizing symptoms (CBCL), or overall dimensions of behavior and personality (BASC).

Such dimensional measures have two major advantages; they capture a wide range of functioning and are very well normed. With regard to the first of these features, symptom scales such as the CBCL and BASC characterize children in terms of varying severity of dysfunction as opposed to simply the presence or absence of diagnoses. From a research standpoint, this is a major advantage because the greater the variance on a particular dimension, the more likely it is that it will show statistical links with other constructs (such as potential causes or ramifications of the symptoms). The issue of norms, similarly, is critical in gauging children's adjustment levels relative to those of the average child of the same age. Instruments such as the CBCL have been administered to thousands of children from all over the country (and world) and as a result, we know the average symptom levels on these. Typically, average levels of problems correspond to a T score of 50 with a standard deviation of 10. Thus, if a child were to obtain a score of over 65 on the YSR, this would represent "much above average" dysfunction and a T score of 70 or more would indicate problems "very much above average."

Making such judgments about functioning vis-à-vis the average child is much more complicated with psychiatric disorders. There have been several large-scale epidemiological studies on children's diagnoses, but there is some disagreement on rates of different disorders, with variations, for example, with the particular structured interview used. To illustrate, an NIMH study using the DISC reported that about 6% of adolescents suffer from depression (24), whereas a study using the K-SADS found the point prevalence to be 2.9% (25). At the same time, structured interviews remain the method of choice when the goal is specifically to assess the incidence of actual psychiatric diagnoses, rather than severity of symptoms.

A thorny problem in assessing childhood disorders—regardless of whether the approach involves diagnoses or symptom levels—is that there is considerable disagreement among respondents. The kappa statistic is commonly used to assess agreement across raters, with values above .75 representing high levels of agreement, values in the range of .40 to .75 representing moderate levels of agreement, and values below .40 representing low levels of agreement (26). In studies involving psychiatric diagnoses, agreement rates between parents and children have ranged from $k = .32$ for diagnoses of separation anxiety to $k = .22$ on diagnoses of general anxiety disorder to as low as $k = .17$ on ADHD (27, 28). Further demonstrating the disconnect between the child's and parents' understanding of the child's functioning, Roberts and colleagues (29) found that in measuring overall mental health, life satisfaction, happiness, and role strain, parent–child agreement was never above .20. On dimensional measures, similarly, the correlation between parents' reports and children's reports has ranged from k = .02 for anxious/depressed symptoms to k = .14 for delinquent behavior (30); there is generally more agreement among mother and father, but again, low consensus between parents and teachers (31).

Researchers have dealt with this disagreement in various ways. In the case of psychiatric diagnoses, a common approach is to use the "either/or" rule, assuming the child does in fact have a diagnosis if either the parent or the child indicates this is the case (32). An alternative strategy is by prioritizing adults' reports for some domains (conduct problems) and children's for others (depression), with the rationale that children are likely to underreport their own oppositional behavior, for example, or that parents are likely to know less about their child's inner life (33, 34). Still others have separately considered parents' and children's reports, with the rationale that each reveals information not captured by the other (35–37).

A final comment about measurement of disorder: What is considered abnormal in one setting may be normative or even adaptive in another. This point is well illustrated in a paper by Richters and Cicchetti (38) entitled Mark Twain meets DSM-III-R: Conduct disorder, development, and the concept of harmful dysfunction, with regard to definitions of conduct disorders. The authors argue that many inner city youth might meet DSM criteria for conduct disorders but in their own subculture, being able to defend themselves physically can be quite adaptive. Accordingly, they exhort additional consideration of the notion of "harmful dysfunction," put forth by Wakefield (39–41). Wakefield argued that the DSM definition of mental disorders fails to distinguish adequately an individual's negative reactions to his problematic environment from a "true" mental disorder, and that a mental disorder is best conceptualized as a harmful dysfunction, where harm is a value judgment regarding the undesirability of a condition, and dysfunction is the failure of a system to function as designed by natural selection. Anchored in notions of evolutionary design, Wakefield specifically defines a harmful dysfunction as the "harmful failure of an internal mechanism to perform a natural function for which it was biologically designed" (42).*

RESILIENCE

A salient construct in developmental psychopathology is resilience: a phenomenon or process reflecting relatively positive adaptation despite experiences of significant adversity or trauma. Inherent in this definition lie two fundamental conditions: significant risk (or adversity) and positive adaptation. Thus, resilience is never directly measured, but is indirectly inferred based on evidence of the two subsumed constructs.

The notion of risk has already been discussed; positive adaptation, the second element in the construct of resilience, is defined as an outcome that is substantially better than what would be expected with respect to the risk circumstance being studied. In past studies of resilience across diverse risk circumstances, positive adaptation has been defined in terms of behaviorally manifested social competence, or success at meeting stage-salient developmental tasks (5, 14, 43). Among young children, for example, competence was operationally defined in terms of the development of a secure attachment with primary caregivers (44), and among older children, in terms of aspects of school-based functioning such as good academic performance and positive relationships with classmates and teachers (43, 45).

In addition to being developmentally appropriate, indicators used to define positive adaptation must also be conceptually of high relevance to the risk examined in terms of both domains assessed and stringency of criteria used (46). When communities carry many risks for antisocial problems, for example, the degree to which children are able to maintain socially conforming behaviors is an appropriate indicator of success (47), whereas among children of depressed parents, the absence of depressive diagnoses would be of special significance (48, 49). With regard to stringency of criteria, similarly, decisions must depend on the seriousness of the risks under consideration. In studying children facing major traumas, it is entirely appropriate to define risk-evasion simply in terms of the absence of serious psychopathology (psychiatric diagnoses) rather than superiority or excellence in everyday adaptation (50).

Regardless of whether competence is described as risk evasion or positive adaptation, competence must be defined across multiple spheres. The multilevel measurement of competence, therefore, differs from the measurement of risk, which may legitimately involve one or multiple negative circumstances. However, doing well in only one domain cannot be conceptualized as connoting resilience, as overly narrow definitions can fallaciously convey a picture of "success in the face of adversity." Adolescents, for example, might be viewed very positively by their peers but at the same time, perform poorly academically, or even demonstrate conduct disturbances (51, 52), such that peer popularity by itself cannot be seen as an indicator of overall risk evasion.

The major focus of resilience researchers is to identify vulnerability and protective factors that might modify the negative effects of adverse life circumstances, and having accomplished this, to identify mechanisms or processes that might underlie associations found (5, 53–55). While researchers have debated how to delineate such factors statistically (see 14, 56), the conceptual definitions are fairly straightforward. Vulnerability factors or markers encompass those indices that exacerbate the negative effects of the risk condition while protective factors modify the effects of risk in a positive direction.

In some instances, it is more appropriate to define positive adaptation in terms of the family or community rather than necessarily of the child him- or herself. As Seifer (57) has argued, because infants' and toddlers' functioning is often regulated by their caregivers, it can be more logical to operationalize positive adjustment in terms of the mother–child dyad or family unit rather than in terms of the young child's behavior. Similarly, there are times when the label resilience is most appropriate for communities of well functioning at-risk youth. Research on neighborhoods, for example, has demonstrated that some low-income urban neighborhoods reflect far higher levels of cohesiveness, organization, and social efficacy than others (58, 59), with the potential, therefore, to serve as important buffers against negative socializing influences.

FACTORS AFFECTING RESILIENCE AND VULNERABILITY

In discussions that follow, we overview major factors that contribute to relatively positive or negative outcomes among at-risk children. These factors fall into three broad categories: aspects of families, features of communities, and attributes of the children themselves.

*Subsequently, this notion has been criticized by some others. Lilienfield and Marino (1995), for example, argue that many mental disorders are not, as Wakefield claims, evolutionary adaptations but rather neutral byproducts of adaptation; they believe that Wakefield's sociobiological definition of disorder is too narrow in its conceptualization. Murphy and Woolfolk (2000) critique Wakefield's view from a different angle, arguing that it fails to account for those disorders that are not a result of malfunction and those disorders whose causes have no adaptive function.

Familial Factors in Resilience and Vulnerability

The critical importance of strong family relationships has been emphasized in various studies of resilience; a plethora of studies identify supportive and responsive parenting as being among the most robust predictors of resilient adaptation (5, 8, 54, 56, 60–64). In particular, early family relationships are extremely important in shaping long-term resilient trajectories. In their comprehensive review of the early childhood literature, Shonkoff and Phillips (65) emphasized that "[relationships] that are created in the earliest years ... constitute a basic structure within which all meaningful development unfolds." Early experience places people on probabilistic trajectories of relatively good or poor adaptation, shaping the lens through which subsequent relationships are viewed and the capacity to utilize support resources in the environment. Thus, if early attachments are insecure in nature, at-risk children tend to anticipate negative reactions from others and can eventually come to elicit these; these experiences of rejection further increase feelings of insecurity (66–68). Conversely, at-risk children with at least one good relationship are able to take more from nurturing others subsequently encountered in development (44, 65, 67, 69). The protective potential of strong family relationship has been demonstrated for mothers, fathers, and siblings (70, 71).

Whereas early relationships are fundamental in shaping the lens through which people view their subsequent interactions, a "faulty lens" can be corrected to some degree. In general, developmental psychopathologists maintain that there is continuity and coherence in development so that positive adaptation in early years determines, in a probabilistic rather than determinative fashion, the likely success at later stages (44, 72, 73). At the same time, scholars recognize that lawful discontinuities often do occur, and in the context of attachment status, such changes frequently derive from modifications in the caregiving environment (73–76). Intervention studies provide consistent evidence with regard to the possibility of shifting attachment status, as seen in work by Heinicke and Dozier. In both sets of studies, children's insecure early attachments were remediated to some degree by intervention services that fostered caregivers' positive qualities including nurturance, responsiveness, and their own attachment states of mind (77–79).

In terms of what defines "good parenting," warmth and appropriate control are the two core constructs that are most important in children's relationships with their primary caregivers. Each factor has protective functions and the benefits of each depend to some degree on levels of the other: Both high warmth with lax discipline and strict discipline without affection can be linked with poor adjustment. The authoritative parenting style, characterized by the appropriate balance of parental warmth and control (80), is generally optimal; authoritative parents are defined as those who "... are warm, supportive, communicative, and responsive to their children's needs, and who exert firm, consistent, and reasonable control and close supervision." (81)

In addition to warmth and control, limit-setting and monitoring are critical for resilient adaptation. Limit-setting refers to the use of appropriate rules and expectations in shaping socially desirable behavior in the child; the degree to which parents clearly define limits and consistently enforce rules is crucial in shaping the child's future compliance (82, 83). Related to limit-setting and also important for resilient adaptation is the construct of parental monitoring, which is defined as a "set of correlated parenting behaviors involving attention to and tracking of the child's whereabouts, activities, and adaptations." (84) The salutary effects of consistent parental monitoring across various high-risk circumstances have been demonstrated from the elementary school years onward (85). The benefits of consistent parental monitoring are particularly pronounced among preadolescents and adolescents, who have increasing independence from parents and thus growing exposure to a host of risks in the peer and community environments. For example, a study of sixth graders with deviant peers showed that firm parental control inhibited the development of externalizing problems in later years (86–88).

Links between parent monitoring and adolescent adjustment are not always simple linear ones, but can depend on coexisting risks in the environment. To illustrate, Mason, Cauce, Gonzales, and Hiraga (89) showed that in terms of ramifications for children's problem behaviors, optimal levels of control exerted by African-American parents varied according to negative influences in the community. When adolescents reported relatively high problem behaviors in their peer groups, for example, optimal levels of parental control tended to be higher than when children's peer problem behaviors were low. Regardless of circumstance, however, parental monitoring has emerged as a powerful construct in resilience research; in fact, among low-income 8- to17-year-olds, Buckner et al. (85) found that of several variables external to the child, only parental monitoring significantly differentiated resilient from nonresilient youths.

A relatively new construct related to limit-setting is parental "containment." Timothy Cavell (82) has emphasized the importance of an appropriate balance of warmth and discipline within the notion of parental containment, which is "any behavior that fosters in children a sense of restraint while not threatening their relationship security." (82) Recent studies have pointed to the protective potential of this construct. Building upon Cavell's (82) arguments on the significance of children's beliefs about the likelihood of being disciplined, Schneider et al. (83) defined perceived containment as the child's beliefs concerning the parent's capacity to enforce firm limits, and the likelihood that the parent will prevail in conflict. They found that children with a particularly strong sense of containment had mothers who applied effective discipline within the context of an emotionally positive relationship. Furthermore, high perceived containment was protective against externalizing behaviors as rated by parents and teachers (83).

The Importance of Genetic Factors

An exciting set of new development in the field of resilience is inquiry into the role of genetic contributions to vulnerability and protective mechanisms in the family, as is seen in research by Caspi and his colleagues. Two studies by this group identified specific genes implicated in protecting some maltreated children from developing psychopathology in adulthood. The first of these showed reduced likelihood of antisocial behavior in the presence of a genotype that confers high levels of the monoamine oxidase A enzyme (90), while the second study demonstrated that the likelihood of developing depression was lower in the presence of a genotype conferring the efficient transport of serotonin (91). Although the specific processes underlying the protective effects of such genetic factors are unknown, it is possible that they operate by shaping aspects of children's social–cognitive reactions to life stressors, as in their propensity to attributional biases, for example, or capacities for emotion recognition (92).

Further explicating the relationship between genetic factors and positive adaptation, a study by Kim-Cohen and colleagues (92) examined both genetic and environmental processes specifically within the resilience framework. The study involved an epidemiological cohort of 1,116 twin pairs from low SES families. Two aspects of resilience were examined—behavioral and cognitive—and results of quantitative genetic models showed that additive genetic effects accounted for approximately 70% of the variation in children's behavioral resilience and 40% of the variation in cognitive resilience. Further analyses established protective effects of both maternal warmth and child's outgoing temperament, with each factor operating through both genetically and environmentally mediated effects.

A particularly critical conclusion drawn by these researchers, however, surrounds the implications for interventions: Heritability does not imply untreatability (93, 94). As Kim-Cohen et al. (92) note, their study entailed "a genetically sensitive design (which demonstrated) that environmental effects can make a positive difference in the lives of poor children ... Even child temperament promoted resilience through environmental processes." Of vital importance is their conclusion that if families confronting the myriad stresses of poverty are helped to move toward bestowing warm, supportive parenting, and providing stimulating learning materials, children can be helped to achieve greater behavioral and cognitive resilience.

Rutter (54, 55) has outlined several important directions for future work involving gene–environment influences in resilience. Twin and adoptee studies of at-risk children can be used to 1) examine the relative contributions of genetic versus environmental influences in the ways that different protective and vulnerability factors operate; 2) uncover the mechanisms entailed in each of these (passive or active G–E mechanisms and critical influences underlying the environmental component); and 3) identify genetic markers that confer protection or vulnerability and better understand processes underlying their effects. Also needed are sibling studies illuminating the relative contributions of shared versus nonshared, extrafamilial environments on different outcomes. Finally, genetics research can also contribute to new developments in the study of resilience through precise quantification of risk. As noted in the first section of this chapter, risk is generally inferred based on statistical links between aspects of the environment (maltreatment or poverty) and children's maladjustment, but this "measure" of risk is imprecise at best. With knowledge that some children have genes conferring liability to particular disorders, examining factors in the lives of those who do not succumb could contribute vastly to our understanding of processes in resilience.

Community Factors in Resilience and Vulnerability

In addition to family-level protective and vulnerability markers, community-level factors can mitigate the effects that risks have on a child's development. Mentors and informal support networks can serve critical protective functions. Evidence in this regard is seen in the Big Brothers Big Sisters of America (BBBSA) movement, where volunteers interact regularly one on one with youth from single-parent homes, and supervision is provided on a monthly basis for the first year, then subsequently on a quarterly basis. Compared to their nonparticipating peers, BBBSA youth reported more positive academic behaviors, had better relationships with their parents and peers, and were 46% less likely to initiate illegal drug use, 27% less likely to initiate alcohol use, and 52% less likely to skip school (95). Other studies have demonstrated that salutatory experiences can derive from religious affiliations (96–98) and other forms of social support (99, 100), demonstrating the powerful potential that community-level factors can have in promoting resilience in adolescents.

Additionally, there are several studies corroborating the protective functions of supportive relationships with teachers (101–103). Assessing more than 3,000 teacher–child relationships, Howes and Ritchie (104) found that in a sample of toddlers and preschoolers with difficult life circumstances, the quality of attachment with teachers was significantly related to measures of behavior problems as well as social competence with peers. Among a group of aggressive second and third graders, African-American and Hispanic students benefited more than did Caucasian students from supportive relationship with their teachers (105). Noting that minority group students typically have lower access to positive relationships with school teachers, the authors suggested that they could be more responsive than Caucasians to supportive teachers when they are encountered (see also 106). Finally, there are substantial benefits when classrooms reflect organized, predictable environments in which students participate in procedures governing their behaviors. Among African-American 7- to 15-year-olds from low-income, mother-headed households, Brody et al. (87) demonstrated protective-stabilizing effects among children in such classrooms. Furthermore, positive classrooms were beneficial even when parent–child relationships were compromised as well as vice versa, indicating unique, significant contributions from both contexts in which children and adolescents spend appreciable amounts of time (87, 107).

Individual Factors in Resilience and Vulnerability

Salient protective and vulnerability processes affecting at-risk children can occur not only at the familial and community level, but at the child level. For example, male gender can be a vulnerability marker among youth living in the ecology of urban poverty, as boys are typically more reactive than girls to negative community influences (108, 109). In addition, lower levels of intelligence can act as a vulnerability factor in that among children experiencing severe and chronic life adversities, those with low intelligence are more vulnerable to adjustment difficulties over time than are others (5). Similarly, some personal attributes are linked with relatively positive outcomes among children facing adversities, such as internal locus of control (beliefs that events in one's life are largely determined by one's own efforts rather than by luck or chance) or feelings of self-efficacy (5, 110–112). Recent studies have suggested the protective potential of emotional intelligence, the ability to perceive and express emotions, to understand and use them, and to manage them to foster personal growth (113, 114). Among adolescents, emotional intelligence is linked with relatively low likelihood of smoking cigarettes and drinking alcohol (115) and following the major life transition to beginning college, with greater likelihood of attaining high academic grades (116).

A critical caveat regarding "protective individual attributes" such as internal locus of control or intelligence is that they themselves are not fixed or immutable, but are highly influenced by the external environment. To consider intelligence as an example, Koenen and colleagues (117) have shown that even after controlling for genetic factors and externalizing and internalizing problems, exposure to domestic violence accounted for significant variation in children's IQs. Therefore, individual factors in resilience and vulnerability must be considered in relation to the environments in which they originate and operate.

Acknowledging the continued malleability of individual traits (especially among younger children), Luthar and Zelazo (56) argued that in considering the triad of protective and vulnerability factors in resilience, children's own attributes should be considered after aspects of their families and communities for three major reasons. From a basic research perspective, numerous studies have shown that many positive child attributes are themselves often dependent on processes in the proximal and distal environments. From an applied perspective, it is logical that interventions to foster resilience should focus less on what young children are able to do for themselves, and more on what adults must do to bolster the children's own efforts. From a policy perspective, finally, to place primary emphasis on child attributes could carry the risk that public debate will shift away from the major environmental risks that affect children, leading to decreased allocation of resources to ameliorate these risks (14, 56).

Biological Factors

The previous examples—like most of resilience research thus far—generally encompass psychological variables; there is a critical need for scientists to increase consideration of biological indices, again, both as mediators of risk itself and as processes underlying vulnerability and protective factors (118, 119). In terms of protective processes, the capacity to regulate or modulate negative emotions in the face of threats is of obvious importance for managing well in inauspicious situations (e.g., (85, 120, 121)) and here again, biological processes can be salient. First, the capacity to recover relatively quickly from negative events experienced may be gauged by studying the startle reflex, which is a biological and involuntary response (a fast twitch of facial and body muscles) to a sudden and intense visual, tactile, or acoustic stimulus (122). Studies have shown that adverse environmental influences not only affect the startle reflex, but the neural network that underlies this response (123). A second biological mechanism that might be implicated is neuroendocrine in nature. Chronic exposure to stressful experiences tends to lead to excessive activation of the hypothalamic-pituitary-adrenal (HPA) axis, causing hypercortisolism, or elevations in the stress hormone cortisol. Hypercortisolism can result in pathogenic effects on neurons (124, 125) and changes in the synthesis and reuptake of neurotransmitters and density of sensitivity of receptors (126, 127). These findings point to the possibility that resilient individuals can be described in a neuroendocrine manner as those who, in the face of various stressors, tend to return relatively quickly to baseline levels of neuroendocrine functioning, and thus avoid the damage conferred by hypercortisolism.

SUMMARY OF EVIDENCE AND IMPLICATIONS FOR THE FUTURE

In concluding a review of almost half a century of work on resilience, Luthar (in press) summarized the major take-home message thus: "Resilience rests, fundamentally, on relationships. The desire to belong is a basic human need and positive connections with others lie at the very core of psychological development; strong, supportive relationships are critical for achieving and sustaining resilient adaptation." The childhood years have emerged as especially significant, as a child's relationship with his or her primary caregiver forms a lens through which future interactions are interpreted. As a result, early attachments influence numerous nascent psychological attributes and the negotiation and resolution of major developmental tasks, and in turn, the likelihood of success at future tasks. Thus, serious disruptions in the early relationships with caregivers, whether in the form of physical, sexual, or emotional abuse, severely impair the chances of resilient adaptation later in life. On a more positive note, secure and healthy relationships with those in one's proximal circle act as invaluable protective processes, for children as well as adults. Over the years, "good relationships" have been conceptualized in terms of two broad components—warmth and support on the one hand, and appropriate control or discipline on the other. A central direction for interventions, therefore, is to foster the development and sustenance of positive parenting patterns among parents in high-risk circumstances. Additionally, there must be attention to the specific relationship ingredients that are particularly influential or important within the context of particular types of risk; in neighborhoods rife with community violence, for instance, strategies to ensure physical safety are clearly of unique importance.

In the community domain, a primary conclusion from extant research is that ongoing exposure to community violence is highly inimical not only for children but also their parents and other adults. Among those who fear for their very lives, it is unrealistic to expect psychological robustness: When physical survival is threatened, all developmental tasks and processes are jeopardized. In the case of such risks, therefore, there must be priority on eradicating these experiences in whatever ways possible.

While resilience research has labeled various community-level risk factors, the community can also be an important source of support when the child's own parents are constrained in this regard. High-quality child care is particularly valuable for children in the most at-risk families, as strong, supportive relationships with teachers can be highly beneficial for school-age children and adolescents. There is great potential to use K–12 schools as venues to foster resilient adaptation. Thus far, several school-based interventions based in social control and social learning theories—involving teachers as well as parents—have shown some success in randomized trials. Attachment-based interventions, where the emphasis is on developing close, supportive bonds with the teacher, have been insufficiently examined in school settings, though the positive effects of such programs are potentially far reaching. In addition to school-based initiatives, support provided by informal mentors (as in Big Brothers, Big Sisters) can serve important protective functions, especially when the relationships are of relatively long duration. Involvement in religion, similarly, can confer benefits via the availability of a stable support network and the promotion of relatively positive coping strategies. At the neighborhood level, cohesion and shared supervision of children are important positive influences, as is high participation in local and voluntary organization. Children benefit from participation in structured extracurricular activities, but unstructured settings (as in youth recreation centers) can exacerbate risks.

In terms of children's personal attributes, resilience researchers must make a concerted effort to examine the biological processes that might confer significant vulnerability. Just as the environment sets confidence limits within which biology determines functioning, biology sets limits within which the environment determines adaptation levels. If a chemical imbalance in the brain predisposes a child or adolescent to depression, the threshold of tolerance to environmental stressors becomes considerably lower so that even stressors of moderate severity could precipitate a debilitating depression; awareness of such biological vulnerabilities, therefore, is essential in gaining complete understandings of risk exposure and positive adaptation. Even as we strive to promote the quality of children's family and community environments, careful pharmacological interventions targeting the biology involved in psychiatric disorders—particularly among youth at high genetic risk by virtue of parent mental illness—will be critical in maximizing resilient adaptation among children and adolescents at high risk.

References

1. Cicchetti D: Fractures in the crystal: Developmental psychopathology and the emergence of the self. *Developmental Review* 11:271–287, 1993.
2. Luthar SS, Burack JA, Cicchetti D, Weisz JR, eds: *Developmental psychopathology: Perspectives on adjustment, risk and disorder*, Cambridge, Cambridge University Press; 1997.

3. Rutter M: The developmental psychopathology of depression: Issues and perspectives. In: Rutter M, Tizard C, Read P, (eds): *Depression in young people: Developmental and clinical perspectives* New York, Guilford, 3–30 1986.
4. Sroufe LA, Rutter M: The domain of developmental psychopathology. *Child Development.* 55:1184–1199, 1984.
5. Masten A: Ordinary magic: Resilience processes in development. *American Psychologist* 56:227–238, 2001.
6. Margolin G, Gordis EB: The effects of family and community violence on children. *Annual Review of Psychology.* 51:445–479, 2000.
7. Wickramaratne PJ, Weissman MM. Onset of psychopathology in offspring by developmental phase and parental depression. *Journal of the American Academy of Child & Adolescent Psychiatry* 37:933–942, 1998.
8. Rutter M: Protective factors in children's responses to stress and disadvantage. In: Kent MW, Rolf JE, (eds): *Primary prevention in psychopathology: Social competence in children.* Vol. 8. Hanover, NH: University Press of New England; 49–74, 1979.
9. Gutman LM, Sameroff AJ, Cole R: Academic growth curve trajectories from 1st grade to 12th grade: Effects of multiple social risk factors and preschool child factors. *Developmental Psychology.* 39:777–790, 2003.
10. Sameroff AJ, Gutman L, Peck SC: Adaptation among youth facing multiple risks: Prospective research findings. In: Luthar SS (ed): *Resilience and vulnerability: Adaptation in the context of childhood adversities*, New York, Cambridge, 364–391, 2003.
11. Masten AS, Morison P, Pellegrini D, Tellegen A.: Competence under stress: Risk and protective factors. In: Rolf J, Masten A, Cicchetti D, Neuchterlein K, Weintraub S (eds): *Risk and protective factors in development of psychopathology*, New York, Cambridge, 236–256, 1990.
12. Martinez CR Jr, Forgatch, MS: Preventing problems with boys' noncompliance: Effects of a parent training intervention for divorcing mothers. *Journal of Consulting and Clinical Psychology*, 69:416–428, 2001.
13. Sandler I, Wolchik S, Davis C, Haine R, Ayers T: Correlational and experimental study of resilience for children of divorce and parentally bereaved children. In: Luthar SS (ed): *Resilience and vulnerability: Adaptation in the context of childhood adversities*, New York, Cambridge, 213–240, 2003.
14. Luthar SS, Cicchetti D, Becker B.: The construct of resilience: A critical evaluation and guidelines for future work. *Child Development.* 71:543–562, 2000.
15. Ceballo R, McLoyd VC: Social support and parenting in poor, dangerous neighborhoods. *Child Development*, 73:1310–1321, 2002.
16. Dearing E: The developmental implications of restrictive and supportive parenting across neighborhoods and ethnicities: Exceptions are the rule. *Journal of Applied Developmental Psychology* 25:555–575, 2004.
17. Gonzales NA, Cauce AM, Friedman RJ, Mason CA: Family, peer, and neighborhood influences on academic achievement among African American adolescents: One year prospective effects. *American Journal of Community Psychology* 24:365–388, 1996.
18. Lansford JE, Deater-Deckard K, Dodge KA, Bates JE, Pettit, GS: Ethnic differences in the link between physical discipline and later adolescent externalizing behaviors. *Journal of Child Psychology and Psychiatry* 45:801–812, 2004.
19. Kaufman J, Birmaher B, Brent D, et al.: Schedule for Affective Disorders and Schizophrenia for School-Age Children—Present and Lifetime Version (K-SADS-PL): Initial reliability and validity. *Journal of the American Academy of Child and Adolescent Psychiatry* 36:980–988, 1997.
20. Shaffer D, Fisher PS, Lucas CP, et al.: NIMH Diagnostic Interview Schedule for Children Version IV (NIMH DISC-IV): Description, differences from previous versions, and reliability of some common diagnoses. *Journal of the American Academy of Child and Adolescent Psychiatry* 39:28–38, 2000.
21. Reynolds CR, Kamphaus RW: *Behavior assessment system for children.* Circle Pines, American Guidance Services, 1992.
22. Achenbach TM: *Manual for the Child Behavior Checklist/4–18 and 1991 Profile*, Burlington, University of Vermont Department of Psychiatry, 1991.
23. Achenbach TM, Rescorla LA: *Manual for the ASEBA School-Age Forms & Profiles.* Burlington, VT, University of Vermont, Research Center for Children, Youth, & Families, 2001.
24. Shaffer D, Fisher P, Dulkan MK, et al.: The NIMH Diagnostic Interview Schedule for Children version 2.3 (DISC-2.3): Description, acceptability, prevalence rates and performance in the MECA study. *Journal of the American Academy of Child and Adolescent Psychiatry.* 35:865–77, 1996.
25. Lewinsohn PM, Hops H, Roberts RE, et al.: Adolescent psychopathology: I. Prevalence and incidence of depression and other DSM-III-R disorders in high school students. *Journal of Abnormal Psychology.* 102:133–144, 1993.
26. Fleiss JL: *Statistical methods for rates and proportions*, New York, John Wiley & Sons, 1981.
27. Grills AE, Ollendick TH: Multiple informant agreement and the Anxiety Disorders Interview Schedule for Parents and Children. *Journal of the Academy of Child and Adolescent Psychiatry.* 42:30–40, 2003.
28. Williams RJ, McDermitt DR, Bertrand LD: Parental awareness of adolescent substance use. *Addictive Behaviors.* 28:803–809, 2003.
29. Roberts RE, Alegria M, Roberts CR, Chen IG: Concordance of reports of mental health functioning by adolescents and their caregivers: A comparison of European, African and Latino Americans. *The Journal of Nervous and Mental Disease.* 193:528–534, 2005.
30. Yeh M, Weisz JR: Why are we here at the clinic? Parent–child (dis)agreement on referral problems at outpatient treatment entry. *Journal of Consulting and Clinical Psychology.* 69:1018–1025, 2001.
31. Grietens H, Van Assche V, Prinzie P, et al.: A comparison of mothers', fathers' and teachers' reports on problem behavior in 5-to-6-year-old children. *Journal of Psychopathology and Behavioral Assessment.* 26:137–146, 2004.
32. Angold A, Costello EJ: The Child and Adolescent Psychiatric Assessment (CAPA). *Journal of the American Academy of Child & Adolescent Psychiatry.* 39:39–48, 2000.
33. Loeber R, Green SM, Lahey BB: Mental health professionals' perception of the utility of children, mothers, and teachers as informants on childhood psychopathology. *Journal of Clinical Child Psychology.* 19:136–143, 1990.
34. Loeber R, Green SM, Lahey BB, Stouthamer-Loeber M. Differences and similarities between children, mothers, and teachers as informants on disruptive child behavior. *Journal of Abnormal Child Psychology.* 19:75–95, 1991.
35. Achenbach TM, McConaughy SH, Howell CT: Child/adolescent behavioral and emotional problems: Implications of cross-informant correlations for situational specificity. *Psychological Bulletin.* 101:213–232, 1987.
36. Grills AE, Ollendick TH: Issues in parent–child agreement: The case of structured diagnostic interviews. *Clinical Child and Family Psychology Review.* 5:57–83, 2002.
37. Hawley KM, Weisz JR: Child, parent, and therapist (dis)agreement on target problems in outpatient therapy: The therapist's dilemma and its implications. *Journal of Consulting and Clinical Psychology.* 71:62–70, 2003.
38. Richters JE, Cicchetti D: Mark Twain meets DSM-III-R: Conduct disorders, development, and the concept of harmful dysfunction. *Development and Psychopathology.* 5:5–29, 1993.
39. Wakefield JC: The concept of mental disorder: On the boundary between biological facts and social values. *American Psychologist.* 47:373–388, 1992.
40. Wakefield JC: Disorder as harmful dysfunction: A conceptual critique of DSM-III-R's definition of mental disorder. *Psychological Review.* 99:232–247, 1992.
41. Wakefield JC: Limits of operationalization: A critique of Spitzer and Endicott's (1978) proposed operational criteria for mental disorder. *Journal of Abnormal Psychology.* 102:160–172, 1993.
42. Wakefield JC, Horwitz AV, Schmitz M: Social disadvantage is not mental disorder: Response to Campbell-Sills and Stein. *Canadian Journal of Psychiatry.* 50:324–326, 2005.
43. Masten A, Coatsworth JD: The development of competence in favorable and unfavorable environments: Lessons from research on successful children. *American Psychologist.* 53:185–204, 1998.
44. Yates TM, Egeland B, Sroufe LA. Rethinking resilience: A developmental process perspective. In: Luthar SS (ed): *Resilience and vulnerability: Adaptation in the context of childhood adversities.* New York, Cambridge, 243–266, 2003.
45. Wyman PA, Cowen EL, Work WC, et al.: Caregiving and developmental factors differentiating young at-risk urban children showing resilient versus stress-affected outcomes: A replication and extension. *Child Development* 70:645–659, 1999.
46. Luthar SS: Annotation: Methodological and conceptual issues in the study of resilience. *Journal of Child Psychology and Psychiatry* 34:441–453, 1993.
47. Seidman E, Pedersen S: Holistic, contextual perspectives on risk, protection, and competence among low-income urban adolescents. In: Luthar SS (ed): *Resilience and vulnerability: Adaptation in the context of childhood adversities*, New York, Cambridge, 318–342, 2003.
48. Beardslee WR: *Out of the Darkened Room: When a Parent is Depressed—Protecting the Children and Strengthening the Family*, New York, Little, Brown and Company, 2002.
49. Hammen C: Risk and protective factors for children of depressed parents. In: Luthar SS (ed): *Resilience and vulnerability: Adaptation in the context of childhood adversities.* New York, Cambridge, 50–75, 2003.
50. Masten AS, Powell JL: A resilience framework for research, policy, and practice: Contributions from Project Competence. In: Luthar SS (ed): *Resilience and Vulnerability: Adaptation in the Context of Childhood Adversities.* New York, Cambridge, 1–25, 2003.
51. Luthar SS, Burack JA: Adolescent wellness: In the eye of the beholder? In: Cicchetti D, Rappaport J, Sandler I, Weissberg R (eds): *The promotion of wellness in children and adolescents.* Washington, DC, Child Welfare League of America, 29–57, 2002.
52. O'Donnell DA, Schwab-Stone ME, Muyeed AZ: Multidimensional resilience in urban children exposed to community violence. *Child Development*, 73:1265–1282, 2003.
53. Luthar SS, Cicchetti D: The construct of resilience: Implications for interventions and social policies. *Development and Psychopathology.* 12:857–885, 2000.
54. Rutter M. Resilience reconsidered: Conceptual considerations, empirical findings, and policy implications. In: Shonkoff JP, Meisels SJ eds. *Handbook of early childhood intervention.* 2nd ed. New York: Cambridge, 651–682, 2000.

55. Rutter M: Genetic influences on risk and protection: Implications for understanding resilience. In: Luthar SS (ed): *Resilience and vulnerability: Adaptation in the context of childhood adversities.* New York, Cambridge, 489–509, 2003.
56. Luthar SS, Zelazo LB: Research on resilience: An integrative review. In: Luthar SS (ed): *Resilience and vulnerability: Adaptation in the context of childhood adversities.* New York, Cambridge, 510–549, 2003.
57. Seifer S: Young children with mentally ill parents: Resilient developmental systems. In: Luthar SS (ed): *Resilience and vulnerability: Adaptation in the context of childhood adversities.* New York, Cambridge, 29–49, 2003.
58. Leventhal T, Brooks-Gunn J: The neighborhoods they live in: The effects of neighborhood residence on child and adolescent outcomes. *Psychological Bulletin.* 126:309–337, 2000.
59. Sampson RJ, Raudenbush SW, Earls F: Neighborhoods and violent crime: A multilevel study of collective efficacy. *Science.* 277:918–924, 1997.
60. Anthony EJ, Koupernik C (eds): *The child in his family: Children at psychiatric risk—III.* New York, Wiley, 3–10, 1997.
61. Garmezy N: The study of competence in children at risk for severe psychopathology. In: Anthony EJ, Koupernik C (eds): *The child in his family: Children at psychiatric risk—III.* New York, Wiley, 547, 1974.
62. Murphy LB, Moriarty A: *Vulnerability, coping, and growth: From Infancy to Adolescence.* New Haven, Yale University Press, 1976.
63. Werner EE. Protective factors and individual resilience. In: Meisells R, Shonkoff J (eds): *Handbook of early intervention.* Cambridge, Cambridge, 115–132, 2000.
64. Werner EE, Smith R: *Kauai's children come of age.* Honolulu, University of Hawaii Press, 1977.
65. Shonkoff JP, Phillips DA (eds): *From neurons to neighborhoods: The science of early childhood development.* Washington, DC National Academy Press, 2000.
66. Allen JP, Hauser ST, Borman-Spurrell E: Attachment theory as a framework for understanding sequelae of severe adolescent psychopathology: An 11-year follow-up study. *Journal of Consulting and Clinical Psychology.* 64:254–263, 1996.
67. Sroufe LA: From infant attachment to promotion of adolescent autonomy: Prospective, longitudinal data on the role of parents in development. In: Borkowski JG, Ramey SL, (eds), *Parenting and the child's world: Influences on academic, intellectual, and social-emotional development—Monographs in parenting.* Mahwah, Lawrence Erlbaum, 187–202, 2002.
68. Weinfield NS, Sroufe LA, Egeland B: Attachment from infancy to early adulthood in a high-risk sample: Continuity, discontinuity, and their correlates. *Child Development.* 71:695–702, 2000.
69. Conger RD, Cui M, Bryant M, Elder GH: Competence in early adult romantic relationships: A developmental perspective on family influences. *Journal of Personality and Social Psychology.* 79:224–237, 2000.
70. Black MM, Dubowitz H, Starr RH Jr.: African American fathers in low income, urban families: Development, behavior, and home environment of their three-year-old children. *Child Development.* 70:967–978, 1999.
71. Brody GH: Siblings' direct and indirect contributions to child development. *Current Directions in Psychological Science.* 13:124–126, 2004.
72. Carlson EA, Sroufe LA, Egeland B: The construction of experience: A longitudinal study of representation and behavior. *Child Development.* 75:66–83, 2004.
73. Sroufe LA, Carlson EA, Levy AK, Egeland B: Implications of attachment theory for developmental psychopathology. *Development and Psychopathology.* 11:1–13, 1999.
74. Egeland B, Sroufe LA: Attachment and early maltreatment. *Child Development.* 52:44–52, 1981.
75. Thompson RA: The legacy of early attachments. *Child Development.* 71:145–152, 2000.
76. Waters E, Weinfield NS, Hamilton CE: The stability of attachment security from infancy to adolescence and early adulthood: General discussion. *Child Development.* 2000; 71:703–706.
77. Dozier M, Albus K, Fisher P, Sepulveda S: Interventions for foster parents: Implications for developmental theory. *Development and Psychopathology.* 14:843–860, 2002.
78. Dozier M, Stovall KC, Albus KE, Bates B: Attachment for infants in foster care: The role of caregiver state of mind. *Child Development.* 72:1467–1477, 2001.
79. Heinicke CM, Rineman NR, Ponce VA, Guthrie D: Relation-based intervention with at-risk mothers: Outcome in the second year of life. *Infant Mental Health Journal.* 22:431–462, 2001.
80. Baumrind D: Rearing competent children. In: Danon W (ed): *Child development today and tomorrow.* San Francisco, Jossey-Bass, 349–378, 1989.
81. Hetherington EM, Elmore AM: Risk and resilience in children coping with their parents' divorce and remarriage. In: Luthar SS, ed. *Resilience and vulnerability: Adaptation in the context of childhood adversities.* New York, Cambridge, 182–212, 2003.
82. Cavell TA: *Working with Parents of Aggressive Children: A Practitioner's Guide.* Washington, DC, American Psychological Association, 27–47, 2000.
83. Schneider WJ, Cavell TA, Hughes JN: A sense of containment: Potential moderator of the relation between parenting practices and children's externalizing behaviors. *Development and Psychopathology.* 15:95–117, 2003.
84. Dishion TJ, McMahon RJ: Parental monitoring and the prevention of child and adolescent problem behavior: A conceptual and empirical formulation. *Clinical Child & Family Psychology Review.* 1:61–75, 1998.
85. Buckner JC, Mezzacappa E, Beardslee WR: Characteristics of resilient youths living in poverty: The role of self-regulatory processes. *Development and Psychopathology.* 15:139–162, 2003.
86. Galambos NL, Barker ET, Almeida DM: Parents do matter: Trajectories of change in externalizing and internalizing problems in early adolescence. *Child Development.* 74:578–594, 2003.
87. Brody GH, Murry VM, Kim S, Brown AC: Longitudinal pathways to competence and psychological adjustment among African American children living in rural single-parent households. *Child Development.* 73:1505–1516, 2002.
88. Lloyd JJ, Anthony JC: Hanging out with the wrong crowd: How much difference can parents make in an urban environment? *Journal of Urban Health: Bulletin of the New York Academy of Medicine.* 80:383–390, 2003.
89. Mason CA, Cauce AM, Gonzales N, Hiraga Y: Neither too sweet nor too sour: Problem peers, maternal control, and problem behavior in African American adolescents. *Child Development.* 67:2115–2130, 1996.
90. Caspi A, McClay J, Moffitt TE, et al.: Role of genotype in the cycle of violence in maltreated children. *Science.* 297:851–854, 2002.
91. Caspi A, Sugden K, Moffitt TE, et al.: Influence of life stress on depression: Moderation by a polymorphism in the 5-HTT gene. *Science.* 301:386–389, 2003.
92. Kim-Cohen J, Moffitt TE, Caspi A, Taylor A: Genetic and environmental processes in young children's resilience and vulnerability to socioeconomic deprivation. *Child Development.* 75:651–668, 2004.
93. Plomin R, Rutter M: Child development, molecular genetics, and what to do with genes once they are found. *Child Development.* 69:1223–1242, 1998.
94. Rutter M. Nature, nurture, and development: From evangelism through science toward policy and practice. *Child Development.* 73:1–21, 2002.
95. Tierney JP, Grossman JB, Resch NL. *Making a difference: An impact study of Big Brothers Big Sisters.* Philadelphia, Public/Private Ventures, 1995.
96. Elder GH, Conger RD: *Children of the land: Adversity and success in rural America.* Chicago, University of Chicago Press, 2000.
97. Miller L, Gur M: Religiosity, depression and physical maturation in adolescent girls. *Journal of the American Academy of Child & Adolescent Psychiatry.* 41:206–214, 2002.
98. Pearce MJ, Jones SM, Schwab-Stone ME, Ruchkin V: The protective effects of religiousness and parent involvement on the development of conduct problems among youth exposed to violence. *Child Development.* 74:1682–1696, 2003.
99. Burchinal MR, Follmer A, Bryant DM: The relations of maternal social support and family structure with maternal responsiveness and child outcomes among African-American families. *Developmental Psychology.* 32:1073–1083, 1996.
100. McLoyd VC, Jayaratne TE, Ceballo R, Borquez J: Unemployment and work interruption among African-American single mothers: Effects on parenting and adolescent socioemotional functioning. *Child Development.* 65:562–589, 1994.
101. Hamre BK, Pianta RC: Early teacher–child relationships and the trajectory of children's school outcomes through eighth grade. *Child Development.* 72:625–638, 2001.
102. NICHD Early Child Care Research Network. Social functioning in the first grade: Associations with earlier home and child care predictors and with current classroom experiences. *Child Development.* 74:1639–1662, 2003.
103. Reddy R, Rhodes JE, Mulhall P: The influence of teacher support on student adjustment in the middle school years: A latent growth curve study. *Development and Psychopathology.* 15:119–138, 2003.
104. Howes C, Ritchie S. Attachment organizations in children with difficult life circumstances. *Development and Psychopathology.* 11:251–268, 1999.
105. Meehan BT, Hughes JN, Cavell TA: Teacher–student relationships as compensatory resources for aggressive children. *Child Development.* 74:1145–1157, 2003.
106. Hughes JN, Cavell TA, Jackson T: Influence of the teacher–student relationship on childhood conduct problems: A prospective study. *Journal of Clinical Child Psychology.* 28:173–184, 1999.
107. Way N, Robinson MG: A longitudinal study of the effects of family, friends, and school experiences on the psychological adjustment of ethnic minority, low-SES adolescents. *Journal of Adolescent Research.* 18:324–346, 2003.
108. Luthar SS: *Poverty and children's adjustment.* Thousand Oaks, Sage, 1999.
109. Spencer MB: Social and cultural influences on school adjustment: The application of an identity-focused cultural ecological perspective. *Educational Psychologist.* 34:43–57, 1999.
110. Luthar SS, Zigler E: Vulnerability and competence: A review of research on resilience in childhood. *American Journal of Orthopsychiatry.* 61:6–22, 1999.
111. Rutter ML: Psychosocial adversity and child psychopathology. *British Journal of Psychiatry.* 74:480–49, 1999.
112. Werner EE, Smith RS: *Overcoming the odds: High risk children from birth to adulthood.* Ithaca, Cornell University Press, 1992.
113. Mayer JD, Salovey P, Caruso DR, Sitarenios G: Measuring emotional intelligence with the MSCEIT V2.0. *Emotion.* 3:97–105, 2003.

114. Salovey P, Mayer JD, Caruso D, Lopes PN: Measuring emotional intelligence as a set of abilities with the Mayer-Salovey-Caruso Emotional Intelligence Test. In: Lopez SJ, Snyder CR (eds): *Positive psychological assessment: A handbook of models and measures.* Washington, DC, American Psychological Association, 251–265, 2003.
115. Trinidad DR, Johnson CA: The association between emotional intelligence and early adolescent tobacco and alcohol use. *Personality and Individual Differences.* 32:95–105, 2002.
116. Parker JDA, Summerfeldt LJ, Hogan MJ, Majeski SA: Emotional intelligence and academic success: Examining the transition from high school to university. *Personality and Individual Differences.* 36:163–172, 2004.
117. Koenen KC, Moffitt TE, Caspi A, et al.: Domestic violence is associated with environmental suppression of IQ in young children. *Development and Psychopathology.* 15:297–311, 2003.
118. Cicchetti D: Experiments of nature: Contributions to developmental theory. *Development and Psychopathology.* 15:833–835, 2003.
119. Rutter M: The interplay of nature, nurture, and developmental influences: The challenge ahead for mental health. *Archives of General Psychiatry.* 59:996–1000, 2002.
120. Aspinwall LG, Taylor SE: A stitch in time: Self-regulation and proactive coping. *Psychological Bulletin.* 121:417–436, 1997.
121. Eisenberg N, Champion C, Ma Y: Emotion-related regulation: An emerging construct. *Merrill-Palmer Quarterly.* 50:236–259, 2004.
122. Davidson RJ: Affective style, psychopathology, and resilience: Brain mechanisms and plasticity. *American Psychologist.* 55:1196–1214, 2000.
123. Curtis WJ, Cicchetti D: Moving research on resilience into the 21st century: Theoretical and methodological considerations in examining the biological contributors to resilience. *Development & Psychopathology.* 15:773–810, 2003.
124. McEwen BS, Sapolsky RM: Stress and cognitive function. *Current Opinion in Neurobiology.* 5:205–216, 1995.
125. Sapolsky RM: Glucocorticoids and hippocampal atrophy in neuropsychiatric disorders. *Archives of General Psychiatry.* 57:925–935, 2000.
126. McEwen BS: Steroid hormone actions on the brain: When is the genome involved? *Hormones and Behavior.* 28:396–405, 1994.
127. Watson C, Gametchu B: Membraine-initated steroid actions and the proteins that mediate them. *Proceedings of the Society for Experimental Biology and Medicine.* 220:9–19, 1999.

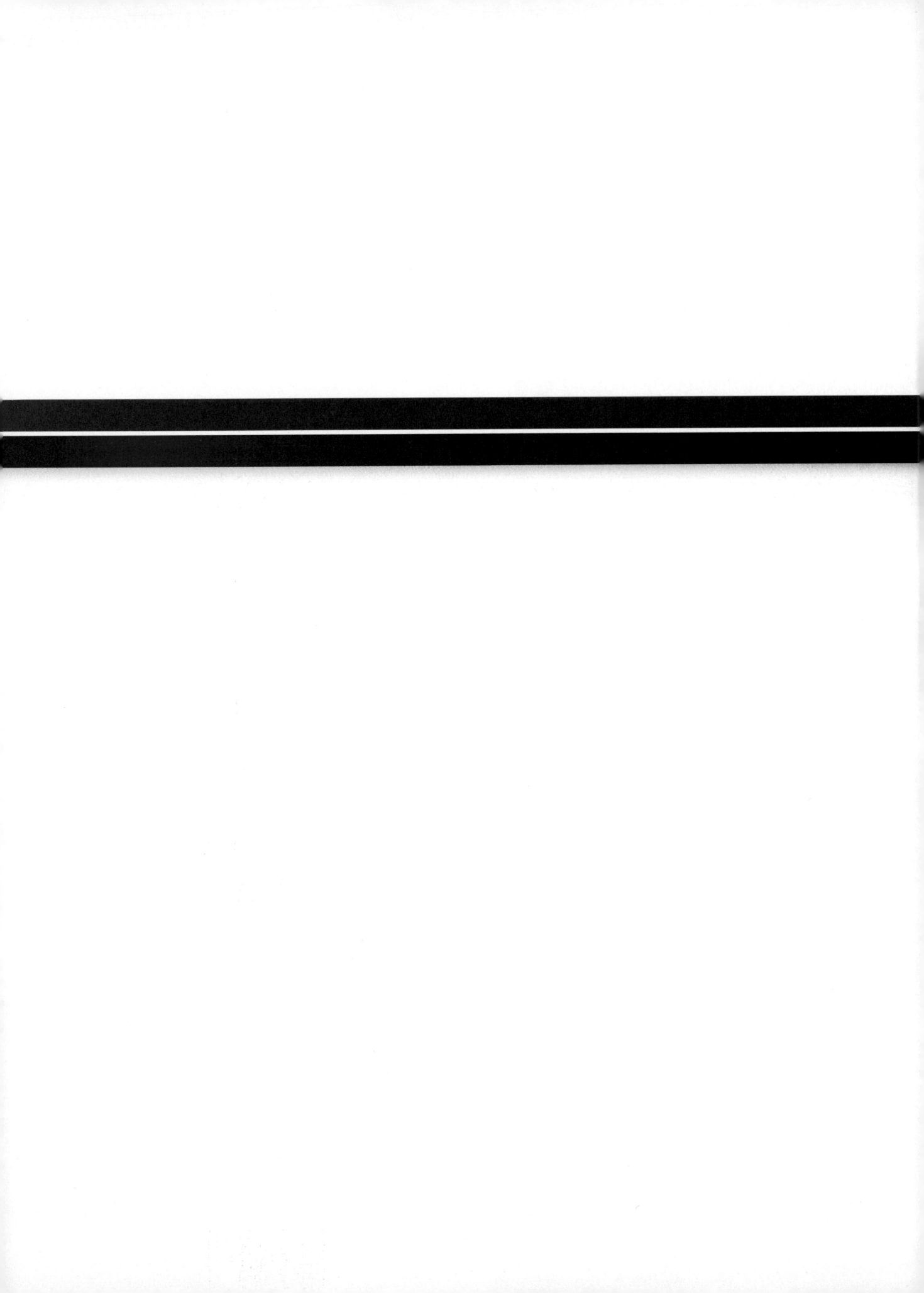

SECTION IV

NOSOLOGY, CLASSIFICATION, AND DIAGNOSTIC ASSESSMENT

CHAPTER 4.1 ■ CLASSIFICATION

FRED R. VOLKMAR, MARY SCHWAB-STONE, AND MICHAEL FIRST

PRINCIPLES OF CLASSIFICATION

The ability and the urge to classify are unique aspects of human experience. They provide us with the capacity to observe, to order our observations, and to formulate general principles and hypotheses. Classification enables us to make use of information for purposes of communication, prediction, and explanation. At the present time in child and adolescent psychiatry, classification systems have their greatest role in facilitating communication for both clinical and research purposes; their role in prediction is somewhat more limited, and their explanatory value is often quite limited. The process of assigning a label may itself be associated with some sense of relief on the part of the patient or the patient's parents (1). Sometimes this reflects the misconception that having a label implies having an explanation (2). Like all human constructions, classification schemes can be abused or ill used (3). This chapter provides an overview of classification in child and adolescent psychiatry and an overview of the current official systems, that is, the tenth edition of the *International Classification of Diseases* (ICD-10) (4) and the fourth edition of the *Diagnostic and Statistical Manual of Mental Disorders* (DSM-IV) (5). (Specific criteria for each disorder are discussed in detail in the respective chapters.)

Various authors (2, 6–11) discuss criteria for psychiatric classification systems. There is no single "right" way to classify disorders in childhood. Classification systems vary, depending on the purpose of classification and what is being classified. As described later, "official" diagnostic systems have tended to adopt, on the whole, a categorical approach, but a dimensional approach would be equally as applicable, if perhaps less useful for clinical purposes.

The goals of classification include facilitating communication among professionals, providing information about given disorders that is relevant to treatment or to prevention, and providing information useful for research aimed at understanding the pathogenesis of disorders. To achieve these goals, classification schemes must be readily and reliably used by clinicians and researchers; hence the need for systems that are readily comprehensible. The disorders should be described, so they can be differentiated from one another. Disorders should differ in important ways, such as associated features and course. The classification system must be applicable over the range of development and must be comprehensive and logically consistent (12). A classification of disorders implies that some clinically significant patterns of symptoms, behaviors, and signs are observed and comprise a source of significant distress or impairment (5). Deviant behavior itself does not necessarily constitute a disorder unless it is a manifestation of dysfunction within the individual person (e.g., conflicts over political beliefs do not constitute a mental disorder). Although it is often assumed that mental disorders must have a biological basis, this need not be the case; for example, maladaptive, enduring personality patterns can readily be classified as disorders (13).

Development of a general classification system for psychiatric disorders inevitably involves various tradeoffs. General classification systems must cover the entire range of disorders in a logically consistent fashion; classification systems developed for a highly specific purpose do not share this concern. The need for reasonable parsimony must be balanced with the need for adequate coverage (1, 9). The needs for a clinically relevant system differ somewhat from those for a research system; for example, highly detailed criteria may be useful for research purposes but are cumbersome in clinical practice. Different diagnostic systems address these issues in different ways. Thus, the DSM-IV (5) is intended to be useful for *both* clinical work and research, whereas the ICD-10 (4) system provides *separate* clinical and research descriptions.

ISSUES IN CLASSIFICATION

Developmental Aspects

Developmental considerations assume major importance in the provision of a classification scheme for children and adolescents, and, indeed, for adults as well (14). Some disorders such as autism have their origin in a specific developmental period, whereas others are frequently associated with developmental problems (Tourette syndrome may be associated with attentional difficulties). At other times, the child's overall level of development may have a major impact on the ways in which various disorders can be expressed (the child with mental retardation who also exhibits conduct problems). Classification systems must be able to encompass such issues without simultaneously making the disorder so developmentally specific that the utility of the category is compromised.

The developmental approach to classification is used whenever disorders are viewed in the context of the unfolding of basic developmental processes. The use of standard, developmentally based assessment instruments such as tests of intelligence or communication skills exemplifies this approach. In contrast, many categorical and dimensional classification systems rely on assessment of deviant behavior. The use of such an approach is often complicated because issues of how deviant behavior is to be evaluated and how instruments are to be "normed" become quite important, and reliability among examiners can be low. Both the ICD-10 and the DSM-IV systems include some categories in which the definition is fundamentally developmental (mental retardation, articulation disorders), whereas in others the deviant nature of the disorder predominates (autism, schizophrenia of childhood onset).

Role of Theory

Theoretical models of psychological disturbance have developed from rather diverse historical traditions; they have considerable value for the individual clinician in understanding and treating children with emotional and behavioral problems. For example, Anna Freud proposed a developmental profile based on and applicable to psychoanalytic assessment of children (15). More phenomenologically based classification systems can be traced to Kraeplin's delineation of schizophrenia and bipolar disorder (16). In the early "official" classifications, theoretical concerns were reflected in terms such as "schizophrenic reaction of childhood" or "obsessional neurosis." Classification schemes that are driven by theory are limited because, by their nature, they are based on a set of assumptions and hypotheses not usually generally shared and may give rise to different terms used to describe the same clinical phenomena; for example, a learning theorist may invoke principles of conditioning to explain a child's phobia, whereas a psychoanalytically oriented theorist may be more concerned with the child's level of psychosexual organization. Particularly following the work on development of research diagnostic criteria (17), the phenomenologic approach to classification has predominated in the various "official" diagnostic systems. The more robust diagnostic concepts have typically emerged from clinical experience rather than from theory (18). In some instances, a theory has been invoked to account for a given set of phenomena, but it is the set of phenomena rather than the theory that has endured. For example, Langdon Down provided a complex theoretical explanation for children with the condition now known as Down syndrome. His theory, based on obsolete racial stereotypes (mongolism), was incorrect, but his observation of some element of commonality among a large group of children with mental retardation has proved enduring.

For clinicians with pronounced theoretical views, the more phenomenon-based approach can be a source of frustration. It is sometimes incorrectly assumed that in such an approach matters as history, course, and outcome, and, for that matter, etiology and theory are irrelevant to classification. Information on course and outcome may provide important data relative to external validation of diagnostic categories, and information on the development of the disorder may be highly relevant to differential diagnosis regardless of how similar, at one point, two different disorders may appear to be. For example, the syndrome of childhood disintegrative disorder clearly appears to resemble autistic disorder once it is established; however, patterns of early development and outcome differ in these conditions (19). Theoretical views of conditions and mechanisms remain highly relevant for both clinical work and research because they are more likely to generate truly testable hypotheses.

Etiology and Classification

It is often assumed that classification systems are developed to approximate some ideal diagnostic system in which the cause could be directly related to clinical condition. This is not, in fact, the case, in that no single ideal system is waiting to be discovered and that cause need not be included in classification systems (12). Similarly, classification need not reflect a "disease" model (12). Different etiologic factors may result in rather similar conditions, and the same etiologic factor may be associated with a range of clinical conditions. Aspects of intervention may be more directly related to the clinical condition than to the cause. Remedial services for children with mental retardation are, for example, much more likely to be oriented around aspects of developmental level than around the precise origin of the specific mental retardation syndrome. With a few exceptions (reactive attachment or posttraumatic stress disorders in the DSM-IV), etiologic factors are not generally included in official diagnostic systems.

Contextual Factors

In certain situations and populations, contextual variables such as family, school, or cultural setting pose major complications to diagnosis. The attentional problems of a child whose difficulties arise only as a result of an inappropriate school placement would not, for example, merit a diagnosis of attention deficit disorder. Contextual variables are particularly problematic in disorders of infancy and early childhood in which the infant exerts effects on the parents, who, in turn, exert effects on the child; attributions of causality may be particularly difficult to make (20). A few of the traditional categorical disorders can be readily observed in infants and young children (autism), but generally clinical complaints in this age group are centered around problems that encompass the infant in the context of the family or life situation. These issues are particularly relevant for diagnosis of disorders in infancy—an area that remains somewhat controversial so that, for example, a diagnosis of autism can often be made in very young children (21), although in some cases not all features are exhibited until around age 3 (22). Although research on disorders of infancy is limited (23), it is clear that infants exhibit a tremendous ability to react, even over relatively short periods, to their environment, and change, rather than stability, is often the rule (24). Clinical problems often relate more to issues of *goodness of fit* between parents and the infant than to a disorder in the infant (25). As children become slightly older, traditional diagnostic groupings become more readily applicable (26). Issues of developmental level also become important in specifying inclusion and exclusion criteria for diagnostic categories; for example, a diagnosis of pica may be appropriate for a 12-year-old child with profound retardation but is less appropriate for a normally developing 10-month-old infant. These will be important issues to consider for DSM-V and ICD-11.

Cultural differences may also affect diagnostic concepts and practice (27). Clearly, certain sociocultural factors are associated with certain types of problems (e.g., economic disadvantage is associated with conduct and attentional problems), but the meanings of such relationships often remain unclear (28).

What Is Classified?

It is particularly important that clinicians and researchers alike bear in mind that disorders, rather than children, are classified. This is a source of considerable confusion. Concerns have been raised about the possible effects of labeling children (3), and to some extent these concerns are valid. It is, of course, also the case that having an adequate label for a child's disorder may be helpful, for example, in securing needed services. Thus, a diagnosis of mental retardation or learning disability may be associated with social stigma or other untoward effects, or it may be associated with more realistic expectations on the part of parents and teachers and provision of potentially more appropriate services. These tensions are also exemplified in the debate between those who advocate broad and encompassing definitions (to maximize clinical and educational service provision) and those who advocate narrow definitions (by defining more homogenous groups of research subjects).

Similar debates arise about aspects of social stigma related to mental illness and behavioral and developmental problems. In this regard, it is always important to refer to the child's disorder, *not to the child as the disorder*. The term *diagnosis* refers both to the notion of assigning a label to a given problem and to the act of evaluation. In important respects, it is the diagnostic process (29) that is the most important of the two. Although diagnostic labels have considerable value, they do not provide information specifically about the individual person, who is unique and uniquely related to intervention.

VALIDATION AND STATISTICAL ISSUES

As official classification systems have become more complex and sophisticated, issues of reliability and validity have assumed increasing importance. For example, both the DSM-IV and the ICD-10 use results of large national or international field trials in providing definitions of disorders. Categorical and dimensional approaches to classification share certain statistical concerns (6).

Validity

Validity is the extent to which a classification system does what it purports to do in terms of facilitating communication, intervention, and research. Various types of validity have been identified, for example, *face validity* (a judgment about whether the description of a category appears to represent the diagnostic construct reasonably), *predictive validity* (whether some aspect of subsequent course or response to treatment is predicted), and *construct validity* (whether the category has meaning in terms of what it purports to assess). Generally, such concepts are most useful in measuring the validity of psychometric assessment instruments; their applicability to classification systems is somewhat different. In general, childhood psychiatric disorders have face validity but not necessarily predictive or construct validity (11). The validity of a given diagnostic category can be established on the basis of its association with various features other than those incorporated in the definition (response to treatment, natural history in the absence of treatment, family pattern, biological correlates, and developmental correlates such as age at onset and intelligence quotient).

The sensitivity and specificity of a given categorical diagnostic instrument can be assessed relative to the true presence or absence of a specific disorder. However, a general problem for both categorical and dimensional classification systems is the nature of the standard against which a given category or criteria set is to be judged. Given the usual absence of an unequivocal diagnostic marker for the various conditions, clinical judgment is often used as the standard against which new instruments or definitions are assessed. The issues of "caseness" and diagnostic thresholds are particularly important in the derivation and validation of diagnostic systems (30, 31).

Reliability

In addition to validity, classification systems should exhibit *reliability;* that is, users in different locations seeing rather similar disorders should be able to agree on the applicability of a specific category or criterion (32). Various kinds of reliability have been identified: interrater, test-retest, and internal consistency. If a given category is not used reliably, it has little value for purposes of communication. Some disorders, almost by definition, have limited test-retest reliability over a relatively short time period (adjustment disorder), whereas other highly stable disorders tend to have better test-retest reliability (profound mental retardation). Sources of unreliability in psychiatric diagnosis include differences in the kinds of information clinicians collect, theoretical biases in the clinician, and differences in internalized diagnostic thresholds, as well as, of course, the true differences that persons with disorders will exhibit at various points over the course of their condition.

High reliability does not guarantee validity. It is possible for a disorder to be reliably defined but have little or no validity. Conversely, a disorder may have validity, but criteria and diagnostic instruments designed to detect its presence may have little or no reliability. In providing diagnostic criteria and descriptions, there is often a tradeoff between the level of detail of a definition and its reliability. What appear to be relatively minor changes in the wording of a criterion can produce major changes in the way in which a diagnosis or diagnostic criterion is applied.

Statistical Analyses

Various *statistical techniques* have been applied to data derived from assessment methods (8, 33, 34). These techniques are theoretically of great interest in that they can provide more rational and empirical approaches to the derivation of diagnostic schemes. The fundamental assumption of such techniques is that the variables of interest lie along some dimension of function and dysfunction that all persons exhibit to some degree. For many types of problems, this assumption is probably justified, such as relative to anxiety or depression. However, the usefulness of such techniques is limited in important ways (12). In the first place, these methods are highly dependent on both the sample and the type of data entered in the analysis. For example, *factor analysis* of an instrument designed to detect conduct problems would not likely produce a factor related to eating disturbance. Similarly, cluster analysis of even a very large normative sample would not likely produce a cluster that corresponded to autism, given the low base rate of this disorder in the population. For rare disorders, other statistical approaches may be useful. Other relevant statistical procedures include *signal detection analysis* (35), which can be used to establish which symptoms and symptom combinations are more strongly related to a particular diagnosis. Similarly, *latent trait analysis* and *latent class analysis* (36, 37) provide other approaches.

MODELS OF CLASSIFICATION

Werry delineated three general approaches to classification of disorders: categorical, dimensional, and ideographic (1985). The *categorical approach,* sometimes referred to as the medical model of classification, views disorders as either present or absent (the patient does or does not have appendicitis). This approach assumes that patients exhibiting a given disorder display certain similarities, that these similarities outweigh differences, and that this knowledge has certain implications for understanding pathophysiology, course, treatment, and so on. Unlike the categorical approach, which views disorders as dichotomous, the *dimensional approach* to classification relies on assessment of dimensions of function or dysfunction by reducing phenomena to various dimensions along which a child can be placed. Various sources of data can be used for this approach, such as behavioral ratings, parental reports, yes–no criteria, developmentally based test scores, and the like. Although the dimensional approach is more commonly used in nonmedical settings, many medical phenomena also exhibit continuous (dimensional) characteristics (stature, blood pressure). For some purposes, categorical diagnoses (levels of mental retardation) are derived from what is essentially a continuous variable, whereas some dimensional assessment instruments can similarly be used to generate categorical diagnoses. *Ideographic classifications* reject simple labels and focus on the total context of the individual person; this approach may be theory driven (by psychoanalytic or behavioral theories) or may be used eclectically. Ideographic approaches are commonly used in clinical work; that is, the child or adolescent is viewed in the totality of life circumstance, and various disorders, problems, and psychosocial situations may be viewed as worthy of notation and treatment.

Categorical Approaches

The most widely used "official" systems are those developed by the World Health Organization (ICD-10) and the American Psychiatric Association (DSM-IV). Both systems have their historical origins in medicine in the ninteenth and twentieth centuries as advances in diagnosis and public health concerns necessitated more systematic approaches to record keeping (Table 4.1.1). During the ninteenth century, many advances in the taxonomy of adult psychiatric disorders were made, and this led Kraepelin to attempt a comprehensive classification system (38). By the mid-twentieth century, certain psychiatric disorders were generally recognized. The second edition of the DSM (DSM-II) (39) includes only a handful of diagnostic categories specific to children: mental retardation, childhood schizophrenia, adjustment, and other "reactions" (hyperkinetic, withdrawing, overanxious, runaway, unsocialized aggressive, group delinquent, and "other"). By the time the DSM-III appeared (40), the number of disorders first evidenced in infancy, childhood, or adolescence had increased more than fourfold to include the following major classes of disorder, each of which included some specific diagnostic categories: mental retardation, specific developmental disorders, attention deficit disorder, conduct disturbance, eating disorders, stereotyped movement disorders, pervasive developmental disorders, other disorders with physical manifestations, and other disorders of infancy, childhood, or adolescence (16). Similar, although not precisely corresponding, changes occurred in the revision of the ICD (10). In the DSM-III, for example, disorders generally specific to childhood were grouped together, and there were many more DSM-III subcategories (40). The DSM-III and its successor, the DSM-III-R (41), differ from the ICD-9 in terms of their greater diagnostic reliance on explicit (if not always truly operationalized) diagnostic criteria (42, 43). Both the DSM and the ICD incorporate a multiaxial framework, although the specific systems adopted differ from each other in some respects. Both systems are hierarchically organized, although the DSM-III and the DSM-III-R encourage multiple diagnoses.

Changes in the DSM-III-R and DSM-IV are generally less dramatic than in the DSM-III (44). Work on the DSM-IV began in 1988 (45), stimulated, in part, by a treaty obligation that mandated terminology compatible with the ICD, which was also undergoing revision at that time. As part of the process of producing the DSM-IV, steps were undertaken to ensure that changes made were based on solid data and thorough documentation (45). This task was somewhat facilitated because it was clear that the DSM-III and III-R had stimulated considerable research of relevance to the DSM-IV (46). Other issues for the DSM-IV relate to clinical utility and compatibility with ICD-10.

TABLE 4.1.1

LANDMARKS IN THE DEVELOPMENT OF PSYCHIATRIC TAXONOMIES*

Kraepelin (1883): Proposal for a comprehensive classification system
ICD-6 (1948): Psychiatric disorders included
DSM-I (1952): First U.S. official classification system
Group for the Advancement of Psychiatry (1966): Diagnostic system for children
DSM-II (1968): Some child disorders, emphasis on theory and Meyer's concept of reaction types
DSM-III (1980): Fourfold increase in child psychiatric disorders, greater diagnostic precision, multiaxial
DSM-III-R (1987): Refinements in criteria, categories
ICD-10 (1992): Separation of research diagnostic criteria from clinical descriptions
DSM-IV (1994): More emphasis on data based modifications in categories and criteria
DSM-IV-TR (2000): Generally minor revisions in text (not criteria)
DSM-V
(2002): Research agenda and white papers
(2012): Anticipated publication date

*DSM, *Diagnostic and statistical manual of mental disorders*; ICD, *International classification of diseases.*

As part of the revision process, extensive literature reviews were conducted, datasets were aggregated and analyzed or reanalyzed, and working groups of experts convened to evaluate the available data and, in some cases, to generate new data. For the child disorders section, field trials were conducted for disruptive behavior disorders (47) and for autism and related conditions (48).

The *International Classification of Causes of Death* was adopted by the International Statistical Institute in 1893 (49). By the 1960s, the ICD had been revised six times, and the deficiencies of the ICD-7 for psychiatric disorders (10) were particularly clear. Many changes were made in eighth edition of the ICD in 1968. Even when this edition was adopted, however, it was clear that further revision would be needed, and a process was instituted for further revision. An important part of this work was the development of a multiaxial classification system for child disorders (10).

The ICD-9 was published in 1977, and work on its revision began shortly thereafter (50–52). As part of the extensive revision process, the number of categories increased substantially (53), and a decision was made to have several versions of the system—one for primary health care providers, another for specialty-based researchers, and one for psychiatric practitioners. The ICD-10 draft generally had good clinical utility and good, although variable, reliability (the latter being less optimal for disorders with more subtle symptoms such as personality disorders) (51).

Comparison of the ICD-10 and the DSM-IV

Although, on balance, the two categorical systems are more alike than different, there are some differences between the two systems, some more and others less explicit. The ICD system has rather more constraints than the DSM, given its international nature and the fact that the psychiatric section is but one part of a large body of diagnostic coding. The systems also differ in the degree to which diagnoses are operationalized. The ICD-10 provides a comprehensive description of the clinical construct, followed by a discussion of differential diagnosis and major symptoms that should be present. In contrast, the DSM-IV is much more truly operationalized but is also accordingly somewhat less flexible for clinicians. Although both systems allow for multiple diagnostic codes, the ICD-10 also gives the option of applying some combination categories (depressive conduct disorder). Rutter discusses the pros and cons of this approach (54–56). Although there are some issues relative to certain disorders (the anxiety disorders), in general the trend has been toward convergence of the DSM and ICD classification systems. The remaining differences largely stem from the emphasis of clinical-diagnostic guidelines in the ICD and the greater specificity for research of the DSM. The more recent text revision of the DSM-IV (DSM-IV-TR) (57) updated the accompanying text but generally did not make any changes in the diagnostic criteria. With regard to children, probably the most extensive revision in the text is that for Asperger's disorder, which was expanded. There were two changes in definitions of childhood disorders. The description of the "subthreshold" category "Pervasive Developmental Disorder Not Otherwise Specified" was corrected: changed from requiring severe and pervasive impairment of reciprocal social interaction or verbal and nonverbal communication skills, or the presence of stereotyped behavior, interests, and activities (any one of the three areas) to requiring impairment in social interaction and *either* impairment in verbal and nonverbal communication skills or the presence of stereotyped behavior, interest and activities (impairment in social interaction is required in all cases). The diagnostic criteria for tic disorders were also corrected by removing the requirement for distress or impairment in social, academic or other activities, given that many children with tics do not experience either distress or impairment (58).

DSM-V is anticipated to be published in 2012. Prior to starting formal work on DSM-V, a research planning effort was initiated with the goal of stimulating research in advance of starting the DSM-V process. The first phase of the effort produced a series of white papers, which were published in 2002 in *A research agenda for DSM-V* (59). One of the white papers (60) reviewed advances in the developmental sciences and proposed a research agenda for the next decade focusing on six areas of research that have the potential to refine the classification of developmental psychopathology. These included 1) developmental neuroscience and genetics, such as studies in animals to determine associations between maternal behavior and hypothalamic-pituitary-adrenal axis regulation; 2) prevention, including studies of early intervention for children and adolescents; (3) improved diagnostic classification of disorders of infancy and early childhood; (4) improvements in the multiaxial system; (5) approaches to psychiatric assessment: integration of information from different assessment approaches; and (6) developmental epidemiology, entailing large-scale population-based samples of children studied from birth, or even earlier, through adulthood.

Detailed critiques of the various diagnostic approaches have appeared (8, 61–63). Criticisms have been made of both the overarching framework and its specifics. In the DSM-III in particular, certain categories were introduced on the basis of rather limited data. The reliability and validity of at least some of the various categories proposed were questionable. Reliability is generally best for the more common and more broadly defined disorders. Information on the stability of the various childhood diagnoses has been limited.

Dimensional Approaches

In contrast to the more clinically oriented (categorical) approach, multivariate (dimensional) approaches to diagnosis offer several potential advantages in that various behaviors and dimensions of behavior are assessed, rather than single, presumably pathognomonic, features (8, 33, 34). Similarly, the dimensional approach can encompass symptom coding in other than a dichotomous fashion; for example, "never," "sometimes," and "always" could be coded, rather than simply presence or absence, to rate specific diagnostic features. Various rating scales, checklists, and so forth can be used for multivariate classification schemes based on self, parent, or teacher report or on direct observation; many such instruments are described in subsequent chapters. As noted previously, various statistical techniques such as factor and cluster analysis may be used to derive relevant clinician patterns or profiles. These patterns may, in turn, be used to derive categorical diagnoses. Given the inherent problems in sample selection and instrument development, issues of replication are particularly important (12).

Jenkins and Glickman (64) and Hewitt and Jenkins (65) were among the first to examine patterns of relationships (correlations) between variables to derive syndrome groupings. A large series of case records was studied, and the presence or absence of specific behaviors was noted in each case. Clusters of deviant behavior were noted, and broad patterns of disturbance (socialized delinquent, overinhibited, unsocialized aggressive) were identified. Subsequently, more sophisticated methods have been applied to a range of children using a variety of assessment instruments (33). Studies done using this approach generally identify several factors with relative consistency; factors identified have included conduct disturbance, overactivity, and emotional disturbance (12, 66).

Not surprisingly, the stability of more narrowly defined factors is less robust. Similarly, as would be expected, such techniques have limited usefulness in detecting children with disorders of very low prevalence.

Reliability of dimensions derived from multivariate studies has been assessed and is generally satisfactory (8). Stability of dimensions or profiles is somewhat more complex to assess, in that some change is, of course, expected, but short-term stability appears to be within acceptable limits (8). The use of dimensional assessment instruments clearly avoids certain of the pitfalls inherent in the categorical approach, for example, in terms of the loss of information inherent in application of dichotomous categories, in increasing reliability, and in issues of "caseness." These issues are relevant to medicine in general and not just to psychiatry.

For some purposes, dimensional assessment instruments are particularly valuable. For such assessments to be clinically useful, their validity must be demonstrated, for example, in terms of some associated features, such as familial pattern or course. The assumption that characteristics have the same meaning throughout their distribution is often questionable (e.g., severe mental retardation differs in a host of ways from normal intelligence) (55). Certain disorders clearly do *not* shade off into normality.

RELATIONSHIP OF CATEGORICAL AND DIMENSIONAL APPROACHES

There are major areas of agreement between both the categorical and dimensional approaches; this is particularly true for the more common disorders. Analysis of data from dimensional assessment instruments has proved useful in the development of categorical systems, for example, in supporting division of conduct disorder into various types. Probably the greatest drawback to the use of such assessments in clinical practice arises from the difficulty in using such instruments in a simple way for purposes of communication; for clinical purposes, it is more helpful to know that a child has attention deficit hyperactivity disorder and learning problems than to know his or her factor or profile scores on a dimensional assessment instrument. Dimensional and categorical approaches need not be used in mutually exclusive ways; the multiaxial classification used in the DSM-III-R, for example, employs both approaches in that although disorders are categorically defined, assessments of severity of psychosocial stressors and global assessment of functioning are dimensional.

IDEOGRAPHIC APPROACHES

Ideographic approaches to diagnosis are common in clinical practice. In the broader sense of diagnosis (as diagnostic process) (29), most clinicians target certain problems or issues for intervention that relate only in part to categorical or even dimensional diagnosis. In some ways, such approaches are more practical in certain situations (family therapy), although again they can be used in conjunction with categorical approaches. They are less useful for certain purposes (in considering pharmacological intervention) (1). Past the level of the individual cases, the utility of ideographic approaches is limited. Such approaches make it very difficult to communicate information for clinical and research purposes in a concise and readily understood fashion. Chapter 4.2.6 suggests efficient ways of incorporating the various classification systems into a meaningful understanding of the patient, in order to institute a balanced and informed treatment plan.

MULTIAXIAL CLASSIFICATION IN CHILD AND ADOLESCENT PSYCHIATRY

Multiaxial classification offers considerable potential advantages for child and adolescent psychiatric disorder (10, 12, 29). In important ways, it parallels the diagnostic process in that different kinds of information are collected and coded independently. Given that the diagnostic picture is often complex and that different conditions and kinds of conditions are associated with one another, the use of a multiaxial system, at least theoretically, should help clinicians by directing their attention to the major relevant areas of diagnosis. In actual practice, clinicians vary considerably in their use of multiple axes, although the use of such a system would be expected, generally, to increase reliability. Putting developmental disorders on a separate axis would, for example, emphasize their developmental, as opposed to "psychiatric," nature and would remind clinicians to look for such disorders in the course of their regular clinical work. Conversely, the placement of certain disorders within a multiaxial framework is problematic; enuresis, for example, clearly has developmental correlates but is generally included as a psychiatric, as opposed to developmental, disorder.

In the absence of a multiaxial system, certain conditions are particularly likely to be overlooked, such as the developmental learning disorders of a child with conduct disorder. Similarly, coding of medical syndromes is helpful in alerting the clinician to potential problems that contribute to the mental or developmental disorder, are associated with it, or should be considered in the provision of a remedial plan. Theoretically, many different kinds of information could be incorporated within a multiaxial framework (intellectual level, adequacy of school placement, associated psychosocial problems). One of the dilemmas, particularly for disorders in adolescence, relates to the problem of comorbidity; often children have more than one diagnosis. This comorbidity may be more apparent than real or may represent a more substantive problem in which, for example, having one disorder predisposes to the second or in which the risk factors for one disorder are also risk factors for the second. Artifactual comorbidity adds little to the classification system; for example, for a child with autism to also receive a diagnosis of stereotypy-habit disorder seems redundant because stereotypies are commonly observed in autism and are included as one of the potential defining features of the condition. In other instances, such as conduct disorder with depression, the particular comorbid pattern does appear to provide important distinguishing features (67). In ICD-10, the general approach is to provide a special code for such conditions, whereas in DSM-IV, the usual diagnoses would be made with no special notation of the concomitant occurrence of the condition. Despite this difference, the general difference in approach to clinical and research diagnosis, and some differences around a few categories, these two systems have tended toward convergence.

SUMMARY

Classification in child and adolescent psychiatry has multiple meanings and functions. Complications for classification of child and adolescent disorders are myriad: The child is often not the person complaining; different kinds of data may be used in making a diagnosis; developmental factors may have a major impact on the expression of disorders; and certain features (e.g., beliefs in fantasy figures) are normative at certain ages but not at others. Additional complications are posed by the unintended, but no less real, uses to which diagnostic concepts are put, such as their inclusion in legislation and their use as mandates for services in educational programs or for purposes of insurance reimbursement for services. Different kinds and levels of classification are needed for different purposes.

The past 20 years witnessed tremendous advances in the area of diagnosis and classification of child and adolescent psychopathology. These advances are particularly welcome because work in this area had lagged behind that in the adult psychiatric disorders. Various approaches to classification have been employed; each has its advantages and limitations. Issues of reliability and validity remain to be addressed for many categories and classification systems; the attempt to address these issues through examining empirical data rather than theorizing is perhaps the greatest accomplishment of these efforts.

Tensions between clinical and research utility will continue to exist. As classification systems become more complex, they are less readily used; conversely, simplistic systems fail to capture important aspects of clinical experience. The likely ability, over the next decade, to identify more clearly the role of genetic factors for at least a few conditions and the growing sophistication of statistical approaches to aspects of classification and diagnosis represent important areas for future work.

A classification scheme is best used by persons with considerable training who take the task of diagnosis (in its broadest sense) seriously. Although categorical systems increasingly use diagnostic criteria, these are often not truly operationalized, although they are often abstracted and reified for specific purposes (development of interview schedules administered by lay interviewers, or the use of simple frequency counts or symptom duration that obscures the more central aspects of the underlying clinical construct). Although the various "official" systems present areas of disagreement, the areas of agreement are even more noteworthy. Certain issues, such as classification of combination categories versus use of multiple diagnoses, remain to be resolved. Specific issues arise with respect to inclusionary and exclusionary rules and aspects of comorbidity. Although much has been accomplished, considerable work remains to be done.

References

1. Werry JS: ICD 9 and DSM III classification for the clinician. *J Child Psychol Psychiatry* 26:1–6, 1985.
2. Jaspers K: *General psychopathology* (Hoenig J, Hamilton M, trans.). Manchester, University Press, 1962.
3. Hobbs N (ed): *Issues in the classification of children.* San Francisco, Jossey-Bass, 1975.
4. World Health Organization: Mental and behavioral disorders, clinical descriptions and diagnostic guidelines. In: *International classification of diseases*, 10th ed. Geneva, World Health Organization, 1992.
5. American Psychiatric Association: *Diagnostic and statistical manual of mental disorders*, 4th ed. Washington, DC, American Psychiatric Association, 1994.
6. Blashfield RG, Draguns JG: Evaluative criteria for psychiatric classification. *J Abnorm Psychol* 85:140–150, 1976.
7. Hempel CG: Problems of taxonomy. In: Zubin J (ed.): *Field studies in the mental disorders.* London, Grune & Stratton 1961, pp. 3–22.
8. Quay HC: Classification. In: Quay HC, Werry JS (eds.): *Psychopathological disorders of childhood*, 3rd ed. New York, Wiley, 1986, pp 1–34.
9. Rutter M: Classification and categorization in child psychiatry. *J Child Psychol Psychiatry* 6:71–83, 1965.
10. Rutter M, Shaffer D, Shepherd M: *A multiaxial classification of child psychiatric disorders.* Geneva, World Health Organization, 1975.
11. Spitzer RL, Cantwell DP: The DSM-III classification of the psychiatric disorders of infancy, childhood, and adolescence. *J Am Acad Child Psychiatry* 19:356–370, 1980.
12. Rutter M, Gould M: Classification. In: Rutter M, Hersov L (eds): *Child and adolescent psychiatry: Modern approaches*, 2nd ed. Oxford, Blackwell Scientific, 1985, pp. 304–321.
13. Morey LC: Personality disorders in DSM-III and DSM-III-R: Convergence, coverage, and internal consistency. *Am J Psychiatry* 145:573–577, 1988.
14. Zigler E, Glick M: *A developmental approach to psychopathology.* New York, Wiley, 1986.
15. Freud A: *Normality and pathology in childhood.* New York, International Universities Press, 1965.
16. Mattison RE, Hooper SR: The history of modern classification of child and adolescent psychiatric disorders: An overview. In: Hooper SR, Hynd GW, Mattison RE (eds): *Assessment and Diagnosis of Child and Adolescent Psychiatric Disorders. Vol 1: Psychiatric Disorders.* Hillsdale, NJ, Erlbaum, 1992.
17. Feighner J, Robbins E, Guze DB, Woodruff RA, Winokur G, Munoz R: Diagnostic criteria for use in psychiatric research. *Arch Gen Psychiatry* 26:57–63, 1972.
18. Weber AC, Scharfetter C: The syndrome concept: History and statistical operationalizations. *Psychol Med* 14:315–325, 1984.
19. Volkmar FR, Cohen DJ: Disintegrative disorder or "late onset" autism. *J Child Psychol Psychiatry* 30:717–724, 1989.
20. Bell RQ, Harper LV: *Child effects on adults.* Hillsdale, NJ, Erlbaum, 1977.
21. Klin A, Chawarska K, Paul R, Rubin E, Morgan T, Wiesner L, Volkmar F: Autism in a 15-month-old child. *Am J of Psychiatry* 161(11):1981–1988, 2004.
22. Lord C: Follow-up of two-year-olds referred for possible autism. *J Child Psychol Psychiatry* 36(8):1365–1382, 1995.
23. Zeanah C (ed): *Handbook of Infant Mental Health.* New York, Guilford, 1993, pp 236–249.
24. Kagan J: *Change and Continuity in Infancy.* New York, Wiley, 1971.
25. Chess S, Thomas A: *Temperament in Clinical Practice.* New York, Guilford, 1986.
26. Earls FR: Application of DSM-III in an epidemiological study of preschool children. *Am J Psychiatry* 139:242–243, 1982.
27. Mezzich JE, von Cranach M: *International Classification in Psychiatry: Unity and Diversity.* Cambridge, Cambridge University Press, 1988.
28. Ozonoff S, Rogers S J, Hendren RL (eds.): *Autism spectrum disorders: A research review for practitioners.* Washington, DC: American Psychiatric Publishing, Inc, 2003.
29. Cohen DJ, Leckman JF, Volkmar FR: The diagnostic process and classification in child psychiatry: Issues and prospects. In: Mezzich JE, von Vranach M (eds.): *International Classification in Psychiatry: Unity and Diversity.* Cambridge, Cambridge University Press, 1988, pp. 284–297.
30. Swets JA: Measuring the accuracy of diagnostic systems. *Science* 240:1285–1292, 1988.
31. Valliant GE, Schnurr P: What is a case? *Arch Gen Psychiatry* 45:313–319, 1988.
32. Grove WM, Andreasen NC, McDonald-Scott P, Keller MB, Shapiro RW: Group for the Advancement of Psychiatry, 1966. Reliability studies of psychiatric diagnosis: Theory and practice. *Arch Gen Psychiatry* 38:408–413, 1981.
33. Achenbach TM: Integrating assessment and taxonomy. In: Rutter M, Tuma H, Lann IS (eds): *Assessment and Diagnosis in Child Psychopathology.* New York, Guilford, 1988, pp. 300–339.
34. Achenbach TM, Edelbrock CS: The classification of child psychopathology: A review and analysis of empirical efforts. *Psychol Bull* 85:1275–1301, 1978.
35. Kraemer HC: Assessment of 2X2 associations: Generalization of signal detection methodology. *Am Statist* 42:37–49, 1988.
36. Szatmari P, Volkmar F, Walter S: Latent class models and the evaluation of diagnostic criteria for autism. *J Am Acad Child Adolesc Psychiatry* 34:216–222, 1995.
37. Zoccolillo M, Pickes A, Quinton D, et al.: The outcome of conduct disorder: Implications for defining adult personality disorder and conduct disorder. *Psychol Med* 22:971–986, 1992.
38. Kraepelin E: *Compendium der Psychiatrie.* Leipzig, Abel, 1883.
39. American Psychiatric Association: *Diagnostic and Statistical Manual of Mental Disorders*, 2nd ed. Washington, DC, American Psychiatric Association, 1968.
40. American Psychiatric Association: *Diagnostic and Statistical Manual of Mental Disorders*, 3rd ed. Washington, DC, American Psychiatric Association, 1980.
41. American Psychiatric Association: *Diagnostic and Statistical Manual of Mental Disorders*, 3rd ed., rev. Washington, DC, American Psychiatric Association, 1987.
42. Puig-Antich J: The use of RDC criteria for major depressive disorder in children and adolescents. *J Am Acad Child Psychiatry* 21:291–293, 1982.
43. Spitzer RL, Endicott JE, Robins E: Research diagnostic criteria. *Arch Gen Psychiatry* 35:773–782, 1978.
44. Schwab-Stone M, Towbin KE, Tarnoff GM: Systems of classification: ICD-10, DSM-III-R, and DSM-IV. In: Lewis M (ed.): *Child and Adolescent Psychiatry: A Comprehensive Textbook.* Baltimore, Williams & Wilkins, 1991, pp. 422–434.
45. Frances AJ, Widiger TA, Pincus HA: The development of DSM-IV. *Arch Gen Psychiatry* 46:373–375, 1989.
46. Widiger TA, Frances AJ, Pincus HA, et al.: Toward an empirical classification for the DSM-IV. J *Abnorm Psychol* 100:280–288, 1991.
47. Lahey BB, Applegate B, McBurnett K, Biederman J, Greenhill L, Hynd GW, Barkley RA, Newcorn J, Jensen P, Richters J: DSM-IV field trials for attention deficit hyperactivity disorder in children and adolescents. *Am J Psychiatry* 151:1673–1685, 1994.
48. Volkmar FR, Klin A, Siegel B, Szatmari P, Lord C, Campbell M, Freeman B, Cicchetti D, Rutter M, Kline W: Field trial for autistic disorder in DSM-IV. *Am J Psychiatry* 151:1361–1367, 1994.
49. Kramer M: The history of the efforts to agree on an international classification of mental disorders. In: *Diagnostic and Statistical Manual*

of *Mental Disorders*, 2nd ed. Washington, DC, American Psychiatric Association, 1968, pp. xi–xx.
50. Brämer G: Tenth revision of the *International Classification of Diseases*: In progress. *Br J Psychiatry* 152[Suppl]:29–32, 1988.
51. Sartorius N: International perspectives of psychiatric classification. *Br J Psychiatry* 152[Suppl]:9–14, 1988.
52. World Health Organization: *International Classification of Diseases*, 9th ed. Geneva, World Health Organization, 1977.
53. Cooper JE: The structure and presentation of contemporary psychiatric classifications with special reference to ICD-9 and 10. *Br J Psychiatry* 152[Suppl]:21–28, 1988.
54. Rutter M: Annotation: Child psychiatric disorders in ICD-10. *J Child Psychol Psychiatry* 30:499–513, 1989.
55. Rutter M, Tuma AN: Diagnosis and classification: Some outstanding issues. In: Rutter M, Tuma H, Lann IS (eds): *Assessment and diagnosis in child psychopathology*. New York, Guilford, 1988, pp. 437–445
56. Volkmar FR, Woolston JL: Comorbidity of psychiatric disorders in children and adolescents. In: Wexler S (ed.): *Comorbidity in psychiatry*. New York, Wiley, 1997, pp. 307–322.
57. American Psychiatric Association: *Diagnostic and statistical manual of mental disorders*, 4th ed, text rev. Washington, DC, American Psychiatric Association, 2000.
58. First MB, Pincus HA: The DSM-IV text revision: Rationale and potential impact on clinical practice. *Psych Services* Mar:53(3):288–92, 2002.
59. Kupfer DA, First MB, Regier DA: *A research agenda for DSM-V*. Washington, DC: American Psychiatric Publishing, 2002.
60. Pine DS, Alegria M, Cook EH, Costello EJ, Dahl RE, Koretz D, Merikangas KR, Reiss AL, Vitiello B: Advances in developmental science and DSM-V. In: Kupfer DA, First MB, Regier DA (eds.). *A research agenda for DSM-V*, Washington, DC: American Psychiatric Publishing, 2002, pp. 85–122.
61. Achenbach TM: DSM-III in light of empirical research on the classification of child psychopathology. *J Am Acad Child Psychiatry* 19:395–412, 1980.
62. Garmezy N: Never mind the psychologists: Is it good for children? *Clin Psychol* 31:1–6, 1978.
63. Rutter M, Shaffer D: DSM-III: A step forward or back in terms of the classification of child psychiatric disorder. *J Am Acad Child Psychiatry* 10:371–394, 1980.
64. Jenkins RL, Glickman S: Common syndromes in child psychiatry. *Am J Orthopsychiatry* 16:244–261, 1946.
65. Hewitt LE, Jenkins RL: *Fundamental patterns of maladjustment: The dynamics of their origin*. Springfield, IL, State of Illinois, 1946.
66. Achenbach TM, Conners CK, Quay HC, et al.: Replication of empirically derived syndromes as a basis for taxonomy of child/adolescent psychopathology. *J Abnorm Child Psychol* 17:299–323, 1989.
67. Angold A, Rutter M: Effects of age and pubertal status on depression in a large clinical sample. *Dev Psychopathol* 4:5–28, 1992.

4.2 ■ DIAGNOSTIC ASSESSMENT

CHAPTER 4.2.1 ■ CLINICAL ASSESSMENT OF INFANTS AND TODDLERS

WALTER S. GILLIAM AND LINDA C. MAYES

Why perform infant assessments? It is perhaps easier to state definitively what infant assessments cannot provide. They do not provide a measure of fixed or immutable intelligence, a trajectory for future development, or a window on future adjustment, nor can they typically partial out the various potential causal factors. Results are descriptive, with only limited application for etiological understanding or detailed prognosticating. Questions such as "How much of this infant's delay comes from his environment, versus how much from his prematurity?" or "What will be the eventual extent of this child's developmental disability?" are not definitively answerable by a developmental assessment. Developmental assessments, however complete and skillfully done, cannot provide sure predictions of long-term outcome or parcel out the complex contributions of endowment, experience, and maturational forces.

Despite the above caveats, assessment of infant development can be highly useful, and in many cases essential to proper clinical treatment. Skillfully done, these assessments can help create a picture of the child's current developmental level and environmental context that can be invaluable to sound clinical decisionmaking and treatment planning. Essentially, developmental assessment results help provide a lens through which we might be better able to perceive the world from the child's perspective. Indeed, Bagnato and Neisworth (1) have pointed out that the word *assidere* (the Greek origin of *assessment*) literally means "to sit beside," and hence to get to know someone.

Clinical assessment of infants and toddlers is a subspecialty area of clinical practice. Not all psychiatrists, psychologists, pediatricians, and other professionals will possess the training and degree of closely supervised practice necessary to competently and independently conduct such evaluations. Those professionals who do possess these specialized skills typically have acquired them through formal subspecialization near the end of their professional training.

A BRIEF HISTORY OF INFANT DEVELOPMENTAL ASSESSMENT

A brief discussion of the history of infant assessment may provide an illustration of the evolving aims and technological advances in this field. (A more complete history is provided by Gilliam & Mayes (2), and the more ambitious readers are referred to Brooks & Weinraub (3) and Wyly (4).)

The Late 1800s: Enlightenment and Curiosity

In the late nineteenth century, the European scientific community was consumed with a fervor and creativity best characterized by the studies of evolution, theories about the unconscious mind, and a growing concern for the mentally deficient and insane. The field of experimental psychology was largely concerned with the measurement of various perceptual abilities, and the science of child development was dominated by single-child case studies—often the children of the scientists. Although these "baby biographies" were insufficient for benchmarking normal child development, they provided the basis for the creation of development tests during the twentieth century.

1900–1920: The Birth of Intelligence Testing

The concept of measuring infant capacities grew out of the concern of scientists of the time to find a metric for human intelligence that would permit the creation of criteria for schools for children with intellectual deficiencies (5). In 1904 the minister of public education in Paris appointed Binet and Simon to be members of a commission studying the question of special education. In response to their charge, Binet and Simon developed the concept of mental age and a test, published in 1905, for measuring it (3). Terman (6) created an adaptation of the Binet-Simon test for use in the United States and revised the concept of mental age by creating the intelligence quotient (IQ), a ratio between mental age and chronological age multiplied by 100.

1920–1940: "Infant IQ" versus "Developmental" Models

In the decades that followed the development of Terman's IQ test, two basic approaches were used in exploring intellectual development in infants. One approach, the infant IQ model, sought to extend downward the IQ assessment model to children younger than school age, eventually including infants. A second approach, the Gesellian model, sought to create a new model of assessment that began with the newborn and extended upward. In contrast to the "baby biographers" of the previous century, the more behaviorally empirical scientists of the 1920s and '30s relied on direct observation of child behavior across several children under highly structured conditions.

The best example of an infant IQ or infant cognition test is the *Cattell Infant Intelligence Scale* (7). Cattell's test was conceptualized as a downward extension of the 1937 Stanford-Binet Intelligence Scale, the much-revised American version of the Binet-Simon test. Although some initial studies were encouraging, the ability of the Cattell and other infant IQ tests to predict an infant's later IQ was weak (8). Overall, "infant IQ tests" were found to be inadequate at meaningfully extending the IQ assessment model into infancy and are now all but extinct in use.

At about the same time that first "infant IQ tests" were being developed, Arnold Gesell began his groundbreaking work at Yale University on systematically documenting normal maturational development in infants and toddlers, leading to the creation of the *Gesell Developmental Schedules* (GDS), first published in 1925. Several aspects of Gesell's work distinguish it from those of his predecessors and contemporaries. First, whereas the infant IQ tradition grew from an interest in identifying deviant patterns of development, Gesell's interest was mostly in documenting normal developmental trends. Second, Gesell's model supported the conceptualization of development occurring simultaneously in many distinct but interrelated domains (9), as opposed to a singular factor of intellectual ability. Third, Gesell's model of developmental maturation supported an understanding of the effects of the child's environment in altering the course of development, as opposed to viewing IQ as a stable and static trait, opening the way for the more transactional and dynamic understanding of developmental processes that would later prevail.

Gesell's work was farreaching, and subsequent researchers relied heavily on the developmental tasks and techniques he pioneered. Most notable was Nancy Bayley of the Berkley Institute of Child Welfare. Bayley applied testing concepts more familiar to the infant IQ model to the assessment techniques developed by Gesell. The result was the development of two scales of infant development that would later revolutionize and dominate the field of infant assessment: the *California First-Year Mental Scale* (10, 11) and the *California Infant Scale of Motor Development* (12, 13).

1940–1960: The Fall of the "Infant IQ" Model

In the 1940s and 1950s, the science of infant developmental assessment gained greater international attention, through the publishing of the *Griffiths Mental Development Scale* (14) in London. At that time, infant assessment techniques were used primarily for diagnosis and categorization purposes, e.g., preadoptive screening, testing for admission to special schools, or evaluating physical handicaps (15). The assessments for diagnosis and categorization were predicated on clinicians' continuing adherence to the belief that intelligence is fixed from infancy. This belief in a fixed IQ still was so well rooted that evidence to the contrary (findings documenting an increase in IQ in high-risk infants after nursery school attendance) was being dismissed and attributed to poor standardization of the scales (3). In the context of this debate, American developmentalists first began to consider seriously the stage theory of Jean Piaget, which clearly favored the view of qualitative, rather than simply quantitative, differences in the abilities of children of various ages. It was largely on the basis of Bayley's longitudinal work with her developmental instruments (16) that the concept of an immutable IQ that was fixed at birth was discredited. The use of infant IQ tests continued for a while, but are now all but extinct in use.

The 1960s and 70s: Breakthroughs in Infant Test Development

The 1960s and 1970s brought a new wave of infant development tests, more rigorously standardized on larger numbers of infants, with careful testing of interobserver agreement and test-retest reliability. The *Bayley Scales of Infant Development* (BSID) (17) consolidated Bayley's original two scales into one assessment instrument with norms based on a nationally representative sample of infants. The BSID set a new and enduring standard of sophistication for the development and standardization of infant developmental assessment tools. Thoughtful research led to far more caution about the predictive validity of early assessment and to important conceptual revisions. Concomitant interest in newborn capacities and the rapidly emerging field of newborn sensory perception also led to the development of a number of scales to measure competency in newborns.

1980–Present: New Directions in Infant Developmental Assessment

The 1980s and 1990s were dominated by increasing psychometric improvements; a renewed interest in diagnostic functionality, again primarily driven by the needs of public education; and the application of information-processing theory to the study of infant development. Federal mandates for the special education of young children created the need for an arsenal of assessment tools that encompassed all of the qualifying areas of delay, utilized information from both direct assessment of the child and parent report, and facilitated early intervention treatment planning and program accountability. Also, a plethora of brief developmental screening instruments also were developed for use by professionals with relatively little training in formal assessment.

The advent of information-processing theories of human intelligence led to more elaborate models of infant cognition. Several studies have shown measures of infant information-processing (e.g., attention, recognition, stimulus habituation, and memory) to be significantly related to later IQ scores (several excellent reviews are available (18, 19)). However, these measures can be difficult to administer under usual clinical assessment conditions, and the model has not been translated to clinical assessment tools. Regardless, measures of information-processing may play an important role in the next generations of developmental assessment instruments.

SOURCES OF INFORMATION IN AN INFANT ASSESSMENT

The developmental assessment of infants involves more than the simple administration of a set of developmental test protocols. Assessments performed in the first three years of life require the clinician to function simultaneously as a generalist and a specialist, to blend quiet observation with active probing, to synthesize information from caregivers with that gathered through direct observation of the child, and to be involved in a curious blend of searching for specifically defined responses from a child with inferences based on behavior. This set of skills is indeed important for adequate clinical assessment of children of all ages. However, the need is even greatest for those providing clinical services to these youngest of patients, since development during the early years is the most rapid, context-dependent, and intersystemic.

Next we discuss general sources of information and three techniques that are central for the clinician doing infant assessments: interviewing skills, observation of children and of caregiver-child interactions (apart from formal structured testing), and synthesis of the information gathered during the evaluation. (See Table 4.2.1.1 for a summary of some of the information obtained during an infant assessment.) While interviewing, observation, and synthesis are the skills of medical diagnosis in general, there are unique aspects to each in the process of assessing infants.

Interviewing

It is axiomatic that skillful interviewing is central to a complete developmental assessment, since much of the data about infants' daily functioning and their relationships with others come from interviews with the caregivers. Skillful interviewing techniques include letting caregivers begin their story wherever they choose; using directed, information-gathering questions in such a way as to clarify but not disrupt the parents' account; and listening for affect as much as content. Importantly, nearly every step of the assessment process requires an alliance between clinician and caregiver, since infants usually perform better when they are in the company of familiar adults, and the initial interview between clinician and family is crucial in setting the tone for such an alliance. Moreover, establishing an alliance is central to evaluating infants' interactions with the adults in their world. Indeed, infant assessments are quite compromised when there are no familiar adults available to meet with the clinician and be with the infant. Parenthetically, it is often in cases involving the most severe environmental disturbance that clinicians do not have access to caregivers that are able to describe the infant's history.

Addressing Caregiver Fears Regarding the Assessment

When parents, foster parents, or other caregivers are available, skillful interviewing is also critical in helping parents follow through with the assessment process. Coming for a developmental evaluation or participating in one while their infant is hospitalized is enormously stressful and often frightening for caregivers. Clinicians working with infants and their families need to understand that, regardless of what caregivers have been told about the assessment, caregivers' fears and fantasies about the process are as potent as the facts of the presenting problem. Not uncommonly, caregivers have begun to see the infant as damaged or defective in some way and are afraid and

TABLE 4.2.1.1

SOME OF THE INFORMATION OBTAINED DURING AN INFANT ASSESSMENT

Caregiver Interview	Observation or Formal Evaluation of Child

■ Family history
■ Genetic influences
■ History of pregnancy, delivery, perinatal period
■ Developmental history (developmental milestones, previous assessments)
■ Medical history
■ Child care and extended family arrangements
■ Child's psychological role in family
■ Caregiver perceptions and expectations of child
■ Stability of home/family environment
■ Family social support systems
■ Family functioning, stress and coping (alcohol and drug abuse, domestic violence, etc.)
	■ Physical health, appearance and growth parameters
	■ Sensory development (vision, hearing, tactile, etc.)
	■ Gross motor development
	■ Fine motor development
	■ Communication development
	  ■ Receptive communication
	  ■ Expressive communication
	  ■ Speech clarity and fluency
	■ Cognitive problemsolving
	■ Developing sense of self
	■ Social relatedness and interest in environment
	■ Capacity for affect regulation and coping skills
	■ Emerging mastery motivation
	■ Capacity for symbolic representation and play

Observation of Caregiver and Infant ■ Infant's use of caregiver for support and reassurance ■ Caregiver's attunement and responsiveness to child's affective state ■ Elicitation and receipt of positive interactions ■ Security of attachment between caregiver and infant ■ Caregiver affective response to child's efforts during assessment	

guilty about the effect of their own behavior on the infant. Their fears of what the infant's problems signify may be expressed in many ways. They may anticipate that their infant has a serious developmental disability, such as autism or mental retardation, or that the infant will have serious emotional difficulties in school, or that they themselves will be, or already are, inadequate caregivers. It is always a vulnerable time for caregivers, and clinicians should keep in mind that what seem inconsequential moments and statements to them may be memorable and powerful for many caregivers. Furthermore, the stress of coming for an assessment affects the caregivers' abilities to report about the infant's development. Often, the "facts" start to change as the alliance between caregivers and clinician develops.

Active Listening

When first interviewed, caregivers may be reluctant to be candid or may not themselves be fully aware of their own perceptions and beliefs about the infant. Open-ended questions, allowing caregivers to begin their story wherever they feel most comfortable, and conveying a nonjudgmental attitude are crucial beginning points in establishing the working alliance. Also, at the risk of stating the obvious, such "interviews" involve considerably more listening than active questioning. Indeed, the type of active listening involved in this type of interview requires the clinician to do much more than passively collect and record requested information, it involves forming numerous connections between "factual" information, observational information (the reactions of the caregivers and their affective responses), and an appreciation of the context of the relationship between the caregiver and the clinician.

The Content of the Interview

Practically, the purpose of interviews with parents, foster parents, or other caregivers is to gather information about the infant. Highlighted above is the affective atmosphere in which such datagathering best occurs. The important areas to cover in terms of the infant's development are the medical history and major developmental milestones; the history of the mother's pregnancy, delivery, and immediate perinatal period; the number, ages, and health of family members; and how the infant fits in the family's daily life (20). The meaning of the individual child for all caregivers is an important window on the infant's place in the family. Many infants and toddlers attend child care or early intervention programs, and the perception of those teachers, as well as their relationship with the infant's primary caregivers at home, also is important.

More specifically, the interviewer should try to get a picture of the caregivers' perceptions of the infant's level of functioning in several areas. These include motor development and activity level, speech and communication, problemsolving and play, self-regulation (ease of comforting, need for routines), relationships with others, and level of social responsiveness. Questions about whether or not the pregnancy was planned or came at a good time for the family and what expectations the parents had for the infant provide important information about perceptions, disappointments, and stresses. Similarly, asking the caregivers of whom the infant reminds them or what traits in their infant they like best and least may be useful avenues for learning about how the parents view both the infant's problem and his or her place within their family.

Techniques of Organizing Information

Provence (21) has suggested that a productive method of gathering developmental and family data is to ask the caregivers to describe a day in the life of their child. Provence outlines how this question can be the framework for learning about daily activities, how the infant and caregivers interact throughout the day, and about interactions around mealtime, bedtime, or times of distress. When all major caregivers are present for the interview, this question provides a time for each of them to present descriptions of his or her time with, and perceptions of, the child. Additionally, clinicians may use structured interviews, such as the *Vineland Adaptive Behavior Scales* (22) currently under revision, in order to collect both quantitative developmental data and provide an opportunity to open new areas of clinical discussion. Also, the *Infant-Toddler Developmental Assessment* (IDA) (23), appropriate for infants from birth to 36 months, is particularly useful in providing schemata for organizing important information from caregiver interviews, medical/developmental records, and behavioral observations.

Implicit in this overview of interviewing caregivers as a part of the clinical assessment is the assumption that such assessments require several sessions. Minimally, one meeting with caregivers, two or more with the child and caregivers together, and another to present the results to the caregivers are necessary. The sessions with the infant also provide an opportunity to gather more interview information, as other questions will occur in the context of the child's behavior and performance. For example, asking whether the child's response to a particular situation within the evaluation context is usual for him or her may open up another area of information from the caregivers. As is likely clear from these suggestions, in our view, infant assessment is a process of constantly gathering information, revising impressions, and testing hypotheses—and that requires time.

On the other hand, clinicians asked to evaluate infants and young children will not always have the ideal situation outlined above. At times, consultants, caregivers, or both may insist that the evaluation be done in one session, or the clinician may have limited access to the child, as with many evaluations done in a hospital setting. It is important at these times for the clinician to be clear about the limitations of the evaluation findings. Another situation that occurs increasingly commonly and does not fit the ideal model just outlined is when no parents, family members, or other caregivers are available. Situations of severe abuse, abandonment, multiple placements, or seriously ill parents are examples of times in which the clinician will not have available certain critical sources of information. In these instances, certain hypotheses suggested by the child's presentation and status may be left unconfirmed. As in situations where the time for the evaluation is brief, it is most important for clinicians to acknowledge which aspects of their diagnostic formulation are relatively certain, which are not, and what information would likely be clarifying, were it available.

Observing

Observation is the fundamental skill needed for measuring infants' development. After all, most diagnostic evaluations are based on observation of physical signs and/or behavioral responses. However, what distinguishes the observational skill necessary for developmental assessment is that it occurs on many levels simultaneously and is perhaps the area in which the developmentalist's dual role as both generalist and specialist is most evident. Moreover, the observational skills inherent in assessments of infants require a blend of free-floating attention bounded by a structure. In other words, while the clinician must be comfortable enough in the setting to attend to whatever occurs, he or she must also have a mental framework by which to organize the observations collected during the session. Such a framework entails at least four broad areas: a) predominant affective tone of the participants, b) involvement in the situation (curiosity and interest), c) use of others (child's use of the caregivers or examiner), and d) reactions to transitions (initial meetings, end of sessions, changes in amount of structure).

What to Observe

There are several opportunities for careful observation during the course of a clinical assessment. Clinical observation begins from the very first contact with the caregivers and infant, including the caregiver interview addressed above. Many important observations of the infant and infant–caregiver and familial interactions can be obtained during the course of formal developmental assessment. Recently, Benham (24) has provided an elaborated framework for structuring observations of infants and toddlers that may be useful during clinical assessment. In many cases, however, the formal developmental evaluation alone may not provide sufficient opportunity to observe all of the important behaviors of the infant and caregiver. Infants may behave differently with different caregivers and in varying contexts. For this reason, both naturalistic and structured analogue procedures can often be used to gather additional observational data that can be useful for both clinical and research purposes (25). Play-based assessment allows the clinician the opportunity to observe the infant and caregivers in a less structured format than provided by the formal developmental assessment. Also, play observations can be very useful in gaining additional information about the infant's cognitive, symbolic/linguistic, social, and motor development, as well as in assessing internal emotional states and conflicts and the infant's internal dynamic representations of the world (26).

Levels of Observation during Assessment

Within the four broad areas of observation described earlier, the clinician makes observations continuously on at least three levels. Perhaps the most obvious level is the observations of how the child responds to the structured assessment items administered during formal testing. As already stated above, observations during formal testing should not be confined to whether or not the child passes or fails a given item, but to how the child approaches the task. The second level of observation during an infant assessment is how the child reacts to the situation apart from the formal testing structure. Does the child approach toys, initiate interactions, refer to the examiner or his caregivers? How does the child react in the beginning of the evaluation versus later, when the situation and the examiner are more familiar?

The third observational level is a specific focus on the interactions between caregivers and infant. The clinician makes these observations throughout the evaluation process and revises hypotheses as both caregivers and infant become familiar with the process. How to interpret the behaviors one observes between caregivers and child in terms of their ongoing relationship is learned partially by experience and requires time to gather many observational points. However, several general areas may provide important descriptive clues. Does the child refer to the caregivers for both help and reassurance? Similarly, does the child show his successes to the caregivers, and do the caregivers respond? Another important observation for toddlers is whether or not the child leaves his caregivers' immediate company to work with items or explore. For infants, how caregivers hold, feed, and comfort their baby may be windows in the emerging dyadic and familial relationships. A caregiver participates with his or her child during such sessions in varying ways, and the clinician continuously will be assessing qualitative aspects of that participation—how intrusively involved, withdrawn, or comfortably facilitative the caregivers are. One of the most important lessons when learning how to observe interactions between infants and caregivers is that clinical observations, even when based in a naturalistic setting, may or may not be an adequate reflection of what is typical for that particular family. Adults may appear very different as individuals in their own right, compared to when they are interacting with their children. Also, the assessment context where one's child (and by implication, one's self as a person and as a caregiver) observed by another is anxiety provoking in varying degrees for all parents, and may profoundly alter their parenting style.

Formal quantitative developmental evaluation is only part of the overall clinical assessment of infants. Indeed, in some ways, formal testing is the least critical of the clinical assessment tasks and serves more as a frame for clinicians to guide their observations (27). It is not sufficient in assessing infants simply to say that the infant is either developmentally delayed or age adequate. For very young children, assessing development involves elaborating a more complex view of the child and his or her environment, and at this age, every developmental evaluation must include descriptions of behavior and the qualitative aspects of the child's behavior in the structured setting. For example, *when* the infant first turned to a voice or successfully retrieved a toy in a manner appropriate for age may be less important than *how* he or she responded to these tasks (with excitement, positive affect, and energy versus slowly, deliberately, and with little affective response). Such qualitative observations are often the best descriptors of those capacities for which we have few standardized assessment techniques but that are absolutely fundamental to fueling the development of motor, language, and problemsolving skills. Through observing how infants do what they do, the clinician gains information about how infants cope with frustration and how they engage the adult world, as well as about their emotional expressiveness, their capacity for persistence and sustained attention, and the level of investment and psychological energy given to their activities.

Synthesis

The process of synthesizing all the data gathered from the different sources during an assessment is a technique and skill unto itself. Moreover, how this synthesis, with its attendant recommendations, is conveyed to caregivers and other professionals is another essential step in the assessment process, and the assessment is not complete until the therapeutic alliance among all stakeholders is brought to fruition in a collaborative formulation. Infant assessments often involve referring pediatricians and other clinicians, all of whom need to be included individually in the clinician's datagathering interviews and in the final synthesis.

The synthesis of information from an infant assessment differs from the synthesis involved in other medical diagnostic processes in that there are very few specific diagnostic categories that encapsulate all the findings of an infant assessment. The synthesis involved in an infant assessment requires a bringing together of all the data gathered from interviews, observations, and testing into a qualitative description of that infant's capacities in different functional areas (motor, problemsolving, language and communication, and social) and of the infant's current strengths and weaknesses. It also involves integrating the assessment information in the context of the infant's individual environment. For example, an infant who has experienced multiple foster placements may be socially delayed, but such a finding may assume a different significance for an infant who has had a stable home environment.

Synthesizing the large amount of data obtained from a comprehensive clinical infant assessment can be quite daunting. As stated in the introduction, in performing the infant assessment the clinician must be both generalist and specialist. The clinician must draw upon and synthesize knowledge from child psychiatry, pediatrics, neurology, developmental psychology, speech/language therapy, physical and occupational therapy, and often genetics and endocrinology (28). Increasingly, clinicians evaluating young children need also know about early childhood education programs and early intervention, as well as laws regarding child abuse, neglect, and domestic violence. Knowledge from these diverse fields allows a clinician to place the results of a developmental assessment in a meaningful context for the individual child and leads to a better conceptualization of treatment options. For example, understanding the physiological effects of prolonged malnutrition and episodic starvation in infancy (29, 30) helps the clinician evaluate the relatively greater gross motor delays of a child with failure to thrive who has no other neurological signs. Similarly, understanding the effects of a parent's affective disorder on a child's responsiveness to the external world (31) adds another dimension to understanding the infant's muted or absent social interactiveness, babbling, and smiling.

Finally, it is often during the synthesis process that the therapeutic effect for caregivers participating in the assessment is most evident. At the very least, caregivers often change their perceptions of their infant's capacities. They may see strengths in their infant they had not previously recognized or become deeply and painfully aware of weaknesses and vulnerabilities that they may or may not have feared before the assessment. Any of these changes in perceptions may affect the caregivers' view of themselves and of their role as caregivers. Also, infants often change during the assessment process, as their caregivers become more involved in the alliance with the clinician, and they experience, at least temporarily, another adult's concern and interest in their family. Emphasizing the potentially therapeutic value of an assessment underscores that the synthesis process is not simply wrapping up the assessment and conveying information, but is also a time to explore with the caregivers the meaning of the process for them and their infant.

FORMAL DEVELOPMENTAL ASSESSMENT TOOLS

A large array of formal developmental assessment tools for infants and toddlers exists. In this section, we discuss the types of quantitative data obtained from these tests and offer basic considerations for choosing an appropriate evaluation tool. Later, we describe some of the most commonly used developmental instruments.

Types of Quantitative Data

Besides the vast amount of qualitative data obtained by careful observation during testing, most developmental assessment procedures provide several methods of quantifying results. As described later in this chapter, most developmental tests have been standardized and normed on a sample of children selected to represent the performance of typically developing children. It is by comparing an individual infant's performance against this set of norms that most test scores are derived. These scores are then used to convey something about the infant's level of developmental skills acquisition, relative to other presumably typical infants.

Of the several different types of scores available, standard scores and age equivalents are the most commonly used. *Standard scores* are the most robust scores obtainable and represent the infant's performance in relation to other infants of about the same chronological age. Common forms of standard scores include *Z*-scores, deviation scores, and *T*-scores, the latter two being linear transformations of the former. Most tests provide some guidance on how to describe an infant's standard score by placing the scores in descriptive bands (average, below average, mildly delayed). Often, in order to increase the interpretability of these scores, they are converted to percentile ranks. Table 4.2.1.2 presents one common method for descriptively banding standard scores, although many other methods also are used.

Age equivalent scores represent an estimate of the chronological age (usually expressed in months) at which the typically developing infant would demonstrate the skills observed in the infant being assessed. This type of score is often appealing to many caregivers and others with little or no training in psychometric tests, since the interpretation is seemingly straightforward. However, age equivalent scores are notoriously easy to misinterpret and may lead to erroneous conclusions. First, age equivalent scores on infant developmental tests tend to be highly unstable, with the infant's performance on only one or two items largely affecting the age equivalent. Second, age equivalent scores may imply too much about an infant's development, especially when their skills are highly scattered. Because of the way in which age equivalent scores are computed, the score may greatly over- or underestimate an infant's developmental level. Due to the way in which tests are scored, infants who are very consistent in their ability to do tasks typical for their age often receive an age equivalent score much higher than their chronological age, even though they are not yet developmentally ready to do the things associated with that age equivalent. Conversely, infants who, for whatever reason, struggle with some less developmentally mature tasks likely will receive an age equivalent score much below their chronological age, even if they are able to do many things typical of their chronological age or older. In cases such as these, age equivalents are best expressed as a range, if expressed at all. Third, developmental delay expressed in age equivalents does not adequately address the frequency or severity of the delays. Clearly, a 6-month delay in development is different for a 12-month-old versus a 30-month-old. Standard scores, with associated percentile ranks, better express this delay in terms that are less dependent on the chronological age of the infant. Finally, the type of data used to compute age equivalents is too weak statistically to support the calculation of confidence intervals that are useful in placing the score within the context of appropriate bands of error. This lack of confidence intervals further exacerbates the preceding limitations. Of course, there are times when age equivalents may be the best or only option

TABLE 4.2.1.2

DESCRIPTIVE RANGES FOR STANDARD SCORES AND THEIR CORRESPONDING PERCENTILE RANKS

Range	*Z*-Score	Deviation Quotient	*T*-Score	Percentile Rank
Significantly delayed	Below − 2	Below 70	Below 30	2 and below
Mildly delayed	−2 to −1	70 to 84	30 to 39	2 to 15
Average	−1 to +1	85 to 114	40 to 59	16 to 83
Above average	+1 and above	115 and above	60 and above	84 and above

available for expressing an infant's performance (when the extent of developmental delay is so great that standard scores cannot be easily calculated and percentile ranks below the first percentile are obtained).

Considerations for Selecting a Formal Developmental Assessment Tool

Below are some basic guidelines for choosing an infant developmental test that best meets the clinician's specific needs. These guidelines also help provide a framework for evaluating the usefulness of some of the various tests currently in use. Four areas of consideration are presented: purpose, sources of data, standardization, and psychometric properties.

Purpose

A developmental test may be useful for one or more of several different purposes: diagnosis, screening, and early intervention planning. Tests designed for these three purposes are quite different, and selecting the correct tests to match the stated purpose is essential. First, *diagnostic tests* are used to provide information necessary for either clinically or eligibility oriented diagnoses. Clinically oriented diagnoses are used by clinicians in order to capture succinctly the infant's overall presentation and in order to provide a common nomenclature for communicating that information to other clinicians. Eligibility oriented diagnoses, however, are used to identify which infants have levels of developmental delay significant enough to establish eligibility for publicly funded early intervention programs. Often the infant must demonstrate a particular degree of developmental delay (performance that is two standard deviations below the mean) in order to "qualify" for these services. Second, *screening tests* are used when it is desirable to use a relatively brief instrument to identify infants who may be "at risk" for delayed development and would benefit from further diagnostic testing. Usually screening tests are used when relatively many children need to be assessed, and a full diagnostic assessment for all children would be too costly or cumbersome. Third, *intervention-planning tests* are used to plan an individualized early intervention program once children have been diagnosed. These instruments help identify important programmatic goals and objectives or track an infant's achievement of these goals over time in order to document the effects of the intervention.

Sources of Data

Developmental assessment instruments, like all psychometric tests, are methods of collecting and organizing data. Developmental tests for infants use one or more of at least three different types of data: direct assessment, incidental observation, and caregiver report. It is important to acknowledge the strengths and limitations of each data source. Direct assessment has the strength of being potentially very standard in its presentation, so that an infant's performance may be directly compared to other infants with the assumption that the material was presented in a similar standard method. The limitation of direct assessment, however, is that it represents only a small sample of the infant's developmental repertoire that will be influenced greatly by current issues regarding the infant's motivation, mood, comfort, and responsiveness to the examiner and the evaluative process. Caregiver report surveys are a useful addition to formal assessment, in particular to document behaviors that occur too infrequently to be observed in a clinical evaluation, or to assess the caregivers' individual perspectives of their infant. However, caregiver reports should not be the sole measure of the infant's development, since they are highly subject to rater bias (32). Given the strengths and limitations of each of these sources of data, a comprehensive assessment should utilize multiple sources of data across multiple contexts.

Standardization

Test standardization involves the process of developing a consistent method of administration and collecting normative data regarding children's typical performance on the test. It is by this normative data that evaluators determine a specific infant's standing relative to the normative group. This relative standing can then be expressed in terms of either standard scores of age equivalents, as described earlier. It is the responsibility of the test user, however, to decide whether a given test's standardization sample is representative of the type of infants the test user plans to assess. For instance, it clearly would be inappropriate to compare the developmental performance of an infant raised in a large city in a highly developed nation to a normative sample of infants living in a small village in a less developed nation, unless one knew a priori that infants from both of these settings scored very similarly on the test. Most decisions regarding the representativeness of a test's standardization are not this apparent, however. Also, standard scores and age equivalents are norm sample dependent. In other words, scores derived from a nationally standardized test indicate an infant's standing relative to other infants throughout that nation, and not necessarily to other infants of the same specific locality, gender, ethnicity, or economic status. Of course, the inverse is true as well. Some tests are normed on very specific populations of children, such as children from a specific city or state or a particular economic status. The use of standard scores derived from these tests with infants from other localities or economic backgrounds, without specific empirical evidence to justify their generalization, is generally not recommended. Furthermore, in order to yield reliable results, normative data should be no more than about a decade old in order to keep pace with intergenerational escalation in test performance (33). Grossly outdated norms often yield inflated scores that may lead to erroneously disqualifying infants for needed services.

Psychometric Properties

The soundness of a psychometric test is judged based on its reliability (the ability to produce similar results under differing conditions) and validity (the collection of evidence that suggests that the test measures what it is supposed to measure). Several forms of reliability exist. *Test-retest reliability* is a measure of a test's stability over time. Test-retest coefficients are often lower for infant tests as compared to tests designed for older children, due in part to the rapidity of early development. *Inter-rater reliability* refers to the degree to which test scores are not dependent on individual differences between test examiners, but reflect the infant's abilities regardless of who is administering the test. Finally, *internal consistency* refers to the correlation between various test items and provides evidence as to the degree to which a test measures a single unitary construct, as opposed to representing an unrelated collection of test items. As a guideline, reliability coefficients of at least .90 for diagnostic tests and .80 for screening tests are recommended in each of these three areas of reliability (34). Besides their use in evaluating the psychometric soundness of a test, reliability coefficients also serve a clinically relevant purpose. Since no test can be completely reliable, scores are often presented within a given *confidence interval*, which bands the infant's obtained score within a certain range of error (e.g., 100 ± 8). This presentation acknowledges the error inherent in all tests, as opposed to presenting a single score, as if it were an exact measurement. *Validity*, in comparison to reliability, is even more multifaceted. There is no single or preferred way to establish a test's validity. Rather, validity represents an accumulation of evidence that together builds a case for the accuracy of that test. Specifically, infant developmental tests are expected to correlate significantly with other similar tests, to reflect developmental changes that result from expected maturation, and to be sensitive to the presence of diagnosable disorders with clear developmental manifestations.

Psychometric reliability and validity are based on a test's properties as demonstrated with groups of test takers. However, psychometric properties that are more individually relevant are also important. For example, it is important that developmental tests have adequate floors and ceilings. In other words, there should be enough lower level items that significant developmental delays can be detected in even the youngest infants for which the test is to be used (floor). Likewise, there should be enough upper level items that significant developmental precocity can be detected in the oldest children for whom the test is to be used. Since standard scores are obtained by comparing an infant's performance to that of similar age peers, the degree to which the normative data approximates the infant's age also is important. The current standard in infant developmental tests is normative bands of 1 month for infants up to 12 or 18 months old, and 1- to 2-month bands for infants up to 36 months old. In other words, infant tests typically compare an infant's performance to other infants no more than 1 month older or younger, whereas a toddler's performance might be compared to other toddlers 1 to 2 months older or younger. Of course, normative bands that are narrow are preferable to those that are wider.

REVIEW OF SELECTED DEVELOPMENTAL TESTS

A few of the more widely used developmental tests are presented in Table 4.2.1.3, and some of the most common examples are further described below, organized under three basic headings: neonatal, infant/toddler development, and screening.

Neonatal Assessment Tests

Several specific procedures exist for assessing infants during the neonatal period (birth to 4 weeks). Previous studies had shown the well known *Apgar Screening Test* (35) to be an inconsistent predictor of subsequent infant development (36), and neonatal tests were created to focus more expressly on describing the range of neurobehavioral differences in normal newborns and highlighting areas of newborn competency. By the early 1960s, newborns and young infants were seen as more active participants in their environment (37). Not only were they seen as developing intrinsic perceptual-cognitive competencies, but they were viewed also as possessing an individualized repertoire of behaviors, known as temperament, that elicited different responses from others. Although clinicians assessing infants are not often asked to evaluate neonates, the conceptual point inherent in these instruments—combining an assessment of innate capacities with attention to individual variability and responsivity—is relevant to all assessments of infants and young children.

Brazelton Neonatal Behavioral Assessment Scale

Although the predecessor scale to the *Graham/Rosenblith Behavioral Test for Neonates* (38) was the first neonatal development test, the *Brazelton Neonatal Behavioral Assessment Scale* (NBAS), currently in its second edition (39), dominates the field today. The NBAS-2 is intended to assess the neonate's current level of neurobehavioral organization, capacity to respond to the stress of labor and delivery, and adjustment to the ex-utero environment. It is designed for use with neonates of 37 to 44 weeks' gestational age who do not currently need mechanical supports or supplemental oxygen. Though it is recommended that neonates be at least 3 days old before testing, it has been used on neonates during the first day of life. It takes about 20 to 30 minutes to administer, followed by about 15 minutes to record and score the neonate's performance. Although the NBAS was originally designed for use with full-term healthy newborns, it has been used extensively with premature and otherwise medically fragile newborns.

The NBAS-2 is used to describe the range of behavioral responses to social and nonsocial stimuli, as the neonate moves from sleeping to alert states. Items assess the neonate's neurological intactness, behavioral organization (state regulation and autonomic reactivity), and interactiveness and responsiveness with both animate and inanimate stimuli on the basis of 27 behavioral items and 20 reflexes. Relative to preceding neonatal development tests, the NBAS-2 places a greater emphasis on assessing the neonates's social competencies, as opposed to assessing only perceptual capacities or behaviors that were presumed to be related to cognitive functioning (3). The NBAS-2 is begun, optimally, when the neonate is sleeping and completed as the neonate is brought to an alert, interactive state. Each behavioral observation is scored along a seven- to nine-point continuum.

The NBAS-2 does not yield a single score, although Als et al. (40) have proposed an a priori four-factor solution. The four-factor scores describe interactiveness, motoric behavior, state control, and physiological response to stress. Lester et al. (41) have summarized the behavioral items as six factors (habituation, orientation, motor, range of state, regulation of state, and autonomic regulation) and use the neurological reflex behaviors to define a seventh factor. Each of the seven factors can be used to yield a numerical score describing the infant's performance in that area. Higher scores on the six behavioral factors indicate more mature newborn performance, while higher scores on the reflex factor indicate a more deviant neurological examination result. However, methods to derive factor scores are somewhat complicated, requiring recoding items to a continuous scale in order to derive meaningful summative scores.

With training, interrater reliability for the 27 items has been shown to be adequate (42, 43), although a considerable degree of judgment is required of the examiner for assigning a rating to the neonate's responses. Although interrater reliability for the NBAS is quite high, studies of the test-retest reliability of the NBAS suggest poor temporal stability for most items (43). The validity of the NBAS is supported by research that has demonstrated its ability to correctly identify neonates who are underweight or who have experienced in-utero drug and alcohol exposure, maternal malnutrition and gestational diabetes. Additionally, the NBAS has been used in a number of studies examining the effect of maternal general anesthesia, withdrawal from methadone, and interventions aimed at teaching mothers and fathers about their newborns' capacities (44). In fact, the NBAS-2 has been shown to be an effective intervention tool for increasing the maternal involvement and responsiveness of low-SES and adolescent mothers (45). Furthermore, the NBAS has been shown to predict infant–parent attachment and subsequent infant development. Unfortunately, research has not consistently shown the NBAS to be a good predictor of infant development much beyond the first year of life (46, 47). Of the dimensions assessed by the Brazelton, state control appears the most stable and predictive (48), possibly speaking to the fundamental importance of early state regulatory capacities for other more

TABLE 4.2.1.3

SELECTED FORMAL TESTS OF INFANT/TODDLER DEVELOPMENT

	Age	Domains†	Norm Sample	Reliability/Validity	Comments
Neonatal Assessment Tests					
Graham/Rosenblith Behavioral Test for Neonates (38)		M, TA, V, A, MT	Not applicable	Encouraging early findings	Currently seldom used
Brazelton Neonatal Behavioral Assessment Scale—2 (39)	37–44 weeks GA	NI, B, PS	Not applicable	High interrater reliability, weak test-retest, poor predictor beyond first year	Most widely used neonatal test
Infant/Toddler Development Tests					
Bayley Scales of Infant Development—II (55)	1–42 months	Mental, M, B	Large, representative	Excellent for mental, adequate for psychomotor, varied for behavior	Most widely used and validated infant test
Mullen Scales of Early Learning (66)	0–68 months	GM, FM, VR, RC, EC	Large, representative	Adequate to exceptional	Mostly useful for toddlers and preschoolers
Battelle Developmental Inventory (67)	0–95 months	PS, Ad; GM; FM; EC; RC; Cg (and sub-domains)	Small, representative	Numerous psychometric concerns cast significant doubts (see text)	Used considerably, despite many test flaws
Griffiths Abilities of Babies (14)	0–24 months	Lm, PS, HS, EH, P	Small, all from London	Mixed results	Mostly used in Europe
Infant Psychological Development Scales (54)	NA	See text	Not applicable	Adequate to exceptional reliability	Most popular Piagetian infant test
Screening Tests					
Battelle Developmental Inventory Screening Test (67)	6–95 months	PS, Ad; GM; FM; EC; RC; Cg	Small, representative	Strong correlation with full BDI	Suffers same limitations as full BDI
Bayley Infant Neurodevelopmental Screen (87)	3–24 months	N; RC; EC/M; Cg	Large; representative	Excellent reliability; promising validity	
Birth to Three Developmental Scale (88)	0–36 months	EC/RC; Cg; PS; M	Small; questionable representation	Strong interrater reliability, but little evidence of validity	
Child Development Inventory (89)	15–72 months	GM; FM; EC; RC; Ad; PS; L; N	Small; from St. Paul, MN	Little evidence of reliability and validity	300 parent report items
Denver Developmental Screening Test-II (81)	0–72 months	GM; FM/Cg; PS; EC/RC	Large, all from Denver area	See text	See text
Developmental Activities Screening Inventory—II (90)	0–60 months	15 sensory and problemsolving areas	>200 disabled children	Little evidence of reliability; valid for severely delayed	Can be used with language and visual impaired children
Developmental Indicators for the Assessment of Learning—Revised (91)	24–72 months	M; AS; EC/RC; B	Large; representative	Acceptable reliability and validity	One of better screeners for age level
Diagnostic Inventory for Screening Children—4 (92)	0–60 months	FM; GM; RC; EC; AM; VM; Ad; PS	Small; all from southwest Ontario	Excellent reliability; limited validity	
Developmental Observation Checklist System (93)	0–72 months	Cg; EC/RC; PS; FM/GM; Adj; PS&S	Adequate; representative	Sound reliability and concurrent validity	Parent report only

(continued)

TABLE 4.2.1.3

(CONTINUED)

	Age	Domains†	Norm Sample	Reliability/Validity	Comments
Developmental Profile—II (94)	0–114 months	M; Ad; PS; AS; EC/RC	Large	Adequate reliability and validity	Parent report only
Early Screening Profile (86)	24–72 months	Cg; EC/RC; M; Ad/PS; Ar	Adequate; representative	Good reliability; exceptional validity	One of better screeners for age level
Kent Infant Development Scales (95)	0–12 months	Cg; M; EC/RC; Ad; PS	All from Northeast Ohio	Adequate reliability and validity	Primarily parent report

†A = Auditory responsiveness; Adj = Adjustment; Ad = Adaptive, self-help or daily living; AM = Auditory attention and memory; Ar = Articulation; AS = Academic or pre-academic skills; B = Behavior; Cg = Cognitive or problemsolving; EC = Expressive communication/language; EH = Eye-hand coordination; FM = Fine motor; GM = Gross motor; HS = Hearing and speech; L = Letters; Lm = Locomotor; M = Motor or physical; MT = Muscle tone; N = Numbers; NI = Neurological intactness; P = Performance; PS = Personal-social; PS and S = Parental stress and support; RC = Receptive communication/language; TA = Tactile-adaptive; V = Visual responsiveness; VM = Visual attention and memory; VR = Visual reception. A slash mark (/) indicates that multiple domains are assessed in the same scale or subtest.

complex functions, such as attention and social interactiveness, that emerge in the first year.

Infant/Toddler Development Tests

Of the various models of infant developmental tests, the norm-referenced multidomain model is arguably the most enduring. Based on the work of Gesell and Bayley, development is assessed in multiple distinct yet interrelated domains. The most commonly used examples of these tests (each described below) are the *Bayley Scales of Infant Development-II, Mullen Scales of Early Learning, Battelle Developmental Inventory*, and *Griffiths Mental Development Scales*. As discussed later, the Bayley and Mullen scales are two of the most common choices for developmental tests for infants and toddlers. Although both are marketed for use throughout the infant and toddler years, for most clinical applications, the Bayley is a better choice for infancy, while the Mullen may be preferable for young children older than 2 1/2 or 3 years (49).

Additionally, criterion-referenced instruments are also popular among professionals who wish to compare an infant's development to expectations based either on a particular model of development (e.g., Piaget's model of infant cognitive development) or expected programmatic outcomes. Though not typically useful for diagnostic or screening purposes, criterion-referenced tests may be quite useful when planning intervention programs. To accomplish this goal, criterion-referenced tests are designed to sample extensively the universe of skills that a child is expected to have mastered at various ages. The infant's performance on these tests can then be translated directly into an individualized intervention plan by targeting those skills that the infant was expected to have mastered but as of yet had not.

One of the most popular criterion-referenced tests for use with young children is the *Brigance Diagnostic Inventory of Early Development-Revised* (50), useful for children birth to 7 years, and surveying skills in 12 different developmental domains (e.g., social/emotional, communicative, motor, pre-academic skills). Other similar tests specifically for infants include the *Hawaii Early Learning Profile* (HELP) (51) and the *Early Learning Accomplishment Profile for Infants* (52). The *Rossetti Infant-Toddler Language Scale* (53) is a popular scale that is designed to assess specifically an infant's verbal and nonverbal communication and level of caregiver–infant interaction. One of the most commonly used Piagetian model instruments is the *Infant Psychological Developmental Scale* (described below), which assesses an infant's ability to grasp object permanence, understand means–ends and cause–effect relationships, imitate vocalizations and gestures, and manipulate objects in space (54).

Bayley Scales of Infant Development-II

The *Bayley Scales of Infant Development-II* (BSID-II) (55) is the most widely used measure of the development of infants and toddlers in both clinical and research settings. The BSID's extensive history of test development and validation makes it the most psychometrically sophisticated infant test on the market. As previously mentioned, the BSID-II is predicated on the early tests developed by Bayley in the 1930s. During the 1960s, these tests were substantially revised and subjected to a level of psychometric standardization and validation previously only attempted with IQ tests, resulting in the original *Bayley Scales of Infant Development* (17). The current BSID-II, a substantial revision and renorming of the original scale, is applicable to children from 1 through 42 months of age. Administration time is about 25 to 35 minutes for infants under 15 months and up to 60 minutes for children over 15 months.

There are three main components of the BSID-II: the Mental Development Index (MDI), Psychomotor Development Index (PDI), and Behavior Rating Scale (BRS). The MDI provides information about the child's language development and problemsolving skills, while the PDI assesses the child's gross and fine motor development. The BRS is a form that evaluators may use to rate the child's behaviors during the assessment. Items on the BRS assess attentional capacities, social engagement, affect and emotion, and the quality of the child's movement and motor control. The BSID-II provides a method for obtaining age equivalence scores for four facets of development: cognitive, language, social, and motor. Unfortunately, little empirical evidence exists to support the reliability and validity of these facet scores. Also, determining the correct facet age equivalent score is often difficult, since several months of development is often determined on the basis of passing only one item. Therefore, considerably more research is needed before clinicians and researchers can have confidence in these facet scores.

The BSID-II is administered in item sets, determined based on the age of the infant. This represents a substantial revision from the original BSID, which, like most tests, used a continuous series of items. This change has created some confusion among infant examiners in terms of which item set to use for infants born prematurely (56). Indeed, the choice of which item set to use as a starting point can significantly impact the infant's final score (57). For testers that use the corrected age procedure, the test developers recommend using the same item set that corresponds to the normative group used for determining that child's standard score (58).

The BSID-II is normed on 1,700 infants (an exceedingly large normative sample by infant assessment standards) representative of 1988 U.S. Census data as stratified by gender, ethnicity, regionality, and parental education. Test-retest reliability for 1 to 16 days ranges from .83 to .91 for the MDI and from .77 to .79 for the PDI. Stability for the BRS varies greatly depending on the age of the child, ranging from .55 to .90. Because the BRS samples behaviors as observed during a given testing session, it may be more subject to state variation than items contributing to either the mental or the motor scales. Interrater reliability for the BSID-II is reported to be .96 for the MDI, .75 for the PDI, and .70 for the total BRS. Across BRS domains, interrater reliability varies, with the lowest agreement being for ratings of attention and arousal in younger children (.57). Agreement among observers for the behavioral ratings improves for children older than 12 months. These stability coefficients approach adequacy for the MDI, but fall somewhat short of optimal for a diagnostic test on the PDI and BRS (34). Concurrent validity of the MDI, as correlated with other measures of general cognitive ability, typically falls in the .70 range, whereas the PDI correlated best with the motor score of the McCarthy at .59. In general, the BSID appears to have some ability to predict which infants will score very poorly on intelligence tests in their preschool years, but shows limited ability to accurately predict specific IQ scores, especially in average developing infants (59, 60).

It is important to note that Bayley did not intend that the MDI or PDI scores be interpretted as intelligence quotients. Correlations between BSID performance and subsequent IQ assessments are variable. In her 1933 sample of 61 infants, Bayley found no relation between the mental scale administered before 24 months and the Stanford-Binet administered from 5 to 13 years of age (16). For the 24-month mental age scale with another sample of infants, she reported a correlation of .53 with the Stanford-Binet. Others have investigated the relation between performance on the 1969 version of the Bayley Scales and subsequent IQ tests and have found modest correlations between MDI and PDI measures collected through 24 months with 30- to 36-month Stanford-Binet scores (61–63). In the 1993 version, more robust correlations were found between the MDI and subscales of both the *Wechsler Preschool and Primary Scale of Intelligence* and the *McCarthy Scales of Children's Abilities* (64), suggesting that items added to the 1993 version may tap constructs more similar to measures of information processing (55). However, for the most part, performance on the BSID does not consistently predict later cognitive measures, particularly when socioeconomic status and level of functioning are controlled (65).

Mullen Scales of Early Learning

A relatively recent addition is the *Mullen Scales of Early Learning* (66). This revision of the original Mullen Scales combined earlier versions of the test designed for infants and preschoolers into one test with continuous norms from birth through 68 months. The Mullen takes about 15 to 60 minutes to administer, depending on the age of the child (15 minutes at 1 year old, 30 minutes at 3 years, and 60 minutes at 5 years). The Mullen assesses child development in five separate domains: gross motor, visual reception (primarily visual discrimination and memory), fine motor, receptive language, and expressive language. The gross motor scale is only applicable to children birth through 33 months old and does not contribute to the overall early learning composite score.

Normative data for the Mullen is based on a sample of 1,849 children from across America, somewhat overrepresentative of children from the Northeast. Internal reliability ranges from .75 to .83 for Mullen subtests and is .91 for the overall developmental score. Median 1- to 2-week test-retest reliability coefficients range from .78 to .96 across subtests, and interrater reliability coefficients range from .94 to .98. The Mullen receptive and expressive language scales show acceptable correlation with similar scales from the Preschool Language Assessment Scale, .85 and .80 respectively. The gross motor scale correlates with the Bayley MDI at .76, and the fine motor scale correlates with the Peabody Fine Motor Scale at .70. These correlations for the motor scales also are acceptable. Overall, these validation studies are quite promising. However, additional studies are warranted of the Mullen's concurrent and predictive validity, particularly with specific subpopulations.

Battelle Developmental Inventory

The *Battelle Developmental Inventory* (BDI) (67) is exceedingly popular, especially among professionals working in publicly funded early intervention and special education programs. It is intended to measure development in children ages birth through 7 years old. Five domains are measured by the BDI, including personal-social, adaptive, motor, communication, and cognitive. Each of the five domains of the BDI are divided into subdomains that finely assess the components of each domain, and all domains contribute to a total developmental score. The assessment time required by the BDI is quite long compared to other similar tests, ranging from about 1 to 2 hours depending on the age of the child.

The standardization sample for the BDI consists of 800 children, stratified to match the 1980 U.S. Census data based on geographic region, race, and gender. In a review of the technical merits of the BDI, McLinden (68) raised several concerns. First, although the test authors reported exceptionally strong test-retest and interrater reliability for the BDI, a general lack of procedural details in the manual makes it difficult to evaluate these data adequately. No information regarding the BDI's internal reliability is provided. Second, the concurrent validity of the various domains is based on findings from exceptionally small studies, ranging from only 10 to 37 subjects. Furthermore, resulting correlations for the BDI's cognitive domain were much less than optimal ($r = .44$; $N = 13$ for the Full Scale IQ from the *Wechsler Intelligence Scale for Children-Revised*; $r = .50$; $N = 23$ for the *Stanford-Binet Intelligence Scale*) (67).

Third, a potentially more detrimental limitation of the BDI exists in its normative data (69). For the first 2 years, normative data are presented in 6-month bands, and in 12-month bands thereafter. Therefore, an infant's performance is compared to other infants that can be as many as 6 to 12 months older or younger. Obviously, standard scores for infants who are old for their normative group will be inflated, whereas standard scores for infants who are young for their normative group will underestimate their true development. Due to these normative discontinuities, children could theoretically score solidly in the average range just before their birthday, and a day or so later, with the exact same performance, score in the range suggestive of serious developmental delay or mental retardation. For this reason, age equivalent score may be more stable on the BDI than standard scores (70). This limitation greatly reduces the diagnostic utility of the BDI and may even lead to grossly distorted results when BDI standard scores are used for longitudinal research or for tracking the development of individual infants. For these reasons, diagnostic use of the BDI for infants and toddlers in general is not recommended, and BDI results administered by others should be interpreted very cautiously.

Griffiths Mental Development Scales

Although the *Griffiths Mental Development Scales* are seldom used in America, they warrant a brief description due to their continued use in Europe and early influence on extending infant developmental testing internationally. The Griffiths consists of two tests: *The Abilities of Babies* (14), designed for infants birth to 24 months, and *The Abilities of Young Children* (71), for children 24 months to 8 years. The infant scale consists of five domains, modeled closely after Gesell's early work: locomotor, personal and social, hearing and speech, eye and hand coordination, and performance. The test is normed on 571 infants from London, England, but oddly stratified to match the 1940 U.S. Census figures. Reliability studies for the Griffiths have yielded mixed results, and validity studies have indicated relatively weak predictive ability for later IQ test scores (8). Despite its outdated and questionable standardization, the Griffiths scales apparently remain rather popular in Europe and Quebec.

Uzgiris-Hunt Infant Psychological Development Scales

Piaget presented a view of the child that was quite different from Gesell's and that reflected, at the least, their different theoretical backgrounds (72). Gesell, the essential pragmatist, presented development as the steady march forward of increasingly complex behaviors and capacities that were relatively unaffected by environmental contingencies. Piaget, the essential epistemologist, described development as a hierarchical series of qualitatively different stages that cut across observable behaviors and that are closely linked to environmental influence. For Gesell, children unfolded on a maturational timetable. For Piaget, children grew to understand the world and themselves, and development was the process of "knowing" in ever more complex ways. Maturation of motor skills and other capacities was the vehicle that would lead to such knowing, and progress depended on previous achievements in all functional areas. It was not until the 1950s that American psychologists became seriously interested in Piaget's work (73), and this was long after the infant assessment field was well established in the tradition of Gesell and Bayley. Thus, the assessment techniques based on Piagetian theories are even now far less widely used or considered, but these techniques are available and present a useful contrast to the norm-referenced multidomain tools described earlier. Of the two most widely known examples, the *Einstein Scales of Sensorimotor Intelligence* (74) and the *Uzgiris-Hunt Infant Psychological Development Scales* (54), the latter is used more often.

The Uzgiris-Hunt is based on Piaget's theory of the sensorimotor period of development, and consists of six subscales. The first scale, visual pursuit and permanence of objects, deals with infants' increasing awareness of objects outside their immediate perceptual field. Behaviors involving searching for a hidden object fall within this subdomain. The second subscale, development of means for achieving desired ends, covers such activities as using a tool to obtain an object. Development of imitation, the third subscale, is divided into vocal and gestural imitation and includes not only repetition of words but different sounds for distress and pleasure. The fourth subscale, development of operational causality, includes anticipatory behaviors, such as attempting to start a mechanical toy or, in younger infants, watching one's own hand movements. Object relations in space, the fifth subscale, describes the infant's capacity to discriminate dimensionality, to track and locate objects, or to localize perceptual cues. Finally, the sixth subdomain involves the development of schemas for relating to objects (e.g., how the infant's use of toys changes) and how exploratory behaviors with objects become increasingly differentiated and complex. The position of an item in the Uzgiris-Hunt Scales is determined a priori by the theory, not by the chronological age at which most children complete the item, as in the Gesell-based tests described earlier. There is also an ordinal assumption in the Piagetian-based scales; that is, success on an item at one level presumes success at all previous levels because of the hierarchical assumptions in the theory.

The Uzgiris-Hunt Scales are administered using a series of situations and materials that elicit children's responses in the various subdomains. The procedures for administering the situations are quite flexible. The six scales are not presented in a specified sequence, nor does the examiner need to cover all the scales. Specific directions for types of items, number of presentations, and types of expected responses are given, but judging success is more flexible because of the more conceptual nature of the tasks. The scales were tested and revised in three samples of infants drawn exclusively from middle-class families. Interrater agreement percentages and test-retest reliability were adequate in the three original samples, ranging from 92% to 97% and .70 and .85, for the six subscales respectively. The subscales were also highly intercorrelated ($r \geq .80$), and each subscale was highly correlated with chronological age ($r \geq .88$). Although Uzgiris and Hunt did present mean ages for the achievement of each scale stage, they emphasized that their samples were not selected to provide normative data for different ages. Subsequently, Dunst (75) has estimated norms for age equivalent scores based on performance in the various subdomains. However, these age equivalent scores tend to average about 2 months lower than Bayley MDI age equivalents (76, 77). In terms of concurrent and predictive validity, there appears to be little correlation with current Bayley scores but moderate correlation with later Stanford-Binet scores (78, 79). Wachs, followed a sample of infants between 12 and 24 months and correlated their performance with the Stanford-Binet at 31 months. By 24 months, all scales except *Means for Obtaining an End* were significantly correlated with performance on the Stanford-Binet IQ test.

Infant/Toddler Screening Tests

Screening tests are brief assessments of a child's current level of functioning, used to determine which children may be developmentally at risk, requiring further diagnostic assessment. In order to fulfill their goal, screening tests should yield scores that are predictive of scores from more comprehensive diagnostic assessments (e.g., the Bayley) but require substantially less time to administer and score. Screening tests are intended to be used routinely when a comprehensive assessment for all children would be either too costly or unwarranted. These instruments usually are not as reliable or valid as comprehensive assessment tools, due largely to their brevity.

The goal of all screening tests is to identify correctly those children who would likely score poorly on a more comprehensive assessment and to reduce two possible sources of error: false positives and false negatives. The ability of a screener to reduce false negative rates is referred to as the test's *sensitivity*, its ability to accurately detect children with delays or disabilities. Conversely, the ability of a screener to reduce false positives is referred to as its *specificity*, its ability to avoid mislabeling a child as delayed or disabled, when in fact that child is not. Though it is desirable to reduce the percentage of both types of error, sensitivity may be more important than specificity with screening tests, since it is assumed that followup assessment will correct any false positives. Meisels (80) recommends that developmental screeners possess both sensitivity and specificity levels of at least 80%. Unfortunately, too many developmental screeners do not provide these data. Several of the more common screening tests are presented in Table 4.2.1.3. All screening tests presented use direct assessment or observation of the child, unless otherwise stated. Most also allow for caregiver report of information in order to gain additional data about behaviors that may be difficult to elicit in the brief assessment period. Some, however, are based solely on caregiver report (e.g., the *Developmental Profile-II* and the *Developmental Observation Checklist System*). In addition, two specific screening tests are further described below.

Denver Developmental Screening Test-II

The *Denver Developmental Screening Test-II* (81) is one of the most popular developmental screening tests, especially in medical settings. This may be due at least in part to its brevity, as it can be administered in as little as 15 to 20 minutes. It is applicable for children birth to 6 years. Items are scored based on a combination of caregiver report, direct assessment of the child, and observation. The Denver produces one overall score, placing children in one of four descriptive categories: pass, questionable, abnormal, or untestable. Since the Denver-II was normed exclusively on children living in Colorado, caution should be used when employing this screener in other localities. The original edition of the Denver (82) had been criticized for not being sensitive enough, missing as many as 80% of children with delays or disabilities (83). Although the Denver-II is a clear improvement over the original Denver, there is evidence that it now significantly overidentifies as many as 72% of children (84). As a result, child-find personnel in both Kentucky and Tennessee reportedly have requested that evaluators use a different screening instrument before referring children for developmental services, in order to reduce costly false positives (85).

Early Screening Profiles

The *Early Screening Profiles* (ESP) (86) is applicable for children 2 through 6 years. It screens for cognitive, language, speech, physical, and social disabilities or delays that may interfere with a child's learning and warrant further diagnostic assessment. Children complete three different subtests: cognitive/language (assessing children's visual discrimination, logical reasoning, verbal concepts, basic school readiness skills), motor (assessing both fine and gross motor skills), and speech articulation. Total testing time per child is only 15 to 30 minutes, depending on the child's age. Additionally, the person who administers the test completes a 2–3 minute Behavior Survey documenting the child's behaviors during the assessment (e.g., activity level, attention span, cooperativeness, independence). Caregivers, or sometimes teachers, complete three different rating forms: the self-help/social profile (which provides a rating of the child's adaptive behaviors), the home survey (regarding the caregiver's perception of the child's home environment and caregiver–child interaction), and the health history survey (which provides information regarding immunizations, health problems, and prenatal health and delivery). Each of these rating forms can be completed in about 5 minutes. The ESP provides a wide variety of scores for all domains and subdomains, including age equivalents, standard scores, percentile ranks, and easy-to-use six-point screening categories. Screener cut-points can be set at several different levels in order to manipulate the false-positive to false-negative ratio. The primary drawback of the ESP is that it has no Spanish version. Psychometrically, the ESP is quite sound and represents one of the very best screening tests on the market.

CONCLUSION

Infant assessments are in part clinical explorations involving a fair amount of uncertainty and inference. While the medical diagnostic process always involves some element of uncertainty, the assessments made in infancy require of the clinician a particular comfort with uncertainty and the unknown. Though the latter half of the last century brought a veritable explosion of knowledge about infancy and the neonatal period, the more we learn, the greater we understand how inexplicably woven are the forces of development. As emphasized throughout this chapter, infant assessment involves far more than the infant and is as much a measure of the infant's environment as it is of his or her functional status. Thus clinicians assessing infants are always dealing more with what they cannot know than with what they can, ever exploring the limits of predictive capabilities and constantly mindful of those distinctions.

References

1. Bagnato SJ and Neisworth JT: Collaboration and teamwork in assessment for early intervention. *Child and Adolescent Psychiatric Clinics of North America*, 1999. 8:347–363.
2. Gilliam WS and Mayes LC: Clinical assessment of infants and toddlers, In: Lewis M (eds): *Child and Adolescent Psychiatry: A Comprehensive Textbook* Philadelphia: Lippincott, Williams & Wilkins. 2002, 507–525.
3. Brooks J. Weinraub J: *A history of infant intelligence testing*, In: Lewis M (eds): *Origins of Intelligence: Infancy and Early Childhood*. New York: Plenum. 19–58, 1976.
4. Wyly MV: *Infant assessment*. Westview Press. Boulder, CO: 1997.
5. Esquirol JD: *Des Maladies Mentales Considerees Sous Les Rapports Medical, Hygienique, and Medicolegal*, Paris, Bailliere, 1938.
6. Terman LM: *The Measurement of Intelligence*, Boston: Houghton-Mifflin, 1916.
7. Cattell P, *The measurement of intelligence in young children*. New York, Psychological Corporation, 1940.
8. Thomas H: Psychological assessment instruments for use with human infants. *Merrill-Palmer Quarterly*, 16: 1970, 179–223.
9. Gesell, A: *The First Five Years of Life: A Guide to the Study of the Preschool Child*. New York: Harper, 1940.
10. Bayley N, *Mental Growth During the First Three Years*, Genetic Psychology Monographs, 14: 1933. 1–92.
11. Bayley N: *The California first-year mental scale*. Berkeley: University of California Press, 1933.
12. Bayley N: The development of motor abilities during the first three years: A study of sixty-one infants tested repeatedly. *Monographs of the Society for Research in Child Development*, 1:1–26, 1935.
13. Bayley N, *The California Infant Scale of Motor Development*, Berkeley, University of California Press, 1936.
14. Griffiths R: *The Abilities of Babies*, London: University of London Press, 1954.
15. Stott, LH and Ball RS: Evaluation of infant and pre-school mental tests. *Monograph of the Society for Research in Child Development*, 30:1–151, 1965.
16. Bayley N: *Consistency and variability in growth and intelligence from birth to eighteen years*. Journal of Genetic Psychology, 75:165–196, 1949.
17. Bayley N, *Bayley Scales of Infant Development*, New York: Psychological Corporation, 1969.
18. Bornstein MH and Sigman MD: Continuity in mental development from infancy. *Child Development*, 57:251–274, 1986.
19. McCall RB and Carriger MS: *A meta-analysis of infant habituation and recognition memory performance as predictors of later IQ*. *Child Development*, 64:57–79, 1993.
20. Cox, CE: Obtaining and formulating a developmental history. *Child and Adolescent Psychiatric Clinics of North America*, 8:271–279, 1999.
21. Provence, S: *Developmental assessment*, in *Ambulatory pediatrics*, M. Green and R. Haggarty, ed.: Philadelphia: Saunders. 374–383, 1977.
22. Sparrow SS, Balla, DA and Chicchetti DV: *Vineland Adaptive Behavior Scales*. Circle Pines American Guidance Service, 1984.
23. Provence, S, et al.: *Infant-Toddler Developmental Assessment*. Chicago, Riverside Publishing, 1995.
24. Benham AL: The observation and assessment of young children including use of the Infant-Toddler Mental Status Exam, In: *Handbook of Infant Mental Health*, CH Zeanah, Editor. New York, Guilford Press, 2000, 249–265.
25. Zeanah CH, et al.: Relationship assessment in infant mental health. *Infant Mental Health Journal* 18: 1997, 182–197.
26. Close N: Diagnostic play interview: Its role in comprehensive psychiatric evaluation. *Child and Adolescent Psychiatric Clinics of North America*, 1999. 8:239–255.
27. Gilliam, WS: Developmental assessment: Its role in comprehensive psychiatric assessment of young children. *Child and Adolescent Psychiatric Clinics of North America*, 8: 1999, 225–238.
28. Mayes LC and WS Gilliam, eds.: Comprehensive psychiatric assessment of young children. *Child and Adolescent Psychiatric Clinics of North America*. 1999, Philadelphia: Saunders.

29. Dickerson JWT: Nutrition, brain growth and development, In: *Maturation and development: Biological and psychological perspectives*, KJ Connolly and HR Prechtl, ed. Philadelphia: JB Lippincott. 1981, 110–130.
30. Shonkoff JP and Marshall PC: *Biological bases of developmental dysfunction*, in *Handbook of early childhood intervention*, SJ Meisels and JP Shonkoff, eds. New York: Cambridge University Press 1990, 35–52.
31. Seifer R, and Dickstein S: *Parental mental illness and infant development*, in *Handbook of infant mental health*, CH Zeanah, ed. New York: Guilford Press, 2000, 145–160.
32. Meisels SJ Waskik BA: *Who should be served? Identifying children in need of early intervention*, In: Meisels SJ, Shonkoff JP (eds): *Handbook of early childhood intervention*, New York, Cambridge University Press, 1990, 605–632.
33. Flynn JR: The mean IQ of Americans: Massive gains 1932 to 1978. *Psychological Bulletin* 95: 1984, 29–51.
34. Salvia J and Ysseldyke JE: *Assessment*. 5th ed. Boston: Houghton Mifflin, 1991.
35. Apgar, V: A proposal for a new method of evaluation of the newborn infant. *Anesthesia and Analgesia: Current Research* 32: 1953, 260–267.
36. Francis PL, Self PA, Horowitz FD: The behavioral assessment of the neonate: An overview, In: Osofsky JD ed. *Handbook of infant development*, 1987, New York: Wiley.
37. Bullowa M: *Before Speech*. New York: Cambridge University Press, 1979.
38. Rosenblith JF: *The Graham/Rosenblith behavioral examination for newborns: Prognostic value and procedural issues*, In: Osofsky, J (ed): *Handbook of infant development*, Ed. 1979, New York: Wiley.
39. Brazelton TB, *Neonatal behavioral assessment scale* (2nd ed.), In: *Clinics in Developmental Medicine (No. 88)*. Philadelphia: Lippincott, 1984.
40. Als H, et al.: The Brazelton Neonatal Behavior Assessment Scale (BNBAS). *Journal of Abnormal Child Psychology* 5:215–231, 1977.
41. Lester B, Als, H, Brazelton TB: Regional obstetric anesthesia and newborn behavior: A reanalysis toward synergistic effects. *Child Development*, 53: 1982, 687–692.
42. Lancione E, Horowitz FD, Sullivan JW: The NBAS-K 1: A study of its stability and structure over the first month of life. *Infant Behavior and Development* 3: 1980, 341–359.
43. Sameroff AJ: Organization and stability of newborn behavior: A commentary on the Brazelton Neonatal Behavioral Assessment Scale. *Monographs of the Society for Research in Child Development* 43: 1978.
44. Sostek AM: Annotated bibliography of research using the neonatal behavior assessment scale. *Monographs of the Society for Research in Child Development* 43: 1978, 124–131.
45. Worobey J, Brazelton TB: Newborn Assessment and Support for Parenting. In: Gibbs ED, Teti DM (eds): *Interdisciplinary assessment of infants: A guide for early intervention professionals*, Baltimore, Brookes, 1990.
46. Horowitz FD, Linn LP: The Neonatal Behavioral Assessment Scale. In: Wolraich M, Routh DK (eds): *Advances in developmental pediatrics, 3*, Greenwich, CT: JAI, 1982, 223–256.
47. Vaughn BE, et al.: Relationships between neonatal behavioral organization and infant behavior during the first year of life. *Infant Behavior and Development*, 3: 1980, 47–66.
48. Als H, et al. Specific neonatal measures: The Brazelton Neonatal Behavior Assessment Scale. In: Osofsky J (ed): *Handbook of Infant Development*, New York, Wiley, 1979, 185–215.
49. Gilliam WS, Mayes LC: Integrating clinical and psychometric approaches: Developmental assessment and the infant mental health evaluation. In: DelCarmen-Wiggins R, Carter A (eds): *Handbook of infant, toddler, and preschool mental health assessment*, New York: Oxford University Press, 2004, 185–203.
50. Brigance AH: *Brigance Diagnostic Inventory of Early Development: Revised*, North Billerica, MA: Curriculum Associates, 1991.
51. Furuno S, et al.: *Hawaii Early Learning Profile (HELP): Activity Guide*. Palo Alto, VORT, 1987.
52. Sanford A: *Learning Accomplishment Profile for Infants (Early LAP)*. Winston-Salem, Kaplan School Supply, 1981.
53. Rossetti LM: *Infant-toddler Assessment: An Interdisciplinary Approach*, Boston, College Hill, 1990.
54. Uzgiris I, Hunt JM: *Assessment in Infancy: Toward Ordinal Scales of Psychological Development in Infancy*, Champaign-Urbana, University of Illinois Press, 1975.
55. Bayley N: *Bayley Scales of Infant Development*. 2nd ed. San Antonio, Psychological Corporation, 1993.
56. Ross G, Lawson K: *Commentary*. Using the Bayley-II: Unresolved issues in assessing the development of prematurely born children. *Developmental and Behavioral Pediatrics* 18:109–111, 1997.
57. Gauthier SM, et al.: The Bayley Scales of Infant Development-II: Where to start? *Journal of Developmental and Behavioral Pediatrics*, 20(2), 1999, 75–79.
58. Matula K, Gyurke JS, Aylward GP: Response to commentary. Bayley Scales-II. *Developmental and Behavioral Pediatrics* 18:112–113, 1997.
59. Gibbs ED: Assessment of infant mental ability: Conventional tests and issues of prediction, In: Gibbs ED, Teti D (eds): *Interdisciplinary Assessment of Infants: A Guide for Early Intervention professionals*, Baltimore, Brookes, 1990, 77–90.
60. Whatley J: *Bayley scales of infant development*, In: Keyser D Sweetland R, eds. *Test Critiques*, Kansas City: Westport, 1987, 38–47.
61. McCall RB: *The development of intellectual functioning in infancy and the prediction of later IQ*, In: Osofsky, J (eds): *Handbook of infant development*, New York: Wiley, 1979, 707–741.
62. Ramey CT: Campbell FA, Nicholson JE The predictive power of the Bayley Scales of Infant Development and the Stanford-Binet Intelligence Test in a relatively constant environment. *Child Development*, 44, 1973, 790–795.
63. Siegel LS: Infant perceptual, cognitive, and motor behaviors as predictors of subsequent cognitive and language development. *Canadian Journal of Psychology* 33, 1979, 382–394.
64. McCarthy D: *McCarthy Scales of Children's Abilities*. San Antonio: Psychological Corporation, 1972.
65. Rubin RA, Balow B: Measures of infant development and socio-economic status as predictors of later intelligence and school achievement. *Developmental Psychology*, 5, 1979, 225–227.
66. Mullen EM: *Mullen Scales of Early Learning: AGS Edition*. Circle Pines: American Guidance Service, 1995.
67. Newborg J, et al.: *Battelle Developmental Inventory (BDI)*, Allen: DLM/Teaching Resources, 1984.
68. McLinden SE: An evaluation of the Battelle Developmental Inventory for determining special education eligibility. Journal of Psychoeducational Assessment, 7, 1989, 66–73.
69. Boyd RD: What a difference a day makes: Age-related discontinuities and the Battelle Developmental Inventory. *Journal of Early Intervention*, 1989 114–119.
70. Boyd RD, et al.: Concurrent validity of the Battelle Developmental Inventory: Relationship with the Bayley Scales in young children with known or suspected disabilities. *Journal of Early Intervention*, 13: 1989, 14–23.
71. Griffiths R: *The abilities of young children*. 1979, London: Child Development Research Center.
72. Yang RK: *Early infant assessment: An overview*, In: Osofsky J (eds): *Handbook of infant development*, New York: Wiley, 1979, 165–184.
73. Baldwin AL: *Theories of Child Development*. New York, Wiley, 1967.
74. Corman HH, Escalona S: *Stages of sensorimotor development: A replication study. Merrill-Palmer Quarterly*, 15: 1969, 351–361.
75. Dunst CJ: *A Clinical and Educational Manual for use with the Uzgiris and Hunt Scales of Infant Psychological Development*, Baltimore: University Park Press, 1980.
76. Dunst CJ, Rheingrover RM, Kistler ED: *Concurrent Validity of the Uzgiris-Hunt Scales: Relationship to Bayley Scale Mental Age, Behavioral Science Documents*, 16: 1986, 65.
77. Sexton D et al.: *Concurrent validity data for the Uzgiris and Hunt Scales and the Bayley mental scale: Additional evidence on the Dunst age norms. Journal of the Division for Early Childhood*, 12: 1988, 368–374.
78. King WL, Seegmiller B: Performance of fourteen- to twenty-two-month-old black, firstborn male infants on two tests of cognitive development: The Bayley Scales and the Infant Psychological Development Scale. *Developmental Psychology*. 8: 1973, 317–326.
79. Wachs TD: Relation of infants' performance on Piaget scales between twelve and twenty-four months and their Stanford-Binet performance at thirty-one months. *Child Development*, 46: 1975, 929–935.
80. Meisels SJ: Can developmental screening tests identify children who are developmentally at risk? *Pediatrics*. 83: 1989, 578–585.
81. Frankenburg WK et al.: *Denver II: Technical manual*, Denver, Denver Developmental Materials, 1990.
82. Frankenburg WK, Dodds J, Fandal A.: *Denver Developmental Screening Test*, Denver: LADOCA, 1975.
83. Greer S, Bauchner H, Zuckerman B.: The Denver Developmental Screening Test: How good is its predictive validity? *Developmental Medicine and Child Neurology*, 31: 1989, 774–781.
84. Glascoe FP, Byrne KE: The accuracy of three developmental screening tests. *Journal of Early Intervention*. 17: 1993, 368–379.
85. Johnson KL et al.: Does Denver II produce meaningful results? *Pediatrics*, 90: 1992, 477–478.
86. Harrison PL: *Early screening profiles (ESP): Manual*, Circle Pines, American Guidance Service, 1990.
87. Aylward GP: *Bayley Infant Neurodevelopmental Screener*. San Antonio, Psychological Corporation, 1995.
88. Bangs, TE, Dodson S.: *Birth to Three Developmental Scale*. Allen, DLM Teaching Resources, 1979.
89. Ireton H: *Child Development Inventory*, Minneapolis, Behavior Science Systems, 1992.
90. Fewell RR, Langley MB: *Developmental Activities Screening Inventory-II*, Austin, Pro-Ed, 1984.
91. Mardell-Czudnowski CD, Goldenberg D: *DIAL-R (Developmental indicators for the assessment of learning-revised)*, Edison, Childcraft Education, 1990.
92. Amdur JR, Mainland, MK, Parker KCH: *Diagnostic inventory for screening children (DISC) manual*: Fourth edition, Kitchner, ON: Kitchner-Waterloo Hospital, 1996.
93. Hrescko WP, et al.: *Developmental Observation Checklist System*, Austin, Pro-Ed, 1994.
94. Alpern GD, Boll TJ, Shearer M: *Developmental Profile-II*, Aspen, Psychological Development Publications, 1986.
95. Reuter J Bickett L: *Kent Infant Development Scale (KIDS)*, Kent, Developmental Metrics, 1985.

CHAPTER 4.2.2 ■ CLINICAL ASSESSMENT OF CHILDREN AND ADOLESCENTS: CONTENT AND STRUCTURE

JEFF Q. BOSTIC AND ROBERT A. KING

The goal of the clinical psychiatric assessment of a child or adolescent is to identify the presence of psychopathology and to guide the planning of appropriate interventions, if indicated (1). The child (except as noted in identified sections, "child" will refer to "child and adolescent") is evaluated in the context of his or her functioning in the family, the school, and with peers, with sensitivity to cultural or community influences. The clinical assessment seeks to detect any developmental aberrations and maladaptive psychodynamic patterns, while casting a wide net to identify the patient's miscellaneous symptoms, as well as protective and resilience factors that may affect treatment outcomes. Many symptom constellations will respond to established treatments, so the clinician must prioritize intervention targets to devise a treatment plan that will address multiple problems, including comorbid disorders (2). A thoughtfully conducted interview provides the clinician with sufficient information to identify not only intervention targets, but those relevant environmental variables, such as family or school factors, which will influence adherence to any treatment efforts.

The purposes of clinical assessment of the child or adolescent vary, and outcome is often contingent on the alignment among the family's, child's, and clinician's acknowledged goals in pursuing a given assessment. The most common purposes of psychiatric assessment are: 1) to determine if psychopathology is present, and if so, to establish target symptom priorities; 2) to determine what treatments, if any, might address the target symptoms; 3) to evaluate with the family and patient the relative benefits and risks of any proposed treatment. A given clinician's assessment of a child or adolescent may focus on any (or all) stages of this process, such as clarification of diagnoses, or consultation regarding benefits or risks of treatment options. Less frequently, clinical assessment may occur for more circumscribed purposes, such as to determine safety issues or potential need for hospitalization; to consult regarding school placement or pedagogical interventions; to advise about custody decisions; to consult in a pediatric setting; to serve as a component of family or other modes of treatment; or for research purposes (3).

DISTINCTIVE ASPECTS OF THE PSYCHIATRIC ASSESSMENT OF CHILDREN

The psychiatric assessment of the child differs from the assessment of adults in several respects. First, children rarely initiate psychiatric assessment or treatments themselves; rather, in most cases their parents or other adults provide the impetus for seeking treatment for the child. The child's behavior may cause greater distress to these adults than it does to the child. In some situations, the adult's expectations for the child may exceed the child's abilities, or the adult's own parenting or teaching style may be a poor fit with this child, yet these adults may seek means to alter the child to remedy this poor fit. On the other hand, children may not recognize their behaviors as problematic for others, or may not be receptive to changing these behaviors. Often these misbehaviors have "worked" by getting parents or teachers to avoid requesting the child to complete chores or tasks, or have culminated in others giving in to the child's requests. Children also may attribute problems to others and be unable or unwilling to accept their personal contribution to an identified problem. The psychiatric assessment of children thus requires consideration of both adult and child contributions to the distressing behaviors for which evaluation is being sought. In addition, the assessment requires explicit attention to the child's perceptions of the problems and what the child desires to change.

Second, the child and the clinician are at different developmental levels, such that they may essentially speak different languages. The school-age child may lack the maturity to abstract "patterns" from isolated events, while the adolescent may perceive the clinician's questions as another inquisition resembling that of parents or school staff. Moreover, phase-specific developmental features may further impede communication. For example, young children may not trust unfamiliar adults, while adolescents may perceive the clinician as simply another adult imposing expectations or judgments.

Third, the child may function differently in different settings. The child may function relatively well in multiple domains (with family, at school or work, with peers), function poorly in only one domain, or may function poorly across multiple domains. This underlines the necessity of multiple informants (4), not only to discern accurately the child's overall functioning, but also to identify the child's areas of strength on which the clinician can build, and to identify others (peers or adults) effective with the child and potentially able to introduce or reinforce more adaptive skills or behaviors.

Fourth, the child's presenting problems must be examined in a developmental context. The child may have a delay in skill development, such as delay in speaking or in areas of self-care, such as toileting. The child may not yet possess the skills necessary to interact appropriately with age-similar peers, and thus require interventions to introduce skills not yet present. The child's problems may also emanate from an inability to select appropriate skills from an existing repertoire. A child with depression or anxiety may have the necessary skills, but not be able to apply them, causing distress. For example, a child may overgeneralize that all animals are dangerous, and fear going outside, or an adolescent may stalk or threaten a classmate when threatened with a breakup. Finally, the child's problems may follow the loss of previously attained skills, often consequent to serious medical and psychiatric disorders, loss, or trauma. For example, a medically hospitalized school-age child may transiently regress with immature behaviors or loss of bowel or bladder control; adolescents developing schizophrenia may lose previously effective interaction skills (Chapter 5.3).

Further complicating this developmental context are developmental differences in presentation of mental illnesses. DSM-IV-TR diagnoses were primarily defined among adult samples. Although some disorders, such as obsessive-compulsive disorder look quite similar in children and adults, other disorders, such as major depression or bipolar disorder present notably differently in younger patients as compared to adults (Chapter 5.4.2). Hence, extrapolating the DSM-IV-TR criteria to children and adolescents can often be difficult or invalid. For example, in major depression, school-age children may be less likely than adults to manifest self-accusatory feelings and more likely to manifest somatic symptoms. Discerning "categories" of mental disorders in children is thus much more difficult, since numbers of symptoms in children predict psychosocial function (5). Efforts to consider where a particular child fits on the depressed mood axis, the inattention spectrum, and the impulsive axis, for example, may ultimately prove fruitful for prioritizing intervention targets.

Finally, an underestimated but critical facet of the psychiatric assessment of children is the necessity for forming alliances with the multiple parties, including among the clinician and the child, the parent, and outside agencies. A breach or rupture in any of these relationships can dramatically impair treatment efforts. Careful attention is required to establish effective alliances not only with the child, but with those adults who can serve as resources in facilitating the child's progress. It is during the assessment phase that efforts must begin to identify and align the agendas of these various treatment "partners" to enhance any intervention efforts. Parental permission should be obtained to contact and elicit information and collaboration from the various relevant parties who may have important information or who play an important role in the child's progress; such contacts include step- and noncustodial parents, teachers (by phone and via school records and requested rating scales), and primary medical care providers. Following the initial evaluation, followup contacts with parents living apart from the child, school staff, and other health providers can often help clarify obstacles to treatment and can help invest others in the child's improvement.

CONTENT OF THE CLINICAL INTERVIEW

Core contents of the clinical assessment of children and adolescents are common across purposes; these components are summarized in Table 4.2.2.1. They illuminate the need for a consistent, thorough assessment of the multiple variables that may contribute to the child's presentation, and the importance of synthesizing the input from multiple informants to derive an accurate picture of each child's unique predicament.

Reason for Referral

Clarity about who actually initiated this referral, their motivations, and what changes they seek is essential to the success of any evaluation. While parents may schedule an evaluation, opening questions about who suggested it, who recognized a need for an evaluation, or who is most uncomfortable with the child's behavior may all help clarify the impetus for the evaluation. More important, clarifying the circumstances and concerned individuals driving the evaluation request may

TABLE 4.2.2.1

CONTENT COMPONENTS OF THE PSYCHIATRIC ASSESSMENT OF CHILDREN AND ADOLESCENTS

Content Component	Primary Informant	Additional Resources
Reason for referral	Usually parent, guardian; sometimes school or legal agency	Letter from school or other agency seeking evaluation
History of problem(s)	Child and parent	Referral source; contact from primary care provider
Past problems	Child and parent	Structured interviews; screening scales
Comorbid symptoms	Child and parent	Structured interviews; screening scales
Substance use	Child, parent	Laboratory screening (as relevant)
Previous assessment/treatment(s)	Child, parent, clinicians	Mental health records
Child's development (includes psychomotor, cognitive, interpersonal, emotional, moral, trauma), harm (to self and others) development	Parents; school staff	School records, including special education evaluations; home video (as relevant)
Family history	Parent	Genogram
Medical history	Parent; health care provider(s)	Review of symptoms checklist; laboratory tests (as relevant)
Child's strengths	Parent; child; teachers; coaches; peers	Activity video (sports, music); cognitive, school, neuropsychological testing
Child's media diet	Parent; child; caregivers; siblings	Media diary; "Tivo" records; DVD/CD collections; magazine subscriptions
Environmental supports	Parent; child; adults familiar to child	Activity schedules (scouting, teams); afterschool/summer programs; mentorships/Big Brother or Sister relationships
Mental status exam	Child	Mini-Mental Status Examination

reveal the expectations of relevant parties and their willingness to implement treatment recommendations. For example, a parent may indicate the school or a grandparent identified distressing behaviors in the child. The parent may be required to obtain an evaluation for the child to return to school. The expectations of these various parties may in fact be in conflict and must be reconciled if effective treatments are to be implemented and for adherence to occur. For example, the school may seek to have parents manage the child differently, or to consider medication treatments, while the parents may be wishing for the evaluation to validate their current parenting efforts, or for diagnoses or recommendations which would yield additional school services. Similarly, grandparents may wish for different parenting approaches, while the parents may seek confirmation that their current approach is appropriate.

History of Problem(s)

The evolution of the child's problem should be elicited by the clinician mindful of the pain most parents encounter while recounting the deterioration or anguish of their child. To minimize this distress, and to obtain a full description, clinicians should provide parents some opportunity to chronicle this history in their own words. Moreover, the more treatments that can be framed within the parents' own description and understanding, by using the parents' words or concepts, the greater the probability parents will feel heard and collaborate in treatment. Parents diverge widely in terms of their own experience with and views of psychiatry, how they understand people's behaviors, and in their acceptance of alternatives to their current responses. Attention throughout the interview to these parent variables allows the clinician to explain behaviors and select interventions in terms acceptable to these particular parents.

As the parent describes the history of the problem, the clinician attends to the context in which the behavior emerged and occurs, changes in frequency and intensity of the behaviors, and the current progression of the problem. Since parents are rarely familiar with medical history taking, they usually will not detail the history as a clinician would. Permitting the parents to tell their own version of the problem for at least several minutes is usually necessary to allow them to articulate the problem or to discern what truly most concerns them, to feel heard or understood by the clinician, and to begin to feel allied with the clinician.

The clinician ultimately needs to inquire directly about specific instances of the child's problematic behaviors, parental responses to these behaviors, and the child's response to current parental interventions.

Since any given symptom (anxiety, inattention, arguing, theft, hallucinations) may have quite different meanings, functions, and clinical implications in different children, it is important not to jump immediately from symptom to diagnosis. The clinician may need to inquire directly about the *functions* of the problem behavior, including any secondary gains for the behavior (tantrums diminish parental expectations of chore completion, complaining of headaches every morning decreases time spent in a painful school class, running away causes parents to unite in efforts to find the child). Identifying specific antecedents and precipitants of the problem behavior and its consequences, both for the child and for others (including the family or classroom) may provide valuable insights into the functions of the problem behavior. In addition, the clinician should clarify the impact of the problem on the patient's quality of life, with particular attention as to whether the problem is specific to one functional domain or whether the behavior pervades multiple or all areas of the child's functioning, such as home, school, and with peers.

Problem behaviors may reflect an underlying disorder within the child, but may also reveal a problem within the child's environment (6). For example, a particular teacher, peer, or adult may contribute to the child's distress, although it is the child's symptom that is being labeled as the problem behavior. Perhaps most commonly, the *fit* between the child and a particular teacher, peer, or adult may culminate in expression or exacerbation of the child's symptoms. Accordingly, even when the child's symptoms occur pervasively across multiple domains of life (home, school/work, peers), attention to changes in school circumstances and peer and adult/parent networks may clarify forces fueling the symptoms.

Past Problems

Significant past problems, which have impaired the child, should be identified, as this provides a historical context for understanding the current problem. It is especially important to understand whether a problem has been persistent since early childhood, is intermittent, or represents a deterioration from a previously better level of functioning. (If the latter, the inquiry naturally leads to the questions of what events and circumstances have accompanied this deterioration). Identification of significant past problems which have interfered substantially with functioning at home, school, or with peers can also be facilitated through the use of screening instruments (see Chapter 4.2.3).

Comorbid Problems

Parents usually do not organize their descriptions of their child's difficulties according to DSM criteria. Rather, they describe the symptoms that appear most prominently in their child. As they do so, the clinician begins thinking implicitly about what diagnostic categories (or other means of conceptualizing the symptoms syndromically) might apply. Symptom constellations may be described by a parent in such a way as to suggest one particular diagnostic category, particularly when parents have heard from other parents, books, or Internet resources about potential diagnoses. However, it is important to recall that psychiatric symptoms are often diagnostically equivocal in that they may often overlap between various disorders, so consideration of disorders that may share similar symptoms should be considered. For example, inattention may occur in children with ADHD, but also among children with bipolar disorder, posttraumatic stress disorder or other anxiety disorders, or autism spectrum disorders, as well as in children who may be preoccupied with obsessions that distract them from focusing on what others are discussing.

Comorbidity is extremely common in childhood psychiatric disorders. Hence, clinicians should inquire about evidence of disorders often seen in tandem. For example, bipolar disorder in children is often associated with previous attention deficit hyperactivity disorder. Similarly, when depressed, many children will manifest symptoms of inattention, oppositionality, or irritability. Screening instruments can be useful to provide comprehensive information about less conspicuous conditions. This may be particularly important in detecting *internalizing* disorders, such as anxiety or mood disorders, which may be difficult for children to articulate, or which may be less troublesome or apparent to adults than disruptive *externalizing* disorders.

Substance Use History

Some symptom patterns, such as substance use, are particularly worrisome, both in terms of the direct hazards they pose to the child's development and as markers for a broader constellation of risk behaviors (7). Hence, it is particularly important to inquire regarding the child's exposure to and use of substances, including tobacco, alcohol, and illicit substances and how they may contribute to current symptoms. Previous exposures (including prenatal), contexts surrounding use, and effects of substances may impact treatment. Some children identify specific reasons for taking certain substances, while others proceed through many substances with diverse motives for taking or continuing use of these agents. For example, some children perceive that substances temporarily alleviate some of their symptoms (anxiety, depression) and so "self-medicate." In such cases, clarifying what impact these substances have on symptoms can clarify symptom priorities of the child, as well as possible intervention points more likely to be embraced by the child.

Previous Treatment(s)

Chronological assessment of past treatment efforts may reveal seasonal patterns, or escalation of a disorder, or may identify past strategies effective with this child which might be useful or adaptable for the current problem. In addition, past treatment history may suggest which treatment modalities have been tolerable (or not) to this patient (and family), signaling adherence issues or approaches that will be important in this case. Previous treatments including medications employed, counseling, hospitalizations, or alternative treatments may all provide useful information about the evolution of a child's problems.

Developmental History

The developmental history is a detailed accounting of the child's development from birth forward. This history includes bodily function regulation, psychomotor development, language development, cognitive growth, social development, emotional regulation, moral development, and exposure to trauma. Parents vary widely in their recollection of precise timing of developmental milestones. However, comparisons with other siblings or children, comparative recollections by different adults, and review of earlier videotapes of the child by the parents may improve the reliability and completeness of parent reports regarding the sequence of the child's growth.

Bodily, or basic, functions include sleeping, eating, and toileting. The child's development in regulating sleep, eating, and toileting may reveal episodes of difficulty. Similarly, previously attained skills may suddenly be lost, sometimes signaling the importance of emotional events at particular times and association with regression. Eating behavior has become complicated as the availability of various types of food, and times to eat, have increased. While hunger remains a risk factor for psychopathology (8), obesity particularly has become more common among younger people, and markedly increases both physical and mental illness (9, 10).

Psychomotor development includes milestones such as standing, walking, throwing, running, hopping, skipping, and playing sports or musical instruments whose timing may reveal uneven periods in development. Inquiry as to how the child enjoys or fares at sports may suggest treatment options through nonverbal modalities. Fine motor and gross motor skills may not be congruent and graphomotor (handwriting skills) may be an area in which some children need classroom accommodation. The ease of toileting, and persisting difficulties with bedwetting or soiling, should be investigated. In addition, medical history from parents may clarify periods when the child could not employ skills or became frustrated in attempting preferred activities.

Cognitive development usually begins with the child's verbal and attentional skills. The history of the child's language development (including higher order social language, prosody, and conversational rules) is important in identifying pervasive developmental disorders. The child's progression in preschool and school often reveal cognitive weaknesses, which may contribute to the current problem, or potential strengths to be harnessed to ameliorate the current problem. Specific inquiry concerning reading, writing, and math skill progression may reveal global difficulties or uneven skills in development. History by grade level can be helpful in discerning environmental changes that ameliorated or exacerbated symptoms. Report cards, behavioral concerns, absences, and retentions can be important in understanding the evolution of the child's development. It is important to bear in mind that adequate progress in school requires more than adequate innate cognitive abilities. It is also reflects the child's motivation, freedom from distraction, attitudes toward authority, capacity for peer relations, tolerance for frustration and delayed gratification, and degree of parental support for learning.

Interpersonal development assesses how the child interacts with others, particularly family members and other children and adults. Early interactions, especially with parents, provide important information about this child's unique temperament and comfort around others and the environment. Early aloofness, disinterest in others, absence of interactive play with parents or attention to objects pointed out by parents may be early markers of pervasive developmental disorder. The child's (and parents') reactions to significant changes in the social environment of the home are often important precipitants for the child's symptoms, particularly births/deaths of family members, marital changes (separations or conflicts, divorce, remarriages), and changes in caretaking arrangements (parent returning to work, or custody/visitation changes).

Exploring the child's compliance with family rules and expectations, the consequences for noncompliance, and the child's reaction to parental interventions in response to noncompliance often provide opportunities for behavioral interventions to diminish symptom expression. It is important to identify parents' style of limit setting in a variety of areas. For school-age children these concern hygiene; sleep; diet; TV, Internet, and video game use; and the expression of aggression. For adolescents, it is additionally important to know what sort of expectations parents do or do not set regarding curfew, dress, leisure activities, and choice of friends. Effective parental monitoring of an adolescent's activities, whereabouts, and peers is an important determinant of problem behaviors and usually reflects not only parents' efforts at active, close surveillance, but also a close parent–child relationship that encourages open communication and child disclosure (11).

The child's interactions with peers and adults outside the family are also important. How the child interacts with other children and preferences in play activities and friends (gender, age, interests) are important data for assessing the child's social skills and interest in relating to others. Stability of relationships, numbers of friends, types of activities shared, and expectations of peers ("plays with me when I want," "plays what I want to play," "helps me out if I need it," etc.) often reveal sources of difficulty or persistent maladaptive clashes where only the names of the antagonists change.

Emotional development and *temperament* is a key component in the evaluation of every child. A child's capacity to recognize his or her own mood state and to self-soothe or regulate negative affect should be investigated. Prevailing moods can be described by parents, as well as past suicidality, irritability, specific fears and anxieties, and conditions associated with the child's happiness and pleasure. Whether the child can recognize when a mood is mild or severe, and what steps the child will take when anxious, sad, or when encountering change or disappointment provide insight into vital coping mechanisms. Circumstances which provoke aggression or anger and the child's responses and capacity to accept input or direction from others may clarify intervention options such as parenting or behavioral treatments. These traits commonly exist along a spectrum, so that bullying, for example, may have started as assertiveness and progressed to exploitation or intimidation of others.

Assessment of the child's *moral development* provides an important gauge of whether the child's conscience or moral values are too lax, too harsh, overly focused on particular areas, or uneven and out of proportion to daily events. The child's religious and cultural/ethical views and practices and how those fit with those of the family also provide helpful information guiding potential treatment interventions. Similarly, the child's ability to recognize the plight of others, to recognize impacts of decisions of others, to reconcile principles with mistakes the child makes, and to acknowledge and correct mistakes often provides clarity about the child's strengths and limitations.

At any stage of the child's development, children may experience *trauma* which has substantially impacted or even arrested development. Investigation of not only actual events (such as documented physical or sexual abuse), but of events perceived traumatic by the child and the vicissitudes of these events for the child and family shed important light on the child's behaviors and patterns of relating to others. Identifying episodes of abuse (physical, sexual, verbal), the events surrounding the trauma, the child's role in disclosing such abuse to others, and the reactions of adults to such disclosures are also important for the clinician to recognize and address.

Harmful behavior, toward self or others, should always be investigated. Past episodes of harmful comments or acts may reveal important developmental progressions or patterns that warrant intervention. Headbanging or self-injurious behaviors may reveal underlying sensory disturbances, sometimes seen in developmental disorders; thoughts or comments about death may reveal suicidality; and self-harmful acts such as self-mutilation or cutting may reveal primitive coping mechanisms (12), and may increase risk for subsequent psychopathology such as eating disorders (13). Harmful acts toward others, animals as well as people, may reveal safety or monitoring issues required to preserve the safety of others while other diagnostic or treatment interventions occur.

Family History

Parental variables may impact the child's problems and warrant examination. First, family conflict, or differences in parenting style, may culminate in the child manifesting symptoms; however, the converse is equally true, in that disturbed behavior by a child may stress otherwise adequate parental coping skills or provoke conflict between parents. Parents may have grown up themselves with different parenting practices in their families of origin that they wish to employ, or avoid, and these influences are important to understand in assessing the consistencies and discrepancies within and between each parent's style. In the face of a child's distressing behaviors, parents may attempt a wide variety of approaches, some uncharacteristic of their usual parenting style, poorly conceived, and enacted at inopportune times (e.g., unenforceable threats during a tantrum); such responses may not improve the problem but do increase parental guilt and hopelessness. Accordingly, the clinician must be mindful that the approach parents ordinarily employ may not be described if it did not work with this child. Clarifying the evolution of the approaches parents have attempted for this child's problems, and how these approaches may have differed from approaches employed with their other children, may help the clinician disentangle child and parent contributions to the current problem.

Second, parents may have problems with the child at particular developmental periods. Certain developmental stages may have particularly challenged the parent's skills or coping responses, or may have reminded the parent of a painful time in his or her own childhood. Discussion with parents about how they navigated past difficulties with this child, their rationales for certain parenting practices, and their expectations (and fears) during this given developmental phase of the child often provide clues about potential parental contributions to the problem. Similarly, information about parents' cultural, ethnic, education, occupation, and religious background may reveal not only sources of adversity or conflict between parents or family members, but sources of pride and resilience that inform interventions to enhance treatment adherence among parents and children.

Third, parental genetic contributions remain an important variable to consider, particularly since some parents perceive that the child's psychopathology may be attributed to one or the other parent based on that parent's personal or family history. Few if any common psychiatric disorders appear exclusively through genetic transmission alone, although increased vulnerabilities to various disorders are likely. In addition, the child's experience of growing up with a parent who has struggled with depression, anxiety, psychosis, or substance abuse is likely to have an impact on the child, over and above any genetically transmitted vulnerability. Tactful but thorough investigation into psychopathology in each parent and among the extended family may suggest which disorders or general conditions (mood, anxiety) may be more probable. Patterns can also be visualized by constructing a genogram, particularly in complex families with multiple psychopathologies. Although unspoken during psychiatric evaluations, many parents fear that their other children may be destined to suffer psychopathology when one sibling manifests a disorder, so clarification of genetic contributions to expression of disorders can often be helpful in reducing unwarranted fear, guilt, and distress among parents.

Divorce, separation, and single-parent family circumstances may stress all family members, including the children. Even when parents part amicably, children may have difficulty with change from what has been familiar. Similarly, even in circumstances where parents and children experience reduced conflict after parents separate, children sometimes exhibit symptoms which coincide with marital changes. The child's symptoms may reveal overwhelming stress or fear, but also may reveal efforts to reunite family members. In addition, children may exhibit symptoms months or years after separations as difficulty adjusting to new roles or environments occurs or as they enter a new developmental phase (14).

Adoption may be a positive event for the child and for the adoptive parents, and the circumstances of the adoption warrant tactful attention by the clinician, including age of the child and biological parents, the degree of ongoing contact with or interest in biological parents, the child's understanding of the adoption and attitudes about the biological and the adoptive parents, and how the adoption is discussed at home. In addition, adoptive parent expectations and feelings about the adoption, particularly as their child now undergoes a psychiatric evaluation, may reveal underlying parental fears, guilt, or disappointments.

However the family system is currently configured, the clinician should inquire about how the family system functions, with whom the child spends time, and the nature of the relationships between the various household members and the child. Boundaries and alliances, conflicts, and the child's affinities or resentments of other family members should be determined. Family communication and problemsolving, including how issues of disagreement are handled, should be assessed. The emotional tone of families vary widely from constricted to overly expressive and dramatic, and should be examined both by observation of family interactions during the interview, as well as by direct inquiry. Clarification of family stressors that are chronic family stressors (family member illness or disability) or acute (sudden illness, job loss/change, financial or legal difficulties) may identify determinants of the child's current problems as well as potential targets for intervention.

Medical History

Medical conditions experienced by the child should be identified beginning with conception (as well as any difficulties the mother had in conceiving or the use of assisted reproductive technologies). Pregnancy complications, birth difficulties, extended hospital stays, and medical illnesses requiring recurrent or ongoing treatments (asthma, diabetes) should be investigated, since these appear to increase the child's risk for psychopathology (15). In addition, inquiry into hospitalizations, emergency room visits, or surgeries can help shed light on the child's fears, or parental over/underprotectiveness. Allergies, particularly to medications, should be ascertained, as well as responses or side effects to previous medications, especially psychotropics, and including naturopathic or homeopathic agents.

Age of menarche and stage of pubertal development should be inquired about when relevant. If the child's weight and/or stature is out of the normal range for age (as plotted on a standard growth chart), a detailed review of the child's growth history and eating habits should be made.

Accidents or illnesses with a potential for central nervous system impact, such as lead exposure, seizures, head trauma, loss of consciousness, deserve specific inquiry.

Child Strengths/Weaknesses

In addition to clarifying the child's problems, the evaluation simultaneously elicits the child's areas of strength so that interventions can build on these existing strengths and assets rather than focusing exclusively on areas of weakness.

Interests, hobbies, and talents of the child should be obtained from both the child and the parents, since these accounts may not match or may even be in conflict.

Parents may have aspirations for their children that the child does not share, or the child may have fantasies beyond apparent abilities. In most cases, though, the child will have some identifiable interests or abilities that serve as potential points of connection with peers and adults (including the therapist) and may serve to facilitate therapy. Exploration of the child's interests, including newly emerging ones, may allow the interviewer to anchor recommendations or treatment metaphors to language or subjects familiar to or valued by the patient. Similarly, the child's and parents' accounts of time spent in an activity (10 years of ballet and modern dance) or perceived fruits of the child's labor ("I won trophies twice," vs. "I've lost most games I've played in") illuminate what effect the activity has had on the child, including pride or disappointment, as well as the parents' and the child's own expectations.

The Child's Media Diet

In an information-processing society, children are exposed to immense doses of media, including television, music, videos, electronic games, cell phones, e-mail and instant messaging, and personal digital assistants. These media, which may provide exposure of the child to much violent and sexually provocative material, may have positive or negative effects. It is important to clarify which media the child uses, how much time each day is spent with these various media, and what consequences these media have on the child (e.g., in response to watching action TV shows the child becomes more violent vs. has developed interest in Asian food through watching cooking programs, or listening to an MP3 player at school serves to distract the child from classroom instruction vs. helps the child calm down on the bus or ignore other disruptions) (16). E-mail, instant messaging, chatrooms, and bulletin boards such as *MySpace* or *Facebook*, can be used to multiple ends, which may be adaptive (maintaining friendships with camp friends), problematic (bullying, harassment, or dangerous exhibitionism), or both (permitting a socially anxious child to maintain a modicum of electronic social contacts, but at the cost of avoiding more face-to-face relationships) (17). Evidence suggests that frequent watching of television during childhood is associated with violent behaviors decades later (18). As with other aspects of parental monitoring, the degree of parental awareness and appropriate limit setting regarding TV, video games, and instant messaging is important to determine, in part as an indicator of parental structure and expectations. As with other of the child's interests, preferred television show, favorite movies, favored musicians or bands provide a common language to examine topics, as well as clues about the child's aspirations and behavioral self-expectations ("[Music idol] swears at adults all the time, so why can't I?") (19). Asking a child to describe an episode of a favorite TV show or movie also provides a convenient picture of the quality of the child's social language and grasp of others' motives and feelings.

Environmental Supports

Although many children must contend with moves or changes in the family constellation, other environmental supports and buffers often provide stability and even sanctuary and warrant investigation. Adults other than the parents (such as grandparents and other relatives, coaches, teachers) may play significant, ongoing roles in the lives of children, while community involvements, such as church groups, athletic team participation, outdoor clubs, musical ensembles, or even preferred places to convene may provide opportunities for intervention or support in natural settings on a regular basis.

Mental Status Examination

The mental status examination is an essential part of any psychiatric interview, as it provides direct information about how the child presents and interacts with the clinician. The mental status examination includes a clinical description of the child's appearance, mood, sensorium, apparent intelligence,

TABLE 4.2.2.2

THE MENTAL STATUS EXAMINATION IN CHILDREN

Category	Components	What to Assess
Appearance	Physical appearance	Gender; ethnicity; age (actual and apparent); cleanliness and grooming, hair/clothing style, presence of physical anomalies, indicators of self-care and parental attentiveness; jewelry, cosmetics, adornments
	Manner of relating to clinician and parents	Ease of separation from each parent, guardedness/warming up to clinician, eagerness to please, defiance, flirtatiousness, reactions to meeting the clinician
	Activity level	Psychomotor retarded to hyperactive, sustained or episodic, goal-oriented or erratic; coordination, unusual postures or motor patterns (tics, stereotypies, compulsions, catatonia, akathisia, dystonia, tremors)
	Speech	Fluency (including stuttering, cluttering, speech impediments), rate, volume, prosody
Mood	Current affect	Predominant emotion and range (constricted to labile) during the interview, and appropriateness to content (giggles while talks about sibling's illness); intensity; lability
	Persisting mood	Predominant emotion over days/weeks; whether current affect unusual or consistent with mood; whether mood reactive to situations or same across range of situations
	Coping mechanisms and regulation of affect	How child manages conflict or distress, age-appropriateness of responses to and dependency on parents; sexual interests, impulses, aggression; control or modulation of urges (finding alternative or socially appropriate means of satisfying urges); how deals with frustration or when anxious
Sensorium	Orientation	Self (name), place (town, state), time (awareness of morning, day of week, month, year varies by age), situation (why at this appointment)
Intellect	Attention	Eye contact, need for redirection/repeating, how long sustained on activity, degree to which child shifts from activity to activity, distractibility (to outside noises, etc.)
	Memory	Immediate (repeat numbers, names back), short-term (recall three objects at 2 and 5 minutes), long-term (recall events of past week)
	Intelligence; fund of knowledge	Age-appropriate recognition of letters, vocabulary, reading, counting, computational skills; age-appropriate knowledge of geography, history, culture (celebrities, sports, movies); concrete to abstract thinking, ability to classify and categorize
	Judgment	Especially concerning the current problems (best assessed after rapport established, as initial responses may be minimization or denial); what do if found stamped envelope next to mailbox, fire started in theater, say if saw man with big feet
	Insight	Ability to see alternative explanations, others' points of view; locus of control (internal vs. external); defense mechanisms
Thought	Form: *Coherence*	Logical, goal-directed, circumstantial or tangential (consider age-appropriateness), looseness of associations, word salad (incoherent, clanging, neologisms)
	Form: *Speed*	Mutism, poverty of thought (long latency, thought blocking), poverty of content (perseveration), racing thoughts, flight of ideas
	Perceptions	Altered bodily experiences (depersonalization, derealization), misperception of stimulus (illusion), no stimulus (hallucination: auditory [psychosis >PTSD >Organic causes], visual [dementia >delirium]), olfactory (neurological, seizure [disorder] gustatory [from medicine side effects])
	Content	Obsessions (ego-dystonic), delusions (ego-syntonic), thoughts of harm to self or others (magical thinking, or fears at night often age appropriate)

and thought content and process. Although often conceptualized as a separate component that is distinct from the history-taking interview, in reality much of the mental status examination takes place implicitly as the clinician interacts and observes the child during the child and family interviews. Although some components of the exam will require specific inquiry or examination (such as orientation, memory, fund of knowledge, and mental contents), most will be noted as the clinician organizes his or her ongoing observations of the child according to the elements of the mental status exam. A format for the child mental status examination is provided in Table 4.2.2.2.

In addition, the mental status examination provides an opportunity for further screening of organic or neurological contributions to the child's symptoms. A mini-mental status examination (MMSE) (Table 4.2.2.3) can provide more detailed assessment of an older child's higher order mental functions, including orientation, attention, memory, language, and constructional ability (20). This MMSE contains items appropriate for older children, although some modified versions provide questions for younger patients (21). However, such scales are best used for screening. More reliable and detailed assessment of a child's speech, language, intellectual, academic achievement, attention and executive functioning, memory, and complex thinking requires standardized psychometric testing (Chapters 4.24 and 4.25).

STRUCTURE OF THE CLINICAL INTERVIEW

While the steps in the process of the psychiatric assessment of the child may unfold in multiple ways, a step-wise approach, individualized by the clinician for the requirements of each specific case, helps ensure thoroughness. More importantly, the quality of the information obtained from which all

TABLE 4.2.2.3

MINI-MENTAL STATUS EXAMINATION

		Score	Points
Orientation			
1. What is the	Year?	____	1
	Season?	____	1
	*Date?	____	1
	Day?	____	1
	Month?	____	1
2. Where are we?	Country	____	1
	State or territory	____	1
	Town or city?	____	1
	*Hospital or suburb?	____	1
	Floor or address?	____	1
Registration			
3. Name three objects, taking 1 second to say each. Then ask the patient all three after you have said them. (Tree, clock, boat, or body parts for children <7 years.) Give one point for each correct answer. Repeat the answers until patient learns all three.		____	3
Attention and Calculation			
4. Serial sevens. Give one point for each correct answer. Stop after five answers. For children <age 7, have them repeat 2–5 digit strings (e.g., "4–7," then 3-5-8," and score one point for each digit string repeated forward correctly).		____	5
5. Spell "world" backwards. For children <7, have them repeat 2–4 digit strings backwards (e.g., examiner says "5–2" and child repeats back "2–5," etc.).		____	5
Recall			
6. Ask for names of three objects learned in 3 above. Give one point for each correct answer.		____	3
Language			
7. Point to a pencil and a watch or to body parts. Have the patient name them as you point.		____	2
8. Have the patient repeat, "No ifs, ands, or buts."		____	1
9. Have the patient follow a three-stage command. "Take a piece of paper in your right hand. Fold the paper in half. Put the paper on the floor."		____	3
10. Have the patient read and obey the following: "CLOSE YOUR EYES." (Write it in large letters.) For children <7, have them read their name.		____	1
11. Have the patient write a sentence of his or her choice. (The sentence should contain a subject and an object and should make sense. Ignore spelling errors when scoring.) For children <7, have them write their name.		____	1
12. Have the patient copy the design printed below. (Give one point if all sides and angles are preserved and if the intersecting sides form a diamond shape.) For children under age 7, have draw a circle or oval.		____	1
TOTAL:		____	(35)

(From Ouvrier RA, Goldsmith RF, Ouvrier S, Williams IC: The value of the Mini-Mental State Examination in childhood: A preliminary study. *J Child Neurol* 1993;8:145, and Jain M, Passi GR: Assessment of a Modified Mini-Mental Scale for Cognitive Functions in Children. Indian Peds 2005; 42:907–912, both with permission.)

diagnoses and treatment planning will follow is contingent on the approach the clinician employs, and how well this approach fits the particular patient. A sample checklist for the preparatory stage of the psychiatric assessment of children is summarized in Figure 4.2.2.1. The clinician, or staff, may begin completing such a checklist during the initial phone contacts with the child's family, although the entire checklist may not be completed until after the assessment.

Preparatory Phase of the Child Interview

Preparation is paramount in child psychiatry interviews. Families are often unfamiliar with what occurs during such an assessment, and concern by the child or the parent that they will be "judged" is almost universal. Unlike routine well-child visits with a pediatrician, a child psychiatry interview is rarely perceived by parents as a mental health checkup for their child, but rather as potentially indicative of their failures as parents. Invocation of a psychiatric diagnosis may help exonerate some parents from feelings of guilty (but sometimes spurious) responsibility for the child's presenting difficulties and, indeed, some parents may seek evidence of a "chemical imbalance" outside their control as responsible for the child's symptoms. Accordingly, interactions prior to the actual interview can help clarify parental fears and expectations. For example, parents may report, "I did toilet training wrong, and now my child—..." as they search for the root of the child's current problems. Similarly, parent anxieties often emerge, as some parents report, "My child only acts badly toward me—I bring out the worst in my child," fearing they uniquely cause the child's symptoms. The parent interview also provides clues as to what difficulties may be encountered in trying to change parental behavior, such as how overwhelmed a parent may become when even basic interventions are suggested for them to enact (e.g., in response to questions such as "What would happen if you were to simply turn the TV off and tell him it is bedtime?"). At the other extreme, some parents may have hopes or expectations that the clinician cannot fulfill, for example, "You [the child psychiatrist] need to tell him how good he has it at home" or "Tell him if he is gay I will disown him and throw him out of the house." Such expectations may require clarifying what expectations the child psychiatrist can or cannot fulfill. Parents may come with other preconceived agendas, such as that their child is bipolar or that they are determined that under no condition will their child ever receive any medication. Preparing parents for what to expect during the assessment diminishes parent and child anxieties, and initiates a process for shared goals and appropriate parent and child expectations. Sample letters clarifying the assessment are provided in Appendixes 1 and 2.

Children also usually have little idea of what occurs in a psychiatric assessment, and may fear being hospitalized, or otherwise punished, especially if their difficulties have been a source of recrimination in the family. A child who harbors a family secret or concerns about a parent's behavior may fear punishment, relocation, or loss of contact with that parent if he or she speaks openly. Other children only know they are being expected to articulate explanations for behaviors that may not make sense to them, let alone to adults.

Similarly, interested others (such as school staff or other healthcare providers) may have diverse (or unrealistic) expectations of what a psychiatric assessment can provide or how it might be implemented (such as a month-long inpatient observation).

In order to diminish unreasonable fears and to encourage more honest, accurate reporting, the clinician will seek, even prior to the first interview, to cultivate a partnership with the parents and interested others to support the child. A brief (under 15 minute) initial phone call can help clarify how parents and teachers perceive the identified problem and introduce potential areas of exploration (e.g., specific patient strengths or interests) that may facilitate the family's and child's functioning and comfort with the assessment. If such calls are not possible or feasible, trained office staff may make these initial inquiries. Finding out the child's favorite toys, games, musical interests, etc., may help diminish resistance and expedite the interview (Figure 4.2.2.1).

During this same initial phone contact, clarification of preferred contact numbers where the parents can be reached without embarrassment, billing information, consent to speak with others familiar with the child can often be accomplished in advance of the actual interview. Some parents are reluctant to consent to contact between the clinician and others (such as the school) until they feel more comfortable with the clinician. Parental preferences for e-mail correspondence can also be discussed before the actual interview, so that efficient methods for data acquisition from others can be determined. Finally, special needs of the child (for example, visual difficulties) can be discussed in a less embarrassing context than in front of the patient. Similarly, ideas from the parents for making the assessment flow more comfortably, such as allowing the child to bring and demonstrate favored toys or music (MP3 or iPod) players with headphones, or preferred discussion topics for teenagers, enhance the initial alliance, crucial in any later treatment efforts.

The Parent Interview

In the initial face-to-face parent interview, the clinician seeks to understand the parents' perspective on the problems leading to this referral. The clinician endeavors to identify the "why now?" reasons that this evaluation is occurring, how parents understand the evolution of their child's symptoms, what current priorities each parent or other party (such as the school or court) describes for this evaluation, what impact the child's difficulties now have on the family, and how the child's symptoms impact his or her functioning with peers and at school or work. Throughout each component of the interview, the clinician remains alert to the potential functions or benefits the current symptoms carry for the child, the apparent attunement of the parents to the child's needs, and available resources; these resources include special skills or talents the child may possess and the presence of other individuals who exert a positive influence on this child. The clinician will also be attentive to any relevant cultural factors that may affect the child's symptoms. The goal is to obtain as full a picture as possible of the child's current developmental trajectory given the totality of these circumstances. Sample questions for eliciting each component of this interview are provided in Table 4.2.2.4.

Special Techniques for the Developmentally Sensitive Parent Interview

The parent interview can be complicated by multiple factors, including parental ambivalence about having a child evaluated by a psychiatrist, by divergent perceptions among parents and adults about the origin of the child's problems, fears of loss of control or criticism, or parental shame or embarrassment about perceived parenting faults or personal past history. Just as the child's level of development will impact the content of the interview, so too do adults vary in their sophistication about parenting techniques or understanding their child's developmental needs. To understand parents' descriptions about the child in their proper context, the clinician will remain attentive throughout the interview to the parents' own vulnerabilities and concerns about parenting. Parents may have their own past experiences rekindled when they see their child in distress, and may seek to prevent outcomes they experienced (22). Clinicians may detect reflexive inclinations in some parents to revert, when stressed, to doing what their parents did to them, and clinicians may detect distressing parental recollections about their own childhood adversities brought back through their child's problems. Multiple techniques may be required for the clinician to help parents overcome such obstacles during the course of the interview. These are summarized in Figure 4.2.2.2.

The Developmentally Sensitive Clinical Interview of the Child

The interview of the child allows the clinician 1) to gather additional history, from the child's point of view, and 2) to examine how the child attributes meaning to this. Although the reliability of information from the child on any given point will vary with the topic and with the individual child, the clinical information derived from direct observation of and interaction with the child is essential. The child's description of feelings, moods, levels of distress, and significant events contribute to a complete understanding of the child, and to matching and framing viable treatments with the individual child. In addition, symptoms such as compulsions, urges, obsessive or suicidal thoughts, hallucinations, tics, or a thought disorder

_____ 1. Child's Name: ____________________ Preferred Name: ____________________

_____ 2. Parents/Guardians: ____________________

_____ 3. Contact Information:

Home Phone: ____________________ Cell Phone: ____________________

Billing Address: ____________________

____

_____ E-mail: ____________________

_____ E-mailp arameters, including privacy caveats, discussed/acceptable to family: YESN O

_____ 4. Reasons for Referral: ____________________

____

____

_____ 5. Expectations from This Assessment: ____________________

____

____

_____ 6. Consents Given to Speak with:

_____ Family _____ School _____ Other Providers

Names/Contact Numbers: ____________________

____

____

____

_____ 7. Taping/Video/Recording: ____________________

_____ 8. Special Needs: _____ Language _____ Audiovisual

(Doest he family have videotapeso f the child's early years? If yes, reviewing these with attention to when thec hild walked, talked, playedw ith otherc hildren, showeda ny concerning behaviors or mannerism, mayb eh elpful during discussions of the child's developmental history.)

_____ 9. Parent Preparation of Child for Clinical Interview

_____ 10. Making Comfortable at Ofce:

_____ Preferred Toys/Games/Activities: ____________________

_____ Interests (Sports, Music, Extracurricular): ____________________

_____ 11. Condentiality (HIPAA, e-mail) Discussed: ____________________

FIGURE 4.2.2.1. Preparatory checklist for clinical assessment.

TABLE 4.2.2.4

PARENT INTERVIEW: SAMPLE CLINICIAN QUESTIONS

Component	Example Parent Questions to Elicit ("Yes" responses warrant followup questions to clarify acts, context, intentions, and consequences.)	Example Child Questions ("Yes" responses warrant followup questions to clarify acts, context, intentions, consequences, and learnings from these events.)
Reason for referral	Whose idea was it that [child] might need this evaluation? Who is most concerned about [child's] behavior? Has anyone else, such as other family members, school staff, or other agencies, encouraged this evaluation? What do you/they hope this evaluation will accomplish?	What did your parent(s) tell you about coming here today? Who wanted you to meet with me today? What did they say to you about us meeting? How do you feel about being here?
History of problem(s)	When did you first notice [child's] problem? How did the problem develop over time? How did you understand [child's] behavior?	What do you wish would be different? What is not going well for you? What do you think is making this such a hard time?
Functional—assessment of problem behaviors	Where does the problem behavior occur most often? How does the problem impact [child] at home? At school? With peers? Is the problem behavior worse in one of these places? What usually occurs right before the problem behavior? What happens after [child] does [problem behavior]? How do [parent, teacher, peers, friends] respond? Has anything changed to make the behavior worse/better?	When/Where does the problem occur? What happens when you [exhibit symptoms]? What usually happens right before you [exhibit symptom]? How does your [parent, teacher, friend] respond when you [exhibit symptom]? How do you feel after you [exhibit symptom]?
Past problems	Did [child] have any problems this severe at an earlier point? What other significant difficulties has [child] had in the past?	Have there ever been any times when things were difficult? Have you had any times before where things were difficult? Has anyone ever been worried about you?
Comorbid symptoms	Does [child] have any other symptoms that trouble you? Does [child] have any other symptoms that interfere at home, school, or with friends? Have others identified any other problems they've noticed with [child]?	Is there anything else going on that you wish were different? Do you feel bad in any other ways? Do you have any difficulty sleeping/eating/going to the bathroom? Is there anything you worry about? How often do you feel sad? Do you wish anything were different with peers/family members/teachers?
Substance use history	Has your child done anything to suggest use of substances? Have you detected your child to be drunk/high/stoned/on drugs? Have you seen or found any drug paraphernalia that might be your child's? Has your child spoken about drinking, smoking, or substance use?	Have you ever been around any substances (alcohol, tobacco, marijuana, etc.)? Have you ever tried tobacco? Alcohol? Any other drugs? Do they help in any way? Have you ever been high/stoned/intoxicated? Has that ever led to any problems for you? Have you ever tried to stop? How did that go?
Previous treatment(s)	What has been attempted to address this in the past? Has [child] received any treatment(s) in the past for emotional or behavioral concerns?	Has anyone tried to help you with ______? Have you talked with anyone about these difficulties before? Have you ever taken any medicines for these difficulties?
Developmental history		
Basic functions	How did [child] progress with sleep? Did [child] always sleep through the night? How has [child's] appetite been? Has [child] ever been overweight? How do you feel about [child's] size/weight? What do you tell [child] about his weight/appearance? How did toilet training progress with [child]? Has [child] had periods of wetting or soiling?	Do you have any trouble falling asleep? Staying asleep? How do you sleep through the night? Do you need/use a nightlight? Do you like it better when someone sleeps with you? How is your appetite? How do you feel about the way you look? What do others (peers, parents) say about your appearance? Do you have any difficulties going to the bathroom?

(continued)

TABLE 4.2.2.4

(CONTINUED)

Component	Example Parent Questions to Elicit ("Yes" responses warrant followup questions to clarify acts, context, intentions, and consequences.)	Example Child Questions ("Yes" responses warrant followup questions to clarify acts, context, intentions, consequences, and learnings from these events.)
Psychomotor development	When did [child] start walking? What sports/activities has [child] participated in? Which ones have gone well? Not so well?	How do you do in sports? How do you do when you play with friends your age? Do you have any problems playing games/sports/ music/dancing?
Cognitive development	Did [child] show interest in things you pointed to? Did [child] point things out to you? When did [child] begin preschool/school? How did that go? How did [child] do with reading? With math? With writing? In which subjects did [child] do particularly well? Which subjects were more difficult? How did [child] do each year in school? Did [child] ever receive any special educational services? Has [child] ever been suspended, expelled, or asked to leave as school? Did [child] ever have any periods of excessive absences? Did [child] ever fail in subjects or grades? Has [child] even had any summer school or after-school tutoring? Is there anything [child] particularly enjoys or does well at in school?	Which subjects do you like best at school? Which subjects do you do best in at school? How do you like reading? Math? Writing? Is anything at school really hard for you to do? Is there anything you have trouble understanding? How do you get along with the other kids in your class? With your teacher? Has anyone ever helped you with school work? What do they do? Have you ever had to take any classes over? Have you ever done any grades over? Have you ever gone to school during the summer?
Interpersonal development	How did [child] relate to you as a child? How did [child] respond to your requests or directions? When did [child] start interacting with other children? How did that go? Did [child] have any significant attachments or relationships to others that ended? What kind of friends does [child] have at this point? How does [child] get along with these children? Does [child] get invited to play dates, birthday parties, sleepovers?	Who are some of your good friends now (when/where met, what do together, how often)? How often do you and _____ play together? How long do you stay at [friend's house]? Do you spend the night at [friend's house]? How does that go (What do you do?)? Any rough spots between you and other kids? How come? Have you lost any good friends (because of moves, misunderstandings.)?
Emotional development	Does [child] recognize when he or she is sad, really happy, etc.? How does [child] soothe him/herself when unhappy or in a bad mood? What is the child's prevailing/most common mood? How does the child respond to unexpected changes? Disappointments? Frustrations? Anxieties or depression moods?	How often do you feel sad? Mad? Worried? Does anything in particular make you sad/ mad/worried? What do you do when you are feeling that way? Can you do anything to stop yourself from getting sad/mad/worried? How do you calm yourself down?
Moral development	Does [child] recognize right from wrong? Does [child] describe any "principles" that guide his/her actions? How does [child] contend with mistakes or when confronted about doing something wrong? Has [child] ever deliberately hurt any animals or other kids? Bullied or been bullied by other kids? Does [child] show remorse after hurting someone? Does [child] anticipate consequences of his or her decisions? Does [child] consider consequences of decisions on others? Is [child] either too perfectionistic or morally rigid?	Do you ever do things that you wish you hadn't? Do you ever hurt others? Even if it's not on purpose? What do you wish will happen when you [hit other, say something really mean, break/steal someone's toy]? What does happen when you do something that hurts or upsets [someone else]? Can you keep yourself from hitting/getting back at someone if you want to?
Trauma history	Has [child] ever been hurt/injured? Has [child] ever witnessed anything really bad or frightening? Has [child] described frightening dreams/nightmares? Has [child] ever made unusual comments about sex? Have you [parent] had any traumatic experiences that remind you of what [child] is going through?	Have you ever been hurt? Injured? Have you ever seen anything really bad? Frightening? Have you ever seen anyone get hurt badly? Do you ever have scary dreams or nightmares? Do you ever see or hear something that reminds you of something really scary? Has anyone ever tried to hurt you? Who did/would you tell if someone tried to hurt you?

TABLE 4.2.2.4

(CONTINUED)

Component	Example Parent Questions to Elicit ("Yes" responses warrant followup questions to clarify acts, context, intentions, and consequences.)	Example Child Questions ("Yes" responses warrant followup questions to clarify acts, context, intentions, consequences, and learnings from these events.)
Harm to self or others history	Has [child] ever talked about hurting himself? Others? Has [child] ever done things to inflict pain on himself? To hurt others? Has [child] ever hurt any animals? What happened? Has [child] ever been involved with school officials or police because of threats or harm toward others?	Have you ever thought about hurting yourself? Others? Have you every deliberately hurt yourself? How did you feel after you did ____? Have you ever hurt anyone else on purpose? How did you feel about that? How do you feel about that now? Have you ever hurt a pet or an animal? How did that feel? Have you ever gotten into trouble with anyone for talking about hurting yourself or someone else?
Family history	What were the circumstances surrounding the conception and pregnancy with [child]? Do [parents] agree on how to respond to [child]? Do you treat him or her differently than you were treated by your parents? Did [parents] grow up in similar type families? Is there anything [one parent] does quite differently from [other parent], or from your own parents? Has anyone on father's (mother's) side of the family had depression, anxiety, problems with attention or learning, tics, substance abuse problems, or any other mental illness? Has anyone in the family had serious medical problems? Has anyone in the family ever been psychiatrically or medically hospitalized? Incarcerated? [If relevant] what was that like for [the child]? What do you think [child] has inherited from [all parents, biological, and adoptive]?	Are you like anyone else in your family? Do you know if anyone in your family has ever felt like you do? How do your parents understand you?
Family constellation history	Have there been any times when [child's parents] were separated/together? Have any changes in the family [loss/addition of parent, loss/addition of sibling or other in the home] contributed to [child's] symptoms? What kind of contact does [child] have with [parents, grandparents, primary caregiving relatives]? What does [child] say about [other parent, caregivers]?	Have either of your parents ever been away very long? Do you miss anyone from your family? Whom do you get along best with in your home? Whom do you have the hardest time with (Why?)?
Medical history	Has [child] ever had any medical illnesses or serious injuries? Been hospitalized? Had any operations? Was [child] physically ill before these symptoms started? Has [child] had any physical symptoms that occur with/since the emotional symptoms? Has [child] ever been allergic to anything?	Have you ever been really sick? Have you ever had to go to the hospital (what happened?) Have you ever had any surgeries (what was that like?)? Have you been physically sick since you have had problems with ____?
Child's strengths	What is [child] good at? What does [child] do for fun? What does [child] do during the day? What does [child] want to do/wish he could do?	What do you most like to do? What are you really good at? What do your friends/other students think you are really good at? What would you like to be better at? Do you feel special in any way? What do you want to do when you grow up?
Child's media diet	What does [child] watch/read/listen to? How much time does [child] spend watching television/movies? Listening to music? Reading magazines? How does television influence [child]? What effects do you think [child's] musical choices have on him? What impacts do you think those magazines have on [child]?	How much do you watch TV every day? Listen to music? Read for fun? What about [TV show, music, magazine] most appeals to you? How do you feel after watching/listening/reading ____? Do you ever get into trouble after watching/listening/reading ____?

(continued)

TABLE 4.2.2.4

(CONTINUED)

Component	Example Parent Questions to Elicit ("Yes" responses warrant followup questions to clarify acts, context, intentions, and consequences.)	Example Child Questions ("Yes" responses warrant followup questions to clarify acts, context, intentions, consequences, and learnings from these events.)
Community and environmental supports	What is your neighborhood like? Do kids play outside much in your neighborhood? Any neighborhood problems or tensions? Is a language other than English spoken at home? If so, by whom, and does [child] also speak/understand that language? [If family is of recent immigrant origins], does [the child] still have close relatives there? Does he or she visit there often? What is the family's religious tradition? Does [the child] attend services regularly or have strong religious identifications? What activities does [child] participate in? Are there others who work with [child]? Do you have any help/support managing these problems with [child]? How do your family members view [child's problems]? Does [child] benefit from interactions/participation with neighbors/scouting/hobbies/shared interests with others?	Outside of your home, where are you most happy? Are there any other adults who are special to you/work with you? Can you tell me about your best friends? Are there any kids that bother you or make you uncomfortable? Is there a group you feel a part of? Who do you "hang out" with? Is there a group you would rather be a part of? Are there particular others you'd like to hang out with? Is there any place you really like to go to feel better? How have your symptoms affected your family?

may not be recognized or acknowledged by the adults in the child's life, and children are often more reliable reporters of internalizing symptoms such as anxiety (23). Similarly, the child may be the only informant with knowledge of traumatic events (e.g., sexual abuse of the child), delinquent acts, or the child's idiosyncratic interpretation of certain events.

For the psychiatric interview of the child to yield accurate, clinically useful information, the interview process and wording of questions must be tailored to fit with the child's understanding (24). The child may simply not understand what the interviewer is seeking, or comprehend terms necessary to answer the questions accurately. In addition, the interviewer must be attuned to the child's efforts with current developmental tasks. The child may provide misleading answers to shield other family members, to protect self-esteem against acknowledging some perceived failing, or to avoid changes even in painful circumstances if the child fears it will entail placement out of the home. The adolescent may not trust the interviewer and may provide evasive or misleading answers for fear that the clinician will see him or her as "weird" or "crazy" or might collude with the parents against the teen.

The Child's Understanding of the Psychiatric Interview

Even if the parents have previously been seen alone, the child and parent are often seen together at the beginning of the child psychiatric interview in order to help put the child at ease. Allowing the child to become sufficiently comfortable before parents depart can cultivate an environment where the child is less guarded. Children can often indicate an acceptable point for the parents to leave the room, usually within a matter of minutes, and transitional objects (from blankets to handheld computer game devices) may ease these transitions.

Once parents have departed, inquiring what the child has been told or understands about the purpose of this interview to be often provides initial information on the relationship and openness of communication between the child and parent(s). The child's description of what he or she has been told regarding the evaluation may further reveal the child's priorities for intervention.

In addition to the purpose of this evaluation generally, the clinician should inquire about what the child believes parents, teachers, or other adults want to be different as a result of this interview. While the child may not know what others seek, this approach helps elucidate what the child recognizes about others' perspectives, and also facilitates the child projecting thoughts or fantasies about this evaluation.

Adolescents sometimes require additional modifications for this interview (25). First, adolescents sometimes fear parents will skew the interview by getting to tell their "version" first and the clinician, as an adult, will side with the parents against the adolescent. To prevent this, the clinician may want to speak over the phone initially with the parent about their concerns and about any information they consider important for the clinician to know prior to meeting with the adolescent. This also affords an opportunity for parents to identify information they do not want shared with the adolescent (e.g., finding drug paraphernalia in the adolescent's room, previous marriages of parents). Meeting briefly for a few minutes with the parent and adolescent to clarify objectives and the format of the evaluation, and then meeting with the adolescent alone at length is more likely to enhance an alliance with an adolescent. Clarifying during this initial segment that the clinician and the parents will later meet alone to review birth history, developmental milestones, and family history usually is acceptable to adolescents.

Adolescents may articulate that they do not want to participate in this evaluation or may resist answering questions. In such situations, the clinician may attempt to encourage the adolescent's cooperation by trying to identify goals the

1. Forming a Clinical Alliance with Parents

   a. Facilitating Narrative History
   Usually open-ended questions allow parents control, and these can be followed by more narrowly focused questions. Using the parent's actual words can help ensure that parents feel heard.

   b. Finding Common Themes/Patterns
   Parents sometimes fear that they alone have a problem with their child. Inquiry into similar problems or conicts the child has with other adults, peers, or unfamiliar others may illuminate patterns of the child's behavior that play out in a variety of settings, decreasing parents' anxiety that they alone provoke the child's problem.

   c. Finding Good Intentions Gone Awry
   Parents may feel ashamed of past parenting efforts done in desperation. Acknowledging the good intention leading to a misguided parenting effort can diminish parental self-reproach. For example, for parents who scream or become verbally abusive to their child, it may be helpful to acknowledge the parent's positive intention ("I guess you really wanted to get through to him") as well as the feelings of helplessness that led to the maladaptive response ("and couldn't think of anything else that would get him to listen").

   d. Partnering with Parents (Clinician as "partner" in decisionmaking process)
   Parents are often well informed and eager to take the lead in making decisions about their child's health. Accordingly, clinicians increasingly serve as partners, outlining several appropriate treatments, risks, and side effects, and helping parents to choose and invest in preferred treatments. If parents are eager to pursue treatments the clinician regards as unhealthy or unproven, the clinician may have to clarify potential risks of such treatments to minimize risks to the child.

   e. Clarifying Expectations of the Evaluation
   Having never participated in a psychiatric evaluation, parents may sometimes have unrealistic fantasies about what the evaluation will accomplish. For example, a parent may believe the evaluation can de nitively prove or rule out that the child had been abused by someone. At the other extreme, some parents are afraid that the clinician will tell them that their child will never be normal, will require institutionalization, or ultimately commit suicide. Inquiring early about what the parent hopes will be accomplished by this evaluation can reveal such expectations and fantasies, which the clinician can address realistically.

2. Eliciting Sensitive Information

   a. Providing the Parent with Opportunities to Convey Sensitive Information with the Child Not Present
   Apprising parents of times and methods to convey information apart from the child can occur before the interview, or can be identi ed and set aside within the interview time. In addition, identifying means for parents to communicate with the clinician via mail, e-mail, or con dential voice mail may allow parents additional opportunities to convey sensitive information forgotten or otherwise omitted during the initial interview.

   b. Revisiting Sensitive Information at Safer Points
   Sensitive information may need to be revisited during the interview as parents become more comfortable with the clinician. If parents resist disclosing information, the clinician should not force answers (as they are more likely to be inaccurate or incomplete), but rather proceed to less distressing information.

   c. Explaining the Purpose of Sensitive Information
   Some parents may need to understand the underlying purpose for inquiring about personal information. For example, parents may have uncomfortable memories of other relatives with mental illness and be reluctant to discuss family members. Explaining the need to gather basic information about relatives so that genetic (and environmental) contributions to the child's dif culties can be considered may allay parental anxieties.

   d. Describing How Sensitive Information Will Be Reported
   Parents are sometimes fearful that details of past histories of substance abuse or embarrassing personal problems of their own may be included in reports to be seen by others. Similarly, parents may fear that marital conict information might be used to alter custody arrangements, or unusual symptoms might appear in a report that could jeopardize their child's future educational or occupational pursuits. Clarifying that general information will be provided ("history of substance abuse on maternal side") rather than speci cs and that parents will be able to review reports whose release they authorize can diminish resistance to sharing sensitive information.

3. Handling Discrepant Reports

   a. Contextualizing Points of View
   Differences between observers' descriptions of a child's behavior have several potential sources. Differing contexts of observation may elicit different behaviors in the child. For example, teachers sometimes report very different presentations than parents, often because the demands of school exceed the coping skills of the child, while home does not stress the child's abilities quite so far. Or, a mother who has the task of getting the child organized and off to school in the morning may report quite a different set of behaviors than a father whose interactions with the child are less structured and more recreational. Examining what precipitates the child's problem, and how it expresses itself in different environments, may allow clinicians to borrow effective strategies across environments without "blaming" disagreeing adults.
   In addition, adult observers may employ differing standards of judgment about the child's behavior. A seasoned teacher will often have seen hundreds of children at a given age or grade level to serve as a basis of comparison, in contrast to the parent of an only child. A depressed parent will sometimes report more negatively about a child's behavior than a parent who is not depressed. Or parents may have unrealistically high demands of a child in a given area for reasons of their own.

   b. Finding Common Ground (Before Stories Diverge)
   When divergent perspectives arise, the clinician may need to examine the circumstances leading to the difference in each person's point of view. For example, one parent may believe the other parent is too lenient, while the other parent may believe his or her partner is too punitive. Examining the circumstances in which each parent responds in his or her respective style may allow the clinician to clarify the underlying child behaviors or symptoms requiring intervention, their meaning to each parent, and the circumstances in which a given response style is likely to be most helpful.

   c. Aligning Different Perspectives
   When parents or adults continue their mutual conicts during the psychiatric evaluation, the clinician may continue to refocus on the needs of the child. Even though parents may disagree vehemently, examining how each parent's efforts help achieve a common goal may help align parents/adults in a more productive direction. For example, each parent may argue for extreme differences in responding to disrespectful behavior, yet the clinician may encourage middle ground approaches to increase consistency between environments and to decrease different sets of behaviors working in one environment and not the other.

FIGURE 4.2.2.2. Parent interview techniques.

adolescent may wish to be advanced by the assessment and siding with those. For example, the adolescent minimizing or resisting psychiatric involvement may respond to clinician efforts to help identify what the adolescent needs to do to satisfy parents that the adolescent no longer needs to see a psychiatrist. In addition, clinicians can decrease resistance by beginning the history taking by inquiring first about the adolescent's interests, strengths, and musical preferences, rather than a too-exclusive focus on "problems." Adolescents are often exquisitely sensitive to feeling that they are being perceived or judged as vulnerable, "weird," or "different" from peers; hence it is generally best to begin with strengths before introducing areas of difficulty. In the same spirit, it is best to try to use lay terms, rather than technical terms or those laden with implications of pathology or transgression.

DEVELOPMENTALLY SENSITIVE TECHNIQUES FOR THE PSYCHIATRIC INTERVIEW

The choice of developmentally appropriate techniques to elicit information from children and adolescents is not strictly dictated by chronological age. As part of their presenting difficulties, some children may have delayed or aberrant development in some realms that impact the conduct of the interview, such as social language. For other children, regression in the face of stress or anxiety may lead to refusal to speak, oppositionality, tantrums, or retreating to other immature behaviors, either in the context of the interview or as an aspect of the child's more general functioning. Distressing content may similarly require interviewer techniques (drawing, puppets, or play therapy) ordinarily used for younger patients. With some children, once they are at ease with the interview situation, more explicit discussion may be able to take the place of play. The optimal combination of techniques, most likely to place the child at ease and to obtain useful information, will depend on where a given child is on the developmental (cognitive, emotional, interpersonal) spectrum. The choice and timing of techniques further depend on the emotional valence or difficulty of the issue being addressed, and the fluctuations in the rapport between the child and the clinician. In child psychiatric interviews, the clinician continuously monitors the usefulness of a technique at a particular moment and shifts between techniques as the interview unfolds, according to the waxing or waning of the child's anxiety, lability, and engagement.

Four categories of techniques are generally employed in the child psychiatric interview. First, *engagement* techniques are often required to help put the child at ease and elicit the child's engagement in the psychiatric interview so that the child will provide accurate and meaningful clinical information. Second, *projective* techniques are used to allow the child to reveal underlying themes or issues which the child may be unable to verbalize directly and to assess the child's unique ways of thinking and responding to stimuli. Third, *direct questioning* techniques are required to clarify particular points or elicit specific information needed to distinguish disorders, contributions to the child's problems, and intervention options. Fourth, *interactive* techniques are needed to clarify how the child relates to, as well as accepts or integrates input from, others. Throughout the psychiatric interview, opportunities for the child to express content in his or her own way must be balanced with the clinician retaining enough control of the interview to ensure sufficient information is obtained to allow effective clinical assessments and treatment planning.

Techniques to Engage the Child

Engaging the child is often challenging, particularly since the child is in an unfamiliar setting with unfamiliar adults involved in an unfamiliar task. Accordingly, making the setting, staff, and tasks more familiar often helps put the child at ease and accelerates engagement. To make the setting more attractive, many child psychiatrists will provide toys in both the waiting room and clinical office. In addition, child-friendly art or even movie posters may simultaneously make the setting more appealing and provide a stimulus for the child to describe reactions to the poster, characters, or movie preferences that may provide important information about the child's underlying concerns or perceptions. Similarly, toy figures, puppets, and similar relationship-oriented toys may ease the child into the interview. Generic toy figures are usually preferable, since they are more likely to evoke the child's specific themes and concerns rather than the prefabricated scripts associated with specific toy characters based on TV shows or movies. Tasks that are framed as games or that involve activities (drawing a house or family) familiar to the child often help the child transition into the psychiatric interview.

In addition to making the child feel comfortable, engagement techniques facilitate the child's presentation of information. Imaginative play with puppets, toys, or the interviewer provides useful inferential material about the child's concerns, perceptions, and characteristic modes of regulating affect, impulses, and transitions. By allowing the child to direct the content, the interviewer can follow the sequence of the child's concerns, note themes that emerge, and observe the points at which a child backs away from the story line, shifts to a new activity or topic, or falls into a repetitive loop. The form of the child's play further provides mental status information about the child's coordination and motor skills, speech and language development, attention span, readiness to engage the interviewer, capacity for complex thought, and affective state. Absence of imaginative play or concrete, repetitive, noninteractive play may suggest a pervasive developmental disorder.

To help put younger children at ease, some child psychiatrists wear ties with children or friendly animals and opt for clothing that permits them to play on the floor if indicated.

Adolescents can be difficult to engage. Efforts to indicate familiarity with contemporary adolescent tastes (music, movies, terms) can be perceived as not genuine by the adolescent. Instead, clinicians may engage the adolescent by inquiring about current interests, musical preferences, and adherence to current adolescent values, but rather from a curious, "just help me understand it" perspective, rather than from one of "trying to be hip." Adolescents often are ambivalent about the talking relationship, so manipulable items (squeeze balls, modeling clay, finger cuffs, cards) allow a socially acceptable option for keeping their hands busy during the interview and make the interview feel less like an interrogation. Complex games, such as chess or video games, require such focus that the interview may become subordinate to the game itself, impeding the clinical interview.

Projective Techniques

In addition to imaginative play, projective techniques may help the child express concerns indirectly, so that anxiety about significant fears, telling family secrets, or betraying loyalties is minimized. Among the most common projective techniques is picture drawing. Commonly, the child is asked to draw a picture of him- or herself or family doing something. The clinician's complimenting the picture close to its completion and to expressing curiosity about what is happening in the drawing can help ensure that the content of the picture, rather than its artistic quality, remains the focus of the interview. For pictures of the child, body details including sizes of appendages or body parts and articulation (fingers, toes), relative size of the figure to the page, and frequent erasures can all reveal underlying issues of anxiety, perceived agency to address difficulties, or needs to control the environment. Depictions of the self as nonhuman, grotesque, imbued with super powers, or of the opposite gender may provide clues about the child's self-image and underlying wishes. The relative size and placement or omission of family members in a family drawing may illuminate the child's feelings about family relationships. Aggressive or sexual themes may be revealed more readily in drawings than in words.

Verbal projective techniques can similarly yield important information. Asking what animal or character (TV/movie star, cartoon, superhero) the child would most like to be, or whom the child would take along to a deserted island, or asking what the child would do with three magic wishes often allow underlying issues to emerge. For example, children may describe wishes to be dominant predator animals to avoid being harmed, or to be gentle animals so that their rage might become less of a problem. Wishes may reveal basic needs, such as food or a safe place to live, or longings for parents to reunite or for the return of a departed friend. Wishes sometimes reveal specific desires, such as "not to have tics anymore," or "never to get teased." Very general or altruistic wishes, such as "world peace" or "to live in a big house with lots of money" warrant further exploration, such as "Are there particular fights you would especially like to stop?" or "Who else would live there?" and "What would you do first with lots of money?"

Open-ended interactive techniques require the child to respond to changes introduced by the clinician. The squiggle game described by Winnicott (26) consists of the clinician drawing a "squiggle," or curvy line, and asking the child to turn it into a picture of something. The resulting picture can then be described and discussed between the child and clinician. The child may also produce a squiggle for the clinician to develop, and the clinician can draw pictures of subjects or topics suspected significant to the child. Incomplete, affectively evocative beginnings of stories or fables can be described to the child, who then elaborates or completes the story (1).

Projective techniques may help adolescents to reveal and share emotionally significant concerns with the clinician despite the developmentally expectable suppression of fantasy in favor of more realistic discourse and reluctance to reveal vulnerabilities or anxieties to adults. Inquiries into favorite, or most disliked, movies, television characters, political or historical figures, musicians or artists, or sports figures all allow elaboration of the teenager's ideas (and ideals) in displacement. The more the adolescent resists direct discussion of his or her own concerns, the greater the displacement that may be required between the projective figure and the adolescent's real life. For example, adolescents less distrustful of the clinician may readily speak about their own social longings or anxieties regarding friends at school, while those adolescents more suspicious of the clinician's motives or wary of self-revelation may be more likely to reveal personal concerns or feelings as projected on or embodied in celebrities or other characters distant from the adolescent's real life. Adolescent resistances are often revealed by reluctance to divulge names of friends, or even questions about why the clinician needs to know this information. If resistance is detected, questions about what the adolescent most admires about a character, or what the adolescent imagines this character would do in given situations, may reveal the adolescent's perceptions or repertoire of response options through projection onto the character.

Since one of the developmental tasks of the adolescent is to find a place among peers, the vicissitudes of joining, rejecting, or being rebuffed by various groups of peers is an essential part of the adolescent's process of social self-definition. Amidst this preoccupation with ingrouping/outgrouping, adolescents are very sensitive to being included or excluded, and issues of fairness, justice, and revenge. Asking the adolescent about the different cliques or groups at school and his or her relationship to them provides useful information about the teen's self-image. Similarly, questions about what the adolescent sees as fair or not fair and what he or she would most like to change about his or her school or the world often reveals underlying concerns and issues.

Older adolescents may be able to respond to second-order or circular questions about what others think someone else's motives or thoughts were. For example, the clinician might ask what the adolescent thinks his best friend was thinking when the friend skipped school. Again, if the adolescent finds a topic too emotionally charged or fears betraying a peer, the clinician may need to ask about those more distant. For example, the clinician might ask what the adolescent thought a celebrity or movie character was thinking or trying to accomplish (motive) when the movie star wore certain clothes or made certain comments.

Additional projective techniques are appropriate for all age levels and provide another vehicle to elicit significant information unique to that child. Asking the child or adolescent about favorite books, magazines, music, television shows, movies, or video games may provide important information and help cultivate bonds of common interest between the child and clinician. Particularly if the evaluation is to extend over multiple sessions, or if treatment with the clinician is anticipated, the clinician's exploration of the child's preferred media may help convey interest in the child's world, as well as help illuminate important concerns on the child's part. While the clinician has to be careful not to impose ideas or judgments of characters important to the child, such figures often provide a vehicle or mechanism for discussing difficult content.

Direct Questioning

The goal of direct questioning is to clarify the presence or chronology of symptoms or events, to explore how the child sees the world and functions within it, and to follow up on themes suggested by the history or through play and other interactions with the clinician. Direct questioning can help fill in gaps not revealed by the child, and may help focus attention if responses become circumstantial or tangential. Direct questions may seem to children to benefit clinician needs more than the concerns of the child, so children may resist answering direct questions, particularly if the child imputes a critical or intrusive intent to the question or an effort to label him or her in some way as crazy, weird, or otherwise deviant. Tact, timing, and the phrasing of the question; appreciation of the child's cognitive and linguistic development; and regard for the impact of the question on the child's self-esteem all influence the effort the child will make to respond to a direct question. In addition, the structure of the question will markedly affect the quality of the child's response.

Questions that allow the child control of the depth of the response are usually preferred early in the interview, and more focused questions can be employed later as needed. Asking the child to describe friends ("Tell me about your best friend."), siblings, or parents, is preferable to "Do you get along with your brother?" which may invite only a "yes" or "no" response. Open-ended questions such as "What sorts of things make you mad/afraid/happy?" and "What do you daydream about?" are similarly preferable to "Do you get mad?" or "Do you ever daydream?" Early in the interview, less anxiety-provoking questions are preferred ("What is your school like?"), as momentum can be generated for the more difficult questions about family relationships or why others are distressed by the child's symptoms or behaviors.

For younger children, anchoring direct questions chronologically to major events may help children provide more accurate answers. For example, "Did that happen before or after your birthday?" or "How has that (problem) been since school ended?" allow greater precision by the respondent. At the same time, direct questions should continue to elicit feelings rather then "just the facts," since the child's affective narrative history is usually more important than the actual chronicle of events.

Direct questioning in adolescents may require particular tact and attention to positives or strengths before questions about the adolescent's negative behaviors can be addressed. For example, inquiries into the adolescent's best school subjects or what avocations the adolescent is good at may need to occur before inquiries about troublesome school subjects, or the adolescent's current problems. "No fault" phrasing of sensitive questions can help diffuse defensiveness on teens' parts. For example, "Are there ever any rough spots between you and other kids?" is a preferable starting point for inquiring about social difficulties rather than "Do you ever have trouble getting along with other kids?"

Substance abuse, sexuality, and risky behaviors are, by necessity, often assessed through direct questions. However, more general questions initially may make these topics more comfortable and thus the information obtained more accurate. The clinician can often use a simple question, such as "Substance use?" that allow substantial latitude, and then focus in further, contingent on the child's responses. For example, the clinician may hear "No, I don't do any of that anymore," which could then be followed by "What led to that decision?" and then proceed backward to when and what substances were used. Similarly, sexuality can be assessed by gentle direct questions such as "Have you ever had romantic feelings toward another? How did that go?" (instead of "Have you had a boyfriend yet?"). Children and adolescents are often very cautious about discussing sexual urges, even more so if they fear the interviewer will be disapproving; hence, non–gender-specific grammar is useful initially ("romantic feelings toward anyone" rather "Are there any girls you like?" (1) to indicate, at least implicitly, that one is open to hearing about homoerotic, as well as heterosexual, attractions. Finally, direct inquiries into risky behaviors (stealing, vandalism, assaults, gambling) often require general questions such as "Have you done anything that you now look back on and think 'that was pretty dangerous'?" "Have you ever done anything that would have gotten you in trouble if your parents or other grown-ups knew about it?" before proceeding to specific questions ("Have you ever stolen anything? Have you ever been beat up? Beat up someone else?"). Suicidal risk behaviors may be minimized or trivialized, particularly in adolescents, so additional questions to examine the adolescent's historical "genogram" of connections to others, fantasies about impacts of the suicide on family and friends, and value contradictions may be needed to clarify suicidality risks (27).

Interactive Techniques

During the interview, the clinician is uniquely positioned to observe firsthand how the child relates to another person and what feelings or reactions this elicits. How the child initially reacts to a new person, how the child sustains interaction throughout the interview, and how the child terminates the interview often reveal patterns important in the child's larger social life. Social rules of conduct, forced transitions, and game playing all allow the clinician to evaluate the child's ways of relating to others. The clinician can employ normal social conventions such as smiling, bending down to the child's level to obtain eye contact, and offering to shake hands to discern the child's initial reactions to unfamiliar others. The clinician can assess how the child negotiates social situations even in small interactions such as determining who will sit in which chair. The clinician can evaluate more complex social interactions during transitions ("It's time to put these toys up in the box.") and during games. Short games (tic tac toe) are useful since the clinician can quickly detect how the child responds to winning, tying, and losing.

Adolescents rely on more complex patterns of relating, often specific to a subgroup to which they now belong. For example, dress or language may be imbued with special meaning within adolescent subgroups, so clarifying what clothing symbols represent, idiosyncratic meanings of confusing terms, and values espoused by any identified subgroup the adolescent appears to embrace can all clarify the adolescent's patterns of relating and values. For example, an adolescent may wear a shirt with Bob Marley's picture on it, and inquiry may reveal the adolescent's commitment to equality. Similarly, the child may describe being "Goth," "punk," "straight-edge," "hip-hop," or other terms. Rather than attempting to be "with it" or assuming one knows what these imply to the patient, it is helpful to inquire what that term or ethos means to this adolescent. In addition, the adolescent may employ gestures or language ordinarily offensive or off-putting to the clinician. The clinician should observe whether these appear to be efforts to provoke the clinician, to titrate space between the clinician and the adolescent, or to be the adolescent's customary idiom, which the adolescent may not realize alienates others.

Asking about future aspirations ("What would you like to do once you've finished with school?") also often provides a useful window into the adolescent's ideals, interests, quality of self-appraisal, and degree of identification with his or her family's values.

Concluding the Interview

Allowing the interview to end in a collaborative fashion increases the likelihood that the child will feel positive about the interview and any subsequent encounters with clinicians, including other evaluations or treatments. The clinician may wind up the interview by empowering the child with some degree of ownership of this interview. Questions which turn the interview topics over to the child such as "Are there other things that would be important for me to know about what you're like or how things have been for you?" or "What else have I not asked about that is important?" facilitate this process. Similarly, questions such as "I've asked you lots of questions—do you have any questions for me?" demonstrate respect for the child.

The child may be curious about what the clinician thinks about the child and with whom the clinician will share findings. Most often, the clinical interview is but one piece of a larger evaluation, so the clinician may need to clarify that additional laboratory or paper-pencil testing, conversations with teachers or family members, or additional meetings may be needed for the clinician to have a fuller or more accurate impression. Discussing findings (including treatment recommendations) with parents first before discussing them with the child is usually advisable so that additional conflict is not generated if parents should disagree with the clinician's conclusions or resist certain suggested interventions (medication, individual therapy, changes in school placement).

Confidentiality is one of the most challenging issues surrounding child psychiatric interviews, especially with adolescents who may be particularly concerned about who might hear what from the clinician. Parents and children should be informed of the confidential nature of the doctor–patient relationship so that the clinician is not seen as a parental spy. However, findings such as diagnoses often must be reported to parents, to insurance companies (for reimbursement), and to schools for classroom or curricular modifications to occur. Describing to the adolescent what will be told to specific others is usually sufficient, as well as what information will not be revealed (e.g., specific details about substance abuse or sexual behaviors). Parents and child should be told explicitly that confidentiality does *not* extend to situations that pose a clear danger to the child or others. In cases where this emerges (the child describes hoarding pills in a drawer to commit suicide, or obtaining bullets to threaten a student at school), the clinician should clarify with the child how they will tell appropriate others, and participate in the disclosure to others. However, state laws vary and change regarding what information must be shared or kept confidential between clinicians and patients, even minors, about substance use, pregnancy/abortion, and weapons possession, so clinicians should remain familiar with local legal standards of confidentiality. While treatment may not be possible with some children unless certain information remains confidential, confidentiality should not become collusion.

LABORATORY EVALUATION IN THE CHILD PSYCHIATRIC EVALUATION

New techniques of molecular genetics, neurobiology, functional and structural imaging, and neuroendocrinology are deepening our understanding about the pathogenesis and biological underpinnings of developmental psychopathology. Still, at this time, few, if any, definitive clinical tests exist to identify specific child psychiatric disorders. In the child psychiatry evaluation, laboratory testing remains a vehicle to identify a small number of specific etiologies of certain psychiatric symptoms, as suggested by history or physical findings that warrant such testing, rather than a widely applicable method of screening for specific psychiatric disorders.

Pediatric Collaboration in the Laboratory Evaluation

Close collaboration with the child's pediatrician, or primary care provider, remains important throughout the child psychiatry evaluation. These providers are familiar with the child's medical and developmental trajectory, as well as family background, and are often positioned to provide essential input on the emergence or progression of a child's symptoms. In addition, the pediatrician or other primary care provider may serve as an invaluable collaborator in the child's ongoing care.

The pediatric examination is a useful complement to the child psychiatric evaluation. The pediatric review of systems may clarify other physical changes important in the evolution of the child's symptoms. In addition, growth charts may reveal changes in head circumference relevant to pervasive developmental disorders, abnormalities in weight suggestive of an eating disorder or failure to thrive, or changes in stature relevant to hormonal or mood changes. Similarly, the pediatric physical examination may identify visual or hearing problems that explain learning, language, social, attentional, or oppositional problems, as well as pubertal precocity or delays which have important psychosocial consequences. The pediatric exam may also reveal emerging complications associated with treatment (such as weight gain or metabolic dysregulation associated with atypical antipsychotic use). The pediatrician may also identify congenital anomalies or other developmental physical features suggestive of specific developmental disorders or other medical disorders accompanied by psychiatric symptoms.

Collaboration with the primary pediatric care provider may help guide decisions about possible further medical consultations (audiometric, genetic, neurological, speech) or other diagnostic tests (blood tests, electroencephalograms, neuroimaging, sleep studies).

Testing in Specific Childhood Disorders

Laboratory evaluation is warranted when other history or physical findings suggest a particular potential medical diagnosis, such as hyperthyroidism. Routine use of laboratory testing yields findings which alter the working diagnosis in approximately 1% of cases, and the yield for laboratory abnormalities, without the presence of other supportive signs or symptoms, remains less than 5% (28). Laboratory tests commonly considered, particularly when history or other symptoms accompany the psychiatric symptoms, are summarized in Table 4.2.2.5. More specialized technologies, such as positron emission tomography (PET), single photon emission computerized tomography (SPECT), functional MRI (fMRI), and brain electrical activity mapping (BEAM) remain attractive research tools, but currently have no routine clinical or diagnostic usefulness in child and adolescent psychiatric populations.

Highlights relevant to laboratory testing in key forms of childhood psychopathology are provided in this section; the interested reader is also referred to the related chapters elsewhere in this volume.

Mental Retardation and Pervasive Developmental Disorders

The more severe the child's disability, the more likely an identifiable (albeit not necessarily treatable) medical cause will be detected. Chromosomal abnormalities, such as trisomy 21 (Down syndrome) or fragile X syndrome, are found in approximately half of cases of mental retardation. Lead testing may be appropriate in children with retardation, since pica can lead to lead ingestion, causing or exacerbating retardation.

In addition to relatively high rates of mental retardation, the incidence of seizure disorders in children with autism increases

TABLE 4.2.2.5

LABORATORY TESTS TO CONSIDER IN CHILDHOOD PSYCHIATRIC DISORDERS

Lab Test	Disorder MR/PDD	Mood	Psychosis	OCD Tics	Substance Abuse	Eating Disorders
Chromosomal testing	X		X			
Wood's (UV) lamp	X					
Monospot		X				
Thyroid		X	X			X
Lyme titer		X				
CBC	X	X	X		X	X
Serum chemistry	X	X	X		X	X
Lead level	X					
Throat culture Antistreptolysin O Antibody (ASO), Antideoxyribonuclease B titers				X		
Urine drug screen		X	X		X	
Cerebrospinal fluid Analysis		X	X			
Neuroimaging			X			
EEG	X					

through adolescence. Tuberous sclerosis is present in up to 5% of cases of children with autism. Accordingly, chromosomal testing to detect fragile X syndrome, EEG to detect comorbid seizures, and Wood's lamp examination to identify tubers all warrant consideration in children with autism.

Mood Disorders

Although uncommon, medical causes of mood disorders include infectious diseases (mononucleosis, Lyme disease, human immunodeficiency virus [HIV], thyroid abnormalities) as well as substance abuse. Sudden onset, severe fatigue, cognitive changes, and physical symptoms such as sore throat, fever, headache, nausea, and weight changes all increase the probability of an organic basis for the mood disturbance.

Psychotic Disorders

New onset psychosis warrants consideration of underlying organic disease, although most cases are not attributable to an identifiable organic cause. Cognitive decline is not uncommon in schizophrenia, but altered level of consciousness, abnormal neurological examination, altered vital signs, or new-onset seizures all suggest the need for further clinical and laboratory workup, including cerebrospinal fluid (CSF) studies, EEG, and neuroimaging.

Characteristic facial features or cardiac anomalies may suggest velo-cardio-facial syndrome, and the need for specialized testing for microdeletions on chromosome 22. Genetic testing is not a routine part of the child psychiatric workup, but this is likely to change over the coming years as more sensitive, reliable, and cost-effective measures become available.

Obsessive-Compulsive Disorder (OCD) and Tics

Acute onset of OCD and/or tics, particularly following pharyngitis, may provide evidence for the proposed syndrome of PANDAS (pediatric autoimmune neuropsychiatric disorder associated with streptococcal infection). Although this proposed mechanism appears to explain only a minority of cases of OCD or tic disorder, in acute onset cases associated with pharyngitis, a throat culture and serological studies for group A beta-hemolytic streptococcus (GABHS) infection, including antideoxyribonuclease B and antistreptolysin O antibody titers may be indicated (29).

Substance Use Disorders

Substance abuse and dependence can cause a wide range of neurological and neuropsychiatric symptoms. Toxicology screens have been recommended for adolescents who have psychiatric symptoms and who exhibit acute behavioral changes, as well as those juveniles at high risk for substance abuse such as runaways or those with conduct disorder symptoms or exposure/access to substances, and those with recurrent accidents or unexplained somatic symptoms.

Eating Disorders

Eating disorders often culminate in physical changes detectable through laboratory testing. Anemia evidenced through a complete blood count, electrolyte imbalances, and electrocardiographic (EKG) changes may be present in patients with eating disorders and warrant consideration.

Attention-Deficit Hyperactivity Disorder (ADHD)

While initial studies suggested thyroid abnormalities in approximately 5% of children with ADHD, subsequent studies failed to support this finding, and thyroid testing is now indicated in children with ADHD when other symptoms of hyperthyroidism are present. Quantitative EEG and neuroimaging have been encouraged by proprietary entities, but currently lack empirical support to be considered part of standard clinical practice. Similarly, allergy testing has not yielded specific findings in sufficient cases of ADHD to support routine use.

APPENDIX 1

SAMPLE LETTER FOR PARENTS DESCRIBING THE CHILD PSYCHIATRIC ASSESSMENT

Dear [Parent],

We look forward to seeing [child's name] on [date]. This assessment will last approximately [time allotted]. Unless your child is very young, or uncomfortable separating from you, usually [clinician's name] will meet briefly with the parent or adults alone to understand their primary concerns, to obtain relevant medical and family history, and to review any sensitive information important to the assessment, but which may not have been discussed with your child. Bringing toys or activities (books, mazes) to occupy your child during this part of the assessment can be helpful in making him or her comfortable. Report cards, reports from school, prior clinicians, or others involved in the child's care (daycare, courts), or educational or psychological testing reports can be very helpful, so we encourage you to bring these.

[Clinician's name] will usually then meet with your child alone for [allocated time], as well as, perhaps, with all of you together. This interview will include questions about how he or she interacts with friends, parents, and teachers; your child does not need to prepare for this interview. [Clinician's name] may measure your child's height, weight, and pulse and blood pressure, but the child will not need to change clothes or to expect to be examined like during a pediatric visit. No needles or shots are given during psychiatric interviews.

After interviews with you, and with your child, [clinician's name] will finish up the meeting by discussing "next steps" with you, and depending on the recommendations, with your child present as well. Commonly, additional input from teachers or other adults familiar with your child may be needed, so your giving consent to speak/interact with them may be discussed. In some situations, [clinician's name] may recommend certain types of treatment, and discuss options, including risks and benefits of these treatments. In some cases, rating scales may be provided for you and others to describe or rate symptoms, or to measure changes as interventions are implemented.

At all times, please feel encouraged to clarify any concerns or advance any questions you may have about any part of this assessment or proposed treatment. We are eager to collaborate with you throughout this process.

Sincerely,

[Clinician's name]

APPENDIX 2

SAMPLE LETTER FOR PARENTS DESCRIBING THE ADOLESCENT PSYCHIATRIC ASSESSMENT

Dear [Parent],

We look forward to seeing [adolescent's name] on [date]. This assessment will last approximately [time allotted]. Usually [clinician's name] will meet briefly with both you and your adolescent to clarify the purpose of this assessment, and then meet for [allocated time] with your adolescent. This interview will include questions about how your teenager interacts with friends, parents, and teachers; he or she does not need to prepare for this interview. [Clinician's name] may measure your adolescent's height, weight, and pulse and blood pressure, but the adolescent will not need to change clothes or to expect to be examined like a regular medical visit. There will not be any needles or shots.

[Clinician's name] usually will then meet with the parent or guardian to review primary concerns, to obtain relevant medical and family history, and to review any sensitive information important to the assessment, but which may not have been discussed with the adolescent. Report cards, reports from school, prior clinicians, or others (daycare, courts), or educational or psychological testing reports can be very helpful, so bringing these is encouraged.

After interviews with you and with your adolescent, [clinician's name] will conclude the meeting by discussing "next steps" with the adults, and depending on the recommendations, with your teenager present as well. Commonly, additional input from teachers or other adults familiar with the adolescent may be needed, so consents to speak/interact with them may be discussed.

Confidentiality can be very important to adolescents, and issues of safety or danger are usually the only circumstances where confidentiality cannot be preserved. Often, however, sensitive subjects may warrant discussion with either the adolescent and parents/guardians alone, so our normal approach is to discuss and decide with adolescents how any sensitive information will be discussed with parents.

In some situations, following this initial evaluation, [clinician's name] may recommend certain types of treatment, and discuss options, including risks and benefits of these treatments. Rating scales may be provided for you and others to describe symptoms, or to measure changes as interventions are implemented.

At all times, please feel encouraged to clarify any concerns or advance any questions you may have about any part of this assessment or proposed treatment. We are eager to collaborate with you throughout this process.

Sincerely,

[Clinician's name]

References

1. King RA. Practice parameters for the psychiatric assessment of children and adolescents. American Academy of Child and Adolescent Psychiatry. *J Am Acad Child Adolesc Psychiatry* 36(10 Suppl):4S–20S, Oct 1997.
2. Bostic JQ, Rho Y: Target-symptom psychopharmacology: Between the forest and the trees. *Child Adolesc Psychiatr Clin N Am* 15(1):289–302, Jan 2006.
3. King RA. Psychiatric examination of the infant, child, and adolescent. In: Sadock BS, V (ed): *Comprehensive textbook of psychiatry*. 8th ed. Philadelphia: WB Saunders; 3044–3075, 2004.
4. Ferdinand RF, Hoogerheide KN, van der Ende J, et al.: The role of the clinician: Three-year predictive value of parents', teachers' and clinicians' judgment of childhood psychopathology. *J Child Psychol Psychiatry* 44(6):867–876, Sep 2003.
5. Pickles A, Rowe R, Simonoff E, Foley D, Rutter M, Silberg J. Child psychiatric symptoms and psychosocial impairment: Relationship and prognostic significance. *Br J Psychiatry* 179:230–235, Sep 2001.
6. Johnson JG, Cohen P, Gould MS, Kasen S, Brown J, Brook JS: Childhood adversities, interpersonal difficulties, and risk for suicide attempts during late adolescence and early adulthood. *Arch Gen Psychiatry* 59(8):741–749, Aug 2002.
7. King RA, Schwab-Stone M, Flisher AJ, et al.: Psychosocial and risk behavior correlates of youth suicide attempts and suicidal ideation. *J Am Acad Child Adolesc Psychiatry* 40(7):837–846, Jul 2001.
8. Weinreb L, Wehler C, Perloff J, et al.: Hunger: Its impact on children's health and mental health. *Pediatrics* 110(4):e41, Oct 2002.
9. Vila G, Zipper E, Dabbas M, et al.: Mental disorders in obese children and adolescents. *Psychosom Med* 66(3):387–394, May–Jun 2004.
10. Erermis S, Cetin N, Tamar M, Bukusoglu N, Akdeniz F, Goksen D. Is obesity a risk factor for psychopathology among adolescents? *Pediatr Int* 46(3):296–301, Jun 2004.
11. Stattin H, Kerr M: Parental monitoring: A reinterpretation. *Child Dev* 71(4):1072–1085, Jul–Aug 2000.
12. King RA, Ruchkin VV, Schwab-Stone M: Suicide and the "continuum of adolescent self destructiveness": Is there a connection? In: King RA, Apter A, (eds): *Suicide in Children and Adolescents*, Cambridge: Cambridge University Press, 2003.
13. Mangweth B, Hausmann A, Danzl C, et al.: Childhood body-focused behaviors and social behaviors as risk factors of eating disorders. *Psychother Psychosom* 74(4):247–253, 2005.
14. Wallerstein JS, Blakeslee S: *The unexpected legacy of divorce: A 25 year landmark study*, New York:Hyperion, 2000.
15. Indredavik MS, Vik T, Heyerdahl S, Kulseng S, Fayers P, Brubakk AM. Psychiatric symptoms and disorders in adolescents with low birth weight. *Arch Dis Child Fetal Neonatal Ed* 89(5):F445–450, Sep 2004.
16. Pataki C, Bostic JQ, Schlozman S: The functional assessment of media in child and adolescent psychiatric treatment. *Child Adolesc Psychiatr Clin N Am* 14(3):555–570, x, Jul 2005.
17. Daley ML, Becker DF, Flaherty LT, et al.: Case study: The Internet as a developmental tool in an adolescent boy with psychosis. *J Am Acad Child Adolesc Psychiatry* 44(2):187–190, Feb 2005.
18. Johnson JG, Cohen P, Smailes EM, Kasen S, Brook JS: Television viewing and aggressive behavior during adolescence and adulthood. *Science* 295(5564):2468–2471, Mar 29, 2002.
19. Bostic JQ, Schlozman S, Pataki C, Ristuccia C, Beresin EV, Martin A: From Alice Cooper to Marilyn Manson: The significance of adolescent antiheroes. *Acad Psychiatry* 27(1):54–62, Spring 2003.
20. Ouvrier RA, Goldsmith RF, Ouvrier S, Williams IC: The value of the Mini-Mental State Examination in childhood: A preliminary study. *J Child Neurol* 8(2):145–148, Apr 1993.
21. Jain M, Passi GR: Assessment of a modified mini-mental state scale for cognitive functions in children. *Indian Pediatrics* 42:907–912, 2005.
22. Shemesh E, Newcorn JH, Rockmore L, et al.: Comparison of parent and child reports of emotional trauma symptoms in pediatric outpatient settings. *Pediatrics* 115(5):e582–589, May 2005.
23. Wren FJ, Bridge JA, Birmaher B: Screening for childhood anxiety symptoms in primary care: Integrating child and parent reports. *J Am Acad Child Adolesc Psychiatry* 43(11):1364–1371, Nov 2004.
24. Lewis M, (ed): Psychiatric assessment of infants, children, and adolescents. In: Lewis M, (ed): *Child and adolescent psychiatry: A comprehensive textbook*. Baltimore: Williams and Wilkins, 1991.
25. King RA, Schowalter JE. The clinical interview of the adolescent. In: Wiener JA, Dulcan MK, (eds): *Textbook of Child and Adolescent Psychiatry*. 3rd ed. Washington, DC: American Psychiatric Publishing, 2004:113–116.
26. Winnicott DW: *Therapeutic consultations in child psychiatry*, London: Hogarth Press, 1971.
27. Galvin MR, Fletcher J, Stilwell BM: Assessing the meaning of suicidal risk behavior in adolescents: Three exercises for clinicians. *Journal of the American Academy of Child & Adolescent Psychiatry* 45(6):745–748, June 2006.
28. Challman TD, Barbaresi WJ, Katusic SK, Weaver A: The yield of the medical evaluation of children with pervasive developmental disorders. *J Autism Dev Disord* 33(2):187–192, Apr 2003.
29. King 2006.

CHAPTER 4.2.3 ■ STRUCTURED INTERVIEWING

ADRIAN ANGOLD, ELIZABETH JANE COSTELLO, AND HELEN EGGER

INTRODUCTION

Interviews are necessary tools for all forms of clinical medical diagnosis, and they have a singularly prominent position in psychiatry because of the lack of other "tests" for psychiatric disorders. All structured interviews used in psychiatry have their roots in the phenomenological clinical interview, although different interviews take rather different routes in the standardization of the collection of phenomenological data relevant to diagnosis. The questioning strategies involved now represent a mature technology, and the sometimes acrimonious methodological debates that once characterized the field have been replaced by the recognition that each approach has advantages and disadvantages that must be weighed in selecting a structured interview for each individual application.

The Limitations of Unstructured Diagnostic Interviews

It has been known for a long time that clinical training is sufficiently varied that colleagues of the same discipline, working in the same establishment, are often unable to agree about an individual's diagnosis, even when presented with exactly the same information (1–4). An apparent difference in rates of schizophrenia between New York and London proved to be almost entirely due to differences in diagnostic criteria applied to observed phenomenology (5). Observations such as these motivated the development of the formalized sets of diagnostic criteria familiar to us today from the DSM-IV and ICD-10.

The literature on medical decision-making had already shown that clinicians suffer from a number of information collection biases: 1) They tend to come to diagnostic determinations before they have collected all the relevant information, 2) they tend then to focus on collecting information to *confirm* that diagnosis (confirmatory bias), 3) they tend to ignore disconfirmatory information, 4) they combine information in idiosyncratic ways, and 5) they tend to make judgments based on the most readily available cognitive patterns (the availability heuristic). Further problems arise because of a tendency to see correlations where none exist (illusory correlation), and to miss real correlations (6).

Added to all these problems is the fact that, even today, standard diagnostic manuals do not provide very detailed descriptions of how to assess psychopathology at the symptom level. All of the criteria for oppositional defiant disorder, for instance, begin with the word "often." But "how often is often?" There is a great deal of room for clinicians to adopt very different decision rules about when to regard such symptoms as being present.

In the face of all these difficulties it became apparent that methods were required to standardize the collection, quantification, and combination of diagnostic information. As a result, all structured interviews aim to:

1. Structure information coverage, so that all interviewers will have collected all relevant information (both confirmatory and disconfirmatory) from all subjects.
2. Define the ways in which relevant information is to be collected.
3. Structure the process by which relevant confirmatory and disconfirmatory information is combined to produce a final diagnosis.

Early Structured Diagnostic Interviews

In the early days of structured interviews, it was supposed that *clinicians* would be using them, because it was felt that only they had the necessary training and experience to be able to decide about the presence or absence of symptoms, even when quite detailed definitions were provided. The interview schedule served as a tool to guide the clinician interviewer in determining whether symptoms were present, but the interviewer made the decisions, on the basis of information provided by the child or adult. Interviews of this sort, like the Present State Examination (7) and the Reynard (8) for adults, and the Isle of Wight interview for children (9, 10), were the first to be developed, since they sprang naturally from clinical practice. They were called *semi*-structured because the interviewer was allowed latitude in the specific form of the questions used.

Although the PSE and Isle of Wight interviews were used extensively in community surveys, it was clear that the use of clinician interviewers created both logistic and budgetary problems. Large scale epidemiological studies, such as the Epidemiologic Catchment Area (ECA) studies (11) mandated the use of nonclinician ("lay") interviewers. Some felt that such interviewers would be incapable of making the judgments about symptoms, so, following methodologies used by political and marketing surveys, interviews were developed that required only that the interviewer ask a set of fixed questions in a preset order, and collect the simple answers to those questions. In such interviews, it is the *questions* put to the subject that are structured, and the interviewer makes no decisions about the presence of symptoms. Hence they came to be called *highly* or *fully* structured. The Diagnostic Interview Schedule (DIS) was the paradigmatic example of this sort of interview in adult psychiatry (12), while the original Diagnostic Interview Schedule for Children and Adolescents (DICA) was the first child-oriented example (13, 14).

Emergence of the Diagnostic Interview with the Child

Until the late 1960s interviews and questionnaires directed to a parent or teacher about a child's behavior and *observation* of the child's behavior were the predominant methods of assessment in child and adolescent psychiatry. Verbal information from the child was typically regarded as being only supplemental, or material for psychodynamic interpretation (15). More attention was paid to playing with the child than to the collection of information through direct questioning. In 1968, a key transitional paper reported on the reliability and validity of the Isle of Wight interview with the child (9). Here the behavior of the child in a face-to-face interview was examined directly, but little was made of the factual content of the child's reports. In 1975, Herjanic and her colleagues asked "are children reliable reporters" of factual information, and presented evidence that they are (16). Since then, a great deal of work has confirmed the importance of children's self-reports as a source of factual information, with the result that fact-finding (as opposed to interpretative) interviews with both parents and children are now regarded as being of equal weight in the diagnostic process, at least from late childhood (prior to about age 9 children are incapable of completing such "adult-style" interviews). The one exception is in the evaluation of attention deficit hyperactivity disorder (ADHD) symptoms, where child reports have been found to be of little help (17, 18). Even here, however, the recent growth of interest in ADHD in adolescence and adulthood has led to the development of new measures in this area (e.g., Conners, 1997) (19).

Disagreement among Informants and Its Implications

Until the 1980s, agreement between child and parent reports of symptomatology was widely regarded as being a test of the *validity* of *child* reports (9, 14). However, it soon became apparent that only low levels of agreement among informants (correlation coefficients around 0.3 for agreement among children, parents and teachers) could be expected (20, 21). It is now considered that low levels of agreement among different informants about the child's clinical state are to be expected and do not invalidate the reports of any of them. Rather, each key informant presents a particular view of the child's problems. Indeed, it is precisely because agreement among informants is low that multiple informants are needed. Were agreement very high, taking the history from more than one informant would be redundant.

The problem is that disagreement among informants means that one has to decide how to weight the information from each informant in arriving at a diagnosis. Since it is uncommon for informants to invent fictitious symptoms, the simple rule of regarding a symptom as being present if any informant reports it usually suffices. When symptoms are combined to make diagnoses, the usual procedure is to ignore the source, and to add up all positive symptoms from any source. Thus, a diagnosis of a major depressive episode (which requires the presence of at least five symptoms) might be made on the basis of three relevant symptoms being reported by the child (say depressed mood, anhedonia and excessive guilt), with two other relevant symptoms (perhaps sleep and appetite disturbances) being reported by another informant (typically a parent and/or teacher). Although some interview developers have recommended "reconciliation" discussions involving the interviewer, the parent and the child to clear up discrepancies between their reports (22), such a discussions are problematic. Reconciliation requires one informant to modify his or her story, but that means admitting being wrong, or at least uninformed. The knowledge that such a discussion will occur could cause informants (e.g., drug-using adolescents) to withhold important information that they did not wish other informants (such as their parents) to hear about. Finally, in most research applications, one wishes to assure informants that what they say will not be revealed to anyone else, in which case a reconciliation interview is ruled out.

The remainder of this chapter is concerned with the description of key points relating to general psychiatric diagnostic interviews, that is, those that cover a broad range of the common disorders of childhood and adolescence. A number of interviews and observational systems exist for more specialized tasks (for instance the Autism Diagnostic Interview and the Autism Diagnostic Observation Schedule (23, 24)), but such instruments will not be considered further here.

A TYPOLOGY OF INTERVIEWS

As we have already seen, a distinction between semistructured and highly structured interviews has found its way into the description and discussion of diagnostic interviewing techniques. However, these terms are not very helpful for two reasons. First, they imply that the key difference between different types of interview concerns the *amount* of structure they impose. The problem is that the real issue is not one of amount of structure, but rather who makes the final decision as to whether a symptom is present.

Respondent-Based Interviews

In interviews where the questions are absolutely prespecified, it is the respondent who makes the final decision (typically by answering yes or no to each question). The interviewer makes no such decisions, but merely reads the questions. Since the decisions as to the presence or absence of psychopathology lie with the respondent in such interviews, we refer to them as being *respondent-based*. The Diagnostic Interview Schedule for Children (DISC (25)) and the computer-assisted version of the Diagnostic Interview Schedule for Children and Adolescents (DICA (26)), and the Dominic-R (27) are the three representatives of this approach.

Interviewer-Based Interviews, and Glossary-Based Interviews

We call interviews that require the interviewer to make an informed decision based on what the respondent says *interviewer-based*. The interviewer is expected to question until s/he can decide whether a symptom meeting the definitions provided by the interview (or known to them from their training) is present. This group of interviews includes the Anxiety Disorders Interview Schedule (ADIS (28)), the Child and Adolescent Psychiatric Assessment (CAPA (29)), the Child Assessment Schedule (CAS (30, 31)), the paper and pencil (not the computerized) versions of the Diagnostic Interview Schedule for Children and Adolescents (DICA (26)) and its close relative the Missouri Assessment of Genetics Interview for Children (MAGIC), the Interview Schedule for Children and Adolescents (ISCA (32)), the various versions of the Kiddie Schedule for Affective Disorders and Schizophrenia (K-SADS (33)), and the Pictorial Instrument for Children and Adolescents (PICA-IIIR (34)). Three of these interviewer-based interviews (the K-SADS-P IVR, the DICA, and the CAPA) provide extensive sets of definitions of symptoms and/or detailed guidance on the conduct of the interview, and we call these *glossary-based*. Such glossaries are particularly important when an interviewer-based interview is to be used by nonclinician interviewers because they provide detailed guidance as to what the interviewer is supposed to be looking for in making symptom ratings. Nonclinician interviewers have been shown to be able to make such "clinical" judgments with high reliability when they have received adequate training with such glossaries (35).

The distinction between interviewer- and respondent-based interviews is not hard and fast in actual practice, because there has been considerable cross-fertilization between these approaches. For instance, the Child and Adolescent Psychiatric Assessment (CAPA), which has its roots in the interviewer-based tradition, includes a subset of questions that are to be asked verbatim of all subjects, as in a respondent-based interview, but then allows further questioning for clarification. On the other hand, the DICA, which had previously been a respondent-based interview, now requires interviewers to question much more flexibly, and is now an interviewer-based instrument (26). Though the distinction between interviewer- and respondent-based interviews provides a useful rough-and-ready typology, it is really better to consider interviews as lying at various locations along three dimensions: 1) Degree of specification of questions, 2) degree of definition of symptom concepts and 3) degree of flexibility in questioning permitted to the interviewers. Interviews that provide extensive definitions and require interviewers to make judgments lie in the interviewer-based region of that three-dimensional space, while those that specify every question and allow no interviewer deviation from those questions lie in the respondent-based region.

Pictorial Interviews

More recently respondent-based child self-report interviews that add *pictorial* cues have been added to the assessment armamentarium. The most developed pictorial interview at this time is the Dominic-R (27, 36, 37) which is intended for use with 6–11-year-olds. Pictures representing psychopathology relevant to seven diagnoses are shown to the child, and questions about whether each symptom is present are read at the same time. Because no frequency, duration, or onset data are collected, it is not yet clear how such information should be combined with diagnostic information from other sources. This is, however, a general problem for interviews with younger children, because before the age of 8 or 9, they simply cannot provide all the frequency, dating and timing information that full diagnostic interviews require. Although diagnostic test-retest reliabilities cannot be reported for the Dominic-R, its item reliabilities are respectable in comparison with those reported from studies of older children with other interviews.

The Pictorial Instrument for Children and Adolescents (PICA-IIIR), for children aged 6–16, adopts a somewhat similar approach, but the questions to be asked with the pictures are more loosely specified, and it is intended to be used by clinicians. It covers a broader range of diagnoses than the Dominic-R, but no test-retest reliability data are yet available (34).

Parent-Only Interviews for Younger Children

Standard practice in adult psychiatry is to rely upon a single key informant for structured diagnostic interviews. The person who is the subject of the interview alone is interviewed. Parent and teacher interviews are added in child and adolescent psychiatry because the child him- or herself is regarded as being a limited informant. The point is that, at any age, interviews need to be conducted with whoever is needed to provide adequate reliable information coverage. We have already noted that younger children cannot provide all the information necessary for making DSM-style diagnoses, but there is no reason why the child's lack of capacity in this regard should invalidate the use of the available best informants (parents and sometimes teachers) for diagnostic purposes. After all, in clinical practice diagnosis for young children is very largely based on parent reports of the child's behavior supplemented by office observations and teacher reports. Following this logic, several groups have modified interviews originally developed for use with parents of older children to allow structured diagnostic assessments down to age 2 (38–40). A test-retest study of one of these (the Preschool Age Psychiatric Assessment (PAPA)) suggests that preschoolers' diagnoses assessed in this way are just a reliable as those of older children (38).

Screened Interviews

The Children's Interview for Psychiatric Syndromes (ChIPS (41)) was designed as a *screening* tool covering 20 DSM-IV Axis 1 disorders. "Cardinal questions" concerning symptoms most often seen in children with a particular disorder are asked at the beginning of each section. If the answers to these screening questions are in the negative, then the rest of that section is skipped. No test-retest reliability data are yet available for the ChIPS. A similarly screened version of the CAPA is also available, but in practice it has been found to save only about 10 minutes of interview time, so the loss of information resulting from not asking about all symptoms may not really be worth the time saving.

Computerized Interviews

Computer-*assisted* psychiatric interviews (CAPI) employ an interviewer to read questions from the screen and enter the appropriate codes into the computer as the interview progresses. The machine takes the interviewer to the appropriate stem questions, and stores the responses in a database. There is no need for bulky interview schedules to be copied and carried around, and data entry is completed during the interview (or during coding of the interview later in the office with some interviews). Furthermore, the computer will not accidentally skip parts of the interview, or accidentally vary the order of its presentation. On the other hand, computerized interviews can be programmed to vary the order in which sections are presented deliberately, so as to reduce the order of presentation effects observed when respondents learn that saying no tends to shorten the interview. However, interviews for use with children do not currently incorporate this potential feature. Recent advances in programming technology for structured interviews mean that even the most "interviewer-based" interviews can now be produced in CAPI formats. For instance, the CAPI version of the Preschool Age Psychiatric Assessment (PAPA) allows interviewers to write and store text notes with a stylus on a tablet PC; similar versions of the CAPA and YAPA are also available. When some interview schedules run to over 300 pages, the costs of buying computers can soon be offset against savings on schedule reproduction and data entry. The DISC has become progressively more complex over the last 20 years (largely because of the ever-increasing complexity of the DSMs), and, except as discussed below, the DISC-IV is now supposed always to be completed in its CAPI format, because it is really too difficult to administer it effectively in a paper-and-pencil format. There is also a CAPI version of the DICA, but this differs from the paper-and-pencil version of the interview in being fully respondent based (42). Given the advantages of CAPI administration, we predict that paper and pencil will soon disappear as a means of interview administration.

The next level of computerization is referred to as *audio* computer-*administered* survey interviewing (ACASI). Here no interviewer is used at all. Rather, digitized audio recordings of the questions (sometimes even with digitized video of an interviewer) are played back by the computer as the written form of the question is displayed. The respondent enters a response to the question, which is saved to the database. Obviously, such an approach can only be adopted with a respondent-based interview, and the DISC provides the paradigmatic example of this approach (43).

INTRODUCTION TO THE INTERVIEWS

Here we present a brief introduction to each of the diagnostic interviews, with a focus on their characteristic *response formats*.

The Schedule for Affective Disorders and Schizophrenia for School-Age Children (Kiddie-SADS, K-SADS)

The K-SADS "family" of interviews consists of a group of very diverse assessments. Indeed, the only features that all of the current versions of the K-SADS share in common are the name, the ability to make DSM-IV diagnoses, and the fact that all were designed to be administered *by clinicians*. The original version of the K-SADS (the K-SADS-P (44)) was a downward extension of the adult Schedule for Affective Disorders and Schizophrenia (SADS) and focused on the Research Diagnostic Criteria (45). Note that the "P" in its title stands for *present* (not parent). It was designed for use with children aged 6–17, but covered only a relatively limited range of symptoms and diagnoses. It was revised to cover DSM-IIIR (46) and DSM-IV.

K-SADS-P IVR

The version of the K-SADS-P most recently developed by Ambrosini and colleagues is called the K-SADS-P IVR (46). This version is closest conceptually to the original K-SADS-P in including quite detailed definitions of severity codings for each symptom. The modal form for these symptom codings is a six-point scale, involving judgments about various combinations of intensity, duration, frequency, environmental responsiveness, psychosocial impairment and observed behavior.

K-SADS-E

The K-SADS-E (47) (E for epidemiologic) collects ratings of the present episode of any disorder *and* the *worst* past episode. This interview was never even remotely similar in format to the K-SADS-P, because it rated only the presence or absence of symptoms, rather than employing the carefully defined severity codings of the K-SADS-P. The latest edition is DSM-IV compatible, and allows the current *episode* (not individual symptoms) to be rated as mild, moderate or severe.

K-SADS-PL

A group in Pittsburgh have developed the K-SADS-PL (present and lifetime), as a sort of cross between the K-SADS-P and the K-SADS-E (48, 49). Symptom ratings have been reduced to three-point scales (typically not at all, subthreshold, threshold), and fairly minimal anchoring definitions of each point are provided. An initial 82-item screen interview, which allows skipping of substantial symptom areas, is also available.

WASH-U-KSADS

Rather brief definitions of symptoms are given, and level of severity is coded, but the severity codings are idiosyncratic, and bear little relation to those in other versions of the K-SADS.

Columbia K-SADS

The symptom "definitions" provided are often simply restatements of the DSM-IV criteria. Sometimes (particularly in relation to depression) a little more guidance is given. Symptom severity is typically rated on what appears to be a 6-point scale like the K-SADS-P and K-SADS-P IVR, but closer inspection reveals that two of the points are usually defined only as being intermediate between two other points. Thus, only four points (one being symptom absence) are really defined.

Although K-SADS interviews were developed for use by clinicians, some have also have been used with lay interviewers (31).

The K-SADS family differs from most interviews (but not the ISCA) in directing that the parent should be interviewed first and then the child should be seen by the same interviewer, who is then expected to resolve any discrepancies between the child's reports and those of the parent. The interviewer then completes a record representing his/her summation of the two interviews. This procedure is highly dependent on clinical judgment, and means that the process of combining the information is not structured. It also seems likely to bias the results of the interview in favor of the parental reports, and some workers have instead scored the interviews with the parent and the child separately (50).

The Child and Adolescent Psychiatric Assessment (CAPA) and Its Congeners

The CAPA is one of an integrated group of instruments developed to assess a variety of risk factors for, manifestations of, and outcomes of child and adolescent psychiatric disorders. In addition to the usual symptom and impairment assessments, it also includes extensive ratings of the family environment and relationships, family psychosocial problems, and life events (including traumatic events and physical and sexual abuse). A separate module called the Child and Adolescent Impact Assessment (CAIA (51)) measures the impact of the child's problems on the family, while the Child and Adolescent Services Assessment (CASA (52, 53)) covers service use for mental health problems in multiple sectors and settings. Psychosocial impairment in 17 domains of functioning is measured at both the syndromic level and overall. In the interview with the child, 62 items reflecting the child's observed behavior during the interview are also coded. In order to facilitate completion of the interview by nonclinicians, the CAPA provides a more molecular approach to symptom codings. Extensive symptom definitions are given in a glossary and on the schedule, and rules are specified to allow nonclinicians make separate codings of the intensity, frequency, duration, date of onset of symptoms, and psychosocial impairment resulting from them. The CAPA emphasizes getting descriptions and examples of possible pathology to ensure that codings are not based on the informant's misunderstanding of what was being asked about (35, 54, 55).

A version of the CAPA has been developed for use with *young adults* (the Young Adult Psychiatric Assessment, YAPA), and a substantially modified version is now available for use with the parents of preschool children (The Preschool Age Psychiatric Assessment, PAPA (38)). The latter includes assessment of a number of areas of particular relevance to preschoolers that are not included in any other diagnostic interview. In addition, a version of the CAPA with empirically derived screen items is available, which allows sections to be skipped if screen symptoms are absent. A streamlined version of the CAPA for collecting data for twin studies has also been developed (56).

Diagnostic Interview for Children and Adolescents (DICA)

The DICA started out as a respondent-based interview over 20 years ago (16, 42, 57, 58). Since then it has been progressively modified so that its paper and pencil version is now an interviewer-based interview (26, 59, 60). However, there is also a computer-based version of the DICA that remains fully respondent based (26, 60). In addition, the group responsible for the development of the DICA has produced a modification called the Missouri Assessment for Genetics Interview for Children (MAGIC). The major difference between the DICA and the MAGIC is that the MAGIC has a specifications manual, which includes a great deal of guidance on how to elicit key features of symptoms, and a variety of clarifications of coding instructions (26).

The DICA and the MAGIC provide alternate versions for self-reports from children aged 6 (or 7)–12 and 13–17, which have differently worded questions. The DICA has also been used with even younger children, but special training is required for its administration in those under 6 or 7, and the instructions to interviewers essentially tell them to ignore the usual questioning format laid out in the schedule and use their own questions.

Symptoms are typically coded on a three-point scale (no, sometimes/somewhat, yes) for items about emotional symptoms, and a two-point scale (no, yes) for disruptive behaviors with additional information on frequency sometimes being added. Impairment is measured at the syndrome level by three items asking about symptoms making it hard to "get along" with the family, friends, and at school, rated on four-point scales (not at all, not too much, somewhat, quite a bit).

Child Assessment Schedule (CAS)

The CAS is organized around thematic topics and provides ratings of many items that are not required if all one wants to do is make ratings of the DSM criteria for disorders (61–65). The CAS now exists in child (7–12), adolescent, and parent report versions. Although originally developed for use by experienced clinicians, the CAS has now been used by lay interviewers in several studies. Symptoms are scored on a four-point scale (yes; no; ambiguous; not scored). This is followed by questioning about the onset and duration of positive symptoms. The items to be coded are defined in brief sentences which outline each symptom concept. The interviewer is expected to make a judgment about the coding based on the answer to the questions on the schedule (plus any additional questions that may be thought necessary).

The CAS also has a 56-item section for recording observations of the child's behavior during the interview. Diagnoses can be generated manually by interviewers using algorithms provided by the developer of the interview, but computerized scoring is recommended. The algorithms also generate symptom scales pertaining to a number of areas of psychopathology.

Psychosocial impairment is measured using a separate measure, the Child and Adolescent Functional Assessment Scale (CAFAS), which can also be used alone or with another diagnostic interview (66–68).

The Anxiety Disorders Interview Schedule (ADIS)

Notwithstanding its title, the ADIS also provides brief ratings of symptoms pertinent to other disorders, but its coverage of the anxiety disorders is more thorough (69–74). The interview is designed for clinician use, and was derived from the adult ADIS (75). Questions that *should* be asked are provided, and guidance is given about when to use additional questions. Most symptoms are scored on a simple three-point scale (yes, no, other). However, in the anxiety section a good deal of use is also made of nine-point scales (represented by a thermometer) ranging from not at all to very, very much. Similar scales are used to rate "interference," which is the ADIS term for psychosocial impairment resulting from disorders. Skip structures are frequently employed, so many individuals will not be asked about all symptoms.

The Interview Schedule for Children and Adolescents (ISCA)

The ISCA mandates administration by experienced clinicians with extensive structured interviewing training, and full understanding of the principles of diagnosis and its application to children with psychopathology. Interviewers must be able to combine the symptom information from both parent and child into diagnoses themselves, since formal algorithms for this process (other than the official diagnostic manual itself) do not appear to be available (32). Questions are clearly specified, but much additional clarification is expected of interviewers, who are not expected slavishly to stick to the written questions. Sixty-nine "major" symptoms plus 10 "mental status" items are covered, and typically coded on a nine-point severity scale that incorporates judgments about associated distress, functional impairment, and the amount of effort required to counteract symptoms. "Subsidiary information" about many symptoms is also collected, typically in a yes/no format. In addition, 17 intra-interview behavioral observation items are assessed.

A version of the interview for use with young adults (the Follow-up Interview Schedule for Adults, FISA) has also been developed.

The Diagnostic Interview Schedule for Children (DISC)

As already indicated, the questions on a respondent-based instrument are designed in a fixed, ordered sequence, and require very simple responses (typically yes/no, or picking one from a set of multiple choices for frequencies and durations of symptoms). Symptom severity is defined by similar yes/no answers on subsidiary questions (asked only if a positive response was obtained to a superordinate question) and forced choices from short sets of frequency ranges. All data combination is performed by computerized algorithms. The DISC covers a wide range of childhood and adolescent disorders and is suitable for use with 9–18-year-olds (76). A version for use with the parents of preschoolers is currently under development. CAPI and ACASI versions are available.

INTERVIEW TIME FRAMES

The K-SADS interviews, the ADIS, the CAS, the Dominic, the PICA-IIIR and the ISCA all focus on the child's current status or the current episode of disorder, though the definition of "current" is largely unspecified, except in the case of the ISCA, where the assessment period is specified (e.g., 2 weeks for irritability). The Columbia K-SADS adds a past 2-week time frame to the current frame. The K-SADS-PL, the Columbia K-SADS and K-SADS-E also explore lifetime histories of "worst" episodes, while the ISCA also provides for assessment of lifetime disorder, and an interim version provides an assessment of current status plus the child's status in the interim between the current assessment and the last assessment for use in followup studies. The DICA and MAGIC focus on the whole lifetime, but for some disorders an additional shorter time frame is also included. For instance, in the depression section, the MAGIC asks about the past month as well as whether the child has "ever" had symptoms. The CAPA covers a "primary period" of three months, but also notes whether certain uncommon symptoms (such as suicide attempts) have ever occurred, and a version that provides lifetime coverage of major episodes of certain syndromes is also available (56). The full DISC-IV can be used to assess either the last month or the last year, and also offers a module to determine whether certain syndromes that did not occur during the preceding year had occurred at any point since the age of 5.

SPECIFICATION OF QUESTIONS, INTERVIEWER FLEXIBILITY, AND DEFINITION OF SYMPTOMS

In a fully respondent-based interview like the DISC, or the computerized version of the DICA, all questions are completely specified and no others may be used. There is no interviewer flexibility, and no need to provide definitions of symptoms. All variability in these features concerns the interviewer-based interviews.

The ADIS, CAPA, DICA, and MAGIC all contain questions that, under most circumstances, should be asked as written in the schedule. Additional questions are then asked as necessary to allow the interviewer to determine exactly whether the symptom is present. Many such questions are provided on the schedule of the CAPA, a smaller number are provided by the CAS schedule (but it is not clear to what extent the "set" questions of the CAS are mandated for use). Most guidance on this process for the DICA and MAGIC is provided in the MAGIC's specifications manual. All these interviews provide at least some additional instructions about when to probe further. The K-SADS group of interviews provides a range of suggested questions, but no formal rules about when they are to be used or skipped. Interviewers are also expected to ask any additional followup questions that may be necessary to clarify responses.

By interviewer flexibility, we mean the degree to which the interviewer is expected or encouraged to use judgment in asking additional clarifying questions. In this respect, the K-SADS and ISCA (and perhaps the ADIS) interviews may be seen as providing most flexibility because they demand that judgments based on clinical experience be made, and in the case of the K-SADS do not mandate the use of any particular questions. The problem question is "flexible to do what?" The answer is relatively clear in the case of the K-SADS-P IV and the CAPA, where detailed coding rules are provided for each symptom. The task of the interviewer is to determine whether those coding criteria are met. With the other interviewer-based instruments it often seems that the interviewer's job is to get the answer *to the original question*. Variable amounts of guidance on how to do so are provided; in considerable detail in the MAGIC specifications manual, with brief symptom definitions in the CAS, but little or no guidance in the K-SADS-E or ADIS.

The K-SADS-P IV and the CAPA provide detailed *definitional* glossaries covering each symptom, which means that the task of the interviewer is quite clearly specified at the level of the definition of symptoms. The CAPA glossary also contains many procedural instructions relating both to questioning in general and questioning about specific symptoms; but these are presented as being secondary to the definitional issues. The MAGIC specifications manual can also be seen as being a glossary, but it is, first and foremost, a *procedural* manual. It is primarily about how to collect the information. In the course of this discussion of procedure, it also includes a good deal of definitional material, but does not provide formal definitions of items in the way that the K-SADS-P IV or CAPA do.

RELIABILITY OF STRUCTURED DIAGNOSTIC INTERVIEWS

A difficulty with the literature on "reliability" is that the term is applied to several very different sorts of design and statistical approaches. Three of these are commonly seen in the literature on structured interviews, but only one presents a useful test of what one ultimately requires in a diagnostic interview. For instance, one often sees reports of *interrater* reliabilities in the interview literature. However, interrater reliability is not a very useful index of interview performance. With respondent-based interviews it tests nothing but whether one interviewer can read aloud adequately while another codes a schedule. With such interviews, if interrater reliability is not in the high .9s, one should retrain or fire one's interviewers! In an interviewer-based interview the questions are not fixed, and so different interviewers could use different questions to elicit the same information. Since the interrater reliability paradigm uses multiple raters to score the same interview, this major source of potential unreliability is eliminated, with the result that the interrater reliability is likely to substantially overestimate the reliability of the interview in actual use. However, if interrater reliabilities fall below about .8 that is an indication that something is either wrong with interviewer training, or that the interview needs to be revised to provide greater clarity about what is supposed to be rated. The point is that, if very high interrater reliability coefficients cannot be obtained, we can be certain that test-retest reliability will be poor.

"Internal reliability" is sometimes reported for scales resulting from diagnostic interviews. Typically the statistic given is Cronbach's alpha. This statistic provides a measure of the degree to which the items in the scale are correlated with one another. There are two problems with the use of such a statistic here. First, it has nothing to do with whether *raters* are coding items "reliably"; it concerns the degree to which the items in a scale are all measuring the same thing. Second, a perfectly good diagnosis could be associated with low correlations among the symptoms that signal the presence of that diagnosis. Most medical (and psychiatric) diagnoses are more concerned with pattern recognition than with scalar values. For instance, in the general population it is unlikely that dry eyes, dry mouth, and arthritis are very highly correlated with one another, but that does not mean that Sjörgren's syndrome is a bad diagnosis. Of course, if the task is to develop a scalar measure of some construct then the scale's alpha is important information. However, from the perspective of a diagnostic interview, low alphas are not necessarily a bad thing, nor are high alphas necessarily a good thing. It is entirely possible to have a perfect measure of a diagnostic entity where Cronbach's alpha for the symptoms constituting that entity was close to zero.

Table 4.2.3.1 shows the results of studies of the *test-retest* reliabilities (Kappas) of diagnoses measured by the instruments considered in this chapter. Test-retest reliability is what is needed in judging an instrument. In the absence of reasonable test-retest reliability, all other reliabilities are moot. It can be seen that all the interviews that have been tested do a reasonably good job, and that there is not much to choose between them. These reliability coefficients are similar to those reported for psychiatric interviews with adults.

TABLE 4.2.3.1

DIAGNOSTIC TEST-RETEST RELIABILITIES (KAPPAS) OF INSTRUMENTS

	MDD*	Dysthy/ Minor D	Any Depress	GAD/ OAD	Sep Anx	Specific Phobia	Social Phobia	Any Anx	PTSD	ADHD	CD	ODD	SA/D
K-SADS-P	.54	.70						.24					
K-SADS-P IIIR	.77	.89						.72		.91		.46	
K-SADS-PL current	.90			.78				.80	.67	.63		.74	
K-SADS-PL lifetime	1.0			.78				.60	.60	.55	.83	.77	
CAS	1.0	.85	.83	.38				.72		.43			
DICA			.90					.76		1.0		.61	
CAPA child only	.90	.85	.82	.79				.64	.64		.55		1.0
PAPA			.72	.39	.60	.36	.54	.49	.73	.74	.60	.57	
ISCA child only				.82	.81								
ADIS - combined P & C. DSM-IIIR				.64		.84	.73	.75					
ADIS—combined P & C. DSM-IV. Clinic sample.				.80	.84	.81	.92			1.0		.62	
DISC-IV - combined P & C. Clinic sample.	.65			.58	.51	.86	.48			.62	.55	.59	
DISC-IV combined P & C. Clinic sample. Chinese	.61				.53					.75		.56	
DISC 2.3 - combined P & C. Community sample	.45			.52	.49		.44	.47		.48	.66	.59	

*MDD = Major depressive disorder/episode; Dysthy = dysthymia; Minor = minor depression; GAD = Generalized anxiety disorder, OAD = overanxious disorder; Sep Anx = separation anxiety disorder; Any Anx = any anxiety disorder; PTSD = post traumatic stress disorder; ADHD = attention deficit hyperactivity disorder; CD = conduct disorder; ODD = oppositional defiant disorder; SA/D = substance abuse or dependence.

Reliabilities for scale scores derived from the interviews are typically rather higher than they are for diagnosis, but that is nearly always true of comparisons between scale score reliabilities and the reliabilities of categories generated by imposing cut points on the same scales. It is also important to remember that some of the unreliability of diagnostic measures is the product of the diagnostic system itself, thanks to its requirement that numerous unmemorable details about past psychopathology be considered. Particular problems have been identified with the reliability of responses concerning the duration of symptoms and the dates of their onsets (77, 78).

Despite enormous efforts on the part of interview developers, it cannot be said that the reliability of diagnostic interviews has increased much over the years. We now have a fairly mature interview technology which has been repeatedly refined in the hope of increasing the reliability of assessments. The current arsenal of diagnostic interviews probably offers as good reliability as can be achieved until quite different means of arriving at psychiatric diagnoses appear.

A problem with the test-retest assessment of reliability is that it requires that the interview be repeated within a short period of time. With both questionnaires and interviews one typically finds that fewer symptoms are endorsed at the second interview than at the first (79, 80). There are many possible explanations for this effect (81), but some evidence suggests that the results of the first interview are probably the most accurate representation of reality. The usual interpretation of test-retest reliability statistics such as Cohen's Kappa for categorical data (such as diagnoses) and the intraclass correlation coefficient (ICC) for continuous data (such as scale scores) involves the supposition that the relationship between scores at the first interview and those at the second involves two components, agreement and random error. The presence of a *consistent difference* between first interviews and second interviews indicates that such statistics underestimate the "true" (and ultimately unmeasurable) reliability of both interviews and psychopathology scales.

VALIDITY OF STRUCTURED DIAGNOSTIC INTERVIEWS

The problem with trying to assess the validity of psychiatric interviews is that there is no noninterview test for most psychiatric disorders. The structured interview itself is now the closest approximation we have to a gold standard. So how are we to validate the diagnoses obtained from such interviews? This is a version of a problem that psychologists have been grappling with for decades, one that led to the concept of *construct validity*. The central idea here is that the validity of an instrument for the measurement of a psychological construct inheres not in some single agreement coefficient with one external standard, but in the instrument's performance within the *nomological net* of theory and data concerning the construct or constructs that the instrument purports to measure (82–90). As Gulliksen (85) pointedly remarked over half a century ago, "at some point in the advance of psychology it would seem appropriate for the psychologist to lead the way in establishing good criterion measures, instead of just attempting to construct imperfect tests for attributes that are presumed to be assessed more accurately and more validly by the judgment of experts."

Structured interviews were developed because of the dismal psychometric properties of unaided clinical diagnosis, so comparisons with unstructured clinical judgment (as might be found for instance in chart diagnoses) are hopelessly flawed tests of diagnostic interview validity. That has been obvious to interview developers for a long time, so "validity" studies have sometimes provided the clinicians with all the information from the interviews to be validated, in addition to allowing them to collect further information should they wish to. In such a circumstance it will often be the case that *most* of the information available to the clinician comes from the interview under test. It will hardly be surprising, then, if there is good agreement between clinician and interview, but no real test will have been done.

In considering the validity of any interview we should take a construct validation approach, and describe what we currently know about it in relation to the nomological net pertaining to child and adolescent psychiatric diagnosis. So far, only the developers of the CAPA have explicitly laid out the evidence for the validity of the CAPA using this approach, but most of the interviews considered here can point to similar chains of evidence. To give a flavor of the sort of evidence relevant to construct validation, the following findings have been adduced as construct validators of the CAPA: (29)

1. Diagnostic rates and age and gender patterns of disorder given by the CAPA are consistent with those found using other interviews.
2. Patterns of diagnostic comorbidity are consistent with those found by other interviews.
3. Symptomatic diagnoses are associated with psychosocial impairment.
4. Parent and child reports of psychopathology on the CAPA are related to parent and teacher reports of problems on well established scales for detecting psychopathology.
5. Children with CAPA-identified disorders use more mental health services than children without diagnoses
6. CAPA-diagnosed children tend to come from families with a history of mental illness.
7. There is genetic loading for a number of CAPA scales scores and diagnoses.
8. CAPA diagnoses show consistency over time.
9. CAPA diagnoses predict negative life outcomes.
10. Different CAPA diagnoses are differentially related to the physiologic changes of puberty.

There is, of course, a big drawback to this approach. No new interview will be able to point to such chains of evidence until it has been in use for quite a time. How then is any new instrument ever to be developed? The answer lies in the application of common sense and well established assessment principles. When a new assessment is needed, it is perfectly proper to use the best available information about the nature of the phenomena to be measured to design what seems, on the face of it, to be an adequate measure. Attention needs to be given to keeping questions short, and focused on single constructs; to defining the task of the interviewer clearly; and to providing good definitions of the constructs to be studied in the case of interviewer-based interviews. If initial test-retest reliability is adequate, then in general, it is unlikely that the interview will prove to be completely "invalid." Since it is very unusual to be trying to assess a construct that has been utterly unmeasured before, or about which nothing whatever is known, it will also usually be possible to include in the test-retest study other measures that will give some indication of the concurrent, predictive, or divergent validity of the new instrument.

ADVANTAGES AND DISADVANTAGES OF INTERVIEWER- AND RESPONDENT-BASED INTERVIEWS

Neither interviewer- nor respondent-based interviews are ideal tools, and there is simply no answer to the question "Which type is best?" In this section, we list the general advantages of each type of interview, and the lack of each advantage can be regarded as a disadvantage of the other type. However, it is worth noting here that it has sometimes been said that respondent-based interviews are more appropriate for general population studies. Since it has now been shown that lay interviewers can provide reliable and valid ratings using interviewer-based interviews, this position is no longer tenable. Indeed a number of larger scale longitudinal general population studies have used (and are still using) interviewer-based interviews (for instance) (91, 92).

Advantages of Interviewer-Based Interviews

Interviewer-based interviews have four theoretical and practical advantages: 1) If the interview has been conducted and coded properly, the meaning of the ratings is precisely known; 2) they provide opportunities to crosscheck discrepant or confusing information; 3) they enable the use of efficient open-ended questioning strategies, and allow the use of redundant questioning, which has been shown in adults to improve the quality of responses; and 4) they appear to be less prone to overdiagnosis on the basis of symptom reports, so arbitrary impairment scale cutoffs do not have to be employed to produce reasonable diagnostic rates in unselected community samples.

What Do the Codings Mean?

In an interviewer-based interview, a positive coding for a symptom means that it has been determined that the symptom as defined in the schedule is present. In a respondent-based interview one knows only that a child or parent responded positively to a particular question. One does not know exactly what the child or parent understood the question to mean. This problem has been documented with unusual symptoms that most children never experience, such as obsessive-compulsive or psychotic symptoms. Such symptoms were greatly overreported using early versions of the DISC (93). When clinicians reviewed what the children said, it was obvious that what was being reported was not obsessive-compulsive disorder or psychosis. However, if an unstructured clinician review is added to the diagnostic process, one no longer knows exactly what factors went into the final rating, and one great advantage of the respondent-based interview is lost.

Crosschecking Information

It is common in clinical practice to find that certain answers appear to contradict previously given information, or lead to uncertainty about whether a symptom is present. In an interviewer-based interview one simply attempts to clarify the contradiction or confusion. The respondent-based approach provides no mechanism for resolving such difficulties, since interviewers are not allowed to exercise their judgment about such matters.

Use of Open-Ended and Redundant Questions

The distinction between open and closed questions is not absolute, but open questions are those that offer the chance to provide a wide range of answers or free-recall descriptions of phenomena, while closed questions call for one of a limited set of responses. For example, an open question in response to being told by a child that he had received a bad school report might be "How did you feel about your bad grades?," whereas "Did your bad grades make you feel unhappy?" would be a closed question. If a child had just admitted to stealing, responding with "Tell me more about that," involves an open question, whereas "What did you steal?" is a closed question. Basically, closed questions call for a yes/no answer or a date, frequency, duration, or other quite specific piece of information, while open questions give the opportunity for the child to provide a description of his feelings, which might or might not involve sadness or hostility. The work of Rutter and Cox and their colleagues offers some direct guidance on the best ways to use these different sorts of questions with adults, and in the light of the literature on children's memory, there is little reason not to use a similar approach with children (94–98). They concluded that, in general, most factual information was collected when a systematic approach that relied heavily on open questions was used. This approach was also conducive to parental expressions of emotion, since it involved less talking on the part of the interviewer and gave more time for parents to discuss their concerns. On the other hand, a noninterventionist approach resulted in the provision of less relevant information, while challenging interpretations and a confrontational style proved less effective in eliciting emotions. Thus, open questions can be effective in collecting information efficiently, but, of necessity, respondent-based interviews must rely on closed questions. On the other hand, closed questions are necessary to elicit information that is otherwise not forthcoming, and respondent-based interviews have been a substantial help to the developers of interviewer-based interviews in establishing well thought-out logical structures for series of closed questions.

A redundant question is one that is asked more than once in different ways; that is, questions that contain two presentations of the same item, as in "Have you been more irritable than usual?," followed by "or made angry more easily?" The adult survey literature (99) suggests that such redundancy is actually helpful in providing both additional time for thought and a second chance to pick up symptoms. If the answer to one question is positive and the other negative, that is no problem for an interviewer-based interview, where followup questions can be used to clarify the situation. However, this cannot be done in a respondent-based interview, where specific chains of questions in response to initially discrepant information would be required. Collapsing the two questions into one is no help because this generates a "multiple question" which requires the respondent to remember and process the two parts of the question simultaneously.

Reasonable Rates of Disorder

Rates of diagnosis based only on symptom reports were found to be unreasonably high with early versions of the DISC. To correct this tendency it is now usual to require that a diagnosis only be allocated when the score on the Child Global Assessment Scale (CGAS) is less than 60 (or sometimes 70; i.e., when notable psychosocial impairment is present). However, in most cases the DSM-IV requires that *either* impairment *or* distress be present, not that significant impairment always be present. Furthermore, the typical impairment cutpoint of 60 was established because it generated what appeared to be sensible rates of diagnosis, not because anyone with a score over 60 is necessarily unimpaired. Since the K-SADS-P and the CAPA employ exacting definitions at the individual symptom level, community studies using these instruments do not need to apply additional rules about impairment to generate sensible rates of diagnosis.

Advantages of Respondent-Based Interviews

We can also identify three advantages of respondent-based interviews: 1) Less intensive training need be provided to interviewers, 2) a lesser degree of quality control is required, and 3) computer-administered (ACASI) interviews offer the prospect of providing a "preclinical" screening for use in clinical settings.

Intensity of Training

There is no doubt that an interviewer-based interview makes greater demands on an interviewer than does a respondent-based interview. For instance, training on the full CAPA package takes a month, compared with a few days for the DISC.

Quality Control

"Interviewer drift" occurs with respondent-based interviews, necessitating continuing quality control throughout a study, but it is unarguable that there is much more to check with an interviewer-based interview. Care must be taken, not only that the interview is being conducted and coded properly, but mechanisms must also be in place to ensure that interviewers continue to interpret the responses of interviewees correctly. Whether this additional burden is worth the effort depends on the situation in which the interview is being used.

Preclinical Screening

We have reached the point where it is feasible to have parents and children complete a computer administered diagnostic interview like the DISC-IV before they see a clinician at all. The possible output from the DISC-IV is almost infinitely flexible, and requires only programming to allow the production of reports tailored to particular clinical needs that can be generated as soon as the interview is finished. Equipped with such a report, a clinician familiar with one of the interviewer-based interviews would then be starting with a very respectable initial diagnostic formulation to guide further elucidation of the clinical status of the child. For instance, the ACASI version of the DISC has also been found suitable for use in juvenile justice settings where staff are rarely available to conduct diagnostic interviews.

SELECTING A STRUCTURED INTERVIEW

As we have already seen, reliability and validity quotients are little help in selecting the "best" interview, because there is little to choose between interviews in this regard. Similarly, all the interviews considered here take quite a long time to complete, and their length is proportional to the amount of symptomatology manifested by a child. None has been shown to be notably shorter than any other in practice, and so reported mean interview durations are also no help in selecting and interview for any particular application. Rather, the key to selecting an interview is to be very clear about what that application demands. This means having thought through what the ideal interview for that application would be like, so that the characteristics of each can be matched against those criteria. It is also worthwhile to prioritize these demand characteristics in advance. It may not be possible to have everything, so it is a big help to have thought through the relative impact of different tradeoffs. In the following sections, we consider some questions that prospective interview users should ask themselves as part of the process of selecting an interview.

1: *What content areas need to be covered?* All interviews do not cover all diagnoses (indeed, none covers all possibly relevant diagnoses). It is essential in the first instance to decide what areas must be covered, and what additional areas would be nice to have, but not essential.

2: *What assessment time frame is needed?* The addition of a lifetime frame involves either compromises in the assessment of current or recent symptomatology (as with the K-SADS-PL) or combining a short time-frame interview with a separate lifetime interview, which results in a very long assessment. If one is conducting a three-month followup assessment following treatment, an interview that focuses on diagnostic status over the last year will not be very helpful.

3: *What sort of interviewers will be available?* In general, clinicians are not enthusiastic about using a respondent-based interview because they have to follow a fixed schedule of questions, and it provides no means to collect more detailed information that may be relevant to a variety of treatment decisions. So it makes sense for them to use one of the interviewer-based interviews. Such interviews can also be very useful clinical training tools, since they provide excellent models for the clinical interviewing process.

If lay interviewers are to be used, then the K-SADS family of interviews may not be the best choice because these interviews have all been developed for use by clinicians and provide less guidance for the training of lay interviewers. No reliability data on their use with lay interviewers are available. On the other hand, the CAS, CAPA, DICA, and ADIS were all developed for use with trained lay interviewers and have been shown to have acceptable reliability in their hands; all of these interviews are also acceptable to clinicians.

4: *What is the age and developmental level of the children to be assessed?* It is clear that "adult-style" diagnostic interviews (all of the interviews considered in this chapter fall into this category) with preschool children are a waste of time, because they are cognitively incapable of providing all the information required by the DSM-IV or ICD-10 diagnostic criteria. Several groups are working on this problem at present, but none of the instruments reviewed here is of any use for interviewing very young children directly. The K-SADS and DICA are said to be suitable for face-to-face use with children down to the age of 6, but others doubt that a *full* diagnostic interview really works with children under the age of 8 or 9, unless the interviewer simply "goes off interview" to get a relatively impressionistic view of the child's symptomatology. Even the interview with the parent requires substantial modification for preschoolers. We would not recommend the use of any of these instruments in face-to-face interviews with children under the age of 8 or 9. Picture-enhanced interviews like the Dominic-R may be suitable down to the age of 6, but even here, reliability appears to be somewhat lower with younger children, and such interviews do not generate full diagnoses. The same problem applies to older individuals with substantial intellectual deficits. When an individual's IQ is much below 70, it becomes very difficult to complete a full diagnostic interview. Interviews with parents and teachers may still be conducted, but we know little about their performance characteristics in such circumstances.

At the other end of the juvenile age range (late adolescence and early adulthood), the researcher or clinician has the choice of shifting to an adult measure, or using an age-appropriate modification of a child interview (such as the YAPA).

5: *How much can I afford to spend on training and quality control?* "Spend" here refers to both time and money. If less than a week is available, then none of the interviewer-based interviews is suitable, because good training for them demands a greater time investment. However, DISC training can be provided in as short a time as this, because the DISC requires far less of interviewers. On the other hand, when amortized over the life of a study or clinical program, initial costs for training usually turn out to be only a small percentage of total costs, so training on an interviewer-based interview may constitute a good investment.

Once each interview is completed, the DICA and CAPA both expect that it will be reviewed for appropriateness of codings. In addition, regular (both recommend weekly) continuing training sessions for interviewers are required to prevent interviewer drift. Are funds and personnel available to support such continuing quality control and training procedures? The CAS and K-SADS interviews do not appear to have standard recommendations for quality control and continuing training, but there is no reason to suppose that data quality and consistency are any easier to maintain with these instruments. Since the DISC-IV is computerized, and the DISC interviewer's task is much less arduous than that required of interviewers using any of the interviews considered in this chapter, it demands less effort to control interviewer drift. However, interviewer monitoring is still necessary to ensure that interviewers are following the questioning rules exactly, and to ensure that they are actually conducting interviews and not simply falsifying them (yes, this does happen!)

6: *What needs and resources do I have for data entry and manipulation of the data?* The K-SADS family of interviews produces diagnoses through the medium of score sheets completed by the interviewer and scored by that person to produce diagnoses. The CAS provides formal algorithms for making diagnoses that can be implemented either by the interviewer or a computer. The CAPA offers only computerized algorithms because its developers (like those of the DISC) believe that the process of producing a final diagnosis from a large array of symptom data is of such complexity that errors are bound to occur if humans do it unaided. These different approaches to producing a final diagnostic formulation have very different implications for data entry and manipulation. If the computer is to make the diagnoses then all the symptom information must be entered (this task easily runs to hundreds or thousands of variables per case), and diagnostic algorithms must be available. If the clinician makes the final diagnosis, then one could simply enter only that information (or not computerize any data at all in a clinical setting where the interview is being used just as a clinical assessment whose results appear only in the medical record). CAPI interviews reduce the need to budget for data entry per se, but consideration still has to be given to data management over the course of an interviewing project.

Once these demand characteristics have been determined one can begin the task of actually selecting an interview:

1. *Review the available instruments and make a shortlist.* It may seem surprising that we place a review of available measures so late in the process. There are two reasons for doing this. First, the choice of measure should be dependent on the nature of the application, not the other way around, so until the application has been well defined the issue of instrumentation is moot. Second, once one has answered questions 1–6, a brief review of instruments may indicate that only one is even remotely suitable. To put it another way, it is more efficient to decide which interview to use relatively late in the process, because one may be able to save a lot of time that would otherwise have been spent in considering instruments that cannot meet the needs of the study. If there seem to be several possibilities at hand, one has at least reduced the number of instruments that need to be considered to a shortlist for further evaluation.

2. *Get copies of the instruments on the shortlist and conduct a detailed evaluation.* Unfortunately, there is absolutely no substitute for getting copies of the instruments still left on the shortlist and reviewing them in detail. The manifold differences between instruments make it impossible to provide more than a flavor of what an interview is like in a review chapter such as this. It is worth remembering that you will be asking the interview developers to send several hundred pages of schedules, glossaries, instruction manuals, and the like, and that these will need to be paid for. At this stage, it should be possible to make a final choice, but if there are still questions that have not been answered in all these materials, a telephone call to someone in the relevant interview development group can be very helpful. If the "homework" outlined above has been done, it is also likely to be well received.

3. *Plan training well ahead of time.* It is not unknown for an interview developer to receive a request like the following: "Hello, I put the . . . in a grant proposal, and the funding has just come through. I need you to train my interviewers next month." Interview developers have busy research and clinical lives, and they cannot provide training programs at a moment's notice. The time to be setting a hopeful date for training is *before the grant proposal is submitted*, not after it has been reviewed and funded.

FUTURE DIRECTIONS

A great deal of work has gone into producing the interviews we have today, and there is little sign that recent efforts to further "improve" such measures have had much effect on their reliability. Of course, as we learn more about psychopathology we will need to modify our measures' content to reflect what we need to measure, but the basic principles used to design new or revised modules will not change in the foreseeable future (and will work just as well or poorly as they do today). What is needed now is to extend the range of structured assessments down to younger ages. There is astonishingly little research on preschool psychopathology, for instance, and it was only in 2000 that the first structured parent-report diagnostic interview specifically designed for use with this age group became available. It remains to be seen how information from the child and caretakers other than parents can usefully be integrated into diagnostic assessments, but work has begun in this area. Newer "self-report" assessments of the mental status of the child that do not tie themselves rigidly to current diagnostic criteria show great promise for the future. For instance, with the MacArthur Story-Stem Battery (100–102) the interviewer uses toys to act out the beginnings of stories which the child is then asked to complete. The videotapes of these interactions are then scored to provide indices of a variety of internal states. The Berkeley Puppet Interview (103) employs two puppets to express two moods/states, and the child indicates the puppet most like him- or herself, thereby providing self-report assessments of perceived academic functioning, social relationships, depression, anxiety, and aggression/hostility. Some simpler "questionnaires with pictures" have also shown promise with preschoolers in relation to the assessment of depression and anxiety (104, 105). Observational assessments, such as the Disruptive Behaviors Diagnostic Observational Schedule (DB-DOS), a structured observational measure to identify clinically significant disruptive behaviors in preschoolers (106), will also likely play a role in the diagnosis of preschool psychiatric symptoms and impairment in the future.

Now that many diagnostic measures are available, it is likely that they will move progressively into ordinary clinical practice. It seems strange that the unstructured clinical interview has been almost entirely supplanted for research purposes because of its well documented inadequacies as a diagnostic procedure, but continues to be the main assessment tool in clinical practice, where good phenomenological assessment is surely of the greatest importance. All clinicians dealing with psychopathology can benefit from training on an interviewer-based structured interview (particularly one of the glossary-based interviews), and it is to be hoped that such training will soon become part of all training programs for psychiatric clinicians. However, it must be admitted that the time to conduct a full psychiatric assessment is not always available, and when that is the case it would be helpful to have shorter interviews available to serve as screening tools. Here, a good start has been made with the DISC predictive scales (107), which have been shown to have good screening properties in relation to DSM-IIIR diagnoses. The idea here is not to force slavish dependence on any particular structured interview on clinicians, but to use the strengths of standardized interviews to underpin their explorations of the nature and meaning of psychopathology. Our understanding of psychopathology and its measurement has have come a long way, and it is time to bring the benefits of what are still typically regarded as being research assessment methods to all of our patients and clients.

References

1. Cantwell DP: DSM-III studies. In M. Rutter TAH & LIS (eds): *Assessment and diagnosis in child psychopathology* New York: Guilford Press, pp. 3–36, 1988.
2. Gould MS, Shaffer D, Rutter M, & Sturge C: UK/WHO study of ICD-9. In M Rutter, AH Tuma & IS Lann (eds.), *Assessment and diagnosis in child psychopathology* pp. 37–65, New York: Guilford Press, 1988.
3. Remschmidt H: German study of ICD-9. In: M Rutter, AH Tuma & IS Lann (eds), *Assessment and diagnosis in child psychopathology* pp. 66–83. London: Guilford Press, 1988.
4. Prendergast M, Taylor E, Rapoport JL, Bartko J, Donnelly M, Zametkin A, et al.: The diagnosis of childhood hyperactivity a U.S.-U.K. cross-national study of DSM-III and ICD-9. *Journal of Child Psychology and Psychiatry* 29, 289–300, 1988.
5. Cooper JE, Kendell RE, Gurland BJ, Sharpe L, & Copeland JRM: *Psychiatric diagnosis in New York and London: A comparative study of mental hospital admissions* (20 ed) London, Oxford University Press, 1972.
6. Achenbach TM: *Assessment and taxonomy of child and adolescent psychopathology*. Beverly Hills, Sage Publications, 1985.
7. Wing JK: *Measurement and classification of psychiatric symptoms*. Oxford, Oxford University Press, 1974.
8. Guze SB, Goodwin DW, & Crane JB: Criminality and psychiatric disorders. *Archives of General Psychiatry* 20:583–591, 1969.
9. Graham P, & Rutter M: The reliability and validity of the psychiatric assessment of the child: II. Interview with the parent. *British Journal of Psychiatry* 114:581–592, 1968.
10. Rutter M, Graham P: The reliability and validity of the psychiatric assessment of the child: I. Interview with the child. *British Journal of Psychiatry* 114:563–579, 1968.
11. Regier DA, Myers JK, Kramer M, Robins LN, Blazer DG, Hough RL, et al.: The NIMH Epidemiological Catchment Area Program: Historical context, major objectives, and study population characteristics. *Archives of General Psychiatry* 41(10):934–941, 1984.
12. Robins LN, Helzer J, Croughan J, Williams JBW, & Spitzer RL: *The NIMH Diagnostic Interview Schedule (DIS): Version II*. National Institutes of Mental Health, 1979.
13. Herjanic B, & Campbell W: Differentiating psychiatrically disturbed children on the basis of a structured interview. *Journal of Abnormal Child Psychology* 5:127–134, 1977.
14. Herjanic B, Herjanic M, Brown F, & Wheatt T: Are children reliable reporters? *Journal of Abnormal Child Psychology* 3(1):41–48, 1975.
15. Lapouse R: The epidemiology of behavior disorders in children. *American Journal of Dysfunctional Children* 111:594–599, 1966.
16. Herjanic B, Reich W: Development of a structured psychiatric interview for children: Agreement between child and parent on individual symptoms. *Journal of Abnormal Child Psychology* 10(3):307–324, 1982.
17. Loeber R, Green SM, Lahey BB, Stouthamer-Loeber, M: Differences and similarities between children, mothers, and teachers as informants on disruptive child behavior. *Journal of Abnormal Child Psychology* 19(1):75–95, 1991.
18. Lahey BB: *Validity of informants and combinations of informants in assessing Childhood Psychopathology*, 1990.
19. Conners CK: *Conners' Rating Scales revised: Instruments for use with children and adolescents*, North Tonawanda, NY, Multi-Health Systems, Inc, 1997.
20. Reich W, Herjanic B, Welner Z, Gandhy PR: Development of a structured psychiatric interview for children: Agreement on diagnosis comparing child and parent interviews. *Journal of Abnormal Child Psychology* 10:325–336, 1982.
21. Stanger C, Lewis M: Agreement among parents, teachers, and children on internalizing and externalizing behavior problems. *Journal of Clinical Child Psychology* 22(1):107–115, 1993.
22. Chambers WJ, Puig-Antich J, Hirsch M, Paez P, Ambrosini PJ, Tabrizi MA, et al.: The assessment of affective disorders in children and adolescents by semistructured interview: Test-retest reliability of the Schedule for Affective Disorders and Schizophrenia for School-age Children, Present Episode Version. *Archives of General Psychiatry* 42:696–702, 1985.
23. Lord C, Rutter M, Goode S, Heemsbergen J, Jordan H, Mawhood L, et al.: Autism diagnostic observation schedule. A standardized observation of communicative and social behavior. *Journal of Autism and Developmental Disorders* 19(2):185–212, 1989.
24. Lord C, Rutter M, LeCouteur A: Autism diagnostic interview—revised: A revised version of a diagnostic interview for caregivers of individuals with possible pervasive developmental disorders. *Journal of Autism and Developmental Disorders* 24(5):659–685, 1994.
25. Shaffer D, Fisher P, Lucas CP, Dulcan MK, & Schwab-Stone ME: NIMH diagnostic interview schedule for children version IV (NIMH DISC-IV): Description, differences from previous versions, and reliability of some common diagnoses. *Journal of the American Academy of Child and Adolescent Psychiatry* 39:28–38, 2000.
26. Reich W: Diagnostic interview for children and adolescents (DICA). *Journal of the American Academy of Child and Adolescent Psychiatry* 59–66, 2000.
27. Valla J-P, Bergeron L, & Smolla N: The Dominic-R: A pictorial interview for 6- to 11-year-old children. *Journal of the American Academy of Child and Adolescent Psychiatry* 39:85–93, 2000.
28. Silverman WK, Rabian B: Test-retest reliability of the DSM-III-R childhood anxiety disorders symptoms using the anxiety disorders interview schedule for children. *Journal of Anxiety Disorders* 9(2):139–150, 1995.
29. Angold A, Costello EJ: The Child and Adolescent Psychiatric Assessment (CAPA). *Journal of the American Academy of Child and Adolescent Psychiatry* 39:39–48, 2000.
30. Hodges K: Structured interviews for assessing children. *Journal of Child Psychology and Psychiatry* 34(1):49–68, 1993.
31. Hodges K, McKnew D, Cytryn L, Stern L, & Kline J: The Child Assessment Schedule (CAS) diagnostic interview: A report on reliability and validity. *Journal of the American Academy of Child Psychiatry* 21(5):468–473, 1982.
32. Sherrill JT, & Kovacs M: Interview schedule for children and adolescents (ISCA). *Journal of the American Academy of Child and Adolescent Psychiatry* 39:67–75, 2000.
33. Ambrosini PJ: Historical development and present status of the schedule for affective disorders and schizophrenia for school-age children (K-SADS). *Journal of the American Academy of Child and Adolescent Psychiatry* 39:49–58, 2000.
34. Ernst M, Cookus BA, & Moravec BC: Pictorial instrument for children and adolescents (PICA-III-R). *Journal of the American Academy of Child and Adolescent Psychiatry* 39:94–99, 2000.
35. Angold A, Costello EJ: A test-retest reliability study of child-reported psychiatric symptoms and diagnoses using the Child and Adolescent Psychiatric Assessment (CAPA-C). *Psychological Medicine* 25:755–762, 1995.
36. Murphy DA, Cantwell C, Jordan DD, Lee MB, Cooley-Quille MR, Lahey BB: Test-retest reliability of Dominic anxiety and depression items among young children. *Journal of Psychopathology and Behavioral Assessment* 22:257–270, 2000.
37. Valla JP, Kovess V, Chan Chee C, Berthiaume C, Vantalon V, Piquet C, et al.: A French study of the Dominic Interactive. *Social Psychiatry and Psychiatric Epidemiology* 37(9):441–448, 2002.
38. Egger HL, Erkanli A, Keeler G, Potts E, Walter B, Angold A (in press): The test-retest reliability of the Preschool Age Psychiatric Assessment. *Journal of the American Academy of Child and Adolescent Psychiatry*.
39. Luby J, Heffelfinger A, Mrakotsky C, Brown K, Hessler M, Wallis J, et al.: The clinical picture of depression in preschool children. *Journal of the American Academy of Child and Adolescent Psychiatry* 42:340–348, 2003.
40. Wakschlag LS, Keenan K: Clinical significance and correlates of disruptive behavior in environmentally at-risk preschoolers. *Journal of Clinical Child Psychology* 30(1):262–275, 2001.
41. Weller EB, Weller RA, Fristad MA, Rooney MT, Schecter J: Children's interview for psychiatric syndromes (ChIPS). *Journal of the American Academy of Child and Adolescent Psychiatry* 39:76–84.
42. Reich W, Cottler L, McCallum K, Corwin D, VanEerdewegh M: Computerized interviews as a method of assessing psychopathology in children. *Comprehensive Psychiatry* 36(1):40–45, 1995.
43. Wasserman GA, McReynolds LS, Ko SJ, Katz LM, Carpenter JR. Gender differences in psychiatric disorders at juvenile probation intake. *American Journal of Public Health*, 95:131–137, 2005.
44. Puig-Antich J, Chambers W: The schedule for affective disorders and schizophrenia for school-aged children (K-SADS). (Unpublished interview schedule): New York State Psychiatric Institute, 1978.
45. Spitzer RL, Endicott J, Robins E: Research diagnostic criteria: Rationale and reliability. *Archives of General Psychiatry* 35:773–782, 1978.
46. Ambrosini P, Metz C, Prabucki K, Lee J-C: Videotape reliability of the third revised edition of the K-SADS. *Journal of the American Academy of Child and Adolescent Psychiatry* 28:723–728, 1990.
47. Orvaschel H, Puig-Antich J., Chambers W., Tabrizi MA, Johnson R: Retrospective assessment of prepubertal major depression with the Kiddie-SADS-E. *Journal of the American Academy of Child Psychiatry* 21:392–397, 1982.
48. Kaufman J, Birmaher B, Brent D, Rao U, Flynn C, Moreci P, et al.: Schedule for affective disorders and schizophrenia for school-age children—Present and Lifetime Version (K-SADS-PL): Initial reliability and validity data.

Journal of the American Academy of Child and Adolescent Psychiatry 36(7):980–988, 1997.
49. Shanee N, Apter A, Weizman A. Psychometric properties of the K-SADS-PL in an Israeli adolescent clinical population. *Israel Journal of Psychiatry and Related Sciences* 34(3):179–186, 1997.
50. Weissman MM, Wickramaratne P, Warner V, John K, Prusoff BA, Merikangas KR, et al.: Assessing psychiatric disorders in children: Discrepancies between mothers' and children's reports. *Archives of General Psychiatry* 44:747–753, 1987.
51. Messer SC, Angold A, Costello EJ, Burns BJ: The Child and Adolescent Burden Assessment (CABA): Measuring the family impact of emotional and behavioral problems. *International Journal of Methods in Psychiatric Research* 6:261–284, 1996.
52. Ascher BH, Farmer EMZ, Burns BJ, Angold A: The Child and Adolescent Services Assessment (CASA): Description and psychometrics. *Journal of Emotional and Behavioral Disorders* 4:12–20, 1996.
53. Farmer EMZ, Angold A, Burns BJ, Costello EJ: Reliability of self-reported service use: Test-retest consistency of children's responses to the Child and Adolescent Services Assessment (CASA). *Journal of Child and Family Studies* 3(3):307–325, 1994.
54. Angold A, Prendergast M, Cox A, Harrington R, Simonoff E, Rutter M: The Child and Adolescent Psychiatric Assessment (CAPA). *Psychological Medicine* 25:739–753, 1995.
55. Costello EJ, Angold A, March J, Fairbank J: Life events and post-traumatic stress: The development of a new measure for children and adolescents. *Psychological Medicine* 28:1275–1288, 1998.
56. Simonoff E, Pickles A, Meyer JM, Silberg JL, Maes HH, Loeber R, et al.: The Virginia Twin Study of adolescent behavioral development: Influences of age, sex and impairment on rates of disorder. *Archives of General Psychiatry* 54:801–808, 1997.
57. Welner Z, Reich W, Herjanic B, Jung KG, Amado H: Reliability, validity, and parent–child agreement studies of the Diagnostic Interview for Children and Adolescents (DICA). *Journal of the American Academy of Child and Adolescent Psychiatry,* 26:649–653, 1987.
58. Reich W, Earls F. Rules of making psychiatric diagnoses in children on the basis of multiple sources of information: Preliminary strategies. *Journal of Abnormal Child Psychology* 15:601–616, 1987.
59. de la Osa N, Ezpeleta L, Domenech JM, Navarro JB, Losilla JM: Convergent and discriminant validity of the structured diagnostic interview for children and adolescents (DICA-R). *Psychology in Spain* 1(1):37–44, 1997.
60. Ezpeleta L, de la Osa N, Júdez J, Doménech JM, Navarro JB, Losilla JM: Diagnostic agreement between clinician and the Diagnostic Interview for Children and Adolescents—DICA-R in an outpatient sample. *Journal of Child Psychology and Psychiatry and Allied Disciplines* 38(4):431–440, 1997.
61. Hodges K, Cools J, McKnew D: Test-retest reliability of a clinical research interview for children: The child assessment schedule. *Journal of Consulting and Clinical Psychology* 1(4):317–322, 1989.
62. Hodges K, Kline J, Stern L, Cytryn L, McKnew D: The development of a child assessment interview for research and clinical use. *Journal of Abnormal Child Psychology* 10:173–189, 1982.
63. Hodges K, & Saunders W: Internal consistency of a diagnostic interview for children: The child assessment schedule. *Journal of Abnormal Child Psychology* 17:691–701, 1989.
64. Hodges K, McKnew D, Cytryn L, Stern L, Kline J: The Child Assessment Schedule (CAS) diagnostic interview: A report on reliability and validity. *Journal of the American Academy of Child Psychiatry* 21(5):468–473, 1982.
65. Hodges K, Saunders W, Kashani J, Hamlett K, Thompson RJ, Jr.: Internal consistency of DSM-III diagnoses using the symptom scales of the child assessment schedule. *Journal of the American Academy of Child and Adolescent Psychiatry* 29:635–641, 1990.
66. Hodges K, Wong MM: Psychometric characteristics of a multidimensional measure to assess impairment: The Child and Adolescent Functional Assessment Scale. *Journal of Child and Family Studies* 5(4):445–467, 1996.
67. Hodges K, Wong MM: Use of the child and adolescent functional assessment scale to predict service utilization and cost. *Journal of Mental Health Administration* 24(3):278–290, 1997.
68. Hodges K, Wong MM, Latessa M: Use of the child and adolescent functional assessment scale (CAFAS) as an outcome measure in clinical settings. *Journal of Behavioral Health Services and Research* 25(3):325–336, 1998.
69. Grills A, Ollendick T: Multiple informant agreement and the anxiety disorders interview schedule for parents and children. *Journal of the American Academy Child and Adolescent Psychiatry* 42(1):30–40, 2003.
70. Silverman W, Saavedra LM, & Pina AA: Test-retest reliability of anxiety symptoms and diagnoses with the anxiety disorders interview schedule for DSM-IV: Child and parent versions. *Journal of the American Academy Child and Adolescent Psychiatry* 40(8):937–944, 2001.
71. Silverman WK: Diagnostic reliability of anxiety disorders in children using structured interviews. *Journal of Anxiety Disorders* 5:105–124, 1991.
72. Silverman WK, and Eisen AR: Age differences in the reliability of parent and child reports of child anxious symptomatology using a structured interview. *Journal of the American Academy of Child and Adolescent Psychiatry* 31:117–124, 1992.
73. Silverman WK, Nelles WB: The anxiety disorders interview schedule for children. *Journal of the American Academy of Child and Adolescent Psychiatry* 27(6):772–778, 1988.
74. Wood J, Piacentini JC, Bergman RL, McCracken J, and Barrios V: Concurrent validity of the anxiety disorders section of the anxiety disorders interview schedule for DSM-IV: Child and parent versions. *Journal of Clinical Child & Adolescent Psychology* 31(3):335–342, 2002.
75. di Nardo PA, Moras K, Barlow DH, Rapee RM, and Brown TA: Reliability of DSM-III—R anxiety disorder categories: Using the anxiety disorders interview schedule—revised (ADIS–R). *Archives of General Psychiatry* 50(4):251–256, 1993.
76. Ho T-p, Leung PW-l, Lee C-c, Tang C-p, Hung S-f, Kwong S-l, et al.: Test-retest reliability of the Chinese version of the Diagnostic Interview Schedule for Children-Version 4 (DISC-IV). *Journal of Child Psychology and Psychiatry* 46(10):1135–1138, 2005.
77. Angold A, Erkanli A, Costello EJ, and Rutter M: Precision, reliability and accuracy in the dating of symptom onsets in child and adolescent psychopathology. *Journal of Child Psychology and Psychiatry* 37:657–664, 1996.
78. Breton J-J, Bergeron L, Valla J-P, Lepine S, Houde L, and Gaudet N: Do children aged 9 to 11 years understand the DISC version 2.25 questions? *Journal of the American Academy of Child and Adolescent Psychiatry* 34:946–956, 1995.
79. Angold A, Erkanli A, Loeber R, Costello EJ, Van Kammen W, and Stouthamer-Loeber M: Disappearing depression in a population sample of boys. *Journal of Emotional and Behavioral Disorders* 4:95–104, 1996.
80. Piacentini J, Roper M, Jensen P, Lucas C, Fisher P, Bird H, et al.: Informant-based determinants of symptom attenuation in structured child psychiatric interviews. *Journal of Abnormal Child Psychology* 27:417–428, 1999.
81. Jensen PS, Shaffer D, Rae D, Canino G, Bird HR, Dulcan MK, et al.: Attenuation of the Diagnostic Interview Schedule for Children (Disc 2.1): Sex, age and IQ relationships. Paper presented at the 39th Annual Meeting of the AACAP, Washington, DC, October 1992.
82. Anastasi A: The concept of validity in the interpretation of test scores. *Journal of Psychology and Educational Measures* 10:67–78, 1950.
83. Anastasi A: Evolving concepts of test validation. *Annual Review of Psychology* 37:1–15, 1986.
84. Cronbach LJ, and Meehl PE: Construct validity in psychological tests. *Psychological Bulletin* 52(4):281–302, 1955.
85. Gulliksen H: Intrinsic validity. *American Psychologist* 5:511–517, 1950.
86. Jenkins JG: Validity for what? *Journal of Consulting and Clinical Psychology* 10 93–98, 1946.
87. Novick MR: *Standards for educational and psychological testing.* Washington: American Psychological Association, 1985.
88. Peak H: Problems of objective observation. In: L. Festinger and Katz D. (eds): *Research methods in the behavioral sciences.* New York: Dryden Press, pp. 243–300.
89. Wallace SR: Criteria for what? *American Psychologist* 20:411–417, 1965.
90. Weitz J: Criteria for criteria. *American Psychologist* 16:228–231, 1961.
91. Costello EJ, Mustillo S, Erkanli A, Keeler G, and Angold A: Prevalence and development of psychiatric disorders in childhood and adolescence. *Archives of General Psychiatry* 60:837–844, 2003.
92. Lewinsohn PM, Hops H, Roberts RE, Seeley JR, and Andrews JA: Adolescent psychopathology: I. Prevalence and incidence of depression and other DSM-III-R disorders in high school students. *Journal of Abnormal Psychology* 102:133–144, 1993.
93. Breslau N: Inquiring about the bizarre: False positives in Diagnostic Interview Schedule for Children (DISC) ascertainment of obsessions, compulsions, and psychotic symptoms. *Journal of the American Academy of Child and Adolescent Psychiatry* 26:639–644, 1987.
94. Cox A, Holbrook D, and Rutter M: Psychiatric interviewing techniques: VI. Experimental Study: Eliciting Feelings. *British Journal of Psychiatry* 139:144–152, 1981.
95. Cox A, Hopkinson K, Rutter M: Psychiatric interviewing techniques: II. Naturalistic study—Eliciting factual information. *British Journal of Psychiatry* 138:283–291, 1981.
96. Cox A, Rutter M, Holbrook D: Psychiatric interviewing techniques: V. Experimental Study—Eliciting factual information. *British Journal of Psychiatry* 139:27–37, 1981.
97. Rutter M, Cox A: Psychiatric interviewing techniques: I. Methods and measures. *British Journal of Psychiatry* 138:273–282, 1981.
98. Rutter M, Cox A, Egert S, Holbrook D, Everitt B: Psychiatric interviewing techniques: IV. Experimental study—Four contrasting styles. *British Journal of Psychiatry* 138:456–465, 1981.
99. Cannell CF, Marquis KH, Laurent A: A summary of studies of interviewing methodology: 1959–1970. *Vital and Health Statistics, Series* 2 26:1–78, 1977.
100. Emde R, Wolfe DP, Oppenheim D: *Revealing the inner worlds of young children: The MacArthur Story Stem Battery and parent–child narratives.* New York: Oxford University Press, 2003.
101. Warren SL, Emde RN, Sroufe A: Internal representations: Predicting anxiety from children's play narratives. *Journal of the American Academy of Child and Adolescent Psychiatry* 39:100–107, 2000.

102. Warren SL, Oppenheim D, Emde RN: Can emotions and themes in children's play predict behavior problems? *Journal of the American Academy of Child and Adolescent Psychiatry* 35:1331–1337, 1996.
103. Measelle JR, Ablow JC, Cowan PA, Cowan CP: Assessing young children's views of their academic, social, and emotional lives: An evaluation of the self-perception scales of the Berkeley Puppet Interview. *Child Development* 69:1556–1576, 1998.
104. Ialongo N, Edelsohn G, Werthamer-Larsson L, Crockett L, Kellam S: Are self-reported depressive symptoms in first-grade children developmentally transient phenomena? A further look. *Development and Psychopathology* 5:433–457, 1993.
105. Martini DR, Strayhorn JM, Puig-Antich J: A symptom self-report measure for preschool children. *Journal of the American Academy of Child and Adolescent Psychiatry* 29:594–600, 1990.
106. Wakschlag LS, Leventhal B, Briggs-Gowan, Danis B, Keenan K, Hill C, et al.: Defining the "disruptive" in preschool behavior: What diagnostic observation can teach us. *Clinical Child and Family Psychology Review* 8(3):183–201, 2005.
107. Lucas CP, Zhang H, Fisher PW, Shaffer D, Regier DA Narrow, WE, et al.: The DISC Predictive Scales (DPS): Efficiently screening for diagnoses. *Journal of the American Academy of Child & Adolescent Psychiatry* 40:443–449, 2001.

CHAPTER 4.2.4 ■ PSYCHOLOGICAL AND NEUROPSYCHOLOGICAL ASSESSMENT OF CHILDREN

KATHLEEN D. TSATSANIS

NATURE AND USE OF PSYCHOLOGICAL AND NEUROPSYCHOLOGICAL ASSESSMENT

The broad aims of a psychological and/or neuropsychological assessment are two-fold: i) to provide a more complete description and understanding of the child, and ii) to inform strategies for intervention. This is accomplished in part through the use of psychological tests that offer an objective and standardized measure of a sample of behavior, one that allows performance to be evaluated on the basis of empirical data (1). However, it must be emphasized that psychological or neuropsychological tests and resulting test scores are but one part of the assessment process. Test selection and administration are important factors, as is above all test interpretation. The final analysis is formed from multiple lines of converging evidence and takes into consideration the developmental and environmental context.

Psychological Assessment

Psychological tests were developed as a means to measure individual differences. Although diverse with regard to content, such measures shared a common use, which was to categorize and classify individuals based on observations of their behavior under uniform conditions (1). At the outset such measures were applied toward educational, personnel, and military classification. Differential diagnosis was also identified as a concern in the context of changes taking place in the nineteenth century in institutional care, and as test development was intended to aid in the educational placement of children, specifically in the study and instruction of children with mental retardation. Experimental psychology was concerned with universal descriptions of human behavior, in the physiology of sensory responses at this time; however, the general emphasis on the need for controlled conditions when making observations has remained at the heart of the standardization of procedures (uniform conditions) in psychological testing (1).

Early interest in educational testing led to the development of more sophisticated principles and measurement techniques that are now used to assess a wide variety of domains of functioning, including social, emotional, neuropsychological, and adaptive behavior. However, it is intellectual assessment that holds a place of notoriety in the history of psychology. Two of the more fundamental issues that have beset intelligence testing are the definition of intelligence, and the use and interpretation of measures of intelligence. As illustrated in Table 4.2.4.1, theories of intelligence abound. More than this, each theorist posits multiple components or abilities as part of his account of intelligence. As such, it is worth keeping in mind that intelligence is a construct that is neither unitary nor fixed. Additionally, there is a distinction to be made between theories of intelligence and psychometric intelligence. Whereas the former provides conceptualizations of the nature of intelligence, the latter represents the measurement of general mental ability using standardized tests. The global scores yielded from these measures are usually stable and have general predictive value for educational, social, and job outcome. The instruments are limited to what they are measuring and their interpretation is contingent on valid use, and are of course subject to misuse.

The use and interpretation of IQ scores is an important matter and a lengthy subject. In brief, from a psychometric perspective, early approaches to psychometric intelligence focused on quantifying a general level of intelligence as represented by a single number (the IQ score) and assignment to a descriptive classification (e.g., "dull" or "very bright"). Subsequent methods have involved profile analysis or a consideration of individual areas of strength and weakness. This approach may be most powerful when integrated with theories of cognitive abilities (13). Indeed, the cross battery assessment approach (14) that has emerged of late in the arena of psychological assessment emphasizes the usefulness of identifying

TABLE 4.2.4.1

FACTOR ANALYTIC THEORIES OF INTELLIGENCE

Thurstone's Primary Mental Abilities

Thurstone (2) identified 13 factors of which a subset was considered to represent primary mental abilities. These included: spatial visualization, perceptual speed, numerical facility, verbal meaning, word fluency, memory, and inductive reasoning.

Cattell–Horn Theory of Cognitive Abilities

Cattell (3–4) proposed two distinct general factors: fluid and crystallized intelligence. Fluid intelligence refers to reasoning ability that is not dependent on prior experience, whereas crystallized intelligence represents learned or stored information. Hence, a distinction is made between those abilities needed in novel problem solving conditions versus rote or familiar learning strategies. Horn (5, 6) modified this theory to include nine abilities: crystallized ability, fluid ability, visual and auditory processing, short-term and long-term memory, processing speed, decision speed, and quantitative knowledge.

Guilford's Structure of Intellect Model

The three dimensions of this model are operations, contents, and products. Content refers to the kind of information that is being processed (figural, symbolic, semantic, and behavioral). Guilford (7) also identifies five types of mental operations or procedures (evaluation, convergent production, divergent production, memory, and cognition), and six products (units, classes, relations, systems, transformations, implications).

Sternberg's Triarchic Theory of Intelligence

Sternberg (8) proposes a systems approach or integrative theory in which different aspects of intelligence are interrelated. The three main parts of the triarchic theory are: componential, experiential, and contextual. In more recent accounts, Sternberg (9) expands his theory and examines the relationship between intelligence and the internal world, experience, and external world of the individual.

Gardner's Multiple Intelligence Theory

Gardner (10) proposes multiple types of intelligence or competencies, including: linguistic, musical, logical-mathematical, spatial, bodily kinesthetic, intrapersonal, interpersonal, and naturalist. Although not easily supported, each of the intelligences is viewed as unrelated or separate in their determination.

Carroll's Three-Stratum Factor Analytic Theory of Cognitive Abilities

Carroll's (11) account of intelligence is based on an impressive metaanalysis of test-based research datasets. From this factor analysis of the data, three levels were identified: narrow (65 ability areas), broad (8 factors), and general (a single general factor, g). The second broad stratum includes: fluid intelligence, crystallized intelligence, general memory and learning, broad visual perception, broad auditory perception, broad retrieval ability, broad cognitive speediness, and processing speed (reaction time/decision speed).

Das, Naglieri, & Kirby's Planning-Attention-Simultaneous-Successive Processing Model of Intelligence (PASS)

The PASS theory (12) is based on the seminal work of A.R. Luria in neuropsychology, but is also consistent with information processing models of more recent development. Three fundamental and related functional units of the brain are considered to represent four basic psychological processes of attention and arousal, simultaneous processing (organization of information into a coherent whole), successive processing (sequential processing or processing of information in a specific order), and planning (developing the plans or strategies to arrive at a solution or complete tasks).

cognitive *processes* versus, for example, reporting cognitive functioning in the context of a single IQ number. This represents a shift in thinking of cognitive activity in terms of a single function—intelligence—to a multifaceted entity.

Psychological Assessment Goals

A fundamental first step toward treatment planning is gaining a full understanding of the individual child. As noted, the psychological/neuropsychological examination is considered to be an integral part of this process. The psychologist/neuropsychologist is also in a unique position to consider the influence of the child's cognitive functioning on academic and social emotional functioning. One purpose for seeking an assessment is that of diagnosis and/or differential diagnosis. The referral question may focus on a diagnostic ambiguity or the question may be one of level of functioning or development of a specific skill. A second major purpose for an evaluation is to gain information about a child's cognitive and academic profile and/or an augmented understanding of his/her behavioral and emotional functioning. Diagnosis is often emphasized, but what may be needed to design educational as well as treatment objectives is a more detailed assessment of the child's strengths and weaknesses in several areas. For example, language deficits may interfere with the child's ability to form a personal narrative; memory deficits may account for challenges in learning or treatment gains; a child's learning strengths/difficulties may inform the best modality for presenting information. Third, clinically and in research, assessment measures may be used for pre- and post-comparisons (in the case of brain trauma, in the evaluation of medication or a treatment program). Measurement through well constructed tests further serves an important function in research toward the identification of environmental and biological factors associated with behavioral differences (e.g., gene–brain–behavior relationships).

Neuropsychological Assessment

The traditional neuropsychological assessment is distinguished by its emphasis on producing a description and understanding of the relationship between brain and behavior. A fundamental approach to neuropsychological assessment is measurement of multiple ability domains sufficient to i) represent the principal areas of functioning thought to be mediated by the brain and ii) gather the information needed to address the clinical problems presented by the child (15). The assessment is typically quite comprehensive, as it is designed to sample a broad range of skills and abilities in the child. Given the emphasis on brain and behavior, it has been the longstanding practice of neuropsychologists to consider cognitive functioning as multidimensional. In describing the brain–behavior relationship, there is the implicit recognition that cognition as an operation of the brain is complex and any inferences that are made about behavior conceptualized in terms of cognition should reflect this complexity (16).

The basic neuropsychological framework for understanding dimensions of behavior reflects the functional systems of the brain. These divisions may be represented broadly as cognitive, emotional, and control processes, and as connected systems in the brain they can be thought to have reciprocal influence. The domains for assessment include: i) alertness/arousal; ii) sensory perception; iii) attention; iv) memory or the encoding, storage, and retrieval of information; v) information processing, such as analysis and synthesis of information, problem solving, concept formation, etc.; vi) motor activity; and vii) intentional or goal-directed activity, i.e., the organizational programs of behavior, sometimes referred to as executive functions. Alterations in motivation and emotional capacity are also evidenced in brain injury or disease and should be considered for their impact on these other systems.

A neuropsychological assessment specifically may be sought to: i) ascertain the likelihood that the child's problems in adaptation are the result of compromised brain functioning (versus, for example, the result of a psychiatric disturbance); ii) enhance understanding of the child's psychosocial behavior by examining cognitive and control processes, such as how information is received, processed, and expressed by the child; and ultimately iii) identify the pattern or constellation of neuropsychological assets and deficits displayed by the child toward developing strategies for behavioral or educational intervention.

THE ASSESSMENT PROCESS

The psychological/neuropsychological assessment involves: i) clarifying the referral question, ii) selection and administration of psychological tests, iii) observation, iv) interpretation, and v) diagnostic formulation and recommendations.

Referral Question and Background History

The referral question(s) are initially identified by the parents and/or referring professional involved in the child's care. They are further refined by obtaining information from multiple sources, including interviews with key people in the child's life (parents, teachers, and other professionals), a review of past records (school reports, previous testing, and medical information), thorough history-taking, and talking with the child.

Selection and Administration of Psychological Tests

The types of assessment methods used and the breadth of the battery formed are key to test selection. Typically, a comprehensive evaluation will make use of a variety of assessment methods and assess a range of domains of functioning. One reason for sampling a range of functions lies in the fact that most psychological measures are not "pure"—that is, they do not assess one ability domain alone. It is important to discern whether, for example, on a timed task in which the child is asked to copy figures, poor performance is related to a motor, visual perceptual, attentional, and/or speed of processing issue. Difficulty on a measure of math skills may reflect limits in understanding numerical concepts, remembering math facts, understanding the *language* of mathematics (symbol use), knowing which operations to apply when sequencing (e.g., performing the correct steps in the correct order), copying errors, and/or attending to meaningful visual details (operational sign, place, columns of numbers). Test selection is guided by evaluation of the test itself and related constructs such as norm groups, reliability, and validity (see Table 4.2.4.2 and discussion below).

TABLE 4.2.4.2

CRITICAL VARIABLES IN TEST SELECTION

Evidence of reliability
Evidence of validity
Representativeness of standardization group
Up-to-date norms
Ample sample (size) of normative group
Difficulty gradients (3 raw score points or more per standard deviation [SD])
Floors and ceilings (the test is sensitive enough to discriminate the lowest and highest scorers)
Clear presentation of instructions, administration, and scoring
Cost and administration time

Test administration variables include the environmental setting (e.g., quiet, well lit room, free of interruptions), establishing rapport with the child, and engaging the child in a manner so as to obtain the best possible performance. The rationale for creating optimal performance conditions is related to the purpose of the evaluation; that is, to determine if the child has the component cognitive skills or abilities necessary to function adequately (or more than adequately) at home, at school, or with others. Standardization, which refers to the uniformity of procedure in administering and scoring a test, is also a key concept in test administration. The examiner must know and adhere to the test procedures, including presentation of directions, use of materials, response to queries, etc. In all, the assessment must be conducted effectively to obtain information regarding the level of performance that the child is capable of but also in a standardized manner to ensure comparability of the scores obtained.

Observation of Test Behavior

In addition to obtaining test data, the examiner makes qualitative observations of the child's presentation and performance during the test sessions. Clinical observation is an essential aspect of test interpretation. Test scores represent how a child performs on a particular test at a particular time. Qualitative observations must be integrated with the quantitative information or test scores to provide a more complete understanding of the results and conditions under which they were obtained. This includes variables such as attention, motivation, persistence, fatigue, illness, and rapport, as well as observations regarding how the child approached the tasks (e.g. use of verbal mediation, trial and error, slow but accurate style).

Interpretation of Results

Test interpretation typically involves an analysis of levels and patterns of test performance. The clinician engages in a dynamic process of hypothesis testing and information gathering, reasoning deductively and inductively from the data collected. Interpretation of test results also requires taking into consideration the behavior observed during testing and other relevant behavioral data (e.g., suspicions of a primary visual or hearing impairment) and case history information (cultural, economic, family variables).

Summary and Recommendations

Assessment conclusions and recommendations should be based on all sources of information. The comprehensive assessment is designed to identify the child's assets and deficits in a variety of domains of functioning. This approach promotes an understanding of the challenges the child faces and why, but also the strengths he/she possesses and how these can be used to help remediate areas of weakness. Inferences are made from these data to determine the services and strategies that will facilitate the child's social, emotional, and academic functioning.

PRINCIPLES OF ASSESSMENT

The psychometric principles of assessment influence test selection, administration, and interpretation. These measurement issues are outlined below to familiarize the reader with the basic constructs and related issues.

Standardization Sampling/Developmental Norms

The raw scores obtained from tests are for practical purposes meaningless without a basis of comparison. As such, the data obtained from psychological tests are interpreted with reference to a norm group. This aspect of test development and use is fundamental as it permits that evaluation of a child's behavior need not rely on subjective interpretation alone. Rather, such norm-referenced tests offer: 1) quantification of the child's level of performance with reference to his/her peer group 2) an ipsative ("of the self") comparison or analysis of the child's performance across different measures to determine areas of personal asset and deficit, and 3) longitudinal comparison or assessment of gains/loss over time.

Norms are developed empirically on the basis of the performance of the normative sample, also sometimes referred to as the standardization sample. Standardization sampling represents the procedure used; the normative data are obtained under standard conditions with regard to consistency of item content, administration procedures, and scoring criteria. The norm group should be evaluated for representativeness, size, and relevance (17). The norm group should be a representative group of the child's peers and large enough to ensure stability of the test scores. Sattler (17) recommends at least 100 subjects for each age group in the normative sample. In most cases, test developers will draw from U.S. Census Bureau data to determine the composition of this sample based on stratification variables such as age, gender, socioeconomic level, race, geographic region, etc. Many instruments will also offer normative data obtained from special populations to permit comparisons of the child to other children with the same disorder (a peer group as well).

Reliability

The reliability of a test refers to the consistency of measurement; as such, it also speaks to the degree to which test scores are free from random fluctuations of measurement (18). The example of a scale used to measure weight vividly illustrates the importance of the stability of test scores as concerns accuracy or dependability of measurement. Let us say that on one day when you step on the scale it shows a weight of 150 pounds, 100 pounds on the next day, and then 175 pounds the following day. The scale could not be considered a meaningful or accurate measure of your weight. The same could be said for a psychological test that is not reliable. Test results are not interpretable if the test is not reliable, making reliability a fundamental factor in test selection and interpretation.

There are different types of reliability, each of which reflects a different aspect of how a test score is reproducible (Table 4.2.4.3). The reliability coefficient, symbolized by the letter r with two identical subscripts, is used to express the degree of consistency of test scores. It is a particular kind of correlation coefficient with a range of .00 (indicating no association or consistency between scores) to 1.00 (perfect reliability). No assessment measure is 100% reliable, and as such, some error of measurement is to be expected. The reliability coefficient can be used to determine the degree of error variance or random or unsystematic variation in the measurement instrument (1). The error variance of a test is calculated by subtracting the reliability coefficient from 1.00, where 1.00 indicates perfect reliability. Thus, a reliability coefficient of .80 indicates 80% reliability and 20% error variance. Typically, a minimum acceptable level of reliability is .80 (17).

The reliability coefficient is an important number as a measure of consistency, but also as a source of the amount of reliable variance associated with the test. As such, it is used in the calculation of the standard error of measurement (SEM) of a test score and in turn the confidence interval. Scores for a psychological test (e.g., an IQ score) are often reported as falling within a specific range of scores, or within a confidence interval. The psychometric properties of a test are such that although they may aim to quantify level of functioning in a real way, the obtained test score is actually composed of a true score (hypothetical) and an error score (1). The confidence interval represents the range of scores surrounding the obtained score within which the true score is likely to lie. For example, if a child obtains an IQ score of 90, we can state at the 95% confidence level (the usual reported level) that her IQ score on any single administration of the test will lie between 84 and 96. That is, 95 times out of 100, her IQ score will fall within this band of values. The confidence interval is determined by the SEM for the instrument, which in turn is computed from the reliability coefficient.

The major point to underscore here is that the obtained test score is not precise or definitive, as each test inherently contains measurement error that should be taken into consideration when decisions are being made based on a single score (e.g., IQ score for qualification of services). The second and related point is that measurement error must be accounted for when reported scores are compared over time or across instruments. The difference between two test scores may be due to chance factors or the error variance associated with each test. Correspondingly, the reliability coefficient for each test is taken into consideration in the calculation of discrepancy scores.

Validity

Test validity is a term used to represent the meaning or relevance of a test, specifically, whether it measures what it is purported to measure (1). It is a fundamental psychometric concept that can be approached in several ways, as detailed in Table 4.2.4.4. The validity of a test is relevant when assessing what is being measured and how completely, as well as how to use a test appropriately. Validity coefficients are a type of correlation coefficient and accordingly are impacted by the range of attributes being measured (the narrower the range, the lower the value of the validity coefficient). Examinee variables also can impact validity; if an examinee presents with severe test-taking anxiety, extreme fatigue or illness, a hearing or vision impairment (and for example forgets to wear her glasses), or fails to understand the instructions, these factors are likely to render the test scores invalid, as the test is no longer measuring the characteristic it is intended to measure. As such,

TABLE 4.2.4.3

OVERVIEW OF TYPES OF RELIABILITY

Types of Reliability	Description
Test-retest reliability	A measure of temporal stability. The reliability coefficient is expressed as r_{tt} and is the correlation between scores obtained by the same persons taking the same test on two different occasions.
Alternate-form reliability	Consistency of test scores when alternate forms of a test are given to the same person. The tests may be given at different times or on the same occasion. As such, this method may be used to minimize practice effects and also to examine whether two different forms (items and item composition) of the test give the same result.
Split-half reliability	A measure of internal consistency or consistency of the content of the test. This type of reliability is measured from a single administration of a single test form, splitting the test in half (e.g., odd and even items of the test) and comparing the two half-scores, usually by means of the Spearman-Brown formula.
Interitem reliability	Another measure of internal consistency using a single test form and a single administration. In this case, however, reliability is measured based on performance on *each* item relative to the other items of the test and thus gives some indication of the homogeneity of the measure. The usual formula used is Kuder Richardson (when items are scored 0 or 1) or Cronbach's alpha coefficient (for items not scored as right or wrong).
Interrater reliability	Apart from temporal, content, and examinee variables, variance in test scores can arise from examiner factors, such as differences in scoring. Interrater reliability provides a measure of consistency of scores obtained when the same test is scored by two different examiners. This is an especially critical variable when evaluating test forms that leave judgment open to the scorer.

psychological reports include a section on observations of test behavior and a description of any presenting factors that are a threat to validity. Extrinsic or environmental factors such as socioeconomic status, access to quality teaching or textbooks, or cultural experiences can similarly impact validity and are addressed in the interpretation of test scores.

INTERPRETATION OF TEST SCORES

Derived Scores

A basic feature of interpretation of test scores is the comparison of scores to some standard or norm. As mentioned above, raw test scores, whether the number of points earned, items successfully completed, or symptoms endorsed, are meaningless on their own. Rather, the raw test score is evaluated relative to the test performance of the standardization sample. The question that is answered in this process is where this particular child's score falls relative to the distribution of scores produced by the standardization sample, where the mean represents the average and the standard deviation (SD) represents the variability. There are a variety of derived scores or ways in which this comparison can be reported.

Standard Scores. Standard scores are the most typical and often the most suitable kind of score to report. Standard scores are particularly useful for making comparisons across tests, as the mean and SD are set and there are equal units along the scale (18). For all standard scores, a score falling 1 SD below the mean (below the average range) or a score falling 2 SD above the mean (well above average) occupies the same position relative to the group apart from the instrument used. Comparability of scores in this manner is achieved through a transformation of the raw data. The usual types of reported scores are: standard scores, scaled scores, and T-scores (Table 4.2.4.5). The typical standard score has a mean set at 100 and a standard deviation of 15. Most major cognitive and achievement assessment batteries report global scores in this format. Individual subtest scores however may be represented as scaled scores with a mean of 10 and a standard deviation

TABLE 4.2.4.4

OVERVIEW OF TYPES OF VALIDITY

Types of Validity	Description
Construct validity	Examines the extent to which a test measures what it purports to measure, such as a psychological construct or trait. Two constituents of construct validity are *convergent* (measures of related constructs should correlate) and *divergent* (measures of unrelated constructs should not correlate) validity.
Content validity	Refers to the degree to which a test covers the behavior or skill or subject matter being measured. A discussion of the content validity of a test should help to answer whether the test offers representative coverage of the domain assessed, and whether there is influence from other variables.
Face validity	As the name suggests, face validity refers to whether on the surface of things the test appears to be appropriate for its intended use.
Concurrent validity	A form of criterion-related validation in which the current measure is compared to a criterion or outcome to which it is related (e.g., ratings or other test scores).
Predictive validity	Another form of criterion-related validation that examines the degree to which the measure predicts some other criterion in the future (e.g., IQ and later academic success).
Treatment validity	Refers to the clinical utility of an instrument as it relates to the impact of the test results on the examinee's behavior.

TABLE 4.2.4.5

Z-SCORES AND DERIVED SCORE EQUIVALENTS

z-score	Standard Score	T-score	Scaled Score	Percentile Rank
−3	55	20	1	<1
−2	70	30	4	2
−1	85	40	7	16
0	100	50	10	50
+1	115	60	13	84
+2	130	70	16	98
+3	145	80	19	>99

of 3. Some tests and many behavior checklists yield T-scores, which have a mean of 50 and a standard deviation of 10.

Percentile Scores. Percentile scores are a popular means for reporting test performance as they are easy to understand; a percentile rank is a way of positioning the child's performance relative to the norm group in familiar terms (17). For example, a percentile rank of 84 indicates that the child scored as well as or better than 84% of the norm group. There are some caveats. Naïve consumers of these test scores may confuse percentile ranks with percent of items passed (such as an 84% on a test). A major concern also with regard to percentile ranks (versus standard scores) is that the units are unequal. The numbers can be deceptive and may overemphasize or underemphasize differences between standard scores. For example, note that scores between the 25th and 75th percentile are all within the average range.

Age and Grade Equivalent Scores. Test scores in some cases are also reported in terms of age and grade equivalents. An age equivalent score is determined based on the performance of each age group in the norm sample. If the average raw score of the 8-year-olds in the sample is 14, then a raw score of 14 yields an age equivalent of 8 years. Age equivalent scores thus describe the raw score obtained and do not necessarily correspond to the child's level of functioning, nor do they represent equal units.

Grade equivalents are similar in that grade norms are computed from the mean raw score obtained by children in each grade in the standardization sample. Again, if the average raw score on a reading test for single words corresponds to 25 for 4th graders, then a raw score of 25 corresponds to a grade equivalent of 4. Grade units are unequal and do not represent the variability between subject areas at different levels. It is also important to recognize that when a fourth grade child obtains a grade equivalent score of 6.5 on an arithmetic test, it does not necessarily indicate that the child is capable of grade 6 arithmetical processes or should be placed in the seventh grade curriculum (1). Rather, the child's total raw score may reflect superior performance on fourth grade arithmetic. The point is that psychological tests are typically constructed to provide a range of scores. If we consider the standardization sample of children in the fourth grade, there will be a distribution of scores for this group of children; an average raw score for this group will represent the average score on the test at the fourth grade level. The children who perform well above average within this distribution will produce a well above average score on the test for their comparison group and may in turn share a total raw score with the average sixth grader. Additionally, the same raw score yielding the same age or grade equivalent could be obtained in a very different way relative to the individual items of the test and thus have a different meaning.

Although appealing, age and grade equivalent scores are easily subject to misinterpretation; they do not necessarily reflect a particular level of knowledge but are rather another means of indicating where a child falls relative to a particular kind of reference group (18). On the other hand, the advantage of reporting scores in this format is that they are easily understandable and place performance within a familiar developmental context. In this case, correct interpretation is paramount.

Descriptive Levels

In addition to a quantitative representation of performance, classification of ability levels is applied to standard scores, based on whether the score corresponds to the average performance of the normative group or, for example, the upper or lower extreme end of the distribution. These descriptions of performance are widely used to represent how far a child's score deviates above or below the mean (Table 4.2.4.6). In the event that a child's file contains several different reports, one should keep in mind that derived scores can be converted to a uniform metric for comparison. Knowing the child's test score, the mean and SD of the test, and assuming that the scores on the test fit to a normal distribution (which would be true of most major assessment instruments), then it is easy to determine where the child's scores fall relative to the mean. This would be achieved by taking the child's test score, subtracting the mean, and dividing by the SD. Thus, if a child obtained an IQ score of 115 on a test that has a mean of 100 and SD of 15, his or her score would be 1 SD above the mean. Similarly, if the same child obtained a T-score of 60 on a different measure (with a mean of 50 and SD of 10), his or her score would also be 1 SD above the mean. If percentile scores are reported on a given test, these too can represent the child's position relative to the standardization sample (see Table 4.2.4.5). A special note about IQ scores: The traditional means of obtaining an IQ score (or intelligence *quotient*) was to take the ratio of mental age (MA) divided by chronological age (CA) and multiply by 100. The problem with this procedure is that ratio IQ scores at different ages are not comparable and thus not psychometrically sound in practice. Although the term IQ has been retained, current measures of IQ do not derive scores based on the above formula; rather, these so-called deviation IQs are a type of standard score and as described above fit to a distribution with a mean of 100 and SD of 15. However, knowledge of the ratio IQ is handy

TABLE 4.2.4.6

CLASSIFICATION LEVELS

Standard Score	Percentile Rank	Classification/Descriptive Level
69 and below	<2	Intellectual deficiency (MR)/Lower extreme
70 to 79	2 to 8	Borderline/Well below average
80 to 89	9 to 23	Low average/Below average
90 to 109	25 to 73	Average
110 to 119	75 to 90	High average/Above average
120 to 129	91 to 97	Superior/Well above average
130 and above	98 to 99.99	Very superior/Upper extreme

when there is limited information and a need to make a *rough* approximation of the child's ability level.

Significant Difference

Derived scores and classification of ability levels provide a means to compare a child's performance relative to his or her peers as defined by the norm group. However, test interpretation also involves a comparison of the child's different ability levels across domains of functioning and in some cases across time. For example, we may want to know whether Sam is more able on verbal versus visual spatial tasks, whether Alice's reading skills are consistent with expectations given her overall IQ, or whether ratings of Justin's behavior at home and school are significantly different. There are two considerations to keep in mind when comparing whether two scores are different or not: a) statistical significance and b) unusualness or abnormality of difference. The first, statistical significance, answers whether the results differ from what would be expected based on chance alone (17). The usual p-value for this calculation is .05, meaning that, if the difference between two scores is significant (not due to chance factors), we accept a 5 out of 100 chance of being wrong. Test publishers will report domain and subtest score differences in their manuals or computerized printouts. When making comparisons between two different tests, either of the following two calculations can be made, which take into account the error variance of each test:

$$SE_{diff} = \sqrt{(SEM_1)^2 + (SEM_2)^2}$$

$$SE_{diff} = SD\sqrt{2\text{-}r_{11}\text{-}r_{22}}$$

The standard error of the difference (SE_{diff}) is then multiplied by 1.96 to determine how large a score difference could be obtained by chance at the .05 level (1).

In addition to answering whether two scores are significantly different in statistical terms, the second part of interpretation lies in determining whether the difference is clinically significant. One way to address this particular question is to examine base rate frequency, that is, to ask how unusual is it to find this difference in scores. Test publishers of cognitive and achievement test batteries will typically provide this information in supplementary tables. A difference of scores that is found in only 5% of the norm sample can be considered unusual and highly unusual when present in only 1% of the sample.

Sometimes standard scores in a domain of functioning may decline over time. This finding does not necessarily represent a deterioration or regression, but rather, may reflect a failure to make age-appropriate gains (rate of gain slower than rate of change in chronological age). If standard scores on the *same* test are found to be significantly different across time, it would be important to look at the raw scores and pattern of scores obtained on each test before assuming there has been a loss of skill. Additionally, of course, it will be important to consider other variables that might have affected test performance (such as fatigue, illness, compliance). Table 4.2.4.7 lists several other factors to consider when test scores for the same child on (ostensibly) the same kind of test differ (the child scores in the mentally retarded range on one cognitive test but not another). These factors are important to consider, particularly in the interpretation of IQ scores, as they impact diagnosis and the procurement of services.

Levels of Analysis

Interpretation involves the analysis and synthesis of all of the data obtained as part of the assessment. To assure ecologically valid conclusions regarding adaptive behavior, it is necessary to sample a wide variety of abilities and skills that interact for successful accomplishment (15). Test performance is examined for statistically significant discrepancies between observed and expected levels. Expected levels of performance may be based on earlier known levels of functioning, age norms, and/or other abilities. It is also generally expected that test scores will converge around the same level, and when functions are not proportionate, one should consider factors such as uneven brain development or brain disturbance, socialization, educational experience, emotional disturbance, physical illness/fatigue, economics, or primary sensory impairments to account for discontinuities in the child's profile (16). Base rates and contextual factors must be taken into account for those discrepancies that are commonly found in the normal population or those measures that are differentially sensitive to cultural, economic, and educational background (e.g., vocabulary level). The test results are further examined for particular patterns of performance. Comparisons may be made along the following lines as examples: domain of functioning (language, visual spatial, memory, problem solving skills), modality (visual, auditory, tactile), level of task difficulty (simple or complex), speed of processing (speeded versus no time limit), closed or open response structure (forced choice versus generative, recognition versus recall), laterality (right versus left performances), and so on. Strengths and weaknesses in the child's information processing are thus examined according to how the information is represented and processed, as well as the nature of the response that is required.

DOMAINS OF ASSESSMENT

The domains of functioning assessed and the methods used in psychological/neuropsychological testing are far-reaching in their scope, with an overview presented in this section. Individual tests are selected relative to the clinical or research need and developmental capacities of the child or adolescent. Several commonly used assessment instruments organized according to the functional domain assessed are presented in Tables 4.2.4.8 and 4.2.4.9. Additionally, for more detailed information, key resources on psychological assessment as well as test selection and acquisition are identified in Table 4.2.4.10.

Psychological Assessment

General Ability and Intelligence

Broad measures of cognitive ability and intelligence provide an estimate of a child's general ability level at a particular point in time in relation to the given age norms (1). Although most cognitive or intelligence tests yield a single IQ or ability score, this should not be interpreted to suggest that intelligence is a single unitary construct. Rather, such measures are typically composed of a variety of subtests measuring a range of functions. Careful interpretation involves an analysis of domain and subtest scores for areas of relative strength and weakness. It is also worth noting that such tests are developed based on different theories of intelligence. Thus, in spite of assessing a shared construct, intelligence tests may differ greatly in terms of content, including emphasis on verbal versus visual information, extent to which speed of processing is emphasized, the type of response format, and so on. In general, tests of cognitive ability and intelligence assess the extent to which a child has acquired information and is able to think abstractly. IQ scores are generally stable in children 5 years of age and older and are predictive of academic abilities in school-aged children. IQ and cognitive assessments may provide useful information with regard to how the child takes in, processes, and responds to information, useful toward treatment planning and provision of differentiated instruction.

TABLE 4.2.4.7

SOME REASONS WHY TEST SCORES MAY DIFFER

Norms	A difference in the age of the norms could impact test scores. The Flynn effect refers to a finding by J.R. Flynn (19) that there is a continued rise in IQ test performance. The average rate of rise seems to be around three IQ points per decade. The composition of the normative sample used to develop the test scores is different and may represent a less or more able group.
Test Units	The scores are reported in different units of measurement. For example, a score of 115 on one test and a score of 60 on another may in fact represent the same level of performance if in the case of the former the mean is 100 with a SD of 15 and in the case of the latter the mean is 50 with a SD of 10. Alternatively, two tests could both have a mean of 100 but different SDs.
Floor and Ceiling Effects	Floor effects occur when the test lacks enough easy items to discriminate between low scorers, and ceiling effects refer to when the measure lacks enough hard items to adequately assess upper levels of ability. A raw score of 0 on one test may produce an IQ score of 40 but an IQ of 70 on another test as a result of differences in the lower limits of the test items. If the referral includes a question of MR, test selection is paramount to ensure adequate range at the lower levels to make this discrimination.
Correlations between Tests	Two tests may yield score differences because the tests are not correlated or only moderately related.
Reliability	Test scores for children 5 years of age and under are typically less reliable than those obtained in school-age children. Test length can also affect reliability. To determine how large a difference is needed for statistical significance (to be confident that the discrepancy between scores is not due to chance factors alone), a calculation is made that takes into account the reliability of each test.
Item Content Differences	Tests intended to measure the same domain may diverge in content and response despite sharing a similar name. For example, IQ measures may differ in terms of the level of language, memory, and/or speed of processing demands that factor into the overall score. A reading comprehension test may involve reading a sentence or a passage, aloud or silently. Additionally, the response required may be dissimilar between tests, ranging from filling in a missing word, enacting what is read, or responding to oral questions about what was read.
Practice Effects	Scores may improve because of familiarity with the test or test items or prior exposure. Practice effects appear to be most pronounced on nonverbal versus verbal tasks, perhaps because of their novelty. Most tests should not be readministered until after a period of time has passed (typically, 1 year) in order to minimize such effects.
Other Factors	Differences related to variables such as fatigue, illness, medication, motivation. Actual gain, loss, or discrepancy in skill level can be noted.

Achievement

Achievement tests measure educationally relevant skills or acquired knowledge in subject areas such as reading, spelling, mathematics, and written expression. Such tests provide a means of identifying strengths or weaknesses in the acquisition of these skills. Traditionally, learning disability (LD) service eligibility has been determined on the basis of IQ-achievement discrepancy scores. There is a host of problems with this approach, both theoretically and practically, as for example that the magnitude of the difference (typically greater than 1 SD) can vary between school districts. The current approach representing revisions to the Individuals with Disabilities Education Act (IDEA) recognizes the importance of examining various cognitive processes and their impact on school learning (20). For example, phonological awareness, familiarity with words, and ability to retrieve words rapidly are relevant components of reading and spelling competence. Deficits in working memory are likely to impact math learning, and planning and organization problems can affect written expression. Of note, achievement tests differ widely in content, presentation, and response format. Reading comprehension for example may be assessed using written words, sentences, or passages, with responses to oral questions or by filling in the blank. Therefore in interpreting achievement scores, it is also important to understand how the subject matter was assessed.

Behavioral, Social, and Emotional

As a complement to direct behavioral observation and clinical interviewing, behavior rating scales and personality inventories offer a psychometric approach to assessing social emotional problems in children and adolescents (21–23). General purpose rating scales provide information about multiple areas of psychopathology as well as attitudes and interpersonal relationships whereas single domain syndrome measures typically assess specific areas such as depression or anxiety according to DSM criteria. Personality tests or inventories are intended to assess relatively stable characteristics of the individual, but in children usually cover a range of psychological and adjustment problems. Social competence measures focus on the assessment of social skills as well as peer relationships; most behavioral scales and personality inventories include these domains but not to the same extent. Behavioral summaries are based on checklists that use dichotomous ratings and an additive scale; the symptom is rated as present or absent and the number of checked items is summed. Rating scales on the other hand permit an indication as to whether a symptom is present or not and also the degree to which it is present in terms of frequency (never, sometimes, usually).

Through the assessment of behavioral, social and emotional functioning, information is obtained in a systematic and standardized format, producing quantified data, relative to normative-developmental reference groups. In addition, rating scales make use of the judgments and observations of others who are familiar with the child, including the child him/herself, parents, or teachers. In some instances, it is possible (and useful) to compare results between reporters and settings. As with other types of measures, scale names may be similar across behavioral instruments, but item content may differ; also, scales of different names may share content (e.g., when hyperactive behaviors are subsumed under the

TABLE 4.2.4.8

COMMONLY USED CHILD AND ADOLESCENT ASSESSMENT INSTRUMENTS

General Ability/Intelligence Tests	For Ages (years)
Differential Ability Scales, Second Edition (DAS-II) (25)	2:6–17:11
Kaufman Assessment Battery for Children, 2nd ed. (KABC-2) (26)	3:0–18:11
Stanford-Binet, Fifth Edition (SB-5) (27)	2:0–89:11
Wechsler Scales	
Wechsler Preschool and Primary Scale of Intelligence, 3rd ed. (WPPSI-III) (28)	2:6–7:3
Wechsler Intelligence Scale for Children, 4th ed. (WISC-IV) (29)	6:0–16:11
Wechsler Adult Intelligence Scale, 3rd ed. (WAIS-III) (30)	16:0–89:0
Wechsler Abbreviated Scale of Intelligence™ (WASI) (31)	6:0–89:0
Woodcock Johnson Tests of Cognitive Abilities, 3rd ed. (WJ-III) (32)	2–90+ yrs
Achievement Test Batteries	
Kaufman Test of Educational Achievement, 2nd ed. (KTEA-II) (33)	4:6–25 yrs
Peabody Individual Achievement Test—Revised (PIAT-R) (34)	5:0–22:11
Wechsler Individual Achievement Test, 2nd ed. (WIAT-II) (35)	4:0–85:0
Wide Range Achievement Test 4 (WRAT4) (36)	5–94 yrs
Woodcock Johnson Tests of Achievement, 3rd ed. (WJ-III) (37)	2–90+ yrs
Neuropsychological Test Batteries	
Delis-Kaplan Executive Function System (DKEFS) (38)	8–89 yrs
Halstead-Reitan Neuropsychological Test Batteries (39)	5–8, 9–14, 15+ yrs
Luria-Nebraska Neuropsychological Battery—Children's Revision (40)	8–12 yrs
Luria-Nebraska Neuropsychological Battery (LNNB) (41)	15+ yrs
NEPSY: A developmental neuropsychological assessment (42)	3–12 yrs
Reitan-Indiana Neuropsychological Test Battery (43)	5–8 yrs
*Nonverbal Tests**	
Comprehensive Test of Nonverbal Intelligence (C-TONI) (44)	6:0–18:11
Leiter International Performance Scale Revised (Leiter-R) (45)	2:0–20:11
Naglieri Nonverbal Ability Test-Individual Administration (46)	5:0–17:11 yrs
Test of Nonverbal Intelligence (TONI-3) (47)	6:0–89:11 yrs
Universal Nonverbal Intelligence Test (UNIT) (48)	5–17 yrs
Wechsler Nonverbal Scale of Ability (49)	4:0–21:11
Adaptive Behavior	
AAMR Adaptive Behavior Scale-School, 2nd ed. (ABS-S2) (50)	3–21 yrs
AAMR Adaptive Behavior Scales-Residential and Community, 2nd ed. (ABS-RC2) (51)	–79yrs
Adaptive Behavior Assessment System, 2nd ed. (ABAS-II) (52)	0–89 yrs
Scales of Independent Behavior-Revised (SIB-R) (53)	infancy-80+years
Vineland Adaptive Behavior Scales, 2nd ed. (54)	0–90 yrs
Vineland Social-Emotional Early Childhood Scales (SEEC) (55)	0–5:11
Diagnostic Instruments	
Child and Adolescent Psychiatric Assessment (CAPA) (56)	8–17
Children's Interview for Psychiatric Symptoms (ChIPS) (57)	6–18
Diagnostic Interview for Children and Adolescents (DICA) (58)	6–18
Diagnostic Interview Schedule for Children (DISC-IV) (59)	6–17
Schedule for Affective Disorders and Schizophrenia for School-aged Children (K-SADS) (60)	6–18
Structured Clinical Interview for DSM-IV Childhood Diagnoses (KID-SCID) (61)	7–17

*The KABC-2, DAS-II, and SB5 also yield nonverbal composite scores.

conduct domain) (23). Although objective in the sense that information is collected under standard conditions, rating scales are subject to respondent variables. Most behavioral measures include scales to assess the response style of the informant, such as whether the individual is reporting in a manner to create a favorable impression ("faking good"), an unfavorable impression ("faking bad"), a more/less socially acceptable picture, as well as to evaluate consistency of response. It is important to interpret these scales first in order to determine whether the results as a whole are valid.

Projective techniques are another method for accessing the "inner life" of the child or adolescent. This assessment method may in fact be particularly useful for children and adolescents. Tasks such as drawing, completing sentences, and providing narratives to pictures may be more engaging and less confrontational than direct questioning [see Kamphaus & Frick (21) for a discussion]. The projective techniques are based upon the premise that responses to and interpretations of ambiguous stimuli provide insight into the examinee's unconscious mental processes, such as needs, motives, and conflicts. Most projective tasks have been in longstanding use and continue to be widely employed; several have an extensive research literature (such as the Rorschach Inkblot Test and Thematic Apperception Test). Although an understanding of projective techniques is typically embedded in psychodynamic theory, these measures can also be viewed as an additional means of capturing how the child processes and organizes novel, ambiguous, or unstructured information.

TABLE 4.2.4.9

COMMONLY USED CHILD AND ADOLESCENT BEHAVIORAL, SOCIAL, EMOTIONAL MEASURES

Behavior Rating Scales					
	Self	Parent	Teacher	Clinician	Ages (yrs)
Broad Measures					
Adolescent Psychopathology Scale (62)	x				12–19
Behavior Assessment System for Children, 2nd Edition (BASC2) (63)	x	x	x		2:0–21:11
Achenbach System of Empirically Based Assessment (64)					
Child Behavior Checklist (CBCL)		x	x		1:6–18
Youth Self Report (YSR)	x				11–18
Minnesota Multiphasic Personality Inventory for Adolescents (MMPI-A) (65)	x				14–18
Personality Inventory for Children, 2nd Edition (PIC-2) (66)	x				5–19
Personality Inventory for Youth (PIY) (67)	x				10–18
Specialized Measures					
Attention					
ADHD Rating Scale-IV(68)		x	x	x	5–17
Conners Rating Scales—Revised (69)	x	x	x		3–17
SNAP-IV Rating Scale (70)		x	x		6–18
SWAN Rating Scale (71)		x	x		6–18
Anxiety					
Revised Children's Manifest Anxiety Scale (RCMAS) (72)	x				6–19
State-Trait Anxiety Inventory for Children (STAIC) (73)	x				9–12
Beck Anxiety Inventory for Youth (74), Beck Anxiety Inventory (75)	x	x		x	7–18; 18+
Self-Report for Childhood Anxiety Related Disorders (SCARED)(76)	x	x			8+
Depression					
Beck Depression Inventory-II (BDI-II) (77)	x				13–80
Beck Depression Inventory for Youth (BDI-Y) (74)	x				7–18
Children's Depression Inventory (CDI) (78)	x	x	x		6–17
Reynolds Child Depression Scale (RCDS) (79)	x				8–12
Reynolds Adolescent Depressive Scale, 2nd Edition (RADS-2) (80)	x				11–20
Children's Depression Rating Scale-Revised (CDRS-R) (81)				x	6–12
Executive Function					
Behavior Rating Inventory for Executive Function (BRIEF) (82)		x	x		5–18
BRIEF—Preschool Version (BRIEF–P) (83)		x	x		2:0–5:11
BRIEF—Self-Report Version (BRIEF–SR) (84)	x				11–18
Projective Tests:					
Children's Apperception Test (85)					3–10
Draw-a-Person Technique (86–87)					5–17
Kinetic Drawing System for Family and School (88)					5–20
Rorschach Inkblot Test (89)					5-adult
Roberts Apperception Technique for Children:2 (90)					6–18
Sentence Completion Techniques e.g., Hart Sentence Completion Test for Children (91)					children
Rotter Incomplete Sentence Blank (92)					adolescent-adult
Thematic Apperception Test (93)					6-adult

TABLE 4.2.4.10

SOURCES OF INFORMATION ON ASSESSMENT AND ASSESSMENT INSTRUMENTS

Websites
American Psychological Association Testing and Assessment http://www.apa.org/science/testing.html
Resource for guidelines and standards for testing, information about psychological tests, as well as links to other testing websites.
Test Publishers
Publishers provide a description of published tests, age range, administration time, user qualifications, types of scores yielded, cost of purchasing, etc.
American Guidance Service www.ags.net
Pearson Assessments www.pearsonassessments.com
Pro-Ed www.proedinc.com
Psychological Assessment Resources www.parinc.com
Riverside Publishing www.riverpub.com
Stoelting Company www.stoeltingco.com
The Psychological Corporation www.harcourtassessment.com
Western Psychological Services www.wpspublish.com
Major Test Reviews
The *Mental Measurements Yearbook* (94) and *Tests in Print* (95), from the Buros Institute, contain the most recent descriptive information and critical reviews of new and revised tests. Typically available in the reference section/online at most college/university libraries, they can also be accessed for a fee at: http://www.unl.edu/buros/
Tests: A Comprehensive Reference for Assessments in Psychology, Education, and Business (96) and *Test Critiques* (97) also a major source for test descriptions and critical review.
Sample Assessment Texts
Assessment of children: Cognitive applications (4th edition) (Sattler, 2001) (17)
Assessment of children: Behavioral, social, and clinical applications (5th edition) (Sattler, 2005) (98)
Clinical assessment of child and adolescent intelligence (2nd edition) (Kamphaus, 2005) (18)
Clinical assessment of child and adolescent personality and behavior (2nd edition) (Kamphaus & Frick, 2005) (21)
Compendium of neuropsychological tests: Administration, norms, and commentary (Strauss, Sherman & Spreen, 2006) (99)
Handbook of nonverbal assessment (McCallum, 2003) (100)
Practice of child-clinical neuropsychology: An introduction (Rourke, van der Vlugt, & Rourke, 2002) (15)
Neuropsychological assessment (4th edition) (Lezak, Howieson, & Loring, 2004) (16)
The neuropsychological evaluation of the child (Ida Sue Baron, 2004) (101)

Adaptive Behavior

Adaptive behavior scales measure domains related to personal independence and social competence. These are the day-to-day activities necessary to take care of oneself and get along with others, as defined by age and cultural standards. The usual domains assessed include: independent living skills (eating, toileting, simple household chores), functional communication and academic skills, fine and gross motor skills, as well as social behavior such as relations with others, participation in leisure activity, and awareness of community rules. An assessment of adaptive behavior enhances the clinical picture of a child or adolescent by providing information about what the individual *actually* does, as opposed to what he or she is capable of doing in the home, school, or community. It is especially valuable when working with children with developmental disabilities toward treatment planning and toward MR classification. As with other measures, interpretation of the results requires a consideration of the variables that are likely to impact performance, including motivation, family expectations, cultural values, and level of cognitive functioning.

Diagnostic Interviews

The unstructured clinical interview is commonly used in psychology, as in psychiatry. However, several instruments are available for use that offer a more structured and uniform approach to the diagnostic interview, which is of particular relevance in research but may have its place increasingly in the clinical setting (24). These interviews are tied to DSM criteria and provide a set of questions and explicit guidelines for how responses are to be scored. They offer the following advantages when compared to behavior scales: They provide information about symptom duration and onset, intensity and level of impairment, and are tied to diagnostic criteria. The explicit interview format may also be helpful for the interviewer in training. Disadvantages include: The use of these instruments requires more time (60 to 90 minutes), they are not norm referenced, and they are subject to the biases of the reporter, which are not captured in any systematic way (21). There are four other factors to keep in mind when evaluating diagnostic interviews relative to one's research or clinical needs. First, there are usually multiple versions of the same instrument (as they are being constantly updated as DSM criteria change). Second, although the interviews are structured, they vary in their degree of explicit instruction (e.g., the K-SADS provides questions to guide the examiner, whereas the DISC requires the questions to be read as written). Third, most interview responses are scored in a dichotomous fashion (present or absent), although some instruments permit a rating of severity for each symptom, allowing for assessment of subclinical presentations. The last point to be made is that the time frame used to assess symptomatology differs among instruments, for example in terms of how "present episode" is defined, and also whether lifetime diagnosis information is collected [see Kamphaus & Frick, 2005 (21) for a further discussion].

Neuropsychological Assessment

A comprehensive neuropsychological assessment will include measures in one or more of the domains above. The basic test battery will also evaluate cognitive behavior in depth by including measures in each of the following domains and then selecting tests to emphasize one area or another according to initial results of the child's particular pattern of assets and deficits.

Sensory Perception

Measures of tactile, visual, and auditory perception are fundamental to the neuropsychological assessment battery. At a basic level, the individual will be evaluated for evidence of sensory imperception and suppression in each sensory domain, and on each side of the body. Higher level perceptual abilities also are evaluated in each domain. A comparison of performance on the two sides of the body is significant for evidence of lateral or bilateral brain impairment. Each sensory system is also subserved by different regions of the brain and thus yields initial information about areas that are likely to be maximally involved (15). This aspect of the assessment is also relevant to particular types of brain impairment, such as the agnosias. From a developmental perspective, information about the child's sensory and perceptual processes is essential to understanding how the child takes in and assembles information in each of these domains and evaluating the impact on more complex or higher order information processing.

Motor Skills

Motor ability is assessed for basic skills such as force, speed, steadiness, and dexterity; it may also be evaluated in the context of more complex skills such as visual motor coordination, visual motor integration, and constructional abilities. If a deficit in one of these multisystem tasks is obtained, then an analysis of each of the individual component processes is important. Motor function is examined both for overall level as well as laterality. It is relevant to performance of activities of daily living, play, and leisure involvement, classroom tasks, drawing, and handwriting. Assessment of motor and visual motor function is relevant to the question of apraxia.

Attention

Attention is a core capacity that is central to the processes of information reduction, response selection, and preparation for eventual action. The widespread use of the phrase "pay attention," illustrates that attentional resources come at some cost and require effort (we have to "concentrate hard"). Further, there is an implicit notion that attention is selective (we pay attention to one aspect of a complex environment to the exclusion of another). New information arrives in the form of a continuous flow of both internal and external stimuli. Children develop an increasing capacity to override the impulse to attend to what is most striking or novel or desired in order to anticipate, direct, or guide attention, based on prior knowledge and internal goals. Components of attention are distinguished in terms of modality (e.g., tactile, auditory, visual) and process (e.g., focusing or sustaining attention and shifting or dividing attention) assessed. Intact attention is relevant for focused behavior as well as mental tracking (such as following a sequence of ideas or steps in one's head) (16).

Memory

It is important to understand the role of memory, as very few aspects of higher cognitive function and learning could operate successfully without some memory contribution. Memory is often treated as a unitary construct but should be recognized as comprising multiple interrelated systems. Performance may be modality (verbal or visual), task (recall versus recognition), or system (immediate versus long term; semantic versus episodic; implicit versus explicit) specific. Organization has a role in memory, as do other executive control processes. Working memory tasks require the ability simultaneously to attend to, recall, and act upon information held in an on-line state. This aspect of memory function is often considered in the domain of executive function and is fundamental to most aspects of problem solving.

Language

Language is typically assessed for the intactness of the child's ability to discriminate speech sounds, repeat words and phrases, retrieve words rapidly, appreciate word meanings, make verbal associations, express him/herself, as well as comprehend more complex utterances (15). The significance of assessing language abilities is understandable, with regard to the functional lateralization of this system (e.g., left cerebral dominance), evaluation of the aphasias, as well as the importance of language development with regard to reading, spelling, and written expression, concept formation, and the regulation of behavior.

Problem Solving, Concept Formation, and Reasoning

Measures of problem solving ability, concept formation, and reasoning have in common an emphasis on abstract reasoning ability; the task demands are typically complex and require higher order problem solving strategies. The stimuli may be verbal, visual, or tactile in nature, although the child may restructure the task such that a visual task is verbally mediated or a verbal reasoning measure is guided by visual imagery (15). Conceptual and reasoning tasks are likely to represent the integrity of brain functioning, given the need for recruitment of multiple systems in the performance of such tasks. Such tasks provide insights into how the examinee thinks, for example revealing concreteness and/or mental inflexibility to form concepts and logical relationships.

Executive Functions

Executive function (EF) is a term generally used to capture several higher order cognitive functions. It refers to the ability to maintain an appropriate problem solving set to guide future goal-directed behavior, and is composed of a set of abilities including 1) inhibition, 2) set shifting, 3) planning, 4) working memory, and 5) self-monitoring. Most cognitive or intelligence test batteries do not comprehensively assess this domain. Adequate assessment of these areas is relevant to evaluating the child's ability to formulate plans of action, test hypotheses, benefit from feedback, and work toward an end goal. The child who presents with problem solving (as above) and/or EF deficits is likely to require a greater deal of structure and contingent feedback in his or her treatment or educational program.

COGNITIVE AND LEARNING CHALLENGES IN PSYCHIATRIC AND NEURODEVELOPMENTAL DISORDERS

There is consistent evidence that psychiatric and neurodevelopmental disorders of childhood are associated with cognitive and learning challenges, although the pattern is neither uniform nor necessarily diagnostic. The constellation of behavioral deficits that encompasses attention deficit hyperactivity disorder (ADHD) is typically identified relative to real world performance. It would be reasonable to consider that executive function deficits are also consistently associated with ADHD; however, the evidence suggests that the degree and nature of involvement may vary from child to child (e.g., 102). Tourette syndrome (TS) is associated with problems with attention, fine-motor coordination, and visual–motor integration, where fine motor skill deficits may be a predictor of future tic severity and global psychosocial function in children with TS (103). Anxiety and depression may impact attention, memory, and learning. For example, bipolar disorder has been linked to impairments in sustained attention, working memory, and processing speed after controlling for ADHD (104). Neuropsychological studies of childhood onset schizophrenia have revealed deficits in attentional capacities and the processing of information (105–109). When groups of children with childhood-onset schizophrenia and high functioning autism were compared, they did not differ in their Full Scale IQ score or performance on the Perceptual Organization and Verbal Comprehension factors of the WISC-R (105). However, the childhood-onset schizophrenia group did show a significantly lower score on the distractibility factor. Indeed, sustained attention for simple repetitive visual information is generally intact in individuals with autism compared to developmentally matched controls, as measured by continuous performance tasks (110–114). Additionally, conceptual flexibility versus perceptual or attentional flexibility (or simple inhibitory control) appears to be the predominant deficit in higher functioning individuals with autism (115–118).

Several disorders clearly necessitate a psychological or neuropsychological evaluation, such as suspicion of a learning disability (LD) or mental retardation. One specific type of LD, nonverbal learning disability (NLD), is defined by a profile of neuropsychological strengths and weaknesses. The NLD syndrome is so named because the clinical presentation is thought to arise from deficits that are primarily nonverbal in nature (119). These primary deficiencies, which include visual, tactile, and motor functioning, also impact apprehension and use of nonverbal aspects of communication, such as facial expressions, gestures, and general body language. Academically, these children show better reading and spelling skills relative to arithmetic. At present, there is no formal provision for NLD in the DSM-IV, although rules for classification have been developed (120, 121). For the purposes of obtaining services, the needs of these children may be partially captured by diagnostic labels such as mathematics disorder, disorder of written expression, pervasive developmental disorder, or other health impaired.

SUMMARY: INTEGRATED APPROACH

The psychological and neuropsychological assessment represents a systematic process for arriving at a more complete understanding of the child. The determinants of human behavior are many and varied; accordingly, when presented with problem behaviors, thought must be given to factors both intrinsic and extrinsic to the child. Intrinsic factors include: a) cognition, which can be thought of as the information processing aspect of behavior; b) emotional status, including feelings, motivation, regulation; and c) executive functions or execution of purposeful behavior (16). An overly simplistic approach is eschewed in favor of considering the relative contributions of each of the domains, the processes within them, and most interestingly, the interaction between them (the impact of a child's cognitive style on his/her affect, how a child's emotional state impacts information processing). In the final analysis, this information is integrated with extrinsic factors, including past experiences, current environmental demands, and the availability of resources toward future treatment planning.

References

1. Anastasi A: *Psychological Testing*, 6th ed. New York, Macmillan Publishing Company, 1988.
2. Thurstone LL: *Primary Mental Abilities: Psychometric Monographs No. 1*. Chicago: University of Chicago Press, 1938.
3. Cattell RB: Theory of fluid and crystallized intelligence: A critical experiment. *Journal of Educational Psychology* 54:1–22, 1963.
4. Cattell RB: *Intelligence: Its Structure, Growth, and Action*. New York: North-Holland, 1987.
5. Horn JL: Organization of abilities and the development of intelligence. *Psychological Review* 75:242–259, 1968.
6. Horn JL: The theory of fluid and crystallized intelligence. In: Sternberg RJ (ed): *The Encyclopedia of Intelligence*. New York, Macmillan, pp. 443–451, 1994.
7. Guilford JP: *The Nature of Human Intelligence*. New York: McGraw-Hill, 1967.
8. Sternberg RJ: *The Triarchic Mind: A New Theory of Human Intelligence*. New York: Viking, 1988.
9. Sternberg RJ: The triarchic theory of successful intelligence. In: Flanagan DP, Harrison PL (eds): *Contemporary Intellectual Assessment: Theories, Tests, and Issues*. New York: Guilford Press, 103–119, 2004.
10. Gardner H: *Frames of Mind: The Theory of Multiple Intelligences*. New York: Basic Books, 1993.
11. Carroll JB: *Human Cognitive Abilities: A Survey of Factor Analytic Studies*. New York: Cambridge University Press, 1993.
12. Das JP, Naglieri JA, Kirby JR: *Assessment of Cognitive Processes: The PASS Theory of Intelligence*. Needham Heights, MA: Allyn & Bacon, 1994.
13. Kamphaus RW, Winsor AP, Rowe EW, Kim S: A history of intelligence test interpretation. In: Flanagan DP, Harrison PL (eds): *Contemporary Intellectual Assessment: Theories, Tests, and Issues*. New York: Guilford Press, 2004:23–38.
14. Flanagan DP, Ortiz S: *Essentials of Cross-Battery Assessment*. New York, Wiley, 2001.
15. Rourke BP, van der Vlugt H, Rourke SB: *Practice of child-clinical neuropsychology: An introduction*. Lisse: Swets & Zeitlinger, 2002.
16. Lezak M, Howieson DB, Loring DW: *Neuropsychological assessment*, 4th ed. Oxford: Oxford University Press, 2004.
17. Sattler J: *Assessment of children: Cognitive applications*, (4th edition). San Diego: Jerome M. Sattler, Publisher, Inc., 2001.
18. Kamphaus RW: *Clinical assessment of child and adolescent intelligence*, 2nd ed. New York: Springer, 2005.
19. Flynn JR: (1987). Massive gains in 14 nations: What IQ tests really measure. *Psychological Bulletin* 101:171–191,
20. Mather N, & Wendling, BJ: Linking cognitive assessment result to academic interventions for students with learning disabilities. In: Flanagan DP, Harrison, PL, (eds): *Contemporary intellectual assessment: Theories, tests, and issues*. New York: Guilford Press, 2004:269–294.
21. Kamphaus RW, Frick PJ: *Clinical assessment of child and adolescent personality and behavior*, 2nd ed. New York: Springer, 2005.
22. Merrell, KW. *Behavioral, social, and emotional assessment of children and adolescents*, 2nd ed. Mahwah, NJ: Lawrence Erlbaum Associates, 2002.
23. Sattler, J: *Assessment of children: Behavioral and clinical applications*, 4th ed. San Diego: Jerome M. Sattler, Publisher, Inc., 2002.
24. Jensen Doss, A: Evidence-based diagnosis: Incorporating diagnostic instruments into clinical practice. *Journal of the American Academy of Child & Adolescent Psychiatry*, 2005; 44:947–952.
25. Elliott, CD. *Differential Ability Scales*, 2nd ed. San Antonio, TX: Harcourt Assessment, Inc, 2006.
26. Kaufman AS, Kaufman NL: *Kaufman Assessment Battery for Children*, 2nd ed. Circle Pines, MN, AGS Publishing, 2004.
27. Roid, GH. *Stanford-Binet Intelligence Scales*, 5th ed. Itasca, IL: Riverside Publishing, 2003.
28. Wechsler, D. *Wechsler Preschool and Primary Scale of Intelligence*-3rd ed. San Antonio, TX: PsychCorp, A brand of Harcourt Assessment, Inc, 2002.
29. Wechsler, D. *Wechsler Intelligence Scale for Children*-4th ed. San Antonio, TX: PsychCorp, A brand of Harcourt Assessment, Inc, 2003.
30. Wechsler, D. *Wechsler Adult Intelligence Scale*, 3rd ed. San Antonio, TX: PsychCorp, A brand of Harcourt Assessment, Inc, 1997.
31. The Psychological Corporation. *Wechsler Abbreviated Scale of Intelligence*. San Antonio, TX: Harcourt Assessment Inc, 1999.
32. Woodcock, RW, McGrew, KS, Mather, N, Schrank, FA. *Woodcock-Johnson Tests of Cognitive Abilities*, 3rd ed. Itasca, IL: Riverside Publishing, 2001.
33. Kaufman, AS, Kaufman, NL. *Kaufman Test of Educational Achievement*, 2nd ed. Circle Pines, MN: AGS Publishing, 2004.
34. Markwardt Jr, FC. *Peabody Individual Achievement Test—Revised*. Circle Pines, MN: AGS Publishing, 1998.

35. Wechsler, D. *Wechsler Individual Achievement Test*, 2nd ed. San Antonio, TX: PsychCorp, A brand of Harcourt Assessment, Inc, 2001.
36. Wilkinson, GS, Robertson, GJ. *Wide Range Achievement Test 4*. Lutz, FL: Psychological Assessment Resources, Inc., 2006.
37. Woodcock, RW, McGrew, KS, Mather, N, Schrank, FA. *Woodcock-Johnson Tests of Achievement*, 3rd ed. Itasca, IL: Riverside Publishing, 2001.
38. Delis, DC, Kaplan, E, Kramer JH. *Delis-Kaplan Executive Function System*. San Antonio, TX: PsychCorp, A brand of Harcourt Assessment, Inc, 2001.
39. Reitan RM: *Halstead-Reitan Neuropsychological Test Battery*. Tucson, AZ, Reitan Neuropsychology Laboratory/Press, 1979.
40. Golden, CJ. *Luria-Nebraska Neuropsychological Battery, Children's Revision*. Los Angeles, CA: Western Psychological Services, 1987.
41. Golden, CJ, Purisch, AD, Hammeke, TA. *Luria-Nebraska Neuropsychological Battery: Forms I and II*. Los Angeles: Western Psychological Services, 1985.
42. Korkman, M, Kirk, U, Kemp, S. NEPSY: *A Developmental Neuropsychological Assessment*. San Antonio, TX: PsychCorp, A brand of Harcourt Assessment, Inc, 1998.
43. Reitan, RM. *Reitan-Indiana Neuropsychological Test Battery*. Tucson, AZ: Reitan Neuropsychology Laboratory/Press, 1981.
44. Hammill, DD, Pearson, NA, Wiederholt, JL. *Comprehensive Test of Nonverbal Intelligence*. Austin, TX: PRO-ED, Inc., 1996.
45. Roid, GH, Miller, LJ. *Leiter International Performance Scale, Revised*. Wood Dale, IL: Stoelting Co., 1998.
46. Naglieri, JA. *Naglieri Nonverbal Ability Test—Individual Administration*. San Antonio, TX: PsychCorp, A brand of Harcourt Assessment, Inc, 2003.
47. Brown, L, Sherbenou, RJ, Johnson, SK. *Test of Nonverbal Intelligence*, 3rd ed. Austin, TX: PRO-ED, Inc., 1997.
48. Bracken, BA, McCallum, RS. *Universal Nonverbal Intelligence Test*. Itasca, IL: Riverside Publishing, 1998.
49. Wechsler, D., Naglieri, JA. *Wechsler Nonverbal Scale of Ability*. San Antonio, TX: Harcourt Assessment Inc., 2006.
50. Lambert, N, Nihira, K, Leland, H. *AAMR Adaptive Behavior Scale-School*, 2nd ed. Austin, TX: PRO-ED, Inc., 1993.
51. Nihira, K, Leland, H, Lambert, N. *AAMR Adaptive Behavior Scale-Residential and Community*, 2nd ed. Austin, TX: PRO-ED, Inc., 1993.
52. Harrison PL, Oakland T: *Adaptive Behavior Assessment System*, 2nd ed. San Antonio, TX, PsychCorp, A brand of Harcourt Assessment, Inc, 2003.
53. Bruininks, RH, Woodcock, RW, Weatherman, RF, Hill, BK. *Scales of Independent Behavior, Revised*. Itasca, IL: Riverside Publishing, 1997.
54. Sparrow, SS, Cicchetti, DV, Balla, DA. *Vineland Adaptive Behavior Scales*, 2nd ed. Minneapolis, MN: Pearson Assessments, a business of Pearson Education, 2006.
55. Sparrow, SS, Balla, DA, Cicchetti, DV. *Vineland Social Emotional Early Childhood Scales*. Circle Pines, MN: AGS, Inc., 1998.
56. Angold A, Costello EJ: The child and adolescent psychiatric assessment (CAPA). *Journal of the American Academy of Child & Adolescent Psychiatry* 39:39–48, 2000.
57. Weller, EB, Weller, RA, Fristad, MA, Rooney, MT. *ChIPS—Children's Interview for Psychiatric Syndromes*. Arlington, VA: American Psychiatric Publishing, Inc., 1999.
58. Reich, W. Diagnostic interview for children and adolescents (DICA). *Journal of the American Academy of Child and Adolescent Psychiatry* 39:59–66, 2000.
59. Shaffer, D, Fisher, P, Lucas, CP, Dulcan, MK, Schwab-Stone, ME. NIMH Diagnostic Interview Schedule for Children Version IV (NIMH DISC-IV): Description, differences from previous versions, and reliability of some common diagnoses. *Journal of the American Academy of Child and Adolescent Psychiatry* 39:28–38, 2000.
60. Ambrosini, PJ. Historical developments and present status of the schedule for affective disorders and schizophrenia for school age children (K-SADS). *Journal of the American Academy of Child and Adolescent Psychiatry* 39:49–58, 2000.
61. Matzner F, Silva R, Silvan M, Chowdhury M, Nastasi L. Preliminary Test-retest Reliability of the KID-SCID, *Scientific Proceedings, American Psychiatric Association Meeting*, 1997.
62. Reynolds, WM. *Adolescent Psychopathology Scale*. Odessa, FL: Psychological Assessment Resources, Inc., 1998.
63. Reynolds, WM, Kamphaus, RW. *BASC2: Behavior Assessment System for Children*, 2nd ed. Minneapolis, MN, Pearson Assessments, a business of Pearson Education, 2004.
64. Achenbach TM, Rescorla LA, McConaughey S, et al.: *Achenbach System of Empirically Based Assessment*. Burlington, VT, ASEBA, 2006.
65. Butcher JN, Williams CL, Graham, JR, et al.: *MMPI-A (Minnesota Multiphasic Personality Inventory—Adolescent): Manual for Administration, Scoring, and Interpretation*. Minneapolis, MN, University of Minnesota Press, 1992.
66. Wirt RD, Lachar D, Seat PD, Broen Jr., WE: *Personality Inventory for Children*, 2nd ed. Los Angeles, Western Psychological Services, 2001.
67. Lachar D, Gruber CP: *Personality Inventory for Youth (PIY) Manual: Administration and Interpretation Guide*. Los Angeles, Western Psychological Services, 1995.
68. DuPaul GJ, Power TJ, Anastopulos AD, Reid R: *ADHD Rating Scale-IV: Checklists, Norms, and Clinical Interpretation*. New York, Guilford Press, 1998.
69. Conners CK. *CRS-R: Conners' Rating Scales Revised*. Minneapolis, MN, Pearson Assessments, 2000.
70. Swanson JM: The SNAP-IV Teacher and Parent Rating Scale. In: Fine A, Kotkin R (eds): *Therapists Guide to Learning and Attention Disorders*. San Diego, Elsevier Science, 2003, pp. 487–500.
71. Swanson JM: The SWAN Rating Form. In: Fine A, Kotkin R (eds): *Therapist's Guide to Learning and Attention Disorders*. San Diego, Elsevier Science, 2003:501–502.
72. Reynolds CR, Richmond BO: *Revised Children's Manifest Anxiety Scale*. Los Angeles, Western Psychological Services, 1985.
73. Spielberger CD: *State-Trait Anxiety Inventory for Children*. Palo Alto, Consulting Psychologists Press, 1973.
74. Beck JS, Beck AT, Jolly J, Steer R: *Beck Youth Inventories™, Second Edition for Children and Adolescents (BYI-II)*. San Antonio, TX, Harcourt Assessment, Inc, 2005.
75. Beck AT, Steer RA: *Beck Anxiety Inventory*. San Antonio, TX, PsychCorp, A brand of Harcourt Assessment, Inc, 1993.
76. Birmaher B, Khetarpal S, Cully M, Brent D, McKenzie S: *Screen for Child Anxiety Related Disorders (SCARED)*. Western Psychiatric Institute and Clinic, University of Pittsburgh, 1995. Email: birmaherb@msx.upmc.edu.
77. Beck AT, Steer RA, Brown GK: *Beck Depression Inventory—II*. San Antonio. TX, PsychCorp, A brand of Harcourt Assessment, Inc, 1996.
78. Kovacs M: *Children's Depression Inventory*. Minneapolis, MN, Pearson Assessments, 1992.
79. Reynolds WM: *Reynolds Child Depression Scale*. Odessa, FL, Psychological Assessment Resources, Inc., 1989.
80. Reynolds WM: *Reynolds Adolescent Depressive Scale*, 2nd ed. Lutz, FL, Psychological Assessment Resources, Inc., 2002.
81. Poznanski E, Mokros HB: *Children's Depression Rating Scale, Revised*. Los Angeles, Western Psychological Services, 1996.
82. Gioia GA, Isquith PK, Guy SC, Kenworthy L: *Behavior Rating Inventory of Executive Function*. Odessa, FL, Psychological Assessment Resources, Inc., 2000.
83. Gioia GA, Espy KA, Isquith PK: *Behavior Rating Inventory of Executive Function—Preschool Version*. Odessa, FL, Psychological Assessment Resources, Inc., 2003.
84. Guy SC, Isquith PK, Gioia GA: *Behavior Rating Inventory of Executive Function—Self-Report Version*. Lutz, FL, Psychological Assessment Resources, Inc., 2004.
85. Bellak L, Bellak SS: *Children's Apperception Test (1991 Revision)*. Larchmont, NY, C.P.S., Inc., 1991.
86. Koppitz EM: *Psychological evaluation of children's human figure drawings*. New York, Grune & Stratton, 1968.
87. Naglieri JA: *Draw A Person: A quantitative scoring system*. San Antonio, TX, PsychCorp, A brand of Harcourt Assessment, Inc, 1988.
88. Knoff HM, Prout HT: *Kinetic Drawing System for Family and School: A Handbook*. Los Angeles, CA, Western Psychological Services, 1985.
89. Weiner IB: *Principles of Rorschach® Interpretation*, 2nd ed. Odessa, FL, Psychological Assessment Resources, Inc., 2003.
90. Roberts GE, McArthur DS: *Roberts Apperception Test for Children*, 2nd. Odessa, FL, Psychological Assessment Resources, Inc., 2005.
91. Hart DH: *The Hart Sentence Completion Test for Children*. Salt Lake City, Educational Support Systems, 1972.
92. Rotter JB, Lah MI, Rafferty JE: *Rotter Incomplete Sentences Blank*, 2nd ed. San Antonio, TX, PsychCorp, A brand of Harcourt Assessment, Inc, 1992.
93. Murray HA: *Thematic Apperception Test*. Cambridge, MA, Harvard University Press, 1943.
94. *Mental Measurements Yearbook*. Highland Park, NJ, The Mental Measurements Yearbook, 1941–2005.
95. Murphy LL, Impara JC, Plake BS: (eds). *Tests in Print VI: An Index to Tests, Test Reviews, and the Literature on Specific Tests*. Lincoln, NB, Buros Institute of Mental Measurements, University of Nebraska–Lincoln. Distributed by the University of Nebraska Press, 2002.
96. Maddox T: (ed) *Tests: A comprehensive reference for assessments in psychology, education, and business*, 5th ed. Austin, TX, Pro-Ed, 2003.
97. Keyser DJ, Sweetland RC: (eds) *Test Critiques*. Kansas City, MO, Test Corporation of America, 1984-
98. Sattler J: *Assessment of children: Behavioral, social, and clinical applications*, 5th ed. San Diego, Jerome M. Sattler, Publisher, Inc., 2005.
99. Strauss E., Sherman EMS, Spreen O: *A compendium of neuropsychological tests: Administration, norms, and commentary*, 3rd ed. New York, Oxford University Press, 2006.
100. McCallum RS: *Handbook of nonverbal assessment*. New York, Kluwer Academic/Plenum Publishers, 2003.
101. Baron IS: *Neuropsychological Evaluation of the Child*. New York, Oxford University Press, 2004.
102. Willcutt EG, Doyle AE, Nigg JT, et al.: Validity of the executive function hypothesis of ADHD: A meta-analytic review. *Biological Psychiatry* 57:1336–1346, 2005.
103. Bloch MH, Sukhodolsky DG, Leckman JF, et al.: Fine-motor skill deficits in childhood predict adulthood tic severity and global psychosocial

functioning in Tourette's syndrome. *Journal of Child Psychology and Psychiatry* 47:551–559, 2006.
104. Doyle AE, Wilens, TE, Kwon A, et al.: Neuropsychological functioning in youth with bipolar disorder. *Biological Psychiatry* 58:540–548, 2005.
105. Asarnow RF, Asamen J, Granholm E, et al: Cognitive/neuropsychological studies of children with a schizophrenic disorder. *Schizophr Bull* 20:647–669, 1994.
106. Asarnow RF, Brown W, Strandburg R: Children with a schizophrenic disorder: neurobehavioral studies. *Eur Arch Psychiatry Clin Neurosci* 245:70–79, 1995.
107. Karatekin C, Asarnow RF: Working memory in childhood-onset schizophrenia and attention-deficit/hyperactivity disorder. *Psychiatry Res* 80:165–176, 1998.
108. Karatekin C, Asarnow RF: Components of visual search in childhood-onset schizophrenia and attention-deficit/hyperactivity disorder. *Journal of Abnormal Child Psychology* 26:367–380, 1998.
109. Karatekin C, Asarnow RF: Exploratory eye movements to pictures in childhood-onset schizophrenia and attention-deficit/hyperactivity disorder. *Journal of Abnormal Child Psychology* 27:35–49, 1999.
110. Buchsbaum MS, Siegel Jr BV, Wu JC, et al.: Brief report: Attention performance in autism and regional brain metabolic rate assessed by positron emission tomography. *J Autism Dev Disord* 22:115–125, 1992.
111. Casey BJ, Gordon CT, Mannheim GB, et al.: Dysfunctional attention in autistic savants. *Journal of Clinical and Experimental Neuropsychology* 15:933–946, 1993.
112. Garretson HB, Fein D, Waterhouse L: Sustained attention in children with autism. *Journal of Autism and Developmental Disorders* 20:101–114, 1990.
113. Minshew N J, Goldstein G, Siegel DJ: Neuropsychologic functioning in autism: Profile of a complex information processing disorder. *Journal of the International Neuropsychological Society* 3:303–316, 1997.
114. Pascualvaca DM, Fantie BD, Papageorgiou M, et al.: Attentional capacities in children with autism: Is there a general deficit in shifting focus? *Journal of Autism and Developmental Disorders* 28:467–478, 1998.
115. Goldstein G, Johnson CR, Minshew NJ: Attentional processes in autism. *Journal of Autism and Developmental Disorders* 31:433–440, 2001.
116. Minshew NJ, Meyer J, Goldstein G: Abstract reasoning in autism: A dissociation between concept formation and concept identification. *Neuropsychology* 16:327–334, 2002.
117. Ozonoff S, Cook I, Coon H, et al.: Performance on Cambridge Neuropsychological Test Automated Battery subtests sensitive to frontal lobe function in people with autistic disorder: Evidence from the Collaborative Programs of Excellence in Autism Network. *Journal of Autism and Developmental Disorders* 34:139–150, 2004.
118. Ozonoff S, McEvoy RE: A longitudinal study of executive function and theory of mind development in autism. *Development and Psychopathology* 6:415–431, 1994.
119. Rourke BP: *Nonverbal Learning Disabilities: The Syndrome and the Model*. New York, Guilford Press, 1989.
120. Drummond CR, Ahmad SA, Rourke BP: Rules for the classification of younger children with nonverbal learning disabilities and basic phonological processing disabilities. *Archives of Clinical Neuropsychology* 20:171–182, 2005.
121. Pelletier PM, Ahmad SA, Rourke BP: Classification rules for basic phonological processing disabilities and nonverbal learning disabilities: Formulation and external validity. *Child Neuropsychology* 7:84–98, 2001.

CHAPTER 4.2.5 ■ ASSESSING COMMUNICATION

RHEA PAUL AND MOIRA LEWIS

This chapter provides a brief outline of the process involved in assessing how children use speech and language for communication. We describe clinical assessment as a process that involves *screening, evaluation*, or deciding upon the degree of disability and the diagnosis that best fits the child's condition, and *assessment*, the use of diagnostic information to detail the aspects of disability and to formulate the most appropriate treatment plan. Evaluation, ideally, is conducted by a team of professionals from multiple disciplines who contribute their expertise in identifying the child's disorder and needs. Teams can take several forms, depending on how the professionals interact. The typical structures of assessment teams appear in Table 4.2.5.1. A speech-language pathologist is the member of the team who specializes in the assessment and treatment of disorders of communication. Qualified speech-language pathologists (SLPs) are certified by the American Speech-Language Hearing Association, and usually licensed by the state, as well.

Screening involves the collection of data to decide whether there is a strong likelihood that an individual has a problem that will require more in-depth assessment. An appropriate speech-language screening measure is one that meets high levels of psychometric criteria, including well established reliability, validity, sensitivity, and specificity, as well as assessing relevant areas of communication. A screening measure should not simply look at one area of concern; for example, looking at a child's ability to comprehend language forms, while ignoring his ability to express language. Failure to achieve a criterion level on a screening measure should result in a child's referral for evaluation and more in-depth assessment. Some examples of language screening measures appear in Table 4.2.5.2.

EVALUATION

The evaluation process usually begins with a gathering and review of historical information about the child. Historical information can be gathered from parent interviews, previous clinical information, and standard questionnaires. This information may include reasons for referral, results from previous testing or treatment, as well as pertinent developmental information about the child. When gathering this information, the team must determine what is known about the child versus what needs to be learned in the current evaluation to establish the presence and type of disorder, and to contribute to the development of a treatment plan. Basic questions to consider when gathering this initial information regarding a child's communication include:

1. Did the child attain normal milestones of speech development (babbling by 10 months, first words by 18 months, two-word combinations and following simple directions by 24 months, sentences by 3 years) and feeding (solid food by 6 months, using a cup by 18 months, drinking from a straw by 30 months)?
2. What does the family see as the child's most important problem in communication?
3. When did the problem begin?
4. Does this problem vary in terms of its severity or occurrence?
5. Can the child's speech be understood by people outside the family?

TABLE 4.2.5.1

ASSESSMENT TEAM STRUCTURES

Multidisciplinary
The team is made up of professionals from different disciplines. Each completes an independent evaluation of the patient and comes up with a separate set of recommendations which are reported to the team and the client's family.
Interdisciplinary
The team consists of professionals from different disciplines, but formal communication channels are established between them. A case manager coordinates services among all disciplines. Some professionals may be involved in the assessment on a consultant basis, providing suggestions to those who work directly with the child, but do not interact directly themselves.
Transdisciplinary
Team members are encouraged to share information and skills across disciplines. Assessment is collaborative in that one individual may do all or most of the interaction with the child, whereas others observe or make suggestions for the interactor to use during the assessment process. Team members work together whenever possible. They train and receive training from each other in reciprocal interactions. *Role release* (1) is employed; this involves sharing information and having team members help each other perform activities traditionally reserved within disciplines.

6. Can the child follow verbal directions at home? At school?
7. How does this problem influence the child across various environments, including school and within social settings?

A common method for gathering this case history information is to ask families to fill out a questionnaire with queries like the above, prior to the evaluation session, and to conduct an interview with the parent at the time of the assessment to clarify and supplement the written information. *Caregiver information* gained through questionnaire and interview procedures can supplement results gathered from direct interaction between the clinician and child. Caregivers can provide information about the child's communicative functioning among a variety of contexts, including home, school, and with peers. Caregivers can describe their own concerns by outlining the child's communication performance across these natural contexts. Parent report can give the clinician a better sense of the child's everyday communication challenges and areas of weakness. Tyler and Tolbert (2) describe other advantages to caregivers as partners in the assessment process, including the tendency for young children to be reluctant to interact with a clinician or in an unfamiliar environment.

TABLE 4.2.5.2

EXAMPLES OF SPEECH-LANGUAGE SCREENING MEASURES

Test (Name/Author(s)/Date/Publisher)	Developmental Range
Bankson Language Screening Test—2nd ed. Bankson, NW (1977). Baltimore: University Park Press	4–7 yrs
Battelle Development Inventory Screening Test Newborg, J, Stock, J, Wnek, L, Guidubaldi, J, and Svinicki, J (2004). Itasca, IL: Riverside Publishing	Birth–8 yrs
Clinical Evaluation of Language Fundamentals—4 Screening Test Semel, E, Wiig, EH, and Secord W (2004). San Antonio: Harcourt Assessment	5–21 yrs
Denver II Frankenburg, WK, et al. (1990). Denver: Denver Developmental Materials	2 wks–6 yrs
Developmental Indicators for the Assessment of Learning—3rd ed. Mardell-Czudnowski, C and Goldenberg, DS (1998). Circle Pines, MN: American Guidance Service	3–6:11 yrs
Diagnostic Evaluation of Language Variation—Screening Test (DELV-Screening Test) Seymour, HN, Roeper, TW, and de Villiers, J (2003). San Antonio: Harcourt Assessment	4–9 yrs
Coston-Reidenbach Articulation/Language Quick Screen Coston, GN, and Reidenbach, ED (1978). Columbia, SC: Columbia Educational Resources	3–7 yrs
Early Screening Profiles (ESP) Harrison, P, Kaufman, A, Kaufman, N, Bruininks, R, Rynders, J, Ilmers, S, Sparrow, S, and Cicchetti D (1990). Circle Pines, MN: American Guidance Service	2–6:11 yrs
Hodson Assessment of Phonological Patterns–Preschool Phonological Screening Hodson, BW (2004). Austin: Pro-Ed	Preschool
Fluharty Preschool Speech and Language Screening Test—2nd ed. Fluharty, NB (2000). Circle Pines, MN: AGS Publishing	3–6:11 yrs
Joliet 3-Minute Speech and Language Screen (Revised) Kinzler, MC, and Johnson, CC (1993). San Antonio: Harcourt Assessment	K, 2nd and 5th grades
Kindergarten Language Screening Test–2nd ed. (KLST–2) Gauthier, S, and Madison, C (1998). Austin: Pro-Ed	3:6–6:11 yrs
Screening Test for Developmental Apraxia of Speech, 2nd ed. Blakely, R (2000). Austin: Pro-Ed	4–12 yrs
Adolescent Language Screening Test Morgan, DL, and Guilford, AM (1984). Austin: Pro-Ed	11–17 yrs

Allowing a child to play or converse with a parent, for example, provides a way for the clinician to observe the child's communication and interaction style indirectly, and may put the child and parent at ease. Additionally, parents may be reluctant or anxious to raise certain of their concerns or reveal specific information in direct conversation with an unfamiliar clinician. In order to decrease both caregiver and child stress, to minimize additional testing sessions, and to obtain a representative sample of the child's skills, gathering information from parents and caregivers as they both describe and interact with their child, can increase the efficiency of an assessment, as well as decrease the stress induced by long testing sessions. Some examples of parent report instruments appear in Table 4.2.5.3.

Once sufficient information about the history and the problem has been gathered, the team will determine the child's general developmental level to begin the evaluation process. Assessment of general developmental level, usually through psychological testing of cognitive and motor function, will help to establish the level of communication skills that might be expected, and help to select instruments that will target skills at the appropriate level.

Communication evaluation will usually include a battery of standardized assessments that provide an answer to the question of whether this child is significantly different from other children in terms of the ability to speak, understand language, and use speech and language to communicate with family, teachers, and peers. For this purpose, again, tests with strong psychometric properties must be chosen in order to answer the question in a fair and valid way. Some examples of tests often used for evaluation at various stages of development are listed in Table 4.2.5.4.

If testing confirms the observations of parents and teachers and corroborates the screening result that the child is showing difficulty with communication skills relative to others at his/her developmental level, the child can be identified as having a disorder in this area. However, not every child who tests low on a standardized test will be able to receive services for a communication deficit. Local, state, and federal regulations determine what level of impairment is necessary for eligibility for educational services of various kinds, including communication services. Thus, one outcome of evaluation will be a determination as to whether a child's disability is severe or pervasive enough to qualify for publicly funded services. Clinicians, then, need to be aware of local requirements for eligibility. If a child fails to meet eligibility criteria, parents may opt to obtain services privately.

In addition to establishing eligibility for services, the evaluation process is aimed at integrating data from the various professionals on the team in order to arrive at a diagnostic label that best describes the child's conditions. Communication disorders are very frequently associated with a variety of conditions, as Chapter 3.1.4 explains. So although failure to talk or poor speech development is frequently a child's presenting problem, it is often the case that evaluation uncovers deficits in other areas of development, such as cognition, hearing, motor or social skills that contribute to the choice of diagnostic label. When this happens, the child may receive a diagnosis of mental retardation, autism, etc. The conferring of one of these diagnoses, however, does not mean that the child's need for communication assessment and intervention diminishes. Even when a child's primary diagnosis is something other than a specific speech or language disorder, assessment of communication strengths and needs remains important in order to develop an intervention program that will address all of the child's developmental concerns.

One additional issue explored by the evaluation team concerns the nonspeaking child. Children may fail to acquire expressive language function for a variety of reasons, primarily because of neuromotor deficits that affect vocal function, such as cerebral palsy. However, some children without diagnosable neuromotor disorders may also fail to begin speaking during early childhood; children with Down syndrome and autism can sometimes show this pattern, for example. When this is the case, the SLP will be charged with deciding whether the child should be taught to use an alternative or augmentative communication (AAC) modality, such as sign language, a picture board, or an electronic speech aid. Although the considerations that go into this decision are beyond the scope of this discussion [see (9) for fuller information], in general, SLPs will attempt to ensure that the child has some way to communicate with others if speech is not an accessible modality for the child. AAC may be provided on a short-term basis, until more useable speech emerges, or may be part of the child's long-term communication program. The SLP will attempt, in investigating AAC usage for a particular child, to identify the best match of a system to a child's developmental level and communication needs. This investigation may continue into the assessment portion of the team's activities.

TABLE 4.2.5.3

EXAMPLE OF PARENT REPORT INSTRUMENTS FOR COMMUNICATION

Instrument	Developmental Level
Autism Diagnostic Interview—Revised (3)	2–21 years
Communication and Symbolic Behavior Scales—Caregiver Questionnaire (CSBS) (4)	8–36 mo.
Children's Communication Checklist–2 (5)	4–16 years
Language Development Survey (6)	8–24 mo.
MacArthur-Bates Communication Development Inventory (7)	8–36 mo.
Vineland Adaptive Behavior Scales—2 (8)	Birth–80 years

ASSESSMENT

Once it has been determined that the child has a disorder that includes communication deficits, a detailed assessment of the child's functioning is undertaken. This process has three main goals: to establish the child's *baseline function*, to identify *goals for intervention*, and to *monitor progress* within the therapy program. To achieve these aims, SLPs typically use a range of methods that include not only standardized tests, but criterion-referenced, observational, and dynamic procedures.

Norm-referenced tests, or standardized instruments, are, as we have discussed, used to compare a child's skills to those of other children of similar age and background. These formal instruments have specific statistical properties that allow meaningful comparisons among children to determine if their functioning is significantly different from typical performance. Standardized tests are particularly useful in determining the existence of a communication disorder, and for establishing eligibility for speech and language services. *Criterion referenced* assessments do not provide statistical comparisons among similar children's abilities, but rather determine whether the child can perform particular tasks deemed to be important for communication. These may examine specific forms of speech and language in more informal ways, without standardized rules and methods. Instead, the clinician can predetermine criteria according to the child and his communication goals. Criterion-referenced assessments allow the clinician to individualize the

TABLE 4.2.5.4

EXAMPLES OF COMMONLY USED LANGUAGE TEST BATTERIES

Test Name, Author(s)/Date, Publisher	Developmental Level
Clinical Evaluation of Language Fundamentals—Preschool, 2nd ed. (CELF-Preschool) Wiig, EH, Secord, W, and Semel, E (2004). San Antonio: Harcourt Assessment	3–6 yrs
Clinical Evaluation of Language Fundamentals—4 Semel, E, Wiig, EH, and Secord, W (2003). San Antonio: Harcourt Assessment	5–21 yrs
Comprehensive Assessment of Spoken Language Carrow-Woolfolk, E (1999). Circle Pines, MN: AGS Publications.	7–21 yrs
Detroit Tests of Learning Aptitude—Primary 2 Hammill, DD, and Bryant, BR (1991). Austin: Pro-Ed	3–9:11 yrs
Diagnostic Evaluation of Language Variation (DELV—Criterion Referenced) Seymour, HN, Roeper, TW, and de Villiers, J (2003). San Antonio: Harcourt Assessment	4–9 yrs
Oral and Written Language Scales (OWLS): Written Expression Scale Carrow-Woolfolk, E (1996). Circle Pines, MN: American Guidance Service	5–21 yrs
Porch Index of Communicative Ability in Children (PICA) Porch, BE (1981—revised edition in preparation). Albuquerque: PICA Programs	3–12 yrs
Preschool Language Scale—4 (PLS-4) Zimmerman, IL, Steiner, V, and Pond, R (2002). San Antonio: Harcourt Assessment	Birth–6:11 yrs
Sequenced Inventory of Communication Development—Revised (SICD-R) Hedrick, DL, Prather, EM and Tobin, AR (1984). Seattle: University of Washington Press	4 mos–4 yrs
Test of Adolescent and Adult Language—3 Hammill, DD, Brown, VL, Larsen, SC, and Wiederholt, JL (1994). Austin: Pro-Ed	12–24:11 yrs
Test of Early Language Development—3rd ed. (TELD-3) Hresko, WP, Redi, K, and Hammill, DD (1999). Austin: Pro-Ed	2:7–11 yrs
Test of Language Development—3: Primary (TOLD-3:P) Newcomer, PL, and Hammill, DD (1997). Austin: Pro-Ed	4–8:11 yrs
Test of Language Development-Intermediate (TOLD-I:3) Newcomer, PL, and Hammill, DD (1997). Austin: Pro-Ed	8:6 yrs–12:11 yrs
Test of Early Written Language—2 Herron, S, Hresko, W, and Peak, P (1996). Austin: Pro-Ed	3–11 yrs
Utah Test of Language Development—4 Mecham, MJ (2003). Austin: Pro-Ed	3–9:11 yrs
Woodcock Language Proficiency Battery—Revised Woodcock, RW (1991). Chicago: Riverside Publishing	2–95 yrs

assessment to examine particular behaviors and are ideal for evaluating whether intervention methods have been successful. These methods can be developed by the clinician to answer particular questions, such as whether a child understands past tense forms, whether a child can understand vocabulary related to a school curricular unit, or whether a child can participate in language arts assignments given by a particular teacher.

The assessment of communication, of necessity, involves some observation of what a child's communication is like in natural situations. It is important to supplement standardized measures with real-life measures for a reliable index of the child's communication in everyday interactions. Observational, or *authentic*, assessment allows for a closer look at a child's communication, by examining the child's spontaneous language use and understanding in familiar contexts. Merrel and Plante (10) demonstrated the importance of supplementing standardized measures with authentic assessment by showing that norm-referenced testing, even when high sensitivity and specificity were present, nonetheless was inconsistent in identifying actual errors made in a child's spontaneous speech. Thus, to get a realistic perspective of a child's expressive functioning, and to determine appropriate goals for expressive language use, sampling spontaneous communication is an important part of assessment.

In contrast to these methods that assess the child's current level of functioning in a relatively static setting, *dynamic assessment* is designed to take a closer look at what factors, supports, or modifications enhance the child's communication performance. Dynamic assessment is used to manipulate the linguistic context through the use of prompts, cues, or various scaffolds to determine what best supports positive changes in communication. In turn, dynamic assessment provides important initial information about what techniques or teaching styles may be appropriate for treatment.

Having examined the range of methods available for assessing communication skills, we can now discuss the three major aims of the assessment process.

Establishing Baseline Function. The purpose of this phase of assessment is not merely to show that the child scores below other children on tests, but to document in detail the child's communicative strengths and weaknesses. Typically, a thorough assessment will include measures of both understanding and production of sounds, words, sentence structures, conversation, and storytelling. Profiles of relative strengths and weaknesses among these communicative skills will be used to decide on the child's overall level of communication, which will determine the goal level for areas that are less well developed. When determining the child's baseline level of communicative functioning, standardized tests can, again, be useful, especially those that focus more narrowly on specific areas of function, rather than the broadbased batteries in Table 4.2.5.4. Some examples of more focused tests appear in Table 4.2.5.5.

In addition to testing, though, SLPs often employ more observational methods to round out their picture of the child's ability to communicate in real settings. Frequently, they collect

TABLE 4.2.5.5

EXAMPLES OF STANDARDIZED TESTS FOR FOCUSED ASSESSMENT

Test	Developmental Level
Boehm Test of Basic Concepts—3rd ed. Boehm, AE (2000). San Antonio: Harcourt Assessment	K–2nd grade
Expressive Vocabulary Test Williams, KT (1997). Circle Pines, MN: AGS	2:6-adult
Expressive One-Word Picture Vocabulary Test—2000 Edition Brownell, R, ed. (2000). Novato, CA: Academic Therapy	2–18 yrs
Lindamood Auditory Conceptualization Test—3rd ed. Lindamood, CH, and Lindamood, PC (2004). Austin: Pro-Ed	5–18:11 yrs
Peabody Picture Vocabulary Test—3rd ed. (PPVT-III) Dunn, L, and Dunn, L (1997). Circle Pines, MN: American Guidance Service	2:6 yrs-adult
Receptive One-Word Picture Vocabulary Test—2000 Edition Brownell, R, ed. (2000). Novato, CA: Academic Therapy Publications	2:11–12 yrs
Rice/Wexler Test of Early Grammatical Impairment Rice, ML, and Wexler, K (2001). San Antonio: Harcourt Assessment	3–8 yrs
Structured Photographic Expressive Language—Test 3 (SPELT-3) Dawson, J, Eyer, J, and Stout, C (2003). DeKalb, IL: Janelle Publications	4–9:11 yrs
Test of Adolescent/Adult Word Finding German, DJ (1990). Austin: Pro-Ed	12–80 yrs
Test for Auditory Comprehension of Language (TACL03) Carrow-Woolfolk, E (1999). Austin: Pro-Ed	3–9:11 yrs
Test of Narrative Language (TNL) Gillam, RB, and Pearson, NA (2004). Austin: Pro-Ed	5–11:11 yrs
Test of Pragmatic Skills (Revised) Shulman, BB (1986). Tucson: Communication Skill Builders	3–8 yrs
Test of Pragmatic Language (TOPL) Phelps-Terasaki, D and Phelps-Gunn, T (1992). Austin: Pro-Ed	5–13:11 yrs
Test of Problem Solving—Revised—Elementary Bowers, L, Barrett, M, Huisingh, R, Orman, J, LoGiudice, C (1994). East Moline, IL: LinguiSystems	6–11 yrs
Test of Word Finding—2nd ed. German, DJ (2000). Austin: Pro-Ed	4:4–12:11 yrs
Test of Word Knowledge Wiig, EH, and Secord, W (1992). San Antonio: Harcourt Assessment	Level 2: 8–17 yrs
Test of Written Language—3 (TOWL-3) Hammill, DD, and Larsen, SC (1996). Austin: Pro-Ed	2nd–12th grades (7:6 yrs–17:11 yrs)

a sample of the child's communication as s/he engages in play or other age-appropriate activities with family or peers. These observations are aimed at discovering how the child uses the communication skills available to him/her to interact socially. Some children with very limited language can show strengths in using gesture, facial expression, and tone of voice to convey a range of meanings, while others at the same level of language show few of these abilities. Conversely, some children with nearly age-appropriate vocabulary and sentence structures who score well on standardized tests are nonetheless severely lacking in social communication skills, and this deficit would not be documented unless data from natural observation were collected. To that end, SLPs often collect samples of spontaneous communication in dyadic conversation. They may also sample the child's ability to construct a coherent narrative about a set of pictures or by discussing a personal experience or retelling a favorite movie or TV show plot. Narrative abilities are known to be highly related to success in the school curriculum (11), and have been documented to represent weaknesses in children with various kinds of language problems (12, 13). Thus, assessment of narrative skill is often an aspect of the communication assessment for school-aged children.

One additional aspect of the communication assessment deals with the issue of variability of performance. Assessment for baseline functioning can also involve answering questions such as, Does this child communicate better with adults than peers? In structured or informal settings? In familiar environments? To answer these questions, a child's communication may be observed in several settings and among different partners. The SLP may, for example, collect language samples of the preschool child playing with a parent and then with a peer, of a toddler playing with a parent and then with a clinician, or of a school-aged child having a conversation with a clinician and then telling her a story. By taking several observations in varying contexts, the SLP derives a fuller picture of the child's relative strengths and needs.

Identifying Goals for Intervention. The completion of a comprehensive communication assessment leads to the identification of appropriate targets for a child's intervention program. Criterion-referenced, dynamic, and observational assessments are central to this aim. The SLP uses these methods to determine for a particular child what skills are next in the normal developmental sequence of language acquisition, and what components and subcomponents of the language system the child has mastered, is using inconsistently, or is not using at all. Observation and language sampling will be used to identify aspects of communication that are most troublesome in preventing the child from effectively communicating with parents, teachers, and peers. Criterion-referenced assessment will be used to fill out the picture of strengths and needs. Dynamic assessment will help to determine what kinds of supports, cues, prompts and materials will be most facilitating for the acquisition of new forms. The end result of this phase of the assessment will be a set of long-term goals that state the desired changes in communication to be targeted over the next 1–3-year period (depending on the child's current age). Each long-term goal will be broken down into a sequence of short-term objectives, which state the steps the child will be led through in order to attain the long-term goal. Short-term objectives typically follow a three-part format:

1. "Do" statement: What the child will do to demonstrate achievement of the goal (James will produce sentences with "I want" and an object ["cookies"])
2. A context: Under what circumstances the child will be able to perform the behavior at this phase of the therapy (when shown a desired object and prompted with "Tell me what you want")
3. A criterion: How frequently the child must perform the activity correctly in order to move on to the next step in the sequence (in 90% of trials)

Monitoring Change in Intervention. Once the basic plan of the intervention program has been designed, the SLP proceeds through each of the short-term objectives. In order to move on to the next step, however, the SLP must show that the child has achieved the criterion level stated in the short-term objective. Further, the SLP will need to document when the long-term goal has been acquired. These require tracking the degree to which the client is producing correct responses within therapy sessions. SLPs routinely record and analyze client responses to therapy activities in order to document these changes. Monitoring change in intervention, however, not only requires that SLPs show their clients can get, for example, 90% correct responses in a treatment activity; they also need to show that these changes generalize to real conversation and interaction. To demonstrate these broader changes, SLPs often use criterion-referenced assessments, as well as language sampling. These assessment methods allow the demonstration of change not only in structured activities, but also in the real-world situations that determine a child's communicative competence.

SUMMARY

The assessment of communication is part of the larger process of diagnostic evaluation and educational planning that goes into determining the strengths and needs of children with disabilities. In conducting these assessments, professionals from a variety of disciplines collaborate to determine a child's diagnostic classification and eligibility for publicly funded services, to describe in detail the child's needs in all areas of functioning, to identify the most appropriate goals for an intervention program, and to monitor the program as it proceeds to ensure it is efficient and effective. SLPs play an integral role as members of the assessment team whose primary responsibility is to evaluate the child's use of communication. They use a variety of methods to achieve these goals, including standardized tests, criterion-referenced assessments, observations of authentic communication, and dynamic methods to identify effective supports for learning.

References

1. Woodruff, G McGonigel, M: Early intervention team approaches: The transdisciplinary model. In: J Jordon, J Gallagher, P Hutinger, & M Karnes (eds): Early childhood special education: Birth to three (pp. 164–181). Reston, Council for Exceptional Children, 1998.
2. Tyler, AA, Tolbert, LC: Speech-language assessment in the clinical setting. *American Journal of Speech-Language Pathology* 11:215–220, 2002.
3. Lord, C, Rutter, M, Le Couteur, A: Autism diagnostic interview—revised: A revised version of a diagnostic interview for caregivers of individuals with possible pervasive developmental disorders. *Journal of Autism and Developmental Disorders* 24(5):659–685, 1994.
4. Wetherby, AM, Prizant, BM: *Communication and symbolic behavior scales: Developmental profile*, 1st normed ed. Baltimore: Paul H. Brookes Publishing Co., 2002.
5. Bishop, DVM: *Children's communication checklist—2*. London: Harcourt Assessment, 2003.
6. Rescorla, L: The language development survey: A screening tool for delayed language in toddlers. *Journal of Speech and Hearing Disorders* 54:587–599, 1989.
7. Fenson, L, Dale, P, Reznick, J, Thal, D, Bates, E, Hartung, JP, et al.: *The Macarthur-Bates communicative development inventories*. Baltimore: Paul H. Brookes, 2002.
8. Sparrow, S, Cicchetti, D, Balla, D: *The Vineland adaptive behavior scales—2*, Circle Pines, American Guidance Service, 2005.
9. Beukelman, D, Mirenda, P: *Augmentative and alternative communication: Supporting children and adults with complex communication needs*, 3rd ed. Baltimore: Paul H. Brookes Publishing, 2005.
10. Merrell, AW, Plante, E: Norm-referenced test interpretation in the diagnostic process. *Language Speech and Hearing Services in the Schools* 19(3):223–233, 1997.
11. Paul, R, Hernandez, R, Taylor, L, Johnson, K: Narrative development in late talkers: Early school age. *Journal of Speech and Hearing Research* 39(6):1295–1303, 1996.
12. Liles, B: Cohesion in the narratives of normal and language-disordered children. *Journal of Speech and Hearing Research* 28:123–133, 1985.
13. Norbury, C, Bishop, DVM: Narrative skills of children with communication impairments. *International Journal of Language and Communication Disorders* 38:287–314, 2003.

CHAPTER 4.2.6 ■ FORMULATION AND INTEGRATION

SCHUYLER W. HENDERSON AND ANDRÉS MARTIN

... (she) took refuge in formulation, presumably in the hope that it would carry her past ambivalence and confusion.

Robert Boyers, 2005 (1)

FORMULATION: PURPOSE AND PLACE

The formulation in child and adolescent psychiatry distills clinical encounters with a child and his or her family into a manageable and meaningful synopsis. It arranges the child's symptoms and circumstances into a specific format and establishes a set of hypotheses about the child, which can then be adapted depending on further clinical encounters and collateral information. The formulation need not be the condensation of a child's life into a single, perfect narrative. Rather, it can be seen as an evolving appraisal and an iterative process, accommodating further information as it is elicited from the child and family. In parallel with an appreciation for the complexities of the process of development itself, the clinician need not view the formulation as static, but as a format that can be adjusted and expanded over time, taking into account the processes of maturation and growth through which the child and family are going. The flexibility of this format reflects the clinician's emerging understanding of a child.

Because treatment options comprise the full spectrum of interventions, including decisions *not* to treat, the formulation must be able to communicate the important information about the child leading to these decisions; explain the rationale for treatment in a clear and concise way; and incorporate new information, new hypotheses, and ongoing assessments of the severity of the child's condition.

The rich history of psychiatric formulations runs the gamut from fragmentary allusions in clinical anecdotes to the most elaborate case studies of Freud and Jaspers. A contemporary clinical formulation would likely avoid some of the more ornamental terms of a classic case study, but the composition would follow a similar trajectory. Throughout the history of the psychiatric formulation, the path has remained fairly steady, signposted by referral source, identifying information, history of present illness, and significant past psychiatric and medical histories (Table 4.2.6.1; see also Chapter 4.2.2). This consistency not only allows for communication between the generations, but permits clinicians to follow a familiar route while attuned to important details and nuances.

Although there is a historical precedent for the overall shape of the formulation, we ought not to be naive about the theoretical work a formulation performs. Tauber notes that in science "observations assume their meanings within a particular context, for facts are not just products of sensation or measurement, as the positivists averred, but rather they reside within a conceptual framework that places the fact into an intelligible picture of the world" (2). The formulation is not a value-neutral format containing dispassionately arranged facts. The choice as to which facts to include and which to reject and the subsequent ordering and presentation of the facts collude to produce a value-laden product.

An obvious example of this is how formulations vary according to clinical circumstances. Certain situations and clinical locations require specific formulations. Encompassing everything from the haiku-like précis and the SOAP note to lengthy descriptive discussions of a patient's life, the formulation mirrors a set of clinical priorities. It can range from the no-nonsense focus of a crisis service where the severity and acuity of a patient's needs must be brought into focus and where biomedical perspectives are prominent, to the developing working model of the inpatient unit, and through to the gradual blossoming of relationships, defenses, and cathexes cultivated and analyzed in a psychodynamic formulation. What each clinical milieu values is reflected in how the child's assessment and treatment will be formulated.

What can a formulation accomplish? It organizes the clinician's interaction with patients into a communicable form that should justify and explain further investigation and intervention. We will examine several formats that can be used to do this, from the biopsychosocial model and the 4 Ps to pluralistic and integrationist critiques of these models. There are, however, two distinct goals of the formulation: *understanding* the patient and *explaining* the patient's symptoms, conditions and concerns (3). We must guard against confusing the one for the other (see Pruett, Chapter 1). In some cases, the depth of our understanding of a patient's experience may not help explain the etiology of a symptom in a way conducive to treatment, and likewise a model of behavior may not adequately impart the patient's experience of that behavior. The various models approach these two goals with different degrees of clarity and transparency.

In this chapter, we cover four ways of conceptualizing the formulation—the biopsychosocial model, the 4 Ps, the pluralist approach, and the integrationist approach. The models are not all mutually exclusive, and the strengths, weaknesses, and compatibility of each will be noted. None of the models was specifically created for child and adolescent psychiatry. Issues such as a youth's rapid, tumultuous, and uneven development (which spans all domains of a child's life) and the centrality of family, school, and peer milieu deserve fuller recognition and integration than originally afforded in these models.

THE BIOPSYCHOSOCIAL MODEL

Developed over the past three decades, the biopsychosocial model is probably the most common formulation used in psychiatry. With its roots deep in the history of medical practice, based on the understanding that the clinician is treating a person and not just a pathology, the model has

TABLE 4.2.6.1

CORE COMPONENTS TOWARD A FORMULATION

Component	Details
Source	Patient, collaterals
Chief complaint	What brought the patient in
History of present illness	Symptoms, course, severity, pertinent negatives
Past psychiatric history	Previous evaluations, therapies, hospitalizations, medications, and treatments; substance abuse history
Past medical history	Treatments, illnesses, hospitalizations/surgeries, medications (including home remedies, homeopathy)
Family history	Pertinent positives and negatives in the family's psychiatric and medical history
Social history	Family constellation, peer relations, interactions with the law, and social services
Education history	Schools, grades, report cards, special or regular education
Developmental history	Mother's pregnancy and labor, delivery, milestones during infancy; stages of motor, cognitive, social, and behavioral development
Psychological testing	IQ, tests of adaptive functioning, speech and language evaluation
Mental status exam	
Assessment	Diagnoses, hypotheses of causality
Plan	Treatment goals and options, collaterals to contact

been successfully adopted throughout medicine. The model is often attributed to Engel, who deserves credit for developing it, naming it, and advocating effectively for it as a "way of thinking that enables the physician to act rationally in areas now excluded from a rational approach" (4). Meyer also merits citation for his "psychobiological" approach (5). Both Engel and Meyer were responding to biomedical advances in medicine and psychiatry—Meyer to the influence of Kraepelin, and Engel to the blossoming of neuropsychiatry in the 1970s—and both sought a balance between what was commonly seen as two warring factions in psychiatry: the psychoanalytic and the biological.

The biopsychosocial model concentrates on three realms of a patient's experience, presenting symptoms and circumstances: the biological, psychological, and social (Table 4.2.6.2). Questions are geared toward eliciting information about each of these domains, and the subsequent formulation is constructed from each one. The biological domain circumscribes neuropsychiatric, genetic, and physiological concerns, focusing on, but not limited to, the functional operations of the brain and what might be directly affecting it. The psychological dimension includes an evaluation of the child's psychological makeup, including strengths and vulnerabilities. It offers the opportunity to note psychodynamic principles like defense structures; consciously and unconsciously driven patterns of behavior; characterization of wishes and desires; responses to trauma and conflict; and strategies the patient has used to resolve these; transference and countertransference (6). The social dimension situates the child in his or her communities, exploring relationships with family and friends, as well as larger collective cultural organizations like schools, religion, socioeconomic class, and ethnicity.

TABLE 4.2.6.2

THE COMPONENTS OF THE BIOPSYCHOSOCIAL MODEL

Biological	Psychological	Social
Genetics	Emotional development	Family constellation
Family history	Response to stressors	Peer relationships
Physical development	Self-esteem	School
Comorbidities	Insight	Neighborhood
Constitution	Defenses	Ethnic, religious influences
Intelligence	Patterns of behavior	Socioeconomic issues
Inborn temperament	Patterns of cognition	Culture(s)

The formulation brings the three domains together into a narrative, arranged according the core components described above. Although the biopsychosocial model may appear to be a neutral mediator between the three domains, it quite specifically is not: It is a considered response to biomedical, psychological, and social reductionism. Regardless of anatomical lesions, or clear psychological or social etiologies, this model insists that all three be accounted for, and in doing so has been a powerful and successful model for physicians in all fields of medicine.

Advocates for the biopsychosocial model argue convincingly that the "broad approach [is] essential to avoid premature closure of our efforts to understand the patient's needs, tunnel vision or an overly narrow approach to treatment" (7). Furthermore, psychiatrists are in a unique position within medicine to minister to the biological, psychological, and social needs of the patient (8), and so are responsible for being attuned to each.

Nevertheless, critics of the model, also convincingly, note that the biopsychosocial model is, as Ghaemi puts it, "silent as to how to understand those aspects under different conditions and in different circumstances" (9). While insisting that medical materialism or psychological and social dogmatism cannot suffice, this model does not guide the clinician on how to weigh or measure the relative contributions of each in any given patient. This results in the so-called "eclectic error," in which the neutrality of the model implies that what works in one area of psychiatry can be applied to all areas.

In addition, the biopsychosocial model does not *blend* the various dimensions as much as loosely knit them together: The model offers very little direction as to how to bring together three conceptually different areas of a patient's life other than through proximity in the formulation. Thus, how the social, biologic and psychological are integrated is left unanswered (10). Some have noted that those who prefer one particular realm can pursue that course while paying lip service to the others in a few short sentences (11). Nevertheless, treating the biopsychosocial formulation as a way of rethinking reductionism and as an opportunity for generating hypotheses about multiply determined etiologies may lead to improved capacity for further synthesis and understanding (12).

A final comment about this model is that even when it is used, the tailing "social" domain is often the least explored (13), either by necessity or by choice. Virchow said that "medicine is a social science," and although psychiatry has a history of collaborating with sociology (14), the intersection of psychiatry and sociology is still underexplored. This is especially true in regard to children, many of whom present to child and adolescent psychiatrists due to some fundamentally social concern, such as impulsivity and hyperactivity in the classroom, conflict with parents, truancy, and school refusal, or other concerns in the realm of externalizing disorders (15). Including the social factors that may be influencing a child's life and symptoms in the formulation is an important contribution of the biopsychosocial model, and it is not necessarily a flaw of the model itself that this dimension is often not given the prominence it deserves.

THE 4 Ps: PREDISPOSING, PRECIPITATING, PERPETUATING, AND PROTECTIVE FACTORS

The second model is the 4 Ps (16). This model organizes the patient's condition into *predisposing, precipitating, perpetuating* and *protective* factors, and with each one comes a mnemonic or trigger question (Table 4.2.6.3). *Predisposing* factors are the constellation of features that render the child vulnerable to the presenting symptoms, such as family history, genetics, medical and psychiatric history, and chronic social stressors. *Precipitating* factors identify current symptoms, diagnostic reasoning about the role of inciting events, and concurrent illness. *Perpetuating* factors are those that make the condition endure, such as the severity of the condition, compliance issues, and unresolved predisposing and precipitating factors. The feature of the 4 Ps that is unusual and exciting is the fourth, *protective*, which looks to describe a patient's strengths, resilience, and supports. Although other models have space for this facet of the evaluation, this is the only one that foregrounds it.

A sample formulation based on the 4 Ps might look like this:

> *A 14-year-old boy presents to an emergency room from school, having been referred by his teacher first to a counselor and then to the ER after writing an essay in which he expressed suicidal ideation.* Predisposing *factors include a mother with a long history of depression treated with psychotherapy, a paternal uncle who committed suicide, and his parent's divorce, with lengthy and often bitter custodial disputes.* Precipitating *factors include three weeks of poor sleep, decreased appetite, rumination about his guilt and helplessness in the context of his parents' divorce, as well as several recent stressors, including a test in school, which he is scared he might fail.* Perpetuating *factors include a desire not to engage in any sort of treatment due to stigma, his parents' denial that their conflicts affect their son, and a depression that has reached such depths that the patient is considering suicide. In his case, though, several* protective *factors can be identified, including the boy's popularity at school as a secretary of the student assembly and as catcher on the baseball team; his willingness to talk with a therapist once he comes in; his parents' care for his wellbeing despite their conflict; and the family's willingness to work together to help the boy through depression.*

Biological, psychological, and social elements can fall under each category. The limitations of this approach include its nonstandard format and an uneasy overlap between categories. There is little consolidation of the many factors except as to how they affect the patient's symptomatology. Nevertheless, it does provide a useful means of organizing a child's symptoms and concerns, and it does so with explicit acknowledgment of its values, such as what in a child's constitution is considered perpetuating and what is considered protective.

The 4 Ps can easily be used in conjunction with other models. For example, they can be blended with the biopsychosocial model (see Table 4.2.6.3). As a framework, they can also be used to organize a psychodynamic formulation, beginning with *predisposing* vulnerabilities, personality structure, and history; *precipitating* trauma or life events; *perpetuating* maladaptive behaviors and resistances; and *protective* facets of the identity.

The 4 Ps can also be used, for example, with the Collaborative Problem Solving (CPS) model (17). The CPS model comprehensively assesses cognitive deficits around frustration tolerance, flexibility, and problemsolving, and it exemplifies a collaborative approach to the formulation, with numerous caregivers coming together to understand the child and then working with the child to prevent dangerous or aggressive behaviors. As the child is also involved in formulating the plan, the 4 Ps provide a concrete way of organizing the different factors that lead to problematic behaviors in a manner comprehensible to staff and patients alike. The CPS approach expands on the precipitating and perpetuating factors, especially the ones pertaining to the child's learning (including social learning). They then allow the staff to formulate appropriate, testable and patient-specific interventions based on observed behaviors and analysis of triggers (precipitating events), continued stresses (perpetuating factors), and strengths that can be tapped into (protective factors). This combination of the 4 Ps formulation and the CPS model may be particularly apt on inpatient units (18).

For the most part, the biopsychosocial model and the 4 Ps are agnostic when it comes to diagnosis: Either can be used to explain and justify a particular diagnostic bent, from biological and psychological to interpersonal and existential. The 4 Ps in

TABLE 4.2.6.3

EXAMPLES OF WHERE THE BIOPSYCHOSOCIAL MODEL MEETS THE 4Ps

P Characteristic *and trigger question*	Biological	Psychological	Social
Predisposing *Why me?*	Genetic vulnerability	Immature defensive structure	Poverty and adversity
Precipitating *Why now?*	Toxic reaction	Recent loss or trauma	School stressors
Perpetuating *Why does it continue?*	Poor response to medication	Poor compliance	Unable to attend therapy sessions because of parents' work schedule
Protective *What can I rely on?*	Family or past history of treatment response	Engaged, insightful	Caring parents and good friends, community and faith as sources of support

particular asks "Why?" but it does not ask "How?" While the models demonstrate that the richness of a child's life may be better captured in a narrative form than a diagnostic category, they nevertheless do not direct the narrative toward a specific treatment plan.

THE FOUR PERSPECTIVES OF PSYCHIATRY

Attempting to provide an alternative to the biopsychosocial model, the four perspectives provide a means of distinguishing psychiatric conditions based not on the conglomerative biopsychosocial model, but on etiology and treatment options (19). The concept of pluralism, defined by Havens as a process of "refining methods, not mixing them," has deeply informed the four perspectives (20).

The four perspectives each come with a treatment paradigm. *Disease*, the keystone of the biomedical perspective, is a clinical entity, a pathological condition with a specific etiology and with a likely prognosis. The treatment for disease necessitates prevention and cure, by interventions that directly or indirectly affect the pathological process and/or symptom relief. *Dimensions* are based on vulnerabilities due to a person's position within ranges of psychological domains (such as mental retardation or temperament). They are addressed with guidance. *Behaviors*, maladaptive or undesirable goal-directed activities, need to be ameliorated, stopped or interrupted, through social, psychological, and/or medical means. The fourth perspective is the *life story*, based on the reconstruction of narratives through talk therapy. Treatment is usually sought due to emotional states of distress and proceeds through interpretation.

Slavney and McHugh point to an essential concern with each perspective: In short, they note the potential adverse effects of each intervention. As they note, all medications can be toxic (have adverse effects); guidance can be paternalistic; stopping can be stigmatizing; and interpretations can be hostile. In so doing, they neatly categorize and foreground matters of continuing importance to child and adolescent psychiatry. In highlighting these concerns and by making the assessment and acknowledgment of potential adverse effects a cornerstone of the formulation, psychiatrists can collaborate more fully with the patient and family, in a transparent and compassionate way (21).

We add to this another category, a "requirement," which we suggest ought also to be included in the formulation (Table 4.2.6.4). For a biomedical cure to be effective, there must be an assessment of compliance: Without adherence to treatment, the intervention cannot succeed. With guidance, there must be a location of patient strength, which the guidance can develop: For example, in working with a patient with mental retardation, intellectual, vocational, and occupational strengths must be assessed. Changing behavior requires a will to change, whether this is intuitive, as in the case of a boy who wishes to stop smoking marijuana and has moved from precontemplation into contemplation, or cultivated through a system of positive and negative reinforcement. And for interpretations to be effective, the patient's insight needs to be appraised.

A formulation based on the four perspectives would take as its conceptual point of origin a conviction about the patient's presentation, which would remain adaptable within the overall formulation, and which would then guide the formulation toward specific interventions. One advantage of the four perspectives is that they make "explicit aspects of reasoning about patients that are often left implicit or vague" (22). The formulation would seek to replicate this. The pluralistic formulation would proceed as the child and adolescent psychiatrist ascertains which categories, perspectives, or dimensions best describe the child's condition; the formulation would then explain how the child and adolescent psychiatrist engages in appropriate, directed treatment, having assessed the requirements and acknowledged the concerns.

The child and adolescent psychiatrist has an array of different diagnoses and treatments, analogous to a quiver full of various arrows: The formulation is a way of choosing the right arrow for each target, whether diagnostic or therapeutic. Which is the best approach for any given situation and which is the worst? For example, the biological approach (the disease model) has a better fit with bipolar disorder, schizophrenia and Rett syndrome than it does with grief. The behavioral approach, which targets known harmful behaviors, may be best for substance abuse (although, of course, medical interventions directed toward addiction as a disease can be countenanced as supplemental). The life story model is geared toward understanding and narrativizing stresses, and so would be more helpful for bereavement after loss or despair associated with stressors or stagnation in life's journey.

Pluralism accepts that there are multiple levels of explanation, and acknowledges that there are currently not enough integrative scientific paradigms (23). As children are multidimensional, it may be appropriate to use several or all of these perspectives with each child: The point is not that they are exclusive, but that each perspective is applied to a specific condition in a thoughtful manner. The question as to how and when to synthesize these various perspectives requires clinical judgment. The ideal is that symptoms and conditions would be targeted with confident refinement and commitment to appropriate treatment options, provided by a clinician with relevant expertise (24). The tools of the trade—whether psychotherapy,

TABLE 4.2.6.4

THE FOUR PERSPECTIVES, ADAPTED FROM MCHUGH AND SLAVNEY

Perspective	Treatment	Problem/Critique	Requirement
Disease What a patient *has*	Cure/Prevention	Medicines can be toxic	Compliance
Dimension What a patient *is*	Guide	Guidance can be paternalistic	Identification of strength
Behavior What a patient *does*	Interrupt	Stopping can be stigmatizing	Will to change
Life story What a patient *wants*	Rescript	Interpretations can be hostile	Insight

pharmacology, or others—ought to be applied in a conscientious and directed way based on appropriate evidence and geared specifically to the condition: One doesn't simply prescribe a course of therapy and a low dose of a medication for every child because of fuzzy notions that psychotherapy and medications tend to augment one another.

Although these assertions are not always practical, the pluralists' insistence on how the formulation should lead to specific, defendable treatment plans is valuable, and a useful corrective to billowing formulations that invariably lead to the clinician's preferred treatment modality.

FROM FORMULATION TO INTEGRATION

The formulation is essentially an integrative process: First, it provides an opportunity for the child and adolescent psychiatrist to consolidate his or her expertise with an understanding of the child; second, it is a format for integrating diagnoses with treatment plans. As the crystallization of the child psychiatrist's understanding of the child, the formulation reveals certain contentious core issues in the field of psychiatry. The formulation also provides the opportunity to integrate some of these longstanding and challenging conflicts, operating in the mode of what Kandel called "complementarity" (25). As one particularly challenging example, the mind–brain problem has not been put to rest, and remains visible in some of the fissures in the formulation (those hinges where psychological and biological and social do not quite fit together). Pluralism accepts this fissure, and insists that we do the best we can, allowing for "differences in understanding mental and brain phenomena [while] not committed to seeking to integrate an understanding of mind and body" (26). Others accept that although there may be different approaches (such as a disease approach or a life story approach), these approaches need not be predicated on the acceptance of dualism (such that disease approaches are for the brain, life story approaches are for the mind, etc.): They seek a nonreductionistic, antidualistic understanding of integration, without being limited to one approach (27).

The field has not reached a point where this can be adequately expressed in the formulation. The roles of brain morphology, neuroplasticity, neuronal pruning, synaptic connection, and genetic expression cannot yet be adequately correlated with complex behaviors, even if current evidence suggests that brain development both results in, and is caused by, behaviors and learning (28). The formulation, however, will be able to reflect this knowledge as it accrues. As such, it does not just reflect the evolution of descriptive powers in the field, but can actually drive that development and play a role in improved classification (29).

UNDERSTANDING AND EXPLAINING

The formulation, as previously alluded to, offers the opportunity to explore the clinician's understanding of the patient and provide an explanation of the patient's concerns. An important difference here between "understanding" and "explaining" is that they require separate tasks and skills. *Understanding* a patient requires an intersubjective appreciation of the patient's experiences, hopes, and concerns, and is acquired through listening, talking, and interacting with the patient (as well as his or her family and others occupying important roles in his or her world). It is these skills that, along with kindness and trust-building, generate an empathic relationship. *Explaining* a patient's symptoms and conditions itself has two dimensions: The *interpretative* task, where psychological, sociological, and neurobiological theories are used, ideally in an explicit and evidence-based manner, in order to locate the contributing factors; and the *explanatory* task, which connects these factors with the patient's experience. Understanding and explanation work in concert. A richer, fuller understanding guides the clinician towards the techniques that will be used for explanation.

There are other areas where the formulation offers reconciliation (if not resolution) between conflicting paradigms, and serves an integrating function. The formulation can be used to bring together the population-based determinants of evidence-based medicine with the individual (30). For example, the formulation may organize the patient's story in such a way as to lead to questions that may be answered in the literature and can expressly articulate how and why the evidence relates to the patient or fails to include the patient (see Chapter 1.7).

The richness of the field of child and adolescent psychiatry, with all its variables, can be reflected in the formulation. In addition to the main theories discussed, the formulation can draw numerous different points of view into the clinical understanding of the child for both explanation and understanding. For example, it would be possible to note and expand upon such diverse ideas as evolutionary perspectives, which seek to organize the patient's experience in a time frame that covers millennia (31). Narrative medicine perspectives seek to prevent reductionism and a cookbook treatment plan by eliciting and recording the patient's own narrative, in order to ensure that the clinician recognizes each patient as a unique person whose story is the most important guide for both understanding and explaining (32); it is an angle that has a healthy history in psychiatry.

Last, but by no means least, the formulation can integrate the individual with his or her cultural context, without which it may not be possible to understand fully the patient (see Chapter 1.8.1). The cultural formulation itself has several core components: the cultural identity of the individual (including self-identified cultural affiliations, languages spoken, and levels of involvement with cultures of origin and host/dominant cultures); cultural explanations of illness (such as local meanings, cultural explanations for symptoms, and idioms to describe illness); cultural adaptations to the environment and stresses (such as specific stresses in the community as well as areas of support in the community, including possible sources of collaboration); and cultural areas of convergence and divergence between the clinician and the individual (33). Attending to this allows for culturally valid assessments on the part of the clinician, but can also be essential in formulating subsequent plans that are acceptable to the patient (34). Culture is everywhere, and children are usually exploring it with vigor. Of all the cultures children participate in, few are more important than the culture of childhood itself. A good formulation will include the child's relationship to this rich culture, including the child's interactions with peers and participation in childhood rituals, and his or her engagement with television, video games, sports, movies, and books.

PARTICULAR ADAPTATIONS TO CHILD AND ADOLESCENT PSYCHIATRY

Although everybody changes over time through experience and with an aging body, most children are caught in a speedy whirlwind of growth and maturation, accumulating language and skills, experimenting with their expanding world, and gaining mastery over various tasks while being introduced to more complicated ones on a daily basis. This process is not straightforward and may be better viewed as a punctuated evolution than as a smooth and even progression; the course charted by the developing child depends on biological factors, family constellation and social circumstances. Nevertheless, a basic appreciation of expected norms can help situate the child and can alert the clinician to delays and disorders.

In light of this, a useful tool for the formulation can be an assessment of the child's tasks in terms of motor, cognitive, and social development, based on models including Piaget's stages of cognitive development or Erikson's tasks (see Chapter 3.1.3). Expressing the child's development in these terms in the formulation will have additional longitudinal value, just as growth charts map a child's physical trajectory.

It is particularly important to note that although child and adolescent psychiatry has offered much to adult psychiatry, and vice versa, the mantra that children are not simply "little adults" is nowhere more true than in the mental health and experience of youngsters. Terminology that is complicated enough with adult patients—for example, "ideas of reference" or "hallucinations"—is even more so with children. The formulation is the venue in which each symptom and each label should be rigorously interrogated. Just as "tummy pain" requires an assessment of location, intensity, quality, duration, radiation, and ameliorating and exacerbating factors, so every psychiatric symptom requires an adequate assessment of quality, duration, severity, mitigating or exacerbating factors (see Chapter 4.2.2). The formulation gives the clinician the opportunity to explain in detail what is meant by these terms.

CONCLUSION

The formulation can be an exciting confluence of ideas, where the philosophy of psychiatry and the values of child and adolescent psychiatrists come together with the patient's experience to create a narrative about that patient leading to treatment. An iterative and adaptive format, the formulation can accommodate different theories and perspectives to explain what is happening to our patients, while we strive better to understand them. Despite all these variables, the formulation need not be either intimidating or cumbersome. The science of the formulation is its hypothesis-generating format, modifiable with new information, in service of causal explanations. The art of the formulation is not instantaneously pinning down the right diagnosis, but rather providing a thoughtful, sympathetic portrait of the child.

ACKNOWLEDGMENTS

The authors would like to thank Vinod Srihari for his helpful comments on an earlier draft manuscript.

References

1. Boyers, R: Many types of ambiguity: The enigma of Ingeborg Bachmann. *Harper's Magazine* April: p. 92, 2005.
2. Tauber, AA: Medicine and the call for a moral epistemology. *Perspectives in Biology and Medicine* 48(1):42–53. p. 44, 2005.
3. Jaspers, Karl: *General psychopathology, volume 1*. Translated J. Hoenig and Marian W. Hamilton. Baltimore: The Johns Hopkins University Press, 1997 [1913].
4. Engel, GL: The clinical application of the biopsychosocial model. *American Journal of Psychiatry* 137:535–544, 1980.
5. Meyer, A: *The commonsense psychiatry of Dr. Adolf Meyer*. New York: McGraw-Hill, 1948.
6. Summers, RF: The psychodynamic formulation updated. *American Journal of Psychotherapy* 57(1):39–42, 2003.
7. Jellinek, MS, McDermott, JF: Formulation: Putting the diagnosis into a therapeutic context and treatment plan. *Journal of the American Academy of Child and Adolescent Psychiatry* 43(7):913–916, 2004.
8. Gabbard, GO, Kay, J: The fate of integrated treatment: Whatever happened to the biopsychosocial psychiatrist? *American Journal of Psychiatry* 158(12):1956–1963, 2001.
9. Ghaemi, SN: *The concepts of psychiatry: A pluralistic approach to the mind and mental illness*, Baltimore: The Johns Hopkins University Press; p. 9, 2003.
10. McLaren, N: A critical review of the biopsychosocial model. *Australian and New Zealand Journal of Psychiatry* 32:86–92, 1998.
11. Jellinek and McDermott, 2004.
12. Freedman, AM: The biopsychosocial paradigm and the future of psychiatry. *Comprehensive Psychiatry* 36(6):397–406.
13. Grunebaum, H: Letter to the editor. *American Journal of Psychiatry* 160(1):186, 2003.
14. Bloom, SW: The relevance of medical sociology to psychiatry: A historical view. *The Journal of Nervous and Mental Diseases* 193(2):77–84, 2005.
15. Centers for Disease Control and Prevention. Mental health in the United States: Health care and well being of children with chronic emotional, behavioral, or developmental problems—United States, 2001. *Morbidity and Mortality Weekly Report* 7;54(39):985–989, Oct 2005.
16. Kline, S, Cameron, PM: Formulation. *Canadian Psychiatric Association Journal* 23:39–42, 1978.
17. Greene RW, Ablon JS: *Treating explosive kids: The collaborative problem solving approach*. New York: Guilford Press, 2005.
18. Greene, RW, Ablon, JS and Martin, A: Use of collaborative problem solving to reduce seclusion and restraint in child and adolescent inpatient units. *Psychiatric Services* 57(5):610–612, 2006.
19. McHugh, PR, Slavney, PR: *The perspectives of psychiatry*. 2nd ed. Baltimore: The Johns Hopkins University Press, 1998.
20. Havens, L: *Psychiatric movements: From sects to science*. Transaction Publishers: New Brunswick, 2005.
21. McHugh, PR: *The mind has mountains*. Baltimore: The Johns Hopkins University Press. 2005.
22. McHugh, PR, Slavney, PR: *The perspectives of psychiatry*. 2nd ed. Baltimore: The Johns Hopkins University Press. P. 293, 1998.
23. Kendler, KS: Toward a philosophical structure for psychiatry. *American Journal of Psychiatry* 162(3):433–440, 2005.
24. Ghaemi, SN: *The concepts of psychiatry: A pluralistic approach to the mind and mental illness*. Baltimore: The Johns Hopkins University Press, 2003.
25. Kandel, ER: Psychotherapy and the single neuron. *New England Journal of Medicine* 301(19):1028–1037.
26. Ghaemi, SN: *The concepts of psychiatry: A pluralistic approach to the mind and mental illness*. Baltimore: The Johns Hopkins University Press. p. 16.
27. Ghaemi, SN: *The concepts of psychiatry: A pluralistic approach to the mind and mental illness*. Baltimore: The Johns Hopkins University Press. p. 292, 2003.
28. Schwartz, JM Begley, S: *The mind and the brain: Neuroplasticity and the power of mental force*. New York: Regan Books, 2002.
29. McHugh, PR: Striving for coherence: Psychiatry's efforts over classification. *Journal of the American Medical Association* 293:2526–2528, 2005.
30. Srihari, V: Evidence-based medicine, clinical expertise and the "tasks" of psychiatry, submitted to *Academic Psychiatry*, 2006.
31. Jensen, PS, Mrazek, D, Knapp, PK, Steinberg, L, Pfeffer, C, Showalter, J, Shapiro, T: Evolution and revolution in child psychiatry: ADHD as a disorder of adaptation. *Journal of the American Academy of Child and Adolescent Psychiatry* 36(12):1672–1679, 1997.
32. Charon, R: Narrative and medicine. *The New England Journal of Medicine*. 350:862–864, 2004.
33. American Psychiatric Association: *Diagnostic and statistical manual of mental disorders*, 4th ed. (DSM-IV). Washington, DC, 1994.
34. Lewis-Fernández, R Díaz, N: The cultural formulation: A method for assessing cultural factors affecting the clinical encounter. *Psychiatric Quarterly* vol. 73: 4, Winter 2002.

SECTION V

SPECIFIC DISORDERS AND SYNDROMES

5.1 ■ DEVELOPMENTAL DISORDERS

CHAPTER 5.1.1 ■ AUTISM AND THE PERVASIVE DEVELOPMENTAL DISORDERS

FRED R. VOLKMAR, CATHERINE LORD, AMI KLIN, ROBERT SCHULTZ, AND EDWIN H. COOK

The pervasive developmental disorders (PDDs) comprise a group of neuropsychiatric disorders characterized by specific delays and deviance in social, communicative, and cognitive development, with an onset typically in the first years of life. Although commonly associated with mental retardation, these disorders differ from other developmental disorders in that their behavioral features are distinctive and do not simply reflect developmental delay (1). Although better definitions of the syndrome continue to be needed, the validity of autism as a diagnostic category is now well established. In addition to autism, various other disorders are included with the PDD class in DSM-IV. These include Asperger's disorder, Rett disorder, childhood disintegrative disorder (CDD), and the "subthreshold" concept of pervasive developmental disorder not otherwise specified (PDD-NOS) (2), The validity of these other proposed PDDs has been more controversial (3). Collectively, these conditions are also often referred to as the autism spectrum disorders (ASDs).

AUTISTIC DISORDER

Definition

The DSM-IV (2) definition of autism was developed on the basis of a very large, international, multisite field trial. This definition retains historical continuity with previous definitions of autism but differs from its immediate predecessor in that age of onset (before age 3 years) is included as a necessary diagnostic feature and criteria are more conceptually framed. Diagnostic criteria are presented in Table 5.1.1.1.

The characteristic social and communicative deficits are believed to be aberrant relative to the person's developmental level (1); consistent with Kanner's original report and subsequent research, social difficulties in autism are a key diagnostic feature (4–6). Complexities for definitions of autism have included the broad range of syndrome expression, changes in syndrome expression with age, and differentiation from other psychiatric and developmental disorders (3, 6).

History

Kraeplin's description of dementia praecox was rapidly extended to children, and the terms childhood schizophrenia and childhood psychosis became synonymous. Early assumptions that all severe childhood disturbance must be a form of schizophrenia were based, in large part, on severity. Kanner's 1943 (4) description of 11 cases of "early infantile autism" noted various ways in which this disorder appeared to be distinctive. These cases exhibited an apparently congenital inability to relate to other people (in contrast to an apparent ability and overconcern with the nonsocial environment); their language (when it developed at all) was remarkable for echolalia, pronoun reversal, and concreteness. Behaviorally, these children engaged in repetitive, apparently purposeless activities (stereotypy), and were intolerant of change. Kanner's use of the term autism was meant to convey the unusual, self-centered quality that his cases exhibited, but it was also suggestive of the autism associated with schizophrenia. Although Kanner's description has been remarkably enduring, early speculations about certain aspects of the condition (e.g., normal levels of intelligence, lack of association with other medical conditions, unusual levels of parental education) proved incorrect (3). The validity of autism was established over the next several decades only, as various lines of evidence became available (3). Autism was included in the landmark third edition of the DSM (DSM-III) (7). The initial definition of the condition in DSM-III lacked an appreciation of developmental change and was modified

TABLE 5.1.1.1

DSM-IV CRITERIA FOR AUTISTIC DISORDER (299.0)

A. A total of at least six items from 1), 2), and 3), with at least two from 1), and one each from 2) and 3):

1) Qualitative impairment in social interaction, as manifested by at least two of the following:
   a) Marked impairment in the use of multiple nonverbal behaviors such as eye-to-eye gaze, facial expression, body postures, and gestures to regulate social interaction
   b) Failure to develop peer relationships appropriate to developmental level
   c) A lack of spontaneous seeking to share enjoyment, interests, or achievements with other people (e.g., by a lack of showing, bringing, or pointing out objects of interest to other people)
   d) Lack of social or emotional reciprocity

2) Qualitative impairments in communication as manifested by at least one of the following:
   a) Delay in, or total lack of, the development of spoken language (not accompanied by an attempt to compensate through alternative modes of communication, such as gestures or mime)
   b) In individuals with adequate speech, marked impairment in the ability to initiate or sustain a conversation with others
   c) Stereotyped and repetitive use of language or idiosyncratic language
   d) Lack of varied spontaneous make-believe play or social imitative play appropriate to developmental level

3) Restricted repetitive and stereotyped patterns of behavior, interests, and activities, as manifested by at least one of the following:
   a) Encompassing preoccupation with one or more stereotyped and restricted patterns of interest that are abnormal either in intensity or focus
   b) Apparently compulsive adherence to specific, nonfunctional routines or rituals
   c) Stereotyped and repetitive motor mannerisms (e.g., hand or finger flapping or twisting, or complex whole body movements)
   d) Persistent preoccupation with parts of objects

B. Delays or abnormal functioning in at least one of the following areas, with onset prior to age three:
   1) Social interaction,
   2) Language as used in social communication, or
   3) Symbolic or imaginative play.

C. Not better accounted for by Rett disorder or childhood disintegrative disorder.

Reprinted, with permission, from American Psychiatric Association: *Diagnostic and statistical manual* (4th ed). Washington, DC: American Psychiatric Association Press, 1994.

in DSM-III-R (8). Unfortunately, while DSM-III-R was more developmentally organized, it proved problematic as it appeared that the diagnostic construct was overly broadened (3). As a result, substantial revisions were made in the DSM-IV (6). Table 5.1.1.2 summarizes historical highlights in the development of the concepts of childhood psychosis and autism.

Epidemiology

More than 40 epidemiological studies have been published; in his review, Fombonne (9) reports prevalence estimates in studies conducted since 1987 ranging from 2.5 to 72.6 per 10,000 with a median rate of 11.3 per 10,000. There does appear to be an increase in reported prevalence over time, although several factors complicate the interpretation of this observation. For example, there is more public awareness of autism, and criteria for the condition have been changed and probably effectively broadened the concept. Furthermore, the lay press and public often equate the notion of "autism spectrum disorder" with more strictly defined autism (10). Other factors accounting for discrepancies include differences in screening and ascertainment procedures, and the size of target populations (with higher rates generally reported in studies with smaller samples). Although an increase in reported rates might reflect an actual increase in incidence, other factors, such as case definition and recognition, are important. Thus, newer studies are more likely to adopt broader definitions of autism. Selected epidemiological reports are summarized in Table 5.1.1.3.

TABLE 5.1.1.2

DEVELOPMENT OF DIAGNOSTIC CONCEPTS: CHILDHOOD "PSYCHOSIS"

Diagnostic Concept	Current Terminology	Originator
Dementia praecocissima	Childhood schizophrenia	DeSanctis, 1906
Dementia infantilis	Childhood disintegrative disorder	Heller, 1908
Early infantile autism	Autistic disorder	Kanner, 1943
Autistic psychopathy	Asperger's disorder	Asperger, 1944
Atypical personality development	PDD-NOS	Rank, 1949
Rett syndrome	Rett disorder	Rett, 1966

TABLE 5.1.1.3

SELECTED EPIDEMIOLOGICAL STUDIES OF AUTISM

Study	Location	Diagnostic Criteria	Prevalence/ 10,000	Gender Ratio (M:F)
Lotter, 1966	U.K.	Rating scale	4.1	2.6
Bohman, et al., 1983	Sweden	Rutter's criteria	5.6	1.6
Ritvo, et al., 1989	U.S.	DSM-III	2.47	3.73
Gillberg, et al., 1991	Sweden	DSM-III-R	9.5	2.7
Baird et al., 2000	U.K.	ICD-10	30.8	15.7
Chakrabarti and Fombonne	U.K.	ICD-10 DSM-IV	22.0	3.8

Data adapted from Fombonne, Epidemiological studies of pervasive developmental disorders, pp. 46–9, in *Handbook of autism,* 3rd Ed, vol. 1, F Volkmar, R Paul, A Klin, & D Cohen, eds. New York: Wiley & Sons, 2005.

Consistent with gender proportion found in clinically referred samples (11), Fombonne (9) reported an average gender ratio across studies of 4.3 males for every female. However, this ratio varies with level of associated intellectual disability, as females are more likely to exhibit associated intellectual disability.

Etiology

Kanner's initial report of the autistic syndrome emphasized the apparently congenital nature of autism, but also noted the remarkable degrees of occupational success observed in the parents of these first patients, as well as evident deficits in parent–child interaction (4). These latter observations were subsequently taken to suggest some role of parental psychopathology in syndrome pathogenesis. During the 1950s and 1960s, considerable efforts were made to remediate the effects of deviant caregiving practices of cold ("refrigerator") parents through, for example, extensive child and parent psychotherapy. Various lines of evidence now make it clear that deviant childrearing practices do not account for autism. Parents of children with autism resemble parents of children with other developmental problems; they do not exhibit specific deficits in childrearing practice. Similarly, early studies showing an association of autism with higher social class appear to be artifacts introduced by ascertainment bias; for example, more successful and well educated families are more likely to seek treatment (9). It is clear that the parents of children with autism may be understandably stressed by the experience of caring for a severely impaired child and may suffer from depression and anxiety.

As the validity of autism became more established, various lines of evidence converged to suggest the importance of neurobiological factors in the pathogenesis of this and similar conditions (3). Although the variety and consistency of this evidence are impressive, neither specific biological markers for autism, nor precise pathogenic mechanisms, have been identified. As summarized in Table 5.1.1.4, individuals with autism exhibit an increased frequency of physical anomalies, persistent primitive reflexes, and various neurologic soft signs, as well as increased abnormalities on electroencephalograms (EEGs) (12).

Neurobiological theories in autism have focused on diverse brain regions (12). Theories have also emphasized various brain systems, with differences in emphasis depending on the focus of the research, e.g., those who emphasize difficulty with complex information processing postulate widespread cortical abnormalities with sparing of early sensory and emotional processes, while those focusing on emotional deficits and social difficulties often highlight the role of the limbic system (12, 13). Clearly, the severity and pervasiveness of difficulties across multiple areas of development suggest that a functionally diverse and widely distributed set of neural systems is impacted (12, 13). However, these affected systems must be discrete, because autism spares certain perceptual and cognitive systems and may, for example, sometimes be observed in individuals with normal IQ or even highly superior skills and talents. Although it is likely that the condition ultimately involves multiple systems, it remains quite possible that the initial insult is relatively circumscribed, with subsequent implications for other aspects of development. Although much work remains to be done, currently available data, including those from postmortem and neuroimaging studies, strongly implicate abnormalities of the limbic system, and circuitry within the temporal and frontal lobes (13, 14).

Neuroimaging techniques have become increasingly sophisticated, with improved resolution and measurement precision, and more functional MRI (fMRI) studies have been conducted (13). Structural MRI studies have suggested a possible role of the amygdala, with most studies suggesting that persons with autism have underactive amygdala activity when performing social perceptual and social-cognitive experimental tasks (13, 14). This is of interest given the connections and functional relationships of the amygdala to both earlier and later sensory processing systems, as well as to areas of the frontal lobe.

One of the best replicated and more intriguing findings to emerge from the structural MRI literature in the past few years is that overall brain size appears to be increased in autism (by 2 to 10%) (15). Brain size is probably normal at birth and it is not

TABLE 5.1.1.4

NEUROBIOLOGICAL FINDINGS IN AUTISM

Increased (peripheral) serotonin levels
Persistent "primitive" reflexes
Increased head size (macrocephaly)
Changes in brain morphology/cytoarchitecture
Failure to activate fusiform face region
High rates of EEG abnormality/seizure disorder

until the later part of the first year of life that brain size becomes abnormally large. By age 2 to 4 years, brain size is 5 to 10% larger than normal, but after this time, growth may decelerate so that by adulthood brain size may be only slightly larger than normal. It remains unclear whether the increase in brain size is generalized or selective, although recent data suggest that enlargement is greatest in the temporal and frontal lobes, and somewhat greater in the white matter than in the gray (14). One theory suggests that white matter volume increases in autism are caused by overgrowth of short-distance pathways, and that there is actually a decrease in longer-range connections. This abnormal balance of connections is believed to contribute in important ways to the autism neuropsychological phenotype, which includes an inordinate focus on details and difficulties with conceptual understanding. Thus, increased brain size might come at the expense of long-range interconnectivity between specialized neural systems, giving rise to a more fragmented processing structure. Consistent with this theory, several functional neuroimaging studies have now shown abnormal patterns of "functional connectivity." This type of reduction in neural integration is consistent with one influential theory that attributes autistic symptoms to a lack of "central coherence," a cognitive processing style that makes the integration of parts into wholes problematic (16).

The best replicated functional neuroimaging finding concerns underactivation during face perception tasks of a region on the ventral surface of the temporal lobe during face perception tasks—the fusiform gyrus (17). Because of the specificity of this area for faces, it has come to be known as the fusiform face area (FFA). (Figure 5.1.1.1)

Nearly a half a dozen studies by different groups have shown that older children, adolescents, and adults with autism have reduced levels of responsivity to the human face in the FFA, especially in the right hemisphere. These data are consistent with an extensive psychology literature documenting performance deficits in face and facial expression recognition in autism (18), and they provide an important key to understanding the core social deficits in autism. Studies now show that this cortical tissue processes a wider range of person-related information, and thus it might more accurately be

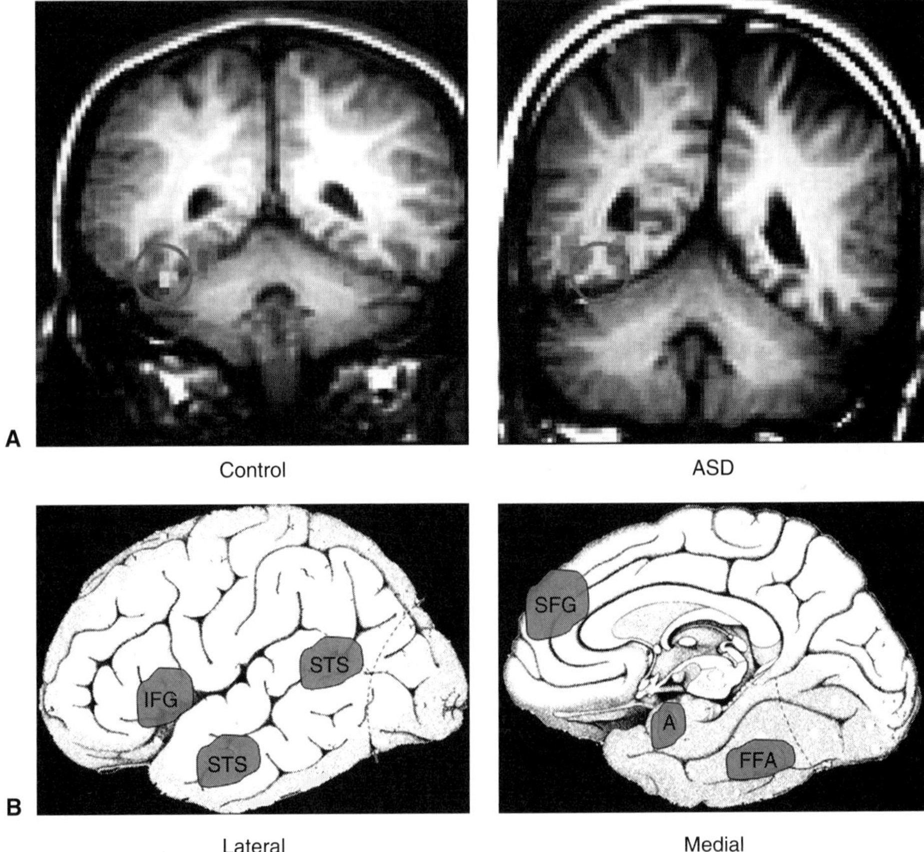

FIGURE 5.1.1.1. Functional MRI abnormalities observed in ASD. **A.** These coronal MRI images show the cerebral hemispheres above, the cerebellum below, and a circle over the fusiform gyrus of the temporal lobe. The examples illustrate the frequent finding of hypoactivation of the fusiform gyrus to faces in an adolescent male with ASD (right) as compared to an age- and IQ-matched healthy control male (left). The red/yellow signal shows brain areas that are significantly more active during perception of faces; signals in blue show areas more active during perception of nonface objects. Note the lack of face activation in the boy with ASD, but average levels of nonface object activation. **B.** Schematic diagrams of the brain from lateral and medial orientations illustrating the broader array of brain areas found to be hypoactive in ASD during a variety of cognitive and perceptual tasks that are explicitly social in nature. Some evidence suggests that these areas are linked to form a "social brain" network. IFG = inferior frontal gyrus (hypoactive during facial expression imitation); pSTS = posterior superior temporal sulcus (hypoactive during perception of facial expressions and eye gaze tasks); SFG = superior frontal gyrus (hypoactive during theory of mind tasks, i.e., when taking another person's perspective); A = amygdala (hypoactive during a variety of social tasks); FG = fusiform gyrus, also known as the fusiform face area (hypoactive during perception of personal identity) (13, 14). (See color insert.)

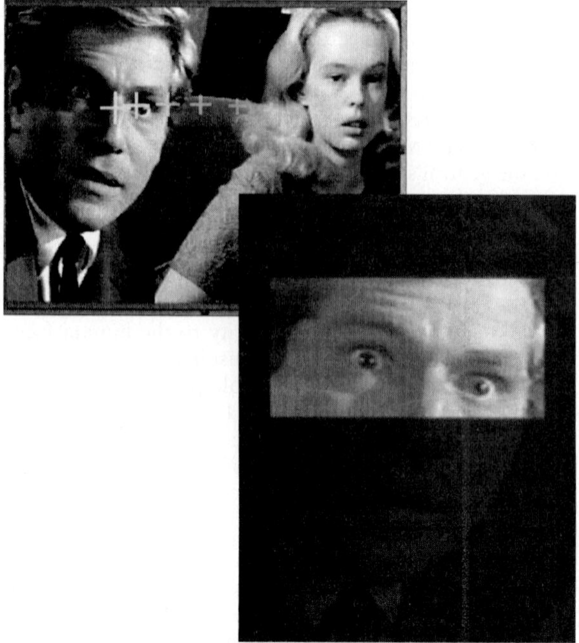

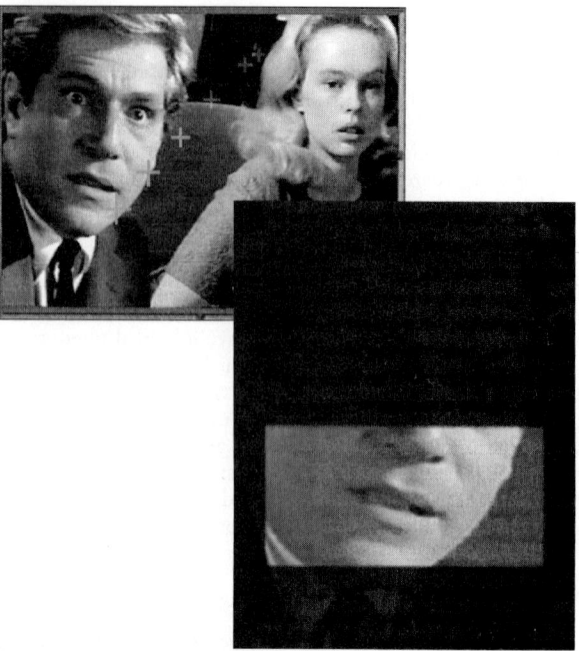

FIGURE 5.1.1.2. Successice visual focus of a typically developing individual (top left) and a person with autism (top right) shown a film clip of a young couple observing a frightening event. The individual who is typically developing focuses on the upper half of the face while the individual with autism is drawn to the mounth region. (Adapted and reprinted with permission from A Klin, W Jones, R Schultz, F Volkmar, and D Cohen. Defining and quantifying the social phenotype in autism. *Am. J. Psychiatry*, 2002. 159:895–908.)

called the fusiform "person" area. This observation may also be relevant to the observation that individuals with autism have particular difficulties in processing certain facial features/information, e.g., the tendency of more able individuals with autism to focus on mouths rather than eyes when they observe social interaction (Figure 5.1.1.2) (19).

Although relatively few in number and sample size, postmortem studies have revealed various abnormalities, including a significant decrease in the number of Purkinje cells and granule cells in the cerebellum, likely of prenatal origin (12). However, early reports of decreases in the midsagittal area of cerebella vermal lobules VI and VII have not been independently replicated in studies that control for age and IQ (13). Postmortem studies also have implicated the limbic system, with decreased neuronal size, decreased dendritic arborization, and increased neuronal packing density of neurons in the amygdala, hippocampus, septum, anterior cingulate, and mammillary bodies (12, 13). These regions are strongly interconnected, and comprise much of the limbic system—a system that supports social and emotional functioning. Orbital and medial prefrontal cortices have dense reciprocal connections with the amygdala, providing the architecture for a system that can regulate social-cognitive processes. A parallel set of amygdala-cortical circuitry in the temporal lobes focuses on social-perceptual processes. One hypothesis is that autism is largely caused by abnormalities in both of these amygdala-cortical loops. These abnormalities are believed to cause faulty social orientation during early infancy (a failure to attend adequately to interpersonal interactions), which in turn cause failures in social and emotional learning, leading to the hallmark symptoms of autism (13).

Animal models of autism have been attempted. For example, lesion studies of the amygdala in nonhuman primates reveal that lesions made just after birth to the amygdala and/or the hippocampus produce some of the cardinal features of autism over the first year of life, including social isolation, lack of eye contact, expressionless faces, and motor stereotypes. However, the specificity of these findings remains unclear, since the lesions are intrinsically relatively crude and the lesioned animals are also deprived of normal social interactions, since they are reared in isolation. Finally, similar lesions in adulthood fail to produce autistic-like sequellae, strongly suggesting that these circuits may only have a critical early role in social learning (12–14).

The role of genetic mechanisms in autistic disorder is suggested by the observation that siblings of affected persons are at a 22-fold or greater risk of autism than the general population and are at higher risk of developing various language and cognitive problems; studies of monozygotic and dizygotic twins have shown an increased concordance for autism in monozygotic twin pairs (20, 21). There presently are promising leads on several chromosomes. It appears that multiple genes are likely implicated.

Although considerable interest has centered on the possible role of environmental agents, e.g., heavy metals or MMR immunization, the available evidence is highly limited (9, 10). Some work has centered on investigation of potential models of autism based on effects of teratogens, e.g., thalidomide (22).

Diagnosis and Clinical Features

Age of Onset. In most cases, the apparent onset of autism occurs within the first or second year of life. Common presenting concerns include delayed language development, social unrelatedness, or unusual sensitivities to the environment. Although Kanner (4) believed that autism was present from, or shortly after, birth, subsequent work has suggested that the disorder sometimes can be observed after some months, or even a few years, of relatively normal development (23). The study of developmental regression in autism has been complicated by several issues, including variables that complicate

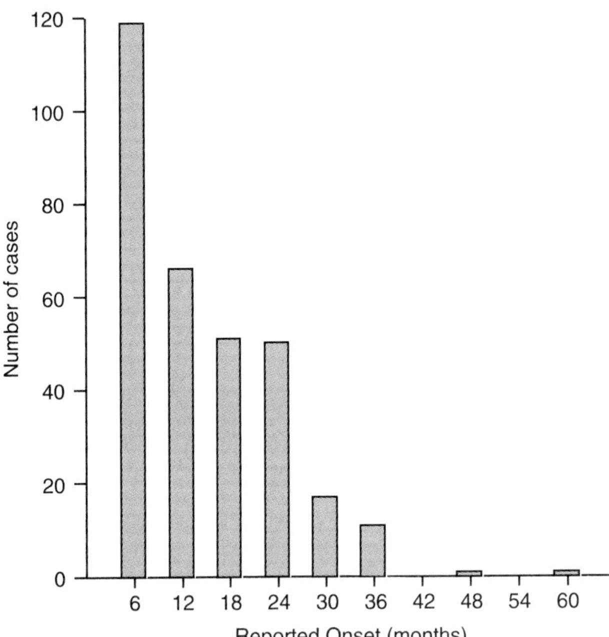

FIGURE 5.1.1.3. Age of onset (cases with clinical diagnosis of autism in DSM-IV field trial). (Reprinted, with permission, from F Volkmar and A Klin, Issues in the classification of autism and related conditions, *Handbook of autism and pervasive developmental disorders*. New York: Wiley, vol. 1, p. 20.)

interpretation of parental reporting. About one-fourth of parents of children with autism spectrum disorders report that their child had a few meaningful words and then stopped talking and/or regressed in social abilities (3). The area of early diagnosis is an important topic for research, since good data indicate that for many children outcome improves with early detection. Figure 5.1.1.3 depicts the onset of cases with clinical diagnoses of autism in the DSM-IV field trial.

Social Disturbance. Autism was initially described by Kanner as a disturbance of affective contact. Social dysfunction in autism is distinctive; it is not explicable in terms of cognitive delay alone and is a, if not the, central defining feature of the disorder (18). Social and adaptive abilities, language level, and nonverbal intelligence are important predictors of independence and long-term prognosis (24). As Kanner emphasized, normally developing infants are remarkably social, even in the first few weeks of life (18). They exhibit an apparent predisposition to form social relationships; this predisposition appears to be an important foundation for the development of other skills. The social development of children with autism is distinctive in many ways. The human face holds little interest for many autistic infants; lack of eye contact, fewer socially directed behaviors such as facial expressions, vocalizations, or pointing, and a lack of interest in other children are typical (18). Early difficulties seen in children with autism include absence or diminution of babbling, failure to respond to their names, and delayed pointing to express interest (not just to request). Deficits in social interaction in autism change somewhat over the course of development but remain an area of great disability even for the highest functioning adults with autism.

Communication. Deficits in the development of expressive language are one of the more frequent sources of initial concern for parents of children later diagnosed with autism. Communication problems appear to be a central aspect of the syndrome. Previous studies have indicated that approximately half the patients with autism never used speech as their primary method of communication, although this number may be decreasing with earlier, more effective intervention (25). Those who do speak exhibit language that is distinctive in several ways, including for use of stereotyped phrases and immediate and delayed echolalia, idiosyncratic language (e.g., saying, "Time for bed, honey" as a request to leave the office), pronoun reversal, lack of usual prosody, impaired semantic development, literalness, and failure to use language for social interaction (26). Immediate echoing (i.e., repeating right back what someone just said) is also observed in normally developing children who are acquiring language and in autism may represent an area that can be used to help build the child's language. Deficits in pragmatic communication, particularly the ability to have a back-and-forth conversation, are typical. The language and communicative deficits in autism differ from those seen, for example, in the developmentally language-disordered child (25, 26).

Cognitive Development. Kanner's initial impression that children with autism exhibited normal levels of intelligence was based on their intelligent appearance and the observation that they performed quite well on certain parts of traditional tests of intelligence; this proved incorrect and many individuals with autism, probably about half, exhibit some degree of intellectual deficiency (mental retardation). IQ scores are relatively stable and predictive of outcome (27), although it is again important to note that with earlier detection and intervention, rates of associated mental retardation may be decreasing (24). Marked scatter in performance on tests of intelligence is common and differs from the usual pattern observed in nonretarded children with autism. Islets of unusual ability (e.g., rote memory or block design) may be present (28). A few persons with autism exhibit truly remarkable, isolated abilities or "splinter skills," for example, in musical or drawing talent, or in exceptional feats of memory, such as the ability to name days of the week corresponding to dates several years in advance ("calendar calculators") (28). In autism, deficits in abstract thinking and in sequencing and processing information are common. Lower levels of intelligence are associated both with a greater risk of developing a seizure disorder in adolescence and with a worse outcome (24). The pattern of verbal and nonverbal (performance) IQ (VIQ and PIQ, respectively) may help differentiate persons with autism (VIQ<PIQ) from those with Asperger's disorder (VIQ>PIQ) (27).

Cognitive deficits may begin to become apparent in infancy (29), and scatter in developmental examination during the preschool years (30). In general, children with autism do best with tasks that involve motor and perceptual–motor skills and worst with tasks that involve symbolic information and verbal skills (28).

Behavioral Features. The contrast between the response of a child with autism to the inanimate environment (seeing the credits flash by on television) and the lack of response to social cues (the voice of a parent) is often quite striking (30). A child may show relatively little differentiation of his sibling from other children, but be particularly attached to an unusual object, such as a spongy puzzle piece. Although parents may initially be concerned that their child with autism is deaf, often the child is quite sensitive to certain nonspeech sounds (the vacuum cleaner or a jingle on the radio). Interest in nonfunctional aspects of objects (taste or feel) and stereotyped (purposeless and repetitive) movements are common and include hand flapping, toe walking, spinning objects, and the like. These observations are quite consistent with Kanner's original report, which contrasted the relative lack of social interest with the overconcern with environmental (nonsocial) change. Such activities appear to be preferred modes of behavior and can consume much of the child's time. Unusual affective responses are also common; a child may become panicked in response to new situations, such as having to walk across a porch to a door, or by regularly recurring stimuli such as singing in church. Play skills are typically quite deviant, accompanied by deficits in imaginative play. These aspects of the disorder are shared with many children without autism who have severe or profound mental retardation, but they appear to be more common in autism and occur even in affected children who have normal intelligence (3).

Physical Characteristics, Pathology, and Laboratory Examination

Over the years, a number of potentially causal medical associations have been reported for autism (31). However, on close examination, many such associations appear weak (32). The strongest connection appears to be with epilepsy; about 20% of individuals develop recurrent seizures, with a bimodal pattern of onset with peaks in early childhood and adolescence (33) (Figure 5.1.1.4). There are also higher than expected proportions of individuals with autism and with fragile X syndrome or tuberous sclerosis (9). Other potential associations include other genetic disorders such as phenylketonuria, maternally inherited deletions (Angelman's syndrome), and duplications of chromosome 15q11–q13 (21). As noted above, overall brain size appears to be increased in autism in toddlerhood, although by adulthood brain size may be only a few percentile fractions larger than normal (15).

As part of a comprehensive examination, it is important to conduct a careful medical and family history (34). Genetic screening, chromosome analysis, and possibly genetic consultation are indicated in the presence of mental retardation or signs of inherited disorders such as dysmorphic features (35). Hearing tests have often already been conducted by the time a child is referred for specialized evaluation; when usual audiologic assessment procedures cannot be employed, brain stem auditory evoked response testing is indicated. Neurologic consultation should be obtained if the child has signs suggestive of overt seizure disorder or other evidence of gross neurologic dysfunction, or if unusual features are present (late disease onset). EEGs may be helpful in such cases (12). Neuroimaging studies may be indicated based on examination and history, and sometimes reveal disorders such as tuberous sclerosis or degenerative CNS disease.

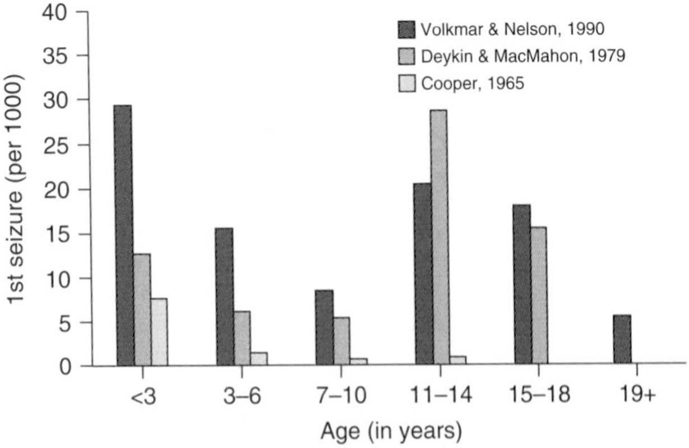

FIGURE 5.1.1.4. Rates of epilepsy (recurrent seizures) in two samples of individuals with autism/PDD (Volkmar and Nelson, 1990 and Deykin and MacMahon, 1979) and a normative British sample (Cooper, 1965). (Data from Volkmar, F and Nelson, D Seizures disorders in autism. Journal of the American Academy of Child and Adolescent Psychiatry, 29, 127–29, 1990.)

By definition, persons with autism have developmental problems in multiple areas of functioning. Level of cognitive functioning establishes the framework for the understanding of other developmental areas, including social, communication, imagination, and adaptive skills, and is critical in differential diagnosis since individuals with autism will display difficulties in social competence that are greatly in excess of what should be expected on the basis of any intellectual impairments (3, 27). Ideally, evaluation should be conducted by a transdisciplinary team of expert clinicians (a psychologist, a speech pathologist, a child psychiatrist, or pediatrician) (27) in order to address essential aspects of the child's developmental skills (cognitive, communication, psychiatric, and real-life skills), as well as other aspects of functioning impacting on learning and quality of life (behavioral challenges and comorbid symptomatology) (36–38). Challenges to assessment include difficulties in engaging affected individuals, the need to employ developmentally appropriate assessment instruments, and the scatter of relative strengths and deficits typically exhibited by individuals with autism. Occupational or physical therapy recommendations can contribute to issues relative to gross and fine motor difficulties and arousal regulation. It is particularly important to approach aspects of psychological assessment, as broadly defined, in a systematic fashion (34). Problems in assessment are often posed by the difficulties in engaging affected persons, by the need to employ developmentally appropriate assessment methods, and by the degree of developmental scatter commonly associated with these conditions.

Intellectual functioning can be assessed by the administration of various standard tests of intelligence or development, with special attention to adequate sampling of the child's cognitive profile (27). Both verbal and nonverbal problem solving skills should be assessed given the frequent discrepancy between the two (typically favoring nonverbal skills in the lower functioning individuals, and at times favoring verbally mediated learning in higher functioning individuals). Typically in autism, nonverbal skills are less severely impaired than more abstract verbal skills, which involve sequencing and coding of information. Given the typical weaknesses in integrative, conceptual, and time-sensitive performance tests, a thoughtful approach to the evaluation is important in order to maximize validity and reliability of results. For very low-functioning persons, administration of tests developed for infants and very young children may be appropriate (27). The assessment of adaptive skills is critical given the virtually universal, large discrepancy between a child's intellectual level and the ability to translate cognitive potential into real-life skills even among those individuals with no intellectual impairment (27). The measurement of adaptive skills is relevant both in terms of documenting degrees of associated mental retardation and for program planning. Speech, language, and communication assessment should include not only formal language skills (such as vocabulary or syntax use) but also language use (25, 26). In very young children, preverbal communicative skills (such as gaze and joint-attention behavior) should be important elements of the assessment (29). Psychiatric assessments should include both direct observations of the child (focusing on presentation of core symptoms of autism) and consultation with parents and schools in order to obtain a broader understanding of the child, as well as of the family and the educational environment (34).

Various rating scales and checklists may aid the diagnostic process but do not replace the need for careful and thoughtful thorough clinical assessment; comprehensive standardized diagnostic instruments are now available that integrate direct observations of the child with historical and other information obtained from parents or caregivers (39). Associated behavior problems and comorbid features are best evaluated in light of

TABLE 5.1.1.5

EVALUATION PROCEDURES: AUTISM AND PERVASIVE DEVELOPMENTAL DISORDERS

1. Historical information
   Early development and characteristics of development
   Age and nature of onset
   Medical and family history
2. Developmental and psychological assessment
   Evaluation of intellectual level and profile of learning
   Communicative assessment (receptive and expressive language skills, use of nonverbal communication, pragmatic use of language)
   Adaptive behavior (ability to generalize skills to real world settings)
   Occupational/Physical therapy assessments as appropriate
3. Psychiatric examination
   Nature of social relatedness (eye contact, attachment behaviors reciprocity, insight)
   Behavioral features (stereotypy/self-stimulation, resistance to change, unusual sensitivities to the environment)
   Language/Communication difficulties (echolalia, presence of communicative speech)
   Play skills (nonfunctional use of play materials, symbolic play and imagination)
4. Medical evaluations
   Associated medical conditions, genetic abnormalities, presence of seizures, additional tests as needed
   Hearing test (if indicated)
   Additional consultation (neurologic/pediatric/genetic) as indicated by history and current examination (e.g., EEG, CT/MRI scan, chromosome analysis)

careful developmental assessments. Table 5.1.1.5 summarizes evaluation procedures.

Differential Diagnosis. Autism and related disorders must be differentiated from other conditions, such as language and other developmental disorders and sensory impairments, particularly deafness (3). Intellectual deficiency (mental retardation) often coexists with autism, and the frequency of autistic-like symptoms increases with more severe retardation (40). Disagreements regarding diagnosis are most pronounced at both ends of the IQ distribution, that is, among very low-functioning and high-functioning persons (3). Discrepancies in abilities (e.g., between verbal and nonverbal skills) should be documented. Because of the multiple areas of impairment, a multiaxial, developmentally based approach of the type advocated in DSM-IV is particularly useful. Specific behavioral features are best viewed in the context of measures of both intellectual and communicative capacities (Table 5.1.1.6). Individual tests and assessment instruments should be selected as appropriate to the individual patient; measures of adaptive skills in communication and socialization can be viewed in relation to overall cognitive

TABLE 5.1.1.6

DIFFERENTIAL DIAGNOSTIC FEATURES OF AUTISM AND NONAUTISTIC PERVASIVE DEVELOPMENTAL DISORDERS

Feature	Autistic Disorder	Asperger Disorder	Rett Disorder	Childhood Disintegrative Disorder	Pervasive Developmental Disorder-NOS
Age at recognition (months)	0–36	Usually >36	5–30	>24	Variable
Sex ratio	M > F	M > F	F (?M)	M > F	M > F
Loss of skills	Variable	Usually not	Marked	Marked	Usually not
Social skills	Very poor	Poor	Varies with age	Very poor	Variable
Communication skills	Usually poor	Fair	Very poor	Very poor	Fair to good
Circumscribed Interests	Variable (mechanical)	Marked (facts)	NA	NA	Variable
Family history—similar problems	Sometimes	Frequent	Not usually	No	Sometimes
Seizure disorder	Common	Uncommon	Frequent	Common	Uncommon
Head growth decelerates	No	No	Yes	No	No
IQ range	Severe MR to normal	Mild MR to normal	Severe MR	Severe MR	Severe MR to normal
Outcome	Poor to good	Fair to good	Very poor	Very poor	Poor to good

Adapted, with permission, from Lippincott-Raven Publishers, Nonautistic pervasive developmental disorders, F. R. Volkmar & D. Cohen, in *Psychiatry*, R. Michaels, et al., eds., Chapter 27.2, p. 4.

skills and also serve a valuable function in guiding remedial programs.

Provision of historical information aids the diagnostic process. The diagnosis of autism is more straightforward when the parents report no history of apparently normal development and when the behavioral deviation is long standing. Less commonly, some period of apparently normal development precedes the apparent onset of the illness. The use of observation scales, parent interviews, and rating scales may be helpful in clarifying diagnostic issues (39).

Course and Prognosis

As with other children, significant changes occur over the course of development (24). However, sometimes not all the required diagnostic features are exhibited until age 3 years; many children with autism do not show clear repetitive behaviors at the age of 2 years (21). By around 3 to 4 years of age, preschool children with autism do exhibit the more classic syndrome picture (41). Delays in case detection unfortunately remain relatively frequent, but greater awareness and better screening and diagnostic instruments have fortunately facilitated early identification of the condition (41). By school age, many children with autism become more responsive socially, develop some response to joint attention (become able to follow a point), and, in some cases, become more socially directed to familiar people (42). Language skills and simple gestures may improve considerably, although other skills may be quite deviant (42). Self-stimulatory and other problematic behaviors, such as self-abuse, also become more common and may be more difficult to manage. In adolescence, a few persons with autism make marked developmental gains; another subgroup shows very problematic deterioration in behavior (44).

Numerous methodologically sound follow-up studies of autism have been conducted (24). With earlier intervention more adults are able to function independently and self-sufficiently, although many continue to require high levels of support. As adults, a majority of persons with autism exhibit significant limitations in the ability to care for basic personal needs, whereas about one-third of these patients achieve some level of personal and occupational independence, with a smaller number of persons becoming able to live fully independently. The two most important predictors of adult outcome are level of intellectual functioning and communicative competence, even though these do not guarantee a positive outcome (24). Persons with IQs in the moderately and severely retarded range and with greater deficits in adaptive skills are more likely to have worse outcomes as adults as are those with very limited expressive language. However, an important trend has been observed: In post-1980 studies, the percentage of persons with better outcomes has significantly increased, whereas the percentage of persons with the poorest outcomes (e.g., living in long-stay institutions) has markedly decreased (24). This observation apparently reflects, to some degree, improved outcome as a result of earlier identification. However, curative claims made by proponents of unestablished forms of intervention on the basis of anecdotal or very small studies are unwarranted, and at this time autism is generally likely to continue to be a lifelong disorder, with an increasing number of children having better outcomes.

Follow-up studies have illustrated some intriguing aspects of autism that remain poorly understood. For example, it is clear that persons with autism are at higher risk of seizures throughout childhood and particularly in adolescence, a pattern quite unlike that of the normal population, in whom the risk of seizures decreases with age (33). A few persons with autism exhibit a pattern of behavioral deterioration during adolescence, whereas another small group appears to improve during this period (24).

Treatment

Given the severity of these conditions and their relatively poor prognoses, it is not surprising that many treatments have been used, including various pharmacologic and somatic treatments, behavior modification, educational intervention, psychotherapy, dietary change, and the like. Unfortunately, until relatively recently, problems in study design and in sample description or selection have made it difficult to assess many treatments systematically (34). Short-term changes may reflect nonspecific effects and be neither sustained nor clinically significant. It is just such changes, which may be associated with various novel and unproven treatments, that are reported, on average, approximately every 6 months in the lay press. Sadly, such reports, usually of amazing successes, are hardly ever rigorously conducted or evaluated (34, 44). One of the few exceptions is the series of studies of the gut-hormone secretin; following initial case and media reports of potential efficacy, a series of well controlled trials failed to show significant improvement relative to placebo (45, 46). The relatively robust placebo response rate in these studies underscores the importance of controlled research in this area.

Alternative treatments are used by many parents—particularly parents of younger children. It is important that parents feel able to discuss these treatments with their physician and health care providers, and that these providers be reasonably informed about these treatments. Potential risks and benefits and the scientific basis (or lack thereof) of such treatments can be discussed with parents (47). These treatments should not replace behavioral and educational programs, which have been shown to be effective. Potential problems, e.g., nutritional deficiencies with restrictive diets (48) should be discussed as appropriate.

At present, the best available evidence points to the importance of appropriate educational interventions to foster the acquisition of basic social, communicative, and cognitive skills (44). Such treatments appear to be improving long-term outcome (24). Appropriate intervention should also provide support and training for parents (44). Behavior modification procedures may be helpful in increasing appropriate and decreasing inappropriate behaviors and may facilitate involvement in educational programming (36, 37). It is clear that early and continuous intervention is highly desirable and has measurable effects on later intellectual and communicative functioning. Educational interventions are best provided on an intensive and continuous basis; the usual pattern of summer school vacations is typically not well tolerated by children with autism and can lead to skill loss (44). Professionals should work with parents to advocate the availability of appropriate educational placements and ancillary services, such as respite care. Because there are often many professionals involved in an evaluation, it is vital that fragmentation of effort be avoided by ensuring that information among professionals and parents is conveyed in a timely and responsible fashion (34). Engagement with persons with autistic spectrum disorders and their families can be lifelong and entails attention to educational interventions, group living situations, and involvement in community-based day and vocational programs, as well as to aspects of family support. Advocacy groups such as the Autism Society of America and similar groups in the United States and other countries have been helpful in this regard; these groups may offer important sources of support to parents as well. Psychotherapy is not usually indicated for children with autism, although it may be useful in higher functioning adolescents or adults with fluent language; in such cases, therapy should be carefully focused on specific goals, whether behavioral or emotional and supportive (34). Cognitive-behavioral therapy that is specifically tailored to the individual strengths and difficulties of the person with an autistic spectrum disorder may be helpful with adolescents and adults, as may social groups that provide opportunities for learning and practice of social skills with peers and relevant to work.

Although none of the pharmacologic agents used in the treatment of autism and related conditions has proven curative, certain medications, particularly the major tranquilizers, have been shown to have an important, if limited role in the management of certain cases (38). The atypical antipsychotics can improve behavioral adaption and significantly reduce problem behaviors and thus increase accessibility to remediation programs (49). Depending on the clinical context and associated comorbidities, other pharmacological treatments may be indicated (50). Patients who receive pharmacologic treatments should be carefully monitored for side effects and sedation should particularly be avoided. Reports suggest the potential usefulness in autism and related conditions of other agents, such as those used in treatment of compulsive behavior (50). Pursuit of unproven treatments at the expense of educational interventions should be avoided (34).

RETT DISORDER

Definition

This progressive condition emerges after some period (months) of normal development. Head circumference is normal at birth and early development is unremarkable. Between about 5 and 48 months (usually before the first birthday), head growth begins to decelerate. As purposeful hand movements are lost, the characteristic handwashing stereotypies develop. Language skills (both receptive and expressive) become severely impaired and marked mental retardation develops. Diagnostic criteria for the disorder are presented in Table 5.1.1.7.

History

The condition was first reported by Rett in 1966 (51), who initially suggested that the condition might be a form of autism. Subsequently others (e.g., Hagberg) collected a series of other cases and it became apparent that the more "autistic-like" phase was generally during the preschool years; after that time the course of the disorder was distinctive (52, 53).

Epidemiology

Studies of prevalence suggest that the condition is observed in between 1 in 15,000 and 1 in 22,000 females (53). Although males exhibit the condition, it likely proves lethal in utero in most cases. An international registry has enrolled several thousand cases.

Etiology

This condition has been shown to be associated with a specific genetic defect in MECP2, a regulator gene on the X chromosome; this defect is present in most cases (54). Rett's original speculation that the condition related to high peripheral ammonia levels proved incorrect.

Diagnosis and Clinical Features

As noted above, early development is normal. Onset may be insidious, following a period of developmental stagnation. As time goes on, the severe developmental delay, head growth deceleration, and lack of interest in the environment become striking. Previously acquired abilities are lost, such as purposeful hand movements. The clinical presentation varies considerably depending on the age of the individual and stage of the illness (53).

Physical Characteristics, Pathology, and Laboratory Examinations

The EEG is frequently abnormal and seizures are common. EEG abnormalities correlate with clinical stages of the illness. Characteristic breathing, movement, and orthopedic problems develop. Cortical atrophy may develop with decreased brain weight and cell loss. Growth problems are common, as are feeding issues (54).

TABLE 5.1.1.7

DSM-IV CRITERIA FOR RETT DISORDER (299.80)

A. All of the following:

1) Apparently normal prenatal and perinatal development
2) Apparently normal psychomotor development through the first 6 months
3) Normal head circumference at birth

B. Onset of all of the following between 5 and 48 months:

1) Deceleration of head growth
2) Loss of previously acquired purposeful hand movements, with the development of stereotyped hand movements (handwringing or handwashing)
3) Loss of social engagement early in the course (although often social interaction develops later)
4) appearance of poorly coordinated gait or trunk movements
5) marked delays and impairment of expressive and receptive language with severe psychomotor retardation

Reprinted, with permission, from American Psychiatric Association: *Diagnostic and statistical manual* (4th ed.). Washington, DC: American Psychiatric Association Press, 1994.

TABLE 5.1.1.8

CLINICAL STAGES OF RETT DISORDER

Stage	Approximate Age	Clinical Profile
1. Onset	6–18 months	Motor growth slows, onset of hypotonia
2. Rapid destructive	1–4 years	Loss of acquired abilities, loss of purposeful hand movements, decline in social communication skills, ataxia/apraxia, breathing difficulties
3. Plateau	2–10 years	Autistic-like features diminish, seizure onset, communication skills may improve, scoliosis and truncal ataxia and apraxia
4. Late motor deterioration	10+ years	Progressive muscle wasting, scoliosis, decreased mobility, cognitive functioning stable, seizures may decrease

Adapted with permission from R. Van Acker, J. Loncola, and E. Van Acker, Rett Syndrome: A pervasive developmental disorder, Chapter 5 in *Handbook of autism and pervasive developmental disorders*, vol. 1, F. Volkmar, R. Paul, A. Klin, D. Cohen, eds. New York: John Wiley and Sons, 2005, pp. 128–129.

Course and Prognosis

The lack of social interest presents some potential for confusion with diagnosis in the preschool years. Typically by the time the child has reached school age the autistic-like features are much less striking and severe mental retardation, motor difficulties, and seizures are observed, even when development stabilizes to some extent. During this "pseudo-stationary" phase, other difficulties include respiratory problems (apneic episodes alternating with hyperventilation), and continued motor difficulties, early scoliosis, and bruxism may be noted. Most individuals remain quite impaired but ambulatory until a final period of motor deterioration. There is an increased risk of sudden death. Clinical stages are summarized in Table 5.1.1.8.

Treatment

At this time there are no specific treatments. Various supportive treatments are used, including special education, occupational, physical and respiratory therapies (54). Caution should be used in terms of medications that may lower the seizure threshold. Support for family members is important.

ASPERGER'S DISORDER

Definition

This condition is characterized by impairments in social interaction and restricted interests and behaviors of the type seen in autism, but it differs from autism in that there is no clinically significant delay in spoken or receptive language, cognitive development, self-help skills, or curiosity about the environment. All-absorbing and intense circumscribed interests as well motor clumsiness, are typical of the condition, but are not required for diagnosis.

Criteria for Asperger's disorder are given in Table 5.1.1.9. It should be noted that these criteria have been criticized as problematic in various ways, and it is likely that changes will be made in future versions of the DSM (2, 3, 55, 56).

History

The condition was described by Asperger in 1944 (57) to describe a group of boys who were verbally precocious but socially quite impaired. Unaware of Kanner's description of early infantile autism just the year before, he referred

TABLE 5.1.1.9

DSM-IV CRITERIA FOR ASPERGER'S DISORDER (299.80)

A. Qualitative impairment in social interaction of the type described for autism
B. Restricted, repetitive, and stereotyped patterns of behavior, interests, and activities of the type described for autism
C. Lack of any clinically significant general delay in language (e.g., single words used by age 2, communicative phrases used by age 3).
D. Lack of any clinically significant delay in cognitive development, as manifested by the development of age-appropriate self-help skills, adaptive behavior (other than in social interaction), and curiosity about the environment.
E. Does not meet criteria for another specific pervasive developmental disorder.

Adapted and reprinted, with permission, from American Psychiatric Association: *Diagnostic and statistical manual* (4th ed.). Washington, DC: American Psychiatric Association Press, 1994.

to the condition as "autistic psychopathy" (perhaps better translated as autistic personality disorder). Although seemingly very intelligent, the boys were quite socially isolated, tended to intellectualize their feelings, and engaged in long-winded conversations about topics of special interest only to them. Asperger (57) made the important point that the latter not only interfered with the child's learning but also intruded on family life (e.g., as the family found itself revolving around the child's special interest). In addition these boys were motorically clumsy and there seemed to be a familial-genetic component, as Asperger noted similar traits in some fathers.

Asperger's report was largely ignored in the English-speaking world until 1981, when Lorna Wing published an influential review of the concept along with a case series (58). Since Wing's paper, various studies have attempted to show the validity of Asperger syndrome apart from autism although controversies, and inconsistencies regarding definition have complicated the interpretation of such studies (59, 60)

Epidemiology

Comparatively few studies on the epidemiology of Asperger's disorder have been published. In his review, Fombonne (9) cautiously suggests a rate of about 4.3 cases per 10,000 children. Boys are clearly more commonly affected than girls.

Etiology

The cause of Asperger's disorder remains unknown, although it is of interest that in his original description Asperger highlighted the familiality of the condition (57). A small body of case reports has supported such associations, as have a few larger studies (59). Differences in method, particularly in definition, seem important in this regard, as the highest rates of family comorbidity are reported if the most stringent definition of Asperger is used; (59) in such instances, perhaps one-third of immediate family members (usually males) have significant social difficulties, and there is an increased risk for both depression and anxiety disorder in other members of the family as well.

There is a possibility that autism and Asperger's are etiologically related (58). This is suggested not only by obvious phenotypic similarities, but by case studies reporting both conditions in different family members (59). There appears to be a strong association of Asperger's with the nonverbal learning disabilities (NVLD) profile, and various etiological speculations have centered on changes in cerebral white matter (61, 62). Overlap with the concept of right hemisphere syndrome/developmental disabilities has also been suggested, i.e., in contrast to autism, where presumed language difficulties are generally left-cortically based (63). The explication of etiological mechanisms in Asperger's disorder and its relation to autism remains the topic of lively debate and research.

Diagnosis and Clinical Features

A diagnosis of Asperger's disorder requires the presence of significant impairments in social interaction (defined in the same way as for autism). These social problems are associated with restricted patterns of interest and activities (often taking the form of highly circumscribed interests). In contrast to autism, by definition there should be no clinically significant delay in language acquisition, or in cognitive and self-help skills.

Although individuals with Asperger's disorder have significant social impairment and are often socially isolated, they often are interested in social interaction but unable to engage appropriately with others because of their one-sided, eccentric social style (56). For example, a child may approach another child and engage in a highly one-sided conversation about a topic of interest. For the older individuals, lack of social sensitivity may lead to innumerable social gaffes, e.g., as the individual makes true, but highly inappropriate comments, about their conversational partner's appearance of vulnerabilities. As a result, individuals with Asperger's disorder are often chronically frustrated and appear to be at increased risk for depression in adolescence (64). Asperger noted the "professorial" and "pedantic" style that often characterizes social interaction (57). Often an attempt to apply rigid rules for social interaction leads to behavioral rigidity and a rather formal, perfectionistic style (56).

By definition, early language in Asperger's disorder is not delayed. In his original description, Asperger emphasized that often children with the condition talked before they walked, or that words were the child's lifeline (57). On the other hand, major difficulties in *communication* are typical, i.e., even though vocabulary and syntax are spared, the child has major problems with the social use of language. In addition, differences in prosody (the musical aspects of speech) are common, with a restricted intonation pattern (65). There may be failure to modulate volume to the situation, or the person may speak too quickly. In addition, there may be little censoring of speech, i.e., what is thought becomes what is said—this leads to major difficulties in adolescence (e.g., relative to sexuality) and may suggest the presence of a thought disorder. For example, the adolescent may make an explicit sexual request to a peer, not understanding the many social (and nonverbal) steps leading up to physical intimacy. The one-sided monologue the person engages in, e.g., about their special interest, may give an eccentric and distinctly odd quality to conversation, as there is a failure to adopt the needs of the conversational partner or respond to social cues. As Asperger emphasized, marked verbosity is often present as the person focuses in great detail and at great length on their topic of special interest.

Although not technically required for the diagnosis, the usual form of restricted interest in Asperger disorder centers around collecting a body of information about a specific, sometimes very esoteric, topic, e.g., weather, the stock market, the operas of Wagner, telegraph line pole insulators, deep fat fryers. Although the topic may change over time, it tends to dominate the individual's life and conversation; Asperger pointed out that often the family discovers that the family's life begins to revolve around the special interest. In childhood it may sometimes be difficult to distinguish such interests from more normal developmental phenomena; the key issue in such instances is whether the interest interferes with functioning and/or is disruptive of the child's development (66). An example of such an interest is presented in Table 5.1.1.10 and Figure 5.1.1.5.

Physical Characteristics, Pathology, and Laboratory Examinations

Although not required for a diagnosis in DSM-IV, motor delays and clumsiness are often present, involving both gross and fine motor activities. The individual may be late in walking and in mastering motor milestones. Handwriting, drawing and fine-motor and visual-motor tasks may be difficult. There may be an unusual posture and gait (56).

In contrast to autism, psychological testing often indicates a pattern in which verbal skills are much stronger than nonverbal, and the nonverbal learning disabilities profile is more frequent (67), with relative strengths in auditory and verbal skills and rote learning, and significant deficits in visual-motor, visual-perceptual skills and conceptual learning. Case reports

TABLE 5.1.1.10

AUTOBIOGRAPHICAL STATEMENT OF A 10 YEAR OLD BOY WITH ASPERGER DISORDER*

My name is Robert Edwards. I am an intelligent, unsociable but adaptable person. I would like to dispel any untrue rumors about me. I cannot fly. I cannot use telekinesis. My brain is not large enough to destroy the entire world when unfolded. I did not teach my long haired guinea pig, Chronos, to eat everything in sight (that is the nature of the long haired guinea pig).
*Name changed. Reprinted, with permission, from Volkmar, Klin, Schultz, Rubin, & Bronen, Asperger's disorder: Clinical case conference. *American Journal of Psychiatry, 157*(2), 262–67, 2000.

have appeared in which Asperger disorder has been associated with specific abnormalities in the right hemisphere (66).

Course and Prognosis

Given the relative recency with which this condition has been included in DSM, it is not surprising that followup and longitudinal data are relatively limited. Clearly, most individuals with the condition can attend regular school and profit from supports around social and communication skills. Asperger's original report (57) was relatively optimistic about longer term outcome, partly because he emphasized the apparent familiarity of the condition. It does appear that in comparison to autism, outcome in Asperger disorder is significantly better, e.g., in terms of adult capacity for personal independence, self-sufficiency, and for marriage (56).

The issue of comorbidity of Asperger's disorder with other conditions has been repeatedly raised. In childhood, significant attentional problems may be present (68). Overactivity, sometimes associated with verbosity, may sometimes lead incorrectly to a diagnosis of bipolar disorder. In adolescents and adults there has been a suggestion, based on case reports, of increased risk of psychosis, particularly schizophrenia (64). However, there is clear potential for misdiagnosis, and it remains unclear whether this risk is greater than that in the general population (56). Depression appears to be the most frequent comorbid condition in adolescents and adults (56).

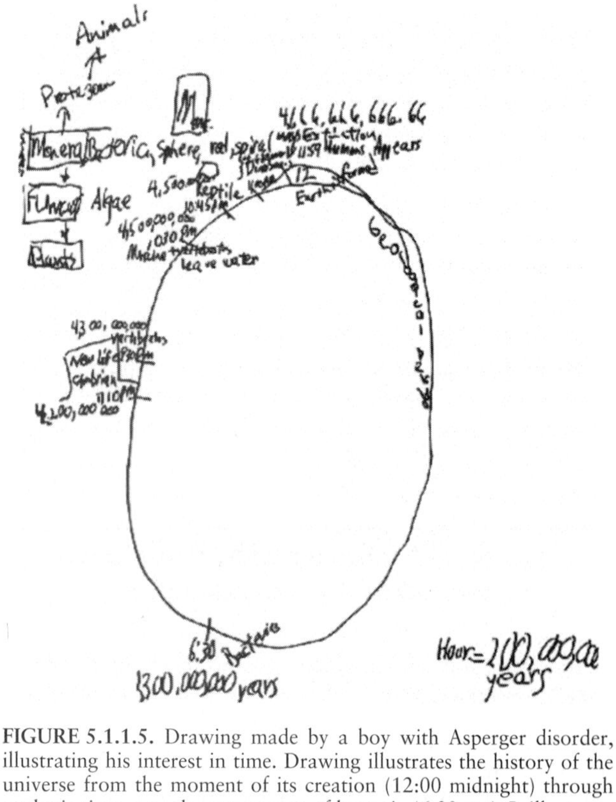

FIGURE 5.1.1.5. Drawing made by a boy with Asperger disorder, illustrating his interest in time. Drawing illustrates the history of the universe from the moment of its creation (12:00 midnight) through geologic time, e.g., the appearance of bacteria (6:30 AM). It illustrates the patient's profound interest (and knowledge) regarding this topic, which tended to be all-encompassing, as well as his less developed fine motor abilities. (Reprinted, with permission, from F Volkmar, A Klin, R Schultz, E Rubin, and R Bronen. Asperger's Disorder. Clinical Case Conference. *American Journal of Psychiatry*, 157(2), 262–67, 2000.)

Treatment

Treatment is symptomatic and shares many similarities with that used for individuals with autism. One major point of exception has to do with the relative (or quite marked) preservation of verbal abilities in Asperger's disorder. Given such sparing, often verbal mediation can be extremely helpful as a modality for intervention through specific teaching, counseling, and so forth (56). Academic strengths can be capitalized on as well, whenever possible. Areas of weakness (social skills, fine motor and gross motor problems) should be addressed (56).

The individual's pattern of strengths and weaknesses should inform the intervention program. For example, use of verbal scripts and routines may be helpful in conjunction with explicit teaching. The tendency to rely rigidly on rules and routines can be used adaptively in programs. Specific strategies in dealing with problem situations can be taught verbally. Teaching should emphasize a parts-to-whole approach, with explicit teaching of social nuance; nothing should be taken as assumed. Role-playing, homework, and supportive psychotherapy can be extremely helpful (56).

Despite what appear to be good verbal abilities, the support of a speech-communication specialist can be extremely helpful. Similarly, use of laptops and organization aids can help individuals circumvent fine motor difficulties and problems with organization and forward planning (executive function). Many individuals with Asperger's disorder can be helped to attend college and achieve vocational independence (56).

CHILDHOOD DISINTEGRATIVE DISORDER

Definition

This rare condition is characterized by development of an "autistic-like" picture and a marked regression following some

TABLE 5.1.1.11

DSM-IV CRITERIA FOR CHILDHOOD DISINTEGRATIVE DISORDER (299.10)

A. Apparently normal development for at least the first 2 years, as manifested by the presence of age-appropriate verbal and nonverbal communication, social relationships, play, and adaptive behavior
B. Clinically significant loss of previously acquired skills in at least two of the following areas:
   1) Expressive or receptive language
   2) Social skills or receptive language
   3) Bowel or bladder control
   4) Play
   5) Motor skills
C. Abnormalities of functioning in at least two of the following areas:
   1) Qualitative impairment in social interaction (e.g., impairment in nonverbal behaviors, failure to develop peer relationships, lack of social or emotional reciprocity);
   2) Qualitative impairments in communication (e.g., delay or lack of spoken language, inability to initiate or sustain a conversation, stereotyped and repetitive use of language, lack of varied make-believe play);
   3) Restricted repetitive and stereotyped patterns of behavior, interests and activities, including motor stereotypes and mannerisms.
D. Not better accounted for by another specific pervasive developmental disorder or by schizophrenia

Reprinted, with permission, from American Psychiatric Association: Diagnostic and statistical manual (4th ed.). Washington, DC: American Psychiatric Association Press, 1994.

period (years) of normal development (69). Criteria for the condition are presented in Table 5.1.1.11.

History

The condition was first described by Heller in 1908. The term has also been described as disintegrative psychosis or Heller's syndrome. Although quite rare, the condition also has been underrecognized. The condition was not included in either DSM-III or DSM-III-R, on the assumption that the condition was almost always the function of some identifiable medical condition, but review of cases has not supported this (3, 69). Furthermore, in general, the child loses skills and then development stabilizes and the outcome appears to be significantly worse than for autism (69).

Epidemiology

The condition is clearly rare. In their recent review, Volkmar and colleagues report data from 173 cases reported since 1908 (69). Prevalence estimates in the range of approximately 1 per 100,000 children have been suggested. Males are more likely to be affected.

Etiology

Various lines of evidence suggest the importance of neurobiological factors in pathogenesis. There are high rates of EEG abnormality, and seizure disorders are sometimes observed. The condition has been associated with various general medical conditions (Table 5.1.1.12), and while an intensive search for such conditions is always indicated, they are not usually found. Given the highly distinctive pattern of onset, a search for potential genetic factors is clearly indicated.

Diagnosis and Clinical Features

By definition, early development is normal up to at least age 2 years. The onset of the condition can be either gradual or more acute, usually with an onset between ages 3 and 4 years. Skills must be lost in at least two areas (usually more than two are affected), including communication, social interaction,

TABLE 5.1.1.12

GENERAL MEDICAL CONDITIONS ASSOCIATED WITH REGRESSION

Landau-Kleffner syndrome (acquired aphasia with epilepsy)	Hypothyroidism
Neurolipidoses	Addison-Schilder disease
Angelman syndrome	Lipofuscinoisis
Mitochondrial deficitis (Leigh disease)	Seizure disorder
Metachromatic leukodystrophy	Gangliosidoses
Aminoacidopathies (e.g., PKU)	Subacute sclerosising panencephalitic
CNS infection	

Adapted from Volkmar, et al., Childhood Disintegrative Disorder, Table 3.2, page 76, in vol. 1 *Handbook of autism*, 3rd ed., Volkmar, Paul, Klin, & Cohen, Eds., 2005. For additional disorders see Neurodegenerative diseases of infancy and childhood, Dyken and Krawiecki, *Annals of Neurology*, 13, 351–64, 1983.

TABLE 5.1.1.13

CHARACTERISTICS OF DISINTEGRATIVE DISORDER CASES*

Variable	Cases 1908–1975	Cases 1977–1995	Cases 1996–2004
	N = 48	N = 58	N = 67
Sex ratio	Male/Female	Male/Female	Male/Female
	35/12	49/9	53/14
Age at onset (years)	X s.d.	X s.d.	X s.d.
	3.42 1.12	3.32 1.42	3.21 0.97
Age at followup	X s.d.	X s.d.	X s.d.
	8.67 4.14	10.88 5.98	10.25 4.81
Symptoms	% of N cases	% of N cases	% of N cases
Speech deterioration/loss	100 47	100 58	100 54
Social disturbance	100 43	98 57	100 54
Stereotypy/resistance to change	100 38	85 54	68 54
Overactivity	100 42	77 37	59 54
Affective symptoms/anxiety	100 17	78 38	55 54
Deterioration self help skills	94 33	82 49	66 54

* Reprinted from Volkmar et al., Childhood disintegrative disorder, Table 3.1 p. 74, *Handbook of autism,* 3rd ed, vol. 1, 2005. Data adapted, with permission, from Volkmar FR: Childhood Disintegrative Disorders: Issues for DSM-IV, *J Aut Devel Dis* 22:625–642, 1992 and Volkmar FR et al.: Childhood disintegrative disorder, in *Handbook of autism*, 2nd ed. Additional cases based on case series reported by Kurita et al. 1994; Malhotra and Gupta, 2002; Mourdisen et al., 2000 with additional cases supplied by Christopher Gillberg and Fred Volkmar.

toileting, or motor abilities. Parents may report a period of anxiety or agitation prior to onset. Once the condition is established it closely resembles autism. Characteristic social and communication problems (of the type seen in autism) are universal. Stereotyped movements and overactivity are common features, as are loss of adaptive/self-help abilities and nonspecific anxiety/overactivity—see Table 5.1.1.13 for a summary of clinical features.

Physical Characteristics, Pathology, and Laboratory Examinations

A careful search for associated medical conditions is always indicated (34, 35, 69), although typically this is negative. Some of the medical conditions associated with developmental loss are listed in Table 5.1.1.12. In the syndrome of acquired aphasia with epilepsy (Landau-Kleffner syndrome) social interest is preserved and an aphasia is present; nonverbal skills are typically present. Findings on physical examination or history (including family history) may be helpful in guiding additional assessments.

Course and Prognosis

In about 75% of cases the child's behavior deteriorates and then stabilizes—with no further deterioration but minimal recovery (69). Sometimes significant recovery occurs, although this is uncommon. In instances associated with a general medical condition or progressive neuropathological process, deterioration continues. Unless associated with such a condition, life expectancy is presumed normal. Unfortunately the outcome appears to be worse than that in autism (70).

Differential diagnosis: Usually children with autism exhibit delayed speech and/or social difficulties with no clear history of regression. Occasionally children with autism exhibit some regression (or period of developmental stagnation) after some limited verbal skills develop (23). For CDD, early development should be clearly normal through at least two years of age. In some instances differentiation from autism may be difficult and it is possible that some cases with very early regression may be difficult to differentiate. In contrast to Rett disorder, head growth does not slow and the unusual hand washing/wringing movements are not present. There may be some potential for confusion with early onset childhood schizophrenia, although in the latter condition the more frequent autistic features do not usually develop (69).

Treatment

Behavioral and educational interventions of the type used in autism are indicated (69). The focus should be on helping the child relearn basic skills. Pharmacological treatments may help with specific symptoms but are not curative.

PERVASIVE DEVELOPMENTAL DISORDER NOT OTHERWISE SPECIFIED

The term pervasive developmental disorder not otherwise specified (PDD-NOS) and the equivalent term, atypical autism, in ICD-10 (71), refers to a residual category for individuals with difficulties suggestive of an autism/autism spectrum diagnosis but who do not meet specific criteria for autism or another more explicitly defined condition in this group.

Historically this concept has some overlap with Rank's term "atypical personality development" (72). As a practical matter, the term refers to a relatively large group (probably about 1 in 150 children) of individuals with problems in social interaction and either communication or restricted interests and behaviors (3, 9). By definition in DSM-IV-TR, some problem should be present in the social area.

There is clearly considerable heterogeneity within this condition. Various attempts have been made to define specific subgroups/subtypes, e.g., individuals with greater attentional difficulties (73) or with social problems associated with complex profiles of affective symptoms (74). As noted in a recent review (75), the lack of research on this condition and its subtypes is unfortunate and, given their frequency, somewhat paradoxical. In at least some instances the disorder presumably reflects some manifestation of the broader phenotype of autism and related conditions (76) and hence may be important to study relative to genetic mechanisms. It is likely that the study of genetic mechanisms in autism will shed some light on potential subgroups/subtypes in PDD-NOS in the future.

Children with PDD-NOS often exhibit unusual sensitivities and atypical affective responses (of the type often seen in autism), but with better cognitive and language abilities. Although some clinicians tend to equate the concept of Asperger disorder and PDD-NOS data from the DSM-IV field trial noted, there are important areas of difference, e.g., with more severe social difficulties in individuals with Asperger disorder (6). As a practical matter, many of the interventions appropriate to individuals with autism readily can be applied. Although it can be a source of frustration from parents to learn that their child has PDD-NOS (rather than autism) it is the case that outcome is almost certainly better (24).

SUMMARY AND DIRECTIONS FOR FUTURE RESEARCH

Considerable progress in understanding the biological bases of autism has occurred over the past decade. As a result of increased interest, research funding and productivity have significantly increased (77). As a result of early diagnosis and treatment, the outcome for autism is improving. While research on autism is well established, knowledge regarding the other PDDs remains more limited.

Longitudinal studies have made it clear that the term infantile autism was, in many ways, a misnomer, since infants grow up to be adults. Studies of adults with all the PDDs remain relatively uncommon; an entire generation or two of individuals with Asperger's disorder were, essentially, missed. Studies of special groups are needed (e.g., children with regression and those who fail positively to treatment) (77).

Newer diagnostic techniques, such as positron emission tomography and functional magnetic resonance imaging scanning, may help to elucidate underlying pathophysiologic mechanisms. The study of specific subgroups (e.g., childhood disintegrative disorder) may be particularly appropriate to for such research. Genetic studies remain an area of very high priority (77). It is quite possible that the final behavioral syndrome known as autism may well represent the effects of multiple insults on the developing CNS acting through different pathways, and it will be critical to consider genetic work on specific endophenotypes in this regard. The explication of underlying CNS substrates for social behavior is a very active area of current work (78). The development of testable hypothesized mechanisms of CNS dysfunction will significantly advance our understanding of these complex disorders; the discovery of specific genes holds the promise for developing better animal models and increasing our understanding of how genetic risk is expressed in the developing brain and in behavior (78).

References

1. Rutter M: Diagnosis and definition of childhood autism. *J Autism Child Schizophr* 8(2):139–61 1978.
2. American Psychiatric Association, (2000): *Diagnostic and statistical manual.* (4th ed.) (Text revision). Washington, DC: APA Press.
3. Volkmar F, Klin A: Issues in classification of autism and related conditions, In: *Handbook of autism and pervasive developmental disorders*, vol. 1. Volkmar F, Klin A, Paul R, Cohen D (eds): New York, Wiley, 2005, pp. 5–41.
4. Kanner L: Autistic disturbances of affective contact. *Nervous Child* 1943; 2:217–250.
5. Siegel B, Vukicevic J, Elliott GR, Kraemer HC: The use of signal detection theory to assess DSM-III-R criteria for autistic disorder. *J Am Acad Child Adolesc Psychiatry* 28(4):542–8, 1989.
6. Volkmar FR, Klin A, Siegel B, Szatmari P, Lord C, Campbell M, et al.: Field trial for autistic disorder in DSM-IV. *American Journal of Psychiatry* 151(9):1361–7, 1994.
7. American Psychiatric Association (1980): *Diagnostic and statistical manual.* Washington, DC: APA Press.
8. American Psychiatric Association (1987): *Diagnostic and statistical manual.* Washington, DC: APA Press.
9. Fombonne E: Epidemiological studies of pervasive developmental disorders, In: *Handbook of autism and pervasive developmental disorders*, vol. 1. Volkmar FR, Klin A, Paul R, Cohen DJ (eds): Hoboken, Wiley, 2005, pp. 42–69.
10. Wing L, Potter D: The epidemiology of autistic spectrum disorders: Is the prevalence rising? *Mental Retardation & Developmental Disabilities Research Reviews* 8(3):151–61, 2002.
11. Lord C, Schopler E, Revicki D: Sex differences in autism. *J Autism Dev Disord* 12(4):317–30, 1982.
12. Minshew NJ, Sweeney JA, Bauman ML, Webb SJ: Neurologic aspects of autism, in *Handbook of autism and pervasive developmental disorders*, vol. 1. Volkmar FR, Klin A, Paul R, Cohen DJ. (eds): Hoboken, Wiley, 2005, pp. 453–72.
13. Schultz RT, Robbins DL: Functional neuroimaging studies of autism: Spectrum disorders, in *Handbook of autism and pervasive developmental disorders*, vol. 1. Volkmar FR, Klin A, Paul R, Cohen DJ (eds): Hoboken, Wiley, 2005, pp. 515–33.
14. Schultz RT: Developmental deficits in social perception in autism: The role of the amygdala and fusiform face area. *International Journal of Developmental Neuroscience* 23(2–3):125–41, 2005.
15. Courchesne E, Redcay E, Kennedy DP: The autistic brain: Birth through adulthood. *Current Opinion in Neurology* 17(4):489–96, 2004.
16. Happe F: The weak central coherence account of autism, in *Handbook of autism and pervasive developmental disorders*, vol. 1. Volkmar FR, Klin A, Paul R, Cohen DJ (eds): Hoboken, Wiley, 2005, pp 640–49.
17. Schultz RT, Gauthier I, Klin A, Fulbright RK, Anderson AW, Volkmar F: Abnormal ventral temporal cortical activity during face discrimination among individuals with autism and Asperger syndrome. *Archives of General Psychiatry* 57(4):331–40, 2000.
18. Carter AS, Davis NO, Klin A, Volkmar FR: Social development in autism, in *handbook of autism and pervasive developmental disorders*, vol. 1. Volkmar FR, Klin A, Paul R, Cohen DJ. (eds): Hoboken, NJ, Wiley, 2005, pp. 312–34.
19. Klin A, Jones W, Schultz R, Volkmar F, Cohen D: Defining and quantifying the social phenotype in autism. *American Journal of Psychiatry.* 2002; 159(6):895–908.
20. Rutter M: Genetic influences and autism, in *Handbook of autism and pervasive developmental disorders*, vol. 1. Volkmar FR, Klin A, Paul R, Cohen DJ (eds): Hoboken, Wiley, pp. 425–52, 2005.
21. Veenstra-VanderWeele J, Cook EH, Jr.: Molecular genetics of autism spectrum disorder. *Molecular Psychiatry* 9(9):819–32, 2004.
22. Filipek, P: Medical conditions associated with autism. In: *Handbook of Autism and Pervasive Developmental Disorders*, F. R. Volkmar, R. Paul, A. Klin, & D. Cohen (Eds.), 3rd edition, (pp. 534–581). Hoboken: Wiley (2005).
23. Luyster R, Richler J, Risi S, Hsu W-L, Dawson G, Bernier R, et al.: Early regression in social communication in autism spectrum disorders: A CPEA study. *Developmental Neuropsychology* 27(3):311–36, 2005.
24. Howlin P: Outcomes in autism spectrum disorders, in *Handbook of autism and pervasive developmental disorders*, vol. 1. Volkmar FR, Klin A, Paul R, Cohen DJ (eds): Hoboken, Wiley, 2005, pp. 201–22 23. 23. Lord C: Follow-up of two-year-olds referred for possible autism. *J Child Psychol Psychiatry* 1995; 36(8):1365–82.
25. Tager-Flusberg H, Paul R, Lord C: Language and communication in autism, In: *Handbook of autism and pervasive developmental disorders*, vol. 1. Volkmar FR, Klin A, Paul R, Cohen DJ (eds): Hoboken, Wiley, 2005, pp. 335–64.
26. Paul R, Sutherland D: Enhancing early language in children with autism spectrum disorders, in *Handbook of autism and pervasive developmental disorders*, vol 2. Volkmar FR, Klin A, Paul R, Cohen DJ (eds): Hoboken, Wiley, 2005, pp. 946–76.
27. Klin A, Saulnier C, Tsatsanis K, Volkmar FR: Clinical evaluation in autism spectrum disorders: Psychological assessment within a transdisciplinary framework, In: *Handbook of autism and pervasive developmental disorders*, vol. 2. Volkmar FR, Klin A, Paul R, Cohen DJ (eds): Hoboken, Wiley, 2005, pp. 772–98.
28. Hermelin B: *Bright splinters of the mind: A personal story of research with autistic savants*, London, Jessica Kingsley, 2001.
29. Chawarska K, Volkmar F: Autism in infancy and early childhood. In: *Handbook of autism and pervasive developmental disorders.* Volkmar F, Klin A, Paul R, Cohen DJ (eds): New York, Wiley, 2005, in press.
30. Klin A, Chawarska K, Paul R, Rubin E, Morgan T, Wiesner L, Volkmar F: Autism in a 15-month-old child. *American Journal of Psychiatry* 161(11):1981–8, 2004.
31. Gillberg C, Coleman M: *The biology of the autistic syndromes* (2nd ed.). (1992). viii,317pp., 1992.
32. Rutter M, Bailey A, Bolton P, Le Couteur A: Autism and known medical conditions: Myth and substance. *J Child Psychol Psychiatry* 35(2):311–22, 1994.

33. Volkmar FR, Nelson DS: Seizure disorders in autism. *J Am Acad Child Adolesc Psychiatry* 29(1):127–9, 1990.
34. Volkmar F, Cook EH, Jr., Pomeroy J, Realmuto G, Tanguay P: Practice parameters for the assessment and treatment of children, adolescents, and adults with autism and other pervasive developmental disorders. American Academy of Child and Adolescent Psychiatry Working Group on Quality Issues. *Journal of the American Academy of Child & Adolescent Psychiatry.* 38(12 Suppl):32S–54S, 1999.
35. Moeschler, JB, Shevell M, and the Committee on Genetics: Clinical genetic evaluation of the child with mental retardation or developmental delays. *Pediatrics* 117(6)2304–16.
36. Powers MD: Behavioral assessment of individuals with autism: A functional ecological approach, in *Handbook of autism and pervasive developmental disorders*, vol. 2. Volkmar FR, Klin A, Paul R, Cohen DJ (eds): Hoboken, Wiley, pp. 817–30, 2005.
37. Bregman JD, Zager D, Gerdtz J: Behavioral interventions. In: *Handbook of autism and pervasive developmental disorders*, vol. 2. Volkmar FR, Klin A, Paul R, Cohen DJ (eds): Hoboken, Wiley, pp. 897–924, 2005.
38. Scahill L, Martin A: Psychopharmacology, in *Handbook of autism and pervasive developmental disorders*, vol. 2. Volkmar FR, Klin A, Paul R, Cohen DJ (eds): Hoboken, Wiley, pp. 1102–22, 2005.
39. Lord C, Corsello C: Diagnostic instruments in autism spectrum disorders, in *Handbook of autism and pervasive developmental disorders.* Volkmar F, Klin A, Paul R, Cohen DJ (eds): New York, Wiley, 2005.
40. Wing L, Gould J: Severe impairments of social interaction and associated abnormalities. *Journal of Autism & Developmental Disorders* 9(1):11–29, Mar 1979.
41. Coonrod EE, Stone WL: Screening for autism in young children, in *Handbook of autism and pervasive developmental disorders.* Volkmar F, Klin A, Paul R, Cohen DJ (eds): New York, Wiley, in press, 2005.
42. Loveland KA, Tunali-Kotoski B: The school-age child with an autistic spectrum disorder, in *Handbook of autism and pervasive developmental disorders*, vol. 1. Volkmar FR, Klin A, Paul R, Cohen DJ (eds): Hoboken, Wiley, pp. 247–87, 2005.
43. Shea V, Mesibov GB: Adolescents and adults with autism, in *Handbook of autism and pervasive developmental disorders*, vol. 1. Volkmar FR, Klin A, Paul R, Cohen DJ (eds): Hoboken, Wiley, 2005, pp. 288–311.
44. National Research C: *Educating Young Children with Autism.* Washington, DC, National Academy Press, 2001.
45. Owley T, McMahon W, Cook EH, Laulhere T, South M, Mays LZ, Shernoff ES, Lainhart J, Modahl CB, Corsello C, Ozonoff S, Risi S, Lord C, Leventhal BL, Filipek PA: Multisite, double-blind, placebo-controlled trial of porcine secretin in autism. *Journal of the American Academy of Child & Adolescent Psychiatry.* 40(11):1293–9, 2001.
46. Unis AS, Munson JA, Rogers SJ, Goldson E, Osterling J, Gabriels R, Abbott RD, Dawson G: A randomized, double-blind, placebo-controlled trial of porcine versus synthetic secretin for reducing symptoms of autism.[comment]. *Journal of the American Academy of Child & Adolescent Psychiatry.* 41(11):1315–21, 2002.
47. Jacobson JW, Foxx RM, Mulick JA (eds): *Controversial therapies for developmental disabilities: Fad, fashion and science in professional practice.* Mahwah, Lawrence Erlbaum Associates, Publishers, 2005.
48. Arnold GL, Hyman SL, Mooney RA, Kirby RS: Plasma amino acids profiles in children with autism: Potential risk of nutritional deficiencies. *Journal of Autism & Developmental Disorders* 33(4):449–54, 2003.
49. McCracken JT, McGough J, Shah B, Cronin P, Hong D, Aman MG, Arnold LE, Lindsay R, Nash P, Hollway J, McDougle CJ, Posey D, Swiezy N, Kohn A, Scahill L, Martin A, Koenig K, Volkmar F, Carroll D, Lancor A, Tierney E, Ghuman J, Gonzalez NM, Grados M, Vitiello B, Ritz L, Davies M, Robinson J, McMahon D, Research Units on Pediatric Psychopharmacology Autism N: Risperidone in children with autism and serious behavioral problems. *New England Journal of Medicine.* 347(5):314–21, 2002.
50. McDougle CJ, Naylor ST, Cohen DJ, Volkmar FR, Heninger GR, Price LH: A double-blind, placebo-controlled study of fluvoxamine in adults with autistic disorder. *Arch Gen Psychiatry* 53(11):1001–8, 1996.
51. Rett, A: Uber ein eigenartiges hirntophisces Syndroem bei hyperammonie im Kindersalter. *Wein Medizinische Wochenschrift* 118: pp. 723–26, 1966.
52. Hagberg, B: The Rett syndrome: An introductory overview 1990. *Brain Dev*, 14(Suppl): pp. S5–8, 1992.
53. VanAcker R, JA Loncola, and EYV Acker: Rett syndrome: A pervasive developmental disorder, in *Handbook of autism and pervasive developmental disorders*, F. R. Volkmar, et al., (eds). 2005, Wiley: Hoboken, NJ. pp. 126–64.
54. Lam CW, et al.: Spectrum of mutations in the MECP2 gene in patients with infantile autism and Rett syndrome. *Journal of Medical Genetics* 37(12): p. E41, 2000.
55. Miller JN and S Ozonoff: Did Asperger's cases have Asperger disorder? A research note. *J Child Psychol Psychiatry* 38(2): pp. 247–51, 1997.
56. Klin A, J McPartland, and FR Volkmar: Asperger syndrome, in *Handbook of autism and pervasive developmental disorders*, F. R. Volkmar, et al. (eds): Hoboken, Wiley: pp. 88–125, 2005.
57. Asperger H: Die "autistichen Psychopathen" im Kindersalter. *Archive fur psychiatrie und Nervenkrankheiten* 117: pp. 76–136, 1944.
58. Wing L: Asperger's syndrome: A clinical account. *Psychol Med* 11(1): pp. 115–29, 1981.
59. Klin A et al.: Three diagnostic approaches to Asperger syndrome: Implications for research. *Journal of Autism & Developmental Disorders* 35(2): pp. 221–34, 2005.
60. Woodbury-Smith M, A Klin, and F Volkmar: Asperger's syndrome: A comparison of clinical diagnoses and those made according to the ICD-10 and DSM-IV. *Journal of Autism & Developmental Disorders* 35(2): pp. 235–40, 2005.
61. Tsatsanis KD: Neuropsychological characteristics in autism and related conditions, in *Handbook of autism and pervasive developmental disorders*, F. R. Volkmar, et al. (eds): Hoboken, Wiley. pp. 365–81, 2005.
62. Volkmar FR and A Klin: Asperger syndrome and nonverbal learning disabilities, In: *Asperger Syndrome or High-functioning Autism? Current issues in autism*, E Schopler and GB Mesibov, eds. New York: Plenum Press: p. 107–21, 1998.
63. Weintraub S and MM Mesulam: Developmental learning disabilities of the right hemisphere. Emotional, interpersonal, and cognitive components. *Archives of Neurology*, 11: pp. 463–8, 1983.
64. Tantam D: Psychological disorder in adolescents and adults with Asperger syndrome. *Autism*, 4(1): pp. 47–62, 2000.
65. Paul R, et al.: Perception and production of prosody by speakers with autism spectrum disorders. *Journal of Autism & Developmental Disorders*, 35(2): pp. 205–20, 2005.
66. Volkmar FR, Klin A, Schultz R, Rubin R, and Bronen R: Asperger's disorder. Clinical case conference. *American Journal of Psychiatry*, 157(2),262–67, 2000.
67. Rourke BP, Tsatsanis KD: Nonverbal learning disabilities and Asperger syndrome, In: *Asperger syndrome.* Klin A, Volkmar FR (eds): New York: Guilford Press, 2000, pp. 231–53.
68. Martin A, et al.: Higher-functioning pervasive developmental disorders: Rates and patterns of psychotropic drug use. *Journal of the American Academy of Child & Adolescent Psychiatry*, 38(7): pp. 923–31, 1999.
69. Volkmar FR, K Koenig, and M State: Childhood disintegrative disorder. In: Volkmar FR et al., (eds): *Handbook of autism and pervasive developmental disorders*, (eds). 2005, Hoboken, NJ: Wiley. pp. 70–8.
70. Volkmar FR and DJ Cohen: Disintegrative disorder or "late onset" autism. *Journal of Child Psychology & Psychiatry & Allied Disciplines* 30(5): pp. 717–24, 1989.
71. World Health Organization: *Diagnostic Criteria for Research.* Geneva, World Health Organization, 1994.
72. Rank B and D. MacNaughton: A clinical contribution to early ego development. In: Freud A (ed.), Hartmann H (ed.) et al.: *The psychoanalytic study of the child*, vol. 3/4. Oxford: International Universities Press. pp. 53–65, 1949.
73. Landgren M, et al.: ADHD, DAMP and other neurodevelopmental/psychiatric disorders in 6-year-old children: Epidemiology and co-morbidity. *Developmental Medicine & Child Neurology* 38(10): pp. 891–906, 1996.
74. Cohen DJ, et al.: Developmental psychopathology of multiplex developmental disorder, in *Developmental follow-up: Concepts, domains, and methods*, SL Friedman and HC Haywood, eds. San Diego: Academic Press, Inc. pp. 155–79, 1994.
75. Towbin KE: Pervasive developmental disorder not otherwise specified, in *Handbook of autism and pervasive developmental disorders*, F. R. Volkmar, et al., (eds). Hoboken, NJ: Wiley. pp. 165–200, 2005.
76. Piven J et al.: Broader autism phenotype: Evidence from a family history study of multiple-incidence autism families. *Am J Psychiatry*, 154(2): pp. 185–90, 1997.
77. Volkmar FR, Lord C, Bailey A, Schultz RT, Klin A: Autism and pervasive developmental disorders. *Journal of Child Psychology & Psychiatry & Allied Disciplines* 45(1):135–70, 2004.
78. Insel TR, Fernald RD: How the brain processes social information: Searching for the social brain. *Annual Review of Neuroscience Vol* 27,697–722, 2004.

CHAPTER 5.1.2 ■ MENTAL RETARDATION

FRED R. VOLKMAR, ELISABETH M. DYKENS, AND ROBERT M. HODAPP

DEFINITION

In DSM-IV-TR (1), *mental retardation* (MR) is defined on the basis of three essential features: subnormal intellectual functioning, commensurate deficits in adaptive functioning, and onset before 18 years. Of these three criteria, the first two are most often discussed. Subnormal intellectual functioning is characterized by an intelligence quotient (IQ) lower than 70, based in most cases on the administration of an appropriate standardized assessment of intelligence. Deficits in adaptive skills, which involve one's social and personal sufficiency and independence, are generally measured on instruments such as the recently re-revised Vineland Adaptive Behavior Scales (2) or a similar scale. DSM-IV-TR criteria for mental retardation are summarized in Table 5.1.2.1.

Various levels of MR are specified in the DSM-IV-TR: mild (IQ 50 to 70), moderate (IQ 35 to 49), severe (IQ 20 to 34), and profound (IQ <20). Borderline MR can be noted as a V code. Some flexibility is allowed for clinical judgment. Most persons with MR in childhood are those with mild MR (about 85% of cases); the remainder of cases comprise those with moderate (about 10%), severe (about 4%), and profound (1% to 2%) MR (Figure 5.1.2.1). In the past, the distinction was made between educable (IQ 50 to 70) and trainable (IQ <50). Although no longer commonly used, this distinction is important. Persons with mild MR often have psychiatric difficulties that are fundamentally similar (if generally more frequent) to those seen in the general population; this is not true for more severely impaired persons. Similarly, specific medical conditions associated with MR are more likely in the group with an IQ lower than 50, whereas lower socioeconomic status is more frequent in the group with mild MR (3). The proportion of persons with severe and profound MR is higher than would be expected given the normal curve, reflecting the impact of genetic disorders and severe medical problems on development (4).

The tests chosen for assessment of intellectual functioning should be appropriate to the patient, have reasonable reliability and validity, and be administered in a standardized way by appropriately trained examiners (see Chapter 4.2.4 for a discussion of psychological assessment.) Unfortunately, in some situations, the selection of an appropriate test can be difficult, such as for a very low-functioning person. Other aspects of assessment can also be problematic, such as when some modification must be made in terms of administration given the specific circumstance. Such modifications may limit the validity of the results obtained. The examiner must then make an informed decision depending on the nature of the issue at hand, for example, determination of eligibility for services versus information on levels of functioning that can guide remediation. Particularly in terms of eligibility for services, it is critical that the examiner administer the test in exactly the standardized fashion. Measures of adaptive skills are generally based on parent or caregiver report, although, in some cases, the person may be interviewed directly. In essence, the conceptual notion is that the term *adaptive skills* refers to the performance of day-to-day activities required for personal or social self-sufficiency.

The inclusion of adaptive skills in the definition of MR rests on the observation that some persons with IQ scores below 70 may, as adolescents or adults, have learned sufficient adaptive skills that they are able to function totally or largely independently. Technically, then, such individuals would not meet criteria for MR. This situation is more typical of persons who, as children, score in the mildly retarded range (5).

The approach to the definition of MR is fundamentally the same in the tenth edition of the *International Classification of Diseases* (ICD-10) (6). However, the definition of MR promulgated by the American Association of Mental Retardation (AAMR)—first in its 1992 manual (7) and later (in revised form) in its 2002 manual (8)—discards the use of IQ levels in favor of a "needs-based" nosology that identifies the intensity of supports that persons require to function best within multiple adaptive domains. This definition also gives the clinician leeway to extend the upper IQ bound to 75; this seemingly small increase would actually considerably broaden the diagnostic concept of MR, potentially doubling the total number of cases (9). The AAMR definition has been much criticized and has had very little empirical support. Partly as a result, the AAMR definition (particularly its 1992 version) has not been widely used either in research (10) or in state guidelines (11).

HISTORICAL NOTE

Interest in MR can be traced to antiquity (12, 13). Modern interest in MR began at the time of the Enlightenment and increased greatly during the nineteenth century; this emphasis occurred at the time of great social upheaval and as infant and child mortality began to decline. There was increased interest in children, in education, and in the role of experience (nurture) versus endowment (nature). The interest in the "nature–nurture problem" is exemplified in Itard's work with Victor, a child who was thought to be wild or "feral" but who may have had autism (14, 15).

Subsequently, educators such as Seguin began to develop specific educational methods for stimulating children's development. By the latter half of the nineteenth century, many facilities had been developed for the care of persons with mental retardation. Although the initial goal of such facilities was to provide a period of treatment before the child was returned to the family, these institutions gradually became places for custodial care (12). This problem has led to a strong counterreaction in recent years and to a renewed emphasis of caring for persons with MR in their homes and communities (16).

During the nineteenth century, various distinctions were made between levels of MR by using what now would be seen as rather pejorative terms (imbecile, cretin, idiot). Originally, the etiologic basis of any such distinctions was quite limited. On one hand, there was little systematic information on intellectual functioning that could be used for purposes of

TABLE 5.1.2.1

DSM-IV DIAGNOSTIC CRITERIA FOR MENTAL RETARDATION

A. Significantly subaverage intellectual functioning: an IQ of approximately 70 or below on an individually administered IQ test (for infants, a clinical judgment of significantly subaverage intellectual functioning)
B. Concurrent deficits or impairments in present adaptive functioning (i.e., the person's effectiveness in meeting the standards expected for his or her age by his or her cultural group) in at least two of the following areas: communication, self-care, home living, social/interpersonal skills, use of community resources, self-direction, functional academic skills, work, leisure, health, and safety
C. Onset before age 18 years

Code based on degree of severity reflecting level of intellectual impairment:

317	Mild Mental Retardation	IQ level 50–55 to ~70
318.0	Moderate Retardation	IQ level 35–40 to 50–55
318.1	Severe Mental Retardation	IQ level 20–25 to 35–40
318.2	Profound Mental Retardation	IQ level <20 or 25
319	Mental Retardation, Severity Unspecified:	when there is a strong presumption of mental retardation but the person's intelligence is untestable by standard tests

Data from American Psychiatric Association: *Diagnostic and Statistical Manual of Mental Disorders*, 4th ed. (DSM-IV). Washington, DC, American Psychiatric Association, 1994.

categorization. On the other, there were few known etiologic causes of MR.

Toward the end of the nineteenth and the beginning of the twentieth centuries, both these limitations began to be addressed. Binet developed the first test of intelligence, which was translated into English and adapted in the United States by Terman (18, 27). As a model psychometric assessment instrument for many years, the Stanford-Binet test allowed much more precise characterization of levels of intellectual disability. In addition, Terman had the brilliant notion of taking the mental age, dividing it by the child's chronological age, and multiplying this quotient by 100. The resulting IQ score allowed for comparisons across children of different ages. Although Binet had originally developed his scale to identify children who were delayed in order to help them, the IQ score quickly became the object of much study.

Faith in the IQ as a predictor variable led to several extensions. First, developmental testing began to be performed on infants and young children (19). Second, proponents of the new tests believed that, when the test was properly administered, the resulting score from an IQ test was fixed and reflected a person's genetic endowment. This proved incorrect.

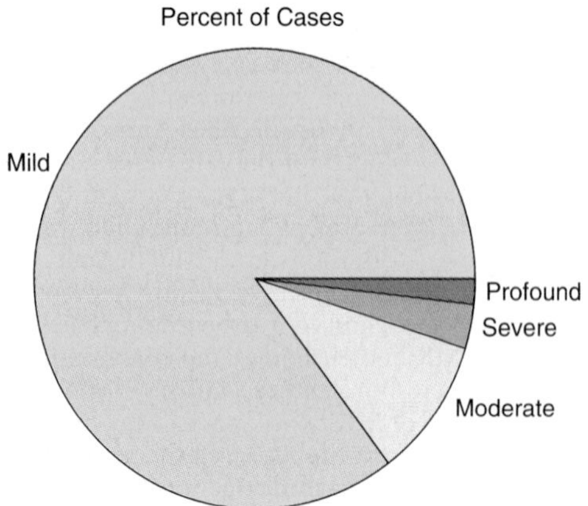

FIGURE 5.1.2.1. Levels of mental retardation.

In a classic study, Skeels and Dye (20) demonstrated this practically by transferring infants and young children from an orphanage to a home for the "feeble-minded" to make the children normal. This fantastic plan had been prompted by clinical observation that children in the home for the feeble-minded received considerably more stimulation than those in the orphanage. Skeels later (21) reported major differences in outcomes for these better cared-for children, both in childhood and in later adult life. By the 1940s and 1950s, there was increased awareness that the IQ score was indeed the product of both experience and endowment, and therapeutic optimism again increased for improving the functioning of children with mental retardation.

In addition to the focus on intellectual functioning, it also became apparent that the person's capacities to engage in appropriate self-care or "adaptive" skills was a major aspect of MR. In the 1930s, the psychologist Edgar Doll developed the Vineland Social Maturity Scale in an attempt to quantify such skills. Originally revised two decades ago (22), the Vineland Adaptive Behavior Scales have recently been re-revised (2). The Vineland Scales, now published in several versions, continue to serve as an important tool in the assessment of children with MR. Along with lower IQs, deficits in adaptive skills are now required as part of the diagnosis of MR. In contrast to IQ, however, adaptive skills can be readily taught.

Another major line of work centers on the origin of MR syndromes. In the nineteenth century, Dr. Langdon Down reported on a syndrome (which now bears his name) that is currently recognized as being the result of a trisomy of chromosome 21. At the time of his report, Dr. Down, of course, had no notion of chromosomes. Indeed, though his theoretical understanding was fundamentally flawed, Down's clinical observation has been remarkably robust. As time went on, more and more syndromes of MR were identified. It became clear that MR could result from a range of risk factors, including problems related to the developing fetus, and ranging from genetic factors (Down syndrome) to exposure to toxins in utero (fetal alcoholism) to maternal infections (congenital rubella). As noted subsequently, advances in genetics have led to an explosion in the recognition of such syndromes, often with a very precise understanding of their cause (3, 23).

In recent years, several developments have substantially changed the approach to treatment and prevention of MR in the United States. Beginning in the 1960s, there has been increased emphasis on the care of persons in their homes and communities. The trend toward deinstitutionalization reflects various concerns about the effects of prolonged institutionalization and has led to creation of many community services. This movement has been further stimulated by the mandate of the federal government that schools provide appropriate education for all children with disabilities, within integrated settings when possible. In the United States, many students with mental retardation are largely or entirely integrated into classrooms with typically developing age mates, although there are marked state-to-state variations (24), and the benefits of mainstreaming are the focus of some debate (25). It is clear that students with more severe disabilities are most likely to spend their school time in more restricted settings.

One unfortunate aspect of current practice has been the often complete separation of services for those who are mentally ill from those who are mentally retarded. Although administratively useful, this approach has made provision of high-quality psychiatric care even more difficult to obtain for many persons with MR. With renewed interest in the field of "dual diagnosis" of MR and psychiatric disorders (26), we can only hope that this separation will soon be ending.

PREVALENCE AND EPIDEMIOLOGY

The use of both subnormal intellectual functioning and deficits in adaptive behavior in the definition of MR has important implications for epidemiology. If only the IQ criterion is used, the expectation, based on the normal curve, would be that about 2.3% of the population should exhibit the condition. This number is significantly decreased, particularly in adulthood, if the adaptive criterion is included.

For example, in the Isle of Wight study, Rutter and colleagues (27) noted that, in 9- to 11-year-old children, about 2.5% would be classified as mentally retarded if IQ were the sole criterion. But if the prevalence were based only on those receiving services, this rate would be cut almost in half (1.3%) (Figure 5.1.2.2). The drop in cases based on inclusion of IQ and adaptive skills is more common among those with mild MR; (28, 29) these children (and adults) may, however, need services and support at times of stress (30, 31). As children, such persons are more likely to have academic and behavioral problems (27).

Additional findings have also recently been reported from large-scale epidemiological studies (32). For individuals with severe MR, prevalence levels mostly converge on 3–4 children per 1,000; for mild MR, rates range wildly from 5.4 to 10.6 children per 1,000 (29, 30). Studies also examine such correlates as gender, age, and SES. More boys than girls have mental retardation, and rates of MR are generally low in the early years, peak at around 10–14 years, and decrease slightly in the late-school years and markedly during adulthood. Individuals of lower SES and of ethnic minority groups (in several cultures) (13) also show higher than expected rates of mental retardation.

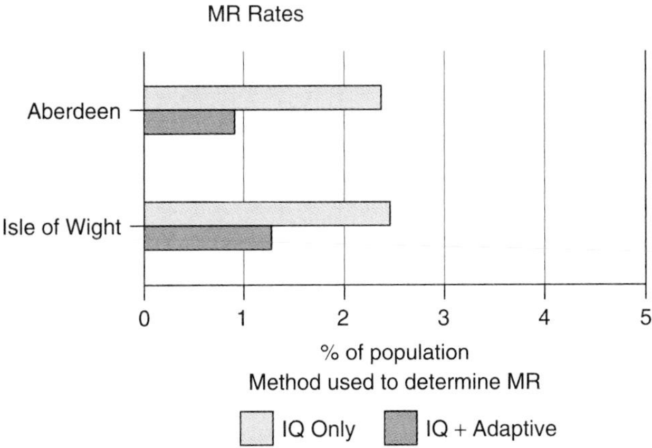

FIGURE 5.1.2.2. Isle of Wight study.

CLINICAL DESCRIPTION

Clinical Features

Associated clinical features vary depending on several factors, most important the level of retardation. Persons with severe and profound MR come to diagnosis at a younger age, more often exhibit related medical conditions, may exhibit dysmorphic features, and have a range of behavioral and psychiatric disturbances. In contrast, persons with mild MR often come to diagnosis much later (typically when academic demands become more prominent in school), are less likely to have medical conditions that could account for the MR, and usually are of normal appearance without dysmorphic features. In this latter group, although rates of psychopathology are increased relative to nondisabled populations, the range and nature of problems seen are fundamentally similar to those in normative samples (3). Persons with moderate levels of MR are intermediate between these two extremes. It is well recognized that the nature of associated psychiatric and behavioral disorders undergoes a marked shift between the mild and more severe levels of MR (33).

ASSOCIATED PSYCHIATRIC AND BEHAVIORAL PROBLEMS

A growing body of work focuses on psychiatric and behavioral difficulties relative to specific genetic causes (34, 35). Features have been identified that are highly frequent to specific syndromes, such as hyperphagia and compulsivity in Prader-Willi syndrome (36), attentional and social problems in fragile X syndrome (37), inappropriate laughter in Angelman's syndrome (38), the unusual cry in 5p- syndrome (39), and the self-hug in Smith-Magenis syndrome (40). In some instances, aspects of syndrome expression have even been related to the genetic features of the syndrome, such as the severity of MR in fragile X syndrome (41, 42) and the type and severity of maladaptive behaviors in Prader-Willi syndrome (43–45). Furthermore, some of these connections between genetic disorder and behavioral outcome appear unique to a single syndrome, whereas others are "shared" between two or more syndromes (46–48). Thus, in some instances, features are relatively syndrome-specific, such as the unusual handwashing stereotypies of Rett syndrome (49), or the extreme hyperphagia in Prader-Willi syndrome (50). More often, however, features are shared in two or more conditions. Thus, attentional problems are frequent in fragile X, Williams, and 5p- syndromes (51, 52).

Somewhat paradoxically, for many years the diagnosis of MR tended to cause clinicians and researchers to overlook the presence of associated psychiatric and behavioral problems; such difficulties, when noted at all, were assumed to be a function of the MR. This "diagnostic overshadowing" (53) remains a problem in clinical practice (54). Although more clinicians and researchers are being specifically trained to work with this population, the separation of MR and mental health services in most states is a further obstacle to appropriate identification and treatment of mental disorders.

Although rates vary, as many as 25% of persons with MR may have significant psychiatric problems; these rates are much higher if persons with salient behavior disorders are included (55). Problems are invariably seen in children who present clinically (56), whereas rates are lower, from 10% to 15%, in more population-based studies, including two large-scale medical record surveys of all clients served in New York and California (57, 58). Rates that fall between these two extremes, from 30% to 40%, are found in other studies based on informant checklists of behavior problems of children or adults in nonreferred samples (59).

Persons with MR experience the same range of psychiatric problems as seen in the general population (60), but prevalence rates for specific disorders vary widely. Some of this variability may be associated with different methods for determining "caseness," with common approaches including record reviews, behavioral checklists, and, to a lesser extent, direct interviews (61–64). An additional concern is that although some researchers assess DSM- or ICD-based diagnoses, others identify maladaptive features commonly seen in the general population (inattention or sadness), whereas still others focus on a narrow range of behaviors seen primarily in persons with MR (stereotypies or self-injury) (47).

For example, rates of schizophrenia or psychosis in persons with MR range from 1% to 9% among nonreferred samples and 2.8% to 24% in referred samples. Although variable, these rates are much higher than the 0.5% to 1% of the general population with schizophrenia (1). Rates for depression vary from 1.1% to 11% across nonreferred and clinic samples of persons with MR, and rates of attention deficit hyperactivity disorder range from 7% to 15% in children with MR, a finding that contrasts with the 3% to 5% estimate among children in general (1). Patterns of psychopathology also differ across persons with or without MR. Relative to the general population, for example, people with MR are more likely to show psychosis, autism, and behavior disorders and are less apt to be diagnosed with substance abuse and affective disorders (35, 36).

ASSESSMENT OF PSYCHIATRIC DISORDERS

As researchers increasingly began to appreciate the scope of problems in persons with MR, they also developed various ways of assessing these problems. Some work has been devoted to the development of specialized rating scales and surveys; most of these measures are geared specifically for persons with MR and have well developed psychometric properties (65). Among the more widely used are the Aberrant Behavior Checklist (66), Reiss Screen (67), and Developmental Behaviour Checklist (62). A tradeoff in using these scales is that, although they are sensitive to the unique concerns of those with MR, they are not necessarily compatible with DSM or ICD psychiatric diagnoses. Further, because each scale has a different set of items and factor structures, these differences may ultimately contribute to inconsistent findings across studies (61).

At the same time, other researchers have taken issue with the applicability of traditional DSM or ICD diagnoses for persons with MR (33). Many of these concerns relate to the psychiatric interview itself, including acquiescence bias, and the limited abilities of many persons with MR to answer questions about the onset, duration, frequency, and severity of symptoms (36). In response to these challenges, several groups have adapted traditional DSM or ICD criteria for persons with developmental delay (3, 60), whereas others have designed interview schedules specifically for those with MR, including the Psychiatric Assessment Schedule for Adults with Developmental Disability (68). Direct interviews with both respondents and informants result in fewer cases of missed diagnoses (69). Still others advocate a more functional analysis of challenging behavior (70).

CAUSES OF INCREASED PSYCHOPATHOLOGY

Although the field has done well with assessment and diagnostic issues, less progress has been made in advancing theories on why persons with MR are at heightened risk of psychopathology in the first place. Many reasons have been discussed over the years and most fall within the "biopsychosocial" spectrum. Yet a comprehensive model of "dual diagnosis" is lacking, in part because researchers cannot simply apply existing risk factors for psychopathology in the general population to the unique characteristics of those with MR (71). In addition, the causal direction of most risk factors is unclear. Poor peer or social relations, for example, may be a precursor of psychopathology or a consequence of disruptive behavior.

Even so, some advances have been made, and heightened psychopathology in persons with MR has now been linked to specific biopsychosocial problems. Biologically, these include increased rates of seizure disorders (72, 73), abnormal neurologic functioning that in most cases is undetected (74, 75), high rates of sensory or motor impairments among persons with MR (76), biochemical or neurologic anomalies associated with unusual behaviors such as severe self-injury (77), and genetic causes that carry higher than usual risks of certain maladaptive or psychiatric vulnerabilities (78).

Psychological risk factors include the following: aberrant personality styles, including an outer-directed orientation and being too wary or disinhibited with others (79, 80); atypical motivational styles or abnormal levels of sensitivity to basic human drives such as the need for attention or acceptance (81); increased risk of failure experiences, which may lead to learned helplessness, low expectancies for success, and depression (80, 81); more global and less differentiated self-concepts that may lead to more sweeping negative evaluations of the entire self instead of not liking just one aspect of one's self (82); and reinforcement of negative behaviors, leading to more entrenched maladaptive behavior or interactions (83).

Finally, specific social risk factors include the following: poor communication or assertiveness skills, which may lead to increased frustration and acting-out behavior (84); social strain or stressful social interactions, more strongly correlated with psychopathology than low levels of social support (85); social stigma, with a subsequent negative impact on daily living, adjustment, and esteem (30); peer rejection and ostracism and, among children, atypical patterns of friendship with nonretarded children (86); compromised "social intelligence," or inappropriate responses to social cues, that may exacerbate stigma and isolation from others (87); heightened risks of exploitation and abuse, which may worsen behavioral or emotional problems (88, 89); and family stress, including low levels of emotional, service, or financial support to families (90).

GENETIC RISK AND PSYCHOPATHOLOGY

As previously noted, a comprehensive model has yet to be developed that identifies the relative importance of these many risk factors. To date, research aimed at doing so has generally relied on heterogeneous groups with MR. Yet each of the factors listed earlier can just as easily apply to those with a genetic diagnosis, and syndrome-specific studies may shed new light on genetic or other mechanisms associated with certain psychopathologic conditions (47, 63).

ETIOLOGY AND PATHOGENESIS

Historically, researchers have used two broad categories to classify persons with MR (13, 91). One group has "organic" causes of their MR and consists of people with known prenatal, perinatal, and postnatal insults. Estimates suggest that approximately one-half of people with MR have known "organic" causes (92). The second group has no clearly identifiable organic cause and is postulated to account for most persons with mild MR. In years past, the terms sociocultural or cultural-familial retardation reflected the view that nonorganic MR stemmed from environmental deprivation. Although impoverished, chaotic environments may indeed be implicated in a few cases, this theory has generally fallen out of favor as an explanation for the population as a whole. Even so, a complicating factor is that disproportionately more persons with sociocultural MR are poor, from minority backgrounds, and of low-IQ parents (92).

With increased diagnostic precision and with the discovery of new genetic disorders, many workers speculate that more persons with nonspecific delay will receive specific genetic diagnoses in the years ahead. The complex interplay of organic and genetic (including polygenic) factors with sociocultural and environmental factors has been increasingly recognized (93). Progress has been slower in identifying clear neurologic causes in persons with unspecified MR, because most neuroimaging research is conducted with persons with known genetic or other causes (75). However, some persons with nonorganic causes may simply represent the lower end of the normal, Gaussian distribution of intelligence (94, 95). Assuming that nonorganic MR is the extreme end of the normal IQ distribution, then some persons will always belong to this group, even as progress is made in uncovering genetic or neurologic causes for other persons at the same IQ levels (Figure 5.1.2.3).

In the "organic" group as well, many unresolved issues remain. Early researchers grouped people together who had different types of organic causes and often compared these heterogeneous groups with those with familial or nonspecific MR. Even today, mixed or heterogeneous groups, consisting of those with known and unknown causes for their delay, predominate in behavioral MR research (23). Yet with the remarkable progress in molecular genetics, and improved diagnostic accuracy, researchers are now much better positioned to examine people with specific genetic causes. Indeed, there are now nearly 1,000 known genetic causes of MR (96), and as many as one-third of all persons with MR have already been diagnosed with a known genetic disorder (97). Further, although genetic and other organic causes are typically seen in persons with severe and profound delay, high-functioning persons with Down, fragile X, Prader-Willi, Williams, and other syndromes may comprise 10% to 50% of persons with mild MR (93).

With these advances, research on so-called behavioral phenotypes is gaining momentum, including both between-syndrome and within-syndrome designs (23, 34, 94). Between-group studies help to identify possible unique syndromic behaviors that may accelerate our understanding of gene or brain function. Further, and as shown in Table 5.1.2.2, some syndromes feature unique psychiatric vulnerabilities, including increased rates of obsessive–compulsive symptoms in Prader-Willi syndrome (43), as well as anxiety, fears, and phobias in Williams syndrome (95). Groups without these syndromes can also have these vulnerabilities, albeit much less often. As such, studies on these syndromes hold much promise for differentiating genetic from other pathways to these psychiatric endpoints.

Cognitively as well, some syndromes show distinctive profiles of relative strength or weakness that are not typically seen in studies of persons with mixed or nonspecific causes of MR. As summarized in Table 5.1.2.2, persons with Williams, Prader-Willi, Down, and other syndromes often show distinctive patterns of cognitive strength or weakness. Many people with Williams syndrome, for example, show relative strengths in specific aspects of expressive language, along with pronounced deficits in visual-spatial functioning. Despite visual-spatial deficits, however, many persons with Williams syndrome have a remarkable sparing of facial recognition and memory. Many, although not all, persons with Prader-Willi syndrome show remarkable skills solving jigsaw puzzles, with performances that exceed those of their chronologic agemates (96).

However, most syndromic behavior appears to be "partially specific" or shared across one or more conditions (46). For example, persons with both fragile X and Prader-Willi syndromes appear to have relative weaknesses in certain short-term memory and sequential processing tasks (50), and inattention and hyperactivity are seen in Williams, fragile X, and 5p-syndromes (51, 52, 62). These disorders, however, show qualitative differences in symptoms. Inattention in Williams syndrome, for example, may be associated with heightened anxiety and social disinhibition, whereas in fragile X syndrome, these difficulties may be related to hyperarousal and anomalies in the size of the posterior cerebellar vermis and caudate nucleus (98).

Although between-group studies help to identify distinctive syndromic behaviors, within-syndrome studies help to explain

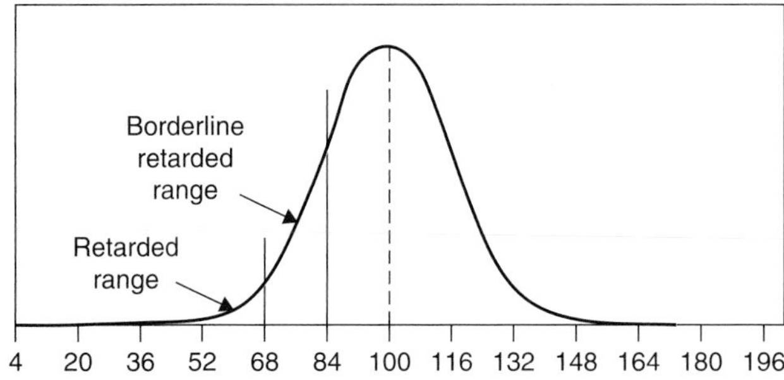

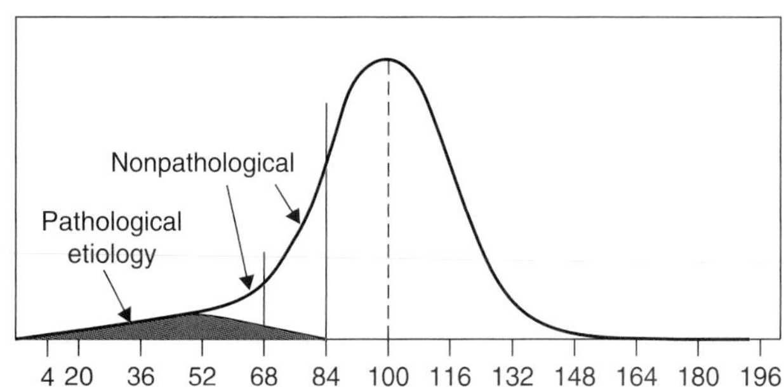

FIGURE 5.1.2.3. **A.** Distribution of Stanford-Binet IQ expected from the normal curve. **B.** Approximate distribution of IQs actually found, with persons having signs of pathologic origin separated from those not having signs of pathologic origin. (From Achenbach T: Developmental Psychopathology, 2nd ed. New York, Wiley, 1974, with permission.)

TABLE 5.1.2.2

EXAMPLES OF COGNITIVE AND BEHAVIORAL PROFILES IN SELECTED MENTAL RETARDATION SYNDROMES

Syndrome	Cognitive Weakness	Cognitive Strengths	Behavioral Profiles
Fragile X	Sequential processing, auditory STM, planning	Verbal LTM acquired information	Social anxiety, shyness, gaze aversion, inattention, hyperactivity, autism/PDD
Prader-Willi	Sequential processing	Verbal LTM, visual-spatial processing	Hyperphagia, nonfood obsessive-compulsive symptoms, skin picking, tantrums
Williams	Spatial organization, visual-motor coordination	Facial recognition, auditory STM, expressive language	Social disinhibition, anxiety, fears, inattention, hyperactivity, hyperacusis
Down	Auditory processing	Visual-spatial processing, expressive language	Noncompliance, stubbornness, inattention, depression and dementia in adults

LTM, long-term memory; PDD, pervasive developmental disorder; STM, short-term memory.

individual variation in these behaviors. Researchers now need to identify the genetic, environmental, developmental, and psychosocial factors that help to explain individual behavioral differences in people with the same genetic disorder. For example, the level of cognitive delay in fragile X syndrome is associated with both age and molecular genetic status (42). Similarly, in Prader-Willi syndrome, the frequency and severity of maladaptive behaviors such as skin picking appear to vary across genetic subtypes of this disorder (36).

Whereas research on heterogeneous groups is still necessary, both between-syndrome and within-syndrome studies offer many advantages (35, 47). In the long term, work on behavioral phenotypes facilitates the search for gene–brain–behavior relationships, as well as contributing toward a more precise science of MR. In the short term, phenotypic data refine intervention and treatment (99, 100). Although many syndrome-specific recommendations for interventions have now been made, the efficacy of these approaches needs to be evaluated, including how they fare relative to more generic interventions.

DIFFERENTIAL DIAGNOSIS

The diagnosis of MR is based on the appropriate assessment of cognitive abilities and adaptive skills; clinical assessment also includes a careful developmental and family history, physical examination, and laboratory studies as appropriate. The clinician should be alert to any medical or environmental conditions that may be associated with developmental disability. For example, a strong family history or certain dysmorphic features in the child should raise the possibility of an inherited condition; a history of significant birth trauma, exposure to environmental toxins, or exposure to marked psychosocial adversity are some of the factors that should be considered.

As noted, the age of diagnosis often varies depending on the severity of the disability, so persons with more severe MR present for clinical assessment earlier than those with mild, or borderline, MR. Careful psychological assessment of the child (Chapter 4.2.2) is obviously critical. Various other developmental difficulties, notably language and other specific developmental disorders and autism and related conditions, may be associated with some degree of mental disability or may be confused with it. Diagnosis can be complicated because persons with MR can exhibit other developmental problems that can complicate the tasks of both diagnosis and assessment. For example, children with a marked expressive language disorder often do poorly on a test of intelligence that is highly verbal. In autism and related disorders, social abilities tend to be the area of greatest weakness (Chapter 5.1.1).

TREATMENT

In most developed countries, the treatment of MR has undergone a marked shift over the past few decades. More persons with MR now reside with their families and in their communities. More children now receive services within regular educational settings, and more services are available to support them and their families. At the same time, it is clear that placement in the community is not sufficient in and of itself, and the provision of adequate and appropriate support is critical. This is particularly important for the growing numbers of older persons with MR, many of whom still reside with their aging parents.

In general, treatment planning begins with a consideration of the underlying cause, if one is known, of the intellectual disability. In many instances, knowing the cause can guide both medical and psychosocial interventions; indeed, many syndrome-specific parent and professional organizations have published "best practice" guidelines across the lifespan (Prader-Willi, Williams, and Down syndromes.). However, for disorders that are more rare, such data are lacking.

Medical Treatment

Medically, laboratory studies should be based on the results of a careful history (including family history) and evaluation. Physical examination should include assessment of growth and developmental status as well as observation for facial features or other physical findings that could suggest a specific medical condition. It is sometimes the case that the evolution of the condition provides important clues to its cause, such as in Rett syndrome. Depending on the clinical circumstance, hearing or visual testing may be indicated as are, at times, specific metabolic studies, chromosome analysis (including fragile X testing), neuroimaging or neurologic assessment, skeletal radiography, screening for organic acidurias, and so forth (101, 102).

Persons with MR may be at increased risk for certain medical conditions (103). In their review of the Aberdeen cohort of cases, Goulden and colleagues noted that at least 15% of patients developed epilepsy by adulthood; the risk was increased when associated disabilities were present or when there was a history of postnatal injury (104).

To some extent, associated medical conditions vary depending on the cause of the MR. Consider Down syndrome, the most common genetic (chromosomal) cause of mental retardation. Although the median age of death among individuals with Down syndrome has increased from 25 to 49 years over the period from 1983 to 1997 (105), specific medical problems persist for these individuals throughout their lifetimes. Congenital heart defects occur in approximately 50% of newborns with Down syndrome (106, 107), and the large majority of these children are hospitalized for heart or other problems (mostly pneumonia, bronchitis, or other respiratory problems), often within the first few months of life (108). Later, children with Down syndrome are more likely than other children to have leukemia, and, by age 40, the plaques and tangles of Alzheimer's disease strike virtually all adults with the syndrome (109). Other genetic disorders, notably Prader-Willi syndrome, also show particularly high rates of etiology-related health problems and higher death rates in the young adult and middle-aged years (110).

Cognitive and Adaptive Intervention

Regardless of the origin of MR, accurate assessment of each person's intellectual and adaptive strengths and weaknesses is essential, because specific recommendations for intervention depend on the overall level and profiles of cognitive functioning. Although there are many different models of intelligence (111), investigators generally agree about such basic features of intelligence as the ability to use conceptual thinking in solving problems and in acquiring knowledge (112). Various IQ tests are now available, and they differ in certain dimensions, such as the degree to which they emphasize language-based problem solving or short-term memory. Tests differ in other ways as well. Some tests include timed tasks, whereas others provide the opportunity for demonstration of tasks by the examiner. As part of the standard administration of test items, the examiner is also able to collect considerable amounts of qualitative information that may be particularly important for treatment.

Some special considerations are involved in assessing persons with MR. To the extent possible, tests should be appropriate for the person's chronological age as well as her or his levels of receptive and expressive language. In some cases, cultural and other factors also need to be considered. The behavioral problems sometimes associated with MR may pose special problems, particularly if they arise around times of change or frustration.

Assessment of adaptive functioning has the goal of providing a representative picture of the person's typical abilities in home, school, and community environments. In this regard, the goal is somewhat different from that of the intellectual assessment, in which the aim is to obtain optimal performance in a structured and standardized situation. Large discrepancies between intellectual level and adaptive skills suggest that the treatment should include a major focus on acquisition and generalization of adaptive skills.

Various measures of adaptive functioning have been proposed. The most widely used instrument is the Vineland Adaptive Behavior Scales (2), which assess capacities for self-sufficiency in various domains of functioning, including communication (receptive, expressive and written language), daily living skills (personal, domestic and community skills), socialization (interpersonal relationships, play and leisure time and coping skills), and motor skills (gross and fine). The Vineland scales are available as a survey interview, an expanded interview for use in more detailed program planning, an informant-administered rating form, and a teacher rating form.

Psychiatric Treatment

As previously described, persons with MR are at increased risk of psychiatric problems, and these are often a major source of distress to the individual and family, and may severely limit opportunities for self-sufficiency and independence (102). Yet these mental and physical heath problems are frequently overlooked. Ryan and Sunada (103) report that up to 75% of persons with MR who are referred for psychiatric assessment have undiagnosed or undertreated medical conditions, and nearly 50% receive nonpsychotropic mediations that could have behavioral side effects.

Even though associated psychiatric problems can severely limit personal and social sufficiency, there is often a tendency to neglect or overlook the mental health needs of this population (59). Although some of the many rating scales, checklists, and other instruments for assessment of psychopathology in the general population are applicable, other instruments have been developed that are specific for persons with MR. Psychiatric assessment may entail some modification in usual procedures, particularly for persons with more severe MR, in whom the psychiatric assessment must be comprehensive and multifocal. The presence of associated difficulties (seizures, motor impairments, sensory problems) may further complicate accurate psychiatric diagnosis.

Other Psychosocial Treatment

General quality-of-life issues are receiving renewed attention in the MR field, with particular emphasis on improving how people with MR live, work, and play in inclusive, community-based settings. Most persons with MR benefit from employment or from structured programs that emphasize vocational, adaptive, or socialization skills, long after formal schooling. Indeed, the transition from school to work is a vulnerable point for many persons and their families. Unlike the school years, when special education and related services (occupational, physical, and speech and language therapies) are typically provided under one roof, the services for adults risk being more fragmented. These young adults may particularly benefit from *case coordination,* to avoid becoming isolated or lost between various cracks in services (113).

A particularly troublesome outgrowth of adult service needs concerns residential placements. As individuals with mental retardation live longer lives, our society increasingly needs to deal with who will take care of these individuals when aging parents can no longer do so. Currently in the United States, 526,000 individuals with disabilities are 60 years and over; by the year 2030, that number is expected to triple, to 1.5 million (114). Since over 60% of these individuals live in their parents' home, who will take care of these aging individuals? Such concerns have recently led to a call from more research on adult siblings of individuals with mental retardation (115), as these adult siblings (116) are likely to become tomorrow's caregivers for aging brothers and sisters with disabilities.

OUTCOME AND FOLLOWUP DATA

As expected, the course and outcome of MR vary considerably, depending on various factors. These include the level of severity of the MR, associated biological or other vulnerabilities, and aspects of the individual's psychological functioning, family support, and other factors (3). Levels of ability to cope with the demands of daily life (adaptive skills) are critical in determining adult outcome. It is also clear that the expectations of caregivers and the provision of intervention services and environmental supports are also important. For persons with known medical causes of MR, certain risks may be present, such as the risk of early development of Alzheimer's dementia in persons with Down syndrome (117). Conversely, even when the specific biomedical cause is known, there may be a wide range in ultimate outcome. To simplify the discussion of outcome, we focus the discussion on levels of MR but again emphasize that the outcome in a given individual patient varies considerably, depending on a host of factors.

In mild MR, many children with the condition go on, as adolescents and adults, to make major gains in adaptive functioning and thus may "lose" the diagnosis as they become older. Such persons may be self-supporting, may marry, and may raise families. At the same time, such persons are not without difficulties, because several studies (27, 31) show that persons with intellectual deficits who have not required special services in school have higher rates of educational and behavioral problems. In their followup study of the Aberdeen cohort of children first seen at 9 to 11 years of age and then followed up at the age of 22 years, Richardson and Koller (118) report that more than 75% no longer require services as adults, although only about 25% of the entire group are judged to be functioning adequately in all areas. Mild MR is likely to be diagnosed only at the time of school entry, that is, when academic demands increase. As discussed previously, persons from backgrounds of social disadvantage or adversity and from certain minority groups are more likely to be represented in these cases.

As adults, persons with moderate levels of MR (IQ 40 to 55) typically have more serious impairment. It is common for such persons to need services as adults. Moderate MR is often identified in the preschool years. At this, and lower, levels of cognitive functioning, specific medical causes are more likely to be identified, and minority group membership and psychosocial adversity in the family are less frequent. The prognosis for adult self-sufficiency is more guarded, although many persons can live semiindependently or with partial support (119).

For persons with severe or profound retardation, case identification may occur in infancy or early childhood. Generally, high levels of supervision and support are required during the person's life. Goals for these patients include facilitating self-care and independence as far as possible. Associated medical problems and behavioral difficulties are frequent. Communication skills may be impaired and are a further source of disability.

Legislation, legal decisions, and some important social policy changes have markedly changed the provision of remedial programs. The provision of early diagnosis and intervention and the availability of community-based resources and educational interventions within public schools have dramatically improved the care of persons with MR as well as overall outcome.

PREVENTION

Estimates of recurrence risk vary depending on the situation, ranging from instances in which a clear genetic origin can be identified (fragile X syndrome) to those in which the difficulties appear to be of nongenetic origin (congenital rubella). When no specific cause is identified, estimates of recurrence risk vary considerably, such as between 3.5% and 14% for the siblings of a boy with MR (120). For some disorders, such as autism, there has been a growing appreciation of genetic factors, and it now appears that, for parents who have one child with autism, the risk of having a second child with autism is between 2% and 10% (121). Siblings of children with MR who are not themselves affected may be at increased risk of other difficulties, due to increased family and personal stress, although data are sorely needed on the range of both positive and negative outcomes in these siblings (122). Support for siblings, and for their parents, is an important element of long-term treatment planning (3).

RESEARCH DIRECTIONS

Several issues will likely dominate the research agenda for the coming decade. They include the interplay between genetic and environmental (including psychosocial) risk factors in the origin of MR as well as the study of basic neural mechanisms (94). Understanding of basic processes that underlie phenotypic expression, including various forms of psychopathology, offers the opportunity to advance knowledge more generally about mechanisms of disorder. Although many advances in the care and treatment of persons with mental retardation have been made, studies of treatment methods remain an important priority.

References

1. American Psychiatric Association: *Diagnostic and Statistical Manual of Mental Disorders*, 4th ed. Washington, DC, American Psychiatric Association, 1994.
2. Sparrow S, Balla, D, Cicchetti D: *Vineland Adaptive Behavior Scales*, Circle Pines, American Guidance Service, 2005.
3. Szymanski L, King BH: Practice parameters for the assessment and treatment of children, adolescents, and adults with mental retardation and comorbid mental disorders: American Academy of Child and Adolescent Psychiatry Working Group on Quality Issues. *J Am Acad Child Adolesc Psychiatry* 38[Suppl]:5S–31S, 1999.
4. Dingman H. G, Tarjan G: Mental retardation and the normal distribution. *Am J Ment Defic* 64:991–994, 1960.
5. Edgerton RB, Bollinger M, Herr B: The cloak of competence: After two decades. *Am J Ment Defic* 88:345–351, 1984.
6. World Health Organization: Mental and behavioral disorders, clinical descriptions and diagnostic guidelines. In: *International Classification of Diseases*, 10th ed. Geneva, World Health Organization, 1992.
7. American Association on Mental Retardation (AAMR): *Mental Retardation: Definition, Classification, and Systems of Support*. 9th ed. Washington, DC, 1992.
8. American Association on Mental Retardation. *Mental retardation: Definition, classification, and systems of supports*. 10th ed. Washington, DC, Author, 2002.
9. MacMillan DL, Gresham FM, Siperstein GN: Heightened concerns over the 1992 AAMR definition: Advocacy vs. precision. *Am J Ment Retar* 100:87–95, 1995.
10. Polloway EA, Smith JD, Chamberlain J, Denning CB, Smith TEC: Levels of deficits or supports in the classification of mental retardation: Implementation practices. *Education and Training in Mental Retardation* 34:200–206, 1999.
11. Denning CB, Chamberlain JA, Polloway EA: An evaluation of state guidelines for mental retardation: Focus on definition and classification practices. *Education and Training in Mental Retardation* 35:226–232, 2000.
12. Trent JW: *Inventing the Feeble Mind: A History of Mental Retardation in the United States*, Berkeley, University of California Press, 1994.
13. Zigler E, Hodapp R: *Understanding Mental Retardation*, New York, Cambridge University Press, 1986.
14. Candland DK: *Feral children and clever animals: Reflections on human nature*, Oxford, Oxford University Press, 1993.
15. Simon N: Kaspar Hauser's recovery and autopsy: A perspective on neurological and sociological requirements for language development. *J Autism Child Schizophr* 8:209–217, 1978.
16. Anderson LL, Lakin KC, Mangan TW, Prouty RW: State institutions: Thirty years of depopulation and closure. *Mental Retardation* 36:431–443, 1998.
17. Binet A, Simon T: *The Development of Intelligence in Children*. [E. S. Kit, trans.] Baltimore, Williams & Wilkins, 1916.
18. Terman LM: The Binet-Simon Scale for measuring intelligence: Impressions gained by its application. *Psychol Clin* 5:199–206, 1911.
19. Bayley N: Consistency and variability in the growth of intelligence from birth to eighteen years. *J of Gen Psychology* 75:165–196, 1949.
20. Skeels A, Dye HB: A study of the effects of differential stimulation on mentally retarded children. *Proceeding of the American Association of Mental Deficiency* 44:114–136, 1939.

21. Skeels HM: Adult status of children with contrasting early life experiences. *Monogr Soc Res Child Dev* 31:1–56, 1966.
22. Sparrow S, Balla, D, Cicchetti D: *Vineland Adaptive Behavior Scales*, Circle Pines, American Guidance Service, 1984.
23. Dykens EM, Hodapp RM, Finucance BM: *Genetics and Mental Retardation Syndromes: A New Look at Behavior and Interventions*, Baltimore, Paul H. Brookes Pub. Co., 2000.
24. Hallahan DP, Kauffman JM: *Exceptional Children: Introduction to Special Education* (10th ed.). Boston, Allyn & Bacon, 2006.
25. Burack JA, Kurtz L, Derevensky JL: Services for persons with mental retardation: A debate for all seasons. *McGill J Educ* 27:275–278, 1992.
26. Bouras N, Holt G (eds.): *Psychiatric and Behavioural Disorders in Developmental Disabilities* 2nd ed. Cambridge, Cambridge University Press, 2006
27. Rutter M, Tizard J, Yule W, Graham P, Whitmore K: Research report: Isle of Wight studies, 1964–1974. *Psychol Med* 6:313–332, 1976.
28. McLaren J, Bryson SE. Review of recent epidemiological studies of mental retardation: Prevalence, associated disorders, and etiology. *Am J Ment Retard* 92(3):243–54, Nov 1987.
29. Leonard H, Wen X: The epidemiology of mental retardation: Challenges and opportunities in the new millennium. *Ment Retard and Dev Dis Res Rev* 8:117–134, 2002.
30. Roeleveld N, Zielhus GA, Gabreels F: The prevalence of mental retardation: A critical review of recent literature. *Dev Med Child Neurol* 39:125–132, 1997.
31. Granat K, Granat S: Adjustment of intellectually below-average men not identified as mentally retarded. *Scand J Psychol* 19:41–51, 1978.
32. Yeargin-Allsopp M, Boyle C: Overview: The epidemiology of neurodevelopmental disorders. Special Issue on The Epidemiology of Neurodevelopmental Disorders (M. Yeargin-Allsopp & C. Boyle, eds.), *Mental Retardation and Developmental Disabilities Research Reviews* 8(3):113–116, 2002.
33. Sovner R: Limiting factors in the use of DSM-III with mentally ill/mentally retarded persons. *Psychopharmacol Bull* 22:1055–1059, 1986.
34. Hodapp RM, Dykens EM: Strengthening behavioral research on genetic mental retardation syndromes. *Am J Ment Retard* 160:4–15, 2001.
35. Hodapp RM, Dykens EM: Measuring behavior in genetic disorders of mental retardation. *Mental Retardation and Developmental Disabilities Research Reviews* 11:340–346, 2005.
36. Dykens EM, Cassidy SB: Prader-Willi syndrome. In: Goldstein S, Reynolds CR (eds): *Handbook of Neurodevelopmental and Genetic Disorders in Children*, New York, Guilford Press, pp. 525–554, 1999.
37. Hagerman RJ, Jackson AW, Levitas A, Rimland B, Braden M: An analysis of autism in 50 males with the fragile X syndrome. *Am J Med Genet* 23:359–374, 1986.
38. Williams CA, Zori RT, Hendrickson J, et al.: Angelman syndrome. *Curr Probl Pediatr* 25:216–231, 1995.
39. Gersh M, Goodard SA, Pasztor LM, Harris DJ, Weiss L, Overhauser J: Evidence for a distinct region causing a cat-cry in patients with 5p deletions. *Am J Hum Gen* 56:1404–1410, 1995.
40. Finucane BM, Konar D, Haas-Givler B, Kurtz MB, Scott CI, Jr: The spasmodic upper body squeeze: A characteristic behavior in Smith-Magenis syndrome. *Dev Med Child Neurol* 36:78–83, 1994.
41. Dykens EM, Hodapp RM, Leckman JF: *Behavior and Development in Fragile X Syndrome*, Thousand Oaks, Sage, 1994.
42. Tassone FI, Hagerman RJ, Ikle D, Dyer PN, Lampe M: FMRP expression as a potential prognostic indicator in fragile X syndrome. *Am J Med Genet* 84:250–261, 1999.
43. Dykens EM, Leckman JF, Cassidy SB: Obsessions and compulsions in Prader-Willi syndrome. *J Child Psychol Psychiatry* 37:995–1002, 1996.
44. Verhoeven WMA, Tuinier S, Curfs L: Prader-Willi syndrome: Cycloid psychosis in a genetic subtype? *Acta Neuropsychiatrica* 15:32–37, 2003.
45. Vogels A, De Hert M, Descheemaeker MJ, Govers V, Devriendt K, Legius E, Prinzie P, Fryns JP: Psychotic disorders in Prader-Willi syndrome. *American J of Med Gen* 127:238–243, 2004.
46. Hodapp RM: Direct and indirect behavioral effects of different genetic disorders of mental retardation. *Am J Ment Retard* 102:67–79, 1997.
47. Dykens EM: Measuring behavioral phenotypes: Provocations from the new genetics. *Am J Ment Retard* 99:522–532, 1995.
48. Dykens EM: Direct effects of genetic mental retardation syndromes: Maladaptive behavior and psychopathology. *Int Rev Res Ment Retard* 22:1–26, 1999a.
49. VanAcker R: Rett's Syndrome. In: Cohen DJ, Volkmar FR (eds): *Handbook of Autism and Pervasive Developmental Disorders*, 2nd ed., New York, Wiley, 1997, pp. 60–93.
50. Dykens EM, Cassidy SB, King BH: Maladaptive behavior differences in Prader-Willi syndrome due to paternal deletion versus maternal uniparental disomy. *Am J Ment Retard* 104:67–77, 1999.
51. Baumgardner TL, Reiss AL, Freund LS, Abrams MT: Specification of the neurobehavioral phenotype in males with fragile X syndrome. *Pediatrics* 95:744–752, 1995.
52. Dykens EM, Clarke DJ: Correlates of maladaptive behavior in individuals with 5p̄ (cri du chat) syndrome. *Dev Med Child Neurol* 39:752–756, 1997.
53. Reiss S, Levitan GW, Szyszko J: Emotional disturbance and mental retardation: Diagnostic overshadowing. *Am J Ment Retard* 86:567–574, 1982.
54. White MJ, Nichols CN, Cook RS, Spengler PM, Walker BS, Look KK: Diagnostic overshadowing and mental retardation: A meta-analysis. *Am J Ment Retard* 100:293–298, 1995.
55. Jacobson JW: Dual diagnosis services: history, progress and perspectives. In: Bouras N (ed): *Psychiatric and Behavioural Disorders in Developmental Disabilities and Mental Retardation*. Cambridge, Cambridge University Press, 1999, pp. 329–35865.
56. Philips I, Williams N: Psychopathology and mental retardation: A study of 100 mentally retarded children I: Psychopathology. *Am J Psychiatry* 132:1265–1271, 1975.
57. Borthwick-Duffy SA, Eyman RK: Who are the dually diagnosed? *Am J Ment Retard* 94:586–595, 1990.
58. Jacobson JW: Problem behavior and psychiatric impairment within a developmentally delayed population. I. Behavioral frequency. *Appl Res Ment Retard* 3:121–139, 1982.
59. Einfeld SL, Tonge BJ: Population prevalence of psychopathology in children and adolescents with intellectual disability. II. Epidemiological findings. *J Intellect Disabil Res* 40:99–109, 1996.
60. King BH, DeAntonia C, McCracken JT, Forness SR, Ackerland V: Psychiatric consultation in severe and profound mental retardation. *Am J Psychiatry* 151:1802–1808, 1994.
61. Dykens EM: Psychopathology in children with intellectual disabilities. *J Child Psychol Psychiatry* 41:407–417, 2000.
62. Einfeld SL, Tonge BJ: *Manual for the Developmental Behavioural Checklist: Primary Carer Version*. Sydney, Australia, School of Psychiatry, University of New South Wales, 1992.
63. Holland AJ, Koot HM: Conference report: Mental health and intellectual disabilities. *J Intellect Disabil Res* 42:505–512, 1998.
64. Moss SC: Assessment: Conceptual issues. In: Bouras N (ed): *Psychiatric and Behavioural Disorders in Developmental Disabilities and Mental Retardation*. Cambridge, Cambridge University Press, 1999, pp. 18–37.
65. Aman MG: *Assessing Psychopathology and Behavior Problems in Persons with Mental Retardation: A Review of Available Instruments*. Rockville, U.S. Department of Health and Human Services, 1991.
66. Aman MG, Singh NN: *Aberrant Behavior Checklist: Community Supplementary Manual*. East Aurora, Slosson Educational Publications, 1994.
67. Reiss S: The Reiss Screen for Maladaptive Behavior. Worthington, IDS Publishing, 1988.
68. Moss SC, Ibbotson B, Prosser H, Goldberg D, Patel P, Simpson N: Validity of the PAS-ADD for detecting psychiatric symptoms in adults with learning disability. *Soc Psychiatric Epidemiol* 32:344–354, 1997b.
69. Moss SC, Prossner H, Ibbotson B, Goldberg D: Respondent and informant accounts of psychiatric symptoms in a sample of patients with learning disability. *J Intellect Disabil Res* 40:457–465, 1996.
70. Sturmey P: Classification: Concepts, progress, and future. In: Bouras N (ed): *Psychiatric and Behavioural Disorders in Developmental Disabilities and Mental Retardation*. Cambridge, Cambridge University Press, 1999, pp. 3–17.
71. Reiss S: Prevalence of dual diagnosis in community-based day programs in the Chicago metropolitan area. *Am J Ment Retard* 94:578–588, 1990.
72. Bird J: Epilepsy and learning disabilities. In: Russell O (ed): *Seminars in the Psychiatry of Learning Disabilities*. London, Gaskell 1997, pp. 223–244.
73. Caplan R, Arbelle S, Magharious W, Guthrie D, Komo S, Shields WD, Chayasirisobhon S, Hansen R: Psychopathology in pediatric complex partial and primary generalized epilepsy. *Dev Med Child Neurol* 40:805–811, 1998.
74. Peterson BS: Neuroimaging in child and adolescent neuropsychiatric disorders. *J Am Acad Child Adolesc Psychiatry* 34:1560–1576, 1995.
75. Robertson D, Murphy D: Brain imaging and behavior. In: Bouras N (ed.): *Psychiatric and Behavioural Disorders in Developmental Disabilities and Mental Retardation*. Cambridge, Cambridge University Press, 1999, pp. 49–70.
76. Hodapp RM: *Development and Disabilities: Intellectual, Sensory and Motor Impairments*, New York, Cambridge University Press, 1998.
77. King BH: Self-injury by people with mental retardation: A compulsive behavior hypothesis. *Am J Ment Retard* 98:93–112, 1993.
78. Dykens EM: Personality-motivation: New ties to psychopathology, etiology, and intervention. In: Zigler E, Bennett-Gates D (eds.): *Personality Development in Individuals with Mental Retardation*. New York, Cambridge University Press, 1999b, pp. 249–270.
79. Bybee J, Zigler E: Outerdirectedness in individuals with mental retardation: A review. In: Burack J, Hodapp RM, Zigler E (eds.): *Handbook of Mental Retardation and Development*. New York, Cambridge University Press, 1998, pp. 434–461.
80. Zigler E, Bennett-Gates D (eds.): *Personality Development in Individuals with Mental Retardation*, New York, Cambridge University Press, 1999.
81. Reiss S, Havercamp SH: Toward a comprehensive assessment of functional motivation: Factor structure of the Reiss profiles. *Psychol Assess* 10:97–106, 1998.
82. Evans DW: Development of the self-concept in children with mental retardation: Organismic and contextual factors. In: Burack J, Hodapp RM, Zigler E (eds.): *Handbook of Mental Retardation and Development*, New York, Cambridge University Press, 1998, pp. 462–480.
83. Reiss S, Havercamp SH: The sensitivity theory of motivation: Why functional analysis is not enough. *Am J Ment Retard* 101:553–566, 1997.

84. Nezu CM, Nezu AM: Outpatient psychotherapy for adults with mental retardation and concomitant psychopathology: Research and clinical imperatives. *J Consult Clin Psychol* 62:34–42, 1994.
85. Lunsky Y, Havercamp SM: Distinguishing low level of social support and social strain: Implications for dual diagnosis. *Am J Ment Retard* 104:200–204, 1999.
86. Siperstein GH, Leffert JS, Wenz-Gross M: The quality of friendships between children with and without learning problems. *Am J Ment Retard* 102:111–125, 1997.
87. Greenspan S, Granfield JM: Reconsidering the construct of mental retardation: Implications of a model of social competence. *Am J Ment Retard* 96:442–453, 1992.
88. Ammerman RT, Hersen M, Van Hasselt VB, Lubstsky MJ, Sieck WR: Maltreatment in psychiatrically hospitalized children and adolescents with developmental disabilities: Prevalence and correlates. *J Am Acad Child Adolesc Psychiatry* 33:567–576, 1994.
89. Sullivan PM, Knutson JF: Maltreatment and disabilities: A population-based epidemiological study. *Child Abuse & Neglect* 24:1257–1273, 2000.
90. Minnes P: Mental retardation: The impact on the family. In: Burack JA, Hodapp RM, Zigler E (eds.): *Handbook of Mental Retardation and Development*. New York, Cambridge University Press, 1998, pp. 693–712.
91. Zigler E: Developmental versus difference theories of retardation and the problem of motivation. *Am J Ment Defic* 73:536–556, 1969.
92. Hodapp RM: Cultural-familial mental retardation. In: Sternberg R (ed.): *Encyclopedia of Intelligence*. New York, Macmillan, 1994, pp. 711–717.
93. Rutter M, Simonoff E, Plomin R: Genetic influences on mild mental retardation: Concepts, findings, and research implications. *J Biosoc Sci* 28:509–526, 1996.
94. Simonoff E, Bolton P, Rutter M: Mental retardation: Genetic findings, clinical implications, and research agenda. *J Child Psychol Psychiatry* 37:259–280, 1996.
95. Zigler E: Familial mental retardation: A continuing dilemma. *Science* 155: 292–298–, 1967.
96. Opitz JM: Vision and insight in the search for gene mutations causing nonsyndromal mental deficiency. *Neurol* 55:335–340, 2000.
97. Matalainen R, Aiaksinen E, Mononen T, Launiala K, Kaariainen R: A population-based study on the causes of severe and profound mental retardation. *Acta Pediatr* 84:261–266, 1995.
98. Mostofsky SH, Mazzocco MM, Aakalu G, Warsofsky IS, Denckla MB, Reiss AL: Deceased cerebellar posterior vermis size in fragile X syndrome: Correlation with neurocognitive performance. *Neurology* 50:121–130, 1998.
99. Dykens EM, Hodapp RM: Treatment issues in genetic mental retardation syndromes. *Profess Psychol Res Pract* 28:263–270, 1997.
100. Hodapp RM, Fidler DJ: Special education and genetics: Connections for the 21st century. *J of Special Ed* 33:130–137, 1999.
101. Curry CJ, Stevenson RE, Aughton D, Byrne JC: Evaluation of mental retardation: Recommendations of a consensus conference: American College of Medical Genetics. *Am J Med Genet* 72:468–477, 1997.
102. Szymanski LS, King BH, Goldberg B, et al.: Diagnosis of mental disorders in people with mental retardation. In: Reiss S, Aman MG (eds): *Psychotropic Medications and Developmental Disabilities: The International Consensus Handbook*. Columbus, Ohio State University Press, 1998, pp. 3–17.
103. Ryan R, Sunada K: Medical evaluation of persons with mental retardation referred for psychiatric assessment. *Gen Hosp Psychiatry* 19:274–280, 1997.
104. Goulden KK, Shinnnar S, Koller K, Katz M, Richardson SA: Epilepsy in children with mental retardation: A cohort study. *Epilepsia* 32:690–697, 1991.
105. Yang Q, Rasmussen SA, Friedman JM: Mortality associated with Down's syndrome in the USA from 1983 to 1997: A population-based study. *Lancet* 359:1019–1025, 2002.
106. Cohen WI (ed.): Health care guidelines for individuals with Down syndrome (Down syndrome preventive medical check list). *Down Syn Quarterly* 1 (2), 1996.
107. Roizen NJ: The early interventionist and the medical problems of the child with Down syndrome. *Infants and Young Children* 16:88–95, 2003.
108. So SA, Urbano RC, Hodapp RM: Hospitalizations for infants and young children with Down syndrome: Evidence from person-records from a statewide administrative database. Submitted 2005.
109. Zigman WB, Silverman W, Wisniewski HM: Aging and Alzheimer's disease in Down syndrome: Clinical and pathological changes. *Ment Retard and Dev Dis Res Rev* 2:73–79, 1996.
110. Whittington JE, Holland AJ, Webb T, Butler J, Clarke D, Boer H: Population prevalence and estimated birth incidence and mortality rate for people with Prader-Willi syndrome in one UK Health Region. *J Med Genet*. 38 (11):792–8, Nov 2001.
111. Sternberg RJ (ed): *Handbook of Intelligence*, Cambridge, Cambridge University Press, 2000.
112. Sparrow SS, Davis SM: Recent advances in the assessment of intelligence and cognition. *J Child Psychol Psychiatry* 41:117–131, 2000.
113. Rusch FR, Chadsey JG (eds): *Beyond High School: Transition from School to Work*, Boston, Allyn & Bacon, 1998.
114. National Center for Family Support: Aging family caregivers: Needs and policy concerns. Family support policy brief #3. National Center for Family Support @ HSRI. Winter, 2000.
115. Hodapp RM, Glidden LM, Kaiser AP: Siblings of persons with disabilities: Toward a research agenda. *Ment Retard* 43:334–338, 2005.
116. Orsmond GI, Seltzer MM: Brothers and sisters of adults with mental retardation: Gendered nature of the sibling relationship. *Am J on Ment Retard* 105:486–508, 2000.
117. Aylward EH, Burt DB, Thorpe LV, Lai F, Dalton A: Diagnosis of dementia in individuals with intellectual disability. *J Intellect Disabil Res* 41:152–164, 1997.
118. Richardson S, Koller H: Vulnerability and resilience of adults who were classified as mildly mentally handicapped in childhood. In: Tizard B, Varma V (eds.): *Vulnerability and Resilience in Human Development*. London, Jessica Kingsley, 1992, pp. 102–119.
119. Ross TT, Begab MK, Dondis EH, Giampiccolo JS, Meyers CE: Lives of the Mentally Retarded: A Forty-Year Follow-Up Study. Stanford, CA, Stanford University Press, 1985.
120. Crow YJ, Tolmie JL: Recurrence risks in mental retardation. *J Med Genet* 35:177–182, 1998.
121. Fombonne E, Bolton P, Prior J, et al.: A family study of autism: Cognitive patterns and levels in parents and siblings. *J Child Psychol Psychiatry* 38:667–683, 1997.
122. Hodapp RM, Glidden LM, Kaiser AP: Siblings of persons with disabilities: Toward a research agenda. *Ment Retard* 43:334–338, 2005.

CHAPTER 5.1.3 ■ LEARNING DISABILITIES

ELENA L. GRIGORENKO

Fundamentally, the concept of learning disabilities (LDs) has to do with society's capacity "to monitor (and recruit) children for unexplained school failure in a way that was not possible before the LD category was reified and passed into law in 1969 (1)". The LD category replaced a variety of loose definitional references to previously used qualifiers such as slow learner, backward children (2) and minimal brain dysfunction (3).

In terms of its realization in the context of current practices, the LD label typically assumes the presence of the following process. Under normal circumstances, LDs are not diagnosable prior to the child's engagement with schooling and the opportunity to master key academic competencies. While in school, a child is assumed to be assigned tasks that are grade appropriate. These tasks assume some degree of variability in children's performance; these theoretical ranges constrain the definitions of acceptable and worrisome variability in performance. It is when the child's performance consistently falls out of the acceptable range in one or more academic subjects that the child becomes the focus of intense observation and documentation and is referred for evaluation to appropriate professionals (educational psychologists, neuropsychologists, and clinicians such as pediatricians, clinical psychologists, or psychiatrists). An important qualifier here is that such observation, documentation, and evaluation are considered only for children whose performance is below that expected based on their general capacity to learn; thus, the concept of "unexpected" school failure is central to the definition of LD. When reports on the child's performance in the classroom, testing results, and clinical evaluations are compiled, the child and his or her family are referred to a special education committee, which determines eligibility for individualized special education services. If eligibility is established, an individualized education program (IEP) is created. The IEP refers to a specific diagnostic label carried by the child and cites a proper category of public laws that guarantees services for an individual with such a diagnosis.

DEFINITION

The definition that currently drives federal regulations was produced by the National Advisory Committee on Handicapped Children in 1968 and subsequently adopted by the U.S. Office of Education in 1977 (4). According to this definition,

> *Specific learning disability* means a disorder in one or more of the basic psychological processes involved in understanding or in using language, spoken or written, which may manifest itself in an imperfect ability to listen, think, speak, read, write, spell, or to do mathematical calculations. The term includes such conditions as perceptual handicaps, brain injury, minimal brain dysfunction, dyslexia, and developmental aphasia. The term does not include children who have learning problems which are primarily the result of visual, hearing, or motor handicaps, of mental retardation, or emotional disturbance, or of environmental, cultural, or economic disadvantage (5).

DSM-IV does not use the term learning disabilities, but makes a reference to the term learning disorders (6). According to DSM-IV, a learning disorder can be diagnosed "...when the individual's achievement on individually administered, standardized tests in reading, mathematics, or written expression is substantially below that expected for age, schooling, and level of intelligence." Of interest here is that this is one of the very few categories of DSM-IV where a reference is made explicitly to psychological tests, although, as stated, DSM-IV does not provide specific guidelines as to what "substantially below" means. Thus, DSM-IV implicitly refers to evidence-based practices (3) as they exist in the field. The problem, of course, is that there are multiple interpretations of these best practices (see discussion following). Yet, assuming there are consistent and coherent guidelines in place for establishing the diagnosis of LD, DSM-IV classifies types of LDs by referencing the primary academic areas of difficulty. The classification includes three specific categories and a residual diagnosis: Reading Disorder, Mathematics Disorder, Disorder of Written Expression, and Learning Disorder NOS. A common practice in the field is to view a diagnosis of a learning disorder as established by DSM-IV as an equivalent to "specific learning disability," which qualifies a child for special services under federal regulations (7).

HISTORY

The introduction of the concept of LD is typically credited to Samuel Kirk (then a professor of special education at the University of Illinois), who, while presenting at a parent meeting in Chicago on April 6, 1963, proposed the term *learning disabled* to refer to "children who have disorders in development of language, speech, reading, and associated communication skills" (ref, http://www.audiblox2000.com/book2.htm). The category was well received by parents and promoted shortly thereafter by an established parent advocacy group known as the Association for Children with Learning Disabilities. Prior to the formal introduction of this concept, the literature had accumulated numerous descriptions of isolated cases and group analyses of children with specific deficits in isolated domains of academic performance (e.g., reading and math) whose profiles were later reinterpreted as those of individuals with specific LDs (e.g., specific reading and math disabilities). It is those examples in the literature and the experiences of many distressed parents who could not find adequate educational support for their struggling children that, in part, resulted in the creation of the field of LDs as a social reality and professional practice (8). Subsequent accumulation of research evidence and experiential pressure led to the formulation of legislation protecting the rights of children with LDs.

Congress enacted the *Education for All Handicapped Children Act* (Public Law 94–142) in 1975 to support states and educational institutions in protecting the rights of, meeting the individual needs of, and improving the results of schooling for infants, toddlers, children, and youth with disabilities, and their families. This landmark law is currently enacted as the *Individuals with Disabilities Education Act* (IDEA, Public Law 105-17), as amended in 2004. The importance of this law is difficult to overstate given that, prior to its enactment, in 1970, U.S. schools provided education to only one in five children with disabilities (9). By 2003–2004, the number of children served under IDEA aged 3–21 was 6,633,902 (http://nces.ed.gov/programs/digest/d04/tables/dt04_054.asp). Specific learning disabilities make up 50% of all special education students served under IDEA.

In its 2004 amendment, IDEA[1] recognized 13 categories under which a child can be identified as having a disability: autism; deaf–blindness; deafness; emotional disturbance; hearing impairment; mental retardation; multiple disabilities; orthopedic impairment; other health impairment; specific learning disability; speech or language impairment; traumatic brain injury; and visual impairment, including blindness. It is of note that LDs as described above in IDEA are referred to as "specific learning disabilities" to emphasize the difference between children with SLD and those with general learning difficulties characteristic of other IDEA categories (e.g., autism and mental retardation). The consensus in the field is that children with LDs possess average to above-average levels of intelligence across many domains of functioning, but demonstrate specific deficits within a narrow range of academic skills. Finally, as stated above, exclusionary factors have been central to diagnoses of LDs since the authoritative definition of LD was introduced in 1977. As per these exclusionary criteria, a child cannot be diagnosed with an LD unless other factors such as other disorders or lack of exposure to high-quality age-, language-, and culture-appropriate educational environments have been ruled out. It is the desire to rule out the exclusionary factor of lack of exposure to high-quality environments that prompted the introduction of the concept of

[1]Although the precise title of the law in its 2004 amendment is "Individuals with Disabilities Education Improvement Act," it is still referred to as IDEA.

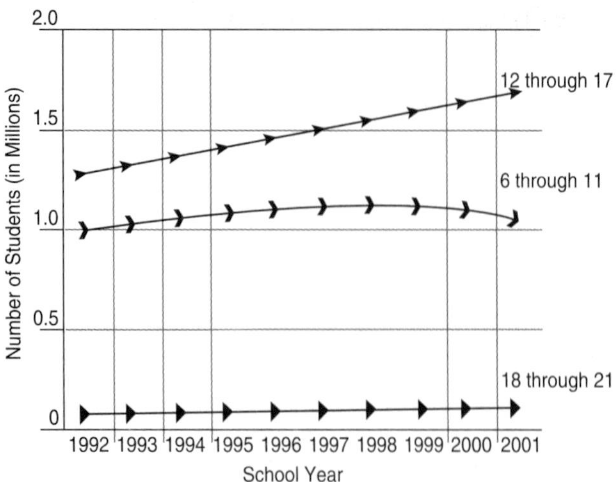

FIGURE 5.1.3.1. Recent dynamics of estimates for prevalence rates of LDs in different age groups. (U.S. Department of Education, 25th Annual Report to Congress, 2003.)

Response to Treatment Intervention [RTI[2] (10)] in the 2004 amendment of IDEA (see more detail on RTI[3] below).

EPIDEMIOLOGY

There are two main sources for obtaining estimates for prevalence rates of LDs. The first and most obvious one is linked to the number of children served under this category of IDEA. Figure 5.1.3.1 provides relevant data. When these data are mapped on the total number of school-aged children in the United States, although the number fluctuates from year to year, the average estimates of prevalence rates for LDs are around 5% to 6% of the total school-age population. To illustrate, in 2003, 2.72 million children were identified as having LDs. This represents a 150% to 200% increase in the number of students with LDs aged 6–17 compared with that number in 1975.

Yet it is important to note that prevalence rates very substantially from district to district and from state to state. For example, in 2004, under the specific learning disabilities category, in Kentucky, 1.8% of all students aged 6–21 received special education services compared with 5.9% in Iowa. Thus, based on these numbers, the prevalence rates of LDs in Iowa are about 3.3 times as high as in Kentucky, two states not very far apart geographically! This observation stresses the mosaic-like situation of LD diagnosis—there is no unified approach to these diagnoses across different local education agencies in the United States.

When IDEA-related prevalence rates are considered, LDs are observed more frequently in boys than in girls (64.5% vs. 33.5% for boys and girls aged 6–17, respectively) and more frequently in underrepresented minority groups than in Asian Americans or whites (the risk ratios[4] are 1.5, 0.4, 1.3, 1.1, 0.9 for American Indian, Asian American, African American, Hispanic American, and white students, respectively).

The second source for these rates is research studies. Per results from these studies, it is assumed that although up to 10% to 12% of school-age children show specific deficits in selected academic domains, high-quality classroom instruction and supplemental intensive small-group activities can reduce this number to ~6% of children. It is assumed that these 6% will meet strict criteria for LDs and will need special education intervention.

It is important to note that most of the research in the field of LDs is currently conducted with reading and, correspondingly, specific reading disability (SRD). There is little established evidence that reliably points to prevalence rates of disorders of math and writing.

To illustrate, according to the results of current research on early reading acquisition, 2% to 6% of children do not show expected progress even in the context of the highest quality evidence-based reading instructions. Based on U.S. national data, the risk for reading problems as defined through failure to reach age- and grade-adequate milestones ranges from 20% to 80%. Specifically, data from the National Assessment of Educational Progress 2005 shows that 36% of fourth graders do not possess the adequate reading skills required for completion of grade-appropriate educational tasks (http://nces.ed.gov/nationsreportcard/pdf/main2005/2006451.pdf). However, it is clear that far from all of these children have SRD. The majority of these children underachieve, mostly likely, because of inadequate educational experiences and causes other than SRD.

Some changes in the 2004 version of IDEA were invoked directly because of concerns regarding the overidentification of students as learning disabled. The category of LDs has often been the largest single category of children served under IDEA (for latest relevant statistics, see https://www.ideadata.org/PartBReport.asp). The reality of everyday practices in school districts was such that most diagnoses prior to the 2004 reauthorization were based on so-called aptitude–achievement discrepancy criteria, which required a severe discrepancy between IQ and achievement scores (e.g., 2 standard deviations, 2 years of age equivalence), although IDEA had never specifically required a discrepancy formula (11). Correspondingly, it has been argued that these discrepancy-based approaches are flawed (12) and might have led to overidentification. In light of this hypothesis, IDEA 2004 emphasizes that there is *no* explicit IQ–achievement discrepancy requirement for diagnosis of LDs. As a possible alternative approach for identification and diagnosis, IDEA 2004 states that local educational agencies may use a child's RTI in lieu of the classification processes (13). A local educational agency (e.g., a school) may choose to administer to the child in question an evidence-based intervention program and, depending on the child's response to this program, determine his or her eligibility for special education services under IDEA.

Specifically, the statutory language of the IDEA 2004 (Public Law 108–446) states:

> *(6) Specific Learning Disabilities.*
>
> **(A) In general.**
>
> Notwithstanding section 607(b), when determining whether a child has a specific learning disability as defined in section 602, a local

[2]RTI signifies "... individual, comprehensive student-centered assessment models that apply a problem-solving framework to identify and address a student's learning difficulties (10)."

[3]It is important to note that RTI might appear counterintuitive at first: How can a disorder be defined through treatment if treatment is prescribed for a particular disorder? This "circularity" of RTI, however, is only superficial. An implicit assumption behind RTI is that teaching is inadequate and that is why schools "produce" such a high level of LDs. A closer analogy would not be with treatment, but with prevention with vitamins; if vitamins are delivered properly, then many deficiencies can be avoided. Thus, if all children get preventive extensive instruction, the frequencies of LDs will diminish.

[4]Risk ratios compare the proportion of a particular racial/ethnic group served to the proportion of all other racial/ethnic groups combined. A risk ratio of 1.0 indicates no difference between the racial/ethnic groups.

educational agency shall not be required to take into consideration whether a child has a severe discrepancy between achievement and intellectual ability in oral expression, listening comprehension, written expression, basic reading skill, reading comprehension, mathematical calculation, or mathematical reasoning.

(B) Additional authority.

In determining whether a child has a specific learning disability, a local educational agency may use a process that determines if the child responds to scientific, research-based intervention as a part of the evaluation procedures described in paragraphs (2) and (3). [§614(b)(6)]

As a consequence of this language, although aptitude–achievement discrepancy has been and continues to remain the common, although not required, practice for local educational agencies, there is a new "entry point" for RTI. Needless to say, these changes are of great theoretical and practical importance. The tradition and system of specific LD identification in the United States is fluid now, and rather few specific recommendations exist to help local educational agencies smoothly transition into the implementation of IDEA 2004.

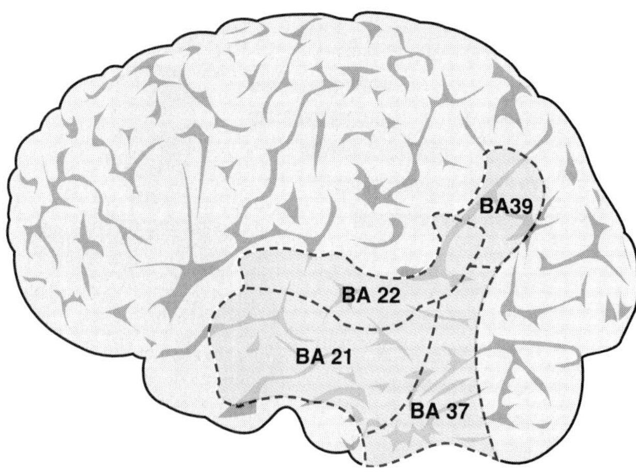

FIGURE 5.1.3.2. Areas of the brain that reportedly form the brain circuitry for reading.

ETIOLOGY

There is a consensus in the field that LDs arise from intrinsic factors and have neurobiological bases, specifically atypicalities of brain maturation and function. There is a substantial body of literature convincingly supporting this consensus and pointing to genetic factors as major etiological factors of LDs. The working assumption in the field is that these genetic factors affect the development, maturation, and functional structure of the brain, which in turn, influences cognitive processes associated with LDs. Yet, the field is acutely aware that a number of external risk factors, such as poverty and lack of educational opportunities, affect patterns of brain development and function and, correspondingly, might worsen the prognosis for biological predisposition for LDs or act as a trigger in LD manifestation.

Although this model, in main strokes, appears to be relevant to all LDs, far more research on relevant genes and brain structure and function is available for children with SRD than for any other LDs. Thus, here illustrative findings are presented from SRD [for a more comprehensive review, see (14)].

Multiple methodological techniques (e.g., EEG, ERP, fMRI, MEG, PET, TMS,[5] to name a few) have been used to elicit brain–reading relationships [for recent reviews, see (15–17)]. When data from multiple sources are combined, it appears that a developed, automatized skill of reading engages a wide, bilateral (but predominantly left-hemispheric) network of brain areas passing activation from occipitotemporal, through temporal (posterior), toward frontal (precentral and inferior frontal gyri) lobes. Clearly, the process of reading is multifaceted and involves evocation of orthographical, phonological, and semantic representations that, in turn, call for the activation of brain networks participating in visual, auditory, and conceptual processing. Correspondingly, it is expected that the areas of activation serve as anatomic substrates supporting all these types of representation and processing.

However, possibly somewhat surprisingly, per recent reviews, there appear to be only four areas of the brain of particular, specific interest with regard to reading (Figure 5.1.3.2). These areas are the fusiform gyrus (the occipitotemporal cortex in the ventral portion of Brodmann's area 37, BA 37), the posterior portion of the middle temporal gyrus (roughly BA 21, but possibly more specifically, the ventral border with BA 37 and the dorsal border of the superior temporal sulcus), the angular gyrus (BA 39), and the posterior portion of the superior temporal gyrus (BA 22).

It is also important to note the developmental changes in patterns of brain functioning that occur with increased mastery of reading skill: progressive, behaviorally modulated development of left-hemispheric "versions" of these areas and progressive disengagement of right-hemispheric areas. In addition, there appears to be a shift of regional activation preferences: The frontal regions are used by fluent more than by beginning readers, and readers with difficulties activate the parietal and occipital regions more than the frontal regions.

In an attempt to understand the mechanism of the "deficient" pattern of brain activation while engaged in reading, researchers are looking for genes that might be responsible, at least partially, for these observed differences in functional brain patterns. This search is supported by a set of convergent lines of evidence [for reviews, see (18–20)]. First, SRD has been considered a familial disorder since the late nineteenth century. This consideration is grounded in years of research into the familiarity of SRD (similarity on the skill of reading among relatives of different degree), characterized by studies that have engaged multiple genetic methodologies, specifically twin (21–23), family (24–26) and sib-pair designs (27, 28). Although each of these methodologies has its own resolution power with regard to explaining similarities among relatives by referring to genes and environments as sources of these similarities and obtaining corresponding estimates of relative contributions of genes and environments, all methodologies have produced data that unanimously point to genetic similarities as the main source of familiarity of SRD.

Today, it is assumed that multiple genes contribute to the biological risk factor that runs in families and forms the foundation for the development of SRD (Figure 5.1.3.3). Specifically, nine candidate regions of the human genome have been implicated (20). These regions are recognized as SRD candidate regions; they are abbreviated as DYX1–9 (DYX for dyslexia, a term often used to refer to SRD) and refer to the regions on chromosomes 15q, 6p, 2p, 6q, 3cen, 18p, 11p, 1p, and Xq, respectively. Each of these regions harbors dozens of genes, so, clearly, the field offers empirical validation that multiple genes contribute to the manifestation of SRD. A number of different research groups are actively at work on these genetic regions in an attempt to identify plausible candidate genes. Four successful attempts have been

[5]EEG: electro-encephalogram; ERP: event-related potentials; fMRI: functional resonance imaging; MEG: magnetoencephalography; PET: positron emission tomography; TMS: transcranial magnetic stimulation.

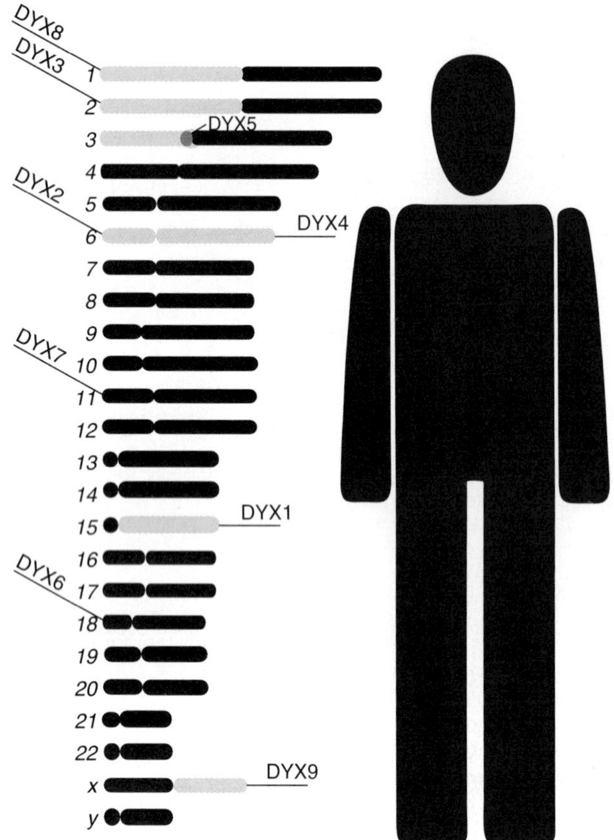

FIGURE 5.1.3.3. Genomic regions of interest for specific reading disability (SRD).

announced in the literature: one for the 15q region—the candidate gene known as *DYX1C1*; (29) two for the 6p region—the candidate gene known as *KIAA0319* (24, 27) and the candidate gene knows as *DCDC2* (30, 31), and one for the 3cen region, *ROBO1* (32). Although the field has not yet converged on "firm" candidates, it is remarkable and of great scientific interest that all four current candidate genes for SRD are involved with biological functions of neuronal migration and axonal crossing. Thus, all these genes are plausible candidates for understanding the pattern of brain functioning in SRD described above.

DIAGNOSIS AND CLINICAL FEATURES

As stated earlier, it is crucially important in a diagnosis of LD to establish "typical" intellectual performance of the child and to document that the child's performance in the area of difficulty (e.g., reading or mathematics) does not correspond to what would be expected given average intellectual functioning. Although this general principle is relatively easy to grasp, the field of LDs has, since its inception in the early 1960s, struggled with establishing specific steps that prescriptively should lead to the establishment of the diagnosis.

As mentioned earlier, prior to the 2004 reauthorization of IDEA, the most common way of establishing an LD diagnosis was the discrepancy criterion. Historically, the introduction of the discrepancy between ability and achievement criteria in the 1977 law was not based on empirical research, but rather driven by a need for a more objective approach to the diagnoses than those commonly used and largely discredited at the time (33). Two decades of research and practical explorations of the discrepancy model resulted in it being discredited from points of view of theory (34), reliability of diagnosis and classification (12), robustness of implementation (35), and treatment validity (36). In response to the overwhelming amount of evidence for the inadequacy of the discrepancy model, however realized (through psychometric indices, age equivalences, regression approaches, or expert opinions), a number of alternative models have been proposed. The major dividing line between these new models and previous discrepancy-based models is in their theoretical orientation. Previous diagnostic models attempted to identify children diagnosable with LDs by looking for characteristic cognitive deficits, so that an intervention could be delivered to children with such deficits (37), whereas the modern models argue for the need to deliver best pedagogical practices to all children and then best remediational-intervention approaches to those children who do not respond as well to good teaching (37).

As per the 2004 reauthorization of IDEA, local educational agencies have some choice in selecting diagnostic models. At this point, the most widely discussed and evidence-supported model of LD identification is the responsiveness to intervention (RTI) model (38). The RTI model has a number of features. First, the performance of the student in question is compared with the performance of his/her immediate peers on academic tasks. Specifically, the RTI assumes tracking the academic performance and rate of its growth for all students within a given class, with a goal of identifying those students in a class whose performance differs from that of their peers both in absolute (level) and relative (rate of growth) terms. Second, the model is structured primarily by intervention, so students identified by these means are offered individualized accommodations and interventions with a goal of maximizing the effectiveness of the learning environment for a given student in need. Third, the model is multilayered, so that each layer offers an opportunity for further differentiation and individualization of education for students who need it. Typically, three layers are recommended, starting with the first tier, which covers regular classroom environment, and going through the second tier, which is characterized as "supplemental" to tier 1, and arriving at tier 3, which is "intensive," "individualized," and "strategic." Fourth, only if these multilayered attempts to modify the regular classroom pedagogical environment are unsuccessful is the prospect of establishing an LD diagnosis considered. In summary, a child could be identified as having an LD if he or she consistently failed to perform at a level and progress at a rate comparable with the child's peers in general education after having experienced and participated in an evidence-based intervention.

Although there is considerable agreement in the field on the promise of RTI as a diagnostic paradigm, there is a variety of opinions regarding how, specifically, RTI should be quantified. Currently, the following paradigms are on trial: 1) Administer norm-referenced assessment batteries at the beginning and end of every school year to quantify the growth in response to intervention—students whose growth rate is below "appropriate" should receive additional intervention, and 2) administer norm-referenced assessment batteries with a particular performance threshold (25th percentile)—students whose performance is below this threshold should receive intensive interventions and their performance should be monitored at least four times a year. There is also significant theoretical and experimental evidence suggesting the need for and importance of continuous progress monitoring with frequent (e.g., weekly) assessments of improvement. Currently, however, there are concerns about both approaches because of a lack of trained educational and practical professionals equipped to translate and implement research-based interventions into the everyday life of American schools. Since the 2004 reauthorization of IDEA, local education agencies have been in search of new robust solutions for identifying LDs that will meet the regulations of federal laws. RTI-based approaches to LD diagnosis present considerable challenges for all professionals involved in the realization of IDEA: general and special education teachers, diagnosticians (psychologists and psychiatrists), and school psychologists. The heart of this challenge is the lack of operationalization and practical guidelines that can be easily implemented at the "frontiers" of diagnosing and treating children with LDs.

RELEVANT THEORETICAL MODELS AND CONSIDERATIONS

As mentioned earlier, the literature on LDs is uneven, with the vast majority of it relating to SRD. Although psychological models of other LDs have been developed, here only those for SRD are exemplified for illustration purposes.

So far, there have been only generic references to the disruption of both the acquisition and mastery of reading skills that constitutes the texture of SRD. When this generic reference is closely considered, another massive body of literature materializes: 1) cognitive psychology literature on types of representation of information involved in reading (reading involves the translation of meaningful symbolic visual codes [orthographical representation] into pronounceable and distinguishable sounds of language [phonological representation] so a meaning [semantic representation] arises); (39) 2) developmental psychology literature on when these representations develop and what might cause the development of a dysfunctional representational system; (40) and 3) educational psychology literature on how the formation of functional representations can be aided or corrected when at risk for malfunction (41). Schematically, the theoretical framework for studying SRD (as presented in 1) above) is shown in Figure 5.1.3.4.

Here only brief commentaries relevant to these literatures are offered. Today, given the predominance of the phonology-based connectionist account of SRD, behavioral manifestation of SRD is captured through a collection of highly correlated psychological traits. Although different researchers use different terms for specific traits, these can be loosely structured into groups aimed at capturing different types of information

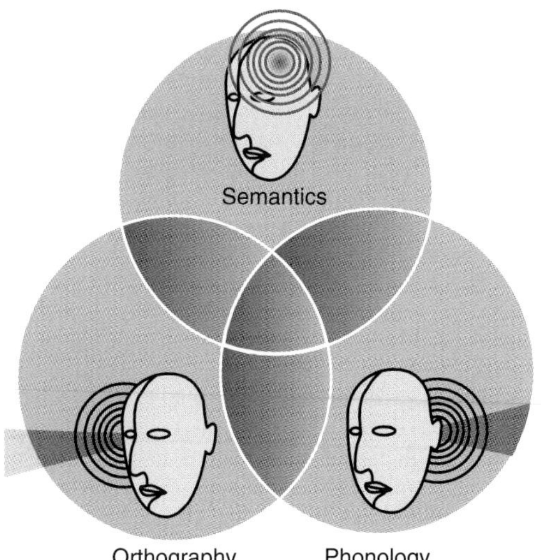

FIGURE 5.1.3.4. Theoretical model grouping psychological processing and types of representations studied in specific reading disability (SRD).

representation, for example: 1) performance on orthographic choice or homonym choice judgment tasks for quantifying parameters of orthographical representation; 2) phonemic awareness, phonological decoding, and phonological memory for quantifying phonological representation; and 3) vocabulary and indices of comprehension at different levels of linguistic processing for quantifying semantic representation. Correspondingly, in studies of the etiology, development, and educational malleability of SRD, the quantification of the disorder is carried out through these various traits (or components of SRD). Thus, many studies attempt to subdivide SRD into its components and explore their etiological bases, developmental trajectories, and susceptibility to pedagogical interventions separately as well as jointly.

DIFFERENTIAL DIAGNOSIS

The majority of students with LDs are identified in middle and high school; this occurrence can be explained by the fact that early years of schooling might simply be insufficient for exposing and making evident a deficit in a particular academic domain. As mentioned, the core conceptual piece of the LD definition is that the deficit could have not been predicted reliably prior to the child's school entry because a child with LDs demonstrates otherwise typical levels of cognitive functioning.

Previously, when the discrepancy criteria were applied, the diagnosis of LD was different from other forms of learning difficulties because of its stress on the specificity of the deficit (i.e., a discrepancy was expected not in *all* academic domains, but in a *specific* academic domain). The introduction of RTI-based approaches to diagnosis makes the question of differential diagnosis somewhat difficult to address. In fact, students with mental retardation, emotional or behavior disorders, ADHD, and other childhood and adolescent disorders might also exhibit low responsiveness to intervention. Yet their nonresponsiveness will occur for reasons very different from those experienced by students with LDs. In other words, if RTI cannot differentiate LDs from other diagnoses where learning difficulties are present but nonspecific, can RTI even be considered as a classification/diagnostic instrument (42)?

Although this question has been raised, it has not yet been answered. The pre-2004 conceptualization of LDs assumed that the texture of LDs was in deficient (or different, atypical) psychological processing of information. In other words, the field was driven by the assumption that LDs were likely to represent a dysfunction in one or more basic psychological processes (phonological processing, sustained attention, different types of memory, executive functioning). These deficient processes, in turn, can slow down or inhibit mastery of a particular academic domain (reading or mathematics). Under this assumption, intensive academic instruction could improve performance in specific academic domains, but could not treat the disorder. Even if reading improves as a result of intervention, in this paradigm, the disorder might remanifest as a deficiency in a bordering domain (writing). In other words, although reading skills might be enhanced, the deficient psychological skills might impede some other academic domain of functioning.

Throughout the existence of the category of specific LDs, there has been a consistent and strong drive from parents, researchers, and educators for differentiating these disorders from generic learning difficulties. In its current iteration, RTI does not differentiate nonspecific and specific learning difficulties, because nonresponsiveness to intervention can occur with a variety of developmental disorders. In sum, because IDEA preserved the category of specific LDs, there is a huge new task to differentiate specific and nonspecific learning difficulties by the means of RTI and possibly other methods in the field.

One of these "other" methods has to do, of course, with psychological testing. Many researchers argue for the necessity of maintaining the role of psychoeducational and neuropsychological tests on a variety of indicators, including IQ, in establishing LD diagnosis (42, 43).

COURSE AND PROGNOSIS

There is an accepted understanding in the field that LDs are typically lifelong disorders, although their manifestations might and often do vary depending on developmental stage and demands of the environment (school, work, retirement) imposed on an individual at a particular time. This understanding assumes that LDs do not manifest themselves exclusively in academic settings. In fact, the assumption here is that, although it might be successfully remediated during years of schooling, a particular LD might need further assistance and remediation in later years of functioning (as a part of the workforce). Although the literature on adults with LDs is still somewhat limited, there is an accumulation of evidence that LDs constitute a serious public health problem even after the schooling years. Such evidence is particularly rich in the field of studies of SRD.

LDs are comorbid with a number of other disorders typically diagnosed in childhood or adolescence, especially attention deficit (44) and disruptive behavior disorders (45). LDs also often co-occur with anxiety and depression (46). Correspondingly, individuals with LDs are at higher risk for developing other mental health problems.

Yet the main drawback for individuals with specific LDs has to do with their educational achievement. On average, only ~50% of students aged 14 and older diagnosed with LDs graduate with regular high school diplomas. Correspondingly, the dropout rate among these students is very high (~45%), and even higher for underrepresented minority students. The employment prospect of these students is also troublesome—only about 60% of student ages 14 and older diagnosed with LDs have paid jobs outside the home.

Thus, it is important to realize that the impact of LDs is not limited to any one academic domain (reading or mathematics); these are lifetime disorders with wide-ranging consequences.

TREATMENT

Currently, there are no approved medical treatments for children with LDs. There is a consensus in the field that children with LDs should be provided special education and related services upon establishing their eligibility and determining the necessity, content, duration, and desired outcomes of such education and services.

Yet, in much of the literature, many educators have expressed concern with the possible presence of faulty identification procedures in states and districts across the country, which has resulted in the possible abuse of the classification and service systems. The ever-growing number of children identified with LDs (Figure 5.1.3.1) might indicate that this category has become a "trap" for lower performing students irrespective of an LD diagnosis.

In response to this concern, the 2004 reauthorization of IDEA makes reference to a set of prevention mechanisms intended to establish a better classification strategy for identifying children with LDs. By law, schools need to implement systemic models of prevention that address 1) primary prevention: the provision of high-quality education for all children; 2) secondary prevention: targeted, scientifically based interventions for children who are not responding to primary prevention; and 3) tertiary prevention: the provision of intensive individualized services and interventions for those children who have not responded to high-quality instruction or subsequent intervention efforts. Per new regulations, it is assumed that this third group of children, those children who have failed to respond to age-, language-, and culture-appropriate, evidence-based, domain-specific instruction (in reading or mathematical cognition), can be identified as eligible for special education services. Of importance here is that these prevention mechanisms are also assumed to be used as diagnostic mechanisms (see the earlier discussion of RTI). This circular system of an outcome of intervention being also an entry point to diagnosis is currently creating significant turmoil in the literature and in practice.

In general, RTI approaches are conceived as a twofold simultaneous realization of high-quality, domain-specific instruction and continuous formative evaluation of students' performance and learning (47, 48). In other words, RTI refers to ongoing assessment of students' response to evidence-based pedagogical interventions in particular academic domains. Thus, it is assumed that LDs can be identified *only* when underachievement related to poor instruction is ruled out.[6] Although present in a number of alternative forms, RTI includes eight central features and six common attributes. Among the central features linking all forms of RTI are: 1) high-quality classroom instruction; 2) research-based instruction; 3) classroom performance measures; 4) universal screening; 5) continuous progress monitoring; 6) research-based intervention; 7) progress monitoring during intervention; and 8) fidelity measures. Among common attributes of different RTI models, there are concepts of 1) multiple tiers; 2) transition from instruction for all to increasingly intense interventions; 3) implementation of differentiated curricula; 4) instruction delivered by staff other than the classroom teacher; 5) varied duration, time, and frequency of intervention; and 6) categorical or non-categorical placement decisions (49). Clearly, the concept of RTI is centered on the field's consensus of what high-quality, research-validated instruction is. It is important to note that, although there is growing consensus with regard to critical elements for effective reading instruction [e.g., (50)], other domains of teaching for academic competencies are far from being consensus-driven.

There are numerous examples of RTI-based treatment of LDs; two often-cited ones are the Minneapolis Public School's Problem Solving Model, which has been in action since 1994 (51), and the Heartland (Iowa) Area Education Association's (AEA) Model, implemented in 1986 (52). The Minneapolis model is a three-tier intervention model where the referral to special education is made only after consecutive failures to benefit from instruction throughout all three tiers of pedagogical efforts. The Iowa model originally include four tiers, where the third tier was subdivided into two related steps, but was then collapsed into one tier, similar to the Minneapolis model. Unfortunately, neither model has published empirical data on its effectiveness. Yet, years of implementations resulted in appreciation from the communities they serve and in a stable, relatively low special education population.

Currently, the concept of RTI is under careful examination by researchers supported by both the U.S. Department of Education and the National Institute of Child Health and Development. The future of RTI and its role in diagnosing and treating specific LDs is dependent on answers to critical questions: 1) whether an RTI model can be implemented on a large scale; 2) how an RTI model can be used for LD eligibility

[6]It is also important to note that the primary diagnosis of LD is established only in absence of other neuropsychiatric conditions.

determination; 3) whether an RTI is an effective prevention system; and 4) whether RTI enhances LD determination and minimizes the number of false positives.

CONCLUSION

Currently, students with specific LDs constitute about half of all students served under IDEA. Effective identification of such students and their efficacious and efficient remediation are crucial steps to address their individual educational needs and to provide them with adequate and equal life opportunities.

Given changes in IDEA 2004, it is of no surprise that RTI is central to current discourse on specific LDs. RTI is central to professional discussions of educators, diagnosticians, and policymakers because of its promise to alleviate many longstanding concerns with the IQ/aptitude–achievement discrepancy model predominant in the field of LDs for the last 30 years. At this point, however, RTI is still to deliver on its promise. If RTI succeeds, numerous benefits to educational systems and individuals might be obtained (49). Specifically, as for the system, many inappropriate referrals might be eliminated to increase the legitimacy and fair nature of "true" referrals; the costs of special education services might be reduced; various gender and ethnicity biases might be minimized; and accountability for student learning might be increased. As for individuals, because the labeling criteria will change, there will be less time for a student to demonstrate a "true" failure in achieving the stipulated discrepancy value—prevention and remediation efforts are expected to start as early as possible; the instruction will be individualized; the identification will be focused on achievement rather than on aptitude–achievement discrepancy; and minimizing labeling should result in reducing social stigma.

Yet, these are only expectations for now, and the immediate future will show whether RTI is a viable replacement to the discrepancy criteria.

AUTHOR NOTE

Preparation of this chapter was supported by grants REC-9979843 from the National Science Foundation, R206R00001 from the Javits Act Program administered by the Institute for Educational Sciences, U.S. Department of Education, and TW006764 from the National Institutes of Health. Grantees undertaking such projects are encouraged to express freely their professional judgment. This article, therefore, does not necessarily represent the position or policies of the NSF, the IES, or the NIH, and no official endorsement should be inferred. The author expresses sincere gratitude to Ms. Robyn Rissman for her editorial assistance, and Ms. Beata Moryl and Mr. Philip Lique for preparing the figures.

References

1. Namjou B, et al.: Stratification of pedigrees multiplex for systemic lupus erythematosus and for self-reported rheumatoid arthritis detects a systemic lupus erythematosus susceptibility gene (SLER1) at 5p15.3. *Arthritis & Rheumatism* 2002. 46: p. 2937–2945.
2. Franklin BM: The first crusade for learning disabilities: The movement for the education of backward children. In: Popkewitz T (ed): *The foundation of the school subjects*, (ed): ed. London, Falmer. 1987 pp. 190–209.
3. Fletcher JM, et al.: Classification of learning disabilities: An evidence-based evaluation, In: Bradley R, Danielson L, Hallahan DP (eds): *Identification of Learning Disabilities: Research to Practice*, Mahwah, NJ: Lawrence Erlbaum Associates, Publishers 2002, pp. 185–250.
4. Mercer CD, et al.: Learning disabilities definitions and criteria used by state education departments. *Learning Disability Quarterly* 1996. 19: pp. 217–232.
5. U.S. Office of Education: Assistance to states for education for handicapped children: Procedures for evaluating specific learning disabilities. *Federal Register*, 1977. 42: pp. 65082–65085.
6. American Psychiatric Association, *Diagnostic and statistical manual of mental disorders*. 4th ed. 1994, Washington, DC: APA.
7. Snowling MJ and J Stackhouse: Spelling performance of children with developmental verbal dyspraxia. *Developmental Medicine and Child Neurology*, 1983. 25: p. 430–437.
8. Hallahan DP and CR Mercer: Learning disabilities: Historical perspectives, In: Bradley R, Danielson L, Hallahan DP (eds): *Identification of learning disabilities: Research to practice*. Mahwah: Lawrence Erlbaum 2002, pp. 1–67.
9. U.S. Office of Special Education Programs: *History: Twenty-five years of progress in educating children with disabilities through IDEA*. Washington, DC: U.S. Department of Education, 2000.
10. Deshler DD, et al.: Research topics in responsiveness to intervention: Introduction to the special series. *Journal of Learning Disabilities* 38: 2005. pp. 483–484.
11. Mandlawitz M: *What Every Teacher Should Know about IDEA 2004*, Boston, Allyn & Bacon, 2006.
12. Francis DJ, et al.: Psychometric approaches to the identification of LD: IQ and achievement scores are not sufficient. *Journal of Learning Disabilities* 38: 2005. pp. 98–108.
13. Council of Parent Attorneys and Advocates, H. R. 1350 Individuals with Disabilities Education Improvement Act of 2004 compared to IDEA 97. Warrenton, Author, 2004.
14. Grigorenko EL: Triangulating developmental dyslexia: Behavior, brain, and genes, In: Coch D, Dawson G, Fischer K (eds): *Human behavior and the developing brain*. In press, New York: Guilford Press.
15. Price CJ, Mechelli A: Reading and reading disturbance. *Current Opinion in Neurobiology*. 15: 2005. pp. 231–238.
16. Shaywitz SE, Shaywitz BA: Dyslexia (specific reading disability). *Biological Psychiatry* 57: 2005, pp. 1301–1309.
17. Simos PG, et al.: Single-word reading: Perspectives from magnetic source imaging, In: *Single-word reading: Cognitive, behavioral and biological perspectives*, EL Grigorenko and A. Naples, eds. In press, Mahwah: Lawrence Erlbaum.
18. Barr CL, Couto JM: Molecular genetics of reading, In: Grigoronko EL, Naples A (eds): *Single-word reading: Cognitive, behavioral and biological perspectives*, In press, Mahwah, NJ: Lawrence Erlbaum.
19. Fisher SE, DeFries JC: Developmental dyslexia: Genetic dissection of a complex cognitive trait. Nature Reviews: *Neuroscience* 3: 2002 pp. 767–780.
20. Grigorenko EL: A conservative meta-analysis of linkage and linkage-association studies of developmental dyslexia. *Scientific Studies of Reading* 9: 2005. pp. 285–316.
21. Byrne B, et al.: Longitudinal twin study of early literacy development: Preschool and kindergarten phases. *Scientific Studies of Reading* 9: 2005. p. 219–235.
22. Cardon LR, et al.: Quantitative trait locus for reading disability on chromosome 6. *Science*, 226: 1994 pp. 276–279.
23. Cardon LR, et al.: Quantitative trait locus for reading disability: Correction. *Science*, 268: 1995. pp. 1553.
24. Cope N, et al.: Strong evidence that KIAA0319 on chromosome 6p is a susceptibility gene for developmental dyslexia. *American Journal of Human Genetics*, 76: 2005. pp. 581–591.
25. Grigorenko EL, et al.: Susceptibility loci for distinct components of developmental dyslexia on chromosomes 6 and 15. *American Journal of Human Genetics*, 60: 1997. pp. 27–39.
26. Wolff PH, Melngailis I: Family patterns of developmental dyslexia. *American Journal of Medical Genetics (Neuropsychiatric Genetics)*. 54: 1994. pp. 122–131.
27. Francks C, et al.: A 77-kilobase region on chromosome 6p22.2 is associated with dyslexia in families from the United Kingdom and from the United States. *American Journal of Human Genetics*. 75(1046–1058), 2004.
28. Ziegler A, et al.: Developmental dyslexia—Recurrence risk estimates from a German bi-center study using the single proband sib pair design. *Human Heredity*. 59: 2005. pp. 136–143.
29. Taipale M, et al.: A candidate gene for developmental dyslexia encodes a nuclear tetratricopeptide repeat domain protein dynamically regulated in brain. *Proceedings of the National Academy of Sciences of the United States of America*. 100: 2003. pp. 11553–11558.
30. Meng H, et al.: DCDC2 is associated with reading disability and modulates neuronal development in the brain. *Proceedings of the National Academy of Sciences of the United States of America*. 102: 2005. pp. 17053–17058.
31. Schumacher J, et al.: Strong genetic evidence of DCDC2 as a susceptibility gene for dyslexia. *American Journal of Human Genetics* 78: 2006. pp. 52–62.
32. Hannula-Jouppi K, et al.: The axon guidance receptor gene ROBO1 is a candidate dene for developmental dyslexia. *PLoS* 1: 2005. pp. e50.
33. Gresham FM, et al.: Comprehensive evaluation of learning disabilities: A response to intervention perspective. *The School Psychologist*, 59: 2004. pp. 26–29.
34. Sternberg RJ, Grigorenko EL: Difference scores in the identification of children with learning disabilities: It's time to use a different method. *Journal of School Psychology* 40: 2002. pp. 65–83.
35. Haight SL, Patriarca LA, Burns MK: A statewide analysis of eligibility criteria and procedures for determining learning disabilities. *Learning Disabilities: A Multidisciplinary Journal*. 11: 2002. pp. 39–46.

36. Joshi RM, and PG, Aaron (eds.) *Handbook of orthography and literacy*. In press, Mahwah: Lawrence Erlbaum Associates.
37. Reschly DJ, Tilly WD, Grimes JP: *Special education in transition: Functional assessment and noncategorical programming*. Longmont, Sopris West, 1999.
38. Vaughn S, and LS, Fuchs, Redefining learning disabilities as inadequate response to instruction: The promise and potential problems. *Learning Disabilities Research & Practice* 18: 2003. pp. 137–146.
39. Harm MW, Seidenberg MS: Computing the meanings of words in reading: Cooperative division of labor between visual and phonological processes. *Psychological Review* 111: 2004. pp. 662–720.
40. Karmiloff-Smith A: Development itself is the key to understanding developmental disorders. *TRENDS in Cognitive Sciences* 2: 1998 pp. 389–398.
41. Blachman BA, et al.: Effects of intensive reading remediation for second and third graders and a 1-year follow-up. *Journal of Educational Psychology* 96: 2004. pp. 444–461.
42. Mastropieri MA, and TE, Scruggs, Feasibility and consequences of response to intervention: Examination of the issues and scientific evidence as a model for the identification of individuals with learning disabilities. *Journal of Learning Disabilities*, 38: 2005. pp. 525–531.
43. Semrud-Clikeman M, Neuropsychological aspects for evaluating learning disabilities. *Journal of Learning Disabilities* 38: 2005. pp. 563–568.
44. Semrud-Clikeman M, et al.: Comorbidity between ADDH and learning disability: A review and report in a clinically referred sample. *Journal of the American Academy of Child & Adolescent Psychiatry* 31: 1992. pp. 439–448.
45. Grigorenko EL: Learning disabilities in juvenile offenders. *Child and Adolescent Psychiatric Clinics of North America* 15: 2006. pp. 353–371.
46. Martinez RS, Semrud-Clikeman M, Emotional adjustment and school functioning of young adolescents with multiple versus single learning disabilities. *Journal of Learning Disabilities* 37: 2004. 37: pp. 411–420.
47. Mellard DF, et al., Foundations and research on identifying model responsiveness-to-intervention sites. *Learning Disability Quarterly*, 27: 2004. pp. 243–256.
48. Mellard DF, Deshler DD, Barth A.: LD identification: It's not simply a matter of building a better mousetrap. *Learning Disability Quarterly*, 274: 2004. pp. 229–242.
49. Graner PS, Faggetta-Luby MN, Fritschmann NS.: An overview of responsiveness to intervention: What practitioners ought to know. *Topics in Language Disorders* 25: 2005. pp. 93–105.
50. Foorman BR, Breier JI, Fletcher JM.: Interventions aimed at improving reading success: An evidence-based approach. *Developmental Neuropsychology* 24: 2003. pp. 613–639.
51. Marston D, et al.: Problem-solving model for decision making with high-incidence disabilities: The Minneapolis experience. *Learning Disabilities Research & Practice*, 18: 2003. pp. 187–200.
52. Ikeda MJ, Gustafson JK: *Heartland AEA 11′ problem solving process: Impact on issues related to special education*. Johnston, IA: Heartland Area Educational Agency 11 2002.

CHAPTER 5.1.4 ■ DISORDERS OF COMMUNICATION

RHEA PAUL

Language, a unique and characteristic capacity of the human mind, is also one of its most vulnerable faculties. Virtually any disruption in cognitive function, particularly during early development, can affect language acquisition. For this reason, disorders of language development typically accompany a variety of conditions, but they can occur in relative isolation as well. It is also true that language is just one form of communication. The term *communication* refers to all forms of sending and receiving messages, not only with language, but in other ways, such as with gestures, body language, even the way we dress. Animals can also communicate; by means, for example, of their vocalizations to alert others to danger. Figure 5.1.4.1 depicts the relationships among speech, language, and communication. Within the realm of communication, *language* represents one specific type, which involves generating a potentially infinite set of never-before conveyed messages through the combination of words in rule-governed ways that allow the formation of sentences to express meaning to others. Only humans are truly creative users of language; animals may communicate a limited range of messages, but only humans can express ideas through utterances they create anew without having heard or learned them previously. Speech, on the other hand, is a particular mode of language, its expression through the use of sounds produced by oral movements and gestures. There are other ways to express ideas in language, through writing, for example, that are not speech. It will be helpful to keep these distinctions in mind as we discuss the disorders addressed in this chapter.

DEFINITIONS

Communication disorders include any difficulty that affects an individual's ability to engage in reciprocal social interactions. Thus, communication disorders are defined quite broadly. They can include the problems high-functioning individuals with autism have in engaging in conversation, the deficits in reading and writing seen in children with language-based learning disabilities, or the lack of access to language input seen in people who are deaf. Thus, the term *communication disorder* subsumes the many kinds of difficulties of speech, language, and social interaction that can affect one's ability to participate in conversation and social intercourse.

The American Speech-Language-Hearing Association (ASHA) has defined *language disorder* as an impairment in "comprehension and/or use of a spoken, written, and/or other symbol system. The disorder may involve (1) the form of language (phonologic, morphologic, and syntactic systems) (2), the content of language (semantic system), and/or (3) the function of language in communication (pragmatic system), in any combination (1)". This definition essentially means that a language disorder can be seen as a disruption in any aspect of verbal communication, whether oral or written. It is important to note that this impairment is not necessarily defined only in relation to cognitive level or mental age. Current practice dictates that any child whose language is inadequate for communication can be diagnosed as having a language disorder, even a child who is mentally retarded with a mental age commensurate with his current level of language function. Since

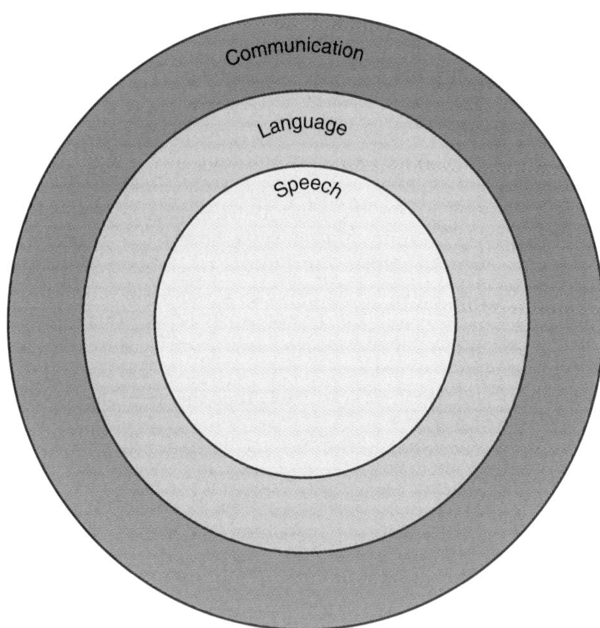

FIGURE 5.1.4.1. Domains of communication.

language is a primary and essential form of communication, it is held that all children who have difficulty with understanding or using linguistic communication should have access to services to improve their language function.

Speech disorders are more limited difficulties. These refer to problems with the production of oral language, although comprehension may be intact. Speech disorders can affect the fluency of speech (e.g., stuttering), the perceived quality of production (e.g., voice disorders), or the pronunciation of particular sounds (e.g., articulation disorders).

HISTORY

Descriptions of the syndrome of disorders of language learning in children date back to at least the early 19th century. Gall (2) was perhaps the first to describe children with poor understanding and use of speech and to differentiate them from the mentally retarded. Subsequently, discoveries about the relations between the brain and language behavior were made by neurologists such as Broca (3) and Wernicke (4). The disorders Gall first identified were thought to be parallel to the aphasias these neurologists were studying in adults. For the first century of the existence of the study of language learning and its disorders, neurologists dominated the field, focusing attention on the physiological substrate of language behavior.

The neurologist Samuel T. Orton (5) can perhaps be thought of as the father of the modern practice of child language disorders. He emphasized the importance not only of neurological but also of behavioral descriptions of the syndrome and pointed out the connections between disorders of language learning and difficulties in the acquisition of reading and writing. In the 1940s and 1950s, other medical professionals, such as psychiatrists and pediatricians, took an interest in children who seemed to be unable to learn language but did not have mental retardation or deafness. Gesell and Amatruda (6) were pioneers in developmental pediatrics and devised innovative techniques for evaluating language development and recognized the condition they called "infantile aphasia." Benton (7, 8) provided us with the fullest descriptions of children with this syndrome and is credited with evolving the concept of a specific disorder of language learning that is structured by excluding other syndromes, rather than by parallels to adult aphasia.

At about the same time as these medical practitioners were refining notions of language disorders, another group of workers was also advancing concepts about children who failed to learn language. Ewing; (9) McGinnis, Kleffner, and Goldstein; (10) and Myklebust (11, 12) were all educators of the deaf and, as such, had developed a variety of techniques for teaching language to children who did not talk or hear. They all noticed that some deaf children's language skills were worse than could be expected on the basis of their hearing impairment alone. This observation led them to focus more interest on the language impairment itself and to attempt to develop more effective methods of remediation for children who did not succeed with the standard approaches that were used to teach language to other children with hearing impairments.

However, until the 1950s, no unified field of endeavor addressing the problems of the language-learning child considered these problems to be disorders of language itself, rather than as a result of some other syndrome ("infantile aphasia" or deafness, for example), or treated language disorders in children regardless of whether the disorder was caused by deafness, mental retardation, or presumed neurological dysfunction. Aram and Nation (13) give credit to three individuals for developing this new field: Mildred A. McGinnis, Helmer R. Myklebust, and Muriel E. Morley. These pioneers integrated the information then available on language disorders in deaf and "aphasic" children and devised educational approaches that could be used to remediate the language dysfunctions demonstrated by these children.

Myklebust (11) perhaps went the furthest in establishing a new and distinct field of study and practice, which he dubbed language pathology. He developed schemes for classifying language disorders in children, which he called auditory disorders, and for differentiating them from deafness and mental retardation. But Myklebust, like Orton, also was concerned with the continuities between disorders of oral language acquisition and their consequences for the acquisition of literacy skills. In founding the new discipline of language pathology, Myklebust pointed the way toward considering language disorders in this broad context, including not only difficulties in producing and comprehending oral language but in the use of written forms of language.

At about the same time that the field of language pathology was being established, the study of language itself was being revolutionized by the introduction of Chomsky's (14) theory of transformational grammar. This innovation led to an explosion in research and interest in child language acquisition, on which the new discipline of language pathology could draw. This evolving database on normal acquisition provided a blueprint of the language development process that could serve as a curriculum guide for planning intervention.

EPIDEMIOLOGY

Accurate estimates of prevalence of specific language disorders are difficult to come by, because of methodological differences across studies (e.g., in the subclassifications and definitions; in the cutoffs and inclusionary criteria; and in the age, sex, and other characteristics of the children sampled). However, delays in language development are the most common presenting symptom in preschool children (15). Estimates of the prevalence of language difficulty in preschool children vary between 7% and 15% (16–18), with an overall median prevalence of 5.9% (19). The prevalence estimate is 8% for boys and 6% for girls (20).

At school age, the prevalence of primary language disorders is thought to be about 4–7% (21), although again there is overlap with related disorders, because some preschoolers with language disorders "grow into" school-age learning disabilities and dyslexia (22). Specific language disorders and learning disabilities combined are some of the most prevalent disorders of school-age children (23). Although disorders of language expression are thought to be more common than those involving comprehension, Bishop (24) has argued that almost all children with language impairments do have receptive difficulties, although they may be subtle in some cases.

ETIOLOGY

Again, etiological discussions are complicated by the fact that language disorders can exist as circumscribed syndromes, but also accompany a range of other developmental disorders. For this reason, we will restrict our discussion of etiology to specific language impairments (SLI). Although biological markers of SLI have not been identified, neurobiological factors are clearly implicated. There is evidence of genetic factors in SLI (25), including higher concordance in monozygotic than dizygotic twins (26) and higher than normal risk in family members for language and learning problems if a child has SLI (27–29). The role of environmental factors in these disorders has long been at issue. Although aberrant parental linguistic input has often been suspected as a cause, numerous researchers (30–33) have concluded that linguistic input to children with language disorders is adequately matched to the children's language level. Some environmental factors appear to be associated with risk for language delay, however. These include lower socioeconomic status, larger family size, recurrent otitis media, neglectful home environment, and later birth order (34). It appears that the operative mechanism behind these factors is deprivation of enriching linguistic input (35), occurring at a critical stage in language development.

Just how specific are specific language disorders? Children with SLI are at greatly increased risk for attention and activity problems (36). Other "soft" neurologic signs are also frequently present in children with SLI (8, 37). The involvement of a variety of nonverbal cognitive skills in SLI also has been indicated (38, 39). These findings have led to the hypothesis that children with SLI may have not just a language problem, but also a general representational deficit, affecting a variety of kinds of symbolic functioning. Tallal (40) cautioned, however, that in each of these studies there were children with SLI who could perform the nonverbal cognitive tasks adequately, and that sometimes the differences between groups were not qualitative, but a matter of speed of response. Leonard (41) pointed out that, although some children with SLI fall below age mates on such tasks, they still do better than younger children with comparable language skills.

Leonard (41, 42) provided an alternative explanation for SLI. He contended that children who score low on language tests, relative to their scores on other areas of cognition, may no more have a "disorder" than children who cannot learn to play the violin. He argued that some children are just "limited" in their ability to learn language, falling (as some must) at the low end of the normal distribution of language ability. If this were the case, in his view, it would not be surprising that such children would also be limited in other abilities that related to symbolic function. He referred to Gardner's (43) notion of "multiple intelligences," which proposes that there is a variety of somewhat independent spheres of intellectual functioning and that some people have greater abilities in some than others. The tendency to call a language limitation a "handicap" stems, in Leonard's view, from the importance of linguistic skills for academic and vocational success in our society, not from any significant neurological or neuropsychological pathology in people limited in this way. The fact that language problems tend to aggregate in families (see 39, 44 for review) could be taken to support the view that some people just have fewer optimal "language genes," and therefore less talent in language areas, than others.

Many would contest this view, however. They would hold that the frequent cooccurrence of SLI with attention and activity problems and other "soft" neurologic signs raises questions about its relation to normal development. Aram (45) argued that children with nearly age-appropriate comprehension but expression limited to single words could not be seen as functioning simply at the low end of the normal range, nor could a 3-year-old who can read but can not produce spontaneous speech (46). Clearly, some children with SLI do have pathologic factors involved. The question for researchers and theoreticians is whether these children are the exception or the rule.

An alternative explanation has been offered by Bishop (24) and Tallal and associates (47). These writers discuss the possibility that SLI is related to deficits in the processing of auditory information, particularly the rapid, short-lived information contained in speech. Tallal and associates have developed an intervention program, known as Fast ForWord, based on this theory. The program trains children to discriminate auditory stimuli on the basis of increasingly brief acoustic cues. Although they have claimed dramatic success in their program, controversy still surrounds these claims at the present writing (48, 49).

Newly emerging imaging techniques have demonstrated some differences in brain function between children with and without specific language disorders. Typically, individuals have asymmetrical brains; language structures (such as the planum temporale) tend to be bigger in the left hemisphere. However, children with SLI have generally smaller and more symmetrical brain hemispheres (50). Studies of adults with language difficulties have revealed that they were more likely than individuals with no history of language impairment to have an extra sulcus in Broca's area, in either brain hemisphere (51). But it is important to realize that no one pattern of brain architecture has been consistently shown in all individuals with language impairment. Instead, these structural differences appear to act as risk factors for language difficulty.

In summary, there is evidence for a genetic component in specific speech and language disorder. However, there are few biological markers of specific language impairment. Although several newly emerging methods have demonstrated differences in the neural structure and auditory functioning of children with SLI, reliable clinical markers have not yet emerged.

SYNDROMES INVOLVING COMMUNICATION DISORDERS

Mental Retardation

Limitation in communicative skill is often one of the first signs of mental retardation. Children with retardation are often first recognized because of their failure to begin talking at the normal time. The sequence of language acquisition in children with retardation follows, in general, the sequence of normal acquisition, although some differences can be identified (52). Many children with mental retardation (MR) show communicative skills that are commensurate with their developmental level, but more than half have language skills that are less than what would be expected for mental age (53). Productive deficits are common, with some children with MR showing deficits relative to mental age in this area only. Others have both receptive and expressive limitations relative to mental age. Phonologic errors are prevalent in children with

MR. These children make similar errors to those seen in normal development, but errors are more frequent (54). Pragmatic skills are usually similar to those seen in children at similar developmental levels (55). The two most prevalent syndromes of MR, Down syndrome (DS) and fragile X syndrome, are both very frequently associated with various problems in language development (56, 57). About a third of children with fragile X also exhibit symptoms of autism, whereas social communication skills in children with DS tend to be relatively preserved. Other syndromes, such as Prader-Willi, also exhibit language deficits (52). Even in Williams syndrome, in which it was previously thought that language was stronger than nonverbal ability, recent research has shown that language is preserved relative to nonverbal skills, but does not typically exceed developmental level (58).

Hearing Impairment

Children with impaired hearing are vulnerable to language disorders because of their lack of access to the linguistic information in the auditory signal. Still, children with hearing impairments vary greatly in their oral language ability. With amplification via hearing aids, children can be moved from greater to lesser levels of severity of hearing loss. Cochlear implants and tactile aids are also used to provide auditory information to children who would otherwise be considered deaf (59). In recent years, cochlear implants are being used more routinely at earlier ages to facilitate language development in children born with severe hearing loss, and research (60) suggests this results in very good outcomes in terms of speech and understanding language.

Language acquisition in children with hearing impairment (HI) who do not receive cochlear implants follows the same general sequence as it does in children with normal hearing, although it is greatly delayed, and the delays affect all modalities: articulation, receptive and expressive communication, and oral and written language (61). Use of language for communication is not a major problem area for children with HI. Rather, most of their difficulties lie in acquiring the conventional verbal forms of communication. Reading and writing present particular problems, primarily because of the language basis necessary for acquiring these skills. Average reading comprehension level for adolescents with HI without cochlear implants is third to fourth grade (61–63). Language and reading outcomes for children who receive cochlear implants are generally higher (60).

Some children with HI, especially those who come from families in which one or more parent is deaf, can be taught to bypass the auditory channel through the use of manual sign language. Using this method, children can develop fluency and eloquence in Sign that would never be available to them through the modality of speech. There is controversy within the community of the hearing impaired as to the role of Sign language versus oral language instruction for children with severe hearing losses. In general, nonimplanted deaf children taught sign develop higher level language skills than those taught speech, although their communication may be limited to those in the deaf community who use sign as their mode of communication. The widespread use of cochlear implantation has had an effect on the prevalence of the use of Sign, since many implanted children can learn adequately through the auditory channel.

Psychiatric Disorders

There is a very high coincidence of sociobehavioral and communicative disorders (64). Benner, Nelson, and Epstein (65) found, in a metaanalysis, that over 70% of children diagnosed with emotional-behavioral disorders (EBD) had clinically significant language deficits. The deficits were broad based and included expressive, receptive, and pragmatic aspects of language. This finding has been confirmed in studies of bilingual children as well (66). In addition, over 50% of children diagnosed with language deficits also had diagnosable EBD. Further, the number of children who have both communicative and behavioral-socioemotional disorders increases as children with language disorders get older (67). It may be impossible to know the source of this connection. Some writers (68) hold that a communication problem leads to frustration, creating behavioral or emotional disorders. It may, alternatively, be the case that a behavioral/socioemotional problem leads to decreased motivation to communicate or an inability to "tune in" to learn the rules of communication or use language for self- and other-regulation; (69) or, perhaps some other underlying factor affects both aspects of development. Whatever the answer to these questions, children with language problems are vulnerable to socioemotional difficulties, and children with psychiatric diagnoses show a higher than normal prevalence of language disorders. The psychiatric problems that most commonly co-occur with language disorders include attention deficit hyperactivity disorder, conduct and oppositional, and anxiety disorders. One particular form of anxiety disorder, *selective mutism,* has the most obvious communicative concomitants. DSM-IV (70) defines selective mutism as a persistent refusal to talk in one or more major social situations, including school, despite the ability to comprehend and use spoken language (71). The problem has been recognized for at least a century (72) and is relatively rare, with prevalence rates of 0.3 to 0.8 per 1,000 (70). Selective mutism is most often seen in school settings, where the child refuses to speak despite being verbal at home. Cultural and linguistic differences (CLDs) can exacerbate the problem, especially when the child has limited English proficiency (LEP) and feels uncomfortable using the language of the classroom (73). Although most children with CLD eventually overcome their reluctance to talk in school, some, as well as up to 50% of monolingual English speakers who experience selective mutism along with other kinds of school-related anxiety, remain selectively mute for extended periods of time (74). The condition shows a 2:1 ratio in favor of girls (74). In spite of the fact that children with this diagnosis must be known to have the ability to use language in some situations, a high incidence of speech and language difficulties has been reported in this population. Seventy-five percent of selectively mute children have been found to have articulation disorders and expressive language problems; 60% show significant deficits in receptive language (75). Speech-language pathologists often work in collaboration with mental health professionals to address the needs of the selectively mute child. Several recent reports have given examples of effective intervention to deal with selective mutism. These include providing inviting, tempting opportunities to interact with familiar peers, first in small, safe environments within the school setting before attempting speech in the classroom or other public environments. McInnes and Manassis (71) argued that intervention should take into account the child's social anxiety and begin by encouraging children to answer simple, factual questions (What color is this?) and avoiding questions that require any self-disclosure (What is your favorite color?).

Autism Spectrum Disorders

The psychiatric disorder most consistently associated with communication deficits is pervasive developmental disorder (PDD), or *autism spectrum disorder* (ASD). Communication problems—including severe delays in language, inability to communicate nonverbally, inability to sustain conversation, stereotyped and repetitive use of idiosyncratic language, and abnormal ability to use language for social communication—are included in the diagnostic criteria for ASD (70). Virtually all children with autism have some form of communication disorder that presents as part of their syndrome. What differentiates autism from a more circumscribed language disorder is the global nature of the child's communication problem. Not only is language affected, but the ability and motivation to send messages by any means, verbal or nonverbal, is severely impaired. Although Sign and other alternative forms of communication are often tried with autistic patients, it is their underlying deficit in communicative skill and motivation that impedes their use of language; therefore, providing an alternate channel does not usually result in dramatic improvement (76).

From early in development, children with ASD show differences in intentional communication. Major differences seen in 1-year-olds later diagnosed with ASD include a lack of joint attentional behavior and an abnormal response to human faces and voices. These babies use gestures to show and point less often than language-matched controls, although they do use gestures to request, protest, and regulate others' behavior (77). In general, they do not communicate in order to share focus as normal infants do, but only to express wants and needs (78). Some children with ASD do not develop speech, although the proportion who do not is declining as earlier identification and intervention is being implemented (79, 80). When speech is absent, it is not spontaneously replaced by communicative gestures, as it is in children with HI, for example. Furthermore, children with ASD may develop maladaptive means for expressing requests and protests. They may begin head-banging, for example, to express rejection of an activity. In children with ASD who do develop speech, some expansion of communicative intentions occurs, along with an elaboration of more socially acceptable means of communicating (76).

Children with ASD who do talk begin speaking late and develop speech at a significantly slower rate than other children (76). About 25% of children with ASD appear to acquire a few words by 12 or 18 months, and then lose them or fail to acquire more (81). When children with ASD begin talking, aspects of language form, including phonology, syntax, and morphology, are relatively spared. These children generally show skills in language form that are at or close to those of mental-age mates (76), although a subgroup of children with ASD show deficits in language form that are similar to those of children with specific language impairment (82). Vocabulary skills also are usually on par with developmental level. Meaning and pragmatic aspects are disproportionately impaired, though (77). When they talk, children with ASD show sparse verbal expression and a lack of spontaneity. They have trouble adapting what they say to the needs and status of the listener, distinguishing given from new information, following politeness rules, making relevant comments, maintaining topics outside their own obsessive interests, and giving listeners their fair share of conversational turns (76).

Children with ASD who talk may use nonreciprocal speech—that is, speech not directed or responsive to others (83). The classic example is from Kanner (84). He told the story of his patient with autism who would scream, "Don't throw the dog off the balcony" at odd times. The remark was incomprehensible until the boy's parents explained that he had once been told not to throw a toy dog off the balcony of a hotel in which the family was staying. Ever after this event, he used the statement as an admonition to himself when he had an impulse to do something he shouldn't do. Such use of language that is "stuck" in its original context, and that cannot be interpreted with only the knowledge that is normally shared among conversational partners, is a classic characteristic of autistic communication. Similarly, speaking children with ASD show extreme literalness in their use of language (76). They have trouble accepting that words can have synonyms or multiple meanings or that there can be different interpretations of the same utterance in contexts such as jokes.

Another classic characteristic of autistic language is *echolalia*, either immediate or delayed (77, 84). Although echolalia was long thought to be a dysfunctional language behavior, investigators such as Fay (85) and Prizant and Duchan (86) have shown that children with ASD often use echolalia for communicative purposes. Echolalia in ASD is selective, as it is in normal development (87). Children with ASD who echo tend to do so when they do not understand what has been said to them or when they lack the language skills to generate an original reply (88). Although echolalia is a "classic" symptom of autistic disorders, not all verbal children with ASD use it. Fay (89) estimated that it appears, at least briefly, in about 75% of autistic children who speak. Also, echolalia is used by children with other syndromes, such as blindness and fragile X syndrome. As language skill in children with ASD improves, echolalia decreases, as it does in normal development.

Kanner (84) also identified *pronoun reversals* as characteristic of autistic language. Fay (90) pointed out, though, that what children with ASD are doing is not reversing pronouns, but *failing* to reverse them: saying the same "you" as the speaker used, rather than changing it to "I." The problem is likely to be related to the autistic child's tendency to echo and to the *deictic* nature of pronoun reference; that is, the fact that in word pairs like *I/you* the referent shifts, depending on the point of view of the speaker: *I* is always the current speaker, not a particular person; similarly, *you* is the term for the currently listener, not for one unchanging individual. This shifting reference is particularly difficult for children with ASD because of their literalness and lack of flexibility.

Paralinguistic aspects of communication also are affected in verbal children with ASD. Intonation is often monotonous and machinelike, and stress, vocal quality, rate, rhythm, prosody, and loudness deviances also have been reported for approximately half of higher functioning speakers with ASD (91). The reasons for these paralinguistic differences are not known. Paralinguistic aspects of communication do, though, carry some of the pragmatic and emotional information in the message. The deficits in affective development seen in children with ASD may, then, form some part of the explanation.

Borderlands of the Autism Spectrum

As a spectrum disorder, autism can be difficult to distinguish from conditions that share some of its features. Since there is no laboratory test to determine whether a child's condition falls within the autism spectrum, it can be hard to decide whether a given constellation of symptoms fall on or off of this continuum. Bishop and Norbury (92) talked about the "borderlands" of the autism spectrum; generally three additional conditions would be considered to reside in these borderlands: Asperger syndrome (AS), Nonverbal Learning Disability (NLD), and Pragmatic Language Impairment (PLI). Much controversy surrounds these classifications: whether there is any real distinction among them; whether they should all be considered part of the autism spectrum; whether some are more closely connected to specific language impairment than ASD; whether they have different genetic and biological roots that provide a justification for keeping them as separate categories even when the behavioral presentation is similar. One clinician may see a child as having AS, while another may feel NLD or PLI is the more appropriate label. Only AS is listed as an "official" diagnosis in the DSM-IV; NLD and PLI are categories that may be used for educational services in some areas. Children with these borderland disorders tend to be relatively high functioning, to have fluent language abilities, and to show deficits primarily in the areas of appropriate conversation and social interaction.

ACQUIRED DISORDERS OF COMMUNICATIVE FUNCTION

Language disorders acquired during the developmental period can be broadly categorized as those related to focal lesions; and those in which more widespread damage is sustained, usually in association with seizure disorders or traumatic brain injury.

Focal Lesions

Lesions that are focal, or localized to a specific area of the brain, are usually caused by cerebrovascular accidents (CVAs) such as strokes and are relatively rare in children; however, children with congenital heart problems are particularly vulnerable to CVAs, and premature babies may suffer focal damage as a result of intracranial bleeding during their first weeks of life outside the womb. Recent research (93, 94) suggests that children with very early focal lesions show delays in the acquisition of language, particularly if the lesion is on the left side of the brain, and some atypical lateralization of language functions in the brain. Delays continue to be shown through early development in children with early-acquired lesions, particularly for those with left-lateralized damage, although in general delays are mild. Children who acquire damage before age 10 usually go through a mute period immediately following the injury, but generally regain most functional language use, with mild deficits in efficiency of language processes. For children with right hemisphere damage, development may appear normal after initial recovery, but there may be difficulty with some higher level language abilities for those over 10 years. Thus, most children who suffer focal lesions make more or less complete recovery in terms of communication, although when seizures persist after the injury, prognosis is more guarded.

Acquired Aphasia Secondary to Seizure Disorders

Some children go through a period of normal development, then suddenly or gradually lose language skills in association with a seizure disorder. The affected child usually stops paying attention to speech, although audiological testing shows normal hearing; the child may stop talking, or regress in language ability, although nonverbal skills are preserved. The seizure disorder itself is often of unknown origin. This condition is known as Landau-Kleffner syndrome (LKS), named after a paper by Landau and Kleffner (95) that first described it. LKS usually has its onset between 3 and 6 years of age, although it can occur any time between 2 and 13 years (96). In general, prognosis is worse the earlier the onset of the syndrome, which is more common in boys than in girls. Cognitive functioning is usually impaired as well. Unlike aphasias associated with focal lesions, LKS may result in a permanent aphasia. Another difference between LKS and aphasias arising from focal lesions is that comprehension is more severely affected in LKS, and reading and writing may be relatively spared (46, 97). Some children can successfully use sign language as a form of communication. Clinical seizures are not always apparent (98, 99), but abnormal EEG activity is one of the two diagnostic criteria for the syndrome, the other being a loss of previously acquired language function. Communication deficits persist in many subjects with LKS (96), although recently developed treatments have shown some potential to limit chronic effects. Both surgical and pharmacological management have been used, but even when these treatments are effective, recovery is not immediate. It can take months or years for a child to regain functional communication skills, and delays in some areas may persist. Educational and speech-language services are usually indicated. Long-term outcomes are generally unknown, due to the relatively recent application of new medical and surgical approaches.

Disorders with Environmental Components

Communication disorders can be associated with prenatal exposure to substances such as drugs and alcohol, or with parental behavior disorders such as abuse and neglect. It can be difficult to separate these types of effects, however. Communication development can also be influenced through the effects of substance abuse on the caregiving environment. A parent who is frequently drunk, high on drugs, or driven to get drugs by any means necessary is not a person who can devote much energy to childrearing. These parents often have difficulty understanding their children's communications and interpret the children's communicative bids as demands, often rejecting or criticizing their efforts (100). If other significant figures are not present in the child's life to mitigate the parent's neglect, the child's development will suffer. Moreover, people who abuse one drug tend to drink, smoke, and abuse other drugs, as well. This section will examine the effects on communication of parental substance abuse and child maltreatment.

Fetal Alcohol Syndrome

Communication disabilities are almost universal in this population (101) and are related to the level of intellectual impairment. These disorders include delayed development, poor receptive vocabulary and comprehension, and pragmatic difficulties. Perseveration and echolalia are often present in children with more severe impairments (100).

Drug Exposure

Although prenatal drug exposure is a developmental risk, Sparks (100, 102) pointed out that fewer than one half of children exposed to drugs prenatally experience low birth weight, prematurity, intrauterine growth retardation, or small head circumference. Sparks (102) reported that drug-exposed newborns are often irritable and stiff and show arousal and attention problems, but these traits do not appear to last past the first year. In general, cognition is not impaired, except when reduced head size is seen. Still, catch-up head growth is a marker of good prognosis for long-term development (100). Several studies (101, 103–105) have found that children with a history of cocaine exposure show delays in language acquisition, particularly in the area of expressive language, with exposure to higher doses prenatally resulting in higher levels of impairment. However, these studies also find that effects are modified by an enriched environment; children placed in foster or adoptive homes show higher levels of communicative skill than those who remain with biological mothers.

Child Abuse and Neglect

Children with communicative and other developmental disorders are, as Knutson and Sullivan (106) pointed out, more likely than normally developing children to experience maltreatment. Fox and colleagues (107) suggested that a child with a communication disorder might be less satisfying for a parent to care for and provide less rewarding interactions. These difficulties might predispose a child to abuse.

Maltreatment itself also constitutes a risk for language disorder. Culp, Watkins, Lawrence, Letts, Kelly, and Rice (108) argued that language development is particularly vulnerable in the maltreatment situation, because of the disruption in social interaction it entails. Coster, Gersten, Beeghly, and Cicchetti (109) showed that maltreated toddlers used shorter sentences and more limited vocabularies during play with their mothers than peers from nonabusing homes. Both Allen and Oliver (110) and Eigsti and Cicchetti (111) found that preschoolers with a history of maltreatment had significantly lower language scores than peers of similar socioeconomic level, with impairments in both vocabulary and sentence production. Lynch and Roberts (112) showed that these children scored significantly lower on verbal IQ relative to nonverbal scores. Fox, Long, and Anglois (107) found that maltreated children had receptive language deficits, with neglected children suffering greater lags than those shown by children who were abused.

SPECIFIC SPEECH AND LANGUAGE DISORDERS

Communication disorders can, as we have seen, be associated with a variety of conditions. They can also occur in relative isolation. These more specific disorders of speech and language development can still have broad effects on a child's ability to succeed in social and academic pursuits because communication is so central to human interaction and the development of the intellect. We will examine the types of specific speech and language disorders discussed in the DSM-IV-R: (70) stuttering, phonologic disorders, and specific language impairments.

Specific Speech Disorders

Stuttering

This syndrome, often referred to in older literature as *stammering*, involves abnormal and persistent dysfluencies that result in deviations in the continuity, smoothness, rhythm, and/or effort with which phonologic, lexical, morphologic, and/or syntactic language units are spoken; (113) these are often accompanied by affective and behavioral reactions. Several types of speech dysfluencies also may be involved, including blocking of sounds, hesitations, and tense pauses. Incidence of childhood stuttering is highest between a child's second and fourth birthdays, ultimately affecting 4% to 5% of the population. Although many children go through periods of dysfluency during the developmental period, these "normal dysfluencies" tend to occur in the larger linguistic units (word, phrases, and sentences). For children who tend to persist in stuttering over time, dysfluencies are more likely to occur in repetitions of syllables ("vi-vi-vi-vi-video") and sounds ("g-g-g-g-ot"). Other red flags for persistent stuttering include sound prolongations ("WWWWWait!"), silent blocks in which the child attempts to speak but no sound comes out, and visible struggle behaviors during speech, such as blinks or grimaces (22). If dysfluencies continue to be relatively effortless, there is a good chance of recovery. In addition, Yairi and associates (114) reported that children who recover from stuttering begin to show reductions in their number of dysfluencies within the first year, whereas those who persist in stuttering are relatively stable in their rate of dysfluency.

When recovery occurs, it usually does so by adolescence, often around the time of puberty. About 1 in 30 children goes through a period of stuttering, but by adolescence, the prevalence drops to 1% (113). Although the ratio of boys to girls who begin to stutter between the ages of two and four is approximately equal, girls are more likely to experience unassisted recovery. The ratio of boys to girls who persist in stuttering increases to approximately three to one by adolescence. When recovery occurs, it is likely to do so from 6 to 36 months after onset, with most children recovering within the first 1 to 2 years after their stuttering was first noted. Boys are more likely to exhibit cooccurring speech disorders than girls, especially in articulation and phonology (114, 115).

For individuals with chronic stuttering, the severity of the disturbance varies from situation to situation and is more severe when there is pressure to communicate. Stress or anxiety have been shown to exacerbate stuttering, but are not thought to play a role in the etiology. Reducing stress during speaking can reduce stuttering episodes (116), but general treatments for anxiety, including the use of tranquilizing medication, have not been found to be effective treatments (117). In general, speech therapy is used both to shape fluent speech and help the patient to stutter with less tension, avoidance, and interruption of the flow of communication (118). Psychotherapy alone has not been shown to be an effective treatment for stuttering, but counseling is often helpful for overcoming the secondary effects of stuttering on self-concept, thoughts, and feelings (119).

Although stuttering has, at times, been thought to be a learned behavior, most researchers today consider stuttering to have a biological component. People who stutter have been found to show laryngeal behavior different from that in normal speakers, even when their speech is apparently fluent (120). Elements of both the central and peripheral nervous system may be involved in stuttering behaviors (22). There also appears to be a familial component in stuttering (114). The risk of stuttering among first-degree relatives is more than three times the population risk (70). Stuttering is believed by most researchers today to have a complex multiplicity of causes that include biological vulnerability, environmental demands and expectations, and temperamental characteristics of the speaker (121).

Phonological Disorders

These difficulties with speech articulation are characterized by impaired production of developmentally expected speech sounds. To diagnose a specific phonologic disorder, it is necessary to ascertain that the problem is not attributable to deficits or abnormalities in intelligence, hearing, or the structure and physiology of the speech mechanism. So a phonologic disorder is one in which, although there is no organic reason for the disability, the child's speech is marked by misarticulations, including distortions of sounds (e.g., /s/is produced with a lisp), omissions of sounds (e.g., *up* is pronounced "uh," *play* is pronounced "pay"), and incorrect substitutions of one sound for another (e.g., *cat* is pronounced "dat"). Many of these misarticulations represent processes that are typical in the speech of young normal children (e.g., deletions of final consonants, simplifications of consonant clusters), but in phonologic disorders more of them are used, they are used more often, and their use persists beyond the normal developmental period. There may also be idiosyncratic preferences for and/or avoidances of certain sounds or sound simplification processes (122–124), and/or reversals or misordering of sounds in words (125). The age of recognition/onset of the disorder is related to severity. Typically, the disorder becomes apparent around the age of 4 years, when normal children become fully intelligible and eliminate almost all of their normal developmental sound change patterns (126). Children as young as 3 years can be diagnosed with this disorder, if their speech is unintelligible even to family members. Milder cases may not be identified until the child is in school.

Phonologic disorders are the most prevalent type of communication problem. Edwards (127) reported that 80% of speech clinic referrals were for articulation disorder. Six percent of school-age children have phonologic disorders. The prevalence is higher for preschoolers, with estimates ranging from 10% to 15% (128).

Phonologic disorders can, of course, occur with many of the syndromes discussed in the preceding. They can also occur in isolation, and are commonly associated with specific language disorders. Shriberg and Kwiatkowski (129) found that over 50% of children with phonologic disorders have delays in expressive language, and 10% to 40% have delays in language comprehension. Shriberg and Kwiatkowski (129) reported that a significant minority of these children, with either speech-only or speech/language delays as preschoolers, required continuing special services throughout their elementary school years. Although most of these children do "outgrow" their unintelligible speech, some continue to require services for other aspects of language and academic development.

Childhood Apraxia of Speech

A subset of children with severe, persistent speech disorders accompanied by certain language and behavioral features are sometimes said to have a *childhood apraxia of speech (CAS)* (130–132). Characteristics most commonly attributed to this syndrome (130, 133, 134) include:

- Limited repertoires of speech sounds
- Predominant use of simple syllable shapes
- Frequent sound omission errors
- Slow rate of speech
- Difficulties with imitating sounds and speech
- Production in single words better than in connected speech
- Stress and pausing unusually equal across words, with loss of normal intonation quality

Davis (135) discussed some of the controversies surrounding this disorder. CAS was originally defined as an analogue to an adult acquired neurological disorder: apraxia of speech, or a neurologically based difficulty in programming speech movements, thought to take place at a prearticulatory motor planning level. Intensive investigation, however, has not been able to document any consistent neuropathology in children who show this speech pattern, even with sophisticated new techniques. Partly as a result of this failure to identify a neurological lesion similar to the one that causes apraxia in adults, some authors (136) have suggested that CAS is not a clinically definable entity. The fact that the behavioral symptomatology associated with CAS overlaps so much with other conditions, such as developmental phonological disorders and expressive language delays, contributes to this view, and makes the diagnostic process difficult. In general, it is best to be conservative about the diagnosis of CAS, and to reserve it for children who have demonstrated some speech production but fail to make progress in articulation after an intensive trial of traditional speech therapy. Since the result of this diagnosis is often that children receive training in using alternative means of communication, such as picture boards, rather than speech, direct speech therapy should be tried before this more radical solution is adopted.

Specific Language Impairment

Some kinds of language disorders have no known concomitants. These disorders have been traditionally defined by exclusion, that is, by the absence of the other factors—mental retardation, sensory disorders, neurologic damage, emotional problems, or environmental deprivation. The terms *childhood aphasia* or *congenital aphasia* were used in the past to describe these disorders. The use of these terms grew out of the conviction of the early neurologists that difficulties in children's learning language were analogous to the loss of language seen in adults who suffered acquired aphasias. This notion evolved from observations that "aphasic" children often appeared bright in other ways and were clearly not retarded. They seemed also to have normal affective bonds to the people around them and were not emotionally disturbed. Their inability to acquire language normally was attributed to some sort of neurologic dysfunction, thought to be comparable to localized brain lesions that resulted in aphasia in adults.

Rescorla and Lee (18) have argued on the basis of recent evidence regarding the development of very young children with delayed speech (137, 138) that it is not appropriate to make the diagnosis of SLI until age 4. Research suggests that younger children with delayed language have a good chance of "outgrowing" their slow start, although their language functioning may seem very similar to children with SLI at earlier ages (139) and they frequently retain subtle weaknesses when compared to social-economic peers (140–143).

Children with SLI are late to begin talking. They may not say their first word until well into their second year. When they do begin to talk, they add new words slowly. They may continue to use single words or telegraphic utterances into their third year. In general, communication patterns of children with SLI are similar to those of younger children at comparable levels of language development. While this pattern holds true when looking at one specific feature of development at a time, Leonard (42) pointed out that children may be 1 year below age level in one set of features, $1\frac{1}{2}$ years below in another, 6 months below in a third, and so on. The result will be that the overall profile of language skills in a child with SLI may not resemble that of a child with normal language function at any point in development. This does not mean that language development is deviant, but rather that it is in some ways asynchronous (52).

Early lexical usage in children with SLI is very much like that of normally developing children at similar language levels but is acquired at a slower pace. Vocabulary sizes of normally developing 2-year-olds are more than 200 words, whereas those of children with SLI are in the range of 20 words (138, 144–146). Moreover, children with SLI talk and communicate less often than same-age peers (18). While these children acquire sounds and make speech errors that are similar to those of peers, their repertoires of consonant sounds are smaller, and they take longer to acquire basic word forms (147–150).

Although vocabulary deficits are the first sign of language delay, these typically resolve by age 3 to 4 (144, 146). Use of early semantic relations appears similar to that of language-matched peers (31). Vocabulary in school aged children with SLI lags behind that of peers (52), perhaps because of reduced experience through reading (which is often problematic for these children).

The first delay to be seen in the syntax of children with SLI is a failure to combine words spontaneously at 18 to 24 months (138, 144, 151, 152). Followup studies indicate that these children continue to lag behind in syntactic development through the preschool period (138, 153). They appear to acquire grammatical structures in roughly the same order as normally speaking children do, although they make more errors for longer periods and use higher rates of ungrammatical sentences (18, 152). They also have special difficulties learning morphological endings for words in English (such as the past tense-ed form), although this differs in children learning other languages (71).

Pragmatic skills are generally better than skills in language form, and this is one of the characteristics that differentiates SLI from ASD (154). While children with SLI have been reported to be less interactive than age-matched peers, they are often similar to younger language-matched children (18), and pragmatic deficits seen are usually in the mild range (52). Still, Marton et al. (155) report finding significant deficits in social knowledge in children with SLI.

For children with chronic mild to moderate language disorders, problems in the school years tend to narrow in their focus and to be concentrated in subtle difficulties of language organization and efficiency, rather than frank errors (140, 141). Word retrieval or "word finding" difficulties are common. Instead of using correct words (e.g., "chair"), a child with SLI may substitute an incorrect word of related meaning (e.g., "table"); or use functional descriptors (e.g., "thing to sit on"), vague or general terms (e.g., "thing"), or his or her own made-up jargon. Storytelling and discourse problems often persist and affect both oral and written modes of expression (144, 156). These children may lack the ability to elaborate and/or self-correct when needed for clarity in conversation (125, 157). There may be tangential or inappropriate responses to questions, a limited range of communicative functions (e.g., requests, imperatives, questions) expressed, difficulty maintaining and/or changing topics, and difficulty initiating interactions (158). These children may sound abrupt, rude, or impolite simply because they do not have access to the full and diverse range of linguistic forms used in normal conversation to encode pragmatic nuance and make language sound appropriate to the social context. In addition, some mild social deficits may also be seen (24). Academic problems tend to involve primarily reading and writing. Despite their persistent problems, however, most of these children do finish high school, some go on to college, and most live independent lives (141, 142, 159).

Prognosis is more guarded for children with severe SLI. Paul and Cohen (160) studied long-term outcomes in children diagnosed as SLI as preschoolers who were not speaking in full sentences by the time they were 6. By the time they were adolescents, these subjects with severe impairments were likely to score in the retarded range on IQ tests, even if they had scored in the normal range at the preschool level. Given intensive intervention, all made steady progress in language skills throughout their school years. Still, 90% of these subjects were significantly below the normal range in both areas by adolescence, and all required intensive special education, with most in special classrooms, schools, or residential facilities.

DIFFERENTIAL DIAGNOSIS

When seeing children suspected of having specific speech and language disorders, the main diagnostic task is to rule out other syndromes with which speech and language problems are frequently associated. These syndromes include the ones discussed in the early section of this chapter, that is, deafness or significant hearing loss, mental retardation, autism spectrum disorder, psychiatric disorder, and organically based communication disorders (cleft palate, apraxia, cerebral palsy, or childhood-acquired aphasia), or a disorder associated with maternal substance abuse or maltreatment.

The absence of significant hearing impairment or deafness must be established by audiometric testing by a certified audiologist. Because subtle deficits in hearing can affect language acquisition, it is important to get complete and accurate results in order to assure that hearing deficits do not play a role in the disorder. Although chronic middle ear pathology is sometimes associated with speech and language problems, research (161) suggests that chronic otitis media alone does not significantly increase the risk of language disorder in otherwise normal children. If parents report chronic otitis in a child who presents with a communication disorder, attributing the problem entirely to the middle ear problem is not justified, and treatment for the otitis will not necessarily alleviate the language disorder.

Mental retardation must be diagnosed by means of an individually administered, standardized test of intelligence, as well as by a standardized measure of adaptive behavior. For children suspected of language disorders, it is necessary to use nonverbal intelligence tests to assess intellectual ability, so as not to penalize the child for the language deficit and to get an estimate of intelligence unbiased by language performance. It is not, however, necessary to show that a child has language skills that are lower than expected for IQ in order for the child to receive communication services through the public schools. Children with MR can qualify for these services if their communication is found to be a significant handicap to their social and academic adjustment.

Organic disorders that can affect the speech mechanism, such as dyspraxia, dysarthria, and motor deficits associated with cerebral palsy, can be ruled out by physical and functional assessment of the speech mechanism (oral peripheral examination). A speech-language pathologist typically examines the morphology, symmetry, and alignment of the facial features. The functional integrity of the larynx, lips, tongue, and velopharyngeal structures, as well as the respiratory support for speech are also assessed. The quality of oral volitional movements also may be examined if an apraxia is suspected. If physical limitations to speech production are identified in this examination, an alternative system of communication—such as a picture board or electronic communicative device—may be indicated (162, 163). However, it is important to note that difficulties in imitation and cognition can affect a child's ability to participate in these assessments. Finding normal speech motor performance can rule out neuromotor involvement, but a finding of poor performance is more difficult to interpret, especially in developmentally young children.

Psychiatric/behavioral assessment can rule out ASD and other psychiatric disorders. Features associated with ASD include lack of (nonverbal) social interactions, absence of imaginative activity, stereotypic behaviors, self-injurious behaviors, odd responses to sensory input, and mood abnormalities. Formal measures, such as the Autism Diagnostic Interview (164) and the Autism Diagnostic Observation Scale (165), as well as checklists such as the Childhood Autism Rating Scale (CARS) (166) can assist in differential diagnosis.

The differential diagnosis among stuttering, phonologic disorder, expressive language disorder, mixed receptive-expressive language disorder, and selective mutism requires detailed speech/language testing. To diagnose stuttering, a clinician should ascertain, by means of standardized testing, that phonologic, receptive, and expressive language skills are age-appropriate. Many children go through periods of developmental dysfluency, and children with language disorders may persist in developmental dysfluency longer than normal because their developmental period is longer than normal. If dysfluency coexists with other speech and language disorders, it may be appropriate to delay making a diagnosis of stuttering until some of the other problems resolve, then reevaluate to determine whether the dysfluency has persisted. For young children, too, dysfluency may be transient. If the preschool dysfluent child is not showing any signs of struggle or self-consciousness about speech, it may be wise to "watch and see," and reevaluate the child in six months before initiating a course of speech therapy.

Phonologic disorders are diagnosed by means of standardized testing of phonologic production, usually using procedures that ask children to name pictures or objects and transcribing the child's rendition of the target word for comparison with adult production standards. Because phonologic disorders typically coexist with other language disorders, it is acceptable to confer a concurrent diagnosis of phonologic disorder even if other language disorders are present. However, it is necessary to rule out hearing impairment, mental retardation, and speech mechanism limitations before diagnosing a specific speech disorder.

To diagnose a specific expressive language disorder, it is necessary to demonstrate—by means of individually administered, standardized tests—that both nonverbal intelligence and receptive language skills are significantly better than expression. Again, because phonologic disorders so frequently coexist with expressive language deficits, both conditions can be diagnosed concurrently.

To make a diagnosis of mixed receptive-expressive (R/E) language disorder, it is must be shown—again using individually administered, standardized tests—that nonverbal intelligence is significantly higher than *both* expression and comprehension of language. As with expressive disorder, phonologic deficits can coexist with R/E disorders and would be diagnosed according to the criteria given earlier.

TREATMENT OF SPEECH AND LANGUAGE DISORDERS

It is important to make a careful differential diagnosis of any communication disorder in order to decide whether the problem is specific to speech and language or is part of a larger syndrome. In the case of communication disorders associated with syndromes such as hearing impairment, mental retardation, and autism, treatment must address all aspects of the child's problem, not just those of speech and language.

Still, once a communication problem has been identified and the broad range of interventions necessary to address all the child's needs has been instigated, treatment for the communicative aspect of the disorder is quite similar, regardless of whether the problem is specific to speech and language or part of a bigger picture of developmental disorder.

The treatment of choice for all the disorders discussed here, except for selective mutism, is individual or small group therapy administered by a certified speech/language pathologist (SLP). Because associated educational and/or psychiatric problems are common with these disorders, educational tutoring, social skills training, and/or psychiatric intervention also may be indicated, even if the disorder is specific to communication.

Methods of intervention are essentially behavioral and educational. Some clinicians use strict operant procedures, whereas others favor more child-centered approaches such as indirect language stimulation, which involves a rich communicative environment with opportunities for incidental learning. Many SLPs take a middle ground between these extremes, using structured play opportunities and focused stimulation to provide examples of desired forms and elicit language targets. Although all these methods have been shown to be effective in small studies (167–169), much more research is needed on the efficacy and effectiveness of particular approaches to intervention and variables that can be used to best match the method to the child.

Because selective mutism is seen more as an anxiety disorder than a developmental disorder, treatment methods differ somewhat for this syndrome. Although some authors have suggested psychodynamic therapy for selective mutism, the most convincing literature pertains to behavioral modification approaches (75). Contingency management (positive reinforcement of verbalizations and nonreinforcement for nonverbal responses), stimulus fading (gradually extending the number of people with whom and environments wherein verbalization is rewarded), shaping (rewarding gradual approximations to speech, such as mouthing and whispering), and response cost procedures (losing money or tokens for not speaking) have all been reported to be successful in eliciting and maintaining speech in selectively mute children (170). Medication management with antidepressant agents may also have an ancillary role in the treatment of selective mutism (171).

Caution should be exerted when treatments make claims of dramatic improvement, particularly when the improvement is claimed for a broad range of disorders. In recent years, several "miracle cures" have been advanced for communication disorders. Facilitated communication (172), Fast ForWord (47), and auditory integration training (173) are just a few examples. Clinicians who work with families of children with communication disorders need to maintain a healthy skepticism regarding these programs that make extravagant claims. If a treatment sounds too good to be true, it probably is. Any intervention, whether familiar or innovative, must be shown to meet the particular needs of the patient receiving it. Communicative interventions need to be evaluated with the same kind of rigor that would be used to evaluate the efficacy of a medical or surgical treatment. Although double-blind, placebo- controlled, randomized assignment trials are difficult to design for behavioral interventions, clinicians must strive to achieve some degree of objective evaluation before deciding that a treatment is appropriate for a given individual.

ACKNOWLEDGMENTS

Preparation of this chapter was supported by Research Grant P01-03008 funded by the National Institute of Mental Health (NIMH); by the STAART Center grant U54 MH66494 funded by the National Institute on Deafness and Other Communication Disorders (NIDCD), the National Institute of Environmental Health Sciences (NIEHS), the National Institute of Child Health and Human Development (NICHD), the National Institute of Neurological Disorders and Stroke (NINDS); by a MidCareer Development grant to Dr. Paul, K24 HD045576 funded by NIDCD; as well as by the National Alliance for Autism Research.

References

1. American Speech-Language-Hearing Association. Guidelines for caseload size and speech-language service delivery in the schools. *American Speech-Language-Hearing Association* 35 (suppl. 10):33–39, 1993.
2. Gall F: *On the Function of the Brain and each of its Parts* (vols. 1–6). Phrenological Library. Boston: Capen & Lyon, March 1825.
3. Broca P: Nouvelle observation d'aphémie produite par une lésion de la mortié posterieure des deuxième et troisième circonvolutions frontales. *Bulletin de la Société Anatomique* 398–407, 1861.
4. Wernicke K: The symptom-complex of aphasia. In: Church A. (ed): *Diseases of the Nervous System*. New York: Appleton-Century-Crofts, 1874.
5. Orton S: *Reading, writing and speech problems in children: A presentation of certain types of disorders in the development of the language faculty*. New York W. W. Norton, 1937.
6. Gesell A, Amatruda C: *Developmental Diagnosis* (ed. 2). New York, Hoeber, 1947.
7. Benton A: Aphasia in children. *Education* 79:408–412, 1959.
8. Benton A: Developmental aphasia and brain damage. *Cortex* 1:40–52, 1964.
9. Ewing A: *Aphasia in children*. London: Oxford University Press, 1930.
10. McGinnis M, Kleffner F, Goldstein R: Teaching aphasic children. *Volta Review* 58:239–244, 1956.
11. Myklebust H: *Auditory disorders in children: A manual for differential diagnosis*. New York, Grune & Stratton, 1954.
12. Myklebust H: Childhood aphasia: An evolving concept. In: Travis L. (ed): *Handbook on speech pathology and audiology*, pp. 1181–1202 Englewood Cliffs, Prentice Hall, 1971.
13. Aram D, Nation J: *Child Language Disorders*, St. Louis, Mosby, 1982.
14. Chomsky N: *Syntactic structures*, Cambridge, MIT Press, 1957.
15. Van Dyke DC, Holte L: Communication disorders in children. *Pediatric Annals* 32 (7):436, (2003, July).
16. Laing G, Law W, Levin A. et al.: Evaluation of a structured test and a parent led method for screening for speech and language problems: Prospective population based study. *British Medical Journal* 325:1152–1156, 2002.
17. Law J, Boyle J, Harris F et al.: Screening for speech and language delay: A systematic review of the literature. *Health Technology Assessment* 2:1–184, 1998.

18. Rescorla L, Lee E: Language impairment in young children. In Layton T. Crais E. Watson L. (eds.), *Handbook of early language impairment in children: Nature* (pp. 1–55). Albany, New York: Delmar Publishers, 2001.
19. National Institute on Deafness and Other Communication Disorders: (2002, December 12). *Statistics and human communication*. Retrieved August 31, 2003, from http://www.nidcd.nih.gov/health/statistics/index.asp.
20. Tomblin JB, Records NL, Buckwalter P et al.: Prevalence of specific language impairments in kindergarten children. *Journal of Speech, Language, & Hearing Research* 40:1245–1260, 1997.
21. Bartlett CW, Flax JF, Logue MW et al.: A major susceptibility locus for special language impairment is located on 13q21. *American Journal of Human Genetics* 71 (1):45–55, July 2002.
22. Plante E, Beeson P: *Communication and communication disorders*. Boston: Allyn & Bacon, 1999.
23. Pore S, Reed K: *Quick reference to speech-language pathology*. Gaithersburg, MD: Aspen, 1999.
24. Bishop D: *Uncommon understanding: Development and disorders of language comprehension in children*. East Sussex, U.K.: Psychology Press, 1997.
25. Bishop DVM, Adams C, Norbury CF: Distinct genetic influences on grammar and phonological short-term memory: Evidence from 6-year-old twins. *Genes, Brain & Behavior* in press, 2005.
26. Bishop DVM, North T, Donlan C: Genetic basis of specific language impairment: Evidence from a twin study. *Dev Med Child Neurol* 37:56, 1995.
27. Tallal P, Ross R, Curtiss S: Familial aggregation in specific language impairment. *Journal of Speech and Hearing Disorders* 54:167–173, 1989.
28. Tomblin JB: Familial concentration of developmental language impairment. *Journal of Speech and Hearing Disorders* 54:587–595, 1989.
29. Viding E, Spinath FM, Price TS, Bishop DVM, Dale PS, Plomin R: Genetic and environmental influence on language impairment in 4-year-old same-sex and opposite-sex twins. *Journal of Child Psychology & Psychiatry* 45 (2):315–325, 2004.
30. Conti-Ramsden G: Maternal recasts and other contingent replies to language-impaired children. *Journal of Speech & Hearing Disorders* 55:262–274, 1990.
31. Leonard L: Language learnability and specific language impairment in children. *Applied Psycholinguist* 10:179–202, 1989.
32. Paul R, Elwood, T: Maternal linguistic input to toddlers with slow expressive language development. *Journal of Speech and Hearing Research* 34:982–988, 1991.
33. Whitehurst G, Falco F, Lonigan C, et al: Accelerating language development through picture-book reading. *Developmental Psychology* 24:552–558, 1988.
34. Nelson N: *Childhood Language Disorders in Context: Infancy Through Adolescence*, 2nd ed. Columbus, OH, Merrill, 1998.
35. Bishop D: (1987). The causes of specific developmental language disorders. *Journal of Child Psychology and Psychiatry* 28:1–8, 1987.
36. Tetnowski J: Attention deficit hyperactivity disorders and concomitant communicative disorders. *Seminars in Speech and Language* 25:215–224, 2004.
37. Eisenson J: *Aphasia in children*, New York, Harper & Row, 1972.
38. Johnston J: Cognitive abilities of children with language impairment. In Watkins R. Rice M. (eds): *Specific language impairments in children (vol. 4)*, Baltimore: Paul H. Brookes, pp. 107–121.
39. Ullman M, Pierpont, E: Specific language impairment is not specific to language: The procedural deficit hypothesis. *Cortex* 41:399–433, 2005.
40. Tallal, P: Developmental language disorders. In: Kavanagh JF, Truss Jr. TJ, (eds): *Learning disabilities: Proceedings of the national conference* Parkton, York Press, 1986, pp. 181–272.
41. Leonard L: *Children with specific language impairment*, Cambridge: MIT Press, 1997.
42. Leonard L 1991: Specific language impairment as a clinical category. *Language, Speech, and Hearing Services in Schools* 22:66–68, 1991.
43. Gardner H: *Frames of Mind: The Theory of Multiple Intelligences*, New York, Basic Books, 1983.
44. Newbury D, Monaco, A: Molecular genetics of speech and language disorders. *Current Opinion in Pediatrics* 14:696–701, 2002.
45. Aram D: Comments on specific language impairment as a clinical category. *Language, Speech, & Hearing Services in Schools* 22:84–87, 1991.
46. Aram D, Healy J: Hyperlexia: A review of extraordinary word recognition. In: Obler LK Fein D. (eds): *The exceptional brain: Neuropsychology of talent and special abilities* New York: Guilford Press, 1988, pp. 70–102.
47. Tallal, P, Miller, S, Bedi, G, et al.: Language comprehension in language learning impaired children improved with acoustically modified speech. *Science* 271:81–84, 1996.
48. Bishop, D, McArthur, G 2005: Individual differences in auditory processing in specific language impairment: A follow-up study using event-related potentials and behavioural thresholds, *Cortex* 41:327–341, 2005.
49. Gillam R, Frome Loeb D, Friel-Patti S: Looking back: A summary of five exploratory studies of Fast ForWord. *American Journal of Speech-Language Pathology* 10:269–273, 2001.
50. Leonard C, Lombardino L, Walsh K, Eckert M, Mockler J, Rowe L, Williams S, DeBose C: Anatomical risk factors that distinguish dyslexia from SLI predict reading skill in normal children. *Journal of Communication Disorders* 35:501–531, 2002.
51. Clark MM, Plante E: Morphology of the inferior frontal gyrus in developmentally language-disordered adults. *Brain and Language* 61:288–303.
52. Rice M, Warren, S, Betz, S: Language symptoms of developmental language disorders: An overview of autism, Down syndrome, fragile X, specific language impairment, and Williams syndrome. *Applied Psycholinguistics* 26:7–27, 2005.
53. Abbeduto L, Boudreau D. 2004: Theoretical influences in research on language development and intervention in individuals with mental retardation. *Mental Retardation & Developmental Disabilities Research Reviews* 10:184–192, 2004.
54. Shriberg L, Widder C: Speech and prosody characteristics of adults with mental retardation. *Journal of Speech and Hearing Research* 33:627–653, 1990.
55. Lahey M: *Language disorders and language development*, New York, Macmillan, 1988.
56. Dykens E, Hodapp R, Leckman, J: *Behavior and development in fragile X syndrome*, London, Sage Publications, 1994.
57. Abbeduto L, Murphy M: Language, social cognition, maladaptive behavior and communication in Down syndrome and fragile X syndrome. In: Rice, M Warren S. (eds): *Developmental language disorders: From phenotypes to etiology* pp. 77–98. Mahwah, Erlbaum, 2004.
58. Laws G, Bishop DVM: Pragmatic language impairment and social deficits in Williams syndrome: A comparison with Down's syndrome and specific language impairment. *Journal of Language & Communication Disorders* 39:45–64, 2004.
59. Roeser R. (1998): Cochlear implants and tactile aids for the profoundly deaf student. In: Roeser RJ, Downs MP (eds): *Auditory disorders in school children*. New York: Thieme, 1998, pp. 260–280.
60. Peng S, Spencer L, Tomblin JB: Speech intelligibility of pediatric cochlear implant recipients with 7 years of device experience. *Journal of Speech, Language, and Hearing Research* 47 (6):1227–1236, 2004.
61. Paul P, Quigley S: *Language and deafness*. San Diego, Singular Publishing Group, 1994.
62. King, C, Quigley S: *Reading and Deafness*, San Diego, College-Hill Press, 1985.
63. Trybus R, Karchmer M: School achievement scores of hearing impaired children: National data on achievement status and growth patterns. *American Annals of Deaf Directory Programs and Services* 122:62–69, 1977.
64. Giddan J, Milling, L, Comorbidity of psychiatric and communication disorders in children. *Child and Adolescent Psychiatry in Clinics in North America* 8:19–36, 1999.
65. Benner G, Nelson J, Epstein M: Language skills of children with EBD: A literature review. *Journal of Emotional & Behavioral Disorders* 10:43–57, 2002.
66. Toppelberg C, Medrano L, Pena Morgens L, Nieto-Castanon A: Bilingual children referred for psychiatric services: Associations of language disorders, language skills, and psychopathology. *Journal of the American Academy of Child & Adolescent Psychiatry* 41:712–722, 2002.
67. Baltaxe C: Emotional, behavioral, and other psychiatric disorders of childhood associated with communication disorders. In: T. Layton, E. Crais, L. Watson (eds), *Handbook of early language impairment in children: Nature* Albany, Delmar Publishers, pp. 63–125, 2001.
68. Redmond S, Rice M: The socioemotional behaviors of children with SLI: Social adaption or social deviance? *Journal of Speech and Hearing Research* 41:688–700, 1988.
69. Paul R, Cohen D, Klin A, et al.: Multiplex developmental disorders: The role of communication in the construction of a self. *Child and Adolescent Psychiatry in Clinics in North America* 8:189–202, 1999.
70. American Psychiatric Association. 2000: *Diagnostic & Statistical Manual of Mental Disorders*. 4th rev. ed. Washington, American Psychiatric Press, 2000.
71. McInnes A, Manassis K 2005: When silence is not golden: An integrated approach to selective mutism. *Seminars in Speech & Language* 26:201–210, 2005.
72. Kussmaul A: *Die Stoerungen der Sprache*, ed. 1 Disturbances in linguistic function. Basel, Germany, Benno Schwabe, 1877, p. 211.
73. Elizur Y, Perednik M: Prevalence and description of selective mutism in immigrant and native families: A controlled study. *Journal of the American Academy of Child & Adolescent Psychiatry* 42:1451–1459, 2003.
74. McInnes A, Fung D, Manassis K, Fiksenbaum L, Tannock R: Narrative skills in children with selective mutism: An exploratory study. *American Journal of Speech-Language Pathology* 13:304–315, 2004.
75. Giddan J, Ross G, Sechler L, Becker B: Selective mutism in elementary school: Multidisciplinary interventions. *Language, Speech, & Hearing Services in Schools* 28:127–133, 1997.
76. Tager-Flusberg H, Paul R, Lord C 2005: Language and communication in autism. In: Volkmar R., Paul R., Klin A., Cohen D. (eds): *Handbook of autism and pervasive developmental disorders* New York: Wiley, 2005, pp. 335–364.
77. Tager-Flusberg H: Dissociations in form and function in the acquisition of language in autistic children. In: Tager-Flusberg H. (ed): *Constraints*

on language acquisition: Studies of atypical children. Hillsdale, Erlbaum, 1995, pp. 175–194.
78. Wetherby A, Woods J, Allen L Cleary J, Dickinson H, Lord C: Early indicators of autism spectrum disorders in the second year of life. *Journal of Autism & Developmental Disorders* 34:473–493, 2004.
79. Paul R, Chawarska K, Klin A, Volkmar F: Dissociations in communication development in children with ASD. In Paul R. (ed): *Language disorders from a developmental perspective: Essays in honor of Robin Chapman*. Mahwah: Erllbaum (in press), 2006.
80. Rogers S: Evidence-based intervention for language development in young children with autism. In: Charman T. Stone W (eds): *Social and communication development in autism spectrum disorders: Early identification, diagnosis, and intervention* NY, Guilford Press. In press, 2006.
81. Lord C, Shulman C, DiLavore P: Regression and word loss in autistic spectrum disorders. *Journal of Child Psychology & Psychiatry* 45:936–955, 2004.
82. Tager-Flusberg H, Joseph R: Identifying neurocognitive phenotypes in autism. *Philosophical Transactions of the Royal Society Series, B* 358:303–314, 2003.
83. Dewey M, Everard P: The near normal autistic adolescent. *Journal of Autism and Childhood Schizophrenia* 4:348–356, 1974.
84. Kanner L: Autistic disturbances of affective contact. *Nervous Child* 2:416–426, 1943.
85. Fay W 1969: On the basis of autistic echolalia. *Journal of Communication Disorders* 2:38–47, 1969.
86. Prizant B, Duchan J: The functions of immediate echolalia in autistic children. *Journal of Speech and Hearing Disorders* 46:241–249, 1981.
87. Carr, E., Schriebman I Lovaas, O.: Control of echolalic speech in psychotic children. *Journal of Abnormal Child Psychology* 3:331–351, 1975.
88. Prizant B: Communication, language, social, and emotional development. *Journal of Autism and Developmental Disorders* 26:173–178, 1996.
89. Fay W.: Infantile autism. In: Bishop D. Mogford K. (eds): *Language development in exceptional circumstances*. Hillsdale,: Erlbaum, 1992, pp. 190–202.
90. Fay W (1971): On normal and autistic pronouns. *Journal of Speech & Hearing Disorders* 36:242–249, 1971.
91. Shriberg L., Paul R., McSweeney J, Klin A., Cohen D, Volkmar F: Speech & prosody characteristics of adolescents and adults with high functioning autism and Asperger syndrome. *Journal of Speech, Language and Hearing Research* 44:1097–1115, 2001.
92. Bishop D, Norbury C: Exploring the borderlands of autistic disorder and specific language impairment: A study using standardised diagnostic instruments. *Journal of Child Psychology & Psychiatry & Allied Disciplines* 43:917–930, 2002.
93. Chilosi, A., Pecini, C., Cipriani, P., Brovedani, P. Brizzolara, D., Ferretti, G. et al.: Atypical language lateralization and early linguistic development in children with focal brain lesions. *Developmental Medicine & Child Neurology* 27:725–730, 2005.
94. Wulfeck B, Bates E, Krupa-Kwiatkowski M, Saltzman, D. 2004: Grammaticality sensitivity in children with early focal brain injury and children with specific language impairment. *Brain & Language* 88 (2):215–228, 2004.
95. Landau W, Kleffner F 1957: Syndrome of acquired aphasia with convulsive disorder in children. *Neurology* 7,523–530, 1957.
96. Miller J, Campbell T, Chapman R, Weismer S: Language behavior in acquired childhood aphasia. In: Holland A. (ed): *Language disorders in children* San Diego, College-Hill Press, 1984. pp. 57–99.
97. Glos J., Jariabkova K., Szabova I: Landau-Kleffner syndrome: A case of a dissociation between spoken and written language. *Bratislavské lekárske listy* 102 (12):556–561, 2001.
98. Harrison M.: Landau-Kleffner syndrome: Acquired childhood aphasia. In: T. Layton, E. Crais, L. Watson (eds.), *Handbook of early impairment in children: Nature* Albany, Delmar Publishers, 2001, pp. 418–450.
99. Robinson R: Landau-Kleffner syndrome: Current issues. *Neurology* 19:53–56, 2003.
100. Sparks S.: Prenatal substance use and its impact on young children. In: Layton, T. Crais, E. Watson L. (eds): *Handbook of early language impairment in children: Nature*. Albany, New York: Delmar Publishers, 2001, pp 451–487.
101. Cone-Wesson B: Prenatal alcohol and cocaine exposure: Influences on cognition, speech, language, and hearing. *Journal of Communication Disorders* 38:279–302, 2005.
102. Sparks S: *Children of prenatal substance abuse*. San Diego, Singular Publishing Group, 1993.
103. Bandstra E, Vogel A, Morrow C, Anthony J, Lihua Xue J: Severity of prenatal cocaine exposure and child language functioning through age seven years: A longitudinal latent growth curve analysis. *Substance Use & Misuse* 39:25–59, 2004.
104. Morrow C, Vogel A, Anthony J, Ofir A, Dausa A, Bandstra, E.: Expressive and receptive language functioning in preschool children with prenatal cocaine exposure. *Journal of Pediatric Psychology* 29:543–554, 2004.
105. Lewis B, Singer L, Short E, Minnes S, Arendt R, Weishampel P, Klein N, Min M: Four-year language outcomes of children exposed to cocaine in utero. *Neurotoxicology & Teratology* 26:617–627, 2004.
106. Knutson J, & Sullivan P: Communicative disorders as a risk factor in abuse. *Topics in Language Disorders* 13:1–14, 1993.
107. Fox L, Long S, Anglois A: Patterns of language comprehension deficit in abused and neglected children. *Journal of Speech and Hearing Disorders* 53:239–244, 1988.
108. Culp R, Watkins R, Lawrence H, et al.: Maltreated children's language and speech development: Abused, neglected, and abused and neglected. *First Language* 11:377–390, 1991.
109. Coster W, Gersten M, Beeghly M, et al.: Communicative functioning in maltreated toddlers. *Developmental Psychology* 25:1020–1029, 1989.
110. Allen R, Oliver J: The effects of child maltreatment on language development. *Child Abuse & Neglect* 6:299–305, 1982.
111. Eigsti I, Cicchetti D: The impact of child maltreatment on expressive syntax at 60 months. *Developmental Science* 7:88–102, 2004.
112. Lynch M, Roberts J: *The consequences of child abuse*. New York, Academic Press, 1982.
113. American Speech-Language-Hearing Association: *Incidence and Prevalence of Communication Disorders and Hearing Loss in Children*. Rockville, Author, 2006.
114. Yairi E, Ambrose N, Cox N: Genetics of stuttering: A critical review. *Journal of Speech and Hearing Research* 40:49–58, 1996.
115. Zebrowski PM: Developmental stuttering. *Pediatric Annals* 32 (7): 453–458, July 2003.
116. Van Riper C: *The Treatment of Stuttering*, Englewood Cliffs, Prentice Hall, 1973.
117. Ham R: *Therapy of stuttering: Preschool through adolescence*, Englewood Cliffs, Prentice Hall, 1990.
118. Gregory H: Analysis and commentary. *Language, Speech, and Hearing Services in Schools* 26:196–200, 1995.
119. Cooper E, Cooper C: Treating fluency disordered adolescents. *Journal of Communication Disorders* 28:119–135, 1995.
120. Conture E, Schwartz H, Brewer D: Laryngeal behavior during stuttering: A further study. *Journal of Speech and Hearing Research* 28:233–240, 1985.
121. Adams M: The demands and capacities model. I: Theoretical elaborations. *Journal of Fluency Disorders* 15:135–141, 1990.
122. Dunn C, Davis B: Phonologic process occurrence in phonologically disordered children. *Applied Psycholinguist* 4:187–207, 1983.
123. Ingram D: *Phonologic Disability in Children*, New York, Elsevier, 1976.
124. Weiner F: Systematic sound preference as a characteristic of phonologic disability. *Journal of Speech and Hearing Disorders* 46:281–286, 1981.
125. Trantham C, Pedersen J: *Normal language development: The key to diagnosis and therapy for language disordered children*, Baltimore, Williams & Wilkins, 1976.
126. Bernthal J, Bankson N: *Articulation and phonologic disorders*, 5th ed. Englewood Cliffs, Prentice Hall, 2003.
127. Edwards M: Speech disability in children: Some general considerations. *International Rehabilitative Medicine* 6:114–116, 1984.
128. Office of Scientific and Health Reports: *Developmental speech and language disorders: Help through research* (NIH Publication No. 88–2757). Washington, DC: National Institute of Neurologic Communication Disorders and Stroke, 1988.
129. Shriberg L, Kwiatkowski J: Developmental phonologic disorders. I: A clinical profile. *Journal of Speech and Hearing Research* 37:1100–1126, 1994.
130. Shriberg L, Kwiatkowski J: A follow-up study of children with phonologic disorders of unknown origin. *Journal of Speech and Hearing Disorders* 53:144–155, 1988.
131. Rosenbek J, Wertz R: A review of 50 cases of developmental apraxia of speech. *Language, Speech, and Hearing Services in Schools* 3:23–33, 1972.
132. Yoss K, Darley F: Developmental apraxia of speech in children with defective articulation. *Journal of Speech & Hearing Research* 17:399–416, 1974.
133. Davis B, Velleman S: Differential diagnosis and treatment of developmental apraxia of speech in infants and toddlers. *Infant–Toddler Intervention: The Transdisicplinary Journal* 10:177–192, 2000.
134. Shriberg L, Campbell T, Karlsson B, Brown R, McSweeny J, Nadler C: A diagnostic marker for childhood apraxia of speech: The lexical stress ratio. *Clinical Linguistics and Phonetics* 17:549–556, 2003.
135. Davis B: Differential diagnosis of developmental apraxia. *Perspectives on Language Learning & Education*, October 1998.
136. Guyette T Dietrich W: A critical review of developmental apraxia of speech. In N. Lass (ed): *Speech and language: Advances in basic practice* vol. 5. London: Academic Press, 1981, pp. 1–49.
137. Paul R: Ethical implications of the natural history of slow expressive language development. In: Bishop D Leonard L (eds): *Proceedings of the Third International Symposium for Aphasic and Speech Impaired Children*, London, Psychology Press, 2000.
138. Rescorla L, Roberts J, Dahlsgaard K: Late talkers at 2: Outcome at age 3. *Journal of Speech and Hearing Research* 40:556–566, 1997.

139. Bishop D, Price T, Dale P, Plomin R: Outcomes of early language delay: II. Etiology of transient and persistent language difficulties. *Journal of Speech, Language, & Hearing Research* 46:561–575, 2003.
140. Rescorla L: Language and reading outcomes to age 9 in late-talking toddlers. *Journal of Speech, Language, and Hearing Research* 45:360–371, 2002.
141. Rescorla L. Age 13 language and reading outcomes in late-talking toddlers. *Journal of Speech, Language, and Hearing Research* 48:459–472, 2005.
142. Snowling M, Adams J, Bishop D, Stothard S: Educational attainments of school leavers with a preschool history of speech-language impairments. *International Journal of Language & Communication Disorders* 36:173–183, 2001.
143. Weismer S, Evans J: The role of processing limitations in early identification of specific language impairment. *Topics in Language Disorders* 22 (3):15–29, 2002.
144. Paul R: Clinical implications of slow expressive language development. *American Journal of Speech-Language Pathology* 5:5–21, 1996.
145. Rescorla L, Alley A: Validation of the Language Development Survey (LDS): A parent report tool for identifying language delay in toddlers. *Journal of Speech, Language, and Hearing Research* 44:434–445, 2001.
146. Rescorla L, Mirak J, Singh L: Vocabulary growth in late talkers: Lexical development from 2.0 to 3. *Journal of Child Language* 27:293–311., 2000.
147. Paul R, Jennings P: Phonological behavior in toddlers with slow expressive language development. *Journal of Speech and Hearing Research* 35 (1):99–107, 1992.
148. Pharr A, Ratner N, Rescorla L: Syllable structure development of toddlers with expressive specific language impairment. *Applied Psycholinguistics* 21:429–449, 2000.
149. Rescorla L, Bernstein Ratner N: Phonetic profiles of typically developing and language-delayed toddlers. *Journal of Speech Language, and Hearing Research* 39:153–165, 1996.
150. Roberts J, Rescorla L, Giroux J, Stevens L: Phonological skills of children with specific expressive language impairment (SLI-E): Outcome at age 3. *Journal of Speech, Language, and Hearing Research* 41:374–384, 1998.
151. Rescorla L, Dahlsgaard K, Roberts J: The relationship of MLU to Index of Productive Syntax (IPSyn) in late talkers and comparison children at ages 3 and 4. *Journal of Child Language* 27:643–664, 2000.
152. Rescorla L, Roberts J: Nominal vs. verbal morpheme use in late talkers at ages 3 and 4. *Journal of Speech, Language, and Hearing Research* 45:1219–1231, 2002.
153. Rescorla L, Mirren L: Communicative intent in late-talking toddlers. *Applied Psycholinguistics* 19:393–411, 1998.
154. Caparulo B, Cohen D: Developmental language studies in the neuropsychiatric disorders of children. In: KE Nelson (ed): *Children's language* 4: Hillsdale, Erlbaum, pp. 423–463. 1983.
155. Marton K, Abramoff B, Rosenzweig, S: Social cognition and language in children with specific language impairment (SLI). *Journal of Communication Disorders* 38:143–162, 2005.
156. Reilly J, Losh M, Bellugi U, Wulfeck B: "Frog, where are you?" Narratives in children with specific language impairment, early focal brain injury, and Williams syndrome. *Brain & Language* 88:229–247, 2004.
157. Graham J, Bashir A, Stark R: Communicative disorders. In: Levine M, Carey W, Crocker A, et al: (eds): *Developmental-behavioral pediatrics* Philadelphia: W.B. Saunders, 1983, (pp. 847–864).
158. Kuder J: *Teaching students with language and communication disabilities*, Boston, Allyn & Bacon, 1997.
159. Hall, P, Tomblin J: A follow-up study of children with articulation and language disorders. *Journal of Speech and Hearing Disorders* 43:227–241, 1978.
160. Paul R, Cohen D: Outcomes of severe disorders of language acquisition. *Journal of Autism and Developmental Disorders* 14:405–421, 1984.
161. Roberts J, Wallace, I, Henderson, F: *Otitis media in young children*. Baltimore, Paul H. Brookes, 1997.
162. Beukelman D, Mirenda P: *Augmentative and Alternative Communication: Supporting Children and Adults with Complex Communication needs*, 3rd ed. Baltimore, Paul H. Brookes Publishing, 2005.
163. Glennen S, DeCoste D: *Handbook of Augmentative & Alternative Communication*. San Diego, Singular Publishing Group, 1997.
164. Lord C, Rutter M, Le Couteur A: *Autism diagnostic interview*. Los Angeles: Western Psychological Services, 2002.
165. Lord C, Risi S, Lambrecht L, Cook E, Leventhal B, DiLavore P, Pickles A, Rutter M: The Autism Diagnostic Observation Schedule—Generic: A standard measure of social and communication deficits associated with the spectrum of autism. *Journal of Autism & Developmental Disorders* 30:205–223, 2000.
166. Schopler E, Reichler RJ, Renner BR: *Childhood Autism Rating Scale*. Circle Pines, AGS, 2006.
167. Fey M, Windsor J, Warren S: *Language Intervention: Preschool through Elementary Years*, Baltimore, Paul H. Brookes, 1995.
168. McCauley R, Fey M (eds): *Treatment of Language Disorders in Children*, Baltimore, Paul H. Brookes, 2006.
169. Paul R: *Language Disorders from Infancy through Adolescence*, 3rd ed. St. Louis, Elsevier Science, 2007.
170. Labbe E, Williamson D: Behavioral treatment of elective mutism: A review of the literature. *Clinical Psychology Review* 4:273–292, 1984.
171. Black B Uhde T: Treatment of elective mutism with fluoxetine: A double-blind, placebo-controlled study. *Journal of the American Academy of Child & Adolescent Psychiatry* 33:1000–1006, 1994.
172. Biklen D: Communication unbound: Autism and praxis. *Harvard Education Review* 60:291–314, 1990.
173. Tharpe A: Auditory integration training: The magical mystery cure. *Language Speech and Hearing Services in Schools* 30:378–382, 1999.

5.2 ■ ATTENTION AND DISRUPTIVE DISORDERS

CHAPTER 5.2.1 ■ ATTENTION-DEFICIT/HYPERACTIVITY DISORDER

LACRAMIOARA SPETIE AND EUGENE L. ARNOLD

DEFINITION

Attention deficit/hyperactivity disorder (ADHD) is a syndrome of inattention, distractibility, restless overactivity, impulsiveness and other deficits of executive function. It involves impairment of the ability to "plan your work and work your plan." It can be manifested in any of 18 official DSM-IV symptoms (Table 5.2.1.1) and can be full-expression (combined type) or partial expression (inattentive or hyperactive-impulsive types). It is not necessary to have all the symptoms to qualify for the diagnosis. Six of the nine inattentive symptoms are required for diagnosis of inattentive type and six of the hyperactive-impulsive for diagnosis of hyperactive/impulsive type, with six of each list for combined type (1). Thus, it is possible for two patients to meet diagnostic criteria with no symptoms in common and it is even possible to have the same subtype with only half the symptoms in common. This leads to wide variability in presenting problems and severity, which is further complicated by common associated symptoms such as irritability, boredom, and impaired social skills, and by psychiatric comorbid diagnoses.

TABLE 5.2.1.1

DSM-IV DIAGNOSTIC CRITERIA FOR ATTENTION DEFICIT HYPERACTIVITY DISORDER

A. Either (1) or (2):

(1) Six (or more) of the following symptoms of inattention have persisted for at least 6 months to a degree that is maladaptive and inconsistent with developmental level:

Inattention

(a) often fails to give close attention to details or makes careless mistakes in schoolwork, work, or other activities
(b) often has difficulty sustaining attention in tasks or play activities
(c) often does not seem to listen when spoken to directly
(d) often does not follow through on instructions and fails to finish schoolwork, chores, or duties in the workplace (not due to oppositional behavior or failure to understand instructions)
(e) often has difficulty organizing tasks and activities
(f) often avoids, dislikes, or is reluctant to engage in tasks that require sustained mental effort (such as schoolwork or homework)
(g) often loses things necessary for tasks or activities (e.g., toys, school assignments, pencils, books, or tools)
(h) is often easily distracted by extraneous stimuli
(i) is often forgetful in daily activities

(2) Six (or more) of the following symptoms of hyperactivity/impulsivity have persisted for at least 6 months to a degree that is maladaptive and inconsistent with developmental level:

Hyperactivity

(a) often fidgets with hands or feet or squirms in seat
(b) often leaves seat in classroom or in other situations in which remaining seated is expected
(c) often runs about or climbs excessively in situations in which it is inappropriate (in adolescents or adults, may be limited to subjective feelings of restlessness)
(d) often has difficulty playing or engaging in leisure activities quietly
(e) is often "on the go" or often acts as if "driven by a motor"
(f) often talks excessively

Impulsivity

(g) often blurts out answers before questions have been completed
(h) often has difficulty awaiting turn
(i) often interrupts or intrudes on others (e.g., butts into conversations or games)

B. Some hyperactive-impulsive or inattentive symptoms that caused impairment were present before age 7 years.
C. Some impairment from the symptoms is present in two or more settings [e.g., at school (or work) and at home].
D. There must be clear evidence of clinically significant impairment in social, academic, or occupational functioning.
E. The symptoms do not occur exclusively during the course of a pervasive developmental disorder, schizophrenia, or other psychotic disorder and are not better accounted for by another mental disorder (e.g., mood disorder, anxiety disorder, dissociative disorder, or a personality disorder).

Code based on type:
314.01 Attention deficit hyperactivity disorder, combined type: If both criteria Al and A2 are met for the past 6 months
314.00 Attention deficit/hyperactivity disorder, predominantly inattentive type: If criterion Al is met but criterion A2 is not met for the past 6 months
314.01 Attention deficit hyperactivity disorder, predominantly hyperactive-impulsive type: If criterion A2 is met but criterion Al is not met for the past 6 months
Coding note: For individuals (especially adolescents and adults) who currently have symptoms that no longer meet full criteria, In partial remission should be specified.
314.9 Attention deficit hyperactivity disorder
Not otherwise specified
This category is for disorders with prominent symptoms of inattention or hyperactivity-impulsivity that do not meet criteria for attention deficit hyperactivity disorder.

(Reprinted with permission from *Diagnostic and Statistical Manual of Mental Disorders*, Fourth Edition (DSM-IV). Copyright 1994, American Psychiatric Association.)

THE ATTENTION DEFICIT HYPERACTIVITY DISORDER CONCEPT AND TERMINOLOGY

As early as the mid-nineteenth century, the problems of inattentiveness and overactivity in children were recognized by Heinrich Hoffman (2) in the moralistic children's book *Slovenly Peter*, which featured the characters Fidgety Phil and Harry Who Looks in the Air. In the early twentieth century Still's disease was recognized as the behavioral sequelae of viral encephalitis. The behavioral constellation, particularly the overactivity and impulsiveness, were therefore considered "minimal brain damage," which morphed over time into "minimal brain dysfunction" as diagnosticians realized it was not possible to find evidence of actual brain damage in most cases (at least not with the technology available through the 1970s). Other descriptive terms used by the second half of the twentieth century included hyperkinesis, hyperkinetic syndrome, hyperactivity, hyperactive-impulse disorder, psychoneurologic integration deficit, and pseudoneurosis.

The second edition of the Diagnostic and Statistical Manual (3) recognized the syndrome for the first time as an official diagnosis, calling it "hyperkinetic reaction," based on the then-prevailing psychodynamic philosophy that mental disorders were always reactions to some stressor. The term "hyperkinetic disorder" is still used in the current International Code of Diseases (4). Recognizing that the cause of most mental disorders is more complex than a reaction to stress, the DSM III (5) changed in 1980 to descriptive phenomenological terms without causal implication. By that time the importance of inattentive symptoms had been recognized, leading to the appellation "attention deficit disorder," which could be diagnosed either without (ADD) or with hyperactivity (ADDH). The term ADD is still used by many to refer to the inattentive subtype, and is preserved in the names of such support/advocacy groups as Attention-Deficit Disorder Association (ADDA) (6) and Children and Adults with ADD (ChADD) (7). DSM-III-R (8) added overactivity back to the name of the disorder via the term "attention deficit/hyperactivity disorder (ADHD)." This name was retained by DSM-IV (1), although the symptom list changed somewhat, being expanded from 14 to 18 symptoms and being split into two lists of nine each (Figure 5.2.1.1).

The ICD 10 criteria for Hyperkinetic Disorder (HD) are more restrictive than the DSM IV criteria in that all three symptom clusters of inattention, hyperactivity and impulsivity should be present and pervasive across settings and that the presence of anxiety or mood disorder is in itself an exclusion criterion. ICD 10 also includes the diagnosis of hyperkinetic conduct disorder (HKD), which would be roughly the same as the DSM equivalent of ADHD combined type with comorbid conduct disorder.

EPIDEMIOLOGY

Attention deficit hyperactivity disorder (ADHD) is one of the most common childhood onset psychiatric disorders, affecting 5–12% of children worldwide. ADHD is a costly public health concern (9) since it can cause significant impairment in functioning that interferes with normal development and all areas of functioning in patients of all ages.

Epidemiological studies of ADHD addressing issues of frequency, distribution, determinants, comorbidity, long-term outcome, and impact of treatment have been complicated by several problems. The first is integrating the different types of information from various sources required to make the diagnosis. A related problem is how to correct for the subjective nature of the information provided by the informants. The diagnosis could be easily overestimated if the information obtained does not include the level of impairment caused by the symptoms reported (10). Another problem is the difficulty integrating epidemiological information obtained over time due to the ongoing refinement in the diagnostic criteria for ADHD. The current DSM IV criteria allow the inclusion of more females, preschoolers, and adults presenting with significant impairment but who would have been otherwise excluded (11). The definition of ADHD may continue to flux over time, as experts now consider more age-specific thresholds for symptom counts.

Further, there are differences between the DSM IV criteria used to make the diagnosis in the United States and the ICD-10 criteria ordinarily used to make the diagnosis in Europe and other parts of the world, although many investigators worldwide use the DSM-IV system. Because of the difference in stringency of definition, DSM IV ADHD is more prevalent than ICD HKD, a finding that could be easily misinterpreted to show that ADHD is more common in countries using DSM criteria than in countries using ICD-10 criteria (12). A recent reanalysis of the data of the National Institute of Mental Health (NIMH) Multimodal Treatment Study of children with ADHD (the MTA) found that only 145 of the 579 children who had DSM-IV combined type ADHD also met criteria for ICD-10 HKD (13). A further complication is whether all the inattentive type cases are detected in a given study.

However, when DSM-IV criteria are applied to the epidemiological information obtained in various international studies, the prevalence in the United States and worldwide is similar, 5–12%, including fairer representation of females and inattentive type, which may have been underappreciated in earlier lower estimates, such as in the DSM-IV (1) estimate of 3–5%. The male to female ratio is about 2:1 in epidemiologically discerned samples, in contrast to 3–5:1 and even up to 9:1 in mental-health clinic samples. Females present more often with less disruptive symptoms, more attention problems and more internalizing problems such as depression and anxiety (14), while boys present with more

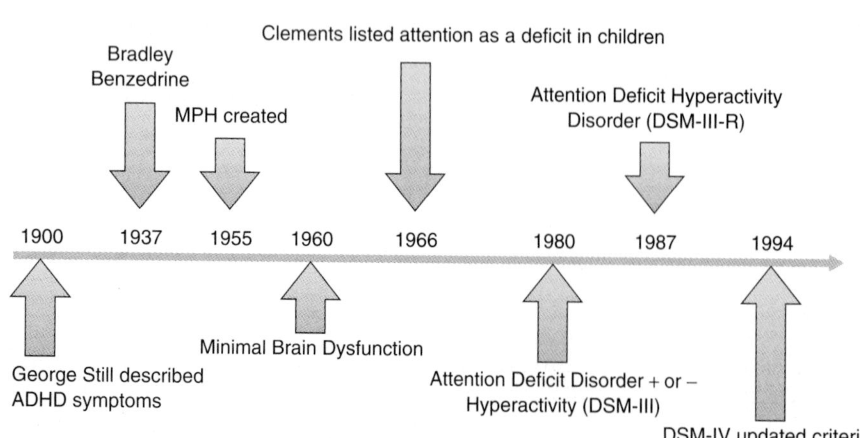

FIGURE 5.2.1.1. Timeline of names from industry set. (Courtesy of Novartis Pharmaceuticals.)

disruptive behavior leading to clinical referral. Male sex, low socioeconomic status, and young age are associated with a higher prevalence of ADHD.

In preschoolers the hyperactive subtype is more common and the prevalence may vary from a low of 2% in the primary care setting to a high of 59% in a child psychiatry clinic (15). The symptoms related to hyperactivity tend to decrease with age. In intermediate elementary school-age children the combined type has been more frequently diagnosed, while the inattentive type was more common in middle and high school. As many as 60% of the childhood cases continue to have some symptoms as adults.

ETIOLOGY

The etiology of ADHD is complex and most likely includes genetic and environmental factors.

Genetics

ADHD is a genetically predisposed disorder that does not follow the Mendelian patterns of inheritance and that is also phenotypically complex. The early genetic studies relied on a categorical diagnosis of ADHD without taking into account differences in the manifestation of the various components of the illness and the currently recognized subtypes, making their results difficult to interpret. Recent studies have shown that ADHD is strongly genetically influenced and is transmitted in families. Extensive data gathered by twin and adoption studies have consistently yielded an estimated heritability of about 75% that has not changed over the past 30 years (Figure 5.2.1.2) (16a-f).

Developments in human genetics, including the completion of the sequencing of the human genome, the availability of powerful technology for genomic analysis, and the generation of new analytical and bioinformatics tools, have led to significant progress in understanding the genetics of many neurodevelopmental disorders, including ADHD. Recent genetic studies have been using endophenotypes as tools to detect the effects of individual genes. Endophenotypes are phenotypes that are assumed to be less complex in presentation and etiology than signs and symptoms of the clinical disorder but are still influenced by one or more of the same susceptibility genes as the disorder. Neuropsychological measures of inhibitory control, impairments in state regulation, and delay aversion are considered potential candidates for ADHD endophenotypes (17, 18). Other methods focus on distinct components or clusters of symptoms of the complex phenotypes that may be heritable and may characterize phenotypically homogenous groups of individuals.

So far there have been three genome-wide linkage studies, and each of them identified different chromosomal regions shared more often than expected by chance among ADHD family members. These regions have included 5p12, 10q26, 12q23 and 16p13 (19); 15q15, 7p13 and 9q33 (20); and 8q12, 11q23, 4q13, 17p11, 12q23, and 8p23 (21).

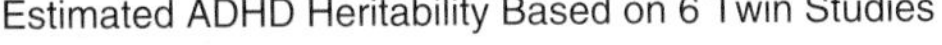

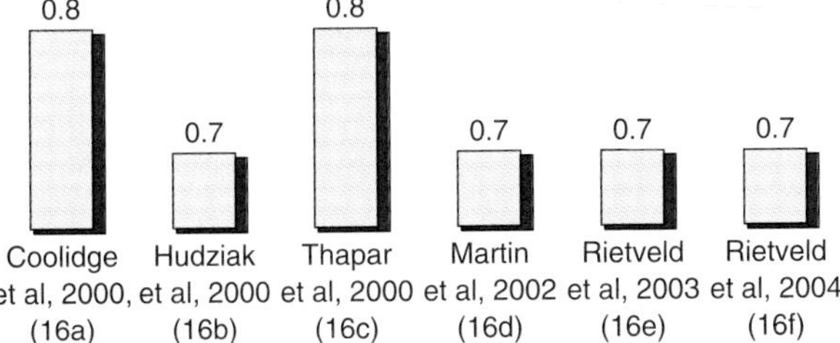

FIGURE 5.2.1.2. Estimated ADHD heritability based on 6 studies.

Association studies of candidate genes have looked for evidence that certain biologically relevant candidate genes may influence the susceptibility to ADHD. Case-control designs compare allele frequencies between patients with ADHD and non-ADHD control subjects, while family-based designs compare the alleles that parents transmit to ADHD children with those they do not transmit. If an allele increases the risk for ADHD, it should be more common among the transmitted alleles than the nontransmitted alleles. The data obtained in both study designs can be analyzed to derive odds ratio (OR) or relative risk (RR) statistics that assess the magnitude of the association between the risk alleles and the diagnosis of ADHD. An OR or RR of 1.0 indicate no association, greater than 1.0 indicates that the allele increases the risk for ADHD, and those less than 1.0 indicate that the allele decreases the risk for ADHD. The most studied candidate genes for ADHD are listed in Table 5.2.1.2.

Structural, Functional, and Electrophysiological Findings in the Brain

Structural Findings in ADHD

Similarities between the symptoms of attention deficit hyperactivity disorder and symptoms observed in certain neurological patients following damage to the prefrontal cortex (22) have prompted researchers to theorize that brain structural abnormalities may be at the root of ADHD symptomatology. Furthermore, neurocognitive studies of patients with ADHD also identified patterns of executive dysfunction in patients with ADHD that are thought to reflect abnormalities in the functioning of the prefrontal cortex, therefore supporting the hypothesis of an alteration of the prefrontal cortex neuroanatomy in ADHD (23–25). The robust symptom response to psychostimulant drugs that target the dopaminergic system that is very well represented in the prefrontal cortex further supported this theory (26). With the introduction of totally automated imaging methods it has been possible to identify more widespread volumetric and cortical changes.

The most consistent structural brain imaging findings in children with ADHD have been significantly smaller volumes in the dorsolateral prefrontal cortex, caudate, pallidum, corpus callosum, and cerebellum (Table 5.2.1.3). There is only one structural brain imaging study in adults (27). Most of the studies to date have had low power (using rather small samples) and have differed widely in the way they address other confounding factors such as the influence of gender, comorbidity, medication status, perinatal complications, DSM subtype, etc. One of the most comprehensive longitudinal case-control imaging studies was of 152 children and adolescents with ADHD (age range 5–18 years) and 139 age- and sex-matched controls (age range 4.5–19 years) completed at the National Institute of Mental Health (NIMH) from 1991 to 2001. The patients with ADHD had significantly smaller brain volumes on the initial scan in all regions (total cerebrum; cerebellum; gray and white matter for the four major lobes: frontal, temporal, parietal and occipital); unmedicated children with ADHD had significantly smaller total cerebral volumes and significantly smaller total white matter; the volumetric abnormalities persisted with age in total and regional cerebral measures and in the cerebellum, except for the caudate nucleus volumes that were initially abnormal for patients with ADHD but lost the diagnostic difference from controls during adolescence; developmental trajectories for all structures except the caudate remained roughly parallel for patients and controls during childhood and adolescence and are unrelated to stimulant treatment (28).

TABLE 5.2.1.2

CANDIDATE GENES FOR ADHD

Gene	Reference	Summary findings
Dopamine Transporter Gene (DAT; SLC6A3)	Cook et al., 1995 (71); Waldman et al., 1998 (72); Dougherty et al., 1999 (73); Krause et al., 2000 (74); Todd et al., 2001 (75); Payton et al., 2001 (76); Muglia et al., 2002 (77); van Dyck et al., 2002 (78); Chen et al., 2003 (79); Smith et al., 2003 (80)	Pooled OR = 1.13
	Metaanalysis: Curran et al., 2001 (81)	Pooled OR = 1.16
D2 Dopamine Receptor Gene (DRD2)	*Case control studies*: Comings, 1991 (82); Comings, 1996 (83) *Family-based studies*: Rowe et al., 1999 (84); Kirley et al., 2002 (85); Huang et al., 2003 (86)	No conclusive results
D4 Dopamine Receptor Gene (DRD4-7)	Faraone SV et al., 2001 (87)—metaanalysis of case studies (CS) and family-based studies (FB)	Found a significant association between 7-repeat allele CR studies—pooled OR = 1.9 FB studies—pooled OR = 1.4
	Other positive case control studies: Payton et al., 2001 (32) *Other positive family-based studies*: Holmes et al., 2002 (88); Grady et al., 2003 (89); Arcos Burgos et al., 2004 (21) *Negative case control studies*: Qian et al., 2003 (90) *Negative family-based studies*: Mill et al., 2001 (91); Manor et al., 2002 (92); Kustanovich et al., 2003 (93); Smith KM et al., 2003 (80)	
Other DRD4 polymorphisms (120 bp repeat 1.2 kb; 240 allele FspI- 521 C to T and Ava- II—616 C to G; 5'120-bp repeat)	McCracken et al., 2000 (94); Todd et al., 2001 (95); Barr et al., 2001 (96); Rowe et al., 2001 (97); Kustanovich et al., 2003 (93); Arcos Burgos et al., 2004 (21) Barkley et al., 2006 (18)	No conclusive results
D5 Dopamine Receptor Gene (DRD5)	*Case control studies*: Comings et al., 2000 (98) *Family-based studies*: Daly et al., 1999 (99); Barr et al., 2000 (100); Tahir et al., 2000 (101); Payton et al., 2001 (76); Kustanovich et al., 2003 (93); Mill et al., 2004 (102)	Minimum association (probably due to study low statistical power)
	Metaanalysis of family-based studies: Maher et al., 2002 (103); Lowe et al., 2004 (104); Manor et al., 2004 (105)	Significant association: pooled OR 1.2
D3 Dopamine Receptor gene (DRD3)	Barr et al., 2000 (106); Payton et al., 2001 (76); Muglia et al., 2002 (107); Coming et al., 2000 (98); Retz et al., 2003 (108)	Pooled OR 1.2
Serotonin Transporter Gene (5-HTT; SLC6A4)	*Case control studies*: Retz et al., 2002 (109); Seeger et al., 2001 (110); Zoroglu et al., 2002 (111); Beitchman et al., 2003 (112) *Family studies*: Manor et al., 2001 (113); Kent et al., 2002 (114); Cadoret et al., 2003 (115)	Pooled OR = 1.31
Norepinephrine Receptor Gene (SLC6A2)	*Case report studies*: Comings et al., 2000 (98) *Family-based studies*: Barr et al., 2002 (116); McEvoy et al., 2002 (117); DeLuca et al., 2004 (118)	No conclusive results
Dopamine Beta Hydroxylase Gene (DBH)	*Case control*: Smith KM, 2003 (119) *Family studies*: Daly et al., 1999 (99); Payton et al., 2001 (76); Roman et al., 2002 (120); Wigg et al., 2002 (121); Hawi et al., 2003 (122); Barkley et al., 2006 (18)	Pooled OR 1.33
Synaptosomal Associated Protein 25 Gene (SNAP 25)	*Family-based studies*: Hess et al., 1992 (123); Hess et al., 1995 (124); Barr et al., 2000 (125); Brophy et al., 2002 (126); Kustanovich et al., 2003 (93); Mill et al., 2002 (127); Kirley, 2002 (128)	Pooled OR 1.19
Tyrosine Hydroxylase Gene (TH)	*Case control*: Comings et al., 1995 (129) *Family studies*: Barr et al., 2000 (125); Payton et al., 2001 (76)	All studies negative

TABLE 5.2.1.2

(CONTINUED)

Gene	Reference	Summary findings
Catechol O COMT, Val108Met)	*Family studies*: Syvanen et al., 1997 (130); Barr et al., 1999 (131); Hawi et al., 2000 (132); Manor et al., 2000 (133); Tahir et al., 2000 (134); Payton et al., 2001 (76); Qian et al., 2003 (135)	No significant association (pooled OR 1.0)
Monoamine Oxidase A (MAO-A)	*Case control*: Manor et al., 2002 (136) *Family studies*: Payton et al., 2001 (76); Manor et al., 2002 (136); Lawson et al., 2003 (137)	All studies but one (Payton, et al., 2001) found a significant association
Noradrenergic Receptors ADRA2A	Comings et al., 1999 (138); Xu et al., 2001 (139); Comings et al., 2003 (140); Roman et al., 2003 (141)	No conclusive results
ADRA1C and ADRA2C	Comings et al., 1999 (138); Barr et al., 2001 (142); De Luca et al., 2004 (118)	No conclusive results
Serotonin Receptors HTR1B (G861C SNP)	*Family studies*: Hawi et al., 2002 (143); Quist et al., 2003 (144)	Pooled OR 1.44
HTR2A (T102C; G1438A; His438Tyr)	*Case control*: Zoroglu et al., 2002 (111) *Family studies*: Quist et al., 2000 (144); Hawi et al., 2002 (143)	No significant association (pooled OR 1.1)
Tryptophan Hydroxylase (TPH-SNP's A218C; 6526G)	*Family studies*: Tang et al., 2001 (145); Li et al., 2003 (146)	No conclusive results
Acetylcholine Receptors CHRNA4 and CHRNA7	*Case control*: Comings et al., 2000 (98) *Family studies*: Kent et al., 2001 (147); Todd et al., 2003 (148)	No conclusive results
Glutamate Receptors GRIN2A	*Family studies*: Turic et al., 2004 (149); Adams, et al., 2004 (150)	Contradicting results

TABLE 5.2.1.3

STRUCTURAL BRAIN ABNORMALITIES IN ADHD

Brain Region	Reference	Summary Findings
Prefrontal Cortex	Castellanos et al., 1996 (151); Filipek et al., 1997 (152); Overmeyer et al., 2001 (153); Castellanos et al., 2002 (28); Mostofsky et al., 2002 (154); Hill et al., 2003 (155); Durston et al., 2004 (156)	General findings in ADHD subjects: smaller volumes in various areas, especially in the dorsolateral prefrontal and orbitofrontal regions and anterior cingulate?
Caudate	Hynd et al., 1993 (157); Semrud-Clickeman et al., 1994 (158); Castellanos et al., 1994 (159); Castellanos et al., 1996 (160); Filipek et al., 1997 (152); Mataro et al., 1997 (161); Castellanos et al., 2001 (162); Castellanos et al., 2002 (28); Pineda et al., 2002 (163); Bussing et al., 2002 (164); Hill et al., 2003 (155); Castellanos et al., 2003 (165)	General findings in ADHD subjects: smaller total caudate volume and/or smaller caudate head, but difference from normal lost with age
Pallidum	Aylward et al., 1996 (166); Castellanos et al., 1996 (151); Overmeyer et al., 2001 (167); Castellanos et al., 2001 (162)	General findings in ADHD subjects: smaller pallidum volume
Corpus Callosum	Hynd et al., 1990 (168); Hynd et al., 1991 (169); Semrud-Clickeman et al., 1994 (158); Giedd et al., 1994 (170); Baumgardner et al., 1996 (171); Lyoo et al., 1996 (172); Castellanos et al., 2001 (162); Mostofsky et al., 2002 (154); Kates et al., 2002 (173); Hill et al., 2003 (155)	General findings in ADHD subjects: smaller volumes especially in the posterior regions linked to temporal and parietal cortices
Cerebellum	Castellanos et al., 1996 (151); Filipek et al., 1997 (152); Berquin et al., 1998 (174); Mostofsky et al., 1998 (175); Castellanos et al., 2001 (162); Bussing et al., 2002 (164); Hill et al., 2003 (155)	General findings in ADHD subjects: smaller volumes in various regions, including vermis

Twin studies using structural neuroimaging suggest that the volume of brain regions relevant to ADHD (subcortical and cortical volumes, left and right neocortex, variation of cerebellar volume) is under significant genetic control and might be used to define neuroimaging ADHD endophenotypes (17).

Brain Functional Abnormalities

New brain imaging techniques, including single photon emission computed tomography (SPECT); positron emission tomography (PET); functional MRI (fMRI) and proton magnetic resonance spectroscopy (PMRS), have made it possible to obtain dynamic measures of brain metabolism at rest and during certain cognitive tasks. Most studies have found abnormalities in cerebral activation in ADHD, with a hypoperfusion of frontal and possibly striatal areas (Table 5.2.1.4). The studies looking at brain function during tasks that challenge the brain inhibitory control also show deficits in the activation of the brain inhibitory control area in the frontal and striatal regions. Because of the important role dopamine (DA) and the dopamine transporter (DAT) seem to have in the pathophysiology and response to treatment in ADHD, several imaging studies using ligands highly selective for the dopamine transporter sites have studied their density in ADHD subjects compared to controls. These studies consistently found an increase in the DAT binding in the striatum of ADHD subjects compared to controls. Several studies also showed a normalization of this brain function following treatment with methylphenidate.

Such functional investigative tools have opened a window on the dynamic nature of ADHD and started to elucidate the flexible and bidirectional causal relationship between brain structure, its neurochemistry, and brain function. Multiple lines of evidence support the role of dopamine in the etiology and the response to treatment (Figure 5.2.1.3). The dopamine circuits are influenced by inputs from multiple areas of the brain involving other neurotransmitter systems, including norepinephrine and serotonin.

Table 5.2.1.5 (30, 39) presents one of the theories explaining the abnormal dopamine transporter density in ADHD subjects and the response to methylphenidate.

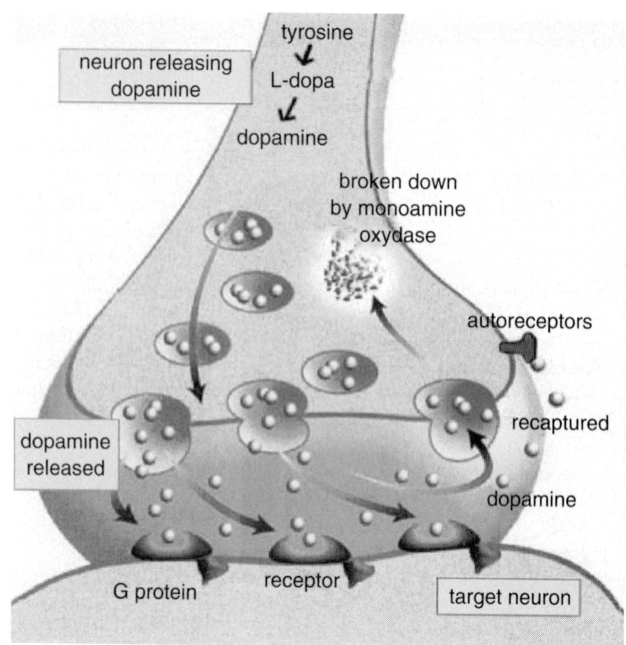

FIGURE 5.2.1.3. Dopamine synapse. Genetic studies indicate that patients with ADHD have a higher rate of certain polymorphisms for the dopamine and other receptors and for the dopamine transporter, resulting in either lower sensitivity of the receptor or faster re-uptake of dopamine molecules. Stimulant drugs inhibit reuptake, keeping each dopamine molecule longer in the synaptic cleft so that it is available to stimulate the receptors longer. Similar considerations apply also to norepinephrine, another neurotransmitter believed to be involved in ADHD.

Electrophysiological Studies

Electroencephalograms (EEG) provide information about the background electrical activity of the brain with good temporal resolution but poor spatial resolution. EEG studies of patients with attention deficit hyperactivity disorder (ADHD) were first done as early as 1938 (31) when they included mostly qualitative EEG studies that used visual evaluation of paper recordings of the EEG. With the advance of computer-aided spectral analysis, new approaches have been used to evaluate EEG characteristics, including quantitative EEG studies; waveform amplitude studies; power studies; ratio coefficients studies; and coherence studies. Most studies consistently found elevated levels of slow wave activity in comparison to normal children, with the most reliable measure being the relative theta power and reduced amounts of relative alpha and beta waves.

Several studies have looked at EEG as a diagnostic tool and reported that the theta/beta ratio could discriminate ADHD subjects from control subjects with sensitivity and specificity (32–35). Several models of ADHD and ADHD subtypes have been proposed based on the EEG studies: the Maturational Lag Model; the Developmental Deviation Model; and the Hypoarousal Model (Table 5.2.1.6). All models fail to account for the complex clinical presentation in ADHD.

Event-Related Potentials

Event related potentials (ERPs) provide information about the brain electrical activity underlying sensory and cognitive brain processes in response to stimuli. The small subject numbers, the use of different types of task performance indicators and reward systems, and other methodological flows have made the results of most of the studies to date difficult to interpret (36).

With the development of molecular genetics, attempts have been made to identify electrophysiological endophenotypes of ADHD. A metaanalytic review of twin studies of electrophysiological measures indicates that genetic factors contribute significantly to both EEG and ERP measures, with significant heritability scores for the EEG alpha power and alpha peak frequency and ERP P3 amplitude (37). More studies are needed to refine such endophenotypes.

Special Etiological Subgroups

Because ADHD is a phenomenological diagnosis rather than etiologic, there can be various causes manifested through the same symptom constellations. Genetic predisposition, of course, is a major cause, but genes can exert their influence only through interaction with the environment (and other genes). The pathogenetic mechanisms for expression of various genes in interaction with various environments—physical, chemical, nutritional, familial, social—can vary widely from one individual to another. The multiple allele polymorphisms described above allow for multiple environmental sensitivities or special environmental needs, and there are probably further polymorphisms not yet discovered. For example, there appears to be a small subgroup of children with ADHD who have some kind of food or food additive sensitivity demonstrated in placebo-controlled studies (38–40). Another very small subgroup has thyroid abnormality intimately linked to ADHD symptoms (41, 42). Heavy metal poisoning can cause ADHD symptoms, and at least one study suggested that in cases of

TABLE 5.2.1.4

FUNCTIONAL NEUROIMAGING STUDIES OF ADHD

Imaging Technique	Reference	Summary Findings
SPECT Studies	Lou et al., 1984 (176), 1989 (177), 1990 (178), 1998 (179); Sieg et al., 1995 (180); Amen et al., 1997 (181); Gustaffson et al., 2000 (46); Langleben et al., 2001 (182), 2002 (183); Spalletta et al., 2001 (184); Kim et al., 2001 (185), 2002 (186)	General findings in ADHD subjects: hypoperfusion in various cortical areas, especially in the frontal and prefrontal cortex, striatum and cerebellum
fMRI Studies	Sunshine et al., 1997 (187); Vaidya et al., 1998 (188); Bush et al., 1999 (189); Rubia et al., 1999 (190); Teicher et al., 2000 (191); Anderson et al., 2002 (192); Durston et al., 2003 (193); Schulz et al., 2004 (195); Tamm et al., 2004 (196)	General findings in ADHD subjects: decreased cerebral blood flow to the frontal, prefrontal, and the basal ganglia; decreased activation of frontal/prefrontal regions and basal ganglia during certain cognitive tasks; atypical increase in activity in other brain areas possibly to compensate for hypoactivation; normalization of cerebral blood flow to frontal/prefrontal areas following administration of methylphenidate
PET Studies	Zametkin et al., 1990 (197), 1993 (198); Matochik et al., 1993 (199), 1994 (200); Ernst et al., 1994 (201), 1997 (202), 1998 (203), 2003 (204); Schweitzer et al., 2000 (205), 2003 (206), 2004 (207)	General findings in ADHD subjects: decreased glucose metabolism in prefrontal/frontal and other cortical areas and reduced metabolic rate in same areas during cognitive tasks
Positive DAT Binding SPECT Studies	Dougherty et al., 1999 (208); Dresel et al., 2000 (209); Cheon et al., 2003 (210)	Elevated DAT binding in ADHD subjects compared to controls
Negative DAT Binding SPECT Studies	Van Dyke et al., 2002 (211)	No difference in striatum binding in ADHD subjects compared with controls
Positive DAT Binding PET Studies	Spencer et al., 2005 (212, 213)	Elevated binding in striatum in ADHD subjects compared to controls
Negative DAT Binding PET Studies	Jucaite et al., 2005 (214)	No difference in DAT binding or D2 receptor binding in the striatum and decreased DAT binding in the midbrain between ADHD subjects and controls Significant correlation between DAT and D2 binding in the striatum and measures of hyperactivity
	Pedro Rosa-Neto et al., 2005 (215)	Estimated binding potential for D2/3 receptors in the striatum in ADHD subjects within range of estimates obtained in healthy subjects; significant correlation between binding in the right striatum and severity of inattention and impulsivity; significant decrease in binding potential following administration of methylphenidate
PMRS Studies	Jin et al., 2001 (216)	Low N-acetyl aspartate/creatine ration in globus pallidus in ADHD subjects
	MacMaster et al., 2003 (217)	Elevated glutamate in the right prefrontal cortex and left striatum
	Yeo et al., 2003 (218)	Lower N-acetyl aspartate levels in girls with ADHD
	Courvoisie et al., 2004 (219)	Significantly higher ratios of N acetyl aspartate; glutamate and choline/creatine in the frontal lobes of ADHD subjects
	Moore et al., 2006 (220)	Glutamatergic dysfunction in the anterior cingulated cortex in ADHD subjects compared to healthy controls and subjects with bipolar disorder

lead toxicity, ADHD symptoms improve as much (or more) with deleading as with a stimulant drug (43). It is possible that because of genetic differences in enzymes and other metabolic features, some individuals may be more sensitive to heavy metal poisoning than others. Some anticonvulsants can make ADHD symptoms worse. Many authors believe that thresholds of vitamin and mineral requirements vary from person to person, so that some may be more susceptible to borderline deficiency symptoms.

DIAGNOSIS AND CLINICAL FEATURES

Importance of History

ADHD is a diagnosis primarily made by history, by caregiver report (or in the case of some adolescents and adults, by self-report) of a chronic pattern of inattentiveness, overactivity,

TABLE 5.2.1.5

THE DOPAMINE TRANSPORTER AND ADHD

Theory	Rationale
Abnormal DAT binding as a "trait"	"Hypertrophy" of the dopaminergic neurons as a result of inadequate pruning during neurodevelopment genetic abnormalities
Abnormal DAT binding as a "state"	Result of processes compensating for abnormal (increased or decreased) dopamine transmission an attempt to increase efficiency of dopamine clearing resulting from abnormalities at the dopamine synapse level (excess dopamine production and/or release; decreased vesicular storage; increased activity of D1-D5 receptors; abnormal receptor–effector coupling)

and/or impulsiveness. Rarely is a short sampling of behavior in an office visit adequate to detect the symptoms, and even then the diagnostician needs caregiver confirmation of their chronicity and pervasiveness. Often a child with ADHD in a novel setting with an adult one on one, especially a strange one, can appear calm and attentive. Therefore, careful collection of the observations of parents, teachers, and other caregivers (bus drivers, coaches, sitters) is the most essential diagnostic strategy.

Parent and Teacher Rating Scales. An excellent way to collect caregiver observations is by using one of the many standardized rating scales. Probably the best ones are those that use the actual DSM-IV symptoms rated on a standard metric, usually 0–3, from no symptom to severe. Examples include the ADHD Rating Scale (44) and the SNAP (Swanson, Nolan & Pelham, adhd.net), which have only DSM symptoms, and the Conners revised long forms (45) which have the DSM-IV symptoms embedded in a longer scale. When counting symptoms, a rating of 2 or 3 on the 0–3 scales is usually considered as presence of the symptom. Numerous other scales are also useful and have been used in research and clinical practice.

Family History. Additional diagnostic information can come from family history, both positive and negative. For example, relatives with ADHD help to confirm the diagnosis. On the other hand, absence of relatives with ADHD, coupled with either history of traumatic stress or family history of bipolar disorder, thyroid disorder, or severe anxiety may alert the diagnostician to the possibility that the patient's symptoms may be another disorder mimicking ADHD and point the direction for further investigation.

Mental Status Exam

The main value of mental status exam is to rule out other mental disorders that might better explain the symptoms (Criterion E of DSM-IV). These include psychosis, bipolar disorder, depression, pervasive developmental disorder, and severe anxiety—especially posttraumatic stress disorder—as well as mental retardation. A reasonable mental status exam for this purpose would include appearance/demeanor, orientation, alertness, speech clarity and content, ability to develop

TABLE 5.2.1.6

EEG-BASED MODELS OF ATTENTION DEFICIT HYPERACTIVITY DISORDER

Model	Rationale	EEG Characteristics	Reference
Maturational Lag	1) ADHD results from a developmental lag in central nervous system functioning. 2) EEG measures in the ADHD subject would be considered normal in a younger child and EEG findings mature in a normal fashion.	Increased centroposterior relative delta; increased relative theta across the scalp; decreased frontocentral relative beta; decreased relative alpha across the scalp	Kinsbourne et al., 1973 (221); Satterfield et al., 1973 (222); Matsuura et al., 1993 (223); John et al., 1987 (224); Clarke et al., 1998 (225); Lazzaro et al., 1998 (226)
Developmental Deviation	1) ADHD results from an abnormality in central nervous system functioning. 2) EEG measures in the ADHD subject are not normal at any age and EEG findings are not likely to mature in a normal fashion.		Klinkerfuss et al., 1965 (227); Wikler et al., 1970 (228); John et al., 1983 (229); Clarke et al., 2001 (230, 231)
Hypoarousal	1) ADHD results from cortical hypoarousal. 2) EEG measures in the ADHD subject indicate lower levels of beta activity during cognitive tasks. 3) EEG findings of hypoarousal in the ADHD subject should correlate with other functional measures of the brain activity showing decreased cortical activation.	Reduced frontal relative delta; increased frontal relative theta; decreased relative beta across the scalp; normal alpha activity	Satterfield and Cantwell, 1974 (232); Satterfield et al., 1973 (233), 1974 (234); Grunewald–Zuberbier et al., 1975 (235); Ackerman et al., 1994 (236); Lubar et al., 1995 (237)
Overaroused		Excess beta activity	

rapport, relevance and logic of thought processes, some estimate of cognitive ability, queries about depressive symptoms, worries, fears, obsessions, compulsions, hallucinations, and traumatic events, and some projective elicitation such as drawing, three wishes, or fable completion.

Physical Exam and Medical History

Although there are no diagnostic physical signs in ADHD (when abnormalities occur, they usually reflect a comorbid disorder such as mental retardation, cerebral palsy, or genetic syndromes), a physical exam and medical history can be useful in ruling out other mimicking disorders and in discovering or confirming the common comorbidity of developmental coordination disorder. Also, the presence of soft neurological signs and/or minor physical anomalies may somewhat increase confidence in the ADHD diagnosis, even though there is no 1:1 link. *Soft neurological signs* are nonfocal motor deficits that in children with ADHD consistently include deficits in balance, motor planning, and control, and deficits in sensory integration (46, 47) (Table 5.2.1.7). Gustaffson et al., 2000 also found a significant correlation between the soft neurological signs and decreased cerebral blood flow measures in the frontal lobes bilaterally in children with ADHD. At this time, functional imaging is not a part of the routine workup of ADHD. Physical exam would note hyperdynamics or hypodynamics, abnormal deep tendon reflexes, fine or coarse skin or hair, and any other signs of endocrine disorder, as well as allergic stigmata (swollen eyes, darkened lids, nasal congestion, allergic salute) and pallor of nailbeds or conjunctivae. Positive findings should, of course, prompt appropriate laboratory tests. The diagnostician should inquire about things like food sensitivities (especially in younger children), dietary imbalance, cardiac problems, and heat or cold intolerance. Prominent allergic signs suggest a possible etiological or exacerbating condition (e.g., food intolerance, atopy).

Subtypes

The distinction among subtypes is more dimensional than categorical. For example, someone with six inattentive symptoms and five hyperactive-impulsive symptoms would have predominantly inattentive type, while someone with six symptoms of each kind would have combined type ADHD. Further, the type does not even firmly predict the ratio of the two kinds of symptoms. For example, six inattentive and five hyperactive-impulsive would make inattentive type, but nine inattentive and six hyperactive-impulsive symptoms would make combined type despite having a greater excess of inattentive symptoms than the first symptom profile. Despite this threshold-definition problem, some experts believe that a substantial proportion of inattentive type, those who are sluggishly hypoactive, may actually constitute a distinct disorder with different etiology. In any event, the inattentive type tends to be referred less often for treatment and tends to be missed diagnostically more often, especially if of high enough intelligence to get by in school without using full potential.

TABLE 5.2.1.7

SOFT NEUROLOGICAL SIGNS IN ADHD

Clinical Finding	Putative Explanation
Difficulties performing repetitive motor tasks (such as hand flipping; foot rocking; serial thumb to finger opposition)	Impaired ability to use cognitive control to alternately inhibit and excite motor activity to maintain a regular cadence
Difficulties performing sequential timed tasks (such as foot rocking; hand flipping; serial finger)	Impaired ability to use cognitive control to adjust motor performance flexibly in a multistep task
Difficulties maintaining gait and balance (sustained motor stance; tandem balance)	Difficulties maintaining balance; integrating proprioceptor input/body position sense; abnormal vestibular function; etc

Comorbidity

ADHD has a high rate of comorbid psychiatric disorders. Half of clinical samples have oppositional-defiant disorder or conduct disorder, 25–30% have anxiety disorder, and 20–25% have a learning disorder (48, 49). There is increased risk for mood disorders (which may develop later). Although the rate of comorbid Tourette's is low (about 2%), it is much higher than in the random population or in other psychiatric disorders. Comorbidity can introduce some diagnostic challenges because the comorbid disorders can mimic ADHD, with overlapping symptoms, so the diagnostician must differentiate between comorbidity and primary diagnosis. Table 5.2.1.8 presents some comparisons and differences.

NEUROPSYCHOLOGICAL TEST RESULTS

A great deal of research has been done within the past 30 years to clarify the neuropsychological profile of attention deficit hyperactivity disorder. Neuropsychological tests have consistently identified deficits in the executive functions (EF) of patients with ADHD. Executive functions are neurocognitive processes that maintain an appropriate problemsolving set to attain a future goal (50). Executive function tasks include response inhibition and execution; working memory and updating; set shifting and task switching; interference control; planning and organization; vigilance; visuospatial orienting; and verbal and spatial working memory. Executive functions employ multiple neural networks that involve the thalamus, basal ganglia and the prefrontal cortex. The most common neuropsychological test results measuring different aspects of executive functioning in ADHD are listed in Table 5.2.1.9.

Several theories have been developed based on the neuropsychological profile of children with ADHD.

1. *The deficit in inhibitory control theory* suggests that the general pattern of executive impairment is caused by developmental abnormalities in inhibitory control processes (51). A metaanalysis of neuropsychological studies in adults found a somewhat different profile of neurocognitive deficits compared to children and adolescents, with deficits related mostly to impairment in measures of verbal memory, focused attention, sustained attention, and abstract verbal problemsolving with working memory. Simple alertness tasks were less impaired than more complex attention tasks (52).
2. *The delay aversion theory* posits a biologically based impairment in the ability to tolerate delay and its consequences on behavior and cognitive style (53, 54). A test used to measure ability to tolerate delay is the Choice Delay Task (55).
3. *In the cognitive energetic model* (56), neurocognitive performance deficits in ADHD are determined by information processing abnormalities at the computational (encoding, search, decision, and motor organization) and state levels (effort, arousal, and activation). The model proposes the existence of three energetic pools: effort (necessary energy to meet the demands of the

TABLE 5.2.1.8

SOME MENTAL DISORDERS THAT CAN MIMIC ADHD: THEIR OVERLAPPING OR SIMILAR SIGNS/SYMPTOMS

ADHD Symptoms	Depression	Bipolar (Manic)	Anxiety, Including PTSD	Psychosis	Autism/PDD
Inattentiveness, distractibility, forgetfulness, losing things, careless mistakes	Impairment of concentration and memory; preoccupation with mood	Flight of ideas, thought racing, distraction by delusions or grandiosity	Preoccupation with worry; intrusive memories; flashbacks, psychic numbing, hypervigilance	Withdrawal from reality, preoccupation, loose association, "distraction" by hallucinations	Disregard of people, decreased responsiveness to attempted communication
Failure to finish tasks or activities; reluctance to start if needs sustained mental effort	Fatigue, anergia, loss of interest	Flight of ideas/activities; grandiosely above common tasks	Fear-induced paralysis of function; afraid to try, expecting failure; avoiding of reminders	As above; abrupt change of activity	Abrupt change of activity, resistance to instructed activity, adherence to preferred activity
Difficulty organizing	Anergia, cognitive impairment	Flightiness		Psychotic fragmentation	
Hyperactivity, fidgeting/squirming restlessness, always on the go	Agitation	Hyperactivity, driven quality	Panic, agitation, anxiety-driven restlessness, "nervousness"	Psychotic agitation, response to hallucinations	Hyperactivity, twirling, pacing, flapping
Excessive talking	Agitated complaining	Pressured speech	Anxious verbosity, obsessions, verbal rituals	Talking to hallucinations	Compulsive stereotyped repetitions
Impulsive blurting of answers, interrupting, intruding	Preoccupied complaining (pain, worry)	Pressured speech, flight of ideas, impulsive poor judgment	Anxious eagerness; reenactments	Responding to hallucinations	Obliviousness of personal space of others
Impatience, easy frustration, difficulty waiting	Easy frustration	Pressured hyperactivity and impulsiveness	Intolerance of delay that builds suspense or reminds of trauma	Lack of social orientation	Easy frustration
Irritability	Irritability	Irritability	Anger when rituals frustrated	Paranoid irritability	Irritability, tantrum when rituals, interrupted routine
Restless sleep	Insomnia	Insomnia	Insomnia or nightmares	Nocturnal agitation	Insomnia
Lability, instability (emotional and physiological)		Labile affect	Physiological instability, nervousness	Psychotic unpredictability	Lability, unpredictability
Distinguishing from ADHD	Depressed mood, anorexia, weight loss, suicidal ideation, guilt feelings, psychomotor slowing, mutism, fatigue	F.H. of mood disorder; extreme driven quality; sometimes episodic; prominent mood: irritable, grandiose; possible appetite change, weight change	Phobias, worries, stress-induced onset, obsessions, compulsions, perfectionism, tremor, physiological symptoms (palpitations, SOB, sweating), posttraumatic play	Delusions, poverty of thought, disorientation, command hallucinations, inappropriate affect	Impaired nonverbal/verbal communication, lack of social relatedness, fantasy, or social or imaginative play

(Table adapted with permission from Arnold LE, Contemporary Diagnosis and Management of ADHD. *Handbooks in Health Care*, Newtown, PA, 2004. Reproduced with permission.)

task); arousal (time locked to stimulus processing), and activation (tonic changes in physiological activity in significant brain areas, including the basal ganglia and corpus striatum), and the existence of a management or evaluation mechanism associated with planning, monitoring, detection and correction of errors that overlaps with the concept of executive functions in other theories.

4. *The sluggish cognitive tempo theory* proposes that inattention presents differently in ADHD without hyperactivity compared with combined type (57), the main features including slow retrieval and information processing; low levels of alertness; and mild problems with memory and orientation. Further studies are needed to answer the question of whether the group of sluggish cognitive tempo children may represent a distinct category of ADHD with a different pathophysiology or may represent a different disorder altogether.
5. *The multiple pathway model* emphasizes the parallels between the core deficits in ADHD as defined by major theories of ADHD and relevant temperament domains, in particular effortful control and regulation (58).

COURSE AND PROGNOSIS

Estimates are that up 60% of childhood cases continue symptomatic into adulthood (59). The ratio of males to females in adult samples approximates 2:1 or even close to 1:1, much more equal than in childhood, where it is more likely 4 or 5 to 1 in clinical samples. The manifestations of ADHD change over the course of life (Figure 5.2.1.4). Just as normal children develop better impulse control, attentional focus, other executive function, and ability to remain calm as they mature, so do those with ADHD, just at a slower pace, lagging behind their age mates. Childhood ADHD severity and childhood

TABLE 5.2.1.9

NEUROPSYCHOLOGICAL TESTS OF EXECUTIVE FUNCTIONING

Test Stop Signal Reaction Time (SSRT)	Executive Function Assessed Response inhibition
Continuous Performance Test commission errors	Response inhibition
Continuous Performance Test omission errors	Vigilance
Wisconsin Card Sorting Test	Set shifting
Trailmaking test part B	Set shifting
Tower of Hanoi/London	Planning ability
Porteus Mazes	Planning ability
Rey–Osterreith complex figure test	Planning/organization
Working Memory Sentence Span test	Working verbal memory
Digits Backward test	Working verbal memory
Self-Ordered Pointing test	Spatial working memory
CANTAB Spatial Working Memory test	Spatial working memory

treatment significantly predict the persistence of ADHD in adulthood in the recent National Comorbidity Survey Replication Study (60). ADHD symptoms in adults are more heterogeneous and subtle, leading some researchers to suggest the need for different diagnostic ADHD criteria in adults.

Hyperactivity is the most likely symptom to be outgrown. Adolescents and adults with ADHD, even those who started with combined type, may have only an inner feeling of restlessness. The most persistent symptom cluster involves inattention, distractibility, disorganization, and failure to finish things. Males with a childhood history of significant hyperactivity, impulsivity, and comorbidity with other disruptive behavior

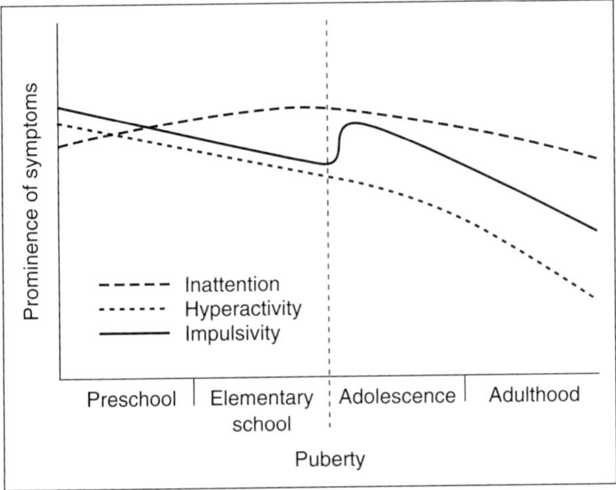

FIGURE 5.2.1.4. Course of different ADHD symptoms over the life span. Hyperactivity tends to wane with maturity, being replaced by a feeling of restlessness. Impulsivity also tends to wane except for a possible blip in adolescence under the influence of "raging hormones." The most persistent cluster of symptoms is inattentiveness, with the main adult manifestations being disorganization, difficulty managing money, keeping schedules, and sticking with a relationship or job. (Reproduced from Arnold LE, Contemporary Diagnosis and Management of ADHD. Newtown, PA: *Handbooks in Health Care*, 2004, with permission.)

disorders are more likely to develop polysubstance abuse and adult antisocial behavior. Adults with ADHD may struggle with frequent job changes, frequent partner changes, divorce, difficulty with schedules and money management, and driving accidents. Girls and women with ADHD have a higher rate of unwed pregnancy than those who do not have ADHD. Adults with ADHD may present with significant self-esteem issues and feelings of hopelessness and helplessness related to ongoing difficulties in managing everyday life. Several follow-up studies have found a high rate of major depression in adult patients with ADHD. Studies show that effective treatment significantly improves quality of life. Intense controversy over the existence of an adult ADHD diagnosis and concerns over prescribing psychostimulants that have a high potential for abuse have made it difficult for adults with ADHD to receive treatment. Minority status, female sex, and low income were found in several studies to predict failure to diagnose and treat the disorder (61, 62).

TREATMENT

Because ADHD is a chronic and pervasive disorder, affecting all areas of function, the treatment plan must be farsighted, comprehensive, and flexibly adapted over time to changing needs. The commitment of patient and family to the plan must be cultivated. This implies that treatment must be not only effective, but also feasible, palatable, and affordable for the particular patient. Therefore treatment planning has to be individualized, with consideration for family preferences. From the beginning, the child, as star of the therapeutic team, should be involved in planning, with an eye toward the day when he or she has to assume responsibility for his or her own treatment as an adult. Other members of the team—physician, teacher, psychologist, and other professional—can come and go; even parents are eventually outgrown; but the patient is permanently involved.

The necessary gradual assumption of personal responsibility for managing the disorder should be discussed periodically with the child and adolescent. For the younger child, this can involve parents. For example, for a 10-year-old, lay out the fact that in 8 years the child will have to assume responsibility for self and discuss how parents can coach and support in gradual assumption of responsibility. A 14-year-old can be seen alone briefly and reminded that he or she has only 4 years to prepare for personal responsibility; it may be useful to inquire if the idea scares them before asking how they plan gradually to take more responsibility. Attention to such psychosocial and psychodynamic aspects of management is important especially for patients who are treated mainly with medication. See also Psychoeducation below.

Established Treatments

Two treatment modalities have been endorsed by both the American Academy of Child and Adolescent Psychiatry (63) and American Academy of Pediatrics (64). They are behavioral treatment and the FDA-approved sympathomimetic agents (stimulants and atomoxetine). Additional drugs are expected to be added to the list of agents with an approved indication for ADHD. The flow chart of evaluation and treatment recommendations published by the American Academy of Pediatrics is reproduced in Figure 5.2.1.5. In acute and medium-length studies medication generally outperforms behavioral treatment for symptom suppression, but 3/4 of children with ADHD can be managed with intensive behavioral treatment alone, and the combination offers several advantages, including equal or better results with a lower medication dose (48, 65, 66).

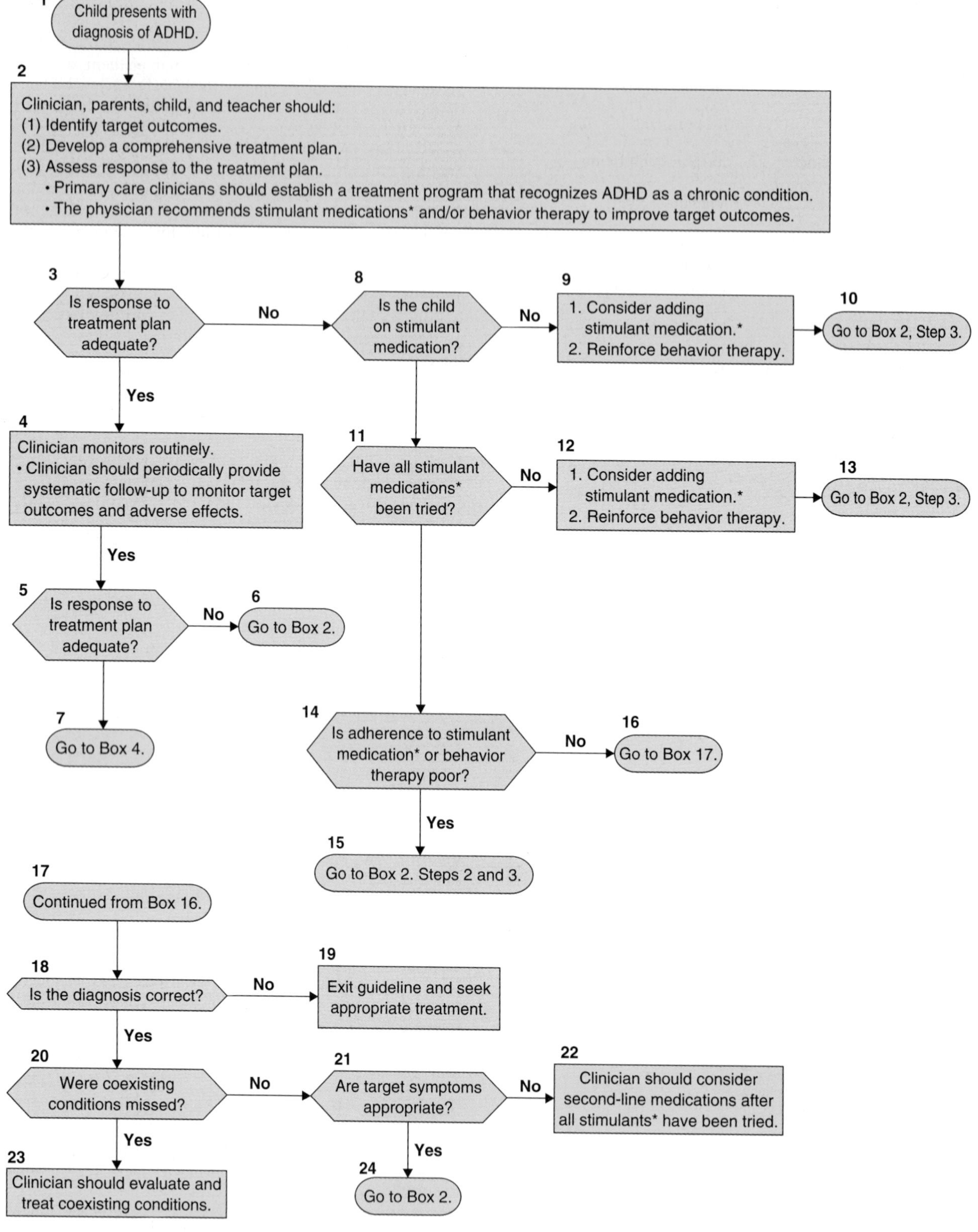
1
Child presents with diagnosis of ADHD.
2
Clinician, parents, child, and teacher should:
(1) Identify target outcomes.
(2) Develop a comprehensive treatment plan.
(3) Assess response to the treatment plan.
• Primary care clinicians should establish a treatment program that recognizes ADHD as a chronic condition.
• The physician recommends stimulant medications* and/or behavior therapy to improve target outcomes.
3
Is response to treatment plan adequate?
No
8
Is the child on stimulant medication?
No
9
1. Consider adding stimulant medication.*
2. Reinforce behavior therapy.
10
Go to Box 2, Step 3.
Yes
4
Clinician monitors routinely.
• Clinician should periodically provide systematic follow-up to monitor target outcomes and adverse effects.
11
Have all stimulant medications* been tried?
No
12
1. Consider adding stimulant medication.*
2. Reinforce behavior therapy.
13
Go to Box 2, Step 3.
Yes
5
Is response to treatment plan adequate?
No
6
Go to Box 2.
7
Go to Box 4.
14
Is adherence to stimulant medication* or behavior therapy poor?
No
16
Go to Box 17.
Yes
15
Go to Box 2. Steps 2 and 3.
17
Continued from Box 16.
18
Is the diagnosis correct?
No
19
Exit guideline and seek appropriate treatment.
Yes
20
Were coexisting conditions missed?
No
21
Are target symptoms appropriate?
No
22
Clinician should consider second-line medications after all stimulants* have been tried.
Yes
23
Clinician should evaluate and treat coexisting conditions.
Yes
24
Go to Box 2.

* Excluding pemoline. Another FDA-approved option is atomoxetine (Strattera©), approved since the guideline was published. Used with the permission of the Academy of Pediatrics. From: Clinical practice guideline: treatment of the school-aged child with attention deficit/hyperactivity disorder. Pediatrics 2001:108:1033-1044

FIGURE 5.2.1.5. Clinical Guidelines by American Academy of Pediatrics, which were written before availability of atomoxetine, which, as an FDA-approved treatment for ADHD, should be considered after a stimulant before resorting to off-label drugs (From American Academy of Pediatrics: Clinical Practice Guideline for the School-Age Child with ADHD. *Pediatrics 2001*; 108:1033–1048, with permission.)

For some comorbid subgroups, such as ADHD combined with both anxiety and oppositional defiant disorder (ODD)/conduct disorder (CD), the combination is impressively more effective (67, 68). Behavioral treatment appears especially effective in the presence of comorbid anxiety.

Behavioral Treatment

Behavioral treatments are based on social learning theory, particularly that behaviors that are reinforced increase in frequency and those that are not reinforced in some way (or are punished) tend to extinguish. A number of practical behavioral treatments can be implemented from first contact. These include star charts for target behaviors, clear house rules, written or pictorial instructions making use of the visual channels if auditory instructions seem unattended to, and contingencies for doing various things. With more time and effort, more refined interventions can be set up, such as a home token economy or a daily report card to tie school behavior to home reinforcement. More specific information and instructions can be downloaded from http://wings.buffalo.edu/adhd. There are several programs for providing parent training in behavioral management, now called parent management training (PMT). For younger children and milder cases, these may provide sufficient intervention, but once diagnosed, a case should be monitored over time. Sometimes additional need for treatment emerges as the child progresses to more challenging academic stresses.

Pharmacological Treatment

Most psychiatric drugs have some evidence of benefit in ADHD (notable exceptions being the selective serotonin reuptake inhibitors), but only a few have a Food and Drug Administration (FDA)–approved indication (Table 5.2.1.10A). The evidence for many of the others, such as tricyclic antidepressants, bupropion, monoamine oxidase inhibitors, modafinil, and alpha-2 agonists is nevertheless rather good, with multiple placebo-controlled trials (Table 5.2.1.10B). However, some have only open trials or a single controlled trial. Table 5.2.1.10 shows approximate relative effect sizes (the number of standard deviations by which active drug differs from placebo).

With any of the drugs, it is important to start low and titrate, preferably weekly, to individual optimal effect. Generally for school-age children, the smallest size stimulant dosage marketed is a good place to start. Because of wide individual variability in sensitivity, size of the patient is only a rough guide to dose: One 30-kg child may require and tolerate 30 mg/day of amphetamine while another 30-kg child has an optimal response to 5 mg/day, with severe side effects above 10 mg. Clinical art is required to optimize the benefit and minimize side effects by size of dose, timing, and management of time-action effects such as "evening rebound" with stimulants. Generally the new extended-release preparations, including the methylphenidate patch, and the new molecule atomoxetine yield a smoother effect with fewer ups and downs. They also avoid the necessity of taking pills at school, which some children find stigmatizing. For such reasons, extended-release formulations of stimulants are preferred, and titration can be

TABLE 5.2.1.10A

DRUGS WITH FDA APPROVAL FOR ADHD

Generic Name	Brand Name	Usual Daily Dose[c] mg [mg/kg]
Stimulants (ES 0.7-1.8)		
Amphetamine, racemic (dextro-levo)[a] dextroamphetamine[a,b]	Benzedrine® (withdrawn)	10-40 (0.3-1)
	Dexedrine® DextroStat®	5-30 (0.2-0.7)
levoamphetamine[a]	Cydril® (withdrawn)	14-42 (0.3-1)
mixture 3/4 d-, 1/4 J-amphetamine[a,b]	Adderall®	5-40 (0.2-1)
	Adderall® XR	5-40 (0.2-1)
methamphetamine[b,d]	Desoxyn®	5-25 (0.2-0.7)
Methylphenidate, racemic threo[a,b]	Ritalin®,	10-60 (0.3-1.5)
	Methylin®	10-60 (0.3-1.5)
	Ritalin® LA	20-60 (0.6-1.5)
	Metadate®	10-60 (0.3-1.5)
	Metadate® CD	20-60 (0.6-1.5)
osmotic release[a,b]	Concerta®▲	18-72 (0.4-1.8)
dextro-threomethylphenidate[a,b]	Focalin™	5-30 (0.2-0.7)
	Focalin XR™	5-30 (0.2-0.7)
Pemoline[a,b*]	Cylert®	37.5-112.5 (1-3)
Nonstimulant With FDA-approved Indication (ES 0.5-1.4)		
Atomoxetine[a,b]	Strattera®	18-100 (0.7-1.4)

[a]Supported by controlled studies
[b]FDA-approved indication for ADHD
[c]Usual daily dose should not be interpreted as either a cap or a minimal effective dose if a higher or lower dose is clinically indicated in individual cases. Actual patient doses must be individually titrated using direct teacher and parent information.
[d]Although it carries an FDA-approved indication for ADHD, methamphetamine, in contrast to other forms of amphetamine, is not favored by many experts because of suspected neurotoxicity in animal data.
▲Because only 5/6 of the MPH in the osmotic-release form is released, 72 mg = 60 mg of other MPH preparations.
*Pemoline, though a stimulant with FDA-approved indication, is not a first-line choice.
ES = effect size, the number of standard deviations different from placebo or from pre-drug measure. It is a measure of clinical significance. An ES of 1 is considered large, 0.5 medium.
(From Arnold LE, Contemporary Diagnosis and Management of ADHD. Newtown, PA: *Handbooks in Health Care*, 2004. Reproduced with permission.)

TABLE 5.2.1.10B

OTHER DRUGS USED FOR ADHD

Generic Name	Brand Name	Usual Daily Dose[b] mg (mg/kg)
Not all of the following drugs have been documented as effective by well-controlled studies, let alone approved by the FDA for ADHD.		
Antidepressants (ES 0.5–1.5)[c]		
Imipramine (TCA)[a]	Tofranil®	20-100 (0.7-3)
Desipramine (TCA)[a]	Norpramin®, Pertofrane®	20-100 (0.7-3)
Amitriptyline (TCA)[a]	Elavil®, Endep®	20-100 (0.7-3)
Nortriptyline (TCA)	Pamelor®	10-50 (0.4-2)
Bupropion[a] [19]	Wellbutrin®	75-300 (3-6)
Clomipramine (TCA)[a]	Anafranil®	25-100
Tranylcypromine (MAOI A + B)[c]	Parnate®	5-15
Clorgyline (MAOI A)[a]		5-20
Pargyline (MAOI)	Eutonyl®	
Venlafaxine[d]	Effexor®	25-100 (1.4)
SSRIs (eg. fluoxetine[d])	Prozac®	5-40
α_2-Agonists (ES 0.3–5.0, depending on patient selection)		
Guanfacine[a]	Tenex®	0.5–4.0 (0.02-0.06)
Clonidine (also patch)[a] [20]	Calapres®	0.05-0.3 (0.002-0.005)
Miscellaneous (ES variable)		
Buspirone (ES<1)	BuSpar®	5-30 (0.2-0.6)
Diphenhydramine	Benadryl®	75-150
Nicotine (adults only, ES>1)[a]	(lower dose for nonsmokers)	7-21 mg patch
Modafinil (ES~1)[a]	Provigil®	50-400
Anticonvulsants (ES up to 1.0)		
Carbamazepine[a] [21]	Tegretol®	50-800, serum level
Valproate	Depakote®, Depakene®	serum level
Phenytoin	Dilantin®	50-300
Antipsychotics (ES usually about half of stimulants)[f]		
Thioridazine[a]	Mellaril®	25-150 (1-6)
Haloperidol[a,e]	Haldol®	0.5-5.0 (0.03-0.075)
Chlorpromazine[a,e]	Thorazine®	25-150 (1-6)
Risperidone	Risperdal®	0.25-2.0 (0.01-0.1)
Precursors (ES <0.6, short term)[g]		
Deanol (possible precursor of acetylcholine)	Deaner®	≥500
Tryptophan (precursor of serotonin)		(70-100)
Tyrosine (precursor of dopamine and norepinephrine)		(100-140)
Phenylalanine (precursor of dopamine and norepinephrine)		(100-140)
Levo-DOPA (precursor of dopamine and norepinephrine)		
Others		
β-Blockers, (eg, propranolol)	Inderal®	10-300
Caffeine		100-450

TCA = tricyclic antidepressant; MAOI = monoamine oxidase inhibitor; SSRI = selective serotonin reuptake inhibitor
[a]Supported by controlled studies
[b]Usual daily dose should not be interpreted as either a cap or a minimal effective dose if a higher or lower dose is clinically indicated in individual cases. Actual patient doses must be individually titrated, using direct teacher and parent information.
[c]No antidepressants are FDA-approved for ADHD, despite well-controlled studies demonstrating efficacy for many of them. In fact, some (but not all) studies show imipramine, desipramine, amitriptyline, and tranylcypromine equal to stimulants, although with worse side effects. For adults, they may equal stimulants despite not seeming to benefit attention as much as behavior.
[d]Despite a report of a positive open trial of fluoxetine, most experts do not consider selective serotonin reuptake inhibitors (SSRIs) generally effective for ADHD core symptoms, in contrast with the documented effectiveness of other antidepressant classes. The newer antidepressants, with both serotonin and catecholamine action (such as venlafaxine, minazapine, and nefazodone) are expected to be effective. ES = effect size, the number of standard deviations different from placebo or from pre-drug measure. It is a measure of clinical significance. An ES of 1 is considered large, 0.5 medium.
[e]FDA-approved for short-term treatment of hyperactive children
[f]Although haloperidol and chlorpromazine have FDA-approved indications for short-term treatment of hyperactive children, antipsychotics should be a last resort because of the risk of tardive dyskinesia. Newer ones, such as risperidone, olanzapine, and quetiapine, may carry less risk.
[g]The precursors of neurotransmitters are nutrients found in the normal diet. They are included because they are used like drugs in supplemental dosage. Deanol (dimethylaminoethanol [DMAE]) was formerly marketed as Deaner®, but initial FDA approval was withdrawn as "possibly effective."
Not ordinarily used: most minor tranquilizers, benzodiazepines Contraindicated: barbiturates (aggravate hyperactivity; can even cause it) ES = effect size, the number of standard deviations different from placebo or from pre-drug measure. It is a measure of clinical significance. An ES of 1 is considered large, 0.5 medium. Adapted with permission from Arnold LE, Jensen PS: Attention-deficit hyperactivity disorder. In: Kaplan H, Sadock B, eds. *Comprehensive Textbook of Psychiatry*. Baltimore, Williams and Wilkins. 1995. pp 2295–2311.
(From Arnold LE, Contemporary Diagnosis and Management of ADHD. Newtown, PA: Handbooks in Health Care, 2004. Reproduced with permission.)

initiated directly with one of them without any need to first establish dose with immediate-release tablets.

Labeled and Off-Label Drugs. The drugs with currently approved FDA (Food and Drug Administration) indications for ADHD are the stimulants and atomoxetine, with others being developed for that indication. Some antipsychotics also have an indication for "childhood hyperactivity" grandfathered from previous use in the 1970s, and there is no doubt that antipsychotics have a moderate benefit for hyperactive symptoms. However, because of their greater risk and less impressive benefit, they would usually be a last resort, logically used mainly when a stimulant worsens the symptoms. Some off-label drugs with good evidence would be preferred to antipsychotics early in the search for an effective medication. Antidepressants other than Selective Serotonin Reuptake Inhibitors (SSRIs) have many placebo-controlled studies supporting their use. These include tricyclics, monoamine oxidase inhibitors (MAOIs), and bupropion. For children the effect is not on average as good as for stimulants, but some individuals may respond better, and comorbid depression or anxiety might point toward considering one of them. The danger of interaction with food amines would limit the feasibility of MAOIs for children. Another class with reasonable evidence is the alpha-agonists, mainly clonidine and more recently guanfacine, which has the advantages of longer half-life and less sedation. They may be good for severely overaroused agitation and comorbid aggression. Clonidine is often used at bedtime alone to promote sleep, although the practice has been questioned on safety grounds if used in conjunction with daytime stimulants. Diphenhydramine, an antihistamine which has some dopamine effect, was an arcane treatment before more modern drug development; for a few patients, especially those whose behavior fluctuates with allergy, it may have considerable benefit. Table 5.2.1.11 lists some of the advantages and disadvantages of the main drugs.

Educational Plan and Psychoeducation about Disorder

Education is important in two ways in ADHD: as a problem area that needs to be addressed and as a treatment modality. Most children with diagnosed ADHD have some problem with academic performance; in fact, that is often what brings them to clinical attention. Although most are able to function in a regular classroom with appropriate treatment and support, some will need an individual educational plan (IEP) or even a special class or resource room. This is particularly so for the 20–25% with comorbid learning disorders. Parents may need some coaching in obtaining appropriate educational services for the child, such as is required by PL 94–142 (Education for All Handicapped Act), IDEA (Individuals with Disabilities Education Act) or section 504 of the Civil Rights Act. Children with learning disorders are likely to be covered by the first two mandates, and those without a specific learning disorder are usually covered by section 504, which provides for "other health impaired."

This brings us to the other side of educational considerations: the education of patient and family (and other caregivers) about ADHD, its symptoms, course, chronicity, treatments, and services available. Some "talking points" for this are listed in Table 5.2.1.12. Referral to a support/advocacy organization, such as Children and Adults with ADD (ChADD) or Attention-Deficit Disorder Association (ADDA) for further peer education may also be useful. There are also numerous explanatory books written for both children and adults, such as *A Family Guide to ADHD* (69). The local support group may have a lending library of these. Such psychoeducation is important in cementing a commitment to enduring treatment for a chronic disorder.

Other Treatments

Treatments other than medication, behavioral treatment, psychoeducation, and special educational services are often called "alternative." Unfortunately, the term alternative implies substitution for proven standard treatment. A better name for most alternative treatments would be complementary treatments because they can theoretically be used in combination with standard treatments (analogous to combining two standard treatments such as medication and behavioral treatment), either to enhance benefit of the standard treatment or to address a problem not covered by the standard treatment. For example, mirror feedback might be used to ease evening homework angst at a time when the daytime stimulant is wearing off.

Unfortunately, the evidence base for most such treatments is rather thin. For example, the mirror feedback mentioned has only one published small randomized controlled trial, which showed a medium effect compared to the control condition. Some other treatments are supported only by open trials or clinical observation. The reported improvement for some is likely due to nonspecific effects (placebo, maturation, history, regression to the mean). However, others have multiple placebo-controlled trials showing medium to large effects, often for only a small subgroup. Objective assessment of the evidence is complicated by unsubstantiated claims and assumptions made by some advocates of such treatments. The task of understanding them is discouraging enough to induce many busy practitioners to discard the lot as not worth the effort. Nevertheless, impatient rejection of such treatments without examining the evidence is as unscientific as uncritical acceptance. Most important, surveys indicate that a high proportion of patients use such treatments on their own, without professional guidance. Therefore it behooves the practitioner to know enough about them and their varying evidence bases to advise and guide the families about likelihood of benefit, possible risks, and risk–benefit ratio. (Summaries of evidence for various treatments may be found in the references for Table 5.2.1.13.)

The following points may be useful in guiding families:

1. The easier, cheaper, and safer a treatment is, the less evidence is needed to justify an individual trial, especially if it can be done along with a proven standard treatment. Risky treatments need controlled convincing evidence. Difficult or expensive treatments risk diverting family emotional and financial resources from better proven treatments.
2. Look for controlled trials in well characterized samples, not anecdotes or testimonials. A major flaw in many published alternative/complementary treatment studies is lack of diagnostic rigor, second only to lack of controls.
3. Herbs are crude drugs (if they work) and can have interactions with other drugs, either prescription or over the counter. Most families do not realize this because herbs are peddled as "nutritional" and "natural" or "dietary supplements," which most people mistakenly interpret as perfectly safe. Some herbs, with further research, may indeed be found useful for treatment of ADHD, and may contain psychoactive chemicals, such as nicotine from tobacco leaf, that can be refined into useful drugs. For now, the unknown risk appears to exceed any proven benefit. To prevent herb–drug interactions, physicians should inquire about herbs or "dietary" supplements containing herbs before prescribing, and explain the risk.
4. Remember that delay of proven treatment is a risk, varying in seriousness with the urgency of the presenting clinical picture. This is a consideration where the family wishes to substitute an alternative they have heard about for standard treatment.

TABLE 5.2.1.11

RELATIVE ADVANTAGES AND DISADVANTAGES/SIDE EFFECTS OF ADHD DRUG CLASSES

Drug Class	Advantages	Side Effects, Disadvantages
Stimulants (FDA indication)	Specifically treat ADHD core symptoms of inattention, overactivity, and impulsiveness Largest and most rapid effect on ADHD of any drug class, especially for children Significant benefit in 85%–90% of ADHD if two or more tried in succession and titrated carefully Calms comorbid aggression and oppositional-defiant behavior Except for pemoline, medically safer than most psychoactive drugs Results of given dose seen immediately; relatively easy titration	Appetite, weight loss Sleep disturbance (if taken late in day) Cramps (first few weeks) Headaches Mild BP and pulse increase Evening crash 'Zombie' appearance (amphetamine look): constricted affect and spontaneity, emotional blunting Depression Tics Hallucinations (skin crawling, visions) Mild growth slowing first 2 years (26) Dose for behavior may not be optimal for attention Nuisance of schedule II Rx
Atomoxetine (Strattera®) (FDA indication)	Specifically treats ADHD core symptoms of inattention, overactivity, and impulsiveness FDA indication for ADHD, like stimulants, but not Schedule II Refills by phone Nearly as effective as stimulants (slower onset), better for some; may help stimulant failures Continuous duration of effect Little or no insomniac side effect Can be given any time of day No tic side effect (good choice with comorbid tics) Some benefit for comorbid oppositional-defiant symptoms May help comorbid depression Smooth action over time (long pharmacodynamic half-life), cumulative benefit	Appetite, weight loss Gastrointestinal Sx (nausea, vomiting, diarrhea, constipation) Fatigue, dizziness Probable, mild growth slowing Allergic reactions In adults: dry mouth, urinary retention, sexual dysfunction Irritating to skin if capsules opened Possibly longer time than stimulants to flush out if adverse effect Slower attainment of full effect than stimulants
Antidepressants Tricyclics, bupropion (Wellbutring), MAOIs (27), probably newer antidepressants with both serotonin action and dopamine	Treat both ADHD and comorbid depression and anxiety Helps some stimulant non-responders Third most effective drug class for ADHD (except for SSRIs, which are not very effective) Some patients/families who are prejudiced against stimulants will accept antidepressants May equal stimulant effectiveness for adults	Sedation BP changes (down or up) Dizziness (especially on standing) Dry mouth Cardiac conduction block: TCAs require ECG monitoring in children Constipation, urinary retention (rare in children) Headache (deserves evaluation) Overdose lethal, and sudden deaths at therapeutic dose (DMI) Response delayed, especially bupropion Dietary restrictions for MAOIs Not as good as stimulants for attention
α_2-Agonists	Treat both hyperactivity-impulsiveness and comorbid tic disorder or comorbid aggression Helps some nonresponders to stimulants and antidepressants Good for those overaroused, possibly with comorbid anxiety	Response delayed Sedation Hypotensive dizziness (especially postural) Dry mouth Rare hallucinations Hypertensive rebound if dose missed Sudden deaths (when used with stimulant) Not as helpful for attention as stimulants
Buspirone	Good for comorbid anxiety and aggression, possibly depression Relatively safe (similar to stimulants) Smooth effect Relatively free of side effects	Possible paradoxic excitation Several weeks needed to see full effect of a given dose, therefore hard/slow to titrate

TABLE 5.2.1.11

(CONTINUED)

Drug Class	Advantages	Side Effects, Disadvantages
Antihistamines (older)	Safe, cheap, over-the-counter Especially good in patients with possible allergic etiology (but not restricted to those)	Sedation Risk of seizures in high doses Not as effective as stimulants, atomoxetine, or antidepressants: unsatisfactory in many patients
Antipsychotics	May work when stimulant or atomoxetine does not, especially if stimulant makes worse Good for comorbid anxiety, aggression, tic disorder, or bipolar disorder	Sedation Extrapyramidal side effects Endocrine effects Tardive dyskinesia Paradoxical agitation (akathisia) Weight gain Not specific. generally less effective than stimulants or atomoxetine Riskiest drug, last resort
Anticonvulsants	Good for comorbid mood disorder, aggression, explosiveness, impulsiveness May work when stimulant, atomoxetine, or antidepressant does not	Blood tests for levels and safety monitoring Liver toxicity Blood dyscrasia Sedation or agitation Ataxia

TCA = tricyclic antidepressant.
MAOI = monoamine oxidase inhibitor.
*Although some antipsychotics (haloperidol and chlorpromazine) have an FDA-approved indication, they should not be preferred to unapproved drugs higher on the list unless for a specific reason, such as comorbid bipolar disorder.
DMI = desipramine
SSRIs = selective serotonin reuptake inhibitors
(From Arnold LE, Contemporary Diagnosis and Management of ADHD. *Handbooks in Health Care*, Newtown, PA, 2004. Reproduced with permission.)

TABLE 5.2.1.12

POINTS FOR EXPLANATION AND CLARIFICATION TO PATIENT AND FAMILY

Talking Point	Reason
Acknowledge what they already know.	Shows respect and attention to their story. Imparts feeling of cognitive familiarity, a base on which to hook the new information.
Give them the current name of the disorder, indicating there are numerous other names.	Defines and clarifies the disorder.
ADHD has many symptoms, and not every patient with ADHD has all of them. Some have partial expressions of the syndrome.	Prevents confusion from having symptoms that are different from those of an acquaintance with ADHD.
Three main symptoms are inattention, hyperactivity, and impulsivity.	Focuses the targets of treatment. Prevents assumption the patient needs to be aggressive.
Other symptoms are frequent and often disabling, though not important for the diagnosis.	Puts all symptoms in perspective.
Symptoms are just excess amounts of normal behavior.	Implies need to control symptoms, not eliminate them.
Symptoms are not the patient's fault, but the patient can improve with help.	Breaks up the blame game, prevents giving up. Promotes teamwork in fighting ADHD.
ADHD lasts a long time, perhaps a lifetime, although it tends to get better with age.	Prepares for long-term treatment.
Important not to give up or neglect treatment.	Giving up allows secondary problems, dropping farther behind.
Treatment helps prevent secondary problems.	So they don't just wait for things to get better.
Many different treatments are available, relative advantages/disadvantages, and scientific basis of each (Chapters 3 to 7).	So they'll know the options, be involved in choice of treatment, and, therefore, commit to it.

(From Arnold LE, Contemporary Diagnosis and Management of ADHD. *Handbooks in Health Care*, Newtown, PA, 2004. Reproduced with permission.)

TABLE 5.2.1.13

SCIENTIFIC STATUS OF TREATMENT ALTERNATIVES FOR ATTENTION DEFICIT HYPERACTIVITY DISORDER (ADHD)

Treatment	Etiology or Mechanism	Type of Data	Effect Size d and/or p	Rating* (0–6); Recommendation and/or Need	Risks, Discomforts, Disadvantages
Sympathomimetic Meds: stimulants, atomoxetine	Catecholamine, esp. dopamine	>100 placebo XOs and RCTs in 1000s	ES 0.5–1.8 p. 01–.0001	6; Use if no cause found	Side effects; doubt neurotoxic
Antidepressants, other psychotropic medications	Catecholamine? serotonin	Multiple placebo-controlled RCTs	ES 0.5–1.5 p. 05–.005	6; When stimulants fail	Cardiotoxicity, other side effects
Behavioral Tx: BM, contingency	Social learning theory, shaping	ABAB, random wait list controls	ES 0.5–1.2 p. 05–.005	6; Selective use (severe, or comorbid anxiety)	Nuisance, time
Few foods diet (oligoantigenic)	Food or additive sensitivity	Controlled trial; placebo challenges	ES 0.5–1.0 p. 05–.001	5; Define subgroup (profile; % ADHD)	Nuisance, expense, nutrition balance
Enzyme-potentiated desensitization	Food or additive sensitivity	Controlled comparison to placebo injections	p. 001	4; Replication Define subgroup	Injection
Elimination of sugar alone	Sugar malaise	Placebo-controlled challenges	p >.1	0; Take FH of diabetes	Delay standard Tx
Amino acid supplementation	Precursors of neuro-transmitters	Placebo-controlled comparisons	ES up to 0.6, p. 01	0; Despite short-lived effect of little utility	Eosinophilia, neurotoxicity
Essential fatty acid supplement	Prostaglandins neural membrane	Serum level in controls five placebo-controlled trials	ES 0.5 p. <05 to >.1	3; trials of specific n-3 or n-6 by serum profile	Upsetting balance
L-carnitine	Promotes EFA anabolism	1 published placebo trial ADHD	ES ~0.5, p<0.05	2; Better placebo trial	Upsetting balance
Glyconutritional supplementation	Need for glycoconjugates	3 open trials, SNAP-IV	2 positive, 1 negative	0; Unless placebo trials	Upsetting balance
Dimethylaminoethanol (DMAE)	Acetylcholine precursor?	Many open and DB trials	ES 0.1–0.6; .1>p>.05	3; Rigorous PBO trial in ADHD	Modest effect, SE, expense
Vitamins	Deficiency vs. idiopathic need for higher dose	Placebo-controlled trials megavitamin combo, not RDI	Megadose combo no benefit	0; For mega-combo; 1 for RDI, specific megavit; pilot trials	Hepatotoxicity, neuropathy in megadose
Iron supplementation	Co-factor make catecholamine	Open trial; ferritin levels cf. controls; r ferritin & P rating	ES 1.0 p< .05 – .001 r = –.34	3 **; controlled trials	Hemochromatosis from excess
Zinc supplementation	Co-factor for many enzymes	2 DB RCT, flawed, high-dose	ES 1 p<.002	3 **; Better trials	WBC aplasia from excess
Magnesium supplementation	Deficiency cf. to controls	Open trial with control group	ES 1.2–1.4 p. <.05	3 **; placebo trials	Aggression from excess
Chinese herbals	Clinical experience	Open trials, one w. MPH control	p<. 05; no diff. MPH	3; placebo trials	Delay of other Tx
Other herbals	Clinical experience	No data	N.A.	1; pilot trials	Delay Tx
Homeopathic prep	Clinical experience	No data	N.A.	1; pilot trials	Delay Tx
Laser acupuncture	Stimulate foci for calming	Open trial	ES 1.0	2; controlled trial	Burn
EEG biofeedback	Suppress theta, increase beta	Open and randomized wait list control trials	p<0.05	3; sham-controlled trial	Expense, time
EMG biofeedback, relaxation, hypnosis	Lower arousal, muscle tone	Randomized trials with controls	ES 1.0–1.3 p<0.01	0 for hypnosis; 4 for EMG/relaxation; cf. med	Delay other Tx
Meditation	Autonomic effect focused attention	cf. relaxation, wait list ctrl, med	p<.05	3; Rigorous replication, sham ctrl	Delay other Tx
Mirror feedback	Improve deficiency in self-focus	Randomized crossover w. and w/o cf. controls	E.S. 0.5 p<. 05	3; Replication, instr.look	May impair non-ADHD children
Channel-specific perceptual training	Basic readiness skills, focus	Randomized previous trial with 2 control groups	ES 0.9 p<0.01	3; Controlled Tx trials	Delay other Tx
Vestibular stimulation	Modulate behavior, attention, perception	Open and single-blind trials rotary stimulation	ES 0.4–1.2 p ns-0.001	3; Randomized sham-controlled trials	Nausea, accident
Cerebellar training	Patterning of behavior, organization of perceptions	Open trials, not well diagnosed, one with waitlist control	p<. 05	1; Controlled trials with comparison Tx of equal duration and intensity	Nuisance, expense, delay of other Tx

(Adapted from: Arnold, LE: Contemporary Diagnosis and Management of ADHD, third Edition. Newtown, PA: *Handbooks in Health Care Co.*, 2004. Reproduced with permission.)

TABLE 5.2.1.13

(CONTINUED)

Treatment	Etiology or Mechanism	Type of Data	Effect Size d and/or p	Rating* (0–6); Recommendation and/or Need	Risks, Discomforts, Disadvantages
Massage	Vagal tone, 5HT, soothing	Single-blind comparison to relaxation	ES med-large $p<0.05$	3; Replication, better assessments	Bruising if too hard
Antifungal Tx	GI yeast toxin; breach mucosa	No data in ADHD; other placebo trials	(ES 1.1–3; $p<0.003$)	1; Trials in ADHD	Medium risk
Thyroid Tx	Thyroid function affects ADHD Sx	Placebo trial: 5/8 GRTH, 1/9 other	n.s. If thyroid function not abnormal	0 If thyroid normal; 6 if thyroid abnormal	Thyroid toxicity
Deleading	Lead toxicity causes ADHD Sx	Placebo-control trial of chelation (= MPH)	ES 0.7–1.6 p. 05–.001	4 if blood Pb>20; 2 if Pb<20; ctrl trial	Toxicity of chelator

*Ratings: 0 = not worth considering further (despite, in the case of amino acids, some evidence of short-lived effect); 1 = credible hypothesis or collateral support or wide clinical experience, needs pilot data; 2 = promising systematic data, but not prospective trial; 3 = promising prospective data (perhaps with random assignment to control or objective/blind measures) lacking some important control OR controlled trial(s) with trends suggesting further exploration; 4 = one significant double-blind controlled trial needing replication OR multiple positive controlled trials in a treatment not easily blinded; 5 = convincing double-blind controlled evidence but needs further refinement (e.g., define target subgroup) for clinical application; 6 = should be considered established Tx for the appropriate subgroup.
**The rating would be 6 for patients showing frank deficiency of vitamins, iron, zinc, or other nutrients.
ES = Effect size, Cohen's d (number of standard deviations difference between means): small ES <0.3; moderate ES = 0.5; large ES = 1.0; p = probability
DB = Double-blind; DO = dropout rate; MPH = methylphenidate; RCT = randomized clinical trial; RDI = recommended dietary intake; Sx = symptoms;
Tx = treatment; XO = crossover trial.

5. Rather than merely advising against an unproven treatment, it is more useful to discuss what is known about it and help the family reach a considered decision. If the treatment is easy, cheap, and safe, there would seem little harm in accepting a trial and providing some guidance about how to monitor the results (baseline and followup measures, log of observed behavior), and the clinician's openmindedness may help the family accept the recommended standard treatment.
6. When any treatment (including standard treatments) is tried, it is important to document the effect. Some rating scale or behavior count at baseline can be repeated periodically to see if there is reasonable progress. If there is, a trial of stopping the treatment can test whether the benefit was nonspecific (e.g., placebo benefit) or specific to the treatment. Lack of progress after a reasonable trial would seem prima facie evidence that it is not working for this patient.

Each family must find its own palatable and effective combination of treatment with professional guidance. The recently presented 36-month Multimodal Treatment Study of children with ADHD results (70) demonstrated that with treatment, symptoms abate significantly by the end of a year for most patients, and at 3 years continue to be significantly better than baseline, even though a substantial minority were able to terminate treatment by that time.

References

1. *Diagnostic and Statistical Manual of Mental Disorders, Fourth Edition (DSM IV).* Washington, DC, APA (American Psychiatric Association), c1994.
2. *Struwwelpeter: Fearful stories and vile pictures to instruct good little folks/Stories by Heinrich Hoffman.* Venice, CA, Feral House, 1999.
3. *Diagnostic and Statistical Manual of Mental Disorders, Second Edition (DSM II).* Washington, DC, APA (American Psychiatric Association), c1970.
4. *The ICD 10 Classification of Mental and Behavioural Disorders: Diagnostic Criteria for Research.* Geneva, World Health Organization (WHO), 1993.
5. *Diagnostic and Statistical Manual of Mental Disorders, Third Edition (DSM III).* Washington, DC, APA (American Psychiatric Association), c1980.
6. Attention Deficit Disorder Association—www.add.org.
7. Children and Adults with Attention Deficit Hyperactivity Disorder—www.chadd.org.
8. *Diagnostic and Statistical Manual of Mental Disorders, Third Edition—Revised (DSM III R).* Washington, DC, APA (American Psychiatric Association), c1987.
9. Rowland AS, Lesesne CA, Abramowitz AJ: The epidemiology of ADHD—A public health view. *Mental Retardation and Dev Disabilities Res Rev* 8:162–170, 2002.
10. Faraone SV, Biederman J, Zimmerman BA: Correspondence of parent and teacher reports in medication trials. *Eur J Child Adolesc Psychiatr* 14:20–27, 2005.
11. Faraone SV, Sergeant J, Gillberg C, Biederman J: The worldwide prevalence of ADHD—Is it an American condition? *World Psych* 2:104–113, 2003.
12. Lahey BB, Applegate B, McBurnett K, et al.: DSM IV field trials for ADHD in children and adolescents. *Am J Psychiatry* 151:1673–1685, 1994.
13. Santosh P, Taylor E, Swanson J, et al.: Refining the diagnoses of inattention and overactivity syndromes: A reanalysis of the Multimodal Treatment study of attention deficit hyperactivity disorder (ADHD) based on ICD-10 criteria for hyperkinetic disorder. *J Clinical Neuroscience Research* 5–6:307–314, 2005.
14. Biederman J, Monuteaux MC, Mick E, et al.: Adolescent outcome of females with ADHD: A controlled 5 year prospective study of girls into adolescence. Presented at the NIMH Pediatric Bipolar Conference, Coral Gables, FL (April 2005).
15. Connor D: Preschool ADHD: A review of prevalence, diagnosis, neurobiology and stimulant treatment. *Developmental and Behavioral Pediatrics* Vol 23, No 1S 2002.

16a. Coolidge F, Thede L, Young S: Heritability and the Comorbidity of Attention Deficit Hyperactivity Disorder With Behavioral Disorders and Executive Function Deficits: *A Preliminary Investigation—Developmental Neuropsychology* 17(3):273–287, 2000.

16b. Hudziak JJ, Rudiger LP, Neale MC, Heath AC, Todd RD: A twin study of inattentive, aggressive, and anxious/depressed behaviors. *J Am Acad Child Adolesc Psychiatry* 39:469–476, 2000.

16c. Thapar A, Harrington R: Does the Definition of ADHD Affect Heritability? *Journal of the American Academy of Child & Adolescent Psychiatry* 39(12), p1528, 9p, 5 charts 1 diagram, Dec 2000.

16d. Martin N, Scourfield J, McGuffin P: Observer effects and heritability of childhood attention-deficit hyperactivity disorder symptoms. *Br J Psychiatry* 180:260–265, 2002.

16e. Rietveld MJ, Hudziak JJ, Bartels M, Van Beijsterveldt CE, Boomsma DI: Heritability of attention problems in children: I. cross-sectional results from a study of twins, age 3–12 years. *Am J Med Genet B Neuropsychiatr Genet* 117:102–113, 2003.

16f. Rietveld M, Hudziak J, Bartels M, Van Beijsterveldt C, Boomsma D: Heritability of attention problems in children: longitudinal results from a study of twins, age 3 to 12. *Journal of Child psychology & Psychiatry* 45(3):577–588, 2004.

17. Doyle AE, Seidman LJ, Biederman J, Chourinard VA, Silva J, Faraone SV: Attention Deficit Hyperactivity Disorder Endophenotypes. *Biol Psychiatry* 57:1313–1323, 2005.
18. Barkley R, Smith K, Fischer M, Navia B: An examination of the behavioral and neuropsychological correlates of three ADHD candidate

gene polymorphisms (DRD4 7+, DBH TaqI A2, and DAT1 bp VNTR) in hyperactive and normal children followed to adulthood. *American Journal of medical Genetics Part B (Neuropsychiatric genetics)* 141B:487–498, 2006.
19. Fisher SE, Francks C, McCracken JT, McGough JJ, Marlow AJ, Macphil IL, et al.: A genomewide scan for loci involved in ADHD. *Am J Hum Gen* 70:1183–1196, 2002.
20. Bakker SC, Van der Maulen EM, Buitelaar JK, Sandkuije LA, Pauls DL, Monsuur AJ, et al.: A whole genome scan in 164 Dutch sib pairs with ADHD: Suggestive evidence for linkage on chromosome 7p and 15q. *Am J Hum Genet* 1251–1260, 2003.
21. Arcos Burgos M, Castellanos FX, Konecki D, Lopera F, Pineda D, Palacio JD, et al.: Pedigree disequilibrium test (PDT) replicates association and linkage between DRD4 and ADHD in multigenerational and extended pedigrees from a genetic isolate. *Mol Psychiatry* 9:252–259, 2004.
22. Mattes JA: The role of frontal lobe dysfunction in childhood hyperkinesis. *Compr Psychiatry* 21:358–369, 1980.
23. Pennington BF, Ozonoff S: Executive functions and developmental psychopathology. *J Child Psychol Psychiatry* 37:51–87, 1996.
24. Barkley RA: Behavioral inhibition, sustained attention, and executive function: Constructing a unified theory of ADHD. *Psychol Bull* 121:65–94, 1997.
25. Seidman LJ, Doyle A, Fried R, Valera E, Crum K, Matthews L: Neuropsychological function in adults with attention deficit hyperactivity disorder. *Psychiatr Clin North Am* 27:261–282, 2004.
26. Volkow ND, Fowler JS, Wang GJ, Ding YS, Gatley SJ: Role of dopamine in the therapeutic and reinforcing effects of methylphenidate in humans: Results from imaging studies. *Eur Neuropsychopharmacol* 12:557–566, 2002.
27. Hesslinger B, Tebartz van Elst L, Thiel T, Haegele K, Hennig J, Ebert D: Frontoorbital volume reductions in adult patients with attention deficit hyperactivity disorder. *Neurosci Lett* 328:319–321, 2002.
28. Castellanos FX, Lee PP, Sharp W, Jeffries NO, Greenstein DK, Clasen LS, et al.: Developmental trajectories of brain volume abnormalities in children and adolescents with attention deficit hyperactivity disorder. *JAMA* 288:1740–1748, 2002.
29. Madras BK, Miller GM, Fischman AJ: The dopamine transporter: Relevance to attention deficit hyperactivity disorder (ADHD). *Behavioural Brain Research* vol. 130, no. 1–2; 57–63, 2002.
30. Madras BK, Miller GM, Fischman AJ: The dopamine transporter and attention-deficit/hyperactivity disorder. *Biological Psychiatry* Jun; vol. 57, no. 11; 1397–409, 2005.
31. Jasper H, Solomon P, Bradley C: Electroencephalographic analyses of behaviour problem children. *Am J Psychiatry* 95:641–658, 1938.
32. Mann C, Lubar J, Zimmerman A, Miller C, Muenchen R: Quantitative analysis of EEG in boys with attention deficit hyperactivity disorder—Controlled study with clinical implications. *Pediatr Neurol* 8:30–36, 1992.
33. Chabot R, Merkin H, Wood L, Davenport T, Serfontein G: Sensitivity and specificity of QEEG in children with attention deficit hyperactivity disorder or specific developmental learning disorders. *Clin Electroencephalogr* 27:26–34, 1996.
34. Monastra V, Lubar J, Linden M, VanDeusen P, Green G, Wing W, Phillips A, Fenger T: Assessing attention deficit hyperactivity disorder via quantitative electroencephalography: An initial validation study. *Neuropsychology* 13:424–433, 1999.
35. Kovatchev B, Cox D, Hill R, Reeve R, Robeva R, Loboschefski T: A psychophysiological marker of attention deficit hyperactivity disorder—Defining the EEG consistency index. *Appl Psychophysiol Biofeedback* 26:127–140, 2001.
36. Barry R, Johnstone SJ, Clarke AR: A review of electrophysiology in attention deficit hyperactivity disorder—Event related potentials. *Clin Neurophysiol* 114:184–198, 2003.
37. van Beijsterveldt CE, van Baal GC: Twin and family studies of the human electroencephalogram: A review and a meta-analysis. *Biol Psychol* 61:111–138, 2002.
38. Arnold LE: Treatment alternatives for attention-deficit/hyperactivity disorder (ADHD). *Journal of Attention Disorders* 3:30–48, 1999.
39. Arnold LE: Treatment alternatives for attention-deficit/hyperactivity disorder. In: Jensen, PS & Cooper, J (eds.). *Attention Deficit Hyperactivity Disorder: State of the Science; Best Practices.* Kingston, NJ: Civic Research Institute, 2002.
40. Rojas NL, Chan E (2005). Old and new controversies in the alternative treatment of attention-deficit/hyperactivity disorder. *Mental Retardation and Developmental Disabilities Research Reviews* 11:116–130.
41. Rovet J & Alvarez M (1996). Thyroid hormone and attention in school-age children with congenital hypothyroidism. *Journal of Child Psychology and Psychiatry* 37:579–585, 1996.
42. Hauser P, Soler R, Brucker-Davis F, & Weintraub BD (1997). Thyroid hormones correlate with symptoms of hyperactivity but not inattention in ADHD. *Psychoneuroendocrinology* 22:107–114, 1997.
43. David OJ, Hoffman SP, Clark J, Grad G, & Sverd J: (1983). The relationship of hyperactivity to moderately elevated lead levels. *Archives of Environmental Health* 38:341–B 346, 1983.
44. DuPaul GJ, Power TJ, Anastopoulos AD, Reid R (1998). *ADHD Rating Scale-IV: Checklists, Norms, and Clinical Interpretations.* New York. Guilford Press.
45. Conners, CK (2001) *Manual for Conners' Rating Scales Toronto*, Canada: Multi-Health Systems.
46. Gustaffson P, Thernlund G, Ryding E, Rosen I, Cederblad, M. Associations between cerebral blood-flow measured by single photon computed tomography (SPECT), electro-encephalogram (EEG), behaviour symptoms, cognition and neurological soft signs in children with attention deficit hyperactivity disorder. *Acta Paediatr* 89(7):830–835, 2000.
47. Dickstein DP, Garvey M, Pradella AG, Greenstein DK, Sharp WS, Castellanos XF, Pine DS, Leibenluft E: Neurologic examination abnormalities in children with attention deficit hyperactivity disorder. *Biol Psychiatry* 58:517–524, 2005.
48. The MTA Cooperative Group. A 14-Month randomized clinical trial of treatment strategies for attention-deficit/hyperactivity disorder. *Archives of General Psychiatry*, 56:1073–1086, and Dec 1999a.
49. Hechtman L, Etcovitch J, Platt R, et al.: Does multimodal treatment of ADHD decrease other diagnoses?. *Clinical Neuroscience Research* 5(5/6), 273–282, 2005.
50. Welsh MC, Pennington BF: Assessing frontal lobe functioning in children: Views from developmental psychology. *Dev Neuropsychol* 4:199–230, 1988.
51. Barkley RA. Behavioral inhibition, sustained attention, and executive function: Constructing a unified theory of ADHD. *Psychol Bull* 121:65–94, 1997.
52. Schoechlin C, Engel RR. Neuropsychological performance in adult attention deficit hyperactivity disorder: Meta-analysis of empirical data. *Arch Clin Neuropsychol* 20:727–744, 2005.
53. Sonuga-Barke EJS. On dysfunction and function in psychological accounts of childhood disorder. *J Child Psychol Psychiat* 35:801–815, 1994.
54. Sonuga-Barke EJS. The dual pathway model of ADHD: An elaboration of neuro-developmental characteristics. *Neuroscience and Biobehavioral Reviews* 27:593–604, 2003.
55. Solanto MV, Abikoff H, Sonuga-Barke E, Schachar R, Logan GD, Wigal T, et al.: The ecological validity of delay aversion and response inhibition as measures of impulsivity in ADHD: A supplement to the NIMH multimodal treatment study of ADHD. *J Abnorm Child Psychol* 29:215–228, 2001.
56. Sergeant J: The cognitive energetic model: An empirical approach to attention deficit hyperactivity disorder. *Neuroscience and Biobehavioral Reviews* 24:7–12, 2000.
57. McBurnett K, Pfiffner LJ, Frick PJ: Symptom properties as a function of ADHD type: An argument for continued study of sluggish cognitive tempo. *J Abnorm Child Psychol* 29:207–213, 2001.
58. Nigg JT, Goldsmith HH, Sachek J: Temperament and attention deficit hyperactivity disorder: The development of a Multiple Pathway Model. *J Clin Child Adolesc Psychol* 33, No 1:42–53, 2004.
59. Biederman J, Mick E, Faraone SV: Age dependent decline of symptoms of attention deficit hyperactivity disorder: Impact of remission definition and symptom type. *Am J Psychiatry* 157:816–818, 2000.
60. Kessler RC, Lenard AA, Barkley R, Biederman J, Conners CK, Faraone SV, Greenhill LL, Jaeger S, Secnik K, Spencer T, Bedirhan Ustun T, Zaslavsky AM: Patterns and predictors of attention deficit hyperactivity disorder persistence in adulthood: Results from the National Comorbidity Survey Replication. *Biol Psychiatry* 57:1442–1451, 2005.
61. Brownell MD, Yogendran MS: Attention Deficit Hyperactivity Disorder in Manitoba children: Medical diagnosis and psychostimulant treatment rates. *Can J Psychiatry* 46:264–272, 2001.
62. Pastor P, Reuben C: Racial and ethnic differences in ADHD and learning disorders in young school age children: Parental reports in the National Health Interview Survey. *Public Health Reports* July/August; Vol 120:383–392, 2005.
63. American Academy of Child & Adolescent Psychiatry: Practice parameters for the assessment and treatment of children, adolescents and adults with ADHD. *J Am Acad Child Adolesc Psychiatry* 36(10S) Supplement 85S–121S, October, 1997.
64. American Academy of Pediatrics: Clinical Practice Guideline: Treatment of the school-age child with attention-deficit/hyperactivity disorder. *Pediatrics* 108:1033–1044, 2001.
65. Conners CK, Epstein JN, March JS, et al.: Multimodal treatment of ADHD in the MTA: An alternative outcome analysis. *J Amer Acad Child & Adolesc Psychiatry* 40:159–167, 2001.
66. Swanson JM, Kraemer HC, Hinshaw SP, et al.: Clinical relevance of the primary findings of the MTA: Success rates based on severity of ADHD and ODD symptoms at the end of treatment. *J Amer Acad Child & Adolesc Psychiatry* 40:168–179, 2001.
67. The MTA Cooperative Group: Moderators and mediators of treatment response for children with attention-deficit/hyperactivity disorder. *Archives of General Psychiatry* 56:1088–1096, Dec. 1999b.
68. Jensen PS, Hinshaw SP, Kraemer HC, et al.: ADHD comorbidity findings from the MTA study: Comparing comorbid subgroups. *J Amer Acad Child & Adolesc Psychiatry* 40:147–158, 2001.
69. Arnold LE: *A Family Guide to ADHD.* Newtown, PA: Handbooks in Health Care Co., 2004.
70. "36-month MTA follow-up and other new insights into ADHD treatment." Symposium at 51st Annual Meeting American Academy of Child and Adolescent Psychiatry, October 19–24, 2004, Washington, DC.
71. Cook EH, Stein MA, Krasowski MD, Cox NJ, Olkon DM, Kieffer JE, et al.: Association of ADHD and the dopamine transporter gene. *Am J Hum Genet* 56:993–998, 1995.

72. Waldman ID, Rowe DC, Abramowitz A, Kozel ST, Mohr JH, Sherman, SL: Association and linkage of the dopamine transporter gene and attention deficit hyperactivity disorder in children: Heterogeneity owing to diagnostic subtype and severity. *Am J Hum Genet* 63:1767–1776, 1998.
73. Dougherty DD, Bonab AA, Spencer TJ, Rausch SL, Madras BK, Fischman AJ: Dopamine transporter density is elevated in patients with ADHD. *Lancet* 354:2132–2133, 1999.
74. Krause K, Dresel SH, Krause J, Kung HF, Tatsch K: Increased striatal dopamine transporter in adult patients with ADHD: Effects of methylphenidate as measured by single photon emission computed tomography. *Neurosci Lett* 285:107–110, 2000.
75. Todd RD, Jong YG, Lobos EA, Reich W, Heath AC, Neumann RJ: No association of the dopamine transporter gene 3′VNTR polymorphism with ADHD subtypes in a population sample of twins. *Am J Med Genet* 105:745–748, 2001.
76. Payton A, Holmes J, Barrett JH, Hever T, Fitzpatrick H, Trumper AL, et al.: Examining for association between candidate gene polymorphisms in the dopamine pathways and ADHD: A family based study. *Am J Med Genet* 105:464–470, 2001.
77. Muglia P, Jain U, Iukster B, Kennedy JL: A quantitative trait locus analysis of the dopamine transporter gene in adults with ADHD. *Neuropsychopharmacology* 27:655–662, 2002.
78. VanDyck CH, Quinlan DM, Cretella LM, Staley JK, Malison RT, Baldwin RM: Unaltered dopamine transporter availability in adult attention deficit hyperactivity disorder. *Am J Psychiatry* 159:309–312, 2002.
79. Chen CK, Chen SL, Mill J, Huang YS, Lin SK, Curran S, et al.: The dopamine transporter gene is associated with ADHD in a Taiwanese sample. *Mol Psychiatry* 8:393–396, 2003.
80. Smith KM, Daly M, Fischer M, Yiannoutsos CT, Bauer L, Barkley R, et al.: Association of the dopamine beta Hydroxylase gene with attention deficit hyperactivity disorder: Genetic analysis of the Milwaukee longitudinal study. *Am J Genet* 119:77–85, 2003.
81. Curran S, Mill J, Tahir E, Kent L, Richards S, Gould A, et al.: Association study of a dopamine transporter polymorphism and ADHD in UK and Turkish samples. *Mol Psychiatry* 6:425–428, 2001.
82. Comings DE, Comings BG, Muhleman D, Dietz G, Shahbahrami B, Tast D, et al.: The dopamine D2 receptor locus as a modifying gene in neuropsychiatric disorders. *JAMA* 266:1793–1800, 1991.
83. Comings DE, Wu H, Chiu C, Ring RH, Gade R, Ahn C, et al.: Polygenic inheritance of Tourette Syndrome, stuttering, ADHD, conduct and oppositional defiant disorder: The additive and subtractive effect of the three dopamine genes—DRD2, DBH and DAT1. *Am J Genet* 67:264–288, 1996.
84. Rowe DC, den Oord EJ, Stever C, Giedinghagen LN, Gard JM, Cleveland HH, et al.: The DRD2 Taq1 polymorphism and symptoms of ADHD. *Mol Psychiatry* 4:580–586, 1999.
85. Kirley A, Hawi Z, Daly G, McCarron M, Mullins C, Millar N, et al.: Dopaminergic system genes in ADHD: Toward a biological hypothesis. *Neuropsychopharmacology* 27:607–619, 2002.
86. Huang YS, Lin SK, Wu YY, Chao CC, Chen CK: A family based association study of ADHD and dopamine D2 receptor Taq1A alleles. *Chang Gung Med J* 26:897–903, 2003.
87. Faraone SV, Doyle AE, Mick E, Biederman J: Metaanalysis of the association between the 7-repeat allele of the dopamine D4 receptor gene and ADHD. *Am J Psychiatry* 158:1052–1057, 2001.
88. Holmes J, Payton A, Barrett J, Harrington R, McGuffin P, Owen, M, et al.: Association of DRD4 in children with ADHD and comorbid conduct problems. *Am J Med Genet* 114:150–153, 2002.
89. Grady DL, Chi HC, Ding YC, Smith M, Wang E, Schuck S, et al.: High prevalence of rare dopamine D4 alleles in children diagnosed with ADHD. *Mol Psychiatry* 8:536–545, 2003.
90. Qian Q, Wang Y, Zhou R: Association studies of dopamine D4 receptor gene and dopamine transporter gene polymorphisms in Han Chinese patients with ADHD. *Beijing Da Xue Xue Bao* 35:412–418, 2003.
91. Mill J, Curran S, Kent L, Richards S, Gould A, Virdee V, et al.: ADHD and the dopamine D4 receptor gene: Evidence of association but no linkage in a UK sample. *Mol Psychiatry* 6:440–444, 2001.
92. Manor I, Tyano S, Mel E, Eisenberg J, Bachner-Melman R, Kotler M, et al.: Family based and association studies of MAO-A and attention deficit hyperactivity disorder: Preferential transmission of the long-promoter region repeat and its and its association with impaired performance on a continuous performance test (TOVA). *Mol Psychiatry* 7:626–632, 2002.
93. Kustanovich V, Ishii J, Crawford L, Yang M, McGough JJ, McCracken JT, et al.: Transmission disequilibrium testing of dopamine-related candidate gene polymorphisms in ADHD: Confirmation of association of ADHD with DRD4 and DRD5. *Mol Psychiatry* 9:711–717, 2003.
94. McCracken JT, Smalley SL, McGough JJ, Crawford L, Del'Homme M, Cantor RM, et al.: Evidence for linkage of a tandem duplication polymorphism upstream of the dopamine D4 receptor gene (DRD4) with attention deficit hyperactivity disorder (ADHD). *Mol Psychiatry* 5:531–536, 2000.
95. Todd RD, Neuman RJ, Lobos EA, Jong YJ, Reich W, Heath AC: Lack of association of dopamine D4 receptor gene polymorphisms with ADHD subtypes in a population sample of twins. *Am J Med Genet* 105:432–438, 2001.
96. Barr CL, Wigg KG, Bloom S, Schachar R, Tannock R, Roberts W, et al.: Further evidence from haplotype analysis for linkage of the dopamine D4 receptor gene and attention-deficit hyperactivity disorder. *Am J Med Genet* 96:244–250, 2000.
97. Rowe DC, Stever C, Chase D, Sherman S, Abramowitz A, Waldman ID: Two dopamine genes related to reports of childhood retrospective inattention and conduct disorder symptoms. *Mol Psychiatry* 6:429–433, 2001.
98. Comings David E, Gade-Andavolu Radhika,Gonzalez Nancy, Wu Shijuan, Muhleman Donn, Blake Hezekiah, Dietz George, Saucier Gerard, P MacMurray, James: Comparison of the role of dopamine, serotonin, and noradrenaline genes in ADHD, ODD and conduct disorder: Multivariate regression analysis of 20 genes. *Clinical Genetics* March, 2000.
99. Daly G, Hawi Z, Fitzgerald M, Gill M: Mapping susceptibility loci in ADHD: Preferential transmission of parental alleles of DAT1; DBH; and DRD5 to affected children. *Mol Psychiatry* 4:192–196, 1999.
100. Barr CL, Wigg KG, Feng Y, Zai G, Malone M, Roberts W, et al.: Attention-deficit hyperactivity disorder and the gene for the dopamine D5 receptor. *Mol Psychiatry* 5:548–551, 2000.
101. Tahir E, Yazgan Y, Cirakoglu OF, Waldman I, Asherson PJ: Association and linkage of DRD4 and DRD5 with attention deficit hyperactivity disorder. *Mol Psychiatry* 5:396–404, 2000.
102. Mill J, Richards S, Knight J, Curran S, Taylor E, Asherson P: Haplotype analysis of SNAP 25 suggests a role in the aetiology of ADHD. *Mol Psychiatry* 9:801–810, 2004.
103. Maher BS, Marazita ML, Ferrell RE, Vanuykov MM: Dopamine system genes and ADHD: A meta-analysis. *Psychiatr Genet* 12:207–215, 2002.
104. Lowe N, Kirley A, Hawi Z, et al.: Joint analysis of DRD5 marker concludes association with ADHD confined to the predominantly inattentive and combined types. *Am J Hum Genet* 74:348–356, 2004.
105. Manor I, Corbex M, Eisenberg J, Gritsenkso I, Bachner-Melman R, Tyano S, et al.: (2004): Association of the dopamine D5 receptor with attention deficit hyperactivity disorder (ADHD) and scores on a continuous performance test (TOVA). *Am J Med Genet*:127.
106. Barr CL, Wigg KG, Wu J, Zai C, Bloom S, Tannock R, et al.: Linkage study of two polymorphisms at the dopamine D3 receptor gene and attention-deficit hyperactivity disorder. *Am J Med Genet* 96:114–117, 2000.
107. Muglia P, Jain U, Kennedy JL: A transmission disequilibrium test of the Ser 9/Gly dopamine D3 receptor gene polymorphism in adult attention deficit hyperactivity disorder. *Behav Brain Res* 130:91–95, 2002.
108. Retz W, Rosler M, Supprian T, Retz-Junginger P, Thome J: Dopamine D3 receptor polymorphism and violent behavior: relation to impulsiveness and ADHD related psychopathology. *J Neural Transm* 110:561–572, 2003.
109. Retz W, Thome J, Blocker D, Baaden M, Rosler M: Association of ADHD related psychopathology and personality traits with the serotonin transporter promoter region polymorphism. *Neurosci Lett* 319:133–136, 2002.
110. Seeger G, Schloss P, Schmidt MH: Functional polymorphism within the promoter of the serotonin transporter gene is associated with severe hyperkinetic disorders. *Mol Psychiatry* 6:235–238, 2001.
111. Zoroglu SS, Erdal ME, Alasehirli Erdal N, Sivasli E, Tutkun H, et al.: Significance of serotonin transporter gene 5-HTTLPR and variable number of tandem repeat polymorphism in attention deficit hyperactivity disorder. *Neuropsychobiology* 45:176–181, 2002.
112. Beitchman JH, Davidge KM, Kennedy JL, Atkinson L, Lee V, Shapiro S, et al.: The serotonin transporter gene in aggressive children with and without ADHD and nonaggressive matched controls. *Ann N Y Acad Sci* 1008:248–251, 2003.
113. Manor I, Eisenberg J, Tyano S, Sever Y, Cohen H, Ebstein RP, et al.: Family based association study of the serotonin transporter promoter region polymorphism (5-HTTLPR) in ADHD. *Am J Med Genet* 105:91–95, 2001.
114. Kent L, Doerry U, Hardy E, Parmar R, Gingell K, Hawi Z, et al.: Evidence that variation at the serotonin transporter gene influences susceptibility to ADHD: Analysis and pooled analysis. *Mol Psychiatry* 7:908–912, 2002.
115. Cadoret RJ, Langbehn D, Caspers K, Troughton EP, Yucuis R, Sandhu HK, et al.: Association of the serotonin transporter promoter polymorphism with aggressivity, attention deficit, and conduct disorder in an adoptee population. *Compr Psychiatry* 44:88–101, 2003.
116. Barr CL, Kroft J, Feng Y, Wigg K, Roberts W, Malone M, et al.: The norepinephrine transporter gene and attention-deficit hyperactivity disorder. *Am J Med Genet* 114:255–259,.
117. McEvoy B, Hawi Z, Fitzgerald M, Gill M: No evidence of linkage or association between the norepinephrine transporter (NET) gene polymorphisms and ADHD in the Irish population. *Am J Med Genet* 114:665–666, 2002.
118. De Luca, V, Muglia P, Vincent J, Lanktree M, Jain U, Kennedy JL: Adrenergic alpha 2C receptor genomic organization: association study in adult ADHD. *Am J Med Genet* 127:65–67, 2004.
119. Smith KM, Daly M, Fischer M, Yiannoutsos CT, Bauer L, Barkley R, et al.: Association of the dopamine beta Hydroxylase gene with attention deficit hyperactivity disorder: genetic analysis of the Milwaukee longitudinal study. *Am J Genet* 119:77–85, 2003.
120. Roman T, Schmitz M, Polanczyk G, Eizirik M, Rohde LA, Hutz MH: Further evidence for the association between attention deficit hyperactivity disorder and the dopamine beta Hydroxylase gene. *Am J Med Genet* 114:154–158, 2002.

121. Wigg K, Zai G, Schachar R, Tannock R, Roberts W, Malone M, et al.: Attention deficit hyperactivity disorder and the gene for dopamine beta Hydroxylase. *Am J Psychiatry* 159:1046–1048, 2002.
122. Hawi Z, Lowe N, Kirley A, Gruenhage F, Nothen M, Greenwood T, et al.: Linkage disequilibrium mapping at DAT1, DRD5, and DBH narrows the search for ADHD susceptibility alleles at these loci. *Mol Psychiatry* 8:299–308, 2003.
123. Hess EJ, Jinnah HA, Kozac CA, Wilson MC: Spontaneous locomotor hyperactivity in a mouse mutant with a deletion including the SNAP gene on chromosome 2 - *J Neurosci* 12:2865–2874, 1992.
124. Hess EJ, Rogan PK, Domoto M, Tinker DE, Ladda RL, Ramer JC: Absence of linkage of apparently single gene mediated ADHD with the human synterric region of the mouse mutant coloboma. *Am J Med Genet* 60:573–579, 1995.
125. Barr CL, Feng Y, Wigg K, Bloom S, Roberts W, Malone M, et al.: Identification of DNA variants in the SNAP-25 gene and linkage study of these polymorphisms and attention-deficit hyperactivity disorder. *Mol Psychiatry* 5:405–409, 2000.
126. Brophy K, Hawi Z, Kirley A, Fitzgerald M, Gill M: Synaptosomal-associated protein 25 (SNAP-25) and attention deficit hyperactivity disorder (ADHD): Evidence of linkage and association in the Irish population. *Mol Psychiatry* 7:913–917, 2002.
127. Mill J, Curran S, Kent L, Gould A, Huckett L, Richards S, et al.: Association study of a SNAP-25 microsatellite and attention deficit hyperactivity disorder. *Am J Med Genet* 114:269–271, 2002.
128. Kirley A, Brophy K, Hawi Z, Fitzgerald M, Gill M: Synaptosomal-associated protein 25 (SNAP 25) and ADHD: evidence of linkage and association in the Irish population. *Mol Psychiatry* 7:913–917, 2002.
129. Comings D, Gade R, Muhleman D, Sverd J: No association of a tyrosine Hydroxylase gene tetranucleotide polymorphism in autism, Tourette syndrome, or ADHD. *Biol Psychiatry* 37:484–486, 1995.
130. Syvanen AC, Tilgmann C, Rinne J, Ulmanen I: Genetic polymorphism of COMT; correlation of genotype with individual variation of S-COMT activity and comparison of the allele frequencies in the normal population and parkinsonian patients in Finland. *Pharmacogenetics* 7:65–71, 1997.
131. Barr CL, Wigg K, Malone M, Schachar R, Tannock R, Roberts W, et al.: Linkage study of COMT and attention deficit hyperactivity disorder. *Am J Med Genet* 88:710–713, 1999.
132. Hawi Z, Millar N, Daly G, Fitzgerald M, Gill M: No association between COMT gene polymorphism and ADHD in an Irish sample. *Am J Med Genet* 96:241–243, 2000.
133. Manor I, Kotler M, sever Y, Eisenberg J, Cohen H, Ebstein RP: Failure to replicate an association between the COMT polymorphism and attention deficit hyperactivity disorder in a second, independently recruited Israeli cohort. *Am J Med Genet* 96:858–860, 2000.
134. Tahir E, Curran S, Yazgan Y, Ozbay F, Cirakoglu Asherson PJ: No association between low and high activity COMT and attention deficit hyperactivity disorder in a sample of Turkish children. *Am J Med Genet* 96:285–288, 2000.
135. Qian Q, Wang Y, Zhou R, Li J, Wang, Glatt S, et al.: Family based and case control association studies of COMT in attention deficit hyperactivity disorder suggest genetic sexual dimorphism. *Am J Med Genet* 118:103–109, 2003.
136. Manor I, Tyano S, Mel E, Eisenberg J, Bachner-Melman R, Kotler M, et al.: Family based and association studies of MAO-A and attention deficit hyperactivity disorder: Preferential transmission of the long-promoter region repeat and its and its association with impaired performance on a continuous performance test (TOVA). *Mol Psychiatry* 7:626–632, 2002.
137. Lawson DC, Turic D, Langley K, Pay HM, Govan CF, Norton N, et al.: Association analysis of monoamine Oxidase A and attention deficit hyperactivity disorder. *Am J Med Genet* 116:84–89, 2003.
138. Comings D, Gade-Andavolu R, Gonzales N, Blake H, MacMurray J: Additive effect of three noradrenergic genes (ADRA2A, ADRA2C, DBH) on attention deficit hyperactivity disorder and learning disabilities in Tourette syndrome subjects. *Clin Genet* 55:160–172, 1999.
139. Xu C, Schachar R, Tannock R, Roberts W, Malone M, Kennedy JL, et al.: Linkage study of the alpha2A adrenergic receptor in attention deficit hyperactivity disorder families. *Am J Med Genet* 105:159–162, 2001.
140. Comings DE, Gonzales NS, Cheng Li SC, MacMurray J: A line item approach to the identification of genes involved in polygenic behavioral disorders: The adrenergic alpha2A (ADRA2A) gene. *Am J Med Genet* 118:110–114, 2003.
141. Barr CL, Wigg K, Zai G, Roberts W, Malone M, Schachar R, et al.: Attention deficit hyperactivity disorder and the adrenergic receptors alpha1C and alpha2C. *Mol Psychiatry* 6:334–337, 2001.
142. Roman T, Schmitz M, Polanczyk GV, Eizirik M, Rohde LA, Hutz MH: Is the alpha - 2A adrenergic receptor gene (ADRA2A) associated with attention deficit hyperactivity disorder? *Am J Med Genet* 120:116–120, 2003.
143. Hawi Z, Dring M, Kirley A, Foley D, Kent L, Craddock N, et al.: Serotonergic system and attention deficit hyperactivity disorder (ADHD): a potential susceptibility locus at the 5-HT (1B) receptor gene in 273 nuclear families from a multi-center sample. *Mol Psychiatry* 7:718–725, 2002.
144. Quist JF, Barr CL, Schachar R, Roberts W, Malone M, Tannock R, et al.: Evidence for the serotonin 5-HTR2A receptor gene as a susceptibility factor in attention deficit hyperactivity disorder (ADHD). *Mol Psychiatry* 5:537–541, 2000.
145. Tang G, Ren D, Xin R, Qian Y, Wang D, Jiang S: Lack of association between the Tryptophan hydroxylase gene A218C polymorphism and attention deficit hyperactivity disorder in Chinese Han population. *Am J Med Genet* 105:485–488, 2001.
146. Li J, Wang YF, Zhou RL, Yang L, Zhang HB, Wang B: Association between the tryptophan hydroxylase gene polymorphisms and attention deficit hyperactivity disorder with or without learning disorder. *Zhong-hua Yi Xue Za Zhi* 83:2114–2118, 2003.
147. Kent L, Middle F, Hawi Z, Fitzgerald M, Gill M, Feehan C, et al.: Nicotinic Acetylcholine receptor alpha4 subunit gene polymorphism and attention deficit hyperactivity disorder. *Psychiatr Genet* 11:37–40, 2001.
148. Todd RD, Lobos EA, Sun LW, Neumann RJ: Mutational analysis of the nicotinic acetylcholine receptor alpha 4 subunit gene in attention deficit hyperactivity disorder: Evidence for association of an intronic polymorphism with attention problems. *Mol Psychiatry* 8:103–108, 2003.
149. Turic D, Langley K, Mills S, Stephens M, Lawson D, Govan C, et al.: Follow up of genetic linkage findings on chromosome 16p13: Evidence of association of N-methyl-D-aspartate glutamate receptor 2A gene polymorphism with ADHD. *Mol Psychiatry* 9:169–173, 2004.
150. Adams J, Crosbie J, Wigg K, Ickowicz A, Pathare T, Roberts W, et al.: Glutamate receptor, ionotropic, N-methyl D-aspartate 2A (GRIN2A) gene as a positional candidate for attention deficit hyperactivity disorder in the 16p13 region. *Mol Psychiatry* 9:494–499, 2004.
151. Castellanos FX, Giedd JN, Marsh WL, Hamburger SD, Vaituzis AC, Dickstein DT, et al.: Quantitative brain magnetic resonance imaging in attention deficit hyperactivity disorder. *Arch Gen Psychiatry* 53:607–616, 1996.
152. Filipek PA, Semrud-Clickeman M, Steingard R, Kennedy D, Biederman J: Volumetric MRI analysis: Comparing subjects having attention deficit hyperactivity disorder with normal controls. *Neurology* 48:589–601, 1997.
153. Overmeyer S, Bullmore ET, Suckling J, Simmons A, Williams SC, Santosh PJ, Taylor E: Distributed gray and white matter deficits in hyperkinetic disorder: MRI evidence for anatomical abnormality in an attentional network. *Psychol Med* 31:1425–1435, 2001.
154. Mostofsky S, Cooper K, Kates W, Denckla M, Kaufmann W: Smaller pre-frontal and premotor volumes in boys with attention deficit hyperactivity disorder. *Biol Psychiatry* 52:785–794, 2002.
155. Hill DE, Yeo RA, Campbell RA, Hart B, Vigil J, Brooks W: Magnetic resonance imaging correlates of attention deficit hyperactivity disorder in children. *Neuropsychology* 17:496–506, 2003.
156. Durston S, Hulshoff Pol HE, Schnack HG, Buitelaar JK, Steenhuis MP, Minderaa RB, et al.: Magnetic resonance imaging of boys with attention deficit hyperactivity disorder and their unaffected siblings. *J Am Acad Child Adolesc Psychiatry* 43:332–340, 2004.
157. Hynd GW, Hern KL, Novey ES, Eliopulos D, Marshall R, Gonzales JJ, Voeller KK: Attention deficit hyperactivity disorder and asymmetry of the caudate nucleus. *J Child Neurol* 8:339–347, 1993.
158. Semrud-Clickeman MS, Filipek PA, Biederman J, Steingard R, Kennedy D, Renshaw P, Bekken K: Attention deficit hyperactivity disorder: Magnetic resonance imaging morphometric analysis of the corpus callosum. *J Am Acad Child Adolesc Psychiatry* 33:875–881, 1994.
159. Castellanos FX, Giedd JN, Eckburg P, Marsh WL, Vaituzis AC, Kaysen D, et al.: Quantitative morphology of the caudate nucleus in attention deficit hyperactivity disorder. *Am J Psychiatry* 151:1791–1796, 1994.
160. Castellanos FX, Giedd JN, Marsh WL, Hamburger SD, Vaituzis AC, Dickstein DP, et al.: Quantitative brain magnetic resonance imaging in attention deficit hyperactivity disorder. *Arch Gen Psychiatry* 53:607–616, 1996.
161. Mataro M, Garcia-Sanchez C, Junque C, Estevez-Gonzales A, Pujol J: Magnetic resonance imaging measurement of the caudate nucleus in adolescents with attention deficit hyperactivity disorder and its relationship with neuropsychological and behavioural measures. *Arch Neurol* 54:963–968, 1997.
162. Castellanos FX, Giedd JN, Berquin PC, Walter JM, Sharp W, Tran T, et al.: Quantitative brain magnetic resonance imaging in girls with attention-deficit/hyperactivity disorder. *Arch Gen Psychiatry* 58:289–295, 2001.
163. Pineda DA, Restrepo A, Sarmiento RJ, Gutierrez JE, Vargas SA, Quiroz YT, Hynd GW: Statistical analyses of structural magnetic resonance imaging of the head of the caudate nucleus in Colombian children with attention deficit hyperactivity disorder. *J Child Neurol* 17:97–105, 2002.
164. Bussing R, Grudnick J, Mason D, Wasiak M, Leonard C: ADHD and conduct disorder: An MRI study in a community sample. *World J Biol Psychiatry* 3:216–220, 2002.
165. Castellanos FX, Sharp WS, Gottesman RF, Greenstein DK, Giedd JN, Rapoport JL: Anatomic brain abnormalities in monozygotic twins discordant for attention deficit disorder. *Am J Psychiatry* 160:1693–1696, 2003.
166. Aylward EH, Reiss AL, Reader MJ, Singer HS, Brown JE, Denckla MB: Basal ganglia volumes in children with attention deficit hyperactivity disorder. *J Child Neurol* 11:112–115, 1996.
167. Overmeyer S, Simmons A, Santosh J, Andrew C, Williams SCR, Taylor A, et al.: Corpus callosum may be similar in children with ADHD and siblings of children with ADHD. *Dev Med Child Neurol* 42:8–13, 2000.

168. Hynd GW, Semrud-Clickeman MS, Lorys AR, Novey ES, Eliopulos D: Brain morphology in developmental dyslexia and attention deficit hyperactivity disorder. *Arch Neurol* 47:919–926, 1990.
169. Hynd GW, Semrud-Clickeman MS, Lorys AR, Novey ES, Eliopulos D, Lytinen H: Corpus callosum morphology in attention deficit hyperactivity disorder: Morphometric analysis of MRI. *J Learn Disabilities* 24:141–146, 1991.
170. Giedd JN, Castellanos FX, Casey BJ, Kozuch P, King AC, Hamburger SD, Rapoport JL: Quantitative morphology of the corpus callosum in attention deficit hyperactivity disorder. *Am J Psychiatry* 151:665–669, 1994.
171. Baumgardner TL, Singer HS, Denckla MB, Rubin MA, Abrams MT, Colli MJ, Reiss AL: Corpus callosum morphology in children with Tourette syndrome and attention deficit hyperactivity disorder. *Neurology* 47:1–6, 1996.
172. Lyoo I, Noam G, Lee H, Kennedy B, Renshaw P: The corpus callosum and lateral ventricles in children with attention deficit hyperactivity disorder: A brain magnetic resonance imaging study. *Biol Psychiatry* 40:1060–1063, 1996.
173. Kates WR, Frederikse M, Mostofsky SH, Folley BS, Cooper K, Mazur-Hopkins P, et al.: MRI parcellation of the frontal lobe in boys with attention deficit hyperactivity disorder or Tourette syndrome. *Psychiatry Res* 116:63–81, 2002.
174. Berquin PC, Giedd JN, Jacobsen LK, Hamburger SD, Krain AL, Rapoport JL, Castellanos FX: Cerebellum in attention deficit hyperactivity disorder: A morphometric MRI study. *Neurology* 50:1087–1093, 1998.
175. Mostofsky SH, Reiss AL, Lockhart P, Denckla MB: Evaluation of the cerebellar size in attention deficit hyperactivity disorder. *J Child Neurol* 13:434–439, 1998.
176. Lou HC, Henricksen L, Bruhn P: Focal cerebral hypoperfusion in children with dysphasia and/or attention deficit hyperactivity disorder. *Arch Neurol* 41(8):825–829, 1984.
177. Lou HC, Henricksen L, Borner H, Nielsen JB: Striatal dysfunction in attention deficit and hyperkinetic disorder. *Arch Neurol* 46(1):48–52, 1989.
178. Lou HC, Henricksen L, Bruhn P: Focal cerebral dysfunction in developmental learning disabilities. *Lancet* 335(8680):8–11, 1990.
179. Lou HC, Andresen J, Steinberg B, McLaughlin T, Friberg L: The striatum in a putative cerebral network activated by verbal awareness in normals and in ADHD children. *Eur J Neurol* 5(1):67–74, 1998.
180. Sieg KG, Gaffney GR, Preston DF, Hellings JA: SPECT brain abnormalities in attention deficit hyperactivity disorder. *Clin Nucl Med* 20(1):55–60, 1995.
181. Amen DG, Carmichael BD: High resolution brain SPECT imaging in ADHD. *Ann Clin Psychiatry* 9(2):81–86, 1997.
182. Langleben DD, Austin G, Krikorian G, Ridlehuber HW, Goris ML, Strauss HW: Interhemispheric asymmetry of regional cerebral blood flow in prepubescent boys with attention deficit hyperactivity disorder. *Nucl Med Commun* 22(12):1333–1340, 2001.
183. Langleben DD, Acton PD, Austin G, et al.: Effects of methylphenidate discontinuation on cerebral blood flow in prepubescent boys with attention deficit hyperactivity disorder. *J Nucl Med* 43(12), 2002.
184. Spalletta G, Pasini A, Pau F, Guido G, Menghini L, Caltagirone C: Prefrontal blood flow dysregulation in drug naive ADHD children without structural abnormalities. *J Neurol Transm* 108(10):1203–1216, 2001.
185. Kim BN, Lee JS, Cho SC, Lee DS: Methylphenidate increased regional cerebral blood flow in subjects with attention deficit hyperactivity disorder. *Yonsei Med J* 42(1):19–29, 2001.
186. Kim BN, Lee JS, Shin MS, Cho SC, Lee DS: Regional cerebral perfusion abnormalities in attention deficit hyperactivity disorder: Statistical parametric mapping analysis. *Eur Arch Psychiatry Clin Neurosci* 252(5):219–225, 2002.
187. Sunshine JL, Lewis JS, Wu DH, et al.: Functional MR to localize sustained visual activation in patients with attention deficit hyperactivity disorder: A pilot study. *AJNR Am J Neuroradiol* 18(4):633–637, 1997.
188. Vaidya CJ, Austin G, Kirkorian G, et al.: Selective effects of methylphenidate in attention deficit hyperactivity disorder: A functional magnetic resonance study. *Proc Natl Acad Sci USA* 95(24):14494–14499, 1998.
189. Bush G, Frazier JA, Rauch SL, et al.: Anterior cingulated cortex dysfunction in attention deficit hyperactivity disorder revealed by fMRI and the Counting Stroop. *Biol Psychiatry* 45(12):1542–1552, 1999.
190. Rubia K, Overmeyer S, Taylor E, et al.: Hypofrontality in attention deficit hyperactivity disorder during higher-order motor control: A study with functional MRI. *Am J Psychiatry* 156(6):891–896, 1999.
191. Teicher MH, Anderson CM, Polcari A, Glod CA, Maas LC, Renshaw PF: Functional deficits in basal ganglia of children with attention deficit hyperactivity disorder shown with functional magnetic resonance imaging relaxometry. *Nat Med* 6(4):470–473, 2000.
192. Anderson CM, Polcari A, Lowen SB, Renshaw PF, Teicher MH: Effects of methylphenidate on functional magnetic resonance relaxometry of the cerebellar vermis in boys with ADHD. *Am J Psychiatry* 159:1322–1328, 2002.
193. Durston S: A review of the biological bases of ADHD: What have we learned from imaging studies? *Ment Retard Dev Disabil Res Rev*; 9:184–195, 2003.
194. Durston S, Tottenham NT, Thomas KM, Davidson MC, Eigsti IM, Yang Y, et al.: Differential patterns of striatal activation in young children with and without ADHD. *Biol Psychiatry* 53:871–878, 2003.
195. Schulz KP, Fan J, Tang CY, Newcorn JH, Buchsbaum MS, Cheung AM, et al.: Response inhibition in adolescents diagnosed with attention deficit hyperactivity disorder during childhood: An event-related FMRI study. *Am J Psychiatry* 161:1650–1657, 2004.
196. Tamm L, Menon V, Ringel J, Reiss AL: Event-related FMRI evidence of frontotemporal involvement in aberrant response inhibition and task switching in attention-deficit/hyperactivity disorder. *J Am Acad Child Adolesc Psychiatry* 43:1430–1440, 2004.
197. Zametkin AJ, Nordahl TE, Gross M, King AC, Semple WE, Rumsey J, et al.: Cerebral glucose metabolism in adults with hyperactivity of childhood onset. *N Engl J Med* 323:1361–1366, 1990.
198. Zametkin AJ, Liebenauer LL, Fitzgerald GA, King AC, Minkunas DV, Herscovitch P, et al.: Brain metabolism in teenagers with attention-deficit hyperactivity disorder. *Arch Gen Psychiatry* 1993; 50:333–340, 1993.
199. Matochik JA, Nordahl TE, Gross M, Semple WE, King AC, Cohen RM, et al.: Effects of acute stimulant medication on cerebral metabolism in adults with hyperactivity. *Neuropsychopharmacology* 8:377–386, 1993.
200. Matochik JA, Liebenauer LL, King AC, Szymanski HV, Cohen RM, Zametkin A: Cerebral glucose metabolism in adults with attention deficit hyperactivity disorder after chronic stimulant treatment. *Am J Psychiatry* 151:658–664, 1994.
201. Ernst M, Liebenauer LL, King AC, Fitzgerald GA, Cohen RM, Zametkin A: Reduced brain metabolism in hyperactive girls. *J Am Acad Child Adolesc Psychiatry* 33:858–868, 1994a.
202. Ernst M, Zametkin AJ, Matochik JA, Liebenauer L, Fitzgerald GA, Cohen RM: Effects of intravenous dextroamphetamine on brain metabolism in adults with attention-deficit hyperactivity disorder (ADHD). Preliminary findings. *Psychopharmacol Bull* 30:219–225, 1994b.
203. Ernst M, Zametkin AJ, Phillips RL, Cohen RM: Age-related changes in brain glucose metabolism in adults with attention-deficit/hyperactivity disorder and control subjects. *J Neuropsychiatry Clin Neurosci* 10:168–177, 1998.
204. Ernst M, Kimes AS, London ED, Matochik JA, Eldreth D, Tata S, et al.: Neural substrates of decision making in adults with attention deficit hyperactivity disorder. *Am J Psychiatry* 160:1061–1070, 2003.
205. Schweitzer JB, Faber TL, Grafton ST, Tune LE, Hoffman JM, Kilts CD: Alterations in the functional anatomy of working memory in adult attention deficit hyperactivity disorder. *Am J Psychiatry* 157:278–280, 2000.
206. Schweitzer JB, Lee DO, Hanford RB, Tagamets MA, Hoffman JM, Grafton ST, et al.: Positron emission tomography study of methylphenidate in adults with ADHD: Alterations in resting blood flow and predicting treatment response. *Neuropsychopharmacology* 28:967–973, 2003.
207. Schweitzer JB, Lee DO, Hanford RB, Zink CF, Ely TD, Tagamets MA, et al.: Effect of methylphenidate on executive functioning in adults with attention-deficit/hyperactivity disorder: Normalization of behavior but not related brain activity. *Biol Psychiatry* 56:597–606, 2004.
208. Dougherty DD, Bonab AA, Spencer TJ, Rauch SL, Madras BK, Fischman AJ: Dopamine transporter density in patients with attention deficit hyperactivity disorder. *Lancet* 354:2132–2133, 1999.
209. Dresel S, Krause J, Krause KH, LaFougere C, Brinkbaumer K, Kung HF, et al.: Attention deficit hyperactivity disorder: Binding of [99mTc] TRODAT-1 to the dopamine transporter before and after methylphenidate treatment. *Eur J Nucl Med* 27:1518–1524, 2000.
210. Cheon KA, Ryu YH, Kim YK, Namkoong K, Kim CH, Lee JD (2003): Dopamine transporter density in the basal ganglia assessed with [123I] IPT SPECT in children with attention deficit hyperactivity disorder. *Eur J Nucl Med Mol Imaging* 30:306–311, 2003.
211. van Dyck CH, Quinlan DM, Cretella LM, Staley JK, Malison RT, Baldwin RM, et al. (2002): Unaltered dopamine transporter availability in adult attention deficit hyperactivity disorder. *Am J Psychiatry* 159:309–312, 2002.
212. Spencer T: *In vivo* neuroreceptor imaging of attention-deficit/hyperactivity disorder: A focus on the dopamine transporter. *Biol Psychiatry* 57:1293–1300, 2005.
213. Spencer TJ, Biederman J, Ciccone PE, Madras BK, Dougherty DD, Bonab AA, Livni El, Parasrampuria DA, Fischman AJ: PET study examining pharmacokinetics, detection and likeability, and dopamine transporter receptor occupancy of short- and long-acting oral methylphenidate. *American Journal of Psychiatry* 163:3; 387–395, 2006.
214. Jucaite A, Fernell E, Halldin C, Forssberg H, Farde L: Reduced midbrain dopamine transporter binding in male adolescents with attention-deficit/hyperactivity disorder: Association between striatal dopamine markers and motor hyperactivity. *Biol Psychiatry* 57:229–238, 2005.
215. Rosa-Neto P, Lou H, Cumming P, Pryds O, Karrebaek H, Lunding J, Gjedde A—Methylphenidate evoked changes in striatal dopamine correlate with inattention and impulsivity in adolescents with attention deficit hyperactivity disorder. *NeuroImage* 25:868–876, 2005.
216. Jin Z, Zang YF, Zeng YW, Zhang L, Wang YF: Striatal neuronal loss or dysfunction and choline rise in children with attention-deficit hyperactivity disorder: A 1H-magnetic resonance spectroscopy study. *Neurosci Lett* 315:45–48, 2001.
217. MacMaster FP, Carrey N, Sparkes S, Kusumakar V—Proton spectroscopy in medication free pediatric attention deficit hyperactivity disorder. *Biol Psychiatry* 53:184–187, 2003.

218. Yeo RA, Hill DE, Campbell RA, Vigil J, Petropoulos H, Hart B, et al.: Proton magnetic resonance spectroscopy investigation of the right frontal lobe in children with attention-deficit/hyperactivity disorder. *J Am Acad Child Adolesc Psychiatry* 42:303–310, 2003.
219. Courvoisie H, Hooper SR, Fine Camille, Kwock L, Castillo M—Neurometabolic functioning and neuropsychological correlates in children with ADHD-H: Preliminary findings. *J Neuropsychiatry Clin Neurosci* 16:63–69, 2004.
220. Moore CM, Biederman J, Wozniak J, Mick E, Aleardi M, Wardrop M, Dougherty M, Harpold T, Hammerness P, Randall E, Renshaw PF: Differences in brain chemistry in children and adolescents with attention deficit hyperactivity disorder with and without comorbid bipolar disorder: A proton magnetic resonance spectroscopy study. *Am J Psychiatry* 163:316–318, 2006.
221. Kinsbourne M: Minimal brain dysfunction as a neurodevelopmental lag. *Ann N Y Acad Sci* 205:268–273, 1973.
222. Satterfield J, Lesser M, Saul R, Cantwell D: EEG aspects in the diagnosis and treatment of minimal brain dysfunction. *Ann N Y Acad Sci* 205:274–282, 1973.
223. Matsuura M, Ojubo Y, Toru M, Kojima T, He Y, Hou Y, Shen Y, Lee C: A cross national EEG study of children with emotional and behavioural problems: A WHO collaborative study in the Western Pacific region. *Biol Psychiatry* 34:52–58, 1993.
224. John E, Princhep L, Easton P: Normative data banks and neurometrics: Basic concepts, method and results of norm construction. In: Gevins A, Remond, A (ed.): Handbook of Electroencephalography and Clinical Neurophysiology 1. Amsterdam, Elsevier, 1987, pp. 919–923.
225. Clarke A, Barry R, McCarthy R, Selikowitz M: EEG analysis in attention deficit hyperactivity disorder: A comparative study of two subtypes. *Psychiat Res* 81:19–29, 1998.
226. Lazzaro I, Gordon E, Whitmont S, Plahn M, Li W, Clarke S, Dosen A, Meares R: Quantitative EEG activity in adolescent attention deficit hyperactivity disorder. *Clin Electroencephalogr* 29:37–42, 1998.
227. Klinkerfuss G, Lange P, Weinberg W, O'Leary J: Electroencephalographic abnormalities of children with hyperkinetic behaviour. *Neurology* 15:883–891, 1965.
228. Wikler A, Dixon J, Parker J: Brain function in children and controls: Psychometric, neurological and electroencephalographic comparisons. *Am J Psychiatry* 127:634–645, 1970.
229. John E, Princhep L, Ahn H, Easton P, Fridman J, Kaye H: Neurometric evaluation of cognitive dysfunctions and neurological disorders in children. *Prog Neurobiol* 21:239–290, 1983.
230. Clarke A, Barry R, McCarthy R, Selikowitz M: EEG differences in two subtypes of attention deficit hyperactivity disorder. *Psychophysiology* 38:212–221, 2001.
231. Clarke A, Barry R, McCarthy R, Selikowitz M: EEG defined subtypes of children with attention deficit hyperactivity disorder. *Clin Neurophysiol* 112:2098–2105, 2001.
232. Satterfield J, Cantwell D: CNS function and response to methylphenidate in hyperactive children. *Psychopharmacol Bull* 10:36–37, 1974.
233. Satterfield J, Cantwell D, Saul R, Lesser M, Podsin R: Response to stimulant drug treatment in hyperactive children: Predictions from EEG and neurological findings. *J Autism Child Schizophr* 3:36–48, 1973.
234. Satterfield J, Cantwell D, Satterfield B: Pathophysiology of the hyperactive child syndrome. *Arch Gen Psychiatry* 31:839–844, 1974.
235. Grunewald-Zuberbier E, Grunewald G, Rasche A: Hyperactive behaviour and EEG arousal reactions in children. *Electroenceph Clin Neurophysiol* 38:149–159, 1975.
236. Ackerman P, Dykman R, Oglesby D, Newton J: EEG power spectra of children with dyslexia, slow learners, and normally reading children with ADD during verbal processing. *J Learn Disabil* 27:619–630, 1994.
237. Lubar J, Swartwood J, O'Donnell P: Evaluation of the effectiveness of EEG neurofeedback training for ADHD in a clinical setting as measured by changes in T.O.V.A. scores, behavioral ratings, and WISC-R performance. *Biofeedback Self Regul* 20:83–99, 1995.

CHAPTER 5.2.2 ■ OPPOSITIONAL DEFIANT AND CONDUCT DISORDERS

JOSEPH M. REY, GARRY WALTER, AND CESAR A. SOUTULLO

> ... His academic performance declined, he became more sullen and argumentative, was occasionally truant or caught lying about his whereabouts, did not adhere to curfews, and had joined in with other troubled teenagers. His mother was sure that he had been stealing money from her purse, possibly to buy cigarettes. The teachers at school had also become concerned about his increasingly unruly behavior and advised his parents to seek professional help.

Young people with the kind of problems described in this brief vignette represent the largest single group of patients seen in child and adolescent mental health settings; they are usually labeled as suffering from oppositional defiant disorder (ODD), conduct disorder (CD), or disruptive behavior disorder (DBD). The cost of these conditions to the individuals themselves, their families, and society is high (1, 2). Leaving aside personal and family suffering and the burden to health services, most juvenile delinquent acts are perpetrated by individuals with CD (3). The number of publications dealing with DBDs is enormous and growing exponentially.

Some professionals describe these children as having a "behavior disorder," which often has negative connotations or implies that the condition is nonpsychiatric, that is, that children are "bad" rather than "mad." However, the DBDs have diagnostic validity because i) symptoms intercorrelate highly, suggesting coherent syndromes rather than an aggregate of various types of deviance; ii) a genetic component is increasingly being documented; iii) these problems are recognized in every society and historical period; and iv) although prevalence may vary with time and place, this also applies to almost all mental and physical disorders (4). While a categorical diagnosis is useful to facilitate communication and clinical decisionmaking, evidence suggests that a dimensional understanding of these disorders might be more helpful, particularly in research.

These "bad kids" have a particularly negative outcome in adulthood. They are more likely to have psychiatric disorders, to show difficulties at work, and to be involved in violent relationships and marriages (5–8). In turn, these behaviors increase the chances of similar problems in their offspring, often abused or neglected by them, thus perpetuating the disorder (9). The challenge lies in finding ways to break this unfortunate cycle.

A pioneer in this area already suggested in 1935 of the children in question that "a strict definition or delimitation of the [component] groups is difficult because they tend to merge with each other" (10). Indeed, individuals with ODD and CD share many characteristics. For example, their conduct is socially unacceptable, they cause disruption or distress to others more than to themselves (i.e., they "externalize" their problems), and they are more likely to be male and to find it difficult to learn from experience. Yet, they also differ widely from one another: They may be aggressive or not, break the law or not, feel guilt and empathy or not, may be sensation-seeking or not. Although ODD and CD represent well characterized, reliable behavioral syndromes, they do not fit easily into a traditional "illness" model because children with these problems are heterogeneous in relation to etiology, natural history, response to treatment, and outcome. This is similar to what happens with heart disease, where multiple factors contribute to the pathology and other illness characteristics, but the construct has heuristic value. Because of their heterogeneity, the usefulness of a diagnosis of ODD or CD for treatment planning is limited; an emphasis on identifying each child's problems and modifying the individual risk factors is likely to be the best way of managing these disorders, as is the case with heart disease.

Although the issue of whether these diagnoses represent independent conditions is unresolved (11, 12), ODD and CD are described together to highlight their similarities and differences and to avoid unnecessary repetitions. The content of this chapter overlaps and should be read in conjunction with topics discussed in other parts of the book, particularly those on Aggression in Children (Chapter 5.2.3), Fire Behavior in Children and Adolescents (Chapter 5.2.4), and the section on Juvenile Delinquency (included in Chapter 6.3.3).

HISTORICAL NOTE

Understanding of the DBDs has been closely linked to the study of delinquency, largely conceptualized in the past as a failure in moral development or "moral insanity." Lombroso, an Italian psychiatrist, gained prominence at the end of the 19th century with his theory that some individuals were born criminal. About 50 years later Cleckley (13) coined the concept of "psychopathy." According to him, psychopaths lacked remorse, were unable to have close relationships, were egocentric, and showed poverty of affect but, contrary to the prevailing opinion, were not necessarily aggressive or criminal. Although this concept of psychopathy was initially applied to antisocial adults, it was soon extended to young people. Psychoanalytic theories were postulating that the behavior had its origins in childhood and was the result of a poorly developed superego, thus opening the way to therapeutic interventions. Interest in juvenile delinquents, which had begun with Aichhorn's *Wayward Youth* (10), impelled Bowlby (14) to examine these youth's early experiences and ultimately led to the development of attachment theory. Robins (5) demonstrated the continuity between childhood conduct problems and adult antisocial personality, stressing their long-term implications. Levy (15) first described the syndrome of childhood oppositionality, which he characterized as the refusal to conform to the ordinary requirements of authority, or willful contrariness. The second half of the twentieth century saw the inclusion of these disorders in the psychiatric taxonomies, their splitting off from attention deficit hyperactivity disorder (ADHD), growing elucidation of their determinants and comorbidity, their implications for public health, and the development of preventive measures.

CLASSIFICATION

Definition

DSM-I (16) included no childhood disorders. DSM-II (17) listed a category of Unsocialized Aggressive Reaction of Childhood (or Adolescence), Group Delinquent Reaction and Runaway Reaction as the closest equivalents to CD. The category of CD was officially introduced in DSM-III (18) to describe children who showed a persistent pattern of behavior in which the basic rights of others or major age-appropriate societal norms or rules are violated, the definition still used in both DSM-IV (19) and ICD-10 (20). DSM-III also listed Oppositional Disorder to characterize children who show persistently disobedient, negativistic and provocative opposition to authority figures, manifested by violations of minor rules, temper tantrums, argumentativeness, provocative behavior and stubbornness. This description remains in DSM-IV (19) as Oppositional Defiant Disorder.

DSM-IV and ICD-10 Diagnostic Criteria

Diagnostic criteria for ODD and CD according to DSM-IV TR (21) and ICD-10 (20) are summarized in Table 5.2.2.1. Both taxonomies require the absence of CD to allow a diagnosis of ODD (i.e., implying a hierarchical relationship). ICD-10 explicitly conceptualizes ODD as part of the same dimension as CD, the former being a milder version of the latter (thus, the term conduct disorder often means ODD *and* CD in countries where ICD-10 terminology is used). In spite of the efforts made to homogenize the main classification systems, a conceptual divide remains. Yet, diagnostic criteria are very similar (Table 5.2.2.1) and differences largely reflect the time requirements for symptoms to be present, exclusion criteria, and the way both taxonomies deal with comorbidity. Using ICD-10 criteria seems to result in more children qualifying for ODD than when using DSM-IV criteria (40% more cases in one study) (22). This is because many children have symptoms of both ODD and CD but not enough to meet criteria for either diagnosis according to DSM-IV (for example two symptoms of each). Children diagnosed as suffering from ODD by ICD-10 but not by DSM-IV do not seem to differ in any respect from those diagnosed by DSM-IV, suggesting that DSM-IV criteria may be too strict or too narrow (22).

Empirical Approaches to Taxonomy

Empirical classifications (23) based on statistical analysis of symptoms have found an aggressive syndrome, which comprises symptoms of both ODD and CD, like destroying objects, bullying, fighting, and vandalism, and a delinquent or rule-breaking syndrome, characterized by stealing, lying, and truancy, which entails features of CD alone. Several types of aggressive behavior have also been identified (see Chapter 5.2.3) Dimensional taxonomies overlap with categorical diagnoses and are widely used to supplement each other and for research (23). The pros and cons of each are discussed in Chapter 4.1.

Subtypes of CD

Subtyping is important given the heterogeneity of CD. Subgroups may have implications for prevention, treatment, and prognosis. However, much disagreement still exists, exemplified by changes to the subtypes of CD listed in each edition of the DSM. DSM-III (18) divided CD into four subgroups according to whether children were socialized or undersocialized, and aggressive or nonaggressive. This was changed in DSM-III-R to "solitary type" and "group type." DSM-IV (21) classifies CD according to age of onset (childhood or adolescent onset type, depending on whether there were symptoms prior to the age of 10 years). ICD-10 (20) describes three subtypes of CD: confined to the family context, unsocialized, and socialized.

Some researchers have emphasized the importance of overt (characterized by confrontation and fighting) and covert

TABLE 5.2.2.1

DIAGNOSTIC CRITERIA FOR OPPOSITIONAL DEFIANT DISORDER (ODD) AND CONDUCT DISORDER (CD) ACCORDING TO DSM-IV (TR) (21) AND ICD-10 (20)

Symptoms*
1. Often loses temper [ICD-10: *Unusually frequent or sever temper tantrums for developmental level*] 2. Often argues with adults 3. Often actively defies or refuses to comply with adults' requests or rules 4. Often deliberately annoys people 5. Often blames others for his or her mistakes or misbehavior 6. Is often touchy or easily annoyed by others 7. Is often angry and resentful 8. Is often spiteful and vindictive
9. Often bullies, threatens or intimidates others 10. Often initiates physical fights [ICD-10: *This does not include fights with siblings*] 11. Has used a weapon that can cause serious physical harm to others 12. Has been physically cruel to people 13. Has been physically cruel to animals 14. Has stolen while confronting a victim (including purse-snatching, extortion, mugging) 15. Has forced someone into sexual activity 16. Has deliberately engaged in fire setting with the intention of causing serious damage 17. Has deliberately destroyed others' property (other than fire setting) 18. Has broken into someone's house, building or car 19. Often lies to obtain goods or favors or to avoid obligations 20. Has stolen items of nontrivial value without confronting a victim [ICD-10: *Within the home or outside*] 21. Often stays out at night despite parental prohibitions, beginning before age 13 years 22. Has run away from home overnight at least twice while living in parental or parental surrogate home (or once without returning for a lengthy period) [ICD-10: *Or has run away once for more than a single night (this does not include leaving to avoid physical or sexual abuse)*] 23. Often truants from school, beginning before age 13 years
■ *DSM-IV ODD*: Four or more of symptoms from 1 to 8, lasting at least 6 months, symptoms do not occur exclusively during a psychotic or mood disorder episode. ■ *ICD-10 Oppositional Defiant Conduct Disorder*: four or more symptoms must be present during 6 months, but no more than two must be from symptoms 9 to 23. ■ Symptoms must be developmentally inappropriate in both DSM-IV and ICD-10.
■ *DSM-IV CD*: Three or more of symptoms from 9 to 23 in the last 12 months (at least one present in last 6 months) ■ *ICD-10 CD*: three or more symptoms must be present, and at least three must be from 9 to 23. At least one symptom from 9 to 23 must be present for 6 months. Symptoms 11, 12, 14, 15, 16, 17, and 18 need only have occurred once for the criterion to be fulfilled. ■ *Impairment*: Symptoms must cause significant functional impairment in both taxonomies.
*Symptom descriptions are summarized slightly. When description is different between DSM-IV and ICD-10, relevant ICD-10 wording is added. Shaded areas refer to ODD.

(typified by deception, such as stealing and lying) symptoms (24), which overlaps with the aggressive–nonaggressive distinction. There are data showing that two different types of covert antisocial behavior may exist: property violations (e.g., stealing) and status offenses (truancy, running away) (24, 25). Other scholars suggest that life-course persistent (beginning during childhood and persisting past adolescence) and adolescence limited may be a useful distinction (26).

Comorbidity

The vexatious issue of comorbidity (27), which presents numerous, still unresolved theoretical and practical questions (discussed in Chapter 4.1) is highly relevant for ODD and CD since both often cooccur with other diagnoses. The most frequent comorbidities are with ADHD [about 10 times more often than expected (27)], major depression [about seven times (27)], and substance abuse [in adolescents, about four times (28)]. According to ICD-10 (20), CD is not diagnosed if ADHD is present (it would warrant a diagnosis of hyperkinetic conduct disorder), or if CD is associated with emotional disorders (mixed disorder of conduct and emotions). In similar circumstances, DSM-IV (21) requires multiple diagnoses to be made (e.g., ODD *and* ADHD, CD *and* major depression). Evidence about the best way of conceptualizing these problems (e.g., ODD and ADHD: two coexisting disorders vs. one condition different from both ODD and ADHD) is lacking. Boys with CD and ADHD have an earlier age of onset of disruptive behavior symptoms and worse outcome than those without ADHD (27), and ADHD symptoms in children with ODD may increase the likelihood of progression to CD. Less is known about individuals with DBDs and comorbid emotional disorders besides depression, but anxiety and somatoform disorders also appear to be more frequent than expected (29).

Reliability

The diagnoses of ODD and CD have acceptable interrater and test-retest reliability, comparable to the reliability of most psychiatric diagnoses in young people (30–32). Agreement varies according to the informant and age of the child, being usually higher when parent or teacher reports or multiple informants are used, for aggressive than nonaggressive behaviors, and in older children or adolescents (33). Reliability is also higher in clinic than in community samples due to base rate issues. For example, test-retest agreement of CD using the NIMH Diagnostic Interview Schedule for Children Version IV in a clinic sample was κ 0.70 for parents as informants, 0.86 for children, and 0.71 when using data from both. The parallel results in a community sample were 0.56, 0.64, and 0.66 (32). Reliability of ODD is lower, in the range of $\kappa = 0.4 - 0.6$ (30, 32).

Validity

Developmental Considerations

Children's prosocial impulses already become apparent in the first year of life, for example through cooperative interactions and sharing. Learning how to deal with and tolerate frustration are important aspects of the socialization process. A degree of defiance and noncompliance is normal in toddlers, probably reflecting the child's assertiveness and search for autonomy or ignorance of what parents are prepared to tolerate. Notwithstanding this, toddler's behavior may already be indicative of problems when it is too intense, persistent, or pervasive. However, there are considerable individual variations and distinguishing behaviors that are within the normal range from problematic defiance or noncompliance is difficult at that age. Prosocial behaviors usually increase up to the age of three years; a temporary decline then begins to emerge. Defiance and noncompliance, particularly in boys, may also increase about the age of two or three years. For the development of aggression, please see Chapter 5.2.3.

ODD symptoms appear earlier than CD symptoms (e.g., stubbornness at a median age of 3 years, defiance and temper tantrums at 5, argumentativeness at 6, compared with lying at 8, bullying at 9, and stealing at 12 years) (34). Aggressive behavior (hitting, biting, smashing objects) is common in 4- to 8-year-olds and decreases with age, although severely aggressive acts typically start after puberty. Covert antisocial actions such as property and status violations (stealing, truancy, running away) increase as children become older, being more prevalent during adolescence. Early adolescence is often associated with an increase in rebellious behavior. Teachers' reports indicate that most oppositional symptoms, such as arguing, screaming, disobedience, and defiance peak between 8 and 11 years and then decline in frequency (35).

Stability and Change

Disruptive behaviours are quite prevalent in children but often extinguish as they grow older. However, many data show that CD symptoms are more enduring than changeable. Research corrected for measurement error, which is considerable, suggests that stability may be even greater than previously thought (36). This may be partly explained by symptoms of conduct disorder becoming increasingly varied with the passage of time while showing a growing resistance to change (37).

ODD and CD

The relationship between ODD and CD is complex. In some children, ODD symptoms begin in infancy, persist during childhood, and evolve into CD, often after puberty. Other young people show noncompliance and defiance for short periods or do not progress to CD; this may occur more often in females than in males (38). Oppositional behavior is present only at home in some children, while symptoms occur in most settings in others. ODD often starts in the family context and generalizes to other settings over time.

Adult Outcomes

The continuity between childhood CD and adult antisocial personality disorder (ASPD) has long been known (5, 6, 39), so much so that DSM-IV (21) requires evidence of CD prior to the age of 15 years for a diagnosis of ASPD. The validity of this requirement, particularly in females, has been questioned (40). A diagnosis of ASPD is only allowed after the age of 18 years (DSM-IV) (36), but there is support for the view that such a diagnosis may be appropriate in some adolescents (41).

Data are mounting showing that childhood DBDs are associated not only with ASPD but with a wide range of other psychiatric disorders in adulthood (e.g., substance abuse, major depression, psychosis), as well as with many adverse outcomes such as suicidal behavior, delinquency, educational difficulties, unemployment, and teenage pregnancy (7, 8, 42–47). The association, which applies equally to males and females (8), reflects not only the already noted stability of disruptive behaviors, but also the fact that childhood DBDs often trigger a chain of events that increase the likelihood of such unfavorable outcomes (for example, early defiance may lead to harsh parental discipline, aggressiveness, and peer rejection, which may in turn be followed by association with deviant peers, antisocial acts, substance use, conflict with the law, and mental illness). It has been argued that much of the research on which these findings are based has significant limitations because studies tend to focus on one specific outcome, such as psychiatric disorder or substance use, and because they often examine consequences over a limited followup period. However, when these weaknesses are circumvented, childhood DBDs are still associated with a wide range of unfavorable adult outcomes, which attests to the robustness of the links (8). Further, studies by and large show a dose–response relationship: The higher the number and variety of disruptive behaviors, the worse the adult outcomes. This said, most adolescents with CD do not develop ASPD in adulthood. A large decline in delinquent and antisocial activities is a commonly reported phenomenon in early adulthood (3, 48). It is not clear if this parallels a reduction in DBDs or if their manifestations change with age (e.g., whether behaviors extinguish, mutate into other psychiatric problems, or delinquent acts become more covert). This decline may reflect the existence of a desisting adolescent-limited—as opposite to a life-course persistent—CD (26). Early onset, severity, and exposure to risk factors would predict the latter group (48).

Most epidemiological studies in adults have neglected to examine the prevalence of childhood-onset disorders, the exception being a recent survey of people older than 18 years in the United States, which reported a 12- month prevalence of 1% each for ODD and CD (49). This shows DBDs can be found in adults although it is not clear whether they appear *de novo* or are a continuation of childhood problems.

There is little information about the adult consequences of children with ODD who do not develop CD. Passive-aggressive personality disorder has been hypothesized as one of the outcomes but there are no data supporting this (6).

EPIDEMIOLOGY

Prevalence

Estimates of the prevalence of ODD and CD vary depending on the population, diagnostic criteria, instrument, period considered (point or lifetime), and informant. Recent surveys using DSM-IV criteria have produced reasonably consistent results, summarized in Table 5.2.2.2. Overall, about 5% of children aged 6 to 18 years met DSM-IV criteria for ODD or CD in the previous 3 or 6 months, slightly lower rates than those reported in earlier studies using DSM-III or DSM-IIIR criteria (50).

TABLE 5.2.2.2

POINT PREVALENCE (PERCENT) OF DSM-IV OPPOSITIONAL DEFIANT DISORDER (ODD) AND CONDUCT DISORDER (CD) IN RECENT EPIDEMIOLOGICAL STUDIES USING DSM-IV CRITERIA

	ODD					CD				
Sample	Male	Female	Children	Adolescents	TOTAL	Male	Female	Children	Adolescents	TOTAL
3171 Australian children aged 6 to 17 years (55)						4.4	1.6	4.4[1]	2.4[2]	3.0
1420 children from North Carolina aged 9 to 13 years (51)	3.1	2.1	2.0[1]	3.0[2]	2.7	4.2	1.2	2.4[1]	2.7[2]	2.7
10438 British 5 to 15 year olds (56)	3.2	1.4	2.6[3]	1.4[4]	2.3	2.1	0.8	0.9[3]	3.3[4]	1.5
1886 children aged 4 to 17 years from Puerto Rico (57)					2.0					5.5
1251 children aged 7 to 14 years attending school in Southeastern Brazil (58)					3.2					2.2
Average across studies	3.2	1.8	2.3	2.2	2.6	3.4	1.2	2.6	2.8	3.0

[1]9 to 12 years of age;
[2]13 to 16 years of age;
[3]5 to 12 years of age;
[4]13 to 15 years of age;

However, the proportion that has met criteria for either ODD or CD at any time before 16 years of age (lifetime rate) is higher respectively for girls and boys; ODD: 9.1%, 13.4%; CD: 3.8%, 14.1% (51). As noted, prevalence of ODD is elevated when using ICD-10 compared with DSM-IV criteria (22).

Epidemiological surveys in the developing world are few and have methodological shortcomings. A recent study in Bangladesh reported prevalence of ODD ranging from 5.2% (slum dwellers) to 6.7% (urban dwellers) and of CD from 6.0% (slum) to 0.4% (urban) (52), while a survey in Bangalore found much lower rates (0.9% for ODD and 0.2% for CD) (53). An examination of questionnaire data of 6- to 17-year-olds from nine cultures showed that cultural differences had a small effect on the delinquent behavior (1%) and aggressive behavior (5%) syndromes (54). ODD and CD are two to three times more prevalent in males than females, though this may vary according to age. Earlier studies suggested that ODD was more prevalent in children (this was incorporated in ICD-10, where diagnosis of ODD is discouraged after the age of 10 years) while CD was more prevalent in adolescents. Epidemiological data is inconsistent with this view; prevalence across studies is similar in both age groups (Table 5.2.2.2).

Secular Changes

It has been suggested that children, particularly females, born later in the twentieth century show higher rates of antisocial behavior than those born earlier (59). This is difficult to verify given the limitations of epidemiological surveys (e.g., changes in diagnostic criteria over time). Indirect approaches, such as variations in juvenile delinquency rates or arrests, are also hazardous because of legal and law enforcement changes over time. However, it is likely that rates may fluctuate. For example, U.S. data suggest an increase in externalizing problems from the late 1970s to the early 1990s, subsequently followed by a fall (60), while a study in the U.K. examining trends in adolescent behavioral and emotional problems between 1974 and 1999 reported a substantial increase in adolescent conduct problems for both genders in that period (61). The pioneering Isle of Wight study (62) conducted in the 1960s showed a prevalence of conduct disorder (which would have included children later diagnosed with ODD and CD) among 10–11 year olds of 4.2%, not dissimilar to the rates reported in recent studies (Table 5.2.2.2).

ETIOLOGY

The literature on etiologic and risk factors for disruptive disorders is voluminous and compelling, but rather nonspecific; it makes reference to ODD, CD, aggression, juvenile offending, and disruptive behaviors defined in a variety of ways (e.g., 63–71); data specific to ODD are scarce. This is not necessarily a major issue given the nature and heterogeneity of ODD/CD. Dodge and Pettit (72) note that the model used to study and treat or prevent heart disease is equally applicable to disruptive behavior problems. Both are vaguely defined, heterogeneous constructs but with easily identifiable outcomes, such as a myocardial infarction or, in the case of disruptive behaviors, an assault. While the traditional goal in medicine is to identify a cluster of symptoms and then to seek a single causal agent, this is not appropriate for heart disease or DBDs, where a single causal agent does not exist. Multiple risk factors or vulnerabilities contribute to the development of heart disease and CD, and their recognition has allowed the implementation of successful preventive interventions.

Heritability of antisocial behavior has been estimated at about 50%, though it is not diagnosis specific (73). It ought to be kept in mind that "heritability is a statistic that applies to population variance and not to individuals or to traits as a fixed feature. A high heritability means that genetic factors account for much of the variation in the liability to show a particular trait in a particular population at a particular point in time. It does not mean that genetic factors play a major role in the causation of that trait in any one individual" (71).

Well known risk factors are listed in Table 5.2.2.3. It is important to emphasize that a large component of the association between risk factors, DBDs, and poor outcomes is probably noncausal, but these factors make the prognosis worse than it should have been. Risk factors include, among others, socioeconomic disadvantage, exposure to dysfunctional family environments, lower IQ, and attentional difficulties (8, 63–71). Absence of these circumstances or attributes can be positively conceptualized as "resilience" or "protective" factors (e.g., comfortable background, a supportive and caring family, higher intelligence).

Interactions between etiological and risk factors are complex. First, the accumulation of risk may not only act additively, but also multiplicatively; for example, impulsivity may convey a small risk for a child developing CD, but in combination with other factors (e.g. poor socializing experiences, harsh discipline) the risk for antisocial outcomes becomes quite high. Second, while genes are important, they interact with, and are modified by environmental variables in complex ways (71) (See also Chapter 3.2.) Thus, it has been shown that genetic influences are stronger in children from poor families than in those from affluent backgrounds (74), and that heritability of problem behavior is significantly lower in children with very low birth weight in relation to gestational age than in those with a normal birth weight (75). Third, genetic factors influence individuals' choice and shaping of their own environment (71). In this line, active children tend to participate in sports and energetic activities; antisocial individuals are more likely to find problematic partners (assortative mating) (76). Fourth, the same risk factor may have different consequences depending on other circumstances. For example, while parental separation increases the risk of DBDs in the children, it may actually reduce that risk if separation means losing contact with an antisocial father (66).

It is firmly established that CD is more prevalent among disadvantaged families, though this applies to relative deprivation; the risk seems to flow from being worse off than other people rather than from the absolute level of poverty (77). An ingenious natural experiment in North Carolina confirmed this but also showed that reducing poverty among American Indian families resulted in a reduction in behavior problems in their children (78). The mechanisms by which this occurred do not seem directly monetary. Rather, higher incomes resulted in more parents working, fewer single parents, fewer demands on parents' time, and ultimately better parental supervision, which probably led to the change.

Low resting heart rate, probably reflecting autonomic underarousal, is the best replicated biological correlate of

TABLE 5.2.2.3

SUMMARY OF FACTORS ASSOCIATED WITH THE DEVELOPMENT OF DISRUPTIVE BEHAVIOR DISORDERS AND OPPORTUNITIES FOR PREVENTION

Risk Factor	Potential Prevention Interventions
Biological	
■ Genetic ■ Low birth weight ■ Antenatal, and perinatal complications ■ Brain injury, brain disease ■ Male sex	■ Improved antenatal, prenatal, and obstetric care. ■ Quit smoking and drug treatment programs targeted to intending parents ■ Programs to reduce domestic violence
Individual	
■ Below average IQ ■ Difficult temperament ■ Aggressiveness ■ Impulsivity and hyperactivity ■ Attentional problems ■ Language impairment ■ Reading problems	■ Early identification, adequate support and services for families and individuals with mental retardation ■ Quality home visiting programs which aim to facilitate attachment and enhance parenting skills ■ Parent management training programs ■ Head Start–type programs ■ Early speech and reading remediation programs
Family	
■ Parental antisocial behavior or substance use ■ Domestic violence ■ Single parent, divorce ■ Harsh discipline, maltreatment, or neglect ■ Parent–child conflict ■ Lack of parental supervision ■ Excessive parental control ■ Maternal depression and anxiety ■ Early motherhood	■ Quality home visitation programs ■ Parent management training programs ■ Programs to reduce domestic violence ■ Drug-treatment programs ■ Child protection initiatives ■ Early identification and treatment of maternal depression ■ Prevention of teenage pregnancy ■ Support programs for teenage mothers
Social and School	
■ Poverty ■ Association with deviant peers/siblings ■ Rejection by peers ■ History of victimization or of being bullied ■ Disorganized, disadvantaged, or high crime neighborhoods ■ Dysfunctional or disorganized schools ■ Intense exposure to media violence	■ Measures to reduce poverty and provide a social safety net ■ Enhance the quality of schools ■ School programs to reduce bullying and prevent behavior problems ■ Initiatives to reduce access to firearms, and gang activities ■ Programs to reduce school truancy ■ Initiatives to enhance neighborhood cohesion ■ Law enforcement initiatives to reduce crime targeted to high-crime areas ■ Public campaigns to reduce media violence and education about how to monitor and prevent children's exposure to it

antisocial behavior in children and adolescents, although its meaning is still poorly understood (79). Studies using a range of imaging techniques have enabled speculation about the brain regions that may be involved in ODD and CD. The frontal lobe in particular has been a focus of attention. Thus, it has been suggested that atypical frontal lobe activation, as detected on EEG, is a basis for negative affective style in children with ODD (80). Positron emission tomography has shown violence to be associated with decreased glucose metabolism in the prefrontal cortex (81), and orbitofrontal lobe damage has been linked to impulsive aggression (82). In a sample of boys with conduct problems, those with a history of rule violations failed to exhibit the normal maturational increase in frontal P300 amplitude that was found among boys without such a history (83). Research has also focused on the role of various neurotransmitters, with serotonin having received most attention; there is a suggested link between aggression and low levels of serotonin in the CNS (e.g., 84) (see Chapter 5.2.3).

DIAGNOSIS

Diagnostic Assessment

An evaluation performed by an experienced clinician based on information from multiple sources and supplemented by questionnaire data should allow making a diagnosis of ODD or CD quite reliable. Diagnostic assessment is discussed in detail in Section 4.2.2. Given the type of problems shown by children with DBDs, it is important to clarify to all concerned the purpose of the evaluation from the outset. Assessment may be requested by parents, schools, courts, children's lawyers, or social services. The purpose will influence how the assessment is conducted and the tone of the interviews. This may also pose limitations to confidentiality, which should be explained to the relevant parties. Building rapport with and achieving cooperation from these children is often problematic because of their difficulty accepting ownership of their actions and hostility to authority figures. Often they do not see a distinction between mental health professionals, parents, teachers, and police. Thus, noncooperation and resistance to disclose information are to be expected, so much so that patients who are too forthcoming with details of their deeds should raise concern (85). Because referral is often triggered by a disciplinary or legal crisis after months or, more often, years of discord, clinicians are usually confronted with stressed, angry families who are unable to see anything positive in one another.

Reports from children, parents, or teachers may disagree but these sets of information often complement each other. Since sexual abuse, inconsistent parenting, maternal depression, and parental drug use are not uncommon in these children's backgrounds, these areas need to be explored carefully. Learning as much as possible about the parenting style, parent–child interactions, and the child's strengths and relationships with peers will be valuable when planning and delivering treatment.

Normality and Disorder

The developmental issues noted raise the question of the boundaries between disorder and extremes of normal behavior. ICD-10 states that judgments concerning the presence of ODD/CD should take into account the child's developmental level. Temper tantrums, for example, are a normal part of a 3-year-old's development and mere presence would not be grounds for diagnosis. While there is much evidence that children who display symptoms of ODD or CD persistently and intensely are significantly impaired (e.g., 86), it is also clear that a continuum of symptoms exist and that children with a subsyndromal level of diagnostic criteria can be equally impaired (22).

Gender and Age

Rather than physical attack, females are more prone to use indirect, verbal, and relational violence such as ostracism and character defamation (87). These behaviors can be difficult to document, are not clearly described as CD symptoms, and may result in underdiagnosis of CD in girls (50).

The age at which a valid diagnosis of ODD or CD can be made is unresolved. For example, ICD-10 states that a violation of other people's civic rights (such as by violent crime) is not within the capacity of most 7-year-olds and so it is not a necessary diagnostic criterion for that age group. Nevertheless, a valid diagnosis of ODD or CD may be made in preschoolers (88, 89). Conversely, the ICD-10 statement warning about diagnosing ODD after the age of 10 years is without foundation, since as many young people qualify for ODD in adolescence as in childhood (Table 5.2.2.2). Further, even some adults may meet criteria for ODD or CD (49).

Social and Cultural Context

DSM-IV highlights that a diagnosis of CD should be made only when the behavior in question is symptomatic of an underlying dysfunction within the individual and not simply a reaction to the immediate social or cultural context. This is to circumvent concerns that a diagnosis of CD may at times be misapplied to individuals in particular settings (threatening, impoverished, high-crime, war) where patterns of undesirable behavior could be protective. This does not necessarily imply an absence of CD in those settings; after all, antisocial behaviors are largely environmentally caused. It only means that the context in which symptoms occur needs to be taken into consideration. Although the difference appears theoretically difficult, clinicians seem able to make such a distinction in practice (90).

Comorbidity and Differential Diagnosis

Assessment must cover all symptom domains to ensure that comorbid disorders are not overlooked. It is common for parents, teachers, and clinicians to focus on the more obvious and annoying behaviors and neglect mentioning or inquiring about less conspicuous symptoms and disorders, which nevertheless may be important for treatment and prognosis. As noted, the most frequent are ADHD, mood disorders, and in adolescents, substance abuse (27, 28, 91). Conditions such as anxiety disorders, tic disorders, specific developmental and learning disorders, Asperger syndrome, and mental retardation ought to be considered also. Antisocial behavior is not uncommon in the prodromal stage of schizophrenia (92).

It is well established that patients with bipolar disorder have a high prevalence of DBDs and vice versa (93, 94). Comorbidity between DBDs and bipolar disorder in prepubertal children, important for its therapeutic implications, has recently received much attention and created controversy, but remains unresolved. It has been suggested that some children with severe impulsivity, hyperactivity, unstable mood, irritability, defiance, and conduct problems may suffer from bipolar disorder, resulting in a higher prevalence of bipolar disorder in this age group than previously thought (95, 96). Results of other prospective and prevalence studies are inconsistent with this view (97–99). An alternative explanation is that this clinical picture may be a manifestation of the severity of the disruptive disorder in these children.

A diagnosis of ODD should not be made when defiance, grouchiness and noncompliance occur only in the course of major depression or if ODD symptoms appear when parents try to force anxious children, for example with a phobia, to confront their fears. Deciding whether a concurrent diagnosis of ODD should or should not be made can be difficult. The opposite scenario, ignoring ODD symptoms when making a diagnosis of depression or ADHD may also occur. ODD may be present if the child has shown symptoms of defiance, temper tantrums, etc. prior to the onset of the other disorder or if oppositionality persists after symptoms of the comorbid condition have lessened.

Clinical Assessment

Questionnaires and checklists provide quantifiable data, reliably supplement information obtained at interview, and are useful to measure progress and outcome (see Chapter 4.2.3). Besides general questionnaires such as the Child Behavior Checklist (100), a variety of specific rating scales are available (101), including the Eyberg Child Behavior Inventory (102), the New York Teacher Rating Scale for Disruptive and Antisocial Behavior (103), and the Home and School Situations Questionnaire (104).

Psychometric and educational assessment is often valuable as part of the initial assessment; it should always be performed when children show difficulties at school or if learning problems are suspected. A careful medical history and review of systems is mandatory in all cases. Routine biochemical, EEG, or radiological investigations are unnecessary (105), with the exception of urine drug screen in adolescents. Laboratory investigations should be conducted when the clinician uncovers symptoms suggestive of a physical illness (e.g., epilepsy), or for sexually transmitted diseases when sexual abuse has occurred, or there is suspicion of unprotected sexual activity.

TREATMENT

In practice, children with DBDs are treated with a variety of psychological, behavioral, or pharmacological approaches, alone or in combination, targeting the child and/or the family. Professionals largely believe that therapy is of limited effectiveness, particularly in the patients with CD typically seen in mental health settings (more chronic, more disturbed, and usually with comorbid conditions). While there have been considerable advances in the last 25 years, effective treatments are few and no great breakthroughs have occurred. Moreover, treatment research, though vast, is hampered by poor definition of target symptoms, mixed populations, small sample sizes, and poor randomization and blinding, among other limitations. Few trials specifically focus on participants with ODD or CD and it is often difficult to translate findings to the complex circumstances of individual patients. This is compounded by psychosocial treatments being less efficacious when delivered in the average clinic than in academic research settings (106, 107). Most studies in adolescents with CD use a decrease in rates of reoffending, aggressive outbursts, or time spent in institutions as measures of treatment success, while in children they use a reduction in the number of disruptive behavior symptoms (108). That is, although trials may report a statistically significant improvement, symptoms and impairment may still remain in the clinical range, and studies often do not assess outcomes in other important domains (109).

General principles to keep in mind when treating these disorders are:

- DBDs tend to be chronic conditions, more similar to heart disease than pneumonia, and treatment should be tailored accordingly.
- Most guidelines concur that structured psychosocial interventions should be the first line of treatment for ODD and CD, and should be continued even if medications are subsequently initiated.
- Treatment is more likely to be effective when administered early in the course of the disorder. Typically, maladaptive behaviors are continually reinforced; over time, negative perceptions, emotions, and patterns of relating become deeper and more entrenched. Once CD is established, it becomes more resistant to intervention.
- Treatment should involve the parents. In almost all instances, improving parenting skills and parent–child interactions are core goals.
- Comorbid conditions (ADHD, depression) ought to be identified and, if appropriate, treated.
- Parental depression, psychosis, or substance abuse should also be noted and treated.
- It is very useful to ascertain children's and families' strengths and build on them in addition to focusing on their problems.
- Dealing with the stress, anger, and hopelessness that many of these families experience and achieving some calm and control is often a necessary initial step.
- The goals of treatment need to be realistic and modified as progress occurs. For example, preventing or minimizing drug use or involvement in delinquent activities in adolescents with CD may be a more appropriate initial step than seeking symptom resolution.
- Because these young people usually show disturbance in a variety of settings (e.g., school, home) and impairment in several aspects of functioning, addressing their multiple needs in the various domains is likely to increase effectiveness (multimodal treatment).
- Association with deviant peers is a well established factor that increases the likelihood of conduct problems, delinquency, and drug use, particularly in adolescence. A goal should be to enhance participation in activities with well functioning peers.
- In the case of ODD, the main goal of treatment is to increase compliance and reduce conflict. Therefore, the treatment plan should include ways of helping the young person become more cooperative, less argumentative, and be better accepted by peers, often in a family therapy context.

Emergencies

Presentation of young people with DBDs to emergency services is not uncommon. For example, 16% of all the child and adolescent presentations to a psychiatric emergency service in Albany, New York, between 1990 and 1995 were due to DBDs (110). Emergencies usually occur following conflict, legal or disciplinary crises that result in the child losing control and becoming aggressive towards the self, others, or property. Differentiating DBDs from other psychiatric problems in the emergency room is reasonably straightforward, but establishing whether ODD or CD is the diagnosis is harder because a comprehensive evaluation is often difficult in that context. Children with DBDs who present to emergency services tend to have more severe disorders, more aggression, more comorbid conditions, and fewer family and social supports than those without DBDs. Police or mobile psychiatric services involvement is often required (110). A detailed discussion of psychiatric emergencies can be found in Chapter 6.4. However, some of the management principles to be followed in these cases are (111):

- Crisis intervention strategies should be employed before resorting to the use of medication to control behavior.
- Physical and mechanical restraints and locked seclusion should be used only as a last resort, when all other approaches have failed.
- The choice to use emergency ("stat" or "p.r.n.") pharmacological management should correspond to the risk for potential injury.
- Emergency staff should be aware of the risks and side effects of acute sedation and follow the appropriate protocols.
- When antipsychotic "p.r.n." or "stat" medications are used several times per day to manage agitation or aggression, clinicians should reevaluate the diagnosis and the adequacy of behavioral and environmental interventions and then readjust the treatment plan and medication regimen. In most cases, physicians should consider using standing antipsychotic medications rather than frequent "stat" medications.

Acute situations similar to the ones seen in emergency settings also occur during inpatient treatment or in institutions. In these settings, crises usually build up over days or hours and can often be predicted. While their management follows the principles listed above, clinicians working in these services need to be skilled in detecting the early symptoms of loss of control and preventing the crisis.

Psychosocial Treatments

Evidence supporting the efficacy of psychosocial treatments is summarized in Table 5.2.2.4. Only treatments for which there is some evidence of effectiveness are mentioned.

Parent Management Training

Parent management training (PMT) is based on the principles of operant conditioning and social-learning theory. In PMT parents are encouraged to use positive reinforcement, to adopt more effective discipline strategies, and to learn how to negotiate with their children (112). PMT has been the most extensively researched therapy in this field. It has the potential to produce improvements in child behavior to within the nonclinical range at home and, sometimes, at school (113–115). Further, these effects can be maintained, together with indirect improvement in other areas such as sibling behavior, maternal psychopathology, marital satisfaction, and family cohesion (109, 116). Key limitations of PMT include the substantial number of parents who do not complete the program, their frequent ineffectiveness in the most dysfunctional families, and that it has been targeted to younger children.

The National Institute for Health and Clinical Excellence in the U.K. has recently recommended PMT as the first line treatment for conduct problems (117). There is a variety of prepackaged PMT programs, which are flexible (five to 15 sessions; may provide for followup telephone contact) and can be administered to groups or individually (e.g., 118, 119). It is believed that to be effective, PMT programs should: i) be structured and have a curriculum informed by principles of social-learning theory; ii) include relationship-enhancing strategies; iii) offer a sufficient number of sessions;

TABLE 5.2.2.4

SUMMARY OF TREATMENTS FOR OPPOSITIONAL DEFIANT AND CONDUCT DISORDERS

Treatment	Strength of Recommendation[1]	Quality of Evidence[2]	Comments
Psychosocial			
Parent management training	333	A	Limited empirical data for adolescents
Multisystemic therapy	33	A	Usually target severely disordered or delinquent youth, resource intensive
Families and Schools Together (FAST Track)	3	B	Children starting school
Problem solving skills training	3	B	
Therapeutic foster care	3	A	Usually target severely disordered or delinquent youth
Anger management programs	37	C	
Wilderness programs, boot camps, and similar	37	C	Usually target severely disordered or delinquent youth
Pharmacological			
Antipsychotic drugs	3	B	Uncertain evidence; good short-term results with risperidone for individuals with mental retardation
Mood stabilizers and anticonvulsants	37	B	Heterogeneous participants (e.g., aggressive adolescents, conduct disorder with various comorbidities); inconsistent results; somewhat better data for lithium
Stimulants	37	B–	In children with comorbid ADHD
Atomoxetine	37	B–	In children with comorbid ADHD
Clonidine	37	B–	In children with comorbid ADHD
SSRIs	37	E	In children with comorbid major depression

[1] 333 (good supporting evidence) through 37 (uncertain evidence).
[2] A (supported by metaanalysis of several, sound, randomized controlled trials) through C (systematic open studies) to E (expert opinion).

iv) enable parents to identify their own parenting objectives; v) incorporate role-play during sessions as well as homework between sessions to achieve generalization of newly rehearsed behaviors to the home situation; vi) be delivered by appropriately trained and skilled facilitators who are supervised, have access to professional development, and are able to engage in a therapeutic alliance with parents; and vii) adhere to the program developer's manual and employ all the necessary aids to ensure consistent implementation (117). Because some parents might find it difficult to access these programs, it is essential to ensure that practical assistance (e.g. transport, childcare) is available to facilitate attendance.

Multimodal Interventions

Given the variety of symptom and impairment domains, it is thought that multimodal interventions may optimize the chances of success. For example, PMT alone often does not generalize to the school context, and antisocial behavior at school is a predictor of poor outcomes. Also, PMT does not necessarily influence the child's capacity to make friends, when having well functioning friends is a protective factor. Hence, adding to PMT a component that addresses the child's problemsolving abilities or a teacher-training element may enhance efficacy (120). This multimodal approach has been shown to produce better results than PMT alone (121). Examples of multimodal programs are Multisystemic Therapy (MST) and Families and Schools Together (FAST Track). The former predominantly targets adolescents with severe conduct problems and delinquency, while the latter focuses on conduct disordered children starting school.

The FAST Track program provides early and sustained interventions involving the school and parents (using PMT strategies) to prevent problems from worsening. Early results suggested that, after the first year of FAST Track, children in the treatment group show better social-coping skills, more positive peer relations, and improved academic performance compared to controls (122). A more recent study reported a significant but modest influence on fourth- and fifth-graders' rates of social competence and social cognition problems, involvement with deviant peers, and conduct problems in the home and community, compared to children in the control condition (123).

MST (See Chapter 6.3.2) also draws on a range of interventions, is home based, goal oriented and intensive—it provides therapy seven days a week for about 4 months (124). A metaanalysis reported that MST is moderately effective in reducing offending, but this appears to be very dependent on the skills of the treatment team (effect sizes ranging from 0.26 to 0.81) (107). Although it is resource intensive, MST seems to be cost effective (125).

Therapeutic foster care is another multimodal approach in which adolescents are placed with specially trained, intensely supervised foster parents who are supported by a team. Placement lasts about 6 months. There is some evidence this reduces these youths' criminal activities (120). Project TEAM is a further manualized multimodal treatment program incorporating parent training, child intervention groups, and parent–child "together time"; at 5 months, parents and teachers reported significant improvements in child behaviors (126).

Evidence for the effectiveness of wilderness programs, boot camps, and other residential treatments is conflicting and studies are of poor quality. The main concern about these interventions is that they provide opportunities to associate and identify with deviant peers, and that gains may not generalize outside the treatment setting.

Individual Interventions

Problemsolving skills training is the best studied and it results in a clinically significant improvement (127). In this therapy, children are taught to understand interpersonal problems and find adaptive solutions using various techniques including games, structured activities, stories, modeling, role play, and reinforcement. Studies have also demonstrated at least modest benefits for other individual interventions (e.g., 127–129). A review of 82 controlled trials found that individual assertiveness training, anger control/stress inoculation, and rational emotive therapy were "probably efficacious" (at least two studies showed the treatment to be better than a control condition) (127). Child CBT-based interventions showed a small to moderate effect in decreasing antisocial behavior (128).

Pharmacotherapy

Pharmacotherapy is *not* the mainstay of treatment of ODD and CD, and research in this area suffers from most of the shortcomings already noted. Psychotropic drugs may be used for the treatment of ODD or CD symptoms only when psychosocial and educational interventions have failed and as a part of a comprehensive management plan, although medication is often used for those individuals who have coexisting conditions, such as ADHD, and in emergency situations.

The rational use of medications is discussed in Chapter 6.1.1. However, some principles should be followed when prescribing medication for DBDs besides those already highlighted in the section on emergencies, which largely follow the guidelines contained in the treatment recommendations for the use of antipsychotic drugs for aggressive youth (TRAAY): (111)

- The dosing strategy of "start low, go slow, taper slowly" should be followed, particularly when using antipsychotic drugs.
- Caution and careful monitoring should be exercised when prescribing stimulants to adolescents with CD, given the high rate of substance abuse in this population.
- Adherence, side effects, and drug interactions should be monitored routinely and systematically. In particular, it is important to ascertain whether patients are concurrently using psychoactive substances or complementary therapies that may interact with prescribed drugs.
- Before switching, augmenting, combining, or discontinuing medications because of a lack of response, it should be ensured that patients have received adequate trials (dose and duration) as well as psychosocial interventions.
- Polypharmacy should be avoided whenever possible.

More in hope than based on evidence, all known psychotropic medications have been tried in the treatment of DBD symptoms. The evidence for the various types of drugs is summarized in Table 5.2.2.4.

Antipsychotic drugs (atypical antipsychotics are to be preferred initially) are often prescribed to reduce aggressive symptoms. However, studies are small and show inconsistent results (e.g., 130, 131). Antipsychotic drugs have often been prescribed to manage disruptive behavior in individuals with mental retardation. Recent controlled trials suggest these medications, particularly risperidone, are beneficial in this population, at least in the short term (132–134). Careful consideration of benefits and risks is required before deciding long-term (longer than 6 months) use of antipsychotics for DBDs because of the side effects (see Chapter 6.1). Mood stabilizing and antiepileptic drugs (lithium, valproate, carbamazepine) have been used to treat aggression, but results of trials are inconsistent (131, 135–137). There are controlled studies suggesting that stimulants (138), clonidine (139), and atomoxetine (140) are of assistance, particularly in children with comorbid ADHD or hyperkinetic conduct disorder, but these results need to be replicated before drawing definite conclusions.

PREVENTION

There is no reason to believe the incidence of DBDs can not be reduced, since that has been achieved with other scourges such as heart disease, but doing so will require a concerted effort and substantial resources. Child and adolescent mental health professionals have a critical role in educating the community and political leaders on the advantages of prevention over treatment and retribution, notwithstanding that treatment and law enforcement are important also. Reducing DBDs is one of the challenges for child mental health in the twenty-first century. Yet simply addressing conduct problems without tackling the social, family, and individual factors associated with these conditions will lead to disappointment. Little may be achieved in communities that fail to protect the disadvantaged and to ensure that all its citizens, particularly women and families with children, are treated with dignity and afforded access to a minimum of resources and life opportunities, as well as having developmental difficulties such as attention and learning problems addressed (8). Schools can play a key role in this endeavor (e.g., 141).

Table 5.2.2.3 lists some of the opportunities for prevention and the range of potential interventions. Many prevention programs already exist (142), often implemented *ad hoc* and without much data about their effectiveness; finding that evidence should be a priority for research. Home visitation is one of the most widespread, though with many variations. Evaluations show that home visitation is no silver bullet, but results of the better programs are encouraging. Participation can improve children's cognitive, social, and linguistic development, and reduce child maltreatment and behavioral problems (143, 144).

Most of the therapies used to treat DBDs can be adapted for prevention purposes. For example, there are packages based on PMT principles, such as Triple-P (145), designed for use at several levels: i) in broad community education (e.g., through media campaigns); ii) for children at risk in a group format; iii) for children with a full-blown syndrome in group or individual format. There is limited data on the effectiveness of these programs outside preschool or early primary school-age children.

References

1. Foster, EM, Jones, DE: The high costs of aggression: Public expenditures resulting from conduct disorder. *Am J Public Health* 95:1767–1772, 2005.
2. Scott S, Knapp M, Henderson J, et al.: Financial cost of social exclusion: Follow up study of antisocial children into adulthood. *BMJ* 323:191–194, 2001.
3. Rutter M, Giller H, Hagell A: *Antisocial Behavior by Young People*. New York, Cambridge University Press, 1998.
4. Robins LN: Sturdy childhood predictors of adult outcomes. Replication from longitudinal studies. *Psychol Med* 8:611–622, 1978.
5. Robins LN: *Deviant Children Grown Up*. Baltimore, Williams & Wilkins, 1966.
6. Rey JM, Morris-Yates A, Singh M, et al.: Continuities between adolescent disorder and personality disorder in young adults. *Am J Psychiatry* 152:895–900, 1995.
7. Kim-Cohen J, Caspi A. Moffitt TE, et al.: Prior juvenile diagnoses in adults with mental disorder: Developmental follow-back of a prospective-longitudinal cohort. *Arch Gen Psychiatry* 60:709–717, 2003.
8. Fergusson DM, Horwood LJ, Ridder EM: Show me the child at seven: The consequences of conduct problems in childhood for psychosocial functioning in adulthood. *J Child Psychol Psychiatry* 46:837–849, 2005.
9. Mofitt TE, Caspi A: Annotation: Implications of violence between intimate partners for child psychologists and psychiatrists. *J Child Psychol Psychiatry* 39:137–144, 1998.
10. Aichhorn A: *Wayward Youth*. New York, Viking Press, 1935.
11. Rey JM, Bashir MR, Schwarz M, et al.: Oppositional disorder: Fact or fiction? *J Am Acad Child Adolesc Psychiatry* 27:157–162, 1988.
12. Sondeijker FEPL, Ferdinand RF, Oldehinkel AJ, et al.: Classes of adolescents with disruptive behaviors in a general population sample. *Social Psychiatry and Psychiatric Epidemiology* 40:93–938, 2005.
13. Cleckley H: *The Mask of Sanity*. St Louis, CV Mosby, 1941.
14. Bowlby J: Forty-four juvenile thieves: Their character and home-life. *Int J Psychoanalysis* 25:1–57, 1994.
15. Levy DM: Oppositional syndromes and oppositional behavior. In: Hoch P, Zubin J (eds.): *Psychopathology of Childhood*. New York: Grune & Stratton, 1955.
16. American Psychiatric Association: *Diagnostic and Statistical Manual: Mental Disorders*. Washington, DC, American Psychiatric Association, 1952.
17. American Psychiatric Association: *Diagnostic and Statistical Manual of Mental Disorders*, 2nd ed. Washington, DC, American Psychiatric Association, 1968.
18. American Psychiatric Association: *Diagnostic and Statistical Manual of Mental Disorders*, 3rd ed. Washington, DC, American Psychiatric Association, 1980.
19. American Psychiatric Association: *Diagnostic and Statistical Manual of Mental Disorders*, 4th ed. Washington, DC, American Psychiatric Association, 1994.
20. World Health Organisation: *The ICD-10 Classification of Mental and Behavioural Disorders: Diagnostic Criteria for Research*. Geneva, World Health Organization, 1993.
21. American Psychiatric Association: *Diagnostic and Statistical Manual of Mental Disorders*, 4th ed., Text Revision. Washington, DC, American Psychiatric Association, 2000.
22. Rowe R, Maughan B, Costello EJ, et al.: Defining oppositional defiant disorder. *J Child Psychol Psychiatry* (in press).
23. Achenbach TM: Challenges and benefits of assessment, diagnosis, and taxonomy for clinical practice and research. *Aust N Z J Psychiatry* 35:263–271, 2001.
24. Frick PJ, Lahey BB, Loeber R, et al.: Oppositional defiant disorder and conduct disorder: A meta-analytic review of factor analyses and cross validation in a clinical sample. *Clin Psychol Rev* 13:319–340, 1993.
25. Rey JM, Morris-Yates A: Are oppositional and conduct disorders of adolescents separate conditions? *Aust NZJ Psychiatry* 27:281–287, 1993.
26. Moffitt TE: Adolescence-limited and life-course-persistent antisocial behavior: a developmental taxonomy. *Psychol Rev* 100:674–701, 1993.
27. Angold A, Costello EJ, Erkanli A: Comorbidity. *J Child Psychol Psychiatry* 40:57–87, 1999.
28. Armstrong TD, Costello EJ: Community studies on adolescent substance use, abuse, or dependence and psychiatric comorbidity. *J Consult Clin Psychol* 70:1224–1239, 2002.
29. Essaue CA: Epidemiology and comorbidity. In: Essau CA. (ed.): *Conduct and Oppositional Defiant Disorders: Epidemiology, Risk Factors and Treatment*. Mahwah, NJ: Lawrence Erlbaum, 2003, pp. 33–59.
30. Rey JM, Plapp JM, Stewart GW: Reliability of psychiatric diagnosis in referred adolescents. *J Child Psychol Psychiatry* 30:879–888, 1989.
31. Ezpeleta L, de la Osa N, Domenech JM, et al.: Diagnostic agreement between clinicians and the diagnostic interview for children and adolescents—DICA-R—in an outpatient sample. *J Child Psychol Psychiatry* 38:431–440, 1997.
32. Shaffer D, Fisher P, Lucas CP, et al.: NIMH Diagnostic Interview Schedule for Children Version IV (NIMH DISC-IV): Description, differences from previous versions, and reliability of some common diagnoses. *J Am Acad Child Adolesc Psychiatry* 39:28–38, 2000.
33. Romano E, Baillargeon RH, Wua HX, et al.: A new look at inter-informant agreement on conduct disorder using a latent class approach. *Psychiatry Research* 129:75–89, 2004.
34. Lahey BB, Loeber R: Framework for a developmental model of oppositional defiant disorder and conduct disorder. In: Routh DK (ed.): *Disruptive Behavior Disorders in Childhood*. New York: Plenum Press, 1994, pp. 139–180.
35. Achenbach TM, Edelbrock CS: *Manual for the Teacher's Report Form and Teacher Version of the Child Behavior Profile*. Burlington VT, University of Vermont Department of Psychiatry, 1986.
36. Fergusson DM: Stability and change in externalising behaviors. *European Archives of Psychiatry & Clinical Neuroscience* 248:4–13, 1998.
37. Loeber R: Antisocial behavior: More enduring than changeable? *J Am Acad Child Adolesc Psychiatry* 30:383–397, 1991.
38. Rowe R, Maughan B, Pickles A, et al.: The relationship between DSM-IV oppositional defiant disorder and conduct disorder: Findings from the Great Smoky Mountains Study. *J Child Psychol Psychiatry* 43:365–373, 2002.
39. Helgeland MI, Kjelsberg E, Torgersen S: Continuities between emotional and disruptive behavior disorders in adolescence and personality disorders in adulthood. *Am J Psychiatry* 162:1941–1947, 2005.
40. Marmorstein NR, Iacono WG: Longitudinal follow-up of adolescents with late-onset antisocial behavior: A pathological yet overlooked group. *J Am Acad Child Adolesc Psychiatry* 44:1284–1291, 2005.
41. Rutter M: What is the meaning and utility of the psychopathy concept? *J Abnorm Child Psychol* 33:499–503, 2005.
42. Brook JS, Newcomb MD: Childhood aggression and unconventionality: Impact on later academic achievement, drug use, and workforce involvement. *Journal of Genetic Psychology* 156:393–410, 1995.
43. Beautrais AL, Joyce PR, Mulder RT: Youth suicide attempts: A social and demographic profile. *Aust N Z J Psychiatry* 32:349–357, 1998.

44. Caspi A, Wright BRE, Moffitt TE, et al.: Early failure in the labor market: Childhood and adolescent predictors of unemployment in the transition to adulthood. *American Sociological Review* 63:424–451, 1998.
45. Fergusson DM, Lynskey MT: Conduct problems in childhood and psychosocial outcomes in young adulthood: A prospective study. *Journal of Emotional and Behavioral Disorders* 6:2–18, 1998.
46. Woodward LJ, Fergusson DM: Early conduct problems and later risk of teenage pregnancy in girls. *Development and Psychopathology* 11:127–141, 1999.
47. Flory K, Milich R, Lynam DR, et al.: Relation between childhood disruptive behavior disorders and substance use and dependence symptoms in young adulthood: Individuals with symptoms of attention-deficit/hyperactivity disorder and conduct disorder are uniquely at risk. *Psychology of Addictive Behaviors* 17:151–158, 2003.
48. Stouthamer-Loeber M, Wei E, Loeber R, et al.: Desistance from persistent serious delinquency in the transition to adulthood. *Development & Psychopathology* 16:897–918, 2004.
49. Kessler RC, Chiu WT, Demler O, et al.: Prevalence, severity, and comorbidity of 12-month DSM-IV disorders in the national comorbidity survey replication. *Arch Gen Psychiatry* 62:617–627, 2005.
50. Loeber R, Burke JD, Lahey BB, et al.: Oppositional defiant and conduct disorder: A review of the past 10 years, part I. *J Am Acad Child Adolesc Psychiatry* 39:1468–1484, 2000.
51. Costello EJ, Mustillo S, Erkanli A, et al.: Prevalence and development of psychiatric disorders in childhood and adolescence. *Arch Gen Psychiatry* 60:837–844, 2003.
52. Mullick MSI, Goodman R: The prevalence of psychiatric disorders among 5–10 year olds in rural, urban and slum areas in Bangladesh. *Social Psychiatry and Psychiatric Epidemiology* 40:663–671, 2005.
53. Srinath S, Girimaji SC, Gururaj G, et al.: Epidemiological study of child & adolescent psychiatric disorders in urban and rural areas of Bangalore, India. *Indian Journal of Medical Research* 122:67–79, 2005.
54. Crijnen A, Achenbach TM, Verhulst FC: Problems reported by parents of children in multiple cultures: The Child Behavior Checklist syndrome constructs. *Am J Psychiatry* 156:569–574, 1999.
55. Sawyer M, Arney F, Baghurst P, et al.: The mental health of young people in Australia: Key findings from the child and adolescent component of the national survey of mental health and well-being. *Aust NZ J Psychiatry* 35:806–814, 2001.
56. Ford T, Goodman R, Meltzer H: The British child and adolescent mental health survey 1999: The prevalence of DSM-IV disorders. *J Am Acad Child Adolesc Psychiatry* 42:1203–1211, 2003.
57. Canino G, Shrout PE, Rubio-Stipec M, et al.: The DSM-IV rates of child and adolescent disorders in Puerto Rico. Prevalence, correlates, service use, and the effects of impairment. *Arch Gen Psychiatry* 61:85–93, 2004.
58. Fleitlich-Bilyk B, Goodman R: Prevalence of child and adolescent psychiatric disorders in Southeast Brazil. *J Am Acad Child Adolesc Psychiatry* 43:727–734, 2004.
59. Rutter M, Smith DJ: *Psychosocial Disorders in Young People: Time Trends and Their Causes*. Chicester, Wiley, 1995.
60. Achenbach TM, Dumenci L, Rescorla LA: Are American children's problems still getting worse? A 23-year comparison. *J Abnorm Child Psychol* 31:1–11, 2003.
61. Collishaw S, Maughan B, Goodman R, et al.: Time trends in adolescent mental health. *J Child Psychol Psychiatry* 45:1350–1362, 2004.
62. Rutter M, Tizard J, Whitmore K: *Education, Health and Behavior*. London, Longman, 1970.
63. Dionne G, Tremblay R, Boivin M, et al.: Physical aggression and expressive vocabulary in 19-month-old twins. *Dev Psychol* 39:261–273, 2003.
64. Fergusson D, Swain-Campbell N, Horwood J: How does childhood economic disadvantage lead to crime? *J Child Psychol Psychiatry* 45:956–966, 2004.
65. Hack M, Taylor G, Drotar D, et al.: Chronic conditions, functional limitations, and special health care needs of school-aged children born with extremely low birth-weight in the 1990s. *JAMA* 294:318–325, 2005.
66. Jaffee SR, Moffitt TE, Caspi A, et al.: Life with (or without) father: The benefits of living with two biological parents depend on the father's antisocial behavior. *Child Development* (in press).
67. Kim-Cohen J, Moffitt TE, Taylor A, et al.: Maternal depression and children's antisocial behavior. *Arch Gen Psychiatry* 62:173–181, 2005.
68. Lansford JE, Dodge KA, Pettit GS, et al.: Long-term effects of early child physical maltreatment on psychological, behavioral and academic problems in adolescence: A 12 year prospective study. *Archives of Pediatrics and Adolescent Medicine* 156:824–830, 2002.
69. Broidy LM, Nagin DS, Tremblay RE, et al.: Developmental trajectories of childhood disruptive behaviors and adolescent delinquency: A six-site, cross-national study. *Developmental Psychology* 39:222–245, 2003.
70. Maughan B, Pickels A, Hagell A, et al.: Reading problems and antisocial behaviour: Developmental Trends in Comorbidity. *J Child Psychol Psychiatry* 37:405–418, 1996.
71. Rutter M, Moffitt TE, Caspi A: Gene–environment interplay and psychopathology: Multiple varieties but real effects. *J Child Psychol Psychiatry* (in press).
72. Dodge KA, Pettit GS. A biopsychosocial model of the development of chronic conduct problems in adolescence. *Dev Psychol* 39:349–371, 2003.
73. Moffitt TE: The new look of behavioral genetics in developmental psychopathology: Gene–environment interplay in antisocial behaviors. *Psychol Bull* 131:533–544, 2005.
74. Tuvblad C, Grann M, Lichtenstein P: Heritability for adolescent antisocial behavior differs with socioeconomic status: Gene–environment interaction. *J Child Psychol Psychiatry* (in press)
75. Wichers M, Purcell S, Danckaerts, et al.: Prenatal life and post-natal psychopathology: Evidence for negative gene–birth weight interaction. *Psychol Med* 32:1165–1174, 2002.
76. Rutter M: Commentary: Causal processes leading to antisocial behavior. *Developmental Psychology* 39:372–378, 2003.
77. Wilkinson R, Marmot M: *Social Determinants of Health: The Solid Facts*, 2nd ed. Copenhagen, WHO, 2003.
78. Costello EJ, Compton SN, Keeler G, et al.: Relationships between poverty and psychopathology: A natural experiment. *JAMA* 290:2023–2029, 2003.
79. Ortiz J, Raine A: Heart rate level and antisocial behavior in children and adolescents: A meta-analysis. *J Am Acad Child Adolesc Psychiatry* 43:154–162, 2004.
80. Baving L, Laucht M, Schmidt MH: Oppositional children differ from healthy children in frontal brain activation. *J Abnorm Child Psychol* 28:267–275, 2000.
81. Pliszka SR: The psychobiology of oppositional defiant disorder and conduct disorder. In: Quay HC, Hogan AE (eds): *Handbook of Disruptive Behavior Disorders*. New York: Kluwer Academic/Plenum, 1999, pp. 371–395.
82. Brower MC, Price BH: Neuropsychiatry of frontal lobe dysfunction in violence and criminal behavior: A critical review. *J Neurol Neurosurg Psychiatry* 71:720–726, 2001.
83. Bauer LO, Hesselbrock VM: Brain maturation and subtypes of conduct disorder: Interactive effects on P300 amplitude and topography in male adolescents. *J Am Acad Child Adolesc Psychiatry* 42:106–115, 2003.
84. Kruesi MJP, Keller S, Wagner MW: Neurobiology of aggression. In: Martin A, Scahill L, Charney D, Leckman JF (eds.): *Pediatric Psychopharmacology. Principles and Practice*. New York: Oxford University Press, 2003 pp. 210–223.
85. Steiner H, Wilson J. Conduct disorder. In: Hendren R (ed.): *Disruptive Behavior Disorders in Children and Adolescents*. Review of Psychiatry vol 18. Washington, DC, American Psychiatric Press, 1999.
86. Vostanis P, Meltzer H, Goodman R, et al.: Service utilization by children with conduct disorders—Findings from the GB national study. *Europ Child Adolesc Psychiatry* 12:231–128, 2003.
87. Crick NR, Grotpeter JK: Relational aggression, gender, and social psychological adjustment. *Child Dev* 66:710–722, 1995.
88. Keenan K, Wakschlag LS: Can a valid diagnosis of disruptive behavior disorder be made in preschool children? *Am J Psychiatry* 159:351–358, 2002.
89. Kim-Cohen J, Arseneault L, et al.: Validity of DSM-IV conduct disorder in 4 1/2–5-year-old children: A longitudinal epidemiological study. *Am J Psychiatry* 162:1108–1117, 2005.
90. Wakefield JC, Pottick KJ, Kirk SA: Should the DSM-IV diagnostic criteria for conduct disorder consider social context? *Am J Psychiatry* 159:380–386, 2002.
91. Sung M, Erkanli A, Angold A, et al.: Effects of age at first substance use and psychiatric comorbidity on the development of substance use disorders. *Drug and Alcohol Dependence* 75:287–299, 2004.
92. Gosden NP, Kramp P, Gabrielsen G, et al.: Violence of young criminals predicts schizophrenia: A 9-year register-based follow-up of 15- to 19-year-old criminals. *Schizophrenia Bulletin* 31:759–768, 2005.
93. Kovacs M, Pollock M: Bipolar disorder and comorbid conduct disorder in childhood and adolescence. *J Am Acad Child Adolesc Psychiatry* 34:715–723, 1995.
94. Kutcher S: Adolescent onset bipolar illness. In: Marneros A, Angst J (eds.): *Bipolar Disorders: 100 Years after Manic Depressive Insanity*. Dordrecht: Kluwer Academic, 2000, pp. 139–152.
95. Wozniak J, Biederman J, Kiely K, et al.: Mania-like symptoms suggestive of childhood onset bipolar disorder in clinically referred children. *J Am Acad Child Adolesc Psychiatry* 34:867–876, 1995.
96. Kennedy N, Boydell J, Kalidindi S, et al.: Gender differences in incidence and age at onset of mania and bipolar disorder over a 35-year period in Camberwell, England. *Am J Psychiatry* 162:257–262, 2005.
97. Hazell PL, Carr V, Lewin TJ, Sly K: Manic symptoms in young males with ADHD predict functioning but not diagnosis after 6 years. *J Am Acad Child Adolesc Psychiatry* 42:552–260, 2003.
98. Soutullo CA, Chang KD, Díez-Suárez A, et al.: Bipolar disorder in children and adolescents: International perspective on epidemiology and phenomenology. *Bipolar Disorders* 7:496–506, 2005.
99. Shaw JA, Egeland JA, Endicott J, et al.: A 10-year prospective study of prodromal patterns for bipolar disorder among Amish youth. *J Am Acad Child Adolesc Psychiatry* 44:1104–1111, 2005.
100. Achenbach TM: *Integrative Guide to the 1991 CBCL/4-18, YSR, and TRF Profiles*. Burlington, VT, University of Vermont, Department of Psychology, 1991.
101. Collett BR, Ohan JL, Myers K: Ten-year review of rating scales. VI: Scales assessing externalizing behaviors. *J Am Acad Child Adolesc Psychiatry* 42:1143–1170, 2003.

102. Eyberg SM, Pincus D: *Eyeberg Child Behavior Inventory and Sutter-Eyberg Student Behavior Inventory-Revised, Professional Manual.* Odessa, FL, Psychological Assessment Resources, 1999.
103. Miller LS, Klein RG, Piacentini J, et al.: The New York teacher rating scale for disruptive and antisocial behavior. *J Am Acad Child Adolesc Psychiatry* 34:359–370, 1995.
104. Barkley RA: *Defiant Children: A Clinician's Manual for Assessment and Parent Training*, 2nd ed. New York, Guilford, 1997.
105. Zametkin AJ, Ernst M, Silver R: Laboratory and diagnostic testing in child and adolescent psychiatry: A review of the past 10 years. *J Am Acad Child Adolesc Psychiatry* 37:464–472, 1998.
106. Weisz JR, Weiss B, Donenberg GR: The lab versus the clinic: Effects of child and adolescent psychotherapy. *Am Psychol* 47:1578–1585, 1992.
107. Curtis NM, Ronan KR, Borduin CM: Multisystemic treatment: A meta-analysis of outcome studies. *J Fam Psychol* 18:411–419, 2004.
108. Woolfenden SR, Williams K, Peat J: Family and parenting interventions in children and adolescents with conduct disorder and delinquency aged 10–17. The Cochrane Collaboration, 2005.
109. Barton J: Conduct disorder: Intervention and prevention. *International Journal of Mental Health Promotion* 5:32–41, 2003.
110. Breslow RE, Klinger BI, Erickson BJ: The disruptive behavior disorders in the psychiatric emergency service. *General Hospital Psychiatry* 21:214–219, 1999.
111. Pappadopulos E, Macintyre II JC, Crismon ML, et al.: Treatment recommendations for the use of antipsychotics for aggressive youth (TRAAY). Part II. *J Am Acad Child Adolesc Psychiatry* 42:145–161, 2003.
112. Patterson GR: *Coercive Family Process.* Eugene, OR, Castalia, 1982.
113. Kazdin AE: Parent management training: Evidence, outcomes and issues. *J Am Acad Child Adolesc Psychiatry* 36:1349–1356, 1997.
114. Scott S, Spender Q, Doolan M, et al.: Multicentre controlled trial of parenting groups for childhood antisocial behavior in clinical practice. *BMJ* 323:194–197, 2001.
115. Hutchings J, Lane E, Kelly J: Comparison of two treatments for children with severely disruptive behaviors: A four year follow-up. *Behavioural and Cognitive Psychotherapy* 32:15–30, 2004.
116. Scott S: Do parenting programs for severe child antisocial behavior work over the longer term, and for whom? One year follow-up of a multi-centre controlled trial. *Behavioural and Cognitive Psychotherapy* 33:403–421, 2005.
117. National Institute for Health and Clinical Excellence: *Parent-Training/Education Programs in the Management of Children with Conduct Disorders.* 22 December 2005. Available at <http://www.nice.org.uk/page.aspx?o=285478> (accessed January 14, 2006).
118. Webster-Stratton C, Hancock L: Training for parents of young children with conduct problems: Content, methods, and therapeutic processes. In: Briesmeister JM, Schaefer CE (eds.): *Handbook of Parent Training*, 2nd ed. New York: Wiley, 1998.
119. Sanders MR: Triple P-Positive parenting program: Towards an empirically validated multilevel parenting and family support strategy for the prevention of behavior and emotional problems in children. *Clin Child Fam Psychol Rev* 2:71–90, 1999.
120. Woolgar M, Scott S: Evidence-based management of conduct disorders. *Current Opinion in Psychiatry* 18:392–396, 2005.
121. Webster-Stratton C, Reid M, Hammond M: Treating children with early-onset conduct problems: Intervention outcomes for parent, child, and teacher training. *J Clin Child Adolesc Psychol* 33:105–124, 2004.
122. Conduct Problems Prevention Research Group: Initial impact of the FAST Track prevention trial for conduct problems:1. The high risk sample. *J Consult Clin Psychol* 67:631–647, 1999.
123. Bierman KL, Coie JD, Dodge KA, et al.: The effects of the Fast Track program on serious problem outcomes at the end of elementary school. *J Clin Child Adolesc Psychol* 33:650–661, 2004.
124. Henggeler SW, Scoenwald SK, Borduin CM, et al.: *Multisystems Treatment of Antisocial Behavior in Children and Adolescents.* New York, Guilford Press, 1998.
125. Aos S, Phipps P, Barnoski R, et al.: *The Comparative Costs and Benefits of Programs to Reduce Crime.* Washington State Institute for Public Policy. 2001. Available at <http://www.wsipp.wa.gov/rptfiles/costbenefit.pdf> (accessed January 14, 2006).
126. Feinfield KA, Baker BL: Empirical support for a treatment program for families of young children with externalizing problems. *J Clin Child Adolesc Psychol* 33:182–195, 2004.
127. Brestan EV, Eyberg SM: Effective psychosocial treatment of conduct disordered children and adolescents: 29 years, 82 studies and 5272 kids. *J Clin Child Psychol* 27:180–189, 1998.
128. Bennett DS, Gibbons TA: Efficacy of child cognitive behavior interventions for antisocial behaviour; a meta-analysis. *Child and Family Behaviour Therapy* 22:1–15, 2000.
129. Sheldrick RC, Kendall PC, Heimberg RG: The clinical significance of treatments: a comparison of three treatments for conduct disordered children. *Clinical Psychology: Science and Practice* 8:418–430, 2001.
130. Findling RL, McNamara NK, Braniky LA, et al.: A double-blind pilot study of risperidone in the treatment of conduct disorder. *J Am Acad Child Adolesc Psychiatry* 39:509–516, 2000.
131. Burke JD, Loeber R, Birmaher B: Oppositional defiant disorder and conduct disorder: A review of the past ten years, Part 2. *J Am Acad Child Adolesc Psychiatry* 41:1275–1293, 2002.
132. Aman MG, De Smedt G, Derivan A, et al.: Double-blind, placebo-controlled study of risperidone for the treatment of disruptive behaviors in children with subaverage intelligence. *Am J Psychiatry* 159:1337–1346, 2002.
133. Snyder R, Turgay, A, Aman M, et al.: The Risperidone Conduct Study Group. Effects of risperidone on conduct and disruptive behavior disorders in children with subaverage IQs. *J Am Acad Child Adolesc Psychiatry* 41:1026–1036, 2002.
134. Croonenberghs J, Fegert JM, Findling RL, et al.: Risperidone in children with disruptive behavior disorders and subaverage intelligence: A 1-year, open-label study of 504 patients. *J Am Acad Child Adolesc Psychiatry* 44:64–72, 2005.
135. Ryan ND, Bhatara VS, Perel JM: Mood stabilizers in children and adolescents. *J Am Acad Child Adolesc Psychiatry* 38:529–536, 1999.
136. Donovan S, Stewart J, Nunes EV, et al.: Divalproex treatment for youth with explosive temper and mood lability: A double-blind, placebo-controlled crossover design. *Am J Psychiatry* 157:818–820, 2000.
137. Steiner H, Petersen ML, Saxena K, et al.: Divalproex sodium for the treatment of conduct disorder: A randomized controlled clinical trial. *J Clin Psychiatry* 64:1183–1191, 2003.
138. Klein RG, Abikoff H, Klass E, et al.: Clinical efficacy of methylphenidate in conduct disorder with and without attention deficit hyperactivity disorder. *Arch Gen Psychiatry* 54:1073–1080, 1997.
139. Hazell PL, Stuart JE: A randomized controlled trial of clonidine added to psychostimulant medication for hyperactive and aggressive children. *J Am Acad Child Adolesc Psychiatry* 42:886–894, 2003.
140. Newcorn JH, Spencer TJ, Biederman J, et al.: Atomoxetine treatment in children and adolescents with attention deficit hyperactivity disorder and comorbid oppositional defiant disorder. *J Am Acad Child Adolesc Psychiatry* 44:240–248, 2005.
141. van Lier PAC, Vuijk P, Crijnen AAM: Understanding mechanisms of change in the development of antisocial behavior: The impact of a universal intervention. *J Abnorm Child Psychol* 33:521–553, 2005.
142. Bor W: Prevention and treatment of childhood and adolescent aggression and antisocial behavior: A selective review. *Aust N Z J Psychiatry* 38:373–380, 2004.
143. Gomby DS, Culross PL, Behrman RE: Home visiting: Recent program evaluations—Analysis and recommendations. *The Future of Children* 9:4–26, 1999.
144. Lyons-Ruth K, Melnick S: Dose-response effect of mother-infant clinical home visiting on aggressive behavior problems in kindergarten. *J Am Acad Chil Adolesc Psychiatry* 43:699–707, 2004.
145. Sanders MR: Parenting interventions and the prevention of serious mental health problems in children. *Med J Australia* 177:S87–S92, 2002.

CHAPTER 5.2.3 ■ AGGRESSION IN CHILDREN: AN INTEGRATIVE APPROACH

JOSEPH C. BLADER AND PETER S. JENSEN

INTRODUCTION

Aggressive and Prosocial Behavior

A central goal of every human community is the mitigation of aggression between its members. The seventeenth century English philosophers who articulated today's Western concepts of liberty and democracy considered the restraint of unsanctioned aggressive behavior the *only* justification for the state to intrude on personal freedom (1, 2). Hobbes wrote about the necessity of a "common power to keep them all in awe." That power (i.e., the state) exists to constrain the antagonisms that flow from three drives: 1) to acquire resources, 2) to protect those resources and personal safety, and 3) to enhance and defend one's prestige. He memorably portrayed the downside of the perpetual conflict that would otherwise result (1):

> In such condition there is no place for Industry because the fruit thereof is uncertain ... no commodious Building; ... no Arts; no Letters; no Society; and which is worst of all, continuall feare, and danger of violent death; And the life of man, solitary, poore, nasty, brutish, and short.

When Charles Darwin considered these issues within a biological framework some 200 years later, these predecessors who depicted life as a struggle for existence influenced his work (3). Natural selection involves competition for the resources that are essential to survival and successful reproduction. Scarcity of these resources means that some creatures inevitably deprive others within their species of access to them, often through aggressive behavior. However, Darwin also devoted much attention to the adaptive benefits of the "social instincts," such as sympathy, cooperation, altruism, and the desire to maintain the approval of one's group, which exert an equally natural countervailing force on intraspecific aggression. After all, when danger is at hand humans tend to seek safety in one another's company. Potential procreative partners may also favor these prosocial characteristics, which would hasten their proliferation through the process of sexual selection (4).

> As man is a social animal, it is almost certain that he would inherit a tendency to be faithful to his comrades, and obedient to the leader of his tribe; for these qualities are common to most social animals. He would consequently possess some capacity for self-command. He would from an inherited tendency be willing to defend, in concert with others, his fellow men; and would be ready to aid them in any way, which did not too greatly interfere with his own welfare or his own strong desires (5).

Since then, behavioral research has supported the overall view that a combination of affective, cognitive, and social factors disincline the majority of people from harming others most of the time (6, 7). We also know a fair amount about when these factors could lose their potency to inhibit aggressive behavior. For instance, aggressive behavior becomes more likely when one perceives that a potential target belongs to a different social grouping; when one believes that another person unjustifiably threatens his or her prerogatives and well being; when one believes that others will approve of or encourage aggressive acts; and when one believes that the benefits of aggression will exceed its probable cost.

Under normal circumstances, then, human interaction has a default value of relative congeniality. Numerous affective, social-cognitive and experiential factors, however, can tip the balance toward disharmony. In effect, then, most peacekeeping and law enforcement activities do not depend entirely on the external displays of might that Hobbes wrote about, but rather seem to take place chiefly within the human skull.

Consequently, many psychiatric conditions have aggressive behavior as a major complication. High negative emotionality may predispose to a low threshold for anger or frustration, so that one reacts forcefully to situations others would find only mildly bothersome. Distorted cognitive processes may lead to unwarranted alarm about environmental threats, to feeling impelled by some force to hurt others, or to erroneous beliefs about entitlement to impose one's will on others. High anxiety may trigger avoidance or escape behaviors that can injure others who get in the way. Inadequate impulse control can disrupt response selection so that aggression has precedence over alternatives. Abnormal development may impair the acquisition of coping behaviors and self-regulatory capabilities that ordinarily suppress dyscontrolled outbursts. In addition, some highly prevalent diagnoses have aggressive behavior as a cardinal feature, such as conduct disorder, antisocial personality disorder, or intermittent explosive disorder.

Certain experiential factors can contribute to persistent aggression and therefore have psychiatric significance. Early severe maltreatment may disrupt the development of empathy. Socialization that promotes violence and threats as vehicles for self-preservation may lead to aggression that persists even in new social contexts that disapprove of such behavior.

Persistent aggressive behavior most often originates in childhood. In particular, aggressive behavior among school-age children confers high risk for unfavorable outcomes not just during youth but also throughout later life (8–10). Aggressive dyscontrol is also the concern that most often motivates families to obtain mental health care for their preadolescent children. Nevertheless, aggressive behavior still eludes consistently effective intervention. The combined force of troubling outcomes, adverse community impact, high prevalence, and uncertain treatment prospects propels childhood-onset aggression to the forefront of challenges in mental health today.

AGGRESSION AND VICTIMIZATION AMONG YOUTH

Community-Based and Clinically Based Estimates

Cross-sectional and longitudinal studies both indicate that physically aggressive behavior among preschoolers is common but diminishes upon school entry and during the elementary school years. Tremblay and colleagues (11) found that only a minority (28%) of 3-year-olds were said to display little or no aggression. Parents of 27% of 3-year-old boys report their child "hits, pushes, or trips" others at least "sometimes" (12). The comparable rate for girls is 19%. Parents reported "modest aggression" was reported for 58%, with equal gender representation (11). Parents reported quite high aggressive behavior among 14%, of whom 57% were male.

In elementary school samples, larger gender differences emerge for "starts fights," with parent reports indicating that fighting is present among about 12% of boys and 6% of girls (13). However, the prevalence of "bullies, threatens, or intimidates" are relatively similar between genders (boys 13%, girls 10%).

Several longitudinal studies have tracked teacher-reported conduct problems through elementary school. Some also had initial assessments from infancy and some had followups through young adulthood. Data from six of these studies found that 8% of boys consistently obtain the highest physical aggression ratings time after time (14). Estimates may be biased toward the higher end, since two of the samples sought to recruit a high-risk cohort. The finding that children appear to show considerable stability in how teachers rate their aggressive behavior across many school years is even more striking than the continuity of parent report, because teachers and classmates change annually for most children. There is also a subgroup representing 10% of girls who also have high, stable levels of physical aggression, though overall severity is lower than that for the boys.

Aggressive behavior, regardless of diagnostic context, is among the most prevalent chief complaints for youth seen in inpatient, outpatient, and residential treatment services (15–19). Among preadolescents, aggressive dyscontrol may be the most frequent reason for treatment in specialty mental health services. By adolescence, rising prevalence of mood disorders and self-injurious behavior, particularly among females, eclipses aggressive behavior as a chief complaint. However, new-onset aggressive behavior among girls in early to middle adolescence seems rather frequent, and in clinical samples may be an associated feature of mood disorders (20). Therefore, despite a shift from "externalizing" to "internalizing" diagnoses with age, aggression may remain as a formidable cotraveller.

The majority of youngsters who fight seem to do so in some settings and not others. Aggressive behavior at home only is especially common: About half of boys who fight show physical aggression within the family exclusively. Only 20% were reported to display physical aggression at both home and school (21).

Crime and Victimization Surveys

Violent crime among juveniles in the United States crested in 1995, and declined steadily until at least 2003 (22). Nevertheless, adolescence remains a dangerous period of life in the United States. Those 12 to 15 years old experienced assaults at a rate of 45.3 per 1,000 during 2003, and the rate for 16- to 19-year-olds was slightly higher, 46.6 per 1,000. Violent victimization decreases with age, dropping by 24% among 20- to 24-year-olds (35.5 per 1,000), with a further 33% decline among those 25 to 34 years of age (22.3 per 1,000). Other youth were most often the perpetrators.

Victims aged 12 to 20 identified their assailant as under 20 in 73.6% of crimes. Overall, 30% percent of victims of all ages in 2003 identified the offender as between the ages of 12 and 20 (23).

Violence among youth is more likely to be a group phenomenon than that perpetrated by adults. In 2003, 54% of violent crimes by juveniles involved more than one assailant (22). During the same period, far fewer of those by adults (18% to 22%) involved multiple offenders (23).

The period between the end of the school day and early evening is the time of greatest risk for youth-on-youth violence during school days. On nonschool days, timing of violent crime better resembles the adult-offender pattern: Incidents gradually ascend to their peak numbers at 11PM, then decline until 6AM, when they begin to rise again (22).

APPROACHES TO CHARACTERIZING AND SUBTYPING AGGRESSION

By Motivation

There is a long tradition of distinguishing aggressive behavior by whether an act's motivation is mainly a) to repel a perceived threat or annoyance, or b) to acquire something desirable. The former often defines *affective, frustrative, impulsive*, or *defensive* aggression. The latter is associated with terms like *proactive* or *instrumental aggression.* In general, psychometric and psychobiological evidence supports such a distinction between these behaviors. As an approach to categorizing *people*, rather than behaviors, it may have some shortcomings, since many individuals display aggressive behaviors characteristic of both types at various times (24–32).

Impulsive, Affective, or Reactive Aggression

Affective or impulsive aggression refers to dyscontrolled reactions, which have the potential or the intent to hurt others, that occur upon exposure to events perceived as noxious. The provocations are usually things that one might agree are annoyances but within a level of intensity that most other children handle with composure. Triggers may appear quite trivial, such as not getting the right cereal for breakfast. Directions to comply with an adult request or the need to end a preferred activity to transition to something else are very frequent antecedents to full-blown rage episodes. Hitting, kicking, destruction of property, and self-abusive behavior are common. A verbal onslaught of screaming, vulgarity, threats, and hurtful insults often provides soundtrack. Since the behavior is most often reactive and nearly instantaneous, it tends to be overt and unplanned. These events can also show a self-defeating character. That is, youngsters in their explosive rage may end up hurting themselves by, for instance, punching walls or glass, damaging their own prized possessions, or escalating when it is obvious, or should be, that doing so only worsens their plight. They may go after people much larger and stronger than themselves. A few children do regain composure when placated, but it is also common for these outbursts, once kindled, to have to run their course before the child regains control. The onset of these difficulties is most often in early childhood, especially among boys, and their risk for persistence into adulthood is great (11, 33, 34).

Proactive, Instrumental, or Appetitive Aggression

Proactive or instrumental aggression includes assaultive or coercive behavior purposefully used to achieve a goal such as material goods or social status. Willful property destruction is also included by some. Descriptions of proactive/instrumental aggression sometimes liken it to hunting, but for many species predation and intraspecific aggression have quite different underpinnings and phenomenology (35). A few features of proactive aggression make plain that the actor is in control. For instance, proactive aggression stops once the goal is achieved or when it becomes clear that it has become unobtainable. Victims are chosen to make success likely. The aggressor may take protective measures to avoid getting hurt and evasive action to avoid apprehension. While planning and premeditation are certainly consistent with proactive aggressive behavior, it is probably not a requirement. A number of "acquisitive" violent acts, such as certain robberies and sexual assaults, are often opportunistic and not necessarily performed with much forethought.

Among youth whose aggressive behavior is principally of the proactive/instrumental type, we can also discriminate two important subgroups.

Adolescent-Onset, Peer-Facilitated Proactive Aggression. First, a group of proactively aggressive youth show adolescent onset of antisocial behavior. Aggressive acts in this context are on the whole less violent, rely on peer encouragement, and seem likely to diminish by adulthood (33, 36). This pattern of antisocial behavior seems practically normative in many Western countries (33), and social mores and penal codes have been relatively tolerant of the milder transgressions. However, the boundary between obnoxious pranksterism and major violations that cause serious injury or damage is fortified by common sense and restraint. The group dynamics of adolescents behaving recklessly do not promote these qualities, often with tragic results. In these situations, a young person may become ensnared by the consequences of delinquent participation. School expulsion, increased wariness of other peers, and involvement with law enforcement or correctional facilities can promote further identification and involvement with delinquent peers, and deflect what had hitherto been a pathway of overall positive adjustment.

Callous-Unemotional ("Psychopathic") Proactive Aggression. Another important subgroup of proactively aggressive youth is profoundly indifferent to the consequences that their misbehavior has upon others. Displays of genuine remorse are rare, and a current descriptor for this group's salient personality features, "callous-unemotional traits," is highly evocative of their lack of empathy, self-centeredness, and shallowness (37). If we can consider eruptive, volatile reactive aggression as "hotheaded," we might regard this conduct, by contrast, as "coldhearted." These youth are responsible for a large number of violent offenses, their aggressive behavior is often persistent, and development of these characteristics may be early in childhood (28, 37–40).

This description bears obvious similarity to some affective features of *psychopathic* or *sociopathic* personality, which has been a topic of study in adult criminology and personality psychology for many years, and more recently, a topic of some interest in cognitive and affective neuroscience (41–43).

As it happens, though, a great many individuals exhibit *both* the angry overreactivity of affective/impulsive aggression and the deliberate, calculated injury to others characteristic of psychopathy. Indeed, some definitions of psychopathy include both impulsive hotheadedness along with the capacity to trample calmly upon the rights of others when it suits the purpose. A majority of aggressive individuals, in both clinical and forensic settings, seem best typified by the affective/impulsive designation. The next largest group comprises a mixed group, and least common are aggressive psychopathic individuals who are not especially impulsive or volatile. Indeed, it has been suggested that some of the latter group may be quite capable of channeling their calm fearlessness and ambition to aggrandize themselves in more socially acceptable ways.

There are interesting findings bearing on possible neuroaffective and neurocognitive substrates of psychopathy. However, the significant overlap between psychopathy's steely emotionality with impulsivity, cognitive or learning deficits, low frustration tolerance, etc. precludes clear interpretation of many studies that compare psychopathic individuals with normal controls. Nonetheless, one rather consistent finding is that psychopathic individuals show significantly less emotional arousal in experimental paradigms that ordinarily elicit differential cognitive, autonomic or CNS responses to neutral or emotionally laden stimuli (29, 42, 44–47). Classic and recent studies of psychopathic adults also found they were more tolerant of pain and less conditionable (45) but are rather more sensitive to monetary cues (48).

A robust neuroendocrine finding is that while many impulsively aggressive individuals do not show elevations in prolactin following acute administration of *d*-fenfluramine (49, 50) (a common phenomenon among depressed patients, attributed to reduced sensitivity for the serotonin-stimulating properties of *d*-fenfluramine that would ordinarily lead to enhanced prolactin release), violent psychopathic individuals show the hyperprolactinemia seen among normal controls (51). On the whole, these data tend to support the value of distinguishing between "dysphoric" aggression and the reward-motivated aggression of those with callous-unemotional traits.

Imperviousness to pain and low conditionability may have etiological significance. One hypothesized process by which people might internalize rules is through the avoidance of unpleasant consequences that might follow transgressions. Low susceptibility to adverse consequences might impair avoidance learning, and thus impede development of the almost instinctual recoil from doing vicious things to others (44, 52).

There are very little data on preadolescents that bear on how much additional risk such factors might have on the development and course of aggressive behavior. Parents very often report that aggressive children do not seem to feel guilty (53), but there may be a difference between lack of remorse when one perceives, even incorrectly, that aggression was justifiable retribution, compared to the lack of remorse when one feels entitled to violate the rights of others to satisfy a personal desire. It is also unclear whether affective psychopathic features may develop over time among certain impulsive, labile individuals, perhaps as a result of environmental effects. For instance, one may become inured to punishment and the negative judgment of others when these are meted out in great abundance or inconsistently, and impulsive, difficult behavior certainly increases the likelihood of such interactions with others over lengthy periods. It is also possible that affective/impulsive aggression is indeed reinforced intermittently, increasing the odds that an individual will utilize it in a volitional manner to gain advantage.

By Behavioral Features

Overt/Covert and Destructive/Nondestructive Dimensions

Frick and colleagues (54) reported that specific forms of antisocial behavior tend to aggregate. Put another way, antisocial youngsters seem to display some degree of "specialization."

Their analysis identified two relatively independent dimensions, which, if dichotomized and crossed, yields quadrants that can categorize most antisocial behavior. One continuum is an overt–covert dimension and the other a destructive–nondestructive dimension. If the destructive dimension roughly corresponds to aggressive behavior, the result is that a certain number of youngsters show mainly overtly aggressive behavior, while another group's aggressive misconduct is chiefly covert. Overt aggression, as mentioned earlier, is confrontative and may or may not be affectively charged. Covert aggression involves property vandalism, arson, and other damage that may well lead to the physical injury of others in addition to the obvious economic harms. The planning and effort needed to conceal one's involvement indicates that covert aggressive behavior is volitional.

In this framework, overt aggression is motivated largely by interpersonal conflict, anger, or to establish dominance (55). Meanwhile, covert misconduct serves mostly acquisitive purposes, is attended by neutral affect, and is thought to be on the whole less violent, although it is not clear what material gain one derives by gratuitous damage to property.

There is evidence that persistent overt and covert antisocial behaviors have distinct developmental pathways (56). Overt aggressors proceed from minor aggression to fighting to major acts of violence. The covert pathway leads from shoplifting and lying to property damage to fraud and burglary. The implication is that while only a minority progress to the most severe forms of misconduct, those who do had progressed through the earlier stages of the respective pathway.

Direct and Indirect Aggression

In addition to unjustified, injurious behaviors directly applied to a victim or property, another form of interpersonal harm occurs when one seeks to undermine the relationships or social standing of another person. Examples of this so-called indirect, or "relational," aggression include ostracism and rumor-mongering. This form of antagonistic behavior seems to be most prevalent among girls and young women. Study of this topic has proliferated in social developmental psychology (57) involving mainly community samples, and to a far lesser degree in psychiatry. One obvious reason is that these behaviors are in themselves unlikely to be the chief complaint that leads to clinical referral or criminal justice involvement. The more common scenario in clinical settings is that child patients are the *victims* of these peer-inflicted adversities. Their attempts at retaliation in kind are prone to backfire, since their lack of social savoir-faire and popularity often leads to poor selections of rumor topics, rebuttals, or audiences. It is therefore unclear how much harm relational aggressors seen in clinical settings actually cause, since effective attacks of this kind seem to require "social capital"—status, credibility, and influence in a peer network (58)—that children seen for mental health care seldom enjoy. Nonetheless, youth whose peers report they display relational *and* physically aggressive behavior receive teacher ratings of behavioral problems that are somewhat higher than physical-only aggressors (59). Even if relational aggression is not currently on the radar as a strong clinical concern by itself, it seems useful to consider such behavior at least for its usefulness as a marker of impaired peer relationships among youth seen in psychiatric care.

A contemporary wrinkle on this issue is the potential for youth to use the Internet to defame peers with anonymity or even impersonating another individual. Schools take this type of misbehavior very seriously, especially when they include threats, even very oblique ones (e.g., "Better watch out"). School suspensions and requests for mental health consultation have grown for such conduct.

By Longitudinal Course

Setting out to explain how antisocial behavior can show great temporal consistency, while at the same time antisocial behavior is far more prevalent from midadolescence through young adulthood, a highly influential paper by Moffitt (33) distinguished two trajectories of antisocial behavior among youth, both of which include aggressive conduct to differing degrees. Aggressive behavior during the early school years tends to persist and signals a risk for delinquent behavior that continues through adulthood. For a much larger group, antisocial behavior emerges in adolescence, only to show a slow but steady decline by the mid-20s. The former comprises a pattern termed "life-course-persistent," the latter a trajectory called "adolescence-limited."

Among early-onset antisocial children, problem behaviors unfold in a fairly well accepted sequence. Early noncompliance, poor rule adherence, and low frustration tolerance are problems at both home and school. While some aggression is common among preschoolers, children whose fighting does not diminish in the early school years are at high risk for persistent violent behavior. As parents themselves, childhood-onset antisocial individuals are more likely to aggress against their offspring and mates, to act irresponsibly, and their behavior or their incarceration burdens their families with hardship.

Adolescence-limited misbehavior, by contrast, usually occurs in a group context and is not pervasive. The earlier discussion about proactive aggression among such "late starters" elaborated on their characteristics. Moffitt suggested that this conduct reflected an antiauthoritarianism derived from frustration over being denied the perquisites of full adulthood despite their physical maturity. However, this group is more likely to sustain productive participation in activities preparatory to adulthood, such as schooling and job training. Delinquent behavior trails off as adulthood finally affords them the opportunity to have the autonomy they craved, but through prosocial means.

INFLUENCES ON AGGRESSIVE BEHAVIOR: PSYCHOPATHOLOGY AND PROCESSES

Overview

We sort a number of risk factors into four overarching categories, shown in the left portion of Figure 5.2.3.1 Four categories of specific deficits and experiential factors that we distinguish are: impulse control deficits, affective instability, experiences to environments that can promote antisocial behavior, and sensory and cognitive abnormalities. Naturally, one vulnerability can give rise to another, and the linkages on the left acknowledge the interdependence of these factors. To the right are several psychiatric disorders and psychosocial processes from which aggressive behavior often springs, and for which the specific vulnerabilities on the left are diatheses or contributors. Finally, severely disruptive behavior itself has sequelae that can abate (interventions) or increase (social marginalization) persistence and impairments; some of these "impact outcomes" appear on the far right.

The overarching idea is that in high enough titers any of these influences may increase risk for problems with aggressive behavior, but it is more often admixtures of these factors that are pertinent in most clinical situations. In the prototypic case, persistent aggression develops in the context of a wider pattern of chronic disruptive behavior problems, whose chief ingredients are impulse control deficits and affective instability.

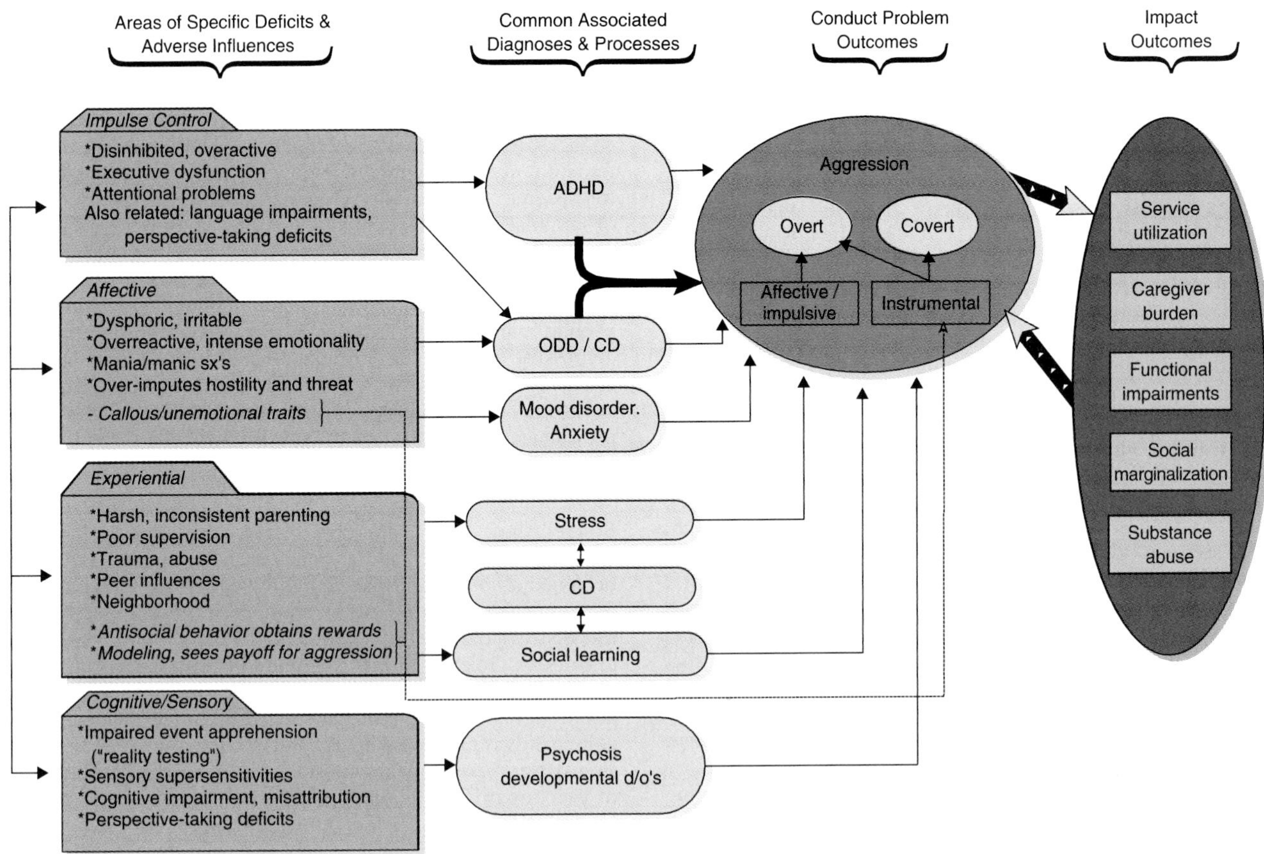

FIGURE 5.2.3.1. Influences on the development of aggressive behavior.

Added to these diatheses, experiences can exert a strong moderating influence.

Impulse Control Deficits

Individuals whose conduct is highly reactive to momentary stimuli and desires often show generalized deficits in their modulation of conduct, cognition, and affect. These deficits are generalized because affected children often show undercontrol of many functions, including self-restraint of *conduct* and activity level, volitional control over *cognition* (sustaining attention, problemsolving) and self-regulation of *affect,* or at least displays of affect. Youngsters whose self-control in these areas deviates markedly from age-typical development usually fulfill diagnostic criteria for attention-deficit hyperactivity disorder (ADHD).

ADHD is the disorder most frequently comorbid with disruptive behavior disorders, oppositional defiant disorder (ODD) and conduct disorder (CD), especially before adolescence (60–65). Disruptive disorders accompanied by ADHD feature much more aggression and persistence than when ADHD is absent (38, 39, 66–69). Children with ODD alone and ODD with ADHD are equally likely to develop CD eventually; however, comorbid youth display this progression much *earlier*, an onset that predicts worse outcomes, including sustained aggression. Dimensional measures of impulsivity also correlate with aggression and self-harming behavior (24, 70). Early hyperactivity predicts subsequent aggression (71, 72) and, in tandem with early aggressive conduct problems, strongly predisposes to persistent antisocial behavior (73).

Problems with language development are prevalent among children with ADHD (74, 75). In particular, weaknesses in the organization of age-appropriate discourse and the comprehension of more complex language seem common, and differ from the sort of lower level phonological processing difficulties characteristic of reading disabilities (76, 77). It is not entirely clear yet if such language difficulties increase the risk for aggression and other conduct problems independent of ADHD. Until more data address this issue, it seems worthwhile to consider that impairments in self-expression plus weak impulse control could make nonaggressive means of conflict resolution more difficult, and that misperceptions of others' attempts to communicate can contribute to disagreements and misunderstandings of others' intentions.

We should also note briefly that *acquired* problems in self-control, such as that following traumatic brain injury, may also contribute to the onset of aggressive behavior (78, 79).

Impairments of Mood, Affect Reactivity and Anxiety

"Hotheadedness"

Evidence from several sources implicates affect disturbances in aggression. The correlation between negative affective features (irritability, lability, anger, dysphoria, frustrability) and disruptive behavior is well established (54, 80). The correlation between emotional instability and aggression in particular is extremely high among youth (81). Studies of comorbidity substantiate the cooccurrence of disruptive disorders and mood and anxiety disorders (61, 63, 64, 82, 83).

One shortcoming of cross-sectional studies of affective features and aggression is lingering uncertainty about which gives rise to which. However, longitudinal studies of temperament show that persistent negative affect early in life, seen as unconsolability, low adaptability, and irritability, predicts subsequent aggression (84, 85). Parental reactions to these difficult characteristics may moderate the ultimate impact of difficult temperament (86, 87). From a diagnostic standpoint, longitudinal studies also indicate that early ODD confers heightened risk for adolescent mood disorder (88). This is not a surprising finding because, despite its frequent alignment with conduct disorder, half the symptoms of ODD describe hostility arising from negative affect.

Among youth with conduct problems, those with negative affect symptoms tend to be more aggressive and to experience worse functional outcomes. Unfavorable outcomes include more hospitalizations, police contacts, impaired social relations, substance abuse, and less improvement with treatment (89–93).

As noted earlier, serotonergic functioning in depressed patients and many aggressive individuals without a primary mood disorder shows similar deviations from controls (94). Findings among children have been less consistent, though, and seem moderated by age, family history, degree of irritability, abuse history, and perhaps ethnicity (30, 95, 96). One recent report indicated that among children with disruptive behavioral problems, those who had normal prolactin elevation to *d,l*-fenfluramine had fewer conduct problems in adolescence than children who showed the blunted response more typical of depressed patients (50).

Affective disturbances may influence aggression through both abnormalities of *sustained* mood and more *momentary* emotional dysregulation. Rageful episodes are common among adults with major mood disorders (97, 98). Similarly, irascibility and explosiveness develop often in the context of posttraumatic stress disorder (PTSD). Aggressive behavior therefore can arise as a complication of mood and anxiety disorders.

In addition, emotion regulation can be disturbed episodically, with or without persistent problems in prevailing mood, hedonic tone, or anxiety (99, 100). Aspects of emotion regulation that are relevant to aggression include high emotional reactivity, poor emotion modulation, lability, and slow recovery from upset (101–103). Vulnerability to hot temper has been also associated with possible defects in social information processing, whereby children too readily impute bad intentions to others who may have unintentionally caused some annoyance for them (104). However, depressed children show a similar phenomenon (105), raising the possibility that negative affect distorts appraisals of threat.

Among aggressive children, these features often do not always summate to clear mood disorder diagnoses based on traditional criteria. The result is that similar phenomenology attracts a variety of diagnostic designations. So, prominent lability and irritability that comes and goes may signify a form of mania to some clinicians, while to others the same features manifest emotional impulsivity thought to accompany ADHD. Intermittent explosive disorder strikes others as an appropriate characterization, though outbursts are usually more than intermittent, and interepisode functioning more impaired, than IED usually connotes. Vulnerability to easy emotional upset leads yet others to emphasize inflexibility that can be characteristic of pervasive developmental disorders. And in many settings, the high defensive reactivity that accompanies affective/impulsive aggression suggests sequelae of trauma. All of these can be very accurate and clinically useful characterizations that explain the context in which aggressive behavior emerges, but it is not certain to what extent clinician predilections, in contrast to patient history, inform such decisions. The coming years should bring greater clarity to this topic, accompanied, hopefully, by advances in our basic understanding of how emotion arises, changes, and become perturbed to produce psychiatric illness.

Anxiety

With the possible exception of posttraumatic stress disorder, discussed later, anxiety disorders by themselves seldom increase the liability for aggressive behavior. The situation changes, though, when comorbid conditions enter the picture. Anxious children with ADHD and ODD are more likely to become behaviorally unmanageable, perhaps by virtue of impulse control problems, making it more difficult for them to tolerate anxious discomfort. For instance, efforts to interrupt compulsive rituals for a child with obsessive-compulsive disorder or to enforce school attendance with a child who has separation anxiety can at times provoke aggressive dyscontrol. A frequent comorbidity with anxiety and with ADHD is chronic tic disorders, including Tourette syndrome, a particularly difficult combination that has a high prevalence of rage attacks and destructive behavior (106).

"Coldhearted"

Besides these "hot" affective features, callousness and *under*emotionality may, as mentioned earlier, influence aggressive behavior used for instrumental goals (38, 107). These individuals appear to display rather blunted emotional reactivity to the distress of others, a stimulus that is thought to inhibit gratuitous violence in most people (44). Similarly, the disapproval of others appears to carry little significance for them and it seems they are more interested in asserting control and gaining advantage over others than in companionship. Perhaps as a partial result of this indifference, the antisocial behavior of psychopathic individuals is especially refractory to current treatments.

Environmental Influences

Stress-Related

Diminished Positive Parental Interactions; Harsh and Inconsistent Discipline. Childrearing practices probably affect the development of children's aggressive behavior through both stress-related and social learning processes; the next section will focus on the latter. It is obvious that children with early onset conduct problems often make difficult housemates, and those with frequent aggressive behavior still more so because family members are the most common targets (108–111). Even when the behavior is not particularly harmful, many aspects of family life that are normally almost effortless are fraught with the prospect that a meltdown or a "scene" will disrupt otherwise enjoyable activities, draw attention and resources away from siblings, and complicate relations with schools.

The compound effects are to corrode the quality of parent–child relationships, particularly when parents believe misbehavior to be volitional (112). Family stress and discord and frequent repercussions (113–116) may further degrade a parent's capacity to apply measured discipline consistently and with composure (87, 115, 117–119). The mutual antagonism that results, and the child's own unpredictability, may incline a parent toward disengagement or involvement that depends on the parent's own energy and mood, than on the child's behavior.

Of course, the child's own characteristics are not the only cause for problematic parent–child relationships. Parental psychopathology and substance abuse can lead to suboptimal interactions with their children (120–122). It remains unclear just how influential deficiencies in parent–child relationship quality would be if one statistically adjusted for other risk factors "intrinsic" to the child. Adoption and twin studies indicate that both are environmental effects for development of antisocial behavior are significant, but even these have not controlled for more specific temperamental vulnerabilities and their interaction with environment (e.g., impulsivity, negative affect) (123).

Poor quality of a child's primary relationships, however it comes about, may independently aggravate behavioral volatility and aggression. There is some evidence that parenting stress and relationship quality are particularly important to the outcomes of aggressive youth, after statistical adjustment for severity of behavioral problems and disciplinary practices (124, 125). Interestingly, it has been suggested that among children with callous-unemotional traits, quality of parenting may play a diminished role in the development of their conduct problems (126), which would comport with the apparent indifference of psychopathic individuals to others' feelings.

Trauma, Abuse, Frequent Endangerment. Maltreatment by caregivers during childhood significantly increases one's liability for lifetime psychopathology, particularly among girls and women. The largest effect sizes of child abuse for both genders is the increase in antisocial behavior (127). A connection between living helplessly with frequent, random infliction of pain and development of defensive hyperreactivity to even minimal threat is both intuitive and supported by recent studies indicating abnormalities in the structures and processes that subserve fear and affect regulation (128). One would also suppose that reactive forms of aggression would predominate among maltreated youth, but abuse correlates equally well with measures of reactive and proactive aggression (129), and abuse was slightly more prevalent among youth categorized as proactively aggressive than reactively aggressive (130).

Caregivers and other adults are not the only sources of endangerment in children's lives. Peers and siblings can also serve as tormentors, though highly proactive children may be less vulnerable (131–133).

Community Factors. Neighborhood socioeconomic disadvantage increases the risk for violent behavior among young people, but which specific adversities most promote antisocial behavior is unclear. Multivariate analyses can adjust for confounding factors, such as poverty and school quality, and attempts to identify a few variables that best account for the association. One variable that may be pivotal is the proportion of households with children that are headed by single adults (134). While single-parent homes are not inherently pathogenic, communities where they predominate have fewer adults providing supervision and those present are more likely to be busy with the burdens of raising children, with fewer resources than would be typical in childrearing homes with at least two adults.

Social Learning

Benefits for One's Own Aggressive Behavior. If aggressive behavior has a payoff, basic learning theory would predict that it will be more likely in the future. Therefore, if a conflict involving the child's aggression ends with the child prevailing in getting his or her way, escaping from an undesirable situation, or gaining some other reward, aggressive behavior is in effect reinforced.

Likewise, victim acquiescence to one's aggressive behavior offers further incentive to attack or intimidate others. Some bullies may also attain high status among peers at least for brief periods (33). In addition, peer encouragement can also provide powerful inducement toward antisocial behavior that outweighs adult-imposed consequences for it. For instance, aggressing against authority figures or tormenting disliked youngsters may provide fine entertainment for behaviorally deviant onlookers who make up the peer groups to which many aggressive youth either aspire or are relegated. Vicarious enjoyment of a peer's antisocial conduct, and reinforcement for the performer, may be related to the findings that outpatient group treatments for youth with severe conduct problems may do more harm than good (135). A similar process may also occur by which a youth with severe conduct problems may enlist the collusion of a sibling to erode the authority structure within the home (136).

There is some evidence that children acquire "display rules" for emotion rather early in life, and can dampen or amplify affective displays to suit context and audience (137, 138). One consequence is that some children may indeed accentuate angry displays if they develop the expectation that it will yield some advantage, so the nature of how others respond to tantrums and bluster are of course an important aspect of assessment.

Modeling, Observed Benefits for Aggression. The phenomenon of learning by observing the consequences that accompany behaviors modeled by others is called social or vicarious learning (139). Therefore, the perception that benefits accrue to those who control others by coercive means would tend to make such coercive behavior seem more desirable, or perhaps even necessary to maintain a minimal degree of social standing and respect that deter would-be assailants.

The weight of the current evidence seems to indicate that very high exposure to depictions of violence in mass media may contribute to the risk of aggressive behavior, particularly among young children (140). One recent study demonstrated an association among young adults between exposure to violent videogames and reduced event-related P300 EEG waveforms when presented with violent images, suggesting that high-exposure individuals are more inured to such stimuli (141).

Cognitive or Sensory Impairments

We can briefly note a few other major psychiatric illnesses and developmental problems that may have aggression as a complication because the illness itself distorts one's information processing or the capacity to communicate and handle distress.

Aggressive behavior frequently accompanies schizophrenia among adolescents and adults (142, 143). The few children who develop the disorder are more typically terrified, disorganized or perplexed souls, rather than bellicose. Several factors that seem to augment the risk of violence include severity of positive symptoms, paranoid delusions, male gender, and premorbid history of aggressive behavior. Following stabilization of acute psychotic symptoms, violence does not seem especially characteristic of residual phase schizophrenia among adults, and indeed increased belligerence, suspiciousness and lashing out would ordinarily warn of relapse, or perhaps of alcohol and drug use. The situation for younger afflicted patients is less clear.

Several major developmental disorders pose significant risk for aggressive behavior. Some developmental disabilities carry higher liability for dyscontrolled behavior than others, being quite common, for instance, within pervasive developmental disorders, moderately high in, say, Prader-Willi syndrome, and less of a complication in Down or Williams syndromes (144). Within any given syndrome, as well as idiopathic mental retardation in general, severity of aggression seems to correlate with lower IQ and male gender. Certain periods of life are more likely to feature cantankerous behavior, notably midchildhood and early adolescence or puberty. Self-injurious behavior is an aspect of several developmental syndromes, also more or less in proportion to the extent of cognitive handicap. Difficulties communicating the nature and cause of discomfort, and a limited repertoire of behaviors to gain the attention of others, mandates that qualified clinicians perform careful assessments to ascertain the triggers for aggressive outbursts and consider environmental changes that can redress factors that provoke problem behavior. Such assessment may reveal a link between problem behavior and a desire to escape a situation, to gain attention, and, particularly for self-directed aggression, to provide sensory stimulation. Complicating matters is that the offending stimuli can be idiosyncratic, such as the supersensivity to sound or touch seen at times among persons with autism (hyperacusis) or difficulties handling changes in routine or environment that may be barely perceptible to others.

Behavioral Pharmacotoxicity

Prescription Drugs: Complications of Therapeutic Use, Overdose

Medication regimens for many aggressive children these days involves coadministration of multiple agents (145, 146). This presents the possibility that medications could contribute to behavioral dyscontrol in ways that may not be obvious. Most of the attention for such escalations in aggression has focused on SSRIs and, less often, atypical antipsychotics, implicating serotonergic mechanisms. Compounds used principally for nonpsychiatric illness also deserve consideration. For instance, higher doses of corticosteroids can precipitate aggressive behavior (147). Of course, any other drug may potentially cause idiosyncratic, untoward behavioral reactions.

Drugs of Abuse

In children and adolescents, it is difficult to ascribe any specific amount of aggressive behavior to the effects of alcohol and other substances. The chief confound, naturally, is that deviant behavior and other psychiatric problems associated with aggression are major risk factors for consuming these products. We have chosen to depict substance abuse in Figure 5.2.3.1 as a sequela of aggressive behavior that may in turn make things worse, even though it may really be a concomitant. A stronger contributory connection may occur when drug use aggravates an existing or latent psychiatric illness, such as cocaine, cannabinoid, or hallucinogen use by psychosis-prone individuals, triggering a period of behavioral dyscontrol that does not taper quickly with usual offset of the drug's action.

ASSESSMENT

The previous section indicates that while aggressive behavior is a common chief complaint when children present for mental health care, it manifests in many psychiatric conditions. We identified some of the chief influences and contexts for aggressive behavior that warrant assessment. This section, however, focuses on some tools for the evaluation of aggressive behavior.

Aggression-Relevant Components of Multidomain Tools

Widely used behavioral rating instruments for youth include subscales that pertain to aggressive behavior, including the Child Behavior Checklist and its related devices (148), and the Behavior Assessment System for Children (149). Items constituting these subscales often include some nonaggressive conduct problems. Multidimensional scales offer a gauge of severity relative to national norms for parent, teacher, and, in some instances, self-report ratings.

Aggression-Specific Measures

For clinical and research purposes, it is useful to obtain finer grained discrimination between specific forms of aggressive behavior. Various versions of the Overt Aggression Scale (150–152) query the frequency over a defined period of specific aggressive acts, categorized as verbal, physical, self-directed and property damage. The item score is the frequency multiplied by weights for the category and the severity of the behavior, so that more harmful behaviors are amplified in the total score that results. Raw frequencies, however, risk skewed distributions. One published adaptation of the OAS approach asks the responded to estimate frequencies over a more limited range of scores, and initial psychometric data are favorable (153).

At least two other assessment devices, the Interview for Antisocial Behavior (154, 155) and the New York Teacher Rating Scale (156), enable assessment of a broader range of antisocial behaviors along with a subscale that quantifies physical aggression specifically. A parent analogue to the latter contains similar content, and was sensitive to change in both an outpatient controlled clinical trial (157) and as a predictor (125) and outcome (145) of psychiatrically hospitalized children postdischarge functioning.

Particularly among older antisocial youth, self-reports of delinquent behaviors are an important complement to other sources that may have high specificity (positives are likely to be valid) but much lower sensitivity (likely to omit serious misconduct unknown to adult informants or official records). One often-used instrument to obtain information on self-reported delinquency inquires about an array of covert, overt, violent and nonviolent antisocial behaviors, as well as substance use (158).

Measuring Facets of Aggressive Behavior

A few scales endeavor to characterize to what extent youngsters' aggressive behavior seems proactive versus reactive (31, 159, 160). Despite high correlations between the dimensions and difficulty extracting "pure" groups, it seems important to clarify whether indeed these two qualities of aggression respond differentially to treatment (161, 162).

The leading method for the assessment of callous-unemotional factor of psychopathy, along with separate measures for an impulsive behavior factor rather generic to those with conduct problems, and a self-centeredness factor, is the Antisocial Process Screening Device (163). The approach facilitates both youth self-report and completion of a parallel form by an adult informant.

TREATMENT

Treatment Planning

Psychopathology and Context

The breadth of clinical scenarios that include aggression as a concern seems to militate against a single treatment protocol for aggression. An alternate view is that aggression may be the final common pathway of these diverse influences. The mechanism that generates aggressive behavior, regardless of how it is activated, might be amenable to some specific antiaggressive, or "serenic," treatment. The latter has some appeal for developing pharmacological treatment, whereby aggression is a target symptom regardless of psychopathological context, and for crisis management that has to train people in managing the "general case," with less opportunity to calibrate it based on individualized assessment.

At this point, the burden of proof probably rests with the latter position. There is ample evidence that effective treatment of a primary disorder can diminish aggressive behavior considerably, and that is the approach taken by most algorithms for aggression among young people. Psychosocial treatments that take a one-size-fits all approach may be ineffective, and in some instances trigger further behavioral dyscontrol.

Multiple impairments in several settings are the rule

Aggression often seems, justifiably, to be the most pressing problem during evaluation. However, it is common for a child to exhibit aggressive behavior in one setting and other problems in other venues. For example, loss of control may be most prominent at home, but school problems can feature frustration and low achievement, and social problems may involve benign neglect by peers accompanied by brushoffs when the patient makes social overtures. Aggressive behavior at home may relate to these other stresses in less than obvious ways, and the latter should be noted in a treatment plan.

Prioritizing and Sequencing Treatments

When psychosocial treatments should precede medications or vice versa is a common issue. Discussion of it often reflects an ethos that pharmacotherapy should be a treatment of last resort. In the developmental disabilities area, there is a strong preference for ecological interventions and some impressive successes applying behavioral analysis to pinpoint the factors to modify. In some instances, out-of-control behavior strikes one as clearly a derivative of timid limit-setting or a dysfunctional parent–child relationship, so it's tempting to focus nonpharmacologically on those facets of the situation. However, in the modal case of aggression in the context ADHD and ODD, there is a case to be made the other way, that for the typical consequence-based treatments to gain traction, impulsivity should decrease, and stimulant treatment is a highly efficacious vehicle for doing so. Family preference is a pivotal factor, and the pros and cons of each approach should be discussed openly along with an agreement about how to monitor an outcome and when to change course.

Pharmacotherapy

Algorithmic Approach

Current practice guidelines for the pharmacological treatment of aggression emphasize the need to address the key underlying syndrome first (164–166). To the extent that this is unsuccessful, these guidelines suggest algorithms based on available data and expert consensus on sequencing and selection of further medication trials. The overarching concept is that pharmacotherapy, when called for, should be judicious, and one should resist knee-jerk responses to add something when improvement is not evident before an adequate trial of the current regimen has been completed. Another major challenge is daring to discontinue medications, to avoid the accretion of agents whose benefits are uncertain and whose risks, particularly in combination with other compounds, are far from clear (145).

A common view is that medication affects only affective/impulsive aggression (167, 168), but data are inconclusive. M. Campbell et al. (168). found that lithium had its greatest impact on "bullying," a proactive/instrumental form of aggression. Malone also (161) found that high instrumental aggression did not predict diminished lithium response: Two of three lithium responders had high instrumental aggression scores, as did one of two lithium nonresponders. Klein et al. (157). and Hinshaw et al. (169). reported benefits for MPH on several proactive/instrumental conduct problems. Among adults, though, Barratt et al. (170). found reductions in aggression with phenytoin treatment only for inmates with impulsive, not premeditated, aggression.

Of the diatheses discussed earlier, impulsivity and affective instability may be amenable to psychopharmacological treatments. We organize our discussion around these problems, focusing on studies that specifically measure aggressive behavior as an outcome.

Treatments Oriented toward Improved Impulse Control

Placebo-controlled trials have repeatedly shown the efficacy of stimulants in treating the core symptoms of ADHD (171). The impact of stimulant treatment on *aggressive and other disruptive behavior* among ADHD youth is also appreciable (172, 173). MPH reduced oppositional and hostile behaviors in numerous controlled trials in school, inpatient, summer treatment, and home settings; some studies suggest that medication must be active through the evening to improve late-day behavior (174–176). Placebo response is uncommon, and when it occurs is rarely durable (171, 177–180, but *cf* 181).

Klein et al. (157). suggested that MPH might ameliorate CD independently of ADHD. MPH reduced conduct problems in a sample of youth with CD (DSM-III) while the placebo-treated group got worse; 70% had comorbid ADHD. MPH remained superior when a composite of baseline ADHD ratings was used as a covariate. The responses of ADHD and non-ADHD subjects to MPH were not directly compared.

Comparisons of stimulants and psychosocial treatments show the overall superiority of medication; (182–185) parent training alone yields improvements for school-age children, but effect sizes are smaller than for medication in studies of children with ADHD (177, 185, 186).

Augmentation of stimulant treatment with behavioral interventions has also been examined. Klein and Abikoff (183) reported better outcomes in some areas for combined treatment over medication alone, but subjects were selected to have generally noncomorbid ADHD, and had low rates of conduct problems. A larger study by this group, which included attention-control conditions as a comparator for their psychosocial treatments, also showed no additional benefit over the substantial effects of stimulant medication over a range of outcomes (187) C. L. Carlson et al. (188) reported that the addition of behavioral treatment did not improve outcomes over stimulant treatment, but it may enable lower dosages. Other studies also found no significant benefits for combined over medication-only treatment (178, 182, 189). For the MTA sample as a whole, combined treatment yielded some improvement in ODD *symptoms* over medication alone (190). However, when subjects comorbid for ADHD and ODD/CD were considered, no significant advantage was apparent for combined treatment over medication alone (191) (those who also had an anxiety disorder did benefit from combined treatment).

Nonstimulant treatments for ADHD, such as bupropion, atomoxetine, and modafinil, have not yet been shown to affect aggressive behavior.

While the overall clinical benefit for stimulant treatment is significant, many children show unsatisfactory reductions of aggressive and other disruptive behaviors. Barkley et al. (192). found that aggressive youth treated with MPH still had much more aggressive behavior than other children with ADHD, despite meaningful improvements on attention ratings. Pelham et al. (193). reported that marked social impairment persisted with stimulant treatment accompanied by intensive psychosocial treatment. Smithee et al. (194). also found limited benefits for MPH on overt aggression, despite significant effects on attention and hyperactivity. "Retaliatory behavior" among children with ADHD and other conduct problems was still markedly higher after MPH treatment relative to MPH-treated children with "pure" ADHD (195). Over one-third of adolescent day treatment patients in a controlled trial of MPH showed no improvement on observed defiance (196). Recent subgroup analyses of the MTA study showed that medication-treated ADHD youth with disruptive disorders were far less likely to show good response to any treatment than other medication-treated subjects (191), even when intensive psychosocial treatments were provided. Indirect evidence for suboptimal stimulant response comes from pharmacoepidemiologic and clinical studies that show high rates of multidrug treatment of children with comorbid disorders (145, 197, 198).

In the context of other primary disorders, the benefits of stimulant treatment on aggressive behavior are less well studied. Youngsters with major developmental disorders, autism in particular, have more variable responses to stimulant therapy, which at times may worsen aggression and irritability (199, 200).

Antipsychotics, Mood Stabilizers, and Other Pharmacotherapy for Affective Disturbance

Antipsychotics. Other medications to treat aggression in youth may help to improve affective stability. Antipsychotics have long held a prominent place in treating aggression in nonpsychotic individuals. Their broad spectrum of effects includes mood stabilizing effects. Early studies suggested the efficacy of antipsychotic medications among nonpsychotic aggressive youth (201, 202), but concerns about their potential to produce extrapyramidal symptoms not only acutely but also after prolonged use (tardive onset), and other side effects, restrained their use. The past decade has witnessed a tremendous increase in the rates of pharmacotherapy for children with severe behavioral disturbances that involves second generation antipsychotics (SGAs) (203, 205, 206). Children so treated initially seemed to tolerate these medicines with lower incidence of acute neuromotor side effects. However, the propensity for these agents to cause adiposity and associated alterations to lipid and glucose metabolism, which pose liabilities for cardiovascular and other morbidities, has raised concerns about their proliferative use (207, 208). The effects of rapid fat deposition on growing bodies, in particular, is now a widespread concern, and it seems that children may be more susceptible to SGA-induced weight gain (209–212).

Risperidone currently has the most extensive data from controlled trials supporting its efficacy as monotherapy among children with aggressive behavior, involving, with one exception (213), children with severe to mild developmental handicaps (214–217). These studies show marked reductions relative to placebo in parent or clinician ratings of aggression and in some instances improvements in the asociality associated with pervasive developmental disorders. Significant weight gain, though in the midrange relative to other SGAs, and hyperprolactinemia are frequently reported.

Published support for other most SGAs (olanzapine, quetiapine, ziprasidone, aripiprazole) as beneficial for aggressive behavior among nonpsychotic youth comes mainly from naturalistic studies, such as retrospective chart reviews or small open-label trials. More data from controlled trials that are appropriate to the patient group of widest use, nonpsychotic aggressive children with ADHD without major developmental impairments, are essential.

Mood Stabilizing Agents. Despite the ascendancy of SGA use, most of the controlled trial data in developmentally typical preadolescents with disruptive behavior disorders involve lithium. Seven double-blind placebo-controlled trials evaluated lithium's efficacy. Only two treated outpatients. Campbell and her colleagues (201) compared lithium, haloperidol, and placebo in the treatment of 61 CD (per DSM-III) inpatient preadolescents, with the primary target symptom of explosive aggression. Clinician ratings showed both drugs' superiority to placebo; lithium had fewer side effects and surpassed haloperidol on some measures. A replication trial (168) was less robust, but still supported lithium's efficacy on consensus ratings by inpatient staff. Another inpatient study (218) reported a significant effect for lithium over placebo among 10- to 17-year-old aggressive inpatients.

Other studies yielded less encouraging findings. Another inpatient study (219) examined response to lithium followed by placebo substitution among seven explosively aggressive children. Aggression improved but the change was said to have meager clinical significance, and was maintained during placebo substitution. A relatively short (2-week) trial (220) found no benefit for lithium over placebo among 33 12- to 17-year-old inpatients with CD and aggression. A prospective followup of 18 lithium-responsive inpatients after discharge, treated half with continued lithium and half with placebo substitution (167). Of the 11 completing the trial, lithium- and placebo-treated children showed comparable aggression scores, though global ratings showed a modest benefit for lithium. Finally, another outpatient study (221) found no benefit for lithium over placebo on any measure during a 5-week trial involving boys with conduct disorder.

Studies using divalproex (DVPX) showed marked effects in reducing aggression and self-reported irritable mood in an open trial with adolescents (222), a double-blind placebo-controlled crossover trial with a somewhat younger sample (223), and a controlled trial with adjudicated adolescents (224). In Donovan et al (222)., 10 patients (average age 16 years) with CD or ODD received a 5-week DVPX trial; patients were selected for significant explosiveness, had histories of school suspensions, half had prior treatment with stimulants, and many abused substances. Significant reductions in overt aggression ratings and improvements in global functioning and self-reported mood occurred. In a subsequent controlled trial (223), eight of 10 aggressive labile outpatients (mean 13.8 years old) treated with DVPX showed marked reductions in aggression and hostile mood; 75% of these youth relapsed following crossover into a placebo phase. Six of seven youth showed significant response after crossover from placebo to active drug after no improvement during the placebo phase. Twenty percent met criteria for ADHD. A controlled trial of DVPX with 16 conduct-disordered adolescents also showed improvements in subjective "distress" and ratings of behavioral restraint in high vs. low (blood levels <50 ml/L) conditions (224).

Although an open pilot trial of carbamazepine appeared to reduce aggression among hospitalized preadolescents with conduct disorder (225), a randomized controlled trial at the same facility showed no benefit of carbamazepine over placebo (226).

Other Agents. There is only one published open trial of the alpha$_2$-agonist clonidine in the treatment of aggression (227). Randomized controlled trials suggest its benefit as monotherapy for ADHD, but its effect is well below that of stimulants (228). Connor et al. (229). found that MPH combined with clonidine afforded no benefit over MPH alone for a sample with conduct problems. Open (230, 231) and controlled (232) trials of guanfacine showed benefits for ADHD symptoms but effects on aggression are not reported. The opposing autonomic effects of alpha-agonists and MPH are also of concern (233), more exactly, whether hypertensive rebound as the former wear off might augment the sympathomimetic effects of stimulants (234). There are no controlled studies of beta blockers for childhood aggressive behavior. The preponderance of case reports and open trials (using mainly propranolol and nadolol) involved developmentally disabled youth (235).

Not all drugs for affective disturbances are helpful for aggression in youth. Antidepressants do not have a major role now in treating childhood aggression outside of depression or anxiety disorders. Benzodiazepines may increase disinhibition and aggression (236) and are disfavored for treating childhood aggression outside of acute use in psychosis or mania.

One intriguing double-blind controlled trial conducted in a British penitentiary showed marked reductions in violent incidents among inmates randomized to receive a combination of vitamins, minerals and omega-3 fatty acid pills compared to those who received matching placebo pills (237). The fact that this study effectively standardized all other aspects of environment and diet appears to strengthen the potential significance of micronutrients in violence-prone populations.

Psychosocial Treatments

Overview

Interventions to alleviate aggressive behavior endeavor to alter the ecological context that seems to promote the behavior or to help individuals develop alternatives to aggression that serve the same function more adaptively. Descriptions of specific therapies [consequence-based approaches, anger control, multisystemic therapy (238)] for these purposes appear elsewhere in this volume. Rather than cataloguing psychosocial interventions, it might be more useful to identify some avenues of approach through which treatments may reduce aggressive behavior. Borrowing from the framework of functional behavior assessment (239), we organize the discussion around the premise that psychosocial interventions aim to make *aggressive* behavior, to varying degrees, *irrelevant, ineffective or inefficient* (Figure 5.2.3.2).

Making Aggression "Irrelevant"

Aggressive behavior is generally not a random event. Certain situations, or antecedents, are more apt to provoke it than others are for a particular youngster. If one identifies these antecedents, then decreased aggressive behavior might result from interventions to reduce or mitigate exposure to these precipitants (240). From a functional viewpoint, if aggression is the child's "solution" to a situation, minimizing exposure to that situation renders aggression irrelevant. If a child frequently fights with a sibling when they're both in their shared bedroom together in the morning, then it seems sensible to have one child eat breakfast while the other is getting dressed, then switch. A simple inquiry or prompt about getting homework finished might precipitate an argument, mutual antagonism and escalation, and finally an explosion. One might avert this simply by enrolling the youngster in an after-school program that includes homework help. The same idea applies not only to reducing stimuli that are aversive for the child, but to reducing exposure to situations that actively encourage antisocial and aggressive behavior. Eliminating a youth's exposure to behaviorally deviant peers exemplifies this approach (238).

Combining the avoidance of situations that often culminate in aggressive behavior with increased prompting to perform behaviors that often culminate in compliance is another way in which altering antecedents can render problem behavior irrelevant. After securing high rates of compliance by asking the child to do only things he or she would want to do anyway, one approach to improve cooperativeness is to then move on to requests that the child had hesitated to do before. When moving onto situations that formerly had a lower likelihood of cooperation fast on the heels of several days of lots of apparent cooperativeness, Ducharme has shown that greater compliance and composure can result (241).

Antecedents that influence behavior also include contextual factors that are not necessarily stimuli immediately present in the situation. Behavioral analysts refer to these as *setting*

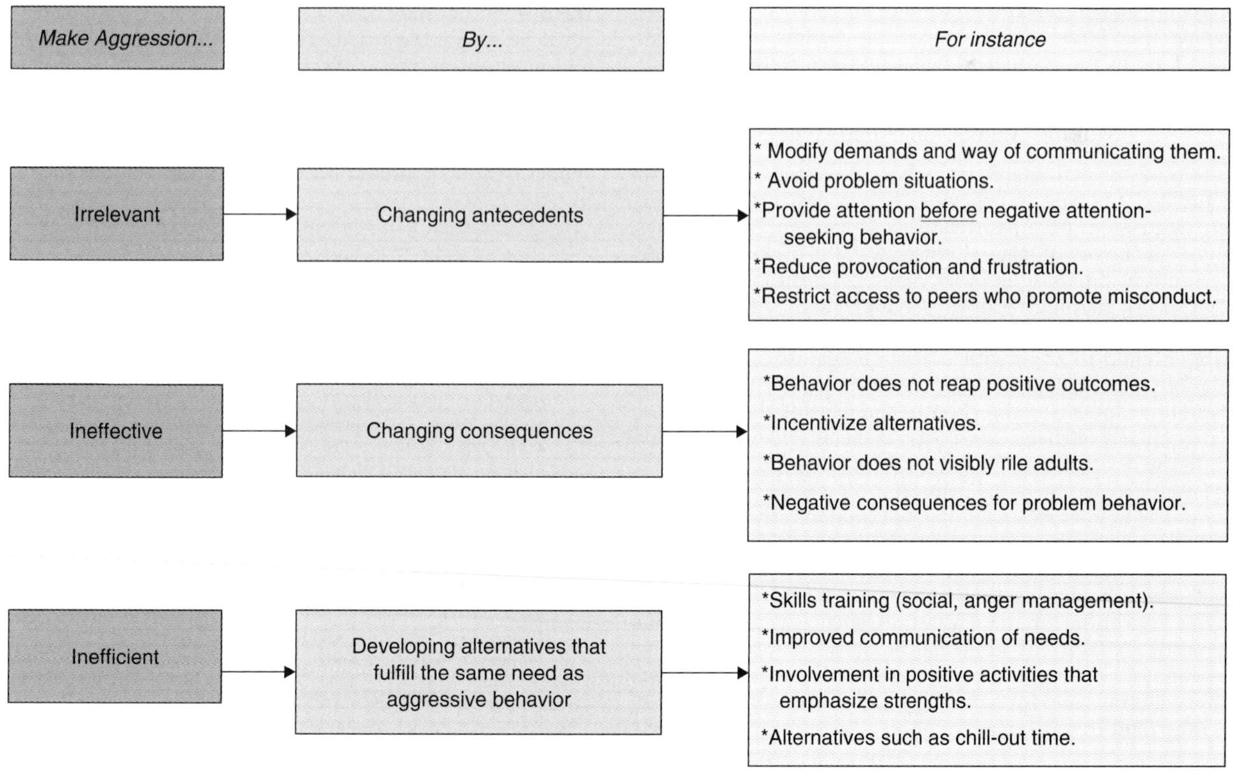

FIGURE 5.2.3.2. Goals and approaches of psychosocial treatment.

events, that is, they set the stage for how the observable stimuli affect the respondent (the child). One such contextual factor involves the quality of the relationship between the adult and the child, which also seems significant for outcome even after adjusting for level of behavior disorder (124, 242). Several common behavioral interventions emphasize positive time and warmth between parent and child (243, 244). By increasing the number of positive interchanges, the goal is to reduce the proportion of the acrimonious ones that tend to dominate among children with severe behavioral dyscontrol and poor rule adherence. If this goal is achieved, the child is more apt to perceive the parent as a source of positive attention, affection and affirmation, and not just an agent of coercion. In this "revised" relational context, the expectation is that children will be more responsive to parents' authority and the consequences that parents can dispense.

Making Aggression "Ineffective"

The reactions of others that accompany aggressive behavior might maintain or reinforce it. Aggression may, for instance, elicit their acquiescence, their giving up trying to gain compliance, or even their barring the child from school if that is a desired result for a child. Approaches that modify the usual consequences of aggressive behavior would therefore make it ineffective in achieving the goal that apparently sustains it. Moreover, the application of consequences one would ordinarily seek to avoid (time outs, loss of privileges, other sanctions) may hasten the learning that aggression is unlikely to provide an effective means of fulfilling a particular wish. Most contingency management approaches and those that employ systematic ignoring of milder misbehavior might be described as interventions that aim to make aggressive behavior less effective by diminishing the "payoff" that previously reinforced it. Such limit-setting and manipulation of consequences are at the core of several interventions for conduct problems, and aggressive behavior may also be affected by these treatments (244–247).

Similarly, bullying and intimidation become ineffective if the social milieu galvanizes around intolerance for the behavior. This often means supporting victims, rather than denigrating them, in order to undermine the secrecy and fear on which such behavior thrives.

Making Aggression "Inefficient"

If the purpose that aggressive behavior seemed to serve can be fulfilled utilizing a behavior that is easier to perform, then aggression becomes relatively inefficient, and should reduce in favor of the alternative. Many skills training interventions discussed in other chapters (anger management, social skills training, problemsolving) (248, 249) seek to develop proficiency in alternatives to aggressive behavior that enable a child to cope with otherwise aggression-provoking situations more adaptively. However, if these end up being far more arduous for the child to implement, they may not be particularly efficient. Moreover, if the alternative does not obtain the desired "payoff," the child may not perceive it as a very useful replacement behavior. It is all well to teach a child how to ask to borrow something, but limited verbal skills may make it harder rather than easier relative to grabbing, and the altercation that follows. Likewise, if the other child does not oblige, the behavior may not be reinforced. Bridging behavior may be appropriate in these instances, such as where the child can easily signal to an adult that he or she wants something from another child and the adult can facilitate the exchange, and reward the child for handling a rebuff with composure. At the other end of the age range, if an adolescent had obtained some social esteem by being antisocial, one would consider exploiting the youngster's prosocial talents and interests as a vehicle to gaining prestige.

A range of psychosocial interventions exists for children and adolescents with various conduct and oppositional-defiant behaviors, often including aggression. Treatment studies targeting aggression per se have been somewhat less common. Nonetheless, various psychosocial treatment strategies have yielded significant reductions in aggressive behaviors, both in prevention trials and clinical treatment settings (155, 246, 250–252). Thus, parent management training (PMT) is an efficacious strategy for treating aggression and related conduct problems (155, 186, 250, 253). Some evidence suggest that PMT may yield durable improvements in behavioral problems across various settings (254). Parent–child interaction training (PCIT) has also been found to reduce aggressive symptoms; by acquiring noninvasive play skills and learning to give clear instructions, reward compliance, and provide consequences for noncompliance, parents can improve interactions with their children and manage their aggression (243). Likewise, school- and community-based programs have been shown to yield improvements in aggressive behavior in youth (255), although research also shows that peer-group interventions can reinforce deviant behavior (135). Individual cognitive-behavioral treatments, including anger management training and problemsolving skills training, have also had some success in improving aggressive behavior (186, 251, 252).

This area of study, while of major importance, has generally lacked sophistication about the causes/precursors of aggression. In our view, development of more effective psychosocial treatments for aggression are likely to depend upon more sophisticated understanding of the motivational and environmental factors contributing to depression, described earlier.

CONCLUSIONS

Aggressive behavior remains a complex and stubborn, yet highly prevalent, clinical problem in the practice of child and adolescent psychiatry. However, one's efforts to grapple with this complexity and persist in supporting families through treatments that may have a long latency to yield benefits will often be amply rewarded. Timely and thoughtful assessment and intervention may deflect a child from a spiral of chronic conflict, social maladjustment, and marginalization. The child psychiatrist has an especially privileged position because the complications that arise from chronic antisocial behavior may render treatment later in life a day late and a dollar short.

References

1. Hobbes T: *Leviathan; or the Matter, Forme, and Power of a Commonwealth Ecclesiaticall and Civil*, M. Oakeshott, ed. Oxford, U.K., Blackwell (originally published 1651), 1960.
2. Locke J: *Two Treatises of Government*, I. Shapiro, ed. New York, Cambridge University Press (originally published 1689), 1988.
3. Malthus TR: *An Essay on the Principle of Population*, G. Gilbert, ed. New York, Oxford University Press (originally published 1798), 1993.
4. Miller G: *The Mating Mind: How Sexual Choice Shaped the Evolution of Human Nature*. London, Heineman, 2000.
5. Darwin C: *The Descent of Man, and Selection in Relation to Sex*. Princeton, NJ, Princeton University Press (originally published 1871), 1981.
6. De Waal FBM: *Good Natured: The Origins of Right and Wrong in Humans and Other Animals*. Cambridge, MA, Harvard University Press, 1996.
7. Ridley M: *The Origins of Virtue: Human Instincts and the Evolution of Cooperation*. New York, Viking, 1996.
8. Moffitt TE, Caspi A, Rutter M, et al.: *Sex Differences in Antisocial Behaviour: Conduct Disorder, Delinquency, and Violence in the Dunedin Longitudinal Study*. New York, Cambridge University Press, 2001.
9. Lahey BB, Loeber R, Burke JD, et al.: Predicting future antisocial personality disorder in males from a clinical assessment in childhood. *J Consult Clin Psychol* 73:389–399, 2005.
10. Tremblay RE: Why socialization fails: The case of chronic physical aggression. In: Lahey BB, Moffitt TE, Caspi A (eds.): *Causes of Conduct*

Disorder and Juvenile Delinquency. New York: Guilford Press, 2003, pp. 182–224.
11. Tremblay RE, Nagin DS, Seguin JR, et al.: Physical aggression during early childhood: trajectories and predictors. *Pediatr* 114:e43–50, 2004, (online edition).
12. Gadow KD, Sprafkin J: *Early Childhood Inventory 4: Norms Manual*. Stony Brook, NY, Checkmate, 1997.
13. Gadow KD, Sprafkin J: *Child Symptom Inventory 4: Screening and Norms Manual*. Stony Brook, NY, Checkmate, 2002.
14. Broidy LM, Nagin DS, Tremblay RE, et al.: Developmental trajectories of childhood disruptive behaviors and adolescent delinquency: A six-site, cross-national study. *Dev Psychol* 39:222–245, 2003.
15. Pottick KJ, Lynn A. Warner LA, Isaacs M, et al.: Children and adolescents admitted to specialty mental health care programs in the United States, 1986 and 1997. In: Manderscheid RW, Henderson MJ (eds.): *Mental Health, United States, 2002*. Rockville, MD: Substance Abuse and Mental Health Services Administration (DHHS Pub. No. SMA04–3938), 2004, pp. 314–26.
16. Leon SC, Uziel-Miller ND, Lyons JS, et al.: Psychiatric hospital service utilization of children and adolescents in state custody. *J Am Acad Child Adolesc Psychiatry* 38:305–310, 1999.
17. Nicholson J, Young SD, Simon LJ, et al.: Privatized Medicaid managed care in Massachusetts: Disposition in child and adolescent mental health emergencies. *J Beh Health Srv Res* 25:279–292, 1998.
18. Gutterman EM: Is diagnosis relevant in the hospitalization of potentially dangerous children and adolescents? *J Am Acad Child Adolesc Psychiatry* 37:1030–7, 1998.
19. Gutterman EM, Markowitz JS, LoConte JS, et al.: Determinants for hospitalization from an emergency mental health service. *J Am Acad Child Adolesc Psychiatry* 32:114–122, 1993.
20. Keenan K, Loeber R, Green S: Conduct disorder in girls: A review of the literature. *Clin Child Fam Psychol Rev* 2:3–19, 1999.
21. Loeber R, Stouthamer-Loeber M: Juvenile aggression at home and at school. In: Elliott DS, Hamburg BA, Williams KR (eds.): *Violence in American Schools*. New York: Cambridge University Press, 1998, pp. 94–126.
22. Snyder HN, Sickmund M: *Juvenile Offenders and Victims: 2006 National Report*. Washington, DC, U.S. Department of Justice, Office of Juvenile Justice and Delinquency Prevention, 2006.
23. Bureau of Justice Statistics: Criminal Victimization in the United States—Statistical Tables. <www.ojp.usdoj.gov/bjs/abstract/cvusst.htm> Accessed May 15, 2006.
24. Barratt ES, Stanford MS, Dowdy L, et al.: Impulsive and premeditated aggression: A factor analysis of self-reported acts. *Psychiatry Res* 86:163–73, 1999.
25. Brennan PA, Raine A: Biosocial bases of antisocial behavior: Psychophysiological, neurological, and cognitive factors. *Clin Psychol Rev* 17:589–604, 1997.
26. Brown K, Atkins MS, Osborne ML, et al.: A revised teacher rating scale for reactive and proactive aggression. *J Abnorm Child Psychol* 24:473–480, 1996.
27. Davidson RJ, Putnam KM, Larson CL: Dysfunction in the neural circuitry of emotion regulation—A possible prelude to violence. *Science* 289:591–4, 2000.
28. Dodge KA, Lochman JE, Harnish JD, et al.: Reactive and proactive aggression in school children and psychiatrically impaired chronically assaultive youth. *J Abnorm Psychol* 106:37–51, 1997.
29. Patrick CJ: Emotion and psychopathy: Startling new insights. *Psychophysiology* 31:319–330, 1994.
30. Pliszka SR: The psychobiology of oppositional defiant disorder and conduct disorder. In: Quay HC, Hogan AE (eds): *Handbook of Disruptive Behavior Disorders*. New York: Kluwer Academic/Plenum Publisher, 1999, pp. 371–395.
31. Vitiello B, Behar D, Hunt J, et al.: Subtyping aggression in children and adolescents. *J Neuropsychiatry Clin Neurosci* 2:189–92, 1990.
32. Vitiello B, Stoff DM: Subtypes of aggression and their relevance to child psychiatry. *J Am Acad Child Adolesc Psychiatry* 36:307–315, 1997.
33. Moffitt TE: Adolescence-limited and life-course persistent antisocial behavior: A developmental taxonomy. *Psychol Rev* 100:674–701, 1993.
34. Barker ED, Tremblay RE, Nagin DS, et al.: Development of male proactive and reactive physical aggression during adolescence. *J Child Psychol Psychiatry* (in press).
35. Gendreau PL, Archer J: Subtypes of aggression. In: Tremblay RE, Hartup WW, Archer J (eds): *Developmental Origins of Aggression*. New York: Guilford, 2005, pp. 25–46.
36. Loeber R, Green SM, Lahey BB, et al.: Physical fighting in childhood as a risk factor for later mental health problems. *J Am Acad Child Adolesc Psychiatry* 39:421–428, 2000.
37. Frick PJ, Ellis M: Callous-unemotional traits and subtypes of conduct disorder. *Clin Child Fam Psychol Rev* 2:149–68, 1999.
38. Christian RE, Frick PJ, Hill NL, et al.: Psychopathy and conduct problems in children: II. Implications for subtyping children with conduct problems. *J Am Acad Child Adolesc Psychiatry* 36:233–241, 1997.
39. Lynam DR: Early identification of the fledgling psychopath: Locating the psychopathic child in the current nomenclature. *J Abnorm Psychol* 107:566–575, 1998.
40. Steiner H, Cauffman E, Duxbury E: Personality traits in juvenile delinquents: Relation to criminal behavior and recidivism. *J Am Acad Child Adolesc Psychiatry* 38:256–262, 2000.
41. Kiehl KA: A cognitive neuroscience perspective on psychopathy: Evidence for paralimbic system dysfunction. *Psychiatry Res* 142:107–28, 2006.
42. Verona E, Patrick CJ, Curtin JJ, et al.: Psychopathy and physiological response to emotionally evocative sounds. *J Abnorm Psychol* 113:99–108, 2004.
43. Raine A, Lencz T, Taylor K, et al.: Corpus callosum abnormalities in psychopathic antisocial individuals. *Arch Gen Psychiatry* 60:1134–1142, 2003.
44. Blair RJR: Responsiveness to distress cues in the child with psychopathic tendencies. *Pers Individ Dif* 27:135–45, 1997.
45. Birbaumer N, Veit R, Lotze M, et al.: Deficient fear conditioning in psychopathy: A functional magnetic resonance imaging study. *Arch Gen Psychiatry* 62:799–805, 2005.
46. Blair RJR: Neurocognitive models of aggression, the antisocial personality disorders, and psychopathy. *J Neurol Neurosurg Psychiatry* 71:727–731, 2001.
47. Loney BR, Frick PJ, Clements CB, et al.: Callous-unemotional traits, impulsivity, and emotional processing in adolescents with antisocial behavior problems. *J Clin Child Adolesc Psychol* 32:66–80, 2003.
48. Forth AE, Hare RD: The contingent negative variation in psychopaths. *Psychophysiology* 26:676–682, 1989.
49. Soloff PH, Kelly TM, Strotmeyer SJ, et al.: Impulsivity, gender, and response to fenfluramine challenge in borderline personality disorder. *Psychiatry Res* 119:11–24, 2003.
50. Halperin JM, Kalmar JH, Schulz KP, et al.: Elevated childhood serotonergic function protects against adolescent aggression in disruptive boys. *J Am Acad Child Adolesc Psychiatry* 45:833–840, 2006.
51. Dolan MC, Anderson IM: The relationship between serotonergic function and the Psychopathy Checklist: Screening Version. *J Psychopharmacol* 17:216–222, 2003.
52. Kochanska G, Thompson RA: The emergence and development of conscience in toddlerhood and early childhood. In: Grusec JE, Kuczynski L (eds): *Parenting and Children's Internalization of Values: A Handbook of Contemporary Theory*. New York: John Wiley & Sons, 1997, pp. 53–77.
53. Loeber R, Farrington DP, Stouthamer-Loeber M, et al.: Male mental health problems, psychopathy, and personality traits: Key findings from the first 14 years of the Pittsburgh Youth Study. *Clin Child Fam Psychol Rev* 4:273–297, 2001.
54. Frick PJ, Lahey BB, Loeber R, et al.: Oppositional defiant disorder and conduct disorder: A meta-analytic review of factor analyses and cross-validation in a clinic sample. *Clin Psychol Rev* 13:319–340, 1993.
55. Loeber R, Stouthamer-Loeber M: Development of juvenile aggression and violence: Some common misconceptions and controversies. *Am Psychol* 53:242–259, 1998.
56. Loeber R, Hay DF: Key issues in the development of aggression and violence from childhood to early adulthood. *Ann Rev Psychol* 48:371–410, 1997.
57. Archer J, Coyne SM: An integrated review of indirect, relational, and social aggression. *Pers Soc Psychol Rev* 9:212–230, 2005.
58. Cillessen AHN, Mayeux L: From censure to reinforcement: Developmental changes in the association between aggression and social status. *Child Dev* 75:147–163, 2004.
59. Crick NR, Ostrov JM, Werner NE: A longitudinal study of relational aggression, physical aggression, and children's social-psychological adjustment. *J Abnorm Child Psychol* 34:131–142, 2006.
60. Abikoff H, Klein RG: Attention-deficit hyperactivity and conduct disorder: Comorbidity and implications for treatment. *J Consult Clin Psychol* 60:881–92, 1992.
61. Angold A, Costello EJ, Erkanli A: Comorbidity. *J Child Psychol Psychiatry* 40:57–87, 1999.
62. Hinshaw SP, Lahey BB, Hart EL: Issues of taxonomy and comorbidity in the development of conduct disorder. *Dev Psychopathol* 5:31–49, 1993.
63. Jensen PS, Martin D, Cantwell DP: Comorbidity in ADHD: Implications for research, practice, and DSM-V. *J Am Acad Child Adolesc Psychiatry* 6:1065–1079, 1997.
64. Loeber R, Keenan K: Interaction between conduct disorder and its comorbid conditions: Effects of age and gender. *Clin Psychol Rev* 14:497–523, 1994.
65. Pliszka SR: Patterns of psychiatric comorbidity with attention-deficit/hyperactivity disorder. *Child Adolesc Psychiatr Clin N Am* 9:525–540, 2000.
66. Biederman J, Newcorn J, Sprich S: Comorbidity of attention deficit hyperactivity disorder with conduct, depressive, anxiety, and other disorders. *Am J Psychiatry* 564–577, 1991.
67. Fergusson DM, Lynskey MT, Horwood LJ: Attentional difficulties in middle childhood and psychosocial outcomes in young adulthood. *J Child Psychol Psychiatry* 38:633–644, 1997.
68. Greene RW, Biederman J, Faraone SV, et al.: Adolescent outcome of boys with attention-deficit/hyperactivity disorder and social disability: Results from a 4-year longitudinal follow-up study. *J Consult Clin Psychol* 65:758–767, 1997.

69. Taylor E, Chadwick O, Heptinstall E, et al.: Hyperactivity and conduct problems as risk factors for adolescent development. *J Am Acad Child Adolesc Psychiatry* 35:1213–1226, 1996.
70. Mann JJ, Waternaux C, Haas GL, et al.: Toward a clinical model of suicidal behavior in psychiatric patients. *Am J Psychiatry* 156:181–189, 1999.
71. Campbell SB: Hard-to-manage preschool boys: Externalizing behavior, social competence, and family context at two-year followup. *J Abnorm Child Psychol* 1994; 22.
72. Tremblay RE, Pihl RO, Vitaro F, et al.: Predicting early onset of male antisocial behavior from preschool behavior. A test of two personality theories. *Arch Gen Psychiatry* 51:732–738, 1994.
73. Simonoff E, Elander J, Holmshaw J, et al.: Predictors of antisocial personality. Continuities from childhood to adult life. *Br J Psychiatry* 184:118–127, 2004.
74. Jonsdottir S, Bouma A, Sergeant JA, et al.: The impact of specific language impairment on working memory in children with ADHD combined subtype. *Arch Clin Neuropsychol* 20:443–456, 2005.
75. Cohen NJ, Menna R, Vallance DD, et al.: Language, social cognitive processing, and behavioral characteristics of psychiatrically disturbed children with previously identified and unsuspected language impairments. *J Child Psychol Psychiatry* 39:853–864, 1998.
76. Cohen NJ, Vallance DD, Barwick M, et al.: The interface between ADHD and language impairment: An examination of language, achievement, and cognitive processing. *J Child Psychol Psychiatry* 41:353–362, 2000.
77. Purvis KL, Tannock R: Language abilities in children with attention deficit hyperactivity disorder, reading disabilities, and normal controls. *J Abnorm Child Psychol* 25:133–144, 1997.
78. Geraldina P, Mariarosaria L, Annarita A, et al.: Neuropsychiatric sequelae in TBI: A comparison across different age groups. *Brain Inj* 17:835–846, 2003.
79. Max JE, Robertson BA, Lansing AE: The phenomenology of personality change due to traumatic brain injury in children and adolescents. *J Neuropsychiatry Clin Neurosci* 13:161–170, 2001.
80. Lahey BB, Applegate B, Barkley RA, et al.: DSM-IV field trials for oppositional defiant disorder and conduct disorder in children and adolescents. *Am J Psychiatry* 151:1163–1171, 1994.
81. Pastorelli C, Barbaranelli C, Cermak I, et al.: Measuring emotional instability, prosocial behavior and aggression in pre-adolescents: A cross-national study. *Pers Individ Dif* 23:691–703, 1997.
82. Pliszka SR, Sherman JO, Barrow MV, et al.: Affective disorder in juvenile offenders: A preliminary study. *Am J Psychiatry* 157:130–132, 2000.
83. Zoccolillo M: Co-occurrence of conduct disorder and its adult outcomes with depressive and anxiety disorders: A review. *J Am Acad Child Adolesc Psychiatry* 31:547–556, 1992.
84. Sanson A, Smart D, Prior M, et al.: Precursors of hyperactivity and aggression. *J Am Acad Child Adolesc Psychiatry* 32:1207–1216, 1993.
85. Eisenberg N, Fabes RA, Guthrie IK, et al.: Dispositional emotionality and regulation: Their role in predicting quality of social functioning. *J Pers Soc Psychol* 78:136–157, 2000.
86. Lytton H: Child and parent effects in boys' conduct disorder: A reinterpretation. *Dev Psychol* 26:683–697, 1990.
87. Stoolmiller M: Synergistic interaction of child manageability problems and parent-discipline tactics in predicting future growth in externalizing behavior for boys. *Dev Psychol* 37:814–825, 2001.
88. Burke JD, Loeber R, Lahey BB, et al.: Developmental transitions among affective and behavioral disorders in adolescent boys. *J Child Psychol Psychiatry* 46:1200–1210, 2005.
89. Biederman J, Faraone SV, Hatch M, et al.: Conduct disorder with and without mania in a referred sample of ADHD children. *J Affect Disord* 44:177–188, 1997.
90. Biederman J, Mick E, Bostic JQ, et al.: The naturalistic course of pharmacologic treatment of children with manic-like symptoms: A systematic chart review. *J Clin Psychiatry* 59:628–637, 1998.
91. Carlson GA, Kelly KL: Manic symptoms in psychiatrically hospitalized children—What do they mean? *J Affect Disord* 51:123–135, 1998.
92. Wozniak J, Biederman J, Kiely K, et al.: Mania-like symptoms suggestive of childhood-onset bipolar disorder in clinically referred children. *J Am Acad Child Adolesc Psychiatry* 34:867–876, 1995.
93. Wu P, Hoven CW, Bird HR, et al.: Depressive and disruptive disorders and mental health service utilization in children and adolescents. *J Am Acad Child Adolesc Psychiatry* 38:1081–1090, 1999.
94. Markowitz PI, Coccaro EF: Biological studies of impulsivity, aggression, and suicidal behavior. In: Hollander E, Stein DJ, Zohar J (eds.): *Impulsivity and Aggression*. Chichester, U.K.: John Wiley & Sons, 1995, pp. 71–90.
95. Snoek H, van Goozen SHM, Matthys W, et al.: Serotonergic functioning in children with oppositional defiant disorder: A sumatriptan challenge study. *Biol Psychiatry* Feb 2002:51:319–325.
96. Pfeffer CR, McBride PA, Anderson GM, et al.: Peripheral serotonin measures in prepubertal psychiatric inpatients and normal children: Associations with suicidal behavior and its risk factors. *Biol Psychiatry* 44:568–577, 1998.
97. Fava M, Rosenbaum JF, Pava JA, et al.: Anger attacks in unipolar depression: I. Clinical correlates and response to fluoxetine treatment. *Am J Psychiatry* 150:1158–1163, 1993.
98. Posternak MA, Zimmerman M: Anger and aggression in psychiatric outpatients. *J Clin Psychiatry* 63:665–672, 2002.
99. Gross JJ: Emotion regulation: Past, present, future. *Cognition and Emotion* 13:551–573, 1999.
100. Thompson RA: Emotion and self-regulation. In: Thompson RA (ed.): *Nebraska Symposium on Motivation, 1988: Socioemotional Development. Current Theory and Research in Motivation*, Vol. 36. Lincoln, NE: University of Nebraska Press, 1990, pp. 367–467.
101. Cole PM, Zahn-Waxler C, Fox NA, et al.: Individual differences in emotion regulation and behavior problems in preschool children. *J Abnorm Psychol* 105:518–529, 1996.
102. Sanson A, Prior M: Temperament and behavioral precursors to oppositional defiant disorder and conduct disorder. In: Quay HC, Hogan AE (eds): *Handbook of Disruptive Behavior Disorders*. New York: Kluwer Academic/Plenum Publishers, 1999, pp. 397–417.
103. Shields A, Cicchetti D: Emotion regulation among school-age children: The development and validation of a new criterion Q-sort scale. *Dev Psychol* 33:906–916, 1997.
104. Lochman JE, Dodge KA: Social-cognitive processes of severely violent, moderately aggressive, and nonaggressive boys. *J Consult Clin Psychol* 62:366–374, 1994.
105. Quiggle NL, Garber J, Panak WF, et al.: Social information processing in aggressive and depressed children. *Child Dev* 63:1305–1320, 1992.
106. Stephens RJ, Sandor P: Aggressive behaviour in children with Tourette syndrome and comorbid attention-deficit hyperactivity disorder and obsessive-compulsive disorder. *Can J Psychiatry* 44:1036–1042, 1999.
107. Viding E: Annotation: Understanding the development of psychopathy. *J Child Psychol Psychiatry* 45:1329–1337, 2004.
108. Glaser BA, Kronsnoble KM, Forkner CBW: Parents and teachers as raters of children's problem behaviors. *Child Fam Behav Ther* 19:1–13, 1997.
109. MacLeod RJ, McNamee JE, Boyle MH, et al.: Identification of childhood psychiatric disorder by informant: Comparisons of clinic and community samples. *Can J Psychiatry* 44:144–150, 1999.
110. Nock MK, Kazdin AE: Parent-directed physical aggression by clinic-referred youths. *J Clin Child Psychol* 31:193–205, 2002.
111. Baillargeon RH, Boulerice B, Tremblay RE, et al.: Modeling interinformant agreement in the absence of a "gold standard." *J Child Psychol Psychiatry* 42:463–473, 2001.
112. Johnston C, Ohan JL: The importance of parental attributions in families of children with attention deficit/hyperactivity and disruptive behavior disorders. *Clin Child Fam Psychol Rev* 8:167–82, 2005.
113. Angold A, Messer SC, Stangl D, et al.: Perceived parental burden and service use for child and adolescent psychiatric disorders. *Am J Public Health* 88:75–80, 1998.
114. Burt SA, McGue M, Krueger RF, et al.: How are parent–child conflict and childhood externalizing symptoms related over time? Results from a genetically informative cross-lagged study. *Dev Psychopathol* 17:145–65, 2005.
115. Barry TD, Dunlap ST, Cotten SJ, et al.: The influence of maternal stress and distress on disruptive behavior problems in boys. *J Am Acad Child Adolesc Psychiatry* 44:265–273, 2005.
116. Stormshak EA, Speltz ML, DeKlyen M, et al.: Observed family interaction during clinical interviews: A comparison of families containing preschool boys with and without disruptive behavior. *J Abnorm Child Psychol* 25:345–357, 1997.
117. Baker BL, Heller TL, Henker B: Expressed emotion, parenting stress, and adjustment in mothers of young children with behavior problems. *J Child Psychol Psychiatry* 41:907–915, 2000.
118. Crouch JL, Behl LE: Relationships among parental beliefs in corporal punishment, reported stress, and physical child abuse potential. *Child Abuse Negl* 25:413–419, 2001.
119. Rodriguez CM, Green AJ: Parenting stress and anger expression as predictors of child abuse potential. *Child Abuse Negl* 21:367–377, 1997.
120. Stanger C, Dumenci L, Kamon J, et al.: Parenting and children's externalizing problems in substance-abusing families. *J Clin Child Adolesc Psychol* 33:590–600, 2004.
121. Cassidy B, Zoccolillo M, Hughes S: Psychopathology in adolescent mothers and its effects on mother–infant interactions: A pilot study. *Can J Psychiatry* 41:379–384, 1996.
122. Frick PJ, Lahey BB, Loeber R, et al.: Familial risk factors to oppositional defiant disorder and conduct disorder: Parental psychopathology and maternal parenting. *J Consult Clin Psychol* 60:49–55, 1992.
123. Rhee SH, Waldman ID: Genetic and environmental influences on antisocial behavior: A meta-analysis of twin and adoption studies. *Psychol Bull* 128:490–529, 2002.
124. Blader JC: Which family factors predict externalizing behavior after discharge from inpatient psychiatric treatment? *J Child Psychol Psychiatry* 41:1133–1142, 2006.
125. Blader J: Symptom, family, and service predictors of children's psychiatric rehospitalization within one year of discharge. *J Am Acad Child Adolesc Psychiatry* 43:440–451, 2004.
126. Wootton JM, Frick PJ, Shelton KK, et al.: Ineffective parenting and childhood conduct problems: The moderating role of callous-unemotional traits. *J Consult Clin Psychol* 65:292–300, 1997.

127. MacMillan HL, Fleming JE, Streiner DL, et al.: Childhood abuse and lifetime psychopathology in a community sample. *Am J Psychiatry* 158:1878–1883, 2001.
128. Teicher MH, Andersen SL, Polcari A, et al.: The neurobiological consequences of early stress and childhood maltreatment. *Neurosci Biobehav Rev* 27:33–44, 2003.
129. Connor DF, Steingard RJ, Cunningham JA, et al.: Proactive and reactive aggression in referred children and adolescents. *Am J Orthopsychiatry* 74:129–136, 2004.
130. Dodge KA, Lochman JE, Harnish JD, et al.: Reactive and proactive aggression in school children and psychiatrically impaired chronically assaultive youth. *J Abnorm Psychol* 106:37–51, 1997.
131. Perren S, Alsaker FD: Social behavior and peer relationships of victims, bully–victims, and bullies in kindergarten. *J Child Psychol Psychiatry* 47:45–57, 2006.
132. Veenstra R, Lindenberg S, Oldehinkel AJ, et al.: Bullying and victimization in elementary schools: A comparison of bullies, victims, bully/victims, and uninvolved preadolescents. *Dev Psychol* 41:672–682, 2005.
133. Wolke D, Samara MM: Bullied by siblings: Association with peer victimisation and behaviour problems in Israeli lower secondary school children. *J Child Psychol Psychiatry* 45:1015–1029, 2004.
134. Laub JH, Lauritsen JL: The interdependence of school violence with neighborhood and family conditions. In: Elliott DS, Hamburg BA, Williams KR (eds): *Violence in American Schools*. New York: Cambridge University Press, 1998, pp. 127–155.
135. Dishion TJ, McCord J, Poulin F: When interventions harm. Peer groups and problem behavior. *Am Psychol* 54:755–764, 1999.
136. Bullock BM, Dishion TJ: Sibling collusion and problem behavior in early adolescence: Toward a process model for family mutuality. *J Abnorm Child Psychol* 30:143–153, 2002.
137. Shipman KL, Zeman J, Nesin AE, et al.: Children's strategies for displaying anger and sadness: What works with whom? *Merrill-Palmer Quarterly* 49:100–122, 2003.
138. Saarni C, von Salisch M, Lewis M, et al.: The socialization of emotional dissemblance. *Lying and Deception in Everyday Life*. New York: Guilford Press, 1993, pp. 106–125.
139. Masia CL, Chase PN: Vicarious learning revisited: A contemporary behavior analytic interpretation. *J Beh Ther Exp Psychiatry* 28:41–51, 1997.
140. Browne KD, Hamilton-Giachritsis C: The influence of violent media on children and adolescents: A public-health approach. *Lancet* 365:702–710, 2005.
141. Bartholow BD, Bushman BJ, Sestir MA: Chronic violent video game exposure and desensitization to violence: Behavioral and event-related brain potential data. *J Exp Soc Psychol* 42:532–539, 2006.
142. Swanson JW, Swartz MS, Van Dorn RA, et al.: A national study of violent behavior in persons with schizophrenia. *Arch Gen Psychiatry* 63:490–499, 2006.
143. Arseneault L, Cannon M, Murray R, et al.: Childhood origins of violent behaviour in adults with schizophreniform disorder. *Br J Psychiatry* 183:520–525, 2003.
144. Graham JM, Jr., Rosner B, Dykens E, et al.: Behavioral features of CHARGE syndrome (Hall-Hittner syndrome) comparison with Down syndrome, Prader-Willi syndrome, and Williams syndrome. *Am J Med Genet* 133A:240–247, 2005.
145. Blader JC: Pharmacotherapy and postdischarge outcomes of child inpatients admitted for aggressive behavior. *J Clin Psychopharmacol* 26:419–25, 2006.
146. Martin A, Van Hoof T, Stubbe D, et al.: Multiple psychotropic pharmacotherapy among child and adolescent enrollees in Connecticut Medicaid managed care. *Psychiatr Serv* 54:72–77, 2003.
147. Kayani S, Shannon DC: Adverse behavioral effects of treatment for acute exacerbation of asthma in children: A comparison of two doses of oral steroids. *Chest* 122:624–628, 2002.
148. Achenbach TM: *The Manual for the ASEBA School-Age Forms and Profiles*. Burlington, VT, ASEBA, University of Vermont, 2001.
149. Reynolds CR, Kamphaus RW: *Behavior Assessment System for Children*. 2nd ed. Bloomington, MN, Pearson Assessments, 2004.
150. Alderman N, Knight C, Morgan C: Use of a modified version of the Overt Aggression Scale in the measurement and assessment of aggressive behaviours following brain injury. *Brain Inj* 11:503–523, 1997.
151. Malone RP, Luebbert J, Pena-Ariet M, et al.: The Overt Aggression Scale in a study of lithium in aggressive conduct disorder. *Psychopharm Bull* 30:215–218, 1994.
152. Coccaro EF, Harvey PD, Kupsaw-Lawrence E, et al.: Development of neuropharmacologically based behavioral assessments of impulsive aggressive behavior. *J Neuropsychiatry Clin Neurosci* 3:S44–S51, 1991.
153. Halperin JM, McKay KE, Newcorn JH: Development, reliability, and validity of the Children's Aggression Scale—Parent Version. *J Am Acad Child Adolesc Psychiatry* 41:245–252, 2002.
154. Kazdin AE, Esveldt-Dawson K: The Interview for Antisocial Behavior: Psychometric characteristics and concurrent validity with child psychiatric inpatients. *J Psychopathol Behav Assess* 8:289–303, 1986.
155. Kazdin AE, Siegel T, Bass D: Cognitive problem-solving skills training and parent management training in the treatment of antisocial behavior in children. *J Consult Clin Psychol* 60:733–747, 1992.
156. Miller LS, Klein RG, Piacentini J, et al.: The New York Teacher Rating Scale for Disruptive and Antisocial Behavior. *J Am Acad Child Adolesc Psychiatry* 34:359–370, 1995.
157. Klein RG, Abikoff H, Klass E, et al.: Clinical efficacy of methylphenidate in conduct disorder with and without attention deficit hyperactivity disorder. *Arch Gen Psychiatry* 54:1073–1080, 1997.
158. Elliott DS, Ageton SS: Reconciling race and class differences in self-reported and official estimates of delinquency. *Am Sociol Rev* 45:95–110, 1980.
159. Atkins MS, Stoff DM, Osborne ML, et al.: Distinguishing instrumental and hostile aggression: Does it make a difference? *J Abnorm Child Psychol* 21:355–365, 1993.
160. Dodge KA, Coie JD: Social information-processing factors in reactive and proactive aggression in children's playgroups. *J Pers Soc Psychol* 53:1146–1158, 1987.
161. Malone RP, Bennett DS, Luebbert JF, et al.: Aggression classification and treatment response. *Psychopharm Bull* 34:41–45, 1998.
162. Waschbusch DA, Willoughby MT, Pelham WE, Jr: Criterion validity and the utility of reactive and proactive aggression: Comparisons to attention deficit hyperactivity disorder, oppositional defiant disorder, conduct disorder, and other measures of functioning. *J Clin Child Psychol* 27:396–405, 1998.
163. Frick PJ, Hare RD: *The Antisocial Process Screening Device*. Toronto, Multi-Health Systems, 2001.
164. Pappadopulos E, Macintyre II JC, Crismon ML, et al.: Treatment recommendations for the use of antipsychotics for aggressive youth (TRAAY). Part II. *J Am Acad Child Adolesc Psychiatry* 42:145–61, 2003.
165. Schur SB, Sikich L, Findling RL, et al.: Treatment recommendations for the use of antipsychotics for aggressive youth (TRAAY). Part I: A review. *J Am Acad Child Adolesc Psychiatry* 42:132–144, 2003.
166. Pliszka SR, Crismon ML, Hughes CW, et al.: The Texas Children's Medication Algorithm Project: Revision of the algorithm for pharmacotherapy of attention-deficit/hyperactivity disorder (ADHD). *J Am Acad Child Adolesc Psychiatry* 45:642–647, 2006.
167. Campbell M, Kafantaris V, Cueva JE: An update on the use of lithium carbonate in aggressive children and adolescents with conduct disorder. *Psychopharm Bull* 31:93–102, 1995.
168. Campbell M, Adams PB, Small AM, et al.: Lithium in hospitalized aggressive children with conduct disorder: A double-blind and placebo-controlled study. *J Am Acad Child Adolesc Psychiatry* 34:445–453, 1995.
169. Hinshaw SP, Heller T, McHale JP: Covert antisocial behavior in boys with attention-deficit hyperactivity disorder: External validation and effects of methylphenidate. *J Consult Clin Psychol* 60:274–281, 1992.
170. Barratt ES, Stanford MS, Felthous AR, et al.: The effects of phenytoin on impulsive and premeditated aggression: A controlled study. *J Clin Psychopharmacol* 17:341–349, 1997.
171. Greenhill LL, Halperin JM, Abikoff H: Stimulant medications. *J Am Acad Child Adolesc Psychiatry* 38:503–512, 1999.
172. Hinshaw SP, Lee SS: Ritalin effects on aggression and antisocial behavior. In: Greenhill LL, Osman BB (eds.): *Ritalin: Theory and Practice*, 2nd ed. Larchmont, NY: Mary Ann Liebert, 2000, pp. 237–51.
173. Connor D, Glatt S, Lopez I, et al.: Psychopharmacology and aggression. I: A meta-analysis of stimulant effects on overt/covert aggression–related behaviors in ADHD. *J Am Acad Child Adolesc Psychiatry* 41:253–261, 2002.
174. Gadow KD, Sverd J, Sprafkin J, et al.: Efficacy of methylphenidate for attention-deficit hyperactivity disorder in children with tic disorder. *Arch Gen Psychiatry* 52:444–455, 1995.
175. Murphy DA, Pelham WE, Lang AR: Aggression in boys with attention deficit-hyperactivity disorder: Methylphenidate effects on naturalistically observed aggression, response to provocation, and social information processing. *J Abnorm Child Psychol* 20:451–466, 1992.
176. Klorman R, Brumaghim JT, Fitzpatrick PA, et al.: Clinical and cognitive effects of methylphenidate on children with attention deficit disorder as a function of aggression/oppositionality and age. *J Abnorm Psychol* 103:206–221, 1994.
177. Hinshaw SP, Klein RG, Abikoff H: Childhood attention-deficit hyperactivity disorder: Nonpharmacologic and combination treatments. In: Nathan PE, Gorman JM (eds.): *A Guide to Treatments that Work*. New York: Oxford University Press, 1998, pp. 26–41.
178. MTA Cooperative Group: A 14-month randomized clinical trial of treatment strategies for attention-deficit/hyperactivity disorder. *Arch Gen Psychiatry* 56:1073–1086, 1999.
179. Pelham WE, Kipp HL, Gnagy EM, et al.: Effects of methylphenidate and expectancy on ADHD children's performance, self-evaluations, persistence, and attributions on a cognitive task. *Exp Clin Psychopharmacol* 5:3–13, 1997.
180. Vitiello B, Severe JB, Greenhill LL, et al.: Methylphenidate dosage for children with ADHD over time under controlled conditions: Lessons from the MTA. *J Am Acad Child Adolesc Psychiatry* 40:188–196, 2001.
181. Pliszka SR: Effect of anxiety on cognition, behavior, and stimulant response in ADHD. *J Am Acad Child Adolesc Psychiatry* 28:882–887, 1989.
182. Kolko DJ, Bukstein OG, Barron J: Methylphenidate and behavior modification in children with ADHD and comorbid ODD or CD: Main and incremental effects across settings. *J Am Acad Child Adolesc Psychiatry* 38:578–586, 1999.

183. Klein RG, Abikoff H: Behavior therapy and methylphenidate in the treatment of children with ADHD. *J Atten Disord* 2:89–114, 1997.
184. Ialongo NS, Horn WF, Pascoe JM, et al.: The effects of a multimodal intervention with attention-deficit hyperactivity disorder children: A 9-month follow-up. *J Am Acad Child Adolesc Psychiatry* 32:182–189, 1993.
185. Pelham WE, Carlson CL, Sams SE, et al.: Separate and combined effects of methylphenidate and behavior modification on boys with attention deficit-hyperactivity disorder in the classroom. *J Consult Clin Psychol* 61:506–515, 1993.
186. Brestan EV, Eyberg SM: Effective psychosocial treatments of conduct-disordered children and adolescents: 29 years, 82 studies, and 5,272 kids. *J Clin Child Psychol* 27:180–189, 1998.
187. Abikoff H, Hechtman L, Klein R, et al.: Symptomatic improvement in children with ADHD treated with long-term methylphenidate and multimodal psychosocial treatment. *J Am Acad Child Adolesc Psychiatry* 43:802–811, 2004.
188. Carlson CL, Pelham WE, Milich R, et al.: Single and combined effects of methylphenidate and behavior therapy on the classroom performance of children with attention-deficit hyperactivity disorder. *J Abnorm Child Psychol* 20:213–232, 1992.
189. Horn WF, Ialongo NS, Pascoe JM, et al.: Additive effects of psychostimulants, parent training, and self-control therapy with ADHD children. *J Am Acad Child Adolesc Psychiatry* 30:233–240, 1991.
190. Swanson JM, Kraemer HC, Hinshaw SP, et al.: Clinical relevance of the primary findings of the MTA: Success rates based on severity of ADHD and ODD symptoms at the end of treatment. *Journal of the American Academy of Child & Adolescent Psychiatry* 40:168–179, 2001.
191. Jensen PS, Hinshaw SP, Kraemer HC, et al.: ADHD comorbidity findings from the MTA study: Comparing comorbid subgroups. *J Am Acad Child Adolesc Psychiatry* 40:147–158, 2001.
192. Barkley RA, McMurray MB, Edelbrock CS, et al.: The response of aggressive and nonaggressive ADHD children to two doses of methylphenidate. *J Am Acad Child Adolesc Psychiatry* 28:873–881, 1989.
193. Pelham WE, Schnedler RW, Bender ME, et al.: The combination of behavior therapy and methylphenidate in the treatment of attention deficit disorders: A therapy outcome study. In: Bloomingdale LM (ed.): *Attention Deficit Disorder.* Vol 3: New Research in Attention, Treatment, and Psychopharmacology. Elmsford, NY: Pergamon, 1988, pp. 29–48, 1988.
194. Smithee JAF, Klorman R, Brumaghim JT, et al.: Methylphenidate does not modify the impact of response frequency or stimulus sequence on performance and event-related potentials of children with attention deficit hyperactivity disorder. *J Abnorm Child Psychol* 26:233–245, 1998.
195. Cunningham CE, Siegel LS, Offord DR: A dose–response analysis of the effects of methylphenidate on the peer interactions and simulated classroom performance of ADD children with and without conduct problems. *J Child Psychol Psychiatry* 32:439–452, 1991.
196. Smith BH, Pelham WE, Evans S, et al.: Dosage effects of methylphenidate on the social behavior of adolescents diagnosed with attention-deficit hyperactivity disorder. *Experimental and Clinical Psychopharmacology* 6:187–204, 1998.
197. Connor DF, Ozbayrak KR, Kusiak KA, et al.: Combined pharmacotherapy in children and adolescents in a residential treatment center. *J Am Acad Child Adolesc Psychiatry* 36:248–254, 1997.
198. Safer DJ: Changing patterns of psychotropic medications prescribed by child psychiatrists in the 1990s. *J Child Adolesc Psychopharmacol* 7:267–274, 1997.
199. Stigler KA, Desmond LA, Posey DJ, et al.: A naturalistic retrospective analysis of psychostimulants in pervasive developmental disorders. *J Child Adolesc Psychopharmacol* 14:49–56, 2004.
200. Handen BL, Johnson CR, Lubetsky M: Efficacy of methylphenidate among children with autism and symptoms of attention-deficit hyperactivity disorder. *J Autism Dev Disord* 30:245–255, 2000.
201. Campbell M, Small AM, Green WH, et al.: Behavioral efficacy of haloperidol and lithium carbonate: A comparison in hospitalized aggressive children with conduct disorder. *Arch Gen Psychiatry* 41:650–656, 1984.
202. Greenhill L, Solomon M, Pleak R, et al.: Molindone hydrochloride treatment of hospitalized children with conduct disorder. *J Clin Psychiatry* 46:20–25, 1985.
203. Patel NC, Crismon ML, Hoagwood K, et al.: Trends in the use of typical and atypical antipsychotics in children and adolescents. *J Am Acad Child Adolesc Psychiatry* 44:548–556, 2005.
204. Zito JM, Safer DJ, dosReis S, et al.: Psychotropic practice patterns for youth: A 10-year perspective. *Arch Pediatr Adolesc Med* 157:17–25, 2003.
205. Patel NC, Crismon ML, Shafer A: Diagnoses and antipsychotic treatment among youths in a public mental health system. *Ann Pharmacother* 40:205–211, 2006.
206. Patel NC, Crismon ML, Hoagwood K, et al.: Unanswered questions regarding atypical antipsychotic use in aggressive children and adolescents. *J Child Adolesc Psychopharmacol* 15:270–284, 2005.
207. Elias M: New antipsychotic drugs carry risks for children. *USA Today.* May 2, 2006.
208. Correll CU, Carlson HE: Endocrine and metabolic adverse effects of psychotropic medications in children and adolescents. *J Am Acad Child Adolesc Psychiatry* 45:771–791, 2006.
209. Correll CU, Penzner JB, Parikh UH, et al.: Recognizing and monitoring adverse events of second-generation antipsychotics in children and adolescents. *Child Adolesc Psychiatr Clin N Am* 15:177–206, 2006.
210. Kelly DL, Love RC, MacKowick M, et al.: Atypical antipsychotic use in a state hospital inpatient adolescent population. *J Child Adolesc Psychopharmacol* 14:75–85, 2004.
211. Safer DJ: A comparison of risperidone-induced weight gain across the age span. *J Clin Psychopharmacol* 24:429–436, 2004.
212. Sikich L, Hamer RM, Bashford RA, et al.: A pilot study of risperidone, olanzapine, and haloperidol in psychotic youth: A double-blind, randomized, 8-week trial. *Neuropsychopharmacology* 29:133–145, 2004.
213. Findling RL, McNamara NK, Branicky LA, et al.: A double-blind pilot study of risperidone in the treatment of conduct disorder. *J Am Acad Child Adolesc Psychiatry* 39:509–516, 2000.
214. Aman MG, De Smedt G, Derivan A, et al.: Double-blind, placebo-controlled study of risperidone for the treatment of disruptive behaviors in children with subaverage intelligence. *Am J Psychiatry* 159:1337–1346, 2002.
215. McCracken J, McGough J, Shah B, et al.: Risperidone in children with autism and serious behavioral problems. *N Engl J Med* 347:314–321, 2002.
216. Snyder R, Turgay A, Aman M, et al.: Effects of risperidone on conduct and disruptive behavior disorders in children with subaverage IQs. *J Am Acad Child Adolesc Psychiatry* 41:1026–1036, 2002.
217. Troost PW, Lahuis BE, Steenhuis M-P, et al.: Long-term effects of risperidone in children with autism spectrum disorders: A placebo discontinuation study. *J Am Acad Child Adolesc Psychiatry* 44:1137–1144, 2005.
218. Malone RP, Delaney MA, Leubbert JF, et al.: A double-blind placebo-controlled study of lithium in hospitalized aggressive children and adolescents with conduct disorder. *Arch Gen Psychiatry* 57:649–654, 2000.
219. Carlson GA, Rapport MD, Pataki CS, et al.: Lithium in hospitalized children at 4 and 8 weeks: Mood, behavior and cognitive effects. *J Child Psychol Psychiatry* 33:411–425, 1992.
220. Rifkin A, Karajgi B, Dicker R, et al.: Lithium treatment of conduct disorders in adolescents. *Am J Psychiatry* 154:554–555, 1997.
221. Klein RG, Abikoff H, Klass E, et al.: Preliminary findings from a controlled trial of lithium, placebo, and methylphenidate in children and adolescents with conduct disorder. Paper presented at: 29th Annual Meeting of the New Clinical Drug Evaluation Unit; May, 1989; Key Biscayne, FL.
222. Donovan SJ, Susser ES, Nunes EV, et al.: Divalproex treatment of disruptive adolescents: A report of 10 cases. *J Clin Psychiatry* 58:12–15, 1997.
223. Donovan SJ, Stewart JW, Nunes EV, et al.: Divalproex treatment for youth with explosive temper and mood lability: A double-blind, placebo-controlled crossover design. *Am J Psychiatry* 157:818–820, 2000.
224. Steiner H, Petersen ML, Saxena K, et al.: Divalproex sodium for the treatment of conduct disorder: A randomized controlled clinical trial. *J Clin Psychiatry* 64:1183–1191, 2003.
225. Kafantaris V, Campbell M, Padron-Gayol MV, et al.: Carbamazepine in hospitalized aggressive conduct disorder children: An open pilot study. *Psychopharm Bull* 28:193–199, 1992.
226. Cueva JE, Overall JE, Small AM, et al.: Carbamazepine in aggressive children with conduct disorder: A double-blind and placebo-controlled study. *J Am Acad Child Adolesc Psychiatry* 35:480–490, 1996.
227. Kemph JP, DeVane CL, Levin GM, et al.: Treatment of aggressive children with clonidine: Results of an open pilot study. *J Am Acad Child Adolesc Psychiatry* 32:577–581, 1993.
228. Connor DF, Fletcher KE, Swanson JM: A meta-analysis of clonidine for symptoms of attention-deficit hyperactivity disorder. *J Am Acad Child Adolesc Psychiatry* 38:1551–1559, 1999.
229. Connor DF, Barkley RA, Davis HT: A pilot study of methylphenidate, clonidine, or the combination in ADHD comorbid with aggressive oppositional defiant or conduct disorder. *Clin Pediatr* 39:15–25, 2000.
230. Hunt RD, Arnstein AFT, Asbell MD: An open trial of guanfacine in the treatment of attention-deficit hyperactivity disorder. *J Am Acad Child Adolesc Psychiatry* 34:50–54, 1995.
231. Chappell PB, Riddle MA, Scahill L, et al.: Guanfacine treatment of comorbid attention-deficit hyperactivity disorder and Tourette's syndrome: Preliminary clinical experience. *J Am Acad Child Adolesc Psychiatry* 34:1140–1146, 1995.
232. Scahill L, Chappell PB, Kim YS, et al.: A placebo-controlled study of guanfacine in the treatment of children with tic disorders and attention deficit hyperactivity disorder. *Am J Psychiatry* 158:1067–1074, 2001.
233. Cantwell DP, Swanson J, Connor DF: Case study: Adverse response to clonidine. *J Am Acad Child Adolesc Psychiatry* 36:539–544, 1997.
234. Regino R, Baren M, Connor DF, et al.: Patterns of use of clonidine alone and in combination with methylphenidate. In: Greenhill LL, Osman BB (eds.): *Ritalin: Theory and Practice*, 2nd ed. Larchmont, NY: Liebert, 2000, pp. 401–404.
235. Arnold LE, Aman MG: Beta blockers in mental retardation and developmental disorders. *J Child Adolesc Psychopharmacol* 1:361–373, 1991.
236. Bond AJ: Pharmacological manipulation of aggressiveness and impulsiveness in healthy volunteers. *Prog Neuropsychopharmacol Biol Psychiatry* 16:1–7, 1992.

237. Gesch CB, Hammond SM, Hampson SE, et al. Influence of supplementary vitamins, minerals and essential fatty acids on the antisocial behaviour of young adult prisoners. *Br J Psychiatry* 181:22–28, 2002.
238. Henggeler SW, Schoenwald SK, Borduin CM, et al.: *Multisystemic Treatment of Antisocial Behavior in Children and Adolescents.* New York, Guilford, 1998.
239. O'Neill RE, Horner RH, Albin RW, et al.: *Functional Assessment and Program Development for Problem Behavior: A Practical Handbook*, 2nd ed. Pacific Grove, CA, Brooks/Cole Publishing, 1997.
240. Greene RW, Ablon JS: *Treating Explosive Kids: The Collaborative Problem-Solving Approach.* New York, Guilford Press, 2006.
241. Ducharme JM, Atkinson L, Poulton L: Success-based, noncoercive treatment of oppositional behavior in children from violent homes. *J Am Acad Child Adolesc Psychiatry* 39:995–1004, 2000.
242. Wells KC, Epstein JN, Hinshaw SP, et al.: Parenting and family stress treatment outcomes in attention deficit hyperactivity disorder (ADHD): An empirical analysis in the MTA study. *J Abnorm Child Psychol* 28:543–553, 2000.
243. Schuhmann EM, Foote RC, Eyberg SM, et al.: Efficacy of parent–child interaction therapy: Interim report of a randomized trial with short-term maintenance. *J Clin Child Psychol* 27:34–45, 1998.
244. Kazdin AE: Parent management training: Evidence, outcomes, and issues. *J Am Acad Child Adolesc Psychiatry* 36:1349–1356, 1997.
245. Barkley RA, Shelton TL, Crosswait C, et al.: Multi-method psycho-educational intervention for preschool children with disruptive behavior: Preliminary results at post-treatment. *J Child Psychol Psychiatry* 41:319–332, 2000.
246. Kellam SG, Ling X, Merisca R, et al.: The effect of the level of aggression in the first grade classroom on the course and malleability of aggressive behavior into middle school. *Dev Psychopathol* 10:165–185, 1998.
247. Barkley RA: *Defiant Children: A Cinician's Manual for Assessment and Parent Training*, 2nd ed. New York, Guilford Press, 1997.
248. Lochman JE, Lenhart LA: Anger coping intervention for aggressive children: Conceptual models and outcome effects. *Clin Psychol Rev* 13:785–805, 1993.
249. Sukhodolsky DG, Kassinove H, Gorman BS: Cognitive-behavioral therapy for anger in children and adolescents: A meta-analysis. *Aggression and Violent Behavior* 9:247–269, 2004.
250. Kazdin AE, Bass D, Siegel T, et al.: Cognitive-behavioral therapy and relationship therapy in the treatment of children referred for antisocial behavior. *J Consult Clin Psychol* 57:522–535, 1989.
251. Lochman JE, Curry JF: Effects of social problem-solving training and self-instruction training with aggressive boys. *J Clin Child Psychol* 15:159–164, 1986.
252. Lochman JE, Lampron LB: Cognitive-behavioral interventions for aggressive boys: 7-month follow-up effects. *Journal of Child and Adolescent Psychotherapy* 5:15–23, 1988.
253. Burke JD, Loeber R, Birmaher B: Oppositional defiant disorder and conduct disorder: A review of the past 10 years, part II. *J Am Acad Child Adolesc Psychiatry* 41:1275–1293, 2002.
254. Kazdin AE: Practitioner review: Psychosocial treatments for conduct disorder in children. *J Child Psychol Psychiatry* 38:161–178, 1997.
255. Farmer EMZ, Dorsey S, Mustillo SA: Intensive home and community interventions. *Child Adolesc Psychiatr Clin N Am* 13:857–884, 2004.

CHAPTER 5.2.4 ■ FIRE BEHAVIOR IN CHILDREN AND ADOLESCENTS

STEVEN J. BARRETO, KAREN R. ZEFF, JOHN R. BOEKAMP, AND MARGARET PACCIONE-DYSZLEWSKI

INTRODUCTION

All children will naturally be exposed to fire during the early years of life. It is part of the normal course of development that they acquire knowledge that is linked both to mastery over fire and its potential for destruction and harm. In contrast to the development of fire interest, the emergence of fire behavior in children and adolescents carries with it the potential for death, injury, and property loss of striking proportions. Children who become involved with fire early in life, and those who use fire in an unsafe and destructive manner, are at risk, not only for continued involvement with fire, but for psychopathology and behavioral problems. The challenge for clinicians therefore becomes identifying children at risk and helping parents and supervising adults curb maladaptive forms of fire activity that may lead a child down a maladaptive developmental pathway.

In this chapter, we summarize the literature on juvenile fire behavior, presenting a foundation for assessment and intervention. In child psychiatric settings, the behavioral health clinician occupies a critical role in adequately identifying children at risk, and offering treatment options that decrease the likelihood of maladaptive developmental outcomes. We will present an ecological transactional model (Figure 5.2.4.1) of the development of fire behavior that can serve as a foundation for research, but also a heuristic for clinical practice. We view this model as more accurately capturing the complexity of the developmental nature of fire behavior when compared with dominant motivational typology models. The ecological model will suggest characteristics of both maladaptive and adaptive pathways of fire behavior. Throughout the chapter, we will stress that fire behavior carries both short- and long-term risks, ranging from more immediate concerns including property damage, risk for human injury, behavioral problems, and psychopathology to more destructive forms of fireplay potentially emerging at a later point in development. We will review important considerations in the clinical evaluation of fire behavior and follow with a contemporary selection of the empirically supported educational and psychosocial interventions.

PREVALENCE, RISK, AND DANGER

Of all individuals arrested for arson during the middle 1990s, over half were under the age of 18, and a third were younger than 15 years old (1). Although prevalence rates vary considerably, it is clear that juvenile firesetting remains an issue of significant clinical concern. Among child and adolescent psychiatric samples, incidence of firesetting has ranged from 2.3% to 15% for outpatients, and 14.3% to 34.7% for inpatients (2, 3). Statistics from community samples have been somewhat more variable, with estimates ranging from as low as 3% (4). as high as 45% (5). with over 80% of males noted to be interested in fire and fireplay. As these data suggest, firesetting is a problem affecting boys more frequently than girls (6). In a review of 22 descriptive studies, Kolko (2). found that 82% of identified firesetters were male and the age of these children was on average 10 years, with older children having more extensive firesetting histories. Although prevalence estimates have focused primarily on U.S. samples, juvenile firesetting is thought to be a problem in other countries as well (7).

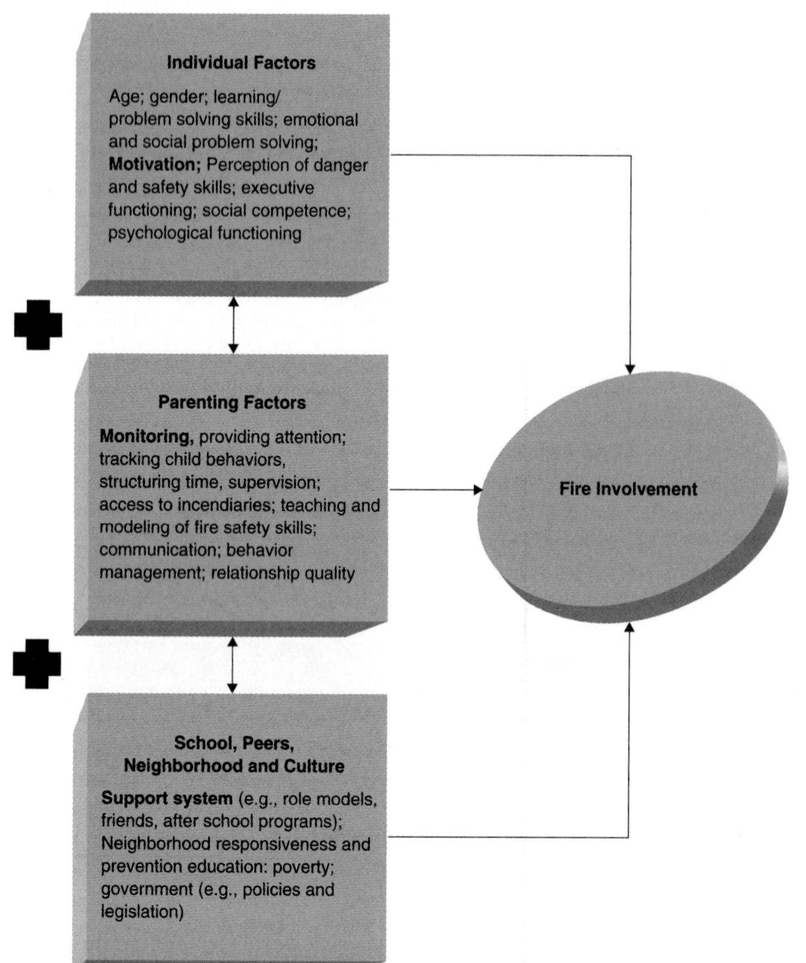

FIGURE 5.2.4.1. The ecological-transactional model of juvenile firesetting.

According to data collected from the Melbourne (Australia) Metropolitan Fire Brigade, nearly 20% of all reported fires are started by children (6).

These statistics are alarming and underscore the seriousness of juvenile firesetting. Fireplay among children annually accounts for thousands of uncontrolled fires, millions of dollars in property damage, severe injury, and death (1, 6, 8–10). In fact, fires and burns have been documented as the fourth most common cause of unintentional injury related death, resulting in more than 4,000 deaths each year (1, 11). In 1997, statistics documented that 8% of deaths from residential fires occurred as a result of children's fireplay, most often the result of the unsupervised use of lighters and matches. Furthermore, a survey conducted by the National Association of Fire Marshals determined that children were responsible for nearly 100,000 fires annually causing more than $250 million in property damage (10). This research clearly highlights the substantial role that children play in fire-related damages, injuries, and deaths. Making these numbers even more concerning is that the damages resulting from fires set by children are likely much larger than estimates suggest, as many fires set by children are never reported to fire departments. One study indicates that as few as 10% of all fires set by children are ever reported to the appropriate authorities (6, 12).

ETIOLOGY AND DEVELOPMENTAL PATHWAYS

Although most descriptive studies have focused on dangers immediate to juvenile firesetting (e.g., property loss, injury, death), enduring developmental outcomes associated with early fire experimentation are of integral importance to correction and prevention efforts. Interest in and attraction to fire is a common feature of childhood (13–17). Early fire curiosity and activity that is ignored or dismissed by supervising adults can lead a child down several possible maladaptive pathways. In a study of males ages 5 through 9 years, researchers found that interest in fire was almost universal across the sample, with one-half of the boys actually engaging in fireplay (5). Some children become involved in early fire activity that leads to continued experimentation and heightened interest and fascination in later childhood and adolescence. Other children remain interested in fire but cease to engage in fire behavior. Still others remain interested and engage in planned and deliberate fire behavior with the intention of causing damage or harm. The present section will serve to explore the etiology and developmental pathways associated with early firesetting. Recognizing risk may be the first step for parents and supervising adults in altering maladaptive developmental outcomes.

We present an ecological-transactional model that integrates theory and empirical findings (Figure 5.2.4.1). This model describes the individual, family, social and ecological factors associated with the onset and perpetuation of juvenile fire activity. Elements of these factors may combine to place a child on one of several pathways associated with dangerous fire behavior. As children mature, their cognitive and emotional development may place them at risk, or protect them against, engagement in destructive or dangerous fire behavior as well. Broadly, risk factors include the child's individual characteristics and motivational repertoire, parental and family features, as well as school, peers, and the community (18). It is important for clinicians to identify early distinguishing characteristics of juvenile firesetters so that intervention efforts can build upon strengths, target problem behaviors, and broaden the child and family's problem solving repertoire, to protect against deviant developmental pathways and long-term maladaptive outcomes (19, 20). In the present discussion, a focus will be placed on elements of the model that may contribute to the development of fire competency in children, despite exposure to conditions of adversity or the experience of failures at early points in development.

As the ecological-transactional model highlights, individual risk factors include age, gender, cognitive ability, fire-safety knowledge, social competence, executive functioning, as well as covert and delinquent behavior (21–23). Males, particularly those in the elementary and middle school years, are at high risk for fire experimentation. Furthermore, younger children (ages 3–8) may be at an increased risk for firesetting behavior due to cognitive developmental status or a limited understanding of the consequences associated with firesetting. Others have found juvenile firesetting samples to be socially immature, isolated, and overall socially incompetent (2). Children who have firesetting histories have also exhibited a higher incidence of other emotional and behavioral disturbances (14, 24). In one pathway, limited social competence and diminished learning capacities can be associated with noncompliant, impulsive, hyperactive and reactive-aggressive behavior, creating a constellation of elements placing the child at risk of firesetting behavior. In another pathway, individual factors may combine to place a child at risk of antisocial, covert and delinquent activities including destruction of property, stealing, lying, running away, and truancy (2). These externalizing problems are thought to be developmental antecedents to fire behavior by some researchers (21), with others suggesting that firesetting behavior is an extreme form of conduct disorder (25).

In addition to the learning capacities and the frequency and intensity of disruptive behaviors, the child's emotion regulation skills play a significant role in early fire behavior. This construct has been subsumed under the domain of motivation (26); however, we think it is important to examine self-regulation skills separately to clarify a child's capacity for self-soothing, self-control, responsiveness to emotional stimuli and the capacity for self-monitoring emotional status. We have suggested elsewhere that curiosity and anger may be emotional triggers for firesetting behavior (12). Curiosity has demonstrated strong associations to parent reports of internalizing and externalizing behavior problems in clinical samples of children who have engaged in fire behavior. Some children who display excessive curiosity may be more emotionally dysregulated and display more frequent, earlier, or more significant forms of fire involvement (27). Compared to firesetting children scoring high on curiosity or interest, children reporting elevated anger have lower levels of psychopathology by parent report, and may engage in more deliberate and destructive involvement with fire (27). These findings highlight the possibility that difficulties regulating intense emotion (e.g., curiosity, fascination, or anger) influence the child's development of maladaptive strategies or skills that lead to potentially more destructive forms of fireplay. It will be fruitful for future studies to examine more closely the effects of emotional dysregulation and its relationship to juvenile firesetting.

The child's individual characteristics need to be considered in his/her environmental context to clarify risk of firesetting when evaluating developmental pathways toward firesetting. Cognitive behavioral models emphasize how children's behavioral repertoires develop through observation, modeling, and conditioning processes. Researchers have noted that early fire experiences, access to incendiary materials, family members who smoke, and siblings and peers who have had a history of firesetting all contribute to the child's development of maladaptive strategies which may increase risk of firesetting (12, 14, 15, 18). In an early study of childhood fireplay, firesetting was found to be more frequent among boys whose fathers' occupations directly or indirectly involved the use of fire when compared with those children whose fathers' occupations were unrelated to fire (28). Furthermore, child and adolescent firesetters have reported more frequent observation of friends and family members who smoke and use fire regularly (22). Kolko and Kazdin (18). report that access to firesetting materials alone can provide the conditions sufficient for children to become involved in fire-related activities (a child who uses a candle to light paper on a stove). Accessibility may be facilitated by peers or adults who model smoking or other fire behaviors or who carelessly leave materials accessible to children. Observation and modeling appear to be an important mechanism in the development of fire behavior.

Fire-related learning, behavioral, and emotional dysregulation are influenced by the family context. Additional familial risk factors for trajectories leading toward firesetting behaviors include parental psychopathology, emotional distance and communication, harsh disciplinary strategies, limited supervision, and stressful life events (22, 27, 29). For example, parents of juvenile firesetters have been found to demonstrate a significantly greater incidence of psychological disturbance including schizophrenia, other psychotic disorders, depression, and substance abuse. Others have reported parents of firesetters to be less nurturing, unresponsive, and at times rejecting (21, 27). These relationships have been described as conflict laden and unaffectionate (27) and frequently involve limited communication between parent and child. A prospective study found a link between marital violence, paternal abuse of animals, paternal alcohol use and children's firesetting behavior (30). Additional work has documented a significant relationship between parental disciplinary strategies and fire behavior. In particular, research suggests that juvenile firesetters tend to come from families who either use unduly harsh punishment practices (31), or mild, less effective, forms of discipline (22). Related to this finding, researchers report that prolonged absence and insufficient supervision from parental figures can also lead to engagement in antisocial behavior (27). Left to their own, children are more likely to participate in covert behaviors and may even act out in an effort to engage otherwise inattentive parents. Moreover, stressful events such as a death in the family, divorce, or the introduction of a new step-parent may also be associated with firesetting among children and adolescents (21). Taken together, these findings suggest that ineffective parenting patterns are both directly and indirectly linked to firesetting.

As the ecological-transactional model suggests, children's developmental pathways are also linked to other social and ecological factors including peers, school, neighborhood, and culture. The presence or absence of a support system, the community's response to fire behavior, and government policies and regulations are all factors that can contribute to a child's risk of continued fire involvement. For example, exposure to peers who smoke or engage in fire activity themselves may contribute to a child's risk for early fire experimentation. Moreover, peer support and attention can serve as significant reinforcers for juvenile firesetters (32), particularly because these children tend to grapple with social skills deficits and often are not accepted by the peer group. However influential the peer group, community response to a child's early fire behavior has significant impact on continued involvement with fire as well. For example, educational intervention and awareness programs provided by fire departments and other community organizations may be effective in reducing the frequency and severity of children's firesetting behavior (6, 11). Over the past several years, major insurance companies have sponsored training opportunities for parents and providers working with juvenile firesetters and associated intervention coalitions (33). The juvenile justice system plays a role in the diversion of youth who are charged with arson (34) and, in many cases, coordinates or provides behavioral health treatment (35). Delinquent youth may be at risk of firesetting but charged with other crimes. The continued allocation of public and private resources in support of interagency collaborations and networks that support fire-specific intervention efforts is crucial.

The influence of cultural values regarding fire use and the level of assimilation of families is an unexplored, but potentially significant, factor in firesetting behavior. Less industrialized societies expose children more regularly to fire use for instrumental purposes (cooking, heating, agriculture/crop maintenance). In one case anecdote, a child referred for firestarting, whose family had recently immigrated from the Dominican Republic, was receiving inconsistent messages regarding fire safety from his mother and grandfather. While his mother emphasized the importance of never using fire without proper supervision and responded with firm prohibition and consequences for this behavior, his grandfather disregarded this approach to home fire safety, noting that in their country of origin, he would be encouraged to use fire without supervision at an early age to meet developmental expectations.

PSYCHOPATHOLOGY AND FIRE BEHAVIOR

As our discussion of risk factors implies, the pathways to juvenile firesetting are multiple and interactive. For example, there is no clear evidence that early fire experimentation and activity causes later fire behavior. Some of the complex factors that influence an early firestarter's later fire behavior include: 1) the individual child's developmental maturation, together with impulse control and behavioral inhibition, emotion regulation skills particularly pertaining to fire fascination/curiosity, anger and loneliness, and the development of social competence, 2) parenting practices including warmth, attention, monitoring, behavior control and discipline, communication, and modeling of fire behavior, and 3) peer modeling and expectations, an active and constructive response of the neighborhood and the availability of ongoing prevention and intervention collaborative efforts in the community through fire service, juvenile justice, and behavioral health networks.

Studies of juvenile firesetting have focused on the association of psychopathology to early fire experimentation and activity that are related to individual risk factors. Although over the years an emphasis has been placed on externalizing symptoms, likely because these features are more observable and intrusive to adults, research has also shown internalizing problems to be significantly related to early fire activity.

Externalizing problems including aggression and covert behavior such as lying and stealing are the most frequently cited correlates of early firesetting (13, 23, 26). A great deal of empirical work has associated firesetting diagnostically with conduct disorder (25, 29, 36–38). For example, when compared to a group of children who had committed murder, firesetters ages 10 through 17 were found to have higher rates of previous violent offenses, and they also were more likely than the homicidal group to carry a diagnosis of conduct disorder (36). Among clinical populations, several authors have noted that the primary reason for referral among firesetters was not for fire activity per se, but rather other externalizing symptomology (e.g., hyperactivity, truancy, running away, destructiveness, aggression) (18, 21). As noted previously, some theorists suggest a developmental framework for understanding firesetting amid other kinds of disruptive behavior. Specifically, early fire activity is conceptualized as part of a deviant pathway characterized by stealing, lying, and other kinds of antisocial behaviors, only eventually ending in fire activity or arson (21). Alternatively some have suggested that fire behavior signifies an extreme form of conduct disorder (25). A recent prospective study of six 12-year-old children found that reports of firesetting increased the likelihood of delinquent behavior within the following 10 years by as much as two- to ten-fold (30).

We view conduct disorder as a much larger and heterogeneous group than children at risk of firesetting. For example, in several comparative studies of firesetting, delinquency, and other kinds of violent offenders, researchers have found no notable behavioral differences between the two groups (29, 39, 40). These authors determined that firesetters tended to demonstrate the same kinds of behavioral problems as children who had no previous history of fire experimentation, but who were classified as delinquent for other reasons.

Although externalizing behaviors tend to be the most widely cited and observed correlates of early fire activity, internalizing problems should not be overlooked or dismissed. Researchers have found some significant associations between fire behavior and the presence of depressive and anxious characteristics. For example, in an investigation of the personality profiles of adolescent firesetters, investigators found that these teens scored significantly higher than nonfiresetters on scales of depression, alienation, and on symptoms such as fear, worry, and withdrawal (41). In the prospective study mentioned earlier, firesetting and cruelty to animals were shown to be related to depression as well as conduct disorder, ADHD, and ODD (30). Furthermore, it has been noted that juvenile arsonists tend to have heightened suicidal thinking and an increased risk of suicide attempts (42). These children frequently have been involved in recent stressful life events including separations, divorces, and deaths in the family (13, 21), all of which tend to heighten internalizing symptomology such as anxiety and depression. In an investigation of female firesetters, depression and low self-esteem were cited as significant antecedents to fire activity (43). Nevertheless, depression and anxiety are reviewed much less often in the firesetting literature than aggression and antisocial kinds of behaviors. It should be noted, however, that assessment information is frequently gleaned from parental reports, which tend to be rich in the endorsement of externalizing over internalizing behaviors. As such, while the majority of research suggests firesetting is mostly associated with disruptive behaviors, anxious and depressive symptomology should remain a clinical consideration. Of particular interest are children with a mixed constellation of externalizing and internalizing psychopathology. These are children who may have multiple diagnoses over their lifetime (e.g. ADHD, mood or anxiety disorder) who are at risk for a variety of behavioral problems (e.g. impulsivity, noncompliance, self-injury or reactive-aggression toward others). Such children may not be as likely to endorse anger as a primary motivation for firesetting and they may struggle with family environments lacking in critical parenting practices of monitoring, structured and responsive behavior management, warmth, and attention.

Two additional clinical considerations are social skill deficits, briefly reviewed in our discussion of etiology and developmental pathways, and substance abuse. Both are strongly associated with psychopathology as well as firesetting among children and adolescents. Kolko, Kazdin, and Meye (23) conducted a comparative study of firesetters and nonfiresetters, and found that firesetters demonstrated significantly lower social ability than their counterparts. In followup work, this same finding has been consistently reported (18, 26, 43). Some have suggested that firesetters are averse to social interaction, and therefore are less likely to develop solutions to problems via socially acceptable routes (26). This aversion may lead to acting out aggressively, and indirectly, in the form of fireplay, when a child's limited problem solving repertoire leads to the aversion of assertive social confrontation and the expression of aggression through covert fire behavior. Another maladaptive pathway is through fire experimentation as a method by which to gain the attention and, potentially, admiration of peers, by children who are unable to do so by more skillful methods.

In addition to social skills deficits, substance abuse has also been implicated in the constellation of psychiatric difficulties observed in young firesetters. Specifically, this population is noted to have difficulties including alcohol dependence (44), and inhalant abuse (42). We view substance abuse as likely linked to increased impulsivity through disinhibition contributing to poor decision making in critical areas of fire competence (e.g., fire safety knowledge and reasoning). The combination of social skills deficits and substance abuse may be associated with deviant peer socialization that may place a child at greater risk of the development of conduct disorder without intensive intervention.

FIRESETTING TYPOLOGIES AND CATEGORIZATIONS

Our discussion of developmental pathways from an ecological-transactional perspective demonstrated that there are several different mechanisms by which juvenile firesetting can emerge. Over the last half-century, clinical theorists have attempted to identify a typology of firesetters in which different motivations (such as curiosity or anger) are thought to influence recidivism or severity of fire behavior (26). To date, no specific classification system has been empirically validated. Nonetheless, it has been suggested that children's motivation for becoming involved in fireplay is predictive of continued involvement with fire as well as other forms of antisocial behavior (26). Several taxonomies have been suggested (32, 45–47). For purposes of integrating these categories and typologies into the ecological transactional model, we organize these into three domains: curiosity, psychopathology and family functioning, and delinquency.

By far, the most well known category is that of the child who is motivated by curiosity (13, 42). Retrospective studies of incidents reported to fire departments over the span of several years have demonstrated that a clear majority of fires and fireplay were the result of curiosity (48, 49). In retrospective incident report studies, the term curious refers to a child who has few to no behavioral difficulties and is in the early stages of fire experimentation (46). These studies, and the broader definition of curiosity continue to influence strongly the firefighter literature that has driven much of the continuing education and training, particularly among fire education specialists. This literature describes children in the curious category as unlikely to set fires again after receiving fire safety education with less intensive intervention assumed to be warranted. In the past, research reported the curious firesetter to be less pathological, younger, and generally only involved in one serious fire incident across the lifespan (13).

The curious firesetting categorization, however, may be evolving and has been challenged by more recent empirical findings. Specifically, Kolko and Kazdi (26) found that children motivated to set fires by curiosity were also found to demonstrate elevations on measures of psychopathology including internalizing and externalizing dysfunction, overt and covert antisocial behaviors, expressed hostility and social skills deficits. These children also had more early experiences with fire and reported to be more interested in, exposed to and in contact with fire over the previous year. This was in contrast to children scoring high on anger, who did not show more psychopathology than those low in anger, but had greater exposure to models of fire interest, elicited more community complaints about fire behavior, and were more frequently hiding matches or incendiary materials. One proposed explanation, which has yet to be tested, is that curiosity is a less transient motive for firesetting (26). At the very least, these findings suggest that curiosity, when compared with anger among firesetters, is more strongly associated with a different constellation of risk factors that combine into distinct maladaptive pathways. The findings also suggest that the broader type of curiosity, associated with one-time fire experimentation, and thought to be developmentally common in children, may be distinct from the construct of curiosity as measured by the Firesetting Risk Interview (FRI) or the Children's Firesetting Inventory (CFI) (14, 15). The comparatively smaller group of children described by these measures may show more psychopathology, hostility, social skills deficits and engage in more disruptive behaviors than those children in the more broadly curious category. High levels of curiosity, as measured by the FRI/CFI, particularly in school-aged children and adolescents, may increase the risk of further engagement in dangerous fire play.

However, even the broader construct of curiosity carries some degree of risk. While this type of curiosity about fire tends to be considered a common developmental feature of early childhood, single-incident fire experimentation, particularly in early childhood and without proper supervision and modeling of fire safety skills, can carry significant risk of harm or destruction. Whereas the broadly curious firesetter tends to become affiliated with fires that spread out of control unintentionally, children scoring high in the narrow construct of curiosity may set fires with a specific intention to harm (26). They may also set fires as an individual expression of family dysfunction or a response to overwhelming life or family stress. This stress may be related to deficits in family functioning such as parental modeling around fire, communication, monitoring, behavior control, or parental psychiatric illness. In this category, children are thought to be inadvertently using fire as way of calling out for help (13). Several researchers have indeed found firesetting to be intimately tied to family and life stressors (13, 21, 29). We term this second category psychopathology and family functioning.

A third, and likely smaller category, refers to children who become involved with fire as part of the development of a pervasive pattern of antisocial behavior. This category can be termed delinquency (13). and may represent a distinctive maladaptive pathway (25). This category may also include many children scoring high in anger and thought to be engaging in firesetting that is more purposive or deliberate than children in the psychopathology and family functioning category. However, this relationship has yet to be tested.

It has been speculated that enuresis, cruelty to animals, and firesetting are not only highly correlated to one another, but also predictive of violent crimes later in adulthood (13, 21). Two studies have failed to identify a relationship between firesetting and enuresis (40, 50). However, juveniles reported to be cruel to animals have been shown to be more likely to engage in repeat firesetting when compared with children not cruel to animals (50). It is possible that the behavior of cruelty to animals when combined with firesetting will increase the likelihood of subsequent delinquent behaviors (30), thus signifying a distinctive maladaptive antisocial pathway that may be included in the category of delinquency.

A fourth category of children and adolescents accounts for a very small portion of child and adolescent fire behavior. This category includes children who set fires as a result of extreme psychopathology including compulsive behaviors and psychotic ideation that may be specifically related to the firesetting (13, 51).

The DSM-IV diagnosis of pyromania represents another category of firesetting that is extremely rare in children. Pyromania describes fire behavior that is deliberate, purposeful, involving an obsession with fire, with children showing tension or affective excitement before the act, and pleasure or gratification during the act (52).

ASSESSMENT

Prior to any evaluation of children's fire behavior it must be determined whether the purpose is to assess for treatment or to evaluate the risk of recidivism. There is currently no empirical support for the predictive validity of risk categories as they primarily rely upon the clinical expertise of individual practitioners (12, 42, 52). In some states, risk assessments are requested by the courts to inform placement decisions. Such assessments can provide useful information that can guide treatment decisions and should be obtained prior to beginning treatment. In this section, we will restrict our discussion to treatment assessment using the ecological-transactional model (53).

Information from referral sources and other outside agencies may be obtained prior to the assessment. Many referrals of firesetting are initially screened through the fire department or juvenile diversion programs. This interdisciplinary involvement has influenced the development of standardized screening measures, which in some states are widely used, but have yet to be validated (54). Examples of screenings/assessments are the Oregon Screening Tool, Maine Screening Tool, and the Federal Emergency Management Tool (54). The evaluating clinician can identify whether any screening measures are being administered in their region and follow up by requesting a copy of the measure prior to interviewing the child and the family. These screenings provide a basis for further inquiry into the nature of the firesetting incident and the existence of other behavior problems or delinquent activities at home or school. In addition, there may be a written report summarizing the fire investigation that rests with the fire department or a law enforcement agency. Reviewing this "cause and origin" or fire/arson investigation report (47, 55). from the fire department can be particularly helpful with preteens and adolescents, who may be less inclined to be truthful regarding the nature of the incident. The report can provide a foundation for confronting the child with inconsistencies in their narrative and promote accountability as well as provide a basis for assessment of the complexity of the fire behavior (e.g., the use of accelerants, covert hiding of materials, deliberation). Finally, prior to the assessment, older children, adolescents, and parents must also be informed about the limits of confidentiality and protections of disclosure within the larger community or juvenile justice system, particularly whether or not disclosure of firesetting may lead to criminal justice involvement.

Once these initial steps are taken, child assessment should proceed with a thorough understanding of firesetting behavior both past and present. Recognizing when fire behavior deviates from normative development requires an understanding of the child's fire involvement, including what was used to start the fire, the location, if others were present, the child's response to the event and how the fire was extinguished (21, 51, 55). Several preliminary questions may precede more structured assessment methods. For example, children are generally asked if they have ever played with matches or lighters and if they have ever "set a fire," or "set a fire in order to burn something" (see Wilcox and Kolko (55) for a more thorough discussion of unstructured interview techniques).

Prior to the assessment, the evaluator should consider modifying the interview format to match the developmental level of the child. In general, preschool-aged children will require visual stimuli (e.g., "PlaySafe; Be Safe" drawings, empty match boxes) (56). and less inquiry into motivational states. Elementary school–aged children, particularly those with learning disabilities and attentional/concentration difficulties can benefit from these methods and techniques as well. Wilcox and Kolko (55), noted several questions that capture important nuances of the child's degree of planning and learning from the experience that may be particularly helpful for elementary school–aged children ("How did you get the idea to start the fire?" What did you think would happen when you actually started the fire?" Did the fire act the way you thought it would?" "Did you learn anything from what happened?"). The latter questions can be helpful in linking assessment to educational or psychosocial interventions. With adolescents, the interviewer may need to confront denial or avoidance directly by using collateral reports and discussion of the context and purpose of the interview in the larger system (57). Self-monitoring techniques have been popular among evaluators in helping children to report accurately on thoughts, feelings, and behavior related to the firesetting incident; however, they may be beneficial in the interview process as well (58). One study has simplified this method using vignettes to introduce the relationship among thoughts, feelings, and actions (12), which can help children become acquainted with the concepts before applying them to their own firesetting incidents. One area that has received very little attention is the assessment of fire behavior among developmentally disabled populations. As with younger children, the interview will likely focus less on motivation and more on curiosity or fascination, use more visual cues and prompts, and include more inquiry on fire safety skills awareness, as well as family and ecological factors that may be contributing to lapses in supervision or monitoring.

Multisource (parent, child, and teacher report) and multimethod assessment protocols are recommended across at least two settings (e.g., home and school environments) to identify the scope and intensity of firesetting or associated behavioral disturbance. Some instruments have been validated in general clinical populations, but clinical utility in firesetting populations is less well established. Other fire-specific instruments have been developed for research purposes, but have not been as well examined in clinical populations.

Both structured interviews and behavioral rating scales have been developed for use with juvenile firesetters. These tools include questions about how materials were obtained, the site of fire, type of property damage, fire competence, exposure to fire models, fire involvement (hiding of matches/lighters), curiosity/fascination with fire (15). The domain of learning and exposure relates to how the child acquired exposure and knowledge of fire in his/her family. Attempts should be made to identify: 1) the current and past adult or peer models of fire behavior, 2) the age of exposure to fire and to models of fire safety, 3) the nature of the exposure (whether unsupervised, supervised or guided with developmentally appropriate explanations), 4) the consistency of the caregiver or peer modeling, 5) child fire competence (knowledge) and fire safety skill (both child report and parental perception).

One important domain is that of fire competence, skill, and understanding. Firesetters (6–13 years old), when compared with nonfiresetters with similar behavioral health profiles, have been shown to be more knowledgeable about types of things that burn, more curious, less fire competent (lacking in both fire safety skills awareness and an understanding of the properties of fire). In addition, exposure to fire activities in the home and community should also be assessed (e.g., individuals in home who smoke or have been burned, fires in neighborhood, or friends who smoke) (14).

Assessment of problems in family functioning is the next important domain for assessment. This may include an evaluation of the quality of the parent-child relationship/communication, the degree of parental involvement, warmth and nurturance, disciplinary practices, as well as parental psychiatric distress and exposure to stressful life events. Generally, the parenting process can be organized into three dimensions: 1) motivation (parental belief systems including norms, values, and parent goals), 2) parental monitoring, or the tracking and structuring of the child's activities, social-ecology or environments, and 3) behavior management (the parent's active attempt to shape positive outcomes by using incentives, reinforcement, limit setting and negotiation). Parental monitoring is thought to be the common denominator within this process and is associated strongly with both parenting practices and measures of the parenting relationship/communication. In this way, parental monitoring may act as a protective factor for children living in high-risk settings and can provide a foundation for brief interventions for child and adolescent problem behavior and child injury prevention (59). One promising area of study is application of these dimensions of parenting as they pertain specifically to fire behavior.

The FRI contains sections assessing parenting regarding both fire-specific issues and more general concerns. Fire-specific domains in the FRI include parental fire awareness (parental safety instruction in the home, fire safety instruction in the home, practicing fire-escape drills), as well as general parenting practices (use of mild vs. harsh punishment, parental supervision). In Table 5.2.4.1 we list several measures of family functioning and stressful life events that are used in the assessment of disruptive behavior disorders and may be useful in the assessment of family functioning among juvenile firesetters specifically (14). Assessment may also include parental psychiatric history/distress, as this is more commonly found among firesetters when compared with nonfiresetters (18).

Finally, the evaluator should be sure to obtain information regarding the range of delinquent behaviors that may be associated with firesetting behavior. In particular, cruelty to animals, violence toward others or property, a history of exposure to domestic violence and to paternal cruelty toward animals are all activities that may increase risk for maladaptive outcomes including delinquency and court involvement (30) and may require interventions targeting a broader range of antisocial behaviors.

TREATMENT

A thorough assessment of fire behavior guided by the ecological transactional model yields information that corresponds with skill-based, multimodal approaches that can stand alone or be used to supplement ongoing treatment such as fire-safety skills training, self-monitoring, parent–child communication, parental psychoeducation, promoting emotion regulation and alternative coping strategies, and restitution for damages (6, 12, 69, 70). Treatment outcome studies for juvenile firesetting are few and yield limited, if promising, results. Samples are heterogeneous, making it difficult to identify whether subgroups based on severity or breadth of dysfunction would benefit from a specific element of treatment (e.g., children vs. adolescents; matchplayers vs. repeat firesetters). Treatment protocols are also varied, making it difficult to identify specific elements of treatment that are more or less effective. There is a relative lack of randomized controlled studies when compared with other areas of child behavioral health (e.g., depression, aggression). Reductions in recidivism may reflect change over time following treatment, additional behavioral health treatment for other problems, or change due to a nonspecific factor in fire treatment. Yet there is accumulating evidence that fire safety skills training (FSST) and cognitive behavioral therapy (CBT) are promising interventions, particularly when combined or

TABLE 5.2.4.1

ASSESSMENT TOOLS FOR USE IN EVALUATION OF JUVENILE FIRESETTING*

Name of Measure	Brief Description	Reporter
The Firesetting Incident Analysis—Parent and Child Version** (FIA-P, FIA-C) (60)	Structured interview that obtains information regarding specific fire incidents	Parent and Child Report
The Firesetting Risk Interview** (FRI) (14)	Structured interview used to assess several domains related to fire involvement	Parent Report
Children's Firesetting Inventory** (CFI) (15)	Structured interview used to assess several domains related to fire involvement, administered to children	Child Report
Child Behavior Checklist (CBCL) (61)	Rating scale used to assess several dimensions of children's emotional and behavioral functioning	Parent Report (Teacher Report Form also available)
IOWA/Conners (IOWA/C) (62)	Rating scale used to determine the presence of hyperactivity, impulsivity, and inattention in children	Parent Report
Children's Hostility Inventory (CHI) (63) and Children's Inventory of Anger (CHIA (64).	Questionnaires used to assess aggression and hostility among children	Parent or Child Report
Children's Depression Inventory (CDI) (65)	Brief rating scale used to measure children's level of depressive symptoms	Child Report
Trauma Symptom Checklist for Children (TSCC) (66)	Rating scale measuring psychological distress and related symptomology	Child Report
The Parent–Child Conflict Tactics Scales (CTSPC) (67)	Assesses parental disciplinary strategies during child conflicts (nonviolent discipline, psychological aggression, physical assault)	Parent Report
Parent–Child Relationship Inventory (PCRI) (68)	Assesses parent–child communication strategies	Parent Report

*This table is not an exhaustive battery, but reflects an array of tools that have been clinically useful and often incorporated into empirical investigations of juvenile firesetting. For a more extensive review of measures, see Kolko (2002).
**These instruments can be solicited from the first author upon request.

delivered in a collaborative format (6, 8). FSST has been shown to be more effective than a general discussion of the fire incident with inpatient children age 4–8 years (26). Another study compared one-time fire-safety discussion/pamphlet with a combined educational and home-based psychosocial intervention delivered by fire educators (satiation, response cost, self-monitoring/graphing of antecedents and associated emotions and cognitions). Of the children, 67% demonstrated improved fire behavior, with 42% setting no fires in the 12 months following the intervention. Thirty percent of the families were not assessed because they could not be located. In this study, even the very brief fire safety intervention had an impact on reducing recidivism, with a one-time pamphlet shown to effectively reduce repeated fire activity (6).

Fire safety education remains a core component of most interventions for juvenile firesetters. One classroom-style fire safety education program included tours of a burn unit, fire knowledge and safety awareness, and lectures from returning veterans of the program. There are innovative programs being developed that involve collaboration with fire departments (71) and more standard group treatment models for disruptive behaviors. In fact, there appears to be a variety of fire-specific psychosocial interventions and/or safety education/skills training that can reduce recidivism from 6 months up to 2-year followup (6, 26); Given findings that a significant percentage of firesetters will repeat if untreated (15), it seems imperative that intervention efforts be early and swift.

The most rigorous outcome study to date shows that when fire safety skills training and psychosocial treatment are administered in a highly standardized format, they can be superior to a one-time pamphlet and safety contract (72), although not superior to each other. This study set the standard for multimodal and collaborative treatment of juvenile firesetters by integrating self-monitoring techniques (identifying the personal and environmental context of the firesetting) into a treatment including relaxation, cognitive restructuring, assertion skills training, problem solving, and parental skills training (selective attention, reinforcement, contingency management). The average number of sessions was 5.5 (8).

Influenced by Kolko's work, other innovative and cost-effective fire-specific interventions for parents and families have been developed that include clearly defined treatment objectives that can lead to standardization of administration and some evaluation of recidivism. One intervention effort has offered classes to 247 families of firesetters from 2000 to 2005 through the Washington County Fire Academy (53), with estimates of 3–6% recidivism. These classes meet two times per week for 6 weeks with parents and children attending concordant programs. Children receive fire safety education with their peers, while parents meet with one another and identify the ecological factors contributing to their child's firesetting (Oregon "Cycles" Model) (53), learn myths and facts about firesetting behavior, are instructed in contingency management, positive praise techniques and response-cost techniques, and identify areas of psychopathology that may need attention (e.g., untreated ADHD, parental conflict, or other family stressors).

Similarly, in an ongoing treatment study through Bradley Hospital in Rhode Island, families of firesetters receive 4 weeks of 1.5-hour concordant sessions. Children meet with their peers prior to working directly with their parents in Multiple Family Group Intervention (MFGT). This model focuses on improving the quality of family communication about fire and uses group and individual exercises (e.g., affect identification, self-monitoring) to facilitate children's experience of mastery over fire behavior. Children learn to identify and monitor both emotions and thoughts associated with fire behavior and identify coping strategies through four exercises: group discussion designed to destigmatize fire communication, vignette and game activities, review of firesetting incidents, and coping strategy contracts. These strategies are then refined with children and parents in a MFGT session. Parents receive psychoeducation about the ecological model and cyclical nature of firesetting (53) combined with experiential discussion related to fire communication in the family (e.g., how parents first learned about the fire behavior, the quality of the family communication around fire behavior/safety, the parent's history of modeling safe fire behavior, and development of a home fire safety checklist and escape plan).

In a third example developed in Ontario, Canada and operating for over 10 years, fire-safety education and parent–child intervention are delivered simultaneously by a trained local behavioral health clinician (73). Content of the protocol is described in a detailed manual with fire-specific exercises and worksheets for caregivers and children. The protocol is conduced in five sessions (total of 7.5 hours) and includes modules on fire safety (attitudes, high risk situations and behaviors) in and out of the home, rewarding fire-safe behavior, parental supervision and monitoring access to ignition materials, understanding antecedents to fire involvement, and teaching a systematic approach to consequences of future fire involvement. Follow-up of over 200 families receiving the intervention indicate that approximately 75% had no further fire involvement over 1 to 2 years (74). Interestingly, this is the only program to evaluate the adoption and implementation of the protocol through a survey of approximately 700 community professionals trained over 8 years. Findings indicated that although 89% of the clinicians made a commitment to use the protocol, only 29% implemented the protocol on a routine basis. Factors such as the compatibility of the protocol with existing practice, ease of use, and adopter self-efficacy may have influenced implementation (75).

Remarkably, there has been little empirical evaluation of the specific treatment needs of preschool or adolescent firesetters, given that preschool fire behavior may be associated with some of the greatest danger for loss of life and adolescent fire behavior can lead to the most costly treatments (i.e., residential and juvenile justice incarceration). Existing fire safety education program curriculums that are directed toward preschoolers can be incorporated into daycare programming for children (56, 71). Parental participation is critical to any systematic approach to treatment of preschoolers and two of the four psychosocial interventions previously described have been used with preschoolers (69, 76).

Many adolescents come to the attention of behavioral health providers through the criminal justice system, and may be engaging in a broad range of delinquent behaviors. Some may be charged with arson and then referred to intervention programs that specialize in working with delinquent adolescents engaging in fire behavior. Several models have been developed, ranging from those offering individually supervised restitution or community service activities to more structured fire safety and CBT skill-based group interventions (77). These court diversion intervention programs designed specifically for children convicted of arson have yet to be evaluated using more rigorous experimental designs, although some conform to best practice guidelines for youth offender programs established by the Office of Juvenile Justice and Delinquency Prevention programs (77). However, many of the studies and treatment models previously reviewed in this chapter included children referred by the court system and may have been influential in reducing or eliminating dangerous fire behavior among these court-referred youth. For group or residential treatments, there is a potential for negative impact for modestly deviant or delinquent adolescents, if these teens are exposed to deviant older youth. Such deviant peer exposure effects may detract from the overall positive impact of the intervention and are in need of rigorous evaluation (78).

There have been calls for clearer standards of care in residential settings for evaluation and placement of firesetters (71). Recently, one study comparing 17 adolescent firesetters in residential treatment with 30 adolescents with first-time fire histories demonstrated no differences in psychopathology, delinquent personality characteristics, and surprisingly, fire-specific characteristics (e.g., number of fires set, use of accelerants, location of the fire, injuries caused by the fire). Instead, a greater proportion of residential teens came from single-parent homes and had higher scores of aggression (79), suggesting that lack of safety, supervision, and monitoring in the home environment, coupled with aggressive behavior, may be the primary factors leading to out of home placement. There has been a call for better integration of fire-specific treatment with residential facilities, making fire safety skills training a treatment objective that is actively monitored in clinical care meetings throughout placement along with coordination of resources outside of the residential program as necessary to provide fire safety skills training (80).

The treatment of specific populations, such as children diagnosed with mental retardation or significant learning limitations (e.g., Asperger's disorder, impaired attention/concentration, reading and writing challenges, limited reasoning capacities) has received little attention. There is need for specialized delivery of fire safety skills training or CBT techniques for these groups. One case study describes the use of a multicomponent behavioral treatment approach with a hospitalized 6-year-old developmentally disabled boy including negative practice with correction from his mother, token reinforcement, and routine discipline instruction (81). Another study used a virtual reality computer game to teach fire safety skills to children diagnosed with fetal alcohol syndrome. The games were administered without direct assistance from parents or observers (82). We have found the use of educational videotapes and testimonials useful for children with limited cognitive abilities who are resistant to fire safety skills training. We have adapted and simplified techniques by avoiding discussions of motivations of firesetting or past experiences (beyond the initial assessment) and adapting workbooks and curriculum available online to create structured learning sequences. The sequences maintain a focus on understanding "how things work" and reinforce a sense of mastery and competence with fire for these youngsters.

Children repeatedly lighting matches to satiate interest under the supervision of an adult is one of the earliest behavioral interventions reported to be effective in decreasing a child's interest in fire and firesetting behaviors (83). This practice, however, is rarely encouraged, due to the risks of the potential negative effects of modeling fire behavior and reports of the large number of sessions required to be effective. Given the prominent association of curiosity or fascination and psychopathology, further development of behavioral interventions that target fire fascination are warranted, perhaps through the specification of overt or covert sensitization techniques (i.e., use of stories, narratives, testimonials, or visual stimuli to discourage contact with fire). If such programs were systematically evaluated and included measures related to specific treatment components, we may better understand the cognitive and behavioral change processes that make both fire safety education and psychosocial treatment effective.

As noted earlier, fire safety education delivered in a classroom, combined with experiential format, has been shown to reduce recidivism significantly (84), and fire safety skills training delivered to children individually has been shown to be as effective as CBT (85). The modality of delivering of fire safety education, however, may differ considerably between local communities and service providers. Guidelines for fire safety education are broad, and the availability of fire safety education intervention will depend upon community resources. Thus, it is incumbent upon the behavioral health clinician to have some knowledge of exactly what is being delivered in the community to facilitate clinical treatment objectives, to avoid duplication of services, and to assess and monitor the child's generalization of fire safety skills. Fire safety education can include the following topics: fire facts (e.g., fuel, how fire grows/spreads and how is it extinguished/controlled, smoke inhalation dangers), fire safety awareness (i.e., "matches are tools and not toys," safe distance, home fire safety "projects" such as identifying common fire safety hazards in the home or collecting information regarding the causes and consequences of fire in the community), fire survival (e.g., smoke detectors, home fire escape plan and strategies, "stop, drop, and roll"), fire consequences (potential criminal justice involvement, burns, damages to community both direct and indirect) (11, 22).

Fire behavior crosses over the boundaries of several disciplines (fire service, juvenile justice, behavioral health, pediatric injury prevention and child protection), with many of these disciplines using public health prevention education techniques (86). Basic fire safety education principles (stop, drop and roll; use of 911; and match/lighter safety slogans) are delivered in many elementary school classrooms around the country. Unfortunately, the efficacy of these education programs has yet to be established. For example, many children do not effectively generalize simple fire safety instruction following a single classroom exposure. Two examples of preschool prevention programs are the "Learn Not to Burn Program" and the "Play Safe; Be Safe" curricula. A middle school curriculum has recently been designed (69). Many of the tools and exercises in these prevention education curricula can be adapted for use in clinical therapies with individuals, families or groups.

Psychopharmacological techniques for treatment of juvenile firesetting populations has largely been neglected in the empirical literature. To date, no specific medications are used to treat firesetting behavior per se. Instead, juvenile firesetters are treated for associated difficulties such as disruptive behavior problems, ADHD, or internalizing distress. In many cases, and as suggested by the ecological-transactional model, risk for future firesetting will decrease secondary to the improvement of associated psychological and behavioral difficulties, as these factors increase vulnerability for repeated fire activity. Improvement in these areas, in turn, provides opportunity for more adaptive developmental outcomes.

As noted earlier, juvenile arson is not merely a clinical concern, but a public health and safety problem of large proportions. Inter-agency collaborative relationships among city departments, community-based organizations, city residents, and state law enforcement and fire prevention agencies are needed to develop multilayered community prevention programs (87). In Detroit (a metropolitan area of over 500,000), one such collaborative effort successfully reduced the incidence of fires set in the community on Halloween night from record numbers of fires set in 1984 (810 fires over a 3-day period) to levels consistent with incidence at other times of the year. Many of these fires were suspected to be set by youth; the intervention included after-school and evening programs as well as a curfew to monitor more effectively children's whereabouts and limit access to dumpsters and abandoned buildings. Moreover, the intervention included the deployment of public safety personnel, the elimination of arson targets through community cleanup, volunteer mobilization and training, public media and communications campaigns, and prohibitions on the safe use of fuel (87).

CONCLUSION

Fire behavior in children and adolescents is a problem of surprising scope, carrying with it the potential for death, injury, and property loss of striking proportions. The problem spans all ages, is particularly prevalent among children in psychiatric settings, and often does not come to the attention of the clinician without specific inquiry. The complexity of the development of juvenile firesetting behavior is best captured by an ecological-transactional model that includes factors related to individual functioning, parental processes, peer socialization, neighborhood and school safety, and cultural socialization. Assessment should be fire specific, but correspond with accepted practices in the general treatment of disruptive behavior disorders (multimodel, parent and child report, developmentally sensitive methods). When child and adolescent fire behavior is associated with externalizing and internalizing disorders, families may benefit from promising collaborative treatment programs combining fire safety education with cognitive-behavioral treatment and/or parent–child treatments. While children without associated emotional disorders will likely benefit from fire safety education alone, some children with behavioral disorders may also see a reduction in repeat fire behavior, without any additional psychosocial treatment.

ACKNOWLEDGEMENT

This research was supported through grants from the Providence Mutual Fire Insurance Agency and the Shriner's Foundation. The authors are grateful to the contributions of Beth Hollander, James Leverone, LCMHC; Julie Lucier, Psy.D.; and Peter Gillen, Psy.D.

References

1. American Academy of Pediatrics, Committee on Injury and Poison Prevention: Reducing the number of deaths and injuries from residential fires. *Pediatrics* 105:1355–1357, 2000.
2. Kolko DJ: Juvenile firesetting: A review and methodological critique. *Clinical Psychol Rev* 5:345–376, 1985.
3. Kolko DJ, Kazdin AE: Parent-child correspondence in identification of firesetting among child psychiatric patients. *J Child Psychol Psyc* 29:175–184, 1988.
4. Achenbach TM, Edelbrock CS: Behavior problems and competences reported by parents of normal and disturbed children aged four through sixteen. *Monogr Soc Res Child* 46:1–82, 1981.
5. Kafry D: Playing with matches: Children and fire. In: Canter D (ed): *Fires and Human Behavior*. New York, Wiley and Sons, 1980, pp. 47–62.
6. Adler R, Nunn R, Northam E, Lebnan V, Ross R: Secondary prevention of childhood firesetting. *J Am Acad Child Psy* 33:1194–1202, 1994.
7. *Juvenile Firesetting Intervention Practices*, National Association of State Fire Marshals International Conference, January 24–25, 2003.
8. Kolko DJ: Efficacy of cognitive-behavioral treatment and fire safety education for children who have set fires: Initial and follow-up outcomes. *J Child Psychol Psyc* 42:359–369, 2001.
9. Kolko DJ, Kazdin AE: The emergence and recurrence of child firesetting: A one-year prospective study. *J Abnorm Child Psych* 20:17–37, 1992.
10. National Association of State Fire Marshals. *Juvenile Firesetter Intervention Research Project: Final Report*. Office of Juvenile Justice and Delinquency Prevention, 2001.
11. Pinsonneault IL: Fire safety education and skills training. In: Kolko DJ (ed): *Handbook on Firesetting in Children and Youth*. San Diego, Academic Press, 2002, pp. 219–260.
12. Barreto SJ, Boekamp JR, Armstrong LM, Gillen P: Community-based interventions for juvenile firestarters: A brief family-centered model. *Psychol Serv* 1:158–168, 2004.
13. Cole R, Grolnick W, Schwartzman P: Firesetting. In: Ammerman R, Hersen M, Last C (eds): *Prescriptive Treatment for Children and Adolescents*. Boston, Allyn & Bacon, 1999, pp. 293–307.
14. Kolko DJ, Kazdin AE: Assessment of dimensions of childhood firesetting among patients and nonpatients: The Firesetting Risk Interview. *J Abnorm Child Psych* 17:157–176, 1989.
15. Kolko DJ, Kazdin AE: The Children's Firesetting Interview with psychiatrically referred and nonreferred children. *J Abnorm Child Psych* 17:609–624, 1989.
16. Simonsen B, Bullis M: *Fire Interest Survey: Final Report*. Salem, Oregon Office of the State Fire Marshal, 2001.
17. Cotterall A, McPhee B, Plecas D: *Fireplay Report—A Survey of School-Aged Youth in Grades 1 to 12*. British Columbia, University College of the Fraser Valley, 1999.
18. Kolko DJ, Kazdin AE: A conceptualization of firesetting in children and adolescents. *J Abnorm Child Psych* 14:49–61, 1986.
19. Rutter M, Sroufe LA: Developmental psychopathology: Concepts and challenges. *Dev Psychopathol* 12:265–296, 2000.
20. Sroufe LA: Psychopathology as an outcome of development. *Dev Psychopathol* 9:251–268, 1997.
21. Fineman KR: Firesetting in childhood and adolescence. *Psychiat Clin N Am* 3:483–500, 1980.
22. Kolko DJ: Education and counseling for child firesetters: A comparison of skills training programs with standard practice. In: Hibbs ED, Jensen PS (eds): *Psychosocial Treatments for Child and Adolescent Disorders: Empirically Based Strategies for Clinical Practice*. Washington, DC, American Psychological Association, 1996, pp. 187–206.
23. Kolko DJ, Kazdin AE, Meyer EC: Aggression and psychopathology in childhood firesetters: Parent and child reports. *J Consult Clin Psych* 53:377–385, 1985.
24. Stickle TR, Blechman EA: Aggression and fire: Antisocial behavior in firesetting and nonfiresetting juvenile offenders. *J Psychopathol Behav* 24:177–193, 2002.
25. Forehand R, Wierson M, Frame CL, Kemptom T, Armistead L: Juvenile firesetting: A unique syndrome or an advanced level of antisocial behavior? *Behav Res Therapy* 29:125–128, 1991.
26. Kolko DJ, Kazdin AE: Motives of child firesetters: Firesetting characteristics and psychological correlates. *J Child Psychol Psyc* 32:535–550, 1991.
27. Kolko DJ, Kazdin AE: Matchplay and firesetting in children: Relationship to parent, marital, and family dysfunction. *J Clin Child Psychol* 19:229–238, 1990.
28. Macht LB, Mack JE: The firesetter syndrome. *Psychiatr* 31:277–288, 1968.
29. Stewart MA, Culver KW: Children who set fires: The clinical picture and a follow-up. *Brit J Psychiat* 140:357–363, 1982.
30. Becker K, Stuewig J, Herrera V, McCloskey L: A study of firesetting and animal cruelty in children: Family influences and adolescent outcomes. *J Am Acad Child Psy* 43:905–912, 2004.
31. Sakheim GA, Vigdor MG, Gordon M, Helprin LM: A psychological profile of juvenile firesetters in residential treatment. *Child Welfare* 64:453–476, 1985.
32. Fineman KR: A model for the qualitative analysis of child and adult fire deviant behavior. *Am J Forensic Psy* 13:31–61, 1995.
33. Doherty J: Parent and community fire education: Integrating awareness in public education programs. In: Kolko DJ (ed): *Handbook on Firesetting in Children and Youth*. San Diego, Academic Press, 2002, pp. 283–303.
34. Schwartzman P, Stambaugh H, Kimball J: *Arson and juveniles: Responding to the violence*. Emmitsburg: United States Fire Administration, 1998.
35. Elliott EJ: Juvenile justice diversion and intervention. In Kolko DJ (ed): *Handbook on firesetting in children and youth*. San Diego, Academic Press, 2002, pp. 383–394.
36. Bailey S, Smith C, Dolan M: The social background and nature of "children" who perpetrate violent crimes: A UK perspective. *J Community Psychol* 29:305–317, 2001.
37. Heath GA, Hardesty VA, Goldfine PE, Walker AM: Diagnosis and childhood firesetting. *J Clin Psychol* 41:571–575, 1985.
38. Sakheim GA, Osborn E: A psychological profile of juvenile firesetters in residential treatment: A replication study. *Child Welfare* 65:495–503, 1986.
39. Hanson M, Mackay-Soroka S, Staley S, Poulton L: Delinquent firesetters: A comparative study of delinquency and firesetting histories. *Can J Psychiat* 39:230–232, 1994.
40. Ritvo E, Shanok SS, Lewis DO: Firesetting and nonfiresetting delinquents: A comparison of neuropsychiatric, psychoeducational, experiential, and behavior characteristics. *Child Psychiat Hum D*. 13:259–267, 1983.
41. Moore JM Jr, Thompson-Pope SK, Whited RM: MMPI—A profile of adolescent boys with a history of firesetting. *J Pers Assess* 67:116–126, 1996.
42. Kolko DJ: Research studies on the problem. In: Kolko DJ (ed): *Handbook on Firesetting in Children and Youth*. San Diego, Academic Press, 2002, pp. 33–52.
43. Stewart LA: Profile of female firesetters: Implications for treatment. *Brit J Psychiat* 163:248–256, 1993.
44. Repo E, Virkkunen M: Young arsonists: History of conduct disorder, psychiatric diagnoses and criminal recidivism. *J Forensic Psychiatr* 8:311–320, 1997.
45. Sakheim GA, Osborn E: *Firesetting child: Risk, assessment, and treatment*. Washington, DC, Child Welfare League of America, 1994.
46. Wooden WS, Berkey ML: *Children and arson*. New York: Plenum Press, 1984.
47. Gaynor J, Hatcher C: *The psychology of child firesetting: Detection and intervention*. New York: Brunnel/Mazel, 1987.

48. Cole R, Grolnick W, Laurenitis L, McAndrews M, Matkowski K, Schwartzman P: *Children and Fire: Rochester Fire-Related Youth Project Progress Report*. Rochester: University of Rochester, 1986.
49. Porth D: *Juvenile Firesetting: A Four Year Perspective*. Portland: SOS Fire Youth Intervention Program, 1997.
50. Slavkin ML: Enuresis, firesetting, and cruelty to animals: Does the ego triad show predictive validity? *Adolescence* 36:461–466, 2001.
51. Stadolnik RF: *Drawn to the Flame: Assessment and Treatment of Juvenile Firesetting Behavior*. Sarasota: Professional Resource Press, 2000.
52. American Psychiatric Association. *Diagnostic and statistical manual of mental disorders*, 4th ed., text revision. Arlington, VA, American Psychiatric Association, 2000.
53. Kolko DJ, Nishi-Strattner L, Wilcox DK, Kopet T: Clinical assessment of juvenile firesetters and their families: Tools and tips. In: Kolko DJ (ed): *Handbook on Firesetting in Children and Youth*. San Diego, Academic Press, 2002, pp. 177–212.
54. DiMillo J: Screening and triage tools. In Kolko DJ (ed): *Handbook on firesetting in children and youth*. San Diego, Academic Press, 2002, pp. 141–159.
55. Wilcox DK, Kolko DJ: Assessing recent firesetting behavior and taking a firesetting history. In Kolko DJ (ed): *Handbook on firesetting in children and youth*. San Diego, Academic Press, 2002, pp. 161–175.
56. Bic Corporation. Play safe! Be safe! *Teacher's Manual and Resource Book for Children's Fire Safety Education Program, Ages 3–5*. Milford, Bic Corporation, 1994.
57. Slavkin ML, Fineman K: What every professional who works with adolescents should know about firesetters. *Adolescence* 35:759–774, 2000.
58. Kolko DJ: Child, parent, and family treatment: Cognitive-behavioral interventions. In Kolko DJ (ed): *Handbook on firesetting in children and youth*. San Diego, Academic Press, 2002; pp. 305–336.
59. Dishion TJ, McMahon RJ: Parental monitoring and the prevention of child adolescent problem behavior: A conceptual and empirical formulation. *Clin Child Fam Psych* 1:61–75, 1998.
60. Kolko DJ, Kazdin AE: Children's descriptions of their firesetting incidents: Characteristics and relationship to recidivism. *J Am Acad Child Psy* 33:114–122, 1994.
61. Achenbach TM: *Manual for the Child Behavior Checklist/4-18 and 1991 Profile*. Burlington: University of Vermont Department of Psychiatry, 1991.
62. Pelham WE, Milich R, Murphy DA, Murphy HA: Normative data on the IOWA Conners teacher rating scale. *J Clin Child Psy* 18:259–262, 1989.
63. Kazdin AE, Rodgers A, Colbus D, Siegel T: Children's Hostility Inventory: Measurement of aggression and hostility in psychiatric inpatient children. *J Clin Child Psy* 16:320–328, 1987.
64. Nelson WM, Finch AJ: *Children's Inventory of Anger: Manual*. Los Angeles, Western Psychological Services, 2000.
65. Kovacs M: *The Children's Depression Inventory (CDI)*. North Tonawanda, NY, Multi-Health Systems, 1992.
66. Briere J: *Trauma Symptom Checklist for Children (TSCC): Professional Manual*. Odessa: Psychological Assessment Resources, 1996.
67. Straus MA, Hamby SL, Finkelhor D, Moore DW, Runyan D: Identification of child maltreatment with the Parent-Child Conflict Tactics Scales: Development and psychometric data for a national sample of American parents. *Child Abuse Neglect* 22:249–270, 1998.
68. Gerard AB: *Parent–Child Relationship Inventory: Manual*. Los Angeles: Western Psychological Services, 1994.
69. Nishi-Strattner L: Are first-time firesetters different from repeat firesetters? *Hot Issues*. 2005; Winter:1–4.
70. Bumpass ER, Brix RJ, Preston D: A community-based program for juvenile firesetters. *Hosp Community Psych* 36:529–533, 1985.
71. Massachusetts Coalition for Juvenile Firesetter Intervention Programs. *Expanding the Circles of Care*. Fall River, Author, 2002.
72. Kolko DJ: ed. *Handbook on Firesetting in Children and Youth*. San Diego, Academic Press, 2002.
73. MacKay S, Hanson M, Dickens S, Henderson J: *Fire Involvement Interview (FII): TAPP-C*. Toronto, Arson Prevention Program for Children, 1999.
74. MacKay S, Henderson J, Root C, Warling D, Gilbert KB, Johnstone J: *TAPP-C: Clinician's Manual for Preventing and Treating Juvenile Fire Involvement, Version 1.0*. Toronto, Centre for Addiction and Mental Health, 2004.
75. Henderson JL, MacKay S, Peterson-Badali, M: Closing the research-practice gap: Factors affecting adoption and implementation of a children's mental health program. *J Clin Child Psy* 35:2–12, 2006.
76. Hanson M, MacKay S, Atkinson L, Staley S, Pignatiello A: Firesetting during the preschool period—Assessment and intervention issues. *Can J Psychiat* 40:299–303, 1995.
77. Elliott EJ: Juvenile justice diversion and intervention. In Kolko DJ (ed): *Handbook on Firesetting in Children and Youth*. San Diego, Academic Press, 2002, pp. 383–395.
78. Dodge KA, Dishion TJ, Lansford JE: Deviant peer influences in intervention and public policy for youth. *Social Policy Report*. 2006; 1–19.
79. Pollinger J, Samuels L, Stadolnik R: A comparative study of the behavioral, personality, and fire history characteristics of residential and outpatient adolescents (ages 12–17) with firesetting behaviors. *Adolescence* 40:345–353, 2005.
80. Richardson JP: Jr. Secure residential treatment for adolescent firesetters. In Kolko DJ (ed): *Handbook on Firesetting in Children and Youth*. San Diego, Academic Press, 2002, pp. 353–381.
81. Kolko DJ: Multicomponent parental treatment of firesetting in a six-year-old boy. *J Behav Ther Exp Psy* 56:628–630, 1983.
82. Padgett LS, Strickland D, Coles CD: Case study: Using a virtual reality computer game to teach fire safety skills to children diagnosed with fetal alcohol syndrome. *J Pediatr Psychol* 31:65–70, 2006.
83. Wolff R: Satiation in the treatment of inappropriate fire setting. *J Behav Ther Exp Psy* 15:337–340, 1984.
84. Franklin GA, Pucci PS, Arbabi S, Brandt M, Wahl WL, Taheri PA: Decreased juvenile arson and firesetting recidivism after implementation of a multidisciplinary prevention program. *J Trauma* 53:260–266, 2002.
85. Kolko DJ, Swenson CC: *Assessing and Treating Physically Abused Children and their Families*. Thousand Oaks, CA, Sage Publications, 2002.
86. Pinsonneault IL, Richardson JP Jr, Pinsonneault J. Three models of educational interventions for child and adolescent firesetters. In Kolko DJ (ed): *Handbook on Firesetting in Children and Youth*. San Diego, Academic Press, 2002, pp. 261–282.
87. Maciak BJ, Moore MT, Leviton LC, Guinan ME: Preventing Halloween arson in an urban setting: A model for multisectoral planning and community participation. *Health Educ Behav* 25:194–211, 1998.

CHAPTER 5.3 ■ CHILDHOOD ONSET SCHIZOPHRENIA AND OTHER EARLY-ONSET PSYCHOTIC DISORDERS

NITIN GOGTAY AND JUDITH RAPOPORT

BACKGROUND

Psychotic disorders are rare in children although transient psychotic phenomena are more common in healthy and mildly disturbed children than generally recognized (1–3). As is often the case with other very early onset illnesses, psychotic disorders in children are usually more severe than their adult counterparts (4), and the disruption of cognitive and social development and the burden to the family can be devastating. Systematic research in this area has been limited by diagnostic uncertainty and the general lack of knowledge about the psychotic processes in children (5).

History of Very Early Onset Psychoses

Although the existence of childhood schizophrenia was recognized early in the twentieth century (6), the term psychosis was used so broadly in children that a spectrum of behavioral disorders and autism were grouped together under the category of childhood schizophrenia (7). The landmark studies of Kolvin (1971) first established the clinical distinction between autism and other psychotic disorders of childhood (8). However, even today high rates of initial misdiagnosis remain due to symptom overlap, particularly for mood disorders, and the presence of relatively fleeting hallucinations and delusions in nonpsychotic pediatric patients (9, 10). Anxiety and stress are probably the most common causes of hallucinations in preschool children, and the prognosis of these phenomena is usually benign (11). On the other hand, psychotic phenomena in school age children generally tend to be more persistent, and are more likely to be associated with drug toxicity or significant mental illness (2, 3, 12, 13). Moreover, recent data from large birth cohort studies suggest that self-reported psychotic symptoms at age 11 years predicted a very high risk (odds ratio 16.4, confidence interval 3.9–67.8) of schizophreniform diagnosis at age 26 years, suggesting that psychotic symptoms probably exist as a continuous phenotype rather than an all-or-none phenomenon (14).

Childhood Schizophrenia—Diagnosis, Clinical Presentation, and Differential Diagnoses

Kolvin's work established that children can be diagnosed with unmodified criteria for schizophrenia, although such cases are rare (15, 16). Childhood-onset schizophrenia (COS) shows a pattern similar to that of poor outcome adult cases, and the psychosis of COS can usually be distinguished by its severe and pervasive nature and its nonepisodic, unremitting course (5). Additionally, these children show poorer premorbid functioning in social, motor, and language domains, learning disabilities, and disruptive behavior disorders (17–19), and although not reported in studies of the premorbid history of adult-onset schizophrenia (20, 21), transient autistic symptoms such as hand flapping and echolalia in toddler years are common (17, 22), probably reflecting more compromised early brain development.

Childhood-onset schizophrenia is rare and must be distinguished from several childhood conditions that can manifest with psychotic symptoms and/or deterioration in function:

1. Affective disorders: Hallucinations are relatively common in pediatric bipolar disorder and major depression (23, 24). However, the psychotic symptoms in these conditions tend to be mood congruent and followup studies on this population generally suggest a stable clinical outcome (25–28).
2. Psychosis due to medical conditions, and substance abuse disorders should be carefully ruled out (29, 30).
3. Pervasive developmental disorders and childhood disintegrative disorder can often be mistaken for psychosis, as they show severe impairment in reciprocal communication, social interactions, and odd stereotyped behaviors.
4. Conduct disorder and various other behavioral disturbances can be associated with hallucinations (28, 29).
5. Atypical psychosis [provisionally labeled as Multi Dimensionally Impaired (MDI) by the NIMH group] is an important differential diagnosis and is described in detail below.

The Multi Dimensionally Impaired (MDI) Group

A sizeable, heterogeneous group of children referred to the NIMH childhood onset schizophrenia study over the past 15 years had transient psychotic symptoms and multiple developmental abnormalities, but were not adequately characterized by existing DSM-IV categories (31–33). In the DSM nosology these patients might be considered as having either psychosis NOS or mood disorder NOS.

The MDI group, although showing similarities with childhood onset schizophrenia, has distinct features which were used as the operational diagnostic criteria by the NIMH group, as listed below (31, 32):

1. Brief, transient episodes of psychosis and perceptual disturbance, typically in response to stress (as opposed to the pervasive hallucinations/delusions in COS)
2. Nearly daily periods of emotional lability disproportionate to precipitants
3. Impaired interpersonal skills despite the desire to initiate peer friendships (distinction from childhood onset schizophrenia)
4. Cognitive deficits as indicated by multiple deficits in information processing
5. No clear thought disorder (although this can be difficult to define clinically, particularly in the presence of a communication disorder)
6. Comorbid ADHD

These children somewhat resemble syndromes such as the borderline syndrome of children, or a behavioral syndrome of affective dysregulation and impairments in social behavior but with more prominent autistic spectrum characteristics labeled as the multiplex developmental disorder (MCDD) (33–36). However, these syndromes have more predominant symptoms of pervasive developmental disorder; greater evidence of a formal thought disorder; and onset before age 5 (as opposed to about age 8 for the MDI group) (33, 37–39).

Initially, the neuropsychological test profiles, smooth pursuit eye movement abnormalities, and familial risk factors suggested that some of the MDI children fell within the schizophrenia *spectrum* (32), but our MDI cohort appears to have a distinct long-term clinical course (described later), while none have progressed to schizophrenia (40).

THE NIMH COS AND MDI EXPERIENCE

The NIMH childhood onset schizophrenia (COS) study has been ongoing since 1990. Inclusion criteria for the study are: onset of psychosis before 12, premorbid IQ of 70 or above, and absence of significant neurological disorder. In the last 15 years, about 2,000 charts have been reviewed, of which 80% are rejected from further consideration as they fail to meet our stringent criteria for childhood onset schizophrenia. Over 250 children have been screened in person, of whom about 60% receive other psychiatric diagnoses, such as affective disorders, anxiety, or behavioral disorders. About 150 children who appeared likely to meet criteria for COS have been admitted to the research unit and undergone a complete medication washout followed by 1 to 3 weeks' drug-free inpatient observation. An additional 20% did not meet criteria for childhood onset schizophrenia, most frequently because a diagnosis of affective disorder was made (5, 31, 41). A recent 4- to 6-year followup study of 33 of the ruled out cases indicated good stability of the alternative diagnoses and confirmed their nonschizophrenic status (42). To date, 32

TABLE 5.3.1

DEMOGRAPHICS OF NIMH COS AND MDI SAMPLES

	COS	("MDI")	T-Test or Chi-Square	COS Parents	MDI Parents	T-Test or Chi-Square
Subject number	89	33	NA	141	53	NA
Age of onset	10.0 ± 2.1	7.7 ± 2.1	p <.0001	N/A	N/A	NA
Years ill (for probands)	3.7 ± 2.2	3.6 ± 2.2	ns	N/A	N/A	NA
Age at first contact	13.6 ± 2.7	12.0 ± 2.7	p = .004	47.6 ± 8.1	43.7 ± 12.6	ns
Gender (males)	52 (58%)	27 (84%)	p = .016,	70 (50%)	25 (47%)	ns
Caucasian	43 (48%)	26 (82%)	p = .022	72 (51%)	45 (85%)	p = .0008
African American	25 (28%)	2 (6%)		37 (26%)	5 (9%)	
Hispanic	8 (9%)	1 (3%)		14 (10%)	2 (4%)	
Asian	4 (5%)	0 (0%)		9 (5%)	0 (0%)	
Other	9 (10%)	3 (9%)		9(5%)	1 (2%)	
Parental SES	2.7 ± 1.2	2.8 ± 1.2	ns	N/A	N/A	NA

children have been given the provisional diagnosis of MDI after the medication washout period and have been followed prospectively along with the COS group. Demographics of the NIMH COS and MDI cohorts are summarized in Table 5.3.1.

PHENOMENOLOGY AND NEUROBIOLOGY OF COS

Premorbid Development

A striking phenomenological feature of COS relative to adult onset schizophrenia appears to be the higher rates of early language, social, and motor developmental abnormalities, possibly reflecting greater impairment in early brain development. In the NIMH sample, premorbid development (defined as development prior to 1 year before psychosis onset and assessed using the Cannon-Spoor Premorbid Adjustment Scale (PAS) (43) and the Hollis premorbid development scale (19)) and social and speech and language impairments were clearly impaired in COS, as has been previously observed by four other independent research centers (17–19, 22, 44–47).

Risk Factors

Since COS represents a more severe phenotype of schizophrenia than the adult onset illness, our initial hypothesis was that most risk factors identified in adult studies would be more striking in our very early onset cases.

Parental Age and Obstetric Complications

Adult schizophrenia studies suggest that association of the illness with advanced paternal age, raising the possibility of increased de novo mutations in the paternal germ cells, and also increased rates of maternal/fetal obstetric complications (48–50). The NIMH COS cohort showed no correlation with maternal or paternal age (51). In a recent analysis, we compared the obstetric records of 60 children with COS and 48 healthy siblings using the Columbia Obstetrics Complication Scale (52), a comprehensive measurement scale consisting of 37 variables. Contrary to our hypothesis, the incidence of obstetric complications in COS patients did not differ from that for the healthy sibling control group (53).

Eye Tracking

Smooth pursuit eye movement (SPEM) abnormalities have been reported in 25–40% of first-degree relatives of schizophrenic probands (54). Other studies have suggested more striking abnormalities in COS than in AOS, with a bilineal pattern of inheritance (55). In a recent analysis we compared 70 COS parents, 64 AOS parents, and 20 COS siblings to separate matched control groups and found that the effect sizes for SPEM abnormalities were higher for COS than for AOS relatives, indicating that genetic factors underlying eye-tracking dysfunction may be more salient for COS (56).

Familial Schizophrenia Spectrum Disorders

Schizophrenia spectrum disorders consist of schizophrenia and schizoaffective disorders on Axis I, and schizotypal, paranoid, and schizoid personality disorders on Axis II (44). A prior study by Asarnow et al. showed higher rates of schizophrenia spectrum diagnoses for COS relatives than for relatives of probands with attention deficit hyperactivity disorder or community controls (57). Similarly, as expected in our recent analyses of parental diagnosis in 97 parents of COS probands, 97 parents of AOS probands and matched community controls, also found that rate of familial schizophrenia spectrum disorders was higher for COS than AOS, and both were higher than community controls, supporting the continuity between COS and AOS, and the particularly salient familial/genetic risk in COS (58).

Familial Neurocognitive Functioning

It is well documented that subtle cognitive deficits, including abnormalities of attention (59, 60), executive functioning (61), spatial working memory (62), and verbal memory (63) are seen in healthy relatives of patients with AOS (64). Deficits in auditory attention, verbal memory and executive functioning are generally considered consistent (65, 66), although it is unclear whether these represent an underlying global cognitive deficit or each deficit represents a discrete endophenotype transmitted in families of patients with schizophrenia (66). When we compared neuropsychological deficits in 67 parents and 24 full siblings of COS probands to matched community controls in the Trail Making Tests A and B and the Wechsler Intelligence Scale-Revised Digit Span and Vocabulary, COS siblings had significantly poorer performance than community controls, although the rates of neuropsychological abnormalities for COS were not significantly higher than for AOS (67).

Pervasive Developmental Disorder and COS

The diagnosis of autism or pervasive developmental disorder (PDD) has been raised early in the development in our cases (n = 19, 25%) and several studies have claimed that autism per se might be a risk factor for later psychosis (68–70). Premorbid

PDD may be a nonspecific manifestation of impaired neurodevelopment, and also may provide an independent additive risk factor for COS. We ascertained the premorbid diagnosis of past or current autism or PDD in 75 COS probands in whom the diagnosis of PDD was made according to DSM-IV criteria (American Psychiatric Association, 1994) based on early chart reviews and clinical interviews of patients and parents. The diagnosis of PDD was made in cases when per history there were clear symptoms of autistic/PDD spectrum present prior to the onset of psychosis that were still observable at the time of the NIH evaluation.

Nineteen (25%) of our COS probands had a lifetime diagnosis of PDD: One met criteria for autism, two for Asperger disorder, and 16 for PDD not otherwise specified. Premorbid social impairment was the most common feature for COS-PDD subjects; the PDD group did not differ from the rest of the COS sample with respect to age of onset, IQ, response to medications, and rate of familial schizotypy. Furthermore, there was no difference between PDD and non-PDD groups with respect to initial brain magnetic resonance imaging (MRI) measures, although the rate of gray matter loss appeared to be greater for PDD ($n = 12$) than for the non-PDD ($n = 27$) subgroup (-19.5 ± 11.3 mL/year vs. -9.6 ± 15.3 mL/year; $p = .05$). These results may indicate that PDD in COS may be a nonspecific marker of more severe early abnormal neurodevelopment. However, siblings of the PDD-COS probands had significantly higher scores on the autism screening questionnaires, and two of 12 (17%) siblings of PDD probands were diagnosed with autism, a total rate similar to that seen for sibling of autistic probands (4.9%) (71), which may still imply a familial–genetic connection between COS and autism (47).

Neurocognitive Functioning in COS Probands

Neuropsychological function in COS outpatients has been studied by Asarnow and colleagues (72–74). While rote language skills and simple perceptual processing are not impaired, these children perform poorly on tasks involving fine motor coordination, attention, short-term and working memory (75). Evoked-potential studies show diminished amplitude of brain electrical activity during these tasks, suggesting that allocation of necessary attentional resources is deficient, which is also shared by adults with schizophrenia (74). It is generally established for adult schizophrenia that cognitive function deteriorates at onset of psychosis but remains stable afterwards (76, 77). Our earlier study had shown that children with COS ($n = 27$) as well as those with MDI ($n = 24$) share similar deficits in attention, learning and abstraction, resembling the pattern in adult patients with schizophrenia (78). In a recent analyses of 71 COS probands where preadmission IQ data were also available from medical and school records for a subgroup ($n = 27$), pre–post psychosis decline in IQ was noted as for adults, but post-psychotic cognitive function for up to 8+ years did not show continued decline (Figure 5.3.1). Thus, in spite of greater severity and generally poor clinical outcome, there was no evidence for a longer term degenerative cognitive process in COS, at least through early adulthood (79).

Comorbid Disorders

Comorbid psychiatric disorders, particularly DSM defined mood and anxiety disorders, often coexist with schizophrenia and can significantly alter the presentation, clinical course, or prognosis of the illness (80, 81). As the symptom manifestations of these disorders can also be part of (or masked by) the symptoms of the primary illness, the diagnoses of independent Axis I conditions are often ignored (82–84). We analyzed the rate of coexistent Axis I diagnoses for 76 COS cases at the time of first NIMH admission, and correlated the comorbid diagnoses with age of onset, ratings of illness severity, familiarity, and premorbid development.

As seen with AOS, the most frequent comorbid diagnosis at NIMH screening was depression (54%), followed by obsessive-compulsive disorder (OCD; 21%), generalized anxiety disorder (GAD; 15%), and attention deficit hyperactivity disorder (ADHD; 15%) (see Table 5.3.2). The rate of "any" anxiety disorder (GAD, OCD, separation anxiety, PTSD, and panic disorder combined) at screening was 42%. In general, comorbid diagnoses were independent of other illness indices, but comorbid depression correlated with poorer global assessment of severity (GAS) scores ($p = 0.01$), and presence of an anxiety disorder only predicted anxiety at four year followup ($p = 0.05$). No other axis I diagnoses showed correlations with any clinical measures, and there were no significant associations between comorbid diagnoses and IQ, familiarity, medication status, premorbid functioning, or age of onset at psychosis. Interestingly, no "current" comorbid depression was seen at the four-year followup for a subgroup of 28

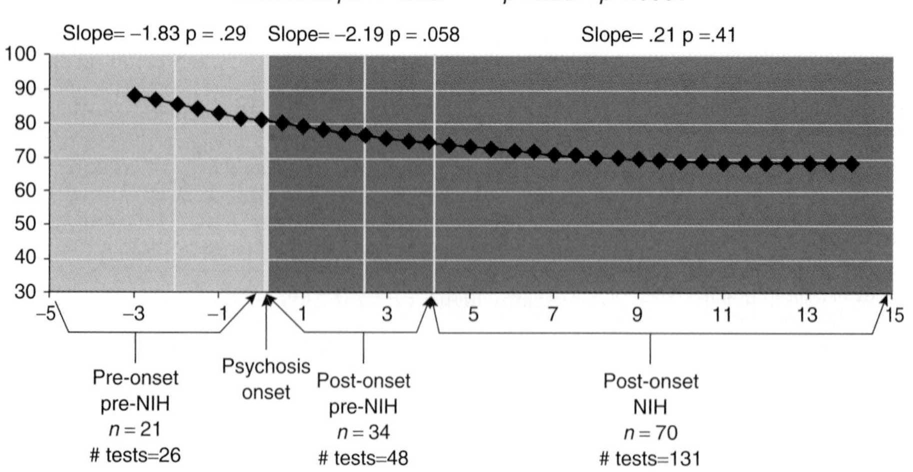

FIGURE 5.3.1. Full-scale IQ measures for 70 COS children plotted before ($n = 21$) and after ($n = 70$) the onset of psychosis, and also before ($n = 56$; obtained from prior charts) and after ($n = 70$) the children were admitted to the NIMH study. Although the children show significant decline in full scale IQ after the onset of psychosis, there is no significant long-term decline over next 14 years.

TABLE 5.3.2

CANDIDATE GENES SHOWING SIGNIFICANT ASSOCIATION WITH COS

Gene	Location	snp Name	T/NT	P Value
G72	13q33.1	P3206	32/17	0.031
		P2311	30/16	0.037
GAD1	2q31	P3017	16/7	0.057
		P3789	23/10	0.022
		M07	24/12	0.043
DTNBP1	6p22.3	P3521	21/9	0.026
MRDS1	6p24	P2139	12/3	0.016
COMT	22q11.21	P3218	26/11	0.012
AKT1	14q32	M000	15/5	0.022
		M002	31/17	0.042
NRG1	8p12	420M9-1395		0.010

snp = single nucleotide polymorphism;
T/NT = transmitted/nontransmitted.

subjects for whom there was complete diagnostic information available, possibly due to our high use of antidepressant treatment (45%). In contrast, anxiety disorders remained highly comorbid despite adjuvant anxiety medication use, suggesting either the refractory nature of these conditions, or a close association with core schizophrenia pathology.

BRAIN IMAGING: STRUCTURAL, FUNCTIONAL AND PET

Brain Development in COS

Imaging studies of childhood onset schizophrenia are scarce and most come from the NIMH sample, with more recent contributions from other groups (85–88). There is general agreement that children with schizophrenia show increased lateral ventricular volume, decreased gray matter volume, and increased basal ganglia volume (probably secondary to medication effect) (89–91), but less agreement with respect to reduced volumes of temporal lobe structures (87, 88, 92).

Prospective longitudinal brain MRI studies of the NIMH childhood schizophrenia population have been uniquely informative. Early analyses using whole-lobe volume measures showed increasing ventricular volume and decreasing total cortical, frontal, medial temporal, and parietal gray matter volumes at 2, 4, and 6 years after initial scan (90, 93). Although some adult schizophrenia studies show some progression in ventricular increase and regional cortical gray matter loss, effect size comparison indicates that such changes are more striking during adolescence (Figure 5.3.2) (94).

Until recently, analyses were limited to whole lobar volumes, but recent advances in computational image analysis permit regional gray matter density or cortical thickness measurements. When automated, these measurements can be applied to large samples, thereby increasing statistical power (95–97), and provide unprecedented anatomic detail of cortical GM change across the entire cortex, and for longitudinal samples, provide 3-D dynamic maps of cortical development across time (98).

Using both cross-sectional and longitudinal data, and with these state of the art cortical brain mapping methods, we have been able to address some broad questions about brain development in COS.

What is the Pattern of GM Loss in COS and its Relationship with Normal Development?

Using the novel cortical pattern matching technique, our initial analyses on 12 adolescent patients with schizophrenia using three prospective scans over 5 years compared to their temporally matched controls showed a unique "wave" of back to front tissue loss, with early parietal gray matter loss followed by frontal and temporal gray matter loss later in adolescence (99), and in a top-down fashion on the medial surface. A similar pattern of GM maturation was seen in our recent analyses of 13 healthy children with three to five scans over a 10-year period (98), suggesting that GM loss in COS may reflect an exaggeration of normal maturational process of synaptic/dendritic pruning during adolescence (Figure 5.3.3) (100, 101).

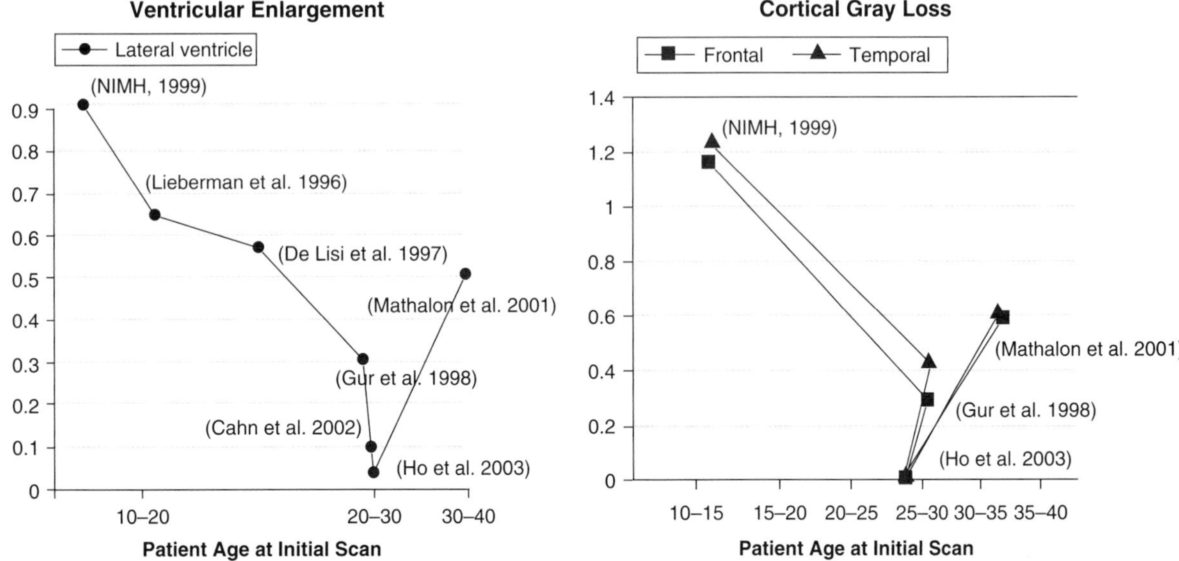

FIGURE 5.3.2. Effect size comparison of progressive ventricular expansion and cortical GM loss between NIMH COS cohort and published structural brain MRI studies in AOS plotted against patient age at the initial scan.

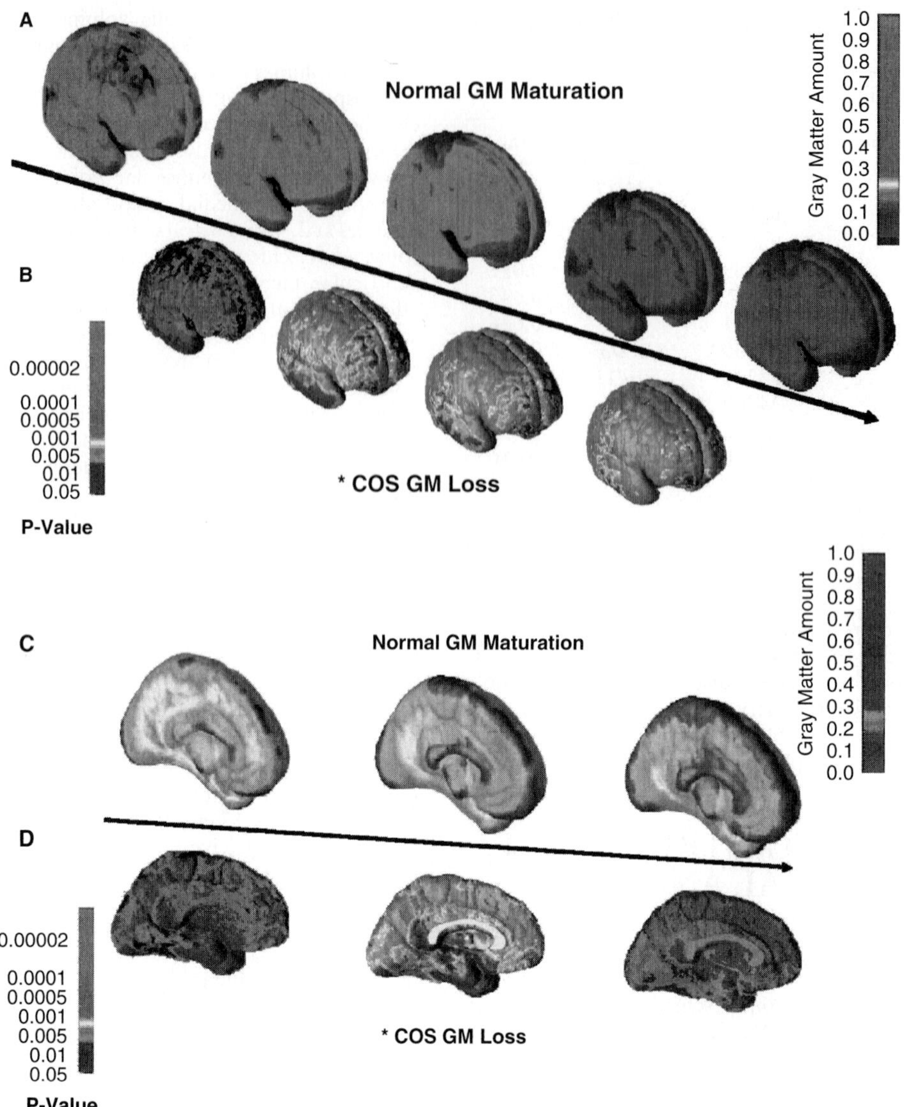

FIGURE 5.3.3. Comparison of the patterns of cortical GM loss in COS (between ages 12 to 16) to that seen in normal cortical maturation (between ages 4 to 22). (**A, C**) Lateral and medial views of the dynamic sequences of cortical GM maturation in healthy children between ages 4 and 22 (n = 13; 54 scans) rescanned every 2 years. Scale bar shows GM amount at each of the 65,536 cortical points across the entire cortex represented using a color scale (red to pink—more GM; blue—GM loss). Cortical GM maturation appears to progress in a back to front (parieto-temporal) manner on the lateral surface and in a top-down fashion on the medial surface. (**B, D**) Lateral and medial views of the dynamic sequence of cortical GM maturation in COS between ages 12 to 16 compared with ages and sex matched healthy controls (n = 12, 36 scans in each group), where children are rescanned every 2 years. Dynamic maps represent p-values for the difference in GM amount between COS and controls at each of the 65,536 cortical points, and p-values are represented using a color scale (e.g., pink $p < 0.00002$). Cortical GM loss in COS also appears to follow in a back to front direction on the lateral surface and in top down direction on medial surface, thus suggesting that the COS pattern is an exaggeration of the normal GM maturation. (Adapted from Gogtay, N., J. N. Giedd, et al. (2004). Dynamic mapping of human cortical development during childhood through early adulthood. Proc Natl Acad Sci USA 101(21): 8174-9; Thompson, P. M., C. Vidal, et al. (2001). Mapping adolescent brain change reveals dynamic wave of accelerated gray matter loss in very early-onset schizophrenia. *Proc Natl Acad Sci USA* 98(20):11650-5.) (See color insert.)

Does the Cortical GM Loss in COS Eventually Resemble the Adult Onset Pattern when Subjects Mature?

Cortical thickness analyses in adult onset schizophrenia document GM loss mostly in prefrontal and temporal cortices (95, 102). We analyzed prospective GM development in 70 COS subjects from age 6 through 26 years, using prospectively acquired anatomic brain scans (one to five scans per subject; total scans = 330) using fully automated cortical thickness analyses and mixed effect regression model statistics and comparing them to 72 matched healthy controls (total scans = 330). The analyses show that as COS subjects mature, the robust and global GM loss during the adolescent years becomes limited to prefrontal and superior temporal cortices by age 24, thus mimicking a pattern seen in adult patients (Greenstein et al., in press).

Is the GM Loss in COS a Medication Effect?

An important question about the GM loss in schizophrenia has been whether it is a medication effect (103, 104). It is not possible to obtain medication naive COS subjects because of the severity of their illness, but the MDI cases provide age, sex, IQ, and treatment matched nonschizophrenia comparison subjects. The GM findings in COS appeared to be due to schizophrenia and not due to medications as quantitative analysis of matched COS (n = 23), MDI (n = 19) and healthy community control (n = 38) groups showed the GM loss to be limited only to the COS group (105).

Is the GM Loss in COS Diagnostically Specific?

At 4- to 8-year followup a subgroup of children with MDI (n = 12, 38%) have converted to bipolar I diagnosis and had scans before and after their first manic episode. The time lapse sequence of cortical development tracked before and after the onset of bipolar illness shows a left lateralized gain in GM density and GM reduction on the right lateral and bilateral anterior cingulate cortices (Gogtay et al., submitted). Thus, the developmental trajectories for COS and pediatric bipolar illness appear diagnostically distinct.

Is the Increased GM Loss in COS a Trait Marker?

A pilot cross-sectional analysis with 15 healthy full siblings of subjects with COS (mean age 19.4+/5.9 years) using whole-lobe volumetric measures showed GM reduction in siblings relative to 32 healthy controls (mean age 18.7+/−6.2), where the difference was most significant in the parietal GM (106). Recent analysis of data from an expanded sample comparing 56 healthy COS siblings with 56 matched controls using cortical thickness analyses and mixed effect regression models that included total 100 scans for each group showed the healthy COS siblings to have smaller prefrontal and superior temporal GM thickness in early ages, which appeared to normalize by age 24 years (Figure 5.3.4) (Gogtay et al., unpublished data).

Given that none of the siblings have had medication exposure, these results show that the GM changes in COS are a trait marker.

Other Imaging Studies

Thomas and colleagues conducted a proton magnetic resonance spectroscopy study of 10 children with schizophrenia and 12 healthy children (107). They found that the ratio of N-acetylaspartate (NAA) to creatine was significantly lower in the frontal lobes of children with schizophrenia. Similarly, lower NAA signals were also seen in hippocampal and dorsolateral prefrontal cortical regions for a small subgroup of the NIMH childhood schizophrenia population (108). Although the role of N-acetylaspartate has not been firmly established, it is thought to be a marker of neuronal density or neuronal volume (109).

Few functional imaging studies have been conducted in childhood-onset schizophrenia, quite possibly because functional imaging modalities demand that patients be immobile for a fixed period of time and/or that they carry out cognitive tasks. PET studies involve exposure to radiation, thus limiting their use in the pediatric population.

Cerebral glucose metabolism was examined in 16 adolescent subjects from the NIMH childhood-onset schizophrenia sample and 26 healthy adolescents matched for age, sex, and handedness (but not task performance) using positron emission tomography (PET) and ^{18}F-fluorodeoxyglucose (FDG). PET findings indicated mild hypofrontality and abnormal neural circuitry that involved cerebellum in childhood-onset schizophrenia (110, 111).

GENETIC STUDIES

Numerous chromosomal abnormalities have been reported in schizophrenia (112, 113). Observations across pediatrics and medicine suggest that early onset cases may have more salient and fewer genetic causes (4, 114, 115), and as with breast cancer and Alzheimer's disease, the familial risk for schizophrenia spectrum disorders appears higher for COS than in AOS contrast groups (57, 58). As summarized in Tables 5.3.2 and 5.3.3, candidate gene association studies and cytogenetic studies show increased rates of abnormalities for the COS population. For the cytogenetic abnormalities, these are clearly higher rates than seen for the AOS. For candidate genes, the high variance in adult studies results in inadequate statistical power to compare with COS results.

Cytogenetic Abnormalities

High-resolution banding karyotype and fluorescent in situ hybridization (FISH) analyses are done routinely on all COS and MDI patients to look for fragile X, 22q11 deletions, Smith-Magenis (17p11.2del), and 15q11–q13 deletions/duplications. As seen in Table 5.3.3, our cohorts show a rate of almost 10% for 120 (COS and MDI) probands with chromosomal abnormalities. The 22q11 deletion syndrome (22q11DS), manifest as velocardio-facial syndrome (VCFS), is estimated to occur 1 in 4,000 live births (116), and is a known risk factor for schizophrenia (117, 118). Four out of 90 (4.4%) of our unselected COS patients have velocardio-facial syndrome (VCFS) with spontaneous 22q11 deletion, a rate significantly higher than 0.46% found for the available reports on a total of 870 adult-onset cases (p = 0.002). Similarly, 2 out of 38 (5.2%) females have mosaic Turner syndrome, a rate about 500 times higher than expected for this particular subtype of Turner syndrome.

Candidate Genes

With an initial hypothesis that there may be more detrimental/penetrant mutations in known schizophrenia susceptibility genes in COS, to date we have examined a total of 15 genes previously reported positive for AOS and also nine putative autism genes given the higher rates of comorbid PDD with our sample (47, 119). As seen in Table 5.3.2, polymorphisms in seven genes previously implicated in AOS samples show significant association with COS, using a family-based design. In contrast, none of the nine putative autism risk genes showed evidence of association with COS.

In addition to supporting the genetic continuity between COS and AOS, these data suggest that the very early onset COS population, with more pronounced neurobiological abnormalities and a more homogeneous phenotype, may turn out to be a relatively efficient population to target for the identification of genetic risk of schizophrenia more generally. However, statistical comparison with the AOS results remains underpowered.

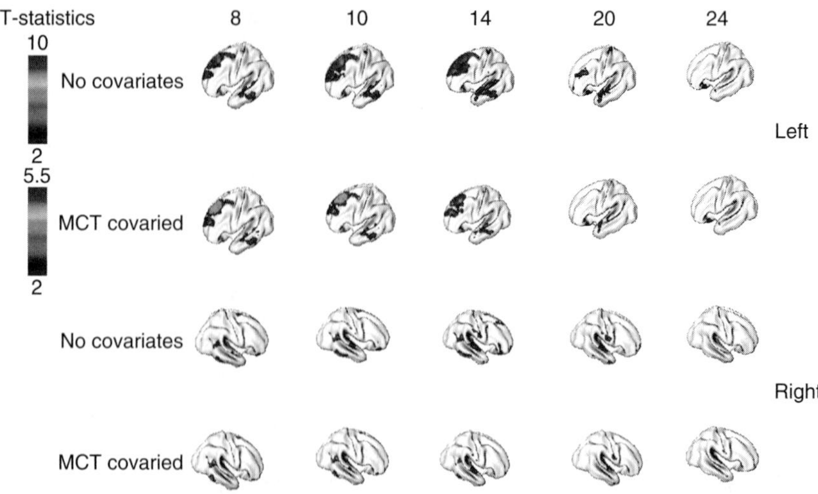

FIGURE 5.3.4. Cortical GM development in healthy COS siblings (n = 56; 100 scans) compared with age and sex matched normal volunteers (n = 56; 100 scans) between 6 to 30 years. Analyses were done using automated cortical thickness measure across 40,000 cortical points over the entire cortex using mixed-effect regression model analyses which allowed using cross-sectional as well as longitudinal scans. Color bars represent t-statistics where t >2 (adjusted for multiple comparisons, using false discovery rate at t = 2) indicate significant loss of GM in healthy siblings compared to controls at that cortical point. GM differences at various ages were obtained by age-recentering the data at that age. Healthy siblings showed GM loss in prefrontal and temporal cortices in early ages, but the GM differences were normalized by age 24 years. Images are shown both with and without adjusting for mean cortical thickness (MCT). (From N Gogtay, D Greenstein, M Lenane, L Clasen, W Sharp, P Gochman, P Butler, A Evans, and J Rapoport. 'Cortical Brain Development in Non-Psychotic Siblings of Patients with Childhood Onset Schizophrenia' (*in Press*) Archives of General Psychiatry.) (See color insert.)

TREATMENT STUDIES IN CHILDHOOD PSYCHOSES

Although rare, childhood-onset schizophrenia is a devastating disorder, frequently resistant to treatment, and with an unfortunately narrow evidence base to guide treatment, particularly as there are no trials comparing atypical antipsychotics, which have become the mainstay of current treatment (120). Two prior randomized controlled trials established the superiority of typical antipsychotics over placebo in COS (121, 122). A single trial in a small group of treatment refractory COS patients had demonstrated the efficacy of clozapine over the typical antipsychotic haloperidol (123). However, as there was no placebo arm in the study, it is hard to assess the true effect size for clozapine. A more recent double-blind randomized control trial of comparing clozapine ($n = 12$) with olanzapine ($n = 13$) showed a significant advantage for clozapine in the alleviation of negative symptoms of schizophrenia, which was not correlated with improvement in mood or extrapyramidal side effects. As anticipated, clozapine was associated with more overall side effects, including enuresis, tachycardia, hypertension, and significant weight gain by 2 years (Dr. Philip Shaw, unpublished data). The results of our prior study and studies in AOS patients (124, 125) show that clozapine has the greatest antipsychotic efficacy, particularly in a pediatric population, although its toxicity limits its use in all but the most severe treatment-refractory patients.

TABLE 5.3.3

CYTOGENETIC ABNORMALITIES IN THE COS AND MDI COHORTS

Diagnosis	Sex	Race	Abnormality
COS	F	W	VCFS
COS	F	W	VCFS
COS	M	W	VCFS
COS	F	W	VCFS
COS	M	W	46,xy,t(1:7)(p22:q22)
COS	F	W	Mosaic Turner 45, XO
COS	F		Mosaic Turner 45, XO
MDI	M	H	47, XYY
MDI	M	W	47, XXY
MDI	M	W	Mosaic Klinefelter 47, XXY
MDI	M	W	9p23 deletion

VCFS = velo-cardio-facial syndrome.

Adverse Effects of Clozapine

In spite of its unique efficacy for some COS patients, clozapine is associated with several side effects, in particular agranulocytosis, weight gain, cardiovascular changes such as postural hypotension and tachycardia, and incontinence. The NIMH study has started addressing the questions of how to manage these side effects so that these children can continue to stay on clozapine.

Neutropenia and Akathisia. Children and adolescents treated with clozapine have increased susceptibility to neutropenia. This can be successfully managed by addition of lithium (126). Similarly, akathisia, seen only rarely in adults on clozapine, appears more common in children (six out of 15 children recently treated with clozapine had developed akathisia) and can frequently manifest as worsening of psychotic symptoms or agitation in children, which frequently results in dosage increment. This side effect is responsive to adjunctive propranolol (127) treatment.

Weight Gain. Weight gain is a significant effect of atypical antipsychotics and appears more pronounced in pediatric patients (128, 129). Clozapine particularly has been noted to cause significant weight gain during childhood (130). Although the mechanism of weight gain in poorly understood, genetic risks (polymorphism in Beta3 and alpha 1A adrenergic, 5HT-2C, TNF-alpha and histamine receptors) and a number of biochemical correlates (e.g., leptin, prolactin, triglyceride and HDL levels) of weight gain have been reported in the literature (131). In our recent analysis of 23 patients treated with clozapine, children with COS showed increases in BMI ($p = 0.001$) and Leptin levels ($p = 0.01$) after 6 weeks of treatment. For COS patients, BMI at baseline and week 6 correlated with insulin level ($r = 0.5, p = 0.004$) and BMI was positively correlated with clinical improvement in CGI, SAPS and SANS rating scales ($p<0.05$) (132). Based on these correlations, a double blind, and placebo controlled trial of antidiabetic medication metformin (which improves peripheral insulin sensitivity) is currently underway.

References

1. Caplan R: Thought disorder in childhood. *J Am Acad Child Adolesc Psychiatry* 33(5):605–615, 1994.
2. Schreier HA: Hallucinations in nonpsychotic children: More common than we think? *J Am Acad Child Adolesc Psychiatry* 38(5):623–625, 1999.
3. McGee R, Williams S, Poulton R: Hallucinations in nonpsychotic children. *J Am Acad Child Adolesc Psychiatry* 39(1):12–13, 2000.
4. Childs B, Scriver CR: Age at onset and causes of disease. *Perspect Biol Med* 29(3 Pt. 1):437–460, 1986.
5. Nicolson R, Rapoport JL: Childhood-onset schizophrenia: Rare but worth studying. *Biol Psychiatry* 46(10):1418–1428, 1999.
6. Kraepelin E: In: *Dementia Praecox and Paraphrenia.* Huntington, NY: Robert E Krieger 1919.
7. Volkmar FR: Childhood and adolescent psychosis: A review of the past 10 years. *J Am Acad Child Adolesc Psychiatry* 35(7):843–851, 1996.
8. Kolvin I: Studies in the childhood psychoses. I. Diagnostic criteria and classification. *Br J Psychiatry* 118(545):381–384, 1971.
9. McKenna K, Gordon CT, Rapoport JL: Childhood-onset schizophrenia: Timely neurobiological research. *J Am Acad Child Adolesc Psychiatry* 33(6):771–781, 1994.
10. Lukianowicz N: Hallucinations in non-psychotic children. *Psychiatr Clin (Basel)* 2(6):321–337, 1969.
11. Rothstein A: Hallucinatory phenomena in childhood. A critique of the literature. *J Am Acad Child Psychiatry* 20(3):623–635, 1981.
12. Abramowicz M: Drugs that cause psychiatric symptoms. *Med Lett Drugs Ther* 35:65–70, 1993.
13. Davison K: Schizophrenia-like psychoses associated with organic cerebral disorders: A review. *Psychiatr Dev* 1(1):1–33, 1983.
14. Poulton R, et al.: Children's self-reported psychotic symptoms and adult schizophreniform disorder: A 15-year longitudinal study. *Arch Gen Psychiatry* 57(11):1053–1058, 2000.
15. Werry JS: Child and adolescent (early onset) schizophrenia: A review in light of DSM-III-R. *J Autism Dev Disord* 22(4):601–624, 1992.
16. Gordon CT, et al.: Childhood-onset schizophrenia: An NIMH study in progress. *Schizophr Bull* 20(4):697–712, 1994.
17. Alaghband-Rad J, et al.: Childhood-onset schizophrenia: The severity of premorbid course. *J Am Acad Child Adolesc Psychiatry* 34(10):1273–1283, 1995.
18. Green WH, et al.: Schizophrenia with childhood onset: A phenomenological study of 38 cases. *J Am Acad Child Adolesc Psychiatry* 31(5):968–976, 1992.
19. Hollis C: Child and adolescent (juvenile onset) schizophrenia. A case control study of premorbid developmental impairments. *Br J Psychiatry* 166(4):489–495, 1995.
20. Done DJ, et al.: Childhood antecedents of schizophrenia and affective illness: Social adjustment at ages 7 and 11. *BMJ* 309(6956):699–703, 1994.
21. Jones P, et al.: Child development risk factors for adult schizophrenia in the British 1946 birth cohort. *Lancet* 344(8934):1398–1402, 1994.
22. Russell A, Bott, L. Sammons C: The phenomena of schizophrenia occurring in childhood. *Journal of the American Academy of Child and Adolescent Psychiatry* 28:399–407, 1989.
23. Chambers WJ, et al.: Psychotic symptoms in prepubertal major depressive disorder. *Arch Gen Psychiatry* 39(8):921–927, 1982.
24. Varanka TM, et al.: Lithium treatment of manic episodes with psychotic features in prepubertal children. *Am J Psychiatry* 145(12):1557–1559, 1988.
25. Ulloa RE, et al.: Psychosis in a pediatric mood and anxiety disorders clinic: Phenomenology and correlates. *J Am Acad Child Adolesc Psychiatry* 39(3): 337–345, 2000.
26. McClellan J, et al.: Early-onset psychotic disorders: Course and outcome over a 2-year period. *J Am Acad Child Adolesc Psychiatry* 38(11):1380–1388, 1999.
27. McClellan J, McCurry C: Early onset psychotic disorders: Diagnostic stability and clinical characteristics. *Eur Child Adolesc Psychiatry* 8 Suppl 1:113–119, 1999.
28. Garralda ME: Hallucinations in children with conduct and emotional disorders: II. The follow-up study. *Psychol Med* 14(3):597–604, 1984.
29. Garralda ME: Hallucinations in children with conduct and emotional disorders: I. The clinical phenomena. *Psychol Med* 14(3):589–596, 1984.
30. Caplan R, et al.: Middle childhood onset of interictal psychosis. *J Am Acad Child Adolesc Psychiatry* 30(6):893–896, 1991.
31. McKenna K, et al.: Looking for childhood-onset schizophrenia: The first 71 cases screened. *J Am Acad Child Adolesc Psychiatry* 33(5):636–644, 1994.
32. Kumra S, et al.: "Multidimensionally impaired disorder": Is it a variant of very early-onset schizophrenia? *J Am Acad Child Adolesc Psychiatry* 37(1):91–99, 1998.
33. Towbin KE, et al.: Conceptualizing "borderline syndrome of childhood" and "childhood schizophrenia" as a developmental disorder. *J Am Acad Child Adolesc Psychiatry* 32(4):775–782, 1993.
34. Dahl EK, Cohen DJ, Provence S: Clinical and multivariate approaches to the nosology of pervasive developmental disorders. *J Am Acad Child Psychiatry* 25(2):170–180, 1986.
35. Petti TA, Vela RM: Borderline disorders of childhood: An overview. *J Am Acad Child Adolesc Psychiatry* 29(3):327–337, 1990.
36. Van der Gaag RJ, et al.: A controlled multivariate chart review of multiple complex developmental disorder. *J Am Acad Child Adolesc Psychiatry* 34(8):1096–1106, 1995.
37. Cohen DJ, Paul R, Volkmar FR: Issues in the classification of pervasive and other developmental disorders: Toward DSM-IV. *J Am Acad Child Psychiatry* 25(2):213–220, 1986.
38. Ad-Dab'bagh Y, Greenfield B: Multiple complex developmental disorder: The "multiple and complex" evolution of the "childhood borderline syndrome" construct. *J Am Acad Child Adolesc Psychiatry* 40(8):954–964, 2001.
39. Kumra S, et al.: "Multidimensionally impaired disorder": Is it a variant of very early-onset schizophrenia? *J Am Acad Child Adolesc Psychiatry* 37(1):91–99, 1998.
40. Nicolson R, et al.: Children and adolescents with psychotic disorder not otherwise specified: A 2- to 8-year follow-up study. *Compr Psychiatry* 42(4):319–325, 2001.
41. Kumra S, et al.: Including children and adolescents with schizophrenia in medication-free research. *Am J Psychiatry* 156(7):1065–1068, 1999.
42. Calderoni D, et al.: Differentiating childhood-onset schizophrenia from psychotic mood disorders. *J Am Acad Child Adolesc Psychiatry* 40(10):1190–1196, 2001.
43. Cannon-Spoor HE, Potkin SG, Wyatt RJ: Measurement of premorbid adjustment in chronic schizophrenia. *Schizophr Bull* 8(3):470–484, 1982.
44. Asarnow JR, Ben-Meir S: Children with schizophrenia spectrum and depressive disorders: A comparative study of premorbid adjustment, onset pattern and severity of impairment. *J Child Psychol Psychiatry* 29(4):477–488, 1988.
45. Watkins JM, Asarnow RF, Tanguay PE: Symptom development in childhood onset schizophrenia. *J Child Psychol Psychiatry* 29(6):865–878, 1988.
46. Nicolson R, et al.: Premorbid speech and language impairments in childhood-onset schizophrenia: Association with risk factors. *Am J Psychiatry* 157(5):794–800, 2000.
47. Sporn AL, et al.: Pervasive developmental disorder and childhood-onset schizophrenia: comorbid disorder or a phenotypic variant of a very early onset illness? *Biol Psychiatry* 55(10):989–994, 2004.
48. Malaspina D, et al.: Advancing paternal age and the risk of schizophrenia. *Arch Gen Psychiatry* 58(4):361–367, 2001.
49. Lewis SW, Murray RM: Obstetric complications, neurodevelopmental deviance, and risk of schizophrenia. *J Psychiatr Res* 21(4):413–421, 1987.
50. Cannon M, Jones PB, Murray RM: Obstetric complications and schizophrenia: historical and meta-analytic review. *Am J Psychiatry* 159(7):1080–1092, 2002.
51. Nicolson R, et al.: Obstetrical complications and childhood-onset schizophrenia. *Am J Psychiatry* 156(10):1650–1652, 1999.
52. Malaspina D: Columbia Obstetrics Complication Scale. In: *Diagnostic Center for Schizophrenia Linkage Studies.* New York: New York State Psychiatric Institute, 2003.
53. Ordonez AE, et al.: Lack of evidence for elevated obstetric complications in childhood-onset schizophrenia. *Biol Psychiatry* 58(1):10–5, 2005.
54. Holzman PS: Eye movements and the search for the essence of schizophrenia. *Brain Res Brain Res Rev* 31(2–3):350–356, 2000.
55. Ross RG, et al.: Evidence for bilineal inheritance of physiological indicators of risk in childhood-onset schizophrenia. *Am J Med Genet* 88(2):188–199, 1999.
56. Sporn A, et al.: Childhood-onset schizophrenia: Smooth pursuit eye-tracking dysfunction in family members. *Schizophr Res* 73(2–3):243–252, 2005.

57. Asarnow RF, et al.: Schizophrenia and schizophrenia-spectrum personality disorders in the first-degree relatives of children with schizophrenia: The UCLA family study. *Arch Gen Psychiatry* 58(6):581–588, 2001.
58. Nicolson R, et al.: Parental schizophrenia spectrum disorders in childhood-onset and adult-onset schizophrenia. *Am J Psychiatry* 160(3):490–495, 2003.
59. Harris JG, et al.: Neuropsychological dysfunction in parents of schizophrenics. *Schizophr Res* 20(3):253–260, 1996.
60. Chen WJ, Faraone SV: Sustained attention deficits as markers of genetic susceptibility to schizophrenia. *Am J Med Genet* 97(1):52–57, 2000. [record as supplied by publisher].
61. Faraone SV, et al.: Neuropsychological functioning among the nonpsychotic relatives of schizophrenic patients: A 4-year follow-up study. *J Abnorm Psychol* 108(1):176–181, 1999.
62. Park S, Holzman PS, Goldman-Rakic PS: Spatial working memory deficits in the relatives of schizophrenic patients. *Arch Gen Psychiatry* 52(10):821–828, 1995.
63. Gold JM, et al.: Memory and intelligence in lateralized temporal lobe epilepsy and schizophrenia. *Schizophr Res* 17(1):59–65, 1995.
64. Egan MF, et al.: Relative risk for cognitive impairments in siblings of patients with schizophrenia. *Biol Psychiatry* 50(2):98–107, 2001.
65. Faraone SV, et al.: Neuropsychologic functioning among the nonpsychotic relatives of schizophrenic patients: The effect of genetic loading. *Biol Psychiatry* 48(2): p. 120–126, 2000.
66. Krabbendam L, et al.: Single or multiple familial cognitive risk factors in schizophrenia? *Am J Med Genet* 105(2):183–188, 2001.
67. Gochman PA, et al.: Childhood Onset Schizophrenia: Familial Neuropsychological Measures. *Schizophr Res*, 2003, In press.
68. Cantor S, et al.: Childhood schizophrenia: Present but not accounted for. *Am J Psychiatry* 139(6):758–762, 1982.
69. Clarke DJ, et al.: Pervasive developmental disorders and psychoses in adult life. *Br J Psychiatry* 155:692–699, 1989.
70. Petty LK, et al.: Autistic children who become schizophrenic. *Arch Gen Psychiatry* 41(2):129–135, 1984.
71. Jorde LB, et al.: Complex segregation analysis of autism. *Am J Hum Genet* 49(5):932–938, 1991.
72. Asarnow RF: Neurocognitive impairments in schizophrenia: A piece of the epigenetic puzzle. *Eur Child Adolesc Psychiatry* 8 Suppl. 1:15–18, 1999.
73. Asarnow RF, et al.: Cognitive/neuropsychological studies of children with a schizophrenic disorder. *Schizophr Bull* 20(4):647–669, 1994.
74. Asarnow RF, Brown W, Strandburg R: Children with a schizophrenic disorder: Neurobehavioral studies. *Eur Arch Psychiatry Clin Neurosci* 245(2):70–79, 1995.
75. Karatekin C, Asarnow RF: Working memory in childhood-onset schizophrenia and attention-deficit/hyperactivity disorder. *Psychiatry Res* 80(2):165–176, 1998.
76. Russell AJ, et al.: Schizophrenia and the myth of intellectual decline. *Am J Psychiatry* 154(5):635–639, 1997.
77. Goldberg TE, et al.: Course of schizophrenia: Neuropsychological evidence for a static encephalopathy. *Schizophr Bull* 19(4):797–804, 1993.
78. Kumra S, et al.: Neuropsychological deficits in pediatric patients with childhood-onset schizophrenia and psychotic disorder not otherwise specified. *Schizophr Res* 42(2):135–144, 2000.
79. Gochman PA, et al.: IQ decline and stabilization in Childhood-Onset Schizophrenia. Submitted, 2003.
80. Fenton WS, McGlashan TH: The prognostic significance of obsessive-compulsive symptoms in schizophrenia. *Am J Psychiatry* 143(4):437–441, 1986.
81. Huppert JD, et al.: Quality of life in schizophrenia: Contributions of anxiety and depression. *Schizophrenia Research* 51(2–3):171–180, 2001.
82. Bermanzohn PC, et al.: Hierarchical diagnosis in chronic schizophrenia: A clinical study of co-occurring syndromes. *Schizophr Bull* 26(3):517–525, 2000.
83. Green AI, et al.: Detection and management of comorbidity in patients with schizophrenia. *Psychiatr Clin North Am* 26(1):115–139, 2003.
84. Huppert JD, Smith TE: Anxiety and schizophrenia: The interaction of subtypes of anxiety and psychotic symptoms. *CNS Spectr* 10(9):721–731, 2005.
85. Sowell ER, Toga AW, Asarnow R: Brain abnormalities observed in childhood-onset schizophrenia: A review of the structural magnetic resonance imaging literature. *Ment Retard Dev Disabil Res Rev* 6(3):180–185, 2000.
86. Sowell ER, et al.: Brain abnormalities in early-onset schizophrenia spectrum disorder observed with statistical parametric mapping of structural magnetic resonance images. *Am J Psychiatry* 157(9):1475–1484, 2000.
87. Matsumoto H, et al.: Superior temporal gyrus abnormalities in early-onset schizophrenia: Similarities and differences with adult-onset schizophrenia. *Am J Psychiatry* 158(8):1299–1304, 2001.
88. Matsumoto H, et al.: Structural magnetic imaging of the hippocampus in early onset schizophrenia. *Biol Psychiatry* 49(10):824–831, 2001.
89. Rapoport JL, et al.: Childhood-onset schizophrenia. Progressive ventricular change during adolescence. *Arch Gen Psychiatry* 54(10):897–903, 1997.
90. Rapoport JL, et al.: Progressive cortical change during adolescence in childhood-onset schizophrenia. A longitudinal magnetic resonance imaging study. *Arch Gen Psychiatry* 56(7):649–654, 1999.
91. Frazier JA, et al.: Brain anatomic magnetic resonance imaging in childhood-onset schizophrenia. *Arch Gen Psychiatry* 53(7):617–624, 1996.
92. Jacobsen LK, et al.: Temporal lobe morphology in childhood-onset schizophrenia *Am J Psychiatry* 153(3):355–361, 1996. [published erratum appears in *Am J Psychiatry* 1996 Jun:153(6):851].
93. Rapoport JL, et al.: Imaging normal and abnormal brain development: New perspectives for child psychiatry. *Aust N Z J Psychiatry* 35(3):272–281, 2001.
94. Gogate N, et al.: Brain imaging in normal and abnormal brain development: New perspectives for child psychiatry. *Clinical Neuroscience Research* 1:283–290, 2001.
95. Luders E, et al.: Mapping cortical gray matter in the young adult brain: Effects of gender. *Neuroimage* 26(2):493–501, 2005.
96. Thompson PM, et al.: Detecting disease specific patterns of brain structure using cortical pattern matching and a population-based probabilistic brain atlas, IEEE Conference on Information Processing in Medical Imaging (IPMI), UC Davis 2001. In: Insana M, Leahy RM (ed.) *Lecture Notes in Computer Science (LNCS)*, Vol. 2082. Springer-Verlag. 2001, pp. 488–501.
97. Thompson PM, et al.: Growth patterns in the developing brain detected by using continuum mechanical tensor maps. *Nature* 404(6774):190–193, 2000.
98. Gogtay N, et al.: Dynamic mapping of human cortical development during childhood through early adulthood. *Proc Natl Acad Sci USA* 101(21):8174–8179, 2004.
99. Thompson PM, et al.: Mapping adolescent brain change reveals dynamic wave of accelerated gray matter loss in very early-onset schizophrenia. *Proc Natl Acad Sci USA* 98(20):11650–11655, 2001.
100. Huttenlocher PR: Synaptic density in human frontal cortex: Developmental changes and effects of aging. *Brain Res* 163(2):195–205, 1979.
101. Huttenlocher PR, Dabholkar AS: Regional differences in synaptogenesis in human cerebral cortex. *J Comp Neurol* 387(2):167–178, 1997.
102. Kuperberg GR, et al.: Regionally localized thinning of the cerebral cortex in schizophrenia. *Arch Gen Psychiatry* 60(9):878–888, 2003.
103. Narr K, et al.: Mapping cortical thickness and gray matter density in first episode schizophrenia. Submitted, 2004.
104. Narr KL, et al.: Mapping cortical thickness and gray matter concentration in first episode schizophrenia. *Cereb Cortex* 15(6):708–719, 2005.
105. Gogtay N, et al.: Comparison of progressive cortical gray matter loss in childhood-onset schizophrenia with that in childhood-onset atypical psychoses. *Arch Gen Psychiatry* 61(1):17–22, 2004.
106. Gogtay N, et al.: Structural brain MRI abnormalities in healthy siblings of patients with childhood-onset schizophrenia. *Am J Psychiatry* 160:569–571, 2003.
107. Thomas MA, et al.: Preliminary study of frontal lobe 1 H MR spectroscopy in childhood-onset schizophrenia. *J Magn Reson Imaging* 8(4):841–846, 1998.
108. Bertolino A, et al.: Common pattern of cortical pathology in childhood-onset and adult-onset schizophrenia as identified by proton magnetic resonance spectroscopic imaging. *Am J Psychiatry* 155(10):1376–1383, 1998.
109. Renshaw PF, et al.: Temporal lobe proton magnetic resonance spectroscopy of patients with first-episode psychosis. *Am J Psychiatry* 152(3):444–446, 1995.
110. Jacobsen LK, et al.: Cerebral glucose metabolism in childhood onset schizophrenia. *Psychiatry Res* 75(3):131–144, 1997.
111. Jacobsen LK, Rapoport JL: Research update: Childhood-onset schizophrenia—Implications of clinical and neurobiological research. *J Child Psychol Psychiatry* 39(1):101–113, 1998.
112. Bassett AS: Chromosomal aberrations and schizophrenia. Autosomes. *Br J Psychiatry* 161:323–334, 1992.
113. Demirhan O, Tastemir D: Chromosome aberrations in a schizophrenia population. *Schizophr Res* 65(1):1–7, 2003.
114. St George-Hyslop PH: Genetic factors in the genesis of Alzheimer's disease. *Ann N Y Acad Sci* 924:1–7, 2000.
115. Bishop DT: BRCA1 and BRCA2 and breast cancer incidence: A review. *Ann Oncol* 10 Suppl 6:113–119, 1999.
116. Papolos DF, et al.: Bipolar spectrum disorders in patients diagnosed with velo-cardio-facial syndrome: Does a hemizygous deletion of chromosome 22q11 result in bipolar affective disorder? *Am J Psychiatry* 153(12):1541–1547, 1996.
117. Pulver AE, et al.: Psychotic illness in patients diagnosed with velo-cardio-facial syndrome and their relatives. *J Nerv Ment Dis* 182(8):476–478, 1994.
118. Murphy KC, Jones LA, Owen MJ: High rates of schizophrenia in adults with velo-cardio-facial syndrome. *Arch Gen Psychiatry* 56(10):940–945, 1999.
119. Rapoport JC, Addington AM, Frangou S: The neurodevelopmental model of schizophrenia: Update 2005. *Mol Psychiatry* 10(6):614, 2005.
120. Campbell M, et al.: The use of atypical antipsychotics in the management of schizophrenia. *Br J Clin Pharmacol* 47(1):13–22, 1999.
121. Pool D, et al.: A controlled evaluation of loxitane in seventy-five adolescent schizophrenic patients. *Curr Ther Res Clin Exp* 19(1):99–104, 1976.
122. Spencer EK, Campbell M: Children with schizophrenia: Diagnosis, phenomenology, and pharmacotherapy. *Schizophr Bull* 20(4):713–725, 1994.

123. Kumra S, et al.: Childhood-onset schizophrenia. A double-blind clozapine-haloperidol comparison. *Arch Gen Psychiatry* 53(12):1090–1097, 1996.
124. Davis JM, Chen N, Glick ID: A meta-analysis of the efficacy of second-generation antipsychotics. *Archives of General Psychiatry* 60(6):553–564, 2003.
125. Moncrieff J: Clozapine v. conventional antipsychotic drugs for treatment-resistant schizophrenia: A re-examination. [see comment]. *British Journal of Psychiatry* 183:161–166, 2003.
126. Sporn A, et al.: Clozapine-induced neutropenia in children: Management with lithium carbonate. *J Child Adolesc Psychopharmacol* 13(3):401–404, 2003.
127. Gogtay N, et al.: Clozapine-induced akathisia in children with schizophrenia. *J Child Adolesc Psychopharmacol* 12(4):347–349, 2002.
128. Ratzoni G, et al.: Weight gain associated with olanzapine and risperidone in adolescent patients: A comparative prospective study. *J Am Acad Child Adolesc Psychiatry* 41(3):337–343, 2002.
129. Sikich L, et al.: A pilot study of risperidone, olanzapine, and haloperidol in psychotic youth: A double-blind, randomized, 8-week trial. *Neuropsychopharmacology* 29(1):133–145, 2004.
130. Taylor DM, McAskill R: Atypical antipsychotics and weight gain—A systematic review. *Acta Psychiatr Scand* 101(6):416–432, 2000.
131. Basile VS, et al.: Genetic dissection of atypical antipsychotic-induced weight gain: Novel preliminary data on the pharmacogenetic puzzle. *J Clin Psychiatry* 62 Suppl 23:45–66, 2001.
132. Sporn AL, et al.: Hormonal correlates of clozapine-induced weight gain in psychotic children: An exploratory study. *J Am Acad Child Adolesc Psychiatry* 44(9):925–933, 2005.

5.4 ■ MOOD DISORDERS

CHAPTER 5.4.1 ■ DEPRESSIVE DISORDERS

DAVID A. BRENT AND V. ROBIN WEERSING

In this chapter, we describe the nosology and epidemiology of unipolar depressive disorders in youth, risk factors for depression onset and recurrence, and the evidence base for psychosocial and pharmacological treatments. We conclude with suggested areas for future inquiry.

CLINICAL PICTURE

Depressive disorders in childhood and adolescence are characterized by core persistent and pervasive sadness, anhedonia, boredom or irritability that is functionally impairing, and relatively unresponsive to usual experiences that might usually bring relief, such as pleasurable activities and interactions and attention from other people. The single most important distinction between depression as an illness and the "normal ups and downs" of childhood and adolescence is that depression is associated with functional impairment, mediated through the intensity, duration, and lack of responsiveness of depressed mood and associated symptoms.

Depressive disorders exist on a continuum, and are classified on the basis of severity, pervasiveness, and presence or absence of mania (1). At the mildest end of the spectrum are adjustment disorders with depressed mood, which are mild, self-limited, and occur in response to a clear stressor. Depression not otherwise specified (NOS), also referred to as "minor" or subsyndromal depression, is diagnosed in the presence of depressed mood, anhedonia, or irritability, and up to three symptoms of major depression (2). Dysthymic disorder is a chronic condition with fewer symptoms than major depression, but lasts a minimum of one year. Major depression is the most severe condition, with either sad or irritable mood, or anhedonia, along with at least five other symptoms, such as social withdrawal, worthlessness, guilt, suicidal thoughts or behavior, sleep increase or decrease, decreased motivation and/or concentration, and increased or decreased appetite. Minor depression and dysthymic disorder are functionally impairing and are often precursors to major depression (2, 3). Furthermore, dysthymia and major depression can coexist in a state referred to as "double depression," which is associated with a particularly chronic course (3). Rarely, young patients with major depression also have psychotic symptoms such as auditory hallucinations or delusions, usually with self-derogatory, paranoid, or depressive content.

Comorbidity is the rule rather than the exception in depressed children and adolescents, especially in clinical samples (4). Anxiety is frequently a precursor of mood disorder and may also occur simultaneously with depression. ADHD and depression are also often comorbid and the two disorders may be cotransmitted in families (5). Alcohol, drug, and tobacco abuse are associated with depression, and longitudinal studies suggest a bidirectional causality, with substance abuse both leading to, and occurring as a consequence of, depression (6–8). Conduct disorder is frequently comorbid with depression, particularly in prepubertal samples (9). Comorbidity with depression may arise because sharing of risk factors that are common to both conditions. For example, the comorbidity of mood disorders and behavioral disorders and substance abuse may be due to common factors, such as parental substance abuse and criminality, exposure to family violence, and family discord (10). Comorbidity may also arise because a condition is either a precursor or a consequence to depression, in the cases of anxiety and tobacco use, respectively.

DESCRIPTIVE EPIDEMIOLOGY

Estimates of Population Prevalence. The point prevalence of depressive disorders is 1–2% of prepubertal children and 3–8% of adolescents, with a lifetime prevalence by the end of adolescence of around 20% (11–13).

Gender Distribution and the Onset of Puberty. The 3:1 female predominance in mood disorders first emerges in adolescence (13). The higher female than male rate of depression after the onset of puberty may be due to: 1) increases in estradiol and testosterone associated with the onset of puberty in females, 2) higher rates of anxiety disorder and a tendency to rumination in females, which in turn predispose to depressive disorders, and 3) adolescent increases in interpersonal conflict that seem to be driven by genetic self-selection into risky environments and maladaptive responses to stress (14–16).

Age and Developmental Factors. Most typically, prepubertal depression has a set of risk factors and course similar to conduct disorder, with comorbid behavioral problems; family adversity such as family discord, parental criminality and parental substance abuse; and increased risk of antisocial disorder, but not depression in adult life (17–19). Less commonly, prepubertal depression is highly familial, with multigenerational loading for depression, with high rates of anxiety and bipolar disorder, and recurrences of mood disorder in adolescence and adulthood (18, 20). Adolescent-onset depression is more likely to result in recurrent episodes in adult life (18, 21). Recent work with structured diagnostic assessments has demonstrated the existence of depression even in preschool children, with the most prominent symptoms being sad or irritable mood, anhedonia, low energy, and change in level of activity (22).

Early-onset of puberty increases the risk of depression in girls (23). Other developmental factors that may contribute to an increased risk of depression after puberty include experimentation with tobacco, drugs and alcohol, decreased adult supervision and contact, and a greater physiological need for sleep, along with a tendency to actually obtain less sleep (6–8, 24, 25).

RISK FACTORS FOR DEPRESSION ONSET AND RECURRENCE

Genetic. Twin studies demonstrate that depressive symptoms have a greater concordance among monozygotic than among dizygotic twins, and a heritability of around 40–65%, with higher estimates of heritability in adolescent vs. prepubertal children (26–30). Both "bottom-up" and "top-down" family studies have shown a 2–4-fold increased risk of depression in first-degree relatives (31, 32). Twin studies suggest a greater genetic component in adolescent vs. pre-pubertal onset depression, supportive of the view that very early onset depression may often be a response to a chaotic environment (30).

There is evidence that liability to depression is cotransmitted along with anxiety symptoms, with a heritability of 61–65% (32–34). Genes that influence the risk of anxiety may in turn lead to a higher rate of postpubertal depression by increasing sensitivity to life events, and also by increasing the likelihood of *exposure* to depressogenic life events (35, 36). This formulation is consistent with the results of longitudinal studies (37, 38), as well as with evidence that stressful life events and genetic diatheses (e.g., shorter allelic form of the serotonin transporter) interact to result in early-onset depression (39).

Cognitive Factors. Depressed individuals have been shown to have a negative view of self, future, and the world. Nondepressed individuals with these biases are more likely than those without these biases to develop depressive symptomatology when confronted with stressful life events (40–42). Cognitive distortions are associated with depression in both prepubertal children and adolescents, but only in adolescents is there some evidence that the distortions persist after the episode resolves (43). Depressed youth also exhibit "performance-based" disruptions in cognitive processes, such as greater difficulty than controls in remembering fearful faces (44), difficulty in inhibiting negative affect in response to distressing stimuli (45), and more global and less specific recall in tests of categorical autobiographical memory (46).

Familial/Environmental Risk Factors. Twin studies show that the effect of shared environment is at least as potent as are heritable factors (30). Parental depression may exert its deleterious effect on child mood disorder not only through genetic mechanisms, but also via modeling of cognitive distortions, and through either passive and withdrawn or hostile interactions (47, 48). Family environmental risk factors for child depression, such as parental criminality, parental substance abuse, lack of family cohesion, and parent-child discord, may be most relevant in the absence of a family history of depression (49). However, in some studies, family discord and expressed emotion interact with a depressive diathesis to predict onset and recurrence (48, 50). Greater chronicity and severity of maternal depression has been related to greater liability for child cognitive distortions and parent–child conflict, both of which increase liability and persistence for child depressive symptoms (48, 51–53). Longitudinal studies show reciprocal interrelationships between maternal and child interpersonal difficulties, child behavior symptoms, cognitive distortions, and depressive outcome (40, 48, 54).

Neglect and child maltreatment increases the risk not only for depression, but also for substance abuse, disruptive disorder, posttraumatic stress disorder, and suicide attempt (55–58) The deleterious effects are strongest for more severe and chronic abuse, such as sexual abuse resulting in intercourse (55, 56). Abuse may be associated with an earlier age of onset of depression (59). The effects of abuse may be long lasting, resulting in a lower rate of response to treatment and a higher risk for recurrent depression (60). However, it is difficult to isolate the effects of abuse from the other interrelated adverse aspects of parental functioning and home environment such as parental mood disorder, substance abuse, and criminality; lower education and income; marital discord; and association with deviant peers (56). The relationship between depression and abuse is much stronger in the presence of other family-genetic risk factors such as a family history of depression or the short form of the serotonin transporter gene (39, 61, 62).

Bereavement due to the loss of a sibling, parent, or close friend is associated with an increased risk for depression, especially if there is a positive family history for mood disorder (63–65).

Connection to family and to school, parental behavioral and academic expectations, and nondeviant peer group are all protective against several key health risk behaviors, including depression and suicidality (66).

Neuroendocrine. Provocative challenges that are putative measures of noradrenergic and serotonergic neurotransmission find differences in depressed children, both during episode and recovery, and in nondepressed children at high risk for depressive disorder (67–70). This pattern of finding suggests that these changes may be trait markers for early-onset depression. However, similar neuroendocrine responses to provocative serotonergic challenge may be found in those with adverse or abusive home environments, and with high levels of aggression (61, 71).

Sleep. Subjective sleep complaints are a very prominent component of early-onset depression, although subjective complaints and objective observations of sleep in a sleep laboratory are not closely correlated (72). Increased cortisol secretion at the time of sleep onset may be related to adolescent depression (73). Decreased REM latency and increased latency of sleep onset were found more often in adolescents compared to prepubertal depressed children, and may be associated with greater severity, onset, and recurrence, although these findings may emerge only after a strict sleep/wake schedule has been imposed (74–79). Decreased sleep efficiency and delayed sleep onset have been reported to be associated with depressive episode persistence and recurrence (78–80).

Neuroimaging Studies. Structural imaging studies of adult subjects with early-onset, familial depression as well as in adolescents with depression have found reduced volume of the left subgenual prefrontal cortex (81–83). Preliminary studies of female adolescent depressed twins suggest that this structural difference is genetically transmitted and may partially mediate the heritability of depression (26). Steingard et al. (84) reported decreased prefrontal cortex and increased third and fourth ventricular volume in depressed adolescents, although these findings may be a marker for the effects of chronicity. MacMillan (85) reported an increased pituitary and amygdala: hippocampal ratio size in depressed subjects compared to nondepressed controls, with amygdala: hippocampal ratio size correlated with the severity of anxiety symptoms. In line with these findings, Thomas and colleagues found, in response to fearful faces, increased amygdala activation in anxious children, and decreased amygdala activation in depressed children (86).

COURSE AND OUTCOME

Episode Length and Recovery. The duration for depressive episodes ranges between 3 and 6 months for community samples, and between 5 and 8 months for referred samples (3, 87). Factors associated with a longer episode duration include comorbid dysthymic disorder, comorbidity with anxiety disorder or substance abuse, greater initial severity of the depressive condition, current or past suicidal ideation or behavior, chronicity and number of episodes of parental depression, and family discord (51, 88–90). In both clinical and community samples, around 20% of adolescents have a persistent depression of 2 or more years' duration (11, 88).

Risk for Recurrence. In one meticulously conducted study of the course of depressive disorder in children age 8 to 13 years old, the risk of recurrence was 40% in 2 years, and 72% in 5 years (89, 91). Other longitudinal studies have shown that the risk for recurrent depression in adolescent depression followed forward is extremely high, with the rate of relapse or recurrence ranging between 30–70% in 1–2 years of follow-up (3, 11, 88, 92, 93). Risk factors for recurrence include early onset of mood disorder in parent, lack of complete recovery, defined as either subsyndromal depression or return to a dysthymic baseline, preexisting social dysfunction, history of sexual abuse, and family discord (3, 11, 50, 60, 88, 90, 94).

Risk for Bipolar Disorder. The risk of bipolar disorder in early-onset depression is estimated to be around 10-20%, and is higher in patients who present with hypomania in response to antidepressant medication, psychotic features, hypersomnia (in some studies), and a family history of bipolar disorder (95, 96). Children and younger adolescents exposed to antidepressants may be at particularly high risk for manic switch (97).

Other Sequelae. Depressed youth are at increased risk for conduct disorder, personality disorders, alcohol, tobacco, and drug abuse, and suicidal behavior, as well as obesity, social adaptation, such as interpersonal problems, unfulfilling social relationships, and educational and occupational underachievement (6–8, 10, 11, 98, 99). These "sequelae" may be attributable to common factors that also contribute to risk for depression, such as parental criminality, parental substance abuse, physical or sexual abuse, and family discord (10). Alternatively, these negative sequelae may be residua of incomplete depressive symptom resolution (100).

CLINICAL MANAGEMENT

There are currently three treatments for adolescent depression with varying levels of empirical support, namely, antidepressant treatment, cognitive behavior therapy (CBT), and interpersonal therapy (IPT) (101). There has been considerably less research on treatment of prepubertal children with depression, although there is some support for the efficacy of antidepressants. Each of these three approaches will be discussed, followed by a recommendation for current "best practice" treatment of youth depression (102, 103).

Antidepressant Medication

Evidence of Efficacy. Both the single largest placebo-controlled comparison study of tricyclic antidepressants (TCAs) and placebo, and a subsequent metaanalysis showed no difference between drug and placebo (104, 105), while several studies have demonstrated efficacy with selective serotonin reuptake inhibitors (SSRI) antidepressants, especially using fluoxetine (106). This may be reflective of an overall developmental difference insofar as adolescents and younger adults may respond better to serotonergic agents, whereas older adults respond equally as well to serotonergic and to noradrenergic agents (107).

Fluoxetine is the best-studied antidepressant with the strongest efficacy data, and consequently is the only antidepressant to receive FDA and MHRA approval for use for the treatment of depression in children and adolescents (108–110). In these three studies of fluoxetine, a higher proportion of those treated with fluoxetine were "much or very much improved" compared to those treated with placebo (52–61% vs. 33–37%), for a median number needed to treat (NNT) of five. In the TADS study, fluoxetine was more efficacious than both placebo and cognitive behavior therapy (proportion "significantly" improved, 61% vs. 43% vs. 35%, respectively) (110). However, combined treatment resulted in the highest rate of symptomatic remission (37% vs. 20% on fluoxetine alone) (111).

A metaanalysis of all available clinical trials, both published and unpublished, shows that SSRIs are superior to placebo, with the average response rate for antidepressant vs. placebo of 60% vs. 49%, for an overall NNT of 9 (95% confidence interval, 7 to 14) (112) The relatively low effect size of SSRIs vs. placebo for child and adolescent depression is due to the high placebo response rate. The drug-placebo difference was inversely proportional to the number of study sites involved in the trial, suggesting that some studies with large numbers of sites may have been less selective in recruitment (112). Other explanations for the relative modest effects of antidepressants include use of inadequate dosage, duration of treatment too short to achieve the full effect, and aggregation of results of children and adolescents, when, in some studies there were significant effects for adolescents, but not for children.

Besides fluoxetine, other drugs for which there are published studies that have demonstrated efficacy are citalopram, paroxetine, and sertraline (105, 113, 114), although the effect sizes were relatively small and there are other negative studies for these agents that have not yet been published. A review of the published and unpublished studies indicates that, for paroxetine, and for venlafaxine, the response to medication was superior to placebo for adolescents, but not for children. In some studies, such as those for venlafaxine, the doses used appeared to be substantially below those recommended for clinical practice.

Adverse Events in Antidepressant Treatment. The FDA conducted a metaanalysis that found a higher rate of suicide-related, spontaneously reported adverse events on drug than on placebo (4% vs. 2%) (115). There were relatively few suicide attempts, no completions, and most suicidal events occurred early in treatment. The increased risk for suicidality was found regardless of indication, in subjects with depression, OCD, and anxiety. A more recent metaanalysis that included additional studies not included in the FDA and using random rather than fixed effects models reported rates of suicidal adverse events for drug and placebo of 2.5% vs. 1.7%, respectively, for a risk difference of 0.8%, and a number needed to harm (NNH) of 125 (95% confidence interval 56 to ∞). Thus, the number of those who benefit from SSRIs (NNT = 9) to those who become suicidal (NNH = 125) is around 14 times higher, which seems to be an acceptable risk benefit ratio (112).

In addition to the concern over suicide and self-injurious behavior, antidepressants are associated with increased incidence of sleep disruption, vivid dreams, nausea and gastrointestinal distress, increase in agitation, akathisia, anxiety, headache, serotonin syndrome (particularly in combination with other serotonergic agents) and bruising (due to a prolongation of clotting time) (116). The latter side effect is usually not clinically significant, but can become so in patients with intrinsic coagulation disorders or who are undergoing surgery. One pharmaco-epidemiological study found that the risk of SSRI-treatment-associated mania was greatest in patients under the age of 14 (97).

Predictors of Antidepressant Response. One report has examined predictors of antidepressant response, finding that poorer outcome was predicted by family discord, comorbidity, and greater severity and impairment at intake (92). One naturalistic study suggests that comorbid ADHD predicted poor outcome (117). In data from the TADS study that have been reported but not published, predictors of poor outcome, regardless of treatment assignment were: age greater than 16, greater functional impairment, high levels of hopelessness, anxiety, melancholic features, and suicidal ideation. Also, a higher dose may predict better outcome in those patients who fail to respond to a lower dose of SSRI (118). There is evidence that adolescents metabolize sertraline, citalopram, and paroxetine (but not fluvoxamine) faster than do adults (119–122), so that higher doses than typically recommended for adults may need to be utilized.

Mechanisms of Action. Two small studies found a correlation between percent reuptake of serotonin in platelet receptors and clinical response (123–125). One study found an association between upregulation of glucocorticoid type II receptors and response to sertraline (125). Several studies found that the short variant of the serotonin transporter (SLC6A4) is associated with a poorer response to SSRIs in adults (126), and this was also found in a mixed population of children and adolescents with anxiety and depression treated with citalopram (127).

Role in Continuation, Maintenance, and Prevention. In patients who have been successfully treated with fluoxetine for the acute phase, continuation treatment with fluoxetine resulted in a much lower rate of relapse than continuation with placebo (128). Since SSRI treatment is much more efficacious for anxiety than for depression (NNT of 3 for anxiety vs. 9 for depression) (112), and since anxiety is often a precursor for depression, the successful treatment of anxiety may reduce the risk for subsequent depression (129, 130).

Cognitive Behavior Therapy

Theory and Techniques. Cognitive behavior therapy (CBT) is predicated on the observation that depressed individuals show "distortions" in their thinking and information processing, tending to emphasize the negative aspects of a situation and to underemphasize the positive (131). These negative thoughts are presumed to play a causal role in the genesis of depressive episodes during times of stress and the maintenance of negative mood states (40–42).

CBT treatments for depression focus on interrupting this cycle of negative thinking, mood, and maladaptive action, through a variety of cognitive techniques and behavioral skill-building exercises. Central to the model is *cognitive restructuring*—an effort to make the patient aware of negative distortions and to teach the individual how to counteract them, relieving depression as a result. Also key to the application of CBT is the use of *behavioral activation* techniques, such as encouraging patients to normalize their routine and engage in rewarding activities, even if they do not feel like it at the time. This technique is based on the observation that depressed individuals tend to withdraw from activities that are potentially reinforcing.

While these two techniques appear to be core to the theory and practice of CBT, the content of CBT treatment manuals, tested in clinical trials, varies greatly in the emphasis on each of these techniques and the inclusion of other, adjunctive skill building elements (e.g., problem solving, relaxation, assertiveness training). In addition, CBT approaches are heterogeneous with regard to the overall number of sessions, the number of sessions devoted to each CBT technique, degree of structure, and therapy format (group or individual), differences that make it difficult to interpret the varying effects of CBT reported across clinical trials.

Efficacy of CBT. Many of the studies using CBT for depression involved symptomatic volunteers (132). In order to allow comparability to the above-noted medication trials, we focus our review on studies enrolling samples that meet formal diagnostic criteria for a depressive disorder. Notably, all of these investigations are with adolescents, and there is yet to be a published CBT efficacy trial in a diagnosed sample composed primarily of prepubertal youth.

The most well studied intervention for depressed adolescents is the CBT-based Coping with Depression for Adolescents (CWD-A) course. This is a group-administered, structured program that includes psychoeducation, pleasant activity scheduling, social skills training, problemsolving, and cognitive restructuring. In two of the first studies of CWD-A, a multisession parent curriculum was tested in addition to CWD-A, which in turn was compared to wait-list control (133, 134). In both of these investigations, CWD-A with and without the parent intervention were superior to wait list at the end of treatment, with regard to diagnosed depression and dimensional measures of depression. However, the addition of the parent group had no additive effect to the group CBT alone. In the second study, one to two booster sessions were provided, which did not reduce the rate of depressive recurrence, but did seem to be helpful to those who had not yet recovered from their depressive episode (134).

Subsequently, the program has been employed with depressed, conduct-disordered youth and adapted for depressed incarcerated youth (135, 136). The success rate was more modest for these more clinically complex youth, but the effect sizes for reduction in rates and severity of depression between the experimental treatment and wait-list control are comparable to the initial studies.

Although the above-noted studies of CWD-A involved diagnosed subjects, participants were not patients, but recruited volunteers. To date, there have been five studies to test the efficacy of CBT in depressed adolescents who are presenting for treatment through standard clinical referral routes. Two of these investigations used similar (but not identical) brief CBT treatment protocols (137, 138). Vostanis et al. (137) compared CBT to supportive treatment and found no difference between treatment groups (86% vs. 75% no longer depressed). Treatment was very brief (around six sessions) and offered over an extended time frame (1 to 5 months). In contrast, Wood et al. (138), who delivered five to eight sessions of CBT over 12 weeks, found that brief CBT was superior to relaxation therapy in depressed adolescents; improvements were also noted in functional impairment, anxiety, and dimensional measures of depression. Upon followup, there was a tendency for those treated with CBT to relapse so that differences were not statistically significant.

Utilizing a treatment closely following Beck's approach (131), Brent et al. (139) compared 12–16 sessions of CBT to family therapy and to supportive treatment, all delivered by therapists who were trained in and adherents of their treatment model. At posttreatment, CBT produced outcomes superior to the alternate intervention, with regard to decline in depressive symptoms, achievement of remission, and speed of response. Upon 2-year followup, there were no statistically significant differences between the three randomized groups, although the results favored CBT (94%) over family therapy (77%) and supportive therapy (74%) (88, 140).

The final CBT efficacy trial in a diagnosed sample is the *Treatment of Adolescents with Depression Study (TADS)* (110). TADS is the only published study to compare CBT, fluoxetine, their combination, and placebo. In this large, well powered investigation, CBT (43% significantly improved) was not superior to placebo (35%), whereas both combination (71%) including fluoxetine, and fluoxetine alone (61%), were markedly superior to both CBT and to placebo. The combination treatment (CBT + fluoxetine) showed a faster recovery than any of the other treatments, although fluoxetine alone had as favorable outcomes with respect to the Clinical Global Impression Improvement (CGI-I) and baseline-adjusted endpoints and in more severely depressed patients. Combined treatment was superior to fluoxetine alone with regard to remission (37 vs. 20%).

Given the generally positive effects of CBT in other investigations, why did CBT fail to outperform placebo in TADS? The authors posit that subjects were more severely ill and more comorbid than in other studies, but other studies found stronger effects with cases of comparable severity and comorbidity, with comorbid anxiety actually being a positive prognosticator (141, 142). Another possible explanation for the relatively weak performance of CBT in this study could be the type of treatment delivered. The TADS treatment package, which itself had never been extensively tested, attempted to deliver, in a relatively brief treatment, a large number of accepted approaches: problemsolving, behavior activation, cognitive restructuring, emotion regulation, relaxation training, and parent–child sessions, whereas some of the more successful interventions have mainly focused on cognitive restructuring or on behavior activation and problemsolving. It is possible that in the TADS manual's attempt to be inclusive of a variety of successful techniques, subjects never received an adequate "dose" of any one of these specific CBT techniques (143).

Combined CBT and Medication. In addition to the TADS study, there have been two other investigations of the impact on combined CBT and antidepressant management compared to antidepressant alone, which in aggregate do not make a strong case for the use of combined treatment, counterintuitive as this seems. Clarke and colleagues (144) studied the addition of the CWD-A treatment to antidepressant management in primary care. This combined treatment resulted in some modest improvement in quality of life, but improvement in depressive symptoms never reached statistical significance; moreover, patients in the combined treatment were more likely to stop their antidepressants. A study conducted in the U.K. compared combination treatment, using the CBT model that had been used successfully by Wood et al. (138) to fluoxetine alone, for moderate to severely ill depressed adolescents (145). CBT did not add to medication alone with regard to global functioning, quality of life, or depressive symptomatology.

Effectiveness. Three published investigations have produced findings relevant to the effectiveness of CBT in practice. One study compared quality improvement to usual care for adolescent depression managed in primary care (146). Subjects were randomized to either clinical monitoring and usual care or clinical monitoring plus on-site specialty mental health care, with the latter consisting of the patient's choice of CBT, medication, or both. The quality improvement (QI) arm, which most often consisted of CBT, was superior to treatment as usual in increasing teens' access to depression care (number of sessions) and on improving depression symptoms and quality of life, similar to parallel studies in adults (147). As noted above, Clarke and colleagues found in their primary care investigation that adding CBT to high-quality medication management provided only modest benefits on measures of symptoms and functioning (144). However, these very small improvements occurred as youths significantly reduced their use of psychotropic medication in the CBT + SSRI arm—an unintended consequence of the CBT intervention. As a final piece of evidence, relevant to effectiveness, a benchmarking study compared CBT delivered in a research study to CBT delivered in a tertiary care clinic with an unselected, clinically complicated sample of depressed adolescents (148). Results of clinic-based CBT were quite similar to the published effects of CBT in the Pittsburgh Study, once symptom trajectories in the research subjects were adjusted for the difference in the proportion of subjects who came by advertisement, as the latter tended to respond more favorably to treatment (141, 148).

Predictors of Outcome. Greater intake severity, older age of onset, low involvement in pleasurable activities, greater hopelessness and other cognitive distortions, history of sexual abuse, and parental depression were found to be predictive of poor response in CBT clinical trials (11, 60, 141, 142, 149, 150). Parental depressive symptoms moderated treatment response to CBT insofar as in the absence of maternal depression CBT was superior to alternative treatments, whereas in its presence, CBT was no better than the alternatives (11, 141). Family discord, and substance abuse, predicted a slower response to treatment, overall (88, 142). In contrast, referral by advertisement as compared to clinical referral predicted a good response in all conditions, and comorbid anxiety disorder predicted a particularly positive response to CBT (141, 142). In some studies, changes in cognitive distortions or improvements in involvement in pleasurable activities are associated with improvement (151–153).

Prevention of Onset, Relapse, or Recurrence. An adaptation of the CWD-A program reduced the risk of onset of major depression in two groups of at-risk adolescents, those with subsyndromal depression (posttreatment rates of major depression 15% in CBT vs. 26% control) (154) and in at-risk adolescent offspring of depressed parents (9% CBT versus 28% control) (150). A metaanalysis of CBT prevention packages has found that interventions that focus on youth with subsyndromal symptoms show more positive effects than universal programs (155), in part because at-risk youth continue to become more symptomatic over time.

With regard to the prevention of relapse, CBT does not appear to produce significantly greater benefit than other interventions at intermediate or long-term followup (88, 138). While the addition of up to six individual CBT monthly booster sessions reduced the rate of relapse from 50% to 20%, the addition of one or two group or individual booster sessions did not, suggesting a dose effect (133, 156).

INTERPERSONAL THERAPY (IPT)

Theory and Techniques. IPT for adolescents (IPT-A) is an adaptation of IPT, a well established, efficacious treatment for adult unipolar depression (157, 158). IPT-A is discussed in detail in Chapter 6.2.3. Briefly, in this treatment depression is conceptualized as occurring within an interpersonal matrix and targets resolution of interpersonal stress that seems to be associated with the adolescent's depression. IPT-A begins by taking an interpersonal inventory of important relationships in order to determine appropriate treatment targets. The types of problems typically targeted by IPT-A are loss, role disputes, role transitions, interpersonal skills deficits, or adjustment to a single-parent family. The goal of treatment is to replace conflictual, unfulfilling relationships with meaningful, lower conflict relationships.

IPT formulation and techniques are not fundamentally incompatible with the cognitive view of depression. In fact, there are several similarities, including encouragement of the individual to resume normal activities, problemsolving, and skill-building. However, IPT tends to look from the outside in, whereas CBT tends to look at inner experience and how it relates to the interpersonal. IPT-A is a very developmentally appropriate treatment, since adolescence is a time of role changes, conflicts with parents, and investing more emotional capital in peer relationships.

Evidence of IPT Efficacy. Mufson et al. (158) conducted the first efficacy trial of IPT-A in a patient population of depressed adolescents. Forty-eight adolescents were randomized to either IPT-A or monthly clinical management. A much higher proportion of adolescents met recovery criteria (Hamilton Depression Scale-Depression ≤ 6) in the IPT-A group (75% vs. 46%). There was a much higher attrition rate in the clinical monitoring group. Analyses of dimensional measures of depressive symptomatology, functional status, and social adaptiveness also favored IPT-A.

In an independent investigation, Rossello and Bernal (159) compared the efficacy of IPT, "culturally adapted" CBT, and a wait-list control condition in a sample of depressed Puerto Rican adolescents. Attrition was a significant problem, as only 68% and 52% of IPT and CBT-treated subjects completed the 12-session intervention. Using a clinical cutoff on the CDI in completer analyses, 59% of those in the CBT condition, and 82% of those treated with IPT achieved a clinically significant improvement by posttreatment. Thus, on some measures of depression and functional status, IPT was superior to CBT.

Effectiveness. Mufson et al. (160) tested IPT-A vs. usual care in school-based mental health clinics. School social workers delivered both interventions, but had a brief training in IPT-A and weekly supervision. IPT-A was superior to usual care on dimensional measures of depression, global function, social adjustment, and global clinical status (50% vs. 33% symptomatically improved). This strongly supports the transportability of IPT-A into community sites.

Predictors of Response and Adverse Events. Relatively little information is available, but Mufson et al. (158) found that IPT-A was differentiated from clinical monitoring only in those subjects who had moderate or severe depression. Improvements in social functioning and problemsolving were associated with IPT-A treatment (158, 160). Little information is available, but rate of suicidal events was similar in one trial in IPT-A vs. clinical management (158).

Prevention of Onset, Relapse, or Recurrence. Thus far, there have been no prevention or continuation studies conducted, but one open study showed a high rate of sustained recovery one year after receipt of IPT-A (161).

Other Available Interventions

Although one initial study did not show efficacy of family therapy (139), the involvement of family factors in the pathogenesis and recurrence of early-onset depression suggests that some targeted family interventions aimed at reducing criticism, facilitating treatment of parental depression, and increasing protective factors such as support and time spent together may prove to be efficacious. One small randomized treatment study suggested that a family intervention that focused on interpersonal attachment, when compared to a minimal contact wait-list control, resulted in reductions in both depression and anxiety, with sustained improvement on 6-month followup (162).

With regard to somatic treatments, light therapy has been shown to be beneficial for pediatric season affective disorder (163). Although electroconvulsive therapy (ECT) has not been rigorously studied in adolescent depression, there is general clinical consensus that it has a role in the management of early-onset depression that is refractory to pharmacological and psychosocial management, particularly for adolescents without significant personality disorder traits (164).

Recommendations for Current Best Practice Treatment

Since there is a relatively high response rate to placebo or brief supportive treatment and education in many of the published treatment studies, the first approach for mild depression should be family education, supportive counseling, case management, and problemsolving (112, 145, 165). For more persistent or severe depression, one of the three empirically validated treatments, SSRI medication, CBT, or IPT, is indicated. Initial treatment with any of the three treatments for moderate depression is reasonable, with the choice informed primarily by patient preference and the availability of local expertise. Given current data, it seems advisable to chose a defined time point, such as 6–8 weeks, to assess treatment response to treatment, and in the case of nonresponse, after which to consider combination of psychotherapy and medication, a switch in medication, or an augmentation strategy. In many communities, there are no clinicians trained in CBT or IPT-A, and the evidence suggests that more generic psychotherapies practiced in the community may not be helpful in the treatment of youth depression (138, 139, 166). In the absence of available specialized psychotherapy, or in the face of a patient's disinclination to engage in psychotherapy, use of an antidepressant as a first-line intervention is indicated. Some evidence suggests that for more severely depressed adolescents, particularly those with difficulties with motivation, concentration, sleep, and appetite, medication should be a first-line treatment. In adults, combination of psychotherapy and medication is superior to either monotherapy in chronic and severe depression, although the support for the use of combined treatment in younger populations is more modest (110, 144, 145, 167, 168). Relative contraindications for use of antidepressant medication are a history of mania or hypomania, for whom mood stabilization should be undertaken prior to the use of antidepressants, and for those with a strong family history of bipolar disorder, for whom it may be safer to begin with psychotherapy for the same reasons.

Given that the most evidence for efficacy exists for fluoxetine, this should be the first-line medication. For those who have failed to respond to fluoxetine, cannot tolerate it, or for some reason do not wish to take it, use of one of the other SSRIs for which there is some evidence of efficacy is warranted. Current clinical recommendations are to begin with half the usual initial target dose (e.g., 10 mg fluoxetine) for 1 week, to determine if the patient can tolerate the medication, and then increase to 20 mg for the next 3 weeks. If the patient is still depressed, then one can continue to increase the dosage around every 4 weeks (because it takes around that amount of time to tell if an increase is going to be helpful). Most patients who respond to fluoxetine achieve symptomatic relief at 20–80 mg of fluoxetine.

If a patient fails to respond to a fluoxetine at an adequate dose and duration (around 40–80 mg), then it is reasonable to switch to another SSRI. However, it is important to rule out reasons for continued depression such as rapid drug metabolism, noncompliance, severe family conflict, parental depression, covert substance abuse, or the influence of other comorbid conditions, such as obsessive-compulsive disorder, ADHD or anxiety, an undiagnosed mixed state, psychosis, or medical illness, such as hypothyroidism. There are no empirical studies in adolescents to guide clinicians for patients who have failed to respond to an SSRI, although clinical guidelines based upon expert consensus exist (101, 169). However, based on clinical consensus and some studies in adults, if one has obtained a partial response, it is reasonable to augment with lithium, another antidepressant, or psychotherapy. If one has obtained no response, a reasonable second step is to switch to a second SSRI, or to add psychotherapy. If after treatment with a second SSRI there is still complete nonresponse, most clinicians recommend using a different class of medication, such as venlafaxine, bupropion, or lamotrigine.

FUTURE CHALLENGES

Depression in childhood and adolescence is a complex and debilitating disease that frequently has a lifelong, chronic course. In this concluding section, we focus on the unknowns of youth depression and suggest several key areas for future investigation.

1. *A better understanding of the neurobiology of depression.* Neuroimaging shows promise at being able to delineate brain regions and circuitry most closely implicated in depressive onset and recovery, thereby helping to classify both the clinical phenotype and potential targets for prevention and treatment.
2. *Genetic, developmental, and environmental determinants of unipolar depression.* Genetic studies of early-onset depression and related endophenotypes such as anxiety or neuroticism may help to identify genetic factors in depressive onset and course, which in turn may aid in identification of individuals at risk and development of more precise targets of treatment. Studies that help to clarify how development and environmental protective and risk factors affect genetic expression are necessary complements to genetic studies.
3. *Mechanisms of action of current treatment.* We also have very little information on how current empirically validated treatments actually work. A better understanding of mechanisms can lead to improvement in treatment outcome and better matching of patients to treatment. On the psychosocial side, there is only weak evidence for cognitive mediation of CBT effects and no investigations of mechanisms of action in interpersonal therapy. For the antidepressants, remarkably, no studies have examined the relationship between drug level and metabolites and treatment outcome in any pediatric pharmacological clinical trial, and there is only preliminary work on potential biomarkers that may mediate drug response (123–125). Affective neuroscience may provide other markers of response or imminent relapse, such as amygdala activation in response to fear-inducing stimuli, task interference to sad stimuli, or cortical and subcortical activation to stimuli associated with pleasurable experiences. These potential markers of pathogenic processes may be used to track response, and even to guide the content and focus of psychotherapy.
4. *Incomplete recovery, adverse events, and boosting treatment response and functional outcome.* Despite some success in treating depression in youth, approximately 40% of youth remain ill at the end of clinical trials and a much higher proportion have achieved incomplete recovery within the "successful" portion of the sample. Since the most common sequela of incomplete recovery is sustained impairment followed by another episode (11, 170), the identification of sequences and combinations of treatment approaches that lead to complete symptomatic remission is important. There are also many related adverse outcomes associated with depression, varying from interpersonal difficulties, educational underachievement, to substance abuse, obesity and suicide. There appear to be some common family and social factors that protect against most of these outcomes. Can a parsimonious treatment package be developed to improve overall functional outcome for depressed youth that increases these protective factors?
   The most serious correlate of depressive disorder is suicidal ideation and behavior, which in depressed patients is associated with greater severity, chronicity, and comorbidity (11, 171, 172). It is an open question as to whether treatment of depression is sufficient to prevent suicidality or whether additional types of interventions are required, since reductions in depression and in suicidality do not always occur together (173–176). However, patients with serious suicidality are often excluded from clinical trials, and suicidal outcomes are not often reported. Our ability to predict and influence suicidality is particularly pressing, given current concerns about suicidal adverse events with SSRI treatment. It is important to better understand the clinical, pharmacokinetic, pharmacogenetic, and neurocognitive predictors of suicidal adverse events in youth treated with SSRIs.
5. *Prevention, early intervention, and public health.* Two extreme views with regard to depression were well articulated by Harrington and Clarke (177). One focuses the bulk of resources on a relatively small number of youths with moderate to severe disease, and a second emphasizes the provision of preventive interventions to those who are at risk or are mildly depressed. From a public health point of view, the impairment burden on the population is mostly from "subsyndromal depression," so that a small reduction in depressive symptoms in a large number of people may indeed benefit more people. Clarke et al. (150, 154) has shown that a group CBT (CWD-A) can reduce the risk of major depression in adolescents at increased risk through subsyndromal depression and/or parental depression. Through linkages between adult and child services, one could potentially offer such treatments, but, based on research experience, many will decline to participate. Harrington and Clarke (177) argue that a more acceptable approach is one that enhances protective factors like problemsolving, interpersonal skills, family connection, and school connection. Can promising, cost-effective interventions to prevent the onset of depression be identified, such as by focusing on youth with anxiety disorder, or those with a parental or prior history of depression?
   Another key factor in reducing the public health burden of depression likely will be the efficient dissemination of our best practice models to the youth health and education systems. As discussed in the section on clinical management, there are still very few data on the effectiveness of SSRIs, CBT, and IPT when delivered in actual practice settings. The data that are available on CBT and IPT are promising, suggesting that bringing these research-based psychosocial interventions to the community may substantially improve on current models of depression care. Similar data are not available for the SSRIs, despite the fact that SSRI prescriptions are dramatically more prevalent and available in community settings than either of

the empirically based psychosocial interventions. In the adult literature, there is a growing evidence base on the efficacy and cost effectiveness of relatively brief psychosocial, antidepressant, and combined treatments for mild to moderate depression, delivered in public health contexts such as primary care and which may serve as models for future investigations in younger populations (178).

References

1. *Diagnostic and Statistical Manual of Mental Disorders (DSM-IV-TR)*, 4th ed. Washington, DC, American Psychiatric Association, 2000.
2. Fergusson DM, Horwood LJ, Ridder EM, Beautrais AL: Subthreshold depression in adolescence and mental health outcomes in adulthood. *Arch Gen Psychiatry* 62:66–72, 2005.
3. Kovacs M: Presentation and course of major depressive disorder during childhood and later years of the life span. *J Am Acad Child Adolesc Psychiatry* 35:705–715, 1996.
4. Angold A, Costello EJ, Erkanli A: Comorbidity. *J Child Psychol Psychiatry* 40:57–87, 1999.
5. Biederman J, Faraone SV, Keenan K, Benjamin J, Krifcher B, Moore C et al.: Further evidence for family-genetic risk factors in attention deficit hyperactivity disorder: Patterns of comorbidity in probands and relatives in psychiatrically and pediatrically referred samples. *Arch Gen Psychiatry* 49:728–738, 1992.
6. Rohde P, Lewinsohn PM, Brown RA, Gau JM, Kahler CW: Psychiatric disorders, familial factors and cigarette smoking: I. Associations with smoking initiation. *Nicotine Tobacco Research* 5:85–98, 2003.
7. Rohde P, Kahler CW, Lewinsohn PM, Brown RA: Psychiatric disorders, familial factors, and cigarette smoking: II. Associations with progression to daily smoking. *Nicotine Tobacco Research* 6:119–132, 2004.
8. Rohde P, Kahler CW, Lewinsohn PM, Brown RA: Psychiatric disorders, familial factors, and cigarette smoking: III. Associations with cessation by young adulthood among daily smokers. *Nicotine Tobacco Research* 6:509–522, 2004.
9. Harrington R, Rutter M, Fombonne E: Developmental pathways in depression: Multiple meanings, antecedents, and endpoints. *Development and Psychopathology* 8:601–616, 1996.
10. Fergusson DM, Woodward LJ: Mental health, educational, and social role outcomes of adolescents with depression. *Arch Gen Psychiatry* 59:225–231, 2002.
11. Lewinsohn PM, Rohde P, Seeley JR: Major depressive disorder in older adolescents: Prevalence, risk factors, and clinical implications. *Clinical Psychology Review* 18:765–794, 1998.
12. Costello EJ, Mustillo S, Erkanli A, Keeler G, Angold A: Prevalence and development of psychiatric disorders in childhood and adolescence. *Arch Gen Psychiatry* 60:837–844, 2003.
13. Reinherz HZ, Giaconia RM, Pakiz B, Silverman AB, Frost AK, Lefkowitz ES: Psychosocial risks for major depression in late adolescence: A longitudinal community study. *J Am Acad Child Psychiatry* 32:1155–1163, 1993.
14. Angold A, Costello EJ, Erkanli A, Worthman CM: Pubertal changes in hormone levels and depression in girls. *Psychol Med* 29:1043–1053, 1999.
15. Rudolph KD, Hammen C: Age and stress determinants of stress exposure, generation, and reactions in youngsters: A transactional perspective. *Child Development* 70:660–677, 1999.
16. Nolen-Hoeksema S, Larson J, Grayson C: Explaining the gender difference in depressive symptoms. *J Pers Soc Psychol* 77:1061–1072, 1999.
17. Harrington R, Fudge H, Rutter M, Pickles A, Hill J: Adult outcomes of childhood and adolescent depression I. Psychiatric status. *Arch Gen Psychiatry* 47:465–473, 1990.
18. Harrington R, Rutter M, Weissman M, Fudge H, Groothues C, Bredenkamp D et al.: Psychiatric disorders in the relatives of depressed probands I. Comparison of prepubertal, adolescent and early adult onset cases. *J Affect Disord* 42:9–22, 1997.
19. Weissman MM, Wolk S, Wickramaratne P, Goldstein RB, Adams P, Greenwald S et al.: Children with prepubertal onset major depressive disorder and anxiety grown up. *Arch Gen Psychiatry* 56:794–801, 1999.
20. Wickramaratne P, Greenwald S, Weissman MM: Psychiatric disorders in the relatives of probands with prepubertal-onset or adolescent-onset major depression. *J Am Acad Child Adolesc Psychiatry* 39:1396–1405, 2000.
21. Weissman MM, Wolk S, Goldstein RB, Moreau D, Adams P, Greenwald S et al.: Depressed adolescents grown up. *J Am Med Assoc* 281:1707–1713, 1999.
22. Luby JL, Mrakotsky C, Heffelfinger A, Brown K, Hessler M, Spitznagel E: Modification of DSM-IV criteria for depressed preschool children. *Am J Psychiatry* 160:1169–1172, 2003.
23. Graber JA, Seeley JR, Brooks-Gunn J, Lewinsohn PM: Is pubertal timing associated with psychopathology in young adulthood? *J Am Acad Child Adolesc Psychiatry* 43:718–726, 2004.
24. Dahl RE, Spear L: Adolescent brain development: A period of vulnerabilities and opportunities. *New York Academy of Sciences* 1021:1–22, 2004.
25. Wolfson A, Carskadon MA: Sleep schedules and daytime functioning in adolescents. *Child Development* 69:875–887, 1998.
26. Todd RD, Botteron KN: Family, genetic, and imaging studies of early-onset depression. *Child Adolesc Psychiatric Clinics North America* 10:375–390, 2001.
27. Thapar A, McGuffin P: A twin study of depressive symptoms in childhood. *Br J Psychiatry* 165:259–265, 1994.
28. Glowinski AL, Madden PAF, Bucholz KK, Lynskey MT, Heath AC: Genetic epidemiology of self-reported lifetime DSM-IV major depressive disorder in a population-based twin sample of female adolescents. *J Child Psychology Psychiatry Allied Disciplines* 44:988–986, 2003.
29. O'Connor TG, Neiderhiser JM, Reiss D, Hetherington EM, Plomin R: Genetic contributions to continuity, change, and co-occurrence of antisocial and depressive symptoms in adolescence. *J Child Psychology Psychiatry Allied Disciplines* 39:323–336, 1998.
30. Scourfield J, Rice F, Thapar A, Harold GT, Martin N, McGuffin P: Depressive symptoms in children and adolescents: Changing aetiological influences with development. *J Child Psychol Psychiatry* 44:968–976, 2003.
31. Kovacs M, Devlin B: Internalizing disorders in childhood. *J Child Psychol Psychiatry* 39:47–63, 1998.
32. Weissman MM, Wickramaratne P, Nomura Y, Warner V, Verdeli H, Pilowsky DJ et al.: Families at high and low risk for depression: A 3-generation study. *Arch Gen Psychiatry* 62:29–36, 2005.
33. Thapar A, McGuffin P: Anxiety and depressive symptoms in childhood: A genetic study of comorbidity. *J Child Psychol Psychiatry* 38:651–656, 1997.
34. Hudziak JJ, Rudiger LP, Neale MC, Heath AC, Todd RD: A twin study of inattentive, aggressive, and anxious/depressed behaviors. *J Am Acad Child Adolesc Psychiatry* 39:469–476, 2000.
35. Eaves L, Silberg J, Erkanli A: Resolving multiple epigenetic pathways to adolescent depression. *J Child Psychol Psychiatry* 44:1006–1014, 2003.
36. Silberg J, Rutter M, Meyer J, Maes H, Hewitt J, Simonoff E et al.: Genetic and environmental influences on the covariation between hyperactivity and conduct disturbance in juvenile twins. *J Child Psychology Psychiatry Allied Disciplines* 37:803–816, 1996.
37. Daley SE, Hammen C, Davila J, Burge D: Axis II symptomatology, depression, and life stress during the transition from adolescence to adulthood. *J Consult Clin Psychol* 66:595–603, 1998.
38. Daley SE, Hammen C, Burge D, Davila J et al.: Predictors of the generation of episodic stress: A longitudinal study of late adolescent women. *J Abnorm Psychol* 106:251–259, 1997.
39. Caspi A, Sugden K, Moffitt TE, Taylor A, Craig IW, Harrington H et al.: Influence of life stress on depression: Moderation by a polymorphism in the 5-HT gene. *Science* 301:386–389, 2003.
40. Garber J, Keiley MK, Martin NC: Developmental trajectories of adolescents' depressive symptoms: Predictors of change. *J Consult Clin Psychol* 70:79–95, 2002.
41. Hammen C: Self-cognitions, stressful events, and the prediction of depression in children of depressed mothers. *J Abnorm Child Psychol* 16:347–360, 1988.
42. Lewinsohn PM, Joiner TE, Rohde P: Evaluation of cognitive diathesis-stress models in predicting major depressive disorder in adolescents. *J Abnorm Psychol* 110:203–215, 2001.
43. Nolen-Hoeksema S, Seligman MEP, Girgus JS: Predictors and consequences of childhood depressive symptoms: A 5-year longitudinal study. *J Abnorm Psychol* 101:405–422, 1992.
44. Pine DS: Face-memory and emotion: Associations with major depression in children and adolescents. *J Child Psychol Psychiatry* 45:1199–1208, 2004.
45. Goodyer IM: Social adversity and mental functions in adolescents at high risk of psychopathology. *Br J Psychiatry* 181:383–386, 2002.
46. Park RJ, Goodyer IM, Treasdale JD: Categoric overgeneral autobiographical memory in adolescents with major depressive disorder. *Psychol Med* 32:267–276, 2002.
47. Hammen C, Shih JH, Brennan PA: Intergenerational transmission of depression: Test of an interpersonal stress model in a community sample. *J Consult Clin Psychol* 72:511–522, 2004.
48. Frye AA, Garber J: The relations among maternal depression, maternal criticism, and adolescents' externalizing and internalizing symptoms. *J Abnorm Child Psychol* 33:1–11, 2005.
49. Nomura Y, Wickramaratne PJ, Warner V, Mufson L, Weissman MM: Family discord, parental depression, and psychopathology in offspring: Ten-year follow-up. *J Am Acad Child Psychiatry* 41:402–409, 2002.
50. Asarnow JR, Goldstein MJ, Tompson M, Guthrie D: One-year outcomes of depressive disorders in child psychiatric in-patients: Evaluation of the prognostic power of a brief measure of expressed emotion. *J Child Psychol Psychiatry* 34:129–137, 1993.
51. Kaminski KM, Garber J: Depressive spectrum disorders in high-risk adolescents: Episode duration and predictors of time to recovery. *J Am Acad Child Adolesc Psychiatry* 41:410–418, 2002.
52. Garber J, Flynn C: Predictors of depressive cognitions in young adolescents. *Cog Ther Res* 25:353–376, 2001.

53. Hammen C, Burge D, Stansbury K: Relationship of mother and child variables to child outcomes in a high-risk sample: A causal modeling analysis. *Dev Psychol* 26:24–30, 1990.
54. Garber J, Robinson NS: Cognitive vulnerability in children at risk for depression. *Cog and Emot* 11:619–635, 1997.
55. Fergusson DM, Horwood LJ, Lynskey MT: Childhood sexual abuse and psychiatric disorder in young adulthood: II. Psychiatric outcomes of childhood sexual abuse. *J Am Acad Child Adolesc Psychiatry* 35:1365–1374, 1996.
56. Fergusson DM, Lynskey MT, Horwood LJ: Childhood sexual abuse and psychiatric disorder in young adulthood: I. Prevalence of sexual abuse and factors associated with sexual abuse. *J Am Acad Child Adolesc Psychiatry* 35:1355–1364, 1996.
57. Molnar BE, Berkman LF, Buka SL: Psychopathology, childhood sexual abuse and other childhood adversities: Relative links to subsequent suicidal behavior in the U.S. *Psychol Med* 31:965–977, 2001.
58. Brown J, Cohen P, Johnson JG, Smailes EM: Childhood abuse and neglect: Specificity of effects on adolescent and young adult depression and suicidality. *J Am Acad Child Adolesc Psychiatry* 38:1490–1496, 1999.
59. Molnar BE, Buka SL, Kessler RC: Child sexual abuse and subsequent psychopathology: Results from the National Comorbidity Survey. *Am J Public Health* 91:753–760, 2001.
60. Barbe RP, Bridge J, Birmaher B, Kolko DJ, Brent DA: Lifetime history of sexual abuse, clinical presentation, and outcome in a clinical trial for adolescent depression. *J Clin Psychiatry* 65:77–83, 2004.
61. Kaufman J, Birmaher B, Perel J, Dahl R, Stull S, Brent D et al.: Serotonergic functioning in depressed abused children: Clinical and familial correlates. *Biol Psychiatry* 44:973–981, 1998.
62. Kaufman J, Yang BZ, Douglas-Palumberi H, Houshyar S, Lischitz D, Krystal JH et al.: Social supports and serotonin transporter gene moderate depression in maltreated children. *Proc Natl Acad Sci USA* 101:17316–17321, 2004.
63. Brent DA, Perper JA, Moritz G, Allman C, Schweers J, Roth C et al.: Psychiatric sequelae to the loss of an adolescent to suicide. *J Am Acad Child Adolesc Psychiatry* 32:509–517, 1993.
64. Brent DA, Perper JA, Moritz G, Liotus L, Schweers J, Roth C et al.: Psychiatric impact of the loss of an adolescent sibling to suicide. *J Affect Disord* 28:249–256, 1993.
65. Weller RA, Weller EB, Fristad MA, Bowes JM: Depression in recently bereaved prepubertal children. *Am J Psychiatry* 148:1536–1540, 1991.
66. Borowsky IW, Ireland M, Resnick MD: Adolescent suicide attempts: Risks and protectors. *Pediatrics* 10:485–493, 2001.
67. Birmaher B, Dahl RE, Williamson DE, Perel JM, Brent DA, Axelson DA et al.: Growth hormone secretion in children and adolescents at high risk for major depressive disorder. *Arch Gen Psychiatry* 57:867–872, 2000.
68. Dahl RE, Birmaher B, Williamson DE, Dorn L, Perel J, Kaufman J et al.: Low growth hormone response to growth hormone-releasing hormone in child depression. *Biol Psychiatry* 48:981–988, 2000.
69. Birmaher B, Kaufman J, Brent DA, Dahl RE, Perel JM, Al-Shabbout M et al.: Neuroendocrine response to L-5-hydroxytryptophan in prepubertal children at high risk for major depressive disorder. *Arch Gen Psychiatry* 54:1113–1119, 1997.
70. Ryan ND, Birmaher B, Perel JM, Dahl RE, Meyer V, Al-Shabbout M et al.: Neuroendocrine response to L-5-hydroxytryptophan challenge in prepubertal major depression. *Arch Gen Psychiatry* 49:843–851, 1992.
71. Pine D, Coplan J: Neuroendocrine response to fenfluramine challenge in boys: Associations with aggressive behavior and adverse rearing. *Arch Gen Psychiatry* 54:839–846, 1997.
72. Bertocci MA, Dahl RE, Williamson DE, Isof AM, Birmaher B, Axelson DA et al.: Subjective sleep complaints in pediatric depression: A controlled study and comparison with EEG measures of sleep and waking. *J Am Acad Child Adolesc Psychiatry* 44:1158–1166, 2005.
73. Dahl RE, Ryan ND, Puig-Antich J, Nguyen NA, Al-Shabbout M, Meyer VA et al.: 24-hour cortisol measures in adolescents with major depression: A controlled study. *Biol Psychiatry* 30:25–36, 1991.
74. Dahl RE, Ryan ND, Matty MK, Birmaher B, Al-Shabbout M, Williamson DE et al.: Sleep onset abnormalities in depressed adolescents. *Biol Psychiatry* 39:400–410, 1996.
75. Rao U, Dahl RE, Ryan ND, Birmaher B, Williamson DE, Rao R et al.: Heterogeneity in EEG sleep findings in adolescent depression: Unipolar versus bipolar clinical course. *J Affect Disord* 70:273–280, 2002.
76. Rao U, Dahl RE, Ryan ND, Birmaher B, Williamson DE, Giles DE et al.: The relationship between longitudinal clinical course and sleep and cortisol changes in adolescent depression. *Biol Psychiatry* 40:474–484, 1996.
77. Rao U, Ryan ND, Dahl RE, Birmaher B, Rao R, Williamson DE et al.: Factors associated with the development of substance use disorder in depressed adolescents. *J Am Acad Child Adolesc Psychiatry* 38:1109–1117, 1999.
78. Emslie GJ, Armitage R, Weinberg WA, Rush AJ, Mayes TL, Hoffmann RF: Sleep polysomnography as a predictor of recurrence in children and adolescents with major depressive disorder. *Int J Neuropsychopharm* 4:159–168, 2001.
79. Armitage R, Hoffmann RF, Emslie GJ, Weinberg WA, Mayes TL, Rush AJ: Sleep microarchitecture as a predictor of recurrence in children and adolescents with depression. *Int J Neuropsychopharm* 5:217–228, 2002.
80. Goetz RR, Wolk SI, Coplan JD, Ryan ND, Weissman MM: Premorbid polysomnographic signs in depressed adolescents: A reanalysis of EEG sleep after longitudinal follow-up in adulthood. *Society of Biol Psychiatry* 49:930–942, 2001.
81. Drevets WC, Price JL, Simpson Jr JR, Todd RD, Reich T, Vannier M et al.: Subgenual prefrontal cortex abnormalities in mood disorders. *Nature* 386:824–827, 1997.
82. Nolan CL, Moore GJ, Madden R, Farchione T, Bartoi M, Lorch E et al.: Prefrontal cortical volume in childhood-onset major depression. *Arch Gen Psychiatry* 59:173–179, 2002.
83. Botteron KN, Raichle ME, Drevets WC, Heath AC, Todd RD: Volumetric reduction in left subgenual prefrontal cortex in early onset depression. *Biol Psychiatry* 51:342–344, 2002.
84. Steingard R, Renshaw PF, Hennen J, Lenox M, Bonella Cintron C, Young AD et al.: Smaller frontal lobe white matter volumes in depressed adolescents. *Society of Biol Psychiatry* 52:413–417, 2002.
85. MacMillan S, Szeszko PR, Moore GT, Madden R, Lorch E, Ivey J et al.: Increased amygdala: Hippocampal volume ratios associated with severity of anxiety in pediatric major depression. *J Child Adolesc Psychopharm* 13:65–73, 2003.
86. Thomas KM, Drevets WC, Dahl RE, Ryan ND, Birmaher B, Eccard CH et al.: Amydgala response to fearful faces in anxious and depressed children. *Arch Gen Psychiatry* 58:1057–1063, 2001.
87. Birmaher B, Arbelaez C, Brent D: Course and outcome of child and adolescent major depressive disorder. *Child Adolesc Psychiatric Clinics North America* 11:619–637, 2002.
88. Birmaher B, Brent DA, Kolko D, Baugher M, Bridge J, Iyengar S et al.: Clinical outcome after short-term psychotherapy for adolescents with major depressive disorder. *Arch Gen Psychiatry* 57:29–36, 2000.
89. Kovacs M, Feinberg TL, Crouse-Novak MA, Paulauskas SL, Finkelstein R: Depressive disorders in childhood: I. A longitudinal study of characteristics and recovery. *Arch Gen Psychiatry* 41:229–237, 1984.
90. Warner V, Weissman MM, Fendrich M, Wickramaratne P, Moreau D: The course of major depression in the offspring of depressed parents: Incidence, recurrence and recovery. *Arch Gen Psychiatry* 49:795–801, 1992.
91. Kovacs M, Feinberg T, Crouse-Novak M, Paulauskas S, Pollock M, Finkelstein R: Depressive disorders in childhood: II. A longitudinal study of the risk for a subsequent major depression. *Arch Gen Psychiatry* 41:643–649, 1984.
92. Emslie GJ, Rush AJ, Weinberg WA, Kowatch RA, Carmody T, Mayes TL: Fluoxetine in child and adolescent depression: Acute and maintenance treatment. *Depression and Anxiety* 7:32–39, 1998.
93. McCauley E, Myers K, Mitchell J, Calderon R, Schloredt K, Treder R: Depression in young people: Initial presentation and clinical course. *J Am Acad Child Adolesc Psychiatry* 32:714–722, 1993.
94. Wickramaratne P, Warner V, Weissman MM: Selecting early-onset MDD probands for genetic studies: Results from a longitudinal high-risk study. *Am J Med Genetics* 96:93–101, 2000.
95. Strober M, Carlson G: Bipolar illness in adolescents with major depression—Clinical, genetic, and psychopharmacologic predictors in a three- to four-year prospective follow-up investigation. *Arch Gen Psychiatry* 39:549–555, 1982.
96. Geller B, Zimerman B, Williams M, Bolhofner K, Craney JL: Bipolar disorder at prospective follow-up of adults who had prepubertal major depression disorder. *Am J Psychiatry* 158:125–127, 2001.
97. Martin A, Young C, Leckman JF, Mukonoweshuro C, Rosenheck R, Leslie D: Age effects on antidepressant-induced manic conversion. *Archives of Pediatrics and Adolescent Medicine* 158:773–780, 2004.
98. Resnick MD, Bearman PS, Blum RW, Bauman KE, Harris KM, Jones J et al.: Protecting adolescents from harm: Findings from the National Longitudinal Study on Adolescent Health. *J Am Med Assoc* 278:823–832, 1997.
99. Pine DS, Goldstein RB, Wolk S, Weissman MM: The association between childhood depression and adulthood body mass index. *Pediatrics* 107:1049–1056, 2001.
100. Lewinsohn PM, Rohde P, Seeley JR, Klein DN, Gotlib IH: Psychosocial functioning of young adults who have experienced and recovered from major depressive disorder during adolescence. *J Abnorm Psychol* 112:353–363, 2003.
101. Birmaher B, Brent D, Work Group on Quality Issues: Practice parameters for the assessment and treatment of children and adolescents with depressive disorders. *J Am Acad Child Adolesc Psychiatry*. in press.
102. Brent DA: Antidepressants and pediatric depression: The risk of doing nothing. *N Engl J Med* 351:1598–1601, 2004.
103. Brent DA, Birmaher B: Adolescent depression. *N Engl J Med* 347:667–671, 2002.
104. Hazell P, O'Connell D, Heathcote D, Robertson J, Henry D: Efficacy of tricyclic drugs in treating child and adolescent depression: A meta-analysis. *Br Med J* 310:897–901, 1995.
105. Keller M, Ryan ND, Strober M, Klein RG, Kutcher SP, Birmaher B et al.: Efficacy of paroxetine in the treatment of adolescent major depression: A randomized, controlled study. *J Am Acad Child Adolesc Psychiatry* 40:762–772, 2001.
106. Bridge JA, Salary CR, Birmaher B, Asare AG, Brent DA: The risks and benefits of antidepressant treatment for youth depression. *Annals of Medicine* 37:404–412, 2005.

107. Mulder RT, Watkins WGA, Joyce PR, Luty SE: Age may affect response to antidepressants with serotonergic and noradrenergic actions. *J Affect Disord* 76:143–149, 2003.
108. Emslie G, Rush JA, Weinberg WA, Kowatch RA, Hughes CW, Carmody T et al.: A double-blind, randomized placebo-controlled trial of fluoxetine in depressed children and adolescents. *Arch Gen Psychiatry* 54:1031–1037, 1997.
109. Emslie G, Heiligenstein JH, Wagner KD, Hoog SL, Ernest DE, Brown E et al.: Fluoxetine for acute treatment of depression in children and adolescents: A placebo-controlled, randomized clinical trial. *J Am Acad Child Adolesc Psychiatry* 41:1205–1215, 2002.
110. March JS, Silva S, Petrycki S, Curry J, Wells K, Fairbank J et al.: Fluoxetine, cognitive-behavioral therapy, and their combination for adolescents with depression. Treatment for Adolescent Depression Study (TADS) randomized controlled trial. *J Am Med Assoc* 292:807–820, 2004.
111. March J: The Treatment of Adolescents with Depression Study (TADS).
112. Bridge J, Iyengar S, Salary CB, Barbe RP, Birmaher B, Pincus H et al.: Efficacy and suicidality risks of treatment: A meta-analysis of randomized controlled antidepressant trials for pediatric major depressive, obsessive-compulsive, and non-OCD anxiety disorders. In preparation.
113. Wagner KD, Ambrosini P, Rynn M, Wohlberg C, Yang R, Greenbaum MS et al.: Efficacy of sertraline in the treatment of children and adolescents with major depressive disorder: Two randomized controlled trials. *J Am Med Assoc* 290:1033–1041, 2003.
114. Wagner KD, Robb AS, Findling RL, Jin J, Gutierrez MM, Heydorn WE: A randomized, placebo-controlled trial of citalopram for the treatment of major depression in children and adolescents. *Am J Psychiatry* 161:1079–1083, 2004.
115. Hammad TA, Laughren T, Racoosin J: Suicidality in pediatric patients treated with antidepressant drugs. *Arch Gen Psychiatry* 63:332–339, 2006.
116. Goldstein BJ, Goodnick PJ: Selective serotonin reuptake inhibitors in the treatment of affectives disorders: III. Tolerability, safety and pharmacoeconomics. *J Psychopharm* 12:S55–S87, 1998.
117. Hamilton JA, Bridge J: Outcome at 6 months for 50 adolescents with major depression treated in a health maintenance organization. *J Am Acad Child Adolesc Psychiatry* 38:1340–1346, 1999.
118. Heiligenstein J, Hoog SL, Wagner KD, Findling RL, Galil N, Kaplan S et al.: Fluoxetine 40–60 mg versus fluoxetine 20 mg in the treatment of children and adolescents with a less-than-complete response to nine-week treatment with fluoxetine 10–20 mg: A pilot study. *J Child Adolesc Psychopharm* 16:207–217, 2006.
119. Axelson D, Birmaher B, Brent D: Pediatric pharmacokinetics and dynamics of R,S-citalopram. In preparation.
120. Axelson D, Perel J, Birmaher B, Rudolph G, Nuss S, Brent D: Sertraline pharmacokinetics and dynamics in adolescents. *J Am Acad Child Adolesc Psychiatry* 41:1037–1044, 2002.
121. Findling RL, Reed MD, Myers C, Riordan MA, Fiala S, Branicky L et al.: Paroxetine pharmacokinetics in depressed children and adolescents. *J Am Acad Child Adolesc Psychiatry* 38:952–959, 1999.
122. Labellarte MJ, Biederman J, Emslie G, Ferguson J, Khan A, Ruckle J et al.: Multiple-dose pharmacokinetics of fluvoxamine in children and adolescents. *J Am Acad Child Adolesc Psychiatry* 43:1497–1505, 2004.
123. Axelson DA, Perel JM, Birmaher B, Rudolph G, Nuss S, Yurasits L et al.: Platelet serotonin reuptake inhibition and response to SSRIs in depressed adolescents. *Am J Psychiatry* 162:802–804, 2005.
124. Sallee FR, Hilal R, Dougherty D, Beach K, Nesbitt L: Platelet serotonin transporter in depressed children and adolescents: 3H-paroxetine platelet binding before and after sertraline. *J Am Acad Child Adolesc Psychiatry* 37:777–784, 1998.
125. Sallee FR, Nesbitt L, Dougherty D, Hilal R, Nandagopal VS, Sethuraman G: Lymphocyte glucocorticoid receptor: Predictor of sertraline response in adolescent major depressive disorder. *Psychopharmacol Bull* 31:339–345, 1995.
126. Lerer B, Macciardi F: Pharmacogenetics of antidepressant and mood-stabilizing drugs: A review of candidate-gene studies and future research. *Int J Neuropsychopharmacology* 5:255–275, 2002.
127. Kronenberg S, Apter A, Brent D, Schirman S, Melhem N, Pick N et al.: Serotonin transporter (5HTT) polymorphism and citalopram effectiveness and side effects in children with depression and anxiety disorders. In preparation.
128. Emslie GJ, Heiligenstein JH, Hoog SL, Wagner KD, Findling RL, McCracken JT et al.: Fluoxetine treatment for prevention of relapse of depression in children and adolescents: A double-blind, placebo-controlled study. *J Am Acad Child Adolesc Psychiatry* 43:1397–1405, 2004.
129. Hayward C, Varady S, Albano AM, Thienemann ML, Henderson L, Schatzberg A: Cognitive-behavioral group therapy for social phobia in female adolescents: Results of a pilot study. *J Am Acad Child Adolesc Psychiatry* 39:721–726, 2000.
130. Stein MB, Fuetsch M, Muller N, Hofler M, Lieb R, Wittchen H: Social anxiety disorder and the risk of depression. *Arch Gen Psychiatry* 58:251–256, 2001.
131. Beck AT, Rush AJ, Shaw BF, Emery G: *Cognitive Therapy of Depression.* New York, Guilford Press, 1979.
132. Compton SN, March JS, Brent D, Albano AM, Weersing VR, Curry J: Cognitive behavioral psychotherapy for anxiety and depressive disorders in children and adolescents: An evidence based medicine review. *J Am Acad Child Adolesc Psychiatry* 43:930–959, 2004.
133. Clarke GN, Lewinsohn PM, Rohde P, Hops H, Seeley JR: Cognitive-behavioral group treatment of adolescent depression: Efficacy of acute group treatment and booster sessions. *J Am Acad Child Adolesc Psychiatry* 38:272–279, 1999.
134. Lewinsohn PM, Clarke GN, Hops H, Andrews J: Cognitive-behavioral treatment for depressed adolescents. *Behavior Therapy* 21:385–401, 1990.
135. Rohde P, Clarke GN, Mace DE, Jorgensen JS, Seeley JR: An efficacy/effectiveness study of cognitive-behavioral treatment for adolescents with comorbid major depression and conduct disorder. *J Am Acad Child Adolesc Psychiatry* 43:660–668, 2004.
136. Rohde P, Jorgensen JS, Seeley JR, Mace DE: Pilot evaluation of the coping course: A cognitive-behavioral intervention to enhance coping skills incarcerated youth. *J Am Acad Child Adolesc Psychiatry* 43:669–676, 2004.
137. Vostanis P, Feehan C, Grattan E, Bickerton W: A randomised controlled out-patient trial of cognitive-behavioural treatment for children and adolescents with depression: 9-month follow-up. *J Affect Disord* 40:105–116, 1996.
138. Wood A, Harrington R, Moore A: Controlled trial of a brief cognitive-behavioural intervention in adolescent patients with depressive disorders. *J Child Psychol Psychiatry* 37:6:737–746, 1996.
139. Brent DA, Holder D, Kolko D, Birmaher B, Baugher M, Roth C et al.: A clinical psychotherapy trial for adolescent depression comparing cognitive, family, and supportive treatments. *Arch Gen Psychiatry* 54:877–885, 1997.
140. Weersing VR, Brent DA: Cognitive-behavioral therapy for adolescent depression: Comparative efficacy, mediation, moderation, and effectiveness. In: Kazdin AE, Weisz JR (eds.): *Evidence Based Psychotherapies for Children and Adolescents.* New York: Guilford Press, 2003, pp. 135–147.
141. Brent DA, Kolko D, Birmaher B, Baugher M, Bridge J, Roth C. et al.: Predictors of treatment efficacy in a clinical trial of three psychosocial treatments for adolescent depression. *J Am Acad Child Adolesc Psychiatry* 37:906–914, 1998.
142. Rohde P, Clarke GN, Lewinsohn PM, Seeley JR, Kaufman NK: Impact of comorbidity on a cognitive-behavioral group treatment for adolescent depression. *J Am Acad Child Adolesc Psychiatry* 40:795–802, 2001.
143. Hollon SD, Garber J, Shelton RC: Treatment of depression in adolescents with cognitive behavior therapy and medications: A commentary on the TADS project. *Cognitive Behavioral Practice* 12:149–155, 2005.
144. Clarke GC, Debar L, Lynch F, Powell J, Gale J, O'Connor E et al.: A randomized effectiveness trial of brief cognitive-behavior therapy for depressed adolescents receiving antidepressant medication. *J Am Acad Child Adolesc Psychiatry* 44:888–898, 2005.
145. Goodyer IM: *A randomised controlled trial of SSRIs with and without cognitive behaviour therapy in adolescents with major depression.* NHS Technology Assessment Programme. Cambridge, U.K., 2006.
146. Asarnow JR, Jaycox LH, Duan N, LaBorde AP, Rea MM, Murray P et al.: Effectiveness of a quality improvement intervention for adolescent depression in primary care clinics: A randomized controlled trial. *J Am Med Assoc* 293:311–319, 2005.
147. Wells KB, Sherbourne CD, Schoenbaum M, Duan N, Meredith L, Unutzer J et al.: Impact of disseminating quality improvement programs for depression in managed primary care: A randomized controlled trial. *J Am Med Assoc* 283:212–220, 2000.
148. Weersing, VR, Iyengar, S, Birmaher, B, Kolko, DJ, Brent, DA: Effectiveness of cognitive-behavioral therapy for adolescent depression: A benchmarking investigation. *Behavior Therapy* 37:36–48, 2006.
149. Clarke G, Hops H, Lewinsohn PM, Andrew J, Williams J: Cognitive-behavioral group treatment of adolescent depression: Prediction of outcome. *Behavior Therapy* 23:341–354, 1992.
150. Clarke GN, Hornbrook M, Lynch F, Polen M, Gale J, Beardslee W et al.: A randomized trail of a group cognitive intervention for preventing depression in adolescent offspring of depressed parents. *Arch Gen Psychiatry* 58:1127–1134, 2001.
151. Kaufman NK, Rohde P, Seeley JR, Clarke GN, Stice E: Potential mediators of cognitive-behavioral therapy for adolescents with comorbid major depression and conduct disorder. *J Consult Clin Psychol* 73:38–46, 2005.
152. Kolko DJ, Brent DA, Baugher M, Bridge J, Birmaher B: Cognitive and family therapies for adolescent depression: Treatment specificity, mediation, and moderation. *J Consult Clin Psychol* 68:603–614, 2000.
153. Ackerson J, Scogin F, McKendree-Smith N, Lyman RD: Cognitive bibliotherapy for mild and moderate adolescent depressive symptomatology. *J Consult Clin Psychol* 66:685–690, 1998.
154. Clarke GN, Hawkins W, Murphy M, Sheeber LB, Lewinsohn PM, Seeley JR: Targeted prevention of unipolar depressive disorder in an at-risk sample of high school adolescents: A randomized trial of group cognitive intervention. *J Am Acad Child Adolesc Psychiatry* 34:312–321, 1995.
155. Horowitz JL, Garber J: The prevention of depressive symptoms in children and adolescents: A meta-analytic review. *J Consult Clin Psychol*, in press.

156. Kroll L, Harrington R, Jayson D, Fraser J: Pilot study of continuation cognitive-behavioral therapy for major depression in adolescent psychiatric patients. *J Am Acad Child Adolesc Psychiatry* 35:1156–1161, 1996.
157. Klerman G, Weissman MM, Rounsaville BJ, Chevron E: *Interpersonal Psychotherapy of Depression*. New York, Basic Books, 1984.
158. Mufson L, Weissman MM, Moreau D, Garfinkel R: Efficacy of interpersonal psychotherapy for depressed adolescents. *Arch Gen Psychiatry* 56:573–579, 1999.
159. Rossello J, Bernal G: The efficacy of cognitive-behavioral and interpersonal treatments for depression in Puerto Rican adolescents. *J Consult Clin Psychol* 67:734–745, 1999.
160. Mufson L, Dorta KP, Wickramaratne P, Nomura Y, Olfson M, Weissman MM: A randomized effectiveness trial of interpersonal psychotherapy for depressed adolescents. *Arch Gen Psychiatry* 61:577–584, 2004.
161. Mufson L, Fairbanks J: Interpersonal psychotherapy for depressed adolescents: A one-year naturalistic follow-study. *J Am Acad Child Adolesc Psychiatry* 35:1145–1155, 1996.
162. Diamond GS, Reis BF, Diamond GM, Siqueland L, Isaacs L: Attachment based family therapy for depressed adolescents: A treatment development study. *J Am Acad Child Adolesc Psychiatry* 41:1190–1196, 2002.
163. Swedo SE, Allen AJ, Glod CA, Clark CH, Teicher MH, Richter D et al.: A controlled trial of light therapy for the treatment of pediatric seasonal affective disorder. *J Am Acad Child Adolesc Psychiatry* 36:816–821, 1997.
164. Walter G, Rey JM: Has the practice and outcome of ECT in adolescents changed? Findings from a whole-population study. *J ECT* 19:84–87, 2003.
165. Renaud J, Brent DA, Baugher M, Birmaher B, Kolko DJ, Bridge J: Rapid response to psychosocial treatment for adolescent depression: A two-year follow-up. *J Am Acad Child Adolesc Psychiatry* 37:1184–1190, 1998.
166. Weersing VR, Weisz JR: Community clinic treatment of depressed youth: Benchmarking usual care against CBT clinical trials. *J Consult Clin Psychol* 70:299–310, 2002.
167. Keller MB, McCullough JP, Klein DN, Arnow B, Dunner DL, Gelenberg AJ et al.: A comparison of nefazodone, the cognitive behavioral-analysis system of psychotherapy, and their combination for the treatment of chronic depression. *N Engl J Med* 342:1462–1470, 2000.
168. Thase ME, Greenhouse JB, Frank E, Reynolds III CF, Pilkonis PA, Hurley K et al.: Treatment of major depression with psychotherapy or psychotherapy-pharmacotherapy combinations. *Arch Gen Psychiatry* 54: 1009–1015, 1997.
169. Hughes CW, Emslie GJ, Crismon L, Wagner KD, Birmaher B, Geller B et al.: The Texas children's medication algorithm project: Report of the Texas consensus conference panel on medication treatment of childhood major depressive disorder. *J Am Acad Child Adolesc Psychiatry* 38:1442–1454, 1999.
170. Brent DA, Birmaher B, Kolko D, Baugher M, Bridge J: Subsyndromal depression in adolescents after a brief psychotherapy trial: Course and outcome. *J Affect Disord* 63:51–58, 2001.
171. Ryan ND, Puig-Antich J, Ambrosini P, Rabinovich H, Robinson D, Nelson B et al.: The clinical picture of major depression in children and adolescents. *Arch Gen Psychiatry* 44:854–861, 1987.
172. Lewinsohn PM, Rohde P, Seeley JR: Adolescent suicidal ideation and attempts: Prevalence, risk factors, and clinical implications. *Clin Psychol Sci Prac* 3:25–46, 1996.
173. Harrington R, Kerfoot M, Dyer E, McNiven F, Gill J, Harrington V et al.: Randomized trial of a home-based family intervention for children who have deliberately poisoned themselves. *J Am Acad Child Adolesc Psychiatry* 37:512–518, 1998.
174. Wood A, Trainor G, Rothwell J, Moore A, Harrington R: Randomized trial of a group therapy for repeated deliberate self-harm in adolescents. *J Am Acad Child Adolesc Psychiatry* 40:1246–1253, 2001.
175. Khan A, Warner HA, Brown WA: Symptom reduction and suicide risk in patients treated with placebo in antidepressant clinical trials: An analysis of the Food and Drug Administration database. *Arch Gen Psychiatry* 57:311–317, 2000.
176. Linehan MM, Armstrong HE, Suarez A, Allmon D, Heard HL: Cognitive-behavioral treatment of chronically parasuicidal borderline patients. *Arch Gen Psychiatry* 48:1060–1064, 1991.
177. Harrington R, Clark A: Prevention and early intervention for depression in adolescence and early adult life. *Eur Arch Psychiatry Clin Neurosci* 248:32–45, 1998.
178. Katon WJ, Unutzer J, Simon G: Treatment of depression in primary care: Where we are, where we can go. *Med Care* 42:1153–1157, 2004.

CHAPTER 5.4.2 ■ BIPOLAR DISORDER

BORIS BIRMAHER, DAVID AXELSON, AND MANI PAVULURI

INTRODUCTION

Consistent with Kraepelin's early descriptions (1921) (1), it is now recognized that bipolar disorder (BP) occurs in children and adolescents. However, many children and adolescents with BP have very short and frequent periods of syndromal or subsyndromal mania, hypomania, or depression, making their diagnosis especially difficult.

Pediatric BP severely affects the normal development and psychosocial functioning of the child and increases the risk for suicide, psychosis, substance abuse, as well as for behavioral, academic, social, and legal problems. However, it takes on average of 10 years to identify and begin treatment of BP (2), indicating the need for timely detection and treatment of this serious illness.

The goal of this chapter is to review the clinical picture, epidemiology, differential diagnosis, course and prognosis, risk factors, and pharmacological and psychosocial treatment of pediatric BP.

For the purposes of this chapter the word youth, unless specified, denotes children and adolescents.

CLINICAL CHARACTERISTICS

Research into the phenomenology of pediatric bipolar disorder is relatively new and has led to substantial debate about how BP presents in children and adolescents. Clear consensus does not exist on key issues such as: 1) the necessity of cardinal symptoms (e.g., elated mood and/or grandiosity) for a bipolar diagnosis; 2) the role of irritable mood in pediatric BP; 3) the requirement of clearly demarcated mood episodes; 4) the temporal relation between manic and depressive symptoms and mood cycling patterns; 5) the validity and importance of manic symptoms that do not meet the DSM-IV symptom or duration thresholds for a manic, hypomanic, or mixed episode; and 6) the best way to attribute potential symptoms of mania that also commonly present in other pediatric psychiatric disorders. Though the diagnostic features of BP in youth has provoked considerable controversy, it is important to note that many of these issues have not been settled in the adult bipolar literature and the conceptualization of BP will continue to evolve as more research becomes available.

Applying the DSM-IV Criteria

It is clear from the work of several groups that some children and adolescents meet the full DSM-IV criteria for BP (Tables 5.4.2.1 and 5.4.2.2), despite the fact that the criteria were not specifically adapted for use in the pediatric population (3–5). When examining the DSM-IV criteria for a manic or hypomanic episode, it is obvious that normal children can exhibit many of these features to some degree, especially in certain situations or environments. It is of utmost importance to evaluate whether the mood and symptoms are abnormal or clearly different from the child's usual mood and behavior given the context and developmental level. For instance, elevated mood, high activity level and rapid speech would not be considered evidence of mania in a 7-year-old at a birthday party, an amusement park or on Christmas morning.

Consideration of how manic symptoms may manifest differently across development can facilitate accurate diagnosis. For instance, in contrast with an adult who is in a manic episode, a school-age child is not likely to exhibit behaviors such as engaging in risky business ventures, driving recklessly, going on spending sprees, or having sexual relations with multiple partners. However, they can exhibit inappropriate sexual behavior (touching others inappropriately, frequent public masturbation or drawing sexually provocative pictures) or engage in uncharacteristically dangerous, risk-taking play such as jumping from high places or performing frequent and exaggerated daredevil stunts on a bicycle (6).

The distinction between a manic and hypomanic episode can be difficult, but also must be taken in a developmental context. Beyond the differences in minimum duration, manic episodes require marked impairment, which should be measured against what would be the expected level of functioning for a child given his/her chronological age and intellectual capabilities, in the psychosocial domains that are relevant to youth (school, family, peers). A hypomanic episode does not require impairment, although there must be an unequivocal positive or negative change from usual functioning and the mood and functional changes must be observable by others. Given that lack of insight can be associated with mania or hypomania, it is imperative to obtain information from caregivers or other significant adults in the child's or adolescent's life in order to accurately assess symptoms and potential change in functioning.

TABLE 5.4.2.1

DSM-IV CRITERIA FOR A MANIC EPISODE

A. A distinct period of abnormally and persistently elevated, expansive, or irritable mood for at least 1 week (or any duration if hospitalization is necessary).
B. During the period of mood disturbance, three (or more) of the following symptoms have persisted (four if the mood is only irritable) and have been present to a significant degree:
   1) Inflated self-esteem or grandiosity
   2) Decreased need for sleep (e.g., feels rested after only 3 hours of sleep)
   3) more talkative than usual or pressure to keep talking
   4) flight of ideas or subjective experience that thoughts are racing
   5) distractibility (i.e., attention too easily drawn to unimportant or irrelevant external stimuli)
   6) increase in goal-directed activity (either socially, at work or school, or sexually) or psychomotor agitation
   7) excessive involvement in pleasurable activities that have a high potential for painful consequences (engaging in unrestrained buying sprees, sexual indiscretions, or foolish business investments)
C. The symptoms do not meet criteria for a mixed episode.
D. The mood disturbance is sufficiently severe to cause marked impairment in occupational functioning or in usual social activities or relationships with others, or to necessitate hospitalization to prevent harm to self or others, or there are psychotic features.
E. The symptoms are not due to the direct physiological effects of a substance (a drug of abuse, a medication, or other treatment) or a general medical condition (hyperthyroidism).

Note: Manic-like episodes that are clearly caused by somatic antidepressant treatment (medication, electroconvulsive therapy, light therapy) should not count toward a diagnosis of Bipolar I Disorder.

TABLE 5.4.2.2

DSM-IV CRITERIA FOR A HYPOMANIC EPISODE

A. A distinct period of persistently elevated, expansive, or irritable mood lasting throughout at least 4 days, that is clearly different from the usual nondepressed mood
B. Same as B criterion for manic episode
C. The episode is associated with an unequivocal change in functioning that is uncharacteristic of the person when not symptomatic.
D. The disturbance in mood and the change in functioning are observable by others.
E. The episode is not severe enough to cause marked impairment in social or occupational functioning, or to necessitate hospitalization, and there are no psychotic features.
F. The symptoms are not due to the direct physiological effects of a substance (a drug of abuse, a medication, or other treatment) or a general medical condition (hyperthyroidism).

Note: Hypomanic-like episodes that are clearly caused by somatic antidepressant treatment (medication, electroconvulsive therapy, light therapy) should not count toward a diagnosis of Bipolar II Disorder.

Symptoms of Mania

A recent metaanalysis of seven published phenomenology studies of pediatric mania determined weighted rates and confidence intervals for 11 symptoms of mania that were measured across most of the studies (Table 5.4.2.3) (4). Increased energy and distractibility were the most common symptoms, while hypersexuality was the least frequent. Elated/euphoric mood and irritability were the two symptoms with the most variability in rates across studies, though there was also significant heterogeneity in the rates of decreased need for sleep, racing thoughts, poor judgment, pressured speech, and distractibility. Sampling issues and methodological differences among the studies, such as the average subject age, or the use of the child in addition to the parent as informants, may have accounted for much of the variability in symptom rates (4). However, differences in how groups conceptualized symptoms may also have contributed to the variability. Though it is not a symptom of mania per se, psychosis frequently occurs in BP youth. The weighted rate of psychosis was 42% (95% CI 24-62%) in the metaanalysis, but again there was significant heterogeneity among the studies.

TABLE 5.4.2.3

SYMPTOMS OF MANIA FROM METAANALYSIS OF PEDIATRIC BP STUDIES

Symptom	Weighted Rate	95% Confidence Interval
Increased energy	89%	76–96%
Distractibility	84%	71–92%
Pressured speech	82%	69–90%
Irritability	81%	55–94%
Grandiosity	78%	67–85%
Racing thoughts	74%	51–88%
Decreased need for sleep	72%	53–86%
Euphoria/elation	70%	45–87%
Poor judgment	69%	38–89%
Flight of ideas	56%	46–66%
Hypersexuality	38%	31–45%

[From Kowatch et al. (4)].

The rate of psychosis was 35% in a report of a large BP-I sample published subsequently (3).

One factor that may contribute to the difficultly of diagnosing BP in youth is that the most common symptoms of pediatric mania from the metaanalysis also happen to be frequently present in other pediatric psychiatric disorders. A recent study comparing the phenomenology of bipolar disorder and ADHD found that there were no significant differences between the BP vs. the ADHD subjects in rates of irritability (98% BP vs. 72% ADHD), accelerated speech (97% vs. 82%), distractibility (94% vs. 96%) or unusual energy (100% vs. 95%) (7). Thus, the lack of specificity makes it problematic to diagnose mania by simply counting the presence or absence of symptoms.

Cardinal Symptoms

The overlap of manic symptoms with features of other psychiatric illnesses emphasizes the diagnostic importance of symptoms that tend to be more specific to mania. Some authors have advocated that two of these mania-specific symptoms, elated/elevated mood and grandiosity, are core features of the manic syndrome so that they should be considered cardinal or hallmark symptoms (6–8). As shown in the metaanalysis above, these two symptoms are present in most manic youth, though there was considerable heterogeneity among studies in the rates of euphoria/elation, and one of the largest studies in the analysis required the presence of either elevated mood or grandiosity as an inclusion criterion for the BP subjects. However, a subsequently published large study of BP-I youth that did not require either of these symptoms also had high rates of elated/elevated mood (86%) and grandiosity (57%) (3). Long-term longitudinal studies of youth meeting the DSM-IV criteria for mania with or without cardinal symptoms have not been completed. Although the cardinal symptom approach has the potential to improve diagnostic accuracy, additional research such as the Longitudinal Assessment of Manic Symptoms (LAMS) and the Course and Outcome of Bipolar Youth (COBY) studies are necessary before elated/elevated mood or grandiosity can be required for a diagnosis of mania.

Irritability in Pediatric BP

Irritability has been defined as "... an emotional state characterized by having a low threshold for experiencing anger in response to negative emotional events" (9). Irritability can encompass multiple temporal features of abnormal emotional reactivity, including a lower threshold to anger, a faster increase in anger, a higher "peak" level of anger, and a longer duration of anger.

As noted above, irritability is present in nearly all manic children and adolescents, so it is a sensitive marker for pediatric BP. However it is also part of the DSM-IV diagnostic criteria for disorders such as disruptive, major depressive, generalized anxiety, and posttraumatic stress disorders. In addition, it is frequently present in youth with other psychiatric diagnoses (e.g. ADHD; pervasive developmental disorders). Therefore irritability has low specificity for BP. The DSM-IV criteria for a manic episode explicitly allows for the presence of irritable mood alone to satisfy the "A" criterion, though it qualifies this by requiring an additional symptom criterion. Some reports have prompted substantial controversy by stating that chronic presentations of irritability alone, particularly when the irritability is severe and accompanied by aggression and volatility, is the primary mood disturbance in bipolar youth and that elevated or expansive mood is uncommon (10–12). However, the high prevalence of elated/expansive mood in most cross-sectional pediatric BP samples stands in contrast to these reports. Prospective evaluations of the phenomenology of new manic episodes in youth have not been published, so it is difficult to assess how frequently pediatric mania presents with only irritable mood.

Episodic vs. Chronic Mania

Some groups have emphasized that BP youth present with chronic manic symptoms and have reported mean durations of 3–4 years for manic or mixed episodes (13, 14). Others have noted that although BP youth may have chronic symptomatology and prolonged symptom-free periods are uncommon, it is an episodic illness and the duration of full threshold manic and mixed episodes are considerably shorter than 3–4 years in most cases (15, 16). The DSM-IV criteria for manic, mixed or hypomania episode require a distinct period of abnormal mood and accompanying symptoms and some authors have advocated that an episodic course is a key feature that should be present for a definitive diagnosis of BP (8). As noted below, BP youth have high rates of comorbid ADHD, rapid mood fluctuations, and complex admixtures of manic and depressive symptoms. These features can make it difficult to identify distinct episodes that are embedded in this "mixed" presentation. However, a strict application of the "distinct period" of abnormal mood and symptoms criterion has certain advantages. The adult bipolar phenotype has an episodic component. In addition, nonspecific symptoms of mania (irritability, rapid speech, psychomotor agitation, distractibility) usually do not present with distinct episodes in other pediatric psychiatric disorders. Though there is no definitive evidence that mania in youth must have an episodic presentation, the presence of distinct periods of manic symptoms in a child or adolescent likely increases the probability of bipolarity and is a reasonable requirement for a conservative approach to the BP diagnosis in youth.

Depression in Pediatric BP

Depressive symptoms are noted to be prominent features in most phenomenological studies of pediatric BP, and BP adults frequently recall having significant depressive symptoms in childhood or adolescence (2, 17, 18). BP youth can have clear periods of depression that meet the full criteria for a major depressive episode (MDE) (see Chapter 5.4.1 for the DSM criteria for MDE). Over 50% of BP youth had a prior history of a MDE in a recent report (3). As described in the differential diagnosis section following, major depression may precede the onset of mania, so that some children and adolescents who appear to have unipolar depression may actually have BP with depression as their initial presentation. Mild or transient manic symptomatology that does not meet the diagnostic threshold for mania or hypomania may also precede an MDE, although the presentation of full DSM-IV criteria BP-II (MDE plus at least one hypomanic episode) does not appear to be common in youth with bipolar spectrum illness (3). All of these factors highlight the need to carefully probe for a history of manic symptoms in youth presenting with depression.

Temporal Relation of Manic and Depressive Symptoms

Many researchers have reported that BP youth present with mixed states and complex cycling patterns between depression and mania. Some groups have reported chronic mixed states lasting years in duration and rapid cycling between mania and depression as frequently as several times per day (10, 19). The issue is complicated by the fact that there are no clear boundaries that delineate a mixed state from an actual switch in episode polarity, or from mood lability and/or transient dysphoria occurring in the midst of mania. The DSM-IV criteria for a mixed episode require that the criteria for both a manic episode and a major depressive episode be met nearly every day during at least a 1-week period. This could be satisfied by an episode consisting of: 1) an amalgamation of manic and depressive symptoms that present concurrently (expansive, irritable, and depressed mood, high energy, racing thoughts, rapid speech, hopelessness, guilt and suicidality); 2) cycling between distinct short periods of predominantly manic symptoms and predominantly depressive symptoms; or 3) or some combination of both types of presentations. Overlapping criteria and features plus the symptoms of other comorbid psychiatric disorders can make it difficult to determine whether symptoms should be attributed to depression or mania. For example, irritability, racing thoughts, and psychomotor agitation can occur in both mood states and it sometimes can be challenging to differentiate decreased need for sleep from insomnia occurring in an agitated depression. Published studies have used the recall of interviewees from over a long time interval, which limits reliable evaluation of symptom patterns. It is not clear whether the reports of multiple mood cycles in a day represent periods where the child switches from meeting the full criteria of the manic syndrome to a period where they are completely depressed or whether they are manifestations of mood lability within the manic state. However, the evidence does indicate that the majority of BP youth have symptoms of depression interspersed in some manner with manic symptoms.

Subthreshold Presentations

Some children and adolescents present in clinical and research settings with what appears to be significant manic symptomatology, but do not meet full DSM-IV criteria for BP-I or BP-II disorders. Reasons for this include: 1) The manic symptoms are not present for sufficient time to meet the DSM-IV duration criteria for a manic, hypomanic or mixed episode; 2) the mood disturbances and symptoms do not occur in distinct episodes; 3) the potential manic symptoms are not clearly temporally associated or do not intensify with the abnormal mood; or 4) it cannot be reliably determined whether the abnormal mood and symptoms are attributable to BP or better accounted for by another psychiatric diagnosis. The diagnosis and management of these children and adolescents is controversial, though many present for mental health treatment with significant impairment and are frequently assigned a diagnosis of bipolar disorder not otherwise specified (BP-NOS) (3, 5). Empirical research in subthreshold presentations of bipolarity in youth is in its early stages. One large study comparing the presentation of youth with an operationalized diagnosis of BP-NOS with those who met full criteria for BP-I found that BP-NOS subjects differed from those with BP-I primarily on duration and severity of manic symptomatology, but not on the fundamental phenomenology of manic symptoms, comorbid disorders, or family psychiatric history (3). The majority of BP-NOS youth fulfilled the mood and symptom criteria for mania and/or hypomania, but did not meet the 4-day duration criteria for a hypomanic episode or the 7-day duration criteria for a manic/mixed episode. Nevertheless, these cases of BP-NOS uniformly presented with histories of significant impairment and nearly all had some form of psychiatric treatment prior to assessment. Preliminary results indicate that some of these BP-NOS cases progress to meet the DSM-IV criteria for BP-I or BP-II disorders within 2 years of followup (15). However it is currently unknown how many will eventually become bipolar adults or which subthreshold presentations predict development of BP-I or BP-II disorder versus those that are not truly bipolar.

Attributing Symptoms to Bipolar Disorder vs. other Pediatric Psychiatric Disorders

As described later in more detail under Differential Diagnosis, clinicians must be cautious about attributing symptoms to mania or hypomania unless they show a clear temporal association with the abnormally elevated, expansive, and/or irritable mood. The manic syndrome exists as a collection of concurrent symptoms and mood abnormalities, not a list of symptoms that occur in temporal isolation. Chronic symptoms such as hyperactivity or distractibility generally should not be considered evidence of mania unless they clearly intensify with the onset of abnormal mood. Prolonged presentations of nonspecific manic-like symptoms that do not change in overall intensity should raise the possibility of an alternative psychiatric diagnosis.

EPIDEMIOLOGY

Due to the difficulties and controversies regarding the diagnosis of pediatric BP, it is not clear what the real prevalence of this disorder is in youth. Retrospective studies in adults with BP have consistently reported that up to 60% had the onset of their mood symptoms before age 20 years (2, 17, 18, 20). Moreover, it appears that there are secular trends in the incidence of unipolar and BP in successive birth cohorts, with ages at first onset of the disorder occurring earlier in later cohorts (21–23).

Some epidemiological studies (24–26), but not all (27) have reported that the combined occurrence of BP is approximately 1%–2% (mainly BP-II, BP-NOS, and cyclothymia), and as high as 6% when including "soft" subsyndromal symptoms (24). However, these results need to be interpreted with caution because of methodological limitations associated with these studies (28). In clinical populations the prevalence of BP has been reported between 0.6% and 15% depending on the setting, the referral source, and the methodology used to ascertain BP (28).

COMORBIDITY

Pediatric BP is usually accompanied by other psychiatric disorders. Depending on the population studied, approximately 50%–80% have ADHD, 20% to 60% disruptive disorders, and 30% to 70% anxiety disorders (28). Beginning in adolescence, the rate of comorbid substance abuse progressively increases (29). In lesser degree, other psychiatric disorders, such as obsessive-compulsive disorder, as well as medical conditions, can accompany BP. The presence of these disorders affects the child's response to treatment and prognosis, indicating the need to identify and treat them effectively (30).

DIFFERENTIAL DIAGNOSIS

As noted above, it is difficult to diagnose pediatric BP because the variability in the clinical presentation (severity, subtype of BP disorder, phase of the illness), high comorbidity and overlap in symptom presentation with other psychiatric disorders, effects of development in symptom expression, children's problems expressing their symptoms, the context where the BP is developing (family conflicts), and if the child is on medications, their potential effects on the child's mood.

The main psychiatric conditions that can be challenging to differentiate from youth with BP are attention deficit hyperactivity disorder (ADHD), disruptive behavior disorders (ODD and conduct disorder), unipolar depression, pervasive developmental disorders (PDD), schizophrenia, substance abuse disorders, and borderline personality disorder. Medical and neurological illnesses (head trauma, brain tumors, hyperthyroidism), and side effects of medications (corticosteroids, antidepressants, and stimulants) may be accompanied by mood fluctuations that may mimic BP. Also normal mood variability sometimes may be misinterpreted as symptoms of hypomania.

In daily practice, severe behavior disruptive disorders and ADHD are the most frequent conditions that may be confused with BP (Tables 5.4.2.4 and 5.4.2.5). There are some symptoms that mainly occur in BP youth and may help to differentiate between BP and these disorders, such as clinically relevant euphoria, grandiosity, decreased need for sleep, hypersexuality (without history of sexual abuse or exposure to sex), and hallucinations (7). Some of the symptoms shared between BP, ADHD, and disruptive disordered children, such as irritability and aggression, are much more severe in BP youth (11). The course of the symptoms over time, the presence of family history for BP disorder, and other issues described in Tables 5.4.2.4 and 5.4.2.5 also may help distinguish between BP and these disorders.

Most depressed youth seen at psychiatric clinics are experiencing their first episode of depression (31). Some of these subjects may develop BP, but so far it is almost impossible to know who will develop BP at the time of first assessment. Thus, a careful assessment for history of manic or hypomanic symptoms is indicated. Also, the presence of psychosis, family history of BP, and pharmacologically induced mania/hypomania may indicate susceptibility to develop BP (32–36).

Schizophrenia is rare in children and sometimes BP may manifest with psychosis and bizarre behaviors. Therefore, mood disorders need to be ruled out in any child with psychosis. Youth with PDD-NOS or Asperger's disorder may have mood lability, aggression, and agitation and be misdiagnosed as having BP. Substance abuse may also induce severe mood changes that may be difficult to differentiate from BP. Moreover, youth with mood disorders are at higher risk for using illicit drugs or alcohol as a way to deal with their mood and daily problems (29).

The use of medications such as antidepressants may unmask or trigger a manic or hypomanic episode in a susceptible individual (37). However, not every child that becomes agitated or giddy and excited with these or other medications has BP. Family history, the severity, length, and quality of manic symptomatology may help to differentiate between BP or agitation induced by these or other medications (38).

Finally, although there is controversy about the validity of borderline personality disorder in youth, some BP teens, particularly those with BP-II, may be misdiagnosed as having this condition.

TABLE 5.4.2.4

BIPOLAR DISORDER VS. ATTENTION DEFICIT HYPERACTIVE DISORDER (ADHD)

Suspect the presence of Bipolar Disorder in a child with ADHD if:

- The ADHD symptoms appeared later in life (e.g., at age 10 years old or older).
- The symptoms of ADHD appeared abruptly in an otherwise healthy child.
- The ADHD symptoms were responding to stimulants and now are not.
- The ADHD symptoms come and go and tend to occur with mood changes.
- A child with ADHD begins to have periods of exaggerated elation, grandiosity, depression, no need for sleep, inappropriate sexual behaviors.
- A child with ADHD has recurrent severe mood swings, temper outbursts, or rages.
- A child with ADHD has hallucinations and/or delusions.
- A child with ADHD has a strong family history of bipolar disorder in his or her family, particularly if the child is not responding to appropriate ADHD treatments.

Note: A child may have both ADHD and BP. Moreover, the noted clinical situations may also be due to other psychiatric disorders (unipolar depression, substance abuse), medical problems (thyroid problems, seizures, tumors), use of medications (prednisone), and environmental stressors (family conflict, chaotic environment, sexual or physical abuse) that may coexist with ADHD.
(Reprinted from Birmaher B: *New Hope for Children and Adolescents with BP Disorders.* New York, Three Rivers Press, a division of Random House, Inc., 2004, with permission.)

ASSESSMENT

This section briefly describes instruments and rating scales used to assess BP symptoms in youth. For further information regarding these scales and for the description of instruments related to the assessment of depressive, suicidal, and other psychiatric conditions, see Chapter 4.2 (28, 39, 40).

Psychiatric Interviews

There are several structured and semistructured interviews that can be used for the diagnosis of BP. The most widely used interviews in BP studies are two similar instruments: the Kiddie Schedule for Affective Disorders and Schizophrenia for School Age Children—Present and Lifetime version (K-SADS-PL) (41) and the Washington University KSADS (WASH-U-KSADS) (42). However, these interviews are lengthy and time-consuming and are mainly used for research purposes. Thus, symptom checklists based on the DSM criteria for BP as well as depressive disorders are also useful.

For any of the interview methods noted above, when assessing mood episodes it is important to evaluate their frequency, intensity, number, and duration (FIND) (30).

Clinician-Based Rating Scales

Two clinician-based rating scales are currently used for the assessment of manic symptoms and their severity in youth, the Young Mania Rating Scale (YMRS) (43, 44) and the KSADS

TABLE 5.4.2.5

BIPOLAR DISORDER VS. DISRUPTIVE BEHAVIOR DISORDER

- If the behavior problems *only* occur while the child is in the midst of an episode of mania or depression, and the behavior problems disappear when the mood symptoms improve, the diagnoses of oppositional or conduct disorder should not be made.
- If a child has "off and on" oppositional or conduct symptoms or these symptoms only appear when the child has mood problems, the diagnosis of BP (or other disorders such as recurrent unipolar depression or substance abuse) should be considered.
- If the child had oppositional behaviors before the onset of the mood disorders, both diagnoses may be given.
- If a child has severe behavior problems that are not responding to treatment, consider the possibility of a mood disorder (bipolar and nonbipolar depressions), other psychiatric disorder (ADHD, substance abuse), and/or exposure to stressors.
- If a child has behavior problems and a family history of BP disorder, consider the possibility that the child has a mood disorder (unipolar major depression or BP disorder).
- If a child has behavior problems and is having hallucinations and delusions consider the possibility of BP disorder. Also consider the possibility of schizophrenia, use of illicit drugs/alcohol, or medical/neurological conditions.

(Reprinted from Birmaher B: *New Hope for Children and Adolescents with BP Disorders*. New York, Three Rivers Press, a division of Random House, Inc., 2004, with permission.)

Mania Rating Scale that was derived from the KSADS-P mania module (KSADS- MRS) (45). However, further studies to evaluate the validity of these rating scales are necessary.

Youth, Parent, and Teacher Rating Scales

It appears that parental reports are more effective in identifying mania than youth or teacher reports (46). The General Behavior Inventory (GBI) (47, 48), the parent version of the YMRS (P-YMRS) (49), and more recently the Child Mania Rating Scale for Parents about their children (CMRS-P) (50) have been shown to have appropriate psychometric properties and be useful for the screening of BP symptoms in youth, but further studies to evaluate the specificity of these instruments for BP are warranted.

Other parent-report instruments have been used to screen for BP in youths, but these instruments were not designed specifically for mania. For example, the CBCL has been used to identify a pattern of psychopathology associated with mania (42, 51–54). A consistent pattern of elevated scores was noted on Aggressive Behavior, Attention Problems, Delinquent Behavior, and Anxious/Depressed profile (55–57). However, the sensitivity of the CBCL for identifying mania was substantially lower than that of the mania-specific instruments cited above (57, 58). Low scores are helpful in "ruling out" mania (or any psychopathology) while high scores are not useful for "ruling in" mania (57, 58). For this reason, mania-specific scales are preferable in screening, over a more general scale such as the CBCL.

Mood Timelines or Diaries

Mood timelines or diaries using school years, birthdays, and holidays as anchors are very helpful in the assessment of the onset and course of mood disorders. These instruments use colors or ratings from 0 to 10 to chart daily changes in mood along with any corresponding significant stressors, illnesses, and treatments. These instruments can help children, parents, and clinicians to visualize the course of their mood, and identify events that may have triggered the depression, hypomania/mania, or irritability and examine the relationship between treatment and response.

Other Assessments

Clinicians should always evaluate for psychosocial functioning, family psychopathology, ongoing negative life events (family conflicts, abuse), child's functioning in several areas (peer relationships, school functioning), and for the presence of psychiatric and medical conditions and suicidal and homicidal ideation (for instruments to evaluate these domains, see the respective chapters). If necessary, once the child's mood is stable, psychoeducational testing is warranted (Chapter 4.2.4).

Also, the clinician together with the child and parents should evaluate the appropriate intensity and restrictiveness of care (hospitalization). The decision for the level of care will depend on factors such as the severity of mood symptoms, presence of suicidal and/or homicidal symptoms, psychosis, substance dependence, agitation, child's and parents' adherence to treatment, parental psychopathology, and family environment.

At the present time, no biological or imaging tests are clinically available for the diagnosis of BP.

COURSE AND OUTCOME

Although there are methodological differences among the current pediatric prospective naturalistic studies, they have consistently shown that 70% to 100% of children and adolescents with BP will eventually recover (e.g., no significant symptoms for 2 months) from their index episode (Table 5.4.2.6) (14, 15, 25, 59–62). However, of those who recover, up to 80% will experience one or more recurrences in a period of 2–5 years. These studies as well as retrospective reports (63–70) have shown high rates of hospitalizations and health service utilization, psychosis, suicide attempts and completion, switch from BP-NOS to BP-I or II, and from BP-II to BP-I, substance abuse, unemployment, legal problems, and poor academic and psychosocial functioning. The ongoing BP symptoms also have negative impact on the family, marital, and sibling relationships, as well as on family economics. The considerable impairment in psychosocial functioning reported in these studies is not only due to the fact that most of them were carried out in clinical samples, because similar findings have been reported in BP adolescents never referred for treatment (24, 25).

Recent studies have shown that BP is not only manifested by punctuated recovery and recurrences, but by ongoing fluctuating syndromal and subsyndromal symptomatology (14–16). In fact, in a recent 2-year follow-up study, for approximately 60% of the observation time, BP youth experienced syndromal and subsyndromal BP symptoms, particularly depressive and mixed symptoms (15) (Figure 5.4.2.1). In addition, pediatric BP frequently manifests with repeated changes in symptom polarity (10, 14–16, 28). These rapid fluctuations in mood appear to be more accentuated than in adults with BP (71) and may

TABLE 5.4.2.6

PROSPECTIVE NATURALISTIC STUDIES OF YOUTH WITH BP

Study	BP Diagnoses/Origin of Most of the Sample	Mean Age (Years)	Sample Size	Frequency and duration of Follow-Up (Months)	% of Remission/ Recovery*	% Relapse/ Recurrence*
Strober et al., 1995	BP-I, inpatients	16	54	Every 6 months for 60 months	98%	44%
Lewinsohn et al., 1995	BP-I, II, NOS community	16	18	Once after 14 months	?	?
Lewinsohn et al., 2000	BP-I, II, NOS community	17	17	Once at age 24	65% by age 19 88% by age 24	27%
Srinath et al., 1998	BP-I, outpatients	14	30	Once after 4–5 years	100%	67%
Birmaher, 2004	BP-I outpatients	17	73	Every 6 months for 19 months	68%	59%
Geller et al., 2004	BP-I, mania outpatients	11	86	Every 6 months for 3 years and then at 1 year for 48 months	87%	70%
Jairam et al., 2004	BP-I outpatients	14	25	Every 6 months for 52 months	100%	64%
Birmaher et al., 2006	BP-I, II, NOS outpatients	13	263	Every 6 months for 24 months	70%	50%

*Some investigators did not differentiate between the terms remission/recovery or relapse/recurrences.
BP = bipolar disorder; NOS = not otherwise specified.

explain, at least in part, the difficulties encountered diagnosing and treating BP symptoms in youth (15) (Figure 5.4.2.2).

Across the extant studies, early age of onset, long duration, low SES, mixed or rapid cycling episodes, psychosis, subsyndromal symptoms, comorbid disorders, exposure to negative life events, and family psychopathology are associated with worse course and outcome.

RISK FACTORS

Twin, Adoption, and Family Studies

Twin and adoption studies have demonstrated that BP runs in families (28, 72–74). The prevalence of BP in first-degree relatives of adults with BP is increased eight- to ten-fold over the expected prevalence of BP in community samples of adults, making BP one of the most familial psychiatric disorders (28, 73–75). However, the rates of BP in relatives of BP subjects may be underestimated because most BP high-risk studies included only offspring of BP parents older than 18 years (73, 76, 77), without considering that many adults with BP experienced their first symptoms of BP early in life (2, 17, 18).

A metaanalysis of the high-risk child BP ("top-down") literature reported that offspring of BP parents had on average a 5.4% lifetime prevalence of BP as compared to 0.0% in offspring of healthy parents (77). More recent studies reported a rate of up to 15% (78, 79). Moreover, preliminary analyses of a large high-risk BP study that included as controls offspring of healthy as well as parents with non-BP psychiatric

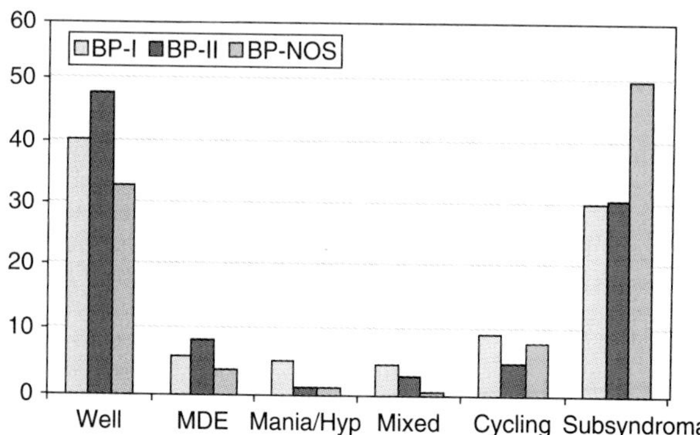

FIGURE 5.4.2.1. Comparison of weekly symptom status (the percentage of followup weeks spent asymptomatic or symptomatic in different mood categories during a 2-year prospective followup) between youth with BP-I, II and NOS. BP = bipolar disorder; NOS: not otherwise specified. (Birmaher B, Axelson D, Strober M, et al.: Clinical course of children and adolescents with bipolar spectrum disorders. *Arch Gen Psychiatry* 63:175–183, 2006.)

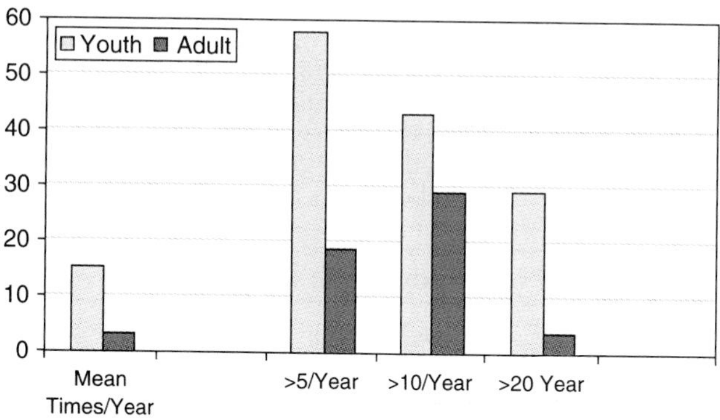

FIGURE 5.4.2.2. Change in polarity: Switch between depression and mania/hypomania or vice versa with or without intervening weeks at the asymptomatic status. Comparison between youth with BP-I vs. adults with BP-I. All comparisons are significant at $p < .001$. (Data from Birmaher B, Axelson D, Strober M, et al.: Clinical course of children and adolescents with bipolar spectrum disorders. *Arch Gen Psychiatry* 63:175–183, 2006; and Judd LL, Akiskal HS, Schettler PJ, et al.: The long-term natural history of the weekly symptomatic status of bipolar I disorder. *Arch Gen Psychiatry* 59:530–537, 2002.

disorders and raters blind to parental diagnosis, showed that in comparison with children of community controls, children of BP parents had a seven-fold higher risk to develop BP (20). However, it is important to note that children of BP parents are not only at high risk to develop BP, but depression, anxiety, ADHD, and behavioral problems as well (20, 76, 77).

In addition to high risk family investigations, "bottom-up" studies of childhood-onset BP also provide further evidence of the familial nature of BP (28). These studies have shown increased risk for BP and depression in first-degree relatives of children and adolescents with BP when compared with relatives of adolescents with other disorders (24, 80). Further, the first-degree relatives of youth whose BP started early in life, adolescents with subsyndromal symptoms of BP, and BP children with comorbid ADHD showed a significantly increased risk for mood disorders when compared with youth without these factors (24, 81).

Genetic Studies

Extant literature has demonstrated a genetic etiology for BP with an estimated heritability at over 80% (72, 75, 82, 83). There has been an intensive search for susceptibility genes and recent metaanalyses of linkage studies have identified several plausible regions on chromosomes 13q, 22q, 9p22.3–21.1, 10q11.21–22.1, and 14q24.1–32.12 (72, 84, 85). Variation in ascertainment, phenotype definition, control selection, limited power, and possible confounding by population substructure have lead to inconsistent results. Nevertheless, current studies suggest that multiple (interacting) loci may contribute to BP liability.

Neuroimaging Studies

Preliminary structural and functional imaging studies have shown changes in several areas of the brain, such as white matter hyperintensities (WMH) in both cortical and subcortical regions, smaller volumes of the amygdala, hippocampus and cingulate gyrus, and reduced gray matter volume in the dorsolateral prefrontal cortex (DLPFC) (86–92).

Preliminary proton magnetic resonance spectroscopy (^{1}H-MRS) studies have also suggested that substances that serve as markers for neuronal integrity such as N-acetyl-aspartate (NAA), choline, myo-inositol, and creatine/phosphocreatine (Cr) are affected in the fronto-striatal region, cingulate cortex, DLPFC and other areas of the brain (93–97). These markers have also been found altered in offspring of bipolar parents (98, 99). These results need to be taken with caution because they include small samples in various phases of illness (depressed, hypomanic, euthymic) and subjects had factors that may confound findings, such as the presence of comorbid disorders and medications.

Neurocognitive Function

Preliminary investigations have found several cognitive deficits, such as difficulties in attentional set-shifting, visuospatial memory, verbal memory and executive function in BP youth (100–103). These studies have limitations similar to those described under neuroimaging studies above, but a recent study suggested that some cognitive deficits appear to be independent of state of the illness or medication status (104).

Psychosocial Factors

Very few studies have evaluated the effects of psychosocial factors on the onset and maintenance of BP in youth. These studies have suggested that low socioeconomic status (SES), exposure to negative events, and high "expressed-emotion" (EE) are associated with poor prognosis (14, 15, 105). In BP adults, high EE, negative events, poor sleep hygiene, and poorly daily routines have been associated with increased risk for recurrences (73, 106).

TREATMENT

Phases of Treatment

The treatment of BP is usually divided into acute, continuation, and maintenance phases. The main goal of the acute treatment is to control or ameliorate the acute BP symptoms that are affecting the child's psychosocial functioning and wellbeing or endangering the child's life. Continuation treatment is required to consolidate the response during the acute phase and avoid relapses and maintenance treatment to avoid recurrences. Pharmacological and psychosocial treatment strategies for each one of these three treatment phases is discussed below. In general, the choice of treatment depends on the severity, phase of illness, subtype of BP, chronicity, comorbid disorders, subject's age, family and patient preference and expectations, availability of experts in psychotherapy, family and environmental circumstances, and family psychopathology.

During each of the three treatment phases noted above, if a child does not respond to treatment, factors associated with nonresponse need to be considered, such as misdiagnosis, poor adherence to treatment, presence of comorbid psychiatric and medical conditions, and ongoing exposure to negative events (family conflict, abuse).

Psychoeducation and Support

At any phase of treatment, basic elements of support are always indicated, including active listening, restoration of hope and reversal of demoralization for the child and his/her parents, and case management (negotiation with school and/or parents about reasonable expectations) (107–110). In addition, family members and the patient should be educated about the causes, symptoms, course, and different treatments of BP and the risks associated with these treatments as opposed to no treatment at all. The patient and family should be prepared for what is likely to be a recurrent and often chronic illness with frequent fluctuations in the child's mood and the importance to have good adherence to treatment.

To assist with psychoeducation, dedicated associations (www.bpkids.org) and several books are now available (109, 110).

As described below, psychoeducation is a common component of most psychosocial treatments and seems to improve treatment adherence and reduce the mood symptoms (111–114). It is critical to help parents understand that the negativity and rapid mood swings are not a reflection of oppositionality in misbehaving children, but symptoms of BP with secondary emotional conflict accruing from a chronic illness. Often, it is hard to accept the illness and therefore, to adhere to treatment. A great deal of time is needed to impress upon the families the need for medication and accompanying psychological treatment. Sleep hygiene and routine are important, especially in view of sleep deprivation leading to worsening of symptoms. Ensuring a stable circadian rhythm is meant to have a positive effect on physiology and daily functioning. School personnel also need education to help them understand the disease model of BP, and to advocate along with the family for adequate accommodations (schedule, workload) to the patient's current difficulties.

Acute Treatment

In this chapter, the term mood stabilizer refers to lithium and anticonvulsants such as valproate, carbamazepine and lamotrigine. However, the extant literature seems to indicate that the atypical antipsychotics also operate as mood stabilizers.

Most of the current treatment evidence is derived from open-label, retrospective analyses, case reports, and small randomized controlled trials (RCTs) and are summarized in more detail in the 10-year review of BP (28) and treatment guidelines for children with BP (30). Until the results of ongoing large RCTs are available, recommendations regarding the acute treatment of pediatric BP disorder should be considered preliminary.

In general, and until further studies are available, doses of mood stabilizers and atypical antipsychotics and blood levels of mood stabilizers are similar to those used in adults with BP. It appears that the pharmacokinetics of these medications is similar across age (e.g., Dutta) (115). However, children have shown lower brain-to-serum lithium concentration ratios than adults, suggesting that youth may need higher serum lithium concentrations (116).

In any case, to avoid unnecessarily high dosages and increase the risk of side effects and poor adherence to treatment, unless the child is too agitated, it is recommended to start at low dosages and increase slowly according to response and side effects.

PHARMACOTHERAPY

Mania/Mixed Episodes

Current studies suggest that monotherapy with lithium, valproate, or carbamazepine are comparable in treating nonpsychotic mania/mixed episodes, with responses ranging from 40% to 50% (28, 30, 117–121). Further, recent studies have suggested that the atypical antipsychotics are equally efficacious as the common mood stabilizers, and appear to yield a quicker response (122–124). Moreover, combination of two mood stabilizers such as lithium and valproate or a mood stabilizer with an atypical antipsychotic appears to be superior to mood stabilizer monotherapy for the acute treatment of manic or mixed episodes, with responses ranging between 60% and 90% (122, 125–129).

In general, monotherapy with lithium, an atypical antipsychotic, or valproate is preferable as the first line of treatment for acute manic/mixed episodes (30). For subjects who do not respond to the initial monotherapy trial or who do not tolerate the medication's side effects, treatment with one of the other mood stabilizers or an atypical antipsychotic not previously tried is recommended (30). For subjects with severe agitation or a partial response to monotherapy with a mood stabilizer, the combination of two mood stabilizers, or of a mood stabilizer with an atypical antipsychotic is indicated (30).

For patients with mania/mixed mania with psychosis, a mood stabilizer combined with an atypical antipsychotic is the first choice (30, 127, 128). However, atypical antipsychotic monotherapy may serve as an alternative choice. For adolescents with severe illnesses that are resistant to these treatments, electroconvulsive therapy (ECT) should be considered (130).

Hypomania

There are no studies in children and adolescents that specifically address the treatment of hypomania. Therefore, until research is available, for those youth whose hypomanic symptoms significantly impair their function, similar treatments to those described for mania are recommended.

Depression

Despite that youth with BP spend substantial amounts of time on syndromal or subsyndromal depressive symptoms that significantly impair their psychosocial functioning and increase their risk for suicide (3, 15), there are no RCTs and very few open-label studies for children and adolescents with BP depression.

In adults, monotherapy with lithium, valproate, atypical antipsychotics, or lamotrigine, and the combination of mood stabilizers or atypical antipsychotics with the serotonin reuptake inhibitors (SSRIs) or bupropion have been found efficacious for the acute treatment of BP depression (131, 132). Using similar treatments, open-label studies and case reports in small samples of depressed BP youth suggest that these medications may be efficacious, but RCTs are needed to confirm these findings (133–138).

In youth, a retrospective study suggested that the selective serotonin reuptake inhibitors (SSRIs) may be helpful for the treatment of depression (139), but the SSRIs or other antidepressants may trigger mania, hypomania, mixed episodes or rapid cycling, particularly when used without concomitant mood stabilizer treatment. When using lamotrigine, gradual titration of the dose is essential, particularly if the child is also taking valproate, to avoid serious rash. The SSRIs or other antidepressants should be prescribed with caution and in small doses, after stabilization of manic or hypomanic symptoms with mood stabilizers or atypical antipsychotic agents. Also, attention should be paid to possible increase or onset of agitation, suicidality, and serotonin syndrome (see Chapter 5.4.1).

Until these studies become available, and taking into account the limitations of extrapolating from the adult literature, it is recommended to use lamotrigine, lithium, valproate or the atypical antipsychotics as first-line medications for BP depression. For partial or non-responders, combinations of these medications with atypical antipsychotics, SSRIs, or bupropion is indicated.

As described below, specific psychosocial treatments designed for BP patients appear to be efficacious for the treatment of BP symptoms, particularly depression. Psychosocial treatments found efficacious for the treatment of unipolar depression such as cognitive-behavioral therapy (CBT) (140, 141) or interpersonal psychotherapy (IPT) (142) and dialectic behavior therapy (DBT) (143, 144) may also be utilized for the treatment of BP depression, but studies for BP youth are needed.

For subjects with recurrent seasonal depression, light therapy should be considered (145). For adolescents with severe and treatment resistant disorders, electroconvulsive treatment (ECT) may be indicated (130). Other treatments such as transcranial magnetic therapy (TMS) (146), or augmentation with omega-3 fatty acids (132) are yet to be evaluated for the treatment of BP depression in youth.

Rapid Cycling

There are no specific studies for the treatment of rapid cycling in youth. Until these studies become available, the same treatments as for mania or mixed episodes are recommended (28, 30, 120)

Adjunctive Medications

Almost all studies use short-term adjuvant medications or rescue paradigms during the acute phase of treatment with monotherapy or combination regimes. This strategy, in fact, becomes inevitable in managing breakthrough symptoms of mania in BP disorder. Lorazepam and clonazepam sometimes are temporarily used for the management of acute agitation or insomnia.

Psychosocial Treatments

In addition to supportive psychotherapy, specific psychosocial treatments have been developed to manage acute manic and depressive symptoms and prevent recurrences, improve adherence to treatment, and manage comorbid conditions. A central feature encompassing all psychosocial treatment models includes education, problem solving, and coping skills. Parents are closely engaged in their children's therapy and referred to treatment if they have any significant psychiatric disorders.

Thus far, there are three lines of overlapping psychosocial therapies, designed to fit specific age groups and methods of delivery, for example group versus individual treatment. First, child and family focused cognitive behavior therapy (CFF-CBT) was specifically designed for 8–18 year olds with BP (147). It integrates the principles of reward-based CBT with interpersonal psychotherapy, with an emphasis on empathic validation. This model attempts to address parental cognitions and prepares them to cope as well as improve their relationship with affected offspring. Second, Fristad et al. (112, 113) employed a multiple family group treatment for youths aged 8 to 12 years with bipolar and depressive spectrum disorders. This method confers a heavy emphasis on psychoeducation around the role of medications and coping strategies. Third, Miklowitz et al. (2004) (108), developed a manualized version of family focused therapy (FFT) specifically for adolescents with BP that addresses their concerns about having this serious illness, the need for mood stabilizing medications, and building resources to manage stress and lower expressed emotions within the family. A preliminary study using FFT for adolescents with BP showed symptomatic improvement in mania, depression, and behavior problems at the end of 1 year of follow-up (108).

Finally, psychosocial treatments that have been found efficacious for the treatment of comorbid conditions such as oppositional behaviors, substance abuse, and anxiety disorder are indicated (see respective chapters).

CONTINUATION AND MAINTENANCE TREATMENTS

Randomized controlled trials in adults have established the efficacy of lithium, lamotrigine, and atypical antipsychotics as compared to placebo for prevention of new mood episodes in stable BP adults, and some data support the use of valproate as maintenance therapy (148, 149). The literature examining ongoing treatment for pediatric BP is limited. An 18-month naturalistic followup study of BP adolescents who were stable on lithium therapy found a relapse rate of 92% in adolescents who stopped lithium treatment, compared to 38% to those who continued with lithium (150). Two controlled studies have been published examining how pediatric BP patients who remitted from acute manic symptoms while taking combination treatment, responded to a switch to monotherapy. In the first, six out of 14 BP adolescents who were stabilized from an acute psychotic manic episode after 4 weeks of treatment with lithium and an antipsychotic relapsed within 1 week of discontinuation of the antipsychotic (127, 128). In the second, subjects stabilized on lithium and valproate combination therapy were switched to either drug alone as monotherapy (126). There was no difference between the two drugs and the majority of subjects had relapsed within 4 months of switching to monotherapy. Fortunately, an extended followup phase of this study found that approximately 90% of the subjects who had a mood relapse responded to restarting the combination treatment (151).

The most current consensus recommendations from experts in pediatric BP suggest that medication taper may be considered once remission has been maintained for 12–24 months (30). However, it may be reasonable to consider shorter treatment in cases when the diagnosis is not clearly established or the illness has been relatively mild. Conversely, severe and recurrent illness may merit more prolonged maintenance pharmacotherapy. The optimal duration of psychosocial treatments for pediatric BP has not been established. Given that bipolar disorder may be best viewed as a chronic disease, it is reasonable to provide some level of ongoing psychosocial support, crisis management, and formal therapy booster sessions when appropriate.

ACUTE AND LONG-TERM PHARMACOTHERAPY SIDE EFFECTS

For a comprehensive review of these and other psychotropics used in the treatment of BP, refer to Chapter 6.1.2. In this section we highlight practical aspects of the pharmacological management of BP.

Lithium

The most serious problem associated with acute and long-term lithium therapy is that of toxicity due to elevated lithium blood levels. Lithium has a low therapeutic index, and severe lithium toxicity can cause permanent renal and neurological damage, as well as death. Though initial signs and symptoms of toxicity usually do not manifest until blood levels are above 1.5 mEq/L, tolerability varies among patients and some individuals will be symptomatic at lower blood levels. The risk of lithium toxicity can be reduced by a number of basic steps. Patients and family members must be aware of the signs of lithium toxicity: dizziness, clumsiness, unsteady gait, slurred speech, coarse tremors, abdominal pain, vomiting, sedation, confusion, and blurry vision. Basically, the subject intoxicated with lithium looks and acts like a "drunk" person and in these cases a stat lithium level is indicated. If a patient has difficulty with taking fluids or has excessive fluid loss (nausea, vomiting, diarrhea, febrile illness), lithium doses should be reduced or temporarily held until regular fluid intake is maintained. If other symptoms of lithium toxicity occur in addition to gastrointestinal distress, referral for immediate evaluation is necessary. Dose escalation should be conservative, especially in outpatient settings, and blood levels should be obtained as early as 4 days after each dose increase, and immediately if clinical symptoms of toxicity occur. Patients should be counseled to maintain adequate hydration during vigorous exercise or on hot days, and avoid major changes in salt, caffeine, or fluid intake. In addition, they must notify physicians and pharmacists that they are taking lithium, and do not take substances that interact with lithium. Common nonprescription drugs and substances that can elevate lithium levels include most nonsteroidal antiinflammatory drugs (not acetaminophen), alcohol, and marijuana. Caffeine tends to lower lithium levels. The list of prescription drugs that interact with lithium is long and should be checked prior to prescribing any new medication.

Lithium has a number of different potential side effects associated with short and long-term treatment, which may be particularly bothersome to youth (acne, increased weight,

TABLE 5.4.2.7

LITHIUM SIDE EFFECTS

Common	Polyuria, polydipsia, tremor, weight gain, nausea, diarrhea, hypothyroidism, cognitive dulling, sedation, leukocytosis
Uncommon	New onset or exacerbation of acne or psoriasis, bradycardia, hair loss, ECG changes (T-wave flattening)
Rare	Kidney, brain damage and death (due to acute toxicity), decreased renal function, pseudotumor cerebri, extrapyramidal symptoms, movement abnormalities, nystagmus, seizure, hyperparathyroidism, sinus node dysfunction, arrhythmias

and polyuria) (see Table 5.4.2.7). Patients have a wide range of tolerability to lithium, with some having minimal or manageable side effects while others will have significant problems. Sometimes side effects can be ameliorated by dose reduction or by switching between extended release and immediate release preparations.

Two issues that require ongoing monitoring are the potential for kidney damage and hypothyroidism. Lithium inhibits the renal tubular response to antidiuretic hormone, which decreases the ability to concentrate urine and leads to polyuria. Evidence from biopsy studies in adults indicate that is some cases lithium can lead to chronic interstitial nephritis (152). However, selection bias and the fact that similar changes have been found in adult psychiatric patients who have not been treated with lithium make it difficult to determine how much lithium treatment elevates the risk of kidney damage (152). Studies of the effects of lithium on glomerular function have generally showed minimal to mild reductions associated with long-term treatment. These data have made it difficult to know how to monitor for the undetermined but likely low risk of developing clinically significant kidney damage. A conservative monitoring approach is noted in Table 5.4.2.8. The decision to refer for renal consultation and/or discontinue lithium treatment remains one of clinical judgment, though a significant change in serum creatinine should trigger a thorough evaluation.

Lithium frequently inhibits the thyroid gland. Approximately 25% of youth developed elevated thyroid stimulating hormone (TSH) levels within 3 months of initiating lithium treatment (153). The long-term effects on the thyroid have not been determined in a pediatric population, and TSH levels can be just transiently elevated in bipolar adults initiating lithium treatment (154). Given the developmental implications, clear hypothyroidism induced by lithium in children and adolescents will require intervention. Whether to treat or discontinue lithium in patients with subclinical hypothyroidism is less clear. However, if lithium is clearly helping the individual, thyroid replacement treatment is indicated.

Preliminary evidence of subtle neuropsychiatric problems associated with elevated TSH levels and reduced mood stability in bipolar adults associated with lower levels of free T4 or higher levels of TSH indicate that intervention may be reasonable (154–156).

Valproate

Valproate has gastrointestinal, neurological, and cognitive side effects that usually can be minimized by careful titration or

TABLE 5.4.2.8

ROUTINE LABORATORY MONITORING BEFORE AND DURING PHARMACOTHERAPY

Medication	Baseline Tests	Follow-up	Test Frequency*	Comments
Lithium	BUN, creatinine, TSH, free T4, urinalysis, CBC, electrolytes, calcium, albumin, height, weight, BMI	Lithium level	Each dose change and q 3–6 months	24-hour urine for protein and creatinine clearance if marked polyuria, proteinuria, or change in serum creatinine
		BUN, creatinine, TSH, free T4, urinalysis, calcium, albumin, height, weight BMI	q 3–6 months	
Valproate	CBC with differential & platelet count, AST, ALT, lipase, height, weight, BMI menstrual history	Valproate level and platelet count, AST, ALT	q 2weeks × 2, then q month × 2, then q 3–6 months and with each dose change	Risk of hepatic failure is highest in first 6 months of treatment
		Height, weight, BMI, menstrual history	Each appointment	Repeat lipase if pancreatitis suspected
Carbamazepine	CBC with differential & platelet count, AST, ALT, sodium	Carbamazepine level, CBC with differential and platelet count, AST, ALT, sodium	1 and 3–4 weeks after dose change and then q 3–6 months	Check labs if unexplained fever, sore throat, lymphadenopathy or severe fatigue
Antipsychotics	Glucose, triglycerides, total cholesterol, HDL, LDL, AIMS, height, weight, BMI	Glucose, triglycerides, total cholesterol, HDL, LDL	3 months after start, then q 6–12 months	Check metabolic status if substantial weight gain
		AIMS	q 3–6 months	
	For ziprasidone EKG	Height, weight, BMI EKG as necessary	Every appointment	

Note: A pregnancy test should be performed in all post-menarchal females at baseline and whenever pregnancy is a possibility over followup.
*Follow-up tests should be performed whenever clinical symptoms of serious side effects occur. Abbreviations: BMI—body mass index; BUN—blood urea nitrogen; TSH—thyroid-stimulating hormone; AST—aspartate aminotransferase; ALT—alanine aminotransferase; CBC—complete blood count; HDL—high-density lipoprotein; LDL—low-density lipoprotein; AIMS—Abnormal Involuntary Movement Scale. EKG—electrocardiogram.

TABLE 5.4.2.9

VALPROATE SIDE EFFECTS

Common	Weight gain, tremor, nausea, diarrhea, cognitive dulling, sedation, fatigue, ataxia, dizziness
Uncommon	Serum transaminase elevations, alopecia, elevated testosterone, polycystic ovarian syndrome, rash, hair loss
Rare	Hepatic failure, thrombocytopenia, pancreatitis, severe dermatological reactions, myelosuppression, anticonvulsant hypersensitivity syndrome

dose reduction. (Table 5.4.2.9) Periodic blood tests are often performed in order to monitor for the rare but serious side effects (hepatic failure, pancreatitis, thrombocytopenia), although it is controversial as to whether this reduces the risk of serious adverse events and it may be justified to perform followup lab tests only when patients show symptoms (157). It is very important that patients and family members are aware of the initial symptomatic presentations of these side effects and know to obtain an urgent assessment if they occur. For instance, hepatotoxicity can present with symptoms of vomiting, nausea, anorexia, lethargy, drowsiness and facial edema. Mild elevations of serum transaminases do occur during treatment and are of questionable clinical significance unless they are more than three times the normal level. The risk of hepatic failure is most elevated in children under the age of 3, in those who have metabolic or neurological disorders, and those who are taking multiple anticonvulsants.

Although uncertain, valproate has been associated with polycystic ovarian syndrome. Thus, baseline menstrual history an a gynecological consultation of any female who develops significant changes in her menstrual cycle and/or hirsutism while on this medication is warranted.

Carbamazepine

As with valproate, carbamazepine has neurological, cognitive, and gastrointestinal side effects that can usually be managed by dose adjustment, as well as rare serious side effects that are difficult to prevent via routine blood monitoring (Table 5.4.2.10). Decreases in platelet and white blood cell counts are not uncommon during carbamazepine treatment, but they do not necessarily predict subsequent development of aplastic anemia or agranulocytosis. Carbamazepine does induce its own metabolism, as well as other drugs that are metabolized by the hepatic cytochrome P450 1A2 and 3A4 isoenzymes. Therefore blood levels must be repeated several weeks after dose changes and care must be taken when other medications are coadministered (such as oral contraceptives), as they may not reach therapeutic levels.

TABLE 5.4.2.10

CARBAMAZEPINE SIDE EFFECTS

Common	Nausea, vomiting, clumsiness, dizziness, nystagmus, sedation, blurred vision, diplopia, cognitive dulling, ataxia, photosensitivity CYP450 enzyme-induction (increased clearance of drugs metabolized by hepatic cytochrome system, including oral contraceptives)
Uncommon	Hyponatremia, rash, confusion, leukopenia
Rare	Serious dermatological reactions, agranulocytosis, aplastic anemia, atrioventricular block, arrhythmias, hepatitis, renal dysfunction, anticonvulsant hypersensitivity syndrome

TABLE 5.4.2.11

LAMOTRIGINE SIDE EFFECTS

Common	Dizziness, ataxia, headache, tremor, blurred vision, diplopia
Uncommon	Rash, nausea, vomiting, ataxia, cognitive dulling, confusion
Rare	Serious dermatological reactions, anemia, anticonvulsant hypersensitivity syndrome

Lamotrigine

The neurological and cognitive side effects of lamotrigine are similar to other anticonvulsants, and are usually managed by dose adjustment (see Table 5.4.2.11). The most concerning problem with lamotrigine treatment is the development of serious dermatological reactions such as Stevens-Johnson syndrome (SLS) or toxic epidermal necrolysis (TEN). Though rare, these reactions are more common in children than adults, and it is difficult to predict whether a rash will progress to SJS or TEN. Therefore, unless a new rash is clearly attributable to something other than lamotrigine, treatment should be suspended. The rate of serious dermatological reactions may be reduced by current dosing recommendations that prescribe small and gradual dose escalation, in particular with the concomitant use of valproate.

Atypical Antipsychotics

The atypical antipsychotics have some differences in side effect profiles, though there are some side effects that are common to all of them in varying degrees (Table 5.4.2.12). In general, there has been increasing concern about the metabolic effects (e.g., increased weight, glucose, and lipids) of some of these medications, which is of substantial concern when these agents are used in children and adolescents over extended periods of time. Routine monitoring parameters have not been established, but it is recommended to measure the child's body mass index (BMI), and fasting glucose and lipids before and routinely (every 6 months and whenever clinical symptoms indicate) while taking these medications. If a patient exhibits significant weight gain, it should prompt a more thorough investigation of metabolic status and a reevaluation of the risk–benefit ratio of continuation of the current atypical antipsychotic.

Although much less often than the typical antipsychotics, the atypical antipsychotics may cause extrapyramidal symptoms, tardive dyskinesia, and neuroleptic malignant syndrome; thus, the need to evaluate the child at baseline and routinely for abnormal movements. Finally, the long-term side effects including chronic hyperprolactinemia associated with the atypicals have not been well studied.

MONITORING PHARMACOTHERAPY

Although the medications that are used to treat bipolar disorder have the potential for significant side effects, there

TABLE 5.4.2.12

ATYPICAL ANTIPSYCHOTIC SIDE EFFECTS

Common	Weight gain,* postural hypotension, extrapyramidal symptoms,* dizziness, sedation*
Uncommon	Hyperglycemia, diabetes, hypercholesterolemia, increased triglycerides, hyperprolactinemia,* rash, photosensitivity, nausea, diarrhea, dyspepsia, constipation, elevated serum transaminases, urinary difficulties, sexual dysfunction, cognitive dulling
Rare	Tardive dyskinesia, neuroleptic malignant syndrome, seizure, hepatic failure

*Rate of side effect may vary substantially among the different atypical antipsychotics.

is no evidence whether routine laboratory monitoring reduces the risk of adverse events. Table 5.4.2.8 gives general monitoring guidelines based on recommendations from FDA package inserts and typical practice from our BP research centers. It does not have empirical support and is not a substitute for clinical judgment. In many cases, the benefits of treatment outweigh potential risks even if regular laboratory monitoring is not feasible for a patient. Laboratory tests are not a replacement for clinical evaluation and it is important to review signs and symptoms of potential adverse events with patients and their families as well as emphasize the need to contact the prescribing physician if these symptoms occur.

MANAGEMENT OF COMORBID DISORDERS

It is crucial to treat accompanying comorbid disorders, because they may worsen the prognosis of BP. However, with the exception of a recent controlled study showing the benefits of adding stimulants for the treatment of ADHD in children with BP (158), almost all the existent literature is anecdotal or open-label studies (28, 30).

If the child's comorbid symptoms (hyperactivity, behavior problems) appear to be secondary to the mood disorder (mania, depression, or both), it is recommended first to optimize treatment of the BP. If the comorbid conditions cannot be attributed to BP or do not improve after the symptoms of mania/hypomania subside, treatment for both the BP and the comorbid conditions is indicated. However, in general, before treating the comorbid disorder(s), it is recommended first to stabilize the symptoms of BP.

Once the BP symptoms are stabilized, if it is still necessary to treat the comorbid conditions, it is recommended to use the best available medications and/or psychosocial treatments for each specific comorbid disorder (see respective chapters in this book and the American Academy of Child and Adolescent Psychiatry treatment parameters for each condition). It is important to begin treatment for each comorbid disorder sequentially. Also, since some medications may cause mood dysregulation, if appropriate, psychosocial treatments should be tried before adding new medications (e.g., cognitive behavior therapy for anxiety disorders). For youths with BP and certain psychiatric or medical conditions, sometimes the use of medications for BP may also target the other disorder (valproate for BP and seizures).

SUMMARY AND FUTURE DIRECTIONS

BP is a recurrent familial disorder that frequently emerges early in life and is associated with significant morbidity and sometimes mortality due to suicide. Pediatric BP usually follows an ongoing changeable and sinuous course, with patients having a wide spectrum of mood symptoms that can range from mild to severe depression, mania, and/or hypomania. These results explain, at least in part, the difficulties encountered when treating subjects with BP-spectrum disorders. Furthermore, it is likely that the very rapid fluctuation in mood symptoms, combined with the developmental issues influencing the clinical picture of BP in youth, the difficulties children and sometimes adolescents have verbalizing their emotions, and the high rates of comorbid disorders, account for the complexity and current controversies in diagnosing children and adolescents with BP.

As reviewed in this chapter, it is clear that youth may manifest classical symptoms of BP. However, most children and adolescents do not fulfill the current DSM BP-I or II criteria for the diagnoses mainly because they lack the required duration of symptoms. Moreover, most children and adolescents referred to be evaluated for BP have severe mood lability, "affective storms", irritability, verbal and/or physical aggression, and ODD- and ADHD-like symptoms. These youth may have BP, but results from prospective studies such as LAMS and COBY are necessary to ascertain whether these symptoms are the way BP manifests in youth, particularly in young children, prodromal symptoms for more classical manifestations of BP, or only the indication that these youth have severe problems regulating their mood.

The enduring and rapid changeability of symptoms of this illness in children and adolescents from very early in life and at crucial stages of their lives deprive them of the opportunity for normal emotional, cognitive, and social development (10, 14–16, 24, 25, 28, 159). Moreover, this illness negatively affects parents' and siblings' relationships and family economics. Thus, early recognition and acute and maintenance treatment of BP in children and adolescents is of utmost importance to ameliorate ongoing syndromal and subsyndromal symptomatology and to reduce or prevent the serious psychosocial morbidity that usually accompanies this illness (28).

The few existent pharmacological studies have suggested that the mood stabilizers and atypical antipsychotics alone or in combination may be helpful for the acute treatment of this disorder. However, randomized controlled pharmacological and psychosocial acute and maintenance studies to reduce the risk of recurrences as well as the effects of maturity, family environment, and parental psychopathology on treatment response, and the long-term side effects of pharmacological treatments in youth are urgently needed. Also, there is a need to tease out the longitudinal effects of these comorbid disorders above and beyond the effects of the BP disorder and the correct treatment of these comorbid conditions.

Algorithms for the acute treatment of youth with BP have been developed and the reader is encourage to examine them (20, 120). However, due the scarcity of RCTs, these recommendations need to be taken as preliminary.

Future studies evaluating possible preventative strategies for youth at high risk for BP disorder are indicated. Also, studies to evaluate and analyze the positive or negative contributions to the child's outcome of factors such as the child's cognitive development, social, and coping skills and the environment where the child lives are warranted. Regarding this last factor, important issues such as parental lifetime and current psychopathology, support, exposure to negative events (abuse, poor school or neighborhoods, ongoing family conflicts) should be considered.

Finally, genetic and other biological studies including pharmacogenetic and further studies correlating the effects of treatment and biochemical changes on the brain are warranted (160, 161).

ACKNOWLEDGMENTS

This work was supported in part by NIMH grants MH59929 and MH60952. The authors would like to thank Carol Kostek for her assistance with manuscript preparation and Andrès Martin for carefully reviewing the manuscript.

References

1. Kraepelin E: *Manic Depressive Insanity and Paranoia*. London, E & S Livingstone, 1921.
2. Egeland JA, Shaw JA, Endicott J, et al.: Prospective study of prodromal features for bipolarity in well Amish children. *J Am Acad Child & Adolesc Psychiatry* 42:786–796, 2003.
3. Axelson D, Birmaher B, Strober M, et al.: Phenomenology of children and adolescents with bipolar spectrum disorders. *Arch Gen Psychiatry* 63:1139–1148, 2006.
4. Kowatch RA, Youngstrom EA, Danielyan A, et al.: Review and meta-analysis of the phenomenology and clinical characteristics of mania in children and adolescents. *Bipolar Disord* 7:483–496, 2005.
5. National Institutes of Mental Health. Research Roundtable on Prepubertal Bipolar Disorder. *J Am Acad Child Adolesc Psychiatry* 40:871–878, 2001.
6. Geller B, Zimerman B, Williams M, et al.: Phenomenology of prepubertal and early adolescent bipolar disorder: Examples of elated mood, grandiose behaviors, decreased need for sleep, racing thoughts and hypersexuality. *J Child Adolesc Psychopharmacol* 12:3–9, 2002.
7. Geller B, Zimerman B, Williams M, et al.: DSM-IV mania symptoms in a prepubertal and early adolescent bipolar disorder phenotype compared to attention-deficit hyperactive and normal controls. *J Child Adolesc Psychopharmacol* 12:11–25, 2002.
8. Leibenluft E, Charney DS, Towbin KE, et al.: Defining clinical phenotypes of juvenile mania. *Am J Psychiatry* 160:430–437, 2003.
9. Leibenluft E, Blair RJR, Charney DS, et al.: Irritability in pediatric mania and other childhood psychopathology. *Annals of the New York Academy of Sciences* 1008:201–218, 2003.
10. Biederman J, Faraone SV, Wozniak J, et al.: Further evidence of unique developmental phenotypic correlates of pediatric bipolar disorder: Findings from a large sample of clinically referred preadolescent children assessed over the last 7 years. *J Affect Disord* 82S:S45–S58, 2004.
11. Mick E, Spencer T, Wozniak J, et al.: Heterogeneity of irritability in Attention-Deficit Hyperactivity Disorder subjects with and without mood disorders. *Biol Psychiatry* 58:576–582, 2005.
12. Wozniak J, Biederman J, Kiely K, et al.: Mania-like symptoms suggestive of childhood-onset bipolar disorder in clinically referred children. *J Am Acad Child Adolesc Psychiatry* 34:867–876, 1995.
13. Biederman J, Faraone SV, Chu MP, et al.: Further evidence of a bidirectional overlap between juvenile mania and conduct disorder in children. *J Am Acad Child Adolesc Psychiatry* 38:468–476, 1999.
14. Geller B, Tillman R, Craney JL, et al.: Four-year prospective outcome and natural history of mania in children with a prepubertal and early adolescent bipolar disorder phenotype. *Arch Gen Psychiatry* 61:459–467, 2004.
15. Birmaher B, Axelson D, Strober M, et al.: Clinical course of children and adolescents with bipolar spectrum disorders. *Arch Gen Psychiatry* 63:175–183, 2006.
16. Findling RL, Gracious BL, McNamara NK, et al.: Rapid, continuous cycling and psychiatric co-morbidity in pediatric bipolar I disorder. *Bipolar Disord* 3:202–210, 2001.
17. Chengappa KN, Kupfer DJ, Frank E, et al.: Relationship of birth cohort and early age at onset of illness in a bipolar disorder case registry. *Am J Psychiatry* 160:1636–1642, 2003.
18. Lish JD, Dime-Meenan S, Whybrow PC, et al.: The National Depressive and Manic-depressive Association (DMDA) survey of bipolar members. *J Affect Disord* 31:281–294, 1994.
19. Geller B, Williams M, Zimerman B, et al.: Prepubertal and early adolescent bipolarity differentiate from ADHD by manic symptoms: Grandiose delusions; ultra-rapid or ultradian cycling. *J Affect Disord* 51:81–91, 1998.
20. Birmaher B: Offspring of bipolar parents. Presented at the 52nd Annual Meeting of the American Academy of Child and Adolescent Psychiatry, Toronto, Canada, October 2005.
21. Gershon ES, Hamovit JH, Guroff JJ, et al.: Birth cohort changes in manic and depressive disorders in relatives of bipolar and schizoaffective patients. *Arch Gen Psychiatry* 44:314–319, 1987.
22. Klerman GL, Lavori PW, Rice JP, et al.: Birth-cohort trends in rates of major depressive disorder among relatives of patients with affective disorder. *Arch Gen Psychiatry* 42:689–693, 1985.
23. Ryan N, Williamson DE, Iyengar S, et al.: A secular increase in child and adolescent onset affective disorder. *J Am Acad Child Adolesc Psychiatry* 31:600–605, 1992.
24. Lewinsohn P, Klein D, Seeley J, et al.: Bipolar disorders in a community sample of older adolescents: Prevalence, phenomenology, comorbidity, and course. *J Am Acad Child Adolesc Psychiatry* 34:454–463, 1995.
25. Lewinsohn PM, Klein DN, Seeley JR.: Bipolar disorder during adolescence and young adulthood in a community sample. *Bipolar Disord* 2:281–293, 2000.
26. Verhulst F, vanderEnde J, Ferdinand R, et al.: The prevalence of DSM-III-R diagnoses in a national sample of Dutch adolescents. *Arch Gen Psychiatry* 54:329–336, 1997.
27. Angold A, Costello EJ, Erkanli A: Comorbidity. *J Child Psychol Psychiatry* 40:57–87, 1999.
28. Pavuluri MN, Birmaher B, Naylor M: Pediatric bipolar disorder: Ten year review. *J Am Acad Child Adolesc Psychiatry* 44:846–871, 2005.
29. Wilens TE, Biederman J, Millstein RB, et al.: Risk for substance use disorders in youths with child- and adolescent-onset bipolar disorder. *J Am Acad Child Adolesc Psychiatry* 38:680–5, 1999.
30. Kowatch RA, Fristad M, Birmaher B, et al.: and The Child Psychiatric Workgroup on Bipolar Disorder. Treatment guidelines for children and adolescents with bipolar disorder. *J Am Acad Child Adolesc Psychiatry* 44:213–235, 2005.
31. Birmaher B, Ryan ND, Williamson DE, et al.: Childhood and adolescent depression: A review of the past ten years. *Part I, J Am Acad Child Adolesc Psychiatry* 35:1427–1439, 1996.
32. Geller B, Zimerman B, Williams M, et al.: Bipolar disorder at prospective follow-up of adults who had prepubertal major depressive disorder. *Am J Psychiatry* 158:125–127, 2001.
33. Kovacs, M: Presentation and course of major depressive disorder during childhood and later years of the life span. *J Am Acad Child Adolesc Psychiatry* 35:705–715, 1996.
34. Strober M, Carlson G: Bipolar illness in adolescents with major depression. *Arch Gen Psychiatry* 39:549–555, 1982.
35. Weissman MM, Wolk S, Goldstein RB, et al.: Depressed adolescents grown up. *JAMA* 281:1707–1713, 1999.
36. Weissman MM, Wolk S, Wickramaratne P, et al.: Children with prepubertal-onset major depressive disorder and anxiety grown up. *Arch Gen Psychiatry* 56:794–801, 1999.
37. Martin A, Young C, Leckman JF, et al.: Age effects on antidepressant-induced manic conversion. *Arch Pediatr Adolesc Med* 158:773–780, 2004.
38. Wilens TE, Wyatt D, Spencer TJ: Disentangling disinhibition. *J Am Acad Child Adolesc Psychiatry* 37:1225–1227, 1998.
39. American Academy of Child and Adolescent Psychiatry. Practice parameter for the psychiatric assessment of children and adolescents. King RA and the Work Group on Quality Issues. *J Am Acad Child Adolesc Psychiatry* 36(10 Suppl):4S–20S, 1997.
40. Myers K, Winters NC: Ten-year review of rating scales. II: Scales for internalizing disorders. *J Am Acad Child Adolesc Psychiatry* 41:634–659, 2002.
41. Kaufman J, Birmaher B, Brent D, et al.: (1997). Schedule for Affective Disorders and Schizophrenia for School-Age Children—Present and Lifetime Version (K-SADS-PL):Initial reliability and validity data. *J Am Acad Child Adolesc Psychiatry* 36:980–988, 1997.
42. Geller B, Warner K, Williams M, et al.: Prepubertal and young adolescent bipolarity versus ADHD: Assessment and validity using the WASH-U-KSADS, CBCL, and TRF. *J Affect Disord* 51:93–100, 1998.
43. Young RC, Biggs JT, Ziegler VE, et al.: A rating scale for mania: reliability, validity and sensitivity. *Br J Psychiatry* 133:429–435, 1978.
44. Fristad MA, Weller EB, Weller RA: The Mania Rating Scale: Can it be used in children? A preliminary report. *J Am Acad Child Adolesc Psychiatry* 31:252–257, 1992.
45. Axelson D, Birmaher B, Brent D, et al.: A preliminary study of the Kiddie Schedule for Affective Disorders and Schizophrenia for School-Age Children mania rating scale for children and adolescents. *J Child Adolesc Psychopharmacol* 13:463–470, 2004.
46. Youngstrom E, Findling R, Calabrese J, et al.: Comparing the diagnostic accuracy of six potential screening instruments for bipolar disorder in youth aged 5 to 17 years. *J Am Acad Child Adolesc Psychiatry* 43:847–858, 2004.
47. Findling R, Youngstrom E, Danielson C, et al.: Clinical decision-making using the General Behavior Inventory in juvenile bipolarity. *Bipolar Disord* 4:34–42, 2002.
48. Danielson CK, Youngstrom EA, Findling RL, et al.: Discriminative validity of the general behavior inventory using youth report. *J Abnorm Child Psychol* 31:29–39, 2003.
49. Gracious BL, Youngstrom EA, Findling RL, et al.: Discriminative validity of a parent version of the Young Mania Rating Scale. *J Am Acad Child Adolesc Psychiatry* 41:1350–1359, 2002.
50. Pavuluri MN, Henry D, Devineni B, et al.: Child Mania Rating Scale: Development, reliability and validity. *J Am Acad Child Adolesc Psychiatry* 45:550–560, 2006.
51. Biederman J, Wozniak J, Kiely K, et al.: CBCL clinical scales discriminate prepubertal children with structured interview-derived diagnosis of mania

from those with ADHD. *J Am Acad Child Adolesc Psychiatry* 34:464–471, 1995.
52. Carlson GA, Kelly KL: Manic symptoms in psychiatrically hospitalized children—What do they mean? *J Affect Disord* 51:123–135, 1998.
53. Dienes K, Chang K, Blasey C, et al.: Characterization of children of bipolar parents by parent report CBCL. *J Psychiatr Res* 36:337–345, 2002.
54. Hazell PL, Lewin TJ, Carr VJ: Confirmation that Child Behavior Checklist clinical scales discriminate juvenile mania from attention deficit hyperactivity disorder. *J Paediatr Child Health* 35:199–203, 1999.
55. Mick E, Biederman J, Pandina G, et al.: A preliminary meta-analysis of the Child Behavior Checklist in pediatric bipolar disorder. *Biol Psychiatry* 53:1021–1027, 2003.
56. Kahana SY, Youngstrom EA, Findling RL, et al.: Employing parent, teacher, and youth self-report checklists in identifying pediatric bipolar spectrum disorders: An examination of diagnostic accuracy and clinical utility. *J Child Adolesc Psychopharmacol* 13:471–488, 2003.
57. Youngstrom EA, Findling RL, Youngstrom JK, et al.: Toward an evidence-based assessment of pediatric bipolar disorder. *J Clin Child Adolesc Psychol* 34:433–448, 2005.
58. Youngstrom EA, Meyers OI, Demeter C, et al.: Comparing diagnostic checklists for pediatric bipolar disorder in academic and community mental health settings. *Bipolar Disord* 7:507–517, 2005.
59. Birmaher B: Bipolare und Depressive Storungen im Kindes—und Jugendalter. In: Maneros A (ed): *Das Neue Handbuch der Bipolaren und Depressiven Erkrankungen*. Stuttgart, Germany, George Thieme Verlag Publications, 2004, pp. 573–590.
60. Jairam R, Srinath S, Girimaji SC, et al.: A prospective 4–5 year follow-up of juvenile onset bipolar disorder. *Bipolar Disord* 6:386–394, 2004.
61. Strober M, Freeman R, Bower S, et al.: Recovery and relapse in adolescents with bipolar affective illness: a five-year naturalistic, prospective follow-up. *J Am Acad Child Adolesc Psychiatry* 34:724–731, 1995.
62. Srinath S, Janarolha N, Reddy YC, et al.: A prospective study of bipolar disorder in children and adolescents from India. *Acta Psychiatrica Scandinavica* 98:437–442, 1998.
63. Bashir M, Russell J, Johnson G: Bipolar affective disorder in adolescence: A 10-year study. *Aust N Z J Psychiatry* 21:36–43, 1987.
64. Carlson G, Davenport Y, Jamison K: A comparison of outcome in adolescent- and late-onset bipolar manic-depressive illness. *Am J Psychiatry* 134:919–922, 1977.
65. Carlson GA, Bromet EJ, Driessens C, et al.: Age at onset, childhood psychopathology, and 2-year outcome in psychotic bipolar disorder. *Am J Psychiatry* 159:307–309, 2002.
66. Jarbin H, Ott Y, Von Knorring AL: Adult outcome of social function in adolescent-onset schizophrenia and affective psychosis. *J Am Acad Child Adolesc Psychiatry* 42:176–183, 2003.
67. McGlashan TH: Adolescent versus adult onset of mania. *Am J Psychiatry* 145:221–223, 1988.
68. Rajeev J, Srinath S, Reddy Y, et al.: The index manic episode in juvenile-onset bipolar disorder: The pattern of recovery. *Can J Psychiatry* 48:52–55, 2003.
69. Welner A, Welner Z, Fishman R: Psychiatric adolescent inpatients: Eight- to ten-year follow-up. *Arch Gen Psychiatry* 36:698–700, 1979.
70. Werry JS, McClellan JM: Predicting outcome in child and adolescent (early onset) schizophrenia and bipolar disorder. *J Am Acad Child Adolesc Psychiatry* 31:147–150, 1992.
71. Judd LL, Akiskal HS, Schettler PJ, et al.: The long-term natural history of the weekly symptomatic status of bipolar I disorder. *Arch Gen Psychiatry* 59:530–537, 2002.
72. Althoff RR, Faraone SV, Rettew DC, et al.: Family, twin, adoption, and molecular genetic studies of juvenile bipolar disorder. *Bipolar Disord* 7:598–609, 2005.
73. Goodwin F, Jamison K: *Manic Depressive Illness*. New York, Oxford University Press, 1990.
74. Neuman RJ, Geller B, Rice JP, et al.: Increased prevalence and earlier onset of mood disorders among relatives of prepubertal versus adult probands. *J Am Acad Child Adolesc Psychiatry* 36:466–473, 1997.
75. Tsuang MT, Faraone SV: *The Genetics of Mood Disorders*. Baltimore, Johns Hopkins University Press, 1990.
76. DelBello MP, Geller B: Review of studies of child and adolescent offspring of bipolar parents. *Bipolar Disord* 3:325–334, 2001.
77. Lapalme M, Hodgins S, LaRoche C: Children of parents with bipolar disorder: A metaanalysis of risk for mental disorders. *Can J Psychiatry* 42:623–631, 1997.
78. Chang KD, Steiner H, Ketter TA. Psychiatric phenomenology of child and adolescent bipolar offspring. *J Am Acad Child Adolesc Psychiatry* 39:453–460, 2000.
79. Henin A, Biederman J, Mick E, et al.: Psychopathology in the offspring of parents with bipolar disorder: A controlled study. *Biol Psychiatry* 58:554–561, 2005.
80. Strober M, Morrell W, Burroughs J, et al.: A family study of bipolar I disorder in adolescence. Early onset of symptoms linked to increased familial loading and lithium resistance. *J Affect Disord* 15:255–268, 1988.
81. Faraone S V, Biederman J, Mennin D, et al.: Attention-deficit hyperactivity disorder with bipolar disorder: A familial subtype? *J Am Acad Child Adolescent Psychiatry* 36:1378–1387, 1997.
82. McGuffin P, Rijsdijk F, Andrew M, et al.: The heritability of bipolar affective disorder and the genetic relationship to unipolar depression. *Arch Gen Psychiatry* 60:497–502, 2003.
83. NIMH Genetics Workgroup Report: Genetics and mental disorders. *Biol Psychiatry* 45:559–602, 1999.
84. Badner, JA, Gershon ES: Meta-analysis of whole-genome linkage scans of bipolar disorder and schizophrenia. *Mol Psychiatry* 7:405–411, 2002.
85. Segurado R, Detera-Wadleigh SD, Levinson DF, et al.: Genome scan meta-analysis of schizophrenia and bipolar disorder. Part III: Bipolar disorder. *Am J Hum Genet* 73:49–62, 2003.
86. Botteron KN, Vannier MW, Geller B, et al.: Preliminary study of magnetic resonance imaging characteristics in 8- to 16-year-olds with mania. *J Am Acad Child Adoles Psychiatry* 34:742–749, 1995.
87. Blumberg H, Kaufman J, Martin A, et al.: Amygdala and hippocampal volumes in adolescents and adults with bipolar disorder. *Arch Gen Psychiatry* 60:1201–1208, 2003.
88. DelBello MP, Zimmerman ME, Mills NP, et al.: Magnetic resonance imaging analysis of amygdala and other subcortical brain regions in adolescents with bipolar disorder. *Bipolar Disord* 6:43–52, 2004.
89. Dickstein DP, Milham MP, Nugent AC, et al.: Fronto-temporal alterations in pediatric bipolar disorder: results of a voxel-based morphometry study. *Arch Gen Psychiatry* 734–741, 2005.
90. Frazier JA, Chiu S, Breeze JL, et al.: Structural brain magnetic resonance imaging of limbic and thalamic volumes in pediatric bipolar disorder. *Am J Psychiatry* 162:1256–65, 2005.
91. Kaur S, Sassi RB, Axelson D, et al.: Cingulate cortex anatomical abnormalities in children and adolescents with bipolar disorder. *Am J Psychiatry* 162:1637–1643, 2005.
92. Pillai JJ, Friedman L, Stuve TA, et al.: Increased presence of white matter hyperintensities in adolescent patients with bipolar disorder. *Psychiatry Res Neuroimaging* 114:51–56, 2002.
93. Castillo M, Kwock L, Courvoisie H, et al.: Proton MR spectroscopy in children with bipolar affective disorder: Preliminary observations. *Am J Neuroradiol* 21:832–838, 2000.
94. Cecil KM, DelBello MP, Sellars MC, et al.: Proton magnetic resonance spectroscopy of the frontal lobe and cerebellar vermis in children with a mood disorder and a familial risk for bipolar disorders. *J Child Adolesc Psychopharmacol* 13:545–555, 2003.
95. Chang K, Adleman NE, Dienes K, et al.: Anomalous prefrontal-subcortical activation in familial pediatric bipolar disorder: A functional magnetic resonance imaging investigation. *Arch Gen Psychiatry* 61:781–792, 2004.
96. Davanzo P, Yue K, Thomas MA, et al.: Proton magnetic resonance spectroscopy of bipolar disorder versus intermittent explosive disorder in children and adolescents. *Am J Psychiatry* 160:1442–1452, 2003.
97. Sassi RB, Stanley JA, Axelson D, et al.: Reduced NAA levels in the dorsolateral prefrontal cortex of young bipolar patients. *Am J Psychiatry* 162:2109–15, 2005.
98. Chang K, Karchemskiy A, Barnea-Goraly N, et al.: Reduced amygdalar gray matter volume in familial pediatric bipolar disorder. *J Am Acad Child Adolesc Psychiatry* 44:565–573, 2005.
99. Chang K, Adleman N, Dienes K, et al.: Decreased N-acetylaspartate in children with familial bipolar disorder. *Biol Psychiatry* 53:1059–1065, 2003.
100. Dickstein DP, Treland JE, Snow J, et al.: Neuropsychological performance in pediatric bipolar disorder. *Biol Psychiatry* 55:32–39, 2004.
101. McClure E, Pope K, Hoberman A, et al.: Facial expression recognition in adolescents with mood and anxiety disorders. *Am J Psychiatry* 160:1–3, 2003.
102. Rich BA, Schmajuk M, Perez-Edgar, et al.: The impact of reward, punishment and frustration on attention in pediatric bipolar disorder. *Biol Psychiatry* 58:532–539, 2005.
103. Olvera RL, Semrud-Clikeman M, Pliska SR, et al.: Neuropsychological deficits in adolescents with conduct disorder and cormorbid bipolar disorder: a pilot study. *Bipolar Disord* 6:1–11, 2005.
104. Pavuluri MN, Schenkel LS, Aryal S, et al.: Neurocognitive function in unmedicated manic and medicated euthymic pediatric bipolar patients. *Am J Psychiatry* 163:286–93, 2006.
105. Miklowitz DJ, Goldstein MJ, Nuechterlein KH, et al.: Family factors and the course of bipolar affective disorder. *Arch Gen Psychiatry* 45, 225–231, 1988.
106. Hlastala SA, Frank E, Kowalski J, et al.: Stressful life events, bipolar disorder, and the "kindling model". *J Abnorm Psychol* 109:777–786, 2000.
107. Colom F, Vieta E: A perspective on the use of psychoeducation, cognitive-behavioral therapy and interpersonal therapy for bipolar patients. *Bipolar Disord* 6:480–486, 2004.
108. Miklowitz DJ, George EL, Axelson DA, et al.: Family-focused treatment for adolescents with bipolar disorder. *J Affect Disord* 82:113–128, 2004.
109. Birmaher B: *New Hope for the Treatment of Children and Teens with Bipolar Disorder*. New York, Three Rivers Press, 2004.
110. Fristad MA, Goldberg JS: *Raising a Moody Child: How to Cope with Depression and Bipolar Disorder*. New York, Guilford, 2003.
111. Brent DA, Poling K, McKain B, et al.: A psychoeducational program for families of affectively ill children and adolescents. *J Am Acad Child Adolesc Psychiatry* 32:770–774, 1993.

112. Fristad MA, Gavazzi SM, Mackinaw-Koons B: Family psychoeducation: An adjunctive intervention for children with bipolar disorder. *Biol Psychiatry* 53:1000–1008, 2003.
113. Fristad MA, Goldberg-Arnold JS, Gavazzi SM: Multi-family psychoeducation groups in the treatment of children with mood disorders. *Marital Fam Ther* 29:491–504, 2003.
114. Renaud J, Brent DA, Baugher M, et al.: Rapid response to psychosocial treatment for adolescent depression: A two-year follow-up. *J Am Acad Child Adolesc Psychiatry* 37:1184–1190, 1998.
115. Dutta S, Zhang Y, Conway JM, et al.: Diavalproex-ER pharmacokinetics in older children and adolescents. *Pediatr Neurol* 30:330–337, 2004.
116. Moore CM, Demopulos CM, Henry ME, et al.: Brain-to-serum lithium ratio and age: An *in vivo* magnetic resonance spectroscopy study. *Am J Psychiatry* 159:1240–2, 2002.
117. Geller B, Cooper TB, Sun K, et al.: Double-blind and placebo-controlled study of lithium for adolescent bipolar disorders with secondary substance dependency. *J Am Acad Child Adolesc Psychiatry* 37:171–178, 1998.
118. Kowatch RA, Suppes T, Carmody TJ, et al.: Effect size of lithium, divalproex sodium, and carbamazepine in children and adolescents with bipolar disorder. *J Am Acad Child Adolesc Psychiatry* 39:713–720, 2000.
119. Kafantaris V, Coletti DJ, Dicker R, et al.: Lithium treatment of acute mania in adolescents: A large open trial. *J Am Acad Child Adolesc Psychiatry* 42:1038–1045, 2003.
120. Pavuluri MN, Henry DB, Devineni B, et al.: A pharmacotherapy algorithm for stabilization and maintenance of pediatric bipolar disorder. *J Am Acad Child Adolesc Psychiatry* 43:859–867, 2004.
121. Wagner KD, Weller EB, Carlson GA, et al.: An open-label trial of divalproex in children and adolescents with bipolar disorder. *J Am Acad Child Adolesc Psychiatry* 41:1224–1230, 2002.
122. DelBello MP, Schwiers ML, Rosenberg HL, et al.: A double-blind, randomized, placebo-controlled study of quetiapine as adjunctive treatment for adolescent mania. *J Am Acad Child Adolesc Psychiatry* 41:1216–1223, 2002.
123. DelBello MP, Kowatch RA, Adler CM, et al.: A double-blind randomized pilot study comparing quetiapine and divalproex for adolescent mania. *J Am Acad Child Adolesc Psychiatry* 45:305–313, 2006.
124. Strakowski SM, DelBello MP, Kowatch R, et al.: A single-blind prospective study of quetiapine for the treatment of mood disorders in adolescents who are at high risk for developing bipolar disorder. *Am College Neuropsychopharmacol* 30:240, 2005.
125. Findling RL, McNamara NK, Gracious BL, et al.: Combination lithium and divalproex sodium in pediatric bipolarity. *J Am Acad Child Adolesc Psychiatry* 42:895–901, 2003.
126. Findling RL, McNamara NK, Youngstrom EA, et al.: Double-blind 18-month trial of lithium versus divalproex maintenance treatment in pediatric bipolar disorder. *J Am Acad Child Adolesc Psychiatry* 44:409–17, 2005.
127. Kafantaris V, Coletti DJ, Dicker R, et al.: Adjunctive antipsychotic treatment of adolescents with bipolar psychosis. *J Am Acad Child Adolesc Psychiatry* 40:1448–1456, 2001.
128. Kafantaris V, Dicker R, Coletti DJ, et al.: Adjunctive antipsychotic treatment is necessary for adolescents with psychotic mania. *J Child Adolesc Psychopharmacol* 11:409–413, 2001.
129. Pavuluri MN, Henry D, Naylor M, et al.: A prospective trial of combination therapy of risperidone with lithium or divalproex sodium in pediatric mania. *J Affect Disord* 82 (Suppl 1):103–11, 2004.
130. Ghaziuddin N, Kutcher SP, Knapp P and the Work Group on Quality Issues: Practice parameter for the use of ECT with adolescents. *J Am Acad Child Adolesc Psychiatry* 43:1521–1539, 2004.
131. Goldberg JF, Ghaemi SN: Benefits and limitations of antidepressants and traditional mood stabilizers for the treatment of bipolar depression. *Bipolar Disord* 7:3–12, 2005.
132. Gao K, Calabrese JR: Newer treatment studies for bipolar depression. *Bipolar Disord* Suppl 5:13–23, 2005.
133. Carandang CG, Maxwell DJ, Robbins DR, et al.: Lamotrigine in adolescent mood disorders. *J Am Acad Child Adolesc Psychiatry* 42, 750–751, 2003.
134. Chang K, Kirti S, Meghan H: An open-label study of lamotrigine adjunct or monotherapy for the treatment of adolescents with bipolar depression. *J Am Acad Child Adolesc Psychiatry* 45:298–304, 2006.
135. Kusumakar V, Yatham LN: An open study of lamotrigine in refractory bipolar depression. *Psychiatry Res* 72:145–8, 1997.
136. Patel NC, DelBello MP, Bryan HS, et al.: Open-label lithium for the treatment of adolescent bipolar depression. *J Am Acad Child Adolesc Psychiatry* 45:289–297, 2006.
137. Swope GS, Hoopes SP, Amy LS, et al.: An open-label study of lamotrigine in adolescents with bipolar mood disorder [abstract]. Presented at the 157th Annual Meeting of the American Psychiatric Association, New York, NY, May 1–6, 2004.
138. Saxena K, Howe M, Chang K: Lamotrigine adjunct or monotherapy for adolescent bipolar depression or mixed mania [abstract]. Presented at the 158th Annual Meeting of the American Psychiatric Association, Atlanta, GA, May 21–26, 2005.
139. Biederman J, Mick E, Spencer TJ, et al.: Therapeutic dilemmas in the pharmacotherapy of bipolar depression in the young. *J Child Adolesc Psychopharmacol* 10:185–192, 2000.
140. Brent DA, Holder D, Kolko D, et al.: A clinical psychotherapy trial for adolescent depression comparing cognitive, family, and supportive therapy. *Arch Gen Psychiatry*, 54:877–885, 1997.
141. Lam DH, Hayward P, Watkins ER, et al.: Relapse prevention in patients with bipolar disorder: Cognitive therapy outcome after 2 years. *Am J Psychiatry* 162:324–329, 2005.
142. Mufson L, Weissman MM, Moreau D, et al.: Efficacy of interpersonal psychotherapy for depressed adolescents. *Arch Gen Psychiatry* 56:573–579, 1999.
143. Linehan M: *Skills Training Manual for Treating Borderline Personality.* New York, Guilford, 1993.
144. Miller AL, Rathus JH, Linehan MM, et al.: Dialectical behavior therapy adapted for suicidal adolescents. *J Practical Psychiatry and Behavioral Health*, 3:78–86, 1997.
145. Swedo SE, Allen AJ, Glod CA, et al.: A controlled trial of light therapy for the treatment of pediatric seasonal affective disorder. *J Am Acad Child Adolesc Psychiatry* 36:816–821, 1997.
146. Quintana H: Transcranial magnetic stimulation in persons younger than the age of 18. *J ECT.* 21:88–95, 2005.
147. Pavuluri, MN, Graczyk PA, Henry DB, et al.: Child- and family-focused cognitive-behavioral therapy for pediatric bipolar disorder: development and preliminary results. *J Am Acad Child Adolesc Psychiatry* 43:528–537, 2004.
148. Muzina DJ, Calabrese JR: Maintenance therapies in bipolar disorder: Focus on randomized controlled trials. *Aust N Z J Psychiatry* 39:652–661, 2005.
149. Vieta E, Goikolea JM: Atypical antipsychotics: newer options for mania and maintenance therapy. *Bipolar Disord* 7 Suppl 4:21–33, 2005.
150. Strober M, Morrell W, Lampert C, et al.: Relapse following discontinuation of lithium maintenance therapy in adolescents with bipolar I illness: a naturalistic study. *Am J Psychiatry* 147:457–461, 1990.
151. Findling RL, McNamara NK, Stansbrey R, et al.: Combination lithium and divalproex sodium in pediatric bipolar symptom restabilization. *J Am Acad Child Adolesc Psychiatry* 45:142–148, 2006.
152. Gitlin M: Lithium and the kidney: An updated review. *Drug Safety* 20:231–243, 1999.
153. Gracious BL, Findling RL, Seman C, et al.: Elevated thyrotropin in bipolar youths prescribed both lithium and divalproex sodium. *J Am Acad Child Adolesc Psychiatry* 43:215–220, 2004.
154. Kleiner J, Altshuler LL, Hendrik V, et al.: Lithium-induced subclinical hypothyroidism: Review of the literature and guidelines for treatment. *J Clin Psychiatry* 60:249–255, 1999.
155. Cole DP, Thase ME, Mallinger AG, et al.: Slower treatment response in bipolar depression predicted by lower pretreatment thyroid function. *Am J Psychiatry* 159:116–121, 2002.
156. Frye MA, Denicoff KD, Bryan AL, et al.: Association between lower serum free T_4 and greater mood instability and depression in lithium-maintained bipolar patients. *Am J Psychiatry* 156:909–1914, 1999.
157. Pellock JM, Willmore LJ: A rational guide to routine blood monitoring in patients receiving antiepileptic drugs. *Neurology* 41:961–964, 1991.
158. Scheffer RE, Kowatch RA, Carmody T, et al.: Randomized, placebo-controlled trial of mixed amphetamine salts for symptoms of comorbid ADHD in pediatric bipolar disorder after mood stabilization with divalproex sodium, *Am J Psychiatry* 162:58–64, 2005.
159. Geller B, Bolhofner K, Craney J, et al.: Psychosocial functioning in a prepubertal and early adolescent bipolar disorder phenotype. *J Am Acad Child Adolesc Psychiatry* 39:1543–1548, 2000.
160. Chang K, Gallelli K, Howe M, et al.: Prefrontal neurometabolite changes following lamotrigine treatment in adolescents with bipolar depression. *Neuropsychopharmacol* 30:102–103, 2005.
161. Davanzo P, Thomas MA, Yue K, et al.: Decreased anterior cingulate myo-inositol/creatine spectroscopy resonance with lithium treatment in children with bipolar disorder. *Neuropsychopharmacol* 24:359–369, 2001.

CHAPTER 5.4.3 ■ SUICIDAL BEHAVIOR IN CHILDREN AND ADOLESCENTS: CAUSES AND MANAGEMENT

CYNTHIA R. PFEFFER

INTRODUCTION

Progress has been made in many areas related to youth suicide prevention, an important mental health problem in the United States and worldwide. This chapter will discuss features of youth suicidal behavior to assist clinicians in recognizing those children and adolescents who are most at risk for suicide and to intervene to prevent fatalities and morbidities arising from suicidal acts. The information reported in this chapter is based on empirical investigations to identify risk factors for youth suicidal behavior. Treatment is discussed with regard to empirical research on efficacy to reduce risk factors for youth suicidal behavior.

Guidelines for a national initiative to prevent youth suicide, published by the Surgeon General of the United States, stimulated renewed intensive efforts for suicide prevention (1). Issues highlighted in this initiative included awareness, intervention, and methodology. Awareness that suicide is a public health problem focused on the reduction of stigma and the enrichment of community resources for suicide prevention. Recommendations included development of a National Strategy for Suicide Prevention involving public and private resources aimed to improve the recognition and treatment of suicide risk by primary care providers, to eliminate barriers in insurance coverage for treatment, to educate families about suicide risk, to implement effective crisis and peer support programs in schools, to use schools and workplaces as referral and access points, and to provide support to those who lose a loved one to suicide. Scientific advances in suicide prevention were considered possible through research on the identification of risk factors, evaluation of suicide prevention interventions, promotion of interagency collaborations to improve identification and treatment of suicidal youth, and reduction of access to lethal suicide methods.

The Surgeon General's report built on the aggressive efforts to eradicate youth suicidal behavior that began in the 1980s with the initiation of innovative research methodologies involving epidemiologic, cross-sectional, psychological autopsy, and longitudinal approaches. Numerous scientific papers published in the 1990s have educated health care professionals and the community about the characteristics of this profound mental health problem.

The definitions of the spectrum suicidal behavior are important to clarify so that a common approach of communicating about youth suicidal risk is possible. The concept of suicidal behavior in children and adolescents includes thoughts about causing intentional self-injury or death (suicidal ideas) and acts that cause intentional self-injury (suicide attempt) or death (suicide) (2, 3). Based on research suggesting that the severity of depression, death preoccupations, and general psychopathology are directly proportional to the severity of suicidal behavior, researchers concluded that suicidal behavior among children and adolescents involves a continuum from nonsuicidal behavior to suicidal ideas, suicide attempts, and suicide (3, 4). These concepts are complicated by cognitive and emotional developmental variations among children and adolescents.

HISTORICAL NOTE

In the early nineteenth century, when Goethe's classic *The Sorrows of Young Werther* was published, an epidemic of youth suicide occurred. This epidemic was attributed to imitation of the book's hero, who shot himself after the breakup of a love relationship. Subsequently, the book was banned in Europe. Issues of imitative suicidal behavior have been empirically studied in the 1980s (5). In 1910, the Vienna Psychoanalytic Society convened a special meeting to evaluate risk factors for youth suicidal behavior (3). Similar to our modern-day concerns, this historic meeting was organized to discuss and understand the causes of the significant rise in youth suicide and to propose means of preventing this tragic problem. Among the participants at this meeting were Federn, Freud, Rank, Steckel, and Tausk. Sigmund Freud, for example, suggested that the most significant influence on youth suicide was conflict with loved persons. He proposed that intensive study of specific suicidal individuals would elucidate dynamic aspects of childhood suicidal behavior. Others offered suggestions about how to decrease stresses, such as school pressure, that may enhance risk of youth suicidal behavior. Many advocated the need to develop systematic techniques to study youth suicidal behavior. These propositions continue to be main foci for prevention of youth suicide in modern times.

A rapid rise in suicide among male 15- to 24-year-olds in the United States began in the late 1960s, peaked in 1977, and has decreased in recent years. Clusters of youth suicide were recognized in the 1980s. This phenomenon stimulated extensive public demands to develop effective suicide prevention strategies. Among methods implemented were programs in schools to increase student awareness about the characteristics of youth suicide and to promote treatment seeking among youth at risk for suicide. Research of such school suicide prevention programs redirected the thinking about the most effective and safe strategies for such suicide prevention efforts (6) and refocused school-based suicide prevention efforts toward identification of youth at risk.

The importance of developing well conceptualized approaches to decrease youth suicide was highlighted in the 1986 Health and Human Services–National Institute of Mental Health Task Force Conferences on Youth Suicidal Behavior. Participants at these conferences included international research experts on youth suicidal behavior.

Recommendations made at the close of these conferences (7) included the need to:

1. Define the term suicide and other aspects of suicidal behavior and to report suicide in national databases more consistently.
2. Develop research to identify the multifaceted elements of youth suicidal behavior.
3. Evaluate the efficacy of treatments for suicidal youth and those at risk.
4. Support and plan appropriate suicide prevention strategies.
5. Educate those providing health care about identification, treatment, and prevention of youth suicidal behavior.
6. Collaborate in the public and private sectors to prevent youth suicide.
7. National attention to this major mental health problem was stimulated by the publication of the Surgeon General's guidelines to prevent youth suicide (1).

EPIDEMIOLOGY

The most recent year for complete death records of the United States Vital Statistics is 2003 (8). The age-adjusted rate of suicide for 15- to 24-year-olds was 9.5 per 100,000, a rate lower than that of 10.5 per 100,000 for all ages. In recent years, the rates of youth suicide have decreased. For example, the rate of suicide for 15- to 24-year-olds in 2003 was less than that of 11.1 per 100,000 in 1998 (9) and 12.4 per 100,000 in 1979. The age-adjusted suicide rate for 15- to 24-year-olds in 2003 is significantly higher than the age-adjusted suicide rate of 0.6 per 100,000 for 5- to 14-year-olds in 2003 (8). Suicide among 15- to 24-year-olds was the third leading cause of death, and in 5- to 14-year-olds the fifth leading cause in 2003. In 2003, there were 3,921 suicides among 15- to 24-year olds and 255 suicides among 5- to 14-year-olds. The recent decrease in youth suicide rates may be related to better identification of youth at risk and more effective treatments.

Suicide rates in the United States in 2003 were highest among white males of all ages.

The age-adjusted suicide rates for white males were followed by those for nonwhite males, white females, and nonwhite females. From 1986 to 1991, suicide among black youths increased more rapidly than among white youths (10). This trend may be attributed to assimilation and loss of traditional cultural support among black youths, as well as higher risk that is associated with increases in social class (11). Rates of suicide are highest among Native Americans (12) and especially among those with high rates of loss of traditional cultural values, unemployment, and alcohol abuse (13).

Compliance of relatives in removing firearms from the home is problematic and a challenge to strategies for suicide prevention (14). Rates of suicide caused by firearms for all ages in 2003 were 5.9 per 100,000 (8). This is the leading cause of completed suicide among youth. Other leading causes of suicide among youth are hanging and poisoning (15).

Reliable national data for suicide attempts do not exist because there is no national registry for suicide attempts. Information about youth nonsuicidal behavior has been derived from the Youth Risk Behavior Surveillance System (16). A nationally representative sample of 1,270 high school students in ninth through twelfth grades in the United States completed this survey (16). Approximately 20% of the students had serious suicidal ideation, with rates of approximately 25% for females and approximately 14% for males in 1999 (16). In the year prior to completing this survey, approximately 8% of the students attempted suicide at least once, with females (10.8%) attempting more than males (5.7%). Approximately 3% of the students sustained serious injury when they attempted suicide. Other reports indicated that approximately 1% of preadolescents living in the community carried out a recent suicide attempt (17) and approximately 34% of adolescent psychiatric inpatients were psychiatrically hospitalized due to a recent suicide attempt (18). Suicide among children and adolescents who had a history of psychiatric hospitalization occurs approximately nine times more often than among children and adolescents in the community (19).

CLINICAL DESCRIPTION

Suicidal ideation and acts are episodic events that have discrete onsets and durations (3). Intent to harm oneself is an essential defining characteristic of suicidal behavior. Suicidal intent may be explicit and strong or it may be ambiguous. Evaluating intentionality often is a difficult clinical task, especially among preadolescents. For example, a 9-year-old boy who was seriously despondent after his dog died threatened to stab himself with a knife during an argument with his mother. He denied that he had thoughts of wanting to kill himself, but stated that he wanted to upset his mother. In this case, the intent was not clear, but the overt behavior was potentially life threatening. In contrast, a 15-year-old girl ingested 127 aspirin tablets after she broke up with her boyfriend. She wanted to kill herself because she felt she "had nothing to live for." In this case, suicidal intent was clearly stated.

Because intentionality often is difficult to identify in children and adolescents, it is helpful for clinicians to consider that self-injurious acts in children and adolescents are potentially suicidal and make efforts to protect such youths from self-harm. In this way, clinicians can be more focused on administering life-sparing interventions rather than to limit their intervention strategies.

It is essential to appreciate that young children will not know that death is final and that it is not until adolescence that comprehension of the finality of death is fully realized. Therefore, in evaluating suicidal behavior in children and adolescents the understanding that death is final is not an essential ingredient in determining whether children or adolescents are suicidal. Concepts about death develop in parallel with children's advancing development (3). Although appreciation of the finality of death may not occur until adolescence, some suicidal adolescents do not have mature concepts of death. Additionally, children's concepts of death may vary. For example, a 7-year-old may understand that because his pet bird has died, it will no longer be alive. However, this child may not understand that if he dies he will never be alive again. Children's understanding of death also may fluctuate. Children may realize that death is final at one time but when severely stressed—for example, by the divorce and arguments of their parents—children may believe that death is reversible. Therefore, it is quite evident that young children, such as preschoolers who do not appreciate the finality of death, can be considered to be suicidal if they wish to carry out a self-destructive act with the goal of causing death.

Children and adolescents, like adults, can plan and carry out suicidal acts using a variety of potentially lethal methods that include shooting, hanging, ingestion, and other suicidal methods involving suffocation, stabbing, running into traffic, burning, and drowning. Females attempt suicide more frequently and use less violent methods than males. Gender differences for suicide methods may account for why suicide rates are higher among males.

ETIOLOGY AND PATHOGENESIS

Suicidal ideation and suicide attempts are psychiatric symptoms whose pathogenesis involves psychiatric disorders, stressful life events, problems in social adjustment, and

TABLE 5.4.3.1

MULTI-AXIAL RISK FACTORS FOR YOUTH SUICIDE

Epidemiological Characteristics
Age, gender, race/ethnicity
Lethal means for suicidal acts
Axis I: Primary Psychiatric Disorders
Presence of a psychiatric disorder
Comorbidity of psychiatric disorders
Mood disorders, disruptive, and substance abuse disorders
Axis II: Developmental and Personality Disorders
Cluster B: Narcissistic, borderline, and antisocial personality disorders
Systems related to personality disorders: aggression, impulsivity, neuroticism
Axis III: Neurobiological Factors
Serotonin neurotransmitter function
Gene × environment interactions: The serotonin transporter gene
Axis IV: Environmental Stress Factors
Family adversity: Losses, violence, abuse, psychiatric disorders, suicidal behavior
Axis V: Psychosocial Functioning
Social maladjustment
Hopelessness, coping mechanisms
Social support, cultural affiliation

sociocultural factors. In addition, the role of genetic factors in suicidal behavior has increasingly become a focus of attention.

A multi-axial approach, similar to that of the *Diagnostic and Statistical Manual of Mental Disorders* (DSM-IV), can be utilized to conceptualize the multiple pathogenic and etiological features of youth suicidal behavior. Factors involved in the incidence and prevalence of youth suicidal behavior may be outlined according to five axes: 1) primary psychiatric disorders, 2) developmental and personality disorders, 3) biological factors, 4) environmental stress factors, and 5) social functioning or coping mechanisms. Table 5.4.3.1 shows risk factors for youth suicide conceptualized within such a multi-axial framework.

Primary Psychiatric Disorders among Youth Suicide Victims

Psychological autopsy studies have provided the most important information about psychosocial characteristics of youth suicide victims. The largest of these studies included 119 youth suicide victims who were younger than 20 years old (20). The methods of these studies involve systematic assessments via interviews of the suicide victim's relatives to determine the psychosocial features of the deceased youth. Because the age of onset of certain psychiatric disorders occurs in late adolescence or young adulthood, risk of suicide associated with these psychiatric disorders, such as schizophrenia, were not evaluated in such studies.

A notable finding in all psychological autopsy studies is that approximately 90% of children and adolescents who committed suicide had a psychiatric disorder at the time of death (20–23). The relative risk for suicide imparted by having a psychiatric disorder varied with each study: approximately 5% (20), 14% (24) and 22% (23). An important implication of this finding is that clinicians should evaluate suicidal risk during *all* evaluations of children and adolescents.

Psychological autopsy studies also documented a high rate of comorbid psychiatric disorders, with rates above 70% (20, 23). This implies that treatment planning may be complex because of the need to provide multiple interventions to address the outcomes related to each psychiatric disorder.

The strongest risk factor for youth suicide is a prior history of a suicide attempt. Prior suicide attempts increase risk for suicide from 51-fold to 89-fold (20, 24). The clinical implication is that inquiry about prior suicide attempts is necessary in evaluating suicidal risk, and such youth should be monitored for new signs of suicidal thinking.

The majority (61%–76%) of youth suicide victims suffered from mood disorders (4, 20, 23). The likelihood of committing suicide is increased 8- to 13-fold in the presence of a current episode of a mood disorder (20, 23, 24). Rates of major depressive disorders among youth suicide victims ranged from 32% to 54% (4, 20, 23, 25). The likelihood of committing suicide was increased 27-fold by the presence of a current episode of major depressive disorder (21). Approximately one-fifth of youth suicide victims were diagnosed as suffering from bipolar disorder, which increased risk for suicide nine-fold (4, 21).

The second most common group of psychiatric disorders was any type of substance abuse disorder, which occurred in approximately 27% to 62% of youth suicide victims (4, 20–23). The likelihood of committing suicide was increased 8.5-fold with a current substance abuse disorder (21). Approximately 43% of suicide victims suffered from comorbid mood and substance abuse disorders (23), a combination that increased risk for suicide 17-fold (21). Substance abuse among suicide victims appears to be a specific characteristic of youth suicide victims as noted in the San Diego Suicide Study, which compared suicide victims older than age 30 years to suicide victims who were younger (26, 27). The youth suicide victims had a higher prevalence of drug abuse, and substance abuse was chronic and prevalent for approximately 9 years among these younger suicide victims. The most frequently abused substances were alcohol, marijuana, and cocaine. The younger suicide victims had a lower prevalence of mood disorders. Another psychological autopsy study highlighted that older adolescent suicide victims, particularly those who were older than 16 years, compared to younger adolescent suicide victims, had higher rates of substance abuse (24). A clinical implication of this report is that specific attention to identifying and treating substance abuse is an important youth suicide prevention strategy.

The New York Psychological Autopsy Study described gender-specific suicide risk factors among youth suicide victims (20). Among males, the likelihood of committing suicide was increased approximately 23-fold with a history of a prior suicide attempt, nine-fold with current major depressive disorder, and seven-fold with current substance abuse disorder. Among females, the likelihood of committing suicide was increased approximately 49-fold with current major depressive disorder and nine-fold with a history of a prior suicide attempt. Implications of these results are that clinicians should be aware to evaluate and plan treatments for gender-specific risk factors for youth suicide.

Psychological autopsy studies of youth suicide victims reported relatively low rates of anxiety disorders (27%), eating disorders (4%), and schizophrenia (4%) (20). Nevertheless, youth suffering from these disorders should be evaluated for suicide risk factors, such as suicidal ideation.

Among youth suicide victims without diagnosed psychiatric disorders, high rates of prior suicidal ideation or suicide attempts, low suicide intent, increased availability of firearms, and disciplinary problems were identified (20, 25, 28).

Primary Psychiatric Disorders among Youth with Nonfatal Suicidal Behavior

Reports of youth at risk for nonfatal suicidal behavior are important to guide clinicians in evaluating and treating risk factors for suicidal ideation and suicide attempts. However, there are few studies of community samples of children and adolescents who attempted suicide and were systematically compared to youth who died as a result of suicide.

Studies of nonfatal suicidal behavior suggest that rates and types of psychiatric disorders are similar for suicide victims and those youth with nonfatal suicidal acts. Approximately 80% of youth who attempted suicide had a psychiatric disorder (29–32). Rates of comorbid mood, substance abuse, and disruptive disorders approximate 80% among adolescents who attempt suicide (33, 34). A high correlation was identified among serious suicide attempts and cannabis abuse or dependence among adolescents in the community (33).

Research with psychiatric patients and youths in the community provided validating information about the significant association of mood disorders and youth suicidal behavior (35). Among child and adolescent psychiatric outpatients with a diagnosis of major depressive disorder, more than 70% reported suicidal ideation or attempts (36). Future suicidal tendencies were best predicted by irritability or anger, past history of suicidal thinking or behavior, and older age.

Prevalence of moderate to severe suicidal ideation in a community sample of 1,542 adolescents was 4% in males and 8.7% in females (37). Prevalence of suicide attempts was 1.9% in males and 1.5% in females. Presence of major depressive disorder imparted a seven-fold increased risk for suicidal ideation and an almost 10-fold increased risk for suicide attempts. Although most studies of community samples included adolescents who attended school, 37% of runaway youths reported a history of a suicide attempt (38). Although females were more likely to have attempted suicide, depression was significantly associated with suicide attempts in males and females.

Complexities exist in relating risk factors for suicide to those youth who actually will attempt or commit suicide. For example, differences between suicidal depressed youth and nonsuicidal depressed youth are difficult to identify (39). A study of adolescent psychiatric inpatients that aimed to identify which aspects of major depressive disorder were associated with suicidal behavior reported that suicidal ideation or acts were significantly associated with severity of depressed mood, intensity of negative self-evaluation, increased level of hopelessness, poor concentration, and high levels of anhedonia (40). The seriousness of suicidal intent was associated with increased degree of depressed mood and elevated degrees of negative self-evaluation. The lethality of suicide attempts was found to be correlated with increased level of depressed mood, elevated negative self-evaluation, intense states of anhedonia, presence of psychomotor agitation, and presence of alcohol or substance abuse. Gender differences have been identified in suicide risk among adolescents with major depressive disorder, with hopelessness being more frequent among females (41).

Reports of population-based studies of adolescents indicated that for males, but not for females, sexual orientation was associated with suicidal intent and suicide attempts (42). Bisexual and homosexual adolescents had higher risk of suicide attempts. Data from 1,007 young adults followed for 21 years in the New Zealand Birth Cohort Study documented that 2.8% who were classified as being gay, lesbian, or bisexual exhibited more suicidal ideation and suicide attempts, as well as more severe symptoms of depression, generalized anxiety, and conduct disorder than the other young adults in this longitudinal study (43).

Follow-up investigations suggest risk factors for youth suicidal behavior. Prospective research indicates that child psychiatric inpatients who attempted suicide are at six-fold increased risk to attempt suicide in adolescence and those who report suicidal ideation are at four-fold increased risk for a suicide attempt in adolescence (44, 45). Adolescent psychiatric inpatients who attempt suicide are at significant risk for a repeat suicide attempt within 6 months of followup (46), and for suicide in less than 10 years (3). Approximately 25% of adolescent psychiatric inpatients were reported to have attempted suicide during the 5 years after psychiatric hospital discharge, but no adolescent committed suicide during this followup period (47). The first year after psychiatric hospital discharge was the period of highest risk. The strongest predictor of a suicide attempt was the number of prior suicide attempts. Mood disorder alone was not a predictor of a posthospitalization suicide attempt, but in conjunction with a history of a suicide attempt, mood disorder predicted a future suicide attempt.

Prepubertal children who have a major depressive disorder are at risk for suicide attempts in adolescence (48) and suicide in young adulthood (49). A 10-year longitudinal followup of children and adolescents suggested that major depressive disorder was related to a seven-fold increased risk for a suicide attempt (50). Clinical implications of these findings are that comprehensive monitoring is warranted for adolescents who were psychiatrically hospitalized after a suicide attempt.

Developmental and Personality Disorders

Although there is evidence that youth with specific developmental disorders are at heightened risk for suicidal behavior, research suggests that IQ per se is not a predictor of youth suicidal behavior. Psychological autopsy studies indicate that approximately one-third of youth suicide victims suffered from a personality disorder, especially antisocial and borderline (21, 51, 52). Some reports indicate higher rates for borderline personality disorders (41%) among youth suicide victims (52). Additionally, narcissistic or schizoid traits have been identified to be frequent among youth suicide victims (25). It is important that clinicians evaluating suicide risk among children and adolescents be aware of symptoms, such as chronic aggression, impulsivity, odd thinking, mood instability, and poor interpersonal relationships, that may suggest the development of a personality disorder.

Borderline personality disorder is associated with nonfatal suicidal acts among adolescents (18, 21, 33, 53). Impulsivity and aggression have been documented as correlates of youth suicidal acts (33, 54–57). Prepubertal children who report both suicidal and violent behaviors were observed to have significant deficits in impulse control (3). Features of violence, suicidal behavior, and impulsivity may be ingredients for future development of personality disorders. Neuroticism, which is a personality trait associated with prolonged negative affects in response to stressful conditions, also has been identified among suicidal youth (33, 58).

Neurobiological Factors

Although there has been extensive research on the neurobiology of suicidal behavior in adults, few studies have focused on neurobiological correlates of youth suicidal behavior (59). Positive correlations in adults between suicidal and violent behaviors, impulsivity, and dysregulation of neurotransmitter systems, especially those involved with serotonin metabolism and regulation, have been described (59, 60). Dysregulation in the serotonergic neurotransmitter system involves the findings of low levels of 5-hydroxyindoleacetic acid (5-HIAA) in cerebrospinal fluid (CSF) of violent suicidal adults (60). These results were validated in numerous other studies, suggesting associations between aberrant serotonin system functioning and α_2-adrenoceptors in postmortem brain samples, especially frontocortical regions, and low levels of 5-HIAA in CSF samples of suicidal adults (59). Dysregulation in the serotonin neurotransmitter system were identified as low levels of CSF 5-HIAA (61) in adolescent suicide attempters, and low levels of whole-blood tryptophan among prepubertal suicide attempters (62). Lower levels of homovanillic acid, a dopamine neurotransmitter metabolite, in the CSF of suicidal compared with nonsuicidal adults have been reported (59). Brain regions of depressed suicide victims have an altered density of the serotonin 2A (5-HT2A) receptors and research suggests that there is an association between suicidal ideation and the 102C allele in the 5-HT2A receptor gene (63). However, the presence of the 102C allele alone is not sufficient to increase risk for youth suicide (64). Neuroimaging techniques applied to youth indicated that those with major depressive disorder and history of suicide attempt had high white matter hyperintensities in the brain (65). This study provides a potential new lead about neurobiological deficits among suicidal youth.

Although no association between the allele frequencies of the serotonin transporter gene and adolescent suicidal behavior have been identified (66). significant associations between the short (s) allele of the promoter region of the serotonin transporter gene and suicidal acts were identified in adolescents and young adults who experienced severe stress (67). This finding of a gene–environment interaction has vast implications for suicide prevention strategies. While vulnerability to suicidal behavior is greater for those youth with the short allele of the promoter region of the serotonin transporter region, this vulnerability enhances risk only in the presence of severe, stressful situations. Prevention strategies can be developed to support those vulnerable youth who may be experiencing severe stress.

Neuroendocrine functioning, especially that of the hypothalamic–pituitary–adrenal (HPA) axis, which is the principal stress response system, has been shown to be dysregulated among suicidal youths. Elevated levels of plasma cortisol have been observed during the dexamethasone suppression test among suicidal children (68), and among adolescent suicide attempters, elevated plasma cortisol levels have been documented before sleep onset (69).

Chronobiological studies of adolescent suicide attempters who suffer from major depressive disorder documented disordered sleep architecture before the onset of sleep (69). Followup assessments of neuroendocrine functioning in depressed adolescents suggest that sleep-related growth hormone secretion may predict future episodes of major depression and suicide attempts (70).

The clinical implications of identifying neurobiological correlates of youth suicidal behavior is that this information may point toward new treatment options for suicidal youth.

Effects of Stress

Children and adolescents who reported suicidal ideation or suicide attempts experience high rates of cumulative stresses, including family losses due to deaths and separations, illness, hospitalization, multiple family moves, family discord involving arguments, overt violence, and parental psychiatric disorders (34, 45, 71, 72).

Adolescent suicide victims have high rates of family suicidal behavior (22). Sixty percent of youth suicide victims, compared with 12% of nonsuicidal adolescents, had parents or adult relatives with suicidal acts, emotional problems, absence from the home, and abusive behavior toward their children (22). An important clinical implication of these results is to identify youth who may suffer from psychological problems after the suicidal behavior of a relative. Family history of suicide imparted a five-fold greater risk of suicide on adolescent boys, and an almost three-fold greater risk for suicide on adolescent girls (73). Youth suicide victims and youth who reported suicidal ideation or suicide attempts have high rates of family mood disorders, antisocial personality disorders, substance abuse, and suicidal and violent behavior (4, 22, 71, 72). Risk for youth suicide has been documented to be transmitted in families, independent of psychiatric disorders (74), and mediated by the transmission of impulsive aggression (75). Children of mothers who attempted suicide are more likely to attempt suicide in adolescence than are youth whose mothers are not suicidal (76). Relatives of adolescent suicide victims have been reported to have a two- to six-fold increased rate of suicidal behavior (11, 77–79).

Violence, especially physical and sexual abuse, is strong risk factor for youth suicidal behavior (80–84). Approximately 12% of youth suicide attempts are associated with family abuse (81). Longitudinal research of a community sample of children and adolescents who were followed up for 17 years documented that a history of childhood maltreatment increased risk for depression or suicide attempts by three-fold (85). The effects of sexual abuse conferred an eight-fold greater risk for repeated suicide attempts in adolescents and young adults (85). A 21-year longitudinal study of a community sample followed from childhood into late adolescence and young adulthood reported the risk for suicidal behavior in late adolescence and young adulthood was related to severe family adversity during childhood, including economic strain, marital disruption, poor parent–child attachment, and exposure to sexual abuse (58). This risk was mediated by mental health problems and stresses in adolescence.

Physical problems near the time of birth, including respiratory distress for more than an hour after birth, no antenatal care before 20 weeks of pregnancy, and chronic maternal physical disease have been associated with increased risk for youth suicide (86). An implication of these findings is that early physical stress may enhance vulnerability to suicide at future times, especially in adolescence. Inquiry about prenatal and birth problems is an essential aspect of the clinical assessment of youth suicide risk. Chronic medical illnesses, such as diabetes and epilepsy, and impairments in functioning during childhood and adolescence are associated with increased risk for suicidal behavior (34, 88).

Exposure to suicide increases risk for youth suicide. For example, a small number of youth suicides and nonfatal suicidal acts occur in the context of time-space clusters that are stimulated by mechanisms of contagion and imitation (89, 90). Exposure to media presentations that include news reports or fictional accounts of suicide increases rates of youth suicide and nonfatal suicidal acts (5, 91–93). Lower risk for suicide is associated with presentations that are factual and not romanticized (93). The risk for such imitative suicidal behavior occurs for only a short time after exposure (5, 91, 92). Clinical implications are that mental health professionals can make significant contributions to educating the community about suicide prevention strategies after a community suffers a suicide of a child or adolescent.

Psychosocial Functioning

Social maladjustment involving interpersonal relations with family, peers, and others are important characteristics of suicidal children and adolescents (3). It accounts for long-term vulnerability of children and adolescents to suicidal acts (45). During the assessment of suicide risk, clinicians should focus on evaluating aspects of youths' daily interactions, perceptions of others, sense of competence, and self-esteem.

Social adjustment in children and adolescents is enhanced by the presence of adequate social supports and predictability of the environmental milieu (11). Suicidal children and adolescents frequently lack available empathic individuals who could offer guidance and an avenue to vent distressing ideas and feelings. An unpredictable social support network combined with a suicidal youth's perceptions of inadequacies in mobilizing social support intensify isolation, anxiety, poor self-esteem, rejection, and hopelessness (31, 94). Perceived hopelessness is among the significant factors that intensify youth suicidal risk (20, 95, 96). Hopeless feelings impair the ability to be motivated to solve problems and to cope with adversity (97). Social support derived from attending school may protect against suicide risk (80, 98). Notably, among adolescents who drop out of school and thereby lack consistent social support and school routines, suicide risk increases (99, 100).

Specific styles of coping among suicidal children and adolescents limit their flexibility and resourcefulness when faced with intense emotions and the need for problemsolving (3, 101–103). Ego mechanisms of defense, empirically studied among suicidal children and adolescents, involve denial of affects or events, turning painful affects and distressing thoughts into the opposite by means of reaction formation, and compensation that involves risk-taking behaviors or exaggeration of one's skills (3, 104).

The role of cultural affiliation is associated with youth suicide risk. For example, a study of 3,094 Native Hawaiian adolescents indicated that problems with cultural affiliation, rather than ethnicity, were significantly predictive of adolescent suicide attempts (105). Similar concerns have been observed for African Americans, in whom increased suicide rates may be related to migration, cultural affiliation, and changing social supports (10, 11).

RISK ASSESSMENT

Assessment of youth suicidal behavior involves comprehensive interviews with youths and their parents to identify presence of current and past suicidal ideation or acts, suicidal intent, accessibility of suicidal methods, and other risk factors, including psychopathology, cognitive distortions (e.g., hopelessness), impulsivity, problematic coping styles, and environmental stress factors involving family psychopathology and discord. Assessment of a suicide attempt should focus on the type of method used, its potential for lethality, the degree of planning, and the likelihood that discovery of the act is possible (the so called "risk—rescue" assessment). Some of the aspects that influence the information obtained in a clinical interview are the youth's cognitive and emotional state and the degree of parental psychopathology (106). It is important that clinical interviews be conducted at the time of maximum suicidal risk and repeated subsequently until the risk of suicidal behavior is diminished. The most important aspect of the assessment is to determine the degree of immediate danger and to determine if safety will be better assured if psychiatric hospitalization is recommended. An important clue for an impending suicide attempt is preoccupation with death (107). Suicidal risk is lower if children and adolescents have good judgment, high impulse control, low levels of hopelessness and helplessness, future-oriented thinking, and ability to communicate openly and honestly about feelings, worries, and thoughts of suicide. However, the status of these factors may change. Therefore, repeated discussions with children and adolescents who are at risk for suicide is necessary.

It is important to determine whether a family can provide a consistent and stable environment or whether there is high degree of stress, violence, and psychopathology, and no relatives available to provide support. Positive social supports are crucial in diminishing youths' suicidal risk (84). The lack of sufficient family support may be a clue to the need to plan for psychiatric hospitalization.

Clinical assessment may be aided by the use of specialized rating scales that measure suicidal risk factors. They can be administered in a brief period by questionnaire format and are reliable and valid (108–110). Another method that focuses on nonverbal indicators of suicide risk is the use of human figure drawings (111). This may be especially helpful with young children. All such screening measures should be used in conjunction with in person interviews to evaluate if the screening risk assessment indicated that a youth was falsely positive for suicide risk.

DIFFERENTIAL DIAGNOSIS

The two most significant issues in a differential diagnosis of youth suicidal behavior are to:

1. Identify whether the destructive act is self-intended rather than accidental, and
2. Identify whether there is a high or low level of risk for an injury to occur.

The first issue is a qualitative one and involves a systematic assessment of intent and the specific circumstances in which a self-destructive act occurred. The second issue is a quantitative one and involves a comprehensive evaluation of the intensity and types of risk factors, such as severity of depressive symptoms, presence of hypomania or manic symptoms, and mixed or rapid cycling states, severity of irritability, agitation, delusional symptoms, poor reality testing and hallucinations.

TREATMENT

The most salient acute issue in treatment is to decrease the likelihood that self-inflicted injury or death could occur. Availability of psychiatric services involving outpatient and emergency services and inpatient or residential programs is important in lowering suicidal risk. Psychiatric hospitalization may be recommended if observation and intensive therapeutic intervention are warranted when a child or adolescent manifests an unpredictable condition. The hospital offers an environment with structure and a consistent high-availability of staff to provide immediate, around-the-clock interventions. Hospitalization also is a way of removing a youngster from an environment that may be too stressful or disorganized. In contrast, outpatient or partial hospitalization should be used when there is a low likelihood for imminent suicidal acts and if there is adequate family support.

Emergency treatment involves certain key principles. Suicidal youths should not be discharged from an emergency service without explicit discussion regarding their clinical condition and assurance that there is limited access to lethal suicidal methods (112–115). Family compliance with planned treatments will be enhanced by positive family experience with the emergency service staff (116).

Psychotherapeutic intervention involves developing a trusting and empathic atmosphere for truthful communication. Discussion that may support effective coping strategies may be accomplished by utilizing a cognitive orientation into the treatment process.

Delineation of the motivations for a suicidal act is an important feature of treatment. Common motives that elevate suicide risk involve despair and guilt over causing the loss of a special person, such as a breakup with a boyfriend or girlfriend or separation of parents. Other motivations involve anger or feelings of revenge in response to frustrations, deprivations, or perceived wrongdoing. Some psychotic youths feel so demoralized and pained that they impulsively plan suicide as a means of decreasing their emotional upset.

Treatment of suicidal children and adolescents is complex and often requires simultaneous use of multiple modalities. At present, there are few systematic controlled studies of treatment efficacy for suicidal youths. Thus, various treatments have been utilized, including dynamic, supportive, and cognitive-behavioral therapy, and psychopharmacologic modalities. Controlled treatment studies exist for risk factors of suicide, such as the treatment of major depressive disorder. However, these studies have excluded youths who are at high risk for suicide.

Cognitive-behavioral therapy for depressed adolescents has been more effective than family or supportive therapy for decreasing depressive symptoms, but there were no treatment type differences in reducing suicidal ideation or acts (117). However, the longer term followup at 2 years after instituting treatment indicated that there were no differences in depressive symptom outcomes with cognitive-behavioral, family, or supportive treatment (118). Interpersonal psychotherapy, which addresses interpersonal conflicts involving loss, interpersonal role disputes, role transitions, and interpersonal deficits, has been found to be more effective in reducing depressive symptoms among adolescents than a control treatment (119). Its efficacy with suicidal adolescents has not been studied.

Dialectical-behavioral therapy is the only psychotherapy that has been effective in reducing suicidal behavior in adults (120), and it has promising results in treatment of suicidal adolescents (121, 122). While family therapy may be useful to decrease family discord and enhance effective family problemsolving and conflict resolution, a time-limited, home-based family intervention had only limited efficacy in reducing suicide attempts, specifically among youths without major depressive disorder (123).

Studies of the efficacy of psychopharmacologic treatment specifically for suicidal children and adolescents are rare. Among adults, lithium has been found to decrease recurrence of suicide attempts in adults with major depression or bipolar disorder by almost nine-fold (124). Discontinuation of lithium was associated with a seven-fold increase in suicide attempts and a nine-fold increase in rates of suicide (124). Use of lithium with suicidal children or adolescents requires careful monitoring by a responsible adult because an overdose may be lethal.

A comparative controlled study, the Treatment of Adolescent Depression Study (TADS) aimed to evaluate among adolescents with major depressive disorder the efficacy of four forms of treatment: combined cognitive-behavioral treatment (CBT) and fluoxetine, fluoxetine alone, CBT alone, and placebo (125). Adolescents with high risk for suicide were excluded from this study. The results indicated that 71% of adolescents improved with the combined treatment, 60.6% with fluoxetine alone, 43.2% with CBT, and 34.8% with placebo. As was true for treatments of youth major depressive disorder with antidepressant medications, such as the selective serotonin reuptake inhibitors (SSRIs), the fluoxetine-treated adolescents in the TADS study had an approximate two-fold increase in adverse effects manifest as suicidal thinking and acts (126).

Due to the adverse effects of increased rates of suicidal ideation and suicide attempts reported in a FDA metaanalysis of clinical treatment trials with depressed children and adolescents (126), black box warnings are included in all manufacturer statements about all classes of antidepressant medications used for depressed children and adolescents. Additionally, guidelines were recommended by the FDA to increase clinical monitoring of adverse effects when antidepressant medications are used to treat depressed children and adolescents. Psychopharmacologic treatment to reduce the risk of underlying conditions associated with suicidal behavior involves use of medications specific to the diagnosis or symptomatology. Caution in use of medications that may disinhibit some children and adolescents, such as psychostimulants, benzodiazepines, or phenobarbital, is required.

Treatment of parents and other relatives may be indicated to improve family functioning and communication. Collaborative efforts with other professionals, such as school professionals, are important in monitoring youths who are at risk for suicide.

STRATEGIES FOR PREVENTION

Suicide prevention efforts should focus on identifying high-risk children and adolescents and monitoring them repeatedly for early signs of suicidal risk. An important issue is to develop community case-finding approaches by means of screening procedures and referral of those children and adolescents found to be at risk for suicidal behavior. Educating mental health, medical, and school professionals, clergy, and others who are in contact with children and adolescents to identify children and adolescents at risk for suicidal behavior is an important suicide prevention strategy.

Efforts to prevent youth suicidal behavior require public health model strategies in school settings. These may focus on encouraging adolescents to seek help if they recognize symptoms of suicidal risk. New approaches for school-based suicide prevention programs are needed because evaluations of prior school programs concluded that their efficacy was not adequate to prevent suicide, change adolescents' attitudes about suicide, or enhance help-seeking behavior (6, 127). Some reports suggested that adolescents who had a history of suicidal behavior were especially upset and had negative feelings about suicide prevention curricula (6).

Comprehensive screening may be a more effective method to identify youth at risk for suicide and to promote their referral to and compliance with treatment (110). Recent research indicates that there are no adverse effects of using direct screening of adolescents for suicidal behavior (128).

Guidelines for media coverage have been developed and may be useful in decreasing risk for suicide after media presentations (129). This may be especially important to reduce the potential for suicide that has been documented to occur within 2 weeks after media presentations of actual or fictional suicide.

Guidelines have been proposed for community response to youth suicide. They focus on organizing community networks that include school professionals, mental health professionals, police, religious leaders, and parents to respond to the needs of peers and family of a youth suicide victim. Organized liaison approaches with the media are essential to promote helpful media coverage of the event and to prevent confusion, fear, and risk for other youth suicidal acts stimulated by the presence of news reports and presentations of the story of a youth suicide. Focus on other vulnerable youths is another aspect of responding to a suicide crisis. Discussions with friends and acquaintances of the adolescent who committed suicide are helpful. Research on risk for suicidal behavior among peers and friends of youth suicide victims has varied results. Some studies suggest suicidal behavior may be low among friends and acquaintances of an adolescent suicide victim within 6 months of the suicidal death, but the risk for a major depressive episode and posttraumatic stress disorder is high among such friends and acquaintances (130, 131). One report of a national representative sample of 5,852 adolescents suggested that youth who are exposed to peer suicide are significantly more likely to have suicidal ideation or suicide attempts as well as to abuse substances and engage in aggressive behavior (132). Community support is necessary to identify youth who are most exposed to peer suicide and to offer acute interventions to assist them with their responses to the loss of their friend.

Suicidal behavior involves a legacy that runs in families. Psychiatric morbidity is significantly greater among youths who suffered the suicide of a parent or other close relative (132–136). Programs are needed to identify such bereaved children and adolescents and to offer them targeted intervention to prevent adverse outcomes, such as traumatic grief, resulting from the sequelae of suicide in the family or peers (136–138).

Finally, strong evidence suggests that availability of guns and firearms is significantly associated with youth suicide risk (139). Efforts to prevent youth suicide require a national focus to advocate for better restrictions on the availability of guns and firearms and other lethal methods, as well as implementation of child access prevention laws to restrict purchase and possession of firearms (140, 141). Clinical assessments of youth suicide risk should determine whether there are available lethal means for suicide in the home.

CONCLUSION

With the recent decrease in youth suicide rates, there is a sense of hopefulness that youth suicide may be prevented. New effective prevention efforts may be identified by translation of new research findings into clinical practice. For example, the interaction effects between environmental factors and constitutional and biological factors that increase youth suicide risk are relevant for developing effective treatments to lower youth suicide risk. Greater understanding of sociocultural factors associated with suicide risk and determination of methods to protect youth from risk is necessary. Efforts to educate the general public and health care professionals about the youth suicide can reduce stigma and enhance seeking treatment when suicide occurs in families.

References

1. U.S. Public Health Service: *The Surgeon General's Call to Action to Prevent Suicide*. Washington, DC, 1999.
2. O'Carroll PW, Berman AL, Maris RW, et al.: Beyond the Tower of Babel: A nomenclature for suicidology. *Sui Life-Threat Behavior* 1996; 26:237–252.
3. Pfeffer CR: *The Suicidal Child*. New York, Guilford Press, 1986.
4. Brent DA, Perper JA, Goldstein CE, et al.: Risk factors for adolescent suicide: A comparison of adolescent suicide victims with suicidal inpatients. *Arch Gen Psychiatry* 1988; 45:581–588.
5. Phillips DP, Carstensen L: Clustering of teenage suicides after television news stories about suicide. *N Engl J Med* 1986; 315:685–689.
6. Shaffer D, Garland A, Vieland V, et al.: The impact of curriculum-based suicide prevention programs for teenagers. *J Am Acad Child Adolesc Psychiatry* 1991; 30:588–596.
7. Alcohol, Drug Abuse, and Mental Health Administration: Report of the Secretary's Task Force on Youth Suicide. DHHS no. (ADM) 1989; 89-1621. Washington, DC, U.S. Government Printing Office.
8. Hoyert DL, Kung HC, Smith BL: Deaths: Preliminary data for 2003. *National Vital Statistics Reports* 2005; vol. 53, no. 15. Hyattsville, MD: National Center for Health Statistics.
9. Murphy SL: Deaths: Final data for 1998. *National Vital Statistics Reports* 2000; vol. 48, no. 11. Hyattsville, MD, National Center for Health Statistics.
10. Shaffer D, Gould M, Hicks RC: Worsening suicide rate in black teenagers. *Am J Psychiatry* 1994; 151:1810–1812.
11. Gould MS, Fisher P, Parides et al.: Psychosocial risk factors of child and adolescent completed suicide. *Arch Gen Psychiatry* 1996; 53:1155–1162.
12. Anderson RN: Deaths: Leading causes for 2000. *National Vital Statistics Reports* 2002; vol. 50, Hyattsville, MD: National Center for Health Statistics.
13. Berlin IN: Suicide among American Indian adolescents: An overview. *Sui Life-Threat Behavior* 1987; 17:218–232.
14. Brent DA, Baugher M, Birmaher B, et al.: Compliance with recommendations to remove firearms in families participating in a clinical trial for adolescent depression. *J Amer Acad Child Adolesc Psychiatry* 2000; 39:1220–1226.
15. Centers for Disease Control: Methods of suicide among persons aged 10–19 years—United States, 1992–2001. *MMWR Morbidity Weekly Report* 2005; 53:471–474.
16. Kann L, Kinchen SA, Williams BI, et al.: Youth Risk Behavior Surveillance—United States, 1999. *J Sch Health* 2000; 70:271–285.
17. Pfeffer CR, Zuckerman S, Plutchik R, et al.: Suicidal behavior in normal school children: A comparison with child psychiatric inpatients. *J Amer Acad Child Psychiatry*, 1984; 23:416–423.
18. Pfeffer CR, Newcorn J, Kaplan G, et al.: Suicidal behavior in adolescent psychiatric inpatients. *J Am Acad Child Adolesc Psychiatry* 1988; 27:357–361.
19. Kuperman, S, Black DW, Burns TL: Excess mortality among formerly hospitalized child psychiatric patients. *Arch Gen Psychiatry* 1988; 45:227–282.
20. Shaffer D, Gould MS, Fisher P et al.: Psychiatric diagnosis in child and adolescent suicide. *Arch Gen Psychiatry* 1996; 53:339–348.
21. Brent DA, Johnson B, Bartle S, et al.: Personality disorder, tendency to impulsive violence and suicidal behavior in adolescents. *J Am Acad Child Adolesc Psychiatry* 1003a; 32:69–75.
22. Shafii M, Carrigan S, Whittinghill JR, et al.: Psychological autopsy of completed suicide in children and adolescents. *Am J Psychiatry* 1985; 142:1061–1064.
23. Shafii M, Steltz-Lenarsky J, Derrick et al.: Comorbidity of mental disorders in the postmortem diagnosis of completed suicide in children and adolescents. *J Affect Disorders* 1988; 15:227–233.
24. Brent DA, Baugher M, Bridge J, et al.: Age- and sex-related risk factors for adolescent suicide. *J Am Acad Child Adolesc Psychiatry* 1999; 38:1497–1505.
25. Apter A, Bleich A, King RA, et al.: Death without warning? A clinical postmortem study of suicide in 43 Israeli adolescent males. *Arch Gen Psychiatry* 1993; 50:138–142.
26. Fowler RC, Rich CL, Young D: San Diego Suicide Study: Substance abuse in young cases. *Arch Gen Psychiatry* 1986; 43:962–965.
27. Rich CL, Young D, Fowler RC: San Diego Suicide Study: Young versus old subjects. *Arch Gen Psychiatry* 1986; 43:577–582.
28. Brent DA, Perper J, Moritz G et al.: Suicide in adolescents with no apparent psychopathology. *J Amer Acad Child Adolesc Psychiatry* 1993 c; 32:494–500.
29. Andrews JA, Lewinsohn PM: Suicidal attempts among older adolescents: Prevalence and cooccurrence with psychiatric disorders. *J Amer Acad Child Adolesc Psychiatry* 1992; 31:655–662.
30. Beautrais AL, Joyce PR, Mulder RT: Psychiatric illness in a New Zealand sample of young people making serious suicide attempts. *New Zealand Med Journal* 1998; 111:44–48.
31. Fergusson DM, Lynskey MT: Childhood circumstances, adolescent adjustment, and suicide attempts in a New Zealand birth cohort. *J Amer Acad Child Adolesc Psychiatry* 1995; 34:612–622.
32. Gould MS, King R, Greenwald S et al.: Psychopathology associated with suicidal ideation and attempts among children and adolescents. *J Amer Acad Child Adolesc Psychiatry* 1998; 37:915–923.
33. Beautrais AL, Joyce PR, Mulder RT: Cannabis abuse and serious suicide attempts. *Addiction* 1999; 94:1155–1164.
34. Lewinsohn PM, Rohde P, Seeley JR: Adolescent suicidal ideation and attempts: Prevalence, risk factors, and clinical implications. *Clin Psychology Science and Practice* 1996; 3:25–36.
35. Lewinsohn PM, Rohde P, Seeley JR: Psychosocial characteristics of adolescents with a history of suicide attempt. *J Am Acad Child Adolesc Psychiatry* 1993; 32:60–68.
36. Myers K, McCauley E, Calderon R et al.: The 3-year longitudinal course of suicidality and predictive factors for subsequent suicidality in youths with major depressive disorder. *J Am Acad Child Adolesc Psychiatry* 1991; 30:804–810.
37. Garrison CZ, Jackson KL, Addy CL, et al.: Suicidal behaviors in young adolescents. *Am J Epidemiol* 1991; 133:1005–1014.
38. Rotheram-Borus MJ: Suicidal behaviors and risk factors among run away youths. *Am J Psychiatry* 1993; 150:103–107.
39. De-Wilde EJ, Kienhorst IC, Diekstra RF, et al.: The specificity of psychological characteristics of adolescent suicide attempters. *J Am Acad Child Adolesc Psychiatry* 1993; 32:51–59.
40. Robbins DR, Alessi NE: Depressive symptoms and suicidal behavior in adolescents. *Am J Psychiatry* 1985; 142:588–592.
41. Barbe RP, Williamson DE, Bridge JA et al.: Clinical differences between suicidal and nonsuicidal depressed children and adolescents. *J Clin Psychiatry* 2005; 66:492–498.
42. Remafedi G, French S, Story M, et al.: The relationship between suicide risk and sexual orientation: Results of a population-based study. *Am J Public Health* 1998; 88:57–60.
43. Fergusson DM, Horwood LJ, Beautrais AL: Is sexual orientation related to mental health problems and suicidality in young people? *Arch Gen Psychiatry* 1999; 56:876–880.
44. Pfeffer CR, Klerman GL, Hurt SW, et al.: Suicidal children grow up: Demographic and clinical risk factors for adolescent suicide attempts. *J Am Acad Child Adolesc Psychiatry* 1991a; 30:609–616.
45. Pfeffer CR, Klerman GL, Hurt SW, et al.: Suicidal children grow up: Rates and psychosocial risk factors for suicide attempts during follow-up. *J Am Acad Child Adolesc Psychiatry* 1993; 32:106–113.
46. Brent DA, Kolko DJ, Wartella ME, et al.: Adolescent psychiatric inpatients' risk of suicide attempt at 6 month follow-up. *J Am Acad Child Adolesc Psychiatry* 1993b; 32:95–105.

47. Goldston DB, Sergent DS, Reboussin DM, et al.: Suicide attempts among formerly hospitalized adolescents: A prospective naturalistic study of risk during the first 5 years after discharge. *J Am Acad Child Adolesc Psychiatry* 1999; 38:660–671.
48. Kovacs M, Goldston D, Gatsonis C: Suicidal behaviors and childhood-onset depressive disorders: A longitudinal investigation. *J Am Acad Child Adolesc Psychiatry* 1993; 32:8–20.
49. Rao U, Weissman MM, Martin JA, et al.: Childhood depression and risk of suicide: A preliminary report of a longitudinal study. *J Am Acad Child Adolesc Psychiatry* 1993; 32:21–27.
50. Weissman MM, Wolk S, Goldstein RB, et al.: Depressed adolescents grown up. *JAMA* 1999; 281:1701–1713.
51. Marttunen MJ, Aro HM, Henriksson MM, et al.: Mental disorders in adolescent suicide: DSM-III-R axis I and II diagnoses in suicides among 13 to 19 years old in Finland. *Arch Gen Psychiatry* 1991; 48:834–839.
52. Rich, CL, Runeson BS: Similarities in diagnostic comorbidity between suicide among young people in Sweden and the United States. *Acta Psychiatr Scand* 1992; 86:335–339.
53. Friedman RC, Aronoff MS, Clarkin JF, et al.: History of suicidal behavior in depressed borderline inpatients. *Am J Psychiatry* 1983; 140:1023–1026.
54. Apter A, Bleich A, Plutchick R, et al.: Suicidal behavior, depression and conduct disorder in hospitalized adolescents. *J Am Acad Child Adolesc Psychiatry* 1998; 27:696–699.
55. Arie M, Haruvi-Catalan L, Apter A: Personality and suicidal behavior in adolescence. *Clin Neuropsychiatr J Treat Evaluation* 2005; 2:37–47.
56. Kingsbury S, Hawton K, Steinhardt K et al.: Do adolescents who take overdoses have specific psychological characteristics? A comparative study with psychiatric and community controls. *J Amer Acad Child Adolesc Psychiatry* 1999; 38:1125–1131.
57. Pfeffer CR, Plutchik R, Mizruchi MS, et al.: Suicidal behavior in child psychiatric inpatients and outpatients and in nonpatients. *Am J Psychiatry* 1986; 143:733–738.
58. Fergusson DM, Woodward LJ, Horwood LJ: Risk factors and life processes associated with the onset of suicidal behaviour during adolescence and early adulthood. *Psychol Med* 2000; 30:23–39.
59. Mann JJ: Neurobiology of suicidal behavior. *Nature Reviews Neuroscience* 2003; 4:819–828.
60. Asberg M, Thoren P, Traskman L: Seratonin depression: A biochemical subgroup within the affective disorders? *Science* 1976; 191:478–480.
61. Greenhill L, Wasliek B. Paricles M, et al.: Biological studies in suicidal adolescent patients. *Proceedings of the 42nd Annual Meeting of the American Academy of Child and Adolescent Psychiatry*, New Orleans, LA, October 17–22, 1995.
62. Pfeffer CR, McBride PA, Anderson GM, et al.: Peripheral serotonin measures in prepubertal psychiatric inpatients and normal children: Associations with suicidal behavior and its risk factors. *Biol Psychiatry* 1998a; 44:568–577.
63. Du L, Bakish D, Lapierre YD, et al.: Association of polymorphism of serotonin 2A receptor gene with suicidal ideation in major depressive disorder. *Am J Med Genet* 2000; 96:56–60.
64. Zalsman G, Frisch A, Baruch M, et al.: Family-based association study of 5-HT-sub(2A) receptor T102C polymorphism and suicidal behavior in Ashkenazi inpatient adolescents. *Internat J Adol Med Health* 2005; 17:231–238.
65. Ehrlich S, Noam GG, Lyoo IK, et al.: White matter hyperintensities and their associations with suicidality in psychiatrically hospitalized children and adolescents. *J Amer Acad Child Adolesc Psychiatry* 2004; 43:770–776.
66. Zalsman G, Frisch A, Bromberg M et al.: Family-based association study of serotonin transporter promoter in suicidal adolescents: No association with suicidality but possible role in violence traits. *Am J of Med Genetics* 2001; 105:239–245.
67. Caspi A, Sugden K, Moffitt TE, et al., Influence of life stress on depression: Moderation by a polymorphism in the 5-HTT gene. *Science* 2003; 301:386–389.
68. Pfeffer CR, Stokes P, Shindledecker R: Suicidal behavior and hypothalamic-pituitary-adrenocortical axis indices in child psychiatric inpatients. *Biol Psychiatry* 1991b; 29:909–917.
69. Dahl RE, Puig-Antich J, Ryan ND, et al.: EEG sleep in adolescents with major depression: The role of suicidality and inpatient status. *J Affect Disord* 1990; 19:63–75.
70. Coplan JD, Wolk SI, Goetz RR, et al.: Nocturnal growth hormone secretion studies in adolescents with or without major depression re-examined: Integration of adult clinical follow-up data. *Biol Psychiatry* 2000; 47:594–604.
71. Pfeffer CR, Normandin L, Kakuma T: Suicidal children grow up: Suicidal behavior and psychiatric disorders among relatives. *J Am Acad Child Adolesc Psychiatry* 1994; 33:1087–1097.
72. Pfeffer CR, Normandin L. Kakuma T: Suicidal children grow up: Relations between family psychopathology and adolescents' lifetime suicidal behavior. *J Nerv Ment Dis* 1998b; 186:151–157.
73. Shaffer D: The epidemiology of teen suicide: An examination of risk factors. *J Clin Psychiatry* 1988; 49:36–41.
74. Brent DA, Mann JJ: Family genetic studies, suicide, and suicidal behavior. *Am J Med Genetics Part C(Semin. Med. Gen)* 2005; 133C:13–24.
75. Brent DA, Oquendo M, Birmaher B, et al.: Peripubertal suicide attempts in offspring of suicide attempters with siblings concordant for suicidal behavior. *Am J Psychiatry* 2003; 160:1486–1493.
76. Lieb R, Bronisch T, Hofler M, et al.: Maternal suicidality and risk of suicidality in offspring: Findings from a community study. *Am J Psychiatry* 2005; 162:1665–1671.
77. Borowsky IW, Ireland M, Resnick MD: Adolescent suicide attempts: Risks and protectors. *Pediatrics* 2001; 107:485–493.
78. Brent DA, Bridge J, Johnson BA, et al.: Suicidal behavior runs in families. A controlled family study of adolescent suicide victims. *Arch Gen Psychiatry* 1996; 53:1145–1152.
79. Fergusson DM, Beautrais AL, Horwood LJ: Vulnerability and resilience to suicidal behaviors in young people. *Psycholog Medicine* 2003; 33:61–73.
80. Borowsky IW, Resnick MD, Ireland M, et al: Suicide attempts among American Indian and Alaska Native youth: Risk and protective factors. *Arch Ped Adol Medicine* 1999; 153:573–580.
81. Deykin, EY, Alpert JJ, McNamarra JJ: A pilot study of the effect of exposure to child abuse or neglect on adolescent suicidal behavior. *Am J Psychiatry* 1985; 142:1299–1303.
82. Evans E, Hawton K, Rodham K: Suicidal phenomena and abuse in adolescents: A review of epidemiological studies. *Child Abuse Neglect* 2005; 29:45–58.
83. Fergusson DM, Horwood LJ, Lynskey MT: Childhood sexual abuse and psychiatric disorder in young adulthood: II. Psychiatric outcomes of childhood sexual abuse. *J Amer Acad Child and Adolesc Psychiatry* 1996; 35:1365–1374.
84. Wagner BM, Cole RE, Schwartzman P: Psychosocial correlates of suicide attempts among junior and senior high school youth. *Sui Life-Threat Behavior* 1995; 25:358–372.
85. Brown J, Cohen P, Johnson JG, et al.: Childhood abuse and neglect: Specificity and effects on adolescent and young adult depression and suicidality. *J Am Acad Child Adolesc Psychiatry* 1999; 38:1490–1496.
86. Salk L, Lipsitt LP, Surner WQ, et al.: Relationship of maternal and perinatal conditions to eventual adolescent suicide. *Lancet* 1985; 1:624–627.
87. Brent DA: Overrepresentation of epileptics in a consecutive series of suicide attempters seen at a children's hospital, 1978–1983. *J Amer Acad Child Psychiatry* 1986; 25:242–246.
88. Goldston DB, Kovacs M, Ho VY, et al.: Suicidal ideation and suicide attempts among youth with insulin-dependent diabetes mellitus. *J Amer Acad Child Adolesc Psychiatry* 1994; 33:240–246.
89. Gould MS, Wallenstein S, Kleinman M: Time-space clustering of teenage suicide. *Am J Epidemiology* 1990; 131:71–78.
90. Gould Ms, Petrie K, Kleinman MH, et al.: Clustering of attempted suicide: New Zealand national data. *Internat J Epidemiology* 1994; 23:1185–1189.
91. Gould MS: Suicide and media. *Ann NY Acad Sciences* 2001; 932:200–221.
92. Schmidtke A, Schaller S: The role of mass media in suicide prevention. In K Hawton and K van Herringen (eds.), *The International Handbook of Suicide and Attempted Suicide*. New York, Wiley, 2000.
93. Stack S: Suicide in the media: A quantitative review of studies based on nonfictional stories. *Sui Life-Threat Behavior* 2005; 35:121–133.
94. Overholser JC, Adams DM, Lehnert KL, et al.: Self-esteem deficits and suicidal tendencies among adolescents. *J Amer Acad Child Adolesc Psychiatry* 1995; 34:919–928.
95. Goldston DB, Daniel SS, Reboussin BA, et al.: Cognitive risk factors and suicide attempts among formerly hospitalized adolescents: A prospective naturalistic study. *J Amer Acad Child Adolesc Psychiatry* 2001; 40:91–99.
96. Spirito A, Overholser J, Hart K: Cognitive characteristics of adolescent suicide attempters. *J Amer Acad Child Adolesc Psychiatry* 1991; 30:604–608.
97. Lewinsohn PM, Rohde P, Seeley JR: Psychosocial risk factors for future adolescent suicide attempts. *J Consult Clin Psychology* 1994; 62:297–305.
98. Resnick MD, Bearman PS, Blum RW, et al.: Protecting adolescents from harm: Findings from the National Longitudinal Study on Adolescent Health. *JAMA* 1997; 278:823–832.
99. Beautrais AL, Joyce PR, Mulder RT: Risk factors for serious suicide attempts among youths aged 13 through 24 years. *J Amer Acad Child Adolesc Psychiatry* 1996; 35:1174–1182.
100. Eggert LL, Thompson EA, Herting JR, et al.: Reducing suicide potential among high-risk youth: Tests of a school-based prevention program. *Sui Life-Threat Behavior* 1995; 25:276–296.
101. Gould MS, Velting D, Kleinman M, et al.: Teenagers' attitudes about coping strategies and help-seeking behavior of suicidality. *J Am Acad Child Adolesc Psychiatry* 2004; 43:1124–1133.
102. Schwartz JAJ, Kaslow NJ, Seeley J, et al.: Psychological, cognitive, and interpersonal correlates of attributional change in adolescents. *J Clin Child Psychol* 2000; 29:188–198.
103. Speckens AEM, Hawton K: Social problem solving in adolescents with suicidal behavior: A systematic review. *Sui Life-Threat Behavior* 2005; 35:365–387.
104. Apter A, Gothelf D, Offer R, et al.: Suicidal adolescents and ego defense mechanisms. *J Amer Acad Child Adolesc Psychiatry,* 1997; 36, 11:1520–1527.
105. Yuen NC, Nahulu LB, Hishinuma ES, et al.: Cultural identification and attempted suicide in native Hawaiian adolescents. *J Am Acad Child Adolesc Psychiatry* 2000; 39:360–367.

106. Jacobsen LK, Rabinowitz I, Popper MS, et al.: Interviewing prepubertal children about suicidal ideation and behavior. *J Am Acad Child Adolesc Psychiatry* 1994; 33:439–452.
107. Gothelf D, Apter A, Brand-Gothelf A, et al.: Death concepts in suicidal adolescents. *J Am Acad Child Adolesc Psychiatry* 1998; 37:1279–1286.
108. Larzelere RE, Andersen JJ, Ringle JL, Jorgensen DD: The child suicide risk assessment: A screening measure of suicide risk in pre-adolescents. *Death Studies* 2004; 28:809–827.
109. Pfeffer CR, Jiang H, Kakuma T: Child-Adolescent Suicidal Potential Index (CASPI): A screen for risk for early onset suicidal behavior. *Psychol Assess* 2000a; 12:304–318.
110. Shaffer D, Scott M, Wilcox H, et al.: The Columbia Suicide Screen: Validity and reliability of a screen for youth suicide and depression. *J Amer Acad Child Adolesc Psychiatry* 2004; 43:71–79.
111. Zalsman G, Netanel R, Fischel T, et al.: Human figure drawings in the evaluation of severe adolescent suicidal behavior. *J Am Acad Child Adolesc Psychiatry* 2000; 39:1024–1031.
112. Brent DA, Perper J, Moritz G, et al.: Firearms and adolescent suicide: A community case-control study. *Am J Dis Children* 1993d; 147:1066–1071.
113. Grossman DC, Mueller BA, Riedy C, et al.: Gun storage practices and risk of youth suicide and unintentional firearm injuries. *JAMA* 2005; 293:707–714.
114. Kruesi MJ, Grossman J, Pennington JM, et al.: Suicide and violence prevention: Parent education in the emergency department. *J Am Acad Child Adolesc Psychiatry* 1999; 38:250–255.
115. McManus BL, Kruesi MJ, Dontes AE, et al.: Child and adolescent suicide attempts: An opportunity for emergency departments to provide injury prevention education. *Am J Emerg Med* 1997; 15:357–360.
116. Rotheram-Borus MJ, Piacentini J, Van Rossem R, et al.: Enhancing treatment adherence with a specialized emergency room program for adolescent suicide attempters. *J Am Acad Child Adolesc Psychiatry* 1996; 35:654–663.
117. Brent DA, Holder D, Kolko D, et al.: A clinical psychotherapy trial for adolescent depression comparing cognitive, family, and supportive therapy. *Arch Gen Psychiatry* 1997; 54:877–885.
118. Birmaher B, Brent DA, Kolko D, et al.: Clinical outcome after short-term psychotherapy for adolescents with major depressive disorder. *Arch Gen Psychiatry* 2000; 57:29–36.
119. Mufson L, Weissman MM, Moreau D, et al.: Efficacy of interpersonal psychotherapy for depressed adolescents. *Arch Gen Psychiatry* 1999; 56:573–579.
120. Linehan MM: *Cognitive-Behavior Therapy of Borderline Personality Disorder*. 1993; New York, Guilford Press.
121. Katz LY, Cox BJ, Gunasekara S, Miller AL: Feasibility of dialectical behavior therapy for suicidal adolescent inpatients. *J Am Acad Child Adol Psychiatry* 2004; 43:276–282.
122. Miller AL, Rathus JH, Linehan MM, et al: Dialectical behavior therapy adapted for suicidal adolescents. *J Practical Psychiatry Behavioral Health* 1997; 3:78–86.
123. Harringtom R, Kerfoot M, Dyer E, et al.: Randomized trial of a home-based family intervention for children who have deliberately poisoned themselves. *J Am Acad Child Adolesc Psychiatry* 1998; 37:512–518.
124. Tondo L, Jamison KR, Baldessarini RJ: Effect of lithium maintenance on suicidal behavior in major mood disorders. *Ann NY Acad Sci* 1997; 836:339–351.
125. Treatment for Adolescents with Depression Study (TADS)-Team-US: Fluoxetine, Cognitive-behavioral therapy, and their combination for adolescents with depression: Treatment for Adolescents with Depression Study (TADS) randomized controlled trial. *JAMA* 2004; 292:807–820.
126. U.S. Food and Drug Administration (FDA): Relationship between psychotropic drugs and pediatric suicidality. http://www.fda.gov/ohrms/dockets/ac/04/briefing/2004-4065b1-10-TAB08-Hammads-Review.pdf., 2004.
127. Vieland V, Whittle B, Garland A, et al.: The impact of curriculum-based suicide prevention programs for teenagers: An 18-month follow-up. *J Amer Acad Child Adolesc Psychiatry* 1991; 30:811–815.
128. Gould MS, Marrocco FA, Kleinman M, et al.: Evaluating iatrogenic risk of youth suicide screening programs: A randomized controlled trial. *JAMA* 2005; 293:1635–1643.
129. Gould MS, Kramer R: *Reporting a Suicide* [brochure]. 1999; New York, American Foundation for Suicide Prevention.
130. Brent DA, Perper J, Moritz G, et al.: Psychiatric effects of exposure to suicide among friends and acquaintances of adolescent suicide victims. *J Am Acad Child Adolesc Psychiatry* 1992; 31:629–639.
131. Hazell P, Lewin T: Friends of adolescent suicide attempters and completers. *J Am Acad Child Adolesc Psychiatry* 1993; 32:76–81.
132. Cerel J, Roberts TA, Milsen WJ: Peer suicidal behavior and adolescent risk behavior. *J Nerv Ment Disease* 2005; 193:237–243.
133. Cerel J, Fristad MA, Weller EB, et al.: Suicide-bereaved children and adolescents: A longitudinal examination. *J Am Acad Child Adolesc Psychiatry* 1999; 38:672–679.
134. Cerel J, Fristad MA, Weller EB, et al.: Suicide-bereaved children and adolescents: II. Parental and family functioning. *J Am Acad Child Adolesc Psychiatry* 2000; 39:437–444.
135. Pfeffer CR, Martins P, Mann J, et al.: Child survivors of suicide: Psychosocial characteristics. *J Am Acad Child Adolesc Psychiatry* 1997; 36:65–74.
136. Pfeffer CR, Karus D, Siegel K, et al.: Child survivors of parental death from cancer or suicide: Depressive and behavioral outcomes. *Psychooncology* 2000b; 9:1–10.
137. Melhem KN, Day N, Shear, et al.: Traumatic grief among adolescents exposed to peer's suicide. *Am J Psychiatry* 2004; 161:1411–1416.
138. Pfeffer CR, Jiang H, Kakuma T, Hwang J, Metsch M: Group intervention for children bereaved by the suicide of a relative. *J Amer Acad Child Adolesc Psychiatry* 2002; 41:505–513.
139. Shah S, Hoffman RE, Wake L, et al.: Adolescent suicide and household access to firearms in Colorado: Results of a case-control study. *J Adolesc Health* 2000; 26:157–163.
140. Grossman DC, Mueller BA, Riedy C, et al.: Gun storage practices and risk of youth suicide and unintentional firearm injuries. *JAMA* 2005; 293:707–714.
141. Webster DW, Vernick JS, Zeoli AM, Manganello JA: Association between youth-focused firearms laws and youth suicides. *JAMA* 2004; 292:594–601.

5.5 ■ ANXIETY DISORDERS

CHAPTER 5.5.1 ■ ANXIETY DISORDERS

AMY L. KRAIN, MANELY GHAFFARI, JENNIFER FREEMAN, ABBE GARCIA, HENRIETTA LEONARD, AND DANIEL S. PINE

Anxiety disorders are among the most common conditions affecting children and adolescents, with prevalence in the 4% to 20% range (1–4). They adversely impact self-esteem, social relationships, and academic performance (5). Moreover, pediatric anxiety disorders represent strong predictors of anxiety disorders during adulthood, and they confer strong risk for other forms of psychopathology, both concurrently as well as later in life (6). These observations highlight the importance of understanding and treating pediatric anxiety.

Most pediatric anxiety disorders are diagnosed using criteria identical to those applied in adults (7). One exception to this rule concerns the diagnosis of separation anxiety disorder, which remains a disorder classified in DSM-IV as "usually first diagnosed in infancy, childhood, or adolescence." Another exception concerns the diagnosis of generalized anxiety disorder, which uses more liberal thresholds in youth relative to adults. While broad comparability of criteria across ages encourages attempts to identify early risks for chronic anxiety, such consistency might minimize identification of potential developmental differences in the expression of anxiety. This point is particularly salient considering the presence of nonpathological developmental manifestations of anxiety.

Considerable controversy surrounds nosological distinctions among the specific pediatric anxiety disorders. From some perspectives, pediatric anxiety disorders have been considered as a group, as each of the disorders share many core features. From other perspectives, pediatric anxiety disorders have been considered as unique, individual disorders. The current chapter adopts both perspectives as to provide a concise summary of research on pediatric anxiety disorders.

The first two sections of the chapter provide a review of the clinical and epidemiological features of pediatric anxiety disorders, broadly conceptualized. This is followed in a third section by a summary of key characteristics of five specific anxiety disorders: separation anxiety disorder (SAD), social phobia/social anxiety disorder, generalized anxiety disorder (GAD), specific phobias, and panic disorder with and without agoraphobia. (See Chapters 5.5.2 and 5.15.2 for discussions of obsessive compulsive disorder [OCD] and posttraumatic stress disorder [PTSD]). Fourth, a review is provided of comorbidity issues and longitudinal findings. A fifth section reviews etiological theories, emphasizing supporting data from genetic and neuroimaging studies. Finally, we provide a brief discussion of therapeutics.

CLINICAL FEATURES OF ANXIETY, BROADLY CONCEPTUALIZED

In the current chapter, we use the term fear to label the brain state elicited by a threat, a stimulus for which an organism will extend effort to avoid. We use the term anxiety to label a brain state that is highly similar to fear but that occurs in the absence of a threatening stimulus. While these definitions derive from research in experimental psychology and neuroscience, they apply equally well to clinical phenomena. Fear and anxiety represent normal reactions to danger; both exhibit well documented age-related fluctuations with strong crosscultural similarity. These fluctuations typically begin with increases in stranger and separation anxiety in toddlers, followed by fears of physical harm in early school-age years. Anxiety about competence, abstract threats, and social situations typically increases during adolescence. Relatively brief periods of anxiety related to these issues represent a normal aspect of human development (8, 9). As a result, major questions arise concerning boundaries between "normal," or developmentally appropriate, and abnormal expressions of anxiety, as manifest in anxiety disorders.

One critical differentiation between normal fears or anxiety and an anxiety disorder derives from the so-called impairment criterion: To receive an anxiety disorder diagnosis there must be significant impairment or interference in the child's everyday functioning. Behavioral avoidance is a primary area of impairment that might lead children to avoid many typical experiences enjoyed by peers. Anxiety or fear is also considered abnormal when the level of distress evoked by danger is considered extreme, relative to a child's peers. However, this "distress" criterion typically has been more difficult to apply than the "impairment" criterion. Such difficulty arises from the fact that fewer guidelines are available for determining when "distress," relative to "impairment," appears "clinically significant."

PREVALENCE AND EPIDEMIOLOGY

Definitive data on prevalence and demographics of common syndromes derive from epidemiological studies randomly selecting subjects from the community. Available data suggest that 2.8%–27% of children and adolescents might be afflicted with some form of pediatric anxiety disorder, broadly conceptualized (10). Rates vary based on the definition used, assessment methods, specific disorders considered, and age ranges of the subjects. In terms of demographic correlates, the strongest findings document an excess of anxiety in females relative to males. This gender difference is found both in studies that rely on self-report scales and in studies that rely on diagnostic interviews for virtually all anxiety diagnoses (6, 11). Interestingly, female preponderance in anxiety emerges before puberty, which is earlier than in depression, which typically first manifests in females at puberty. An exception to this rule may be found in GAD, which appears to follow a pattern similar to depression, becoming more common in girls during adolescence (12, 13).

Some demographic data document distinctions among the anxiety disorders. For example, SAD has an earlier age of onset than the other anxiety disorders (14), and it shows dramatic reductions in prevalence with age. Social phobia, in contrast, typically exhibits an increase in prevalence during adolescence, which is consistent with normative developmental trajectories (6, 15).

The strongest evidence concerning an association between socioeconomic status (SES) and pediatric anxiety pertains to specific fears. Low SES has been linked both to typical fears as well as the diagnosis of specific phobia (6, 16). Data for other forms of pediatric anxiety appear less consistent. Additionally, data concerning crosscultural differences in prevalence are inconsistent (15, 17, 18).

CLINICAL FEATURES OF ANXIETY: INDIVIDUAL DISORDERS

Separation Anxiety Disorder

Definition and Clinical Description. Separation anxiety disorder (SAD) is defined in the DSM-IV as "developmentally inappropriate and excessive anxiety concerning separation from home or from those to whom the individual is attached" (7). The essential clinical feature of separation anxiety is excessive worry about losing or being permanently separated from a major attachment figure. Manifestations of this anxiety include recurrent excessive distress and/or repeated somatic complaints when separation from home or major attachment figures occurs or is anticipated. SAD may also include nightmares involving the theme of separation, and a persistent refusal to go to sleep or be alone without having a major attachment figure nearby (7). School refusal and excessive somatic complaints in the context of actual or anticipated separations are the most common reasons for parents and children to seek treatment for SAD (Table 5.5.1.1).

Further criteria for a diagnosis of separation anxiety are that the "disturbance" must last at least 4 weeks and cause clinically significant impairment in social, academic, and occupational arenas. The onset must occur before 18 years of age, and it is generally not expected to occur below 6 years of age. If the onset occurs before the child is 6 years old, it is labeled as early onset separation anxiety disorder (7). The lower age boundary is established to account for the fact that such anxiety is age-appropriate from 7 months to 6 years of age, and therefore should not necessarily be viewed as unusual or a problem below the age of 6 (19–21).

Specific Features. It has been suggested that childhood SAD is a risk factor for the development of panic disorder or agoraphobia as an adolescent or adult (22–25). This is supported by physiological studies demonstrating an increased

TABLE 5.5.1.1

ANXIETY DISORDERS KEY CHARACTERISTICS

DSM-IV Disorder	Key Characteristics*
Separation anxiety disorder (SAD)	■ Excessive anxiety concerning separation from loved one ■ Possible risk factor for development of panic disorder or agoraphobia in adulthood
Social phobia (social anxiety disorder)	■ Persistent fear of social or evaluative situations ■ Behavioral inhibition may be a temperamental predictor of social phobia in childhood or adulthood
Generalized anxiety disorder (GAD)	■ Excessive and uncontrollable worry about multiple issues ■ At least one somatic complaint ■ Close genetic link with depression
Specific phobia	■ Extreme fear of a specific situation or object ■ Five types of phobias, some corresponding to evolutionary dangers (snakes, blood)
Panic disorder with or without agoraphobia	■ Unexpected panic attacks accompanied by worry about future attacks ■ Agoraphobia is diagnosed if individual avoids places in which escape would be difficult or embarrassing ■ Panic attacks can be caused by medical conditions (hyperthyroidism, cardiac abnormalities)

*All DSM-IV anxiety disorder diagnoses require clinically significant distress or impairment in social, academic, or other areas of functioning.

sensitivity to carbon dioxide exposure in children with SAD similar to that seen in panic disorder patients (26). Such increased sensitivity to carbon dioxide, as well as other manifestations of respiratory dysfunction, occurs selectively in pediatric SAD but not in pediatric social phobia. This emphasizes the validity of nosological distinctions between SAD and social phobia. However, longitudinal studies of children with SAD have not necessarily supported this relationship with panic disorder (27). Similarly, family-based studies provide mixed support for the association between SAD in children and panic disorder in their parents (28, 29).

Social Phobia/Social Anxiety Disorder

Definition and Clinical Description. Social phobia, or social anxiety disorder, is defined in the DSM-IV as a persistent fear of one or more social situations in which a person is exposed to unfamiliar persons or to scrutiny by others. The term social anxiety disorder was added to this diagnosis in DSM-IV to emphasize the distinction between social phobia and other forms of phobias, which are classified as specific phobias. In social phobia/social anxiety disorder, the threat of exposure to such situations provokes anxiety, and even panic attacks. Feared social situations include public speaking and performance, attending social gatherings, and speaking to strangers. Social phobia interferes with daily functioning because sufferers try to avoid anxiety-provoking situations or endure them with intense distress (7). Children and adolescents with social phobia tend to focus excessively on concerns about embarrassment, negative evaluation, and rejection. They often experience increased heart rate, blushing, lightheadedness, gastrointestinal distress, and tremulousness when faced with a feared situation (30). Untreated, social phobia may result in school refusal, premature termination of formal education, and failure to enter the workforce. In older adolescents, social phobia can interfere with occupational development and dating relationships, which creates later relationship difficulties and dysfunction (31).

Specific Features. The development of social phobia in adolescence or adulthood has been significantly associated with the temperamental characteristic of behavioral inhibition to the unfamiliar, seen in infants as young as 21 months (31, 32). Behavioral inhibition is described as a tendency to exhibit withdrawal and excessive autonomic arousal to challenge or novelty (33). Moreover, some evidence suggests that children and adolescents with social phobia, unlike children and adolescents with SAD, exhibit increased fear when challenged in the laboratory with social stressors (34).

Differential diagnosis of social phobia is often complicated by social skills deficits and anxiety characteristic of pervasive developmental disorders (PDD) such as high-functioning autism and Asperger disorder. Evidence of some relationship between these classes of disorders emerges from family studies, where PDD in children has been linked to social phobia in parents (35). On the other hand, these disorders do represent distinct conditions. Social skills deficits in children with social phobia result from delayed learning and refinement of social skills due to anxiety, whereas deficits found in children with PDD are more likely due to neuropsychiatric impairment (31). If the child has the capacity for social relationships with familiar people, the diagnosis of social phobia is made, rather than PDD.

Generalized Anxiety Disorder

Definition and Clinical Description. Generalized anxiety disorder (GAD) is characterized by a pattern of excessive and uncontrollable worry that causes impairment in daily functioning. To meet diagnostic criteria, this pattern of extreme worry must be accompanied by at least one associated symptom and must last for at least six months. The worry associated with GAD is not confined to one topic area and is often focused on competence, approval, future events, and new or unfamiliar situations. These children frequently seek reassurance from others, although this reassurance usually provides only fleeting relief from the oppressive worries (36, 37). Somatic complaints such as headaches, stomach distress, sleep difficulties, and muscle aches are common. Patients also may report feeling on edge and unable to relax, and often seem irritable when worrying. As a result of these physical symptoms, these children often see their pediatrician rather than a mental health professional (38). Prior to DSM-IV, children and adolescents presenting with these symptoms typically were classified as suffering from overanxious disorder, a condition that was replaced by GAD in DSM-IV. Despite this nosological convention, symptoms for the two conditions exhibit only moderate overlap, and it remains unclear the degree to which these two constructs identify overlapping or distinct populations of children.

Specific Features. The results of a multivariate genetic analysis show a close genetic link between GAD and depression, suggesting that they are influenced by the same genetic factor (39). These findings are indicative of a more general predisposition toward anxiety and depression than specific to GAD. In light of findings that demonstrate that adolescent GAD precedes later depression (6), these genetic factors may predispose children or adolescents to develop GAD that in turn leads to depressive symptoms. Additional prospective studies of children with GAD are needed to tease apart this complex genetic linkage. This association may reflect the impact of broad personality factors, such as neuroticism or negative emotionality, on risk for both GAD and major depressive disorder. Such personality constructs have been linked to specific genetic factors, such as a functional polymorphism in the promoter for the serotonin transporter gene (see following).

Specific Phobia

Definition and Clinical Description. Specific phobia is defined as a marked and persistent fear that is excessive or unreasonable and interferes in daily life, which is cued by the presence or anticipation of a specific object or situation (flying, animals, heights, sight of blood) (7). Exposure to the phobic stimulus will almost always provoke an immediate anxiety response, such as a panic attack. In children, this response may appear as tantrums, crying, freezing, or clinging. Anxious symptoms can also include increased heart rate, sweating, hyperventilating, and upset stomach. Unlike adults with specific phobia who are usually aware that the fear is abnormal and maladaptive, children often do not recognize that their fear is excessive or unreasonable. For adolescents and children under 18 the phobia must have persisted for at least 6 months.

Specific Features. Specific phobias are grouped into five categories. In animal-type, the fear is cued by animals or insects. For natural-environment-type, the fear is cued by objects in the natural environment (storms, heights, water). Blood-injection-injury type involves a fear of seeing blood or an injury, or of receiving an injection. This type of specific phobia may involve feelings of disgust and a vasovagal response to feared stimuli. Situational type is cued by a specific situation (flying, using elevators, going over bridges). There is a fifth category, "other type," which encompasses all other objects or situations, such as choking or costumed characters (7, 40–42). Evolutionary theorists speculate that these five types of phobias correspond to evolutionary dangers that have become embedded in the genetic code. Fear of spiders, snakes, and blood are thus a product of innate survival tendencies. The fear is not a rational process, but rather a genetically coded reaction (41).

Panic Disorder with or without Agoraphobia

Definition and Clinical Description. Panic disorder refers to the experience of unexpected panic attacks accompanied by persistent apprehension about their recurrence or behavioral modifications in daily routine as a result of the attacks. While panic attacks can occur in many conditions, including phobias and social anxiety disorder, the panic attack associated with panic disorder is unique in that it occurs spontaneously without an environmental trigger. For example, panic disorder is uniquely associated with nocturnal panic attacks, which spontaneously awaken a patient from sleep.

A panic attack is a discrete period of intense fear or discomfort that is characterized by the presence of at least four somatic and/or cognitive symptoms. The most commonly reported symptoms among adolescents with panic attacks appear to be trembling, dizziness/faintness, pounding heart, nausea, shortness of breath, and sweating (43, 44). Cognitive symptoms, such as a fear of going crazy or dying, are reported less frequently than somatic ones (44). A diagnosis of panic disorder with agoraphobia is indicated if the patient avoids places or situations in which escape might be difficult or embarrassing. The most commonly avoided settings include those involving large groups of people unknown to the patient, such as restaurants, crowds, and auditoriums (43).

Specific Features. The most difficult distinction to make when diagnosing panic disorder in youth is the difference between an unexpected panic attack, as required for a diagnosis of panic disorder, and situationally cued attacks that are typical of other anxiety disorders. This task becomes especially challenging given the cognitive predisposition of children to attribute their experiences to external, identifiable, situational factors. Careful attention to the circumstances surrounding attacks will help with this distinction, as panic attacks occurring in the context of another anxiety disorder will occur primarily in the presence of the target stimulus. Additionally, presence of pervasive apprehension about having a panic attack, as opposed to facing a feared stimulus, supports the diagnosis of panic disorder rather than another anxiety disorder.

Panic attacks can also be caused by a variety of medical conditions, including hyperthyroidism, hyperparathyroidism, vestibular dysfunction, seizure disorders, and cardiac abnormalities. Appropriate laboratory tests and physical examinations should be used to rule out these causes prior to assigning a diagnosis of panic disorder. In particular, when panic is accompanied by cardiac symptoms, a discussion with a pediatrician as to the need for EKG and cardiac consultation is encouraged.

COMORBIDITY

As in adults, anxiety disorders in youth are frequently comorbid with each other and with other types of psychopathology. Rates of comorbidity among anxiety disorders tend to be somewhat lower in the general population—39% in children (45, 46) and 14% in adolescents (47)—than in clinic samples (50%) (48). This likely reflects a referral bias; children with multiple disorders, and consequently greater impairment, are more likely to seek treatment.

A recent community-based study found panic attacks and social phobia to be highly comorbid with other anxiety disorders. Social anxiety was found to be highly associated with any anxiety disorder (odds ratio [OR] = 14.2) (49). After adjusting for differences in age and gender, the presence of panic attacks was associated with increased likelihood of any anxiety disorder (OR = 4.6), social anxiety (OR = 2.3), specific phobia (OR = 3.4), agoraphobia (OR = 2.9), generalized anxiety disorder (OR = 4.8), overanxious disorder (OR = 3.7), and separation anxiety disorder (OR = 3.1) (50). In clinic samples, SAD is found to be more highly comorbid with other anxiety disorders than GAD and social phobia (51). Children with SAD are more likely to have comorbid specific phobia than children with GAD or social phobia. In contrast, children with GAD and social phobia were more likely to have comorbid mood disorders as compared to children with SAD. With respect to gender differences, in a nonreferred sample, having more than one anxiety disorder during childhood and adolescence was observed almost exclusively in females (52).

After comorbidity with another anxiety disorder, depression is the most commonly reported comorbid condition among youth with anxiety disorders (53, 54). Depression is 8.2 times as likely in children with anxiety disorders than in children without anxiety disorders (55). Specifically, there is a significant link between GAD and depression that persists into adulthood (6). Children and adolescents with GAD and comorbid MDD report significantly more anxiety symptoms and demonstrate greater functional impairment than GAD youth without MDD (56).

Approximately 20% of children with an anxiety disorder also meet criteria for an externalizing disorder (14, 45, 57, 58). In a selective review of attention deficit/hyperactivity disorder (ADHD), Biederman noted that about 30% of children and adolescents with ADHD also have an anxiety disorder (59). Interestingly, the prevalence of comorbid anxiety disorders increases in adults with ADHD to approximately 50%. In both children and adults with ADHD, females have a higher rate of comorbid anxiety disorders. Girls with the inattentive subtype of ADHD have higher rates of comorbid SAD, while those with the combined type have increased comorbidity with GAD (60). This is in contrast to males with ADHD who have a higher prevalence of oppositional defiant and conduct disorders.

Two additional conditions/disorders require mention when discussing comorbidity of pediatric anxiety disorders. First, selective mutism, a disorder characterized by persistent failure to speak in specific settings (school) despite full use of language at home or with family, may be found in younger children with social phobia. Approximately 68% of children with selective mutism also meet diagnostic criteria for social phobia (61). Second, while school refusal is not a DSM-IV diagnosis, it is a condition that often cooccurs with anxiety disorders, specifically SAD, specific phobia, and social phobia (62). School refusal is characterized by significant difficulty attending school, resulting in a prolonged absence and/or severe emotional upset. These children often display excessive fearfulness, temper outbursts, or complaints of feeling ill when faced with the prospect of going to school (62). The nature of the anxiety associated with school refusal behavior is likely to change with age, as is the nature of the precipitating events. For example, fear of separation is more common in younger school refusers, while social-evaluative fears, such as fears of teachers or peers, are more common in older children.

COURSE OF PEDIATRIC ANXIETY DISORDERS

Most prospective epidemiological studies examine the longitudinal outcome of anxiety disorders, broadly conceptualized, as opposed to specific conditions (63, 64). These studies find a statistically robust association between pediatric anxiety and a range of adult conditions, including both mood and anxiety disorders. However, from the standpoint of effect sizes, these associations are best characterized as modest: Odds ratios tend to fall between 2.0 and 4.0, varying as a function of severity and length of followup. This magnitude of association is somewhat weaker than typically found in longitudinal studies of stability in behavior disorders, such as conduct disorder. In terms of specific anxiety disorders, relatively few longitudinal data examine outcome for any one condition, compared with other conditions. Pine et al. (63) and Poulton et al. (65) provide two of the few examples in community-based samples. While few consistent associations emerge across these studies, data from both suggest that GAD exhibits a robust association with a range of adult conditions, including anxiety disorders and major depression. Data for other conditions, such as SAD or social phobia, appear more variable. Some studies document specific outcomes in these disorders (6), whereas other studies do not (65). Finally, similar conclusions derive from longitudinal studies of pediatric anxiety disorders based in the clinic. As with epidemiological studies, this research finds statistically robust associations with medium effect sizes. While more evidence emerges in these studies to support specificity of outcome, such as an association between SAD and panic disorder, the evidence is far from compelling (22, 24, 25).

ETIOLOGICAL/BIOLOGICAL THEORIES

Anxiety disorders, like most common psychiatric disorders, represent complex conditions that result from interactions among multiple risk factors and underlying predispositions. The majority of proposed etiological theories recognize the complexity of causal pathways, leading to a general, comprehensive model. As illustrated in Figure 5.5.1.1, this comprehensive model of anxiety disorders focuses on four factors: 1) genetic and environmental influences, 2) neural circuitry underlying emotion processing, 3) core psychological processes, and 4) broad behavioral tendencies, including temperament. Each of these components and their influences on the rest of the model will be discussed briefly in turn (Figure 5.5.1.1).

In terms of primary causes, this model implicates significant genetic and environmental influences. Family and twin studies consistently note a strong association between anxiety in parents and their children (29, 66). Moreover, twin studies among both children and adults document a statistically significant genetic component to various forms of anxiety (66–68). These genetic and environmental influences are unlikely to directly predispose toward anxiety disorders per se. Rather, they are likely to shape more basic psychological processes which in turn influence risk for anxiety. For example, there is evidence

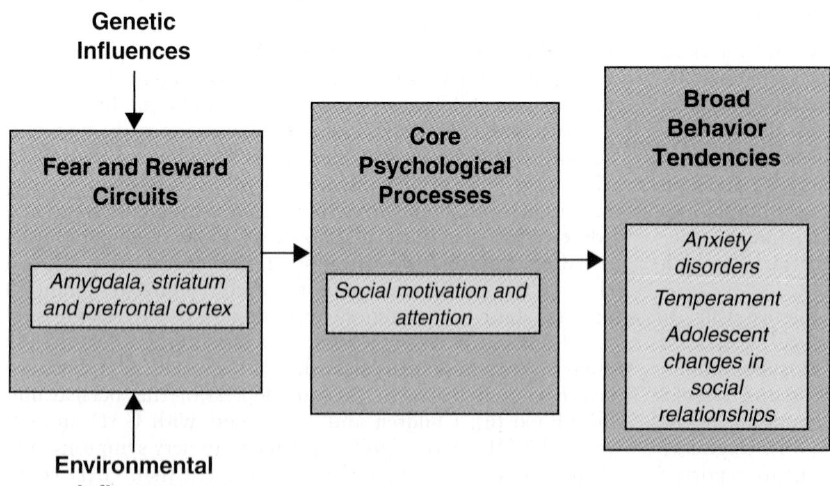

FIGURE 5.5.1.1. Etiological model of pediatric anxiety disorders.

for genetic influences on fear conditioning, the process by which an association is formed between a neutral stimulus, such as a tone or a light, and a noxious stimulus, such as an electric shock (69). Elements of this process are believed to underlie anxiety disorders, although the precise nature of the relationship between fear conditioning and anxiety remains ill specified (70).

In terms of specific genetic contributions, recent studies have focused on a polymorphism in the promoter region of the serotonin transporter gene (5HTT) involving a 44-bp insertion or deletion. As noted above, in the discussion of GAD, individuals with the short form of the gene (*ss* or *sl*) have been shown to have higher neuroticism, harm avoidance, and anxiety than individuals homozygous for the long variant (*ll*) (71, 72). A polymorphism of the variable-number-tandem-repeat in the second intron of the serotonin transporter gene has also been associated with increased risk of anxiety disorders, including OCD and GAD (73).

Despite such evidence of a genetic contribution, anxiety disorders generally involve a large environmental component. From an environmental perspective, parents with anxiety disorders may use distinctive child rearing practices that affect risk for anxiety (66, 74). For example, parents of anxious youth have been shown indirectly and directly to encourage maladaptive patterns of responding to ambiguous situations (75), exhibit overcontrolling and intrusive behaviors (76–78), and model anxious behavior themselves (79). As such, familial associations between parent and child anxiety may result through direct effects of these parenting behaviors, or through interactions between parent–child relationships and a genetically predetermined diathesis. Similar to genetic effects, these influences are unlikely to directly predispose towards anxiety. Rather, they are likely to shape core psychological processes, which in turn give rise to anxiety disorders.

There is increasing interest in understanding the interaction between genetic and environmental factors in the development of anxiety disorders. One recent report found an interaction between maternal reports of social support and child 5-HTT status in predicting behavioral inhibition at age 8 (80). Further research on similar interactions will allow for more comprehensive pathophysiologic models of anxiety disorders.

As noted above, the primary causes of anxiety, as reflected in genetic and environmental risk factors, influence the development of anxiety by shaping core psychological processes, such as fear conditioning. These psychological processes reflect the influence of genes and the environment on functional aspects of brain regions involved in fear and reward circuits. These regions include structures of the striatum as well as limbic and paralimbic systems, including the amygdala, orbitofrontal cortex (OFC), and anterior cingulate cortex (ACC) (81–86). These areas are highly interconnected and play a significant role in the integration of internal and external experience of emotion.

Animal and human studies provide indisputable evidence that the amygdala plays an important role in fear conditioning, a basic process by which fear toward a previously neutral stimulus develops. As a result, it has been implicated as a critical element of the neural circuitry underlying anxiety disorders (87). This is supported by neuroimaging findings that show that anxiety-disordered adults and children demonstrate greater amygdala activity in response to face stimuli than controls (88–90). In children, the magnitude of the signal change between fearful and neutral faces has been shown to be positively correlated with child self-report ratings of anxiety (90). A recent study found that this anxiety-related amygdala response to fearful faces is greater when the child attends to his/her internal emotional state than to the features of the face itself (91).

Structural imaging studies also document abnormalities in the amygdala among children and adolescents with anxiety disorders. For example, recent voxel-based morphometry findings show decreased left amygdala volume in children with anxiety disorders (92). These results, together with the functional neuroimaging findings, suggest an excitotoxic process may occur in the anxiety disorders, through which amygdala volume is reduced and responsivity increased. This theory of excitotoxicity as a risk factor for psychopathology was first introduced as a model for MDD (93). In light of the association between childhood anxiety disorders and MDD, it is a plausible model for these disorders as well. Nevertheless, relatively few studies examine amygdala volume in the anxiety disorders, and findings appear inconsistent: At least one group has reported an increased amygdala volume in pediatric GAD (94).

Beyond the amygdala, the orbitofrontal cortex (OFC) represents a second structure directly implicated in aspects of emotion processing that are perturbed in anxiety disorders. This includes the flexible representation of both negative and positive reinforcers (95). As such, it is likely a critical element of the neural circuitry of anxiety and anxiety disorders. In support of this theory, anxiety induction studies have demonstrated increased activation in areas of the right prefrontal cortex (96, 97) and left OFC (98). Pooling data across three groups of anxiety-disordered adults, Rauch and colleagues found consistent activation of the right medial OFC during symptom provocation (99). Magnetic resonance spectroscopy (MRS) studies demonstrate anxiety-related alterations in chemical composition of the OFC that are suggestive of changes in neuronal viability (100, 101). Monk et al. (102) report comparable perturbations in pediatric anxiety disorders.

Through its connections to the OFC and amygdala, the anterior cingulate cortex (ACC), particularly the rostral-ventral portion, serves to regulate emotional responses, and therefore is likely to be involved in the neural circuitry of anxiety. Studies of healthy adults using anxiety induction have demonstrated a decrease in activity in ACC (103, 104). A similar result has been found in patients with posttraumatic stress disorder (PTSD) who fail to demonstrate normal activation of the rostral ACC when shown combat-related stimuli (105). Through connections with the PFC, this dampening of the rostral ACC signal might serve to lessen cognitive control over threat-related information, which likely leads to the distress characteristic of patients with PTSD when exposed to trauma-related stimuli. In contrast, Rauch et al. (106) used PET to examine regional cerebral blood flow changes in patients with specific phobias during symptom provocation and found significant increases in the ACC, as compared to a control condition. These conflicting results suggest that specific phobias may rely on a different neural mechanism than other anxiety disorders.

According to this general model, perturbations in this core circuitry contribute to anxiety disorders through their effects on anxiety-related biases in information-processing functions. These functions can be conceptualized as core psychological processes, such as attention and motivation. Independent of research on brain imaging or neural circuitry function, a wealth of research examines the association between variations in anxiety and various core psychological processes. In experimental work, the most consistent cognitive feature associated with fear and anxiety in humans represents an attention bias for stimuli associated with danger (107–111). This bias resembles the high degree of vigilance that animals show for feared scenarios or objects. In human studies, it is most often measured using the dot probe and Stroop paradigms.

In the dot probe task, individuals monitor two stimuli presented on a computer screen: One is either a threatening word or picture and the other is a neutral word or picture.

Subjects must press a button when a target appears in place of one of the stimuli, and reaction times to these targets are influenced in individuals with high levels of anxiety by proximity between the threat cue and the target. Studies using dot probe tasks demonstrate a bias toward threatening stimuli in adults and children with anxiety disorders that is not seen in nonanxious controls (112–116). Recording of eye movements during a face dot probe task confirmed that patients are more likely than normal controls to initially look toward a threatening face than a neutral one (117). Interestingly, this orienting toward threat is more likely to occur with brief stimulus presentations (500 ms), suggesting cognitive mechanisms early in information processing (116).

The Stroop task requires subjects to name the color of potentially threatening words, such as "coronary" or "snake." Prolonged latency for naming such color-words is presumed to be the result of interference, such that reactions elicited by a fear word interfere with attention to the color of the word. This effect has been demonstrated in both adults (118–121) and children (122) with anxiety disorders. While similar degrees of attention bias are found across anxiety disorders, the particular stimuli that cause this bias differ. For example, panic disorder patients may show a particularly prolonged latency to panic-related words, such as "smother," while subjects with social phobia may show greater latencies to relevant words such as "embarrass."

This bias toward threat is also evident in interpretations of ambiguity. Children with anxiety disorders have been shown to be more likely to interpret ambiguous stimuli as threatening. When performing a homophone task during which the subject is asked to write down words he hears on an audiotape, GAD patients display a greater tendency to write down the word associated with the more negative interpretation (pain vs. pane) (123). In a homograph study where children were shown a list of words with neutral and threatening meanings, youth with GAD showed a greater tendency to produce sentences using threatening interpretations than control participants (124). Similar results are found in studies when children diagnosed with anxiety disorders are presented with ambiguous situations and asked to interpret them (75, 125). Anxiety-disordered youth are more likely to make a threatening interpretation of these situations than their nonanxious peers.

Finally, these core psychological processes are believed to underlie broad behavioral tendencies such as early temperament and later development of anxiety disorders. Behavioral inhibition is a temperamental factor measurable during the first years of life that has been shown to predict later onset of anxiety disorders (126, 127). Children with temperaments characterized by behavioral inhibition react to novel situations with signs of reticence or withdrawal. Based on peripheral physiologic data, behavioral inhibition is thought to result from an underlying hypersensitivity within amygdala-based neural circuits (126). While most children with behavioral inhibition do not develop clinical anxiety disorders, behavioral inhibition does predict an elevated risk for childhood anxiety disorders, particularly social phobia (32).

Clearly, the development of anxiety and its disorders is a complex process that likely involves biological vulnerabilities as well as environmental influences. Significant advances in basic research have provided a neurobiological framework on which to base hypothesized etiological models. Additionally, advanced research technologies in genetics and neuroimaging have allowed us to test these models with ever increasing sophistication and detail. Continued translation of basic research findings to clinical studies will be essential to the further advancement of our understanding of anxiety disorders.

TREATMENT OF PEDIATRIC ANXIETY DISORDERS

Over the past two decades, significant advances have been made in the treatment of pediatric anxiety disorders. Cognitive-behavioral and pharmacological interventions have emerged as effective treatments for these disorders. While a few trials have evaluated these treatments for a specific anxiety disorder, most have included children and adolescents with a primary diagnosis of GAD, SAD, or social phobia. In light of the high comorbidity among these disorders, this approach improves the feasibility and generalizability of these studies. The most widely used interventions and their empirical support will be discussed here.

Cognitive-Behavioral Interventions

Cognitive-behavioral treatments (CBT) have proven to be effective at treating anxiety disorders in children and adolescents (128–130). Most cognitive-behavioral interventions were initially developed for adult anxiety and phobic disorders, so the techniques for children are conceptually and structurally similar but modified according to developmental level. For example, to introduce cognitive restructuring, these treatments use cartoons and thought bubbles to help children learn to identify and then change their thoughts. In addition to cognitive techniques, these treatments include behavioral strategies such as modeling, relaxation skills training, homework, contingency management, and most importantly, exposure to feared situations. The aim of exposures, either imaginal or in vivo (real life), is to provide the patient with opportunities to practice newly learned coping skills in a safe, controlled environment. Feared stimuli or situations are presented in a graduated fashion, beginning with the easiest and ending with the most difficult, so that the child experiences early success in using these new skills. The pace at which the child and therapist move up the hierarchy is determined by these successes.

Empirical evidence supports the use of these cognitive-behavioral interventions for pediatric anxiety disorders. Kendall et al. conducted two randomized-controlled trials demonstrating the efficacy of a 16-week individual CBT for children with social phobia, GAD, and SAD (129, 130). Treatment gains were maintained at 1, 3 (131), and 7 years post-treatment (132). Barrett and colleagues modified Kendall's CBT and added a family-based component that teaches parents how to be effective models for their children and how to encourage coping with feared situations, rather than avoidance. Individual CBT plus the family component was shown effectively to reduce anxiety symptoms and may have had some added benefits, particularly for younger, female children (128). Treatment gains were maintained at 6-year follow-up (133). Group cognitive-behavioral interventions have been shown to be effective for the treatment of socially phobic children and adolescents (134–136). Conducting treatment in a group setting provides these children with greater opportunities for in vivo exposures.

While this work clearly documents the benefits of CBT in pediatric anxiety disorders, major questions remain concerning the mechanism of these effects. Such questions emerge given limitations in the available studies. In particular, the majority of controlled trials compare CBT to relatively crude comparison conditions, such as a wait-list control. A few trials have used more rigorous designs, whereby a credible attention-control condition is used. Results in these trials are less consistent than in the trials comparing CBT to a wait-list (137, 138). Nevertheless, at least one study in pediatric social anxiety disorder demonstrated a superior response to

CBT relative to a credible attention-control intervention. Moreover, ongoing studies are comparing CBT for pediatric anxiety disorders to placebo control. Findings in pediatric MDD using this same contrast recently generated considerable questions on efficacy of CBT in this condition. Results from the comparison of CBT with placebo in the anxiety disorders are thus eagerly anticipated. A more detailed discussion of CBT appears in Chapter 6.2.2.

Pharmacological Interventions

Advances in psychopharmacology and the design and implementation of large placebo-controlled studies have led to significant improvement in the treatment of pediatric anxiety disorders. As with CBT, pharmacological agents that have been shown effectively to treat adult anxiety disorders, such as antidepressants and anxiolytics, are now being used to treat children. Benzodiazepines have shown mixed results (31, 139) and are not indicated as a first-line treatment in children due to their potential adverse effects. There is also little or no evidence for the efficacy of other anxiolytics, such as buspirone or beta-blockers. While tricyclic antidepressants have demonstrated some efficacy, they have not been shown convincingly to treat pediatric anxiety disorders, beyond the data documenting the efficacy of clomipramine for pediatric OCD. In addition, their side effect profiles do not make them a viable first-line treatment option for children. Overall, efficacy and safety data support the use of selective serotonin reuptake inhibitors (SSRIs) to treat childhood social phobia, SAD, and GAD. In light of this, this section will review only current findings regarding the treatment of pediatric anxiety disorders using SSRIs. A greater discussion of psychopharmacologic agents appears in Chapter 6.1.

Early open trials of SSRIs showed promising results for children with mixed anxiety disorders (140, 141). Following from these results, the Research Unit on Pediatric Psychopharmacology (RUPP) conducted the largest medication trial of children (ages 6–17) with a primary diagnosis of SAD, GAD, or social phobia (142). Following a 3-week supportive psychoeducational treatment lead-in, 128 children were assigned to either fluvoxamine or placebo for 8 weeks. The children in the fluvoxamine group had greater reductions in symptoms of anxiety and higher rates of clinical response than the children in the placebo group. On the Clinical Global Impression scale, 48 of 63 (76%) children in the fluvoxamine group were classified as treatment responders, in comparison to only 19 of 65 (29%) children in the placebo group ($p < 0.001$). In a somewhat smaller randomized placebo-controlled study of 74 children with GAD, social phobia, and/or SAD, fluoxetine was found to be superior to placebo in decreasing symptoms of anxiety (143).

Recent studies have demonstrated the efficacy of SSRIs for specific anxiety disorders. For example, Rynn et al. conducted a placebo-controlled study of sertraline with children and adolescents with GAD (144). Beginning at 4 weeks, the sertraline-treated group showed significantly reduced scores on the Hamilton anxiety scale and the Clinical Global Impression (CGI) severity and improvement scales. Recently a multicenter, randomized, double-blind, placebo-controlled trial of children and adolescents with social anxiety disorder concluded that paroxetine is an effective, generally well tolerated treatment for social phobia (145). A total of 322 children and adolescents age 8–17 either received placebo or paroxetine (10–50 mg/day) for 16 weeks. As measured by the CGI-Improvement scale, the odds of responding were significantly greater for paroxetine versus placebo.

There have been no placebo-controlled, double-blind trials of the treatment of panic disorder in children. A small, open label study of 12 children and adolescents with panic disorder showed improvement on SSRIs with minimal side effects (146). In a preliminary naturalistic study, 15 of 18 children and adolescents with panic disorder were considered responders to paroxetine (147). In adults, SSRIs have become the pharmacotherapeutic treatment of choice, and several SSRIs have approved indications for the treatment of panic.

Questions have been raised about the safety of SSRIs in children and adolescents. In particular, the Food and Drug Administration (FDA) issued a "black box" warning in the fall of 2004 concerning the use of SSRIs in this age group. This warning cautioned physicians about the possible adverse behavioral side effects of SSRIs. Specifically, analyses performed by the FDA demonstrated a higher rate of suicidal thoughts and acts in a metaanalysis of randomized controlled trials. These trials had examined approximately 4,000 children and adolescents with various forms of psychopathology, including anxiety. While the overall rate of clinically significant suicidal thoughts or acts was less than 5%, the rate was statistically greater for individuals randomized to SSRIs as compared to placebo. As a result, prescribing clinicians need to be very careful to assess for signs of behavioral activation and/or suicidality when using these treatments. It is also especially important to take a careful history before prescribing that includes signs of mood instability in the patient or family members.

Future Directions/Research Challenges

Over the past 20 years, significant strides have been made in the development of effective treatments of pediatric anxiety disorders. Cognitive-behavioral treatments and SSRIs have proven to be first-line interventions. However, we have little information about which is more effective, and for whom. The next step is to conduct a study examining these issues. Are medications more effective than CBT; is CBT more effective than medication? Is the combination of CBT plus medications more effective than either alone? Such a study is currently underway and we will have to await the results.

In conclusion, this chapter has provided a review of pediatric anxiety disorders, including current findings regarding their prevalence, etiology, and treatment. The study of these disorders is relatively new, as compared to other psychiatric conditions (schizophrenia, major depressive disorder). As a result, our understanding of underlying developmental and neurobiological mechanisms is limited. Continued advances in basic science research, genetics, and neuroscience will allow for further refinement of current models and subsequent development of new interventions for the prevention and treatment of pediatric anxiety disorders.

References

1. Marmorstein NR: Generalized versus performance-focused social phobia: Patterns of comorbidity among youth. *J Anxiety Disord* 2005.
2. Achenbach TM, Howell CT, McConaughy SH, Stanger C: Six-year predictors of problems in a national sample of children and youth: I. Cross-informant syndromes. *J Am Acad Child Adolesc Psychiatry* 34:336–347, 1995.
3. Gurley D, Cohen P, Pine DS, Brook J: Discriminating depression and anxiety in youth: A role for diagnostic criteria. *J Affect Disord* 39:191–200, 1996.
4. Costello EJ, Mustillo S, Erkanli A, Keeler G, Angold A: Prevalence and development of psychiatric disorders in childhood and adolescence. *Arch Gen Psychiatry* 60:837–844, 2003.
5. Klein RG, Last CG: *Anxiety Disorders in Children.* Newbury Park, CA: Sage, 1989.
6. Pine DS, Cohen P, Gurley D, Brook J, Ma Y: The risk for early-adulthood anxiety and depressive disorders in adolescents with anxiety and depressive disorders. *Archives of General Psychiatry* 55:56–64, 1998.

7. American Psychiatric Association. *Diagnostic and Statistical Manual of Mental Disorders* 4th ed. Washington, DC, Author, 1994.
8. Bell-Dolan DJ, Last CG, Strauss CC: Symptoms of anxiety disorders in normal children. *J Am Acad Child Adolesc Psychiatry* 29:759–765, 1990.
9. Bernstein GA, Shaw K: Practice parameters for the assessment and treatment of children and adolescents with anxiety disorders. American Academy of Child and Adolescent Psychiatry. *J Am Acad Child Adolesc Psychiatry* 36:69S–84S, 1997.
10. Costello EJ, Egger HL, Angold A: The developmental epidemiology of anxiety disorders: Phenomenology, prevalence, and comorbidity. *Child Adolesc Psychiatr Clin N Am* 14:631–48, vii, 2005.
11. Lewinsohn PM, Gotlib IH, Lewinsohn M, Seeley JR, Allen NB: Gender differences in anxiety disorders and anxiety symptoms in adolescents. *Journal of Abnormal Psychology* 107:109–117, 1998.
12. Cohen P, Cohen J, Kasen S, Velez CN, Hartmark C, Johnson J et al.: An epidemiological study of disorders in late childhood and adolescence: I. Age- and gender-specific prevalence. *J Child Psychol Psychiatry* 34:851–867, 1993.
13. Werry JS: Overanxious disorder: A review of its taxonomic properties. *J Am Acad Child Adolesc Psychiatry* 30:533–544, 1991.
14. Last CG, Perrin S, Hersen M, Kazdin AE: DSM-III-R anxiety disorders in children: Sociodemographic and clinical characteristics. *J Am Acad Child Adolesc Psychiatry* 31:1070–1076, 1992.
15. Compton SN, Nelson AH, March JS: Social phobia and separation anxiety symptoms in community and clinical samples of children and adolescents. *J Am Acad Child Adolesc Psychiatry* 39:1040–1046, 2000.
16. Gullone E: The development of normal fear: A century of research. *Clin Psychol Rev* 20:429–451, 2000.
17. Dong Q, Yang B, Ollendick TH: Fears in Chinese children and adolescents and their relations to anxiety and depression. *J Child Psychol Psychiatry* 35:351–363, 1994.
18. Neal AM, Lilly RS, Zakis S: What are African-American children afraid of? A preliminary study. *Journal of Anxiety Disorders* 7:129–139, 1993.
19. Bernstein GA, Borchardt CM: Anxiety disorders of childhood and adolescence: A critical review. *J Am Acad Child Adolesc Psychiatry* 30:519–532, 1991.
20. Chorpita BF, Albano AM, Heimberg RG, Barlow DH: A systematic replication of the prescriptive treatment of school refusal behavior in a single subject. *J Behav Ther Exp Psychiatry* 27:281–290, 1996.
21. Silverman WK, Rabian B: Test-retest reliability of the Dsm-III-R Childhood Anxiety Disorders symptoms using the Anxiety Disorders Interview Schedule for Children. *Journal of Anxiety Disorders* 9:139–150, 1995.
22. Battaglia M, Bertella S, Politi E, Bernardeschi L, Perna G, Gabriele A et al.: Age at onset of panic disorder: Influence of familial liability to the disease and of childhood separation anxiety disorder. *Am J Psychiatry* 152:1362–1364, 1995.
23. Biederman J, Petty C, Faraone SV, Hirshfeld-Becker DR, Henin A, Rauf A et al.: Childhood antecedents to panic disorder in referred and nonreferred adults. *J Child Adolesc Psychopharmacol* 15:549–561, 2005.
24. Gittelman R, Klein DF: Relationship between separation anxiety and panic and agoraphobic disorders. *Psychopathology* 17 Suppl 1:56–65, 1984.
25. Moreau D, Follet C: Panic disorder in children and adolescents. *Child and Adolescent Psychiatric Clinics of North America* 2:581–602, 1993.
26. Pine DS, Klein RG, Coplan JD, Papp LA, Hoven CW, Martinez J et al.: Differential carbon dioxide sensitivity in childhood anxiety disorders and nonill comparison group. *Archives of General Psychiatry* 57:960–967, 2000.
27. Aschenbrand SG, Kendall PC, Webb A, Safford SM, Flannery-Schroeder E: Is childhood separation anxiety disorder a predictor of adult panic disorder and agoraphobia? A seven-year longitudinal study. *J Am Acad Child Adolesc Psychiatry* 42:1478–1485, 2003.
28. Biederman J, Petty C, Faraone SV, Hirshfeld-Becker DR, Henin A, Dougherty M et al.: Parental predictors of pediatric panic disorder/agoraphobia: A controlled study in high-risk offspring. *Depress Anxiety* 22:114–120, 2005.
29. Pine DS: Pathophysiology of childhood anxiety disorders. *Biol Psychiatry* 46:1555–1566, 1999.
30. Beidel DC, Christ MG, Long PJ: Somatic complaints in anxious children. *J Abnorm Child Psychol* 19:659–670, 1991.
31. Mancini C, Van Ameringen M, Bennett M, Patterson B, Watson C: Emerging treatments for child and adolescent social phobia: A review. *Journal of Child and Adolescent Psychopharmacology* 15:589–607, 2005.
32. Schwartz CE, Snidman N, Kagan J: Adolescent social anxiety as an outcome of inhibited temperament in childhood. *J Am Acad Child Adolesc Psychiatry* 38:1008–1015, 1999.
33. Rosenbaum JF, Biederman J, Hirshfeld DR, Bolduc EA, Faraone SV, Kagan J et al.: Further evidence of an association between behavioral inhibition and anxiety disorders: results from a family study of children from a non-clinical sample. *J Psychiatr Res* 25:49–65, 1991.
34. Pine DS, Klein RG, Roberson-Nay R, Mannuzza S, Moulton JL, III, Woldehawariat G et al.: Response to 5% carbon dioxide in children and adolescents: Relationship to panic disorder in parents and anxiety disorders in subjects. *Arch Gen Psychiatry* 62:73–80, 2005.
35. Piven J, Palmer P: Psychiatric disorder and the broad autism phenotype: Evidence from a family study of multiple-incidence autism families. *Am J Psychiatry* 156:557–563, 1999.
36. Kearney CA, Albano AM: *Therapist's Manual for the Prescriptive Treatment of School Refusal in Youth*. The Psychological Corporation, 2000.
37. Kendall PC, Krain AL, Treadwell KR: Generalized anxiety disorder. In: Ammerman RT, Hersen M, Last CG (eds): *Handbook of Prescriptive Treatments for Children and Adolescents*. Boston, Allyn & Bacon, 1999, pp. 155–171.
38. Bell-Dolan D, Brazeal TJ: Separation anxiety disorder, overanxious disorder, and school refusal. *Child and Adolescent Psychiatric Clinics of North America* 2:563–580, 1993.
39. Kendler KS, Walters EE, Neale MC, Kessler RC, Heath AC, Eaves LJ: The structure of the genetic and environmental risk factors for six major psychiatric disorders in women: Phobia, generalized anxiety disorder, panic disorder, bulimia, major depression, and alcoholism. *Arch Gen Psychiatry* 52:374–383, 1995.
40. Fredrikson M, Annas P, Fischer H, Wik G: Gender and age differences in the prevalence of specific fears and phobias. *Behav Res Ther* 34:33–39, 1996.
41. Merckelbach H, Dejong PJ, Muris P, vandenHout MA: The etiology of specific phobias: A review. *Clinical Psychology Review* 16:337–361, 1996.
42. Muris P, Schmidt H, Merckelbach H: The structure of specific phobia symptoms among children and adolescents. *Behav Res Ther* 37:863–868, 1999.
43. Kearney CA, Albano AM, Eisen AR, Allan WD, Barlow DH: The phenomenology of panic disorder in youngsters: An empirical study of a clinical sample. *J Anxiety Disord* 11:49–62, 1997.
44. King NJ, Ollendick TH, Mattis SG: Nonclinical panic attacks in adolescents: Prevalence, symptomatology, and associated features. *Behavior Change* 13, 1997.
45. Anderson JC, Williams S, McGee R, Silva PA: DSM-III disorders in preadolescent children. Prevalence in a large sample from the general population. *Arch Gen Psychiatry* 44:69–76, 1987.
46. Kashani JH, Orvaschel H: A community study of anxiety in children and adolescents. *Am J Psychiatry* 147:313–318, 1990.
47. McGee R, Feehan M, Williams S, Anderson J: DSM-III disorders from age 11 to age 15 years. *J Am Acad Child Adolesc Psychiatry* 31:50–59, 1992.
48. Last CG. Developmental considerations. In: Last CG, Hersen M (eds): *Issues in Diagnostic Research*. New York, Plenum, 1987, pp. 201–216.
49. Marmorstein NR: Generalized versus performance-focused social phobia: Patterns of comorbidity among youth. *J Anxiety Disord* 2005.
50. Goodwin RD, Gotlib IH: Panic attacks and psychopathology among youth. *Acta Psychiatr Scand* 109:216–221, 2004.
51. Verduin TL, Kendall PC: Differential occurrence of comorbidity within childhood anxiety disorders. *J Clin Child Adolesc Psychol* 32:290–295, 2003.
52. Lewinsohn PM, Zinbarg R, Seeley JR, Lewinsohn M, Sack WH: Lifetime comorbidity among anxiety disorders and between anxiety disorders and other mental disorders in adolescents. *J Anxiety Disord* 11:377–394, 1997.
53. Costello EJ, Mustillo S, Erkanli A, Keeler G, Angold A: Prevalence and development of psychiatric disorders in childhood and adolescence. *Archives of General Psychiatry* 60:837–844, 2003.
54. Brady EU, Kendall PC: Comorbidity of anxiety and depression in children and adolescents. *Psychol Bull* 111:244–255, 1992.
55. Angold A, Costello EJ, Erkanli A: Comorbidity. *Journal of Child Psychology and Psychiatry and Allied Disciplines* 40:57–87, 1999.
56. Masi G, Favilla L, Mucci M, Millepiedi S: Depressive comorbidity in children and adolescents with generalized anxiety disorder. *Child Psychiatry Hum Dev* 30:205–215, 2000.
57. Last CG, Strauss CC, Francis G: Comorbidity among childhood anxiety disorders. *Journal of Nervous and Mental Disease* 175:726–730, 1987.
58. McGee R, Feehan M, Williams S, Partridge F, Silva PA, Kelly J: DSM-III disorders in a large sample of adolescents. *Journal of American Academy of Child and Adolescent Psychiatry* 29:611–619, 1990.
59. Biederman J: Attention-deficit/hyperactivity disorder: A selective overview. *Biological Psychiatry* 57:1215–1220, 2005.
60. Levy F, Hay DA, Bennett KS, McStephen M: Gender differences in ADHD subtype comorbidity. *J Am Acad Child Adolesc Psychiatry* 44:368–376, 2005.
61. Kristensen H: Selective mutism and comorbidity with developmental disorder/delay, anxiety disorder, and elimination disorder. *J Am Acad Child Adolesc Psychiatry* 39:249–256, 2000.
62. King NJ, Ollendick TH, Tonge BJ: School Refusal: *Assessment and Treatment*. Boston, Allyn and Bacon, 1995.
63. Pine DS: Treating children and adolescents with selective serotonin reuptake inhibitors: How long is appropriate? *J Child Adolesc Psychopharmacol* 12:189–203, 2002.
64. Costello EJ, Egger HL, Angold A: In: Ollendick TH, March JS (eds): *Developmental Epidemiology of Anxiety Disorders*. New York, Oxford University Press, 2004, pp. 61–91.
65. Poulton R, Pine DS, Harrington H: Are anxiety disorders and their etiologies stable across the lifecourse? In: Andrews G, Charney DS, Sirovatka PJ, Regier DA (eds): *Stress-Induced and Fear Circuitry Disorders: Refining the Research Agenda for DSM-V*. Washington, DC, American Psychiatric Press, 2006.
66. Klein RG: Anxiety disorders. In: Rutter M, Taylor E, Hersov L (eds): *Child and Adolescent Psychiatry: Modern Approaches*. London, Blackwell Scientific Publications, 1995, pp. 351–374.

67. Hettema JM, Prescott CA, Myers JM, Neale MC, Kendler KS: The structure of genetic and environmental risk factors for anxiety disorders in men and women. *Arch Gen Psychiatry* 62:182–189, 2005.
68. Fyer AJ, Mannuzza S, Chapman TF, Martin LY, Klein DF: Specificity in familial aggregation of phobic disorders. *Arch Gen Psychiatry* 52:564–573, 1995.
69. Hettema JM, Annas P, Neale MC, Kendler KS, Fredrikson M: A twin study of the genetics of fear conditioning. *Arch Gen Psychiatry* 60:702–708, 2003.
70. Lissek S, Powers AS, McClure EB, Phelps EA, Woldehawariat G, Grillon C et al.: Classical fear conditioning in the anxiety disorders: A meta-analysis. *Behav Res Ther* 43:1391–1424, 2005.
71. Schinka JA, Busch RM, Robichaux-Keene N: A meta-analysis of the association between the serotonin transporter gene polymorphism (5-HTTLPR) and trait anxiety. *Mol Psychiatry* 9:197–202, 2004.
72. Mazzanti CM, Lappalainen J, Long JC, Bengel D, Naukkarinen H, Eggert M et al.: Role of the serotonin transporter promoter polymorphism in anxiety-related traits. *Arch Gen Psychiatry* 55:936–940, 1998.
73. Ohara K, Suzuki Y, Ochiai M, Tsukamoto T, Tani K, Ohara K: A variable-number-tandem-repeat of the serotonin transporter gene and anxiety disorders. *Prog Neuropsychopharmacol Biol Psychiatry* 23:55–65, 1999.
74. Ginsburg GS, Siqueland L, Masia-Warner C, Hedtke KA: Anxiety disorders in children: Family matters. *Cognitive and Behavioral Practice* 11:28–43, 2004.
75. Barrett PA, Rapee RM, Dadds MR, Ryan SM: Family enhancement of cognitive style in anxious and aggressive children. *Journal of Abnormal Child Psychology* 24:187–203, 1996.
76. Dumas JE, LaFreniere PJ, Serketich WJ: "Balance of power": A transactional analysis of control in mother–child dyads involving socially competent, aggressive, and anxious children. *J Abnorm Psychol* 104:104–113, 1995.
77. Hudson JL, Rapee RM: Parent-child interactions and anxiety disorders: An observational study. *Behav Res Ther* 39:1411–1427, 2001.
78. Siqueland L, Kendall PC, Steinberg L: Anxiety in children: Perceived family environments and observed family interaction. *Journal of Clinical Child Psychology* 25:225–237, 1996.
79. Whaley SE, Pinto A, Sigman M: Characterizing interactions between anxious mothers and their children. *J Consult Clin Psychol* 67:826–836, 1999.
80. Fox NA, Nichols KE, Henderson HA, Rubin K, Schmidt L, Hamer D et al.: Evidence for a gene–environment interaction in predicting behavioral inhibition in middle childhood. *Psychol Sci* 16:921–926, 2005.
81. Davis M: Neurobiology of fear responses: The role of the amygdala. *J Neuropsychiatry Clin Neurosci* 9:382–402, 1997.
82. Davis M: Are different parts of the extended amygdala involved in fear versus anxiety? *Biol Psychiatry* 44:1239–1247, 1998.
83. Gray TS, Bingaman EW: The amygdala: Corticotropin-releasing factor, steroids, and stress. *Crit Rev Neurobiol* 10:155–168, 1996.
84. LeDoux J: Emotional networks and motor control: A fearful view. *Prog Brain Res* 107:437–446, 1996.
85. LeDoux J: Fear and the brain: Where have we been, and where are we going? *Biol Psychiatry* 44:1229–1238, 1998.
86. Maren S: Long-term potentiation in the amygdala: A mechanism for emotional learning and memory. *Trends Neurosci* 22:561–567, 1999.
87. Rauch SL, Shin LM, Wright CI: Neuroimaging studies of amygdala function in anxiety disorders. *Annals of the New York Academy of Sciences* 985:389–410, 2003.
88. Birbaumer N, Grodd W, Diedrich O, Klose U, Erb M, Lotze M et al.: fMRI reveals amygdala activation to human faces in social phobics. *Neuroreport* 9:1223–1226, 1998.
89. Stein MB, Goldin PR, Sareen J, Zorrilla LT, Brown GG: Increased amygdala activation to angry and contemptuous faces in generalized social phobia. *Arch Gen Psychiatry* 59:1027–1034, 2002.
90. Thomas KM, Drevets WC, Dahl RE, Ryan ND, Birmaher B, Eccard CH et al.: Amygdala response to fearful faces in anxious and depressed children. *Archives of General Psychiatry* 58:1057–1063, 2001.
91. McClure EB, Monk C, Nelson EE, Schweder AE, Roberson-Nay R, Zarahn E et al.: Attention-modulated neural engagement to emotional facial expressions in adolescents with anxiety disorders. Presented at the Annual Meeting of the Society for Biological Psychiatry, 2004.
92. Milham MP, Nugent AC, Drevets WC, Dickstein DP, Leibenluft E, Ernst M et al.: Selective reduction in amygdala volume in pediatric anxiety disorders: A voxel-based morphometry investigation. *Biol Psychiatry* 57:961–966, 2005.
93. Drevets WC: Neuroimaging abnormalities in the amygdala in mood disorders. *Ann N Y Acad Sci* 985:420–444, 2003.
94. De Bellis MD, Casey BJ, Dahl RE, Birmaher B, Williamson DE, Thomas KM et al.: A pilot study of amygdala volumes in pediatric generalized anxiety disorder. *Biological Psychiatry* 48:51–57, 2000.
95. Rolls ET: The functions of the orbitofrontal cortex. *Brain Cogn* 55:11–29, 2004.
96. Davidson RJ: Anxiety and affective style: Role of prefrontal cortex and amygdala. *Biol Psychiatry* 51:68–80, 2002.
97. Rauch SL, Savage CR, Alpert NM, Fischman AJ, Jenike MA: The functional neuroanatomy of anxiety: A study of three disorders using positron emission tomography and symptom provocation. *Biol Psychiatry* 42:446–452, 1997.
98. Chua P, Krams M, Toni I, Passingham R, Dolan R: A functional anatomy of anticipatory anxiety. *Neuroimage* 9:563–571, 1999.
99. Rauch SL, Savage CR, Alpert NM, Fischman AJ, Jenike MA: The functional neuroanatomy of anxiety: A study of three disorders using positron emission tomography and symptom provocation. *Biol Psychiatry* 42:446–452, 1997.
100. Grachev ID, Apkarian AV: Anxiety in healthy humans is associated with orbital frontal chemistry. *Molecular Psychiatry* 5:482–488, 2000.
101. Mathew SJ, Mao X, Coplan JD, Smith EL, Sackeim HA, Gorman JM et al.: Dorsolateral prefrontal cortical pathology in generalized anxiety disorder: A proton magnetic resonance spectroscopic imaging study. *Am J Psychiatry* 161:1119–1121, 2004.
102. Monk CS, Nelson EE, McClure EB, Mogg K, Bradley BP, Leibenluft E et al.: Ventrolateral prefrontal cortex activation and attentional bias in response to angry faces in adolescents with generalized anxiety disorder. *American Journal of Psychiatry* 163: 1091–1097, 2006.
103. Kimbrell TA, George MS, Parekh PI, Ketter TA, Podell DM, Danielson AL et al.: Regional brain activity during transient self-induced anxiety and anger in healthy adults. *Biol Psychiatry* 46:454–465, 1999.
104. Bishop S, Duncan J, Brett M, Lawrence AD: Prefrontal cortical function and anxiety: Controlling attention to threat-related stimuli. *Nat Neurosci* 7:184–188, 2004.
105. Shin LM, Whalen PJ, Pitman RK, Bush G, Macklin ML, Lasko NB et al.: An fMRI study of anterior cingulate function in posttraumatic stress disorder. *Biol Psychiatry* 50:932–942, 2001.
106. Rauch SL, Savage CR, Alpert NM, Miguel EC, Baer L, Breiter HC et al.: A positron emission tomographic study of simple phobic symptom provocation. *Arch Gen Psychiatry* 52:20–28, 1995.
107. Lang PJ, Davis M, Ohman A: Fear and anxiety: Animal models and human cognitive psychophysiology. *J Affect Disord* 61:137–159, 2000.
108. McNally RJ: Information-processing abnormalities in anxiety disorders: Implications for cognitive neuroscience. *Cognition and Emotion* 12:479–495, 2003.
109. McNally RJ: Cognitive bias in the anxiety disorders. *Nebr Symp Motiv* 43:211–250, 1996.
110. Mineka S: *Evolutionary Memories, Emotional Processing, and the Emotional Disorders*. The Psychology of Learning and Motivation. 1992.
111. Vasey MW, MacLeod C: Information-processing factors in childhood anxiety: A review and developmental perspective. In: Vasey MW, Dadds MR (eds): *The Developmental Psychopathology of Anxiety*. London, Oxford University Press, 2001, pp. 253–277.
112. Bradley BP, Mogg K, White J, Groom C, de Bono J: Attentional bias for emotional faces in generalized anxiety disorder. *Br J Clin Psychol* 38 (Pt 3):267–278, 1999.
113. Mogg K, Bradley BP, Williams R: Attentional bias in anxiety and depression: The role of awareness. *Br J Clin Psychol* 34 (Pt 1):17–36, 1995.
114. Vasey MW, Daleiden EL, Williams LL, Brown LM: Biased attention in childhood anxiety disorders: A preliminary study. *J Abnorm Child Psychol* 23:267–279, 1995.
115. Taghavi MR, Neshat-Doost HT, Moradi AR, Yule W, Dalgleish T: Biases in visual attention in children and adolescents with clinical anxiety and mixed anxiety-depression. *J Abnorm Child Psychol* 27:215–223, 1999.
116. Mogg K, Philippot P, Bradley BP: Selective attention to angry faces in clinical social phobia. *J Abnorm Psychol* 113:160–165, 2004.
117. Mogg K, Millar N, Bradley BP: Biases in eye movements to threatening facial expressions in generalized anxiety disorder and depressive disorder. *J Abnorm Psychol* 109:695–704, 2000.
118. Mogg K, Bradley BP, Millar N, White J: A follow-up study of cognitive bias in generalized anxiety disorder. *Behav Res Ther* 33:927–935, 1995.
119. Mathews A, MacLeod C: Selective processing of threat cues in anxiety states. *Behav Res Ther* 23:563–569, 1985.
120. Bradley BP, Mogg K, Millar N, White J: Selective processing of negative information: Effects of clinical anxiety, concurrent depression, and awareness. *J Abnorm Psychol* 104:532–536, 1995.
121. Mathews A, Mogg K, Kentish J, Eysenck M: Effect of psychological treatment on cognitive bias in generalized anxiety disorder. *Behav Res Ther* 33:293–303, 1995.
122. Taghavi MR, Dalgleish T, Moradi AR, Neshat-Doost HT, Yule W: Selective processing of negative emotional information in children and adolescents with Generalized Anxiety Disorder. *Br J Clin Psychol* 42:221–230, 2003.
123. Mathews A, Richards A, Eysenck M: Interpretation of homophones related to threat in anxiety states. *J Abnorm Psychol* 98:31–34, 1989.
124. Taghavi MR, Moradi AR, Neshat-Doost HT, Yule W, Dalgleish T: Interpretation of ambiguous emotional information in clinically anxious children and adolescents. *Cognition & Emotion* 14:809–822, 2000.
125. Chorpita BF, Albano AM, Barlow DH: Cognitive processing in children: Relationship to anxiety and family influences. *Journal of Clinical Child Psychology* 25:170–176, 1996.
126. Kagan J: *Galen's Prophecy*. New York, Basic Books, 1995.
127. Biederman J, Rosenbaum JF, Chaloff J, Kagan J: Behavioral inhibition as a risk factor for anxiety disorders. In: March J (ed): *Anxiety Disorders in Children and Adolescents*. New York, Guilford Press, 1995, pp. 61–81.

128. Barrett PA, Dadds MR, Rapee RM: Family treatment of childhood anxiety: A controlled trial. *Journal of Consulting and Clinical Psychology* 64:333–342, 1996.
129. Kendall PC: Treating anxiety disorders in children: Results of a randomized clinical trial. *J Consult Clin Psychol* 62:100–110, 1994.
130. Kendall PC, Flannery-Schroeder E, Panichelli-Mindel SM, Southam-Gerow M, Henin A, Warman M: Therapy for youths with anxiety disorders: A second randomized clinical trial. *J Consult Clin Psychol* 65:366–380, 1997.
131. Kendall PC, Southam-Gerow MA: Long-term follow-up of a cognitive-behavioral therapy for anxiety-disordered youth. *J Consult Clin Psychol* 64:724–730, 1996.
132. Kendall PC, Safford S, Flannery-Schroeder E, Webb A: Child anxiety treatment: Outcomes in adolescence and impact on substance use and depression at 7.4-year follow-up. *J Consult Clin Psychol* 72:276–287, 2004.
133. Barrett PM, Duffy AL, Dadds MR, Rapee RM: Cognitive-behavioral treatment of anxiety disorders in children: Long-term (6-year) follow-up. *J Consult Clin Psychol* 69:135–141, 2001.
134. Beidel DC, Turner SM, Morris TL: Behavioral treatment of childhood social phobia. *J Consult Clin Psychol* 68:1072–1080, 2000.
135. Hayward C, Varady S, Albano AM, Thienemann M, Henderson L, Schatzberg AF: Cognitive-behavioral group therapy for social phobia in female adolescents: Results of a pilot study. *J Am Acad Child Adolesc Psychiatry* 39:721–726, 2000.
136. Albano AM, Marten PA, Holt CS, Heimberg RG, Barlow DH: Cognitive-behavioral group treatment for social phobia in adolescents. A preliminary study. *J Nerv Ment Dis* 183:649–656, 1995.
137. Silverman WK, Kurtines WM, Ginsburg GS, Weems CF, Rabian B, Serafini LT: Contingency management, self-control, and education support in the treatment of childhood phobic disorders: A randomized clinical trial. *J Consult Clin Psychol* 67:675–687, 1999.
138. Last CG, Hansen C, Franco N: Cognitive-behavioral treatment of school phobia. *J Am Acad Child Adolesc Psychiatry* 37:404–411, 1998.
139. Fedoroff IC, Taylor S: Psychological and pharmacological treatments of social phobia: A meta-analysis. *J Clin Psychopharmacol* 21:311–324, 2001.
140. Birmaher B, Waterman GS, Ryan N, Cully M, Balach L, Ingram J et al.: Fluoxetine for childhood anxiety disorders. *J Am Acad Child Adolesc Psychiatry* 33:993–999, 1994.
141. Fairbanks JM, Pine DS, Tancer NK, Dummit ES, III,Kentgen LM, Martin J et al.: Open fluoxetine treatment of mixed anxiety disorders in children and adolescents. *Journal of Child and Adolescent Psychopharmacology* 7:17–29, 1997.
142. Walkup JT, Labellarte MJ, Riddle MA, Pine DS, Greenhill L, Klein R et al.: Fluvoxamine for the treatment of anxiety disorders in children and adolescents. *New England Journal of Medicine* 344:1279–1285, 2001.
143. Birmaher B, Axelson DA, Monk K, Kalas C, Clark DB, Ehmann M et al.: Fluoxetine for the treatment of childhood anxiety disorders. *J Am Acad Child Adolesc Psychiatry* 42:415–423, 2003.
144. Rynn MA, Siqueland L, Rickels K: Placebo-controlled trial of sertraline in the treatment of children with generalized anxiety disorder. *Am J Psychiatry* 158:2008–2014, 2001.
145. Wagner KD, Berard R, Stein MB, Wetherhold E, Carpenter DJ, Perera P et al.: A multicenter, randomized, double-blind, placebo-controlled trial of paroxetine in children and adolescents with social anxiety disorder. *Arch Gen Psychiatry* 61:1153–1162, 2004.
146. Renaud J, Birmaher B, Wassick SC, Bridge J: Use of selective serotonin reuptake inhibitors for the treatment of childhood panic disorder: A pilot study. *J Child Adolesc Psychopharmacol* 9:73–83, 1999.
147. Masi G, Toni C, Mucci M, Millepiedi S, Mata B, Perugi G: Paroxetine in child and adolescent outpatients with panic disorder. *J Child Adolesc Psychopharmacol* 11:151–157, 2001.

CHAPTER 5.5.2 ■ OBSESSIVE-COMPULSIVE DISORDER

KENNETH E. TOWBIN AND MARK A. RIDDLE

INTRODUCTION

Obsessions are among the oldest mental symptoms for which there are detailed descriptions. Obsessions and compulsions were depicted as possession by the devil in 1467 in *Malleus Malficarum* (1) and described in the "Obsessi" of Paracelsus. In the 1600s, pious texts tell of extremes of religious doubting and "scrupulosity," or excessive devotion (2). Pioneers of psychiatry like Esquirol (3), Maudsley (4), Freud (5), and Janet (6) took up this troubling and fascinating disorder and their writings reflect the prevailing philosophy of thought, motivation, and free will.

Two discoveries promoted OCD research in the last three decades. First, there was the discovery that medications that inhibit serotonin reuptake are effective for many OCD patients. Subsequently, powerful techniques for observing structures and measuring regional brain activity were applied to learn about brain function during performance of tasks tapping specific regions of interest. The effort to understand OCD has deepened our understanding of the prevalence, course, etiology, and pathology of these symptoms and along the way, broadened our knowledge of the neuroanatomy of voluntary cognitive functions and behavior.

DEFINITIONS

Obsessions are unwanted thoughts, images, or impulses that are recognized as senseless or unnecessary, intrude into consciousness involuntarily, and cause functional impairment and distress. Despite this lack of control, a person with obsessions is aware that these thoughts originate in his or her own mental activity. Since they arise in the mind, obsessions can take the form of any mental event—simple repetitive words, thoughts, fears, memories, pictures, or elaborate dramatic scenes.

Compulsions are actions that are responses to a perceived internal obligation to follow certain rituals or rules; they too cause functional impairment. Compulsions may arise as direct consequences of obsessions or indirectly through efforts to ward off certain thoughts, impulses, or fears. Children often report that their compulsions do not have a preceding mental component. Like obsessions, compulsions are often viewed as being unnecessary, excessive, senseless, involuntary, or forced. Individuals suffering from compulsions will often elaborate a variety of precise rules for the chronology, rate, order, duration, and number of repetitions of their acts.

These definitions reflect three critical concepts that are relevant to the differential diagnosis. An essential criterion is functional impairment as a consequence of symptoms. Two others draw on classic definitions (4, 7): Individuals feel that they are being forced or controlled by the symptoms, while they possess insight into the senselessness or excessiveness of their thoughts or acts. Although most patients see their compulsions as unnecessary or their thoughts as senseless, some have this only intermittently. Consequently, some investigators have reservations about the criterion that patients possess insight about their illness. Insel and Akiskal (8) and Lelliott and coworkers (9) reported on severely impaired patients who at times doubted the need to perform their rituals or thought their behaviors were senseless and, at others, were convinced of their necessity to the point of near or actual psychotic proportions. DSM-IV criteria for obsessive-compulsive disorder (OCD) (Table 5.5.2.1) have been modified such that awareness of the senselessness or excess of the symptoms only must be present at *some* phase of the illness. For children, this criterion is set aside altogether.

Few studies differentiate between participants with childhood- and adolescent-onset OCD. Therefore, in this chapter, "child," "childhood," or "children" will be used to signify children *and adolescents*. There are studies that have sampled adolescent subjects only. When this is so, the more exclusive term will be employed.

PREVALENCE AND EPIDEMIOLOGY

The prevalence of OCD in childhood should be understood in the context of the high prevalence of subclinical obsessions or compulsions in the population. Evans and coworkers (10) sent out mailings to parents of children less than 6 years old and found that urges to make things "just right" and preoccupations with symmetry and rules were very common in this unselected population. It was notable that these concerns declined as children entered grade school age. To learn about the prevalence of obsessive and/or compulsive symptoms and compare prevalences across development, Zohar and Bruno (11) used self-report measures for a study of 1,083 children attending grades four, six, and eight. As predicted, a large segment of the pediatric population confirmed experiencing these features. Sixty percent of fourth graders reported preoccupations with guilt about lying and engaging in checking behaviors and 50% reported contamination and germ fears. By eighth grade, rates for these concerns declined to 40%, but 60% of eighth graders reported worries about cleanliness and 50% noted intrusive rude thoughts. Mean scores across the age range on the Maudsley Obsessive Compulsive Inventory were 11–12.5/30 in this population; like Evans and coworkers' (10) finding from a younger population, rates of behaviors and symptoms declined over time. A subgroup of eighth graders had high symptom scores (greater than 2 standard deviations from the mean) and reported high levels of anxiety. The authors suggest that this small group (4%) represented a clinically at-risk group because the large number of symptoms and elevated state and trait anxiety were such a contrast to the decline in both in their age-mates.

Twenty years after the Epidemiologic Catchment Area (ECA) survey (12), there continue to be important disagreements over the most reliable prevalence rate for OCD. Significant disparities and varied methods have yielded figures between 0.5 and 3%. It is useful to place these figures in the context of adult epidemiological reports.

TABLE 5.5.2.1

DSM-IV CRITERIA FOR OCD

A. Either obsessions or compulsions:
   Obsessions: as defined by 1), 2), 3), and 4):
   1) Recurrent and persistent ideas, thoughts, impulses, or images that are experienced at some time during the disturbance as intrusive and inappropriate and cause marked anxiety or distress.
   2) The thoughts, impulses, or images are not simply excessive worries about real-life problems.
   3) The person attempts to ignore or suppress such thoughts, impulses, or images to neutralize them with some other thought or action.
   4) The person recognizes that the obsessional thoughts are the product of his or her own mind (not imposed from without, as in thought insertion).

   Compulsions: as defined by 1) and 2):
   1) Repetitive behaviors or mental acts that the person feels driven to perform in response to an obsession, or according to rules that must be applied rigidly.
   2) The behaviors or mental acts are aimed at preventing or reducing distress or preventing some dreaded event or situation; however, these behaviors or mental acts either are not connected in a realistic way with what they are designed to neutralize or prevent or are clearly excessive.
B. At some point, the person has recognized that the obsessions or compulsions are excessive or unreasonable. *Note*: This does not apply to children.
C. The obsessions or compulsions cause marked distress, are time consuming (take more than 1 hour a day), or significantly interfere with the person's normal routine, occupational (or academic) functioning, or usual social activities or relationships.
D. If another Axis I disorder is present, the content of the obsessions or compulsions is not restricted to it (e.g., preoccupation with food in the presence of an eating disorder; hair pulling in trichotillomania; concern with appearance in the presence of body dysmorphic disorder; preoccupations with having a serious illness in the presence of hypochondriasis; or guilty ruminations in the presence of a major depressive disorder).
E. Not due to the direct effects of a substance (e.g., a drug of abuse, a medication) or a general medical condition.

(Adapted from American Psychiatric Association: *Diagnostic and Statistical Manual of Mental Disorders-TR* (4th ed.). Washington, DC, American Psychiatric Association, 2001.)

The early work (13), using weak methods by current standards, reported a prevalence of 0.05% for adult OCD. The scarcity of OCD was predominant until 1984, when the ECA survey reported surprising prevalences of 1.2–3.29% (12). Subsequent examination of these high rates uncovered weak concordances for OCD. Among all the diagnoses in the ECA study, the concordance between diagnoses derived from lay interviewers and trained clinicians for OCD were the poorest (14–16). Lay interviews employing the Diagnostic Interview Schedule (DIS) rely on simple yes or no responses to queries about the presence of broadly defined obsessions or compulsions. These are not reliable measures for actual clinical cases of obsessive-compulsive disorder. Helzer and coworkers (15) went on to say that results from community surveys, where many subjects cluster at the "threshold of the diagnostic definition," will be unreliable because the response to a single probe carries too much weight. Karno and coworkers (17) reanalyzed ECA data, and prevalence rates were sustained despite the flawed methodology. False negatives balanced false positives.

In an effort to learn more about this problem, Nelson and Rice (18) used ECA methods and interviewed a community sample at two intervals separated by 12 months. The 1-year stability of the diagnosis of OCD was "very low." Only 20% of those responding to "ever having symptoms" at Time 1 reported, "ever having symptoms" at Time 2. They concluded that "the DIS diagnosis of obsessive-compulsive disorder possesses extremely limited validity."

Stein and coworkers (19) employed a different measure (the Comprehensive International Diagnosis Interview) and DSM-IV criteria. Again, rates derived from lay interviews revealed 22–25% of adults expressed having obsessions or compulsions. However, when clinicians reviewed lay interviews, the rates dropped seven-fold (to 0.7%). They also examined rates of "subclinical OCD" in which criteria were met for symptoms, but not impairment in DSM-IV. Rates for this subclinical syndrome were roughly equivalent to clinical OCD (0.6%). Stein and coworkers (19) concluded, like Karno (17) and Nestadt (16), that lay interviews led to many false-positive diagnoses.

The first prevalence rates reporting childhood data ranged from 0.2% (20, 21) to 1.2% (22). Flament and coworkers (23) conducted a rigorous study of children and adolescents to discover a general adolescent population prevalence. Screening employed a modified Leyton Obsessional Inventory (LOI); this was followed by direct clinical interviews of subjects with a high score. This produced a point prevalence of 0.35% and a lifetime prevalence of 0.40%. Weightings, such as those used in the ECA study, gave hypothetical point and lifetime prevalence rates of 1% and 1.9%, respectively (23). Of the 18 adolescents diagnosed with OCD, 12 (67%) reported that symptoms resulted in high subjective interference, yet global assessment (CGAS) scores averaged 67 ("generally functioning pretty well"). To ascertain prevalence in a nonclinical population, Zohar and coworkers (24) performed detailed clinician-rated evaluations of 562 consecutive 16- to 17-year-old male and female inductees to the Israeli army. The OCD prevalence rate was 3.6%. Fifty percent of cases were identified as having "obsessions only." This latter figure was substantially higher than that reported from clinical populations and casts doubt on the validity of the diagnoses generated by this method. However, rates for compulsions compared favorably to those of Flament and coworkers (23).

Overall, the prevalence of OCD is greater than that reported in the 1950s, but is not as great as reported in the ECA (17). Current valid studies place the prevalence closer to 0.6–1% (19, 25, 26). Adult epidemiological studies have reported prevalence from 0.5 to 3%. However, these figures may be erroneous because of unreliable diagnostic methods using nonclinician interviews, the DIS, or similar highly structured instruments (18, 26, 27). Also, it is obvious that rates will change as different diagnostic criteria are employed (19, 26, 27).

Valid epidemiological studies suggest that OCD shows an equal sex distribution. Males appear to have an earlier age of onset (28, 29). Noshirvani and coworkers (30) reported that males and females were equally represented in their sample, but 35% of male subjects had their onset between the ages of 5 and 15, compared to 20% of cohort females. Generally, symptoms exist an average of 7–8 years before reaching clinical attention (23). Noshirvani and coworkers (30) suggested that males tend to have a longer duration of illness prior to seeking treatment, yet the ECA study (17) showed that subjects with OCD had rates of medical and mental health service utilization roughly equal to persons with other disorders.

CLINICAL DESCRIPTION

The variety of obsessions and compulsions match the unlimited capacity of the human mind and body. Typically, patients experience obsessions and compulsions. A few individuals have one or the other exclusively (28, 31) and when this arises, having only obsessions appears to be the more common (24). At any one time, most patients experience multiple obsessions or compulsions. Over time, the objects and contents of symptoms change (32). The content of obsessions can show a wide range, but some themes are more frequent and influenced by the individual's level of development. Adolescents' obsessions typically focus on dirt and germs, fears of an ill fate befalling loved ones, exactness or symmetry, and religious scrupulousness (28). Bodily functions, lucky numbers, sexual or aggressive preoccupations, and fear of harm to oneself are less common. In adults, these remain frequent, but aggressive and sexual obsessions are more common (29, 33, 34).

Although any action can become a compulsion, some actions are more common. An adolescent clinical cohort (28) displayed (in descending order of frequency) cleaning rituals, repeating actions (doing and undoing), and checking rituals most commonly. Many fewer subjects reported rituals to protect themselves from illness or injury, ordering maneuvers, and counting behaviors. In adults, the most common compulsions are checking and cleaning (29, 34, 35). Slowness (34), counting (29), or doing things by numbers (35) each have been reported as third most common.

Several investigators (36–38) suggest that obsessions and compulsions should no longer be viewed as separate entities. These investigators used factor analysis to reconfigure Children's Yale–Brown Obsessive Compulsive Scale (CY–BOCS) symptom categories and found a four-factor model that they believed was more meaningful (39). Rather than just one homogeneous entity or as "two factors" (obsessions or compulsions), there are strong reasons to consider that OCD might be better viewed as composed of four or more subtypes. A number of investigators have now identified four-factor subtypes: 1) aggressive, sexual, religious and somatic obsessions with checking compulsions, 2) symmetry obsessions with counting, arranging, ordering, and repeating compulsions, 3) contamination obsessions with cleaning and washing and 4) hoarding obsessions with hoarding and collection compulsions (36–38, 40–44). Mataix Cols and coworkers (41) found a five-factor model that has been replicated as well: 1) aggressive-checking, 2) symmetry-ordering, 3) contamination-cleaning, 4) sexual and religious obsessions, and 5) hoarding. These solutions are close to one another and it is not yet clear which will be the most predictive.

Subsequent research, using factor analyses of symptoms without starting with Y-BOCS categories, argues for a yet more meaningful, "multidimensional" way of grouping symptoms and thinking about OCD symptom patterns and subtypes (45). Using latent class analysis of symptoms, Mataix-Cols and coworkers (45) and Nestadt and co-workers (46, 47) identified symptom groupings that were more meaningful when placed in the context of age of onset and comorbid diagnoses. From this work there is evidence for factors 1 and 2 (above) that are associated with early onset OCD, and a factor 4 (hoarding) that does not associate with other disorders. Furthermore, these factors show some association with comorbid disorders. Factor 2, described above, has been associated with earlier age of onset and tic disorders (37, 41, 48). Hoarding was associated with more Axis II psychopathology [particularly obsessive-compulsive personality disorder (49)], social disability and social anxiety disorder (45). Subsequent work looking more closely at comorbid diagnoses also relying on latent class analysis suggests greater likelihood of comorbid diagnostic groupings, such that OCD occurs with recurrent major depression and generalized anxiety (46, 48), and another that associates OCD with agoraphobia, panic disorder, and tic disorders (46).

There is mounting evidence that these factors correlate with treatment response (41), neuroimaging results (45, 50), neuropsychological function (51), and genetics (52, 53). The evidence suggests that the course, genetic risk, neuropathology, and treatment might be different among these subgroups. For example, Alsobrook and coworkers (54) found that a major gene locus model was more strongly supported in families ascertained where the probands had symmetry/ordering symptoms (factor grouping II), than in probands with other symptom groupings. Alonso and coworkers (49) found that those scoring highly on the religious-sexual obsessions dimension fared more poorly over two years. Nevertheless, a serotonin reuptake inhibitor treatment study failed to support differences in response among three of these five subtypes (41). Several other caveats were suggested by Summerfeldt and coworkers (38), including the possibility that "more-than-four" factor models might also be viable, that a variety of items have been excluded in the analyses performed to date that use categories from the YBOCS, and problems with using "lifetime" ratings as these are subject to recall bias.

Last, longitudinal studies suggest that symptoms are likely to change over time. One study suggested that individuals are not confined to one subgroup exclusively over the course of their illness (32). However, in several longitudinal studies of adults, symptoms change but remain within the same symptom-groupings that have been identified by latent class analysis (55). Thus, adults with OCD show a high two-year symptom-grouping stability (41, 55). It remains to be shown whether this is true for children.

Children with OCD might be described as more selectively impaired than children with other psychiatric disorders. Academic achievement and extracurricular functioning are often preserved, although the quality of peer relationships may be variable (56). Studies with adults point to significant impairment in social and role function (57). In Koran and coworkers' study (57), moderate to severe illness was correlated in a linear way with social impairment. Clinical studies of children entering treatment programs have consistently demonstrated average intellectual quotients, although the selection bias of these cohorts must be considered in interpreting these data.

It is hard to convey how limiting OCD can be. On the surface children and adolescents appear to function well and seem relatively well adapted to their lives. However, severe symptoms often envelop the patient and his or her family completely (57, 58). It is common to learn of washing rituals that consume 4 hours of scrubbing daily, dissolve an entire bar of soap each session, leave the patient's hands worn raw and macerated, and raise monthly water bills dramatically. Counting or ordering compulsions can waste half a day and lead to complete obstruction. Rituals repetitively executed from night to early morning may curtail sleep to a few hours. Checking or cleansing rituals can produce physical injury such as skin lacerations, ulcers, and chemical burns.

The family's reaction to the patient's symptoms is crucial. Several common response patterns may produce delays in evaluation and treatment of childhood OCD. Although patients are embarrassed and secretive about the content of, and the limitations imposed by, their symptoms, serious impairments rarely elude family members. Parents may delay obtaining treatment as a result of a false hope that symptoms will extinguish if everyone acquiesces and aids in performing the activities or out of fear of stigmatization (58, 59). This kind of family assistance does not relieve the child's anxiety. Many times, parents cannot extricate themselves once they involve themselves in the rituals. Their children force assistance from them and implore them to continue. Over time, the child and parent may become pathologically entangled in rituals. When a child has sturdy development in other domains, parents find it hard to believe that he or she suffers from a serious disorder. In addition, the child's claims that the thoughts or acts are ridiculous or unnecessary can instill false security, leading parents to think that "its just a phase." Parents with subclinical obsessive or compulsion-like behaviors may be unable to recognize symptoms in their child and unwittingly minimize the child's impairment. Reassurance from clinicians and pediatricians who are unfamiliar with OCD may lead to mistaking severe symptoms for "normal" reactions. It is a frightening and painful moment when parents recognize that their child is ill and has lost control of his or her thoughts and actions.

ETIOLOGY AND PATHOGENESIS

Genetic Studies

There is ever-stronger evidence that genetic transmission confers vulnerability to OCD. Elevated concordance rates are observed among monozygotic compared to dizygotic twins (29, 60) and higher rates for OCD are seen among first-degree relatives of clinically ascertained individuals (61–63).

The initial family studies did not find elevated rates in first-degree relatives (64–66). However, after the ECA study (12), methods changed and rates began to climb. Lenane and coworkers (67) reported that 30% of 46 adolescent probands had a first-degree relative with OCD. OCD was reported in 17% of parents and the age-corrected rate for siblings was 35%. Riddle and co-workers (31) reported that 10% of parents from a cohort of 21 clinic patients with OCD were diagnosed with OCD. Twenty-five percent had subthreshold symptoms of obsessions or compulsions. In contrast to studies that relied on questionnaires or telephone inquiry, Pauls and coworkers (61) directly examined relatives of 100 individuals with OCD and of a control group of 33 psychiatrically unaffected individuals. The rate of DSM-III-R OCD among OCD relatives was 10% versus 2% of the unaffected probands' relatives. There were also significant differences in rates of OC traits (or subclinical OCD), with 8% of OCD probands' relatives being affected and 2% of the relatives of those in the control group. Combining the subclinical and clinical threshold groups, 18% of OCD probands relatives were affected, compared to 4% of the control relatives. Like Pauls and coworkers (61), Nestadt and coworkers (62) blindly evaluated 343 relatives of adults with OCD and obtained a control sample of 300 relatives of 73 individuals ascertained by random number dialing. OCD patients were obtained from clinic rosters. Most family members were interviewed directly and all family members were required to participate for a family to be included. Using a threshold of "definite" DSM-IV criteria, 11.7% of relatives of persons with OCD were affected, compared to 2.7% of control relatives. If "probable and definite" OCD were included, then the rates climbed to 16% versus 6%. An additional finding from this group (62) was that earlier age of onset was associated with greater "familiality" (greater likelihood of OCD among relatives). This finding was later replicated in a separate study by another group (69). Nestadt, Lan, and coworkers (68) performed an elaborate study employing segregation analysis of 80 families and a control group. The model of an autosomal dominant pattern of transmission provided the best fit to the data by both groups (68, 69).

Reports of elevated rates of OCD among patients with Tourette syndrome (70) and of tics and a family history of tics among OCD probands (63, 71–73) suggest that some OCD may arise from the same genetic etiology as Tourette syndrome (74). Reevaluation of the National Institute of Mental Health (NIMH) cohort and their relatives in a 2–7-year followup lends support to this hypothesis (75). Fifty-seven percent of 54 probands had a lifetime history of tics, 15% met criteria for Tourette syndrome, and 22% had chronic multiple tics. Among their relatives, 14% had lifetime diagnoses of tics. Using a control group, Grados and coworkers (73) and Hanna and coworkers (63) found that tics and OCD were significantly more likely in relatives of probands ascertained for OCD. Even more provocative were findings that "any tic disorder" was equally likely in relatives of probands with OCD, whether the proband had a lifetime history of tics or not. An additional finding from both studies (63, 73) was that those relatives with tics plus OCD had an earlier age of onset when compared to those relatives with only OCD.

Neuropsychological Functions

There is good evidence from neuropsychological investigations that OCD is associated with impairment in prefrontal lobe functions. The evidence is strongest for impairments in executive functions of set-shifting and motor inhibition, and in nonverbal memory, visual motor integration, and visual-spatial memory (76–78). The most robust findings for pediatric OCD point to deficits in set motor inhibition and response suppression (76). These data point to deficits in dorsolateral prefrontal cortex, orbitofrontal cortex, cingulate, and parietal lobes (77). Also, the data suggest that attention, planning, working memory, and decisionmaking are not particularly weak in those with OCD (77). There appear to be significant problems in frontal lobe functions affecting visual-spatial integration, reasoning, and memory in studies performed on adults with chronic OCD (79). This does not hold true for adolescents or children, however. Flor-Henry and coworkers (80) studied 11 subjects with adult-onset OCD employing age- and sex-matched controls to find frontal deficits, especially in the dominant lobe. They proposed that associated dominant temporal and parietal dysfunction stemmed from the failure of frontal inhibitory responses. Others (81) could not confirm frontal lobe findings. Behar and coworkers (82) found signs of immaturity among 16 adolescent subjects on two measures reflecting frontal lobe function and visual-spatial tasks. The performance of six subjects on another test suggested "neurodevelopmental immaturity." Neurological soft signs, such as synkinesia, were seen in five of the seven adolescents. Cox and coworkers (83) suggested deficits in regulatory functions localized to the frontal lobe, although they did not confirm dominance of the frontal hemisphere. Few measures supported right–left hemispheric differences. The group underscored that findings were independent of impairment from OCD, implying a stable deficit that was unrelated to severity. Beers and coworkers (84) examined 21 drug-naïve children with new onset OCD using a neuropsychological battery and found no abnormalities.

Imaging Studies

Structural Imaging Studies

Mataix-Cols and coworkers (50, 51) employed an entirely novel approach when they posed aversive experiences to patients based on symptom profiles in an fMRI environment. The profiles were based on factor-analytic subgroups as discussed above. The results showed symptom-specific significant activation in brain regions based on clinical phenotype (50, 51). Individuals with washing/contamination symptoms showed activation in ventromedial prefrontal cortex, left middle temporal gyrus, and anterior cingulate, while those with checking/aggression symptoms activated basal ganglia structures (globus pallidus, putamen) and dorsolateral prefrontal cortex (50). Individuals with hoarding symptoms showed activation in the left precentral, frontal gyrus, fusiform gyri, and right orbital-frontal regions (50). These studies show that employing undifferentiated groups would have failed to identify differences. The investigators went on to suggest that the findings lend support to a concept of OCD as multiple conditions with separate, overlapping abnormalities in neuropsychological function (45).

Imaging studies suggest that the function of the anterior cingulate gyrus (ACC) may have particular bearing on OCD. Van Veen and coworkers (85) and Ursu and coworkers (86) offered new insights when they proposed that the ACC is activated in response to incoming streams of information that are in conflict with other information or in response to errors. In an fMRI study, Ursu and coworkers (86) reported increased activation in ACC regions in persons with OCD compared to controls in response to conflicting information and when given a task that forced increased error rates. Participants with OCD performed as well as controls on the task, but there were substantial between group differences in ACC activation. In addition, levels of ACC activation were correlated with OCD severity (86).

Magnetic Resonance Imagining and Computerized Tomography (CT). Overall, morphometric findings lend support to the hypothesis of impairments in cortico-striato-thalamo-cortical circuitry, with increased volumes in frontal regions (cingulate gyrus) and decreased volumes in striatal regions (especially globus pallidus) and increased volumes in thalamic regions (87). However, as will be seen below, the implication that OCD can be explained on the basis of a generic impairment in a single network of circuits has been challenged by fMRI studies (88).

Computerized Axial Tomography (CAT)

Views of patients with OCD or OCD whose onset was in adolescence suggested ventricular enlargement independent of sex, age, duration, and types of symptoms (82). Luxenberg and coworkers (89) employed quantitative scanning in males with adolescent-onset OCD and a never-ill control group. In the OCD cohort, decreased mean volumes were seen in caudate nuclei bilaterally. Values of subjects with OCD and healthy controls overlapped considerably, but pooled mean differences were consistent with a hypothesis of basal ganglia changes in OCD.

Structural MRI. Jenike and coworkers (90) studied 10 female patients with OCD and a control group using structural magnetic resonance imaging (MRI). Increased opercular and whole cortex volumes were noted, as well as a decrease of total white matter. In a parallel study, Alward and coworkers (91) failed to find any differences between 24 adults with OCD when compared to a control group. Garber and coworkers (92) compared MRI scans of adults with OCD and healthy controls and reported abnormalities in frontal cortex, cingulate gyrus, and lenticular nuclei. Past medication treatment or family history did not significantly influence findings. Kellner and coworkers (93) did not discover significant structural differences between OCD subjects and normal controls, but Calabrese and coworkers (94) reported increases in the size of the caudate nuclei. A subsequent study reported left caudate nuclei volumes exceeded those on the right.

Rosenberg and Keshavan (95) proposed a neurodevelopmental view of OCD and performed MRI morphometric studies of drug-naïve children and age-matched healthy volunteers. They observed increased volumes only in the anterior cingulate and not in posterior cingulate, amygdala, dorsolateral prefrontal cortex, hippocampus, or temporal lobe. In addition, unlike healthy volunteers, the anterior cingulate volume did not increase with age (95). The investigators suggested that increased anterior cingulate volume might be an early marker for OCD.

Szeszko and coworkers (96) reported increased gray matter in the left cingulate gyrus and decreased volume in the left globus pallidus when they compared 23 drug-naïve children with OCD to pediatric healthy volunteers. OCD patients and healthy participants showed no between-group differences in caudate nucleus volumes (96). Also, drug naïve children with OCD treated with paroxetine, a highly selective serotonin reuptake inhibitor, showed reductions in caudate nucleus volumes after successful treatment (87). The decrement in caudate nucleus volume was correlated with clinical improvement (87).

Functional Studies Using Radioligands

Cerebral Blood Flow, Single Photon Emission Computed Tomography and Positron Emission Tomography (PET). The general consensus is that exposing children to radioactivity for research that does not benefit them directly is unethical and thus there is only adult research data making use of this technology. These are powerful techniques that allow visualization of highly specific dopamine and serotonin transporter proteins and the specific regions in which they are active. These agents also can be measured rapidly, allowing for close temporal association to functional activity. These techniques have become more powerful when scanning is performed in conjunction with provocation maneuvers in populations that are stratified according to symptom dimensions, noted above. Taken together, these studies support findings of abnormalities in left orbital-frontal cortex and bilateral caudate nuclei. Data from more recent studies suggest different pathways of impairment based on symptom profiles with frontal-striatal regions being involved with ritualistic activity, the insula relating to disgust, and medial temporal regions being involved with anxiety.

Zohar and coworkers (97) employed cerebral blood flow and *Single Photon Emission Computed Tomography* (SPECT). They observed changes in regional cerebral blood flow (rCBF) with [^{133}Xe] xenon inhalation. Subjects who were stressed specifically to increase anxiety displayed *decreased* temporal rCBF. This pattern was sustained as the stressful stimuli were changed to induce higher levels of anxiety.

There are no published studies of SPECT in children with OCD. Van der Wee and coworkers (98), using 123-I-labeled 2-β-carbomethoxy-3-β-(4-iodophenyl)-tropane ([123-I]β-CIT), found increased dopamine transporter density in the left basal ganglia of drug-naïve adult patients with OCD compared to healthy volunteers. No differences in serotonin transporter densities were observed (98). Also, Stengler-Wenzke and coworkers (99) measured serotonin transporter density with SPECT using the same agent in adult patients with OCD and healthy volunteers. Patients with OCD had 30% reduction in binding to serotonin transporter in mid-brain and brainstem structures.

Other adult studies with SPECT report increases in medial-frontal rCBF (100, 101). Rubin and coworkers (102) examined regional cerebral blood flow with xenon inhalation and technetium uptake. Xenon studies did not reveal differences between adults with OCD and normal controls, but with technetium uptake increased activity in the orbito-frontal cortex was observed, with significantly decreased bilateral activity in the head of the caudate (102), a phenomenon previously noted by others (101). Using SPECT, McGuire and coworkers (103) found increased orbital-frontal, striatum, putamen, globus pallidus, and thalamus rCBF among four patients with OCD when urges to perform rituals were the greatest. They also reported that hippocampus and posterior cingulate showed greater blood flow in response to anxiety surrounding these urges.

Cottraux and coworkers (104) studied patients with predominant checking and washing compulsions using SPECT. Compared to controls, those with OCD showed diminished rCBF at baseline in the putamen and thalamus and greater rCBF in the ACC. In response to provocation, there were substantial increases in rCBF in orbital-frontal and superior temporal regions.

Positron Emission Tomography (PET) has emerged as one of the most powerful tools to learn about OCD. The first wave of studies examined persons with OCD compared to controls (105–110). Taken together, these studies replicate findings of increased activity in orbital-frontal cortex (OFC) and caudate nuclei when patients with OCD are compared to healthy volunteers (111). Some, though not all, of these studies also measured increased activity in the anterior cingulate gyrus and thalamus (111).

The technology has expanded to include PET scanning but ascertaining or stratifying by dimensional subtypes and employing tasks that provoke symptoms. Rauch and coworkers (112) scanned individuals with OCD while they were provoked with a feared stimulus and found increased activation in the right caudate, orbital, thalamic and anterior cingulate gyrus. Similarly, Saxena and coworkers (113) compared individuals with symptoms of hoarding to OCD patients without hoarding and to healthy volunteers. Those with hoarding showed a differential pattern of lower glucose metabolism in posterior cingulate and cuneus regions, while individuals with nonhoarding OCD had elevated glucose metabolism in the thalamus and caudate nuclei bilaterally. Unique, large differences between those with OCD plus hoarding and OCD without hoarding were noted in the dorsal anterior cingulate (113).

Initial comparisons of OCD and depressed adults suggested bilateral increased metabolism in the orbital gyri (105–107) and the head of the caudate nuclei. Baxter and colleagues proposed that the orbital gyri might be specific for tension and anxiety in OCD (114). Swedo and coworkers (108) scanned adults with both current OCD and documented adolescent onset; they found increased bilateral prefrontal and anterior cingulate gyri activity. Other observations of elevated caudate nuclei activity (106) were not confirmed. Increased metabolism in premotor and mid-frontal regions were reported in patients with obsessional slowness (115).

Some work has examined regional brain metabolic changes following behavioral or pharmacological treatment. Benkelfat and coworkers (116) reported that medication decreased left caudate and orbital frontal activity. Baxter and coworkers (117) studied adults before and after treatment with fluoxetine or behavior therapy. Responders displayed decreased right caudate nucleus glucose metabolism; no changes appeared in treatment nonresponders and never-ill controls. Swedo and coworkers (118) found that adults with childhood onset OCD exhibited decreased OFC metabolism associated with medication-related or spontaneous improvement in OCD severity ratings. Conversely, Brody and coworkers (119) found left OFC glucose metabolism was increased in behavioral treatment responders. Using provocation techniques and PET, Rauch and coworkers (120) found that decreased rCBF in orbital-frontal cortex and elevated rCBF in posterior cingulate cortex predicted responses to fluvoxamine. This is in line with findings of decreased antero-lateral orbital-frontal cortex glucose metabolism noted in responders to paroxetine in a study by Saxena and coworkers (121), although for this study patients with OCD were not characterized according to subtype.

Functional Magnetic Resonance Imaging (fMRI)

An important frontier in OCD research is the use of fMRI to learn about the function of specific brain regions in OCD. The safety of fMRI allows investigators to compare function across development and to compare earlier and later onset patients. There is a close relationship between findings from neuropsychological dysfunction and validation of these findings using fMRI, SPECT, and PET. As above, the findings strongly implicate OFC and the head of the caudate nuclei (111). In addition, there may be deficits in hippocampal activation during specific learning tasks (122). Increasingly, the effort has turned toward seeking correlations between specific symptom-dimensions and fMRI findings. The push is also to discover brain circuits that relate to specific functional impairments. At this very early point in these investigations, it appears that a generic model of neuropsychiatric/regional-anatomical impairment in OCD is unlikely. Future studies will require correlations with symptom groupings if we are to elucidate the interplay of mechanisms within neural networks that lead to this disorder.

Parallel to work with PET, investigations have turned to employing fMRI scanning during execution of tasks that provoke symptoms in those with OCD. Breiter and coworkers (123) used functional MRI in 10 subjects who were studied during provocation of symptoms. Their results pointed to elevated activity in the medial orbito-frontal, lateral frontal, and anterior cingulate gyri, and in insular cortex, the caudate nucleus, lenticular nuclei (putamen and globus pallidus), and amygdala. Adler and coworkers (124) examined seven patients with diverse symptom patterns and reported increased activation in OFC, dorsolateral, and superior frontal cortex, temporal cortex, and anterior cingulate gyrus. Rauch and coworkers (122) extended these studies and reported specific increased regional activity during a serial reaction task in fMRI based on the symptom dimensions defined by Mataix-Cols and coworkers (50). The findings point to symptom-groups 2 (symmetry, ordering) and 3 (washing, contamination) having decreased activation in the right inferior caudate and ventral striatum, while symptom-grouping 1 (aggressive, sexual, checking) was associated with increased left OFC activation.

A consistent focus in adult studies has been on the anterior cingulate cortex (ACC). There is mounting evidence to suggest that ACC is sensitive to conflicting information as well as control and attention (85, 86, 125). Ursu and coworkers (86) found very significant differences in ACC activation when they compared 11 OCD participants to healthy volunteers on a task that introduced conflict and error rates. A similar finding was reported in children by Viard and coworkers (126).

Van der Wee and co-workers (127) sought to learn about working memory frontal lobe functions in OCD. They reported that despite similar behavioral performance, drug-free participants with OCD showed significantly higher activation in cortical regions linked to the "n-back" working memory task when compared to healthy volunteer controls, particularly the anterior cingulate (127).

Emerging work in neurophysiology and fMRI suggests the role of the ACC in monitoring the success of responses or strategies to solve tasks (128–130). This is a logical connection to symptoms in OCD in which the appraisal of success is distorted leading to doubt and repetition. It is also possible that there are differences in ACC activation among child subjects who demonstrate resistance to symptoms and those who do not (126).

Diffusion Tensor Imaging

Diffusion tensor imaging (DTI) is a technique of observing connections between white matter regions based on principles of water diffusion within tissues in MRI. In the first DTI study of OCD, Szeszko and coworkers (131) studied the anterior cingulate gyrus in adults with OCD and compared them to healthy volunteers. As predicted, their findings suggested bilateral abnormalities in fiber tracts in the anterior cingulate gyri. Results also revealed abnormalities in tract coherence in posterior cingulate and parietal regions.

Magnetic Resonance Spectroscopy

Magnetic Resonance Spectroscopy (MRS) is a noninvasive technique using magnetic fields. It measures the effects on unbalanced elements of specific perturbations generated by a magnetic field. In particular, MRS measures the influence of tiny local magnetic forces exerted by nearby nuclei on elements subsequent to magnetic perturbation. It has been applied to learn the density and activity of glutamate and N-acetyl-aspartate (NAA) (a measure of neuronal destruction or injury) in the brain. One study explored the density of NAA in 11 drug-naïve pediatric subjects and reported decreased NAA levels in the medial thalamus (132). A subsequent study of the same 11 subjects found elevated glutamate levels in the caudate nucleus bilaterally (133). Furthermore, after paroxetine treatment, levels of glutamate in the caudate nuclei were equivalent to those in normal controls (133). A subsequent study of 20 drug-naïve pediatric patients with OCD compared to healthy volunteers revealed a 15% decrease in anterior cingulate glutamate (134). This may suggest inverse relationship between activity in the cingulate and caudate nuclei.

Neurochemistry: Serotonin, Dopamine and Glutamate

Serotonin

Several lines of evidence lend support to the importance of serotonin (5-HT) in the pathophysiology of OCD. Agents that affect serotonin reuptake inhibition (SRIs) have been the most effective medication treatments for persons with OCD. Decreased cerebrospinal fluid concentrations of 5-hydroxyindoleacetic acid (5-HIAA) have correlated with clinical response to SRIs. Substances that increase serotonergic transmission, such as L-tryptophan and lithium, also have been successful in augmenting serotonergic medication in unresponsive patients.

However, studies of serotonin in patients with OCD have produced equivocal findings. Adolescents with OCD were found to have normal 5-HT platelet levels when compared to healthy volunteers (135), and adults with OCD showed tritiated imipramine binding and 5-HT uptake similar to normals (136). A cohort composed of adolescents and adults with OCD displayed a substantial decrease in tritiated imipramine binding but no differences in 5-HT uptake (137). Also, when patients who are successfully treated with SRIs for depression or OCD undergo tryptophan depletion, depression reemerges in depressed patients, but OC symptoms do not reappear in those with OCD (138).

"Pharmacological probes" that are putatively specific for 5-HT, such as metachlorophenyl-piperazine (MCPP), tryptophan, fenfluramine, and metergoline yield contradictory results (139). MCPP elevated temperature, obsessive-compulsive symptoms, and anxiety in one study (140) did not affect OCD symptoms or create physiologic responses in another (141). In yet another study (142), oral MCPP reportedly increased symptoms in 55% of subjects. Symptom exacerbation with MCPP predicted nonresponse to a selective serotonin reuptake inhibitor (142). MCPP administered after 3 months of clomipramine treatment did not evoke acute elevations in obsessive-compulsive symptoms that initially were seen in the untreated OCD subjects (143). Metergoline, a specific 5-HT agonist, decreased symptoms only slightly (140). Fenfluramine did not produce increased symptoms (139). Unresponsiveness to tryptophan depletion, MCPP, and metergoline administration implies that other transmitter systems are relevant in OCD (141).

Dopamine

A contributing role also has been proposed for dopamine (139, 144). There are several lines of support for this. First, increased metabolism in basal ganglia regions, which are rich in dopaminergic neurons, is observed on PET scanning in persons with OCD. Second, OCD symptoms are often observed in disorders affecting basal ganglia (e.g., Sydenham's chorea, toxic agents, trauma). Third, dopaminergic blocking agents (such as pimozide, haloperidol, risperidone, and olanzapine) have been used with some success to augment treatment in patients who are unresponsive to SRIs (145). There is also evidence that fluoxetine, paroxetine, and clomipramine exert dopaminergic and serotonergic activity (146, 147).

Glutamate

There are substantive reasons to consider the role of glutamate in OCD (148). Glutamate is an excitatory neurotransmitter that mediates activity in regions that are thought to be important in OCD (95, 149, 150). Glutamate efferents from the thalamus are particularly dense in the orbital frontal and anterior cingulate cortex (151, 152) and influence aversive reactions (153, 154). Some investigators have hypothesized that aversion reactions, particularly in the subgroup of OCD patients with contamination fears, are particularly applicable to the neurophysiology of OCD (154). Chakrabarty and coworkers (148) examined cerebrospinal fluid in drug-naïve adults with OCD and healthy volunteers and found significantly elevated levels. Result of MRS studies, reviewed above, reported significant decreased glutamate in the ACC in drug-naïve children with OCD prior to treatment with paroxetine (134). These changes may have been associated with paroxetine treatment, as they were not observed in a replication study of children with OCD who were CBT treatment-responders (155). Nevertheless, intriguing possibilities have been raised about the prospect of applying glutamatergic agents such as riluzole as augmentation agents for the treatment of OCD (156, 157).

Neuroendocrine Studies

When compared to a matched sample of normal controls and subjects with Tourette syndrome (TS), a cohort of adults with OCD, who did not have a personal or family history of tic disorders, displayed significantly elevated CSF levels of oxytocin (OT) (158, 159). This is all the more interesting in view of findings of low CSF OT in TS subjects who exhibit OCD (158). Leckman and coworkers (158, 159) point out that cognitive and behavioral symptoms of OCD are similar to the behavioral effects of OT (e.g., cognitive, grooming, affiliative, and reproductive behaviors) that have been observed in animals. However, a subsequent trial of intranasal OT (160) to treat OCD did not produce discernible effects. However, the investigators acknowledge that only small amounts of OT cross the blood–brain barrier.

Pediatric Autoimmune Neuropsychiatric Disorders Associated with Streptococcal Infections (PANDAS)

Some children appear to develop obsessive-compulsive symptoms associated with streptococcal infection. Swedo and coworkers (161) termed this specific syndrome PANDAS and offered an autoimmune hypothesis to explain it. Estimates are that this may be an important mechanism in some children developing OCD. Typically, symptoms arise along with tics and this phenomenon may be related to obsessive-compulsive symptoms seen in Sydenham's chorea (162–164). Swedo and coworkers proposed that this represents an autoimmune disorder caused by the crossreaction of streptococcal bacteria and basal ganglia structures (161). Several lines of evidence support this hypothesis. Scanning data suggest that increased basal ganglia volumes are associated with PANDAS, just as they are in OCD, tic disorders and Sydenham's chorea (165). Also, investigators reported on the efficacy of immunoglobulin or plasmapheresis treatments in patients carefully diagnosed with PANDAS (166). Furthermore, Hallett and coworkers (167) infused rat basal ganglia with sera from boys who had both a PANDAS history and the presence of antineuronal antibodies or with sera from healthy boys without antineuronal antibodies. Only rats infused with sera from affected boys were observed to have stereotyped behaviors. A survey of children with new-onset OCD and/or tics also reported beta-hemolytic streptococcal infection in the 3 months prior to onset of symptoms compared to a matched cohort (168).

However, some investigators doubt the hypothesis and validity of PANDAS (169). A multisite collaborative effort to replicate the Hallett study showed no differences in rats given high or low antibody sera (170) and cast doubt on any hypotheses proposing an animal model for PANDAS. Singer and coworkers (171) looked at antineuronal antibodies and found them in boys with TS and in normal control subjects. Although TS subjects had higher median levels, they did not find any correlation between mean levels of antibodies, clinical severity, symptom types, history (age of onset or suddenness), or evidence of streptococcal infection (171). Also, there was no correlation between symptom severity or duration and basal ganglia size in a study of children diagnosed with PANDAS (165). A criticism of survey studies is that participants are subject to recall bias (168). Furthermore, an autoimmune mechanism would predict particularly high rates of illness among relatives, but a careful family study did not show rates greater than those seen for all OCD and the number of first-degree relatives with childhood-onset symptoms was the same as in studies of ordinary OCD probands and their families (172).

Therefore, caution is in order when considering clinical intervention for a child who might have PANDAS. First, it is very common for children with tic disorders (and perhaps OCD) to report an abrupt onset and experience exacerbation of symptoms with infection. Singer and coworkers (173) reported that over 50% of clinic patients with tic disorders reported this finding and that 11% reported exacerbation of illness within 6 months of streptococcal infection. It appears that considering an autoimmune mechanism is only relevant when the highly specific pattern of acute onset and associated symptoms are observed. When Peterson and coworkers (174) compared a cohort of children with "ordinary" OCD to normal controls, children with ADHD, and children with tic disorders, they found no correlation with antistreptolysin O, anti-DNAase B, or basal ganglia volumes and OCD. In addition, therapeutic applications of immunoglobulin or plasmapheresis are not helpful for patients with OCD who do not exhibit the pattern of infection-related onset and exacerbation of PANDAS (175).

The Cortico-Striato-Thalamo-Cortical Circuit

There is a reinforcing relationship between learning about serious mental disorders and our understanding of the neural networks operating in the central nervous system. From the study of disorders we learn about the development, functional interconnections, and neurotransmitter circuitry of the central nervous system. In turn, this new knowledge about the brain further extends our understanding of the pathophysiology of brain disorders, our ability to treat symptoms, and our understanding of the relationship between disorders. Obsessive-compulsive disorder is a paradigm of this reverberating process. Once it was shown that medication could improve OCD (176), the way was opened to identifying biological mechanisms that predispose to it, precipitate it, and maintain it. In turn, this has advanced our general understanding of neural networks.

The current understanding of OCD integrates neuropsychological, anatomical, neurochemical, and electrophysiological findings (117, 149–151, 177, 178). It posits the existence of somatotopically organized connections between distant brain structures arranged into cortico-striato-thalamo-cortical circuits that subserve planning, execution, and termination of voluntary movements. In 1990, Alexander and coworkers (179) and Delong (180) proposed the existence of "basal ganglia-thalamocortical circuits." They suggested that a "lateral orbito-frontal circuit" projecting to ventromedial sectors of the caudate, the substantia nigra, and the globus pallidus might be impaired in OCD. There were doubts about how separate these circuits might be. Subsequent PET findings led investigators (117, 177) to propose an "orbital-basal ganglia-thalamic circuit" similar to Alexander's.

This "basic model" (149, 150) puts forth that frontal cortical and limbic structures have excitatory effects on striatal structures via glutamatergic efferents. These striatal structures, including the caudate nucleus, putamen, nucleus accumbens, and olfactory tubercle, project to the internal and external globus pallidus. From the internal globus pallidus, inhibitory efferents using gamma amino butyric acid (GABA) have tonic activity at the thalamus. Consequently, *increased* striatal activity *decreases* inhibitory activity (or creates disinhibition) at the thalamus. Increased activation of thalamic nuclei produces excitatory transmission to cortical structures and then movement.

However, this basic model has required modification in two ways. The first modification introduces separate "direct" and "indirect" pathways between the striatum and the thalamus. The direct pathway is so termed because efferents pass directly from the striatum to the thalamus, exerting a disinhibiting (activating) effect. Conversely, the indirect pathway sends a variety of efferents to subthalamic nuclei, which in turn send efferents to both the globus pallidus externa and globus pallidus interna. The indirect pathway moderates activity in the thalamus (149, 150, 177).

The second modification proposes two parallel systems from the striatum, one related to the dorsolateral region and the other the ventromedial region. Input to the ventromedial region is largely from limbic structures, whereas dorsolateral regions receive input from the dorsal cortex. From the striatum, both direct and indirect systems send information to the thalamus. Activation of the dorsolateral system can produce either disinhibition or inhibition of the dorsal thalamus via the direct or indirect system, respectively. Activation of the ventromedial pathway only results in inhibition of the dorsal thalamus (149, 177). Balance in the activity between the dorsolateral and ventromedial striatal systems is crucial in maintaining control. In OCD, increased tone in the pathway from limbic cortex to ventromedial striatum excessively activates the direct pathway, decreasing inhibition, and producing symptoms (overactivation) (149, 177). With treatment using serotonin reuptake inhibitors, afferents to the ventromedial pathway are attenuated at the level of the striatum; direct pathway tone decreases relative to the dorsolateral system and equilibrium is restored. Baxter (177) hypothesizes that behavioral treatment works by increasing tone in the dorsolateral system relative to the ventromedial system; increasing tone in dorsolateral system restores the balance.

This model is compatible with the variety of neurochemical findings. First, it accounts for the efficacy of serotonin reuptake inhibitors. Serotonin selectively activates GABA and reduces glutamatergic output from limbic efferents to the ventromedial caudate. Consequently, serotonergic augmentation substantially reduces activation in the ventromedial system.

The relationship between serotonin and dopamine adds another important dimension. Parent and Hazrati (149, 150) and Baxter (177) proposed that dopaminergic inputs distributed throughout the caudate nucleus have downstream effects on the thalamus. There is a gradient of D1 and D2 receptors across the caudate. Higher concentrations of D2 receptors are observed in the dorsolateral caudate and decrease as one moves toward the ventromedial region. Conversely, a lower concentration of D1 receptors in the dorsolateral caudate increases as one moves toward the ventromedial region. Blockade of D2 receptors would have a greater effect on dorsolateral circuitry and produce a decrease in both direct and indirect pathway activity. This too would change the balance in activity between the dorsolateral and ventromedial regions.

Differential Diagnosis

Table 5.5.2.2 offers a partial list of disorders in which obsessions or compulsions are seen. Though rare, OCD can

TABLE 5.5.2.2

DISORDERS MANIFESTING OBSESSIONS AND/OR COMPULSIONS

Anorexia nervosa
Body dysmorphic disorder
Delusional disorder (all types)
Depression
Hypochondriasis
Obsessive-compulsive personality disorder
Organic mental disorder[a]
Panic disorder
Pervasive developmental disorder
Phobias
Posttraumatic stress disorder
Schizophrenia
Schizotypal personality
Somatization disorder
Somatoform disorders
Trichotillomania
Tourette syndrome

[a] Specifically arising from CNS trauma, tumors, toxins.

arise as a consequence of specific brain disorders ("organic brain syndromes") (181).

The DSM-IV handles disorders comorbid with OCD by requiring that the content of the obsessions not be restricted to any coexistent disorder. Although this eliminates some difficulties, it creates others; it can be difficult to discern how related or unrelated a symptom may be. DSM-IV combines a heterogeneous group of disorders and comorbid features (28, 75) under the term OCD on the basis of presence of a single symptom. Many disorders and comorbid symptoms from different etiologies are subsumed under this one label. Therefore, clinicians are obligated to conduct thorough diagnostic assessments in order to detect all active comorbid conditions (182). Neglecting to do so will lead one to miss findings that are relevant to treatment and prognosis (183). Similarly, if research studies are to be generalizable and valid, investigators are obligated to provide comprehensive descriptions of their sample subjects (182). Care should be taken not to equate subclinical obsessions or compulsions with threshold OCD, especially in adolescents. Subclinical phenomena appear to be stable features that do not interfere with development and functioning (23) and are seen in as much as 80% of the population (184).

Inexperienced clinicians mistake obsessive-compulsive personality disorder (OCPD) for OCD. Most patients with OCD do not have OCPD, although they may be at higher risk than others for developing OCPD later in adulthood (as will be discussed below). In distinguishing OCD from OCPD, it is important to note that in either condition, a person may have rigid routines, needs for orderliness, hoarding behaviors, and indecisiveness, but in OCPD these symptoms are not troubling to the individual or cause him/her distress. Compulsive behaviors in persons with OCPD typically do not generate anxiety or impairment. In OCPD, impairment is a product of patterns of interpersonal interactions and detached, inflexible behavior toward others, not isolated, private symptoms. OCPD typically shows phases of exacerbation and remission; there is escalation under stress. Conversely, patients with OCD generally are not emotionally cold, unexpressive, stingy, or especially rigid about moral or ethical matters. Furthermore, hoarding, list making, and rigidity about schedules and time are uncommon among compulsions reported by patients with OCD (29).

It can be difficult to differentiate psychosis from the overvalued ideas in patients with OCD. Some patients with OCD balance precariously between delusional conviction and insight. At some moments their compulsive behaviors seem logical and necessary to them and, at others, these same behaviors are viewed as senselessness, excessive, or grossly distorted. Unlike DSM-III-R, DSM-IV permits the diagnosis of OCD when schizophrenia or delusional disorders are present. Comorbid combinations like these can complicate attempts to discover whether the patient possesses insight (the ability to understand that their obsessions originate in their minds and are not imposed by external sources). Lack of insight in OCD is associated with a poorer prognosis and should influence treatment strategies (126). Clinicians should carefully search for comorbid diagnoses when patients have little or no insight.

EVALUATION

Clinical Evaluation

The critical first step in the treatment of children with OCD is evaluation. Children usually feel embarrassed about their symptoms and minimize impairment and underreport their symptoms to their parents (185). Frequently, children fear that their symptoms are bizarre and "crazy." They are most likely to describe symptoms to a clinician who resists confrontation, conveys acceptance, and respects privacy; it takes time for the patient to reveal his or her fears fully. Consequently, assessment usually cannot be completed in one meeting (AACAP, 1998).

An adequate evaluation of OCD samples multiple sources. It is desirable to gather history from the patient alone, from his or her parents alone, and from the family together. Helpful information can be obtained from teachers on academic performance, peer relationships, areas of impairment, and tasks presenting special challenges. Siblings may provide valuable information on family responses to the patient.

The objectives of individual meetings are to ascertain the patient's developmental level, extent of impairment, and associated diagnoses and symptoms. The clinician should discover the patient's strengths and weaknesses, fears and aspirations, achievements and disappointments. Symptoms often ruin life at home, school, and work; they damage peer relations and self-image. Therefore each of these domains should be assessed. Although one may feel pressure to overpower denial, root out secrets, and unmask obsessions, fostering a relationship is crucial. A clinician can become so entangled in unearthing symptoms and penetrating concealment that he or she loses the relationship.

Information from family members can allow one to learn the extent to which symptoms interfere with the patient's life and if there are ways the family is unwittingly facilitating symptoms (58, 59). The family evaluation should yield information about family dynamics and how the patient's illness influences the family. It is helpful to learn the significance of the patient's symptoms to the parents, how the parents understand their child, and what the family's responses to the patient's behaviors have been. These aims are most readily accomplished by direct observation and interaction with the family. A critical question is whether concomitant family treatment may be needed to change patterns of communication, patterns of interaction, and other sources of conflict. It is valuable for parents to obtain treatment when their psychopathology is exacerbating the patient's condition.

Meeting with parents alone is pivotal for gathering sensitive information and educating them about OCD. Personal information about each parent and their marriage, medical and psychiatric history, disappointments, concerns, and frustrations, and confidential information about the history in extended family members should be obtained without the patient. Meeting with parents alone is important for teaching and reassuring them about their child's illness. A parent may fear that their child is psychotic or untreatable, feel guilty that they have caused their child's condition, fear that the clinician is going to blame them for their child's difficulties or compete with them for their child's affection (59). Parent-only meetings are opportunities to reassure and solidify a collaborative relationship.

Although a comforting atmosphere fosters discussion of symptoms and stresses and assists in monitoring progress, it may not yield a thorough overview of strengths and difficulties. Standardized instruments do not convey the quality of difficulties or the impact of symptoms on the patient and others, but they are more effective for general assessment and screening. They also permit the clinician to assess severity in comparison with clinical populations. Two instruments have been used with children and may assist a general clinician in this way: the Leyton Obsessional Inventory—Children's Version (LOI-CV) (186, 187) and the Children's Yale–Brown Obsessive Compulsive Scale (CY–BOCS) (188–190).

Laboratory Studies

There are no pathognomonic laboratory findings in OCD. Appropriate laboratory evaluation follows from the findings of the history, physical, mental status, and psychological examination. An electrocardiogram, complete blood count with differential and baseline blood chemistries, including electrolytes, as well as liver function tests, blood urea nitrogen, and creatinine may be necessary before commencing somatic treatment. Measures of serum copper for Wilson's disease are unnecessary in the absence of psychotic symptoms or physical findings of tics or chorea. CT or MRI scanning is warranted only when focal neurological findings are discovered. Electroencephalography is indicated only when other features suggest a seizure disorder.

Psychological tests can provide a detailed picture of intellectual function, severity of acute stressors, and characteristic defensive structures in patients with OCD. Standardized Intelligence tests, such as the Wechsler Intelligence Scales for Children edition III or IV (WISC-III or- IV) or the Differential Abilities Scale (DAS) for younger children, are appropriate. The role of projective tests, such as the Rorschach, Thematic Apperception Test, or Draw-a-Person Test to identify sources of stress is more equivocal. The Adolescent Multiphasic Personality Inventory may be useful in identifying current characteristic defense patterns.

Severity measures of obsessions and compulsions are discussed below. In addition, the parents-on-child version of the Child Behavior Checklist (CBCL) (191) or the BASC can help discover other maladaptive behaviors.

TREATMENT

A variety of treatments have been applied to children with OCD, although only behavioral approaches and medications have been systematically studied. Adjunctive family treatment is often necessary. There is a role for inpatient hospitalization under some circumstances.

Family Support and Illness Education

Whichever modalities will be used, the clinician's relationship with the patient is paramount. First, most children with OCD are apprehensive and secretive. They are anxious about treatment and their symptoms. The relationship with the clinician can reassure and absorb much of the anxiety in a way that promotes discussion and treatment. Second, many patients are uneasy discussing their thoughts or rituals because the content is scatological or sexual. Patients must feel that the clinician will understand the distress they experience and can be trusted with the unacceptable content of their symptoms. Third, when treatments require a lengthy trial period or cause increasing anxiety, the relationship with the clinician must be a sturdy one if treatment is to be sustained. Fourth, since treatment usually does not produce a cure, most patients have a chronic course. The relationship established with a clinician may be a long one and must be capable of sustaining both parties over years.

After the diagnosis is established, it is critical to sit with the patient and his or her parents to review the causes, nature, and course of illness. The clinician should explain the relevance of comorbid features for interventions and prognosis. This may need repetition at other times during the course of treatment. It is helpful to the family and patient to understand that the course of OCD is likely to be chronic and that the objectives of treatment are to reduce the interference symptoms generate in the patient's life and to support optimal development. It may be unrealistic to expect that symptoms will disappear. Furthermore, there is an important role to explaining how the family can best support the patient and to sort out what sorts of support they need to sustain themselves for the long haul. At the same time, clinicians have every reason to be encouraging and optimistic that symptoms can be reduced.

Behavioral Therapy

There is a sturdy consensus that behavioral treatments, particularly cognitive-behavioral therapy, are the first line of intervention for children and in adolescents when symptoms are mild to moderate (192). Behavioral treatments have been systematically investigated for adults (193, 194) and children (192, 195, 196) with OCD. There are now several studies in children and adolescents that support the efficacy of CBT (196–198). Graduated exposure with response prevention is a less aversive modification of "flooding with response prevention" (195, 199). March and coworkers (195) employed a cognitive-behavioral method plus exposure and response prevention to treat 15 children of whom nine (60%) achieved at least a 50% reduction in symptoms that was sustained for 18 months. DeHaan and coworkers (196) found exposure with response prevention to be as effective as clomipramine. Barrett and coworkers (197) performed 14 weeks of "individual with family" or groups of "individuals plus families" CBT with children with OCD and compared them to one another and a waitlist control sample. Active treatment was successful in 75–90% of patients and there were no statistically significant differences in rates between the family-group and individual-family modalities. Rates of symptom reduction were 60–65%.

The most rigorous test to date of CBT in children with OCD was performed in the Pediatric OCD Treatment Study (POTS) (198). The design emphasized an adequately sized treatment cohort, standardized assessments, random assignment, control groups, and strict fidelity to treatment techniques. CBT response was 40%, significantly lower than that reported in less rigorous studies. Nevertheless, response rates to sertraline were not different than to CBT (198).

Despite many continued design shortcomings, there is suggestive evidence that behavioral interventions can be at least as useful as medication in the treatment of OCD. Those who are trained and experienced in applying these techniques achieve the best results.

Pharmacological Treatment

Single Drug Treatment

Treatment with a single agent has been shown to be effective in nearly 50% of patients with OCD. Early systematic investigations of medication were plagued by problems in diagnosis and measurement that made it difficult to generalize and interpret the findings (182). Today it is widely known that a variety of agents that inhibit serotonin reuptake appear to be useful in the treatment of OCD. Although the claims for efficacy are ubiquitous in advertisements and media, they may mislead patients to conclude that everyone with OCD will be healed by medication. It is helpful to inform patients at the outset that reliable studies have shown 40–50% of drug naïve patients experience a reduction of 25 to 40% severity in symptoms. This is important when obtaining consent prior to treatment and in helping patients understand why they may continue to experience symptoms after a course of treatment.

The choice of agents should consider not only OCD, but also whether other psychopathology is present. The choice of medication for OCD should be influenced by the presence of coexisting panic disorder, psychotic or schizotypal features, depression, or Tourette disorder.

In order to determine whether a patient has responded to a medication, it is crucial that sufficient doses be given for a sufficient duration. A majority of studies suggest that an adequate trial has been offered when the patient receives either the maximum allowable dose or the maximum dose that a patient can tolerate for no less than 12 weeks. Gradual dose reductions are necessary to avert withdrawal reactions when discontinuing those medications with shorter half-lives such as fluvoxamine, paroxetine, and sertraline.

The most studied medications in the treatment of OCD are potent serotonin reuptake inhibitors (SRIs), which also affect other neurotransmitter systems. Blinded, placebo-controlled trials in children have been conducted with clomipramine (200–202), fluoxetine (56, 203, 204), fluvoxamine (205–207), sertraline (198, 208–210) and paroxetine (211). Open trials with citalopram (212, 213) have also been reported.

Mataix-Col and coworkers (41) attempted to predict the outcome to placebo or active agents by stratifying the cohort according to factor analyzed subgroups (see above). Their results suggested that the hoarding group was less likely than other subtypes to respond to SRIs. The other factor groups were not different from one another in their responsiveness to SRIs.

In adolescent patients, clomipramine has been studied most (201). Initial studies reported an average 46% symptom reduction. Response rates were noted in 74% of patients (200). These results correlated with the findings from adult trials, where an average 30% reduction occurred (202). The improvement occurred in a broad variety of patients in both studies and was independent of symptom type, age of onset, or response to previous medications. Flament and coworkers (135) found that response correlated with platelet 5-HT concentration and MAO activity; lower 5-HT concentration was associated with greater symptom severity, and high 5-HT concentrations appeared to predict clinical response to clomipramine. The specificity of serotonergic effects of clomipramine in the treatment of OCD symptoms was suggested by two studies. In a double-blind, placebo-controlled investigation of desipramine versus clomipramine (214), desipramine was no more effective than placebo in reducing OCD symptoms in adolescents. Later, a double-blind substitution study (215) suggested substantially higher relapse rates on desipramine compared to clomipramine.

Side effects from clomipramine can be problematic. Anticholinergic side effects, including dizziness, xerostomia, blurred vision, postural hypotension, tachycardia, sedation, and constipation can occur and generate noncompliance. Side effects are less likely when one starts with very low doses and gradually increases medication until symptoms decline. The maximum recommended dose is 5 mg/kg/day, or 250 mg/day. One should obtain electrocardiograms and liver function studies at 3-month intervals for the first year of treatment, and then at 6-month intervals.

Compared to clomipramine, fewer side effects are reported with fluoxetine (216). Double-blind, placebo-controlled trials with children suggest that it is effective in controlling OCD symptoms (217). Doses beginning with 5 mg/day and increasing gradually to a maximum of 60 mg/day are most commonly used. Of the reported side effects, the most frequent are agitation, insomnia, anorexia, dizziness, xerostomia, and increased anxiety. Fluoxetine also may cause a disturbing akathisia. Concerns about suicidal ideation and aggression have also been raised (218) and are now an important focus of monitoring for all children and adolescents on these agents (219).

Sertraline was reported to be safe and useful in an open trial (210), and then superior to placebo in a multisite, double blind, placebo-controlled trial of 187 patients (209). Doses up to 200 mg/day were provided via a flexible strategy. Using a definition of 25% or greater reduction in symptoms, 42% of patients on sertraline were judged to be "responders." The response rate on placebo was 26%. Thirteen percent of patients on medication discontinued treatment subsequent to the trial because of side effects. The most common ill effects were insomnia, nausea, agitation, and tremor. There were no effects on vital signs or cardiac function.

Fluvoxamine has a single ring structure. Side effects resemble fluoxetine and include nausea, lethargy, and insomnia (206). Doses beginning at 25 mg/day and increasing gradually up to a maximum of 5 mg/kg/day or 300 mg/day have been employed (205, 220). Apter and coworkers (220) conducted an open trial in 14 adolescents. Riddle and coworkers (206) performed a multisite, double-blind placebo-controlled trial of fluvoxamine employing doses up to 200 mg/d in 136 children and adolescents with OCD, which produced a mean 25% (or greater) decline in CYBOCS scores over 10 weeks. Overall, 42% of patients were deemed responders.

A metaanalysis of 12 studies of pediatric OCD employing SSRIs or clomipramine concluded that response rates among the SRRIs were comparable, and clomipramine was superior by a significant margin (221). Nevertheless, the side effect profile and tolerance for clomipramine continue to place it outside consideration as the first-line pharmacological treatment for pediatric OCD (222).

Augmentation Strategies

It can be readily seen that between 40 and 50% of individuals with OCD without associated diagnoses may not respond to adequate trials of SRIs. The response to one SRI agent does not predict the response to another, and side effects from one agent do not predict side effects on another. For this reason, it is important to offer adequate doses for a sufficient period of at least two and possibly three agents before moving on to augmentation strategies. When combining agents with selective SRIs, particular attention should be directed to the metabolic pathways of the agents employed. Drug–drug interactions based on inhibition of the cytochrome P450 system can lead to toxicity and side effects. There are excellent and reliable Website resources that can be consulted prior to adding any prescription medication to an SSRI agent, such as the one maintained by David Flockhart at Indiana University School of Medicine (http://medicine.iupui.edu/flockhart).

Although the use of polypharmacy is generally to be avoided, when adequate trials of two agents fail, an augmentation strategy may be necessary. McDougle and coworkers (145) found that patients with Tourette syndrome, tics, or a family history of tics who are refractory to single drug SRI treatment may benefit from the addition of dopaminergic blocking agents, such as haloperidol or pimozide. In addition, a small minority of SRI-refractory OCD patients who did not have tics or a family history of tics also improved with addition of dopaminergic blocking agents. This work was recently extended to risperidone in blinded placebo-controlled trials (223, 224) and olanzapine in open trials (225). This step was conceptually important, too. Dopaminergic inhibition in the cortico-striato-thalamo-cortical circuit may be critical to successful serotonin facilitation.

There are only scanty data on adding lithium (226) or triiodothyronine. Buspirone can increase serotonergic activity in conjunction with SRIs, but there was no evidence of benefit using buspirone augmentation in OCD (227). (228) Small-scale studies suggest that addition of clomipramine to an SSRI may be warranted (229). Care must be taken to monitor ECG changes and cardiovascular side effects closely. Clonazepam has been useful to add for high levels of comorbid anxiety or panic, but sedation and memory problems may be encountered. Serious toxicity result from taking fluoxetine with L-tryptophan and this combination is discouraged (230).

Comparing CBT to Pharmacological Treatment

A rigorously designed trial comparing an SSRI, sertraline, to CBT in a pediatric population yielded nuanced results (POTS)

(198). One hundred twelve patients from three sites were randomly assigned to one of four groups: CBT plus sertraline (CBT + S), CBT alone (CBTA), sertraline alone (SerA), or pill placebo. Improvement was observed in all the active treatment arms compared to placebo (CBT + S > CBTA = SerA > placebo). Comparing *symptom remission rates* by treatment, CBT + S (54%) was not superior to CBTA (40%), but it was superior to SerA (21%) and placebo (4%). CBTA was not superior to SerA, but it was superior to placebo. The SerA symptom remission rate was not superior to placebo. Site differences complicated interpretation of the findings. Despite similar CBT manuals, experience, and application, CBT was superior at one site (U. Penn) over another (Duke). Reciprocally, SerA treatment at Duke was superior to SerA at U. Penn. CBT + S treatment yielded similar response rates at both sites. The investigators concluded that the first-line intervention for OCD should be CBT alone with addition of medication if CBT was not successful.

Partial Hospital and Inpatient Treatment

Hospitalizing patients in order to evaluate their symptoms thoroughly is appropriate for only a small minority of patients. However, acute hospital care may be useful for patients and families in crisis. Examples are when symptoms spiral completely out of everyone's control, the family's capacity to support the patient is thoroughly depleted, symptoms are dangerous, or there is ongoing severe impairment following a course of adequate treatment. Clinicians may feel pressure to initiate additional interventions quickly, but usually crises emerge from the accumulation of chronic stressors. Initiating hospitalization before obtaining sufficient understanding of these strains may undermine subsequent therapy.

In a crisis, partial (or day treatment) hospitalization can be a constructive alternative to precipitous changes in outpatient treatment. Furthermore, should partial hospital treatment fail, inpatient treatment may be more acceptable. Partial or inpatient hospitalization can reduce the burden on parents and the patient to manage and contain uncontrolled symptoms. The primary objectives of hospitalization are to provide rapid, objective assessment of the severity of the patient's impairment outside the home, to facilitate simultaneous initiation of psychological, family, and pharmacological treatments, and to diminish symptoms by reducing stresses and anxiety.

OUTCOME AND FOLLOWUP DATA

Outcome from an episode of OCD can range from complete, permanent remission to relentless decline. Points along this continuum include complete remission with discrete recurrent episodes, partial remission (chronic low to moderate symptoms), and partial remission punctuated by severe flare-ups (231). Studies of patients who are self-referred for treatment do not provide conclusions about outcome that are generalizable to other patient groups. Rasmussen and Tsuang (29) suggested that, in adults, "continuous" illness with fluctuating severity is most common (84%) and a deteriorating course is next most common (15%). Others (34) reported 2-year spontaneous remission rates of 65%. Mawson and coworkers (232) followed their treatment cohort of 40 patients over 2 years and discovered greater than 80% improvement on all measures for the 37 subjects available. But when hospitalized patients are sampled, the rates of those who are rated "greatly improved" declines to 30% (35, 231).

It has been challenging to obtain reliable longitudinal clinical data. This gap shrank with the study of Skoog and Skoog (233) on the natural history of 251 adult patients over 30 years. In this sample 29% had their onset before age 20, 40% between ages 20 and 29 years, and 32% after age 30. This corresponds to Black's (1974) report of 40% with onset before age 20, and an average age of onset in the early 20s. The ECA data also reflect this; the mean onset was 20.9–25.4 years of age (17). But this does not correspond to several more recent reports. Nestadt (62) found age of onset of OCD to be almost exclusively before age 18.

Departing from reports of others (34), Skoog and Skoog (233) reported that intermittent illness (periods of OCD interspersed with completely symptom-free periods) was the most common course of illness, occurring in 56% of patients. Chronic illness (continuous, unremitting severity lasting over 5 years) was noted in 27%, and an episodic course (one episode of illness lasting < 5 years) was reported in 17%. In this 40-year longitudinal study, 83% of patients improved, 48% improved clinically, and 20% recovered completely (233).

There is one prospective study of a nonclinical adolescent cohort. Berg and coworkers (234) resampled a public high school adolescent cohort of 46 subjects two years after they were first identified with either OCD (n = 16) or "sub-clinical" obsessions or compulsions (n = 10). Initially, of the students with elevated LOI scores, only one had sought treatment. Two findings emerged at followup. First, those with "subclinical" obsessions and compulsions did not worsen; only one of 10 developed OCD. Second, only five of 16 (31%) initially diagnosed with OCD met criteria 2 years later. Furthermore, the mean LOI interference scores of those diagnosed OCD diminished by 30%, beneath the cutoff for clinically significant impairment. The authors suggested that this could reflect actual improvement or methodological unreliability. The most likely predictors of an OCD diagnosis after 2 years were previous diagnosis of OCD and presence of another psychiatric diagnosis with OC features. This supports the concept of OCD as a heterogeneous disorder with waxing and waning symptoms, and a relatively more benign, nondeteriorating course. The 69% recovery rate approaches the spontaneous adult remission rate proposed by Rachman and Hodgson (34) and Goodwin and others (231).

In a prospective study of an adolescent clinical cohort Leonard and coworkers (75) evaluated adolescents who participated in clinical trials of clomipramine at the NIMH. Two to 5 years after successful clinical trials, 25 subjects (92%) continued to have depression or anxiety, despite improvement in OCD. Bolton and coworkers (235) reviewed the outcomes of 15 adolescent in- and outpatients 9 to 48 months following family and behavioral treatment. A "good" response to treatment occurred in 66%. Leonard and coworkers (1993) reviewed records of 54 adolescents at 3.5 (range 2–7) years after treatment. Although 94% had some symptoms, 57% did not meet criteria for OCD; only 19% were worse than on initial evaluation. Seventy percent remained on medication. Poor response to medication, presence of tics, and parental psychopathology predicted a poorer outcome (72). Similarly, Wewetzer and coworkers (236) followed up a cohort of 55 children (mean age 12) an average of 11 years following initial treatment. In these now young adults, 36% continued to have OCD and roughly an equal number had some other Axis I psychiatric disorder; 25% had at least one personality disorder. Finally, in a large metaanalysis of 16 studies of pediatric OCD, Stewart and coworkers (237) found that 41% of children or adolescents continued to have full-fledged OCD while an additional 20% had subthreshold continuation of OC symptoms.

Taken together for pediatric OCD, the general prognosis that emerges is of a less severe disorder than was reported in early studies. Sixty percent of children will improve to a level that they no longer meet criteria for the disorder and roughly two-thirds of those will recover (40% overall). Although this is certainly encouraging for the large majority, those with cooccurring disorders, earlier onset, longer duration of symptoms, initial treatment resistance, and poor psychosocial functioning are not as likely to recover.

FUTURE RESEARCH

OCD research reflects many exciting possibilities. Already we have come a great distance. We now know the prevalence of this disorder, have learned the limitations of screening instruments for ascertaining internalizing disorders, demarcated a boundary between ordinary defenses and pathology, and discovered meaningful subtypes. New imaging techniques have illuminated structural relationships and linked neurochemical and anatomical findings in meaningful ways. Family study methodology has provided important clues to patterns of transmission, and genetic linkage studies are underway.

OCD continues to hold out opportunities to discover answers to basic, far-reaching questions. Among these are the basic relationships between genetic endowment and environmental experience (238). Purer agonists and antagonists, and radioligands that act at specific subtype sites, may uncover more details of serotonin and glutamate physiology, relationships between brain structures, and complex frontal, basal ganglia, and thalamic pathways. The lines of inquiry in genetics are already charted. Products of these genes can reveal the molecular biology of OCD and provide clues about the relationship between physiology and psyche. While learning about these genetic sites, risk and protective factors contributing to severity and outcome can be studied and understood.

We continue to be optimistic about clinical care. Interest in OCD has produced well informed clinicians with greater diagnostic and treatment skills. Self-help organizations, such as the OC Foundation (P.O. Box 9573, New Haven, CT 06535), have informed the public and are lessening the isolation and embarrassment of many persons with OCD. As organizations and clinicians educate the public, persons who fear treatment or have been disappointed in previous efforts are now receiving treatment and achieving some relief. The use of specific cognitive-behavioral therapies and family treatments, and medications offer improvement for a majority of seriously ill patients. Nevertheless, pharmacological treatments, even with augmentation, are still not sufficiently effective for up to 40% of OCD sufferers. Psychotherapies fail in 40–50% of cases (239). Failure rates are as high as 70% in those with disabling hoarding symptoms (240).

It is apparent that many persons with OCD continue to suffer in secrecy. Epidemiological studies remind us that the majority of persons with OCD have not sought consultation or treatment. There are too few clinicians schooled in the specific techniques of cognitive behavioral treatment and there is a tendency to neglect this intervention (241). Continued vigorous effort to inform the public and assist primary care clinicians in recognition of OCD is still needed. As we learn more about neural circuitry and brain chemistry there is a realistic basis to be hopeful that new and better treatments will become available. Moreover, preventative measures can reduce the risk of developing OCD and severity of symptoms once genetic factors are known.

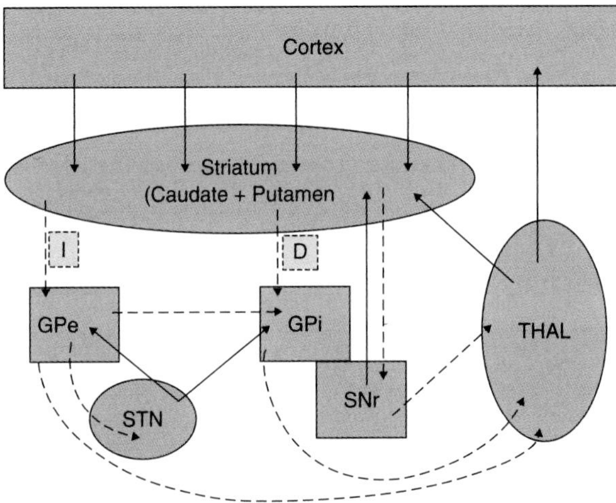

Legend:
D = Direct pathway
I = Indirect pathway
GPe = Globus Pallidus externa
GPi = Globus Pallidus interna
SNr = Substantia Nigra pars reticulata
STN = Subthalamic nucleus
THAL = Thalamus

Solid lines indicate excitatory activity (usually glutamatergic).
Dotted lines are inhibitory (GABAergic).

FIGURE 5.5.2.1. Frontal cortex excites the striatum (caudate nucleus, putamen, nucleus accumbens, and olfactory tubercle) via glutamatergic efferents. The striatum projects to the internal and external globus pallidus. From the internal globus pallidus, inhibitory GABA efferents have tonic activity on the thalamus. Increased activation (by decreased inhibition) of thalamic nuclei produces excitation of cortex. The direct pathway passes efferents "directly" from the striatum to the thalamus, generating a disinhibiting (activating) effect. The "indirect pathway" sends efferents to the subthalamic nuclei, which in turn send efferents to both the globus pallidus externa and globus pallidus interna. Thus, the indirect pathway is able to "moderate" activity in the thalamus. The striatum has dorsolateral and ventromedial output. Input to the ventromedial region is largely from limbic structures, whereas dorsolateral regions receive input from the dorsal cortex. Activation of the striatal dorsolateral system can produce either disinhibition or inhibition of the dorsal thalamus via the direct or indirect system respectively. Activation of the ventromedial pathway by limbic cortical structures results only in inhibition of the dorsal thalamus. Balance in the activity between the dorsolateral and ventromedial striatal systems is crucial in maintaining control equilibrium. (Adapted from Gilbert DL: Motor cortex inhibitory function in Tourette syndrome, attention deficit hyperactivity disorder and obsessive compulsive disorder: Studies using transcranial magnetic stimulation. *Adv in Neurology*, 99: 107–114, 2006.)

References

1. Kramer H, Sprenger J: *Malleus Maleficarum*. London, Pushkin Press, 1928.
2. Hunter R, MacAlpine I: *Three Hundred Years of Psychiatry*. London, Oxford University Press, 1963.
3. Esquirol JED: *Des maladies mentales*. Paris, Ballière, 1845.
4. Maudsley H: *Pathology of the Mind*. London, Macmillan, 1895.
5. Freud S: *Notes upon a case of obsessional neurosis*. London, Hogarth Press, 1953.
6. Pitman RK: Pierre Janet on obsessive-compulsive disorder (1903). Review and commentary. *Arch Gen Psychiatry* 44(3):226–232, 1987.
7. Jaspers K: *General Psychopathology*. Chicago, University of Chicago Press, 1963.
8. Insel TR, Akiskal HS: Obsessive-compulsive disorder with psychotic features: A phenomenologic analysis. *Am J Psychiatry* 143(12):1527–1533, 1986.
9. Lelliott PT, Noshirvani HF, Basoglu M, Marks IM, Monteiro WO: Obsessive-compulsive beliefs and treatment outcome. *Psychol Med* 18(3):697–702, 1988.
10. Evans DW, Leckman JF, Carter A, Reznick JS, Henshaw D, King RA et al.: Ritual, habit, and perfectionism: The prevalence and development of compulsive-like behavior in normal young children. *Child Dev* 68(1):58–68, 1997.
11. Zohar AH, Bruno R. Normative and pathological obsessive-compulsive behavior and ideation in childhood: A question of timing. *J Child Psychol Psychiatry* 38(8):993–999, 1997.

12. Robins LN, Helzer JE, Weissman MM, Orvaschel H, Gruenberg E, Burke JD, Jr. et al.: Lifetime prevalence of specific psychiatric disorders in three sites. *Arch Gen Psychiatry* 41(10):949–958, 1984.
13. Rudin E: [On the problem of compulsive disease with special reference to its hereditary relations.] *Arch Psychiatr Nervenkr Z Gesamte Neurol Psychiatr* 191(1):14–54, 1953.
14. Anthony JC, Folstein M, Romanoski AJ, Von Korff MR, Nestadt GR, Chahal R et al.: Comparison of the lay Diagnostic Interview Schedule and a standardized psychiatric diagnosis. Experience in eastern Baltimore. *Arch Gen Psychiatry* 42(7):667–675, 1985.
15. Helzer JE, Robins LN, McEvoy LT, Spitznagel EL, Stoltzman RK, Farmer A et al.: A comparison of clinical and diagnostic interview schedule diagnoses: Physician reexamination of lay-interviewed cases in the general population. *Arch Gen Psychiatry* 42(7):657–666, 1985.
16. Nestadt G, Samuels JF, Romanoski AJ, Folstein MF, McHugh PR: Obsessions and compulsions in the community. *Acta Psychiatr Scand* 89(4):219–224, 1994.
17. Karno M, Golding JM, Sorenson SB, Burnam MA: The epidemiology of obsessive-compulsive disorder in five U.S. communities. *Arch Gen Psychiatry* 45(12):1094–1099, 1988.
18. Nelson E, Rice J: Stability of diagnosis of obsessive-compulsive disorder in the Epidemiologic Catchment Area study. *Am J Psychiatry* 154(6):826–831, 1997.
19. Stein MB, Forde DR, Anderson G, Walker JR: Obsessive-compulsive disorder in the community: An epidemiologic survey with clinical reappraisal. *Am J Psychiatry* 154(8):1120–1126, 1997.
20. Berman L: Obsessive compulsive neurosis in children. *J Nerv Ment Disease* 95:26–39, 1942.
21. Hollingsworth CE, Tanguay PE, Grossman L, Pabst P: Long-term outcome of obsessive-compulsive disorder in childhood. *J Am Acad Child Psychiatry* 19(1):134–144, 1980.
22. Judd LL: Obsessive compulsive neurosis in children. *Arch Gen Psychiatry* 12:136–143, 1965.
23. Flament MF, Whitaker A, Rapoport JL, Davies M, Berg CZ, Kalikow K et al.: Obsessive compulsive disorder in adolescence: An epidemiological study. *J Am Acad Child Adolesc Psychiatry* 27(6):764–771, 1988.
24. Zohar AH, Ratzoni G, Pauls DL, Apter A, Bleich A, Kron S et al.: An epidemiological study of obsessive-compulsive disorder and related disorders in Israeli adolescents. *J Am Acad Child Adolesc Psychiatry* 31(6):1057–1061, 1992.
25. Bebbington PE: Epidemiology of obsessive-compulsive disorder. *Br J Psychiatry Suppl* (35):2–6, 1998.
26. Crino R, Slade T, Andrews G: The changing prevalence and severity of obsessive-compulsive disorder criteria from DSM-III to DSM-IV. *Am J Psychiatry* 162(5):876–882, 2005.
27. Nestadt G, Bienvenu OJ, Cai G, Samuels J, Eaton WW: Incidence of obsessive-compulsive disorder in adults. *J Nerv Ment Dis* 186(7):401–406, 1998.
28. Swedo SE, Rapoport JL, Leonard H, Lenane M, Cheslow D: Obsessive-compulsive disorder in children and adolescents: Clinical phenomenology of 70 consecutive cases. *Arch Gen Psychiatry* 46(4):335–341, 1989.
29. Rasmussen SA, Tsuang MT: Clinical characteristics and family history in DSM-III obsessive-compulsive disorder. *Am J Psychiatry* 143(3):317–322, 1986.
30. Noshirvani HF, Kasvikis Y, Marks IM, Tsakiris F, Monteiro WO: Gender-divergent aetiological factors in obsessive-compulsive disorder. *Br J Psychiatry* 158:260–263, 1991.
31. Riddle MA, Scahill L, King R, Hardin MT, Towbin KE, Ort SI et al.: Obsessive compulsive disorder in children and adolescents: Phenomenology and family history. *J Am Acad Child Adolesc Psychiatry* 29(5):766–772, 1990.
32. Rettew DC, Swedo SE, Leonard HL, Lenane MC, Rapoport JL: Obsessions and compulsions across time in 79 children and adolescents with obsessive-compulsive disorder. *J Am Acad Child Adolesc Psychiatry* 31(6):1050–1056, 1992.
33. Dowson JH: The phenomenology of severe obsessive-compulsive neurosis. *Br J Psychiatry* 131:75–78, 1977.
34. Rachman SL, Hodgson RJ: *Obsessions and Compulsions*. Prentice Hall Inc, 1980.
35. Welner A, Reich T, Robins E, Fishman R, Van Doren T: Obsessive-compulsive neurosis: Record, follow-up, and family studies: I. Inpatient record study. *Compr Psychiatry* 17(4):527–539, 1976.
36. Baer L: Factor analysis of symptom subtypes of obsessive compulsive disorder and their relation to personality and tic disorders. *J Clin Psychiatry* 55 Suppl:18–23, 1994.
37. Leckman JF, Grice DE, Boardman J, Zhang H, Vitale A, Bondi C et al.: Symptoms of obsessive-compulsive disorder. *Am J Psychiatry* 154(7):911–917, 1997.
38. Summerfeldt LJ, Richter MA, Antony MM, Swinson RP: Symptom structure in obsessive-compulsive disorder: A confirmatory factor-analytic study. *Behav Res Ther* 37(4):297–311, 1999.
39. Leckman JF, Zhang H, Alsobrook JP, Pauls DL: Symptom dimensions in obsessive-compulsive disorder: Toward quantitative phenotypes. *Am J Med Genet* 105(1):28–30, 2001.
40. Leckman JF, Zhang H, Alsobrook JP, Pauls DL: Symptom dimensions in obsessive-compulsive disorder: Toward quantitative phenotypes. *Am J Med Genet* 105(1):28–30, 2001.
41. Mataix-Cols D, Rauch SL, Manzo PA, Jenike MA, Baer L: Use of factor-analyzed symptom dimensions to predict outcome with serotonin reuptake inhibitors and placebo in the treatment of obsessive-compulsive disorder. *Am J Psychiatry* 156(9):1409–1416, 1999.
42. Mataix-Cols D, Marks IM, Greist JH, Kobak KA, Baer L: Obsessive-compulsive symptom dimensions as predictors of compliance with and response to behaviour therapy: Results from a controlled trial. *Psychother Psychosom* 71(5):255–262, 2002.
43. Foa EB, Huppert JD, Leiberg S, Langner R, Kichic R, Hajcak G et al.: The Obsessive-Compulsive Inventory: Development and validation of a short version. *Psychol Assess* 14(4):485–496, 2002.
44. Feinstein SB, Fallon BA, Petkova E, Liebowitz MR: Item-by-item factor analysis of the Yale–Brown Obsessive Compulsive Scale Symptom Checklist. *J Neuropsychiatry Clin Neurosci* 15(2):187–193, 2003.
45. Mataix-Cols D, Rosario-Campos MC, Leckman JF: A multidimensional model of obsessive-compulsive disorder. *Am J Psychiatry* 162(2):228–238, 2005.
46. Nestadt G, Addington A, Samuels J, Liang KY, Bienvenu OJ, Riddle M et al.: The identification of OCD-related subgroups based on comorbidity. *Biol Psychiatry* 53(10):914–920, 2003.
47. Nestadt G, Samuels JF, Riddle MA, Bienvenu OJ, Liang KY, Grados MA et al.: Obsessive-compulsive disorder: Defining the phenotype. *J Clin Psychiatry* 63 Suppl 6:5–7, 2002.
48. Hasler G, LaSalle-Ricci VH, Ronquillo JG, Crawley SA, Cochran LW, Kazuba D et al.: Obsessive-compulsive disorder symptom dimensions show specific relationships to psychiatric comorbidity. *Psychiatry Res* 135(2):121–132, 2005.
49. Alonso P, Menchon JM, Pifarre J, Mataix-Cols D, Torres L, Salgado P et al.: Long-term follow-up and predictors of clinical outcome in obsessive-compulsive patients treated with serotonin reuptake inhibitors and behavioral therapy. *J Clin Psychiatry* 62(7):535–540, 2001.
50. Mataix-Cols D, Wooderson S, Lawrence N, Brammer MJ, Speckens A, Phillips ML: Distinct neural correlates of washing, checking, and hoarding symptom dimensions in obsessive-compulsive disorder. *Arch Gen Psychiatry* 61(6):564–576, 2004.
51. Phillips ML, Mataix-Cols D: Patterns of neural response to emotive stimuli distinguish the different symptom dimensions of obsessive-compulsive disorder. *CNS Spectr* 9(4):275–283, 2004.
52. Cavallini MC, Albertazzi M, Bianchi L, Bellodi L: Anticipation of age at onset of obsessive-compulsive spectrum disorders in patients with obsessive-compulsive disorder. *Psychiatry Res* 111(1):1–9, 2002.
53. Miguel EC, Leckman JF, Rauch S, do Rosario-Campos MC, Hounie AG, Mercadante MT et al.: Obsessive-compulsive disorder phenotypes: Implications for genetic studies. *Mol Psychiatry* 10(3):258–275, 2005.
54. Alsobrook II JP, Leckman JF, Goodman WK, Rasmussen SA, Pauls DL: Segregation analysis of obsessive-compulsive disorder using symptom-based factor scores. *Am J Med Genet* 88(6):669–675, 1999.
55. Mataix-Cols D, Rauch SL, Baer L, Eisen JL, Shera DM, Goodman WK et al.: Symptom stability in adult obsessive-compulsive disorder: Data from a naturalistic two-year follow-up study. *Am J Psychiatry* 159(2):263–268, 2002.
56. Riddle MA, Hardin MT, King R, Scahill L, Woolston JL: Fluoxetine treatment of children and adolescents with Tourette's and obsessive compulsive disorders: Preliminary clinical experience. *J Am Acad Child Adolesc Psychiatry* 29(1):45–48, 1990.
57. Koran LM, Thienemann ML, Davenport R: Quality of life for patients with obsessive-compulsive disorder. *Am J Psychiatry* 153(6):783–788, 1996.
58. Stengler-Wenzke K, Trosbach J, Dietrich S, Angermeyer MC: Coping strategies used by the relatives of people with obsessive-compulsive disorder. *J Adv Nurs* 48(1):35–42, 2004.
59. Stengler-Wenzke K, Trosbach J, Dietrich S, Angermeyer MC: Experience of stigmatization by relatives of patients with obsessive compulsive disorder. *Arch Psychiatr Nurs* 18(3):88–96, 2004.
60. Carey G, Gottesman II: Twin and family studies of anxiety, phobic and obsessive disorders. In: Klein DF RJ, ed. *Anxiety: New Research and Changing Concepts*. New York: Raven Press, 117–136, 1981.
61. Pauls DL, Alsobrook JP, Goodman W, Rasmussen S, Leckman JF: A family study of obsessive-compulsive disorder. *Am J Psychiatry* 152(1):76–84, 1995.
62. Nestadt G, Samuels J, Riddle M, Bienvenu OJ, III, Liang KY, LaBuda M et al.: A family study of obsessive-compulsive disorder. *Arch Gen Psychiatry* 57(4):358–363, 2000.
63. Hanna GL, Himle JA, Curtis GC, Gillespie BW: A family study of obsessive-compulsive disorder with pediatric probands. *Am J Med Genet B Neuropsychiatr Genet* 134(1):13–19, 2005.
64. Hoover CF, Insel TR: Families of origin in obsessive-compulsive disorder. *J Nerv Ment Dis* 172(4):207–215, 1984.
65. McKeon P, Murray R: Familial aspects of obsessive-compulsive neurosis. *Br J Psychiatry* 151:528–534, 1987.
66. Black DW, Noyes R, Jr., Goldstein RB, Blum N: A family study of obsessive-compulsive disorder. *Arch Gen Psychiatry* 49(5):362–368, 1992.

67. Lenane MC, Swedo SE, Leonard H, Pauls DL, Sceery W, Rapoport JL: Psychiatric disorders in first degree relatives of children and adolescents with obsessive compulsive disorder. *J Am Acad Child Adolesc Psychiatry* 29(3):407–412, 1990.
68. Nestadt G, Lan T, Samuels J, Riddle M, Bienvenu OJ, III, Liang KY et al.: Complex segregation analysis provides compelling evidence for a major gene underlying obsessive-compulsive disorder and for heterogeneity by sex. *Am J Hum Genet* 67(6):1611–1616, 2000.
69. Hanna GL, Fingerlin TE, Himle JA, Boehnke M: Complex segregation analysis of obsessive-compulsive disorder in families with pediatric probands. *Hum Hered* 60(1):1–9, 2005.
70. Pauls DL, Towbin KE, Leckman JF, Zahner GE, Cohen DJ: Gilles de la Tourette's syndrome and obsessive-compulsive disorder: Evidence supporting a genetic relationship. *Arch Gen Psychiatry* 43(12):1180–1182, 1986.
71. Green RC, Pittman RK: Tourette's syndrome and obsessive compulsive disorder. In: Jenike MA BLMW, ed. *Obsessive Compulsive Disorders: Theory and Management*. Littleton, MA: PSG Publishing, 1986.
72. Leonard HL, Lenane MC, Swedo SE, Rettew DC, Gershon ES, Rapoport JL: Tics and Tourette's disorder: A 2- to 7-year follow-up of 54 obsessive-compulsive children. *Am J Psychiatry* 149(9):1244–1251, 1992.
73. Grados MA, Riddle MA, Samuels JF, Liang KY, Hoehn-Saric R, Bienvenu OJ et al.: The familial phenotype of obsessive-compulsive disorder in relation to tic disorders: The Hopkins OCD family study. *Biol Psychiatry* 50(8):559–565, 2001.
74. Pauls DL, Leckman JF: The inheritance of Gilles de la Tourette's syndrome and associated behaviors: Evidence for autosomal dominant transmission. *N Engl J Med* 315(16):993–997, 1986.
75. Leonard HL, Swedo SE, Lenane MC, Rettew DC, Hamburger SD, Bartko JJ et al.: A 2- to 7-year follow-up study of 54 obsessive-compulsive children and adolescents. *Arch Gen Psychiatry* 50(6):429–439, 1993.
76. Schultz RT, Evans DW, Wolff M: Neuropsychological models of childhood obsessive-compulsive disorder. *Child Adolesc Psychiatr Clin N Am* 8(3):513–31, viii, 1999.
77. Chamberlain SR, Blackwell AD, Fineberg NA, Robbins TW, Sahakian BJ: The neuropsychology of obsessive compulsive disorder: The importance of failures in cognitive and behavioural inhibition as candidate endophenotypic markers. *Neurosci Biobehav Rev* 29(3):399–419, 2005.
78. Evans DW, Lewis MD, Iobst E: The role of the orbitofrontal cortex in normally developing compulsive-like behaviors and obsessive-compulsive disorder. *Brain Cogn* 55(1):220–234, 2004.
79. Hollander E, Schiffman E, Cohen B, Rivera-Stein MA, Rosen W, Gorman JM et al.: Signs of central nervous system dysfunction in obsessive-compulsive disorder. *Arch Gen Psychiatry* 47(1):27–32, 1990.
80. Flor-Henry P, Yeudall LT, Koles ZJ, Howarth BG: Neuropsychological and power spectral EEG investigations of the obsessive-compulsive syndrome. *Biol Psychiatry* 14(1):119–130, 1979.
81. Insel TR, Donnelly EF, Lalakea ML, Alterman IS, Murphy DL: Neurological and neuropsychological studies of patients with obsessive-compulsive disorder. *Biol Psychiatry* 18(7):741–751, 1983.
82. Behar D, Rapoport JL, Berg CJ, Denckla MB, Mann L, Cox C et al.: Computerized tomography and neuropsychological test measures in adolescents with obsessive-compulsive disorder. *Am J Psychiatry* 141(3):363–369, 1984.
83. Cox C, Fedio P, Rapoport JL: Neuropsychological testing of obsessive compulsive adolescents. In: Rapoport JL, ed. *Obsessive Compulsive Disorder in Children and Adolescents*. Washington, DC: American Psychiatric Press, 73–85, 1989.
84. Beers SR, Rosenberg DR, Dick EL, Williams T, O'Hearn KM, Birmaher B et al.: Neuropsychological study of frontal lobe function in psychotropic-naive children with obsessive-compulsive disorder. *Am J Psychiatry* 156(5):777–779, 1999.
85. van V, V, Carter CS: The anterior cingulate as a conflict monitor: fMRI and ERP studies. *Physiol Behav* 77(4–5):477–482, 2002.
86. Ursu S, Stenger VA, Shear MK, Jones MR, Carter CS: Overactive action monitoring in obsessive-compulsive disorder: Evidence from functional magnetic resonance imaging. *Psychol Sci* 14(4):347–353, 2003.
87. Gilbert AR, Moore GJ, Keshavan MS, Paulson LA, Narula V, Mac Master FP et al.: Decrease in thalamic volumes of pediatric patients with obsessive-compulsive disorder who are taking paroxetine. *Arch Gen Psychiatry* 57(5):449–456, 2000.
88. Rauch SL, Wedig MM, Wright CI, Martis B, McMullin KG, Shin LM et al.: Functional magnetic resonance imaging study of regional brain activation during implicit sequence learning in obsessive-compulsive disorder. *Biol Psychiatry* 2006.
89. Luxenberg JS, Swedo SE, Flament MF, Friedland RP, Rapoport J, Rapoport SI: Neuroanatomical abnormalities in obsessive-compulsive disorder detected with quantitative X-ray computed tomography. *Am J Psychiatry* 145(9):1089–1093, 1988.
90. Jenike MA, Breiter HC, Baer L, Kennedy DN, Savage CR, Olivares MJ et al.: Cerebral structural abnormalities in obsessive-compulsive disorder: A quantitative morphometric magnetic resonance imaging study. *Arch Gen Psychiatry* 53(7):625–632, 1996.
91. Aylward EH, Harris GJ, Hoehn-Saric R, Barta PE, Machlin SR, Pearlson GD: Normal caudate nucleus in obsessive-compulsive disorder assessed by quantitative neuroimaging. *Arch Gen Psychiatry* 53(7):577–584, 1996.
92. Garber HJ, Ananth JV, Chiu LC, Griswold VJ, Oldendorf WH: Nuclear magnetic resonance study of obsessive-compulsive disorder. *Am J Psychiatry* 146(8):1001–1005, 1989.
93. Kellner CH, Jolley RR, Holgate RC, Austin L, Lydiard RB, Laraia M et al.: Brain MRI in obsessive-compulsive disorder. *Psychiatry Res* 36(1):45–49, 1991.
94. Calabrese G, Colombo C, Bonfanti A, Scotti G, Scarone S: Caudate nucleus abnormalities in obsessive-compulsive disorder: Measurements of MRI signal intensity. *Psychiatry Res* 50(2):89–92, 1993.
95. Rosenberg DR, Keshavan MS: A.E. Bennett Research Award. Toward a neurodevelopmental model of of obsessive compulsive disorder. *Biol Psychiatry* 43(9):623–640, 1998.
96. Szeszko PR, MacMillan S, McMeniman M, Chen S, Baribault K, Lim KO et al.: Brain structural abnormalities in psychotropic drug-naive pediatric patients with obsessive-compulsive disorder. *Am J Psychiatry* 161(6):1049–1056, 2004.
97. Zohar J, Insel TR, Berman KF, Foa EB, Hill JL, Weinberger DR: Anxiety and cerebral blood flow during behavioral challenge: Dissociation of central from peripheral and subjective measures. *Arch Gen Psychiatry* 46(6):505–510, 1989.
98. van der Wee NJ, Stevens H, Hardeman JA, Mandl RC, Denys DA, van Megen HJ et al.: Enhanced dopamine transporter density in psychotropic-naive patients with obsessive-compulsive disorder shown by [123I]{beta}-CIT SPECT. *Am J Psychiatry* 161(12):2201–2206, 2004.
99. Stengler-Wenzke K: MUAMSOHS. Reduced serotonin transporter-availability in obsessive-compulsive disorder (OCD). *Eur Arch Psychiatry Clin Neurosci* 254(4):252–255, 2004.
100. Hoehn-Saric R, Pearlson GD, Harris GJ, Machlin SR, Camargo EE: Effects of fluoxetine on regional cerebral blood flow in obsessive-compulsive patients. *Am J Psychiatry* 148(9):1243–1245, 1991.
101. Machlin SR, Harris GJ, Pearlson GD, Hoehn-Saric R, Jeffery P, Camargo EE: Elevated medial-frontal cerebral blood flow in obsessive-compulsive patients: A SPECT study. *Am J Psychiatry* 148(9):1240–1242, 1991.
102. Rubin RT, Villanueva-Meyer J, Ananth J, Trajmar PG, Mena I: Regional xenon 133 cerebral blood flow and cerebral technetium 99m HMPAO uptake in unmedicated patients with obsessive-compulsive disorder and matched normal control subjects: Determination by high-resolution single-photon emission computed tomography. *Arch Gen Psychiatry* 49(9):695–702, 1992.
103. McGuire PK, Bench CJ, Frith CD, Marks IM, Frackowiak RS, Dolan RJ: Functional anatomy of obsessive-compulsive phenomena. *Br J Psychiatry* 164(4):459–468, 1994.
104. Cottraux J, Gerard D, Cinotti L, Froment JC, Deiber MP, Le Bars D et al.: A controlled positron emission tomography study of obsessive and neutral auditory stimulation in obsessive-compulsive disorder with checking rituals. *Psychiatry Res* 60(2–3):101–112, 1996.
105. Baxter LR, Jr., Phelps ME, Mazziotta JC, Guze BH, Schwartz JM, Selin CE: Local cerebral glucose metabolic rates in obsessive-compulsive disorder: A comparison with rates in unipolar depression and in normal controls. *Arch Gen Psychiatry* 44(3):211–218, 1987.
106. Baxter LR, Jr., Schwartz JM, Mazziotta JC, Phelps ME, Pahl JJ, Guze BH et al.: Cerebral glucose metabolic rates in nondepressed patients with obsessive-compulsive disorder. *Am J Psychiatry* 145(12):1560–1563, 1988.
107. Nordahl TE, Benkelfat C, Semple WE, Gross M, King AC, Cohen RM: Cerebral glucose metabolic rates in obsessive compulsive disorder. *Neuropsychopharmacology* 2(1):23–28, 1989.
108. Swedo SE, Schapiro MB, Grady CL, Cheslow DL, Leonard HL, Kumar A et al.: Cerebral glucose metabolism in childhood-onset obsessive-compulsive disorder. *Arch Gen Psychiatry* 46(6):518–523, 1989.
109. Martinot JL, Allilaire JF, Mazoyer BM, Hantouche E, Huret JD, Legaut-Demare F et al.: Obsessive-compulsive disorder: A clinical, neuropsychological and positron emission tomography study. *Acta Psychiatr Scand* 82(3):233–242, 1990.
110. Perani D, Colombo C, Bressi S, Bonfanti A, Grassi F, Scarone S et al.: [18F]FDG PET study in obsessive-compulsive disorder: A clinical/metabolic correlation study after treatment. *Br J Psychiatry* 166(2):244–250, 1995.
111. Whiteside SP, Port JD, Abramowitz JS: A meta-analysis of functional neuroimaging in obsessive-compulsive disorder. *Psychiatry Res* 132(1):69–79, 2004.
112. Rauch SL, Jenike MA, Alpert NM, Baer L, Breiter HC, Savage CR et al.: Regional cerebral blood flow measured during symptom provocation in obsessive-compulsive disorder using oxygen 15-labeled carbon dioxide and positron emission tomography. *Arch Gen Psychiatry* 51(1):62–70, 1994.
113. Saxena S, Brody AL, Maidment KM, Smith EC, Zohrabi N, Katz E et al.: Cerebral glucose metabolism in obsessive-compulsive hoarding. *Am J Psychiatry* 161(6):1038–1048, 2004.
114. Baxter LR, Jr., Schwartz JM, Guze BH, Bergman K, Szuba MP: PET imaging in obsessive compulsive disorder with and without depression. *J Clin Psychiatry* 51 Suppl:61–69, 1990.

115. Sawle GV, Hymas NF, Lees AJ, Frackowiak RS: Obsessional slowness. Functional studies with positron emission tomography. *Brain* 114 (Pt 5):2191–2202, 1991.
116. Benkelfat C, Nordahl TE, Semple WE, King AC, Murphy DL, Cohen RM: Local cerebral glucose metabolic rates in obsessive-compulsive disorder: Patients treated with clomipramine. *Arch Gen Psychiatry* 47(9):840–848, 1990.
117. Baxter LR, Jr., Schwartz JM, Bergman KS, Szuba MP, Guze BH, Mazziotta JC et al.: Caudate glucose metabolic rate changes with both drug and behavior therapy for obsessive-compulsive disorder. *Arch Gen Psychiatry* 49(9):681–689, 1992.
118. Swedo SE, Pietrini P, Leonard HL, Schapiro MB, Rettew DC, Goldberger EL et al.: Cerebral glucose metabolism in childhood-onset obsessive-compulsive disorder. Revisualization during pharmacotherapy. *Arch Gen Psychiatry* 49(9):690–694, 1992.
119. Brody AL, Saxena S, Schwartz JM, Stoessel PW, Maidment K, Phelps ME et al.: FDG-PET predictors of response to behavioral therapy and pharmacotherapy in obsessive compulsive disorder. *Psychiatry Res* 84(1):1–6, 1998.
120. Rauch SL, Shin LM, Dougherty DD, Alpert NM, Fischman AJ, Jenike MA: Predictors of fluvoxamine response in contamination-related obsessive compulsive disorder: A PET symptom provocation study. *Neuropsychopharmacology* 27(5):782–791, 2002.
121. Saxena S, Brody AL, Maidment KM, Dunkin JJ, Colgan M, Alborzian S et al.: Localized orbitofrontal and subcortical metabolic changes and predictors of response to paroxetine treatment in obsessive-compulsive disorder. *Neuropsychopharmacology* 21(6):683–693, 1999.
122. Rauch SL, Wedig MM, Wright CI, Martis B, McMullin KG, Shin LM et al.: Functional magnetic resonance imaging study of regional brain activation during implicit sequence learning in obsessive-compulsive disorder. *Biol Psychiatry* 2006.
123. Breiter HC, Rauch SL. Functional MRI and the study of OCD: From symptom provocation to cognitive-behavioral probes of cortico-striatal systems and the amygdala. *Neuroimage* 4(3 Pt 3):S127–S138, 1996.
124. Adler CM, McDonough-Ryan P, Sax KW, Holland SK, Arndt S, Strakowski SM: fMRI of neuronal activation with symptom provocation in unmedicated patients with obsessive compulsive disorder. *J Psychiatr Res* 34(4–5):317–324, 2000.
125. Bush G, Luu P, Posner MI: Cognitive and emotional influences in anterior cingulate cortex. *Trends Cogn Sci* 4(6):215–222, 2000.
126. Viard A, Flament MF, Artiges E, Dehaene S, Naccache L, Cohen D et al.: Cognitive control in childhood-onset obsessive-compulsive disorder: A functional MRI study. *Psychol Med* 35(7):1007–1017, 2005.
127. van der Wee NJ, Ramsey NF, Jansma JM, Denys DA, van Megen HJ, Westenberg HM et al.: Spatial working memory deficits in obsessive compulsive disorder are associated with excessive engagement of the medial frontal cortex. *Neuroimage* 20(4):2271–2280, 2003.
128. Carter CS, Macdonald AM, Botvinick M, Ross LL, Stenger VA, Noll D et al.: Parsing executive processes: Strategic vs. evaluative functions of the anterior cingulate cortex. *Proc Natl Acad Sci USA* 97(4):1944–1948, 2000.
129. Macdonald AW, III, Cohen JD, Stenger VA, Carter CS: Dissociating the role of the dorsolateral prefrontal and anterior cingulate cortex in cognitive control. *Science* 288(5472):1835–1838, 2000.
130. Botvinick M, Nystrom LE, Fissell K, Carter CS, Cohen JD: Conflict monitoring versus selection-for-action in anterior cingulate cortex. *Nature* 402(6758):179–181, 1999.
131. Szeszko PR, Ardekani BA, Ashtari M, Malhotra AK, Robinson DG, Bilder RM et al.: White matter abnormalities in obsessive-compulsive disorder: A diffusion tensor imaging study. *Arch Gen Psychiatry* 62(7):782–790, 2005.
132. Fitzgerald KD, Moore GJ, Paulson LA, Stweart CM, Rosenberg DR: Proton spectroscopic imaging of the thalamus in treatment-naive pediatric obsessive-compulsive disorder. *Biol Psychiatry* 47(3):174–182, 2000.
133. Rosenberg DR, MacMaster FP, Keshavan MS, Fitzgerald KD, Stewart CM, Moore GJ: Decrease in caudate glutamatergic concentrations in pediatric obsessive-compulsive disorder patients taking paroxetine. *J Am Acad Child Adolesc Psychiatry* 39(9):1096–1103, 2000.
134. Rosenberg DR, Mirza Y, Russell A, Tang J, Smith JM, Banerjee SP et al.: Reduced anterior cingulate glutamatergic concentrations in childhood OCD and major depression versus healthy controls. *J Am Acad Child Adolesc Psychiatry* 43(9):1146–1153, 2004.
135. Flament MF, Rapoport JL, Murphy DL, Berg CJ, Lake CR: Biochemical changes during clomipramine treatment of childhood obsessive-compulsive disorder. *Arch Gen Psychiatry* 44(3):219–225, 1987.
136. Insel TR, Mueller EA, Alterman I, Linnoila M, Murphy DL: Obsessive-compulsive disorder and serotonin: Is there a connection? *Biol Psychiatry* 20(11):1174–1188, 1985.
137. Weizman A, Carmi M, Hermesh H, Shahar A, Apter A, Tyano S et al.: High-affinity imipramine binding and serotonin uptake in platelets of eight adolescent and ten adult obsessive-compulsive patients. *Am J Psychiatry* 143(3):335–339, 1986.
138. Barr LC, Goodman WK, McDougle CJ, Delgado PL, Heninger GR, Charney DS et al.: Tryptophan depletion in patients with obsessive-compulsive disorder who respond to serotonin reuptake inhibitors. *Arch Gen Psychiatry* 51(4):309–317, 1994.
139. McDougle CJ: The neurobiology and treatment of OCD. In: Charney DL, Nessler E, Bunney BS, eds. *Neurobiology of Mental Illness*. London: Oxford University Press, 1999: 518–533.
140. Zohar J, Insel TR: Obsessive-compulsive disorder: Psychobiological approaches to diagnosis, treatment, and pathophysiology. *Biol Psychiatry* 22(6):667–687, 1987.
141. Charney DS, Goodman WK, Price LH, Woods SW, Rasmussen SA, Heninger GR: Serotonin function in obsessive-compulsive disorder. A comparison of the effects of tryptophan and m-chlorophenylpiperazine in patients and healthy subjects. *Arch Gen Psychiatry* 45(2):177–185, 1988.
142. Hollander E, Decaria CM, Nitescu A, Gully R, Suckow RF, Cooper TB et al.: Serotonergic function in obsessive-compulsive disorder: Behavioral and neuroendocrine responses to oral m-chlorophenylpiperazine and fenfluramine in patients and healthy volunteers. *Arch Gen Psychiatry* 49(1):21–28, 1992.
143. Zohar J, Insel TR, Zohar-Kadouch RC, Hill JL, Murphy DL: Serotonergic responsivity in obsessive-compulsive disorder: Effects of chronic clomipramine treatment. *Arch Gen Psychiatry* 45(2):167–172, 1988.
144. Rapoport JL, Wise SP: Obsessive-compulsive disorder: Evidence for basal ganglia dysfunction. *Psychopharmacol Bull* 24(3):380–384, 1988.
145. McDougle CJ, Goodman WK, Leckman JF, Lee NC, Heninger GR, Price LH: Haloperidol addition in fluvoxamine-refractory obsessive-compulsive disorder: A double-blind, placebo-controlled study in patients with and without tics. *Arch Gen Psychiatry* 51(4):302–308, 1994.
146. Baldessarini RJ, Marsh E: Fluoxetine and side effects. *Arch Gen Psychiatry* 47(2):191–192, 1990.
147. Austin LS, Lydiard RB, Ballenger JC, Cohen BM, Laraia MT, Zealberg JJ et al.: Dopamine blocking activity of clomipramine in patients with obsessive-compulsive disorder. *Biol Psychiatry* 30(3):225–232, 1991.
148. Chakrabarty K, Bhattacharyya S, Christopher R, Khanna S: Glutamatergic dysfunction in OCD. *Neuropsychopharmacology* 30(9):1735–1740, 2005.
149. Parent A, Hazrati LN: Functional anatomy of the basal ganglia: I. The cortico-basal ganglia-thalamo-cortical loop. *Brain Res Brain Res Rev* 20(1):91–127, 1995.
150. Parent A, Hazrati LN: Functional anatomy of the basal ganglia. II. The place of subthalamic nucleus and external pallidum in basal ganglia circuitry. *Brain Res Brain Res Rev* 20(1):128–154, 1995.
151. Modell JG, Mountz JM, Curtis GC, Greden JF: Neurophysiologic dysfunction in basal ganglia/limbic striatal and thalamocortical circuits as a pathogenetic mechanism of obsessive-compulsive disorder. *J Neuropsychiatry Clin Neurosci* 1(1):27–36, 1989.
152. Rowland LM, Bustillo JR, Mullins PG, Jung RE, Lenroot R, Landgraf E et al.: Effects of ketamine on anterior cingulate glutamate metabolism in healthy humans: A 4-T proton MRS study. *Am J Psychiatry* 162(2):394–396, 2005.
153. Husted DS, Shapira NA, Goodman WK: The neurocircuitry of obsessive-compulsive disorder and disgust. *Prog Neuropsychopharmacol Biol Psychiatry* 2006.
154. Johansen JP, Fields HL: Glutamatergic activation of anterior cingulate cortex produces an aversive teaching signal. *Nat Neurosci* 7(4):398–403, 2004.
155. Benazon NR, Moore GJ, Rosenberg DR: Neurochemical analyses in pediatric obsessive-compulsive disorder in patients treated with cognitive-behavioral therapy. *J Am Acad Child Adolesc Psychiatry* 42(11):1279–1285, 2003.
156. Coric V, Taskiran S, Pittenger C, Wasylink S, Mathalon DH, Valentine G et al.: Riluzole augmentation in treatment-resistant obsessive-compulsive disorder: An open-label trial. *Biol Psychiatry* 58(5):424–428, 2005.
157. Pittenger C, Krystal JH, Coric V: Glutamate-modulating drugs as novel pharmacotherapeutic agents in the treatment of obsessive-compulsive disorder. *NeuroRx* 3(1):69–81, 2006.
158. Leckman JF, Goodman WK, North WG, Chappell PB, Price LH, Pauls DL et al.: Elevated cerebrospinal fluid levels of oxytocin in obsessive-compulsive disorder: Comparison with Tourette's syndrome and healthy controls. *Arch Gen Psychiatry* 51(10):782–792, 1994.
159. Leckman JF, Goodman WK, North WG, Chappell PB, Price LH, Pauls DL et al.: The role of central oxytocin in obsessive compulsive disorder and related normal behavior. *Psychoneuroendocrinology* 19(8):723–749, 1994.
160. Epperson CN, McDougle CJ, Price LH: Intranasal oxytocin in obsessive-compulsive disorder. *Biol Psychiatry* 40(6):547–549, 1996.
161. Swedo SE, Leonard HL, Garvey M, Mittleman B, Allen AJ, Perlmutter S et al.: Pediatric autoimmune neuropsychiatric disorders associated with streptococcal infections: Clinical description of the first 50 cases. *Am J Psychiatry* 155(2):264–271, 1998.
162. Leonard HL, Swedo SE, Garvey M, Beer D, Perlmutter S, Lougee L et al.: Postinfectious and other forms of obsessive-compulsive disorder. *Child Adolesc Psychiatr Clin N Am* 8(3):497–511, 1999.
163. Swedo SE, Leonard HL, Schapiro MB, Casey BJ, Mannheim GB, Lenane MC et al.: Sydenham's chorea: Physical and psychological symptoms of St Vitus dance. *Pediatrics* 91(4):706–713, 1993.
164. Garvey MA, Giedd J, Swedo SE. PANDAS: The search for environmental triggers of pediatric neuropsychiatric disorders. Lessons from rheumatic fever. *J Child Neurol* 13(9):413–423, 1998.
165. Giedd JN, Rapoport JL, Garvey MA, Perlmutter S, Swedo SE: MRI assessment of children with obsessive-compulsive disorder or tics associated with streptococcal infection. *Am J Psychiatry* 157(2):281–283, 2000.

166. Perlmutter SJ, Leitman SF, Garvey MA, Hamburger S, Feldman E, Leonard HL et al.: Therapeutic plasma exchange and intravenous immunoglobulin for obsessive-compulsive disorder and tic disorders in childhood. *Lancet* 354(9185):1153–1158, 1999.
167. Hallett JJ, Harling-Berg CJ, Knopf PM, Stopa EG, Kiessling LS: Anti-striatal antibodies in Tourette syndrome cause neuronal dysfunction. *J Neuroimmunol* 111(1–2):195–202, 2000.
168. Mell LK, Davis RL, Owens D: Association between streptococcal infection and obsessive-compulsive disorder, Tourette's syndrome, and tic disorder. *Pediatrics* 116(1):56–60, 2005.
169. Kurlan R, Kaplan EL. The pediatric autoimmune neuropsychiatric disorders associated with streptococcal infection (PANDAS) etiology for tics and obsessive-compulsive symptoms: Hypothesis or entity? Practical considerations for the clinician. *Pediatrics* 113(4):883–886, 2004.
170. Singer HS, Mink JW, Loiselle CR, Burke KA, Ruchkina I, Morshed S et al.: Microinfusion of antineuronal antibodies into rodent striatum: Failure to differentiate between elevated and low titers. *J Neuroimmunol* 163(1–2):8–14, 2005.
171. Singer HS, Giuliano JD, Hansen BH, Hallett JJ, Laurino JP, Benson M et al.: Antibodies against a neuron-like (HTB-10 neuroblastoma) cell in children with Tourette syndrome. *Biol Psychiatry* 46(6):775–780, 1999.
172. Lougee L, Perlmutter SJ, Nicolson R, Garvey MA, Swedo SE: Psychiatric disorders in first-degree relatives of children with pediatric autoimmune neuropsychiatric disorders associated with streptococcal infections (PANDAS). *J Am Acad Child Adolesc Psychiatry* 39(9):1120–1126, 2000.
173. Singer HS, Giuliano JD, Zimmerman AM, Walkup JT: Infection: A stimulus for tic disorders. *Pediatr Neurol* 22(5):380–383, 2000.
174. Peterson BS, Leckman JF, Tucker D, Scahill L, Staib L, Zhang H et al.: Preliminary findings of antistreptococcal antibody titers and basal ganglia volumes in tic, obsessive-compulsive, and attention deficit/hyperactivity disorders. *Arch Gen Psychiatry* 57(4):364–372, 2000.
175. Nicolson R, Swedo SE, Lenane M, Bedwell J, Wudarsky M, Gochman P et al.: An open trial of plasma exchange in childhood-onset obsessive-compulsive disorder without poststreptococcal exacerbations. *J Am Acad Child Adolesc Psychiatry* 39(10):1313–1315, 2000.
176. Thoren P, Asberg M, Cronholm B, Jornestedt L, Traskman L: Clomipramine treatment of obsessive-compulsive disorder. I. A controlled clinical trial. *Arch Gen Psychiatry* 37(11):1281–1285, 1980.
177. Baxter L: Functional imaging of brain systems mediating obsessive compulsive disorder. In: Charney DL, Nessler E, Bunney B (eds): *Neurobiology of Mental Illness*. London, Oxford Press, pp. 534–547, 1999.
178. Insel TR, Winslow JT: Neurobiology of obsessive compulsive disorder. *Psychiatr Clin North Am* 15(4):813–824, 1992.
179. Alexander GE, Crutcher MD, DeLong MR: Basal ganglia-thalamocortical circuits: Parallel substrates for motor, oculomotor, "prefrontal" and "limbic" functions. *Prog Brain Res* 85:119–146, 1990.
180. DeLong MR: Primate models of movement disorders of basal ganglia origin. *Trends Neurosci* 13(7):281–285, 1990.
181. Coetzer BR: Obsessive-compulsive disorder following brain injury: A review. *Int J Psychiatry Med* 34(4):363–377, 2004.
182. Towbin KE, Leckman JF, Cohen DJ: Drug treatment of obsessive-compulsive disorder: A review of findings in the light of diagnostic and metric limitations. *Psychiatr Dev* 5(1):25–50, 1987.
183. Samuels J, Bienvenu OJ, III, Riddle MA, Cullen BA, Grados MA, Liang KY et al.: Hoarding in obsessive compulsive disorder: Results from a case-control study. *Behav Res Ther* 40(5):517–528, 2002.
184. Salkovskis PM, Harrison J: Abnormal and normal obsessions—A replication. *Behav Res Ther* 22(5):549–552, 1984.
185. Rapoport JL, Inoff-Germain G: Treatment of obsessive-compulsive disorder in children and adolescents. *J Child Psychol Psychiatry* 41(4):419–431, 2000.
186. Berg CJ, Rapoport JL, Flament M: The Leyton Obsessional Inventory-Child Version. *J Am Acad Child Psychiatry* 25(1):84–91, 1986.
187. Cooper J: The Leyton Obsessional Inventory. *Psychol Med* 1:48–64, 1970.
188. Goodman WK, Price LH, Rasmussen SA, Mazure C, Fleischmann RL, Hill CL et al.: The Yale–Brown Obsessive Compulsive Scale. I. Development, use, and reliability. *Arch Gen Psychiatry* 46(11):1006–1011, 1989.
189. Goodman WK, Price LH, Rasmussen SA, Mazure C, Delgado P, Heninger GR et al.: The Yale–Brown Obsessive Compulsive Scale: II. Validity. *Arch Gen Psychiatry* 46(11):1012–1016, 1989.
190. Scahill L, Riddle MA, McSwiggin-Hardin M, Ort SI, King RA, Goodman WK et al.: Children's Yale–Brown Obsessive Compulsive Scale: Reliability and validity. *J Am Acad Child Adolesc Psychiatry* 36(6):844–852, 1997.
191. Achenbach TM: *Manual for the Child Behavior Checklist and Revised Behavior Profile*. Burlington, VT: Thomas Achenbach, 1983.
192. March JS: Cognitive-behavioral psychotherapy for children and adolescents with OCD: A review and recommendations for treatment. *J Am Acad Child Adolesc Psychiatry* 34(1):7–18, 1995.
193. Foa EB, Steketee GB, Ozarow B, I: Behavior therapy with obsessive compulsives. In: Mavissakalian M TSML (ed): *Obsessive Compulsive Disorder: Psychological and Pharmacological Treatment*. New York, Plenum Press, 1985, pp. 49–131.
194. Marks IM, Stern RS, Mawson D, Cobb J, McDonald R: Clomipramine and exposure for obsessive-compulsive rituals: i. *Br J Psychiatry* 136:1–25, 1980.
195. March JS, Mulle K, Herbel B: Behavioral psychotherapy for children and adolescents with obsessive-compulsive disorder: An open trial of a new protocol-driven treatment package. *J Am Acad Child Adolesc Psychiatry* 33(3):333–341, 1994.
196. de Haan E, Hoogduin KA, Buitelaar JK, Keijsers GP: Behavior therapy versus clomipramine for the treatment of obsessive-compulsive disorder in children and adolescents. *J Am Acad Child Adolesc Psychiatry* 37(10):1022–1029, 1998.
197. Barrett P, Healy-Farrell L, March JS: Cognitive-behavioral family treatment of childhood obsessive-compulsive disorder: A controlled trial. *J Am Acad Child Adolesc Psychiatry* 43(1):46–62, 2004.
198. March JS: Pediatric Obsessive-Compulsive Treatment Study Group. Cognitive-behavior therapy, sertraline, and their combination for children and adolescents with obsessive-compulsive disorder: The Pediatric OCD Treatment Study (POTS) randomized controlled trial. *JAMA* 292(16):1969–1976, 2004.
199. Wolff RP, Wolff LS: Assessment and treatment of obsessive-compulsive disorder in children. *Behav Modif* 15(3):372–393, 1991.
200. Flament MF, Rapoport JL, Berg CJ, Sceery W, Kilts C, Mellstrom B et al.: Clomipramine treatment of childhood obsessive-compulsive disorder. A double-blind controlled study. *Arch Gen Psychiatry* 42(10):977–983, 1985.
201. DeVeaugh-Geiss J, Moroz G, Biederman J, Cantwell D, Fontaine R, Greist JH et al.: Clomipramine hydrochloride in childhood and adolescent obsessive-compulsive disorder—A multicenter trial. *J Am Acad Child Adolesc Psychiatry* 31(1):45–49, 1992.
202. Insel TR, Murphy DL, Cohen RM, Alterman I, Kilts C, Linnoila M: Obsessive-compulsive disorder: A double-blind trial of clomipramine and clorgyline. *Arch Gen Psychiatry* 40(6):605–612, 1983.
203. Fontaine R, Chouinard G: Fluoxetine in the treatment of obsessive compulsive disorder. *Prog Neuropsychopharmacol Biol Psychiatry* 9(5–6):605–608, 1985.
204. Geller DA, Hoog SL, Heiligenstein JH, Ricardi RK, Tamura R, Kluszynski S et al.: Fluoxetine treatment for obsessive-compulsive disorder in children and adolescents: A placebo-controlled clinical trial. *J Am Acad Child Adolesc Psychiatry* 40(7):773–779, 2001.
205. Price LH, Goodman WK, Charney DS, Rasmussen SA, Heninger GR: Treatment of severe obsessive-compulsive disorder with fluvoxamine. *Am J Psychiatry* 144(8):1059–1061, 1987.
206. Riddle MA, Reeve EA, Yaryura-Tobias JA, Yang HM, Claghorn JL, Gaffney G et al.: Fluvoxamine for children and adolescents with obsessive-compulsive disorder: A randomized, controlled, multicenter trial. *J Am Acad Child Adolesc Psychiatry* 40(2):222–229, 2001.
207. Riddle M: Obsessive-compulsive disorder in children and adolescents. *Br J Psychiatry Suppl* (35):91–96, 1998.
208. Chouinard G, Goodman W, Greist J, Jenike M, Rasmussen S, White K et al.: Results of a double-blind placebo controlled trial of a new serotonin uptake inhibitor, sertraline, in the treatment of obsessive-compulsive disorder. *Psychopharmacol Bull* 26(3):279–284, 1990.
209. March JS, Biederman J, Wolkow R, Safferman A, Mardekian J, Cook EH et al.: Sertraline in children and adolescents with obsessive-compulsive disorder: A multicenter randomized controlled trial. *JAMA* 280(20):1752–1756, 1998.
210. Alderman J: Sertraline treatment of children and adolescents with obsessive-compulsive disorder or depression: Pharmacokinetics, tolerability, and efficacy. *Journal of the American Academy of Child & Adolescent Psychiatry* 37(4):386–394, 1998.
211. Geller DA, Wagner KD, Emslie G, Murphy T, Carpenter DJ, Wetherhold E et al.: Paroxetine treatment in children and adolescents with obsessive-compulsive disorder: A randomized, multicenter, double-blind, placebo-controlled trial. *J Am Acad Child Adolesc Psychiatry* 43(11):1387–1396, 2004.
212. Mukaddes NM, Abali O, Kaynak N: Citalopram treatment of children and adolescents with obsessive-compulsive disorder: A preliminary report. *Psychiatry Clin Neurosci* 57(4):405–408, 2003.
213. Thomsen PH: Child and adolescent obsessive-compulsive disorder treated with citalopram: Findings from an open trial of 23 cases. *J Child Adolesc Psychopharmacol* 7(3):157–166, 1997.
214. Leonard HL, Swedo SE, Rapoport JL, Koby EV, Lenane MC, Cheslow DL et al.: Treatment of obsessive-compulsive disorder with clomipramine and desipramine in children and adolescents: A double-blind crossover comparison. *Arch Gen Psychiatry* 46(12):1088–1092, 1989.
215. Leonard HL, Swedo SE, Lenane MC, Rettew DC, Cheslow DL, Hamburger SD et al.: A double-blind desipramine substitution during long-term clomipramine treatment in children and adolescents with obsessive-compulsive disorder. *Arch Gen Psychiatry* 48(10):922–927, 1991.
216. Pigott TA, Pato MT, Bernstein SE, Grover GN, Hill JL, Tolliver TJ et al.: Controlled comparisons of clomipramine and fluoxetine in the treatment of obsessive-compulsive disorder: Behavioral and biological results. *Arch Gen Psychiatry* 47(10):926–932, 1990.
217. Riddle MA, Scahill L, King RA, Hardin MT, Anderson GM, Ort SI et al.: Double-blind, crossover trial of fluoxetine and placebo in children and adolescents with obsessive-compulsive disorder. *J Am Acad Child Adolesc Psychiatry* 31(6):1062–1069, 1992.
218. King RA, Riddle MA, Chappell PB, Hardin MT, Anderson GM, Lombroso P et al.: Emergence of self-destructive phenomena in children

and adolescents during fluoxetine treatment. *J Am Acad Child Adolesc Psychiatry* 30(2):179–186, 1991.
219. Jick H, Kaye JA, Jick SS: Antidepressants and the risk of suicidal behaviors. *JAMA* 292(3):338–343, 2004.
220. Apter A, Ratzoni G, King RA, Weizman A, Iancu I, Binder M et al.: Fluvoxamine open-label treatment of adolescent inpatients with obsessive-compulsive disorder or depression. *J Am Acad Child Adolesc Psychiatry* 33(3):342–348, 1994.
221. Geller DA, Biederman J, Stewart SE, Mullin B, Martin A, Spencer T et al.: Which SSRI? A meta-analysis of pharmacotherapy trials in pediatric obsessive-compulsive disorder. *Am J Psychiatry* 160(11):1919–1928, 2003.
222. March JS. Review: Clomipramine is more effective than SSRIs for paediatric obsessive compulsive disorder. *Evid Based Ment Health* 7(2):50–, 2004.
223. Fitzgerald KD, Stewart CM, Tawile V, Rosenberg DR: Risperidone augmentation of serotonin reuptake inhibitor treatment of pediatric obsessive compulsive disorder. *J Child Adolesc Psychopharmacol* 9(2):115–123, 1999.
224. McDougle CJ, Epperson CN, Pelton GH, Wasylink S, Price LH: A double-blind, placebo-controlled study of risperidone addition in serotonin reuptake inhibitor-refractory obsessive-compulsive disorder. *Arch Gen Psychiatry* 57(8):794–801, 2000.
225. Weiss EL, Potenza MN, McDougle CJ, Epperson CN: Olanzapine addition in obsessive-compulsive disorder refractory to selective serotonin reuptake inhibitors: An open-label case series. *J Clin Psychiatry* 60(8):524–527, 1999.
226. Rasmussen SA: Lithium and tryptophan augmentation in clomipramine-resistant obsessive-compulsive disorder. *Am J Psychiatry* 141(10):1283–1285, 1984.
227. Grady TA, Pigott TA, L'Heureux F, Hill JL, Bernstein SE, Murphy DL: Double-blind study of adjuvant buspirone for fluoxetine-treated patients with obsessive-compulsive disorder. *Am J Psychiatry* 150(5):819–821, 1993.
228. Markovitz PJ, Stagno SJ, Calabrese JR: Buspirone augmentation of fluoxetine in obsessive-compulsive disorder. *Am J Psychiatry* 147(6):798–800, 1990.
229. Figueroa Y, Rosenberg DR, Birmaher B, Keshavan MS: Combination treatment with clomipramine and selective serotonin reuptake inhibitors for obsessive-compulsive disorder in children and adolescents. *J Child Adolesc Psychopharmacol* 8(1):61–67, 1998.
230. Steiner W, Fontaine R: Toxic reaction following the combined administration of fluoxetine and L-tryptophan: Five case reports. *Biol Psychiatry* 21(11):1067–1071, 1986.
231. Goodwin DW, Guze SB, Robins E: Follow-up studies in obsessional neurosis. *Arch Gen Psychiatry* 20(2):182–187, 1969.
232. Mawson D, Marks IM, Ramm L: Clomipramine and exposure for chronic obsessive-compulsive rituals: III. Two year follow-up and further findings. *Br J Psychiatry* 140:11–18, 1982.
233. Skoog G, Skoog I: A 40-year follow-up of patients with obsessive-compulsive disorder. *Arch Gen Psychiatry* 56(2):121–127, 1999.
234. Berg CZ, Rapoport JL, Whitaker A, Davies M, Leonard H, Swedo SE et al.: Childhood obsessive compulsive disorder: A two-year prospective follow-up of a community sample. *J Am Acad Child Adolesc Psychiatry* 28(4):528–533, 1989.
235. Bolton D, Collins S, Steinberg D: The treatment of obsessive-compulsive disorder in adolescence: A report of fifteen cases. *Br J Psychiatry* 142:456–464, 1983.
236. Wewetzer C, Jans T, Muller B, Neudorfl A, Bucherl U, Remschmidt H et al.: Long-term outcome and prognosis of obsessive-compulsive disorder with onset in childhood or adolescence. *Eur Child Adolesc Psychiatry* 10(1):37–46, 2001.
237. Stewart SE, Geller DA, Jenike M, Pauls D, Shaw D, Mullin B et al.: Long-term outcome of pediatric obsessive-compulsive disorder: A meta-analysis and qualitative review of the literature. *Acta Psychiatr Scand* 110(1):4–13, 2004.
238. Hyman SE. The millennium of mind, brain, and behavior. *Arch Gen Psychiatry* 57(1):88–89, 2000.
239. Fisher PL, Wells A: How effective are cognitive and behavioral treatments for obsessive-compulsive disorder? A clinical significance analysis. *Behav Res Ther* 43(12):1543–1558, 2005.
240. Abramowitz JS, Khandker M, Nelson CA, Deacon BJ, Rygwall R: The role of cognitive factors in the pathogenesis of obsessive-compulsive symptoms: A prospective study. *Behav Res Ther* 2005.
241. Lewin AB, Storch EA, Adkins J, Murphy TK, Geffken GR: Current directions in pediatric obsessive-compulsive disorder. *Pediatr Ann* 34(2):128–134, 2005.

CHAPTER 5.5.3 ■ TRICHOTILLOMANIA

KENNETH E. TOWBIN

Franciose Henri Hallopeau coined trichotillomania (TTM) from the Greek words for "hair + pulling + madness" in 1889 (1, 2). TTM and OCD share an obvious similarity of repetitive behavior and this has led some investigators to consider whether there is more than a surface relationship between them (3–6). Some have proposed that both are part of a larger obsessive-compulsive spectrum disorder (4, 7). The concept of an obsessive-compulsive spectrum disorder draws on shared characteristics of impulsive and repetitive behaviors and encompasses a wide range of conditions—obsessive-compulsive disorder, all impulse control disorders (kleptomania, pyromania, trichotillomania, intermittent explosive disorder), all the paraphilias, sexual and gambling addictions, autism, Tourette disorder, and all the DSM Cluster B (antisocial, borderline, narcissistic, histrionic) personality disorders (4, 7). The merits and problems of an obsessive-compulsive spectrum disorder are beyond the scope of this chapter, but the association of TTM and OCD demand that one considers whether it is appropriate to place them together and appreciates their similarities and dissimilarities. This is especially the case for child psychiatry, since there is evidence to suggest that childhood-onset OCD is a risk factor for TTM (8, 9) and that TTM often has its onset in childhood and adolescence (8–11).

The formal diagnosis of TTM in DSM-IV-TR (12) requires both behavioral and psychological components—hair pulling to the point of conspicuous hair loss accompanied by rising tension prior to hair pulling and gratification during or after it. Some investigators consider the DSM criteria to be excessively restrictive (10, 13–16). The prevalence of hair pulling (HP) without psychological components is nearly 4% in the general population (13, 15), compared to the 0.6–1% prevalence reported for TTM (13, 15). Generally females are more common in clinical samples. The age of onset is bimodal, with incident peaks in early childhood and adolescence. Forty-five to 55% of TTM/HP patients report a childhood (before age 18) onset (17). Demonstrating that HP shows a similar course, prognosis, genetic risk, and treatment response to TTM convincingly would establish that they have a close relationship.

It appears that TTM and HP are often comorbid with OCD (15, 18, 19). Four to 35% of patients with OCD report lifetime histories of TTM/HP (16, 19–22), while 13–16% of those with TTM/HP report lifetime histories of OCD (17, 23, 24). TTM and HP also are commonly associated with tic disorders (8, 10, 19, 21, 22, 25). As with tics, TTM/HP appears to be particularly associated with early-onset OCD (10, 19, 21). TTM/HP are also associated with hoarding (26). Most studies have relied exclusively on clinical populations at risk, producing an erroneous, biased association (27). However, two studies drawing on nonreferred, more epidemiological populations suggest an association may in fact exist (13, 15).

There are some indications that TTM/HP may be genetically associated with OCD (10, 22, 28) though the evidence gives mixed results. In an uncontrolled observational cohort study, 15% of 60 adults with TTM/HP interviewed by Christenson and coworkers (17) reported lifetime histories of OCD. Lenane and coworkers (28) interviewed 65 of 69 first degree relatives of 16 girls with OCD and similar number of parents of healthy volunteer control group. Three of 16 (19%) girls with TTM had a first-degree relative with a lifetime history of OCD, and there was overall a 6.4% lifetime prevalence rate of OCD in the first-degree relatives of girls with TTM. King and coworkers (10) described 15 clinic-referred children with TTM/HP who were assessed for comorbid diagnoses and whose parents were also assessed for lifetime histories of tics and OCD. Seven participants had comorbid disruptive behavior disorders, three had a current or past history of chronic motor tics and three had comorbid anxiety disorders. Only two participants had OCD. For the family study, 11 participants had both parents interviewed and four had only one parent directly interviewed; one participant was adopted and another was in the care of his/her father and stepmother. Among the parents, two met criteria for OCD and six had OC symptoms that were subthreshold. Two fathers had Tourette disorder and one had chronic multiple tic disorder. In contrast, a controlled family study of 88 adults with rigorously diagnosed OCD and 343 of their first degree relatives was conducted by Bienvenu and coworkers (22). Individuals were included if they has YBOCS severity scores greater than 15, and individuals with Tourette disorder were excluded. Among probands, 4% had current or past histories of TTM, but this was not statistically significant in comparison to controls, where one case was identified. Similarly, two cases (1%) of first degree relatives gave a history for TTM and this was not statistically different from controls. The scope of the Bienvenu and coworkers (22) study was wider than just TTM and included other "pathological grooming behaviors" such as pathological skin picking and nail biting. When probands were compared to healthy volunteers, the rate for TTM was not elevated, but the rates for the other pathological grooming behaviors were (25% for nail picking and 24% for skin picking, compared to 14% and 6% respectively in healthy volunteers). However, only skin picking was statistically significantly greater, and rates for all grooming behaviors were not elevated in first-degree relatives of OCD patients compared to relatives of controls (22).

Characterization of neuropsychological features in TTM is only preliminary. However, this work suggests that deficits in TTM do not appear to be the same as in persons with OCD (29–31). Similar to genetic studies, the evidence in support of a relationship with OCD is mixed. Bohne and coworkers (29) examined "executive functions" of age- and IQ-matched groups of patients with OCD, TTM, and healthy volunteers (HVs) on measures of organizing, planning, set shift, attention, mental flexibility, and on visual spatial tasks. The TTM group was predominantly female. There were no differences between groups on measures of attention, memory, organization (verbal and nonverbal), visual spatial abilities, and concept learning (29). Only two differences emerged in this study. Patients with TTM showed increased perserveration errors, suggesting cognitive inflexibility, compared to those with OCD and HVs. Furthermore, patients with OCD showed impaired learning from feedback based on the Wisconsin Card Sort (29). Chamberlain and coworkers considered endophenotypes for OCD and proposed that the primary neuropsychological deficits in OCD were in strategy implementation (31), which integrates cognitive functions, and in motor inhibition (30), as measured by the Stop Signal Task, which is linked to internal suppression. Both are closely tied to the orbitofrontal striatal circuitry described for OCD (Chapter 5.5.2). In a series of studies comparing matched patients and controls with only OCD to those with only TTM and HVs, Chamberlain and coworkers found that patients with TTM displayed abilities in strategy implementation equal to those in HVs (31), but very significant deficits in motor inhibition compared to patients with OCD and HVs (30).

Morphometric MRI studies support findings of decreased volumes in the left frontal cortex in women with TTM. Stein and coworkers (32) compared women with OCD ($n = 13$), TTM ($n = 17$) and HVs ($n = 12$) and found no differences in caudate nuclei or ventricular brain ratio. O'Sullivan and coworkers (33) performed a morphometric MRI study of 10 women with TTM who had no comorbid diagnoses with 10 healthy volunteers. Comparisons showed decreased volumes in TTM patients in the left lenticulate nucleus and left putamen. There were no differences in the caudate or in white matter structures; this is a significant departure from findings in OCD. The investigators did remark on the similarity between these findings and morphometric studies of Tourette disorder. Similarly, Grachev (34) performed a study of 10 women with TTM using voxel-based morphometry and found decreased left inferior frontal gyrus volumes.

The relative rarity of TTM has made it difficult to develop a database for the course and treatment of this condition. As with many rare disorders, the patients who come to clinical attention are more likely to be severely impaired and suffer from comorbid conditions like depression or anxiety disorders. At this point the literature suggests that the course of TTM is chronic. Lerner and coworkers (35) reviewed the course of 14 participants in a study of Cognitive Behavioral Therapy (CBT) at mean followup period of 3 years 9 months. Upon completion of CBT 12 of 14 individuals were considered responders. At followup only four of 13 were still considered responders, and when this was compared to a group of 10 individuals who initially refused treatment, there was no difference in overall response rates between treated and untreated groups (35). Keuthen and coworkers (36) reviewed the course of 63 individuals who had participated in a "state-of-the-art" treatment study a mean of 42 months earlier. At followup 51% were still in treatment and 27% were not. At this followup point, 33 (52%) of participants were considered themselves treatment responders; 16 (25%) improved with CBT alone. The investigators found that higher rates of depression correlated with better outcome (36). However, in a subsequent followup of the same cohort (37) some 30 months later, 61% were still in active treatment for TTM and only 37% considered themselves treatment responders. Although initial gains in self-esteem, depression, and anxiety were noted at the first followup, these had diminished by the second followup time, such that there were no longer differences in depression, anxiety, or self-esteem from initial evaluation to second followup period, despite improvements in hair-pulling (37).

Pharmacotherapy has offered only modest results for trichotillomania and among all agents, serotonin reuptake inhibitors have been the most studied (36, 38–45). Few randomized controlled studies have been conducted and rates of improvement have been disappointing. Open-label studies report rates of improvement of 30 to 60%, but the two placebo-controlled trials showed no significant improvement over placebo (39, 46). Generally, pharmacological response appears to be less in TTM than what is observed in patients with OCD (43, 45). A number of small case reports also suggest that augmentation with dopamine antagonists, such as pimozide (42), risperidone (47, 48), or olanzapine (49, 50) may be helpful but have not been systematically studied in randomized, blinded trials.

The most persuasive treatment studies point to the efficacy of cognitive behavioral interventions. Two studies examined randomized treatment to CBT or medication (40, 51, 52) and demonstrated superiority of CBT. Ninan and coworkers (40) randomly assigned 23 patients to 6 weeks of CBT, clomipramine (mean dose 116 mg/d; up to 250 mg/d) or placebo. Sixteen of 23 participants completed treatment and CBT was superior to clomipramine and placebo; clomipramine was not statistically different from placebo (40). Van Minnen and coworkers (52) randomly assigned 15 patients to 12 weeks of behavioral therapy, 13 patients to 12 weeks of fluoxetine (60 mg/d) and 15 patients remained on a wait list as controls. Behavioral therapy was superior to fluoxetine and the wait-list condition. Behavioral therapy showed a large effect size, with 64% of behavior therapy participants improved, compared to 9% in the fluoxetine group and 20% in the wait-list group (52). In order to explore whether these gains could be maintained, Keijsters and coworkers (51) performed a 3-month and then 2-year followup on 28 participants, some of whom were in the van Minnen study, and others who were treated with open behavioral study subsequently. Initial treatment effects, again showing large effect sizes, rivaled those observed in the van Minnen study (52) but deteriorated at 3 months and at 2 years (51). Pretreatment depression was a significant predictor of poor outcome, and the ability to cease hair pulling by the end of behavioral treatment was associated with a greater likelihood of improvement (51).

Overall, manualized cognitive behavioral treatment appears to be superior to pharmacological treatment for TTM. At best the initial gains made in CBT are difficult to maintain and comorbid depression makes them even harder to sustain. At this point there are no specific indicators to suggest which patients will be more likely to respond to CBT or medication and there are no augmentation strategies that have been studied with sufficient rigor to permit one to recommend them.

Many more questions remain to be answered before we will understand the genetics, neurobiology, course, and treatment of TTM. Although the last decade has seen very significant gains, particularly in understanding the cognitive underpinnings of TTM, it is likely that the larger majority of children with TTM remain to be identified and offered treatment. Clearly without treatment the majority of patients with TTM have very severe impairment in function (53). Some individuals develop severe gastrointestinal complications from trichobezoars (54–58). At this juncture, half to two-thirds of those who enter into CBT will find their symptoms improve, but only about 50% of those for whom treatment is successful will be able to maintain those gains over 2 years and most require ongoing treatment for many years.

References

1. Christenson GA, Mansueto CS: Trichotillomania: Descriptive characteristics and phenomenology. In: Stein DJ, Christenson GA, Hollander E (eds): *Trichotillomania*. Washington, DC, American Psychiatric Publishing, Inc., 1999, pp. 1–41.
2. Hallopeau M: Alopécia par grattage (trichomanie ou trichotillomanie). *Ann Dermatol Venereol* 10:440–441, 1889.
3. Stein DJ, Hollander E: Dermatology and conditions related to obsessive-compulsive disorder. *J Am Acad Dermatol* 26(2 Pt 1):237–242, 1992.
4. Hollander E, Rosen J: Impulsivity. *J Psychopharmacol* 14(2 Suppl 1):S39–S44, 2000.
5. Stein DJ, Simeon D, Cohen LJ, Hollander E: Trichotillomania and obsessive-compulsive disorder. *J Clin Psychiatry* 56 Suppl 4:28–34, 1995.
6. Stein DJ, Lochner C: Obsessive-compulsive spectrum disorders: A multidimensional approach. *Psychiatr Clin North Am* 29(2):343–351, 2006.
7. Hollander E, Benzaquen SD: The obsessive-compulsive spectrum disorders. *International Review of Psychiatry* 9(1):99–109, 1997.
8. Diniz JB, Rosario-Campos MC, Shavitt RG, Curi M, Hounie AG, Brotto SA et al.: Impact of age at onset and duration of illness on the expression of comorbidities in obsessive-compulsive disorder. *J Clin Psychiatry* 65(1):22–27, 2004.
9. Hanna GL: Trichotillomania and related disorders in children and adolescents. *Child Psychiatry Hum Dev* 27(4):255–268, 1997.
10. King RA, Scahill L, Vitulano LA, Schwab-Stone M, Tercyak KP, Jr., Riddle MA: Childhood trichotillomania: Clinical phenomenology, comorbidity, and family genetics. *J Am Acad Child Adolesc Psychiatry* 34(11):1451–1459, 1995.
11. Reeve EA, Bernstein GA, Christenson GA: Clinical characteristics and psychiatric comorbidity in children with trichotillomania. *J Am Acad Child Adolesc Psychiatry* 31(1):132–138, 1992.
12. American Psychiatric Association. *Diagnostic and Statistical Manual of Mental Disorders-IV-TR*. IV-TR ed. Washington, DC: American Psychiatric Press, Inc, 2000.
13. Christenson GA, Pyle RL, Mitchell JE: Estimated lifetime prevalence of trichotillomania in college students. *J Clin Psychiatry* 52(10):415–417, 1991.
14. Woods DW, Flessner C, Franklin ME, Wetterneck CT, Walther MR, Anderson ER et al.: Understanding and treating trichotillomania: What we know and what we don't know. *Psychiatr Clin North Am* 29(2):487–501, ix, 2006.
15. King RA, Zohar AH, Ratzoni G, Binder M, Kron S, Dycian A et al.: An epidemiological study of trichotillomania in Israeli adolescents. *J Am Acad Child Adolesc Psychiatry* 34(9):1212–1215, 1995.
16. du Toit PL, van Kradenburg J, Niehaus DJ, Stein DJ: Characteristics and phenomenology of hair-pulling: An exploration of subtypes. *Compr Psychiatry* 42(3):247–256, 2001.
17. Christenson GA, Mackenzie TB, Mitchell JE: Characteristics of 60 adult chronic hair pullers. *Am J Psychiatry* 148(3):365–370, 1991.
18. Fontenelle LF, Mendlowicz MV, Versiani M: Impulse control disorders in patients with obsessive-compulsive disorder. *Psychiatry Clin Neurosci* 59(1):30–37, 2005.
19. Jaisoorya TS, Reddy YC, Srinath S: The relationship of obsessive-compulsive disorder to putative spectrum disorders: Results from an Indian study. *Compr Psychiatry* 44(4):317–323, 2003.
20. Richter MA, Summerfeldt LJ, Antony MM, Swinson RP: Obsessive-compulsive spectrum conditions in obsessive-compulsive disorder and other anxiety disorders. *Depress Anxiety* 18(3):118–127, 2003.
21. Stewart SE, Jenike MA, Keuthen NJ: Severe obsessive-compulsive disorder with and without comorbid hair pulling: Comparisons and clinical implications. *J Clin Psychiatry* 66(7):864–869, 2005.
22. Bienvenu OJ, Samuels JF, Riddle MA, Hoehn-Saric R, Liang KY, Cullen BA et al.: The relationship of obsessive-compulsive disorder to possible spectrum disorders: Results from a family study. *Biol Psychiatry* 48(4):287–293, 2000.
23. Cohen LJ, Stein DJ, Simeon D, Spadaccini E, Rosen J, Aronowitz B et al.: Clinical profile, comorbidity, and treatment history in 123 hair pullers: A survey study. *J Clin Psychiatry* 56(7):319–326, 1995.
24. Swedo SE, Leonard HL: Trichotillomania. An obsessive compulsive spectrum disorder? *Psychiatr Clin North Am* 15(4):777–790, 1992.
25. Hemmings SM, Kinnear CJ, Lochner C, Niehaus DJ, Knowles JA, Moolman-Smook JC et al.: Early- versus late-onset obsessive-compulsive disorder: Investigating genetic and clinical correlates. *Psychiatry Res* 128(2):175–182, 2004.
26. Samuels J, Bienvenu OJ, III, Riddle MA, Cullen BA,Grados MA,Liang KY et al.: Hoarding in obsessive compulsive disorder: Results from a case-control study. *Behav Res Ther* 40(5):517–528, 2002.
27. Cohen P, Cohen J: The clinician's illusion. *Arch Gen Psychiatry* 41(12):1178–1182, 1984.
28. Lenane MC, Swedo SE, Rapoport JL, Leonard H, Sceery W, Guroff JJ: Rates of obsessive compulsive disorder in first degree relatives of patients with trichotillomania: A research note. *Journal of Child Psychology and Psychiatry and Allied Disciplines* 33(5):925–933, 1992.
29. Bohne A, Savage CR, Deckersbach T, Keuthen NJ, Jenike MA, Tuschen-Caffier B et al.: Visuospatial abilities, memory, and executive functioning in trichotillomania and obsessive-compulsive disorder. *J Clin Exp Neuropsychol* 27(4):385–399, 2005.
30. Chamberlain SR, Fineberg NA, Blackwell AD, Robbins TW, Sahakian BJ: Motor inhibition and cognitive flexibility in obsessive-compulsive disorder and trichotillomania. *Am J Psychiatry* 163(7):1282–1284, 2006.
31. Chamberlain SR, Blackwell AD, Fineberg NA, Robbins TW, Sahakian BJ: Strategy implementation in obsessive-compulsive disorder and trichotillomania. *Psychol Med* 36(1):91–97, 2006.
32. Stein DJ, Coetzer R, Lee M, Davids B, Bouwer C: Magnetic resonance brain imaging in women with obsessive-compulsive disorder and trichotillomania. *Psychiatry Res* 74(3):177–182, 1997.
33. O'Sullivan RL, Rauch SL, Breiter HC, Grachev ID, Baer L, Kennedy DN et al.: Reduced basal ganglia volumes in trichotillomania measured via morphometric magnetic resonance imaging. *Biol Psychiatry* 42(1):39–45, 1997.
34. Grachev ID: MRI-based morphometric topographic parcellation of human neocortex in trichotillomania. *Psychiatry Clin Neurosci* 51(5):315–321, 1997.

35. Lerner J: Effectiveness of a cognitive behavioral treatment program for trichotillomania: An uncontrolled evaluation. *Behavior Therapy* 29(1):157–171, 1998.
36. Keuthen NJ, O'Sullivan RL, Goodchild P, Rodriguez D, Jenike MA, Baer L: Retrospective review of treatment outcome for 63 patients with trichotillomania. *Am J Psychiatry* 155(4):560–561, 1998.
37. Keuthen NJ, Fraim C, Deckersbach T, Dougherty DD, Baer L, Jenike MA: Longitudinal follow-up of naturalistic treatment outcome in patients with trichotillomania. *J Clin Psychiatry* 62(2):101–107, 2001.
38. Streichenwein SM, Thornby JI: A long-term, double-blind, placebo-controlled crossover trial of the efficacy of fluoxetine for trichotillomania. *Am J Psychiatry* 152(8):1192–1196, 1995.
39. Christenson GA, Mackenzie TB, Mitchell JE, Callies AL: A placebo-controlled, double-blind crossover study of fluoxetine in trichotillomania. *Am J Psychiatry* 148(11):1566–1571, 1991.
40. Ninan PT, Rothbaum BO, Marsteller FA, Knight BT, Eccard MB: A placebo-controlled trial of cognitive-behavioral therapy and clomipramine in trichotillomania. *J Clin Psychiatry* 61(1):47–50, 2000.
41. Potenza MN, Wasylink S, Epperson CN, McDougle CJ: Olanzapine augmentation of fluoxetine in the treatment of trichotillomania. *Am J Psychiatry* 155(9):1299–1300, 1998.
42. Stein DJ, Hollander E: Low-dose pimozide augmentation of serotonin reuptake blockers in the treatment of trichotillomania. *J Clin Psychiatry* 53(4):123–126, 1992.
43. Stein DJ, Bouwer C, Maud CM: Use of the selective serotonin reuptake inhibitor citalopram in treatment of trichotillomania. *Eur Arch Psychiatry Clin Neurosci* 247(4):234–236, 1997.
44. Swedo SE, Leonard HL, Rapoport JL, Lenane MC, Goldberger EL, Cheslow DL: A double-blind comparison of clomipramine and desipramine in the treatment of trichotillomania (hair pulling). *N Engl J Med* 321(8):497–501, 1989.
45. Walsh KH, McDougle CJ: Pharmacological strategies for trichotillomania. *Expert Opin Pharmacother* 6(6):975–984, 2005.
46. Streichenwein SM, Thornby JI: A long-term, double-blind, placebo-controlled crossover trial of the efficacy of fluoxetine for trichotillomania. *Am J Psychiatry* 152(8):1192–1196, 1995.
47. Epperson CN, Fasula D, Wasylink S, Price LH, McDougle CJ: Risperidone addition in serotonin reuptake inhibitor-resistant trichotillomania: Three cases. *J Child Adolesc Psychopharmacol* 9(1):43–49, 1999.
48. Stein DJ, Bouwer C, Hawkridge S, Emsley RA: Risperidone augmentation of serotonin reuptake inhibitors in obsessive-compulsive and related disorders. *J Clin Psychiatry* 58(3):119–122, 1997.
49. Srivastava RK, Sharma S, Tiwari N, Saluja B: Olanzapine augmentation of fluoxetine in trichotillomania: Two cases. *Aust N Z J Psychiatry* 39(1–2):112–113, 2005.
50. Ashton AK: Olanzapine augmentation for trichotillomania. *Am J Psychiatry* 158(11):1929–1930, 2001.
51. Keijsers GP, van Minnen A, Hoogduin CA, Klaassen BN, Hendriks MJ, Tanis-Jacobs J: Behavioural treatment of trichotillomania: Two-year follow-up results. *Behav Res Ther* 44(3):359–370, 2006.
52. van Minnen A, Hoogduin KA, Keijsers GP, Hellenbrand I, Hendriks GJ: Treatment of trichotillomania with behavioral therapy or fluoxetine: A randomized, waiting-list controlled study. *Arch Gen Psychiatry* 60(5):517–522, 2003.
53. Diefenbach GJ, Tolin DF, Hannan S, Crocetto J, Worhunsky P: Trichotillomania: Impact on psychosocial functioning and quality of life. *Behav Res Ther* 43(7):869–884, 2005.
54. Ciampa A, Moore BE, Listerud RG, Kydd D, Kim RD: Giant trichophytobezoar in a pediatric patient with trichotillomania. *Pediatr Radiol* 33(3):219–220, 2003.
55. Frey AS, McKee M, King RA, Martin A: Hair apparent: Rapunzel syndrome. *Am J Psychiatry* 162(2):242–248, 2005.
56. Lynch KA, Feola PG, Guenther E: Gastric trichobezoar: An important cause of abdominal pain presenting to the pediatric emergency department. *Pediatr Emerg Care* 19(5):343–347, 2003.
57. Ramadan N, Pandya NA, Bhaduri B: A Rapunzel with a difference. *Arch Dis Child* 88(3):264, 2003.
58. Salaam K, Carr J, Grewal H, Sholevar E, Baron D: Untreated trichotillomania and trichophagia: Surgical emergency in a teenage girl. *Psychosomatics* 46(4):362–366, 2005.

CHAPTER 5.6 ■ TIC DISORDERS

MICHAEL H. BLOCH AND JAMES F. LECKMAN

Tic disorders are transient or chronic conditions associated with difficulties in self-esteem, family life, social acceptance or school or job performance that are directly related to the presence of motor and/or phonic tics. Tic disorders have been noted since antiquity. The first identified case of TS in historical literature was recounted in *Malleus Maleficarium* (*The Witches' Hammer*), a 1482 treatise on recognizing and curing demonic possession. Sprenger and Kraemer, the authors of *Malleus Maleficarium*, provide a detailed description of a young priest with motor and vocal tics, who is saved from a fiery death at the stake only by successful treatment with exorcism (1). In later French historical archives, there is a chilling account of one Prince de Conde, a seventeenth century French nobleman in the court of Louis XIV, who resorted to stuffing objects in his mouth to prevent an involuntary bark when in the presence of his royal highness (2).

Although reported since antiquity, recognition of TS as a distinct neuropsychiatric syndrome, and systematic study of individuals with tic disorders, began only with the reports of French neurologists Itard (1825) and Gilles de la Tourette (1885) in the nineteenth century. Gilles de la Tourette, in his classic study of 1885, described nine cases characterized by motor "incoordinations" or tics, "inarticulate shouts accompanied by articulated words with echolalia and coprolalia (3)." In addition to identifying the cardinal features of severe tic disorders, his report noted an association between tic disorders and obsessive-compulsive symptoms, as well as the hereditary nature of the syndrome in some families.

Since the case series presented by Gilles de la Tourette, we have learned that TS typically has a much more benign course than initially suggested in his account. We have also developed some effective pharmacological, psychological, and now, even surgical, treatments for individuals with TS. With increasing longitudinal assessment of children with tic disorders we have learned that many present or develop a broad array of behavioral difficulties, including disinhibited speech or conduct, impulsivity, distractibility, motoric hyperactivity, and obsessive compulsive symptoms (4). In this chapter, a presentation of the phenomenology and classification of tic disorders precedes a review of the epidemiology, clinical course, neurobiological substrates, assessment and management of tic disorders and their associated comorbidities.

DEFINITION

Tics are sudden, repetitive movements, gestures, or phonic productions that typically mimic some aspect of normal behavior. Usually of brief duration, individual tics rarely last more than a second. Many tics tend to occur in bouts, with brief inter-tic intervals of less than one second (5). Individual tics can occur singly or together in an orchestrated pattern. They vary in their intensity or forcefulness. Motor tics, which can be viewed as disinhibited fragments of normal movement, can vary from simple, abrupt movements such as eye blinking, nose twitching, head or arm jerks, or shoulder shrugs to more complex movements that appear to have a purpose, such as facial or hand gestures or sustained looks. These two phenotypic extremes of motor tics are classified as simple and complex motor tics respectively. Similarly, phonic tics can be classified into simple and complex categories. Simple vocal tics are sudden, meaningless sounds such as throat clearing, coughing, sniffing, spitting, or grunting. Complex phonic tics are more protracted, meaningful utterances, which vary from prolonged throat clearing to syllables, words or phrases, to even more complex behaviors such as repeating one's own words (palalalia) or those of others (echolalia) and, in rare cases, the utterance of obscenities (coprolalia) (6). Clinicians typically characterize tics by their anatomical location, number, frequency, duration, forcefulness and complexity as outlined above. Each of these elements has been incorporated into clinician rating scales that have proven to be useful in monitoring tic severity (7).

Many individuals with tics, especially those above the age of ten, are aware of premonitory urges that may either be experienced as a focal perception in a particular body region where the tic is about to occur (like an itch or a tickling *sensation*) or as a mental awareness (8, 9). A majority of patients also report a fleeting sense of relief after a bout of tics has occurred, and most individuals are able to suppress their tics for short intervals of time (9, 10).

DIAGNOSTIC CLASSIFICATION

The currently accepted diagnostic criteria for TS as defined in the *Diagnostic and Statistical Manual of Mental Disorders Text-Revision (DSM-IV-TR)* include: 1) presence of multiple motor tics, 2) presence of one or more vocal tics, 3) onset before age 18, 4) tics that may appear many times a day, either everyday or intermittently, 5) presence of tics for a period longer than 1 year, 6) change in anatomic location and character of tics over time and 7) occurrence of tics not attributable to CNS disease (Huntington disease or postviral encephalopathies) or psychoactive medication or substance usage (Table 5.6.1).

Tics that appear in childhood are often ephemeral. When a patient exhibits motor and/or vocal tics for less than a year, a diagnosis of a transient tic disorder is made, regardless of tic frequency or severity. If either motor or phonic tics (but not both) are present for a year or more, then a diagnosis of chronic motor or phonic tic disorder, respectively, can be made, according to DSM-IV-TR. Chronic tics are viewed by experts

TABLE 5.6.1

DSM-IV-TR TIC DISORDER CLASSIFICATION

Diagnostic criteria for 307.23 TS

A. Both multiple motor and one or more vocal tics have been present at some time during the illness, although not necessarily concurrently. (A *tic* is a sudden, rapid, recurrent, nonrhythmic, stereotyped motor movement or vocalization.)
B. The tics occur many times a day (usually in bouts) nearly every day or intermittently throughout a period of more than 1 year, and during this period there was never a tic-free period of more than 3 consecutive months.
C. The onset is before age 18 years.
D. The disturbance is not due to the direct physiological effects of a substance (e.g., stimulants) or a general medical condition (e.g., Huntington's disease or postviral encephalitis).

Diagnostic criteria for 307.22 Chronic Motor or Vocal Tic Disorder

A. Single or multiple motor or vocal tics (sudden, rapid, recurrent, nonrhythmic, stereotyped motor movements or vocalizations), but not both, have been present at some time during the illness.
B. The tics occur many times a day nearly every day or intermittently throughout a period of more than 1 year, and during this period there was never a tic-free period of more than 3 consecutive months.
C. The onset is before age 18 years.
D. The disturbance is not due to the direct physiological effects of a substance (stimulants) or a general medical condition (Huntington's disease or postviral encephalitis).
E. Criteria have never been met for Tourette's Disorder.

Diagnostic criteria for 307.21 Transient Tic Disorder

A. Single or multiple motor and/or vocal tics (sudden, rapid, recurrent, nonrhythmic, stereotyped motor movements or vocalizations).
B. The tics occur many times a day, nearly every day for at least 4 weeks, but for no longer than 12 consecutive months.
C. The onset is before age 18 years.
D. The disturbance is not due to the direct physiological effects of a substance (stimulants) or a general medical condition (Huntington's disease or postviral encephalitis).
E. Criteria have never been met for Tourette's Disorder or Chronic Motor or Vocal Tic Disorder.

Diagnostic criteria for 307.20 Tic Disorder Not Otherwise Specified

This category is for disorders characterized by tics that do not meet criteria for a specific Tic Disorder. Examples include tics lasting less than 4 weeks or tics with an onset after age 18 years.

(From the American Psychiatric Association: *Diagnostic and Statistical Manual*, Text Revision (DSM-IV-TR, Washington DC, 2000.)

as a milder phenotypic expression of TS, while transient tic disorders are generally viewed as a separate entity (4).

CLINICAL COURSE OF TS

The onset of TS is usually characterized by the appearance of simple, transient motor tics that affect the face (typically eye blinking) around the age of 5–7 (11). Over time these simple motor tics generally progress in a rostrocaudal direction affecting other areas of the face, followed by the head, neck, arms and last and less frequently, the lower extremities (12). Phonic tics usually appear several years after the onset of motor tic symptoms, at 8–15 years of age. Phonic tics seldom appear in isolation without the prior onset of motor tics—fewer than 5% of all patients with tic disorders have isolated phonic tic disorder, whereas the vast majority of children afflicted with tic disorders have isolated motor symptomatology (10). Tic complexity, also, generally evolves with age. During the first years of TS onset there is a steady unfolding of symptoms with single, rapid motor tics evolving into stereotyped, complex movements and nonsense sounds developing into elaborate words and phrases. The character of these complex phonations and movements are highly unique to the individual. Due to the rapid progression of symptoms during childhood, the vast majority of TS cases are diagnosed by age 11 (10).

Typically, as they grow older, children with TS gain an increasing ability to recognize when tics will ultimately strike and gain control over them. The first transient motor tics TS patients experience in the latency years are usually sudden, involuntary, unconscious movements. Often the afflicted individual is only made aware of the presence of these movements through the reactions of others around him. By the age of 10 or 11, however, many children report premonitory urges: feelings of tightness, tension, or itching that are accompanied by a mounting sense of discomfort or anxiety that can be relieved only by the performance of a tic (9). These premonitory urges are similar to the sensation preceding a sneeze or an itch. Premonitory urges cause many TS patients to suffer from an endless cycle of rising tension and tic performance because the relief provided by tic performance is ephemeral. Thus, soon after tic performance the tension of the premonitory urge again rises to a crescendo (13).

With increasing awareness of premonitory urges, TS patients begin to exhibit a variable degree of voluntary control over tic performance. Ninety-two percent of TS subjects in one study reported that the tics they exhibited were either partially or totally voluntary (9). However, this voluntary control should be likened to that governing control of eye blinking. Eye blinking and tics can both be inhibited voluntarily, but only for a limited period of time and only with mounting discomfort. Thus, some adult TS patients are able to demonstrate nearly complete control over the situation when expression of their tics will occur. However, when complete or near complete control of tics is present, resistance to the mounting tension of premonitory urges can produce mental and physical exhaustion even more impairing and distracting than the tics themselves (12).

The severity of tics in TS waxes and wanes throughout the course of the disorder. The tics of TS and other tic disorders are highly variable from minute to minute, hour to hour, day to day, week to week, month to month and even year to year (5). Tic episodes occur in bouts, which in turn also tend to cluster. Tic symptoms, however, can be exacerbated by stress, fatigue, extremes of temperature and external stimuli (in echolalia tics) (14). Intentional movements attenuate tic occurrence over the affected area and intense involvement and concentration in activities tends to dissipate tic symptoms. The power of this effect in many patients with TS is illustrated beautifully in Oliver Sacks' short story, *A Surgeon's Life*. As Sacks writes:

> And, indeed, whenever the stream of attention and interest was interrupted, Bennett's (the surgeon) tics and iterations immediately reasserted themselves—in particular, obsessive touchings of his mustache and glasses. His mustache had constantly to be smoothed and checked for symmetry, his glasses had to be "balanced"—up and down, side to side, diagonally, in and out—with sudden, ticcy touchings of the fingers, until these, too, were exactly "centered." There were also occasional reachings and lungings with his right arm; sudden, compulsive touchings of the windshield with both forefingers ("the touching has to be symmetrical," he commented); sudden repositionings of the knees, or the steering wheel ("I have to have the knees symmetrical in relation to the steering wheel. They have to be *exactly* centered"); and sudden, high-pitched vocalizations, in a voice completely unlike his own, that sounded like "Hi, Patty," "Hi, there," and, on a couple occasions, "Hideous!"

Sacks keenly observes that Dr. Bennett's tics and tic-related compulsive behavior are noticeably absent in two situations: 1) in the morning when he is conducting preparatory reading for his later surgeries while simultaneously riding an exercise bike and 2) when performing surgery (15).

Tic severity, however, typically dissipates with the onset of adolescence. TS symptoms generally peak in severity between the ages of 8 and 12 (11, 16). Reduction in TS severity generally ends by the early 20s. Although a small minority of TS patients does experience catastrophic outcomes in adulthood, on the whole, individuals rarely experience either a sustained worsening or improvement of their symptoms after the third decade of life. One-half to two-thirds of individuals with TS experience a marked reduction of symptoms by their late teens and early 20s, with one-third to one-half becoming virtually asymptomatic in adulthood (11, 17). Figure 5.6.1 diagrams the general course of tic severity of TS patients through the first two decades of their illness (11, 16).

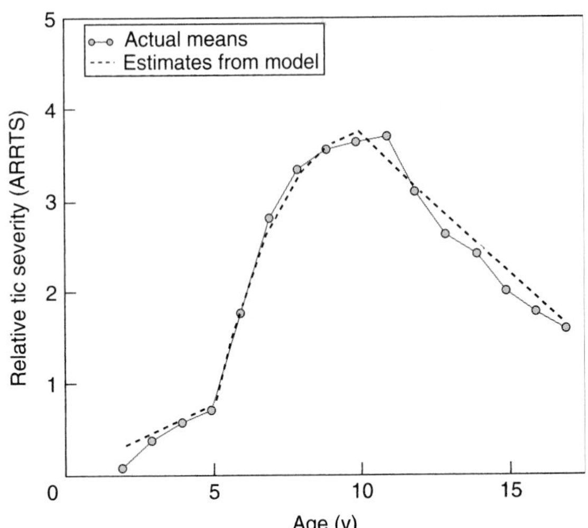

FIGURE 5.6.1. Plot of mean tic severity, ages 2 to 18 years. The solid line connecting the small circles plots the means of the annual rating of relative tic severity scores (ARRTS) recorded by the parents. The dashed line represents a mathematical model designed best to fit the clinical data. Two inflection points are evident that correspond to the age of tic onset and the age at worst-ever tic severity, respectively. (Adapted from Leckman JF, Zhang H, Vitale A, et al. Course of tic severity in Tourette syndrome: the first two decades. *Pediatrics*. Jul 1998;102(1 Pt 1):14–19.)

PREVALENCE

Transient tic behaviors are commonplace among children. Studies have estimated that 4–24% of school-age children experience tics (18–21). The upper end of this estimate was based on a study by Snider et al. (2002) that assessed a community sample of 553 children ages 5–12 years in a suburban elementary school (19). Assessment was obtained by direct observations by trained observers on each child over multiple occasions over an 8-month period. Snider et al. estimated that 18% of the children (n = 101) experienced a single tic or transient tics. A much smaller portion (n = 34), 6%, had multiple or persistent tics. A similar study by Khalifa and von Knorring examined the prevalence of tic disorders in an epidemiologic sample of 4,479 Swedish children ages 7–15 using a three-stage evaluation procedure including screening, parental interview, and clinical assessment. This study estimated the prevalence of chronic motor tics at 0.7% and transient tics at 4.5% in this sample (20). The difference in prevalence measurements of transient and persistent motor tic disorders reported in these studies is likely due to their different ascertainment methods (parent interview vs. direct observation). Nonetheless, the relative commonness of transient tics in the school-age population is evident in both these studies and the difference in prevalence between transient and multiple tic disorders is relatively conserved across studies.

Although boys are more commonly affected with tic behaviors than girls, the male–female ratio in most community surveys is less than 2 to 1. For example, in the Isle of Wight study of 10 to 11 year olds, approximately 6% of boys and 3% of girls were reported by their parents to have "twitches, mannerisms, tics of face or body (18)." Similar estimates have been reported from Quebec and from North Carolina (22, 23).

There exists drastic variation in estimates of prevalence of TS in the published medical literature. Once thought to be rare, current estimates vary 100 fold, from 2.9 per 10,000 to 299 per 10,000 (24, 25). There are three main reasons for this variation in the measurement of the estimation of TS prevalence: 1) The prevalence and severity of tic disorders varies drastically as a function of age (with highest prevalence and greatest severity taking place late in the first decade and early in the second decade of life, and decreasing roughly with the onset of puberty), 2) assessment method of individual studies has varied (patient registries, parent interview, direct observation vs. clinically ascertained cases) and 3) the diagnostic criteria of TS has changed with time—specifically, whether the diagnosis of TS requires an impairment criteria. DSM-III included a requirement that tic symptoms need to "cause marked distress of significant impairment in social, occupational or other important areas of functioning" in order to qualify as TS. By contrast, the impairment criteria was removed in DSM-IV-TR and ICD-10. Estimates of TS prevalence since 1990 among school-age children have estimated a prevalence somewhere between 10 to 100 per 10,000 (20, 26–30). Studies incorporating the older DSM-III definition of TS have estimated the prevalence of TS around the lower end of this range, while studies relying on the newer DSM-IV definition of TS not incorporating an impairment criteria have estimated TS prevalence toward its higher end. Estimates of older teenagers and adults with TS is considerably lower, at approximately 4.5 per 10,000 and this result is not surprising since many cases of TS improve drastically or remit completely during the course of adolescence (31).

COEXISTING CONDITIONS

Tics, which are the most prominent feature of TS, are often neither the first nor the most impairing psychological disturbance endured by patients. It has become apparent that children with TS have higher rates of obsessive-compulsive disorder (OCD), attention deficit hyperactivity disorder (ADHD), and disinhibited speech and behavior compared to individuals in the general population. In one study, 65% of TS patients in late adolescence regarded their behavioral problems (including ADHD and OCD) and learning difficulties to have had an equal or greater impact on their life function than did the tics themselves (32). In the natural course of comorbid psychiatric illness in TS, ADHD symptoms, when they occur, typically precede the onset of tic symptoms by a couple of years, whereas OC symptoms typically present around the age of 12–13 after tics have reached their peak severity (11, 16) (Figure 5.6.2).

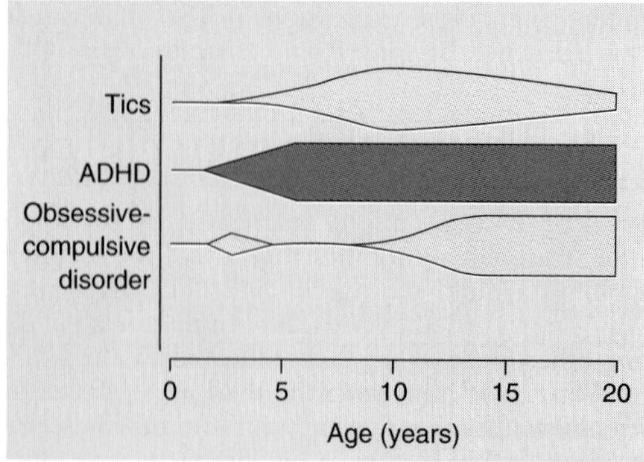

FIGURE 5.6.2. Age at which tics and coexisting disorders affect patients with TS. Width of bars shows schematically the amount the disorder affects a patient at a particular age. (Adapted from Leckman JF. Tourette's syndrome. *Lancet.* Nov 16 2002;360(9345):1577–1586.)

Attention Deficit Hyperactivity Disorder

Clinical and epidemiological studies sharply differ on rates of ADHD seen among individuals with TS (33). Clinical studies vary according to setting and established referral patterns, but it is not uncommon to see reports of 50% or more of referred children with TS diagnosed with comorbid ADHD. In contrast, epidemiological studies typically indicate a much lower rate of comorbidity (31). Although the etiological relationship between TS and ADHD is in dispute, it is clear that those individuals with both TS and ADHD are at a much greater risk for a variety of untoward outcomes (34). Uninformed peers frequently tease individuals with TS and ADHD. They are often regarded as less likeable, more aggressive, and more withdrawn than their classmates (35). These social difficulties are amplified in a child with TS who also has ADHD (36). In such cases, their level of social skill is often several years behind their peers (37).

Negative appraisal by peers in childhood is a strong predictor of global indices of psychopathology (38). This appears to be particularly true for children with TS and ADHD. Children with TS and comorbid ADHD are at much greater risk for disruptive behavior disorders and functional impairment from psychiatric illness than children with TS alone (39). Longitudinal studies confirm that these individuals are at high risk for anxiety and mood disorders, oppositional defiant disorder, and conduct disorder (34, 40). Much of this negative impact appears to be due to the ADHD, as children who only have TS tend to fare better (34, 39, 41). Surprisingly, levels of tic severity are less predictive of peer acceptance than is the presence of ADHD (36). Furthermore, the rates of subsequent psychiatric morbidity seen in TS plus ADHD subjects are nearly identical to those seen in prior cross-sectional and longitudinal studies of ADHD subjects who do not have tics (42, 43).

Obsessive-Compulsive Symptoms

Clinical and epidemiological studies indicate that more than 40% of individuals with TS experience recurrent obsessive-compulsive (OC) symptoms (16, 44, 45). Genetic, neurobiological, and treatment response studies suggest that there may be qualitative differences between tic-related forms of OCD and cases of OCD in which there is no personal or family history of tics. Tic-related OCD tends to have an earlier age of onset, prior to the age of 12–13, compared to non–tic-related OCD, which usually appears during late adolescence or early adulthood. Patients with OCD and comorbid tics have a significantly higher rate of intrusive violent or aggressive thoughts and images; sexual and religious preoccupations; concerns with symmetry and exactness; hoarding and counting rituals; and touching and tapping compulsions compared to patients with non-tic OCD, who often suffer primarily from contamination worries and cleaning compulsions (44, 46). Compulsions designed to eliminate a perceptually tinged mental feeling of unease, coined in the literature as "Just Right" perceptions, are particularly typical of patients with OCD and comorbid tics (45). A new rating scale, the Dimensional Yale–Brown Obsessive-Compulsive Scale (DY–BOCS), was designed to measure the presence and severity of OCD symptoms within six thematically related dimensions and should aid in further discriminating the OCD experienced by patients with TS compared to those with comorbid tics (47, 48). In addition, tic-related OCD is significantly less responsive to pharmacological therapy with SRIs than non–tic-related OCD and appears to be more responsive to augmentation with antipsychotic agents (49, 50).

In a previous prospective longitudinal study the presence of tics in childhood and early adolescence predicted the future development of OCD (30). Similarly, in a recent followup study of adult outcomes in children with TS, 41% of TS patients experienced at least moderate obsessive-compulsive symptoms in adulthood, with these symptoms reaching their worst-ever severity between the ages of 12–13 years, an average of 2 years later than tics (16). Also, obsessive-compulsive symptoms, when present in children with TS, appear more likely to persist into adulthood than the tics themselves (16). Higher intelligence may also herald a higher risk of developing more severe OCD symptoms in adulthood (16).

ETIOLOGY

Genetic Factors

TS and other closely related disorders clearly have a strong genetic component. The overall risk of an offspring of a parent with TS developing TS is approximately 10–15%; the risk of their offspring developing a tic disorder (20–29%) or OCD (12–32%) is slightly higher (51–54). The risk of developing tic disorders in male offspring is higher, while the risk of developing OCD is less. Twin and family studies provide evidence that genetic factors are involved in the vertical transmission within families of a vulnerability to TS and related disorders (55). The concordance rate for TS among monozygotic twin pairs is greater than 50 percent, while the concordance of dizygotic twin pairs is about 10 percent (56, 57). If cotwins with chronic motor tic disorder are included, these concordance figures increase to 77 percent for monozygotic and 30 percent for dizygotic twin pairs. Differences in the concordance of monozygotic and dizygotic twin pairs indicate that genetic factors play an important role in the etiology of TS and related conditions. These figures also suggest that nongenetic factors are critical in determining the nature and severity of the clinical syndrome.

Several studies involving segregation analysis of large multigenerational families have implicated the possible importance of single gene(s) inherited with an autosomal dominant pattern in the pathogenesis of TS (53, 55, 58). Unfortunately, genetic linkage studies that have screened the entire genome have eliminated the possibility of a single gene being responsible for TS (59). More recently, nonparametric approaches using families in which two or more siblings are affected with TS have been undertaken (60). This sib-pair approach is suited for diseases with an unclear mode of inheritance and has been used successfully in studies of other complex disorders such as diabetes mellitus and essential hypertension. In this study, two areas are suggestive of linkage to TS, one on chromosome 4q and another on chromosome 8p. Currently, this international consortium of researchers is actively completing high-density maps of several genomic regions in an effort to refine and extend their preliminary results. In addition, a new sample of sibling pairs is being ascertained to determine if the linkage results on 4q and 8p can be replicated.

It is also noteworthy that none of the chromosomal regions (e.g., 3 [3p21.3], 8 [8q21.4], 9 [9pter], and 18 [18q22.3]) in which cytogenetic abnormalities have been found to co-segregate with TS showed any convincing evidence for linkage in the sib-pair study. It is still possible that rare susceptibility genes may be found in one or more of these regions using molecular cytogenetic techniques. Furthermore, none of the regions associated with candidate genes, such as DRD2 [11q22] and DRD4 [11p15], were supported by the results of the sib-pair study.

Recently, using a candidate gene approach identified by chromosomal anomalies in patients with TS, Abelson et al. (61) identified and mapped a de novo chromosome 13 inversion in a patient with TS. The gene SLITRK1 was identified as a brain-expressed candidate gene mapping approximately 350 kilobases from the 13q31 breakpoint (61). Mutation screening of 174 patients with TS was undertaken, with the resulting identification of a truncating frame-shift mutation in a second family affected with TS. In addition, two examples of a rare variant were identified in a highly conserved region of the 3′ untranslated region of the gene corresponding to a brain-expressed micro-RNA binding domain. None of these anomalies were demonstrated in 3,600 controls. In vitro studies showed that both the frame-shift and the miRNA binding site variant had functional potential and were consistent with a loss-of-function mechanism. Studies of both SLITRK1 and the micro-RNA predicted to bind in the variant-containing 3′ region showed expression in multiple neuroanatomical areas implicated in TS neuropathology, including the cortical plate, striatum, globus pallidus, thalamus, and subthalamic nucleus.

Perinatal Factors

The search for nongenetic factors that mediate the expression of a genetic vulnerability to TS and related disorders has also focused on the role of adverse perinatal events. This interest dates from the report of Pasamanick and Kawi, who found that mothers of children with tics were 1.5 times more likely to have experienced a complication during pregnancy than the mothers of children without tics (62). Other investigations have reported that among monozygotic twins discordant for TS, the index twins with TS had lower birth weights than their unaffected cotwins (57, 63). Severity of maternal life stress during pregnancy, severe nausea and/or vomiting during the first trimester have also emerged as potential risk factors in the development of tic disorders (64). In 1997, Whitaker and coworkers reported that premature and low birth weight children are at increased risk of developing tic disorders and ADHD. This appears to be especially true of children who had ischemic parenchymal brain lesions. More recently, Burd and colleagues (1999) presented the results of a case control study in which low Apgar scores at 5 minutes and *more* prenatal visits were associated with a higher risk of TS (65). Finally, there is limited evidence that smoking and alcohol use, as well as forceps delivery, can predispose individuals with a vulnerability to TS to develop comorbid OCD (66). Investigations into the effects of perinatal complications into the later development of TS are severely hampered by 1) the possibility that recall bias likely influences results in the retrospective case-control studies addressing this question and 2) multiple hypothesis testing without appropriate statistical correction. The only nested case-control study to date that examined TS cases arising in a Swedish community sample (rather than a clinically referred sample) found a higher rate of pre-, peri- and neonatal adverse events between TS patients and controls, but this difference was not significant (67).

Neuroanatomical Factors

Strong evidence implicates the basal ganglia and cortico-striatal thalamacocortical (CSTC) abnormalities as central to the pathogenesis of tics. Indirect evidence for the involvement of the basal ganglia in the pathogenesis of TS comes from the association of other movement disorders, such as Huntington's disease, hemiballismus, and Parkinson's disease, with basal ganglia pathology. Direct evidence supporting CSTC abnormalities in TS comes from neuroimaging, neuropathological, and neurosurgical studies.

CSTC loops are multiple, parallel, but occasionally interacting, neuroanatomical circuits, which relay information from most regions of the cortex to subcortical areas, particularly the striatum and thalamus, which in turn project to a subset of the original cortical areas (Figure 5.6.3). In CSTC loops, the basal ganglia can be viewed as a waystation between intent and action (thought, affect and movement). Tics, repetitive and stereotyped movements, are believed to form imbalances in focal populations of basal ganglia circuits. A tic may arise when a focal population of striatal neurons becomes

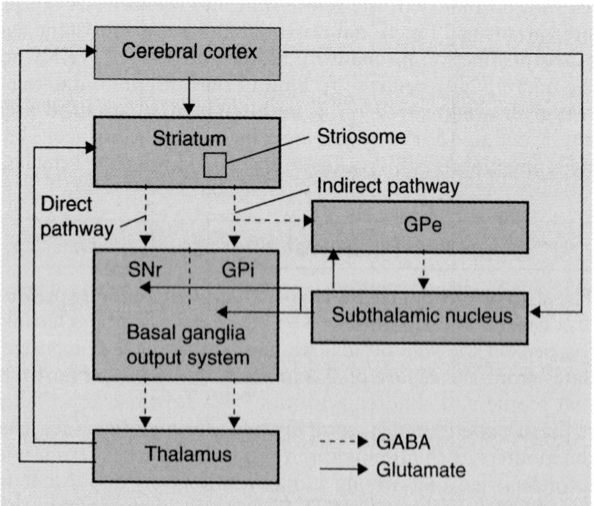

FIGURE 5.6.3. Schematic diagram of the major connections of the basal ganglia. GPe = globus pallidus, pars externa; GPi = globus pallidus, pars interna; SNr = substantia nigra, pars reticulata. (Adapted from Leckman JF. Tourette's syndrome. *Lancet*. Nov 16 2002;360(9345):1577–1586.)

abnormally active and causes an unwanted inhibition of a group of tonically active, inhibitory thalamic projection neurons, activating a cortical motor pattern generator so that an unintended movement is triggered. If striatal neurons became overactive in discrete, repeated episodes, the result would be multiple, stereotyped movements—tics (68, 69).

Support for this hypothesis of tic generation comes from experiments conducted by Anderson et al. (1992), which demonstrated that microstimulation at numerous sites of the putamen produced tic-like stereotyped movements in awake monkeys (70). Furthermore, microstimulation of discrete striatal zones produced characteristic stereotyped movements of individual body parts and, stunningly, even stereotyped movements of multiple body parts reminiscent of complex tics (71).

Human postmortem specimens in humans have fairly consistently demonstrated abnormalities in basal ganglia development or function in the pathogenesis of TS. In a recent postmortem study of three adult patients with severe TS, a markedly higher total neuron number was found in the globus pallidus pars interna (GPi) of TS. In contrast, a lower neuron number and density was observed in the globus pallidus pars externa and in the caudate nucleus. An increased number and proportion of the GPi neurons were positive for the calcium-binding protein parvalbumin in tissue from TS subjects, whereas lower densities of parvalbumin-positive interneurons were observed in both the caudate and putamen of TS subjects. This loss of parvalbumin-positive fast-spiking interneurons in the striatum has been hypothesized to cause somatotopically arranged clusters of medium-spiny interneurons to become disengaged from their normal high-voltage spindle activity. The result could be a disturbance in discrete CSTC loops through thalamocortical dysrhythmia, (a disturbance in the normal rhythmic τ-band activity by the thalamus, in conjunction with ectopic γ-band activity thought to be due to hyperpolarization of thalamic cells), resulting in the premonitory urges and tics characteristic of TS (72). Earlier postmortem studies of TS patients have also reliably demonstrated an association between abnormalities in basal ganglia anatomy, development, and function, and TS (73, 74). Abnormalities of the dopaminergic system within the CSTC loops has also been demonstrated in previous postmortem studies. For example, a postmortem study of four adults with intractable TS revealed 1) an increased number of presynaptic dopamine uptake sites in their striatum, 2) increased striatal dopamine levels compared to controls, and 3) similar D2 receptor affinity between TS subjects and controls (73, 75).

Neuropharmacological support for the involvement of CSTC and basal ganglia abnormalities in TS comes from the effectiveness of dopamine-depleting agents (tetrabenazine and alpha-methyl-para-tyrosine) and dopaminergic receptor antagonists (pimozide, haloperidol) in the suppression of tics and from the exacerbation of tics caused by administration of dopamine agonists (L-DOPA) and stimulants, such as methylphenidate, amphetamines, and cocaine (76). Additionally, the application of stimulants directly to specific regions of the basal ganglia can produce tic-like stereotypic movements (77).

Perhaps the strongest evidence implicating basal ganglia pathology in TS is from neuroimaging studies. An MRI study assessing MRI volumetric differences between 10 pairs of monozygotic twins differing in tic severity revealed that right caudate volume was reduced an average of 6% in the more severely affected twin compared to that of the less severely affected one (78). A structural neuroimaging study comparing 154 children and adults with TS to 130 normal controls demonstrated smaller caudate volumes in TS patients compared to healthy controls (79). Furthermore, a recent study associated decreased childhood caudate volume in children with TS with increased tic severity in adulthood (80).

Early functional neuroimaging studies of TS demonstrated hypometabolism and reduced cerebral blood flow to the ventral striatum of TS patients compared to normal controls. Positron emission tomography (PET) studies examining striatal dopamine metabolism in adults with TS have found increased right ventral striatal dopamine receptor density and increased amphetamine-induced dopamine release in the putamen compared to normal controls (81, 82). Single-photon-emission computed tomography (SPECT) studies have demonstrated increased striatal dopamine transporter (DAT) density in children and adults with TS compared to normal controls (83, 84).

A functional neuroimaging study examining circuits activated when patients with TS were asked to willfully suppress their tics illustrates the importance of cortical input in the pathogenesis of TS. Peterson et al. (1998) reported significantly increased activation in the right frontal cortex and in the right caudate nucleus during tic suppression (85). Increased activity of the right caudate nucleus was in turn associated with decreases in the activity of the globus pallidus, putamen, and thalamus. Thus, increased right frontal cortex activity was associated with inhibition of the basal ganglion motor loop during willful tic suppression. Volumetric neuroimaging studies have also shown larger dorsal prefrontal cortical volumes in children with TS but smaller volumes in adults with the disorder (86). This same volumetric study indicated that volumes of the orbitofrontal and the parieto-occipital regions were inversely associated with worst-ever tic severity (86). Despite the extensive and diverse neuroimaging studies conducted in TS, it is still a matter of substantial debate whether caudate, thalamic, or cortical dysfunction is primary to the pathogenesis of this disorder. Prospective, longitudinal neuroimaging studies of children with TS are necessary to determine whether the functional and structural abnormalities observed in patients with TS are causes or consequences of the disorder.

Post-Infectious Autoimmune Mechanisms

It is well established that group A beta hemolytic streptococci (GABHS) can trigger immune-mediated disease in genetically predisposed individuals (87). Speculation concerning a post-infectious (or at least a post-rheumatic fever) etiology for tic disorder symptoms dates from the late 1800s (88). Acute rheumatic fever (RF) is a delayed sequela of GABHS, occurring approximately three weeks following an inadequately treated upper respiratory tract infection. RF is characterized by inflammatory lesions involving the heart (rheumatic carditis), joints (polymigratory arthritis), and/or central nervous system (Sydenham's chorea [SC]). SC and TS, OCD, and ADHD share common anatomic targets—the basal ganglia of the brain and the related cortical and thalamic sites (89). Furthermore, SC patients frequently display motor and vocal tics, obsessive-compulsive, and ADHD symptoms suggesting the possibility that at least in some instances these disorders share a common etiology (90, 91).

It has been proposed that pediatric autoimmune neuropsychiatric disorder associated with streptococcal infection (PANDAS) represents a distinct clinical entity, and includes SC and some cases of TS and OCD (92). The most compelling evidence of an etiological link between TS and OCD and GABHS infection comes from a recently published case-control study that found an increased proportion of GABHS infections (odds ratio = 3.1) within the preceding 3 months in children newly diagnosed with TS compared to well matched controls (93). A larger odds ratio (OR = 12.1 for TS) was demonstrated when subjects were required to have multiple GABHS infections in the previous year, suggesting a dose-dependent effect of exposure. There was also a statistically significant positive association between preceding streptococcal infection and a new diagnosis of OCD and tic disorders.

Evidence that acute exacerbations of TS and OCD could also be triggered by GABHS comes from three independent reports demonstrating that the majority of patients with childhood-onset TS or OCD have elevated expression of a stable B-cell marker (94–96). The D8/17 marker identifies close to 100% of RF patients (with or without SC) but is present at low levels of expression in healthy control populations. The identity of the D8/17 epitope is not yet known, but it can be expressed by several non–B-cell types (97). Further suggestive evidence comes from Swedo and her colleagues (1998), who reported that in children who met PANDAS criteria, GABHS infection was likely to have preceded neuropsychiatric symptom onset for 44% of the children, whereas pharyngitis (no culture obtained) preceded onset for another 28% of the children (92). There were 144 episodes of symptom exacerbation among these 50 children. In addition to tic and obsessive-compulsive symptoms, cognitive deficits, oppositional behaviors, and motor hyperactivity were reported to be "particularly common" during periods of exacerbation. Thirty-one percent of these exacerbations were associated with documented GABHS infection, and 42% with symptoms of pharyngitis or upper respiratory infection (no throat culture obtained). While these results are intriguing, they are preliminary. Since individuals were selected for having a recent or recurrent history of GABHS infections, the magnitude of some of the reported associations may have been biased upward. Furthermore, a recent longitudinal study found no greater temporal relationship between GABHS infection and symptom exacerbations than would be expected by chance alone among 40 children with TS and/or OCD (95). Among this study sample there was no consistent change in D8/17-reactive cells with symptom exacerbation. Another prospective cohort study failed to demonstrate any increase in the occurrence of *de novo* PANDAS symptoms in the three months following a pediatric visit among 411 children ages 4–11 who experienced a GABHS infection and 403 uninfected controls (98).

In summary, a substantial body of circumstantial evidence exists that links postinfectious autoimmune phenomena with some cases of TS, OCD, and ADHD. However, these cases likely represent a small subgroup of all pediatric TS and OCD cases. The PANDAS data are also not compelling with regard to specific immunological mechanisms, nor do they establish where in the sequence of causal events these immune changes occur (99).

Psychological Factors

Tic disorders have long been identified as "stress-sensitive" conditions (100, 101). Typically, symptom exacerbations follow in the wake of stressful life events. Children with TS on average experience higher levels of psychosocial stress compared to matched controls (14). As noted by Shapiro and colleagues (1988), these events need not be adverse in character (102). Clinical experience suggests that in some unfortunate instances a vicious cycle can be initiated in which tic symptoms are misunderstood by the family and teachers, leading to active attempts to suppress the symptoms by punishment and humiliation. These efforts can lead to a further exacerbation of symptoms and further increase in stress in the child's interpersonal environment. Unchecked, this vicious cycle can lead to the most severe manifestations of TS and dysthymia, as well as maladaptive characterological traits. Although psychological factors are insufficient to cause TS, the intimate association of the content and timing of tic behaviors and dynamically important events in the lives of children make it difficult to overlook their contribution to the intramorbid course of these disorders (34, 40). The interaction of TS symptom exacerbation and comorbid depressive symptoms is an area that warrants further investigation. Short-term symptom exacerbation in TS is also influenced by sleeplessness and fatigue, so proper sleep hygiene is also advisable in children with TS.

DIAGNOSTIC ASSESSMENT

Differential Diagnosis

The differential diagnosis of simple motor tics includes a variety of hyperkinetic movements: myoclonus, tremors, chorea, athetosis, dystonias, akathitic movements, paroxysmal dyskinesias, and ballistic movements (103). These movements may be associated with genetic conditions such as Huntington's chorea or Wilson's disease; structural lesions, as in hemiballismus (associated with lesions to the contralateral subthalamic nucleus); infectious processes as in Sydenham's chorea; idiopathic functional instability of neuronal circuits, as in myoclonic epilepsy; and pharmacological treatments such as acute akathisia and dystonias associated with the use of neuroleptic agents. Differentiation between these conditions and tic disorders is usually accomplished on clinical grounds and is based on the presentation of the disorder and its natural history. For example, although aspects of tics such as their abruptness, their paroxysmal timing, or their suppressible nature may be similar to symptoms seen in other conditions, it is rare for all of these features to be combined in the absence of a *bona fide* tic disorder. Occasionally diagnostic tests are needed to exclude alternative diagnoses.

Complex motor tics can be confused with other complex repetitive behaviors such as stereotypies or compulsive rituals. Differentiation among these behaviors may be difficult, particularly among retarded individuals with limited verbal skills. Stereotypies, as opposed to tics, tend to have an earlier age of onset (2–3 as opposed to 6), tend to be bilateral rather than unilateral in nature, the individual movements stay more consistent over time in stereotypies, and stereotypies usually do not have a waxing-and-waning course (104). In other settings where these symptoms are closely intertwined, as in individuals with both TS and obsessive-compulsive disorder, efforts to distinguish between complex motor tics and compulsive behaviors may be futile. In cases of a tic disorder, it is unusual to see complex motor tics in the absence of simple tics. Involuntary vocal utterances are uncommon neurological signs in the absence of a tic disorder. Examples include sniffing and brief sounds in Huntington's disease and involuntary moaning in Parkinson's disease, particularly as a result of l-dopa toxicity. Complex phonic tics characterized by articulate speech typically can be distinguished from other conditions, including voluntary coprolalia. Because of their rarity in other syndromes, phonic tics can play an important role in differential diagnosis.

Clinical history, family history, observation, and neurological examination are usually sufficient to establish the diagnosis of a tic disorder. There are no confirmatory diagnostic tests. Neuroimaging studies, EEG-based studies, and laboratory tests are usually noncontributory except in atypical cases.

Assessment

Once the diagnosis has been established, care should be taken to focus on the overall course of an individual's development, not simply on tic symptoms. This may be a particular problem in the case of TS, where the symptoms can be dramatic and there is the temptation to organize all of an individual's behavioral and emotional difficulties under a single, all-encompassing rubric.

The principal goal of an initial assessment is to determine the individual's overall level of adaptive functioning and to identify areas of impairment and distress (4). Close attention to the strengths and weaknesses of the individual and the family is crucial. Relevant dimensions include the presence of comorbid mental, behavioral, developmental or physical disorders; family history of psychiatric and/or neurological disease; relationships with family and peers; school and/or occupational performance; and the history of important life events. Medication history is important, particularly if the disorder is longstanding or if medications have been prescribed for physical disorders. It may be necessary to evaluate the adequacy of the prior trials with pharmacological agents used to treat tic disorders. Table 5.6.2 demonstrates all the components that are important in the initial evaluation of a patient suspected of having TS (105).

Inventories such as the *Yale Child Study Center: TS Obsessive-Compulsive Disorder Symptom Questionnaire* (4) completed by the family prior to their initial consultation can be valuable ancillary tools to gain a long-term perspective of the child's developmental course and the natural history of the tic disorder. In addition, valid and reliable clinical rating instruments that have been developed to inventory and quantify recent tic symptoms, such as the Yale Global Tic Severity Scale, are particularly useful in judging an individual's current level of tic severity and monitoring changes in tic severity over time (7).

The Yale Global Tic Severity Scale (YGTSS) is a clinician-rated, semistructured scale that begins with a systematic inventory of tic symptoms that the clinician rates as present or absent over the past week. Current motor and phonic tics are then rated separately according to number, frequency, intensity, complexity, and interference on a 6-point ordinal scale (0 = absent; 1 through 5 for severity) yielding three scores: total motor, total phonic and total tic score. The scale concludes with an overall impairment rating. The YGTSS has shown excellent inter-rater agreement as well as other desirable psychometric properties (7). Because the YGTSS permits the clinician to incorporate direct observation with historical information, it requires both training with the instrument and clinical experience with tic disorders. At present most investigators consider the YGTSS to be the state of the art with regard to clinician ratings of tic severity.

Direct observational methods include videotape tic counting procedures (106, 107) or in vivo evaluation of tic symptoms (108). These direct observational methods would appear to be the most objective measure of tic severity; however, the frequency of tics varies according to setting and activity. In addition, many individuals with TS can suppress their symptoms for brief periods of time. In practice, videotaped tic counting appears to be most useful for acute research procedures that take place over several hours. Clinically, videotaping can be quite valuable when the diagnosis is in doubt or when tics are not observed in the consultation room.

TREATMENT

Tic disorders are frequently chronic, if not lifelong, conditions. Continuity of care is desirable and should be considered before embarking on a course of treatment. Usual clinical practice focuses initially on the educational and supportive interventions. Pharmacological treatments are typically held in reserve. Given the waxing and waning course of the disorders, it is likely that whatever is done (or not done) will lead in the short term to some improvement in tic severity. The decision to employ psychoactive medications is usually made after the educational and supportive interventions have been in place for a period of months, and it is clear that the tic symptoms are persistently severe and are themselves a source of impairment

TABLE 5.6.2

CLINICAL EVALUATION OF TIC DISORDERS AND CLOSELY RELATED CONDITIONS

1. Tics:

Anatomic location and symmetry, number, frequency, intensity, complexity, degree of interference (family and clinician ratings of current and worst-ever severity).

Onset—Age, characteristics (sudden, gradual, associated with stressful life events, infections—particularly recurrent streptococcal infections).

Course—Bout-like occurrence, waxing or waning course, and changing repertoire (most occurring in the eyes, face, head, and shoulders); tic complexity likely to increase with increasing age; momentary suppressibility, reduction during fine motor or vocal tasks that require mental effort, marked diminution during sleep, and usual improvement during the second half of the second decade of life; intramorbid factors associated with worsening or improvement (stress, fatigue, recent infections); current treatment regimen; history of response to medications (efficacy, side effects, adequacy of trials); history of other interventions.

Associated Perceptual Phenomena and Disinhibited Behavior—Premonitory sensory urges, mental tics, site sensitization, trigger stimuli; socially inappropriate urges or behaviors (calling out in libraries or other quiet public places, urges to do prohibited actions).

Comorbidity—Obsessive-compulsive symptoms; attention deficit hyperactivity disorder; mood and anxiety disorders.

Impairment—Impact on self-esteem, family function, social acceptance, educational or job performance; risk of physical injury to self or others.

2. Obsessive-Compulsive Symptoms and Behaviors:

Range of obsessive worries and thoughts with aggressive, sexual, or religious content, need for symmetry or exactness, a need for things to look, feel or sound "just right," contamination fears, thoughts about saving or hoarding; simple compulsive rituals ("evening-up," ordering behaviors); full-fledged obsessive-compulsive disorder (time-consuming ego-dystonic obsessive thoughts and compulsive rituals that are "resisted" and interfere with normal cognitive function); pathologic doubting; family and clinician ratings of current and worse-ever severity and assessment of obsessive-compulsive symptom dimensions.

Onset—Age, characteristics (associated with recurrent streptococcal infections or the onset of puberty, recent moves, separations, or losses).

Course—Time spent and types of obsessions and compulsions, level of autonomic arousal and anxiety; level of control and resistance; perceived distress if prevented from performing compulsions; role of environmental cues and avoidance behaviors; progression from ego-neutral to ego-dystonic compulsions; changing repertoire of obsessions and compulsions; intramorbid factors associated with worsening or improvement (stress, fatigue, recent infections); current treatment regimen; history of response to cognitive behavioral interventions, medications (efficacy, side effects, adequacy of trials); history of other interventions.

Comorbidity—Depression and other mood and anxiety disorders; obsessive-compulsive personality; schizophrenia; developmental disorders (autism, Prader-Willi syndrome).

Impairment—Impact on self-esteem; subjective distress; pervasive slowness and getting stuck in routine behaviors; impact on family function (level of involvement of the family in the performance of compulsions); effect on social adaptation, educational or job performance; risk of physical injury to self or others.

3. Attention Deficit Hyperactivity Disorder.

Distractibility and impulsive behavior; poor sustained attention, motoric hyperactivity and fidgetiness; associated disruptive behaviors; need for multiple sources of information, especially teachers and other school personnel.

Onset—Age, timing (before or after onset of tic syndrome).

Course—Context dependence: settings where these difficulties are less apparent versus settings of greatest difficulty; history of tutoring and other special educational services; current treatment regimen; history of response to stimulants (efficacy, side effects, adequacy of trials); history of other nonsomatic interventions.

Comorbidity—Oppositional and defiant disorder, conduct disorder, and substance abuse disorders; specific learning disabilities; depression and other mood and anxiety disorders; developmental disorders (fragile X syndrome and other mental retardation syndromes).

Impairment—Impact on self-esteem; impact on family function especially difficulties with siblings; effect on peer relationships; school underachievement; job performance.

4. Comorbid Developmental, Behavioral, Emotional, Personality, or Substance Abuse Problems:

Presence of pervasive developmental disorders (autism, Asperger's syndrome, and pervasive development disorder [PDD] not otherwise specified), specific developmental disorders, mood liability and increased irritability, major depression, bipolar disorder, and anxiety disorders (panic disorder, phobias including social and agoraphobia, generalized anxiety disorders), perfectionism and other obsessive-compulsive personality traits, other personality disorders as well as any history of substance abuse.

5. Prenatal and Birth History:

Prenatal events (severe nausea and vomiting, maternal emotional stress during pregnancy, history of smoking and alcohol use, other drug and hormonal exposures); birth history (hypoxic episodes, prolonged labor, use of forceps).

6. Developmental, Neurologic, and Pediatric Histories.

Developmental delays; exposure to toxins (lead); medication exposures; infectious diseases (streptococcal pharyngitis and other infections such as varicella), rheumatic fever, rheumatic carditis, or Sydenham's chorea; head injuries; seizures; asthma; allergies; migraine; disorders of arousal (night terrors, sleep walking).

(continued)

TABLE 5.6.2

(CONTINUED)

7. Family and Social Environment, Stress and Adaptive Function, Awareness of Advocacy Organizations.
Premorbid history; family environment—stability of family life, coping skills and social supports; relationship of life events (major losses or moves, changes in family circumstances) to onset and exacerbations of symptoms; current adjustment (patient's general knowledge and attitude toward tics, obsessive-compulsive symptoms, and problems with impulsivity and attention, willingness to teach others about symptoms, and the level of understanding and acceptance of the symptoms by close family members); existence of close and lasting friendships; marital status. How aware is the patient and family of the existence of national and local advocacy organizations such as the TS Association (TSA), Obsessive Compulsive Foundation (OCF), and the Children and Adults with Attention Deficit Disorder (CHADD)?
8. School Status.
Cognitive level, special talents or gifts, specific learning problems, adequacy of placement, level of understanding and acceptance of the symptoms by school personnel and classmates.
9. Employment Status.
Current occupation, job difficulties associated with tic behaviors or related phenomena, adequacy of placement given patient's native abilities, level of understanding and acceptance of the symptoms by employer and coworkers.
10. Family History of Developmental, Autoimmune, Behavioral, and Emotional Disorders.
Review of family pedigree with regard to tics, Sydenham's chorea, other movement disorders; rheumatic fever; attentional problems and hyperactivity; learning problems; developmental disorders; obsessive-compulsive behaviors; personality disorders; major depression and other mood and anxiety disorders; schizophrenia; alcoholism and other substance abuse disorders.
11. Neuropsychological Assessment.
Estimate of cognitive ability, visual motor integration.
12. Physical and Neurological Evaluations.
Health history; evidence of recent physical examinations; throat culture and titers for antistreptolysin 0 and anti-DNAse B (if requested); presence of soft, nonlocalizing neurological signs; consider more extensive workup (EEG and structural MRI scan) in atypical cases (negative family history, positive seizure history, history of severe hypoxia, head trauma, marked symptom severity, atypical pattern of response to medication).

(Adapted from Leckman JF, Zhang H, Vitale A, et al. Course of tic severity in Tourette syndrome: The first two decades. *Pediatrics*. Jul 1998; 102(1 Pt 1):14–19.)

in terms of self-esteem, relationships with the family or peers, or the child's ability to perform at school.

Educational and Supportive Interventions

Educational activities are among the most important interventions available to the clinician. They should be undertaken first, not only with patients with severe TS, but with patients with milder presentations. Although the efficacy of these educational and supportive interventions has not been rigorously assessed, they appear to have positive effects by reshaping familial expectations and relationships (109). This is particularly true when the family and others have misconstrued the tic symptoms as being intentionally provocative. Families also find descriptions of the natural history comforting in that the disorders tend not to be relentlessly progressive and usually improve during adulthood. This information often contradicts the impressions gained from the available lay literature on TS that typically focuses on the most extreme cases. Armed with this knowledge, patients and family members and others can begin to understand why waiting before beginning medical treatment makes good sense. If a patient is in the midst of a bad period of tics, it is likely that whether or not a new medication is prescribed, the tics will probably get significantly better in the near future. This insight will also help patients and their families realize why at times in the past their medications have suddenly stopped working. These dialogues can be relieving and can interrupt a vicious cycle of recrimination that leads to further tic exacerbation, and it can help aggravated parents shift the focus from blame to problem solving.

For children, contact with their teachers can be enormously valuable. By educating the educators, clinicians can make significant progress toward securing for the child a positive and supportive environment in the classroom. If possible, teachers need to respond to outbursts of tics with grace and understanding. Repeatedly scolding a child for his tics can be counterproductive. The child may develop a negative attitude toward authority figures and may be reluctant to attend school; classmates may feel freer to tease the child. If tics interfere with a student's ability to receive information in the classroom, it is imperative to find alternative ways to present the material. By helping the student find a way to function even during periods of severe tics, teachers model problem solving skills that will foster future self-esteem. It is also important for teachers to know that unstructured settings such as the cafeteria, gym, playground, and school bus tend to be very difficult. In these situations, peers who tease or taunt tend to take advantage of the lack of adult supervision. The assignment of a paraprofessional aide to accompany the student can be remarkably beneficial—particularly in situations where there is a history of teasing. Other useful strategies that teachers may consider include: providing short breaks out of the classroom to let the tics out in private, allowing students with severe tics to take tests in private so that a child does not have the pressure to suppress tics during the test period, and being flexible with regard to the scheduling of oral presentations so that the child is not expected to make an oral presentation at a point when his tics are severe (110). A useful compendium of educational accommodations is available on the World Wide Web at http://www.tourettesyndrome.net/TouretteSyndrome_Plus/.

Educated peers are equally important. Many clinicians actively encourage patients, families, and teachers to help educate peers and classmates about TS. It is remarkable what can be tolerated in the classroom and on the playground when teachers and peers simply know what the problem is and learn to disregard it.

Finally, it is important for clinicians to determine the family's awareness and potential interest in advocacy organizations such as the TS Association, Obsessive Compulsive Foundation, and the Children and Adults with Attention Deficit Disorder. In the United States of America, these organizations have made a positive contribution to the lives of many patients and their families by providing support and information. They can also be a valuable outlet for families, to advance research and raise the general level of awareness among health care professionals, educators, and the public at large. Readers are referred to their respective Web sites for additional information: TS Association: http://tsa.mgh.harvard.edu; Obsessive-Compulsive Foundation: http://www.ocfoundation.org/; and Child and Adults with Attention Deficit: http://www.chadd.org/.

Psychological Interventions

Habit reversal training (HRT) is the first behavioral intervention that has shown promise in reducing tic severity in patients with TS (111). HRT consists of two main focuses: 1) awareness training and 2) competing response practice. Awareness training consists of four components designed to increase an individual's awareness of his own tics. These components include: 1) response description, in which an individual learns how to describe tic movements and reenacts them into a mirror; 2) response detection, in which the therapist aids the patient in tic detection by pointing out each tic immediately after it occurs in the session; 3) early warning procedure, in which an individual learns how to identify the earliest signs of tic occurrence and 4) situational awareness training, in which an analysis is conducted to identify the high-risk situations where tics are most likely to occur. Competing response practice involves teaching individuals to produce an incompatible physical response (isometric contraction of tic-opposing muscles) contingent upon the urge to perform a tic (112).

HRT in its current form, originally developed by Azrin and Nunn (1973), and refined by many others over the intervening years, has recently been demonstrated to significantly reduce tic symptoms in adults with TS, as compared to supportive therapy in randomized controlled clinical trials (113, 114). Unblinded studies in children with TS have shown similar efficacy (115). Further studies are needed to replicate these current findings at other sites. Assuming these studies are equally promising, the next challenge will be effectively to disseminate this behavioral therapy available only at a few academic institutions to more therapists out in the community.

Pharmacological Interventions

The decision to begin medication is based on the level of symptoms and the clinical presentation of the individual case. Given the waxing and waning of tic symptoms, it is best to withhold psychotropic medications until the tics, even at their best, are a significant source of impairment. Many cases of TS can be successfully managed without medication. When patients present with coexisting ADHD, OCD, depression, or bipolar illness, it is often better to treat these comorbid conditions first, as successful treatment of these disorders often will diminish tic severity.

A variety of therapeutic agents are now available to treat tics (116). Each medication should be selected on the basis of expected efficacy and potential side effects. Dopamine D_2 receptor antagonists remain the most predictably effective tic-suppressing agents in the short term. Documentation of haloperidol's effectiveness in the early 1960s was a landmark in the history of TS, as it called into question the prevailing view that tics were psychogenic in nature (88). The most widely used typical D_2 receptor antagonists are haloperidol, pimozide, fluphenazine, and tiapride (not presently available in the United States). Favorable data from double-blind clinical trials are available for haloperidol, pimozide, and tiapride (117–120). The U.S. Food and Drug Administration has approved TS as an indication for haloperidol and pimozide use. Long-term experience has been less favorable, and the "reflexive" use of these agents should be avoided (121, 122). Typically, treatment is initiated with a low dose (0.25 mg of haloperidol or 1 mg of pimozide) given before sleep. Further increments (0.5 mg of haloperidol or 1 mg of pimozide) may be added at 7 to 14 day intervals if the tic behaviors remain severe. In most instances, 0.5 to 6.0 mg per day of haloperidol or 1.0 to 10.0 mg per day of pimozide administered over a period of 4 to 8 weeks is sufficient to achieve adequate control of tic symptoms. Common potential side effects include tardive dyskinesia, acute dystonic reactions, sedation, depression, school and social phobias, and/or weight gain. In many instances, by starting at low doses and adjusting the dosage upward slowly clinicians can avoid these side effects. The goal should be to use as little of these medications as possible to render the tics "tolerable." Efforts to stop the tics completely often risk overmedication.

Due to the extrapyramidal side effects associated with typical neuroleptics, atypical neuroleptics, such as risperidone, olanzapine and ziprasidone have been used to treat tic symptoms. These agents have potent 5-HT2 blocking effects as well as more modest blocking effects on dopamine D2. Initial favorable double-blind clinical trials have now been reported for risperidone (123), olanzapine (124) and ziprasidone (125). Risperidone and olanzapine use is often associated with weight gain and sedation. Ziprasidone use can be associated with QT prolongation in children so serial monitoring with electrocardiograms may be necessary (126).

Clonidine and Guanfacine are potent $\alpha 2$-receptor agonists that are thought to reduce central noradrenergic activity. Initial open label studies of clonidine were favorable, subsequent double-blind clinical trials have had mixed results (127, 128). Clinical trials indicate that subjects can expect on average a 25 to 35% reduction in their symptoms over an 8 to 12 week period. Motor tics may show greater improvement than phonic symptoms. The usual starting dose is 0.05 mg on arising. Further 0.05 mg increments at 3 to 4 hour intervals are added weekly until a dosage of 5 mcg per kg is reached, or the total daily dose exceeds 0.25 mg. Although clonidine is clearly less effective than haloperidol and pimozide for immediate tic suppression, it is considerably safer. The principal side effect associated with its use is sedation, which occurs in 10 to 20 percent of subjects and which usually abates with continued use. Other side effects include dry mouth, transient hypotension, and rare episodes of worsening behavior. Clonidine should be tapered and not withdrawn abruptly, to reduce the likelihood of symptom or blood pressure rebound (128). Guanfacine is another $\alpha 2$-receptor agonist that has been demonstrated in double-blind studies to be effective in the treatment of TS and TS with comorbid ADHD (129). Guanfacine is generally preferred to clonidine because it is less sedating and not associated with rebound hypertension following withdrawal. Guanfacine is generally started at a dose of 0.5 mg at night and then gradually increased by 0.5 mg roughly weekly to TID dosing, with a maximum dose of 4 mg daily (129).

The use of botulinum toxin injections to weaken temporarily muscles associated with severe motor or vocal tics also appears effective (130–133). Botulinum toxin injections also appear to significantly reduce the premonitory urges associated with both motor and vocal tics in the regions injected (131–133).

Pharmacotherapy of Coexisting ADHD

The stimulants methylphenidate, d-amphetamine, and Adderall are first-line agents for the medical management of ADHD (134). However, the use of stimulants in ADHD associated with a tic disorder is controversial (135). While many patients with both ADHD and a preexisting tic disorder will do well on stimulants, data from clinical case reports and controlled studies indicate that some children with ADHD will exhibit tics *de novo* when exposed to a stimulant. In other cases tics may increase to a level that warrants discontinuation of the stimulant. Commonly used nonstimulants for ADHD include the antidepressants nortriptyline and atomoxetine and bupropion, and the α_2-agonists clonidine and guanfacine (134). Compared to clonidine, guanfacine is less sedating and has a longer duration of action as well as being more specific for α_2-receptors in the prefrontal cortex (136). Double-blind clinical trials with guanfacine in subjects with both ADHD and coexisting tics has demonstrated efficacy (129).

Pharmacotherapy of Coexisting OCD

Cognitive behavioral therapies, particularly exposure and response prevention alone or in combination with serotonin reuptake inhibitors (SRIs), are the standard interventions for OCD (137). Unfortunately, many patients with OCD and a coexisting tic disorder respond less well to these interventions (138). Investigators in controlled clinical trials have found that addition of small doses of the neuroleptic haloperidol, or the atypical neuroleptic risperidone, increases the response to SRIs (49, 50). OCD patients with comorbid tics seem to be particularly responsive to SRI augmentation with traditional or atypical neuroleptics (49, 50).

Neurosurgical Interventions

Neurosurgical interventions for TS have been appropriately reserved for adults with intractable tics that severely affect social functioning. Many neurosurgical sites have been targeted for tics in previous lesioning studies—the frontal cortex (139), limbic cortex (140, 141), thalamus (142), infrathalamic area (143, 144) and cerebellum (145). Increasingly, with the successful use of deep brain stimulation—a relatively reversible, stereotactic technique to treat other movement disorders—DBS has been looked to as the preferred method of neurosurgical treatment for medically intractable tics. The original electrode placement for DBS surgery was placed in the medial part of the thalamus, based on the results of previous lesioning studies. All four patients, who received bilateral medial thalamic DBS surgery, experienced a substantial improvement in tic severity following the procedure (146, 147). Two subsequent case reports demonstrated comparable efficacy in bilateral palladial stimulation compared with bilateral medial thalamic stimulation (147). Likewise, the joint activation of both pairs of electrodes did not lead to a further reduction in tic severity (147). DBS has several advantages over previous neurosurgical lesioning procedures in that it lacks many of the permanent complications typically associated with lesioning procedures (the electrodes can be removed), lends access to many surgically inaccessible sites, and allows for bilateral stimulation and thus holds great promise for adult patients with intractable tics (145). However, currently in DBS for tics, neither the appropriate site of electrode placement nor the electrode stimulation parameters have been examined in carefully controlled clinical studies and differ markedly in the few sites willing to engage in this procedure. Therefore DBS is currently not advisable for all but the most severely affected adults with TS (as children with tics will likely get better with time) and even those most severely affected with TS will likely benefit more from the procedure as the protocol is refined over the upcoming years. Any patient considering this intervention should be very discerning regarding the neurosurgical team, especially regarding experience in this area, as no one has much, and should exhaust every possible medical option to treat tics beforehand and conclude that the tics are unbearable despite these interventions. Any DBS team attempting such surgeries should minimally consist of a neurosurgeon specialized in the stereotactic technique, a neurologist and a psychiatrist trained in movement disorders and their comorbidities, and a specially trained nursing staff (68). The utmost caution is warranted from everyone when engaging in this intervention, especially until the surgical method is improved and this refined method bears the test of more rigorous scientific testing.

FUTURE DIRECTIONS

Recent research efforts have uncovered the first gene, SLTRK1, associated with TS. HRT is the first psychotherapeutic invention proven effective in double-blind studies for TS. DBS, although in its infancy, as applied to TS seems to show some promise in helping the most medically refractory adult patients with TS. Although significant advances in TS treatment have been made, our major challenge over the next few years remains to perfect them and disseminate them to the general public effectively. Despite these advances, our current best available therapies are far from optimum in treating this disorder. With improved understanding of TS—other genes involved in its pathogenesis, prognostic factors to determine which children with TS will improve and which will not, a further understanding of the neurocircuitry involved in TS—future treatment advances will come.

References

1. Sprenger J, Kraemer H: *Malleus Maleficarum* (1489). London, Pushkin Press, 1948.
2. Stevens H. Gilles de la Tourette and his syndrome by serendipity. *Am J Psychiatry* 128:489–492, 1971.
3. Gilles de la Tourette G: Étude sur une affection nerveuse caractérisée par de l'incoordination motrice accompagnée d'echolalie et de copralalie. *Archive Neurologie* 9:19–42, 158–200, 1885.
4. Leckman JF, King RA, Scahill L, Findley D, Ort S, Cohen DJ: Yale approach to assessment and treatment. In: JF Leckman, Cohen DJ (eds): *Tourette's Syndrome—Tics, Obsessions, Compulsions—Developmental Psychopathology and Clinical Care.* New York, John Wiley and Sons, pp. 285–309, 1998.
5. Peterson BS, Leckman JF: The temporal dynamics of tics in Gilles de la Tourette syndrome. *Biol Psychiatry* 44(12):1337–1348, 1998.
6. Leckman JF, Cohen DJ. Evolving models of pathogenesis. In: JF Leckman, Cohen DJ (eds.) *Tourette's Syndrome—Tics, Obsessions, Compulsions—Developmental Psychopathology and Clinical Care.* New York, John Wiley and Sons, pp. 156–175, 1999.
7. Leckman JF, Riddle MA, Hardin MT, et al.: The Yale Global Tic Severity Scale: Initial testing of a clinician-rated scale of tic severity. *J Am Acad Child Adolesc Psychiatry* 28(4):566–573, 1989.
8. Lang A: Patient perception of tics and other movement disorders. *Neurology* 41(2 [Pt 1]):223–228, 1991.
9. Leckman JF, Walker DE, Cohen DJ. Premonitory urges in Tourette's syndrome. *Am J Psychiatry* 150(1):98–102, 1993.
10. Robertson MM: The Gilles de la TS: The current status. *Br J Psych.* 154:147–169, 1989.
11. Leckman JF, Zhang H, Vitale A, et al.: Course of tic severity in Tourette syndrome: The first two decades. *Pediatrics* 102(1 Pt 1):14–19, 1998.
12. Peterson BS, Leckman JF, Cohen DJ. TS: A genetically predisposed and an environmentally specified developmental psychopathology. In: Cichetti D, Cohen DJ (eds): *Developmental Psychopathology: Vol. 2. Risk, Disorder and Adaption.* New York, Wiley, pp. 213–241, 1985.
13. Bliss J: Sensory experiences of Gilles de la TS: *Archives of General Psychiatry.* 37:1343–1347, 1980.
14. Findley DB, Leckman JF, Katsovich L, et al.: Development of the Yale Children's Global Stress Index (YCGSI) and its application in children and

adolescents with Tourette's syndrome and obsessive-compulsive disorder. *J Am Acad Child Adolesc Psychiatry* 42(4):450–457, 2003.
15. Sacks O: A surgeon's life. In: *An Anthropologist on Mars: Seven Paradoxical Tales*. New York, Random House, pp. 77–107, 1995.
16. Bloch MH, Peterson BS, Scahill L, et al.: Adulthood outcome of tic and obsessive-compulsive symptom severity in children with Tourette syndrome. *Arch Pediatr Adolesc Med* 160(1):65–69, 2006.
17. Pappert EJ, Goetz CG, Louis ED, Blasucci L, Leurgans S: Objective assessments of longitudinal outcome in Gilles de la Tourette's syndrome. *Neurology* 61(7):936–940, 2003.
18. Rutter M, Tizard J, Whitmore K: *Education, Health, and Behaviour*. Longman, London; 1970.
19. Snider LA, Seligman LD, Ketchen BR, et al.: Tics and problem behaviors in schoolchildren: Prevalence, characterization, and associations. *Pediatrics* 110(2 Pt 1):331–336, 2002.
20. Khalifa N, von Knorring AL: Prevalence of tic disorders and Tourette syndrome in a Swedish school population. *Dev Med Child Neurol* 45(5):315–319, 2003.
21. Gadow KD, Nolan EE, Sprafkin J, Schwartz J: Tics and psychiatric comorbidity in children and adolescents. *Dev Med Child Neurol* 44(5):330–338, 2002.
22. Costello EJ, Angold A, Burns BJ, et al.: The Great Smoky Mountains Study of Youth: Goals, design, methods, and the prevalence of DSM-III-R disorders. *Arch Gen Psychiatry* 53(12):1129–1136, 1996.
23. Breton JJ, Bergeron L, Valla JP, et al.: Quebec child mental health survey: Prevalence of DSM-III-R mental health disorders. *J Child Psychol Psychiatry* 40(3):375–384, 1999.
24. Caine ED, McBride MC, Chiverton P, Bamford KA, Rediess S, Shiao J: Tourette's syndrome in Monroe County school children. *Neurology* 38(3):472–475, 1988.
25. Mason A, Banerjee S, Eapen V, Zeitlin H, Robertson MM: The prevalence of Tourette syndrome in a mainstream school population. *Dev Med Child Neurol* 40(5):292–296, 1998.
26. Comings DE, Himes JA, Comings BG: An epidemiologic study of Tourette's syndrome in a single school district. *J Clin Psychiatry* 51(11):463–469, 1990.
27. Kadesjo B, Gillberg C: Tourette's disorder: Epidemiology and comorbidity in primary school children. *J Am Acad Child Adolesc Psychiatry* 39(5):548–555, 2000.
28. Kurlan R, McDermott MP, Deeley C, et al.: Prevalence of tics in schoolchildren and association with placement in special education. *Neurology* 23 57(8):1383–1388, 2001.
29. Landgren M, Pettersson R, Kjellman B, Gillberg C.: ADHD, DAMP and other neurodevelopmental/psychiatric disorders in 6-year-old children: Epidemiology and co-morbidity. *Dev Med Child Neurol* 38(10):891–906, 1996.
30. Peterson BS, Pine DS, Cohen P, Brook JS.: Prospective, longitudinal study of tic, obsessive-compulsive, and attention-deficit/hyperactivity disorders in an epidemiological sample. *J Am Acad Child Adolesc Psychiatry* 40(6):685–695, 2001.
31. Apter A, Pauls DL, Bleich A, et al.: An epidemiologic study of Gilles de la Tourette's syndrome in Israel. *Arch Gen Psychiatry* 50(9):734–738, 1993.
32. Erenberg G, Cruse RP, Rothner AD.: The natural history of Tourette syndrome: A follow-up study. *Ann Neurol* 22(3):383–385, 1987.
33. Walkup JT, Khan S, Schuerholz L, Paik Y-S, Leckman JF, Schultz RT: Phenomenology and natural history of tic-related ADHD and learning disabilities. In: JF Leckman, Cohen DJ (eds): *Tourette's Syndrome—Tics, Obsessions, Compulsions—Developmental Psychopathology and Clinical Care*. New York, John Wiley and Sons, pp. 63–79, 1998.
34. Carter AS, O'Donnell DA, Schultz RT, Scahill L, Leckman JF, Pauls DL.: Social and emotional adjustment in children affected with Gilles de la Tourette's syndrome: Associations with ADHD and family functioning. Attention Deficit Hyperactivity Disorder. *J Child Psychol Psychiatry* 41(2):215–223, 2000.
35. Stokes A, Bawden HN, Camfield PR, Backman JE, Dooley JM.: Peer problems in Tourette's disorder. *Pediatrics* 87(6):936–942, 1991.
36. Bawden HN, Stokes A, Camfield CS, Camfield PR, Salisbury S: Peer relationship problems in children with Tourette's disorder or diabetes mellitus. *J Child Psychol Psychiatry* 39(5):663–668, 1998.
37. Dykens E, Leckman J, Riddle M, Hardin M, Schwartz S, Cohen D.: Intellectual, academic, and adaptive functioning of Tourette syndrome children with and without attention deficit disorder. *J Abnorm Child Psychol* 18(6):607–615, 1990.
38. Hinshaw SP.: *Attention Deficits and Hyperactivity in Children*. London, Sage, 1994.
39. Sukhodolsky DG, Scahill L, Zhang H, et al.: Disruptive behavior in children with Tourette's syndrome: Association with ADHD comorbidity, tic severity, and functional impairment. *J Am Acad Child Adolesc Psychiatry* 42(1):98–105, 2003.
40. Carter AS, Pauls DL, Leckman JF, Cohen DJ.: A prospective longitudinal study of Gilles de la Tourette's syndrome. *J Am Acad Child Adolesc Psychiatry* 33(3):377–385, 1994.
41. Spencer T, Biederman J, Harding M, et al.: Disentangling the overlap between Tourette's disorder and ADHD. *J Child Psychol Psychiatry* 39(7):1037–1044, 1998.
42. Greene RW, Biederman J, Faraone SV, Sienna M, Garcia-Jetton J.: Adolescent outcome of boys with attention-deficit/hyperactivity disorder and social disability: Results from a 4-year longitudinal follow-up study. *J Consult Clin Psychol* 65(5):758–767, 1997.
43. Mannuzza S, Klein RG, Bessler A, Malloy P, LaPadula M.: Adult psychiatric status of hyperactive boys grown up. *Am J Psychiatry* 155(4):493–498, 1998.
44. Leckman JF, Grice DE, Boardman J, et al.: Symptoms of obsessive-compulsive disorder. *Am J Psychiatry* 154(7):911–917, 1997.
45. Leckman JF, Walker DE, Goodman WK, Pauls DL, Cohen DJ. "Just right" perceptions associated with compulsive behavior in Tourette's syndrome. *Am J Psychiatry* 151(5):675–680, 1994.
46. Baer L: Factor analysis of symptom subtypes of obsessive compulsive disorder and their relation to personality and tic disorders. *J Clin Psychiatry* 55 Suppl:18–23, 1994.
47. Rosario-Campos MC, Miguel EC, Quatrano S, et al.: The Dimensional Yale–Brown Obsessive-Compulsive Scale (DY-BOCS): An instrument for assessing obsessive-compulsive symptom dimensions. *Mol Psychiatry* 11(5):495–504, 2006.
48. Mataix-Cols D, Rosario-Campos MC, Leckman JF: A multidimensional model of obsessive-compulsive disorder. *Am J Psychiatry* 162(2):228–238, 2005.
49. McDougle CJ, Goodman WK, Leckman JF, Lee NC, Heninger GR, Price LH: Haloperidol addition in fluvoxamine-refractory obsessive-compulsive disorder. A double-blind, placebo-controlled study in patients with and without tics. *Arch Gen Psychiatry* 51(4):302–308, 1994.
50. Bloch MH, Landeros-Weisenberger A, Kelmendi B, Coric V, Bracken MB, Leckman JF: A systematic review: Antipsychotic augmentation with treatment refractory obsessive-compulsive disorder. *Mol Psychiatry*. In press.
51. Hebebrand J, Klug B, Fimmers R, et al.: Rates for tic disorders and obsessive compulsive symptomatology in families of children and adolescents with Gilles de la Tourette syndrome. *J Psychiatr Res* 31(5):519–530, 1997.
52. McMahon WM, Carter AS, Fredine N, Pauls DL: Children at familial risk for Tourette's disorder: Child and parent diagnoses. *Am J Med Genet B Neuropsychiatr Genet* 121(1):105–111, 2003.
53. Pauls DL, Raymond CL, Stevenson JM, Leckman JF: A family study of Gilles de la Tourette syndrome. *Am J Hum Genet* 48(1):154–163, 1991.
54. Walkup JT, LaBuda MC, Singer HS, Brown J, Riddle MA, Hurko O: Family study and segregation analysis of Tourette syndrome: Evidence for a mixed model of inheritance. *Am J Hum Genet* 59(3):684–693, 1996.
55. Pauls DL, Leckman JF: The inheritance of Gilles de la Tourette's syndrome and associated behaviors. Evidence for autosomal dominant transmission. *N Engl J Med* 16 315(16):993–997, 1986.
56. Price RA, Kidd KK, Cohen DJ, Pauls DL, Leckman JF: A twin study of Tourette syndrome. *Arch Gen Psychiatry* 42(8):815–820, 1985.
57. Hyde TM, Aaronson BA, Randolph C, Rickler KC, Weinberger DR: Relationship of birth weight to the phenotypic expression of Gilles de la Tourette's syndrome in monozygotic twins. *Neurology* 42(3 Pt 1):652–658, 1992.
58. Hasstedt SJ, Leppert M, Filloux F, van de Wetering BJ, McMahon WM: Intermediate inheritance of Tourette syndrome, assuming assortative mating. *Am J Hum Genet* 57(3):682–689, 1995.
59. Barr CL, Sandor P: Current status of genetic studies of Gilles de la Tourette syndrome. *Can J Psychiatry* 43(4):351–357, 1998.
60. The Tourette Syndrome Association International Consortium for Genetics. A complete genome screen in sib pairs affected by Gilles de la Tourette syndrome. *Am J Hum Genet* 65(5):1428–1436, 1999.
61. Abelson JF, Kwan KY, O'Roak BJ, et al.: Sequence variants in SLITRK1 are associated with Tourette's syndrome. *Science* 310(5746):317–320, 2005.
62. Pasamanick B, Kawi A: A study of the association of prenatal and paranatal factors with the development of tics in children; A preliminary investigation. *J Pediatr* 48(5):596–601, 1956.
63. Leckman JF, Price RA, Walkup JT, Ort S, Pauls DL, Cohen DJ: Nongenetic factors in Gilles de la Tourette's syndrome. *Arch Gen Psychiatry* 44(1):100, 1987.
64. Leckman JF, Dolnansky ES, Hardin MT, et al.: Perinatal factors in the expression of Tourette's syndrome: An exploratory study. *J Am Acad Child Adolesc Psychiatry* 29(2):220–226, 1990.
65. Burd L, Severud R, Klug MG, Kerbeshian J: Prenatal and perinatal risk factors for Tourette disorder. *J Perinat Med* 27(4):295–302, 1999.
66. Santangelo SL, Pauls DL, Goldstein JM, Faraone SV, Tsuang MT, Leckman JF: Tourette's syndrome: What are the influences of gender and comorbid obsessive-compulsive disorder? *J Am Acad Child Adolesc Psychiatry* 33(6):795–804, 1994.
67. Khalifa N, von Knorring AL: Tourette syndrome and other tic disorders in a total population of children: Clinical assessment and background. *Acta Paediatr* 94(11):1608–1614, 2005.
68. Mink JW, Walkup JT, Frey KA, et al.: Recommended guidelines for deep brain stimulations in Tourette syndrome movement disorders. In press.
69. Mink JW: Neurobiology of basal ganglia circuits in Tourette syndrome: Faulty inhibition of unwanted motor patterns? *Adv Neurol* 85:113–122, 2001.
70. Anderson GM, Polack ES, Chatterjee D, Leckman JF, Riddle MA, Cohen DJ: Postmortem analysis of subcortical monoamines and aminoacids in Tourette syndrome. In: Chase TN, Friedhoff AJ, Cohen DJ (eds): *Tourette*

Syndrome: Genetics, Neurobiology, and Treatment. New York, Raven Press, pp. 253–262, 1992.

71. Alexander GE, DeLong MR: Microstimulation of the primate neostriatum: II. Somatotopic organization of striatal microexcitable zones and their relation to neuronal response properties. *J Neurophysiol* 53(6):1417–1430, 1985.
72. Leckman JF, Vaccarino FM, Kalanithi PS, Rothenberger A: Tourette syndrome: a relentless drumbeat—driven by misguided brain oscillations. *J Child Psychol Psychiatry* 47:537–550, 2006.
73. Singer HS: Neurochemical analysis of postmortem cortical and striatal brain tissue in patients with Tourette syndrome. *Adv Neurol* 58:135–144, 1992.
74. Richardson EP: Neuropathological studies of *Toutette's Syndrome*. In: Friedhoff AJ, Chase TN (eds.) *Advances in Neurology*, vol. 35: Gilles de la *Toutette's Syndrome*. New York, Raven Press, pp. 83–87, 1982.
75. Haber SN: The primate basal ganglia: Parallel and integrative networks. *J Chem Neuroanat*. 26(4):317–330, Dec 2003.
76. Peterson BS: Neuroanatomical circuitry. In: Leckman JF, Cohen DJ, eds. *Toutette's Syndrome—Tics, Obsessions, Compulsions—Developmental Psychopathology and Clinical Care*. New York: Wiley; 230–260: 1999.
77. Kelley AE, Lang CG, Gauthier AM: Induction of oral stereotypy following amphetamine microinjection into a discrete subregion of the striatum. *Psychopharmacology* (Berl). 95(4):556–559, 1988.
78. Hyde TM, Stacey ME, Coppola R, Handel SF, Rickler KC, Weinberger DR: Cerebral morphometric abnormalities in Tourette's syndrome: A quantitative MRI study of monozygotic twins. *Neurology* 45(6):1176–1182, 1995.
79. Peterson BS, Thomas P, Kane MJ, et al.: Basal ganglia volumes in patients with Gilles de la Tourette syndrome. *Arch Gen Psychiatry* 60(4):415–424, 2003.
80. Bloch MH, Leckman JF, Zhu H, Peterson BS: Caudate volumes in childhood predict symptom severity in adults with Tourette syndrome. *Neurology* 65(8):1253–1258, 2005.
81. Albin RL, Koeppe RA, Bohnen NI, et al.: Increased ventral striatal monoaminergic innervation in Tourette syndrome. *Neurology* 61(3):310–315, 2003.
82. Singer HS, Szymanski S, Giuliano J, et al.: Elevated intrasynaptic dopamine release in Tourette's syndrome measured by PET. *Am J Psychiatry* 159(8):1329–1336, 2002.
83. Serra-Mestres J, Ring HA, Costa DC, et al.: Dopamine transporter binding in Gilles de la Tourette syndrome: A [123I]FP-CIT/SPECT study. *Acta Psychiatr Scand* 109(2):140–146, 2004.
84. Cheon KA, Ryu YH, Namkoong K, Kim CH, Kim JJ, Lee JD: Dopamine transporter density of the basal ganglia assessed with [123I]IPT SPECT in drug-naive children with Tourette's disorder. *Psychiatry Res* 130(1):85–95, 2004.
85. Peterson BS, Skudlarski P, Anderson AW, et al.: A functional magnetic resonance imaging study of tic suppression in Tourette syndrome. *Arch Gen Psychiatry* 55(4):326–333, 1998.
86. Peterson BS, Staib L, Scahill L, et al.: Regional brain and ventricular volumes in Tourette syndrome. *Arch Gen Psychiatry* 58(5):427–440, 2001.
87. Bisno AL: Group A streptococcal infections and acute rheumatic fever. *N Engl J Med* 325(11):783–793, 1991.
88. Kushner HI: *A Crusing Brain? The Histories of Tourette Syndrome*. Cambridge, MA: Harvard University Press; 1999.
89. Husby G, van de Rijn I, Zabriskie JB, Abdin ZH, Williams RC, Jr.: Antibodies reacting with cytoplasm of subthalamic and caudate nuclei neurons in chorea and acute rheumatic fever. *J Exp Med* 144(4):1094–1110, 1976.
90. Mercadante MT, Campos MC, Marques-Dias MJ, Miguel EC, Leckman J: Vocal tics in Sydenham's chorea. *J Am Acad Child Adolesc Psychiatry* 36(3):305–306, 1997.
91. Swedo SE, Rapoport JL, Cheslow DL, et al.: High prevalence of obsessive-compulsive symptoms in patients with Sydenham's chorea. *Am J Psychiatry* 146(2):246–249, 1989.
92. Swedo SE, Leonard HL, Garvey M, et al.: Pediatric autoimmune neuropsychiatric disorders associated with streptococcal infections: Clinical description of the first 50 cases. *Am J Psychiatry* 155(2):264–271, 1998.
93. Mell LK, Davis RL, Owens D. Association between streptococcal infection and obsessive-compulsive disorder, Tourette's syndrome, and tic disorder. *Pediatrics* 116(1):56–60, 2005.
94. Murphy TK, Goodman WK, Fudge MW, et al.: B lymphocyte antigen D8/17: A peripheral marker for childhood-onset obsessive-compulsive disorder and Tourette's syndrome? *Am J Psychiatry* 154(3):402–407, 1997.
95. Luo F, Leckman JF, Katsovich L, et al.: Prospective longitudinal study of children with tic disorders and/or obsessive-compulsive disorder: Relationship of symptom exacerbations to newly acquired streptococcal infections. *Pediatrics* 113(6):e578–585, 2004.
96. Swedo SE, Leonard HL, Mittleman BB, et al.: Identification of children with pediatric autoimmune neuropsychiatric disorders associated with streptococcal infections by a marker associated with rheumatic fever. *Am J Psychiatry* 154(1):110–112, 1997.
97. Kemeny E, Husby G, Williams RC, Jr., Zabriskie JB. Tissue distribution of antigen(s) defined by monoclonal antibody D8/17 reacting with B lymphocytes of patients with rheumatic heart disease. *Clin Immunol Immunopathol* 72(1):35–43, 1994.
98. Perrin EM, Murphy ML, Casey JR, et al.: Does group A beta-hemolytic streptococcal infection increase risk for behavioral and neuropsychiatric symptoms in children? *Arch Pediatr Adolesc Med* 158(9):848–856, 2004.
99. Singer HS, Giuliano JD, Hansen BH, et al.: Antibodies against human putamen in children with Tourette syndrome. *Neurology* 50(6):1618–1624, 1998.
100. Silva RR, Munoz DM, Barickman J, Friedhoff AJ: Environmental factors and related fluctuation of symptoms in children and adolescents with Tourette's disorder. *J Child Psychol Psychiatry* 36(2):305–312, 1995.
101. Jagger J, Prusoff BA, Cohen DJ, Kidd KK, Carbonari CM, John K: The epidemiology of Tourette's syndrome: A pilot study. *Schizophr Bull* 8(2):267–278, 1982.
102. Shapiro AK, Shapiro ES, Young JG, Freinberg TE: *Gilles de la Tourette Syndrome*. 2nd ed. New York, Raven Press, 1988.
103. Towbin KE, Peterson BS, Cohen DJ, Leckman JF: Differential diagnosis. In: JF Leckman, Cohen DJ (eds): *Tourette's Syndrome—Tics, Obsessions, Compulsions—Developmental Psychopathology and Clinical Care*. New York, John Wiley and Sons, pp. 118–139, 1998.
104. Mahone EM, Bridges D, Prahme C, Singer HS: Repetitive arm and hand movements (complex motor stereotypies) in children. *J Pediatr* 145(3):391–395, 2004.
105. Leckman JF: Tourette's syndrome. *Lancet*. 360(9345):1577–1586, 2002.
106. Chappell PB, McSwiggan-Hardin MT, Scahill L, et al.: Videotape tic counts in the assessment of Tourette's syndrome: Stability, reliability, and validity. *J Am Acad Child Adolesc Psychiatry* 33(3):386–393, 1994.
107. Goetz CG, Pappert EJ, Louis ED, Raman R, Leurgans S: Advantages of a modified scoring method for the Rush Video-Based Tic Rating Scale. *Mov Disord* 14(3):502–506, 1999.
108. Nolan EE, Gadow KD, Sverd J: Observations and ratings of tics in school settings. *J Abnorm Child Psychol* 22(5):579–593, 1994.
109. Cohen DJ, Ort SI, Leckman JF, Riddle MA, Hardin MT: Family functioning and Tourette's Syndrome. In: Cohen DJ, Bruun RD, JF Leckman, eds. *Tourette's Syndrome and Tic Disorders*. New York: John Wiley and Sons; 179: 1988.
110. Bronheim S: An educator's guide to Tourette syndrome. *J Learn Disabil* 24(1):17–22, 1991.
111. Woods DW: Habit reversal treatment manual for tic disorders. In: Woods DW, Miltenberger RM (eds): *Tic Disorders, Trichotillomania, and Other Repetitive Behavior Disorders: Behavioral Approaches to Analysis and Treatment*. Boston, Kluwer Academic Publishers, pp. 97–132, 2001.
112. Piacentini JC, Chang SW: Behavioral treatments for tic suppression: Habit reversal training. *Adv Neurol* 99:227–233, 2006.
113. Deckersbach T, Rauch S, Buhlmann U, Wilhelm S: Habit reversal versus supportive psychotherapy in Tourette's disorder: A randomized controlled trial and predictors of treatment response. *Behav Res Ther* 2005.
114. Wilhelm S, Deckersbach T, Coffey BJ, Bohne A, Peterson AL, Baer L: Habit reversal versus supportive psychotherapy for Tourette's disorder: A randomized controlled trial. *Am J Psychiatry* 160(6):1175–1177, 2003.
115. Woods DW, Twohig MP, Flessner CA, Roloff TJ: Treatment of vocal tics in children with Tourette syndrome: Investigating the efficacy of habit reversal. *J Appl Behav Anal* 36(1):109–112, 2003.
116. Scahill L, Erenberg G, Berlin CM Jr, Budman C, Coffey BJ, Jankovic J, Kiessling L, King RA, Kurlan R, Lang A, Mink J, Murphy T, Zinner S, Walkup J: Tourette Syndrome Association Medical Advisory Board: Practice Committee. Contemporary assessment and pharmacotherapy of tourette syndrome. *NeuroRx* 32:192–206, 2006.
117. Eggers C, Rothenberger A, Berghaus U: Clinical and neurobiological findings in children suffering from tic disease following treatment with tiapride. *Eur Arch Psychiatry Neurol Sci* 237(4):223–229, 1988.
118. Sallee FR, Nesbitt L, Jackson C, Sine L, Sethuraman G: Relative efficacy of haloperidol and pimozide in children and adolescents with Tourette's disorder. *Am J Psychiatry* 154(8):1057–1062, 1997.
119. Shapiro E, Shapiro AK, Fulop G, et al.: Controlled study of haloperidol, pimozide and placebo for the treatment of Gilles de la Tourette's syndrome. *Arch Gen Psychiatry* 46(8):722–730, 1989.
120. Tourette Syndrome Study Group. Short-term versus longer-term pimozide therapy in Tourette's syndrome: A preliminary study. *Neurology* 52:874–877, 1999.
121. Kurlan R: Treatment of tics. *Neurologic Clinics* 15:403–409, 1997.
122. Silva RR, Munoz DM, Daniel W, Barickman J, Friedhoff AJ: Causes of haloperidol discontinuation in patients with Tourette's disorder: Management and alternatives. *J Clin Psychiatry* 57(3):129–135, 1996.
123. Bruggeman R, van der Linden C, Buitelaar JK, Gericke GS, Hawkridge SM, Temlett JA: Risperidone versus pimozide in Tourette's disorder: A comparative double-blind parallel-group study. *J Clin Psychiatry* 62(1):50–56, 2001.
124. Stephens RJ, Bassel C, Sandor P: Olanzapine in the treatment of aggression and tics in children with Tourette's syndrome—A pilot study. *J Child Adolesc Psychopharmacol* 14(2):255–266, 2004.
125. Sallee FR, Kurlan R, Goetz CG, et al.: Ziprasidone treatment of children and adolescents with Tourette's syndrome: A pilot study. *J Am Acad Child Adolesc Psychiatry* 39(3):292–299, 2000.
126. Blair J, Scahill L, State M, Martin A: Electrocardiographic changes in children and adolescents treated with ziprasidone: A prospective study. *J Am Acad Child Adolesc Psychiatry* 44(1):73–79, 2005.

127. Goetz CG, Tanner CM, Wilson RS, Carroll VS, Como PG, Shannon KM: Clonidine and Gilles de la Tourette's syndrome: Double-blind study using objective rating methods. *Ann Neurol* 21(3):307–310, 1987.
128. Leckman JF, Hardin MT, Riddle MA, Stevenson J, Ort SI, Cohen DJ: Clonidine treatment of Gilles de la Tourette's syndrome. *Arch Gen Psychiatry* 48(4):324–328, 1991.
129. Scahill L, Chappell PB, Kim YS, et al.: A placebo-controlled study of guanfacine in the treatment of children with tic disorders and attention deficit hyperactivity disorder. *Am J Psychiatry* 158(7):1067–1074, 2001.
130. Jankovic J: Botulinum toxin in the treatment of dystonic tics. *Mov Disord* 9(3):347–349, 1994.
131. Kwak CH, Hanna PA, Jankovic J: Botulinum toxin in the treatment of tics. *Arch Neurol* 57(8):1190–1193, 2000.
132. Marras C, Andrews D, Sime E, Lang AE: Botulinum toxin for simple motor tics: A randomized, double-blind, controlled clinical trial. *Neurology* 56(5):605–610, 2001.
133. Porta M, Maggioni G, Ottaviani F, Schindler A: Treatment of phonic tics in patients with Tourette's syndrome using botulinum toxin type A. *Neurol Sci* 24(6):420–423, 2004.
134. Dulcan M: Practice parameters for the assessment and treatment of children, adolescents, and adults with attention-deficit/hyperactivity disorder. American Academy of Child and Adolescent Psychiatry. *J Am Acad Child Adolesc Psychiatry* 36(10 Suppl):85S–121S, 1997.
135. Castellanos FX: Stimulants and tic disorders: From dogma to data. *Arch Gen Psychiatry* 56(4):337–338, 1999.
136. Arnsten AF, Steere JC, Jentsch DJ, Li BM: Noradrenergic influences on prefrontal cortical cognitive function: Opposing actions at postjunctional alpha 1- versus alpha 2-adrenergic receptors. *Adv Pharmacol* 42:764–767, 1998.
137. Practice parameters for the assessment and treatment of children and adolescents with obsessive-compulsive disorder. AACAP. *J Am Acad Child Adolesc Psychiatry* 37(10 Suppl):27S–45S, 1998.
138. McDougle CJ, Goodman WK, Leckman JF, Barr LC, Heninger GR, Price LH: The efficacy of fluvoxamine in obsessive-compulsive disorder: Effects of comorbid chronic tic disorder. *J Clin Psychopharmacol* 13(5):354–358, 1993.
139. Baker EFW: Gilles de la TS treated by medial frontal leucotomy. *Can Med Assoc J* 86:746–747, 1962.
140. Kurlan R, Kersun J, Ballantine HT, Jr.,Caine ED: Neurosurgical treatment of severe obsessive-compulsive disorder associated with Tourette's syndrome. *Mov Disord* 5(2):152–155, 1990.
141. Sawle GV, Lees AJ, Hymas NF, Brooks DJ, Frackowiak RS: The metabolic effects of limbic leucotomy in Gilles de la Tourette syndrome. *J Neurol Neurosurg Psychiatry* 56(9):1016–1019, 1993.
142. Hassler R, Dieckmann G: Relief of obsessive-compulsive disorders, phobias and tics by stereotactic coagulations of the rostral intralaminar and medial-thalamic nuclei. In: Laitinen L, Livingston K (eds): *Surgical Approaches in Psychiatry: Proceedings of the Third International Congress of Psychosurgery*. Cambridge, Garden City Press, pp. 206–212, 1973.
143. Leckman JF, de Lotbiniere AJ, Marek K, Gracco C, Scahill L, Cohen DJ. Severe disturbances in speech, swallowing, and gait following stereotactic infrathalamic lesions in Gilles de la Tourette's syndrome. *Neurology* 43(5):890–894, 1993.
144. Babel TB, Warnke PC, Ostertag CB: Immediate and long term outcome after infrathalamic and thalamic lesioning for intractable Tourette's syndrome. *J Neurol Neurosurg Psychiatry* 70(5):666–671, 2001.
145. Singer HS. Tourette's syndrome: From behaviour to biology. *Lancet Neurol* 4(3):149–159, 2005.
146. Visser-Vandewalle V, Temel Y, Boon P, et al.: Chronic bilateral thalamic stimulation: A new therapeutic approach in intractable Tourette syndrome. Report of three cases. *J Neurosurg* 99(6):1094–1100, 2003.
147. Ackermans L, Temel Y, Cath D, et al.: Deep brain stimulation in Tourette's syndrome: Two targets? *Mov Disord* 21(5):709–713, 2006.

5.7 ■ EATING DISORDERS

CHAPTER 5.7.1 ■ EATING AND GROWTH DISORDERS IN INFANTS AND CHILDREN

JOSEPH L. WOOLSTON AND SHARON M. HASBANI

Although eating disorders are frequently assumed to be synonymous with adolescent-onset anorexia and bulimia nervosa, a panoply of eating and growth disorders occurs earlier in life. This clinical myopia is reflected in DSM-IV (1), which recognizes only three eating disorders of early childhood: pica, rumination, and feeding disorder of infancy or early childhood. The lack of official diagnostic recognition of many eating disorders is reflective of their extraordinary complexity and resulting problems in nosological definition. Eating and growth disorders are unique in medicine and psychiatry in their position at the dynamic interface of the somatopsychic boundary of developmental neuropsychiatric disorders, emotional/behavioral disturbances, and physical changes, all of which interact in a complex fashion over time. Unfortunately, this complex interaction has not been sufficiently recognized. For example, the two most common eating and growth disorders of infancy and childhood, failure to thrive syndrome (FTT) and obesity, are both currently categorized as medical conditions in DSM-IV and ICD-10 (2). The rationale for this approach is that both syndromes are defined by caloric nutritional status regardless of etiology. Therefore, some infants and children may have failure to thrive or obesity but not actually have an eating disorder.

Until recently understanding, and even categorization, of such disorders has been hampered by a reductionistic approach relying on deterministic, linear causality (3) in which each disorder or developmental disturbance was viewed as having a single cause. This approach has gradually been replaced by the concept of a multifactorial, transactional model of development (4–6). Despite this more sophisticated theoretical approach of developmental psychopathology, advancement in the understanding of early growth disorders has been hampered by a variety of controversies that actually arise from the complexity of the phenomena. Two such controversies are in phenomenology and etiology. The phenomenology of eating disorders has been plagued by a paucity of data and by persistent diagnostic confusion. For example, FTT and psychosocial dwarfism are frequently used synonymously (7); the distinctions among rumination, gastroesophageal reflux, and psychophysiological vomiting are rarely delineated; and subtypes of such disorders as FTT (8, 9), obesity (10), and rumination (11) have proliferated. Furthermore, controversy about etiology has frequently focused upon a rigid dichotomy between an intrinsic, organic cause ("sick baby") versus an external, environmental disturbance ("bad mother") (12). The counterproductive effect of such a dichotomous approach has been best demonstrated by research in FTT, in which the organic/nonorganic differentiation has not held up to scrutiny (13, 14).

A fundamental obstacle to progress in the understanding and treatment of eating and growth disorders is lack of understanding of the basic mechanisms of hunger and satiety.

The first major advancement in this field occurred with the identification and coding of the ob gene, as well as its protein product, leptin (15–17). Experimental evidence suggests that leptin, produced in adipocytes, acts as a hormonal feedback signal to regulate fat cell size through hypothalamic mechanisms controlling food intake and metabolic rate (18–20). Leptin levels are highly correlated with body mass index in normal children, but not in children with eating disorders resulting in a significantly elevated or reduced body mass index (21). These findings provide the first steps in elucidating the physiological mechanisms of hunger and satiety. Other mechanisms involved in the control of hunger and satiety, both normal and derailed, are covered in detail in the adjacent chapter on obesity (Chapter 5.7.3).

PICA

Definition and Clinical Description

Pica would appear to be without the nosological problems that beset other eating and growth disorders of infants and children. In fact DSM-IV, which lists pica as the first feeding/eating disorder, defines it as the persistent eating of nonnutritive substances for at least 1 month in such a fashion that such eating is inappropriate to developmental level and is not part of culturally sanctioned practice. The two dependent clauses in this definition disqualify the two largest populations described in the centuries-old literature about pica: toddlers who ingest paint chips and young pregnant women who eat starch and clay (22). This artificial clarity in definition attempts to solve the confusion that bedevils all aspects of the understanding of this disorder. Rather than being a narrowly homogenous phenomenon, pica represents an eating disorder of enormously differing populations, including normally developing toddlers mouthing lead paint chips, rural pregnant women eating clay or starch, severely retarded adults eating feces, and normally developed adults chewing pencil erasers, fingernails, and ice. As if to create an aura of scientific understanding, pica as defined in the literature before DSM-IV was subtyped according to the substance ingested. These terms include geophagia (eating clay), pagophagia (eating ice), plambophagia (eating lead), amylophagia (eating starch), coprophagia (eating feces), cautopyreiophagia (eating burnt matches), tricophagia (eating hair), lithophagia (eating stones), geomelophagia (eating raw potatoes). Aside from a review of Greek root words, such subtyping is most useful at documenting the extraordinary range of substances that people may ingest.

In many ways, the heterogeneity of pica precludes a coherent statement about age of onset, developmental outcome, etiology, or treatment. Because the pediatric literature has paid great attention to the phenomenology of lead poisoning, pica has become synonymous with children eating paint chips. For these children, pica has been reported to be more common in situations of relative environmental deprivation (23) or parental psychopathology. In this population, pica begins in the second or third year of life and may continue into childhood. In a second population, young pregnant women, the onset of pica begins with the first pregnancy in late adolescence or early adulthood and may continue intermittently for several decades. Pica in mentally retarded individuals begins in childhood and may diminish after middle age (24). In this population, the risk of pica appears to be related to the degree of retardation so that the most severely retarded are most likely to have the disorder (25). Pica in chronically anxious children or adults has never been studied or described in the literature. In this last group, a possible relationship among pica, trichotillomania, and other compulsive behavior disorders has never been investigated.

Prevalence and Epidemiology

Incidence and prevalence figures for such a heterogenous disorder are difficult to interpret. However, among specific at-risk populations, pica has been reported to be quite common. Halstead (26) summarized findings from research studies that indicated that pica occurred in 25–33% of young children and 40–50% of poor black pregnant women. Pica among institutionalized retarded adults has been reported to range from 9% (24) to 25% (25).

Numerous studies have documented that the eating of specific substances such as clay and starch has been strongly influenced by cultural and family factors (27) because various social groups, especially poor and rural people, regard the eating of certain nonnutritive substances as acceptable. In addition, toddlers who are poorly supervised and understimulated are at high risk for ingesting inappropriate materials like paint chips.

Biology and Pathogenesis

Except as mediated by mental retardation, there are no known genetic factors in the etiology of pica. Boredom, anxiety, and depression may exacerbate pica, but little has been reported about such associated psychopathology. Iron deficiency is sometimes associated with pica, but the direction of the causal association is unclear (28).

Laboratory Studies and Differential Diagnosis

While the extraordinary diversity of this disorder makes any useful classification schema unlikely, the remarkable prevalence and seriousness of its medical complications require a thoughtful, vigorous approach. These medical complications include heavy metal poisoning, mineral/vitamin deficiency, parasite ingestion, and intestinal obstruction. For toddlers and young children with a history of pica, a careful evaluation of the home environment and family functioning is required. In addition, these children should be evaluated for cognitive and psychiatric impairments. Pregnant women with pica presumably have more voluntary control over their eating. A careful assessment of their cultural and nutritional beliefs is essential so that nutritional counseling can be helpful. Severely retarded individuals presenting with pica should be assessed for access to noxious materials and provided with sufficient supervision to prevent pica.

Treatment, Natural History, and Outcome

Because of the extreme heterogeneity of the disorder, few comments are germane about treatment and natural history for the wide spectrum of people who meet the criteria for pica. For toddlers and young children, proper supervision is the most important intervention. In addition, careful scrutiny of the environment to remove toxic substances is crucial. In mentally retarded and developmentally delayed individuals both pharmacological and behavioral approaches have been used to treat pica. Most treatments focus on behavioral techniques such as response blocking, redirection, and differential reinforcement. There have been two cases in the literature of the use of antidepressants in the treatment of this disorder (29, 30). However, this treatment is in need of further investigation. In anemic individuals both zinc and iron supplementation have been used with some success (31). Older adolescents and young adults should be provided with psychoeducation and counseling about the medical risks associated with ingestion of nonnutritive substances.

RUMINATION DISORDER

Definition

Similar to pica, rumination disorder has the superficial appearance of a homogenous, unitary disorder. DSM-IV defines rumination as 1) repeated regurgitation and rechewing of food (in the absence of associated gastrointestinal illness) for a period of at least 1 month following a period of normal functioning, and 2) not due to an associated gastrointestinal or other general medical condition (e.g., esophageal reflux).

Prevalence and Epidemiology

Very little is known about the incidence and prevalence of rumination, although the most severely affected cases, which are the ones that have been reported, are rare. The sex ratio of the disorder is also unclear. One case series (11) reported a male predominance, while another, larger series (32) reported a female predominance in the school age population.

Clinical Description

Rumination appears to require three factors: an impaired ability of the infant or retarded person to regulate his or her internal state of satisfaction, a physical propensity to regurgitate food, and a learned association that regurgitation helps relieve the internal state of dissatisfaction. The assessment of the child must include an evaluation of each of these factors as well as the medical sequelae of rumination, such as malnutrition and aspiration. Obviously, these medical sequelae will influence the vigor of the intervention as well as serving as a baseline by which to measure the child's response to treatment.

Biology and Pathogenesis

Unfortunately the clinical reality of this phenomenon is more complex than portrayed by DSM-IV. Some infants and retarded adults may vomit the stomach contents rather than rechewing and reswallowing it. Although this phenomenon is called psychophysiological (33) or operant (34) vomiting, its differentiation from rumination is problematic. Furthermore, the requirement that rumination not be associated with gastrointestinal disorders such as gastroesophageal reflux is overly restrictive since it implies that rumination has no underlying physiological contributions. Indeed the relationship, if any, between gastroesophageal reflux, rumination, and operant vomiting has not been investigated.

Because rumination is apparently a relatively rare disorder, virtually all of the information about the phenomenology must be derived from single case reports or small case series (e.g., (11, 35, 36)) without comparison groups. In otherwise normally developing infants, the age of onset is in the first year of life, whereas in mentally retarded individuals, the age of onset can extend into adulthood (11). Rumination has been reported to occur in nonretarded adults, many of whom have an additional comorbid eating disorder (37). In some unknown proportion of cases, the disorder remits spontaneously, while in others, the course may be malignant, marked by aspiration, severe malnutrition, growth failure, developmental delay, and death. Some authors (11) have proposed two diagnostic subgroups, self-stimulatory and psychogenic, to capture the difference in the course of retarded and nonretarded individuals, respectively. However, the relatively small sample size appears to make diagnostic subtyping premature.

Several authors have proposed that an adverse psychosocial environment is central to the development of rumination in otherwise normal infants (e.g., (11, 38, 39)). The most common environmental factor cited in the genesis of rumination is an unsatisfactory mother–infant relationship that causes the infant to seek an internal source of gratification. This turning inward by the infant has been proposed to occur because the environment is more stimulating than the infant can tolerate, or because the environment is not gratifying enough (39), or because the environment is too stimulating with negative effects (33, 38). Aside from these proposed contradictory environmental factors, no information has been reported about more general sociodemographic features. Similarly, the role of genetic factors is unknown.

Learning theorists have explained rumination in terms of the reinforcing response that it elicits (34). These proposed feedback mechanisms include positive reinforcement when a desired event such as pleasure or attention follows rumination and negative reinforcement when an undesired event such as anxiety is reduced or removed. A more sophisticated theory involves combining the concept of positive and negative reinforcement by proposing a change in the valence of the behavioral consequences. For example, consequences that are normally behavior-suppressing may acquire behavior-reinforcing characteristics if other, usually positive, consequences are lacking (36). These concepts of the operant conditioning psychogenic factors in rumination are useful as the theoretical underpinnings of certain behavioral treatments of rumination.

The role of organic factors in rumination remains obscure, but some authors have argued that rumination is totally the result of physical disorders, including hiatal hernia and other esophageal abnormalities (40). The relationship between the syndromes of rumination and gastroesophageal reflux (GER) is unknown, although high rates of association have been reported (41). GER, or chalasia, is the syndrome of regurgitation of the stomach contents into the mouth and esophagus, apparently as a result of hypomotility of the gastric fundus and delayed gastric emptying rather than a weakened esophageal sphincter (42). A possible but untested hypothesis is that GER is the physiological substrate upon which various psychosocial disruptions or deviant operant conditioning act so that rumination develops.

The assessment of the infant's capacity to regulate his or her internal state must include a general developmental assessment to evaluate for serious developmental delay as well as hyperirritability states. In addition, the mother–infant relationship must be carefully examined for clues to stimuli that are noxious or disruptive to the infant.

Laboratory Studies

The child's propensity to regurgitate can be best evaluated by procedures developed for GER, including esophageal pH monitoring, scintigraphic gastroesophageal reflux scan, endoscopy, and gastric emptying studies. In addition, various radiological procedures that evaluate esophageal abnormalities should be considered.

Treatment and Natural History

Similar to other eating disorders of early childhood, the extraordinary heterogeneity precludes specific treatments for all persons with this disorder. The learned aspect of rumination, especially in retarded individuals, may be crucial to modify. After careful evaluation of this factor, various behavioral interventions must be considered, especially if there are serious medical complications. These interventions include aversive techniques in which a noxious stimulus is paired with rumination (43), and nonaversive techniques such as differential reinforcement of other incompatible responses. Indeed, in one large study (32) the nonaversive technique of habit reversal showed a greater than 80% success rate.

FAILURE TO THRIVE AND FEEDING DISORDER OF INFANCY OR EARLY CHILDHOOD

Definition

Failure to thrive (FTT) is a disorder of infancy and early childhood characterized by a marked deceleration of weight gain and a slowing or disruption of acquisition of emotional and social developmental milestones. Deceleration of linear growth and head circumference growth are associated but not primary phenomena.

Historical Note

DSM III (44) focused on the developmental delays presumably caused by psychosocial deprivation and virtually ignored the disordered growth and feeding. For this reason DSM III described FTT as a reactive attachment disorder. DSM IV (1) sought to redress this lack of recognition of the feeding disorders by introducing a new diagnosis of feeding disorder of infancy and early childhood. Although creating a new diagnostic category has the advantage of freeing it from a long history of misconception and controversy, it has the disadvantage of losing a long, rich history of research. Despite a 45-year history of study, the understanding of FTT has been marked by confusion and controversy about such basic issues as the definition and the name of the disorder. The plethora of syndromic names provides a glimpse into the confused literature: hospitalism, anaclitic depression, institutionalism, environmental retardation, maternal deprivation syndrome, psychosocial deprivation dwarfism, deprivational dwarfism, deprivation syndrome, failure to thrive, environmental failure to thrive, and nonorganic failure to thrive syndrome. This blizzard of interchangeably used but nonsynonomous terms, which frequently represented the mistaken or oversimplified underlying conceptions of the investigators, has created a major obstacle to the course of research. These misconceptions arose out of the multifaceted nature of the syndrome. At different times the three components of FTT—weight gain deceleration, linear growth delay and developmental delays—were separated so that each was perceived as the central aspect to the exclusion of other parts. In fact, depending upon the focus of the definition, FTT has been reported as consisting of only one component rather than a triad. For example, when the diagnosis of FTT is made on the basis of primary weight gain deceleration, developmental deficits are less evident (45), and indeed, in one study using age-matched controls, there were no differences in development test scores between FTT and normally growing infants (46). A second aspect of this confusion in the understanding of FTT has been the controversy between the contribution of emotional deprivation and that of malnutrition. From the earliest observers to present-day clinicians, the correlation between emotional misery and growth problems has been obvious. Perhaps too simplistically, some investigators argued that such disorders were directly caused by misery, mediated by some effect on the mind acting directly upon the body, without requiring such external factors as altered caloric intake.

The starkest presentation of the argument has been the theoretical debate of the importance of love versus food in the etiology of FTT (47). Early clinical experience indicated that some infants with FTT who were given a normal caloric intake did not gain weight at their expected rate. These observations were used to bolster the argument that calories alone were not sufficient for weight gain. However, studies of malnourished children have demonstrated that they have supracaloric requirements before catch-up growth is possible (48). In addition, Whitten et al. (49) reported that even grossly understimulated infants with FTT gained weight rapidly if given enough food.

Prevalence and Epidemiology

FTT is a common disorder, occurring at a rate of 1–5% of pediatric hospital admissions (50). Surveys of low income children in primary care suggest that nearly 10% show weight or length below the fifth percentile for age (51). Approximately 5–10% of all children 2 to 5 years of age in the United States exhibit poor growth that is unrelated to a medical disorder (52). This common condition is of great concern because FTT is associated with increased risk for lasting deficits in growth, cognition, and socioeconomic functioning (e.g., 53). Despite the clinical importance of FTT in pediatric populations, the heterogeneity of etiology and phenomenology has impeded research efforts (54).

Clinical Description, Etiology, and Pathogenesis

The persistence of this debate about love versus food has several origins. First, FTT is a syndrome with physical (weight gain and growth deceleration) and behavioral/emotional (developmental delays) components. The overwhelming evidence indicates that inadequate caloric intake is the primary cause of growth deceleration, while emotional and socioeconomic deprivation is the primary cause of the developmental delays (55). However, the depression-like symptoms associated with FTT probably reduce the infant's interest in feeding, rendering the infant harder to feed. Similarly, the significant malnutrition associated with FTT can produce a state of apathetic withdrawal. To further complicate matters, a small group of severely deprived and abused young children has a disruption of pituitary function even in the presence of adequate nutrition. Although these children represent a clearly defined and distinct diagnostic syndrome of psychosocial dwarfism (PSD) (56), their conditions are persistently confused with FTT.

FTT is a disorder with an onset in the first 3 years of life. Typically, infants who have the onset of FTT before the end of 1 year of life are more likely to have been actively deprived of food or to have primary physiological disorders that interfere with caloric intake. When the initial onset of FTT occurs in older infants and toddlers, there are more likely to be active interactional difficulties between the child and primary caregiver, which manifest as an eating disorder. Frequently, a young infant who presents with FTT will respond rapidly to adequate feeding. However, the same social/familial conditions that are associated with such acute malnutrition may also be associated with chronic emotional and physical deprivation and poor infant–caregiver relationships. Therefore, infants whose initial episode of FTT is rapidly ameliorated by refeeding may develop a second episode of FTT that is characterized by a more chronic and internalized eating disorder. These toddlers and young children resist ingestion of adequate caloric intake and show secondary stunting of linear growth and head circumference as a result of chronic malnutrition.

The developmental outcome of children with FTT is remarkably varied, perhaps because of the heterogeneity of the syndrome. Significant variables that influence outcome include general factors such as socioeconomic status, maternal education, parental mental illness, and family social functioning. Since these are risk factors for both FTT and poor developmental outcome, they probably mediate their influence somewhat independently of FTT per se. Risk factors that are more directly linked to FTT include degree and chronicity of malnutrition, degree and chronicity of developmental delay, severity and duration of the dysfunction in the infant–caretaker relationship, and severity of major medical disorder. Problems associated with FTT such as physical abuse, medical neglect, educational neglect, and social isolation interact with the general and specific risk factors to influence developmental outcome. Nonetheless, it has been shown that with the appropriate interventions and therapies both attachment styles and parenting styles of these children can normalize.

As indicated above, FTT is a common disorder, ranging from 1 to 3% of inpatient pediatric admissions to 10–15% of some outpatient populations. Few data exist on historical trends for shifting prevalence of FTT. Sex ratio is reported to be approximately equal, although studies of older infants indicate a slighter preponderance of boys.

Although FTT occurs in children of all social strata, it is more common in families where functioning is compromised by poverty, unemployment, social dislocation and isolation, and parental mental illness (57). As with any complex, multifactorial disorder, most infants develop relatively normally in conditions characterized by many of these risk factors, while a minority develop an eating/growth disorder such as FTT. On the other hand, some infants develop FTT despite the apparent absence of any of these risk factors. Thus, social and family risk factors are just that: risk factors rather than specific etiological agents.

Virtually nothing is known about what, if any, genetic factors exist in various forms of FTT. Obviously, there are important genetic contributions to various mental disorders that can influence caretaker adequacy.

Since the etiology of FTT is a multifactorial process, virtually any temperament or psychological factor that interferes with somatic homeostasis and/or attunement between infant and caretaker may well disrupt feeding and cause inadequate caloric intake. In young infants, the two most common such difficulties are marked irritability and apathy. Both of these states are themselves the result of multiple underlying factors including basic psychophysiological temperament, nutritional state, physical health, and affective interaction with the primary caregiver. This last factor has been the focus of considerable research as the major etiological factor in the development of FTT. Investigators have postulated that any emotional and/or behavioral disturbance in the primary caretaker that causes her or him to be physically and/or emotionally absent will result in the state of apathetic depression in the infant. Alternatively, emotional disturbance in the caregiver that results in the infant's experiencing constant anger, rejection, irritability, or hatred will cause the infant to be irritable, difficult to soothe, and/or withdrawn.

Laboratory Studies

Clinicians in the past have sometimes overemphasized the importance of the search for occult organic factors, as has been demonstrated by the low yield from exhaustive testing (58). A major impetus for this excessive use of laboratory testing has been the misconception of the organic/nonorganic dichotomy. To be sure, the number of primary medical illnesses that can be associated with FTT is extensive. However, a thorough pediatric history, physical examination, and minimal screening laboratory tests usually identify physical illnesses that are contributing to FTT. These screening tests include complete blood count, lead level and free erythrocyte protoporphyrin, tuberculosis skin test (PPD), urinalysis and urine culture, and a sweat test in populations predisposed to cystic fibrosis (59).

Some organic factors may be caused by the malnutrition associated with FTT as well as aggravating its course. Malnutrition suppresses immune functions so that children with FTT are at risk for chronic respiratory and gastrointestinal infections. The illnesses that these infections produce interfere with the infant's ability to ingest adequate calories, which exacerbates the infant's state of malnutrition. Similarly, infants with FTT are at risk for vitamin and mineral deficiencies, especially of calcium, iron, and zinc. These deficiencies result in blood dyscrasias and metabolic disturbances, which worsen the infant's clinical state. In addition, the mineral deficiencies and malnutrition increase the risk of lead toxicity, since lead absorption is significantly increased in these deficiency states. Perhaps most important in evaluation of organic factors is the concept that illnesses that coexist with FTT belong in a continuum, from those that actually cause malnutrition (malabsorption) at one end to those that are caused by malnutrition (immunosuppression) (60) at the other.

More recently, studies have pointed specifically to the infant's premorbid disposition. Prospective studies have demonstrated that infants' sucking ability (61), poor response to hunger (62), increased episodes of food refusal, and decreased episodes of self-feeding (63) may all play a role in the interaction between mother and child and be a part of the picture that leads to a child's failing to thrive.

Treatment

As with other eating disorders that have associated malnutrition, ensuring adequate caloric intake is the most important intervention. Obviously the clinician must identify the major reason for such inadequate caloric intake and remediate it. For infants who primarily are severely neglected, this simply means providing enough appropriate food. For older infants, toddlers, and children who have developed a more active pattern of food refusal, a more careful assessment of the triggers for food refusal must be performed to guide the intervention.

Natural History and Outcome

The crucial axes on which to evaluate an infant with FTT include age of onset and duration of FTT, degree of malnutrition, degree of linear growth and head circumference stunting, presence of other physical illness, developmental delay, and level of family functioning.

Age of onset is important both in understanding the genesis of the FTT as well as in its prognosis. FTT with onset in the first 12 months of life in the absence of any concurrent medical illness is almost always a feeding disturbance resulting from either the infant's being deprived of adequate caloric intake or being so fussy and irritable that feeding is nearly impossible. In the former situation, the infant will rapidly gain weight when offered enough food. Thus, if the factors that contributed to the inadequate caloric intake can be ameliorated, infants with this pattern of FTT have an excellent prognosis. Similarly, most infants who have severe problems with establishment of basic physiological homeostasis will develop more effective state regulation by the second and third years of life. However, the presence of other risk factors on the multiaxial approach to FTT put such infants at high risk for poor developmental outcome. Some authors have been very specific in the linkage between developmental stage and etiology. For example, Chatoor and colleagues (64) have proposed three distinct forms of FTT based upon developmental stage of onset: 1) feeding disorder of homeostasis, in the newborn period; 2) feeding disorder of attachment, between 2 and 8 months of age, usually associated with maternal deprivation; 3) feeding disorder of separation, between 6 months and 3 years of age, during the transition to self-feeding.

Calculation of degree of malnutrition is crucial in all aspects of the clinical management of FTT, including diagnosis, prognosis, and treatment. Frequently the severity of the malnutrition is associated with the severity of the other risk factors that are influencing the FTT. The degree of malnutrition affects the severity of medical complications associated with FTT, ranging from acute immunosuppression to permanent interference with brain growth. Calculation of degree of malnutrition is essential for the correct nutritional treatment required for compensatory catch-up growth. There are numerous indices for assessing serious malnutrition. Among these are ideal body weight, height for age, BMI, and mid–upper arm circumference (65). A child who is more than two standard deviations below the mean might be malnourished. As a simple screen, one can use the cutoff of 60% of ideal body weight as indicative of serious malnutrition (66). In addition, any physiologic symptoms such as hypothermia, low pulse rate, or low blood pressure point to a more severe form of malnutrition (67).

The degree of height and head circumference growth stunting provides important data about the chronicity and severity of malnutrition (68). Generally such stunting is associated with a poorer growth prognosis, because such growth arrest is both difficult to overcome as well as is strongly associated with longstanding psychosocial deprivation. Stunting of head circumference growth is especially ominous because it reflects structural alterations in brain size. If nutritional interventions are delayed or inadequate, deficits in head circumference may be lifelong, even if weight and length deficits may be largely restored.

Beyond growth stunting, cognitive development may also be affected. Studies have shown mixed results thus far. Problems with methodology and matching cohorts abound. What is clear, however, is that at diagnosis these infants and children will have developmental delays. Numerous studies have shown that in terms of height and weight, children typically will not reach their expected centiles. It is also clear that with appropriate treatment, the children's cognitive development will improve over time; how much is currently in debate. Though a recent metaanalysis found that these children had an average IQ that was around 4 points lower (95% CI 2–6) than their matched cohorts (69), others have shown nearly complete catching up by age 4 in both physical growth and cognitive level for those whose poor physical state was treated before the age of 6 months (70).

An important caveat in the calculation of growth stunting is the consideration of intrauterine growth retardation (IUGR) and prematurity. IUGR is defined as both weight and height less than the 10th percentile for gestational age (59). The growth prognosis for children with a history of IUGR varies with the nature of the prenatal insult. Infants with IUGR who are underweight as compared with their length or head circumference (the so called asymmetric or head-sparing IUGR) have the best prognosis for later growth. Presumably such infants have been poorly nourished during the end of gestation and can regain adequate weight-for-height after appropriate caloric intake. In contrast, infants with IUGR whose weight and length are equally delayed (symmetric or non–head-sparing IUGR) frequently remain small despite intervention. These infants have often suffered a variety of systemic intrauterine pathological events, including exposure to teratogens, infections, and chromosomal abnormalities (59).

Infants who were born prematurely may appear to be growth delayed simply because they are being evaluated by chronological age of birth rather than by gestational age. The age used to evaluate height and weight should be calculated by subtracting the number of weeks since (premature) birth (59). Such corrections should be made for head circumference until 18 months after birth, for weight until 24 months, and for height until 40 months. Obviously children with IUGR and prematurity may develop FTT in addition to their preexisting conditions. In fact, since both conditions are commonly associated with such risk factors for FTT such as maternal substance and alcohol abuse, family dysfunction, and maternal mental illness or poor competence, infants with prematurity or IUGR are at higher risk for developing FTT than are full-term, normally developed neonates. Thus, while the diagnosis of either of these conditions by no means precludes the diagnosis of FTT, prematurity and IUGR must be taken into account when assessing the infant's degree of growth delay.

The presence of other medical disorders associated with FTT is a complex phenomenon that covers the continuum from illnesses like malabsorption, which directly cause malnutrition, to recurring infections secondary to malnutrition-induced immunosuppression (59). At one time, researchers and clinicians alike attempted rigidly to dichotomize children who were "only" malnourished (so-called nonorganic failure to thrive) and children who had a presumably etiological medical illness (organic failure to thrive). This rigid dichotomy served to obscure both evaluation and treatment (59). Rather than focusing only on a disorder that causes the malnutrition, the clinician must evaluate a child with FTT as being at high risk for chronic infectious illnesses, elevated blood levels of heavy metals, and mineral deficiencies.

As with the other factors in the multiaxial approach to diagnosis and assessment of FTT, developmental delay is an important, multiply determined, and transactional risk factor. Both malnutrition and emotional deprivation are independently associated with developmental delay (59). Obviously, when they are combined, they are potent risk factors. In addition, developmental delays themselves may contribute to the infant's feeding problems.

Level of family functioning is a crucial variable in assessment and treatment of FTT. The clinician must come to understand which of a myriad of family dysfunctions is contributing to the infant's failure to ingest adequate caloric intake. Earlier researchers had wondered about a specific type of family and especially maternal problem. No such specific dysfunctions have been found for children with FTT as a group. However, many reports have described specific family-related problems that appear to be directly related to specific infants with FTT. Thus, the absence of a prototypical family dysfunction that is related to most cases of FTT should not discourage the clinician from the search for sources of family problems for a specific child with FTT. Such an exploration is crucial because the ongoing nutritional supplementation and emotional stimulation must be done in the context of the child's family. Frequently the family problems that contributed to the infant's FTT will serve as roadblocks to effective treatment.

Feeding Disorder of Infancy or Early Childhood and the DSM

Definition. DSM-IV addressed the complex and controversial issues associated with failure to thrive (FTT) syndrome by creating a new diagnostic category, feeding disorder in infancy or early childhood. DSM-IV defined this disorder as: 1) a feeding disturbance as manifested by persistent failure to eat adequately with a significant failure to gain weight or significant loss of weight over at least 1 month; 2) not due to an associated gastrointestinal or other general medical condition (e.g., esophageal reflux); 3) not better accounted for by another mental disorder or lack of available food; and 4) onset before age 6. Although this new diagnostic category has provided a rational basis for the development of a nosology for eating and growth disorders in early childhood, there are a number of problems with the current definition. First, DSM-IV did not quantify "significant" failure to gain weight. Hopefully, future iterations of DSM will provide some quantification of this in terms of percentage of ideal body weight or shift in percentile on weight and length growth curves. Second, DSM-IV ignored the proven lack of validity of the organic/nonorganic dichotomy implied by the criteria of the absence of a general medical condition (13, 14, 71). Perhaps most important, this new diagnostic category makes no provision for subtyping. The likelihood that a single general diagnosis will cover two developmental epochs is very small. As described in the section on FTT, Chatoor and colleagues have proposed three distinct feeding disorders of infancy and early childhood that are well defined and have preliminary empirical support as valid and separate disorders within the broad diagnostic category (72, 73).

FUNCTIONAL DYSPHAGIA

Definition

Functional dysphagia is an eating disorder characterized by a subjective experience of difficulty or discomfort associated with the act of swallowing that is not primarily due to an organic medical condition.

Clinical Description

The two most commonly described variations are conversion dysphagia and posttraumatic dysphagia (74). Functional dysphagia and its variants have a variety of alternate names, including posttraumatic feeding disorder (75); food aversion (76); food phobia (77); feeding resistance (78); food refusal (79, 80); phagophobia (74); and globus hystericus (81). Although functional dysphagia can occur throughout the life cycle, its onset is most commonly in preschool and school-aged children (74). Problems associated with functional dysphagia include total or partial food refusal, food selectivity, adipsia or polydipsia, rumination and/or vomiting, failure to gain weight or weight loss, dehydration. Functional dysphagia frequently has a variety of initiators and maintainers. These include organic factors such as esophageal irritation or hyperactive gag reflex; psychosocial factors such as abuse related to feeding, dysfunctional family meal time culture and social reinforcement; emotional and behavioral factors such as an actual or vicarious choking event, anxious/intense temperament, anxiety disorders, and distorted body image (74).

Treatment

Treatment of functional dysphagia has included cognitive-behavioral therapy (81), hypnobehavioral therapy (74), as well a multimodal approach that integrates cognitive behavioral, individual, family, and pharamacotherapies (82).

Natural History and Outcome

The prognosis of patients with functional dysphagia is variable. Given the variety of etiologies of this disorder, and the lack of reporting of the developmental outcome of functional dysphagia, it is difficult to ascertain the prognosis for all forms of this disorder. In the case of globus hystericus, which is a conversion disorder, there is evidence that the prognosis is fairly good regardless of treatment modality used. The reported outcomes vary from two-thirds of patients improving with time (83), to 85% recovering completely with an additional 5% having some improvement (84), though this last study looked at patients with a variety of conversion symptoms. However, all studies report an overall improvement in symptoms over time. Finally, as in all these disorders it is important to treat possibly comorbid depressive and anxiety disorders in order to achieve full remission.

PSYCHOSOCIAL DWARFISM

Definition

Psychosocial dwarfism (PSD), also called deprivational dwarfism or hyperphagic short statue (HSS), is a syndrome of deceleration of linear growth combined with characteristic behavior disturbances (sleep disorder and bizarre eating habits), both of which are reversible by a change in the psychosocial environment (7, 56, 85, 86).

Prevalence and Epidemiology

PSD apparently is a rare disorder, so that virtually all of the available literature consists of case reports or small case series. Incidence, prevalence, sex ratio, and sociodemographic features are unknown.

Clinical Description

The deceleration of linear growth is remarkable in that it occurs in the absence of weight gain deceleration. In this way, PSD is quite distinct from growth stunting secondary to malnutrition (FTT), but rather resembles primary hypopituitarism (56, 87). Recently investigators have highlighted some of the clinical similarities between Prader-Willi syndrome and hyperphagic short stature, such as hyperphagia, short stature, learning difficulties, and psychosocial disturbance. One study of this hypothesis confirmed these clinical commonalities but did not find any genetic lesion in the 5q11-13 region (88). The most common characteristic abnormal eating behaviors include polyphagia, gorging, vomiting, stealing and hoarding food, and eating from garbage pails and animal food dishes. Other behaviors reported include polydipsia, including drinking stagnant water, toilet bowl water, and dishwater. Various sleep disorders have been described, such as initial onset insomnia and night wandering. These sleep disturbances may be related to growth delay since they interfere with the major nocturnal pulsatile release of growth hormone. Children with PSD may exhibit a variety of unusual patterns of relatedness and problems with behavior, including aggressiveness, impulsivity, and hyperactivity. Both specific language delays and delays in general intellectual development have been reported (89). The age of onset is unclear but reportedly occurs between 18 and 48 months. Blizzard (87) argued that the onset must occur after 24 months in order to reliably distinguish it from FTT.

Etiology and Pathogenesis

The literature is virtually unanimous in describing parental psychopathology that results in maltreatment of the child (56), including overt abuse and/or neglect (89). Several reports have indicated that both the parental psychopathology and maltreatment of the child may be obscured in initial interviews. The parents have been reported to withhold clinical information and be uncooperative with treatment. The frequent association of parental psychopathology and the reversal of the associated features with change in environment appear to be quite convincing. However, since no studies have been reported that control for such basic variables as socioeconomic class, the validity of these findings should be viewed as preliminary.

Laboratory Studies

Much of the research on PSD has focused on neuroendocrine abnormalities found in the syndrome in an attempt to unravel the relationship between growth rate and neuroendocrine changes. Unfortunately, these investigations have led to the discovery of no pathognomonic or consistently abnormal findings, with the possible exception of depressed somatomedin levels (7). The abnormalities in hormonal levels and hypothalamic functioning have been found to normalize partially or completely following subjects' removal from their inimical environments. However, Gilmour et al. (88) point out that in their experience, after an initial honeymoon period, the children's growth would often reduce or cease altogether. At this time, however, there have been no published data to support this assertion. This normalization may occur in several weeks or require as long as 2 years, depending on the specific endocrine disturbance and the type of specific medical, hormonal, or psychiatric treatment (7). In addition to this great variability in the normalization of endocrine abnormalities, none of the abnormal hormonal findings correlate specifically with growth failure. Growth failure has occurred with normal endocrine values, and catch-up growth has occurred with subnormal values (7). The mechanisms causing the growth failure in PSD are thus, as yet, unknown.

Natural History and Outcome

Developmental outcome appears to be highly variable, although limited outcome data are available. Outcome appears to be highly contingent upon the adequacy of the child's psychosocial environment. Hospitalization or removal to a less noxious home environment is presumed to be ameliorative since it is associated with reversal of some of the neuroendocrine, growth, and behavioral concomitants of the disorder (56). If the child is returned to the noxious home environment, the various gains that have been achieved may be arrested or reversed. Behavioral disturbance, developmental delays, and short stature are possible long-term sequelae. In addition, delayed puberty may occur (90).

The explanation for the rarity of PSD, even among children exposed to severe maltreatment, is a mystery. Possible factors may include genetic vulnerability, the disruption in the rate or rhythm of growth hormone production, or some specific type of psychosocial deprivation that causes such neuroendocrine dysfunction. A putative genetic vulnerability has been hypothesized to be the primary stress that leads to the HSS phenotype. It is this HSS phenotype that then leads to the secondary stress of managing the features of HSS. However, the unraveling of these mysteries awaits better designed studies with larger sample sizes and matched controls.

Treatment

The treatment and evaluation of PSD must include the three cardinal factors associated with the disorder: a reversible neuroendocrine and growth dysfunction, behavioral disturbances and developmental delays, and presumably a noxious psychosocial environment. The evaluation of the neuroendocrine and growth dysfunction is important in the differential diagnosis of other disorders that are associated with short stature as well as in monitoring the response to treatment. Other such disorders involving short stature include primary dwarfism, IUGR with persistent small size, hypopituitarism from a variety of etiologies, constitutionally delayed growth, Turner's syndrome (XO chromosomal pattern), osteochondrodystrophies, and growth stunting secondary to chronic malnutrition, with or without chronic disease. PSD is unique in being reversible with a change in living situations and in its absence of any signs of physical illness except growth delay.

The behavioral disturbances and developmental delays found in PSD serve as important factors to help monitor response to treatment as well as to represent serious aspects of the disorder that must be addressed. A careful psychiatric evaluation of the child is required that assesses for the presence of bizarre and disruptive behaviors as well as for problems in normal social relatedness. A developmental assessment must evaluate for both specific delays, especially in language, and general developmental delays. In older children, psychoeducational testing is helpful to assess specific intellectual, academic, and adaptive functioning. Psychotherapeutic and educational interventions should be guided by these findings.

The evaluation and intervention to ameliorate the psychosocial adversity is both the most important as well as most difficult task. According to all reports, caretakers of a child with PSD may be actively uncooperative in the assessment and treatment phases. Ideally, the caretakers can be engaged in the appropriate individual and family psychotherapies. In addition, they can use various social supports such as home aides and support groups. In the event of active treatment refusal, which may result in permanent damage to the child, the treaters must consider removal of the child from the home. If, however, PSD turns out to be an illness that is more akin to Prader-Willi syndrome, what is going to be most important is early diagnosis and support. Clearly the stress that the caregivers experience in raising a child with such behavioral difficulties worsens and complicates the clinical picture.

References

1. American Psychiatric Association: *Diagnostic and Statistical Manual* (4th ed.). Washington, DC, American Psychiatric Association, 1994.
2. World Health Organization: *International Classification of Diseases* (10th ed.). Criteria for Research (Draft). Geneva, World Health Organization, 1990.
3. Woolston JL: Theoretical considerations of the adjustment disorders. *J Am Acad Child Adolesc Psychiatry* 27:280–287, 1988.
4. Sameroff AJ, Chandler M: Reproductive risk and the continuum of caretaking causality. In: Horowitz F (ed.): *Review of Child Development Research* (vol 4). Chicago, University of Chicago Press, pp. 197–244, 1975.
5. Sameroff AJ, Fiese BH: Conceptual issues in prevention. In: Shaffer D, Philips I, Enzer N (eds.): *Prevention of Mental Disorders, Alcohol and Other Drug Use in Children and Adolescents*. Rockville, MD, U.S. Department of Health and Human Services, Public Health, Alcohol, Drug Abuse and Mental Health Administration, pp. 23–53, 1989.
6. Woolston JL: Transactional risk model for short and intermediate term psychiatric inpatient treatment of children. *J Am Acad Child Adolesc Psychiatry*, 28:38–41, 1989.
7. Green WH, Campbell M, David R: Psychosocial dwarfism: A critical review of the evidence. *J Am Acad Child Psychiatry* 23:39–48, 1984.
8. Egan J, Chatoor I, Rosen G: Nonorganic failure to thrive: Pathogenesis and classification. *Clin Proc Child Hosp Natl Med Cent* 34:173–182, 1980.
9. Woolston JL: Eating disorders in infancy and early childhood. *J Am Acad Child Psychiatry* 22:114–121, 1983.

10. Woolston JL: Obesity of infancy and early childhood. *J Am Acad Child Adolesc Psychiatry* 26:123–126, 1987.
11. Mayes SD, Humphrey FJ, Handford HA, et al.: Rumination disorder: Differential diagnosis. *J Am Acad Child Adolesc Psychiatry* 27:300–302, 1988.
12. Woolston JL: Eating and growth disorder in infants and children. In: Kazdin AE (ed.): *Developmental Clinical Pathology* (vol 24). Newbury Park, CA, Sage Publications, 1991.
13. Bell LS, Woolston JL: The relationship of weight gain and caloric intake in infants with organic and non-organic failure to thrive syndrome. *J Am Acad Child Adolesc Psychiatry* 24:447–452, 1985.
14. Polan HJ, Kaplan MD, Kessler DB, et al.: Psychopathology in mothers of children with failure to thrive. *Infant Mental Health J* 12:55–64, 1991.
15. Zhang Y, Proenca R, Maffei M, et al.: Positional cloning of the mouse gene and its human homologue. *Nature* 372:425–432, 1994.
16. Considine RV, Consinine EL, Williams CJ, et al.: Evidence against either a premature stop codon or the absence of obese gene mRNA in human obesity. *J Clin Invest* 95:2986–2988, 1995.
17. Green ED, Maffei M, Braden VV, et al.: The human obese (OB) gene: RNA expression pattern and mapping on the physical, cytogenetic, and genetic maps of chromosome 7. *Genome Res* 5:5–12, 1995.
18. Lonnqvist F, Arner P, Nordfors L, Schalling M: Overexpression of the obese (ob) gene in adipose tissue of human obese subjects. *Nat Med* 1:953–959, 1995.
19. Considine RV, Sinha MK, Helman ML, et al.: Serum immunoreactive-leptin concentrations in normal-weight and obese humans. *N Engl J Med* 334:292–295, 1996.
20. Woods AJ, Stock MJ: Leptin activation in hypothalamus. *Nature* 381:745, 1996.
21. Argente J, Barrios V, Chowen JA, Sinba MK, Considine RV: Leptin plasma levels in healthy Spanish children and adolescents, children with obesity, and adolescents with anorexia nervosa and bulimia nervosa. *J Pediatr* 131:833–838, 1997.
22. Lacey EP: Phenomenology of pica. In: Woolston JL (ed.): *Child and Adolescent Psychiatric Clinics of North America. Vol 2: Eating and Growth Disorders*. Philadelphia, Saunders, 1993; pp. 75–91.
23. Madden NA, Russo DC, Cataldo MF: Environmental influences on mouthing in children with lead intoxication. *J Pediatr Psychol* 5:207–216, 1980.
24. McAlpine C, Singh NW: Pica in institutionalized mentally retarded persons. *J Ment Defic Res* 30:171–178, 1986.
25. Danforth DE, Huber AM: Pica among mentally retarded adults. *Am J Ment Defic* 87:141–146, 1982.
26. Halstead JA: Geophagia in man: Its nature and nutritional effects. *Am J Chem Nutr* 21:1384–1393, 1968.
27. Lacey EP: Broadening the perspective of pica: Literature review. *Public Health Rep* 105:29–35, 1990.
28. Vyas D, Chandra RK: Functional implications of iron deficiency. In: Stekel A, Nestle V (eds.): *Iron Nutrition in Infancy and Childhood*. New York, Raven Press, 1984, pp. 45–59.
29. Jawed SH, Krishnan VH, Prasher VP et al.: Worsening of pica as a symptom of depressive illness in a person with severe mental handicap. *British Jnl Psych* 162:835–837, 1993.
30. Bashir, A, Loschen EL, Baluga J, Kirchner L: A case of pica in a patient with mental retardation treated with venlafaxine extended release. *Ment Health Aspects of Developmental Disabilities* 5:87–89, 2002.
31. Stiegler LN: Understanding pica behavior: A review for clinical and education professionals. *Focus on Autism and Other Developmental Disabilities* 20:27–38, 2005.
32. Chial HJ, Camilleri M, Williams DE, et al.: Rumination syndrome in children and adolescents: Diagnosis, treatment, and prognosis. *Pediatrics* 111:158–162, 2003.
33. Ferholt J, Provence S: Diagnosis and treatment of an infant with psychophysiological vomiting. *Psychoanal Study Child* 31:439–461, 1976.
34. Johnston JM: Phenomenology and treatment of rumination. In: Woolston JL (ed.): *Child and Adolescent Psychiatric Clinics of America, Vol 2: Eating and Growth Disorders*. Philadelphia, Saunders, 1993, pp. 93–107.
35. Sauvage D, Leddet L, Hameur L, et al: Infantile rumination: Diagnosis and follow-up of twenty cases. *J Am Acad Child Psychiatry* 24:97–203, 1985.
36. Winton ASW, Singh NN: Rumination in pediatric populations: A behavioral analysis. *J Am Acad Child Psychiatry* 22:269–275, 1983.
37. Eckern M, Stevens W, Mitchell J: The relationship between rumination and eating disorders. *J Eat Disord* 26:414–419, 1999.
38. Hollowell JG, Gardner LI: Rumination and growth failure in male fraternal twin: Association with disturbed family environment. *Pediatrics* 36:565–571, 1965.
39. Richmond JB, Eddy E, Green M: Rumination: A psychosomatic syndrome of infancy. *Pediatrics* 22:49–55, 1958.
40. Herbst J, Friedland GW, Zboralske FF: Hiatal hernia and rumination in infants and children. *J Pediatr* 78:261–265, 1971.
41. Shepherd RW, Wren J, Evans S, et al: Gastroesophageal reflux in children: Clinical profile, course, and outcome with active therapy in 126 cases. *Clin Pediatr* 26:55–60, 1987.
42. Papaila JG, Wilmont D, Grosfeld JL, et al.: Increased incidence of delayed gastric emptying in children with gastroesophageal reflux. *Arch Surg* 128:933–936, 1989.
43. Glasscock SG, Friman PC, O'Brien S, et al.: Varied citrus treatment of ruminant gagging in a teenager with Batten's disease. *J Behav Ther Exp Psychiatry* 17:129–133, 1986.
44. American Psychiatric Association: *Diagnostic and Statistical Manual of Mental Disorders* (3rd ed., rev). Washington, DC, American Psychiatric Association, 1987.
45. Field T: Follow-up developmental status of infant hospitalized for nonorganic failure to thrive. *J Pediatr Psychol* 9:241–256, 1984.
46. Mitchell WG, Gorrell RW, Greenberg RA: Failure to thrive: A study in a primary care setting: Epidemiology and follow-up. *Pediatrics* 65:971–976, 1980.
47. Widdowson EM: Mental contentment and physical growth. *Lancet* 1:1316–1318, 1951.
48. Casey PH, Arnold WC: Compensatory growth in infants with severe failure to thrive. *South Med J* 78:1057–1060, 1985.
49. Whitten CF, Pettit MG, Fischoff J: Evidence that growth failure from maternal deprivation is secondary to undereating. *JAMA* 209:1675–1682, 1969.
50. Berwick DM: Nonorganic failure to thrive. *Pediatr Rev* 1:265–270, 1980.
51. Koumjian LL, Marks R: *Catching up! Annual Report for Failure to Thrive Program in Massachusetts, 1985*. Boston, Massachusetts Department of Public Health, Division of Family Health Services, Statistics and Evaluation Unit, 1985.
52. Drotar D, Sturm L: Prediction of intellectual development in young children with early histories of nonorganic failure to thrive. *J Dev Behav Pediatr* 13:281–296, 1998.
53. Oates RK, Peacock A, Forrest D: Long-term effects of nonorganic failure to thrive. *Pediatrics* 75:36–40, 1985.
54. Benoit D: Phenomenology and treatment of failure to thrive. *Child Adolesc Clinics North Amer* 2:61–73, 1993.
55. Casey PH, Bradley R, Worthham B: Social and nonsocial home environment of infants with organic failure to thrive. *Pediatrics* 73:348–353, 1984.
56. Powell R, Brasel JA, Raiti S, et al.: Emotional deprivation and growth retardation simulating idiopathic hypopituitarism: I. Clinical evaluation of the syndrome. II. Endocrinological evaluation of the syndrome. *N Engl J Med* 276:1271–1283, 1967.
57. Kessler DB, Dawson P (eds.): *Failure to Thrive and Pediatric Undernutrition: A Transdisciplinary Approach*. Baltimore, MD, Paul H Brookes Publishing Co., 1999.
58. Sills RH: Failure to thrive: The role of clinical and laboratory evaluation. *Am J Dis Child* 132:967–969, 1978.
59. Frank DA, Zeisel SA: Failure to thrive. *Pediatr Clin North Am* 35:1187–1206, 1988.
60. Woolston JL: Diagnostic classification: The current challenge in failure to thrive syndrome research. In: Drotar D (ed.): *New Directions in Failure to Thrive: Implications for Research and Practice*. New York, Plenum, 1985, pp. 225–233.
61. Ramsey M, Gisel EG, McCusker J et al.: Infant sucking ability, non-organic failure to thrive, maternal characteristics, and feeding practices, and feeding practices: A prospective cohort study. *Developmental Med Child Neurol* 44:405–414, 2002.
62. Kasese-Hara M, Wright C, Drewett R: Energy compensation in young children who fail to thrive. *Jnl Child Psychol Psych* 43:449–456, 2002.
63. Drewett RF, Kasese-Hara M, Wright C: Feeding behaviour in young children who fail to thrive. *Appetite* 40:55–60, 2002.
64. Chatoor I, Dickon L, Schaefer S, Egan J: A developmental classification of eating disorders associated with failure to thrive: Diagnosis and treatment. In: Drotar D (ed.): *New Directions in Failure to Thrive: Research and Clinical Practice*. New York, Plenum, 1985, pp. 235–258.
65. Berkley J, Mwangi I, Griffiths K, et al.: Assessment of severe malnutrition in hospitalized children in rural Kenya: Comparison of weight for height and mid upper arm circumference. *JAMA* 294:591–597, 2005.
66. Gomez F, Galvan RR, Frenk S, et al.: Mortality in second and third degree malnutrition. *J Trop Pediatr* 2:77–83, 1956.
67. Shah MD: Failure to thrive in children. *J Clin Gastroenterol* 35:371–374, 2002.
68. McLaren DS, Reed WE: Classification of nutritional status in early childhood. *Lancet* 2:146–148, 1972.
69. Corbett SS, Drewett RF: To what extent is failure to thrive in infancy associated with poorer cognitive development? A review and meta-analysis. *Jnl Child Psychol Psych* 45:641–654, 2004.
70. Rutter M: Developmental catch-up, and deficit, following adoption after severe global early privation. *J Child Psychol Psychiatr* 4:465–476, 1998.
71. Polan HJ, Leon A, Kaplan M, et al.: Disturbances of affect expression in failure to thrive. *J Am Acad Child Adolesc Psychiatry* 30:897–903, 1991.
72. Chatoor I, Hirsch R, Ganban J, et al.: Diagnosing infantile anorexia: The observation of mother–infant interactions. *J Am Acad Child Adolesc Psychiatry* 37:959–967, 1998.
73. Chatoor I, Ganiban J, Colin V, et al.: Attachment and feeding problems: A reexamination of nonorganic failure to thrive and attachment insecurity. *J Am Acad Adolesc Psychiatry* 37:1217–1224, 1998.
74. Culbert TP, Kajander RL, Kohen DP, Reaney, JB: Hypnobehavioral approaches for school-age children with dysphagia and food aversion: A case series. *Devel Behav Pediatrics* 17:335–341, 1996.
75. Chatoor C, Conley C, Dickson L: Food refusal after an incident of choking: A post-traumatic eating disorder. *J Am Acad Child Adolesc Psychiatry* 27:105–110, 1988.

76. Siegel L: Classical and operant procedures in the treatment of a case of food aversion in a young child. *J Clin Child Psychology* 11:167–172, 1982.
77. Singer LT, Ambuel B, Wade S, Jaffe AC: Cognitive-behavioral treatment of health-impairing food phobias in children. *J Am Acad Child Adolesc Psychiatry* 31:847–852, 1992.
78. Geerstma MA, Huams J, Pelletier JM, et al.: Feeding resistance after parenteral hyperalimentation. *Am J Dis Child* 139:225–256, 1985.
79. Linscheid TR, Tarnowski KJ, Rasnake LK, et al.: Behavioral treatment of food refusal in a child with short-gut syndrome. *J Pediatr Psychol* 12:451–459, 1987.
80. Ramsey M, Zelazo P: Food refusal in failure to thrive infants: Nasogastric feeding combined with interactive behavioral treatment. *J Pediatr Psychol* 13:329–347, 1988.
81. Koon R: Conversion dysphagia in children. *Psychosomatics* 24:182–184, 1983.
82. Atkins DL, Lundy MS, Pumariega AJ: A multimodal approach to functional dysphagia. *J Amer Acad Child Adolesc Psychiatry* 33:1012–1016, 1994.
83. Moloy P, Charter R: The globus symptom. *Arch Otolaryngol* 108:740–744, 1982. Morgan HG, Russell GFM: Value of family background and clinical features as predictors of long-term outcome in anorexia nervosa: Four-year follow-up study of 41 patients. *Psychol Med* 5:355–372, 1975.
84. Pehlivanturk B, Unal F: Conversion disorder in children and adolescents: A 4-year follow-up study. *Jnl Psychosomatic Res* 52:187–191, 2002.
85. Gilmour J, Skuse D: A case-comparison study of the characteristics of children with a short stature syndrome induced by stress (hyperphagic short stature) and a consecutive series of unaffected "stressed" children. *J Child Psychol Psychiat* 40:969–978, 1999.
86. Skuse D, Albanese A, Stanhope R, Gilmour J, Voss L: A new stress-related syndrome of growth failure and hyperphagia in children, associated with reversibility of growth-hormone insufficiency. *Lancet* 348:353–358, 1996.
87. Blizzard RM: Discussion: Plasma somatomedin activity in children with growth disturbances. In: Raiti S (ed.): *Advances in Human Growth Hormone Research*. Washington, DC, Department of Health Education and Welfare Publication, NIH, No. 74–612, 1973, pp. 124–125.
88. Gilmour J, Skuse D, Pembrey M: Hyperphagic short stature and Prader-Willi syndrome: A comparison of behavioural phenotypes, genotypes and indices of stress. *Brit Jnl Psych* 179:129–137, 2001.
89. Drash PW, Greenberg NE, Mooney J: Intelligence and personality in four syndromes of dwarfism. In: Cheek DB (ed.): *Human Growth: Body Composition, Cell Growth, Energy and Intelligence*. Philadelphia, Lea & Febiger, 1986.
90. Howse PM, Rayner, PH, Williams JW, et al.: Secretion of growth hormone in normal children of short stature and in children with hypopituitarism and intrauterine growth retardation. *Clin Endocrinol* 6:347–359, 1977.

CHAPTER 5.7.2 ■ ANOREXIA NERVOSA AND BULIMIA NERVOSA

KATHERINE A. HALMI

DEFINITION

Anorexia nervosa and bulimia nervosa are the two major eating disorders. They are complex syndromes with considerable psychiatric and medical comorbidities. Current diagnostic criteria for anorexia nervosa and bulimia nervosa from DSM-IV (1) are shown in Tables 5.7.2.1 and 5.7.2.2. For those patients who have serious problems with eating behavior but do not fall into the diagnostic categories of anorexia nervosa or bulimia nervosa, the DSM-IV has designated a category of "Eating Disorder Not Otherwise Specified" (EDNOS). Most cases of eating disorders have an onset during adolescence.

There are four major criteria which define anorexia nervosa. The first criterion is a guideline for defining weight loss, since there is no specific amount of weight loss associated with the other symptoms that constitute anorexia nervosa. Therefore, an adult is considered "underweight" if the individual weighs less than 85% of a weight that is considered normal for that person's age and height. For children up to the age of 18, pediatric growth charts should be used. Some children may not have weight loss but still weigh less than expected weight because they have failed to make weight gains during a growth in height.

There is no consensus on how weight loss should be calculated, especially with adolescent patients. Some clinicians calculate weight loss below a normal weight for age and height and others figure the amount loss from an original baseline. Body mass index (BMI) is height in meters squared divided by weight in kilograms. This measure is a standard score that somewhat corrects for height and different body build. This index has the advantage of not being subjected to cultural influences. Generally, a BMI of less than 17.5 is regarded as being underweight. A BMI between 25 and 30 is considered overweight and over 30 is labeled obesity.

The second criterion, "intense fear of gaining weight," is present even during emaciated states. Anorectic patients often deny this fear since they are resistant to treatment and thus, their fear of gaining weight must often be inferred by reports of their behavior which reveal rigorous attempts to prevent weight gain such as severe food restriction and exercising.

The third criterion, pertaining to body image disturbance, has evolved into a more complex concept. The significance of body weight and shape are greatly distorted in these individuals. Some feel globally overweight and others realize they are thin but feel certain parts of their body, especially the abdomen and thighs, are too fat. The distorted significance of body weight and shape is related to a feeling of being very ineffective. Losing weight and being thin is one area in which these individuals can be effective and in control. The latter undoubtedly influences their denial of the serious medical complications of their malnourished state.

The fourth criterion for diagnosis of anorexia nervosa in the DSM-IV is amenorrhea. In some adolescents who have never menstruated, the amenorrhea is primary and menarche is delayed by the anorexia nervosa. Amenorrhea can appear before noticeable weight loss has occurred (2). Because it is difficult to obtain an accurate history of menses and because of the great variation associated with weight loss in menses, some academicians are advocating abolishing this criterion.

There are two subtypes of anorexia nervosa: the restricting type and the binging-purging type. Studies have consistently demonstrated that impulsive behaviors including stealing, drug abuse, suicide attempts, self-mutilation and promiscuity are more prevalent in anorectic—bulimics compared with

TABLE 5.7.2.1

DIAGNOSTIC CRITERIA FOR ANOREXIA NERVOSA

A. Refusal to maintain body weight at or above a minimally normal weight for age and height (e.g., weight loss leading to maintenance of body weight less than 85% of that expected; or failure to make expected weight gain during period of growth, leading to body weight less than 85% of that expected).
B. Intense fear of gaining weight or becoming fat, even though underweight.
C. Disturbance in the way in which one's body weight or shape is experienced, undue influence of body weight or shape on self-evaluation, or denial of the seriousness of the current low body weight.
D. In postmenarcheal females, amenorrhea, i.e., the absence of at least three consecutive menstrual cycles.

(From American Psychiatric Association: *Diagnostic and Statistical Manual of Mental Disorders* (4th ed). Washington, DC, American Psychiatric Association, 1994.)

anorectic restrictors. Those with anorexia binge-purge type also have a higher prevalence of premorbid obesity, familial obesity, debilitating personality traits, and specific medical complications compared with those anorexia restrictive type (3–5).

The criteria for bulimia nervosa are more arbitrary and less specific than the criteria for anorexia nervosa. There is no consensus on what constitutes a binge and how frequently bingeing must occur to warrant a diagnosis of this disorder. In the first criterion for bulimia nervosa in DSM-IV, binge eating is defined as eating more food than most people eat in similar circumstances and in a similar period of time. The sense of losing control is a significant subjective aspect that needs to be present. The second criterion, which is the recurrent use of inappropriate compensatory behaviors to avoid weight gain, usually means self-induced vomiting. However, bulimic patients often use cathartics for weight control and have an eating pattern of alternate binges and long fasting periods. The third criterion designed to address chronicity and frequency is not based on specific research but rather clinicians' consensus for obvious impairment of functioning. The fourth criterion acknowledges that bulimia nervosa patients are also concerned about their body shape and weight and tend to place excessive estimation of their worth in terms of appearance. The fifth criterion of bulimia nervosa differentiates the latter from the binge-purge subtype of anorexia nervosa. The diagnosis of bulimia nervosa is also subtyped into a purging type for those who regularly engage in self-induced vomiting or use of laxatives or diuretics and a nonpurging type for those who use strict dieting, fasting, or rigorous exercise but do not engage in purging behaviors. Bulimia nervosa patients who do not purge tend to have less body image disturbance and less anxiety concerning eating compared with those who do (6).

Binge eating disorder is listed in the "Not Otherwise Specified" category of the DSM-IV for eating disorders. People with this disorder lack the compensatory weight-control behaviors and the overconcern with weight and shape (7). Field trials are being conducted to provide evidence as to whether binge eating disorder should be a specific diagnostic category.

Other examples of persons who are given an EDNOS diagnosis are those who vomit after eating small amounts of food but maintain a weight within a normal weight range and menstruate.

TABLE 5.7.2.2

DIAGNOSTIC CRITERIA FOR BULIMIA NERVOSA

A. Recurrent episodes of binge eating. An episode of binge eating is characterized by both of the following:
   1. Eating, in a discrete period of time (e.g., within any 2-hour period), an amount of food that is definitely larger than most people would eat during a similar period of time and under similar circumstances
   2. A sense of lack of control over eating during the episode (e.g., a feeling that one cannot stop eating or control what or how much one is eating)
B. Recurrent inappropriate compensatory behavior in order to prevent weight gain, such as self-induced vomiting; misuse of laxatives, diuretics, enemas, or other medications; fasting; or excessive exercise
C. The binge eating and inappropriate compensatory behaviors both occur, on average, at least twice a week for 3 months.
D. Self-evaluation is unduly influenced by body shape and weight.
E. The disturbance does not occur exclusively during episodes of anorexia nervosa.

(From American Psychiatric Association: *Diagnostic and Statistical Manual of Mental Disorders* (4th ed). Washington, DC, American Psychiatric Association, 1994.)

HISTORICAL CONTEXT

Disturbances of eating behavior were described in the Middle Ages. Well documented case reports of anorexia nervosa are found in the literature describing early Christian saints. Monastery documents record the severe starving behavior and binging episodes of Saint Catherine of Siena, along with the kind of reed she used to induce vomiting and the herbal cathartics she used for purging (8). Another example of this irreversible self-starvation in a fasting female saint is Princes Margaret of Hungary, who lived from 1240 to 1271 (9). She was the daughter of a king and was raised in a Dominican convent where she excelled in all of her studies and in the undesirable chores of the monastery. It is likely that biological vulnerability factors are similar in those dieting for sainthood during the Middle Ages and those dieting for thinness (attractiveness) in the twentieth century. In the seventeenth century both John Reynolds (10) and Richard Morton (11) described cases of typical anorexia nervosa symptomatology and distinguished them from consumption. In the nineteenth century Marcé (12), Sir William Gull (13) and Laséque (14) described additional cases of anorexia nervosa and recommended treatment. In the twentieth century the first major publication on anorexia nervosa was a book by Bliss and Branch (15) that presented endocrine studies as well as psychological descriptions of the disorder. A decade later Hilda Bruch (16) further articulated the psychology of anorexia nervosa in her phrase "the relentless pursuit of thinness" and "the paralyzing sense of ineffectiveness, which pervades all thinking and activities." In 1979 Russell identified bulimia nervosa as a separate entity from anorexia nervosa (17). Subsequently it became apparent that there were young women who had the full syndrome of bulimia nervosa without a history of anorexia nervosa.

EPIDEMIOLOGY AND DEMOGRAPHIC CHARACTERISTICS

Most of the studies of incidence and prevalence of eating disorders have been conducted on limited populations and countries. Thus, the true incidence and prevalence of anorexia nervosa and bulimia nervosa within various countries is not likely truly accurate. Some may be a closer approximation to reality. A recent incidence study conducted in Northeastern Scotland showed that between 1965 and 1991, there was almost a six-fold increase in the incidence of anorexia nervosa, from 3 per 100,000 per year to 17 per 100,000 per year (18). In a large representative sample of the Dutch population in Holland, Hoek (19) reported the incidence of bulimia nervosa as 9.9/100,000 per year during the period 1985/1886 and 11.4 during the period 1986–1989. In Rochester, MN, a study covering a 50-year span found an overall adjusted incidence for females of 14.6 per 100,000 per year; for men the corresponding figure was 1.8 (20). This study showed no change in the rates for females 20 years and older. Among 10- through 19-year-old girls, the incidence rates increased substantially from 1950 to 1984. In summary, when estimates are based on the population at large, the incidence of anorexia nervosa in industrialized countries is estimated at 8.1 per 100,000 per year.

Soundy et al. (21) found the community-based incidence of bulimia nervosa rose sharply from 1980 to 1983 and then remained relatively constant through 1990. The incidence rates of Rochester, MN during that decade were 26.5 per 100,000 per year for females and 0.8 per 100,000 per year for males. The mean age of onset for females is 23 years. Among 15- through 24-year-old adolescent girls and young women, it had become at least twice as common as anorexia nervosa.

Prevalence studies of eating disorders are more abundant and are easier to conduct. An average prevalence of anorexia nervosa in England, Sweden, and Scotland using strict diagnostic criteria was 0.28% of young females (18).

Over 50 prevalence studies of bulimia nervosa conducted between 1981 and 1989 had a fairly consistent prevalence rate of 1% for bulimia nervosa in adolescent and young adult women (22).

The male to female ratio for eating disorders in clinical samples lies consistently between 1:10 and 1:20 (19). The onset of anorexia nervosa is usually between the ages of 10 and 30, with 85% of all anorectic patients developing the illness between the ages of 13 and 20 (23). In one large sample study a bimodal distribution of age onset was found, with peaks at 14 and a half and 18 years (24). The stress of dieting may be greater at these times, during mid-puberty and at age 18, when adolescents are preparing to leave home for a job or attend college. Since attractiveness is equated with better acceptance, young women may be more concerned about their appearance when they are preparing to leave the safe and dependent home environment.

CLINICAL DESCRIPTION

Two hallmark characteristics of patients with anorexia nervosa are denial of the seriousness of their illness and resistance to treatment, both of which make obtaining an accurate history and producing an effective treatment result a challenge. Anorectic individuals demonstrate their intense fear of gaining weight by their intense preoccupation with thoughts of food and irrational worries about fatness. They frequently look in mirrors to make sure they are thin and incessantly express concern about their appearance. They will take a great deal of time cutting up food into small pieces and rearranging food on their plates in order to eat less. An overwhelming feeling of inadequacy and ineffectiveness is a core symptom of all anorectics. Their success at losing weight is an impressive accomplishment and boosts their self-confidence. Obsessive compulsive behaviors often develop or become worse as their anorexia nervosa becomes more severe. Obsessions with cleanliness and an increase in cleaning activities and compulsive studying are commonly observed. Perfectionistic traits are common in the restricting type of anorexia nervosa patient.

TABLE 5.7.2.3

COMPLICATIONS OF BINGEING AND PURGING BEHAVIOR

1. Dental enamel erosion and caries
2. Perioral dermatitis
3. Periodontitis
4. Subconjunctival hemorrhage
5. Esophageal or gastric rupture
6. Metabolic alkalosis with hypokalemia
7. Cardiac arrhythmias
8. Cardiomyopathy and cardiac failure secondary to ipecac abuse
9. Renal failure
10. Seizures

Many adolescent anorectics have delayed psychosocial development and adults often have a markedly decreased interest in sex with the onset of anorexia nervosa.

There are important physiological differences between the two subtypes of anorectic patients. Most of the physiological and metabolic changes in anorexia nervosa are secondary to the starvation state or to purging behavior. These changes revert to normal with nutritional rehabilitation and the cessation of purging behavior.

In the patients with anorexia nervosa who engage in self-induced vomiting or abuse laxatives and diuretics, hypokalemic alkalosis may develop (Table 5.7.2.3). These electrolyte disturbances are associated with physical symptoms of weakness, lethargy and at times cardiac arrhythmias. The latter condition may result in sudden cardiac arrest, a cause of death in patients who purge. Mild elevation of serum liver enzymes may occur both in the emaciated anorectic phase and during refeeding. This reflects some fatty degeneration of the liver. Elevated serum cholesterol levels tend to occur more frequently in younger patients and return to normal with weight gain. Other common laboratory findings in emaciated anorexia nervosa patients are listed in Table 5.7.2.4. Laboratory findings present with bingeing and purging behavior are listed in Table 5.7.2.5.

Patients with bulimia nervosa should not be below 15% of the normal weight range. If they are, in most circumstances the correct diagnosis will be anorexia nervosa binge-purge subtype. Bulimia nervosa patients can be overweight. The sense of losing control of eating is a significant subjective aspect that occurs during binge eating. Abdominal pain or discomfort, self-induced vomiting, sleep, or social interruption usually terminate the bulimic episode, which is followed by feelings of guilt, depression, or self-disgust. Bulimic patients have a fear of not being able to stop eating voluntarily. Thus, ironically they may fast for long periods of time, lose control because of severe hunger, and then binge eat. Thus, they completely forgo a normal eating pattern and establish a routine of alternate binges and fasts. The food consumed during a binge usually has a high dense caloric content and a texture that facilitates rapid eating. Frequent weight fluctuations occur in bulimia nervosa but without the severity of weight loss present in anorexia nervosa. Most bulimic patients have difficulty feeling satiety at the end of a normal meal. They usually prefer to eat alone and at their homes. About one-fourth to one-third of these patients will have had a previous history of anorexia nervosa.

The majority of bulimia nervosa patients have depressive signs and symptoms. They have problems with interpersonal relationships, self-concept, impulsive behaviors, and also show

TABLE 5.7.2.4

COMMON LABORATORY FINDINGS IN EMACIATED ANOREXIA NERVOSA

1. Hematologic
   - Anemia
   - Leukopenia with relative lymphocytosis
2. Serum and Plasma
   - Hypercarotenemia
   - Hypoproteinemia
   - Hypercholesterolemia
3. Endocrine
   - Decreased estrogens
   - Decreased testosterone (in males)
   - Immature secretion pattern of luteinizing hormone
   - Decreased or blunted luteinizing hormone-releasing hormone
   - Decreased triiodothyronine
   - Increased corticotropin releasing hormone
   - Increased fasting and impaired growth hormone secretion responses
   - Blunted diurnal cortisol levels
   - Uncoupled vasopressin secretion from osmotic challenge
   - Low basal metabolic rate
   - Reduced bone density

high levels of anxiety and compulsivity. Alcohol abuse and other drug dependency are not uncommon in this disorder. Bulimics will abuse amphetamines to reduce their appetite and lose weight. As is present in the binge-purge type anorectic patient, bulimia nervosa patients can have severe erosion of the enamel of their teeth, pathologic pulp exposures, loss of integrity of dental arches, diminished masticatory ability, and an obvious unaesthetic appearance of their teeth.

Parotid gland enlargement is associated with elevated serum amylase in bulimics who binge and vomit. Other complications of bingeing and purging behavior are listed in Table 5.7.2.3. Severe abdominal pain in the bulimic patients should alert the physician to a diagnosis of gastric dilatation and a need for nasal gastric suction, x-rays, or surgical consultation.

Cardiac failure may be caused by a cardiomyopathy from ipecac abuse. This is a medical emergency that usually results in death. Symptoms of pericardial pain, dyspnea, and generalized muscle weakness associated with hypotension, tachycardia, and electrocardiogram abnormalities should alert one to possible ipecac intoxication.

ETIOLOGY AND PATHOGENESIS

The development of anorexia nervosa and bulimia nervosa is best conceptualized within the framework of a multidimensional model, which states that these disorders begin with dieting behavior. Antecedent conditions such as social cultural influences, family environment, psychological or personality characteristics, and biological vulnerabilities impact on the dieting behavior to produce the full-blown disorders of anorexia nervosa and bulimia nervosa. As fasting behavior, weight loss, and binge/purge behavior continue, significant psychological and physiological changes occur. Some of these changes are strong secondary reinforcers that allow the process of fasting, weight loss, and binge/purge behavior to continue.

Secondary psychological reinforcement occurs when the young women initially receive compliments for their weight loss and later realize this is one area of their life in which they can be extremely effective and in control. Binge eating patients soon achieve a relief of anxiety during their binge eating even though that is followed by unpleasant feelings of guilt and depression. The physiological reinforcements are less precisely defined. For example, with the period of only 8 hours of fasting, there is an increased secretion of corticotrophin releasing hormone, which is a potent anorectic agent. This may be effective in assisting some anorectics to continue their decreased calorie intake. Exercising causes a release of norepinephrine and endogenous opioids, which may also reinforce a feeling of exhilaration.

TABLE 5.7.2.5

COMMON LABORATORY FINDINGS WITH BINGEING AND PURGING BEHAVIOR

- Hypokalemia
- Hypochloremic alkalosis
- Elevated serum amylase
- Electrocardiogram—QT and Twave changes
- Photon absorptionmetry—reduced bone density

SOCIAL AND CULTURAL INFLUENCES

Anorexia nervosa and bulimia nervosa seem to be predominately a "Western" disorder in that they are largely associated with the effects of industrialization and its resulting affluence. The Japanese health care system has been facing increasing numbers of patients with anorexia nervosa since World War II and the greater influence of Western values (25). Transcultural studies show that anorexia nervosa is rare in non-Western and poorly industrialized countries (26). When non-Westerners are exposed to Western ideals of thinness, they are significantly affected by the exposure. For example, Fichter et al. (27) found the prevalence of anorexia nervosa in Greek girls who are living in Germany and exposed to Western ideals of thinness was twice that of Greek girls who remained in Greece and were not exposed to Western values of body image. There have been suggestions that cultural differences in dietary habits, patterns of parent—child interactions, value orientation, and family structure may reveal more about the societal impact on the development of eating disorders (28).

The contributions of ethnicity to the development of eating disorders have been evaluated mainly by self-answering questionnaires rather than structured interviews. In a large cross-sectional study no differences among Asians, African Americans, Hispanics and Caucasians were found in mean levels of any eating disorder symptoms (29). The authors suggested the homogenization of cultural influences on body image and eating disturbances may account for the findings. Another study found no differences among Asian, Latino, and white adolescent girls and boys in dieting and restraint scores (30). However, a metaanalysis of 18 published studies from 1987 through 2001 found African-American women have fewer eating disturbances than do white women (31).

Ethnic variations in body image and self-perceptions, which are an integral part of some eating disorders, were found in several studies. In a comparison of African-American with Caucasian adolescent girls, a study by White et al. (32) showed the African-American girls had more favorable attitudes about physical appearance, reported less social pressures for thinness, and less tendency of basing self-esteem on body-related factors. In two other studies African Americans perceived a significantly different and larger body ideal for themselves than did Caucasians (33) and African-American men preferred significantly larger body size for women than Caucasian men (34).

In a study by Iyer and Haslam (35) racial teasing was found in women of South Asian decent to be associated with body dissatisfaction and disturbed eating. It is possible that the social and economic disadvantage present in non-Caucasian girls may sensitize them toward the culturally dominant body ideals and thus instill a risk factor for developing eating disorders. For example, a study of anorexia nervosa in Curacão found cases in only mixed ethnicity women who reported that thinness allowed them greater acceptance in the more affluent white community (36).

Feminist theories emphasize that women are indoctrinated into a belief system that overvalues feminine beauty, and in particular thinness. Women cannot achieve satisfactory self-esteem without attaining ideals that are impossible to fulfill. Eating disorders then become the adaptive response to the stress of demands that women conform to an impossible and oppressive social expectation. Some support for this hypothesis comes from a study done in Japan, which suggested eating pathology there may be linked to a conflict between traditional and modernizing roles for women (37).

Peer groups that tout slimness contribute to the risk for the development of eating disorders. In a study of 9- to 11-year-old girls, Wardell and Watters (38) found that greater exposure to older peers in school was associated with increased weight concern, dieting, and thinner size ideals. In another study sorority women were found to maintain a more rigorous dietary control than nonsorority women (39). Peer groups transmit and reinforce social values that perpetuate risk for body dissatisfaction and eating disorders (40). Higher rates of eating disorders are reported in sport activities in which leanness is valued, such as dance, gymnastics, and among jockeys (41). A study in England showed that girls from a higher social economic status environment reported greater exposure to weight loss and dieting by family and friends and the higher SES girls indicated a greater awareness of ideals of thinness (42).

Several studies have found an adverse effect of the media on body image, eating attitudes and behaviors. In one study magazine exposure to thin body images found the resulting body dissatisfaction was mediated by internalization of thin ideals (43). In another study of college women Low et al. (44) found internalization of the thin ideal was associated with increased eating and weight concerns. An increased desire to emulate unrealistic body standards was found in grade school girls and boys who were exposed to pictures of "ideal men and women" (45). Adolescent girls exposed to commercials depicting thin, attractive models reported feeling more dissatisfied with their bodies and expressed a greater drive for thinness two years later in a study by Hargreaves and Tiggeman (46).

STRESSFUL LIFE EVENTS

Studies investigating the role of sexual abuse as a risk factor in the initiation of an eating disorder have produced contradictory results (47). Overall, approximately 30% of eating disordered patients have been sexually abused in childhood and this figure is comparable to rates found in the normal population. Studies have shown that abuse in multiple forms increases the likelihood of lifetime comorbid Axis I disorders and personality pathology among bulimic patients' (48). It is probably most reasonable to suggest that for some patients there may be a direct link between sexual trauma and eating pathology, but that in general, sexual abuse may best be considered a risk factor for developing a wide range of psychological and psychiatric problems.

In the premorbidly vulnerable individual, normative developmental events such as the onset of puberty, leaving home, beginning school, and the start of new relationships have been precipitating events for the onset of an eating disorder (49). Adverse life events such as the death of a close relative, the breakup of a relationship, or an illness have also been related as precipitant of eating disorder problems.

BIOLOGICAL FACTORS

Genetic Factors

A genetic vulnerability may be direct, through the inheritance of genes that are directly associated with the development of anorexia nervosa or bulimia nervosa. An indirect genetic predisposition on the other hand could become manifest under adverse conditions such as inappropriate dieting or emotional stress. These predispositions could be a particular personality type, a tendency to susceptibility to psychiatric instability (especially affective or anxiety disorders), or a hypothalamic dysfunction. There are six controlled studies that have found familial aggregation of anorexia nervosa and bulimia nervosa in the first-degree relatives of anorexia nervosa and bulimia nervosa probands (50). In a series of 67 twin probands, Treasure and Holland (51) found that the concordance for restricting anorexia nervosa was markedly higher for monozygotic (66%) than for dyzygotic twins (0%). In a large population-based twin registry study, Kendler et al. (52) showed that concordance for bulimia nervosa was significantly higher in monozygotic than in dyzygotic twin pairs. In the first large uncontrolled study of siblings of anorectics, Theander (1970) (53) found in a sample of 94 anorectic patients a risk of 6.6% for female siblings to be diagnosed with anorexia nervosa.

Recent twin studies have examined the influence of genetic and environmental factors on eating disorder related attitudes and behaviors. Klump et al. (54) studied a prepubertal and postpubertal 11-year-old twin girl cohort and compared them with a 17-year-old twin cohort. In prepubertal twins common environmental factors were important on eating disorder related attitudes and behaviors but no influence of additive genetic factors was evident. For the postpubertal 11-year-old and 17-year-old girls, genetic effects were significant and shared environment was not associated with eating disorder attitudes and behaviors. These results suggests that genes relevant to eating disorders are activated during puberty in young women.

The tendency to place undo importance on weight as an indicator of self evaluation was studied with a Norwegian twin panel. Common environmental factors were associated with this trait, which had no genetic contribution (55). Another twin study by Neale et al. (56) showed the restraint subscale on the Three Factor Eating Questionnaire was associated with environmental factors and the disinhibition scale was influenced significantly by additive genetic factors. These studies suggest both genetic factors and environmental factors make important contributions to certain features of the eating disorder phenotype. The assessment of eating disorder traits at the symptom level may provide more information about genetic and environmental structure of these disorders than the diagnostic level assessment.

Molecular genetic studies have rapidly increased in the past decade. Those involving eating disorders have used either a linkage or association method of analysis. In linkage analyses, variation in the paternal and maternal contribution to the genome of the offspring is used to localize genes that influence a trait. In the association study cases that display a trait of interest are compared to controls who do not have the trait. Candidate genes are genotyped and the allele and genotype frequencies are compared in cases vs. controls. An association study can also be done in an affected individual in both biological parents. This is called a transmission disequilibrium test (TDT). In the TDT approach, the transmission versus nontransmission of marker alleles to affected offspring is compared. A large collaborative multisite group found significant linkage on chromosome 1 for anorexia nervosa (57). Two candidate genes, the serotonin 1D receptor (HTR1D) and the opioid delta receptor (OPRD1) located at the chromosome 1 area of disequilibrium were evaluated for sequence variation and for linkage in an association of this sequence variation to AN and family and case-control data sets. Significant genotypic, allelic, and haplotypic association to anorexia nervosa and the case-control design was observed for both of these candidate genes. The genotype data on parents and AN probands showed a significant transmission disequilibrium. This same collaborative group conducted a genome-wide linkage analysis for bulimia nervosa and found a significant linkage on chromosome 10 with a suggestive linkage on chromosome 14.

Other studies have simply examined specific candidate genes without total genome linkage studies. Most of these studies have yielded conflicting results. A more promising consistent association is that of BDNF polymorphism, the Met 66 variant, which appears to be associated with the restricting type of anorexia nervosa. This was confirmed with both a case-control design and a TDT approach (58).

Neuroendocrine Factors

Under stress such as severe dieting, vulnerability for destabilization of some of the endocrine and metabolic mechanisms affecting eating behavior may influence the development of a full-blown eating disorder. Most of the neuroendocrine changes in the eating disorders are directly related to dieting behaviors, weight loss, and reduced caloric intake. These changes revert to normal with resumption of normal eating behavior and nutritional rehabilitation. For example, increased corticotrophin-releasing hormone (CRH) secretion occurs in underweight anorectic patients and in normal weight dieting individuals but returns to normal with weight restoration. However, CRH is a potent anorectic hormone and may have a role in maintaining anorectic behaviors and initiating a relapse.

It is well established that pituitary cells producing leutinizing hormone are understimulated in patients with anorexia nervosa because of hyposecretion of GnRH by the hypothalamus. A dysfunction may be present in the neurotransmitter systems that influence GnRH release and secretion. The considerable difference in patterns of severe dieting and fasting in bulimia nervosa patients probably explains the variability in the function of the hypothalamic-pituitary-ovarian axis as measured in various studies of bulimia nervosa patients. Some anorectic women remain amenorrheic for long periods of time (several years) after weight restoration. Studies have shown these women to be more psychologically disturbed compared to those who have a rapid resumption of menses (59).

The neurotransmitter serotonin is inhibitory to feeding, exploratory, and sexual behaviors, all of which are inhibited in anorexia nervosa. Studies of the serotonin receptor polymorphisms have been contradictory. Both serotonin agonists and antagonists have been found useful as an adjunct treatment of anorexia nervosa. Cyproheptadine, a serotonin antagonist, was shown to facilitate weight gain in anorectic restrictor patients. This drug most likely acts on hypothalamic appetite centers to decrease satiety and hence, increase food intake. Clomipramine and fluoxetine (serotonin reuptake inhibitors) have been useful in preventing weight relapse in anorexia nervosa and may specifically target the characteristic of obsessive-compulsive behaviors that are seen with food and weight control. Decreased serotonergic turnover in the cerebral spinal fluid has been associated with impulsive, suicidal, and aggressive behavior. Animal studies have shown that impaired serotonergic function leads to overeating and obesity. The bingeing and purging behaviors of bulimia nervosa patients are suggestive of impulse control and satiety-regulation problems. Several studies have reported impaired serotonergic function in bulimic patients. Bulimia nervosa patients have lower cerebral spinal fluid 5-HIAA levels compared to control subjects and blunted prolactin responses to the pharmacological challenge of m-CPP and to the serotonin agonist fenfluramine (60, 61).

Regional decreases in brain serotonin transporter availability (62) and increases in 5-HT$_{1A}$ receptor binding (63) but no apparent alteration in binding to the 5-HT$_{2A}$ receptor (64) were found in bulimia nervosa with functional imaging studies using single-photon emission computed tomography (SPECT) or positron emission tomography (PET). Studies in anorexia nervosa have consistently shown reduced serotonin function. Regional cortical reduction in 5-HT$_{2A}$ binding was found in a brain imaging study using SPECT (65). Individuals who recovered from the binge-eating/purging subtype of anorexia nervosa showed a persistent alteration of serotonin function demonstrated in regional 5HT$_{2A}$ receptor binding (66).

The abnormal pleasure-reward response to food seen in both anorexia and bulimia nervosa patients could be related to a dysfunction of the dopaminergic system and its role in self-stimulating or addictive behaviors. This is an area that needs to be further studied. The neurotransmitters, norepinephrine, dopamine, and serotonin all interact and affect secretions of neuropeptides which in turn can have appetite stimulating or satiety-producing effects. At the present time there is no definitive evidence that any of the neuropeptides are actually the cause of initiating an eating disorder (67).

Serum levels of leptin, a product of an obesity gene, were shown to correlate significantly with body mass index (BMI) and the amount of adipose tissue in anorexia nervosa patients. Thus, emaciated anorectics have extremely low levels of leptin, which increase as the patients gain weight (68). Baseline serum leptin levels in bulimia nervosa patients compared with controls have shown variable results (69). A compounding factor is that leptin levels decreased during short periods of caloric deficit. It is unlikely that leptin is a causal agent for producing eating disorders. Adiponectin is another adipokine protein that is released from adipose tissue and has an effect of enhancing insulin sensitivity. An inverse correlation between adiponectin and body mass index (BMI) is consistent with the increased adiponectin levels found in anorexia nervosa and variable findings in bulimia nervosa (70).

Ghrelin is a peptide released from endocrine cells in the stomach which acts in the hypothalamus to increase meal size (71). Fasting baseline plasma ghrelin levels were not different in BN patients compared with controls (72). However, the ghrelin response to standardize meals was significantly attenuated in patients with BN compared to controls (73). This suggests an impairment of postingestive satiety in bulimia nervosa with abnormal ghrelin regulation possibly contributing to the binge-eating episodes. In anorexia nervosa patients' plasma ghrelin levels are elevated in comparison to healthy controls, and these levels decrease toward normal values as patients regain their weight (74). The relationship of these peptide levels to various clinical symptom patterns needs to be clarified.

Crisp (75) espoused the theory that anorexia nervosa reflects an attempt to cope with maturational problems through the mechanism of avoidance of biological maturity. He found that females who have an early menarche and who are mildly overweight are at greater risk for developing eating disorders.

PSYCHOLOGICAL FACTORS

Assessing psychological factors as risk factors in the development of eating disorders is fraught with the problem that it is retrospective research. In a study of recovered anorexia nervosa patients, both Casper (76) and Strober (77) found that compared to controls and compared to their sisters, anorectics with long-term recovery had greater obsessive-compulsive life personality disorder traits. More recently a multinational collaborative study showed perfectionism and obsessive-compulsive characteristics to be robust traits in anorexia nervosa patients (78). Restricting anorectics tend to receive Cluster C (anxious-fearful) diagnoses such as avoidant or dependent personality disorder. By contrast, anorectic bulimics have an equal likelihood of receiving Cluster B (dramatic-erratic personality diagnoses such as borderline or a Cluster C diagnosis). There appears to be no fundamental personality trait identified as the risk factor for the development of bulimia nervosa.

FAMILY FACTORS

Since family interactions are studied during or after the development of an eating disorder, it is impossible to determine specific interactions as risk factors. There is also the problem of valid instruments by which to assess family interactions. In bulimic families studies have uncovered deficits such as lack of parental affection; negative, hostile, and disengaged interactions within the family; parental impulsivity; and family alcoholism and obesity (79). Anorexia nervosa patients perceive their families as stable, nonconflictive, cohesive, with adequate nurturance (80). In contrast, bulimic patients rate their families as conflictive, badly organized, noncohesive and lacking in nurturance (81). Undoubtedly, family factors have a role in the development, maintenance, and relapse of eating disorders but what percent of the "variance" can be attributed to family factors is unknown.

DIFFERENTIAL DIAGNOSIS

In making a diagnosis of anorexia nervosa it is important to be certain the patient has no medical illness that can account for weight loss. Occasionally, a patient may have both anorexia nervosa and a medical illness contributing to weight loss. In this situation the diagnosis of anorexia nervosa is made by the positive criteria for the disorder, and both the underlying medical condition and the anorexia nervosa are diagnosed and treated as such. Weight loss frequently occurs in depressive disorders. However, in the latter the patient usually has a decreased appetite, whereas an anorectic patient denies the existence of an appetite. The hyperactivity seen in anorexia nervosa differs from the agitated activity seen in depressive disorders in that the anorectic's activity is planned and ritualistic, such as exercising programs of jogging and cycling. The preoccupation with the calorie content of food, collecting recipes, and preparing meals for others is typical of the anorectic patient but not present in those with a depressive disorder. The latter do not have a fear of becoming fat or a disturbance in their body image, as is characteristic in anorexia nervosa.

Delusions about food in schizophrenia are rarely concerned with the calorie content of food. A fear of becoming obese and hyperactivity is also uncommon in the schizophrenic but is typical of the anorectic patient.

Chronic medical illnesses frequently associated with weight loss are Crohn's disease, hyperthyroidism, Addison's disease and diabetes mellitus. Overeating episodes may occur in the Klüver-Bucy syndrome, which consists of visual agnosia, compulsive licking and biting, inability to ignore any stimulus, and hypersexuality. Another uncommon syndrome associated with hyperphasia is the Kleine-Levin syndrome, which is characterized by periodic hypersomnia lasting for several weeks.

TREATMENT

Anorexia Nervosa

Three publications on guidelines on the treatment of anorexia nervosa were published in 2004. The British National Institute for Clinical Excellence (NICE) developed a grading scheme for which all treatment was classified according to an accepted hierarchy of evidence (82). A summary of the NICE guidelines is as follows: 1) Patients should be managed on an outpatient basis whenever possible with psychological treatment given by an experienced and competent service that also assesses physical risks. 2) Inpatient treatment should be in an experienced setting that can implement refeeding with careful physical monitoring and give psychosocial intervention. 3) Family intervention that directly addresses the eating disorder should be offered to children and adolescents.

Practice guidelines from the Australian and New Zealand Royal College of Psychiatrists (83) acknowledge that the recommendations rely on expert opinion and not on controlled trials. They recommend a multidimensional approach with close attention to medical manifestations and weight restoration. Family therapy is mentioned as a valuable part of treatment for children and adolescents. Dietary advice should be a part of all treatment programs, antidepressants may have a role in patients with depressive symptoms, and olanzapine may be useful in attenuating hyperactivity.

The Cochrane Review of six small outpatient psychotherapy trials concluded that no specific psychotherapy approach can be recommended (84).

There are fewer than 10 randomly assigned controlled treatment studies in anorexia nervosa. This is most likely due to the fact that these patients are resistant to and disinterested in treatment as well as the problem of developing serious medical complications, which requires withdrawal from research treatment protocols. Open studies have indicated that a multidimensional treatment approach that includes medical management, psychoeducation, and individual therapy utilizing both cognitive and behavioral principles is the most effective treatment. Controlled studies have shown that children under the age of 18 do better if they have family therapy or counseling. Nutritional counseling and pharmacological intervention can also be useful components in the treatment plan.

The severity of illness will determine the intensity of treatment required for anorexia nervosa patients. Treatment levels can range from a medical intensive care unit to a specialized eating disorder inpatient unit to a general psychiatric hospital unit to a day program to outpatient care. Outpatient therapy as an initial approach has the best chance of success in anorectic patients who have had the illness for less than 6 months, are not bingeing and vomiting, and have parents who are likely to cooperate and effectively participate in family therapy.

Cognitive and behavior therapy principles can be applied in both inpatient and outpatient settings. Although there have been controlled inpatient studies of the effectiveness of behavior therapy for inducing weight gain (85), there have been no satisfactory controlled studies of any other type of individual psychotherapy in the treatment of anorexia nervosa. An in-depth discussion of cognitive behavioral therapy (CBT) for anorexia nervosa can be found in articles by Garner and Bemis (86) and Kleifield et al. (87). Alliance building with the patient is essential since anorexia nervosa patients find it extremely difficult to participate honestly in any therapeutic relationship. At best they are ambivalent about any treatment attempt or therapeutic relationship that may change their behavior. It is important to foster the patient's cooperation in the treatment program; this can be done by conveying respect for the patient's dependence on anorexia as a means of coping. Weight restoration and nutritional rehabilitation are extremely important since the state of being underweight is associated with depression, difficulty concentrating, irritability, and preoccupation with food. Also, cognitive impairment is present during this state of calorie restriction. In order to accomplish necessary changes with psychotherapy the patient must be in a condition where she can actually concentrate on the issues of psychotherapy. Monitoring is an important part of CBT. In an outpatient setting the patient is taught to record not only her food intake but stressful circumstances during the day and her emotional responses to them. Cognitive restructuring is a method in which patients are taught to identify their disturbing cognitions and challenge their core beliefs. In this process they become aware of specific negative thoughts and present arguments and evidence both to support their validity and to cast doubt on their validity. From this they try to form a reasoned conclusion based on the evidence. Problemsolving is another method whereby patients learn to reason through difficult food-related and/or interpersonal situations. Adolescents from age 12 on are fully capable of participating in this type of therapy.

A family analysis should be done on all anorectic patients who are living with their families. From this analysis a clinical judgement should be made as to what type of family therapy or counseling is clinically advisable. There will be some cases in which family therapy is not possible, and in those instances family relationships can be addressed in individual therapy. In other situations brief counseling sessions with the immediate family members may be the best manner of dealing with family issues. A controlled family therapy study (88) has shown that anorectic patients under the age of 18 benefited from this whereas patients over age 18 did worse in family therapy compared with the control therapy. In another randomized controlled treatment trial 40 adolescent patients with anorexia nervosa were randomly assigned to conjoint family therapy or to separated family therapy with one therapist conducting both forms of treatment. On a global measure of outcome, the two forms of therapy had equivalent end of treatment results. For those patients with high levels of maternal criticism toward the patient the separated family therapy was shown to be superior to the conjoint family therapy (89). In actual practice many clinicians provide individual therapy and some sort of family counseling in managing anorexia nervosa.

Medications can be useful adjuncts in the treatment of anorexia nervosa. There have been many large sample open studies in Europe concerning the use of chlorpromazine in the treatment of anorexia nervosa. Unfortunately, there are no controlled double-blind studies to prove definitely the efficacy of this drug for inducing weight gain. However, this medication on an observational basis is especially effective in the severely obsessive-compulsive and overwhelmed anorectic patient in that it helps reduce their preoccupations and makes them more amenable for therapy. It may be necessary to start at a low dose of 10 mg three times a day and gradually increase the dosage. An open label study of olanzapine 10 mg/day showed that of the 14 patients who completed the study, 10 gained an average of 8.75 lbs. and three of those obtained their ideal body weight. This was conducted in an outpatient setting over a 10-week period (90). There have been several double-blind studies to show that cyproheptadine—especially in high doses, up to 24 mg/day—is effective in facilitating weight gain and reducing depressive symptomatology. This drug has the advantage of very few side effects, which make it attractive for use in emaciated anorectic patients. Unlike the tricyclic antidepressants it does not reduce blood pressure and increase heart rate. There is some indication that fluoxetine may be effective in preventing relapse in weight-restored anorexia nervosa patients (91).

Medical management, a necessary part of the treatment of anorexia nervosa patients, is based on the experience of clinicians and not randomized controlled trials. Nutritional rehabilitation programs should establish healthy target weights with a weight gain of two to three pounds per week for inpatient and one pound per week for outpatient treatment programs. Patients must be monitored for discarding food, vomiting, or exercising frequently. Medical monitoring during refeeding includes assessment of vital signs, food and fluid intake and output, assessment of electrolytes (including phosphorous), observation for edema, rapid weight gain with fluid overload, congestive heart failure, constipation, and bloating. Physical activity should be adapted to the food intake and energy expenditure of the patient. Liquid food supplements may be very helpful in the initial stages of treatment. Forceful intervention should be considered only when patients are unwilling to cooperate with oral feedings and their physical safety is in danger. Nasal gastric feedings may be required in life-threatening circumstances. During hospitalization the use of liquid formula in the early stages of weight gain with gradual exposure to food and gradual increase in activity can be very effective for inducing weight gain (92). It should be noted that estrogen replacement in anorexia nervosa patients with chronic amenorrhea has not been shown to prevent or reverse bone loss (93, 94). Specialized eating disorder units yield better outcome than general psychiatric units because of the specific nursing expertise and more effective protocols (95). A study by Watson et al. (96) showed that short-term outcomes for involuntarily hospitalized patients are similar to those voluntarily admitted.

Anorexia nervosa is a complex disorder which responds best to a multifaceted treatment approach that includes medical rehabilitation with weight restoration, individual cognitive psychotherapy, and family therapy or counseling for patients under the age of 18. At times specific medication such as chlorpromazine, olanzapine, fluoxetine, or cyproheptadine can be useful as adjuncts in the treatment of anorexia nervosa.

Bulimia Nervosa

CBT is the first-line treatment for bulimia nervosa. It has been found to be the most effective treatment in over 35 controlled studies. In these studies the treatment program was usually 16–20 weeks, after which 40–50% of the patients were abstinent from both bingeing and purging. A reduction of bingeing and purging occurred in 70–95% of patients. Another 30% of those who did not show improvement immediately after treatment did show improvement to full recovery one year after treatment. In bulimia nervosa, CBT interrupts the self-maintaining cycle of bingeing and purging and alters the individual's dysfunctional cognitions and beliefs about food, weight, body image and overall self-concept. It should be noted that in order for therapists to be effective in using CBT for the treatment of bulimia nervosa, they need to be trained in these specific manuals available for this purpose. Wilson and Fairburn (97) have written an excellent review of these studies.

Although there are no family studies of bulimia nervosa, it is common practice for most clinicians to include the family either in counseling sessions or a form of family therapy in the program of those patients under the age of 18.

Over a dozen double-blind, placebo-controlled trials of antidepressants, including desipramine, imipramine, amitriptyline, nortriptyline, phenelzine and fluoxetine, have been conducted in normal-weight outpatients with bulimia nervosa. The dosage of antidepressant medication used was similar to that used for the treatment of depression. In all trials, antidepressants were significantly more effective than placebo in reducing binge eating. These medications also improved mood and reduced eating disorder symptoms such as preoccupation with shape and weight. However, the abstinence rate from bingeing and purging on the average was only 22%. An excellent review of these studies is available in Mitchell and DeZwaan (98). There is some indication that combining antidepressant medication with CBT is helpful in some individuals (99).

More recently topiramate, an antiepileptic drug associated with appetite suppression and weight loss, was investigated as a treatment for bulimia nervosa in a randomized control trial involving 69 patients treated for 10 weeks. The median dose was 100 mg daily (range 25 to 400 mg daily). Topiramate was more effective than placebo in its effects on binge eating and purging and on measures of psychosocial impairment (100, 101).

Although group therapy has not been studied in a controlled manner, in practice many clinicians are conducting group CBT for patients with bulimia nervosa. This seems to be especially effective and popular with college students and young adults. Furthermore, it is a cost-effective treatment modality for both patients and therapist.

Adolescents from age 12 on are fully capable in participating in CBT therapy for bulimia. This treatment has been widely investigated and consistently shown effective in reducing binge eating and purging, improving mood and self-esteem, improving interpersonal functioning, and reducing concerns about shape and weight. These results are generally well maintained. Interpersonal psychotherapy also shows promise as an alternative treatment but requires further investigation. When CBT is not available or possible most clinicians opt to use a serotonin reuptake inhibitor in treating bulimic patients, since this class of drugs has fewer side effects than the tricyclic antidepressants.

OUTCOME AND COURSE OF ILLNESS

Long-term outcome studies have been conducted only on patients who have presented for treatment, and therefore a generalization cannot be made about the course of all eating disorder patients. Long-term followup research (10 years or longer for all patients) indicates that the majority of patients with anorexia nervosa have ongoing problems with the illness (102–104). About one-fourth recover, one-fourth stay chronically ill with no improvement, and about one-half will have partial improvement. Mortality rates at 10 years are 6.6% and at 30 years are 18–20% after presentation for treatment. Predictors of outcome in younger patients with AN have shown that those with purging subtype tend to do better than those with the restricting subtype, which is opposite to that reported in many adult studies (105). The same study found premorbid asociality and exercise compulsion predicted poor outcome. The majority of followup studies for bulimia nervosa have had a 6-month to 2-year posttreatment followup. A review of 88 articles on the naturalistic and treatment followup studies on bulimic patients (106) summarizes mortality rates between 0 and 3%. For those patients who were followed between 5 and 10 years, about 50% recovered fully, while 20% continued to meet criteria for bulimia nervosa. Relapse poses a serious threat for bulimics, as about one-third of recovered bulimics relapse within 4 years after treatment. About 20% of bulimics seem to sustain an unremitting bulimic illness.

For anorexia nervosa, predictors of outcome have varied from study to study. Most studies however, have shown that age onset between 12 and 18 portends a better outcome than onset before age 12 and after age 18. Repeated hospitalizations, purging behavior, long duration of illness, and very low weight at presentation for treatment are also predictors of worse outcome in most studies (102). For bulimia nervosa larger patient samples and longer term followups are needed to obtain more accurate predictors of outcome in this disorder. A review of research studies on bulimia nervosa (106) concluded that personality disorders marked by problems with impulse control were associated with a worse prognosis in these patients.

RESEARCH DIRECTIONS

Since the advent of new and efficient techniques in genetic research, this is an area that is currently developing in eating disorders. Several multinational collaborative studies are underway using a variety of methodologies. The search is on for identification of genetic markers, clusters of genes associated with anorexia and bulimia nervosa, and receptor polymorphisms of specific neurotransmitters in these disorders. Although it will be many years before any clinical meaningful application can be derived from these studies, nonetheless it is an important and essential undertaking in the next decade.

Improving treatment strategies is another extremely important area for further research. Strategies for motivation of eating-disorder patients are necessary to keep them in treatment. Treatment studies conducted over the course of a year invariably show high dropout rates, with less than half of the patients actually being completely cured from the illness. Thus, more immediately effective treatment strategies need to be developed as well as effective means of giving those patients who need more time to deal with a greater number of complex problems the motivation to stay in treatment. Valid assessments for evaluating family interaction need to be developed to better ascertain the family's effect on the course of eating disorders. Cost efficacy studies are necessary to present evidence for adequate insurance coverage for the treatment of eating disorders.

Many patients who are significantly impaired with eating disorders do not meet criteria for either anorexia nervosa or bulimia nervosa. Call for a revision of the existing classification of eating disorders should be recognized (107, 108). Recommendations from a National Institutes of Health workshop on overcoming barriers to treatment research in anorexia nervosa included the need to improve early recognition of anorexia nervosa in adolescence, to facilitate early treatment when outcomes are most likely to be favorable, and to encourage supporting innovative treatment approaches with pilot research efforts that can guide larger scale studies (109).

References

1. American Psychiatric Association: *Diagnostic and Statistical Manual of Mental Disorders*, 4th ed. Washington, DC, American Psychiatric Association, 1994.
2. Halmi KA and Falk JR: Common physiological changes in anorexia nervosa. *Int J Eat Dis* 1:16–27, 1981.
3. Eckert E, Halmi KA and Marchi P: Comparison of bulimic and nonbulimic anorexia nervosa patients during treatment. *Psychol Med* 17:891–898, 1987.
4. Halmi KA and Falk JR: Anorexia nervosa: A study of outcome discriminators in exclusive dieters and bulimics. *J Acad Child Psychiat* 21:4–7, 1982.
5. Strober M, Salkin B and Burroughs J: Validity of the bulimia–restrictor distinctions in anorexia nervosa: Parental personality characteristics and familial psychiatric morbidity. *J Nevr Men Dis* 170:345–351, 1982.
6. Davis CG, Williamson DA and Gorecmy T: Body image distortion in bulimia: An important distinction between binge purgers and binge eaters. *Paper Annu Conv Assoc Adv Behav Ther*, Chicago, 1997.
7. Devlin MJ, Walsh BT and Spitzer RL: Is there another binge eating disorder? A review of the literature on overeating in the absence of bulimia nervosa. *Int J Eat Disord* 11:341–350, 1992.
8. Bell RM: *Holy Anorexia*. Chicago, University of Chicago Press, 1985.
9. Halmi KA: Images in psychiatry. *Am J Psychiat* 151:1216, 1994.
10. Reynolds JA: *Discourse upon Prodigious Abstinence Occasioned by the 12 Months Fasting of Martha Taylor, the Famed Derbyshire damosell.* London, RW, 1669.
11. Morton R: *Phthisiologia Seu Exercitationes de Phtisi*. London, S. Smith, 1689.
12. Marcé LV: On a form of hypochondriacal delirium occurring consecutive to dyspepsia and characterized by refusal of food. *J Psychol Med Ment Pathol* 13:264–266, 1860.

13. Gull W: *Anorexia nervosa. Lancet* 1:516–517, 1888.
14. Lasèque EC: On hysterical anorexia. *Med Times Gaz* 2:265–266, 1873.
15. Bliss EL and Branch CH: *Anorexia Nervosa: Its History, Psychology and Biology*. Hoeber, NY, 1960.
16. Bruch AH: *Eating Disorders: Obesity, Anorexia Nervosa, and the Person Within*. New York, Basic Books, 1973.
17. Russell GFM: Bulimia nervosa: An ominous variant of anorexia nervosa. *Psychol Med* 9:492–448, 1979.
18. Hoek HW: Review of the epidemiological studies of eating disorders. *Int Rev Psychiat* 5:61–74, 1993.
19. Hoek HW: The incidence and prevalence of anorexia nervosa and bulimia nervosa in primary care. *Psychol Med* 21:455–460, 1991.
20. Lucas AR, Berd CM, O'Fallon WN, et al. 50 year trend in the incidence of anorexia nervosa in Rochester, Minn.: A population–base study. *Am J Psychiat* 148:917–922, 1991.
21. Soundy TJ, Lucas AR, Suman VJ et al. Bulimia nervosa in Rochester, Minnesota, 1980–1990. *Psychol Med* 25:1065–1071, 1995.
22. Fairburn CG, Beglin SJ: Studies of the epidemiology of bulimia nervosa. *Am J Psychiat* 147:401–408, 1990.
23. Halmi KA: Anorexia nervosa: Demographic and clinical features in 94 cases. *Psychosom Med* 36:18–24, 1974.
24. Halmi KA, Casper RC, Eckert ED et al.: Unique features associated with age onset of anorexia nervosa. *Psychiat Res* 3:209–215, 1979.
25. Suematsu H, Ishikawa H, Quboki T and Ito T: Statistical studies on anorexia nervosa in Japan: Detailed clinical data on 1,011 patients. *Psychotherapy and Psychosom* 43:96–103, 1985.
26. Lee S, Chiu HFK, and Chen CN: Anorexia nervosa in Hong Kong: Why not more in Chinese? *Brit J Psychiat* 154:683–688, 1989.
27. Fichter MM, Elton M, Sourdi L et al.: Anorexia nervosa in Greek and Turkish adolescents. *European Arch Psychiat and Neurol Sciences* 237:200–208, 1988.
28. Pate JDE, Pumariega AJ, Hester C. and Gerner DM: Cross-cultural patterns in eating disorders: A review. *J Amer Acad Child and Adol Psychiat* 31:802–809, 1992.
29. Shaw H, Ramirez L, Trost A. et al.: Body image and eating disturbances across ethnic groups: More similarities than differences. *Psychol of Add Beh* 18:12–18, 2004.
30. Cachelin FM, Weiss JW and Garbanati JA: Dieting and its relationship to smoking, acculturation, and family environment in Asian and Hispanic adolescents. *Eat Dis* 11:51–61, 2003.
31. O'Neill SK: African-American women and eating disturbances: A meta-analysis. *J Black Psychol* 29:3–16, 2003.
32. White MA, Kohlmaier JR, Varnado-Sullivan T et al.: Racial/Ethnic differences in weight concerns: Protective and risk factors for the development of eating disorders and obesity among adolescent females. *Eat and Weight Dis* 8:20–25, 2003.
33. Perez M and Joiner TE: Body image dissatisfaction and disordered eating in black and white women. *Int J Eat Dis* 33:342–350, 2003.
34. Freedman R, Carter MM, Sbrocco T et al.: Ethnic differences in preferences for female weight and waist to hip ratio: A comparison of African-American and white American college and community samples. *Eat Beh* 5:191–198, 2004.
35. Iyer DS and Haslam N: Body image and eating disturbance among South Asian-American women: A role of racial teasing. *Int J Eat Dis* 34:142–147, 2003.
36. Katzman MA, Hermans KME, Van Koeken D et al.: Not your typical island woman: Anorexia nervosa is reported only in subcultures in Curacão. *Culture Med and Psychiat* 28:463–492, 2004.
37. Pike KM and Borovoy A: The rise of eating disorders in Japan: Issues of culture and limitations of the model of westernization. *Culture Med and Psychiat* 28:493–531, 2004.
38. Wardle J, and Watters R: Sociocultural influences on attitudes on weight and eating: Results of a natural experiment. *Int J Eat Dis* 35:589–596, 2004.
39. Allison KC and Park CL: A prospective study of disordered eating among sorority and non-sorority women. *Int J Eat Dis* 35:354–358, 2004.
40. Presnell K, Bearman SK and Stice E: Risk factors for body dissatisfaction in adolescent boys and girls: A prospective study. *Int J Eat Dis* 36:389–401, 2004.
41. Thompson SH and Digsby S: A preliminary survey of dieting, body dissatisfaction, and eating problems among high school cheerleaders. *J. School Health* 74:85–90, 2004.
42. Wardel J, Robb KA, Johnson F et al.: Social economic variation and attitudes to eating and weight in female adolescence. *Health Psychol* 23:275–282, 2004.
43. Tiggeman NM: Media exposure, body dissatisfaction and disordered eating: Television and magazines are not the same. *Eur Eat Dis Rev* 11:418–430, 2003.
44. Low KA, Charanasomeoon S, Brown C et al.: Social behavior and personality. 31:81–90, 2003.
45. Murnen SK, Smolak L, Mills JA et al.: Thin, sexy women and strong, muscular men: Grade school children's responses to objectified images of women and men. *Sex Roles* 49:427–437, 2003.
46. Hargreaves D and Tiggeman M: Younger-term implications of responsiveness to thin-ideal television: Support for a cumulative hypothesis of body image disturbance. *Eur Eat Dis Rev* 11:465–477, 2003.
47. Connors ME and Morce W: Sexual abuse and eating disorders: A review. *Int J Eat Dis* 13:1–11, 1993.
48. Rorty M, Yager J, and Rossotto E: Childhood sexual, physical and psychological abuse and their relationship to comorbid psychopathology in bulimia nervosa. *Int J Eat Dis* 16:317–334, 1994.
49. Cooper Z: The development and maintenance of eating disorders. In: KD Brownell and CG Fairburn (eds.). *Eating Disorders and Obesity: A Comprehensive Handbook*. New York and London, Guilford Press, 1995, pp. 199–206.
50. Kaye W, Lilenfeld L, Berrettini W, et al.: A search for susceptibility loci for anorexia nervosa: Methods and sample description. *Biol Psychiat* 47:794–803, 2000.
51. Treasure J, Holland AJ: Genetic vulnerability to eating disorders: Evidence from twin and family studies. In Remschmidt H, Schmidt MH (eds.). *Child and Use Psychiatry: European Perspectives*. New York, Hogrefe and Hubert, 1989, pp. 59–68.
52. Kendler KS, MacLean C, Neal M et al.: The genetic epidemiology of bulimia nervosa. *Am J Psychiatr* 148:1627–1637, 1991.
53. Theander S: Anorexia nervosa: A psychiatric investigation of 94 female cases. *Acta Psychiat Acand* Suppl 214:1–94, 1970.
54. Klump KL, McGue M and Iacono WG: Differential heritability of eating attitudes and behaviors in prepubertal versus pubertal twins. *Int J Eat Dis* 33:287–292, 2003.
55. Reichborn-Kjennerud T, Bulik CM, Kendler KS et al.: On the influence of weight on self-evaluation: A population-twin study of gender differences. *Int J Eat Dis* 35:123–132, 2004.
56. Neale BM, Mazzeo SE and Bulik CM: A twin study of dietary restraint, disinhabitation and hunger: An examination of the eating inventory. *Twin Research*, 6:471–478, 2003.
57. Grice DE, Halmi KA, Fichter MM et al.: Evidence for a susceptibility gene for anorexia nervosa on chromosome 1. *Am J Hum Gen* 70:787–792, 2002.
58. Ribases M, Gratacos M, Armengol L et al.: Met. 66 in the brain-derived neurotrophic factor (BDNF) precursor is associated with anorexia nervosa restrictive type. *Mrl Psychiat* 8:745–751, 2003.
59. Halmi KA and Falk JR: Behavioral and dietary discriminators of menstrual function in anorexia nervosa. In: Darby, Garner and Garfinkel (eds.): *Anorexia Nervosa: Recent Development*. New York, Allen R. Liss, pp. 323–329, 1983.
60. Levitan RD, Kaplan AS, Joffery T: Hormonal and subjective responses to intravenous method-chlorophneyl piperazine in bulimia nervosa. *Arch Gen Psychiat* 54:521–587, 1997.
61. Jimmerson DC, Wolfe BE, Metzger ED et al.: Decreased serotonin function in bulimia nervosa. *Arch Gen Psychiat* 54:529–534, 1997.
62. Tauscher J, Pirker W, Willeit M et al.: I^{123} B-CIT and single photon emission computed tomography reveal reduce brain serotonin transporter availability in bulimia nervosa. *Biol Psychiat* 49:326–332, 2001.
63. Tiihonen J, Keski-Rahkonen A, Lipponen M, et al.: Brain serotonin 1A receptor binding in bulimia nervosa. *Biol Psychiat* 55:871–873, 2004.
64. Goethals I, Vervaet M, Audenaert K et al.: Comparison of cortical 5-HT2A receptor binding in bulimia nervosa patients and healthy volunteers. *Am J Psychiat* 161:1916–1918, 2004.
65. Audenaert K, Van Laere K, Dumont F: Decreased 5-HT2A receptor binding in patients with anorexia nervosa. *J Nucl Med* 44:163–169, 2003.
66. Bailer UF, Price JC, Meltzer CC et al.: Altered 5-HT2A receptor binding after recovery from bulimia-type anorexia nervosa: Relationships to harm avoidance and drive for thinness. *Neuropsychopharmacology*, 89:1143–1155, 2004.
67. Halmi KA: Basic biological overview of eating disorders. In: Bloom FE, Kuper DJ (eds.): *Psychopharmacology; The Fourth Generation of Progress*. New York, Raven Press, 1995, pp. 1609–1616.
68. Eckert E, Pomeroy C, Raymond N et al.: Leptin in anorexia nervosa. *J Clin Endocrinol Metab* 83:791–795, 1998.
69. Monteleone P, Di Lieto A, Castaldo E et al.: Leptin functioning in eating disorders. *CNS Spectr* 9:523–529, 2004.
70. Monteleone P, Fabrazzo M, Martiadis Z. et al.: Opposite changes in circulating adiponectin in women with bulimia nervosa or binge eating disorder. *J Clin Endocrin Metad* 88:5387–5391, 2003.
71. Chen HA, Trumbauer ME, Chen AS et al.: Orexigenic action of peripheral ghrelin is mediated by neuropeptide Y and agouti-related protein. *Endocr* 145:2607–2612, 2004.
72. Monteleone P, Fabrazzo M, Tortorlly A. et al.: Circulating ghrelin is decreased in non-obese and obese women with binge eating disorder was well as in obese non-binge eating women, but not in patients with bulimia nervosa. *Psychoneuroendocrinology*, 30:243–250, 2005.
73. Monteleone P, Martiadis V, Fabrazzo M et al.: Ghrelin and leptin responses to food ingestion in bulimia nervosa: Implications for binge eating and compensatory behaviors. *Psychol Med* 33:1387–1394, 2003.
74. Otto B, Cuntz U, Fruhauf E.: Weight gain decreased elevated plasma ghrelin concentrations of patients with anorexia nervosa. *Eur J Endocrin* 145:66–673, 2001.
75. Crisp AH: Premorbid factors in adult disorders of weight, with particular reference to primary anorexia nervosa (weight phobia). *J Psycholsom Res* 14:1–22, 1984.
76. Casper RC: Personality features of women with good outcome from restricting anorexia nervosa. *Psychosom Med* 52:156–170, 1990.

77. Strober M: Personality and symptomalogical features in young, nonchronic anorexia nervosa patients. *J Psychosom Res* 24:353–359, 1980.
78. Halmi KA: Obsessive compulsive traits and behaviors in anorexia nervosa. In: Bellodi L, Brambilla F (eds.): *Eating Disorders and Obsessive Compulsive Disorder: An Etiopathogenic Link*. Centro Scientifico Edet. pp. 4–10, 1999.
79. Strober M, Humphrey LL: Familial contributions to the etiology and course of anorexia nervosa and bulimia. *J Consult Clin Psychol* 55:654–659, 1987.
80. Vandereycken W, Koge L, Vanderlinden J: *The Family Approach to Eating Disorders: Assessment and Treatment of Anorexia Nervosa and Bulimia*. New York, PMA, 1989.
81. Wonderlich SA, Swift WJ, Slotnick HB and Goodman S: DSM-III-R personality disorder in eating disorder subtypes. *Int J Eat Dis* 9:607–616, 1990.
82. NICE (National Institute for Clinical Excellence) Core interventions in the treatment and management of anorexia nervosa, bulimia nervosa and related eating disorders. *Clinical Guidelines* 9. London, 2004, pp. 1–15.
83. Royal Australian and New Zealand College of Psychiatrist. Clinical practice guidelines for anorexia nervosa. *Australian and New Zealand Journal of Psychiatry*, 38:659–670, 2004.
84. Hay P, Bacaltchuk J, Caludino A, et al.: Individual psychotherapy in the outpatient treatment of adult with anorexia nervosa. In: *Cochran Library*, Issue 3. Chichester, U.K., John Wiley & Sons Ltd., 2003.
85. Wulliemier F, Rossel F, Sinclair K: La therapie compartamentale de l'anorexie nerveuse, behavior therapy and anorexia nervosa. *J Psycholsom Res* 19:267–272, 1995.
86. Garner DM and Bemiss KN: A cognitive-behavioral approach to anorexia nervosa. *Cog Ther and Res* 6:1223–1250, 1982.
87. Kleifield EI, Wagner W, and Halmi KA: Cognitive-behavioral treatment of anorexia nervosa. *Psychiat Clin In Amer* 19:715–737, 1996.
88. Russell GFM, Szmukler GI, Dare C. et al.: An evaluation of family therapy and anorexia nervosa and bulimia nervosa. *Arch Gen Psychiat* 44:1047–1056, 1987.
89. Eisler I, Dare C, Hodes M et al.: Family therapy for adolescent anorexia nervosa: The result of a control comparison of two-family intervention. *J Child Psychol and Psychiat* 41:727–736, 2000.
90. Powers PS, Santana CA and Bannon YS: Olanzapine in the treatment of anorexia nervosa: An opened label trial. *Int J Eat Dis* 32:146–154, 2002.
91. Kaye W, Nagata T, Weltzin T: Double-blind placebo-control administration of fluoxetine in restricting and restricting-purging type anorexia nervosa. *Biol Psychiat* 49:644–652, 2001.
92. Okamoto A, Yamachita T, Nagoshi H: A behavior program combined with liquid nutrition designed for anorexia nervosa. *Psychiat and Clinical Neuroscience* 56:516–520, 2002.
93. Golden N: Osteopenia and osteoporosis in anorexia nervosa. *Adol Med* 14:97–108, 2003.
94. Grinspoon S, Thomas L, Miller K et al.: Effects of recombinant human IGH-I and oral contraceptive administration on bone density and anorexia nervosa. *J Clin Endocr Met* 87:2883–2891, 2002.
95. Wolfe BE, Gimby LB: Caring for the hospitalized patient with an eating disorder. *Nursing Clinics N Am* 38:75–99, 2003.
96. Watson TL, Bowers W, Anderson AE: Involuntary treatment of eating disorders. *Am J Psychiat* 157:1806–1810, 2000.
97. Wilson CG and Fairburn CG: Cognitive treatment for treating eating disorders. *J Cons and Clin Psychol* 61:261–269, 1993.
98. Mitchell JE and DeZwaan M: Pharmacological treatments of binge eating. In: CG Fairburn and GT Wilson (eds). *Binge Eating: Nature, Assessment and Treatment*. New York, Guilford Press, 1993.
99. Agras WS, Rossiter EN, Arnow B. et al.: Pharmacologic and cognitive-behavioral treatment for bulimia nervosa: A control comparison. *Amer J Psychiat* 149:82–87, 1992.
100. Hedges DW, Renherr FW, Hoops SP et al.: Treatment of bulimia nervosa with Topiramate in a randomized-double-blind, placebo-controlled trial, part 2: Improvements in psychiatric measures. *J Clin Psychiat* 64:1449–54, 2003.
101. Hoopes SP, Riemherr FW, Hedges DW et al.: Treatment of bulimia nervosa with Topiramate in a randomized-double-blind placebo-controlled trial, part 1: Improvement in binge and purge measures. *J Clin Psychiat* 64:1335–1341, 2003.
102. Eckert ED, Halmi KA, Marchi EP et al.: Ten year follow-up of anorexia nervosa: Clinical course and outcome. *Psychol Med* 25:143–156, 1995.
103. Theander S: Outcome and prognosis in anorexia nervosa and bulimia: Some results of previous investigations compared with those with a Swedish long-term study. *J Psychiat Res* 19:493–500, 1985.
104. Hsu H, Crisp A: Outcome of anorexia nervosa. *Lancet* 1:61–65, 1979.
105. Rome E, Ammerman S, Rosen D: Children and adolescents with eating disorders: The state of the art. *Pediatrics* 111:98–108, 2003.
106. Keel P, Mitchell JE: Outcome in anorexia nervosa. *Am J Psychiat* 154:31–321, 1997.
107. Fairburn C and Harrison P: Eating disorders. *Lancet* 361:407–416, 2003.
108. Hebebrand J, Casper R, Treasure T et al.: The need to revise the diagnostic criteria for anorexia nervosa. *J Neuraltransmission* 111:827–840, 2004.
109. Agras S, Brandt H, Bulik C et al.: Report on the National Institutes of Health workshop on overcoming barriers to treatment of research in anorexia nervosa. *Int J Eat Dis* 35:509–521, 2004.

CHAPTER 5.7.3 ■ OBESITY

JOHANNES HEBEBRAND

DEFINITION AND DIAGNOSIS

Overweight is present if body weight adjusted for height exceeds a specified cutoff; obesity implies an excessive fraction of total body weight comprised of fat mass. In theory at least, obesity can only be diagnosed if fat and fat-free mass are determined. Various models and indirect methods for estimation of body composition have been developed, all of which are imperfect and require a number of assumptions, including age-specific considerations. For research purposes, body composition in children has been determined using techniques such as total body water, dual energy X-ray absorptiometry (DEXA), total body electrical conductivity, and total body potassium. By contrast, in clinical studies bioelectrical resistance and skinfold measurements have been employed instead (1).

In clinical practice, however, the BMI, defined as weight in kilograms divided by height in meters squared (kg/m^2), has become widely accepted as the optimal weight-height index throughout childhood and adolescence and as a surrogate measure of adiposity (2). Indeed, the correlations between BMI and percent body fat as determined by DEXA are high (3, 4). Nevertheless, a high fat free mass can, as in the case of some athletic individuals, also entail a high BMI.

The developmental pattern of BMI is similar to that of fat mass. Typically BMI increases steeply during the first 6 months of life primarily due to an increase of fat mass, to then decline until age 6 to 8 years as a result of a strong relative increase in height (Figure 5.7.3.1a,b). The time point during childhood at which BMI again increases has been termed adiposity rebound; the earlier it occurs, the higher the risk of subsequent development of obesity and vice versa (5). BMI rises throughout the

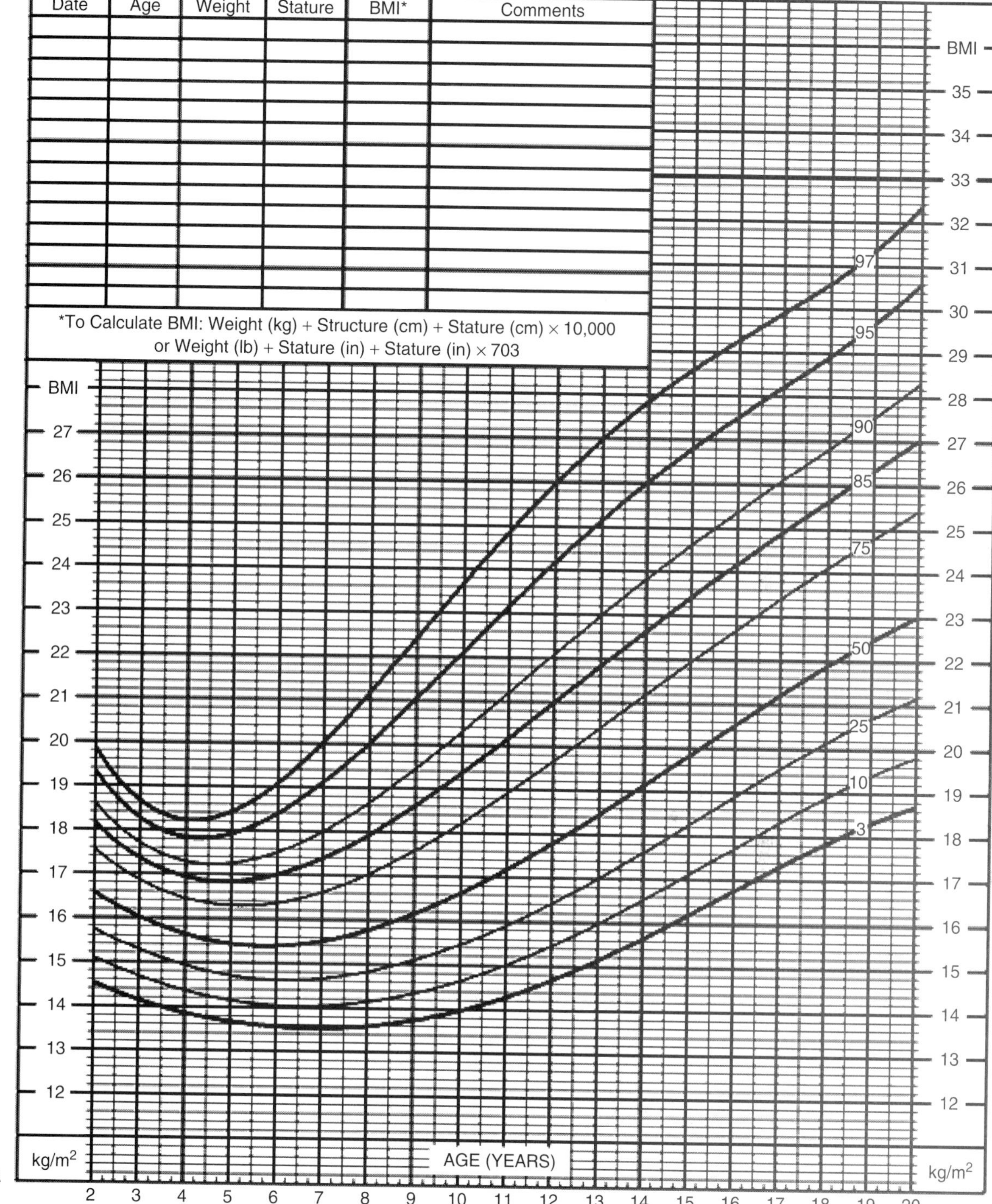

Published May 30, 2000 (modified 10/16/00),
SOURCE: Developed by the National Center for Health Statistics in collaboration with the National Center for Chronic Disease Prevention and Health Promotion (2000).
http://www.cdc.gov/growthcharts

CDC
SAFER • HEALTHIER • PEOPLE™

FIGURE 5.7.3.1. Body mass index-for-age percentiles for boys (A) and girls (B) for the U.S. population (http://www.cdc.gov/growthcharts).

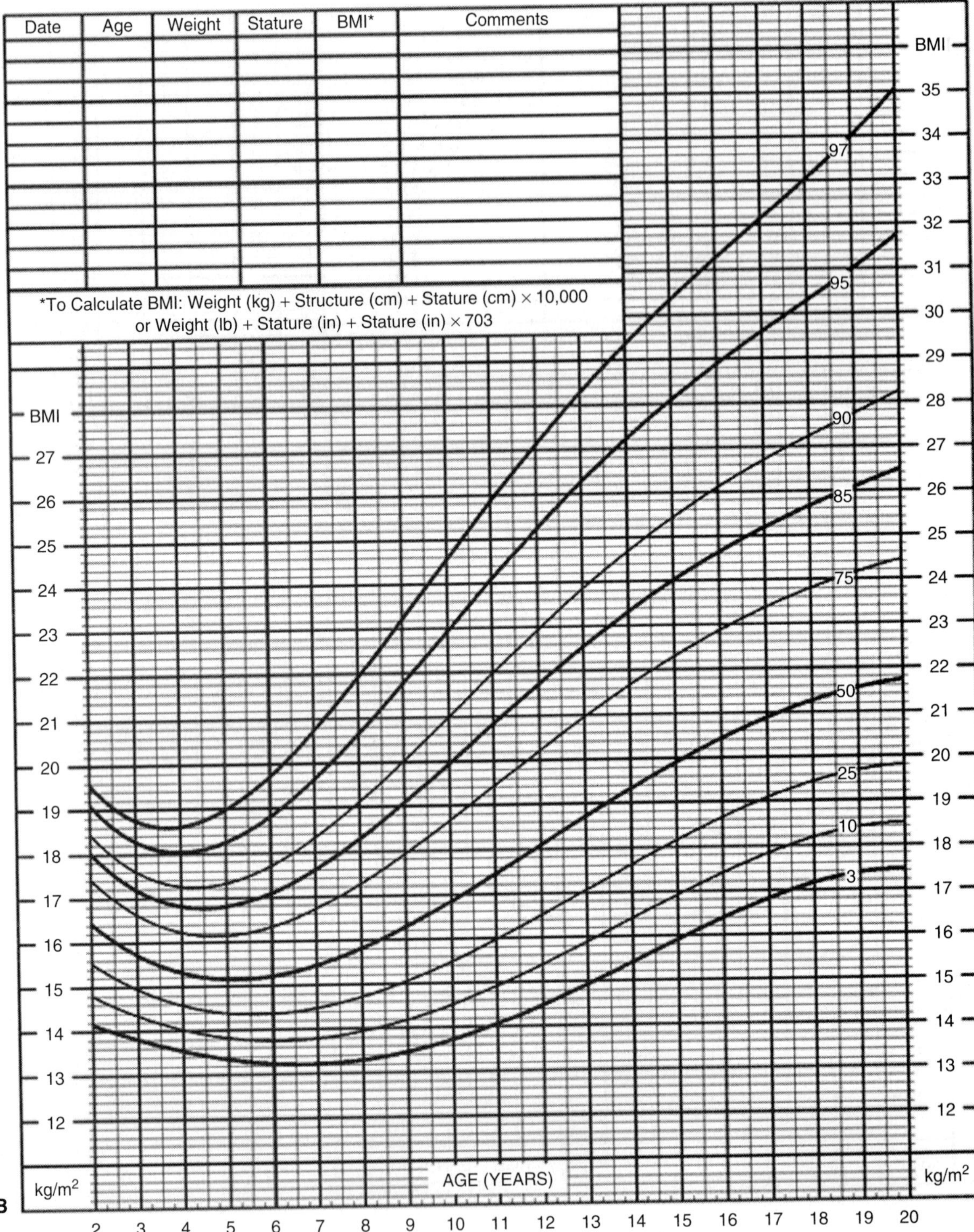

Published May 30, 2000 (modified 10/16/00),
SOURCE: Developed by the National Center for Health Statistics in collaboration with the National Center for Chronic Disease Prevention and Health Promotion (2000).
http://www.cdc.gov/growthcharts

CDC
SAFER • HEALTHIER • PEOPLE™

FIGURE 5.7.3.1. *(Continued)*

rest of childhood and adolescence; this rise continues—albeit more slowly—during adulthood. In males the rise during adolescence is on average largely due to an increase in fat-free mass; percent body fat remains stable at approximately 15 to 18%, whereas in females percent body fat increases from a prepubertal value similar to that of boys to a value of 20 to 25% after puberty (6).

Birth weight is minimally correlated with BMI at age 35 ($r = 0.1$). Accordingly, an overweight infant is only at a minimally elevated risk for obesity in adulthood provided that parental obesity is not present (Figure 5.7.3.2). The greatest variation in rates of weight gain is seen in the first 1 to 2 years of life, when infants may show significant "catch-up" or "catch-down" growth as a consequence of intrauterine restraint or enhancement of fetal growth. By age two, growth usually follows the genetic trajectory (7). Small-for-date babies who rapidly gain weight after birth (catch-up growth) are at an elevated risk for adult obesity and cardiovascular disorders (8). At age 10 BMI is correlated with BMI at age 35 in the magnitude of 0.35; during late adolescence BMI tracks well into adulthood ($r = 0.7$) (9). If a child is obese the risk of persistence into adulthood increases with the degree of adiposity (10), age of the child, and parental obesity (Figure 5.7.3.2).

The strong age dependency of BMI implies that an adequate interpretation of the index of an individual child requires knowledge of the BMI distribution of same aged and sexed children. Frequently, centile curves are based on BMI values of a large and ideally representative sample; older children and parents are readily able to grasp this epidemiological concept as having good face value for educatory purposes. BMI standard deviation scores (BMI-SDS) or Z-scores are commonly employed to further differentiate extreme overweight or underweight (> 99th and < 1st centile).

In adults, overweight, obesity and extreme obesity are diagnosed if BMI is ≥ 25, ≥ 30 and ≥ 40 kg/m^2, respectively; (11) these cutoffs were chosen because they mark increments in risks for complications of elevated BMI. For children and adolescents, however, there is no clear-cut consensus as to what cutoff should be used to define overweight and obesity; all existing definitions are statistically rather than risk-based. Himes and Dietz (12) have suggested use of the 85th and 95th centiles; in other countries the 90th and 97th centiles serve as the respective cutoffs. The 85th and 95th centiles, based on nationally representative data from the 2000 growth curves of the Centers for Disease Control and Prevention (CDC) (13) have been recommended for classification of persons as being overweight or at risk of overweight in the United States (Figure 5.7.3.1a,b; CDC; http://www.cdc.gov/growthcharts). However, these cutoffs are not consistent with those used in adulthood; for example, the centile of an 18-year-old female with a BMI of 30.1 kg/m^2—thus fulfilling the adult criterion for obesity—is below the 95th centile.

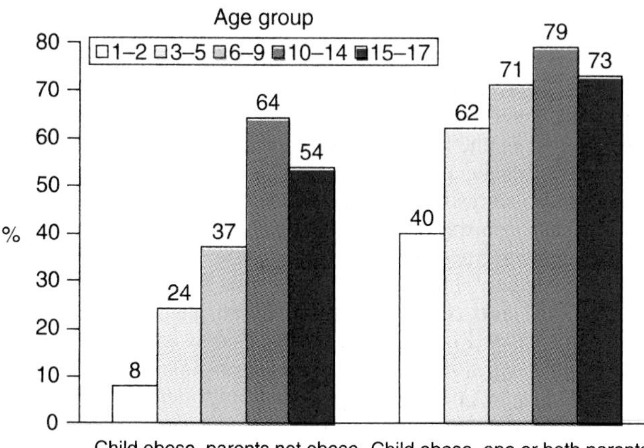

FIGURE 5.7.3.2. Risk of persistence of childhood obesity into adulthood. Obesity in childhood and young adulthood (21–29 years of age) was defined via a BMI ≥85th centile for age and sex and a BMI at or above 27.8 kg/m^2 for men and 27.3 kg/m^2 for women, respectively. (From Whitaker RC, Wright JA, Pepe MS, Seidel KD, Dietz WH: Predicting obesity in young adulthood from childhood and parental obesity. *New England Journal of Medicine*; 337:869–873, 1997.)

Use of specific centiles as cutoffs for the definition of obesity additionally requires a consensus as to the reference population. International comparison of the absolute BMI values constituting centiles in the lower to middle range typically reveals only a slight degree of divergence among different Western countries. However, large differences exist in the upper centile range; BMI values corresponding to the 90th or 97th centile are for example substantially higher in the United States of America in comparison to most European countries. Because of secular trends for both height and weight, centiles based on a formerly representative population-based survey usually do not reflect the true BMI distribution of the current population. For instance, the measurement data used to construct the nationally representative CDC Growth Charts were obtained from a series of national health examination surveys conducted by the National Center for Health Statistics from 1963 to 1994 and from supplemental data sources; more recent data were excluded to avoid an upward shift in the BMI-for-age curves (http://www.cdc.gov.growthcharts; see link *interactive training modules*).

In an attempt to define internationally acceptable centile cutoffs for overweight and obesity, the International Obesity Task Force (IOTF) averaged the national curves from six different countries passing through BMIs of 25 and 30 kg/m^2 at age 18 years (14). It remains to be seen if the cutoffs are adopted sufficiently to indeed reach an international consensus of the definition of childhood obesity.

EPIDEMIOLOGY

Physical growth and development are sensitive indicators of the quality of the psychosocial, economic, and political environment. Child growth in terms of height, weight and body composition are widely used indicators of nutritional and health status for both the individual child and the community (15). Three major secular trends have consistently emerged at the population level in industrialized countries: Mean height and BMI have increased, and mean age at puberty has decreased. Increments in height and decrements in age at menarche can be dated back several decades; the increment in BMI roughly began three decades ago. Both body height and age at menarche have recently reached plateaus in several industrialized countries; within a society the achievement of these plateaus typically occurred first among individuals with a higher socioeconomic status (16). These plateau effects indicate that the full genetic potential has been realized under an advantageous environment, or that social conditions have ceased to improve.

Obesity has only recently reached epidemic proportions in several countries worldwide. Currently, approximately 66%, 31%, and 5% of adults over 20 in the United States are overweight, obese, and extremely obese, respectively; (17) it has been estimated that if the recent secular trend continues unabated, obesity prevalence will reach 50% by 2025. Similar trends have been observed in other countries in Asia, Europe, North and South America (18). However, it should be pointed out that slight increments in mean BMI of a population can translate into substantial elevations of prevalence rates for overweight and obesity.

Children and adolescents have also been affected strongly by this secular trend. The National Health Examination Surveys have revealed a four-fold increase in the prevalence of overweight among children aged 6 to 11 and a three-fold increase for adolescents aged 12 to 19 between the 1960s and the most recent survey, conducted between 1999 and 2002 (17). In the 1999–2002 survey 16% of the children aged 6 through 19 years were overweight as defined via a BMI $\leq$ 95th centile of the surveys in the 1960s. An additional 16% of children were classified as at risk of overweight. In the United States of America, African Americans and Mexican Americans are bearing the brunt of the obesity epidemic (19). Worldwide mean BMI and, as a consequence, prevalence rates for overweight and obesity in children and adolescents have been on the rise in both industrialized and developing countries (20). The most pronounced secular increments in absolute BMI have been detected in the overweight and obese range (21).

A detailed review of the medical consequences of childhood and adolescent obesity is beyond the scope of this chapter (22–24). In brief, cardiovascular disorders including hypertension, type 2 diabetes mellitus, dyslipidemia and metabolic syndrome are becoming increasingly prevalent during adolescence as a consequence of the obesity epidemic [e.g., 25]. Childhood and adolescent obesity has been associated with increased mortality even after adjustment for adult BMI (24). Child and adolescent psychiatrists need to be aware of medical complications associated with obesity, including nocturnal enuresis and sleep apnea, both of which can occur in up to 16% of obese children and adolescents (23). Although far less common, pseudotumor cerebri can occur in young obese subjects.

ETIOLOGY

Obesity is a truly complex disorder that is caused by several genetic and nongenetic risk factors. In historic terms, the etiology of childhood obesity has been perceived differently over the past 100 years; the pendulum has swung from biological to psychological explanations and back. In the early part of the 20th century, pituitary/hypothalamic dysfunction was assumed to underlie obesity (26). From the 1940s through to the 1970s psychological and psychodynamic aspects were thought to play the most prominent role (27, 28). Prader, Labhart and Willi delineated the first syndromal form of obesity in 1956. As of the 1970s the relevance of (psycho)social factors has been discussed (29–32). At the end of the 1980s and 1990s milestone twin and adoption studies substantiated that genetic factors play a prominent role in body weight regulation (33–35). The cloning of the leptin gene in 1994 (36) led to a virtual explosion of biomedical research and marked the introduction of large-scaled molecular genetic studies. The detection of children with leptin deficiency (37) and their successful treatment with recombinant leptin (38) for the first time proved that mutations in a single gene can lead to hyperphagia and obesity in individuals of normal intelligence. The most recent years have viewed a strengthening of the hypothesis that obesity is a neuroendocrine disorder, which results if "obesogenic" environmental factors and a polygenic predisposition act in concert. The genetic predisposition is thought to affect both metabolic and behavioral features. Both public and scientific interest in obesity has witnessed an unparalleled boom over the past 20 years, reflecting the obesity epidemic, the discovery of novel pathways involved in body weight regulation, greater health concerns, the perception of social inequality, and a stronger awareness of the societal norms for body weight.

Genetic Factors

There is a general consensus that parental obesity is by far the strongest risk factor for childhood and adolescent obesity. The risk is influenced by the degree of parental obesity (39) and is further elevated if both parents are obese (Table 5.7.3.1) (40). Several studies have found a stronger effect of maternal than paternal obesity (41). Formal genetic studies have led to the conclusion that the strong predictive value of parental BMI mainly stems from genetic rather than environmental factors (42). Accordingly, older studies that failed to include parental weight as a variable are seriously flawed. For example, the well known finding that parental neglect during childhood predicts obesity in young adulthood (30) was not controlled for parental obesity.

Twin studies (42, 43) have produced the most consistent and highest heritability estimates, in the range of 0.6 to 0.9 for BMI. These high estimates apply to twins reared both together and apart. However, only single and comparatively small studies exist for twins reared apart, in contrast to the vast amount of studies pertaining to twins reared together, some of which included thousands of twin pairs; in addition, a substantial number of reared apart twin pairs were not separated immediately after birth.

Except for the newborn period, for which a lower heritability of 0.4 has been calculated (44), age does not affect heritability estimates of body weight to a substantial degree. The influence of the intrauterine environment on birth weight is strong; it is well known that particularly in monozygotic (MZ) twins other anthropometric measurements, such as body height, also correlate less well in infancy than in childhood. The feto-fetal transfusion syndrome observed only in MZ twins contributes to this phenomenon, as it substantially reduces the effect of genetic factors at birth and during infancy. Genetic factors are subsequently able to exert their influence; in school-age children high heritability of BMI already applies. Possibly, the heritability of BMI is maximal (≈ 0.9) during late childhood and adolescence (45).

Adoption and family studies have mostly derived considerably lower heritability estimates of 0.25 to 0.7 (42, 46). Twin studies have the advantage of a better control for age effects on BMI and are more valid if nonadditive genetic factors play a larger role in body weight regulation. For an adequate interpretation of the heritability estimates it is noteworthy to point out that both direct and indirect genetic effects are subsumed under the genetic component. If for example both infant twins of a MZ pair are frequently irritable due to a biologically driven hunger (direct genetic effect), frequent feedings by the caretaker ensue (indirect genetic effect); even if the twins are separated at birth, the respective caretakers can be expected to respond similarly.

Another interesting and important aspect of formal genetic studies has been the observation that nonshared environment explains considerably more variance of the quantitative phenotype (BMI) than shared environment. In the large twin study of Stunkard and coworkers (35), which encompassed adult twin pairs reared together or apart, shared environment did not explain variance at all; instead nonshared environment totally explained the environmental component, estimated at 30%. Accordingly, only genetic factors would account for a familial loading with obesity. However, more recent studies indicate that the shared environment might play a more substantial role after all (46); past research may have underestimated common environmental effects on BMI because the designs lacked the power or ability to detect them. Finally, the environment of modern-day societies (easy access to a large variety of cheap and tasty foods, a lifestyle promoting physical inactivity) is quite similar for basically all children, irrespective of the family in which they grow up.

TABLE 5.7.3.1

ASSOCIATION OF RISK FACTORS AND OBESITY AT AGE 7 YEARS. THE AVON LONGITUDINAL STUDY OF PARENTS AND CHILDREN, USING MULTIVARIABLE BINARY LOGISTIC REGRESSION MODELS. OBESITY WAS DEFINED AS A BMI ≥95TH CENTILE RELATIVE TO THE 1990 BRITISH REFERENCE POPULATION

Risk Factor	Prevalence (%) of Childhood Obesity (n = 7,758)	Final Model Adjusted Odds Ratio (95% Confidence Interval; n = 5,493)*
Birth weight, continuous (100 g increments)	8.4	1.05 (1.03–1.07)
Maternal smoking during pregnancy		
None	7.5	1.00
1–9	11.5	1.76 (1.21–2.52)
10–19	11.3	1.59 (1.08–2.34)
≥20	13.8	1.80 (1.01–3.39)
Parental obesity		
Both parents: <30 kg/m^2	6.2	1.00
Father >30	16.2	2.54 (1.72–3.75)
Mother >30	23.6	4.25 (2.86–6.32)
Both parents >30	43.8	10.44 (5.11–21.32)
Time spent watching TV (hours per week)		
≤4	5.2	1.00
4.1–8	8.3	1.37 (1.02–1.83)
>8	10.3	1.55 (1.13–2.12)
Duration of night time sleep (hours)		
First quartile	10.3	1.45 (1.10–1.89)
Second quartile	8.8	1.35 (1.02–1.79)
Third quartile	6.4	1.04 (0.76–1.42)
Fourth quartile	6.8	1.00

*Odds ratio is adjusted for maternal education, energy intake at 3 years and sex; all listed variables significant at the p <0.01 level.
Nonsignificant variables: infant feeding (breast feeding, age at introduction of solids), dietary patterns (junk food, healthy food, traditional, fussy).
Variables that did not enter the model: Parity, season of birth, gestational age, number of fetuses, number of siblings, ethnicity of child, age of mother at delivery, time in car per day. (From Reilly JJ, Armstrong J, Dorosty AR, Emmett PM, Ness A, Rogers I, Steer C, Sherriff A, *Avon Longitudinal Study of Parents and Children Study Team: Early life risk factors for obesity in childhood*: Cohort study. BMJ 330:1357, 2005.)

The complexity of the genetic basis of obesity applies both from a metabolic and behavioral perspective (46): Behavioral genetic research has convincingly demonstrated that approximately 50% of the variance of diverse complex quantitative behaviors is genetically determined (47). Both macronutrient intake (48) and activity levels (49) have been shown to be genetically codetermined. Restrained eating, drive for thinness, and other eating behaviors show heritability estimates in the range of 20 to 55% (46). It appears that television viewing may have a heritable component, albeit a small one (50).

Because the gene pool of a population cannot have changed within the past generation, environmental changes affecting both energy intake and expenditure are assumed to underlie the obesity epidemic (18). These changes are presumed to have a major impact because according to the thrifty genotype hypothesis (51) many common genotypes render humans obesity prone: Gene variants facilitating energy deposition as fat have accumulated over time in different species to enhance survival during periods of famine. Put simplistically, "the genetic background loads the gun, but the environment pulls the trigger" (52).

A small genetic contribution to the obesity epidemic cannot be dismissed. For one, overweight females have more children (53). Secondly, the recent rise of social stigmatization of obese individuals (see following) might actually have led to an increase of assortative mating (43). This mechanism could conceivably contribute to epidemic obesity, particularly by affecting the uppermost tail of the BMI distribution via both genetic and environmental factors.

Epigenetic phenomena have also been invoked to contribute to the obesity epidemic. Indeed, it is conceivable that modern-day living might affect methylation patterns of specific genes, which in turn increase the risk of obesity. In line with these considerations young monozygous twins are epigenetically indistinguishable from each other during the early years of life, whereas remarkable differences in their overall content and genomic distribution of 5-methylcytosine DNA and histone acetylation with an effect on gene-expression become evident with increasing age (54). Such environmentally induced changes could have an influence on BMI.

Over the past 10 years mutations in the genes for leptin, leptin receptor, prohormone convertase 1 (PC1), and pro-opiomelanocortin (POMC) (46, 55) have been shown to lead to autosomal recessive forms of obesity in humans. All of the mutations are rare and lead to early onset extreme obesity induced by an increased energy intake. Each of these mutations leads to additional phenotypical manifestations, including adrenal insufficiency (POMC), red hair (POMC), reduced or impaired fertility (PC1, leptin and leptin receptor) and impaired immunity (leptin gene). Whereas they seemingly do not affect intelligence, the pleiotropic effects warrant the consideration that these recessive disorders are classified as syndromal forms of obesity—similar to the Bardet-Biedl, Prader-Willi and other genetic syndromes associated with reduced intelligence. The pleiotropic Bardet-Biedel syndrome, of which obesity is a feature, has been shown to have an oligogenic basis (55).

As of 1998, over 60 functionally relevant mutations have been detected in the melanocortin-4 receptor gene (*MC4R*) (46), which result in a codominantly inherited form of obesity; 2–4% of extremely obese children and adolescents harbor such mutations. Relevant mutations lead to a reduced or total loss of function; the endogenous ligand alpha-melanocyte–stimulating hormone is not able to induce its satiating effect. Adult male and female mutation carriers are 15 and 30 kg heavier than their sex matched wildtype relatives (56); estimates for children are not available. The effect sizes of these mutations are lower than those of the leptin or leptin receptor gene mutations. Phenotypical effects of *MC4R* mutations other than obesity have been shown to encompass hyperinsulinemia, elevated growth rate and higher bone density (57). Whether or not these mutations induce binge eating is viewed controversially (58–60). Children with *MC4R* mutations have been shown to eat more at a test meal than obese controls (57).

A large number of association and linkage studies have been performed in "normal" obesity (46). Whereas many associations have been reported, it is largely unclear which of these represent truly positive findings. Presumably, the power of many of these studies is too low to detect minor genes; false positive findings can result from not correcting for multiple testing. Over 30 genome linkage scans pertaining to obesity and related phenotypes have been performed; as yet unequivocal evidence for the contribution of a specific gene to one of these peaks has not been provided.

Presumably, the effect sizes of most gene variants predisposing to obesity are quite small (polygenic inheritance). Interestingly, the V103I polymorphism in the MC4R, which occurs in 2–7% of individuals of different populations, is associated with a reduced body weight (61, 62). Adult carriers are on average 0.5 kg/m^2 less heavy than wildtype carriers; the variant also exerts an as yet unquantified small effect in children. To identify and confirm gene variants with minor effect sizes, several thousands of probands need to be assessed.

Genetic, biological, physiological, and pharmacological research over the past 15 years has tremendously broadened our understanding of the mechanisms involved in body weight regulation. It has become evident that body weight is tightly regulated via both peripheral and central mechanisms; numerous hormones including leptin and ghrelin, anorexigenic, orexigenic neuropeptides, their respective receptors and intracellular signalling pathways underlie this regulation (63, 64). One of the main functions of these pathways is to enable adaptation to semistarvation.

Environmental Factors

Secular changes in both energy intake and expenditure are assumed to underlie the obesity epidemic (18). However, attempts to pinpoint unequivocally the relevant mechanisms even within a single country or society have been largely futile. For example, the relationship between TV viewing and obesity has been studied repeatedly in cross-sectional studies (Table 5.7.3.1). Several, but by no means all, studies have shown a clearcut association; however, only two longitudinal studies have been performed which allow a causal inference. Gortmaker et al. (65) observed a dose-dependent effect of the daily hours spent watching TV on obesity rates; a five-fold higher rate applied to those children and adolescents who watched TV for more than 5 hours per day as compared to those who watched less than 2 hours. Over the 4-year study period 60% of the obesity incidence was attributed to watching TV. More recently, a longitudinal study of 980 children followed up biannually from age 3 to 15 and at ages 21 and 26 revealed that the population attributable fraction for overweight at age 26 due to viewing between ages 5 and 15 was 17% after adjustment for potential confounders (66).

Inactivity is prominent among children and adolescents of industrialized countries. According to a recent Scottish study (67) mean time spent in sedentary behavior was 79% and 76% of monitored hours of children at ages 3 and 5, respectively. Children spent only 2% of their time pursuing moderate to vigorous activity. According to a representative survey conducted in 2002, 61.5% of U.S. children aged 9–13 did not participate in any organized physical activity during nonschool hours (CDC, 2003). Overweight and obesity are associated with a poorer body gross motor development and endurance performance (68). Comparisons of motor skills, such as a 6-minute-long run, a 50-meter sprint and the number of pushups within 30 seconds using the same test procedure in German children, who were 10 years old in 1976 and 1996, revealed a significantly poorer performance in the later study group (69).

Dietary changes including increased energy intake and portion sizes (70, 71), elevations in fat and/or carbohydrate intake (72), reduced intake of fruits and vegetables, and increased consumption of soft drinks (73) have all been implicated in the obesity epidemic. Consumer trends and food marketing strategies, including advertisement, have also been deemed important (74–76). Most of these factors are viewed controversially, and unequivocal data casually linking the obesity epidemic to any one of these factors are virtually absent.

Maternal smoking during pregnancy is associated with an increased risk of childhood obesity (Table 5.7.3.1) (40, 77). A minor protective effect of breast feeding has been observed repeatedly, which according to some studies is still detectable in adolescence (78). However, as yet undetected confounding variables cannot be excluded as underlying the associations (79). Cross-sectional studies have revealed that a shorter duration of sleep is associated with obesity during childhood (40, 80) and adulthood (81). In adults with a short sleep duration, serum levels of the anorexigenic hormone leptin were reduced, whereas those of the orexigenic hormone ghrelin were elevated, thus suggesting a mechanism for the elevated BMI (81).

Psychological and Behavioral Factors

Recently, longitudinal studies have revealed a predictive value of depressive symptoms in childhood and adolescence for obesity in later childhood, adolescence and adulthood (82–87); these findings remained stable after adjustment for potential confounders. Whereas both design and results of these studies differed, the findings linking depression to subsequent weight gain are remarkably consistent. In their large study encompassing 9,374 adolescents in grades 7 through 9, depressed mood assessed with a depression scale was not related to baseline BMI (85). The odds ratio for obesity at the 1-year followup for those with a depressed mood was 2.05 (95% CI: 1.04–4.06) after controlling for BMI at baseline, age, race, gender, parental obesity, number of parents in the home, socioeconomic status, smoking, physical activity, conduct disorder, self-esteem and delinquent behavior. Causality is implied by the fact that the duration of depression between childhood and adulthood also emerged as a predictor of adult BMI (84); even among the children with obesity at baseline the depression scale score predicted BMI 1 year later (85). These studies suggest that rates of obesity can potentially be reduced by successful treatment of depression in children and adolescents.

Other psychological and behavioral variables have been associated with subsequent weight gain. Self-reported dietary restraint, radical weight-control behaviors, and perceived parental obesity—but not high-fat food consumption, binge eating, or exercise frequency—predicted obesity onset among 496 11–15 year old girls, who were followed up after 4 years (87). Parental overcontrol of children's feeding behavior, particularly for those at high risk of developing overweight, may lead to overweight (88). However, a large study based on almost 800 third-grade children revealed that counter to the hypothesis, parental control over children's intake was inversely associated with overweight in girls. No relationship between parental control of children's intake and their children's degree of overweight was found in boys (89).

Medications

Several different kinds of medication can induce weight gain; for psychiatrists it is important to realize this side effect is particularly common and potentially prominent with atypical antipsychotics, lithium and valproate (90, 91). In adults, clozapine and olanzapine have been associated with the greatest weight gain, the individual extent of which is apparently genetically codetermined (92). In children and adolescents, weight gain, obesity, and related metabolic complications can ensue upon use of atypical neuroleptics (92–95). Overeating and in some cases binge eating attacks have been observed in adolescent patients receiving clozapine or olanzapine (93, 96).

PSYCHOLOGICAL AND PSYCHIATRIC ASPECTS OF OBESE CHILDREN

The quality of life of obese children and adolescents is reduced. 106 children and adolescents (age range 5–18) with a mean BMI of 34.7 ± 9.3 kg/m^2 scored 67 ± 16.3 in comparison to 83 ± 14.8 for controls on a pediatric quality of life (QOL) inventory (range 0–100). The cases were more likely (odds ratio 5.5) to have impaired health-related QOL; the mean value was similar to that of young cancer patients (97).

Stigmatization of obese children and adolescents is a common event. Fifth and sixth graders who ranked six drawings of same-sexed children with obesity, various physical disabilities, or no disabilities ("healthy") in 1961 and 2001 liked the drawing of the obese child least at both time periods; in 2001 the obese child was rated even lower than in 1961, suggesting an increase in stigmatization over this 40-year period (98).

Self-esteem specific to physical appearance has been shown to be inversely associated with BMI in both male and female adolescents. The magnitude of the association, however, was modest. Low self-esteem did not predict the development of obesity over time (99). In an independent study of clinically ascertained obese children and adolescents, self-esteem and depression were inversely related (100).

Single studies have assessed psychiatric symptomatology in obese children and adolescents using both dimensional and categorical diagnostic evaluations. For an appropriate understanding of the respective results it is crucial to distinguish between clinical and population-based samples. Furthermore, differences in age, gender, the severity of obesity, psychiatric classification schemes (DSM vs. ICD), interviews, questionnaires, and rating scales need to be taken into account.

In clinical samples, i.e., among children and adolescents who seek weight reduction, higher rates of anxiety and mood disorders have repeatedly been reported (101, 102). In a clinical study encompassing 54 children and adolescents with a mean age of 12.1 years who participated in a weight management program, 32% of the study group fell in the depressed group as defined by a score of ≥ 13 on the Children's Depression Inventory (CDI) (100); within the study group no correlation was found between CDI score and BMI. 42.6% of the participants were classified as mildly obese ($20 < \text{BMI} < 30$ kg/m^2), 44.4% as moderately obese ($30 < \text{BMI} < 39$ kg/m^2) and 13% as severely obese (BMI >40 kg/m^2). In a clinical study group of 47 (30 female) extremely obese adolescents with a mean BMI of 42.4 kg/m^2 only 14 (29.8%) did not receive a lifetime DSM-IV diagnosis; 16 (34%) fulfilled criteria for three or more diagnoses (101). Lifetime rates for mood, anxiety, substance abuse/dependence, somatoform, and eating disorders were 42.6%, 40.4%, 36.2%, 14.9%, and 17.0%, respectively. Most of these patients retrospectively predated their obesity to the development of their psychiatric disorders.

In contrast, epidemiologically based studies have not revealed an elevated rate of psychopathology in obese children and adolescents. For example, 393 tenth grade female adolescents (mean age: 15.8 ± 0.3 years) revealed no differences in anxiety (State-Trait Anxiety Inventory) and depression (Children's Depression Inventory) between underweight, average and overweight females (103). The 47 most obese adolescents (mean BMI of 29.8 kg/m^2) out of a representative sample of 1,655 adolescents did not show elevated rates of psychiatric disorders (101). These 47 adolescents formed a subgroup of 3,021 German subjects aged 14 to 21 in whom obesity was also not associated with increased rates of psychiatric disorders (104).

Both childhood and parental obesity are risk factors for bulimia nervosa (105); in contrast, overweight and obesity are not a risk factor for anorexia nervosa; (106) furthermore, patients with anorexia nervosa only rarely become obese after recovery (107). Approximately 2% of 6-year-old children show binge eating, which at this age is already associated with obesity (108). Clinically relevant binge eating is common among obese adolescents seeking weight reduction; however, only a subgroup fulfills the DSM-IV research criteria for binge eating disorder (101, 109).

The elevated rates of psychopathology of obese children and adolescents seeking weight reduction are reminiscent of findings in adults (110). Alternatively, or additionally, treatment-seeking young obese patients might have higher BMIs than obese children and adolescents detected in school or population-based surveys (101). A very large population-based sample would for instance be required to ascertain a sufficient number of adolescents with a BMI ≥ 40 kg/m^2. Irrespective of these considerations, current data imply that psychiatric screening of obese children and adolescents seeking weight reduction, and of young subjects with extreme obesity, should be part of their diagnostic assessment.

PREVENTION AND TREATMENT

Despite the fact that obesity has a strong behavioral component, the field of child and adolescent psychiatry/psychology has only recently begun to view obesity as a behavioral disorder on its own; the inclusion of a stand-alone chapter on obesity in this textbook illustrates this change. Based on 1) the recent identification of depression in the development of obesity (see earlier), 2) the frequent comorbid psychiatric disorders in young subjects seeking weight loss, and 3) our tradition and expertise in the management of behavioral disorders, including motivational aspects, we strongly support a more prominent role for child and adolescent psychiatry in the prevention and treatment of obesity. Finally, because the central pathways relevant in weight regulation overlap with pathways involved in regulation of stress, mood, and anxiety, psychiatric expertise is required to adequately address potential effects and side effects of centrally active antiobesity drugs.

In light of the obesity epidemic and its dire health consequences the need for successful programs for treatment of childhood and adolescent obesity is immense. Age, degree of adiposity, and length of followup are crucial variables for an adequate interpretation of the results of treatment studies; potential side effects require close monitoring. Furthermore, the degree of interference with everyday life of a child and its family needs to be considered.

Expectations of the young subjects and their parents should be realistic. In contrast to adults, a growing child can achieve a BMI reduction by maintaining weight; a reduction in SDS or z-scores for BMI can be accomplished even if BMI increases over time. Such progress frequently does not fulfill the expectations of children and adolescents with obesity, who wish to lose substantial amounts of weight. Children and their parents need to learn that treatment effects are usually rather small and that ongoing efforts are required to prevent further or renewed weight gain. Some physicians require that children and adolescents participate in a sports group prior to their admittance to a treatment program; (111) dropout during the treatment program can thus be reduced. Motivation is of paramount importance; treatment of unmotivated and uninformed subjects and their parents frequently results in frustration.

Currently, routine screening and interventions for overweight children and adolescents are viewed as controversial by physicians and public health experts (2, 112–115). Some experts have advocated specific recommendations (2, 114, 115) which pertain to screening, treatment, and prevention; political measures to counter the "obesogenic" environment are frequently called upon (Table 5.7.3.2). However, other experts conclude that interventions in clinical settings have not been shown to have clinically significant benefits and are not widely available (113). Evidence of effectiveness was deemed insufficient to recommend for or against routine screening for overweight in children and adolescents as a means to prevent adverse health outcomes (112). The evidence for the effectiveness of behavioral counseling or other preventive interventions that can be conducted in primary care settings has been deemed insufficient.

In line with these latter experts, many physicians are skeptical of behaviorally oriented treatment programs. Some believe that the development of novel antiobesity drugs represents the only effective strategy. Indeed, from a psychiatric point of view a comparison with attention deficit/hyperactivity disorder is of interest, for the treatment of which (long-term) medications are considerably more effective than psychotherapy (116). Others favor political measures to combat the obesity epidemic (see following).

In the following sections we briefly review lifestyle, pharmacological, and surgical interventions.

Lifestyle Interventions

As of today, only a very limited number of randomized controlled trials (RCT) of lifestyle interventions have been completed (117). In their Cochrane analysis based on 18 RCTs with 975 participants aged < 18 years, Summerbell et al. concluded that the respective studies were very small and included only homogeneous motivated groups in hospital settings. As such, generalizable evidence was limited and no direct conclusions for treatment of childhood obesity could be drawn. The studies had focused on changes in physical activity and sedentary behavior (n = 5), problemsolving with usual care versus behavioral therapy (n = 2), behavioral therapy at varying degrees of family involvement versus no treatment, usual care or mastery criteria and contingent reinforcement (n = 9), and cognitive behavioral therapy versus relaxation (n = 2).

The most recent RCTs have focused on changing dietary habits (118), gym class (119), dietary habits, and physical activity levels (120). According to Van Horn et al. (118)

TABLE 5.7.3.2

RECOMMENDATIONS FOR PREVENTION OF PEDIATRIC OBESITY ACCORDING TO THE AMERICAN ACADEMY OF PEDIATRICS COMMITTEE ON NUTRITION

1. Health supervision
   a. Identify and track patients at risk by virtue of family history, birth weight, or socioeconomic, ethnic, cultural, or environmental factors.
   b. Calculate and plot BMI once a year in all children and adolescents.
   c. Use change in BMI to identify rate of excessive weight gain relative to linear growth.
   d. Encourage, support, and protect breastfeeding.
   e. Encourage parents and caregivers to promote healthy eating patterns by offering nutritious snacks, such as vegetables and fruits, low-fat dairy foods, and whole grains; encouraging children's autonomy in self-regulation of food intake and setting appropriate limits on choices; and modeling healthy food choices.
   f. Routinely promote physical activity, including unstructured play at home, in school, in childcare settings, and throughout the community.
   g. Recommend limitation of television and video time to a maximum of 2 hours per day.
   h. Recognize and monitor changes in obesity-associated risk factors for adult chronic disease, such as hypertension, dyslipidemia, hyperinsulinemia, impaired glucose tolerance, and symptoms of obstructive sleep apnea syndrome.
2. Advocacy
   a. Help parents, teachers, coaches, and others who influence youth to discuss health habits, not body habitus, as part of their efforts to control overweight and obesity.
   b. Enlist policy makers from local, state, and national organizations and schools to support a healthful lifestyle for all children, including proper diet and adequate opportunity for regular physical activity.
   c. Encourage organizations that are responsible for health care and health care financing to provide coverage for effective obesity prevention and treatment strategies.
   d. Encourage public and private sources to direct funding toward research into effective strategies to prevent overweight and obesity and to maximize limited family and community resources to achieve healthful outcomes for youth.
   e. Support and advocate for social marketing intended to promote healthful food choices and increased physical activity.

(From Krebs NF, Jacobson MS, American Academy of Pediatrics Committee on Nutrition. Prevention of pediatric overweight and obesity. *Pediatrics* 112:424–430, 2003.)

the intervention group showed positive changes of intake of dairy foods, desserts, and fats/oils, but intake of fruits and vegetables was low in both the intervention and the control groups (118). In addition, despite the intervention snacks, desserts, and pizza still contributed heavily to the diet. Carrel et al. (119) randomized 50 overweight middle-school children with a BMI >95th percentile to lifestyle-focused, fitness-oriented gym classes (cases) or standard gym classes (controls) for 9 months. Cases showed greater loss of body fat, increase in cardiovascular fitness, and improvement in fasting insulin levels than controls. A 3-month, combined dietary-behavioral-physical activity intervention (24 cases, 22 controls) resulted in a lower BMI at both 3 and 12 months after the intervention. Leisure-time physical activity increased significantly among the intervention participants, compared with a decrease among the control subjects. It appears that treatment directed at the parents of children in the age range of 7 to 12 years can be more effective than targeting the child. Random assignment of the intervention in 60 obese young patients to a parent-only group and child-only group resulted in a better outcome at the 7-year followup in the parent-only group (121).

122 children and adolescents with a mean age of 12.7 and a mean BMI of 32.5 kg/m^2 on average lost 49% of their body weight during a 10-month-long inpatient treatment program (122). At the 14-month followup average weight loss was still 39%. In a second inpatient program, 40 consecutively admitted adolescents with a mean age and BMI of 14.2 years and 39.7 kg/m^2 achieved a mean BMI of 31.3 kg/m^2 upon discharge from an on average 6-month-long inpatient program; 12 months later their mean BMI was 40.1 kg/m^2 (Mieg et al., unpublished data).

In many conventional treatment studies the assessment of potential medium and long-term side effects is ignored. Frequently, data only on successful completers are presented (percentage of subjects who have lost 5% or 10% of their body weight) at the end of a relatively short treatment episode. However, treatment of children and adolescents should entail that data on adverse outcomes be reported in detail; Obviously medium- and long-term followups should be attempted. Conventional obesity treatment can result in transient curtailment of height growth velocity (123). Sensible weight loss practices do not entail an elevated risk for the development of eating disorders (124). Dieting has been associated with increased weight gain (125, 126). Thus, dieting frequency was predictive of larger relative weight change during 3 years of followup in the prospective study of Field and coworkers (126); even after statistical adjustment for age, Tanner stage of development, and age-specific *z* score of BMI in the previous year, the effect of dieting on weight gain remained significant. The investigators discussed a dieting-induced increase in metabolic efficiency, intermittent bouts of overeating and binge eating and/or metabolic effects of a carbohydrate-rich diet as underlying mechanisms. Alternatively, the weight gain associated with dieting may be because restrictive diets are rarely maintained for an extended period of time. If adolescents engage in unhealthy dieting behaviors, such as vomiting, use of laxatives, diuretics, and diet pills, they are at an increased risk of a host of other problematic behaviors, including alcohol, nicotine and marijuana use, risky sexual contacts, delinquency, and suicide attempts (127).

Elevated mortality rates have been associated with weight cycling in adults (128, 129). However, this association has been attributed to disadvantageous lifestyle factors and preexisting disease. Wannamethee et al. (129) conclude that weight loss and weight fluctuation (cycling) do not directly increase the risk of death. In a recent study (130), intentional weight loss was linked to increased mortality: Compared with a group not intending to lose and able to maintain stable weight, the hazard ratios (with 95% confidence intervals) in the group intending to lose weight were 0.84 (0.49–1.48) for those with stable weight, 1.86 (1.22–2.87) for those losing weight, and 0.93 (0.55–1.56) for those gaining weight. The authors concluded that deliberate weight loss in overweight individuals without known comorbidities may be hazardous in the long term. Obviously, the health effects of weight loss are complex and need more research. This particularly holds true for children and adolescents.

Pharmacological Interventions

RCTs in adolescents exist for the two current major antiobesity drugs sibutramine (131, 132) and orlistat (133). The centrally active norepinephrine reuptake inhibitor sibutramine in combination with behavior therapy resulted in a 8.5% BMI reduction 6 months after initiation of treatment as compared to 4% in controls who received placebo and behavior therapy (132). Sibutramine had to be reduced or discontinued in a substantial number of adolescents to manage increases in blood pressure, pulse rate, or other symptoms. In the second double-blind RCT of sibutramine (131) adverse effects leading to withdrawal were not observed; pulse and blood pressure were similar in cases and controls; no echocardiographic abnormalities were detected. In this trial, all patients initially received placebo and a hypocaloric diet plus exercise orientation during the first month. For the next 6 months, participants received either sibutramine or placebo. The mean body mass index reduction was significantly greater in the sibutramine group (3.6 ± 2.5 kg/m^2) than in the placebo group (0.9 ± 0.9 kg/m^2). Orlistat is a lipase inhibitor and suppresses the breakdown of triglycerides in the intestine. A year-long double-blind RCT of 539 obese adolescents revealed that BMI reduction in the orlistat group was greater than in the control group (−0.55 versus 0.31 kg/m^2). Mild to moderate gastrointestinal tract adverse events (e.g., steatorrhea) occurred in 9% to 50% of the orlistat group and in 1% to 13% of the placebo group (133).

In conclusion, for the time being drug treatment of adolescent obesity is at an experimental stage only; only off-label prescription of the currently available antiobesity drugs is possible. Clearly, further safety and efficacy data are required. Because the upcoming years will witness the introduction of novel antiobesity drugs in adults, further RCTs in adolescents are to be expected. Irrespective of the type of drug, long-term treatment will most likely be required, if the weight loss is to be maintained. Safety issues are thus pertinent.

Surgical Interventions

Bariatric surgery is increasingly being performed on extremely obese adolescents (BMI >40 kg/m^2) who have not been able to lose weight through conventional treatment. Nevertheless, use of surgery must be viewed as experimental (134, 135). To avoid adverse physical and psychosocial outcomes, the application of the principles of growth and development is essential; generally, bariatric surgery should not be applied to girls and boys younger than 13 and 15 years, respectively. The decisional capacity of the patient, family structure, and barriers to adherence must be considered. Multidisciplinary programs should meet the guidelines for surgical treatment outlined by the American Society of Bariatric Surgery and should ensure optimal preoperative decisionmaking and postoperative management and long-term followup. Laparoscopic Roux-en-Y gastric bypass is a promising procedure, which justifies a clinical trial to confirm the safety and efficacy of bariatric surgery in the adolescent population. Obviously, treatment centers need to collect long-term data on the clinical outcomes of young bariatric patients.

Prevention

22 prevention studies were included in the recent Cochrane analysis by Summerbell and coworkers (117), thus indicating an improvement of the scientific basis in comparison to only seven studies that were included in the 2001 analysis (136). Of the 22 studies, less than half lasted for at least one year. 19 were school/preschool-based interventions, one was a community-based intervention targeting low-income families, and two were family-based interventions targeting nonobese children of obese or overweight parents. Six of the 10 long-term studies combined dietary education and physical activity interventions; five resulted in no difference in overweight status between groups; and one resulted in improvements for girls receiving the intervention, but not boys. Two studies focused on physical activity alone. Of these, a multimedia approach appeared to be effective in preventing obesity. Two studies focused on nutrition education alone; both were ineffective in preventing obesity. Of the 12 short-term studies 10 did not have a significant impact on obesity prevention. Two of the four studies that focused on interventions to increase physical activity levels resulted in minor reductions in overweight status in favor of the intervention. Nearly all of the 22 studies resulted in some improvement in diet or physical activity.

Whereas only 15 to 30% of the modern population is obese, prevention programs affect everyone. Societies in many countries worldwide will need to determine if and how prevention programs should be initiated. Children are particularly affected by the obesity epidemic; as a result their health is compromised early in life. The environment for children has become unfavorable. Recent research indicates that within the context of our current obesogenic environment, an obesity prone individual stands only a limited chance of avoiding a body weight in the upper range. The high socioeconomic costs of obesity have become evident. Even small reductions in mean BMI of a population translate into large effects in terms of obesity prevalence rates. On the other hand, we are seemingly resistant to lifestyle changes; we are incapable of or reluctant to give up our relative physical inactivity and overeating.

It seems that structural changes involving political action are required if we indeed want to stem the rising tide. The first step is to educate society that such changes are necessary to achieve this objective. In parallel we need to debate if we as a society are willing indeed to tackle the obesity epidemic. Despite the fact that overweight directly affects "only" 50% of the population, prevention entails that potentially every member of a society is involved. Preventive measures could require that we for instance impose regulations on the food industry, systematically curtail television viewing, and/or walk instead of taking the car for short distances. Such changes may sound trivial, but their enforcement would exert a dramatic effect on our norms and in particular of our perception of self-responsibility. Because from a scientific point of view we cannot in advance estimate the effect of the introduction of such changes on obesity rates, the necessity to reach a societal consensus is all the more important.

References

1. Goran MI: Measurement issues related to studies of childhood obesity: Assessment of body composition, body fat distribution, physical activity and food intake. *Pediatrics* 101:505–518, 1998.
2. Barlow SE, Dietz WH: Obesity evaluation and treatment: Expert committee recommendations. *Pediatrics* 102:E29, 1998.
3. Mei Z, Grummer-Strawn LM, Pietrobelli A, Goulding A, Goran MI, Dietz WH: Validity of body mass index compared with other body-composition screening indexes for the assessment of body fatness in children and adolescents. *Am J Clin Nutr* 75:978–985, 2002.
4. Dietz WH, Robinson TN: Use of the body mass index (BMI) as a measure of overweight in children and adolescents: Periods of risk in childhood for the development of adult obesity—What do we need to learn? *J Pediatr* 132:191–193, 1998.
5. Rolland-Cachera MF: Rate of growth in early life: A predictor of later health? *Adv. Exp Med Biol* 569:35–39, 2005.
6. Gray DS: Diagnosis and prevalence of obesity. *Medical Clinics of North America* 73:1–13, 1989.
7. Ong KKL, Ahmed ML, Emmett PM, Preece MA, Dunger DB: The Avon Longitudinal Study of Pregnancy and Childhood Study Team. Association between postnatal catch-up growth and obesity in childhood: Prospective cohort study. *BMJ* 320:967–971, 2000.
8. Eriksson JG, Forsen R, Tuomilehto J, Winter PD, Osmond C, Barker DJP: Catch-up growth in childhood and death from coronary heart disease: A longitudinal study. *BMJ* 318:7–11, 1999.
9. Guo SS, Roche AF, Chumlea WC, Gardner JD, Siervogel RM: The predictive value of childhood body mass index values for overweight at age 35 yr. *Am J Clin Nutr* 59:810–19, 1994.
10. Serdula MK, Ivery D, Coates RJ, Freedman DS, Williamson DF, Byers T: Do obese children become obese adults? A review of the literature. *Prev Med* 22:167–177, 1993.
11. World Health Organization: *Obesity: Preventing and Managing the Global Epidemic*. Geneva, 1998.
12. Himes JH, Dietz WH: Guidelines for overweight in adolescent preventive services: Recommendations from an expert committee. The Expert Committee on Clinical Guidelines for Overweight in Adolescent Preventive Services. *Am J Clin Nutr* 59:307–316, 1994.
13. Centers for Disease Control and Prevention: Physical activity levels among children aged 9–13 years—United States, 2002. *Morb Mortal Wkly Rep* 52:785–788, 2003.
14. Cole TJ, Bellizi MC, Flegal KM, Dietz WH: Establishing a standard definition for child overweight and obesity worldwide: International survey. *BMJ* 320:1–6, 2000.
15. Tanner JM: Introduction: Growth in height as a mirror of the standard of living. In Komlos J (ed.). *Stature, living standards, and economic development*. Chicago/London University of Chicago Press, 1994.
16. Weber G, Seidler H, Wilfing Hauser G: Secular change in height in Austria: An effect of population stratification? *Ann Hum Biol* 22:277–288, 1995.
17. Hedley AA, Ogden CL, Johnson CL, Caroll MD, Curtin LR, Flegal KM: Prevalence of overweight and obesity among U.S. children, adolescents, and adults, 1999–2002. *JAMA* 291:2847–50, 2004.
18. Taubes G: As obesity rates rise, experts struggle to explain why. *Science* 280:1367–1368, 1998.
19. Kimm SY, Glynn NW, Kriska AM, Fitzgerald SL Aaron DJ, Similo SL, McMahon RP, Barton BA: Racial divergence in adiposity during adolescence: The NHLBI Growth and Health Study. *Pediatrics* 107:E34, 2001.
20. Ebbeling CB, Pawlak DB, Ludwig DS: Childhood obesity: Public health crisis, common sense cure. *Lancet* 360:473–482, 2002.
21. Herpertz-Dahlmann B, Geller F, Böhle C, Khalil C, Troost-Brinkhues G, Hebebrand J: Secular trends in body mass index measurements in German preschool children. *European Journal of Pediatrics* 162:104–109, 2003.
22. Dietz WH: Health consequences of obesity in youth: Childhood predictors of adult disease. *Pediatrics* 101 (Suppl):518–525, 1998.
23. Slyper AH: Childhood obesity, adipose tissue distribution, and the pediatric practitioner. *Pediatrics* 102:e4, 1998.
24. Must A, Strauss RS: Risks and consequences of childhood and adolescent obesity. *Int J Obes Relat Metab Disord* Suppl 2:2–11, 1999.
25. Weiss R, Dziura J, Burgert TS, Tamborlane WV, Taksali SE, Yeckel CW, Allen K, Lopes M, Savoye M, Morrison J, Sherwin RS, Caprio S: Obesity and the metabolic syndrome in children and adolescents. *NEJM* 350:2362–2374, 2004.
26. Fröhlich A: Ein Fall von Tumor der Hypophysis cerebri ohne Akromegalie. *Wiener Klinische Rundschau* 15:833–836; 906–908, 1901.
27. Bruch H: Obesity in childhood and personality development. 1941. *Obes Res* 5:157–161, 1997.
28. Bruch H: Psychological aspects of overeating and obesity. *Psychosomatics* 5:269–274, 1964.
29. Garn SM, Clark D: Nutrition, growth, development, and maturation: Findings of the Ten State Nutritional Survey of 1968–70. *Pediatrics* 56:306–19, 1975.
30. Lissau-Lind I, Sörensen TIA: Parental neglect during childhood and increased risk of obesity in young adulthood. *Lancet* 343:324–327, 1994.
31. Sobal J, Stunkard AJ: Socioeconomic status and obesity: A review of the literature. *Psychol Bull* 105:260–275, 1989.
32. Strauss RS, Knight J: Influence of the home environment on the development of obesity in children. *Pediatrics* 103:e85, 1999.
33. Bouchard C, Tremblay A, Despres JP, Nadeau A, Lupien PJ, Theriault G, Dussault J, Moorjani S, Pinault S, Fournier G: The response to long-term overfeeding in identical twins. *N Engl J Med* 322:1477–1482, 1990.
34. Stunkard AJ, Sorensen TI, Hanis C, Teasdale TW, Chakraborty R, Schull WJ, Schulsinger F: An adoption study of human obesity. *N Engl J Med* 314:193–198, 1986.
35. Stunkard AJ, Harris JR, Pedersen NL, McClearn GE: The body mass index of twins who have been reared apart. *N Engl J Med* 222:1483–1487, 1990.

36. Zhang Y, Proenca R, Maffei M, Barone M, Leopold L, Friedman JM: Positional cloning of the mouse obese gene and its human homologue. *Nature* 372:425–432, 1994.
37. Montague CT, Farooqi IS, Whitehead JP, Soos MA, Rau H, Wareham NJ, Sewter CP, Digby JE, Mohammed SN, Hurst JA, Cheetham CH, Earley AR, Barnett AH, Prins JB, O'Rahilly S: Congenital leptin deficiency is associated with severe early-onset obesity in humans. *Nature* 387:903–908, 1997.
38. Farooqi IS, Jebb SA, Langmack G, Lawrence E, Cheetham CH, Prentice AM, Hughes IA, McCamish MA, O'Rahilly S: Effects of recombinant leptin therapy in a child with congenital leptin deficiency. *N Engl J Med* 341:879–884, 1999.
39. Whitaker RC: Predicting preschooler obesity at birth: The role of maternal obesity in early pregnancy. *Pediatrics* 114:e29–36, 2004.
40. Reilly JJ, Armstrong J, Dorosty AR, Emmett PM, Ness A, Rogers I, Steer C, Sherriff A: Avon Longitudinal Study of Parents and Children Study Team: Early life risk factors for obesity in childhood: Cohort study. *BMJ* 330:1357, 2005.
41. Magnusson PK, Rasmussen F: Familial resemblance of body mass index and familial risk of high and low body mass index: A study of young men in Sweden. *Int J Obes Relat Metab Disord* 26:1225–1231, 2002.
42. Maes HH, Neale MC, Eaves LJ: Genetic and environmental factors in relative body weight and human adiposity. *Behav Genet* 27:325–351, 1997.
43. Hebebrand J, Wulftange H, Görg T, Ziegler A, Hinney A, Barth N, Mayer H, Remschmidt H: Epidemic obesity: Are genetic factors involved via increased rates of assortative mating? *Int J Obes Relat Metab Disord* 24:345–353, 2000.
44. Vlietinck R, Derom R, Neale MC, Maes H, van Loon H, Derom C, Thiery M: Genetic and environmental variation in the birth weight of twins. *Behav Genet* 19:151–161, 1989.
45. Pietilainen KH, Kaprio J, Rissanen A, Winter T, Rimpela A, Viken RJ, Rose RJ: Distribution and heritability of BMI in Finnish adolescents aged 16y and 17y: A study of 4884 twins and 2509 singletons. *Int J Obes Relat Metab Disord* 23:107–115, 1999.
46. Hebebrand J, Wemter A, Hinney A: Genetic aspects. In: Kiess W, Marcus C, Wabitsch M (eds.). *Obesity in Childhood and Adolescence* (vol 9). Basel Karger, 2004a pp. 80–90.
47. Plomin R, DeFries JC, McClearn GE, Rutter M: *Behavioral Genetics*. New York: WH Freeman, 1997.
48. Reed DR, Bachmanov AA, Beauchamp GK, Tordoff MG, Price RA: Heritable variation in food preferences and their contribution to obesity. *Behav Genet* 27:373–387, 1997.
49. Pérusse L, Tremblay A, Leblanc C, Bouchard C: Genetic and environmental influences on level of habitual physical activity and exercise participation. *Am J Epidemiol* 129:1012–1022, 1989.
50. Plomin R, Corley R, Carey G, DeFries JC, Fulker DW: Individual differences in television viewing in early childhood: Nature as well as nurture. *Psychological Science* 1:371–377, 1990.
51. Neel JV, Weder AB, Julius S: Type II diabetes, essential hypertension, and obesity as "syndromes of impaired genetic homeostasis": The "thrifty genotype" hypothesis enters the 21st century. *Perspect Biol Med* 42:44–74, 1998.
52. Bray GA: The epidemic of obesity and changes in food intake: The fluoride hypothesis. *Physiol and Behav* 82:115–121, 2004.
53. Ellis L, Haman D: Population increases in obesity appear to be partly due to genetics. *J Biosoc Sci* 36:547–559, 2004.
54. Fraga MF, Ballestar E, Paz MF, et al.: Epigenetic differences arise during the lifetime of monozygotic twins. *Proc Natl Acad Sci USA* 102(30):10604–10609, 2005.
55. Farooqi IS, O'Rahilly S: Monogenic obesity in humans. *Annu Rev Med* 56:443–458, 2005.
56. Dempfle A, Hinney A, Heinzel-Gutenbrunner M, Raab M, Geller F, Gudermann T, Schafer H, Hebebrand J: Large quantitative effect of melanocortin-4 receptor gene mutations on body mass index. *J Med Genet* 41:795–800, 2004.
57. Farooqi IS, Yeo GS, Keogh JM, Aminian S, Jebb SA, Butler G, Cheetham T, O'Rahilly S: Dominant and recessive inheritance of morbid obesity associated with melanocortin 4 receptor deficiency. *J Clin Invest* 106:271–279, 2000.
58. Branson R, Potoczna N, Kral JG, Lentes KU, Hoehe MR, Horber FF: Binge eating as a major phenotype of melanocortin 4 receptor gene mutations. *N Engl J Med* 348:1096–1103, 2003.
59. Herpertz S, Siffert W, Hebebrand J: Binge eating as a phenotype of melanocortin 4 receptor gene mutations. *N Engl J Med* 349:606–609, 2003.
60. Hebebrand J, Geller F, Dempfle A, et al.: Binge-eating episodes are not characteristic of carriers of melanocortin-4 receptor gene mutations. *Mol Psychiatry* 9:796–800, 2004b.
61. Geller F, Reichwald K, Dempfle A, et al.: Melanocortin-4 receptor gene variant I103 is negatively associated with obesity. *Am J Hum Genet* 74:572–581, 2004.
62. Heid IM, Vollmert C, Hinney A, et al.: KORA Group—Association of the 103I MC4R allele with decreased body mass in 7937 participants of two population based surveys. *J Med Genet* 42:e21, 2005.
63. Friedman JM: A war on obesity, not the obese. *Science* 299:856–858, 2003.
64. Friedman JM: Modern science versus the stigma of obesity. *Nat Med* 10:563–569, 2004.
65. Gortmaker SL, Must A, Sobol AM, Peterson K, Colditz GA, Dietz WH: Television viewing as a cause of increasing obesity among children in the United States, 1986–1990. *Arch Pediatr Adolesc Med* 150:356–362, 1996.
66. Hancox RJ, Milne BJ, Poulton R: Association between child and adolescent television viewing and adult health: A longitudinal birth cohort study. *Lancet* 364:257–262, 2004.
67. Reilly JJ, Jackson DM, Montgomery C, Kelly LA, Slater C, Paton JY: Total energy expenditure and physical activity in young Scottish children: Mixed longitudinal study. *Lancet* 363:211–212, 2004.
68. Graf C, Koch B, Kretschmann-Kandel E, Falkowsiki G, Christ H, Coburger S, Lehmacher W, Bjarnason-Wehrens B, Platen P, Tokarski W, Predel HG, Dordel S: Correlation between BMI, leisure habits and motor abilities in childhood (CHILT-project). *Int J Obes Relat Metab Disord* 28:22–26, 2004.
69. Hebebrand J, Boes K: Umgebungsfaktoren—Körperliche Aktivität. In: Wabitsch M, Zwieauer K, Hebebrand J, Kiess W (hrsg.): *Adipositas bei Kindern und Jugendlichen*. Berlin, Springer, 2005, pp. 50–60.
70. Nielsen SJ, Siega-Riz AM, Popkin BM: Trends in energy intake in U.S. between 1977 and 1996: Similar shifts seen across age groups. *Obes Res* 10:370–378, 2002.
71. Nielsen SJ, Popkin BM: Patterns and trends in food portion sizes, 1977–1998. *JAMA* 289:450–453, 2003.
72. Slyper AH: The pediatric obesity epidemic: Causes and controversies. *JCEM* 89:2540–2547, 2004.
73. Ludwig DS, Peterson KE, Gortmaker SL: Relation between the consumption of sugar-sweetened drinks and childhood obesity: A prospective, observational analysis. *Lancet* 358:505–508, 2001.
74. Schlosser E: *Fast Food Nation*. Houghton Mifflin Books, 2001.
75. Nestle M: *Food Politics*. University of California Press, 2003.
76. Lobstein T, Dibb S: Evidence of a possible link between obesogenic food advertising and child overweight. *Obes Rev* 6:203–208, 2005.
77. Toschke AM, Koletzko B, Slikker W Jr, Hermann M, von Kries R: Childhood obesity is associated with maternal smoking in pregnancy. *Eur J Pediatr* 161:445–448, 2002.
78. Arenz S, Ruckerl R, Koletzko B, von Kries R: Breast feeding and childhood obesity—A systematic review. *Int J Obes Relat Metab Dis* 28:1247–1256, 2004.
79. Nelson MC, Gordon-Larsen P, Adair LS: Are adolescents who were breast-fed less likely to be overweight? Analyses of sibling pairs to reduce confounding. *Epidemiology* 16:247–253, 2005.
80. Von Kries R, Toschke AM, Wurmser H, Sauerwald T, Koletzko B: Reduced risk for overweight and obesity in 5- and 6-y-old children by duration of sleep—A cross- sectional study. *Int J Obes Relat Met Dis* 26:710–716, 2002.
81. Taheri S, Lin L, Austin D, Young T, Mignot E: Short sleep duration is associated with reduced leptin, elevated ghrelin, and increased body mass index. *PLOS Medicine* 1:e62, 2004.
82. Hasler G, Pine DS, Klaghofer R, Gamma A, Ajdacic V, Eich D, Rossler W, Angst J: The associations between psychopathology and being overweight: A 20-year prospective community study. *Psychol Med* 34:1047–1057, 2004.
83. Franko DL, Striegel-Moore RH, Thompson D, Schreiber GB, Daniels SR: Does adolescent depression predict obesity in black and white young adult women? *Psychol Med* 35:1505–1513, 2005.
84. Pine DS, Goldstein RB, Wolk S, Weissman MM: The association between childhood depression and adulthood body mass index. *Pediatrics* 107:1049–1057, 2001.
85. Goodman E, Whitaker RC: A prospective study of the role of depression in the development and persistence of adolescent obesity. *Pediatrics* 110:497–504, 2002.
86. Richardson LP, Davis R, Poulton R, McCauley E, Moffitt TE, Caspi A, Connell F: A longitudinal evaluation of adolescent depression and adult obesity. *Arch Pediatr Adolesc Med* 157:739–745, 2003.
87. Stice E, Presnell K, Shaw H, Rohde P: Psychological and behavioral risk factors for obesity in adolescent girls: A prospective study. *J Consult Clin Psychol* 73:195–202, 2005.
88. Birch LL, Davison KK: Family environmental factors influencing the developing behavioral controls of food intake and childhood overweight. *Pediatr Clin North Am* 48:893–907, 2001.
89. Robinson TN, Kiernan M, Matheson DM, Haydel KF: Is parental control over children's eating associated with childhood obesity? Results from a population-based sample of third graders. *Obes Res* 9:306–312, 2001.
90. Schwartz TL, Nihalani N, Jindal S, Virk S, Jones N: Psychiatric medication-induced obesity: A review. *Obes Rev* 5:115–121, 2004.
91. Zimmermann U, Kraus T, Himmerich H, Schuld A, Pollmacher T: Epidemiology, implications and mechanisms underlying drug-induced weight gain in psychiatric patients. *J Psychiatr Res* 37:193–220, 2003.
92. Theisen FM, Linden A, Geller F, Schafer H, Martin M, Remschmidt H, Hebebrand J: Prevalence of obesity in adolescent and young adult patients with and without schizophrenia and in relationship to antipsychotic medication. *J Psychiatr Res* 35:339–345, 2001.
93. Gothelf D, Falk B, Singer P, Kairi M, Phillip M, Zigel L, Poraz I, Frishman S, Constantini N, Zalsman G, Weizman A, Apter A: Weight gain associated with increased food intake and low habitual activity levels

in male adolescent schizophrenic inpatients treated with olanzapine. *Am J Psychiatry.* 159:1055–1057, 2002.
94. Martin A, Scahill L, Anderson GM, Aman M, Arnold LE, McCracken J, McDougle CJ, Tierney E, Chuang S, Vitiello B: Weight and leptin changes among risperidone-treated youths with autism: 6-month prospective data. *Am J Psychiatry* 161:1125–1127, 2004.
95. McConville BJ, Sorter MT: Treatment challenges and safety considerations for antipsychotic use in children and adolescents with psychoses. *J Clin Psychiatry* 65 Suppl 6:20–29, 2004.
96. Theisen FM, Linden A, Konig IR, Martin M, Remschmidt H, Hebebrand J: Spectrum of binge eating symptomatology in patients treated with clozapine and olanzapine. *J Neural Transm* 110:111–121, 2003.
97. Schwimmer JB, Burwinkle TM, Varni JW: Health-related quality of life of severely obese children and adolescents. *JAMA* 289:1813–1819, 2003.
98. Latner JD, Stunkard AJ: Getting worse: The stigmatization of obese children. *Obes Res* 11:452–456, 2003.
99. French SA, Perry CL, Leon GR, Fulkerson JA: Self-esteem and change in body mass index over 3 years in a cohort of adolescents. *Obes Res* 4:21–27, 1996.
100. Wallace W, Sheslow D, Hassink S: Obesity in children: A risk for depression. *Ann NY Acad Sci* 699:301–303, 1993.
101. Britz B, Siegfried W, Ziegler A, Lamertz C, Herpertz-Dahlmann BM, Remschmidt H, Wittchen HU, Hebebrand J: Rates of psychiatric disorders in a clinical study group of adolescents with extreme obesity and in obese adolescents ascertained via a population based study. *Int J Obes Relat Metab Disord* 24:1707–1714, 2000.
102. Vila G, Zipper E, Dabbas M, Bertrand C, Robert JJ, Ricour C, Mouren-Simeoni MC: Mental disorders in obese children and adolescents. *Psychosom Med* 66:387–394, 2004.
103. Wadden TA, Foster GD, Stunkard AJ, Linowitz JR: Dissatisfaction with weight and figure in obese girls: Discontent but not depression. *Int J Obes* 13:89–97, 1989.
104. Lamertz CM, Jacobi C, Yassouridis A, Arnold K, Henkel AW: Are obese adolescents and young adults at higher risk for mental disorders? A community survey. *Obes Res* 10:1152–1160, 2002.
105. Fairburn CG, Welch SL, Doll HA, Davies BA, O'Connor ME: Risk factors for bulimia nervosa: A community based case-control study. *Arch Gen Psychiatry* 54:509–517, 1997.
106. Coners H, Remschmidt H, Hebebrand J: The relationship between premorbid body weight, weight loss, and weight at referral in adolescent patients with anorexia nervosa. *Int J Eat Disord* 26:171–178, 1999.
107. Hebebrand J, Himmelmann GW, Herzog W, Herpertz-Dahlmann B, Steinhausen HC, Amstein M, Seidel R, Deter HC, Remschmidt H, Schäfer H: Prediction of low body weight at long-term follow-up in acute anorexia nervosa by low body weight at referral. *Am J Psychiatry* 154:566–569, 1997.
108. Lamerz A, Kuepper-Nybelen J, Bruning N, Wehle C, Trost-Brinkhues G, Brenner H, Hebebrand J, Herpertz-Dahlmann B: Prevalence of obesity, binge eating, and night eating in a cross-sectional field survey of 6-year-old children and their parents in a German urban population. *J Child Psychol Psychiatry* 46:385–393, 2005.
109. Berkowitz R, Stunkard AJ, Stallings VA: Binge-eating disorder in obese adolescent girls. *Ann NY Acad Sci.* 29;699:200–206, 1993.
110. Friedman MA, Brownell KD: Psychological correlates of obesity: Moving to the next research generation. *Psychol Bull* 117:3–20, 1995.
111. Reinehr T, Brylak K, Alexy U, Kersting M, Andler W: Predictors to success in outpatient training in obese children and adolescents. *Int J Obes Relat Metab Disord.* 27:1087–1092, 2003.
112. Moyer VA, Klein JD, Ockene JK, Teutsch SM, Johnson MS, Allan JD, Childhood Obesity Working Group: Screening for overweight in children and adolescents: Where is the evidence? A commentary by the childhood obesity working group of the U.S. Preventive Services Task Force. *Pediatrics* 116:e125–144, 2005.
113. Whitlock EP, Williams SB, Gold R, Smith PR, Shipman SA: Screening and interventions for overweight: A summary of evidence for the U.S. Preventive Services Task Force. *Pediatrics* 116:e125–144, 2005.
114. Fowler-Brown A, Kahwati LC: Prevention and treatment of overweight in children and adolescents. *Am Fam Physician* 69:2591–2598, 2004.
115. Krebs NF, Jacobson MS, American Academy of Pediatrics Committee on Nutrition: Prevention of pediatric overweight and obesity. *Pediatrics* 112:424–430, 2003.
116. Abikoff H, Hechtman L, Klein RG, Weiss G, Fleiss K, Etcovitch J, Cousins L, Greenfield B, Martin D, Pollack S: Symptomatic improvement in children with ADHD treated with long-term methylphenidate and multimodal psychosocial treatment. *J Am Acad Child Adolesc Psychiatry* 43:802–811, 2004.
117. Summerbell CD, Waters E, Edmunds LD, Kelly S, Brown T, Campbell KJ. Interventions for preventing obesity in children. *Cochrane Database Syst Rev* (3):CD001871, 2005.
118. Van Horn L, Obarzanek E, Friedman LA, Gernhofer N, Barton B: Children's adaptations to a fat-reduced diet: The Dietary Intervention Study in Children (DISC). *Pediatrics* 115:1723–1733, 2005.
119. Carrel AL, Clark RR, Peterson SE, Nemeth BA, Sullivan J, Allen DB: Improvement of fitness, body composition, and insulin sensitivity in overweight children in a school-based exercise program: A randomized, controlled study. *Arch Pediatr Adolesc Med* 159:963–968, 2005.
120. Nemet D, Barkan S, Epstein Y, Friedland O, Kowen G, Eliakim A: Short- and long-term beneficial effects of a combined dietary-behavioral-physical activity intervention for the treatment of childhood obesity. *Pediatrics* 115:e433–439, 2005.
121. Golan M, Crow S: Targeting parents exclusively in the treatment of childhood obesity: Long- term results. *Obes Res* 12:357–361, 2004.
122. Braet C, Tanghe A, Decaluwe V, Moens E, Rosseel Y. (2004) Inpatient treatment for children with obesity: Weight loss, psychological well-being, and eating behavior. *J Pediatr Psychol* 29:519–529, 2004.
123. Epstein LH, McCurley J, Valoski A, Wing RR: Growth in obese children treated for obesity. *Am J Dis Child* 144:1360–1364, 1990.
124. Butryn ML, Wadden TA: Treatment of overweight in children and adolescents: Does dieting increase the risk of eating disorders? *Int J Eat Disord* 37:285–293, 2005.
125. Stice E, Cameron RP, Killen JD, Hayward C, Taylor CB: Naturalistic weight-reduction efforts prospectively predict growth in relative weight and onset of obesity among female adolescents. *J Consult Clin Psychol* 67:967–974, 1999.
126. Field AE, Austin SB, Taylor CB, Malspeis S, Rosner B, Rockett HR, Gillman MW, Colditz GA: Relation between dieting and weight change among preadolescents and adolescents. *Pediatrics* 112:900–906, 2003.
127. Neumark-Sztainer D, Story M, French SA: Covariations of unhealthy weight loss behaviors and other high-risk behaviors among adolescents. *Arch Pediatr Adolesc Med* 150:304–308, 1996.
128. Jeffery RW: Does weight cycling present a health risk? *Am J Clin Nutr* 63(3 Suppl):452S–455S, 1996.
129. Wannamethee SG, Shaper AG, Walker M: Weight change, weight fluctuation, and mortality. *Arch Intern Med* 162:2575–2580, 2002.
130. Soerensen TI, Rissanen A, Korkeila M, Kaprio J: Intention to lose weight, weight changes, and 18-y mortality in overweight individuals without co-morbidities. *PLoS Med* 2:e171, 2005.
131. Godoy-Matos A, Carraro L, Vieira A, Oliveira J, Guedes EP, Mattos L, Rangel C, Moreira RO, Coutinho W, Appolinario JC: Treatment of obese adolescents with sibutramine: a randomized, double-blind, controlled study. *J Clin Endocrinol Metab* 90:1460–1465, 2005.
132. Berkowitz RI, Wadden TA, Tershakovec AM, Cronquist JL: Behavior therapy and sibutramine for the treatment of adolescent obesity: A randomized controlled trial. *JAMA* 289:1805–12, 2003.
133. Chanoine JP, Hampl S, Jensen C, Boldrin M, Hauptman J: Effect of orlistat on weight and body composition in obese adolescents: A randomized controlled trial. *JAMA* 293:2873–83, 2005. Erratum in: *JAMA* 294:1491, 2005.
134. Inge TH, Krebs NF, Garcia VF, Skelton JA, Guice KS, Strauss RS, Albanese CT, Brandt ML, Hammer LD, Harmon CM, Kane TD, Klish WJ, Oldham KT, Rudolph CD, Helmrath MA, Donovan E, Daniels SR: Bariatric surgery for severely overweight adolescents: Concerns and recommendations. *Pediatrics* 114:217–223, 2004.
135. Warman JL: The application of laparoscopic bariatric surgery for treatment of severe obesity in adolescents using a multidisciplinary adolescent bariatric program. *Crit Care Nurs Q* 28:276–287, 2005.
136. Campbell K, Waters E, O'Meara S, Kelly S, Summerbell C: Interventions for preventing obesity in children. *Cochrane Database Syst Rev* (2):CD001871, 2002.
137. Whitaker RC, Wright JA, Pepe MS, Seidel KD, Dietz WH: Predicting obesity in young adulthood from childhood and parental obesity. *New England Journal of Medicine* 337:869–873, 1997.

CHAPTER 5.8 ■ SUBSTANCE USE DISORDERS

CHRISTIAN HOPFER AND PAULA RIGGS

DEFINITION

Substance use disorders (SUDs) encompass two major categories: substance abuse (SA) and substance dependence (SD). In addition, there are intoxication and withdrawal states related to specific substances. This chapter will limit its discussion to SA and SD, as these are the most common conditions encountered in child and adolescent clinical practice. SA, generally thought of as a more limited and less severe syndrome, is defined as a maladaptive pattern of substance use leading to clinically significant impairment. The diagnosis of abuse cannot be made if the criteria for dependence are met. SD encompasses a cluster of cognitive, behavioral, and physiological symptoms that indicate a persistent pattern of substance use despite adverse consequences. If either of the criteria of withdrawal or tolerance to a substance is met, the diagnosis of SD is made, with the qualifier of "with physiological dependence." Thus, to contrast the two categories, abuse involves psychosocial impairment due to substance use, but does not include physiological symptoms, persistent drug-seeking in the face of adverse consequences, or cognitive features such as being preoccupied with obtaining or using drugs. The criteria for these diagnoses are described in Table 5.8.1.

HISTORY

Use and abuse of substances have been documented throughout history and date back to ancient times. The active ingredients in substances of abuse were initially identified and extracted during the nineteenth century, leading to an increase in the purity of substances available for consumption as more concentrated formulations were made. Initially, when substances such as opiates or cocaine were first identified, they were either freely available or prescribed widely by physicians and made available through many tonics. The liability of certain substances to result in "addiction" was recognized in the late nineteenth and early twentieth centuries, when laws regulating abusable substances were introduced. The 1914 Harrison Narcotic Act, which forbade the sale of cocaine or opiates except by licensed physicians or pharmacists, was one of the first laws introduced to regulate substances seen as having a liability for abuse. Also, the widespread perception that alcohol created societal problems led to the Prohibition Amendment of 1919 to the American Constitution, which made alcohol an illegal substance. This amendment, however, was overturned in 1933.

With the creation of the U.S. Federal Bureau of Narcotics (now the Drug Enforcement Administration) in 1930 the federal government took a more active role in regulating drugs and also defining which drugs could be legally purchased, could be available only by prescription, or would be completely banned. Throughout the latter half of the twentieth century, major societal changes occurred in the acceptance and use of various substances—including marijuana, tobacco, cocaine, amphetamines, and more recently, "designer" drugs such as Ecstasy.

Along with changes in societal views and consumption of various substances came an increased scientific understanding of the mechanisms of actions of most addictive compounds, including the realization that these were binding to specific brain receptor sites. Animal models of addiction established the neurobiological basis for understanding addiction as a psychiatric illness.

The psychiatric nosology of the two major substance use disorders of abuse and dependence largely evolved from epidemiological studies of adults with alcohol problems. An important question in the development of the nosology of SA or SD was whether most patients who met the criteria for abuse would go on to develop dependence and thus, whether, in effect, abuse represented a prodromal state. However, studies of adults with alcohol problems did not confirm this view, as the majority of subjects who met the criteria for abuse either continued in that category, or reported no alcohol

TABLE 5.8.1

CRITERIA FOR SUBSTANCE ABUSE AND DEPENDENCE

Substance Abuse 1 out of 4 Criteria within 1 Year	Substance Dependence 3 out of 7 Criteria within 1 Year
Recurrent substance use resulting in failure to fulfill major role obligations	Tolerance
Recurrent substance use in situations which are physically hazardous	Withdrawal
Recurrent substance-related legal problems	Substance taken in larger amounts and/or for a longer period than was intended
Continued substance use despite having persistent social problems due to use	Unsuccessful efforts to cut down or control use
Exclusion: Does not meet dependence criteria	Great deal of time spent in activities necessary to obtain the substance or recover from its effects
	Important social, occupational, or recreational activities given up because of use
	Substance use continues despite knowledge that medical or psychological problems are due to use

(Adapted from DSM IV TR. Reprinted with permission from the *Diagnostic and Statistical Manual of Mental Disorders*, Fourth Edition, Text Revision, American Psychiatric Association, 2000.)

problems at followup, with only 11% going on to develop dependence (1–3). Studies of the category of SD demonstrated that it represented a more chronic relapsing condition, with the majority of adult subjects with alcohol dependence continuing to meet dependence criteria at follow-up (3, 4).

For adolescents with SUDs, the question of whether those with abuse usually develop dependence remains currently unanswered. What is known is that SA is reported more commonly than SD by approximately 2:1 in adolescents (5); that in adolescence abuse and dependence may represent a single unidimensional construct (6); that polysubstance abuse is very common for adolescents with SUDs (5); and that the severity of dependence, as measured by number of dependence symptoms, predicts a poorer clinical outcome (7). Thus, the history of the development of the separate categories of abuse and dependence derives largely from studies of adults, with only limited information being available about the predictive value of these categories for adolescents.

EPIDEMIOLOGY

Annual surveys of U.S. adolescents' drug use are conducted by the Monitoring the Future Survey (8). The prevalence of adolescents reporting experimenting with substances has changed over the last decade. Trends in the consumption of alcohol, marijuana, tobacco, and other illicit substances as reported by U.S. twelfth graders are shown in Figure 5.8.1. While experimentation with alcohol and tobacco declined somewhat, marijuana experimentation increased from 35% in 1991 to a peak of 50% in 1997, and then drifted down again to approximately 45% in 2004. What has remained consistent is that the most commonly used substances among adolescents are alcohol, tobacco, and marijuana, with roughly a third of twelfth graders reporting lifetime experimentation with an illicit substance besides marijuana.

The frequency of substances used by general population adolescents is mirrored in admissions to substance abuse treatment facilities. Table 5.8.2 shows the substances that are listed as most common upon admission to publicly funded substance abuse treatment programs in the United States, by age category. This data is collected annually by the Treatment Episode Data Set for all publicly funded substance abuse treatment programs (9). For the youngest age group (12–14), marijuana constitutes the most frequently cited primary admitting substance of abuse. For the older (18–20) age group, marijuana and alcohol continue to represent a large portion of treatment admissions, but other illicit substances such as cocaine, methamphetamine, and heroin are more commonly cited as reasons for admission compared with younger adolescents.

General population surveys of adolescent substance use disorders indicate clear marked age trends. The prevalence of substance use and SUDs increases almost linearly from early to late adolescence. Approximately one in four older adolescents meets criteria for abuse for at least one substance, and one in five meets criteria for SD. Nearly one in three adolescents reports daily smoking and 8.6% meet criteria for tobacco dependence by age 18. Although alcohol is the most commonly abused substance (10%), a slightly larger proportion of adolescents meet criteria for dependence on marijuana (4.3%) than alcohol (3.5%) (10). Additionally, there are gender differences, as males report more substance use than females, and more frequently meet criteria for dependence on alcohol and marijuana in late adolescence, while females are more often nicotine dependent (10). In clinical settings rates of SUDs are high. Aarons et al. (2001) (11) reported that 62.1% of youth in juvenile justice and 40.8% of youth in mental health settings met criteria for lifetime substance use disorders.

TABLE 5.8.2

PRIMARY ADMITTING SUBSTANCE OF ABUSE (% OF TOTAL ADMISSIONS), BY AGE, FROM THE TREATMENT EPISODE DATA SET

Substance	Age 12–14,%	Age 15–17,%	Age 18–20,%
None	8.3	2.2	0.9
Alcohol	17.7	19.9	30.6
Crack/cocaine	1.2	2.4	6.3
Marijuana/hashish	66.7	66.9	37.9
Heroin	0.2	1.2	9.8
Nonprescription methadone	0	0	0.1
Other opiates and synthetics	0.4	0.6	2.5
PCP	0.1	0.1	0.4
Hallucinogens	0.1	0.3	0.4
Methamphetamine	2.1	4	8.4
Other amphetamines	0.6	0.9	1.4
Other stimulants	0.2	0.1	0.1
Benzodiazapines	0.2	0.2	0.4
Other tranquilizers	0.1	0.1	0
Barbiturates	0	0	0
Other sedatives or hypnotics	0.2	0.1	0.2
Inhalants	0.9	0.2	0.1
Over-the-counter medications	0.2	0.2	0.1
Other	0.9	0.6	0.5
Total percent	100	100	100
(Total N)	(24,911)	(123,496)	(119,138)

(From TEDS: *Treatment Episode Data Set: 2003 Highlights. National Admissions to Substance Abuse Treatment Services*, DASIS Series: S-27. Rockville, MD; Services DoHaH, ed.; 2005. DHHS Publication No. SMA 05–4043, with permission.)

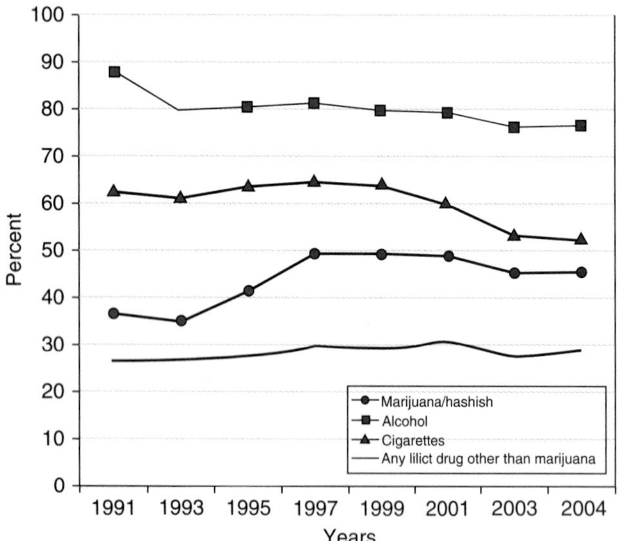

FIGURE 5.8.1. Trends in prevalence of twelfth grade lifetime drug use. (Adapted from Johnston, LD, O'Malley, PM, Bachman, JG, Schulenberg, JE: *Monitoring the Future: National Survey Results on Drug Use, 1975–2004. Volume I: Secondary School Students.* Bethesda, MD: National Institute on Drug Abuse; 2005; 680. NIH Publication No. 05–5727.)

Recent Trends in Substance Use among U.S. Adolescents

Recent surveillances of U.S. adolescents in 2004 indicate changes in patterns of substance use: Drugs that are declining in use among adolescents include marijuana and ecstasy, and amphetamine use to a lesser extent. Steroid use declined slightly from a previous peak. Drugs whose use patterns were fairly unchanged include LSD, heroin, cocaine, GHB (gamma hydroxy butyrate), and Rohypnol (flunitrazepam), as well as tranquilizers. Prescription opiates and inhalants have shown marked increases, with abuse of prescription opiates by adolescents increasing markedly over the past decade. Remarkably, roughly 10% of U.S. twelfth graders reported nonmedical use of hydrocodone, making it the third most widely abused illicit substance (after marijuana and amphetamine) among that age group (8).

ETIOLOGY

Substance use disorders can only develop if substances are available for experimentation to occur. However, despite widespread availability of many substances, only a portion of youth experiment, and only a smaller percentage of those who do experiment go on to become regular users or to develop SUDs. Thus, the etiology of SUDs lies in those factors that predispose an individual to experiment with substances, and to progress to regular use and the development of abuse or dependence.

A range of risk factors has been associated with the development of adolescent SUDs. Although a comprehensive review is beyond the scope of this chapter, major theories about the etiology of adolescent SUDs will be covered. See Whitmore and Riggs (2006) (12) for a more complete review.

Genetic and Environmental Influences

Twin and adoption studies have demonstrated that considerable shared environmental influences exist for the initiation of substance use, and that genetic influences become more apparent when environments allow for their expression (13). Thus, for example, Koopmans et al. (14) demonstrated that there were no genetic influences on the liability to initiate alcohol use when adolescents were raised in a religious household, but that 40% of the variation in initiation could be explained by genetic factors when adolescents were raised in a nonreligious household. Genetic influences on the development of adolescent SUDs may act through a direct effect on psychophysiological reactions to substances or their metabolism, or indirectly through genetic effects on personality traits such as behavioral disinhibition, which leads to substance experimentation (15). Thus, genetic factors influence individual risk, but do not account for population-wide shifts in patterns of substance use. A strong family history of SA or SD is a strong predictor for who goes on to initiate substance use or develop SUDs.

Externalizing Disorders

Externalizing disorders have been shown to be major risk factors predicting the initiation of substance use and the development of abuse and dependence [reviewed by Crowley and Riggs, 1995 (7)]. Many of the risk factors associated with the development of externalizing disorders similarly predispose to the development of substance use disorders. Conduct disorder has consistently been shown to be a predictor of substance use initiation and progression toward SUDs. Oppositional defiant disorder (ODD) and attention-deficit hyperactivity disorder (ADHD) appear to increase risk for developing SUDs somewhat, although there is controversy about the magnitude of the effect of ODD or ADHD due to their comorbidity with CD. Externalizing disorders and SUDs can also be thought of as influenced by a single underlying factor, as posited by problem behavior theory (16).

Stage Theory and the "Gateway" Theory

Stage theory posits that there is a temporal ordering of substance experimentation in which lower order substances, which are more commonly used, precede the use of higher order substances. Thus, typically a licit substance, such as alcohol or cigarettes, is used first in a sequence, followed by marijuana, which is usually the first illicit substance before progressing on to use of other illicit substances (17). Related to stage theory is the gateway hypothesis as it relates to marijuana: This posits that the use of marijuana facilitates the entry into other illicit substance use.

A review of the available literature about the effect of marijuana use on other drug use concluded that there is a relationship between marijuana use and progression to other drugs. This effect can be explained by 1) the selective recruitment to heavy cannabis use of persons with preexisting traits that predispose to the use of a variety of different drugs (i.e., that marijuana use is a marker for a tendency to use multiple drugs); 2) the affiliation of cannabis users with drug-using peers in settings that provide more opportunities to use other illicit drugs at an earlier age; and 3) that marijuana use results in socialization into an illicit drug subculture which creates favorable attitudes toward the use of other illicit drugs (18).

Early Onset of Use

Early onset of substance use has been shown to be a strong predictor for the development of substance use disorders over the lifetime (2). Whether this is due to early use being a marker for other risk factors that predict substance involvement or whether it has a causal effect is unknown. Recent animal work has suggested that the adolescent brain may be particularly vulnerable to the effects of drug sensitization, providing a possible neurobiological explanation for the increased incidence of substance use disorders among those who begin drug use early (19).

Family and Peer Effects

Substance use disorders tend to aggregate in families. This may be in part due to some common genetic influences within families; however, there is substantial evidence of environmental mediation. Parental drug use, as well as drug use by older siblings, is a significant risk factor for the development of adolescent substance use. However, the mechanism of transmission is complex, with individual personality dimensions mediating the effect of sibling and parent influences (20, 21).

Association with delinquent peers has been one of the hallmarks of the development of adolescent substance use disorders. However, while the common notion has been that peers create "peer pressure" to consume substances, most studies support the notion that there exists a complex process by which individuals select peer groups, and then in turn influence these, as well as are influenced by them (22).

Biological Mechanisms in the Etiology of Substance Use Disorders

A large body of animal work has shown that repeated exposure to substances leads to neural adaptations altering the hedonic "tone" of individuals. This tone is reset by substance use so that it is lower over time, resulting in dysphoria and craving when not using, and driving the substance dependence cycle (23). This animal work has been key in demonstrating that all substances of abuse, although acting at different receptors, create a common downstream pathway resulting in neural adaptations that perpetuate the addictive cycle.

Substance-Specific Risks

Although all substances share common neurologic pathways that are involved in the development of substance use disorders, there are differences between substances in terms of their addictive potential. The time course toward the development of dependence varies by individual, by substance, and by route of administration. Some substances, such as cocaine, are characterized by a rapid onset of the development of dependence, as for example 6% of cocaine users develop dependence within one year of experimenting with cocaine (24). In a longitudinal study, Wagner and Anthony (25), for example, demonstrated that whereas some 15–16% of cocaine users had developed cocaine dependence within 10 years of first use, the corresponding values were about 8% for marijuana users, and 12–13% for alcohol users.

DIAGNOSIS AND CLINICAL FEATURES

The diagnosis of SA or SD is made primarily through the clinical interview with the adolescent, as well as through obtaining collateral information from parents and teachers. Adolescents are likely to be in a "precontemplative" stage of change and may thus minimize the extent of their substance involvement (26). Establishing rapport with the adolescent is critical in order to increase the chance of self-disclosure of drug use. Early strong therapeutic alliance is facilitated by use of motivational interviewing (MI) style which is characterized by a nonjudgmental, collaborative approach.

Of primary clinical concern is the extent or severity of substance involvement, the specific substances that the patient is abusing or dependent on, and the length of time that the pattern has persisted. When an MI approach is taken and the limits of confidentiality are carefully explained to adolescents and parent/guardians, clinicians are much more likely to get an honest history of substance severity along with other behavioral problems.

When conducting an initial assessment with an adolescent for substance use disorders, the parents or caretakers should ideally be present at the initial interview. This allows the establishment of the rules of confidentiality (including that reports of abuse, neglect, or threats of harm to self or others must be disclosed). In order to optimize therapeutic alliance with adolescent patients and to enhance validity of clinical information, it is recommended that the adolescent's confidentiality be honored, unless specific permission and release is obtained or unless the patient is clinically judged to be a danger to self or others. Adolescents may be more willing to self-disclose if the rules of confidentiality are clearly established at the beginning of treatment. But the exceptions to confidentiality should be specified at the beginning of treatment.

The interview with the parents or caretakers can also be used to obtain a history of the presenting complaint, early development history, and assess family dynamics. Subsequently, a private interview with the adolescent is important in facilitating a strong treatment alliance and eliciting candid information about substance abuse and behavior problems that the patient may not be comfortable disclosing with parents present.

The interviewing technique should have an empathic, nonjudgmental, supportive, and motivation-enhancing style with adolescent patients. This approach can be integrated into most treatment modalities. This approach is particularly useful and developmentally appropriate when working with adolescents because they often resist adult authority figures mandating behavior changes. In addition, the use of MI helps the adolescent internalize motivation to reduce or discontinue using drugs as opposed to doing so in response to external pressures and contingencies; for clinicians unfamiliar with MI approaches, resources for training are available at http://www.motivationalinterview.org/. Adolescents' self-reports of drug use have been shown to be reliable when confidentiality is assured (27). In general the substance use history should be obtained with a similar style and sensitivity to obtaining medical/clinical information for any other disorder or evaluation of a medical review of systems. For each substance, clinicians should inquire about age of onset of first use or experimentation, age of progression to regular use; peak use, current use (past month); and last use. Following that, for those that are endorsed, DSM-IV diagnostic criteria for SA and SD should be assessed. Other important information includes triggers for craving and use; context of use (for example, with particular peers, or at or before school); perceived motivation for using; positive and negative consequences of use; and current motivation and goals for treatment (28).

Since it is quite important to obtain development factors/history as well as gather other longitudinal information about developmental risk factors, onset and progression of psychiatric symptoms, as well as onset and progression of substances, a lifetime timeline to anchor this information is useful. It also helps build trust and empathic alliance if the initial clinical interview shifts focus away from drug abuse to developmental history. Thus, one can spend 15 minutes gathering a developmental history in order to build alliance/trust by gathering less sensitive information. This establishes the necessary trust so that the drug interview is more reliable, and the adolescent is more comfortable telling the clinician the truth.

SPECIFIC LABORATORY TESTING OF SUBSTANCES

Detection of substances is a key component of SUD diagnosis and treatment. While the technologies to detect specific substances are changing, urinalysis remains the most commonly used method (for the detection of substances). There are a number of substances where urinalysis is ineffective or inefficient: detection of alcohol use by urinalysis is limited by the quick elimination time of alcohol; similarly, detection of inhalants by urinalysis is ineffective. Most commercial labs offer standard "panels" that may include the "NIDA 5." These are commonly abused substances that are detected by urinalysis. The NIDA 5 include marijuana, cocaine, methamphetamine, heroin, and PCP. Detection of alcohol is usually done via breathalyzer. If inhalant abuse is suspected, a commercial product is a Tox-Trap that will detect the presence of residual volatile organic compounds. If there is a clinical suspicion of the abuse of hallucinogens, MDMA, or GHB, usually specific lab tests for these must be ordered. Table 5.8.3 shows the detection time of commonly tested substances by urinalysis. If laboratory testing is going to be used in a legal proceeding, the laboratory must

TABLE 5.8.3

DETECTION PERIODS (TYPICAL)

Substance	Urine Detection Time
Alcohol	After absorption, decreases by −.02gm%/hr
Amphetamine	24–72 hrs
Barbiturates	1–2 days
Benzodiazepines	3 days for therapeutic dose
Cannabis (single use)	1–3 days
Cannabis (moderate use)	3–5 days
Cannabis (heavy use)	10 days
Cocaine	24–96 hours
Codeine/morphine	24–72 hours
Heroin	24–72 hrs
Methamphetamine	24–72 hours
PCP	14–30 days
LSD	1.5–5 days

meet certain standards defined in federal law as the Clinical Laboratory Improvement Amendments (CLIA). In addition, for youth with chronic Δ-9 tetrahydrocannabinol (THC) use, a quantitative test is available that will show a decline in use over time, and thus can distinguish current from past use.

SUBSTANCE SPECIFIC CLINICAL FEATURES

While all substance use disorders have common features that are characterized by the criteria for abuse and dependence, there are substance-specific issues of clinical relevance.

Alcohol

Alcohol is one of the first substances that adolescents usually experiment with, and alcohol use disorders constitute a major proportion of adolescent SUDs. Six percent of 12–17-year-olds met criteria for past year alcohol abuse or dependence in a large national household survey (29). The acute effects of alcohol intoxication include sedation, loss of balance, restlessness, slurred speech, decreased heart rate, and lowered blood pressure. Tolerance to alcohol develops with repeated ingestion, and withdrawal symptoms, although rare in adolescents, can be observed. These may include increased heart rate, elevated blood pressure, elevated temperature, vomiting and diarrhea, sweating, and possibly confusion, seizures, delirium, or psychosis. Withdrawal from alcohol can be medically life threatening and may need to be managed in a medically supervised setting. Detection of alcohol use is usually accomplished via breathalyzer, as its detection time in a urinalysis is limited.

Tobacco

The addictive ingredient in tobacco is nicotine, which has been shown to produce dependence in a substantial proportion of users (30). The primary concern with tobacco dependence is the long-term medical sequelae of use, as well as evidence that consumption of tobacco may facilitate the use of other substances. Nicotine is rapidly absorbed through either smoking or chewing and results in CNS stimulation, followed by withdrawal symptoms. It binds to the nicotinic acetylcholine receptors. Blood and brain levels of nicotine increase with each puff of a cigarette, and nicotine accumulates throughout the day. The half-life of nicotine is usually about 2 hours. Withdrawal symptoms from nicotine typically include craving, irritability, difficulty concentrating, and possibly anxiety and depressed mood.

Marijuana

Marijuana is the most commonly used illicit drug by adolescents and marijuana abuse or dependence accounts for the greatest number of admissions to substance abuse treatment facilities for adolescents (9). Approximately 4% of 12–17-year-olds meet criteria for past year marijuana abuse or dependence (29). Over the past decade, much has been learned about marijuana's effect on the brain and development. The active ingredient in marijuana is Δ-9 tetrahydrocannabinol (THC). THC binds to the cannabinoid receptor (CNR1), which is broadly distributed throughout the central nervous system. The endogenous cannabinoid system is an important neurotransmitter system involved in memory formation, appetite regulation, and coordinated movement. Marijuana has a range of effects on the user, consistent with the widespread distribution of the CNR1 receptor. It may have sedative, analgesic, hallucinogenic, appetite-enhancing, and anxiolytic properties for the user. It usually results in a relatively short-lived intoxication state, often characterized as euphoria. THC-intoxication impairs cognitive and psychomotor performance, although it is unclear currently if these effects persist after abstinence. There is also increasing evidence that marijuana use may be a causal factor in the development of other psychiatric disorders. In particular, evidence points to marijuana use increasing the risk for developing psychosis, as well as other psychiatric disorders (31, 32). Finally, DSM-IV TR does not recognize a cannabis withdrawal syndrome; however, a substantial recent body of research clearly demonstrates that such a syndrome exists (33).

Opiates

Heroin use and abuse of prescription opiates has risen during the past decade. Heroin use by twelfth graders was reported by 0.5% of U.S. high school seniors for years until 1993, when use began to rise and roughly doubled by 2001, having held steady since then. Abuse of prescription opiates by adolescents has increasingly become a major concern, as recent epidemiological surveys report that one in 20 U.S. high school seniors reported using the prescription opiate OxyContin illicitly (8). Past year heroin abuse or dependence is reported by 0.1% and past year opiate abuse or dependence by 1.5% of 12–17-year-olds (29). The increasing purity of heroin has made it possible to smoke or snort it, and this has led to an increase in its use over the past decade among adolescents. Heroin dependence in adolescents is typically associated with a rapid psychosocial decline, school failure, criminal behaviors, and family problems (34). The intense pleasurable effects of heroin are largely responsible for the addictive potential of heroin and tolerance may develop rapidly.

Cocaine

Cocaine abuse or dependence is reported by 0.4% of 12–17-year-olds (29). Cocaine use may quickly lead to the development of dependence. Approximately 6% of users who experiment with cocaine become dependent within 1 year (24). Physical effects of cocaine use include constricted blood vessels, dilated pupils, and increased temperature, heart rate, and blood pressure. The duration of cocaine's euphoric effects, which include hyperstimulation, reduced fatigue, and mental clarity, depends on the route of administration. The faster the absorption, the more intense the high and the shorter the duration. The high from snorting may last 15 to 30 minutes, while that from smoking may last 5 to 10 minutes.

Amphetamines

Nonmedical use of stimulants is reported by approximately 2% of 12–17-year-olds, with 0.6% reporting methamphetamine use (29). Methamphetamine is known by a variety of street names including ice, speed, crystal, glass, and crank. It is an addictive stimulant that can be smoked, injected, or inhaled. Its use is associated with major health consequences, including memory loss, aggression, violence and psychotic behavior, and neuropsychological deficits (35). Similar to cocaine, dependence can develop quickly and be associated with rapid psychosocial decline. The physical effects of acute intoxication include increased wakefulness, increased physical activity, decreased appetite, increased respiration, hyperthermia, and euphoria. Convulsions and seizures may occur.

MDMA

Approximately 1.2% of 12–17-year-olds report that they used (3,4-methylenedioxymethamphetamine) (MDMA) or ecstasy within the past year (8). MDMA is a synthetic drug with both psychedelic and stimulant effects. In the past, some therapists in the United States used the drug to facilitate psychotherapy. In 1988, however, MDMA became a Schedule I substance under the Controlled Substances Act. MDMA is a stimulant usually taken orally in pill form and whose psychedelic effects can last between 4 and 6 hours. The psychological effects of MDMA include confusion, depression, anxiety, sleeplessness, and paranoia. Physical effects may include muscle tension, involuntary teeth clenching, nausea, blurred vision, feeling faint, tremors, rapid eye movement, and sweating or chills. In rare cases, severe hyperthermia may develop. The epidemiological evidence suggests that most users do not develop dependence upon MDMA and that its use spontaneously remits in the early 20s. However, a minority of users, primarily those who meet dependence symptoms, will continue to use MDMA (36).

GHB

Approximately 2% of U.S. high school seniors reported using gamma hydroxy butyrate (GHB) within the past year (8). GHB is known by such street names such as "grievous bodily harm," "G," or "liquid ecstasy." It is a central nervous system depressant originally sold in health food stores as a muscle growth agent. The effects of GHB have been described as being similar to those of alcohol, except that periods of unconsciousness appear to be more frequent and unpredictable. Effects usually last about 4 hours. Some users report developing dependence upon GHB and experience rebound symptoms, with features similar to benzodiazepine withdrawal.

Inhalants

Roughly one in six U.S. high school students reports having tried inhalants at least once (8); however, rates of inhalant abuse or dependence are much lower, as only 0.1% of adolescents report abuse or dependence upon inhalants (37). Inhalants are volatile organic compounds that include many gases and fumes that are deliberately taken in order to achieve intoxication. Their abuse is more common among young adolescents, since these are some of the first substances available to them. Inhalants may be taken by directly spraying them into the mouth, "huffed"—meaning that the substance is held in a cloth and several breaths are taken, or "bagged"—meaning that the vapors are inhaled from a bag. The acute effects of inhalant intoxication resemble alcohol intoxication in that the youth often experiences acute euphoria and disorientation, which may be followed by a period of drowsiness, as inhalants are CNS depressants. Because inhalants encompass a wide range of possible compounds, it is not possible to cover all aspects of their presentation. However, inhalant use may quickly result in neurological sequelae and persistent use has been associated with white matter changes and loss of cognitive performance. Due to the neurotoxicity of inhalants, any use must be taken seriously.

Steroids

Approximately 3% of male U.S. high school students report having used anabolic steroids within the past year (8). Steroids are used generally not in order to achieve an immediate pleasurable effect, but in order to increase muscle mass, and thereby body image. Thus, the abuse of steroids differs from abuse of other substances, which are usually taken because of their immediate, rewarding effects. Steroids are typically taken in order to achieve a long-term goal: improved body image or physical performance. Anabolic steroids are usually taken in "cycles" and typically combined with weight-lifting regimens. There are numerous medical consequences of administering exogenous steroids, including premature growth stoppage and either shrinking testicles for men or the development of male sexual characteristics for women. In addition, mood swings or psychotic episodes may result from steroid abuse. Details of the medical and psychiatric sequelae are described by Brown (38).

DIFFERENTIAL DIAGNOSIS AND COMORBIDITY

The primary differential diagnosis is establishing whether SA or SD exists for each substance and to what extent relevant comorbid conditions are present, as adolescent SUDs typically present with comorbid conditions. The most frequent of these are externalizing disorders, but internalizing disorders are also more prevalent than in the general population (39). Lewinshohn et al. (40) reported 60% of 14–18-year-olds with substance use disorders had another psychiatric disorder. Similarly, the Methods for the Epidemiology of Child and Adolescent Mental Disorders (MECA) study found past 6-month prevalence for comorbid psychiatric disorders with an adolescent SUD sample to be 76% for any comorbid disorder, 68% for any disruptive behavior disorder, 32% for any mood disorder, and 20% for any anxiety disorder (41). Thus, comorbidity is the rule rather than the exception among adolescents in treatment for SUDs (11).

COURSE AND PROGNOSIS

The course and prognosis of SUDs is varied. Earlier onset, more severe substance use, and comorbid conditions predict a more severe course and outcome (7). In general, substance dependence implies a chronic, relapsing condition.

Treatment

Treatment for adolescent SUDs involves recognizing that these are chronic relapsing conditions. Patients may need multiple episodes of treatment over time. Treatment typically involves initial attempts to create abstinence or markedly reduced drug use, a period of addressing the biopsychosocial aspects of SUDs, and a maintenance or "relapse prevention" phase. Adolescents usually do not self-refer for treatment, but are often pressured into treatment by family, school, or court. They often present as defiant, or minimizing of their drug use. The primary initial goals of treatment are to engage the adolescent and the family in processes that interrupt drug-seeking and -using behaviors and to replace these with prosocial behaviors. A variety of evidence-based approaches have been shown to be successful. Typically, effective treatments are multimodal and address individual, family, peer, and other social environment domains simultaneously. Pharmacotherapy may be an important component for certain SUDs, as well as comorbid conditions.

Specific Therapeutic Approaches

Motivational Interviewing

Motivational enhancement techniques have been demonstrated to promote treatment engagement and can be used to establish a strong treatment alliance and to elicit patient-generated treatment goals (42). These empirically based psychotherapy techniques focus on increasing the patient's motivation to change by increasing the frequency and strength of "change talk," which in turn is positively correlated with making behavioral changes. Adolescents are generally resistant to more directive, confrontational approaches and are often ambivalent and relatively unmotivated for treatment, making motivational approaches critical (43, 44). Motivational interviewing principles can be effectively used in conjunction with another of the empirically supported treatment modalities, such as individual and/or family-based treatment (45–48).

Cognitive-Behavioral Therapy

Cognitive-behavioral therapy (CBT), based on learning theory, also has been shown to be effective in treating adolescent substance use disorders (43, 47). There is more empirical support for individual CBT; however, preliminary data indicate that group CBT may also reduce adolescent SA and improve related problem behaviors (49). Treatment manuals have been developed for courses of weekly CBT treatment ranging from 5 to 16 weeks. CBT typically relies on a "functional analysis" that identifies reinforcers of substance use as well as competing behaviors, skills deficits, and specific cognitive distortions associated with substance use. A "skills training" approach is then used to enhance coping strategies to deal effectively with drug cravings and negative affects, to strengthen problemsolving and communication skills, and to identify and avoid high-risk situations. Riggs et al. (2005) (50), in a randomized controlled trial, demonstrated that engaging adolescents with SUDs and depression with CBT as a background therapy resulted in a high rate of compliance, retention, and treatment response for drug and depression. Thus, individual CBT is a viable therapeutic option for youth with SUDs. An important feature of CBT is its emphasis on identifying and developing new skills and behaviors that are enjoyable, but incompatible with drug use. Typically, the patient has daily "homework," receives regular feedback, and reviews successes and setbacks weekly with a therapist (43, 47). Interestingly, Riggs et al. (2005) also demonstrated that when treatment was free or incentivized, many adolescents voluntarily entered treatment when referred by counselors, teachers, friends, or family.

Family and Multisystemic Therapies

A range of family-based therapies have been shown to be successful in treating adolescent SUDs. Family and multisystemic therapies all treat adolescents within the context of their environment, and try to modify multiple environmental factors contributing to SUDs (51). These approaches have been widely studied and shown to be effective for adolescent SUDs. Multisystemic therapy is an approach that addresses social and family influences of drug use and associated antisocial behaviors. Therapists make frequent home visits and are available on a full-time basis to families. Henngeler et al. (1996) (52) demonstrated that over 98% of youth receiving MST remained in treatment, compared to very few youth in a control group accessing treatment. Other approaches include brief strategic family therapy, which is a less intensive approach and can be delivered through weekly office visits (53). Other family therapies include multidimensional family therapy (54), which has also reported positive outcomes in controlled, randomized trials.

Community Reinforcement and Behavioral Approaches

Community reinforcement therapy is a skills-based approach to treatment that focuses largely on changing environmental factors in the community in order that nonusing behaviors be rewarded. A manual has been developed for the treatment of adolescent cannabis use (the most common presentation for adolescents with substance use disorders), and is available from the Substance Abuse and Mental Health Services Administration. This approach, and similar ones that focus on altering environmental rewards for drug use and non–drug-using behaviors, has been shown to be superior to a supportive model (55). The primary goal of these approaches is to promote abstinence by altering the conditions that promote substance use. Typically, therapists conduct a functional analysis of substance use that identifies antecedents to drug use, actual behaviors, and positive and negative consequences of substance use. Therapists aim to promote positive social activities that are not compatible with drug use and improve relationships with family members. The primary goal with parents is to motivate them to participate in the community reinforcement process and to teach the family members skills to promote abstinence and discourage drug use. Furthermore, other systems such as school or probation may be engaged in order to affect their behavior to promote adolescent abstinence. Waldron et al. (2005) (56) recently demonstrated that it was possible to engage 71% of treatment-resistant youth in treatment using a community-reinforcement family therapy model. Both parents and youth showed significant improvements in multiple domains of functioning and significant reduction in drug use for the youth who participated in treatment.

Pharmacotherapies

For many substance use disorders, there are no effective pharmacotherapies. However, for the abuse of alcohol, nicotine, and opioids, there are effective pharmacotherapies. In addition, comorbid conditions may often be the target of pharmacotherapy. These are described in Tables 5.8.4 and 5.8.5.

TABLE 5.8.4

COMMON COMORBID DISORDERS PHARMACOTHERAPY FOR ADOLESCENTS WITH A SUBSTANCE USE DISORDER

Comorbid Disorder	Effective Treatment for Adolescents without SUD	Impact of Treatment on Adolescents with SUD
Attention-deficit/hyperactivity disorder (ADHD)	■ First line: pharmacotherapy (generally; psychostimulants) ■ Medication options with low abuse potential: pemoline, bupropion, atomoxetine	**One controlled trial of pemoline (Riggs et al., 2004 (57); n = 69) suggests:** ■ Efficacy for ADHD despite nonabstinence ■ Good safety profile in 12-week trial; potential for hepatotoxicity, relative contraindication for pemoline ■ No decrease (or increase) in drug use in the absence of specific behavioral intervention for SUD ■ Potential for hepatoxicity relative contraindication for pemoline given other current options ■ Clonidine relatively contraindicated
Bipolar disorder	■ First line: pharmacotherapy ■ Mood stabilizers (lithium, valporic acid, carbamazepine)	**One randomized controlled trial of lithium in adolescents with SUD and comorbid bipolar (Geller et al. 1998 (58); n = 25) suggests:** ■ Efficacy and reasonable safety for bipolar disorder despite nonabstinence ■ Not adequate as an effective treatment for SUD in the absence of specific behavioral treatment for SUD
Depression	■ First line: combined pharmacotherapy and psychotherapy ■ Pharmacotherapy: SSRIs (> support, fluoxetine) in adolescents without SUD ■ Psychotherapy: cognitive behavioral therapy (CBT) and interpersonal psychotherapy, combined with medication for severe depression fluoxetine + CBT > efficacy than either alone (TADS study March/TADS team 2005, JAMA) (59)	**One randomized controlled trial of fluoxetine in adolescents with SUD and comorbid MDD + CBT for SUD (Riggs et al., 2005 (50); n = 126) suggests:** ■ Efficacy for depression despite nonabstinence (16-week trial) ■ Good safety profile, fluoxetine (? other SSRIs) ■ High rate of depression remission in both fluoxetine and placebo-treated subjects suggests that CBT also + impact on depression despite focus on drug abuse, not depression ■ Remission of depression, regardless of medication assignment, was a more important predictor of decreased drug use than fluoxetine vs. placebo ■ Remitters drug use decreased significantly; nonremitters had no change in drug use ■ Tricyclics relatively contraindicated in adolescents with SUD (e.g., arrhythmias; anticholinergic adverse effects)
Anxiety disorder (often comorbid with depressive disorders)	■ First line: combined psychotherapy (CBT) and pharmacotherapy (> evidence, SSRIs)	**40% of adolescents in aforementioned controlled trial of fluoxetine for MDD in adolescents with SUD (Riggs et al., 2005 (50)) suggests:** ■ Fluoxetine (? other SSRIs) efficacy and safety in reducing symptoms of anxiety in depressed, substance-dependent adolescents with significant anxiety symptoms and/or anxiety disorders (GAD, SAD, PTSD) ■ No difference in depression and drug use outcomes comparing those with and without anxiety disorders

TABLE 5.8.5

PHARMACOTHERAPIES FOR ADOLESCENT SUBSTANCE USE DISORDER

Substance	Medication	Dose	Comments
Alcohol	Disulfiram	250 mg po qd or 500 mg po qod	FDA approved for alcohol dependence in adults Carroll et al. (2000) (60) showed that, in adults, it was also effective for cocaine dependence when alcohol involved
	Acamprosate	1–4 g per day given in a tid dosing schedule	FDA approved for alcohol dependence in adults One study (Niederhofer and Steffan, 2003 (61); N = 26) suggests similar efficacy in adolescents as for adults
	Naltrexone	50 mg po qd, also available in injection form	FDA approved for alcohol dependence in adults Deas et al. (2005) (62) showed in open-label trial (N = 5) that it was safe and well tolerated
	Topiramate	25–300 mg po qd	Not FDA approved yet. Review by Johnson (2005) (63) indicates effectiveness for adults
Nicotine	Buproprion	100–300 mg po qd	FDA approved for smoking cessation in adults
	Nicotine patch	Varies depending upon product	
Opiates	Methadone	Varies	For adolescents under 18 must have two documented failures at drug-free detoxification Needs to be prescribed at a certified clinic. See Hopfer et al. (2003) (64)
	Buprenorphine	Varies	Marsch et al. (2005) (65) showed effectiveness for adolescent detoxification in first randomized controlled trial
	Naltrexone	50 mg po qd	Low compliance without monitoring. Recently an injectable form has been approved and is available.

References

1. Hasin DS, Grant B, Endicott J: The natural history of alcohol abuse: Implications for definitions of alcohol use disorders. *Am J Psychiatry* 147:1537–41, 1990.
2. Grant BF, Dawson DA: Age at onset of alcohol use and its association with DSM-IV alcohol abuse and dependence: Results from the National Longitudinal Alcohol Epidemiologic Survey. *J Subst Abuse* 9:103–10, 1997.
3. Schuckit MA, Smith TL, Landi NA: The 5-year clinical course of high-functioning men with DSM-IV alcohol abuse or dependence. *Am J Psychiatry* 157:2028–35, 2000.
4. Culverhouse R, Bucholz KK, Crowe RR, et al.: Long-term stability of alcohol and other substance dependence diagnoses and habitual smoking: An evaluation after 5 years. *Arch Gen Psychiatry* 62:753–60, 2005.
5. Harrison PA, Fulkerson JA, Beebe TJ: DSM-IV substance use disorder criteria for adolescents: A critical examination based on a statewide school survey. *Am J Psychiatry* 155:486–92, 1998.
6. Fulkerson JA, Harrison PA, Beebe TJ: DSM-IV substance abuse and dependence: Are there really two dimensions of substance use disorders in adolescents? *Addiction* 94:495–506, 1999.
7. Crowley TJ, Riggs PD: Adolescent substance use disorder with conduct disorder and comorbid conditions. *NIDA Res Monogr* 156:49–111, 1995.
8. Johnston LD, O'Malley PM, Bachman JG, Schulenberg JE: *Monitoring the Future: National Survey Results on Drug Use, 1975–2004. Volume I: Secondary School Students*. Bethesda, MD, National Institute on Drug Abuse, 2005, p. 680. NIH Publication No. 05–5727.
9. TEDS: *Treatment Episode Data Set: 2003 Highlights*. National Admissions to Substance Abuse Treatment Services, DASIS Series: S–27. Rockville, MD, Services DoHaH (ed.) 2005. DHHS Publication No. SMA 05–4043.
10. Young SE, Corley RP, Stallings MC, Rhee SH, Crowley TJ, Hewitt JK: Substance use, abuse and dependence in adolescence: Prevalence, symptom profiles and correlates. *Drug Alcohol Depend* 68:309–22, 2002.
11. Aarons GA, Brown SA, Hough RL, Garland AF, Wood PA: Prevalence of adolescent substance use disorders across five sectors of care. *J Am Acad Child Adolesc Psychiatry* 40:419–26, 2001.
12. Whitmore EA, Riggs PD: Developmentally informed diagnostic and treatment considerations in comorbid conditions. In: HA Liddle and CL Rowe (eds.): *Adolescent Substance Abuse: Research and Clinical Advances*. Cambridge, U.K., Cambridge University Press, pp. 264–83, 2006.
13. Hopfer CJ, Crowley TJ, Hewitt JK: Review of twin and adoption studies of adolescent substance use. *J Am Acad Child Adolesc Psychiatry* 42:710–19, 2003.
14. Koopmans JR, Slutske WS, van Baal GC, Boomsma DI: The influence of religion on alcohol use initiation: Evidence for genotype X environment interaction. *Behav Genet* 29:445–53, 1999.
15. Young SE, Stallings MC, Corley RP, Krauter KS, Hewitt JK: Genetic and environmental influences on behavioral disinhibition. *Am J Med Genet* 684–95, 2000.
16. Jessor RT, Jessor SL: *Problem Behavior and Psychosocial Development: A Longitudinal Study of Youth*. New York: Academic Press; 1977.
17. Kandel DB, Yamaguchi K, Chen K: Stages of progression in drug involvement from adolescence to adulthood: Further evidence for the gateway theory. *J Stud Alcohol* 53:447–57, 1992.
18. Hall WD, Lynskey M: Is cannabis a gateway drug? Testing hypotheses about the relationship between cannabis use and the use of other illicit drugs. *Drug Alcohol Rev* 24:39–48, 2005.
19. Chambers RA, Taylor JR, Potenza MN: Developmental neurocircuitry of motivation in adolescence: A critical period of addiction vulnerability. *Am J Psychiatry* 160:1041–52, 2003.
20. Brook DW, Brook JS, Rubenstone E, Zhang C, Singer M, Duke MR: Alcohol use in adolescents whose fathers abuse drugs. *J Addict Dis* 22:11–34, 2003.
21. Brook JS, Whiteman M, Brook DW, Gordon AS: Sibling influences on adolescent drug use: older brothers on younger brothers. *J Am Acad Child Adolesc Psychiatry* 958–66, 1991.
22. Schulenberg JE, Maggs JL: A developmental perspective on alcohol use and heavy drinking during adolescence and the transition to young adulthood. *J Stud Alcohol Suppl* 54–70, 2002.
23. Koob GF, Le Moal M: Drug abuse: Hedonic homeostatic dysregulation. *Science* 278:52–8, 1997.
24. O'Brien MS, Anthony JC: Risk of becoming cocaine dependent: Epidemiological estimates for the United States, 2000–2001. *Neuropsychopharmacology* 30:1006–18, 2005.
25. Wagner FA, Anthony JC: From first drug use to drug dependence; developmental periods of risk for dependence upon marijuana, cocaine, and alcohol. *Neuropsychopharmacology* 26:479–88, 2002.
26. Prochaska JO, DiClemente CC, Norcross JC: In search of how people change: Applications to addictive behaviors. *Am Psychol* 47:1102–14, 1992.
27. Winters KC, Stinchfield RD, Henly GA, Schwartz RH: Validity of adolescent self-report of alcohol and other drug involvement. *Int J Addict* 25:1379–95, 1990–1991.
28. Riggs PD, Davies RD: A clinical approach to integrating treatment for adolescent depression and substance abuse. *J Am Acad Child Adolesc Psychiatry* 41:1253–5, 2002.
29. Substance Abuse and Mental Health Services Administration. *Results from the 2004 National Survey on Drug Use and Health: National Findings*. Rockville, MD, Office of Applied Studies, NSDUH Series H-28, 2005. DHHS Publication No. SMA 05–4062.
30. Colby SM, Tiffany ST, Shiffman S, Niaura RS: Are adolescent smokers dependent on nicotine? A review of the evidence. *Drug Alcohol Depend* 59 Suppl 1:S83–95, 2000.

31. Lynskey MT, Glowinski AL, Todorov AA, et al.: Major depressive disorder, suicidal ideation, and suicide attempt in twins discordant for cannabis dependence and early-onset cannabis use. *Arch Gen Psychiatry* 61:1026–32, 2004.
32. Henquet C, Krabbendam L, Spauwen J, et al.: Prospective cohort study of cannabis use, predisposition for psychosis, and psychotic symptoms in young people. *BMJ* 330:11, 2005.
33. Budney AJ, Hughes JR, Moore BA, Vandrey R: Review of the validity and significance of cannabis withdrawal syndrome. *Am J Psychiatry* 161:1967–77, 2004.
34. Hopfer CJ, Khuri E, Crowley TJ, Hooks S: Adolescent heroin use: A review of the descriptive and treatment literature. *J Subst Abuse Treat* 23:231–37, 2002.
35. Monterosso JR, Aron AR, Cordova X, Xu J, London ED: Deficits in response inhibition associated with chronic methamphetamine abuse. *Drug Alcohol Depend* 79:273–7, 2005.
36. von Sydow K, Lieb R, Pfister H, Hofler M, Wittchen HU: Use, abuse and dependence of ecstasy and related drugs in adolescents and young adults—A transient phenomenon? Results from a longitudinal community study. *Drug Alcohol Depend* 66:147–59, 2002.
37. Sakai JT, Hall SK, Mikulich-Gilbertson SK, Crowley TJ: Inhalant use, abuse, and dependence among adolescent patients: Commonly comorbid problems. *J Am Acad Child Adolesc Psychiatry* 43:1080–8, 2004.
38. Brown JT: Anabolic steroids: What should the emergency physician know? *Emerg Med Clin North Am* 23:ix–x 815–26, 2005.
39. Whitmore EA, Mikulich SK, Thompson LL, Riggs PD, Aarons GA, Crowley TJ: Influences on adolescent substance dependence: Conduct disorder, depression, attention deficit hyperactivity disorder, and gender. *Drug Alcohol Depend* 47:87–97, 1997.
40. Lewinsohn PM, Hops H, Roberts RE, Seeley JR, Andrews JA: Adolescent psychopathology: I. Prevalence and incidence of depression and other DSM-III-R disorders in high school students. *J Abnorm Psychol* 102:133–44, 1993.
41. Kandel DB, Johnson JG, Bird HR, et al.: Psychiatric disorders associated with substance use among children and adolescents: Findings from the Methods for the Epidemiology of Child and Adolescent Mental Disorders (MECA) Study. *J Abnorm Child Psychol* 25:121–32, 1997.
42. Monti PM, Barnett NP, O'Leary TA, Colby SM: Motivational enhancement for alcohol-involved adolescents. In: Monti PM, Colby SM (eds): *Adolescents, Alcohol, and Substance Abuse: Reaching Teens through Brief Interventions*. New York, Guilford Press, pp. 145–82, 2001.
43. Drug Strategies. *Treating Teens: A Guide to Adolescent Drug Programs*. Washington, DC: Drug Strategies; 2002.
44. National Institute on Drug Abuse. *Principles of Drug Addiction Treatment: A Research-Based Guide*. Rockville, MD: National Institute on Drug Abuse; 1999. NIDA Publication No. 99–4180.
45. Muck R, Zempolich KA, Titus JC, Fishman M, Godley MD, Schwebel R: An overview of the effectiveness of adolescent substance abuse treatment models. *Youth & Society* 33:143–68, 2001.
46. Riggs PD, Whitmore EA: Substance use disorders and disruptive behavior disorders. In: Hendren RL (ed): *Review of Psychiatry, Vol 18: Disruptive Behavior Disorders in Children and Adolescents*. Washington, DC, American Psychiatric Press, Inc, pp. 33–174, 1999.
47. Wagner EF, Brown SA, Monti PM, Myers MG, Waldron HB: Innovations in adolescent substance abuse intervention. *Alcohol Clin Exp Res* 23:236–49, 1999.
48. Waldron HB, Slesnick N, Brody J, Turner C, Peterson T: Treatment outcomes for adolescent substance abuse at 4- and 7-month assessments. *J Consult Clin Psychol* 69:802–13, 2001.
49. Kaminer Y, Blitz C, Burleson JA, Kadden RM, Rounsaville BJ: Measuring treatment process in cognitive-behavioral and interactional group therapies for adolescent substance abusers. *J Nerv Ment Dis* 186:407–13, 1998.
50. Riggs PD, Lohman M, Davies R, et al.: Randomized controlled trial of fluoxetine/placebo and CBT in depressed adolescents with substance use disorders. Paper presented at: 2005 Annual Meeting, American Academy of Addiction Psychiatry, Scottsdale, AZ, December, 2005.
51. Liddle HA: Theory development in a family-based therapy for adolescent drug abuse. *J Clin Child Psychol* 28:521–32, 1999.
52. Henggeler SW, Pickrel SG, Brondino MJ, Crouch JL: Eliminating (almost) treatment dropout of substance abusing or dependent delinquents through home-based multisystemic therapy. *Am J Psychiatry* 153:427–8, 1996.
53. Robbins MS, Bachrach K, Szapocznik J: Bridging the research–practice gap in adolescent substance abuse treatment: The case of brief strategic family therapy. *J Subst Abuse Treat* 23:123–32, 2002.
54. Liddle HA, Rowe CL, Quille TJ, et al.: Transporting a research-based adolescent drug treatment into practice. *J Subst Abuse Treat* 22:231-43–, 2002.
55. Azrin NH, McMahon PT, Donohue B, et al.: Behavior therapy for drug abuse: A controlled treatment outcome study. *Behav Res Ther* 32:857–66, 1994.
56. Waldron HB, Turner CW, Ozechowski TJ: Profiles of drug use behavior change for adolescents in treatment. *Addict Behav* 30:1775–96, 2005.
57. Riggs PD, Hall SK, Mikulich-Gilbertson SK, Lohman M, Kayser A: A randomized controlled trial of pemoline for attention-deficit/hyperactivity disorder in substance-abusing adolescents. *J Am Acad Child Adolesc Psychiatry* 43:420–9, 2004.
58. Geller B, Cooper TB, Sun K, et al.: Double-blind and placebo-controlled study of lithium for adolescent bipolar disorders with secondary substance dependency. *J Am Acad Child Adolesc Psychiatry* 37:171–8, 1998.
59. March J, Silva S, Petrycki S, et al.: Treatment for Adolescents With Depression Study (TADS) Team. Fluoxetine, cognitive-behavioral therapy, and their combination for adolescents with depression: Treatment for Adolescents With Depression Study (TADS) randomized controlled trial. *JAMA* 292:807–20, 2004.
60. Carroll KM, Nich C, Ball SA, McCance E, Frankforter TL, Rounsaville BJ: One-year follow-up of disulfiram and psychotherapy for cocaine-alcohol users: Sustained effects of treatment. *Addiction* 95:1335–49, 2000.
61. Niederhofer H, Staffen W: Acamprosate and its efficacy in treating alcohol dependent adolescents. *Eur Child Adolesc Psychiatry* 12:144–8, 2003.
62. Deas D, May MP, Randall C, Johnson N, Anton R: Naltrexone treatment of adolescent alcoholics: an open-label pilot study. *J Child Adolescent Psychopharmacol* 15:723–8, 2005.
63. Johnson BA: Recent advances in the development of treatments for alcohol and cocaine dependence: focus on topiramate and other modulators of GABA or glutamate function. *CNS Drugs* 19:873–96, 2005.
64. Hopfer CJ, Khuri E, Crowley TJ: Treating adolescent heroin use. *J Am Acad Child Adolesc Psychiatry* 42:609–11, 2003.
65. Marsch LA, Bickel WK, Badger GJ, et al.: Comparison of pharmacological treatments for opioid-dependent adolescents: A randomized controlled trial. *Arch Gen Psychiatry* 62:1157–64, 2005.

CHAPTER 5.9 ■ SLEEP DISORDERS

THOMAS F. ANDERS

INTRODUCTION

Our understanding of clinical sleep disorders has advanced significantly since the 1950s, when polysomnographic (PSG) recordings first described the rapid eye movement (REM) and nonrapid eye movement (NREM) sleep states. Aserinsky and Kleitman (1) first described the electrophysiological differences between the two states of sleep. Today, standards of practice, official nosologies, and certification processes are all in place. The American Academy of Sleep Medicine certifies clinical laboratories and the technicians who record sleep, and the American Boards of Internal Medicine, Pediatrics, and Psychiatry/Neurology have collectively agreed to certify board-eligible clinicians in a new subspecialty, sleep disorders medicine. A pediatric section of the Associated Professional Sleep Societies, the national professional organization of sleep specialists, held its first organizing and scientific meeting in 2005 and is planning a second meeting in 2006. Unfortunately, child and adolescent psychiatrists continue to be underrepresented in all of these groups.

How are sleep disorders defined and diagnosed? A number of psychophysiological systems are routinely recorded in a sleep laboratory: peripheral muscle tone (electromyogram, EMG) from submental muscles, horizontal and vertical eye movements (electrooculogram, EOG) from electrodes placed peri-orbitally, the electroencephalogram (EEG) from an array of scalp electrodes, and cardiac, respiratory, and peripheral motor activity from thermistors placed around the chest, airway, and limbs. Eye movement, muscle tone, and EEG patterns are the primary parameters used to score REM and NREM sleep states. Patterns of obstructed breathing, heart rate irregularity, and episodic behaviors, including limb movements, are associated features useful in diagnosing specific sleep disorders.

PSG studies are largely confined to nighttime recordings in a sleep laboratory. However, sleeping in an unfamiliar sleep laboratory disrupts normal sleep architecture and often requires recording over several nights to eliminate the "first night" stress effect. The need for multiple nights of recording has made sleep research with young subjects difficult as both children, wired with an array of electrodes and thermistors in an unfamiliar sleep laboratory, and their parents are reluctant to sleep away from home for even one night. Ambulatory polysomnography, actigraphy, and time-lapse video recording have greatly expanded the scope of sleep evaluations by providing opportunities for home recording and for 24-hour recording.

NEUROPHYSIOLOGY OF SLEEP STATES

The EEG pattern during REM sleep is low voltage, fast, resembling the EEG of wakefulness; the EMG pattern is inhibited and the EOG is characterized by bursts of vertical and horizontal saccadic eye movements. Heart and respiratory rates are rapid and irregular. Neuronal firing, neurotransmitter release and uptake, and metabolic rates also resemble patterns of waking. Mental activity during REM sleep is present and is reported as dreams. Thus, during REM sleep, an individual appears asleep, but for the most part the central nervous system is highly activated. In infants, REM sleep has been called active sleep.

In contrast to the psychophysiological activation of REM sleep, NREM sleep is characterized by more basal, organized patterns of physiological inhibition. Both respiratory and heart rates are slowed and more regular. The EEG is synchronized with specific slower frequency wave forms. In infants NREM sleep is also called quiet sleep. The EEG of stage 1 NREM sleep resembles the tracing of REM sleep; however, respiratory and heart rate patterns are regular, and saccadic eye movements are absent. The EEG of stage 2 NREM sleep contains K complexes and sleep spindles. Stages 3 and 4 NREM sleep have varying amounts of slow, high-voltage synchronized delta waves. In newborns, only two sleep states—REM sleep and NREM sleep—can be distinguished. By 6 months of age, the specific EEG waveforms that are used to subclassify the four stages of NREM sleep have emerged.

DEVELOPMENT OF SLEEP-WAKE STATE ORGANIZATION

The characteristics of the electrophysiologic patterns and the proportions of sleep-wake states change with development.

TABLE 5.9.1

SLEEP-WAKE STATE CHANGES WITH AGE

	Infants	Adults
REM / NREM %	50/50	20/80
Ultradian cycle	50–60 min.	90 min.
Circadian cycle	Polyphasic	Diurnal
Temporal	Equi-distributed	First Third/Last Third
Sleep stages	States only	4 Stages NREM

Proportionally in adults, REM sleep occupies about 20% and NREM sleep about 80% of total sleep time each night. Stages 3 and 4 NREM sleep account for approximately 20% of all NREM sleep. In newborns, REM sleep occupies 50% of total sleep time (2). REM and NREM sleep states alternate with each other in sleep cycles that recur periodically through the sleep period. In adults, the REM-NREM sleep cycle length averages 90 minutes; in infants the cycle length is approximately 50 minutes. Adult sleep organization is achieved by adolescence (Table 5.9.1).

In adults, sleep typically begins with NREM stage 4 sleep, and the first third of the sleep period has most of the total night's stage 4 NREM sleep. That is, although REM-NREM cycles recur at 90-minute intervals throughout the night, the percentage of stage 4 NREM sleep in a single cycle is greater during the early part of the night than later in the night. The proportion of REM sleep in a single sleep cycle is greater during the latter part of the night.

In infants, sleep begins with an initial REM period, and sleep cycles throughout the night include as much REM sleep as NREM sleep. No early- and late-night differences in REM–NREM proportions are found. The shift in the temporal organization of states during the course of a night's sleep, which begins in the first month of life, reflects the maturation of internal central nervous system timing mechanisms. That is, biological clocks mature to regulate both the ultradian and circadian control mechanisms to achieve sleep-wake state consolidation. These changes are depicted schematically in Figures 5.9.1 and 5.9.2.

An understanding of these developmental changes is important for understanding the presentation of specific sleep disorders that affect infants, children, and adolescents.

FROM DYADIC REGULATION TO SELF-REGULATION: A TRANSACTIONAL MODEL

During early development, transitions between sleep and waking at bedtime and during the middle of the night offer multiple opportunities for parent–infant interaction (3). Sensitive responses during these interactions facilitate the development of self-regulation. An assessment of sleep disturbances in the infant, toddler, and preschool child, therefore, necessarily involves assessment of the parent–child interactions and the psychosocial factors that impact that relationship. Figure 5.9.3 schematically depicts a transactional model useful in the evaluation of sleep disorders in young children (4).

Proximal influences on the relationship include the primary caregiver's current state of physical and psychological well being, the primary caregiver's own childhood experiences of being parented, including their experiences around sleep, current social support networks, the family's economic and household condition, and the infant's temperament and physical health. More distal factors in the transactional

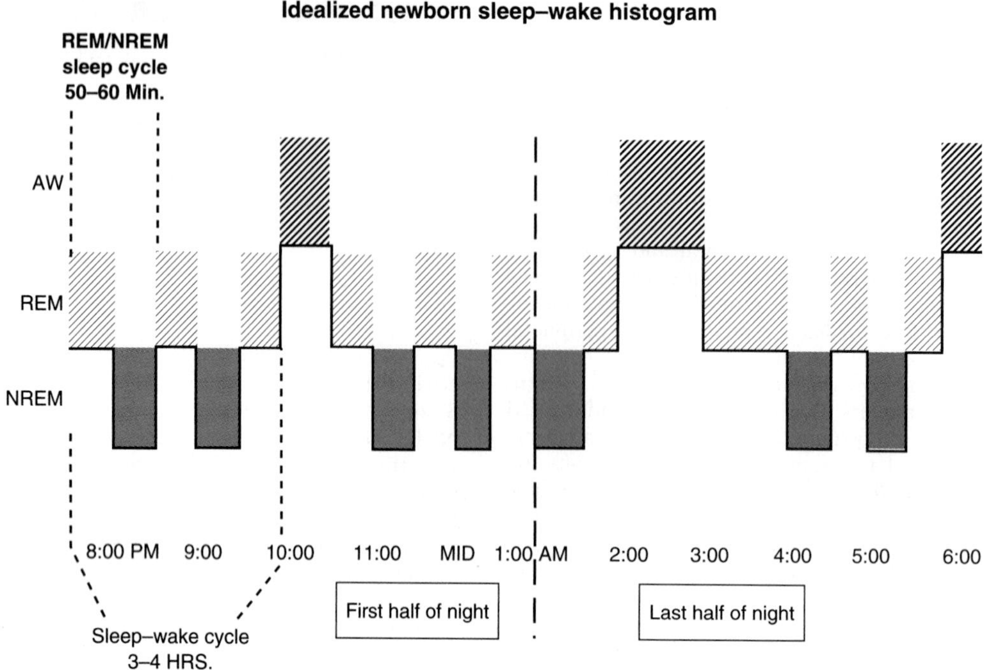

FIGURE 5.9.1. Note the regular distribution (~50:50) between REM and NREM sleeps throughout the sleep cycle and the initial REM sleep period at sleep onset.

model include the broader cultural context and belief systems of the family and more indirect environmental influences. Stressors, such as infant physical illness or maternal depression, serve as proximate factors that directly impact parent–child interaction. At bedtime and during the night, if parental sensitivity and consistency are affected, the regulation of sleep may become disrupted. In turn, when the infant's sleep becomes disorganized, the entire family is impacted, which in turn affects infant sleep-wake regulation.

In early childhood, a sleep problem may be specific to a particular relationship or setting. A child may nap at the daycare center but not at home (or vice-versa), or a child may fall asleep more easily when the babysitter puts the infant to bed

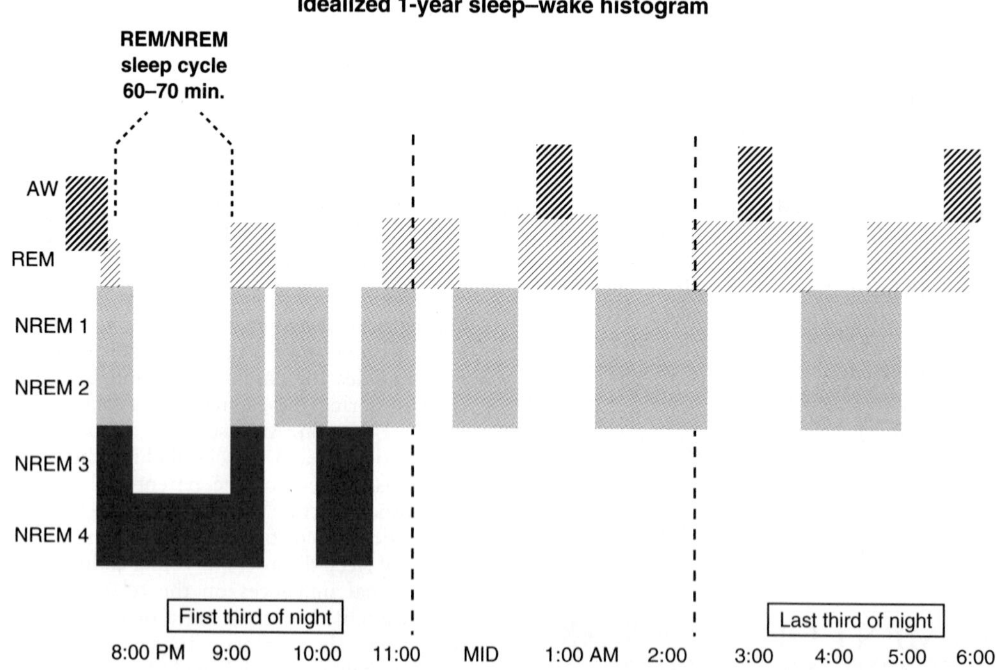

FIGURE 5.9.2. Note that the majority of NREM 3 and 4 occurs during the first third of the night, and that REM periods progressively lengthen during the middle and last third of the sleep cycle. The initial REM sleep bout is brief and sometimes absent. The descent to NREM stage 3–4 is rapid.

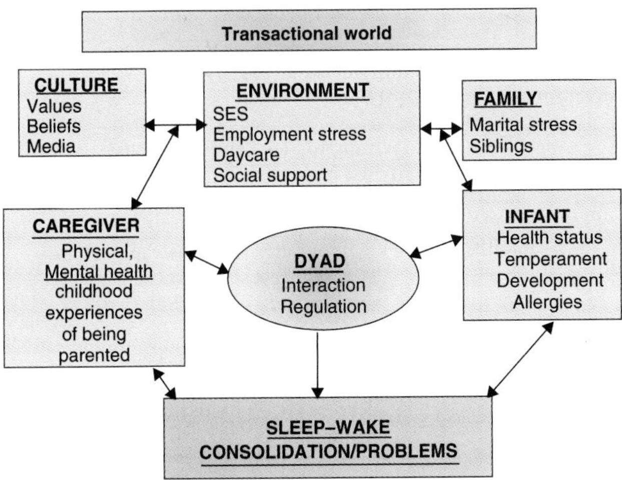

FIGURE 5.9.3. Transactional world.

than when the parent does (or vice-versa). Sometimes, infants and young children's sleep problems present differentially with mothers and fathers.

CLASSIFICATION OF SLEEP DISORDERS IN CHILDHOOD

Several nosologies for classifying pediatric sleep disorders are currently available, although none adequately present criteria for the night waking and sleep resistance problems that are such prevalent concerns of parents of young children. They are *The International Classification of Sleep Disorders: Diagnostic and Coding Manual, 2nd Edition (ICSD-DCM2)* (5), the *Diagnostic and Statistical Manual of Mental Disorders (DSM-IV-TR)* (6) and *Diagnostic Classification: Zero to Three, Revised (DC 0-3R)* (7). Table 5.9.2 compares their principal similarities and differences.

All three nosologies define major categories of disordered sleep: 1) dysomnias; 2) parasomnias; and 3) sleep disorders associated with medical/psychiatric conditions. Each of the systems then subclassifies the major categories slightly differently. Dysomnias are defined as disruptions of sleep-wake state organization, i.e., the disruption of the REM-NREM pattern. Parasomnias are defined as intrusions of events upon a normally organized sleep-wake process.

ICSD-DCM2 lumps together the disorders of night waking and sleep resistance, so common in early childhood, as *behavioral sleep disorders*. Cut points are not specified, especially as they pertain to differentiating disorder from typical age-appropriate behaviors. Similarly, the DSM-IV-TR diagnostic criteria for dysomnias in young children often are not easily met, especially for the primary insomnias and hypersomnias.

New quantitative and more developmentally appropriate research diagnostic criteria (RDC) for disorders of initiating and/or maintaining sleep (dysomnias) for younger children have been proposed (8) (Tables 5.9.3 and 5.9.4). Because they do not meet full adult criteria of DSM-IV-TR for functional impairment, the disorders are referred to as "protodysomnias." *Perturbations* refer to age-appropriate temporary disruptions of sleep patterns, such as the behavioral sleep response related to an acute respiratory infection. Perturbations are time limited and self correcting. *Disturbances* suggest potentially more significant risk conditions that warrant monitoring and, perhaps, parent guidance. *Disorders* are persistent and severe and require treatment. Further research with large, ethnically diverse populations, focused on age-related prevalence, natural course and efficacy of guidance and treatment programs, is necessary before these criteria can be officially adopted.

DC 0-3R, like DSM-IV-TR, is a multiaxial nosology of mental disorders developed specifically for use in infancy and early childhood. DC 0-3R provides several opportunities to classify sleep problems, either as a primary entity or as a symptom of another Axis 1 disorder such as traumatic stress disorder, adjustment disorder, regulatory disorder, anxiety disorder or mood disorder. For the primary sleep disorder category, DC 0-3R has adopted the research diagnostic criteria for sleep onset and night waking protodysomnias described next.

A DEVELOPMENTAL APPROACH TO DIAGNOSIS

Infants, Toddlers, and Preschoolers

Night Waking and Sleep Onset Protodysomnias

"My infant is not sleeping through the night" is one of the most common concerns of parents at the time of well baby

TABLE 5.9.2

SLEEP DISORDERS NOSOLOGIES

	ICSD-DCM2	DSM IV-TR	DC 0-3R
DYSOMNIAS (Disruptions)	Intrinsic disorders Extrinsic disorders Circadian disorders	Primary Insomnia Primary Hypersomnia Narcolepsy Breathing Related (OSA) Circadian Rhythm Disorder RLS / PLMD	RDC-INFANT
PARASOMNIAS (Intrusions)	Arousal Disorders Sleep-Wake Trans. REM Parasomnias	Nightmare Disorder Sleep Terror Dis. Sleep Walking Dis.	DSM-IV-TR
MED/PSYCH DISORDERS	Mental Disorders Neurological Dis. Other Medical Dis.	Mental Disorders General Medical Dis. Substance Induced	Regulatory Dis. with Sleep Prob.

OSA, Obstructive Sleep Apnea; RLS, restless legs syndrome; PLMD, periodic limb movement disorder.

TABLE 5.9.3

NIGHT-WAKING DYSOMNIA IN TODDLERS AND PRESCHOOLERS (OCCURS AFTER INFANT HAS BEEN ASLEEP FOR >10 MINUTES)

	Frequency and Duration of Nighttime Awakenings**
Perturbation *(1 episode/week for at least 1 month)*	
12–24 months of age	≥3 awakenings/night totaling ≥30 minutes
>24 months of age	≥2 awakenings/night totaling ≥20 minutes
>36 months of age	≥2 awakenings/night totaling ≥10 minutes
Disturbance *(2–4 episodes/week for at least 1 month)*	
12–24 months of age	≥3 awakenings/night totaling ≥30 minutes
>24 months of age	≥2 awakening/night totaling ≥20 minutes
>36 months of age	≥2 awakenings/night totaling ≥10 minutes
Disorder (307.42.1) *(5–7 episodes/week for at least 1 month)*	
12–24 months of age	≥3 awakenings/night totaling ≥30 minutes
>24 months of age	≥2 awakening/night totaling ≥20 minutes
>36 months of age	≥2 awakenings/night totaling ≥10 minutes

**Awakenings that require parental intervention.
In the Gaylor et al. paper, the criteria for night waking disorder were:
12–23 mos: ≥2 awakenings/night, totaling ≥20 min
≥24 months of age: ≥1 awakening/night, totaling ≥20 min.

TABLE 5.9.4

SLEEP ONSET DYSOMNIA IN TODDLERS AND PRESCHOOLERS

	Settling to Sleep and Reunions** (Must meet any 2 of the 3 criteria)
Perturbation *(1 episode/week for at least 1 month)*	
12–24 months of age	1) >30 minutes to fall asleep, 2) parent remains in room for sleep onset, 3) more than three reunions
>24 months of age	1) >20 minutes to fall asleep, 2) parent remains in room for sleep onset, 3) more than two reunions
Disturbance *(2–4 episodes/week for at least 1 month)*	
12–24 months of age	1)>30 minutes to fall asleep, 2) parent remains in room for sleep onset, 3) more than three reunions
>24 months of age	1) >20 minutes to fall asleep, 2) parent remains in room for sleep onset, 3) more than two reunions
Disorder (307.42.2) *(5–7 episodes/week for at least 1 month)*	
12–24 months of age	1)>30 minutes to fall asleep, 2) parent remains in room for sleep onset, 3) more than three reunions
>24 months of age	1) >20 minutes to fall asleep, 2) parent remains in room for sleep onset, 3) more than two reunions

**Reunions reflect resistances going to bed (e.g., repeated bids, protests, struggles).

visits. Some parents expect their infants to sleep through the night shortly after birth. Others complain that their infant "resists falling asleep" and must be rocked or nursed to sleep for prolonged periods. Occasionally, health professionals prescribe hypnotics or antihistamines for 6- to 12-month-old infants with these problems, or they may counsel parents to let their babies cry.

During the second year of life, toddlers commonly resist bedtime and separating from their parents. Infants with significant problems have severe and intractable battles at bedtime associated with frequent and prolonged bouts of night waking that begin shortly after sleep onset and persist until morning rise time. These more serious disorders become a major source of family tension and are usually associated with significant parental conflict about managing the infant's sleep.

Preschoolers, especially if there are older siblings in the family, enjoy participating in the family's evening activities. Since many families have irregular schedules, time with parents may be a precious commodity that the child wishes to prolong. Young children fervently deny being tired when asked. When daytime experiences for preschoolers are too exciting or overstimulating, calming down at bedtime may be difficult. The role of television in overstimulation and fear arousal has also been posited. Whatever the causes, the preschool child may protest vigorously, attempting to delay bedtime. Examples of protestation include requesting bedtime stories to be repeated, returning for more good-night hugs and kisses, asking for another glass of water or snack, and pleading for "five more minutes" until bedtime. A child may also insist on falling asleep in the parents' bed or while lying next to and holding the parents.

Nightmares

Dreams are normally reported by children after age 3 years (9) and nightmares shortly thereafter. Nightmares occur during REM sleep and result in a fully awake and oriented child who remembers and recounts the content of the dream. Because REM sleep occurs most commonly in the latter third of the night, nightmares generally are noted in the early morning hours, after 2:00 A.M. Nightmares must be distinguished from night terrors. A nightmare is frightening. Its content often involves being injured, lost, or abandoned. For preschool children, nightmares often include images of monsters and frightening animals; for older school-age children, nightmares typically include more comprehensible human imagery. If nightmares are frequent, they can be another source of the child's reluctance to go to bed. Nightmares are associated with both acute and posttraumatic stress disorders.

In treating frequent, recurrent nightmares and nightly prolonged struggles at bedtime, the clinician must explore sources of anxiety and suggest interventions that can address, as best as possible, the child's needs for comfort, security, regularity of sleep habits, and protection from overstimulation.

Night Terrors (Pavor Nocturnus)

A relatively rare but dramatic group of disorders, the parasomnias, may appear during this age period. The two most common parasomnias in childhood are night terrors (pavor nocturnus) and sleepwalking (somnambulism). Night terrors are characterized by a sudden arousal, accompanied by screaming and thrashing uncontrollably in bed. The child may appear glassy-eyed and may stare without seeing, unresponsive to visual or verbal cues. In the laboratory, such an episode is characterized by continuous high-voltage delta waves on the EEG, characteristic of NREM stage 4 sleep. During a night terror attack, the child is not awake but may appear to be highly agitated. Autonomic arousal characterized by tachypnea, tachycardia, and diaphoresis is obvious. Consolation by parents is not effective. The attack terminates spontaneously after approximately 3–5 minutes, as the transition to REM sleep occurs. Occasionally, an attack may last 30 minutes. If parental intervention is sustained and vigorous, the child may awaken but then is confused, disoriented, and unable to relate dream material. The child quickly returns to sleep and does not remember the episode on the following morning.

These NREM sleep parasomnias generally occur at a particular point in the sleep cycle, at the end of a NREM stage 4 sleep period, just prior to a transition to REM sleep. Physiologically, NREM stage 4 sleep is the deepest stage of sleep. Sensory thresholds are highest, and it is difficult to arouse individuals. Thus, when aroused from a NREM parasomnia, subjects are generally disoriented, their thinking is confused, and there is no verbal recounting of mental activity. Other common features of NREM parasomnias are a predominance of males to females (6–8:1), and a strongly positive family history (along male lines).

The clinical presentation of night terrors is distinct from that of nightmares. Nightmares are associated with vivid dream imagery; a fully alert, frightened, and oriented youngster; and recollection of the episode in the morning. Night terrors occur in the first third of the night when NREM Stage 4 sleep predominates and are not associated with mental content. Amnesia for the event is present in the morning.

The most parsimonious treatment for parasomnias is reassuring the child and family that the problem is transient, not serious, and requires no specific pharmacological or psychotherapeutic intervention. Since overexertion and stress may be associated with an increased need for NREM stage 4 sleep, these two daytime conditions may predispose a susceptible child to an increase in the frequency and intensity of NREM parasomnias. Parents should be advised of the importance of regular sleep habits, particularly sufficient amounts of nighttime sleep. An after-school nap also may reduce any NREM stage 4 sleep deficit.

When a parasomnia is so frequent that the child becomes too embarrassed to sleep at a friend's house, or becomes inhibited in other usual daytime social activities, a benzodiazepine may be tried at bedtime. These drugs are usually effective, but termination of pharmacotherapy often results in a recurrence of the parasomnia. When parasomnias persist into adolescence, or present initially in adolescence, neurological evaluation is warranted to rule out sleep-related seizures. Parasomnias frequently resemble seizures, and an EEG with nasopharyngeal electrodes may be warranted for persistent, intractable cases before prescribing benzodiazepines in adolescents (10).

Obstructive Sleep Apnea (OSA)

OSA is a disorder that most often affects adults. However, it may occur in toddlers and preschoolers, often secondary to enlarged tonsils and adenoids. OSA is characterized by expiratory snoring and mouth breathing. OSA should be suspected in any child who snores. In older children and adolescents, excessive obesity that reduces airflow during sleep may be present. Finally, some congenital birth defects of the oro-nasopharynx may result in narrowing or collapse of the airway during sleep (11).

OSA is classified as a disorder of excessive somnolence because a brief awakening is required to restore breathing, and the multiple arousals that occur each night following the many brief apnea episodes, fragment sleep, and lead to daytime fatigue and sleepiness. Since young children rarely complain of sleepiness or feeling tired, they may present with inattention or even "hyperactivity" as they fidget to fight off their sleepiness. On occasion the multiple awakenings significantly interfere with the secretion of growth hormone, which normally occurs during NREM stage 4 sleep. A young, growing child with OSA may, thus, present with mild growth retardation or, in extreme cases, a full-blown failure-to-thrive syndrome (12).

To aid in diagnosing OSA, an audiocassette recorder at the bedside can record snoring, mouth breathing, and the "stopped" breathing episodes that signify apnea. However, sleep apnea should be investigated by polysomnography in a sleep laboratory in order to identify its specific cause and severity, and prescribe an appropriate intervention.

School-Age Children

Sleepwalking (*Somnambulism*) and Sleep Talking (*Somniloqy*)

Sleepwalking, like night terrors, occurs approximately 90–120 minutes after sleep onset. The child sits up in bed and may fidget for a time or may leave the bed and walk to another location. The child generally does not scream, so he or she may be found in a new location in the morning. If sitting up or moving around the bed is the only manifestation of the parasomnia, then no one may be aware of the episode in the morning. The child does not recall the episode.

A popular misconception is that sleepwalking is purposeful. In general, sleepwalkers are poorly coordinated and are unable to carry out complex behaviors. In fact, sleepwalkers are in danger of injuring themselves, and parents should be advised to safe-proof their child's sleeping environment to protect their child from harm. Securing windows, locking doors and setting alarms may be necessary. It is highly unlikely that a child or adolescent who leaves the house and takes a drive in the family car or who wanders to the kitchen to consume a midnight snack is sleepwalking. Sleepwalkers are unable to perform such complex behaviors.

Sleep talking, like sleepwalking and night terror attacks, generally is confined to NREM stage 4 sleep. Short cries or garbled utterances can be heard; usually, the sleep utterances are unintelligible. The episode is short and not remembered in the morning.

Adolescence

Narcolepsy

Narcolepsy, the only sleep disorder that is a disorder of REM sleep, has its onset in adolescence. The disorder is attributed to dysfunction of brain-stem mechanisms associated with sleep-wake regulation (13, 14). Except for the first few months of a newborn infant's life, REM sleep never follows a period of wakefulness; rather the transition from wakefulness to sleep is characterized by NREM sleep (Figures 5.9.4 and 5.9.5). Individuals with narcolepsy are exceptions to this rule. All the manifestations of REM sleep may intrude upon wakefulness in a REM sleep or narcoleptic "attack."

Full-blown narcolepsy is characterized by the narcoleptic tetrad: 1) irresistible attacks of REM sleep intruding upon wakefulness; 2) cataplexy characterized by sudden loss of bilateral peripheral muscle tone, often provoked by strong affect. This condition reflects the peripheral muscle inhibition of REM sleep. Cataplectic attacks are brief, rarely more than several

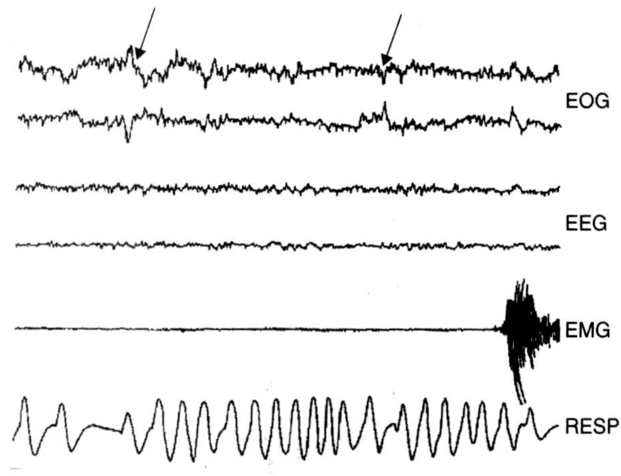

FIGURE 5.9.4. Polygraphic recording of REM sleep. An epoch of REM sleep in a newborn infant characterized by a low voltage, fast EEG, active rapid eye movements (arrows), an inhibited EMG, and rapid irregular respirations.

minutes, with immediate and complete recovery. Attacks may occur only several times a year or as frequently as many times in one day. Consciousness and memory remain intact. Both 3) hypnagogic hallucinations (vivid dream-like mentation at sleep onset) and 4) sleep paralysis (immobility of limbs as sleep begins) similarly represent REM sleep EMG inhibition and dreaming, occurring during sleep onset, when REM sleep normally is not prominent. Although cataplexy, hypnagogic hallucinations, and sleep paralysis diminish in frequency over time, narcolepsy, once present, is a lifelong, chronic condition.

The peak age at onset is in adolescence and young adulthood, although cases of childhood onset have been reported (15, 16). Genetic factors are important. First-degree probands of narcoleptic patients are at eight times greater risk of having some disorder of excessive sleepiness than are individuals in the general population. Recently, speculation regarding pathophysiology has focused on genetically mediated dysfunction in cholinergic-dopaminergic interactions (17). Epidemiological studies have reported the prevalence of narcolepsy at 0.04% to 0.07%, making narcolepsy twice as common as multiple sclerosis and half as common as Parkinson's disease.

Human leukocyte antigen (HLA) testing is essentially 85% positive for the HLA-DQB1*0602 and HLA-DR2 alleles for patients with narcolepsy, compared with 12–38% of the general population. Genetic factors other than HLA are also likely to be involved. In narcoleptic dogs, a specific narcolepsy gene has been identified, and it is likely that the discovery of the human gene(s) is soon to follow (18–20). Nevertheless, environmental factors are also important, as evident by the reported concordance rates of only 25–30% for monozygotic twins (21).

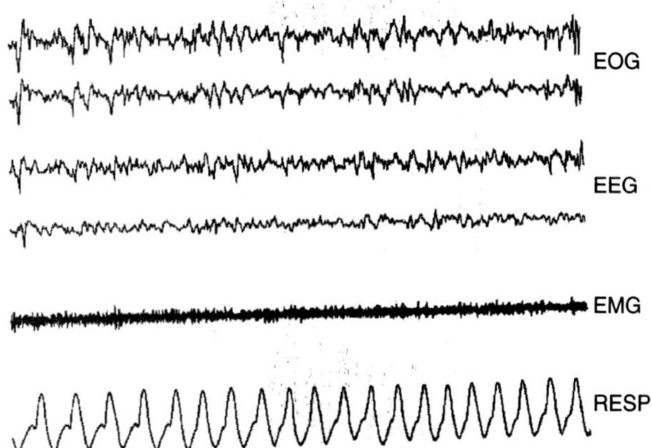

FIGURE 5.9.5. Polygraphic recording of NREM sleep. An epoch of NREM sleep characterized by high voltage, slow waves in the EEG, an absence of rapid eye movements, a tonic EMG pattern, and slowed, regular respirations.

The narcoleptic adolescent naps for 20- to 40-minute periods, awakening refreshed. The cycle is repeated again within 2–3 hours. This refreshed feeling contrasts with the disorientation and persistent fatigue associated with disorders of excessive somnolence secondary to other causes.

The definitive diagnosis of narcolepsy requires polysomnographic evaluation in a sleep laboratory. To assess quantitatively the amount of excessive daytime sleepiness that patients with disorders of excessive somnolence experience, the Multiple Sleep Latency Test should be performed (22). The test is done in a sleep laboratory and uses polysomnography to measure the amount of sleep that is obtained during five 20-minute trials, from midmorning to early evening. At each 20-minute period, the subject tries to fall asleep, and the latency to sleep onset for each attempted nap represents how sleepy the individual is. The test, standardized for use with adults and for adolescents, has been a sensitive indicator of sleepiness and is significantly correlated with the performance decrement associated with sleepiness.

The treatment of narcolepsy is symptomatic and must be individualized depending on the severity of specific symptoms (23). Stimulant medications are used most commonly for the treatment of excessive daytime sleepiness, and tricyclic antidepressant medications for the treatment of cataplexy.

In a retrospective study of adult patients with narcolepsy, a significant number had been misdiagnosed as having ADHD in adolescence but had been treated appropriately with amphetamines or methylphenidate, with good symptom improvement (24). Although narcolepsy is a rare disorder, occurring in only 4 in 10,000 (0.04%) individuals, and hyperactivity is a more common disorder, estimated to occur in 7%–10% of school-age children, in all children who present with attention-deficit/hyperactivity disorder or other hyperactivity syndromes, a careful sleep history should be obtained. The therapist should ask specific questions that focus on symptoms of the narcoleptic tetrad and on a family history of sleep disorders.

Clomipramine 10 to 20 mg/day in divided doses has been used successfully to manage cataplexy. Monoamine oxidase inhibitors may be used to manage both cataplexy and the REM sleep onset symptoms of sleep paralysis and hypnagogic hallucinations. A new wake-promoting drug, Modafinil (Provigil), which activates orexin-containing neurons, is reported to be more effective and have fewer side effects than the traditional stimulants (25, 26).

Patients with narcolepsy usually adjust poorly to their disorder. They exhibit problems in school and in social relationships. Associated psychiatric disorders include major depression, generalized anxiety, and substance abuse. Behavioral management with psychosocial support and counseling is an essential component of treatment. Patients must be encouraged to follow regular bedtimes and rise times. Regularly scheduled naps for 20 to 30 minutes, two to three times daily, should be encouraged. School and work schedules need to be designed to accommodate the sleep needs of the patient. Patients are advised to attend self-help support groups. The American Narcolepsy Association publishes a newsletter that keeps members informed of recent advances.

Circadian Rhythm Sleep Disorder

A much more common sleep disorder that occurs in adolescence meets criteria for circadian rhythm sleep disorder (27).

A sleep debt occurs as the adolescent stays up late each night and then arises early for school. Typically, adolescents begin to complain of feeling tired and frequently "sleep in" on weekends to catch up. A circadian rhythm sleep disorder results as the sleep debt accumulates with awakenings later in the morning, especially on weekends and holidays. As the body's timing mechanisms shift, it becomes more difficult physiologically to fall asleep and wake up at the usual hours. Adolescents thus find themselves in a perpetual condition of jet lag. Sufficient sleep—at least 9–10 hours each night—at regular, socially acceptable times, is particularly important during adolescence. When sleep debts accumulate by force of circumstances, napping should be encouraged.

Narcolepsy usually can be diagnosed from the history alone. Occasionally, however, adolescents are poor reporters and misrepresent both the degree of their sleepiness and the phase disturbances of their sleep. Multiple Sleep Latency Test evaluations and spending a night in the sleep laboratory may clarify confusing pictures. Once a phase delay syndrome is chronic and persistent, phase advance methods of resetting the biological clock may be necessary (28).

Disordered Sleep in Medical and Psychiatric Conditions

Less information about sleep disorders in children and adolescents who have medical and psychiatric conditions is available than there is for adults. However, a recent book provides an excellent summary of what is known. (12) Even the disruptions of sleep presumably associated with common childhood illnesses are, in general, anecdotal reports not supported by systematic research.

Children who live in institutions are reported to have short sleep periods, repeated nighttime awakenings, and phase delay disorders. Children with neurodevelopmental disorders such as autism and children with developmental delay also experience frequent night awakenings and phase shifts (12, 29). In general, disorganization of REM and NREM sleep structure, however, is associated only with profound syndromes of brain damage (30).

Sleep disruption in children with psychiatric disorders remains controversial. Although it has been clearly demonstrated that adults with major depressive disorder have characteristic indicators of disturbed sleep, including disruptions of sleep-related endocrine regulation, these indicators are not regularly present in the sleep of children and adolescents with major depressive disorder (31–33).

Similarly, in the few studies of children with attention-deficit disorder, despite complaints from parents about disturbed sleep, the children's sleep-wake state organization in a sleep laboratory was unaffected (34, 35). Again, the paucity of studies, characterized by small samples and heterogeneous diagnostic groupings, contributes to the lack of definitive conclusions. The waking behavioral fidgeting and restlessness, associated with "fighting" sleepiness, either associated with narcolepsy or OSA, has been mentioned earlier in this chapter.

Finally, studies examining the effects of alcohol and other chemicals on sleep generally report two patterns of sleep-wake state disorganization: (36) 1) decreased REM sleep and fragmented sleep resulting from multiple arousals during agitated states of hallucinosis and withdrawal and 2) periods of prolonged atypical "drugged" sleep during states of intoxication. However, these results are difficult to interpret. The pharmacological effects of chemicals, both prescription and nonprescription, vary by dose, chronicity of use, and chemical structure of the compound. Initially, most sedatives lead to increased sleep; habituation and tolerance then develop, leading to chronic sleep deprivation, particularly REM deprivation.

Both hypnotic drugs and alcohol are frequently misused for insomnia that masks underlying disorders of anxiety and depression. After periods of drug misuse, it is often unclear whether inappropriate drug use led to disordered sleep or whether disordered sleep precipitated the course of self-medication. Careful studies of the effects of substance abuse on sleep-wake state organization in children and adolescents have not been done.

TAKING A SLEEP HISTORY

It is important to obtain a careful sleep history in all children with behavior problems, as well as in children with a specific sleep disorder. Obtaining a reliable sleep history requires a detailed description of all sleep-related symptoms in the child and a thorough history of sleep problems and patterns in other family members. What is the age at onset of the problem? What is the frequency of the symptom in terms of events per week or per night, and what has been its course (stable, worsening, improving)? What time during the night or day does the symptom occur, in terms of both clock time and time since falling asleep? For example, parasomnias are related to sleep onset and not to clock time. They generally occur 90–120 minutes after falling asleep. Phase delay syndromes are related to clock time. Sleep onset usually occurs at times that are later than usual.

The child's customary sleep habits are important to establish. What is the usual bedtime and rise time? How regular are sleep habits? What are the sleeping arrangements? With whom does the child share a room or bed? Do the child's symptoms disturb others? Are bedtime rituals present? How common are dreams and nightmares? How common are night waking and bed-wetting? All sleep histories need to gather data about breathing during sleep. In the absence of colds, is breathing labored? Are pauses in breathing audible? Is snoring prominent, regular? Is mouth breathing common, regular? Finally, it is important to assess the effects of a nighttime sleep problem on daytime functioning. Is the child sleepy during the day, or is the child alert and active? Does the child nap regularly? Do the nighttime symptoms encroach on normal social functions? For example, is the child embarrassed to sleep at a friend's house or away at camp because of the sleep problem?

Monitoring Sleep and Waking Behavior

A sleep diary or log should be maintained for one to two weeks prior to a formal evaluation. The diary measures night-to night stability of the problem(s) and includes information about sleeping, waking and interactional behaviors. Parental report measures include the Child Sleep Habits Questionnaire (CSHQ) (37) and the Pediatric Sleep Questionnaire (PSQ) (38), both of which are dimensional scales of problem sleep behaviors (bedtime problems, sleep-disordered breathing, etc.). These questionnaires have demonstrated reliability and validity with respect to identifying both behaviorally based and medically based sleep disorders in children ages 2 to 18 years (39) and 4 to 10 years (40). The CHSQ has been adapted for use in parental interviews in a younger population (1 to 4 years), although psychometric data from the interview format have not been calculated (41, 42).

Screening tools are available to detect problem sleep in normative populations (e.g., BEARS) (39, 40, 43, 44) and can help health practitioners who are in a position to identify sleep problems in children and implement education and intervention.

CONCLUSIONS

Researchers have learned a great deal about sleep-wake state maturation, regulation, and organization in children and adolescents. Many disorders, such as parasomnias and disorders of excessive somnolence, previously overlooked or misdiagnosed, can now be treated effectively. Although the pathogenesis of most of the sleep disorders remains uncertain, the ability to diagnose them better and to prescribe more specific treatments provides reassurance to children and their families and prevents the stigma of inappropriate or inaccurate diagnoses.

We clearly need more information about sleep disorders in preschool-aged children and in children with physical and psychiatric disorders. These studies need to be designed with sufficient numbers of subjects and with special sensitivity to the cultural contexts and family values and beliefs that are so important in establishing the household sleep environment.

References

1. Aserinsky E, Kleitman N: A motility cycle in sleeping infants as manifested by ocular and gross bodily activity. *J Appl Physiol* 8:11–13, 1955.
2. Roffwarg HP, Muzio JN, and Dement WC: Ontogenetic development of the human sleep-dream cycle. *Science*, 152, 604–619, 1966.
3. Anders TF, Goodlin-Jones BL, and Sadeh A: Sleep disorders. In: JCH Zeanah (ed), *Handbook of Infant Mental Health* (2nd ed). New York, Guilford Publications, (2000) pp. 326–338.
4. Goodlin-Jones B, Burnham M, and Anders T: Sleep and sleep disturbances: Regulatory processes in infancy. In: A Sameroff, M Lewis and S Miller (eds): *Handbook of Developmental Psychopathology* (2nd ed). New York, Kluwer Academic/Plenum Publishers, pp. 309–325, 2000.
5. American Academy of Sleep Medicine: *The International Classification of Sleep Disorders, Diagnostic and Coding Manual* (ICSD-DCM2) (2nd ed). American Academy of Sleep Medicine, MN, 2005.
6. American Psychiatric Association: *Diagnostic and Statistical Manual of Mental Disorders-TR* 4th ed. Washington, DC, 2004.
7. Zero to Three, Revised: *Diagnostic Classification of Mental Health and Developmental Disorders of Infancy and Early Childhood (DC–0-3R)*. Washington, DC, Zero to Three/National Center for Clinical Infant Programs, 2005.
8. Anders T and Dahl R: Classifying sleep disorders in infants and toddlers. In: I. Chatoor and D. Pine (eds). *A Research Agenda for DSM-V*, Washington DC, APPI Press, in press, 2006.
9. Foulkes D: A cognitive-psychological model of REM dream production. *Sleep* 5:169–187, 1982.
10. Zucconi M, Ferine-Strambi L: NREM parasomnias: Arousal disorders and differentiation from nocturnal frontal epilepsy. *Clin Neurophysiology* 111: (Suppl 2) S129–S135, 2000.
11. Guilleminault C, Stoohs R: Obstructive sleep apnea syndrome in children. *Pediatrician* 17:46–51, 1990.
12. Stores G and Wiggs L. (eds): *Sleep Disturbance in Children and Adolescents with Disorders of Development: Its Significance and Management, Clinics in Developmental Medicine, No. 155.* Mac Keith Press, 2001.
13. Guilleminault C: Narcolepsy and its differential diagnosis. In: C Guilleminault (ed) *Sleep and Its Disorders in Children*. New York, Raven, 1987, pp. 181–194.
14. Broughton RJ: The treatment of narcolepsy. *Suppl Clin Neurophysiol* 53:371–374, 2000.
15. Guilleminault C, Pelayo R: Narcolepsy in prepubertal children. *Annals of Neurology* 43:135–142, 1998.
16. Wise, M: Childhood narcolepsy. *Neurology* 50: (Suppl.1) S37–S42, 1998.
17. Guilleminault C, Heinzer R, Mignot E, et al.: Investigations into the neurologic basis of narcolepsy. *Neurology* 50:(Suppl.1) S8–S15, 1998.
18. Takahashi, J: Narcolepsy genes wake up the sleep field. *Science* 285:2076–2077, 1999.
19. Honda Y, Juji T, Matsuki K, et al.: HLA-DR2 and Dw2 in narcolepsy and in other disorders of excessive somnolence without cataplexy. *Sleep* 9:133–242, 1986.
20. Matsuki K, Honda Y, Juji T: Diagnostic criteria for narcolepsy and HLA-DR2 frequencies. *Tissue Antigens* 30:155–160, 1987.
21. Mignot E: Genetic and familial aspects of narcolepsy. *Neurology* 50: (Suppl. 1) S16–S22, 1998.
22. Carskadon M, Dement W: Sleepiness in normal adolescents. In: C Guilleminault (ed) *Sleep and Its Disorders in Children*. New York, Raven, 1987, pp. 53–66.
23. Thorpy M: Current concepts in the etiology, diagnosis and treatment of narcolepsy. *Sleep Med* 2:5–17, 2001.
24. Navalet Y, Anders T, Guilleminault C: Narcolepsy in children. In: C Guilleminault, Dement W, Passouant P. Holliswood (eds):, *Narcolepsy: Advances in Sleep Research*, Vol 3., New York, Spectrum, pp. 171–177, 1976.
25. Fry, J. Treatment modalities in narcolepsy. *Neurology* 50 (Suppl.1), S43–S48, 1998.
26. Chemelli R, Willie J, Sinton C et al.: Narcolepsy in orexin knockout mice: Molecular genetics of sleep regulation. *Cell* 98:47–51, 1999.
27. Thorpy M, Korman E, Spielman A, et al.: Delayed sleep-phase syndrome in adolescents. *Journal of Adolescent Health Care* 9:22–27, 1988.
28. Ferber R: *Solve Your Child's Sleep Problems*. New York, Simon & Schuster, 1985.
29. Okawa M, Sasaki H: Sleep disorders in mentally retarded and brain impaired children. In: C Guilleminault (ed) *Sleep and Its Disorders in Children*. New York, Raven, pp. 171–177, 1987.
30. Feinberg I: Sleep in organic brain conditions. In: Kales A (ed.) *Sleep: Physiology and Pathology*. Philadelphia, JB Lippincott, 1969, pp. 131–147.
31. Dahl R, Puig-Antich J: Sleep disturbances in child and adolescent psychiatric disorders. *Pediatrician* 17:32–37, 1990.
32. Dahl RE, Ryan ND, Perel J et al.: Cholinergic REM induction test with arecoline in depressed children. *Psychiatry Res* 51:269–282, 1994.
33. Waterman G, Dahl R, Birmaher B, et al.: The 24-hour pattern of prolactin secretion in depressed and normal adolescents. *Biol Psychiatry* 35:440–445, 1994.
34. Greenhill L, Puig-Antich J, Goetz R, et al.: Sleep architecture and real sleep measures in prepubertal children with attention-deficit disorder with hyperactivity. *Sleep* 6:91–101, 1983.
35. Kaplan B, McNicol J, Conte R, et al.: Sleep disturbances in preschool-aged hyperactive and nonhyperactive children. *Pediatrics* 80:839–844, 1987.
36. Lumley M, Roehrs T, Askel D, et al.: Ethanol and caffeine effects on daytime sleepiness/alertness. *Sleep* 10:306–312, 1987.
37. Owens J, Maxim R, Nobile C, McGuinn M, and Msall, M: Parental and self-report of sleep in children with attention-deficit/hyperactivity disorder. *Archives of Pediatric and Adolescent Medicine*, 154:549–555, 2000.
38. Chervin RD, Aldrich MS, Pickett R, and Guilleminault C: Comparison of the results of the Epworth Sleepiness Scale and the Multiple Sleep Latency Test. *Journal of Psychosomatic Research*, 42:145–155, 1997.
39. Chervin R, Hedger K, Dillon J, and Pituch KJ: Pediatric Sleep Questionnaire (PSQ): Validity and reliability of scales for sleep-disordered breathing, snoring, sleepiness, and behavioral problems. *Sleep Medicine*, 1(1):21–32, 2000.
40. Owens J, Spirito A, and McGuinn M: The Children's Sleep Habit Questionnaire (CSHQ): Psychometric properties of a survey instrument for school-aged children. *Sleep*, 23(8):1043–1051, 2000.
41. Gaylor EE, Burnham MM, Goodlin-Jones BL, and Anders TF: A longitudinal follow-up study of young children's sleep patterns using a developmental classification system. *Behavioral Sleep Medicine*, 3:44–61, 2005.
42. Gaylor EE, Goodlin-Jones BL, and Anders TF: Classification of young children's sleep problems: A pilot study. *Journal of American Academy of Child and Adolescent Psychiatry*, 40(1):61–67, 2001.
43. Bruni O, Ottaviano S, Guidetti V, Romoli M, Innocenzi M, Cortesi F, Giannotti F: The Sleep Disturbance Scale for Children (SDSC). Construction and validation of an instrument to evaluate sleep disturbances in childhood and adolescence. *Journal of Sleep Research*, 5:251–261, 1996.
44. Sadeh, A: A brief screening questionnaire for infant sleep problems: Validation and findings for an internet sample. *Pediatrics*, 113(6):e570–e577, 2004.

CHAPTER 5.10 ■ SOMATOFORM DISORDERS

JOHN V. CAMPO AND GREGORY K. FRITZ

INTRODUCTION

The biomedical model central to many of the triumphs of Western medicine maintains that the subjective suffering of our patients, most commonly described as *illness*, can best be understood as consequent to demonstrable biophysical or biochemical processes characterized as *disease*. It is nevertheless well known that many patients presenting with physical symptoms and associated disability in general medical settings do not suffer from explanatory disease in the traditional sense. Such patients are ubiquitous and are seen across all branches of medicine, in both primary and specialty care, and in both traditional medical and mental health settings. Conceptual problems associated with presumably "unexplained" symptoms are peculiar to the Western medical tradition (1), where a psychological model of illness causation developed alongside the biomedical model, with its own analogous terminology (psychopathology) and a separate system for reimbursement and care delivery (mental health). While it is increasingly well accepted that physical and mental health are inextricably linked and that health is a unitary construct, a practical dualism continues to influence our conceptualizations, attitudes, behaviors, and the structure of modern health care. The goal of this chapter is to introduce the clinical problems posed by youth presenting for the evaluation and management of somatic symptoms in the absence of discernible tissue damage or pathology, to place these problems into cultural and epidemiological context, to describe modern attempts at classification, and then to outline a practical approach to management that avoids mistakes rooted in dualistic thinking and professional bias.

There are cultural expectations associated with illness. Being "sick" implies that the affected individual suffers, is not responsible for the illness, and will seek competent medical help (2). Furthermore, cultural sanctions associated with the sick role such as exemptions from usual duties and obligations (school attendance), are dependent on whether a physician has evaluated, diagnosed, and thus legitimized the patient's illness. While illness associated with disease is readily accepted as "legitimate," otherwise subjectively real symptoms and sufferings in the absence of "proper" objectified disease may be stigmatized as somehow "illegitimate," and considered due to individual weakness or sociomoral failure. It takes little imagination to appreciate how individuals with medically unexplained or "functional" somatic symptoms are viewed similarly to those with other common mental disorders. Indeed, the term "neurosis" was initially applied to patients with "nervous symptoms" that did not appear to be associated with explanatory pathology in the brain or nervous system. The term *somatization* has been used descriptively to refer to the experience of physical symptoms where standard medical evaluation reveals no disease or biophysical process sufficient to explain the symptoms or their impact; such symptoms have commonly been referred to as *functional* (3, 4). A variety of related descriptive terms for presumably medically unexplained symptoms include "psychogenic," "nonorganic," and "hysterical," each typically falling out of favor with ongoing use, generally after acquiring a pejorative connotation and becoming viewed as problematically dualistic.

This chapter builds on several prior reviews of the limited available research literature addressing pediatric somatoform illness and specific functional somatic symptoms and syndromes (5–8). Given the demands of space and the reality that this chapter at best will provide an overview of the problem, considerable license will be taken in bundling findings about youth with a variety of different sorts of unexplained physical symptoms (e.g., chronic pain, fatigue, conversion symptoms). The reader should nevertheless appreciate the very real insufficiencies of the knowledge base and understand that existing approaches to one sort of somatoform problem may or may not prove to be applicable to others over time.

NOSOLOGY

Not surprisingly, efforts to classify the problems suffered by patients with medically unexplained or functional somatic symptoms diverge depending on whether they were initiated in general medicine, where the approach has been to develop criteria for functional somatic syndromes based on the organ system of interest, or in the mental health sector, where such problems have been incorporated into the existing classification system for mental disorders.

Somatoform disorders are defined by the presence of physical symptoms that suggest a physical disorder but are not fully explained by the presence of a general medical condition, the direct effects of a substance, or another mental disorder (9); the symptoms must cause distress or functional impairment and should not appear to be voluntarily or intentionally produced. Seven specific somatoform disorders are described in the DSM-IV: somatization disorder; undifferentiated somatoform disorder; conversion disorder; pain disorder; hypochondriasis; body dysmorphic disorder (BDD); and somatoform disorder, not otherwise specified (9). *Somatoform disorders* were introduced into modern psychiatric classification as a speculative diagnostic category in order to account for physically ill patients who do not suffer from an explanatory general medical condition or disease.

In order to diagnose a somatoform disorder, the clinician must make a judgment about whether a particular physical symptom is caused by a physical disease or general medical disorder, and whether that disease is sufficient to account for the patient's functional impairment and distress. This clearly can be quite subjective, raising questions about the diagnostic reliability of somatoform disorders as a category. In the case of a child who has been diagnosed with a functional somatic illness such as irritable bowel syndrome, clinicians might struggle to determine whether it is reasonable to consider that such a diagnosis "explains" the patient's symptoms. Different diagnosticians may conceptualize particular symptom constellations such as irritable bowel syndrome, chronic fatigue, or fibromyalgia differently, with some considering such syndromes representative of a bona fide, explanatory general medical condition and others considering the associated physical symptoms medically unexplained. Similarly, if a physical disease is present, the clinician might attempt to judge if the patient's impairment is greater than what might be "expected" based on objective pathology. Furthermore, the examiner must also infer the patient's sense of control over the production of the symptom.

Pediatric somatoform disorders are distinguished from *factitious disorders* and *malingering*, both disorders where physical symptoms are voluntarily fabricated, feigned, or intentionally produced (9). Another distinction is made from *psychological factors affecting medical condition,* in which psychological factors have an adverse effect on a general medical condition that would be coded on Axis III (9). Physical symptoms are also included in some of the criteria used to diagnose specific anxiety and depressive disorders, and the diagnostic manual notes that the clinician must determine whether the somatic symptoms are "better explained" by a "comorbid" emotional disorder. Diagnosis may thus be influenced by clinician training and experience, as well as by the site of initial presentation (10), findings suggesting that the diagnosis of somatoform disorder in children and adolescents is likely to be relatively unreliable in its current form. Unfortunately, studies addressing the reliability or validity of the diagnosis of somatoform disorder per se in children and adolescents have not been performed.

The somatoform disorder category remains the subject of intensive debate, with several authorities in favor of abolishing the category altogether, coding functional somatic symptoms and syndromes (e.g., fibromyalgia, irritable bowel syndrome) on axis III, and redistributing some of the disorders currently grouped within the somatoform disorders to other diagnostic categories (11). They argue persuasively that: 1) The category is inherently dualistic and culturally limited; 2) the diagnoses are unreliable, in part because of poorly defined symptom thresholds and ambiguities in the exclusionary criteria; 3) the included subgroupings are not coherent; and 4) the diagnoses have not been well accepted by patients or adopted by our colleagues in general medicine (11). Such revisions could help avoid false dichotomies in determining whether a particular symptom is "physical" or "mental," and are more consistent with current approaches in general medicine.

Currently accepted specific somatoform disorders are described below.

Somatization Disorder

The diagnosis of *somatization disorder* is rooted historically in early diagnostic conceptualizations of "Briquet's syndrome" or "hysteria" and refers to a recurrent disorder beginning before the age of 30 years that is characterized by multiple and diverse somatic complaints associated with medical help seeking and/or significant functional impairment. The French physician Briquet described patients with multiple medically unexplained physical symptoms and suggested that most of these patients developed symptoms and associated disability before the age of 20 years; early onset was associated with an especially poor prognosis (12). Diagnostic criteria for somatization disorder are quite specific yet may appear to be somewhat arbitrary, with the diagnosis requiring a history of pain in at least four different body sites, at least two gastrointestinal symptoms, one sexual or reproductive symptom, and one pseudoneurologic symptom other than pain (9). The criteria are based on the work of psychiatric researchers in the Midwest, and earlier editions of the DSM employed elaborate symptom counts from an extensive list of physical symptoms (13). Current DSM-IV criteria are an empirically based simplification aimed at addressing the core features of the disorder. Given the requirement for at least one sexual or reproductive symptom, the diagnosis is unusual in children, but not unheard of (14, 15).

Undifferentiated Somatoform Disorder

Children and adolescents with multiple somatic complaints across numerous different body locations who do not meet criteria necessary to justify a diagnosis of somatization disorder are likely to meet diagnostic criteria for *undifferentiated somatoform disorder,* a somatoform disorder characterized by the presence of one or more physical complaints (e.g., individual symptoms of fatigue, urinary, or gastrointestinal distress) lasting at least 6 months (9). *Neurasthenia* is a diagnosis with a long tradition in Western medicine that is sometimes made in Europe, but not included in the DSM-IV. Neurasthenia is characterized by persistent and troubling complaints of fatigue after mental effort or minimal physical effort, as well as at least two symptoms from a list that includes muscular aches and pains, dizziness, headache, sleep disturbance, inability to relax, irritability, and dyspepsia (16). Children with so-called neurasthenic symptoms of sufficient duration would be diagnosed with undifferentiated somatoform disorder.

Conversion Disorder

Conversion disorder is the somatoform diagnosis made when the clinician is confronted by one or more deficits or symptoms affecting voluntary motor or sensory function that suggest a neurologic or other general medical condition, and psychological factors are judged to be associated with the symptoms or deficits (9). The presence of psychological factors is inferred from an association of the symptom with a significant psychosocial stressor such as family conflict, bereavement, or trauma. Presenting symptoms classically resemble neurologic dysfunction (paralysis, paresis, anesthesia, paresthesia), follow the psychological stressor by hours to weeks, and may cause more distress for parents or physicians than for the patient *(la belle indifferénce)*. Symptoms frequently reported in children and adolescents include nonepileptic seizures, paralysis or paresis, sensory symptoms such as paresthesias, and gait disturbances (17–20). Symptoms are usually self limited but may be associated with chronic sequelae such as contractures or iatrogenic injury (8). There are four subtypes of conversion disorder in the DSM-IV, based on whether the symptoms presented are primarily motor, sensory, nonepileptic seizures, or mixed.

Pain Disorder

Pain disorder is diagnosed when there is pain in one or more anatomic sites of sufficient severity to warrant clinical attention and to cause significant distress or functional impairment (9). The three subtypes are: *pain disorder associated with psychological factors,* in which psychological factors are judged to play the predominant role in the causation or persistence of the pain; *pain disorder associated with both psychological factors and a general medical condition,* in which psychological factors and a general medical condition are judged to interact significantly in the development or maintenance of pain; and *pain disorder associated with a general medical condition,* in which psychological factors appear to play no more than a minimal role. The third subtype is not considered a mental disorder and is coded on Axis III. The pain disorder diagnoses are considered *acute* if less than 6 months in duration and *chronic* when lasting 6 months or more.

Hypochondriasis

Hypochondriasis is diagnosed when an individual fears or believes that they suffer from a serious physical disease, and these fears or beliefs persist for at least 6 months despite the reassurance of a physician (9). Such illness fears or disease convictions may be rooted in misinterpretation or exaggeration of the threat associated with one or multiple physical sensations, a process sometimes referred to as somatosensory amplification (21). In hypochondriasis, the patient's disease conviction is not of delusional intensity, as in a delusional disorder, somatic type. Hypochondriasis is also not diagnosed when the belief or preoccupation is limited to an imagined defect in appearance, as in body dysmorphic disorder (see following). Hypochondriasis may overlap with obsessive-compulsive disorder, and there is good reason to consider grouping hypochondriasis among the anxiety disorders as a health anxiety disorder or phobia (11).

Body Dysmorphic Disorder

Body dysmorphic disorder (BDD) is defined in the DSM-IV as a preoccupation with an imagined or slight defect in physical appearance causing clinically significant distress or impairment in functioning (9). The psychiatric literature on BDD in children and adolescents is limited and consists primarily of case reports (22), though approximately 10% of a recent large case series were age 18 or younger (23). BDD is distinguished from common developmental preoccupations with appearance by the presence of clinically significant distress and/or impairment in functioning. Excessive concerns about the skin are probably the most common manifestation of BDD in adolescents, with preoccupations focusing on scars or facial acne, but any body area can be a focus of concern. Patients may sometimes cause self-injury as a consequence of attempts to "fix" the perceived flaw (e.g., compulsively picking at the skin), and some patients may even deliberately self-mutilate or attempt to perform surgical procedures on themselves. Insight is often poor, and patients are more likely to present in general medical settings, where they may seek costly and potentially dangerous dermatologic and surgical treatments. Because BDD can be associated with considerable shame and the need for secrecy, the diagnosis may be missed unless clinicians ask directly about symptoms. Parents of children with BDD report excessive mirror checking, grooming, attempts to "camouflage" a particular body area, and reassurance seeking by the child. BDD may prove to be quite time consuming as a result of efforts to examine the perceived defect and/or conceal it. BDD may be related to obsessive-compulsive disorder (24), and it has been suggested that BDD would be better classified in the same category as that disorder (11) given a rather low likelihood of other comorbid somatoform disorders (23).

Somatoform Disorder, Not Otherwise Specified

Somatoform disorder, not otherwise specified is diagnosed when symptoms consistent with a somatoform disorder are present, but criteria for a specific disorder are not met (9). Examples include unexplained physical symptoms such as fatigue or hypochondriacal concerns of less than 6 months' duration.

EPIDEMIOLOGY

Prevalence

Medically unexplained physical symptoms and complaints (functional somatic symptoms) are exceptionally common in children and adolescents, yet most available studies are not comprehensive, relying on self- or parent-report checklists, focusing on some physical symptoms but not others, and failing to include independent medical assessments to determine if the reported symptoms are truly "medically unexplained" (5, 8, 25). Furthermore, with rare exception (26), most available studies have not assessed the prevalence of specific somatoform disorders, and standardized research interviews for pediatric somatoform disorders have yet to be widely used. With these caveats aside, all manner of functional somatic symptoms have been reported by youth in clinical and community based studies. Approximately half of preschool and school aged children will report at least one somatic complaint in the previous 2 weeks (27–29), and approximately 15% endorse at least four symptoms (27, 29).

Although individuals presenting for medical evaluation typically focus on a single symptom, the presence of one type of somatic complaint predicts another (30). Empirical support for a "somatic complaints syndrome" is provided by principal components analysis of parent ratings for over 8,000 youth referred for mental health services (31). The Ontario Child Health Study (32) found recurrent distressing somatic symptoms in 11% of girls and 4% of boys ages 12 to 16 years, and other studies have reported multiple and frequent somatic complaints in 10 to 15% of adolescents (33). Groups of somatic symptoms tend to cluster, with examples including pain/weakness, gastrointestinal symptoms, conversion/pseudoneurological symptoms, and cardiovascular symptoms (29, 34, 35).

Chronic complaints of pain are particularly common in children and adolescents. A 3 month prevalence of 25% has been reported, with over half of affected children taking medication and over 40% seeking medical help for the pain over a 3 month period (36). Pain can be defined as an unpleasant sensory and emotional experience that is associated with tissue damage or perceived as representative of such damage (37). Pain and nociception are not identical. Pain is essentially subjective, and must be assessed by self-report. While typically considered a sign of tissue damage, pain can arise spontaneously in the absence of nociceptor activity; conversely, pain can be minimal or absent in the presence of great nociceptor activation. The experience of subjective pain and peripheral nociception can be modified by central nervous system mechanisms, and prior tissue damage can also sensitize peripheral nociceptors, with resultant hyperalgesia at the site or in surrounding, presumably undamaged areas.

Headache appears to be the most common type of pain reported by school aged children and adolescents, with 10 to 30% endorsing "frequent" headaches or headaches on an at least weekly basis (28, 38–41). Headache is cited as the reason for 1 to 2% of pediatric ambulatory visits (42). The classification system currently in use for headaches is descriptive in nature, since most headaches are considered "primary" and not attributable to an underlying physical disease (43). The primary headaches of greatest relevance are *migraine* and *tension type headache (TTH)*. Migraine may be diagnosed when: a child or adolescent presents with a history of at least 5 headache attacks where the headache lasts 1 to 72 hours (4 to 72 hours in adults); the headache has at least two of the following characteristics—unilateral location, pulsating quality, moderate to severe pain intensity, and/or is aggravated by routine physical activity; and the headache is accompanied by nausea and/or vomiting or photophobia and phonophobia. Migraine may be accompanied by aura, defined as focal neurological features that may precede or accompany the headache such as visual scintillating scotoma, sensory symptoms such as numbness, tingling, or paresthesias, and motor symptoms such as motor weakness or dysphasia. TTH may be episodic or chronic, with the main features being bilateral location, nonpulsatile quality, mild to moderate intensity, and lack of aggravation by routine physical activity (43).

Functional abdominal pain (FAP) is also quite common, with a prevalence of 7 to 25% in school aged youth (44–46), and is responsible for 2 to 4% of pediatric visits (42). It is the most common somatic symptom reported by preschool children (27). Gastrointestinal (GI) symptoms such as nausea, vomiting, and bowel related complaints are also common, often in association with abdominal pain. Gastrointestinal symptoms are commonly associated with headache, particularly with migraine (44, 47). *Cyclical vomiting syndrome* refers to recurrent and stereotyped episodes of intense, unexplained vomiting that appears to be related to migraine (48). Interestingly, dizziness is another common symptom reported by up to 15% of children in surveys (29, 39) that may also be related to migraine. Most cases of pediatric abdominal pain are considered functional, particularly in the absence of clues to serious physical disease such as weight loss, bleeding, fever, other systemic symptoms, or laboratory abnormalities (49). Gastroenterologists apply symptom based diagnostic criteria that have been developed for pediatric functional gastrointestinal disorders (FGID), with the best known FGID associated with pain being *irritable bowel syndrome (IBS)* (i.e., FAP with at least two of the following: relief with defecation; change in bowel frequency; change in bowel character) (50).

Chest pain is reported by approximately 10% of school aged children and adolescents (5, 29), and is a frequent presentation in pediatric emergency rooms and in pediatric cardiology (51, 52). Other common pains include musculoskeletal pains such as limb pain and back pain (5). Approximately one-third of Finnish youth reported musculoskeletal pain at least once per week in a community study, with 7.5% endorsing widespread musculoskeletal pains in a number of sites and approximately 1% meeting criteria for *fibromyalgia* (a functional somatic syndrome characterized by at least 3 months of multiple musculoskeletal aches and pains and pain to palpation on physical examination in at least 11 of 18 "tender point" sites) (53). Other varieties of musculoskeletal complaints may present in pediatric settings. Although more commonly seen among adults, *complex regional pain syndrome type I*, formerly known as *reflex sympathetic dystrophy*, may also occur in children and adolescents (54). The condition typically presents following a history of immobilization or trauma to the limb (injury, venipuncture, intramuscular injection), though there is no correlation between the severity of the injury and the ensuing syndrome. Clinical features include: pain disproportionate to any inciting event such as allodynia (pain from innocuous tactile stimulation) and/or hyperalgesia (an exaggerated response to painful stimulation), as well as swelling, changes in skin blood flow, or changes in skin temperature at some stage of the illness, and limitation of functioning. The pathophysiology of complex regional pain syndrome type I is still undetermined, and though psychological mediators have been proposed, scientific support is limited (55).

Fatigue is among the most common physical symptoms reported by youth, with up to one-half of adolescents complaining of at least weekly fatigue and 15% reporting daily fatigue (33, 39, 56). *Chronic fatigue syndrome (CFS)* more specifically refers to a condition characterized by severe, disabling fatigue of at least 6 months' duration that is associated with self-reported limitations in concentration and short-term memory, sleep disturbance, and musculoskeletal aches and pains, and where alternative medical and psychiatric explanations (e.g., hypothyroidism, malignancy, hepatitis, narcolepsy, obstructive sleep apnea, medication side effects, major mood disorder, schizophrenia, or eating disorder) have been excluded (56). Available studies are limited, but CFS appears to be rare in childhood and uncommon in adolescence, with prevalence likely below 1%. Onset typically follows an acute febrile illness in approximately two-thirds of cases (57).

A variety of respiratory symptoms may appear to be medically unexplained or somatoform in nature, including complaints of cough and shortness of breath or dyspnea (58). *Vocal cord dysfunction (VCD)* is an often-unrecognized condition in which presumed vocal cord spasm leads to symptoms that can mimic acute asthma. Affected youth may present with a history of "asthma" unresponsive to aggressive medical management. VCD may be differentiated from asthma by the absence of nocturnal symptoms, localization of wheezing to the upper chest and throat, normal blood gases despite extreme symptoms, and significant adduction of the vocal cords when visualized on laryngoscopy (59, 60). The prevalence of VCD in children's hospitals is unknown, and clinicians are often unaware of its existence (61).

Conversion symptoms (those suggestive of a neurologic illness in the absence of neurological disease) have generated considerable interest in the psychiatric literature, but are unusual in community samples of Western youth (5, 41, 62, 63). Presentations with conversion symptoms become increasingly common in tertiary referral centers and pediatric neurology services, where nonepileptic seizures, unresponsiveness, faints, falls, and abnormalities of gait or sensation are the most commonly reported symptoms (17–19, 64–67). *Nonepileptic seizures*, sometimes described as "pseudoseizures," resemble epileptic seizures but are not associated with the electroencephalographic abnormalities or clinical course characteristic of true epilepsy, though affected individuals may also suffer from concomitant epilepsy. Relatively little definitive is known about course, though the outcome is favorable in the majority of cases (68), with most resolving within 3 months of diagnosis (18, 69). Though past clinical teaching has emphasized that symptoms considered to be representative of conversion disorder are commonly found to be caused by unrecognized physical disease (70), a systematic review found that the rate of misdiagnosis of conversion symptoms averaged 4% across the studies conducted since 1970 (71).

A prospective epidemiologic study of somatoform disorders and symptoms in a sample of 3021 German youth aged 14 to 24 year olds found the lifetime prevalence of any specific somatoform disorder to be 3% at baseline, and clinically meaningful somatoform illness that did not meet diagnostic criteria for a specific somatoform disorder was reported by an additional 10% of the sample (26). Pain disorder was the most common specific diagnosis, with most affected youth falling into the nonspecific, "undifferentiated," or "subsyndromal" category. Somatization disorder and hypochondriasis both appear to be quite rare in children and adolescents, as no cases of either were identified, and the lifetime prevalence of conversion disorder was only 0.3%. Somatoform illness was relatively stable and persistent over time, as about half of subjects with a specific somatoform disorder or nonspecific somatic complaints reported persistent symptoms over the next four years. There was nevertheless considerable fluidity in the overall symptom profile of individual subjects. Onset of somatoform illness was predicted by female gender, lower socioeconomic status, a history of sexual trauma or physically threatening events, and premorbid anxiety, depressive, or substance abuse disorder, whereas symptom persistence was predicted by female gender, history of a serious accident, and the presence of an affective, substance abuse, or eating disorder (26).

The community prevalence of BDD has been reported to be 0.7% (72). A somewhat higher prevalence has been reported in youth, with one study finding BDD prevalence to be 2% in a community sample of adolescents (73).

Demographics and Sociocultural Factors

Age appears to be an important variable in the presentation of functional somatic symptoms and syndromes. In general, somatic symptom reporting appears to increase with increasing age into adolescence (40, 74). Unfortunately, there are few methodologically sound longitudinal studies (5). Though headache appears to be the most common type of pain reported across childhood and adolescence, FAP appears to be the most common complaint in early childhood, with headache peaking at approximately age 12 (27, 40). Polysymptomatic presentations become more common in adolescence (32, 75, 76). Conversion disorder is especially rare in very young children, and clinicians are advised to be skeptical of the diagnosis in children younger than age 6 years (17, 18, 67, 77) Body dysmorphic disorder is similarly more common during adolescence than early childhood (73).

In general, recurrent complaints of pain occur equally in boys and girls until late childhood and puberty, after which female symptom reporting predominates (29, 40, 76). Chronic fatigue is also more common in females (57), and conversion symptoms appear to be more common among girls than boys across all age groups (19, 64, 66). Girls may be more likely to use health services for functional symptoms than are boys (36), and appear to be more consistent in reporting somatic symptoms over time (78). Female gender has been associated with both the onset and persistence of somatoform symptoms and disorders in adolescents (26).

Low socioeconomic status and low levels of parental education have been associated with somatic symptom reporting in childhood and adolescence in some studies (26, 66, 79, 80), as well as with symptom stability (26), but not in others (76, 81). The impact of race/ethnicity and the role of social and cultural factors have been inadequately studied. Cultural influences may nevertheless be influential. Conversion symptoms have been reported to be common presentations of psychiatric disorder in non-Western clinical settings, including Turkey and India (69, 82), and cultural differences in pain expression and behavior have been suggested, but existing studies may confound ethnicity, socioeconomic status, and acculturation (83).

Family, Genetic, and Temperamental Factors

There is growing evidence that youth with a variety of different medically unexplained physical symptoms are more likely to have parents and family members who perceive their own health more negatively and report more somatic symptoms and complaints than those of unaffected peers (14, 40, 67, 75, 76, 84–88). Somatization disorder, though relatively uncommon, appears to cluster in the family members of affected patients (89), and children of parents with somatization disorder are more likely to report medically unexplained physical symptoms than children of controls (90). Chronic fatigue also appears to cluster in families of affected children (56).

Exposure to illness in a parent has been associated with the experience of functional somatic symptoms in adulthood, and the offspring of adults with functional somatic symptoms are more likely to suffer from health anxieties and higher levels of health service use for functional somatic symptoms than those of controls (91). Parents may encourage illness related behaviors and particular coping styles in youth with functional somatic symptoms, and thus behaviorally influence the experience of somatic symptoms by the child and the associated level of disability (92–95). A number of observers suggest that there is often a family "model" for the child's symptoms (17, 18, 65, 67). Parents of youth with functional somatic symptoms have been described as overprotective (17, 77, 86) and prone to view their children as particularly vulnerable (96), which may increase the degree to which the child's symptom are viewed as threatening.

Family systems theorists have sometimes understood pediatric somatoform illness as serving a specific function within the family system, with the child's symptoms potentially allowing the family to avoid conflict, most notably parental marital conflict, and thus preserving family homeostasis (97, 98). Families of youth with medically unexplained physical symptoms are more likely than those of peers to be described as low in perceived support (99), and affected children are more likely to come from nonintact families (100) and those characterized by parental marital conflict (65, 88, 101). Some observers have also called attention to how a particular child's somatic symptoms may serve a communicative function in the family on the order of body language or a plea for help (102, 103).

Functional pain syndromes, anxiety, and depression have been associated with temperamental traits such as behavioral inhibition, harm avoidance, neuroticism, and negative affect (104–109). These traits share associations with pessimistic worry, fear of uncertainty, and a tendency to respond to environmental challenge at lower thresholds (110, 111). FAP may be the best studied variety of pediatric chronic pain, and is more likely to be reported by the family members of affected youth than by those of controls (40, 75, 78, 88, 100). The same is true for nongastrointestinal symptoms such as headache, including migraine (100, 112), raising questions as to whether these are pain prone families (45). Mothers of youth with chronic pain in clinical (75, 84, 100) and community settings (88, 112), also report higher levels of anxiety and/or depressive symptoms than mothers of unaffected children, but do not differ from mothers of psychiatrically referred children (84, 113, 114). In a multivariate regression model, maternal history of anxiety and depression was significantly associated with childhood FAP, while maternal somatic symptoms dropped out of the model once psychiatric symptoms were entered (100). Physiologic responses of youth with FAP to a social stressor also appear more akin to those of anxiety disordered youth than of healthy controls (115).

The contribution of genetics to familiality in somatoform illness is not especially well studied, though there is some evidence suggesting a prominent heritable component (116). Most available studies suggest that genetic and environmental factors play an interactive role in the development of functional somatic symptoms and complaints (93, 117–119). A functional polymorphism in the promoter region of the serotonin transporter gene has been associated with trait neuroticism and anxiety (120, 121), a vulnerability to react to life adversity or threat with higher levels of emotional arousal and distress (122), as well as with FAP in adults (123). Interestingly, Walker and colleagues (2001) have reported that youth with chronic abdominal pain who report higher levels of negative affect or neuroticism are more likely to complain of abdominal pain in the face of day to day stressors or "daily hassles." Other polymorphisms in genes important to the metabolism of specific neurotansmitters have been related to susceptibility for somatoform illness, including association of a polymorphism in catecholamine-O-methyl transferase (COMT) with pain sensitivity (124) and the association of a polymorphism in the gene coding for tryptophan hydroxylase, the rate limiting enzyme in the biosynthesis of serotonin, with somatic anxiety (125).

Life Events and Trauma

A variety of negative experiences and stressors have been associated with the experience of functional somatic symptoms in both childhood and adolescence (5, 8), most notably child maltreatment (126). Sexual maltreatment appears to predict the onset of functional somatic symptoms and somatoform disorders and syndromes in children and adolescents (26, 127–131), and has also been associated with a variety of different functional somatic syndromes and somatoform disorders in adulthood, including somatization disorder (132). Exposure to parental neglect and the experience of poor care in childhood has been associated with somatic symptom reporting later in life (133, 134). Persistence of somatoform symptoms has also been associated with exposure to other sorts of trauma such as accidents (26), and youth with persistent posttraumatic stress disorder appear to be at increased risk of somatoform disorders (135).

Coping

Compas and colleagues (1999) contrast *coping*—voluntary efforts to regulate emotion, thought, behavior, physiology, and/or environment in response to challenge or adversity—with involuntary responses rooted in inherited or acquired individual physiological differences and/or conditioned patterns of behavior. Vulnerability to chronic pain may be understood as being derivative of individual differences in stress reactivity, stress exposure, threat appraisal, pain tolerance, and coping skills (136, 137). *Active coping* reflects problem-focused strategies focused on making the pain "go away" such as emotional expression, emotional regulation, and problem solving. *Accommodative coping* is characterized by efforts to accept and adjust to the pain, generally by regulating attention or thought patterns via strategies such as acceptance, distraction/ignoring, self-encouragement, and cognitive restructuring. Accommodative strategies are consistently associated with lower levels of pain, other somatic symptoms, and emotional distress in youth with chronic pain. *Passive coping* reflects strategies that avoid confronting pain such as avoidance, denial, and wishful thinking, and is considered maladaptive given strong associations with worsening levels of pain and emotional distress in children with chronic pain and with anxiety disorders (138). Existing research has also highlighted the importance of exaggerated threat appraisal in magnifying and sustaining functional somatic symptoms, including pain and fatigue, and how beliefs about the nature of the illness may influence choice of coping strategy (56, 139). Unchecked fears that the child's illness represents a serious threat to the child and family can provoke maladaptive responses (frenetic efforts to "make it just go away"; despair and a wish to "give up") that are counter to what research recommends (accepting the pain and maximizing activities in spite of it) (139).

PUBLIC HEALTH RELEVANCE

Functional Impact and Service Use

Why are the problems of youth with functional somatic symptoms worthy of attention and concern? As noted above, functional somatic symptoms and disorders are common in children and adolescents, and it should not be forgotten that these children do indeed suffer, and are viewed by parents as being in poorer health than unaffected peers (80, 99). It is also well documented that youth with all varieties of functional somatic symptoms suffer from considerable functional impairment, most notably from school absences and poor school performance (5, 8, 28, 56, 95, 99, 104, 140–143). Children with CFS report more impairment and disability than those with juvenile arthritis or emotional disorders (56). Not surprisingly, youth with medically unexplained physical symptoms use more health services than unaffected peers (80, 99), and are at risk to fall between the cracks in a rigidly polarized health care system that triages care based on whether a disorder is considered to be "physical or mental." While affected youth and their families are commonly reassured that serious physical disease is absent, sometimes with a discussion of the potential impact of stress and/or a referral for psychosocial services, they may also embark on a prolonged quest to rule out unrecognized disease, increasing the likelihood of unnecessary medical investigations and treatments, and potentially putting the child at risk for needless physical suffering and even iatrogenic (physician caused) disease (144). Unnecessary evaluations and testing may have the unintended consequence of increasing the family's conviction that the child is "sickly" and that a serious disease is being overlooked (17, 102). Patients and families may feel profoundly misunderstood or dismissed after hearing that there is "nothing wrong" despite an illness associated with considerable distress and impairment for the child (6). Consultation with a mental health professional who explains away the pain as representative of an anxiety or depressive disorder can generate similar confusion and a sense of empathic failure by the clinician.

Comorbid Psychopathology

Given the lack of a clear biomedical explanation for youth with medically unexplained physical symptoms, the symptoms have most often been considered psychogenic, or a manifestation of emotional distress in response to psychosocial adversity (45). This has been bolstered by the consistent observation of high rates of psychiatric symptoms and disorders in studies comparing affected to unaffected youth (27, 29, 145). High rates of anxiety and/or depressive symptoms and disorders have been reported in youth with recurrent pain, including those with recurrent abdominal pain (84, 95, 104, 146); headache (28, 145–147); musculoskeletal pain (53, 145); and chest pain (51, 148). An anxiety disorder can be diagnosed in approximately three-quarters of youth with FAP presenting in primary care (104) and specialty care (84, 146). Youth suffering from chronic fatigue syndrome also appear to report higher levels of anxiety and depressive symptoms than healthy controls (56, 143). Symptoms of emotional distress, particularly depression, have been associated with the functional impairment so commonly seen in youth with functional somatic symptoms (149). Respiratory symptoms such as cough and dyspnea appear to be associated with the presence of a mental disorder in general, as well as the presence of specific disorders such as depression, panic anxiety, ADHD, and substance abuse (58). Finally, preexisting anxiety, depressive, and substance use disorders have been associated with the new onset of somatoform disorders in adolescents, and persistence of somatoform disorder has been associated with depressive, substance abuse, and eating disorders (26).

Adult Disorder and Impairment

Somatic symptom reporting early in life likely predicts subsequent symptom reporting. Children who complain of stomachaches at the age of 4 years are three times more likely to have similar complaints on follow-up at age 10 than peers (150). Early follow-up studies reported persistence of FAP into adulthood for one-third to one-half of affected children (144, 151, 152). Young adults with a childhood history of abdominal pain not only are more likely to report more functional somatic symptoms than controls with no history of childhood pain, but are also much more likely to experience psychiatric symptoms and disorders in adulthood, particularly anxiety and depressive disorders (74, 85, 153, 154). Adults with multiple functional somatic symptoms are more likely to have experienced physical illness before age 17 years than other ill adults (133), and adults with somatoform disorders tend to report retrospectively that their physical symptoms and sufferings began early in life (3, 12, 155).

ASSESSMENT

Approach to the Patient and Family

The specifics of assessment should be individualized on a case by case basis, and are beyond the scope of this chapter. It is nevertheless important to address some basic principles in each assessment and to realize that assessment is the cornerstone of successful intervention, with both the content and process being critical features (7). Youth with medically unexplained symptoms and their parents have often seen a variety of other health care professionals prior to referral for psychiatric consultation, so it is important to explore prior assessment and treatment experiences. This is especially true for patients and families who feel as if they have been "dismissed" by prior clinicians, and/or who are concerned that the child's symptoms have not been taken seriously. Patients and families may bristle after being reassured by a physician that "nothing is wrong" after weeks or months of symptomatic distress and several hours in a waiting room. Other than in the unusual circumstance of overt factitious illness or malingering, it is both unproductive and presumptuous to challenge the subjective reality of the child's symptom. Empathic acknowledgement of the patient's suffering and the family's very real fears and concerns can aid in establishing a working partnership. Many patients are worried that their symptoms will be viewed pejoratively by others as feigned, imaginary, or shameful, and subjective embarrassment can sometimes be expressed interpersonally as anger and a sense of entitlement.

Families may also have had experiences with health care providers that have generated considerable mistrust of the medical profession in general. For example, stories about a friend or relative who was reassured by a trusted physician only to learn later that a serious physical disease had been missed are uncomfortably common. The child's symptoms may provoke specific patient and family fears, and effort should be made to explore any such concerns since illness worry can worsen existing symptoms and cloud judgment. Concerns experienced by individual patients and their parents can be quite variable in the clinical setting, with some terrified that a serious physical disease has been missed and others unconcerned about serious disease but simply searching for symptomatic relief and functional improvement.

Patients and families may experience the very idea of psychiatric referral as dismissive due to concerns that the child's symptoms have not and will not be taken seriously, and mental health professionals risk a loss of credibility if the child's physical suffering is approached narrowly as being purely "psychological" or as a consequence of emotional distress. Concerns related to stigma can interfere with the willingness of patients and families to engage with mental health professionals, and even motivate patients, families, and clinicians to push for potentially dangerous and unnecessary medical investigations and procedures. Ideally, psychiatric assessment will take place within the context of a relationship with a collaborating primary care physician or specialist.

It is particularly important to explore a particular symptom's timing, context, and characteristics, as well as to examine associated social reinforcements and other potential benefits of the sick role. Parents may inadvertently encourage sick role behaviors by responding to complaints of pain with attention, rewards, or opportunities to avoid unpleasant activities or school (156, 157). Multiple sources of information are helpful, with important resources including parents, other professionals, teachers, and school nurses. Identifying any school difficulties can be especially relevant, since learning problems or peer problems such as bullying can reinforce absenteeism. The child's symptoms may become part of a self-handicapping strategy by becoming a ready "explanation" for the child not performing up to expectations (156).

Differential Diagnosis

The specific components necessary to a competent assessment of the youthful patient with medically unexplained symptoms are best determined on a case by case basis and dictated by clinical judgment and experience, but a practiced approach is best informed by a general differential diagnosis at the outset. Perhaps most important, the thoughtful clinician will remain alert to the possibility of unrecognized physical disease, conduct the assessment with an open mind, and communicate an unwillingness to prejudge the etiology of the symptom (158). It is essential to remember that there are circumstances in which medically unexplained symptoms are just that—unexplained. Previous records should be carefully reviewed, and there should be no reluctance to initiate additional medical evaluation if the assessment generates new concerns about physical disease or if the clinical picture appears to be changing over time. A balanced approach that avoids excessive testing is nevertheless of great importance, since unnecessary medical tests and treatments carry the risk of iatrogenic disease, as well as of miscommunicating physician uncertainty, which can help maintain or worsen somatoform illness (17, 102). There is no simple answer to the question as to when the medical workup is complete, since it may be impossible definitively to rule out unrecognized disease, but unless the treating professionals are reasonably comfortable that serious physical disease has not been missed and are able to communicate this conviction to the patient and family, it is difficult to adequately build a solid foundation for intervention. A given symptom may prove functional despite the presence of a coexisting physical disease, so the simple presence of disease (e.g., epilepsy) does not exclude the possibility of a functional disorder (nonepileptic seizures). Functional symptoms at times develop following an acute physical illness or accident (18, 159).

In addition to unrecognized physical disease, medically unexplained symptoms in a child or adolescent may be functional, meaning that they are quite real and subjectively outside the patient's sense of voluntary control. Functional somatic symptoms and syndromes are generally classified as being representative of a somatoform disorder or understood as a component of an anxiety or depressive disorder. In addition, "psychological factors affecting medical condition" may be the diagnosis on Axis I if the functional somatic syndrome (e.g., chronic fatigue syndrome) is codified by the diagnostician as a general medical condition where emotional or psychological factors are impacting on the illness. As noted previously, the many decision points requiring a clinician to judge "physical vs. mental" or "somatoform vs. part of an established emotional disorder" certainly complicate the diagnostic process and can affect diagnostic reliability. So-called positive findings or clues to a symptom or cluster of symptoms being considered somatoform or functional go beyond simply eliminating or ruling out physical disease (6, 102, 103, 159). Such clues include: contiguity of the symptom with a psychosocial stressor or stressors; the presence of another diagnosable psychiatric disorder; the association of a symptom with some interpersonal, familial, or social gain for the patient (secondary gain), or even a presumed intrapsychic gain (primary gain); existence of a model for the symptom within the child's immediate environment; a communicative or symbolic meaning for the symptom within the family or immediate social milieu; the violation of known anatomic or physiologic patterns by the symptom; and the response of the symptom to placebo, suggestion, or psychological treatment. Clearly, these clues should not be considered to be definitive in any way, since virtually all could be found in association with physical disease, but a constellation of such clues taken together is most persuasive (6, 7). For example, while "la belle indifférence" (an apparent lack of concern in relation to the symptom) has often been considered to be suggestive of conversion disorder, it hardly constitutes proof that a given symptom is functional (67, 103, 159).

In circumstances where the child's physical symptoms are judged to be intentionally produced or feigned, functional disorders are distinguished from factitious disorders and malingering (9). In factitious disorder, physical symptoms are deliberately feigned or self inflicted by the patient, with the patient's goal appearing to be an internal one in the form of the psychological gain presumably associated with the sick role. In factitious disorder by proxy, a parent or caretaker feigns, simulates, or causes disease in a child with the motivation being an internal one for the caretaker. Malingering is the deliberate feigning, simulation, or production of physical symptoms in pursuit of an external incentive, such as the avoidance of a particular responsibility or punishment, or the pursuit of financial gain. Inconsistencies or apparent fabrications in the history should raise concerns about these uncommon but real problems. Medical or psychiatric records hand carried by a parent are certainly not uncommon, yet should provoke at least mild suspicion given that record tampering has been reported in some cases of factitious disorder by proxy.

Careful assessment of the social and family environment is similarly critical. Family history of psychiatric disorder, functional somatic syndromes, chronic physical illness, and disability should be explored, with attention to known risk factors. Because pediatric somatoform illness is commonly associated with separation fears, consideration should be given to experiences which may have led to the family perceiving the child to be especially vulnerable from a physical or emotional perspective (96). Other relevant areas include possible marital conflict and parent–child relational problems, as well as other negative life events. Perhaps the most critical environmental issue to consider is that of maltreatment, which is particularly important to consider in youth suffering from conversion symptoms, genitourinary complaints, and chronic, polysymptomatic somatization (129–131).

MANAGEMENT

There is considerable phenomenological heterogeneity in youth with somatoform illness, even within groups of children with a single type of symptom such as those with FAP, but functional somatic syndromes do appear to share high rates of comorbidity with one another and with anxiety and depressive disorders, leading some to suggest a common pathophysiology (10). One goal of this chapter is to present a management model that builds upon a few core principles distilled from the available pediatric and adult literature with the understanding that well designed trials of specific interventions will be necessary to support any one approach.

Diagnosis and Psychoeducation

The diagnostic impression should be discussed directly with the patient and the family. It is generally wise for the clinician first to review the number and types of physical, emotional, and behavioral symptoms noted during the assessment, as well as the time course and context of the symptoms with the patient and family prior to discussing the diagnosis. This allows for clarification of historical details and can help establish consensus about the symptomatic profile. In circumstances where the diagnostic formulation appears to be clear, it should be discussed clearly, frankly, and directly with the patient and family together (7). In cases where the diagnosis is presumptive or uncertain, truthful acknowledgment of diagnostic uncertainty is superior to feigned certainty or avoidance. Once the diagnosis has been made and reviewed, additional medical workup should be avoided in the absence of new information, a change in clinical status, or a strong conviction that a relatively low-risk investigation is needed to reassure the patient and family in order for treatment to proceed.

Education of the patient and family should provide a solid foundation for treatment, challenge stigma, and instill hope and positive expectations. The clinician should avoid communicating any sense of unease or embarrassment about the diagnosis, since this might contribute to treatment resistance and a wish to perpetuate the search for disease. Patients and families can be educated about how physical symptoms of distress in the absence of serious disease are common and considered to be quite real by physicians and other health care professionals, and should be reassured that although our knowledge base is limited, much practical help is still available. Discussing the relationship between mind and body and the false dichotomy implied by separate systems of care of "physical" and "mental" disorders can also be useful. Too much emphasis on the functional symptoms being reactions to adversity or stress often proves unproductive, since the patient or family may not be aware of such stress, may believe that illness in response to stress implies personal weakness, or may jump to the unhelpful conclusion that avoidance of uncomfortable situations will solve the problem.

Discussions about the nature of functional pain may be helpful, particularly a discussion of how certain individuals may be especially vulnerable to experience bodily sensations as painful and/or as signifying a special threat to health. Pain is thought to be a signal of a potential threat to physical integrity, and is accompanied by a wish to avoid additional distress. Both pain and anxiety can serve defensive neurobehavioral functions, steering the organism away from perceived threats and motivating adaptive behaviors. By analogy, the sensitivity to abdominal pain in youth with FAP represents pain that is inappropriate to the context (pain in the absence of tissue damage), just as an anxiety disorder is characterized by fear inappropriate to context. A few small studies suggest that youth with FAP may be especially sensitive to gut sensations or discomfort (160, 161), and to peripheral physical sensations such as deep muscle pressure as well (162).

The collaborative nature of the treatment process should be discussed early and often, and the importance of a therapeutic partnership or alliance as the foundation for therapeutic success should be emphasized. Patient, family, and professional roles and responsibilities should be delineated, with an emphasis on solid communication and the importance of working together. Determining shared functional goals for the patient, the family, and the treating professionals is an important task, as a focus on functional improvement rather than an unequivocal "cure" is generally most productive.

TREATMENT

Treatment should be individualized on a case by case basis, but therapeutic approaches to somatoform disorders often share common features, and some generic approaches have been described elsewhere (7, 163). It should be kept in mind that the evidence base is spare and that randomized controlled trials of intervention in youth are unusual, so much of what follows is a synthesis of available evidence and what has become relatively accepted practice. An important role for the child and adolescent psychiatrist may be that of a consultant to primary care physicians and general medicine specialists, who are often out front in managing such children. Youth with somatoform illness and their families think and speak in terms of physical illness, medical problems, and somatic dysfunction, and may resist psychiatric referral, either actively or passively. The psychiatric consultant and referring physician must coordinate planning in order to maintain the physician–patient alliance and avoid unnecessary doctor shopping. Though sometimes tempting, particularly to generalists, the use of placebo and/or sham interventions is discouraged for both ethical and practical reasons. Such efforts may inadvertently contribute to patient and family convictions that the symptom is caused by physical disease, and if suggestion or placebo prove unsuccessful, the clinician is then forced to perpetuate new deceptions or must backtrack and attempt to convince the patient that serious physical disease is absent and that symptom removal is not really necessary for functional improvement to take place.

Reassurance

Reassurance that a life threatening or serious physical disease is not present is often a necessary, but rarely sufficient, step in the treatment process. It is often essential that the patient and family view the presenting symptoms as less threatening in that it may be impossible to proceed with intervention until anxiety generated by the symptom has decreased for the patient and/or family. Parents must be helped to understand that the child's quite real subjective distress does not appear to be associated with actual tissue damage. Excessive reassurance may nevertheless prove counterproductive in cases where obsessional illness worry and hypochondriacal fears are prominent (164, 165). In such cases, the illness worry should be addressed directly and framed as a problem to be solved rather than attempting to overcome it by reassurance alone.

Rehabilitative and Psychotherapeutic Treatment

Many authors have discussed the advantages of a *rehabilitative approach* to pediatric somatoform illness (7, 56, 163). By encouraging the patient to return to usual activities and responsibilities prior to definitive symptomatic relief and by discouraging illness related behaviors, the rehabilitative approach directs the patient and family focus away from finding a "cure" to instead finding a way to cope with and overcome a distressing physical problem (18, 103, 159, 166). This approach can empower the patient and family and shift the burden of responsibility for therapeutic success to the patient in the context of professional support and encouragement, directly challenging the notion that symptom resolution is necessary for the child to return to normal function. The metacommunication that the child will not be harmed by activity and effort can help neutralize concerns about the somatoform symptoms and generate meaningful changes in behavior for both child and parents. Achievement of functional goals is then understood as a personal success based on individual courage and hard work, and rightly treated as an accomplishment of which the patient can be proud. The rehabilitative approach has been applied with some success in chronic fatigue syndrome (167–169), producing superior results to "pacing," an energy management strategy that involves accepting the limitations associated with the illness and resting based on subjective need (56, 169). Indeed, there is little evidence that rest alone is helpful in chronic fatigue, and may in fact exacerbate the condition (56). In keeping with a rehabilitative model, the use of physical therapy has sometimes been advocated (170), particularly in conversion disorder (18, 20, 103, 159).

Cognitive factors such as expectations and beliefs that the child's symptoms signal the threat of tissue damage are likely important in youth with somatoform disorders, and such concerns have been associated with enhanced somatic symptom perception and the amplification of somatic symptoms (171). The rehabilitative approach challenges misperceptions about the child's health and capabilities, and serves as the linchpin of a cognitive-behavioral strategy by emphasizing the child's fundamental health, strength, and adaptability. Success largely depends on the clinician's ability to address patient and family anxiety about the child's illness and to successfully challenge patient and family distorted health beliefs. Parents and caretakers must understand that rehabilitative expectations in the face of the child's real distress are not cruel. Instead, a discussion of how kindness demands a firm approach is often indicated. Clinician speech and behavior should communicate that the child is fundamentally strong, competent, and capable of overcoming the challenge presented by the illness. To expect less may actually be counter therapeutic and representative of "misplaced kindness." Specifically, school attendance and performance should be emphasized as critical indicators of developmentally appropriate functioning. Homebound instruction is sometimes sought by youth with somatoform illness and/or their parents, but should almost always be avoided or challenged by treatment professionals. Respect for the importance of school should be communicated by attempting to schedule followup visits outside of regular school hours whenever possible.

Cognitive-behavioral methods have been examined as regular features in a number of multimodal interventions that have been reported to be helpful in the treatment of recurrent pain (172–175), fibromyalgia (176), and chronic fatigue syndrome (167–169). Sanders and colleagues (1989) employed cognitive coping skills training in association with differential reinforcement of healthy behavior and self-monitoring techniques for youth with FAP. Although the sample size was small, the positive results of the study were encouraging, with the treated group of patients doing significantly better than controls. Two studies using a cognitive behavioral family intervention compared to standard pediatric care for children with FAP have extended this research, with both reporting reductions in abdominal pain (173, 175), and the earlier study reporting higher levels of parental satisfaction with treatment, greater functional improvement, and lower levels of relapse at 6 and 12 month followup (175). A recent study found that youth with recurrent pain assigned to Internet-based intervention based on cognitive behavioral principles that included relaxation training were more likely to show clinically significant improvement than those randomized to a wait list control condition (177).

Behavioral and operant interventions are common to most successful interventions, with core features being the reward of health promoting behaviors and the discouragement of illness behaviors and disability. Controlled trials of behavioral interventions for pediatric somatoform disorders are lacking, but several case reports highlight potential benefits (5, 8). Most have emphasized *positive reinforcement* for functional improvement, as well as *extinction* or *withdrawal of reinforcement* for sick role behaviors (77, 159, 178–181). While the use of punishment per se is not advisable, the successful application of a time out procedure in the management of recurrent pain has also been reported (182). *Negative reinforcement*, which produces an increase in the frequency of a desired response by removing an aversive event immediately after the desired response (183), has typically been applied by lifting restrictions theoretically imposed by illness contingent upon functional improvement (18, 178, 184). For example, discharge from the hospital might be allowed only if the patient evidenced sufficient physical improvement (18), or persistent bed rest might be imposed with removal contingent on the patient returning to premorbid function and responsibilities (184). Similarly, the threat of inpatient psychiatric hospitalization can be removed contingent on the child maintaining at least minimally acceptable function (e.g., returning to school). Parents may have difficulty implementing behavioral interventions unless their fears and concerns that their actions might be punitive have been addressed.

Encouraging results have been reported with the use of *self-management strategies* (185), with specific techniques such as self-monitoring, training in coping and relaxation (59, 186–188), hypnosis (189–191), and the use of biofeedback (179) being described as helpful. Such strategies are likely helpful in providing some degree of symptomatic relief, and also encourage more active coping strategies, which may contribute to efforts to improve functioning. Interpersonal and expressive psychotherapies have not been systematically studied in pediatric somatization, but may be useful, particularly in the presence of psychological trauma (192). Though not studied using randomized controlled trials, case reports of the successful treatment of youth with somatoform disorders continue to appear (193).

Family therapy and family based interventions have been advocated (97, 98, 194), but aside from the study of the Sanders group (1994), specific family interventions have not been studied. Since children presenting with medically unexplained physical symptoms are more likely as a group to be viewed as health impaired (80) and have sick role behaviors inadvertently encouraged by parents (157), it is important to respectfully challenge the perceived physical vulnerability of the child and any familial encouragement of illness behavior (142). Group psychotherapy in the treatment of pediatric somatoform illness has not been systematically evaluated.

In summary, psychotherapeutic approaches to pediatric somatoform illness seek to help child and family: 1) diminish the perceived threat associated with the child symptom (158); 2) modulate affective and physiologic reactivity to relevant environmental or physical triggers; 3) promote healthy coping by encouraging accommodative coping strategies such as acceptance, distraction, self-encouragement, and cognitive restructuring, while discouraging passive strategies such as avoidance, denial, and wishful thinking; 4) optimize social reinforcement by using positive reinforcement for healthy behaviors and withdrawal of reinforcement for illness behaviors; and 5) strengthen the child's perceived competence and self-worth.

Psychopharmacologic Treatment

Pharmacological management has the advantage of relative simplicity and acceptability within general medical settings, and is in keeping with traditional office practice. Unfortunately, there have been no large randomized controlled trials of of psychoactive medications in the treatment of pediatric somatoform disorders or functional somatic syndromes, so psychopharmacologic treatment of youth with somatoform disorders has largely been presumptive and based on experience with adults. Psychopharmacologic interventions are nevertheless worthy of consideration in the treatment of persistent medically unexplained pain, gastrointestinal symptoms, or fatigue, particularly in the presence of psychiatric comorbidity or when psychotherapeutic interventions have not been entirely successful. Antidepressant medications have been reported to be of benefit in the treatment of a number of somatoform disorders and functional somatic syndromes in adults (195, 196), including BDD (197, 198), somatoform pain (199), irritable bowel syndrome (200, 201), and a variety of other functional somatic symptoms and syndromes such as fibromyalgia, functional gastrointestinal disorders, and headache (202). St. John's Wort has also been reported to be efficacious for adult somatoform illness (203). Both clomipramine (197) and the selective serotonin reuptake inhibitor fluoxetine (198) have demonstrated efficacy in a few studies in adults with BDD, often in relatively high doses, but other than case reports (204, 205), randomized controlled trials in youth are not available. Because pediatric somatoform disorders and complaints are commonly associated with comorbid internalizing symptoms and disorders, attention to comorbid psychopathology is very much indicated. Evidence from studies of adults suggests that active intervention for comorbid anxiety and depression can ameliorate associated somatic symptoms (206).

The literature on the pharmacologic treatment of FAP was recently reviewed and judged inconclusive and inadequate (207). A recent open trial of citalopram for pediatric FAP found that 21 of 25 (84%) treated youth responded positively based on clinician ratings of much or very much improved, with child and parent ratings of abdominal pain, anxiety, depression, other somatic symptoms, and functional impairment all improving significantly over the course of the study (208). A double-blind placebo controlled study is now in progress. Though pediatric gastroenterologists have often favored the use of tricyclic antidepressants in youth with FAP (209) based in part on adult experience (200), it is difficult to advocate their use given the lack of well controlled trials in youth, the potential for toxicity in households with young children, past reports of sudden death, and the lack of proven efficacy in the treatment of pediatric emotional disorders, particularly depression (210).

With regard to pediatric headache, both acetaminophen and ibuprofen have been shown to be effective in the acute treatment of pediatric migraine, as has been sumatriptan nasal spray (211). Though not well studied in youth, antipsychotic medications such as chlorpromazine, prochlorperazine (212), and haloperidol have been demonstrated to be efficacious in the acute management of adult migraine with effects comparable to sumatriptan (213). Antidepressant medications have been shown to be useful agents to prevent chronic headache in adults (214), and a variety of preventive strategies have been explored in youth, with the goals of reducing attack frequency, severity, and duration, as well as to improve responsiveness to acute treatment and day to day function. Data remain insufficient to draw firm conclusions about agents as diverse as cyproheptadine, beta blockers such as propranolol, the antidepressants amitriptyline (215) and trazodone (216), and a variety of anticonvulsants including divalproex sodium, topiramate (215), and levetiracetam (211). The alpha adrenergic agonist clonidine has not demonstrated efficacy and is most likely ineffective (211). The use of serotonergic antimigraine drugs such as sumatriptan in combination with serotonergic antidepressants had previously been considered to be relatively safe (217), but the U.S. Food and Drug Administration (FDA) issued a warning in 2006 raising concerns about the risk of serotonin syndrome when triptans are used in combination with SSRIs and related antidepressants.

In youth with recurrent pain syndromes such as FAP who do not respond to psychotherapeutic intervention or prefer pharmacological management, our clinical approach has been to initiate treatment with an SSRI at low dose (e.g., citalopram or fluoxetine 10 mg per day), then increase to a potentially therapeutic dose over the next week (20 mg per day), and advance to higher doses at approximately week four in the absence of full improvement (to 40 mg per day). Clinicians considering the use of SSRIs should understand that this represents an off-label use and should review the potential risks and benefits with patients and families in detail, including the recent "black box warning" that antidepressant use can be associated with suicidal thinking and/or behavior in a small proportion of children and adolescents, especially during the early phases of treatment. The Food and Drug Administration (FDA) recommends that "ideal" followup and safety monitoring take place weekly for the first month of treatment, then every other week in the second month, then at 12 weeks, with subsequent followup taking place as appears clinically indicated. There is no available information about the use of other novel antidepressants such as duloxetine in pediatric somatoform disorders, and there is little research addressing the use of psychoactive medications in pediatric chronic fatigue syndrome (56). Given the common association of anxiety and depressive disorders with the symptom profile in chronic fatigue syndrome, consideration might be given to the use of antidepressant medications, including more activating antidepressants such as bupropion, as well as the use of stimulants, though such approaches cannot be recommended as standard practice and would deserve careful study.

Clinical experience suggests that some patients who experience physical symptoms associated with emotional arousal and anxiety may benefit from a short course of a benzodiazepine such as clonazepam or lorazepam, which can sometimes produce rapid symptomatic relief, help reassure the patient and family, and demonstrate the potential contribution of emotional activation to somatic distress (6, 7). For youth with nausea or vomiting, and in the presence of symptoms suggesting acute migraine, the use of an antipsychotic medication or antiemetic may also be worthy of consideration.

Collaborative Care

Successful communication and collaboration with the professionals involved in the child's care, including teachers and school nurses, can prove critical to success over time. Because these disorders commonly present in general medical settings, a close working relationship with the primary care physician or referring specialist is essential. Indeed, our own experience suggests that collaborative models of care that integrate mental health professionals into the primary care setting may be especially helpful for this group of patients and families (218). Poor communication is the most frequent complaint made by pediatricians about child and adolescent psychiatrists (219), and increases the risk that treatment efforts will be misapplied, diluted, or overlooked. A simple consultation letter outlining a general approach to adult somatization disorder patients from a consulting psychiatrist to primary care physicians was shown to be effective in improving patient satisfaction and reducing disability and healthcare expenditures (220). Because absenteeism from school is common in youth with somatoform illness, communication and collaboration with school officials can prove instrumental in developing a rehabilitative plan. The clinician can serve as a bridge to help bring together the school and the patient's family, as tensions frequently develop regarding absences and requests for special treatment of the child. A retrospective excuse for past school absences can be negotiated with the family and school as being contingent upon the child's commitment to a forward looking management plan which will treat subsequent absenteeism for somatoform complaints as inexcusable. It is thus useful to define what constitutes a legitimate, medically excused absence for the child, family, and school, and the physician who will be responsible for legitimizing medical excuses should be specified beforehand in order to prevent doctor shopping in search of medical excuses. Absence from school without the approval of the treatment team should then be viewed as truancy, allowing the school to leverage attendance and benefit overall treatment efforts.

Ideally, coordination of the child's medical care should be consolidated with a single physician or clinician. Regularly scheduled medical visits can prove useful in reassuring the patient and family that their concerns have not been dismissed. The primary physician may serve as a powerful attachment figure for patients and families. Regularly scheduled visits allow the patient and family to see the physician without the requirement that the child be sick (3).

CONCLUSION

The study and management of pediatric somatoform disorders and functional somatic syndromes remain handicapped by problems of conceptualization and classification, and pediatric mental health professionals often feel confused and intimidated by these patients, their sometimes distressed and demanding families, and the general medical colleagues who call on us for help. The existence of parallel systems of care for mental and physical disorders does not help, since these disorders are "neither fish nor fowl." New ways of conceptualizing the problems posed by patients with physical symptoms that defy traditional medical explanations may prove to be important in the future, and well done epidemiologic studies are needed to compare the prevalence, severity, and comorbidity associated with functional somatic symptoms in community and clinical settings. Longitudinal studies of youth with somatoform illness are needed to determine the relationship between childhood presentations and adult disorders and impairment, and a better understanding of the relationship between somatoform disorders and the emotional disorders is likely to be an important development in the future. Well designed and well executed empirical studies will help guide the work of clinicians in addressing these common, but difficult to manage, problems. Future studies should examine not only the efficacy of tested interventions, but whether symptomatic and functional improvements are independent of changes in comorbid anxiety and depressive symptoms. This is an area where efforts to bridge the gap between efficacy and effectiveness research and develop relatively potent, tiered interventions are likely to prove exceptionally important, particularly given the prevalence of presentations with medically unexplained symptoms in primary care and other medical settings.

References

1. Fabrega H: The concept of somatization as a cultural and historical product of Western medicine. *Psychosomatic Medicine* 52:653–672, 1990.
2. Parsons T: *Social Structure and Personality*. New York, Free Press, 1964.
3. Kellner R: *Somatization and Hypochondriasis*. New York: Praeger; 1986.
4. Lipowski Z: Somatization: The concept and its clinical application. *American Journal of Psychiatry* 145(11):1358–1368, 1988.
5. Campo J, Fritsch S: Somatization in children and adolescents. *Journal of the American Academy of Child & Adolescent Psychiatry* 33(9):1223–1235, 1994.
6. Campo JV, Garber J: Somatization. In: Ammerman RT, Campo JV (eds): *Handbook of Pediatric Psychology and Psychiatry*. vol 1. Boston, Allyn and Bacon, 1998, pp. 137–161.
7. Campo J, Fritz G: A management model for pediatric somatization. *Psychosomatics* 42:467–476, 2001.
8. Fritz G, Fritsch S, Hagino O: Somatoform disorders in children and adolescents: A review of the past 10 years. *Journal of the American Academy of Child & Adolescent Psychiatry* 36(10):1329–1338, 1997.
9. American Psychiatric Association. *Diagnostic and Statistical Manual of Mental Disorders* (4th ed.) Washington, DC, American Psychiatric Association, 1994.

10. Barsky A, Borus J: Functional somatic syndromes. *Annals of Internal Medicine* 130:910–921, 1999.
11. Mayou R, Kirmayer L, G S, Kroenke K, Sharpe M: Somatoform disorders: Time for a new approach in DSM-V. *American Journal of Psychiatry.* 162:847–855, 2005.
12. Mai F, Merskey H: Briquet's treatise on hysteria. *Archives of General Psychiatry.* 37:1401–1405, 1980.
13. Cloninger CR: Somatoform and dissociative disorders. In: Winokur G, Clayton PJ (eds.): *The Medical Basis of Psychiatry.* New York, W.B. Saunders, 1994, pp. 169–192.
14. Kreichmanm A: Siblings with somatoform disorders in childhood and adolescence. *Journal of the American Academy of Child and Adolescent Psychiatry* 26:226–231, 1987.
15. Livingston R, Martin-Cannici C: Multiple somatic complaints and possible somatization disorder in prepubertal children. *Journal of the American Academy of Child and Adolescent Psychiatry* 24:603–607, 1985.
16. Wessely S: Old wine in new bottles: Neurasthenia and "ME." *Psychological Medicine* 20:35–53, 1990.
17. Grattan-Smith P, Fairley M, Procopis P: Clinical features of conversion disorder. *Archives of Disease in Childhood* 63:408–414, 1988.
18. Leslie S: Diagnosis and treatment of hysterical conversion reactions. *Archives of Disease in Childhood* 63:506–511, 1988.
19. Spierings C, Poels P, Sijben N, et al.: Conversion disorders in childhood: A retrospective follow-up study of 84 inpatients. *Devel Med Child Neurol* 32:865–871, 1990.
20. Thomson A, Sills J: Diagnosis of functional illness presenting with gait disorder. *Archives of Disease in Childhood* 63:148–153, 1988.
21. Barsky A, Goodson J, Lane R, Cleary P: The amplification of somatic symptoms. *Psychosomatic Medicine* 50:510–519, 1988.
22. Phillips K, Atala K, Albertini R: Body dysmorphic disorder in adolescents. *Journal of the American Academy of Child and Adolescent Psychiatry* 34:1216–1220, 1995a.
23. Phillips K, Menard W, Fay C, Weisberg R: Demographic characteristics, phenomenology, comorbidity and family history in 200 individuals with body dysmorphic disorder. *Psychosomatics* 46:317–325, 2005.
24. Phillips K, McElroy S, Hudson J, et al.: Body dysmorphic disorder: An OCD-spectrum disorder, a form of affective disorder, or both? *Journal of Clinical Psychiatry* 56:41–51, 1995b.
25. Garralda M: A selective review of child psychiatric syndromes with a somatic presentation. *British Journal of Psychiatry* 161:759–773, 1992.
26. Lieb R, Zimmerman P, Friis R, Hofler M, Tholen S, Wittchen H: The natural course of DSMV-IV somatoform disorders and syndromes among adolescents and young adults: A prospective longitudinal community study. *European Psychiatry* 17:321–331, 2002.
27. Domenech-Llaberia E, Jane C, Canals J, Ballespi S, Esparo G, Garralda E: Parental reports of somatic symptoms in preschool children: Prevalence and associations in a Spanish sample. *Journal of the American Academy of Child and Adolescent Psychiatry* 43:598–604, 2004.
28. Fichtel A, Larsson B: Psychosocial impact of headache and comorbidity with other pains among Swedish school adolescents. *Headache* 42:766–775, 2002.
29. Garber J, Walker L, Zeman J: Somatization symptoms in a community sample of children and adolescents: Further validation of the Children's Somatization Inventory. *Psychological Assessment: A Journal of Consulting and Clinical Psychology* 3:588–595, 1991.
30. Alfvén G: The covariation of common psychosomatic symptoms among children from socio-economically differing residential areas. An epidemiological study *Acta Paediatricia.* 82:484–487, 1993a.
31. Achenbach T, Conners C, Quay H, Verhulst F, Howell C: Replication of empirically derived syndromes as a basis for taxonomy of child/adolescent psychopathology. *Journal of Abnormal Child Psychology* 17:299–323, 1989.
32. Offord D, Boyle M, Szatmari P, et al.: Ontario Child Health Study. II. Six-month prevalence of disorder and rates of service utilization. *Archives of General Psychiatry* 44(9):832–836, 1987.
33. Belmaker E, Espinoza R, Pofrund R: Use of medical services by adolescents with nonspecified somatic symptoms. *International Journal of Adolescent Medicine and Health* 1:150–156, 1985.
34. Litcher L, Bromet E, Carlson GA, Gilbert T, Panina N, Golovakha E, et al.: Ukrainian application of the Children's Somatization Inventory: Psychometric properties and associations with internalizing symptoms. *Journal of Abnormal Child Psychology* 29:165–175, 2001.
35. Meesters C, Muris P, Ghys A, Reumerman T, Rooijmans M: The Children's Somatization Inventory: Further evidence for its reliability and validity in a pediatric and a community sample of Dutch children and adolescents. *Journal of Pediatric Psychology* 413–422, 2003.
36. Perquin C, et al.: Pain in children and adolescents: A common experience. *Pain* 87:51–58, 2000.
37. Basbaum A, Jesell T: *The Perception of Pain.* New York, McGraw-Hill, 2000.
38. Aro H: Life stress and psychosomatic symptoms among 14 to 16-year old Finnish adolescents. *Psychological Medicine* 17(1):191–201, 1987.
39. Larsson B: Somatic complaints and their relationship to depressive symptoms in Swedish adolescents. *Journal of Child Psychology and Psychiatry* 32:821–832, 1991.
40. Oster J: Recurrent abdominal pain, headache and limb pains in children and adolescents. *Pediatrics* 50:429–436, 1972.
41. Rutter M, Tizard J, Whitmore K: *Education, Health and Behavior.* London, Longman Group, 1970.
42. Starfield B, Gross E, Wood M, et al.: Psychosocial and psychosomatic diagnoses in primary care of children. *Pediatrics* 66:159–167, 1980.
43. Lipton R, Bigal M, Steiner T, Silberstein S, Olesen J: Classification of primary headaches. *Neurology* 63:427–435, 2004.
44. Abu-Arafeh I, Russell G: Prevalence and clinical features of abdominal migraine compared with those of migraine headache. *Archives of Disease in Childhood* 72(5):413–417, 1995.
45. Apley J, Naish N: Recurrent abdominal pains: A field study of 1,000 school children. *Archives of Disease in Childhood* 33:165–170, 1958.
46. Scharff L: Recurrent abdominal pain in children: A review of psychological factors and treatment. *Clinical Psychology Review* 17(2):145–166, 1997.
47. Mortimer M, Kay J, Jaron A, Good P: Clinical epidemiology of childhood migraine in an urban general practice. *Developmental Medicine* 35:243–248, 1993.
48. Fleischer D: Cyclic vomiting syndrome and migraine. *Journal of Pediatrics* 134:533–535, 1999.
49. Boyle J: Recurrent abdominal pain: An update. *Pediatrics in Review* 18(9):310–320, 1997.
50. Rasquin-Weber A, Hyman PE, Cucchiara S, et al.: Childhood functional gastrointestinal disorders. *Gut* 45 (2):II60–68, 1999.
51. Lipsitz J, Masia-Warner C, Apfel H, et al.: Anxiety and depressive symptoms and anxiety sensitivity in youngsters with noncardiac chest pain and benign heart murmurs. *Journal of Pediatric Psychology* 29:607–612, 2004.
52. Selbst S, Ruddy R, Clark B, et al.: Pediatric chest pain: Prospective study. *Pediatrics* 82:319–323, 1988.
53. Mikkelsson M, Sourander A, Phia J, Salminen J: Psychiatric symptoms in preadolescents with musculoskeletal pain and fibromyalgia. *Pediatrics* 100:220–227, 1997.
54. Raja S, Grabow T: Complex regional pain syndrome I (Reflex sympathetic dystrophy). *Anesthesiology* 96:1254–1260, 2002.
55. Sherry D, Weisman R: Psychologic aspects of childhood reflex neurovascular dystrophy. *Pediatrics* 81:572–578, 1988.
56. Garralda ME, Chalder T: Practitioner review: Chronic fatigue syndrome in childhood. *Journal of Child Psychology and Psychiatry* 46:1143–1151, 2005.
57. Marshall G: Report of a workshop on the epidemiology, natural history and pathogenesis of chronic fatigue syndrome in adolescents. *Journal of Pediatrics* 134:395–405, 1999.
58. Goodwin R, Lewinsohn P, Seeley J: Respiratory symptoms and mental disorders among youth: Results form a prospective, longitudinal study. *Psychosomatic Medicine* 66(6):943–949, 2004.
59. Brugman S, Newman K: Vocal cord dysfunction. *Medical Scientific Update, National Jewish Center for Immunology and Respiratory Medicine* 11:1–5, 1993.
60. Goldman J, Muers M: Vocal cord dysfunction and wheezing. *Thorax* 46:401–404, 1991.
61. McQuaid E, et al.: The pediatric psychologist' role in differential diagnosis: Vocal cord dysfunction presenting as asthma. *Journal of Pediatric Psychology* 22:739–748, 1997.
62. Stefansson J, Messina J, Meyerowitz S: Hysterical neurosis, conversion type: Clinical and epidemiological considerations. *Acta Psychiatric Scand* 53:119–138, 1976.
63. Tomasson K, Kent D, Coryell W: Somatization and conversion disorders: Comorbidity and demographics at presentation. *Acta Psychiatric Scand* 84:288–293, 1991.
64. Goodyer I, Mitchell C: Somatic and emotional disorders in childhood and adolescence. *Journal of Psychosomatic Research* 33:681–688, 1989.
65. Maloney M: Diagnosing hysterical conversion reactions in children. *Journal of Pediatrics* 97:1016–1020, 1980.
66. Steinhausen H, Von Aster M, Pfeiffer E, et al.: Comparative studies of conversion disorders in childhood and adolescence. *Journal of Child Psychology & Psychiatry* 30:615–621, 1989.
67. Volkmar R, Poll J, Lewis M: Conversion reactions in children and adolescents. *Journal of the American Academy of Child and Adolescent Psychiatry* 23:424–430, 1984.
68. Pehlivanturk B, Unal F: Conversion disorder in children and adolescents: A 4-year follow-up study. *Journal of Psychosomatic Research* 52:187–191, 2002.
69. Turgay A: Treatment outcome for children and adolescents with conversion disorder. *Canadian Journal of Psychiatry* 35:585–589, 1990.
70. Rivinus T, Jamison D, Graham P: Childhood organic neurological disease presenting as psychiatric disorder. *Archives of Disease in Childhood* 40:115–119, 1975.
71. Stone J, Smyth R, Carson A, et al.: Systematic review of misdiagnosis of conversion symptoms and "hysteria." *BMJ* 331(7523):989, 2005.
72. Veale D: Body dysmorphic disorder. *Postgraduate Medical Journal* 80:67–71, 2003.
73. Mayville S, Katz R, Gipson M, Cabral K: Assessing the prevalence of body dysmorphic disorder in an ethnically diverse group of adolescents. *Journal of Child and Family Studies* 8:357–362, 1999.
74. Campo J, Di Lorenzo C, Chiappetta L, et al.: Adult outcomes of pediatric recurrent abdominal pain: Do they "just grow out of it"? *Pediatrics* 108:E1, 2001.

75. Walker L, Greene J: Children with recurrent abdominal pain and their parents: More somatic complaints, anxiety, and depression than other patient families? *Journal of Pediatric Psychology* 14(2):231–243, 1989.
76. Walker L, Garber J, Greene J: Somatization symptoms in pediatric abdominal pain patients: Relation to chronicity of abdominal pain and parent somatization. *Journal of Abnormal Child Psychology* 19(4):379–394, 1991.
77. Lehmkuhl G, Blanz B, Lehmkuhl U, et al.: Conversion disorder: Symptomatology and course in childhood and adolescence. *European Archives of Psychiatry & Neurological Sciences* 238:155–160, 1989.
78. Walker L, Greene J: The Functional Disability Inventory: Measuring a neglected dimension of child health status. *Journal of Pediatric Psychology* 16:39–58, 1991.
79. Aro H, Paronen O, Aro S: Psychosomatic symptoms among 14–16 year old Finnish adolescents. *Social Psychiatry* 22(3):171–176, 1987.
80. Campo J, Jansen-McWilliams L, Comer D, Kelleher K: Somatization in pediatric primary care: Association with psychopathology, functional impairment, and use of services.[comment]. *Journal of the American Academy of Child & Adolescent Psychiatry* 38(9):1093–1101, 1999.
81. Stevenson J, Simpson J, Bailey V: Research note: Recurrent headaches and stomachaches in preschool children. *Journal of Child Psychology & Psychiatry* 29:897–900, 1988.
82. Chandrasekaran R, Goswami U, Sivakumar V, et al.: Hysterical neurosis: A follow-up study. *Acta Psychiatric Scand* 89:78–80, 1994.
83. Pfefferbaum B, Adams J, Aceves J: The influence of culture on pain in Anglo and Hispanic children with cancer. *Journal of the American Academy of Child and Adolescent Psychiatry* 29:642–647, 1990.
84. Garber J, Zeman J, Walker L: Recurrent abdominal pain in children: Psychiatric diagnoses and parental psychopathology. *Journal of the American Academy of Child & Adolescent Psychiatry* 29(4):648–656, 1990.
85. Hotopf M: Childhood experience of illness as a risk factor for medically unexplained symptoms. *Scandinavian Journal of Psychology* 43:139–146, 2002.
86. Robinson J, Aleverez J, Dodge J: Life events and family history in children with recurrent abdominal pain. *Journal of Psychosomatic Research* 34:171–181, 1990.
87. Wasserman A, Whitington P, Rivara F: Psychogenic basis for abdominal pain in children and adolescents. *Journal of the American Academy of Child & Adolescent Psychiatry* 27(2):179–184, 1988.
88. Zuckerman B, Stevenson J, Bailey V: Stomachaches and headaches in a community sample of preschool children. *Pediatrics* 79:677–682, 1987.
89. Cloninger C, Reich T, Guze S: The multifactorial model of disease transmission: III. Familial relationship between sociopathy and hysteria (Briquet's syndrome). *British Journal of Psychiatry* 127:23–32, 1975.
90. Livingston R: Children of people with somatization disorder. *Journal of the American Academy of Child and Adolescent Psychiatry* 32:536–544, 1993.
91. Craig T, Cox A, Klein KB: Integration transmission of somatization behavior: A study of chronic somatizers and their children. *Psychological Medicine* 32:805–816, 2002.
92. Dunn-Geier B, McGrath P, Rourke B, et al.: Adolescent chronic pain: The ability to cope. *Pain* 26:23–32, 1986.
93. Levy RL, Jones KR, Whitehead WE, Feld SI, Talley NJ, Corey LA: Irritable bowel syndrome in twins: Heredity and social learning both contribute to etiology. *Gastroenterology* 121(4):799–804, 2001.
94. Osbourne R, Hatcher J, Richtsmeier A: The role of social modeling in unexplained pediatric pain. *Journal of Pediatric Psychology* 14:43–61, 1989.
95. Walker L, Garber J, Greene J: Psychosocial correlates of recurrent childhood pain: A comparison of pediatric patients with recurrent abdominal pain, organic illness, and psychiatric disorders. *Journal of Abnormal Psychology* 102:248–258, 1993.
96. Green M, Solnit A: Reactions to the threatened loss of a child: A vulnerable child syndrome. *Pediatrics* 34:58–66, 1964.
97. Mullins LL, Olson R: Familial factors in the etiology, maintenance, and treatment of somatoform disorders in children. *Family Systems Medicine* 8:159–175, 1990.
98. Wood B: Physically manifested illness in children and adolescents: A biobehavioral family approach. *Child & Adolescent Psychiatric Clinics of North America* 10:543–562, 2001.
99. Campo J, Comer D, Jansen-McWilliams L, Gardner W, Kelleher K: Recurrent pain, emotional distress, and health service use in childhood. *Journal of Pediatrics* 141:76–83, 2002.
100. Campo J, Bridge J, Lucas A, et al.: Physical and emotional health of mothers of youth with functional abdominal pain. *Archives of Pediatrics & Adolescent Medicine* 161(2):131–137, 2007.
101. Aro H, Hanninen V, Paronen O: Social support, life events and psychosomatic symptoms among 14–16-year-old adolescents. *Social Science & Medicine* 29(9):1051–1056, 1989.
102. Goodyer I, Taylor D: Hysteria. *Archives of Disease in Childhood.* 60:680–681, 1985.
103. Maisami M, Freeman J: Conversion reactions in children as body language: A combined child psychiatry/neurology team approach to the management of functional neurologic disorders in children. *Pediatrics.* 80:46–52, 1987.
104. Campo JV, Bridge J, Ehmann M, et al.: Recurrent abdominal pain, anxiety, and depression in primary care. *Pediatrics.* 113(4):817–824, 2004a.
105. Davison I, Faull C, Nicol A: Research note: Temperament and behaviour in six-year-olds with recurrent abdominal pain—A follow up. *Journal of Child Psychology and Psychiatry.* 27(4):539–544, 1986.
106. Manassis K, Bradley S, Goldberg S, Hood J, Price-Swinson R: Behavioural inhibition, attachment and anxiety in children of mothers with anxiety disorders. *Canadian Journal of Psychiatry.* 40:87–92, 1995.
107. Muris P, Meesters C: Children's somatization symptoms: Correlations with trait anxiety, anxiety sensitivity, and learning experiences. *Psychological Rep.* 94:1269–1275, 2004.
108. Watson D, Pennebaker J: Health complaints, stress, and distress: Exploring the central role of negative affectivity. *Psychological Review.* 96:234–254, 1989.
109. Bursch B, Walco GA, Zeltzer L: Clinical assessment and management of chronic pain and pain-associated disability syndrome. *Journal of Developmental & Behavioral Pediatrics.* 19:45–53, 1998.
110. Boyce W, Barr R, Zeltzer L: Temperament and the psychobiology of childhood stress. *Pediatrics* 90:483–486, 1992.
111. Kagan J, Reznick J, Snidman N: Biological bases of childhood shyness. *Science.* 40:167–171, 1988.
112. Mortimer M, Kay J, Jaron A, Good P: Does a history of material migraine or depression predispose children to headache or stomach-ache? *Headache.* 32:353–355, 1992.
113. Hodges K, Kline J, Barbero G, Woodruff C: Anxiety in children with recurrent abdominal pain and their parents. *Psychosomatics.* 26(11):850–866, 1985a.
114. Hodges K, Kline J, Barbero G, Flanery R: Depressive symptoms in children with recurrent abdominal pain and in their families. *Journal of Pediatrics.* 107:622–626, 1985b.
115. Dorn L, Campo JV, Thato S, Dahl RE, Lewin D, Chandra R, et al.: Psychological comorbidity and stress reactivity in children and adolescents with recurrent abdominal pain and anxiety disorders. *Journal of the American Academy of Child and Adolescent Psychiatry.* 42(1):66–75, 2003.
116. Kendler KS, Walters E, Truett K, et al.: A twin-family study of self-report symptoms of panic-phobia and somatization. *Behavior Genetics.* 25:499–515, 1995.
117. Gillespie N, Zhu G, Heath A, HIckie I, Martin N: The genetic aetiology of somatic distress. *Psychological Medicine.* 30:1051–1061, 2000.
118. Morris-Yates A, Talley NJ, Boyce P, Nandurar S, Andrews G: Evidence of a genetic contribution to functional bowel disorder. *American Journal of Gastroenterology.* 93(8):1311–1317, 1998.
119. Torgensen S: Genetics of somatoform disorders. *Archives of General Psychiatry.* 84:288–293, 1986.
120. Greenberg B, Li Q, Lucas F, et al.: Association between the serotonin transporter promoter polymorphism and personality traits in a primarily female sample. *American Journal of Medical Genetics* 96:202–216, 2000.
121. Lesch K, Bengel D, Heils A, et al.: Association of anxiety related traits with a polymorphism in the serotonin transporter gene regulatory region. *Science.* 274:1483, 1996.
122. Hariri AR, Mattay VS, Tessitore A, et al.: Serotonin transporter genetic variation and the response of the human amygdala. [comment]. *Science.* 297(5580):400–403, 2002.
123. Camilleri M, Atanasova E, Carlson P, et al.: Serotonin-transporter polymorphism pharmacogenetics in diarrhea-predominant irritable bowel syndrome. *Gastroenterology.* August 123(2):425–432, 2002.
124. Diatchenko L, Slade G, Nackley A, et al.: Genetic basis for individual variations in pain perception and the development of a chronic pain condition. *Human Molecular Genetics.* 14:135–143, 2005.
125. Du L, Bakish D, Hrdina P: Tryptophan hydroxylase gene 218A/C polymorphism is associated with somatic anxiety in major depressive disorder. *Journal of Affective Disorders.* 65:37–44, 2001.
126. Haugaard J: Recognizing and treating uncommon behavioral and emotional disorders in children and adolescents who have been severely maltreated: Somatization an other somatoform disorders. *Child Maltreatment.* 9:169–176, 2004.
127. Atlas J, Wolfson M, Lipschitz D: Dissociation and somatization in adolescent inpatients with and without history of abuse. *Psychological Reports.* 76:1101–1102, 1995.
128. Friedrich W, Schafer L. Somatic symptoms in sexually abused children. *Journal of Pediatric Psychology* 20:661–670, 1995.
129. Klevan J, DeJong A: Urinary tract symptoms and urinary tract infection following sexual abuse. *American Journal of Diseases in Childhood* 144:242–244, 1990.
130. Livingston R, Taylor J, Crawford S: A study of somatic complaints and psychiatric diagnosis in children. *Journal of the American Academy of Child & Adolescent Psychiatry* 27(2):185–187, 1988.
131. Rimza M, Berg R, Locke C: Sexual abuse: Somatic and emotional reactions. *Child Abuse and Neglect* 12:201–208, 1988.
132. Kinzl J, Traweger C, Biebl W: Family background and sexual abuse associated with somatization. *Psychotherapy & Psychosomatics* 64:82–87, 1995.
133. Craig T, Boardman A, Mills K: The South London Somatization Study. I. Longitudinal course and influence of early life experiences. *British Journal of Psychiatry* 163:579–588, 1993.
134. Craig T, Drake H, Mills K, et al.: The South London Somatization Study. II. Influence of stressful life events and secondary gain. *British Journal of Psychiatry* 165:248–258, 1994.

135. Perkonigg A, Pfister H, Stein M, et al.: Longitudinal course of posttraumatic stress disorder and posttraumatic stress disorder symptoms in a community sample of adolescents and young adults. *American Journal of Psychiatry* 162:1320–1327, 2005.
136. Compas BE, Thomsen AH: Coping and responses to stress among children with recurrent abdominal pain. *Journal of Developmental & Behavioral Pediatrics* 20(5):323–324, 1999.
137. Thomsen AH, Compas BE, Colletti RB, Stranger C, Boyer MC, Konik BS: Parent reports of coping and stress responses in children with recurrent abdominal pain. *Journal of Pediatric Psychology* 27(3):216–226, 2002.
138. Walker L, Smith C, Garber J, Van Slyke D: Development and validation of the Pain Response Inventory for children. *Psychological Assessment* 9(4):392–405, 1997.
139. Walker L, Smith C, Garber J, Claar R: Testing a model of pain appraisal and coping in children with chronic abdominal pain. *Health Psychology* 24(4):364–374, 2005.
140. Bernstein G, Massie E, Thuras P, Perwien A, Borchardt C, Crosby R: Somatic symptoms in anxious-depressed school refusers. *Journal of the American Academy of Child & Adolescent Psychiatry* 36:661–668, 1997.
141. Konijnenberg A, Uiterwaal C, Kimpen MJ, Van Der Hoeven J, Buitelaar J, De Graeff-Meeder E: Children with unexplained chronic pain: Substantial impairment in everyday life. *Archives of Disease in Childhood* 90:680–686, 2005.
142. Palermo T: Impact of recurrent and chronic pain on child and family daily functioning: A critical review of the literature. *Journal of Developmental & Behavioral Pediatrics* 21:58–69, 2000.
143. Smith M, Martin-Herz S, Womack W, Marsigan J: Comparative study of anxiety, depression, somatization, functional disability, and illness attribution in adolescents with chronic fatigue or migraine. *Pediatrics* 111:376–381, 2003.
144. Stickler G, Murphy D: Recurrent abdominal pain. *American Journal of Diseases in Childhood* 133:486–489, 1979.
145. Egger H, Costello E, Erkanli A, Angold A: Somatic complaints and psychopathology in children and adolescents: Stomach aches, musculoskeletal pains and headaches. *Journal of the American Academy of Child & Adolescent Psychiatry* 38:852–860, 1999.
146. Liakopoulou-Kairis M, Alifieraki T, Protagora D, et al.: Recurrent abdominal pain and headache: Psychopathology, life event and family functioning. *European Child & Adolescent Psychiatry*. 11:115–122, 2002.
147. Kowal A, Pritchard D: Psychological characteristics of children who suffer from headache: A research note. *Journal of Child Psychology and Psychiatry* 31:637–649, 1990.
148. Kashani J, Lababidi Z, Jones R: Depression in children and adolescents with cardiovascular symptomatology: The significance of chest pain. *Journal of the American Academy of Child Psychiatry* 21:187–189, 1982.
149. Peterson C, Palermo T: Parental reinforcement of recurrent pain: The moderating impact of child depression and anxiety on functional disability. *Journal of Pediatric Psychology* 29:331–342, 2004.
150. Borge A, Nordhagen R, Moe B, G B, Bakketeig L: Prevalence and persistence of stomach ache and headache among children. Follow-up of a cohort of Norwegian children from 4 to 10 years of age. *Acta Paediatricia* 83:433–437, 1994.
151. Apley J, Hale B: Children with abdominal pain: How do they grow up? *British Medical Journal* 3:7–9, 1973.
152. Christensen M, Mortensen O: Long-term prognosis in children with recurrent abdominal pain. *Archives of Disease in Childhood* 50:110–115, 1975.
153. Hotopf M, Carr S, Mayou R, Wadsworth M, Wessely S: Why do children have chronic abdominal pain, and what happens to them when they grow up? Population based cohort study. *British Medical Journal* 316:1196–1200, 1998.
154. Walker L, Guite J, Duke M, Barnard J, Greene J: Recurrent abdominal pain: A potential precursor of irritable bowel syndrome in adolescents and young adults. *Journal of Pediatrics* 132:1010–1015, 1998.
155. Pilowsky I, Bassett D, Begg M, et al.: Childhood hospitalization and chronic intractable pain in adults: A controlled retrospective study. *International Journal of Psychiatry in Medicine* 12:75–84, 1982.
156. Walker L, Garber J, Van Slyke D: Do parents excuse the misbehavior of children with physical or emotional symptoms? An investigation of the pediatric sick role. *Journal of Pediatric Psychology* 20:329–345, 1995.
157. Walker L, Zeman J: Parental response to child illness behavior. *Journal of Pediatric Psychology* 17:49–71, 1992.
158. Costello E, Costello A, Edelbrock C, et al.: Psychiatric disorders in pediatric primary care: Prevalence and risk factors. *Archives of General Psychiatry* 45:1107–1116, 1988.
159. Dubowitz V, Hersov L: Management of children with non-organic (hysterical) disorders of motor function. *Devel Med Child Neurol* 18:358–368, 1976.
160. Di Lorenzo C, Youssef N, Sigurdsson L, Scharff L, Griffiths J, Wald A: Visceral hyperalgesia in children with functional abdominal pain. *Journal of Pediatrics* 139:838–843, 2001.
161. Ginkel R, Voskuljl W, Benninga M, Taminiau J, Boeckxstaens G: Alterations in rectal sensitivity and motility in childhood irritable bowel syndrome. *Gastroenterology* 120:31–38, 2001.
162. Alfvén G: The pressure pain threshold (PPT) of certain muscles in children suffering from recurrent abdominal pain of non-organic origin. An algometric study. *Acta Paediatricia* 82:481–483, 1993b.
163. Garralda M: Assessment and management of somatization in childhood and adolescence: A practical perspective. *Journal of Child Psychology & Psychiatry* 40:1159–1167, 1999.
164. Warwick H: Provision of appropriate and effective reassurance. *International Review of Psychiatry* 4:76–80, 1992.
165. Warwick H, Salkovskis P: *Hypochondriasis*. London: Helm; 1988.
166. Schulman J: Use of a coping approach in the management of children with conversion reactions. *Journal of the American Academy of Child and Adolescent Psychiatry* 27:785–788, 1988.
167. Stulemeijer M, De Jong L, Fiselier T, Hoogveld S, Bleijenberg G: Cognitive behavior therapy for adolescents with chronic fatigue syndrome: Randomized controlled trial. *BMJ* 330(7481):14, 2005.
168. Viner R, Gregorowski A, Wine C, et al.: Outpatient rehabilitative treatment of chronic fatigue syndrome. *Archives of Disease in Childhood* 89:615–619, 2004.
169. Wright B, Ashby B, Beverley D, et al.: A feasibility study comparing two treatment approaches for chronic fatigue syndrome in adolescents. *Archives of Disease in Childhood* 90:369–372, 2005.
170. Calvert P, Jureidini J: Restrained rehabilitation: An approach to children and adolescents with unexplained signs and symptoms. *Archives of Disease in Childhood* 88:399–402, 2003.
171. Barsky A: Amplification, somatization, and the somatoform disorders. *Psychosomatics* 13:28–33, 1992.
172. McGrath P, Humphreys P, Keene D, Goodman J, et al.: The efficacy and efficiency of a self-administered treatment for adolescent migraine. *Pain* 49:321–324, 1992.
173. Robins P, Smith S, Glutting J, Bishop C: A randomized controlled trial of a cognitive-behavioral family intervention for pediatric recurrent abdominal pain. *Journal of Pediatric Psychology* 30:449–452, 2005.
174. Sanders MR, Rebgetz M, Morrison M, et al.: Cognitive-behavioral treatment of recurrent nonspecific abdominal pain in children: An analysis of generalization, maintenance, and side effects. *Journal of Consulting & Clinical Psychology* 57(2):294–300, 1989.
175. Sanders MR, Shepherd RW, Cleghorn G, Woolford H: The treatment of recurrent abdominal pain in children: A controlled comparison of cognitive-behavioral family intervention and standard pediatric care. *Journal of Consulting & Clinical Psychology* 62(2):306–314, 1994.
176. Kashikar-Zuck S, Swain N, Jones B, Graham T: Efficacy of cognitive behavioral intervention for juvenile primary fibromyalgia syndrome. *Journal of Rhematology* 32:1594–1602, 2005.
177. Hicks D, VonBaeyer C, McGrath P: Online psychological treatment for pediatric recurrent pain: A randomized evaluation. *Journal of Pediatric Psychology* 31(7):724–736, 2006.
178. Delameter A, Rosenbloom N, Conners K, Hertweck L: The behavioral treatment of hysterical paralysis in a ten-year-old boy: A case study. *Journal of the American Academy of Child and Adolescent Psychiatry* 1: 73–79, 1983.
179. Klonoff E, Moore D: "Conversion reactions" in adolescents: A biofeedback-based operant approach. *Journal of Behavior Therapy and Experimental Psychology* 17:179–184, 1986.
180. Mizes J: The use of contingent reinforcement in the treatment of a conversion disorder: A multiple baseline study. *Journal of Behavior Therapy and Experimental Psychology* 16:341–345, 1985.
181. Sank LI, Biglan A: Operant treatment of a case of recurrent abdominal pain in a 10-year-old boy. *Behavior Therapy* 5:677–681, 1974.
182. Miller AJ, Kratochwill RT: Reduction of frequent stomachache complaints by time out. *Behavior Therapy* 10:211–218, 1979.
183. Kazdin A: *Behavior Modification in Applied Settings*. 5th ed. Pacific Grove, CA: Brooks Cole Publishing; 1994.
184. Campo J, Negrini B: Case study: Negative reinforcement and behavioral management of conversion disorder. *Journal of the American Academy of Child & Adolescent Psychiatry* 39:787–790, 2000.
185. Holden E, Deichman M, Levy J: Empirically supported treatments in pediatric psychology: Recurrent pediatric headache. *Journal of Pediatric Psychology* 24:91–109, 1999.
186. Larsson B, Carlsson J, Fichtel A, Melin L: Relaxation treatment of adolescent headache sufferers: Results from a school-based replication series. *Headache* 45:692–704, 2005.
187. Linton S: A case study of the behavioural treatment of chronic stomach pain in a child. *Behaviour Change* 3:70–73, 1986.
188. Masek B, Russo D, Varni J: Behavioral approaches to the management of chronic pain in children. *Pediatr Clin North Am* 31:1113–1131, 1984.
189. Caldwell T, Stewart R: Hysterical seizures and hypnotherapy. *American Journal of Clinical Hypnosis* 23:294–298, 1981.
190. Elkins G, Carter B: Hypnotherapy in the treatment of childhood psychogenic coughing: A case report. *American Journal of Clinical Hypnosis* 29:59–63, 1986.
191. Williams D, Singh M: Hypnosis as a facilitating therapeutic adjunct in child psychiatry. *Journal of American Academy of Child and Adolescent Psychiatry* 15:326–342, 1976.
192. Pennebaker J, Susman J: Disclosure of traumas and psychosomatic processes. *Social Science & Medicine* 26(327–332), 1988.

193. Milrod B: A 9-year-old with conversion disorder, successfully treated with psychoanalysis. *International Journal of Psycho-Analysis* 83:623–631, 2002.
194. Liebman R, Honig P, Berger H: An integrated treatment program for psychogenic pain. *Family Process* 15:397–405, 1976.
195. Fallon B: Pharmacotherapy of somatoform disorders. *Journal of Psychosomatic Research* 56:455–460, 2004.
196. Stahl S: Antidepressants and somatic symptoms: Therapeutic actions are expanding beyond affective spectrum disorders to functional somatic syndromes. *Journal of Clinical Psychiatry* 64:745–746, 2003.
197. Hollander E, Allen A, Kwon J, et al.: Clomipramine vs. desipramine crossover trial in body dysmorphic disorder: Selective efficacy of a serotonin reuptake inhibitor in imagined ugliness. *Archives of General Psychiatry* 56:1033–1039, 1999.
198. Phillips K, Albertini R, Rasmussen S: A randomized placebo-controlled trial of fluoxetine in body dysmorphic disorder. *Archives of General Psychiatry* 59:381–388, 2002.
199. Fishbain DA, Cutler RB, Rosomoff HL, Rosomoff RS: Do antidepressants have an analgesic effect in psychogenic pain and somatoform pain disorder? A meta-analysis. *Psychosomatic Medicine.* 60(4):503–509, 1998.
200. Drossman DA, Toner BB, Whitehead WE, Diamant NE, Dalton CB, Duncan S: Cognitive-behavioral therapy versus education and desipramine versus placebo for moderate to severe functional bowel disorders. [comment]. *Gastroenterology* 125(1):19–31, 2003.
201. Jailwala J, Imperiale T, Kroenke K: Pharmacologic treatment of irritable bowel syndrome: A systematic review of randomized, controlled trials. *Annals of Internal Medicine.* 133:136–147, 2000.
202. O'Malley PG, Jackson JL, Santoro J, Tomkins G, Balden E, Kroenke K: Antidepressant therapy for unexplained symptoms and symptom syndromes. *Journal of Family Practice.* 48(12):980–990, 1999.
203. Muller T, Mannel M, Murck H, Rahlps V: Treatment of somatoform disorders with St. John's wort: A randomized, double-blind and placebo-controlled trial. *Psychosomatic Medicine.* 66:538–547, 2004.
204. El-Khatib H, Dickey T: Sertraline for body dysmorphic disorder. *Journal of the American Academy of Child & Adolescent Psychiatry.* 27:251–260, 1995.
205. Sondheimer A: Clomipramine treatment of delusional disorder, somatic type. *Journal of the American Academy of Child and Adolescent Psychiatry.* 27:188–192, 1988.
206. Simon GE, Katon W, Rutter C, et al.: The impact of improved depression treatment in primary care on daily functioning and disability. *Psychological Medicine.* 28:693–701, 1998.
207. Campo J. Coping with ignorance: Exploring pharmacologic management of pediatric functional abdominal pain. *Journal of Pediatric Gastroenterology & Nutrition.* 41(5):569–574, 2005.
208. Campo JV, Perel J, Lucas A, et al.: Citalopram treatment of pediatric recurrent abdominal pain and comorbid internalizing disorders: An exploratory study. *Journal of the American Academy of Child & Adolescent Psychiatry* 43(10):1234–1242, 2004.
209. Hyams JS, Hyman PE: Recurrent abdominal pain and the biopsychosocial model of medical practice. [comment]. *Journal of Pediatrics.* 133(4):473–478, 1998.
210. Geller B, Reising D, Leonard HL, Riddle MA, Walsh BT: Critical review of tricyclic antidepressant use in children and adolescents. *Journal of the American Academy of Child & Adolescent Psychiatry.* 38(5):513–516, 1999.
211. Lewis D, Ashwal S, Hershey A, Hirtz D, Yonker M, Silberstein S: Practice parameter: Pharmacological treatment of migraine headache in children and adolescents: Report of the American Academy of Neurology Quality Standards Subcommittee and the Practice Committee of the Child Neurology Society. *Neurology.* 63:2215–2224, 2004.
212. Kabbouche M, Vockell A, LeCates S, Powers S: Tolerability and effectiveness of procholorperazine for intractable migraine in children. *Pediatrics.* April 107(4):E62, 2001.
213. Siow H, Young W, Silberstein S: Neuroleptics in headache. *Headache.* 45:358–371, 2005.
214. Tomkins G, Jackson J, O'Malley P, Balden E, Santoro J: Treatment of chronic headache with antidepressants: A meta-analysis. *American Journal of Medicine.* 111:54–63, 2001.
215. Hershey A, Powers S, Vockell A, LeCates S, Kabbouche M: Effectiveness of topiramate in the prevention of childhood headaches. *Headache.* 42:810–818, 2002.
216. Battistella P, Ruffilli R, Cernetti R, et. al.: A placebo controlled crossover trial using trazodone in pediatric migraine. *Headache.* 33:36–39, 1993.
217. Putnam G, O'Quinn S: Bolden-Watson Cea. Migraine polypharmacy and the tolerability of sumatriptan: A large scale, prospective study. *Cephalalgia.* 19:668–675, 1999.
218. Campo J, Shafer S, Lucas A, et al.: Managing pediatric mental disorders in primary care: A stepped collaborative care model. *Journal of the American Psychiatric Nurses Association* 11(5):1–7, 2005.
219. Fritz G, Bergman A: Child psychiatrists seen through pediatricians' eyes: Results of a national survey. *Journal of the American Academy of Child and Adolescent Psychiatry.* 24:81–86, 1985.
220. Smith G, Monson R, Ray D: Psychiatric consultation in somatization disorder. *New England Journal of Medicine.* 314:1407–1413, 1986.

CHAPTER 5.11 ■ DELIRIUM AND CATATONIA

DANIEL T. WILLIAMS

With a growing level of sophistication in recent years, we have come to appreciate important neurophysiological substrates of central nervous system dysfunction inherent in many traditional psychiatric disorders. By virtue of functional neuroimaging studies clarifying that every behavior and subjective experience has a neurophysiologic correlate, it is now well recognized that the organic versus psychiatric distinction is ultimately a semantic one, determined by our current level of neurophysiologic sophistication or lack thereof.

Perturbations of consciousness and motor function that are a byproduct of a significant change in the functional integrity of the central nervous system from its baseline state merit specific clinical consideration by both neurologists and psychiatrists. Two such patterns of perturbation, delirium and catatonia, are classic neuropsychiatric syndromes. We will address here the phenomenology, evaluation and treatment of these disorders in children and adolescents.

DELIRIUM

Delirium may be defined as a transient and usually reversible dysfunction in cerebral activity that has an acute or subacute onset and is manifest clinically by a wide array of neuropsychiatric abnormalities, including impairment of consciousness or cognition, which causes a "confusional state" (1–3). Associated symptoms may include perceptual disturbances, delusions, affective lability, disordered thought processes, sleep disturbances, and psychomotor symptoms. If there is a progression of functional derangement of consciousness from normal alertness through delirium to further impairment, the patient can decline into a state of stupor, coma, and eventually death.

Insofar as there are a variety of underlying causes of delirium in different patients, it is reasonable to consider it as a syndrome rather than a single disorder. Although the term has

TABLE 5.11.1

DIAGNOSTIC CRITERIA FOR DELIRIUM DUE TO . . .* (1–5)

A. Disturbance of consciousness (reduced clarity of awareness of the environment) with reduced ability to focus, sustain, or shift attention.
B. A change in cognition (such as memory deficit, disorientation, language disturbance) or the development of a perceptual disturbance that is not better accounted for by a preexisting, established, or evolving dementia.
C. The disturbance develops over a short period of time (usually hours to days) and tends to fluctuate during the course of the day.
D. There is evidence from the history, physical examination, or laboratory findings that the disturbance is caused by the direct physiological consequences of . . . * (1–5)
 *1) . . . a general medical condition.
 *2) . . . substance intoxication.
 *3) . . . substance withdrawal.
 *4) . . . multiple etiologies.
 *5) . . . not otherwise specified.

(Adapted from American Psychiatric Association. *Diagnostic and Statistical Manual of Mental Disorders, Fourth Edition, Text Revision.* Washington, DC: American Psychiatric Association, 2000.)

been used with differing connotations over the years and has many synonyms in the neurological and psychiatric literature, it seems best for current purposes to define delirium as outlined in DSM-IV-TR (Table 5.11.1).

Predisposing Factors

Children and the elderly reportedly are at higher risk to the development of delirium under circumstances of physiological stress (4–6). While the elderly are thought to be more vulnerable because of diminished cholinergic reserve, children are thought to be more vulnerable because of immature and evolving structural and biochemical brain development. Intrinsic predisposing patient vulnerabilities in addition to age would include a previous delirium episode, preexisting cognitive impairment, a CNS disorder, and increased blood–brain barrier permeability. Environmental risk factors include social isolation, sensory extremes, visual or hearing deficits, immobility, as well as environmental novelty or stress. Other risk factors include medical illness, surgery, and pharmacological influences. Clearly, during hospitalization, there is often a confluence of these predisposing and precipitating factors.

Some of the above risk factors may be modifiable and consequently present opportunities for preventive intervention. Closer observation of patients at high risk for delirium could allow for earlier detection of emergent delirium and allow for attenuation of modifiable risk factors. Probably most readily modifiable is medication exposure, particularly of anticholinergic medications (7). Because of the general acceptance of a tendency for children to regress under stressful circumstances, milder forms of delirium may be mistaken for simply regressive or provocative behavior. As with adults, however, undetected delirium may proceed to the point of self-injury or serious interference with medical treatment.

Paradoxically, children may have a reduced risk of postcardiotomy delirium compared to adults. Kornfeld et al (8). reported on a sample of 119 unselected open heart patients that included 20 children who had surgical procedures for repair of congenital lesions. Only one of the children developed delirium, whereas 30% of the adults operated on for congenital repairs did. It is noteworthy that preoperative psychiatric interviews may reduce postoperative delirium and psychosis by 50% (9). Others have also reported the benefit of using preoperative psychological interventions to reduce anxiety and improve perioperative management in children (10). A clinical consensus suggests that as the severity of pathophysiologic strain increases, so does the probability of developing a delirium (11). This is particularly true for burn patients, as well as for postoperative patients. Additional factors that are considered to foster the development of delirium include sleep deprivation, sensory deprivation, and sensory overload. Thiamine deficiency can be a risk factor for delirium in pediatric intensive care and oncology patients (12). Low serum albumin is another factor, resulting in a greater bioavailability of drugs that are transmitted in the bloodstream, potentially contributing to delirium (13).

Clinical Features

Given that there is a wide variety of etiologies for delirium, it may be most useful to conceptualize delirium as a final common neural pathway that leads to its characteristic symptoms (4). These symptoms often fluctuate in intensity over a 24-hour period and may be associated with shifts between hypoactive and hyperactive states or with disruption of the sleep-wake cycle. Table 5.11.2 outlines symptoms generally associated with delirium that may be variably represented in different patients. Review of studies of delirium in adults with a variety of underlying etiologies shows that some symptoms are reported more often and more consistently than others, suggesting that there may be some core symptoms, irrespective of etiology. Postulated core symptoms include attentional deficits, memory impairment, disorientation, sleep-wake cycle disturbance, thought process abnormalities, motoric alterations, and language disturbances. Associated or noncore symptoms would include perceptual disturbances, (illusions, hallucinations), delusions, and affective changes (14). The associated symptoms might reflect the impact of either specific etiological influences or individual differences in brain circuitry and vulnerability.

Some studies suggest that the motoric profile in delirium is influenced by etiology. Thus, delirium due to drug and alcohol related causes is more commonly hyperactive, whereas delirium due to metabolic disturbances, including hypoxia, is more frequently hypoactive (15, 16). As yet, however, available studies have not provided clear evidence that gross motoric subtypes have discernible neurobiological mechanisms.

Mortality rates during a hospitalization involving delirium for adults have ranged from 1.5% to 65% in different case series (17). Turkel and Tavare (18) retrospectively reviewed 84 children and adolescents with delirium, among 1,027 consecutive inpatient psychiatric consultations during a 4-year period. They found a mortality rate of 20% and a prolonged length of stay when delirium was documented. It is clear therefore that the diagnosis of delirium constitutes a matter of severe medical urgency. Since some of the medical conditions contributing to delirium are potentially reversible, early clarification of diagnosis and aggressive initiation of treatment are clinically imperative.

Etiology

When a diagnosis of delirium is established, a thorough search for causes must be pursued, insofar as correction or amelioration of specific underlying causes is important in reversing the condition. However, this process of investigation should not unduly delay prompt treatment of the delirium itself, since such treatment can reduce symptoms even before

TABLE 5.11.2

SIGNS AND SYMPTOMS OF DELIRIUM ("*PLASTRD*")

Psychosis
Perceptual disturbances (especially visual), including illusions, hallucinations, metamorphopsias
Delusions (usually paranoid and poorly formed)
Thought disorder (tangentiality, circumstantiality, loose associations)
Language impairment
Word-finding difficulty/dysnomia/paraphasia
Dysgraphia
Altered semantic content
Severe forms can mimic expressive or receptive aphasia
Altered or labile affect
Any mood can occur, usually incongruent to context
Anger or increased irritability common
Hypoactive delirium often mislabeled as depression
Lability (rapid shifts) common
Unrelated to mood preceding delirium
Sleep-wake disturbance
Fragmented throughout 24-hour period
Reversal of normal cycle
Sleeplessness
Temporal course
Acute/abrupt onset
Fluctuating severity of symptoms over 24-hour period
Usually reversible
Subclinical syndrome may precede and/or follow the episode
Reactivity Altered
Hyperactive
Hypoactive
Mixed
Diffuse cognitive deficits
Attention
Orientation (time, place, person)
Memory (short- and long-term; verbal and visual)
Visuoconstructional ability
Executive functions

(Adapted from Trzepacz PT, et al. Neuropsychiatric aspects of delirium. In Yudofsky SC, Hales RE, eds. *The American Psychiatric Publishing Textbook of Neuropsychiatry and Clinical Neurosciences, 4th ed.* Washington, DC: American Psychiatric Publishing, 2002; 525–564.)

the underlying medical causes have been reversed. As noted above, from a DSM-IV-TR perspective, delirium is broadly categorized according to etiology into five groups. These include delirium due to a general medical condition, due to substance use or withdrawal, due to multiple causes, and due to no apparent cause that can be identified. It is probably useful to spell out in more detail a list of the wide variety of etiologies that may pertain, either individually or in combination. These are listed in Table 5.11.3.

Delirium in children and adolescents involves the same categories of etiologies as adults, though the relative frequency of specific etiologies differs. Thus, delirium related to illicit drugs is more common in the child and adolescent age group, as is the incidence of delirium from hypoxia due to foreign body inhalation, drowning and asthma, as well as delirium related to head trauma.

Differential Diagnosis

Delirium frequently goes undetected in a variety of therapeutic settings by a variety of medical specialists, including neurologists and psychiatrists (19). Failure of detection may derive from insidious onset and fluctuating course involving multiple symptom constellations that can generate much clinical variability. Thus an agitated, hyperactive delirium, that is more likely to be recognized, contrasts with the more common, mixed or hypoactive symptom pattern that may be more readily overlooked. This is particularly true in a hospital setting, with multiple shift changes of staff, where subtle and gradual changes of mental status may not be discerned. Diagnosis can be improved by routinely assessing cognitive function, by improving staff awareness of the varied presentations of delirium, and by using one of the screening instruments for delirium currently available (4).

Differential diagnosis includes depression, psychosis, anxiety, somatoform disorders, dementia (more commonly in the elderly) and, particularly in children, behavioral disturbance. Because of the general tendency for children to regress under stressful circumstances, milder forms of delirium may be mistaken for simply regressive or provocative behavior. As with adults, however, undetected delirium may proceed to the point of self-injury or serious interference with medical treatment. Effective diagnosis requires close attention to symptom pattern, temporal sequence, and objective clinical test results (laboratory, cognitive, electroencephalographic). Since delirium is often the first indication of serious medical deterioration, any patient manifesting an abrupt decline in attentional or cognitive function should be evaluated for possible delirium.

TABLE 5.11.3

ETIOLOGIES OF DELIRIUM

Drug intoxication	Intracranial infection
Drug withdrawal	Systemic infection
Metabolic/endocrine disturbances	Cerebrovascular disorder
Traumatic brain injury	Organ insufficiency
Seizures	Other CNS etiologies
Neoplastic disease	Other systemic etiologies

(Adapted from: Hales RE and Yudofsky SC: *The American Psychiatric Publishing Textbook of Neuropsychiatry and Clinical Neurosciences*, 3rd ed. Washington, DC: American Psychiatric Press, 2002.)

Assessment

To allow more accurate diagnosis and monitoring, more than 10 different assessment instruments suitable for adults have been developed (20). One of these, the Delirium Rating Scale, has been systematically evaluated retrospectively with 84 children and adolescents diagnosed with delirium (age range 6 months to 19 years) (21). The Delirium Rating Scale is composed of 10 items: Two items ascertain the temporal onset of symptoms and their relationship to a physical disorder; eight other items evaluate major symptoms of delirium. These eight items rate perceptual disturbances, hallucinations, delusions, changes in psychomotor behavior, diffuse cognitive dysfunction, disturbances of sleep-wake cycle, lability of mood, and variability of symptoms. The cognitive dysfunction item includes impairment of attention, concentration, and memory. The results of the Turkel et al. study (21) suggest that the Delirium Rating Scale can be used effectively to evaluate delirium in the pediatric population.

In most cases, electroencephalograms are not needed to make a clinical diagnosis of delirium, but are used when seizures are suspected or when differential diagnosis is difficult. The degree of slowing on EEGs recorded serially over time in children and adolescents correlates with the severity of, and recovery from, delirium (22).

The psychiatrist will clearly not be primarily responsible for diagnosing and managing the underlying medical condition contributing to the delirium. However, supportively maintaining the morale and involvement of family members who can be invaluable observers and informers to the medical staff regarding the patient's mental status can be a vital part of the consulting psychiatrist's function. This, of course, is supplementary to the psychiatrist's own longitudinal assessments of the patient, which should be documented systematically.

Treatment

Prompt treatment is vital because of the substantial morbidity and mortality associated with delirium. Symptomatic treatments include medication, environmental manipulation, as well as patient and family psychosocial support (11). These should be initiated concomitant with the attempts to identify and reverse underlying causes of the delirium.

Pharmacological treatment with a neuroleptic, most commonly haloperidol, is the most commonly reported medical intervention for delirium, despite the absence of double-blind, placebo-controlled trials documenting efficacy. Haloperidol can be given orally, intramuscularly, or intravenously, although haloperidol is not approved by the U.S. Food and Drug Administration for intravenous use. Clinical experience with haloperidol in pediatric delirium supports its beneficial effects, although purely based on uncontrolled case reports (23). Based on such existing clinical experience, one suggested dosage regimen for children younger than 4 years of age is starting with 0.25 mg slowly intravenously over 30 to 45 minutes as a loading dose, and 0.05 to 0.5 mg/kg/24h intravenously as a continuing dose. When using higher doses of IV haloperidol (e.g. > 20mg/day), electrocardiographic tracking of QTc interval prolongation and other relevant parameters should be done daily, as well as monitoring and correction of magnesium, phosphate, and other electrolytes in order to minimize the risks of cardiotoxicity (up to torsade de pointes and other tachyarrhythmias). The oral dose of haloperidol is twice the intravenous dose. Although no fixed dosing schedule based on controlled studies is available for either children or adults, a protocol for haloperidol use in agitated delirium in adults has been proposed (11). Intravenous administration of haloperidol is reportedly associated with fewer extrapyramidal symptoms compared with oral administration (24). The rationale for this neuroleptic treatment intervention is based on clinical evidence suggesting a low cholinergic, excess dopaminergic state as the final common neural pathway for delirium (4).

Benzodiazepines are generally reserved for delirium due to alcohol or sedative-hypnotic withdrawal. Occasionally, lorazepam may be used as an adjunct with haloperidol in cases of delirium where agitation and insomnia persist. Caution is needed, however, to avoid over-sedation or paradoxical disinhibition.

Environmental interventions for delirium are often helpful but are not by themselves adequate treatment. Family members and nurses can help reorient the patient with a clock, calendar, and familiar objects. A room with a window can help with diurnal cues and adequate lighting at night can diminish frightening visual misperceptions. Encouraging a stable parent to stay overnight, with appropriate explanation to the parent about the phenomenon of delirium and about the merits of supportive measures for the patient, can be quite reassuring.

Psychiatrists are often called to evaluate the fluctuating, confusing, and bizarre behaviors that may characterize delirium. Insofar as significant morbidity and mortality can be associated with this condition, it is important for the psychiatrist to help organize a systematic differential diagnosis, collaborate with the primary care physician in identifying the underlying cause(s), and help formulate a plan for monitoring and treating the associated agitation as well as related psychiatric symptomatology in both the patient and family.

CATATONIA

In contrast to delirium, which is defined primarily by alterations in level of consciousness as reflected by attention and cognition, with occasionally accompanying psychomotor symptoms, catatonia is defined by a cluster of *motor* symptoms, including a rigid posture, mutism, fixed staring, stereotypic movements, hyperkinetic movements, or stupor. Implicit in this varied constellation of motor symptoms, however, is the presumption of an underlying neuropsychiatric derangement which presents the clinician with a differential diagnostic and treatment challenge of comparable complexity to that posed by delirium. Like delirium, catatonia is best understood as a syndrome that may be associated with a wide array of psychiatric and medical disorders that lead to the final common path of these motor manifestations. In some patients, the differential diagnostic challenge will include differentiating between delirium and catatonia.

In the current diagnostic classification nomenclature of the American Psychiatric Association, there are three domains in which catatonia is represented and these are represented in Tables 5.11.4, 5.11.5, and 5.11.6. This diverse representation speaks to the multifactorial contributants to this syndrome from diverse etiologies.

Predisposing Factors

By definition in the existing psychiatric nomenclature, predisposing factors to catatonia include the three clinical domains referred to above, namely a variety of medical conditions, a variety of mood disorders, and a particular type of schizophrenia. Although the occurrence of catatonia in children and adolescents is well documented in the clinical literature (25), there are no epidemiologic studies that indicate a relative difference in incidence associated with age (26). It appears that the range of primary diagnoses with which catatonia is associated in

TABLE 5.11.4

DSM-IV-TR CRITERIA FOR CATATONIC DISORDER DUE TO . . . [INDICATE THE GENERAL MEDICAL CONDITION]

A. ***Cat***atonia is manifested by motoric immobility, excessive motor activity (that is apparently purposeless and not influenced by external stimuli), extreme negativism or mutism, peculiarities of voluntary movement, or echolalia or echopraxia.
B. ***Med:*** There is evidence from the history, physical examination, or laboratory findings that the disturbance is the direct physiological consequence of a general medical condition.
C. ***Not Ment:*** The disturbance is not better accounted for by another mental disorder (e.g., a manic episode).
D. ***Not Del:*** The disturbance does not occur exclusively during the course of a delirium.

(Adapted from American Psychiatric Association. *Diagnostic and Statistical Manual of Mental Disorders, Fourth Edition, Text Revision.* Washington, DC: American Psychiatric Association, 2000.)

TABLE 5.11.5

DSM-IV-TR CRITERIA FOR CATATONIC FEATURES SPECIFIER OF A MOOD DISORDER

Specify if:
With Catatonic Features (can be applied to the current or most recent major depressive episode, manic episode, or mixed episode in major depressive disorder, bipolar I disorder, or bipolar II disorder)
The clinical picture is dominated by at least two of the following characteristics (*MUMEE*)
1) *M*otoric immobility as evidenced by catalepsy (including waxy flexibility) or stupor
2) *U*tmost negativism (an apparently motiveless resistance to all instructions or maintenance of a rigid posture against attempts to be moved) or mutism
3) *M*otor hyperactivity (that is apparently purposeless and not influenced by external stimuli)
4) *E*ccentricities of voluntary movement as evidenced by posturing (voluntary assumption of inappropriate or bizarre postures), stereotyped movements, prominent mannerisms, or prominent grimacing
5) *E*cholalia or echopraxia

(Adapted from American Psychiatric Association. *Diagnostic and Statistical Manual of Mental Disorders, Fourth Edition, Text Revision.* Washington, DC: American Psychiatric Association, 2000.)

youngsters broadly overlaps that reported in adults. In addition, there are a significant number of reports of catatonia associated with autism, the Prader-Willi syndrome, and mental retardation (27, 28). As with delirium, catatonia in youngsters may be more difficult to diagnose because of the more limited expressive capacity of children and adolescents, as well as the tendency of observers to ascribe symptomatic behavior to willful regression of an oppositional nature.

Clinical Features

The principal motor signs associated with catatonia are mutism, immobility, negativism, posturing, stereotypy, and echophenomena. Although DSM-IV-TR defines a requirement for two of these to be present in cases of mood disorder or schizophrenia, it does not specify a duration. Some clinicians advocate that these signs be present for at least an hour or be reproducible on at least two occasions (29). Prolonged immobility may generate malnutrition, dehydration, weight loss, muscle wasting, contractures and bedsores. Death may ensue from venous thrombosis and pulmonary emboli. A summary description of clinical features frequently associated with catatonia is presented in Table 5.11.7.

TABLE 5.11.6

CATATONIC TYPE OF SCHIZOPHRENIA

A type of schizophrenia in which the clinical picture is dominated by at least two of the following characteristics (*MUMEE*):
6) *M*otoric immobility as evidenced by catalepsy (including waxy flexibility) or stupor
7) *U*tmost negativism (an apparently motiveless resistance to all instructions or maintenance of a rigid posture against attempts to be moved) or mutism
8) *M*otor hyperactivity (that is apparently purposeless and not influenced by external stimuli)
9) *E*ccentricities of voluntary movement as evidenced by posturing (voluntary assumption of inappropriate or bizarre postures), stereotyped movements, prominent mannerisms, or prominent grimacing
10) *E*cholalia or echopraxia

Etiology

As with delirium, there have been efforts to define a final common neurophysiological pathway, whereby many different pathophysiological conditions may contribute to the clinical features of catatonia. Recent views implicate frontal lobe circuitry dysfunction (29). Disruption of connections from perceptual-integrating brain systems because of thalamic or parietal lobe lesions as well as limbic interference (as occurs in certain mood states) have been postulated to play etiological roles. The neurotransmitters dopamine and GABA have been implicated and this has therapeutic relevance.

As previously noted, conditions in which catatonia is expressed include mood disorders, psychosis, and a variety of medical conditions, including neurological disorders, metabolic disorders, as well as drug intoxication and withdrawal.

Catatonia has been reported in about 15% of manic episodes in adult patients with bipolar mood disorders, with one series of 99 manic patients finding as high as a 27% incidence (30). Bipolar mood disorder is the most common cause of catatonia. Depression is the second most common condition underlying catatonia in adults. Catatonia in depressed patients is often manifest as profound psychomotor retardation, sometimes progressing to stupor or pseudodementia. Delay in diagnostics and treatment intervention for treating catatonia in mood disorder patients clearly can increase morbidity and mortality.

Schizophrenia accounts for about 10% of adult patients with catatonia (31). Catatonic features more commonly encountered in these patients include catalepsy, mannerisms, posturing, and mutism. Historically, this diagnosis has been invoked more frequently than that of mood disorder in patients with catatonia, which is a disservice if it leads to premature or exclusive reliance on neuroleptic medication, with associated increased risks of disabling side effects. (These side effects can include neuroleptic malignant syndrome, an admittedly rare complication that can initially be difficult to differentiate from catatonic schizophrenia.)

Many general medical conditions can manifest with catatonia, including many of the same conditions that are associated with delirium. These include a variety of neurological syndromes, metabolic, autoimmune, and endocrine disorders, infections, burns, and drug-induced states. The latter may include both recreational and prescribed drugs, including neuroleptic malignant syndrome. Neurological conditions and metabolic disorders associated with catatonia are outlined in Tables 5.11.8 and 5.11.9.

A review of the literature regarding catatonia in children and adolescents suggests that signs of catatonia in youngsters are similar to those in adults (29). It appears that catatonia is sufficiently frequent in this age group that children and adolescents with otherwise unexplained motor symptoms should be formally assessed for it.

Differential Diagnosis

The first task in diagnosis is recognizing the constellation of motor symptoms that constitute catatonia. If, after initial evaluation, there is no clear etiology, it is often diagnostically

TABLE 5.11.7

PRINCIPAL FEATURES OF CATATONIA

Feature	Description
Mutism	Verbal unresponsiveness, not always associated with immobility.
Stupor	Unresponsiveness, hypoactivity, and reduced or altered arousal during which the patient fails to respond to queries; when severe, the patient is mute, immobile, and does not withdraw from painful stimuli.
Negativism (Gegenhalten)	Patient resists examiner's manipulations, whether light or vigorous, with strength equal to that applied, as if bound to the stimulus of the examiner's actions.
Posturing (catalepsy)	Maintains postures for long periods. Includes facial postures, such as grimacing or *Schnauzkrampf* (lips in an exaggerated pucker). Body postures, such as *psychological pillow* (patient lying in bed with his head elevated as if on a pillow), lying in a jackknifed position, sitting with upper and lower portions of body twisted at right angles, holding arms above the head or raised in prayer-like manner, and holding fingers and hands in odd positions.
Waxy flexibility	Offers initial resistance to an induced movement before gradually allowing himself to be postured, similar to bending a candle.
Stereotypy	Non–goal-directed, repetitive motor behavior. The repetition of phrases and sentences in an automatic fashion, similar to a scratched record, termed *verbigeration,* is a verbal stereotypy. The neurologic term for similar behavior is *palilalia,* during which the patient repeats the sentence just uttered, usually with increasing speed.
Automatic obedience	Despite instructions to the contrary, the patient permits the examiner's light pressure to move his limbs into a new position (posture), which may then be maintained by the patient despite instructions to the contrary.
Ambitendency	The patient appears "stuck" in an indecisive, hesitant movement, resulting from the examiner verbally contradicting his own strong nonverbal signal, such as offering his hand as if to shake hands with stating, "Don't shake my hand; I don't want you to shake it."
Echophenomena	Includes *echolalia,* in which the patient repeats the examiner's utterances, and *echopraxia*, in which the patient spontaneously copies the examiner's movements or is unable to refrain from copying the examiner's test movements, despite instruction to the contrary.
Mannerisms	Odd, purposeful movements, such as holding hands as if they were handguns, saluting passerby, or exaggerations or stilted caricatures of mundane movements.

(Reprinted from Fink M, Taylor MA. *Catatonia. A Clinician's Guide to Diagnosis and Treatment.* New York: Cambridge University Press, 2003, with permission.)

helpful to administer an intravenous infusion of lorazepam in a medically supervised setting. Because of the possibility of respiratory depression, facilities for assisted respiration should be available. In either adolescents or adults, intravenous infusion of lorazepam, 0.1 mg/kg, with a maximum dose of 1–2 mg, can be infused over two minutes. This is often helpful in alleviating mutism, posturing, and rigidity. The infusion should be accompanied by supportive communication to the patient of the prospect of benefit of this intervention. A positive response, including relaxation of posture, improvement or restoration of speech, diminished mannerisms, and responsiveness to commands would confirm the diagnosis of catatonia (29). There is insufficient data to allow for an advisory on dosage of diagnostic intravenous infusion in children with catatonia, although one may be influenced in this regard by the dose range indicated for treatment of status epilepticus (maximum pediatric dose of 0.32 mg/kg/day, as specified by the Physician's Desk Reference).

When catatonia is ascertained in a child or adolescent, the differential diagnosis regarding underlying etiology in order of decreasing frequency is mood disorder, seizure disorder, pervasive developmental disorder, and schizophrenia, followed by other neurological and metabolic disorders, including the effects of psychoactive substances (29). Although some underlying etiologies can be clarified by laboratory tests, catatonia secondary to a mood disorder or a schizophreniform disorder has no pathognomonic laboratory correlate. In those cases, personal and family history, most often with input from parents or other informants, is crucial in establishing the psychiatric diagnosis.

Electroencephalograms (EEGs) can be diagnostic if an epileptiform disorder is presenting as catatonia. The EEG will be diagnostic in these cases if obtained during the symptomatic episode, but not necessarily if administered interictally. Clearly, if there are indications that there may be nonpsychiatric contributants to the catatonia, it is imperative that a neurologist and often other primary care physicians become involved in the medical workup seeking to define the underlying etiology.

Conditions that can be mistaken for catatonia include elective mutism, involving conscious and volitional withholding of speech. However, elective mutism is generally not accompanied by any of the motor signs needed for the diagnosis of catatonia. Juvenile Parkinson disease (PD) can present in childhood or adolescence with bradykinesia (slowing of movement) and bradyphrenia (slowing of cognition). However, PD will often include tremor, pill-rolling finger movements, a shuffling gait, and does not present with bizarre posturing or mutism. Torsion dystonia may present with seemingly bizarre posturing and indeed is often initially misdiagnosed as a psychiatric disorder, but is generally not associated with mutism and will be readily diagnosable by a neurologist familiar with this movement disorder. Somatoform disorder should also be considered in the differential diagnosis, with a different personal and family history pattern, as well as atypical physical presentations often being helpful in the differential (32).

Delirium and its devolution to stupor will often present with reduced central nervous system arousal that is also a hallmark of catatonia. Indeed, as noted above, some of the neurological and metabolic conditions that can generate

TABLE 5.11.8

NEUROLOGICAL CONDITIONS ASSOCIATED WITH CATATONIA

Encephalitis
Postencephalitic states
Parkinsonism
Subacute sclerosing panencephalitis
Bilateral lesions of the globus pallidus
Bilateral infarction of the parietal lobes
Temporal lobe infarction
Thalamic lesions
Periventricular diffuse pinealoma
Anterior cerebral and anterior communicating artery aneurysms and hemorrhagic infarcts
Frontal lobe traumatic contusions, arteriovenous malformations, neoplasms
Primary frontal lobe degeneration
Traumatic hemorrhage in the region of the third ventricle
Subdural hematoma
General paresis
Tuberous sclerosis
Paraneoplastic encephalopathy
Multiple sclerosis
Pediatric autoimmune neuropsychiatric disorder associated with streptococcal infections (PANDAS)
Familial cerebellar-pontine atrophy
Epilepsy (particularly psychosensory)
Creutzfeldt-Jakob's disease
Alcohol degeneration and Wernicke's encephalopathy
AIDS related dementia and other white matter dementias
Narcolepsy

(Adapted from Fink M, Taylor MA. *Catatonia. A Clinician's Guide to Diagnosis and Treatment.* New York: Cambridge University Press, 2003.)

TABLE 5.11.9

METABOLIC DISORDERS ASSOCIATED WITH CATATONIA

Diabetic ketoacidosis
Hyperthyroidism
Hypercalcemia from a parathyroid adenoma
Pellagra, vitamin B12 deficiency
Acute intermittent porphyria
Endocrinopathies: Addison's disease, Cushing's disease
Syndrome of inappropriate antidiuretic hormone secretion
Hereditary coproporphyria, porphyria
Homocystinuria, uremia, glomerulonephritis
Hepatic dysfunction or encephalopathy
Thrombocytopenic purpura
Lupus erythematosus or other causes of arteritis
Infectious mononucleosis
Bacterial infections: tuberculosis, typhoid, malaria
Langerhans carcinoma
Toxic states secondary to mescaline, amphetamine, phencyclidine, cortisone, disulfiram, aspirin, antipsychotic agents, illuminating gas, organic fluorides

(Adapted from Fink M, Taylor MA. *Catatonia. A Clinician's Guide to Diagnosis and Treatment.* New York: Cambridge University Press, 2003 with permission.)

either delirium or catatonia can also generate the other. The diagnostic distinction between these two syndromes is at this point primarily phenomenological. Delirium is defined by the primary presenting deficits in the areas of consciousness, attention and cognition, while variable alterations in motor function, generally considered to be associated phenomena, are not necessarily present. Catatonia is defined by the primary presenting deficits in motor function, often with preservation of awareness and memory, as demonstrable on resolution of the catatonic state, when patients can often reproduce conversations and observations that occurred during the catatonic state. Undoubtedly there are some patients in which these syndromes may coexist, though the frequency of this is not clearly documented in the clinical literature. The clinician's primary task, after defining and documenting the presenting the presenting phenomenology, is to actively search for the underlying etiology in an effort to delineate routes of treatment intervention and symptomatic resolution.

Assessment

Rating scales have value both for enhancing precision in documenting clinical symptoms as well as for teaching and clinical research purposes. There are several rating scales available for catatonia with good reported interrater reliability (33–35). The Stony Brook scale (33) has a reported interrater reliability of 0.9 and is easy to administer in a simpler version for screening purposes as well as in a more detailed version for rating severity.

Treatment

As with any serious medical condition, early diagnosis and prompt, effective treatment diminishes morbidity and mortality. The clinical literature documents that there have often been unfortunate delays in both of these domains. Insofar as patients with catatonia need protection, intensive treatment, and close monitoring, this is usually best administered in a hospital setting. The number and pattern of catatonic symptoms do not predict response to treatment, but clinical data suggest that most patients respond well to treatment, with prognosis strongly influenced by that of the underlying etiology.

Different treatment algorithms have been outlined for different varieties of catatonia (29). Patients with "retarded catatonia" often present in a stuporous state or with rigid posture. They may become dehydrated and nutrition may be compromised. If untreated for extended periods, bedsores and contractures may develop. Supportively explaining to family members the diagnosis and need for prompt treatment is a top priority. Restoration and maintenance of hydration with intravenous fluid and electrolytes is often necessary, with appropriate EKG monitoring. If antipsychotic drugs have been previously in place without benefit, they are best discontinued to avoid precipitating or perpetuating a neurotoxic effect. If a specific etiology is identified, its treatment takes priority (e.g., nonconvulsive status epilepticus). If no such cause is identified, treatment is started with a benzodiazepine, most often lorazepam, and most often initially by the intravenous route (36, 37). As noted earlier, an intravenous infusion of lorazepam, 0.1 mg/kg, with a maximum dose of 1–2 mg, can be infused over 2 minutes with adolescents or adults. If there is a positive response with symptom attenuation, one shifts to a maintenance dose geared to sustain and enhance improvement, with a maximum pediatric dose of 0.32 mg/kg/day specified by the Physician's Desk Reference (the dose indicated for treatment of status epilepticus). For adolescents, one will often start with a daily dose of 3–4 mg. If improvement is only partial, the dose can be titrated within a few days to 8–16 mg/day (38). If clinical status stabilizes and improves on this benzodiazepine

TABLE 5.11.10

MANAGEMENT FOR MALIGNANT CATATONIA/NEUROLEPTIC MALIGNANT SYNDROME

Goal	Measures to Take
Reverse hyperthermia	Aspirin or acetaminophen suppositories; place patient under cooling blankets or give alcohol bath; gastric lavage with ice water.
Reverse dehydration	Intravenous normal or half normal saline. Ringer's lactate is avoided as it may increase acidosis. Glucose loads may precipitate a Wernicke's encephalopathy in a chronic alcoholic or other persons with chronically low thiamine levels.
Maintain stable blood pressure and cardiac rhythm	Blood pressure and pulse rate are monitored.
	Hyperkalemia from muscle breakdown is prevented or resolved. Hypertensions is controlled with labetalol or esmolol; hypotension by increasing blood volume, and giving vasopressors.
Ensure adequate oxygenation	Continuously monitor oxygen saturation. Maintain airway artificially if rigidity blocks air exchange. Use 100% oxygen if oximetry shows blood saturation less than 95%.
Avoid complications of immobility: thrombosis, embolism, aspiration pneumonia, bedsores	Critical care nursing, moving of limbs, changing of position, skin care.
Avoid renal failure	Frequent monitoring of serum creatinine phosphokinase (as an indicator of muscle necrosis), creatine, and urea nitrogen. Check urine for myoglobinuria to monitor renal function. Dialysis may be required if the syndrome is not promptly and fully resolved.

(Reprinted from Fink M, Taylor MA. *Catatonia. A Clinician's Guide to Diagnosis and Treatment.* New York: Cambridge University Press, 2003. With permission.)

regimen, one addresses further the issues of nutrition, physical rehabilitation, and treatment of the underlying etiological influences. If, however, response remains inadequate after a few days, ECT becomes the treatment of choice (29).

Patients with "excited catatonia," including patients with "delirious mania," are a potential danger both to themselves and to others, frequently requiring not only hospitalization but physical restraints and isolation. If no specific treatable etiology can be identified, aggressive treatment with a benzodiazepine is recommended. A common protocol with adolescents or adults is 1–2 mg of lorazepam IV every 20–30 minutes, up to 10 mg within a few hours (38). If this intervention is not rapidly effective, daily or twice daily ECT for several days may be needed to achieve stabilization.

"Malignant catatonia" is a life-threatening condition with many features of catatonia plus fever and autonomic instability. Some consider neuroleptic malignant syndrome (NMS) to be a variant and the most common current presenting manifestation of malignant catatonia, precipitated by neuroleptics (29). The first treatment interventions for malignant catatonia/NMS should be the stopping of neuroleptics, the physical protection of the patient when agitated, control of temperature and hydration, as well as close medical monitoring of vital signs in a hospital setting (Table 5.11.10). Two alternative treatment approaches have evolved for management of this disorder. The dopaminergic-muscle relaxant approach considers NMS to be an idiosyncratic response to the dopamine blockade that is generated by neuroleptics. This formulation led to a treatment strategy using the presynaptic dopamine agonist amantadine; the postsynaptic dopamine receptor agonist bromocriptine; and the muscle relaxant dantrolene (39). An alternate strategy involves the benzodiazepine/ECT approach which is a variant of that described above in the treatment of excited catatonia (29, 40). Finally, conservative management consisting of stopping potentially offending agents and hydrating vigorously has also been endorsed by some. Controlled studies are needed to clarify the preferred management strategy for NMS.

Once a patient has recovered from an acute episode of catatonia, current advisories call for a maintenance dose of benzodiazepine for at least 6 months. Recurrence of catatonia requires dose augmentation and the possible use of ECT (29). This maintenance recommendation is a supplement to the designated treatment strategy addressed to the patient's underlying clinical condition.

Conclusions

Delirium and catatonia are neuropsychiatric conditions representing perturbations of consciousness and motor function that are byproducts of significant changes in the functional integrity of the central nervous system. It is vital that child and adolescent psychiatrists be familiar with the phenomenology, assessment, differential diagnosis and treatment of these syndromes, insofar as early diagnosis and treatment intervention can have significant impact on the patient's survival and prognosis for future functioning.

References

1. Stewart JT: Behavioral and emotional complications of neurological disorders. In: Noseworthy JH (ed): *Neurological Therapeutics: Principles and Practices.* London, Martin Dunitz, pp. 2855–2870, 2003.
2. Taylor DA, Ashwal S: Impairment of consciousness and coma. In: Swaiman KF, Ashwal S, Ferriero DM (eds): *Pediatric Neurology: Principles and Practice* (4th ed). Philadelphia, Mosby/Elsevier, pp. 1377–1400, 2006.
3. American Psychiatric Association: *Diagnostic and Statistical Manual of Mental Disorders, Fourth Edition, Text Revision.* Washington, DC, American Psychiatric Association, 2000.
4. Trzepacz PT, et al.: Neuropsychiatric aspects of delirium. In Yudofsky SC, Hales RE, eds. *The American Psychiatric Publishing Textbook of Neuropsychiatry and Clinical Neurosciences*, 4th ed. Washington, DC: American Psychiatric Publishing, pp. 525–564, 2002.
5. Inouye SK, Charpentier PA: Precipitating factors for delirium in hospitalized elderly patients: Predictive model and interrelationships with baseline vulnerability. *JAMA* 275:852–857, 1996.
6. O'Keefe S, Lavan J: The prognostic significance of delirium in older hospital patients. *J Am Geriatr Soc* 45:174–178, 1997.
7. Inouye SK, et al.: A multicomponent intervention to prevent delirium in hospitalized older patients. *New Engl J Med* 340:669–676, 1999.
8. Kornfeld DS, Zimberg S, Malm J: Psychiatric complications of open-heart surgery. *New Engl J Med* 273:287–292, 1965.

9. Kornfeld DS, Heller SS, Frank KA, et al.: Personality and psychological factors in postcardiotomy delirium. *Arch Gen Psychiatry* 31:249–253, 1974.
10. Stoddard FJ, Wilens TE: Delirium. In: Jellinek MS, Herzog DB (eds): *Psychiatric Aspects of General Hospital Pediatrics*. Chicago, Yearbook Medical Publishers, pp. 254–259, 1995.
11. Wise MG, Hilty DM, Cerda GM: Delirium due to a general medical condition, delirium due to multiple etiologies, and delirium not otherwise specified. In: Gabbard GO, ed. *Treatment of Psychiatric Disorders* (3rd ed). Washington, DC: American Psychiatric Publishing pp. 387–412, 2001.
12. Seear M, et al.: Thiamine, riboflavin and pyridoxine deficiency in a population of critically ill children. *J Pediatrics* 121:533–538, 1992.
13. Dickson LR: Hypoalbuminemia in delirium. *Psychosomatics* 32:317–323, 1991.
14. Trzepacz PT: Update on the neuropathogenesis of delirium. *Dement Geriatr Cogn Disord* 10:330–334, 1999.
15. Meagher et al.: Use of environmental strategies and psychotropic medication in the management of delirium. *Br J Psychiatry* 168:512–515, 1996.
16. O'Keeffe ST, Lavan J: Clinical significance of delirium subtypes in older people. *Age Ageing* 28:115–119, 1999.
17. Oloffseon et al.: A retrospective study of the psychiatric management and outcome of delirium in the cancer patient. *Support Care Cancer* 4:351–357, 1996.
18. Turkel SB, Tavare CJ: Delirium in children and adolescents. *J Neuropsychiatry Clinical Neuroscience* 15:431–435, 2003.
19. Johnson JC et al.: Prospective versus retrospective methods of identifying patients with delirium. *J Am Geriatrics Society* 40:316–319, 1992.
20. Trzepacz PT: A review of delirium assessment instruments. *General Hospital Psychiatry* 16:394–405, 1994b.
21. Turkel SB, Brazlow K, Tavare CJ, et al.: The delirium rating scale in children and adolescents. *Psychosomatics* 44:126–129, 2003.
22. Montgomery EA et al.: Psychobiology of minor head injury. *Psychosomatic Med* 21:375–384, 1991.
23. Schieveld JN, Leentjens AF: Delirium in severely ill young children in the pediatric intensive care unit. *J Am Acad Child & Adolescent Psychiatry* 44:392–394, 2005.
24. Menza MA, Murray GB, Holmes VF, et al.: Decreased extrapyramidal symptoms with intravenous haloperidol. *J Clinical Psychiatry* 48:278–280, 1987.
25. Fink M, Taylor MA: The many varieties of catatonia. *Eur Arch Psychiatry Clin Neurosci* 8–13, 2001.
26. Thakur A, Jagadheesan K, Dutta S, Sinna VK: Incidence of catatonia in children and adolescents in a paediatric psychiatric clinic. *Aust N Z J Psychiatry* 37:200–203, 2003.
27. Wing L, Shah A. Catatonia in autistic spectrum disorders. *Br J Psychiatry* 176:357–362, 2000.
28. Cohen D: Towards a valid nosography and psychopathology of catatonia in children and adolescents. *Int. Rev. Neurobiol.*, 72:131–47, 2006.
29. Fink M, Taylor MA: *Catatonia. A Clinician's Guide to Diagnosis and Treatment*. New York: Cambridge University Press, 2003.
30. Braunig P, Kruger S, Shugar G: Prevalence and clinical significance of catatonic symptoms in mania. *Compr Psychiatry* 39:35–46, 1998.
31. Kruger S, Braunig P: Catatonia in affective disorder: New findings and a review of the literature. *CNS Spectrums* 5:48–53, 2000.
32. Williams DT: Somatoform disorders. In: Rowland LP (ed): *Merritt's Neurology* (11th ed.). Philadelphia, Lippincott Williams and Wilkins, pp. 1140–1145, 2005.
33. Bush G, Fink M, Petrides G, Dowling F, Francis A: Catatonia: I: Rating scale and standardized examination. *Acta Psychiatr. Scand* 93:129–136, 1996.
34. Braunig P, Kruger S, Shugar G, Hoffler J, Borner I: The catatonia rating scale I: Development, reliability and use. *Compr Psychiatry* 41:147–158, 2000.
35. Northoff G, Kock A, Wenke J, Ecket J, Boker H, Pflug B, Bogerts B: Catatonia as a psychomotor syndrome: A rating scale and extrapyramidal motor symptoms. *Mov Disord* 14:404–416, 1999.
36. Bush G, Fink M, Petrides G, Dowling F, Francis A: Catatonia: II: Treatment with lorazepam and electroconvulsive therapy. *Acta Psychiatr. Scand* 93:137–143, 1996.
37. Ungvari GS, Kau LS, Wai-Kwong T, Shing NF: The pharmacological treatment of catatonia: An overview. *Eur Arch Psychiatry Clin Neurosci* 251 (Suppl 1):31–34, 2001.
38. Ungvari GS, Chiu HFK, Chow LY, Lau BST, Tang WK: Lorazepam for chronic catatonia: A randomized, double-blind, placebo-controlled cross-over study. *Psychopharmacology* 142:393–398, 1999.
39. Davis JM, Caroff SN, Mann SC: Treatment of neuroleptic malignant syndrome. *Psychiatr Ann* 30:325–331, 2000.
40. Slooter AJ, Balk FJ, van Nieuwenhuizen O, van der Hoeven J: Electroconvulsive therapy for malignant catatonia in childhood. *Pediatr Neurol.*, 32:190–2, 2005.

CHAPTER 5.12 ■ ELIMINATION DISORDERS: ENURESIS AND ENCOPRESIS

EDWIN J. MIKKELSEN

ENURESIS

Definition and Historical Note

Enuresis is subclassified into two subtypes, primary and secondary. *Primary enuresis* encompasses children who have never achieved continence, whereas *secondary enuresis* refers to those children who maintain continence for at least one year, only to lose it at some point after that. The term itself is derived from the Greek *enourein*, "to void urine" and has come to imply nocturnal events, although that connotation is not inherent in the derivation of the word itself.

There is a rich literature concerning enuresis and its treatment over the centuries. In retrospect, many of these treatment approaches now appear to have been quite sadistic. This history has been summarized in an excellent review in 1951 by Glicklich (1), which covers material dating back to the Ebers Papyrus of 1550 B.C.

There has been substantial progress in the treatment of enuresis, which in turn has contributed to a greater understanding of the fundamental pathophysiologic processes involved. These advances are reviewed in this chapter.

Prevalence and Epidemiology

Statistics concerning the prevalence of enuresis also must take into account the severity of the disorder. For example, in the Isle of Wight Study, Rutter and colleagues (1989) (2) found that 15.2% of boys were wet less often than once a week, whereas only 6.7% wet at least once a week. The corresponding figures for girls were 12.2% and 3.3%, respectively. By age 14 years, only 1.9% of boys were wet less often than once a week, and 1.1% were wetting at least once a week, with the corresponding figures for girls being 1.2% and 0.5%, respectively (Rutter et al., 1973) (3). Longitudinal data from the Isle of Wight Study have illustrated that wetting develops in many children between the ages of 5 and 7 years. Enuresis also was found in greater frequency in children undergoing psychosocial stress and in those living in socially disadvantaged circumstances (2).

A Scandinavian study of 3,206 7-year-old children found an overall prevalence of 9.8%; 6.4% of this group was accounted for by children with night wetting, 1.8% by day wetters, and 1.6% by those with mixed day and night wetting. This study also showed a strong genetic influence in that the risk of a child having enuresis was 7.1 times greater if the father manifested enuresis after 4 years of age, and 5.2 times greater if the mother did (4).

An 8-year longitudinal study in New Zealand found a prevalence of 7.4% for nocturnal enuresis in 8 year olds. This figure was accounted for by 3.3% with primary enuresis and 4.1% with secondary enuresis (5).

More recent studies have found remarkably similar results. In a group of 392 7-year-old children from the west coast of Sweden, Wille (6) reported a prevalence of 7.3% for monosymptomatic primary enuresis. A questionnaire study involving a large cohort of Australian children in the 5- to 12-year-old range reported an overall incidence of 5.1% for nocturnal enuresis of at least weekly frequency and 1.4% for daytime wetting of similar frequency (7). In a population-based questionnaire study, Soderstrom et al. (8) reported bedwetting at a frequency of at least once per month in 7.1% of first-graders, and 2.7% of fourth-graders.

Clinical Description

As noted, the term *enuresis* itself denotes only the voiding of urine, but over the years, it has acquired both a pathologic and a nocturnal connotation. Daytime wetting is correctly referred to as *diurnal enuresis*, whereas nighttime wetting is referred to as *nocturnal enuresis*.

In the text revision of the fourth edition of the *Diagnostic and Statistical Manual of Mental Disorders* (*DSM-IV-TR*), the American Psychiatric Association (2000) defines functional enuresis as "repeated voiding of urine during the day or at night into bed or clothes, whether involuntarily or intentionally." *DSM-IV-TR* goes on to specify that "the behavior is clinically significant as manifested by either a frequency of at least twice per week for at least three consecutive months or impairment in social, academic (occupational) or other important areas of functioning." The child must also have reached an age at which continence could reasonably be expected. The *DSM-IV-TR* uses a chronologic age of 5 years as a cutoff or a mental age of 5 years for those children with developmental delays. The *DSM-IV-TR* also stipulates that the wetting not be the result of "the direct physiological effects of a substance (e.g., diuretics) or a general medical condition (e.g., diabetes, spina bifida, a seizure disorder)." Three subtypes of enuresis are defined: nocturnal only (nighttime wetting), diurnal only (daytime wetting), and nocturnal and diurnal (mixed day and night wetting). A distinction also is made between primary and secondary enuresis. Primary enuresis refers to those children who have never achieved urinary continence, whereas secondary enuresis refers to those children who have achieved continence and then lost it. The period of continence necessary to differentiate between primary and secondary enuresis had variously been proposed to be 6 months to 1 year. The *DSM-IV-TR* does not specify a precise period of time for the distinction, but instead makes reference to "a secondary type in which the disturbance develops after a period of established urinary continence." A child is not considered to have primary functional enuresis until 5 years of age. Secondary enuresis can begin at any time, once the criterion of initial continence has been fulfilled, but the usual onset is between 5 and 7 years of age (2).

Etiology and Pathogenesis

The physiologic manifestations of this disorder have led to a wide range of etiologic theories. A primary focus of these studies has naturally been the anatomy of the bladder and urinary tract. Shaffer et al. (9) elegantly combined an investigation of bladder anatomy and physiology with the covariable of behavioral disturbance. It might intuitively be expected that children with dysfunctional or abnormal bladders would be those without a concomitant behavioral disorder to explain their enuresis and that those whose enuresis could be explained on the basis of psychopathology would have normal bladders. The results were counterintuitive in that those children who were behaviorally disturbed also had significantly lower functional bladder volumes and more developmental delays. Thus, although not providing a parsimonious explanation to differentiate the etiology of enuretic events between psychiatrically disturbed and nondisturbed children with enuresis, the study did lend further support to a theory of general developmental delay, which would explain both the enuresis and the high frequency of behavioral disturbance. Another study that investigated bladder capacity in children with primary nocturnal enuresis, former enuretic patients, and control subjects, also failed to find any significant difference in bladder capacity between the groups (10). It also has been demonstrated that fluid loading can produce enuretic events in children who do not have a history of enuresis (11, 12). Children with enuresis were found to have developmental delays twice as often as those without in a large longitudinal population study (13) and Touchette et al. (14) have more recently reported an association between bedwetting and related developmental milestones. An investigation of event-related potentials and brain stem auditory-evoked responses found longer latencies in children with enuresis, as compared to controls, which the authors interpreted as evidence of a maturational delay (15). A study that compared 35 otherwise healthy children with enuresis with a control group found that the bone age of the children with enuresis displayed a significant lag behind chronologic age, leading the authors to speculate about delayed maturation of central nervous system regulatory functions (16). However, a more recent investigation found no statistical difference in the bone age of children with enuresis and controls (17).

There is an obvious relationship between enuresis and bladder infection; (18) thus, an infection of the urogenital tract should be ruled out before a diagnosis of functional enuresis is made. This is especially important for girls, who are more prone to urinary tract infections (19). The possibility of urinary tract obstruction as a widespread cause of enuresis has been reported (20) but has been criticized because such a hypothesis can lead to unnecessary surgery (21). After extensively reviewing the literature on this subject, Shaffer (22) concluded, "There is no evidence that urethral dilatation or bladder neck repair are effective treatment for enuresis." The only exception to this would be if there were very specific pathophysiologic findings.

Other investigations into the role of urodynamic abnormalities in the pathogenesis of primary enuresis support Schaffer's conclusion (23). In a large study, Kawauchi et al. (24) found an incidence of urologic abnormalities of 1.8% on intravenous pyelography ($n = 940$), 7.1% on voiding cystourethrography ($n = 695$), 11.5% on cystometry ($n = 487$), and no abnormalities on renal ultrasonography ($n = 58$). Of those who did manifest reflux on voiding cystourethrography, the degree of reflux was assessed as mild in 92.1%.

Yeung et al. (25) utilized noninvasive ultrasound techniques to assess physiological bladder parameters in 514 children with primary enuresis (age 5 to 18 years; mean age 11.2 years), and 339 age-matched controls. Analysis of the data from the entire study group yielded three subtypes: small-capacity bladder with thick wall; normal-capacity bladder with normal wall thickness; and large-capacity bladder with thin wall. There was also a four-week period of treatment with DDAVP for the children with enuresis. The authors found that "poor response to treatment was significantly associated with pathological bladder conditions, that is, small-capacity bladder with thick bladder wall or large-capacity bladder with thin bladder wall."

The nature of the enuretic phenomenon has naturally led to speculation concerning a psychodynamic etiology. These hypotheses have in general evolved from case reports or have been derived from theoretical considerations. There has been one rigorous attempt to define the generalizations derived from the literature regarding enuresis and encopresis and then to determine with what frequency these generalizations were borne out by an analysis of the clinical material. This elegant study by Achenbach and Lewis (26) revealed that "only two of the twenty-four generalizations derived from the literature regarding encopresis and enuresis received support at the conventional level (probability = 0.05) of statistical significance."

Epidemiologic studies have, however, shown a correlation between psychological disturbance and enuresis, which is more pronounced in older children (2). This observation then raises the question of the nature of the relationship: Is it a causal, incidental, or secondary relationship? The aforementioned link between enuresis and developmental delays, which are also linked to psychopathology, would suggest that there is a common underlying maturational factor that predisposes vulnerable children to manifest both behavioral disturbances and enuresis. In further support of this hypothesis are the observations that the nature of the behavioral disturbance in children with enuresis is nonspecific (27) and that no physiologic marker can be found that reliably differentiates psychologically disturbed from nondisturbed children with enuresis (9, 28). Biederman et al. (29) have evaluated the possible linkage between enuresis and attention deficit hyperactivity disorder (ADHD). Their findings indicated that enuresis did not increase the risk for psychopathology in children with or without ADHD but was associated with increased risk for learning disability in normal control children, but not in those with ADHD. Baeyens et al. (30) investigated the prevalence of ADHD in 120 children (age 6 to 12 years) with primary enuresis, utilizing parent and teacher questionnaires as well as diagnostic interviews. Their results indicated that 15% met the criteria for ADHD, and a further 22.5% met the criteria for ADHD Inattentive Type. A two-year follow-up study of the same cohort indicated that 73% of those diagnosed with ADHD had the diagnosis reconfirmed at follow-up (31). The authors also noted that the odds of a child with ADHD still having episodes of nocturnal enuresis at 2-year follow-up were 3.2 times higher than those for a child who did not have comorbid ADHD. The association with behavioral disturbance has been reported as being greater for secondary enuresis (32, 33) and for enuresis persisting into adolescence (34). One study that specifically evaluated risk factors for development of secondary enuresis found that delayed attainment of initial nocturnal continence and exposure to four or more stressful life events in a year were significantly related to the development of secondary enuresis (35). Similar results with regard to the relationship between psychosocial stress and secondary enuresis have been reported by von Gontard et al. (36) However, at least one large study in the Netherlands found no difference in psychopathology between children with primary and secondary enuresis (37). Of interest is an investigation by Van Hoecke et al. (38), that compared the results of the Child Behavior Checklist and the Disruptive Behavior Disorder Rating Scale in 154 children with enuresis and 153 controls. The results indicated that although the children with enuresis scored significantly higher on both scales, when the socioeconomic status of the children was controlled for the relationship was no longer present.

The occurrence of the enuretic episodes during sleep naturally led to a series of studies investigating the relationship between sleep states and the occurrence of enuretic events. The earliest of these studies suggested that the enuretic events occurred in "deep" sleep and led to a theory that enuretic events were dream equivalents (39). This theory was subsequently supplanted by Broughton's (40); (41) view that enuresis was a disorder of arousal. This research suggested that enuretic episodes were preceded by arousal signals and originated in delta sleep. A further elaboration of this theory held that psychiatrically disturbed children with enuresis received normal arousal signals but did not respond to them, whereas those without psychiatric disturbance did not generate arousal signals (42). The largest and most convincing sleep studies indicate that enuretic episodes occur in each sleep stage in proportion to the time spent in that stage, when time of night also is considered (27, 43, 44). There have been three studies that suggested that children with primary enuresis may be more difficult to arouse from sleep than control subjects, although the methodology is somewhat subjective with regard to defining arousability (6, 45, 46). Other research in this area has focused on combining sleep studies with cystometry (47), and may eventually lead to the identification of subtypes of children with enuresis (48, 49).

The development of desmopressin acetate (DDAVP) as a treatment for enuresis (described later) has led to the observation that some children with enuresis do not have the ability to concentrate the urine they produce during the night and reduce urine volume (50). In a further investigation of this hypothesis, Rittig et al. (51) compared the circadian variation of plasma atrial natriuretic peptide (ANP) with the clearance of creatinine and the excretion of sodium and potassium. Subjects in the study consisted of 15 children with nocturnal enuresis and 11 control subjects matched for age, sex, and weight. The children with enuresis did not differ from control subjects with regard to ANP, but during the first hours of sleep, they did manifest significantly more polyuria, natriuresis, and kaliuresis despite normal levels of ANP. The authors concluded that children with enuresis display abnormal diurnal rhythmicity in the urinary excretion of potassium and sodium that is not correlated with plasma levels of ANP. They speculated that the abnormalities in sodium and potassium may be related to abnormal tubular handling. This hypothesis has been further supported by subsequent research (52–54) that used radioimmunoassay to evaluate the circadian rhythmicity of plasma arginine vasopressin (AVP) in 55 children with enuresis and 15 control subjects. The AVP levels were measured under conditions of controlled water intake three times per day for 72 hours. Only 14 of the 55 children with enuresis had a significant decrease in AVP compared with control subjects. Nine of these 14 AVP-deficient children subsequently were found to be totally dry with DDAVP treatment.

The circadian rhythmicity of AVP has continued to be a focus of investigation because it theoretically could explain both the pathophysiology of enuresis and its response to DDAVP. Accordingly, researchers have been particularly interested in any differences that could be detected between DDAVP responders and nonresponders. One study has reported significant differences in morning values of AVP between normal control subjects (n = 7) and children whose enuresis responded to DDAVP (n = 6), as well as between the responders (n = 6) and nonresponders to DDAVP (n = 5). Thus, the morning AVP levels were able to differentiate the children with enuresis from the control subjects, and the responders from the nonresponders (Medel et al., 1998) (55). However, further complicating this line of research has been the finding that AVP is secreted in a "pulsatile pattern," which dictates frequent sampling of plasma levels to be meaningful (56). Studies using frequent measurements of AVP have produced mixed results. Two studies that used more frequent AVP measurements (56, 57) found no differences between responders and nonresponders to DDAVP. Aikawa et al. (58, 59) addressed this question in a series of studies that measured AVP secretion on an hourly basis for 24 hours. The first set of these studies looked at AVP secretion profiles in children with enuresis (n = 9) and control subjects (n = 8). The results did establish that the plasma AVP level was significantly lower in the children with enuresis in the 11 PM to 4 AM time period. They then looked at the secretion dynamics in two phenomenologic subgroups of children with enuresis: those with low urinary osmotic pressure and large nocturnal urine output, as opposed to a group with normal urinary osmotic pressure and small nocturnal urine output. The results showed that the mean nocturnal AVP levels were significantly lower in the first (large nocturnal output) group and that treatment with DDAVP did produce a significant increase in AVP for this group as a whole, but not for every child.

Another area of research has been the role of urine osmolality in the production of nocturnal enuresis. Three separate studies that looked at first morning urinary specific gravity in preschool children have suggested that children who wet the bed tend to have lower mean urinary specific gravity than those who do not, but the findings do not reach statistical significance (60–62). An investigation into nocturnal and daytime urine volume, osmolality, and ion excretion in children with primary enuresis and controls reported a significant decrease in the ratio of nocturnal/daytime urine osmolality, as well as urine chloride and potassium excretion, and urine osmolality in children with enuresis as compared to controls (63). However, these values were not found to be predictive of response to either treatment with DDAVP or behavioral conditioning therapies. Hypercalciuria has also been discussed as a potential pathogenetic factor. However, a study involving DDAVP-responsive children, therapy-responsive children and controls found no difference in urinary excretion between children with enuresis and controls (64). An investigation by Valenti et al. (65) suggested that there may be a subgroup of enuretic children who present with hypercalciuria. Their investigation involved 46 children with enuresis, of whom 26 had hypercalciuria. All of the children received DDAVP, and those with hypercalciuria were also treated with a low calcium diet. In those children who had low AVP levels prior to treatment, the levels were normalized after treatment and the low calcium diet effectively resolved the hypercalciuria.

The effect of fluid restriction on AVP levels and urine osmolality also has been investigated. These studies indicate that AVP levels are increased in both control subjects and in children with enuresis in response to fluid restriction, and that the degree of AVP secretion is related to plasma osmolality (66). When DDAVP responders and nonresponders are compared with control subjects, all three groups manifest an increase in AVP, but the DDAVP responders showed a smaller increase than the other groups (67). Studies involving adolescents and adults with refractory enuresis also have suggested that the primary pathophysiologic mechanism may be an abnormal tubular processing of sodium related to a relative insensitivity to AVP [Hunsballe et al. (68, 69)] that is corrected to some degree by DDAVP. Similar research in children led Eggert and Kuhn (70) to hypothesize that the primary difference between children with enuresis and control subjects may be at the distal tubular AVP receptor level.

Although this line of research has primarily involved DDAVP, it also has led to a reexamination of the therapeutic effect exerted by imipramine. Hunsballe et al. (71) reported a decrease in urine output and reduced osmolar clearance induced by imipramine that was, in part, contributed to by a lower excretion of sodium and potassium.

One of the newest areas of research has been the exploration of genetic linkages. It has long been known that enuresis tends to run in families, and that a positive family history can be related to positive treatment outcome (72). In general, genetic studies involve large numbers of families with multigenerational transmission of primary nocturnal enuresis. The chromosomes that have been identified to date include 13q, 12q, 8, and 22 (73–75). In some families, an autosomal dominant mode of transmission with penetrance above 90% has been identified (76).

Loeys et al. (77) studied 32 families with extensive histories of nocturnal enuresis, which ranged from two to four generations. Linkage to an area on chromosome 22q11 was noted in nine families, to 13q13-14 in six, and to 12q in four. Evidence of linkage to chromosome 8q could not be established. Thus, the findings were heterogeneous with regard to the chromosome sites involved. A genetic investigation of a large, four-generation family with a history of both nocturnal and diurnal enuresis indicated an autosomal dominant pattern with high penetrance. The author concluded that, "The most likely genetical model in this kindred seems to be a gene located on chromosome 4p16.1 causing primary nocturnal enuresis." However, involvement of chromosome 12q24.3 could not be excluded (78).

Deen et al. (79) specifically investigated the aquaporin-2 water channel locus (AQP-2) in six families with a dominant pattern of transmission, as AQP-2 is necessary for concentrating urine and DDAVP enhances AQP2 expression. The authors indicated that they could not locate a mutation in the AQP2 coding sequence and, "The AQP-2 gene is excluded as a candidate for autosomal dominant DNE in these families in which the disease co-segregates with chromosome 12q." The results of this line of research to date would support the view of von Gontard et al. (76) that "Nocturnal enuresis is a common, genetic, and heterogeneous disorder. The association between genotype and phenotype are complex and are susceptible to environmental influences."

Laboratory Studies

The fact that urinary tract infections can precipitate enuretic events in children means that a urinalysis should be performed to rule out this readily treatable cause of enuresis.

The use of more invasive and painful studies remains controversial. Although it is certainly possible that altered bladder physiology may lead to primary enuresis, the yield from these studies does not appear to be of sufficient magnitude to warrant subjecting all children with enuresis to them. A thorough review of this subject by Cohen (80), found the incidence of obstructive lesions in children with enuresis to be 3.7% in a primary care pediatric setting. Accordingly, he suggested that, "contrast studies are indicated only when there is significant evidence of anatomical or functional pathology by history or exam." Subsequent studies have supported this general position (23, 24), while suggesting that those children with daytime wetting and overt symptoms of voiding disturbance are more apt to have urinary tract abnormalities than those who wet solely at night (81). As discussed above, ultrasound bladder measurements may prove useful in the future, but currently this is viewed as a technique utilized in research only (25).

Differential Diagnosis

The differential diagnosis includes the possibility of urinary tract infection and altered bladder physiology. There are scattered case reports of enuresis being secondary to other primary medical problems, such as hyperthyroidism (82), constipation (83), and central hormonal abnormalities (84). Although such reports are infrequent, the clinician should do a thorough physical examination and consider the possibility of underlying organic illness—particularly readily treatable constipation. Brooks and Topol (85) have reported an association between obstructive sleep apnea in children and nocturnal enuresis. They hypothesize that this could be related to the effects of sleep apnea on arousal patterns, and bladder dynamics on urinary hormone production.

There are reports of nocturnal enuresis occurring as a side effect of treatment with selective serotonin reuptake inhibitor antidepressants (SSRIs). Given the frequency with which these agents are prescribed to children, this should be considered. The chronological correlation between the initiation of treatment with an SSRI and the onset of enuretic episodes would tend to substantiate the diagnosis (86–88). Psychological testing in conjunction with structured interviews may provide further insight into the coexistence of psychopathology. However, the studies reviewed previously suggest that any coexisting psychological disorder should be viewed as an accompanying finding rather than as a causal effect.

The distinction between primary and secondary enuresis can be made by history.

Treatment

Although psychotherapy may be helpful for managing the behavioral disorders that accompany enuresis, it appears to have little effect on primary enuresis itself, with studies showing a success rate of 20%, which may largely be accounted for by spontaneous remission (80). Psychotherapy may be more useful for those children with secondary enuresis, especially those whose episodes begin after a traumatic event or parental divorce, or in those cases where a specific parent–child conflict appears to be contributing to the continuation of the enuresis (89) (Table 5.12.1).

It has been shown that having nocturnal enuresis has a negative impact on self-esteem, which can be normalized by effective treatment (90–92). The factors related to negative self-image were male gender, primary enuresis, and a greater frequency of wet nights.

The two primary means of treating children with enuresis fall into the categories of behavioral and psychopharmacologic methods.

TABLE 5.12.1

FACTORS TO CONSIDER WHEN CONSTRUCTING A TREATMENT ALGORITHM FOR PRIMARY NOCTURNAL ENURESIS

- Age of child
- Medical cause has been ruled out
- Rate of spontaneous remission (approximately 14%–16% per year)
- Behavioral conditioning with bell and pad or similar methodology
  - Equally effective as pharmacological treatment
  - Lower rate of relapse than with pharmacological treatment
  - Safer than pharmacological treatment
- Most commonly used pharmacological intervention is Desmopressin acetate (DDAVP)
- Most serious side effect (rare) is hyponatremia, leading to seizures
- Imipramine is no longer first-line choice for pharmacological treatment, but can be used for refractory individuals
- Combination of behavioral and pharmacological treatment can be considered for refractory enuresis

Behavioral Methods

Behavioral treatment should be attempted first because it is usually more innocuous than pharmacologic intervention. The underlying assumption of the behavioral strategy is that it is helping children with enuresis and their families master an affliction rather than tacitly implying that the children are either consciously or unconsciously causing the wetting themselves. One unfortunate consequence of various reward–punishment strategies is that they can subtly imply to children and their families that the disorder is quasivolitional. The bell and pad method of conditioning is a reasonable first approach. A review of this treatment modality indicated that it was first reported in 1904 and has been in routine use since the 1930s (93). In reviewing the results of several studies involving over 1,000 children, Werry (94) found a success rate of 75%, and subsequent studies have been consistent with this (95). There have been two relatively recent systematic reviews of the literature with regard to the efficacy of the alarm method of treatment for nocturnal enuresis. Glazener et al. (96) noted that approximately two-thirds of children treated with the alarm achieved nocturnal continence during treatment and nearly half who complete this form of treatment remained dry after the termination of treatment. In a similar study, Butler and Gasson (97) reviewed 38 studies involving at least 10 children, and found that the success rate ranged from 30% to 87%. However, there were considerable methodological differences, including the definition of success. When they narrowed the review to 20 relatively homogeneous studies, they found an overall 65% success rate and a relapse rate of 42%. There appear to be two subgroups of responders: those who sleep through the night after treatment without wetting, and those who wake up spontaneously to go to the bathroom (98). A psychiatric disorder in the child, and family stress, appear to be negative prognostic factors when predicting outcome with this modality (95). As noted previously, whenever reward–punishment contingencies are considered, it is extremely important to ensure that one is not unwittingly communicating that the disorder is quasivolitional.

An attempt has been made to investigate the relationship between bladder capacity and response to behavioral treatment. A study involving 50 children who were wet at least two nights a week found that children with small pretreatment maximal functional bladder capacities did better with the bell and pad method in conjunction with retention–control training, whereas the children with larger bladder capacities responded to the bell and pad method alone. However, this was a qualitative difference in response, as 92.5% of the 40 children who completed the study met the outcome criteria of 14 consecutive dry nights, regardless of which group they were in (99). A similar study that examined the impact of bladder capacity on response to the bell and pad system found no association with outcome (100). Both of these investigations indicated that behavioral disturbance was related to failure to respond to conditioning techniques (99, 100). Butler and Robinson (101) found low functional bladder capacity and inability to be aroused by the alarm to correlate with lack of success, and a higher pretreatment frequency of enuretic events has been found to correlate with increased success with this form of treatment (102).

Bladder capacity also has been investigated with regard to changes occurring during treatment. Oredsson and Jorgensen (103) measured bladder capacity in 18 children with severe nocturnal enuresis before beginning a 6-week period of treatment with the bell and pad and again after treatment. Ten of the 18 children ceased wetting, but overall there was a significant increase in bladder capacity for the entire group that did not correlate with outcome. Subsequent investigations have also reported an increase in bladder capacity following treatment with the alarm method (104, 105). This may explain why one study found that children whose nocturnal enuresis responded to the alarm also had significant improvement in daytime wetting (106).

Behavioral treatment continues to evolve. In a study involving 125 children, an attempt was made to replace the bell and pad mechanism with a simple alarm clock that was either set to go off at a time when the bladder might be expected to be reaching maximal capacity (group I) or after 2 to 3 hours of sleep (group II). The results were comparable with previously published figures for the bell and pad, with success noted in 77.1% of group I and 61.8% of group II, and respective 6-month relapse rates of 24.1% and 14.7% (107).

Another innovation involves replacing the pad that signals the enuretic event with a small ultrasonic monitor mounted to an elastic abdominal belt that signals the alarm when bladder capacity is reaching a predetermined threshold (108). Results of a clinical trial of this methodology were comparable with those obtained with the traditional bell and pad technique, and increases in nighttime bladder capacity also were noted (109).

An approach using bladder biofeedback has been developed for children with enuresis who are refractory to other forms of treatment, have small bladder capacities, and have evidence of an unstable detrusor. Specifically, the authors noted that of the 24 children who fit these criteria, 17 experienced complete remission (two of these later relapsed), six experienced a decrease, and in one, there was no change (110). A subsequent report by the same group (111) also reported an increase in bladder capacity with biofeedback treatment. As noted earlier, the presence of behavioral or family functioning problems can have a negative impact on the outcome of behavioral treatment. A successful intervention in refractory children with severe wetting who have these issues is to combine traditional alarm therapy with treatment with DDAVP (112, 113).

Glazener and Evans (114) performed a review of studies involving simple behavioral interventions for enuresis. The procedures involved included reward systems, such as star charts, nighttime awakening to urinate, retention-control training, and fluid restriction. They noted that many of the studies were small and poorly controlled, which precluded a metaanalysis. There was some suggestion that star charts and nighttime awakening achieved better outcome than no treatment. A similar review was completed for the more complex behavioral and educational interventions of dry bed training and full spectrum home training (115). Again, there were methodological issues that compromised many of the studies. These modalities were found to be superior to no treatment, but as stand alone treatments were not as effective as alarm treatment. However, there was some indication that combining dry bed treatment with the alarm might provide better results than the alarm alone in some children. Bennett (116) has developed a protocol that utilizes educational and simple behavioral interventions as a prelude to treatment with the bell and pad. He reports a success rate of 85%, and a relapse rate of 15% (many of whom become dry with a repeat of the program) with this methodology. Bennett's book also contains a very useful chapter that describes the advantages and disadvantages of each of the various subtypes of the bell and pad form of treatment that are commercially available.

Psychopharmacologic Methods

The Australian psychiatrist MacLean (117) first described the efficacy of imipramine for nocturnal enuresis in 1960. Since then, there have been over 40 double-blind studies confirming the efficacy of imipramine for nocturnal enuresis. Lack of response to imipramine often can be traced to the reluctance of primary care physicians to exceed dosages of 25 to 50 mg. Nevertheless, it is reasonable to begin at a dose of 25 mg and to titrate up slowly because some children respond to the lower dosages. Allowing 4 to 7 days between dosage increments makes it possible to detect these low-dose responders. Most children respond in the 75- to 125-mg range. The upper range of dosage is determined by the child's weight, with the standard upper limit being 5 mg/kg/day. A baseline electrocardiogram should be obtained before instituting treatment with imipramine, and monitoring is advised above 3.5 mg/kg (27).

The relatively high rate of spontaneous remission in enuresis dictates caution against keeping children on medication for long periods. A practical approach is to taper slowly and discontinue the imipramine every 3 months. If wetting resumes as the dosage is tapered or after it is discontinued, then the dosage can simply be titrated back up to the effective dose for another 3-month period. It has been the author's impression that more children do not experience a reactivation of the enuresis after a 3-month period of imipramine treatment than can be accounted for by spontaneous remission alone, but this has not been statistically proven.

There have been tragic reports of children who reasoned that if three pills would stop the wetting for a night, then taking the whole bottle should stop it permanently. Thus, it is important to warn parents about the magical thinking of children in this regard and the importance of controlling the medication. Younger siblings also are at risk of overdosing with the medication if it is not controlled. In cases of mild to moderate overdose, supportive measures, including the symptomatic management of seizures and cardiac arrhythmias, may be sufficient.

There have been five studies investigating the relationship between blood level of imipramine and clinical response. One study found no correlation between improvement in enuresis and the blood level of imipramine either alone or in conjunction with its metabolites (118). However, three studies have now demonstrated a significant correlation between the diminution of enuretic events and the steady-state concentrations of imipramine plus its metabolite desipramine (119–122). One of these studies found an optimal effect when the combined steady-state imipramine plus desipramine concentrations were above 60 ng/ml (121), and another reported favorable outcomes when steady-state combined levels were greater than 80 ng/mL (119). The most recent study in this line of investigation (123) evaluated the blood level–efficacy equation in 18 children who, after baseline and placebo, received increasing dosages of imipramine at 2-week intervals. The specific dosages used were 1, 1.5, 2, and 2.5 mg/kg/day. They found that efficacy was "moderately but significantly" related to increasing dose. However, there was wide variation (sevenfold) in serum levels between the individual children at every dosage level. There is a good correlation between side effects and blood level, especially dry mouth (122). This may prove clinically useful in monitoring children who are phobic about having their blood drawn.

As might be expected, the advent of treatment with DDAVP has led to a marked decline in new research concerning imipramine.

One multicenter, randomized, double-blind, placebo-controlled study did compare imipramine with the quadricyclic antidepressant mianserin, which does not have significant anticholinergic effects (124). The authors reported that imipramine was statistically significantly superior to both mianserin and placebo, leading them to conclude that imipramine's efficacy was not related to its antidepressant effect. As noted previously, one study has suggested that imipramine may exert a nocturnal antidiuretic effect mediated by effects at the renal tubular level (71). Gepertz and Neveus (125) utilized imipramine in the treatment of 49 children who had been refractory to treatment with DDAVP, the alarm, and anticholinergic treatment. They reported that 31 children (64.6%) achieved a 50% reduction in the frequency of enuresis and 22 of these realized complete cessation of the enuresis. It was also noted that seven children with comorbid attention deficit showed improvement in those symptoms as well. Thus, the authors concluded that it was reasonable to consider imipramine for children who had not responded well to other modalities.

Despite the efficacy of behavioral interventions, survey studies tend to indicate that in clinical practice medication is more apt to be used than behavioral interventions (126). A large population-based study found that only 38% of children with enuresis had seen a physician. Over one-third of this physician-treated group had been prescribed some form of pharmacotherapy, and only 3% had been advised to use the bell and pad conditioning technique. This study also revealed that over half of the children were psychologically distressed by the enuresis, and two-thirds of the parents expressed concern (127). This may be changing, as a subsequent study reported 80% of physicians recommended the bell and pad (128). Boulis and Long (129) have reported that family practitioners are more likely to recommend DDAVP as a first treatment for enuresis than are pediatricians. Throughout the literature there also are reports of novel treatment approaches such as acupuncture (130–132), a prostaglandin synthesis inhibitor (133), an anticholinergic calcium antagonist (134), the oral synthetic androgen mesterolone (135), and hypnosis (136). Although many of these studies are controlled, the use of these approaches in enuresis should still be considered experimental. Systematic reviews of both nonpharmacological alternative interventions (137) and pharmacological treatments other than DDAVP and imipramine (138) have indicated that the studies generally involve small numbers of subjects and many have methodological shortcomings, so that a definite conclusion about efficacy cannot be reached.

Oxybutynin hydrochloride has been reported as effective for children who are refractory to imipramine and also have inadequate bladder storage function (139). The newest research into pharmacotherapy for enuresis involves the use of DDAVP. Moffatt et al. (140) reviewed all of the then-existing controlled studies concerning the use of DDAVP for enuresis. In the process, they located 18 randomized, controlled trials (11 crossover and seven parallel), which included a total of 689 subjects, most of whom had been refractory to prior treatment. The decreased frequency of enuretic events in the study ranged from 10% to 91%. In general, wetting resumes once the medication is discontinued. Those studies that reported long-term followup indicated that 5.7% remained dry after stopping the medication. The most common side effects were nasal stuffiness, headache, epistaxis, and mild abdominal pain. Positive prognostic factors appear to be fewer initial (pretreatment) wet nights and age greater than 9 years. Hogg and Husmann (72) and Terho (141) particularly looked at the efficacy of DDVAP for children who had been refractory to conditioning treatment and imipramine, using a randomized, double-blind, placebo-controlled crossover study. Of the 52 children studied (age range 5 to 13 years), 53% had a complete cessation of wetting, 19% were partial responders, and 28% had no or minimal response. The dosages used ranged from 20 to 40μg (intranasal) and response did not persist after termination of treatment. In a five year retrospective review of 59 children, Key et al. (142) suggested that lower doses may be just as effective. In their series, 5μg at bedtime was the initial starting dose, and 81% improved on less than 10μg.

A study investigating the differential response of children with enuresis to DDAVP and the bell and pad method of conditioning found that 70% improved with the DDAVP and 86% improved with the alarm method, yielding no significant differences (143). A similar experiment that compared the therapeutic benefits of DDAVP in combination with the bell and pad to placebo found that the combination of DDAVP and the alarm resulted in significantly more dry nights (144). Leebeek-Groenewegen et al. (145) found that the combination of the alarm with DDAVP provided a more rapid response than monotherapy with the alarm, but the long-term success rates were comparable. Combining DDAVP with oxybutynin has also been reported to produce quicker results than either DDAVP or imipramine alone (146). However, a recent study by Naitoh et al. (147) found that neither combination treatment with the alarm and imipramine nor the alarm and DDAVP was superior to the alarm alone. There have been reports of hyponatremia (148) and hyponatremic seizures (149–151) with intranasal use of DDAVP. A case report and literature review documented 14 cases in the English language literature with symptomatic hyponatremia involving seizures or mental status changes (152). A similar review noted that excess fluid intake was identified in six of 11 case reports, leading the authors to recommend that patients receiving DDAVP for nocturnal enuresis should not ingest more than eight ounces of fluid on the nights when DDAVP is administered (153). The most comprehensive review of this subsect identified a total of 93 instances of symptomatic hyponatremia in children treated with DDAVP (154). Younger children appeared to be more susceptible and the risk was greater at the beginning stages of treatment.

Sufficient time has now elapsed since the institution of the widespread use of DDAVP to permit more followup studies. A large, multicenter Swedish study used a 4-week observation phase, a 6-week dose titration period (20 to 40 μg DDAVP), and a 1-year long-term treatment period into which a treatment-free week was introduced every 3 months to assess for remission. Subjects were 399 children with primary nocturnal enuresis aged 6 to 12 years. Sixty-one percent (245) experienced a 50% or greater reduction in wet nights during the dose titration phase and then entered the long-term phase. The average number of wet nights decreased from 5.3 during the observation phase to 0.8 during the last 3-month interval. Within 6 months of treatment initiation, 77 children became dry. There were significantly more responders in the older age groups. Overall, long-term treatment at these dosages was found to be safe (155, 156).

Another strategy has been to rapidly titrate the dosage of DDAVP (maximum, 50 μg) until dryness is achieved, maintain this dosage for at least 4 to 6 weeks, then decrease the daily dosage by 10 μg every 4 dry weeks. This strategy resulted in 71% achieving complete dryness with no relapses. A further 7% achieved dryness after relapses, 7% showed partial improvement, and 15% showed little or no response. The mean dose was 20 μg, the mean duration of treatment was 28 weeks, and median followup was 18 months (157).

The formulation of oral DDAVP has made it significantly easier to administer. In an early open 6-week trial involving 33 children with primary nocturnal enuresis, five children responded to 200 μg/day and 17 to 400 μg/day, whereas seven showed no response, and four dropped out. A subsequent 2-week treatment with 40 μg of the nasal spray showed similar efficacy and was able to increase the number of dry nights in two of the nonresponders (158). A multicenter, randomized study compared 200- and 400-μg doses of the oral preparation, as well as a 20-μg dose of the spray. No significant differences were found between any of the treatment conditions. However, there tended to be fewer wet nights when the children who initially received 200 μg of the oral preparation were increased to 400 μg (159). Similar positive results with oral DDAVP have been reported by Schulman et al. (160).

The dose response of oral DDAVP was explored in a randomized, placebo-controlled study that used 200-, 400-, and 600-μg daily doses. The 400- and 600-μg doses were significantly more effective than placebo, and there also was a significant linear trend for decreases in wet nights with increasing dosage (161).

An early oral DDAVP study with adolescents (162) has also provided long-term follow-up data (163). The initial study included two 12-week treatment periods with most of the patients receiving 400 μg/day. The initial studies showed that oral DDAVP was significantly more effective than placebo. The long-term, 7-year follow-up indicated that the "cure rate" at both the 2-year and 7-year follow-ups was greater than would be expected by data on the rate of spontaneous remission.

A large Canadian study found that long-term administration of oral DDAVP was safe and well tolerated (164). As indicated earlier, the success of treatment with DDAVP has led to an increase in research regarding the etiology of enuresis. Related to this are studies that try to elucidate predictors of successful treatment with DDAVP. A consistent finding in this regard is older age, larger bladder capacity, and fewer pretreatment numbers of wet nights (165–171).

Urine osmolality parameters also have been extensively investigated as potential predictors of response to DDAVP. Rushton et al. (172) found that DDAVP treatment is associated with a significant increase in nocturnal urine osmolality, as well as nocturnal diurnal osmolality ratios. Although responders tended to have higher urine osmolality than nonresponders, the differences did not reach statistical significance and the authors concluded that it therefore was not a reliable predictor of response. Similar results have been reported by other investigators (166, 168, 169).

Outcome and Followup

The natural history of primary enuresis must be taken into account in any treatment plan, whether it is primarily behavioral or pharmacologic. There is a high rate of spontaneous remission between the ages of 5 and 7 and again after age 12 years. Accordingly, the clinician might want to wait until after age 7 years before instituting pharmacologic treatment, unless other factors indicate otherwise. Similarly, the strong possibility of spontaneous remission should be considered in any positive treatment response after 10 or 11 years of age. In general, the rate of spontaneous remission from year to year is in the range of 14% to 16% (89).

Pharmacological studies have indicated that treatment with imipramine can result in three subtypes of response. There are true responders who have a sustained response, and there are also true nonresponders. There also is a surprisingly large group of transient responders. These children have an initial response to imipramine and then lose it over 2 to 3 weeks. When the dosage is increased by another 25 mg, they again respond for another 2 to 3 weeks. Eventually, the dosage required to maintain a response becomes prohibitive. Although long-term treatment with imipramine is not an option for these children, imipramine still can be used for brief, socially important periods, such as camp, because the initial response can be recaptured after a medication-free period (122).

There has been one large follow-up study that compared observation, imipramine, DDAVP, and the alarm system. Patients were weaned from therapy after 6 months. Continence was assessed at the 3-, 6-, 9-, and 12-month points of the protocol, so that the 12-month assessment would be 6 months after treatment ceased. Among the observation group (n = 50), only 6% were continent at 6 months and 16% at 12 months. Of the imipramine group (n = 44), 36% were continent at 6 months while still on medication, but this decreased to 16% at the 12-month assessment. The corresponding figures for DDAVP (n = 88) were 68% continent at 6 months, but only 10% at 12 months. The alarm system showed the best long-term effects, with 63% continent at 6 months, and 56% at 12 months (173). A systematic review of the literature with regard to treatment with the alarm, imipramine, and DDAVP indicated that there is less risk of relapse with the alarm (174). The data with regard to treatment outcomes clearly indicate that behavioral interventions should constitute the first line of treatment, as they do not possess the side effect potential of pharmacological interventions. The bell and pad method of conditioning is the most thoroughly researched form of behavioral treatment. The relapse rate after termination of this treatment is also substantially less than that seen with either DDAVP or imipramine. For children who do not respond to the bell and pad, treatment with DDAVP is a reasonable alternative. Treatment with imipramine is now usually reserved for children who have been refractory to other interventions.

Following the introduction of DDAVP, there were significant cost differentials related to the different forms of treatment, as treatment with DDAVP was significantly more expensive than treatment with either the bell and pad or imipramine (175). However, DDAVP is now available in generic form so the large cost differentials no longer exist.

Areas for Future Research

As indicated by the new research reviewed previously, there has been a dramatic increase in research into the etiology and treatment of enuresis. Much of this has been stimulated by the recognition that DDAVP is an effective treatment for the disorder. Despite this new research, a definitive explanation that would link DDAVP efficacy with the pathophysiology of the disorder has yet to be proven, and there is no consistently reliable way to differentiate DDAVP responders from nonresponders, either retrospectively or prospectively.

This and other findings related to bladder physiology and anatomy suggest that we might ultimately be able to differentiate distinct phenomenologic subgroups that relate to treatment outcome. Of particular interest in this regard are the studies involving changes in bladder capacity that result from treatment and correlate with outcome.

The long-standing observation that enuresis has a hereditary basis has been advanced by the elucidation of genetic linkages in some large, multigenerational pedigrees. This research will likely continue to advance and, when coupled with physiological variables that predispose to enuresis, may ultimately provide important information on clinical subtypes. Thus, while it appears increasingly likely that a single etiology for all children with enuresis will not be identified, it may be possible to identify clinically relevant subtypes.

ENCOPRESIS

Definition

Encopresis is defined by *DSM-IV-TR* (American Psychiatric Association, 2000) as the "repeated passage of feces into inappropriate places." There is a notation that the soiling is usually involuntary, but may be intentional in some cases. The manual goes on to note that the soiling must occur at least once a month for at least 3 months and that the mental or chronological age of the child must be at least 4 years. Physical disorders must, of course, be ruled out. If there has been a period of fecal continence preceding the recurrence of soiling, *it is classified as secondary encopresis.*

The DSM-IV-TR also denotes two subtypes of encopresis, which it labels as "with constipation and overflow incontinence" and "without constipation and overflow incontinence." The former category roughly corresponds to what has been referred to in the literature as *retentive encopresis*, whereas the latter corresponds to what has been known as *nonretentive encopresis*.

Prevalence and Epidemiology

A study involving 8,863 children found a prevalence of 1.5% among children between 7 and 8 years of age, with a male to female ratio of over 3:1 (176). In the Isle of Wight Study, Rutter and colleagues (2) found that 1.3% of boys between the ages of 10 to 12 years soiled at least once a month, with the corresponding figure for girls being 0.3%. That study also found a significant relationship between enuresis and encopresis (177). A more recent, large population-based study in the Netherlands investigated the prevalence in a sample of 13,111 5- to 6-year-old children, and 9,780 11- to 12-year-old children. The authors report a prevalence of 4.1% in the 5–6-year age group. The corresponding frequency for the older age (11–12 years) group was 1.6%. Of interest is the finding that 37.7% of the younger age group children and 27.4% of the older age group had not been taken to a physician for evaluation (178). A large population-based questionnaire study reported episodes of fecal incontinence in 9.8% of first-graders, and 5.6% of fourth-graders (8). Of interest was a positive correlation between daytime urinary incontinence and fecal soiling.

Clinical Description

Encopresis has been classified in different ways. As noted, *DSM-IV-TR* makes a distinction between primary and secondary encopresis and has added subtypes that denote the distinction between retentive and nonretentive encopresis. Retentive encopresis is characterized by a cycle of several days of retention, a painful expulsion, and another period of retention. While the fecal mass is growing, there may be leakage around the mass. The category of nonretentive encopresis applies to those children who simply do not control the expulsion of feces on a psychological, physiologic, or combined basis.

Hersov (179) has proposed three categories: a) children who have adequate bowel control and volitionally deposit feces in inappropriate places; b) children who either are unaware that they are soiling or are aware but unable to control the process; and c) situations where the soiling is due to excessive fluid, which may be caused by diarrhea, anxiety, or the retentive overflow process described previously. The last mechanism is responsible for approximately 75% of this category.

The importance of constipation to the development of retentive encopresis has led to the formulation of proposed criteria for functional fecal retention (FFR), which include a history greater than 12 weeks with passage of large diameter stools that are sufficiently large to obstruct the toilet, abdominal pain that is relieved by laxatives or enemas, and fecal soiling (180).

Etiology and Pathogenesis

There have been extensive investigations into the physiologic basis for encopresis. Loening-Baucke (181) found that 56% of children with retentive encopresis were unable to defecate rectal balloons, and most of these children had abnormal contractions of the external anal sphincter. This study also had prognostic significance in that only 14% of those who were unable to defecate the rectal balloons had responded to treatment after 1 year, whereas 64% of those who could defecate the balloons recovered after 1 year. Similarly, only 13% of patients who were unable to relax the anal sphincter at initial evaluation were improved 1 year later, whereas the corresponding figure for those who could relax the sphincter was 70%. Interestingly, none of the patients who presented with an abdominal fecal mass at the time of the initial evaluation showed improvement 1 year later, regardless of ability to defecate the rectal balloons. Constipated children subsequently were compared with control subjects on a wide range of physiologic measures during the act of bearing down (182). These studies revealed that the act of bearing down led to decreased anal sphincter activity in 100% of control children, 58% of constipated children who were able to defecate a rectal balloon, and 7% of those constipated children who were unable to defecate the balloon. The latter group was significantly less likely to respond to conventional laxative treatment, and the authors concluded that the increased external sphincter activity could relate to their chronic fecal retention and encopresis. A companion study (183) investigated the social competence and behavioral profiles of 38 children with encopresis and correlated physiologic variables of anorectal manometric and electromyographic evaluations to treatment outcome. The study found that social competence and behavioral rating scores were not significantly different between those boys who were or were not able to defecate the balloons. The behavioral problem ratings also were similar in both physiologic subgroups of girls. The social competence score of the girls who could not defecate the balloons was lower than that of those who could. The followup data indicated that the behavioral and social competence scores did not correlate with successful outcome at 6-month and 1-year followups, but there was a significant negative correlation between positive outcome in the inability to defecate the balloon and the inability to relax the sphincter. Thus, the physiologic variables were predictive of outcome, and the psychological variables were not. A subsequent study by the same group with a similar design continued to demonstrate some predictive value of the balloon test, in that children with functional constipation and encopresis who were able to defecate the balloon were twice as likely to have recovered at 12-month followup. However, the author concluded that even though these results were statistically significant, the calculation of predictive value indicated that the defecation test could not, in and of itself, reliably predict recovery (184).

A similar study at a different center concluded that a significant number of boys with encopresis have abnormalities of anorectal expulsion dynamics, but the researchers could not find abnormalities of anorectal sensory or motor function (185, 186). They specifically investigated pudendal nerve terminal motor latency in 23 children with encopresis, compared with 23 control subjects, and could find no significant difference. However, anal electromyography did indicate nonrelaxation of the external anal sphincter in 75% of the encopretic children, as opposed to 13% of the control subjects, as well as lower pressures at rest and with squeezing. Complementary abnormalities of anal sphincter function have been reported by others (187, 188).

Another approach has been to investigate potential involvement of hormones that affect gastrointestinal motility. Stern et al. (189) measured plasma levels of gastrin, pancreatic polypeptide, cholecystokinin, motilin, thyroxin, estrogen, and insulin at several intervals after the administration of a standardized meal to 10 children with encopresis and the same number of matched control subjects. The authors reported significant differences for postprandial levels of pancreatic polypeptide, which peaked earlier and remained higher in children with encopresis, as well as a lower motilin response. However, the authors could not entirely rule out that their findings were not the result of chronic constipation, rather than the cause (189).

Environmental factors have been noted for some time and include the observations of Freud and Burlingham (190), who noted a high frequency of soiling and wetting in children separated from their parents during World War II.

At least two studies that revealed no correlation between social class and soiling (177, 191, 192) specifically looked at associated psychopathology in boys with primary encopresis, compared with those with secondary encopresis. They found that the children with primary encopresis were more likely to have experienced developmental delays and to have associated enuresis, whereas those with secondary encopresis had experienced more psychosocial stressors and had higher rates of associated conduct disorder. A study involving 86 children with encopresis and 62 control children found that children with encopresis had more symptoms of anxiety and depression, more attentional difficulties, more disruptive behavior and poorer school performance. However, the differences only reached significant levels for a minority of the children with encopresis (193).

Klages et al. (194) reported higher rates of both enuresis and encopresis in children with a prepubertal and early adolescent bipolar disorder phenotype as compared to controls. An investigation utilizing the Child Behavior Checklist identified significantly more behavioral difficulties in children with functional nonretentive fecal soiling when compared to a Dutch normative sample. Von Gontard and Hollmann (195) have reported elevated Child Behavior Checklist scores and comorbid psychiatric disorders in children who present with both enuresis and encopresis.

Laboratory Studies

The physiologic studies described previously must be considered research investigations and not the representation of a usual and customary workup. However, they do suggest that a more detailed physiologic investigation than usually is done may be warranted. Usually, once the more obvious physiologic problems, such as Hirschsprung disease, are ruled out, the problem is considered to be psychogenic.

The plain abdominal x-ray reveals evidence of fecal retention. In general, a positive rectal examination is sufficient to determine fecal retention, but a negative rectal examination does not rule it out, and in those cases, the abdominal x-ray can be helpful in establishing the diagnosis (196).

One of the most important investigations may well be a thorough history that documents the frequency, nature, and circumstances of the soiling events in great detail. This history should be elicited both from the parents and from the child.

Psychological testing and evaluation are important in providing a thorough picture of the child, but it remains difficult to know if concomitant psychological problems are associated, causal, or secondary.

Differential Diagnosis

The differential diagnosis of encopresis must take into account that the soiling can be either a symptom of another problem or the primary problem itself. For example, historically encopresis and enuresis have been reported to occur under stress in normal children and to remit when the stressor is removed. Similarly, in children who have significant developmental delays, the encopresis may be only one expression of the primary problem. Children who are impulsive and hyperactive may have occasional episodes of encopresis simply because they do not attend to the stimuli until it is too late. Thus, the symptom of encopresis must be viewed in the context of the child's larger psychological and environmental profile. Strictly medical causes, such as Hirschsprung disease, stenosis of the rectum or anus, smooth muscle disease, and endocrine abnormalities, also should be ruled out.

Treatment

The most widely accepted first line of treatment is one that encompasses educational, psychological, and behavioral approaches. As outlined by Levine (197), this approach entails an initial meeting that is designed to educate both the parents and child about bowel function and to diffuse the psychological tension that may have developed in the family around the encopresis. This educational and psychological intervention is then followed by an initial bowel catharsis, after which the child receives daily doses of laxatives or mineral oil. There also is a behavioral component to the treatment, which consists of daily timed intervals on the toilet with rewards for success. A 78% success rate has been reported for this approach, without symptom substitution (198–200). The addition of a behavior management component to the intensive medical treatment provides some additional benefit (Table 5.12.2).

Stark et al. (201) have replicated earlier work reporting the efficacy of group treatment with an educational and behavioral focus in conjunction with medical management for children who had not responded to medical management alone.

The adjunctive use of oral laxatives and conditional rectal cathartics also has been investigated (202). Specifically, the authors compared the results obtained with children who were all treated with a high-fiber diet, initial bowel evacuation, behavior modification program, and random assignment to either oral laxatives (n = 24) or conditioning rectal cathartics

TABLE 5.12.2

FACTORS TO CONSIDER WHEN CONSTRUCTING A TREATMENT ALGORITHM FOR ENCOPRESIS

- Subtypes of encopresis
  - Retentive (most common)
  - Nonretentive
  - Volitional (least frequent)
- A thorough history is essential that documents frequency, nature, and circumstances of event
- First line of treatment for retentive subtype usually includes:
  - Education about bowel functioning with both parents and child
  - Physiological treatment with laxatives or mineral oil
- Behavioral component with time intervals on toilet and positive reinforcement
- Extensive research into biofeedback
  - Not proven to be more effective than traditional interventions
  - May be a consideration in refractory cases
- Case reports of imipramine in the treatment of nonretentive encopresis
- Psychodynamic assessment for those with volitional encopresis

(n = 37). Only 61 of 136 patients evaluated completed treatment, and thus there was a high dropout rate. No significant outcome difference was found between the two groups, and 87% continued in remission at 6- to 12-month follow-up. Nolan et al. (203) used a random allocation design to compare combined treatment with laxatives and behavior modification (n = 83) to behavior modification alone (n = 86). At 12-month follow-up, 51% of the combined therapy group had at least one 4-week period without an encopretic episode, compared with 36% of the behavior modification group. After the authors excluded children with poor compliance, there was no statistical difference between groups, although the authors maintained that from a clinical perspective, use of laxatives combined with behavior modification was superior to behavior modification alone. Laxative therapy is an important component of treatment for children who have encopresis related to chronic constipation. A number of studies have reported success with polyethylene glycol (PEG) 3350 for this group (204–207).

Loening-Baucke (208) has expanded on the pathophysiologic studies described earlier by exploring the utility of biofeedback training in children with abnormal defecation dynamics. Specifically, patients (ages 5 to 16 years) were randomly assigned to traditional medical treatment alone (n = 19) or conventional treatment plus up to six biofeedback sessions. Eighty-six percent of the biofeedback group had learned normal defecation dynamics at the conclusion of biofeedback treatment. At 7-month follow-up, 77% of the biofeedback group had normal defecation dynamics, as opposed to only 13% of the conventionally treated. The improvement in defecation dynamics was correlated with clinical improvement at 12 months (16% with conventional treatment and 50% with biofeedback). Similar successful results were reported in a European study (209).

A longer followup study (4.1 ± 1.5 years) compared the long-term outcome in 129 children with constipation and encopresis, as well as abnormal defecation dynamics, who were treated with conventional treatment, with 63 children who received additional biofeedback training that was directed toward normalizing the defecation dynamics. The results indicated that both groups showed similar rates of improvement (86% of the conventionally treated and 87% of the biofeedback group). At long-term followup, complete recovery was documented in 62% of the conventionally treated, 50% of those who had achieved success with the biofeedback treatment, and 23% of those who had not responded to biofeedback treatment. Length of time at followup was significantly related to recovery for the group as a whole, suggesting that the natural history of the disorder is to move toward continence. The author concluded that biofeedback treatment can not be demonstrated to be statistically superior to conventional treatment (210).

A subsequent study by another group with a somewhat similar design reached the same conclusion (211), and two large literature reviews also failed to demonstrate any benefit from biofeedback as compared to the standard medical treatment (212, 213). However, research into biofeedback treatment continues using a newly developed portable apparatus (214), and as an adjunctive treatment in combination with other behavioral strategies and laxative therapy (215, 216) have reported a significant decrease in soiling frequency and laxative use in a group of 36 patients treated with biofeedback who had a history of constipation and encopresis, and who had not responded to 6 months of conventional treatment.

Pharmacological treatment with imipramine also has been reported as useful for encopresis. There have been 15 reported cases of children with encopresis responding to imipramine, which have been described in six papers (217–222). All but three of the reported subjects are male. In general, the therapeutic effect occurred within a few days to 2 weeks. The doses of imipramine reported are relatively low, in the 25- to 75-mg range. There also is a similar positive case report involving amitriptyline treatment of a 6-year-old (223). There is one double-blind study demonstrating the effectiveness of the prokinetic agent cisapride (Propulside) for encopresis related to constipation (224). However, this agent has been removed from the market in the U.S. by the FDA, due to serious side effects.

Outcome and Followup Data

The 78% success rate described by Levine suggests that most children will respond to a relatively innocuous approach that involves educational, behavioral, and physiologic components, as do the followup data of Loening-Baucke (210). In general, the longer term followup studies consistently indicate that the passage of time is an important contributor to remission of the disorder (210, 225). The epidemiological data also indicate that the effects of maturation will provide a significant number of spontaneous remissions from year to year. The evaluation of any long-term intervention such as psychotherapy should take this factor into account. All but a few children will have either responded to treatment or spontaneously remitted by age 16 years, and persistence beyond that age is quite unusual (226).

Areas for Future Research

This review suggests that encopresis is an excellent paradigm for assessing the relative impacts of biological, psychological, and social factors. For example, do the physiologic findings described previously represent a constitutional vulnerability, or are they the result of the effects of chronic constipation on the bowel? The symptom of encopresis in its various presentations can be a fruitful area of research for those interested in elucidating the interrelation of mind, body, and culture in children.

References

1. Glicklich LB: A historical account of enuresis. *Pediatrics* 8: 859–876, 1951.
2. Rutter M: Isle of Wight revisited: Twenty-five years of child psychiatric epidemiology. *J Am Acad Child Adolesc Psychiatry* 28:633–653, 1989.
3. Rutter ML, Yule W, Graham PJ: Enuresis and behavioural deviance: Some epidemiological considerations. *Clin Dev Med* 48, 49:137–147, 1973.
4. Jarvelin MR, Vikevainen-Tervonen L, Moilanen I, Huttunen NP, Huttunen NP: Enuresis in seven-year-old children. *Acta Paediatr Scand* 77:148–153, 1988.
5. Fergusson DM, Horwood LJ, Shannon FT: Factors related to the age of attainment of nocturnal bladder control: An 8-year longitudinal study. *Pediatrics* 78:884–890, 1986.
6. Wille S: Primary nocturnal enuresis in children: Background and treatment. *Scand J Urol Nephrol* 156:1–48, 1994c.
7. Bower WF, Moore KH, Shepherd RB, Adams RD: The epidemiology of childhood enuresis in Australia. *Br J Urol* 78:602–606, 1996.
8. Soderstrom U, Hoelcke M, Alenius L, Soderling AC, Hjern A: Urinary and faecal incontinence: A population-based study. *Acta Paediatr* 93(3):386–389, 2004.
9. Shaffer D, Gardner A, Hedge B: Behavior and bladder disturbance of enuretic children: A rational classification of a common disorder. *Dev Med Child Neurol* 26:781–792, 1984.
10. Wille S: Functional bladder capacity and calcium-creatinine quota in enuretic patients, former enuretic and non-enuretic controls. *Scand J Urol Nephrol* 28:353–357, 1994a.
11. Kirk J, Rasmussen PV, Rittig S, Djurhuus JC: Provoked enuresis-like episodes in healthy children 7 to 12 years old. *J Urol* 156:210–213, 1996.
12. Rasmussen PV, Kirk J, Rittig S, Djurhuus JC: The enuretic episode: A complete micturition from a bladder with normal capacity? A critical reappraisal of the definition. *Scand J Urol Nephrol* 183:23–24, 1997.
13. Essen J, Peckham C: Nocturnal enuresis in childhood. *Dev Med Child Neurol* 18:577–589, 1976.

14. Touchette E, Petit D, Paquet J, Tremblay RE, Boivin M, Montplaisir JY: Bed-wetting and its association with developmental milestones in early childhood. *Arch Pediatr Adolesc Med* 159(12):1129–1134, 2005.
15. Iscan A, Ozkul Y, Unal D, Soran M, Kati M, Bozlar S, Karazeybek AH: Abnormalities in event-related potential and brainstem auditory evoked response in children with nocturnal enuresis. *Brain Dev* 24(7):681–687, 2002.
16. Mimouni M, Shuper A, Mimouni F, Grunebaum M, Varsan I: Retarded skeletal maturation in children with primary enuresis. *Eur J Pediatr* 144(3):234–235, 1985.
17. Erguven M, Celik Y, Deveci M: Bone age and probable aetiological causes in primary nocturnal enuresis. *Acta Paediatr* 94(10):1416–1420, 2005.
18. Hansson S: Urinary incontinence in children and associated problems. *Scand J Urol Nephrol* 141:47–55, 1992.
19. Hjalmas K: Functional daytime incontinence: Definitions and epidemiology. *Scand J Urol Nephrol* 141:39–44, 1992.
20. Mahony DT: Studies of enuresis: I. The incidence of obstructive lesions and pathophysiology of enuresis. *J Urol* 106:951–958, 1971.
21. Smith DR: Critique on the concept of vesical neck obstruction in children. *JAMA* 207:1686–1692, 1969.
22. Shaffer D: Enuresis. In: Rutter M, Hersov L (eds.): *Child and Adolescent Psychiatry: Modern Approaches*, 2nd ed. London, Blackwell Scientific, 1985, pp. 465–481.
23. McDermott VG, Merrick MV: Isotope renography in childhood enuresis. *Clin Radiol* 49:705–707, 1994.
24. Kawauchi A, Kitamori T, Imada N, Tanaka Y, Watanabe H: Urological abnormalities in 1,328 patients with nocturnal enuresis. *Eur Urol* 29:231–234, 1996a.
25. Yeung CK, Sreedhar B, Leung VT, Metreweli C: Ultrasound bladder measurements in patients with primary nocturnal enuresis: A urodynamic and treatment outcome correlation. *J Urol* 171(6 Pt 2):2589–2594, 2004.
26. Achenbach TM, Lewis M: A proposed model for clinical research and its application to encopresis and enuresis. *J Am Acad Child Psychiatry* 10:535–554, 1971.
27. Mikkelsen EJ, Rapoport JL, Nee L, Gruneau C, Mendelson W, Gillin JC: Childhood enuresis: I. Sleep patterns and psychopathology. *Arch Gen Psychiatry* 37:1139–1144, 1980.
28. Mikkelsen EJ, Rapoport JL: Enuresis: Psychopathology, sleep stage, and drug response. *Urol Clin North Am* 7:361–377, 1980.
29. Biederman J, Santangelo SL, Faraone SV: Clinical correlates of enuresis in ADHD and non-ADHD children. *J Child Psychol Psychiatry* 36:865–877, 1995.
30. Baeyens D, Roeyers H, Hoebeke P, Verte S, Van Hoecke E, Walle JV: Attention deficit/hyperactivity disorder in children with nocturnal enuresis. *J Urol* 171(6 Pt 2):2576–2579, 2004.
31. Baeyens D, Roeyers H, Demeyere I, Verte S, Hoebeke P, Vande Walle J: Attention-deficit/hyperactivity disorder (ADHD) as a risk factor for persistent nocturnal enuresis in children: A two-year follow up study. *Acta Paediatr* 2005; 94(11):1619–1625
32. Feehan M, McGee R, Stanton W, Silva PA: A six-year follow-up of childhood enuresis: Prevalence in adolescence and consequences for mental health. *J Paediatr Child Health* 26(2):75–79, 1990.
33. von Gontard A, Mauer-Mucke K, Pluck J, Berner W, Lehmkuhl G: Clinical behavioral problems in day- and night-wetting children. *Pediatr Nephrol* 13:662–667, 1999b.
34. Fergusson DM, Horwood LJ: Nocturnal enuresis and behavioral problems in adolescence: A 15-year longitudinal study. *Pediatrics* 95:662–668, 1994.
35. Fergusson DM, Horwood LJ, Shannon FT: Secondary enuresis in a birth cohort of New Zealand children. *Paediatr Perinat Epidemiol* 4:53–63, 1990.
36. von Gontard A, Hollmann E, Eiberg H, Benden B, Rittig S, Lehmkuhl G: Clinical enuresis phenotypes in familial nocturnal enuresis. *Scand J Urol Nephrol* 183:11–16, 1997.
37. Hirasing RA, Van Leerdam FJ, Bolk-Bennink LB, Bosch JD: Bedwetting and behavioural and/or emotional problems. *Acta Paediatr* 86:1131–1134, 1997.
38. Van Hoeck E, Baeyens D, Vande Walle J, Hoebeke P, Roeyers H: Socioeconomic status as a common factor underlying the association between enuresis and psychopathology. *J Dev Behav Pediatr* 24(2):109–114, 2003.
39. Pierce CM, Whitman RM, Mass JW, Gay ML: Enuresis and dreaming: Experimental studies. *Arch Gen Psychiatry* 166–170, 1961.
40. Broughton RF: Sleep disorders: Disorders of arousal? *Science* 159:1070–1078, 1968.
41. Gastaut H, Broughton R: A clinical and polygraphic study of episodic phenomena during sleep. In: Wortis J (ed) *Recent Advances in Biological Psychiatry*. New York, Plenum, 1964, pp. 196–221.
42. Ritvo ER, Ornitz EM, Gottlieb F, Poussaint AF, Maron BJ, Ditman KS, Blinn KA: Arousal and nonarousal enuretic events. *Am J Psychiatry* 126(1):77–84, 1969.
43. Kales A, Kales JD, Jacobson A, Humphrey FJ, Soldatos CR: Effects of imipramine on enuretic frequency and sleep stages. *Pediatrics* 60:431–436, 1977.
44. Robert M, Averous M, Besset A, Carlander B, Billiard M, Guiter J, Grasset D: Sleep polygraphic studies using cystomanometry in twenty patients with enuresis. *Eur Urol* 24(1) 97102, 1993.
45. Neveus T, Hetta J, Cnattingius S, Tuvemo T, Lackgren G, Olsson U, Stenberg A: Depth of sleep and sleep habits among enuretic and incontinent children and incontinent children. *Acta Paediatr* 88(7):748–752, 1999a.
46. Wolfish N: Sleep arousal function in enuretic males. *Scand J Urol Nephrol* 202:24–26, 1999.
47. Norgaard JP, Hansen JH, Wildschiotz G, Sorensen S, Rittig S, Djurhuus JC: Sleep cystometries in children with nocturnal enuresis. *J Urol* 141:1156–1159, 1989.
48. Imada N, Kawauchi A, Tanaka Y, Yameo Y, Watanabe H, Takeuchi Y: Classification based on overnight simultaneous monitoring by electroencephalography and cystometry. *Eur Urol* 33(3):45–48, 1998.
49. Watanabe H, Kawauchi A, Kitamori T, Azuma Y: Treatment system for nocturnal enuresis according to an original classification system. *Eur Urol* 25:43–50, 1994.
50. Miller K, Atkin B, Moody ML: Drug therapy for nocturnal enuresis: Current treatment recommendations. *Drugs* 44:47–56, 1992.
51. Rittig S, Knudsen UB, Norgaard JP, Gregersen H, Pedersen EB, Djurhuus JC: Diurnal variation of plasma atrial natriuretic peptide in normals and patients with enuresis nocturna. *Scand J Clin Lab Invest* 51:209–217, 1991.
52. Natochin YV, Kuznetsova AA: Defect of osmoregulatory renal function in nocturnal enuresis. *Scand J Urol Nephrol* 202:40–43, 1999.
53. Vurgun N, Gumus BH, Ece A, Ari Z, Tarhan S, Yeter M: Renal functions of enuretic and nonenuretic children: Hypernatriuria and kaliuresis as causes of nocturnal enuresis. *Eur Urol* 32:85–90, 1997.
54. Steffens J, Netzer M, Isenberg E, Alloussi S, Ziegler M: Vasopressin deficiency in primary nocturnal enuresis: Results of a controlled prospective study. *Eur Urol* 24:366–370, 1993.
55. Medel R, Dieguez S, Brindo M, Ayuso S, Canepa C, Ruarte A, Podesta ML: Monosymptomatic primary enuresis: Differences between patients responding or not responding to oral desmopressin. *Br J Urol* (3):46–49, 1998.
56. Wood CM, Butler RJ, Penny MD, Holland PC: Pulsatile release of arginine vasopressin (AVP) and its effect on response to desmopressin in enuresis. *Scand J Urol Nephrol* 163:93–101, 1994.
57. Lackgren G, Neveus T, Stenberg A: Diurnal plasma vasopressin and urinary output in adolescents with monosymptomatic nocturnal enuresis. *Acta Paediatr* 86:385–390, 1997.
58. Aikawa T, Kashara T, Uchiyama M: The arginine-vasopressin secretion profile of children with primary nocturnal enuresis. *Eur Urol* 33(3):41–44, 1998.
59. Aikawa T, Kashara T, Uchiyama M: Circadian variation of plasma arginine vasopressin concentration, or arginine vasopressin in enuresis. *Scand J Urol Nephrol* 202:47–49, 1999.
60. Kawauchi A, Watanabe H, Miyoshi K: Early morning urine osmolality in nonenuretic and enuretic children. *Ped Nephrol* 10:696–698, 1996b.
61. Mevorach RA, Bogaert GA, Kogan BA: Urine concentration and enuresis in healthy preschool children. *Arch Pediatr Adolesc Med* 149:1400–1401, 1995.
62. Salita M, Macknin M, Medendorp SV: First-morning urine specific gravity and enuresis in preschool children. *Clin Pediatr* 37:719–724, 1998.
63. Unuvar T, Sonmez F: The role of urine osmolality and ions in the pathogenesis of primary enuresis nocturna and in the prediction of responses to desmopressin and conditioning therapies. *Int Urol Nephrol* 37(4):751–757, 2005.
64. Neveus T, Hansell P, Stenberg A: Vasopressin and hypercalciuria in enuresis: A reappraisal. *BJU Int* 90(7):725–729, 2002.
65. Valenti G, Laera A, Gouraud S, Pace G, Aceto G, Penza R, Selvaggi FP, Svelto M: Low-calcium diet in hypercalciuric enuretic children restores AQP2 excretion and improves clinical symptoms. *Am J Physiol Renal Physiol* 283(5):F895–903, 2002.
66. Eggert P, Muller-Schluter K, Muller D: Regulation of arginine vasopressin in enuretic children under fluid restriction. *Pediatrics* 103:452–455, 1999.
67. Hunsballe JM, Rittig S, Pedersen EB, Djurhuus JC: Fluid deprivation in enuresis: Effect on urine output and plasma arginine vasopressin. *Scand J Urol Nephrol* 202:50–51, 1999.
68. Hunsballe JM, Hansen TK, Rittig S, Pedersen EB, Djurhuus JC: The efficacy of DDAVP is related to the circadian rhythm of urine output in patients with persisting nocturnal enuresis. *Clin Endocrinol* 49:793–801, 1998.
69. Robertson G, Rittig S, Kovacs L, Gaskill MB, Zee P, Nanninga J: Pathophysiology and treatment of enuresis in adults. *Scand J Urol Nephrol* 202:36–38, 1999.
70. Eggert P, Kuhn B: Antidiuretic hormone regulation in patients with primary nocturnal enuresis. *Arch Dis Child* 73:508–511, 1995.
71. Hunsballe JM, Rittig S, Pedersen EB, Olesen OV, Djurhuus JC: Single dose imipramine reduces nocturnal urine output in patients with nocturnal enuresis and nocturnal polyuria. *J Urol* 158:830–836, 1997.
72. Hogg RJ, Husmann D: The role of family history in predicting response to desmopressin in nocturnal enuresis. *J Urol* 150:444–445, 1993.
73. Arnell H, Hjalmas K, Jagervall M, Lackgren G, Stenberg A, Bengtsson B, Wassen C, Emahazion T, Anneren G, Pettersson U, Sundvall M, Dahl N: The genetics of primary nocturnal enuresis: Inheritance and suggestion of a second major gene on chromosome 12q. *J Med Genet* 34:360–365, 1997.
74. Eiberg H, Berendt I, Mohr J: Assignment of dominant inherited nocturnal enuresis (ENUR1) to chromosome 13q. *Nat Genet* 10:354–356, 1995.

75. von Gontard A, Eiberg H, Hollmann E, Rittig S, Lehmkuhl G: Molecular genetics of nocturnal enuresis: Linkage to a locus on chromosome 22. *Scand J Urol Nephrol* 202:76–80, 1999a.
76. von Gontard A, Schaumburg H, Hollmann E, Eiberg H, Rittig S: The genetics of enuresis: a review. *J Urol* 166(6):2438–2443, 2001.
77. Loeys B, Hoebeke P, Raes A, Messiaen L, De Paepe A, Vande Walle J: Does monosymptomatic enuresis exist? A molecular genetic exploration of 32 families with enuresis/incontinence. *BJU Int* 90(1):76–83, 2002.
78. Eiberg H, Shaumburg HL, von Gontard A, Rittig S: Linkage study of a large Danish four-generation family with urge incontinence and nocturnal enuresis. *J Urol* 166(6):2401–2403, 2001.
79. Deen PM, Dahl N, Caplan MJ: The aquaporin-2 water channelin autosomal dominant primary nocturnal enuresis. *J Urol* 167(3):1447–1450, 2002.
80. Cohen M: Enuresis. *Pediatr Clin North Am* 22:545–560, 1975.
81. Jarvelin MR, Huttunen NP, Seppanen J, Seppanen U, Moilanen I: Screening of urinary tract abnormalities among day and nightwetting children. *Scand J Urol Nephrol* 24:181–189, 1990.
82. Stoffer SS: Loss of bladder control in hyperthyroidism. *Postgrad Med* 84:117–118, 1988.
83. O'Regan S, Yazbeck S, Hamberger B, Schick E: Constipation a commonly unrecognized cause of enuresis. *Am J Dis Child* 140(3):260–261, 1986.
84. Kikuchi K, Fujisawa I, Ohie T, Yoshioka F, Masutani A, Nakano Y, Konishi J, Sudo M, Mori C: Ectopic posterior lobe of the pituitary gland and intractable nocturnal enuresis in a case with pituitary dwarfism. *Acta Paediatr Scand* 78(3):479–481, 1989.
85. Brooks LJ, Topol HI: Enuresis in children with sleep apnea. *J Pediatr* 142(5):515–518, 2003.
86. Monji A, Yanagimoto K, Yoshida I, Hashioka S: SSRI-induced enuresis: A case report. *J Clin Psychopharmacol* 24(5):564–565, 2004.
87. Kandil ST, Aksu HB, Ozyavuz R: Reversible nocturnal enuresis in children receiving SSRI with or without Risperidone: Presentation of five cases. *Isr J Psychiatry Relat Sci* 41(3):218–221, 2004.
88. Ramadan MI, Khan AY, Weston WE: Response to SSRI-induced enuresis: A case report. *J Clin Psychopharmacology* 26(1):99–100, 2006.
89. Fritz G, Rockney R, Bernet W, Arnold V, Beitchman J, Benson RS, Bukstein O, Kinlan J, McClellan J, Rue D, Shaw JA, Stock S, Kroeger Ptakowski K: Practice parameter for the assessment and treatment of children and adolescents with enuresis. *J Am Acad Child Adolesc Psychiatry* 1540–1550, 2004.
90. Hagglof B, Andren O, Bergstrom E, Marklund L, Wendelius M: Self-esteem in children with nocturnal enuresis and urinary incontinence: Improvement of self-esteem after treatment. *Eur Urol* 33(3):16–19, 1998.
91. Moffatt ME, Kato C, Pless IB: Improvements in self-concept after treatment of nocturnal enuresis: Randomized controlled trial. *J Pediatr* 110:647–652, 1987.
92. Collier J, Butler RJ, Redsell SA, Evans JH: An investigation of the impact of nocturnal enuresis on children's self-concept. *Scand J Urol Nephrol* 36(3):204–208, 2002.
93. Rappaport L. Prognostic factors for alarm treatment. *Scand J Urol Nephrol* 183:55–57, 1997.
94. Werry J: The conditioning treatment of enuresis. *Am J Psychiatry* 123:226–229, 1996.
95. Devlin JB, O'Cathain C: Predicting treatment outcome in nocturnal enuresis. *Arch Dis Child* 65:1158–1161, 1990.
96. Glazener CM, Evans JH, Peto RE: Alarm interventions for nocturnal enuresis in children. *Cochrane Database Syst Rev* (2):CD002911, 2003. Update in *Cochrane Database Syst Rev* (2):CD002911, 2005.
97. Butler RJ, Gasson SL: Enuresis alarm treatment. *Scand J Urol Nephrol* 39(5):349–357, 2005.
98. Bonde HV, Andersen JP, Rosenkilde P: Nocturnal enuresis: Change of nocturnal voiding pattern during alarm treatment. *Scand J Urol Nephrol* 28:349–352, 1994.
99. Geffken G, Johnson SB, Walker D: Behavioral interventions for childhood nocturnal enuresis: The differential effect of bladder capacity on treatment progress and outcome. *Health Psychol* 5:261–272, 1986.
100. Berg I, Forsythe I, McGuire R: Response of bed wetting to the enuresis alarm influence of psychiatric disturbance and maximum functional bladder capacity. *Arch Dis Child* 57:394–396, 1982.
101. Butler RJ, Robinson JC: Alarm treatment for childhood nocturnal enuresis: An investigation of within-treatment variables. *Scand J Urol Nephrol* 36(4):268–272, 2002.
102. Jensen N, Kristensen G: Frequency of nightly wetting and the efficiency of alarm treatment of nocturnal enuresis. *Scand J Urol Nephrol* 35(5):357–363, 2001.
103. Oredsson AF, Jorgensen TM: Changes in nocturnal bladder capacity during treatment with the bell and pad for normosymptomatic nocturnal enuresis. *J Urol* 160:166–169, 1998.
104. Hvistendahl GM, Kamperis K, Rawashdeh YF, Rittig S, Djurhuus JC: The effect of alarm treatment on the functional bladder capacity in children with monosymptomatic nocturnal enuresis. *J Urol* 171(6 Pt 2):2611–2614, 2004.
105. Taneli C, Ertan P, Taneli F, Genc A, Gunsar C, Sencan A, Mir E Onag, A: Effect of alarm treatment on bladder storage capacities in monosymptomatic nocturnal enuresis. *Scand J Urol Nephrol* 38(3):207–210, 2004.
106. Van Leerdam FJ, Blankespoor MN, van der Heijden AJ, Hirasing RA: Alarm treatment is successful in children with day- and night-time wetting. *Scand J Urol Nephrol* 38(3):211–215, 2004. Erratum in: *Scand J Urol Nephrol* 38(4):350. Hiraing, RA [corrected to Hirasing, Remy A].
107. El-Anany FG, Maghraby HA, Shaker SE, Abdel-Moneim AM: Primary nocturnal enuresis: A new approach to conditioning treatment. *Urology* 53:405–408, 1999.
108. Petrican P, Sawan MA: Design of a miniaturized ultrasonic bladder volume monitor and subsequent preliminary evaluation on 41 enuretic patients. *IEEE Trans Rehabil Eng* 6:66–74, 1998.
109. Pretlow RA: Treatment of nocturnal enuresis with an ultrasound bladder volume controlled alarm device. *J Urol* 162:1224–1228, 1999.
110. Hoekx L, Wyndaele JJ, Vermandel A: The role of bladder biofeedback in the treatment of children with refractory nocturnal enuresis associated with idiopathic detrusor. *J Urol* 160:858–860, 1998.
111. Hoekx L, Vermandel A, Wyndaele JJ: Functional bladder capacity after bladder biofeedback predicts long-term outcome in children with nocturnal enuresis. *Scand J Urol Nephrol* 37(2):120–123, 2003.
112. Bradbury M: Combination therapy for nocturnal enuresis with desmopressin and an alarm device. *Scand J Urol Nephrol* 183:61–63, 1997.
113. Bradbury MG, Meadow SR: Combined treatment with enuresis alarm and esmopressin for nocturnal enuresis. *Acta Paediatr* 84:1014–1018, 1995.
114. Glazener CM, Evans JH: Simple behavioural and physical interventions for nocturnal enuresis in children. *Cochrane Database Syst Rev* (2):CD003637, 2004.
115. Glazener CM, Evans JH, Peto RE: Complex behavioural and educational interventions for nocturnal enuresis in children. *Cochrane Database Sys Rev* (1):CD004668, 2004.
116. Bennett HJ: Waking up dry: A guide to help children overcome bedwetting, *American Academy of Pediatrics*:241, 2005.
117. MacLean RE: Imipramine hydrochloride (Tofranil) and enuresis. *Am J Psychiatry* 117:551, 1960.
118. Devane CL, Walker RD III, Sawyer WP, Wilson JA: Concentrations of imipramine and its metabolites during enuresis therapy. *Pediatr Pharmacol* 4:245–251, 1984.
119. de Gatta MF, Garcia MJ, Acosta A, Rey F, Gutierrez JR, Dominquez-Gil A: Monitoring of serum levels of imipramine and desipramine and individualization of dose in enuretic children. *Ther Drug Monit* 6:438–443, 1984.
120. Fernandez de Gatta MM, Galindo P, Rey F, Gutierrez J Tamayo M, Garcia MJ, Dominquez-Gil A: The influence of clinical and pharmacological factors on enuresis treatment with imipramine. *Br J Clin Pharmacol* 30:693–698, 1990.
121. Jorgensen OS, Lober M, Christiansen J, Gram LF: Plasma concentration and clinical effect in imipramine treatment of childhood enuresis. *Clin Pharmacokinet* 5:386–393, 1980.
122. Rapoport JL, Mikkelsen EJ, Zavadil A, Nee L, Gruenau C, Menelson W, Gillen JC: Childhood enuresis: II. Psychopathology, tricyclic concentration in plasma, and antienuretic effect. *Arch Gen Psychiatry* 37:1146–1152, 1980.
123. Fritz GK, Rockney RM, Yeung AS: Plasma levels and efficacy of imipramine treatment for enuresis. *J Am Acad Child Adolesc Psychiatry* 33:60–64, 1994.
124. Smellie JM, McGrigor VS, Meadow SR, Rose SJ, Douglas MF: Nocturnal enuresis: A placebo controlled trial of two antidepressants. *Arch Dis Child* 75:62–66, 1996.
125. Gepertz S, Neveus T: Imipramine for therapy resistant enuresis: A retrospective evaluation. *J Urol* 171(6 Pt 2):2607–2610, 2004.
126. Devlin JB: Prevalence and risk factors for childhood nocturnal enuresis. *Ir Med J* 84:118–120, 1991.
127. Foxman B, Valdez RB, Brook RH: Childhood enuresis: Prevalence, perceived impact, and prescribed treatments. *Pediatrics* 77:482–487, 1986.
128. Vogel W, Young M, Primack W: A survey of physician use of treatment methods for functional enuresis. *J Dev Behav Pediatr* 17:90–93, 1996.
129. Boulis AK, Long J: Variation in the treatment of children by primary care physician specialty. *Arch Pediatr Adolesc Med* 156(12):1210–1215, 2002.
130. Capozza N, Creti G, De Gennaro M, Minni B, Caione P: The treatment of nocturnal enuresis: A comparative study between desmopressin and acupuncture used along or in combination. *Minerva Pediatr* 43:577–582, 1991.
131. Minni B, Capozza N, Creti G, Degennaro M, Caione P, Bischko J: Bladder instability and enuresis treated by acupuncture and electrotherapeutics: Early urodynamic observations. *Acupunc Electrother Res* 15(1):19–25, 1990.
132. Roje-Starcevic M: The treatment of nocturnal enuresis by acupuncture. *Neurologica* 39:179–184, 1990.
133. Metin A, Aykol N: Diclofenac sodium suppository in the treatment of primary nocturnal enuresis. *Int Urol Nephrol* 24:113–117, 1992.
134. Elmer M, Adolfsson T, Norgaard JP, Djurhuus JC: Diurnal enuresis in childhood is effectively treated with terodiline. *Lakartidningen* 88:850–851, 1991.
135. el-Sadr A, Sabry AA, Abdel-Rahman M, el-Barnachawy R, Koraitim M: Treatment of primary nocturnal enuresis by oral androgen mesterolone: A clinical and cystometric study. *Urology* 36:331–335, 1990.

136. Banerjee S, Srivastav A, Palan BM: Hypnosis and self-hypnosis in the management of nocturnal enuresis: A comparative study with imipramine therapy. *Am J Clin Hypn* 36:113–119, 1993.
137. Glazener CM, Evans JH, Cheuk DK: Complementary and miscellaneous interventions for nocturnal enuresis in children. *Cochrane Database Syst Rev* (2):CD005230, 2005.
138. Glazener CM, Evans JH, Peto RE: Drugs for nocturnal enuresis in children (other than Desmopressin and tricyclics). *Cochrane Database Syst Rev* (4):CD002238, 2003.
139. Kosar A, Arikan N, Dincel C: Effectiveness of oxybutynin hydrochloride in the treatment of enuresis nocturna: A clinical and urodynamic study. *Scand J Urol Nephrol* 33:115–118, 1999.
140. Moffatt ME, Harlos S, Kirshen AJ, Burd L: Desmopressin acetate and nocturnal enuresis: How much do we know? *Pediatrics* 92:420–425, 1993.
141. Terho P: Desmopressin in nocturnal enuresis. *J Urol* 145:818–820, 1991.
142. Key DW, Bloom DA, Sanvordenker J: Low-dose DDAVP in nocturnal enuresis. *Clin Pediatr* 31:299–301, 1992.
143. Wille S: Comparison of desmopressin and enuresis alarm for nocturnal enuresis. *Arch Dis Child* 61:30–33, 1986.
144. Sukhai RN, Mol J, Harris AS: Combined therapy of enuresis alarm and desmopressin in the treatment of nocturnal enuresis. *Eur J Paediatr* 148:465–467, 1989.
145. Leebeek-Groenewegen A, Blom J, Sukhai R, van der Heijden B: Efficacy of Desmopressin combined with alarm therapy for monosymptomatic nocturnal enuresis. *J Urol* 166(6):2456–2458, 2001.
146. Lee T, Suh HJ, Lee HJ, Lee JE: Comparison of effects of treatment of primary nocturnal enuresis with oxybutynin plus Desmopressin, Desmopressin alone or imipramine alone: A randomized controlled clinical trial. *J Urol* 174(3):1084–1087, 2005.
147. Naitoh Y, Kawauchi A, Yamao Y, Seki H, Soh J, Yonedan, Mizutani Y, Miki T: Combination therapy with alarm and drugs for monosymptomatic nocturnal enuresis not superior to alarm monotherapy. *Urology* 66(3):632–635, 2005.
148. Kallio J, Rautava P, Huupponen R, Korvenranta H: Severe hyponatremia caused by intranasal desmopressin for nocturnal enuresis. *Acta Paediatr* 82:881–882, 1993.
149. Beach PS, Beach RE, Smith LR: Hyponatremic seizures in a child treated with desmopressin to control enuresis: A rational approach to fluid intake. *Clin Pediatr* 31:566–569, 1992.
150. Schwab M, Wenzel D, Ruder H: Hyponatraemia and cerebral convulsion due to short term DDAVP therapy for control of enuresis nocturna. *Eur J Pediatr* 155:46–48, 1996.
151. Yaouyanc G, Jonville AP, Yaouyanc-Lapalle H: Seizure with hyponatremia in a child prescribed desmopressin for nocturnal enuresis. *J Toxicol* 30:637–641, 1992.
152. Bernstein SA, Williford SL: Intranasal desmopressin-associated hyponatremia: A case report and literature review. *J Fam Pract* 44:203–208, 1997.
153. Robson WL, Norgaard JP, Leung AK: Hyponatremia in patients with nocturnal enuresis treated with DDAVP. *Eur J Pediatr* 155:959–962, 1996.
154. Thumfart J, Roehr CC, Kapelari K, Querfeld V, Eggert P, Muller D: Desmopressin associated symptomatic hyponatremic hypervolemia in children. Are there predictive factors? *J Urol* 174(1):294–298, 2005.
155. Hjalmas K, Hanson E, Hellstrom AL, Kruse S, Sillen U: Swedish Enuresis Trial (SWEET) Group: Long-term treatment with desmopressin in children with primary monosymptomatic nocturnal enuresis: An open multicentre study. *Br J Urol* 82:704–709, 1998.
156. Tullus K, Bergstrom R, Fosdal I, Winnergard I, Hjalmas K: Efficacy and safety during long-term treatment of primary monosymptomatic nocturnal enuresis with desmopressin. *Acta Paediatr* 88:1274–1278, 1999.
157. Riccabona M, Oswald J, Glauninger P: Long-term use and tapered dose reduction of intranasal desmopressin in the treatment of enuretic children. *Br J Urol* 81:24–25, 1998.
158. Matthiesen TB, Rittig S, Djurhuus JC, Norgaard JP: A dose titration, and an open 6-week efficacy and safety study of desmopressin tablets in the management of nocturnal enuresis. *J Urol* 151:460–463, 1994.
159. Janknegt RA, Zweers HM, Delaere KP, Kloet AG, Khoe SG, Arendsen HJ: Oral desmopressin as a new treatment modality for primary nocturnal enuresis in adolescents and adults: A double-blind, randomized, multicenter study. Dutch Enuresis Study Group. *J Urol* 157:513–517, 1997.
160. Schulman SL, Stokes A, Salzman PM: The efficacy and safety of oral desmopressin in children with primary nocturnal enuresis. *J Urol* 166(6):2427–2431, 2001.
161. Skoog SJ, Stokes A, Turner KL: Oral desmopressin: A randomized double-blind placebo controlled study of effectiveness in children with primary nocturnal enuresis. *J Urol* 158:1035–1040, 1997.
162. Stenberg A, Lackgren G: Desmopressin tablets in the treatment of severe nocturnal enuresis in adolescents. *Pediatrics* 94:841–846, 1994.
163. Lackgren G, Lilja B, Neveus T, Stenberg A: Desmopressin in the treatment of severe nocturnal enuresis in adolescents: A 7-year follow-up study. *Br J Urol* 81(3):17–23, 1998.
164. Wolfish NM, Barkin J, Gorodzinsky F, Schwarz R: The Canadian enuresis study and evaluation—short- and long-term safety and efficacy of an oral desmopressin preparation. *Scand J Urol Nephrol* 37(1):22–27, 2003.
165. Butler R, Holland P, Devitt H, Hiley E, Roberts G, Redfern E: The effectiveness of desmopressin in the treatment of childhood nocturnal enuresis: Predicting response using pretreatment variables. *Br J Urol* 81(3): 29–36, 1998.
166. Eller DA, Homsy YL, Austin PF, Tanguay S, Cantor A: Spot urine osmolality, age and bladder capacity as predictors of response to desmopressin in nocturnal enuresis. *Scand J Urol Nephrol* 183:41–45, 1997.
167. Eller DA, Austin PF, Tanguay S, Homsy YL: Daytime functional bladder capacity as a predictor of response to desmopressin in monosymptomatic nocturnal enuresis. *Eur Urol* 33(3):25–29, 1998.
168. Folwell AJ, Macdiarmid SA, Crowder HJ, Lord AD, Arnold EP: Desmopressin for nocturnal enuresis: Urinary osmolality and response. *Br J Urol* 80(3):480–484, 1997.
169. Neveus T, Lackgren G, Tuvemo T, Stenberg A: Osmoregulation and desmopressin pharmacokinetics in enuretic children. *Pediatrics* 103:65–70, 1999b.
170. Rushton HG, Belman AB, Zaontz MR, Skoog SJ, Sihelnik S: The influence of small functional bladder capacity and other predictors on the response to desmopressin in the management of monosymptomatic nocturnal enuresis. *J Urol* 156:651–655, 1996.
171. Kruse S, Hellstrom AL, Hanson E, Hjalmas K, Sillen U: Swedish Enuresis Trial (SWEET) Group: Treatment of primary monosymptomatic nocturnal enuresis with desmopressin: predictive factors. *BJU Int* 88(6):572–576, 2001.
172. Rushton HG, Belman AB, Zaontz M, Skoog SJ, Sihelnik S: Response to desmopressin as a function of urine osmolality in the treatment of monosymptomatic nocturnal enuresis: A double-blind prospective study. *J Urol* 154:749–753, 1995.
173. Monda JM, Husmann DA: Primary nocturnal enuresis: A comparison among observation, imipramine, desmopressin acetate and bed-wetting alarm systems. *J Urol* 154:745–748, 1995.
174. Glazener CM, Evans JH: Desmopressin for nocturnal enuresis in children. *Cochrane Database Syst Rev* (3):CD002112, 2002.
175. Mikkelsen EJ: Enuresis and encopresis: Ten years of progress. *Am Acad Child and Adol Psychiatry* 1146–1158, 2001.
176. Bellman M: Studies on encopresis. *Acta Paediatr Scand* 1996; 170(suppl), 1966.
177. Rutter M, Tizard J, Whitmore K (eds): *Education, Health and Behavior*. New York, Krieger, Huntington, 1981.
178. van der Wal MF, Benninga MA, Hirasing RA: The prevalence of encopresis in a multicultural population. *J Pediatr Gastroenterol Nutr* 40(suppl 3):345–8, 2005.
179. Hersov L: Faecal soiling. In: Rutter M and Sersov L: (eds) *Child and Adolescent Psychiatry: Modern Approaches*, 2nd ed. London, Blackwell Scientific, 1985, pp. 482–489.
180. Loening-Baucke V: Functional fecal retention with encopresis in childhood. *J Pediatr Gastroenterol Nutr* 38(suppl 1):79–84, 2004.
181. Loening-Baucke VA: Factors responsible for persistence of childhood constipation. *J Pediatr Gastroenterol Nutr* 6:915–922, 1987.
182. Loening-Baucke VA, Cruikshank BM: Abnormal defecation dynamics in chronically constipated children with encopresis. *J Pediatr* 108:562–566, 1986.
183. Loening-Baucke V, Cruikshank B, Savage C: Defecation dynamics and behavior profiles in encopretic children. *Pediatrics* 80:672–679, 1987.
184. Loening-Baucke V: Balloon defecation as a predictor of outcome in children with functional constipation and encopresis. *J Pediatr* 128:336–340, 1996.
185. Wald A, Chandra R, Chiponis D, Gabel S: Anorectal function and continence mechanisms in childhood encopresis. *J Pediatr Gastroenterol Nutr* 5:346–351, 1986.
186. Sentovich SM, Kaufman SS, Cali RL: Pudendal nerve function in normal and encopretic children. *J Pediatr Gastroenterol Nutr* 26:70–72, 1998.
187. Catto-Smith AG, Nolan TM, Coffey CM: Clinical significance of anismus in encopresis. *J Gastroenterol Hepatol* 13:955–960, 1998.
188. Sutphen J, Borowitz S, Ling W, Cox DJ, Kovatchev B: Anorectal manometric examination in encopretic-constipated children. *Dis Colon Rectum* 40:1051–1055, 1997.
189. Stern HP, Stroh SE, Fiedorek SC, Kelleher K, Mellon MM, Pope SK, Rayford PL: Increased plasma levels of pancreatic polypeptide and decreased plasma levels of motilin in encopretic children. *Pediatrics* 96:111–117, 1995.
190. Freud A, Burlingham DT: *War and Children*. New York, Medical War Books, 1943.
191. Stein Z, Susser M: Social factors in the development of sphincter control. *Dev Med Child Neurol* 9:692–706, 1967.
192. Foreman DM, Thambirajah MS: Conduct disorder, enuresis and specific developmental delays in two types of encopresis: A case-note study of 63 boys. *Eur Child Adolesc Psychiatry* 5:33–37, 1996.
193. Cox DJ, Morris Jr JB, Borowitz SM, Sutphen JL: Psychological differences between children with and without chronic encopresis. *J Pediatr Psychol* 27(suppl 7):585–591, 2002.
194. Klages T, Geller B, Tillman R, Bolhofner K, Zimerman B: Controlled study of encopresis and enuresis in children with a prepubertal and

early adolescent bipolar-I disorder phenotype. *J Am Acad Child Adolesc Psychiatry* 44(suppl 10):1050–1057, 2005.
195. von Gontard A, Hollmann E: Comorbidity of functional urinary incontinence and encopresis: Somatic and behavioral associations. *J Urol* 71(suppl 6 Pt 2):2644–2647, 2004.
196. Rockney RM, McQuade WH, Days AL: The plain abdominal roentgenogram in the management of encopresis. *Arch Pediatr Adolesc Med* 149:623–627, 1995.
197. Levine MD: Encopresis: Its potentiation, evaluation and alleviation. *Pediatr Clin North Am* 29:315–330, 1982.
198. Levine MD, Bakow H: Children with encopresis: A study of treatment outcome. *Pediatrics* 58:845–852, 1976.
199. Levine MD, Mazonson P, Bakow H: Behavioral symptom substitution in children cured of encopresis. *Am J Dis Child* 134:663–667, 1980.
200. Borowitz SM, Cox DJ, Sutphen JL, Kovatchev B: Treatment of childhood encopresis: A randomized trial comparing three treatment protocols. *J Pediatr Gastroenterol Nutr* 34(suppl 4):378–384, 2002.
201. Stark LJ, Opipari LC, Donaldson DL, Danovsky MB, Rasile DA: Evaluation of a standard protocol for retentive encopresis: A replication. *J Pediatr Psychol* 22:619–633, 1997.
202. Sprague-McRae JM, Lamb W, Homer D: Encopresis: A study of treatment alternatives and historical and behavioral characteristics. *Nurse Pract* 18(suppl 10):52–53, 56–63, 1993.
203. Nolan T, Debelle G, Oberkland F, Coffey C: Randomized trial of laxatives in treatment of childhood encopresis. *Lancet* 31:523–527, 1991.
204. Pashankar DS, Bishop WP: Efficacy and optimal dose of daily polyethylene glycol 3350 for treatment of constipation and encopresis in children. *J Pediatr* 139(suppl 3):428–432, 2001.
205. Loening-Baucke V: Polyethylene glycol without electrolytes for children with constipation and encopresis. *J Pediatr Gastroenterol Nutr* 34(suppl 4):372–377, 2002.
206. Pashankar DS, Bishop WP, Loening-Baucke V: Long-term efficacy of polyethylene glycol 3350 for the treatment of chronic constipation in children with and without encopresis. *Clin Pediatr* 42(suppl 9):815–819, 2003.
207. Voskuijl W, de Lorijn F, Verwijs W, Hogeman P, Heijmans J, Makel W, Taminiau J, Benninga M: PEG 3350 (Transipeg) versus lactulose in the treatment of childhood functional constipation: A double-blind, randomized, controlled, multicentre trial. *Gut* 53(suppl 11):1590–1594, 2004.
208. Loening-Baucke V: Modulation of abnormal defecation dynamics by biofeedback treatment in chronically constipated children with encopresis. *J Pediatr* 116:214–222, 1990.
209. Benninga MA, Buller HA, Iaminiau JA: Biofeedback training in chronic constipation. *Arch Dis Child* 68:126–129, 1993.
210. Loening-Baucke V: Biofeedback treatment for chronic constipation and encopresis in childhood: Long-term outcome. *Pediatrics* 96:105–110, 1995.
211. Nolan T, Catto-Smith T, Coffey C, Wells J: Randomised controlled trial of biofeedback training in persistent encopresis with anismus. *Arch Dis Child* 79:131–135, 1998.
212. Brooks RC, Copen RM, Cox DJ, Morris J, Borowitz S, Sutphen J: Review of the treatment literature for encopresis, functional constipation, and stool-toileting refusal. *Ann Behav Med* 22(suppl 3):260–267, 2000.
213. Brazzelli M, Griffiths P: Behavioural and cognitive interventions with or without other treatments for defecation disorders in children. *Cochrane Database Syst Rev* (4):CD002240, 2001.
214. Griffiths P, Dunn S, Evans A, Smith D, Bradnam M: Portable biofeedback apparatus for treatment of anal sphincter dystonia in childhood soiling and constipation. *J Med Eng Tech* 23(suppl 3):96–101, 1999.
215. Cox DJ, Sutphen J, Borowitz S, Kovatchev B, Ling W: Contribution of behavior therapy and biofeedback to laxative therapy in the treatment of pediatric encopresis. *Ann Behav Med* 20:70–76, 1998.
216. Croffie JM, Ammar MS, Pfefferkorn MD, Hom D, Klipsch A, Fitzgerald JF, Gupta SK, Molleston JP, Corkins MR: Assessment of the effectiveness of biofeedback in children with dyssynergic defecation and recalcitrant constipation/encopresis: Does home biofeedback improve long-term outcomes? *Clin Pediatr* 44(suppl 1):63–71, 2005.
217. Abrahams D: Treatment of encopresis with imipramine. *Am J Psychiatry* 119:891–892, 1963.
218. Connell HM: The practical management of encopresis. *Aust Paediatr J* 8:279–281, 1972.
219. Gavanski M: Treatment of non-retentive secondary encopresis with imipramine and psychotherapy. *CMAJ* 104:46–48, 1971.
220. Geormaneanu M, Voiculescu VP: Treatment of encopresis with imipramine. *Rev Roum Med Neurol Psychiatr* 18:209–210, 1980.
221. Siomopoulos V: Psychogenic encopresis treated with imipramine. *JAMA* 235:1842, 1976.
222. White JH: *Pediatric Psychopharmacology*. Baltimore, Williams & Wilkins, 1977, pp. 109–114.
223. Dossetor D, Stiefel I, Gomes L: A case of predominantly nocturnal soiling treated with amitriptyline. *Eur Child Adolesc Psychiatry* 7:114–118, 1998.
224. Nurko S, Garcia-Aranda JA, Worona LB, Zlochisty O: Cisapride for the treatment of constipation in children: A double-blind study. *J Pediatr* 136:135–140, 2000.
225. Rockney RM, McQuade WH, Days AL, Linn HE, Alario AJ: Encopresis treatment outcome: Long-term follow-up of 45 cases. *J Dev Behav Pediatr* 17:380–385, 1996.
226. Rex DK, Fitzgerald JF, Goulet RJ: Chronic constipation with encopresis persisting beyond 15 years of age. *Dis Colon Rectum* 35:242–244, 1992.

CHAPTER 5.13 ■ GENDER IDENTITY DISORDER

KENNETH J. ZUCKER

GENDER IDENTITY DISORDER

Definition

At a nascent cognitive level, gender identity has been defined as a child's recognition that he or she is a member of one sex but not of the other (1). Four decades ago, Stoller (2) coined the term *core gender identity* to refer to the development of a "fundamental sense of belonging to one sex," the awareness that one is a male or female. At an affective level, this sense of belonging is emotionally valued, so that a child experiences a sense of comfort or security from being a boy or a girl. A child's gender identity is often closely tied to the adoption of culturally defined behavioral markers of masculinity or femininity (*gender roles*).

What does one observe in children and adolescents who meet the DSM-IV-TR criteria for gender identity disorder (GID)? The most salient feature is a strong identification with, and preference for, the gender role characteristics of the other sex. This can be inferred from various age-related behavioral manifestations of gender identification, such as toy interests, fantasy role and activity preferences, and peer affiliation preferences. Cross-gender identification is also expressed through verbal statements that one is, or would like to be, a member of the other sex. Moreover, children with GID often have few positive things to say about their own sex and appear to experience a sense of *gender dysphoria,* or unease, about their own sex. By adolescence, when the clinical picture more closely resembles what one observes in adults with GID, the pervasive sense of gender dysphoria becomes even more salient. Table 5.13.1 shows the DSM-IV-TR diagnostic criteria for GID.

TABLE 5.13.1

DSM-IV DIAGNOSTIC CRITERIA FOR GENDER IDENTITY DISORDER

A. A strong and persistent cross-gender identification (not merely a desire for any perceived cultural advantages of being the other sex).
   In children, the disturbance is manifested by at least four (or more) of the following:
   1. Repeatedly stated desire to be, or insistence that he or she is, the other sex
   2. In boys, preference for cross-dressing or simulating female attire; in girls, insistence on wearing only stereotypical masculine clothing
   3. Strong and persistent preferences for cross-sex roles in make-believe play or persistent fantasies of being the other sex
   4. Intense desire to participate in the stereotypical games and pastimes of the other sex
   5. Strong preference for playmates of the other sex

   In adolescents . . . the disturbance is manifested by symptoms such as a stated desire to be the other sex, frequent passing as the other sex, desire to live or be treated as the other sex, or the conviction that he or she has the typical feelings and reactions of the other sex.

B. Persistent discomfort with his or her sex or sense of inappropriateness in the gender role of that sex.
   In children, the disturbance is manifested by any of the following: in boys, assertion that his penis or testes are disgusting or will disappear or assertion that it would be better not to have a penis, or aversion toward rough-and-tumble play and rejection of male stereotypical toys, games, and activities; in girls, rejection of urinating in a sitting position, assertion that she has or will grow a penis, or assertion that she does not want to grow breasts or menstruate, or marked aversion toward normative feminine clothing.
   In adolescents . . . the disturbance is manifested by symptoms such as preoccupation with getting rid of primary and secondary sex characteristics (e.g., request for hormones, surgery, or other procedures to physically alter sexual characteristics to simulate the other sex) or belief that he or she was born the wrong sex.

C. The disturbance is not concurrent with a physical intersex condition.

D. The disturbance causes clinically significant distress or impairment in social, occupational, or other important areas of functioning.
   Specify if (for sexually mature individuals):
   Sexually attracted to males
   Sexually attracted to females
   Sexually attracted to both
   Sexually attracted to neither

(From the American Psychiatric Association, with permission.)

History

In the 1950s, two clinical developments led to an increased interest in the study of children with potential problems in their gender identity development. First, Money et al's (3) research on children with various types of physical intersex conditions showed that a key milestone in gender identity formation occurred sometime between 18 and 36 months of age, if not earlier. Money et al. reported that, despite an ambiguous sexual biology, children with disorders of sex development (DSD) (4) could develop a stable gender identity if they were reared unambiguously as members of one sex or the other. Second, retrospective clinical reports on the adult syndrome of GID, commonly referred to as *transsexualism* (5), led to the recognition that the behavioral markers of this condition were often expressed during the first few years of life.

In the early 1980s, thinking about children with gender identity problems was influenced by a third development. A series of studies on homosexuality in adults, perhaps peaking with the volume by Bell et al. (6) indicated that a pattern of childhood cross-gender behavior was also a strong developmental predictor of later homosexuality, which was subsequently confirmed in a meta-analytic review by Bailey and Zucker (7). Over the past decade, increasing attention has been given to the identification of variation in the long-term developmental trajectories of children with GID (see Course and Prognosis).

Epidemiology

Prevalence

To my knowledge, none of the numerous contemporary epidemiological studies on the prevalence of psychiatric disorders in children and youth have examined GID. Accordingly, estimates of prevalence have had to rely on less sophisticated approaches. For example, it has been suggested that one estimate of prevalence might be inferred from the number of persons attending clinics for adults that serve as gateways for hormonal and surgical sex reassignment. Because not all gender dysphoric adults may attend such clinics, this method may well underestimate the prevalence of GID; in any case, the number of adult transsexuals is small—one estimate from the Netherlands suggested a prevalence of 1 in 11,000 men and 1 in 30,400 women (8).

More liberal estimates of prevalence can be judged from studies of children in whom specific cross-gender behaviors have been assessed. For example, the standardization study of the Child Behavior Checklist (CBCL) (9), a widely used parent-report questionnaire of childhood behavioral psychopathology, included information on the percentage of mothers of both clinic-referred and nonreferred boys and girls who endorsed two items pertaining to cross-gender identification: "behaves like opposite sex" and "wishes to be of opposite sex."

TABLE 5.13.2

PERCENTAGE OF U.S. NONREFERRED CHILDREN WHOSE MOTHERS ENDORSED CHILD BEHAVIOR CHECKLIST ITEMS RELEVANT TO CROSS-GENDER IDENTIFICATION

Sex of Child Behaves Like Opposite Sex (Item 5)	Age Grouping (in years)								
	4	5	6	7	8	9	10	11	Total
Boys									
Rating of 1	6.1	4.0	6.0	4.0	2.0	2.0	6.0	0.0	3.8
Rating of 2	0.0	0.0	0.0	2.0	2.0	0.0	4.0	0.0	1.0
Girls									
Rating of 1	2.0	12.0	6.1	4.0	12.0	8.0	12.0	10.0	8.3
Rating of 2	4.1	2.0	2.0	8.0	0.0	2.0	0.0	0.0	2.3
Wishes to Be of Opposite Sex (Item 110)									
	4	5	6	7	8	9	10	11	Total
Boys									
Rating of 1	2.0	0.0	0.0	0.0	0.0	0.0	2.0	1.0	1.0
Rating of 2	0.0	0.0	0.0	0.0	0.0	0.0	0.0	0.0	0.0
Girls									
Rating of 1	6.1	2.0	2.0	2.0	2.0	2.0	4.0	0.0	2.5
Rating of 2	2.0	2.0	2.0	0.0	2.0	0.0	0.0	0.0	1.0

Note. Data from Achenbach and Edelbrock (9) and reported in Zucker et al (15). The CBCL raw data were provided on diskette by T. M. Achenbach, Ph.D. For each sex× age cell, N = 50 except in a few cases where there was one missing data point.

Table 5.13.2 shows the percentage of mothers of nonreferred boys and girls, across the age range of 4 to 11 years, who endorsed these two items by giving ratings of either a 1 (somewhat or sometimes true) or a 2 (very true or often true) on a 0- to 2-point scale for frequency of occurrence. For both items, more mothers of girls gave ratings of either a 1 or a 2 than did mothers of boys; however, chi-square tests showed that the differences were significant only for the rating of a 1 for the item "behaves like the opposite sex." By maternal report, the percentage of both boys and girls who wished to be of the opposite sex was quite low (range, 0.0–2.5% by sex and intensity).

These findings were largely replicated in a recent large-scale study of Dutch twins (N = 23,393) at ages 7 and 10 (10). As shown in Table 5.13.3, at both ages and for both sexes, behaving like the opposite sex was more common than wishing to be of the opposite sex (ratings of 1 and 2 combined); in general, more girls than boys were rated as showing these behaviors. Again, the percentage of both boys and girls who wished to be of the opposite sex was quite low (range, 0.9–1.7% by sex and age).

Sex Differences in Referral Rates

Among children between the ages of 3–12, it has been found that boys are referred clinically more often than girls for concerns regarding gender identity. From one speciality clinic in Toronto, Canada, Cohen-Kettenis et al (11) reported a sex ratio of 5.8:1 (N = 358) of boys to girls based on consecutive referrals from 1975 to 2000.* In this study, comparative data were available on children evaluated at the only gender identity clinic for children in Utrecht, The Netherlands. Although the sex ratio was significantly smaller at 2.9:1 (N = 130), it still favored referral of boys over girls.

Among adolescents between the ages of 13–20, however, the sex ratio in the Toronto clinic narrowed considerably, at 1.3:1 (N = 72) of males to females (12). This ratio was remarkably similar to that of 1.2:1 (N = 133) reported by Cohen-Kettenis and Pfäfflin (13) in the Netherlands. Thus, across both clinics, there was a sex-related skew in referrals

TABLE 5.13.3

PERCENTAGE OF DUTCH TWINS (7 AND 10 YEARS) WHOSE MOTHERS ENDORSED CHILD BEHAVIOR CHECKLIST ITEMS RELEVANT TO CROSS-GENDER IDENTIFICATION

Sex of Child Behaves Like Opposite Sex (Item 5)	Age Group (in years)	
Boys	7 N = 7202	10 N = 4266
Rating of 1 or 2	3.4	2.4
Girls	N = 7395	N = 4530
Rating of 1 or 2	5.2	3.4
Wishes to Be of Opposite Sex (Item 110)		
Boys	7 N = 7202	10 N = 4266
Rating of 1 or 2	1.0	1.0
Girls	N = 7395	N = 4530
Rating of 1 or 2	1.7	0.9

Note. Data from van Beijsterveldt et al (10).

*Through early 2006, the number of referred boys to girls (N = 470) was 5.10:1.

during childhood, but this lessened considerably during adolescence.

How might this age-related developmental disparity in the sex ratio best be understood? One possibility is that it reflects accurately the change in prevalence of GID in males and females between childhood and adolescence, but because prevalence data from the general population are lacking, this remains a matter of conjecture. Another possibility is that social factors play a role. For example, in childhood, it is well established that parents, teachers, and peers are less tolerant of cross-gender behavior in boys than in girls, which might result in a sex differential in clinical referral (14).

Two studies provided data that supported this prediction, in which it was shown that girls may need to display more cross-gender behavior than boys before a referral is initiated (11, 15). This higher threshold for referral appeared consistent with the fact that, in both the Toronto and Utrecht clinics, girls were referred, on average, about 10 months later than boys (M age, 8.1 years vs. 7.3 years, respectively), a significant difference, despite the fact that the girls showed, on average, higher levels of cross-gender behavior than the boys (11). However, it is important to note that the sexes did not differ in the percentage who met the complete DSM criteria for GID; thus, there was no gross evidence for a sex difference in false positive referrals.

Another factor that could affect sex differences in referral rates pertains to the relative salience of cross-gender behavior in boys vs. girls. For example, it has been long observed that the sexes differ in the extent to which they display sex-typical behaviors; when there is significant between-sex variation, it is almost always the case that girls are more likely to engage in masculine behaviors than boys are likely to engage in feminine behaviors (16). Thus, the base rates for cross-gender behavior, at least within the range of normative variation, may well differ between the sexes.

In adolescence, the picture may change considerably in that extreme cross-gender behavior is subject to more equivalent social pressures across sex and thus there is a lowering in the bias towards a greater referral of boys. Along similar lines, it is possible that gender dysphoria in adolescent girls is more difficult to ignore than it is during childhood, as the intensification of concerns with regard to physical sex transformation becomes more salient to parents and other adults involved in the life of the adolescent.

Age at Referral

In the Cohen-Kettenis et al (11) study, the age distribution at referral showed some remarkable differences. It can be seen in Figure 5.13.1 that the Toronto sample had a substantially higher percentage of referrals between the ages of 3–4, 4–5, and 5–6 years than did the Utrecht sample (40.5% vs. 13.1%) and these differences were even more pronounced for the age intervals of 3–4 and 4–5 years (22.6% vs. 2.3%).

Cohen-Kettenis et alnoted that the "delay" in referral to the Dutch clinic could not readily be accounted for by differences in natural history, including degree of cross-gender behavior, base rates of cross-gender behavior in the two countries, or financial factors (such as insurance coverage). It was speculated that cultural factors might account for the cross-national difference in age at referral, in that North American parents become concerned about their child's cross-gender behavior at an earlier age than do Dutch parents.

Diagnosis and Clinical Features

The initial behavioral signs (age of onset) of GID most typically appear during the toddler and preschool years (17), the same developmental time period in which more conventional patterns of sex-typed behavior can also first be observed (18). The central clinical issue concerns the degree to which a pattern of behavioral signs is present, because this pattern is the basis for inference on the extent to which a child is cross-gender-identified and meets the DSM-IV-TR criteria for GID (Table 5.13.1).

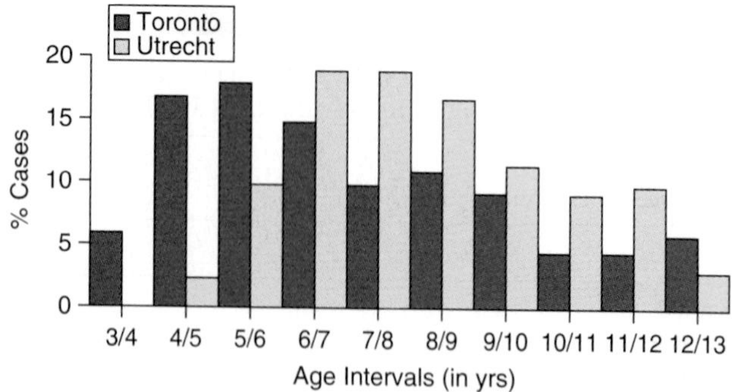

FIGURE 5.13.1. Age at referral by clinic. (Data from Cohen-Kettenis PT, Owen A, Kaijser VG, et al.: Demographic characteristics, social competence, and behavior problems in children with gender identity disorder: A cross-national, cross-clinic comparative analysis. *J Abnorm Child Psychol* 31:41–53, 2003.)

For child patients, both the Toronto and Dutch clinics have reported that about 70% of their probands met the complete DSM criteria for GID at the time of assessment and the remainder were subthreshold for the diagnosis, i.e., they had some symptoms but not enough to meet the criteria for GID (11). In several quantitative studies, it has been shown that the subthreshold probands had patterns of cross-gender behavior that were intermediate between the threshold probands and controls (14, 19), thus providing some validity evidence for clinician-based diagnosis of GID (20).

For patients seen for the first time in adolescence, however, the clinician needs to be aware of two major subgroups. The first subgroup consists of male and female youth who have a very clear childhood onset of GID, which has persisted into adolescence. Almost all of the youth in this subgroup have a homosexual sexual orientation, i.e., they are sexually attracted to members of their own birth sex (21). The second subgroup consists almost exclusively of males. These youth have a relatively "late onset" of GID, i.e., there is no clear indication of a childhood cross-gender history and the desire to be of the opposite sex is voiced only during the beginning of adolescence or even later (22, 23). Many of these adolescent boys have a cooccurring clinical presentation of transvestic fetishism or autogynephilia (sexual arousal at the thought of being a female) (24). These youth often have a heterosexual, bisexual, or asexual sexual orientation.

Associated Behavior Problems

Comorbidity—the presence of two or more psychiatric disorders—occurs frequently among children referred for clinical evaluation. Assuming that the putative comorbid conditions actually represent distinct disorders, it is important to know, for various reasons, whether one condition increases the risk for the other condition or if the conditions are caused by distinct or overlapping factors (25).

Regarding GID, an interesting new example of comorbidity comes from several case reports describing its cooccurrence with Pervasive Developmental Disorders (PDD) (26–28). These case reports mesh with my own clinical experience, having systematically evaluated 10 boys with comorbid GID and PDD

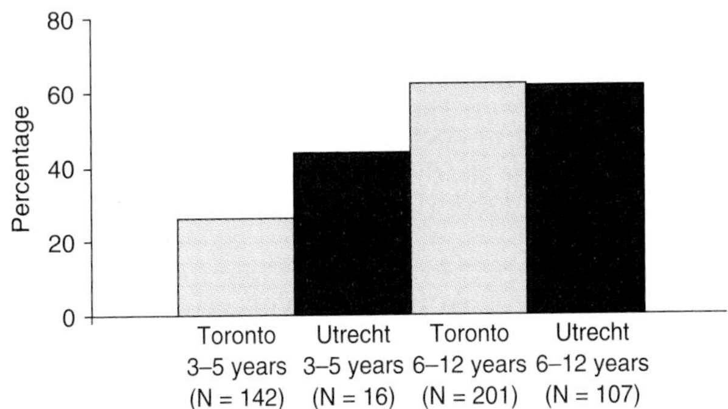

FIGURE 5.13.2. Percentage of CBCL clinical range scores (> 90th percentile) by age group and clinic. (Data from Cohen-Kettenis PT, Owen A, Kaijser VG, et al.: Demographic characteristics, social competence, and behavior problems in children with gender identity disorder: A cross-national, cross-clinic comparative analysis. *J Abnorm Child Psychol* 31:41–53, 2003.)

over the past several years. One 6-year-old boy, for example, who had many of the classic features of PDD, including intense behavioral rigidity and obsessional preoccupations (e.g., with vacuum cleaners), had been insisting that he was a girl for the past 3 years and would introduce himself to other children using a girl's name. He would have catastrophic temper tantrums if reminded that he was really a boy. It is, of course, highly unlikely that GID "causes" PDD or the other way round. Rather, it is conceivable that the relation between GID and PDD is linked by traits of behavioral rigidity and obsessionality.

The most systematic information on general behavior problems in children with GID comes from parent-report data using the CBCL. On the CBCL, clinic-referred boys and girls with GID show, on average, significantly more general behavior problems than do their siblings and nonreferred children (11, 14). Figure 5.13.2 shows the percentage of 3–5- and 6–12-year-olds from the Toronto and Dutch clinics of GID children with clinical range scores on the CBCL.

Patterns and Correlates of Behavior Problems

On the CBCL, boys with GID have a predominance of internalizing, as opposed to externalizing, behavioral difficulties, whereas girls with GID do not (11, 14). Edelbrock and Achenbach (29) used cluster analysis to develop a taxonomy of profile patterns from CBCL data. Intraclass correlations were calculated and then subjected to centroid cluster analysis, from which profile types were identified and labeled. Intraclass correlations can range from −1.00 to 1.00 and a score of .00 represents the mean of the referred sample in the standardization study.

Using this system, we found evidence for a clear internalizing pattern for boys with GID (14). For 3–5-year-old boys, the mean intraclass correlation for *Depressed-Social Withdrawal* was .04. For 6–11-year-old boys, the mean intraclass correlations for *Schizoid-Social Withdrawal* and *Schizoid* were .04 and .16, respectively. For both age groups, there was considerable "distance" from externalizing profile types; for example, for the 4–5-year-old boys, the mean intraclass correlation for *Aggressive-Delinquent* was −.42 and for the 6–11-year-old boys, the mean intraclass correlation for *Hyperactive* was −.33.

Zucker and Bradley (14) found that increasing age was significantly associated with degree of behavior problems in boys with GID (depending on the metric, *r*s ranged from .28–.42, all *p*s $< .001$). This finding was replicated in the cross-national, cross-clinic comparative study by Cohen-Kettenis et al (11).

One explanation for these age effects pertains to the role of peer ostracism. That children with GID experience significant difficulties within the peer group has been noted for some time. Using a composite index of poor peer relations derived from three CBCL items (Cronbach's alpha = .81), Zucker et al (15) showed that children with GID had significantly more peer relationship difficulties than did their siblings, even when controlling for overall number of behavior problems. Cohen-Kettenis et al (11) found that in both Toronto and The Netherlands boys with GID had significantly poorer peer relations than girls with GID, consistent with normative studies, which show that cross-gender behavior in boys is subject to more negative social pressure than is cross-gender behavior in girls. Nonetheless, Cohen-Kettenis et al found that poor peer relations was the strongest predictor of CBCL behavior problems in *both* GID boys and girls, accounting for 32% and 24% of the variance, respectively, suggesting that social ostracism within the peer group may well be a potential mediator between cross-gender behavior and behavior problems.

An observational study by Fridell (30) provided more direct support for the idea that the cross-sex-typed behavior of boys with GID may influence how well they are liked by other children. Fridell created 15 age-matched experimental play groups consisting of one boy with GID and two nonreferred boys and two nonreferred girls (age range, 3–8 years). During these sessions, the children in the play groups had the opportunity to play with masculine, feminine, and neutral toys. After two 60-minute play sessions, conducted a week apart, each child was asked to select their favorite playmate from the group. The nonreferred boys most often chose the other nonreferred boy as their favorite playmate, thus indicating a distinct preference over the boy with GID. The nonreferred girls chose the other girl as their favorite playmate, thus showing a relative disinterest in either the boy with GID or the two nonreferred boys.

In summary, children with GID show, on average, as many other behavioral problems as do other clinic-referred children. Although these general behavior problems may contribute to their difficulties in the peer group, like other children with behavior problems, it is likely the case that their marked cross-gender behavior is particularly salient in eliciting negative reactions from their peers.

Although we have shown that poor peer relations is an important correlate of general behavior problems in children with GID, this is not meant to imply that it is the only source of these difficulties. Other research, for example, has shown that CBCL behavior problems in boys with GID are associated with a composite index of maternal psychopathology, which may reflect generic, nonspecific familial risk factors in producing behavior problems in general (14) and the predominance of internalizing psychopathology may reflect familial risk for affective disorders and temperamental features of the boys (31). Thus, it is likely the case that there are both specific and general risk factors involved in accounting for the general behavioral problems of children with GID.

Laboratory Studies

Biological Assessment

There are no known biomedical tests that can identify children with GID. Various parameters of biological sex, such as the sex chromosomes and the appearance of the external genitalia, are invariably normal; however, children with DSD (physical intersex conditions) may be at some risk for gender dysphoria (32–35). For these youngsters, pediatric endocrinologic and urologic or gynecologic evaluations are warranted, because certain biomedical treatments may be required; however, it is rare that such conditions have not already been identified prior to psychiatric assessment.

Psychological Assessment

A number of parent-report and behavioral measures can be used to assess sex-typed behavior in children with GID (14, 16). From a diagnostic standpoint, it should be recognized that no one psychologic test is a replacement for a diagnosis that is established by a clinical interview that covers the behavioral signs for GID. Nevertheless, these measures have strong discriminant validity and constitute one strong line of evidence that GID is, in fact, a distinct syndrome. As one example of this, Johnson et al (19). provided psychometric data on the Gender Identity Questionnaire for Children, a one-factor parent-report questionnaire consisting of 14 items rated on a 5-point scale that capture the behavioral phenomenology of GID. With specificity set at 95% for the controls (N = 504), proband sensitivity (N = 325) was 86.8%. When only probands who met the complete DSM criteria for GID were used, sensitivity rose to 96.3%.

Differential Diagnosis

When all the clinical signs of GID are present, it is not difficult to make the diagnosis. But the clinician who accepts the notion that there is a spectrum of cross-gender identification must be prepared to identify what Meyer-Bahlburg (36) described as the "zone of transition between clinically significant cross-gender behavior and mere statistical deviations from the gender norm" (p. 682). As noted earlier, the transitional zone is captured by youngsters who did not meet the complete DSM criteria for GID and, on various quantitative measures, fall in between that of threshold cases and controls. For such youngsters, the residual diagnosis of Gender Identity Disorder Not Otherwise Specified may be indicated, particularly if there are clinical reasons for some type of intervention.

Etiology

Biological Mechanisms

As noted earlier, children with GID invariably do not show signs of a gross physical intersex condition, which would rule out a marked prenatal hormonal anomaly (37). Thus, the search for biological influences on the development of GID must focus, therefore, on factors that do not affect the configuration of the external genitalia. Prenatal hormonal influences may play a role, but there would have to be some kind of brain-genital dissociation in their impact (e.g., perhaps due to timing effects) (38). Given that there are no post-mortem studies on brain neuroanatomy in GID children or youth, research has focused either on indirect markers of putative prenatal hormonal influences or on other biological factors.

Molecular and Behavior Genetics

There have been no molecular genetic studies of GID, but several behavior genetic studies have suggested that the liability for cross-gender behavior in the general population has a strong heritable component. At the same time, however, such studies have also identified both shared and nonshared environmental influences (10). Such environmental influences could, of course, pertain to nongenetic biological factors but could also involve postnatal psychosocial factors. In any case, it should be recognized that these studies have not identified the specific genetic and environmental factors, or gene-by-environment interactions, underlying the liability to cross-gender behavior. That genetic factors do not account for all of the variance in the liability to cross-gender behavior is demonstrated quite clearly from detailed clinical case reports of identical twins discordant for GID (39).

Activity Level

Activity level (AL) is a commonly accepted dimension of temperament, with some evidence for a genetic basis and possibly prenatal hormonal influences (40). Regarding children with GID, AL as a predisposing factor is a promising possibility, because it shows a rather strong sex difference, with boys having a higher AL than girls. Rough-and-tumble (RT) play, another sex-dimorphic behavior, bears some similarity to AL, in that it is often characterized by high energy expenditure; however, a distinguishing feature of RT is that it is a social-interactive behavior involving such sequences as "play fighting" and "chasing." Unlike AL, marked avoidance of RT is one of the defining features of GID for boys in the DSM-IV-TR.

Using parent-report measures of AL, two studies found that boys with GID had a lower AL than control boys (14, 41). Zucker and Bradley (14) also found that girls with GID had a higher AL than control girls; indeed, the girls with GID had a higher AL than the boys with GID whereas for the controls, the typical sex difference was observed. In another study, it was shown that a heterogeneous group of intersex girls, all of whom had been exposed to female-atypical levels of prenatal androgen, had an AL that was comparable to that of somatically normal girls with GID (42).

It is possible, therefore, that a sex-atypical AL is a temperamental factor that predisposes to the development of GID. For example, a low-active boy with GID may find the typical play behavior of other boys to be incompatible with his own behavioral style, which might make it difficult for him to integrate successfully into a male peer group; conversely, a high-active girl with GID may find the typical play behavior of girls to be incompatible with her own behavioral style (18).

Handedness

Slightly more males than females show a preference for using the left-hand in unimanual behavioral tasks, such as writing. There is no established consensus for understanding the basis of this sex difference. Genetic factors clearly play a role in determining hand preference. Another line of research implicates adverse prenatal and/or perinatal events that result in an elevation in left-handedness above the approximate gold standard of 10% in the general population.

Zucker et al (43) found that boys with GID (N = 205) had a significantly elevated rate of left-handedness (19.5%) when compared to three separate quasi-epidemiologic samples of boys (11.8%, total N = 13,253) and with a diagnostically heterogeneous sample of clinical control boys (8.3%, N = 205). This finding parallels studies of adult males with GID, who also appear to have an elevated rate of left handedness as well as studies of adult men with a homosexual sexual orientation (44). Although adult females with GID and women with a homosexual sexual orientation appear to have higher rates of left handedness (or nonrighthandedness), one study of girls with GID did not find any indication of a higher rate of left handedness (45). At present, the explanation for the elevation in boys with GID remains unclear, but candidate factors have centered on some type of perturbation in prenatal development that, in some way, affects sex-dimorphic behavioral differentiation.

Sibling Sex Ratio and Birth Order

Boys with GID have an excess of brothers to sisters (sibling sex ratio) and have a later birth order. Some additional evidence shows that boys with GID are born later primarily in relation to the number of older brothers, but not sisters (46, 47). In the Blanchard et al (46) study, clinical control boys showed no evidence for an altered sibling sex ratio or a late birth order. These findings mesh nicely with studies of adult males with GID with a homosexual sexual orientation, who also have an excess of brothers to sisters and a later birth order (48).

One biological explanation that has been offered to account for these results pertains to maternal immune reactions during pregnancy. The male fetus is experienced by the mother as more "foreign" (antigenic) than the female fetus. Based on studies with lower animals, it has been suggested that one consequence of this is that the mother produces antibodies that have the consequence of demasculinizing or feminizing the male fetus, but no corresponding masculinizing or defeminizing of the female fetus (48). This model would predict that males born later in a sibship might be more affected, since the mother's antigenicity increases with each successive male pregnancy, which is consistent with the empirical evidence on sibling sex ratio and birth order among GID probands. At present, however, this proposed mechanism has not been formally tested in humans.

Psychosocial Mechanisms

Psychosocial factors, to truly merit causal status, must be shown to influence the emergence of marked cross-gender behavior in the first few years of life. Otherwise, such factors would be better conceptualized as perpetuating rather than predisposing.

Sex Assignment at Birth

Because most children with GID do not have a cooccurring physical intersex condition, sex assignment at birth is invariably in accordance with the external markers of biological sex. In some physical intersex conditions, sex assignment is delayed and, on occasion, changed from the initial sex assignment. It has been argued that prolonged delay or uncertainty about the child's "true" sex can contribute to gender identity conflict in affected individuals (49). This does not, however, appear to be the situation for children with GID.

Prenatal Gender Preference

It is common for parents to express a prenatal gender preference. Other things being equal, parents will have a child of the nonpreferred sex about 50% of the time. Are parents of children with GID more likely than control parents to report having had a desire for a child of the opposite sex? The simple answer appears to be no, at least with regard to the mothers of boys with GID (50). We did find, however, that the maternal wish for a girl was significantly associated with the sex composition and birth order of the sibship. Among the boys with GID with only older brothers, the percentage of mothers who recalled a desire for a daughter was significantly higher than among the probands with other sibship combinations; however, the same pattern was observed in a control group (50).

Social Reinforcement of Cross-Gender Behavior

Understanding the role of parent socialization in the genesis and/or perpetuation of GID (e.g., via reinforcement principles or modeling) has been influenced by the normative developmental literature on sex-dimorphic sex-typed behavior (18). It should be recognized, however, that some critics are quite skeptical of the role of parent socialization in inducing sex differences in sex-typed behavior among ordinary children or within-sex variations. The literature on GID must be appraised against this backdrop of competing views on the role of socialization.

Clinicians of diverse theoretical persuasions have consistently reported that the parental response to early cross-gender behavior in children with GID is typically neutral (tolerance) or even encouraging (14). Regarding boys with GID, Roberts et al (51) assessed parental recall of such responses taken from clinical and structured interviews at the time of assessment. From this line of research, Green (17) concluded that "what comes closest so far to being a *necessary* variable is that, as any feminine behavior begins to emerge, there is *no* discouragement of that behavior by the child's principal caretaker" (p. 238, italics in original). In a structured interview study, Mitchell (52) found that mothers of boys with GID were more likely to tolerate or encourage feminine behaviors and less likely to encourage masculine behaviors than were the mothers of both clinical and normal control boys.

Of course, the limitations of this kind of interview data need to be recognized. Nonetheless, one aspect of these data deserves special comment. As noted, clinicians of diverse theoretical persuasions have observed the apparent tolerance, or even encouragement, of feminine behavior shown by parents of boys with GID. However, the fact that these parents have sought out a clinical assessment usually means that they are now concerned about their child's gender identity development. From the standpoint of attribution theory (53), one might predict that parents would minimize their encouragement or tolerance of cross-gender behavior, since it has such an obvious bearing on "causality." Yet a majority of the parents whom we have assessed do not recall systematic efforts to limit or redirect their child's cross-gender behavior, particularly during the initial period of symptom onset and for various periods of time thereafter.

The reasons why parents might tolerate, if not encourage, early cross-gender behaviors appear to be quite diverse, suggesting that the antecedents to this "end state" are multiple in origin. Some parents report being influenced by ideas regarding nonsexist child rearing. In other parents, the antecedents seem to be rooted in pervasive conflict that revolves around gender issues. For example, a small subgroup of mothers (about 10%) of boys with GID appear to experience something akin to what we have termed *pathologic gender mourning* (14). During the pregnancy, there is a strong desire for a girl [in all of the cases, the mother had already borne at least one other son, but no daughter—except in three instances in which the daughter was given up for adoption (one case) or had died in infancy (two cases)]. After the birth of the nonpreferred son, this wish seems to color strongly the mother's perception and relationship with her newborn, and there are strong signs of ambivalence about his gender status. Various signs of pathologic gender mourning include severe postpartum depression related to the birth of a son, recurrent night dreams about being pregnant with a girl, delayed naming, and active cross-dressing of the boy (14, 54). The most common psychological trait associated with the strong wish for a daughter appears to be the need to nurture and be nurtured by a female child, which often reflects compensatory needs originating in childhood.

General Psychopathology

The role of maternal psychopathology in the genesis and perpetuation of GID has received a great deal of clinical and theoretical attention but, unfortunately, only limited empirical evaluation. At the outset, it should be noted that the available empirical studies have been delimited to the mothers of boys with GID—comparable studies are not available regarding the mothers of girls with GID (14).

Marantz and Coates (31) found that the mothers of boys with GID showed more signs of psychopathology than did the mothers of demographically matched normal boys, including more pathologic ratings on the Diagnostic Interview for Borderline Personality Disorder and more symptoms of depression on the Beck Depression Inventory.

Figure 5.13.3 shows the percentage of mothers of boys with GID (N = 245) with 0, 1, 2, or 3+ diagnoses on the Diagnostic Interview Schedule (55). It can be seen that almost half of the mothers met DIS criteria for two or more diagnoses and over 30% had three or more diagnoses. The most common diagnoses were major depressive episode and recurrent major depression.

The emerging data on emotional distress and psychiatric impairment in the mothers of boys with GID indicate that it is more common than in the mothers of normal control boys and at least comparable to the mothers of clinical control boys (55). Still, we are left with the problem of specificity (56), in that these maternal characteristics are not unique to the mothers of boys with GID, but common to the mothers of clinic-referred boys in general. Accordingly, maternal emotional distress/impairment functions, at best, only as a nonspecific risk factor in the development of GID. If the mother's emotional state truly is involved in the genesis of GID, then there should be evidence of psychiatric impairment prior to and during the emergence of the child's symptoms. The data are suggestive that this is the case, and that the presence of emotional difficulties in the mothers is not simply a reaction to having a child with GID (14).

Marantz and Coates (31) argued that the presence of psychopathology renders the mothers emotionally unavailable, which results in anxiety and insecurity in the son, and that it is this state of affairs that is partly responsible for symptom onset. Indeed, Coates and Person (57) advanced a very specific hypothesis, namely that the erratic and uneven emotional availability of the mothers activated separation anxiety in the boys, which, in turn, activated the symptoms of GID: "In imitating 'Mommy' [the boy] confuse[s] 'being Mommy' with 'having Mommy.' [Cross-gender behavior] appears to allay, in part, the anxiety generated by the loss of the mother" (p. 708). Indeed, boys with GID appear to have high rates of separation anxiety traits, as judged by maternal report on a structured interview schedule (58) and their own responses on the Separation Anxiety Test (59).

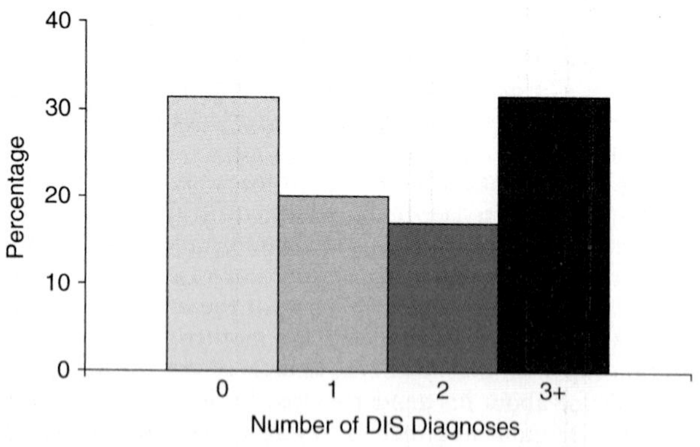

FIGURE 5.13.3. Maternal Diagnostic Interview Schedule diagnoses (in %). (Data from Zucker KJ: Patterns of psychopathology in boys with gender identity disorder. Paper presented at the joint meeting of the American Academy of Child and Adolescent Psychiatry and the Canadian Academy of Child and Adolescent Psychiatry, Toronto, October 2005.)

Because separation anxiety is likely a nonspecific risk factor (i.e., many boys who have these qualities do not have GID), the crucial question that remains is why only a small minority of boys develop the "fantasy solution" of wanting to be a girl. Various predisposing factors have been implicated, including temperamental characteristics of the child, the premorbid relationship with the mother, the position of the father in the family system, that the family psychopathology must occur during the putative sensitive period for gender identity formation (3), and so on. At present, however, the question of specificity remains unanswered in any satisfactory manner.

The role of paternal influences in the genesis and perpetuation of GID has also received a great deal of clinical and theoretical attention but, again, only limited empirical evaluation, which has been delimited to the fathers of boys with GID.

One account implicates the father's role by virtue of his absence from the family matrix. Across 10 samples of boys with GID, the rate of father absence (e.g., owing to separation or divorce) was 34.5% (14). It is unlikely, however, that this rate would differ significantly from the rate found in clinical populations in general, if not the general population. Green (60) found that paternal separations occurred earlier in the families of boys with GID than normal control boys; therefore, it is possible that timing is an additional variable to consider. Green also found that the fathers of boys with GID (both father-present and father-absent) recalled spending less time with their sons than did the fathers of control boys during the second year of life, years 3 to 5, and at the time of assessment. The inclusion of a clinical control group would be helpful in gauging the specificity of this finding.

Course and Prognosis

Followup Studies of Boys

Green's (60) study constitutes the most comprehensive long-term followup of behaviorally feminine boys, the majority of whom would likely have met DSM criteria for GID. His study contained 66 feminine and 56 control boys (unselected for gender identity) assessed initially at a mean age of 7.1 yrs (range, 4–12). Forty-four feminine boys and 30 control boys were available for followup at a mean age of 18.9 yrs (range, 14–24). The majority of the boys were not in therapy between assessment and followup. Sexual orientation in fantasy and behavior was assessed by means of a semistructured interview. Kinsey ratings were made on a 7-point continuum, ranging from exclusive heterosexuality (a Kinsey "0") to exclusive homosexuality (a Kinsey "6"). Depending on the measure (fantasy or behavior), 75–80% of the previously feminine boys were either bisexual or homosexual (Kinsey ratings between 2 and 6) at followup, vs. 0–4% of the control boys. Green also reported on the gender identity status of the 44 previously feminine boys. He found that only one youth, at the age of 18 yrs, was gender-dysphoric to the extent of considering sex-reassignment surgery.

Data from six other followup reports on 55 boys with GID were summarized by Zucker and Bradley (14). At followup (range, 13–26 yrs), five of these boys were classified as transsexual (with a homosexual sexual orientation), 21 were classified as homosexual, one was classified as a (heterosexual) transvestite, 15 were classified as heterosexual, and 13 could not be rated with regard to sexual orientation. If one excludes the 13 "uncertain" cases in these six studies, then 27 (64.2%) of the remaining 42 cases had "atypical" (i.e., homosexual, transsexual, or transvestitic) outcomes. In these studies, the percentage of boys who showed persistent GID was higher than that reported by Green (11.9% vs .2.2%, respectively), but the percentage who were homosexual (62.1%) was somewhat lower.

Zucker and Bradley (14) reported preliminary followup data on their own sample of 40 boys first seen in childhood (M age at assessment, 8.2 years; range, 3–12). At followup, these boys were, on average, 16.5 years (range, 14–23). Gender identity was assessed by means of a semistructured clinical interview and by questionnaire. Sexual orientation (for a 12-month period prior to the time of evaluation) was assessed for fantasy and behavior using the Kinsey scale in a manner identical to Green's study.

Of the 40 boys, eight (20%) were classified as gender-dysphoric at follow-up. The remaining 80% had a "normal" gender identity. Regarding sexual orientation in fantasy, 20 (50%) were classified as heterosexual, 17 (42.5%) were classified as bisexual/homosexual, and three (7.5%) were classified as "asexual" (i.e., they did not report any sexual fantasies). Regarding sexual orientation in behavior, nine (22.5%) were classified as heterosexual, 11 (27.5%) were classified as bisexual/homosexual, and 20 (50.0%) were classified as "asexual" (i.e., they did not report any interpersonal sexual experiences).

Cohen-Kettenis (61) reported preliminary data on a sample of 56 boys first seen in childhood (M age at assessment, 9 years; range, 6–12) and who had now reached adolescence. Of these, nine (16.1%) requested sex-reassignment, and all nine had a homosexual sexual orientation (PT Cohen-Kettenis, personal communication, February 1, 2003). Thus, the rate of GID persistence, at least into adolescence, was higher than that reported by Green (60) and comparable to the rate obtained by Zucker and Bradley, as noted above.

In taking stock of these outcome data, Green's study clearly shows that boys with GID were disproportionately, and substantially, more likely than the control boys to differentiate a bisexual/homosexual sexual orientation. The other followup studies yielded somewhat lower estimates of a bisexual/homosexual sexual orientation. In this regard, at least one caveat is in order. In the Zucker and Bradley followup, for example, the boys were somewhat younger than were the boys followed up by Green, so their lower rate of a bisexual/homosexual sexual orientation outcome should be interpreted cautiously; one would expect, if anything, these youth to underreport an atypical sexual orientation due to social desirability considerations. But even these lower rates of a bisexual/homosexual sexual orientation are substantially higher than the currently accepted base rate of about 2–3% of a homosexual sexual orientation in men that has been identified in recent epidemiological studies (62).

A more substantive difference between Green's study and the other followup reports pertains to the persistence of gender dysphoria. Both Zucker and Bradley and Cohen-Kettenis, for example, found higher rates of persistence than Green. At present, the explanations for this are unclear. One possibility pertains to sampling differences. Green's study was carried out in the context of an advertised research study, whereas the Zucker and Bradley and Cohen-Kettenis samples were clinic referred. Thus, it is conceivable that their samples may have included more extreme cases of childhood GID than in the sample ascertained by Green. Because the Toronto and Dutch groups now have substantially larger samples on which to complete outcome studies, it should be possible to carry out within-group analyses to identify predictor variables (e.g., with regard to persistent GID vs. desistent GID). Such information is urgently needed in order to understand the variation in gender identity and sexual orientation outcomes within a population of children referred for gender identity problems.

Followup Studies of Girls

Unfortunately, the long-term followup of girls with GID remains very patchy. In part, this reflects the comparatively lower rate of referred girls to referred boys with GID in child samples (11). Since the last edition of this volume, the first systematic followup of girls with GID has become available. Drummond (63) evaluated 25 girls, originally assessed in my clinic at a mean age of 8.8 years (range, 3–12), at a followup mean age of 23.2 years (range, 15–36). Of these 25 girls, three (12%) had persistent GID (at followup ages of 17, 21, and 23 years, respectively), two of whom had a homosexual sexual orientation, the third being asexual. The remaining 22 (88%) girls had a "normal" gender identity.

Regarding sexual orientation in fantasy (Kinsey ratings) for the 12 months preceding the followup assessment, 15 (60%) girls were classified as exclusively heterosexual, eight (32%) were classified as bisexual/homosexual, and two (8%) were classified as "asexual" (they did not report any sexual fantasies). Regarding sexual orientation in behavior, 11 (44%) girls were classified as exclusively heterosexual, six (24%) were classified as bisexual/homosexual, and eight (32%) were classified as "asexual" (they did not report any interpersonal sexual experiences).

Although these data are preliminary, it appears that there is a range of outcomes, but it is clear that the rates of GID and a bisexual/homosexual sexual orientation without cooccurring gender dysphoria are likely to be higher than the base rates of these two aspects of psychosexual differentiation in an unselected population of women. For example, using the Bakker et al (8) estimation of GID prevalence in females, the odds of persistent gender dysphoria in Drummond's sample was 4,084 times the odds of gender dysphoria in the general population. Using prevalence estimates of bisexuality/homosexuality in fantasy among biological females (anywhere between 2% and 5%), the odds of reporting bisexuality/homosexuality in fantasy was 8.9–23.1 times higher than in the general population. The odds of reporting bisexuality/homosexuality in behavior was 6.7–15.5 times higher than in the general population.

In another study, Cohen-Kettenis (61) reported preliminary data on a sample of 18 girls first seen in childhood (M age at assessment, 9 years; range, 6–12) and who had now reached adolescence. Of these, eight (44.4%) requested sex reassignment, and all had a homosexual sexual orientation (P. T. Cohen-Kettenis, personal communication, February 1, 2003). Thus, the rate of GID persistence, at least into adolescence, was high (and much higher than the rate of persistence for boys with GID).

GID Persistence and Desistance in a Comparative-Developmental Perspective

A key challenge for developmental theories of psychosexual differentiation is to account for the disjunction between retrospective and prospective data with regard to GID persistence: It is clear that only a minority of children followed prospectively show a persistence of GID into adolescence and young adulthood.

In some respects, the situation is comparable to that which has been found for other child psychiatric disorders. For example, adults with antisocial personality disorder (APD) invariably will have had a childhood history of oppositional defiant disorder (ODD) and conduct disorder (CD), an example of retrospective continuity (64). Yet, the vast majority of children with ODD and the majority of children with CD followed prospectively will not be diagnosed with APD in adulthood (65, 66).

Regarding children with GID, then, we need to understand why, for the majority, the disorder apparently remits by adolescence, if not earlier. One possible explanation concerns referral bias. Green (17) argued that children with GID who are referred for clinical assessment (and then, in some cases, therapy) may come from families in which there is more concern than is the case for adolescents and adults, the majority of whom did not receive a clinical evaluation and treatment during childhood. Thus, a clinical evaluation and subsequent therapeutic intervention during childhood may alter the natural history of GID. Of course, this is only one account of the disjunction and there may well be additional factors that might distinguish those children who are more strongly at risk for the disorder's continuation from those who are not. One possibility is that the diagnostic criteria for GID, at least as they are currently formulated, simply are not sharp enough to distinguish children who are more likely to show a persistence in the disorder from those who are not.

An additional clue comes from consideration of the concepts of developmental malleability and plasticity. It is possible, for example, that gender identity shows relative malleability during childhood, with a gradual narrowing of plasticity as the gendered sense of self consolidates as one approaches adolescence. Some support for this idea comes from followup studies of adolescents with GID, who appear to show a much higher rate of GID persistence as they are followed into young adulthood.

The best data on long-term outcome on adolescents comes from the Dutch group. Cohen-Kettenis and van Goozen (21) reported that 22 (66.6%) of 33 adolescents went on to receive sexual reassignment surgery (SRS).

At initial assessment, the mean age of the 22 adolescents who received SRS was 17.5 years (range, 15–20). Of the 11 who did not receive SRS, eight were not recommended for it because they were not diagnosed with transsexualism (presumably, the DSM-IV diagnosis of GID); the three remaining patients were given a diagnosis of transsexualism but the "real-life test" (i.e., living for a time as the opposite sex prior to the institution of contrasex hormonal treatment and surgery) was postponed because of severe concurrent psychopathology and/or adverse social circumstances. These data suggest a very high rate of GID persistence, which is eventually treated by SRS. It should be noted that the persistence rate could be even higher than 66% since Cohen-Kettenis and van Goozen did not provide followup information on the 11 patients who were not recommended to proceed with the real-life test or were unable to implement it.

In another study, Smith et al (67) reported that 20 (48.7%) of 41 other adolescent patients went on to receive SRS. At initial assessment, the mean age of the 20 adolescents who received SRS was 16.6 years (range, 15–19). Of the 21 who did not receive SRS (M age, 17.3 yrs; range, 13–20), the reasons were similar to that reported in the earlier study. Data from Smith et al suggest that a substantial number of the patients who did not receive SRS were still gender-dysphoric at the time of a followup assessment that occurred, on average, 4.3 years later.

Treatment

Regarding therapeutics, there are two broad issues that need to be considered: a developmental perspective and the debate about GID as disorder (68–70). From a developmental perspective, there is reasonable evidence to see GID in childhood as malleable and thus likely responsive to therapeutics. In contrast, when GID persists into adolescence (or, as in the "late onset" cases, manifests for the first time in adolescence), the evidence appears to favor a narrowing of plasticity and thus, for many youth, it is probably the case that psychological interventions will be less successful and biomedical interventions (e.g., puberty-blocking treatments followed by cross-sex hormonal treatments and surgery) will need to be implemented (13).

Critics who question the legitimacy of the GID diagnosis and favor alternative terminology, such as "gender-variant" children, are much less inclined to consider therapeutic interventions other than to be supportive of the child's cross-gender identity and to guide children and their families in dealing with the social stigma that is encountered.

The conceptual model adopted by such critics is essentialism, the belief that the child is "born this way" and that there are no psychosocial, psychodynamic, or other factors that might be involved in either a causal or perpetuating manner (69). Some parents who adhere to this perspective and locate therapists who share their viewpoint are enacting some rather bold interventions, not practiced by the more traditional approach, such as encouraging the child to transition to the cross-gender identity and role at a very early age (71). In many respects, then, the approach to treatment is going to depend on the conceptual lens adopted by the clinician regarding the origins of GID (and whether or not it is viewed as a condition to be treated or a "variant" to be supported) (69).

For those clinicians who believe that a therapeutic intervention with GID children is viable, he or she will find a variety of approaches in the literature, including behavior therapy, psychotherapy, family therapy, parental counseling, group therapy, and eclectic combinations of these strategies (72, 73). As reviewed elsewhere (72), all of these strategies appear to have some clinical utility; unfortunately, formal comparative studies have not been conducted; therefore, the most efficacious types of treatment remain unclear.

With adolescents, many clinicians will initially explore with their clients alternatives to physical interventions. One area of inquiry pertains to the meaning behind the adolescent's desire for sex-reassignment surgery and if there are viable alternative life-style adaptations. In this regard, the most common area of exploration pertains to the patient's sexual orientation. Although many adolescents with GID recall that they always felt uncomfortable growing up as boys or as girls, for some the idea of a "sex change" did not begin to crystallize until they became aware of homoerotic attractions. For some of these youth, the idea that they might be gay or homosexual is abhorrent. For such adolescents, psychoeducational work can explore their attitudes and feelings about homosexuality. Group therapy, in which such youngsters have the opportunity to meet gay adolescents, can be a useful adjunct in such cases. In some cases, the gender dysphoria will resolve and a homosexual adaptation ensues. For others, however, a homosexual adaptation is not possible and the gender dysphoria does not abate (74).

For adolescents in whom the gender dysphoria appears chronic, the clinician can consider two main options: 1) management until the adolescent turns 18 and can be referred to an adult gender identity clinic or 2) "early" institution of contra-sex hormonal treatment. Regarding the latter, Gooren and Delemarre-van de Waal (75) recommended that one option with gender-dysphoric adolescents is to prescribe puberty-blocking luteinizing hormone-release agonists (e.g., depot leuprolide or depot triptorelin) that facilitate more successful passing as the opposite sex. Thus, for example, in male adolescents, such medication can suppress the development of secondary sex characteristics, such as facial hair growth and voice deepening, which makes it more difficult to pass in the female social role. Although such early hormonal treatment is controversial, it may well be the treatment of choice once the clinician is confident that other options have been exhausted. If the GID persists after this initial phase of hormonal treatment, one can then move to cross-sex hormonal treatments and surgical interventions (13, 76).

References

1. Martin CL, Ruble DN, Szkrybalo J: Cognitive theories of early gender development. *Psychol Bull* 128:903–933, 2002.
2. Stoller RJ: The hermaphroditic identity of hermaphrodites. *J Nerv Ment Dis* 139:453–457, 1964.
3. Money J, Hampson JG, Hampson JL: Imprinting and the establishment of gender role. *Arch Neurol Psychiatry* 77:333–336, 1957.
4. Hughes IA, Houk C, Ahmed SF, et al.: Consensus statement on management of intersex disorders. *Arch Dis Child* 91:554–563, 2006.
5. Benjamin H: Transsexualism and transvestism as psychosomatic somato-psychic syndromes. *Am J Psychother* 8:219–230, 1954.
6. Bell AP, Weinberg MS, Hammersmith SK: *Sexual Preference: Its Development in Men and Women*. Bloomington, Indiana University Press, 1981.
7. Bailey JM, Zucker KJ: Childhood sex-typed behavior and sexual orientation: A conceptual analysis and quantitative review. *Dev Psychol* 31:43–55, 1995.
8. Bakker A, van Kesteren PJM, Gooren LJG, et al.: The prevalence of transsexualism in the Netherlands. *Acta Psychiatr Scand* 87:237–238, 1993.
9. Achenbach TM, Edelbrock CS: Behavioral problems and competencies reported by parents of normal and disturbed children aged four through sixteen. *Monogr Soc Res Child Dev* 46(1, Serial No. 188), 1981.
10. van Beijsterveldt CEM, Hudziak JJ, Boomsma DI: Genetic and environmental influences on cross-gender behavior and relation to behavior problems: A study of Dutch twins at ages 7 and 10 years. *Arch Sex Behav* 35:647–658, 2006.
11. Cohen-Kettenis PT, Owen A, Kaijser VG, et al.: Demographic characteristics, social competence, and behavior problems in children with gender identity disorder: A cross-national, cross-clinic comparative analysis. *J Abnorm Child Psychol* 31:41–53, 2003.
12. Zucker KJ, Owen A, Bradley SJ, et al.: Gender-dysphoric children and adolescents: A comparative analysis of demographic characteristics and behavioral problems. *Clinical Child Psychology and Psychiatry* 7:398–411, 2002.
13. Cohen-Kettenis PT, Pfäfflin F: *Transgenderism and Intersexuality in Childhood and Adolescence: Making Choices*. Thousand Oaks, CA, Sage Publications, 2003.
14. Zucker KJ, Bradley SJ: *Gender Identity Disorder and Psychosexual Problems in Children and Adolescents*. New York, Guilford Press, 1995.
15. Zucker KJ, Bradley SJ, Sanikhani M: Sex differences in referral rates of children with gender identity disorder: Some hypotheses. *J Abnorm Child Psychol* 25:217–227, 1997.
16. Zucker KJ: Measurement of psychosexual differentiation. *Arch Sex Behav* 34:375–388, 2005.
17. Green R: *Sexual Identity Conflict in Children and Adults*. New York, Basic Books, 1974.
18. Ruble DN, Martin CL, Berenbaum SA: Gender development. In: Damon W, Lerner RM (series eds), Eisenberg N (vol ed): *Handbook of Child Psychology*, 6th ed. Vol .3: Social, Emotional, and Personality Development. New York, Wiley, 2006:858–932.
19. Johnson LL, Bradley SJ, Birkenfeld-Adams AS, et al.: A parent-report Gender Identity Questionnaire for Children. *Arch Sex Behav* 33:105–116, 2004.
20. Cohen-Kettenis PT, Wallien M, Johnson LL, et al.: A parent-report Gender Identity Questionnaire for Children: A cross-national, cross-clinic comparative analysis. *Clinical Child Psychology and Psychiatry* 11:397–405, 2006.
21. Cohen-Kettenis PT, van Goozen SHM: Sex reassignment of adolescent transsexuals: A follow-up study. *J Am Acad Child Adolesc Psychiatry* 36:263–271, 1997.
22. Smith YL, van Goozen SH, Kuiper AJ, et al.: Transsexual subtypes: Clinical and theoretical significance. *Psychiatry Res* 137:151–160, 2005.
23. Zucker KJ, Blanchard R: Transvestic fetishism: Psychopathology and theory. In: Laws DR, O'Donohue W (eds): *Sexual Deviance: Theory, Assessment, and Treatment*. New York, Guilford Press, pp. 253–279, 1997.
24. Blanchard R: Early history of the concept of autogynephilia. *Arch Sex Behav* 34:439–446, 2005.
25. Caron C, Rutter M: Comorbidity in child psychopathology: Concepts, issues and research strategies. *J Child Psychol Psychiatry* 32:1063–1080, 1991.
26. Williams PG, Allard AM, Sears L: Case study: Cross-gender preoccupations in two male children with autism. *J Autism Dev Disord* 26:635–642, 1996.
27. Mukaddes NM: Gender identity problems in autistic children. *Child Care Health Dev* 28:529–532, 2002.
28. Perera H, Gadambanathan T, Weerasiri S: 2003. Gender identity disorder presenting in a girl with Asperger's disorder and obsessive compulsive disorder. *Ceylon Med J* 48:57–58, 2003.
29. Edelbrock C, Achenbach TM: A typology of Child Behavior Profile patterns: Distribution and correlates in disturbed children age 6 to 16. *J Abnorm Child Psychol* 8:441–470, 1980.
30. Fridell SR: Sex-typed play behavior and peer relations in boys with gender identity disorder. Unpublished doctoral dissertation, Ontario Institute for Studies in Education of the University of Toronto, 2001.
31. Marantz S, Coates S: Mothers of boys with gender identity disorder: A comparison with matched controls. *J Am Acad Child Adolesc Psychiatry* 30:310–315, 1991.
32. Dessens AB, Slijper FME, Drop SLS: Gender dysphoria and gender change in chromosomal females with congenital adrenal hyperplasia. *Arch Sex Behav* 34:389–397, 2005.
33. Cohen-Kettenis PT: Gender change in 46,XY persons with 5α-reductase-2 deficiency and 17β-hydroxysteroid dehydrogenase-3 deficiency. *Arch Sex Behav* 34:399–410, 2005.
34. Mazur T: Gender dysphoria and gender change in androgen insensitivity or micropenis. *Arch Sex Behav* 34:411–421, 2005.
35. Meyer-Bahlburg HFL: Gender identity outcome in female-raised 46,XY persons with penile agenesis, cloacal exstrophy of the bladder, or penile ablation. *Arch Sex Behav* 34:423–438, 2005.
36. Meyer-Bahlburg HFL: Gender identity disorder of childhood: introduction. *J Am Acad Child Psychiatry* 24:681–683, 1985.
37. Meyer-Bahlburg HFL: Introduction: gender dysphoria and gender change in persons with intersexuality. *Arch Sex Behav* 34:371–373, 2005.
38. Goy RW, Bercovitch FB, McBrair MC: Behavioral masculinization is independent of genital masculinization in prenatally androgenized female rhesus macaques. *Horm Behav* 22:552–571, 1988.
39. Segal NL: Two monozygotic twin pairs discordant for female-to-male transsexualism. *Arch Sex Behav* 35:346–357, 2006.
40. Campbell DW, Eaton WO: Sex differences in the activity level of infants. *Infant Child Dev* 8:1–17, 1999.
41. Bates JE, Bentler PM, Thompson SK: Gender-deviant boys compared with normal and clinical control boys. *J Abnorm Child Psychol* 7:243–259, 1979.
42. Zucker KJ: Gender-related behavior in girls with or without somatic intersexuality. Paper presented at the International Behavioral Development Symposium: Biological Basis of Sexual Orientation, Gender Identity, and Sex-Typical Behavior, Minot, ND, August 2005.
43. Zucker KJ, Beaulieu N, Bradley SJ, et al.: Handedness in boys with gender identity disorder. *J Child Psychol Psychiatry* 42:767–776, 2001.
44. Lalumière ML, Blanchard R, Zucker KJ: Sexual orientation and handedness in men and women: A meta-analysis. *Psychol Bull* 126:575–592, 2000.
45. Zucker KJ: Do girls with gender identity disorder have a natural history? Presidential address, International Academy of Sex Research, Amsterdam, The Netherlands, July 2006.
46. Blanchard R, Zucker KJ, Bradley SJ, et al.: Birth order and sibling sex ratio in homosexual male adolescents and probably prehomosexual feminine boys. *Dev Psychol* 31:22–30, 1995.
47. Zucker KJ, Green R, Coates S, et al.: Sibling sex ratio of boys with gender identity disorder. *J Child Psychol Psychiatry* 38:543–551, 1997.
48. Blanchard R: Fraternal birth order and the maternal immune hypothesis of male homosexuality. *Horm Behav* 40:105–114, 2001.
49. Meyer-Bahlburg HFL, Gruen RS, New MI, et al.: Gender change from female to male in classical congenital adrenal hyperplasia. *Horm Behav* 30:319–332, 1996.
50. Zucker KJ, Green R, Garofano C, et al.: Prenatal gender preference of mothers of feminine and masculine boys: Relation to sibling sex composition and birth order. *J Abnorm Child Psychol* 22:1–13, 1994.
51. Roberts CW, Green R, Williams K, et al.: Boyhood gender identity development: A statistical contrast of two family groups. *Dev Psychol* 23:544–557, 1987.
52. Mitchell JN: Maternal Influences on gender identity disorder in boys: Searching for specificity. Unpublished doctoral dissertation, York University, Downsview, Ontario, Canada, 1991.
53. Weiner B: On sin versus sickness: A theory of perceived responsibility and social motivation. *Am Psychol* 48:957–965, 1983.
54. Zucker KJ, Bradley SJ, Ipp M: Delayed naming of a newborn boy: Relationship to the mother's wish for a girl and subsequent cross-gender identity in the child by the age of two. *J Psychol Hum Sex* 6:57–68, 1993.
55. Zucker KJ: Patterns of psychopathology in boys with gender identity disorder. Paper presented at the joint meeting of the American Academy of Child and Adolescent Psychiatry and the Canadian Academy of Child and Adolescent Psychiatry, Toronto, October 2005.
56. Garber J, Hollon SD: What can specificity designs say about causality in psychopathology research? *Psychol Bull* 110:129–136, 1991.
57. Coates S, Person ES: Extreme boyhood femininity: isolated behavior or pervasive disorder? *J Am Acad Child Psychiatry* 24:702–709, 1985.
58. Zucker KJ, Bradley SJ, Sullivan CBL: Traits of separation anxiety in boys with gender identity disorder. *J Am Acad Child Adol Psychiatry* 35:791–798, 1996.
59. Birkenfeld-Adams AS: Quality of attachment in young boys with gender identity disorder: A comparison to clinic and nonreferred control boys. Unpublished doctoral dissertation, Downsview, Ontario, York University, 1999.
60. Green R: *The "Sissy Boy Syndrome" and the Development of Homosexuality*. New Haven, Yale University Press, 1987.

61. Cohen-Kettenis PT: Gender identity disorder in *DSM*? [Letter]. *J Am Acad Child Adolesc Psychiatry* 40:391, 2001.
62. Laumann EO, Gagnon JH, Michael RT, et al.: *The Social Organization of Sexuality: Sexual Practices in the United States.* Chicago, University of Chicago Press, 1994.
63. Drummond KD: A follow-up study of girls with gender identity disorder. Unpublished master's thesis, Ontario Institute for Studies in Education of the University of Toronto, 2006.
64. Robins LN: Sturdy childhood predictors of adult antisocial behaviour: Replication from longitudinal studies. *Psychol Med* 8:611–622, 1978.
65. Lahey BB, McBurnett K, Loeber R: Are attention-deficit/hyperactivity disorder and oppositional defiant disorder developmental precursors to conduct disorder? In: Sameroff AJ, Lewis M, Miller SM (eds). *Handbook of Developmental Psychopathology*, 2nd ed. New York, Kluwer Academic/Plenum Publishers, 2000, pp. 431–446.
66. Zoccolillo M, Pickles A, Quinton D, et al.: The outcome of childhood conduct disorder: Implications for defining adult personality disorder and conduct disorder. *Psychol Med* 22:971–986, 1992.
67. Smith YLS, van Goozen SHM, Cohen-Kettenis PT: Adolescents with gender identity disorder who were accepted or rejected for sex reassignment surgery: A prospective follow-up study. *J Am Acad Child Adolesc Psychiatry* 40:472–481, 2001.
68. Bartlett NH, Vasey PL, Bukowski WM: Is gender identity disorder in children a mental disorder? *Sex Roles* 43:753–785, 2000.
69. Menvielle EJ, Tuerk C, Perrin EC: To the beat of a different drummer: The gender-variant child. *Contemp Pediatrics* 22(2):38–39, 41, 43, 45–46, 2005.
70. Langer SJ, Martin JI: How dresses can make you mentally ill: Examining gender identity disorder in children. *Child Adolesc Soc Work J* 21:5–23, 2004.
71. Santiago R: 5-year-old "girl" starting school is really a boy. *The Miami Herald*. Retrieved on July 11, 2006 at http://www.miami.com/mld/miamiherald/living/education/15003026.htm.
72. Zucker KJ: Gender identity disorder in children, adolescents, and adults. In: Gabbard GO, (ed). *Treatments of Psychiatric Disorders*, 4th ed. Washington, DC, American Psychiatric Press, in press.
73. Zucker KJ: "I'm half-boy, half-girl": Play psychotherapy and parent counseling for gender identity disorder. In: Spitzer RL, First MB, Williams JBW, et al. (eds). *DSM-IV-TR® Casebook, Volume 2. Experts Tell How They Treated Their Own Patients.* Washington, DC, American Psychiatric Publishing, 2006, pp. 321–334.
74. Zucker KJ: Gender identity disorder. In: Wolfe DA, Mash EJ (eds). *Behavioral and Emotional Disorders in Adolescents: Nature, Assessment, and Treatment.* New York, Guilford Press, 2006, pp. 535–562.
75. Gooren L, Delemarre-van de Waal H: The feasibility of endocrine interventions in juvenile transsexuals. *J Psychol Hum Sex* 8(4):69–84, 1996.
76. Meyer W, Bockting WO, Cohen-Kettenis P, et al.: The Harry Benjamin Gender Dysphoria Association's Standards of Care for Gender Identity Disorders, 6th Version. *J Psychol Hum Sex* 13(1):1–30, 2001.

CHAPTER 5.14 ■ PERSONALITY DISORDERS IN CHILDREN AND ADOLESCENTS

CARLA SHARP AND EFRAIN BLEIBERG

INTRODUCTION

The revised fourth edition of the *Diagnostic and Statistical Manual of Mental Disorders (DSM-IV—TR)* (1) defines personality disorder (PD) as "an enduring pattern of inner experiences and behavior that deviates markedly from the expectations of the individual's culture." This pattern is manifested in two or more of the following areas: cognition; affectivity; interpersonal functioning; and impulse control. The enduring pattern is characterized as "inflexible and pervasive across a broad range of personal and social situations" and as a pattern that leads to "clinically significant distress or impairment in social, occupational or other important areas of functioning." Finally, *DSM-IV-TR* states that the pattern is "stable and of long duration" and that its onset can be traced back "at least to adolescence or early adulthood."

PD represent a staggering burden to society. Surveys document that they affect a significant percentage of the general population, with a prevalence estimated between 10% and 13% (2, 3). Merikangas and Weissman (4) found that approximately half of those receiving mental health treatment suffer from a personality disorder. Yet the significance of the personality disorders extends far beyond the suffering of the affected individuals and their families. Personality disorders involve patterns of maladjustment associated with extraordinary social costs: Individuals with personality disorder experience high rates of divorce, unemployment, and homelessness (5); accidents (6); violence, assaultive behavior, and homicide (7, 8); self-injurious and parasuicidal behavior (9); attempted and completed suicide (10); increased need for medical care and hospitalization and visits to the emergency room (11); and criminality, alcoholism and drug abuse (12). Personality disorders are associated with disability, underachievement, family disruption, child abuse and neglect, illegitimacy, STDs, delayed recovery from medical illness, malpractice suits, medical and judicial recidivism, and dependency on the public (13).

Patients with PD present formidable challenges to clinicians and psychiatric treatment settings as they display characteristically maladaptive patterns of coping and relating in their relationships with their treaters. The presence of a personality disorder accounts for a significant degree of the treatment failures or delayed recoveries in the treatment of comorbid axis I psychiatric disorders such as depression (14), bipolar disorder (15), or obsessive compulsive disorder (16), as well as with dissatisfaction and disruption of psychiatric treatment. Clinicians treating patients with PD struggle with their own emotional reactions as the treatment process strains their competence, sensitivity, integrity and commitment to ethical standards and professional behavior.

Not surprisingly, the study of PD, as Millon and Davis (17) noted, is fraught with more controversy than any other area of psychopathology. The controversies are particularly pronounced regarding the child and adolescent antecedents of the PD of adulthood. Questions can indeed be raised regarding whether we can make the diagnosis of personality disorder in a child or an adolescent. PD is defined as relatively enduring and pervasively maladaptive patterns of coping, thinking, feeling, and relating. Children and adolescents, whether suffering from psychiatric disorders or not, are engaged in dramatic and highly fluid developmental processes in which every aspect of their bodies and personalities affecting their patterns of coping, thinking, feeling, and relating are constantly changing at different rates, creating new equilibriums and disequilibriums within the children and in their relations with the environment.

Such fluidity challenges the categorical approach to PD enshrined in *DSM-IV-TR*, which defines PD as a discrete diagnosis with clear boundaries. Yet, as Cicchetti and Cohen (18), among others, have noted, the developmental trajectories of specific patterns of adjustment and maladjustment, including the patterns of coping, thinking, feeling, and relating that define personality and underlie adjustment or maladjustment, may be categorized and classified just as "disorders" are. Along these lines, Kernberg, Weiner and Bardenstein (19) contend that children exhibit distinctive patterns of perceiving reality and thinking about themselves and the environment that endure across time and situation and that these patterns warrant the designation of personality disorder, regardless of the children's age, when they become inflexible, maladaptive, and chronic; cause significant impairment, and produce severe subjective distress. A developmental approach to the investigation of personality and PD is thus crucial not only conceptually but also as a path to early identification, treatment and prevention. Early intervention appears essential in PD in order to preclude the development of the relatively enduring traits and patterns of maladjustment associated with the enormous personal and family suffering and massive social burden outlined above.

As Shapiro (20) cautions, however, empirical data supporting the validity and reliability of the construct and diagnosis of PD in children and adolescents are largely lacking. Given the significant stigma associated with a diagnosis of personality disorder, particularly in regard to diagnoses such as psychopathy (21) or borderline personality, diagnostic circumspection is clearly warranted, particularly in the absence of solid empirical evidence of diagnostic validity and reliability.

Not surprisingly, there has been growing interest in the empirical investigation of personality disorders in children and adolescents over the last two decades. Most research has focused on Borderline Personality Disorder (BPD) and antisocial personality disorder (22, 23).

This chapter will review BPD, the most extensively studied personality disorder in children, adolescent and adults, as illustrative of the challenges and the importance of understanding PD as it unfolds and becomes organized in childhood and adolescence and as a window into the developmental processes in which biological and psychosocial risk and protective factors interact to shape developmental trajectories and patterns of adjustment and maladjustment.

BORDERLINE PERSONALITY DISORDER (BPD)

Definition

DSM-IV-TR includes BPD in the cluster B of the personality disorders, which also comprises the histrionic, narcissistic, and antisocial personality disorders. *DSM-IV* provides criteria for BPD unmodified by developmental considerations (Table 5.14.1).

However, the fourth edition of the *DSM* suggests, for the first time, that BPD can be diagnosed in children and adolescents when maladaptive traits have been present for at least 1 year (in contrast to 2 years for adult BPD) and the traits are pervasive, persistent, and unlikely to be limited to a particular developmental stage or an episode of Axis I disorder.

TABLE 5.14.1

DSM-IV-TR CRITERIA FOR BORDERLINE PERSONALITY DISORDER

A pervasive pattern of instability of interpersonal relationships, self-image, and affects, and marked impulsivity beginning by early adulthood and present in a variety of contexts, as indicated by five (or more) of the following:

1. Frantic efforts to avoid real or imagined abandonment *Note*: Do not include suicidal or self-mutilating behavior covered in criterion 5.
2. A pattern of unstable and intense interpersonal relationships characterized by altering between extremes of idealization and devaluation
3. Identity disturbance: markedly and persistently unstable self-image or sense of self
4. Impulsivity in at least two areas that are potentially self-damaging (e.g., spending, sex, substance abuse, reckless driving, binge eating) *Note*: Do not include suicidal or self-mutilating behavior covered in criterion 5.
5. Recurrent suicidal behavior, gestures, or threats, or self-mutilating behavior
6. Affective instability due to a marked reactivity of mood (e.g., intense episodic dysphoria, irritability, or anxiety usually lasting a few hours and only rarely more than a few days)
7. Chronic feelings of emptiness
8. Inappropriate, intense anger or difficulty controlling anger (e.g., frequent displays of temper, constant anger, recurrent physical fights)
9. Transient, stress-related paranoid ideation or severe dissociative symptoms

To diagnose a personality disorder in an individual under age 18 years, the features must have been present for at least 1 year.

History

Clinical descriptions of BPD in childhood, beginning in the late 1940s, formulated these children's symptoms within a psychoanalytic framework (24). Margaret Mahler and colleagues (25) suggested the term borderline psychosis to refer to children at the milder end of a proposed continuum that extended to the most severe psychotic conditions of childhood. Ekstein and Wallerstein (26) used the term borderline to describe children who were not mildly or incipiently psychotic but presented, instead, a stable condition, paradoxically defined by its persistent instability, and characterized by rapid and ongoing shifts in levels of ego functioning, including reality testing, relationships with others, and defense mechanisms. Such formulations defined borderline children as less severely disturbed than psychotic children but more seriously impaired than neurotic children. In a similar vein, Kernberg (27) characterized "borderline" as a level of development and organization underlying several personality disorders. This developmental pattern, according to Kernberg, included limitations in the capacity to differentiate self from others, reliance in primitive defenses and attainment of reality testing, without the achievement of object constancy and identity integration.

Such formulations of borderline pathology in children used diverse clinical criteria, and likely described a heterogeneous population (28), but laid the foundation for the development of formal criteria for BPD in children and adolescents, as summarized in Table 5.14.2.

TABLE 5.14.2

EFFORTS TO DESCRIBE FORMAL DIAGNOSTIC CRITERIA OF BPD IN CHILDREN AND ADOLESCENTS

Lofgren, Bemporad, et al. (63)	Vela, Gottlieb, et al. (98)	Golman, D'Angelo, et al. (18)
1. Paradigmatic fluctuation of functioning, with rapid shifts between psychotic-like and neurotic levels of reality testing 2. A lack of "signal anxiety" and a proneness to states of panic dominated by overwhelming concerns of body dissolution, annihilation, or abandonment 3. A disruption in thought processes and content that shifts rapidly into loose, idiosyncratic thinking 4. An impairment in relationships, with much difficulty, when under stress, in distinguishing self from others, in appreciating other people's needs, or in integrating disparate emotional experiences into a coherent relationship 5. A lack of impulse control with an inability to contain intense affects, delay gratification, control rage, or modulate destructive an self-destructive tendencies	1. Disturbances in interpersonal relationships 2. Disturbances in the sense of reality 3. Excessive anxiety 4. Severe impulse problems 5. "Neurotic-like" symptoms 6. Uneven or distorted development	1. A pattern of unstable and intense interpersonal relationships characterized by alternation between extremes of overidealization and devaluation and/or marked distortion of the nature of the relationship *Example:* Describing teacher as a "girlfriend," chronic inability to maintain friendships despite wish to do so 2. Impulsiveness in at least two areas that are potentially self-damaging (e.g., reckless risk taking, running away, stealing, substance abuse, sex, binge eating) *Example:* Walking across railroad bridge railing; sniffing glue 3. Affective instability: marked, rapid shifts from baseline mood to depression, irritability, or anxiety lasting less than a few hours and only rarely more than a few days; episodes may include transient distortions of reality *Example:* Early-afternoon anxiety attached with persecutory delusions, followed by successful participation in soccer game in late afternoon 4. Inappropriate, intense anger or lack of control of anger (e.g., frequent displays of temper, constant anger, recurrent physical fights) *Example:* Easily provoked, frequent fights, threatens and attempts to throw therapist out window 5. Recurrent suicidal threats, gestures, or behavior or self-mutilating or self-endangering acts *Example:* Carves boyfriend's name into arm, multiple episodes of being struck by car 6. Marked and persistent disturbance in self-perception and self-presentation characterized by confusion regarding two of the following: gender identity or roles, friendships, socially appropriate behaviors, school or career plans, self-image *Example:* Chronic cross-dressing, running for class president despite having no friends 7. Chronic feelings of emptiness or boredom *Example:* Chronic complaints of boredom, unable to invest in appropriate activities 8. Frantic efforts to avoid, or major preoccupation with, real or imagined abandonment (do not include suicidal or self-mutilating behavior covered in item 5). *Example:* Continual concern that therapist will not be there at next appointment, refusal to leave house while parent is at work

Goldman and colleagues (29) were the first to adapt standardized adult DSM criteria for BPD in children and adolescents (see third column, Table 5.14.2), thus allowing for the comparison of findings from different studies and the application of adult assessment tools to child and adolescent samples.

Epidemiology

Reliable epidemiological data on prevalence rates of BPD in children and adolescents are limited, with rates varying depending on the population sampled.

Inpatient Settings

Studies that have investigated rates of BPD in adolescents' inpatients with histories of depression and suicide attempts points to higher prevalence rates in adolescents compared to adults (30–32). Similarly, Levy et al. (33) showed a BPD rate of 43% in 165 adolescent inpatients (mean age 15.5 years). Grilo and colleagues (34) demonstrated nonsignificant differences in rates of BPD for adolescents (49%) versus young adults (43%) using the same measures for both samples.

Community Settings

The Toronto Adolescent Longitudinal Study (35) by Korenblum and colleagues pioneered the study of BPD in children and adolescents in community settings in a small community sample (n = 72), where 42% of adolescents showed some degree of personality disturbance, of which 40% fell into a cluster B disorder. In a second community sample (n = 63) the same investigators found that 46% of 13-year old school children met criteria for BPD. The largest community based study of juvenile BPD to date (the Children in the Community Study), assessed a sample of 733 children between the ages of 9 and 19 years, and found a prevalence of 3%.

The inconsistency in prevalence rates likely resulted from variations in the design of the studies, the measures employed and the populations studied. Clearly, large-scale, community-based, epidemiological studies, utilizing reliable measures, are needed in order to ascertain the true prevalence rates of juvenile BPD.

Etiology

Models are emerging that seek to integrate biological and psychosocial factors interacting with one another to generate a developing organization of capacities, attitudes, values and goals, coping strategies, relationship patterns and ways of feeling, processing experience and responding across contexts. A selective review of investigations of genetic-biological and psychosocial factors in the etiology of BPD will be followed by an examination of these emerging interactional models.

Genetic Factors

Studies investigating genetic factors associated with BPD have included family, adoption, and twin studies. Family studies of BPD point to a morbidity risk of 11.5% in first-degree relatives (36). A twin study reported concordances rates for BPD of 35% for dizygotic twins and 7% for monozygotic pairs (37).

Studies taking a dimensional approach have combined phenotypic factor analyses of personality disorder questionnaires with multivariate genetic analyses. Using this methodology, several genetic factors underlying personality disturbance have been identified. One factor includes affective liability and instability in cognitive functioning, sense of self, and interpersonal relationships, a cluster of traits closely resembling the diagnostic criteria for BPD. This factor has shown heritability estimated at 47% (38).

This and other studies point to a genetic role in the etiology of BPD, but verification in child and adolescent samples is lacking. Recent reports confirm the role of genetic factors in psychopathy in children as young as 7 years old (39). Such data are not yet available for other PDs, including juvenile BPD.

Biological Factors

A robust body of evidence supports the linkage between a broad array of neuropsychiatric vulnerabilities and BPD (40). Some authors proposed that at least a subgroup of borderline patients have a vulnerability to affective dysregulation, which gives rise to mood lability and heightened sensitivity to rejection and abandonment (41). Klein hypothesized that manipulative relations result from affective dysregulation rather than causing it.

A number of studies demonstrate significantly higher rates of depression, mood disorders, and substance abuse in first-degree relatives of individuals with personality disorder, but no increase in schizophrenia spectrum disorders (42). The linkage between these disorders and BPD, however, is neither uniform nor strong.

A linkage has also been established between BPD and impulse-control disorders. A clear overlap exists between the disruptive behavior disorders—particularly ADHD, conduct disorder, and BPD (43). Studies of delinquent adolescents document a high prevalence of learning disorders and ADHD in this population. Studies of delinquent and conduct-disordered adolescents suggest that at least a subset of these youngsters present BPD associated with ADHD and learning disorders.

Empirical research (44) has focused on impulsive aggression and affective instability as psychobiologic domains relevant to the ethiopathogenesis of BPD. The last decade has seen an explosion of studies investigating these domains in BPD through structural neuroimaging, positron emission tomography (PET), functional neuroimaging (fMRI), neuropsychological tests, EEG and SPECT (45–50).

Studies of serotonergic metabolites, such as 5-hydroxyindoleaacetic acid (5-HIAA) in cerebrospinal fluid (CSF) have demonstrated serotonergic involvement in impulsive aggression (51–53). Neuroimaging data have confirmed reduced serotonergic neurotransmission in cortical inhibitory areas that are usually associated with regulating or dampening the release of aggression (54). Such studies have paved the way for the search of serotonergic candidates genes (55–57), suggesting that individual genetic differences may contribute to reduced serotoninergic involvement in the impulsive aggression associated with BPD.

Functional neuroimaging of affective processing in BPD have shed light on the psychobiology of affective instability. In response to affective stimuli, BPD patients show bilateral increases in activation of the amygdala, suggesting an increased reactivity to emotionally relevant stimuli (58). BPD patients also display increased left amygdala activation to facial expressions of emotion (59), further supporting the notion of deficient affective processing in BPD. In addition, several studies using structural MRI have demonstrated reduced amygdala and hippocampal volume in BPD.

Taken together, studies of the neurobiological correlates of BPD converge in pointing to a dysfunctional fronto-limbic network that could account for both symptoms of impulsive aggression and affective instability and the characteristic hyperreactivity of BPD individuals to loss, abandonment, or frustration. The neural circuit implicated in such dysfunction includes the anterior cingulate cortex (ACC), the orbitofrontal and dorsolateral prefrontal cortex, the hippocampus, and the amygdala (Figure 5.14.1).

Studies of neurobiological correlates of BPD in adults enhance diagnostic specificity and offer the potential of more reliable predictors of treatment response as well as novel targets for therapeutic interventions. However, its etiopathogenic relevance to childhood and adolescent BPD is unclear, as similar neurobiological correlates have not been demonstrated in children and adolescents, except for studies that show that children with significant precursors of BPD precursors present difficulties in executive functioning similar to those demonstrated in adult BPD (61, 62).

Psychosocial Factors

A large body of research into psychosocial predictors of BPD has suggested a range of adverse and traumatic childhood experienced as etiological factors. Most of the studies have been retrospective in nature, thus calling for cautious interpretation. Adult patients with BPD report higher rates of abuse and neglect during childhood (63–68), experiences of disturbed parental involvement during childhood (69), problems tolerating separations and frustration (70); childhood attachment problems (71); parental separation and loss (72, 73) and symptoms of externalizing disorder combined with abnormal neuropsychological functioning, physical abuse, and separations (74).

Studies examining the concurrent presence of the above correlates and risk factors in children and adolescents demonstrate similar psychosocial risk factors to those described in adult BPD, including trauma, neglect, maltreatment, and separation (75–80), exposure to sexual and physical abuse (31), as well as serious parental psychopathology, including depression, substance abuse, or antisocial personality (81). A finding of sexual abuse, in particular, is more discriminatory between BPD and other personality disorders. Obviously correlation does not prove causality. Most abused children do not grow into adults with BPD (82), and a substantial number of adults with BPD lack a history of maltreatment. The focus of research

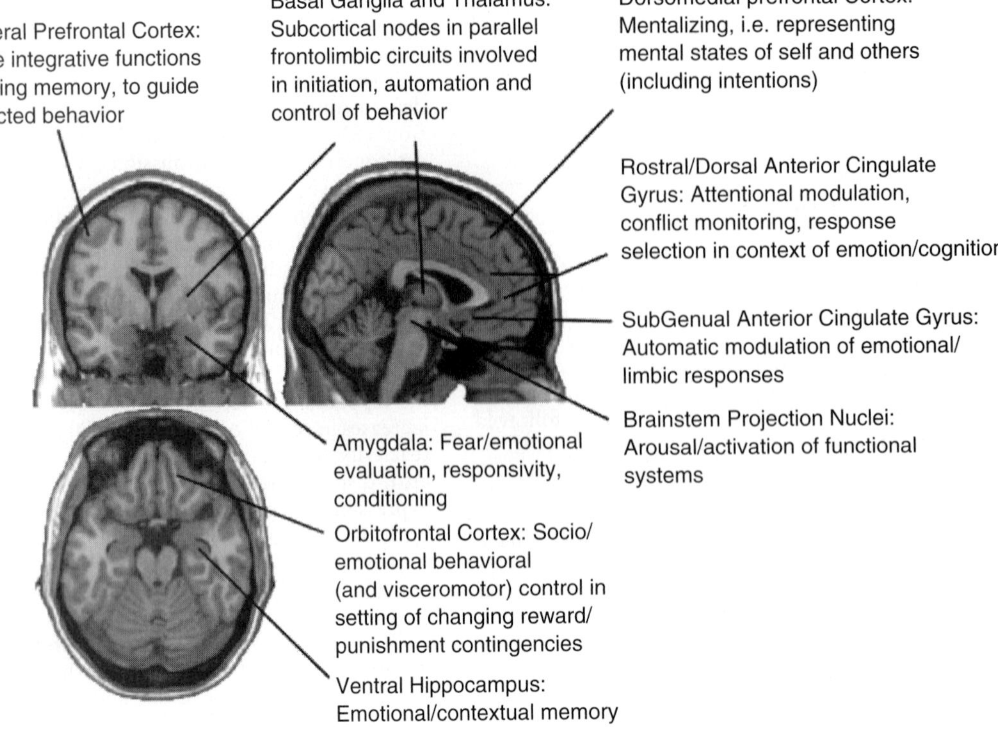
Dorsolateral Prefrontal Cortex: Executive integrative functions and working memory, to guide goal-directed behavior
Basal Ganglia and Thalamus: Subcortical nodes in parallel frontolimbic circuits involved in initiation, automation and control of behavior
Dorsomedial prefrontal Cortex: Mentalizing, i.e. representing mental states of self and others (including intentions)
Rostral/Dorsal Anterior Cingulate Gyrus: Attentional modulation, conflict monitoring, response selection in context of emotion/cognition
SubGenual Anterior Cingulate Gyrus: Automatic modulation of emotional/ limbic responses
Brainstem Projection Nuclei: Arousal/activation of functional systems
Amygdala: Fear/emotional evaluation, responsivity, conditioning
Orbitofrontal Cortex: Socio/ emotional behavioral (and visceromotor) control in setting of changing reward/ punishment contingencies
Ventral Hippocampus: Emotional/contextual memory

FIGURE 5.14.1. The dysfunctional fronto-limbic network underlying the symptoms of Borderline Personality Disorder. (From Brendel GR, Stern E, Silbersweig DA: Defining the neurocircuitry of BPD: functional neuroimaging approaches. *Dev Psychopathol* 17(4):1197–1206, 2005, with permission.)

has thus shifted from whether maltreatment was present or absent to the more nuanced study of the context of relationships and interactions between children and their parents that increase risk or promote resilience in the face of adversity and vulnerability (83).

Psychoanalytic theorists have hypothesized that disruptions in early relationships, particularly in mother–child relationships and in the separation–individuation process, are key factors in the etiology of BPD. Masterson and Rinsley (84) claimed that mothers of future BPD individuals reward passive-dependent, helpless behavior, while ignoring, rejecting, or punishing active striving for mastery, autonomy, and independence, thus thwarting separation and individuation. Adler (85) suggested that the central feature of borderline psychopathology is the patient's inability to evoke the memory of a soothing, comforting parental image when facing distress. Adler attributes this "defect" in internalization to maternal failure in providing a holding environment. The consequence, claimed Alder, is a response to separations and stress characterized by an inner sense of emptiness; reliance on "transitional objects" (86) such as drugs, food, or sex to provide soothing and comfort; and angry, manipulative efforts to force involvement and attention from others.

As the emphasis in maternal responsibility became discredited, greater attention was given to the significance of children's genetically determined strengths and vulnerabilities in shaping their own subjective experience and their parents' response to them. This change in perspective has led to the emergence of integrating perspectives focused on studying the interactive development of biologically prepared appraising and regulating mechanisms, generated in the context of attachment relationships, which in turn underlie adaptive or maladaptive relationships and patterns of coping and experiencing (87).

INTERACTIONAL-INTEGRATING MODELS

Attachment theory has been proposed by a number of authors as a particularly useful framework for conceptualizing the relationship of psychosocial adversity, such as maltreatment and loss, and BPD symptomatology. A review of attachment studies in BPD (71) shows an inverse relationship between adult BPD and security of attachment, with all studies demonstrating an association between BPD and insecure or disorganized attachment.

Fonagy and colleagues (87) suggest that security of attachment is, in turn, linked to the caregiver's mentalizing capacity. Mentalization, the biologically prepared capacity to interpret the mental states that give behavior meaning and intentionality, is proposed by these authors as a fundamental maturational achievement underpinning personality development, particularly the capacity for self-agency and the construction of an autobiographical narrative; the ability for social reciprocity and empathy; the capacity for self-regulation and affect modulation; and the capacity to play and symbolize.

Functional neuroimaging studies provide compelling evidence of brain systems mediating mentalization (88), particularly a neural network including the superior temporal sulcus, the medial prefrontal cortex (including the anterior cingulated cortex) and, to a lesser extent, the amygdala and the orbito-frontal cortex (89, 90).

Secure attachment appears to be the optimal and perhaps the necessary developmental context for the unfolding of the psychobiological capacity to mentalize (87, 91). For Fonagy and colleagues, at the root of the core symptomatology of BPD lies a diminished capacity to mentalize in the context of attachment relationships.

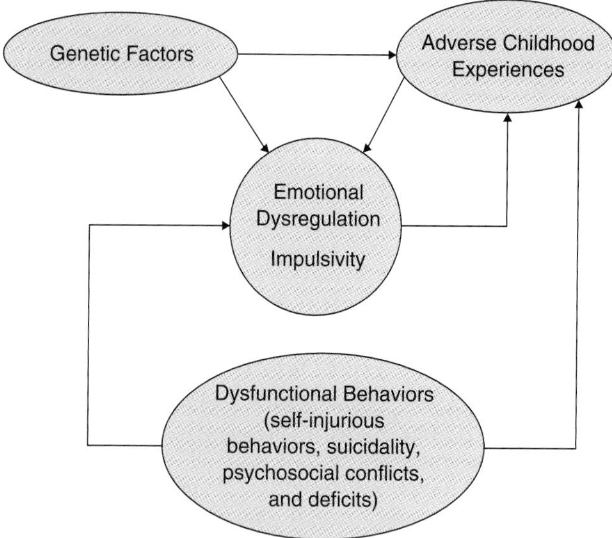

FIGURE 5.14.2. A neurobehavioral model of borderline personality disorder. (Adapted with permission from Lieb K, Zanarini MC, Schmahl C, Linehan MM, Bohus M: Borderline personality disorder. *The Lancet.* 364:453–461, 2004.)

Neurodevelopmental models of BPD have attempted to examine the reciprocal relationship between biological and psychosocial factors underlying the developmental disruptions postulated to account for BPD (Figure 5.14.2).

An example of such models is proposed by Fonagy, Bleiberg, and others (87, 92), who advanced the hypothesis that the developmental trajectory leading to BPD comprises the following elements in various combinations: 1) infants with an exceptional disposition to mentalization (hypersensitivity to social cues); 2) a disposition to increased arousal or affective dysregulation associated to neuropsychiatric vulnerabilities, such as mood disorders or ADHD (37); 3) parents who share similar genetic, neuropsychiatric vulnerabilities or histories of maltreatment; 4) a parental disposition to respond to their children's hyperarousal and signals of distress with hyperarousal and distress of their own and inhibition of their capacity to mentalize, interfering with the capacity to accurately match the children's internal state (87, 93); 5) a corresponding impairment in children's capacity to maintain a stable, mentalized representation of affect and intentionality in self and others in the context of close attachments (94); 6) children's adaptation to stress and relationship trauma with an inhibition of their capacity to deal with mental states, relying instead on prementalistic, coercive maneuvers aiming at achieving self-stability and a sense of attachment (95); and 7) a reinforcement of this psychological and psychosocial adaptation by changes in neural mechanisms of arousal that lead to a low threshold for the triggering of the arousal system with a concurrent inhibition of the frontal and prefrontal structures involved in mentalizing in response to relatively mild emotional stimuli (96). The prototype of such adaptation appears to be the disorganized pattern of attachment.

Such a model may help explain one of the paradoxes of borderline psychopathology of an uncanny sensitivity and reactivity to other people's mental states, accounting for their exquisite capacity to know the right buttons to push to evoke responses from others, and the dramatic intensity of their responses to interpersonal events, incongruously coexisting with remarkable self-centeredness and utter disregard for other people's feelings.

Diagnosis and Clinical Features

Beginning in the early 1980s, a number of authors reported on a substantial consensus among clinicians on the diagnostic criteria for borderline children. These clinical criteria closely parallel the adult criteria for BPD, as defined in *DSM-IV-TR*.

Petti and Vela (27, 97) described the confusion in the clinical literature between children with borderline personality or borderline spectrum disorders and children who, although often referred to as *borderline,* are more appropriately described as falling within the schizotypal personality or schizoid spectrum disorders. Both groups of children present transient psychotic episodes, idiosyncratic fantasies, and magical thinking. Yet only schizotypal children have a family history of schizophrenia spectrum disorder or present constricted, flat, or inappropriate affect; oddness of speech; and discomfort in social situations, which contrast with the intense, dramatic affect and hunger for social response of borderline youths. This differentiation is supported by genetic, epidemiological, and followup studies of adult BPD that discriminate BPD from the schizophrenia–schizotypal spectrum.

Clinical Evaluation

Early manifestations of developmental difficulties are apparent in children who subsequently develop BPD, including a difficult temperament, high activity levels, poor adaptability, negative mood, and problems settling into rhythmic patterns of sleep–wakefulness and feeding. Cranky and hard to soothe, these infants frequently challenge and burden their caretakers.

Hyperactivity and temper tantrums are common in the preschool years of many children on the path to BPD, whereas others are more notable for their clinginess and vulnerability to separations. By school age, these children almost invariably meet diagnostic criteria for an Axis I diagnosis, more commonly ADHD, conduct disorder, separation anxiety disorder, or mood disorder.

Many of these youngsters appear anxious, moody, irritable, and explosive. Minor upsets or frustrations trigger intense affective storms—episodes of uncontrolled emotion wholly out of proportion to the apparent precipitant. The lability of their affect mirrors the kaleidoscopic quality of their sense of self and others. One moment they feel elated and expansive, blissfully connected in perfect love and harmony to an idealized partner. Next, they plunge into bitter disappointment and rage coupled with self-loathing and despair.

On clinical examination, school-age borderline children may appear helpless and vulnerable, provocative and suspicious, or eager to comply and ingratiate themselves with the examiner. These youngsters quickly attempt to establish highly coercive, controlling relationships with their examiners (98). Some show surprisingly little anxiety about meeting alone with the clinician and proceed to take over the office as if they owned it. Even those who seem vulnerable and anxious try vigorously to set the agenda for the meeting. They become anxious and even more desperate and arbitrary when the examiner does not comply with their demands or when they feel that their control is threatened. A distorted sense of reality is a distinctive and puzzling feature of borderline children, as they create a vivid fantasy world in which they become intensely absorbed. They then attempt to coerce others to assume certain roles that fit their particular fantasy. While they can generally recognize the arbitrariness with which they treat reality, they behave as if they must believe their own falsification of reality. When others do not match the prescribed roles, borderline children become desperate, enraged, and transiently psychotic.

Psychological testing reveals rigid and tenuous repressive defenses coexisting with primitive defenses; a highly egocentric, arbitrary interpretation of reality; transitory disturbances in reality testing and impairments in formal thought processes in unstructured tests; constant or recurrent disturbances in ego functions, such as frustration tolerance, attention, and goal-directedness; primitive, unmodulated experience of affects and drives; and marked disturbances in interpersonal relationships and in the experiences of self and others (98).

The developmental and psychosocial pressures of adolescence typically trigger the onset of the full range of borderline psychopathology and allow for greater diagnostic certainty. Adolescence may be the point at which the coping mechanisms, relationship patterns, and modes of organizing experience acquire self-perpetuating rigidity and the capacity to coercively evoke responses from others that maintain and reinforce these youngsters' maladjustment.

Unstable relationships with peers become prominent as transient idealization and clingy overdependence alternate with rage, devaluation, and feelings of abandonment and betrayal. Regardless of whether idealization or anger predominates, all of their interpersonal exchanges have an intense, dramatic quality. Promiscuity is more common in borderline girls, particularly in sexually abused girls, for whom aggressive seductiveness affords the opportunity to turn around and gain control of the helplessness associated with being abused.

Borderline boys are often burdened with intense shyness and fears of rejection. Manipulative efforts to secure attention and prevent abandonment become prominent interpersonal strategies for both boys and girls. Bulimic binges or drugs are relied on for soothing and comfort and become essential regulators of wellbeing and self-esteem (99, 100). Yet the transient nurturance derived from food binges, drug abuse, or promiscuous sex only leads to shame, guilt, and a dreaded feeling of inner deadness or emptiness. Self-mutilation and suicidal gestures result from a wish to "feel something" and relieve the emptiness, an effort to escape unbearable feelings of anxiety and depression, a desire to punish a previously idealized partner, and a manipulative attempt to evoke guilt and involvement. Dissociative episodes appear more commonly in sexually abused borderline adolescents.

A central feature of BPD—and all personality disorders—is the construction of a rigid set of beliefs, mental representations, and coping mechanisms. As Zanarini (64) remarks, individuals with BPD believe that people cannot be loved comfortably or left gracefully and transform anxiety, sorrow, and rage into indirect, dramatic, reproachful attempts to evoke attention. They anticipate experiencing subjective dyscontrol and fragmentation, so they actively provoke these very experiences, thus gaining an illusion of control over themselves and others. Borderline children's rigid and desperate insistence on inducing interpersonal responses that support and validate their own mental representations and expectations turns into one of the most daunting therapeutic challenges facing child and adolescent clinicians.

In contrast to most disorders of childhood, the diagnosis of juvenile BPD has traditionally relied on clinical assessment. More recently, however, structured interviews and questionnaires have been developed or adult measures have been adapted to children and adolescents such as the Personality Disorder Examination (PDE) (34, 101, 102), a child version of the Diagnostic Interview for Borderline patients (C-DIB) (74), and an adaptation for adolescents of the Revised and Structured Clinical Interview for DSM-IV-R Personality Disorders (SCID-II) (103), leading to accumulating evidence of validity of the BPD construct in childhood.

Crick and colleagues (104) developed the Borderline Personality Features Scale for Children and Adolescents (BPFC-C) based on the borderline scale of the Personality Assessment Inventory (PAI (105)). The BPFS-C includes age-appropriate items adapted from the original PAI to reflect the domains of affective instability (e.g., "My feelings are very strong. For instance, when I get mad, I get really, really mad. When I get happy, I get really, really happy"); identity problems (e.g., "I feel that there is something important missing about me, but I don't know what it is"); negative relationships (e.g., "I've picked friends who have treated me badly"); and self-harm (e.g., "I get into trouble because I do things without thinking"). Preliminary evidence is supportive of the validity of this measure.

Differential Diagnosis

Axis I Disorders

Adult BPD is often comorbid with Axis I disorders, including major depression, substance misuse, post-traumatic stress disorder, other anxiety disorders, and eating disorders. Evidence is now accumulating of a similar cooccurrence and both Axis I and Axis II diagnosis should be made when criteria are met in childhood and adolescence. The strongest comorbidity demonstrated for BPD and Axis I is with externalizing disorder (106, 107). In one study (108), conduct disorder was the only Axis I disorder significantly more prevalent in adolescents with BPD than in those without (Table 5.14.3).

Physical and sexual abuse and early losses are common features in BPD and conduct disorders. ADHD uncomplicated by BPD does not include the array of problems with self-destructiveness, unstable relationships, and fragile sense of reality. Conduct disorders can also be associated with other personality disorders—for example, narcissistic personality disorder—as well as with depression and developmental disorders such as dyslexia.

Equally complex is the differentiation between BPD and mood disorders. A vulnerability to affective dysregulation and a proneness to excessive rage may be significant predisposing factors to BPD. Children of bipolar parents present a range of psychiatric difficulties, including conduct disorders, substance abuse, and dysthymia. Clinical descriptions of childhood presentations of bipolar or dysthymic disorders portray moody, irritable, affectively labile children with a low tolerance for frustration and explosive anger. More definite mood

TABLE 5.14.3

COMORBID DIAGNOSES IN BORDERLINE AND NONBORDERLINE CHILDREN

Comorbid Disorder	Borderline (n = 41) (%)	Nonborderline (n = 53) (%)
Major depressive disorder	22.5	23.1
Dysthymia	17.5	11.5
Overanxious	30.0	21.2
Separation anxiety	22.5	11.5
Simple phobia	15.0	9.6
Social phobia	2.5	1.9
Attention deficit	67.5	50.0
Conduct disorder*	55.0	25.0
Oppositional defiant disorder	47.5	63.5

*$\chi^2 = 8.6$; $p < .01$. (From Guzder J, Paris J, Zelkowitz P, Feldman R: Psychological risk factors for borderline pathology in school-age children. *J Am Acad Child Adolesc Psychiatry* 38(2):206–212, 1999 with permission.)

changes in late school-age years or adolescence should point to a diagnosis of mood disorder, particularly exuberant affect, loud giggling, increased activity, disturbed sleep, recent onset of angry outbursts, and decreased attention. Manic adolescents may do poorly in school because of poor concentration or high-flown thinking or end relationships because of irritability or impulsivity. The acute onset of a depressive episode characterized by hypersomnia, psychomotor retardation, and psychosis in a child or adolescent with a family history of two or more generations with mood disorders is predictive of a bipolar course.

A history of trauma, particularly sexual abuse, is common in BPD. PTSD follows exposure to an identifiable, overwhelming stressor. Repeated traumatization can result in a response of reenactment, avoidance, dissociation, and hyperarousal that becomes woven into the child's or adolescent's habitual and pervasive patterns of coping, relating, and experiencing and can contribute to the development of BPD.

The Axis I diagnosis of eating disorders, particularly bulimia nervosa, is often part of the clinical picture of BPD. In younger children, separation anxiety disorder should be differentiated from the clinginess and distress following separations characteristic of borderline youths. Children with an uncomplicated anxiety disorder do not exhibit the impulsivity, rage, self-destructiveness, and impaired sense of reality typical of borderline psychopathology.

The cross-sectional presentation of mood disorders and externalizing disorders (including ADHD and conduct disorder) may mimic BPD. Thus, adequate treatment of the Axis I disorder and a longitudinal perspective is needed before arriving at a dual diagnosis.

Another group of Axis I disorders that must be ruled out is schizophrenia spectrum disorders. Transient psychotic episodes, suspiciousness, and a disturbed sense of reality are typical features of BPD, but delusions, hallucinations, and loose associations are not. A family history of schizophrenia spectrum disorders is suggestive of these disorders.

Axis II Disorders

The most common Axis II disorders occurring with adult BPD include avoidant, dependent, and paranoid personality disorders. The child clinical literature often confuses BPD and schizotypal personality disorder. Schizotypal children present magical thinking, unusual perceptual experiences, idiosyncratic fantasies, and paranoid ideation, all common in borderline children. Schizotypal children, however, have a family history of schizophrenia spectrum disorders and present constricted or inappropriate affect, oddness of speech and behavior, and extreme discomfort in social situations, which contrast with the intense and dramatic affect and hunger for social response of borderline youths.

Children with a schizoid disorder of childhood may become intensely absorbed in a world of fantasy of their own making but are not distressed by their social isolation and do not attempt to coerce caretakers and peers to play roles prescribed by their idiosyncratic fantasies or play themes.

Children in the process of developing narcissistic personality or histrionic personality disorders present significant clinical overlap with children with BPD. Narcissistic or histrionic children are self-centered and self-absorbed, need constant attention, respond with rage to rejection or indifference, alternate between idealization and devaluation, are seductive and manipulative, express affect with undue intensity and drama, and, in the case of narcissistic youngsters, are preoccupied with fantasies of power and control. Borderline children, however, display much greater impulsivity, self-destructiveness, affective instability, disturbances in the sense of reality, and transient psychotic episodes.

Course and Prognosis

The few prospective longitudinal studies conducted to assess the course and prognosis of juvenile BPD have shown inconsistent findings. Some studies provide limited evidence of developmental continuity of BPD symptoms from adolescence into adulthood (109). Others, by contrast, support a developmental trajectory that begins with childhood externalizing disorder and develops into adult BPD. Crawford and colleagues (110) examined the developmental link between Cluster B personality disorder symptoms (borderline, histrionic, and narcissistic) and comorbid internalizing and externalizing symptoms in a community sample of 407 adolescents. Cross-lagged longitudinal models tested the hypothesis that Cluster B symptoms reflect primary disturbances that give rise to cooccurring internalizing and externalizing symptoms, versus the alternative hypothesis that these Axis I symptom clusters reflect primary problems that interfere with normal personality development and lead to dysfunctional patterns of coping and relating. Internalizing and externalizing symptoms each predicted subsequent Cluster B symptoms in girls, although these effects occurred only at specific developmental stages. Cluster B symptoms in boys and girls at ages 10 to 14 years predicted externalizing symptoms two years later. Instead of clearly supporting one hypothesis over the other, longitudinal models suggested gender-specific developmental effects that were partially consistent with both hypotheses. The role for externalizing disorder in the developmental course of juvenile BPD was confirmed in two retrospective studies of BPD (111, 112).

In anticipation of more empirical work on the course and prognosis of juvenile BPD, current evidence supports the conclusion that adolescence and young adulthood of BPD patients are marked by dramatic crises of affective dyscontrol, interpersonal storms, and impulsive and self-destructive behavior, which often require extensive use of health and mental health resources. Family dysfunction and occupational impairment associated with suicide risk and substance abuse are most notable during the late adolescent and young adult years and tend to decrease in intensity during middle age, a time when a significant percentage of patients with BPD "mellow" and are able to gain greater stability in their relationships.

Treatment

The treatment of children and adolescents with BPD remains controversial. Typically, these youths experience repeated crises and become involved in multiple systems and treatment modalities (special education, juvenile justice, private and public hospitals, residential treatment centers, social services, and private practitioners). Data on treatment effectiveness in children and adolescents are virtually nonexistent due to methodological problems and funding restrictions. Under current patterns of reimbursement, services for children and adolescents and their families with protracted problems have often been limited to crisis interventions or short-term treatment. Clinical consensus and emerging research, however, suggests that these youths and their families require extended treatment in which multiple interventions are carefully integrated to address maladaptive patterns of coping and relating, neuropsychiatric problems and vulnerabilities, and dysfunctional cycles of family interaction.

Inpatient and Residential Treatment and the Continuum of Care

Children and adolescents with BPD often require acute inpatient treatment because of suicidality or reckless, impulsive, destructive or self-destructive behavior. Crisis intervention is typically limited to 3 to 5 days of hospitalization and is designed to prevent destructive and self-destructive behavior and stabilize an acute crisis; to help parents establish at least a modicum of safety and control in the family; to foster an alliance with the parents and, if possible, with the youngster; to complete a thorough assessment and treatment plan; to initiate outpatient treatment (individual and family treatment, pharmacotherapy, educational programs, day treatment); or to refer to residential treatment. A critical function of inpatient crisis intervention is the assessment of the services and approaches necessary for effective treatment and the means to ensure coordination and continuity of services (113, 114).

Faced with the empathic yet consistent limits and structure of an inpatient setting, borderline children and adolescents can become enraged or anxious or engage in a variety of maneuvers designed to help them regain a sense of safety and control. These maneuvers create formidable challenges to the treatment team's capacity to communicate, maintain a therapeutic environment, and avoid potentially destructive responses. Some staff members are idealized, while devaluation and rage are directed at other members of the treatment team. The treatment team is also challenged by the patient's seductive and sexualized behavior, defiance, or attempts to run away or commit suicide.

Following short-term inpatient care, some children and adolescents with BPD are referred to residential treatment. Residential treatment, however, is costly and lacks empirical evidence of effectiveness. Research is clearly needed to document which borderline youngsters require residential treatment because outpatient interventions will not suffice. Just as important is a more specific, empirically based definition of which treatment interventions and components of care, in what sequence, are effective for particular youngsters with BPD. Finally, research is needed to demonstrate what continuum of services must be in place to allow for a safe transition to the community as rapidly as possible.

From a clinical standpoint, indications for residential treatment are determined by 1) the capacity of the patients to contain destructive or self-destructive behavior; 2) the extent of the youth's need for containment, which may exceed the capacity of even exceptionally competent parents; and 3) the availability of community resources and services to support the family's containment. Several clinical constellations are common indications for residential treatment: 1) borderline children and adolescents with an intricate combination of neuropsychiatric problems and a traumatic history or current maltreatment who respond to stress with dissociative or self-destructive behavior; 2) borderline children with out-of-control addictive or eating disorder problems; 3) borderline-narcissistic children and adolescents who are severely mistrusting and become destructive or impulsive when their grandiosity or efforts to control and manipulate are challenged.

Residential treatment seeks to interrupt coercive cycles of interaction between parents and children, to interrupt addictive patterns involving drugs, food, promiscuous sex, or self-mutilation; to stabilize symptomatology; and to facilitate the use of outpatient interventions and social supports. As such, these programs optimally integrate daily life structure, family treatment, psychotherapy, pharmacotherapy, group treatment, school and vocational treatment, recreational and life skills programs, religious and spiritual activities, substance abuse programs, and eating disorders interventions. Structured interventions to enhance parental skills or increase the youngster's capacity for affective regulation, such as dialectical behavior therapy, have been integrated in the residential treatment program (115, 116).

Family and Individual Psychotherapy

The clinical literature on psychotherapeutic interventions with BPD children and adolescents, while providing moving descriptions of the efforts to engage these youngsters and their families in a therapeutic process, generally lack specificity regarding the interventions used or empirical evidence of efficacy.

The empirical foundations of both family-based and individual therapy for adult BPD, however, have changed dramatically over the past decade. Efforts are underway to adapt and test out therapeutic interventions with BPD youngsters that are operationally defined and backed by evidence of effectiveness.

Dialectical-behavioral therapy (DPT) developed by Linehan (117) for the outpatient treatment of chronically suicidal and parasuicidal patients with BPD has shown effectiveness in decreasing parasuicidal behavior, "therapy interfering behaviors" (particularly, dropping out of treatment), and behaviors that "interfere with the quality of life", such as repeated visits to the emergency room or rehospitalizations.

DPT involves individual therapy, group skills training, telephone contact and consultation for the therapist. DBT has been eagerly received and extended to substance misuse (118, 119), eating disorders (120) and suicidal adolescents (121), showing promising results.

Mentalization based treatment (MBT), developed by Bateman and Fonagy (122, 123), showed, like DBT, dramatically effective results in diminished hospitalizations, medication usage and suicidal and parasuicidal behavior. MBT, however, showed significant benefits, in randomized controlled trials, in anxiety, depression, and in social and interpersonal functioning, areas in which DBT has not been shown to be effective.

MBT involves individual and group psychotherapy focused on helping patients identify and interpret mental states, both in themselves and in others, in the here-and-now of the therapeutic interaction, in order to promote a sense of the self as the agent of behavior, based on underlying mental states.

DBT and MBT differ in their theoretical perspective, as DBT assumes that the core issue in BPD—and the key therapeutic target—is emotional dysregulation, while MBT sees emotional dysregulation as secondary to a primary impairment in mentalization producing a related disturbance in self-coherence and self-agency.

Both MBT and DBT, however, emphasize cognitive processes and skill building in the here-and-now. DBT's focus on the skills of mindfulness and interpersonal effectiveness may be promoting more similar capacities than those targeted by MBT.

Family interventions have also increasingly focused on improving the cognitive and relationship skills that allow for the resolution in the here-and-now of parent–adolescent conflicts, particularly interactions characterized by negative exchanges, emotional disengagement, and poor problemsolving. Diamond and Liddle (124) illustrate an evidence-based shift in therapeutic focus from behavior management to identifying ruptures in attachment and the feeling states associated with ruptures. As Diamond and Liddle point out, when core relationship conflicts are identified as underlying interpersonal impasses, parents gain a new perspective on their teenager that helps rekindle empathy and the more adaptive expression of emotions and concerns.

Such treatment models can enhance the effectiveness of approaches designed to build a therapeutic alliance and improve parents' effectiveness in setting limits and containing destructive, self-destructive, or otherwise maladaptive behavior. There is empirical evidence that a number of structured approaches designed to improve parental effectiveness—such as "Helping The Noncompliant Child" (125) or The Oregon Social Learning Center Program (126), also decrease destructive and self-destructive behavior and enhance adaptive, prosocial behavior.

In summary, while lacking systematic, empirical research in BPD treatment in children and adolescents, clinical practice can be informed by a set of guidelines derived from the clinical literature and evidence with adults with BPD:

1. Establish a collaborative relationship with the parents aiming at supporting parental competence in general, and parental mindfulness, empathy and mentalizing capacities in particular. Such focus allows parents to identify stressors impacting their caregiving capabilities, to determine how to protect children from the impact of these stressors, and access supportive and therapeutic resources.
2. Form a collaborative relationship with the child in order to create a space in which they can share some aspects of the internal states underlying their behavior with the ultimate aim of enhancing self-control and self-regulation. Transforming the sterility of coercive and unreflective interactions into a sense of mutuality is aided by the therapist promoting verbalization of internal states and conveying a view of the patient as an intentional being.
3. Avoid confronting vulnerabilities, such as linking past and present, or addressing highly conflictive or defended internal states, which tend to exacerbate the use of maladaptive coping mechanisms. Therapists seek instead to enhance children's sense of self-control. To this end, borderline children need first to learn to observe their own internal states without becoming overwhelmed. They need help to understand the relationship between their behavior and internal states, focusing initially on the circumstances that lead them, for example, to become aggressive when they feel misunderstood or anxious. Therapists introduce a mentalizing perspective from which children can observe their own *mental states*, as well as those of others. The aim of introducing this perspective is to create a context in which it is safe to experience internal states as mental states rather than concrete actions. Specific interventions—such as DBT or MBT—seek to enhance the capacity to mentalize, strengthen impulse control, and create awareness of others' mental states, emotional regulation, and interpersonal effectiveness. Stepping back from overwhelming or unmanageable experiences is facilitated by breaking down experiences into more manageable bits and by channeling responses into more adaptive conduct, with increasing control over the expression of feelings in action.
4. The therapy process can incorporate structured behavioral and cognitive-behavioral approaches. These include training in anger management and problemsolving. These approaches include modeling, reinforcement of prosocial behavior, feedback, role-playing, and homework assignments. Behavioral approaches also include support to youngsters to free themselves from maladaptive behavioral patterns by acknowledging both the price they pay for relying on them and the difficulties associated with relinquishing them. Such acknowledgment opens the path to a systematic exploration of the core beliefs that are at the root of maladaptation.
5. Therapists should be aware of their own emotional reactions. One of the greatest challenges facing therapists treating borderline children and adolescents are their own emotional reactions. As Gabbard (127) has pointed out, borderline patients apply interpersonal pressure through specific behaviors that evoke specific clinician responses. Therapists, for example, are vulnerable to experience the coercive pressure to become an idealized rescuer or are threatened with the implicit message, "If I die, it will be because of your failure."
6. Therapists should be aware of countertransference reactions that are shaped by the parent's behavior. Therapists find themselves competing with the parents, devaluing them in overt or subtle ways, or unwittingly seeking to rescue parents from their children's cruelty. Countertransference reactions, however, can become useful windows into the child's and the family's dysfunctional patterns of coping and relating.

Psychopharmacotherapy

The use of medications can powerfully support the parents' competence and the alliance between parents and treaters. Randomized control trials of pharmacological interventions with BPD children and adolescents are very limited (128) and thus, pharmacotherapy is largely based on clinical studies and research with adults. Pharmacotherapy is also grounded in clinical experience with these youths and in studies documenting the effectiveness of medications in a range of related or comorbid child and adolescent problems. The role of pharmacotherapy in the treatment of children and adolescents with BPD is to target dysregulations of arousal, cognition, affect, and impulse.

Pharmacotherapy targets both the symptoms that emerge during episodes of acute psychobiological decompensation and the trait vulnerabilities that represent an enduring diathesis to dysfunction. No one-to-one correspondence has been identified between specific neurobiological vulnerabilities and types of personality disorders. Thus, given the current level of knowledge, pharmacotherapy targets personality dimensions, such as affective dysregulation and impulsive-behavior dysregulation, and Axis I disorders, such as depression, anxiety disorders, ADHD, and mood disorders. By impacting the neurobiological underpinnings of arousal, cognition, affect, and impulse, pharmacotherapy creates optimal conditions for psychotherapy and family treatment.

Children and adolescents can more readily become engaged in treatment when they are not buffeted by subjective distress, anxiety, or hyperarousal, or when their depressed energy level and reduced capacity for concentration have improved. Parents' position as providers of containment and support is enhanced when they collaborate with the treaters in administering medication effectively.

References

1. American Psychiatric Association: *Diagnostic and Statistical Manual of Mental Disorders*, 4th ed. Washington, DC, American Psychiatric Association, 2000.
2. Lenzenweger MF, Loranger, AW, Korfine L, et al.: Detecting personality disorders in a nonclinical population. *Arch. Gen. Psychiatry* 54:345–351, 1997.
3. Weissman MM: The epidemiology of personality disorders: A 1990 update. *J. Personal Disord* 7:44–62, 1993.
4. Merikangas KR, Weissman MM: Epidemiology og DSM-III Axix II personality disorders. In: Frances AJ, Hales RE (eds) Psychiatry update: *American Psychiatric Association Annual Review* (vol 5). Washington, DC, American Psychiatric Press, 1986, pp. 258–278.
5. Caton CL, Shrout PE, Eagle PF, et al.: Risk factors for homelessness among schizophrenia men. A case-control study. *American Journal of Public Health* 84:265–270, 1994.
6. McDonald AS, Davey GLC: Psychiatric disorders and accidental injury. *Clinical Psychological Review* 16:105–127, 1996.
7. Miller RJ, Zadolinnyj K, Harper RJ: Profiles and predictors of assaultiveness for different psychiatric ward populations. *Am J Psychiatry* 150:1368–1373, 1993.
8. Raine, A: Features of borderline personality and violence. *Journal of Clinical Psychology* 49:277–281, 1993.
9. Hillbrand, M, Krystal JH, Swarpe JS, et al.: Clinical predictors of self-mutilation in hospitalized forensic patients. *Journal Nerv Mental Disorders* 5:135–144, 1994.
10. Brent DA, Johnson BA, Perpen, et al.: Personality disorder, personality traits, impulsive violence and completed suicide in adolescents. *J Am Acad Child Adolesc Psychiatry* 33:1080–1086, 1994.

11. Reich JH, Boerstler H, Yates W, et al.: Utilization of medical resources in persons with DSM III personality disorders in a community sample. *Int. J. Psychiatry Med* 19:1–9, 1989.
12. Jordan BK, Schlenger WE, Fairbank JA, et al.: Prevalence of psychiatric disorder among incarcerated women. *Arch. Gen. Psychiatry* 53(6):513–519, 1996.
13. Ruegg R, Francis A: New research in personality disorders. *J Personal Disorders* 9(1):1–48, 1995.
14. Nelson JC, Mazure CM, Jatlow PI: Characteristics of desipramine-refractory depression. *Journal of Clinical Psychiatry* 55:12–19, 1994.
15. Calabrese JR, Woyshville MJ, Kimmel SE, et al.: Predictors of valproate response in bipolar rapid cycling. 13:280–283, 1993.
16. Jenike MA, Baer L, Minichiello WE, et al.: Coexistent obsessive-compulsive disorder and schizotypal personality disorder: A poor prognostic indicator. *Arch Gen Psychiatry* 43(3):296–, 1986.
17. Millon T, Davis AD: *Disorders of Personality: DSM-IV and Beyond*. New York, Wiley, 1996.
18. Cicchetti D, Cohen DJ: *Developmental Psychopathology*. New York, Wiley, 2006.
19. Kernberg PF, Weiner AS, Bardenstein KK: *Personality Disorder in Children and Adolescents*. New York, Basic Books,
20. Shapiro T: Resolved: Borderline personality exists in children under twelve: Negative (Debate Forum). *J. Amer Acad Child Adolesc Psychiatry* 29:480, 1990.
21. Edens JF, Skeem JL, Cruise KR, Cauffman E: Assessment of "juvenile psychopathy" and its association with violence: A critical review. *Behavioural Sciences and the Law* 19:53–80, 2001.
22. Seagrave D, Grisso T: Adolescent development and the measurement of juvenile psychopathy. *Law and Human Behavior* 26(2):219–239, 2002.
23. Frick PJ: Juvenile psychopathy from a developmental perspective: Implications for construct development and use in forensic assessments. *Law and Human Behavior* 26(2):247–253, 2002.
24. Bleiberg E: Borderline disorders in children and adolescents: The concept, the diagnosis, and the controversies. *Bull Menninger Clin* 58(2):169–196, 1994.
25. Mahler M, Ross, JA, de Friess Z: Clinical studies in benign and malignant cases of childhood psychosis. *American Journal of Orthopsychiatry* 1949.
26. Ekstein R, Wallerstein J: Observations on the psychology of borderline and psychotic children. *The Psychoanalytic Study of the Child* 19:344–372.
27. Kernberg OF: Borderline personality organization. *J. of the American Psycholoanal. Assoc* 15:641–685, 1967.
28. Petti TA, Vela RM: Borderline disorders of childhood: An overview. *J Am Acad Child Adolesc Psychiatry* 29(3):327–337, 1990.
29. Goldman SJ, D'Angelo EJ, DeMaso DR, Mezzacappa E: Physical and sexual abuse histories among children with BPD. *American Journal of Psychiatry* 149(12):1723–1726, 1992.
30. Clarkin JF, Widiger TA, Frances A, Hurt SW, Gilmore M: Prototypic typology and the BPD. *Journal of Abnormal Psychology* 92:263–275, 1983.
31. McManus M, Lerner H, Robbins D, Barbour C: Assessment of borderline symptomatology in hospitalized adolescents. *J Am Acad Child Psychiatry* 23(6):685–694, 1984.
32. Marton P, Korenblum M, Kutcher S, Stein B, Kennedy B, Pakes J: Personality dysfunction in depressed adolescents. *Can J Psychiatry* 34(8):810–813, 1989.
33. Levy KN, Becker DF, Grilo CM, et al.: Concurrent and predictive validity of the personality disorder diagnosis in adolescent inpatients. *Am J Psychiatry* 156(10):1522–1528, 1999.
34. Grilo CM, McGlashan TH, Quinlan DM, Walker ML, Greenfeld D, Edell WS: Frequency of personality disorders in two age cohorts of psychiatric inpatients. *Am J Psychiatry* 155(1):140–142, 1998.
35. Korenblum M, Marton P, Golombek H, Stein B: Personality status: changes through adolescence. *Psychiatr Clin North Am* 13(3):389–399, 1990.
36. Nigg JT, Goldsmith HH: Genetics of personality disorders: Perspectives from personality and psychopathology research. *Psychol Bull* 115(3):346–380, 1994.
37. Torgensen S, Lygren S, Oien PA, et al.: A twin study of personality disorders. *Comprehensive Psychiatry* 41:416–425, 2001.
38. Livesley WJ, Jang KL, Vernon PA: Phenotypic and genetic structure of traits delineating personality disorder. *Arch Gen Psychiatry* 55(10):941–948, 1998.
39. Viding E, Blair RJ, Moffitt TE, Plomin R: Evidence for substantial genetic risk for psychopathy in 7-year-olds. *J Child Psychol Psychiatry* 46(6):592–597, 2005.
40. Skodol AE, Siever LJ, Livesley WJ, Gunderson JG, Pfohl B, Widiger TA: The borderline diagnosis II: Biology, genetics, and clinical course. *Biol Psychiatry* 51(12):951–963, 2002.
41. Klein DF. Psychopharmacological treatment and delineation of borderline disorders. In: Hartocollins P (ed): BPD: *The Concept, The Syndrome, The Patient*. New York, International Universities Press, 1977, pp. 365–383.
42. Gunderson J, Zanarini M, Kisiel C: BPD: A review of data on DSM III R descriptions. *J Personal Disorders* 5:340–352, 1991.
43. Andrulonis P: Disruptive behavior disorder in boys and the BPD in men. *Annals of Clinical Psychiatry* 3:23–26, 1991.
44. Schmahl CG, McGlashan TH, Bremner JD: Neurobiological correlates of BPD. *Psychopharmacol Bull* 36(2):69–87, 2002.
45. Gurvits IG, Koenigsberg HW, Siever LJ: Neurotransmitter dysfunction in patients with BPD. *Psychiatr Clin North Am* 23(1):27–40, vi–, 2000.
46. Friedel RO: Dopamine dysfunction in BPD: A hypothesis. *Neuropsychopharmacology* 29(6):1029–1039, 2004.
47. Johnson PA, Hurley RA, Benkelfat C, Herpertz SC, Taber KH: Understanding emotion regulation in BPD: Contributions of neuroimaging. *J Neuropsychiatry Clin Neurosci* 15(4):397–402, 2003.
48. Bohus M, Schmahl C, Lieb K: New developments in the neurobiology of BPD. *Curr Psychiatry Rep* 6(1):43–50, 2004.
49. Siever LJ, Torgersen S, Gunderson JG, Livesley WJ, Kendler KS: The borderline diagnosis III: identifying endophenotypes for genetic studies. *Biol Psychiatry* 51(12):964–968, 2002.
50. Hyman SE: A new beginning for research on BPD. *Biol Psychiatry* 51(12):933–935, 2002.
51. Asberg M, Traskman L, Thoren P: 5-HIAA in the cerebrospinal fluid. A biochemical suicide predictor? *Arch Gen Psychiatry* 33(10):1193–1197, 1976.
52. Brown CS, Kent TA, Bryant SG, et al.: Blood platelet uptake of serotonin in episodic aggression. *Psychiatric Research* 27(5):5–12, 1989.
53. Coccaro EF: Neurotransmitter function in personality disorders. In: Silk KR (ed): *Biology of Personality Disorders*. Washington, DC, American Psychiatric Press, 1998, pp. 1–25.
54. Soloff PH, Meltzer CC, Greer PJ, Constantine D, Kelly TM: A fenfluramine-activated FDG-PET study of BPD. *Biological Psychiatry* 47:540–547, 2000.
55. Lesch KP, Bengel D, Heils A, et al.: Association of anxiety-related traits with a polymorphism in the serotonin transporter gene regulatory region. *Science* 274(5292):1527–1531, 1996.
56. New AS, Gelernter J, Yovell Y, et al.: Tryptophan hydroxylase genotype is associated with impulsive-aggression measures: A preliminary study. *Am J Med Genet* 81(1):13–17, 1998.
57. New AS, Gelernter J, Goodman M, et al.: Suicide, impulsive aggression, and HTR1B genotype. *Biol Psychiatry* 50(1):62–65, 2001.
58. Herpetz SC, Dietrich TM, Wenning B, et al.: Evidence of abnormal amygdala functioning in BPD: A functional MRI. *Biol Psychiatry* 50:292–298, 2001.
59. Donegan NH, Sanislow CA, Blumberg HP, et al.: Amygdala hyperreactivity in BPD: implications for emotional dysregulation. *Biol Psychiatry* 54(11):1284–1293, 2003.
60. Brendel GR, Stern E, Silbersweig DA: Defining the neurocircuitry of BPD: Functional neuroimaging approaches. *Dev Psychopathol* 17(4):1197–1206, 2005.
61. Rogosch FA, Cicchetti D: Child maltreatment, attention networks, and potential precursors to BPD. *Development and Psychopathology* 17:1071–1089, 2005.
62. Zelkowitz P, Paris J, Guzder J, Feldman R: Diatheses and stressors in borderline pathology of childhood: The role of neuropsychological risk and trauma. *J Am Acad Child Adolesc Psychiatry* 40(1):100–105, 2001.
63. Battle CL, Shea MT, Johnson DM, et al.: Childhood maltreatment associated with adult personality disorders: Findings from the Collaborative Longitudinal Personality Disorders Study. *J Personal Disorders* 18(2):193–211, 2004.
64. Zanarini MC, Williams AA, Lewis RE, et al.: Reported pathological childhood experiences associated with the development of BPD. *Am J Psychiatry* 154(8):1101–1106, 1997.
65. Links PS, Steiner M, Offord DR, Eppel A: Characteristics of BPD: A Canadian study. *Can J Psychiatry* 33(5):336–340, 1988.
66. Zanarini MC, Gunderson JG, Marino MF, Schwartz EO, Frankenburg FR: Childhood experiences of borderline patients. *Compr Psychiatry* 30(1):18–25, 1989.
67. Westen D: Towards a revised theory of borderline object relations: Contributions of empirical research. *International Journal of Psychoanalysis* 71(4):661–693, 1990.
68. Shearer SL, Peters CP, Quaytman MS, Ogden RL: Frequency and correlates of childhood sexual and physical abuse histories in adult female borderline inpatients. *Am J Psychiatry* 147(2):214–216, 1990.
69. Goldberg RL, Mann LS, Wise TN, Segall EA: Parental qualities as perceived by BPDs. *Hillside J Clin Psychiatry* 7(2):134–140, 1985.
70. Reich DB, Zanarini MC: Developmental aspects of BPD. *Harv Rev Psychiatry* 9(6):294–301, 2001.
71. Agrawal HR, Gunderson J, Bjarne M, Holmes BM, Lyons-Ruth K: Attachment studies with borderline patients: A review. *Harvard Review of Psychiatry* 12(2):94–104, 2004.
72. Paris J, Zweig-Frank H, Guzder J: Risk factors for borderline personality in male outpatients. *J Nerv Ment Dis* 182(7):375–380, 1994.
73. Paris J, Zweig-Frank H, Guzder J: Psychological risk factors for BPD in female patients. *Compr Psychiatry* 35(4):301–305, 1994.
74. Greenman DA, Gunderson JG, Cane M, Saltzman PR: An examination of the borderline diagnosis in children. *Am J Psychiatry* 143(8):998–1003, 1986.
75. Lofgren DP, Bemporad J, King J, Lindem K, O'Driscoll G: A prospective follow-up study of so-called borderline children. *Am J Psychiatry* 148(11):1541–1547, 1991.
76. Kestenbaum CJ: The borderline child at risk for major psychiatric disorder in adult life: Seven case reports with follow-up. In: Robson KS (ed): *The*

Borderline Child: Approaches to Etiology, Diagnosis and Treatment. New York, McGraw Hill, 1983, pp. 50–81.
77. Ludolph PS, Westen D, Misle B, Jackson A, Wixom J, Wiss FC: The borderline diagnosis in adolescents: Symptoms and developmental history. *Am J Psychiatry* 147(4):470–476, 1990.
78. Famularo R, Kinscherff R, Fenton T: Posttraumatic stress disorder among children clinically diagnosed as BPD. *The Journal of Nervous and Mental Disease* 179(7):428–431, 1991.
79. Rogosch FA, Cicchetti D: Child maltreatment and emergent personality organization: Perspectives from the five-factor model. *J Abnorm Child Psychol* 32(2):123–145, 2004.
80. Johnson JG, Smailes EM, Cohen P, Brown J, Bernstein DP: Associations between four types of childhood neglect and personality disorder symptoms during adolescence and early adulthood: Findings of a community-based longitudinal study. *J Personal Disorders* 14(2):171–187, 2000.
81. Goldman SJ, D'Angelo EJ, DeMaso DR: Psychopathology in the families of children and adolescents with BPD. *Am J Psychiatry* 150(12):1832–1835, 1993.
82. Battle CL, Shea MT, Johnson DM, et al.: Childhood maltreatment associated with adult personality disorders: Findings from the Collaborative Longitudinal Personality Disorders Study. *J Personal Disorders* 18(2):193–211, 2004.
83. Fruzzetti AE, Shenk C, Hoffman PD: Family interaction and the development of BPD: A transactional model. *Development and Psychopathology* 17:1007–1030, 2005.
84. Masterson JF: *Treatment of the Borderline Adolescent: A Developmental Approach*. New York, Wiley, 1972.
85. Adler G: *Borderline Psychopathology and Its Treatment*. New York, Jason Aronson, 1986.
86. Winnicott DW: Transitional object and transitional phenomena: A study of the first not-me possession. *Intl J of Psychoanalysis* 34:89–97, 1953.
87. Fonagy P, Gergely G, Jurist E, Target M: *Affect Regulation, Mentalization and the Development of the Self*. New York, Other Press, 2002.
88. Frith CD, Frith U. Interacting minds—A biological basis. *Science* 286(5445):1692–1695, 1999.
89. Fletcher PC, Happé F, Frith U, Baker SC, et al.: Other minds in the brain: A functional imaging study of "theory of mind" in story comprehension. *Cognition* 57(2):109–128, 1995.
90. Gallagher HL, Frith CD: Functional imaging of 'theory of mind.' *Trends Cogn Sci* 7(2):77–83, 2003.
91. Fonagy P, Redfern S, Charman T: The relationship between belief-desire reasoning and a projective measure of attachment security (SAT). *British Journal of Developmental Psychology* 15(Pt 1):51–61, 1997.
92. Bleiberg E: *Treating Personality Disorders in Children and Adolescents: A Relational Approach*. New York, Guiford Press, 2001.
93. Carndell LE, Patrick MP, Hobson RP: "Still-face" interactions between mothers with BPD and their 2-month-old infants. *British Journal of Psychiatry* 183:239–247, 2003.
94. Posner MI, Rothbart MK, Vizueta N, et al.: Attentional mechanisms of BPD. *Proceeding of the National Academy of Sciences* 99(25)16366–16370, 2002.
95. Fonagy P, Leigh T, Steele M, et al.: The relation of attachment status, psychiatric classification, and response to psychotherapy. *Journal of Consulting and Clinical Psychology* 64:22–31, 1996.
96. Arnsten RF: The biology of being frazzled. *Science* 280:1711–1712, 1998.
97. Vela RM, Gottlieb EH, Gottlieb HP: Borderline syndromes in childhood: A critical review. In: Robson KS (ed): *The Borderline Child: Approaches to Etiology, Diagnosis, and Treatment*. New York, McGraw-Hill, 1983, pp. 31–48.
98. Leichtman M, Nathan S: A clinical approach to the psychological testing of borderline children. In: Robson KS (ed): *The Borderline Child: Approaches to Etiology, Diagnosis, and Treatment*. New York, McGraw-Hill, 1983.
99. Grilo CM, Becker DF, Walker ML, Levy KN, Edell WS, McGlashan TH: Psychiatric comorbidity in adolescent inpatients with substance use disorders. *J Am Acad Child Adolesc Psychiatry* 34(8):1085–1091, 1995.
100. Grilo CM, Levy KN, Becker DF, Edell WS, McGlashan TH: Comorbidity of DSM-III-R axis I and II disorders among female inpatients with eating disorders. *Psychiatr Serv* 47(4):426–429, 1996.
101. Garnet KE, Levy KN, Mattanah JJ, Edell WS, McGlashan TH: BPD in adolescents: Ubiquitous or specific? *Am J Psychiatry* 151(9):1380–1382, 1994.
102. Kutcher SP, Marton P, Korenblum M: Adolescent bipolar illness and personality disorder. *J Am Acad Child Adolesc Psychiatry* 29(3):355–358, 1990.
103. First MB, Spitzer RL, Gibbon M, Williams JBW: *Structured Clinical Interview for DSM-IV TR Axis I Disorders, Research Version, Patient Edition (SCID-I/P)*. New York, Biometrics Research, New York State Psychiatric Institute, 2002.
104. Crick NR, Murray-Close D, Woods K: Borderline personality features in childhood: A short-term longitudinal study. *Dev Psychopathol* 17(4):1051–1070, 2005.
105. Morey L: *Personality Assessment Inventory*. Odessa, FL, Psychological Assessment Resources, Inc., 1991.
106. Eppright TD, Kashani JH, Robison BD, Reid JC: Comorbidity of conduct disorder and personality disorders in an incarcerated juvenile population. *Am J Psychiatry* 150(8):1233–1236, 1993.
107. Myers WC, Burket RC, Otto TA: Conduct disorder and personality disorders in hospitalized adolescents. *J Clin Psychiatry* 54(1):21–26, 1993.
108. Guzder J, Paris J, Zelkowitz P, Feldman R: Psychological risk factors for borderline pathology in school-age children. *J Am Acad Child Adolesc Psychiatry* 38(2):206–212, 1999.
109. Marton P, Connolly J, Kutcher S, Korenblum M: Cognitive social skills and social self-appraisal in depressed adolescents. *J Amer Acad Child Adolesc Psychiatry* 32(4):739–744, 1993.
110. Crawford TN, Cohen P, Brook JS: Dramatic-erratic personality disorder symptoms: II. Developmental pathways from early adolescence to adulthood. *J Personal Disorders* 15(4):336–350, 2001.
111. Goodman G, Hull JW, Clarkin JF, Yeomans FE: Childhood antisocial behaviors as predictors of psychotic symptoms and DSM-III-R borderline criteria among inpatients with BPD. *J Personal Disorders* 13(1):35–46, 1999.
112. Modestin J, Matutat B, Wurmle O: Antecedents of opioid dependence and personality disorder: attention-deficit/hyperactivity disorder and conduct disorder. *Eur Arch Psychiatry Clin Neurosci* 251(1):42–47, 2001.
113. Rosenbluth M, Silver D: The inpatient treatment of BPD. In: Silver D, Rosenbluth M: *Handbook of Borderline Disorders*. Madison, Co, International Universities Press, 1992.
114. Silk K, Eisner, W Allport C, et al.: Focused time-limited inpatient treatment of BPD. *J Personal Disorders* 8(4): 1994.
115. Barley WD, Buie SE, Pererson FW, et al.: Development of an inpatient cognitive-behavioral treatment. *J Personal Disorders* 7(3):232–240, 1973.
116. Bohus M, Maaf B, Stiglmayr C, et al.: Evaluation of inpatient dialectical-behavior therapy for BPD —A prospective study. *Behaviour Research and Therapy* 38:875–887, 2000.
117. Linehan MM, Armstrong HE, Suarez A, et al.: Cognitive-behavioral treatment of chronically parasuicidal borderline patients. *Arch Gen Psychiatry* 48:1060–1064, 1991.
118. Linehan MM, Schmidt HI, Dimeff LA, et al.: Dialectical behavior therapy for patients with BPD and drug dependence. *American Journal on Addiction* 8:279–292, 1999.
119. Linehan MM, Dimeff LA, Reynolds SK, et al.: Dialectical behavior therapy versus comprehensive validation therapy plus 12-step for the treatment of opioid dependent women meeting criteria for BPD. *Drug and Alcohol Dependence* 67:13–26, 2002.
120. Safer DL, Telch CF, Agras WS: Dialectical behavior therapy for bulimia nervosa. *American Journal of Psychiatry* 158:632–634, 2001.
121. Rathus JH, Miller AL: Dialectical behavior therapy adapted for suicidal adolescents. *Suicide and Life-Threatening Behavior* 32:146–157, 2002.
122. Bateman AW, Fonagy PG: The effectiveness of partial hospitalization in the treatment of BPD—A randomized controlled trial. *The American Journal of Psychiatry* 156:1563–1569, 1999.
123. Bateman AW, Fonagy P: *Psychotherapy for BPD: Mentalization Based Treatment*. University Press, Oxford, U.K., Oxford, 2004.
124. Diamond, GS, Liddle H: Transforming negative parent-adolescent interactions: From impasse to dialogue. *Family Process* 38(1):5–26, 1999.
125. Forehand R, Sturgis ET, McMahon A, et al.: Parent behavioral training to modify child noncompliance: Treatment generalization across time and from home to school. *Behavior Modification* 3:3–25, 1979.
126. Patterson CA, Chamberlin P: Treatment process: A problem at three levels. In: Wynne LC (ed): *The State of the Art in Family Therapy Research: Controversies and Recommendations*. New York, Family Process Press, 1988, pp. 189–223.
127. Gabbard GO: Countertransference: The emerging common ground. *Int J Psychoanalysis* 76:475–485, 1995.
128. Nickel M, Muelhbaker M, Nickel C, et al.: A ripiprazole in the treatment of patients with BPD: A double-blind, placebo-controlled study. *American Journal of Psychiatry* 163(5):833–838, 2006.

5.15 ■ NEGLECT, ABUSE, AND TRAUMA-RELATED CONDITIONS

CHAPTER 5.15.1 ■ CHILD ABUSE AND NEGLECT

JOAN KAUFMAN

INTRODUCTION

By all standards of measurement, the problem of child maltreatment is enormous in terms of both its cost to the individual, and its cost to society (1). Child abuse occurs at epidemic rates, with nearly 1,000,000 substantiated reports of child maltreatment each year (2), many reported cases of actual abuse that are not verified (3), and countless other cases which never come to the attention of authorities (4). Victims of abuse comprise a significant proportion of all child psychiatric admissions, with lifetime incidence of physical and sexual abuse estimated at 30% among child and adolescent outpatients (5), and as high as 55% among psychiatric inpatients (6). While not all abused children develop difficulties, many experience a chronic course of psychopathology (7).

This chapter reviews definitions, prevalence, and sequelae of abuse. It then discusses genetic and environmental modifiers of child outcomes, and briefly describes treatment strategies. Problems within the child welfare system are delineated, and the value of utilizing translational approaches in the area of child maltreatment research highlighted. A central tenet of translational research is that preclinical studies—especially animal studies on the effects of early stress—can help to guide hypotheses regarding the etiology, pathophysiology, prevention, and treatment of stress-related disorders. The topics surveyed in this chapter are broad, but together support the following conclusions: 1) Maltreated children are at elevated risk for a whole host of negative outcomes; 2) these bad outcomes can be avoided; 3) multiple genetic and environmental factors modify risk for adversity; 4) the quality of the subsequent caregiving environment is critical in determining the long-term impact of child maltreatment; and 5) research foci that span from neurobiology to social policy are essential to improve the knowledge base necessary to facilitate the development of effective interventions for this vulnerable population.

DEFINITIONS

Definitions of the various maltreatment categories were drafted by the American Academy of Child and Adolescent Psychiatry (8). They are summarized here. As the legal definitions related to child maltreatment vary from one part of the country to the next, clinicians are encouraged to learn the specific definitions used in their state.

Generally, neglect occurs when caretakers fail to appropriately provide for and protect children. It may involve failing to meet the child's nutritional, supervision, or medical needs.

Physical abuse involves the intentional injury of a child by a caretaker. It may take the form of shaking, beating, or other forms of violence that lead to injury, and frequently occurs in the context of discipline.

Sexual abuse of children refers to sexual behavior between a child and an adult or between two children when one of them is significantly older or uses coercion. The perpetrator and the victim may be of the same or opposite sex. The sexual acts may include exhibitionism; nongenital or genital fondling; fellatio; cunnilingus; or vaginal or anal penetration. Pornographic photography is usually considered sexual abuse as well. It is important to think about context and developmental factors in determining whether sexual behaviors between two children are abusive.

Psychological abuse occurs when an adult repeatedly conveys to a child that he or she is worthless, defective, unloved, or unwanted. The child may be isolated and locked in a closet or otherwise restricted. Psychological abuse can also be caused by repeatedly taking a child for unnecessary medical treatment (see Forsyth, 5.15.4, p. 719). It may also involve threatened or actual abandonment. Psychological abuse most often cooccurs with neglect, physical abuse, and/or sexual abuse.

Failure to thrive was previously believed to be due to abuse or neglect. The best available evidence now suggests that child abuse and neglect are implicated in failure to thrive in less than 10% of all cases (9). Child abuse and/or neglect should be ruled out, but not assumed to be of etiological significance, in cases of failure to thrive (see Woolston and Hasbani, 5.7.1).

The maltreatment of children occurs in a wide range of circumstances. It may constitute an isolated incident or represent a chronic pattern of childrearing. Given there are wide variations in acceptable parenting practices, it is important to consider cultural and religious beliefs when evaluating suspected abuse and neglect.

PREVALENCE

Each year there are approximately 3,000,000 reports of child maltreatment, and approximately one-third of these are substantiated (2). Within 4.5 years, however, 50% of all cases will be re-referred to protective services, and 20% will have a new substantiated report of child maltreatment, with no difference in the rate of re-referral or new reports of abuse between cases that are substantiated or unsubstantiated at time of initial referral (10). The process of case substantiation is extremely idiosyncratic, with substantiated *and* unsubstantiated cases at equally high risk of recidivism.

Of the cases that are substantiated, approximately 60% are for neglect, 20% for physical abuse, 10% for sexual abuse, and 10% for other forms of maltreatment (e.g., psychological abuse, abandonment, congenital drug addiction) (2). Over time, however, it is estimated that the average child receiving protective services experiences two or more forms of maltreatment. Comorbidity is the rule, not the exception.

Since a peak in 1993, rates of substantiated cases of child maltreatment have declined more than 20%, with decreases greatest in rates of physical and sexual abuse. The decline is believed to be "real," and has been attributed to prevention efforts, more aggressive criminal prosecution of perpetrators, and increased dissemination of psychiatric medications targeting behaviors that increase risk for abuse (11). Despite the decline in substantiated reports, over a similar time frame child fatalities related to abuse and neglect have increased 35%, with 1,490 child maltreatment–related fatalities documented in the last recorded year (2). There continues to be a long way to go for the eradication of abuse and neglect in this country.

DETECTION AND DISCLOSURE OF CHILD ABUSE

In one study, the rate of sexual abuse in a cohort of child psychiatric outpatients increased from 6% to 31%, when instead of requiring spontaneous independent reporting of these experiences, children were specifically asked about a possible abuse history (5). Clinicians sometimes hesitate to query children about abuse, out of fear of generating "false memories." The potential for suggestibility is greatest in preschoolers (12), but even very young children are capable of recalling much that is forensically relevant and providing reliable reports of abuse experiences. Suggestibility is minimized by promoting free recall and asking open-ended questions (13).

Children are more likely to deny true experiences when initially asked, than fabricate false experiences. For example, in one study of children with sexually transmitted diseases, 43% of the children initially denied sexual contact when queried, and most children required support and time to reveal ultimately their past abuse (8). Given the high prevalence of abuse experiences in child psychiatric populations, maltreatment experiences should routinely be screened in all mental health evaluations.

Mental health providers are mandated reporters. They are required by law to report suspected abuse. There is no systematic research on optimal procedures for handling mandated reporting requirements. In our clinical experience, it is usually best to inform the parent or guardian of one's intention to file a report, and to suggest that the parent or guardian call in the information as well. The parent's response to this fact will provide valuable information in evaluating the parent's capacity to support and protect the child, and determine the safety of the child staying in the immediate custody of the parent. It also gives the parent a sense of control at a very stressful time, and in truth, protective service workers look favorably upon a parent who calls to report a problem independently. Regardless of whether the parent agrees to call in the alleged abuse or not, the mental health professional is obligated to make the report. Given the data discussed above regarding the idiosyncratic nature of case investigation and substantiation, the mental health professional should be prepared to advocate for the child's best interest, and provide ongoing clinical support for the parent and/or child.

For guidelines on forensic evaluation of physical and sexual abuse cases, see the Practice Parameters drafted by the American Academy of Child and Adolescent Psychiatry (8). In addition, the interested reader is referred to the following excellent resources for the medical detection of physical abuse (14, 15) and sexual abuse (16).

COASSOCIATION OF CHILD MALTREATMENT, POVERTY, DOMESTIC VIOLENCE, AND SUBSTANCE ABUSE

Child abuse most often occurs in the context of other risk factors. Child abuse can and does occur across all socioeconomic classes, but is most prevalent among the poor. Families earning $15,000 or less per year are 22 times more likely to abuse or neglect their children than families with annual incomes of $30,000 or more (17). While most poor families do not maltreat their children, poverty is a significant risk factor for child abuse and neglect, with more than half of the families participating in a large-scale representative sample of protective services cases falling below the federal poverty line (18). The association between poverty and child maltreatment does not appear to be merely a reporting or detection bias, as a study of a national probability sample of 6,002 households surveyed via telephone also found the highest rate of abusive violence in families whose annual income is below the poverty line (4).

Substance abuse and domestic violence are two other problems that frequently cooccur in association with child maltreatment. It is estimated that 60% of cases involved with protective services have histories of severe domestic violence (18), and close to 80% of parents who lose custody of their children have a substance use disorder (19). Unfortunately, less than one-quarter of the families involved with protective services who are struggling with these issues receive any services for these problems (20), and there is no evidence that the services being offered decrease risk for re-abuse (21).

SEQUELAE

Indices of Adaptation and the Intergenerational Transmission of Abuse

A history of maltreatment is associated with deficits on numerous indices of adaptation across the lifecycle. When compared to community controls, maltreated children have significantly more disturbances in attachment relations in infancy, delays in autonomous functioning and deficits in frustration tolerance in toddlerhood, and problems with self-esteem and peer relations in later childhood (22, 23). Problems in language development and school performance have also been reported, including below average standardized achievement test scores, frequent repeated grades, low cumulative grade point averages, and significant social and behavior problems in class (24–26). In one study examining resiliency in maltreated children (27), few children could be classified resilient when multiple domains of functioning were considered. Approximately half the children in the maltreated sample had significant academic, social, *and* behavioral problems, and less than 5% of the sample was functioning well in all three domains.

In addition to these indicators of functional impairment, in adolescence (28) and adulthood (29), victims of child maltreatment are more likely than controls to be involved in intimate partner violence. They are also more likely to experience teen parenthood (30), and have difficulties parenting their children. While approximately 80%–90% of abusive parents have a history of child maltreatment, and being abused puts one at risk of experiencing parenting problems, only approximately one in three individuals who were abused as children repeats the cycle in the next generation (31, 32). Most break the cycle (or there would be exponential increases in rates of abuse with each generation), and there are many factors, as will be discussed later, that can help promote positive outcomes in maltreated children.

Psychiatric Diagnoses

Child maltreatment is a nonspecific risk factor for multiple forms of psychopathology (7, 33). Compared to community controls, maltreated children have elevated externalizing and internalizing behavior problems according to parent and teacher report (34). They also have increased rates of posttraumatic stress disorder (35–38); depression diagnoses (39, 40);

reactive attachment disorder (41); dissociative symptoms (42); self-destructive behavior and borderline traits (29, 43); sexually inappropriate behaviors (29, 44); drug and alcohol problems (7, 45, 46); eating disorders (47); oppositional defiant disorder (48, 49); and conduct disorder (48, 49). When compared to psychiatric controls, however, elevated rates of externalizing and internalizing problems (44), and most psychiatric disorders, with the exception of PTSD (50), have not been found.

Sexual Behavior Problems and Sexual Offending Behavior

Sexual behavior problems are frequently utilized as indicators of child sexual abuse. While inappropriate sexual behaviors are strongly related to experiences of sexual abuse, they are also associated with histories of physical abuse, witnessing domestic violence, inappropriate exposure to family sexuality, and child psychiatric illness (51). Table 5.15.1.1 delineates behaviors that are highly suggestive of a possible sexual abuse history, behaviors that are relatively prevalent in abuse victims and psychiatric controls with no history of abuse, and behaviors that are frequently observed in these high risk groups and normal controls (51, 52). Poor personal boundaries, increased sexual interest, and advanced sexual knowledge are reported at elevated rates in child psychiatric outpatients and child sexual abuse victims. These symptoms are not specific indicators of child sexual abuse, and neither are other common sexualized behaviors.

Fecal soiling has also in the past been attributed to a possible history of sexual abuse. In a recent large-scale study of 466 children with documented histories of sexual abuse, 429 psychiatric outpatients, and 641 normal controls, with the latter two groups carefully screened for abuse, there was no evidence that fecal soiling was a sensitive indicator of child sexual abuse (53). Ten percent of the children in both the abuse and the psychiatric control group reported soiling.

The question of whether child abuse victims are at high risk of becoming sexual offenders was addressed in a large prospective study of 908 maltreated children and 667 controls followed to adulthood (54). Victims of sexual abuse were more likely than physically abused, neglected, and control subjects to be arrested for prostitution, but no more likely to be arrested for incest, child molestation, or rape—all of which were relatively rare. Arrests for rape were highest among individuals physically abused as children, and although the rate was five times the rate observed in controls, the rate overall was quite low—2.1% for physically abused individuals, 0.7% for sexually abused individuals, and 0.4% for controls.

While official arrest rates likely underestimate the rate of true sexual offenses, it appears most victims of abuse do not become sexual offenders. Like in the case of the intergenerational transmission of abuse, however, most sexual offenders have a history of some form of child maltreatment. Data from the National Adolescent Perpetrator Network, a representative sample of 1,616 youth sexual offenders, suggest approximately 40% of youth offenders have a history of physical abuse, a similar proportion have a history of sexual abuse, 25% have a history of neglect, and approximately two-thirds have a history of witnessing severe domestic violence (55). The majority of the youth (63%) also had a history of engaging in other antisocial acts (e.g., theft, assault).

Juvenile sex offenses are frequently serious. Within the National Adolescent Perpetrator Network, the average number of victims per offender reported at intake was between seven and eight. In addition, 67% of the assaults involved vaginal penetration, sodomy, and/or oral–genital contact. Despite the seriousness of documented cases, there is preliminary data to suggest these behaviors are not persistent. In a recent longitudinal study of 300 male registered sex offenders who were juveniles at the time of their initial arrest for a sex offense, less than 5% were rearrested for a sex offense by their early to mid-20s. This is in sharp contrast to the arrest rate for nonsexual offenses, which exceeded 50% (56). Although there has been relatively little research on the treatment and longitudinal outcome of juvenile sex offenders, preliminary findings suggest treatment outcomes are good, and few juveniles are repeat offenders in adulthood (57, 58).

Neuroimaging Studies in Maltreated Children

As most of the neuroimaging studies of maltreated children have been limited to children who meet criteria for PTSD, these studies are only briefly discussed in this chapter (see Stover et al, 5.15.2, for further discussion). One of the best replicated findings in adults with PTSD is reduction in hippocampal volume (59–65). Multiple pediatric studies, however, failed to detect hippocampal atrophy in children with PTSD. Instead of hippocampal atrophy, children and adolescents with PTSD have been found to have reduced medial and posterior corpus callosum area (66–68). One recent study of adults with PTSD has similarly detected atrophy in the corpus callosum (69). Emerging preclinical and clinical studies suggest that alteration in corpus callosum and white matter tracts may be more prevalent early in development, although further systematic investigation is warranted.

MODIFIERS

Sensitive Periods

It has been hypothesized that trauma that occurs during the first 3 years of life will have particularly pernicious effects, given the rapid changes that occur in brain architecture during

TABLE 5.15.1.1

DISTINCTIVENESS OF SEXUALIZED BEHAVIORS IN INDICATING ABUSE HISTORY

Moderately Prevalent in Sexually Abused Children, Exceedingly Rare in Psychiatric and Normal Controls	Moderately Prevalent in Sexually Abused Children *and* Psychiatric Controls, Uncommon in Normal Controls	Moderately Prevalent in Sexually Abused Children, Psychiatric Controls, *and* Normal Controls
Puts mouth on sex parts	Stands too close to others	Talks flirtatiously
Asks to engage in sexual acts	Hugs adults they do not know well	Masturbates with hand
Masturbates with an object	Talks about sexual acts	Touches sex parts at home
Inserts objects in vagina or anus	Wants to watch movies that show nudity	Tries to look at nude pictures/undressing people
	Knows more about sex than other children their age	

this developmental period (70–72). There is growing interest, however, in the study of protective factors associated with resilience (73–75), and gaining a better understanding of the mechanisms by which vulnerabilities associated with early traumatic life events can be overcome. Emerging data suggests that while "sensitive" periods clearly exist, with adversity during early childhood associated with a greater propensity for deleterious outcomes (76, 77), negative outcomes are not inevitable. There are no known critical periods associated with indelible bad outcomes.

Emerging findings from preclinical studies suggest the negative effects associated with prenatal and early postnatal stress can be eliminated through environmental enrichment later in the postnatal or peripubertal period. Functional reversal of the behavioral and stress reactivity changes associated with early adversity appear to be mediated by the reversal of some neural changes (70, 78), and the induction of other changes that compensate, rather than reverse, other neural sequalae associated with early life stress (79). The remaining portions of this section delineate genetic and environmental risk and protective factors that can alter the probability of long-term deleterious outcomes in maltreated children.

Foster Care and Multiple Out-of-Home Placements

Recent studies estimate that there are slightly over one-half million maltreated children in out-of-home care nationwide, nearly twice as many children than there were two decades ago (2). It is estimated that 50–75% of children who enter care will return home (80), but 20–40% of these children will reenter care within a year or two (81). Unfortunately, many children who enter out-of-home care experience multiple placements and spend the majority of their lives in "foster-care drift"—moving from one place to the next without ever obtaining a permanent home (3). Nineteen percent of children in out-of-home care, or just under 100,000 children, are living in group homes or institutions (2), and it is estimated that 5% of children in care, or approximately 26,000 children, have experienced 10 or more placements since entering the system (81).

In 1991, Widom reported on the relationship between number of out-of-home placements and antisocial and violent behavior in adulthood. Rates of these problems in individuals maltreated as children were low, approximately 10%, in individuals with zero or one placement. With a second placement, rates of antisocial behavior doubled to 20%, and with three or more placements it more than quadrupled. Forty-five percent of individuals with three or more placements had a criminal record for antisocial behavior, and almost 30% had a history of violent offenses (82).

As the Widom study was a follow forward study with no child behavior assessments at baseline, it is impossible to tell if the greater number of placements was a cause *or* consequence of behavioral problems. Landsverk and colleagues (83) conducted the first prospective longitudinal investigation aimed at disentangling the relationship between problem behaviors and placement number. They assessed 415 children approximately 5 months after entering care, and again 12 months later. While they did find evidence that initial behavior problems was the strongest predictor of placement changes, they also clearly documented that children who showed no evidence of psychopathology at baseline developed significant behavior problems subsequent to multiple changes in placement (Figure 5.15.1.1).

We similarly have followed a cohort of 100 maltreated children prospectively and obtained self-report measures of anxiety within 6 months of initial placement, and again at 1-year followup. We also collected anxiety ratings on a

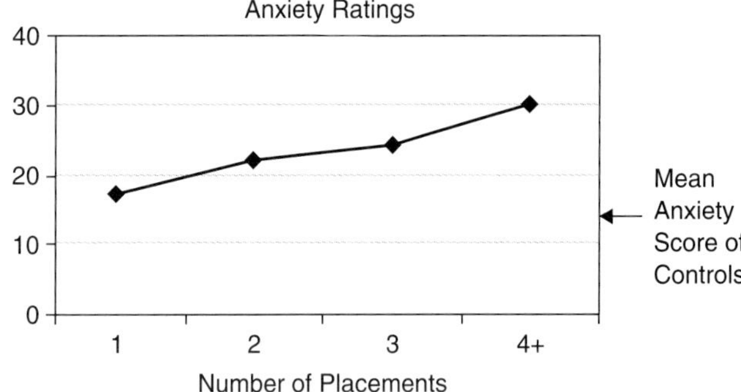

FIGURE 5.15.1.1. Relationship between number of placements and children's anxiety ratings. After covarying for children's baseline anxiety scores, number of placements was a robust predictor of children's anxiety symptoms at 1-year followup.

demographically matched cohort of community controls carefully screened for maltreatment experiences. After covarying for baseline anxiety measures, number of placements was a robust predictor of anxiety symptoms at followup. Children with only one placement over the course of the followup period had anxiety scores that were comparable to controls. With a second placement, children's scores increased 50%, and those children with four or more placements had anxiety scores that were double those of maltreated children who had experienced stable placements.

Multiple out-of-home placements are the rule, not the exception. No "best practices" exist to assure placement stability for children in care. As discussed in the treatment section, preliminary efforts are underway to develop intervention approaches to prevent placement disruption, but to date, support for these efforts are limited.

GENETIC FACTORS

Caspi, Moffitt, and colleagues (84) were the first to examine the role of genetic factors in moderating the outcome of maltreated children. They studied a large sample of 1,037 males from birth to adulthood. The dataset allowed them to address the question of why some children who are maltreated grow up to develop antisocial behavior, and others do not. A functional polymorphism in the gene encoding the neurotransmitter-metabolizing enzyme monoamine oxidase A (MAOA) was found to moderate the relationship between maltreatment and later sociopathy. Maltreated children with a genotype conferring high levels of MAOA expression were less likely to develop antisocial problems. The role of MAOA in moderating the development of sociopathy in maltreated children has now been replicated in several other studies (85).

Caspi, Moffitt, and colleagues then examined gene-by-environment interactions in the development of depression (86). They were the first to report that a functional polymorphism in the promoter region of the serotonin transporter (5-HTTLPR) gene moderated the influence of early child maltreatment and stressful life events on the development of depression. Individuals with a history of abuse with one or two copies of the short allele of 5-HTTLPR exhibited more depressive symptoms and diagnosable depression than individuals homozygous for the long allele. This finding has since been replicated in three independent investigations with child (87), adolescent (88), and young adult (89, 90) populations.

Given that gene by gene interactions have been hypothesized to contribute to the etiology of depression (91, 92), we hypothesized that a polymorphism in brain derived neurotrophic factor (BDNF) gene might interact with 5-HTTLPR to further increase risk for depression in maltreated children. BDNF genetic variation has recently been associated with child onset depression in two independent samples (93, 94). In addition, both BDNF (the protein product of the BDNF gene) and serotonin (5-HT) have been implicated in the etiology of depression, and they are also known to interact at multiple intra- and intercellular levels (95, 96). We studied a sample of 109 maltreated and 87 nonmaltreated demographically matched comparison children. We were able to document a significant three-way interaction between BDNF genotype, 5-HTTLPR, and maltreatment history in predicting depression. As depicted in Figure 5.15.1.2, children with the Met allele of the BDNF gene and two short alleles of 5-HTTLPR had the highest depression scores, but the vulnerability associated with these two genotypes was only evident in the maltreated children (97).

We have also followed a subset of our cohort for 2 years and examined predictors of early alcohol use, including: maltreatment, family loading for alcohol/substance use disorders, and 5-HTTLPR (98). Alcohol use before the age of 14 is a potent predictor of later alcohol problems and is associated with a 40% risk for the development of alcohol dependence (99). Participants were 127 subjects—76 maltreated children and 51 demographically matched community controls. At followup, 29% of the maltreated children reported alcohol use, a rate more than seven times the rate observed in controls. Maltreated children also drank, on average, more than 2 years earlier than controls (11.2 versus 13.5 years). Early alcohol use was predicted by maltreatment, 5-HTTLPR, and a gene-by-environment interaction, with increased risk for early alcohol use associated with the "s" allele.

There is converging evidence that multiple genetic and environmental factors are involved in the etiology of depression and other diagnoses frequently observed in maltreated children (see Luthar, 3.2). Future and ongoing investigations of relevant genetic and environmental risk and protective factors will help to identify the children who are most vulnerable to adverse outcomes, delineate environmental and neural mechanisms to help promote resilience, and facilitate the development of multimodal prevention and intervention efforts.

Social Supports

There are emerging preclinical and clinical data to suggest that the long-term neurobiological and behavioral changes associated with early stress can be modified by the availability of positive supports and optimal subsequent caregiving experiences (100). Several investigators utilizing mother–infant separation paradigms in rodents, one of the most frequently employed preclinical paradigms to examine the effects of early stress, noted that separation resulted in subtle disruptions in the quality of maternal–pup interaction. By providing the mother with a "foster" litter during the period of pup separation, they were able to prevent the deterioration in maternal care behaviors, and subsequently prevent most of the long-term neurobiological changes associated with early separation (101). These findings are consistent with the results of studies examining the effects of prenatal stress. In these studies "adoption" with "optimal parenting" has also been found to reverse the HPA axis alterations typically observed in association with these early stress paradigms (102). Consistent with these preclinical findings, clinical studies of individuals with a history of abuse also suggest that the availability of a caring and stable parent or alternate guardian is one of the most important factors that distinguish abused individuals with good developmental outcomes, from those with more deleterious outcomes (76).

Consequently, we have examined the effect of social supports in moderating genetic and environmental risk for depression in children. Children were asked to name people they 1) talk to about personal things; 2) count on to buy the things they need; 3) share good news with; 4) get together with to have fun; and 5) go to if they need advice. The summary social support measure used was the number of positive support categories listed for the child's top support. The children were most likely to name an adult as their primary support. Sixty-one percent of the maltreated children and 83% of the controls listed their mothers as their top support, and 30% of the maltreated children and 10% of the controls listed alternative parental figures (e.g., father, stepfather, foster mother), grandparents, or other adult relatives as their primary support.

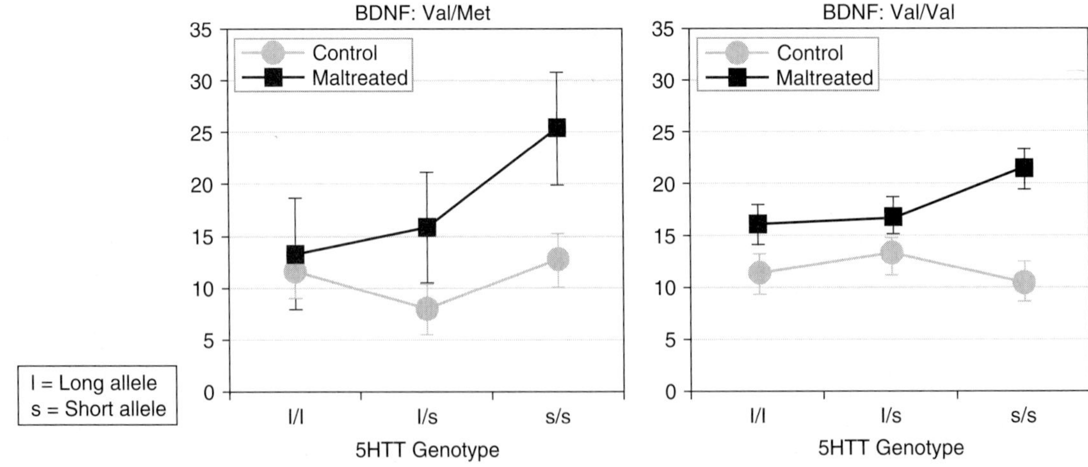

FIGURE 5.15.1.2. Three-way interaction between maltreatment history, BDNF, and 5-HTTLPR genotype. The graphs depict the data of the maltreated and control children. There was a significant three-way interaction between BDNF genotype, 5-HTTLPR genotype, and maltreatment history in predicting children's depression scores. Children with the BDNF gene Val66Met polymorphism and the "s/s" 5-HTTLPR genotype had the highest depression scores, with the vulnerability associated with these two genotypes only elevated in the maltreated children. (Adapted from Kaufman J, Yang BZ, Douglas-Palumberi H, Grasso D, Lipschitz D, Houshyar S, Krystal JH, Gelernter J: Brain-derived neurotrophic factor-5-HTTLPR gene interactions and environmental modifiers of depression in children. *Biological Psychiatry* 59:673–680, 2006, with permission.)

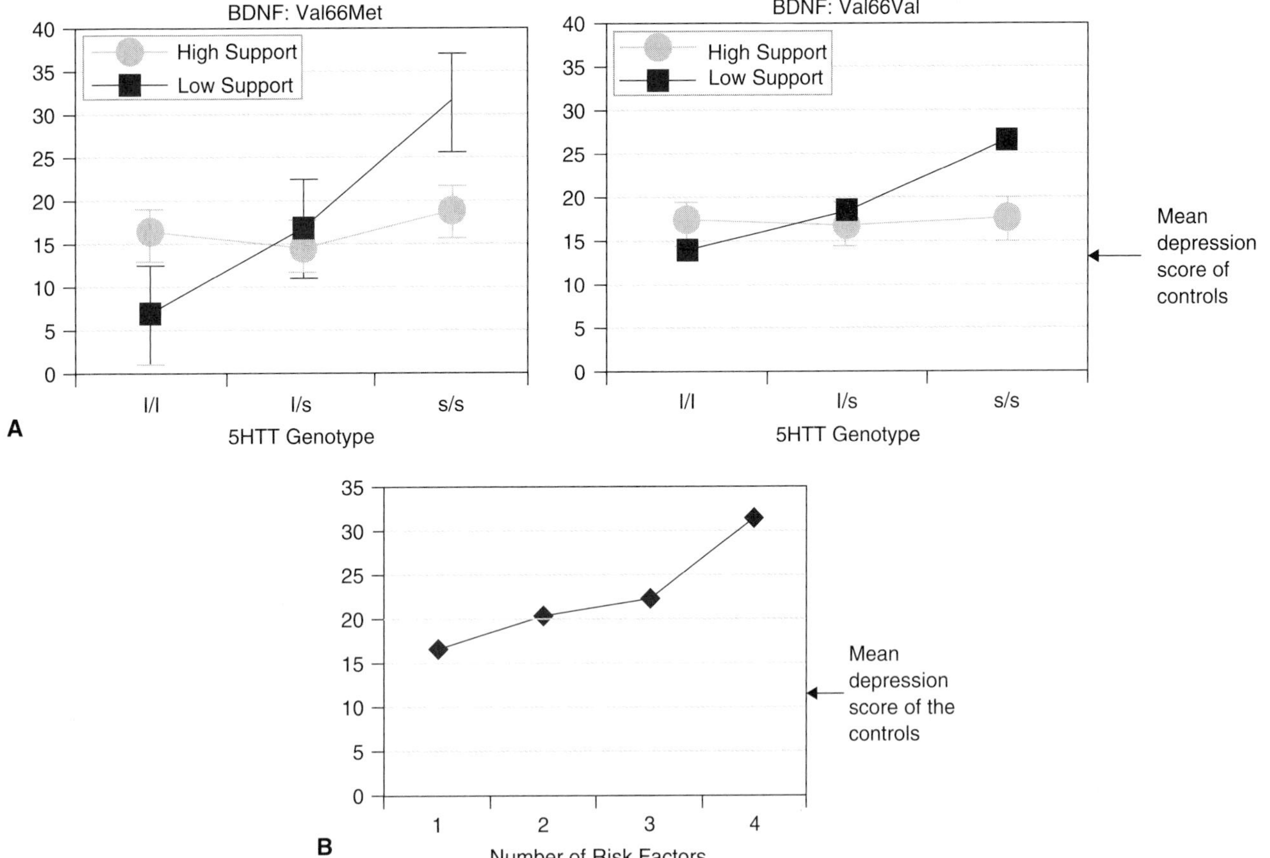

FIGURE 5.15.1.3. (A) **Four-way interaction between maltreatment history, BDNF genotype, and 5-HTTLPR genotype and social supports: Maltreated children's data.** The graphs depict only the data of the maltreated children. The mean score of the controls is indicated on the right as a frame of reference. The depression scores of the maltreated children with high social supports were close to the mean depression score of the controls, regardless of genotype. The "s/s" genotype was associated with an increase in maltreated children's depression scores, which was greatest for the children without positive supports and the additional presence of the met allele of the BDNF polymorphism. (B) **Cumulative effect of each risk factor on children's depression scores.** The mean depression score of the maltreated children (Risk = 1) is depicted in the first column of the current graph. A history of maltreatment is associated with a 33% increase in depression scores, or approximately 4 extra points on the Mood and Feelings Questionnaire. Having the "s/s" genotype on top of a history of maltreatment (Risk = 2) adds on average an additional 4 points to children's depression scores, and the addition of the Met allele of the BDNF Val66Met polymorphism (Risk = 3) adds on average an extra 2 points. When the effect of social supports was examined for the maltreated group as a whole, it had little effect, with maltreated children with high and low supports having very similar depression scores (Maltreated/high supports: 16.6 ± 9.2; Maltreated/low supports: 16.9 ± 11.1). Low social supports, however, contributed significantly to the depression scores of the children with the most vulnerable genotypes (Risk = 4), adding on average an extra nine points to the depression scores of the maltreated children with two "s" alleles and the Met allele of the BDNF Val66Met polymorphism. (Adapted, Kaufman J, Yang BZ, Douglas-Palumberi H, Grasso D, Lipschitz D, Houshyar S, Krystal JH, Gelernter J: Brain-derived neurotrophic factor-5-HTTLPR gene interactions and environmental modifiers of depression in children. *Biological Psychiatry* 59:673–680, 2006.)

As depicted in Figure 5.15.1.3a,b, maltreated children with positive supports had depression scores that were only slightly greater than controls, regardless of genotype. The quality and availability of social supports was extremely potent in reducing risk for depression in maltreated children—with the effect greatest for those maltreated children with the most vulnerable genotypes. Negative sequelae associated with abuse are not inevitable; they can be modified by both genetic and environmental factors.

There are likely multiple mechanisms by which social supports may ameliorate risk. Data from preclinical studies suggest that maternal behavior can produce stable changes in DNA methylation and chromatin structure of the glucocorticoid receptor gene promoter in the hippocampus (103). These epigenetic changes and the subsequent alteration in hypothalamic pituitary adrenal (HPA) axis response to stress may be one important mechanism by which variations in maternal behavior/social supports alter risk for stress-related disorders.

A take-home message from the gene by environment studies is that to help promote resiliency in maltreated children we must: 1) prevent the re-abuse of children; and 2) facilitate the formation of lasting positive relationships with birth parents or alternative caregivers. As is evident from the material discussed in multiple sections of this chapter, we are not yet succeeding in achieving these goals for most maltreated children.

TREATMENT

Service Delivery

Results of a recent national survey suggest that approximately 40% of all confirmed cases of child maltreatment do not receive any therapeutic or supportive services (2). For these families, the investigation is the only "service" provided. The unmet service needs of this clinical population are enormous. While it is estimated that one-half to two-thirds of children involved with protective services have significant developmental or mental health care needs, only approximately one-quarter will receive specialized services to address these issues (26, 104). A similar proportion of parents with mental health and/or substance abuse problems likewise fail to receive services to address these issues (20). Failure to provide needed mental health services for children in care is associated with increased likelihood of placement disruption, and failure to adequately address parents' mental health and substance abuse problems is associated with elevated rates of re-abuse.

Child Focused Interventions

Children involved in the child protective services system are two to three times more likely to be prescribed psychotropic medications than children in the community (105, 106). These medications are often prescribed without adjunctive psychotherapeutic interventions. Over the past decade there has been a marked increase in the number of carefully controlled treatment trials for children with PTSD (see Stover, 5.15.2), and other clinical diagnoses common in maltreated children (107–110). To enhance dissemination, groups are beginning to utilize community-based approaches (e.g., in-home, in-school) to facilitate access to effective evidence-based behavioral and cognitive-behavioral treatments for trauma-related psychopathology (111). Dissemination and access to care, however, remain considerable problems in most areas.

Knowledge that a child has a history of abuse provides only the most rudimentary information necessary for planning interventions. A history of abuse is not an Axis I diagnosis (112). As discussed throughout this chapter, maltreated children represent a very heterogenous group, with varied treatment needs. In planning interventions with maltreated children it is important to conduct a comprehensive psychiatric assessment to identify the unique clinical needs of the child. Axis I diagnoses such as attention deficit disorder, major depression, conduct disorder, and PTSD should be treated using accepted empirically validated approaches as part of a larger more comprehensive intervention that addresses the many other needs of the maltreated child and his or her family. Two key tenets to keep in mind in conducting clinical interventions with this population are: 1) The treatment of maltreated children requires working as part of a larger multidisciplinary team with child protective services workers, adult treatment providers, and others; and 2) assessing the treatment needs of maltreated children requires moving beyond clinical symptomatology and abuse-related issues, to other family (e.g., parental substance use) and environmental (e.g., poverty, social supports) factors. Without addressing a range of foci, risk for placement disruption and revictimization are high.

Permanency Planning Focused Interventions

In light of the negative consequences associated with long stays in care and multiple changes in placements, Congress passed the Adoption and Safe Families Act in 1997 (113). This legislation mandates, with some exceptions, that permanency be achieved for maltreated children who have been in out-of-home care for 15 of the last 22 months. Connecticut and several other states require permanency be achieved if children have been in out-of-home care for only 12 months. Permanency can be attained via: 1) family reunification, 2) child adoption, or 3) long-term placement with kin or nonrelative foster caregivers who are granted legal guardianship. The aim of permanency planning efforts is to maximize the likelihood of children being wanted and having at least one adult that they identify as a psychological parent (114), since, as discussed previously, the availability of a positive relationship with one or more caregivers has been identified as one of the most important factors in ameliorating a host of negative sequelae associated with child maltreatment.

Given the timelines imposed by the Adoption and Safe Families Act (P.L. 105–89, 1997), unless substance abuse treatment is available promptly, the opportunity for intervention may be lost (115). Some intervention approaches currently being utilized to address parent substance abuse problems include: having adult addiction services liaisons work in child welfare offices to facilitate client referral for treatment (115); hiring substance abuse counselors to work in child welfare offices to perform on-site evaluations and identify appropriate resources for clients (116); and establishing family drug courts that provide a highly structured venue within which treatment services are offered, sanctions are applied for noncompliance, and program progress is meticulously monitored, allowing permanency decisions to be made more quickly on the basis of better information (116). Dialectical Behavior Therapy (DBT) programs for substance-abusing parents may be an additional alternative promising approach worthy of evaluation, as DBT programs have been found to be more effective than treatment-as-usual for substance abusing patients with borderline personality disorder (117)—patients who exhibit many of the core difficulties observed among protective service clients (history of early childhood trauma, intense unstable relationships, difficulty tolerating distress, labile affect, impulsiveness).

Interventions targeting adult problems tend to be completely separate from interventions targeting child problems, and vice versa. For example, the Early Intervention Foster Care (EIFC) Program (118), a comprehensive program aimed at promoting permanency for maltreated children in care includes: 1) 20 hours of parent management training for foster parents, 2) daily telephone calls from staff to monitor child behavior, 3) weekly support meetings with program staff and other foster parents, 4) weekly home visits, 5) 24/7 emergency back-up; and 6) a multidisciplinary team that includes a consulting psychiatrist. In a recent evaluation of the EIFC program (118), by 2 years postremoval only approximately half the children had attained permanency. The failure to achieve permanency for more children suggests there is something missing from this comprehensive clinical package, whose efficacy might be enhanced by the inclusion of trauma-focused child interventions and greater attention to birth parents and their clinical needs (119).

Future Directions—Integrated Treatment Models

The Comprehensive Assessment and Training Services (CATS) Project was also developed to promote permanency and prevent children from lingering in foster care (120). The program is designed to assess and facilitate treatment for child (developmental, psychiatric), birth family (substance abuse, domestic violence), socioeconomic (housing), and maltreatment-specific (protective services, criminal justice) issues. Outcome data are currently pending, but the approach appears quite promising.

CLOSING REMARKS

In the closing of its 1990 report, the U.S. Advisory Board on Child Abuse and Neglect concluded that "... the scope of the problem of child maltreatment is so enormous and serious, and the failure of the system designed to deal with the problem so catastrophic, that the crisis has reached the level of a national emergency" (121). In its 1993 report the Board reaffirmed this view stating "... the status of emergency remains in effect and may even be more dire today (in 1993) than it was in 1990." They then went on to describe the child protection system as "broken" (122). While rates of physical and sexual abuse have declined since their peak reached in 1993, by all standards, the child protective services system remains "broken."

Advances in legislation, efficacy of clinical interventions, and translational research approaches offer novel opportunities to make real progress in alleviating the suffering associated with child abuse and neglect. Maltreated children are at elevated risk for a host of negative outcomes, but the cycle of adversity can be broken. We can and must do better.

References

1. Zigler E: Controlling child abuse: Do we have the knowledge and/or the will? In: Gerbner G, Zigler E (eds): In: *Child Abuse: An Agenda for Action*. CR New York, Oxford Press, 1980, pp. 293–304.
2. Children's Bureau AoC, Youth, and Families. U.S. Department of Health and Human Services: *Child Maltreatment 2004*. Washington, DC, U.S. Government Printing Office, 2006.
3. Kaufman J, Zigler E: Child abuse and social policy. In Zigler E, Kagan S, Hall N (eds): *Children, Families and Government: Preparing for the Twenty-First Century*. New York, Cambridge University Press, 1996, pp. 233–255.
4. Wolfner GD, Gelles RJ: A profile of violence toward children: A national study. *Child Abuse Negl* 17(2):197–212, 1993.
5. Lanktree C, Briere J, Zaidi L: Incidence and impact of sexual abuse in a child outpatient sample: The role of direct inquiry. *Child Abuse Negl* 15(4):447–453, 1991.
6. McClellan J, Adams J, Douglas D, McCurry C, Storck M: Clinical characteristics related to severity of sexual abuse: A study of seriously mentally ill youth. *Child Abuse Negl* 19(10):1245–1254, 1995.
7. Molnar BE, Buka SL, Kessler RC: Child sexual abuse and subsequent psychopathology: Results from the National Comorbidity Survey. *Am J Public Health* 91(5):753–760, 2001.
8. Lawson L, Chaffin M: False negatives in sexual abuse interviews: Incidence and influence of caretaker's belief in abuse in cases of accidental abuse discovery by diagnosis of STD. *Journal of Interpersonal Violence* 7:532–542, 1992.
9. Black MM, Dubowitz H, Casey PH, Cutts D, Drewett RF, Drotar D, Frank DA, Karp R, Kessler DB, Meyers AF, Wright CM: Failure to thrive as distinct from child neglect. *Pediatrics* 117(4):1456–1458; author reply 1458–1459, 2006.
10. Drake B, Jonson-Reid M, Way I, Chung S: Substantiation and recidivism. *Child Maltreat* 8(4):248–260, 2003.
11. Jones LM, Finkelhor D, Halter S: Child maltreatment trends in the 1990s: Why does neglect differ from sexual and physical abuse? *Child Maltreat* 11(2):107–120, 2006.
12. Ceci SJ, Bruck M: Suggestibility of the child witness: A historical review and synthesis. *Psychol Bull* 113(3):403–439, 1993.
13. Saywitz K, Goodman GS, Lyon TD: Interviewing Children in and out of court: Current research and practice implications. In: Myers J, Berliner L, Briere J, Hendrix CT, JC, Reid TA (eds): *The APSAC Handbook on Child Maltreatment*. Thousand Oaks, California, Sage Publications, Inc., 2002, pp. 349–378.
14. Thompson S: Accidental or inflicted? *Pediatr Ann* 34(5):372–381, 2005.
15. Hymel KP, Hall CA: Diagnosing pediatric head trauma. *Pediatr Ann* 34(5):358–370, 2005.
16. Kellogg N: The evaluation of sexual abuse in children. *Pediatrics* 116(2):506–512, 2005.
17. DHHS: *Third National Incidence Study of Child Abuse and Neglect (NIS-3)*. Edited by Department of Health and Human Services AfCNCoCAaN. Washington, DC, 1996.
18. Connelly CD, Hazen AL, Coben JH, Kelleher KJ, Barth RP, Landsverk JA: Persistence of intimate partner violence among families referred to child welfare. *J Interpers Violence* 21(6):774–797, 2006.
19. Besinger BA, Garland AF, Litrownik AJ, Landsverk JA: Caregiver substance abuse among maltreated children placed in out-of-home care. *Child Welfare* 78(2):221–239, 1999.
20. Libby AM, Orton HD, Barth RP, Webb MB, Burns BJ, Wood P, Spicer P: Alcohol, drug, and mental health specialty treatment services and race/ethnicity: A national study of children and families involved with child welfare. *Am J Public Health* 96(4):628–631, 2006. Epub 2006 Feb 28.
21. Barth RP, Gibbons C, Guo S: Substance abuse treatment and the recurrence of maltreatment among caregivers with children living at home: A propensity score analysis. *J Subst Abuse Treat* 30(2):93–104, 2006.
22. Cicchetti D, Toth S: A developmental psychopathology perspective on child abuse and neglect. *Journal of the American Academy of Child and Adolescent Psychiatry*. 34(5):541–565, 1995.
23. Myers J, Berliner L, Briere J, Hendrix CT, Jenny C, Reid TA: *The APSAC Handbook on Child Maltreatment*. Thousand Oaks, California, Sage Publications, Inc., 2002.
24. Kendall-Tackett KA, Eckenrode J: The effects of neglect on academic achievement and disciplinary problems: A developmental perspective. *Child Abuse Negl* 20(3):161–169, 1996.
25. Perez CM, Widom CS: Childhood victimization and long-term intellectual and academic outcomes. *Child Abuse Negl* 18(8):617–633, 1994.
26. Stahmer AC, Leslie LK, Hurlburt M, Barth RP, Webb MB, Landsverk J, Zhang J: Developmental and behavioral needs and service use for young children in child welfare. *Pediatrics* 116(4):891–900, 2005.
27. Kaufman J, Cooke A, Arny L, Jones B, Pittinsky T: Problems defining resiliency: illustrations from the study of maltreated children. *Develop and Psychopathology* 6(Special Issue: Child Maltreatment):215–229, 1994.
28. Wolfe DA, Wekerle C, Scott K, Straatman AL, Grasley C: Predicting abuse in adolescent dating relationships over 1 year: the role of child maltreatment and trauma. *J Abnorm Psychol* 113(3):406–415, 2004.
29. Noll JG, Horowitz LA, Bonanno GA, Trickett PK, Putnam FW: Revictimization and self-harm in females who experienced childhood sexual abuse: Results from a prospective study. *J Interpers Violence* 18(12):1452–1471, 2003.
30. Noll JG, Trickett PK, Putnam FW: A prospective investigation of the impact of childhood sexual abuse on the development of sexuality. *J Consult Clin Psychol* 71(3):575–586, 2003.
31. Widom CS: The cycle of violence. *Science* 244(4901):160–166, 1989.
32. Kaufman J, Zigler E: Do abused children become abusive parents? *Am J Orthopsychiatry* 57(2):186–192, 1987.
33. Kendler KS, Bulik CM, Silberg J, Hettema JM, Myers J, Prescott CA: Childhood sexual abuse and adult psychiatric and substance use disorders in women: An epidemiological and cotwin control analysis. *Arch Gen Psychiatry* 57(10):953–959, 2000.
34. Kaplan SJ, Labruna V, Pelcovitz D, Salzinger S, Mandel F, Weiner M: Physically abused adolescents: Behavior problems, functional impairment, and comparison of informants' reports. *Pediatrics* 104(1 Pt 1):43–49, 1999.
35. Kilpatrick D, Ruggiero K, Acierno R, Saunders B, Resnick H, Best C: Violence and risk of PTSD, major depression, substance abuse/dependence, and comorbidity: Results from the National Survey of Adolescents. *J Consult Clin Psychol* 71(4):692–700, 2003.
36. Famularo R, Kinscherff R, Fenton T: Psychiatric diagnoses of maltreated children: Preliminary findings. *J Am Acad Child Adolesc Psychiatry* 31:863–867, 1992.
37. Famularo R, Fenton T, Kinscherff R, Augustyn M: Psychiatric comorbidity in childhood post traumatic stress disorder. *Child Abuse Negl* 20(10):953–961, 1996.
38. Ruggiero K, McLeer S, Dixon J: Sexual abuse characteristics associated with survivor psychopathology. *Child Abuse Negl* 24(7):951–964, 2000.
39. Kaufman J: Depressive disorders in maltreated children. *J Am Acad Child Adolesc Psychiatry* 30(2):257–265, 1991.
40. Pelcovitz D, Kaplan SJ, DeRosa RR, Mandel FS, Salzinger S: Psychiatric disorders in adolescents exposed to domestic violence and physical abuse. *Am J Orthopsychiatry* 70(3):360–369, 2000.
41. Zeanah CH, Scheeringa M, Boris NW, Heller SS, Smyke AT, Trapani J: Reactive attachment disorder in maltreated toddlers. *Child Abuse Negl* 28(8):877–888, 2004.
42. Putnam FW, Helmers K, Horowitz LA, Trickett PK: Hypnotizability and dissociativity in sexually abused girls. *Child Abuse Negl* 19(5):645–655, 1995.
43. Romans SE, Martin JL, Anderson JC, Herbison GP, Mullen PE: Sexual abuse in childhood and deliberate self-harm. *Am J Psychiatry* 152(9):1336–1342, 1995.
44. Cosentino CE, Meyer-Bahlburg HF, Alpert JL, Weinberg SL, Gaines R: Sexual behavior problems and psychopathology symptoms in sexually abused girls. *J Am Acad Child Adolesc Psychiatry* 34(8):1033–1042, 1995.
45. Widom CS, Ireland T, Glynn PJ: Alcohol abuse in abused and neglected children followed-up: Are they at increased risk? *J Stud Alcohol* 56(2):207–217, 1995.
46. Schuck AM, Widom CS: Childhood victimization and alcohol symptoms in women: An examination of protective factors. *J Stud Alcohol* 64(2):247–256, 2003.
47. Ackard DM, Neumark-Sztainer D: Multiple sexual victimizations among adolescent boys and girls: Prevalence and associations with eating behaviors and psychological health. *J Child Sex Abus* 12(1):17–37, 2003.
48. Garland A, Hough R, McCabe K, Yeh M, Wood P, Aarons G: Prevalence of psychiatric disorders in youths across five sectors of care. *J Am Acad Child Adolesc Psychiatry* 40(4):409–418, 2001.

49. Kolko D: Child physical abuse. In Myers J, Berliner L, Briere J, Hendrix CT, JC, Reid TA (eds): *The APSAC Handbook on Child Maltreatment*. Thousand Oaks, California, Sage Publications, Inc., 2002, pp. 21–54.
50. McLeer S, Callaghan M, Henry D, Wallen J: Psychiatric disorders in sexually abused children. *J Am Acad Child Adolesc Psychiatry*. 33:313–319, 1994.
51. Friedrich WN, Fisher JL, Dittner CA, Acton R, Berliner L, Butler J, Damon L, Davies WH, Gray A, Wright J: Child Sexual Behavior Inventory: Normative, psychiatric, and sexual abuse comparisons. *Child Maltreat* 6(1):37–49, 2001.
52. Friedrich WN, Grambsch P, Damon L, Hewitt SK, Koverola C, Lang RA, WOlfe V, Broughton D: Child Sexual Behavior Inventory: Normative and Clinical Comparisons. *Psychological Assessment* 4(3):303–311, 1992.
53. Mellon MW, Whiteside SP, Friedrich WN: The relevance of fecal soiling as an indicator of child sexual abuse: A preliminary analysis. *J Dev Behav Pediatr* 27(1):25–32, 2006.
54. Widom CP, Ames MA: Criminal consequences of childhood sexual victimization. *Child Abuse Negl* 18(4):303–318, 1994.
55. Ryan G, Miyoshi TJ, Metzner JL, Krugman RD, Fryer GE: Trends in a national sample of sexually abusive youths. *J Am Acad Child Adolesc Psychiatry* 35(1):17–25, 1996.
56. Vandiver DM: A prospective analysis of juvenile male sex offenders: Characteristics and recidivism rates as adults. *J Interpers Violence* 21(5):673–688, 2006.
57. Chaffin M, Letourneau E, Silovsky JF: Adults, adolescents, and children who sexually abuse children: Myers J, Berliner L, Briere J, Hendrix CT, JC, Reid TA (eds): *A developmental perspective. In The APSAC Handbook on Child Maltreatment*. Thousand Oaks, California, Sage Publications, Inc., 2002, pp. 205–232.
58. Shaw JA: Summary of the practice parameters for the assessment and treatment of children and adolescents who are sexually abusive of others. American Academy of Child and Adolescent Psychiatry. *J Am Acad Child Adolesc Psychiatry* 39(1):127–130, 2000.
59. Villarreal G, Hamilton DA, Petropoulos H, Driscoll I, Rowland LM, Griego JA, Kodituwakku PW, Hart BL, Escalona R, Brooks WM: Reduced hippocampal volume and total white matter volume in posttraumatic stress disorder. *Biol Psychiatry* 52(2):119–125, 2002.
60. Bernstein D, Ahluvalia T, Pogge D, Handelsman L: Validity of the Childhood Trauma Questionnaire in an adolescent psychiatric population. *J Am Acad Child Adolesc Psychiatry* 36(3):340–348, 1997.
61. Bremner JD, Randall P, Vermetten E, Staib L, Bronen RA, Mazure C, Capelli S, McCarthy G, Innis RB, Charney DS: Magnetic resonance imaging-based measurement of hippocampal volume in posttraumatic stress disorder related to childhood physical and sexual abuse—A preliminary report. *Biol Psychiatry* 41(1):23–32, 1997.
62. Bremner JD, Randall P, Scott TM, Bronen RA, Seibyl JP, Southwick SM, Delaney RC, McCarthy G, Charney DS, Innis RB: MRI-based measurement of hippocampal volume in patients with combat-related posttraumatic stress disorder. *Am J Psychiatry* 152(7):973–981, 1995.
63. Gurvits TV, Shenton ME, Hokama H, Ohta H, Lasko NB, Gilbertson MW, Orr SP, Kikinis R, Jolesz FA, McCarley RW, Pitman RK: Magnetic resonance imaging study of hippocampal volume in chronic, combat-related posttraumatic stress disorder. *Biol Psychiatry* 40(11):1091–1099, 1996.
64. Vythilingam M, Heim C, Newport J, Miller AH, Anderson E, Bronen R, Brummer M, Staib L, Vermetten E, Charney DS, Nemeroff CB, Bremner JD: Childhood trauma associated with smaller hippocampal volume in women with major depression. *Am J Psychiatry* 159(12):2072–2080, 2002.
65. Driessen M, Hermann J, Stahl K, Zwann M, Meier S, Hill A, Osterheider M, Petersen D: Magnetic resonance imaging: volumes of the hippocampus and the amygdala in women with borderline personality disorder and early traumatization. *Arch Gen Psychiatry* 57:1115–1122, 2000.
66. De Bellis MD, Keshavan MS, Clark DB, Casey BJ, Giedd JN, Boring AM, Frustaci K, Ryan ND: Developmental traumatology. Part II: Brain development. *Biol Psychiatry* 45(10):1271–1284, 1999.
67. De Bellis MD, Keshavan MS, Shifflett H, Iyengar S, Beers SR, Hall J, Moritz G: Brain structures in pediatric maltreatment-related posttraumatic stress disorder: A sociodemographically matched study. *Biol Psychiatry* 52(11):1066–1078, 2002.
68. Teicher MH, Dumont NL, Ito Y, Vaituzis C, Giedd JN, Andersen SL: Childhood neglect is associated with reduced corpus callosum area. *Biol Psychiatry* 56(2):80–85, 2004.
69. Villarreal G, Hamilton DA, Graham DP, Driscoll I, Qualls C, Petropoulos H, Brooks WM: Reduced area of the corpus callosum in posttraumatic stress disorder. *Psychiatry Res* 131(3):227–235, 2004.
70. Charmandari E, Tsigos C, Chrousos G: Endocrinology of the stress response. *Annu Rev Physiol* 67:259–284, 2005.
71. Cicchetti D, Cannon TD: Neurodevelopmental processes in the ontogenesis and epigenesis of psychopathology [editorial]. *Dev Psychopathol* 11(3):375–393, 1999.
72. Sanchez MM, Ladd CO, Plotsky PM: Early adverse experience as a developmental risk factor for later psychopathology: Evidence from rodent and primate models. *Dev Psychopathol* 13(3):419–449, 2001.
73. Charney DS, Manji HK: Life stress, genes, and depression: multiple pathways lead to increased risk and new opportunities for intervention. *Sci* STKE 2004; 2004(225):re5
74. Curtis WJ, Cicchetti D: Moving research on resilience into the 21st century: Theoretical and methodological considerations in examining the biological contributors to resilience. *Dev Psychopathol* 15(3):773–810, 2003.
75. Luthar SS, Cicchetti D, Becker B: The construct of resilience: A critical evaluation and guidelines for future work. *Child Dev* 71(3):543–562, 2000.
76. Kaufman J, Henrich C: Exposure to violence and early childhood trauma. In: Zeanah Jr. C (ed): *Handbook of Infant Mental Health*. New York, Guilford Press, 2000, pp. 195–207.
77. McClellan J, McCurry C, Ronnei M, Adams J, Eisner A, Storck M: Age of onset of sexual abuse: Relationship to sexually inappropriate behaviors. *J Am Acad Child Adolesc Psychiatry* 35(10):1375–1383, 1996.
78. Bredy TW, Zhang TY, Grant RJ, Diorio J, Meaney MJ, Humpartzoomian RA, Cain DP, Morley-Fletcher S, Rea M, Maccari S, Laviola G: Peripubertal environmental enrichment reverses the effects of maternal care on hippocampal development and glutamate receptor subunit expression. *Eur J Neurosci* 20(5):1355–1362, 2004.
79. Francis DD, Diorio J, Plotsky PM, Meaney MJ: Environmental enrichment reverses the effects of maternal separation on stress reactivity. *J Neurosci* 22(18):7840–7843, 2002.
80. Barth RP: Adoption research: Building blocks for the next decade. *Child Welfare* 73(5):625–1638, 1994.
81. Wilson D: Research on multiple placements. Seattle, Washington, Children's Administration, 2003.
82. Widom CS: The role of placement experiences in mediating the criminal consequences of early childhood victimization. *Am J Orthopsychiatry* 61(2):195–209, 1991.
83. Newton RR, Litrownik AJ, Landsverk JA: Children and youth in foster care: Disentangling the relationship between problem behaviors and number of placements. *Child Abuse Negl* 24(10):1363–1374, 2000.
84. Caspi A, McClay J, Moffitt TE, Mill J, Martin J, Craig IW, Taylor A, Poulton R: Role of genotype in the cycle of violence in maltreated children. *Science* 297(5582):851–854, 2002.
85. Kim-Cohen J, Caspi A, Taylor A, Williams B, Newcombe R, Craig IW, Moffitt TE: MAOA, maltreatment, and gene-environment interaction predicting children's mental health: New evidence and a meta-analysis. In press.
86. Caspi A, Sugden K, Moffitt TE, Taylor A, Craig IW, Harrington H, McClay J, Mill J, Martin J, Braithwaite A, Poulton R: Influence of life stress on depression: Moderation by a polymorphism in the 5-HTT gene. *Science* 301:386–389, 2003.
87. Kaufman J, Yang BZ, Douglas-Palumberi H, Houshyar S, Lipschitz D, Krystal J, Gelernter J: Social supports and serotonin transporter gene moderate depression in maltreated children. *Proc Natl Acad Sci USA* 101(49):17316–17321, 2004.
88. Eley TC, Sugden K, Corsico A, Gregory AM, Sham P, McGuffin P, Plomin R, Craig IW: Gene-environment interaction analysis of serotonin system markers with adolescent depression. *Mol Psychiatry* 9(10):908–915, 2004.
89. Kendler KS: "A gene for . . .": The nature of gene action in psychiatric disorders. *Am J Psychiatry* 162(7):1243–1252, 2005.
90. Kendler KS, Kuhn JW, Vittum J, Prescott CA, Riley B: The interaction of stressful life events and a serotonin transporter polymorphism in the prediction of episodes of major depression: A replication. *Arch Gen Psychiatry* 62(5):529–535, 2005.
91. Kendler KS, Karkowski-Shuman L: Stressful life events and genetic liability to major depression: Genetic control of exposure to the environment? *Psychol Med* 27(3):539–547, 1997.
92. Holmans P, Zubenko GS, Crowe RR, DePaulo JR, Jr., Scheftner WA, Weissman MM, Zubenko WN, Boutelle S, Murphy-Eberenz K, MacKinnon D, McInnis MG, Marta DH, Adams P, Knowles JA, Gladis M, Thomas J, Chellis J, Miller E, Levinson DF: Genomewide significant linkage to recurrent, early-onset major depressive disorder on chromosome 15q. *Am J Hum Genet* 74(6):1154–1167, 2004.
93. Strauss J, Barr CL, George CJ, King N, Shaikh S, Devlin B, Kovacs M, Kennedy JL: Association study of brain-derived neurotrophic factor in adults with a history of childhood onset mood disorder. *Am J Med Genet B Neuropsychiatr Genet* 131(1):16–19, 2004.
94. Strauss J, Barr CL, Vetro A, King N, Shaikh S, Brathwaite J, Woineskos D, Kovacs M, Kennedy JL: Brain derived neurotrophic factor gene and childhood-onset depressive disorder: Results from a Hungarian sample. In *Collegium International Neuro-Psychopharmacologicum (CINP) Congress*. Paris, 2004.
95. Duman RS, Heninger GR, Nestler EJ: A molecular and cellular theory of depression [see comments]. *Arch Gen Psychiatry* 54(7):597–606, 1997.
96. Malberg JE, Eisch AJ, Nestler EJ, Duman RS: Chronic antidepressant treatment increases neurogenesis in adult rat hippocampus. *J Neurosci* 20(24):9104–9110, 2000.
97. Kaufman J, Yang BZ, Douglas-Palumberi H, Grasso D, Lipschitz D, Houshyar S, Krystal JH, Gelernter J: Brain-derived neurotrophic factor-5-HTTLPR gene interactions and environmental modifiers of depression in children. *Biological Psychiatry* 59:673–680, 2006.
98. Kaufman J, Yang BZ, Douglas-Palumberi H, Crouse-Artus M, Lipschitz D, Krystal JH, Gelernter J: Genetic and environmental predictors of early alcohol use. *Biological Psychiatry*. In press.
99. Grant BF, Dawson DA: Age at onset of alcohol use and its association with DSM-IV alcohol abuse and dependence: Results from the National

Longitudinal Alcohol Epidemiologic Survey. *J Subst Abuse* 9:103–110, 1997.
100. Wiedenmayer CP, Magarinos AM, McEwen BS, Barr GA: Mother lowers glucocorticoid levels of preweaning rats after acute threat. *Ann N Y Acad Sci* 1008:304–307, 2003.
101. Huot RL, Gonzalez ME, Ladd CO, Thrivikraman KV, Plotsky PM: Foster litters prevent hypothalamic-pituitary-adrenal axis sensitization mediated by neonatal maternal separation. *Psychoneuroendocrinology* 29(2):279–289, 2004.
102. Barbazanges A, Vallee M, Mayo W, Day J, Simon H, Le Moal M, Maccari S: Early and later adoptions have different long-term effects on male rat offspring. *J Neurosci* 16(23):7783–7790, 1996.
103. Weaver IC, Cervoni N, Champagne FA, D'Alessio AC, Sharma S, Seckl JR, Dymov S, Szyf M, Meaney MJ: Epigenetic programming by maternal behavior. *Nat Neurosci* 7(8):847–854, 2004.
104. Burns B, Phillips S, Wagner H, Barth R, Kolko D, Campbell Y, Landsverk J: Mental health need and access to mental health services by youths involved with child welfare: A national survey. *J Am Acad Child Adolesc Psychiatry* 43(8):960–970, 2004.
105. Raghavan R, Zima BT, Andersen RM, Leibowitz AA, Schuster MA, Landsverk J: Psychotropic medication use in a national probability sample of children in the child welfare system. *J Child Adolesc Psychopharmacol* 15(1):97–106, 2005.
106. Martin A, Van Hoof T, Stubbe D, Sherwin T, Scahill L: Multiple psychotropic pharmacotherapy among child and adolescent enrollees in Connecticut Medicaid managed care. *Psychiatr Serv* 54(1):72–77, 2003.
107. Cohen JA, Deblinger E, Mannarino AP, Steer RA: A multisite, randomized controlled trial for children with sexual abuse-related PTSD symptoms. *J Am Acad Child Adolesc Psychiatry* 43(4):393–402, 2004.
108. Cohen JA, Mannarino AP, Zhitova AC, Capone ME: Treating child abuse-related posttraumatic stress and comorbid substance abuse in adolescents. *Child Abuse Negl* 27(12):1345–1365, 2003.
109. Henggeler SW, Clingempeel WG, Brondino MJ, Pickrel SG: Four-year follow-up of multisystemic therapy with substance-abusing and substance-dependent juvenile offenders. *J Am Acad Child Adolesc Psychiatry* 41(7): 868–874, 2002.
110. Lieberman AF, Van Horn P, Ozer EJ: Preschooler witnesses of marital violence: predictors and mediators of child behavior problems. *Dev Psychopathol* 17(2):385–396, 2005.
111. De Arellano MA, Waldrop AE, Deblinger E, Cohen JA, Danielson CK, Mannarino AR: Community outreach program for child victims of traumatic events: A community-based project for underserved populations. *Behav Modif* 29(1):130–155, 2005.
112. Kaufman J, Mannarino A: Evaluation of child maltreatment. In: Ammerman RT, Hersen M (eds): *Handbook of Child Behavior Therapy in the Psychiatric Setting*. New York, Wiley, 1995, pp. 73–92.
113. PL105-89: Adoption and Safe Families Act, in P.L. 105–89, 1997.
114. Goldstein J, Solnit A, Goldstein S, Freud A: *The Best Interest of the Child: The Least Detrimental Alternative*. New York, Free Press, 1996.
115. McAlpine C, Marshall CC, Doran NH: Combining child welfare and substance abuse services: A blended model of intervention. *Child Welfare* 80(2):129–149, 2001.
116. Semidei J, Radel LF, Nolan C: Substance abuse and child welfare: Clear linkages and promising responses. *Child Welfare* 80(2):109–128, 2001.
117. Linehan MM, Schmidt H, 3rd, Dimeff LA, Craft JC, Kanter J, Comtois KA: Dialectical behavior therapy for patients with borderline personality disorder and drug-dependence. *Am J Addict* 8(4):279–292, 1999.
118. Fisher PA, Burraston B, Pears K: The early intervention foster care program: Permanent placement outcomes from a randomized trial. *Child Maltreatment* 10(1):61–71, 2005.
119. Kaufman J, Grasso D: The early intervention foster care program: a glass half full. *Child Maltreat* 11(1):90–1; author reply 92–94, 2006.
120. Sprang G, Clark J, Kaak O, Brenzel A: Developing and tailoring mental health technologies for child welfare: The Comprehensive Assessment and Training Services (CATS) Project. *Am J Orthopsychiatry* 74(3):325–326, 2004.
121. DHHS: *Child Abuse and Neglect: Critical First Steps in Response to a National Emergency*. Washington, DC, Department of Health and Human Services, 1990.
122. DHHS: *Neighbors Helping Neighbors: A New National Strategy for the Protection of Children*. Washington, DC, Department of Health and Human Services, 1993.

CHAPTER 5.15.2 ■ POSTTRAUMATIC STRESS DISORDER

CARLA SMITH STOVER, STEVEN BERKOWITZ, STEVEN MARANS, AND JOAN KAUFMAN

INTRODUCTION

Kevin is a 5-year-old boy whose father murdered his mother in a domestic dispute while he was at school. His father was arrested the same day and Kevin initially went to stay with his paternal grandparents who frequently provided care for him while his parents worked. That evening, Kevin sat for several hours on the family couch not reacting to the chaos and upset around him. He was quiet and appeared distant and withdrawn. He refused to speak to anyone and stared off into space. The following day, he was removed from his paternal grandparents' care and placed in a foster home because his grandfather posted bail for his father. Child protective services felt Kevin was at risk due to the grandfather's actions in support of Kevin's father. Kevin's relatives then began a custody battle over who would serve as his guardian. Kevin remained in foster care for several months while protective services assessed which family member was most appropriate. A custody and placement evaluation was conducted over the subsequent months and it was a full year until the guardianship issue was resolved.

This case illustrates several important factors that can increase the likelihood of Posttraumatic Stress Disorder (PTSD) developing following a traumatic event: 1) Kevin evidenced dissociation immediately following the event. Children are more likely to develop severe PTSD symptomatology if they display dissociative symptoms following the trauma (1); 2) Kevin experienced additional stress in the aftermath of the initial loss of his mother by being dislocated to a foster home. He not only lost his mother, but his home with all its familiar surroundings, and several other close family supports. PTSD is more likely when there are additional post event stressors such as dislocation, and loss or separation from significant caregivers (2, 3); and 3) Kevin's other relatives, with whom he had a previous close relationship, were not as available to provide appropriate support given their own grief and subsequent custody battle over his guardianship. If caregivers are distressed and distracted by other issues, children tend to have more difficulties, as caregivers' own psychological problems render them less capable of providing for the children's needs (4).

Intrafamilial violence is the most common precipitant of PTSD in children and adolescents (5–7), yet PTSD can emerge as a consequence of exposure to a wide range of traumas, including terrorism, war, natural disasters, automobile accidents, and community violence. The precipitant may constitute an isolated incident, or as in the case of Kevin, a chronic stressor. Over the past two decades there has been a burgeoning of research in the area of PTSD, and significant advances in its assessment and treatment in children and adolescents.

DEFINITIONS

Formal diagnostic criteria for PTSD were not introduced until 1980, with the publication of the *Diagnostic and Statistical Manual of Mental Disorders, Third Edition* (DSM-III) (8). In 1987, in response to new data suggesting that symptoms and distress were common after severe trauma (9), minimum duration criteria requiring symptoms to be present for at least 30 days were added to the diagnosis of PTSD (10). The minimum duration criteria, however, created a diagnostic dilemma, such that the diagnosis of adjustment disorder was the only possible diagnosis for stress-related symptomatology in the first month after a traumatic event (9). This deficit was addressed with the inclusion of the diagnosis Acute Stress Disorder (ASD) in the DSM-IV (11).

The diagnostic criteria for ASD and PTSD are delineated in Table 5.15.2.1. To receive a diagnosis of ASD, a child must exhibit symptoms for a minimum of 2 days and a maximum of 4 weeks post trauma. If symptoms persist or occur after the 4-week time limit for ASD, then the diagnosis of PTSD is given. An immediate diagnosis of ASD is not required for a child to later be diagnosed with PTSD, and PTSD can be diagnosed with acute onset, or delayed onset, if symptoms emerge 6 or more months after the event.

Criterion A for ASD and PTSD are exactly the same. The diagnosis of either disorder requires the experience of extreme stress and an intense response to the event. In practice, however, it is often quite difficult to elicit information about the child's response to a given trauma.

The diagnoses of ASD and PTSD require the presence of re-experiencing, avoidance and/or dissociation, and hyperarousal symptoms. ASD and PTSD differ in the priority given to the different categories of symptoms, with three or more dissociative symptoms required for the diagnosis of ASD, and fewer if any dissociative symptoms necessary for the diagnosis of PTSD.

The DSM allows for developmental differences in the presentation of symptoms in children. Recurrent thoughts may be evident in children, not only through verbal reports, but also in play themes. A child who underwent a stressful medical procedure may enact doctor and patient themes repeatedly, a child who was physically abused may depict a parent character degrading and harming a child character, and a child who was sexually abused may play out scenes with sexually explicit material. In addition, in children, nightmares need not specifically be related to the trauma to count as a reexperiencing symptom; any frightening dreams with onset after the trauma can count toward the diagnosis of PTSD. Also, instead of reliving the trauma mentally, trauma-specific reenactment can count toward the diagnosis of PTSD in children. In sexually abused children this frequently takes the form of initiating sexual advances toward other children. Additional information about diagnosing PTSD in children, and developmental considerations in diagnosing very young children, are discussed later in the chapter in the Diagnosis and Assessment section.

EPIDEMIOLOGY

The National Comorbidity Study is the most comprehensive epidemiological survey of psychiatric disorders in the United States. Just under 6,000 individuals aged 15–54 participated in the study. The estimated prevalence of PTSD was 7.8% overall, and 10.4% for women, double the rate observed in men. Rape and combat were the most likely events to be associated with PTSD in the National Comorbidity Study (12).

PTSD rates are believed to be similar, if not higher, in children and adolescents (13). Several epidemiological studies estimate trauma exposure rates in children to be between 25% and 45% (14, 15). Of children with a history of traumatic event exposure, rates of PTSD range from 5% to 45% (15–17), with higher rates reported in low income high-risk subjects, and lower rates reported in pediatric emergency room samples. Within juvenile cohorts, as discussed earlier, physical abuse, sexual abuse, and intrafamilial violence are the most common precipitants of PTSD (5–7).

NEUROBIOLOGY

Preclinical studies of the effects of stress provide a valuable heuristic in understanding the pathophysiology of PTSD in *adults* (18, 19), with many of the biological alterations associated with early stress in preclinical studies reported in adults with PTSD. For example, one of the best replicated findings in adults with PTSD is reduction in hippocampal volume (20–26). There has been some suggestion that reduced hippocampal volume represents a preexisting, inherent vulnerability factor, rather than a consequence of trauma exposure, given one study found combat exposed twins with PTSD *and* their unexposed cotwins had smaller hippocampal volumes than combat-exposed twins without PTSD and their unexposed cotwins (27). This interpretation has to be accepted with caution, however, as the combat-exposed veterans who developed PTSD and their unexposed cotwins were more likely to have had a history of childhood physical and/or sexual abuse, suggesting the potential importance of early developmental insults on later hippocampal structure.

Preclinical studies of the effects of stress suggest a minimum of three mechanisms through which hippocampal atrophy may result: neuronal atrophy, neurotoxicity, and disruption of neurogenesis. In animals, 3 weeks of exposure to stress and/or stress levels of glucocorticoids can cause neuronal atrophy in the CA3 region of the hippocampus (28, 29). At this level, glucocorticoids produce a reversible decrease in number of apical dendritic branch points and length of apical dendrites of sufficient magnitude to impair hippocampal-dependent cognitive processes (28). More sustained stress and/or glucocorticoid exposure can lead to neurotoxicity—actual permanent loss of hippocampal neurons through binding of glutamate to N-methyl-D-aspartate (NMDA) receptors. Rats exposed to high concentrations of glucocorticoids for approximately 12 hours per day for 3 months experience a 20% loss of neurons specific to the CA3 region of the hippocampus (30). Evidence of stress-induced neurotoxicity of cells in this region has been reported in nonhuman primates as well (31, 32). Reductions in hippocampal volume may also be affected by decreases in neurogenesis, which results from decreased expression of Brain Derived Neurotrophic Factor (BDNF) caused by elevated glucocorticoids (33). The granule cells in the dentate gyrus of the hippocampus continue to proliferate into adulthood, and neurogenesis in this region is markedly reduced by stress.

Contrary to expectations derived from preclinical studies of the effects of early stress on hippocampus structure (34), and imaging studies of adults (35), multiple pediatric studies have failed to detect hippocampal atrophy in children with PTSD (36–39). While some clinical studies suggest the failure to detect hippocampal atrophy may be due to the low rate of recurrent depressive illness or comorbid alcohol problems in pediatric samples (40, 41), there are emerging findings that suggest multiple developmental factors may be relevant in

TABLE 5.15.2.1

DIAGNOSTIC CRITERIA FOR ASD AND PTSD

Acute Stress Disorder	Posttraumatic Stress Disorder
A. The person has been exposed to a traumatic event in which both of the following were present: 1) The person experienced, witnessed, or was confronted with an event or events that involved actual or threatened death or serious injury or a threat to the physical integrity of self or others 2) The person's response involved intense fear, helplessness, or horror *Note:* In children, this may be expressed instead by disorganized or agitated behavior. B. Either while experiencing or after experiencing the distressing event, the individual has three (or more) of the following dissociative symptoms: 1) a subjective sense of numbing, detachment, or absence of emotional responsiveness 2) a reduction in awareness of his or her surroundings (e.g., "being in a daze") 3) derealization 4) depersonalization 5) dissociative amnesia (inability to recall an important aspect of the trauma) C. The traumatic event is persistently reexperienced in at least one of the following ways: 1) recurrent images thoughts, dreams, illusions, or flashbacks 2) a sense of reliving the experience 3) distress on exposure to reminders of the traumatic event D. Marked avoidance of stimuli that arouse recollections of the trauma (thoughts, feelings, conversations, activities, places, people). E. Marked symptoms of anxiety or increased arousal (difficulty sleeping, irritability, poor concentration, hypervigilance, exaggerated startle response, motor restlessness). F. The disturbance causes clinically significant distress or impairment. G. The disturbance lasts for a minimum of 2 days and a maximum of 4 weeks and occurs within 4 weeks of the traumatic event.	A. The person has been exposed to a traumatic event in which both of the following were present: 1) The person experienced, witnessed, or was confronted with an event or events that involved actual or threatened death or serious injury or a threat to the physical integrity of self or others 2) The person's response involved intense fear, helplessness, or horror *Note:* In children, this may be expressed instead by disorganized or agitated behavior. B. The traumatic event is persistently reexperienced in one (or more) of the following ways: 1) recurrent and intrusive distressing recollections of the event, including images, thoughts, or perceptions. *Note:* In young children, repetitive play may occur in which themes or aspects of the trauma are expressed. 2) Recurrent distressing dreams of the event. *Note:* In young children there may be frightening dreams without recognizable content. 3) acting or feeling as if reliving the traumatic event (illusions, hallucinations, flashbacks). *Note:* In young children, trauma-specific reenactment may occur. 4) intense psychological distress at exposure to internal or external cues. 5) physiological reactivity to internal or external cues. C. Persistent avoidance of stimuli and numbing of general response as indicated by three (or more) of the following: 1) efforts to avoid thoughts, feelings or conversations about trauma 2) efforts to avoid places or people that arouse memories of the trauma 3) inability to recall an important aspect of the trauma 4) markedly diminished interest or participation in significant activities 5) feeling of detachment or estrangement from others 6) restricted range of affect (e.g., unable to have loving feelings) 7) sense of foreshortened future D. Persistent symptoms of increased arousal (not present before the trauma), as indicated by (two or more) of the following: 1) difficulty falling asleep or staying asleep 2) irritability or outbursts of anger 3) difficulty concentrating 4) hypervigilance 5) exaggerated startle response E. Duration of disturbance is more than 1 month. F. Disturbance causes clinically significant distress or impairment.

understanding the absence of hippocampal findings in children and adolescents with PTSD. For example, there are age-dependent changes in sensitivity to NMDA receptor blockade, as in preclinical studies of neurotoxicity in corticolimbic regions, cell death has been reported to be minimal or absent during prepuberty, only reaching its peak in early adulthood (42).

Instead of hippocampal atrophy, children and adolescents with PTSD have been found to have reduced medial and posterior corpus callosum areas in two independent investigations (36, 38). This is a finding that has likewise been reported in psychiatric inpatients with a history of maltreatment when compared to psychiatric and healthy controls without a history of early childhood trauma (43).

To the best of our knowledge, there is only one published structural MRI study in prepubescent nonhuman primates subjected to early stress (44). Most preclinical studies of the effects of early stress have examined the impact of early stress on the neurobiology of *adult* animals. Consistent with the child clinical studies, prepubescent primates subjected to early maternal deprivation failed to show evidence of hippocampal atrophy, and instead had reductions in the medial and posterior portions of the corpus callosum.

The medial and posterior portions of the corpus callosum contain interhemispheric projections from the auditory cortices, posterior cingulate, insula, and somatosensory and visual cortices to a lesser extent. They also include connections from the inferior parietal lobe to the contralateral inferior parietal lobe, superior temporal sulcus, cingulate, retrosplenial cortex, and parahippocampal gyrus (45). Several of the regions with interhemispheric projections through the medial and posterior portions of the corpus callosum have connections with prefrontal cortical areas, and are involved in circuits that mediate the processing of emotional stimuli and various memory functions—core disturbances associated with PTSD.

Given findings in juvenile cohorts in the corpus callosum—the primary white matter tract in the brain—we utilized diffusion tensor imaging (DTI) in a cohort of maltreated children with PTSD. DTI is a relatively new application of MRI technology that measures the extent and direction of diffusion of water in the brain, and can be used to assess the integrity of white matter tracts (see Peterson, 2.4.1). When compared to demographically matched controls, maltreated children with PTSD had reduced fractional anisotropy (FA) in the medial and posterior region of the corpus callosum (46). FA is greatest in axons, and increases with myelination, suggesting the possibility of myelination alterations in association with early traumatic life events.

It is probably premature to conclude that alterations in hippocampal structure are not evident in preadolescents. MRI methodology may just be too crude to identify structural hippocampal changes. In order to better understand the neurobiological effects of stress early in development, additional preclinical studies are needed that systematically examine the effects of stress on prepubertal animals and across development using refined research methodologies to detect subtle changes in hippocampus structure (e.g., cell proliferation and gene expression, to complement MRI findings). Emerging findings from adult studies implicate a range of neuroanatomical structures that are likely relevant in the pathophysiology of PTSD, and additional work in this area in juvenile samples will also help to elucidate structures and circuits relevant early in development.

As was discussed extensively in the previous chapter (see Kaufman, 5.15.1), the negative neurobiological sequelae associated with a history of early trauma are not inevitable. There is a host of environmental and genetic factors that can modify the impact of early trauma. Some of the factors most relevant in modifying the emergence and course of PTSD are delineated in the Course and Prognosis section of this chapter.

DIAGNOSIS AND ASSESSMENT

Multiple Informants and the Assessment of Trauma

In the area of child psychopathology assessment, extensive attention has been paid to the finding that independent raters (parents, teachers, children) often provide discrepant yet important information about children's psychiatric symptomatology (47). Emerging findings suggest the same is true in assessing children's trauma experiences (48, 49).

Multiple informants and multiple measures appear necessary to accurately assess children's trauma histories, a first and critical step in the assessment of PTSD. For example, in one recent study (50), child-, parent-, and protective-services data were used to assess children's traumatic experiences. Each of the data sources missed a number of traumas identified by the other methods. All three sources of information, however, were able to be reliably integrated to provide a "best estimate" of children's maltreatment experiences. Figure 5.15.2.1 shows the proportion of traumas experienced by the children identified after all sources of data were reviewed that were *not* reported by each informant alone. Substantiated incidents of physical and sexual abuse documented in protective service records were denied by parents and children approximately 50% of the time when queried directly about these types of experiences. Of the various types of traumas, parents were most likely to report incidents of domestic violence. In addition, parents occasionally reported incidents of physical and sexual abuse that occurred in the past when the family was living in another state and that their workers did not know about. Utilizing only parent and child interview data, without access to the protective service record, 40% of the children with a history of sexual abuse, 30% of the children with a history of physical abuse, and 16% of the children with a history of witnessing domestic violence would not have been identified. In these cases, PTSD symptoms would not ordinarily be surveyed, and the diagnosis of PTSD would have been missed.

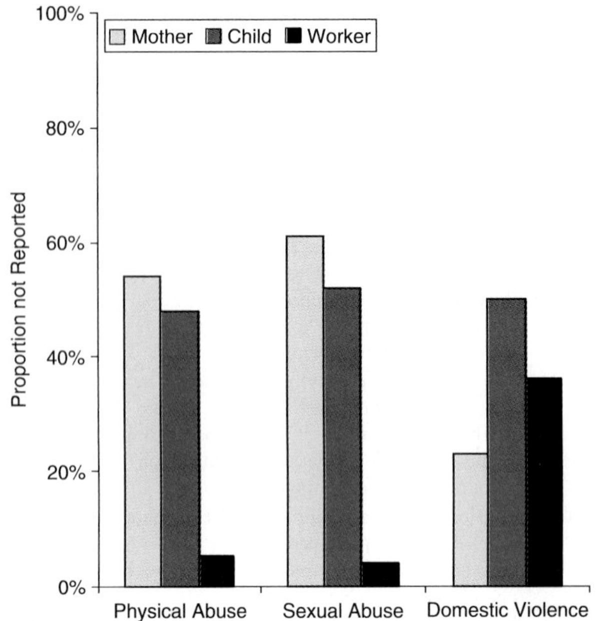

FIGURE 5.15.2.1. Proportion of traumas not reported by each informant. The proportion of traumas experienced by the children identified after all sources of data were reviewed that were *not* reported by each informant alone. Each of the data sources missed a number of traumas identified by the other methods.

The data described above highlight the importance of clinicians obtaining information from multiple sources (child protective services, children, parents) when making psychiatric diagnoses and delineating treatment plans for maltreated children. Comprehensive multi-informant assessment will help to assure proper diagnoses and optimal selection of appropriate clinical interventions, including trauma-focused psychotherapies. Working collaboratively with parents and/or protective service workers is essential in the care of these children.

As reviewed elsewhere (51), there are several good measures of trauma exposure to help clinicians determine if a child has experienced a Criterion A trauma. The Traumatic Events Screening Inventory (TESI) (52) and Violence Exposure Scales (VEX-R) (53) assess a wide variety of childhood traumas, and both have caregiver and child-report versions. Most of the standard semistructured and structured child psychiatric diagnostic interviews also include a survey of a variety of criterion A traumas. Reliable, more detailed measures of domestic violence can be obtained with the Revised Conflict Tactics

Scale (CTS2) (54) or the Partner Violence Inventory (PVI) (55), and the Child Trauma Questionnaire (CTQ) (56) provides an excellent assessment of a range of maltreatment experiences. Reliable methods have also been developed to extract and rate severity of maltreatment experiences from case records (57), and to integrate trauma data from multiple informants (48).

Symptom Assessment

In our clinical and research practice, we aim to have trauma history data from multiple informants prior to assessing psychiatric symptomatology in children. We then query them about various trauma experiences. If children deny a trauma we know they have experienced via other sources, we consider that evidence of "avoidance." We then let them know what we learned about from the other source, let them know that we are not going to ask them too much about those experiences, but want to know if they have any problems a lot kids experience who have been through the type of things they have. We then query them regarding the presence of PTSD symptoms. If children are particularly reticent to talk, we begin by asking the more benign hyperarousal items (sleep difficulties, concentration problems, irritability), progress to ask about the avoidance/numbing symptoms, and then query about the more *stressful reexperiencing items.*

Just as the assessment of trauma requires the collection of data from multiple informants, the assessment of PTSD symptomatology is best achieved with the use of data from multiple informants. If children are living in foster care or with other guardians who do not know them well, obtaining adjunctive information from birth parents and/or school teachers can be enormously helpful. In addition, parents and caretakers are notoriously poor at identifying internalizing (depression, anxiety) symptoms. Children are the best informants of these symptoms. Children are also frequently the best to ask about nightmares and sleeping difficulties. As traumatized children frequently have not received comfort when distressed, many do not seek adult reassurance when they wake up from a nightmare. Rather, they stay in their beds alone, terrified. Their guardians have no idea they are not sleeping through the night.

Several reviews have identified a number of valid and reliable DSM-IV–based measures for the assessment of trauma symptomatology in school-aged children (51, 58). There is only one measure that specifically assesses ASD symptomatology, the 29-item Acute Stress Checklist for Children (ASC-Kids) (59). This measure has been validated with children aged 8–17, is available in English and Spanish, and has an advantage over other PTSD symptom scales in assessing ASD since it surveys the full range of dissociative symptoms required for the diagnosis of ASD.

There are multiple well validated scales to assess PTSD symptomatology, including: the Child Post-Traumatic Stress Disorder Reaction Index (CPTSD-RI) (60), Clinician Administered PTSD Scale for Children and Adolescents (CAPS-CA) (61), Trauma Symptom Checklist for Children (TSCC) (62), Levonn's Cartoon-Based Interview for Assessing Children's Distress (63), and Angie/Andy Cartoon Trauma Scales (ACTS) (64). The CPTSD-RI is probably the most widely used instrument in the field, and has validated clinical cutoffs suggestive of a likely PTSD diagnosis (65). The TSCC, Levonn, and ACTS are child self-report measures developed to assess a range of symptoms, but are not made to specifically diagnose PTSD. The Levonn and ACTS both have cartoon pictures that provide visual cues to help children understand the questions surveyed.

All of the structured and semistructured research child diagnostic interviews also include items to assess PTSD symptomatology (66–69). These interview schedules are comparably reliable in diagnosing PTSD. Given the differential diagnostic issues discussed in the following section, and the high rates of comorbidity between PTSD and other child psychiatric diagnoses, there is an advantage to using more inclusive psychiatric assessment measures when evaluating traumatized children.

Differential Diagnosis and Psychiatric Comorbidity

Approximately three-quarters of individuals with PTSD experience one or more comorbid lifetime diagnosis, and 37% to 48% report a lifetime history of major depression (MDD) (12, 70, 71). In one-half to three-quarter of all cases, the onset of PTSD is primary. The risk for MDD following PTSD is about the same as the risk of MDD following any other anxiety disorder, and 30% to 40% more likely in individuals with a history of a preexisting anxiety disorder (71). PTSD is also highly comorbid with alcohol and substance abuse disorders in adolescents and adults (12, 72), and with mood and behavioral disorders in children.

The diagnosis of PTSD has numerous symptoms in common with multiple other child psychiatric diagnoses. PTSD and MDD have five symptoms in common; concentration difficulties associated with PTSD are frequently misattributed to attention deficit hyperactivity disorder (ADHD); extreme irritability reported in PTSD is sometimes misattributed to mania or oppositional defiant disorder (ODD); and trauma-related hallucinations are sometimes misattributed to a primary psychotic disorder.

Determining the presence of PTSD and potential comorbid diagnoses requires careful assessment of the developmental timing of the onset of symptoms, evaluating the pattern of problem behaviors, the severity of difficulties across different settings, and the association of problem behaviors with trauma triggers. For the diagnosis of PTSD to be given, there must be at least one reexperiencing symptom, a cardinal feature of the disorder. For comorbid MDD to be diagnosed, beyond symptoms which overlap with the diagnosis of PTSD, there should be at least one symptom that is uniquely associated with MDD (depressed mood, suicidality). For concentration problems to be attributed to ADHD, they should have existed prior to age 7, been evident before the trauma, be relatively chronic, and generally worse in a school setting. If they emerged after the trauma and are worse in the home setting or when the child is exposed to trauma triggers, they are likely not related to ADHD. Irritability is a totally nonspecific symptom associated with many of the major child psychiatric diagnoses. Most symptoms of ODD involve some expression of irritability, but for a comorbid ODD diagnosis to be given there should be evidence of a fundamental disregard for social norms and rules. In PTSD, irritability is frequently worse when the child is exposed to trauma triggers and less evident in non–emotionally charged environments. Sleep disturbance is another symptom shared by several child diagnoses. While both PTSD and mania are associated with sleep disturbances, decreased need for sleep is the cardinal feature of mania, and nightmares and insomnia (wanting to sleep, but not being able to) are the sine qua non of PTSD.

Hallucinations have been reported to occur in 9% of abused children recruited from juvenile court or pediatric clinics (73), 20% of child sexual abuse victims on psychiatric inpatient units (74), and 75% to 98% of abused children who meet criteria for a dissociative disorder (75). Differentiating between PTSD, MDD or bipolar disorder with psychotic features, or a primary psychotic disorder has extremely important treatment implications. A number of distinctive features of psychotic-like symptoms in traumatized children facilitate this differential diagnosis. For example, hallucinations in maltreated children are frequently trauma related (hearing the perpetrator's voice), are often nocturnal (76), and frequently resolve with psychotherapeutic intervention and safety reassurances (75). In addition, the presence of hallucinations in traumatized children is not typically associated with other psychotic symptoms that would suggest schizophrenia or another primary psychotic diagnosis. They are less likely to be associated with negative symptoms (withdrawn behavior, blunted affect) or abnormal early development as would be typical in childhood-onset schizophrenia (77). Hallucinations in traumatized children tend to be associated with impulsive, aggressive, and self-injurious behavior, nightmares, and trance-like states, and less likely to be associated with evidence of formal thought disorder (78).

Developmental Considerations

It is only within the past decade that the diagnosis PTSD has been used with infants and toddlers. In a series of studies by Scheeringa and colleagues (79–82), the reliability and validity of the DSM-IV and an alternate set of criteria were evaluated in several cohorts of infants and young children less than 6 years of age. The alternative criteria for PTSD are also composed of the three core types of symptoms used to diagnose PTSD in older children and adults (reexperiencing, avoidance or numbing, increased arousal). However, DSM-IV items which require reports of subjective experience were eliminated from the alternate criteria (foreshortened sense of future), and all remaining items were behaviorally anchored. In addition, a cluster of symptoms assessing loss of previously acquired skills (toilet training), new-onset separation anxiety, new onset of fears unrelated to the trauma, and the onset of aggression following exposure to the traumatic event were added to the alternate PTSD criteria for very young children.

Across the studies (79–82), very few children were found to meet DSM-IV criteria for PTSD, but expected proportions of children met the alternative criteria. In addition, individual raters were able to reliably diagnose PTSD using the alternative criteria. The novel proposed age-specific symptoms (loss of previously acquired skills, new onset separation anxiety) did not add to the diagnostic utility of the alternative PTSD criteria. Scheeringa and colleagues, however, believe they may be useful in dimensional assessment tools of PTSD for purposes of predicting treatment outcome, as they were among the most common symptoms observed in young children across their studies.

The avoidance cluster of symptoms is the set of symptoms least frequently endorsed in young children. Only 2% of highly traumatized children this age endorse sufficient avoidance symptoms for the diagnosis of PTSD according to the DSM-IV criteria (three symptoms). Limiting the number of avoidance symptoms to only one resulted in approximately one-quarter of the highly traumatized children in their studies meeting diagnostic criteria for PTSD, a rate comparable to that reported in other traumatized samples of older children. The alternative criteria recommended by Scheeringa and colleagues for diagnosing PTSD in preschoolers are depicted in Table 5.15.2.2.

Current measures of PTSD for young children (under age 6) are primarily caregiver report forms with little direct assessment of the child. Of the measures available for young children, the Posttraumatic Stress Disorder Semi-Structured Interview and Observation Schedule is the most comprehensive, developmentally appropriate, and well validated (51). An additional measure for preschool children that is showing good early psychometric properties is the Preschool Aged Psychiatric Assessment (PAPA) (83). The PAPA is an interviewer based, structured parental interview for the comprehensive assessment of mental health symptoms in children aged 2 through 5, which includes PTSD. The Trauma Symptoms Checklist for Young Children (TSCYC) is also a good tool for use with young children. It is a parent-report screening checklist that covers a broad range of symptoms, but is not meant as an independent assessment of the diagnosis of PTSD (84). The Levonn cartoon interview was originally developed for preschoolers and has been used extensively with children this age (63).

Course and Prognosis

The likelihood of individuals developing PTSD, and the course of the disorder over time, are influenced by three primary factors: inherent vulnerability factors, the nature of the trauma, and aspects of the recovery environment (85). While ASD is a potent predictor of later PTSD, most children who develop PTSD do not meet criteria for ASD in the first month after trauma exposure (1). In adults, peritraumatic dissociation predicts acute-onset PTSD, but not the longitudinal course of the disorder (86).

Across multiple studies, family history of psychiatric illness and the presence of a preexisting psychiatric disorder uniformly predict the onset of PTSD following trauma exposure (87). Twin studies suggest genetic factors account for approximately 20%–30% of the variance in predicting onset of PTSD, with genetic factors accounting for a greater amount of the variance in predicting avoidance and hyperarousal than reexperiencing symptoms (88). There have been relatively few studies examining candidate genes in patients with PTSD. No association was found between PTSD and variation in the dopamine (89) and glucocorticoid (90) receptor genes. There is one study that reported association between PTSD and variation in the serotonin transporter gene (91), and another that reported an association between PTSD and the dopamine transporter polymorphism (92), but these have yet to be replicated.

Trauma factors, such as unexpectedness, chronicity, severity, and emotional and physical proximity are also significant predictors of PTSD onset and persistence (87, 93). Factors in the post-trauma environment, however, have the greatest contribution in determining the likelihood of PTSD becoming chronic. The absence of social supports and exposure to ongoing psychosocial adversity, as in the case of Kevin depicted at the onset of this chapter, are the most potent predictors of PTSD chronicity (87, 93). Moreover, as discussed previously, PTSD frequently is associated with new onset mood and substance use disorders, with comorbidity of these disorders associated with worse prognosis and greater psychosocial impairment (94). As discussed in the next section, however, promising advances have been made in the treatment of PTSD.

TREATMENT

Several empirically validated treatments have been developed for children with PTSD. Central to the efficacy of each of these treatments is the importance of evaluating the child's current safety and exposure to ongoing risks, delineating strategies to minimize the impact of secondary stressors, working to strengthen and support the child's primary caregivers, and identifying trauma triggers in the environment that exacerbate clinical symptomatology (contact with the perpetrator, reminders around the home). Available treatment strategies are described below.

Trauma-Focused Cognitive Behavior Therapy

The available research strongly supports the efficacy of cognitive behavioral therapy (CBT) for the treatment of PTSD

TABLE 5.15.2.2

ALTERNATIVE PTSD CRITERIA FOR PRESCHOOL CHILDREN

A. The person has been exposed to a traumatic event:
   1) The person experienced, witnessed, or was confronted with an event or events that involved actual or threatened death or serious injury, or a threat to the physical integrity of self or others.
   2) Is not required because preverbal children cannot report on their reaction at the time of the event and an adult may not have been present to witness the child's reaction.

B. The traumatic event is persistently reexperienced in one (or more) of the following ways:
   1) Recurrent and intrusive recollection of the event *(but not necessarily distressing),* including images, thoughts, or perceptions. *Note*: In young children, repetitive play may occur in which themes or aspects of the trauma are expressed.
   2) Recurrent distressing dreams of the event. *Note*: In children, there may be frightening dreams without recognizable content.
   3) Objective, behavioral manifestations of a flashback are observed but the individual may not be able to verbalize the content of the experience.
   4) Intense psychological distress at exposure to internal or external cues that symbolize or resemble an aspect of the traumatic event.

C. Persistent avoidance of stimuli associated with the trauma and numbing of general responsiveness (not present before the trauma), as indicated by *one* (or more) of the following:
   1) Efforts to avoid activities, places, or people that arouse recollections of the trauma
   2) Markedly diminished interest or participation in significant activities. *Note:* In young children, this is mainly observed as constriction of play.
   3) Feeling of detachment or estrangement from others. *Note:* In young children, this is mainly observed as social withdrawal.
   4) Restricted range of affect (e.g., unable to have loving feelings)

D. Persistent symptoms of increased arousal (not present before the trauma), as indicated by *one* (or more) of the following:
   1) Difficulty falling or staying asleep
   2) Irritability or outbursts of anger *or extreme temper tantrums and fussiness*
   3) Difficulty concentrating
   4) Hypervigilance
   5) Exaggerated startle response

(Modified from Scheeringa MS, Zeanah CH, Myers L, Putnam FW: New findings on alternative criteria for PTSD in preschool children. *J Am Acad Child Adolesc Psychiatry* 42(5):561–570, 2003.)
Note: Modifications in wording to *DSM-IV* criteria are noted in italics.
PTSD = posttraumatic stress disorder.

in children and adolescents (95–99). One of the most well validated and widely disseminated treatments for childhood PTSD is Trauma Focused-CBT (TF-CBT) (100). TF-CBT comprises specific modules including: psycho-education; expressing feelings; recognizing the relationship among thoughts, feelings, and behaviors; learning stress management and relaxation skills; gradual exposure; cognitive processing of the abuse experience; joint parent–child sessions; and parent management training to address behavioral problems. As treatment continues, children are encouraged to confront increasingly detailed and distressing abuse-related reminders and memories and to ultimately share them with their caregiver. TF-CBT for children is typically provided in 10–18 sessions and caregiver involvement is important for treatment success (97). TF-CBT has been used successfully with a wide age range of children with a variety of traumatic histories; and a manual and Web-based training are available (www.musc.edu/tfcbt).

Randomized controlled trials have shown that children who received TF-CBT exhibited significantly greater improvements in terms of PTSD, depression, and overall behavior problems than children who receive standard Child-Centered Therapy (CCT). In addition, TF-CBT was more effective than CCT in improving children's self-reported interpersonal trust and decreasing shame. In terms of the clinical significance of the interventions, at the end of treatment, 21% of those who received TF-CBT and 46% of those who received CCT met diagnostic criteria for PTSD. Parents also seemed to benefit more from the trauma-focused intervention; depression, abuse-related distress, parental support, and parenting practices all were reported to be more improved in TF-CBT compared with CCT (100, 101). In addition, benefits associated with TF-CBT have been found to be maintained one year after treatment termination (102).

Relationship-Based Models of Intervention

Another evidence-based treatment has emerged in recent years specifically for preschool children. Child-Parent Psychotherapy (CPP (103)) was developed to address the needs of children exposed to family violence. It is a 52-week dyadic treatment. CPP integrates modalities derived from psychodynamic, attachment, trauma, cognitive-behavioral, and social learning theories. The parent–child relationship is used as a vehicle for improving the child's emotional, cognitive, and social functioning through a focus on safety, affect regulation, the joint construction of a trauma narrative, and engagement in developmentally appropriate goals and activities. CPP is based on the following premises: 1) the attachment system is the main organizer of children's responses to danger and safety in the first years of life; 2) early mental health problems should be addressed in the context of the child's primary attachment relationships; 3) child outcomes emerge in the context of transactions between the child and environmental protective and risk factors; 4) interpersonal violence is a traumatic stressor with pathogenic repercussions on its witnesses as well as its recipients; 5) the therapeutic relationship is a key mutative factor in early mental health treatment; and 6) cultural values must be incorporated into treatment (104). A randomized controlled trail of CPP for young children exposed to domestic violence resulted in significant reductions in both child and parent symptoms post-treatment and at 6-month follow-up compared to standard treatment in the community (103).

Group Treatment

Several models of group therapy have been developed for the treatment of PTSD. Most are based on CBT interventions. Multi-Modality Trauma Treatment (MMTT) (96) is an 18-week, manualized, group CBT intervention for children exposed to single event traumas. The treatment includes: psychoeducation, exposure through trauma narratives, muscle relaxation, breathing exercises, interpersonal problem solving for anger control, development of positive self-talk and relapse prevention. Evaluation of the treatment resulted in a 57% reduction in the diagnosis of PTSD post-treatment and an 86% reduction at 6-month followup. Stein and colleagues (105) studied a shorter 10-session CBT group therapy for PTSD conducted within the school setting. Post-treatment assessments revealed an 86% reduction in PTSD for those in the intervention group. These data suggest that group treatment can be an effective mode of intervention for PTSD secondary to single event traumas.

Community-Based Approaches

The Child-Development Community Policing (CD-CP) program began as a partnership between the New Haven, CT Department of Police Service and the Yale University Child Study Center in 1991 (106–109). The aim of the CD-CP program is to address the psychological consequences of children and families exposed to violence and trauma in their homes and communities in the immediate aftermath of an event. The CD-CP program has been replicated in more than a dozen communities nationwide. The key components include: cross-training for police officers, mental health clinicians and other professionals involved in responding to children and families affected by violence and other potentially traumatic events; a 24-hour consultation and acute crisis response service; and individualized intervention strategies coordinated through an interdisciplinary team. This police/mental health collaboration is unique in the degree to which it engages police officers in addressing the psychological needs of traumatized children as part of their everyday work both at the scene of a traumatic incident and in the days and weeks that follow. The CD-CP model includes an Acute Response Protocol that outlines components of psychological first aid that are important to address the needs of traumatized children within the immediate hours or days following a traumatic event (www.nccev.org). Following a violent incident such as a shooting at a neighborhood block party, police officers on scene will secure the area and page an on-call clinician. A clinical team will meet officers at the scene to jointly canvas the area talking to affected children and families providing psychoeducation to parents about common symptoms they or their children might experience following a traumatic event, talk to children and parents as needed about what they witnessed, and assist with concrete safety planning needs. The police-clinical teams help provide structure at a time of extreme stress and chaos, which in turn can help children and their families cope with the trauma. In addition, the connections made during this acute phase often allow families to seek further needed treatment with the clinical team following the peritraumatic period.

Integrated Treatment Models

In general, significant strides have been made in trauma-focused treatment interventions in the last 10 years. However, as discussed further in an earlier chapter (see Kaufman, 5.15.1), many traumatized children come from families grappling with multiple problems such as substance abuse and domestic violence. Current interventions have not adequately addressed the needs of these families. Treatments for perpetrators, victims, and their children are often segregated without consideration of the overlap between substance abuse, domestic violence, and child abuse, and the reality that many victims and children continue living with violent perpetrators or in unsafe settings following law enforcement and social service interventions. Based on these issues, we are developing a new approach that involves integrating a coordinated substance abuse/domestic violence intervention (110) for parents who have comorbid domestic violence and substance abuse histories with state-of-the-art child trauma treatments (based on principles of the current evidence-based dyadic treatments, TF-CBT and CPP). Continued development of integrated adult- and child-focused, evidence-based treatments is an area of significant need.

Psychopharmacological Intervention

Very few studies have examined the pharmacological treatment of ASD and/or pharmacological prevention of PTSD. One randomized controlled pilot study in children with severe burns and ASD found one week low-dose treatment with the tricyclic antidepressant imipramine (1 mg/kg) produced remission in twice as many children as the control condition in which children were only provided chloral hydrate to assist with sleep (111). In adults there are also two studies, one randomized (112), and the other nonrandomized (113), that suggest treatment with the ß-blocker propranolol immediately after trauma can prevent the onset of PTSD. An earlier pilot study with children with PTSD also suggests some benefit with propranolol. Using a B-A-B (off-on-off) medication design in a clinical setting, children exhibited significantly fewer symptoms when receiving medication (114). In contrast to the potential benefits of these medications, a study with adults found benzodiazepines administered prophylactically shortly after trauma exposure were associated with worse clinical outcomes (115).

There are no randomized controlled treatment trials of children with PTSD, but significant work has been accomplished in adult populations. Multiple studies in adults support the use of selective serotonin reuptake inhibitors (SSRIs) as a first-line therapy for PTSD (115). In adults, SSRIs are effective in reducing all PTSD symptom clusters, although they are sometimes less effective in targeting nightmares and other sleep problems (115). Multiple case reports and one controlled study also provide initial support for prazosin, an α_1-adrenergic antagonist, in the treatment of PTSD in adults. Prazosin treatment is associated with overall symptom improvement and decreases in nightmares and sleep difficulties (116). Preliminary controlled studies also show support for the serotonin norepinephrine reuptake inhibitor (SNRI) venlafaxine in the treatment of adult PTSD. In contrast, one controlled study showed no efficacy for buproprion (115). Atypical antipsychotics have been used in children with PTSD and profound hyperarousal symptoms (117, 118), although in adults these agents are considered second line and mostly used to augment partial response to SSRI treatments (115). The addition of atypical antipsychotics is associated with further reduction in PTSD symptom severity, and improvement on sleep indices. Open trial studies show some efficacy for SSRIs, clonidine, and guanfacine in the treatment of PTSD in children and adolescents (13), but controlled studies are needed. The data to guide the pharmacological treatment of children and adolescents with PTSD is very limited, and as the field has learned from work in child depression, one cannot generalize from studies in adults to determine the optimum pharmacological treatment strategies for children and adolescents (119). More work is needed in this area.

CLOSING REMARKS

PTSD is a common and yet frequently missed diagnosis in children and adolescents. Proper identification requires the collection of trauma history and symptom data from multiple informants. Over the past two decades, significant strides have been made in the assessment and treatment of PTSD in children and adolescents. More work is needed to understand the pathophysiology of early-onset PTSD, determine optimal pharmacological intervention strategies, and devise integrative treatment approaches that can address the range of difficulties commonly experienced by families of children with the disorder.

References

1. Kassam-Adams N, Winston FK: Predicting child PTSD: The relationship between acute stress disorder and PTSD in injured children. *Journal of the American Academy of Child & Adolescent Psychiatry* 43(4):403–411, 2004.
2. Lonigan C, Shannon M, Finch A, Daugherty T, et al.: Children's reactions to a natural disaster: Symptom severity and degree of exposure. *Advances in Behaviour Research & Therapy* 13(3):135–154, 1991.
3. Ajdukovic M: Displaced adolescents in Croatia: Sources of stress and posttraumatic stress reaction, in *Adolescence*, 1998, pp. 209–217.
4. Laor N, Wolmer L, Cohen DJ: Mothers' functioning and children's symptoms 5 years after a SCUD missile attack. *Am J Psychiatry* 158(7):1020–1026, 2001.
5. Kilpatrick D, Ruggiero K, Acierno R, Saunders B, Resnick H, Best C: Violence and risk of PTSD, major depression, substance abuse/dependence, and comorbidity: Results from the National Survey of Adolescents. *J Consult Clin Psychol* 71(4):692–700, 2003.
6. Saunders BE, Villeponteaux LA, Lipovsky JA, Kilpatrick DG, et al.: Child sexual assault as a risk factor for mental disorders among women: A community survey. *Journal of Interpersonal Violence* 7(2):189–204, 1997.
7. Boney-McCoy S, Finkelhor D: Psychosocial sequelae of violent victimization in a national youth sample. *J Consult Clin Psychol* 63(5):726–736, 1995.
8. American Psychiatric Association: *Diagnostic and Statistical Manual of Mental Disorders: DSM-III*. Washington, DC, American Psychiatric Association, 1980.
9. Marshall RD, Spitzer R, Liebowitz MR: Review and critique of the new DSM-IV diagnosis of acute stress disorder. *Am J Psychiatry* 156(11):1677–85, 1999.
10. American Psychiatric Association: *Diagnostic and Statistical Manual of Mental Disorders: DSM-III R*. Washington, DC, American Psychiatric Association, 1987.
11. American Psychiatric Association: *Diagnostic and Statistical Manual of Mental Disorders: DSM-IV*. Washington, DC, American Psychiatric Association, 1994.
12. Kessler R, Sonnega A, Bromet E, Hughes M, Nelson C: Posttraumatic stress disorder in the National Comorbidity Survey. *Arch Gen Psychiatry* 52(12):1048–1060, 1995.
13. De Bellis MD, Van Dillen T: Childhood post-traumatic stress disorder: An overview. *Child Adolesc Psychiatr Clin N Am* 14(4):745–1772, ix, 2005.
14. Costello E, Angold A: Developmental psychopathology and public health: Past, present, and future. *Development & Psychopathology* 12(4):599–618, 2000.
15. McCloskey LA, Walker M: Posttraumatic stress in children exposed to family violence and single-event trauma. *Journal of the American Academy of Child & Adolescent Psychiatry* 39(1):108–115, 2000.
16. Stallard P, Velleman R, Baldwin S: Psychological screening of children for post-traumatic stress disorder. *Journal of Child Psychology & Psychiatry & Allied Disciplines* 40(7):1075–1082, 1999.
17. Daviss WB, Racusin R, Fleischer A, Mooney D, Ford JD, McHugo GJ: Acute stress disorder symptomatology during hospitalization for pediatric injury. *J Am Acad Child Adolesc Psychiatry* 39(5):569–575, 2000.
18. Gorman JM, Mathew S, Coplan J: Neurobiology of early life stress: Nonhuman primate models. *Semin Clin Neuropsychiatry* 7(2):96–103, 2002.
19. Heim C, Owens MJ, Plotsky PM, Nemeroff CB: The role of early adverse life events in the etiology of depression and posttraumatic stress disorder: Focus on corticotropin-releasing factor. *Ann N Y Acad Sci* 821:194–207, 1997.
20. Villarreal G, Hamilton DA, Petropoulos H, Driscoll I, Rowland LM, Griego JA, Kodituwakku PW, Hart BL, Escalona R, Brooks WM: Reduced hippocampal volume and total white matter volume in posttraumatic stress disorder. *Biol Psychiatry* 52(2):119–125, 2002.
21. Bernstein D, Ahluvalia T, Pogge D, Handelsman L: Validity of the Childhood Trauma Questionnaire in an adolescent psychiatric population. *J Am Acad Child Adolesc Psychiatry* 36(3):340–348, 1997.
22. Bremner JD, Randall P, Vermetten E, Staib L, Bronen RA, Mazure C, Capelli S, McCarthy G, Innis RB, Charney DS: Magnetic resonance imaging-based measurement of hippocampal volume in posttraumatic stress disorder related to childhood physical and sexual abuse—A preliminary report. *Biol Psychiatry* 41(1):23–32, 1997.
23. Bremner JD, Randall P, Scott TM, Bronen RA, Seibyl JP, Southwick SM, Delaney RC, McCarthy G, Charney DS, Innis RB: MRI-based measurement of hippocampal volume in patients with combat-related posttraumatic stress disorder. *Am J Psychiatry* 152(7):973–981, 1995.
24. Gurvits TV, Shenton ME, Hokama H, Ohta H, Lasko NB, Gilbertson MW, Orr SP, Kikinis R, Jolesz FA, McCarley RW, Pitman RK: Magnetic resonance imaging study of hippocampal volume in chronic, combat-related posttraumatic stress disorder. *Biol Psychiatry* 40(11):1091–1099, 1996.
25. Vythilingam M, Heim C, Newport J, Miller AH, Anderson E, Bronen R, Brummer M, Staib L, Vermetten E, Charney DS, Nemeroff CB, Bremner JD: Childhood trauma associated with smaller hippocampal volume in women with major depression. *Am J Psychiatry* 159(12):2072–2080, 2002.
26. Driessen M, Hermann J, Stahl K, Zwann M, Meier S, Hill A, Osterheider M, Petersen D: Magnetic resonance imaging volumes of the hippocampus and the amygdala in women with borderline personality disorder and early traumatization. *Arch Gen Psychiatry* 57:1115–1122, 2000.
27. Gilbertson M, Shenton ME, Ciszewski A, Kasai K, Lasko N, Orr SP, Pittman RK: Smaller hippocampal volume predicts pathologic vulnerability to psychological trauma. *Nat Neurosci* 5:1242–1247, 2002.
28. Watanabe Y, Gould E, McEwen BS: Stress induces atrophy of apical dendrites of hippocampal CA3 pyramidal neurons. *Brain Res* 588(2):341–345, 1992.
29. Woolley CS, Gould E, McEwen BS: Exposure to excess glucocorticoids alters dendritic morphology of adult hippocampal pyramidal neurons. *Brain Res* 531(1–2):225–231, 1990.
30. Sapolsky RM, Krey LC, McEwen BS: Prolonged glucocorticoid exposure reduces hippocampal neuron number: Implications for aging. *J Neurosci* 5(5):1222–1227, 1985.
31. Sapolsky RM: Stress, glucocorticoids, and damage to the nervous system: The current state of confusion. *Stress* 1(1):1–19, 1996.
32. Uno H, Eisele S, Sakai A, Shelton S, Baker E, DeJesus O, Holden J: Neurotoxicity of glucocorticoids in the primate brain. *Horm Behav* 28(4):336–348, 1994.
33. Cameron HA, Gould E: Distinct populations of cells in the adult dentate gyrus undergo mitosis or apoptosis in response to adrenalectomy. *J Comp Neurol* 369(1):56–63, 1996.
34. Sapolsky RM: Glucocorticoids and hippocampal atrophy in neuropsychiatric disorders. *Arch Gen Psychiatry* 57(10):925–935, 2000.
35. Bremner JD: Alterations in brain structure and function associated with post-traumatic stress disorder. *Semin Clin Neuropsychiatry* 4(4):249–255, 1999.
36. De Bellis MD, Keshavan MS, Clark DB, Casey BJ, Giedd JN, Boring AM, Frustaci K, Ryan ND: Developmental traumatology. Part II: Brain development. *Biol Psychiatry* 45(10):1271–1284, 1999.
37. De Bellis MD, Hall J, Boring AM, Frustaci K, Moritz G: A pilot longitudinal study of hippocampal volumes in pediatric maltreatment-related posttraumatic stress disorder. *Biol Psychiatry* 50(4):305–9, 2001.
38. De Bellis MD, Keshavan MS, Shifflett H, Iyengar S, Beers SR, Hall J, Moritz G: Brain structures in pediatric maltreatment-related posttraumatic stress disorder: A sociodemographically matched study. *Biol Psychiatry* 52(11):1066–1078, 2002.
39. Carrion VG, Weems CF, Eliez S, Patwardhan A, Brown W, Ray RD, Reiss AL: Attenuation of frontal asymmetry in pediatric posttraumatic stress disorder. *Biol Psychiatry* 50(12):943–951, 2001.
40. Sheline YI, Wang PW, Gado MH, Csernansky JG, Vannier MW: Hippocampal atrophy in recurrent major depression. *Proc Natl Acad Sci USA* 93(9):3908–3913, 1996.
41. Kaufman J, Aikins D, Krystal J: Neuroimaging Studies in PTSD. In *Assessing Psychological Trauma and PTSD*. Keane JPWaTM (ed): New York, Guilford Press, 2004, pp. 389–417.
42. Farber NB, Wozniak DF, Price MT, Labruyere J, Huss J, St. Peter H, Olney JW: Age-specific neurotoxicity in the rat associated with NMDA receptor blockade: Potential relevance to schizophrenia? *Biol Psychiatry* 38(12):788–796, 1995.
43. Teicher MH, Dumont NL, Ito Y, Vaituzis C, Giedd JN, Andersen SL: Childhood neglect is associated with reduced corpus callosum area. *Biol Psychiatry* 56(2):80–5, 2004.
44. Sanchez MM, Hearn EF, Do D, Rilling JK, Herndon JG: Differential rearing affects corpus callosum size and cognitive function of rhesus monkeys. *Brain Res* 812(1–2):38–49, 1998.
45. Pandya DN, Seltzer B: The topography of commissural fibers In: Lepore F, Ptito M, Jasper HH. *Two Hemispheres One Brain: Functions of the Corpus Callosum (vol 17)*. (eds:) New York, Alan R. Liss, Inc., 1986, pp. 47–74.
46. Jackowski AP, Douglas-Palumberi H, Jackowski M, Win L, Schultz RT, Staib LH, Krystal JH, Kaufman J: Corpus callosum in maltreated children

with PTSD: A diffusion tensor imaging study. *Biological Psychiatry*. Submitted for publication.

47. Achenbach T, McConaughy S, Howill C: Child and adolescent behavioral and emotional problems: Implications of cross-informant correlations for situational specificity. *Psychopharmacol Bull* 101:213–232. 1987.
48. Kaufman J, Jones B, Steiglitz E, Vitulano L, Mannarino A: The use of multiple informants to assess children's maltreatment experiences. *Journal of Family Violence*. 9:227–248, 1994.
49. McGee R, Wolfe D, Yuen S, Wilson S, Carnochan J: The measurement of maltreatment: A comparison of approaches. *Child Abuse Negl* 19(2):233–249, 1995.
50. Grasso D, Lipschitz D, Guyer A, Houshyar S, Douglas-Palumberi H, Billingslea E, Crouse-Artus M, Massey J, Kaufman J: PTSD: The Missed Diagnosis. *Child Abuse & Neglect*. Submitted for publication.
51. Stover CS, Berkowitz S: Assessing violence exposure and trauma symptoms in young children: a critical review of measures. *J Trauma Stress* 18(6):707–717, 2005.
52. Ford JD, Racusin R, Ellis CG, Daviss WB, Reiser J, Fleischer A, Thomas J: Child maltreatment, other trauma exposure and posttraumatic symptomatology among children with oppositional defiant and attention deficit hyperactivity disorders. *Child Maltreatment* 5(3):205–217, 2000.
53. Nathan A, *L.A.L. F: The violence exposure scale for children: VEX (preschool version)*. College Park, MD, Department of Human Development, 1995.
54. Straus MA, Hamby SL, Boney-McCoy S, Sugarman DB: The Revised Conflict Tactics Scales (CTS2): Development and preliminary psychometric data. *Journal of Family Issues* 17:283–316, 1996.
55. Bernstein D: A new screening measure for detecting hidden domestic violence. *Psychiatric Times* 15(11):448–453, 1998.
56. Bernstein DP, Ahluvalia T, Pogge D, Handelsman L: Validity of the Childhood Trauma Questionnaire in an adolescent psychiatric population. *J Am Acad Child Adolesc Psychiatry* 36(3):340–348, 1997.
57. Barnett D, Manly J, Cicchetti D: Defining child maltreatment: The interface between policy and research. In (eds): Cicchetti D, Toth S: *Child Abuse, Child Development, and Social Policy: Advances in Applied Developmental Psychology* (vol 8). 1993. pp. 7–74.
58. Hawkins SS, Radcliffe J: Current measures of PTSD for children and adolescents. *J Pediatr Psychol* 31(4):420–430, 2006. Epub 2005 Jun 9.
59. Kassam-Adams N: The Acute Stress Checklist for Children (ASC-Kids): Development of a child self-report measure. *Journal of Traumatic Stress* 19(1):129–139, 2006.
60. Pynoos RS, Frederick C, Nader K, Arroyo W, et al.: Life threat and posttraumatic stress in school-age children. *Archives of General Psychiatry* 44(12):1057–1063, 1987.
61. Newman E, Weathers F, Nader K, Kalouped D, Pynoos R, Blake D: *Clinician-Administered PTSD scale for children and adolescents (CAPS-CA)*. Los Angeles, Western Psychological Services, 2004.
62. Briere J: *Trauma Symptom Checklist for Children (TSCC)*. Odessa, FL, Psychological Assessment Resources, 1996.
63. Richters J, Martinez P, Valla J: *Levonn: A cartoon-based interview for assessing children's distress symptoms*. Washington, DC, National Institutes of Mental Health, 1990.
64. Praver F, DiGiuseppe R, Pelcovitz D, Mandel FS, Gaines R: A preliminary study of a cartoon measure for children's reactions to chronic trauma. *Child Maltreatment: Journal of the American Professional Society on the Abuse of Children* 5(3), 273–285, 2000.
65. Steinberg AM, Brymer MJ, Decker KB, Pynoos RS: The University of California at Los Angeles Post-traumatic Stress Disorder Reaction Index. *Curr Psychiatry Rep* 6(2):96–100, 2004.
66. Angold A, Costello EJ: The Child and Adolescent Psychiatric Assessment (CAPA). *J Am Acad Child Adolesc Psychiatry* 39(1):39–48, 2000.
67. Kaufman J, Birmaher B, Brent D, Rao U, Flynn C, Moreci P, Williamson D, Ryan N: Schedule for Affective Disorders and Schizophrenia for School-Age Children-Present and Lifetime Version (K-SADS-PL): Initial reliability and validity data. *J Am Acad Child Adolesc Psychiatry* 36(7):980–988, 1997.
68. Reich W: Diagnostic interview for children and adolescents (DICA). *J Am Acad Child Adolesc Psychiatry* 39(1):59–66, 2000.
69. Shaffer D, Fisher P, Lucas CP, Dulcan MK, Schwab-Stone ME: NIMH Diagnostic Interview Schedule for Children Version IV (NIMH DISC-IV): Description, differences from previous versions, and reliability of some common diagnoses. *J Am Acad Child Adolesc Psychiatry* 39(1):28–38, 2000.
70. Breslau N, Davis GC, Andreski P, Peterson E: Traumatic events and posttraumatic stress disorder in an urban population of young adults. *Arch Gen Psychiatry* 48(3):216–222, 1991.
71. Breslau N, Davis GC, Andreski P, Peterson EL, Schultz LR: Sex differences in posttraumatic stress disorder. *Arch Gen Psychiatry* 54(11):1044–1048, 1997.
72. Clark DB, Lesnick L, Hegedus AM: Traumas and other adverse life events in adolescents with alcohol abuse and dependence. *J Am Acad Child Adolesc Psychiatry* 36(12):1744–1751, 1997.
73. Famularo R, Kinscherff R, Fenton T: Psychiatric diagnoses of maltreated children: Preliminary findings [see comments]. *J Am Acad Child Adolesc Psychiatry* 31(5):863–867, 1992.
74. Livingston R, Lawson L, Jones JG: Predictors of self-reported psychopathology in children abused repeatedly by a parent. *J Am Acad Child Adolesc Psychiatry* 32(5):948–953, 1993.
75. Hornstein NL, Putnam FW: Clinical phenomenology of child and adolescent dissociative disorders. *J Am Acad Child Adolesc Psychiatry* 31(6):1077–1085, 1992.
76. Putnam FW: Dissociative disorders in children: Behavioral profiles and problems. *Child Abuse & Neglect* 17(1):39–45, 1993.
77. Nurcombe B, Mithchell W, Begtrip R, Tramontaria M, LaBasbera J, Pruitt J: Dissociative hallucinations in allied conditions. In Volkmar F (ed): *Psychoses and Pervasive Developmental Disorders in Childhood and Adolescence*. Washington, DC, American Psychiatric Press, 1996, pp. 107–128.
78. Kaufman J, Birmaher B, Clayton S, Retano A, Wongchaowart B: Case study: Trauma-related hallucinations. *Journal of the American Academy of Child & Adolescent Psychiatry* 36(11), 1602–1605, 1997.
79. Scheeringa MS, Zeanah CH, Myers L, Putnam FW: New findings on alternative criteria for PTSD in preschool children. *J Am Acad Child Adolesc Psychiatry* 42(5):561–570, 2003.
80. Scheeringa MS, Zeanah CH, Myers L, Putnam FW: Predictive validity in a prospective follow-up of PTSD in preschool children. *J Am Acad Child Adolesc Psychiatry* 44(9):899–906, 2005.
81. Scheeringa MS, Wright MJ, Hunt JP, Zeanah CH: Factors affecting the diagnosis and prediction of PTSD symptomatology in children and adolescents. *Am J Psychiatry* 163(4):644–651, 2006.
82. Scheeringa MS, Zeanah CH, Drell MJ, Larrieu JA: Two approaches to the diagnosis of posttraumatic stress disorder in infancy and early childhood. *J Am Acad Child Adolesc Psychiatry* 34(2):191–200, 1995.
83. Egger H, Ascher B, Angold A: The Preschool Age Psychiatric Assessment (PAPA): A structured parent interview for diagnosing psychiatric disorders in preschool children. 1999.
84. Briere J: *Trauma Symptom Checklist for Young Children (TSCYC)*. Odessa, FL, Psychological Assessment Resources, 2004.
85. Ballenger JC, Davidson JR, Lecrubier Y, Nutt DJ, Marshall RD, Nemeroff CB, Shalev AY, Yehuda R: Consensus statement update on posttraumatic stress disorder from the international consensus group on depression and anxiety. *J Clin Psychiatry* 65(Suppl 1):55–62, 2004.
86. Freedman SA, Brandes D, Peri T, Shalev A: Predictors of chronic posttraumatic stress disorder: A prospective study. *Br J Psychiatry* 174:353–9, 1999.
87. Brewin CR, Andrews B, Valentine JD: Meta-analysis of risk factors for posttraumatic stress disorder in trauma-exposed adults. *J Consult Clin Psychol* 68(5):748–766, 2000.
88. True WR, Rice J, Eisen SA, Heath AC, Goldberg J, Lyons MJ, Nowak J: A twin study of genetic and environmental contributions to liability for posttraumatic stress symptoms. *Arch Gen Psychiatry* 50(4):257–264, 1993.
89. Gelernter J, Southwick S, Goodson S, Morgan A, Nagy L, Charney DS: No association between D2 dopamine receptor (DRD2) "A" system alleles, or DRD2 haplotypes, and posttraumatic stress disorder. *Biol Psychiatry* 45(5):620–625, 1999.
90. Bachmann AW, Sedgley TL, Jackson RV, Gibson JN, Young RM, Torpy DJ: Glucocorticoid receptor polymorphisms and post-traumatic stress disorder. *Psychoneuroendocrinology* 30(3):297–306, 2005.
91. Lee HJ, Lee MS, Kang RH, Kim H, Kim SD, Kee BS, Kim YH, Kim YK, Kim JB, Yeon BK, Oh KS, Oh BH, Yoon JS, Lee C, Jung HY, Chee IS, Paik IH: Influence of the serotonin transporter promoter gene polymorphism on susceptibility to posttraumatic stress disorder. *Depress Anxiety* 21(3):135–139, 2005.
92. Segman RH, Cooper-Kazaz R, Macciardi F, Goltser T, Halfon Y, Dobroborski T, Shalev AY: Association between the dopamine transporter gene and posttraumatic stress disorder. *Mol Psychiatry* 7(8):903–937, 2002.
93. Pynoos RS, Steinberg AM, Piacentini JC: A developmental psychopathology model of childhood traumatic stress and intersection with anxiety disorders. *Biological Psychiatry* 46(11):1542–1554, 1999.
94. Kessler RC: Posttraumatic stress disorder: The burden to the individual and to society. *J Clin Psychiatry* 61(Suppl 5):4–12; discussion 13–4, 2000.
95. Deblinger E, AHeflin A: *Cognitive Behavioral Interventions for Treating Sexually Abused Children*. Thousand Oaks, CA, Sage Publications, 1996.
96. March JS, Amaya-Jackson L, Murray MC, Schulte A: Cognitive-behavioral psychotherapy for children and adolescents with posttraumatic stress disorder after a single-incident stressor. *Journal of the American Academy of Child & Adolescent Psychiatry* 37(6):585–593, 1998.
97. Cohen JA, Mannarino AP: Factors that mediate treatment outcome of sexually abused preschool children: Six- and 12-month follow-up. *J Am Acad Child Adolesc Psychiatry* 37(1):44–51, 1998.
98. Saigh PA: The behavioral treatment of child and adolescent posttraumatic stress disorder. *Advances in Behaviour Research & Therapy* 14(4): 247–275, 1992.
99. Kolko D: Treatment and intervention for child victims of violence. In: Trickett PK, Schellenbach CJ (eds): *Violence against Children in the Family and the Community* pp. 213–249 xi, 1998.
100. Cohen JA, Deblinger E, Mannarino AP, Steer RA: A multisite, randomized controlled trial for children with sexual abuse-related PTSD symptoms. *J Am Acad Child Adolesc Psychiatry* 43(4):393–402, 2004.

101. Cohen JA, Mannarino AP: A treatment study for sexually abused preschool children: Outcome during a one-year follow-up. *Journal of the American Academy of Child & Adolescent Psychiatry* 36(9):1228–1235, 1997.
102. Cohen JA, Mannarino AP, Knudsen K: Treating sexually abused children: 1 year follow-up of a randomized controlled trial. *Child Abuse & Neglect* 29(2):135–145, 2005.
103. Lieberman AF, Van Horn, P, Ghosh Ippen, C: Toward evidence based practice: Child–parent psychotherapy with preschoolers exposed to marital violence. *Journal of the American Academy of Child and Adolescent Psychiatry* 44(12):1241–1248, 2005.
104. Lieberman AF, Van Horn, P: *"Don't hit my mommy!": A Manual for Child–Parent Psychotherapy with Young Witnesses of Family Violence.* Washington, DC, Zero to Three Press, 2005.
105. Stein BD, Jaycox LH, Kataoka SH, Wong M, Tu W, Elliott MN, Fink A: A mental health intervention for schoolchildren exposed to violence: A randomized controlled trial. *JAMA* 290(5):603–611, 2003.
106. Marans S: Psychoanalysis on the beat: Children, police, and urban trauma. *Psychoanal Study Child* 51:522–541, 1996.
107. Marans S, Berkowitz SJ, Cohen DJ: Police and mental health professionals: Collaborative responses to the impact of violence on children and families. *Child Adolesc Psychiatri Clin North Am* 7(3):635–651, 1998.
108. Berkowitz SJ, Marans SM: The child development-community policing program: A partnership to address the impact of violence. *Israel Journal of Psychiatry & Related Sciences* 37(2):103–114, 2000.
109. Murphy RA, Rosenheck RA, Berkowitz SJ, Marans SR: Acute service delivery in a police-mental health program for children exposed to violence and trauma. *Psychiatr Q* 76(2):107–121, 2005.
110. Easton C, Mandel DM, Hunkele K, Nich C, Rounsaville BJ, Carroll KM: A cognitive behavioral therapy for alcohol dependent domestic violence offenders: An integrated substance abuse–domestic violence approach (SADV). *American Journal on Addictions*. In press.
111. Robert R, Blakeney PE, Villarreal C, Rosenberg L, Meyer WJ, III: Imipramine treatment in pediatric burn patients with symptoms of acute stress disorder: A pilot study. *Journal of the American Academy of Child & Adolescent Psychiatry* 38(7):873–882, 1999.
112. Pitman RK, Sanders KM, Zusman RM, Healy AR, Cheema F, Lasko NB, Cahill L, Orr SP: Pilot study of secondary prevention of posttraumatic stress disorder with propranolol. *Biol Psychiatry* 51(2):189–192, 2002.
113. Vaiva G, Ducrocq F, Jezequel K, Averland B, Lestavel P, Brunet A, Marmar CR: Immediate treatment with propranolol decreases posttraumatic stress disorder two months after trauma. *Biol Psychiatry* 54(9):947–949, 2003.
114. Famularo R, Kinscherff R, Fenton T: Propranolol treatment for childhood posttraumatic stress disorder, acute type: A pilot study. *Am J Dis Child* 142(11):1244–1247, 1988.
115. Davidson JR: Pharmacologic treatment of acute and chronic stress following trauma: 2006. *J Clin Psychiatry* 67(Suppl 2):34–39, 2006.
116. Raskind MA, Peskind ER, Kanter ED, Petrie EC, Radant A, Thompson CE, Dobie DJ, Hoff D, Rein RJ, Straits-Troster K, Thomas RG, McFall MM: Reduction of nightmares and other PTSD symptoms in combat veterans by prazosin: A placebo-controlled study. *Am J Psychiatry* 160(2):371–373, 2003.
117. Horrigan JP, Barnhill L, Kohli R: Adderall, the atypicals, and weight gain. *Journal of the American Academy of Child & Adolescent Psychiatry* 40(6):620, 2001.
118. Horrigan J: Guanfacine for posttraumatic stress disorder nightmares. *Journal of the American Academy of Child & Adolescent Psychiatry* 32(1077–1085), 1996.
119. Martin A, Kaufman J, Charney D: Pharmacotherapy of early-onset depression: Update and new directions. *Child Adolesc Psychiatr Clin N Am* 9(1):135–57, 2000.

CHAPTER 5.15.3 ■ REACTIVE ATTACHMENT DISORDER

MARY MARGARET GLEASON AND CHARLES H. ZEANAH

INTRODUCTION

Bowlby and Ainsworth

Psychiatry has long acknowledged the importance of a child's caregiving environment for emotional development. Since the mid-twentieth century, the literature has included descriptions of the negative impact of severe emotional deprivation (1). Descriptive studies of young children raised in institutions have described important effects of these caregiving environments on social and emotional development, including descriptions of indiscriminant behavior, which is considered to be part of the clinical syndrome of reactive attachment disorder.

Although disorders of attachment were not described in formal nosologies until the DSM-III (2), attachment theory has been the focus of active investigation for decades. Attachment theory was developed by John Bowlby and refined in collaboration with Mary Ainsworth and others (3, 4). Bowlby proposed that infants are born with a biological predisposition to develop an attachment relationship with a small number of caregiving adults from whom the child seeks comfort, nurturance, support, and protection (Table 5.15.3.1).

Developmental Stages of the Attachment Relationship

In the first few 2 months of life, infants preferentially orient to people's movement, faces, and sounds, although they do not discriminate among people, except in very subtle ways. From ages 2–7 months, children become more socially interactive and do appear to respond differentially to their caregivers, although they continue to engage socially with unfamiliar adults as well. Attachment behavior, characterized by proximity-seeking in times of stress, appears in the second half of the first year of life. The presence of the focused attachment relationship is heralded by the onset of separation protest and stranger anxiety. According to attachment theory, the attachment system works in conjunction with a number of other biologically driven systems, most prominently the exploration system. An equilibrium develops between the attachment and exploration systems. The parent serves as a secure base from which the child can explore the world when the exploration system is more highly activated, and a safe haven to whom s/he can return in times of stress when the attachment behaviors are more prominent.

TABLE 5.15.3.1

DEVELOPMENT OF ATTACHMENT

0–2 months	2–7 months	7–18 months	18–26 months
Bowlby's Characterization			
■ "Orientation and signals without discrimination"	■ "Orientation and signals directed towards >1 or more discriminated figures"	■ "Maintenance of proximity to a discriminated figure"	■ "Formation of a reciprocal relationship"
Social Interaction Patterns			
■ Physical and social attributes attract adults for social interactions ■ Recognition of maternal face ■ Olfactory/auditory recognition ■ Spontaneous smile	■ Able to engage adults in reciprocal social interactions ■ Evidence of differential responses to adults	■ Focused attachment ■ Separation protest ■ Stranger reactions ■ Intersubjectivity evident ■ Social referencing	■ Develop negotiating abilities with caregivers ("goal-corrected partnership") ■ Increased interest in peers; moves toward interactive play and exploration
Communication/Methods of Cueing Adults to Needs			
■ Crying, cooing	■ Eye contact ■ Social smile ■ Responsive cooing, babbling	■ Intentional communication with gestures and then words	■ Able to express needs ■ Rapid vocabulary expansion

Interactions of Attachment, Exploration, and Social Systems

In human infants, attachment formation appears to be an example of *experience expectant* neural development. That is, in species-typical rearing environments, infants are hardwired to form selective attachments to caregiving adults. On the other hand, it appears that environmental and relationship factors play a strong role in the *type* of attachment relationship that the child develops, reflecting *experience dependent* neural processes. Ainsworth demonstrated a relationship between early patterns of parental sensitivity, infant responsiveness, and the development of a secure attachment relationship at age 12 months (5–8).

Different types or patterns of attachment are important because they serve as risk and protective factors for subsequent psychosocial adaptation. Children with insecure attachment patterns are at higher risk for subsequent psychiatric disorders and impairment from emotional and behavioral symptoms than securely attached infants (9–11). Although insecure attachment classifications are not necessarily indicative of psychopathology, the extremes of insecurity may reflect clinically relevant disorders of attachment (12).

DEFINITIONS

While the core features of reactive attachment disorder (RAD) are fairly consistent across diagnostic nosologies, each nosology uses a slightly different focus, as described in Table 5.15.3.2. For the first time in the DSM-III-R, the two subtypes of "inhibited" and "disinhibited" reactive attachment disorder were introduced; these subtypes remain in all extant nosologies. The DSM-IV criteria highlight problems of social relatedness in RAD, and require that a child demonstrate these aberrant patterns across settings. The DSM-IV also requires that there be a known history of "grossly pathogenic care (13)".

More recently, the American Academy of Child and Adolescent Psychiatry convened an expert task force to develop empirically based research diagnostic criteria for the preschool age group using DSM-IV criteria and existing clinical and research data. These Research Diagnostic Criteria—Preschool Age (RDC-PA) explicitly link the diagnosis to disordered attachment behaviors and to a child's lack of use, or misuse, of the primary attachment figure, unlike the DSM, which describes aberrant social behavior patterns (14). The use of these criteria may help to standardize the way in which RAD is studied and described in the literature.

The ICD-10, used primarily in Europe, classifies reactive attachment symptoms into two separate disorders, both with an emphasis on social relatedness. The first, which corresponds to the inhibited form of RAD, is called simply "reactive attachment disorder of childhood" and describes children with inhibited emotional responsiveness and contradictory social responses. In the ICD-10 nosology, "disinhibited attachment disorder of childhood" describes children with diffuse attachments and indiscriminate behaviors (15).

PHENOMENOLOGY OF RAD

While the categorization of RAD differs across diagnostic nosologies, and continues to evolve, there are certain common features that are generally agreed upon. The major nosologies, as well as historical descriptions of RAD (16), consistently describe two categories of attachment disorder behaviors: the inhibited and the disinhibited or indiscriminate types. It remains unclear how these two distinct subtypes relate to one another (17).

Emotionally Withdrawn/Inhibited Reactive Attachment Disorder

In the inhibited form of RAD, children show restriction of affect and behavior in situations that would normally activate the attachment system. In a healthy attachment behavioral

TABLE 5.15.3.2

COMPARATIVE NOSOLOGY OF REACTIVE ATTACHMENT DISORDER

DSM-IV	DSM-IV RDC: PA	ICD-10	DC: Zero to three
Core Criteria			
"Markedly disturbed and developmentally inappropriate social relatedness in most contexts" (p.118)	"A pattern of markedly disturbed and developmentally inappropriate attachment behaviors in which the child rarely or minimally turns preferentially to a discriminated attachment figure for comfort, support, protection, and nurturance" (p.11)	"Persistent abnormalities in the child's pattern of social relationships" (p. 219) and "particular pattern of ... diffuse attachments" from infancy through middle childhood (pp. 220–221)	"A child with RAD will usually fail to initiate social interactions or will manifest ambivalent or contradictory social responses ... A child may also show developmentally inappropriate social relatedness by social indiscriminance" (p. 30)
Age of Symptom Development			
<5 yo	<5 yo	<5 yo	Not specified
Maltreatment Criteria?			
"Grossly pathogenic care"	No requirement	Suggests caution if no known history of abuse or neglect	"Evidence of deprivation or maltreatment" (pp. 29–30)
Subtypes of Disorder			
Inhibited, disinhibited	Inhibited, disinhibited/indiscriminate, mixed	Reactive attachment disorder of childhood Disinhibited attachment disorder of childhood	None
Exclusions			
No PDD Not explained by developmental delay	No PDD Developmental age >= 9 months	Two attachment disorders are mutually exclusive; no PDD, cannot include other abuse syndromes	None Rule out: affective, relationship, adjustment, psychic trauma disorder

system, stressors activate the attachment system and a child seeks comfort from his or her attachment figure, but children with inhibited RAD tend neither to seek comfort from nor to respond to comfort offered by their caregiver. These children also may show contradictory behavioral response patterns, such as approaching and then avoiding a parent during a reunion (2, 18). Children with the inhibited form of RAD tend to demonstrate a constricted range of affect and limited social reciprocity in social situations (19, 20). In addition, emotional dysregulation has been described in clinical populations of children with RAD (15, 19, 21). Although emotional dysregulation may be an important clinical finding in children with histories of maltreatment, concerns have been raised about including it in the diagnostic criteria, as it lacks diagnostic specificity, particularly in the preschool age range (22). The inhibited form of RAD has been described primarily in maltreated or institutionalized children (20, 23).

Indiscriminately Social/Disinhibited Reactive Attachment Disorder

In indiscriminate RAD, children show a different pattern of responses to stressors which would usually activate the attachment system. In novel situations or stressful situations, these children tend to be overly familiar with strangers. Whereas a healthy attachment system counterbalances children's ploratory drive and motivates children to check in with their attachment figure as they explore new places or people, these children may approach strangers and even willingly leave with a stranger. Their proximity-seeking and comfort-seeking behaviors overall are applied indiscriminately. While these children have been described as "overly friendly," their behaviors do not necessarily represent friendliness or reciprocal social interactions. In fact, the approaches may feel empty or shallow to the other person (24, 25).

Other Clinical Forms of Attachment Disorders

Mixed RAD

While the standard nosologies only allow for the presence of inhibited *or* disinhibited RAD, research in maltreated and institutionalized children has found moderate intercorrelations between disinhibited and inhibited RAD (17, 20). The question that remains unanswered is whether there are children who truly manifest features of both types of RAD, or whether there is a spurious problem with measurement. It is possible to imagine that some children with the inhibited type of RAD might passively go off with a stranger, fail to check back with a caregiver and show little reticence with strangers because they are so withdrawn and unresponsive rather because they are actively seeking engagement in a nonselective manner.

Secure Base Distortions

The diagnostic criteria for RAD imply the lack of a focused attachment relationship. However, investigators and clinicians have noted severely disordered attachment behaviors in children who appear to have a focused attachment figure, albeit in the context of a disturbed relationship (22, 26). Zeanah and colleagues have proposed a revised set of alternative diagnostic criteria, which explicitly allow for the diagnosis of a reactive attachment disorder when the child's use of the caregiver as an emotional secure base is distorted (26, 27). The distortions can be of four major types: role-reversed behaviors, provocative self-endangering behaviors, excessive clinginess and restriction in exploration, and excessive vigilance and hypercompliance. In a role-reversed pattern, a child takes on a directive, parent-like role in his or her relationship with a primary caregiver. Provocative self-endangering behaviors, unlike impulsive behaviors, appear to be intended to elicit a response from a parent. While many preschoolers cling to their parent, some children's clinginess increases exponentially in the presence of strangers, as if the child is not sure the parent will protect him or her. Finally, children can become excessively vigilant or show robotic hypercompliance, sometimes in the context of an unpredictable, harsh parenting style. While these criteria have not been incorporated into diagnostic nosologies, these alternative criteria for RAD can be used to reliably diagnose high-risk children (23) and may be valuable constructs in clinical assessments of attachment behaviors.

ASSOCIATED CLINICAL FEATURES

The particular risks and contexts that give rise to RAD also have been associated with other clinical conditions.

Quasi-Autistic Features

Rutter and colleagues described a small subgroup of previously institutionalized children who presented with "quasi-autistic" features, including limited social reciprocity, poor observance of social boundaries and poor social awareness (28). These children, who represented just 6% of the total group of previously institutionalized children, demonstrated several features that distinguished them from typically described autism. The severity of symptoms in these children correlated with the length of time a child spent institutionalized, suggesting an environmental, rather than neurobiological, etiology. Importantly, unlike autism, these symptoms diminished over a course of 2 years following adoption.

Hyperactivity and Inattention

Indiscriminate behavior has been noted to be accompanied by hyperactivity and inattention. While these symptoms are not part of RAD, some have suggested that the inattention and overactivity seen in children with a history of institutionalization and attachment disturbances may reflect an "institutional deprivation syndrome" (29). Rather than invoking traditional ADHD, these investigators suggest this syndrome is directly related to the deprivation of the institutional experience, citing a correlation between attachment disturbances and the levels of the hyperactivity, between duration of institutionalization and inattention/hyperactivity, and the clinical differences in the presentation compared with ADHD.

Failure to Thrive

Failure to thrive has been associated with RAD symptoms since the development of the DSM-III criteria in which growth failure was a criterion. This criterion was dropped subsequently from the DSM because of a lack of face validity as an attachment-related symptom. However, failure to thrive has been shown to be associated with some parental indicators of attachment disturbances (30) and continues to be cited in the clinical guidelines of the ICD-10 (14). While neither necessary nor sufficient as a sign of disordered attachment, it may be an associated finding. Other feeding abnormalities, particularly stuffing or hoarding food, also have been described in maltreated children and may be associated with RAD (21).

EPIDEMIOLOGY

Although believed by most to be a rare disorder, RAD has not been included in population based studies, and the actual prevalence is unknown. Interpretation of estimates in other groups must be limited because of varying application of diagnostic criteria. Nevertheless, experts agree that the disorder is rare in the general population (19).

Rates of RAD in high risk samples have been studied slightly more extensively. In clinics focused on Infant Mental Health, reported rates of RAD range from 1% to 20% (31–33). These differences likely reflect differences in referral patterns and method of diagnosis. In maltreated populations, the prevalence is significantly higher. A single study found that 40% of foster children under 48 months who were assessed within 3 months of placement in care were diagnosed with RAD using a semistructured interview (17). Rates of attachment disorder behaviors in institutionalized or previously institutionalized children are also high, with rates of 22–56% reported (20, 24, 34). In institutionalized samples, rates of indiscriminate behaviors are described as higher in frequency than inhibited attachment disorder behaviors.

ETIOLOGY

Pathogenic care or maltreatment is required to make the diagnosis in DSM-IV-TR and strongly recommended in ICD-10. Nevertheless, it is not clear that it should be a criterion for diagnosis, as it is often difficult to substantiate such a history at the time of presentation to a clinical setting (19, 22). In support of its inclusion, however, is the report that children with excellent caregiving but a microdeletion on one of chromosome 7 typically show indiscriminate behavior (35). No studies have yet explored the phenomenology of indiscriminate behavior in the two conditions to determine if they are clinically distinguishable.

There is evidence to support a dose-dependent effect of pathologic care on attachment behavior disturbances. In a Romanian institution, children placed in a pilot program with a higher staff ratio and staffing schedules more conducive to the development of attachment relationships had lower rates of indiscriminate behaviors than those in the traditional unit, and higher rates than children who had never been institutionalized (36). Within standard institutional care, children who received higher quality caregiving were more likely to have lower rates of disturbed attachment behaviors (34). After adoption, the same dose-dependent relationship has been documented, with length of institutionalization correlating closely with the severity of indiscriminant attachment disorder behaviors (24, 37). Similarly, in the United States, rates of RAD parallel the environmental or family risk of adverse caregiving. Children in foster care had the highest rates of RAD, followed by homeless children and then children in Head Start (23). While there appears to be a dose-dependent relationship, at this time there is no clear evidence to suggest sensitive periods (37–39). Further, being exposed to maltreatment or institutionalization does not create sufficient conditions for the development of RAD. Up to 70% of children post-institutionalization may show no attachment disorder behaviors (39). While the protective mechanisms are not sufficiently understood, being considered a "favorite child" may be one factor favoring a resilient outcome to young children in institutions (34).

DIAGNOSIS

Clinical History and Interview

As with all other psychiatric disorders in young children, evaluation of a child who may have reactive attachment disorder is a multimodal process that should involve more than one appointment, ideally in more than one setting. Interviews with caregivers as well as child–caregiver observations provide the central core of the diagnostic evaluation. An interview focused on reactive attachment disorder should address a child's attachment behavior with the primary caregiver, including the presence of a focused attachment relationship, inhibited or indiscriminate patterns, and secure base distortions.

First, the presence of a focused attachment relationship should be explored. Specifically, an interviewer should assess whether the child has one (or more) adults from whom he or she seeks comfort, reassurance and nurturing, particularly in times of distress. In addition, patterns of inhibited attachment behaviors (not using attachment figure for comfort), and indiscriminate (overly friendly) attachment behaviors should be identified. While the DSM-IV and IDC-10 emphasize the presence of generalized problems with social relationships, a child with RAD should show some flexibility of relationship behaviors and may show relationship specificity of behaviors (27). It is also useful to assess the child's use of parents as a secure emotional base and to explore distortions of this secure base (24, 40). The use of a semistructured interview, such as the Disturbances of Attachment Interview (41), may be helpful to assess these categories of attachment disorder behaviors in a systematic manner.

The context of the child's attachment behaviors and relationships must be investigated during the interview, including details of a child's history of maltreatment. The DSM-IV requires a history of "grossly pathogenic care" in order to meet the RAD criteria (2) and details of the caregiving history, with attention to neglect, changes in caregiving relationships, or significant losses should be investigated during the interview.

Because of the high rates of other psychiatric disorders in children with high risk family or environmental backgrounds, reviewing other areas of disturbance is an essential part of the history. Disruptive behavior disorders, mood disorders, and anxiety disorders are seen at higher rates in maltreated populations. With any child, but particularly one whose history includes a deprived caregiving context, assessment of both developmental and cognitive status is important. In particular, a child who is not developmentally 9 months of age should not be diagnosed with RAD because he or she may not have the developmental capacity for an attachment relationship and therefore cannot have a disorder of such.

Clinical Observations

Clinical practice settings provide opportunities to observe and stimulate attachment behaviors (42). Observing children in the beginning of the assessment when first meeting the interviewer (a stranger) can provide information about how a child references and/or seeks comfort from a caregiver in the context of a new person and setting. In addition, asking a parent to leave the room for a brief separation from the child can activate the child's attachment system and provide valuable information about how a child reconnects with the parent upon reunion. A single observation is insufficient to make a diagnosis of RAD, and serial observations are recommended. Throughout the assessment, it is valuable to compare the child's interactions with a caregiver and the stranger (43). In addition, observations of a child with all important caregivers can help to distinguish between child-specific behaviors and relationship-specific behaviors (44).

Standardized observations of attachment behaviors have primarily been studied for assessment of attachment classification, a qualitatively different categorization of attachment. However, one clinical assessment of attachment involving a stranger, separations, and reunions and the introduction of a robot as a mildly distressing stimulus has also been used reliably to diagnose attachment disorders in a clinical context (24). The use of standardized procedure provides the clinician the opportunity to observe patterns of children's attachment behaviors in a consistent manner in repeated episodes and potentially with different caregivers, reducing the influence of other variables.

The Strange Situation (45), which introduces a stranger and caregiver–child separations, is a research method designed to assess the attachment classification of the relationship. This procedure assumes the existence of a focused attachment, an assumption that is not universally warranted in children with RAD and may make the observations uninterpretable (25). The Strange Situation is not intended to provide a clinical diagnosis and should not be substituted for clinical observations, although the observed interactions between child and caregiver may provide insights into the attachment relationship.

DIFFERENTIAL DIAGNOSIS AND COMORBID DISORDERS

The differential diagnosis of RAD is broad. A child must have a developmental age of at least 9 months to be diagnosed with RAD; a child with mental retardation and a developmental age significantly younger than chronological age will not show the usual patterns of healthy attachment but will also have other findings consistent with developmental delay. The DSM requires that PDD not be present in a child diagnosed with RAD. This differentiation may be hard to assess when a child is first evaluated. The ICD uses the longitudinal course of symptoms as a differentiating feature between PDD and RAD, pointing out that if the symptoms are secondary to RAD, they will improve in a safe caregiving environment. While true, this differentiation may be hard to assess when a patient is first presenting for care. However, while children with quasi-autistic features present with autism behavior scores similar to those of children with autism, several features may help distinguish them: 1) Children with RAD and quasi-autistic features have normal or small (not large) head circumference, 2) they may show more frequent (though socially inappropriate) approaches to others and even indiscriminant behavior, and 3) they use language more than children with typical autism, although again, often in unusual styles (28). While the ICD-10 suggests that children with RAD do not have stereotypical behaviors, Rutter's Romanian subgroup did show significant rates of stereotypies.

Institutionalized and maltreated children are also at risk for other diagnoses related to their early experiences, and RAD must be distinguished from these disorders. Most prominent among them are disruptive behavior disorders, anxiety disorders, particularly posttraumatic stress disorder, and mood disorders (46). PTSD has been described in a child with RAD with a suggestion that inhibited features of RAD might be related to anxiety symptoms (21).

While there may be a high comorbidity rate in children with RAD and disruptive behavior disorders, the nonattachment-related behavioral symptoms should not be considered reflective of the attachment disorder. For example, while children with ADHD may impulsively run from their parent if they see something of interest, they should also use a parent selectively for comfort, a behavior not seen in indiscriminant children. Aggressive behaviors, seen commonly in disruptive behavior disorders, are not reflective of attachment disorder behaviors (36). It is possible that in maltreated children, the pathologic care may be a shared etiological factor in more than one disorder, as has been argued in the case of inattention and hyperactivity, but they remain diagnostically distinct entities.

Posttraumatic stress disorder can occur at rates of up to 40% in abused children 5–10 years old, and it seems likely that the history of abuse also puts this group at increased risk for RAD. For the most part, RAD signs do not overlap with those of PTSD except perhaps for the shared hypervigilance symptom and the need to differentiate frozen watchfulness of a secure base distortion from dissociative episodes in PTSD. Similarly, while mood disorders occur at higher rates in maltreated populations than in the general population, signs or symptoms reflective of a mood disorder should not be interpreted as representing attachment disorders in the absence of other necessary criteria.

COURSE AND PROGNOSIS

In a small study of young children in foster care, nearly all of the dyads showed a distinct pattern of attachment behaviors, most within days of placement, although those patterns were vulnerable to external disruptions like respite placement (47). While this study did not address a clinical diagnosis of RAD, it highlights the rapidity with which infants can develop new attachment relationships, particularly when placed in favorable caregiving settings.

At this time, prospective longitudinal studies of RAD follow children into the early school-aged years. The limitations of diagnosing RAD in infants and preschoolers are magnified in older children; measurements of normal attachment behaviors do not exist, and the application of the infant and preschool definitions of a disorder is likely inappropriate (43). Descriptions of RAD in older children tend to apply criteria that are completely lacking empirical support and should be viewed with skepticism (48, 49).

TREATMENT

Data related to specific interventions for RAD are limited. A commonality on which most infant mental health interventions are based is the inclusion of both child and primary caregiver as participants in the intervention.

Foster Care Placement

While the need to remove a child from pathologic care or the extremes of deprivation seems to be an obvious intervention for RAD, only one study has examined the effect of this process on children's attachment disorder behaviors. The Bucharest Early Intervention Project is a longitudinal intervention study that includes baseline data about the children before their placement into foster care (50). In foster care, these children and families received regular visits and support from social workers who were supervised by foster care experts. The children who were placed in foster homes showed robust improvement in inhibited patterns of attachment disorder behaviors and somewhat less improvement in indiscriminate patterns. Compared to children who had never been institutionalized, children in foster care continue to demonstrate higher levels of indiscriminate behaviors than the community group (34), a result consistent with other studies of Romanian adoptees (37, 38). Young children who remained in the institutional environment continued to demonstrate both forms of attachment disorder behaviors—at least to 42 months of age (34). These results suggest that placement in a safe, family environment is an effective intervention for inhibited attachment disorder behaviors, but is not sufficient to eliminate signs of indiscriminate attachment disorder.

As early as 2 years after adoption, children adopted from institutions show virtually no symptoms of inhibited attachment disorder, suggesting that it is remediated by adoptive placement. Indiscriminate behaviors, on the other hand, tend to persist in adoptive placements up to 5 years later (37, 38, 51). The fact that signs of RAD are reduced or eliminated by enhanced environments does not mean there are no lasting attachment disturbances. Insecure, especially atypical classification patterns of attachment are increased in children after institutionalization (37, 39).

Attachment-Based Therapies

Attachment-focused therapies have not been studied as interventions for reactive attachment disorder. However, given the lack of specific treatments for RAD and the shared theoretical foundations for attachment classifications and attachment disorder behavior, there is reason to consider attachment-based interventions in this discussion. Attachment-based therapies seek, through various mechanisms and points of entry, to strengthen the primary attachment relationship.

A number of caveats must be identified when considering attachment-based therapies in the context of RAD (18). While these attachment-based therapies assume a focused attachment relationship (albeit usually an unsatisfying one), it is not safe to assume the existence of a focused attachment in children with RAD. It is not known whether attachment-based interventions can stimulate development of an attachment relationship where none exists.

It is not even clear that increasing rates of secure attachment classifications is associated with resolution of disinhibited attachment disorder signs. Intuitively, given the distinct patterns of behavior seen in indiscriminate and inhibited attachment disorders, it would seem that they would call for different treatment approaches, which is not a part of these treatment strategies.

In spite of these caveats, there is a theoretical basis for believing that interventions that strengthen the attachment relationship can create an environment in which a child's negative internal representations can be modified and which can interrupt the perpetuation of attachment disorder behaviors (52). Particularly important may be helping the child's caregiver reinterpret the child's behaviors in order to function as a more effective, secure base (53, 54).

Infant–Parent Psychotherapy

Infant–parent psychotherapy (IPP) and Child–parent psychotherapy (CPP) are therapies which draw on psychoanalytic and attachment theory to provide corrective attachment experiences to the parent and infant. IPP identifies targets of change ("mutative factors") as central to the treatment (55). In keeping with its psychodynamic roots, the development of parental insight into her use of the child as a negative transference object is defined as one target of treatment. In addition, through the therapeutic relationship and interventions, IPP provides the dyad with corrective attachment experiences that model and emphasize nurturing, support, protection, and reciprocity. The third mutative factor is the "power of learning and practicing mutually satisfying forms of interaction" (55). IPP and CPP sessions are flexibly structured, and access a parent's current and past experiences to increase awareness and insight into the relationship. Throughout IPP, the therapist provides a nurturing, and supportive experience for both partners in the dyad. The infant's presence in IPP provides an opportunity for the therapist to identify themes and distortions that might not be evident in individual therapy (56). CPP shares the same foundation, but uses play as the modality through which the child and parent together can create joint meaning in their interactions (55).

In a randomized controlled study comparing anxiously attached low-income dyads with the untreated control group, the IPP group showed higher maternal sensitivity and fewer toddler angry behaviors and more evidence of a goal-corrected partnership in a laboratory situation (57). The intervention was not associated with a difference in attachment classification, although the authors suggest that such a change might require more than 1 year to solidify enough to be seen in the laboratory setting.

Circle of Security

Attachment-based intervention can also be provided in a group setting. The circle of security (COS) model integrates attachment theory and object relations theory (54). This therapy initially provides parents with information about children's emotional and attachment needs, and uses a visual aid (the "circle of security") to demonstrate the processes of exploration from a safe base and returning to the safe haven. Using group discussions about video clips of each dyad, this treatment model focuses on enhancing parents' observational skills of their children's exploration and attachment cues, reflective functioning, emotional regulation, and empathy (58). The use of video clips allows parents to observe their interactions in a safe, supportive environment, and gives them an opportunity to consider their children's experiences as well as their own. Like IPP, the COS model encourages parents to identify early relationship experiences that may contribute to their difficulties in effectively responding to their children's exploration and attachment cues. Early assessment of the COS model in Head Start communities has demonstrated improvement in rates of secure attachment, increased organized attachment patterns, and a striking increase in organized caregiving responses to their children (58).

Treatments Not Recommended

Perhaps because of the high intensity clinical needs of children who have experienced severe deprivation or maltreatment, alternative treatments for emotional and behavioral problems in adopted children have proliferated. Some treatments have advocated "holding" a child as a means of eliciting suppressed rage (59). Others advocate holding as a means to provide physical nurturing that the child did not experience as an infant and advise that the child may need to be restrained during the procedure if he or she physically resists the holding (60). These interventions are not empirically supported (61). Coercive restraint, when applied for reasons other than imminent safety, seems more likely to further support a child's negative self-perception and his or her sense that caregivers cannot protect him or her, than to enhance the development of positive relationships with a caregiver and others. In addition, holding therapy and other alternative approaches, including rebirthing, are associated with high risk and deaths (62). Professional organizations, including the American Academy of Child and Adolescent Psychiatry and the American Professional Society on the Abuse of Children, have formal policies against the use of coercive restraint, especially for children with severe emotional problems (63).

SUMMARY AND FUTURE DIRECTIONS

The current state of the literature related to RAD provides a foundation from which further research can be developed. Clinical experience and research have validated two primary forms of reactive attachment disorder, inhibited and disinhibited, both of which seem to be proportionately related to the degree of pathological care a child has experienced. A careful interview focused on a child's attachment behaviors, with particular attention to patterns of inhibition and indiscriminate behaviors, as well as the child's caregiving history, is an important element in establishing the diagnosis. While standardized observational systems have not been developed for clinical use, it is of value to supplement the routine child psychiatry office assessment with a structured separation and reunion to elicit attachment behaviors in a young child suspected of having RAD. Removal from an institution and placement in foster care has been shown to be an effective intervention for the symptoms of inhibited RAD, although most studies show continued indiscriminate behaviors long after placement. After placement in a safe caregiving environment, current treatment recommendations focus on enhancing positive caregiver interactions (43).

Current knowledge leaves us with further questions as well. Children exposed to adverse caregiving can present with a wide range of internalizing and externalizing symptoms in addition to RAD. As described in the case of inattention and hyperactivity, some investigators suggest that these symptoms may represent a qualitatively different form of disorder than that seen in the general population. Careful assessment of these symptoms and study of treatment effects and longitudinal course may help to clarify this question. A second remaining question relates to the timing of an intervention. While all clinicians agree that amelioration of a child's caregiving environment should be accomplished as soon as possible, the presence of critical periods remains unclear. Because of the early childhood focus of current RAD research, little is known about the manifestation of this disorder in middle childhood and adolescence. It seems clear that attachment behaviors, like all behaviors, vary with developmental stages and therefore that disorders of attachment will present differently across different ages. To date, most research specific to RAD has focused on early childhood with followup over the course a few years. Longitudinal studies will provide information about the natural course of this disorder and developmental variations in its presentation.

References

1. Spitz R. Hospitalism: An inquiry into the genesis of psychiatric conditions in early childhood. *Psychoanal Study Child* 1:53–74, 1945.
2. American Psychiatric Association: *Diagnostic and Statistical Manual of Mental Disorders*, 4th ed. (DSM-IV). Washington, DC, American Psychiatric Association, 1999.
3. Bowlby J: *Attachment and Loss: Attachment.* New York, Basic Books, 1962/1982.
4. Ainsworth MDS: Object relations, dependency and attachment: A theoretical review of the infant-mother relationship *Child Dev* (40):969–1025, 1969.
5. Bell SM, Ainsworth M. Infant crying and maternal responsiveness. *Child Dev* 43:1171–1190, 1972.
6. Blehar MC, Lieberman AF, Ainsworth M. Early face-to-face interaction and its relation to later infant–mother attachment. *Child Dev* 48(1):182–194, 1977.
7. Tracy RL, Ainsworth MS. Maternal affectionate behavior and infant–mother attachment patterns. *Child Dev* 52:1341–1343, 1981.
8. Bretherton I. The origins of attachment theory: John Bowlby and Mary Ainsworth. *Dev Psychol* 28:759–775, 1992.
9. Lyons-Ruth K, Easterbrooks MA, Cibelli CD. Infant attachment strategies *Dev Psychol* 33(4):681–692, 1997.

10. Main M., Cassidy J. Categories of response to reunion with the parent at age 6: Predictable from infant attachment classifications and stable over a 1-month period. *Dev Psychol* 24:1–12, 1998.
11. van Ijzendorn MH, Scheungel C, Bakersmans-Kranenburg MK: Disorganized attachment in early childhood: Meta-analysis of precursors, concomminants and sequelae. *Dev Psychopathol* 11:225–249, 1999.
12. Boris NW and Zeanah CH. Disturbances and disorders of attachment: An overview. *Infant Mental Health Journal* 1999; 20:1–9.
13. American Psychiatry Association. *Diagnostic and Statistical Manual* (4th ed.), 1994.
14. AACAP Task Force on Research Diagnostic Criteria: Infancy and Preschool: Research diagnostic criteria for infants and preschool: The process and empirical support. *J Am Acad Child Adolesc Psychiatry* 42(12):1504–1512, 2003.
15. World Health Organization. *The ICD-10 Classification of Mental and Behavioral Disorders: Clinical Descriptions and Diagnostic Guidelines.* Geneva, World Health Organization, 1992.
16. Tizard B, Rees J. The effect of early institutional rearing on the behavior problems and affectional relationships of four-year-old children. *J Child Psychol Psychiatry* 19:99–118, 1975.
17. Zeanah CH, Scheeringa MS, Boris NW, Heller SS, Smyke AT, Trapani J. Reactive attachment disorder in maltreated toddlers. *Child Abuse Negl* 28:877–888, 2004.
18. O'Connor TG, Zeanah CH. Assessment strategies and treatment approaches. *Attach Hum Dev* 5:223–244, 2003.
19. Richters MM. Volkmar FR. Reactive attachment disorder of infancy or early childhood. *J Am Acad Child Adolesc Psychiatry* 33(3):328–332, 2004.
20. Smyke AT, Dumitrescu A, Zeanah CH. Disturbances of attachment in young children: I. The continuum of caretaking casualty. *J Am Acad Child Adolesc Psychiatry* 41:972–982, 2002.
21. Hinshaw-Fuselier S, Boris NW, Zeanah CH: Reactive attachment disorder in maltreated twins. *Infant Mental Health Journal* 20:42–59, 1999.
22. Zeanah CH. Beyond insecurity: A reconceptualization of attachment disorders of infancy. *J Consult Clin Psychol* 64:42–52, 1996.
23. Boris NW, Hinshaw-Fuselier SS, Smyke AT, Scheeringa M, Heller SS, Zeanah CH. Comparing criteria for attachment disorders: Establishing reliability and validity in high-risk samples. *J Am Acad Child Adolesc Psychiatry* 43:568–577, 2004.
24. O'Connor TG, Bredenkamp D, Rutter M. Attachment disturbances and disorders in children exposed to early severe deprivation. *Infant Mental Health Journal* 20, 10–29, 1999.
25. Zeanah CH, Boris NW, Bakshi S, Lieberman A: Attachment disorders of infancy. In: J. D. Osofsky (ed): *WAIMH Handbook of Infant Mental Health.* New York, John Wiley and Sons, Inc., 93–122, 1999.
26. Zeanah CH, Mammen O, Lieberman A. Disorders of attachment. In: Zeanah, CH (ed.): *Handbook of Infant Mental Health.* New York, Guilford Press, pp. 332–349, 1993.
27. Zeanah CH, Boris NW. Disturbances and disorders of attachment in early childhood. In: Zeanah C.H. (ed): *Handbook of Infant Mental Health,* 2nd ed. New York, Guilford Press, pp. 353–368, 2000.
28. Rutter M, Anderson-Wood L, Beckett C, Bredenkamp D, Castle J, Groothues C, Keaveney L, et al. Quasi-autistic patterns following severe early global privation. *J Child Psychol Psychiatry* 40:537–549, 1999.
29. Kreppner JM, O'Connor TG, Rutter M. Can inattention/hyperactivity be an institutional deprivation syndrome? *J Abnorm Child Psychol* 29:513–528, 2001.
30. Coolbear J, Benoit D: Failure to thrive: Risk for clinical disturbance of attachment? *Infant Mental Health Journal* 20:87–104, 1999.
31. Boris NW, Zeanah CH, Larrieu JA, Scheeringa MS, Heller SS. Attachment disorders in infancy and early childhood: A preliminary investigation of diagnostic criteria. *Am J Psychiatry* 155:295–297, 1998.
32. Dunitz M, Scheer PJ, Kvas E, Macari S. Psychiatric diagnoses in infancy: A comparison. *Infant Mental Health Journal* 17(1):12–23, 2000.
33. Frankel KA, Boyum LA, Harmon RJ. Diagnosis and presenting symptoms in infant psychiatry clinics: Comparison of two diagnostic systems. *J Am Acad Child Adolesc Psychiatry* 43(5):578–581, 2004.
34. Zeanah CH, Smyke AT, Koga S, Carlson E, BEIP Core Group. Attachment in institutionalized and community children in Romania. *Child Dev* 76(5):1015–1028, 2005.
35. Tager-Flusberg, H, Plesa-Skwerer, D. Social engagement in Williams Syndrome. In: Marshall PJ, Fox NA (eds): *The Development of Social Engagement: Neurobiological Perspectives.* New York: Oxford University Press Series in Affective Science. In press.
36. Zeanah CH, Smyke AT, Dumitrescu A. Disturbances of attachment in young children: II. Indiscriminate behavior and institutional care. *J Am Acad Child Adolesc Psychiatry* 41, 983–989, 2002.
37. O'Connor TG, Rutter M. Attachment disorder behavior following early severe deprivation: extension and longitudinal follow-up. *J Am Acad Child Adolesc Psychiatry* 39, 703–712, 2000.
38. Chisholm K. A three year follow-up of attachment and indiscriminate friendliness in children adopted from Romanian orphanages. *Child Dev* 69:1092–1106, 1998.
39. O'Connor TG, Marvin RS, Rutter M, Olrick JT, Britner PA: Child–parent attachment following early institutional deprivation. *Dev Psychopathol* 15:19–38, 2003.
40. Boris NW, Hinshaw-Fuselier SS, Smyke AT, Scheeringa M, Heller SS, and Zeanah CH. Comparing criteria for attachment disorders: Establishing reliability and validity in high-risk samples. *J Am Acad Child Adolesc Psychiatry* 43:568–577, 2004.
41. Smyke AT, Zeanah CH. Disturbances of attachment interview. Unpublished manuscript, New Orleans, LA: Tulane University Health Sciences Center; 1999.
42. Boris NW, Fueyo M, and Zeanah CH. The clinical assessment of attachment in children under five. *J Am Acad Child Adolesc Psychiatry* 36(2):291–293, 1997.
43. AACAP Work Group on Quality Issues (Boris NW and Zeanah CH, principal authors). Practice parameters for the assessment and treatment of reactive attachment disorder in children and adolescents. *J Am Acad Child Adolesc Psychiatry* 44:1206–1219, 2005.
44. Zeanah CH, Larrieu JA, Heller SS, Valliere J. Infant-parent relationship assessment. In: Zeanah CH (ed): *Handbook of Infant Mental Health.* New York, Guilford Press, pp. 222–235, 2000.
45. Ainsworth MDS, Blehar MS, Waters E, Wall S. *Patterns of Attachment: A Psychological Study of the Strange Situation.* Hillsdale, NJ, Erlbaum, 1978.
46. Famularo R, Kinscherff R, Fenton T. Psychiatric diagnoses of maltreated children: Preliminary findings. *J Am Acad Child Adolesc Psychiatry* 31(5):863–867, 1992.
47. Stovall KC, Dozier M. The development of attachment in new relationships: Single subject analyses for ten foster infants. *Dev Psychopathol*, 12, 133–156, 2000.
48. Kay Hall SE, Geher G. Behavioral and personality characteristics of children with reactive attachment disorder. *J Psychol* 137:145–162, 2003.
49. www.radkid.com, *accessed 9/27/05.*
50. Zeanah CH, Nelson CA, Fox NA, Smyke AT, Marshall P, Parker S et al.: Studying the effects of institutionalization on brain and behavioral development: The Bucharest early intervention project. *Dev Psychopathol* 15:885–907, 2003.
51. Tizard B, Hodges J. The effect of early institutional rearing on the development of eight year old children *J Child Psychol Psychiatry* 19:99–118, 1978.
52. Lieberman A. The treatment of attachment disorder in infancy and early childhood: Reflections from clinical intervention with later-adopted foster children. *Attach Hum Dev.* 5(3):279–282, 2003.
53. Lieberman AF, Zeanah CH: Contributions of attachment theory to infant–parent psychotherapy and other interventions with infants and young children. In: Cassidy J, Shaver PR (eds): *Handbook of Attachment: Theory, Research and Clinical Applications.* New York, Guilford Press, pp. 555–574, 1999.
54. Marvin R, Cooper G, Hoffman K, Powell B. The circle of security project: Attachment-based intervention with caregiver-preschool child dyads. *Attach Hum Dev* 4:10–124, 2002.
55. Lieberman A: Child parent psychotherapy. In: Sameroff AJ, McDonough SC, Rosenblum KL (eds): *Treating Parent-Infant Relationship Problems: Strategies for Intervention.* New York, Guilford Press, pp. 97–122, 2004.
56. Lieberman A, Silverman R, Pawl JH: Infant–parent psychotherapy: Core concepts and current approaches. In: Zeanah CH, (ed): *Handbook of Infant Mental Health,* 2nd ed. New York, Guilford Press, pp. 353–368, 2000.
57. Lieberman A, Weston DR, Pawl JH. Prevention intervention and outcomes with anxiously attached dyads. *Child Dev* 62:199–209, 1991.
58. Cooper G, Hoffman K, Powell B, Marvin R: The circle of security intervention. In: Berlin LJ, Ziv Y, Amaya-Jackson L, Greenberg MT: *Enhancing Early Attachments.* New York, Guildford Press, pp. 127–151, 2005.
59. Cline FW. Hope for high risk and rage filled children. Evergreen, CO, EC Publications, 1992.
60. Keck GC, Kupecky R. *Adopting the hurt child.* Pinion Press, Colorado Springs, CO, 1995.
61. Mercer J. Attachment therapy: A treatment without empirical support. *Scientific Review of Mental Health Practice* 1:105–112, 2002.
62. Crowder C. Prosecutors add charges for rebirthing therapist. *Denver Rocky Mountain News.* July 29, 2000.
63. American Academy of Child and Adolescent Psychiatry. Policy Statement: Coercive interventions for reactive attachment disorder. Washington, DC, American Academy of Child and Adolescent Psychiatry, 2003.

CHAPTER 5.15.4 ■ MUNCHHAUSEN SYNDROME BY PROXY

BRIAN W.C. FORSYTH AND ANDREA GOTTSEGEN ASNES

HISTORICAL NOTE

In 1951, Asher first used the eponym Munchhausen syndrome to describe adults who consistently fabricate symptoms of illness for themselves, leading to numerous medical investigations and frequently to surgical operations (1). The syndrome was named after Baron von Munchhausen of Hanover, who lived in the eighteenth century and was renowned for telling greatly embellished stories about his adventures in the wars against the Turks (2). In 1976, Sneed and Bell used the term "the dauphin of Munchhausen" to describe a case in which a 10-year-old boy presented with factitious recurrent urinary calculi and in which the mother was suspected of colluding with the child in fabricating the symptoms (3). The following year, Meadow coined the term Munchhausen syndrome by proxy in his report of observations of two cases in which parents repeatedly caused their children to be ill (4). Prior to this time, there had been reports in the literature of cases referred to as "nonaccidental poisoning" in which children repeatedly presented as diagnostic dilemmas and were found to have been poisoned by a parent; such cases are now considered to be variants of Munchhausen syndrome by proxy (5, 6). Subsequent to Meadow's initial report, there were other suggestions for a title for the syndrome; these included the names Meadow's syndrome or Polle syndrome, but these have now given way to the more commonly used Munchhausen syndrome by proxy (7–9).

DEFINITION

Definitional issues in Munchhausen syndrome by proxy have been pivotal in recent years. Initially it was described by Meadow as a disorder in which a person persistently fabricates symptoms of illness on behalf of another, thereby causing that person to be regarded as ill, but more recent efforts have been made to provide a more specific definition of the syndrome (4). Meadow has updated and operationalized the syndrome to include a combination of: 1) an illness fabricated in a child by a parent or someone in loco parentis; 2) the presentation of a child to doctors persistently while the perpetrator denies causing the child's illness; 3) the illness goes away when the child is separated from the perpetrator; and 4) the perpetrator is considered to be acting out of a need to assume the sick role by proxy or as another form of attention seeking-behavior (10).

In 1998 a multidisciplinary group convened by the American Professional Society on the Abuse of Children developed definitional guidelines which have since been refined (11, 12). These guidelines define the disorder as encapsulating two distinct entities: the maltreatment of a child and the motivation of the adult who perpetrates the maltreatment. The term "pediatric condition falsification" is employed to describe the form of child abuse in which an adult fabricates or directly causes symptoms and/or signs of illness in a child, resulting in a perception of that child as sick (12). The severity of the disorder and extent of the fabrication are variable. In the least severe cases mothers only report false symptoms, and the physical harm to the children is only that resulting from the medical investigations carried out in attempting to diagnose the illnesses. At the other end of the spectrum are instances in which mothers have caused severe physical harm to their children or even the death of their children in the continued pursuit of making their children appear ill. Perpetrators who act to either invent or induce illness in children to meet their own, self-serving psychological needs are diagnosed with factitious disorder by proxy, which is listed in Appendix B of *Diagnostic and Statistical Manual of Mental Disorders* (DSM-IV-TR) as a category requiring further study (13). The following criteria are suggested:

1. There is intentional production or feigning of physical or psychological signs or symptoms in another person who is under the individual's care.
2. The motivation for the perpetrator's behavior is to assume the sick role by proxy.
3. External incentives for the behavior (e.g., economic gain) are absent.
4. The behavior is not accounted for by another mental disorder.

The perpetration of pediatric condition falsification by an adult diagnosed with factitious disorder by proxy comprises Munchhausen syndrome by proxy (14, 15).

Of interest is the entity of pediatric condition falsification occurring in the absence of factitious disorder by proxy in the adult. Caretakers may invent or induce illness in children to keep them from attending school or falsely allege sexual abuse as a tool in custody battles. In other forms of pediatric condition falsification the parent falsifies the illness solely to gain help with other problems, such as depression (15). This latter form has been dubbed as "help seeking" and is exemplified by the mother who puts cranberry juice in a child's diaper as a reason to be seen by a doctor, but the behavior ceases once the mother's own psychological needs have been identified and treated (15). In the definition proposed by the American Professional Society on the Abuse of Children, if there is absence of factitious disorder by proxy, that is, the absence of a need by the perpetrator to assume a sick role by proxy to meet his or her own psychological needs, it is not seen as comprising Munchhausen syndrome by proxy. Similarly, according to this definition, a situation in which a parent who abuses a child physically or emotionally and then invents an organic medical or psychological ailment to explain the abuse would not be characterized as Munchhausen syndrome by proxy.

Others attempting to operationalize and define Munchhausen syndrome by proxy have questioned whether the presence of psychopathology in the perpetrator, or even understanding of the perpetrator's motivation at all, is a prerequisite for diagnosis of Munchhausen syndrome by proxy. Rosenberg has wondered if parents who induce illness in their children are ill themselves or if they simply exhibit "nasty, self-serving cruel behavior (16)." Some diagnostic formulations, such as that in DSM-IV, require the desire of the perpetrator to assume the sick role and that other types of external gain be absent. Others point to the perpetrator's desire to outwit medical professionals or others in perceived powerful roles. Rogers has recently addressed this confusion with a call to define carefully the diagnosis in adults by the use of systematic measures and explicit inclusion and exclusion criteria (17). Finally, two other entities that need to be distinguished from Munchhausen syndrome by proxy are those parents of chronically ill children who are perceived as "difficult" or overly demanding by medical staff, and "overanxious" parents who may display exaggerated concern for their children's health when they feel proper medical attention is not bestowed (15).

Definitional issues play an important role in the legal aspects of suspected cases of Munchhausen syndrome by proxy. Controversy has played out in recent years over whether the term may or should be used to prosecute perpetrators of this special form of child abuse. Meadow has suggested that the term Munchhausen syndrome by proxy be used to identify a "collection of features characterizing a particular form of child abuse" and that diagnosing the adult perpetrators is the task of mental health professionals (10). These tensions carry weight when medical professionals are asked to render diagnoses to be used in court. Recent cases would suggest that pediatricians are best able to diagnose child abuse and that mental health professionals are best able to diagnose adult psychopathology. Given that current thinking about Munchhausen syndrome by proxy requires both entities to be present, making a diagnosis may require the cooperation of at least two medical professionals.

EPIDEMIOLOGY

Although the true prevalence remains unknown, Munchhausen syndrome by proxy is almost certainly a rare disorder. Active reporting of cases in a prospective study conducted over a 2-year period in the United Kingdom and Republic of Ireland established an annual incidence of 0.5/100,000 children aged under 16 years, and the peak incidence of 2.8/100,000 children in the first year of life (18).

To date, two comprehensive literature reviews have been published. In the first, published in 1987, Rosenberg conducted a review of the existing literature and summarized all the published reports (19). These included 117 children in 97 families. Of these cases the perpetrator was the mother in every case reviewed (98% birth mother and 2% adoptive mother). In the second, published in 2003, Sheridan conducted a similar review and found 451 cases in which 76.5% of the perpetrators were mothers (20). Fathers have previously been found to be only rarely implicated as being the perpetrator or appearing to be complicit in the fabrication of illness, although Meadow has published a series of 15 such cases occurring over a 10-year period, and in Sheridan's review fathers were the perpetrators in 6.7% of the cases (20–23). In a review of cases published outside the United States, Canada, U.K., Australia, and New Zealand, Feldman and Brown reported on 93 cases, and in these the mother was the sole perpetrator in 86% and the father the sole perpetrator in 4% (24).

The diagnosis has been made in children of all ages from the first month of life to 21 years, with the mean age being reported as 40 months and 49 months in the Rosenberg and Sheridan reviews respectively (19, 20). In the prospective British epidemiologic study, however, the median age of diagnosis was 20 months (18). The mean time interval between the onset of symptoms and time of diagnosis was found by Rosenberg to be 15 months, and by Sheridan to be 22 months. There are reports of instances in which the condition started prior to birth with mothers inducing preterm delivery (25, 26). There is an approximately equal prevalence among male and female children.

CLINICAL DESCRIPTION

Medical Presentation

The variety of medical symptoms in children who present with Munchhausen syndrome by proxy is extensive and includes practically all organ systems. Generally the illness appears to be multisystem, and the children may appear to have different types of illness at different times. The four presentations that were among the most common in both Rosenberg's and Sheridan's reviews were seizures, apnea, diarrhea and fevers. Altogether Rosenberg listed 68 different presentations or pathologic findings, and Sheridan listed 101, highlighting the striking diversity of possible potential presentations of Munchhausen syndrome by proxy cases. The means by which the perpetrators caused the symptoms or abnormal findings are just as diverse and illustrate the severity and horrifying nature of the syndrome: One mother had put bleach in her child's eye, causing the appearance of a periorbital infection; others had repeatedly suffocated their children so as to simulate recurrent apnea or seizures. Other mothers caused sepsis by putting fecal material into their children's intravenous lines (19, 20).

In approximately 40% of cases in Sheridan's review, the perpetrator had simulated an illness but had not actually done anything directly to the child to cause harm (20). These were instances where the perpetrator had done something such as putting drops of her own blood in her child's urine or contaminating the specimen. In these instances, although the perpetrator does not herself physically harm the child, she does continue to collaborate with the physicians as distressing and often painful investigations and procedures are carried out.

Bools and associates have pointed out that there is a significant amount of comorbidity among cases of Munchhausen syndrome by proxy: In a review of 56 cases, 29% had a history of failure to thrive and 25% had a history of either nonaccidental injury or neglect (27). Siblings also might have a history of such findings or might themselves have been the subjects of fabricated illnesses. This appears to be particularly true among cases that have presented as apnea and which, in fact, are owing to suffocation (28–30). Of note, in Sheridan's sample, apnea was the most common presenting symptom, representing 26.8% of all cases reviewed (20). When children present with apnea, Munchhausen syndrome by proxy should always be considered if there is a history of death of a sibling or if episodes of apnea have occurred only in the presence of one person.

Ayoub and colleagues have recently reported on a series of five families in which educational disabilities were the presenting symptom in cases ultimately diagnosed as Munchhausen syndrome by proxy. This diagnostic entity has been called educational condition or disability falsification. These cases, unlike those which present with medical problems, are played out within schools, among teachers, guidance counselors and principals, and especially within the special education system (31). Another recently recognized subcategory of Munchhausen syndrome by proxy is that in which a psychiatric or behavioral problem is the presenting complaint. These cases have involved repeated outpatient visits and hospitalizations for psychotic disorders, multiple personality disorders, attention deficit disorders, temporal lobe epilepsy with rages, Tourette's disorder, and autistic spectrum disorders (32).

Description of the Mother

As noted previously, it is most often mothers who are fabricating illness in their children. These mothers often have had prior extensive exposure to the health care system. This, in some instances, has been from past training and work experience as a nurse, medical receptionist, or other health care professional. In Meadow's description of 17 families, nine of the mothers had such a background, and Rosenberg reported that 27% of 97 mothers had a nursing background and another 3% had worked in medical offices (19, 33). In other cases, the mother herself has had Munchhausen syndrome and therefore has brought to her experience as a mother both her own psychopathology and often a vast knowledge of medicine, hospitals, and medical practice acquired from her experiences prior to her child's birth. In a study of covert deaths in infancy, one-half of the perpetrators had some form of abnormal illness behavior such as somatizing disorder, and 22% were reported to have Munchhausen syndrome and in Sheridan's review, 29% of the perpetrators had some features suggestive of Munchhausen syndrome (20, 34).

A striking characteristic of the mothers is that they are often considered exemplary in all their interactions with medical staff. This is in contrast to adults with Munchhausen syndrome and also to parents who provoke sickness behavior in their children and refuse to accept psychological mechanisms (35, 36). Both of these groups are often described as demanding and difficult. In Munchhausen syndrome by proxy, the mothers often develop close relationships with the nurses and doctors with whom they come in frequent and continued contact. These relationships sometimes traverse the more usual boundaries between parent and medical staff and may include such things as helping the nurses in their duties, eating meals with the doctors, or maintaining social contact with the medical personnel outside of the hospital. However, these mothers tend to be unavailable for genuine interpersonal interactions, and hospital staff often report subjective feelings of uneasiness or feeling intrusive in the mother's presence (37). Some perpetrators are thought to be motivated by a desire to manipulate or control doctors or other professionals perceived to be powerful. In this case it is the deception of medical staff, rather than a desire to somehow join their ranks or be perceived as an ideal mother, that appears to motivate the perpetrator (11).

The quality of the mother's care for her child is also notable; they are often considered model parents who are extremely attentive to their children. They take over the care of their children to a greater degree than is usual in hospitals and often live in the hospital and remain with the child constantly. It has been noted, however, that the care given to the child can be of an excessive nature; for example, the child may be dressed in inappropriately lavish clothing, or the hospital room may be stocked with an outrageous number of toys (37). Prolonged covert videotaped observation of these mothers, however, has often revealed detached or even directly cruel behavior to children when they are not in the public view (14).

One striking quality of the mother that may be important in recognizing the syndrome is her inappropriate affect when given information about the severity of her child's illness or discussing invasive medical investigations. There is a bland acceptance, rather than obvious distress, and she appears to be relatively at ease with medical uncertainties (37). In one report, the mother was even described as appearing euphoric as her child became sicker (38).

Besides fabrication of symptoms of illness, these mothers often fabricate extensively about other parts of their lives. An example of this is a mother who made statements that she had just completed a law degree and was working toward a master's degree in Russian history, both of which were false (39). Certainly an important element of the syndrome is the mother's ability to converse with the medical staff about her child's illness in a very knowledgeable and medically sophisticated manner. The other fabrications often serve to add to the mother's appearance as an intelligent person or as someone who has achieved despite adversity.

Description of the Father

In contrast to the mother's constant presence, the father may have very little involvement in his child's care and sometimes does not even visit the hospital. This is particularly noteworthy considering the severity of the child's illness. In a review of 37 families, 70% of the fathers were described as peripheral or absent from the family system; often the fathers have jobs that keep them away from the family for prolonged periods of time (33, 40). The marital relationship between the parents is often poor, although in some instances the child's apparent illness serves to bring the parents closer together.

In those rare instances where fathers are the perpetrators of Munchhausen syndrome by proxy, their interactions with medical personnel appear quite different than is the case with mothers. Like mothers, the fathers often stay with their children in hospital, but are considered by staff to be demanding, overbearing, and unreasonable, and are often quick to make formal complaints and seek legal redress. It is notable that in Meadow's description of 15 fathers, none were actively employed and 11 had factitious disorders, including five who were considered to have Munchhausen syndrome (23).

Psychiatric Description of the Child

There is little in the literature describing the children in this disorder. The one striking comment, however, is that the children, particularly older children, collude with their mothers in the ongoing deception. In the original report of Sneed and Bell, it was the 10-year-old boy who was presenting the pebbles as renal calculi (3). A 2½-year-old girl at our institution did not cry out when her mother, in what must have been a painful process, produced signs of gastrointestinal bleeding by excoriating her anal canal. Furthermore, these children, like children who have been repeatedly physically abused, quickly learn to tolerate passively medical procedures. A separate diagnostic entity has emerged from these observations, that of child and adolescent illness falsification. Children who induce or fabricate illness are thought to do so either as a continuation of perpetration of Munchhausen syndrome by proxy by a parent or covert parent coaching, or because of a strong attraction to the medical world in themselves (41). Other symptoms that have been described include feeding disorders among infants and toddlers and withdrawn, hyperactive, or oppositional behavior among preschoolers (38).

ETIOLOGY AND PATHOGENESIS

Although reports of Munchhausen syndrome by proxy are largely found in pediatric journals rather than the psychological or psychiatric literature, there is now an expanding literature that has contributed to a greater understanding of the disorder. Most have been individual case reports, but Bools and colleagues have reported the systematic evaluation of a series of cases (5, 27, 42–45). Thus, there is now some understanding of the underlying psychopathology of the condition and knowledge of features that are common to most cases. However, the full extent to which some of the descriptions may be generalized and an understanding of the limits of the spectrum of the disorder remain undefined.

Three major etiologic factors appear to be important in the pathogenesis of the disorder. These include the mother's experience of abuse or rejection in her own childhood, her pathologic relationship with her child, and the rewarding effect of the medical care system on the mother. In addition, associated psychopathology often contributes to the development of the syndrome.

Abuse or Rejection of the Mother

Perpetrators of Munchhausen syndrome by proxy often have experienced abuse in their own childhoods or have felt rejected by one or both parents (38, 44, 46). In a study of 47 cases, they were able to interview 19 mothers at variable intervals after the event. Of these 19, 15 (79%) were described as having suffered emotional neglect or abuse in childhood, four had experienced physical abuse, and five had experienced sexual abuse (47). Twenty-two percent of the perpetrators in Sheridan's review had or claimed a personal history of abuse (20). The experience of rejection continues into adult life, and there is often a poor marital relationship (33). The mothers often feel isolated and have a decreased sense of self-worth.

Pathologic Relationship with Child

Early characterizations of Munchhausen syndrome by proxy describe a typical mother as having an extremely close, symbiotic relationship with her children. The child is viewed as very precious but also as somehow damaged and susceptible to illness or harm. Meadow, in his first description of the syndrome, described a child who had been a "long-awaited baby" and who was born after the mother had taken a fertility medication (4). The child described by Nicol and Eccles was born after a pregnancy in which there had been a threatened miscarriage at 12 weeks' gestation, an antepartum hemorrhage at 36 weeks, and termination of breast-feeding because of cracked nipples when the child was 5 weeks old (43). In this regard, cases of Munchhausen syndrome by proxy are similar to those seen in the vulnerable child syndrome in which the mother develops an abnormally overprotective relationship with the child following a severe illness early in the child's life (48). Obviously, there is the important difference that in the vulnerable child syndrome the mother does not cause her child to be ill, although she views her child as abnormally susceptible to illness. More recently, with the aid of covert surveillance, the close bond between mother and child has been questioned. Review of surveillance videos in one study revealed that mothers witnessed by medical staff and thought to be extremely caring largely ignored their children when alone with them (49, 50). Many have hypothesized that the child in Munchhausen syndrome by proxy is merely a tool through which engagement with medical and other professionals is made possible (14).

Effect of the Medical Care System

Important components in the development of the syndrome are the behavior of the doctors, the hospital environment, and the effect that both have on the mother. In the report by Nicol and Eccles, the mother reported that "she found, in her general practitioner, a source of support and kindness and this reinforced the pattern of very regular attendance at the surgery (43)." Guandolo has commented that "illness is the ticket of admission to a place where understanding and caring relieved the feelings of hopelessness and isolation (39)." The interaction, however, is more complex than just the mothers' feelings of being supported. With the increasing severity of illness of their children, these mothers feel a sense of self-worth and importance that is otherwise lacking in their lives. One mother, after confessing to repeatedly suffocating her child, reported that whenever she did it, she experienced a similar feeling to that which she had felt on her graduation day. This mother, during one of the times her child was being resuscitated in the hospital, was overheard by a nurse calmly telling other mothers on the ward that she had already had a child die from a similar episode. This, in fact, was a fabrication but serves to illustrate the mother's need to make the situation even more dire so as to gain greater sympathy and appear the more heroic. The hospital environment contributes to these feelings of importance. Chan and associates described a mother who would visit the intensive care unit just to talk to other mothers, and Meadow has described another mother who had some nursing training and who would help teach nursing students (22, 42). There obviously becomes an increasing need for the mother to gain admission to the hospital through her child's illness.

Another factor is the pleasure gained from the contact with the doctors. In the case discussed by Nicol and Eccles, the mother reported that she liked to feel that she "was being considered by intelligent people (43)." There appears to be an additional element in which the mother gains pleasure from outwitting the doctors. It becomes a bizarre game in which the mother matches herself against the specialists, and as one problem is resolved, another one is created.

Associated Psychopathology

As Meadow has stated, "Many mothers who have perpetrated Munchhausen syndrome by proxy have been referred to psychiatrists, and many have had detailed psychological testing. Usually the tests are normal and no disorder is apparent to the psychiatrist (51)." This likely speaks to the misdirected focus of these evaluations rather than to a true lack of psychopathology. Sheridan's review found that 23% of perpetrators carried a psychiatric diagnosis, the most common of which were depression and personality disorder (20). In the followup study of 47 mothers conducted by Bools and coworkers, 55% had a history of harming themselves, 21% had a history of abuse of alcohol or drugs (usually prescribed medications), and 72% had a history of somatoform or factitious disorders. For the 19 cases in which there were detailed interviews and completion of the Personality Assessment Schedule, 17 of the 19 were considered to have personality disorders; histrionic and borderline personality disorders were predominant, and many had multiple disorders. Other disorders included avoidant, dependent, narcissistic, schizotypal, and paranoid categories (47). However, the cases evaluated in this study likely represent a biased sample with more severe symptomatology, and it is often true that there is sometimes a surprising lack of associated psychiatric symptoms, considering the severity of the nature of the disorder.

Some of the case reports serve to demonstrate a spectrum of illness rather than a universal picture. Chan and associates described a mother who demonstrated several features consistent with both narcissistic and borderline personality disorders. She was explosive, constantly sought attention, displayed sadomasochistic tendencies, showed marked shifts in attitude and affect, and presented a sense of entitlement. Her primary defenses seemed to be denial and splitting (42). In the report by Nicol and Eccles of a mother's progress in psychotherapy, they describe an important part of the pathogenesis of the abuse as being the mother's affect, which included infantile rage as a central component together with devastatingly low self-esteem (43). In the report by Palmer and Yoshimura of a mother who herself had Munchhausen syndrome, psychological testing "revealed a profoundly needy individual whose reality testing was impaired. She perceived the world as a malevolent place and people as attacking. Thought processes were distorted and interpersonal boundaries were blurred. Coping strategies included extreme forms of denial, projection and paranoid vigilance (44)."

The fabrication of illness and often-continued denial do not have the fixed quality of a delusion, although the mother does not appear to be consciously lying. It has been described as "quasidelusional" and Waller has commented that "the disturbance in thought content and behavior may be a dissociative phenomenon or a form of pseudologia phantastica or pathological lying in which the parent comes to believe, at least intermittently, the fantasy that the child has a primary rather than a factitious illness" (45).

Mothers who have confessed to the perpetration of injury on their children have been able to describe the incident but have little recollection for the details and describe themselves as committing the act in a disassociated-like state.

SPECTRUM OF THE DISORDER

Meadow, in reporting on what he terms mild cases, raises questions regarding the limits of the definition of the disorder. He points out that, at times, parents often exaggerate their children's symptoms or may perceive that a problem is present when it is not apparent to the doctor (51). This is particularly true for some parents who consider their children allergic and limit their exposure to various foods and things in the environment. Certainly some of these parents share a number of the same characteristics as those more severe cases of parents who actually cause their children to be ill (52).

It is also important to ask the question of when Munchhausen syndrome by proxy begins in an individual case, recognizing that some cases start with parental concerns surrounding a real illness and that these concerns, at some stage, overflow into fabricated illness. Also, is it only the lack of the medical knowledge that prevents others from developing Munchhausen syndrome by proxy? In fact, the syndrome has been described as only one end of a spectrum of parental behaviors surrounding chronic and factitious illnesses of children (18, 46, 53). It is important, however, that we recognize the significant differences in the psychopathology of the parent who injures her child or causes her child to appear ill and the parent who repeatedly presents as overly concerned about her child's illness. What appears to set Munchhausen syndrome by proxy apart is the synergistic effect of the mother's prior experience of abuse or rejection, her pathologic symbiotic relationship with her child, and the powerful rewarding effects of her interaction with the medical environment. McKinlay describes the parent "who provokes sickness behavior in the child, refuses to accept psychological mechanism, seeks multiple opinions and insists on repeated investigations," and points out that this type of parent is often combative or has a contemptuous style, which is very different from the at least outwardly exemplary, ingratiating parental style seen in Munchhausen syndrome by proxy (36). The former does not appear to experience the elevation of self-worth and feeling of importance that seem so much a part of Munchhausen syndrome by proxy. There is, however, a striking similarity between these cases and Munchhausen syndrome by proxy in the symbiotic relationship between mother and child and the way in which the child colludes with the mother in continuing the illness (54).

The proposed DSM-IV diagnosis of factitious disorder by proxy requires that external incentives for the production or feigning of symptoms in a child be absent. These criteria would limit the use of the term to cases in which the perpetrator's behavior is motivated by the need to assume the sick role by proxy, which would serve to exclude a number of situations in which the term Munchhausen syndrome by proxy is presently inappropriately used, such as with parents who are overanxious, or "doctor-shopping," or seek opinions from multiple doctors for other reasons (55).

TREATMENT

The management of Munchhausen syndrome by proxy often is extremely difficult. There is a number of reasons why this is true: First, there is the difficulty of making the diagnosis—It often goes unsuspected for a long time, and then, even when suspected, it is often difficult to be sure that one's suspicions are in fact correct. Second, the disbelief that the diagnosis engenders often serves to sabotage overall management. Last, psychotherapy is extremely difficult when the therapist is reliant on the patient telling the truth, which is something that rarely happens in these cases, at least initially.

Medical Management

The warning signals that should alert a physician to the possibility of a factitious illness have previously been identified by Meadow and are shown in Table 5.15.4.1 (56). Once it is suspected that an illness may be fabricated, the physician needs to establish the diagnosis with certainty. This is often an arduous and time-consuming task. Obviously, the safety of the child and protection from further harm are of utmost importance during this time.

The physician should review the medical history in detail and distinguish those complaints that may have been fabricated from those that are definitely real; complaints that occurred when only the mother was present need to be separated from those witnessed by others; details of the medical, psychiatric, personal, and social history, as presented by the mother, need to be verified. This may require careful and detailed histories from other family members.

Detailed descriptions of the mother's behavior and incidents that occurred while in the hospital may provide a profile consistent with Munchhausen syndrome by proxy. A number of laboratory methods have been used to confirm fabricated symptoms. These include biochemical analyses of blood and

TABLE 5.15.4.1

WARNING SIGNALS OF MUNCHHAUSEN SYNDROME BY PROXY

Persistent or recurrent illness that cannot be explained
Discrepancies between the history, clinical findings, and general health of the child
Working diagnosis is a rare disorder, or experienced clinicians have "never seen a case like it before"
Symptoms and signs occur only in the mother's presence
A mother who is extremely attentive and always in the hospital
A child who is frequently intolerant to treatments
A mother who appears less worried about her child's illness than is the medical staff
Seizures that do not respond to appropriate therapy
Families in which sudden unexplained infant death has occurred
A mother with previous medical or nursing experience or who has an extensive history of illness

(Adapted from Meadow R: Munchhausen syndrome by proxy. *Arch Dis Child* 67:92–98, 1982.)

urine samples, typing of blood to determine if it is the child's or the mother's, and analyzing recordings from apnea monitors. Continuous observation of the mother by nursing staff is extremely difficult and usually not possible. Also, it is often not possible to exclude the parents from the hospital for a long enough time to establish a temporal association between the symptoms and the presence of the mother. Video surveillance of the mother and child in the hospital is sometimes necessary. This, like searching a mother's personal belongings, creates ethical and legal problems; however, these need to be weighed against the risks to the child (57, 58). A retrospective review of 41 cases in which covert video surveillance was used to investigate a possible diagnosis of Munchhausen syndrome by proxy in one pediatric hospital found that 23 diagnoses were actually confirmed. Of these 23, covert video surveillance was seen as crucial to making the diagnosis in 13 (56%) and supportive of the diagnosis in five (28%) (59).

Once the diagnosis has been established, the mother needs to be confronted and informed of the doctor's knowledge about what is going on and the course of action that needs to be taken to ensure the safety of the child. Other family members also need to be notified and the diagnosis explained to them. The protective services agency needs to be notified and legal services need to be involved because in most instances the child has been abused and needs continued protection.

The Role of the Psychiatrist

Although the early literature seldom commented on the role of the psychiatrist in the management of Munchhausen syndrome by proxy, more recent reports of cases being successfully managed with psychiatric approaches suggest that child psychiatrists have a very important role to play in ensuring an optimal outcome for these children and parents. One difficulty is that, although it is a psychiatric disorder, the clinical presentation is medical, and often the apparent lack of psychiatric symptoms precludes a reason for the psychiatrist's involvement. Once the diagnosis is suspected, however, the child psychiatrist's contribution can be very important in a number of different ways.

Helping to Establish the Diagnosis

Even though the mother may not herself request psychiatric help, once the diagnosis is suspected, a reason should be sought for the child psychiatrist to meet with the mother. Because care needs to be taken not to sabotage the overall management plan by giving the mother warning that she is under suspicion, the reason might be that the psychiatrist can often be helpful to families of children with chronic illnesses. The history taken at this time should include family, social, and psychiatric information, but the most important focus, and that likely to be most acceptable to the mother, is around the child's illness. In reviewing the details of the child's life and illness, the child psychiatrist may be able to obtain an understanding of the special meaning of this child to the mother and the symbiotic relationship between mother and child. An example of this is a mother's description of how much more worried she had been about her daughter (the child now presenting with illness) than she had been about her older child, a son, although both had been on home monitoring because of concern about apnea. When the daughter, who was named after the mother, was 8 weeks old, the mother heard of another child who had died of sudden infant death syndrome. Since that time, she had feared that her daughter would die and was compulsively careful about the apnea monitor in a way that she described as being very different from when her son was on the monitor. With her son, she had often turned the monitor around so that she could not see all the flashing digital lights and alarms; with her daughter it was intolerable for her not to see these. It is the ability to elicit this quality of the relationship between the mother and child that might be most helpful in the interview. The child psychiatrist, with his or her training and experience in understanding the relationship between mother and child, is likely to be more helpful in assessing this quality of the relationship than would someone without training in child psychiatry (51, 53). During the assessment, the child psychiatrist also may be able to elicit other information that provides evidence of fabrication or is indicative of other psychiatric symptoms associated with Munchhausen syndrome by proxy. The child psychiatrist also should be able to provide an assessment of the degree of psychological disturbance experienced by the child and should be key in planning how this should be addressed.

Developing a Therapeutic Relationship

A potentially important part of the early assessment is to provide an opportunity for the mother to start to develop a therapeutic relationship with the psychiatrist. Because in most of the cases reported in the literature the psychiatrist has only been involved once the mother has been confronted, it is unclear whether an earlier meeting, prior to the confrontation, might be beneficial, or whether the mother's later realization that the psychiatrist was complicit in the suspicion of her might be detrimental to ongoing treatment. It seems likely, however, that the mother could accept reassurance that the psychiatrist is intent on helping her and that she could therefore maintain the trust necessary for ongoing therapy. Therefore, it may be important for the psychiatrist doing the early assessment to continue to provide ongoing treatment, although this is not always possible in some centers.

Confrontation

The aim of the confrontation is to explain to the mother that the clinicians know she is harming her child and the possible consequent effects. She should be informed of the steps that will be taken to protect her child and provide help for her and her family. Meadow has suggested that the pediatrician alone, without other professionals or family members present, best confronts the mother (51). Although this may be true for someone like Meadow, who has such a vast experience with this syndrome, it may not necessarily be true in instances where the pediatrician has had no prior experience of Munchhausen syndrome by proxy. In these cases, it may be helpful to have a child psychiatrist present to help in the process. It is important, however, that the pediatrician be the one who confidently affirms what has been going on. The child psychiatrist then is able to speak of it as a psychiatric problem and outlines what is likely to happen, at the same time being supportive.

At this stage, only a few mothers will confess to what they have been doing, although at times there are remarks that serve as tacit admission of the activity. The majority of mothers continue to deny their activity, often in a very convincing way, although sometimes in a remarkably calm, flat manner. It is not helpful to try to prove to the mother that you are right and she is wrong, nor is it helpful to counter every explanation she provides.

Some mothers have become extremely agitated, acutely psychotic, or depressed and suicidal following the confrontation (44). An assessment may need to be made regarding the need for psychiatric hospitalization. Needless to say, it is critically important that the child be protected from the mother at this time, because she may have a heightened need for the child to be truly sick.

Assisting Staff in Understanding the Dynamics of the Case

This may be an extremely difficult problem to deal with for medical and social services staff, particularly if they have had no prior experience with or knowledge of the syndrome. The emotional responses of the staff are made more complicated by the fact that some might have known the family for a long time and developed close relationships with the mother and child. For some people, there is complete disbelief; for others, there is anger at the mother and feelings of guilt that they have participated in harming the child or have not been more astute in correctly identifying the problem at an earlier time. Group discussions are helpful in both informing staff about the syndrome and providing them an opportunity to express their feelings. It is also helpful to provide written material about the syndrome for staff to read.

The psychiatrist also may play an important role in providing protective services workers and lawyers with an understanding of the syndrome and may even appear as an expert witness in the courts. In this way, the psychiatrist can help to facilitate an appropriate legal course of action. The psychiatrist's role in this may have important ramifications in later treatment: The assertion of the severity of the disorder and the danger to the child, together with an uncritical view of this as a psychiatric disorder, may have therapeutic implications for the mother.

Psychotherapy

As noted, there is limited information available in the literature concerning psychotherapy of mothers and children with Munchhausen syndrome by proxy. Palmer and Yoshimura have emphasized that the following are important determinants of how a case should be managed: the degree and duration of abuse; the parent's psychological state; whether the reaction to the confrontation is denial or acknowledgment of behavior; resistance or willingness to engage in treatment; and whether the child is perceived as part of herself or as a separate entity (44).

Obviously, each of these factors might be an important indicator of the accessibility of the individual to psychotherapeutic intervention, but an adverse factor should not necessarily be considered a contraindication to therapy.

Nicol and Eccles have provided details of their case in which the mother initially denied the allegations but later confessed when faced with the possibility that her children might be placed in foster care. The mother, in this case, continued in therapy on a weekly basis for 6 months and then biweekly for a further 6 months. From early on it was "clear that the mother had a strong wish to understand herself, that she was intelligent, and that she had a capacity to bring active and painful feelings to therapy sessions." General themes of therapy included the complex reasons for the abuse, where a full realization of the danger she had put her child in gradually emerged. Other important themes were her relationship with her parents and fears about her child's health that first originated during her pregnancy (43).

In a report describing outcomes for 13 cases receiving psychiatric intervention, Berg and Jones (60) described an inpatient treatment approach provided in the family unit of a children's hospital by a multidisciplinary psychiatric team experienced in management of child maltreatment. "The theoretical orientation of the team is founded on principles of infant–parent attachment theory" and treatment included "psychological interventions targeted at: the parent-child relationship, the quality of the child's attachment to each parent, the abuser's own childhood experiences, and the current social network and family dynamics, together with work with the parental couple (60).

The length of stay in the family unit varied between 3 days and 4 months, with the average duration being 7½ weeks (60).

OUTCOME

The final outcome for children with Munchhausen syndrome by proxy is very variable and dependent both on the severity of the disorder and treatment provided. The mother who has other psychiatric disorders in addition to Munchhausen syndrome by proxy and the child who has been involved in the fabrication of symptoms for many years are more difficult to treat than those with a simpler presentation. This is likely true for those mothers who have Munchhausen syndrome themselves, which is often very difficult to treat successfully (61). The child whose symptoms of illness has been caused by a more dangerous activity (e.g., suffocation) is obviously at higher risk of dying than the child whose symptom was owing to less dangerous methods (e.g., a mother's putting blood in her child's urine). In Rosenberg's review of the 117 cases reported in the literature, 9% died and 8% of the survivors had permanent disfigurement or impairment of physical function. The leading causes of death were suffocation and poisoning (19). Children have died even after the diagnosis was made and their mothers confronted, and younger siblings have been abused after older siblings died.

The psychiatric sequelae have been less well described both for the mother and child. Certainly, some of these children have continued to fabricate illness for themselves, and the child with Munchhausen syndrome by proxy has grown up to be the adolescent or adult with Munchhausen syndrome (51, 62). Of the 12 children described by McGuire and Feldman, 11 were described as having adverse effects that included immaturity, abnormal relationships with their mothers, separation problems, and aggressive behavior (38). Some children have expressed fears of poisoning and death, and at least two children have required psychiatric hospitalization (6).

In the most comprehensive followup study reported to date, Bools and colleagues described 54 children for whom they obtained information an average of 5.6 years after the event. Thirty of these children continued to live with their biologic mothers, whereas 24 children were with other family members or in substitute care. For 10 of the 30 children living with their mothers there was evidence of further fabrications, and for another eight there were "other concerns," either about the relationship between the mothers and their children, or about other aspects of the mothers' behaviors. Of these 18 children for whom there were continuing concerns about the family, 12 exhibited psychological symptoms, including somatic complaints, emotional disorders, conduct disorder, and poor functioning at school. Among the 24 children who were no longer living with their biologic mothers, eight had persistent psychological symptoms, and another six children had disorders that had shown signs of gradual improvement. Altogether, the authors of the study concluded that half of the children had outcomes that they considered to be unacceptable, but, because of the variability in cases, it was not possible to comment on whether better outcomes were obtained when children remained with their mothers or were separated. However, the authors did conclude that when children remained with their mothers, the outcome appeared improved when there had been a temporary placement in foster care (62). Preliminary findings from investigation of the consequences of separation from the perpetrator suggest that many children are "quite indifferent" to separation when it does occur, and that they go on to embrace their own wellness and engage with others around them (63).

In reporting on the followup of cases enrolled in the intensive, inpatient treatment program described above, Berg and Jones reported greater success. When 16 families were reevaluated an average of 27 months after treatment, there were no ongoing concerns for nine of the families; the mothers had no mental health problems and had insight into their original condition, and the children had no psychological disorders. There continued to be mild concerns for five families in which the mothers continued to have mild to moderate mental health problems, although these did not impact on their relationship with their children or on the children's development. In only two families were there more serious concerns about the mother's mental health, although they were not overtly abusive. However, the authors stressed that these cases had been selected for treatment on their likelihood of achieving success and that cases considered unsuitable for psychiatric treatment were excluded, usually because of persistent parental denial or the severity of the parent's personality disorder (60).

CONCLUSION

In this condition, perhaps more so than any other, there needs to be extensive collaboration between the child psychiatrist and pediatrician, as well as with the other services involved (51, 53, 64). The role of the psychiatrist may be very different from that with other psychiatric diagnoses, particularly when a case is first diagnosed, and although it is recognized as a psychiatric disorder, it needs also to be remembered that it is a serious form of child abuse. It is hoped that with our increased understanding of this syndrome and an appropriate psychiatric approach to management, there will be an improvement in outcome for both the children and their mothers.

References

1. Asher R: Munchhausen syndrome. *Lancet* 1:339–341, 1951.
2. Raspe RE: *Singular Campaigns and Adventures of Baron Munchhausen.* London, Cresset Press, 1948.
3. Sneed RC, Bell RF: The dauphin of Munchhausen: Factitious passage of renal stones in a child. *Pediatrics* 58:127–130, 1976.
4. Meadow R: Munchhausen syndrome by proxy: The hinterland of child abuse. *Lancet* 2:343–345, 1977.
5. Lansky SB, Erickson HM: Prevention of child murder. *J Am Acad Child Psychiatry* 13:691–698, 1974.
6. Rogers D, Tripp J, Bentovim A, et al.: Non-accidental poisoning: An extended syndrome of child abuse. *Br Med J* 1:793–796, 1976.
7. Lazoritz S: Munchhausen by proxy or Meadow's syndrome? *Lancet* 2:631, 1987.
8. Meadow R, Lennert T: Munchhausen by proxy or Polle syndrome: Which term is correct? *Pediatrics* 74:554–556, 1984.
9. Verity GM, Winckworth C, Burman D, et al.: Polle syndrome: Children of Munchhausen. *Br Med J* 2:422–423, 1979.
10. Meadow R: Different interpretations of Munchhausen Syndrome by Proxy. *Child Abuse Negl* 26:501–508, 2002.
11. Ayoub CC, Alexander, R: Definitional issues in Munchhausen Syndrome by Proxy. *American Professional Society on the Abuse of Children* 11:7–10, 1998.
12. Ayoub CC, Alexander R, Beck, D, et al.: Position paper: Definitional issues in Munchhausen Syndrome by Proxy. *Child Maltreatment* 7:105–111, 2002.
13. American Psychiatric Association: *Diagnostic and Statistical Manual of Mental Disorders,* 4th ed. rev. Washington, DC, American Psychiatric Association, 2000.
14. Schreier H: On the importance of motivation in Munchhausen Syndrome by proxy: The case of Kathy Bush. *Child Abuse Negl* 26:537–549, 2002.
15. Libow JA, Schreier HA: Three forms of factitious illness in children: When is it Munchhausen syndrome by proxy? *Am J Orthopsychiatry* 56:602–611, 1986.
16. Rosenberg, DA: Munchhausen Syndrome by Proxy: Medical diagnostic criteria. *Child Abuse Negl* 27:421–430, 2003.
17. Rogers R: Diagnostic, explanatory, and detection models of Munchhausen Syndrome by proxy: Extrapolations from malingering and deception. *Child Abuse Negl* 28:225–238, 2004.
18. McClure RJ, Davis PM, Meadow SR, et al.: Epidemiology of Munchhausen syndrome by proxy, non-accidental poisoning, and non-accidental suffocation. *Arch Dis Child* 75:57–61, 1996.
19. Rosenberg D: Web of deceit: A literature review of Munchhausen syndrome by proxy. *Child Abuse Negl* 11:547–563, 1987.
20. Sheridan MS: The deceit continues: An updated literature review of Munchhausen syndrome by proxy. *Child Abuse Negl* 27:431–451, 2003.
21. Makar AF, Squier PJ: Munchhausen syndrome by proxy: Father as a perpetrator. *Pediatrics* 85:370–373, 1990.
22. Meadow R: Fictitious epilepsy. *Lancet* 2:25–28, 1984.
23. Meadow R: Munchhausen syndrome by proxy abuse perpetrated by men. *Arch Dis Child* 78:210–216, 1998.
24. Feldman MD, Brown RMA: Munchhausen by proxy in an international context. *Child Abuse Negl* 26:509–524, 2002.
25. Goss PW, McDougall PN: Munchhausen syndrome by proxy: A cause of preterm delivery. *Med J Aust* 157:814–817, 1992.
26. Porter GE, Heitsch GM, Miller MD: Munchhausen syndrome by proxy: Unusual manifestations and disturbing sequelae. *Child Abuse Negl* 18:789–794, 1994.
27. Bools CN, Neale BA, Meadow SR: Co-morbidity associated with fabricated illness (Munchhausen syndrome by proxy). *Arch Dis Child* 67:11–19, 1992.
28. Alexander R, Smith W, Stevenson R: Serial Munchhausen syndrome by proxy. *Pediatrics* 86:581–585, 1990.
29. Light MJ, Sheridan MS: Munchhausen syndrome by proxy and apnea (MPBA): A survey of apnea programs. *Clin Pediatr* 29:162–168, 1990.
30. Meadow R: Suffocation, recurrent apnea, and sudden infant death. *J Pediatr* 117:351–357, 1990.
31. Ayoub CC, Schreier HA, Keller, C: Munchhausen by proxy: Presentations in special education. *Child Maltreatment* 7:149–159, 2002.
32. Schreier HA: Factitious disorder by proxy in which the presenting problem is behavioral or psychiatric. *J Am Acad Child Adol Psychiatry* 39:668–670, 2000.
33. Meadow R: Munchhausen syndrome by proxy. *Arch Dis Child* 57:92–98, 1982.
34. Meadow R: Unnatural sudden infant deaths. *Arch Dis Child* 80:7–14, 1999.
35. Kaplan HI, Sadock BJ: *Synopsis of Psychiatry, Behavioral Sciences, Clinical Psychiatry,* 5th ed. Baltimore, Williams & Wilkins, pp. 396–399, 1988.
36. McKinlay I: Munchausen's syndrome by proxy (letter). *Br Med J* 293:1308, 1986.
37. Zitelli BJ, Seltman MF, Shannon RM: Munchausen's syndrome by proxy and its professional participants. *Am J Dis Child* 141:1099–1102, 1987.
38. McGuire TL, Feldman KW: Psychologic morbidity of children subjected to Munchhausen syndrome by proxy. *Pediatrics* 83:289–292, 1989.
39. Guandolo VL: Munchhausen syndrome by proxy: An outpatient challenge. *Pediatrics* 75:526–530, 1985.
40. Gray J, Bentovim A: Illness induction syndrome: Paper I-a series of 41 children from 37 families identified at the Great Ormond Street Hospital for Children, NHS Trust. *Child Abuse Negl* 20:655–673, 1996.
41. Libow JA: Child and adolescent illness falsification. *Pediatrics* 105:336–342, 2000.
42. Chan DA, Salcedo JR, Atkins DM, et al.: Munchhausen syndrome by proxy: A review and case study. *J Pediatr Psychol* 11:1–80, 1986.
43. Nicol AR, Eccles M: Psychotherapy for Munchhausen syndrome by proxy. *Arch Dis Child* 60:344–348, 1985.
44. Palmer AJ, Yoshimura GJ: Munchhausen syndrome by proxy. *J Am Acad Child Psychiatry* 234:503–508, 1984.
45. Waller DA: Case report: Obstacles to the treatment of Munchhausen by proxy syndrome. *J Am Acad Child Psychiatry* 22:80–85, 1983.
46. Krener P, Adelman R: Parent salvage and parent sabotage in the care of chronically ill children. *Am J Dis Child* 142:945–951, 1988.
47. Bools CN, Neale B, Meadow R: Munchhausen syndrome by proxy: A study of psychopathology. *Child Abuse Negl* 18:773–788, 1994.
48. Green M, Solnit AJ: Reactions to the threatened loss of a child: A vulnerable child syndrome. *Pediatrics* 34:58–66, 1964.
49. Southall DP, Stebbens VA, Rees SV et al.: Apnoeic episodes induced by smothering: Two cases identified by covert video surveillance. *Br Med J* 294:1637–1641, 1987.
50. Samuels MP, McClaughlin W, Jacobson RR, et al.: Fourteen cases of imposed upper airway obstruction. *Arch Dis Child* 67:162–170, 1982.
51. Meadow R: Management of Munchhausen syndrome by proxy. *Arch Dis Child* 60:385–393, 1985.
52. Warner O, Hathaway MJ: Allergic form of Meadow's syndrome (Munchhausen by proxy). *Arch Dis Child* 59:151–156, 1984.
53. Eminson DM, Postlethwaite RJ: Factitious illness: Recognition and management. *Arch Dis Child* 67:1510–1516, 1992.
54. Woollcott P, Aceto T, Rutt C, et al.: Doctor shopping with the child as proxy patient: A variant of child abuse. *J Pediatr* 101:297–301, 1982.
55. Meadow R: What is, and what is not, 'Munchhausen syndrome by proxy'? *Arch Dis Child* 72:534–538, 1995.
56. Meadow R: Munchhausen syndrome by proxy. *Arch Dis Child* 67:92–98, 1982.

57. Meadow R: Video recording and child abuse. *Br Med J* 294:1629–1630, 1987.
58. Williams C, Bevan VT. The secret observation of children in hospital. *Lancet* 1:780–781, 1988.
59. Hall DE, Eubanks L, Meyyazhagan S: Evaluation of covert surveillance in the diagnosis of Munchhausen syndrome by proxy: Lessons for 41 cases. *Pediatrics* 105:1305–1312, 2000.
60. Berg B, Jones D: Outcome of psychiatric intervention in factitious illness by proxy (Munchausen's syndrome by proxy). *Arch Dis Child* 81:465–572, 1999.
61. Mayo JP, Haggerty JJ: Long-term psychotherapy of Munchhausen syndrome. *Am J Psychother* 38:571–579, 1984.
62. Bools CN, Neale BA, Meadow R: Follow-up of victims of fabricated illness (Munchhausen syndrome by proxy). *Arch Dis Child* 69:625–630, 1993.
63. Ayoub CC, Deutsch R, Kinscherff R: Munchhausen by proxy: Definitions, identification, and evaluation. In: Reece R (ed): *The Treatment of Child Abuse*. Baltimore, Johns Hopkins University Press, 2000, pp. 213–225.
64. Bentovim A: Munchausen's syndrome and child psychiatrists (letter). *Arch Dis Child* 60:688, 1985.

CHAPTER 5.15.5 ■ CHILDREN EXPOSED TO DISASTER: THE ROLE OF THE MENTAL HEALTH PROFESSIONAL

NATHANIEL LAOR AND LEO WOLMER

INTRODUCTION

Mass disasters, whether natural, technological or human made, take an enormous toll in human life and impose untold physical, psychological, and economic hardships on survivors. Indeed, disasters affect individuals, families, and entire communities. In recent years, we have been witness to significant growth in the mortality associated with nearly all types of disasters, apparently as a result of increased population density, urbanization and climatic changes (1). From 1980 to 2000, about 75% of the world's population lived in areas that had been affected at least once by an earthquake, a tropical cyclone, flooding, or drought (2). Less developed countries account for a considerable proportion (about 40%) of the worst natural disasters, and an even higher proportion of disaster-related deaths. For example, in 2004 the tsunami in the Indian Ocean took an estimated 250,000–300,000 lives (2).

This chapter focuses on the psychological impact of disasters on children. Unlike physical damage, which is usually easy to identify, the internal suffering of children can remain hidden even from the most sensitive observers. Therefore, clinicians and researchers have begun attempting to elucidate the type, extent, and risks of children's maladaptive responses to mass disaster.

Modern empirical methodologies and clinical observations have proven erroneous the statement by Garmezy and Rutter (3) that children show only a mild response to traumatic conditions. Indeed, the adverse psychological effects of such conditions can be severe and long lasting (4–8), and they may persist even in the face of apparently normal social functioning (9). Nevertheless, according to the Task Force Report of the American Psychological Association, "few psychologists have had specific training for working with children after disasters, and discussions of children's responses to disasters have been rare in texts on psychopathology or issues in normal development (7)".

The aims of this chapter are: a) to present a theoretical perspective of disaster as a systemic social phenomenon; b) to clarify the role of child mental health professionals in large-scale preparedness and community reactivation under conditions of disaster; c) to review the major findings on children's responses to disaster from the developmental perspective; and d) to propose models of assessment and intervention for children, families, and communities exposed to mass disaster.

DEFINITIONS

The literature distinguishes between "trauma" and "disaster." *Traumas* are experiences that threaten individual health and well-being, render one helpless in the face of intolerable internal or external danger, overwhelm coping mechanisms, violate basic assumptions about survival, and stress the uncontrollability and unpredictability in the world (10). Traumas may be caused by an isolated, unanticipated event or they may be long lasting, the result of repeated exposure to several extreme external events (11).

Disasters are relatively sudden events that are more or less time delimited. They are public events that cause extensive damage to property and lives and that have a total and ongoing disruptive impact on the social network and on the basic daily routines of children and families (7, 12, 13). During a disaster, the community as a whole is compromised in its capacity to negotiate the recovery of its individual members. Matters are often made worse when resources are overwhelmed (1) and the community's infrastructure is affected, often resulting in unemployment, housing and food shortages, poor health, deficient school and mental health services, job absenteeism, and family dysfunction.

Unlike traumas, disasters are characterized by the immediate, long-lasting and repeated exposure of victims to reminders of the event. Disasters usually involve three interconnected types of experiences: terror due to threats to one's life or exposure to grotesque sights; grief following loss (e.g., human lives, basic trust, self-esteem); and disruption of normal living (14). On the social level, disasters are accompanied by shock, depression and mourning, confusion and social disarray, rage and blame, the collapse of formal leadership, and social disintegration. Children sense that their family, neighborhood, and school have been disrupted (12). The recovery processes continues long after the disastrous event itself is over, even if it was limited to a single point in time. Hence, theoretical, research, and intervention studies should be both all encompassing and long term.

DISASTERS AND THE MENTAL HEALTH SYSTEM

Mass disaster poses a multifaceted challenge to the mental health system (15): a) *Environmental challenge:* Massive needs, routinely defined as pathological, emerge and must be confronted; b) *Systemic challenge:* Multidisciplinary orientation and multisystemic collaboration are required to counter the impact; c) *Practical challenge:* Problems to be faced involve resource allocation, extended deployment, organization, dissemination of information and communications; d) *Theoretical challenge:* The mental health system lacks a comprehensive and integrative "mass disaster theory" with a general social perspective in addition to the public health perspective; (16) and e) *Professional challenge:* Most teaching programs are not committed to disaster intervention training. Hence, professionals have insufficient knowledge and little stamina due to continuous stress.

Mental health professionals operate within multiple social systems: psychiatric, medical, welfare, urban, and national. Each of these systems may be characterized by its degree of adaptability and flexibility under stress. *Static* systems are rigid, indifferent to the environment, and show no adaptive change in structure or function over time. *Chaotic* systems show an anarchic response to the environment (disintegrated, disorganized, and dysfunctional). *Learning* systems respond in a flexible-reactive manner, show sensitivity to the environment and openness to some change in structure or function; however, their range of change is restricted to routine operations, based on past experience. *Meta-adaptive* systems are both flexible and proactive, containing units specializing in forecasting and preparing alternative scenarios for coping with change.

STAGES OF DISASTERS

Different models have been proposed to describe the disaster response, most from the event perspective (warning, threat, impact, inventory, rescue, and recovery) (17). The systemic model allows a formulation of disaster that integrates the event, the individual, and the sociocultural reaction, including the mental health response (18). From this perspective, a disaster consists of three stages, though it may loom long before the expected event actually takes place (e.g., the months of anticipation preceding the outbreak of a war). This *pre-disaster stage* includes warning, alert and alarm signs, and a sense of massive threat to communal and personal security.

The *first stage* consists of the damaging event itself, the primary disaster, and the attempts to alleviate its effects, i.e., rescuing as many victims as possible and providing basic needs (food, water, and shelter) to the affected population. The *second stage* consists of massive changes in societal structure and function (establishment of evacuation centers and tent-cities, movement of refugees), which may lead to a breakdown of norms, structures, and functions. This breakdown, reflected in societal regression, may be viewed as the secondary disaster. Life usually stabilizes in due course, generally after 18 to 36 months. At this point, there may be a *third stage* of disaster wherein the sociocultural losses, the tertiary disaster, threaten the existing collective ideology and identity (the religious identity of generations of Holocaust survivors) (19, 20).

When the severity of the damage evolves gradually and over an extended period of time (AIDS epidemic in Africa), primary, secondary, and tertiary types of disaster coexist. This gradual pattern allows for preparation and short-term adaptation to minor increments of destruction. Yet it may also engender habituation (21), within both the affected and the international communities, hence damaging the capacity for long-term forecasting and proper coping.

CHILDREN'S REACTIONS TO DISASTER: THE DISASTER SYNDROME

A child's protective matrix consists of various dimensions in his or her reality that can be disrupted and rehabilitated, among them political, cultural, social, physical, familial, maternal, and personal dimensions (22). Since disasters affect all these components, the disaster syndrome, unlike posttraumatic syndrome, involves all aspects of a child's developing cognitive structures and capacities and poses a more intricate pathological threat. Children must cope with many different kinds of losses: of people, of support systems, of normal routines, and of basic assumptions of safety and normalcy. Children may become withdrawn and alienated from the reality they perceive as having betrayed them: nature, parents, society, and its technology (23, 24).

Disasters may affect children's ability to regulate the intensity of their impulses and unconscious fantasies, thereby jeopardizing their sense of self-efficacy, security, and autonomy, and the normal maturation of their defensive functioning, object relations, reality testing, and attachment. Structural developments, such as superego consolidation and its behavioral consequences, ego ideal structure formation with its relevance to affiliation and ideology development, and ego functions with their significance in areas of cognition and attention, may also be hampered. Traumatization has a potentially damaging effect on the development of a lasting sense of identity and of the historical continuity of the self that integrates thoughts, images, feelings, and sensations (25).

Preschoolers may exhibit behavioral changes and regressive behaviors, mostly within the normal range. These may include irritability, sleep difficulties, separation problems, fears, nervousness, posttraumatic play, demanding or dependent behavior, whining or temper tantrums (26–28). Older children may report disturbances in conscience functioning, although their moral functioning may seem advanced (29).

Studies suggest that parents and teachers tend to report fewer posttraumatic symptoms in children than the children themselves report (30, 31). Adults may be preoccupied with their own stress and not be attuned to their child's inner emotional states. Children may also be more reliable reporters of internalizing or dissociative symptoms. Thus, clinicians must be careful to assess children's functioning directly and not rely exclusively on external reports. They must bear in mind that while the initial response tends to predict later adjustment, initial symptomatic ratings may not correlate with later assessments (32), and posttraumatic responses may have a delayed onset (33). If a disaster is limited and well controlled, most of the pathological reactions in children will abate within the first year (32). If community functioning is substantially disrupted, however, symptoms may persist for years (4, 9, 33).

TYPES OF POST-DISASTER SYMPTOMS

In response to disasters, children may exhibit a combination of some or many of the following behaviors: posttraumatic stress symptoms, fears, depression and grief, and dissociation (34). Anthony et al. (35) found that anhedonia, inattention and learning problems are the most common symptoms after disasters. But rather than being markers of a pathological reaction, such symptoms reflect the normal disruptive consequences of disasters.

Symptoms of posttraumatic stress disorder (PTSD) are grouped under three domains: intrusion, avoidance/numbing, and arousal. Empirical studies have identified certain symptoms that are specific to children, such as persistent posttraumatic play, omens, and somatic complaints (36). Scheeringa et al. (37) proposed the following diagnostic criteria for this disorder in young children: intrusive reexperiencing of the event, avoidance of reminders, general psychic numbing, and increased arousal.

Intrusive reexperiencing of the event may be observed in thoughts, feelings, or sensations. Children may retell their experiences over and over, report nightmares and exhibit repetitive trauma-related play. They may also describe *vivid* traumatic images: visual (mutilated bodies), auditory (the sound of the earthquake or screams for help), olfactory (odors of burned or decaying bodies) or kinesthetic (feeling as if they were buried under the rubble).

Avoidance of reminders is manifested in the evasion of places, people, thoughts or activities associated with the disaster. Such avoidance can be both a symptom and a defensive maneuver to reduce internal stress. Nevertheless, persistent avoidance coping is associated with negative mental health outcomes (38). The avoidance may be active (purposeful engagement in thoughts unrelated to the trauma to avoid traumatic reminders) or passive (not engaging in social interactions) (35).

General psychic numbing may be considered a mild dissociation response, and is more difficult to detect in children than in adults (31). Children exposed to disasters may lose interest in activities that were significant in the past, feel estranged from others, exhibit constricted affect, lose recently acquired developmental skills, and express a sense of foreshortened future.

Increased arousal symptoms include irritability, angry outbursts, exaggerated startle response, hypervigilance, difficulty in concentrating, and sleep disturbances such as difficulties in falling asleep or in sleeping alone (39). In a study of Armenian children exposed to the 1988 earthquake, 18 months after the event about 90% of those living adjacent to the epicenter met the diagnosis of PTSD, compared to only 30% of children from the periphery of the earthquake zone (40).

Mass disasters typically induce specific *fears and dependent behavior* in children (28, 41). Old fears may be reactivated, current ones may intensify, and new fears with a more or less clear relationship to the event may emerge. Fears may lead to dependent and clingy behavior, difficulty separating from caretakers, or refusal to attend school, thereby interrupting the separation-individuation process. Vogel and Vernberg (7) claimed that disasters challenge children's basic assumption that the world is a secure place, leaving them helplessly vulnerable. Empirical support for this hypothesis was provided by the finding that 5 years after a disaster, young children's symptoms still correlated with the reactions of their mothers (42).

Children exposed to disasters may show symptoms of *depression and grief*, but these are usually of lesser severity than are PTSD symptoms (7). Since grief and posttraumatic stress symptoms may appear independently of one another, separate diagnostic interviews are required for each domain (43). The mood symptoms, which have been suggested to be at least partially secondary to the posttraumatic reactions (44), are the result of different types of loss (of home, family members, personal belongings, basic assumptions). The traumatic grief reaction, recently defined for adults (45), still awaits validation in children.

After the 1999 earthquakes in Turkey, Laor et al. (46) found that children who had seen severely injured or dead people, experienced hunger or lack of sleep after the event, or had undergone more traumatic experiences in the past reported more depressive/grief symptoms.

Disasters may be perceived as an overwhelming interruption of human experience, thereby distorting an individual's basic assumptions, both cognitive ("*What is real and what is imaginary?*") and existential ("*Is it happening to me?*"). To reestablish well being, some people define a different "spatial" arrangement of their position relative to the world: "*I am not affected because I am elsewhere.*" This type of distancing is adaptive. Pathological *dissociation* goes one step further, with manipulation of adverse stimuli through the reconstruction of perception and the splitting up of consciousness: "*What is happening to me is not real*" or "*I, who is experiencing, am not real* (22)".

Dissociative reactions may be manifested by symptoms that reflect a discontinuation of personal experience. Children may have out-of-body experiences, perceive life as a dream or a movie, and "see" or "hear voices" of people who died. Amnesia is apparently less frequent in children than in adolescents. Dissociative mechanisms may provide temporary relief from the overwhelming trauma. If they persist, however, they may engender a long-term alteration in normally integrative functions of identity, memory, and/or consciousness (47).

FACTORS AFFECTING CHILDREN'S RESPONSES TO DISASTERS

Several factors have an impact on the scope of children's symptomatic response to disaster.

Factors Related to the Disaster

Children whose traumatic exposure is more severe tend to react more extremely. This "dose of exposure" effect is apparent, for example, in the child's proximity to the epicenter of an earthquake (40), the impact zone of a hurricane (48), or the site of missile attacks (27). More severe responses have been noted in children who were exposed to the harshest experiences, such as witnessing severely injured people and mutilated bodies, being faced with a direct threat to their own life, or suffering human loss, especially of family members (49, 50), as well as in children who sustained personal injuries (44, 51, 52). Continuous displacement predicts the degree of psychological response (9, 53), with children exposed to several traumatic experiences more likely to exhibit a greater number of posttraumatic symptoms (54, 55).

In cases of severe disaster, children need to cope with a massive range of problems: lack of food, water and shelter; property damage; inadequate housing; violence; lack of medical care; traumatic reminders; bereavement; relocation; separation from parents; and economic crisis. Under such circumstances, their posttraumatic reactions may intensify and interfere with symptomatic recovery, at least during the first year, as well as with their long-term development (25, 40, 49, 56).

Factors Related to the Child

Age

The variations in both subject age and symptom domains that have been examined by different studies make generalizations difficult, even though young children are considered more vulnerable (21, 57). Nevertheless, behavioral problems, specific fears, regressive symptoms and separation problems appear to be more characteristic among young children, whereas depression and anxiety are more characteristic of older children and adolescents (58). Three months after Hurricane Hugo, preadolescent children reported more posttraumatic symptoms than those in early and late adolescence who had similar responses (59).

Gender

Results regarding gender differences are conflicting. Some studies reported no gender differences (9, 27, 48). Others found that girls tend to report more internalizing symptoms (anxiety, depression, fears) and posttraumatic symptoms, while boys exhibit more externalizing behavior (acting out, aggression) (40, 52, 58, 59). Girls tend to be described as more resilient than boys in childhood, but more vulnerable in adolescence (60). The greater readiness among girls to share their concerns may explain some of these gender differences.

Vulnerabilities and Resiliency

Children with prior pathology, particularly anxiety and learning difficulties (38, 52, 53), and children who have suffered more traumatic events in the past (55, 61) are more prone to severe symptoms months after a disaster. By contrast, resilient children are those who have the support of caring adults during and after major stressors, as well as those who are also good learners, good problemsolvers, and engaging to other people. These children have areas of competence and are perceived by themselves or by society to have high efficacy (60, 62). Kassam-Adams et al. (63) found an association between early physiological arousal and the development or persistence of PTSD symptoms in children with traffic-related injuries. Asarnow et al. (38) found that children's reactions to the Northridge earthquake, a mild to moderate stressor, showed that the role of heritable biology was minor compared to the role of the children's subjective appraisals of stress and past psychopathology.

Coping Skills

A child's coping skills also mediate between exposure severity and response. More immature coping/defensive strategies for dealing with stress (blaming others, anger) are associated with greater symptomatic persistence over time (39, 64).

Factors Related to the Family

Reaction of the Parents

The presence of adults caring for a child during and after a major stressor is considered the most important and consistent protective factor (60, 61). Indeed, the reaction of the parents, especially the mother, to the disaster is generally correlated with the severity of the child's responses (65). Researchers found that the reaction of preschool children to the missile attacks during the Gulf War was highly correlated with the reaction of their mothers (9, 27, 42). This was true for 3–4-year olds, but not for 5-year-olds, probably owing to the older children's increasing autonomy and the control of psychological buffering systems for development (60). Five years after the war, poor psychological functioning among mothers was associated with heightened symptoms in their children (66).

The ability of parents to contain the anxiety generated by extreme threats of disasters seems to be the most important factor influencing their children's responses (56, 67). Parents are critical mediators of stress, mainly owing to their roles in social referencing (pooling information and processing of meaning), responding emotionally, and caring for the child (60).

Functioning of the Family System

The family is an important mediatory factor, particularly in young children (9, 27, 68). Families with extreme levels of cohesion—boundaries that are either too loose or too rigid—may not provide the appropriate support or allow the child to withdraw at times in order to process traumatic experiences and reach a constructive resolution of concerns. Caring support, open communication patterns, and sensitivity to the child's needs enable parents and children to regulate dyadic processes and discuss disaster-related issues when necessary. Stressed parents may be preoccupied with their own suffering and may tend to overprotect the child, thus interfering with the healthy process of resolution (56).

Factors Related to the Society and the Culture

Friendships

Friendships are valuable sources of reciprocal affection and attachment, mutual assistance, emotional security and self-esteem, and nonfamilial contexts for intimacy, thereby contributing to the child's ability to cope with stress (69). Natural sources of friendships—the family, the neighborhood, and the school—may be shattered in times of disaster. Friendships may also include supportive relationships with teachers or other adults (30, 52). Even the presence of a single concerned and caring adult may do much to offset the impact of misfortune in the lives of children (62).

Community

Communities mobilize at times of disaster by relying on their inner strength and external backup support. The inner strength of a community under disaster is a result of various factors and processes: effective leadership; social cohesiveness; institutional empowerment; available emergency services; appropriate infrastructure; disaster preparedness plans; and communal hardiness (e.g., education, ideology).

Culture

Cultures define the terms under which symptoms are expressed and set the parameters for expression of personal distress. Some cultures encourage children to express their feelings of distress, while others do not. For example, in some cultures adults may admonish children who were victims of disaster to be prim and proper or to refrain from crying (41, 70). Thus, cultural background, with its strengths and its weaknesses, needs to be taken into account by clinicians when planning treatment interventions. In addition, culture also mediates ideology and identity. As the purveyor of the meaning ascribed to disastrous events and consequences, the culture regulates the individual's capacity to maintain an active and resilient stance. Yet a traumatically grieving culture may succumb to expressions of mourning and aggression, and, when faced with further threats, could fuel a cycle of violence.

ASSESSMENT OF CHILDREN UNDER CONDITIONS OF DISASTER

It is extremely important that children at risk of psychopathology after exposure to disaster be identified and treated as early as possible. Child mental health professionals need to be well informed about the valid assessment tools available. In the first and second stages of a disaster, such professionals must remain sensitive to the setting in which they operate. Efforts must be directed not only to treating the children themselves, but also to reactivating society's childcare systems via existing childcare workers. In a natural setting, assessment may be integrated into normal institutional activity (see "School-Based Interventions" following).

The preferred clinical screening tools are those that directly assess the child rather than relying on external reporters. Such tools should also be simple and quick to administer, accurate, repeatable, sensitive, and specific (71, 72). The criteria for identifying pathological cases should be tempered by consideration of the psychological and economic costs of possible false positives and false negatives. The use of cutoff scores may facilitate the decision making process, but can obscure minor but "real" differences between children with scores slightly above or slightly below threshold. Green (73) suggested that clinicians think in terms of degree of impairment in a given sample rather than in terms of case identification. Moreover, the assessment of a single domain rather than a complex of posttraumatic, dissociative, and grief symptoms may decrease the sensitivity of the battery (71). (For a review of screening tools to assess trauma and its effects, see 74–75.)

Assessment of risk factors deserves special attention. Information should be gathered concerning the child's past functioning (traumatic/stressful experiences such as divorce, hospitalization, birth of a sibling, mental and general health problems) as well as disaster-related events (personal injury, loss of family members or friends, witnessing severely injured or dead people, separation from parents, experiencing hunger or lack of sleep). A risk index may prove a useful guide in identifying symptomatic children as well as those requiring special attention (55).

PRINCIPLES OF CHILD MENTAL HEALTH INTERVENTION

Systemic Perspective

Mass disasters have an impact not only on exposed children, but on their families, their school system, and their entire sociocultural milieu, as well as on peripheral communities (41, 48). To cope with this complex challenge, interventions must be formulated from an integrative perspective, focusing on maximizing well being and self-efficacy and minimizing stress and disorganization; they must help victims find meaning and instill a sense of control.

In their approach to public mental health, Pynoos et al. (16) emphasized the need to resolve institutional conflicts over authority and resource allocation, to address teachers' own disaster experiences, and to properly select and train intervention teams to work with severely traumatized victims. Population screening is useful to pinpoint areas that require specific resources and government support.

The effect of mass disasters is so devastating because of the concomitant loss of sociocultural regulators, leading to the destruction of basic schemes, values, roles, and structures (family and individual) and leaving the community vulnerable to pain, grief, trauma, and anger. Working in such a milieu, professionals may find themselves embroiled in confusion and red tape from the various social/government systems (medicine, education, welfare, nongovernment organizations [NGOs]) and the intervention teams trying to help. Therefore, a systemic perspective is needed to clarify the picture and to help psychiatrists a) formulate the newly established needs of child-oriented institutions, b) transfer knowledge and empower professionals in related fields to resume their role, c) define their own role and carry out specific interventions, and d) be familiar with the system within which they operate.

Mental health interventions for children and families exposed to mass disaster should follow the following five AREST principles, for which specific implementation will differ according to the particular characteristics of each country (18):

Anticipate First and foremost, interventions must provide an integrated vision, foresee different scenarios, and include contingency plans. Professionals and paraprofessionals must be trained, human and economic resources appropriately allocated, and treatment protocols created and exercised. Efficient local, national, and international networks need to be developed, including collaboration among agencies (education, police, health), clear command and control chains and communication channels, and the establishment of sponsorship and legitimacy (76).

Redifferentiate. Child psychiatrists must identify the extent of social loss in terms of institutional and role dysfunction. They must plan the process of context-related redevelopment of professional roles within and between systems (health, welfare, education) with the help of multidisciplinary teams. Particular attention should be addressed to reconstituting the roles of parents and teachers.

Empower. Child psychiatrists need to debrief (if necessary), educate and empower social agents (e.g., teachers) who are in direct contact with children to serve as mental health mediators. They must help these agents restore and adapt their original roles, and delegate some therapeutic responsibilities to them. Furthermore, child psychiatrists must assume a leadership position and supply the team with professional vision and positive expectations.

Supervise and Assess. Psychiatrists must define boundaries, provide knowledge, expertise and support to therapeutic agents, assess program development, and identify needs by feedback mechanisms. As leaders, mental health professionals need to encourage creative initiatives among team members and provide them with individualized consideration.

Treat and Followup. Treatment focuses on the rehabilitation of individuals and families. Delayed responses should also be considered.

Systems and Stages of Disaster

Application of the AREST principles is far from straightforward. Actions taken during routine times differ from those during times of disaster, not only in intensity, speed, and expediency, but primarily in the planned systemic change. The response of mental health professionals is determined by the type of reacting system. Preparedness and flexibility are key factors ensuring response effectiveness.

During the first stage of a disaster, rigid systems tend to remain encapsulated in their normal routines, whereas learning systems may undergo structural modifications and create information centers and outreach programs. Metaadaptive systems may already be in a state of partial readiness and will be able to initiate professional interdisciplinary teaming up with social agencies early in the process of redifferentiation and empowerment.

In the second stage of societal regression, rigid systems treat acute referrals in existing clinics, while learning systems establish field stations and initiate self-training toward the formation of larger trauma centers. Metaadaptive systems concentrate on the rehabilitation of roles and institutions and draw on resources prepared by national and international collaborations.

In the third stage, rigid systems revert to their original constricted outlook and ignore the larger scope of the tertiary disaster (loss of ideology and identity). Such systems deal with suffering individuals as they are referred to their clinics, this time as chronic victims. Learning systems maintain operative trauma centers and may internalize some of the lessons learned from coping with the first two stages into their institutional response pattern. The main focus of metaadaptive systems is the establishment of community-based disaster intervention centers. These address the tertiary disaster by operating on both the sociocultural and the communal clinical levels to enhance resilience, regeneration and growth. Such centers may be planned in advance and developed out of the existing community mental health system, in conjunction with the general public agencies responsible for disaster intervention (see following).

Professional Role Containment and Enhancement in Conditions of Disaster

At times of disaster, the priority is basic survival. Safety, shelter and food, the most immediate and conspicuous needs, are usually within the domain of professional relief teams. Yet team members may themselves suffer from role-related problems because of the disaster-induced collapse of their familiar sociocultural matrix. Therefore, mental health professionals in positions of authority must respond to these needs, both within their own team and in the teams in which they act as mediators (e.g., teachers, school counselors). They must make team members feel cared for and help them develop a sense of belonging and purpose. Professionals may take a leadership position by formulating a vision ("revitalizing our school and prevent suffering"), providing individualized consideration, fostering an atmosphere of creative intellectual coping (supporting initiatives, delegating authority) and transmitting positive expectations (concerning professionals' capacities and end results) (77).

Program Implementation

Studies of mental health interventions after disasters clearly support their effectiveness (78–80). Nevertheless, their ongoing operation requires the constant commitment of professionals, leaders, and local agencies. By endorsing a systemic perspective, mental health professionals may overcome repeated adversities and challenges, inadequate professional training, limited resources, and organizational conflicts that tend to characterize the process.

Because parents and teachers tend to underestimate the extent of children's suffering (31), and given that disaster survivors are also often reluctant to seek professional help (81), *outreach* efforts should be made systematically to screen victims at risk. Optimally this screening should take place 1 to 3 months after the disaster (82). Thereafter, clinical triage protocols can be utilized to match risk groups with intervention programs (14, 50, 82).

Studies have demonstrated the applicability of Western therapeutic programs in non-Western cultures as well (79, 83). The first step in implementing these programs is to train members of the affected community. The local staff may need constant support and supervision. If handled correctly, this process may help reduce the ambivalent resistance of traumatized survivors to what might be perceived as a foreign "intrusion" that threatens the "trauma membrane" protecting them from an overload of psychic tension (14, 82).

INTERVENTION MODELS

Effective treatments for traumatized children should include the psychoeducation of children and parents about the nature of the disorder, some form of work on exposure, and dysfunctional cognitive restructuring (84). Furthermore, treatments need to be implemented within the broader social reality of the disaster (e.g., entire community, neighborhood, peer group) in order to alleviate the sequelae of secondary and tertiary disasters. To this end, the child psychiatry system must collaborate with three additional systems that will provide them with the authority to intervene on all institutional levels: community leadership, school and medical clinics.

Commonly used structured treatment and rehabilitation community programs (e.g., psychotherapy, programs for the disadvantaged, adolescents, and women, as well as school empowerment and class activation) that reinforce enhancement of participants' initiative, activity, empowerment, hardiness, and responsibility may be adapted for disaster conditions. This adaptation is based upon a formulation of disaster as destructive both to external (concrete) reality and to internal functional representations—of stability (predictability and controllability) as well as of effective engagement with the environment (the physical and the communal world). Therefore, child intervention programs should aim to restitute damaged communal institutions and norms as well as communal functioning (to reclaim communal roles: parent, teacher, worker, leader).

In circumscribed mass disasters, effective programs may take 12 to 18 months. The first phase is dedicated to assessing and reactivating the community and its institutions, as well as to introducing clinical intervention programs. This phase may take up to a year, culminating in the ceremony commemorating the first anniversary of the disaster. The second phase is characterized by the community and the individual taking responsibility for the future; it involves development of physical and social infrastructure and job opportunities.

Immediate Interventions

During the acute stage of a disaster, the role of the mental health professional needs to be modified because of the limited number of professionals and the masses of individuals requiring help. Large populations need to be screened to identify children at risk. Other important tasks include initiating telephone crisis hotlines, supplying psychological first aid for children and families in evacuation centers and hospitals, consulting authorities to assess immediate needs, and planning large-scale public health education programs. At this stage, professionals become aware of the need quickly to acquire new disaster-related skills. Despite their experience with technically formulated protocol-based interventions, such professionals soon discover that mastering new therapeutic techniques and implementing them under disaster conditions requires thorough training and ongoing supervision. Such skills can be secured before proceeding with the intervention program.

The mass media can be helpful for confused parents, teaching them about typical reactions to stress and about how to cope and to restore their parental role. Parents should be advised to tolerate regression, encourage children to ask questions and express feelings, assure their children there are no bad thoughts or feelings, assign children appropriate activities, reestablish stability and family rituals, and convey positive expectations for the future (85). Television programs addressing children should cover the same issues. Delegating age-appropriate functions to children as well as allowing them to take responsibility and provide active help may avoid the sense of helplessness and passivity that leads to more severe responses.

Appropriate preparedness of a city/country can significantly reduce the consequences of a disaster. For example, as part of its general Disaster Preparedness Program, the Tel-Aviv Municipality has developed an Emergency Psychosocial Intervention System (EPIS; 86) that focuses on social and psychological welfare in times of emergency. The EPIS is composed of 10 multidisciplinary units: 1) on-site intervention (triage and evacuation), 2) family notification, 3) hospital liaison, 4) information center, 5) crisis hotline, 6) evacuation and absorption centers, 7) community resources (volunteers and donations), 8) special populations, 9) team support, and 10) regional trauma units. The EPIS headquarters coordinates these units and their integrated operation with relevant institutions (e.g., police, army) as well as with the clinical trauma and disaster community center, out of which the child mental health professionals operate.

Interventions During the Second and Third Stages

Debriefing

The disaster syndrome may be viewed as a predictable reaction, akin to the fear response to danger or the mourning process following loss. In the long run, most affected individuals recover their functioning. It was assumed that the recovery of traumatized survivors may be facilitated by a debriefing process that allows them to express traumatic experiences and flooding reactions; facilitate relaxation; promote cognitive organization and self-control; identify and mobilize internal and external resources; set realistic expectations; restore self-esteem and hope; and prepare participants for future experiences (87).

With children, such a structured technique may last one or more meetings and must be carried out by an educated professional. The technique may include play activities, such as individual or group drawing, writing, or imagery games. Participants are given time for self-expression and questions. The tasks of the leader are to protect limits, set rules, provide information, facilitate verbal and physical peer support, and manage containment. The leader may also identify symptomatic children and refer them for further help after the meeting, as well as distribute psychoeducational handouts about symptoms or positive coping strategies for followup.

After reporting their trauma-related experiences, participants are encouraged to focus on thoughts, emotions, images, and sensations related to the event. Special attention should be given to feelings of guilt and anger, since clinical experience shows that these may interfere with the process of working through the trauma. Thereafter, participants explore personal and communal coping resources and use creative imagery to return to the "here and now," fantasize about a positive future, and construct plans of action. Parallel sessions may be held with the parents.

Debriefing may be an efficient tool to help children and adults (87, 88). Yet it is important to be aware that very early exposure to the memory of a traumatic event may in some individuals interfere with the normal affective-cognitive processes that lead to recovery, resulting in neutral effects or even an exacerbation of symptoms (89, 90).

The criticism raised against debriefing addresses not only outcome but the issue of timing of the intervention. Hobbs and Mayou think that a too early intervention may disrupt the adaptive defenses, including those that may look to us pathological, i.e., numbing (91). Therefore, several authors have suggested intervening after the victims' recovery from their initial shock (92). In a recently published randomized control trial with children involved in road traffic accidents, both children who received psychological debriefing 4 weeks after the event and those who did not demonstrated significant improvement at the 8 month followup (93). Since the researchers provided all participants in the study a structured assessment, they could not conclude whether the improvements reported in both groups are better or worse than natural recovery rates. The authors suggest that further studies looking at repeated measures over time would clarify whether the intervention shortens the recovery period.

Given the recent study, we may conclude that in a well supervised context and in the hands of trained clinicians, debriefing may prove a useful tool in the recovery from traumatic events. The specific therapeutic factors of debriefing, and who may benefit from it, remain open questions.

The School Setting

To assist as many children as possible, professionals may need to work with groups rather than individuals. Since teachers have already established relations of trust with children and parents, and since most are ready to be educated and to serve a therapeutic role, intact school environments are appropriate societal recovery centers for early interventions (76, 94, 95).

Support from classmates and teachers is a significant predictor of fewer symptoms after a major disaster and prevents withdrawal and isolation (30, 95). Moreover, the class setting provides a predictable routine, clear expectations, consistent rules, and immediate feedback. It is recognized as the place to apply learning skills for exploring causes and consequences of disasters, and to emphasize that survivors may experience "normal reactions to abnormal events."

Teachers should allocate time to deal with traumatic experiences, model children's responses, reinforce emerging coping skills, provide factual information and dispel rumors, facilitate mutual support, identify suffering children, prepare the class for future experiences, and encourage students to become active contributors to their family, school, and community.

For a program to be effective, mental health professionals should ensure that the teachers a) are not traumatized themselves; b) are capable of mastering disaster-related educational techniques; and c) have adapted their view of their role as teachers/educators to the new and harsh reality. To help regenerate the normal school setting after a disaster, the child psychiatrist needs to meet with teachers, debrief them about their own disaster experiences, and clearly describe the educational task at hand.

Based on these principles, Wolmer et al. (55) implemented a three-stage supervision program for the principal and teachers at one school after the 1999 earthquake in Turkey. First, a group debriefing session was conducted to normalize responses and enable expression of trauma-related affects (anger, guilt, helplessness, hopelessness). Then, an experiential activity was introduced to help the teachers redefine their role vis-à-vis the students as "educators" and "leaders." The authors stressed that in times of disaster, rather than merely covering the regular curricula, teachers were expected to maintain and enhance their role by providing individualized attention, transmitting values, and conveying positive expectations. As part of this role, they were taught to implement a disaster-related classroom activation program (see below). Finally, an ongoing supervision process was begun, led by local professionals, wherein teachers were not only educated but also provided support for each other (79).

School-based interventions include single-session debriefings, small-group programs, and class activation programs.

Targeted *small-group programs* within the school setting may benefit high-risk children or children who are more agitated and need closer attention than can be provided in the classroom (94, 96). Smith et al. (97) formulated a three-session program to teach recovery techniques to small groups of children affected by disaster. The techniques used are psychoeducation, imagery, and cognitive techniques, and exposure practice. Each session is dedicated to one domain of the posttraumatic syndrome: intrusion, avoidance, and arousal. The professional may also offer a fourth session for bereaved children and a session with parents, to provide them with information and suggest ways for them to help their children.

Class activation programs, programs implemented in the classroom itself, may vary in focus, scope and depth, but all are intended to minimize stigma, encourage normalcy, and reinforce the expectation that the children will soon resume their roles as students (5, 76, 94). Nevertheless, because teachers themselves may be struggling with severe posttraumatic symptoms and personal losses, they may feel unable to help their students. Some may try to avoid dealing with reminders of the event by stressing that children have no need to talk about their traumatic experiences (16).

For children who survived an earthquake in Italy, Galante and Foa (78) provided seven monthly sessions to discuss and deal with related feelings, and noted a significant reduction in symptoms. Other models also utilize expert mental health professionals in school settings, with or without the presence of the teacher (94, 98). Direct teacher involvement is, however, encouraged for disasters of large proportions, when expert resources prove insufficient.

Saltzman et al. (99) proposed a public health approach consisting of a screening process and three tiers of mental health school- and community-based interventions after war and terrorism: general and broad-scale psychoeducational activities; manualized trauma/grief focused group psychotherapy for students at risk (see following); and highly specialized traditional treatments in the community for severely distressed and high-risk students.

The class activation described in Wolmer et al., (55) which was led by teachers, began with an initial meeting with the parents to provide information about the program and the children's expected reactions to the disaster, and to engage them in the process. The subsequent eight 2-hour meetings of the whole class focused on various aspects of the recovery process (e.g., establishing a safe place, learning about the earthquake, loss and death, dealing with anger, planning the future). The program combined psychoeducational modules, cognitive-behavioral techniques, play activities, and ongoing documentation in personal diaries. The program yielded significant immediate reductions in posttrauma and dissociation symptoms. In addition, a three-year controlled followup showed that children who had participated in the class intervention adapted better than nonparticipants in terms of academic, social, and behavioral functioning (83).

CLINICAL INTERVENTIONS

Individual Interventions

Although group interventions are efficient and costeffective, they may not be sufficient for those children who are most affected. Controlled and uncontrolled studies have confirmed the effectiveness of brief cognitive behavioral treatment in traumatized children (84). Other modes have been employed, such as play therapy, psychodynamic psychotherapy, or eye movement desensitization and reprocessing (EMDR; 100). Particular attention should be directed to prior and current comorbid pathology, as well as to a thorough differential diagnosis (e.g., mania, ADHD).

Goenjian et al. (79) implemented a brief treatment program combining classroom group psychotherapy and individual sessions that focused on trauma and grief. The sessions, led by therapists, allowed for open discussion of the traumatic experiences and associated feelings, assisted the children in solving intra- and interpersonal problems, and offered effective cognitive-behavioral techniques to manage thought distortions, disturbing images, and stress-related sensations. Five years after the event, the posttraumatic symptoms of treated adolescents had decreased more significantly that those of untreated adolescents (4).

Group Interventions

Parent–Child Groups:

Families have the potential either to protect children and mitigate their post-disaster suffering or to jeopardize their adjustment to and processing of the event, thereby exacerbating their symptoms. After disasters, children and parents tend not to discuss their distress, probably to avoid upsetting each other further (6). Yet studies consistently show a significant association between the symptomatic response of children and their parents (particularly their mothers) (9, 27, 65), which may in turn have a traumatic impact on the whole parent–child dyad (42).

Based on previous successful application of parent–child group psychotherapy in treating child anxiety disorders (101), and as a second stage of class activation, Laor et al. (70) formulated an eight-session protocol for mothers and children (five dyads) with chronic PTSD. The group addressed dynamic, cognitive, and behavioral aspects of the disaster syndrome, and offered techniques to manage anxiety, relieve, control and transform distressing affects, correct thought distortions, and plan for the future. Special attention was paid to identifying and correcting maladaptive family dynamics and helping mothers and children recover their attachment and roles. Preliminary clinical and empirical results showed significant symptomatic alleviation as well as a dramatic improvement in familial communication and mutual support.

Mothers' Groups:

Group interventions with mothers facilitate indirect focusing on preschool children, a population that may not be reached in formal settings yet can display maladaptive behavioral reactions. Providing structured therapeutic interventions, psychoeducation, and practical suggestions for the children as well as strengthening participants' confidence in their maternal role are important objectives for such groups (102).

POSTDISASTER COMMUNITY-BASED INTERVENTIONS

Disasters affect entire communities, threatening social structures and functions. To be effective, interventions require collaborative efforts among NGOs and formal and informal agencies. Developing a local leadership of committed individuals and empowering these leaders to actively meet the short- and long-term needs of the community provide a valuable source of support (103). Child psychiatry relief programs need to respond to disasters on three levels: a) *The family.*

Families may suffer from injury, loss, or death of loved ones; relocation and unemployment; loss of boundaries, routine, and values; and loss of esteem and hope. b) *The neighborhood.* Neighborhoods are subject to physical and economic destruction, loss of routines, boundaries and safety, disintegration of informal networks, and restriction of leisure time activities. c) *The community.* Communities suffer from a lack of proper leadership and resources, frozen initiative, dependence on external resources, destruction of social and cultural institutions (schools, community centers, religious centers) and as a result, a foreshortened sense of communal future.

Through auxiliary social functions and structures introduced from the outside, as well as through professional clinical and social teams, temporary communities of displaced population can be helped to gradually develop coping and functioning mechanisms. The goal of community-based intervention is to transform evacuated fragments of families and singletons into self-governing communities made up of autonomous individuals and families (15) (Table 5.15.5.1). Since children cannot be fully rehabilitated until their parents resume working and regain income, professionals may also help facilitate the creation of new job resources in the community.

Using the intervention principles described above, child mental health professionals together with child community workers and local leadership can help set up community-center programs for young mothers, children and adolescents. Programs for empowerment and enhancing resilience may include the arts, sports, gardening and decorating, continuing education, job clubs, and volunteer recruitment and training in different areas (104). By *empowerment* we mean a process of involvement by which individuals and communities supplant their helpless stance by recovering their dignity and self-esteem, enhancing their critical self-awareness, gaining control over resources and objectives, and regaining a sense of personal and collective responsibility and self-efficacy (103). Individuals are able to identify specific needs and discover hidden leadership qualities, while communities gain a greater sense of interdependence, cohesion and cooperation. In the case of dislocated population groups, communal empowerment is the process by which communities are formed to achieve greater control over their environment.

Interventions at the community level facilitate the integration of community members with the natural and social environment. For example, as part of the Community Reactivation Program after the 1999 earthquake in Turkey, Spirman et al. (102) developed a 2-week summer program for a whole village of displaced individuals. The goal of this program was to transform the community and its habitat from a place where death and alienation had been culturally internalized (withdrawn fathers, unemployment, neglected neighborhood). The method rested on five principles: 1) Teaming up and training international and local youth leaders on site to serve as instructors. 2) Identifying a natural habitat adjacent to the village that would represent "life" for the community, a place for the program's activities (arts, sports) to take place. 3) Enlisting the achieved revitalization and initiative to construct recreation areas and cultivated gardens within the original village habitat. As a result, the artificial prefab neighborhood representing "death and displacement" was turned into a lively community. 4) Designating an area within the village where an artistic commemoration monument would be erected; individuals were invited to contribute treasured personal objects. The event culminated in an anniversary ceremony. This process of collective mourning allowed for an honorable and lively representation of the loss of cherished people and things, as well as the dynamic reconnection with historical identity. 5) Involvement of social and political leaders, both local and international, to facilitate the social integration of the community.

Such interventions provide child mental health professionals entry into the arena of the long-term effects of tertiary disaster, of the sociocultural losses that threaten the collective ideology and identity. Professionals may take part in modifying the school curricula to address group mourning and resilience, collective memorials as well as celebrations of rebirth. The

TABLE 5.15.5.1

THE PROCESS OF RECOVERING FROM A MASS DISASTER IN EVACUATED COMMUNITIES

Disaster	Primary	Secondary			Tertiary
Stage	I	IIa	IIb	IIc	III
Social structures in the affected community	Singletons, fragments of families.	Temporary camps, families, children's tent.	Temporary village, neighborhoods, school.	Community center, religious center.	Self-governing community.
Auxiliary social structures and functions (introduced from the outside)	Rescue teams, evacuation centers, international support.	Tent city, external supply, police, welfare and clinical services, international support.	Prefab housing, village administration, communication, transport, community services.	Social infrastructure, job development.	
Professional child mental health interventions	Field stations, emergency teams, assessment, crisis intervention.	Teaming up, adaptation of protocols, training, planning.	Consultation to community leaders, school reactivation, community-based group programs.	Psychotherapy programs (individual, group), whole community activation.	Consultation to community leaders and educators, psychotherapy programs, job development.
Rehabilitated roles	—	Basic self-care, parent.	Teacher, pupil.	Family, neighborhood.	Communal roles.
Existential orientation	Death panic.	Shock, alienation.	Grief, anger.	Acceptance, hope, revitalization.	Autonomy, initiative.

juxtaposition of commemoration and rebirth ceremonies helps individuals gain a new meaning of life in the face of profound mourning and leads to integration on both the personal and the communal levels, thus offering children an uninterrupted supportive matrix.

BUILDING A CHILD-CENTERED MODEL OF URBAN RESILIENCE

Mobilizing community resources to meet the vast needs following a disaster is a complex and demanding operation. When plans and processes are operational during ordinary times, the chances are greater that such plans will be implemented during emergencies as well. To that end, communities need to 1) foresee which emergency interventions can be developed and practiced routinely by central institutions as part of their regular goals; 2) empower these institutions as mediators of operations in the areas of mental health and rehabilitation; and 3) create a network of collaboration between these institutions to fill in structural and functional lacunae created by systemic gaps, both vertical (federal/state/county/city) and horizontal (institutions/organizations in routine and emergency times). Table 5.15.5.2 summarizes the institutions, routine goals and emergency functions of the Tel-Aviv Network, which has been initiated and coordinated by the Donald J. Cohen and Irving B. Harris Center for Civic Resilience, Trauma and Disaster Intervention to function synergistically during times of disaster and emergency (18).

PHARMACOLOGICAL INTERVENTIONS

It is widely accepted that psychotherapy is the first-choice treatment for posttraumatic states (105). Nonetheless, note that reduction of even one disabling symptom (insomnia, hyperarousal) may have a positive ripple effect on a childs functioning (106). The systematic assessment of pharmacological treatments for traumatized children and adolescents has so far been limited (76, 84). Thus, most proposals for pharmacotherapy with children are based on studies with adults. These studies, too, invite improved controlled design (107). Professionals should be aware that well intentioned donations of medications by drug companies and the urge to reach as many individuals as fast as possible may lead to anarchic management and nonprofessional medication of children.

Even in the early stages of intervention, medications can be administered to children with a known history of psychopathology prior to the disaster; to individuals who do not respond to short-term specific interventions; and to members of families at risk that are overwhelmed by acute symptoms. Even though the empirical data to support their use may be limited, medications can be directed at specific symptoms, such

TABLE 5.15.5.2

THE TEL-AVIV NETWORK OF URBAN RESILIENCE

Routine Function	Preparedness	Post-disaster Function
Cohen-Harris Center for Trauma and Disaster Intervention		
Academic center, research, education, Training		Directorship for Emergency Mental Health in Tel-Aviv and coordination of the following institutions (in collaboration with the Tel-Aviv Mental Health Center)
Tel-Aviv Medical Center		
City's largest hospital, including treatment of trauma victims	Training of resilience teams in 14 wards	Treatment of medical and psychological casualties; referral to Community Trauma Units
Community Trauma Units, Located in Municipal Social Clinics		
Treatment of victims of terrorist attacks	Ongoing training	Treatment of children and adults affected by disaster (in collaboration with the hospital staff, the police department and the Department of Rehabilitation of the Defense Ministry)
Infant Resilience and Development Centers, Located in Municipal and Public Health Well-Baby Clinics		
Infant developmental assessment and treatment	Training in trauma-related protocols of assessment and healing	Treatment of affected infants and their families (in collaboration with the hospital and the HMO)
Primary Care Providers		
Primary care of patients with stress-related conditions	Short-term protocols for trauma and stress-related conditions	Community-based treatment of trauma-related conditions (in collaboration with the Tel-Aviv Mental Health Center)
Tel-Aviv Municipality		
Comprehensive care of its residents	Training 900 members of the Emergency Psychosocial Intervention System	Comprehensive management of human services for disaster victims
School Counselors		
Psychoeducational counseling to schools	Training of leadership teams of counselors as trauma experts	Assessment and school-based interventions following disaster
Tel-Aviv University Sackler Faculty of Medicine		
Education of medical students	Integration of medical students within community-based programs	Incorporation of medical students within community-based intervention programs
Israel Defense Forces		
Coordination and logistics interface with all other parties		

as intrusion, hyperarousal and impulsivity (e.g., clonidine), anxiety (SSRIs, benzodiazepines), depression (SSRIs), psychotic symptoms or severe aggression (antipsychotics) (105).

In a recent comprehensive review, Donnelly proposes that broad-spectrum agents such as SSRIs are a good first choice because they are effective in treating the core symptoms of PTSD and comorbid symptoms (depression, anxiety) (106). In addition, Donnelly suggests that adrenergic agents may be useful in alleviating symptoms of hyperarousal and impulsivity, mood stabilizers may be necessary in severe affective dyscontrol, and atypical neuroleptics may be required in cases of acute self-injurious behavior, dissociation, and aggression.

TAKING CARE OF THE CARETAKER COMPASSION FATIGUE

Professionals engaged in disaster intervention programs are analogous to marathon runners rather than to short-distance sprinters. Project coordinators need to be aware of each worker's strengths and weaknesses, personal losses and vulnerabilities in order to regulate exposure to trauma and to prevent burnout. Program leaders need to help relief workers enhance their own coping mechanisms, tolerate the shock inherent in their work, and maintain high levels of commitment and motivation (14, 108). Therefore, leaders should facilitate adequate training and peer supervision, encourage mutual support, lead debriefing sessions, teach stress management skills, and introduce appropriate work breaks.

DISASTER RESEARCH

While disaster research is of utmost importance, it is extremely hard to carry out. Most disasters occur unexpectedly, and even those that are predictable have such an overwhelming impact that they exhaust all professional and economic resources. Furthermore, even when professional curiosity is maintained, assessment measures are enlisted, and questions are defined, implementation of such research is met by resistance on the part of both victims and clinicians. Research under such conditions tends to be perceived as hostile, foreign, exploitative, and abusive, intended to satisfy an alien agenda that is irrelevant to the priorities of disaster relief. These claims have a kernel of truth: The hands that pass out the questionnaires could have been offering bread instead.

The perspective offered in this chapter enables mental health professionals to deal seriously with these issues rather than simply explaining them away. Research initiatives need to be integrated within the systemic intervention program and to rely on direct assessment of the affected population at every stage. In this way, real risks and needs can serve a basis for rational planning as well as for improvement of existing programs. It is the responsibility of the professional to educate community leaders to take practical advantage of assessment data.

The scene of a disaster as a large-scale natural experiment offers access to communities that constitute different types of research groups and controls. Furthermore, in each community, one may encounter a large number of entire families whose members were simultaneously exposed and affected in different manners (direct/indirect) and degrees, and for different lengths of time, as well as individuals suffering from losses of varying severity. An important issue in studies of children is the phenomenology and biological susceptibility to the disaster syndrome, that is, the interplay of traumatic grief, posttraumatic symptoms and dissociation with psycho-neuro-endocrinological and psychophysiological parameters. This particular setting provides a unique opportunity for genetic studies. Special attention ought also to be directed at partial and delayed onset types of disorder, as well as concurrent psychiatric and medical morbidity.

Another area of interest is the control study and the comparative effectiveness of various interventions (social interventions vs. pharmaco- and psychotherapies, for example), as well as assessment of parameters of community resilience and vulnerability. Other important avenues of research are the long-term sequelae of disaster in terms of the developmental psychopathology of high-risk populations, the transgenerational transmission of trauma and grief, and the development of sociopolitical attitudes. Nevertheless, the search for answers to these intellectual questions cannot at any time violate the privacy of the children being studied, and clinicians must be careful to comply with accepted ethical guidelines. Institutional review boards can facilitate the process by offering a fast track for disaster-related research proposals.

CONCLUSION

Disasters irrevocably destroy the space within which children and families thrive, thereby disrupting normal development. The overwhelming nature of such an event combined with the massive extent of the resulting loss give rise to a complex clinical and social picture that may be termed the disaster syndrome. Children, families, neighborhoods, and whole communities are affected. Immediate damages can only be partially remedied, and therefore the physical, psychological and social effects are long lasting.

For effective intervention, the child mental health professional needs a comprehensive systemic, social, and mental health perspective in order to develop the appropriate program, team up with the proper authorities, proactively assess needs, and implement intervention based on real-time integrated information systems. The best results are achieved when communities are prepared. Some interventions are clinical and specific. They may be mediated by educated professionals who work with children in schools and community centers. Some other interventions are systemic.

The systemic concepts and principles presented in this chapter are reflected in the congressional report investigating the preparation for and response to Hurricane Katrina (109). As the report demonstrates, even when enormous resources are allocated, if authorities do not adhere to theoretical, organizational, and implementation principles of disaster management, disasters exact colossal consequences.

No single community can cope on its own, for adequate coping requires networking in advance on the local, national, and international levels. Thus, the challenge posed by disasters can be met by our vision of the siblinghood of humanity. A global community committed to the cause of children must respond to the challenge.

References

1. Ursano RJ, Fullerton CS, McCaughey BG: Trauma and disaster. In: Ursano RJ, McCaughey BG, Fullerton CS (eds): *Individual and Community Responses to Trauma and Disaster: The Structure of Human Chaos.* Cambridge, Cambridge University Press, 1994, pp. 3–27.
2. Integrated Regional Information Networks: Disaster reduction and the human cost of disaster. http://www.irinnews.org/webspecials/DR (retrieved Dec. 18, 2005).
3. Garmezy N, Rutter M: Acute reactions to stress. In: Rutter M, Hersov L (eds): *Child and Adolescent Psychiatry: Modern Approaches*, 2nd ed. Oxford, Blackwell, 1985, pp. 152–176.
4. Goenjian AK, Walling D, Steinberg AM, et al.: A prospective study of posttraumatic stress and depressive reactions among treated and untreated adolescents 5 years after a catastrophic disaster. *Am J Psychiatry* 162:2302–2308, 2005.

5. Pfefferbaum B: Posttraumatic stress disorder in children: A review of the past 10 years. *J Am Acad Child Adolesc Psychiatry* 36:1503–1511, 1997.
6. Udwin O: Annotation: Children's reactions to traumatic events. *J Child Psychol Psychiatry* 34:115–127, 1993.
7. Vogel JM, Vernberg EM: Children's psychological responses to disasters. *J Clin Child Psychol* 22:464–484, 1993.
8. Yule W, Perrin S, Smith P: Post-traumatic stress reactions in children and adolescents. In: Yule W (ed): *Post-Traumatic Stress Disorders: Concepts and Therapy*. Chichester, John Wiley & Sons, 1999, pp. 25–50.
9. Laor N, Wolmer L, Mayes LC, et al.: Israeli preschoolers under Scuds: A thirty-month follow-up. *J Am Acad Child Adolesc Psychiatry* 36:349–356, 1997.
10. Eisen ML, Goodman GS: Trauma, memory, and suggestibility in children. *Dev Psychopathol* 10:717–738, 1998.
11. Terr LC: Childhood traumas: An outline and overview. *Am J Psychiatry* 148:10–20, 1991.
12. Laor N, Wolmer L: Trauma and emergency in child psychiatry: Clinical theory and innovative, multidisciplinary and multi-modal interventions. Presented at the 11th International Congress of the European Society for Child and Adolescent Psychiatry, Hamburg, 1999.
13. López-Ibor, JJ: What is a disaster? In: López-Ibor JJ, Christodoulou G, Maj M, et al. (eds): *Disasters and Mental Health*. Chichester, John Wiley & Sons, 2005, pp. 1–11.
14. Austin LS, Godleski LS: Therapeutic approaches for survivors of disaster. *Psychiatr Clin North Am* 22:897–910, 1999.
15. Laor N: The role of mental health professionals after mass disasters. Presented at the Congress on the Promised Childhood, Tel Aviv, 2001.
16. Pynoos RS, Goenjian AK, Steinberg AM: A public mental health approach to the postdisaster treatment of children and adolescents. *Child Adol Psychiat Clin North Am* 7:195–210, 1998.
17. Raphael B: *When Disaster Strikes: How Individuals and Communities Cope with Catastrophe*. New York, Basic Books, 1986.
18. Laor N, Wiener Z, Spirman S, et al.: Community mental health procedures for emergencies and mass disasters: The Tel-Aviv model. In: Danieli Y, Brom D, Sills J (eds): *The Trauma of Terrorism: Sharing Knowledge and Shared Care, An International Handbook*. New York, Hawarth Press, 2004, pp. 681–684.
19. Danieli Y (ed): *International Handbook of Multigenerational Legacies of Trauma*. New York, Plenum Press, 1998.
20. Laor N: Saving the Holocaust witness. In: Ariel Y, Biderman S, Rotem O (eds): *Relativism and Beyond*. Leiden, Brill, 1998, pp. 265–298.
21. Solomon Z: *Coping with War-Induced Stress: The Gulf War and the Israeli Response*. New York, Plenum Press, 1995.
22. Laor N: The protective matrix as risk-modifying function of traumatic effects in preschool children: A development perspective. Presented at the 6th International Psychoanalytic Association Conference on Psychoanalytic Research, London, 1996.
23. Krystal H: *Massive Psychic Trauma*. New York, International University Press, 1968.
24. Valent P: Disaster syndrome. In: Fink G (ed): *Encyclopedia of Stress* (vol 1). San Diego, CA, Academic Press, 2000, pp. 706–709.
25. Pynoos RS, Steinberg AM, Wraith R: A developmental model of childhood traumatic stress. In: Cicchetti D, Cohen DJ (eds): *Developmental Psychopathology. Vol 2: Risk, Disorder, and Adaptation*. New York, John Wiley & Sons, Inc, 1995, pp. 72–95.
26. Bingham RD, Harmon RJ: Traumatic stress in infancy and early childhood: Expression of distress and developmental issues. In: Pfeffer C (ed): *Severe Stress and Mental Disturbance in Children*. Washington, DC, American Psychiatric Association Press, 1996, pp. 499–532.
27. Laor N, Wolmer L, Mayes LC, et al.: Israeli preschoolers under Scud missile attacks: A developmental perspective on risk-modifying factors. *Arch Gen Psychiatry* 53:416–423, 1996.
28. Sullivan MA, Saylor CF, Foster KY: Post-hurricane adjustment of preschoolers and their families. *Adv Behav Res Ther* 13:163–171, 1991.
29. Goenjian A, Stillwell BM, Steinberg AM, et al.: Moral development and psychopathological interference in conscience functioning among adolescents after trauma. *J Am Acad Child Adolesc Psychiatry* 38:376–384, 1999.
30. Vernberg EM, La Greca AM, Silverman WK, et al.: Prediction of posttraumatic stress symptoms in children after Hurricane Andrew. *J Abnorm Psychol* 195:237–248, 1996.
31. Yule W, Williams RM: Post-traumatic stress reactions in children. *J Trauma Stress* 3:279–295, 1990.
32. Green BL, Grace MC, Vary MG, et al.: Children of disaster in the second decade: A 17-year follow-up of Buffalo Creek survivors. *J Am Acad Child Adolesc Psychiatry* 33:71–79, 1994.
33. Sack WH, Him C, Dickason D: Twelve-year follow-up study of Khmer youths who suffered massive war trauma as children. *J Am Acad Child Adolesc Psychiatry* 38:1173–1179, 1999.
34. Gordon R, Wraith R: Responses of children and adolescents to disaster. In: Wilson JP, Raphael B (eds): *International Handbook of Traumatic Stress Syndromes*. New York, Plenum Press, 1993, pp. 561–575.
35. Anthony JL, Lonigan CJ, Hecht SA: Dimensionality of posttraumatic stress disorder symptoms in children exposed to disaster: Results from confirmatory factor analyses. *J Abnorm Psychol* 108:326–336, 1999.
36. Terr LC: Chowchilla revisited: The effects of psychic trauma four years after a school-bus kidnapping. *Am J Psychiatry* 140:1543–1550, 1983.
37. Scheeringa MS, Zeanah CH, Drell MJ, et al.: Two approaches to the diagnosis of posttraumatic stress disorder in infancy and early childhood. *J Am Acad Child Adolesc Psychiatry* 34:191–200, 1995.
38. Asarnow J, Glynn S, Pynoos RS, et al.: When the earth stops shaking: Earthquake sequelae among children diagnosed for pre-earthquake psychopathology. *J Am Acad Child Adolesc Psychiatry* 38:1016–1023, 1999.
39. La Greca AM: Posttraumatic stress disorder in children. In: Fink G (ed): *Encyclopedia of Stress* (vol 3). San Diego, CA, Academic Press, 2000, pp. 181–186.
40. Pynoos RS, Goenjian A, Tashjian M, et al.: Post-traumatic stress reactions in children after the 1988 Armenian earthquake. *Br J Psychiatry* 163:239–247, 1993.
41. Goenjian A: A mental health relief programme in Armenia after the 1988 earthquake: Implementation and clinical observations. *Br J Psychiatry* 163:230–239, 1993.
42. Wolmer L, Laor N, Gershon A, et al.: The mother-child facing trauma: A developmental outlook. *J Nerv Ment Dis* 188:409–415, 2000.
43. Pynoos RS, Nader K, Frederick C, et al.: Grief reactions in school age children following a sniper attack at school. *Isr J Psychiatry Relat Sci* 24:53–63, 1987.
44. Goenjian AK, Pynoos RS, Steinberg AM, et al.: Psychiatric comorbidity in children after the 1988 earthquake in Armenia. *J Am Acad Child Adolesc Psychiatry* 34:1174–1184, 1995.
45. Noaghiul S, Prigerson H: Grieving. In: Fink G (ed): *Encyclopedia of Stress* (vol 3). San Diego, CA, Academic Press, 2000, pp. 289–296.
46. Laor N, Wolmer L, Kora M, et al.: Posttraumatic, dissociative and grief symptoms in Turkish children exposed to the 1999 earthquakes. *J Nerv Ment Dis* 190:824–32, 2002.
47. Putnam FW: Development of dissociative disorders. In: Cicchetti D, Cohen DJ (eds): *Developmental Psychopathology. Vol 2: Risk, Disorder, and Adaptation*. New York, John Wiley & Sons, Inc., 1995, pp. 581–608.
48. Shaw JA, Applegate B, Tanner S, et al.: Psychological effects of Hurricane Andrew on an elementary school population. *J Am Acad Child Adolesc Psychiatry* 34:1185–1192, 1995.
49. Husain SA, Nair J, Holcomb W, et al.: Stress reactions of children and adolescents in war and siege conditions. *Am J Psychiatry* 155:1718–1719, 1998.
50. Pfefferbaum B, Nixon SJ, Tucker PM, et al.: Posttraumatic stress responses in bereaved children after the Oklahoma City bombing. *J Am Acad Child Adolesc Psychiatry* 38:1372–1379, 1999.
51. Green BL, Korol M, Grace MC, et al.: Children and disaster: Age, gender, and parental effects on PTSD symptoms. *J Am Acad Child Adolesc Psychiatry* 30:945–951, 1991.
52. Udwin O, Boyle S, Yule W, et al.: Risk factors for long-term psychological effects of a disaster experienced in adolescence: Predictors of posttraumatic stress disorder. *J Child Psychol Psychiatry* 41:969–979, 2000.
53. Lonigan CJ, Shannon MP, Taylor CM, et al.: Children exposed to disaster: II. Risk factors for the development of post-traumatic symptomatology. *J Am Acad Child Adolesc Psychiatry* 33:94–105, 1994.
54. Thabet AA, Vostanis P: Post-traumatic stress disorder in children of war. *J Child Psychol Psychiatry* 40:385–391, 1999.
55. Wolmer L, Laor N, Yazgan Y: School reactivation programs after disaster: Could teachers serve as clinical mediators? *Child Adolesc Psychiatr Clin N Am* 12:363–381, 2003.
56. McFarlane AC: Posttraumatic phenomena in a longitudinal study of children following a natural disaster. *J Am Acad Child Adolesc Psychiatry* 26:764–769, 1987a.
57. Garbarino J, Kostelny K: The effects of political violence on Palestinian children's behavior problems: A risk accumulation model. *Child Dev* 67:33–45, 1996.
58. Gleser G, Green BL, Winget C: *Prolonged Psychosocial Effects of Disaster: A Study of Buffalo Creek*. New York, Academic Press, 1981.
59. Shannon MP, Lonigan CJ, Finch JR AJ, et al.: Children exposed to disaster: I. Epidemiology of post-traumatic symptoms and symptom profiles. *J Am Acad Child Adolesc Psychiatry* 33:80–93, 1994.
60. Masten AS, Best KM, Garmezy N: Resilience and development: Contributions from the study of children who overcome adversity. *Dev Psychopathol* 2:425–444, 1990.
61. Earls F, Smith E, Reich W, et al.: Investigating psychopathological consequences of a disaster in children: A pilot study incorporating a structured diagnostic interview. *J Am Acad Child Adolesc Psychiatry* 27:90–95, 1988.
62. Cohler BM, Stott FM, Musick JS: Adversity, vulnerability, and resilience: Cultural and developmental perspectives. In: Cicchetti D, Cohen DJ (eds): *Developmental Psychopathology. Vol 2: Risk, Disorder, and Adaptation*. New York, John Wiley & Sons, 1995, pp. 753–800.
63. Kassam-Adams N, Garcia-España, JF, Fein JA, et al.: Heart rate and posttraumatic stress in injured children. *Arch Gen Psychiatry* 62:335–340, 2005.
64. Wolmer L, Laor N, Cicchetti DV: Validation of the Comprehensive Assessment of Defense Style (CADS): Mothers' and children's responses to the stresses of missile attacks. *J Nerv Ment Dis* 189:369–376, 2001.
65. Winje D, Ulvik A: Long-term outcome of trauma in children: The psychological consequences of a bus accident. *J Child Psychol Psychiatry* 39:635–642, 1998.

66. Laor N, Wolmer L, Cohen DJ: Mothers' functioning and children's symptoms five years after a Scud missile attack. *Am J Psychiatry* 158:1020–1026, 2001.
67. Bromet EJ, Goldgaber D, Carlson G, et al.: Children's well-being 11 years after the Chernobyl catastrophe. *Arch Gen Psychiatry* 57:563–571, 2000.
68. McFarlane AC: Family functioning and overprotection following a natural disaster: The longitudinal effects of posttraumatic morbidity. *Aust N Z J Psychiatry* 21:210–218, 1987b.
69. Parker JG, Rubin KH, Price JM, et al.: Peer relationships, child development, and adjustment: A developmental psychopathology perspective. In: Cicchetti D, Cohen DJ (eds): *Developmental Psychopathology. Vol 2: Risk, Disorder, and Adaptation.* New York, John Wiley & Sons, 1995, pp. 96–161.
70. Laor N, Wolmer L, Sunar S, et al.: Mother–child short-term group psychotherapy for posttraumatic stress disorder. Presented at the Congress on the Promised Childhood, Tel Aviv, 2001.
71. Cochrane A, Holland W: Validation of screening procedures. *Br Med J* 27:3–8, 1969.
72. Stallard P, Velleman R, Baldwin S: Psychological screening of children for post-traumatic stress disorder. *J Child Psychol Psychiatry* 40:1075–1082, 1999.
73. Green BL: Assessing levels of psychological impairment following disaster: Consideration of actual and methodological dimensions. *J Nerv Ment Dis* 170:544–552, 1982.
74. Ohan JL, Myers K, Collet BR: Ten-year review of rating scales. IV: Scales assessing trauma and its effects. *J Am Acad Child Adolesc Psychiatry* 41:1401–1422, 2002.
75. Strand VC, Sarmiento TL, Pasquale LE: Assessment and screening tools for trauma in children and adolescents. *Trauma, Violence & Abuse* 6:55–78, 2005.
76. Vernberg EM, Vogel JM: Interventions with children after disasters. *J Clin Child Psychol* 22:485–498, 1993.
77. Bass BM, Avolio BJ: *Improving Organizational Effectiveness through Transformational Leadership.* Thousand Oaks, CA, Sage Publications, 1994.
78. Galante R, Foa E: An epidemiological study of psychic trauma and treatment effectiveness after a natural disaster. *J Am Acad Child Adolesc Psychiatry* 25:357–363, 1986.
79. Goenjian AK, Karayan I, Pynoos RS, et al.: Outcome of psychotherapy among early adolescents after trauma. *Am J Psychiatry* 154:536–542, 1997.
80. Wolmer L, Laor N, Kora M: School reactivation after disaster: The case of the Israeli Village. Presented at the Congress on the Promised Childhood, Tel Aviv, 2001.
81. Schwarz ED, Kowalski JM: Malignant memories: Reluctance to utilize mental health services after a disaster. *J Nerv Ment Dis* 180:767–772, 1992.
82. Lindy JD, Grace MC, Green BL: Survivors: Outreach to a reluctant population. *Am J Orthopsychiatry* 51:468–478, 1981.
83. Wolmer L, Laor N, Dedeoglu C, et al.: Teacher-mediated intervention after disaster: A controlled three-year follow-up of children's functioning. *J Child Psychol Psychiatry* 46:1161–1168, 2005.
84. Perrin S, Smith P, Yule W: Practitioner review: The assessment and treatment of post-traumatic stress disorder in children and adolescents. *J Child Psychol Psychiatry* 41:277–289, 2000.
85. Flynn BW, Nelson ME: Understanding the needs of children following large-scale disasters and the role of government. *Child Adolesc Psychiatr Clin North Am* 7:211–227, 1998.
86. Spirman S, Friedman Z, Buchner N: *Mass Emergency Treatment System.* Tel Aviv-Jaffa Municipality, 2001.
87. Stallard P, Law F: Screening and psychological debriefing of adolescent survivors of life-threatening events. *Br J Psychiatry* 163:660–665, 1993.
88. Chemtob CM, Tomas S, Law W, et al.: Postdisaster psychosocial intervention: A field study of the impact of debriefing on psychological stress. *Am J Psychiatry* 154:415–417, 1997.
89. Mayou RA, Ehlers A, Hobbs M: Psychological debriefing for road traffic accident victims. *Br J Psychiatry* 176:589–593, 2000.
90. Wessely S, Rose S, Bisson J: A systematic review of brief psychological interventions ("debriefing") before the treatment of immediate trauma related symptoms and the prevention of post traumatic stress disorder. *Cochrane Library* (vol 4). Oxford, Update Software, 1998.
91. Hobbs M, Mayou R: Debriefing and motor accidents: Interventions and outcomes. In: Raphael B, Wilson JP (eds): *Psychological Debriefing: Theory, Practice and Evidence.* Cambridge, Cambridge University Press, 2000, pp. 145–160.
92. Chemtob CM: Delayed debriefing: After a disaster. In Raphael B, Wilson JP (eds): *Psychological Debriefing: Theory, Practice and Evidence.* Cambridge, Cambridge University Press, 2000, pp. 227–240.
93. Stallard P, Velleman R, Salter E et al.: A randomized controlled trial to determine the effectiveness of an early psychological intervention with children involved in road traffic accidents. *J Child Psychol Psychiatry* 47:127–134, 2006.
94. Klingman A: School-based interventions following a disaster. In: Saylor CF (ed): *Children and Disasters.* New York, Plenum Press, 1993, pp. 187–210.
95. Pynoos RS, Nader K: Psychological first aid and treatment approach to children exposed to community violence: Research implications. *J Trauma Stress* 1:445–473, 1988.
96. Gillis HM: Individual and small group psychotherapy for children involved in trauma and disaster. In: Saylor CF (ed): *Children and Disasters.* New York, Plenum Press, 1993, pp. 165–186.
97. Smith P, Dyregrov A, Yule W et al.: *Children and Disasters: Teaching Recovery Techniques.* Bergen, Norway, Children and War Foundation, 1999.
98. Eth S: Clinical response to traumatized children. In: Austin LS (ed): *Responding to Disaster: A Guide for Mental Health Professionals.* Washington, DC, American Psychiatric Press, 1992, pp. 101–123.
99. Saltzman WR, Layne CM, Sternberg AM, et al.: Developing a culturally and ecologically sound intervention program for youth exposed to war and terrorism. *Child and Adolescent Psychiatric Clinics of North America* 12:319–342, 2003.
100. Lovett J: *Small Wonders: Healing Childhood Trauma with EMDR.* New York, The Free Press, 1999.
101. Toren P, Wolmer L, Rozental B, et al.: Case series: Brief parent–child group therapy for childhood anxiety disorders using a manual-based cognitive-behavioral technique. *J Am Acad Child Adolesc Psychiatry* 39:1309–1312, 2000.
102. Spirman S, Mizrahi C, Refetov, et al.: Development and implementation of a community reactivation program after disasters. Presented at the Congress on the Promised Childhood, Tel-Aviv, 2001.
103. Rappaport J: Terms of empowerment/exemplars of prevention: Toward a theory for community psychology. *Am J Community Psychol* 15:121–145, 1987.
104. Kobasa SC: Stressful life events, personality, and health: An inquiry into hardiness. *J Pers Soc Psychol* 37:1–11, 1979.
105. Shiloh R, Nutt D, Weizman A: *Atlas of Psychiatric Pharmacotherapy*, London, Martin Dunitz, 1999, p. 191.
106. Donnelly CL: Pharmacologic treatment approaches for children and adolescents with posttraumatic stress disorder. *Child Adolesc Psychiatr Clin N Am* 12:251–269, 2003.
107. Marshall RD, Davidson JRT, Yehuda R: Pharmacotherapy in the treatment of posttraumatic stress disorder and other trauma-related syndromes. In: Yehuda R (ed): *Psychological Trauma.* Washington, DC, American Psychiatric Press, Inc., 1998.
108. Cohen RE: The Armero tragedy: Lessons for mental health professionals. *Hosp Community Psychiatry* 38:1316–1321, 1987.
109. Congressional Reports: H. Rpt. 109-377—A Failure of Initiative: Final Report of the Select Bipartisan Committee to Investigate the Preparation for and Response to Hurricane Katrina. Retrieved April 17, 2005 at http://www.gpoaccess.gov/serialset/creports/katrina.html.

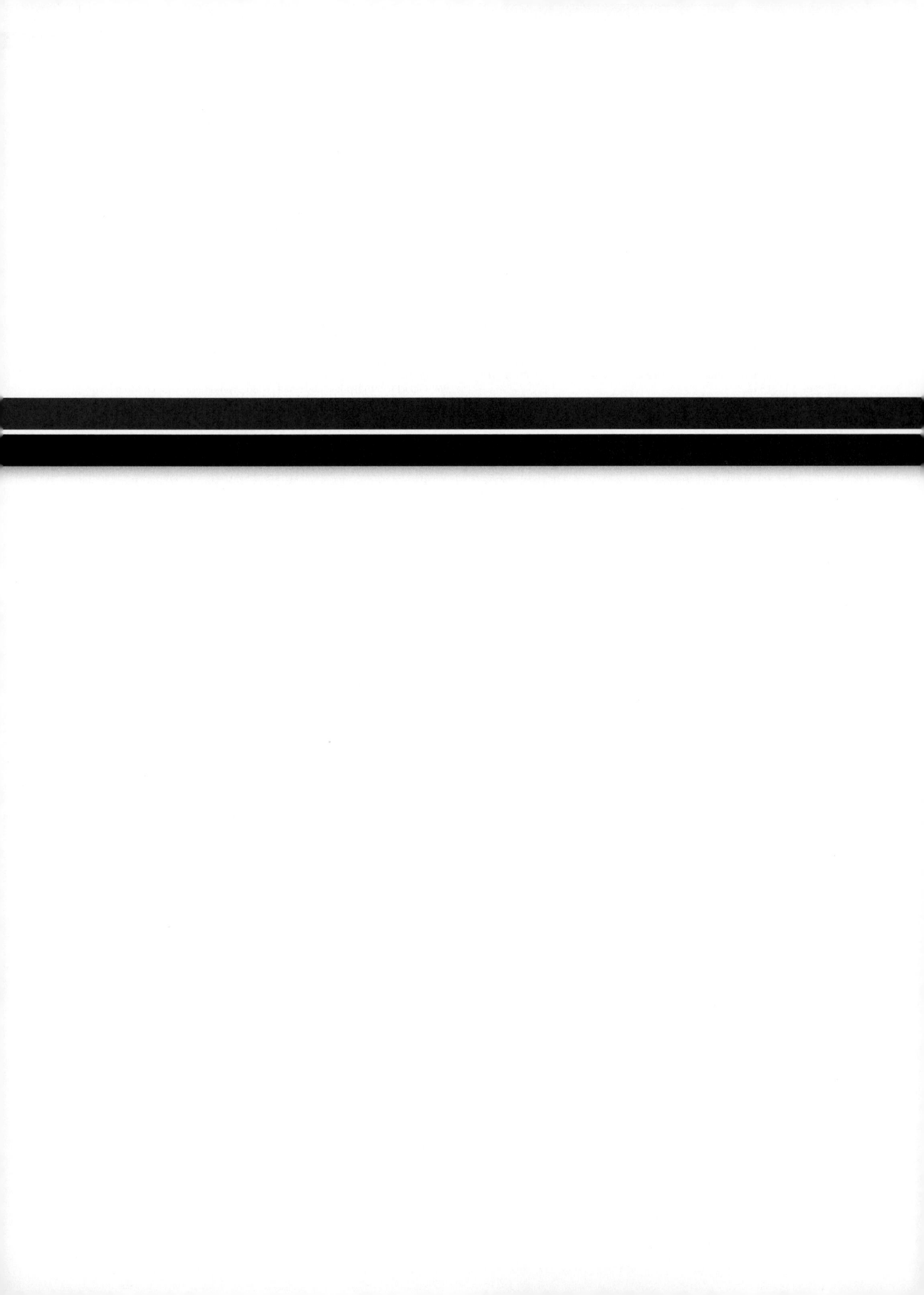

SECTION VI
TREATMENT

CHAPTER 6.1.1 ■ CLINICAL AND DEVELOPMENTAL ASPECTS OF PHARMACOKINETICS AND DRUG INTERACTIONS

JESSICA R. OESTERHELD, RICHARD I. SHADER, AND ANDRÉS MARTIN

OVERVIEW

In the first part of this chapter, the concept of pharmacokinetics is differentiated from pharmacodynamics, and basic clinical pharmacokinetic principles that are shared by children, adolescents, and adults are reviewed, including therapeutic drug monitoring. Next, the pharmacokinetic differences that distinguish pediatric populations from adults are examined, highlighting the ontogeny of individual P450 cytochromes (CYPs), intestinal and hepatic influx and efflux transporters, and UDP-glucuronylsyltransferases (UGTs). Finally, since one of the more clinically relevant applications of pharmacokinetic principles is in helping to understand (and at times to predict) important drug interactions, emphasis has been placed on presenting basic principles that underlie drug interactions and the real-world strategies to prevent them. This chapter serves as a complement to the following and related chapter, in which specific drug classes and individual agents are discussed in detail.

PHARMACOKINETICS AND PHARMACODYNAMICS

Pharmacokinetic principles relate to the handling and disposition of drugs within the body (i.e., those biological processes that lead to changes over time in drug concentration in body tissues and fluids). In general, drug concentration in a target organ determines how long a drug's therapeutic and adverse effects will last. Changes during development in the processes of drug absorption, distribution, metabolism, and excretion may have an impact on the delivery of drug to target tissues. By contrast, pharmacodynamic principles are concerned with the biochemical and physiological effects of drugs at their effect sites, with their specific mechanisms of action. Stated succinctly, pharmacokinetics refers to what the body does to a drug and pharmacodynamics to what a drug does to the body (Figure 6.1.1.1). The effects of a medication may change during development, as brain regions or neurotransmitter systems develop and mature at different rates. These developmental changes in neurochemical systems (pharmacodynamic systems) can influence both therapeutic response and side effect profile. For example: 1) Compared to adults, adolescents have a higher risk of dystonic reactions to conventional antipsychotics agent (1, 2); 2) prepubertal children appear to be at a higher risk for the activating side effects of the SSRIs (3), and 3) developmental differences in the maturation of noradrenergic pathways may explain, at least in part, why tricyclic antidepressants are less effective in children with depression as compared to adults (4). Taken together, these findings suggest that major neurochemical systems that are altered by psychotropic drug treatments (e.g., dopaminergic, serotonergic, and noradrenergic, respectively) are subject to age-related effects.

BASIC PRINCIPLES

An understanding of pharmacokinetic principles is important for safe and effective patient care. Pharmacokinetic factors are often critical in a variety of clinical decisions, such as choosing between agents within a same drug class, switching between different medication preparations, adjusting dosages, preventing drug interactions, or correctly utilizing and interpreting therapeutic drug levels.

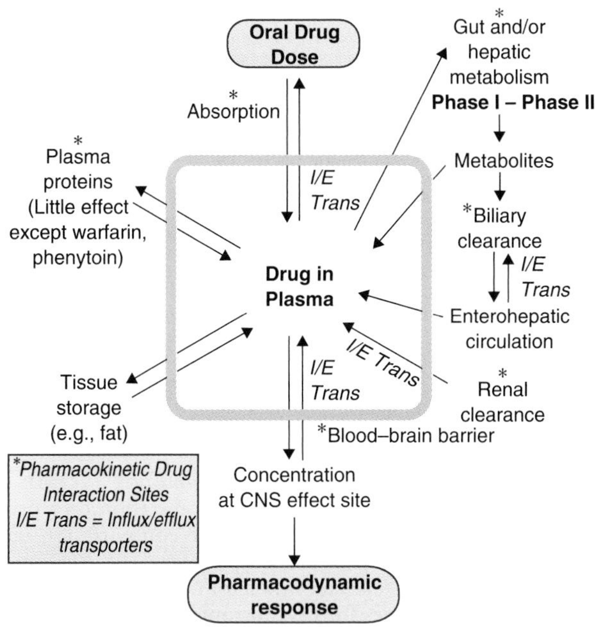

FIGURE 6.1.1.1. Pharmacokinetics and pharmacodynamics of a CNS drug.

Pharmacokinetics can be conceptualized as having four functionally distinct phases: absorption, distribution, metabolism, and excretion. Absorption and distribution are primarily responsible for determining the speed of onset of drug effect, while the processes of metabolism and excretion terminate the action of the pharmacologic agent by removing the active form of the drug from the body. Taken together, these four phases help to determine the duration of drug activity (5).

Once a drug gains entry to the bloodstream, it is diluted in the plasma and bound at varying degrees to plasma proteins. The drug, usually protein-bound, is then either excreted by the kidneys or carried to the liver and transformed to a more water-soluble (and usually inactive) metabolite, which can then be excreted in urine or bile. This complicated and interdependent series of events is designed to reduce the effect of foreign molecules, with the ultimate goal of eliminating the drug from the body (Figure 6.1.1.1). If the dose of a drug is sufficiently large to withstand this "pharmacokinetic assault," then a fraction of a psychoactive drug will cross the blood–brain barrier and endure to produce its pharmacodynamic effect (5). The last step of this process presumes that the drug in question is not a substrate for blood–brain barrier transport proteins that keep certain entities from reaching the brain.

LINEAR AND NON-LINEAR PHARMACOKINETICS

A basic working knowledge of key pharmacokinetics principles is relevant to the clinical practice of pediatric psychopharmacology to understand the fate of administered drugs. Some psychotropic medications follow *first-order* (or *linear) kinetics*, in which the amount of drug eliminated is proportional to its amount circulating in the bloodstream. Once alterations during absorption have taken place, first-order kinetics provide close to a one-to-one relationship between changes in dosage and in plasma concentration. Such a linear association generally allows for clinically relevant predictions of the impact of a dose change on circulating drug levels [bupropion SR (6), oxcarbazepine (7).] By contrast, *zero-order* (or *non-linear) kinetics* prevail when metabolizing or eliminating mechanisms are exceeded or saturated. This results in a fixed amount of drug being eliminated per unit of time, regardless of the plasma level. Certain drugs [paroxetine (8), nefazodone (9)] demonstrate zero-order kinetics at clinically relevant doses, making the relationship between dose changes and subsequent plasma levels much less predictable.

Vignette 1

A 12-year-old boy with a diagnosis of obsessive-compulsive disorder is not responding to 10 mg of paroxetine. Would an increase to 20 mg be appropriate? When the dosing of paroxetine is increased from 10 mg to 20 mg per day in children and teens, the plasma concentration can increase nearly seven-fold instead of a predicted two-fold if the drug's kinetics were linear (8). Paroxetine inhibits its own catabolic pathway (CYP 2D6) and interferes with its own elimination. It could be prudent to increase the dose to 12.5 mg per day.

MULTIPLE DOSING TO AVERAGE STEADY STATE CONCENTRATION

For drugs that follow first-order kinetics, the concepts of elimination half-life and of steady-state concentration are relevant for the practicing clinician. The elimination half-life ($t_{1/2}$) is the time required for the concentration of drug to decrease by one-half. This term is also referred to as the beta-phase half-life or the biologic half-life. We prefer the term elimination half-life since it makes this concept distinct from the half-life of absorption and the half-life of biologic activity. In clinical practice, this parameter is usually assessed by measuring the decay of plasma or serum drug concentration and is referred to as the plasma or serum half-life. Plasma half-life values can be useful when determining dosing intervals. At consistent dosing intervals, it is the plasma half-life that determines the average plasma *steady-state concentration* (C_{SS}). Css is reached when there is an equilibrium between the amount of drug ingested and the amount of drug eliminated, resulting in no net change in plasma concentration over time, and it is attained after four to five half-lives. The same time is necessary for reaching a new Css if daily dosing is increased or decreased or for complete elimination after drug intake is abruptly stopped (Figure 6.1.1.2). Most of the drugs commonly used in child psychiatry reach Css. However, in extensive CYP 2D6 metabolizers, neither psychostimulants nor atomoxetine does because of very short half-lives and therapeutic effectiveness at low concentrations. Carbamazepine, which induces its own metabolism, may take a much greater time to reach Css.

Vignette 2

A 14-year-old girl with major depression has failed a trial of fluoxetine, and she has been treated with 150 mg of twice-daily bupropion SR for 2 weeks. She has developed adverse cognitive effects. The clinician wishes to know if he discontinues the drug, how long before the adverse effects are likely to diminish. The half-life of bupropion SR in youth is approximately 12 hours (6), and in four to five half-lives or 2 to 3 days, it will be eliminated. This is an approximate answer because certain side effects may have a different concentration response relationship from the main therapeutic effects.

THERAPEUTIC DRUG MONITORING

Css is sometimes misunderstood by clinicians to imply an absence of daily peak and trough concentrations. Peak and trough concentrations exist within each dosing interval, and

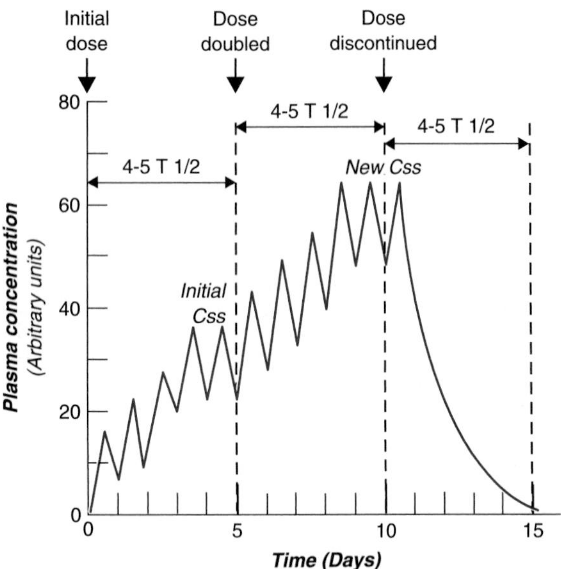

FIGURE 6.1.1.2. Multiple drug dosing leads to steady-state concentration.

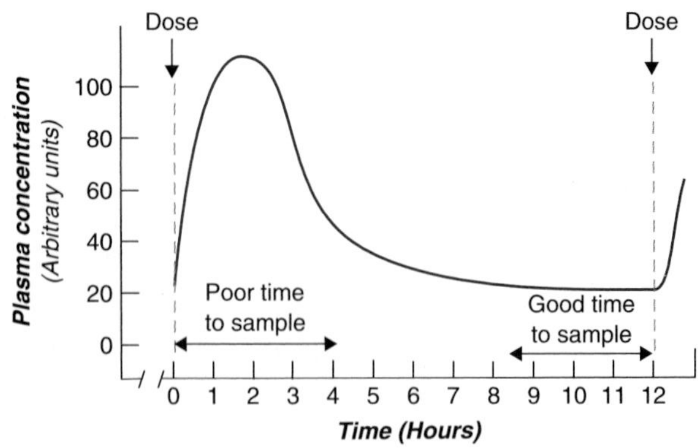

FIGURE 6.1.1.4. Idealized plasma curve.

when maximum and minimum drug concentrations are the same with two or more successive doses, Css is reached (Figure 6.1.1.2. Dosing some drugs once a day because they have a sufficiently long half-life may lead to excessive peak concentrations that can be associated with toxicity or increased adverse effects (e.g., clozapine is dosed twice daily because of potential for seizures at peak concentration). As Figure 6.1.1.3 shows, if the initial dose is doubled and dosed once daily, the peak concentration exceeds the desired concentration to toxicity, but if the original dose is doubled but given twice daily, the concentration is above the plasma concentration that is likely to produce a clinical effect, the minimal effective concentration (MEC), but below toxic levels, the maximal tolerable concentration.

Clinicians must tailor drug dosing and frequency to maximize the probability of drug efficacy and to minimize toxicity. Some drugs (lithium, valproate, carbamazepine, nortriptyline) that have narrow therapeutic indices, significant consequences associated with toxicity, wide interpatient variability, and no clinical endpoint to guide drug dosing, are candidates for therapeutic drug monitoring (TDM). A final requirement must be met: The concentration of a drug must have a proportional relation to the concentration and the pharmacologic action at the receptor site (10). Ranges of concentrations have been established for drugs that meet these requirements, and values for psychotropic drugs used by child psychiatrists are given in Chapter 6.1.2.

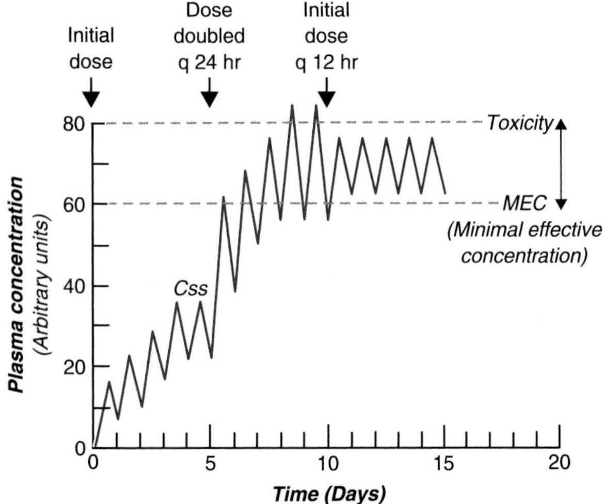

FIGURE 6.1.1.3. Changes in plasma concentration with changes in amount of drug or frequency of dosing.

The range between subtherapeutic and toxic doses, or *therapeutic range* (sometimes called the therapeutic window) is a misnomer of sorts, since even when drug concentration is within the range, not every youth will respond to the drug, and a percentage will experience toxicity. For some drugs, there are data only on the MEC. Therapeutic drug monitoring (TDM) can reveal individuals with unusual metabolism (see the metabolism section), uncover nonadherance, demonstrate increased or decreased concentration with the addition of other drugs (see drug interaction section), and confirm toxicity. TDM provides information that supplements clinical assessment.

There are two common errors in using TDM: not waiting for Css to occur before drawing a blood sample, and not drawing the blood sample at trough level.

As Figure 6.1.1.4 shows, sampling at "trough," or just before the next dose, offers the flattest part of the curve. For drugs given two or three times daily, sampling blood concentration *before the* AM *dose in the morning* is recommended, and for drugs given once daily, sampling *before the next dose* is suggested.

Vignette 3

A 17-year-old girl with bipolar disorder has been maintained on 600 mg of lithium carbonate twice daily. A trough level of lithium of 0.8 mEq/l has been maintained for 8 months, with reduction in her symptoms. Parents phone the clinician because their daughter is nauseated and vomiting. As previously instructed, the teen has not been given her morning medication. The finding of a trough level of 1.4 mEq/l initiates careful inquiry and reveals that friends have been giving her ibuprofen for menstrual cramps. By inhibiting prostaglandins, NSAIDs affect renal blood flow and thus the renal clearance of lithium (11).

PHARMACOKINETICS IN CHILDREN AND ADOLESCENTS

There are many pharmacokinetic similarities between adults and children and adolescents. Indeed, age-independent genetic influences on metabolism can be more salient than those influences attributable to age and developmental change. Nonetheless, children and adolescents do display unique pharmacokinetic parameters. Premature infants, neonates, toddlers, children, and adolescents are not a homogenous group in terms of drug distribution patterns (12). These differences can be especially dramatic both at the neonatal stage and around the time of puberty, when the release of gonadal hormones can strongly influence plasma drug concentrations (13).

FACTORS AFFECTING DRUG DISPOSITION

Absorption and Bioavailability

Drugs gain entry into the body through a variety of portals. The *bioavailability* of a medication in the systemic circulation—the amount of unbound drug available to exert a biological effect on target tissues—is determined by its absorption and, for orally administered medications, by *presystemic clearance (first pass effect)* from intestinal and hepatic transporters, metabolism, and conjugation (see next section) and protein binding. Drugs have variable *first pass effects.* Some drugs are metabolized very efficiently on first pass (60 to 70%) and others less so (less than 30%). Bioavailability measures the completeness of drug absorption, and it is determined in reference to intravenous dosing. Oral administration is by far the most common portal of entry but often the most unpredictable in terms of final bioavailability. Some drugs are given to children as tinctures or in alcohol-based syrups. Although drugs like penicillin G are absorbed in the stomach, most psychotropic medications are absorbed in the proximal small intestine.

Little information is available regarding the effect of age on the absorption of psychotropic medications, although there are several theoretical considerations regarding the influence of this process in children and adolescents. A major factor influencing gastrointestinal absorption is pH-dependent diffusion. In infants, the gastric pH is nearly neutral in the first week after birth. It slowly reaches adult values by age three years (14). In toddlers, stomach contents tend to be less acidic than in adults, causing weakly acidic drugs to be more highly ionized. Because it is the un-ionized fraction that is absorbed from the stomach, weakly acidic drugs may be absorbed more slowly in children. This process theoretically could affect phenobarbital and other anticonvulsants, amphetamines, and antidepressants (15).

Other factors that could reduce overall absorption are gastric and intestinal transit time. Gastric transit time is likely increased in neonates and infants, and the age of maturation is not known (14). Intestinal transit time is increased and the absorptive surface area of the intestine is reduced in young children, suggesting that drugs with a long phase of absorption (e.g., carbamazepine) and some sustained-release preparations may be incompletely absorbed (16). It is important to remember that although the rate at which many drugs are absorbed is slower in neonates and infants, there are no data indicating a generally reduced absorption of orally administered drugs in prepubertal children or teenagers (17).

Intestinal Influx and Efflux Transporters and Intestinal Metabolism

Until 10 to 15 years ago, it was believed that the first-pass effect was limited to the hepatic metabolic enzymes and conjugation, and that diffusion was the only mechanism involved in absorption in the small intestine. It was known that lipid-soluble drugs passively diffuse through the apical membrane of the small intestine, that some small hydrophilic ionized drugs squeeze through intracellular junctions, and that both types of drugs cross the cytosol and exit the basolateral membrane into the portal circulation (18). It is now known that non–lipid-soluble drugs are also actively transported (both imported and exported) across these liminal boundaries by members of the solute carrier family of transporter proteins that currently includes 43 subfamilies and 298 transporter genes (19, 20) (Figure 6.1.1.5). Several names exist for each transporter especially in the earlier literature.

Best characterized of these influx transporters is the peptide transporter 1, PEPT1, SLC15A1. This transporter uses the intestinal-cellular proton gradient as a source of energy to ferry dipeptides and tripeptides across the apical membrane. Hundreds of peptides and other molecules are possible substrates (beta-lactam antibiotics, ACE inhibitors, thrombin inhibitors, acyclovir, sulpiride, and others). After crossing to the cytosol, these drugs are shepherded across to the portal circulation by a second peptide transporter embedded in the basolateral membrane (21) (Figure 6.1.1.5). Although the development of SLC15A1 has been studied in mice and rats, there is no information about when it matures in humans. Targeting the peptide transport system represents a new strategy for drug delivery of poorly absorbed drugs. Acyclovir, a polar antiviral drug, is poorly absorbed from the intestine, but if the L-valyl ester pro-drug valacyclovir is given, it is transported by SLC15A1, and therapeutic levels can be obtained. The ester drugs like methylphenidate are also hydrolyzed by plasma esterases. In the case of methylphenidate, the inactive metabolite ritalinic acid is formed. In the case of acyclovir, an active metabolite is formed.

Efflux transporters are also embedded in both of the intestinal membranes. Members of a superfamily of transporters that use ATP as an energy source (ATP-binding cassette transporters or ABC transporters (20) can flip compounds which have entered the cytosol back into the intestinal lumen on the apical side and from the cytosol into the portal system on the basolateral side (Figure 6.1.1.5). Efflux transporters act not only to limit drug absorption and bioavailability in the intestine, but they efflux compounds into the biliary system and the kidney, protect "sanctuaries" such as the brain (Figure 6.1.1.1), and are responsible in part for resistance to cancer drugs.

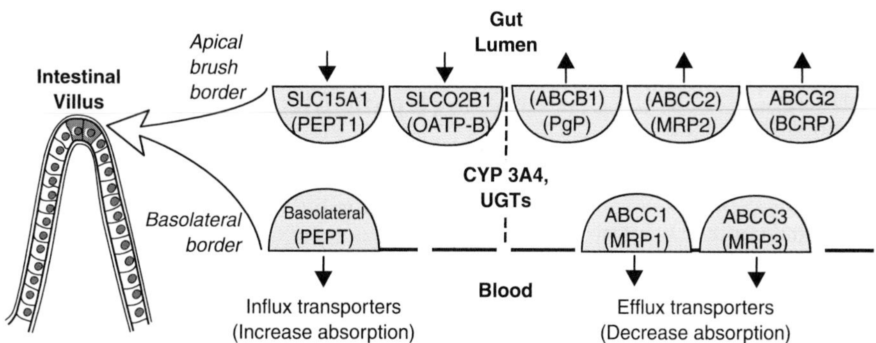

FIGURE 6.1.1.5. Intestinal transporters.

About 30 years ago, Juliano and Ling (22) noted that after initial efficacy, many oncologic drugs stopped being effective at the same time; they named this phenomenon multiple drug resistance (MDR). A gene on chromosome seven (MDR1) was found to encode a glycoprotein (P-glycoprotein, P-gp) that pumps out compounds from cells. Multiple drugs were affected at the same time because all of them were P-gp substrates.

P-gp is now numbered 1 of subfamily B of superfamily ABC (ABCB1). Other members of this family involved in efflux drug transport are in subfamily C (Figure 6.1.1.5). There is an avalanche of *in vitro* data on what compounds are substrates of these transporters, and how other drugs, foods, or genetic variations can affect ABCB1. Since ABCB1 is saturable *in vivo*, only drugs that are therapeutic in low doses can be shown to be affected [digoxin, talinolol, fexofenadine, (23)]. Drugs that affect ABCB1 either through inhibition or induction represent a new form of drug interaction. For example, quinidine, an inhibitor of ABCB1, blocks the efflux of digoxin in the kidney, and more digoxin will be absorbed and enter the circulation [(23); see drug interaction section].

In the intestine, both ABCB1 and CYP 3A4 are located in the endoplasmic reticulum. There is a considerable overlap in compounds that are substrates of both (dexamethasone, diltiazem, vincristine).

ABCB1 and CYP 3A4 act together as an intestinal defense tag-team to protect against exogenous compounds: ABCB1 provides a barrier to absorption and any remaining compound is converted by CYP 3A4 to less active metabolites [(24); see metabolism section and drug interaction section]. Levels of both ABCB1 and CYP 3A4 are higher in the intestine than in the liver, and there is a growing awareness of the importance of these intestinal proteins as compared to hepatic ABCB1/CYP 3A4 in first-pass metabolism. There is no coordination between the duodenal and the hepatic tag-teams, and in each organ there is a different ontogeny of CYPs and ABCB1 [(25); see metabolism section]. ABCB1 is also found in the blood–brain barrier, in the prostate, and in the placenta.

Drug Distribution and Plasma Proteins

Following absorption, drugs are distributed into intravascular and various extravascular spaces. Numerous physical factors can influence the distribution of a drug throughout the body: the size of body water compartments and adipose tissue depots, cardiac output, regional blood flow, organ perfusion pressure, permeability of cell membranes, acid-base balance, and binding to plasma and tissue proteins (13). Each of these factors may change during development, resulting in changes in the distribution of a drug and, subsequently, in its pharmacological effect.

Drugs are transported in the general circulation in two forms that are in dynamic equilibrium with each other: bound to plasma protein (acidic drugs to albumin and basic drugs to alpha 1-acid glycoproteins) and unbound (free). Only the unbound drug is usually available to pass across membranes and to have pharmacological effects. Although albumin and alpha 1-acid glycoproteins are reduced in the neonate and infant, this does not appear to be an important developmental factor in older children and adolescents (14, 17).

Two important factors affecting distribution that change substantially during development are fat stores and the relative proportion of total body water to extracellular water. The relationship between the amount of drug absorbed (D), also referred to as the concentration at time zero, plasma concentration (Cp), and volume of distribution (Vd) can be summarized by the simple equation: $Cp = D/Vd$. Note that the larger the Vd, the smaller the Cp. The proportion of body fat is highest in the first year of life, followed by a steady decrease until an increase occurs prepubertally (12, 26). The adipose tissue of infants has a lower ratio of lipid to water (17). The relative volume of extracellular water is high in children and tends to decrease with development. For example, total body water decreases gradually from about 85% of body weight in a small premature infant to about 70% in the full-term newborn to about 60% in the 1-year-old infant, a level that is generally maintained throughout adulthood. Similarly, extracellular water decreases gradually from about 40 to 50% of body weight in the newborn to about 15 to 20% by age 10 to 15 years (27). Thus, if weight-based drug administration is utilized, infants will tend to have lower drug plasma levels (17). Drugs that are primarily distributed in body water (lithium) can be expected to have a lower plasma concentration in the pediatric population compared with that in adults because the volume of distribution is higher in children and early adolescents.

Another consideration in distribution of drugs in preterm newborns and infants is the relative permeability of the blood–brain barrier when compared with that in children and adults (14). The blood–brain barrier is formed by capillary endothelial cells that have very tight junctions. Paracellular passive diffusion of hydrophilic substances is blocked, and only low molecular weight lipophilic agents can cross the blood–brain barrier. The increased permeability of the blood–brain barrier in infants could result in increased bioavailability of drugs within the central nervous system (CNS), as with anticonvulsants (28).

Compounds can also gain entry into the CNS via solute carrier family transporters [blood to brain, (29)]. Efflux transporters (especially ABCB1 and ABC subfamily C) in astrocytes and brain capillary cells guard entry to the brain by "flipping" out substrates (amitriptyline, quetiapine, and risperidone (30). Although the ontogeny of ABCB1 is incompletely understood, there is a suggestion that premature infants may have reduced levels (31).

HEPATIC INFLUX AND EFFLUX TRANSPORTERS AND METABOLISM

Influx and Efflux Transporters

After absorption, drugs are carried to the liver via the portal system. Many drugs are able to passively enter hepatocytes, but large or ionized drugs need active transport. They are transported across the membrane by a variety of solute family carriers, and they are exposed to cytosol CYPs and glucuronide conjugates. Bile acids are similarly transported via specialized influx transporters (the sodium/bile acid cotransporter, NTCP, SLC10A1).

Drugs can be effluxed from hepatocytes into the bile canniculi via ABC transporters, (ABCB1 and ABCC2 transporters), while bile salts have their own unique carrier (bile salt export pump, BSEP, ABCB11). Other ABC efflux transporters can pump out drugs back into the venous circulation (32).

Hepatic Metabolism

Most psychotropic drugs are lipid soluble, which is usually a necessary requirement for absorption, distribution, and availability at receptor sites. To be effectively excreted, however, *lipophilic* drugs need to be metabolized to more polar or *hydrophilic* forms (having a greater affinity for water). Although some drugs are renally excreted unmetabolized (lithium, gabapentin), most undergo extensive biotransformation in the intestine and the liver (33) (Figure 6.1.1.6).

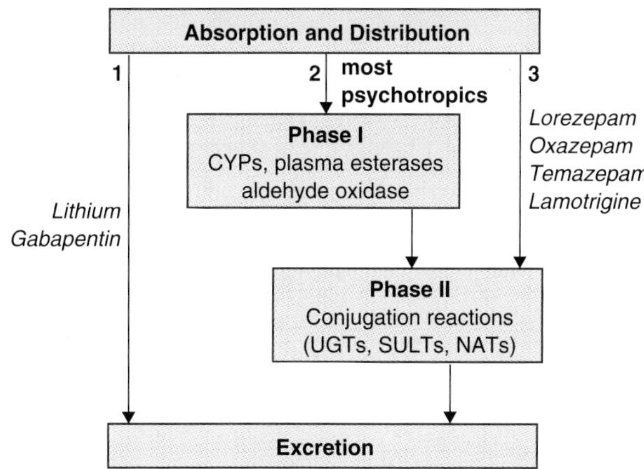

FIGURE 6.1.1.6. Phase 1/2.

Phase 1 metabolic reactions, including *hydroxylation, reduction*, and *hydrolysis*, convert drugs to forms more suitable for elimination. Intestinal and hepatic CYPs are the most important enzyme systems responsible for phase I reactions, and others include plasma esterases that metabolize methylphenidate, flavin-containing monooxygenases, and aldehyde oxidase (Figure 6.1.1.6). The products of phase I reactions, collectively referred to as *metabolites*, are usually less active and less toxic than their parent compounds. Notable exceptions of clinical significance are desipramine, the demethylated active metabolite of imipramine, and norfluoxetine, the demethylated long-lived active metabolite of fluoxetine. These metabolites have comparable toxicities to their parent compounds and comparable therapeutic activity.

In *phase II reactions, conjugation* of metabolites generated in phase I takes place with glucuronic acid, sulfate, or others. Conjugated compounds are then readily excreted in urine or other body fluids. It is clinically important to note that some drugs are never metabolized in a phase I reaction and instead simply undergo conjugation by Phase II enzymes (Figure 6.1.1.6). Drugs such as the 3-hydroxybenzodiazepines (lorazepam, oxazepam, temazepam) are conjugated by glucuronidation, and they are rapidly cleared at equal rates regardless of age as long as renal function is normal (34). These drugs are preferred in instances of liver insufficiency because other benzodiazepines depend on cytochromes for metabolism, which may be more influenced by hepatic dysfunction than is glucuronidation.

Cytochromes (CYPs)

CYPs are heme-containing enzymes, located principally in the intestine and liver, that metabolize two types of substrates: endogenous (the body's own steroids, lipids, fatty acids) and exogenous (toxins, drugs). CYPs that metabolize exogenous compounds are located in the endoplasmic reticulum. The sequencing of CYP amino acids has led to a classification system based on similarity (35): Arabic numbers 1 to 4 designate family members, letters A–E label subfamily members, and Arabic numbers note specific enzymes (isoform, gene). CYP 3A4, for example, is a member of family 3, subfamily A, and enzyme 4. The CYPs that are near each other on the same gene and are related are grouped together (CYP 3A4, CYP 3A5, CYP 3A7) and referred collectively as CYP 3A. It is the major CYP family involved in human hepatic drug metabolism, handling about half of psychotropic drugs. CYP 3A constitutes 30% of total CYP hepatic content and 70% of intestinal CYP content, and it serves as a high-capacity reservoir. The other clinically relevant CYPs include 1A2, 2B6, 2C9, 2C19, 2D6, and 2E1.

Most psychotropic drugs undergo both Phase I and Phase II reactions (Figure 6.1.1.6). A few drugs are metabolized by only one CYP (desipramine via CYP 2D6, triazolam via CYP 3A). Some others undergo Phase II conjugation only (lorazepam, oxazepam, and lamotrigine are glucuronidated only). However, most drugs require multiple CYPs to be completely metabolized. As examples, sertraline is N-demethylated via six different pathways (36), and clomipramine (CMI) demethylated by CYP 1A2, CYP 2C19, and CYP 3A to desmethylclomipramine (DCMI), an active metabolite that is then hydroxylated by CYP 2D6. In addition, CMI is directly hydroxylated by CYP 2D6.

CYP-based metabolism of drugs is influenced by genetic factors. Seven to 10% of Caucasians have a genetic deficiency of CYP 2D6 and are thus less efficient at metabolizing CYP 2D6 substrates, including many psychotropic agents. For these "slow metabolizers," blood levels of drugs metabolized by 2D6 may increase considerably as unmetabolized drug enters the blood. Some Asian individuals have a 2D6 variant that causes them to be "somewhat slow" metabolizers, and they require lower dosing of relevant drugs to achieve therapeutic blood levels. Some African Americans also have an allelic variant of CYP 2D6 that is linked to slow or poor metabolism of CYP 2D6 substrates. CYP 2C9 and CYP 2C19 are also genetically polymorphic. One to 3% of Caucasians are slow metabolizers of CYP 2C9, and 18 to 23% of Japanese and 2 to 3% of Caucasians and African Americans are slow metabolizers of CYP 2C19 (37). Fewer than five Caucasians in 1,000 are slow metabolizers of both CYP 2D6 and CYP 2C19, putting them at particular risk for high levels of substrates that are metabolized by *both* pathways (certain tricyclics, propranolol, citalopram).

It has been possible to ascertain the CYP genetic status of individuals for some time, but in the last year, the FDA has approved a diagnostic DNA chip for CYP 2D6 (27 variants) and CYP 2C19 (two variants) (38). Clinicians can consider testing youth who have adverse effects with substrate CYP 2C19 or CYP 2D6 drugs at usual therapeutic doses (poor metabolizers or intermediate metabolizers) or who have poor responses with substrate CYP 2D6 drugs at usual therapeutic doses (ultrarapid metabolizer) (39).

UDP-Glucuronylsyltransferases (UGTs)

Located close to the CYPs in the endoplasmic reticulum, UGTs are a superfamily of membrane-based enzymes that catalyze the transfer of glucuronic acid to endogenous or exogenous compounds. They are considered to be the principal phase II system by virtue of the number of different types of compounds they conjugate, as well as their superior quantity compared to other phase II enzymes. The nomenclature of UGTs is similar to CYPs, being designated by family, subfamily, and gene (UGT 1A1, UGT 2B7).

There are two families of UGTs, UGT 1, and UGT 2, and three subfamilies (UGT 1A, UGT 2A, and UGT 2B). The subfamily of UGT 1A shares exons two to five in common, and they are distinguished by a unique exon one. UGT 1A1 is the most abundant UGT 1 in the liver (40). UGT 2A and UGT 2B are encoded by separated genes. Like CYPs, individual UGTs have both unique and overlapping substrates (Table 6.1.1.1), and they have tissue-specific patterns of expression and genetic variations.

Unlike CYPs, UGTs handle both endogenous and exogenous compounds. Thus, deficient glucuronidation as a result of genetic polymorphism or UGT inhibition can lead to increased levels of both endogenous and exogenous substrates. For example, UGT 1A1 is the only conjugative pathway for bilirubin. Gilbert's syndrome (in which UGT 1A1 activity is reduced by about 70%) is characterized by a benign fluctuating

TABLE 6.1.1.1

UGT TABLE

	UGT1A1	UGT1A3	UGT1A4	UGT1A6	UGT1A9	UGT2B7	UGT2B15
Chromosome	2	2	2	2	2	4	4
Genetic Variation	yes	yes	yes	yes	yes	yes	yes
Some Endogenous substrates	bilirubin estriol	estrones	androsterone progestins	serotonin	thyroxine	androsterone bile acid	dihyrotestosterone
Some Substrate drugs	acetaminophen buprenorphine ethinyl estradiol ibuprofen irinotecan mb-SN-38 nicotine phenytoin	buprenorphine (chlorpromazine) (clozapine) cyproheptadine diphenhydramine doxepin (ibuprofen) (valproate)	(amitriptyline) chlorpromazine clomipramine clozapine diphenhydramine cyproheptadine diphenhydramine doxepin imipramine lamotrigine loxapine olanzapine phenytoin trifluoperazine	acetaminophen phenytoin valproate	acetaminophen ethinyl estradiol ibuprofen phenytoin valproate	carbamazepine ibuprofen lamotrigine lorazepam morphines propranolol sertraline valproate zidovudine	desloratadine s-oxazepam s-lorazepam
Possible Inducers	dexamethasone phenobarbital phenytoin		carbamazepine ethinyl estradiol (oxcarbamazepine) phenobarbital phenytoin rifampin	dexamethasone	phenobarbital	phenobarbital phenytoin rifampin	
Possible Inhibitors	ketoconazole probenecid	imipramine probenecid	probenecid	probenecid	probenecid ketoconazole valproate	codeine diazepam ketoconazole morphine probenecid valproate	ibuprofen ketoconazole probenecid valproate

() = Minor pathway.

bilirubinemia in association with illness or stress. Individuals with Gilbert's syndrome can also develop toxic levels of SN-38, the active metabolite of the cancer chemotherapy agent, irinotecan, because UGT 1A1 is an important conjugative pathway for SN-38. The influence of polymorphisms of individual UGTs has been shown to correlate with clinical outcomes of psychotropic drugs such as clozapine, imipramine, and cyproheptadine (UGT 1A4, 41), with levels of the active enantiomer of oxazepam (UGT 2B15, 42), and with intolerance to morphine (UGT 2B7, 43). A new rapid genetic test for UGT 1A1 has been approved by the FDA (44).

The clinical application of knowledge about UGTs has lagged at least a decade behind CYPs, but it may become increasingly clinically relevant. At present, clinicians must understand UGT-based drug interactions to appropriately use lamotrigine, olanzapine, and others (see drug interaction section).

Ontogeny of Hepatic CYPs and Phase II Enzymes

In the neonate, activities of hepatic CYP-mediated metabolism and the phase II reactions, UGTs, glutathione conjugation (GST) and acetylation (NAT) are decreased, but some types of sulfate conjugation function efficiently. Since sulfation is a major conjugative pathway of acetaminophen, individuals have speculated that this is the reason why young children are more resistant to the toxic effects of this drug (45).

Neither CYPs nor Phase II enzymes come "on line" at the same time, and each has a unique ontogeny. CYP 3A7 is the predominant fetal CYP. In the first few weeks after birth, CYP 3A4 gradually appears and increases as CYP 3A7 peaks at two weeks and fades (46). CYP 3A5 is variably present in some individuals, and it appears to be under genetic control. CYP 2D6, CYP 2C9, and CYP 2C19 become active in the first weeks of life. CYP 2E1 gradually develops over the first 3 months (47). CYP 1A2 is the last CYP to appear at the fourth or fifth month (48). Clinicians must take account of these changes in dosing premature infants and neonates. For example, clinicians must decrease the dosing of midazolam, a CYP 3A4 and CYP 3A5 substrate, as infants are increasing their ability to metabolize it (49).

Each CYP has a unique development. CYP 2C19 levels are highly variable from 5 months to 10 years, and levels approach adult values by 10 years of age (50). CYP 2D6 matures to adult levels by 10 years or earlier (46). There is some evidence that levels of CYP 3A4 are actually lower in youth aged 5 to 15 years than in adults (51). CYP 2C9 gradually increase over the first 5 months (and as many as half of individuals may reach adult values), exceeds adult activity in youth from 3 to 10 years, and achieves adult activity after puberty (50). CYP 1A2 activity in childhood exceeds adult levels until after puberty (girls, Tanner stage two; boys, Tanner stage four) (52).

There is less known about the development of hepatic Phase II enzymes. The bilirubinemia of premature infants occurs because of the immaturity of hepatic UGT 1A1. Low levels of neonatal UGT 2B7 are responsible for the toxicity of chloramphenical, the so-called *grey-baby syndrome.* Both of these UGTs reach adult values by 3 to 6 months (53), but in some individuals, full maturation may not be reached until 30 months (46). Two UGTs start to develop only after the second year of life: UGT 1A9 and UGT 2B4 (54). It has been speculated that the immaturity of UGTs in young children is partially responsible for their increased risk of valproate hepatotoxicity, and they may produce higher concentrations of a hepatotoxic metabolite of valproate, 4-ene valproic acid (45). Individual enzymes of other phase II proteins [sulfotransferases (SULTs), N-acetyl transferases (NAT's)] have unique stagger-step developments, but most achieve adult levels by 2 to 4 years of age (46).

Plasma Clearances of Liver-Metabolized Drugs by Prepubertal Children

Children under 10 years require larger, weight-adjusted doses of most hepatically metabolized medications than do adults in order to achieve comparable blood levels and therapeutic effects (12, 17). The reason for this is not obvious. Originally, it was proposed that the greater liver to body mass ratio of children compared to adults and other developmental changes in youth were responsible. However, it has been subsequently shown even when liver volume is normalized, that systemic clearance of a nonspecific CYP substrate (antipyrine) is higher in children when compared to adults (55). It also had been speculated that children have more efficient CYPs, but when individual hepatic CYPs were evaluated *in vitro*, no differences in maximal activities were found in children when compared to adults (56). Finally, as outlined above, during development, CYPs and phase II conjugates have *not* been shown to be uniformly increased in prepubertal children.

Renal Excretion

The kidney is an important organ for drug excretion. Three mechanisms are involved in the renal excretion of drugs: glomerular filtration through which drugs not bound to plasma proteins are "filtered," active tubular secretion in the proximal convoluted tubule, and passive reabsorption from the tubule.

Adult values of glomerular filtration are reached by 3 months in full-term infants, and if weight-adjusted, they can exceed adult values thereafter (14). Although in infants, tubular secretion is believed to develop more slowly than glomerular filtration, the efficacy of both mechanisms may be greater in children and teens than in adults (14). There is less information available about the ontogeny of tubular reabsorption, but it may not mature fully until adolescence (14).

Increased glomerular filtration and changes in tubular reabsorption, as well as increased body water in children, are responsible for the fact that children from 9 to 12 years can have greater clearance and shorter elimination half-life of lithium (57). Newer anticonvulsants that are primarily or entirely handled by the kidney (gabapentin, levetiracetam, topiramate) may also require higher weight-adjusted dosing in prepubertal children (58–60).

DRUG INTERACTIONS: FOCUS ON CYPS

Given the increasing recourse to medication combinations, augmentation strategies, and polypharmacy as an accepted and thoughtful (61) or sometimes as a controversial and potentially problematic (62) practice in child psychiatry, astute clinicians need to be aware and clinically suspicious of potential drug interactions. For children concurrently treated with nonpsychiatric drugs (including seemingly innocuous over-the-counter agents), the degree of oversight needs to be particularly heightened.

Time Courses of CYP-Based Drug Interactions

Drugs that interact with CYPs can inhibit, induce, or have no effect on CYP activity. Drugs with a *low presystemic clearance* (little of the drug is metabolized and conjugated in *the first pass* through the intestine and liver) are more susceptible to CYP induction or inhibition because they have *more unused metabolic capacity.* If a CYP is inhibited, more unmetabolized drug will enter the circulation, leading to increased levels of the drug (similar to a phenotypic slow metabolizer). Since inhibition requires blocking *existing* pathways, inhibition occurs rapidly for drugs that have a *high presystemic clearance.* The time course of the occurrence of the drug interaction is not changed if a *victim* drug is added to a *perpetrator* inhibitor drug or if a *perpetrator* inhibitor drug is added to a *victim* drug (see Figure 6.1.1.7). When a *perpetrator* inhibitor drug is added to a victim drug, the time to achieve a new Css is longer than the initial Css because the half-life has been prolonged, and the full effect of the interaction may not be evident until

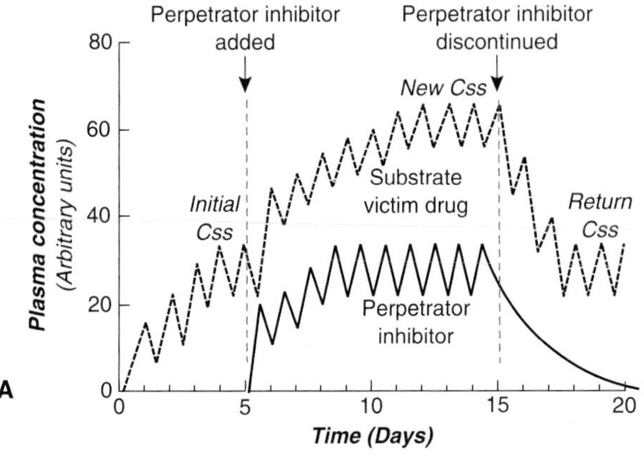

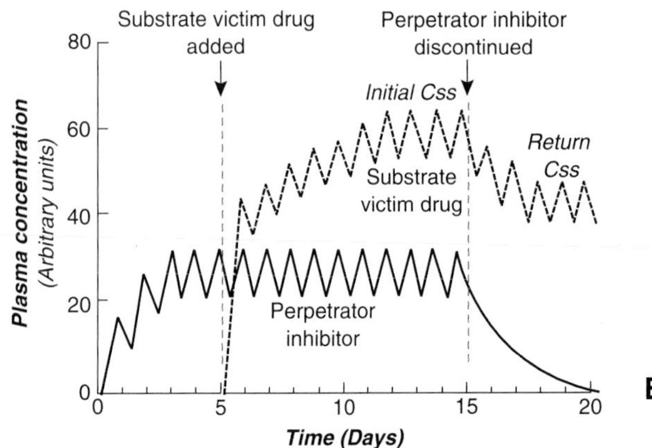

FIGURE 6.1.1.7. (A,B) Pharmacokinetics of substrate to inhibitor and inhibitor to substrate.

the *perpetrator* inhibitor reaches Css. Further, as illustrated by Figure 6.1.1.7, if the *perpetrator* drug is discontinued, the drug interaction will resolve as the concentration of the *perpetrator* drug falls to zero.

By contrast, if a drug has a *low presystemic clearance*, then the drug interaction will be evident only after both drugs have had several passes through the circulation and the *victim* drug reaches Css. Therefore the drug interaction will be clinically evident after some time.

Vignette 4

An 18-year-old woman has generalized anxiety disorder for which she has been prescribed daily triazolam for the past year. She develops a significant bacterial infection and clarithromycin is added. The next day, she develops signs of benzodiazepine toxicity. Triazolam is discontinued, and after 5 days, alprazolam is substituted. The toxicity reemerges 5 days later (63). In this vignette, triazolam has a high presystemic clearance and alprazolam a low presystemic clearance (even though both are CYP 3A substrates).

If a CYP is induced, additional enzyme will be available for metabolism (similar to a phenotypic ultrarapid metabolizer), leading to lower drug levels. Induction takes some time to start (3 to 10 days) or stop (5 to 12 days), as protein synthesis must first occur and then cease.

The time course of the occurrence of the drug interaction is different if a *victim* drug is added to an already present *perpetrator inducer* drug than if *the perpetrator inducer* drug is added to an already present victim drug. In the first example, the drug interaction will take place quickly because the CYPs are already induced, but in the second, it will occur only after new or additional protein synthesis is initiated. In either case, however, if the perpetrator inducer is discontinued, it will take time for protein synthesis to cease and for the concentration of the perpetrator inducer to decrease. The drug interaction will persist over several days despite the absence of the perpetrator inducer. If both drugs are discontinued at the same time, the half-life of the victim drug will determine the persistence of the drug interaction only if it is less than the time necessary for protein synthesis to cease (see Figure 6.1.1.8).

UGT and Transporter Drug Interactions

Although there are significantly less data, UGTs are also susceptible to inhibition and induction (Table 6.1.1.1). For example, lamotrigine is handled only by glucuronidation (probably UGT 1A4 and UGT 2B7), and the addition of valproate (a UGT 2B7 inhibitor) can significantly elevate lamotrigine levels, and increase the likelihood of the development of life-threatening Stevens-Johnson syndrome (64). The prescribing information of lamotrigine details dosage recommendation for this combination and for other anticonvulsants that induce or inhibit UGTs (65). It is less well known that when coadministered with lamotrigine, ethinyl estradiol (present in oral contraceptives), an inducer of glucuronidation, can reduce levels of lamotrigine up to 50% (66). There are only a few drug interactions involving transporters that are unquestionably tied to a specific transporter and are clinically significant because it is difficult to clearly separate out the effects of transporters from phase I and phase II effects and because a drug can have multiple transporters. The best known drug interactions involving efflux transporters are those of digoxin: For example, quinidine inhibits the ABCB1 uptake of digoxin in the kidney, leading to increases in digoxin levels (67). Although the current information about these drug interactions is still meager, as information grows, clinicians will need to keep abreast.

Clinical Aspects of Drug Interactions, Additional Resources

Vignette 5

A 14-year-old girl has diagnoses of major depressive disorder and attention-deficit hyperactivity disorder (ADHD). The depressive symptoms have responded well to fluoxetine at 10 mg per day, but difficulties with attention and impulsivity continue. Because she has had failed trials of methylphenidate and dextroamphetamine, she is begun on nortriptyline. Unaware of a possible drug interaction, the clinician begins treatment with a low dose of nortriptyline and plans to gradually increase dosing. The clinician is surprised to find that after 5 days of 10 mg twice daily of nortriptyline a trough blood level is 85 ng/ml. Fluoxetine is a potent CYP 2D6 inhibitor, and the level of victim CYP 2D6 substrate nortriptyline is already within therapeutic range.

Vignette 6

A 17-year-old youth with a diagnosis of bipolar 1 disorder has failed lithium, valproate, and several atypical antipsychotics. Her manic symptoms are well controlled on carbamazepine. She is sexually active and has been on low-dose oral contraceptives for 1 year without any side effects. The clinician is unaware that carbamazepine is an inducer of CYP 3A4. The patient begins to experience break-through bleeding for the first time.

The six most relevant CYPs and selected common psychotropic and other pediatric drugs and herbs metabolized by them are shown in Table 6.1.1.2. Common potent inhibitors and inducers of CYPs are grouped alphabetically by CYP.

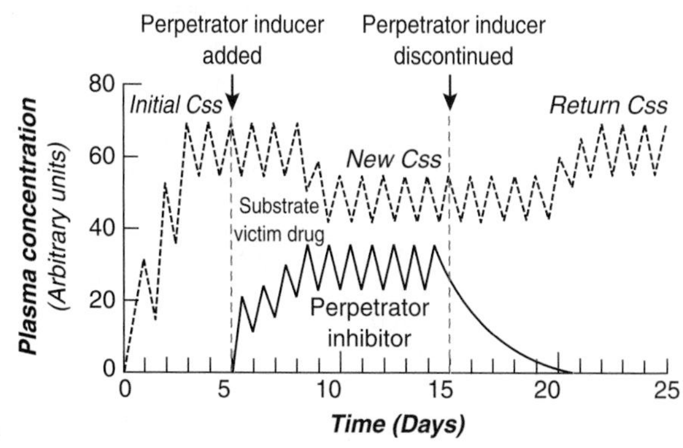

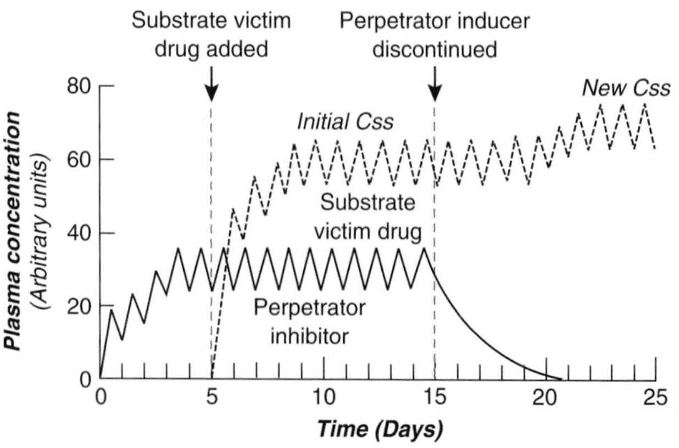

FIGURE 6.1.1.8. (A,B) Pharmacokinetics of substrate to inducer and inducer to substrate.

TABLE 6.1.1.2

P450 CYTOCHROME TABLE

	CYP1A2	CYP2B6	CYP2C19	CYP2C9	CYP2D6	CYP3A4/5/7
Substrates	Psychotropics clozapine duloxetine fluvoxamine imipramine melatonin (mirtazapine) (olanzapine) propafenone (propranolol) ramelteon Others acetaminophen caffeine naproxen (phenacetin) R-warfarin theophylline	bupropion meperidine nicotine methadone sertraline	Psychotropics amitriptyline citalopram clomipramine diazepam (fluoxetine) imipramine (sertraline) Anticonvulsants mephenytoin phenobarbital phenytoin Others progesterone propranolol (ranitidine) R-warfarin	Psychotropics fluoxetine (sertraline) valproate NSAIDS (diclofenac) flurbiprofen ibuprofen indomethacin meloxicam (naproxen) piroxicam suprofen Hypoglycemics glipizide <Glucotrol> glimepiride<Amaryl> glyburide <DiaBeta> nateglinide <Starlix> rosiglitazone tolbutamide Others celecoxib phenobarbital phenytoin progesterone sulfa drugs tetrahydrocannabinol S-warfarin zafirlukast <Accolate>	Psychotropics amitriptyline aripiprazole benztropine chlorpromazine (citalopram) clomipramine desipramine doxepin duloxetine fluoxetine fluvoxamine haloperidol imipramine mirtazapine nortriptyline paroxetine perphenazine risperidone (sertraline) thioridazine venlafaxine Others Antihistamines chlorpheniramine diphenhydramine hydroxyzine <Atarax> Anti- ADHD amphetamines atomoxetine Cough Medicines MDMA <ecstasy> Opiates codeine *pro-drug hydrocodone *pro-drug (oxycodone) tramadol phenacetin propranolol (ranitidine <Zantac>) tolterodine <Detrol>	Psychotropics alprazolam amitriptyline aripiprazole carbamazepine citalopram (clomipramine) (clozapine) (diazepam) estazolam eszopiclone <Lunesta> fluoxetine haloperidol midazolam nefazodone pimozide quetiapine risperidone (sertraline) trazodone triazolam zaleplon <Sonata> (ziprasidone) zolpidem <Ambien> Drugs of abuse/treatment buprenorphine cocaine hydrocodone *pro-drug ketamine methadone oxycodone phencyclidine <PCP> Antibiotics/Antifungal macrolides itraconazole ketoconazole telithromycin Anticonvulsants carbamazepine ethosuximide felbamate tiagabine zonisamide Antihistamines desloratadine<Clarinex> fexofenadine <Allegra> loratadine <Alavert, Claritin> Asthma Medication fluticasone <Flovent> salmeterol <Serevent> zileuton <Zyflo> Calcium Channel Blockers Hormones/Steroids/Immune Modulators cortisols desogestrel (pro-drug) ethinyl estradiol <oral contraceptives> progestins and progesterone Others nateglinide <Starlix> omeprazole pioglitazone <Actos> tolterodine <Detrol>

(continued)

TABLE 6.1.1.2

(CONTINUED)

	CYP1A2	CYP2B6	CYP2C19	CYP2C9	CYP2D6	CYP3A4/5/7
Inhibitors	caffeine cimetidine **ciprofloxacin** echinacea **enoxacin** **fluvoxamine** oral contraceptives zileuton <Zyflo>	**paroxetine** fluoxetine fluvoxamine PCP <phencyclidine> sertraline	cimetidine felbamate fluconazole (fluoxetine) **fluvoxamine** gestodene ketoconazole modafinil omeprazole **oral contraceptives** oxcarbazepine (sertraline) topiramate	cimetidine **fluconazole** fluoxetine isoniazid sulfinpyrazone valproate (zafirlukast)	(amitriptyline) **bupropion** celecoxib chlorpheniramine chlorpromazine cimetidine (citalopram) clomipramine cocaine (desipramine) diphenhydramine doxepin duloxetine (fluvoxamine) haloperidol (hydroxyzine) imipramine methadone metoclopramide **paroxetine** **quinidine** (ranitidine) (sertraline) **terbinafine** thioridazine	(cimetidine) ciprofloxacin **diltiazem** doxycycline echinacea enoxacin **clarithromycin** fluvoxamine **grapefruit juice** **itraconazole** **ketoconazole** **nefazodone** Star fruit **terithromycin** **verapamil**
Inducers	carbamazepine charbroiled meat cigarette smoke cruciferous vegetables insulin marijuana smoke modafinil phenobarbital	carbamazepine phenobarbital phenytoin	carbamazepine glucocorticoids phenobarbital	barbiturates glucocorticoids	dexamethasone rifampin	barbiturates carbamazepine felbamate glucocorticoids modafinil (oxcarbazepine) phenytoin primidone St. John's wort pioglitazone topiramate at >200 mg/d

() = Minor pathways or modest inhibitor or modest inducer; bold = Potent inhibitors.

The table can be used to anticipate CYP-based drug interactions and to prevent some of the unexpected outcomes depicted in the previous vignettes. If one drug is an inducer or inhibitor and it is listed on the same vertical axis as a substrate (the same CYP), a drug interaction is possible. However, *possible* is not the same as *likely* or *clinically significant*. A drug interaction is more likely to be clinically evident when a new drug is added or an existing drug is discontinued. Three other drug characteristics should help raise a clinician's drug interaction antennae. A drug interaction is especially likely to occur and can be significant if the victim drug has *one major* metabolic pathway (nortriptyline, desipramine, ethinyl estradiol). Many of the most serious drug interactions occur when a CYP inhibitor or inducer is added to a substrate with a narrow therapeutic index, as exemplified in Vignette 5. Finally, clinicians should be alert if a *perpetrator* inhibitor or inducer is *potent,* as shown in Vignette 6. Potent inhibitors and inducers are marked in bold in Table 6.1.1.2.

Although clinicians can glean important information from this table and from UGT Table 6.1.1.1 to predict drug interactions, they must utilize additional resources. They should know the metabolic characteristics and common drug interactions of medications they frequently prescribe. Clinicians can research these and other coprescribed over-the-counter and recreational drugs and herbs by using any common search engine on their computer to locate a drug's product insert and to review the "Metabolism" and "Drug Interaction" sections. Alternatively, clinicians can use PubMed to find the metabolic characteristics of a drug by entering the drug name and metabolism. They also can uncover clinical studies or case reports of known drug interactions involving pertinent drugs by entering the names of the drugs and the term drug interaction.

Clinicians need to amass trusted references: books such as Ciraulo's *Drug Interactions in Psychiatry* (68), Cozza's *Drug Interaction: Principles for Medical Practice* (69), articles such as Sandson's *An Overview of Psychotropic Drug–Drug Interactions* (70), Websites such as Flockhart's CYP table (71), or Oesterheld's P-glycoprotein, ABCB1 table (72), and UGT table (73). A collegial relationship with a clinical pharmacologist, especially one who is hospital based, should be treasured, since they have access to pharmaceutical references not readily available to clinicians. A patient's primary medical provider and his/her family should be educated to the common drug interactions with prescribed psychotropics and encouraged to be vigilant for their possibility. Drug interaction computer programs can be useful, but they are rarely complete (lacking influx and efflux transporters and phase II proteins) or up to date. Barron's *Evaluation of personal digital assistant software for drug interactions* (74) places iFacts and Lexi-Interact as the best, and ePocrates Rx as the worst. Although computer programs cannot factor in patient's characteristics such as genetic CYP status or developmental age, some are invaluable because they can sum the effects of multiple drugs if patients are taking many drugs or herbs at the same time (e.g., Genemedrx, 75).

In evaluating *suspected* drug interactions that may have already occurred, clinicians can use these resources to determine the metabolic characteristic of the involved drugs. They also should determine the time course between the initiation of the drugs and the development of adverse effects to help evaluate the likelihood of the suspected interaction. Does it fit the time courses that have been previously described? Does it fit the immediate development of adverse effects, as exemplified by the addition of a perpetrator inhibitor added to triazolam in Vignette 63.4, or the delayed timeline of a perpetrator inducer drug added to an oral contraceptive, as in Vignette 6?

CONCLUSION

Understanding the pharmacokinetic and drug interaction principles discussed in this chapter can be useful in clinical practice. It is hoped that readers will find the information in this chapter useful in improving the quality of care of their patients.

References

1. Aguilar EJ, Keshavan MS, Martinz-Quiles MD, et al.: Predictors of acute dystonia in first-episode psychotic patients. *Am J Psychiatry* 151: 1819–1821, 1994.
2. Rodnitzky RL: Drug-induced movement disorders in children and adolescents. *Expert Opin Drug Saf* 4:91–102, 2005.
3. [No authors listed]: Practice parameters for the assessment and treatment of children and adolescents with obsessive-compulsive disorder. *J Am Acad Child Adolesc Psychiatry* 37(10 Suppl):27S–45S, 1998.
4. Martin A, Kaufman J, Charney D: Pharmacotherapy of early-onset depression: Update and new directions. *Child Adolesc Psychiatr Clin N Am* 9:135–157, 2000.
5. Paxton JW, Dragunow M: Pharmacology. In: Werry JS (ed): *Practitioner's Guide to Psychoactive Drugs for Children and Adolescents.* New York, Plenum, 1993, pp.23–55.
6. Daviss WB, Perel JM, Rudolph GR, et al.: Steady-state pharmacokinetics of bupropion SR in juvenile patients. *J Am Acad Child Adolesc Psychiatry* 44:349–357, 2005.
7. May TW, Korn-Merker E, Rambeck B. Clinical pharmacokinetics of oxcarbazepine. *Clin Pharmacokinet* 42:1023–1042, 2003.
8. Findling RL, Reed MD, Myers C, et al.: Paroxetine pharmacokinetics in depressed children and adolescents. *J Am Acad Child Adolesc Psychiatry* 38:952–959, 1999.
9. Findling RL, Preskorn SH, Marcus RN, et al.: Nefazodone pharmacokinetics in depressed children and adolescents. *J Am Acad Child Adolesc Psychiatry* 39:1008–1016, 2000.
10. Greenblatt DJ, Shader RI: *Pharmacokinetics in Clinical Practice.* Philadelphia, WB Saunders Company, 1985.
11. Ragheb M: The clinical significance of lithium-nonsteroidal anti-inflammatory drug interactions. *J Clin Psychopharmacol* 10:350–354, 1990.
12. Jatlow PI: Psychotropic drug disposition during development. In: Popper C (ed): *Psychiatric Pharmacosciences of Children and Adolescents.* Washington, DC, American Psychiatric Press, 1987, pp.29–44.
13. Morselli PL, Pippenger CE: Drug disposition during development. In: *Applied Therapeutic Drug Monitoring.* Washington, DC, American Association of Clinical Chemistry, 1982, pp.63–70.
14. Benedetti MS, Baltes EL: Drug metabolism and disposition in children. *Fundamental Clin Pharmacol* 17:281–299, 2003.
15. Taylor E: Physical treatments. In: Rutter M (ed): *Child and Adolescent Psychiatry.* Cambridge, Blackwell Scientific, 1994, pp.880–899.
16. Gilman JT, Duchowny M, Campo AE: Pharmacokinetic considerations in the treatment of childhood epilepsy. *Paediatr Drugs* 5:267–777, 2003.
17. Kearns GL, Abdel-Rahman SM, Alander SW, et al.: Developmental pharmacology—Drug disposition, action, and therapy in infants and children. *NEJM* 349:1157–1167, 2003.
18. Chan LMS, Lowes S, Hirst BH: The ABCs of drug transport in intestine and liver: Efflux proteins limiting drug absorption and bioavailability. *Eur J Pharm Sciences* 21:25–51, 2004.
19. Steffansen B, Nielsen CU, Brodin B, et al.: Intestinal solute carriers: An overview of trends and strategies for improving oral drug absorption. *Eur J Pharm Sciences* 21:3–16, 2004.
20. Website of HUGO Genome Nomenclature Committee at University College London (accessed 1/08/06).
21. Terada T and Inui K: Peptide transporters: Structure, function, regulation and application for drug delivery. *Current Drug Metabol* 5:85–94, 2004.
22. Juliano RL, Ling V: A surface glycoprotein modulating drug permeability in Chinese hamster ovary cell mutants. *Biochim Biophys Acta* 455:152–162, 1976.
23. Fischer V, Einolf HJ, Cohen D: Efflux transporters and their clinical significance. *Mini-Reviews in Medicinal Chem* 5:183–195, 2005.
24. Kivisto KT, Niemi M, Fromm MF: Functional interaction of intestinal CYP3A4 and P-glycoprotein. *Fundam Clin Pharmacol* 18:621–626, 2004.
25. Fakhoury M, Litalien C, Medard Y, et al.: Localization and mRNA expression of CYP3A and P-gp in human duodenum as a function of age. *Drug Metab Dispos* 33:1603–1607, 2005.
26. Hattis D, Ginsberg G, Sonawane B, et al.: Differences in pharmacokinetics between children and adults.II. Children's variability in drug elimination half-lifes and in some parameters needed for physiologically-based pharmacokinetic modeling. *Risk Anal* 23:117–142, 2003.
27. Fetner HH, Geller B: Lithium and tricyclic antidepressants. *Psychiatr Clin North Am* 15:223–241, 1992.
28. Painter MJ, Pippenger C, Wasterlain C, et al.: Phenobarbital and phenytoin in neonatal seizures: Metabolism and tissue distribution. *Neurology* 31:1107–1112, 1981.
29. Kusuhara H, Sugiyama Y: Active efflux across the blood–brain barrier: Role of the solute carrier family. *NeuroRx* 2:73–85, 2005.
30. Carson SW, Ousmanou AD, Hoyler SL: Emerging significance of P-glycoprotein in understanding drug disposition and drug interactions in psychopharmacology. *Psychopharmacol Bull* 36:67–81, 2002.
31. Tsai C, Ahdab-Barmada M, Daood MJ, et al.: P-glycoprotein expression in the developing human central nervous system: Cellular and tissue localization. *Pediatr Res* 47:Suppl 436A abstract, 2001.
32. Plass JRM: Function and regulation of the human bile salt export pump. http://dissertations.ub.rug.nl/faculties/medicine/2005/j.r.m.plass/ (accessed 1/03/06).
33. Janicak PG, Davis JM, Preskorn SH, et al.: (eds): Pharmacokinetics. In: *Principles and Practice of Psychopharmacotherapy.* Baltimore, Williams & Wilkins, 1993, pp.59–79.
34. Janicak PG: The relevance of clinical pharmacokinetics and therapeutic drug monitoring: Anticonvulsant mood stabilizers and antipsychotics. *J Clin Psychiatry* 54:9 (suppl):35–41, 1993.
35. Nelson DR, Koymans L, Kamataki T, et al.: P450 superfamily: Update on new sequences, gene mapping, accession numbers and nomenclature. *Pharmacogenetics* 6:1–42, 1996.
36. Greenblatt DJ, von Moltke LL, Harmatz JS, et al.: Human cytochromes mediating sertraline biotransformation: seeking attribution. *J Clin Psychopharmacol* 19:489–493, 1999.
37. Bertilsson L: Geographical/interracial differences in polymorphic drug oxidation: Current state of knowledge of cytochromes P450 (CYP) 2D6 and 2C19. *Clin Pharmacokinet* 29:192–209, 1995.
38. CDRH Consumer Information Website. http://www.fda.gov/cdrh/mda/docs/k042259.html (accessed 1/06/06).
39. de Leon J, Armstrong SC, Cozza KL: Clinical guidelines for psychiatrists for the use of pharmacogenetic testing for CYP450 2D6 and CYP450 2C19. *Psychosomatics* 2006;47:75–85.
40. Wells PG, Mackenzie PI, Chowdhury JR, et al.: Glucuronidation and the UDP-glucuronosyltransferases in health and disease. *Drug Metab Dispos* 32:281–290, 2004.
41. Mori A, Maruo Y, Iwai M, et al.: UDP-glucuronosyltransferase 1A4 polymorphisms in a Japanese population and kinetics of clozapine glucuronidation. *Drug Metab Dispos* 33:672–675, 2005.
42. Court MH, Hao Q, Krishnaswamy S, et al.: UDP-glucuronosyltransferase (UGT) 2B15 pharmacogenetics: UGT2B15 D85Y genotype and gender are major determinants of oxazepam glucuronidation by human liver. *J Pharmacol Exp Ther* 310:656–665, 2004.
43. Ross JR, Rutter D, Welsh K, et al.: Clinical response to morphine in cancer patients and genetic variation in candidate genes. *Pharmacogenomics J* 5:324–336, 2005.
44. Food and Drug Administration: FDA News. http://www.fda.gov/bbs/topics/NEWS/2005/NEW01220.html (accessed 1/06/06).
45. Johnson TN: The development of drug metabolizing enzymes and their influence on the susceptibility to adverse drug reactions in children. *Toxicol* 192:37–48, 2003.
46. Blake MJ, Castro L, Leeder JS, et al.: Ontogeny of drug metabolizing enzymes in the neonate. *Seminars in Fetal and Neonatal Med* 10:123–138, 2005.
47. Johnsrud EK, Koukouritaki SB, Brunengraber DK, et al.: Human hepatic CYP2E1 expression during development. *J Pharmacol Exp Ther* 307: 402–407, 2003.
48. Oesterheld JR: A review of developmental aspects of cytochrome P450. *J Child Adolesc Psychopharmacol* 8:161–174, 1998.
49. de Wildh SN, Kearns GL, Hop WC, et al.: Pharmacokinetics and metabolism of oral midazolam in preterm infants. *Br J Clin Pharmacol* 53:390–392, 2002.

50. Koukouritaki SB, Namro JR, Marsh SA, et al.: Developmental expression of human hepatic CYP2C9 and CYP2C19. *J Pharm and Exp Ther* 307:402–407, 2003.
51. Stevens JC, Hines RN, Gu C, et al.: Developmental expression of the major human hepatic CYP3A enzymes. *J Pharm and Experimental Ther*573–582, 2003.
52. Lambert GH, Schoeller DA, Kotake AN, et al.: The effect of age, gender, and sexual maturation on the caffeine breath test. *Dev Pharmacol Ther* 9:375–88, 1986.
53. de Wildt SN, Kearns GL, Leeder JS, et al.: Glucuronidation in humans. Pharmacogenetic and developmental aspects. *Clin Pharmacokinet* 36:439–452, 1999.
54. Strassburg CP, Strassburg A, Kneip S, et al.: Developmental aspects of human hepatic drug glucuronidation in young children and adults. *Gut* 50:259–265, 2002.
55. Murry DJ, Crom WR, Reddick WE, et al.: Liver volume as a determinant of drug clearance in children and adolescents. *Drug Metab Dispos* 23: 1110–1116, 1995.
56. Blanco JG, Harrison PL, Evans WE, et al.: Human cytochrome P450 maximal activities in pediatric versus adult liver. *Drug Metab and Dispos* 28:379–382, 2000.
57. Vitiello B, Behar D, Malone R, et al.: Pharmacokinetics of lithium carbonate in children. *J Clin Psychopharmacol* 8:355–359, 1988.
58. Armijo JA, Pena MA, Adin J, et al.: Association between patient age and gabapentin serum concentration-to-dose ratio: A preliminary multivariate analysis. *Ther Drug Monit* 26:633–637, 2004.
59. Vigevano F: Levetiracetam in pediatrics. *J Child Neurol* 20:87–93, 2005.
60. Battino D, Croci D, Rossini A, et al.: Topiramate pharmacokinetics in children and adults with epilepsy: A case-matched comparison based on therapeutic drug monitoring data. *Clin Pharmacokinet* 44:407–416, 2005.
61. Wilens TE, Spencer T, Biederman J, et al.: Combined pharmacotherapy: An emerging trend in pediatric psychopharmacology. *J Am Acad Child Adolesc Psychiatry* 34:110–112, 1995.
62. Woolston JL: Combined pharmacotherapy: Pitfalls of treatment. *J Am Acad Child Adolesc Psychiatry* 38:1455–1457, 1999.
63. Greenblatt DJ, Wright CE, von Moltke LL, et al.: Ketoconazole inhibition of triazolam and alprazolam clearance: Differential kinetic and dynamic consequences. *Clin Pharmacol Ther* 64:237–247, 1998.
64. Anderson GD, Yau MK, Gidal BE, et al.: Bidirectional interaction of valproate and lamotrigine in healthy subjects. *Clin Pharmacol Ther* 60:145–156, 1996.
65. GlaxoSmithKline: Prescribing information, Lamictal. http://www.lamictal.com.
66. Sabers A, Ohman I, Christensen J, et al.: Oral contraceptives reduce lamotrigine plasma levels. *Neurology* 61:570–571, 2003.
67. Ding R, Tayrouz Y, Riedel KD, et al.: Substantial pharmacokinetic interaction between digoxin and ritonavir in healthy volunteers. *Clin Pharmacol Ther* 76:73–84, 2004.
68. Ciraulo DA, Shader RI, Greenblatt DJ, Creelman WL: *Drug Interactions in Psychiatry*, 3rd ed. Philadelphia, Lippincott Williams and Wilkins, 2005.
69. Cozza KL, Armstrong SC, Oesterheld JR: *Drug Interaction: Principles for Medical Practice*, 2nd ed. Washington, DC, American Psychiatric Publishing, 2003.
70. Sandson NB, Armstrong SC, Cozza KL: An overview of psychotropic drug–drug interactions. *Psychosomatics* 46:464–494, 2005.
71. Flockhart D: Drug Interactions Website. http://medicine.iupui.edu/flockhart/table.htm (accessed 1/06/06).
72. Oesterheld J: Pgp table. http://www.mhc.com/PGP/PgpTable.HTML (accessed 1/03/06).
73. Oesterheld J: UGT table. http://www.mhc.com//Cytochromes//UGT//UGTTable.HTML (accessed 1/03/06).
74. Barrons R: Evaluation of personal digital assistant software for drug interactions. *Am J Health Syst Pharm* 61:380–385, 2004.
75. Patterson R, Oesterheld J: Genemedrx drug interaction program. http://www.genemedrx.com (accessed 1/06/06).

CHAPTER 6.1.2 ■ GENERAL PRINCIPLES, SPECIFIC DRUG TREATMENTS, AND CLINICAL PRACTICE

LAWRENCE SCAHILL, JESSICA R. OESTERHELD, AND ANDRÉS MARTIN

INTRODUCTION

The now famous clinical trial conducted by Charles Bradley (1) is often cited as the beginning of pediatric psychopharmacology. In that study, the racemic mixture of levo- and dextro-amphetamine (benzedrine) was administered openly to a group of 30 children with mixed behavioral and emotional symptoms. Bradley and his colleagues observed that the children characterized as "noisy, aggressive and domineering" were calmer and more manageable. In the same issue of the *American Journal of Psychiatry*, Molitch and Eccles reported what may be the first placebo-controlled study in child psychiatry (2). Ninety-three boys described as juvenile delinquents were randomly assigned to gradually escalating doses of benzedrine or placebo. The benzedrine group showed dose-related improvements across a range of measures on learning, motor control, and short-term memory that exceeded the improvements in the placebo group. Since this pioneering work, the field of pediatric psychopharmacology has made steady progress.

Despite clear progress in some areas, there are important gaps between research and clinical practice. For example: 1) There have been over 100 placebo-controlled studies on the efficacy of methylphenidate in the treatment of attention deficit hyperactivity disorder (ADHD), yet only a few studies have evaluated its long-term effects (3, 4); 2) for serious psychiatric disorders such as autism, empirical support for the use of medication remains meager, leaving clinicians and families with limited guidance on appropriate treatment of affected children; 3) despite the demonstrated efficacy and safety of selective serotonin reuptake inhibitors (SSRIs) in the treatment of children and adolescents with obsessive-compulsive disorder (OCD), little is known about the appropriate duration of treatment; 4) based on an evaluation of prescribing trends in three large health care systems, methylphenidate use among children 2 to 4 years of age increased from 1–5 per 1,000 in 1991 to 4–11 per 1,000 in 1995 (5). This two- to three-fold increase, depending on the health system under consideration, stands in sharp contrast to the lack of clinical research with methylphenidate for this age group. Clearly, the empirical foundations for pediatric psychopharmacology are not yet fully anchored. Over the past decade, however, there have been several initiatives that are having a substantial impact on the pace of progress in the field.

The purpose of this chapter is to present general principles of clinical psychopharmacology in pediatric populations. Following the discussion of seven overarching principles, this chapter reviews the major classes of psychotropic medications and current approaches to their use in children and adolescents. Drugs within the major classes are considered in terms of their pharmacology, adverse effects, clinical applications and management, and available empirical support. Pharmacokinetic aspects, including drug interactions, as well as mechanisms of action and other pharmacodynamic issues, will be considered only briefly here, as such topics are dealt with in depth in the preceding, and complementary, chapter. Throughout this chapter, the reader is referred to the interspersed tables, in which the most salient information for each drug class and its specific agents are summarized.

Seven Guiding Principles

1. *The Role of Development.* There is general recognition that development can have a major impact on pharmacological effects (6). Thus, children and adults may show divergent responses to psychotropic drugs. The sources of these differences, as elaborated in the preceding chapter, are manifold. First, children often metabolize and eliminate drugs from the body more quickly than adults, resulting in shorter drug half-lives. This is apparently due to a larger liver-to–total body ratio and more efficient glomerular filtration rate in children as compared to adults. One practical implication of these pharmacokinetic differences is that in order to achieve therapeutic serum levels for some drugs when compared to adults, children may require higher weight-adjusted (mg/kg) dosages (see previous chapter on Pharmacokinetics). In addition to pharmacokinetic considerations, because the central nervous system undergoes substantial developmental change during childhood, there can be age effects on drug action as well. For example, activating side effects of selective serotonin reuptake inhibitors (SSRIs) and other antidepressants (7), and developmental differences in the maturation of noradrenergic pathways may explain, at least in part, why tricyclic antidepressants are less effective in children with depression as compared to adults (8). Taken together, these findings suggest that the three major neurochemical systems that are manipulated by psychotropic drug treatments (dopaminergic, serotonergic, and noradrenergic, respectively) are subject to age effects.

In recognition of these developmental influences, federal policy initiatives have been instituted to promote studies specific to pediatric populations. First, in 1997 Congress passed the Food and Drug Modernization Act (FDAMA), which offers pharmaceutical companies an additional 6 months of market exclusivity for products that are evaluated in children. For some drugs, this 6-month extension represents a powerful financial incentive. A second policy initiated by the Food and Drug Administration (FDA) requires pharmaceutical companies to evaluate new products in children if they are likely to be used in this population when released into the marketplace (9). A third and related development has been the commitment of federal funds by the National Institutes of Health to establish research networks capable of conducting large-scale, multisite studies in pediatric populations (3, 10–12). The combined impact of these initiatives has lead to rapid growth in the knowledge base of pediatric psychopharmacology and its incorporation into clinical practice.

2. *The Limits of Categorical Diagnoses and Occurrence of Multiple Disorders as the Norm.* The second principle acknowledges the limitations of psychiatric diagnoses and of the current nosological system of classification. Most psychiatric disorders in childhood are probably heterogeneous with respect to etiology. This presumption is supported by the high co-occurrence of psychiatric disorders in children—both in clinical (13) and in community samples (14). The extent to which these mixed syndromes represent a variant of a given disorder is often unclear, but may be relevant to drug response; for example, tics are a common cooccurring feature in OCD. The presence of tics may signal a different form of OCD and may be associated with a lower probability of positive response to monotherapy with an SSRI in OCD (15, 16). Along the same lines, hyperactivity and impulsiveness are common complaints for children with pervasive developmental disorders (PDDs). Results from a recent multisite study in children with PDDs accompanied by hyperactivity, impulsiveness, and distractibility showed a lower rate of positive response to stimulants compared to what is observed in typically developing children with attention deficit hyperactivity disorder (ADHD). In addition, children with PDDs appear to be at higher risk for adverse events with stimulant treatment (17). Thus, etiological heterogeneity may explain differences in clinical response. These issues underscore the importance of large treatment studies to identify clinically meaningful subgroups and predictors of positive and negative response.

3. *Target Symptoms and the Integration of Data from Multiple Informants.* This principle concerns the importance of pretreatment assessment and the identification of target symptoms. Given the common occurrence of multiple psychiatric disorders in children, the identification of target symptoms for pharmacological intervention may be easier said than done. One of the practical challenges in child psychiatry is the requirement of gathering information from multiple sources, including the child and parents at a minimum, and in many cases, the child's teacher or other caregiver as well. Obtaining data from multiple sources can be aided by the use of behavioral checklists, child self-reports, and clinician ratings. Behavioral checklists completed by parents and teachers permit comparison of the current patient to a normative sample. Clinician-rated instruments can assist with establishing a pretreatment baseline of symptom severity. Some checklists and clinician-rated instruments can also be used to measure change over time. Although checklists and rating instruments can be extremely useful in the evaluation phase and to measure change over time, they cannot replace the clinical interview and direct observation of parent and child. A closely related challenge is the integration of all available information, in order to identify the most pressing target symptoms and select the most appropriate medication in combination with other needed interventions. The joint agreement on relevant target symptoms by caregivers and clinicians can be useful in monitoring therapeutic outcomes, but may also lead to greater consumer satisfaction with treatment (18).

4. *Adverse Effects: Monitoring Risks and Benefits.* The dramatic increase in the availability of new psychotropic drugs, their expanded use in pediatric populations, and their uncertain impact on development underscore the importance of ongoing assessment of adverse effects. At present, there is no clear consensus on the best method of eliciting information about adverse events that occur in the context of pharmacotherapy. This lack of consensus is not limited to child psychiatry; it extends to adult psychiatry as well as other areas of medicine. Three approaches have been described: the use of an open-ended general inquiry; the use of general inquiry augmented by a set of drug-specific queries or checklist; or the use of a detailed review of body systems (19). At the center of this debate are concerns about sensitivity, specificity, and efficiency.

The use of a detailed review of systems by an experienced clinician is unlikely to miss adverse effects of medication (high sensitivity). However, some experts express concern that this method may produce an unacceptably high number of false positive responses. If true, this low specificity would come at a great cost in clinician time.

On the other hand, the open-ended general inquiry gives the parent and child an opportunity to express any concern that may have emerged since starting the medication or since the last visit. Based on the assumption that parents and children will notice important changes in behavior and/or health status, responses to the open-ended inquiry are likely to be clinically meaningful—even if they are not drug-related. Because parents and children may not detect subtle adverse effects, the high specificity may result in missed adverse events (low sensitivity).

A recent multisite study compared general inquiry, drug-specific queries and review of systems approach in 60 children on various medications. The study showed that the review of systems approach did indeed identify adverse effects that the other methods missed. Moreover, in approximately a third of cases, the identified adverse effect from the review of systems interview led to an alteration in dose. Nonetheless, the review of systems used in the study was time consuming and unlikely to be adopted in busy clinical practice (20). Thus, appropriate clinical practice entails the use of open-ended questions, followed by drug-specific queries. In the pages that follow, we list the adverse effects associated with each of the medications presented. Additional safety concerns are also presented in the tables. Other fundamental issues to be covered in contemporary medication management of children include questions about concomitant medications, intercurrent illness, and other medical contacts since the previous visit. The need for vital signs, height, and weight monitoring, for neurological examination, electrocardiogram, laboratory tests and drug levels, are medication specific and described in the appropriate sections below.

5. *The Role of Caregivers and the Meaning of Medication.* Collaboration and successful engagement of the child's family is critical to the success of treatment interventions, pharmacological or otherwise. A detailed discussion with the parents and the child concerning the recommended medication, as well as an examination of the alternative treatments are prerequisites for initiating psychopharmacological treatment. In addition, the family and the child should be (to the extent possible) active partners in the treatment process (21). Once chosen, the dose schedule, potential adverse effects, anticipated magnitude of response on target symptoms as well as the time to effect warrant explicit review. This discussion gives an opportunity to evaluate and temper unrealistic expectations about the medication. Depending on the medication, it may be necessary to establish a contingency plan to manage specific adverse effects prior to their occurrence, such as being prepared to start benztropine for a child who develops dystonia when started on a potent antipsychotic such as haloperidol. Children, and to a lesser extent adolescents, are dependent on their parents to administer medications, so that parental endorsement of the treatment plan is both ethically sound and practical. Failure to involve parents in the decisionmaking process may threaten treatment compliance, which in turn may undermine the success of the intervention. Attention should also be paid to the meaning that taking medication has for the child and family (22). Exploration of these issues may reveal a sense of failure on the part of the child or family. Some children may express concern that having to take medication implies that they are crazy or "weird." These issues should be identified and addressed prior to initiating treatment. Even when handled prior to treatment, however, these issues often reemerge and require attention over the course of treatment.

6. *Psychopharmacology in Context, and the Combination of Therapeutic Modalities.* Psychotropic medications, no matter how effective, are often but one element in a multimodal treatment plan that includes other individually tailored interventions. This guiding principle, which may seem self-evident to clinicians accustomed to using various therapeutic approaches in their practice, has become a focal point for research and practice guidelines. For example, practice parameters often provide guidance of selection and sequence of interventions, such as when to use one modality (behavioral therapy or medication) versus a combined medication approach. To date, it has been difficult to demonstrate the unique and significant contribution of psychotherapy over and above medication. However, several cognitive-behavioral treatments have proven efficacy and should not be overlooked in the treatment of children and adolescents with major psychiatric conditions (23). Three large-scale, NIMH-sponsored, multisite studies in pediatric samples with ADHD (3), depression (12) and OCD (24) have been completed and provide some insight into the use of combined treatments (see following).

7. *Empirically Informed, Evidenced-Based Clinical Decision-Making.* A final principle is that treatment plans should be grounded on available empirical evidence. As the database of pediatric psychopharmacology expands, the value of this principle will become even more pressing and places a higher demand for clinicians to stay apace of research findings. The International Algorithm Project has put forth a simple method for ranking available treatments according to their level of empirical support: (25) *Class A* includes medications with good empirical support, based on consistently positive results in randomized controlled trials (RCTs). *Class B* consists of drugs with fair empirical support showing positive, but inconsistent, results in RCTs or positive results from small sample trials. *Class C* includes drugs with minimal empirical support, based primarily on accumulated clinical experience from case reports and open-label studies. As examples relevant to pediatric psychopharmacology, *A level* of empirical support exists in the case of: stimulants, atomoxetine, and clonidine for ADHD; fluvoxamine for OCD and other anxiety disorders of childhood; sertraline for OCD; fluoxetine for depression; risperidone, haloperidol, and pimozide for tic disorders; and risperidone for autism and disruptive behavior. *B level* of support exists for: clonidine for tics; guanfacine for ADHD; and lithium for aggression and conduct disorder.

This ranking system clearly reflects the state of the science at a particular point in time. Given the rapid pace of development in pediatric psychopharmacology, clinicians have a responsibility to remain up to date with the empirical evidence to ensure the best possible match between target symptoms and treatment options.

SPECIFIC DRUG TREATMENTS

Stimulants

Clinical Applications and Empirical Support. The stimulants, especially the short- and long-acting forms of methylphenidate and amphetamine, are first-line treatments for attention deficit hyperactivity disorder (ADHD). In its classic form, ADHD is characterized by inattention, impulsiveness, and hyperactivity, though current convention includes primarily inattentive and impulsive/hyperactive subtypes (26). Epidemiological studies indicate that ADHD is relatively common in childhood, affecting 2% to 10% of school-aged children (27, 28). Boys are affected more often than girls. It persists into adolescence in a majority of cases (29), and into adulthood in as many as 30% to 40% of cases (30). Studies of clinical populations indicate that the symptoms of ADHD are among the most common reasons for referral of children to mental health agencies (3). Nonetheless, there also is a substantial number of affected children who are not receiving treatment (31). Given the high prevalence of ADHD in school-age children, the potential for long-term functional disability and the high health-related costs associated with the disorder (32), ADHD is a major public health concern.

The most commonly used stimulants for the treatment of ADHD include methylphenidate, dextroamphetamine, and the mixed preparation of D,L-amphetamine (33). Immediate-release methylphenidate has been studied more carefully than the other stimulants and remains the most commonly used agent in clinical practice—though the longer acting preparations are growing in market share. Although less well studied, the amphetamine products and extended-release formulations of methylphenidate have short-term efficacy and safety profiles that are comparable to methylphenidate (34, 35) (Table 6.1.2.1).

The empirical basis for the use of stimulants in children with ADHD rests on findings from hundreds of short-term, randomized, placebo-controlled studies conducted over the past 30 to 40 years (33). Results from controlled studies over the last decade provide additional information about dose response, similarities and differences in response across stimulant preparations, and the importance of regular clinical monitoring to achieve optimal response. Rapport and colleagues (36) conducted a dose-response study in 76 subjects (66 boys and 10 girls) between the ages of 6 and 11 years. The 5-week study used 4 dose levels of methylphenidate (5 mg, 10 mg, 15 mg, and 20 mg given bid) and placebo given in random order in a crossover design. All dose levels of active medication were superior to placebo. In addition, there was a clear linear trend, such that classroom behavior and the number of completed assignments improved with each increase in dose. However, the incremental improvement was smaller as the dose moved above the 10 mg dose level.

In order to compare methylphenidate and d-amphetamine, a placebo-controlled crossover study was conducted in 48 boys between 6 and 12 years of age (37). Subjects were treated with methylphenidate, d-amphetamine, or placebo in random order for 3 weeks in each treatment condition. During each condition the dose was increased on a weekly basis (e.g., methylphenidate doses for children under 30 kg of body weight were 12.5 mg, 20 mg, and 35 mg at breakfast and lunchtime for the respective weeks). Based on a global rating of response, 79% of the subjects showed a positive response to methylphenidate and 88% showed a positive response to d-amphetamine. Only 2 of the 48 subjects failed to respond to one or the other stimulant.

Pelham and colleagues (35) compared the extended methylphenidate release product, Concerta, to immediate release methylphenidate and placebo in a crossover trial. Sixty-eight children between 6 and 12 years old were assigned to receive placebo, immediate release methylphenidate, or the extended release methylphenidate in random order. All children were on methylphenidate prior to enrollment. Thus, each child was assigned to a dosage level that was similar to the pretrial dose. The three dose levels for immediate release methylphenidate were 5 mg three times per day, 10 mg three times per day or 15 mg three times per day. Each dose level of immediate release methylphenidate was matched to a similar, though slightly higher, dose of extended release. Specifically, the dose levels of extended release were: 18 mg, 36 mg and 54 mg given as a single morning dose. Each treatment (immediate release, matching dose of extended release, or placebo) was given in random order for 1 week. Both active treatments were superior to placebo, achieving showed approximately 50% improvement on both parent and teacher measures of ADHD symptoms. There were no detectable differences between immediate release and extended release methylphenidate preparations with respect to efficacy or adverse effects.

To date, only methylphenidate has been evaluated in long-term studies (3). With its sample size of 576 children, the Multimodal Treatment Study of children with attention-deficit/hyperactivity disorder (MTA) provides convincing evidence for the long-term benefits of methylphenidate. In the MTA study, children between 7 and 10 years of age were randomly assigned to one of 4 treatment groups: medication management (N = 144; primarily methylphenidate administered in a systematic fashion with close monitoring); an intensive behavioral treatment program (N = 144); combined medication management and the same behavioral treatment program (N = 145); or community care, which served as the control group (N = 146). The MTA research sites provided treatment to three of these groups, including the medication management group, the behavioral therapy only group, and the combined medication plus behavioral therapy group. The community care group received treatment from self-selected practitioners. In most cases (84 of 146, or 58%), community care consisted of methylphenidate given on a twice-daily schedule. After 14 months of treatment, all four groups showed improvement compared to baseline. Comparisons across the four groups showed that the combined treatment group and the medication management group did significantly better than the community care group and the behavioral treatment only group across a range of outcomes.

Several potentially important differences emerged when community care was compared to medication management provided by the MTA sites. First, community practitioners most often administered methylphenidate on a twice-daily schedule, compared to three times per day in the MTA-treated groups. Among the children randomly assigned to community care, 33% (N = 48) stopped taking medication during the study period. Not surprisingly, this group showed the least improvement on the primary outcome measures. By contrast, only 3% (N = 18) of the research medication management groups (both medication only and medication plus behavioral treatment) discontinued medication during the study. Finally, in the MTA medication management groups, follow-up visits were more frequent and parent and teacher ratings were used in a systematic way to inform clinical decision-making.

Taken together, the results of these studies suggest that stimulants are effective for short- and long-term treatment of children with ADHD. When considering group effects, stimulants appear to be equally beneficial, but individual patients may respond better to one preparation over another. The modest effectiveness of stimulants observed in the community care group of the MTA suggests that close clinical monitoring with dose adjustments based on systematic assessment of therapeutic and side effects contributes to compliance and optimal results.

Mechanism of Action. Although stimulants have become the standard treatment for ADHD, their mechanism of action is not clearly understood. In addition, the mechanism of action for amphetamines and methylphenidate may be slightly different (38). Methylphenidate promotes release of stored dopamine and blocks the return of dopamine at presynaptic dopamine transporter sites. Amphetamines also block dopamine reuptake at the transporter, but appear to promote the release of newly synthesized dopamine more selectively. These combined effects enhance dopamine function in striatum and, at least indirectly, in the prefrontal cortex. It is also clear that both methylphenidate and the amphetamines affect the norepinephrine system (39). For example, both compounds decrease the firing rate in the locus coeruleus (LC),

TABLE 6.1.2.1

STIMULANTS AND STIMULANT ALTERNATIVES

Drug	Mechanism of Action	Main Indications and Clinical Uses	Dosage (mg/d)	Schedule	Adverse Effects	Comments	Select Brand Names and Preparations Available
Methylphenidate	Dopamine presynaptic release and reuptake blockade	ADHD	15–60 (Ritalin) 18–72 mg/d (Concerta)	bid/tid (MPH); qd (Concerta)	Insomnia, decreased appetite, weight loss, dysphoria Possible reduction in growth velocity during long-term use Withdrawal and rebound hyperactivity Unmasking or induction of tics. Possible induction acceleration of mania psychosis	Longer acting preparations may have lower peak and valley effects and less rebound hyperactivity	Ritalin/Methylin: 5, 10, 20 mg t; sustained release t, 20 mg; Concerta: 18, 54 mg t
Dextroamphetamine			10–40	bid/tid			Dexedrine: 5, mg t; sustained release spansules, 5, 10, 15 mg
Amphetamine compound			10–40	qd/bid			Adderall: 5, 10, 20, 30 mg; Adderall XR: 5, 10, 15, 20, 25, 30 c
Atomoxetine	Selective noradrenergic reuptake inhibitor		10–80	qd/bid	Loss of appetite, dizziness, nausea; rare instances of hepatotoxicity have been reported	Technically an antidepressant and not a stimulant, but used only in the treatment of ADHD	Strattera: 10, 18, 25, 40, 60, 80 mg c

Note: Doses are provided as general guidelines only, and are not meant to be definitive. All doses must be individualized and monitored through the appropriate clinical and/or laboratory means.
Abbreviations: c (capsule); t (tablet); FDA (Food and Drug Administration).

though amphetamine appears to be more potent in this action. Whether the effect on the norepinephrine system is facilitory or inhibitory is not clear at present. Nonetheless, these combined effects appear to be essential to the clinical effects of the stimulants, as drugs with more selective action (guanfacine or desipramine) tend to have smaller clinical effects.

Pharmacokinetics. Immediate release formulations of methylphenidate, dextroamphetamine, and the combined levo- and dextroamphetamine preparation are readily absorbed and show behavioral effects 30 to 60 minutes after ingestion. The peak level of immediate release methylphenidate occurs approximately 90 to 150 minutes after ingestion and the clinical effects last 3 to 5 hours. The immediate release amphetamine products achieve peak levels between 1 and 3 hours, with duration of action of 5 to 7 hours. Based on blinded studies in a research classroom setting, the D,L-amphetamine preparation appears to have a slightly longer duration of action than standard D-amphetamine (40). Methylphenidate and amphetamine are metabolized in the liver, but by quite different pathways (see previous chapter for more details). For the immediate release formulations of these stimulants, the parent compound and metabolites are excreted in the urine within 24 hours. Several newly developed sustained release products have been introduced, offering a range of options for clinical management of children and adolescents with ADHD. Individual manufacturer's materials should be reviewed before prescribing these agents and some trial and error may be needed in some cases.

Specific Stimulants and Clinical Management. There has been considerable debate over whether stimulant dose should be weight based or a fixed dose (33, 41). At least in part, this controversy can be traced to early research suggesting that lower doses, such as 0.3 mg/kg/dose, were optimal for enhancing cognitive performance, whereas higher doses (0.6 mg/kg/dose or higher) were more effective for behavioral control (42). Subsequent studies have not supported this view. For example, a convincing linear dose-response was demonstrated across a range of outcomes in a placebo-controlled, crossover study involving 76 children and four dose levels of methylphenidate (36). Nonetheless, individual children may indeed show variability in response across a range of dose levels. Other children may show an orderly dose-response up to a threshold, above which there is little additive benefit. Thus, the mg/kg calculation can be used as a crude guide to calculate the starting dose of 0.3 mg/kg/dose and to a usual ceiling dose (e.g., 0.8 mg/kg/dose).Thereafter, the dose can be increased to establish an optimal response. For example, school-age children can be started on 5 mg tid (just before breakfast, just before lunch and 3 to 4 PM). The dosage may be increased to 10 mg bid (morning and noon) and 5 mg after school after 5 to 7 days. Subsequent increases are based on clinical response and emergence of adverse effects. The third dose typically remains half (or even less) of the first and second doses so as to minimize *rebound* effects and possible interference with sleep (41).

To determine the optimal daily dose of methylphenidate, it is essential to get feedback from both parents and teachers. In the MTA study, children were seen weekly when starting the medication to monitor progress and side effects. The study used daily ratings to assist with the assessment of response. Although this is not always feasible in clinical practice, clinicians may elect to pace dose increases with the collection of parent and teacher ratings. For example, in the first month of treatment, clinicians may increase the dose on a weekly basis. Collection of parent and teacher ratings prior to each increase would allow comparisons across dose levels. This information could be integrated with side effect data in order to select the optimal dose.

A similar approach can be used with D-amphetamine and D,L-amphetamine. The dosing of these two drugs is similar and both have approximately two-fold greater effect compared to methylphenidate. Thus the amphetamines are administered at half the methylphenidate dose. Moreover, due to their slightly longer duration of action, the amphetamines are typically given twice a day—morning and noon. The initial dosage may be a single 2.5-mg dose in younger children or a 5-mg dose in older children. After 5 to 7 days, the medication may be raised 5 mg bid in younger children and 10 mg bid in older children. Thereafter the dosage may be raised every 5 to 7 days to a total of 15 to 20 mg per day in younger children, and 40 mg per day in older children.

Until recently, methylphenidate sustained release, and D-amphetamine spansules (as well as pemoline, which has been taken off the U.S. market) were the only available long-acting formulations. Several new extended release products—formulated with methylphenidate and one with D,L-amphetamine—have entered the marketplace (Concerta, Focalin XR, Meladate CR, Ritalin RA). These longer acting preparations are as effective as the immediate release compounds and show similar side effect profiles (34, 35, 43). The advantage of the long-acting preparations is that children do not need to take a dose in school, which may enhance compliance. The longer duration formulations may minimize the behavioral rebound often seen with immediate release formulations. Originally developed for childern who could not swallow pills, Daytrana (methylphenidate transdermal patch) has been tested clinically on youth from 7 to 16 years with the patch adhered to intact skin only on their hips.

Adverse Effects. Growth retardation, presumed to be secondary to stimulant-induced appetite suppression, has been a common concern among clinicians and families alike. Based on data from a large cohort of clinic cases treated with stimulants, Spencer and colleagues contend that slowed growth may be temporary, and that children with ADHD may be shorter than their age mates before puberty, but "catch up" in adolescence (44). Followup data from the MTA study show that children who remained on medication from the end of the 14-month study to the 24-month followup did not gain as much in height or weight when compared to the children who were never started stimulant medication. The group who did not receive medication (N = 106) was about 1 cm taller and 1 kg heavier at the 24-month followup than the group (N = 222) that was treated with stimulant medication for the entire 2-year period (4). Appetite suppression can often be managed by giving stimulant medications with food, or immediately after meals. Height and weight should be monitored regularly in children treated with stimulants, and tracked during long-term maintenance on population-normed weight- and height-for-age charts.

Other common side effects include sleep disturbance, depressed mood, stomachaches, headaches, overfocusing on details, tics and mannerisms, and picking at skin. Insomnia can be difficult to sort out, as many children with ADHD have sleep difficulties prior to receiving stimulant medications. Rebound effects associated with stimulant withdrawal may compound preexisting sleep problems. Thus, the child's sleep history should be documented prior to treatment and monitored throughout. As noted, it is common practice for the third dose of methylphenidate to be lower than the first two in order to minimize a possible rebound effect. The use of clonidine as an aid for sleep has been proposed, yet remains a controversial practice (45). A multisite trial conducted by the Tourette Syndrome Study Group (46) showed that complaints of insomnia were indeed lower in subjects randomly assigned to combined treatment with methylphenidate and clonidine compared to methylphenidate also.

Results from case reports and controlled studies suggest that exposure to stimulants can be associated with the emergence of tics (47) or the worsening of preexisting tics (48). However, several studies have also shown that tics do *not* invariably worsen when children with ADHD and comorbid tic disorders are treated with stimulants (and if fact about one third get better) (46, 49, 50). Nonetheless, children with tic disorders should be monitored carefully when treated with stimulants. Dose reduction may be sufficient, but discontinuation may be warranted in some cases (48).

Antidepressants

The antidepressants include a group of chemically diverse compounds that have been shown to be effective in the treatment of adults with major depression. More recently, several antidepressants have been used in the treatment of adults with a range of other disorders, including OCD, generalized anxiety disorder (GAD), panic disorder, social phobia, and posttraumatic stress disorder (PTSD). These broader clinical applications are likewise being implemented with increasing frequency in the pediatric population, even though the level of empirical support varies widely, and depends largely on the disorder under consideration. Antidepressants can be classified according to: 1) Chemical similarity (such as tricyclic compounds, and within these, secondary or tertiary amines); 2) primary mode of action (such as the selective serotonin reuptake inhibitors (SSRIs), selective norepinephrine reuptake inhibitors, or monoamine oxidase inhibitors); and 3) miscellaneous, newer antidepressants (such as buproprion, venlafaxine, or mirtazapine). The SSRIs are by far the most extensively used antidepressant class in children and adolescents, and the class with the best empirical support. Because of these facts, and the recent controversy over their potential association with suicidal thoughts, plans, and self-injurious behavior (prompting an FDA warning for all antidepressants), the SSRIs will be discussed first (Table 6.1.2.2a).

Selective Serotonin Reuptake Inhibitors

The SSRIs are a group of chemically unrelated compounds that potently inhibit the return of serotonin into presynaptic neurons. Currently marketed SSRIs include fluoxetine, sertraline, paroxetine, fluvoxamine, citalopram, and l-citalopram. In contrast to the tricyclic agent clomipramine discussed later, and which inhibits the reuptake of both norepinephrine and serotonin, these compounds are more restricted in their reuptake of serotonin, hence their denotation as selective.

Clinical applications. All of the SSRIs in current use are approved for use in the treatment of adults with OCD. With the exception of fluvoxamine, the SSRIs are also approved for use in adults with major depression. More recently, paroxetine and sertraline have been approved for adults with anxiety disorders, and sertraline for PTSD. In pediatric populations, fluvoxamine and sertraline have been approved by the FDA for the treatment of OCD, and fluoxetine for the treatment of depression.

Empirical Support. The introduction of the SSRIs, starting with fluoxetine in the late 1980s, has had a dramatic impact on the practice of pediatric psychopharmacology. Compared to the TCAs, monotherapy with the SSRIs is relatively simple. As a group, these medications are generally well tolerated, can typically be given once a day, and do not require blood level monitoring or ECGs. Following the early clinical trials with clomipramine and fluoxetine in children and adolescents (51–53), several large placebo-controlled clinical trials with sertraline (54) and fluvoxamine (55) in OCD; with fluoxetine (56) and paroxetine (57) in depression; and with fluvoxamine in non-OCD anxiety disorders (10) have been conducted in pediatric populations. In each of these studies, the SSRI was superior to placebo in the primary outcome measure of interest. More recently, trials comparing the relative efficacy of SSRIs, cognitive behavioral therapy (CBT), and their combination, have been completed with fluoxetine for depression (12), and with sertraline for OCD (24).

Obsessive-Compulsive Disorder (OCD). Sertraline and fluvoxamine have been evaluated in randomized, multisite, placebo-controlled trials of parallel groups. Using the Children's Yale–Brown Obsessive-Compulsive Scales (CYBOCS) as the primary outcome measure, both drugs were superior to placebo in improving obsessive-compulsive symptoms. Sertraline was evaluated in 187 subjects ranging from 6 to12 years of age. In that study, sertraline, at an average daily dose of 167 mg, was associated with at least a 25% improvement in the CYBOCS score in 53% of subjects, compared to 37% for placebo ($p = 0.03$) (54). In 120 children between the ages of 8 and 17 years, fluvoxamine at a mean daily dose of 165 mg was effective in 42% of children, compared to 26% among those treated with placebo ($p = 0.06$) (55).

An open-label study of paroxetine in pediatric OCD revealed not only promising results (58), but also interestingly, reductions in thalamic volume (59) and caudate glutamate levels (60), which paralleled clinical response. Two small placebo-controlled studies provide additional support for the efficacy of fluoxetine in OCD (15, 61). Finally, one open-label study with citalopram has been done in children with OCD (62). In that study, 23 subjects were treated with 10 to 40 mg per day of citalopram for 10 weeks in an open-label fashion. Eleven of 23 subjects showed a clinically meaningful positive response (30% improvement or more). Five patients showed little or no response, and the remaining seven showed a partial response.

Taken together, these data suggest that the SSRIs are effective for the treatment of OCD in children and adolescents. However, the magnitude of response may not be large, as has been shown in a metaanalysis of all studies published through 2002 (63). In addition, some children with OCD may show only a partial response to an adequate trial of an SSRI. For example, approximately 40% of the subjects in the multisite sertraline study showed less than a 25% improvement in obsessive-compulsive symptoms (54). This observation indicates that clinicians should remind parents and patients not to have unreasonably high expectations for SSRI treatment. The problem of partial response raises questions about whether to switch to another SSRI or clomipramine, or to embark on one of several augmentation medication strategies. Although not well studied in children (64), two studies have shown that the addition of low-dose haloperidol (65) or risperidone (66) to an SSRI can be effective in adults with refractory OCD. A recent metaanalysis provides support for augmentation of SSRIs with haloperidol and risperidone in the treatment of adults with OCD (67). In view of the inadequate support for combined pharmacotherapy in children with refractory OCD, other interventions should be considered, particularly CBT.

Indeed, the Pediatric Obsessive Compulsive Treatment Study (POTS) (23) showed superiority of CBT over SSRI treatment alone. In that study, 112 children (mean age about 11.5 years, 56 boys and 56 girls) with OCD enrolled across three treatment sites were randomly assigned to sertraline, CBT, their combination, or pill placebo. Statistical analyses on the Children's Yale–Brown Obsessive-Compulsive Disorder Scales (CYBOCS) indicated a significant advantage for CBT alone ($P = .003$), sertraline alone ($P = .007$), and combined treatment ($P = .001$) compared with placebo. Combined treatment showed a 53% improvement on the CYBOCS

TABLE 6.1.2.2A

SSRI ANTIDEPRESSANTS

Drug	Mechanism of Action	Main Indications and Clinical Uses	Dosage (mg/d)	Schedule	Adverse Effects	Comments	Select Brand Names and Preparations Available
A. Selective Serotonin Reuptake Inhibitors (SSRIs)							
Fluoxetine	Serotonin presynaptic reuptake blockade	Obsessive compulsive disorder/Major depression/Other anxiety disorders	2.5–40	qd/FLV = bid	Irritability Akathisia Insomnia Appetite decrease (acute use) or increase (chronic) GI symptoms Headaches/Dizziness Flu-like symptoms during discontinuation Complex drug interactions. All SSRIs have variable degrees of CYP inhibition (see previous chapter). Higher doses often needed for OCD. Exacerbation or new onset of suicidal ideation was initially reported for paroxetine in 2003; careful monitoring recommendations for *all* antidepressants followed a review of all clinical trials for child and adolescent depression (see text for details)	Only SSRI with FDA approval for the treatment of depression. Longest half-life	Prozac: 10 mg t/c 20 mg t, oral solution 20 mg/5 ml
Sertraline			25–200				Zoloft: 25, 50; 100 mg t
Paroxetine			10–30			SSRI originally associated with suicidal ideation; no longer recommended for use in children and adolescents	Paxil: 10, 20, 30, 40 mg t oral suspension 10 mg/5 ml
Fluvoxamine			12.5–200			Short half-life implies bid dosing and greater likelihood of withdrawal syndrome	Luvox: 25, 50, 100 mg t
Citalopram			10–40			Most favorable drug interaction profiles among the SSRIs	Celexa: 20, 40 t
I-Citalopram			10–20				Lexapro: 10, 20 t

Note: Doses are provided as general guidelines only, and are not meant to be definitive. All doses must be individualized and monitored through the appropriate clinical and/or laboratory means.
Abbreviations: c (capsule); t (tablet); FDA (Food and Drug Administration).

compared to 46% for CBT alone, 30% for sertraline alone and 15% for placebo. These results suggest that CBT, if readily available, may be the preferred first treatment for OCD, either alone or in combination with an SSRI. The two groups who were treated with active medication each started on a dose of 25 mg per day with gradual increases to a maximum of 200 mg per day. The combined treatment group received an average of 133 mg per day compared to 170 mg per day for the sertraline only group.

Based on the demonstrated efficacy and safety of the SSRIs in children and adolescents with OCD, these medications are commonly used to reduce repetitive behavior in pervasive developmental disorders (PDDs) (68). Despite their common use in clinical practice, however, the SSRIs have not been well studied in children with PDD. Moreover, the best available evidence indicates that the SSRIs may only be moderately effective. Hollander and colleagues (69) compared fluoxetine to placebo in a crossover trial of 39 subjects age 5 to 17. At an average dose of approximately 10 mg per day, the drug was well tolerated with a low frequency of activation. The low frequency of activation appears to be due the low starting dose and gradual increase.

Although the report notes that the active drug was superior to placebo, fluoxetine showed an average 10% improvement over baseline on a clinician measure of repetitive behavior. Clearly, more study is needed. To address questions of efficacy and safety of the SSRIs for repetitive behavior in PDD, an NIH-sponsored, multisite study by the STAART Group is comparing citalopram to placebo in a 12-week parallel group trial. When completed, the study will enroll 144 subjects, which may provide guidance for clinicians concerning which children with PDD are appropriate for SSRI treatment.

Depression. Fluoxetine, sertraline, paroxetine, and citalopram have each been studied for the treatment of depression in children and adolescents. The landmark fluoxetine study by Emslie and colleagues (56) was the first to show superiority of an antidepressant over placebo for the treatment of depression in children and adolescents and was subsequently followed by a replication study (70). A placebo-controlled, multicenter trial comparing paroxetine, imipramine, and placebo (71) indicated that paroxetine was superior to placebo, achieving a 63% response rate, compared to 46% in the placebo group. By contrast, the response rate in the imipramine group was 50%, which was not statistically different from placebo. Imipramine was associated with common TCA side effects and with a high rate of premature discontinuations. Two identical, industry-sponsored trials of sertraline showed superiority over placebo when combined into a single report (72), but failed to differentiate from placebo when analyzed separately. A randomized clinical trial of citalopram has also shown superiority over placebo (73).

The largest and most important study to date in this area is the Treatment for Adolescents with Depression Study (TADS) (12). In it, 439 adolescents 12–17 of age, were randomly assigned to fluoxetine alone, CBT alone, their combination, or pill placebo. They were followed for 12 weeks in the acute phase and for a 6-month extension. Results of the acute phase (12-week trial) showed that combined treatment had the highest rate of positive response (71% for the combined treatment, compared to 61% for medication alone, 43% for CBT alone, and 35% for placebo). The combined treatment group also had a slightly lower rate of suicidal ideation (5.6%) compared to the fluoxetine-only group (8.3%). Fluoxetine alone and fluoxetine with CBT were both superior to placebo. However, combined treatment with fluoxetine and CBT was not significantly better than medication only and CBT alone was not superior to placebo.

Concerns over safety of the use of the SSRIs in children and adolescents have become paramount, initially garnering substantial attention in the media and lay press, and following extensive review by British and American regulatory agencies, eventually led to the removal (in the U.K.) and the introduction of an FDA-mandated *black-box warning* (in the U.S.). The history and full implications of this series of concerns is explored in detail in a recent review (74) and continues to be a source of controversy, shifting policy, and clinical recommendations. In the context of this general overview of pediatric psychopharmacology, the following are important high points of the discussion to date: 1) A review of all clinical trials (both published and unpublished) using SSRIs in the treatment of children and adolescents with depression and other indications (N>4,400 subjects, across 26 controlled trials, 16 of them for depression) was commissioned by the FDA. It revealed an increase risk in new onset suicidal ideation between SSRI- and placebo-treated individuals (occurring at respective rates of 4% and 2%, for a risk ratio of 1.95 (95% confidence interval, 1.28–2.98) (75); 2) all reported events referred to suicidal *ideation*, rather than suicidal acts or completed suicides; 3) there is compelling pharmacopidemiological data to suggest that paralleling the widespread use of SSRIs in the US, the suicide rate among those ages 15 to 19 fell from about 11 per 100,000 in 1990 to 7.3 per 100,000 in 2003 and synchronous with the FDA Black Box warning on antidepressants and the likely reduction in antidepressant usage in 2004, the suicide rate climbed 18 percent for those younger than 20, from 1,737 deaths to 1,985 (76); and 4) based on these data, it seems most parsimonious to recommend the judicious use of antidepressants in children and adolescents, particularly if other interventions have failed or are not available. When treatment with an SSRI is opted for, fluoxetine may be generally recommended as the first-line agent because of its FDA indication for depression and a lower reported rate of incident suicidal ideation. Guidelines from the FDA and the American Academy of Child and Adolescent Psychiatry (AACAP) call for intensive monitoring during the early phases of treatment: as often as weekly for the first 4 weeks, every other week for the next month, and monthly thereafter. While such recommendations are clinically sensible, such guidelines may potentially lead to the perverse outcome of increased suicide rates in that practitioners may hesitate resorting to these agents if unable to provide monitoring as intense as is being called for. This may become especially problematic in underserved areas, where nonspecialists may be reluctant to prescribe antidepressants.

Non-OCD Anxiety Disorders. To date, only fluvoxamine has been evaluated in the treatment of children and adolescents with non-OCD anxiety disorders. In a multisite study sponsored by the National Institute of Mental Health (10), 128 subjects between the ages of 6 and 17 years were randomly assigned to placebo or fluvoxamine after a 3-week psychoeducational intervention. The primary outcome measure was the Pediatric Anxiety Rating Scale (PARS), a new scale developed specifically for the trial. After 8 weeks of treatment, children in the fluvoxamine group showed a 52% improvement (mean decrease in PARS from 18.7 to 9.0) compared to 16% improvement (mean decrease from 19.0 to 15.9) for the placebo group ($p < 0.001$). The dose began at 25 mg per day, with a planned increase to 25 mg twice a day after 4 days. The dose schedule continued upward in 25 mg increments every 4 to 5 days as tolerated. The findings from this study provide support for the efficacy and large effect size of fluvoxamine in the treatment of generalized anxiety disorder, social phobia, and separation anxiety. This study also paves the way for the study of the other SSRIs and combination treatments (medication and psychotherapy) in non-OCD anxiety disorders. Indeed, the Children and Adolescents Anxiety Multimodal Treatment study (CAMS) is currently underway. With a projected sample size of 320 children and adolescents (ages 7–17), it will compare the efficacy of sertraline, CBT, or their combination in the treatment of generalized or separation anxiety or social phobia (77).

Mechanism of Action. The SSRIs interfere with the return of serotonin into the presynaptic neuron by blocking the serotonin transporter located on presynaptic nerve terminals. Over time, this blockade leads to a desensitization of the serotonin autoreceptors, which typically exert an inhibitory influence on serotonin release. With continued blockade of the transporter, the desensitized autoreceptors do not exert their usual inhibitory influence and serotonergic function is enhanced. Based on a series of animal studies, Blier and colleagues suggest that the main location of the enhanced serotonergic function appears to be the hippocampus in depression, and the orbital frontal cortex in OCD (78).

Pharmacokinetics. All SSRIs have relatively long half-lives, permitting single daily dosing. Fluvoxamine, which has the shortest half-life, is sometimes given on a twice-daily schedule. A recent pharmacokinetic evaluation of paroxetine showed that children metabolize the medication faster than adults (79). Despite the shorter half-life in the pediatric population, these investigators still recommend once-daily dosing for paroxetine. At low doses of sertraline, 50 mg per day or less, children may require bid dosing (80). The pharmacokinetic profiles of the other SSRIs in pediatric populations have not been documented. In adults, fluoxetine and citalopram have the longest half-lives of currently available SSRIs, with estimates of 48 to 72 and of 33 hours, respectively. In addition, fluoxetine has an active metabolite (norfluoxetine) with an elimination half-life of 7 to 14 days. Both fluoxetine (primarily norfluoxetine) and paroxetine are potent inhibitors of CYP 2D6. Because both paroxetine and fluoxetine are 2D6 substrates, they inhibit their own metabolism, resulting in nonlinear kinetics at higher doses. Fluvoxamine also has nonlinear pharmacokinetics, which may be related to its inhibiting its own metabolism.

Clinical Management. *Fluoxetine* (Prozac) is available in a 10-mg scored tablet, a 20-mg capsule and in a liquid preparation (20 mg per 5 ml). A typical starting dose for school-age children is 5 to 10 mg per day; smaller children may start at 2.5 mg per day. Given its long half-life, fluoxetine should be increased slowly (weekly or even at 2-week intervals) to avoid "overshooting" the optimal dose. The usual dose range for children and adolescents is 5 to 40 mg per day, though some children and adolescents may require higher doses (81).

Sertraline (Zoloft) is available in 25-, 50-, and 100-mg tablets that can be easily broken in half; it is also available as an oral suspension in a 20 mg/ml strength. Treatment might start with a 12.5 to 25-mg dose, with similar weekly increments to a range of 50 to 150 mg in children. Higher dosages may be required in older adolescents. Clinicians should review therapeutic response during the dose adjustment phase to determine whether additional increases are needed, rather than using an automatic dose schedule.

Fluvoxamine (marketed under the generic name) is available in 25-, 50-, and 100-mg scored tablets. Treatment usually begins at 12.5 to 25 mg per day and is increased by 25 mg on a weekly basis. The typical dose range is 50 to 200 mg per day. Although the double-blind trial in children and adolescents with OCD used a rapid dose escalation with increases every 3 days (55), the more recent RUPP anxiety study used a slower upward adjustment (10). This study started with 25 per day and increased to 25 mg twice a day within the first week. Thereafter, the dose was increased in 25 mg steps each week as tolerated.

Paroxetine (Paxil) is available in 10-, 20-, and 30-mg tablets that can be broken in half, as well as in an oral suspension (10 mg per 5 ml). The typical starting dose is 5 to 10 mg per day, with weekly increases to a total daily dose of 10 to 40 mg. As noted before, paroxetine is no longer recommended for the routine use of children and adolescents. Exposure to paroxetine during the first trimester of pregnancy may increase the risk for congenital malformations, especially cardiac ones.

Citalopram (Celexa) is available in 10-, 20-, and 40-mg scored tablets, as well as in a liquid preparation. Based on experience with the other SSRIs, a reasonable starting dose would be 5 mg per day, with increases on weekly or 2-week intervals, to a maximum of 40 mg per day.

Escitalopram (Lexapro) is available in 10- and 20-mg scored tablets.

Adverse Effects. As a group, the SSRIs are generally well tolerated, and potentially serious side effects such as alterations in cardiac conduction times or seizures have not been reported in the usual dose range. In addition to their propensity for cytochrome P450-based drug interactions (as reviewed in the preceding chapter), common side effects of the SSRIs in children and adolescents appear to be behavioral activation and GI complaints such as nausea or diarrhea. Signs of behavioral activation include motor restlessness, insomnia, impulsiveness, disinhibited behavior, and garrulousness. It may occur early in treatment, with dose increases (82), or following the addition of drugs that inhibit the metabolism of the SSRIs (e.g., cimetidine). The potential for behavioral activation early in treatment underscores the importance of starting at low doses and moving upward slowly. As with other antidepressants, hypomania and mania have also been reported, and peripubertal children may be at especially heightened risk (7). Other adverse effects include diarrhea, nausea, heartburn, decreased appetite, and fatigue. Sexual side effects, such as erectile dysfunction, delayed ejaculation, or anorgasmia, all of which are relatively common in adults, should also be considered in sexually active adolescents.

The controversy over suicidal ideation is briefly presented above, and in greater detail in a recent review (74). As with all antidepressants, particularly when treating depression, clinicians should monitor suicidal thought and self-injurious potential in any child or adolescent treated with an SSRI.

SSRI Discontinuation Syndrome and Duration of Therapy. A flu-like syndrome characterized by dizziness, moodiness, nausea, vomiting, myalgia, and fatigue occurring in association with the withdrawal or acute discontinuation of shorter acting SSRIs such as paroxetine, fluvoxamine, and sertraline has been described (83). Recently, a controlled discontinuation study in 220 adults compared the withdrawal effects of fluoxetine, paroxetine, and sertraline: Paroxetine and sertraline were associated with irritability, agitation, fatigue, insomnia, confusion, dizziness and nervousness upon abrupt withdrawal, but fluoxetine was not (84). The long half-life of norfluoxetine presumably results in a gradual "auto-taper," even when the oral dose is stopped abruptly. Based on these results, a slow withdrawal of the shorter acting SSRIs is warranted. Citalopram has a 33-hour half-life, but no known active metabolites. In the absence of data on adverse effects following abrupt withdrawal, sudden discontinuation of citalopram should also be avoided.

Another clinical issue that often arises in the course of treating children and adolescents with an SSRI concerns the duration of treatment. Studies of adults with depression suggest that an episode of depression typically lasts 9 months to a year. Based on this evidence, the duration of treatment for depression can be set at a 1-year minimum. For OCD and anxiety disorders, however, there are no data upon which to base duration of treatment. A review on OCD suggests discontinuation after a relatively symptom-free period of 8 to 12 months (85). A long-term followup study of 54 children and adolescents with OCD found that 70% (N = 39) remained on medication for more than 2 years (86), and persistence of OCD through late adolescence and adulthood is estimated to occur in about 40% of subjects (87). Given the potential for chronicity in

OCD, children and parents should be informed that symptoms may return following a planned SSRI discontinuation.

Drug Interactions. Due to their multiple clinical applications, ease of use and perceived safety, the SSRIs are increasingly common in clinical practice. In addition, the use of combined psychotropic medications seems to be on the rise. These trends underscore the importance of monitoring drug–drug interactions in clinical practice. SSRIs vary in their potential for such interactions at particular P450 cytochromes. As illustrated previously, inhibition of the P450 cytochrome responsible for metabolizing an additive drug raises its serum level, thereby enhancing its beneficial or deleterious effects. For example, oculogyric crises and other dystonic reactions have been reported in youngsters when an antipsychotic was added to ongoing treatment with paroxetine, probably the result of the latter's inhibition of CYP2D6, which is a major pathway of risperidone metabolism (88). (For a more detailed discussion of drug interactions, interested readers are referred to the previous chapter).

Tricyclic Antidepressants

Clinical applications and empirical support. Tricyclic antidepressants (TCAs) have been used to treat several psychiatric disorders of childhood over the past three decades, including depression, ADHD, OCD, separation anxiety disorder, and enuresis. Although TCAs have been used frequently in clinical practice, evidence for their efficacy in treating children with these psychiatric disorders is inconsistent. For example, a series of carefully conducted controlled trials have consistently failed to show the superiority of any TCA over placebo in the treatment of child- and adolescent-onset depression (89). This poor track record stands in marked contrast to the more compelling results in adult depression (90). The use of TCAs in non-OCD anxiety is equivocal. One study found imipramine superior to placebo in the treatment of separation anxiety (91), but another failed to replicate an earlier report of efficacy (92). In contrast to these respectively disappointing or inconclusive findings in depression or separation anxiety, double-blind, placebo-controlled studies have demonstrated the efficacy of desipramine in children with ADHD (93–95), and of clomipramine for the treatment of OCD in children and adolescents (51). Tricyclic agents continue to have a limited but important role in the treatment of enuresis and of treatment-refractory ADHD and OCD (Table 6.1.2.2b).

Mechanism of Action. To varying degrees, all TCAs inhibit the reuptake of norepinephrine by presynaptic neurons. Over time, this pharmacologic effect *is presumed* to enhance noradrenergic neurotransmission. Among the TCAs, desipramine is the most selective in its capacity to block norepinephrine reuptake. This highly selective property of desipramine plays a role in its efficacy in ADHD. Based on the favorable effects of desipramine in ADHD, interest developed in other compounds, such as atomoxetine, with highly selective norepinephrine reuptake inhibiting properties (96). Unlike desipramine, however, atomoxetine does not appear to prolong cardiac conduction times. Clomipramine is unique among the TCAs in that it is a potent inhibitor of serotonin reuptake. This property explains its superiority over desipramine for the treatment of OCD.

Tertiary amine TCAs such as imipramine (or amitryptiline, rarely used in psychiatry, but useful in medicine for the treatment of neuropathic pain) have highly anticholinergic profiles. Because of this, they are less often used as a first-line intervention, with the exception of enuresis, for which imipramine continues to be used in clinical practice. By contrast, the secondary amines desipramine and nortriptyline (derived from their patent compounds imipramine and amitryptiline, respectively) are less likely to cause orthostatic hypotension, constipation, or urinary retention, and are thus generally preferred in clinical practice.

Pharmacokinetics. Due to genetic differences in P450 cytochrome enzyme activity, serum levels of TCAs can show wide variation across individuals taking the same oral dose. Thus, therapeutic levels for the TCAs are not well established in pediatric populations. Serum levels may be useful, however, to identify children with low or ultrarapid metabolic activity, to rule out toxicity, and to assess compliance. As a general rule of thumb, blood levels of nortriptyline are close in absolute value to daily oral dosage among normal metabolizers (thus, 75 mg/day would be expected to yield a steady-state trough level of ~ 75 ng/ml). When major discrepancies are seen to this pattern, the clinician can anticipate noncompliance or ultrafast metabolism of CYP2D6 (in the case of low levels), or CYP2D6 inhibition from a medication or another chemical compound or slow metabolism (in the case of high levels).

Clinical Management. An ECG, pulse, and blood pressure should be obtained prior to starting any of the TCAs. A medical and family history that focuses on syncope in the child, as well as in episodes of syncope or sudden death in close relatives may be informative. Evidence of a normal physical examination within the past year should also be documented. The typical dose range for TCAs in children is up to 5 mg/kg/ day for imipramine, and 2.5 mg/kg/day for nortriptyline and perhaps somewhat higher for clomipramine (3 mg/kg/day). Imipramine may be started at a dosage of 25 mg and increased every 4 or 6 days in similar increments to 100 to 150 mg per day. In younger children, nortriptyline is typically introduced with a 10-mg dose, with increases every 4 to 6 days to a range of 50 to 75 mg per day in divided doses. Clomipramine is usually started at a dose of 25 mg, with gradual increases every 4 or 6 days to a maximum of 100 mg per day in younger children and 150 mg in older children. For all of the TCAs, repeat vital signs and ECGs should be obtained during the dose adjustment phase and when the maintenance dose has been achieved. As part of the informed consent process, potential cardiac effects and the reason for repeat ECG monitoring should be discussed with the family and with the child in a developmentally appropriate manner. A corrected QT interval (QTc) above 450 ms, a QRS complex longer than 120 ms, or a PR interval greater than 200 ms (97) warrant dose reduction followed by a repeat ECG. Exceeding these parameters should prompt treatment reevaluation and perhaps discontinuation. For cases showing clinical benefit and persistent ECG abnormalities, consultation with a pediatric cardiologist is in order.

Adverse Effects. The TCAs are associated with a range of adverse effects, including sedation, dizziness, dry mouth, excessive sweating, weight gain, urinary retention, tremor, and agitation. In addition to these largely anticholinergic-based side effects, TCAs can have dose-dependent adverse effects on cardiac conduction (which can be tracked with an expectable dose-dependent prolongation of the QTc) as well as on the seizure threshold. With regard to seizures, clomipramine may have the highest vulnerability to lower the seizure threshold, so that its dose and potential drug interactions need to be monitored closely.

For most adverse effects, lowering the dose, changing dose schedules, or switching from a tertiary to a secondary amine can often help manage symptoms. For example, to deal with sedation, the medication could be given twice a day, with the higher dose in the evening. Switching between TCAs can be helpful at times: For example, imipramine can be changed to nortriptyline in an effort to minimize sedation or constipation. Despite the evidence showing the efficacy of clomipramine for

TABLE 6.1.2.2B

TRICYCLIC ANTIDEPRESSANTS

Drug	Mechanism of Action	Main Indications and Clinical Uses	Dosage	Schedule	Adverse Effects	Comments	Select Brand Names and Preparations Available
B. Tricyclic Antidepressants (TCAs)							
Impiramine Desipramine Nortriptyline	Norepinephrine > dopamine presynaptic reuptake blockade; anticholinergic, antihistamine, alpha-1 postsynaptic effects	MDD Enuresis ADHD ADHD + tic disorders Anxiety disorders	2.5–5.0 mg/kg/d (Impiramine, Desipramine) 1.0–2.5 mg/kg/d (Nortriptyline)	bid/tid	Anticholinergic (dry mouth, constipation, blurred vision) Weight gain Cardiovascular (mild blood pressure and ECG conduction parameters Treatment requires serum levels and ECG monitoring	Serum levels can be useful in adjusting dosage, monitoring potential toxicity, determining metabolizer status	Imipramine hydrochloride: 10, 25 50 mg t Imipramine pamoate: 75, 100, 125, 150 mg c Desipramine: 10, 25, 50, 75, 100, 150 mg t Nortriptyline: 10, 25, 50, 75 mg; elixir (?) Clomipramine: 25, 50, 75 t
Clomipramine	Same as other TCAs; serotonin presynaptic reuptake blockade	Same as other TCAs OCD	2.0–3.0 mg/kg/d				

Note: Doses are provided as general guidelines only, and are not meant to be definitive. All doses must be individualized and monitored through the appropriate clinical and/or laboratory means.
Abbreviations: c (capsule); t (tablet); FDA (Food and Drug Administration).

OCD and desipramine for ADHD, the TCAs appear to be declining in use. This trend is largely due to the side effect profile and the potential for serious adverse effects, with the rare possibilities of sudden death related to tachyarrhythmias such as t*orsade de pointes* being the most ominous. Originally reported in cases treated with desipramine, the series of case reports that accrued over ensuing years has prompted many experts to recommend avoiding TCAs in the pediatric population (98). The combination of: 1) stepwise dosing within clear weight-adjusted margins; 2) careful ECG monitoring; 3) full disclosure of the risk-to-benefit ratio in the treatment planning process; and 4) their selective use in nonresponders to first-line agents provides a rational basis for keeping these compounds as potential treatment options.

Interactions. As with most other psychotropic drugs, the TCAs are metabolized by hepatic enzymes in the cytochrome P450 system (CYP 450). Several psychotropic (fluoxetine, fluvoxamine, paroxetine) and nonpsychotropic drugs (ketoconazole, cimetidine, clarithromycin) inhibit the action of one or more of these hepatic enzymes. Inhibition of the enzyme specific for metabolizing the TCA can result in toxicity. (For a more detailed discussion of drug–drug interactions, see previous chapter).

Other Antidepressant Medications

Bupropion (Wellbutrin)

Bupropion is unrelated to all other available antidepressants. Although its mechanism of action is unclear, it appears to have both dopaminergic and noradrenergic effects. It is approved for the treatment of depression and smoking cessation in adults. Although bupropion has not been studied for depression in children or adolescents, it has been evaluated in controlled studies for the treatment of ADHD. A placebo-controlled trial of bupropion in 72 children with ADHD showed its superiority over placebo, although the treatment effect was smaller than that usually seen with stimulants (99). The dose of bupropion (3–6 mg/kg/day) ranged from 50 to 200 mg per day in divided doses. The findings of this study are consistent with previous placebo-controlled studies, and a direct comparison with methylphenidate (100). In an open-label study conducted in 24 adolescents (ages 11 to 16) with ADHD and depression, sustained release bupropion was associated with improvements in both conditions in 58% (N = 14), in depression only in 29% (N = 7), and in ADHD alone in 4% (N = 1), suggesting that further studies of this monotherapy appear warranted for these commonly co-occurring conditions (Table 6.1.2.2c) (101).

Side effects of bupropion include agitation, insomnia, skin rashes, nausea, vomiting, constipation, and tremor. Bupropion may also reduce the seizure threshold in a dose-dependent fashion. The seizure liability of bupropion was first described in a group of female patients with bulimia nervosa. Because of this, regardless of diagnosis, it is recommended that daily doses not exceed 300 mg in children, and no single dose be higher than 150 mg. Bupropion (Wellbutrin) is available in 75- and 100-mg tablets, in 100- and 150-mg sustained release (SR) tablets, and 150 mg and 300 mg Bupropion XL tablets. Treatment is usually on a tid basis for the immediate release formulation given the agent's short half-life; bid dosing is possible with the SR preparations and once daily is recommended with XL preparations.

Venlafaxine (Effexor)

Venlafaxine is an agent that selectively inhibits serotonin reuptake at lower doses (<150 mg/d) and acts on both norepinephrine and serotonin reuptake at the higher dose range. To date, there is one placebo-controlled trial in children with depression. The study, which included 32 youngsters, found that the drug was no better than placebo in relieving depression (102). The lack of a significant results were replicated in a larger scale, as yet unpublished, industry-sponsored study. These negative results, coupled with the fact that venlafaxine had the single highest association with incident suicidal ideation (75), advise against the routine use of this agent in pediatric psychopharmacology.

Venlafaxine is available in 25-, 37.5-, 50-, 75-, and 100-mg tablets, and in 37.5-, 75-, and 150-mg extended release (XR) capsules. Dosing is started with the smallest dose given at bedtime, and with attention to early sedation and dizziness, before moving to a twice-daily regimen. At higher doses (>150 mg/d), venlafaxine can be associated with diastolic hypertension, an effect that is clearly dose-dependent in nature.

Trazodone (Desyrel) and Nefazodone

These agents are potent $5HT_{2a}$ postsynaptic antagonists and moderate serotonin and norepinephrine reuptake inhibitors. This novel mechanism of action initially raised great interest in these compounds, but lackluster efficacy results among adults, coupled with rare but serious adverse effects (priapism for trazodone, hepatotoxicity for nefazodone) has led to the selective use of trazodone as an adjunct for insomnia in females only. Trazodone is available in 50-,100-, 150-, and 300-mg pills, and is prescribed in HS dosing for insomnia. Due to concern about hepatic toxicity, serzone but not nefazodone has been taken off the market.

Mirtazapine (Remeron)

Several other new antidepressants have entered into the marketplace, including mirtazapine, a combined norepinephrine pre- and serotonin post-synaptic antagonist with a characteristic side effect profile of drowsiness, increased appetite and weight gain, though uncommon in the lower dosage range. Few data on the use of mirtazapine in the pediatric population are available, but an unpublished industry-sponsored randomized clinical trial did not show efficacy in depression in youth (103).

Atomoxetine (Strattera)

Atomoxetine was originally developed for the treatment of depression, but it has never been marketed as an antidepressant. As noted previously, atomoxetine is a selective norepinephrine reuptake inhibitor—a property that it shares in common with desipramine. Unlike desipramine, however, atomoxetine does not appear to prolong cardiac conduction times. Given the efficacy of desipramine for the treatment of ADHD, atomoxetine was evaluated as a treatment for ADHD. Following the completion of several placebo-controlled trials (104, 105), atomoxetine was approved by FDA as a safe and effective treatment of children and adolescents with ADHD. In fact, it is the only approved, nonstimulant medication for the treatment of ADHD. It may also be useful in the treatment of comorbid oppositional defiant disorder (106, 107).

The serum half-life of atomoxetine is approximately 4 hours, which implies that the drug would be given at least twice a day. Indeed, initial studies used a twice daily regimen, but subsequent trials evaluated the efficacy of once a day dosing (104, 105). Although both dosing strategies have been shown to be superior to placebo, twice a day dosing showed a similar magnitude of improvement than once daily dosing (30% improvement on a rating of ADHD symptoms scored by a clinician following a semistructured interview) (104, 105). Improvement in ADHD symptoms are not as robust as stimulants (108). The total daily dose is likely to fall between 0.8 and 1.2 mg/kg. Doses greater than 1.2 mg per kg per day are unlikely to produce greater benefit (107). Based on these data, clinicians might consider starting with once a day dosing

TABLE 6.1.2.2C

OTHER ANTIDEPRESSANTS

Drug	Mechanism of Action	Main Indications and Clinical Uses	Dosage	Schedule	Adverse Effects	Comments	Select Brand Names and Preparations Available
				C. Other Antidepressants			
Bupropion	Unknown. ?Norepinephrine > dopamine presynaptic reuptake blockade	MDD ADHD	3.0–6.0 mg/kg/d	tid	Irritability Insomnia Drug-induced seizures (in doses >6 mg/kg) Contraindicated in bulimia Seizures associated with >300 mg/day or >150 mg/dose	Useful alternative to stimulants in ADHD, but exacerbation of tics has been reported	Wellbutrin: 75, 100 mg t Wellbutrin SR: 100, 150 t Wellbutrin XL: 150, 300 t
Venlafaxine	Serotonin/norepinephrine presynaptic reuptake blockade	MDD	1.0–3.0 mg/kg/d	bid/tid	Similar to selective serotonin reuptake inhibitors Nausea, sleepiness, dizziness Dose-dependent (?) sustained diastolic hypertension Exacerbation of suicidal ideation highest for venlafaxine; careful monitoring especially warranted with its use. Not recommended for routine use in children and adolescents	Under 150 mg/d, similar to an SSRI; noradrenergic effects at higher doses	Effexor: 25, 37.5, 50, 75, 100 mg t Effexor XR: 37.5, 75, 150 mg c
Trazodone	Serotonin presynaptic reuptake blockade/5HT2a postsynaptic antagonism	Insomnia	25–200 mg/d	hs	Nausea, dry mouth, dizziness, constipation Orthostatic hypotension Sedation Priapism	Although the closely related compound, nefazodone, had less alpha antagonism than trazodone (i.e., less risk of hypotension and priapism), it is seldom used because of concerns over liver toxicity.	Trazodone: 50, 100, 150, 300 mg t
Mirtazapine	$Alpha_2$ presynaptic and $5HT_{2A/3}$ postsynaptic antagonism	MDD	7.5–30 mg/d	hs	Drowsiness (greater at low doses?) Appetite/weight gain	Useful alternative to SSRIs leading to activation?	Remeron: 7.5, 15 mg

Note: Doses are provided as general guidelines only, and are not meant to be definitive. All doses must be individualized and monitored through the appropriate clinical and/or laboratory means. Abbreviations: c (capsule); t (tablet); FDA (Food and Drug Administration).

with gradually increasing doses. If the child encounters adverse effects or the benefits are inadequate, a twice a day schedule could be considered.

Common side effects of atomoxetine include dyspepsia, nausea, vomiting, fatigue, decreased appetite, weight loss, mood swings, headache, constipation, difficulty sleeping, and dizziness (109). Decreased appetite, vomiting, and weight loss are more likely early in treatment and may be attenuated by slow upward adjustment. Black box warnings on this drug include: hepatitis, increased aggression and hostility and suicidal thinking (110, 111). Atomoxetine is metabolized by the cytochrome P450 2D6 and thus it is vulnerable to interaction from drugs that inhibit 2D6, such as paroxetine or fluoxetine.

Mood Stabilizers

Background: Bipolar-Spectrum Disorders and Other Indications

There has been a dramatic increase in the prevalence of the diagnosis of bipolar disorder (BP) in youth (112). At the same time, there are ongoing disagreements about the diagnostic criteria. There is no controversy about the diagnosis of teens with full DSM-IV criteria, the "narrow phenotype." (113) The stability of a BD diagnosis of this type of teen-onset BD has been shown to persist into young adulthood. However, this group of teens can be differentiated from those who demonstrate *core positive* symptoms of mania—but fail to meet full criteria (subsyndromal BP). A large-scale followup study of community-identified youth with core positive symptoms showed that these teens were more likely to develop anxiety or depression rather than BD when reevaluated in young adulthood (114). There is considerable controversy about the diagnosis of BP in prepubertal children with nonepisodic, chronic irritability, and "multiple, intense, prolonged mood swings each day," the "broad phenotype." (113, 115) A consensus conference agreed to the designation of bipolar NOS for this group of difficult to treat children (116). Leibenluft has operationalized this "broad phenotype," and using the Great Smoky Mountain database, concluded that like the teen subsyndromal BP group, these children will later develop a depressive diagnosis (117). Because the DSM-IV has no other diagnosis for youth who show some symptoms of mania, but fail to meet full criteria for mania (due to symptom count or duration), BP-NOS has also been applied to these youth. These youngsters would likely fall into Leibenluft's "intermediate phenotype" and their course may be different than those in the "broad phenotype." A followup (average 2 years) of 92 children with BD-NOS revealed that 25% met criteria for bipolar 1 (BP-1) or bipolar 2 (BP-2) (118).

The prototype for the chemically unrelated group of mood stabilizers is lithium, which has been used in the treatment of bipolar illness for over 50 years. It is currently the only FDA-approved drug for the treatment of bipolar disorder in youth (older than 13 years). Other mood stabilizers include valproate, carbamazepine, lamotrigine, oxcarbazepine, and topiramate. Of these, only valproate, carbamazepine and lamotrigine have been carefully studied in adults. By contrast, empirical data for any of the mood stabilizers are scarce in the pediatric population (119, 120). In addition to bipolar-spectrum conditions, the mood stabilizers are commonly used in pediatric psychopharmacology for the management of aggressive outbursts and intense emotional lability. Although the empirical database for these indications (including bipolar disorders) is modest, there is some support for the use of valproate in the treatment of conduct, rather than mood disorders (121, 122).

Treatment guidelines for youth with a diagnosis of only BP-1, mixed, or manic types have been developed (115). The first two-stage trials focus on the use of monotherapy with the traditional mood stabilizers: lithium, valproate, and carbamazepine, or with atypical antipsychotics (AAPs) olanzapine, quetiapine, or risperidone. Stage three has two possible routes, an additional monotherapy trial or combination therapy. Stage four also has two routes: combination therapy for those treated with monotherapy at stage three or use of two mood stabilizers and one of the AAPs for those treated with combined therapy at stage three. At stage five, monotherapy with oxcarbazepine, ziprasidone or aripiprazole is recommended. The recommendation for the use of oxcarbazepine in the treatment of acute mania in teens (but not in prepubertal children) has been challenged by a recent double-blind placebo controlled study that showed negative results in teens (73). At stage six, trials of clozapine for all youth and ECT for teens conclude the algorithm.

Treatment of BP-1 with psychosis skips over the first two stages and begins with combined treatment with an AAP and a mood stabilizer, followed by a combination of two mood stabilizers and an AAP at stage four. Stages five and six are identical to the BP-1 without psychosis algorithm. For the acute treatment of bipolar depression, no specific algorithm is presented. Treatment first with a mood stabilizer, especially lithium, followed by a selective serotonin reuptake inhibitor or bupropion for 8 weeks after remission is suggested. A recently reported open trial of lithium in this population supports this recommendation (123). The presence of a mood stabilizer may protect against manic induction with SSRIs in the most vulnerable, prepubertal age group (7). Lamotrigine may also be useful in the acute treatment of youth bipolar depression (124, 125). A retrospective review of three studies shows preliminary support for quetiapine use in BP depression of youth (123), and ziprasidone and risperidone may also be useful (126). Although no specific recommendations are made for maintenance therapy, there is acknowledgment of the disappointing results of lithium or valproate monotherapy ("50% of youth get 50% better" (73)) and a suggestion to try combination therapies. No suggestions are made for youth with BP-2 or for the variety of presentations that fit BP-NOS.

Each of the best-studied mood stabilizers will be discussed, and the evidence for use of AAPs will be briefly reviewed. The reader is referred to the AAP section of this chapter for further discussion of individual AAPs.

Lithium

Clinical Applications and Empirical Support. The efficacy of lithium in the acute and maintenance treatment of and prophylaxis of children and adolescents with classic bipolar disorder has been demonstrated in case reports, open trials, and retrospective naturalistic studies (127–131). Geller and colleagues conducted the first placebo-controlled study of lithium in youngsters, including 25 adolescents with various forms of bipolar illness and comorbid substance abuse (132). Although lithium was associated with improvements in overall functioning and a lower rate of substance abuse relapse, there was no difference between active and placebo groups on measures of manic or depressive symptoms. The failure of lithium to separate from placebo on the core bipolar symptoms may be due to the small sample size. In an open trial of 100 teens with acute BP-1, 63% responded to lithium treatment at the end of 4 weeks (133). However, in a followup placebo-controlled study of maintenance treatment with lithium compared to placebo after an initial response of 4 weeks, more than 55% of youth failed to show continuing efficacy (134). In children and teens with a BP-1 or BP-2 diagnosis and first treated with a combination of lithium and valproate, maintenance treatment with lithium was equal to valproate (135). In the subgroup of those with acute mania and psychosis, however, treatment with an AAP appears to be necessary (136, 137). Taken together with the studies cited above, these data provide class B support for the use of lithium for the short-term or maintenance treatment of bipolar illness in children and adolescents. The presence of ADHD in children and teens with BD may be a factor that leads to a diminished response either to lithium or valproate (138–140), although this was not shown in another study (141). After relapse on either lithium or valproate of youth with either BP-1 or BP-2, a prospective open study showed that 90% of youth responded to combination treatment (142). The treatment of acute depression in BP-1 in hospitalized teens with lithium is supported by a single open study with a response rate of 50% and a remission rate of about 30% (six youth with psychosis responded to lithium without AAPs) (143).

Other Clinical Applications. Aggression, a study comparing haloperidol, lithium, and placebo in 61 treatment-resistant aggressive children (5 to 13 years) found that after 4 weeks of inpatient treatment, both haloperidol and lithium were superior to placebo in reducing aggressive behavior; and lithium was associated with fewer side effects (144). Lithium was found to be superior (16 out of 20 responders) when compared to placebo (six out of 20) in the treatment of aggressive behaviors in hospitalized children with conduct disorder (145). In contrast, a study of only 2 weeks' duration failed to demonstrate efficacy in teens with conduct disorder (146).

Mechanism of Action. Lithium affects several neurochemical systems, including serotonin, norepinephrine, and dopamine. However, its main actions appear to be mediated by effects on intracellular signaling processes, specifically of the phosphatidylinositol and protein kinase C pathways (147) (Table 6.1.2.3).

Pharmacokinetics and Drug Interactions. Lithium is readily absorbed from the gastrointestinal tract, and peak levels occur 1 to 4 hours after oral ingestion, depending on the formulation. Lithium carbonate is available in tablet and capsule, in two extended-release formulations (Eskalith CR, Lithobid), and a liquid form (lithium citrate). The liquid has the shortest TMax, and the sustained release formulations have slower absorption and lower plasma peaks. Lithium is not metabolized in the liver, nor does it bind to plasma proteins, and approximately 95% of the ingested drug is excreted in the kidneys. The half-life in adults is approximately 24 hours, slightly longer than the 18 hours reported in children (148). This shorter half-life has the practical implication that reliable blood levels can be obtained in children after just 4 days (or approximately 5 × 18 hours), rather than the traditional 5 days required in adults. The shorter half-life in children is due to faster glomerular filtration rates in the young. Because of their higher total body water, prepubertal children require higher weight-adjusted dosage than adults to achieve similar serum levels. Magnetic resonance spectroscopy has revealed that children have lower brain-to-serum concentrations of lithium as compared to adults, and they may require higher serum levels to achieve comparable brain levels (149).

Drug interactions occur at the level of the kidney. When given concomitantly, nonsteroidal antiinflammatory drugs, tetracyclines, and thiazide diuretics can decrease urinary clearance of lithium and increase lithium levels and should therefore be used cautiously. By contrast, theophylline and caffeine promote lithium excretion, resulting in lower serum levels.

Clinical Management. Prior to initiating a trial of lithium, a child should have a physical examination, including screening laboratory tests such as a complete blood count, electrolytes, blood urea nitrogen, creatinine, and thyroid indices. In outpatient settings, dosing may be initiated at 300 mg twice a day for children and 600 mg twice a day for adolescents. Weller has developed a useful guide to approximate daily lithium dosing (150). For children under 12 years of age, dosages in the range of 10 to 30 mg/kg per day are typical. Thus, a 30 kg child would receive 900 mg per day in divided doses. Older adolescents are likely to be treated in the range of 1,200 to 1,800 mg/day during acute mania. Maintenance doses are typically lower.

Due to its narrow therapeutic index, lithium levels should be monitored closely. The optimal serum level range is in the range of 0.6 to 1.1 mEq/L. Serum levels should be drawn on average 4 days after a dose adjustment to ensure that a steady state has been achieved and 12 hours after the previous dose to ensure a trough reading (151). When used to treat bipolar illness, the clinical benefit of lithium may be evident within 10 to 14 days of reaching therapeutic serum level in some cases, although as many as 4 to 6 weeks of treatment may be required (152). Current recommendations include repeat laboratory tests at 6-month intervals. An increased white count in the range of 12–15,000 cells/mm^3 is common and without clinical significance. Thyroid-stimulating hormone (TSH) levels may increase in association with higher lithium levels and a higher baseline TSH (153), but thyroid hormone replacement is not generally recommended unless T4 levels start to decrease, or if clinical symptoms of hypothyroidism appear. Lithium levels should also be obtained when the patient's clinical status changes, if adverse effects occur, and routinely at 3- to 6-month intervals. The FDA has approved an in-office "finger-stick" lithium-testing device that avoids venipuncture, but it has yet to gain widespread use in clinical practice (154).

Adverse Effects and Toxicity. Lithium appears to be generally well tolerated in children and adolescents. Common side effects include fatigue, nausea, diarrhea, abdominal distress, tremor, ataxia, aggravation of acne, cognitive dulling, and weight gain. Because lithium is excreted by the kidneys, it is generally not recommended in children with compromised renal function. The risk of glomerular damage with long-term lithium treatment appears to be minimal, but polyuria and polydipsia are relatively common due to lithium's effect on tubular reabsorption. Lithium-induced polyuria can generally be managed conservatively, either by reducing the total daily dose (when possible), by switching from a short- to a long-acting preparation, or by the addition of a low dose of a potassium-sparing diuretic such as amiloride. In a few cases, nephrogenic diabetes insipidus can occur, which may warrant discontinuation of lithium.

Signs of lithium toxicity can occur even at "normal serum levels." In mild forms symptoms include nausea, diarrhea, impaired concentration, and muscle weakness. At serum levels above 2.5 mEq/L, multiple organs may be affected and toxicity may prove fatal. Because dehydration can increase lithium levels and may induce toxicity, parents and children should be educated about the importance of adequate fluid intake. Lithium has been associated with a small increased occurrence of tricuspid valve abnormalities and transient neurodevelopmental deficits in exposed newborns (155). Contraception should be encouraged in adolescents and treatment of a pregnant mother with lithium should weigh possible fetal effects against the adverse outcomes of an untreated mood disorder (156).

Valproate

Clinical Applications and Empirical Support. Valproate (VPA) is an anticonvulsant that has been shown to be an effective mood stabilizer in adults. Clinicians have utilized VPA in the treatment of a range of problems in children and adolescents, including bipolar illness and aggression associated with conduct disorder or oppositional defiant disorder. There are case reports and open studies that support the use of VPA in youth with conduct disorder, explosive behaviors,

TABLE 6.1.2.3

MOOD STABILIZERS

Drug	Mechanism of Action	Main Indications and Clinical Uses	Dosage	Schedule	Adverse Effects	Comments	Select Brand Names and Preparations Available
Lithium	Inhibition of phosphatidyl inositol and protein kinase C signaling pathways Enhancement of serotonergic transmission	Bipolar disorder, manic Prophylaxis of bipolar disorder MDD Aggressive behavior/ Conduct disorder Adjunct treatment in refractory MDD	10–30 mg/kg/d, dose adjusted to serum levels in the range of 0.6–1.1 mEq/l	bid/tid	Polyuria, polydipsia, tremor, ataxia, nausea, diarrhea, weight gain, drowsiness, acne, hair loss Possible effects on thyroid and renal functioning with long-term administration Children prone to dehydration are at higher risk for acute lithium toxicity Lithium levels >2 mEq/L can be life-threatening	Therapy requires monitoring of lithium levels, thyroid and renal function	Lithium carbonate: 150, 300, 600 mg c sustained release forms: Lithobid 300 mg t, Eskalith 450 mg t/Lithium citrate elixir: 8 mEq (300 mg)/5 ml
Divalproex	Inhibition of catabolic enzymes of GABA, and of protein kinase C signaling	Bipolar disorder Aggressive behavior Conduct disorder Seizure disorders	15–60 mg/kg/d, dose adjusted to serum levels in the range of 50–125 mcg/l	bid/tid	Sedation, nausea, liver toxicity (requires baseline and close monitoring) Thrombocytopenia, pancreatitis	Polycystic ovarian disorder has been reported during long-term use for seizure control	Depakene (valproic acid): 250 mg; elixir Depakote (divalproex): 125, 250, 500 mg t; sprinkles: 125 mg c
Carbamazepine Oxcarbamazepine	Inhibition of glial steroidogenesis Inhibition of alpha 2 receptors Blocks sodium channels Blocks glial calcium influx	Bipolar disorder Complex partial seizures	10–20 mg/kg/d, dose adjusted to serum levels in the range of 4–14 mcg/l Maintenance dose of 18.5–48 mg/kg/day, not to exceed 2100 mg/day	bid	Bone marrow suppression (requires baseline and close monitoring of blood counts) Dizziness, drowsiness, rashes, nausea Liver toxicity, especially under 10 years of age No reports of bone marrow suppression, and more benign drug interaction profile compared to carbamazepine No blood level monitoring necessary	Potent inductor of CYP3A4, leading to auto-induction requiring periodic dose adjustment No empirical data available for children and adolescents	Tegretol: 100 mg chewable t; 200 mg/Elixir: 100 mg/5 ml Tegretol XR: 100, 200, 400 mg t Trileptal: 150, 300, 600 mg t
Lamotrigine	Weak 5HT3 inhibition/?Release of aspartate and glutamate	Seizure disorders	75–300 mg/d	qd	Potentially life-threatening rash Stevens-Johnson syndrome (dose-[direct] and age-[inverse] related event rates)	Slow dose titration (12.5 mg qoWk) may reduce risk of skin reactions	Lamictal: 25, 100, 150, 200 mg t chewable: 2, 5, 25 mg t
Gabapentin	Gabapentin is chemically related to GABA, but GABAergic effects unclear	Seizure disorders	100–1000+ mg/d	tid	Sedation, ataxia at high doses Very high therapeutic index	Excreted renally unchanged No significant drug interactions	Neurontin: 100, 300, 400, 600, 800 mg c
Topiramate	Glutamate release antagonist/GABA reuptake inhibitor	Migranes seizure disorders	50–400 mg/d	bid	Cognitive difficulties (dulling, word retrieval, attention) Dizziness, sedation	Weight loss may be a potentially beneficial side effect	Topamax: 25, 50, 100, 200 mg t 15, 25 mg sprinkle

Note: Doses are provided as general guidelines only, and are not meant to be definitive. All doses must be individualized and monitored through the appropriate clinical and/or laboratory means.
Abbreviations: c (capsule); t (tablet); FDA (Food and Drug Administration).

or impulsive aggression (157–160), and there are two small randomized clinical trials that support VPA efficacy in this population (121). There is less evidence supporting the use of VPA in acute or maintenance therapy of bipolar disorder in youth; two open studies showed a response rate of 50 to 60% (152, 161) and a study in teens with mixed mania showed more than a 70% response (162). Studies involving VPA with atypical antipsychotics have yielded response rates of 80% or higher for the combination therapy (163, 164). Treatment of ADHD after manic symptoms treated with VPA in children and teens showed that a mixed salt amphetamine did not worsen manic symptoms (165). In conclusion, these emerging data provide a modest level of support for the use of VPA in the treatment of children and adolescents with bipolar disorder (class C support).

Mechanism of action. VPA has multiple pharmacological effects (decreased dopamine turnover, decreased N-methyl D-asparate currents, decreased release of asparate (166)), and the details of its therapeutic actions are not fully known. VPA enhances GABA-ergic inhibition through increased synthesis and release. Given the inhibitory role of GABA in the brain, this effect may account for the drug's anticonvulsant and antimanic effects. VPA also directly effect neurons by inhibiting sodium influx and increasing potassium influx (167).

Pharmacokinetics and Drug Interactions. There are three formulations of VPA: valproic acid (Depakene, capsule and syrup), delayed released divalproex (a combination of valproic acid and sodium valproate, Depakote, capsule and sprinkle), and extended released divalproex (Depakote ER). All formulations release the valproate ion in the gastrointestinal tract, and this moiety is responsible for the pharmacologic action. Absorption is more rapid in the liquid form, and it can be delayed in the enteric forms. The sprinkle form has a lower Cmax and may have fewer gastrointestinal side effects. Slightly higher dosing (8 to 20%) is needed when shifting from VPA to the extended release formulation (168). VPA has very complex metabolism. It is therefore not surprising that valproate has been noted to interact with medications of all classes. As monotherapy, VPA is metabolized mostly by beta-oxidation or conjugated via glucuronidation and it produces no toxic metabolites. Only 10 to 20% is metabolized via P450 cytochromes (CYP 2C9 and CYP2 A6). Children under the age of 10 years excrete less VPA-glucuronide and metabolize more VPA through the P450 cytochromes (169). When a potent CYP inducer (carbamazepine, phenobarbital, phenytoin) is added, more VPA shuttles through CYPs and more toxic metabolites are produced. Children under the age of 2 years who are on multiple inducing anticonvulsants, or who have congenital metabolic disease or organic brain syndromes, are more susceptible to developing hepatic failure. VPA is a moderate inhibitor of epoxide hydrolase, CYP 2C9, and some UDP-glucuronylsyltransferases (UGTs). It inhibits the glucuronidation of lamotrigine at UGT 2B7, increasing its blood levels and the risk of developing Stevens-Johnson syndrome (170, 171). In addition, VPA exhibits saturable protein binding (it has nonlinear pharmacokinetics), and it competes with many drugs for protein binding sites (aspirin can displace it, VPA displaces carbamazepine).

Clinical Management. Prior to initiating therapy, a physical examination should be completed and laboratory-screening studies including a complete blood count, liver function tests, and a pregnancy test for female teens should be obtained. Dosing in outpatient adolescents could start with 250 mg twice daily, and increased every 3 to 5 days in 250 to 500 mg increments to a target dose of 20 mg/kg/day in two to three divided doses. Younger children might start with half the starting dose used in adolescents and move up in 125 to 250 mg increments. Trough levels should be checked after steady state is achieved (3 to 5 days), and target serum levels are in the range of 45–125 μg/L. Clinical management involves monitoring weight, appetite, energy level, evidence of bruising or clinical symptoms of pancreatitis, and of androgenism in girls. Liver enzymes and a CBC should be obtained within the first month of treatment and periodically during chronic treatment (172). Reductions in platelets and white blood count can occur and should be carefully evaluated.

Adverse Effects and Toxicity. Gastrointestinal complaints, sedation, and (rarely) transient hair loss may accompany the initiation of treatment and may subside with continued dosing. Other adverse effects include increased appetite and weight gain, postural tremor, dizziness, asthenia, and cognitive dullness. Rare idiosyncratic effects can occur. VPA has also been associated with hepatic failure, and in children under the age of 2, with fatal hepatitis (see Pharmacokinetics and Drug Interactions). Early in treatment there is also a small risk of pancreatitis. Agranulocytosis is extremely rare. In women treated for seizure disorders, there have also been reports of polycystic ovary disease manifested clinically by hyperandrogenism, accelerated weight gain, and menstrual and lipid profile irregularities (173). The role of VPA in these adverse endocrine effects is unclear and a matter of some debate, especially among teenage girls. Studies in adult women with bipolar disorder have shown high rates of preexisting menstrual abnormalities and increased testosterone levels with chronic VPA treatment (174). Clearly, monitoring weight and menstrual cycles is an essential component of clinical care in adolescent and adult females treated with VPA. VPA toxicity can be life threatening and may begin with increased tremor and confusion. It is associated with hyperammonemia, respiratory depression, and multiorgan failure (175).

VPA is associated with a variety of major and minor malformations in babies born to mothers taking VPA during pregnancy, including a twenty-fold increase in neural tube defects, cleft lip and palate, cardiovascular abnormalities, genitourinary defects, and others (176). These effects appear to be dose-dependent (especially evident at doses above 800–1000 mg/day (177). Prior to initiating treatment with VPA in sexually active female adolescents, therefore, a negative pregnancy test and a reliable method of contraception should be documented.

Carbamazepine

Clinical Application and Empirical Support. Carbamazepine (CBZ) is an anticonvulsant that has been used in adults for a variety of neurological and psychiatric disorders, including seizures, trigeminal neuralgia, and bipolar disorder. It has demonstrated efficacy since the 1980s for the treatment of acute mania and prophylaxis of mania and depression in adults, but it was not until 2004 that it received FDA approval for the treatment of acute mania and mixed bipolar states in adults. Case series and open-label studies in children have included bipolar disorder (152, 178, 179), aggression (180), and treatment-resistant ADHD (181). To date, however, the one controlled carbamazepine trial in youngsters failed to show its superiority over placebo for the treatment of aggression among 5- to 12- year-old inpatients diagnosed with conduct disorder (182).

Mechanism of Action. The mood-stabilizing effects of CBZ are not well understood: It decreases sodium influx, and the release of glutamate; it inhibits adenosine A1 and dopaminergic activity, but it may also affect several types of calcium channels (183).

Pharmacokinetics and Drug Interactions. CBZ is available as an immediate release formulation in tablets, chewables, and suspension, as well as in sustained-release formulations: an osmotic pump tablet (Tegretol-XR) and beaded extended-release capsules (Carbatrol, Equetro). CBZ is involved in an innumerable number of drug interactions, both as a victim substrate vulnerable to CYP inhibition and as an active inducer of CYPs and UGTs. As a substrate of CYP 3A4 and CYP 2C8, potent 3A4 inhibitors can affect CBZ (erythromycin). As an inducer of CYP 1A2, CYP 3A4, and glucuronidation, CBZ can induce its own metabolism and perhaps decrease efficacy of the drug. The active metabolite, CBZ 10,11 epoxide, can also be increased or decreased via drug interactions and can contribute to efficacy and toxicity. CBZ's free fraction can be displaced from plasma proteins by aspirin and NSAIDs, leading to toxicity. Valproate can inhibit the epoxidation and glucuronidation of CBZ 10,11 epoxide.

Clinical Management. CBZ is slowly absorbed, and peak plasma concentration is achieved within 2 to 8 hours following oral administration. As an anticonvulsant, the initial dose of the immediate and extended release formulation for children ages 6 to 12 years is 100 mg daily, and it can be increased at weekly intervals by 100–200 mg. The usual maintenance dose is 10–20 mg/kg/day, administered in divided doses (bid for extended, or tid for immediate formulations). Given the drug's short half-life following the induction of its own metabolism, frequent dose adjustments, especially in the first few weeks of treatment, are common. Pretreatment physical examination and laboratory studies should be completed, including complete blood count, liver function tests, and creatinine. Although there is scant evidence for an increase in major congenital anomalies in babies exposed to CBZ monotherapy in the first trimester of pregnancy (184), until further evidence is available, a pretreatment pregnancy test should be obtained in sexually active girls. They should receive counseling about appropriate contraception (as CYP 3A4 substrates, ethinyl estradiol and progestins can be reduced through CBZ's induction of CYP 3A4). The clinical utility of therapeutic plasma levels for children with mood disorders is unclear. Trough plasma concentrations for anticonvulsant effect can be drawn after 4 to 5 days, and they may be maintained in the range of 4–14 μg/ml. These guidelines may be useful during dose adjustment and in order to prevent toxicity. CBCs and LFTs should be followed periodically. Sedation, gastrointestinal effects and rash may occur. Leukopenia is common and rarely progresses to agranulocytosis. Very rarely, other bone marrow toxicities, liver toxicity, and inappropriate antidiuretic secretion syndrome may develop. Given the lack of controlled studies, the multiple drug–drug interactions, and its potentially serious adverse effects, CBZ should be considered as a third-line mood stabilizer in the treatment of children and adolescents and may be particularly useful as an alternative if there is morbid weight gain associated with lithium, VPA, or atypical antipsychotics.

Oxcarbazepine (Trileptal)

Oxcarbazepine (OXC) is a carbamazepine prodrug metabolized through noncytochromal pathways to an active metabolite, monohydroxy derivative (MHD). In turn, MHD is minimally metabolized through CYP 3A4, and it is mostly glucuronidated and subsequently excreted in the urine. As a result, OXC does not show the autoinduction observed with CBZ, nor is it vulnerable to potent 3A4 inhibitors, but like CBZ, it does possess a moderate ability to induce CYP 3A4 and some UGTs and to potently inhibit CYP 2C19. OXC may act through inhibition of voltage-sensitive sodium channels and modulation of potassium conductance and high voltage–activated calcium channels (product insert). A recent study has not shown efficacy in acute mania in bipolar teens but more equivocal results in children (73). In epilepsy trials, common adverse events include somnolence, headache, nausea and vomiting, dizziness and rash (185). Like CBZ, there have been reports of inappropriate secretion of antidiuretic hormone and Stevens-Johnson syndrome. Since OXC can induce CYP 3A4 and there is little information about fetal abnormalities, pretreatment pregnancy testing and appropriate contraceptive counseling is needed. According to the prescribing information, the recommended initial dose for youth 4 to 16 years of age with seizures is 8–10 mg/kg/d bid not to exceed 600 mg daily, and as monotherapy, a maintenance dose of 18.5–48 mg/kg/day not to exceed 2,100 mg/day (see product insert for dosing range by weight).

Lamotrigine (Lamictal)

In adults, lamotrigine has been shown effective in the treatment of BP-1 depression, to stabilize mood in rapid cycling BP-2 patients, and to provide prophylaxis for depression in BP-1 patients (186). In youth, recent retrospective or open-label studies of the acute treatment of BP depression in teens have shown efficacy, although significant depression persisted after treatment (123, 187). Lamotrigine has diverse actions on many neurotransmitters: It inhibits serotonin, norepinephrine, glutamate, and dopamine receptors, blocks calcium ion influx in N- and P-type channels, and stabilizes presynaptic neural membranes through sodium channels (188). Lamotrigine's pharmacokinetics are linear, and most of it is conjugated by the UGTs (UGT 1A4 and UGT 2B7). VPA inhibits its glucuronidation and decreases its clearance by about 50%. Conversely, UGT inducers (carbamazepine, ethinyl estradiol) can lower lamotrigine levels by 50% (188). Lamotrigine is well documented to cause skin rashes that are usually mild and seen within the first months of treatment, but full-blown Stevens-Johnson syndrome (a potentially lethal condition associated with widespread skin sloughing) can develop. Rapid dose escalation and coadministration with VPA are risk factors, especially for children. A 10% rate for all rashes is commonly reported in adults (189). A recent review in adults suggests that slow dose titration and dermatologic precautions (limited antigen exposure) may reduce this rate (189). There is data suggesting a higher risk of major congenital abnormalities in babies exposed to lamotrigine in doses higher than 200 mg per day, and pending further studies, pretreatment pregnancy tests and contraceptive counseling should be made available to sexually active girls (184). Toxicity is associated with lethargy, vomiting, ataxia, vertigo and tachycardia, but only rarely is the outcome serious (190).

Other (Third Generation) Anticonvulsants

New anticonvulsants recently approved for the treatment of epilepsy in adults have become the focus of interest as potential mood stabilizers. Only case reports on their use in pediatrics are available to date.

Gabapentin (Neurontin)

This agent undergoes virtually no hepatic metabolism, and it is excreted largely unaltered by the kidneys. Despite a benign side effect profile among adults, aggressive behavior and worsening hyperactivity have been reported among 12 children receiving gabapentin for the treatment of seizure disorders (172). Studies in adults as monotherapy in bipolar disorder have not demonstrated efficacy. Consequently, its use as a mood stabilizer for children cannot be recommended.

Topiramate (Topamax)

Topiramate is a glutamate release antagonist, a GABA reuptake inhibitor, and it reduces activity at sodium and calcium channels (191). Most of topiramate is excreted unchanged through the kidney, and therefore plasma levels will be lower in younger children because of their higher glomerular filtration rates. About 30% is handled by the CYPs and UGTs, and these pathways can be induced when the potent inducing antiepileptics (carbamazepine) are added, leading to a doubling of topiramate's clearance. Topiramate modestly inhibits CYP 2C19, and when combined with higher doses of phenytoin, the concentration of the latter drug can be significantly increased. At topiramate doses at or above 200 mg/day, the concentrations of ethinyl estradiol and/or progestins in oral contraceptives can be decreased. Topiramate has been shown to be ineffective in acute mania in adults (192), and as a result, a pilot trial in youth with mania was discontinued (191). A chart review of the efficacy of adjunctive topiramate in BP-1 is promising (160). Decreased appetite and nausea appeared as the most common adverse events in this study, as did weight loss, especially in some overweight subjects (191). Topiramate may be associated with cognitive blunting and word retrieval difficulties. Its use in bipolar disorder in youth as monotherapy cannot be endorsed.

Use of AAPs in Mood Disorders

The atypical antipsychotics (AAPs) are used to treat various target symptoms and disorders in children and adolescents (see following), including bipolar disorder. Both as monotherapy and in coadministration with mood stabilizers, the use of the AAPs for adults is commonplace and well supported by research and FDA approval for acute mania, mixed mania, bipolar depression, and maintenance therapy. Although currently there is limited research evidence that supports their use in youth with BP, clinical use of these agents is routine (for example, 77% of youth with bipolar disorder in a community sample have tried AAPs) (193). There are several double-blind, placebo-controlled trials underway or completed, but results are still pending on the efficacy and safety of AAPs in youth with BP. Many authors advocate the use of these agents either as the drug of choice or in combination with mood stabilizers for the treatment of mania (167, 194, 195). Open studies of monotherapy involving risperidone or olanzapine have yielded a reduction in Young Mania Rating Scale scores of 30% in 50 to 70% of subjects with BP-1, BP-2 or BP-NOS (196–198); similar results have been observed with quetiapine and ziprasidone, in 75% (126). Open studies of clozapine as monotherapy have shown encouraging results (199, 200). Studies involving coadministration of AAPs with mood stabilizers have yielded response rates of 80% or higher in acute and maintenance studies (201, 202). Further support for the value of AAPs in maintenance therapy is provided by studies in which attempts to discontinue the antipsychotic was unsuccessful and often resulted in relapse after successful resolution of psychosis with lithium (136, 137). A study of quetiapine in acute onset depression in adolescents with BP has shown statistically significant superiority compared to valproate (143), and quetiapine has shown promise in high-risk adolescents with bipolar depression (123).

Antipsychotics

Clinical Applications and Empirical Support. Antipsychotics were introduced to adult psychiatry in the early 1950s and were used in children shortly thereafter. The antipsychotics can be classified according to chemical family, such as phenothiazines or butyrophenones. Alternatively, they may be classified according to the relative potency of their dopamine blockade. Chlorpromazine and thioridazine are low potency drugs, in that relatively high doses are required to achieve usual therapeutic effects. By contrast, haloperidol and fluphenazine are high potency dopamine blocking drugs. With the introduction of clozapine and a short list of newer compounds, it is becoming commonplace to classify antipsychotics as typical or atypical. Pediatric uses of antipsychotics include the treatment of psychosis, severe behavioral problems associated with autism and other developmental disorders, aggression, tics, bipolar disorders, and as an adjunctive treatment in OCD.

Atypical Antipsychotics

Clozapine (Clozaril)

Clozapine was the first AAP agent to be developed and entered into the marketplace. It is a dibenzodiazepine derivative and chemically unrelated to any of the typical antipsychotic drugs. Soon after it was introduced in 1960, its effectiveness in treatment-resistant patients with schizophrenia was recognized, but initial enthusiasm waned following the report of fatal agranulocytosis in a series of cases in Europe. Two open studies (203, 204) and one controlled comparison with haloperidol (205) have been carried out in pediatric populations. Collectively, these studies included 53 patients from ages 6 to 18 years. Clozapine was effective in 30 of 53 (56%) of these patients. This figure is impressive considering that this was a group of treatment-resistant patients. In the controlled trial, doses ranged from 125 to 525 mg/day given in divided doses. Although there were no reports of EPS, several serious adverse effects were observed, most notably seizures (N = 1) and hematopoetic abnormalities (N = 4). Weight gain was a frequently observed complication of clozapine treatment. Due to differences in the duration of the studies, however, it is not possible to aggregate data across them.

A retrospective comparison of clozapine (N = 20), olanzapine (N = 13) and risperidone (N = 38) in adults indicated that clozapine and olanzapine confer a higher risk for weight gain than risperidone. Using a 10% increase in body weight as a threshold, 40% in the clozapine group and 30% of patients treated with olanzapine had excessive weight gain. These rates were significantly greater than the 10% of patients in the risperidone group. In addition, the absolute increase in weight was significantly greater for the clozapine group compared to the risperidone group. The olanzapine group and the risperidone group were not different in mean weight increase (206).

Risperidone (Risperdal)

Following clozapine, risperidone was the second AAP to be released to the U.S. marketplace. It is a benzisoxazol derivative that has some pharmacologic features in common with clozapine, but has not been associated with agranulocytosis. Large multisite studies in adults with schizophrenia have shown that risperidone is an effective antipsychotic with lower risk of neurological side effects compared to traditional antipsychotics such as haloperidol (207). Unlike clozapine, it is associated with an increase in prolactin, suggesting more potent D_2 blockade. At doses above 6 mg per day, the risk of neurological side effects increases in a dose-dependent manner. This apparent dose threshold effect may be due to protective effects of $5HT_2$ receptors to which the AAPs appear to bind preferentially. In this model, as the dose of the antipsychotic medication increases, $5HT_2$ receptors become saturated, which is followed by an increase in D_2 binding (208). Alternatively, the protective role of $5HT_2$ may be less important than D_2 occupancy. Occupancy is influenced by rate of association (binding to the receptor) and the rate of dissociation (release from the receptor). As pointed out by Kapur and Seeman (209), AAPs have lower affinity to D_2 receptors because they are more easily displaced by endogenous dopamine. The result of this "fast off" property of the AAPs is that at usual doses these drugs remain under the D_2 occupancy threshold that is associated with neurological side effects. For example, 65% D_2 occupancy is the estimated threshold for antipsychotic activity compared to 80% occupancy for neurological side effects (209). At usual doses, risperidone or olanzapine do not exceed the 80% threshold, but haloperidol does (Table 6.1.2.4a) (209).

To date, risperidone is the best studied AAP in pediatric populations. An emerging body of evidence from short-term, placebo-controlled, randomized clinical trials shows that risperidone is safe and effective for serious behavior problems in children with autism (11, 210); severe disruptive behavior (211–214); and Tourette syndrome (216, 217). A few studies have also shown that short-term gains endure over the intermediate term (17, 217).

The RUPP Autism Network (11) completed an 8-week, placebo-controlled study of risperidone in 101 children with autism accompanied by tantrums, aggression, and self-injury. At an average dose of 1.8 mg per day, the risperidone group improved 57% on a parent-rated scale measuring the target symptoms of tantrums, aggression, and self-injury compared to 14% in placebo. Similarly, blinded clinicians rated 75% of children in the risperidone group as much improved or very much improved compared to 12% for the placebo group. Children initially randomized to placebo who showed no improvement were offered treatment in an 8-week open label trial using the same dosing schedule that was used in the double-blind trial. Sixty-three who showed a positive response to risperidone (in the double-blind or the open-label trial) were followed forward for an additional 4 months to evaluate the stability of gains and continued safety (17). Finally, at the 6-month mark, children were randomly assigned to remain on risperidone or to gradual withdrawal from active medication by placebo substitution over a 4-week period. The results of this study show that the short-term gains of risperidone were stable over time and that it was not necessary to increase the dose of medication to maintain the observed benefits. Thirty-two children entered the double-blind, placebo-controlled discontinuation phase. Ten of 16 children assigned to discontinuation showed a return of symptoms compared to two of 16 children who remained on risperidone who met prespecified criteria for relapse.

Aman and colleagues (211) conducted a 6-week, randomized, placebo-controlled risperidone trial in 118 children with disruptive behavior. The subjects ranged in age from 5 to 12 years; many were functioning in the mentally retarded range (IQ 36–84). After 6 weeks of risperidone, the active treatment group showed nearly a 16-point improvement on the parent-rated Nisonger Child Behavior Rating Form compared to a 6-point improvement in the placebo group. The average dose of risperidone was 1.16 mg per day. This finding was replicated in a separate trial (214) using an identical design and similar entry criteria. Both studies included a 12-month extension phase, which showed that gains were stable (217).

In a placebo-controlled study of risperidone that included both children and adults, risperidone was superior to placebo for the treatment of tics in Tourette syndrome (TS) (216). Thirty-four subjects (26 children and 8 adults) were randomly assigned to placebo or risperidone. After 8 weeks of treatment with doses ranging from 1 to 2 mg per day in the pediatric sample, risperidone was associated with a 36% improvement on a clinician-rated measure of tic severity, which was significantly better than the 9% in the placebo group ($p < 0.01$). No neurological side effects were observed in this study. Weight gain averaged 2.8 kg in the active treatment group compared to 0.7 kg in the placebo group ($p < .05$). Treatment emergent social phobia was observed in two cases in the risperidone group, which has been reported by others (218).

Risperidone has also been compared to pimozide in a randomized, double-blind trial (219). In that study, risperidone and pimozide were similar in their positive effects, with reductions in tic severity of 44% and 47%, respectively. Not surprisingly, the pimozide group reported more neurological side effects. Weight gain was greater in the risperidone group (4.5 kg compared to 2.7 kg). Dose ranges were similar, up to 6 mg/day for each drug. The study included 50 subjects in total, but only 17 were in the pediatric age group. Results in the pediatric sample were not reported.

In many of these studies, the drug was initiated at 0.5 mg per day (0.25 in younger children) and increased by 0.5 mg every 5 to 7 days to a range of 1 to 2.5 mg per day in a single dose or two divided doses. Studies by Aman et al. (211); Snyder et al. (214), and Findling et al. (213) used single day dosing. Not surprisingly, the average dose in these studies was lower than the studies that used a twice daily dosing schedule. Taken together, these data suggest that twice a day dosing may be better tolerated, though single day dosing may be considered if the total daily dose is low (less than 1.5 mg per day).

Quetiapine (Seroquel)

Although not chemically related to clozapine, quetiapine resembles clozapine in its receptor occupancy profile. It has low affinity for D_2 receptors. Because it is a relatively low affinity for D_2 receptors, it does not show the dose threshold effect observed with risperidone or olanzapine. Thus, even at high doses, quetiapine is unlikely to produce neurological side effects and shows only transient rises in prolactin. As with the other available atypical antipsychotics, quetiapine has demonstrated safety and efficacy for the treatment of adults with schizophrenia. To date, only limited data are available on its use in children and adolescents. Preliminary results suggest that quetiapine may be useful for the treatment of psychotic symptoms in adolescents (220). Less promising results were reported in an open-label study of six adolescents with pervasive developmental disorder (221). In that study, only two of six subjects showed a positive response on global measures of behavior. The most promising results for quetiapine have been observed in children with bipolar disorders (see earlier).

Olanzapine (Zyprexa)

Olanzapine is another agent with atypical features that are preserved only in the lower dose range (<20 mg per day in adults). The use of olanzapine has been described in two open-label trials in adolescents with schizophrenia (222, 223). As noted previously, olanzapine has also been used as monotherapy or as adjunctive treatment in children or adolescents with bipolar disorders. Two studies involving a total of 31 children with autism or pervasive developmental disorder not otherwise specified have been evaluated in open-label studies. Malone et al. (224) compared olanzapine to haloperidol in 12 children (six per group) in a 6-week study. At an average dose of 8 mg per day, olanzapine showed improvements in aggression and was slightly better than haloperidol. Given the small sample size, this difference was not significant. Using a mean dose of 10 mg per day, Kemner et al. (225) evaluated the efficacy of olanzapine in 25 children and adolescents with PDD and showed modest improvements in aggression and hyperactivity. Across these two studies, the most common adverse effects included increased appetite and weight gain: 4 kg in 6 weeks (224) or 4.7 kg in 12 weeks (225).

Ziprasidone (Geodon)

This atypical antipsychotic medication has also been shown to be effective in adults with schizophrenia (226). Like risperidone, it is a potent blocker at the D_2 and $5\text{-}HT_2$ sites. Compared to risperidone, however, much larger doses are required to achieve an antipsychotic effect. For example, the usual dose of risperidone in adults with schizophrenia is 6 mg

TABLE 6.1.2.4A

ATYPICAL ANTIPSYCHOTICS

Drug	Mechanism of Action	Main Indications and Clinical Uses	Dosage (mg/d)	Schedule	Adverse Effects	Comments	Select Brand Names and Preparations Available
A. Atypical							
Risperidone	Dopamine and 5HT receptor blockade/ Atypical antipsychotics in general have high 5HT2a/D2 affinity ratios: Risperidone 8:1 Olanzapine: 5:1 Quetiapine: 1:1 Aripiprazole: 10:1 Clozapine: 30:1	Psychosis: positive and negative symptoms TS Augmentation in OCD Bipolar disorder Autism and PDDs Aggression and agitation	0.25–4	qd/bid	Sedation Appetite increase Weight gain Metabolic syndrome (glucose intolerance, dyslipidemia) Low incidence of extrapyramidal adverse effects Insomnia, mild activation more likely with Aripiprazole		Risperdal: 0.25, 0.5, 1, 2, 3, 4 mg t/elixir: 1 mg/ml, oral disintegrating tablet: 0.9, 1, 2, 3, 4, mg t, injectable
Olanzapine			2.5–10				Zyprexa: 2.5, 5, 7.5, 10, 15, 20 mg t oral disintegrating tablet: 5, 10, 15, 20, mg t, injectable
Quetiapine			100–600				Seroquel: 25, 50, 100, 200, 300, 400 mg t
Aripiprazole			5–40				Abilify: 2, 5, 10, 15, 20, 30 mg t
Ziprasidone			40–160			Monitoring of QTc interval recommended	Geodon 20, 40, 60, 80 mg c
Clozapine		Treatment—refractory psychosis	50–400	bid/tid	Low incidence of extrapyramidal adverse effects; does not induce dystonia Low risk for tardive dyskinesia Granulocytopenia/ agranulocytosis (treatment requires constant monitoring of blood count) Higher risk of seizures (dose related)	Weekly blood counts mandatory (monitoring for WBC >3000, ANC >2000). Possibility of going to qoWk monitoring by 6 months, qM by 12 months. Seizure prophylaxis (with valproate or gabapentin) recommended at higher doses (>300 mg/d)	Clozaril: 25, 100 mg t

Note: Doses are provided as general guidelines only, and are not meant to be definitive. All doses must be individualized and monitored through the appropriate clinical and/or laboratory means. Abbreviations: c (capsule); t (tablet); FDA (Food and Drug Administration).

per day. By contrast, the dose of ziprasidone is typically in the range of 120 to 160 mg per day or higher, given in two divided doses (227). Two published studies of ziprasidone provide information on the use of ziprasidone in pediatric populations. In the first trial, 28 children (age 7 to 17 years) with TS or chronic motor tic disorder were randomly assigned to placebo (N = 12) or ziprasidone (N = 16) under double-blind conditions. The mean dose of ziprasidone was approximately 30 mg per day given in divided doses. Using the same outcome measure mentioned for the risperidone study in TS, ziprasidone was associated with a 35% improvement in tic severity, compared to a 7% decline in the placebo group ($p < .05$) (228). Common side effects included moderate sedation (one subject), mild sedation (11 subjects), insomnia (four subjects) and akathisia (one subject). There were no changes in laboratory values, cardiac conduction times, or body weight in the ziprasidone group. A second study was an open-label study in 12 subjects with pervasive developmental disorder (PDD) by McDougle and colleagues (229). All subjects had been previously treated unsuccessfully with another antipsychotic for the target symptoms of tantrums, aggression, or self-injurious behavior. At a mean dose of approximately 60 mg per day, six of 12 subjects were rated as much improved. In each of these studies, ziprasidone was not associated with weight gain. Noting that some patients had discontinued treatment with other AAPs, McDougle et al. (229) observed weight loss in five of 12 subjects. The difference in mean dose across these two studies is probably related to when the study was conducted Sallee et al. (228) conducted their study before ziprasidone came to market using 5-, 10-, and 20-mg capsules. McDougle et al. (229) initiated their open trial after the drug came to market. The lowest marketed strength of ziprasidone in 20 mg. Clearly, larger studies are needed to establish the optimal dose schedule and range. Concern about cardiac conduction changes remains with ziprasidone (see Adverse Effects).

Aripiprazole (Abilify)

Aripiprazole is the newest AAP to enter the marketplace. It is approved for the treatment of adults with schizophrenia, but very few studies are currently available for the use of this medication in children and adolescents. This drug has been described as a *third generation* antipsychotic due to its novel mechanism of action. Aripiprazole is classified as a partial dopamine agonist. This term refers to the fact that aripiprazole binds with presynaptic dopamine receptors, which is purported to turn down the dopamine system in brain regions with increased dopaminergic tone. In addition, like the other AAPs, aripiprazole has serotonin blocking properties at the five HT2 receptor sites. It is likely that aripiprazole will be evaluated in pediatric populations for many of the same target symptoms described earlier for risperidone. Thus data on efficacy and safety will be forthcoming.

Typical Antipsychotics (Antipsychotics)

Chlorpromazine (Thorazine)

Chlorpromazine is an aliphatic agent, and was the first antipsychotic used in children with severe behavioral disturbances. With the introduction of newer agents, the use of chlorpromazine has declined, although it is still routinely used for the acute management of agitation or aggression, when it can be administered through either oral or intramuscular (IM) routes. When used IM, careful caution must be paid to vital signs, as significant hypotension can occur even at seemingly low doses (e.g., <25 mg) (Table 6.1.2.4b).

Thioridazine (Mellaril)

Another low potency phenothiazine in the piperidine chemical family, thioridazine had been among the most commonly used antipsychotics in pediatric populations. The recommended dosage for treating psychosis or severe behavioral dyscontrol in 3- to 12-year-old children is 0.5 to 3.0 mg per kg per day, given in two or three divided doses. In addition to the introduction of the atypical antipsychotics, recent case reports indicating that thioridazine can prolong cardiac conduction times, particularly the QTc interval, have led to decline in its use. Indeed, an FDA advisory council has advised against the use of thioridazine.

Haloperidol (Haldol)

A butyrophenone that is structurally unrelated to the phenothiazines, it represents the prototype of a high potency typical antipsychotic. Since its introduction in the early 1960s, it has been used to treat children with psychosis, aggressive behavior, tics, and behavioral dyscontrol associated with autism (230, 231).

Compared to the low potency antipsychotics, haloperidol is much more likely to cause extrapyramidal symptoms (EPS), but it is less sedating. The dose of haloperidol varies according to the target symptoms. For example, in school-age children with tics or severe behavioral dyscontrol associated with autism, the dose is typically in the range of 0.75 mg to 2.5 mg per day (66, 228). By contrast, doses in the range of 10 may be used to deal with an acute psychotic episode (232).

Fluphenazine (Prolixin)

A piperizine phenothiazine, fluphenazine is not approved for children under the age of 12 years, and has not been well studied in pediatric populations. At low dosages (0.04 mg per kg per day) fluphenazine decreased aggression, hyperactivity, and stereotypies in an open-label study of 12 children with PDD (233). At a mean dose of 7 mg per day in divided doses (range, 2 to 15 mg per day) fluphenazine reduced tics and was favored over haloperidol by most patients (234). This open-label trial of 21 patients with Tourette syndrome (TS) included both children and adults, but results were not separately reported by age group.

Thiothixene (Navane)

A thioxanthene derivative, this midpotency agent is structurally unrelated to the phenothiazines or the butyrophenones. It is approved for the treatment of psychosis in children over the age of 12 years. The available evidence in children under age 12 indicates that thiothixene is less sedating than are low potency antipsychotics, and that it may have a lower risk of EPS than high potency antipsychotics such as haloperidol (235).

Pimozide (Orap)

A diphenylbutylpiperidine, pimozide it is not related to the phenothiazines or to haloperidol. It is a potent blocker of dopamine at the D_2 postsynaptic receptors, and it is used to treat tics in TS. In placebo-controlled studies involving both children and adults, pimozide has been shown to be superior to placebo in reducing tics (236). It has also evaluated in head-to-head trials with haloperidol. These studies suggest that pimozide is equivalent to haloperidol with respect to tic suppression, and that it has a more favorable side effect profile (231, 237).

Mechanism of Action. The principal therapeutic action of the traditional antipsychotics is to block postsynaptic D_2 receptors (209). The observed differences across traditional antipsychotics may be related to the regional specificity of

TABLE 6.1.2.4B

TRADITIONAL ANTIPSYCHOTICS

Drug	Mechanism of Action	Main Indications and Clinical Uses	Dosage (mg/d)	Schedule	Adverse Effects	Comments	Select Brand Names and Preparations Available
B. Typical (Traditional), or Neuroleptic							
Phenothiazines: Low Potency							
Chlorpromazine	D2 receptor blockade All agents in this family have similar efficacy, but different potency based on the dosage required to achieve a similar effect. 100 mg of chlorpromazine are equivalent to: Thioridazine: 95 mg Perphenazine: 8 mg Fluphenazine: 2 mg Haloperidol: 2 mg Thiothixene: 5 mg Molindone: 10 mg Pimozide: 1 mg	Psychosis Mania Aggressive behavior Agitation Self-injurious behavior Autism	25–400	qd/bid/tid	Anticholinergic (dry mouth, constipation, blurred vision, hypotension—more common with low potency agents) Weight gain Extrapyramidal reactions (dystonia, rigidity, tremor, akathisia, greater risk with higher potency) Drowsiness Risk for tardive dyskinesia with long-term administration Withdrawal dyskinesia Hypotension, especially when administered IM	A warning label from the FDA was introduced for thioridazine in 2000, advising against its use as a first-line drug, given concerns over QTc interval prolongation Traditional agents are not as effective in treating the negative or affective symptoms of psychosis Low potency agents have high anticholinergic profiles (e.g. sedation, hypotension), whereas high potency agents are likely to cause extrapyramidal side effects (EPS)	Chlorpromazine: 10, 25, 50, 100, 200 mg t; elixir; suppositories; injectable
Thioridazine							Thioridazine: 10, 15, 25, 50, 100, 150, 200 mg t; elixir
Phenothiazines: Medium and High Potency							
Perphenazine			4.0–32.0 (Perphenazine) 0.5–10 (Fluphenazine)				Perphenazine: 2, 4, 8, 16 mg t; elixir, injectable
Fluphenazine							Fluphenazine. 1, 2, 5, 5, 10 mg; elixir, injectable, long acting
Other Traditional Antipsychotics—potency							
Haloperidol—high *(butyrophenone)*			0.5–10		Lowest weight gain liability among traditional agents		Haloperidol: 0.5, 1, 2.5, 10, 20 mg t; elixir, injectable, long acting
Thiothixene—medium *(thioxanthene)*		Same as other antipsychotics/Tourette disorder	1–20		Cardiac arrhythmias (EKG prolonged QTc) Seizures Extrapyramidal reactions Drowsiness Tardive dyskinesia Withdrawal dyskinesia		Thiothixene: 1, 2, 5, 10, 20 mg t; elixir, injectable
Molindone—medium *(indole derivative)*			5–150				Molindone: 5, 10, 25, 50, 100 mg t; elixir
Pimozide—high			1–4				Orap: 1, 2 mg t

Note: Doses are provided as general guidelines only, and are not meant to be definitive. All doses must be individualized and monitored through the appropriate clinical and/or laboratory means.
Abbreviations: c (capsule); t (tablet); FDA (Food and Drug Administration).

the D_2 blockade (striatum vs. limbic structures), and the effects on other neurotransmitter systems. By contrast, the atypical antipsychotics block both dopamine and serotonin postsynaptic receptors to varying degrees. The addition of postsynaptic 5-HT blockade may lower the risk of neurological side effects and perhaps of tardive dyskinesia (TD) as well. It may also contribute to beneficial effects on negative symptoms of schizophrenia, though this remains a matter of controversy. Some investigators argue that the beneficial effects of the atypicals on negative symptoms have yet to be demonstrated in a convincing manner. As noted previously, the protective role of $5HT_2$ may be less important than D_2 occupancy. Occupancy is influenced by rate of association (binding to the receptor) and the rate of dissociation (release from the receptor). Because the AAPs are more easily displaced by endogenous dopamine, the occupancy at D_2 receptors is lower than the traditional antipsychotics of similar potency. The result of this "fast off" property of the AAPs is that at usual doses these drugs remain under the D_2 occupancy threshold and less likely to produce neurological side effects.

Antipsychotic medications may also have anticholinergic and antihistamine effects, as well as adrenergic blocking effects. These additional pharmacologic properties probably do not contribute to the therapeutic effects of the antipsychotic drugs, but do have an impact on side effect profiles. For example, low potency antipsychotics such as chlorpromazine and thioridazine cause more sedation, dry mouth, and constipation, presumably due to antihistamine and anticholinergic effects. Their propensity to cause hypotension may be related to alpha-adrenergic blockade.

Adverse Effects. Neurological side effects such as dystonic reactions, rigidity, and akathisia are more common with the high potency antipsychotics. In addition to these neurological side effects, adverse effects of the typical antipsychotic drugs in children and adolescents can include cognitive blunting, weight gain, depressed mood, social phobia, elevated prolactin levels with possible emergence of gynecomastia in boys and galactorrhea or amenorrhea in girls. Drowsiness is a common side effect with the low potency antipsychotic agents, but may occur in the high potency antipsychotics as well. Anticholinergic side effects such as dry mouth, constipation, and blurred vision should also be monitored. As noted, thioridazine, pimozide, ziprasidone, and other antipsychotics can prolong cardiac conduction times (97). Recommendations on whether to obtain ECGs at baseline and how often to monitor cardiac conduction times when using antipsychotics in children and adolescents are not consistent. For example, electrocardiograms at baseline and during maintenance treatment with antipsychotics are recommended in one guideline (238), but not in others (239). The explanation for this inconsistency is not clear, but may simply reflect the incomplete state of current evidence. Thioridazine has largely fallen out of use. Expert opinion in published guidelines for the use of antipsychotics in TS indicates that when using pimozide or ziprasidone in children and adolescents, an ECG should be obtained prior to treatment, during the dose adjustment phase and periodically thereafter (240). One important difference in considering treatment with pimozide or ziprasidone is their relative vulnerability to drug–drug interaction. Pimozide is a substrate for the CYP 3A4 pathway and will show a dramatic rise in serum level following the addition of a potent 3A4 inhibitor such as erythromycin (241). Case reports indicate that this type of interaction may have serious consequences (242). Ziprasidone, on the other hand, does not appear to be vulnerable to drug–drug interaction due to its use of multiple metabolic pathways (243).

Although the atypical antipsychotics are less likely to cause neurological side effects, they are not free of adverse effects. Clozapine is associated with a low risk of agranulocytosis. For this reason, it is only used in treatment-resistant schizophrenia. Other adverse effects of clozapine include lowered seizure threshold and tachycardia. An adverse effect of the AAPs that has emerged as a clinically important concern is increased appetite and weight gain. Several reports in pediatric samples across several diagnostic groups have shown that clozapine, olanzapine, quetiapine, and risperidone are associated with excessive weight gain (11, 201, 205, 211, 216, 224, 244, 245). For example, in the study by Kumra and colleagues (205) of 21 adolescents with schizophrenia showed no difference in weight gain for clozapine compared to haloperidol with each group gaining approximately 1 kg over a 6-week period. In placebo-controlled studies with risperidone, weight gain was significantly greater in the active treatment group as compared to placebo ranging from to 2 to 3 kg vs. 1 kg over 6 to 8 weeks (11, 211, 213, 216). The weight gain associated with olanzapine reported in two trials ranged from 4 to 5 kg over 6 to 12 weeks' duration (224, 225). Based on available data in pediatric populations, the risk of weight gain appears to follow this order: clozapine, olanzapine, quetiapine, risperidone. The number of pediatric subjects treated with ziprasidone or aripiprazole remains relatively small, making it difficult to assess the risk of weight gain in children and adolescents with these compounds.

Data on the intermediate-term impact on weight gain of AAP treatment in children and adolescents are only available for risperidone. These results suggest that the rate of weight gain is greatest in the first 2 months of treatment, with some leveling thereafter. For example, children in the RUPP Autism Network study with risperidone showed an average weight gain of 1.4 kg per month for the first 2 months and approximately 0.9 kg per month over the subsequent 4 months (7). The mechanism for weight gain appears to be through an increase in appetite, which may be due to interference with the satiety mechanism. The health consequences of obesity can be significant, including increased serum triglycerides and drug-induced Type II diabetes (246).

The risk of *tardive dyskinesia* (TD) increases as a function of dose and duration, but it may occur with brief exposures as well. TD has been reported in pediatric patients, but it does not appear to be common (247). Thus, children and adolescents treated with antipsychotics should be monitored for abnormal movements. The largest systematic study to date (248) raises questions regarding the difficulty in distinguishing between TD and withdrawal dyskinesia (WD). In that study, 30% of children between the ages of 2 and 8 years showed persistent dyskinetic movements for up to 3 months of followup after a planned withdrawal from haloperidol.

Questions of how and when to discontinue antipsychotic medication are critical ones, but data to guide clinical decisions are limited. To minimize TD, dose reductions should be done gradually while evaluating changes in symptom severity. In autism and tic disorders, discontinuation may be considered annually for cases in which good control has been achieved. If symptoms persist, the maintenance dose of the antipsychotic should be reduced to the lowest possible one sufficient to maintain symptomatic control and minimize overall exposure (249). Based on the collective experience with clozapine, the newer atypicals may also have a lower risk of TD. More study, such as long-term followup of clinical samples treated with atypical antipsychotics and careful postmarketing surveillance of these agents in pediatric populations, is needed.

Neuroleptic malignant syndrome (NMS) is a rare adverse effect due to antipsychotic medications. NMS is characterized by high fever, autonomic instability, and muscle breakdown (reflected by elevated CPK titers) and is potentially life threatening. The mortality rate may be as a high as 9% in children and adolescents (250). Discontinuation of the medication is usually all that is required, highlighting the importance of early identification of the condition. In severe

TABLE 6.1.2.5

ANTIHISTAMINE, ANTICHOLINERGIC AGENTS

Drug	Mechanism of Action	Main Indications and Clinical Uses	Dosage (mg/d)	Schedule	Adverse Effects	Comments	Select Brand Names and Preparations Available
Diphenhydramine	Antihistamine	Sleep disorders Agitation, acute dystonic reactions	12.5–100	tid/qid	Sedation, cognitive impairment, anticholinergic (dry mouth, constipation, blurred vision) Delirium (rare, except at higher doses)		Diphenhydramine: 25, 50 mg t; elixir, injectable
Benztropine	Anticholinergic (muscarinic)	Extrapyramidal reactions (dystonia, rigidity, tremor akathisia)	0.5–3	bid/tid			Benztropine: 0.5, 1, 2 mg; elixir, injectable

Note: Doses are provided as general guidelines only, and are not meant to be definitive. All doses must be individualized and monitored through the appropriate clinical and/or laboratory means.
Abbreviations: c (capsule); t (tablet); FDA (Food and Drug Administration).

cases, I.V. fluids are needed, and some authors have advocated the use of dantrolene or bromocriptine to hasten recovery.

Treatment of Antipsychotic-Associated Adverse Effects: Emphasis on Anticholinergic Agents. Among the many potential side effects associated with the traditional antipsychotics, neurological side effects represent some of the most common and ones likely to be treated with additional pharmacotherapy. Acute neurological side effects include dystonia, torticollis, or oculogyric crisis. Chronic side effects include Parkinsonism: tremor, rigidity, mask-like facies or festinant gait. These adverse effects can be prevented or reversed with the judicious use of anticholinergic agents. Given that all of these adverse effects are associated with unchecked D_2 receptor blockade, it follows that they are most common with high potency traditional agents (such as haloperidol or fluphenazine) and least common with low potency compounds (such as chlorpromazine). Although less common with atypical antipsychotics, the risk of neurological side effects increases at higher dose levels of risperidone, olanzapine, or ziprasidone. In most instances, the anticholinergics discussed here are used in combination with high potency agents, and they should rarely (if at all) be used in combination with lower potency drugs. Not only are the low potency agents less likely to cause neurological side effects, the addition of anti-Parkinsonian mediations may exacerbate the inherent anticholinergic properties of low potency antipsychotics. This point is of more than academic interest: The additive effects of combining agents with anticholinergic or antihistaminergic effects can rapidly lead to behavioral toxicity, including paradoxical agitation, confusion, or full-blown delirium (Table 6.1.2.5).

The two most commonly used agents in this category are diphenhydramine (Benadryl) and benztropine (Cogentin). The antihistamine diphenhydramine is best used in acute situations, both given its ready availability (in household medicine cabinets and crash carts alike), as well given its side effect profile. However, the sedation induced by diphenhydramine can be intense, so this agent should be used sparingly as a maintenance intervention. Alternatively, such sedation can be exploited therapeutically in the acutely agitated patient. By contrast, the purely anticholinergic compound benztropine is preferred for longer term management of neurological side effects, as it does not induce somnolence. Diphenhydramine is usually dosed in the 12.5–50 mg range (single or repeat dose, administered orally or by IM injection), while benztropine is used in 0.5-, 1-, or 2-mg doses, usually given orally in a bid regimen. The long-term use (>1 month) of anticholinergic agents should be avoided if at all possible, particularly in younger children, for whom the resulting Sjögren-like iatrogenic syndrome can lead to widespread cavities. The slow upward adjustment of antipsychotics, coupled with time-limited (as opposed to regular) use of these agents can avert unnecessary longer term use.

Alpha-2 Adrenergic Agents

The alpha-2 adrenergic agents (clonidine and guanfacine) are only approved for use in adults with hypertension. Beginning with the early studies of clonidine for the treatment of TS, these drugs have become increasingly common in child psychiatry for treating tics, ADHD, and aggressive behavior in children (251). Indeed, between 1991 and 1995 the largest rise in the rate of psychotropic drugs used in preschoolers was for clonidine, with a 28-fold increase in one large database (Table 6.1.2.6) (5).

Clonidine (Catapres)

Clinical Applications and Empirical Support. There are only two controlled studies of clonidine in the treatment of tics. Both studies included children and adults. In the first of these studies, clonidine was no better than placebo in suppressing tics (252), but a subsequent, slightly larger trial proved it superior to placebo, producing approximately 35% improvement in tic severity (253). Similarly, findings in ADHD have also been inconsistent: In an early study involving 10 children in a placebo-controlled discontinuation study, clonidine provided modest benefit for ADHD (254). These findings were not replicated in a crossover study in which 34 children received desipramine, clonidine, and placebo in random order. Desipramine, but not clonidine, was superior to placebo on a parent measure of ADHD symptoms (94).

Taken together, these findings suggest that clonidine has modestly beneficial effects for ADHD symptoms and tics. These results also point out the potential limitations of small studies—even when a controlled design is used. One study shows benefit, but the next study fails to replicate the findings.

It is in this context that the multisite Treatment of ADHD in Children with Tourette's Syndrome (TACT) study was undertaken by the Tourette Syndrome Study Group (46). In this study, 136 children (age 7 to 14 years) with ADHD and a chronic tic disorder were randomized to one of four treatments: clonidine, methylphenidate, clonidine + methylphenidate, or placebo. All three active treatments were superior to placebo on teacher and parent measures of ADHD. The magnitude of effect for monotherapy with methylphenidate and monotherapy with clonidine was moderate with improvement on teacher ratings of 38% for the methylphenidate only and 40% for the clonidine group. By contrast, teacher ratings showed a 59% improvement for the combined treatment group. At doses averaging 0.25 mg/day for clonidine and approximately 26 mg

TABLE 6.1.2.6

NORADRENERGIC AGENTS

Drug	Mechanism of Action	Main Indications and Clinical Uses	Dosage (mg/d)	Schedule	Adverse Effects	Comments	Select Brand Names and Preparations Available
Alpha Agonists							
Clonidine	Nonspecific alpha-2 presynaptic agonist	Tourette disorder ADHD Aggression/self-abuse Severe agitation Withdrawal symptoms	0.025–0.4	bid/tid/qid	Sedation (very frequent) Hypotension (rare) Dry mouth irritability Dysphoria Rebound hypertension Localized irritation with transdermal preparation	Transdermal absorption can be erratic; limited bioavailability	Clonidine: 0.1, 0.2, 0.3 mg t transdermal patch: Catapres TTS 1, 2, 3 (delivering 0.1, 0.2, 0.3 mg/d/wk)
Guanfacine	Selective alpha-2a agonist	Tourette disorder ADHD	0.5–4	bid/tid	Same as clonidine Less sedation, hypotension		Tenex: 1, 2 mg t
Beta Blockers							
Propranolol	Postsynaptic beta blockade	Akathisia, lithium-induced tremor Aggression self-abuse Severe agitation Alternative to neuroleptics, especially in developmentally delayed individuals	2.0–8.0 mg/kg/d	bid	Similar to clonidine Higher risk for bradycardia and hypotension (dose dependent) and rebound hypertension Bronchospasm (contraindicated in asthmatics) Rebound hypertension on abrupt withdrawal Contraindicated in diabetics		Inderal: 10, 20, 40, 60, 80 mg t Inderal LA: 60, 80, 120, 160 mg t
Nadolol			20–200				Nadolol: 20, 40, 80, 120, 160 mg t

Note: Doses are provided as general guidelines only, and are not meant to be definitive. All doses must be individualized and monitored through the appropriate clinical and/or laboratory means. Abbreviations: c (capsule); t (tablet); FDA (Food and Drug Administration).

for methylphenidate, there were no serious adverse effects and no evidence of cardiac conduction problems with either drug alone or the combination. The results suggest that the combination of clonidine + methylphenidate provided fuller coverage of ADHD symptoms in this population and may have provided some protection against adverse effects. For example, sedation was a problem in 35% for subjects in the clonidine group compared to 21% in the combined treatment group. As noted above, the combined treatment was associated with a lower rate of insomnia compared to the methylphenidate only group. Finally, in 35% (n = 13) of cases in the stimulant alone had their medication dose lowered or a scheduled increased delayed due to the treating clinician's concern about increased tics. These clinical decisions occurred in only 18% of cases in the clonidine only group and in the combined treatment group. This finding is remarkable given that the study was conducted under blinded conditions.

This study has several clinical implications. First, it was the first large-scale study to evaluate a combined pharmacotherapy in children with a psychiatric disorder. Second, it provides valuable efficacy and safety information about a treatment combination that is becoming commonplace in the field. Concern about the safety of this combination heightened following the death of three children being treated with clonidine and methylphenidate. Although a careful review of these cases concluded that neither drug nor the combination was responsible for the deaths of these children, controversy about this drug combination in children continues (45). Given the sample size, this study cannot answer questions concerning the occurrence of rare adverse events, but the results do provide support for the efficacy and safety of this combined treatment approach. The high rate of sedation associated with clonidine in this sample confirms the narrow dose range of the agent.

Third, this study adds to the list of other recent controlled studies showing that tics do not invariably increase when children with TS are treated with stimulants. Nonetheless, this was a dose-limiting side effect in a third of the subjects treated with methylphenidate alone.

Guanfacine (Tenex)

Guanfacine is an alpha-2 agonist that is similar to clonidine and was also developed as an antihypertensive agent. Interest in guanfacine has been prompted by three observations. First, compared to clonidine, it is less sedating. Second, it has longer half-life than clonidine. This longer duration of action could translate into a need for fewer doses per day and a lower risk of rebound effects. Third, accumulated data from a series of animal studies provides compelling evidence that guanfacine is more specific in action than clonidine (255). Until recently, there were only three open-label studies of guanfacine, involving a total of 38 children (256–258). All three studies showed promising results for guanfacine in the treatment of ADHD. The study by Chappell et al. (257) also reported that guanfacine had a modestly beneficial effect on tics.

The first placebo-controlled study of guanfacine in children included 34 subjects (17 in each treatment group) with ADHD symptoms and a tic disorder (259). After 8 weeks of treatment at doses ranging from 1.5 to 3.0 mg per day given in three divided doses, the guanfacine group showed a 37% improvement a teacher rating of classroom behavior compared to an 8% change in the placebo group ($p < .001$). Similar results were observed for teacher ratings of inattention as well as hyperactivity and impulsiveness. Nine of 17 subjects in the guanfacine group were blindly rated as "much improved" or "very much improved," compared to 0 of 17 in the placebo group ($p < 0.001$). The 27% drop in the Conners Parent Questionnaire in the guanfacine group was not significantly different from the 21% drop in placebo. Because the target symptoms in this study were inattention, hyperactivity, and impulsiveness, children with marked tic severity were excluded from the trial. Nonetheless, guanfacine was also associated with a 31% drop in a clinician-rated measure of tic severity, compared with 0% improvement in the placebo group ($p = 0.05$).

Guanfacine was no better than placebo in a trial involving 24 subjects (12 per group) (260). The entry criteria did not require subjects to have ADHD at baseline and indeed behavior rating scores varied widely from the normal to the ADHD range. Thus, the wide variability in the sample and the small sample size renders these results difficult to interpret. Adverse effects were generally mild. One subject withdrew from the study due to moderate sedation. Six other subjects complained of mild sedation, which resolved with continued treatment or dose decrease. Other complaints included midsleep awakening in three subjects, dry mouth (n = 4), constipation (n = 2), loss of appetite in the morning (n = 2). Weight was stable in both groups and there were no alterations in clinical laboratory results, including cardiac conduction parameters. The mean resting diastolic blood pressure showed an 8-point decline at midpoint in the guanfacine group that returned to baseline by the 8-week mark. There was no difference between groups on blood pressure measured from the supine to standing position. In a case by case review, six subjects in the guanfacine group showed a one standard deviation drop (10 mm of Hg) in resting systolic or diastolic blood pressure at one visit, compared to two subjects in the placebo group ($p = 0.11$). No subject showed such a reduction in blood pressure at more than a single visit.

In conclusion, these preliminary results suggest that guanfacine is a safe and effective treatment for children with ADHD and tics. The 37% improvement in teacher-rated behavior is less than the 50% to 60% improvement reported in stimulant trials (261), but is similar to the level of improvement observed in other nonstimulant studies (93, 99, 262). Given that two-thirds of the subjects in the guanfacine trial had failed prior stimulant treatment, the results observed in this sample may not be comparable to the findings of other nonstimulant trials.

Mechanism of Action. The traditional view is that clonidine regulates central noradrenergic activity through its agonist effects on presynaptic alpha-2 receptors in the locus coeruleus (LC). Clonidine is indeed 10 times more potent than guanfacine in reducing LC firing and inhibiting norepinephrine (NE) release. In addition to weaker presynaptic effects, accumulated data from studies in primates show that guanfacine has direct stimulating effects on postsynaptic alpha-2_A receptors located in the prefrontal cortex (PFC) (255, 263). These animal studies have established that this pharmacological mechanism improves PFC function. Given the fundamental role of the PFC in attention and working memory, this action is likely to be relevant for the treatment of ADHD.

Clinical Management. Clonidine comes in 0.1-, 0.2-, and 0.3-mg tablets. In school-age children, the starting dose is typically 0.05 (1/2 of a 0.1 mg tablet) at bedtime. The dose is then increased in 0.05 mg increments every 3 to 5 days as tolerated to a maximum of 0.2 mg per day (0.05 mg qid) in prepubertal children, and 0.3 mg in teenagers. To ensure even behavioral effects and thus blood levels across the entire day, clonidine is typically given three to four times per day. Clonidine transdermal patches (Catapres TTS) delivering 0.1, 0.2, and 0.3 mg per day are available, but they have not been well studied in youngsters, and may have erratic absorption from the skin. The typical starting dose of guanfacine is 0.5 mg at bedtime, with 0.5 mg increases every 3 to 5 days to a total of 1.5 to 3.0 mg per day in two or three divided doses.

The adverse effects of clonidine and guanfacine are similar, though guanfacine appears to be better tolerated. The most common side effects include sedation, dizziness, irritability (especially when the medication wears off), and midsleep awakening. Hypotension is generally not a problem with either drug in children and adolescents, but warrants monitoring, particularly in the dose adjustment phase. A related concern with clonidine is the well documented phenomenon of rebound hypertension following precipitous withdrawal (264). In adults with high blood pressure, however, abrupt discontinuation of guanfacine did not result in rebound hypertension (265). Nonetheless, abrupt discontinuation of either drug should be avoided. There is incomplete consensus in the field regarding the need for electrocardiograms in children and adolescents treated with the alpha-2 agonists. A recent statement from the American Heart Association indicates that no cardiovascular monitoring other than blood pressure and pulse is required for clonidine and guanfacine (238).

Beta Blockers

Beta blockers such as propranolol and nadolol have been explored in child psychiatry. After some initial enthusiasm over their use for the management of aggression, their use has more recently become rare. They are mentioned here, in the context of the other adrenergic agents, although they are rarely used in clinical practice (for example, for the occasional management of akathisia or of lithium-induced tremor).

Anxiolytics

Although SSRIs remain the only empirically proven pharmacologic intervention for the treatment of pediatric anxiety disorders, the benzodiazepines (BZD) remain widely used, particularly in primary care settings, or in medical wards where clinicians may be more familiar and comfortable with their use than with other psychotropics. Thus, the BZDs are often *misused* in pediatrics, as misguided efforts to treat depression, delirium, or agitation, for example. And yet, it would be a mistake to think of these drugs exclusively in that negative light, as they are powerful compounds that can be quite useful, even if the empirical database for their use is very limited in pediatrics.

Of the many available BZDs, the three more commonly used are lorazepam (Ativan), alprazolam (Xanax), and clonazepam (Klonopin). These agents are similarly effective as anxiolytics, although they differ widely in their potency (1 mg lorazepam being roughly equivalent to 0.5 mg of alprazolam, or 0.25 mg of clonazepam) and in their half-life (shorter for lorazepam and alprazolam, longer for clonazepam). All BZDs can cause drowsiness, disinhibition, agitation, and confusion, and clonazepam in particular can lead to dysphoria or depression. Withdrawal reactions can occur if maintenance doses are not slowly weaned down, or even between doses for the shorter acting agents. These medications do carry a potential risk for abuse and dependence, and need to be prescribed cautiously in the context of personal or family history of substance abuse or dependence.

Clonazepam (Klonopin)

Clonazepam is a long-acting benzodiazepine that is approved as an anticonvulsant. In adults it is also used to treat anxiety disorders and as an adjunctive treatment for tics. A study of 15 prepubertal children showed that clonazepam can be useful in anxiety disorders in some children, but side effects including disinhibition, irritability, and drowsiness were common and problematic (266). Given these results, clonazepam does not appear to be a first-line agent for the treatment of anxiety disorders in pediatric populations, although it can be useful as an adjunctive intervention, especially on a time-limited basis. Treatment can begin with 0.25 mg in the morning and increasing to 0.25 mg twice daily after 3 to 4 days. Thereafter the dose may be increased slowly to a maximum of 2 mg per day in divided doses. Clonazepam should be tapered gradually when discontinued. As with other benzodiazepines, long-term use can be associated with dependence, albeit less commonly than with shorter acting agents. Children treated for more than 4 weeks should be gradually tapered when coming off of the drug to limit the rebound anxiety or seizures associated with abrupt withdrawal (Table 6.1.2.7).

Buspirone (BuSpar)

Buspirone is an atypical anxiolytic drug that is unrelated to the benzodiazepines. It acts as a 5-HT1A agonist, which results in a presynaptic release of serotonin (267). In an initial study buspirone, 10 to 20 mg per day in two divided doses, was associated with significant improvement in anxiety symptoms, as measured by a global scale (268). This improvement was evident within 3 to 4 weeks of starting the medication. Adverse effects included tiredness, sleep disturbance, abdominal discomfort, and headache. In a group of 25 hospitalized children with anxiety and aggressive behavior, improvement in anxiety and aggression was noted in about 75% of the cases (269). Approximately 16% (N = 8) worsened and four developed hypomania. Another open-label study was conducted in 22 subjects with pervasive developmental disorders with prominent anxiety symptoms. The subjects, who ranged in age from 6 to 16 years, were treated with 15 to 45 mg per day given on a three times per day schedule. After 8 weeks of treatment, 16 of the 22 subjects showed a clinically significant improvement in a global measure of anxiety (270). Side effects included mild activation in two subjects, nausea in one, and orofacial movements in another, the last of which resolved when the drug was discontinued.

The typical starting dose is 5 mg three times per day, with gradual increases weekly to 45 mg per day (15 mg tid). In younger children, buspirone may be initiated at 2.5 to 5 mg per day and increased thereafter every 3 to 4 days to a total of 20 to 30 mg per day in three divided doses. In the absence of improvement after 8 weeks, buspirone should be discontinued.

Antienuretic Agents

Desmopressin, Oxybutynin, and Tolterodine

Desmopressin (DDAVP) is synthetic antidiuretic hormone (ADH), a powerful inhibitor of the production of urine. It can be administered orally or via intranasal spray. One review suggested that desmopressin helps approximately 25% of children who use it, with minimal risk of adverse effects (271). Although desmopressin is usually well tolerated, the beneficial effects often do not endure over time. The most effective treatment for enuresis is the use of behavioral interventions, such as a "pad and buzzer" or a "moisture alarm." However, DDAVP can be a useful short-term adjunct, as in the facilitation of sleepovers or overnight camp stays. For longer term pharmacological management of enuresis, usually in cases unresponsive or only partially responsive to behavioral interventions, antimuscarinic agents can occasionally be useful. Alternatives to the time-tested use of low (25–50 mg HS) (272) or regular dose imipramine include oxybutynin (Ditropan) or the less sedating tolterodine (Detrol). As is the case of other pharmacologic interventions for enuresis, beneficial effects usually disappear rapidly upon drug discontinuation (Table 6.1.2.8).

ACKNOWLEDGMENTS

This work was supported, in part, by Scientist Career Development Award K01 MH01792-01 to Dr. Martin,

TABLE 6.1.2.7

ANXIOLYTICS

Drug	Mechanism of Action	Main Indications and Clinical Uses	Dosage (mg/d)	Schedule	Adverse Effects	Comments	Select Brand Names and Preparations Available
High Potency Benzodiazepines							
Clonazepam (long-acting)	Enhancement of GABAergic transmission via binding to a specific benzodiazepine site within the GABAa receptor	Anxiety disorders Adjunct in treatment—refractory psychosis Adjunct in mania Severe agitation Severe insomnia MDD + anxiety akathisia	0.25–3	qd/bid	Drowsiness, disinhibition, agitation, confusion Depression Withdrawal reactions Potential risk for abuse and dependence Less risk for rebound and withdrawal reactions		Klonopin: 0.5, 1, 2 mg t
Alprazolam (short-acting)			0.25–4	tid	Same as other benzodiazepines Higher risk for rebound and withdrawal reactions		Xanax: 0.25, 0.5, 1, 2 mg t
Lorazepam (short-acting)			0.5–6	tid		Does not go through phase I reactions: good choice in the context of hepatic failure	Ativan: 0.5, 1, 2 mg t injectable
Atypical Anxiolytic							
Buspirone	Serotonin 1A agonist	Anxiety disorders Adjunct treatment refractory OCD	15–60	tid	Drowsiness, disinhibition	No cross tolerance with benzodiazapines	BuSpar: 5, 10, 15, 30 mg t

Note: Doses are provided as general guidelines only, and are not meant to be definitive. All doses must be individualized and monitored through the appropriate clinical and/or laboratory means. Abbreviations: c (capsule); t (tablet); FDA (Food and Drug Administration).

TABLE 6.1.2.8

ANTIENURETIC AGENTS

Drug	Mechanism of Action	Main Indications and Clinical Uses	Dosage (mg/d)	Schedule	Adverse Effects	Comments	Select Brand Names and Preparations Available
Desmopressin	Antidiuretic hormone analogue	Enuresis	10–40 mcg	qhs/bid	Headache Nausea Hyponatremia and water intoxication at toxic doses	Can be useful for acute situations (e.g., sleepaways)	DDAVP: 0.1, 0.2 mg t; nasal spray: 10 mcg/spray
Oxybutynin	Antimuscarinic agents		5.0–15	bid/tid	Anticholinergic side effects		Ditropan: 5 mg t, elixer 5 mg/5 ml Ditropan XL: 5, 10, 15 t
Tolterodine			1–2	bid	Less anticholinergic effects, less sedation		Detrol: 1 mg t Detrol LA: 2, 4 mg c

Note: Doses are provided as general guidelines only, and are not meant to be definitive. All doses must be individualized and monitored through the appropriate clinical and/or laboratory means.
Abbreviations: c (capsule); t (tablet); FDA (Food and Drug Administration).

by Public Health Service grants M01 RR06022, 5P01 HD1DC35482, and 5P01 HD03008, and by a National Institute of Mental Health Research Unit on Pediatric Psychopharmacology U10 MH66764 (Dr. Scahill).

The authors acknowledge the efforts of Aprna Shyam for assistance in preparing this manuscript.

Dr. Scahill has served as consultant to Janssen Pharmaceuticals, Bristol-Myers Squibb, and Pfizer Pharmaceuticals. Dr. Oesterheld and Dr. Martin have no conflicts of interest to declare.

References

1. Bradley C: The behavior of children receiving benzedrine. *American Journal of Psychiatry* 94:577–585, 1937.
2. Molitch M and Eccles AK: The effect of benzedrine sulfate on the intelligence scores of children. *American Journal of Psychiatry* 94:577–585, 1937.
3. MTA: A 14-month randomized clinical trial of treatment strategies for attention-deficit/hyperactivity disorder. The MTA Cooperative Group. Multimodal Treatment Study of Children with ADHD. *Arch Gen Psychiatry* 56:1073–1086, 1999.
4. MTA Cooperative Group: National Institute of Mental Health Multimodal Treatment Study of ADHD follow-up: Changes in effectiveness and growth after the end of treatment. Pediatrics. 113:762–769, 2004.
5. Zito JM, Safer DJ, dosReis et al.: Trends in the prescribing of psychotropic medications to preschoolers [see comments]. *JAMA* 283:1025–1030, 2000.
6. Vitiello B and Jensen PS: Developmental perspectives in pediatric psychopharmacology. *Psychopharmacol Bull* 31:75–81, 1995.
7. Martin A, Scahill L, Anderson GM, et al.: Weight and leptin changes among risperidone-treated youths with autism: Six-month prospective data. *American Journal of Psychiatry*, 161:1125–1127, 2004.
8. Kaufman J, Martin A, King RA, et al.: Are child-, adolescent-, and adult-onset depression one and the same disorder? *Biological Psychiatry.* 49:980–1001, 2001.
9. Food and Drug Administration: The FDA modernization act of 1997. Available on line: http://www.fda.gov/cder/fdama/default.htm, 1999.
10. RUPP (Research Unit on Pediatric Psychopharmacology) Anxiety Study Group: Fluvoxamine for the treatment of anxiety disorders in children and adolescents. *N Engl J Med* 344:1279–1285, 2001.
11. RUPP (Research Units on Pediatric Psychopharmacology) Autism Network: Risperidone in children with autism for serious behavioral problems. *NEJM*, 347:314–321, 2002.
12. Treatment for Adolescents with Depression Study (TADS) Team. Fluoxetine, cognitive-behavioral therapy, and their combination for adolescents with depression. *Journal of the American Medical Association,* 292,807–820, 2004.
13. Biederman J, Newcorn J and Sprich S: Comorbidity of attention deficit hyperactivity disorder with conduct, depressive, anxiety, and other disorders [see comments]. *Am J Psychiatry* 148:564–577, 1991.
14. Angold A, Costello EJ and Erkanli A: Comorbidity. *J Child Psychol Psychiatry* 40:57–87, 1999.
15. Scahill L, Riddle MA, King RA, et al.: Fluoxetine has no marked effect on tic symptoms in patients with Tourette's syndrome: A double-blind placebo-controlled study. *J Child Adolesc Psychopharmacol* 7:75–85, 1997.
16. Scahill L, Kano Y, King RA, et al.: Influence of age and tic disorders on obsessive-compulsive disorder in a pediatric sample. *J Child Adolescent Psychopharmacol,* 13(S1):7–18, 2003.
17. RUPP (Research Units on Pediatric Psychopharmacology) Autism Network. Risperidone treatment of autistic disorder: Longer term benefits and blinded discontinuation after six months. *Am J Psychiatry,* 162:1361–1369, 2005.
18. Arnold LE, Vitiello B, McDougle C, et al.: Parent-defined target symptoms respond to risperidone in RUPP autism study: Customer approach to clinical trials. Multicenter Study. *J Am Acad Child Adolesc Psychiatry* 42:1443–1450, 2003.
19. Greenhill LL, Vitiello B, Riddle MA, et al.: Review of safety assessment methods used in pediatric psychopharmacology. *J Am Acad Child Adolesc Psychiatry* 42:627–633, 2003.
20. Greenhill LL, Vitiello B, Fisher P, et al.: Comparison of increasingly detailed elicitation methods for the assessment of adverse effects in pediatric psychopharmacology. *J Am Acad Child Adoles Psych* 43:1488–1496, 2004.
21. Joshi P: Marine peptides and related compounds in clinical trial. *Current Medicinal Chemistry—Anti-Cancer Agents* 6:33–40, 2006.
22. Pruett KD and Martin A. Thinking about prescribing: The psychology of psychopharmacology. *Pediatric Psychopharmacology* 33:417, 2003.
23. Kazdin AE, Weisz JR (eds): *Evidence-Based Psychotherapies for Children and Adolescents.* New York, Guilford Press, 2003.
24. Pediatric OCD Treatment Study (POTS) Team. Cognitive-behavior therapy, sertraline, and their combination for children and adolescents with obsessive-compulsive disorder: The Pediatric OCD Treatment Study (POTS) randomized controlled trial. *JAMA* 292(16):1969–1976, 2004.
25. Jobson KO and Potter WZ: International Psychopharmacology Algorithm Project Report: Introduction. *Psychopharmacol Bull* 31:457–459, 1995.
26. American Psychiatric Association: *Diagnostic and Statistical Manual of Mental Disorders, Fourth Edition, Treatment Revised.* Washington, DC, American Psychiatric Association, 2000.
27. Costello EJ, Angold A, Burns BJ, et al.: The Great Smoky Mountains Study of Youth: Goals, design, methods, and the prevalence of DSM-III-R disorders. *Arch Gen Psychiatry* 53:1129–1136, 1996.
28. Wolraich ML, Hannah JN, Baumgaertel A, et al.: Examination of DSM-IV criteria for attention deficit/hyperactivity disorder in a county-wide sample. *J Dev Behav Pediatr* 19:162–168, 1998.
29. Biederman J, Faraone S, Milberger S, et al.: Predictors of persistence and remission of ADHD into adolescence: Results from a four-year prospective follow-up study. *J Am Acad Child Adolesc Psychiatry* 35:343–351, 1996.
30. Faraone SV, Biederman J, Spencer T, Wilens et al.: Attention-deficit/hyperactivity disorder in adults: An overview. *Biol Psychiatry* 48:9–20, 2000.
31. Scahill L, Schwab-Stone M, Merikangas KR, et al.: Psychosocial and clinical correlates of ADHD in a community sample of school-age children. *J Am Acad Child Adolesc Psychiatry.* 38(8):976–984, 1999.
32. Leibson CL, Katusic SK, Barbaresi WJ, et al.: Use and costs of medical care for children and adolescents with and without attention-deficit/hyperactivity disorder. *JAMA* 285:60–66, 2001.
33. Ford RE, Greenhill LL, Posner K: Stimulants. In: Martin A, Scahill L, Charney DS, Leckman JF, (eds): *Pediatric Psychopharmacology.* New York, Oxford University Press, 2003, pp. 255–263.
34. Biederman J, Lopez FA, Boellner SW, et al.: A randomized, double-blind, placebo-controlled, parallel-group study of SL1381 (Adderall XR) in

children with attention-deficit/hyperactivity disorder. *Pediatrics* 110:258–266, 2002.
35. Pelham WE, Gnagy EM, Burrows-Maclean L, et al.: Once-a-day Concerta methylphenidate versus three-times-daily methylphenidate in laboratory and natural settings. *Pediatrics* 107(6):E105–E119, 2001.
36. Rapport MD and Denney C: Titrating methylphenidate in children with attention-deficit/hyperactivity disorder: Is body mass predictive of clinical response? *J Am Acad Child Adolesc Psychiatry* 36:523–530, 1997.
37. Elia J: Stimulants and antidepressant pharmacokinetics in hyperactive children. *Psychopharmacol Bull* 27:411–415, 1991.
38. Solanto MV: Neuropsychopharmacological mechanisms of stimulant drug action in attention-deficit hyperactivity disorder: A review and integration. *Behav Brain Res* 94:127–152, 1998.
39. Biederman J and Spencer T: Attention-deficit/hyperactivity disorder (ADHD) as a noradrenergic disorder. *Biol Psychiatry* 46:1234–1242, 1999.
40. Swanson JM, Wigal S, Greenhill LL, et al.: Analog classroom assessment of Adderall in children with ADHD. *J Am Acad Child Adolesc Psychiatry* 37:519–526, 1998.
41. Greenhill LL, Abikoff HB, Arnold LE, et al: Medication treatment strategies in the MTA Study: Relevance to clinicians and researchers. *J Am Acad Child Adolesc Psychiatry* 35:1304–1313, 1996.
42. Sprague RL and Sleator EK: Methylphenidate in hyperkinetic children: Differences in dose effects on learning and social behavior. *Science* 198:1274–1276, 1977.
43. Greenhill L, Posner K, Freid J, Wigal S, et al.: The use of a laboratory school protocol to evaluate concepts about efficacy and side effects of new formulations of stimulant medications. *Journal of Attention Disorders*. 6,Suppl 1:S73–888, 2002.
44. Spencer T, Biederman J, and Wilens T: Growth deficits in children with attention deficit hyperactivity disorder. *Pediatrics* 102:501–506, 1998a.
45. Wilens TE, Spencer TJ, Swanson JM, et al.: Combining methylphenidate and clonidine: A clinically sound medication option. *J Am Acad Child Adolesc Psychiatry* 38:614–619; discussion 619–622, 1999.
46. Tourette Syndrome Study Group. Treatment of ADHD in children with tics: A randomized controlled trial. *Neurology* 58(4):527–536, 2002.
47. Borcherding BG, Keysor CS, Rapoport JL, et al.: Motor/vocal tics and compulsive behaviors on stimulant drugs: Is there a common vulnerability? *Psychiatry Res* 33:83–94, 1990.
48. Law SF, and Schachar, R. J.: Do typical clinical doses of methylphenidate cause tics in children treated for attention-deficit hyperactivity disorder? *J Am Acad Child Adolesc Psychiatry* 38:944–951, 1999.
49. Castellanos FX, Giedd JN, Elia J, Marsh et al.: Controlled stimulant treatment of ADHD and comorbid Tourette's syndrome: Effects of stimulant and dose. *J Am Acad Child Adolesc Psychiatry* 36:589–596, 1997.
50. Gadow KD, Sverd J, Sprafkin J, et al.: Efficacy of methylphenidate for attention-deficit hyperactivity disorder in children with tic disorder. *Arch Gen Psychiatry* 52:444–455, 1995.
51. DeVeaugh-Geiss J, Moroz G, Biederman J, et al.: Clomipramine hydrochloride in childhood and adolescent obsessive-compulsive disorder—A multicenter trial. *J Am Acad Child Adolesc Psychiatry* 31:45–49, 1992.
52. Leonard HL, Swedo SE, Rapoport JL, et al.: Treatment of obsessive-compulsive disorder with clomipramine and desipramine in children and adolescents: A double-blind crossover comparison. *Arch Gen Psychiatry* 46:1088–1092, 1989.
53. Riddle MA, Scahill L, King RA, et al.: Double-blind, crossover trial of fluoxetine and placebo in children and adolescents with obsessive-compulsive disorder. *J Am Acad Child Adolesc Psychiatry* 31:1062–1069, 1992.
54. March JS, Biederman J, Wolkow R, et al.: Sertraline in children and adolescents with obsessive-compulsive disorder: A multicenter randomized controlled trial. *JAMA* 280:1752–1756, 1998.
55. Riddle MA, Reeve EA, Yaryura-Tobias JA, et al.: Fluvoxamine for children and adolescents with obsessive-compulsive disorder: A randomized, controlled, multicenter trial. *J Am Acad Child Adolesc Psychiatry* 40:222–229, 2001.
56. Emslie GJ, Rush AJ, Weinberg WA, et al.: A double-blind, randomized, placebo-controlled trial of fluoxetine in children and adolescents with depression. *Arch Gen Psychiatry* 54:1031–1037, 1997.
57. Keller MB, Ryan ND, Birmaher B, et al.: Paroxetine and imipramine in the treatment of adolescent depression. In *Program and Abstracts on New Research from the 151st Annual Meeting of the American Psychiatric Association*. Toronto, Ontario, 1998, p. NR206.
58. Rosenberg DR, Stewart CM, Fitzgerald KD, et al.: Paroxetine open-label treatment of pediatric outpatients with obsessive-compulsive disorder. *J Am Acad Child Adolesc Psychiatry* 38:1180–1185, 1999.
59. Gilbert AR, Moore GJ, Keshavan MS, et al.: Decrease in thalamic volumes of pediatric patients with obsessive-compulsive disorder who are taking paroxetine. *Arch Gen Psychiatry* 57:449–456, 2000.
60. Rosenberg DR, MacMaster FP, Keshavan MS, et al.: Decrease in caudate glutamatergic concentrations in pediatric obsessive-compulsive disorder patients taking paroxetine. *J Am Acad Child Adolesc Psychiatry* 39:1096–1103, 2000.
61. Kurlan R, Como PG, Deeley C, et al.: A pilot controlled study of fluoxetine for obsessive-compulsive symptoms in children with Tourette's syndrome. *Clin Neuropharmacol* 16:167–172, 1993.
62. Thomsen PH: Child and adolescent obsessive-compulsive disorder treated with citalopram: Findings from an open trial of 23 cases. *J Child Adolesc Psychopharmacol* 7:157–166, 1997.
63. Geller DA, Biederman J, Stewart SE, et al.: Which SSRI? A meta-analysis of pharmacotherapy trials in pediatric obsessive-compulsive disorder. *American Journal of Psychiatry*. 160(11):1919–128, 2003.
64. Fitzgerald KD, Stewart CM, Tawile V, et al.: Risperidone augmentation of serotonin reuptake inhibitor treatment of pediatric obsessive compulsive disorder. *J Child Adolesc Psychopharmacol*. 1999;9(2):115–123.
65. McDougle CJ, Goodman WK, Leckman JF, et al.: Haloperidol addition in fluvoxamine-refractory obsessive-compulsive disorder: A double-blind, placebo-controlled study in patients with and without tics. *Arch Gen Psychiatry* 51:302–308, 1994.
66. McDougle CJ, Epperson CN, Pelton GH, et al.: A double-blind, placebo-controlled study of risperidone addition in serotonin reuptake inhibitor-refractory obsessive-compulsive disorder. *Arch Gen Psychiatry* 57:794–801, 2000.
67. Bloch MH, Landeros-Weisenberger A, Kelmendi B, et al.: A systematic review: Antipsychotic augmentation with treatment refractory obsessive-compulsive disorder. *Mol Psychiatry* 2006.
68. Aman MG, Buican B, Arnold LE: Methylphenidate treatment in children with borderline IQ and mental retardation: Analysis of three aggregated studies. *J Child Adolesc Psychopharmacol Adolescent Psychopharmacol* 13(1):29–40, 2003.
69. Hollander E, Phillips A, Chaplin W, Zagursky et al.: Placebo controlled crossover trial of liquid fluoxetine on repetitive behaviors in childhood and adolescent autism. *Neuropsychopharmacol* 30:582–589, 2005.
70. Emslie GJ, Heiligenstein JH, Wagner KD, et al.: Fluoxetine for acute treatment of depression in children and adolescents: A placebo-controlled, randomized clinical trial. *J Am Acad Child Adolesc Psychiatry* 41(10):1205–1215, 2002.
71. Keller M, Klein R, Kutchner S, et al.: Efficacy of paroxetine in the treatment of adolescent major depression: A randomized controlled trial. *Journal of the American Academy of Child and Adolescent Psychiatry* 40(7):762–772, (2001).
72. Wagner K, Ambrosini P, Rynn M, et al.: (2003). Efficacy of sertraline in treatment of children and adolescents with major depressive disorder: Two randomized controlled trials. *Journal of the American Medical Association*, 290(8),1033–1041.
73. Wagner KD: American Academy of Child and Adolescent Psychiatry Meetings 2005 (tapes).
74. Rey JM and Martin A: Selective serotonin reuptake inhibitors and suicidality in juveniles: review of the evidence and implications for clinical practice. *Child & Adolescent Psychiatric Clinics of North America* 15(1):221–237, 2006.
75. Hammad TA, Laughren TP, Racoosin JA: Suicide rates in short-term randomized controlled trials of newer antidepressants. *J Clin Psychopharmacol* 26:203–207, 2006.
76. Hamilton BE, Minino AM, Martin JA, et al.: Annual summary of vital statistics: 2005. *Pediatrics* 119:345–60, 2007.
77. Vitiello B, Zuvekas SH, Norquist GS: National estimates of antidepressant medication use among U.S. children, 1997–2002. *J Am Acad Child Adolesc Psychiatry* 45(3):271–279, 2006.
78. Blier P, and de Montigny C: Possible serotonergic mechanisms underlying the antidepressant and anti-obsessive-compulsive disorder responses. *Biol Psychiatry* 44:313–323, 1998.
79. Findling RL, Reed MD, Myers C, et al.: Paroxetine pharmacokinetics in depressed children and adolescents. *J Am Acad Child Adolesc Psychiatry* 38:952–995, 1999.
80. Axelson DA, Perel JM, Birmaher B, et al.: Sertraline pharmacokinetics and dynamics in adolescents. *J Am Acad Child Adolesc Psychiatry* 2002.
81. Heiligenstein JH, Hoog SL, Wagner KD, et al.: Fluoxetine 40–60 mg versus fluoxetine 20 mg in the treatment of children and adolescents with a less-than-complete response to nine-week treatment with fluoxetine 10–20 mg: A pilot study. *J Child Adolesc Psychopharmacol* 16:207–217, 2006.
82. King RA, Riddle MA, Chappell PB, et al.: Emergence of self-destructive phenomena in children and adolescents during fluoxetine treatment. *J Am Acad Child Adolesc Psychiatry* 30:179–186, 1991.
83. Black K, Shea C, Dursun S, et al.: Selective serotonin reuptake inhibitor discontinuation syndrome: Proposed diagnostic criteria. *J Psychiatry Neurosci* 25:255–261, 2000.
84. Rosenbaum JF, Fava M, Hoog SL, et al.: Selective serotonin reuptake inhibitor discontinuation syndrome: A randomized clinical trial. *Biol Psychiatry* 44:77–87, 1998.
85. Grados M, Scahill L, and Riddle MA: Pharmacotherapy in children and adolescents with obsessive-compulsive disorder. *Child Adolesc Psychiatr Clin N Am* 8:617–634, 1999.
86. Leonard HL, Swedo SE, Lenane MC, Rettew, et al.: A 2- to 7-year follow-up study of 54 obsessive-compulsive children and adolescents. *Arch Gen Psychiatry* 50:429–439, 1993.
87. March J, Shapiro M, Andreason PJ, et al.: Child and adolescent psychopharmacology in the new millennium: A workshop for academia,

industry, and government. *J Am Acad Child Adolesc Psychiatry* 45(3):261–270, 2006.
88. Lombroso PJ, Scahill L, King RA, et al.: Risperidone treatment of children and adolescents with chronic tic disorders: A preliminary report. *J Am Acad Child Adolesc Psychiatry* 34:1147–1152, 1995.
89. Hazell P, O'Connell D, Heathcote D, et al.: Tricyclic drugs for depression in children and adolescents. *Cochrane Database of Systematic Reviews* (3):CD002317, 2000.
90. Martin A, Kaufman J, and Charney D: Pharmacotherapy of early-onset depression: Update and new directions. *Child Adolesc Psychiatr Clin N Am* 9:135–157, 2000a.
91. Bernstein GA, Borchardt CM, Perwien AR, et al.: Imipramine plus cognitive-behavioral therapy in the treatment of school refusal. *J Am Acad Child Adolesc Psychiatry* 39:276–283, 2000.
92. Klein RG, Koplewicz HS, and Kanner A: Imipramine treatment of children with separation anxiety disorder. *J Am Acad Child Adolesc Psychiatry* 31:21–28, 1992.
93. Biederman J, Baldessarini RJ, Wright V, et al.: A double-blind placebo controlled study of desipramine in the treatment of ADD: I. Efficacy. *J Am Acad Child Adolesc Psychiatry* 28:777–784, 1989.
94. Singer HS, Brown J, Quaskey S, et al.: The treatment of attention-deficit hyperactivity disorder in Tourette's syndrome: A double-blind placebo-controlled study with clonidine and desipramine. *Pediatrics* 95:74–81, 1995.
95. Spencer T, Biederman J, Coffey B, et al. (2002). A double-blind comparison of desipramine and placebo in children and adolescents with chronic tic disorder and comorbid attention-deficit/hyperactivity disorder. *Archives of General Psychiatry*, 59:649–656.
96. Kratochvil CJ, Vaughan BS, Harrington MJ, et al.: (2003). Atomoxetine: A selective noradrenaline reuptake inhibitor for the treatment of attention-deficit/hyperactivity disorder. *Expert Opinion on Pharmacotherapy* 4(7):1165–1174.
97. Blair J, Taggart B, Martin A: Electrocardiographic safety profile and monitoring guidelines in pediatric psychopharmacology. *Journal of Neural Transmission* 111(7):791–815, 2004.
98. Werry JS, Biederman J, Thisted R, et al.: Resolved: Cardiac arrhythmias make desipramine an unacceptable choice in children. *J Am Acad Child Adolesc Psychiatry* 34:1239–1245; discussion 1245–1248, 1995.
99. Conners CK, Casat CD, Gualtieri CT, et al: Bupropion hydrochloride in attention deficit disorder with hyperactivity. *J Am Acad Child Adolesc Psychiatry* 35:1314–1321, 1996.
100. Barrickman LL, Perry PJ, Allen AJ, et al.: Bupropion versus methylphenidate in the treatment of attention-deficit hyperactivity disorder. *J Am Acad Child Adolesc Psychiatry* 34:649–657, 1995.
101. Daviss WB, Bentivoglio P, Racusin R, et al.: Bupropion sustained release in adolescents with comorbid attention-deficit/hyperactivity disorder and depression. *J Am Acad Child Adolesc Psychiatry* 40:307–314, 2001.
102. Mandoki MW, Tapia MR, Tapia MA, et al.: Venlafaxine in the treatment of children and adolescents with major depression. *Psychopharmacol Bull* 33:149–154, 1997.
103. www.fda.gov/cder/foi/esum/2004/20415 SE5_011_ Mirtazapine%20MO%20ReviewFIN;pdf accessed 4/30/06.
104. Michelson D, Faries D, Wernicke J, et al. (2001). Atomoxetine in the treatment of children and adolescents with attention-deficit/hyperactivity disorder: A randomized, placebo-controlled, dose-response study. *Pediatrics,* 108(5),E83.
105. Michelson D, Allen AJ, Busner J, et al.: Once-daily atomoxetine treatment for children and adolescents with attention deficit hyperactivity disorder: A randomized, placebo-controlled study. *American Journal of Psychiatry,* 159(11),1896–1901, (2002).
106. Hazell P, Zhang S, Wolanczyk T, et al.: Comorbid oppositional defiant disorder and the risk of relapse during 9 months of atomoxetine treatment for attention-deficit/hyperactivity disorder. *Eur Child Adolesc Psychiatry* 15:105–110, 2006.
107. Newcorn JH, Spencer, TJ, Biederman J, et al. Atomoxetine treatment in children and adolescents with attention-deficit/hyperactivity disorder and comorbid oppositional defiant disorder. *J Am Acad Child Adolesc Psychiatry* 44:240–248, 2005.
108. Wigal SB, McGough JJ, McCracken JT, et al.: A laboratory school comparison of mixed amphetamine salts extended release (Adderall XR) and atomoxetine (Strattera) in school-aged children with attention deficit/hyperactivity disorder. *J Atten Disord* 9:275–289, 2005.
109. Wernicke JF, & Kratochvil CJ: (2002). Safety profile of atomoxetine in the treatment of children and adolescents with ADHD. *Journal of Clinical Psychiatry* 63 (Suppl. 12):50–55.
110. www.fda.gov/bbs/topics/ANSWERS/2004/ANS01335.html.
111. www.fda.gov/bbs/topics/ANSWERS/2004/ANS01335.html and www.fda.gov/cder/drug/advisory/atomoxetine.html.
112. Harpaz-Rotem I, Leslie DL, Martin A, et al.: Changes in child and adolescent inpatient psychiatric admission diagnoses between 1995 and 2000. *Soc Psychiatry Psychiatr Epidemiol* 40:642–647, 2005.
113. Leibenluft E, Charney DS, Towbin KE, et al.: Defining clinical phenotypes of juvenile mania. *Am J Psychiatry* 160:430–437, 2003.
114. Lewinsohn PM, Klein DN, and Seeley JR: Bipolar disorders in a community sample of older adolescents: prevalence, phenomenology, comorbidity, and course. *J Am Acad Child Adolesc Psychiatry* 34:454–463, 1995.
115. Kowatch RA, Fristad M, Birmaher B, et al.: Child Psychiatric Workgroup on Bipolar Disorder: Treatment guidelines for children and adolescents with bipolar disorder. *J Am Acad Child Adolesc Psychiatry* 2005; 44:213–235.
116. Carlson GA, Jensen PS, Findling RL, et al.: Methodological issues and controversies in clinical trials with child and adolescent patients with bipolar disorder: Report of a consensus conference. *J Child Adolesc Psychopharmacol*, 13:13–27, 2003.
117. Leibenluft E: American Academy of Child and Adolescent Psychiatry Meetings, 2005 (tapes).
118. Birmaher B, Axelson D, Strober M, Gill MK, Valeri S, Chiappetta L, Ryan N, Leonard H, Hunt J, Iyengar S, Keller M: Clinical course of children and adolescents with bipolar spectrum disorders. *Arch Gen Psychiatry* 63:175–183, 2006.
119. Masi G: Prepubertal bipolar disorder: Available pharmacological treatment options. *Expert Opinion on Pharmacotherapy* 6(4):547–560, 2005.
120. Pavuluri MN, Birmaher B, Naylor MW. Pediatric bipolar disorder: A review of the past 10 years. *J Am Acad Child Adolesc Psychiatry* 44:846–871, 2005a.
121. Donovan SJ, Stewart JW, Nunes EV, et al.: Divalproex treatment for youth with explosive temper and mood lability: A double-blind, placebo-controlled crossover design. *Am J Psychiatry* 157:818–820, 2000.
122. Steiner H: Psychopharmacologic treatment of aggression in children and adolescents. *Pediatric Annals* 33(5):318–327, 2004.
123. Delbello MP: American Academy Child and Adolescent Psychiatry Meetings, 2005b (tapes).
124. DelBello MP, Adler CM, Amicone J, et al.: Parametric neurocognitive task design: A pilot study of sustained attention in adolescents with bipolar disorder. *Journal of Affective Disorders.* 82 (Suppl 1):S79–88, 2004.
125. Chang K, Saxena K, Howe M: An open-label study of lamotrigine adjunct or monotherapy for the treatment of adolescents with bipolar depression. *J Am Acad Child Adolesc Psychiatry* 45(3):298–304, 2006.
126. Biederman J. American Academy of Child and Adolescent Psychiatry Meetings, 2005c (tapes).
127. McKnew DH, Cytryn L, Buchsbaum MS, et al.: Lithium in children of lithium-responding parents. *Psychiatry Res* 4:171–180, 1981.
128. Younes RP, DeLong GR, Neiman G, et al.: Manic-depressive illness in children: Treatment with lithium carbonate. *J Child Neurol* 1:364–368, 1986.
129. DeLong GR. and Aldershof AL.: Long-term experience with lithium treatment in childhood: Correlation with clinical diagnosis. *J Am Acad Child Adolesc Psychiatry* 26:389–394, 1987.
130. Strober M, Morrell W, Lampert C, et al.: Relapse following discontinuation of lithium maintenance therapy in adolescents with bipolar I illness: A naturalistic study. *Am J Psychiatry* 147:457–461, 1990.
131. Carlson GA, Rapport MD, Pataki CS, et al.: Lithium in hospitalized children at 4 and 8 weeks: Mood, behavior and cognitive effects. *J Child Psychol Psychiatry* 33:411–425, 1992.
132. Geller B, Cooper TB, Sun K, et al.: Double-blind and placebo-controlled study of lithium for adolescent bipolar disorders with secondary substance dependency [see comments]. *J Am Acad Child Adolesc Psychiatry* 37:171–178, 1998.
133. Kafantaris V, Coletti DJ, Dicker R, et al.: Lithium treatment of acute mania in adolescents: A large open trial. *J Am Acad Child Adolesc Psychiatry* 42:1038–1045, 2003.
134. Kafantaris V, Coletti DJ, Dicker R, et al.: Lithium treatment of acute mania in adolescents: A placebo-controlled discontinuation study. *J Am Acad Child Adolesc Psychiatry*, 43:984–993, 2004.
135. Findling RL, McNamara NK, Youngstrom EA, et al.: Double-blind 18-month trial of lithium versus divalproex maintenance treatment in pediatric bipolar disorder. *J Am Acad Child Adolesc Psychiatry* 44:409–417, 2005.
136. Kafantaris V, Dicker R, Coletti DJ, et al.: Adjunctive antipsychotic treatment is necessary for adolescents with psychotic mania. *J Child Adolesc Psychopharmacol* 11:409–413, 2001a.
137. Kafantaris V, Coletti DJ, Dicker R, et al.: Adjunctive antipsychotic treatment of adolescents with bipolar psychosis. *J Am Acad Child Adolesc Psychiatry* 40:1448–1456, 2001b.
138. Strober M, DeAntonio M, Schmidt-Lackner S, et al.: Early childhood attention deficit hyperactivity disorder predicts poorer response to acute lithium therapy in adolescent mania. *J Affect Disord* 51:145–151, 1998.
139. State RC, Frye MA, Altshuler LL, et al.: Chart review of the impact of attention-deficit/hyperactivity disorder comorbidity on response to lithium.
140. Masi G, Perugi G, Toni C, et al.: Predictors of treatment nonresponse in bipolar children and adolescents with manic or mixed episodes. *J Child Adolesc Psychopharmacol* 14:395–404, 2004.
141. Kafantaris V, Coletti DJ, Dicker R, et al.: Are childhood psychiatric histories of bipolar adolescents associated with family history, psychosis, and response to lithium treatment? *J Affect Disord* 51:153–164, 1998.
142. Findling RL, McNamara NK, Stansbrey R, et al.: Combination lithium and divalproex sodium in pediatric bipolar symptom re-stabilization. *J Am Acad Child Adolesc Psychiatry* 45:142–148, 2006.
143. DelBello MP, Kowatch RA, Adler CM, et al.: A double-blind randomized pilot study comparing quetiapine and divalproex for adolescent mania. *J Am Acad Child Adolesc Psychiatry* 45:305–313, 2006.
144. Campbell M, Small AM, Green WH, et al.: Behavioral efficacy of haloperidol and lithium carbonate: A comparison in hospitalized aggressive

children with conduct disorder. *Arch Gen Psychiatry* 41:650–656, 1984.
145. Malone RP, Delaney MA, Luebbert JF, et al.: A double-blind placebo-controlled study of lithium in hospitalized aggressive children and adolescents with conduct disorder. *Arch Gen Psychiatry* 57:649–654, 2000.
146. Rifkin A, Karajgi B, Dicker R, et al.: Lithium treatment of conduct disorders in adolescents. *Am J Psychiatry* 154:554–555, 1997.
147. Manji HK, and Lenox, RH: Lithium: A molecular transducer of mood-stabilization in the treatment of bipolar disorder. *Neuropsychopharmacology* 19:161–166, 1998.
148. Vitiello B, Behar D, Malone R, et al.: Pharmacokinetics of lithium carbonate in children. *J Clin Psychopharmacol* 8:355–359, 1988.
149. Moore CM, Demopulos CM, Henry ME, et al.: Brain-to-serum lithium ratio and age: An in vivo magnetic resonance spectroscopy study. *Am J Psychiatry* 159:1240–1242, 2002.
150. Weller EB, Weller RA, Fristad MA: Lithium dosage guide for prepubertal children: A preliminary report. *J Am Acad Child Psychiatry* 25:92–95, 1986.
151. Geller B, and Luby J: Child and adolescent bipolar disorder: A review of the past 10 years. *J Am Acad Child Adolesc Psychiatry* 36:1168–1176, 1997.
152. Kowatch RA, Suppes T, Carmody TJ, et al.: Effect size of lithium, divalproex sodium, and carbamazepine in children and adolescents with bipolar disorder. *J Am Acad Child Adolesc Psychiatry* 39:713–720, 2000.
153. Gracious BL, Findling RL, Seman C, et al.: Elevated thyrotropin in bipolar youths prescribed both lithium and divalproex sodium. *J Am Acad Child Adolesc Psychiatry* 43:215–220, 2004.
154. www.accessdata.fda.gov/scripts/cdrh/cfdocs/cfClia/Detail.cfm?ID=4960.
155. Kozma C. Neonatal toxicity and transient neurodevelopmental deficits following prenatal exposure to lithium: Another clinical report and a review of the literature. *Am J Med Genet A*, 132:441–444, 2005.
156. Eberhard-Gran M, Eskild A, Opjordsmoen S: Treating mood disorders during pregnancy: Safety considerations. *Drug Saf* 28:695–706, 2005.
157. Kastner T, Friedman DL, Plummer AT, et al.: Valproic acid for the treatment of children with mental retardation and mood symptomatology. *Pediatrics* 86:467–472, 1990.
158. Papatheodorou G, Kutcher SP, Katic M, et al.: The efficacy and safety of divalproex sodium in the treatment of acute mania in adolescents and young adults: An open clinical trial. *J Clin Psychopharmacol* 15:110–116, 1995.
159. Donovan SJ, Susser ES, Nunes EV, et al.: Divalproex treatment of disruptive adolescents: A report of 10 cases. *J Clin Psychiatry* 58:12–15, 1997.
160. Barzman DH, McConville BJ, Masterson B, et al.: Impulsive aggression with irritability and responsive divalproex: A pediatric bipolar spectrum disorder phenotype? *J Affect Disord*, 88:279–285, 2005.
161. Wagner KD, Weller EB, Carlson GA, et al.: An open-label trial of divalproex in children and adolescents with bipolar disorder. *J Am Acad Child Adolesc Psychiatry*, 41:1224–1230, 2002.
162. Pavuluri MN, Henry DB, Carbray JA, et al.: Divalproex sodium for pediatric mixed mania: A 6-month prospective trial. *Bipolar Disord* 7:266–273, 2005b.
163. DelBello MP, Kowatch RA, Warner J, et al.: Adjunctive topiramate treatment for pediatric bipolar disorder: A retrospective chart review. *Journal of Child and Adolescent Psychopharmacology* 12(4):323–330, 2002.
164. Kowatch RA, Sethuraman G, Hume JH, et al.: Combination pharmacotherapy in children and adolescents with bipolar disorder. *Biol Psychiatry* 53:978–984, 2003.
165. Scheffer RE, Kowatch RA, Carmody T, et al.: Randomized, placebo-controlled trial of mixed amphetamine salts for symptoms of comorbid ADHD in pediatric bipolar disorder after mood stabilization with divalproex sodium. *Am J Psychiatry* 162:58–64, 2005.
166. Rana M, Khanzode L, Karnik N, et al.: Divalproex sodium in the treatment of pediatric psychiatric disorders. *Expert Rev Neurother* 5:165–176, 2005.
167. Czapinski P, Blaszczyk B, Czuczwar SJ: Mechanisms of action of antiepileptic drugs. *Curr Top Med Chem* 5:3–14, 2005.
168. Dutta S, Zhang Y. Bioavailability of divalproex extended-release formulation relative to the divalproex delayed-release formulation. *Biopharm Drug Dispos* 25:345–352, 2004.
169. Reith DM, Andrews J, Parker-Scott S, Eadie MJ: Urinary excretion of valproate metabolites in children and adolescents. *Biopharm Drug Dispos* 21:327–330, 2000.
170. Kanner AM: When thinking of lamotrigine and valproic acid, think "pharmacokinetically"! *Epilepsy Curr* 4:206–207, 2004.
171. Rowland P, Blaney FE, Smyth MG, et al.: Crystal structure of human cytochrome P450 2D6. *Journal of Biological Chemistry* 281(11):7614–22, 2006.
172. Davanzo PA, McCracken JT: Mood stabilizers: Lithium and anticonvulsants. *Pediatric Psychopharmacology* 25:309, 2003.
173. Isojarvi JI, Laatikainen TJ, Pakarinen AJ, et al.: Polycystic ovaries and hyperandrogenism in women taking valproate for epilepsy. *N Engl J Med* 329:1383–1388, 1993.
174. Rasgon NL, Altshuler LL, Fairbanks L, et al.: Reproductive function and risk for PCOS in women treated for bipolar disorder. *Bipolar Disord* 7:246–259, 2005.
175. Eyer F, Felgenhauer N, Gempel K, et al.: Acute valproate poisoning: Pharmacokinetics, alteration in fatty acid metabolism, and changes during therapy. *J Clin Psychopharmacol* 25:376–380, 2005.
176. Alsdorf R, Wyszynski DF. Teratogenicity of sodium valproate. *Expert Opin Drug Saf* 4:345–353, 2005.
177. Perucca E: Birth defects after prenatal exposure to antiepileptic drugs. *Lancet Neurol* 4:781–786, 2005.
178. Hsu LK: Lithium-resistant adolescent mania. *J Am Acad Child Psychiatry* 25:280–283, 1986.
179. Woolston JL: Case study: Carbamazepine treatment of juvenile-onset bipolar disorder. *J Am Acad Child Adolesc Psychiatry* 38:335–338, 1999.
180. Kafantaris V, Campbell M, Padron-Gayol MV, et al.: Carbamazepine in hospitalized aggressive conduct disorder children: An open pilot study. *Psychopharmacol Bull* 28:193–199, 1992.
181. Silva RR, Munoz DM, and Alpert M: Carbamazepine use in children and adolescents with features of attention-deficit hyperactivity disorder: A meta-analysis. *J Am Acad Child Adolesc Psychiatry* 35:352–358, 1996.
182. Cueva JE, Overall JE, Small AM, et al.: Carbamazepine in aggressive children with conduct disorder: A double-blind and placebo-controlled study. *J Am Acad Child Adolesc Psychiatry* 35:480–490, 1996.
183. Schmidt D, Elger CE. What is the evidence that oxcarbazepine and carbamazepine are distinctly different antiepileptic drugs? *Epilepsy Behav* 5:627–635, 2004.
184. Morrow JI, Russell A, Gutherie E, et al. Malformation risks of antiepileptic drugs in pregnancy: A prospective study from the U.K. Epilepsy and Pregnancy Register. *J Neurol Neurosurg Psychiatry* 2005
185. Bourgeois BF, D'Souza J: Long-term safety and tolerability of oxcarbazepine in children: A review of clinical experience. *Epilepsy Behav* 7:375–338, 2005.
186. Gao K, Calabrese JR: Newer treatment studies for bipolar depression. *Bipolar Disord* 7 (Suppl 5):13–23, 2005.
187. Chang KD, Suppes T: Treatment of rapid-cycling bipolar disorder. *Cns Spectrums*. 9(2):1–11, 2004.
188. Fung J, Mok H, Yatham LN: Lamotrigine for bipolar disorder: Translating research into clinical practice. *Expert Rev Neurother* 4:363–370, 2004.
189. Ketter TA, Wang PW, Chandler RA, et al.: Dermatology precautions and slower titration yield low incidence of lamotrigine treatment-emergent rash. *J Clin Psychiatry* 66:642–645, 2005.
190. Lofton AL, Klein-Schwartz W: Evaluation of lamotrigine toxicity reported to poison centers. *Ann Pharmacother* 38:1811–1185, 2004.
191. Delbello MP, Findling RL, Kushner S, et al.: A pilot controlled trial of topiramate for mania in children and adolescents with bipolar disorder. *J Am Acad Child Adolesc Psychiatry* 44(6):539–547, 2005.
192. Powers PS, Santana C: Available pharmacological treatments for anorexia nervosa. *Expert Opinion on Pharmacotherapy* 5(11):2287–2292, 2004.
193. Bhangoo RK, Lowe CH, Myers FS, et al.: Medication use in children and adolescents treated in the community for bipolar disorder. *J Child Adolesc Psychopharmacol* 13:515–522, 2003.
194. Pavuluri MN, Henry DB, Carbray JA, et al.: Divalproex sodium for pediatric mixed mania: A 6-month prospective trial. *Bipolar Disorders* 7(3):266–273, 2005.
195. Wozniak J: Recognizing and managing bipolar disorder in children. *J Clin Psychiatry* 66 (Suppl 1):18–23, 2005.
196. Frazier JA, Biederman J, Tohen M, et al.: A prospective open-label treatment trial of olanzapine monotherapy in children and adolescents with bipolar disorder. *Journal of Child and Adolescent Psychopharmacology*. 2001.
197. Biederman J, Mick E, Wozniak J, et al.: An open-label trial of risperidone in children and adolescents with bipolar disorder. *J Child Adolesc Psychopharmacol* 15:311–317, 2005a.
198. Biederman J, Mick E, Hammerness P, et al.: Open-label, 8-week trial of olanzapine and risperidone for the treatment of bipolar disorder in preschool-age children. *Biol Psychiatry* 58:589–594, 2005b.
199. Masi G, Mucci M, Millepiedi S. Clozapine in adolescent inpatients with acute mania. *J Child Adolesc Psychopharmacol* 12:93–99, 2002.
200. Kant R, Chalansani R, Chengappa KN, et al.: The off-label use of clozapine in adolescents with bipolar disorder, intermittent explosive disorder, or posttraumatic stress disorder. *J Child Adolesc Psychopharmacol* 14:57–63, 2004.
201. Delbello MP, Schwiers ML, Rosenberg HL, et al.: A double-blind, randomized, placebo-controlled study of quetiapine as adjunctive treatment for adolescent mania. *J Am Acad Child Adolesc Psychiatry* 41:1216–1223, 2002.
202. Pavuluri MN, Henry DB, Carbray JA, et al.: Open-label prospective trial of risperidone in combination with lithium or divalproex sodium in pediatric mania. *J Affect Disord* 82 (Suppl 1):S103–111, 2004.
203. Frazier JA, Gordon CT, McKenna K, et al.: An open trial of clozapine in 11 adolescents with childhood-onset schizophrenia. *J Am Acad Child Adolesc Psychiatry* 33:658–663, 1994.
204. Siefen G and Remschmidt H: Results of treatment with clozapine in schizophrenic adolescents. *Z Kinder Jugendpsychiatr* 14:245–257, 1986.
205. Kumra S, Frazier JA, Jacobsen LK, et al.: Childhood-onset schizophrenia: A double-blind clozapine-haloperidol comparison. *Arch Gen Psychiatry* 53:1090–1097, 1996.
206. Wirshing DA, Wirshing WC, Kysar L, et al.: Novel antipsychotics: comparison of weight gain liabilities. *J Clin Psychiatry* 60:358–363, 1999.

207. Marder SR and Meibach RC: Risperidone in the treatment of schizophrenia. *Am J Psychiatry* 151:825–835, 1994.
208. Kapur S, Remington G, Zipursky RB, et al.: The D2 dopamine receptor occupancy of risperidone and its relationship to extrapyramidal symptoms: A PET study. *Life Sci* 57:L103–107, 1995.
209. Kapur S, and Seeman P: Does fast dissociation from the dopamine D_2 receptor explain the action of atypical antipsychotics?: A new hypothesis. *Am J Psychiatry* 158:360–369, 2001.
210. Shea S, Turgay A, Carroll A, et al.: Risperidone in the treatment of disruptive behavioral symptoms in children with autistic and other pervasive developmental disorders. *Pediatrics* 114(5):e634–641, 2004.
211. Aman MG, De Smedt G, Derivan A, et al.: Risperidone Disruptive Behavior Study Group: Double-blind, placebo-controlled study of risperidone for the treatment of disruptive behaviors in children with subaverage intelligence. *American Journal of Psychiatry* 159(8):1337–1346, 2002.
212. Buitelaar JK, van der Gaag RJ, Cohen-Kettenis P, et al.: A randomized controlled trial of risperidone in the treatment of aggression in hospitalized adolescents with subaverage cognitive abilities. *Journal of Clinical Psychiatry* 62(4):239–248, 2001.
213. Findling RL, McNamara NK, Branicky LA, et al.: A double-blind pilot study of risperidone in the treatment of conduct disorder. *J Am Acad Child Adolesc Psychiatry* 39:509–516, 2000a.
214. Snyder R, et al.: Long-term safety and efficacy of risperidone for the treatment of disruptive behavior disorders in children with subaverage IQs. *Pediatrics* 110(3):e34, 2002.
215. Dion Y, Annable L, Sandor P, et al.: Risperidone in the treatment of tourette syndrome: A double-blind, placebo-controlled trial. *Journal of Clinical Psychopharmacology* 22(1):31–39, 2002.
216. Scahill L, Leckman JF, Schultz RT, et al.: A placebo-controlled trial of risperidone in Tourette syndrome. *Neurology* 60:1130–1135, 2003.
217. Turgay A, Aman M, Binder C, et al.: Risperidone Conduct Study Group: Effects of risperidone on conduct and disruptive behavior disorders in children with subaverage IQs. *J Am Acad Child Adolesc Psychiatry* 41(9):1026–1036, 2002.
218. Hanna GL, Fluent TE, Fischer DJ: Separation anxiety in children and adolescents treated with risperidone. *J Child Adolesc Psychopharmacol* 9:277–283, 1999.
219. Bruggeman R, van der Linden C, Buitelaar JK, et al.: Risperidone versus pimozide in Tourette's disorder: A comparative double-blind parallel-group study. *J Clin Psychiatry* 62:50–56, 2001.
220. McConville BJ, Arvanitis LA, Thyrum PT, et al.: Pharmacokinetics, tolerability, and clinical effectiveness of quetiapine fumarate: An open-label trial in adolescents with psychotic disorders. *J Clin Psychiatry* 61:252–260, 2000.
221. Martin A, Koenig K, Scahill L, Bregman J: Open-label quetiapine in the treatment of children and adolescents with autistic disorder. *Journal of Child and Adolescent Psychopharmacology* 9:99–107, 1999.
222. Findling RL, et al.: *J Am Acad Child Adolesc Psychiatry* 42:170–175, 2003.
223. Kumra S, Jacobsen LK, Lenane M, et al.: Childhood-onset schizophrenia: An open-label study of olanzapine in adolescents. *Journal of the American Academy of Child and Adolescent Psychiatry* 37:377–385, 1998.
224. Malone RP, et al.: *J Am Acad Child Adolesc Psychiatry* 40:887–894, 2001
225. Kemner C, Willemsen-Swinkels SHN, de Jonge M, et al.: Open-label study of olanzapine in children with pervasive developmental disorder. *J Clin Psychopharmacol* 22:455–460, 2002.
226. Bagnall A, Lewis RA, Leitner ML: Ziprasidone for schizophrenia and severe mental illness (Cochrane Review). *Cochrane Database Syst Rev* 21:CD001945, 2000.
227. Tandon R: Introduction. Ziprasidone appears to offer important therapeutic and tolerability advantages over conventional, and some novel, antipsychotics. *Br J Clin Pharmacol* 49 (Suppl 1):1S–3S, 2000.
228. Sallee FR, Kurlan R, Goetz CG, et al.: Ziprasidone treatment of children and adolescents with Tourette's syndrome: A pilot study. *J Am Acad Child Adolesc Psychiatry* 39:292–299, 2000.
229. McDougle CJ, Kem DL, Posey DJ: Case series: Use of ziprasidone for maladaptive symptoms in youths with autism. *J Am Acad Child Adolesc Psychiatry* 41(8):921–927, 2002.
230. Anderson LT, Campbell M, Adams P, et al.: The effects of haloperidol on discrimination learning and behavioral symptoms in autistic children. *J Autism Dev Disord* 19:227–239, 1989.
231. Shapiro E, Shapiro AK, Fulop G, et al.: Controlled study of haloperidol, pimozide and placebo for the treatment of Gilles de la Tourette's syndrome. *Arch Gen Psychiatry* 46:722–730, 1989.
232. Spencer EK, Kafantaris V, Padron-Gayol MV, et al.: Haloperidol in schizophrenic children: Early findings from a study in progress. *Psychopharmacol Bull* 28:183–186, 1992.
233. Joshi PT, Capozzoli JA, Coyle JT: Low-dose neuroleptic therapy for children with childhood-onset pervasive developmental disorder. *Am J Psychiatry* 145:335–338, 1988.
234. Goetz CG, Tanner CM, Klawans HL: Fluphenazine and multifocal tic disorders. *Arch Neurol* 41:271–272, 1984.
235. Realmuto GM, Erickson WD, Yellin AM, et al.: Clinical comparison of thiothixene and thioridazine in schizophrenic adolescents. *Am J Psychiatry* 141:440–442, 1984.
236. Shapiro AK, Shapiro E: Controlled study of pimozide vs. placebo in Tourette's syndrome. *J Am Acad Child Psychiatry* 23:161–173, 1984.
237. Sallee FR, Sethuraman G, Rock CM: Effects of pimozide on cognition in children with Tourette syndrome: Interaction with comorbid attention deficit hyperactivity disorder. *Acta Psychiatr Scand* 90:4–9, 1994.
238. Gutgesell H, Atkins D, Barst R, et al.: AHA scientific statement: Cardiovascular monitoring of children and adolescents receiving psychotropic drugs. *J Am Acad Child Adolesc Psychiatry* 38:1047–1050, 1999.
239. Pappadopulos E, Macintyre Ii JC, Crismon ML, et al.: Treatment recommendations for the use of antipsychotics for aggressive youth (TRAAY). Part II. *J Am Acad Child Adolesc Psychiatry* 42(2):145–161, 2003.
240. Scahill L, Erenberg G, Berlin CM, et al.: Tourette Syndrome Association Medical Advisory Board: Practice Committee: Contemporary assessment and pharmacotherapy of Tourette syndrome. *NeuroRx* 3(2):192–206, 2006.
241. Flockhart DA, Oesterheld JR: Cytochrome P450-mediated drug interactions. *Child and Adolescent Psychiatric Clinics of North America* 9(1):43–76, 2000.
242. Desta Z, Soukhova N, Flockhart DA: *In vitro*inhibition of pimozide N-dealkylation by selective serotonin reuptake inhibitors and azithromycin. *Journal of Clinical Psychopharmacology* 22(2):162–168, 2002.
243. Obach RS, Walsky RL: Drugs that inhibit oxidation reactions catalyzed by aldehyde oxidase do not inhibit the reductive metabolism of ziprasidone to its major metabolite, S-methyldihydroziprasidone: An in vitro study. *Journal of Clinical Psychopharmacology* 2005.
244. Ratzoni G, Gothelf D, Brand-Gothelf A, et al.: Weight gain associated with olanzapine and risperidone in adolescent patients: A comparative prospective study. *J Am Acad Child Adolesc Psychiatry* 41(3):337–343, 2002.
245. Sikich L, Hamer RM, Bashford RA, et al.: A pilot study of risperidone, olanzapine, and haloperidol in psychotic youth: A double-blind, randomized, 8-week trial. *Neuropsychopharmacology*. 29(1):133–145, 2004.
246. American Diabetes Association; American Psychiatric Association; American Association of Clinical Endocrinologists; North American Association for the Study of Obesity. Consensus development conference on antipsychotic drugs and obesity and diabetes. *Journal of Clinical Psychiatry*. 65(2):267–272, 2004.
247. Riddle MA, Hardin MT, Towbin KE, et al.: Tardive dyskinesia following haloperidol treatment in Tourette's syndrome. *Arch Gen Psychiatry* 44:98–99, 1987.
248. Campbell M, Armenteros JL, Malone RP, et al.: Neuroleptic-related dyskinesias in autistic children: A prospective, longitudinal study. *J Am Acad Child Adolesc Psychiatry* 36:835–843, 1997.
249. McClellan J, Werry J: Practice parameters for the assessment and treatment of children and adolescents with schizophrenia: American Academy of Child and Adolescent Psychiatry. *J Am Acad Child Adolesc Psychiatry* 33:616–635, 1994.
250. Silva RR, Munoz DM, Alpert M, et al.: Neuroleptic malignant syndrome in children and adolescents. *J Am Acad Child Adolesc Psychiatry* 38:187–194, 1999.
251. Newcorn JH, Schulz KP, Halperin JM: Adrenergic agonists: Clonidine and guanfacine. In: Martin A, Scahill L, Charney DS, Leckman JF (eds): *Pediatric Psychopharmacology: Principles and Practice*. Oxford, New York, 2003, pp. 264–273.
252. Goetz CG, Tanner CM, Wilson RS, et al.: Clonidine and Gilles de la Tourette's syndrome: double-blind study using objective rating methods. *Ann Neurol* 21:307–310, 1987.
253. Leckman JF, Hardin MT, Riddle MA, et al.: Clonidine treatment of Gilles de la Tourette's syndrome. *Arch Gen Psychiatry* 48:324–328, 1991.
254. Hunt RD, Minderaa RB, Cohen DJ: Clonidine benefits children with attention deficit disorder and hyperactivity: Report of a double-blind placebo-crossover therapeutic trial. *J Am Acad Child Psychiatry* 24:617–629, 1985.
255. Arnsten AFT: Catecholamine regulation of the prefrontal cortex. *J Psychopharm* 11:151–162, 1997.
256. Hunt RD, Arnsten AF, Asbell MD: An open trial of guanfacine in the treatment of attention-deficit hyperactivity disorder. *J Am Acad Child Adolesc Psychiatry* 34:50–54, 1995.
257. Chappell PB, Riddle MA, Scahill L, et al.: Guanfacine treatment of comorbid attention-deficit hyperactivity disorder and Tourette's syndrome: Preliminary clinical experience. *J Am Acad Child Adolesc Psychiatry* 34:1140–1146, 1995.
258. Horrigan JP, Barnhill LJ: Guanfacine for treatment of attention-deficit hyperactivity disorder in boys. *J Child Adolesc Psychopharmacology* 5:215–223, 1995.
259. Scahill L, Chappell PB, Kim YS, et al.: Guanfacine in the treatment of children with tic disorders and ADHD: A placebo controlled study *Am J Psychiatry*, 158:1067–1074, 2001.

260. Cummings DD, Singer HS, Krieger M, et al.: Neuropsychiatric effects of guanfacine in children with mild Tourette syndrome: A pilot study. *Clin Neuropharmacol* 25:325–332, 2002.
261. Rapport MD, Denney C, DuPaul GJ, Gardner MJ: Attention deficit disorder and methylphenidate: Normalization rates, clinical effectiveness, and response prediction in 76 children. *J Am Acad Child Adolesc Psychiatry* 33(6):882–893, 1994.
262. Feigin A, Kurlan R, McDermott MP, et al.: A controlled trial of deprenyl in children with Tourette's syndrome and attention deficit hyperactivity disorder. *Neurology* 46:965–968, 1996.
263. Avery RA, Franowicz JS, Studholme C, van Dyck CH, Arnsten AF: The alpha-2A-adrenoceptor agonist, guanfacine, increases regional cerebral blood flow in dorsolateral prefrontal cortex of monkeys performing a spatial working memory task. *Neuropsychopharmacol* 23(3):240–249, 2000.
264. Leckman JF, Ort SI, Cohen DJ, et al.: Rebound phenomena in Tourette's syndrome after abrupt withdrawal of clonidine: Behavioral, cardiovascular, and neurochemical effects. *Arch Gen Psychiatry* 43:1168–1176, 1986.
265. Wilson MF, Haring O, Lewin A, et al.: Comparison of guanfacine versus clonidine for efficacy, safety and occurrence of withdrawal syndrome in step-2 treatment of mild to moderate essential hypertension. *Am J Cardiol* 57:43E–9E, 1986.
266. Graae F, Milner J, Rizzotto L, et al.: Clonazepam in childhood anxiety disorders. *J Am Acad Child Adolesc Psychiatry* 33:372–376, 1994.
267. Velosa JF, Riddle MA: Pharmacologic treatment of anxiety disorders in children and adolescents. *Child Adolesc Psychiatr Clin N Am* 9:119–133, 2000.
268. Simeon JG, Knott VJ, Dubois C, et al.: Buspirone therapy of mixed anxiety disorders in childhood and adolescence: A pilot study. *J Child Adolesc Psychopharmacology* 4:159–170, 1994.
269. Pfeffer CR, Jiang H, Domeshek LJ: Buspirone treatment of psychiatrically hospitalized prepubertal children with symptoms of anxiety and moderately severe aggression. *J Child Adolesc Psychopharmacol* 7:145–155, 1997.
270. Buitelaar JK, van der Gaag RJ, van der Hoeven J: Buspirone in the management of anxiety and irritability in children with pervasive developmental disorders: Results of an open-label study. *J Clin Psychiatry* 59:56–59, 1998.
271. Thompson S, Rey JM: Functional enuresis: Is desmopressin the answer? *J Am Acad Child Adolesc Psychiatry* 34:266–271, 1995.
272. Werry JS, Dowrick PW, Lampen EL, et al.: Imipramine in enuresis—psychological and physiological effects. *J Child Psychol Psychiatry* 16:289–299, 1975.

6.2 ■ PSYCHOTHERAPIES

CHAPTER 6.2.1 ■ PSYCHOTHERAPY FOR CHILDREN AND ADOLESCENTS: A CRITICAL OVERVIEW

V. ROBIN WEERSING AND MELANIE A. DIRKS

The study of psychotherapy in youth dates back to the dawn of therapy itself—to the anxieties of Little Hans (1) and young Peter (2)—and to the beginning of both psychoanalysis and behaviorism. Since these first, seminal case reports, research in child and adolescent therapy has morphed considerably in form, and the scale of research grown exponentially. Over time, the dominant method for investigating therapy effects has become the clinical trial—in essence, a psychotherapy experiment, with manualization of the "independent variable" of therapy, randomization to treatment conditions, and use of standardized symptom-focused outcome assessments. At last review, over 1,500 of these randomized studies had been conducted (3), and the youth therapy research base grows markedly with every passing year.

In this overview chapter, we aim to provide a brief summary of the main findings across this large literature, focusing on three main questions. First, *can* psychotherapy work? That is, under ideal, experimental conditions, is psychotherapy *efficacious* for youth and families? Second, *does* psychotherapy work? That is, in real world clinical setting and samples, do we have evidence that psychotherapy is, in fact, *effective* in practice? And third, *how* does psychotherapy work? That is, do we have any substantive evidence on the underlying *mechanisms* of action of therapy effects? Our treatment of the questions of efficacy, effectiveness, and mechanism will be necessarily broad and is designed to highlight progress to date and critical areas for further research.

CAN PSYCHOTHERAPY WORK? THE QUESTION OF EFFICACY

A Historical Overview

The first summary review of the effects of youth psychotherapy appeared over 50 years ago. The author, Eugene Levitt, reviewed the existing evidence base of 18 studies treating "neuroses" in youth and came to a startling conclusion. There was little to no empirical evidence to suggest that psychotherapy was beneficial, and, indeed, the recovery rate for child and adolescent psychotherapy might be marginally worse than the simple improvement observed with the passage of time. In combination with the Eysenck (4) review of adult therapy, the Levitt (5) review and followup report (6) produced intense debate in the field. Many of the critiques focused on the methodological weaknesses of the psychotherapy studies that served as a basis for the author's negative conclusions. Early therapy efficacy studies typically: a) failed to randomly assign youths to treatment and control conditions; b) used nonequivalent comparison groups, such as therapy dropouts, as control conditions; c) failed to specify what therapy procedures were used in the intervention being tested; d) allowed therapists or other nonblind raters to assess outcome; and e) enrolled very heterogeneous samples of youth in terms of diagnoses and developmental level (see Kazdin (7) for review). These characteristics of early efficacy research substantially weakened the internal validity of the designs and made it difficult to impossible to interpret results, whether positive or negative.

In response to these critiques, the design of the prototypical therapy efficacy study evolved into that of the experimental *clinical trial*, characterized by explicit inclusion and exclusion criteria, random assignment, blinded and standardized diagnostic assessment, and manualized treatments. Within two decades, the evidence base of 18 studies available to Levitt had expanded to include over 100 clinical trials, and this explosion of therapy research coincided with the advent of modern meta-analytic methods for summarizing research findings. Together, these two developments provided a unique opportunity to revisit the conclusions of Levitt (5, 6), and the 1980s and 1990s were marked by the publication of several major metaanalyses on the efficacy of therapy in youth.

Evidence from Meta-analysis

In *meta-analysis,* traditional narrative reviews of a research area are supplemented by a quantitative analysis of empirical findings across studies. As in a narrative review, meta-analysis begins with an exhaustive, well documented literature search, with predetermined criteria for study inclusion and exclusion (e.g., requiring a minimum sample size). Following this collection of studies, researchers develop a coding scheme to capture the critical characteristics of each study, establish the reliability of the system, and code the findings from each investigation. Next, the empirical results of each investigation are transformed into a common metric of *effect sizes*, and these effect sizes form the unit of analysis for subsequent statistical tests. Statistical analyses range from simple estimates of a population effect size in a set of homogenous studies to multivariate models designed to explain variability in effect sizes across a complex literature.

In psychotherapy meta-analyses, the most common effect size metric is Cohen's d (8). If the relevant summary statistics are reported in the published study, d is very simply calculated by taking the mean of the treated group on a measure of interest (e.g., depression symptoms at post-treatment), subtracting it from the mean of the control group, and then dividing this difference by the standard deviation of the control group (see Smith, Glass, and Miller (9) for other estimation techniques). This process creates a score indicating how "far apart" in outcomes a therapy condition is from a control group, expressed in standard deviation units. By convention, a d of 0.2 is considered a small effect size, while a d of 0.8 is a large effect (10).

Casey and Berman (11) were the first to apply meta-analytic methods of this kind to the child psychotherapy literature. They reviewed and coded 64 controlled studies of therapy for youth (age 12 and under) and found that the average effect size for psychotherapy was a very respectable 0.71. A series of more comprehensive and complex meta-analyses followed the publication of the Casey and Berman (11) report, and the findings told a similar, positive story (12–14). Overall, youth therapy reliably had medium to large effects on symptoms, with results similar in magnitude to effect size evidence from the adult literature (9). Furthermore, the confidence intervals around these population estimates did not cross zero, suggesting that, as a whole, psychotherapeutic interventions for youth were more efficacious than control conditions (typically a wait list or no treatment control).

In addition to supporting the overall benefit of child treatment, meta-analyses examining moderators of efficacy suggested that some youths may profit from therapy more than others, and that some treatments may have larger effects. Notably, type of youth problem did not emerge from these analyses as being significantly related to the magnitude of therapeutic improvement (12, 14). Youths with internalizing problems, such as depression and anxiety, showed the same positive symptom gains as youths with externalizing behavior problems. More recent meta-analyses have added some caveats to this finding (15), but the preponderance of evidence across the literature indicated that therapy "worked" for most major childhood psychiatric problems. Controlling for problem type and other confounding factors, Weisz and colleagues (14) found that adolescent girls were particularly likely to do well in psychotherapeutic treatment, although this analysis was, necessarily, at the level of the study rather than at the level of the individual. Gender was coded as the proportion of youths in the sample who were male, and developmental level keyed in a similar fashion. Thus, as with all meta-analytic findings, results are best interpreted as indicating that studies that include large numbers of adolescent girls have stronger findings than studies that do not. Notably, other theoretically interesting youth predictors of treatment success have been difficult to test, due to their spotty reporting in the clinical trial literature. For example, in a recent review of the methodological characteristics of youth treatment research, it was reported that less than half of investigations provided information on the ethnicity of the study sample and a mere 25% provided any information on socioeconomic status (16).

In terms of treatment factors, it appears that for children and adolescents, behavioral interventions may be more effective, on average, than nonbehavioral psychotherapies (11, 12, 14). In the metaanalyses making this comparison, "behavioral treatments" typically include such direct behavioral techniques as teaching parents more effective discipline styles or developing anxious children's relaxation skills, as well as cognitive-behavioral therapies (CBT), such as helping depressed youth to label and correct unrealistically negative thinking and self-talk. Nonbehavioral psychotherapy has been conceived as a broad category including traditional psychodynamic-based approaches, client-centered therapies, and discussion groups. Notably, this division does not characterize well several treatment programs of recent vintage that have significant empirical support, such as interpersonal therapy (IPT) for adolescents with depression (see Chapter 6.2.3) or multisystemic therapy (MST), a behavioral–family systems approach for juvenile offenders (see Chapter 6.3.2). Also note that some treatment modalities used with youth, such as family (Chapter 6.2.6) or group (Chapter 6.2.5) work, could be coded as either behavioral or nonbehavioral depending on the content of the intervention.

Not surprisingly, the finding of superior outcomes for behavioral treatments has been hotly contested, and a host of alternate explanations proposed (17). However, this result has been robust in analyses controlling for other potentially confounding differences between behavioral and nonbehavioral studies that might spuriously produce this effect, such as differences in problem type, severity of symptoms, or methodology (see Weiss & Weisz (18) for discussion). Two critiques of this effect cannot be tested in the current clinical trial literature base and remain as possible alternate explanations of the superiority of behavioral treatments: a) far more clinical trials of behavioral therapies have been published, and additional research on nonbehavioral therapies may yet yield more positive results; and b) nonbehavioral therapies have been used as control conditions in some studies by investigators, and these treatments may not have been implemented with the same care and vigor as the main behavioral treatment being tested by the study, artificially lowering estimates of nonbehavioral therapy effect sizes (19). These possibilities speak to the central thesis of Chapter 6.2.4 on psychoanalysis and psychodynamically informed psychotherapies, and the growing efforts within the analytic research community to conduct high-quality clinical trials of insight-oriented therapeutic approaches (20, 21). However, psychoanalysis and other nonbehavioral therapies may have a high hill to climb, given the volume of research on behavioral treatments and the consistency of positive effects, particularly for exposure-based treatments for the anxiety disorders (22, 23) and behavioral parent training for child oppositional behaviors (24). The hill also may have been made steeper by the trend in the early 1990s for professional organizations in the mental health field to move beyond broad examination of the efficacy of therapy to begin identifying specific *evidence-based treatment* (EBT) programs for targeted diagnostic clusters (see Chapter 2.1.2).

The Movement toward Evidence-Based Treatment

In the early 1990s, evidence-based medicine was broadly defined as the practice of weighing the available scientific evidence when making decisions regarding clinical care (25). At around the same time, the Society of Clinical Psychology (American Psychological Association [APA] Division 12) formed a task force charged with "educating clinical psychologists, third party payors, and the public about effective psychotherapies" (26). This effort resulted in a series of reports identifying evidence-based psychosocial treatments (EBT) for adults (26–28). Parallel efforts by the Society of Clinical Child and Adolescent Psychology (APA Division 53) and the Society of Pediatric Psychology (APA Division 54) led to the publication of major EBT reviews for children and adolescents (29, 30). In addition to these efforts driven by professional organizations, several other research teams have endeavored to identify EBTs for psychological problems (22, 31–33).

As reviewed by Chambless and Ollendick (34), different groups use varying criteria when evaluating the strength of the support for an intervention's efficacy. In general, however, treatments are considered a well established EBT if they have shown positive effects in a series of carefully controlled, prospective studies by at least two independent teams of investigators. Most often, this is defined as clinical trials in which: a) participants were randomly assigned to conditions, and b) treatment was compared to a placebo or other established treatment. However, some groups consider a large series of well controlled single case studies to be sufficient for this designation. A second class of EBTs, identified as "probably efficacious" (28), is supported by scientific evidence but has been subjected to less rigorous tests (e.g., comparison to a wait-list control group).

Based on these criteria, EBTs have been identified for a wide range of social, emotional, and behavioral difficulties commonly experienced by children and adolescents. To date, well established psychosocial interventions have been developed for conduct disorder, enuresis, and phobias, and probably efficacious EBTs have been identified for other anxiety disorders (e.g., separation anxiety) and depression (34). As discussed in the section on metaanalysis, behavioral treatments are eight to 10 times more likely to be tested systematically than nonbehavioral approaches (16), and it is not surprising that the majority of EBTs identified by the various work groups are behaviorally focused. Although the majority of therapeutic interventions focus on the child, many efficacious programs target the systems in which youths function, such as their families (functional family therapy) or the juvenile justice system [MST (35)].

Currently, the EBT movement has reached beyond the professional exercise of identifying therapies with promising outcomes and moved into the domain of policy, by funding and shaping the content of youth mental health care in practice. Policymakers at the national (36–38) and international (39) levels have endorsed the importance of evidence-based mental health care, and U.S. federal funding has been made available to clinical care providers to support the training of community therapists in EBT programs (40, 41). Family and patient organizations have begun to advocate for access to mental health interventions with demonstrated effectiveness (42), and states have developed initiatives to support the use of EBT services (43). However, while these efforts may be seen as laudable in their attention to findings on the *efficacy* of psychotherapy, they have proceeded, in large part, with very little evidence on the actual *effectiveness* of therapy in practice.

DOES PSYCHOTHERAPY WORK? THE QUESTION OF EFFECTIVENESS

The news, thus far, has appeared good for those concerned with providing quality psychological services to youth and families. Psychotherapy for youth has effects of a reasonable magnitude and progress has been made in identifying specific treatments most likely to be beneficial for particular problems and diagnoses. However, limitations in the conduct of psychotherapy research have left core questions unanswered, including whether the research that supports the benefits of youth therapy and forms the base of the process of identifying EBTs is applicable to everyday clinical practice. As explicated by Weisz and colleagues (44, 45), the majority of therapy clinical trials take place under conditions substantially different from community treatment as usual (TAU). For example, clinical trials typically are based in university clinics, academic medical centers, and research labs with copious resources and support staff. Families are usually recruited to participate in the study and screened to identify the primary target problem under investigation. Therapists in a research study may receive extensive pretherapy training in the treatment protocol, be closely supervised on protocol adherence, and carry a small caseload of homogeneous clients. Psychotherapy may be free, or clients may be paid to participate in the research therapy. And, as discussed earlier, clinical trials are far more likely to utilize behavioral treatments than nonbehavioral therapies, which are heavily used in typical clinical practice (46, 47). These differences between psychotherapy research and community TAU may dim the rosy outlook on the benefit of child and adolescent therapy in two major ways.

The Effects of Community Treatment as Usual (TAU)

First, it may be that current clinical care is not as effective as the psychotherapy clinical trial literature suggests. Very few of the 1,500+ studies of child and adolescent therapy have examined the effectiveness of the therapy program of a functioning service-oriented clinic. In the early 1990s, Weisz and colleagues searched the youth treatment outcome literature for studies of "real world" psychological services (48). They found only nine studies of clinic treatment-as-usual (TAU), but results of this small body of research stood in stark contrast to those of the hundreds of typical psychotherapy clinical trials included in metaanalyses. Whereas clinical trials reported consistently beneficial effects of therapy for youth, the mean effect size of the TAU studies was near zero. Many of the studies included in the Weisz review are now over 40 years old, but modern investigations of community TAU have not produced substantially superior results.

One source of evidence comes from investigations of large mental health service systems, such as the well known Fort Bragg investigation (49). In these studies, efforts to boost the effectiveness of youth mental health care by coordinating services have not led to improved outcomes over uncoordinated care (50–52). One explanation of this finding is that the original community TAU elements were not effective to begin with and, thus, synergies between these services impossible to achieve (53). Similarly, community TAU for children and adolescents does not seem to display the type of dose–response relationships that would be expected in an active intervention (54–57). Indeed, in an investigation of community TAU services for depressed youths, the shape of symptom change was more similar to the trajectories of untreated children than the symptom change seen in clinical trials of CBT for youths with depression (58).

Consistent with this pattern, Weiss, Catron, Harris, and Phung (59) found minimal effects of TAU delivered to disturbed school-aged youths by therapists hired through a local community clinic. TAU therapists were free to use whatever techniques and dose of treatment they viewed as best, and they averaged 60 individual sessions, 18 parent sessions, and 13 school consultations per treated youth. After this substantial dose of therapy, TAU youth outcomes were equivalent to the outcomes of youth who had been randomized to receive only academic tutoring. At 2-year follow-up, the authors were able to contact 95% of their original sample of participants ($N = 112$), and the outcomes of the two groups remained quite similar (60), arguing against a longer term preventive benefit or "sleeper effect" for community TAU.

These sobering findings have reinforced calls by many (61) for a broad effort to reform mental health care practice by exporting EBTs from clinical trials into the community. This prescription relies on the assumption that it is differences in treatment type that account for the superior outcomes of psychotherapy in clinical trials compared to therapy in practice. Certainly, evidence from metaanalyses suggests that this assumption is plausible and that behavioral EBTs may perform robustly in the samples and settings of real-world clinical care. However, this hypothesis is only beginning to be tested, and there are reasons to suspect that the effects of EBT may be attenuated in practice.

The Effectiveness of Research Treatments in Practice

The second implication of the differences between clinical trial research and typical clinical care is that the promising EBTs may not work so well when tested under conditions more closely approximating real life. In addition to difference in treatment type, clinical trials and community care may vary along a number of sample and setting factors. For example, clinical trials for youth depression historically have included: a) youth either "at risk" for depression or exhibiting only mild depression symptoms (62, 63); b) youth recruited from schools and newspaper advertisements rather than ascertained through clinical referral routes (64); and c) youth carefully screened to possess a minimal number of comorbid psychiatric problems (65)—a sample of young patients *not* representative of community mental health practice (66). Preliminary investigations of patient factors related to depression treatment outcome have suggested that these three characteristics of research samples may predict therapy success (67), and, thus, treatment effects for more severe, comorbid clinical samples of depressed youth may not be as positive as clinical trial data would suggest. There may be a similar level of mismatch between the samples of youths enrolled in clinical trials of anxiety disorders compared to anxious youths in community clinics (68). Clinical trial research on disruptive behavior problems may fare better in terms of research–practice sample comparability, in part because of the efforts of many investigators to recruit research patients from settings such as juvenile justice (35) and foster care (69).

Again, metaanalysis has proved a useful tool to generate hypotheses about the "robustness" of EBTs if transported to practice. Shadish and colleagues reanalyzed data from several previously published metaanalyses on the effects of psychotherapy in a megaanalysis of the adult and child literature (70, 71). Studies were coded in terms of "clinical representativeness"—the extent to which the therapists, setting, and sample of the investigation were similar to active clinical practice. The authors clustered studies into tiers of representativeness and explored whether effect sizes for clinical trials decreased, as study characteristics became closer and closer to real-world conditions. Overall, the authors found that effect sizes were constant across levels, but they also found only one study that fulfilled all of their clinically representative criteria. Interestingly, all of the studies included in the Weisz, Weiss, and Donenberg (48) analysis of community TAU were screened out of the Shadish metaanalysis (70) on methodological grounds, further highlighting the paucity of strong research probing the effectiveness of therapy.

A few investigative teams have sought to export and test the effectiveness of research-based interventions in practice. One of the most direct tests was by Laura Mufson and colleagues, who have taken interpersonal psychotherapy (IPT) for adolescent depression into school-based health clinics and conducted a randomized effectiveness trial comparing IPT and school counseling (72). Previously, IPT had shown positive outcomes in a clinical trial by the same research group (73), and one promising replication by an independent team (74). In the effectiveness study, IPT outcomes were not as dramatic as in the clinical trials; however, the intervention did produce clinically and statistically significant effects compared to school-based counseling, an existing TAU mental health service. Notably, Mufson et al. (72) were able to obtain these effects using community therapists in both arms of the study, suggesting that IPT may be "trainable" in conventional settings.

Also in the area of adolescent depression, there is evidence that CBT may show positive effects in practice. A project examining archival medical records data from an active outpatient depression clinic found that youths treated with CBT in general practice had outcomes similar to teens enrolled in a locally based CBT clinical trial (75), when controlling for baseline differences in the two samples (76). In addition, there have been several recent efforts to export CBT for adolescent depression into pediatric primary care settings, mirroring trends in the adult treatment effectiveness literature. To date, there are two, randomized CBT effectiveness studies for depressed adolescents based in primary care: a) a multisite quality improvement (QI) study comparing enhanced care with patient choice of interventions, including a CBT treatment option, to primary care treatment as usual (77); and b) an investigation of CBT plus selective serotonin reuptake inhibitors (SSRIs) compared to standard medication management, embedded in a large health maintenance organization (78). In their QI investigation, Asarnow and colleagues found that enhanced care was superior to treatment as usual in increasing participants' access to depression care (number of sessions) and on improving depression symptoms and quality of life. Results were similar in magnitude to findings in adult primary care depression studies (79) and have been interpreted as evidence that exporting psychosocial EBT treatments for depression can significantly improve general medical TAU for this condition. However, unlike the adult literature, the Asarnow QI intervention did not increase rates of medication use, as, typically, depressed teens chose the CBT treatment option within the QI arm. Clarke and colleagues (78) found a similar result in their CBT + SSRI study. Overall, adding CBT to standard medication management provided only modest added benefit on measures of symptoms and functioning (Cohen's $d = 0.17$ to 0.20); however, these very small improvements occurred as youths significantly reduced their use of psychotropic medication in the CBT + SSRI arm—an unintended consequence of the CBT intervention. In addition, teens in the CBT + SSRI program utilized fewer health care services over one year followup, while maintaining the same level of symptoms as youths in the SSRI arm.

Taken together, results of Mufson et al. (72) and the CBT investigations suggest that it may be possible to improve the care of depressed teens over and above the effects of community TAU. Caution is warranted, as the number of studies is very small, and the primary contribution of research to date is to serve as proof that effectiveness trials in the internalizing disorders are a fruitful area for further research. Efforts to probe the effectiveness of interventions for externalizing behavior problems are significantly more advanced. For many years, treatment researchers interested in disruptive behavior problems have turned to community agencies to ascertain their samples, and randomized effectiveness trials testing the effects of parent management training (PMT) and multisystemic therapy (MST) have been built on this community foundation.

Efforts to test the effectiveness of parent management training (PMT) in practice have been occurring on both the national and international levels, with accumulating evidence for the clinical and cost effectiveness of this EBT compared to clinic TAU (80). In the most ambitious project to date, Marion Forgatch and her colleagues at the Oregon Social Learning Center have partnered with the U.S. National Institute on Drug Abuse and the Norwegian Center for Studies on Behavioral Problems and Innovative Practice to study the adoption, adaptation and implementation of PMT in every community in Norway (81). The project aims to evaluate adherence to the PMT model and assess whether fidelity to the core PMT treatment elements will prevent negative youth outcomes, such as substance abuse. In addition to these within-PMT analyses, agencies that are selected for PMT training will be compared against matched control agencies in terms of therapeutic practices and child outcomes.

In a similar large-scale fashion, Scott Henggeler, Sonja Schoenwald, and the MST research team have conducted a series of community-based effectiveness studies and formed a nonprofit consulting company (MST Services) to aid in the implementation and evaluation of MST in real world service agencies across the United States. MST was developed originally as an ecological treatment for serious juvenile delinquency. Treatment is home based, targeted at the youth, family, and the surrounding environment, and the techniques employed draw heavily from behavioral and family systems theories (35) (see Chapter 6.3.2). Initial efficacy outcomes were very promising, with statistically and clinically significant improvements in "hard outcomes," such as arrests and days in jail, compared to a variety of community TAU control conditions, including traditional juvenile justice services (82–84). In recent years, MST has been adapted and tested by the investigators as an intervention for substance-abusing youth, juvenile sex offenders, maltreated youths, and youths at risk for inpatient hospitalization due to serious emotional disturbance (85, 86). During this time, MST also has been transported into the service systems of 30 states and eight nations (87). The resulting body of program evaluation studies provides a unique dataset in which to examine the generalizability of EBT effects to a wide variety of practice settings and also to probe the sustainability of the intervention, when divorced from the original research team.

In a recent metaanalysis, Curtis, Ronan, and Borduin (88) reviewed seven studies of MST, enrolling a total of 708 youth, and coded the extent to which the investigations more closely resembled efficacy research or a true effectiveness trial, embedded in real-world practice. Again, all youths in these studies were drawn from real-world referral sources, and the major indicator of the efficacy–effectiveness distinction was the identity of therapists and the mode of supervision. Three investigations utilized graduate student therapists, supervised by MST treatment developers, with extensive weekly reviews and feedback on audio or videotapes of sessions. In contrast, the effectiveness studies used community mental health providers who received initial training in MST but little ongoing supervision (by design, as sustainability of the program was a research question under investigation) (87). Effect sizes were significantly larger in studies utilizing graduate students as therapists ($d = 0.81$) than in studies with therapists from the community ($d = 0.26$). This meta-analytic result maps onto work done by the MST team examining the dissemination of the program to 45 sites, 400 therapists, and 2,000 treated youths, in which adherence to the MST model and strong quality assurance procedures are correlated with positive youth outcomes (89–91). In the next generation of MST effectiveness research, emphasis is shifting to investigation of the characteristics of therapists and community organizations (92) that impact adherence to MST, sustainability of the program in practice, and, through these links, youth and family outcomes.

HOW DOES PSYCHOTHERAPY WORK? THE QUESTION OF MECHANISM

In our final section, we turn to the question of mechanism. Given evidence that psychotherapy for youth *can* work and that, under some conditions, it *does* actually work in practice, is there evidence on *how* psychotherapeutic interventions achieve their effects?

The brief answer to this query is no, due in large part to the content of most therapy manuals for youth and the design of most clinical trials. The majority of research therapies consist of multicomponent treatment packages. For example, a CBT manual for youth anxiety likely includes several of the following components: a) teaching the child how to identify and label different emotions; b) working to correct anxious self-talk and thinking; c) teaching relaxation skills; d) guiding desensitization of imagined feared objects; e) participating in role-plays of coping skills; and f) coaching the youth in real-life exposure to anxiety-provoking stimuli. From a design perspective, if a treatment utilizing a package of these techniques is compared to a waiting list control and found to be more effective on global measures of anxiety, it is not clear whether every component of the treatment is necessary to produce therapeutic change. Additionally, in this hypothetical design, underlying pathogenic processes have not been assessed (e.g., shifts in anxious cognitions), nor tests conducted to determine if changes in these mechanisms mediate the impact of treatment on anxious symptomatology.

This example is intended as an illustration, yet it describes a fair proportion of the existing youth clinical trial literature. In 2002, Weersing and Weisz reviewed the psychosocial clinical trials for anxiety, depression, and disruptive behavior cited in the Society of Clinical Child and Adolescent Psychology EBT reports (29). In this review of 67 studies, only 10% included an attempt to measure treatment processes and test whether change in these processes mediated therapy effects (93). Furthermore, these six investigations (94–99) suffered from significant methodological limitations, such as failing to show that change in the proposed treatment mechanism actually occurred before change in outcome, and one of the studies did not demonstrate mediation (95).

While formal tests of mediation were very rare, simple measurement of possible mediators was much more common in the literature. Nearly every study of parent training assessed whether treatment impacted parenting behaviors, and the majority of depression studies included at least one measure of a potential treatment process (79%) (93). Overall, when EBT studies included these measures, investigators found that treatment significantly changed the process, at least when the process was assessed at posttreatment, along with the other general symptom measures of outcome. While this provides only weak and indirect evidence of mechanism, it may be a useful developmental step in the maturation of the youth psychotherapy research literature.

As treatment mechanism research moves forward, it would seem valuable for psychotherapy investigators to employ more rigorous designs and to move beyond the traditional self-report, parent report, and behavioral observation rating scales that have long characterized assessment of youth therapy processes and outcome. For example, it is notable how little the youth psychotherapy literature appears to have been informed by modern advances in developmental psychopathology, including the explosion of research on biological bases of behavior (100). In the Weersing and Weisz review (93), the only studies to include putatively "biological" mediators were early investigations of behavioral treatments for anxiety that measured indices of physiological habituation such as galvanic skin response and heart rate. This is a far cry for mechanism studies assessing shifts in cortisol, brain activation, or the buffering effect of social support programs on genetic vulnerability to acute stress reactions (101). In the next 50 years of youth psychotherapy research, it seems likely that these sorts of tests will move from conjecture to reality and substantially enhance our knowledge of why therapy is therapeutic.

CONCLUSIONS AND FUTURE DIRECTIONS

In sum, the available evidence suggests that a) psychotherapy for youth can produce positive effects and is generally efficacious in research studies; b) there may be a need to improve on the effects of typical community mental health care for youth; and c) we may have the means to do so, through the careful implementation of efficacy-tested EBT programs. However, these general conclusions come with caveats. The number of rigorous studies of community TAU is quite small, and there is still a gap in efficacy research focusing on the insight-oriented and eclectic approaches typically used in practice. The body of EBT effectiveness trials is growing and outcomes appear promising, but coverage of internalizing problems is thin, and results from the better developed externalizing literature suggest that effect sizes of EBTs in practice may be moderated by therapist and organizational factors.

In addition, we still know remarkably little about how psychotherapeutic interventions work. This lack of precision is unsatisfying scientifically and may make the task of transporting these multicomponent research treatments into clinical settings more difficult than need be. If only one or two techniques of a complicated treatment package are producing change, then time spent training and providing the rest of the treatment package is wasted effort. Lack of understanding of mechanism also hampers our ability to develop new treatments that efficiently target core processes of disorder—a critical task, given evidence that the effect sizes for interventions in practice may be halved from efficacy estimates (88). In the next generation of psychotherapy research, a better understanding of why therapy works would seem to be of paramount importance.

References

1. Freud S: Analysis of phobia in a five-year-old boy. In: *Standard Editions of the Complete Psychological Works of Sigmund Freud* (vol 10). London, Hogarth, 1955, pp. 3–149.
2. Jones MC: A laboratory study of fear: The case of Peter. *Pedagog Sem* 31:308–315, 1924.
3. Kazdin AE: Developing a research agenda for child and adolescent psychotherapy. *Arch Gen Psychiat* 57:829–835, 2000.
4. Eysenck HJ: The effects of psychotherapy: An evaluation. *J Consult Psychol* 16:319–324, 1952.
5. Levitt EE: The results of psychotherapy with children: An evaluation. *J Consult Psychol* 21:189–196, 1957.
6. Levitt EE: Psychotherapy with children: A further evaluation. *Behav Res Ther* 1:45–51, 1963.
7. Kazdin AE: *History of Behavior Modification: Experimental Foundations of Contemporary Research.* Baltimore, University Park Press, 1978.
8. Cohen J: *Statistical Power Analysis for the Behavioral Sciences.* New York: Academic Press, 1977.
9. Smith ML, Glass GV, Miller TI: *The Benefits of Psychotherapy.* Baltimore: Johns Hopkins, 1980.
10. Cohen J. A power primer. *Psychol Bull* 112:155–159, 1992.
11. Casey RJ, Berman JS. The outcome of psychotherapy with children. *Psychol Bull* 98:388–400, 1985.
12. Weisz JR, Weiss B, Alicke MD, et al. Effectiveness of psychotherapy with children and adolescents: A meta-analysis for clinicians. *J Consult Clin Psych* 55:542–549, 1987.
13. Kazdin AE, Bass D, Ayers WA, et al.: Empirical and clinical focus of child and adolescent psychotherapy research. *J Consult Clin Psych* 58:729–740, 1990.
14. Weisz JR, Weiss B, Han SS, et al.: Effects of psychotherapy with children and adolescents revisited: A metaanalysis of treatment outcome studies. *Psychol Bull* 117:450–468, 1995.
15. Weisz JR, McCarthy CA, Valeri, SM: Effects of psychotherapy for depression in children and adolescents: A metaanalysis. *Psychol Bull* 132:132–149, 2006.
16. Weisz JR, Doss AJ, Hawley KM: Youth psychotherapy outcome research: A review and critique of the evidence base. *Annu Rev Psychol* 56:337–363, 2005.
17. Shirk SR, Russell RL: A reevaluation of estimates of child therapy effectiveness. *J Am Acad Child Psy* 31:703–709, 1992.
18. Weiss BH, Weisz JR: Relative effectiveness of behavioral and nonbehavioral child psychotherapy. *J Consult Clin Psych* 63:317–320, 1995.
19. Westen D, Novonty CM, Thompson-Brenner H: Empirical status of empirically supported psychotherapies: Assumptions, findings, and reporting in controlled clinical trials. *Psychol Bull* 130:631–663, 2004.
20. Lieberman AF, Van Horn P, Ippen CG: Toward evidence-based treatment: Child-parent psychotherapy with preschoolers exposed to marital violence. *J Am Acad Child Psy* 44:1241–1248, 2005.
21. Toth SL, Maughan A, Manly JT, et al.: The relative efficacy of two interventions in altering maltreated preschool children's representational models: Implications for attachment theory. *Dev Psychopathol* 14:877–908, 2002.
22. Compton SN, March JS, Brent DA, et al.: Cognitive-behavioral psychotherapy for anxiety and depressive disorders in children and adolescents: An evidence-based medicine review. *J Am Acad Child Psy* 43:930–959, 2004.
23. Ollendick TH, King NJ: Empirically supported treatments for children with phobic and anxiety disorders. *J Clin Child Psychol* 27:156–167, 1998.
24. Brestan EV, Eyberg SM: Effective psychosocial treatments of conduct-disordered children and adolescents: 29 years, 82 studies, and 5,272 kids. *J Clin Child Psychol* 27:180–189, 1998.
25. Hamilton J: The answerable question and a hierarchy of evidence. *J Am Acad Child Psy* 44:596–600, 2005.
26. Task Force on Promotion and Dissemination of Psychological Procedures. Training in and dissemination of empirically validated psychological treatments: Report and recommendations. *Clin Psychol* 48, 3–24, 1995.
27. Chambless DL, Sanderson WC, Shoham V, et al.: An update on empirically validated therapies. *Clin Psychol* 49:5–18, 1996.
28. Chambless DL, Baker MJ, Baucom DH, et al.: Update on empirically validated therapies, II. *Clin Psychol* 51:3–16, 1998.
29. Lonigan C, Elbert J: Empirically supported psychosocial interventions for children: An overview. (Special issue on empirically supported psychosocial interventions for children.) *J Clin Child Psychol* 27:138–145, 1998.
30. Spirito A (ed): Special series on empirically supported interventions in pediatric psychology (Series of special issues). *J Pediatr Psychol* 24:2–4, 6, 1999.
31. Roth A, Fonagy P: *What Works for Whom? A Critical Review of Psychotherapy Research.* New York, Guilford, 1996.
32. Farmer EM, Compton SN, Burns JB, et al.: Review of the evidence base for treatment of childhood psychopathology: Externalizing disorders. *J Consult Clin Psych* 70:1267–1302, 2002.
33. Kazdin AE, Weisz JR: *Evidence-Based Psychotherapies for Children and Adolescents.* New York, Guilford Press, 2003.

34. Chambless DL, Ollendick TH. Empirically supported psychological interventions: Controversies and evidence. *Annu Rev Psychol* 52:685–716, 2001.
35. Henggeler SW, Lee T. Multisystemic treatment of serious clinical problems In: (Kazdin AE, Weisz JR (eds): *Evidence-Based psychotherapies for Children and Adolescents* New York, Guilford Press, 2003.
36. National Institute of Mental Health. Blueprint for change: Research on child and adolescent mental health. *Report of the National Advisory Mental Health Council's Workgroup on Child and Adolescent Mental Health Intervention Development and Deployment.* Rockville, MD, Department of Health and Human Services, 2001.
37. Office of the Surgeon General. *Mental Health: A Report of the Surgeon General.* Rockville, MD, Department of Health and Human Services, 1999.
38. President's New Freedom Commission on Mental Health. *Achieving the Promise: Transforming Mental Health Care in America.* Final report. Rockville, MD, Department of Health and Human Services, 2003.
39. National Institute for Health and Clinical Excellence. Published clinical guidelines, 2006. Available at: www.nice.org.uk/page.aspx?o=guidelines. completed. Accessed July 3, 2006.
40. Department of Health and Human Services. National training and technical assistance center for child and adolescent mental health cooperative agreement (SM 04-002), 2004. Available at: http://alt.samhsa.gov/grants/2004/nofa/sm04-002_inf_NTTAC.asp. Accessed March 17, 2006.
41. Department of Health and Human Services (2004b). State implementation of evidence-based practices II—Bridging science and service (RFA-MH-05-004). 2004. Available at http://grants1.nih.gov/grants/fuide/rfa-files/RFA-MH-05-004.html. Accessed June 7, 2006.
42. National Alliance for the Mentally Ill. An update on evidence-based practices in children's mental health. *NAMI Beginnings*. Issue 3, Fall 2003.
43. National Association of State Mental Health Program Directors. NASMHPD Website listings: Available at: www.nasmhpd.org. Accessed July 3, 2006.
44. Weisz JR, Weiss B: Assessing the effects of clinic-based psychotherapy with children and adolescents. *J Consult Clin Psych* 57:741–746, 1989.
45. Weisz JR, Donenberg GR, Han SS, et al.: Bridging the gap between laboratory and clinic in child and adolescent psychotherapy. *J Consult Clin Psych* 63:688–701, 1995.
46. Weersing VR, Weisz JR, Donenberg GR: Development of the Therapy Procedures Checklist: A therapist-report measure of technique use in child and adolescent treatment. *J Clin Child Adolesc Psychol* 31:168–180, 2002.
47. Kazdin AE, Siegel TC, Bass D: Drawing on clinical practice to inform research on child and adolescent psychotherapy: Survey of practitioners. *Prof Psychol—Res Pr* 21:189–198, 1990.
48. Weisz JR, Weiss B, Donenberg GR: The lab versus the clinic: Effects of child and adolescent psychotherapy. *Am Psychol* 47:1578–1585, 1992.
49. Bickman L, Guthrie PR, Foster EM, et al.: *Evaluating Managed Mental Health Services: The Fort Bragg Experiment*. New York, Plenum, 1995.
50. Bickman L: A continuum of care: More is not always better. *Am Psychol* 51:689–701, 1996.
51. Bickman L, Noser K, Summerfelt WT: Long-term effects of a system of care on children and adolescents. *J Behav Health Serv Res* 26:185–202, 1999.
52. Bickman L, Lambert EW, Andrade AR, et al.: The Fort Bragg continuum of care for children and adolescents: Mental health outcomes over 5 years. *J Consult Clin Psych* 68:710–716, 2000.
53. Weisz JR, Han SS, Valeri, SM: More of what?: Issues raised by the Fort Bragg study. *Am Psychol* 52:541–545, 1997.
54. Andrade AR, Lambert W, & Bickman L: Dose effect in child psychotherapy: Outcomes associated with negligible treatment. *J Am Acad Child Psy* 39:161–168, 2000.
55. Bickman L, Andrade AR, Lambert EW: Dose response in child and adolescent mental health services. *Ment Health Serv Res* 4:57–70, 2002.
56. Salzer MS, Bickman L, Lambert EW: Dose-effect relationship in children's psychotherapy services. *J Consult Clin Psych* 67:228–238, 1999.
57. Angold A, Costello JE, Burns BJ, et al.: The effectiveness of non-residential specialty mental health services for children and adolescents in the "real world." *J Am Acad Child Psy* 39:154–160, 2000.
58. Weersing VR, Weisz JR: Community clinic treatment of depressed youth: Benchmarking usual care against CBT clinical trials. *J Consult Clin Psych* 70:299–310, 2002.
59. Weiss B, Catron T, Harris V, et al.: The effectiveness of traditional child psychotherapy. *J Consult Clin Psych* 67:82–94, 1999.
60. Weiss B, Catron T, Harris V: A 2-year follow-up of the effectiveness of traditional child psychotherapy. *J Consult Clin Psych* 68:1094–1101, 2000.
61. Bickman L: The death of treatment as usual: An excellent first step on a long road. *Clin Psychol—Sci Pr* 9:195–199, 2002.
62. Clarke GN, Hawkins W, Murphy M, et al.: Targeted prevention of unipolar depressive disorder in an at-risk sample of high school adolescents: A randomized trial of a group cognitive intervention. *J Am Acad Child Psy* 34:312–321, 1995.
63. Weisz JR, Thurber CA, Sweeney L, et al.: Brief treatment of mild-to-moderate child depression using primary and secondary control enhancement training. *J Consult Clin Psych* 65:703–707, 1997.
64. Butler L, Miezitis S, Friedman R, et al.: The effect of two school-based intervention programs on depressive symptoms in preadolescents. *Am Educ Res J* 17:111–119, 1980.
65. Lewinsohn PM, Clarke GN, Hops H, et al.: Cognitive-behavioral treatment for depressed adolescents. *Behav Ther* 21:385–401, 1990.
66. Hammen C, Rudolph K, Weisz J, et al.: The context of depression in clinic-referred youth: Neglected areas in treatment. *J Am Acad Child Psy* 38:64–71, 1999.
67. Brent DA, Kolko D, Birmaher B, et al.: Predictors of treatment efficacy in a clinical trial of three psychosocial treatments for adolescent depression. *J Am Acad Child Psy* 37:906–914, 1998.
68. Southam-Gerow MA, Weisz JR, Kendall, PC: Youth with anxiety disorders in research and service clinics: Examining client differences and similarities. *J Clin Child Adolesc Psychol* 32:375–385, 2003.
69. Chamberlain P: *Treating Chronic Juvenile Offenders: Advances Made through the Oregon Multidimensional Treatment Foster Care Model.* Washington, DC, American Psychological Association, 2003.
70. Shadish WR, Matt GE, Navarro AM, et al.: Evidence that therapy works in clinically representative conditions. *J Consult Clin Psych* 65:355–365, 1997.
71. Shadish WR, Navarro AM, Matt GE, et al.: The effects of psychological therapies under clinically representative conditions: A metaanalysis. *Psychol Bull* 126:512–529, 2000.
72. Mufson L, Dorta KP, Wickramaratne P, et al.: A randomized effectiveness trial of interpersonal psychotherapy for depressed adolescents. *Arch Gen Psychiat* 61:577–584, 2004.
73. Mufson L, Weissman MM, Moreau D, et al.: Efficacy of interpersonal psychotherapy for depressed adolescents. *Arch Gen Psychiat* 56:573–579, 1999.
74. Rosselló J, Bernal G: The efficacy of cognitive-behavioral and interpersonal treatments for depression in Puerto Rican adolescents. *J Consult Clin Psych* 67:734–745, 1999.
75. Brent DA, Holder D, Kolko D, et al.: A clinical psychotherapy trial for adolescent depression comparing cognitive, family, and supportive therapy. *Arch Gen Psychiat* 54:877–885, 1997.
76. Weersing VR, Iyengar S, Birmaher B, et al.: Effectiveness of cognitive-behavioral therapy for adolescent depression: A benchmarking investigation. *Behav Ther* 37:36–48, 2006.
77. Asarnow JR, Jaycox LH, Duan N, et al.: Effectiveness of a quality improvement intervention for adolescent depression in primary care clinics: A randomized controlled trial. *JAMA* 293:311–319, 2005.
78. Clarke GN, Debar L, Lynch F, et al.: A randomized effectiveness trial of brief cognitive-behavioral therapy for depressed adolescents receiving anti-depressant medication. *J Am Acad Child Psy* 44:888–898, 2005.
79. Wells KB, Sherbourne C, Schoenbaum M, et al.: Impact of disseminating quality improvement programs for depression in managed primary care: A randomized controlled trial. *JAMA* 283:212–220, 2000.
80. van de Weil NMH, Matthys W, Cohen-Kettenis P, et al. Application of the Utrecht Coping Power Program and care as usual to children with disruptive behavior disorders: A comparative study of cost and course of treatment. *Behav Ther* 34:421–436, 2003.
81. CRISP (Computer Retrieval of Information on Scientific Projects). Implementing parent management training in Norway (5R01DA016097). 2006. Available at: http://crisp.cit.nih.gov. Accessed July 3, 2006.
82. Borduin CM, Mann BJ, Cone LT, et al. Multisystemic treatment of serious juvenile offenders: Long-term prevention of criminality and violence. *J Consult Clin Psych* 63:569–578, 1995.
83. Henggeler SW, Melton GB, Smith LA. Family preservation using multisystemic therapy: An effective alternative to incarcerating serious juvenile offenders. *J Consult Clin Psych* 60:953–961, 1992.
84. Henggeler SW, Rowland MD, Pickrel, SG, et al. Investigating family-based alternatives to institution-based mental health services for youth: Lessons learned from the pilot study of a randomized field trial. *J Clin Child Psychol* 26:226–233, 1997.
85. Henggeler SW, Pickrel SG, Brondino MJ. Multisystemic treatment of substance-abusing and dependent delinquents: Outcomes, treatment fidelity, and transportability. *Ment Health Serv Res* 1:171–184, 1999.
86. Henggeler SW, Rowland MD, Randall J, et al. Home-based multisystemic therapy as an alternative to the hospitalization of youth in psychiatric crisis: Clinical outcome. *J Am Acad Child Psy* 38:1331–1339, 1999.
87. Henggeler SW: Decreasing effect sizes for effectiveness studies—implications for the transport of evidence-based treatments: Comment on Curtis, Ronan and Borduin (2004). *J Fam Psychol* 18:420–423, 2004.
88. Curtis NM, Ronan KR, Borduin CM. Multisystemic treatment: A meta-analysis of outcome studies. *J Fam Psychol* 18:411–419, 2004.
89. Schoenwald S, Sheidow AJ, Letourneau EJ. Toward effective quality assurance in evidence-based practice: Links between expert consultation, therapist fidelity, and child outcomes. *J Clin Child Adolesc Psychol* 33:94–104, 2004.
90. Schoenwald S, Sheidow AJ, Letournea EJ, et al. Transportability of multisystemic therapy: Evidence for multilevel influences. *Ment Health Serv Res* 5:223–239, 2003.
91. Henggeler SW, Schoenwald SK, Liao JG, et al. Transporting efficacious treatments to field settings: The link between supervisory practices

and therapist fidelity in MST programs. *J Clin Child Adolesc Psychol* 13:155–167, 2002.
92. Schoenwald S, Hoagwood K. Effectiveness, transportability, and dissemination of interventions: What matters when? *Psychiatr Serv* 52:1190–1197, 2001.
93. Weersing VR, Weisz JR. Mechanisms of action in youth psychotherapy. *J Child Psychol Psyc* 43:3–29, 2002.
94. Treadwell, KRH, & Kendall PC: Self-talk in youth with anxiety disorders: Content specificity and treatment outcome. *J Consult Clin Psych* 64:941–950, 1996.
95. Kolko D, Brent D, Baugher M, et al.: Cognitive and family therapies for adolescent depression: Treatment specificity, mediation and moderation. *J Consult Clin Psych* 68:603–614, 2000.
96. Patterson GR, Forgatch MS: Predicting future clinical adjustment from treatment outcome and process variables. *Psychol Assessment* 7:275–285, 1995.
97. Eddy MJ, Chamberlain P: Family management and deviant peer association as mediators of the impact of treatment condition on youth antisocial behavior. *J Consult Clin Psych* 68:857–863, 2000.
98. Huey SJ, Henggeler SW, Brondino, MJ, et al.: Mechanisms of change in multisystemic therapy: Reducing delinquent behavior through therapist adherence and improved family and peer functioning. *J Consult Clin Psych* 68:451–467, 2000.
99. Guerra NG, Slaby RG: Cognitive mediators of aggression in adolescent offenders: II. Intervention. *Dev Psychol* 26:269–277, 1990.
100. Caspi A, Sugden K, Moffitt TE, et al.: Influence of life stress on depression: Moderation by a polymorphism in the 5-HTT gene. *Science* 301:386–389, 2003.
101. Kaufman J, Yang B, Douglas-Palumberi H, et al.: Brain-derived neurotrophic factor-5-HHTLPR gene interactions and environmental modifiers of depression in children. *Biol Psychiat* 59:673–680, 2006.

CHAPTER 6.2.2 ■ COGNITIVE AND BEHAVIORAL THERAPIES

MENDY A. BOETTCHER AND JOHN PIACENTINI

INTRODUCTION

Cognitive-behavioral therapy (CBT) is the most widely researched and evidence-based form of psychotherapy today. Although CBT technically refers to a group of therapeutic interventions employing an integrated approach to both behavior and cognition, this chapter also covers interventions addressing each of these domains in relatively isolated fashion (behavior therapy and cognitive therapy, respectively; all collectively referred to hereinafter as CBT). CBT can be differentiated from other psychotherapeutic approaches by its historical roots in experimental and learning psychology and ongoing emphasis on experimental validation of efficacy and treatment mechanisms. Over the past decade, CBT has rapidly progressed from a specialized intervention into a mainstream therapeutic approach that is now a mandated part of psychiatric residency training in the United States (1). This widespread acceptance is due in no small part to the fact that CBT is, by design, a problem-based, short-term, and contextually relevant treatment approach.

BACKGROUND AND HISTORY

Cognitive Therapy Foundations

Cognitive therapies are based on the notion that it is not events, but people's interpretations of events, that cause psychological disturbance. As such, therapy from a cognitive perspective focuses on identifying and changing people's cognitions as a way of changing their feelings and reducing psychological distress.

Behavior Therapy Foundations

When working within a purely behavioral framework, overt behavior is typically the primary concern or symptom. "Overt behavior that one can see" (2) is targeted through a variety of intervention strategies, and behavioral changes are thought to influence thoughts and feelings. Setting concrete goals and measuring specific behaviors is an integral part of this approach and is considered the primary means of evaluating progress and outcomes.

When focusing on overt behaviors in behavior therapy, an emphasis is placed on the determinants of or current influences on behavior (2, 3). That is, one does not view the behavior in isolation, rather events leading up to (antecedents) and resulting from (consequences) the behavior are examined and patterns are discerned. This view of behavior is known as the functional perspective and attempts to pinpoint functions that behaviors serve so that intervention can be tailored accordingly. Taking a functional perspective on behavior allows one to understand how certain behaviors are maintained over time. A functional analysis or assessment is performed when variables that maintain a behavior must be identified. This assessment consists of systematically observing or manipulating variables to ascertain antecedents and consequences of specific target behaviors. Analysis of data obtained from a functional analysis/assessment allows one to determine what variables are maintaining the behavior; however, it often does not reveal original causes of behavior. For purposes of behavioral intervention planning, maintaining variables are typically more important than the original cause.

Classical Conditioning

Classical conditioning studies were some of the earliest demonstrations of learned behaviors resulting from manipulation of consequences (4). In these studies, a stimulus (unconditioned stimulus) that elicited a reflexive response (unconditioned response) was paired with a stimulus (conditioned stimulus) that initially would have elicited no response. Over repeated trials, this conditioned stimulus came to elicit the same response as the original unconditioned stimulus. In Pavlov's (4) classic study, meat powder (unconditioned stimulus) was paired with a bell (conditioned stimulus) to elicit a salivating response (unconditioned response) in dogs. Over time, the bell came to elicit this response even when the meat powder was not presented (conditioned response). It is important to note that, unlike operant conditioning, classical conditioning does not entail the acquisition of a new response; rather it establishes the connection of an existing response to a new stimulus.

The cognitive behavioral approach to therapy dates back to early applications of classical conditioning to phobias (5). In classical conditioning of phobias, phobic stimuli (which were previously neutral) were paired at one point in time with a traumatic event, which then lead to avoidance of stimuli related to that event. This avoidance behavior is said to be classically conditioned because it arose when an inherently fear-producing event became paired with an otherwise neutral event in an individual's mind. The subsequent avoidance behavior does not allow extinction to occur, such that the phobia is maintained (the person does not allow him-or herself to be exposed to the feared stimuli, so cannot see that the traumatic event will not occur again). For example, if a person is attacked on a street that they walk every day, a previously neutral stimulus (the street) is then associated with a traumatic event (being attacked). If the person avoids that street in the future as a result, classical conditioning has occurred.

The classical conditioning paradigm is often used to explain other phenomena, such as emotional responses, addictions, and psychosomatic disorders. As a result, many treatments for these disorders are based on the notion of classical extinction. Extinction occurs once the connection between the conditioned stimulus and response has been established and the conditioned stimulus is then presented repeatedly without the unconditioned stimulus (the bell is presented without the meat powder). When this occurs, the conditioned response will decay over time because the reflexively reinforcing stimulus is no longer available. So in the case of Pavlov's dogs, when they are repeatedly presented with the bell without the meat powder, over time their salivating response will decline. Therapy techniques that are associated with classical conditioning and classical extinction include counterconditioning, systematic desensitization, covert sensitization, and exposure and response prevention. These techniques will be discussed in further detail later in this chapter.

Operant Conditioning

Principles of operant conditioning underlie functional analysis and assessment procedures. These techniques are based on the work of B.F. Skinner (6, 7), who demonstrated that new behaviors could be shaped through reinforcement (behavior followed by a positive consequence is likely to occur again) and its subsequent removal (when reinforcement is removed, behavior will decline over time).

Principles of operant conditioning are also often used in behavioral interventions. Operant conditioning has been described in the following way: "Responses are increased or strengthened (and thus shaped) by having consequences that are rewarding (positive reinforcement), or that lead to the avoidance of, or escape from, punishment (negative reinforcement); they are reduced or eliminated by sanctions (fines, penalties, etc.) as outcomes"(8). That is, positive reinforcement is the application of a consequence that the individual finds rewarding. Negative reinforcement is the removal of a negative stimulus that results in a positive outcome for the individual. Similarly, punishment is a consequence that decreases the likelihood that a behavior will occur in the future. Positive punishment is the application of negative consequence and negative punishment is taking away positive consequences.

Schedules of Reinforcement

Reinforcement occurs in multiple schedules, which have different impacts on behavior. Schedules of reinforcement are either continuous or intermittent. A continuous schedule is best for initially teaching a new behavior, because the behavior is reinforced each time it occurs. Once the behavior is established, it is best to then decrease the ratio of reinforcers to responses (called *thinning* the schedule of reinforcement) so that the individual does not become satiated and therefore unmotivated. When thinning a continuous schedule of reinforcement, there are four types of intermittent schedules that can be used. These are: 1) fixed interval (the individual is reinforced on a fixed time interval), 2) variable interval (the individual is reinforced after varying time intervals), 3) fixed ratio (the individual is reinforced after a fixed number of responses), and 4) variable ratio (the individual is reinforced after a variable number of responses). The variable ratio schedule is the most effective schedule when trying to maintain a behavior because it creates relatively high steady rates of responding.

Extinction

Operant extinction occurs when reinforcement that was previously available is withheld in order to decrease or eliminate that behavior. That is, a behavior that was previously followed by positive consequences can be eliminated by withholding those positive consequences. When using extinction as an intervention, it is important to understand the phenomenon of an extinction burst. An extinction burst occurs immediately after removal of a previously available reinforcer. When the reinforcer is initially removed, the individual will engage in the behavior at a higher, more intense rate before learning that the behavior no longer results in reinforcement. Once this learning has occurred, the behavior will gradually decrease. Understanding this characteristic pattern can be very important for intervention, as the initial increase in behavior often leads therapists and patients alike to believe that the intervention is not working. In fact, if the reinforcement is consistently not available during this time, the burst will occur and the behavior will decline.

Many therapy techniques are associated with the principles of operant conditioning. Some common techniques can be found in Table 6.2.2.1.

Therapies that involve multiple techniques based on operant conditioning are applied behavior analysis (ABA) and various

TABLE 6.2.2.1

COMMON THERAPY TECHNIQUES ASSOCIATED WITH PRINCIPLES OF OPERANT CONDITIONING

Type and Technique	Description
Reinforcement to Increase Behaviors	
Token economy	Reinforcing target behavior with tokens (stickers, points, poker chips) that can then be traded in for reinforcers once multiple tokens have been earned
DRO (Differential Reinforcement of Other Behavior)	Reinforcing specific appropriate behaviors while ignoring inappropriate behaviors that serve the same function
Shaping	Reinforcing gradual approximations of a behavior
Punishment to Decrease Behaviors	
Overcorrection	Applied consequence that involves engaging in a series of retribution steps that are related to the inappropriate behavior (washing soiled clothes after toileting accident)
Response cost	Removal of previously earned reinforcers as consequence of negative behavior. Used especially in conjunction with token economy when tokens are removed
Time out	Removing all sources of reinforcement for allotted period of time. Typically involves placing the individual in a location where access to reinforcing activities, including social attention, is not available
Extinction to Decrease Behaviors	Removing previously available reinforcement from an inappropriate behavior to decrease the probability that the behavior will occur in the future

types of behavior management programs, such as parent management training (PMT) (112, 147) and problem solving skills training (PSST (2)). These therapies will be discussed in detail elsewhere in this chapter.

Cognitive-Behavior Therapy Foundations

Behavioral difficulties and other symptoms of disorders often result from a complicated interaction among thoughts, feelings, and behaviors. As such, treatment will often include both cognitive and behavioral techniques. For example, when completing a functional analysis of behavior, it is possible that antecedents and consequences are covert, rather than overt. Covert variables are often internal and consist of cognitions or emotions. As such, thorough analysis of a behavior that involves covert variables will require that the clinician obtain detailed information about the patient's thoughts and feelings before and after the observable behavior. It has also been noted that while traditional behaviorists believed that changes in behavior result in changes in thoughts and feelings, this relationship can be reversed such that changes in thoughts and feelings results in behavioral changes (2). As such, many symptoms and disorders are more thoroughly addressed by the combination of cognitive and behavioral techniques that is known as cognitive behavioral therapy.

COGNITIVE-BEHAVIORAL MODEL

Escape or Avoidance Conditioning

Much of cognitive-behavioral therapy is based on an understanding of why negative thoughts and beliefs persist and why behavioral cycles do not get broken over time. For example, it has been proposed that avoidance, escape and safety-seeking behaviors (5) maintain anxiety because the individual does not have the opportunity to disconfirm beliefs by experiencing that the negative outcome does not occur if they do not avoid or escape. Instead, they are lead to believe that they did not experience danger because they made a good decision to avoid or escape. People who do not avoid situations may engage in other types of behaviors (safety-seeking behaviors) that allow them to believe that danger was avoided. For example, individuals who engage in compulsions in OCD are lead to believe that their obsessive thought did not result in a negative outcome because they engaged in the compulsive behavior. Similarly, individuals who "take it slow" to prevent a heart attack in panic disorder believe that they did not have a heart attack because they modified their activity level. In these examples, individuals erroneously believe they prevented the feared situation from occurring by engaging in certain behaviors. Through this cycle, the preventative behaviors are reinforced, which confirms in the individual's mind that the anxiety was legitimate.

Attention-Related Factors

It has also been proposed that attentional factors play a role in disorders that can be treated using a cognitive-behavioral model. For example, individuals with anxiety disorders, depression, and other disorders that involve disturbance in cognitions often selectively attend to cues that confirm or exacerbate their condition. Individuals with social phobia may be overly attentive to negative cues from others at the expense of positive cues, and individuals with panic disorder may attend closely to bodily sensations, which they then interpret as dangerous.

Cognitive Images

Cognitive images are often examined when viewing a disorder from a cognitive-behavioral perspective. Images of distressing events are common among all individuals; however, in individuals with pathology, these images are interpreted as signs of danger. For example, individuals with OCD may believe that thinking about hurting someone increases the likelihood that it will happen. As a result, they believe that something must be done to prevent the danger. Similarly, in posttraumatic stress disorder (PTSD), intrusive memories may occur frequently and are interpreted as a sign that recurrence of the trauma is likely.

Memory Processes

Similarly, memory processes may play a role as well. For example, anxious individuals may have a tendency to recall situations that confirm their anxiety, such as a person with social phobia who recalls situations in which s/he performed poorly, but not those where s/he performed successfully. Finally, rumination may perpetuate and enhance fear (5). That is, thinking about an event may lead to the interpretation that the event is more likely to occur. Further, selective attention for negative past events may lead to the perception that they are more likely to happen again in the future. In contrast to some forms of cognitive treatment that involve reliving an event through imagery, rumination does not focus on constructive reprocessing of events. Rather it focuses on elaboration that makes the event more abstract and therefore threatening. For example, an individual with PTSD may persistently ruminate about the event, while asking, "What else could I have done?" without realistically considering the limits of what a person is capable of doing.

CLINICAL CONSIDERATIONS IN USE OF CBT WITH CHILDREN AND ADOLESCENTS

Generally speaking, the patient–therapist relationship in CBT treatment has been referred to as one of "collaborative empiricism" (9, 10). This relationship is characterized by a high degree of collaboration and a "scientific attitude" (11) toward testing the validity and accuracy of the patient's cognitions and behaviors. That is, the cognitive-behavioral therapist typically works as a team with the patient to examine and understand thoughts, feelings, and behaviors. This is done by developing hypotheses about thoughts and behaviors, collecting data on those thoughts and behaviors, examining patterns, and generating alternative, more adaptive, ways of thinking and behaving.

When working with children and families, however, certain factors must be taken into consideration with regard to this model. For example, children may have difficulty reporting on their thoughts, feelings, and behaviors. Further, parent and family thoughts, feelings, and behaviors may influence those of the child. As a result, the following areas are briefly examined with regard to engaging in cognitive-behavioral treatments with children and families.

Developmental Perspective

Adopting a developmental perspective when working with children and adolescents is critical for effective intervention planning. Several developmental considerations are suggested for use when doing CBT with children. First, the child's level of autonomy and independence must be taken into consideration. This issue is important both in terms of giving older children and adolescents enough autonomy in setting and following through with their treatment goals, and in making sure that younger children have enough support from parents and other involved individuals. As such, it is also important to consider what other individuals or systems are involved in the child's life and what their role should be in therapy. Further, analysis of how these individuals and other family or systems variables may be maintaining the child's difficulties is an important clinical consideration as well. That is, families, schools, and other systems may have adapted to a child's symptoms in ways that actually maintain, rather than decrease, the difficulties. Parent, teacher, and other adult-focused training is often necessary in addition to individual therapy sessions with the child (2). It may also be important to involve such individuals because treatment in the natural environment often produces more rapid and enduring effects than treatment that only occurs during therapy sessions.

Adapting treatment concepts to children's developmental level is an important part of using CBT with children and adolescents. For example, efforts to address the cognitive biases and distortions underlying a number of psychiatric disorders (e.g., anxiety, depression) can be complicated by the lack of strong abstract thinking skills in most young children. To address this limitation, multiple strategies have been developed to concretize target cognitions and abstract concepts (12). For example, symptoms can be characterized as persona that the child can relate to, such as the "Bad Thought Monster" who must be conquered (13). Similarly, obsessions in OCD can be understood as external and can be blamed on a pesky bug, named "OC Flea" (14), whose ideas must be resisted. Children can also be encouraged to play the role of detective or team up with a detective in testing assumptions and beliefs (13). These types of developmentally appropriate adaptations assist children in understanding concepts that are otherwise verbally explained, which may not be an appropriate treatment vehicle for them.

With very young children, cognitive-behavioral play therapy (CBPT) may be indicated, as it embeds cognitive-behavioral strategies into play-based interactions (15). As young children may have difficulty understanding concepts in CBT, CBPT allows teaching and therapeutic work to occur in play. The primary way in which this happens is through modeling, which has been shown to be effective in teaching new behaviors (16). Many different CBT concepts are modeled with puppets or other toys, such as demonstrating that a puppet gets over his fear gradually the more he enters into a situation. CBPT also involves some adult administration of CBT concepts, such as scheduling activities for a withdrawn child.

Other developmental considerations include the child's age, language level, cognitive ability, and the intensity, duration, and frequency of the symptoms. It has been suggested that younger children benefit more from behavioral techniques than cognitive ones, especially because they often have difficulty reporting cognitions that accompany symptoms and behaviors. Cognitive techniques that younger children have benefited from include relaxation training, imagery, and positive self-talk. Children over the age of 9 are thought to have increased capacity for reporting and understanding cognitions and may begin to benefit from more sophisticated cognitive aspects of treatment. Each child must be individually evaluated, however, as other factors, such as language level, may cause cognitive techniques to be difficult for older children as well.

FAMILY-RELATED FACTORS

The Role of Families and Other Systems in Cognitions and Behaviors

Assessing the child's symptoms within the context of the family is an important part of treatment programming when using CBT. Because CBT interventions place an emphasis on antecedents and consequences of behaviors, avoidance behaviors that maintain symptoms, and other factors that may be affected by the environment, the role of family and other relevant systems is critical in assessment and treatment planning (17). Depending on the nature of the symptoms, it is likely that others in the child's life are making accommodations that support and maintain, rather than discourage, the maladaptive behaviors. For example, in a child with OCD, the family may tolerate extensive rituals that interfere with daily routines to avoid having the child engage in a temper tantrum should the ritual be stopped (18). As such, careful analysis of the child's symptoms within family, school, and other relevant contexts is critical for CBT treatment planning with children and adolescents.

Parent/Family Involvement in Therapy

Families play a pivotal role in therapy for children in several ways. First, it is often important to have information about family context, and parental cognitions, emotions, and behaviors, to better understand the child's symptoms within a cognitive behavioral framework. Changes in family routines, dynamics, and discipline practices may be critical in facilitating changes in individual child-focused symptoms (as discussed earlier). Young children, in particular, may need ongoing assistance from parents and other relevant adults to follow through with treatment goals and homework. Moreover, with older children, families may need to learn to allow the child or adolescent to take responsibility for treatment goals and homework, which may require decreasing their level of involvement. All of these issues are important when deciding whether to work with a child individually, a parent individually, or with the child and other family members. Older children and adolescents often attend therapy sessions individually, and parents are informed during the latter portion of the session about session content and subsequent homework to occur between sessions. It is sometimes necessary to work individually with parents, however, especially with young children who are having behavioral difficulties. Finally, the child's symptoms are often a large source of family stress and parent/child conflict. In these cases, it can be beneficial to work individually with the child and/or the parents. It is sometimes helpful to instruct that parents not remind their child about therapy homework and treatment goals, rather that performance be evaluated by the child and the therapist during sessions. This tactic can be useful in decreasing negative parent–child interactions, especially with adolescents, until symptoms have decreased.

GENERALIZATION AND MAINTENANCE

Three types of generalization are important to consider in CBT interventions with children. These are a) generalization across settings; b) generalization across functional domains (behavior, cognitions); and c) generalization over time, which is termed maintenance. Generalization and maintenance must be considered with regard to intervention strategies as well as improvements in functioning. That is, for successful change, the patient must use the techniques learned in session across settings, learn to apply them to a variety of domains, and continue to use them over time for as long as necessary. Similarly, when change begins to occur it is important that the change is observed across settings (not just in the therapy setting), that change in multiple domains occurs, and that the change is maintained over time.

Kendall and Lochman (19) propose several strategies for promoting generalization and maintenance of improvements in functioning when using CBT strategies with children. First, they propose rewarding behavior change using attainable goals that are applied across an increasing number of settings over time. These goals should be reinforced in each successive setting, and reinforcement should only be faded when the behavioral change appears stable and lasting. Second, they propose that treatment length is an important consideration in programming for maintenance of changes made in therapy. Specifically, it has been suggested that 6 months or longer may be most effective. It has also been suggested that length of treatment over time may be more important than the number of sessions (20); however, intensity may be an important factor as well (148). Use of behavioral rehearsal (e.g., role playing) to emphasize use of techniques in specific situations has also been proposed as an important mechanism for generalization of skills. That is, once a child has learned the concept of a skill, the likelihood that the skill will be used outside therapy in an actual situation is increased if the child has had opportunities to practice it under low demand, low stress circumstances. Role-plays can then be used to assist the child in refining skills to fit increasingly specific situations. Finally, generalization is promoted when the child is taught skills that apply to multiple behaviors and situations, such as problem solving processes rather than specific behaviors. For example, self-instruction training has been proposed as a means of promoting generalization of skills, especially across settings and behaviors. Because self-instruction training involves having the child learn a series of steps in self-instruction of positive decision-making, this skill is considered more flexible than a series of specific steps that apply to a specific situation. In this way, the child can apply the steps to multiple problems in multiple settings.

Although these techniques may be helpful in generalizing skills across settings and over time, long-term data on such procedures are limited, especially with children. The mean duration of followup data is 5 to 7 months posttreatment (21, 22), with little available data to indicate outcomes over longer periods.

COURSE OF THERAPY

General Characteristics of CBT Treatment Plans

Some general aspects of treatment are characteristic of CBT regardless of diagnosis, age, developmental level, or other individual qualities, and are important for the patient to understand at the outset of treatment. According to Friedman, Thase, and Wright (11), these are: 1) The patient will be an active participant in trying new strategies; 2) the patient will be expected to complete homework; 3) therapy outcomes will be measured via data collection, and techniques will be modified if they are unsuccessful; 4) therapy will focus on symptoms and daily functioning; 5) therapy will be time limited; and 6) maintenance of treatment gains and relapse prevention will depend on generalization of techniques into everyday life. When working with children, families may need to be incorporated in these treatment aspects. For example, it may be that the child and the parents must be active participants, rather than the patient alone.

The cognitive-behavioral therapies are generally characterized by three phases of treatment. In the initial stage, the nature of the patient's presenting problem is assessed, rapport is established and psychoeducation (described later) occurs to prepare the patient for the active phase of treatment. Once the symptoms, related variables, and cognitive and emotional characteristics have been identified, a treatment plan is developed. This plan typically begins with psychoeducation of the patient about symptoms, cognitive behavioral understanding of those symptoms, and rationale for treatment. In the middle phase, active treatment occurs, which involves the acquisition, application, and mastery of cognitive-behavioral treatment strategies. This phase involves regular treatment sessions as well as consistent homework. Over the course of treatment, goals and hypotheses about symptoms are reevaluated and modified as necessary on an ongoing basis. The middle phase tapers off when symptomatic relief has occurred and the patient appears ready for maintenance and relapse prevention.

The final phase then focuses on generalization and maintenance of techniques, and relapse prevention. During this phase, the treatment schedule is thinned and the patient assumes greater responsibility for implementation of techniques on an ongoing basis. Finally, as necessary, "booster sessions" may occur after treatment has been completed to ensure that long-term changes are maintained.

Frequency and Duration of Treatment

CBT sessions typically occur once or twice per week in an outpatient setting. Generally speaking, it is important that enough time elapse between sessions for homework exercises to be meaningful. In inpatient settings, sessions may occur as frequently as once per day; however, the severity of illness is generally proportional to the frequency of sessions in such cases (i.e., the child is significantly ill to warrant daily monitoring and practicing of techniques). In general, it is recommended that the therapist decide on a case-by-case basis whether sessions should occur any more than once per week, as with any type of therapeutic intervention.

With some exceptions, CBT typically occurs over a 3- to 6-month period, with some type of tapering period near the final termination of therapy. Using clinical judgment, it is generally recommended that a tapering strategy be used in termination due to the concrete nature of the need for generalization of techniques learned in therapy. That is, once termination has occurred, patients will be required to continue using strategies learned in therapy. Tapering the therapy can be a helpful way to monitor the patient's success in using the techniques on an ongoing basis over increasing periods of time.

It is not uncommon for patients to require a brief "booster" session(s) after termination has occurred. In such cases, patients' use of previously learned CBT techniques may have declined, or new unanticipated situations may have arisen that have resulted in a reoccurrence of symptoms. Frequently, patients do not require an additional full course of therapy; rather, they can benefit from one or several sessions to "refresh" their skills or assist them with application of their skills to new problems.

The phases of treatment outlined here each involve specific areas of focus.

Assessment for Treatment Planning

CBT treatment for any disorder must begin with a thorough assessment of the patient's cognitive, behavioral, and emotional symptoms. Assessments should address detailed information about the patient's symptoms (chief complaint) and identification of maintaining factors. Normalization of the patient's problems can be an important therapeutic aspect of the assessment phase, which may lead to immediate symptomatic relief. The goal of this phase should be to develop a cognitive behavioral model of the presenting problem that can be used to guide treatment. Depending on the chief complaint, the initial assessment may include the following types of information:

- Descriptions of when the symptoms occur (time, place, circumstances, antecedents, consequences)
- Cognitions that accompany each symptom (may be different for different symptoms)
- Behaviors that accompany each symptom (also may be different for different symptoms)
- Emotions that occur with each symptom (also may be different for different symptoms)
- If cognitions and behaviors relieve symptoms, detailed description of how this occurs
- Information about factors that help or exacerbate the symptoms
- Maintaining variables: avoidance, escape, safety behaviors, attention/focus, dysfunctional/faulty beliefs, automatic thoughts
- Overall beliefs (cognitive schemas) that lead to cognitions, behavior, and feelings
- Previous treatment and treatment outcome
- Onset: including any possible causal factors that are not maintaining factors (e.g., traumatic event in PTSD, negative situation paired with stimuli in specific phobias)

One helpful way of eliciting cognitive and behavioral factors can be to have the patient describe a recent event in detail, while asking pointed and specific questions, such as "What were you thinking when that happened?" or "How did your body feel at that moment?" Sometimes it is difficult to elicit enough explicit information from children and homework is required as part of the assessment phase. Such homework might include writing down thoughts, feelings, and behaviors when certain events occur to gain a better understanding of these variables if the patient has difficulty reporting in session. It might also include having the patient or parent self-monitor frequency of symptoms and associated variables. Once this initial assessment is complete, the patient's symptoms can be framed and described in terms of a cognitive-behavioral model and treatment can begin with psychoeducation about this model.

Psychoeducation

Cognitive behavioral interventions typically begin with some form of psychoeducation, which often continues throughout treatment. Psychoeducation is particularly important because many of the techniques utilized in CBT are driven by theoretical or empirical underpinnings that, when understood, allow the patient to better grasp *why* such techniques are being used and *how* change will occur, thus increasing motivation and followthrough. When working with children and adolescents, psychoeducation often occurs separately for children and their parents. This way, parents can have a more in-depth understanding of their child's treatment plan and children's psychoeducation can be developmentally appropriate to their age and cognitive level.

Psychoeducation may be conducted using a variety of procedures. Symptoms and related variables may be explained to individuals, and basic concepts may also be demonstrated. For example, when in the early stages of teaching patients that thoughts do not increase the likelihood of events occurring, *behavioral experiments* to demonstrate this point may be helpful (e.g., have the patient think about making someone else in the room stand up to demonstrate that the thought does not cause the event to occur). Bibliotherapy and CBPT techniques may also be helpful, with young children in particular, to illustrate concepts and educate about symptoms. These techniques may be particularly useful for young children who are resistant to change, as the focus is initially on the symptoms of the characters in the story or play, as opposed to the patient.

Psychoeducation often covers a variety of topic areas as well. For many disorders it is important to educate the individual about *physiological* symptoms, which can lead to an immediate reduction in anxiety as they learn that such symptoms are normal and do not represent serious health or physical risk. Education about *cognitive* symptoms is typically relevant as well, such as teaching a patient with PTSD that intrusive memories are normal reactions to traumatic experiences, or teaching patients with OCD that intrusive thoughts are common in the general population. Education about the *connection between thoughts and events* may also be relevant during this phase. Patients who have specific beliefs about the connection between thoughts and events need to begin to learn that such connections do not exist. Thought–action fusion (TAF), an OCD-related phenomenon that is characterized as the belief that thinking about a despicable act is as morally wrong as actually doing it, is one example of the kinds of irrational cognitions that need to be addressed in treatment (23). Behavioral experiments (discussed above) may be helpful when educating about this topic. Psychoeducation may also include identification of past experiences that disprove the patient's dysfunctional beliefs. Finally, once the patient is educated about symptoms, education about the rationale and plan for treatment must occur. Understanding the connection between the cognitive behavioral model of the symptoms and the rationale for treatment can be particularly important, as it can have an important effect on motivation and followthrough in treatment.

Middle Phase of Treatment

Once assessment and psychoeducation are complete, the middle, and most active, phase of treatment begins. This phase typically involves ongoing active participation in therapy, as well as homework. Homework often must be completed on a daily basis. Goals and content of therapy sessions during this phase will vary widely depending on the chief complaint. Some general CBT techniques commonly utilized during this phase are discussed later in this section. More information about the active phase of treatment can also be found under the discussion of specific disorders. During the active phase of treatment, significant symptom reduction should occur.

Termination and Relapse Prevention

Once symptoms are substantially reduced, therapist and patient must begin planning for termination. This phase of therapy involves concrete planning in several areas when using CBT. First, programming for generalization and maintenance must be considered, as discussed earlier. Ideally, active phase intervention was planned to target generalization of skills. The schedule of therapy sessions is also often thinned during this time to promote maintenance of therapeutic changes with decreasing therapist support. Finally, relapse prevention must be addressed to ensure that changes endure over time. Relapse prevention strategies may include a cognitive framework for thinking about brief relapses (160, 161), such as helping patients to identify antecedents to relapse behaviors and to think about them in ways that do not lead to total loss of treatment gains. Another common relapse prevention strategy is the use of "booster sessions." Should old symptoms return or new ones emerge, one or a small number of sessions is often enough to assist the patient in returning to their termination level of functioning.

CBT TECHNIQUES

Cognitive Restructuring

Cognitive strategies are a primary component of CBT interventions (24). Commonly used cognitive strategies focus on restructuring dysfunctional cognitions and intervening on automatic thoughts and their underlying schemas. Automatic thoughts are defined as "cognitions that stream rapidly through an individual's mind" (25). Such thoughts can be spontaneous or in response to stimuli, a situation, prompt, or other antecedent. Individuals with automatic thoughts typically do not question them for believability. That is, individuals believe that because the thoughts are present they are true or valid. Such thoughts occur with increased intensity and frequency in disorders such as anxiety, depression, and obsessive-compulsive disorder. Automatic thoughts may be valid worries (about events that have or actually could happen) or they may contain cognitive errors or distortions. Common cognitive errors are identified and described in Table 6.2.2.2.

The following cognitive strategies are commonly used to assess and intervene on automatic thoughts and cognitive errors in CBT.

Identifying Automatic Thoughts

Assessment of automatic thoughts does not always rely on interview techniques, especially with children, who may have difficulty understanding and reporting specific thoughts. Techniques such as imagery and role playing can be helpful in identifying automatic thoughts because they set the scene for an event or situation in which specific questions can be asked. For example, when asked to role play a situation, a child can be asked while acting out the scenario what s/he is thinking, feeling, etc. Such exercises are less hypothetical for children, which often helps them generate important information that they cannot report during an interview.

Thought recording is another technique that can be used in a similar fashion. This technique is a form of self-monitoring in which events, thoughts, and feelings are recorded on a daily basis. Self-monitoring is a helpful way to assess automatic thoughts, as it does not rely on recollection of thoughts in a specific situation; rather it requires that the individual record thoughts as they occur or immediately following an event. Although children often require reminders and assistance from adults to keep this type of data on a daily basis, this technique can be developmentally appropriate, as it does not rely on children's memories to assess cognitions.

Socratic Questioning/Examining the Evidence

Socratic questioning is discussed as an important part of CBT, and one of the main components of cognitive restructuring. This technique involves questioning the patient with the goal of eliciting automatic thoughts and calling their validity into question. During this process, thoughts are considered to be hypotheses, rather than truths, and the patient is taught to determine and evaluate evidence for and against automatic thoughts. This technique is an important way to begin teaching children that such thoughts are not true simply because they occur. This technique may be especially helpful with distorted thoughts because rational consideration of evidence increases the patient's awareness that such thoughts are not grounded in reality.

Once automatic thoughts have been called into question, the therapist and patient can begin to revise them based on evidence and reality, and generate new coping thoughts that are more accurate. Examining the evidence can be helpful when combined with self-monitoring because it forces the patient to examine the evidence each time they have a maladaptive thought. This repetition is often helpful in changing a patient's beliefs over time, as s/he is constantly challenging thoughts and generating new coping thoughts throughout the day.

Correct Misinterpretations

Socratic questioning may also be helpful in correcting misinterpretations. Individuals with anxiety and depression

TABLE 6.2.2.2

COMMON COGNITIVE ERRORS TO TARGET IN COGNITIVE RESTRUCTURING

Cognitive Error	Description	Example
Catastrophizing	Placing unrealistic importance on thoughts and events and assuming terrible negative outcomes will occur as a result	"I got a C on my report card, so I will never get into college and I will fail in life."
Magnifying/ minimizing	Placing an inaccurate amount of importance on thoughts, feelings, events (either too much or too little)	Believing getting caught doing drugs is not important because the implications of having a drug problem are too anxiety provoking (minimizing)
Absolutism (black and white thinking)	All events and experiences are thought of in extreme categories, rather than moderately	"I will *never* lose any weight because I just ate a cookie."
Personalization	Attributing responsibility for external events to the self with no basis for the attribution	"It is my fault that my parents are getting divorced."
Selective abstraction	Taking information out of context and ignoring relevant details	"My soccer coach hates me" when s/he did not play you in spite of the fact that you have started the last three games
Arbitrary inference	Making arbitrary conclusions contrary to or without evidence	Believing homework is too hard when in fact the child completed the same work that day in class
Ignoring evidence	Leaving out important information when forming thoughts about events	Believing that werewolves are a danger at night in spite of the fact that multiple adults have told the child they do not exist, and all the doors in the house are locked
Overgeneralization	Believing the outcome of one situation applies in many situations, when it may not	"All my teachers hate me" when one teacher yelled at the child at school
Attending to negative features of events	Placing greater cognitive importance on negative features of events and ignoring positive features	Focusing on one poor grade when all others were good

may in particular misinterpret events, the behavior of others, thoughts, feelings, and other stimuli. Calling into question an individual's interpretation and noting how it impacts thoughts, feelings, and behaviors can be an important aspect of cognitive restructuring as well.

Behavioral Experiments

Many different types of behavioral experiments may be helpful when using CBT, especially during the psychoeducation phase. These "experiments" are exercises that a patient can complete in session, which demonstrate errors in thinking in a concrete manner.

For example, patients are often taught during psychoeducation that attempts at thought suppression actually lead to increased thinking about distressing topics. To demonstrate this principle, the patient may be asked to engage in an exercise where s/he is told to not think of a specific topic (e.g., pink elephants) for a period of 2 minutes. Inevitably, patients find during such an exercise that, in fact, they were unable to avoid thinking about the forbidden topic no matter what it was. This behavioral thought experiment allows patients to learn that an increase in the frequency of a thought is a typical consequence of thought suppression. Instead of trying to suppress thoughts, patients are encouraged to observe their thoughts as they "come and go" without trying to suppress them. This technique typically results in a reduction in intrusive thoughts.

Modification of Imagery

Anxious patients, in particular, often have cognitive imagery associated with their symptoms (e.g., imagery associated with a feared or traumatic event). Such patients may benefit from modification of such imagery, such as by identifying aspects of it that are exaggerated. Patients may also benefit from learning to continue the image through to a positive outcome. That is, negative or anxiety-producing images often stop at the height of the crisis in a patient's mind (5), and never come to a positive or adaptive resolution. For example, the images end when the patient has passed out, embarrassed himself in public, or helplessly experienced the traumatic event. Therefore, helping the patient continue the image to a positive resolution (getting up off the floor after fainting, making statements to others when embarrassed, modifying the outcome of a traumatic event) can be an important exercise in decreasing anxiety and catastrophic thinking. Role-playing exercises may serve a similar role, as they allow the patient an opportunity to understand an event in a new way with the assistance of a therapist and then experience a new, more adaptive, outcome (known as behavioral rehearsal).

Altering Core Beliefs

In addition to identifying automatic thoughts, CBT focuses on the more complex task of identifying the core beliefs, or cognitive schemas, that underlie those thoughts. That is, the thought is typically generated because the individual has an underlying belief about him/herself, which is typically maladaptive. For example, a child who has to complete homework perfectly for fear of being thought stupid may have the automatic thought, "If I don't write that sentence with perfect handwriting everyone will know I am stupid." Core beliefs that may underlie such a thought might be, "I am stupid" or "Stupid kids are unlovable, therefore, no one loves me." Understanding these core beliefs is important for relapse prevention in particular, as modification of automatic thoughts will generally be temporary if the underlying belief or schema is not addressed.

Modification of the child's existing cognitive structures or schemas is an important way to decrease automatic thoughts and cognitive distortions, increase adaptive thoughts, and promote coping (19). Through use of many of the cognitive techniques described in the earlier section, therapy must result in a reduction of support for dysfunctional schemas. As such, a primary goal of CBT when addressing thoughts and schemas is the acquisition and use of a coping template through modification of schemas.

It is important to note that identification of underlying cognitive schemas can be a complicated process, which relies on insight, self-awareness, ability to articulate thoughts, and cognitive ability. As such, this level of cognitive intervention is not always appropriate for all ages and ability levels when working with children. Although adolescents can have difficulty articulating themselves, identifying core beliefs may be more successful with this age group than with younger children.

Physiological Techniques

CBT also relies on many physiological techniques for modifying thoughts, feelings, and behavior. These techniques are particularly useful when treating anxiety disorders, as a core component of such disorders can be misinterpreting and catastrophizing physical symptoms and bodily sensations. These techniques can also be particularly useful with children, as they do not rely on cognitive ability to the same extent as cognitive techniques.

Regulated Breathing

Breathing control exercises are often taught in CBT, especially in the treatment of anxiety. These exercises are helpful in two ways. First, they are physically effective for counteracting hyperventilation, reducing physical tension, and decreasing physical sensations associated with anxiety. Second, uncovering the patient's understanding of the physiology behind them is helpful in decreasing their fears of bodily sensations. This change in perception thereby interrupts the vicious cycle in which patients believe that physical symptoms are a sign of danger, thus increasing anxiety. Although understanding how to physically interrupt this cycle may be beyond the cognitive capacity of young children, learning regulated breathing is nonetheless effective without this understanding. Regulated breathing is most effective when practiced during low stress circumstances on a regular basis to acquire the skill. This technique can then be applied to increasingly more stressful situations.

Relaxation Training

Relaxation training is another commonly taught physiological technique in CBT. This technique incorporates regulated breathing, but also involves progressively tensing and relaxing individual muscle groups in the body until the entire body is relaxed. When doing muscle relaxation with children it may be necessary to focus on large muscle groups (arms, stomach, legs, whole body at once) such that the progression does not take too long and to ensure that children have adequate muscle control (it may be difficult for children to isolate small muscles). It has been suggested that this technique is helpful for treatment of sleep-onset insomnia (26). Relaxation training is also often incorporated into anger management treatment protocols (159) so that children may learn physiological techniques for calming down. The goal of relaxation in this context is often to reduce disruptive behaviors that accompany anger, especially in impulsive children.

Exposure Techniques

Exposure therapy is based on the premise that patients with anxiety symptoms engage in avoidance or "safety behaviors" that do not allow them to experience that their fears will not be realized if they put themselves in feared situations (27). As such, exposure involves developing a progressive hierarchy of feared situations. The patient then engages in a graded series of exercises whereby these situations are experienced or recreated such that anxiety is initially present, but decreases over the course of the exercise until it has diminished completely. Anxiety typically decreases during such exercises, as the patient has the experience that the feared outcome will not occur (e.g., if I think about death, it will not actually cause someone to die). Historically, this type of treatment has been viewed as a habituation process, whereby the anxiety reaction decreases over time with repeated exposure to anxiety-provoking situations. Habituation has been conceptualized within a classical conditioning framework, as the anxiety reaction is thought to extinguish over time. More recently, especially with older children, adolescents, and adults, the cognitive aspects of exposure exercises have been emphasized. For example, rather than just practicing putting oneself in a feared situation and experiencing that the worst does not happen, thus resulting in a decrease of anxiety over time, this exercise might also include specific discussion of what the patient *thought* would happen, whether it actually did happen, reasons for the outcome, etc. With children, this cognitive component may be more difficult depending on developmental level. Exposure therapy is still effective, however, as anxiety reactions extinguish over time with repeated exercises even without this level of insight.

Exposure techniques are often used in treatment of fears and phobias and research indicates their efficacy. For example, children with specific phobias can be gradually and systematically exposed to situations that increasingly resemble or represent their fear. Over time, they come to realize that the feared outcome does not occur and fear diminishes.

In the treatment of obsessive-compulsive disorder, the compulsive behaviors are the "safety behaviors" that prevent bad things from happening as a result of the obsessive thoughts. Therefore, exposure exercises in these cases involve having the patient think about or experience their obsessions, which are often urges accompanied by a worry, without engaging in compulsions. This process facilitates the repeated experience that their feared outcome does not occur (e.g., have the patient experience that if they do not check the door, a robber will not enter the house).

Flooding is similar to exposure, with the exception that it does not utilize a hierarchy, thus, exposure to the target stimuli is not graded and begins by eliciting the full-blown fear response. While flooding typically works more quickly than hierarchical exposure, substantial self-control is required to prevent the individual from engaging in avoidance, escape, or other anxiety-reducing behaviors. As a result, flooding may be very difficult with children and adolescents, who may lack this self-control and therefore engage in extreme behaviors (e.g., tantrums) to avoid the level of anxiety that is required to complete a flooding intervention. It is also questionable from an ethical perspective, as use of this procedure may cause the child significant psychological distress.

Exposure can also be used to challenge core beliefs. When used this way, it is known as cognitive response prevention. Cognitive response prevention entails giving the patient homework assignments that involve behaving in a manner inconsistent with the pathological or problematic belief. This exercise allows the patient a real-life opportunity to cope with thoughts that accompany behavior. For example, a child who has to do homework perfectly or s/he will think "I am stupid and a terrible student" will be assigned to do homework with some imperfections while thinking coping thoughts ("A couple of mistakes does not make me stupid."). Similarly, a girl who must exercise a certain amount of time per day to prevent thoughts such as, "I am fat" will be assigned to exercise for a shorter period of time and see that her pants still fit and her weight has not changed.

SELF-MONITORING/SELF-MANAGEMENT

Self-monitoring was mentioned above as an important part of assessing and intervening on automatic thoughts. This technique can be used in other ways as well, such as to keep track of moods and plan for pleasant events in the treatment of depression, increase awareness and train competing responses in habit disorders (Tourette's disorder, trichotillomania), assess and modify eating and exercise habits in the treatment of eating disorders, and track use of breathing and relaxation procedures in treatment of anxiety disorders.

Extending from self-monitoring techniques are interventions in which the child not only monitors his/her behavior, but is responsible for administration of a behavior intervention plan. Such techniques, known as self-management procedures, are also used to treat a variety of chief complaints (e.g., disruptive behaviors, communication disorders, developmental disabilities, anxiety disorders). These interventions have been successful in improving a variety of skill areas [play skills, on-task responding, social skills; (28–31)] as well as in decreasing undesirable behaviors [off-task responding, disruptive behaviors; (29, 32)].

Activity Scheduling

Activity scheduling is commonly used in the treatment of depression. Models of depression suggest that part of the disorder can be accounted for by a lack of reinforcement in the individual's life (33, 34). Individuals with depression often engage in negative patterns of thinking, including negative evaluations of the self, the world, and the future [Beck's cognitive triad; (33, 34)]. This triad of negative thoughts is believed to be a primary source of cognitive distortions associated with depression. Further, they often cease engaging in previously enjoyed activities due to decreased motivation and interest. As such, treatment typically includes a component to increase the individual's participation in reinforcing daily activities. In activity scheduling, the patient and therapist agree upon homework assignments to engage in activities that result in pleasurable feelings, feelings of competence/mastery, or other similar positive emotional and cognitive outcomes. Using this technique, a change in behavior often results in an improvement in emotional functioning.

ABA/Behavior Modification

Applied behavior analysis (ABA) and behavior modification are techniques used to increase desirable behaviors and decrease undesirable behaviors (35). These techniques primarily rely on use of contingent reinforcers. Specifically, when reinforcement is applied to a positive behavior, it increases the frequency with which that behavior occurs. In contrast, when reinforcement is removed from a negative behavior or when a punishment is applied, it decreases the frequency with which the negative behavior occurs. Many specific therapeutic techniques to treat a variety of disorders are based on these principles.

Counterconditioning

Counterconditioning techniques are used to decrease specific maladaptive behaviors, such as anxiety-related behaviors. Use of such techniques requires pairing a maladaptive behavior with an incompatible behavior in order to eliminate the maladaptive behavior. Counterconditioning techniques are based on the work of Wolpe (36), who stated, "If a response antagonistic to anxiety can be made to occur in the presence of anxiety-evoking stimuli so that it is accompanied by a complete or partial suppression of the anxiety responses, the bond between these stimuli and the anxiety response will be weakened". For example, in one of the earliest demonstrations of counterconditioning, Joes (37) cured a child's phobia of a rabbit by systematically exposing the child to the rabbit while pairing the exposures with the incompatible response of eating food.

Systematic Desensitization

Systematic desensitization (36) is perhaps the most commonly used counterconditioning technique. It involves training relaxation techniques to be used in conjunction with an anxiety hierarchy for the purpose of reducing fear and anxiety over time. The four stages of systematic desensitization are: 1) relaxation training; 2) constructing the anxiety hierarchy; 3) desensitization in imagination; and 4) in vivo desensitization. Specifically, this technique uses an imaginal or in vivo exposure hierarchy (discussed later) paired with progressive muscle relaxation techniques to reduce the anxiety/fear reaction to specific situations. This treatment is typically done first through visualization, followed by in vivo training.

Originally, this technique was based on the premise of counterconditioning, that is, pairing the feared stimulus with relaxation to counter the fear reaction, which results in decreased anxiety. Recent evidence suggests, however, that the exposure exercises may be the active ingredient in this treatment (38), rather than the counterconditioning.

Systematic desensitization is supported in the literature for use with children. However, studies that demonstrated efficacy typically targeted specific, subclinical fears. Little research has been conducted on its use with more generalized anxiety (19) in children. This technique may have limited use with children under age 9 because they have difficulty understanding the notion of a hierarchy and problems using visual imagery (19).

Aversive Counterconditioning

Aversive counterconditioning is another related technique, based on principles of classical conditioning. This technique pairs the target behavior or stimulus associated with it (conditioned stimulus) with a stimulus (unconditioned) that naturally elicits an unpleasant response. As a result, the maladaptive behavior is increasingly avoided in order to avoid the negative outcome. This technique is most commonly used in the treatment of addictions and problematic sexual fetishes. For example, the use of medications such as disulfiram (Antabuse) that cause an individual to be physically ill when consuming alcohol rely on principles of aversive counterconditioning to reduce the patient's drinking behavior. While these techniques may be periodically relevant in the treatment of adolescents, they rarely apply to treatment with children.

Covert Sensitization

Covert sensitization relies on the same principles as aversive counterconditioning; however, the individual *imagines* an aversive condition while imagining engaging in maladaptive behavior, rather than actually experiencing the negative stimuli.

Habit Reversal

Habit reversal procedures are most commonly used in the treatment of habit disorders, such as trichotillomania and skin-picking, and Tourette syndrome and other tic disorders (39). Habit reversal involves three stages: 1) awareness training; 2) training in an incompatible competing response; and 3) social support, which is particularly important when using this technique with children and adolescents.

INDICATIONS AND EFFICACY

A wide variety of disorders are commonly treated using cognitive-behavioral treatment strategies. These are outlined in this section with a cognitive-behavioral model of each disorder, followed by a description of the application of CBT to its treatment.

ANXIETY DISORDERS

Cognitive-Behavioral Model

Cognitive-behavioral therapy for anxiety "focuses on dysfunctional cognitions and their implications for the child's subsequent thinking and behavior" (2).

Similar to adults, cognitive distortions are thought to play a major role in the development of anxiety in children and have been defined as "information processes that lead to misperceptions of oneself or the environment" (2). The primary cognitive distortion in patients with anxiety disorders is overestimation of the danger associated with certain situations, bodily sensations, or even thoughts (40). Distortions or overestimations may include inaccurate estimates of: 1) the likelihood of an event, 2) the severity of an event, or 3) one's coping skills and the availability of help, support, or escape (5). Individuals with anxiety may also tend to interpret events from a negative and therefore inaccurate perspective, especially with regard to beliefs about self. For example, an individual with anxiety may have negative thoughts in specific situations when s/he is anxious (e.g., kids don't want to play with me because I am stupid, versus kids don't want to play with me because they all like soccer and I don't).

The two-factor learning theory (41) has been proposed to explain the development and maintenance of fearful behavior. This theory proposes that an anxiety reaction is initially elicited via *classical conditioning* when a feared stimulus or event is experienced. As a result, the individual avoids the situation in the future to avoid experiencing the anxiety again. The avoidance behavior is then reinforced under an *operant conditioning* paradigm when anxiety is avoided as a result. The individual does not have an opportunity to learn that exposure to the stimuli is unlikely to result in the traumatic outcome again. For example, if a child encounters a scary dog while walking outside, s/he might come to believe that going outside is dangerous (classical conditioning). As a result, staying inside reinforces this notion, as the child does not experience anxiety unless s/he goes outside (operant conditioning). Therefore, until the child can learn that going outside does not result in negative outcomes, the anxiety reaction will continue to be reinforced. Similarly, Clark (5), has proposed that reflexively elicited somatic and cognitive symptoms of anxiety become problematic when they are misinterpreted as indicating danger is present ("I'm going crazy"). Such an interpretation can lead to further increased physiological arousal, which then serves to confirm the initial incorrect hypothesis.

Symptoms of anxiety in children may be physiological, behavioral, and/or cognitive (19, 42). For example, physiological symptoms may include shaky voice, rigid posture, perspiration, abdominal pain, flushed face, need to urinate, trembling, and increased heart rate. Physiological symptoms, especially ongoing somatic complaints, are often the most common anxiety symptoms in children, as their cognitions may not be as clear and identifiable as those of adults. Behavioral symptoms may include nail biting, avoidance, thumb sucking, crying, toileting accidents, and others. Cognitions may include thoughts of being hurt or scared, thoughts of danger, self-critical thoughts, preoccupation with evaluation by self and others, worries about likelihood of severe negative consequences, and intrusive images. These can be difficult to determine in anxious children who may not be accurate reporters or may not have enough self-awareness to understand their thoughts clearly (43). Distorted information processing is another cognitive area that may be involved in anxiety. For example, distorted/biased views of social or environmental cues, preoccupation with evaluation by self and others, preoccupation with likelihood of negative consequences, or misperception of demands in the environment (19) are common distortions.

Treatment

Treatment strategies for anxiety in children must target cognitive, behavioral, physiological, and emotional aspects of the disorder. Kazdin (2) suggested that these strategies must "help the child develop new skills, provide new experiences for the child to test dysfunctional as well as adaptive beliefs, and assist the child in processing new experiences." Treatment strategies can be divided into several categories, based on which symptom area they are addressing.

Physiological Treatment Strategies

In CBT for childhood anxiety, physiological symptoms are typically targeted first, given the high rate with which these symptoms occur in this age group and the difficulty many young children have in identifying and changing cognitions (44). The most common methods for addressing the physiological symptoms of anxiety are relaxation training and systematic desensitization. Relaxation training for children typically involves a combination of progressive muscle relaxation, deep breathing, and pleasant imagery, which the child and therapist develop prior to starting the training. In systematic desensitization, relaxation techniques are paired with a fear hierarchy to countercondition the fear response. Studies of efficacy for systematic desensitization have generally shown efficacy with otherwise nonclinical samples who have specific fears (45). As systematic desensitization requires the child to report levels of anxiety in relation to various stimuli on a hierarchy, it may be difficult for young children (under age 9). Relaxation training, however, has been used with younger children, although they may not acquire the skill as well as older children.

It has been suggested that young children may have more difficulty with systematic desensitization for two reasons. They appear to have difficulty acquiring the skill of muscle relaxation and may not be able to clearly visualize the fear-producing stimuli (46). Therefore, *in vivo* desensitization may be more effective with younger children (47). Using developmentally appropriate imagery may help remediate this difficulty, however, such as in a case example by Jackson and King (48). In this example, a child was taught to imagine that Batman (a preferred cartoon character for this child) was accompanying him to view the feared stimulus (the dark, shadows). After four sessions, the child no longer evidenced fear of the dark.

Behavioral Treatment Strategies

Children may also benefit from strategies that address learning new behaviors, such as coping skills. For example, modeling has been used to demonstrate desired coping behaviors for use in a feared situation. The child is then reinforced for engaging in these behaviors and can be provided with feedback (49). The therapist is often used as the coping model (50). However, in group settings, children may be models for one another as well. For example, the therapist can place him/herself in an anxiety-producing situation and model self-talk in front of the patient. Role-plays have also been used, particularly with younger children who have difficulty describing anxiety-provoking events. The role play itself may allow the therapist to observe when the child becomes anxious and may help facilitate a more *in vivo* discussion about the child's cognitions at that time (19). Role plays may also serve an important behavioral rehearsal function, which allows children to practice new skills under less stressful circumstances before being required to use them in the actual anxiety-provoking situation. Children can also be taught problemsolving steps, such as the ones proposed by Spivak and Shure (51). These include 1) problem identification, definition, and formulation, 2) generation of alternative solutions, 3) choosing a new strategy, 4) implementing the new strategy, and 5) evaluating the new strategy. These types of steps are often the foundation for skills training curriculums for children, both in group and individual therapy.

Cognitive Strategies

Children with anxiety disorders often require assistance in identifying their dysfunctional thoughts and beliefs, which they then must learn to modify. Several strategies are suggested for modification of cognitions and the cognitive and behavioral processes that maintain them. First, psychoeducation is used to increase children's awareness about their cognitive processes and help them understand how their thoughts maintain anxiety symptoms. An extension of psychoeducation is refocusing the child's attention on less negative aspects of situations, less negative self-evaluation, and less negative interpretations of events. Self-talk is also used to to identify maladaptive thoughts and then dispute or correct their misinterpretations or biases (19, 52). Self-talk can also be used to challenge and alter anxiety-provoking thoughts and internal dialogue. For example, children can be taught to think about evidence for and against negative thoughts when they have them. This method of questioning thoughts typically leads the child to the conclusion that the "evidence" does not support their thinking. Similarly, when children have intrusive thoughts or ongoing internal dialogue they can be taught thought-stopping techniques to interrupt the cycle, such as thinking about yelling, "stop!" while picturing a large stop sign in their head.

Combined Strategies

Many CBT treatment plans combine physiology, learning new behaviors, and changing cognitions. For example, *in vivo* exposure and exposure with response prevention combine cognitive and behavioral strategies to reduce anxiety related to specific stimuli or symptoms of OCD. A series of waitlist controlled studies by Kendall and colleagues (53, 54) has demonstrated the efficacy of a combined CBT approach in treating generalized, separation, and social anxiety disorders, with gains maintained up to 7 years posttreatment (54).

OBSESSIVE-COMPULSIVE DISORDER (OCD)

Cognitive-Behavioral Model

The cognitive-behavioral model of OCD involves "intrusive and distressing thoughts, impulses, or images about possible harm coming to oneself or others" (5), which must then be neutralized through counterthoughts or behaviors to prevent harm or negative consequences from occurring. Many people have intrusive thoughts of this nature; however, individuals with OCD are thought to interpret such thoughts differently. That is, they assume that such thoughts are a sign that something terrible will actually happen and they will be responsible for this terrible outcome. As a result, they engage in all types of neutralizing, undoing, and compensatory behaviors (checking, washing, ordering, meaningless rituals, self-statements) in order to prevent these negative outcomes. As the distressing thoughts in OCD typically have a low likelihood of actually occurring, the individual comes to believe that their neutralizing behaviors (compulsions) successfully prevented the feared outcome. As such, the the individual never comes to realize that they are unnecessary. In addition, and perhaps more importantly, reduction in distress and anxiety contingent on performance of the ritual creates a negative reinforcement cycle which serves to further strengthen the perceived benefits of the ritual [the socalled OCD cycle; (55)].

Treatment

Exposure and response prevention (ERP) has substantial empirical support for the treatment of pediatric OCD (56, 57). This intervention is based on models of classical extinction, as the individual learns over the course of treatment that the feared outcome does not occur if they do not engage in their compulsions (18). ERP begins with the development of a hierarchy of obsessions and compulsions, listed in order from least to most distressing (Table 6.2.2.3). Once this hierarchy is developed, exposure begins with the least distressing item on the hierarchy. Depending on the nature of the obsession, exposure involves either exposing the individual to the actual stimuli or having him/her imagine or think about it. As the symptom pattern in OCD involves compulsions that are tied to obsessions, the exposure will elicit a desire to perform the compulsion. The patient's compulsive response must be prevented, however (response prevention), or s/he is not truly being exposed to the anxiety-provoking situation. As the patient is repeatedly exposed to the anxiety (the obsession) without engaging in a neutralizing response (the compulsion), the anxiety about that particular issue will decrease over time until the obsession no longer elicits an anxiety response. Once this decrease in anxiety occurs, the patient moves on to the next item on the hierarchy. Treatment continues in this manner until all obsessions on the hierarchy have been addressed. At times, booster sessions may be required if obsessions begin to provoke anxiety again.

The Pediatric OCD Treatment Study (POTS), (57) the largest pediatric trial of CBT for OCD to date, compared CBT alone, selective serotonin reuptake inhibitor (SSRI) alone, and combined CBT + SSRI to pill placebo in a sample of 128 youngsters drawn from three treatment sites. Overall, CBT + SSRI was found to be the most effective treatment, yielding illness remission in 54% of youngsters, followed by CBT alone (39% remission), SSRI alone (21% remission), and placebo (3% remission). However, CBT alone was found equally efficacious as CBT + SSRI at one site, leading the researchers to conclude that either CBT or CBT + SSRI should be considered

TABLE 6.2.2.3

SAMPLE OCD SYMPTOM HIERARCHY

OCD Ritual	SUDS Rating
Mom needing to say "okay, goodnight" three times at bedtime	9
Washing hands when feel contaminated	8
Turning light switch on/off three times	7
Turning TV on and off three times	6
Erasing and rewriting math homework	6
Rereading sentences in history book until feels right	5
Rereading sentences in pleasure books until feels right	4
Needing to brush teeth at bedtime three times	3
Saving old school homework	2

Note: SUDS = subjective units of distress scale; SUDS rating = degree of distress associated with not being able to complete each listed ritual

the first line of treatment in children with OCD. Group CBT involving other family members has also been shown as effective as individual CBT in one controlled trial (56).

PHOBIAS

Cognitive-Behavioral Model

As noted earlier, the two-factor learning theory (41) has been used to explain the development and maintenance of phobic behavior, in that repeated avoidance of the feared situation or object does not allow for disconfirmation of distorted harm beliefs and, in fact, is reinforced by the patient's belief that such avoidance is keeping him/her safe. As a result, treatment involves breaking this operant conditioning cycle and teaching the individual that the feared situation is unlikely to occur again even when it is not avoided.

Treatment

Several CBT strategies have demonstrated efficacy in the treatment of phobias. Graded exposure, systematic desensitization, and relaxation training (36, 58) have all been effective treatment strategies. However, component analysis of systematic desensitization suggests that exposure may be the key ingredient in this therapy. Exposure treatment of phobias is much like that described above in the treatment of OCD. In the case of phobias, the individual is exposed to increasingly difficult versions of the feared stimuli, and is prevented from escaping contact with the situation or object. Typically, treatment involves both imaginal (initially) and *in vivo* exposure exercises.

Treatment of social phobial may also involve additional components, most notably social skills training (59, 60). This combination was found to be efficacious for children and adolescents with social phobia (59), with gains maintained at 3-year followup (60).

PANIC DISORDER

Cognitive-Behavioral Model

Panic disorder is characterized by a fear of impending disaster, which is confirmed by physiological and cognitive symptoms. Individuals with panic disorder often misinterpret their symptoms as confirmation that their anxiety represents real danger, which results in more anxiety, leading to further symptoms, and so on. This loss of control over those symptoms leads to further anxiety, which is a maintaining factor in panic attacks. Individuals with panic disorder typically quickly come to fear having panic attacks in certain situations and begin altering their behavior as a result. For example, in agoraphobia, individuals may resist leaving the house due to anxiety about the social or interpersonal consequences of having an attack in public. The distinguishing factor between panic disorder and other phobias, however, is that the precipitating factor in the attack is a fear of having one, rather than a fear of a specific stimulus. Therefore, in differential diagnosis of these disorders, an individual who has a panic attack in an elevator because s/he does not like small, enclosed spaces would be diagnosed with a specific phobia, whereas an individual who has a panic attack in an elevator for fear of having one there would be diagnosed with panic disorder.

Treatment

Treatment of panic disorder involves cognitive and physiological strategies as well as exposure therapy (61). The patient must learn to interpret bodily cues more accurately and often may benefit from learning to place less emphasis on such cues altogether. Understanding the physiology of the cycle is critical as well, as the patient can then learn to intervene to decrease physiological anxiety symptoms. Self-control and relaxation exercises (controlled, deep breathing, muscle relaxation) are important in preventing and controlling panic attacks and their associated symptoms. Cognitive strategies are important as well, as patients must learn to decrease their exaggerated thinking patterns. Cognitive restructuring, Socratic questioning, and other related strategies are important in decreasing the catastrophizing and ongoing worry that accompany the panic attacks in this disorder. Exposure therapy is often used in the treatment of panic as well, as the individual has come to avoid certain situations over time due to fear of having an attack. As such, once the individual learns physiological and cognitive strategies for avoiding and reducing the severity of attacks, s/he may require exposure therapy to learn that previously avoided situations can now be managed. Exposure exercises are conducted on a hierarchy as described above, and over time the individual learns that panic attacks will not occur and that situations are therefore no longer to be feared.

POSTTRAUMATIC STRESS DISORDER (PTSD)

Cognitive-Behavioral Model

Posttraumatic stress disorder (PTSD) is diagnosed when a constellation of anxiety-related symptoms manifests after the occurrence of a traumatic event. Many individuals experience intrusive, unwanted distressing thoughts and memories after a traumatic event and many may even experience other PTSD symptoms, such as avoidance, numbing, hypervigilance, and hyperarousal (62). Individuals who then develop PTSD, however, do not adequately cope with these symptoms and they persist or worsen as a result. Over time, many other cognitive aspects of anxiety may then manifest in individuals with PTSD. For example, they may begin to misinterpret the recurrent intrusive thoughts as a sign that something terrible will happen again, as described above in the development of OCD. They may also develop anxiety about their symptoms that perpetuates the anxious state as in panic disorder, such as "I can't control my recurrent memories so I must be going mad." As such, while PTSD has an etiology very different from other anxiety disorders, its treatment is quite similar, as misinterpretation of thoughts, avoidance, and other anxiety symptoms are what must be addressed.

Trauma reactions may appear somewhat different in very young (under age 6) children (63). Scheeringa (63) proposed an alternative set of diagnostic criteria for preschool-aged trauma victims. Modifications to the existing criteria may include 1) the individual does not have to be able to report the anxiety reaction, as many young children are incapable of doing so, 2) recurrent recollection of the event may manifest in repetitive trauma-related play themes, 3) recurrent distressing dreams do not have to include trauma-related content, but must be distressing, 4) flashbacks may be behavioral in nature, with no accompanying verbal description, 5) diminished interest in significant activities may present as constriction of play, 6) a feeling of detachment or estrangement may manifest as withdrawal, 7) loss of developmental skills may occur, 8) increased arousal may manifest as tantrums and fussiness. An additional cluster of symptoms is also proposed, which includes: 1) new separation anxiety, 2) new onset of aggression, 3) new fears (e.g., fear of the dark) without obvious links to the trauma. Although these criteria are not currently part of the *Diagnostic and Statistical Manual of Mental Disorders* [DSM-IV; (62)], they may be helpful in evaluating young children's reactions to trauma.

Treatment

Research suggests that CBT approaches are the most effective treatment for PTSD in children (64–66). Exposure is considered the main component of treatment of PTSD, although other CBT strategies, such as cognitive restructuring and relaxation, are also often used (66–68). The literature proposes that the forced thinking about the traumatic incident involved in imaginal exposure may be especially important because studies have shown that avoidance of thoughts associated with the traumatic event is predictive of persisting PTSD (5, 69, 70).

Studies using CBT to treat PTSD in children and adolescents are somewhat limited; however, several controlled studies have demonstrated clinically significant reductions in symptoms (71–73). Additional randomized controlled trials are available for specific populations, such as victims of sexual abuse (74). Exposure therapy in the treatment of PTSD is also well validated with adults. Therefore, the combination of single-case design studies with children, and randomized controlled trials with children and adults, suggests that these procedures are beneficial in work with children (66, 74). Exposure therapy in PTSD typically involves repeated, imaginal reexperiencing of the traumatic event until the anxiety associated with these exposure exercises diminishes. Therapists coaching their patients through exposure exercises typically try to elicit as much detail as possible about the patient's experience of the event, including thoughts and feelings that were experienced at the time. This level of detail and focus on thoughts and feelings results in decreased anxiety over time (75, 76). Alternative exposure strategies are sometimes used with children, such as having them write or illustrate a book about the event in gradual, systematic steps (74), or having them experience the event via play. In vivo exposure may also be helpful in situations where it is possible for the client to be exposed to the location of the trauma or other related situations.

Individuals with PTSD may also benefit from anxiety management training (66, 75, 77) or stress inoculation techniques (74, 149), which may include cognitive restructuring of their thoughts about the event, relaxation, positive imagery and self-talk, thought stopping, self-monitoring, and other physiological strategies to decrease hyperarousal (68). Cognitive restructuring in PTSD involves altering the distorted cognitions that play a role in the development and maintenance of the disorder. For example, young children often experience serious misattributions about the traumatic event, such as self-blame (74). Anxiety management training may also involve application of learned skills in role-plays and in vivo exposure exercises. Research in this area is limited as well; however, initial studies appear promising (78). Parent participation in treatment is often important when working with children and adolescents. Pine and Cohen (74) suggest that parents may participate in exposure exercises with their children, and that they may benefit from learning behavior management techniques.

DEPRESSION

Cognitive-Behavioral Model

Seligman (79) noted that depression in children and adolescents lends itself to a cognitive-behavioral intervention model (when developmentally appropriate), as these individuals tend to exhibit high rates of intrusive negative thoughts (e.g., selective ruminations about past unpleasant events, hopelessness about the future, and helplessness about improving their situation). Consistent with Beck's model, adolescents have been shown to attribute positive outcomes to external, unstable, and specific factors (80) and to lack self-efficacy with regard to these outcomes. Depressed children and adolescents may also experience cognitive distortions in attributions, self-evaluation, and perception of past and present events (81). Similarly, they may engage in overgeneralization, catastrophizing, taking responsibility for negative outcomes, and attending to negative features of events (82, 83). These distortions can be thought to result from "pathological information processing" (11), which leads to symptoms of depression.

Depressed children also often have low self-esteem, low perceived academic competence, and low perceived social competence (84) and may have poor problem solving skills, especially regarding interpersonal problems (19). Kazdin (2) also noted that depression in children and adolescents is associated with "restricted behavioral repertoires" (limited participation in pleasant activities, few experiences of reinforcement in the environment) as well, thereby lending itself to the behavioral aspects of treatment.

Treatment

CBT has been found effective for the treatment of depression in adults across a variety of studies (11, 150) and treatment delivery models (individual CBT, CBT in conjunction with medication, group CBT, marital CBT). As symptoms of depression are both cognitive and behavioral in nature, a variety of strategies are employed depending on individual patient symptoms.

Cognitive restructuring is often used to address negative thought patterns associated with depression. Socratic questioning, in which the patient examines evidence for and against distorted perceptions, is one strategy for intervening on such thought patterns. Patients may also benefit from self-control strategies, including learning more positive self-consequation (reinforce self more, punish self less), adaptive self-monitoring (increasing attention to positive actions, events, accomplishments), and more accurate and realistic self-evaluation, such as learning to set less perfectionistic standards for one's self. One kind of adaptive self-monitoring includes monitoring pleasant events and associated moods. This type of procedure encourages the child to engage in reinforcing activities, while simultaneously increasing focus on the resulting positive affective change. Charts such as the one in Figure 6.2.2.1 are easily used with older children and adolescents for this type of intervention.

Skills training is also often involved in the treatment of depression, especially for children and adolescents. Types of skills training may include assertiveness training, conflict management skills training, relaxation training, and social skills training. Social skills training in particular may be important for children and adolescents, as poor social relationships are predictive of many psychological and emotional difficulties. Further, interpersonal conflicts with peers are the most common antecedent to adolescent suicide attempts (85). Social skills training involves different components and skill sets depending on the model; however, the focus is generally on teaching skills for initiating and maintaining social interactions (86). Social skills interventions may also focus on handling interpersonal conflicts. Other behavioral interventions, such as activity scheduling/monitoring, and tracking pleasant events and associated moods, are also often part of changing behaviors, gaining skills, and increasing self-administered reinforcement.

The Adolescent Coping with Depression Course (CWD-A) (87, 88, 151, 152) is a classroom-based group treatment program for treating adolescents with depression. This program first involves increasing the patient's awareness of negative cognitions, followed by learning new, more constructive ones. Strategies to increase positive reinforcement in the patient's life are then used, such as increasing activities associated with positive reinforcement and teaching social skills associated with increased reinforcement. The final component of the program is parent education, which is designed to facilitate practicing skills learned in session at home with parental support. Ongoing research has demonstrated the efficacy of this model (88, 151, 152), and further examination of various treatment mediators suggests that a reduction in negative thinking may be the primary mechanism involved in reduction of depressive symptoms (87).

AUTISM AND PERVASIVE DEVELOPMENTAL DISORDERS (PDD)

Cognitive-Behavioral Model

Autism and pervasive developmental disorders are often conceptualized as having a social disability and lack of motivation at their core (89). This inherent difficulty interacting with others combined with a lack of social motivation may result in severe learned helplessness. Children with autism do not naturally learn from observing their peers and interacting with their environment as typically developing children do. As such, many developmental skills that children acquire naturally (language, play skills) are not acquired by children with autism if they are not explicitly taught. Further, the lack of motivation and learned helplessness that children with autism frequently experience require that alternative methods of motivating them be used. As such, treatment of autism is primarily behavioral and focuses on finding ways to motivate socially appropriate language, social skills, and behavior to recruit reinforcement that is meaningful to the child.

Treatment

The treatment of autism and pervasive developmental disorders involves the use of operant procedures in applied settings, otherwise known as applied behavior analysis (ABA). ABA is

Pleasant Events and Mood Monitoring

Name:
Week of (dates):
Chart filled out by:

	Monday	Tuesday	Wednesday	Thursday	Friday	Saturday	Sunday
Pleasant events:							
Mood rating:							

DIRECTIONS:

Note pleasant events for each day.

Give each day a rating of 0–5 to indicate overall mood for that day.

If mood changes significantly within a day, it is fine to give that day two separate ratings.

0 = sad, no energy at all, unmotivated
5 = very happy, nonstop busy, very motivated

FIGURE 6.2.2.1. Mood monitoring chart for treatment of depression.

based on operant conditioning procedures (6, 7), and places an emphasis on developing prosocial, positive, and adaptive social and communicative behaviors. It is also often necessary to focus on the reduction of problem behaviors, which result from a lack of appropriate skills. In ABA therapy, reinforcement is used to teach explicit target behaviors, such as making verbalizations, imitating the actions of others, and making eye contact. Behavioral goals are set for the child at the outset of therapy and progress is tracked throughout by collecting data on the frequency of correct responding. Target behaviors are chosen based on the child's developmental level and current skill set, and are operationally defined for clarity of deciding when reinforcement has been earned and tracking the child's progress. There are many types of ABA treatment models, such as discrete trial training (90), pivotal response training (89), and incidental teaching (91, 92). Some models are structured and require the child to work one-on-one with a therapist [discrete trial training (90), (93)], while others embed behavioral teaching opportunities into developmentally appropriate interactions in the child's natural environment, such as during play-time, while at school, and within family routines (pivotal response training; (28, 94)). Interventions that involve one-on-one work between a therapist and the patient are often criticized for not resulting in successful generalization of the target behaviors. As such, a strong program will address both the need for structured, behavioral teaching interactions as well as the need for opportunities to promote use of skills across settings, behaviors, and social partners (95). This goal is often achieved through training individuals who regularly interact with the child (parents and teachers) in the use of intervention strategies so that target behaviors may be prompted in a variety of natural settings and interactions. Many specific techniques are used in ABA therapy. Some examples of these are outlined in Table 6.2.2.4.

Strategies that are used in the reduction of inappropriate behaviors include reinforcement as well as punishment procedures. Behavior plans may include goals whereby the child can earn reinforcement for not engaging in an inappropriate behavior and/or engaging in an appropriate one. Punishment is also sometimes used, such as time out for inappropriate behavior and removing points or tokens that the child has earned in working toward a larger reinforcer (response cost). Overcorrection is a punishment procedure whereby the child engages in restitution after engaging in a disruptive behavior, such as cleaning up a mess made during a tantrum and then being required to clean other related messes. Similarly, in positive practice, the child is required to practice excessively the adaptive behavior that should have been used in place of a disruptive behavior (having to walk back and forth from the scene of a toileting accident to the toilet five times after wetting occurs). Functional analysis procedures are often used in devising behavior plans for children with autism, as it is necessary to determine the communicative function of the behavior prior to deciding on an intervention plan. Using functional analysis ensures that the disruptive behavior will be reduced and a positive replacement behavior will be taught in its place.

Behavioral treatments for children with autism have substantial empirical support (90, 95). For example, Lovaas (90) provided intensive behavioral programming to young children with autism, including the use of operant techniques in a one-on-one therapy setting as well as across individuals (parents, teachers). After two years of intensive (40 hours per week) therapy the children had made substantial gains, including improvements in IQ and less restrictive school placements, such as mainstream classrooms. Other studies have suggested that 40 hours of one-on-one therapy is not necessary; rather children can be taught throughout the natural course of their day (28, 94) by embedding behavioral trials in natural interactions. Whatever the format for teaching, research clearly supports that behavioral strategies are most effective for teaching children with autism.

EMOTIONAL AND BEHAVIORAL DISTURBANCE

Children with conduct disorder are at risk in a variety of areas, including risk of dropping out of school, juvenile delinquency, adult crime, antisocial personality, alcoholism, drug abuse,

TABLE 6.2.2.4

ABA TECHNIQUES USED IN INTERVENTION FOR CHILDREN WITH AUTISM

Technique	Description	Example
Prompting	Providing the child with a clear command about what behavior is expected	Stating "What is it?" in reference to a toy to practice language
Fading	Making prompts less explicit over time, such that the child more independently engages in a behavior	Move from verbally prompting the child to speak to waiting for the child to initiate language independently
Shaping	Providing reinforcement for successive approximations of a target behavior, rather than initially expecting the child to perform the behavior perfectly	Providing reinforcement for saying, "ba" in reference to a ball and reinforcing better approximations of the word over time until the child can say "ball"
Task analysis	Breaking a complex task down into its simpler parts and reinforcing the child for correctly performing each step individually	Teaching getting dressed by reinforcing the child after each step (e.g., after putting on a shirt, after putting on pants, etc.)
Backwards chaining	Teaching a complex behavior by starting with reinforcement for correct performance of the last step and working successively backwards to the beginning until the child is being reinforced for performing the whole behavior	Teaching putting on your coat by first reinforcing the child for zipping the coat (the final step in the process) while helping with the preceding steps, then requiring the child to pull the coat onto his shoulders, then requiring him to put his arms in the sleeves, then requiring him to complete the sequence from the beginning without help

interpersonal problems, marital disruption, and poor physical health (96, 97).

Cognitive-Behavioral Model

A cognitive-behavioral model of conduct problems suggests that disruptive behavior develops and is maintained by maladaptive parent–child interactions, specifically those that are coercive (98). Coercive interactions involve the child engaging in deviant behavior and the parent reinforcing it via inadequate and misguided discipline practices.

Distortions or deficiencies in cognitive processes are often present in individuals with behavioral and conduct problems as well (2). It has also been suggested that cognitive problem solving skills play a specific role in the prediction of social and behavioral adjustment (2). Other experts in this area (99–102) have suggested that a variety of cognitive distortions may contribute to risk of conduct problems. Specifically, Milich and Dodge's (100) Information Processing Model suggests that aggressive children make cognitive and attributional errors in processing information related to interactions with others. Specifically, they recall high rates of hostile cues present in social stimuli (99, 100), are prone to attribute ambiguous behavior to hostile intentions (99, 101), and ignore some cues in their interpretation of the behavior of others (102). These children also have distorted perceptions of their own behavior, such as perceiving their level of aggression as less than it is and taking less responsibility for conflict than other children (103). Similarly, other models have suggested that children with conduct problems have different outcome expectations and social goals than other children. Specifically, they may expect that aggressive solutions will decrease aversive reactions/behaviors of others and believe that aggressive solutions will result in positive outcomes (104). Adolescents have been shown to believe aggression will increase their self-esteem, decrease negative images, and will not cause suffering in victims (105). Finally, children with conduct problems often value the social goals of dominance and revenge more than affiliation (106). As a result, they tend toward action-oriented and aggressive, rather than verbal, solutions to social problems (107–109).

Treatment

Cognitive-behavioral interventions with aggressive children are indicated to address attributional processes, problemsolving, schemas for social goals, and expectations regarding the outcome of behavior. Further, behavioral contingencies are often used to motivate use of adaptive, rather than maladaptive, skills once alternative strategies have been taught.

It has been suggested that four types of therapeutic change are required in the treatment of conduct and related disorders (8). These are: 1) ecological, 2) operant methods, 3) medication, and 4) behavioral parent training. Specifically, ecological changes include manipulation of environments to reduce antecedents and increase opportunities for learning more appropriate and adaptive behaviors. Operant methods include reinforcing appropriate behaviors across settings, such as home and school. Medication has been suggested as a helpful addition to behavioral programming and other interventions (110, 111). Clinicians are cautioned, however, against using medication alone without engaging in a detailed analysis and behavioral treatment of the child's behavior problems. Finally, behavioral parent training (sometimes called parent management training) (112, 147) is designed to decrease negative and increase positive interactions between parents and children. It also teaches parents behavior management and problem solving techniques to improve parents' skills in managing their children's behaviors.

Other components of intervention that have been used include self-monitoring, self-instruction, perspective-taking, social problem solving, affect-labeling, and relaxation (106). Self-monitoring and self-instruction are used to monitor arousal state, learn to label the accompanying emotions, learn to recognize trigger situations, and learn use of inhibitory self-talk (e.g., "Stop and think!"). Perspective taking and social problem solving are also suggested components of intervention. Perspective taking involves increasing awareness of nonhostile cues in social situations and understanding of the multiple types of intentions that others can have besides negative ones. In social problem solving, children are taught to think of alternative solutions to being provoked, such as use of words and compromising. Skills training often involves practice of these alternatives to promote competent enactment when real situations arise. These skills are often most helpful when children learn to "insert" them between the antecedent and the impulsive behavior. In this way, they become preventive and are effective positive coping strategies.

Parent management training (PMT) (112, 147) is a widely used model of intervention that incorporates many of the above-mentioned components. This model is based on Patterson's (98) coercive model of parent–child interactions. The goal of PMT is to alter the interaction pattern between the child and parent, such that "prosocial, rather than coercive, behavior is directly reinforced and supported within the family" (2). Specific parent behaviors that are shaped in sessions over time include: 1) establishing clear rules for the child to follow, 2) providing positive reinforcement for appropriate behavior, 3) implementing mild punishments to deter inappropriate behavior, and 4) negotiating compromises. These skills are shaped in treatment sessions through practice, feedback, role-plays, and review of in-home implementation with parents on a regular basis. Intervention also sometimes includes coordination with teachers and other service providers.

Problem solving skills training (PSST) (2) is an intervention approach designed to develop interpersonal cognitive problem solving skills in children with conduct problems. PSST begins with a focus on understanding the thought processes involved in how the child approaches situations. Patients are then taught step-by-step processes that guide them through solving interpersonal problems. This process involves making self-statements that cue the child to attend to certain aspects of the problem, which lead to an effective outcome. In PSST, patients are first taught problem solving skills through use of games, stories, and other related approaches. As the child gains mastery, skills are applied to more "real" situations first, through role-playing and practice, before requiring their use in actual interactions with others. The PSST therapist plays an active role in modeling behaviors, cueing and prompting skills, giving feedback, and praising correct use of skills. As skills are correctly displayed they are reinforced.

ATTENTION DEFICIT HYPERACTIVITY DISORDER (ADHD)

Cognitive-Behavioral Model

In addition to the inattentive, hyperactive, and impulsive symptoms that characterize the various forms of this disorder, children with ADHD have poor self-monitoring and self-evaluation skills, may have difficulty with receptive and expressive language, and suffer from associated executive functioning deficits, such as disorganization, poor problem solving skills, and difficulty utilizing the appropriate behavior at the correct time. The symptoms of inattention, hyperactivity, and impulsivity, associated with ADHD require that patients learn self-control strategies to improve functioning. These self-control strategies typically target cognitions that accompany behavior, as well as the behaviors themselves.

Treatment

Treatment with stimulant medications is the most commonly used intervention for ADHD. Studies show, however, that functioning typically returns to premorbid levels when medication is terminated (113, 114). Therefore, combination pharmacological and behavioral treatments are considered more desirable in the treatment of this disorder (115, 116), especially when potential side effects associated with long-term stimulant use (e.g., growth suppression) are considered (114). Behavioral or cognitive behavioral interventions in the treatment of ADHD are warranted, and have demonstrated efficacy in increasing learning, improving academic performance, reducing impulsivity, and improving attention and concentration. A recent randomized controlled trial demonstrated that the most effective way to implement CBT in treating ADHD was to program in the home, the school, and within the individual child (115).

Programming at home involves parent education, which typically consists of psychoeducation around several issues including symptoms of ADHD, behavioral observation and measurement, and behavior management skills (117). Parents are first taught to observe and measure behavior, including basic functional assessment skills. They are also often required to increase awareness of their own parenting behaviors during this time, through exercises such as monitoring statements made to their child during a 15-minute period, or being required to practice making positive statements only to their child for a specified time period. Behavior management skills are taught to reward appropriate behavior and extinguish inappropriate behavior. Specifically, they learn to use positive reinforcement to increase appropriate behaviors (independence in play, compliance, prosocial interactions) and mild punishment to decrease negative behaviors (time out, response cost).

School intervention emphasizes similar techniques, as well as additional techniques specific to this setting. The use of a daily report card on which current goals are evaluated is a recommended component of school-based interventions (115). The daily report card facilitates communication between home and school and allows the child to be reinforced at home for good days at school. Environmental and curricular modifications, such as preferential seating in the classroom and shortened assignments, are also often made for children with ADHD. Coordination of goals across contexts (home, school, other activities) is extremely important to ensure consistency of approach.

A long-term goal in ADHD treatment is gradually to fade the adult control to child-driven self-management. This is one of several key procedures taught to the child individually in ADHD treatment packages. Individuals can learn to self-manage a variety of behaviors such as staying on task, compliance, attention, and suppression of disruptive behaviors. Individuals with ADHD also often need social skills intervention, including instruction in self-evaluation skills, as they have difficulty evaluating whether their behavior is appropriate and understanding how to choose the appropriate behavior given a particular context. Hinshaw et al (115). recommend that these skills be taught in groups so that children may benefit from the inherent social context. They recommend that groups be structured with clear limits and reward systems for appropriate behavior. Further, they suggest that teaching methodologies include discussion of target behaviors and goals, modeling, behavioral rehearsal, rewards for correct performance, and feedback.

It has been suggested that cognitive-behavioral strategies are best for treating impulsivity specifically (19). Teaching step-by-step problem solving skills, including learning to anticipate the consequences of actions, is often key in the treatment of this disorder. Problem solving strategies may be taught in a variety of formats, including coping modeling and role-plays (118). For example, in self-instruction training, children are taught to internalize the steps involved in effective problem solving (119); specifically, they are taught steps such as how to recognize the problem, reflect on solutions, make a decision, and take action (119).

EATING DISORDERS

Cognitive distortions have been described in the literature as the core psychopathology of eating disorders (120), with other symptoms being driven by and secondary to cognitive factors. For example, Bruch (153) noted the "relentless pursuit of thinness" in patients with anorexia, and Russell (154) discussed the bulimic patient's "morbid fear of becoming fat." These patients often judge their self-worth almost solely based on weight and shape, leading to related emotional difficulties, such as low self-esteem, and cognitive distortions, such as perfectionism (especially in anorexia). The cognitive distortions are then thought to underlie all other eating disorder symptoms, such as dieting and compensatory behavior, arbitrary rules imposed upon oneself about eating (e.g., lists of allowed and forbidden foods, times of day that one is allowed to eat), and extreme negative reaction to breaking the rules because of the implications for the patient's dysfunctional belief system ("breaking a rule means I have no self control"). Anorexia and bulimia will be discussed separately below, as their cognitive models and treatment differ from one another.

Bulimia

Cognitive-Behavioral Model

In bulimia, the patient is caught in a vicious cycle of bingeing and purging. This cycle originates and is maintained as a result of the mistaken view that compensatory behaviors (vomiting, laxative use, diuretics, overexercising) are effective means of weight control. This belief causes the barrier against binge eating to be removed and the cycle begins. That is, the individual binges because s/he believes before doing so that there is a means of controlling the outcome. This belief is especially salient with vomiting because it is easier to vomit when the stomach is very full. In this cycle, however, vomiting leads to intense self-hatred, which decreases self-esteem, and exacerbates the notion that weight control will lead to more positive self-evaluation. As a result, the cycle is maintained. This binge-purge cycle is also associated with the antecedent of negative affect, which may lead to overeating and begin the cycle. As a result, cognitive and emotional interpretations of a negative event can significantly exacerbate the bulimic cycle and must be a focus in therapy and relapse prevention.

Treatment

Treatment research for bulimia in children and adolescents is somewhat sparse, with most approaches drawing heavily from the adult literature. The most important issues to address in treatment of this disorder include: binge eating and purging behaviors, dieting behaviors, and concerns about shape and weight (120). Motivation for treatment is typically less a problem in bulimia than anorexia, as bulimic patients are typically distressed by the binge-purge cycle.

Fairburn (120) proposes several stages in the treatment of bulimia. In the first stage, the clinician conducts psychoeducation about the disorder, and attempts to decrease binge eating and increase a stable pattern of eating. This is accomplished using the following steps: 1) teaching the patient self-monitoring of eating and related behaviors, 2) educating the patient about eating and weight (physical effects of binge eating, information about weight fluctuation, ineffectiveness of compensatory strategies, effects of dieting), 3) prescribing a regular pattern of eating (regular, planned meals and snacks), and 4) developing a plan to address post-meal vomiting when this behavior is part of the illness. Normalization of the eating pattern typically leads to a reduction in bingeing, which automatically leads to a reduction in purging. As such, it may not be necessary to separately address purging behavior. As part of this stage of treatment, the patient also contracts to stop using laxatives and diuretics.

Stage two involves a continued emphasis on regular eating. The patient must then begin to address the desire to diet, concerns about weight/shape, and cognitive distortions. Cognitive restructuring and behavioral experiments are often used to identify and question dysfunctional thoughts about eating, weight, and shape. Dieting is eliminated by progressively reintroducing forbidden foods and returning eating to normal quantities. Finally, bulimic patients often have associated behaviors such as body checking and body avoidance that must be eliminated. The patient works progressively toward eliminating checking behaviors and engaging in behaviors they previously avoided (wearing tight clothes, seeing self in mirror).

Stage three focuses on maintenance and relapse prevention. Relapse prevention typically involves having a plan in the event of relapse and viewing it as a temporary lapse, but not total relapse. Antecedent interventions for negative affect may be important in relapse prevention. That is, if the individual learns other coping strategies, s/he will be less likely to binge as a result of stress, anxiety, or other negative feelings.

A recent metaanalysis suggested that while CBT results in a reduction in symptoms, it is not necessarily a reduction into the "normal" range when patients are compared with nonbulimic individuals (155). Further research is warranted in this area, especially in the treatment of children and adolescents.

Anorexia

Cognitive-Behavioral Model

The primary cognitive distortion in anorexia is that most patients do not believe they have a problem (120); rather, they believe that they are fat and truly need to lose weight. Therefore, the restricting behaviors of a patient with anorexia are reinforced when they result in weight loss. This egosyntonic viewpoint differs from the view of patients with bulimia, who view their bingeing and purging behavior as aversive, leading to negative self-evaluation and motivation to change. The interaction of dysfunctional cognitions and starvation are important maintaining factors in anorexia (120). For example, preoccupation with food and eating exaggerates the concerns about eating, and lowering of mood due to starvation intensifies negative self-evaluation, thus leading to increased efforts to restrict food to control weight. An additional cognitive distortion that may exist involves "an extreme need for self-control upon which shape and weight concerns are superimposed" (120). This notion suggests that cognitive distortions regarding perfectionism, need for control, and rigidity need to be addressed in treatment.

Treatment

Issues that must be addressed in treatment include concerns about shape and weight, dieting behavior, and lack of motivation to change (120). The first goal of anorexia treatment is typically weight gain, especially in severe cases. This is accomplished through contingency management in which activities and privileges become contingent on weight gain. Some of the treatment components outlined in the treatment of bulimia may apply; however, several additional components may be necessary (120). Specifically, clinicians treating anorexic patients must address the lack of motivation of the patient. As a result, intervention procedures, such as self-monitoring and meal planning, must be introduced slowly, as the patient is likely to resist them initially. Correcting the patient's state of starvation and family involvement are key components as well, with family involvement being especially important for long-term maintenance of treatment gains. Family members often need guidance in supporting the goals of the program, but other family pathology may need to be addressed as well.

In trying to alter the lack of motivation in anorexia, the patient's viewpoint must be validated, followed by a review of the advantages and disadvantages of the disorder versus change. It may also be helpful to identify clinical features that the patient might view as problematic to increase motivation, which may be accomplished through psychoeducation about the effects of starvation on the patient's health.

The following stages of anorexia treatment are proposed by Garner, Vitousek, and Pike (156) and are similar to the treatment stages outlined for bulimia.

In stage one, immediate priorities are stabilization of the patient's physical health and building a therapeutic alliance. The therapeutic alliance is particularly important, as these patients are typically unmotivated in treatment. Features of the disorder must then be assessed for treatment planning. Treatment then proceeds with psychoeducation regarding issues such as starvation, symptoms of the disorder, and a cognitive rationale for the treatment. Patients then begin to learn self-monitoring, meal planning, and normalized eating patterns, which are initially prescribed until the patient's motivation increases. Cognitive interventions can also begin at this time, especially to increase motivation and explore and challenge cultural values that reinforce the patient's dysfunctional cognitions. Finally, family involvement should be established in this stage.

In stage two, there is a continued emphasis on weight gain and normal eating. Additionally, patient and therapist continue identifying dysfunctional thoughts and schemas and working to restructure them. A primary focus of cognitive restructuring is on modification of self-concept. The interpersonal focus of therapy can begin in this stage as well, as the patient's health is stabilized and s/he is working toward normalization of eating and other age appropriate activities.

In stage three progress is summarized to maintain motivation and the reasons for the progress are emphasized to reinforce continued use of treatment strategies. Coping with relapse and relapse prevention are also addressed in this stage.

TOURETTE SYNDROME AND TRICHOTILLOMANIA (TTM)

Tourette Syndrome

Cognitive-Behavioral Model

Tourette syndrome and other transient tic disorders are characterized by the presence of vocal and/or motor tics.

Although often described as involuntary, research suggests that tics are not analogous to other involuntary movements, such as choreas or dystonias (121). Instead, it appears to be the *urge* to engage in the movement that is involuntary, with the movement behavior itself being "irresistible" as a result of the urge (122). This conceptualization of tics suggests the role of negative reinforcement (dissipation of the urge upon performance of the tic) as a contributing factor in the shaping and maintenance of tic expression (123) and supports the use of cognitive-behavioral treatments aimed at disrupting the urge–tic relationship (124).

Treatment

The treatment of tics is based on the early work of Azrin & Nunn (125) and involves implementation of habit reversal procedures (126, 127). Habit reversal includes multiple components including an assessment phase, awareness training, competing response training, and social support. During the assessment phase tics must be identified, operationally defined, and ranked in order from least to most distressing. It is also helpful to complete a functional analysis to understand maintaining environmental variables. It has been suggested that, although tics are considered to be organic in nature, they may also come under operant control. Therefore, understanding how socially mediated positive reinforcement, socially mediated negative reinforcement, and automatic reinforcement play a role in maintaining tics can be critical to successful treatment (127). A monitoring procedure is then used to establish baseline tic frequency. Ongoing monitoring may include in-home video or audio-taped observation, direct observation by another individual, self-monitoring, or self-report (127).

During awareness training, the patient is trained to identify the occurrence of each tic and the sensations that precede it. This procedure is completed through several steps including: 1) describing the tic and its associated preceding sensations in detail, 2) observing therapist simulations of the tic, 3) observing and acknowledging ones' own simulated or actual tics. These procedures result in a heightened awareness of the tic that is critical for successful implementation of the habit reversal procedures.

After awareness training is complete, competing response training, the primary treatment component for habit reversal, is implemented. Competing responses are incompatible behaviors that can be performed instead of the tic contingent on the urge to tic. Competing response training involves determining the competing behavior, clinician demonstration of the competing response, and patient demonstration of the competing response with feedback from the clinician. The clinician continues to provide feedback until it is clear that the patient is performing the competing response correctly (127).

Social support training is the final component of habit reversal and involves having someone else (usually a parent when working with children and adolescents) support the implementation of the procedures outside the session. The role of the support person involves praising and acknowledging correct use of the competing response, and prompting its use when necessary (when a tic is observed without use of the competing response). The supportive individual should be trained in session through modeling and behavioral rehearsal how to provide both types of feedback. When working with children, it may also be necessary to have a teacher's social support, as the child may spend a substantial period of the day away from parents. Subsequent sessions involve monitoring progress and troubleshooting difficulties that arise until the targeted tic is reduced or eliminated. Once these procedures have been completed for a single tic, the next tic on the hierarchy can be targeted. Each time a tic is reduced or eliminated, a new one can be targeted until the patient's overall symptoms are significantly reduced.

TRICHOTILLOMANIA (TTM)

Cognitive-Behavioral Model

TTM is characterized by chronic hair pulling, which results in noticeable hair loss most commonly on the scalp, eyebrows and lashes, facial hair, and pubic hair (128). Hair loss may result in distress and stigmatization that leads to avoidance of social situations. Similar to tic disorders, the individual typically experiences an urge or increasing sense of tension prior to pulling that is released when the behavior occurs (62). TTM is categorized in the DSM-IV-TR under Impulse Control Disorders Not Elsewhere Classified (62), since the behavioral reaction of pulling hair in response to the urge or tension is considered to be an impulsive one. The cognitive-behavioral conceptualization of TTM suggests that hair pulling behaviors are maintained by a negative reinforcement paradigm similar to OCD and tic disorders, as tension is reduced when the hair-pulling behavior occurs (129, 130).

Treatment

Similar to tic disorders, the most well supported treatment for TTM is habit reversal (125, 131–133). In treatment of TTM, awareness training involves becoming aware of the tension or urge that precedes the pulling as well as becoming aware of the behavior itself. Awareness training is followed by competing response training and social support, as in tic disorders. The most common competing responses involve engaging the child's hands in a manner incompatible with pulling (making a fist, squeezing a soft ball, sitting on hands or putting them in one's pocket). Stimulus control techniques such as putting bandages on the pulling fingers and/or wearing gloves or other hand coverings are also employed. Training aimed at reducing the tension that precedes the pulling is also a common element of treatment (132).

OTHER CLINICAL PROBLEMS

Enuresis

Treatment

The night alarm has often been sighted as the most effective treatment for nocturnal enuresis (134, 135). This device electronically signals the child with an alarm when it becomes wet with urine, thereby providing a prompt to get out of bed and use the bathroom. This procedure has been found to be effective 75–80% of the time (136, 157, 158). Its effectiveness has also been demonstrated when combined with other treatment components, such as waking the child during the night to prompt voiding (positive practice), requiring the child to change the bed and their clothes after a toileting accident (punishment or overcorrection), and reinforcing the child for successful nighttime toileting behaviors. This combination treatment is known as dry bed training (137, 138) and is thought to be more effective than the night alarm alone in relapse prevention (136, 139).

Children who have diurnal enuresis are often treated behaviorally, whereby they are prompted to use the bathroom on a regular schedule (e.g., once per hour) and are then reinforced for trying as well as for actually urinating in the toilet. Over time, prompts can be faded such that the child learns to initiate using the toilet on his/her own. This process may also be accompanied by overcorrection or positive practice. For example, when the child has a toileting accident, s/he may be prompted to return to the scene of the accident and go through all the steps involved in going to the toilet (e.g., walk to the toilet, pull down pants, sit down, wipe, stand up, etc.) multiple times to practice the positive behavior.

Encopresis

Treatment

It has been proposed that the pain of having a bowel movement when constipated is often significant and causes children to become avoidant of doing so (8). Therefore, treatment of encopresis often consists of a combination of laxative prescription, dietary changes, and behavioral methods (140). For example, children are often given laxatives to ensure regular, pain-free bowel movements and are then rewarded for having a movement in the toilet (141–143). Establishing a toileting routine is often an additional component, whereby the child is reinforced for sitting on the toilet for a short period of time on a systematic schedule (in the morning, after school, and before bed). The child is then further reinforced if a bowel movement actually occurs. In this way, adaptive toileting behaviors are taught in addition to training actual bowel movements. These procedures may also be complemented with regular pants checks, with clean pants resulting in reinforcement as well. Overcorrection procedures are sometimes used in conjunction with pants checks, in which the child is required to wash the soiled clothing and take a bath (143). These procedures must be modified developmentally, as they may result in significant resistance from young children, thereby making the training experience more negative than is necessary.

Selective mutism

Treatment

Selective mutism is typically treated using behavioral methods that begin with a functional analysis (144). Based on the observed patterns, shaping is often used to increase the frequency with which the child verbalizes (145, 146). Cunningham (146) proposed two types of fading: situational and individual. In situational fading, the child and a person s/he is willing to talk to are gradually and systematically moved from a location where speech occurs to one where it does not. In individual fading, new individuals are gradually and systematically introduced into situations in which the child already speaks. When these systematic shaping procedures are paired with reinforcement of speaking, the child gradually learns to speak to an increasing number of individuals in an increasing number of settings.

Stuttering

Treatment

Relaxation training is often cited as the most common treatment for stuttering. Often when children are encouraged to slow down their speaking, take deep breaths, and relax, their stuttering decreases. Habit reversal is used to treat stuttering when relaxation training is paired with awareness training and psychoeducation about the nature of the disorder. Contingency management may be helpful as well, whereby a child is reinforced for slowing down and speaking in a more relaxed fashion. Distraction may also be helpful as it can serve to decrease the child's anxiety and take the focus off the stuttering behavior, which can be anxiety provoking in and of itself.

CBT RESOURCES

The following resources may be helpful for practitioners and families using cognitive-behavioral treatment strategies with children and adolescents. As of the printing of the present edition of this text, these resources were a sampling of the most up to date in the field. They were chosen to represent a variety of disorders possibly treated using CBT techniques.

For Practitioners

Barkley RA: *Defiant Children: A Clinician's Manual for Assessment and Parent Training*, 2nd ed. New York, Guilford Press, 1997.

Kendall P (ed): *Child and Adolescent Therapy*, 3rd ed. NY, Guilford Press, 2006.

March JS and Mulle K: *OCD in Children and Adolescents: A Cognitive-Behavioral Treatment Manual.* New York, Guilford Press, 1998.

National Research Council. *Educating Children with Autism*, National Academy Press, Washington, DC, 2001.

Rapee R, Wignall A, Hudson J, Schniering C: *Treating Anxious Children and Adolescents: An Evidence-Based Approach*, Oakland, CA: New Harbinger Publications, Inc. 2000.

Volkmar FR, Paul R, Klin A, Cohen DJ: *Handbook of Autism and Pervasive Developmental Disorders*, Third Edition (2 vols). John Wiley & Sons: Hoboken, NJ, 2005.

Woods DW, Miltenberger RG, (Eds.): *Tic Disorders, Trichotillomania, and Other Repetitive Behavior Disorders: Behavioral Approaches to Analysis and Treatment.* Kluwar Academic Publishers, Norwell, MA, 2001.

For Families

Barkley R: *Taking Charge of ADHD: The Complete, Authoritative Guide for Parents* (rev ed). New York, Guilford Press, 2000.

Barkley RA, Benton CM: *Your Defiant Child: Eight Steps to Better Behavior.* New York, Guilford Press, 1998.

Chansky TE: *Freeing Your Child from Obsessive-Compulsive Disorder.* New York, Crown Publishers, 2000.

Koegel LK, LaZebnik C: *Overcoming Autism.* Viking, Penguin Group, New York, 2004.

Koegel RL, Koegel LK: *Pivotal Response Treatments for Autism: Communication, Social, and Academic Development.* Paul H. Brookes, Baltimore, 2006.

Last CG: *Help for Worried Kids: How Your Child Can Conquer Anxiety and Fear.* New York, Guilford Press, 2006.

Moritz EK, Jablonsky J: *Blink, Blink, Clop, Clop: Why Do We Do Things We Can't Stop?*, Plainview, New York, Childswork/Childsplay, 1998.

Rapee R, Spence S, Cobham V, Wignall A: *Helping Your Anxious Child: A Step-by-Step Guide for Parents.* Oakland, CA, New Harbinger Publications, Inc, 2000.

Taulbee J: *Understanding Children of Special Needs: What Every Parent Needs to Know.* Monrovia, CA, Wayne Publishing, 2005.

Wagner AP: *Up and Down the Worry Hill: A Children's Book about Obsessive-Compulsive Disorder and Its Treatment.* Lighthouse Press, 1999.

References

1. Albano A: Cognitive-behavioral psychotherapy for children and adolescents. In: Sadock B, Sadock V (eds): *Comprehensive Textbook of Psychiatry*, 8th ed. (vol 2). Philadelphia, Lippincott Willams & Wilkins, 2005, pp. 3332–3342.
2. Kazdin AE: Cognitive-behavior modification. In: Weiner JM, Dulcan MK (eds): *Textbook of Child and Adolescent Psychiatry.* Arlington, VA, American Psychiatric Publishing, Inc., 2004, pp. 985–1006.
3. Baldwin JD, Baldwin JI: *Behavior Principles in Everyday Life.* NJ, Prentice Hall, Upper Saddle River, 2001.
4. Pavlov IP: (Translated by GV Anrep): *Conditioned Reflexes.* Oxford, Clarenden Press, 1927.

5. Clark DM: Cognitive-behavior therapy for anxiety disorders. In: Gelder MG, Lopez-Ibor JJ, Andreasen N (eds): *New Oxford Textbook of Psychiatry*. New York, Oxford University Press Inc, 2000.
6. Skinner BF: *The Behavior of Organisms*. New York, Appleton-Century-Crofts, 1938.
7. Skinner BF: *Science and Human Behavior*. New York, Free Press, 1953.
8. Herbert M: Behavioral methods. In: Rutter M, Taylor E, Hersov L (eds): *Child and Adolescent Psychiatry Modern Approaches*, Third Edition. Oxford, Blackwell Scientific Publications, 1994, pp. 858–879.
9. Clark DA, Beck AT, Alford BA: *Scientific Foundations of Cognitive Theory and Therapy of Depression*. New York, John Wiley, 1999.
10. Wright JH, Beck AT: Cognitive therapy. In: Hales RE, Yudofsky SC, Talbott JA (eds): *American Psychiatric Press Textbook of Psychiatry* (vol 13). Washington, DC, American Psychiatric Press, 1994, pp. 1083–1114.
11. Friedman ES, Thase ME, Wright JH: *Cognitive and Behavioral Therapies*: John Wiley and Sons Ltd., 2003.
12. Piacentini J, Bergman RL: Developmental issues in cognitive therapy for childhood anxiety disorders. *Journal of Cognitive Psychotherapy* 15:165–182, 2001.
13. Leahy RL: Cognitive therapy of childhood depression: Developmental considerations. In: Shirk SR, ed. *Cognitive Development and Child Psychopathology*. New York, Plunum, 1988, pp. 187–204.
14. Moritz EK, Jablonsky J: *Blink, Blink, Clop, Clop: Why Do We Do Things We Can't Stop?* Plainview, New York, Childswork/Childsplay, 1998.
15. Knell SM: Cognitive behavioral play therapy. In: Schaefer CE, ed. *Foundations of Play Therapy*. Hoboken, NJ., John Wiley & Sons, Inc., 2003, pp. 177–191.
16. Bandura A: *Social Learning Theory*. Englewood Cliffs, NJ, Prentice Hall, 1977.
17. Kendall PC, Suveg C: Treating anxiety disorders in youth. In: Kendall PC, ed. *Child and Adolescent Therapy*. New York, Guilford Press, 2006, pp. 243–294.
18. Piacentini J, March J, Franklin M: Cognitive-behavioral therapy for youngsters with obsessive-compulsive disorder. In: Kendall P, ed. *Child and Adolescent Therapy: Cognitive-Behavioral Procedures*, 3rd ed. New York, Guilford, 2006, pp. 297–321.
19. Kendall PC, Lochman J: Cognitive-behavioral therapies. In: Rutter M, Taylor E, Hersov L (eds): *Child and Adolescent Psychiatry*. Oxford, Blackwell Scientific Publications, 1994, pp. 844–857.
20. Lochman JE: Modification of childhood aggression. In: Hersen M, Eisler R, Miller PM (eds): *Progress in Behavior Modification* (vol XXV). Newbury Park, CA, Sage, 1990, pp. 47–85.
21. Durlak JA, Wells AM, Cotton JK, et al.: Analysis of selected methodological issues in child psychotherapy research. *Journal of Clinical Child Psychology* 24:141–148, 1995.
22. Kazdin AE, Bass D, Ayers WA, et al.: The empirical and clinical focus of child and adolescent psychotherapy research. *Journal of Consulting and Clinical Psychology* 58:729–740, 1990.
23. Rachman S: Obsessions, responsibility, and guilt. *Behaviour Research and Therapy* 31:149–154, 1993.
24. Kendall P: *Child and Adolescent Therapy: Cognitive-Behavioral Procedures*, 3rd ed. New York, Guilford Press, 2006.
25. Friedman ES, Thase ME, Wright JH: Cognitive and behavioral therapies. In: Tasman A, Kay J, Lieberman J (eds): *Psychiatry*, Second Edition *(vol. 2)*. West Sussex, England, John Wiley & Sons, Ltd., 2003, pp. 1753–1777.
26. Goldfried MR, Davidson GC: *Clinical Behavior Therapy, Expanded Version*. New York, John Wiley, 1994.
27. Piacentini J, Roblek T: Exposure plus response prevention. In: Ollendick T, Schroeder C (eds): *Encylopedia of Pediatric and Child Psychology*. New York, Kluwer Academic, 2003, pp. 222–223.
28. Koegel RL, Frea WD: Treatment of social behavior in autism through the modification of pivotal social skills. *Journal of Applied Behavior Analysis* 26(3):369–377, 1993.
29. Koegel LK, Harrower JK, Koegel RL: Support for children with developmental disabilities in full inclusion classrooms through self-management. *Journal of Positive Behavior Interventions* 1(1):26–34, 1999.
30. Ninness CHA, Fuerst J, Rutherford RD, Glenn SS: Effects of self-management training and reinforcement on the transfer of improved conduct in the absence of supervision. *Journal of Applied Behavior Analysis* 24(3):499–508, 1991.
31. Stahmer AC, Schreibman L: Teaching children with autism appropriate play in unsupervised environments using a self-management treatment package. *Journal of Applied Behavior Analysis* 25(2):447–459, 1992.
32. Gregory KM, Kehle TJ, McLoughlin CS: Generalization and maintenance of treatment gains using self-management procedures with behaviorally disordered adolescents. *Psychological Reports* 80:683–690, 1997.
33. Beck AT: *Depression: Clinical, Experimental, and Theoretical Aspects*. New York, Harper and Row, 1967.
34. Beck AT, Rush AJ, Shaw BF: *Cognitive Therapy of Depression*. New York, Guilford, 1979.
35. Hanley G, Iwata B, McCord B: Functional analysis of problem behavior: A review. *JABA* 36:147–185, 2003.
36. Wolpe J: *Psychotherapy by Reciprocal Inhibition*. Stanford, CA, Stanford University Press, 1958.
37. Jones MC: The elimination of children's fears. *Journal of Experimental Psychology* 7:382–390, 1924.
38. Kazdin AE, Wilcoxin LA: Systematic desensitization and nonspecific treatment effects: A methodological consideration. *Psychological Bulletin* 83:729–758, 1976.
39. Woods DW, Miltenberger RG: *Tic Disorders, Trichotillomania, and Other Repetitive Behavior Disorders: Behavioral Approaches to Analysis and Treatment*. Norwell, MA, Kluwer Academic Publishers, 2001.
40. Beck AT: *Cognitive Therapy and the Emotional Disorders*. New York, International Universities Press, 1976.
41. Mowrer OH: Two-factor learning theory: Versions one and two. In: Mowrer OH (ed): *Learning Theory and Behavior*. Hoboken, NJ, John Wiley & Sons, Inc., 1960, pp. 63–91.
42. Barrios BA, Hartman DB: Fears and anxieties. In: Mash EJ, Terdal LG (eds): *Behavioral Assessment of Childhood Disorders*, 2nd ed. New York, Guildford Press, 1988, pp. 196–264.
43. Francis G: Assessing cognitions in anxious children. *Behavior Modification* 12:115–130, 1988.
44. Kendall P, Suveg C: Treating anxiety disorders in youth. *Child and Adolescent Therapy: Cognitive-Behavioral Procedures* (3rd Ed). New York, Guilford Press, 2006, pp. 243–294.
45. Deffenbacher JL, Kemper CC: Systematic desensitization of test anxiety in junior high students. *School Counselor* 22:216–222, 1974.
46. Rosenstiel SK, Scott DS: Four considerations in imagery techniques with children. *Journal of Behavior Therapy and Experimental Psychiatry* 8:287–290, 1977.
47. Hatzenbuehler LC, Schroeder HE: Desensitization procedures in the treatment of childhood disorders. *Psychological Bulletin* 85:831–844, 1978.
48. Jackson HJE, King N: The emotive imagery treatment of a child's trauma-inspired phobia. *Journal of Behavior Therapy and Experimental Psychiatry* 12:325–328, 1981.
49. Ollendick TH, Francis G: Behavioral assessment and treatment of childhood phobias. *Behavior Modification* 12:165–204, 1988.
50. Kendall P, Chansky T, Kane M, et al.: *Anxiety Disorders in Youth: Cognitive-Behavioral Interventions*. Needham Heights, Allyn and Bacon, 1992.
51. Spivak G, Shure MB: *Social Adjustment of Young Children: A Cognitive Approach to Solving Real-Life Problems*. San Francisco, CA, Jossey-Bass, 1974.
52. Kanfer FH, Karoly P, Newman A: Reduction of children's fear of the dark by competence-related and situational threat-related verbal cues. *Journal of Consulting and Clinical Psychology* 43:251–258, 1975.
53. Kendall P, Flannery-Schroeder E, Panicelli-Mindel S, et al.: Therapy for youths with anxiety disorders: A second randomized clinical trial. *Journal of Consulting and Clinical Psychology* 65:366–380, 1997.
54. Kendall P, Flannery-Schroeder E, Safford S, Webb A: Child anxiety treatment: Outcomes in adolescence and impact on substance use and depression at 7.4-year follow-up. *Journal of Consulting and Clinical Psychology* 72:276–287, 2004.
55. Piacentini J, Langley A: Cognitive behavior therapy for children with obsessive compulsive disorder. *In Session: Journal of Clinical Psychology* 60:1181–1194, 2004.
56. Barrett P, Healy-Farrell L, March J: Cognitive-behavioral family treatment of childhood obsessive-compulsive disorder: A controlled trial. *Journal of the American Academy of Child & Adolescent Psychiatry* 43:46–62, 2004.
57. Pediatric OCD Treatment Study Team. Cognitive-behavior therapy, Sertraline, and their combination for children and adolescents with obsessive-compulsive disorder. *Journal of the American Medical Association* 292:1969–1976, 2004.
58. Wolpe J: *The Practice of Behavior Therapy*. New York, Pergamon Press, 1982.
59. Beidel DC, Turner SM, Morris TL: Behavioral treatment of childhood social phobia. *Journal of Consulting and Clinical Psychology*. 68:1072–1080, 2000.
60. Beidel DC, Turner SM, Young B, Paulson A: Social effectiveness therapy for children: Three-year follow-up. *Journal of Consulting and Clinical Psychology* 73:721–725, 2005.
61. Addis ME, Hatgis C, Krasnow AD, Jacob K, Bourne L, Mansfield A: Effectiveness of cognitive-behavioral treatment for panic disorder versus treatment as usual in a managed care setting. *Journal of Consulting and Clinical Psychology* 72:625–635, 2004.
62. American Psychiatric Association: *Diagnostic and Statistical Manual, Fourth Edition Text Revision (DSM-IVTR)*. Washington, DC, American Psychiatric Association, 2000.
63. Scheeringa MS, Zeanah CH, Myers L, Putnam FW: New findings on alternative criteria for PTSD in preschool children. *Journal of the American Academy of Child and Adolescent Psychiatry* 42:561–570, 2003.
64. American Academy of Child and Adolescent Psychiatry. Practice parameters for the assessment and treatment of children and adolescents with posttraumatic stress disorder. *Journal of the American Academy of Child and Adolescent Psychiatry* 37:4–26, 1998.
65. Cohen JA, Berliner L, March J: Treatment of children and adolescents. In: Foa E, Keane T, Friedman M (eds): *Effective Treatments for PTSD*. New York, Guilford Press, 106–138, 2000.

66. Feeny NC, Foa EB, Treadwell KRH, March J: Posttraumatic stress disorder in youth: A critical review of the cognitive and behavioral treatment outcome literature. *Professional Psychology: Research and Practice* 35:466–476, 2004.
67. Hembree EA, Rauch SAM, Foa EB: Beyond the manual: The insider's guide to prolonged exposure therapy for PTSD. *Cognitive and Behavioral Practice* 10:22–30, 2003.
68. Perrin S, Smith P, Yule W: Practitioner review: The assessment and treatment of posttraumatic stress disorder in children and adolescents. *Journal of Child Psychology and Psychiatry* 41:277–289, 2000.
69. Bryant RA, Harvey AG: Avoidant coping style and posttraumatic stress following motor vehicle accidents. *Behavior Research and Therapy* 33:631–635, 1995.
70. Ehlers A, Mayou RA, Bryant B: Psychological predictors of chronic posttraumatic stress disorder after motor vehicle accidents. *Journal of Abnormal Psychology* 107:508–519, 1998.
71. Cohen JA, Mannarino AP: A treatment outcome study for sexually abused preschool children: Initial findings. *Journal of the American Academy of Child and Adolescent Psychiatry* 35:42–50, 1996.
72. Cohen JA, Mannarino AP: Interventions for sexually abused children: Initial treatment outcome findings. *Child Maltreatment* 3:17–26, 1998.
73. Deblinger E, Lippman J, Steer R: Sexually abused children suffering posttraumatic stress symptoms: Initial treatment findings. *Child Maltreatment* 1:310–321, 1996.
74. Pine DS, Cohen JA: Trauma in children and adolescents: Risk and treatment of psychiatric sequelae. *Biological Psychiatry* 51:519–531, 2002.
75. Foa EB, Rothbaum BO, Riggs DS, Murdock TB: Treatment of posttraumatic stress disorder in rape victims: A comparison between cognitive-behavioral procedures and counseling. *Journal of Consulting and Clinical Psychology* 59:715–723, 1991.
76. Marks I, Lovell K, Noshirvani H, Livanou M, Thrasher S: Treatment of posttraumatic stress disorder by exposure and/or cognitive restructuring: A controlled study. *Archives of General Psychiatry* 55:317–325, 1998.
77. Foa EB, Dancu CV, Hembree EA, Jaycox LH, Meadows EA, Street GP: A comparison of exposure therapy, stress inoculation training, and their combination for reducing posttraumatic stress disorder in female assault victims. *Journal of Consulting and Clinical Psychology* 67:194–200, 1999.
78. Farrell SP, Hains AA, Davies WH: Cognitive behavioral interventions for sexually abused children exhibiting PTSD symptomatology. *Behavior Therapy* 29:241–255, 1998.
79. Seligman MEP. *Helplessness*. San Francisco, CA, Freeman, 1975.
80. Curry JF, Craighead WE. Attributional style in clinically depressed and conduct disordered adolescents. *Journal of Clinical and Consulting Psychology* 58:109–116, 1990.
81. Rehm LP, Carter AS: Cognitive components of depression. In: Lewis M, Miller SM (eds): *Handbook of Developmental Psychopathology*. New York, Plenum Press, 1990, pp. 341–351.
82. Leitenberg H, Yost LW, Carrol-Wilson M. Negative cognitive errors in children: Questionnaire development, normative data, and comparisons between children with and without self-reported symptoms of depression, low self-esteem, and evaluation anxiety. *Journal of Consulting and Clinical Psychology*. 54:528–536, 1986.
83. Kendall PC, Reber M, McLeer S, Epps J, Ronan KR. Cognitive behavioral treatment of conduct disordered children. *Cognitive Therapy and Research*. 14:279–297, 1990.
84. Kaslow NJ, Rehm LP, Siegel AW: Social and cognitive correlates of depression in children: A developmental perspective. *Journal of Abnormal Child Psychology*. 12:605–620, 1984.
85. Hovey J, King C. The spectrum of suicidal behavior. In: Marsh DT, Fristad MA, eds. *Handbook of Serious Emotional Disturbance in Children and Adolescents*. Hoboken, NJ: John Wiley & Sons, Inc.; 2002, pp. 284–303.
86. Frame C, Matson JL, Sonis WA, Fialkov MJ, Kazdin AE: Behavioral treatment of depression in a prepubertal child. *Journal of Behavior Therapy and Experimental Psychiatry* 3:239–243, 1982.
87. Kaufman NK, Rhode P, Seeley JR, Clarke GN, Stice E. Potential mediators of cognitive-behavioral therapy for adolescents with comorbid major depression and conduct disorder. *Journal of Consulting and Clinical Psychology* 73:38–46, 2005.
88. Lewinsohn PM, Clarke GN, Rohde P, et al.: A course in coping: A cognitive-behavioral approach to the treatment of adolescent depression. In: Hibbs ED, Jenson PS (eds): *Psychosocial Treatment Research of Child and Adolescent Disorders: Empirically Based Strategies for Clinical Practice*. Washington, DC, American Psychological Association, 1996, pp. 109–135.
89. Koegel RL, O'Dell MC, Koegel LK: A natural language teaching paradigm for nonverbal autistic children. *Journal of Autism and Developmental Disorders*. 17(2):187–200, 1987.
90. Lovaas OI: Behavioral treatment and normal educational and intellectual functioning in young autistic children. *Journal of Consulting and Clinical Psychology* 5:3–9, 1987.
91. McGee GG. What's incidental about incidental teaching? Part I. *Autism-Asperger's Digest*. Arlington, TX, Future Horizons, 2003a, pp. 10–13.
92. McGee GG: What's incidental about incidental teaching? Part II. *Autism-Asperger's Digest*. Arlington, TX: Future Horizons, 2003b.
93. McEachin JJ, Smith T, Lovaas OI: Long-term outcome for children with autism who received early intensive behavioral treatment. *American Journal on Mental Retardation*. 97:359–372, 1993.
94. Koegel LK, Koegel RL, Carter CM: Pivotal responses and the natural language paradigm. *Seminars in Speech and Language* 19(4):355–372, 1998.
95. National Research Council. *Educating Children with Autism*. Washington, DC, National Academy Press, 2001.
96. Kazdin AE: *Treatment of Antisocial Behavior in Children and Adolescents*. Homewood, IL, Dorsey Press, 1985.
97. Patterson GR, DeBaryshe BD: A developmental perspective on antisocial behavior. *American Psychologist* 44:329–335, 1989.
98. Patterson GR: *Coercive Family Processes*. Eugene, OR, Castalia, 1982.
99. Dodge KA, Pettit GS, McClaskey CL, Brown MM: Social competence in children. *Monographs of the Society for Research in Child Development* 51:2, 213, 1986.
100. Milich R, Dodge KA: Social information processing in child psychiatric populations. *Journal of Abnormal Child Psychology* 12:471–490, 1984.
101. Dodge KA, Price JM, Bachorowski J, Newman JP: Hostile attributional biases in severely aggressive adolescents. *Journal of Abnormal Psychology* 99:385–392, 1990.
102. Dodge KA, Newman JP: Biased decision making processes in aggressive boys. *Journal of Abnormal Psychology* 90:375–379, 1981.
103. Lochman JE: Self and peer perceptions and attributional biases of aggressive and nonaggressive boys in dyadic interventions. *Journal of Consulting and Clinical Psychology* 55:404–410, 1987.
104. Perry DG, Perry LC, Rasmussen P: Cognitive social learning mediators of aggression. *Child Development* 57:700–711, 1986.
105. Slaby RG, Guerra NG: Cognitive mediators of aggression in adolescent offenders: Assessment. *Developmental Psychology* 24:580–588, 1988.
106. Lochman JE, Meyer BL, Rabiner DL, White JJ: Parameters influencing social problem-solving of aggressive children. In: Prinz R (ed): *Advances in Behavioral Assessment of Children and Families* (vol 5). London, Jessica Kingsley Publishers, 1991, pp. 31–63.
107. Richard BA, Dodge KA: Social maladjustment and problem solving in school aged children. *Journal of Consulting and Clinical Psychology* 50:226–233, 1982.
108. Asarnow JR, Callan JW: Boys with peer adjustment problems: Social cognitive processes. *Journal of Consulting and Clinical Psychology* 53:80–87, 1985.
109. Lochman JE, Lampron LB: Situational social problem-solving skills and self-esteem of aggressive and nonaggressive boys. *Journal of Abnormal Child Psychology* 14:605–617, 1986.
110. Barkley RA: *Hyperactive Children: A Handbook for Diagnosis and Assessment*. Chichester, Wiley, 1982.
111. Campbell M, Cohen IL, Perry R, Small M: Psychopharmacological treatment. In: Ollendick TH, Hersen M, eds: *Handbook of Child Psychopathology* New York, Plenum, 1989.
112. Kazdin AE: *Behavior Modification in Applied Settings*, 6th ed. Belmont, CA, Wadsworth, 2001.
113. MTA Cooperative Group. National institute of mental health multimodal treatment study of ADHD follow-up: 24-month outcomes of treatment strategies for attention-deficit/hyperactivity disorder. *Pediatrics*. 113:754–761, 2004a.
114. MTA Cooperative Group. National Institute of Mental Health multimodal treatment study of ADHD follow-up: Changes in effectiveness and growth after the end of treatment. *Pediatrics* 113:762–769, 2004b.
115. Hinshaw SP: Attention-deficit/hyperactivity disorder: The search for viable treatments. In: Kendall PC (ed): *Child and Adolescent Therapy: Cognitive-Behavioral Procedures*, 2nd Ed. New York, Guilford Press, 2000, pp. 88–128.
116. Rapoport JL, Inoff-Germain G: Tourette syndrome: Medical and surgical treatment of obsessive-compulsive disorder. *Neurol Clin*. 15(2):421–428, 1997.
117. Weiss G, Hechtman LT: *Hyperactive Children Grown Up*. New York, Guilford Press, 1986.
118. Kendall PC, Braswell L: *Cognitive Behavioral Therapy for Impulsive Children*. New York, Guilford Press, 1985.
119. Meichenbaum D, Goodman J: Training impulsive children to talk to themselves: A means of developing self-control. *Journal of Abnormal Psychology* 77:115–126, 1971.
120. Fairburn CG: Cognitive-behavior therapy for eating disorders. In: Gelder MG, Lopez-Ibor JJ, Andreasen N (eds): *New Oxford Textbook of Psychiatry*. New York, Oxford University Press, Inc.; 2000, pp. 1388–1393.
121. Leckman J, Block M, King R, Scahill L: Phenomenology and natural history of tic disorders. In: Walkup J, Mink J, Hollenbeck P (eds): *Advances in Neurology: Tourette Syndrome*. Philadelphia: Lippincott, Williams & Wilkins, 2006, pp. 1–16.
122. Lang A: Patient perception of tics and other movement disorders. *Neurology*. 41:223–228, 1991.
123. Piacentini J, Chang S: Behavioral treatments for tic suppression: Habit reversal therapy. In: Walkup J, Mink J, Hollenbeck P (eds): *Advances in Neurology: Tourette Syndrome*. Philadelphia: Lippincott, Williams & Wilkins, 2006, pp. 227–233.
124. Himle M, Woods D, Piacentini J, Walkup J: A brief review of habit reversal training for Tourette syndrome. *Journal of Child Neurology*. In press.

125. Azrin NH, Nunn RG: Habit reversal: A method of eliminating nervous habits and tics. *Behav Res Ther* 11(4):619–628, 1973.
126. Piacentini J, Chang S: Habit Reversal Training for tic disorders in children and adolescents. *Behavior Modification* 29:803–822, 2005.
127. Woods DW: Habit reversal treatment manual for tic disorders. In: Woods DW, Miltenberger RG (eds): *Tic Disorders, Trichotillomania, and Other Repetitive Behavior Disorders: Behavioral Approaches to Analysis and Treatment.* Norwell, MA, Kluwer Academic Publishers, 2001, pp. 97–132.
128. Miltenberger RG, Rapp JT, Long ES: Characteristics of trichotillomania. In: Woods DW, Miltenberger RG (eds): *Tic Disorders, Trichotillomania, and Other Repetitive Behavior Disorders: Behavioral Approaches to Analysis and Treatment.* Norwell, MA, Kluwer Academic Publishers, 2001, pp. 134–150.
129. Hanson DJ, Tishelman AC, Hawkins RP, Doepke KJ: Habits with potential as disorders: Prevalence, severity, and other characteristics among college students. *Behavior Modification* 14:66–80, 1990.
130. Woods DW, Miltenberger RG, Flach AD: Habits, tics, and stuttering: Prevalence and relation to anxiety and somatic awareness. *Behavior Modification* 20:216–225, 1996.
131. Elliot AJ, Fuqua RW: Trichitillomania: Conceptualization, measurement, and treatment. *Behavior Therapy* 31:529–545, 2000.
132. Elliot AJ, Fuqua RW: Behavioral interventions for trichotillomania. In: Woods DW, Miltenberger RG (eds): *Tic Disorders, Trichotillomania, and Other Repetitive Behavior Disorders: Behavioral Approaches to Analysis and Treatment.* Norwell, MA, Kluwer Academic Publishers, 2001, pp. 151–170.
133. Miltenberger RG: Habit reversal treatment manual for trichotillomania. In: Woods DW, Miltenberger RG (eds): *Tic Disorders, Trichotillomania, and Other Repetitive Behavior Disorders: Behavioral Approaches to Analysis and Treatment.* Norwell, MA, Kluwer Academic Publishers, 2001, pp. 172–195.
134. Doleys DM: Behavioral treatment for nocturnal enuresis in children: A review of recent literature. *Psychological Bulletin* 8:30–54, 1977.
135. Mowrer OH, Mowrer W: Enuresis: A method for its study and treatment. *American Journal of Orthopsychiatry* 8:436–447, 1938.
136. O'Leary KD, Wilson GT: *Behavior Therapy: Application and Outcome,* 2nd ed. Englewood Cliffs, NJ, Prentice Hall, 1987.
137. Azrin NH, Sneed TJ, Foxx RM: Dry-bed training: Rapid elimination of childhood enuresis. *Behavior Research and Therapy* 12:147–156, 1974.
138. Said JA, Wilson PH, Hensley VR: Primary versus secondary enuresis: Differential response to urine-alarm treatment. *Child and Family Behavior Therapy* 13:1–13, 1991.
139. Ronen T, Wozner Y, Rahav G: Cognitive intervention in enuresis. *Child and Family Behavior Therapy* 14:1–14, 1992.
140. Doleys DM: Assessment and treatment of enuresis and encopresis in children. In: Hersen M, Eisler RM, Miller PM (eds): *Progress in Behavior Modification* (vol 6). New York, Academic Press, 1978, pp. 85–121.
141. Ashkenazi A: The treatment of encopresis using a discriminative stimulus and positive reinforcement. *Journal of Behavior Therapy and Experimental Psychiatry* 6:155–157, 1975.
142. Wright L, Walker CE: Behavioral treatment of encopresis. *Pediatric Psychology* 4:35–37, 1976.
143. Young IL, Goldsmith AD: Treatment of encopresis in a day treatment program. *Psychotherapy: Theory, Research, and Practice* 10:231–235, 1972.
144. Reed GF: Elective mutism in children: A reappraisal. *Journal of Child Psychology and Psychiatry* 4:99–107, 1963.
145. Bergman RL, Piacentini J: Selective mutism. In: Kaplan H, Sadock B (eds): *Comprehensive Textbook of Psychiatry,* 8th ed. Philadelphia, Lippincott, Williams & Wilkins, 2005, pp. 3302–3306.
146. Cunningham CE, Cataldo MF, Mallion C, Keyes JB: A review and controlled single case evaluation of behavioral approaches to the management of elective mutism. *Child and Family Behavior Therapy* 5:25–49, 1983.
147. Kazdin AE: Parent Management Training: Evicence, outcomes, and issues. *Journal of the American Academy of Child and Adolescent Psychiatry* 36:1349–1356, 1997.
148. Kazdin AE: *Conduct Disorder in Childhood and Adolescence.* Newbury Park, CA, Sage, 1987.
149. Meichenbaum D: *Stress Inoculation Training.* New York, Pergamon Press, 1985.
150. Elkin I, Shea MT, Watkins JT, et al.: National Institutes of Mental Health Treatment of Depression Collaborative Research Program: General effectiveness of treatments. *Archives of General Psychiatry* 46:971–982, 1989.
151. Clarke GN, Lewinsohn PM, Hops H: *Adolescent Coping with Depression Course: Leader's Manual for Adolescent Groups.* Eugene, OR, Castalia, 1990.
152. Clarke GN, DeBar LL, Lewinsohn PM: Cognitive behavioral group treatment for adolescent depression. In: Kazdin AE, Weisz JR (eds): *Evidence-Based Psychotherapies for Children and Adolescents.* New York, Guilford Press, 2003, pp. 120–134.
153. Bruch H. *Eating Disorders: Obesity, Anorexia Nervosa, and the Person Within.* New York, Basic Books, 1973.
154. Russell GFM: Bulimia nervosa: An ominous variant of anorexia nervosa. *Psychological Medicine* 9:429–448, 1979.
155. Lundgren JD, Danoff-Burg S, Anderson DA: Cognitive-behavioral therapy for bulimia nervosa: An empirical analysis of clinical significance. *International Journal of Eating Disorders* 35:262–274, 2004.
156. Garner DM, Vitousek KM, Pike KM: Cognitive behavioral therapy for anorexia nervosa. In: Garner DM, Garfinkel PE (eds): *Handbook of Treatment for Eating Disorders.* New York, Guilford Press, 1997, pp. 94–144.
157. Doleys DM: Behavioral treatments or nocturnal enuresis in children: A review of the recent literature. *Psychological Bulletin* 84:30–54, 1977.
158. Doleys DM: Enuresis and encopresis. In: Kazdin AE, ed. *Handbook of Clinical Behavior Therapy with Children* Homewood, IL, Dorsey Press, 1985, pp. 412–440.
159. Kellner M: *In Control: A Skill-Building Program for Teaching Young Adolescents to Manage Anger.* Champaign, IL, Research Press, 2001.
160. Curry SH, Marlatt GA, Gordon J, Baer JS: A comparison of alternative theoretical approaches to smoking cessation and relapse. *Health Psychology.* 7:545–556, 1988.
161. Curry SH, Marlatt GA, Gordon JR: Abstinence violation effect: Validation of an attributional construct with smoking cessation. *Journal of Consulting and Clinical Psychology.* 55:145–149, 1987.

CHAPTER 6.2.3 ■ INTERPERSONAL PSYCHOTHERAPY

LAURA MUFSON AND JAMI F. YOUNG

INTRODUCTION

Interpersonal psychotherapy (IPT) is a brief, time-limited psychotherapy that was developed in the late 1960s for the treatment of nonbipolar, nonpsychotic, depressed adult outpatients (1). The underlying assumption of IPT is that the quality of interpersonal relationships can cause, maintain, or buffer against depression. This view is similarly articulated in interpersonal theories of depression (2–4). When someone is depressed, it affects his interpersonal relationships, and the quality and stability of his relationships in turn affect his moods. IPT assumes that if one improves the relationships, one can actually change the course of the depressive episode. IPT educates individuals about the link between their mood and problems that are occurring in their relationships, and teaches them how improving their interpersonal skills and addressing these relationship problems can lead to recovery from their depression.

The emphasis on the connection between relationships and mental health has its origin in the work of Adolf Meyer (5) and Harry Stack Sullivan (6). Meyer postulated that mental illness was a result of the difficulties a person had in attempting to adapt to his environment, including his relationships. Sullivan stated that mental disorders were in part affected by inadequate communication and lack of understanding of one's behavior within relationships. In addition to these theories, IPT has its roots in Bowlby's attachment theory, specifically in its emphasis on the importance of relational bonds with other people. When there are conflicts or losses of the important bonds, the outcome is emotional distress, and specifically depression (7). Accordingly, IPT focuses on teaching individuals ways to decrease conflict and to cope with other changes in their relationships, including actual losses of relationships due to death, which can affect a person's mood.

BACKGROUND

Basic Principles

The two main goals of IPT are to: 1) decrease depressive symptoms and 2) improve social functioning within significant relationships. The strategies for achieving these goals include: 1) identifying a specific problem area; 2) identifying effective communication and problemsolving techniques to use with the problem area; and 3) practicing in session, and eventually experimenting outside the session, with the use of these techniques in the context of significant relationships. Clinical depression is conceptualized in IPT as consisting of three components: 1) symptom formation, 2) social functioning and 3) personality (1). IPT is originally conceptualized as intervening in symptom formation and social functioning and less in personality, given its short duration. More recently, colleagues are adapting IPT for the treatment of adults with borderline personality disorders and so the focus may be broadened.

Modifications for Use with Adolescents

IPT has been selected for use with adolescents due to its developmental relevance to the adolescent population. Interpersonal Psychotherapy for Depressed Adolescents (IPT-A) is active, structured, and includes a large psychoeducational component. As treatment progresses, the adolescent takes more control and develops a more active, action-oriented way of problemsolving (8) that is consistent with appropriate developmental changes in their approach to problemsolving (9). IPT-A emphasizes interpersonal competencies and skills training. Treatment works by addressing the difficulties and enhancing the strengths of the individual, with the goal of increasing independence and interdependence. Thus, IPT-A supports the task of individuation and increased autonomy that is so important to adolescents and therefore makes the treatment attractive to them.

Several alterations have been made to the IPT manual to increase the model's appropriateness for the treatment of adolescent depression. Although the overall goals and problem areas of IPT are employed in IPT-A, the latter also includes a discussion, within the specific problem area, of role transitions for adolescents that are due to family structural change (divorce). This separate discussion of a specific transition is included given the frequency with which it occurs for adolescents, the empirically demonstrated connection to depressive symptoms, and the interpersonal challenges and difficulties that are associated with this situation (10). A second adaptation is the addition of a parent component to the treatment protocol. Although IPT-A is an individual treatment, some degree of involvement on the part of the parent or guardian is needed to promote the wellbeing of the adolescent and to facilitate the success of the treatment. Parent involvement in IPT-A is flexible, though it should minimally include involvement in the initial phase of treatment so as to provide education about the disorder and its treatment. The parent may also be involved as needed in the middle phase to work on specific relationship strategies and it is best if the parent attends a final session to review his or her child's progress in treatment and future treatment needs. The role of the parent or guardian in treatment is presented for each phase of the treatment in the manual (11).

The objectives of treatment have been altered slightly to take into account developmental tasks including individuation, establishment of autonomy, development of romantic relationships, coping with initial experiences of death and loss, and managing peer pressure. Second, the techniques employed in the treatment for working toward the goals of decreasing depressive symptoms and improving interpersonal functioning have been geared toward adolescents. Techniques employed specifically with adolescents include giving them a rating scale from 1 to 10 to rate their mood, which is concrete and makes it easier for them to monitor improvement; doing more basic social skills work; conducting explicit work on perspective-taking skills to counteract adolescent black-and-white thinking about solutions to problems; and learning how to negotiate parent–child tensions. Additional strategies have been identified to address special issues that arise in the treatment of adolescents, such as school refusal, physical or sexual abuse, suicidality, aggression, and involvement of a child protective service agency.

Overview of Efficacy

IPT-A meets four conditions that permit its inclusion as an efficacious treatment: 1) the treatment is manual based (1, 11); 2) the sample characteristics are detailed; 3) the treatment has been tested in randomized clinical trials (12–14); and 4) at least two different investigator teams demonstrated the intervention's effects (15, 16). The efficacy work on IPT-A began with an initial open clinical trial (17) that provided preliminary support for the use of IPT with depressed adolescents and for further study of IPT-A in controlled clinical trials. Since that study, the efficacy of IPT-A has been demonstrated in three randomized controlled clinical trials (12–14). The efficacy clinical trial conducted by Mufson and colleagues (12) included adolescents who met DSM-III-R criteria for major depression. The study showed that IPT-A (N = 24) was superior to clinical management (N = 24) (monitoring of symptoms) with respect to decreasing depressive symptoms, rates of recovery from depression, and rates of retention in treatment for depressed adolescents. In addition, adolescents who received IPT-A demonstrated significant improvement in certain areas of social functioning and interpersonal problemsolving skills compared to adolescents who received clinical management.

Rosselló and Bernal (13), who used a different modification of the adult IPT manual (18), similarly provided independent replication in their study that showed that both IPT (N = 23) and CBT (N = 25) were superior to waitlist control (N = 23) for the treatment of depressed adolescents (N = 71) who met DSM-III criteria for major depressive disorder, dysthymic disorder or both. They also found that IPT was significantly better than the waitlist condition at increasing self-esteem and improving social adaptation. They found that 82% of the adolescents receiving IPT compared to 52% of the adolescents receiving CBT met recovery criteria by the end of treatment.

Current empirical investigations of IPT-A aim to reach a broader range of depressed adolescents by providing treatment in community-based practice settings. A recent effectiveness study compared IPT–A to treatment as usual (TAU) in the school-based health clinics in New York City for depressed adolescents with a broader diagnostic picture including major depression, dysthymia, depression disorder NOS, and adjustment disorder with depressed mood (14). In addition, adolescents were included with comorbid diagnoses including anxiety disorders, ADHD, and oppositional defiant disorder. School-based clinicians delivered both treatments. Treatment as usual consisted of the psychological treatment the adolescents would have received had the study not been in place (generally supportive, individual counseling). Adolescents treated with IPT-A compared to TAU showed greater symptom reduction, significantly better social functioning, and greater decrease in clinical severity of depression and improvement in overall functioning. In addition, the study demonstrated the ability to train community clinicians to deliver IPT-A effectively using a streamlined therapy training program, thereby demonstrating the transportability of IPT-A from the university lab setting to the community (19).

Who is Suitable to Treat with IPT-A?

An integral part of the assessment process is determining an adolescent's suitability for IPT-A based upon diagnosis, severity of illness and impairment, as well as on an assessment of the family environment and willingness to engage in treatment. Based on our clinical experience, the following characteristics of an adolescent make IPT-A a good treatment choice: 1) the adolescent's willingness to work in a one-to-one therapeutic relationship in a time-limited therapy; 2) recognition by the adolescent that there seem to be difficulties of an interpersonal nature that may be causing problems at this time; and 3) a family willing to support the therapy or at least allow the adolescent to participate in treatment.

An adolescent is felt to be suitable for treatment first and foremost if he is willing to acknowledge the depression and is willing to discuss the impact the depression is having on his relationships. An adolescent who is willing to discuss feelings and problems, and explore connections among feelings, events and relationships, is a particularly good candidate for IPT-A. IPT-A is probably most effective with adolescents who have had an acute onset of depressive symptoms and historically have not had chronic and severe interpersonal problems with friends or family. The acute onset increases the likelihood of being able to identify an interpersonal precipitant to the depression and/or exacerbation of a longer standing interpersonal problem. IPT-A may also be helpful to adolescents with longstanding interpersonal problems, but the goals for improvement may need to be more circumscribed.

IPT-A is designed for use with adolescents, ages 12 to 18 years, who have an acute onset of major depression or other milder forms of depression such as dysthymia, an adjustment disorder with depressed mood or depression not otherwise specified. Adolescents are suitable for the treatment if they are of normal intelligence, and are not actively suicidal. Many of the treated adolescents report suicidal ideation consisting of passive thoughts about wanting to be dead but they typically do not report an intent to die or a specific plan to harm themselves. The therapist must feel that once-a-week therapy is sufficient and safe for the adolescent's current level of depression. Depressed adolescents with psychotic symptoms or primary diagnoses of manic depression, substance abuse, or conduct disorders have not been treated with IPT-A. However, depressed adolescents with comorbid anxiety disorders, attention deficit disorder, and oppositional defiant disorder have been treated successfully with IPT-A. If the adolescent has comorbid disorders, a decision should be made confirming that the depression is the appropriate disorder upon which to focus treatment initially.

Prior to the initiation of IPT-A, a thorough diagnostic evaluation of the adolescent should be undertaken to gather information on current symptoms as well as previous psychiatric, family, developmental, medical, social, and academic history. The goals of the diagnostic assessment are to: 1) make a current clinical diagnosis using DSM-IV-TR diagnostic criteria; 2) ascertain the adolescent's level of psychosocial functioning and pinpoint areas of interpersonal problems; and 3) assess which treatment would be most appropriate for the adolescent. This evaluation should be conducted by an intake clinician and/or the IPT-A therapist prior to initiating treatment. Such information should be gathered during the evaluation from the adolescent, parents, and other family members, teachers and other school personnel, and other caretakers such as pediatricians and clergy to facilitate an informed decision about the treatment of choice for the teen (11).

INITIAL PHASE OF THERAPY

IPT-A is divided into three phases: initial, middle, and termination. There are three main components of IPT-A that are evident in the three phases of treatment (Table 6.2.3.1). The initial phase focuses primarily on the first component of psychoeducation with some attention to affect identification. The middle and termination phases focus more directly on affect identification and interpersonal skill building techniques and prevention of relapse.

TABLE 6.2.3.1

INTERPERSONAL PSYCHOTHERAPY: PRIMARY COMPONENTS OF TREATMENT

Education	Affect Identification	Interpersonal Skills Building
■ Psychoeducation ■ Limited sick role ■ Treatment contract	■ Labeling emotions ■ Clarification of emotions ■ Facilitating expression of emotions ■ Monitoring emotions	■ Modeling ■ Use of therapeutic relationship as sample of interpersonal interaction ■ Communication analysis ■ Perspective-taking ■ Interpersonal problem solving ■ Role-playing

Psychoeducation about Depression and IPT-A

There are several tasks to be accomplished during the first session of IPT-A. These include: 1) explaining the nature of depression in adolescents; 2) assigning the limited sick role in treatment; and 3) introducing the basic principles of IPT-A. It is preferable to involve the parents in the first session by dividing the initial IPT-A session into a combination of meetings with the adolescent and parent together, adolescent alone, and parent alone as was done in the pretreatment evaluation. At the conclusion of the initial session, the adolescent and parent(s) should know that the depression symptoms are a) time-limited, b) reflective of a disorder which can be treated successfully, and c) that the adolescent will likely be able to function better with treatment.

Explaining the Nature of Depression in Adolescents. An important task of the first session is to impart information about the course of depression and its treatment to both adolescent and family. This should include a discussion about the symptoms of depression, their impact on functioning, and the prevalence rates of depression in adolescents. It is important for the adolescent and family to know that the prognosis for recovery is good. The adolescent and the parent(s) also need to be informed that there are other treatment options available, including other forms of psychotherapy and/or medication if for some reason IPT-A is not sufficiently effective for this adolescent.

Giving the Adolescent a Limited "Sick Role". The purpose of the limited sick role is to allow the adolescent some relief from the pressure of performing his usual social role at the same level as prior to being depressed, and to receive some extra support for his efforts without punishment for the quality of the work while he recovers. The adolescent and his family are encouraged to think of him as in treatment and as having an illness that affects his motivation and the quality of his performance. Nonetheless, the adolescent is encouraged to maintain the usual social roles in the family, at school, and with friends. Specifically, he needs to get up every morning and get to school, participate in his usual school activities, complete homework, and perform his chores around his house to the best of his abilities. The parent is advised to be supportive, less punitive, and to encourage the adolescent to engage in as many normal activities as possible, while recognizing that the adolescent may have difficulty performing up to par. The assignment of the sick role and psychoeducation can help family members to respond more positively toward the adolescent and shift the blame for difficulties in fulfilling his social roles from the adolescent to the illness (11).

Education about IPT-A. At this point in the session, it is a good idea to introduce the basic structure of IPT-A to the adolescent. The therapist restates that the focus of treatment will be on reducing the depression symptoms he is experiencing and improving relationship difficulties that seem most connected to his depression. The therapist and adolescent together will identify and practice strategies and skills to improve the targeted relationships and in turn improve his mood. Most of the sessions will occur with the therapist and adolescent alone, but they may talk about inviting parents or significant others into a session or two in the middle phase if it looks like it might be helpful.

Interpersonal Inventory

In the remainder of the initial phase, the therapist conducts the Interpersonal Inventory, which is a detailed review of the adolescent's significant relationships, both current and past. To conduct the Interpersonal Inventory, it is helpful for the therapist to use the Closeness Circle (Figure 6.2.3.1). This is a series of concentric circles with the adolescent's name in the center. The goal is to place the adolescent's significant relationships within the appropriate circles of closeness/importance in the teenager's life. The result is a picture of the significant people orbiting the adolescent's life and the emotional valence associated with their position in the adolescent's life.

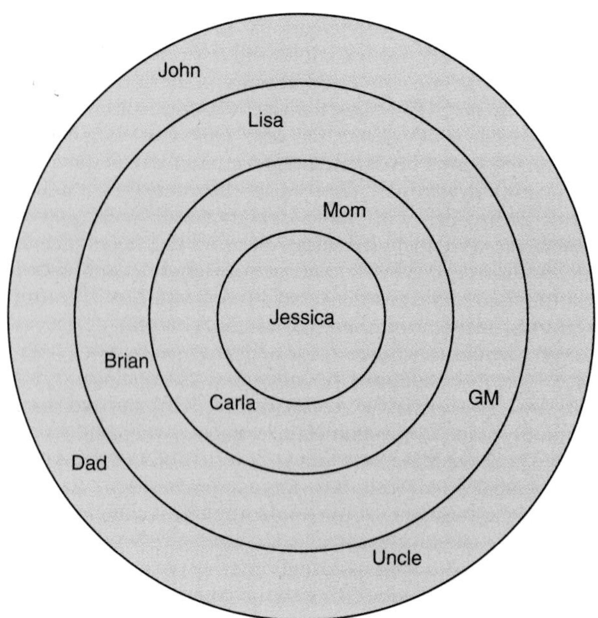

FIGURE 6.2.3.1. Example of a closeness circle.

Once the circle has been completed, the therapist asks detailed questions about each relationship. Examples of questions from the inventory are: "What is your relationship with X like?" "What do you like about X? What don't you like? What types of things do you do with X? Do you ever argue?" The therapist should use these questions to facilitate the adolescent's telling the story of his current life as played out in his significant relationships. It is important when conducting the interpersonal inventory to obtain information about relationships that illustrate interpersonal strengths as well as those that illustrate deficits or areas of weakness.

The Interpersonal Inventory facilitates the adolescent and the therapist's understanding of the interpersonal context of the depression. The therapist gathers information about events that may have precipitated the depressive episode, the reasons for seeking treatment now, and what has been happening in these significant relationships that may be associated with the onset of symptoms. Although the emphasis is on current relationships, obtaining a complete picture of the adolescent's social relationships including some information about past relationships and interpersonal functioning is helpful in understanding his overall patterns of interaction and communication in his relationships. The therapist can think of it as the diagnostic assessment of interpersonal symptoms to parallel the completed assessment of depression symptoms. This inventory provides the necessary interpersonal data to select one of the four problem areas for focus in the middle phase.

Formulation of Problem Area and Making a Treatment Contract

By the end of the fourth session, the therapist will have completed a comprehensive interpersonal assessment and will conclude the session with an interpersonal formulation linking the adolescent's interpersonal situation with his depressed mood and placing the formulation within the framework of one of the four problem areas. The problem area formulation should occur as a natural outgrowth of the recent discussions. It is helpful for the therapist to weave the narratives of each relationship into one larger interpersonal narrative for the adolescent, pointing out any noticeable patterns across relationships. The therapist should seek the adolescent's opinion of the formulation, giving the adolescent the opportunity to acknowledge the issues, show understanding, and have the opportunity to disagree.

Setting the treatment contract involves outlining the adolescent's and parents' roles in the treatment, identifying treatment goals, clarifying expectations for treatment, and outlining the nuts and bolts of treatment. Both the improvement in interpersonal functioning and reduction of symptoms are equally important achievements and most frequently will cooccur. Therapist and adolescent should set goals that are likely to be attainable within the brief treatment so that the adolescent can feel the goals were achieved and can have a sense of progress throughout the treatment. The culmination of this discussion is a specific verbal treatment contract.

MIDDLE PHASE OF THERAPY

Following agreement on the treatment contract and the identified problem area, the middle phase of treatment begins. Typically this occurs by session 5 and continues through session 9. Session 9 is a transitional session in which the work of the middle phase continues while the therapist begins to discuss concluding the treatment in several weeks. The middle sessions focus on the problem area identified in the initial sessions as a means toward achieving recovery from depression. The objectives of the middle phase of treatment for all adolescents include: 1) further clarification of the problem area; 2) identification of effective strategies to attack the problem; and 3) implementation of interventions to bring about resolution of the problem. The therapist's general tasks associated with the middle phase of treatment are as follows: 1) monitoring depression symptoms and the need to consider adjunctive therapy such as medication if there is no improvement or a worsening of symptoms; 2) facilitating the adolescent's self-disclosure of his affective state; and 3) keeping in contact with parents to support and participate in treatment as necessary (11).

During the middle phase of treatment, the therapist and adolescent continually assess the accuracy of the initial formulation of the problem to maximize the amount of change that can be accomplished in the treatment. The therapist must keep the adolescent's discussions relevant to the identified problem areas. The therapist helps generate strategies and suggests the application of techniques that will lead to clarification and resolution of the adolescent's problem. This includes illuminating the process of identifying problems, clarifying the issues, generating strategies, applying strategies for problem resolution, and acquiring skills that result in increased interpersonal self-confidence and improved functioning.

Therapeutic Techniques

During the middle phase of the treatment, the therapist teaches the adolescent specific strategies that can help him deal with his interpersonal difficulties within one or two problem areas. The therapeutic relationship in IPT-A provides a forum in which skills can be practiced and feedback can be given in a nonthreatening environment (11). IPT-A techniques include exploratory techniques, encouragement of affect, communication analysis, behavior change techniques (including decision analysis and role plays), use of the therapeutic relationship and adjunctive techniques such as interpersonal experiments. Exploratory techniques can be either directive or nondirective. Directive exploratory techniques include targeted questioning and interviewing. The nondirective techniques include supportive acknowledgment, and extension of the topic being discussed by the adolescent (11). Encouragement of affect involves facilitating discussion of painful feelings about events or issues and helping the adolescent use his affective experiences to better understand the link between mood and relationships and eventually to make interpersonal change.

Communication analysis is a thorough investigation of a specific dialogue or argument that occurred between an adolescent and another person. Communication analysis identifies ways in which the adolescent's communication is ineffective and fails to achieve the goal of the communication. In conducting the communication analysis, the therapist can illustrate how changing one phrase can change the entire feeling about the interaction and the other person. Decision analysis is employed by the therapist to help the adolescent consider a range of alternative actions that he can take and the possible consequences associated with each of those actions. In role-playing, the therapist and adolescent act out the skills that the adolescent is learning in the treatment in a nonthreatening way. The therapist can model many useful interpersonal skills such as: affective expression, effective communication and decision making strategies. Adjunctive techniques include work assignments to be done at home between the sessions. The assignments usually involve practicing specific skills that were the focus of the sessions. They are referred to as "interpersonal experiments" or "work at home."

Interpersonal Problem Areas

As in the adult version of IPT, there are four identified problem areas in IPT-A upon which the therapy can be focused: 1) grief due to death; 2) interpersonal disputes with friends, teachers, parents and siblings; 3) role transitions such as changing schools (elementary to junior high or junior high to high school), entering puberty, becoming sexually active, birth of another sibling, becoming a parent, parental divorce, illness of a parent; and/or 4) interpersonal deficits such as difficulty initiating and maintaining relationships and communicating about feelings (11). When there seem to be two problem areas, the therapist should identify a primary and possibly a secondary problem area.

1. *Grief* is defined in IPT-A as loss through death. The grieving process can be abnormal by being delayed, distorted, or by becoming a chronic reaction. The IPT-A therapist helps by reconstructing the adolescent's relationship with the deceased, addressing unresolved issues in the relationship, linking the depression to the feelings for the deceased, providing empathic listening to help facilitate the mourning process, and assisting the adolescent in establishing new relationships. The IPT-A therapist can use these strategies to similarly help adolescents who are suffering while in the midst of the normal grieving process.
2. *Interpersonal disputes* for adolescents tend to occur within the context of family, peer or school relationships. They can be conceptualized as a situation in which the adolescent and other parties have diverging expectations of a situation and this conflict is severe enough to lead to significant distress. In these circumstances, IPT-A aims to define how intractable the dispute is, the specific stage of the dispute, and identify sources of misunderstanding

via faulty communication, poor perspective-taking, and invalid or unreasonable expectations. The therapist aims to intervene by using communication training, problemsolving or other techniques that facilitate change in the situation.

3. *Role transitions* are situations in which the adolescent is having difficulty adapting to a change in life circumstances. These may be developmental crises or adaptations following life events or relationship dissolutions. In those who develop depression, these transitions are often experienced as losses and hence contribute to the development of psychopathology. IPT-A aims to help the adolescent to reappraise the old and new roles, to identify sources of difficulty in the new role, identify skills and strategies that would make it easier to adapt to the new role, and to develop skills and implement solutions for these difficulties in their significant relationships.
4. *Interpersonal deficits* are identified as the problem area when an adolescent reports impoverished interpersonal relationships in both number and quality of the relationships. In many cases, the adolescent and therapist will need to focus upon old relationships as well as the relationship with the therapist. In the former, common themes should be identified and linked to current circumstances. In using the therapeutic relationship, the therapist aims to identify problematic processes, such as deficits in initiating or maintaining relationships, and will aim to modify these by practicing approaches to developing new relationships. By practicing the interpersonal skills with the therapist, the therapeutic relationship can serve as a template for other relationships that the adolescent will be striving to develop.

TERMINATION PHASE

A termination date is set with the adolescent and family at the beginning of treatment and the adolescent is reminded of the number of weeks remaining until the end of treatment. Twelve weeks is the time frame chosen for the clinical trials assessing the efficacy of IPT-A. It is a reasonable duration for adolescents who are reluctant to stay in treatment for any significant length of time. The time period can be modified in either direction. The important issue is to retain the treatment's time-limited nature by setting the initial treatment contract for the number of weeks that seem most appropriate for that adolescent.

Tasks of Termination

The termination phase includes clarification of the adolescent's warning symptoms of future depressive episodes, identification of successful strategies that were used in the therapy, generalization of skills to future situations, emphasis on mastery of new interpersonal skills, and discussion of the need for further treatment (11). The therapist needs to balance the tasks of the termination phase with concluding work on the identified problem area. It is crucial to devote a major portion of the termination phase to reviewing interpersonal strategies used during the middle phase and to applying these strategies to ongoing and future situations. This may help reduce relapse and recurrence, which are common in adolescent depression, improve social self-confidence, and enable the adolescent to negotiate successful endings of other relationships at future points in his life.

Throughout the treatment and termination, the therapist should identify the changes that she observes in the adolescent: improved communication and ability to see another person's perspective, attempts made to negotiate a dispute, increased awareness about his own feelings associated with a relationship, successful mourning of the loss and/or the establishment of new relationships. The therapist and adolescent together highlight how specific strategies have enabled him to make improvements within his identified problem area, in specific relationships, and most importantly in his mood.

Terminating treatment with an adolescent also means terminating treatment with the family. Ideally, the therapist will conduct a final termination session with the adolescent alone and then have another joint termination session for the adolescent and family. The therapist also may see the parents alone if necessary or if the adolescent prefers it that way. The goals of the final session for the family are similar to those of the adolescent's final session: a review of the adolescent's presenting symptoms, initial goals for the therapy, achievement of these goals, and a discussion of the changes in the family interactions and functioning as a result of the therapy. The termination phase enables both the adolescent and parent to participate in the review of accomplishments and the identification of areas that would benefit from further treatment. It is important to discuss with the family, the possible recurrence of mild symptoms shortly after termination, the need for further treatment if it is indicated, and management of future recurrent episodes of depression.

There are adolescents for whom there has been some improvement, but who are still moderately symptomatic at the conclusion of treatment. Further treatment may be necessary under certain circumstances when the symptoms have not fully remitted or when there are other more chronic problems contributing to the adolescent's impairment. This information is utilized by the family, adolescent and therapist to make decisions about the need for further treatment and the type of additional treatment that may be needed.

SPECIAL ISSUES

Working with Parents

Due to high divorce rates as well as increases in single-parent families, adolescents often live in nonnuclear families, including homes of other relatives and foster or group homes. As with the parents, these people are important in the adolescent's daily life and must be educated about the nature of depression, ways to support the adolescent's recovery and, if necessary, participate in the treatment to facilitate changes in the home environment that will play a role in the adolescent's recovery.

Awareness and understanding of the mental health status of an adolescent's parent or guardian is critical to understanding the adolescent's depression and developing the most effective treatment plan. In cases where the parent is depressed, it is often necessary for the adolescent's therapist to help the adolescent by first helping the parent find an appropriate referral for his/her own treatment. It is important to explain that in the IPT-A framework, depression affects the parents' as well as the teen's interpersonal functioning. Any alleviation of parental depression is likely to reduce the stress the adolescent is facing.

Depressed parents often model a depressive interpersonal style that can range from ineffective communication and conflict negotiation skills to social withdrawal and helplessness. Therefore, when these adolescents try to practice new interpersonal skills at home, they face an uphill battle. In such cases, the therapist and adolescent will need to do more in-session practice of interpersonal strategies as well as have the adolescent identify others in his life with whom he can practice these skills. Enlisting the parent as a "coach" and "collaborator" in the treatment can foster the parent's willingness to support the adolescent's experiments with new skills, both during and outside of the session. Having a good grasp of the role of parental depression in the family allows the adolescent and therapist to develop realistic treatment goals and focus on the relationships that can have the greatest impact on increasing his feelings of support and decreasing his depressed mood (11).

Not all parents, unfortunately, are open to intervention for themselves or their child. In these situations, the therapist should, with the adolescent's approval, attempt to intervene with the parent during an in-person meeting, or over the phone if the parent is unable to attend a session. The therapist, using an empathic and nonjudgmental psychoeducational approach, can sometimes alter the parent's perspective and enjoin them to support the treatment. If the parent continues to be resistant to collaborating in the treatment, the therapist will need to work with the adolescent on a modified treatment plan.

Use of Medication with IPT-A

The use of IPT-A in combination with medication has not been studied in a clinical trial; however, it is frequently used this way in our general outpatient psychiatry clinics with benefits to the adolescent. Most of the clinical trials have included a homogenous sample of adolescents who typically have a depression disorder with a possible anxiety disorder, excluding adolescents with other disorders such as conduct disorder or substance abuse (19). In the clinics, the adolescents may present with depression and other comorbid disorders that may require a combination of medication and IPT-A. Antidepressant medication is not contraindicated during IPT-A and, in fact, may be a useful adjunctive treatment for severely depressed adolescents whose symptoms do not remit during the initial phase of treatment. The main goal of any acute phase of treatment, medication, or psychotherapy is to achieve a timely treatment response measured by remission of the depressive symptoms. Therefore, if the adolescent is not responding as well as one would like to the therapy, it is advisable to consider adding an adjunctive treatment.

Our guidelines are to consider antidepressants if there is little or no remission of symptoms after four weeks of IPT-A. Experience treating adolescents suffering from a more chronic depression (either dysthymia or chronic major depression) suggests that medication might be beneficial from the outset of treatment to help alleviate the hopelessness and listlessness that often characterize these adolescents and prevent them for more actively engaging in psychotherapy (11). The clinician should discuss with the adolescent and his parents the reasons for considering medication: that the adolescent is still showing significant signs of depression or significant anhedonia and lethargy, and that in such instances medication can often be beneficial. The guidelines for the use of IPT-A in conjunction with medication evolved from our clinical experience using IPT-A to treat depressed adolescents. More research is needed to assess the efficacy of using both medication and IPT-A to treat adolescent depression and its comorbid disorders.

Crisis Management

Crises are not infrequent during the treatment of a depressed adolescent. A crisis is a major change in the adolescent's living situation, interpersonal relationships, family relationships, or emotional wellbeing that jeopardizes the adolescent's psychological health and overwhelms the adolescent's capacity to cope with the situation. Examples of crises include: running away, pregnancy, illness in family or friend, involvement with the law, exposure or involvement in violence (11). The first task facing the IPT-A therapist is to determine the nature and etiology of the crisis by speaking both to the adolescent and other parties involved. In the case of suicidal or homicidal ideation, if an appointment cannot be set up soon enough, the adolescent should be sent to the nearest emergency room to evaluate the need for hospitalization or an increase in the frequency and intensity of the treatment. The therapist's most important decision is whether or not the adolescent can remain in IPT-A or whether the adolescent must receive other types of services either at the same or another facility.

If the adolescent is evaluated as being able to remain in outpatient adolescent treatment, the IPT-A treatment contract should be reexamined and revised as necessary. Such items in the contract that may change include the frequency of the sessions, involvement of the family, frequency of phone calls between therapist and adolescent, and the identified problem area that is the focus of the treatment. At times the crisis may suggest that a significant problem area was overlooked or there may be an interaction between two problem areas, thus requiring a shift in the focus of the sessions. With the new contract, the therapist can move forward to address the new information about the adolescent's interpersonal relationships and the context of the depression.

TRAINING IN IPT-A

In the IPT-A efficacy study, therapists received two days of didactics and then treated three cases for training purposes, videotaping every session and receiving 1 hour of supervision for each session. A random selection of these tapes was rated by experts for therapist competency prior to certifying the therapists to participate in the clinical trial. Such an intensive training program is not feasible in effectiveness research due to constraints on the clinicians' time, nor is it realistic for training clinicians to implement the treatment in their practices. Clinicians in community-based settings routinely have pressing clinical demands competing for their time so that the training program in the effectiveness study was abbreviated to one full day of didactics and the practice cases characteristic of the efficacy trials were eliminated.

Nonetheless, when it comes to training and certifying clinicians as IPT-A therapists, the intensity of the efficacy model of therapist training is still believed to produce the best adherence and competence in IPT-A. In addition, to be considered an IPT-A supervisor of other clinicians in training, at least another two training cases with supervision are typically required, along with consultation on the supervision of several cases to ensure that the therapist feels confident and can competently train others in the use of the IPT-A model. The International Society for Interpersonal Psychotherapy (ISIPT) is currently working to settle upon guidelines for the training and certification of IPT therapists.

CONCLUSIONS

IPT for depressed adolescents (IPT-A) is an evidence-based psychotherapy that is based on the premise that depression occurs in an interpersonal context. The goals of treatment are to improve the adolescent's interpersonal relationships and his depression symptoms. IPT-A is defined in a treatment manual that is adapted to address the developmental needs of adolescents and their families in a time limited approach (11). IPT-A is unique in that it has been demonstrated to be effective both in the laboratory and community setting and when delivered by expert and community clinicians (12–14). Furthermore, IPT-A has been demonstrated to be efficacious with an underserved Latino population that typically has less access to treatment services (12). Research studies and clinical experience point to the utility of IPT-A as a treatment for adolescent depression. Clinical experience further suggests the benefits of combining IPT-A with medication for adolescents with more severe depression. However, a controlled clinical trial is needed to examine this question empirically.

References

1. Weissman MM, Markowitz JC, Klerman GL: *A comprehensive Guide to Interpersonal Psychotherapy*. Albany, Basic Books, 2000.
2. Coyne JC: Toward an interactional description of depression. *Psychiatry* 39(1):28–40, 1976.
3. Hammen C: The emergence of an interpersonal approach to depression. In: Joiner T, Coyne J (eds): *The Interactional Nature of Depression: Advances in Interpersonal Approaches*. Washington, DC, American Psychological Association, 1999, pp. 22–36.
4. Joiner T, Coyne J, Blalock J: On the interpersonal nature of depression: Overview and synthesis. In: Joiner T, Coyne J (eds): *The Interactional Nature of Depression: Advances in Interpersonal Approaches*. Washington, DC, American Psychological Association; 1999, pp. 3–20.
5. Meyer A: *Psychobiology: A Science of Man*. Springfield, IL, Charles C, Thomas, 1957.
6. Sullivan HS: *The Interpersonal Theory of Psychiatry*. New York: W.W. Norton & Co., 1953.
7. Bowlby J: Attachment theory and its therapeutic implications. *Adolesc Psychiatry* 6:5–33, 1978.
8. Mufson L, Dorta KP: Interpersonal psychotherapy for depressed adolescents: theory, practice and research. In: Esman AH (ed): *The Annals of the American Society for Adolescent Psychiatry*, 148–164, 2000.
9. Marx EM, Schulze CC: Interpersonal problem-solving in depressed students. *J Clin Psychol* 47(3):361–370, 1991.
10. Hetherington EM, Bridges M, Insabella GM: What matters? What does not? Five perspectives on the association between marital transitions and children's adjustment. *Am Psychol* 53(2):167–184, 1998.
11. Mufson L, Dorta KP, Moreau D, Weissman MM: *Interpersonal Psychotherapy for Depressed Adolescents*, 2nd ed. New York, Guilford Publications, Inc., 2004.
12. Mufson L, Weissman MM, Moreau D, Garfinkel R: Efficacy of interpersonal psychotherapy for depressed adolescents. *Arch Gen Psychiatry* 56(6):573–579, 1999.
13. Rossello J, Bernal G: The efficacy of cognitive-behavioral and interpersonal treatments for depression in Puerto Rican adolescents. *J Consult Clin Psychol* 67(5):734–745, 1999.
14. Mufson L, Dorta KP, Wickramaratne P, Nomura Y, Olfson M, Weissman MM: A randomized effectiveness trial of interpersonal psychotherapy for depressed adolescents. *Arch Gen Psychiatry* 61(6):577–584, 2004.
15. Chambless DL, Hollon SD: Defining empirically supported therapies. *J Consult Clin Psychol* 66(1):7–18, 1998.
16. Chorpita BF: The frontier of evidence-based practice. In: Kazdin AE, Weisz JR (eds): *Evidence-Based Psychotherapies for Children and Adolescents*. New York: Guilford Press; 42–59.
17. Mufson L, Moreau D, Weissman MM, Wickramaratne P, Martin J, Samoilov A. Modification of interpersonal psychotherapy with depressed adolescents (IPT-A): Phase I and II studies. *J Am Acad Child Adolesc Psychiatry* 33(5):695–705, 1994.
18. Klerman GL, Weissman MM, Rousanaville BJ, Chevron ES: *Interpersonal Therapy of Depression*. New York: Basic Books, 1984.
19. Mufson LH, Dorta KP, Olfson M, Weissman MM, Hoagwood K: Effectiveness research: Transporting interpersonal psychotherapy for depressed adolescents (IPT-A) from the lab to school-based health clinics. *Clin Child Fam Psychol Rev* 7(4):251–461, 2004.

CHAPTER 6.2.4 ■ PSYCHODYNAMIC PRINCIPLES IN PRACTICE

RACHEL Z. RITVO AND SAMUEL RITVO

HISTORY

The monumental work of Sigmund Freud looms so large in the field of dynamic psychiatry that students in the twenty-first century easily equate Freudian psychoanalysis with dynamic psychiatry. However, it is useful to place psychodynamic psychiatry in a broader context both historically and epistemologically. Gabbard (1) describes the several uses of the term *dynamic* in the late nineteenth century by Leibniz, Herbart, Fechner, and the renowned neurologist Hughlings Jackson. In their usage, dynamic was contrasted with static. It referred to changing states of consciousness and physiologic processes, as opposed to anatomic structures. Dynamic included a concept of mental energy. It implied functional rather than fixed organic impairment. In the twentieth century dynamic psychiatry—with its emphasis on the patient's subjective experience, the workings of unconscious psychological processes, and the patient's unique inner life—was contrasted with *descriptive* psychiatry, which strove to categorize patients according to observable behavior.

Psychodynamic psychotherapy of children began with Freud's publication (2) of the case of "Little Hans." Freud's interest was not the treatment of children but the centrality of childhood experience in shaping the adult psyche. Although he sought to "reconstruct" childhood experience from the analysis of adults, he encouraged his students to observe children for "a more direct and less round about proof" of the existence of infantile sexuality. It was in this context that Freud came to supervise the analysis of Little Hans by Hans' father.

Hermine Von Hug-Hellmuth was the first to undertake psychoanalytic therapy of children and adolescents. Her paper "On the Technique of Child-Analysis" (3) surveyed technical aspects of the psychodynamic treatment of children recognized as core issues to this day. She noted that the child does not come of his own accord. She advises against a judgmental stance or the giving of direct commissions and prohibitions. Hug-Hellmuth demonstrated her engagement of the child in "talking over things together." She introduced the role of an educational method founded on psychoanalytic knowledge. She examined the multiple ways in which work with children and adolescents differs from that with adults, including the complexities of the relationship between the analyst and the child's parents. Her observation that the child's spontaneous play could stand in the place of the verbal communications of the adult to reveal unconscious conflict was most significant for the development of psychodynamic therapy with children. Further, she observed that fully conscious avowal of analytic understanding was not a prerequisite for therapeutic effect in children.

Melanie Klein (4) and Anna Freud (5) emerged as the founders of child psychoanalysis. Klein coined the term play analysis, emphasizing the child's play as equivalent to free association in adult analysis. Her methods encouraged early, deep interpretations and minimized the analyst's contact with parents and teachers. Anna Freud's long career, from the 1920s to her death in 1982, allowed for significant evolution in her ideas regarding psychodynamic treatment of children and adolescents. Trained as a teacher, she was interested in the "educative" functions of the analyst in addition to the interpretive functions. Her work on ego mechanisms of defense (6) led to the development of defense analysis of children and adolescents. Her attention to observing the developmental process in children led her to conceptualize interweaving lines of development (7). Emigrant analysts in the wake of World War II brought both Kleinian and Freudian ideas to America. Child analytic training took root in the United States, allowing child psychoanalysts to play a major role in the training of child and adolescent psychiatrists throughout the mid- and late twentieth century.

Two distinctly American therapeutic traditions, admittedly influenced and stimulated by the frisson of psychoanalytic thought, have contributed their own unique emphases to the field of dynamic psychotherapy with children, particularly play therapy. The contributions of the child guidance movement (8) and client-centered therapy (9) to the development of dynamic play therapy reminds one not to equate "psychoanalytic" with "psychodynamic." Homegrown American psychodynamic therapists such as Frederick Allen and Carl Rogers sought to counteract the impact of the American behaviorist tradition. Allen wrote:

> The behaviorists advanced the belief that a child with relatively normal equipment could be made into anything parents wanted him to be if they exercised their power, adequately and intelligently, in the first few years of the child's life. The child was seen as little more than a by-product of another's desire .... This created a distortion of a parent's sense of responsibility ... [and a] failure to appreciate the nature of growth and the participation of both child and parent in the child's development (8).

Allen regarded the child:

> as an individual who could be helped to grow and to become a person in his own right ... the child was included as an active participant in the relationship designed to help him. Instead of being seen as an object to be changed, he was accepted as a human being with the capacity to change (8).

The child's exercise of free expression, a here-and-now focus, and the rapport in the relationship between patient and therapist were emphasized as "nondirective" therapy developed through the work of Axline (10) and Dorfman (11).

John Bowlby (12–14) was a psychoanalyst who broke with the mainstreams of mid-twentieth century child psychoanalysis in Britain and America by taking a strong empirical approach to studying psychoanalytic developmental constructs. His focus was on the direct observation of the behavior of infants and their caregivers through prospective studies of the effects of early attachment on relationships and on personality development. Attachment theory has bridged the gap between clinical psychodynamic theory and general psychology, particularly developmental psychology. In the past decade a rapprochement has occurred between attachment researchers and clinical psychodynamic researchers, with a new interest in empirical validation of psychoanalytic concepts and empirical tools to test the efficacy of therapeutic approaches. Of particular interest has been the elucidation of the impact of attachment history on patients' capacity for mentalization, also referred to as reflective function and defined as "the ability to take account of one's own and others' mental states in understanding why people behave in specific ways (p. 470) (15)." An example of treatments developed by drawing on this research is Bleiberg's relational approach to the treatment of personality disorder in children and adolescents (16).

DEFINITION

Psychotherapy has been defined as a treatment that ameliorates psychopathologic conditions, functional impairments, and developmental disturbances by means of psychological processes and a therapeutic relationship with a trained therapist (17, 18). In the treatment of children and adolescents these three elements—psychopathology, psychological processes, and the therapeutic relationship—should be considered in the context of the patient's social environment and ongoing development (19). Psychodynamic psychotherapy aims at bringing about change in psychological processes that are largely unconscious but can be inferred from observable phenomena, such as actions or speech. The processes determining the inner world of subjective experience are of particular interest. The plethora of unconscious processes of which the human brain is capable allows for great diversity of focus for dynamic psychotherapy.

Psychodynamic therapy capitalizes on the observation that human beings are psychologically changed by relationships with other human beings. Psychodynamic technique utilizes two aspects of human relationships to achieve this mutative effect. Particular attention is paid to *transference,* the unconscious displacement onto the therapist of patterns of feelings, thoughts, and behavior originally experienced in relation to significant figures during childhood. Additionally, the manifest or "real" relationship between the therapist and patient is used to further the aims of the treatment.

The psychodynamic therapist conceptualizes psychopathologic conditions, functional impairments, and developmental disturbances in terms of unconscious psychological processes inferred from the observed symptoms and the patient's history. Similarly, social context and developmental and maturational factors are evaluated for both their role in the etiology of the condition and potential interventions in the social environment that would affect the patient's unconscious, internal psychological functions, e.g., defenses, self-concept, ego ideal, conscience, and reflective function.

PSYCHODYNAMIC THEORY

Psychodynamic therapy requires as a foundation a theory of the functioning of the unconscious mind and the internal experience of the individual as well as a theory of the psychological impact of human relationships. Psychoanalysis provides a rich tradition of observation and theory on which dynamic therapists can draw. Sigmund Freud was a research neuroscientist at the cutting edge of his era before he turned to the clinical practice of neurology and eventually psychiatry. Although he recognized that the research methods of his time did not allow for a full explication of the neuronal base of psychic events, he endeavored to keep his psychological theories consistent with biology. For instance,

Freud conceptualized the mind as the interplay of excitatory (drive) and inhibitory (defense) phenomena. Greatly influenced by the Darwinian theories of the German zoologist Carl Claus, with whom he trained (20), Freud sought to construct a developmental framework for his psychology, an approach that put the psychic phenomena of childhood in the spotlight and paved the way for child psychotherapy. Psychoanalytic psychology as a theory of adaptation of the organism to its environment derived from these Darwinian roots, as did the "libidinal drive" as an aspect of the innate striving for survival and reproduction and the concept of conflicting forces within the mind. Modern neuroscience offers an opportunity to refine psychoanalytic theory. The growing field of neuropsychoanalysis seeks to integrate the latest findings from cognitive neuroscience with psychoanalytic observations to improve our understanding of the brain substrates of psychoanalytic constructs (21).

Freud (22) used the Darwinian concept of a *complemental series* to position himself as a centrist in the nature–nurture controversy over the origins of psychopathology with severe constitutional deficits at one end of the spectrum of pathogenic etiology and severely traumatic experiences at the other. The psychodynamic therapist utilizes these complementary series to evaluate the interaction and impact of nature and nurture on the patient's pathology.

In dynamic theory the mind is not seen as a blank slate at birth but rather as endowed with the biological potential to develop psychic structure given an adequate environment. *Internalization* denotes the process by which experiences with the external world, usually in the realm of relationships, form stable intrapsychic structures or capacities. Once a process is internalized it no longer requires an external stimulus for its function to be executed. *Identification,* the psychological process by which one individual becomes like another, is a familiar mechanism of internalization.

Unconscious psychological processes may be considered as primary determinants of the inner world of subjective experience. The individual's total subjective experiential world, including thoughts, feelings, and fantasies as well as perceptions of the external world, regardless of whether they accurately reflect the external world as viewed by another observer, has been designated *psychic reality.* The dynamic therapist attempts to grasp the patient's psychic reality and convey to the patient an interest in understanding his experience of himself.

A primary tenet of psychoanalysis is *psychic determinism* (23), the principle that nothing in the mind happens by chance or in a random way. All psychic acts and events have meanings and causes and can be understood in terms of earlier psychic events. The mind retains experiences and is shaped by them. Conscious thoughts and overt behaviors provide observable clues to their underlying unconscious psychic determinants. A corollary hypothesis, *overdeterminism* or *multideterminism,* states that a psychic event (e.g., a symptom), is typically caused by more than one factor and may serve more than one purpose in the psychic framework. The multidetermined nature of symptoms provides the psychodynamic therapist with more than one way to approach a symptom. This clinical flexibility is very appealing to the practitioner but frustrating to researchers who seek standardization of method.

The concept of multideterminism is further refined in dynamic theory by the observation that the multiple determinants of a particular observable psychic phenomenon are frequently in opposition or *conflict* with one another. Psychodynamic theorists have identified several types of psychic conflict. *External conflict* denotes the conflicts that arise between the child and the environment, the consequent frustration demanding management by the child's psyche. External conflicts are most evident in early childhood when the infant or toddler has little internal restraint and struggles with the caretaker over such matters as bedtime or playing with an electrical plug. As prohibitions become internalized, the conflicts become *internal.* Not all conflicts are caused by prohibitions. Conflicts may arise between competing urges, thereby creating ambivalence. For example, conflicts arise between urges toward passive-dependence and active-mastery. An external conflict may or may not become a fully *internalized conflict.* An internalized conflict is conceptualized as continuing in the individual's psyche when environmental forces that triggered the initial internal conflict no longer exist.

Freud realized that a conceptual tool was needed to provide an orienting and systematizing framework for clinical data and hypotheses about unconscious phenomena and subjective experience. He termed such a tool "metapsychology" and offered several different models as he strove to find a conceptual frame that accommodated all his data. The most lasting of Freud's metapsychological frameworks was a structural theory, *the tripartite model,* which divides mental functions into *id, ego,* and *superego.* Id is a concept that encompasses the mental representations of the instinctual drives (24). *Drive* is a term applied to a stimulus arising within the individual that arouses the mind and incites mental activity. The term ego encompasses all the capacities of the mind to manage and channel the arousal and activity incited by the drives. Freud, with an apt metaphor, says of ego:

> in its relation to the id it is like a man on horseback, who has to hold in check the superior strength of the horse.... Often a rider, if he is not to be parted from his horse, is obliged to guide it where it wants to go; so in the same way the ego is in the habit of transforming the id's will into action as if it were its own (25).

Superego functions conceptualize the inner voice of conscience, which maintains ideals and values, observing and criticizing any shortfall of the self.

For many students id is difficult to conceptualize and to recognize in the clinical situation. "Id" did not make its way into the vernacular to the extent that "ego" did, nor is "drive" or "internal stimulus" as close to a common usage as "conscience," which makes "superego" more accessible to the untutored ear. The internal stimuli that are most familiar to the average person are feelings. Because emotions arise from genetically endowed, physiologic response patterns, they are an early, although in psychoanalytic theory not primary, step in the pathway to arousal and mental activity. In psychoanalytic parlance affects serve a signal function triggering ego efforts to manage drives. The drives themselves may be thought of as genetically endowed motivational states. Commonly we think of these as urges, needs, wishes, and desires.

Advances in neuroscience have identified at least four basic mammalian instinctual mechanisms that might be correlated with the id of psychoanalytic theory: a seeking/reward/curiosity system, an anger-rage system, a fear-anxiety system, and a panic system (26). The classical Freudian nomenclature works with a dualistic system of an aggressive and sexual drive. The sexual or *libidinal* drive includes affiliative and pleasure-seeking urges. A child who enjoys being bathed by the parent and having his or her naked body admired is displaying a derivative of the libidinal drive. The pleasure the child takes from the sensuous experience of the water would also be a libidinal drive derivative. The aggressive drive in its broad connotation includes impulses toward self-assertion and the desire to prevail in one's wishes. This urge to prevail brings forth the more colloquially recognized aspect of the aggressive drive when in the face of frustration the urge to prevail becomes an urge to subjugate or destroy the perceived source of frustration. Pleasure in motoric or mental activity is an aggressive drive derivative at a basic level. Because pleasures sought in response to libidinal drive inevitably run into some requirement for delay or other frustration in the external world, aggressive and libidinal drives are intimately related; ego mechanisms must develop to regulate aggressive drives if libidinal drives are to be satisfied. In this metapsychological model, a clinical formulation that failed to assess the role of aggressive drive in symptom formation would not be complete.

Many theorists and clinicians have been dissatisfied with Freud's dual drive approach. When using conceptual models other than the tripartite model they postulate other motivating forces within the individual. For example, Miller (27), applying Kohut's *self-psychology* to children, proposes three primary drives: the drive toward internal integration, the will to do, and the need for others. Whichever conceptual framework is utilized, dynamic psychotherapy sees the individual's motivations, impulses, and desires as important determinants of subjective experience, mental functioning, and behavior.

In the tripartite model of the mind, ego includes all the mental capacities available to the individual for regulation of the internal milieu and adaptation to external reality. Ego's task is to optimize pleasure and gratification of wishes and needs while maintaining internal equilibrium, the health of the body, good relations with the external world, and peace with superego. Although ego includes all the mental capacities for engaging with external reality, it also focuses on internal reality. As with id, there is no single psychodynamic approach to describing or organizing all the phenomena that can be subsumed in the concept of ego. One approach divides basic categories of ego functions into reality testing, object relations, regulation of affect, thought, defensive activity, autonomous functions, and synthetic or integrative functions. Work with children requires examining each of these functions in the context of the child's age and developmental accomplishments.

In the broad range of psychological theories, defensive ego activity and the capacity for object relations are conceptualizations of mental functioning most uniquely attributable to psychodynamic theory. *Defense* is a term describing ego efforts to protect against *internal* dangers. From experience with loved persons on whom the child is entirely dependent for survival, the child internalizes the displeasure expressed by the caretaker toward unacceptable drive derivatives, such as biting the nipple when nursing, and identifies with the pleasure expressed toward socially acceptable drive derivatives, such as biting and chewing finger foods. Ego is challenged to restrain prohibited expressions and promote approved expressions of inner urges once this process of internalizing permissions and prohibitions has begun. Psychoanalytic observations reveal how fear of the disappearance or loss of the loved caretaker, the "object" of object relations, generates a need for defensive maneuvers. The psychological maneuver by which the inhibition is accomplished is termed a *mechanism of defense.* The fear shifts from fear of loss of the object itself to fear of loss of the object's love with increasing ego maturity and development in an environment of "good enough" parenting. Fear of loss of body integrity, often referred to as castration anxiety, enters the signaling system with further development. Finally, as superego functions and ego ideals develop, unpleasant affects of shame, guilt, and remorse stimulate restraint. Intense anxiety and mobilization of powerful and often primitive defenses occur when coping capacities are on the verge of being overwhelmed by massive overstimulation or frustration, for example, with acute or chronic trauma or the upsurge of urges associated with the onset of puberty.

Defense mechanisms are typically unconscious, automatic, psychological processes. The individual does not consciously choose to institute a defense; however, an individual can learn to recognize defensive activity as it occurs through dynamic psychotherapy, psychoanalysis, or self-analysis (28). Anna Freud's classic *The Ego and the Mechanisms of Defense* (6) enumerated several patterns of defense already in the analytic literature: regression, repression, reaction formation, isolation, undoing, projection, introjection, turning against the self, reversal, and sublimation. To these she added: turning passive to active, denial, intellectualization, displacement, identification with the aggressor, and altruistic surrender. Following that publication, effort was devoted to developing a comprehensive catalog of defense mechanisms. Clinical observation eventually led to the conclusions that any aspect of ego functioning may be used in the service of defense and the attempt to delineate a comprehensive list of specific mechanisms was impossible and potentially misleading in its reductionism. Nonetheless, children use certain mechanisms with sufficient frequency that it is of value to psychodynamic child therapists to be able to recognize them in the clinical situation (Table 6.2.4.1).

Controversy exists both within dynamic child psychiatry and between dynamic and descriptive psychiatry regarding the degree to which defensive activity and internal conflict involve such "autonomous" ego functions as perception, motility

TABLE 6.2.4.1

DEFENSES COMMONLY EXHIBITED BY CHILDREN IN PSYCHODYNAMIC THERAPY

Denial	The disavowal of intolerable external reality factors or of thoughts, feelings, wishes, or needs that are apparent to an observer
Displacement	The transfer of emotions, ideas, or wishes from the original object to a more acceptable substitute
Externalization	The attribution of internal conflicts to the external environment and a search for environmental solutions. In therapy, the person of the therapist is used to represent one or the other part of the patient's personality structure
Reaction formation	The adoption of affects, ideas, or behaviors that are the opposites of impulses harbored either consciously or unconsciously
Repression	The exclusion of unacceptable ideas, fantasies, affects, or impulses from consciousness or the keeping out of consciousness what has never been conscious. Repressed material emerges in disguised form in thought, speech, and actions
Suppression	The *conscious* effort to control and conceal unacceptable impulses. Suppression is the exception to the rule that defenses are unconscious processes
Somatization	The transfer of tension from drives or affects into disturbances of bodily functions or rhythms
Turning passive to active	The management of affects and impulses stirred by a passive experience with an active, more powerful "other" by playing out in action or story the active "other's" role. This includes the process of identification with the aggressor

From Edgerton J, Campbell RJ (eds): *American Psychiatric Glossary,* Washington, DC, American Psychiatric Press, 1994; (84) Freud A: *The Ego and Mechanisms of Defense,* New York, International Universities Press, 1936; (6) Freud A: *Normality and Pathology in Childhood: Assessments of Development.* New York, International Universities Press, 1965 (7).

(walking, eye–hand coordination), intention, intelligence, logical thought, speech, and language. "Autonomous" ego functions were conceptualized by Heinz Hartmann (29) as relatively resistant to disturbance by intrapsychic conflict. It is clear that many disturbances in this area have their origins in constitutional variations in brain functioning. However, it is also clear from clinical material that in many children and adults these presumed autonomous functions are impacted by conflict and defense; this is no surprise to psychiatrists familiar with the way cognitive function is impaired by defensive denial. The challenge to the child and adolescent psychodynamic therapist is in the differential diagnosis. Psychological testing by a professional skilled in elucidating this distinction can be very useful.

Superego, the moral agency in the tripartite model, encompasses conscience, morality, critical self-observation, self-punishment, and the holding up of ideals (30). Although available to consciousness as moral precepts and ideals, superego functions are predominantly unconscious, out of awareness. Superego is built out of the child's desire to please adults, fear of displeasing adults and thereby losing their approval and affection, experiences of consequences from the physical and social world, and identification with the models of self-control and moral values presented by important adults. There is continuing development of a set of standards, *ego ideal,* epitomizing the individual's beliefs of what is right, good, or desirable. Superego can be effective in controlling behavior in conformance with this ideal only to the degree that ego capacities have developed to be deployed in thwarting and channeling unacceptable impulses. When misbehavior is the presenting complaint about a particular child, the clinician must evaluate whether the behavioral expectations of the adults are "age appropriate." The clinician also pays attention to the meaning of the behavior rooted in the child's anxiety and conflict over drive derivatives.

Superego is a concept that describes an internal, intrapsychic phenomenon derived from relationships, especially with caregivers, and experiences with the external world. The clinician observes superego functions by attending to the affects signaling pleasure and displeasure. When thought and behavior conform to the internalized standards of the developing ego ideal, the child shows pleasure in performance of daily tasks, self-esteem, happiness, or contentment. The child displays signs of humiliation, shame or guilt, and low self-esteem when thought and behavior disappoint the strictures of internalized standards and superego functions. Children frequently externalize blame as a defense against the painful affect when negative affect or a sense of being bad is unbearable. Unfortunately, when the child lies or blames others, adults may assume that the child does not know he was naughty, whereas the child does know but cannot tolerate the knowing. Children frequently express their guilt through enactments in which their behavior brings about a punishment. For example, a child struggling with urges to injure a new sibling may become accident-prone.

An interesting finding from psychoanalysis is that the harshness and rigidity of an individual's superego is not directly proportional to the parent's severity or the child's experiences with the parent but rather to the intensity of the aggressive wishes and relative weakness and immaturity of the individual's ego and defenses. Parental harshness is thought to weaken superego functions because when the parent's aim is to inflict a punishment that hurts the child, either physically or through deprivation, the child becomes focused on the external struggle with the parent and is distracted from the internal struggle with shame, guilt, or remorse.

Although ego psychologists have focused on defensive ego functions, an alternative metapsychology has developed under the rubric of object relations theory. Freud's emphasis on early experience as a source of both psychopathology and transference focused interest on the earliest relationships of the human infant and toddler. This emphasis and the observational studies of young children that it spawned (31–33) have reaped extensive benefit for our understanding of the mental health needs of children. Although loosely anchored in the tripartite model of the mind, psychoanalytic object relations theories as defined by Kernberg are:

> ...those that place the internalization, structuralization, and clinical reactivation (in the transference and countertransference) of the earliest dyadic object relations at the center of their motivational (genetic and developmental), structural, and clinical formulations (34).

Object relations theories use a metapsychology organized around the concept of an *internal representational world,* a world which is only gradually differentiated in the course of development (35). The child constructs representations that enable him or her to perceive sensations arising from various sources, to organize and to structure them in a meaningful way. It is useful to make a distinction between representations and images. A representation is a more or less enduring organization or schema constructed from a multitude of images, each derived from a multitude of experiential impressions. Sandler gives the example of a child who experiences many images of his or her mother—mother feeding, mother talking, mother preparing food, and so on—out of which gradually is created the mother representation encompassing the entire range of mother images, all bearing the label "mother."

The object relations metapsychological construct of the intrapsychic representational world provides a conceptual framework for the processes of internalization. Identification is the coalescence of a self-representation with an object representation, or a change in the self-representation so that the object representation is duplicated. En route to a stable identification are temporary identifications and imitations with transitory changes in self-image. The object representation used as a model in identification may be based to a degree on fantasy rather than wholly on real attributes of the object from which it derived. Identification, with its duplication of the object representation within the self-representation, is seen as a step in the loosening of the dependency tie to the object.

In psychodynamic therapy special attention is given to understanding and manipulating the impact of the patient–therapist relationship on the patient's intrapsychic structures and functions. A basic concept of *transference* "refers to the way in which the patient's view of and relations with his childhood objects are expressed in his current perceptions, thoughts, fantasies, feelings, attitudes, and behavior in regard to the analyst (36)." The therapist can observe the transference by looking for distinctive types: transference of habitual ways of relating, current relationships, and past experiences (36). It is particularly useful to examine and utilize transference onto the therapist of defensive functions. Transference is frequently used as a general term for the patient's attitudes and behavior toward the therapist and as such includes *externalizations,* which Anna Freud specifies as:

> ...processes in which the person of the analyst is used to represent one or the other part of the patient's personality structure.... The child thus re-stages his internal (intersystemic) conflicts as external battles with the analyst, a process which provides useful material (7).

Therapists' interventions differ with each therapist's assessment of transference phenomena. Brenner points out that the phenomenon of transference is not unique to the therapeutic relationship but rather "*every* object relation is a new edition of the first, definitive attachments of childhood (37)." In essence, psychodynamic theory proposes that psychologically significant relationships contribute to the individual's perceptions, thoughts, fantasies, feelings, attitudes, and behavior in all future relationships.

The patient's experience of the therapist is not limited to the transference. A portion of the therapeutic action of psychodynamic therapy is thought to rest in the experience of the *real relationship* with the therapist. The child even more than the adult has receptivity for new experiences. The psychodynamic therapist provides the child or adolescent with a new object with new potentials for internalization. The therapist strives to cultivate specific qualities, some of which may be novel to the child. These include a respectful attitude toward the child, particularly toward the child's thoughts and feelings, as well as the protection of the child's confidences from intrusion by parents or teachers. The therapist strives to be reliable and predictable in the arrangements made for meeting with the child. Most significantly, the psychodynamic therapist establishes a relationship with the child that is largely unilateral in its focus so that the events of the therapy evolve primarily from the child. Unlike the relationship with parents or peers, in which there is a necessary and healthy reciprocity, the focus on the child in the relationship with the psychodynamic therapist allows the internal world of the child to dominate the transactions (38). The therapist as an interested and thoughtful observer becomes a model for the child's development of the capacity for self-observation, a capacity termed *observing ego*. For children who have deficits in reflective function, the therapist's respect for the child's mental life and implied recognition that it is uniquely the child's is important in helping the child to develop this capacity.

Although the primary focus in the patient–therapist relationship is tipped toward the patient, psychodynamic theory does address the therapist's experience of this relationship. *Countertransference* refers specifically to intrapsychic conflicts stirred in the therapist by the patient. Generically, countertransference refers to all the reactions of the therapist to the patient. Detection of countertransference requires a "constant internal vigilance of the psychiatrist, who notes the emergence of powerful positive and negative feelings toward the patient and reflects on the possible origin of those feelings in the context of past relationships (1)." Marshall (39) operationalizes the definition of countertransference into two categories: a) reactions arising from the therapist's unresolved internal conflicts; and b) natural reactions to a patient's provocative behavior. Winnicott (40) dubbed this second type *objective* countertransference, objective in the sense that virtually everyone would find the patient's behavior provocative. The challenge to the therapist when the objective countertransference is recognized is to construct a response that is both honest and therapeutic. Marshall suggests that either type of countertransference may occur consciously or unconsciously. By definition, the therapist, at least initially, is unaware of unconscious self-derived responses. Table 6.2.4.2 lists behaviors that signal the presence of unconscious therapist-derived countertransference. Many of these same factors may be purposefully instituted as adaptations of technique, *parameters*, when clinically warranted. The therapist's task is to prevent countertransferences from distorting the treatment.

Treatment alliance and *working alliance* are terms used to refer to "all the factors that keep a patient in treatment and which enable him to remain there during phases of resistance and hostile transference (36)." *Resistance* is a conceptualization of the psychological mechanisms that cling to the intrapsychic status quo and seek to prevent change. In essence, resistance is a defense against affects, undesirable self-representations, or unwanted drive derivatives that are stirred and moved toward awareness by the therapeutic process. Inherent in the treatment alliance is the patient's awareness of internal difficulties and an acceptance of the need to be helped. Children with very fragile self-esteem may refuse to enter into therapy because they cannot tolerate the recognition of their difficulties.

TABLE 6.2.4.2

CLINICAL CLUES TO UNCONSCIOUS THERAPIST-DERIVED COUNTERTRANSFERENCE

Excessive play with diminution of talk
Quick yielding to requests
Gratification of the child, particularly feeding and gift-giving
Any strong feeling, especially if accompanied by guilt or anxiety
"Lulling": The altering of attention when a child plays out similar fantasies repetitively
Impulsive talk or action
Physical contact
Allowing parents to use child's time
Consultation with parents or others without child's involvement or agreement
Strong, unresolved feelings toward parents
Inability to involve parents appropriately
Preoccupation with changing behavior, especially as desired by parents or school

(From Marshall R: Countertransference in the psychotherapy of children and adolescents. *Contemporary Psychoanalysis* 15(3):595–629, 1979, with permission.)

In child and adolescent treatments the establishment and maintenance of the alliance is more complex than in adults because of the dependence on parents to bring the child to treatment. A positive alliance with the parents sustains the child's engagement in treatment even when the child's resistance is strong. Parents can subtly oppose the child's wish to come to treatment or collude with the child's resistance. The therapist must establish and maintain a working alliance with the parents sufficient to keep the therapy going. Novick and Novick reach beyond this minimum. They view the therapeutic alliance with the parents as a transformative task "designed to help parents gain or regain some feeling of competence as parents and love for their child as a separate person (41)."

CLINICAL APPROACH

The clinical application of psychodynamic theory to the treatment of children and adolescents covers a broad range of settings, participants, intensities, and combinations with other modalities of treatment such as psychopharmacology, educational remedies, family therapy, and environmental change. Individual, intensive, psychodynamic therapy, based largely on psychoanalysis but drawing as well on American client-centered therapy and the child guidance approach to individual therapy, can be used to demonstrate the fundamental techniques and practices of dynamic psychotherapy.

Indications and Goals

Individual psychodynamic therapy formulates the intrapsychic component of the child or adolescent's condition within a developmentally attuned biopsychosocial model of dysfunction. Formulation goes beyond the simple descriptive categories of the *Diagnostic and Statistical Manual of Mental Disorders*, 4th. ed (DSM-IV) or *International Classification of Diseases*, 10th rev. (ICD-10) to include life events and chronology related to the emergence of psychopathology, the pathophysiology of symptoms, signs, and problematic behaviors, and the developmental status, leading conflicts, and coping and adaptive mechanisms of the child (42–44) (see also Henderson and Martin, Chapter 4.2.6). Individual psychodynamic therapy is most clearly indicated in cases where the patient's difficulties are the product of intrapsychic conflict and adherence to defensive solutions or object representations that are developmentally regressive. Frequently, a child's difficult behaviors are externalizations of intrapsychic conflict. Psychodynamic therapy is indicated in cases where the etiologic factors in the social environment, such as mother's pregnancy and birth of a sibling or maternal depression over the death of grandparents, have resolved but the child's defenses have become fixed. Anna Freud (45) proposes two other categories of disturbance that psychoanalysts have attempted to treat that are not generated solely from the past but from significant present circumstances. One such circumstance is the child or adolescent's difficulty coping with a current developmental imperative such as entry into school, the upheaval in self-image at puberty, or the adolescent shift in relationships with the parents. The focus of therapy would still be on the intrapsychic difficulties of the youth. In Anna Freud's second category, the environment or the child's own constitution, such as blindness or multiple learning disabilities, presents a current and ongoing interference with development. In these cases, Anna Freud suggests, intensive individual work may be important but is unlikely to bring the youth to health without environmental interventions.

Intensive, individual psychodynamic therapy is contraindicated in cases of severe constitutional deficits such as autism, severe pervasive developmental disorder, or moderate to severe mental retardation, particularly to the degree that these disorders affect capacity for self-observation and receptive language function. Intensive treatment is contraindicated when circumstances within the family or the treatment facility cannot sustain the continuity and integrity of the therapy, especially if disruption of the therapy repeats previous traumas of loss and unpredictability for the child. Because intensive treatment places considerable strain on family resources and the child and parents' time, it should not be undertaken if a less intensive treatment is adequate.

The goals of therapy extend beyond symptom relief. A primary goal is to restore psychological development to a normal path, including management of anxiety, enhanced affect regulation, improved self-esteem, increased frustration tolerance, age-appropriate autonomy, greater capacity for pleasure and satisfaction in school work and play, and better relationships with peers. Additional goals are to enhance the child's resilience and decrease the likelihood of relapse by developing the child's capacity for understanding his or her own feelings, thoughts, and the connection between feelings and behavior. The child or adolescent comes to a more sophisticated understanding of other people's thoughts, feelings, and behaviors by learning to know and observe his own mental functions. This contributes to improved interpersonal relationships.

Opening Phase

The challenge and gratification provided by the practice of psychodynamic therapy stems in part from the requirement that the practitioner pursue diagnostic and therapeutic goals simultaneously. Thus, the psychodynamic child and adolescent psychiatrist seeks to establish a psychodynamic treatment stance from the very first contact with the adult caretaker and patient. While directing and observing the evaluation process, the clinician acts in a manner that respects the parental functions of the caretaker as well as the developmentally appropriate autonomy and inner experience of the child.

The First Visit

With adolescents, particularly older adolescents, the clinician usually meets with the patient for one or several sessions before meeting with the parents. This allows the adolescent to explore issues of trust with the clinician and demonstrates that the clinician's primary relationship is to the adolescent. For younger children, it is typical for the parents to meet with the psychiatrist to provide background data, but even more importantly to establish their own trust and confidence in the psychiatrist so that they can assure the child of the appropriateness of this undertaking. It is important to explore with parents how they will prepare the child for the first visit. If the child has expressed distress over a particular symptom, the parent may explain that the doctor is there to help with that symptom. In language appropriate to the child's age, the parents ought to tell the child that the doctor is someone who helps children with their feelings and worries by talking and playing with them.

Structuring the Psychodynamic Therapy for the Child or Adolescent

The intention in individual therapy is for the therapist and child to work together separately from the parents. The child may have difficulty leaving the parent, either because for a preschooler this is within the range of age-appropriate behavior or for an older child because of underlying conflicts. Such separation difficulties require an adaptation of technique and preliminary work with the child and parent to understand and work through the issue. The idea behind working with the child without the parent in the room is to create a zone of confidentiality and psychic safety within which the child and therapist can explore feelings, thoughts, and behaviors. If the parent is present, the child's spontaneity is restrained or stimulated in part by the possible reaction from the parent. When the child is seen alone, the therapist is in a better position to see how the child has internalized the authority of the parents.

The psychiatrist should clarify to both the parents and the child that, although he or she meets with the child's parents on a regular basis, the confidentiality in this therapy is a one-way street which allows the psychiatrist to tell the child what the parents have said but precludes the psychiatrist reporting to the parents what the child has said or done. Children, particularly at the beginning of therapy, frequently will not report to the therapist current events that provide a context for understanding the child's talk and play within the session because children are very oriented in the present moment and are defensive against affect. A meeting or phone call from the parents is important if the therapist is to know about these events. The "one-way street" implies that the therapist will share these communications from the parents with the child. The child's understanding of the purpose of the therapist's meetings with parents develops as the therapy continues. It is the therapist's task through word and deed to help the child understand that, although the therapist tries to help the parents understand their role as parents of a child this age and with these problems, the therapist can not control the parents and will not take sides in a specific struggle between the child and parents. On the other hand, particularly with older children and adolescents, it can be pointed out that the parent has a responsibility to the child for assuring that the therapist is doing a responsible job and thus needs some report from the therapist on the progress of the work.

There are several other elements the psychodynamic therapist uses to create a special person, place, and time for dealing with feelings and worries in addition to creating a zone of confidentiality. The therapist deals with the child in a nonjudgmental and nondirective manner such as that described by Virginia Axline (10) in her classic text, *Play Therapy*. In an intensive individual psychodynamic therapy, the therapist strives to relate to the child in the style McConville (46) has described as the "empathic participant" who approaches the child with the wish to know "what's it like to be you." The therapist and child explore together rather than doing something *to* or *for* the child. Eventually the therapist is *with* the child as the child examines and explores his own thoughts, feelings, and conflicts. If doctor–patient relationships are conceived of as either prescriptive, collaborative, or facilitative, the psychodynamic therapist eschews the prescriptive, choosing to be collaborative and facilitative.

The office must be suitably sturdy and equipped in a manner age-appropriate to the patients who will be treated in order to work nondirectively with children. A separate playroom is advantageous when working with young children who are struggling to control intensely messy or aggressive impulses. The toys do not need to be numerous or elaborate. Children's activities in a play therapy tend to fall into the following categories: games with rules, physical activities, creative projects, solo imaginary play, and imaginary play with the therapist as a participant. It is helpful to have a deck of cards, one or two simple board games such as checkers or Trouble, a Nerf or Koosh ball, paper, washable markers or crayons, tape and children's scissors, a set of blocks, puppets, action figures, and dolls or animal figures. A family grouping of animals or small dolls is useful. The child can use a ferocious animal (shark, lion, or dinosaur, either a puppet or animal figure) to express aggressive urges.

The issue of limit setting will arise no matter how appropriately the office or playroom is outfitted. Commonsense limitations are necessary to protect the room, therapist, and child from physical damage. One way to understand the limits is to say, "When we are done I have to be able to clean up and have you, me, and the office/playroom back the way it was." This creates in the child's world of expression through action the same safety from real-world consequences the adult analysand on the couch enjoys when expressing himself or herself verbally. Frequently, the therapist is able to address the impulse toward an unacceptable action while redirecting its aim. Thus one might say, "You may not cut my dress when you feel like attacking but you may cut this paper I will hold. I can see you feel strong and safe when you are doing the cutting. You let me know how scary it feels to have someone attacking." The therapist tries to prevent the dangerous action without creating a physical struggle if the child cannot be redirected. It is important that the therapist not become angry, blaming, and punitive while commenting on the child's struggle over the destructive wish and maneuvering of the therapist into being the "policeman who must keep us and the office safe." It is also appropriate for the therapist to remind the child that "We must try to find words for these feelings so you can tell me about it without things getting broken." The implementation of a set starting and ending time is the most frequently imposed limitation, as Axline (10) points out. The therapist's adherence to routine in keeping the time and dates of appointments on a predictable schedule is a necessary part of creating reliability and boundaries in the therapeutic relationship. The child's reaction to waiting in the waiting room for the appointed starting time and dealing with leaving the therapist at the end of the session can serve to reveal the particular child's conflicts.

The Interpretive Session: Structuring the Therapy for the Parents

Intensive individual psychodynamic therapy is initiated after a period of evaluation, crisis management, or possibly a trial of pharmacotherapy or another psychotherapy that has failed or been incomplete in its effectiveness. It is important that the therapist and parents meet in an interpretive session or two to review the formulation of the child's diagnosis and prognosis in dynamic and developmental terms, and to discuss a possible recommendation for intensive treatment and make the necessary arrangements. Intensive therapy implies two or more sessions per week. Psychoanalysis with sessions four or five times per week is indicated when the pathologic conflicts and maladaptive, regressive defenses are longstanding and pervasive in the child's response to a wide range of circumstances. Parents understand that frequency of practice enhances the outcome and shortens the overall time course in order to acquire a foreign language or master a musical instrument. In intensive psychodynamic therapy the child undertakes to learn a new "psychological language" and develop new skills to master feelings and impulses. The patient must be helped to counteract the resistance to change that is a natural mechanism for maintaining stability. The wise therapist is cautious in predicting the duration of treatment. Much depends on the stability of the environment and degree of current destabilizing stresses. What are the burdens and constraints on the parents in terms of effort and expense that might limit the duration of treatment? Parents should be told that intensive individual psychodynamic therapy is generally measured in years, not weeks or months. The therapist can from the very start work with the parents to generate goals and termination criteria focused on the resumption of progressive development, renewed pleasure in the child's own functioning and in the relationship with the parents (41). Shorter intense treatments are adaptations to specific circumstances undertaken after weighing the risks and benefits over other treatment modalities.

The frequency and purpose of parent sessions also must be discussed. As third-party coverage for intensive psychotherapy has diminished in the past 20 years, the tendency has been to decrease the parent visits in order to maximize the resources available for the child's visits, a short-sighted solution, especially with younger children. The parents and therapist need to meet to maintain an alliance and avoid undermining splits and competition for the child. Helping parents to make changes in daycare, bedtime rituals, family modesty, and discipline facilitates recovery of a healthy developmental trajectory more rapidly in the younger child. Frequently the therapist will need to use his or her dynamic understanding to comprehend the parents' difficulties and conflicts that interfere with their primary parental concern (41).

Beginning the Process of Interpretation

Interpretation is the process whereby the therapist, by expressing in words what he or she has come to understand about the patient's mental life, helps the patient to observe and understand his or her inner life in a new and more complete way (23). The therapist engages the child or adolescent in the act of observation by making *attention statements* (47), comments that draw the patient's conscious attention to the content of his actions or verbalizations (48). Beginning with ego syntonic and nonthreatening content, the therapist provides verbal commentary on the child's play, or enactments within the play, to reflect the child's defenses, judgments, wishes, or anxieties. As the therapeutic alliance develops, the therapist begins to draw the patient's attention to coincidences, paradoxes, and remarkable absences of affects, topics, or persons who ought to be central to the child's experience.

Middle Phase

Whereas the initial and termination phases may last several weeks to months, the middle phase of treatment lasts months to years. Intrapsychic structure is created or remodeled, new defenses are developed, and old patterns of response are relinquished during the middle phase.

The Child in the Middle Phase

The middle phase begins when the patient has taken in the structure of the treatment: the therapist's nonjudgmental attitude, regularity of appointment times, and maintenance of confidentiality. The patient implicitly knows that a goal of the treatment is to understand the way she or he feels and behaves, that everything she or he says or does is to be considered in the therapy. The child's play or the older child's conversation and behavior are part of the associative process revealing the patient's intrapsychic state. It does not meet the criteria of free association in adult psychoanalysis because the child's capacity for introspection is limited and the child is not instructed to say whatever comes to mind. The child or adolescent tends to maintain a consciously goal-directed stance (winning the game of checkers). This goal-directedness creates considerable tension between the child's tendency to become absorbed in the play and the capacity to self-observe. The therapist's verbalizations about the play model the observing function as well as clarify the dynamic functions of the play for the child.

The transition in late childhood and early adolescence from playing in therapy to sitting and talking reflects a developmental move from expression through action to enhanced verbal communication. Superego development contributes to this process with increasing superego autonomy and constriction in primary process expression to meet an increasingly mature ego ideal. Often in this transitional stage the patient will fiddle with objects in the office; draw or play cards; or bring in homework, magazines, books, or a pocket full of gadgets to allow an action outlet or focus that is not threatening in its pull back toward childhood play. In this period the therapist needs to allow the patient to establish a comfortable blend of action and verbal expression while being alert for the ways in which either might be used as a resistance.

Resistance is an inevitable aspect of a psychodynamic therapeutic process. Lewis and Blotcky (49) describe three categories of resistance: active, passive, and compliant. The actively resistant patient expresses overt objections to the treatment, such as opposition to coming to appointments and complaints about interference in his or her life. The passively resistant youth may be stubbornly silent, withholding, and plead boredom. The compliant patient is described as eager to do the right things, to give lip service but without emotional engagement. These may be thought of as "macroresistances," appearing as an overarching response to treatment. One also finds "microresistances," moment-to-moment rejections of the therapist's offered interpretations. The child may demonstrate these by shutting down, a sudden shift of focus or behavior, or an eruption of disinhibited behavior. By observing these microresistances, the therapist can measure the intensity of the superego in opposing awareness of the mental contents the therapist was seeking to bring to the patient's conscious awareness or the weakness of the ego when it loses control of the drive.

The patient continues to develop a relationship with the therapist during this middle phase, in addition to bringing forward the content of his inner experience. A true transference occurs, that is, the patient experiences in the current relationship with the therapist fixated conflicts, superego projections, and object representations that stem from previous experiences with the parents. The transference is affected and modified by the developmental achievements or delays of the patient. The child patient differs from the adult patient because the child is still living with the parents, who continue to exert influence over the patient. The patient may make a simple, current displacement rather than a deep transference to the therapist. The child is not the equal of the therapist because the child is still a child relating to the therapist as a child to an adult (48). In addition to the emerging transference, the child or adolescent experiences the therapist as a new object for identification and satisfaction of developmental needs. The experience with an adult who respects the child or adolescent's inner life and demonstrates an approach to understanding and managing that inner life contributes significantly to the therapeutic outcome of intensive individual psychodynamic therapy.

It is important not to underestimate the contribution to the therapeutic process of the child's play and verbal self-expression. The play and verbalizations, by expressing heretofore-unconscious mental contents in conscious communications of speech and action, make meaning and offer an opportunity for active mastery of components of the patient's problems apart from the effect of the specific interventions of the therapist.

The Therapist's Mental Process

The gap between the therapist's theoretical understanding of the moment-to-moment content of the therapy sessions and what it is possible to do or say at the developmental level of the child is more evident in child psychotherapy than in work with adults. Lewis describes the multistep process by which the therapist, while keeping up the play with the child, takes "mental distance," places the immediate observations into an ongoing formulation, develops an interpretation, brings the interpretation back, and presents it to the child in the context of the play or conversation (48). For many years interpretation was seen as the sine qua non of psychodynamic treatment. Recently attention has been given to ways in which the therapist may offer developmental help or assistance rather than an interpretation (50). The choice of interpretation versus developmental assistance will be made on the basis of the formulation, particularly the assessment of ego development as age appropriate or lagging in development.

The therapist's interest is neither limited to nor primarily focused on the factual content of the patient's productions in the session. Even when a patient in late childhood or adolescence presents a narrative of an external event, the therapist listens for the defensive regulation of affect and drive in the narrative as well as the accuracy or potential distortions in the presentations of relationships. The therapist also assesses the patient's ability or inability to see multiple sides of the story. Referencing earlier material, the therapist considers what patterns emerge. The therapist may begin to formulate a reconstruction by thinking about how these patterns reflect a repetition of defenses and attitudes fixated by past trauma. The psychodynamic therapist continually monitors the patient's utilization of the therapist. Is the transference being manifested or is the patient turning passive to active, letting the therapist know what it feels like to be on the receiving end? Nonnarrative material is as useful in psychodynamic therapy, as is narrative. In nonnarrative play the therapist observes where shifts and disruptions in the play occur in response either to frustration or the emergence of strong emotions or thoughts the child finds unacceptable.

The Therapist's Interventions

The basic process of constructing interpretations was laid out by Loewenstein (51) and is explored comprehensively by Lewis in "The therapeutic relationship and the technique of interpretation: The use of play in psychodynamic therapy (48)." Interpretations may be classified as *clarifications, defense interpretations*, and *reconstructions*. Clarifications bring the patient's attention to bear on his or her characteristic patterns of action and interaction but do not imply a reason for the pattern. A defense interpretation picks up on the drive derivative (rivalry as an aggressive drive derivative) and points out that a defense has been instituted. The drive derivative has been changed in a way that makes it manageable and acceptable to the superego (rivalry becomes the avoidance of competition). The therapist should address the defense before addressing the drive derivative when making a defense interpretation (6). The defense is acceptable to the patient. It is ego-syntonic. Drawing the patient's attention to the defense reminds the patient that he or she has a way to manage the affect or drive derivative. The patient will be more likely to tolerate looking back at the intolerable drive or affect from this position of strength.

A reconstruction is an interpretation that explains current feelings, thoughts, and behaviors in terms of critical past events in the patient's life or fantasies from an earlier stage of development. Reconstructions are only offered late in the therapy process. The clinical decision to offer a reconstruction to a child or adolescent requires weighing the patient's capacity to use it to "make sense" of perplexing feelings and behaviors (52). Lewis (1996) points out that a reconstruction can be helpful to a child when it clarifies an essentially correct perception by the child at the time of the trauma that has subsequently undergone distortion. The therapist must consider whether a reconstruction is premature. A child too close to the trauma will reject the reconstruction in order to defend against the affects and drives the reference stirs. A reconstruction may be intellectualized or rejected because it arouses unmanageable shame or guilt.

Developmental help or assistance is a technique of psychodynamic psychotherapy with children and adolescents that has been used for decades but is only being written about and defined recently. Developmental assistance may be seen as a precursor needed to build ego capacities that will eventually allow the patient to use the play process and interpretation to gain self-understanding. Yanof describes working with 7-year-old Robert, who lacked perseverance and frustration tolerance leading to poor performance in school when he had difficulty learning to read. Through much of the treatment he could use imaginative play to express his feelings of anger and unlovableness. As the summer break in treatment approached Robert had undertaken to build Lego models:

> Whenever Robert came to something difficult, he began to complain that he could not do it—that he was not smart enough to do it. He immediately demanded that I do it for him. I made a technical decision not to do it for him but to support his plan to build the object. I did not interpret conflict, but I told him that learning how to do things was hard work and it made everyone feel like giving up. At times I gave him strategies. Much of the time he was angry at me for not doing enough. However, when he finally finished the project, he was elated (50).

Yanof was aware that Robert was lagging behind in his ability to join in his peers' pursuits and function competently. She used her skills to help him increase his frustration tolerance and experience a new competence.

The psychodynamic therapist must select the optimal context in addition to the level of interpretation. In play therapy, the therapist decides whether to work within the play utilizing the defensive protection displacement affords or to comment more directly to the child. If the child is playing that a tiger makes a preemptive attack on a lion, the therapist may speak about the tiger's wish to protect himself by striking first or the therapist can say to the child, "You are showing me with the tiger that you feel it is sometimes important to protect yourself by attacking first." The relationship between the child and therapist is a context for interpreting transference or externalization, clarifying the real, nontransference, relationship and offering developmental assistance. Working in the play or in the patient–therapist relationship focuses the work on events inside the treatment setting. The focus could be extended to events outside the treatment setting. The patient and therapist can discuss issues or experiences with family, peers, or school. Finally, the temporal focus may be on the past, present, or future.

Work with Parents in the Middle Phase

Success of an intensive individual psychodynamic therapy with a child or adolescent often rests on the therapist's skill in the collateral work with the parents. The therapist must come to understand the parents' fantasies and fears about therapy, their child, and themselves as parents. Parents may come with the attitude that the therapist will redeem them from past transgressions that have affected the child. The parents may hope that the therapist will rescue the child. Alternatively, parents may see the therapist as a rival for the child's affection or as an authority figure seeking to find fault or blame the parent. Even with the most dysfunctional parent, the therapist seeks to ally with the parent's wish to be a good parent and supports the parent in those efforts. Many parents find referral for individual treatment beneficial. Where there is marital conflict the therapist tactfully explores its role in the child's difficulties. If marital therapy is indicated the parents should be referred to an appropriate clinician in order to maximize the parents' effectiveness in their parenting role, minimize the possibility that the marital conflict will disrupt the child's treatment, and protect the therapist's primary relationship with the child.

In "Problems of termination in child analysis," Anna Freud (53) lists parental reasons for terminating treatment sooner than the Hampstead Child-Therapy Clinic recommended. Parents may be satisfied when presenting symptoms have resolved but the therapist is aware that the underlying pathologic conflicts are not stabilized. Or the parents find unacceptable transitory oppositional behaviors of the child whose therapeutic developmental gains lead to a newly achieved autonomy.

Parent work in the middle phase has the tasks of: a) facilitating the flow of information from the parents about the child; b) counseling and educating parents both about sensitive issues in parenting and the particular child's diagnosis, strengths, and vulnerabilities; and c) assisting parents in advocating for the child and in case management (54). The therapist must always plan interventions with parents in the context of what the therapist knows of the parents' own issues and needs. Suggestions must be given with cautious awareness that parents may resist giving up a parenting behavior or pattern of relationship with the child either because it is gratifying for the parent or represents a parental defense against negative or aggressive impulses. If such resistances are present or the parent's own conflicts can be shown to destabilize the child's progress in the therapy, the therapist has the additional task of skillfully counseling and educating the parent (41) or assisting the parent to undertake therapy for herself or himself.

Closing Phase

The closing phase presents two distinct tasks: the decision to conclude the treatment and the *termination process* by which the treatment is ended. The psychiatrist's ability to maintain the working alliance with the patient and parents consolidates the patient's therapeutic gains and enables the patient or family to seek help in the future if needed.

The Decision to Stop Treatment

Because intensive psychodynamic therapy with children and adolescents is a three-way contract (55) between therapist, child, and parents, the conclusion may be initiated by any one, two, or all three of the parties. The optimal situation is for all three to concur that the goals of treatment have been met. A successfully completed case may be said to have "reached termination."

Premature terminations occur when there is a decision to end the therapy before the treatment goals have been met. There are two types of premature termination: disruption and interruption. Disruption refers to the decision to end the treatment because of external factors affecting any of the three parties. For example, the family may be moving or the therapist may be leaving the treatment facility. Interruption refers to a unilateral decision by one of the parties to end the treatment based on intrapsychic factors such as parents' unexamined intrapsychic conflicts aroused by the therapy. In all terminations, and particularly in the case of premature terminations, the therapist must be alert to the patient's fantasies about the reasons for ending the treatment so that they can be worked on during the termination process.

In initiating the termination process, the therapist considers the patient's ability to maintain the gains of treatment and grow in the family despite parental difficulties, the extent to which "developmental forces have been set free again and are ready to take over," (53) and the progress the patient has made in internal consolidation of intrapsychic changes. The process of consolidation of intrapsychic changes is called *working-through* (48, 56). Psychoanalysis strives for a therapeutic process based on self-observation, self-awareness, and insight. Insight, according to Anna Freud, "does not occur without a working-through process," defined as the elaboration and extension into different contexts and directions of relevant interpretations. The tracing of anxieties resulting from the child's infantile perception of the world and correction of distortions of perception that were caused by the immaturity of the child's cognitive apparatus are included in her concept of working-through (36).

The Termination Process

All psychotherapies have a termination phase regardless of theoretical orientation (49). Psychoanalysts give particular attention to this phase of treatment. The understanding gained of the meaning and psychological challenges to the patient inherent in "saying goodbye" are useful to the clinician in managing the conclusion of any doctor–patient relationship.

At the theoretical level, termination is conceptualized as an experience of separation and loss. The patient, parents, and therapist bring their own characteristic approaches to separation and loss to the process. Although the therapist's attention is primarily on the patient, countertransference reactions may be triggered by the loss of the patient as a real-life object. It is essential to evaluate and address the parents' needs in the face of the impending loss of the therapist as an ally.

The intrapsychic tasks for the patient are the resolution of the transference relationship and relinquishing of the real relationship with the therapist. The transference reaction to termination is colored by the patient's previous experiences with separation and loss. Ego functions may regress and symptoms recur. The therapist works to help the child verbalize feelings and ideas about the impending change and work through these reactions in light of the patient's current capacities, those appropriate to the patient's developmental level, and those gained in therapy. As the patient relinquishes the real relationship with the therapist, the therapist aids the patient to internalize the therapist's functions so that the patient may carry on in developing self-understanding, particularly an ability to tolerate and examine internal conflicts and ambivalence.

The technical and practical approaches to termination are designed to promote the theoretical goals. The therapist engages the patient in *active* planning and execution of the termination seeking to avoid repetition of *passive* experiences of loss (loss of parental attention with the birth of a sibling). First, the reasons for concluding the treatment must be acknowledged and the treatment goals, child's achievements, and remaining concerns reviewed, allowing the clinician, patient, and parents to gauge the patient's reaction to the impending loss. Typical reactions of children and adolescents faced with the proposition of ending therapy are: a) fear, anger, aggression, or depression; b) return of symptoms; c) recapitulation of the themes of the therapy; d) adoption of the "plan" presented; and e) a bid not to end the therapy (49).

Next, logistics of termination are addressed. Logistics include setting the date for the last session, deciding whether to make a clean break or a gradual diminution in the frequency of sessions, and clarifying followup plans. General guidelines for these decisions are tailored to the needs of the particular patient.

The clinician works to avoid precipitous endings without enough time to say goodbye and work through the patient's reactions. Optimally, the patient chooses the date by working with the therapist to understand why the patient feels one date is more suitable than another. A date at a natural time of separation, such as the end of the school year or the Christmas vacation, tends to downplay the reality of the termination. This may be desirable in some circumstances but may compromise a full working-through of the termination.

Following the model of adult psychoanalysis, many clinicians assume that therapy should be continued at the established intensity until the final session and stopped with no planned followup or contact. Anna Freud seriously questioned this approach with children and adolescents (36). She observed that, when normal development is achieved, the child detaches himself or herself in the course of time, just as children move on from teachers and even friends. Therefore, she recommended allowing the child to reduce the frequency of visits or schedule a followup visit.

Classical adult psychoanalysis leaves followup contact up to the patient. Early followup is regarded as evidence of the patient's failure to resolve the transference relationship. With children and adolescents who are in psychotherapy, not analysis, one must be aware that one is working two steps removed from classical adult analysis. In conditions of significant ongoing pathology, either constitutional in the child or endemic in the family, one is well advised to establish a followup plan. Even in less severe cases followup offers several potential benefits: reinforcement of treatment gains, assessment of any possible deterioration, maintenance of the therapist–patient relationship, as well as providing valuable communication between parents, clinicians, and teachers (49). Followup is also beneficial for the clinician to learn more about the effectiveness of the treatment. Whether or not the clinician initiates followup contact it is important for the patient to feel free to return.

PSYCHODYNAMIC PSYCHOTHERAPY RESEARCH

Today's psychoanalysis and its offspring, the psychodynamic psychotherapies, face a research crisis, having fallen out of step with developments in research methodology. Child psychotherapy began with the advent of psychoanalysis when analysts turned to the observation of children to clarify the developmental origins of adult psychopathology. As important as this interest in developmental origins was, the research method Freud applied to the study of mental disturbances had important shortcomings by today's standards. Coming out of the nineteenth-century tradition of careful naturalistic observation, a scientific tradition that led Darwin and Wallace to the theory of evolution, Freud developed an observational method that allowed independent observers to study inner life (57). Although by today's research standards psychoanalysis lacks clearly operationalized terms and tests of internal and external reliability and validity, at the time of its development Freud's specification of the approach of free association and his writings on technique permitted independent observers following his specifications to compare their observations and accumulate a remarkable and revolutionary body of observations of mental functions and their connections to behavior and to symptoms.

In the latter quarter of the twentieth century, empirical psychology moved away from the topics of interest to dynamic psychiatry toward behaviorist, cognitivist, and descriptive approaches. In the current era of evidence-based medicine, no medical discipline can afford to ignore the need for a vibrant research community to test its clinical practices and underlying assumptions.

The Case Report

The case report is likely to continue to play a role in the development and dissemination of psychodynamic psychotherapy practice for the treatment of children and adolescents not just because of the deep attachment of psychodynamic psychotherapists to reporting their findings in this manner but also because it is much less expensive than mounting multisubject studies, particularly studies that hope to achieve statistical significance. The strengths of the case report are its ability to portray the subject in all its complexity in a manner that is compelling to clinicians and lends itself to comparison with the clinicians' own cases. In the tradition of medical case reports, the case report is an important first step in filling a gap in the clinical literature.

A major disadvantage of case reports is the difficulty accounting for the bias introduced by the subjectivity of the clinician's perceptions, memory, and interpretation of the clinical data. There is also the concern that the clinician's awareness of an intention to write about the case will influence how the clinical material is heard. Further distortion may be introduced by attempts to disguise the case or otherwise protect the patient's confidentiality. Increasingly, patient permission is sought for publication of case material, but this practice also constrains what the clinician is willing to write.

Outcome Studies

In the 1950s and 1960s researchers reviewing the available studies of psychotherapy questioned whether outcome was affected by treatment at all. Partially in response to this challenge, overall research methodology improved, with better specification of the therapies through manualization and clearer definition of patient characteristics. With these improvements, the data support the basic tenet that psychotherapy improves outcome. Examination of the results of four metaanalyses of youth treatment outcomes published between 1985 and 1995 concluded that "the average treated youth scored better than more than three-fourths of control group youths on outcome measures at the end of treatment (58)." However, very few of the treatments deemed psychodynamic in these studies met basic criteria for that label. Many lacked an established psychodynamic theoretical framework or trained therapists. For the very few that did truly warrant designation as psychodynamic, the effect sizes were comparable with those for cognitive-behavioral treatments (59). Although there are not sufficient youth psychodynamic psychotherapy efficacy trials to allow for a metaanalysis specific to psychodynamic psychotherapy, the adult psychodynamic psychotherapy research has grown sufficiently to allow such a study. Examining studies of short-term psychodynamic psychotherapy between 1970 and 2004, German researchers found 17 that met rigorous inclusion criteria regarding the integrity of the treatment, therapist experience, diagnostic specificity, and randomized controls. Pretreatment-posttreatment effect sizes were calculated for target problems (1.39), general psychiatric symptoms (0.90), and social functioning (0.80). Effect sizes tended to increase at followup (1.57, 0.95, and 1.19, respectively) (60).

The Anna Freud Centre, formerly the Hampstead Clinic, has promoted psychoanalytic research since its founding in 1940. The Hampstead Indexing Project (61) established a charting requirement that had clinicians record the clinical data along several constructs critical to psychoanalysis, producing charts unmatched for their quantity and quality of clinical information. In the early 1990s, Mary Target and Peter Fonagy conducted a retrospective chart review of 763 cases, representing 90% of the cases treated at the Centre. With rigorous attention to interrater reliability they chose to use standardized psychiatric and psychological instruments to describe the outcome of youths treated at the Centre. Although the study is limited by its retrospective design, it is unlikely ever to be matched for the size of its sample. Target and Fonagy conducted three studies on the closed case records.

Clustering internalizing disorders, either anxious or depressive as emotional disorders, they found 352 charts (62). Seventy-two per cent of those youths treated for at least 6 months showed reliable, clinically significant improvement in adaptation. Only 24% of cases had a diagnosable disorder at termination. Phobic and depressive disorders were respectively the most and least likely conditions to remit. Children under the age of 11 were significantly more likely to be well at the end of treatment than were older children. More frequent sessions led to greater improvement, independent of the child's age or length of treatment. Intensive treatment, defined as four or five times per week psychoanalysis, was significantly more helpful for children who presented with more severe disturbance, multiple diagnoses, or pervasive impairment affecting social, emotional, or cognitive functioning. Looking at demographic factors, those who were most likely to improve had: higher IQ, younger age, longer treatment, good peer relations, poor overall adjustment of mother, anxiety symptoms in the mother, and absence of history of maternal antisocial behavior. The heterogeneity of these cases was demonstrated by the finding that within the 352 cases groups of children with depressive, overanxious, or specific anxieties had different predictors of outcome.

Taking a second approach to the 763 cases, Fonagy and Target (63) selected the 135 with a principal diagnosis of disruptive disorder and matched them on demographic, clinical, and treatment variables to individuals suffering from emotional disorders. Overall improvement rates were lower for the youths with disruptive disorder. Many children, nearly one-third, terminated their treatment within 1 year. Early termination was associated with older age, nonintensive treatment, a less wellfunctioning mother, fewer learning difficulties at school, and lack of concurrent parental guidance. Of the youths who stayed in treatment beyond 1 year, 69% were no longer diagnosable at termination. The predictors of improvement included: presence of anxiety disorders, younger age, intensive treatment, longer treatment, maternal anxiety disorder, the subject having been in foster care, and the mother receiving psychotherapy.

In a third study of the Anna Freud Centre, a retrospective chart review by Target and Fonagy (64) examined the way in which the age of the child or adolescent at the time of the treatment in psychoanalytic psychotherapy related to the treatment outcome. The 763 cases were sorted into three broad age bands: under 6, 6 to 12 years, and adolescents. One hundred and twenty-seven cases selected from each of the three bands were matched on broad diagnostic grouping, gender, socioeconomic status, global adaptation, and frequency of sessions. The outcome indicators were diagnostic change and clinically significant change in adaptation. Predictors of good and poor outcome were different for the three age groups. Younger children generally showed more improvement. The children under 12 benefited more from intensive (four to five sessions per week) treatment than from nonintensive treatment, but this was not the case for adolescents.

These studies shed some light on which children might be expected to benefit from long-term psychodynamic psychotherapies. Children with pervasive symptoms and uneven development did well, particularly the younger children in longer and more intensive treatments, whereas children with significant organic difficulties in the pervasive developmental disorder/autism spectrum did not do well even with prolonged intensive treatment (65). This observation has led psychoanalysts to look more carefully at the value of developmental assistance in their treatments. Neurotic patients, those who benefit from recovering threatening ideas and feelings that have been distorted or repressed and whose conflicts and defenses can be transformed by interpretation, did as well in twice per week treatments as in the intensive psychoanalytic treatments. This was particularly true of adolescents.

Prospective efficacy studies of psychoanalytic psychotherapies have been gradually accumulating. In the early 1990s Moran and Fonagy (66) used success of diabetic control, as manifested in HbA_{1C} levels and other physiologic tests, as an outcome measure for the efficacy of a brief, intensive psychoanalytic psychotherapy for adolescents with brittle, insulin-dependent diabetes. The 11 youths in the treatment group received three to four sessions per week for an average of 15 weeks while hospitalized on a medical unit. The 11 youths in the control group were those admitted on a medical unit at a different hospital staffed by the same endocrinologists. They received medical treatment only. Both groups manifested significant psychiatric symptoms on psychological assessment: 73% in the experimental group and 64% in the control group. The two therapists, who had both trained in "classical" psychoanalysis at the Anna Freud Centre, used techniques consistent with those described in a manual by Sandler et al. (36). The focus of the therapy was on the formulation of the unconscious factors underlying poor blood glucose control, as these factors emerged in the assessment and treatment sessions. The treatment group showed considerable improvement in diabetic control on HbA_{1C}, both at the 3-month and 1-year followups, while the control group returned to pretreatment levels. The most interesting aspect of this study from the perspective of psychotherapy efficacy measurement is its use of a physiologic marker for measurement of outcome. In this way the investigators sidestepped debates about the relevance of currently available psychological measurements of change to psychoanalytically oriented treatments.

Like the diabetes study, the work of Trowell et al. (67) on psychodynamic psychotherapy for sexually abused girls focuses on youths struggling with a significant life stress rather than treatment for a specific psychiatric diagnosis. However, psychiatric disorder was common among the total of 81 girls who were assessed at baseline: post-traumatic stress disorder in 73%, major depression in 57%, generalized anxiety disorder in 37%, and separation anxiety disorder in 58%. The Schedule for Affective Disorders and Schizophrenia for School-age Children (K-SADS), the Kiddie Global Assessment Scale (K-GAS) and the Orvaschel PTSD scale, were the assessment instruments used at baseline and followup. Seventy-one girls, ages 6 to 14 years, who had experienced contact sexual abuse, were enrolled as they presented for treatment at two clinics in London. Random assignment was made to the study treatment of an individual psychodynamic psychotherapy or a comparison group therapy that combined psychotherapeutic discussion of relationships with psychoeducational topic-focused sessions. The psychotherapy consisted of weekly sessions of manualized, nondirective, psychodynamic psychotherapy. The therapists did ensure that over time all the topics on the list covered in the psychoeducational group were raised in the individual therapy. Sessions were limited to a maximum of 30, typically distributed as five for engagement, 15 addressing issues identified as relevant for the particular child and 10 sessions focused on separation and ending, as well as reworking any key topics that had emerged in the course of treatment. The child's or adolescent's caregiver was seen about every two weeks for support and guidance. Both treatment groups showed a substantial reduction in psychopathological symptoms and an improvement in functioning, but with no evident difference between individual and group therapy. However, individual therapy led to greater improvement in severity of PTSD and "persistent avoidance of stimuli" measures on the PTSD scales, with effect sizes ranging around 0.6.

The work of Muratori et al. (68) uses an active treatment versus community services model to examine the short- and long-term effects of time-limited psychodynamic psychotherapy for children meeting DSM-IV criteria for depressive or anxiety disorders. Fifty-eight outpatients between the ages of 6 and 9 years were studied at baseline (T_1), 6 months (T_2), and 2-year followup (T_3) with the Child Behavior Checklist (CBCL) and the Children's Global Assessment Scale (C-GAS). Therapy was provided in 11 weekly sessions, of which five were parent–child sessions, five were individual sessions with the child, and one a final parent–child session. The treatment was manualized to include observing defenses and exploring the representational world of the parents, formulating transgenerational conflicts, verbalizing patients' defenses and wishes, and connecting feelings and mental contents to symptoms. The final session addressed the shared, parent–child, core-conflictual theme and its relationship to the child's symptom and the parents' internal representations. Therapists were monitored by means of video recordings and weekly supervision. On the C-GAS there was no difference between the experimental group and the comparison group at baseline (T_1). Both groups improved from T_1 to T_2 with no change from T_2 to T_3. The magnitude of the change was greater in the experimental group, with an effect size on the C-GAS of 0.73. No group differences emerged on the CBCL in the first 6 months, whereas at 2-year followup only the experimental group improved significantly in all summary scales. The authors describe this continued improvement as a sleeper effect, an emerging phenomena in the study of psychodynamic psychotherapies. The authors also noted that between T_2 and T_3 the treatment-condition patients were significantly less likely to seek further treatment than were the community-treated comparison patients. This finding suggests that savings on future treatment may offset costs over time for the psychodynamic therapy group. Limitations of this study included its lack of random assignment and the fact that, although all the children reached full criteria for diagnosis of a psychiatric disorder, the CBCL score means were lower than in many other clinical samples. The authors also questioned whether there were cultural influences particular to these (Italian) families. The percentage of intact families was high, raising the possibility that the findings might not extend to other populations.

It is important to note that the studies reviewed above are all from European research groups, albeit published in the English language literature. In addition to these studies in England and Italy, Trowell is working on a three-center study of psychodynamic psychotherapy for childhood depression that is coordinated from London, with centers in Athens and Helsinki (69). Difficulty thus arises for the dissemination of research findings in psychodynamic psychotherapy to American child and adolescent psychiatrists if literature searches for the development of practice guidelines or metaanalyses is limited to reports in English.

Psychodynamic psychotherapy research is moving forward in America on two fronts. Researchers are developing manualized treatments of classical transference and defense-oriented individual therapies, although few of these manuals are for treatment of children or adolescents. Other North American researchers are building off of the attachment school of psychoanalytic psychology, developing treatments for the parent–child dyad.

Kernberg and Chazan developed a psychotherapy manual for children with conduct disorder (70). There have not been subsequent studies published in which this manual was utilized. Publication of pilot studies is evidence of a more promising start for manualized psychodynamic psychotherapy in the United States evolving around the *Manual of Panic-Focused Psychodynamic Psychotherapy* (PFPP) developed by Milrod et al. at Cornell University Medical College (71). PFPP is a 12-week, 24-session individual psychodynamic psychotherapy emphasizing unconscious thought, free association, and the centrality of transference. The hypothesis underlying PFPP is that common psychodynamic conflicts in panic disorder involve difficulties with separation and independence as well as recognition and management of anger and sexual excitement. These issues are addressed as they arise in the sessions and particularly as they arise in the transference under the pressure of impending termination. Findings from an open trial pilot study in adults are promising, with remission of symptoms sustained at 6 months after completion of treatment (72–74) Looking separately at the results for patients 18 to 21 years of age showed that these late adolescents, or young adults, also did well with PPFP (75). The research team has developed a manual for treatment of adolescents (PFPP-A) (76). The major changes from the adult version focus on a psychodynamic approach to the work with the adolescent's family and the particular countertransference issues adolescents generate.

The dyadic treatment of mothers and their preschool children is an area in which research on psychodynamic interventions is moving forward. This research brings together the work of Bowlby, Ainsworth, and Main on the quality of attachment of infants and toddlers to their caregivers with the work of Selma Fraiberg and her collaborators on the intergenerational transmission of internal representations, aggressive conflicts and negative self-representations. The work of Toth et al. at the University of Rochester testing preschooler–parent psychotherapy (PPP) and of Lieberman, Van Horn, and Ippen at the University of California–San Francisco evaluating child–parent psychotherapy (CPP) are fine examples of this active area of research.

Toth et al. (77) took as their study population maltreated preschoolers and their mothers. The outcome measure of interest to them was the child's internal representation of self and of mother and of the mother–child relationship as tested on the McArthur Story-Stem Battery (MSSB) and the Attachment Story Completion Task (ASCT). Mothers and their preschoolers receiving PPP were seen for weekly, 60-minute, dyadic sessions with a clinical therapist, usually at the treatment center but with occasional home visits. The therapist was sensitive to distortions enacted within the preschooler–parent interactions and other clues to influences of maternal internal representations on parenting. Therapists strove to provide a corrective emotional experience for the parent by providing empathy, respect, and an unfailingly positive regard. Within this holding, therapist–mother relationship, new experiences of self in relationship to others could be internalized. Additionally, new representations of the preschooler could be internalized. Positive representations of the therapist, as they evolved in the therapy, were utilized to contrast with maternal representations of self in relation to her own parents and in relation to her child. In this way PPP addresses the "ghosts in the nursery" so poignantly described by Selma Fraiberg. Within the sessions, the therapist attends to both the interactional and the representational levels manifested in the mother's and child's behaviors. By using observations and empathic comments, the therapist assists the mother in recognizing how her representations are enacted during her interactions with her preschooler. Although the therapist's interactions with the child may provide a model of adult–child interaction, no effort is made to be didactic or explicitly instructive. The therapist seeks to respond to maternal utterances and interactional patterns, linking current maternal conceptualizations of relationships to mothers' own experience of care in childhood.

Study participants included 87 maltreated preschoolers and their mothers and 35 demographically matched, nonmaltreated, normal controls (NC). The 87 dyads in the maltreated group were randomly assigned to PPP (n = 23), psychoeducational home visitation (PHV, n = 34) or community standard care (CS, n = 30). The PHV treatment emphasized a focus on the present and the provision to mothers of didactic information and parenting skills training as well as cognitive-behavioral techniques designed to change mother–child interactional patterns. Additionally these children were enrolled in a 10-month full-day preschool program. The length of treatment for both PPP and PHV was comparable, about 12 months and 32 sessions. Both treatments were manualized. Therapists had comparable levels of professional training in the treatment modality, including mock therapy sessions and review of videotapes.

The results of this study are rich and complex. Change in maladaptive maternal representations over time was dependent on the intervention condition. The PPP group exhibited a highly significant decrease in maladaptive maternal representations over time, whereas for the children in the PHV condition, only a marginally significant decline occurred. On this measure the PPP children were significantly distinguished from the CS and NC groups, whereas the PHV children were not. The PPP group was the only group of children to exhibit a significant decrease in negative self-representation. In regard to positive self-representations over time, PPP, CS, and NC child participants exhibited significant increases in positive self-representation over time, whereas for the PHV group the improvement in positive self-representation was only marginal. Increasingly positive expectations of the mother–child relationship were seen in all four conditions, but were most dramatically positive in the PPP condition. When coupled with the PPP group's more significant decline in negative maternal representations, this finding indicates that the PPP intervention brought an across the board improvement in the child's maternal representation.

By using an outcome measure reflective of internal representations, this study moves in a direction that is meaningful to psychodynamic practitioners. This study begins to develop an evidence base for the aim of psychodynamic psychotherapy to reach beyond behavioral symptoms, to create psychological health and resilience. This study may also suggest lines for investigation of the sleeper effect hinted at in several outcome studies of psychodynamic psychotherapy: Do positive internal representations continue to yield benefits over time?

Lieberman, Van Horn, and Ippen's child–parent psychotherapy (CPP) (78) also takes the mother–child dyad, rather than an individual child patient, as the treatment unit. As with preschooler parent psychotherapy, this treatment developed for preschoolers exposed to marital violence draws on attachment theory and the work of Fraiberg. CPP consists of weekly parent–child sessions for 1 year, during which the therapist's interventions are guided by the unfolding child–mother interactions and by the child's free play with developmentally appropriate toys selected to encourage social interaction and to elicit trauma play. The therapist seeks to guide the mother and child in creating a joint narrative of the traumatic events they experienced. Additionally, the therapist seeks to change maladaptive behaviors and support developmentally appropriate interactions between mother and child. Seventy-five preschoolers and their mothers were enrolled in the study and randomly assigned to the CPP treatment group or to a comparison group receiving monthly case management and individual treatment in the community. At baseline, 6 months, and 1 year, the children were assessed with the Child Behavior Checklist and a clinician-administered caregiver interview using a standardized format to systematize the traumatic stress disorder diagnostic criteria of the *Diagnostic Classification Manual for Mental Health and Developmental Disorders of Infancy and Early Childhood*. Children assigned to CPP improved significantly more than children receiving the community treatment. Children in the test treatment demonstrated decreased total behavioral problems and decreased traumatic stress disorder.

Trends

What conclusions can be drawn from the evidence currently available regarding the intensity and duration of psychodynamic treatments for children and adolescents? In an early study of the impact of intensity and duration on the outcome of psychodynamic psychotherapy for children, Heinicke and Ramsey-Klee (79) studied the impact of frequency of sessions on outcome for children referred for reading retardation associated with emotional disturbance. Their study looked at three groups of children, those treated once per week for 2 years, those treated four times per week for 2 years, and a group that was treated once per week for the first year and four times per week for the second year. While all three treatment groups showed gains in self-esteem, adaptation, and the capacity for relationships, the gains were greater and better sustained in the groups that had been treated four times per week for one or both years. Methodological weaknesses relating to lack of definition of the target disorders and treatment procedures and concerns regarding the validity of the outcome measures require that the results be taken as preliminary.

All the trials of manualized psychodynamic psychotherapy for children and adolescents reviewed in this chapter tested short-term treatments. Except for the intensive, in-hospital intervention for diabetes and the 24-session, twice-weekly panic-focused psychodynamic psychotherapy, all were weekly in intensity. Taken together, these studies suggest that low to moderate intensity, time-limited psychodynamic psychotherapies can be beneficial for some children and adolescents.

The Anna Freud Centre retrospective chart review compared four to five times per week psychoanalysis with one to three time per week psychodynamic psychotherapy. Either intensity of treatment was undertaken with an open-ended approach to length of treatment. Children under 12 benefited more from the four to five times per week treatments than from those of lesser intensity. However, adolescents, particularly neurotic adolescents, did better with the less intense therapy. In this study, 72% of children with emotional disorders who stayed in treatment for more than 6 months showed reliable, clinically significant improvement in adaptation (80). Further study of the effects of intensity and duration of treatment is necessary if we are to apply resources in a cost-effective manner.

Another question generated by research on psychodynamic psychotherapies is whether there is a "sleeper effect." Do patients continue to improve on outcome measures months to years after the cessation of the treatment? The early study by Heinicke and Ramsey-Klee found little difference at the conclusion of treatment between the group seen once per week and those seen four times per week for either 1 or 2 years. However, at 1-year followup, the two groups that had received four times per week treatment showed continued improvement on all outcome measures. Those who were treated just once per week did not show similar improvement. Nearly 20 years later, Muratori and Picchi found that for patients receiving an 11-week psychodynamic psychotherapy for internalizing disorders, improvement in global functioning occurred early and was evident at the 6-month followup, whereas symptom improvement as measured by the CBCL was most significant at the 2-year followup. Patients in the comparison treatment did not show this continued improvement. In fact, patients in the comparison condition sought further mental health services at a significantly higher rate than those who had received the test psychodynamic psychotherapy. Continued accrual of benefit is seen in studies of adults treated with psychodynamic psychotherapy (81, 82).

Psychodynamic researchers and clinicians find in the sleeper effect support for the assumption that addressing underlying psychological processes and moving a patient to a more mature and adaptive level of function will bring lasting benefit, while removing target symptoms may bring only transitory relief. Furthermore, demonstration of continued return on the investment made in a therapy directed at deeper structures can support the cost-effectiveness of treatments that may take considerable investment in therapist training at the front end. It is of note that in Weiss, Catron, and Harris's (83) study of non-manualized, "traditional" psychotherapy provided by masters level clinicians, no sleeper effect was found at 2-year followup.

Under pressure from surrounding disciplines, from the emphasis on empirical research in the evidence based medicine movement, and from an ever-tightening mental health care budget, psychodynamic psychotherapy research is expanding in scope and methods. Yet psychodynamic research retains an emphasis that is true to its underlying theoretical base. Both treatment interventions and outcome measure are designed to change and to measure psychic structure and overall wellbeing rather than symptoms and behaviors. Additionally, the focus of treatment is frequently relational, whether in the child–parent dyad or the patient–therapist dyad. Much of psychodynamic research is aimed at those who struggle with adversity, e.g., diabetes or psychosocial trauma, rather than at specific diagnoses. This is in keeping with the holistic trend in psychodynamic psychiatry that favors a biopsychosocial model over a more narrowly biomedical disease model for clinical formulations. Psychodynamic psychotherapy research also benefits from a rich collaboration with developmental research.

References

1. Gabbard G: *Psychodynamic Psychiatry in Clinical Practice*. Washington, DC, American Psychiatric Press, Inc., 1990.
2. Freud S: Analysis of a phobia in a five-year-old boy. In: Strachey JE (ed): *The Standard Edition of the Complete Psychological Works of Sigmund Freud* (vol X). London, Hogarth Press, 1955, pp. 3–149.
3. Von Hug-Hellmuth H: On the technique of child analysis. *International Journal of Psychoanalysis* 2:287–305, 1921.
4. Klein M: *The Psychoanalysis of Children*. London, Hogarth Press, 1932.
5. Freud A: *The Psycho-Analytical Treatment of Children*. London, Imago Publishing, 1946.
6. Freud A: *The Ego and the Mechanisms of Defense*. Vol II, 1966 ed. New York, International Universities Press, Inc., 1936.
7. Freud A: *Normality and Pathology in Childhood: Assessments of Development*. New York, International Universities Press, Inc., 1965.
8. Allen FH: *Psychotherapy with Children*. New York, Norton, 1942.
9. Rogers CR: The developing character of client-centered therapy. In: Rogers CR (ed): *Client-Centered Therapy: Its Current Practice, Implications, and Theory*. Boston, Houghton Mifflin Company, 1951: pp. 3–18.

10. Axline VM: *Play Therapy*. New York, Ballantine, 1947.
11. Dorfman E: Play therapy. In: Rogers C (ed): *Client-Centered Therapy*. Boston, Houghton Mifflin, 1951: pp. 235–277.
12. Bowlby J: *Attachment and Loss. Vol 1: Attachment*. New York, Basic Books, 1969.
13. Bowlby J: *Attachment and Loss. Vol 2: Separation: Anxiety and Anger*. New York, Basic Books, 1973.
14. Bowlby J: *Attachment and Loss. Vol 3: Loss: Sadness and Depression*. New York, Basic Books, 1980.
15. Weinberger J, Levy KN: Chapter 30: Psychology. In: Person ES, Cooper A, Gabbard G, (eds): *Textbook of Psychoanalysis*. Washington, DC, American Psychiatric Publishing, Inc., 2005:463–477.
16. Bleiberg E: *Treating Personality Disorders in Children and Adolescents: A Relational Approach*. New York, Guilford Press, 2001.
17. Gabbard G, Lazar S, Hornberger J, Spiegel D: The economic impact of psychotherapy: A Review. *American Journal of Psychiatry* 154:147–155, 1997.
18. Werry J, Andrews L: The psychotherapies: A critical overview. In: M. Lewis (ed): *Child and Adolescent Psychiatry: A Comprehensive Textbook*, 2nd ed. Baltimore, Williams and Wilkins, 1996, pp. 878–883.
19. Brent D, Kolko D: Psychotherapy: Definition, mechanisms of action, and relationship to etiologic models. *Journal of Abnormal Child Psychology* 26:17–25, 1998.
20. Ritvo LB: *Darwin's Influence on Freud: A Tale of Two Sciences*. New Haven, Yale University Press, 1990.
21. Solms M: Freud Returns. *Scientific American* 290(5):82–88, 2004.
22. Freud S: Introductory Lectures on Psychoanalysis: Part III. In: Strachey J (ed): *The Standard Edition of the Complete Psychological Works of Sigmund Freud* (vol XVI). London, Hogarth Press, 1963.
23. Moore BE, Fine BD: *Psychoanalytic Terms and Concepts*. New Haven, Yale University Press, 1990.
24. Ritvo S, Solnit AJ: Instinct theory. In: Moore BE, Fine BD (eds): *Psychoanalysis: The Major Concepts*. New Haven, Yale University Press, 1995, pp. 327–333.
25. Freud S: The Ego and the Id (1923). In: Strachey J (ed): *The Standard Edition of the Complete Psychological Works of Sigmund Freud*. Vol XIX. London: Hogarth Press, 1961, pp. 3–66.
26. Solms M: Chapter 36: Neuroscience. In: Person ES, Cooper A, Gabbard G (eds): *Textbook of Psychoanalysis*. Washington, DC, American Psychiatric Publishing, Inc., 2005, pp. 535–546.
27. Miller J: *Using Self Psychology in Child Psychotherapy: The Restoration of the Child*. Northvale, NJ, Jason Aronson, 1996.
28. Gray P: *The Ego and Analysis of Defense*. Northvale, Jason Aronson Inc., 1994.
29. Hartmann H: Comments on the psychoanalytic theory of the ego. *Psychoanalytic Study of the Child* 5:74–96, 1950.
30. Compton A: Objects and object relationships. In: Moore B, Fine B, (eds): *Psychoanalysis: The Major Concepts*. New Haven, Yale University Press, 1995:433–449.
31. Mahler M. Thoughts about development and individualtion. *Psychoanalytic Study of the Child* 18:307–324, 1962.
32. Provence S, Ritvo S: Effects of deprivation on institutionalized infants. *Psychoanalytic Study of the Child* 16:189–205, 1961.
33. Spitz R: Hospitalism: An inquiry into the genesis of psychiatric conditions in early childhood. *Psychoanalytic Study of the Child* 1:53–74, 1945.
34. Kernberg O: Psychoanalytic object relations theories. In: Moore B, Fine B (eds): *Psychoanalysis: The Major Concepts*. New Haven, Yale University Press, 1995, pp. 450–462.
35. Sandler J, Rosenblatt B: The Concept of the Representational World. In: *Psychoanalytic Study of the Child* 17:128–145, 1962.
36. Sandler J, Kennedy H, Tyson R: *The Technique of Child Psychoanalysis: Discussions with Anna Freud*. Cambridge, MA, Harvard University Press, 1980.
37. Brenner C: *The Mind in Conflict*. New York, International Universities Press, 1982.
38. Lewis O: Integrated psychodynamic psychotherapy with children. *Child and Adolescent Psychiatric Clinics of North America* 6(1):53–68, 1997.
39. Marshall R: Countertransference in the psychotherapy of children and adolescents. *Contemporary Psychoanalysis* 15(3):595–629, 1979.
40. Winnicott D: Hate in the counter-transference. *International Journal of Psychoanalysis* 30:69–74, 1949.
41. Novick KK, Novick J: *Working with Parents Makes Therapy Work*. Lanham, MD, Jason Aronson, 2005.
42. Robson K: *Manual of Clinical Child and Adolescent Psychiatry*, rev. ed. Washington, DC, American Psychiatric Press, Inc; 1986.
43. Shapiro T: The psychodynamic formulation in child and adolescent psychiatry. *Journal of the American Academy of Child and Adolescent Psychiatry* 28:675–680, 1989.
44. Jellinek MS, McDermott JF: Formulation: Putting the diagnosis into a therapeutic context and treatment plan. *Journal of the American Academy of Child and Adolescent Psychiatry* 43(7):913–916, 2004.
45. Freud A: Indications and contraindications of child analysis. *Psychoanalytic Study of the Child* 23:37–46, 1968.
46. McConville B: An overview of diagnosis and treatment planning. In: Klykylo W, Kay J, Rube D (eds): *Child Psychiatry*. Philadelphia, W.B. Saunders, 1998, pp. 85–103.
47. Lewis M: Interpretation in child analysis. *Journal of the American Academy of Child Psychiatry* 13:32–53, 1974.
48. Lewis M: Chapter 79: Intensive individual psychodynamic psychotherapy: The therapeutic relationship and the technique of interpretation: The use of play in psychodynamic therapy. In: Lewis M, (ed). *Child and Adolescent Psychiatry: A Comprehensive Textbook*, 3rd ed. Philadelphia: Lippincott Williams & Wilkins, 2003, pp. 984–992.
49. Lewis JM, Blotcky MJ: *Child Therapy: Concepts, Strategies, and Decision Making*. Washington, DC, Brunner/Mazel, 1997.
50. Yanof JA: Technique in child analysis. In: Person ES, Cooper A, Gabbard G, eds. *Textbook of Psychoanalysis*. Washington, DC, American Psychiatric Publishing, Inc.; 2005, pp. 267–280.
51. Loewenstein R: The problem of interpretation. *Psychoanalytic Quarterly* 20:1–14, 1951.
52. Kennedy H: Problems in reconstruction in child analysis. *Psychoanalytic Study of the Child* 26:386–402, 1971.
53. Freud A: Problems of termination in child analysis (1970 [1957]). *The Writings of Anna Freud* (vol VII). New York, International Universities Press, Inc; 1971, pp. 3–21.
54. Sperling E: The collateral treatment of parents with children and adolescents in psychotherapy. *Child and Adolescent Psychiatric Clinics of North America* 6(1):81–95, 1997.
55. Novick J: Comments on termination in child, adolescent, and adult analysis. *Psychoanalytic Study of the Child* 45:419–436, 1990.
56. Freud S: Remembering, repeating and working-through (Further recommendations on the technique of psycho-analysis II) (1914). In: Strachey JE (ed): Strachey J (trans): *The Standard Edition of the Complete Psychological Works of Sigmund Freud* (vol XII). London, Hogarth Press, 1957, pp. 145–156.
57. Gedo JE: The enduring scientific contributions of Sigmund Freud. *Annual of Psychoanalysis* 29:105–115, 2001.
58. Weisz JR, Hawley KM, Doss AJ: Empirically tested psychotherapies for youth internalizing and externalizing problems and disorders. *Child and Adolescent Psychiatric Clinics of North America* 13(4):729–815, 2004.
59. Fonagy P, Target M, Cottrell D, Phillips J, Kurtz Z: *What Works for Whom? A Critical Review of Treatments for Children and Adolescents*. New York, Guilford Press, 2005.
60. Leichsenring F, Rabung S, Leibing E: The efficacy of short-term psychodynamic psychotherapy in specific psychiatric disorders. *Archives of General Psychiatry* 61(12):1208–1216, 2004.
61. Sandler J: Research in psycho-analysis: The Hampstead Index as an instrument of psycho-analytic research. *International Journal of Psychoanalysis* 43:287–291, 1962.
62. Target M, Fonagy P: Efficacy of psychoanalysis for children with emotional disorders. *Journal of the American Academy of Child and Adolescent Psychiatry* 33(3):361–371, 1994.
63. Fonagy P, Target M: The efficacy of psychoanalysis for children with disruptive disorders. *Journal of the American Academy of Child and Adolescent Psychiatry* 33(1):45–55, 1994.
64. Target M, Fonagy P: The efficacy of psychoanalysis in children: Prediction of outcome in a developmental context. *Journal of the American Academy of Child and Adolescent Psychiatry* 33(8):1134–1144, 1994.
65. Target M: The problem of outcome in child psychoanalysis: Contributions from the Anna Freud Centre. In: Leuzinger-Bohleber M, Target M (eds): *Outcomes of Psychoanalytic Treatment: Perspectives for Therapists and Researchers*. New York, Brunner-Routledge, 2002, pp. 240–251.
66. Moran G, Fonagy P, Kurtz A, Bolton A, Brook C: A controlled study of the psychoanalytic treatment of brittle diabetes. *Journal of the American Academy of Child and Adolescent Psychiatry* 30:926–935, 1991.
67. Trowell J, Kolvin I, Weeramanthri T, et al.: Psychotherapy for sexually abused girls: Psychopathological outcome findings and patterns of change. *The British Journal of Psychiatry* 180:234–247, 2002.
68. Muratori F, Picchi L, Bruni G, Patarnello M, Romagnoli G: A two-year follow-up of psychodynamic psychotherapy for internalizing disorders in children. *Journal of the American Academy of Child and Adolescent Psychiatry* 42(3):331–339, 2003.
69. Trowell J, Rhode M, Miles G, Sherwood I: Childhood depression: Work in progress: Individual child therapy and parent work. *Journal of Child Psychotherapy* 29(2):147–169, 2003.
70. Kernberg PF, Chazan SE: *Children with Conduct Disorders: A Psychotherapy Manual*: Basic Books, 1991.
71. Milrod B, Busch F, Cooper A, Shapiro T: *Manual of Panic-Focused Psychodynamic Psychotherapy*. Washington, DC, American Psychiatric Press, Inc., 1997.
72. Busch F, Milrod B, Rudden M, et al.: How treating psychoanalysts respond to psychotherapy research constraints. *Journal of the American Psychoanalytic Association* 49(3):961–984, 2001.
73. Milrod B, Busch F, Leon A, et al.: A pilot open trial of brief psychodynamic psychotherapy for panic disorder. *Journal of Psychotherapy Practice and Research* 10(4):239–245, 2001.
74. Milrod B, Busch F, Leon A, et al.: Open trial of psychodynamic psychotherapy for panic disorder: A pilot study. *American Journal of Psychiatry* 157(11):1878–1880, 2000.
75. Milrod B, Busch F, Shapiro T: A pilot study of psychodynamic psychotherapy for 18 to 21 year old patients with panic disorder. *Annals of the American Society for Adolescent Psychiatry* 29:289–314, 2005.

76. Milrod B, Busch F, Shapiro T: *Psychodynamic Approaches to the Adolescent with Panic Disorder.* Malabar, FL, Krieger Publishing Company, 2004.
77. Toth S, Maughan A, Manly JT, Spagnola M, Cicchetti D: The relative efficacy of two interventions in altering maltreated preschool children's representational models: Implications for attachment theory. *Development and Psychopathology* 14(4):877–908, 2002.
78. Lieberman AF, Van Horn P, Ippen CG: Toward evidence-based treatment: Child–parent psychotherapy with preschoolers exposed to marital violence. *Journal of the American Academy of Child and Adolescent Psychiatry* 44(12):1241–1248, 2005.
79. Heinicke CM, Ramsey-Klee D: Outcome of child psychotherapy as a function of frequency of session. *Journal of the American Academy of Child and Adolescent Psychiatry* 25(2):247–253, 1986.
80. Target M: The problem of outcome in child psychoanalysis: Contributions from the Anna Freud Centre. In: Leuzinger-Bohleber M, Target M (eds): *Outcomes of Psychoanalytic Treatment: Perspectives for Therapists and Researchers.* New York, Brunner-Routledge, 2002, pp. 240–251.
81. Sandell R, Blomberg J, Lazar A, Carlsson J, Broberg J, Schubert J: Varieties of long-term outcome among patients in psychoanalysis and long-term psychotherapy: A review of the findings in the Stockholm Outcome of Psychoanalysis and Psychotherapy Project (STOPPP). *International Journal of Psychoanalysis* 81:921–942, 2000.
82. Bateman A, Fonagy P: Treatment of borderline personality disorder with psychoanalytically oriented partial hospitalization: An 18-month follow-up. *American Journal of Psychiatry* January 158(1):36–42, 2001.
83. Weiss B, Catron T, Harris V: A 2-year follow-up of the effectiveness of traditional child psychotherapy. *Journal of Consulting and Clinical Psychology* 68(6):1094–1101, 2000.
84. Edgerton J, III RC (eds): *American Psychiatric Glossary,* 7th ed. Washington, DC, American Psychiatric Press, Inc., 1994.

CHAPTER 6.2.5 ■ GROUP THERAPY

NANCY E. MOSS, GARY R. RACUSIN, AND CORINNE MOSS-RACUSIN

INTRODUCTION

Group treatment stands as a powerful intervention available to professionals serving the child and adolescent population. The aim of this chapter is to provide an intellectually informed clinical guide to implementation of this modality of treatment. The chapter begins by placing group therapy in a historical context and considering aspects of group development. A theoretical framework for group treatment is then discussed, followed by examination of the many pragmatic issues to be managed in offering a therapeutic group. Parent involvement and leadership functions are then considered. A description follows of special applications of group treatment for HIV-affected youngsters and individuals on the autism spectrum. Indications and contraindications for group treatment, as well as training and supervision needs, are then examined. The chapter concludes with a discussion of the efficacy of group treatment and the status of research in the field.

Group treatment with children and adolescents has a long history (1–6). At the end of the nineteenth and beginning of the twentieth century, early efforts were designed to rehabilitate particular medically affected populations (7). Group homes that included intensive attention to group process were organized to treat adolescents with severe behavior disorders (8). Heavy use was made of psychodrama in treating a variety of problems in a group context (9). Related to the settlement house movement, groups were offered to youngsters from lower socioeconomic strata to expose them to aspects of more affluent, mainstream culture (10). The hope of this last type of group was that such exposure would elevate the group members' overall functioning, improve their behavior, and facilitate their moving into productive adulthood.

As the twentieth century continued, many groups for children and adolescents were offered under the auspices of child guidance centers and community mental health centers. Activity groups for children became prominent, based on the premise that participation in age-appropriate play activity would promote better mental health. Later in the twentieth century, groups based on the principles of behavior modification were conducted to treat numerous psychiatric problems. As the twentieth century closed and the twenty-first century began, social skill groups and manual-based psychoeducational groups designed to impart specific curricula assumed greater prominence (6).

Just as the broad field of group therapy with children and adolescents has developed over time, many clinicians and researchers involved in child and adolescent group therapy have formulated the developmental stages through which each individual group moves over the course of its operation (11–14). Generally, groups move through an initial phase during which the foundation is laid for group cohesion. The group then often has a relatively euphoric period when the members have great hope and feel relief at having become part of the group. This period may then be followed by a more discouraged period as the full impact of the presenting problems becomes more evident. With good leadership, the group is then able to move into a more realistic, hardworking phase of its life. Ultimately, the group must go through the termination phase, during which members need help in internalizing and consolidating the gains made and in preparing to separate from the group.

Stages of group development take on different contours in both open-ended and shorter term, time-limited groups. The relevance of group development to leadership interventions varies greatly depending on the type of group offered. In groups intended to be long term but with a planned ending date, correct interpretations of group behavior should rest on a sound understanding of the stage at which a group is operating. In contrast, in open-ended groups, members are admitted and discharged as dictated by their clinical needs. The group as a whole remains in a hardworking developmental stage as it incorporates new members and disengages from departing ones. Finally, in briefer, time-limited groups, group developmental stages become less relevant. The group tackles its specific tasks, knowing throughout that termination is close.

THEORETICAL UNDERPINNINGS OF GROUP THERAPY

Amid the daily pressures of clinic life and professional practice, therapeutic groups are often designed and implemented without a foundation of theoretical knowledge. Rather than being derived from comprehensive theory, many groups reflect professionals' efforts to manage time and caseload constraints. Such an atheoretical approach limits severely the range and effectiveness of group interventions. Without a theory for guidance, group leaders must rely more purely on intuition and moment-to-moment creativity in responding to the ongoing demands of group life.

Theory-based group practice allows for much more coherent intervention and thereby capitalizes most fully on the potential impact of a group treatment. A theoretical foundation allows group leaders to offer a range of group treatments that address group structure, procedures, and leadership style. When issues of structure, procedure, and essential leadership skills are mastered, they can be applied to any clinical population or specified problem. A guiding theory is also invaluable in navigating any single meeting of a group. Since each group meeting generates a wealth of clinical data and information, myriad decisions face the group leaders regarding intervention choices. A theoretical basis provides a map for leaders to discriminate among levels of information and thereby determine the most appropriate responses and interventions at any point in time.

A variety of theories have been used to guide group practice. Cognitive behavioral, psychodynamic, and gestalt theories are prominent among those that have been mined for group practice (15). Choice of a theoretical guide should be at the discretion of the leaders. Designation of a comprehensive theory and its full utilization are much more important than which particular theory is chosen.

While many theories can be helpful in group leadership, Bion's group-as-a-whole is a powerful theory available to group leaders (16–21). Originated in Britain by Wilfred Bion and his psychiatric/psychoanalytic colleagues to assist the British military during World War II, the theory posits that group structure and strong leadership are critical variables in group practice. Essential features of this body of theory are discussed below.

Consistent with its name, this theory asserts that the group as a whole is greater than the sum of its parts. The group as a whole is the "organism" to be considered. Individuals are believed to participate in the group life as dictated by their singular needs and capacities, in interaction with shared group needs and capacities. Individual behavior is therefore always understood as conveying information not only about that individual but about issues that require the group's attention. Individual behavior displayed in a group context is always believed to be a necessary expression by the group and to have relevance for the group. To have the greatest therapeutic impact, then, interpretations of behavior and interventions should be aimed at the group level.

The theory posits further that a group must be distinguished from a more casual collection of individuals. This distinction rests on identification of the group's shared task. The fundamental task of the group becomes the bedrock on which the group's life is based. As the group proceeds, practice decisions and behavioral interpretations should always be evaluated by their fidelity to the fundamental task of the group.

There is a range of tasks that can be addressed in therapeutic groups for children and adolescents. These tasks fall in roughly five categories. Traditionally, many groups were organized to provide formal, insight-oriented, psychodynamic psychotherapy. The task of such a group is to use both talk and play, as appropriate, to help make the unconscious conscious, presumably leading to greater psychological health characterized by intentionally chosen appropriate behaviors. While such formal psychotherapeutic groups still exist, briefer and more behaviorally oriented types of group work with children are now offered more widely. This broadening of the kinds of groups offered can be understood as a response to increased financial constraints in the mental health field. A second type of group offered to children and adolescents is the social skills group. The task of this type of group is to increase the members' repertoire of age-appropriate social skills, thereby enhancing the members' interpersonal relationships overall and improving their peer relationships, in particular. The task of a third type of group, a support group, is to acknowledge a traumatic experience or set of circumstances common to all group members and to provide clinically informed support aimed at facilitating good coping skills. Some groups are more formally didactic, taking on the task of imparting knowledge and teaching skills relevant to a particular psychoeducational problem. Finally, a fifth type of child/adolescent group is a goal-focused group. This group has the task of marshalling internal and external resources to allow the members to attain a specified, tangible goal or create a tangible product.

For groups to be effective, leaders must begin with a clear conceptualization of the group's task. Leaders must be vigilant about remaining true to the task, carrying out actions relevant to the designated task and foregoing actions that would actually be aimed at an alternate one. To take on task-irrelevant issues essentially makes an offer to the group that can't be delivered fully and thereby threatens the integrity of the leadership and the group as a whole.

Members' conceptualization of the group task operates differently than the leaders'. Members must hear a clear statement of the group's task as they enter group. Otherwise, they would be justifiably confused about the nature of their participation and expectations for them to work would be unfair. It is often true, however, that group members develop a full understanding of the task only as they participate in the life of the group. Many times, the nature of the task is so difficult that the task itself only becomes truly understandable psychologically as the group begins to have some initial success in task accomplishment and develops greater capacity to tolerate the tension involved in group participation.

Once the group begins, its activity can be defined in two ways, rational work and/or basic assumption group life. Rational work is defined as any activity that moves the group further toward accomplishment of its task. For groups of children and adolescents, it is essential to note that rational work will be expressed in developmentally determined forms. For young children, this might be a variety of play activities. For older children and adolescents, more conversation might be used. Thus, a firm grasp of normative child/adolescent development is necessary to allow group leaders to recognize and interpret accurately the members' behavior.

This body of theory presumes, however, that carrying out rational work is extremely arduous. By definition, the task of a therapeutic group is difficult. If the task were an easy one, creation of the therapeutic group and its dedication to ongoing effort would be unnecessary. Formal psychotherapy groups lead members to confront some of their most basic unmet needs and deficits. Social skill groups highlight fundamental interpersonal impairment. Support groups focus on specific traumas that engender significant distress. Didactic groups require substantial cognitive growth, typically regarding emotionally charged topics. Goal-focused groups elicit disturbing emotions about the necessity for reaching the specified goal. In addition to particular group characteristics, group membership itself is understood as a psychologically challenging transaction. Each member must relinquish enough individuality to join fully with the group as a whole. At the same time, each member must retain a firm hold on a singular identity. Balancing of these requirements requires considerable psychological energy and strength.

When the difficulties posed by rational work become too great, groups are assumed to feel that their continued existence is threatened. To defend themselves, they retreat to basic assumption life. Basic assumption life is defined as a variety of defensive postures, each expressing a fundamentally irrational notion of how the group may avoid the perils of rational work and thereby continue to exist. It is incumbent upon the leaders to recognize basic assumption life and to interpret it appropriately. Group-as-a-whole theory states that such interpretation and exploration of the group's reaction are instructive for the group and ease the group back into a rational work mode.

Group-as-a-whole theory was developed as a compelling, comprehensive approach to group operation and leadership primarily appropriate for adults. Considerable group experience has demonstrated that, with appropriate developmental modifications, the theory is equally useful with children and adolescents (21, 22). Embedded as the theory is in group and organizational life, it takes the fullest therapeutic advantage of the group treatment modality.

PRAGMATICS IN THE OPERATION OF GROUP THERAPY

Along with theoretical underpinnings, a number of pragmatic considerations have a significant impact on the usefulness of group treatment. Many of these considerations are explored by Lomonaco, Scheidlinger, and Aronson (3), Schamess (23), Schectman (24), and Slavson and Schiffer (25). Relevant considerations are discussed below.

Recruitment of Members

The main goal of the recruitment phase of group treatment is to identify members who need both to accomplish the designated task of the group and who are able to work together toward that task accomplishment. Such identification requires sufficient clinical knowledge about each prospective group member. Several concrete steps facilitate the identification and recruitment process. First, group leaders must communicate clearly and broadly with all potential referral sources in an enthusiastic and welcoming manner. Referrals should be encouraged by conveying an eagerness and willingness to be helpful to colleagues and potential group members. Once a referral has been suggested, group leaders need to determine whether the child or adolescent has been fully evaluated. If a psychiatric evaluation or psychological assessment has been completed recently, the results of the evaluation should be reviewed carefully to assess compatibility with the designated group. If no recent evaluation has been done, group leaders either need to obtain in-depth clinical information about the prospective member from a clinician with ongoing knowledge about the member, or the leaders need to carry out a relevant evaluation. An in-depth, clinical understanding of each prospective group member is necessary to ensure appropriate group composition. Should the group leaders then determine that the prospective group member is inappropriate for the designated group, alternative treatment options or experiences should be suggested to the child or adolescent and his/her family. Should the group leaders conclude that the referral is appropriate, the leaders should meet with the group member's parents to describe the group in detail, to plan for the child's or adolescent's course in the group treatment, and to answer parent questions. The leaders should then meet with the prospective group member to again describe the group, make certain that the member appears to fit admission criteria, and to answer the child's or adolescent's questions. At times, actually meeting with the prospective group member raises particular concerns about potential group membership. These concerns should be taken up with parents and referring clinicians to allow for confident admission decisions. If all are then agreed and comfortable, a date should be set for entrance into the group.

Diagnostic Composition

The question arises often about the relative merits of diagnostic homogeneity or heterogeneity in a group. This question should be resolved in relation to the proposed task of the group. A group designed to address specific, diagnosis-related issues would clearly demand diagnostic homogeneity. Thus, for example, a psychoeducational group for children with diabetes would, by definition, require that all members have diabetes. Similarly, a support group for HIV-affected youngsters would require that all members had direct experience with HIV infection. In contrast, a group with a developmental or psychotherapeutic task would thrive on diagnostic heterogeneity. Mirroring the diversity to be encountered in naturalistic environments, such group heterogeneity would bring differences in perspective, observational capacity, and interpersonal relatedness that would allow for spirited, mutually beneficial interactions among members and leaders. To illustrate, a social skills group would do best if members all displayed impaired social functioning but did so for widely different reasons. In such a group, a socially inhibited, depressed member might be able to give very age-appropriate social feedback to an idiosyncratic member on the autism spectrum, while an impulsive, acting-out member might be able to challenge the inhibited member toward more vigorous, instrumental interaction.

One important caution should always be considered in regard to diagnostic composition of the group. To the greatest extent possible given real-life contingencies, a group should not contain only one representative of any critical attribute or category. A solitary representative of any salient classification—racial, religious, ethnic, gender, or level of diagnostic severity—invites isolation and hinders significantly the potentially useful interventions implemented by the leaders. For example, a group for psychotic youngsters could be extremely beneficial, offering them evidence that they were not fully alone in their disorganization, and teaching them pragmatic coping strategies. Placement of a single psychotic child or adolescent into a group of more realistically functioning members, however, intensifies the psychotic member's sense of isolation, highlights his/her impairment, deprives that member of appropriate group interventions, and frightens the group as a whole. In forming a group or admitting new members to an ongoing group, then, every effort should be made to include members who share important, relevant attributes with at least one other member.

Group Size

Therapeutic groups for children and adolescents should be big enough to generate multiple, challenging interpersonal interactions and to allow for both dyadic, triadic, and whole-group activities. At the same time, the groups should be small enough to permit a sense of intimacy and close personal attention. Groups composed of 4–6 members are ideal for most therapeutic tasks. While not overwhelming to individuals, groups of this size can continue to work productively even with occasional absences due to member illness, vacation, or other reasons.

Gender

As with the issue of diagnostic consistency, the question of same-sex versus mixed-sex groups is often debated and should be resolved in reference to the group's task. Traditionally, therapeutic groups were offered to single sex populations. More currently, common practice has changed. For most tasks in groups of children and adolescents, mixed-sex groups prove to be most useful, since interacting with others of both sexes again parallels most closely real-life experience. Group members derive benefits directly applicable to the demands and challenges of daily life. There are, however, some groups that should remain single-sex groups. These are the groups designed to address sensitive issues related to sexuality, aggression, and/or sexual abuse. The need for comfort, trust, and empathy in such groups is difficult enough to satisfy but would be even more difficult in a mixed sex group.

Age Range

In actual clinical life, age ranges are rarely absolute. Developmental and school grade levels tend to influence and sometimes extend the age range of a group. Still, a general age range of 2–3 years is most appropriate. It is important, too, that the span of years be contained within one developmental phase of life. This type of clustering allows for the necessary commonality of experience and capacity to benefit from group interventions.

Setting

A space should be dedicated to the group on a consistent, reliable basis. Two conditions are most important in identifying a group setting. First, the setting must be private for the duration of each group meeting. Intrusions by individuals not associated with the group are very destructive of the group process. Second, the setting must be furnished and equipped in a developmentally appropriate manner. While leaders should work hard to limit damage to the physical space, some wear and tear in the environment must be a realistic expectation in working with children and adolescents. It would be too difficult to carry out the work of the group if leaders were faced with constant worry about protecting a more adult-oriented room that contained objects or interior decorations of great value. If these conditions are met, groups can adapt to many different kinds of spaces of varying sizes.

Materials

When embarking on group treatment for children or adolescents, leaders are often tempted to amass a large collection of tempting, exciting, attractive play materials. In actuality, a big, tempting array is usually over stimulating to a group and leads to excessively active, disorganized interactions. A modest amount of developmentally appropriate materials facilitates much more productive group interaction. For adolescents, some decks of cards, a few advanced board games, and some limited art materials would likely be sufficient. Groups at this adolescent level tend to engage more in conversation than activity. Younger groups rely more heavily on activity as the vehicle of their clinical work. Thus, for elementary and middle schoolchildren, it would be best to provide decks of cards, a larger number of simpler board games, limited art materials, some building toys such as Legos, and something that allows the group to engage safely in an indoor large-motor activity, e.g., a soft, inflatable beach ball or a plastic indoor bowling set. Preschool groups do best with a small amount of building toys, some drawing materials, a few very simple board and card games, and materials that promote fantasy play such as a dollhouse or dress-ups. Whatever the age of the group, it would always be best to do with fewer rather than more materials.

Food

In carrying out group treatment with children and adolescents, the challenge of group participation should always be remembered. Management of the self in relation to the group as a whole is daunting, in addition to the difficulty of the actual therapeutic work. In recognition of the challenges faced by group members, it is helpful to provide a snack as a tangible support to the group. In addition to its nurturing aspects, time spent eating together as a group promotes more intimate, relaxed interactions that often help with task accomplishment. The logistics of providing food in the group are important, as well. The exact food and accompanying drink to be provided should be very simple and should be decided by the group leaders. Accommodations should be made to any specific dietary requirements of group members. The group should be told that a set amount of snack will be offered to each member. Group protest should be expected no matter what the designated amount of snack is. Such protest should be understood as part of the group establishing and maintaining its trust in the group leadership. Leaders should adhere to the snack plans set forth at the outset of the group. The only useful exceptions to these snack plans involve either essential dietary restrictions on the part of individual members or special occasions. In regard to dietary restrictions, parental report sometimes indicates that a child cannot tolerate a food or drink for medical reasons. At other times, religious or cultural beliefs dictate acceptable vs. unacceptable food. These specific needs should be accommodated by the entire group, whenever possible. If group as a whole accommodations are impractical or impossible, the individual member should be cared for appropriately with a simple explanation offered to the group. In regard to special occasions, from time to time the group may observe a holiday if such observance is consistent with the task of the group. On these occasions, it is helpful to have the group plan together about food and drink, with the leaders retaining veto powers if the plans get too lavish to be practical.

Duration

Length of each meeting and lifespan of the group should both be considered. Regarding meeting length, 1–1 1/2 hours is an optimal amount of time for a group meeting. Less than one hour deprives the group of sufficient time to enter fully into work on its task. Instead of concentrating on the work, both leaders and members feel the constant pressure of time and spend most of their energy hurrying to finish. More than 1 1/2 hours is simply too exhausting. Many groups meet for 1 1/4 hours and find that duration to be very comfortable. In public school settings, the demands of the school day often dictate that groups must meet for only 20 minutes to 1/2 hour. Under such conditions, leaders should work hard to design group agendas that can be implemented realistically. Regarding group lifespan, professional preference and practical realities of organizational life in many settings lead to decisions to offer time-limited groups. In such settings, constraints on professional availability, organizational resources, theoretical outlook, and regulations of third-party payers may all require a time-limited group. In other settings and under different conditions, long-term, open-ended groups are still offered, as they were more routinely in earlier years. It should be understood that time-limited versus long-term groups offer different possibilities for meaningful work and can accomplish different tasks. Time-limited groups are best for teaching specific, discrete skills, or imparting well specified information. They can also be very useful for individuals who could not tolerate the intensity of long-term interpersonal interaction. Brief groups may also lend themselves more readily to empirical research designs. In contrast, long-term, open-ended groups are best for facilitating more fundamental, broader changes in designated areas of personal functioning. To carry out formal, intensive psychotherapy in a group format, to engender genuine change in naturalistic social functioning, to provide support with some life-threatening situations, there is no substitute for a long-term, open-ended group experience.

MEETING PROTOCOL MODEL

To allow the group members to rely fully on the structure of the group, group meetings should always follow the same protocol. The exact amount of time allotted to each portion of the agenda may vary based on the leaders' appraisal of the group work in any particular meeting. What should never vary is inclusion of each segment of the meeting protocol in each meeting. Omission of any segment, regardless of how justified such an omission might seem by the events of the moment, will always diminish the group's trust in its leaders and in the structure of the group and will, therefore, impede the work of the group. A useful protocol follows.

Gathering of Members

A comfortable place for the group to go to on arrival at the clinic, school, or private therapy office should be designated. It should be communicated clearly that parents or substitute caregivers retain responsibility for behavior management in the arrival area. Exactly at the time for the group to begin, the leaders should go to the arrival area to greet the members and bring them to the group meeting room. Acceptable behavioral standards and full physical safety should be maintained as the group is escorted to the meeting room. In some behaviorally challenging groups, members may need to be escorted in subgroups if moving as a whole group is too stimulating. In public schools, this gathering of members may need to be modified to include bringing the group members from their classrooms. Once in the group meeting room, members should be guided to settle into their designated places, putting away any personal belongings as directed. Overall, the purpose of this period is to welcome the group members and help them settle back into being together.

Talking Time

The group should be seated so that everyone can see each other. In most groups, a circular, square, or rectangular seating arrangement on the floor or single chairs is appropriate. In some groups for more psychologically disorganized individuals, the informality and intimacy of such an arrangement might be overwhelming. Such groups should be seated around a table for more formality and support. The first purpose of talking time is to allow the leaders to make any necessary announcements regarding member absences, upcoming events, or other practical issues. The leaders may also use this time to lead the group in discussion of a particular occurrence or ongoing situation that requires the group's consideration. The second purpose of talking time is to promote sustained, verbal interaction among the group members. Each member is encouraged to tell the group something of significance, if they choose to do so. In older, more mature groups, this part of talking time might be fairly informal. To the extent that the members can manage themselves, the leaders might be able to allow for free conversation. In younger, less mature groups, members' participation in talking time has to be managed much more carefully by the leaders. A helpful model is to have each child/adolescent talk to the group about one or two topics of importance and then turn to the next child/adolescent and elicit a question or comment about what was just related. This model teaches group members about listening to one another, staying on topic, responding to someone else, and about distinguishing between questions and comments. In psychotherapy and clinical support groups, talking time may become quite lengthy as the group moves more deeply into its work. In social skill groups, leaders should limit talking time to approximately 10 minutes to allow for sufficient opportunities to engage the group members in fuller social interaction. Leaders should always be the ones to announce when talking time is completed.

Activity Times

The group activity times are periods of the group meeting devoted to developmentally appropriate board or card games, role-playing, projects, arts and crafts, physically active indoor games, and other forms of play. These activity times are intended to enhance age-appropriate, multifaceted interpersonal interaction aimed at accomplishing the group's task. The activity periods are divided between group activity and free activity or play time. The group activity time is a period during which all the members must engage in a whole group activity. In psychotherapy groups, the groups should be free, within parameters specified by the leaders, to choose this whole group activity. The process of choosing and entering into the activity is as important to the work of the group as the activity itself. In social skill and more didactically oriented support groups, the group activities should be designed by the leaders based on adult observations of areas of need in the group. First and foremost, the leader-designated activities should be enjoyable for group members. Beyond the pleasure of the interaction, each activity should incorporate critical variables that teach aspects of the group task. The free activity time is a period during which members are allowed to choose their own forms of play, again within parameters set forth by the leaders and using acceptable play materials. During this period, the leaders are involved directly only as needed and as invited by the members. When not playing directly, the leaders are active observers, moving among the members to interpret or facilitate interactions. Leaders are able to teach a great deal about adaptive behavior in this relatively naturalistic situation. The free activity period is thus intended as a time for members to learn more about spontaneous interactions and the issues engendered by such informality in relationships. For some very young, very impaired groups of children, a free activity time is too overwhelming and disorganizing. Children with extremely deficient play skills, e.g., severely affected children on the autism spectrum, experience a free choice playtime as painfully bewildering. Such a lack of structure leads mainly to very maladaptive behaviors as group anxiety increases in the face of ambiguity. For such groups, a leader-guided play time is a good substitute. Each coleader leads a separate, developmentally appropriate game or activity for a portion of the group. The group members alternate between the leaders' activities, according to a schedule designated by the leaders. Disorganized youngsters find this type of adult-centered play much more reassuring and enjoyable. As a result, they are able to learn much more than they would otherwise.

Snack Time

Once cleanup from the activity periods is completed, the group should have snack time. Each member should be assigned an ongoing "job" to help with snack, handing out napkins, spreading a tablecloth. The intention of snack time is to provide tangible support to the group, to promote more relaxed interaction and reflection among group members, and to teach members about appropriate informal behavior. Once the food and drink are passed around, the group journal should be brought out. The journal is a written record of the group's work. Members dictate and the leader writes in the journal. Each member is able to contribute what s/he would like to remember about the current group meeting. Leaders are free to add comments. The combined entries are then read back to the group. Afterward, the journal is circulated among members and leaders for each person's signature. In groups too young to write comfortably and quickly, individualized stamps or hand tracings can replace signatures. The journal provides a wonderful written record of the life of the group. Periodically, members refer to earlier entries to answer questions about the chronology of events or the tenure of various members. At other times, members sign nicknames or add comments to express feelings about themselves, previous group members who are missed, or particular occurrences in group. As time permits in the snack period, groups tend to focus back on their task in a variety of ways. A social skills group, for example, might use the time to tell jokes and rate the humorous value and social comedic skill involved in each joke.

Dismissal

Once snack time is cleaned up, it is time to dismiss the group. This period of the group is typically very tense and overwrought. Having participated in the intense interaction of the group meeting, it is difficult for the members to prepare themselves for separation and return to their individual pastimes. Leaders need to be actively involved in helping the members ready themselves, in maintaining order in the group, and in being reassuring about when the group will meet again. Leaders can help members learn more adaptive ways to manage the ending transition by instituting additional group rituals, providing "social scripts," and modeling appropriate departure behavior. When ready, group members should be returned to their parents or caregivers. In particularly active or disorganized groups, it might be necessary to return the members in shifts separated by 1 or 2 minutes rather than all at once. Leaving in subgroups of two to three members is often more manageable for parents/caregivers and less chaotic in a professional office or clinic setting.

BEHAVIOR MANAGEMENT

Leaders must respect the enormous impact of the particular form of psychopathology, trauma, or skill deficit common to the group members. In dedicating the group to work on grappling with fundamental psychopathology, overcoming significant trauma, or building much-needed skills, the leaders must understand the extreme challenge facing the group as a whole. While every effort should be made to create a group structure that can facilitate accomplishment of a challenging group task, the group should still be expected to falter at times. Through inappropriate behavior, child and adolescent groups often manifest not only their possible presenting problems but also their reaction to the demanding nature of task accomplishment. Because inappropriate behavior is so intimately related to the fundamental clinical core of the group, efforts to manage this behavior should likewise be thoughtfully intertwined with sound, clinical reasoning. Without a comprehensive approach to behavior management, no amount of clinical acumen, theoretical sophistication, or leadership skill will be sufficient to ensure the group's safety, organization, and productivity. Crawford-Brolyn and White (26) and Soo (27) supported the need for careful behavior management in groups for children and adolescents. The five-level approach to behavior management discussed below represents an effort to implement both therapeutic understanding and realistic practicality in managing behavior in a child or adolescent group.

Consideration by Leaders

In the face of difficult, inappropriate behavior, leaders should first think carefully about the communicative intent and underlying meaning of the undesirable behavior. Almost invariably, leaders can either link such negative behavior to the basic problems that led to group admission in the first place or can understand the negative behavior as an expression of the difficulty experienced by the group in attempting to respond to leader interventions. Well reasoned understanding of the negative behavior constitutes the best foundation possible for effective response by the leadership. As important as this thoughtful consideration is, it should be understood that, on relatively rare occasions, some negative behavior is displayed in group that demands immediate intervention to maintain safety. Quick action should be taken to protect group members and property. Fuller consideration of the meaning of the behavior should follow.

Structural or Procedural Change

Once the behavior has been understood, the leaders should explore the possibility of a structural or procedural change that could address the need being expressed in the negative behavior. A structural change might involve switching from a free activity period to a leader-guided play activity to help the group feel more supported and secure, thereby containing acting-out behavior among very impaired young children. A procedural change might involve escorting group members to and from group in subgroups, rather than in the group as a whole, to reduce stimulation and allow for more organized behavior under closer leader supervision. In most appropriately constructed outpatient or community-based therapeutic groups, most negative behavior can be contained using these two levels of intervention. Realistically, however, not all inappropriate behaviors can be managed so readily. The remaining intervention levels are intended to address greater levels of need.

Verbal Interpretation

Should negative behavior persist despite clear understanding by the leaders and any appropriate structural or procedural accommodation, it is helpful to interpret aloud the meaning of the unwanted behavior. Such verbal interpretation operates in groups much as it does in a dynamically oriented individual psychotherapy. The verbal clarification of the negative behavior illuminates that behavior's communicative intent and/or significance. That intent or significance can then be discussed or acted upon appropriately, relieving the group of the need for continued negative behavioral acting out. Discussion and decisions for group action have the greatest impact if multiple members are involved. Reactions and opinions from the group as a whole have much more motivational power than input solely from group leaders. Again, in most groups, behavior management usually does not move beyond this level.

Verbal Limit

When undesirable behavior does continue despite taking the above steps, a limit is required. If preliminary levels of intervention have been tried and have been inadequate, leaders should not hesitate to set a verbal limit, reminding the group about appropriate behavior and directing members to remain within acceptable behavioral parameters. It is always most effective to phrase verbal limits in positive terms. Group members will respond best when told what *to do* as opposed to what *not to do*.

Physical Limit

On infrequent occasions, inappropriate behavior persists despite all efforts. On such occasions, a physical limit is mandatory to guarantee the group's safety. For example, unacceptable materials should be taken from members, members may have to move to less desirable physical locations within the group meeting room, or members may have to take a time out. The group should be well informed ahead of time of what limits will be implemented, depending on the need. In the most extreme circumstances, a member might pose such a danger to the group due to uncontrolled acting out or some other condition that s/he must be removed permanently from the group. Such a step should be explained clearly and concisely to the group. This step should be taken only if the danger to the group is pronounced and if no alternative is available. Reluctance in removing a group member is recommended because there is always irreparable damage to the group when a member is removed, regardless of the justifications for the removal. The group usually experiences the loss of a member as an aggressive act by the leaders. Remaining group members worry permanently about potential ramifications and implications of that act. Members scrutinize and inhibit their own behavior because they are afraid that they too will be expelled. Members feel angry toward the leaders and guilty about any negative feelings that they may have had toward the lost member. While explanation and reassurance by the leaders is helpful, the leaders should be prepared to deal with reactions to and memories of the removal of the group member for as long as the group continues to meet.

PARENT INVOLVEMENT

For child and adolescent groups to succeed, parent knowledge and support of the group are essential (28). The nature of parent involvement in group treatment for children and adolescents varies greatly, however, depending on the population served and on whether the group is in an outpatient or inpatient/residential program setting. For inpatient/residential program groups, parent involvement is relatively distant. Parents are typically informed periodically about their youngster's progress in the hospital or residential treatment program as a whole.

In contrast, because attendance in the outpatient group generally requires parent assistance with transportation and because the outpatient group tends to represent a singular investment of family time, effort, and finances, parents are much closer to outpatient group experiences. Various approaches to including parents in the group therapeutic work have been discussed elsewhere (29). It is most useful to consult closely with the parents in making group admission decisions. A thorough understanding of parental concerns and perspective is necessary to ensure that the group experience, as constructed, is capable of addressing those concerns. Following admission to the group, parent involvement should be managed in accord with the developmental level of the group members. As appropriate, periodic meetings should be held with parents to keep them informed about group progress and the progress of their individual child. Written correspondence is a good alternative to face-to-face meetings to keep parents informed about the group's work. Whenever possible, suggestions based on knowledge gained in the group should be offered to parents to enhance functioning in all the spheres of the child or adolescent's life.

In addition, parents should be encouraged to contact the group leaders at any time with questions or concerns. Group members should be fully aware of the parents' access to the leaders. Managed correctly, this parent–group leader communication is very beneficial to the child and adolescent group members. Members will often request or direct specific communications between the adults to address particular issues. Adult communication should occur outside of the group meeting times, however. In line with the discussion below about boundary management regarding information, parents should be helped to see that direct parental input into the group meetings would likely interfere with the ongoing group process.

LEADERSHIP FUNCTIONS

Group leaders' fulfillment of their role requirements is essential for the group to accomplish its task (30). The group should be able to rely as heavily as necessary on the consistent strength and good judgment of the leaders as it engages in rational work and struggles to pull itself out of more defensive, irrational functioning. Several leadership functions are of paramount importance.

Safety

The single most important leadership function is to ensure the safety of the group as it works toward task accomplishment. The group leaders must demonstrate a fundamental commitment to physical and emotional safety in the group. A coherent approach to behavior management, such as the one outlined earlier, should be implemented to ensure group safety. Without such a guarantee, it would be unfair to maintain expectations for intensive therapeutic work of any type.

Primacy of Cotherapy Relationship

From a clinical perspective, to ensure physical safety, mainly in groups of younger or more disturbed individuals, to process adequately the enormous amount of clinical information generated in each group meeting, and to have a dyad within the group that can be used as a model of a functional interpersonal relationship, it is always advisable for a group to be led by two coleaders. Dies (31) underscored, however, that empirical support was lacking for the benefits of group cotherapy. In view of the fact that cotherapy is utilized widely regardless of the status of empirical support, both Dies (31) and Riva,

Wachtel, and Lasky (30) emphasized the need for careful management of the cotherapy relationship to enhance group functioning. If the group is to reap the benefits of the cotherapy relationship, however, this relationship must be fostered and supported carefully.

The coleaders must communicate openly and honestly regarding their work together. This communication should occur both during regularly scheduled formal meetings as well as in more informal moments while the work proceeds. The leaders should choose a mutually acceptable way of sharing the leadership work. There are many possible, equally productive choices available. Leaders should make a choice based on the task of the group, differential leadership skills, individual preferences, interpersonal style, and relative professional status/responsibilities. One commonly made choice is for one leader to assume managerial responsibilities, i.e., setting the agenda, being the most vocal, leading activities, introducing topics, while the other leader remains quieter, focusing intently on emotional reactions within the group and articulating those as appropriate. While no one choice is correct for all coleader pairs, a successful choice must be genuinely acceptable to both leaders and must be made based on leadership strengths rather than weakness or fear of carrying out specific leadership functions.

Leaders should know that they always have the freedom and responsibility to speak directly to one another regarding group matters in the presence of the group. To gain needed support in the face of challenging group interactions, to articulate an issue relevant to the group's work, to ensure full knowledge and cooperation between the leaders regarding a particular intervention, to resolve differences, and to model reciprocity between people, there is no better method than public communication between leaders. Even when the group may appear to be ignoring the leaders' conversation, the group in fact often listens intently and makes productive use of the interaction. Unlike genuine points of disagreement or difficulty in coleading, coleaders will sometimes become embroiled in disagreements or stuck in generalized tension between themselves but be unable to identify the actual source of the problems. Such disagreements and tension should be understood as unspoken, empathic responses to the group. The coleadership relationship often becomes the vehicle for expression of group conflicts, wishes, or needs that the group cannot yet verbalize directly. When the coleader pair finds itself in such a quagmire, first it is best to discuss the problem fully within the pair. Then, it is most useful to offer a developmentally attuned interpretation to the group and go on to help the group identify, understand, and grapple with the issue facing it. Without such exploration between the leaders, it becomes all too easy for the negativity between the coleaders to become so firmly and unpleasantly entrenched that all the work of the group is stalled.

Protection of Group Structure and Boundaries

To provide the group with sufficiently strong support in approaching its task, the third most important function for the leaders is to safeguard the structure within and boundaries around the group (31–34). The members need to be able to rely on predictability and reliability in the group's life if they are to be able to muster the strength to continue with rational work. The leaders must make sure that the group agenda is adhered to at each meeting, that limits are set and implemented in a consistent fashion, and that appropriate material resources are available to the group. The leaders must also maintain firm time, space, informational, and membership boundaries around the group. Group meetings must begin and end promptly, regardless of extraneous demands/events or enticing clinical material that is presented in the last few moments of a group's scheduled meeting. The group must have a dedicated space, in which the group's privacy can be respected for the duration of each group meeting. Leaders should take care to conduct the group's business only within the group's designated space. Entering into group discussion or play in a waiting room or hallway, no matter how critical or tantalizing the material may seem to be, weakens the group's potential reliance on the leader because the work cannot be pursued adequately in a more public and therefore less reliable setting. As the group becomes a meaningful entity for its members, the group should set a policy about how information will flow into and out of the group. Salient facets of this policy include member responsibilities to maintain group confidentiality, procedures for taking up information communicated by parents, and procedures to be followed by leaders in introducing essential issues that members might be uncomfortable about bringing up themselves. In firmly led discussions, groups are usually well able to make rational policy decisions about the flow of information. Leaders always retain veto power should policy decisions be inappropriate. Finally, the leaders must maintain clear distinctions between who belongs to the group and who does not. For both clinically relevant and for defensive reasons, members and their families often invite leaders to allow other people to attend group meetings or to join in group activities. These invitations should be declined politely but firmly in the interests of maintaining the group's integrity and reliability.

Distinction Between Leader and Member Roles

Groups that are led with sufficient strength and reassurance are rarely democracies. To provide adequate support and guidance, leaders should retain authority and responsibility while continuing to convey respect and appropriate clinical sensitivity toward the group members. An important aspect of such authority and responsibility is maintenance of the distinction between the roles of members as opposed to leaders. Leaders should reserve the right to make the physical environment as comfortable as necessary to allow them to concentrate fully on their leadership tasks. Decisions about self-disclosure, participation in activities, and behavioral demands should be made in relation to the task of the group rather than to any notion of "fair play" or assumed obligation to do "themselves" whatever is asked of the group members. While such a distinction between leader and member roles may seem autocratic in the abstract, in clinical practice this type of distinction serves very well the clinical work of the group. Group members understand that they can rely heavily on the leaders; they do not feel oppressed by them.

Management of Relationship Between Group and Organizational Base

Many clinical groups for children and adolescents are offered under the auspices of a clinic, hospital, or child guidance center. In such settings, factors such as billing practices, physical space, interaction with organizational staff and other patients/clients, attendance policies, privacy, personnel, material resources, and the tone of the organizational atmosphere all have a potential impact on the life of the group. It is the responsibility of the leaders to manage this relationship between the group and its surrounding organization. Although the group leaders rarely if ever have the authority to control the larger organization in the interest of their group, the leaders can and should articulate the needs of the group within the larger organization, advocate strongly for the necessary resources of all types, intervene if there are potentially disruptive interactions between group members and/or their parents and representatives of the organization, and facilitate the group members' transactions within the larger organization. When group leaders abdicate this managerial aspect of their leadership responsibilities, premature departure of members and group dysfunction are common outcomes. Fulfillment of these leadership responsibilities, on the other hand, helps to further protect the group and models adaptive behavior for the group members.

Support Through Group Transitions

Some of the most challenging experiences in groups involve major transitions. Changes in coleadership, new members joining a group, either planned or abrupt terminations of an individual's membership in the group, or changes in meeting location are examples of common transitions through which groups must sometimes navigate. At such times, leaders must be very conscious, deliberate, visible, and direct in providing adequate, developmentally attuned information about what the group should expect, reassuring the members about continued leadership and support available to the group, and helping the group articulate their reactions and concerns regarding the transitions. As at all other times in the life of the group, leaders should facilitate the group's movement through any given transition in a manner consistent with the task of the group. The group should be encouraged to marshal skills consistent with its task as it manages the transition.

SPECIAL APPLICATIONS

As discussed throughout this chapter, group treatment can be directed at a wide variety of issues facing children and adolescents. Two particularly useful special applications of this treatment modality involve provision of support for youngsters contending with HIV/AIDS in their families (35, 36) and teaching of social skills to youngsters on the autism spectrum (37).

HIV/AIDS Support Groups

In the early days of the HIV/AIDS pandemic, many children faced the rapidly worsening illness and imminent deaths of parents and other loved ones in their families. As medical treatments improved, many children had to learn to contend with HIV/AIDS as a more chronic illness in their families. At any time, supportive group experiences structured and operated in the manner discussed above offer a great deal to children affected by HIV/AIDS. The basis for admission to such a group has to be some family acknowledgement that HIV/AIDS has touched the family. Group members must be able to tolerate learning that the group is designed for youngsters who are facing HIV/AIDS in one or more loved ones. Almost always, youngsters are already aware of the presence of HIV/AIDS in their families even before direct adult acknowledgement is made. Their awareness and understanding are often covert and incomplete, however. Open recognition and admission to the group help to give an honest name to what has often been a burdensome, quasisecret in the family. Participation in the group facilitates a fuller understanding of the facts and implications of HIV/AIDS in the family. Without the burden of secrecy, children and adolescents can feel less afraid to learn how to cope with their situation.

Beyond naming a previously known but unacknowledged phenomenon, membership in an HIV/AIDS support group challenges the sense of isolation that frequently accompanies dealing with a devastating illness. In the case of HIV/AIDS, this isolation often stems from shame and guilt about the nature of the illness itself. The group's existence testifies to the fact that many individuals share the problems associated with HIV/AIDS. Such testimony diminishes individual shame and guilt, thereby relieving the loneliness of coping with the disease, and assists the members as they tackle each difficult phase of HIV/AIDS with their loved ones.

A third benefit of an HIV/AIDS support group is that it offers the members a set of reliable interpersonal relationships that are not endangered by the disease. The group offers closeness and intimacy that are invaluable for the members' sense of interpersonal relatedness. In so doing, the group provides a framework in which more normative psychosocial development can proceed.

Finally, the group experience also reminds members that there is life beyond HIV/AIDS. The group demonstrates that life events and transitions can relate to a host of factors, both positive and negative, unrelated to HIV/AIDS. One particularly striking example involves leadership changes. As with any clinical endeavor, HIV/AIDS support groups must contend with the departure of leaders from time to time due to career changes, assignment of different responsibilities, pregnancies, etc. In this type of support group, members are often shocked when a farewell is prompted by something other than illness and/or death. Enduring the sadness of a parting but knowing that the missed person is going onto another satisfying life stage opens up countless possibilities for the members themselves as they begin to contemplate their own futures.

HIV/AIDS support groups for children and adolescents present two main challenges to leaders. First, leaders must be able to tolerate extremely sad information. Without resorting to defensive minimization or avoidance, leaders must accept and be comfortable exploring devastation in the lives of the group members. Often, to demonstrate concern and to provide assistance, carefully modulated participation in sad events, such as funerals in the families of group members, is also required as part of full group leadership.

Second, leaders must learn to cope with often dramatic acting-out behavior in the group. In many instances, the family's experience of HIV/AIDS is part of a constellation of psychosocial problems. Together with the stress of HIV/AIDS, this constellation of problems contributes frequently to the development of significant behavior problems that challenge the safe operation of the treatment group. Leaders must learn a variety of strategies to meet such behavioral challenges. Relevant strategies have been discussed in Gossart-Walker and Moss (35, 36).

Autism Spectrum Social Skill Groups

Social, communication, and peer relationship problems are the core deficits of individuals with diagnoses on the autism spectrum. Accordingly, group treatment is an ideal setting in which to teach social, interpersonal skills to be implemented in real-life situations (38). The group serves as a microcosm in which all the social demands of everyday life come into play. Unlike everyday life, however, leaders of the social skills group are present to instruct and to orchestrate helpful peer interactions.

Social skill groups for individuals with autism spectrum disorders are usually one of two types. The first is curriculum based. Such a group is generally time limited and follows a set plan for teaching discrete social skills. Such a group is excellent for lower functioning individuals on the autism spectrum. For such group members, learning such skills as how to greet another person or to say thank you when appropriate is an impressive accomplishment.

The second type of social skill group is more naturalistic. Such a group is generally long term or open ended. While structure remains essential, as discussed above, this type of group capitalizes on the naturally occurring interpersonal interactions within the group as the source and object of instruction. Naturalistic social exchanges are used to teach about more fluid social functioning. Given its more interactive nature, this second type of group is better suited to higher functioning individuals with autism spectrum disorders.

Regardless of level of functioning or type of group, two characteristics are essential if a social skill group is to be useful for autism spectrum members. First, group leadership and instruction have to be concrete, blunt, direct, and down to earth. Subtler, inquiring, insight-oriented forms of leadership and instruction would be far too vague and bewildering for individuals with autism-related disorders. While professional standards demand that leaders refrain from being rude, leaders in this sort of social skill group should understand that their responsibility is to use their own individual behavior, their interaction with one another, judicious self-disclosure, and all of their teaching skill to provide the most direct instruction possible. As a leader in a group for autism spectrum individuals, it is impossible to be too blunt or too concrete.

Second, for the group to be of maximum benefit, it should include exposure to peers who are not on the autism spectrum. Only with some diversity is it possible to provide socially grounded, realistic reactions to and modeling for the members on the autism spectrum. If composed solely of individuals on the autism spectrum, the group risks having no counterbalance to the social idiosyncrasy that characterizes autistic disorders. In turn, those on the spectrum can often bypass defensive behavior on the part of other members and speak directly to the problems that brought them to the group. Exposure to diverse individuals can be accomplished by admitting members with a range of diagnoses to the group. While their diagnostic status can vary, with only some of them on the autism spectrum, all of the group members should have social deficits. This exposure can also be accomplished by admitting only members on the spectrum but incorporating the services of typical peers as role models for the group members. Minimal training should be given to typical peers so as to maximize their capacity to model true-to-life peer behavior rather than pseudoadult, therapist-like behavior. Typical peers should receive enough basic information about the autism spectrum to feel reasonably comfortable, followed by encouragement to behave as naturally as possible.

Social skill groups are capable of facilitating significant improvement among children and adolescents with autism spectrum disorders. Many of the group members are able to fit in much better at school, develop a social life suited to their particular needs and wishes, and display much more socially appropriate general behavior. Enthusiasm about the groups must be realistic, however. Social skill groups are not powerful enough to change the fundamental organization of an autism spectrum disorder. Even successful members may remain idiosyncratic.

INDICATIONS AND CONTRAINDICATIONS FOR GROUP THERAPY

The issue of who would best benefit from group treatment is tied intimately to the identified task of the specific group. Appropriate admissions are those individuals in need of work on the group's task. Beyond this relatively simple statement at the level of group content, however, there are also broader concepts that should guide admission decisions. Group treatment would be indicated for reasons and under conditions such as those discussed directly below.

First, some mental health difficulties and aftereffects of traumatic experience burden affected individuals with a sense of isolation and culpability. Affected individuals may feel somehow to blame for calling down on themselves damaging experiences that paradoxically confirm negative self-assessments. Individual or family treatments in such situations, regardless of how expertly implemented, rely on discussion or other indirect methods to challenge the negative personalization. In contrast, by definition and by its very existence, a treatment group combats the isolation that so often oppresses children and adolescents struggling with developmental, psychological, and behavioral disorders (39). Inclusion in a group with others who are grappling with similar difficulties challenges individual self-blame and invites the individual to join with peers in shared, instrumental attempts to cope and overcome.

Second, whether due to innate personality characteristics, acquired interpersonal experience, or the cumulative effect of multiple therapeutic relationships, some people have the capacity to maintain excessive psychological distance between themselves and an individual therapist. Such individuals can insulate themselves from true consideration of even the best therapeutic overtures, plans, or interpretations. It is much more difficult, however, to ward off the power of an entire group process. Varied input from fellow group members often spurs this type of individual on toward greater therapeutic progress. Conversely, some more psychologically fragile individuals find the intimacy of one-to-one or even family therapy to be overwhelming. The shared relationships of a group treatment dilute the intimacy sufficiently so that therapeutic input becomes tolerable (40).

Third, some problems that are presented to mental health practitioners not only benefit from but require the presence of more than a therapist–patient dyad for the most efficacious intervention. Most prominent among such problems are deficits in social/peer functioning, such as those that afflict individuals on the autism spectrum, and conditions requiring psychoeducational support (chronic medical illness, family disruption). Unlike more intrapsychic problems or personal psychopathology that often play themselves out in a dyadic therapeutic relationship, thereby lending themselves to psychological interpretation and redirection, peer difficulties and psychoeducational support needs may rarely be as evident in a one-to-one setting. As a result, a therapist–patient dyad would be reduced to talking *about* rather than experiencing immediately the most relevant situations. In contrast, tackling problems with peer relationships in the social environment of the group allows for enactment of and immediate intervention in the problems that interfere with the group member's more optimal functioning in the real world. Addressing needs in the group for guidance regarding logistical organization, social embarrassment, and fear about the future offers maximum support to group members in need of coping assistance. Both the fundamental experiences of group membership, as well as the content of the group's work, have a beneficial effect.

There are three main principles that argue against inclusion of an individual in a group. First, while group treatment can be helpful to impulsive children and adolescents, no individual should be permitted to join a therapeutic group if that individual poses a substantial threat to the basic safety or health of the other group members. Thus, impulsive children and adolescents whose poorly controlled acting-out takes the form of extremely aggressive or excessively risk-taking behavior are inappropriate candidates for group therapy. This contraindication needs to be taken very seriously since, as noted earlier, physical and psychological safety is the fundamental guarantee that group leaders must provide to the group if any meaningful work is to occur. Prospective members who pose a safety threat to the group should be referred to other treatment modalities or for consultation, as appropriate. Many times, addition or modification of psychiatric medication can alter sufficiently the troubling behavior and thereby allow for reconsideration of an individual's group admission.

The removal of a group member by the group leaders is a related issue that merits attention in the context of indications and contraindications for group treatment. Often, leaders focus on one child or adolescent as the primary source of difficulty in a group. Typically, this is the group member that presents the greatest challenges in behavior management. Many times, leaders wish or proceed to remove this group member in the interests of more meaningful group work. For two main reasons, such a removal is almost never successful. First, as stated before, remaining members become angry and anxious about the possibility that they, too, will be required to leave. Behavior in the group is impacted as the remaining members enact their angry anxiety in the forms of limit testing, excessive inhibition, or open accusations directed against the leaders. Second, theoretical principles argue that the offending member was carrying out a function or making a communication relevant to the group's work, regardless of how seemingly inappropriate that function or communication seemed. As a result, it is usually the case that a previously well functioning group member takes over the ousted member's more provocative role. The difficult behavior subsides only when the group has dealt with its meaning, in ways discussed above, and then moves onto new aspects of its task.

From time to time, though, the decision to remove a group member is actually clinically indicated. This comes about most often when new, more disturbing diagnostic information becomes manifest as the group proceeds or when an individual's status changes in such a way that poses a risk to the group. Then, the leaders have no choice but to carry out a planned termination in the most open, thoroughly discussed, and fully anticipated way possible. Regardless of the reasons for member removal, the group's negative reaction to removal of a member persists for a substantial amount of time, in some instances for the remainder of the life of the group. Even when the subject is dropped temporarily from discussion, it resurfaces at stressful times in the group's work. Leaders must be prepared to work through the issue of the member's removal on multiple occasions. Partly because removal of a member is so devastating to a group, admission decisions should be made as carefully as possible to do everything possible to avoid the necessity of member removal.

Second, as mentioned previously, groups do not operate effectively if there is only one member representing a key variable (one female in a group of males, one member of a particular race or ethnicity in an other homogenous group, one psychotic individual in a group in which no one else's diagnosis involves impairments in reality testing). A single representative along a key dimension promotes loneliness, isolation, and scapegoating. Should an individual be an appropriate admission on other inclusion criteria, admission should be deferred until a similar member can be admitted at the same time.

Third, there are some children and adolescents who need and would benefit from work aimed at the stated task of a given group but who have never before identified or explored their relevant needs. Abused children and adolescents who have never acknowledged the abuse in any way would be examples of this type of prospective group member. While group participation at some point might be the treatment of choice for such children and adolescents, a group is too large, interpersonally diffuse, and unpredictable to be the setting in which an individual takes the first step toward confronting their traumatic history. These children and adolescents should receive more individualized services first to ready them for group participation, as needed and as appropriate.

TRAINING AND SUPERVISION OF GROUP THERAPISTS

Many authorities have addressed training needs as they relate to group therapy practitioners (3, 41–43). Azima (44) also addressed the impact of group work on the therapist's own functioning. The foundation of training as a child/adolescent group therapist is the same as the foundation of training for any mental health clinician. Regardless of discipline, the practitioner should have thorough knowledge of child/adolescent development, psychopathology, and a range of therapeutic interventions. The therapist should be comfortable with a wide variety of individuals and diagnostic categories. With this type of foundation, an interested mental health professional would be well able to pursue more specialized training in group approaches. Ideally, the training should be three-pronged. Simultaneously, the practitioner should receive didactic training in the history, theory, and practice of group therapy with children and adolescents, colead a group with an advanced group leader, and receive ongoing clinical supervision of the cotherapy. The didactic experience places the group work in an intellectual and historical context that deepens and solidifies the work, distinguishing clinical group endeavors from more casual group experiences for young people. The coleadership provides immersion in and illustrations of the material discussed in the didactic setting. Finally, the ongoing supervision articulates the nuances of the group life and of the cotherapy relationship, enhancing the trainee's learning and extending his/her clinical skills. When ready, the trainee can assume greater independence in group leadership. In this regard, MacLennan (45) delineated specific training required to conduct groups at particular age and developmental levels while Soo (43) called for strengthening fundamental clinical skills to facilitate successful group leadership.

It should be noted that group supervision/consultation is often very helpful even for well established, talented group therapists. The supervision can, of course, assist with therapeutic questions and problematic group issues. Beyond the immediate resolution of treatment problems, however, expert group supervision can elevate the leaders' understanding of the group's life. In the press of day-to-day group management demands and the challenges posed by diverse diagnostic needs among group members, it is often understandably easy for group leaders themselves to lose sight of the group historical context or the theoretical concepts that underlie current group experiences. Consultation and guidance from an expert who is somewhat removed from the meeting-to-meeting stimulation can have a clarifying, instructive effect for the group leaders. Critical variables and best practice recommendations regarding supervision of group leadership are well summarized by DeLucia-Waack and Fauth (46).

EFFICACY AND CURRENT RESEARCH

For a long time, there has been a broad consensus that group treatment is beneficial for specified populations of children and adolescents (47). To a great extent, this consensus rested originally on clinical observations and professional experience. Early research efforts were qualitative, narrative reports. While often rich in clinical insight and technique, such efforts were subject to criticism regarding validity, reliability, relevance to larger populations, and cost effectiveness. Mirroring broader psychotherapy research efforts and to address such criticism, group therapy research attempted to move more in the direction of sound, empirical studies (48). A number of studies and reviews demonstrated comparable effectiveness of group and individual therapies (33, 49–51). Effective application of group therapeutic techniques to a wide variety of populations has been documented (24).

Yet many questions remain. The full potential efficacy of cotherapy needs to be explored (30, 31). The most useful integration and application of theoretical perspectives need to be articulated (6). In addition, the complex interaction among group structure, process, leadership style, and outcome needs further study. Precise linkage of the most curative processes in group therapy with specific populations of children and adolescents stands as most prominent among current research and clinical questions (24, 28). New instruments measuring such variables as group cohesion have been developed to facilitate comparability across more rigorous research studies. Leaders in the field have called for shared use of these new instruments to promote comparability across studies (48). While a great deal remains to be done, strong interest in and need for group therapy with children and adolescents exist throughout the medical and mental health communities (52). It would be reasonable to expect a body of research to emerge that expands greatly our knowledge of group treatment, integrates standards for sound empirical research with recognition of clinical complexity, and thereby guides efforts in efficacious ways.

References

1. Anthony J: Comparison between individual and group psychotherapy. In: Kaplan HI, Sadock BJ (eds): *Comprehensive Group Psychotherapy.* Baltimore, Williams and Wilkins, 1971, pp. 104–117.
2. Barlow SH, Burlingame GM, Fuhrman A: Therapeutic application of groups: From Pratt's "thought control classes" to modern group psychotherapy. *Group Dynamics* 4:115–134, 2000.
3. Lomonaco S, Scheidlinger S, Aronson S: Five decades of children's group treatment: An overview. *Journal of Child and Adolescent Group Therapy* 10:77–96, 2000.
4. Scheidlinger S, Schamess G: Fifty years of AGPA, 1942–1992: An overview. In: MacKenzie MR (ed): *Classics in Group Psychotherapy.* New York, Guilford Press, 1992, pp. 1–24.
5. Scheidlinger S: The group psychotherapy movement at the millennium: Some historical perspectives. *International Journal of Group Psychotherapy* 50:315–339, 2000.
6. Scheidlinger S: Group psychotherapy and related helping groups today: An overview. *American Journal of Psychotherapy* 58:265–280, 2004.
7. Kraft IA, Riester AE: Past as prologue to the future in child group psychotherapy practice. In: Riester AE, Kraft IA, (eds.): *Child Group Psychotherapy: Future Tense.* Madison, Connecticut: International Universities Press, 1986, pp. 3–8.
8. Rachman AW, Raubolt RR: The pioneers of adolescent group psychotherapy. *International Journal of Group Psychotherapy* 34:387–413, 1984.
9. Moreno JL: The ascendancy of group psychotherapy and the declining influence of psychoanalysis. *Journal of Sociopsychopathology & Society* 3:121–141, 1950.
10. Ettin MF: "By the crowd they have been broken, by the crowd they shall be healed": The advent of group psychotherapy. *International Journal of Group Psychotherapy* 38:139–167, 1988.
11. Dies K: The unfolding of adolescent groups: A five phase model of development. In: Kymmissis P, Halperin D (eds): *Group Therapy with Children and Adolescents.* Washington, DC, American Psychiatric Press, 1996.
12. Dies K: Adolescent development and a model of group psychotherapy: Effective leadership in the new millennium. *Journal of Child and Adolescent Group Therapy* 10, 2000.
13. Garland JA: The establishment of individual and collective competency in children's groups as a prelude to entry into intimacy, disclosure, and bonding. *International Journal of Group Psychotherapy* 42:395–405, 1992.
14. Garland J, Jones H, Kolodny R: A model for stages of development in social work groups. In: Bernstein S (ed): *Explorations in Group Work.* Boston: Milford House, 1973, pp. 7–17.
15. Yalom I: *The Theory and Practice of Group Psychotherapy*, 4th ed. New York: Basic Books, 1995.
16. Agazarian Y: Group-as-a-whole systems theory and practice. *Group* 13:131–164, 1989.
17. Agazarian Y: Contemporary theories of group psychotherapy: A systems approach to the group-as-a-whole. *International Journal of Group Psychotherapy* 42:177–203, 1992.
18. Bion WR: *Experiences in Groups and Other Papers.* New York: Basic Books, 1961.
19. Pines M: *Bion & Group Psychotherapy.* London: Routledge & Kegan Paul, 1985.
20. Rioch MJ: The work of Wilfred Bion on groups. *Psychiatry* 33:56–66, 1970.
21. Schamess G: Reflections on a developing body of group-as-a-whole theory for children's therapy groups: An introduction. *International Journal of Group Psychotherapy* 42:351–356, 1992.
22. Racusin GR, Moss NE: Rational work and basic assumption life in a psychotherapy group for preschool victims of abuse: A case study. *Journal of Child and Adolescent Group Therapy* 2:3–15, 1992.
23. Schamess G: Differential diagnosis and group structure in the outpatient treatment of latency age children. In: Riester AE, Kraft I (eds): *Child Group Psychotherapy: Future Tense.* Madison, CT, International Universities Press, 1986, pp. 29–70.
24. Schectman Z: Group counseling and psychotherapy with children and adolescents. In: De-Lucia-Waack JL, Gerrity DA, Kalodner CR, Riva MT (eds): *Handbook of Group Counseling and Psychotherapy.* Thousand Oaks, CA, Sage Publications, Inc., 2004, pp. 429–444.
25. Slavson SR, Schiffer M: *Group Psychotherapy for Children.* Madison, CT, International Universities Press, 1975.
26. Crawford-Brolyn J, White A: A two-stage model for group therapy with impulse-ridden latency age children. In: Riester AE, Kraft I (eds): *Child Group Psychotherapy: Future Tense.* Madison, CT, International Universities Press, 1986, pp. 123–138.
27. Soo ES: Strategies for success for the beginning group therapist with child and adolescent groups. *Journal of Child and Adolescent Group Therapy* 1:95–106, 1991.
28. Slavson SR: *Child Centered Group Guidance for Parents.* New York: International Universities Press, 1950.
29. Arnold LE, Rowe M, Tolbert HA: Parents groups. In: Arnold LE (ed): *Helping Parents Help Their Children.* New York: Brunner-Mazel; 114–125, 1978.
30. Riva MT, Wachtel M, Lasky GB: Effective leadership in group counseling and psychotherapy. In: De-Lucia-Waack JL, Gerrity DA, Kalodner CR, Riva MT (eds): *Handbook of Group Counseling and Psychotherapy.* Thousand Oaks, CA, Sage Publications, Inc., 2004, pp. 37–48.
31. Dies RR: Therapist variables in group psychology research. In: Fuhriman A, Burlingame GM (eds): *Handbook of Group Psychotherapy: An Empirical and Clinical Synthesis.* New York, Wiley, 1994, pp. 114–154.
32. Bednar RL, Melnick J, Kaul TJ: Risk, responsibility, and structure: A conceptual framework for initiating group counseling and psychotherapy. *Journal of Counseling Psychology* 21:31–37, 1974.
33. Burlingame GM, Fuhriman A: Epilogue: In: Fuhriman A, Burlingame GM (eds): *Handbook of Group Psychotherapy: An Empirical and Clinical Synthesis.* New York: Wiley, 1994, pp. 559–562.
34. Gazda GM, Ginter EJ, Horne AM: *Group Counseling and Group Psychotherapy.* Boston, MA, Allyn & Bacon, 2001.
35. Gossart-Walker S, Moss NE: Support groups for HIV-affected children. *Journal of Child and Adolescent Group Therapy* 8:55–69, 1998.
36. Gossart-Walker S, Moss NE: An effective strategy for intervention with children and adolescents affected by HIV and AIDS. *Child and Adolescent Psychiatric Clinics of North America* 9:331–345, 2000.
37. Volkmar F, Klin A, Paul R (eds): *Handbook of Autism and Pervasive Developmental Disorders.* Hoboken, NJ, John Wiley & Sons, 2005.
38. Krasny et al.: Social skills interventions for the autism spectrum: Essential ingredients and a model curriculum. *Child and Adolescent Psychiatric Clinics of North America* 12:107–122, 2003.
39. Mishna F, Muskat B: "I'm not the only one!" Group therapy with older children and adolescents who have learning disabilities. *International Journal of Group Psychotherapy* 54:455–476, 2004.
40. Pfeifer G: Complementary cultures in children's psychotherapy groups: Conflict, co-existence, and convergence in group development. *International Journal of Group Psychotherapy* 42:357–368, 1992.
41. Rosenthal L: Qualifications and tasks of the therapist in group therapy with children. *Clinical Social Work* 5:191–199, 1977.
42. Soo ES: Training and supervision in child and adolescent group psychotherapy. In: Riester AE, Kraft I (eds): *Child Group Psychotherapy: Future Tense,* Madison, CT, International Universities Press, 1986, pp. 157–172.
43. Soo ES: Is training and supervision of children and adolescent group therapists necessary? *Journal of Child and Adolescent Group Therapy* 8:181–196, 1998.
44. Azima F: Countertransference: In and beyond child group psychotherapy. In: Riester AE, Kraft I (eds): *Child Group Psychotherapy: Future Tense.* Madison, CT, International Universities Press, 139–156, 1986.
45. MacLennan BW: Fifty years of training and supervision for group psychotherapy with children and adolescents. *Journal of Child and Adolescent Group Therapy* 8:169–179, 1998.
46. DeLucia-Waack JL, Fauth J: Effective supervision of group leaders. In: DeLucia-Waack JL, Gerrity DA, Kalodner CR, Riva MT (eds): *Handbook of Group Counseling and Psychotherapy.* Thousand Oaks, CA, Sage Publications, Inc., 2004, pp. 136–150.
47. Anthony EJ: The history of group psychotherapy. In: Kaplan HI, Sadock BJ (eds): *Comprehensive Group Psychotherapy.* Baltimore, Williams and Wilkins, 1971, pp. 4–31.

48. Burlingame GM, Fuhriman AJ, Johnson J: Current status and future directions of group therapy research. In: DeLucia-Waack JL, Gerrity DA, Kalodner CR, Riva MT (eds): *Handbook of Group Counseling and Psychotherapy.* Thousand Oaks, CA, Sage Publications, Inc., 2004, pp. 651–660.
49. Dagley JC, Gazda GM, Eppinger SJ, Stewart EA: Group psychotherapy research with children, preadolescents, and adolescents. In: Fuhrman A, Burlingame GM (eds): *Handbook of Group Psychotherapy.* New York, Wiley, 1994.
50. Hoag MJ, Burlingame GM: Evaluating the effectiveness of child and adolescent group treatment: A meta-analysis review. *Journal of Clinical Child Psychology* 26, 234–246.
51. Kulic KR, Dagley JC, Horne AM: Prevention groups with children and adolescents. *Journal for Specialists in Group Work*, 26, 211–218.
52. Taylor NT et al. A survey of mental health care provider and managed care organization attitudes toward, familiarity with, and use of group interventions. *International Journal of Group Psychotherapy* , 51, 243–263.

CHAPTER 6.2.6 ■ FAMILY THERAPY

G. PIROOZ SHOLEVAR

INTRODUCTION

Since the publication of the last volume of this textbook, family therapy has continued to expand its scientific base and theoretical evolution. Evidence-based programs primarily delivered as home-based, family-centered interventions in the community have continued to produce impressive results with adolescents with conduct disorders and substance abuse. Family interventions also have been applied systematically in controlled studies to a very broad range of clinical disorders of children and adolescents.

The fundamental theoretical concepts and technical interventions developed by pioneers in family systems and psychodynamic therapy have been adopted by the contemporary generation of family therapists who apply them in a multidimensional and ecological manner, incorporating the characteristics of the children, their peer group, community, and broader culture. This broad framework has allowed the incorporation of other treatment modalities, such as cognitive behavior therapy (CBT) and pharmacotherapy, which has significantly enhanced treatment effectiveness. A more flexible approach to involving parents has enhanced engagement in treatment, retention, and treatment outcome. Partly in response to these developments, NIMH has encouraged the use of family interventions in investigative projects; more than half of NIMH-funded intervention proposals and programs include a family component (1).

DEFINITION

Family theory focuses on human behavior and psychiatric disturbances in the context of interpersonal relationships (2–4). This theory forms the basis of *family therapy,* which is an umbrella term for a number of clinical practices that treat psychopathology within the context of family systems rather than individuals. Interventions are designed to effect change in family relationships rather than in an individual (2, 5). This approach is based on observations that symptomatic behavior appears in individuals involved in certain dysfunctional processes within their families or with other significant persons. Conversely, positive family interactions such as effective parenting practices, emotionally nurturing family environments and secure attachment relationships are associated with normative child development, healthy functioning and serve as protective factors against emotional disorders (6).

Family theory considers the family as an interpersonal system with cybernetic qualities. The relationships among the components of the system are nonlinear (or circular); the interactions are cyclical rather than causative. Complex interlocking feedback mechanisms and patterns of interaction among the members of the system repeat themselves sequentially. Any *given* symptom can be viewed simply as a behavior functioning as a homeostatic mechanism that regulates family interactions (7).

The family system is nonsummative and includes the assets and dysfunctions of the individuals as well as their interactions (8). A person's problems cannot be evaluated or treated apart from the context in which they occur and the functions that they serve. It is assumed, therefore, that an individual cannot be expected to change unless the family system changes (8). Treatment addresses the behavioral dysfunctions as a manifestation of disturbances within the entire family relational system; the role of the total family in aiding or in sabotaging treatment is the focus even when a distinct diagnosable psychiatric illness is present in one of the family members.

The goals of family therapy as a psychotherapeutic approach are as follows (3)

- Explore the interactional dynamics of the family and their relation to psychopathology.
- Mobilize the family's internal strength and functional resources.
- Restructure the maladaptive interactional family styles.
- Strengthen the family's problemsolving behavior.

The term family therapy has been expanded to include *family intervention*, a broader array of procedures. It subsumes a large number of clinical practices based on a variety of theoretical concepts with explicit focus on altering the interactions among family members and subsystems with the goal of improving the functioning of the family as a unit, its subsystems and members. Treatment of disturbed individuals as well as dysfunctional relationships can be achieved through family interventions (3, 4). Improved functioning in parental and parent/child subsystems is a fundamental goal in treatment of children and adolescents.

HISTORY

Family therapy and conjointed treatment of families emerged in the late 1940s and early 1950s. The towering figures in the field were Nathan Ackerman, Gregory Bateson, Murray Bowen, Bell, Theodore Lidz, Don Jackson, Jay Heley and many others. Family therapy with a focus on children and adolescents was introduced by Carl Whitaker, Salvadore Minuchin and more recently by David and Jill Scharff, Joan Zilbach and others. A detailed description of the history can be found in recent literature (9, 10).

In late 1960s, Minuchin in collaboration with Montalvo and Haley established the Structural School of Family Therapy. The structural approach reached its height in theoretical development by defining the term *psychosomatic families*—the families of patients with anorexia nervosa and other psychosomatic disorders (11). The structural approach has been applied extensively to families of children with behavior disorders (12).

An underappreciated approach to family therapy with adolescents and children was attempted by the Multiple Impact Therapy group (MIT) in Galveston, Texas (13). The novel intervention by this group included 2 days of family therapy by a number of professionals who alternated their work with different family members during the therapeutic encounter. They classified the families according to the disorders of the adolescents and children, mostly oppositional/defiant and conduct disorders.

INDICATIONS AND CONTRAINDICATIONS

An apparent and clear indication for family therapy is open and stressful conflicts among family members, with or without symptomatic behaviors in one or more members. Family therapy also can be applicable when there are covert problems within the family, which can give rise to dysfunctional behavior in one or more family members, or when other family members covertly support and perpetuate the disorder. Recognizing covert family interactional problems coexisting with overt dysfunctions in one or more family members is the specific contribution of the field of family therapy. Recently, family interventions have been used extensively with externalizing adolescent disorders and substance abuse.

Contraindications to family therapy are relative rather than absolute. They include discussing long dormant, charged, or explosive family issues with the whole family before the family commits seriously to treatment. Another relative contraindication is discussing stressful situations with the family when one or more members are severely destabilized and require hospitalization. Insufficient expertise in family therapy relative to a high level of resistance and defensiveness in the family can result in a counterproductive treatment course. Lack of knowledge of child development and psychopathology can render family intervention with children and adolescents equally unproductive and result in missed therapeutic opportunities.

MODELS OF FAMILY THERAPY

The diversity of models of family therapy raises questions about the common ground among family therapies. The pioneers in family therapy focused on different dimensions in the family system, and to some degree, these different focuses reflected unrecognized differences among patient populations treated by the early family therapists. Although family therapists adopted divergent paths, they ignored the likely conclusion that different approaches to family therapy are closely linked to family characteristics commonly observed in different disorders.

Different models of family therapy are applicable to various patient populations. The intergenerational family therapy models are particularly applicable to families whose members have longstanding disorders and have not negotiated adequate separation and differentiation between the generations (14, 15). Structural and strategic family therapies are particularly applicable to families encountering a crisis situation in which there has been adequate separation from previous generations and a reasonably satisfactory precrisis adjustment in the nuclear family. Behavior family therapy is particularly applicable to marital problems and children with chronic conduct disorders. Psychodynamic and experiential family therapies are helpful to family members with narcissistic vulnerability and a broad range of personality and neurotic disorders who have maintained a relatively adequate level of functioning but find little enjoyment in their lives. An emerging array of family-based interventions attempt to reverse the disintegrative processes in chronically and seriously disordered families effected by abuse, neglect, and placement of the children outside of the family.

Each model of family therapy includes different theoretical concepts and techniques. Some models of family therapy can be grouped based on their similarities. The major models of family therapy, their core concepts, goals, and approaches and techniques, are summarized in Table 6.2.6.1.

Structural Family Therapy

Structural family therapy was developed by Minuchin in collaboration with Montalvo and Haley and applied to children and adolescents with acute behavioral problems and eating disorders. The foundational theoretical concept in structural family therapy is boundary. Clear and flexible *boundaries* are characteristic of functional families. *Enmeshed* and *disengaged* boundaries describe families with excessive intrusiveness or unavailability to one another, respectively.

Structural family interventions emphasize establishing boundaries within the family through the decisive and sensitive actions of the therapist. Family tasks and homework assignments further enforce this process. Methods of "joining" the family allow the therapist to join the family and shift family members' positions to disrupt dysfunctional patterns and strengthen parental hierarchies. Clear and flexible boundaries are established in the session, and the family is encouraged to search for alternative interactional patterns.

Structural family therapy has been used to treat eating disorders, particularly anorexia nervosa in children and adolescents. Its effectiveness in treating psychosomatic disorders and behavioral problems has been proven through numerous case reports and observations, as well as family outcome studies (11).

Strategic Family Therapy

Strategic family therapy emphasizes the need for a strategy developed by the family therapist to intervene in a family's efforts to maintain homeostasis by adhering rigidly to dysfunctional family patterns and symptoms. Strategic family therapy, like psychodynamic family therapy, has a well articulated approach to address the resistance within family systems. Dealing with resistance, particularly in the family's response to the therapist's interventions, requires innovative methods. One technique, *paradoxical intervention*, attempts to reduce resistance and enhance change in the family structure and interactions by discouraging change. Paradoxical interventions facilitate the therapist's joining the family with minimal resistance to restructure the family's interactional system.

TABLE 6.2.6.1

MODELS OF FAMILY THERAPY

Model of Family Therapy	Core Concepts	Goal	Strategies/Techniques
Structural Family Therapy Minuchin et al.	■ Generational hierarchy ■ Boundaries and Subsystems ■ Flexibility of system for: a. Autonomy and interdependence b. Continuity and adaptive restructuring to fit changing internal and external demands	■ Symptoms result from Current family structural imbalance: ■ Enmeshed or disengaged styles ■ Maladaptive reaction to changing demands (developmental, environmental) ■ Defuse generational hierarchy and boundaries	■ Intervene in family interactions ■ Reorganize family structure ■ Shift members' relative positions to balance interactional patterns ■ Strengthen parental hierarchy ■ Reinforce clear, flexible boundaries ■ Mobilize more adaptive alternative patterns
Strategic Family Therapy Milton Erickson Jay Haley Cloe Madanes Paul Waltzlawick John Weakland	■ Repeated patterns of interaction ■ Power/control Struggles ■ Flexibility ■ Large behavioral repertoire for: a. Problemsolving b. Life-cycle passage	■ Symptom is a communication embedded in interaction pattern. ■ Problems; symptoms are maintained by: a. Unsuccessful problemsolving attempts b. Impasse at life-cycle transition c. Rigid view; paucity of alternatives	■ Resolve presenting problem through: ■ Specific strategies/objectives ■ Interrupt rigid feedback cycle: change symptom-maintaining sequences ■ Shift perspective to empower positions ■ Paradoxical instructions
Solutions-focused Steve de Shazar et al.	■ Focus on solutions, not problems ■ Disregard "resistance" ■ Inattention to origin of problems	■ Creation of solutions ■ Presolve presenting problems	■ "Exception" questions ■ "Miracle" questions ■ Coping questions ■ Client empowerment
Bowen family systems Murray Bowen, Micheal Kerr, Philip Guerin	■ Differentiation of self ■ Triangulation ■ Transmission of symptoms across generations ■ Family emotional system ■ Emotional cutoffs	■ Increased differentiation ■ Detriangulation ■ Improved ability to manage anxiety ■ Resolution of cutoff	■ Use of genogram ■ Therapist as coach ■ Education about Multigenerational family processes
Psychodynamic-Psychoanalytic Nathan Ackerman David & Jill Scharff Helm Steirlin Emotionally focused Therapy Susan Johnson Leslie Greenburg	■ Projective identification ■ Interlocking conflicts and defenses observation ■ Object relations ■ Projective identification ■ Splitting ■ Scapegoating problem ■ Attachment disorders	■ enhance awareness and self ■ enhance empathy ■ Improve insight ■ Disentangle interlocking alliance pathologies and resistances ■ Interpretation ■ Differentiation of Attachment vs defensive feelings	■ Transference, resistance, and countertransference analysis ■ Creation of holding environment ■ De-emphasize presenting ■ Emphasis on therapeutic alliance
Evidence-Based Family Therapies **Parent Management Training (PMT)** Patterson et al. Forehand, McMahon et al.	■ Negative reinforcement of maladaptive behaviors ■ Ineffective/unskilled Parent management Interventions ■ Coercive family processes	■ Establishment of effective parent management techniques ■ Promotion of prosocial behaviors in children ■ Reduce coercive interactions	■ Parent management training with parents ■ Behavior management training with parents ■ Problemsolving and communication training
Functional Family Therapy (FFT) Alexander et al. Sexton T	■ Defensive interactions ■ Lack of supportive interaction ■ Nonfunctional Dysfunctional/family patterns	■ Address the function of symptoms in family interaction ■ Enhance supportive Interactions ■ Reduce defensive interactions	■ Intensive home-based ■ Enhance support and other functions in the family
Multisystemic Therapy (MST) Henggeler et al.	■ Multisystemic dysfunctions on family, peer group, school and community level	■ Multisystemic problemsolving	■ Intensive home-based intervention ■ Train and empower family to problem solve in multiple systems

TABLE 6.2.6.1

(CONTINUED)

Model of Family Therapy	Core Concepts	Goal	Strategies/Techniques
Multidimensional Family Therapy (MDFT) Liddle et al.	■ Multidimentional/multisystemic dysfunctions on family, individual, school, community levels	■ Multisystemic/multidimensional intervention on family, individual,Peer group and community level	■ Structural, systemic, strategic, group therapy, behavioral intervention techniques ■ Multidimensional/ multicomponent Problemsolving
Behavioral Patterson et al. Forehand et al. Falloon	■ Adaptive behavior is rewarded; maladaptive behavior is not ■ Exchange benefits outweigh costs; reciprocity ■ Communication and problemsolving ability ■ Flexibility	■ Family attention and reward ■ Alter deficient exchanges e.g., coercive,skewed) ■ Correct communication deficits	■ Change contingencies of social reinforcement ■ Reward adaptive behavior, not maladaptive ■ Communication, problemsolving skills training
Psychoeducational McFarlane Carol Anderson	■ Successful coping and mastery of developmental Challenges: a. Caregiving in chronic illness b. Skill in family relationships and community living skills ■ Stress-diathesis model of Biologically based disorders	■ Reduction in normative and nonnormative stresses (e.g., in couples; relationships, parenting, remarriage, adverse life events)	■ Information, coping skills and social support for: a. Family management of chronic illness b. Stress and stigma reduction c. Mastery of family adaptational challenges

Partially adopted and significantly revised from Steinglass (1995) Guman and Lebow (2000).

Strategic interventions are based on identifying a family's "rules"—the metacommunicational patterns that underlie symptomatic behaviors. These interventions are applied through directives and homework assignments practiced between sessions. The homework can be a logical, straightforward approach to the behavior or a seemingly illogical, paradoxical approach such as "prescribing the symptom," a technique requiring family members to do and acknowledge what the family have been doing all along to undermines interactional patterns by supporting the family's communicational pathways. Family life-cycle passages are considered important because they reveal inflexibility in the family's structure that makes the familial response to internal and developmental demands difficult.

The strategic approach of Haley (8) and Madanes (16) emphasizes the importance of strengthening the parental alliance to deal effectively with the symptomatic and challenging behavior of the children. Power struggles between family members and subsequently between the therapist and the family are the focus of treatment.

SOLUTION-FOCUSED THERAPY

Solution-focused therapy concentrates on the "exceptional solution" repertoire already practiced by the patients to deemphasize their problem-saturated outlook and enlarge the application of such solutions. The therapeutic effectiveness is enhanced by shifting the focus to the "solution" rather than the "problems" (10, 17).

PSYCHODYNAMIC FAMILY THERAPY

Psychodynamic family therapy emphasizes individual maturation, personality development, early childhood experiences, and resolution of symptoms and conflicts in the context of the family system. Common theoretical concepts of psychodynamic family therapy include projective identification, shared unconscious conflicts and defenses, intrafamilial transference reactions, dyadic and triadic family transferences in treatment, and a host of object relations psychoanalytic concepts, such as holding environment and empathy.

BEHAVIORAL FAMILY THERAPY

Behavior family therapy applies the principles of positive and negative reinforcement to the family unit with the goal of enhancing reciprocity and minimizing coercive family processes. Coercive family processes generally are in the form of punishment, avoidance, and power play. Enhancing communication and problemsolving skills in the family is emphasized and punishment is discouraged.

Contemporary behavior family therapy is based on social learning theory and has been applied in the form of parent management training (PMT). The parents and children are taught environmental contingencies (positive and negative reinforcement, reward and punishment) which shape behavior. Strong attention is paid to enhancing prosocial behavior.

Behavior family therapy can be combined with communication and problemsolving training.

PSYCHOEDUCATIONAL FAMILY INTERVENTION

Psychoeducational family intervention based on stress–diathesis theory attempts to enhance family adaptation primarily through informing the family and patient about the nature of psychopathology in psychiatric disorders. The family and patient also receive detailed information about the treatment process and outcome. Psychoeducational intervention has been applied extensively in treating major mental illnesses such as schizophrenia, depression, alcoholism, and anxiety disorders. It consists of a series of in-depth and expert instructional sessions on the phenomenology, etiology, and diagnosis of the disorders. Clinical research findings are explained and made user friendly for the family. Information is also provided about social institutions and systems involved in the care of the patient. Psychoeducational family therapy can be easily combined with other treatment modalities, particularly pharmacotherapy and crisis intervention. The psychodynamic and exploratory psychotherapies are postponed to the later phases of treatment, when the patient and the family are stabilized.

Psychoeducational approaches make extensive use of empirical findings on expressed emotion (EE), communication deviance, affective styles, and problemsolving. This reduces the stressful family processes, recurrence in illness and rehospitalization.

The application of psychoeducational model to childhood depression and suicidality has been particularly productive. The model has been applied preventively to a range of stressful and potentially pathogenic situations for the children such as pediatric cancer, death, and dying. A model for prevention of depression in children of depressed parents has been empirically tested by Beardslee et al. (18) in the past decade with positive outcome.

THE FAMILY LIFE CYCLE

The term family life cycle proposes that the family moves through a series of developmental stages. Carter and McGoldrick defined critical emotional issues for the family at different stages of the life cycle (19). Haley (8) applied the family life cycle concept to understanding the clinical problems of families by relating their dysfunctions to the difficulties they have in moving from one developmental stage to another.

Marriage is considered the first stage of family life cycle (20). The expectable seven stages of the family life cycle are 1) beginning family, 2) childbearing family, 3) family with school age children, 4) family with teenagers, 5) family as a launching center, 6) family in its middle years, and 7) aging family. Combrinck-Graham (21) proposed the family life spiral, with overlapping development issues for different generations.

FAMILY THERAPY WITH CHILDREN AND ADOLESCENTS: OVERVIEW

The conceptional and technical differences between the fields of child psychiatry and family therapy can be summarized in the following way. Child psychiatrists have accused systemic family therapists of lack of appreciation for the individual child's unique developmental characteristics and intrapsychic life (22, 23). According to child psychiatrists, family therapists were oblivious to biological vulnerabilities and pharmacotherapy. Conversely, family therapists have accused child psychiatrists of lacking understanding of the interpersonal dimensions of the child's life, the multiple sources of stress in contemporary family life, and preoccupation with minute developmental deviations and past events at the expense of present-life realities.

In the 1980s, the two camps approached reconciliation. Recognition of family therapy's limitations with certain populations forced many family therapists to reach "beyond family therapy" and address peer-group, psychological (intrapsychic and cognitive), and social dimensions of behavior disorders. Teaching family therapy has been a requirement in child and adolescent, as well as general, psychiatric residency programs for the past 20 years. The integrative approach in treating major mental illnesses has resulted in the consolidation of a true field of family psychiatry (10, 24). Psychodynamic and object relations family therapies have demonstrated the many advantages of recognizing the interrelationships between interpersonal and intrapsychic processes (25–27).

We briefly summarize the application of family therapy to multiple disorders of children and adolescents and refer the reader to the references listed for more information.

THEORETICAL CONCEPTS

All schools of family therapy are founded on theoretical concepts that are specifically applicable to family therapy with children and adolescents. In enmeshed families, there is not sufficient distance and objectivity among family members to allow differentiation of the children through the separation and individuation processes. The children have significant difficulties in school and social relationships, further curtailing their maturity. Overinvolvement between a child and a parent, projective family mechanisms, and triangulation as described by Bowen are major impediments to differentiation and maturity, which can transfer across generations.

Projective identification describes the unconscious processes of projection of unresolved parental conflicts onto a child, who assumes an identity based on a historically assigned role. Assumption of this role interferes with the child's appropriate identity formation. Traumatic events such as child neglect and physical or sexual abuse in the early history of the family can result in the repetition of such traumatic situations in subsequent generations. "Parentification," another impediment to the child's development, assigns a parental role to a child and deprives him or her of age-appropriate experiences.

Although many schools of family therapy recognize the significance of the separation-individuation process for adolescent family members, few of them describe the intricate network of developmental failures within the family and the adolescent that undermine the separation-individuation process. Stierlin (28) proposed that binding, delegating, and expulsion are three ways that families negotiate a pathological separation to overcome the fear of prolonged fusion. In the *binding mode*, the excessive binding of the family to the adolescent can force the growing adolescent into psychotic or suicidal behavior to free himself or herself from the family unit. In the intricate *delegating mode*, the family allows the adolescent to depart from the family unit "on a long leash" to return periodically to share the tales of his or her exploits in order to compensate for the restricted life of the parents. In the *expulsion mode*, the adolescent is rejected by and extruded from the family to free him or her from the family unit.

TECHNIQUES

The literature on family therapy with children describes the clinical process and office arrangements that are most welcoming toward the children. The office should be equipped with toys that are conductive to imaginative play; paper and crayons provide unlimited possibilities for drawing and expression of fantasies. A special attempt should be made to include the children in the treatment process by using age-appropriate methods of communication for the child. Long and complex discussions discourage children from participating and should be avoided. The observational data on families with young children are especially significant. Techniques for family therapy with children have been described by Zilbach (29) and Chasen and White (30). Sholevar has described in detail the process of initial and diagnostic family interview (31).

Often, family therapy with children can disclose physical or emotional child neglect. When family support is potentially available, family intervention can mobilize and rehabilitate family resources to provide the necessary nurturance to resume the child's developmental progress. When such resources are not present, enabling the family to search for an alternative living situation with the help of social agencies may be necessary (31, 32).

FAMILY INTERVENTION WITH ATTENTION DEFICIT HYPERACTIVITY DISORDER (ADHD)

Family interventions have been employed to reduce the core symptoms of ADHD. The reduction in negative interaction between the parents and children has been enhanced when parent therapy and family interventions were provided as a primary or adjunctive treatment (33–35). Parent training allows the parents to enhance the capacity of the ADHD child to focus, remain on task, solve problems, act prosocially with peers, and reduce impulsivity and aggression through cognitive processing. These are effective tools to strengthen the positive parent–child bonds and the ADHD child's fragile self-esteem by reducing negative and counterproductive parental behavior and enhancing skillful and goal-directed intervention by parents in potentially conflictual situations.

Multimodal Treatment Study of Children with ADHD is a comprehensive psychosocial treatment package of 30 parent training sessions, school visits, and teacher training with or without medication (33, 36). The combined treatment exhibited the best results in control of ADHD core symptoms.

FAMILY THERAPY AND CONDUCT DISORDERS

Paterson et al. (37) described "coercive family processes" by which the parents, who generally lack management skills, initiate overly punitive and aggressive actions toward their children but withdraw in the face of strong opposition by the children. The coercive processes result in a high level of aggressive and uncontrollable behavior in the children. Subsequent research by Patterson et al. (37) focused on the relationship between aggressive behavior in children and depression in parents, particularly single mothers.

Other researchers also have studied the families of children with conduct disorders. Alexander, Barton, and Parsons (38–40) examined the function of aggressive behavior in the family and attempted to change the family's interactions from defensive to supportive interactions through Functional in order to undermine conduct problems.

Functional family therapy (FFT), parent management training (PMT), and multisystemic therapy (MST) have produced very encouraging therapeutic results with conduct disorders.

Parent Management Training (PMT)

Forehand and McMahon (41) and Patterson et al. in 1982 have produced extensive and empirically based interventions in parent management training (PMT). Their approach has been applied in multiple settings by independent teams of investigators and has proved beneficial in altering oppositional/defiant behavior and conduct disorders, and enhancing prosocial behavior in children at home and in school. The preventive effect on younger siblings of children with conduct disorders also has been noted (37, 41). PMT addresses the deficient parental management skills that are intimately correlated with antisocial behavior and arrested socialization in children. It teaches the parents to interact proactively and more productively with their children by reinforcing prosocial behavior rather than inadvertently rewarding deviant behavior (42–44).

The basic principles of PMT are accurate labeling of the child's behavior, emphasis on prosocial behavior, deemphasis of disruptive behavior, administration of tangible reinforcers, use of nonviolent methods of "punishment" and anticipation/resolution of problems. The keystone targeted behavior of the child is *noncompliance.*

The interventions are based on positive reinforcement of prosocial behavior, use of time out, guidelines for attending/ignoring, shaping the desirable behavior (successive approximation of terminal behaviors), and enhancement of problemsolving, negotiations, and compromise formations. Coercive family processes (37) are identified and resolved through effective reinforcement.

Extensive research by numerous independent investigators in different settings has demonstrated the effectiveness of PMT over the control groups by generalization of therapeutic results in different settings, short-term and long-term beneficial outcome. There has been a lowering of parental (maternal) depression and subsequent referral of younger siblings for antisocial behavior. The treatment has been less effective with "insular mothers" who are socially isolated, depressed, and have economic problems (45). A range of behavioral and cognitive interventions, enlargement of the social network, and medication in the case of parental depression can all help to enhance maternal functioning.

In response to the large number of delinquent children placed out of home, parent management training (PMT) has been applied to children in foster care. Oregon Treatment Foster Care (OTFC) is a family- and home-based treatment model that teaches effective parenting practices through close monitoring and limiting contact with deviant peer groups (46, 47). This intervention has produced a reduction in rearrests, detention center placement, runaway behavior and improved relationships with biological families in comparison to adolescents placed in conventional foster care.

FUNCTIONAL FAMILY THERAPY

Functional family therapy developed by Alexander et al. (38–40) attempts to alter *defensive* family interactions to supportive ones in families of delinquent children through an integration of behavioral, structural/strategic techniques.

MULTISYSTEMIC THERAPY (MST): MOVING BEYOND FAMILY THERAPY

In the past 2 decades, there have been many attempts to broaden the scope of family interventions to include multiple other systems. The multisystemic therapy (MST) of Henggeler and colleagues (48–50) is the most widely recognized and empirically validated intervention system of its kind. The target of the family-based intervention has been chronic, violent, or substance-abusing juvenile offenders at high risk for out-of-home placement. The intervention is based on the premise that the individual with CD is nested within a complex network of interconnected systems that encompass individual, familial, and extra-familial (peer, school, neighborhood) factors. The goal of MST is to empower parents with the skills and resources needed to raise their teenage children and to empower the youth to cope with family, peer, school, and neighborhood problems. The therapeutic approach provides support and skill building in the family and the youth to achieve this goal. It emphasizes building youth and family strength (protective factors) on an individualized and comprehensive basis to attenuate risk factors. The home-based model enhances service access and family retention in treatment. It has been applied with male and female African American and white adolescents between the ages of 12 and 17 years. The therapists have a low caseload and strong system of supervision supplemented by consultation to allow intensive intervention. The approximate length of the treatment is 4 months.

Multisystemic therapy has produced strong evidence for program effectiveness in multiple controlled and randomized clinical trials with violent and chronic juvenile offenders.

They have demonstrated the following findings:

- Reduction in long-term rate of criminal offences
- Reduced rates of out-of-home placement
- Reduced rates of drug use and drug-related offenses
- Improvement in family functioning
- Decrease of other mental health problems
- A lower level of rearrest, reincarceration, and reduction in the days of out-of-home placement.

MST as an alternative to psychiatric hospitalization at the time of crisis has produced an 85% reduction in days of hospitalization.

FAMILY INTERVENTION AND DEPRESSION

Depressed patients tend to be aversive to others and also feel victimized by them. They frequently engage in escalating negative exchanges. Depressed patients and their family members tend to verbalize negative, subjective feelings more frequently than nondepressed couples, whose communications are more task oriented (51–55). The marriages of depressed women (or men) are characterized by friction, poor communication, a lack of affection, withdrawal, and a tendency for the nondepressed spouse to view his or her spouse as accusatory (51, 53).

Children of depressed parents are at risk for many diagnosable psychological problems, a rate as high as 40%–50% (53). The risk to children is increased if 1) the depressed person's spouse becomes depressed or is unavailable to the child, 2) there are marital problems or divorce (53), and 3) there is no supportive relationship with another adult.

Family-based interventions with depressed patients are based on an integration of family systems theory psychoeducational model, psychodynamic theory and attachment theory within a developmental model (54). The role of nondepressed parent in enhancing the coping capacity of the family is crucial (54).

Brent et al. (56) have reported that CBT is more effective than structural family therapy with depressed adolescents at the end of treatment but equally effective in 2-year followup. When methodological issues are put aside, structural family therapy as practiced by the group may not have addressed crucial family issues for depressed adolescents such as poor attachment and low affective involvement between the parents and children. Beardslee's (18) comprehensive preventive model to reduce the likelihood of transmission of depression from the parents to the children remains dominant in the field.

ANXIETY DISORDERS

A number of family variables have been implicated in anxiety disorders. They include overprotective and overly controlling parenting styles, parents modeling or reinforcing anxious and avoidant behaviors, and parental perception of excessive threats (57). Cognitive behavior therapy (CBT) and behavioral family therapy have been compared in treatment of childhood anxiety disorders (58). The family therapy component included communication and problemsolving techniques and anxiety management methods for parents. The combination of CBT and BFT was significantly more effective than CBT alone, particularly with younger children and girls. In addition to a reduction in anxiety, there was an improvement in general functioning and enhancement in parental competence. Cobham et al. (57) have reported that anxious children whose parents were excessively anxious did well in the combined treatment but very poorly with CBT alone (77% vs. 39%).

FAMILY THERAPY AND "PSYCHOSOMATIC" DISORDERS

Minuchin et al. (11) described several common characteristics among families with children and adolescents who have a range of "psychosomatic" disorders such as anorexia nervosa. "Psychosomatic families" were enmeshed, overprotective, rigid; avoided conflict; and used the child's problems to detract attention from parental. The treatment corrects defensive interactional patterns to enhance separation and autonomy in the child. They demonstrated the impressive impact of structural family therapy on families with younger adolescents who have eating disorders and other psychosomatic reactions. However, the utility of the model with older patients who have bulimia has not been established (59).

Behavioral family therapy and psychoeducational also have been applied to eating disorders and anorexia nervosa. They address risk factors for eating disorders such as parental intrusive, critical, and overcontrolling behavior and low family cohesion (60).

Eisler et al. (61) argue that parallel treatment of the parents and anorexic adolescents is highly effective when there is a high level of maternal criticism. Application of family therapies is effective in bringing about weight gain, but has also increased the level of overt family conflict, which supports the observation that conflict avoidance and denial is a significant characteristic of families of adolescents with eating disorders (62).

FAMILY THERAPY AND ADOLESCENT SUBSTANCE ABUSE

Family therapy with adolescent substance abuse has been described by multidimensional family therapy and multisystemic therapy (MST). Liddle and Liddle, et al. (63, 64) have applied multidimensional, multicomponent, and multisystemic comprehensive family intervention to substance abusing adolescents. They have investigated the links between changes in parenting and reductions in adolescents' drug abuse, improving the therapist–adolescent alliance and addressing cultural and gender issues in treatment. Their preliminary findings are supportive of effectiveness of family interventions in comparison with other treatment modalities.

Multisystemic therapy (MST) (48–50, 65) has been applied to treatment of substance abuse in adolescents with very encouraging results. It has been effective in reducing drug use, rearrests, and the number of days in placement.

FAMILY INTERVENTION IN RESIDENTIAL TREATMENT CENTERS

Research has identified the lack of a meaningful conceptual framework guiding intervention with families as the major factor limiting the effectiveness of residential treatment (66). Family intervention in a residential treatment center should be guided by two variables: 1) the state of disintegration of the family unit and 2) the level of availability of the family as a potential care provider or participant in psychiatric treatment. Based on assessment of these variables, families of patients in a residential treatment center can be divided into four groups: 1) available families, 2) potentially available families, 3) partially available families, and 4) totally unavailable families (32, 66).

Available Families

The available family is forced to institutionalize the child after family confrontations at the height of negatively escalated interactions. The family and child are strongly bonded and depend on one another to the point that they cannot live with or without each other. Such families are available for home visits, participation in family sessions, and eventual family reunification.

Potentially Available Families

The potentially available family has lost its immediate ability to care for the child because of a loss of functional capacity in the nuclear or extended family. A history of divorce, remarriage, physical or psychiatric illness, or death should alert the treatment team to the loss of family resources and capacity. The therapeutic task is to recognize the limitations in the functional and caretaking capacity of these families and protect them from any unrealistic and premature demands. The functional capacity of the family should be increased by resolving intergenerational conflicts, improving the functional and economic capacity of the parents, and activating the parents' social networks.

Partially Available Families

The partially available family interacts with the child through erratic telephone calls, occasional visits, or irregular attendance in treatment sessions. A major clinical finding in such families is the extreme nature of parental incapacity in managing life tasks. A realistic treatment strategy is to maintain the family's connection with the child psychologically while making realistic living plans for the child after discharge from residential treatment center. The family can continue to remain as a resource to the group home or foster family after the child's discharge from the residential treatment center.

Totally Unavailable Families

The totally unavailable family is characterized by loss of contact with the child many years before his or her admission to a residential treatment center. There is usually a distorted and unrealistic expectation of a potential reunion between the family and the child. Such distorted fantasies should be discussed immediately and continuously throughout residential treatment. It would be helpful if the families could be located early in the course of residential treatment to verify—either in person or by telephone—their inability to take care of the child. This strategy would help resolve some of the child's dormant fantasies and conflicts and facilitate his or her future adaptation to other living possibilities.

RECENT DEVELOPMENTS IN FAMILY THEORY AND THERAPY

In the past decade, the field of family therapy has moved toward more empirically derived measures, such as expressed emotion, and away from theoretically driven constructs. There has been a close adherence to the stress-diathesis model (67–69) and the Finnish adoption studies (68), particularly in reference to major mental illnesses. This model recognizes the presence of reasonably convincing evidence for a strong genetic predisposition to a number of major mental disorders, such as schizophrenia, bipolar disorders, and alcoholism, which, in interaction with various intercurrent life events within and outside of the family, can affect the risk for emerging or recurring disorder in a family member. Contemporary family therapy also clearly recognizes the efficacy of psychopharmacology in schizophrenia and depression.

Stress-Diathesis Theory

Stress-diathesis or stress-vulnerability theory was first proposed by Rosenthal in 1970 and further refined by Zubin and Spring (69). Stress-diathesis theory regards the disorder as a product of two sets of variables: 1) vulnerability and 2) stressors. Vulnerability can be the result of genetic and psychobiological factors, although psychological and interpersonal vulnerability can function in a similar fashion. Genetic factors have been studied in schizophrenia, depression, and alcoholism. Stress can be caused by external factors or as a result of stressful psychological mechanisms or interpersonal patterns. The perspective of stress-diathesis theory is that illness is the result of heightened vulnerability and stress, and can be best prevented, managed, and treated by altering both sets of factors. Psychotropic medications function by reducing vulnerability, and family interventions focus on lowering interpersonal sources of stress and enhancing coping and problemsolving capacities.

Finnish Adoption Studies

The Finnish adoption studies (68) have produced data supporting the combined and interconnected role of genetic and familial variables in schizophrenia and other mental disorders. Researchers studied the level of family functioning, adaptability, and organization of adoptive families and dividing them into five groups from "optimally functioning" to "inadequately functioning." Although all families adopted children with comparable genetic vulnerability to schizophrenia, the outcome of the children was significantly correlated with level of family functioning. There were no psychotic or borderline children in the two groups of families with optimal or close to optimal functioning. In contrast, there was a preponderance of schizophrenic and borderline patients in the two groups with the lowest level of functioning. The Finnish study strongly supports the notion that genetic risk can be enhanced or decreased according to the level of functioning and adequacy of the family.

FAMILY VARIABLES IN DEVELOPMENTAL PSYCHOPATHOLOGY; SCHIZOPHRENIA

A significant change has occurred in conceptualizing the family dimension of schizophrenia. The family is viewed as a major resource whose availability to the patient can make a crucial difference in positive outcome. Negative interaction between the patient and family now is seen as largely reactive to the patient's symptoms rather than causative. Blaming family interactions (double bind) or the parents (schizophrenogenic mother) has become obsolete.

Family studies based on the stress-vulnerability model have investigated variables that can differentiate families of schizophrenic patients from families of nonschizophrenic patients. Studies of indicators of risk have focused particularly on three variables: 1) expressed emotion, 2) communication deviance, and 3) affective style (70, 71).

Expressed Emotion

In 1962, Brown et al. reported that male patients with chronic schizophrenia who had returned to live with their families following psychiatric hospitalization were more prone to rehospitalization than patients who went to other living arrangements (71). He proposed the term *expressed emotion,* a composite variable with the values of high and low, as an index of the family's criticism of and overinvolvement with the patient. Expressed emotion refers to negative emotional attitude. A number of subsequent British and American studies have indicated that the rate of relapse in schizophrenic and depressed patients in families with high expressed emotion is four times higher than that in families with low expressed emotion (72). The interventions with families having high expressed emotion, with specific goals for reducing familial hostility and over involvement, have provided experimental evidence that a decrease in the level of expressed emotion results in a decrease in the occurrence of relapse (72). Vaughn and Leff (73) have suggested that families who blame the illness rather than the patient for the behaviors typically accompanying psychiatric impairment are likely to be supportive or have low expressed emotion. Families with high expressed emotion, in contrast, seem more inclined to attribute the causes of deviant behavior to the patient.

Communication Deviance

Wynne and Singer (1963) posed the concept of communication deviance to describe nonschizophrenic patients (74, 75). A lack of clarity in communication and disturbances in maintaining attention in the parents of schizophrenic patients in comparison to nonschizophrenic patients Subsequent studies have indicated that communication deviance is related to the severity of psychopathology in the offspring, although some of the disturbances are nonschizophrenic in nature. Communication deviance may represent a cross generational shared vulnerability in the parents and children affecting attention, perception, and information processing. Longitudinal studies of communication deviance have shown a high risk for psychopathology in children of parents with high communication deviance, particularly if there is concomitant high expressed emotion and negative affective style.

FAMILY CLASSIFICATION AND DIAGNOSIS

Family therapists have described different types of families: undifferentiated, enmeshed, disengaged, and psychosomatic. DSM-IV has rekindled the interest in an empirically based family classification and diagnostic system. A family classification system has been proposed by the family committee of the Group for the Advancement of Psychiatry (GAP) (76). They have proposed a document consistent with DSM-IV to specify diagnostic criteria for family and couple relational disorders. The committee's criteria focus on specific family problems such as sexual or physical abuse, divorce, failure to thrive, and separation anxiety (77).

The Global Assessment of Relational Functioning Scale (GARF) developed by Endicott and Spitzer (77) has been used by the GAP committee to evaluate the level of a family's dysfunction, analogous to the Axis V rating of global functioning of the individual DSM-III-R. have proposed a second classification system of family relational disorders (71, 78).

FAMILY INTERVENTION IN PSYCHIATRIC HOSPITALS

The goals of the family-oriented model of inpatient intervention are to prevent rehospitalization, strengthen fragile ties between the family and the patient, and help the family and patient reach the highest functional level. This approach is psychoeducationally oriented, and emphasizes the rehabilitation of the family for a successful reunion when the patient returns home. Inpatient family intervention focuses on treating the patient's illness while recognizing the importance of family variables. It places the relatively causative biological factors in perspective with the familial and environmental influences. Medication is considered a natural ally of family intervention (10, 79, 80).

The multiple functions of the psychiatric hospital in regard to the family include addressing problems that are disturbing the family's homeostasis, assisting other disturbed but resistant family members, and helping the family to regain a "lost," severely dysfunctional family member. The family is considered the most important resource, and as such deserves support and respect rather than criticism and blame (81). The relationship between the family and the psychiatrist should be collaborative on behalf of the patient. A variety of family therapy approaches have been used in treating hospitalized patients. The psychoeducational model of family intervention is most effective for families with a member who has been hospitalized for schizophrenia or an affective disorder.

Sholevar (80) has described an "institutionalization process" by which a dysfunctional family in a crisis situation attempts to extrude a vulnerable adolescent to reestablish homeostasis. A variation of the institutionalization process is a multiple hospitalization syndrome, whereby the family insists on returning the child home prematurely to reinvolve him or her in the family's conflicts. Institutionalization process can be countered through conjoint family therapy evaluation and treatment of the whole family by the hospital staff. The family should be involved in the treatment process before the patient's admission to the hospital.

RESEARCH IN FAMILY THERAPY

Progress in family therapy research has been apparent in the past 2 decades. The question of whether family therapy is effective has been further refined by examining the effect of specific treatment formats and strategies on specific family problems, individual diagnoses, and mediating therapeutic goals. Studies comparing family therapy with other treatment modalities or combining family therapy with other treatment approaches have focused on the level of responsiveness of different problems to different treatment modalities including family therapy (82).

Studies on child and adolescent disorders, particularly the treatment of conduct disorders and delinquency, have produced encouraging results. Parent management training (33, 41) and functional family therapy (38) have proved very effective. In addition to their favorable effect on targeted behaviors of adolescent patients, they have produced beneficial results with siblings and parents. Research on family intervention with substance abuse has demonstrated effectiveness with subgroups of substance abusers, possibly with younger abusers still living at home. There has been surprisingly less interest in the efficacy of family therapy in treating patients with eating disorders. The recent findings (61) suggest that nonchronic eating disorders in young patients who live at home with their parents are amenable to family interventions.

There has been a number of studies that clearly define symptomatic behavioral problems in children. The most impressive result has been reduced aggressive behavior in children and adolescents (83). Family therapy was effective in reducing specific problematic child behaviors, as well as in reducing anxiety and depression in the parents, and contributing to parenting skills.

A very promising recent study by Reiss and colleagues (84) examines the role of genetic and environmental factor in a wide range of family types. The differential impact of shared and nonshared environments on child development can have far-reaching impact on family investigations and treatment in coming decades due to dramatic ongoing changes in family composition.

CONCLUSION

A field of family psychiatry has emerged based on the treatment of disorders with relatively clear genetic components, namely, schizophrenia, depression, and alcoholism. Recent elaboration of stress-diathesis theory has led to new developments in family psychiatry, especially the focus on genetic vulnerability of different family members to stress and on methods for reducing it. Psychoeducational family intervention has been used extensively to enhance family adaptation, without the risk of increasing stresses in the family by stimulating charged conflictual issues.

Family therapy, in collaboration with the broader field of psychiatry, should better define the family variables of different disorders and their responses to single or combined treatment modalities or a particular family therapy approach. Considering the advances made in biological psychiatry and mapping human genomes, the interactional and psychological correlates of biological vulnerability and dysfunction present family therapists with an exciting challenge.

References

1. Hibbs ED, Jensen PS: *Psychosocial Treatments for Child and Adolescent Disorders: Empirically Based Strategies for Clinical Practice.* Washington, DC, American Psychological Association, 1996.
2. Minuchin S: *Families and Family Therapy.* Cambridge, MA, Harvard University Press, 1974.
3. Steinglass P: Family therapy. In: P Kaplan and B Saddack (eds): *Comprehensive Textbook of Psychiatry*, 6th ed. Baltimore, Maryland, Williams & Wilkins Publishers, 1995, pp. 1838–1847.
4. Gurman A, Lebow J: Family and couple therapy. In: B Saddock and V Saddock (eds): *Comprehensive Textbook of Psychiatry*, 7th ed. Lippincott, Williams & Wilkins, Baltimore, 2000, pp. 2157–2167.
5. Shapiro R: Psychodynamic family therapy with children and adolescents. In: *Treatment of Emotional Disorders in Children and Adolescents.* Edited by Sholevar GP. Jamaica, NY, SP Medical and Scientific Books, 1986, pp. 135–159.
6. Cicchetti D, Toth SL: The development of depression in children and adolescents. *Am Psycho* 53:221–241, 1998.
7. Jackson DD: The question of family homeostasis. *Psychiatr Q* 31 (suppl):79–90, 1965.
8. Haley J: *Strategies of Psychotherapy.* New York, Grune & Stratton, 1963.
9. Sholevar GP: Family therapy. In: Jerry Weiner and Mina Dulcan (eds): *Textbook of Child and Adolescent Psychiatry*, 3rd ed. Washington DC APPI Press, ch. 53, 2002, pp. 1001–1027.
10. Sholevar GP: Introduction. In: Sholevar GP, Schwoeri L (eds): *Textbook of Family and Marital Therapy.* Washington, DC, American Psychiatric Press, 2003, pp. 1–33.
11. Minuchin S, Rosman B, Baker L: *Psychosomatic Families: Anorexia Nervosa in Context.* Cambridge, MA, Harvard University Press, 1978.
12. Stanton MD: Systems approaches to family therapy. In: Sholevar GP, Jamaica NY (eds): *Treatment of Emotional Disorders in Children and Adolescents.* SP Medical and Scientific Books, 1986, pp. 159–180.
13. MacGregor R: Multiple impact psychotherapy with families. *Fam Process* 1:15–29, 1962.
14. Bowen M: *Family Theory in Clinical Practice.* New York, Jason Aronson, 1978.
15. Boszormenyi-Nagy I, Spark GM: *Invisible Loyalties.* New York, Harper & Row, 1984.
16. Madanes C: *Strategic Family Therapy.* San Francisco, Jossey-Bass, 1981.
17. Browning S, Green RJ: Constructing therapy. In: GP Sholevar (ed), *Textbook of Family and Marital Therapy*, Washington, DC, APPI Press, 2002, Ch. 3.
18. Beardslee W, Schwoeri LD, Preventive intervention with children of depressed parents. In: GP Sholevar and LD Schwoeri (eds): *Transmission of Depression in Families and Children*, Northvale, NJ, Jason Aronson, Inc., pp 285–318, 1994.
19. Carter E, McGoldrick M (eds): *The Family Life Cycle.* New York, Gardner Press, 1980.
20. Zilbach J: The family life cycle: Framework for understanding children in family therapy. In: Combrinck-Graham L (eds): *Children in Family Context.* New York, Guilford, 1989, pp. 46–68.
21. Combrinck-Graham L: A developmental model for family systems. *Fam Process* 24:131–151, 1985.
22. Malone CA: Observations on the role of family therapy in child psychiatric training. *Journal of the American Academy of Child Psychiatry* 13:437–458, 1974.
23. McDermott JF, Char WF: The undeclared war between child and family therapy. *Journal of the American Academy of Child Psychiatry* 13:422–436, 1974.
24. Malone CA: Child psychiatry and family therapy: an overview. *Journal of the American Academy of Child Psychiatry* 18:4–21, 1979
25. Scharff D, Scharff JS: *Object Relations Family Therapy.* Northvale, NJ, Jason Aronson, 1987.
26. Lansky MR: Family therapy. In: Kaplan HI, Sadock BJ (eds): *Comprehensive Textbook of Psychiatry*, 5th ed. (vol 2). Baltimore, MD, Williams & Wilkins, 1989, pp. 1535–1541.
27. Ravenscroft K: Family therapy. In: Lewis M (eds): *Child and Adolescent Psychiatry.* Baltimore, MD, Williams & Wilkins, 1991, pp. 850–869.
28. Stierlin H: *Separating Parents and Adolescents.* New York, Quadrangle/New York Times Book Company, 1974
29. Zilbach J: *Young Children in Family Therapy.* New York, Brunner/Mazel, 1986
30. Chasin R, White T: Family therapy with children: A model for engaging the whole family. In: Sholevar GP, Schwoeri L (eds): *Textbook of*

Family and Marital Therapy. Washington, DC, American Psychiatric Press, 2002.
31. Sholevar GP: Initial and diagnostic family interview. In: Jerry Weiner, Mina Dulcan (eds): *Textbook of Child and Adolescent Psychiatry*, 3rd ed. Washington, DC, APPI Press, 2004, pp. 125–136.
32. Sholevar GP: Family intervention with conduct disorders. In: *Conduct Disorders in Children and Adolescents*, Washington, DC, APPI Press, 1995, pp. 193–209.
33. Diamond G, Sigueland L: Current status of family intervention science. In: Josephson AM (ed): *Current Prospectives on Family Therapy, Child and Adolescent Psychiatric Clinics of North America*. Philadelphia, WB Saunders Co. (vol. 10, number 3), 2001.
34. Pelham WE, Wheeler T, Chronus A: Empirically supported psychological treatments for attention deficit hyperactivity disorder. *J. Clin Child Psychol* 27:190–205, 1998.
35. Barkley RA: *Hyperactive Children: A Handbook for Diagnosis and Treatment*. New York, Guilford Press, 1981.
36. Hinshaw SP, Owens EB, Wells KC et al.: Family processes and treatment outcomes in the MTA: Negative/ineffective parenting practices in relation to multimodal treatment. *M Abnorm Child Psychol*. 28:555–568, 2000.
37. Patterson GR: *A Social Learning Approach to Family Interventions: III. Coercive Family Process*. Eugene, OR, Castalia, 1982
38. Alexander J, Barton D, Walfron H: Beyond the technology of family therapy: The anatomy of an intervention model. In: *Advances in Clinical Behavior Therapy*. Edited by Craig K, McMahon R. New York, Bronner/Mazel, 1983, pp. 48–73.
39. Alexander, JF, Parsons BV: *Functional Family Therapy*. Monterey, CA, Brooks/Cole, 1982.
40. Sexton TL. Alexander JF Functional family therapy: An empirically supported, family-based intervention model for at-risk adolescents and their families, In: *Comprehensive Handbook of Psychotherapy*: II: *Cognitive-Behavioral Approaches*, Kaslow FW, ed. New York Wiley, pp 117–140 2002.
41. Forehand R, Kotchick BA: Cultural diversity: A wake-up call for parent training. Behavioral Therapy 27:187–206, 1996.
42. Kazdin AE, Siegel TC, Bass D: Cognitive problem-solving skills training and parent management training in the treatment of antisocial behavior in children. *J Consult Clin Psychol* 60:733–747, 1992.
43. Mabe PA, Turner MK, Josephson AM: Parent management training. In: Josephson AM (ed): *Child and Adolescent Psychiatric Clinics of North America: Current Perspectives on Family Therapy*. (vol 10) Philadelphia, WB Saunders Co. 2001, pp. 451–464.
44. Sholevar E: Parent management training. In: Sholevar P (ed): *Textbook of Family and Couples Therapy*, Washington, DC, pp. 403–417.
45. Wahler RG, Cartor PG, Fleishman J, et al: The impact of synthesis teaching and parent training with mothers of conduct-disordered children. *J Abnorm Child Psychol* 21:425–440, 1993.
46. Chamberlain P, Mihalic S: *Blueprints for Violence Prevention: The Study and Prevention of Violence* 1998.
47. Chamberlain P, Reid JB: Comparison of two community alternatives to incarceration for chronic juvenile offenders. *J Consult Clin Psychol* 66:624–633, 1998.
48. Henggeler SW, Schoenwald SK, Borduin CM, et al: *Multisystemic Treatment of Antisocial Behavior in Children and Adolescents*. New York, Guilford Press, 1998.
49. Henggeler SW, Schoenwald SK, Borduin CM, Rowland MD, Cunningham PB: *Multisystemic Treatment of Antisocial Behavior in Children and Adolescents*. New York, Guilford Press, 1998.
50. Henggeler SW, et al: Home-based multisystemic therapy as an alternative to the hospitalization of youth in psychiatric crisis. *J Am Acad Child Adolesc Psychiatry* 38: 1331–1339, 1999.
51. Haas G, Glick I: Inpatient family intervention: A randomized clinical trial. II: Results at hospital discharge. *Arch Gen Psychiatry* 35:1169–1177, 1988.
52. Hinchcliffe M, Hooper D, Roberts F: *The Melancholy Marriage*. New York, Wiley, 1978.
53. Coyne JC: Depression, biology, marriage, and marital therapy. *Fam Process* 24:131–151, 1985.
54. Schwoeri L. Sholevar GP: A social learning family model of depression and aggression: Focus on the single mother. In: Sholevar GP, Schwoeri L (eds): *The Transmission of Depression in Families and Children*, Northvale, NJ, Jason Aranson, 1994, pp. 145–166.
55. Sholevar GP, Schwoeri L, Jardin H: Family therapy with depression. In: P Sholevar (editor), *Textbook of Family and Couples Therapy*, Washington, DC, APPI Press, 2003, pp 619–637.
56. Brent DA, Holder D, Kilko D et al.: A clinical psychotherapy trial for adolescent depression comparing cognitive, family, and supportive therapy. *Arch Gen Psychiatry* 54:877–885, 1997.
57. Siqueland L, Kendall PC, Steinberg L: Anxiety in children: Perceived family environments and observed family interaction. *J Clin Child Psychol* 25:225–237, 1996.
58. Barrett PM, Healy-Farrell L, March JS: Cognitive behavioral family treatment of childhood obsessive-compulsive disorder: A controlled trial *J Am Acad Child Adolescent Psychiatry* 43:46–62, 2004.
59. Russell GFM, Szmukler GI, Dare C, et al: An evaluation of family therapy in anorexia nervosa and bulimia nervosa. *Arch Gen Psychiatry* 44:1047–1056, 1987.
60. Robin AL, Siegel PT, Moye AW, Gilroy M, Dennis AB, Sikand A: A controlled comparison of family versus individual therapy for adolescents with anorexia nervosa. *J A, Acad Child Adolesc Psychiatry* 38:1482–1489, 1999.
61. Eisler I, Dare C, Russell GFM, Szmukler GI, Le Grancge D, Dodge E: Family therapy for adolescent anorexia nervosa: The results of a controlled comparison of two family interventions. *J Child Psychol Psychiatry* 41:727–736, 2000.
62. Berkowitz RI, Lyke JA, Wadden TA: Treatment of child and adolescent obesity. In: *Obesity, Growth and Development*, Johnston FE, Foster GD, eds. London: Smith-Gordon, 2001, pp. 169–184.
63. Liddle HA: Family-based therapies for adolescent alcohol and drug use research contributions and future research needs. *Addiction* 99:76–92, 2004.
64. Liddle HL, Dakof G: Family-based treatment for adolescent drug use: State of the science. In: Rahdert E (ed): *Adolescent Drug Abuse Assessment and Treatment*. Rockville, MD, NIDA, 1995, pp. 218–254.
65. Henggeler SW, Cligempee WG, Brondino MJ, Pickrel SG: Four-year follow-up of multisystemic therapy with substance-abusing and substance-dependent juvenile offenders. *J am Acad Child Adolescent Psychiatry* 41:868–874, 2002.
66. Sholevar, GP: Family intervention with conduct disorders. In: AM Josephson (editor), *Child and Adolescent Psychiatric Clinics of North America: Current Perspectives on Family Therapy*. Philadelphia, W.B. Saunders Co. (vol 10), 2001, pp. 501–518.
67. Rosenthal D: *Genetic Theory and Abnormal Behavior*. New York, Brunner/Mazel, 1970
68. Tienari P, Lahti I, Sorri A, et al: The Finnish adoptive study of schizophrenia: possible joint effects of genetic vulnerability and family interaction. In: *Understanding Major Mental Disorder: The Contribution of Family Interaction Research*. Edited by Halweg K, Goldstein M. New York, Family Process Press, 1987, pp. 33–54.
69. Zubin J, Spring B: Vulnerability: A new view of schizophrenia. *J Abnorm Psychol* 86:103–126, 1977.
70. Goldstein MJ: Family interaction patterns that antedate the onset of schizophrenia and related disorders: A further analysis of data from a longitudinal prospective study. In: Halweg K, Goldstein MJ (eds): *Understanding Major Mental Disorder: The Contribution of Family Interaction Research*. New York, Family Process Press, 1987, pp. 11–32.
71. Miklowitz D, Thompson, M: Family variables in schizophrenia. In: G.P Sholevar (ed): *Textbook of Family and Couples Therapy*, Washington DC, APPI Press, 2003, pp. 585–618.
72. Halweg K, Neuchterlein K, Goldstein MJ, et al: Parental expressed emotion attitudes and intrafamilial communication behavior. In: *Understanding Major Mental Disorder: The Contribution of Family Interaction Research*. Edited by Halweg K, Goldstein MJ. New York, Family Process Press, 1987, pp. 156–175.
73. Vaughn C, Leff J: The influence of family and social factors on the course of psychiatric illness: A comparison of schizophrenic and depressed neurotic patients. *Br J Psychiatry* 129:125–137, 1976.
74. Wynne LC, Singer MT: Thought disorder and family relations of schizophrenics. I: A research strategy. *Arch Gen Psychiatry* 9:191–198, 1963.
75. Wynne LC: Family variables in the University of Rochester Project. In: *Understanding Major Mental Disorder: The Contribution of Family Interaction Research*. Edited by Halweg K, Goldstein J. New York, Family Process Press, 1987, pp 55–73
76. Group for the Advancement of Psychiatry: *The Family, the Patient, and the Psychiatric Hospital: Toward a New Model*. New York, Brunner/Mazel, 1985, p. 24.
77. Endicott J, Spitzer R: Use of research diagnostic criteria for affective disorders and schizophrenia to study affective disorders. *Am J Psychiatry* 136:52–56, 1979.
78. Clarkin J, Miklowitz D: Diagnosis of family relational disorders. In: Sholevar GP, Schwoeri L (eds): *Textbook of Family and Marital Therapy*. Washington, DC, American Psychiatric Press, 2000.
79. Glick I, Clarkin J, Spencer J: A controlled evaluation of inpatient family intervention. I: Preliminary results of the six month follow-up. *Arch Gen Psychiatry* 42:882–886, 1987b.
80. Sholevar GP: Family therapy with hospitalized and disabled patients. In: *Helping Families with Special Problems*. (ed) Trexler M. Northvale, NJ, Jason Aronson, 1983, pp. 15–35.
81. Hatfield A: The family as partner in the treatment of mental illness. *Hosp Community Psychiatry* 30:338–340, 1986.
82. Clarkin J, Carpenter D: Family therapy process and outcome research. In: *Textbook of Family and Marital Therapy*. Sholevar GP, Schwoeri L. (ed) Washington, DC, American Psychiatric Press 2003.
83. Sayger T, Horne A, Walker J, et al: Social learning family therapy with aggressive children: treatment outcome and maintenance. *Journal of Family Psychology* 1:261–285, 1988.
84. Reiss D. Neiderhisser JM, Hetherington, EM, et al. *The Relationship Code: Deciphering Genetic and Social Influences on Adolescent Development*. Cambridge, MA. Harvard University Press, 2000.

6.3 ■ THE CONTINUUM OF CARE AND LOCATION-SPECIFIC INTERVENTIONS

CHAPTER 6.3.1 ■ MILIEU-BASED TREATMENT: INPATIENT AND PARTIAL HOSPITALIZATION, RESIDENTIAL TREATMENT

JOSEPH C. BLADER AND CARMEL A. FOLEY

INTRODUCTION

Because they subordinate nearly all aspects of a physically capable person's life to the practices and rules of an institution, inpatient and residential psychiatric treatments are highly intrusive interventions. Although autonomy and privacy may not be very abundant in childhood, their loss in these treatment settings is still nearly total. Moreover, separation from home under difficult circumstances, curtailed access to family and friends, and the substitution of strangers as caregivers and peers are confusing and frightening experiences. Families too are justifiably wary. While hospital admission is typically a last resort and provides some relief, parents look to clinicians for help with their own misgivings and emotional turmoil.

By the same token, these milieu settings can leverage many otherwise unavailable assets with the potential to profoundly affect the course of illness and functioning for many youth. The leadership roles that child and adolescent psychiatrists assume in these settings therefore entail not just great responsibility for the children now in their physical custody but great opportunity as well. This chapter's goal is to orient the practitioner a) to the contemporary mission of milieu-based services, b) to the development and implementation of the multifaceted psychiatric care and related programming these services provide, and c) to contextual issues pertaining to leadership, administration and quality surveillance unique to the management of these complex settings.

EVOLUTION OF MILIEU-BASED TREATMENTS

Early Models of Treatment and Facilities

Confinement of the Mentally Ill

Centers that provided compassionate and humane care for the mentally ill flourished intermittently in Europe and the Arab world since classical times. Healing temples offered care and serenity for many of the afflicted. In some places priests, perhaps exploiting a person's delusions, impersonated gods to provide patients with reassurance or to command changes in behavior (1). Ancient Greek physicians were probably the first to offer physiological explanations for behavioral disturbances that supplanted supernatural ones, and they devised various somatic therapies to rebalance or promote proper circulation of bodily fluids or "humors." While it is likely that these treatments were availed to only the more privileged strata of these societies, the ancients did have a protoscientific concept of mental disorder.

Nevertheless, for most of Western history the treatment of people with psychiatric illness rates among the more ignominious of human endeavors. One influential Roman, Aulus Cornelius Celsus (25 BC–50 AD), advocated a calm environment and encouragement for the melancholic in addition to specific herbal remedies (2). However, for agitated behavior he called for avowedly punitive measures:

> If however, it is the mind that deceives the madman, he is best treated by certain tortures. When he says or does anything wrong, he is to be coerced by starvation, fetters and flogging ... To be thoroughly frightened is beneficial in this illness.

This strain of thought in effect sanctioned a range of odious practices toward people with severely disordered behavior for centuries. In medieval times, demonic explanations for aberrant behavior and thought resurged and motivated the confinement, persecution, shackles, and harsh and neglectful treatment that dominated to greater or lesser degrees until the late eighteenth century.

The contemporary Euro-American model of the psychiatric hospital originates with reforms during the 1790s in Britain (William Tuke, founding the York Retreat, which in turn influenced Benjamin Rush in America), France (Philippe Pinel at the Bicêtre and Salpêtrière asylums), and Italy (Vicenzo Chiarugi at Florence's Hospital of Bonifazio). All three men's writings contributed to the modern nosological approach to mental illness based on symptom-defined syndromes and observed course. (Honoring Chiarugi's work, the University of Pisa appointed him *Professore di Malattie Afrodisiache e Perturbazioni Intellettuali*, or Professor of Aphrodisiac Diseases and Intellectual Perturbations, a distinction today's psychiatric illuminati might rather forgo.) In the United States and United Kingdom, the establishment and maintenance of facilities for the care of those with chronically debilitating mental illness became a function of local government.

This wave of reform and the infusion of government investment, along with an optimistic view that more humane treatment would also cure patients, helped stimulate a significant growth of institutions for the mentally ill beginning in the early 1800s. Many facilities were set in locations removed from the main population centers from which their residents came. It was almost inevitable, though, that the burdens of increasing urbanization and migration, economic dislocation, and the infectious epidemics of subsequent eras, along with the fact that more humane care was not necessarily curative, combined to strain these resources. Underfunding, public discouragement, and a growing patient population degraded many publicly supported facilities into quite dismal places well into the twentieth century. However, from about 1960 onward, vigorous advocacy, the deinstitutionalization movement, more effective treatments, and a generally prosperous economy led to a major reduction in the census of large long-term hospitals and more community-based treatment. Inpatient psychiatric treatment gradually came to be seen as another health service, and acute units developed in general hospitals and relatively short stays for episodic crises became far more common.

Recent improvements in care and outcomes for mental illness notwithstanding, the larger historical context of psychiatric hospitalization and enduring apprehensions about the people who need it continue to imbue inpatient psychiatry with arguably the most negative stigma among medical treatments today.

Children's Inpatient Treatment

Both before and after the reformation of the early 1800s we know that disturbed children and adolescents were at times placed in these facilities along with adults. Beyond a few scholarly reports whose aim was to document the occurrence of severe mental illness in the young as a source of curiosity in itself, little is known about the care and outcomes of children in asylums. The first dedicated child psychiatric inpatient units as such in the United States were created in the 1920s and '30s, mostly as custodial services for children with postencephalitic brain disorders. The prevailing philosophies of these settings and their successors are discussed later.

By the mid-1980s, inpatient beds for children and adolescents proliferated markedly, chiefly in private sector general and specialty psychiatric hospitals. The U.S. Supreme Court's 1985 decision in *Massachusetts v. Metropolitan* (3) supported mental health coverage by insurance plans, and earlier the *Parham v. J.R.* decision affirmed that parents' could compel admission to psychiatric inpatient care for an unwilling minor, much as any other necessary medical treatment (4). Lengths of stay were extensive, standards for admission were liberal, and many inpatient settings adopted rather high, if subjective, criteria for judging wellness to warrant discharge. Direct-to-consumer advertising by these facilities, aimed at parents worried about their sullen or unruly teenagers, became commonplace. Inpatient care also served an evaluative purpose, with some referrals made for diagnostic clarification.

However, by the early 1990s this trend had rapidly reversed. Scandals plagued certain for-profit facilities. Managed care established increasingly strict criteria to justify inpatient admission. The *Parham* decision was partially blamed for the ease with which parents could have their adolescents psychiatrically hospitalized, often for rebellious or obnoxious behavior alone. The managed care revolution greatly reduced the length of stay, though actual rates of admission have remained mostly unaltered or increased, and perhaps readmissions have increased (5, 6). In the public sector, policymakers also recognized that a disproportionate amount of the mental healthcare dollar was spent on very costly inpatient care to the detriment of less expensive community-based options that were far more appropriate for many children. This line of thought followed naturally from the somewhat earlier deinstitutionalization movement for adults with chronic psychiatric conditions.

Child advocates, who had earlier called attention to the scarcity of community-based resources that might help impaired children to remain at home (7, 8), found that cost concerns were aligning policymakers' interests toward development of a fuller range of supports in the community calibrated to the needs of individual children and families. The espousal of such continuum-of-care principles by federal, state, and county levels of mental health planning increased significantly the array of community-based programming. Such services included in-home and out-of-home respite services, supportive case management, therapeutic after-school programs, innovative programs based on "blended funding" from several agencies—all aimed at avoiding or reducing hospitalizations and optimizing a child's opportunities for successful retention in the community. Localities, though, still vary widely in the availability and quality of these resources. Moreover, some evaluation projects raised the prospect that such enhanced services do not necessarily produce more favorable outcomes, although families do find them preferable to service systems that omit them (9).

At the present time, inpatient psychiatric treatment in the United States is regarded, properly, as an expensive resource to be used sparingly and as a last resort for the most ill of youngsters. Comparatively few children now depend on long-term psychiatric inpatient settings to receive care, and acute-care lengths of stay are shorter. Admissions for evaluative purposes often occur only upon court order. Nonetheless, inpatient treatment remains an important component of the system of care for very ill youngsters. Eligibility for many of the community wraparound services discussed earlier often depends on prior psychiatric hospitalization, or at least on the risk for admission. Moreover, despite the value placed on alternatives to restrictive placements, admissions to acute inpatient settings with a principal diagnosis of psychiatric disorder have increased strikingly between 1996 and 2004 among children (45% population-adjusted increase) and adolescents (25%), greatly outpacing the 11% increase for adults (10).

Evolution of Treatment Philosophy

The first children's units were essentially custodial in emphasis, due to the mostly organic impairments of the patient population (11). Most would be regarded today as fundamentally mentally retarded, whether by congenital or acquired (usually infectious) conditions.

By the mid-twentieth century, psychoanalytic thinking dominated child and adolescent psychiatry. Child psychoanalysis early on emphasized the primacy of interpersonal experience in development and emotional disturbances, and different strains of thought came to converge on a basic notion that early attachment and nurturance, and the promotion of autonomy, formed the template for a person's manner of relating to the world (12). Some features of hospital treatment now considered at best "necessary evils" came to be seen as rather integral elements of the era's psychoanalytically oriented model of inpatient care. In particular, separation of the child from his or her putatively pathogenic home environment was felt "to be the first requirement for successful treatment . . . since he is comparatively helpless to re-order his own surroundings or change them to better suit his needs" (13). Consequently, hospital settings did not seek to redress directly perceived deficiencies in the family. The premise of inpatient and residential settings for quite disturbed children was that in a more capable caregiving environment the child might have corrective experiences that would allay basic insecurities and foster ego development so that better modulated behavior and affect might blossom. Until such time, residential settings also were thought to provide an empathic surrogate "holding environment" (14) that would help the child manage destructive urges or disorganized behavior. There was no expectation that this would be a rapid or easy process and long hospital stays were common.

In the 1960s and 1970s, learning theories from experimental psychology, especially its neobehaviorist schools, acquired steadily greater traction in clinical psychology. Interventions based on environmental manipulation to modify pathological behavior, known broadly as behavior modification or behavior therapy, gained wider application in facilities for developmentally impaired and chronically mentally ill adults. Approaches based on *operant conditioning* principles prioritized the adaptive behaviors that the individual lacked, and sought to promote them by following their appearance with rewards or reinforcers. Likewise, efforts to eliminate (or "extinguish") the problematic behaviors involved withholding the reinforcer that it usually elicited (such as attention or avoidance) or by applying an aversive consequence. Approaches rooted in *classical conditioning* sought to unlink troubling exaggerated emotional responses, such as intense anxiety, from the relatively benign stimuli that had come to elicit them, or to reduce the attraction of a problematic stimulus, such as tobacco, by associating it with something unpleasant. Integrating these and other principles, *applied behavioral analysis* provided some elegant demonstrations of how systematic assessment of antecedents, behaviors, and consequences could lead to interventions that resulted in marked behavior change. Offering patients explicit training and practice in specific behavioral skills, such as assertiveness, anger control, and social interaction, were also undertaken in a variety of formats.

Particularly influential reports showed dramatic improvements in the social engagement and activities of daily living among chronically ill adults, the acquisition of some language by autistic children, and reductions in self-abusive behavior by those with mental retardation (15–18).

Settings that provided round-the-clock care were ideal for the implementation of treatments that required consistent monitoring of behavior and the systematic manipulation of the consequences for that behavior. Moreover, constant supervision by a professional staff facilitated recording that *quantifies* behavior, a methodological necessity of behaviorism and an appealing feature of behavior therapy. "Token economies," in which patients earned chits toward various privileges for prespecified behaviors, became especially widespread, and influenced the rather ubiquitous point or level systems in the inpatient and residential settings of today. The appeal of these systems may derive partly from their implementation on a unit-wide basis, in that many patients will share similar behavioral objectives and thus offer a common template for the whole service. In contrast, classical conditioning and applied behavioral analytic approaches are highly idiographic and the staffing of most psychiatric settings seldom permits such intense staff training and individualized implementation efforts on a routine basis. The obvious availability of a peer group also enables on-the-spot opportunities to develop and practice social and other skills. Behavioral interventions are conceived to yield dividends in weeks, or at least that is the period for evaluating the usefulness of a particular treatment plan.

However, the very intensity of specialized out-of-home settings that facilitates ecological interventions of these types militates against the generalization of behavior changes to other settings once the individual no longer experiences the environmental contingencies that supported them. One potential remedy is to regard the patient's family as a suitable locus for intervention that might enable maintenance of gains after the youngster's return to the community. Outpatient "child guidance" clinics for youth with conduct problems had since the 1920s included parents seeing a social worker as ancillary to the child's psychotherapy (19), and family therapy as an identifiable treatment modality for outpatients had been practiced since at least the 1940s. However, family-focused treatment did not assume a widespread central position in the treatment of hospitalized children's psychiatric disorders until the 1980s. In 1980, the most common type of treatment received across all settings was individual therapy, received by 89%, while family therapy was provided to only 38% (20). At that time, some settings had programs where entire families were admitted and under constant observation.

Family therapy encompasses a range of approaches and theories, so its incorporation into psychiatric inpatient settings displays eclecticism. However, child psychiatry is perhaps unique in that the recognized standards of care for several of its most common disorders explicitly include interventions focused on parent–child interaction. These include parent management training (PMT) for conduct problems, the mainstay of this patient population. The obvious continuity between behavior therapy approaches in the inpatient setting and PMT has led to the latter's becoming a significant component of family intervention in many settings. Moreover, parents can see methods modeled by staff and undertake them with guidance and support during hospitalization. Regardless of the specific disorder and treatment approach, psychoeducation and support to families coping with an ill child are now universally judged as essential to compassionate care by all members of the treatment team. This is obviously a significant philosophical shift from earlier times, when families were at best ancillary to the child's treatment, when not the object of clinicians' reproach as the source of the patient's illness.

As behavioral therapy matured as an influential clinical specialty, a significant development was the view that a person's thoughts and beliefs are behaviors in their own right that could be altered and thereby affect overt behavior or mood. Imparting systematic methods of thinking through problems to suppress disadvantageous "automatic" responses (problem solving), and reevaluating unhelpful beliefs that motivate maladaptive behavior (cognitive restructuring) were melded with learning approaches to yield the area we know today as cognitive-behavioral therapy (CBT). These treatments have had modest impact on the overall inpatient milieu, but are often incorporated into group therapy as befits clinician preference. A few settings have woven some of these approaches, such as dialectical behavior therapy for self-injurious adolescents, into their milieus, such that patients having trouble are prompted and coached *in situ* to utilize these skills. Such milieu-based adjuncts to CBT are probably underutilized, especially with adolescents, but multidisciplinary staff training in these methods requires a substantial commitment that may be the limiting factor in many settings with short stays.

Pharmacotherapy now plays a prominent role in the psychiatric treatment of youth. The 1980 NIMH report (20) indicated that 42% of child and adolescent inpatients were treated with standing psychotropic medication. While the pharmacologic evidence base still has extensive gaps, the use of medication in inpatient settings has increased dramatically. It is now the rare youngster whose inpatient or residential treatment does not include medication (21–23). Greater severity of illness to obtain approval for admission may account for some of this change, but it does mirror data showing a corresponding increase among outpatients. Consequently, youth are more likely to be receiving treatment with psychotropics, often two or more, at the time of admission. Medication trials tend to be a reason for continuing stay most acceptable to managed care reviewers. The combined effect is that the role of the child psychiatrist in these settings has increasingly focused, perhaps to the detriment of other areas, on which preadmission agents were doing any good, which were potentially making things worse, and what to try next, all in the context of constrained lengths of stay with a possibly more treatment-refractory patient population.

Recent Developments and Their Impact

The current ethos prevailing in psychiatric care is that it should be provided in the least restrictive environment possible. Many innovations in psychiatric services for children have therefore aimed at reducing reliance on congregate care settings such as inpatient and residential facilities. These include family support services, such as emergency respite—both in and outside of the home—using trained professional or paraprofessionals, volunteers or other parents. This service may take the form of regular after-school or weekend specialized recreation or therapeutic care programs. Home care programs may include child supervision, instruction in parenting skills, and case advocacy assistance. Home-based crisis intervention programs provide in-home services to families for 4–6 weeks with the goal of avoiding hospitalization. Family-based treatment uses surrogate families who are "professional parents" to care for and treat youth with serious emotional disturbance (24). Some well developed programs have shown benefits compared to "usual care" in the hands of the group that designed them and a major challenge concerns the exportability of such services to other facilities, especially when their adoption represents a marked shift from practitioners' prior mode of functioning (25).

Although an important development, these alternatives remain unevenly available and demand exceeds supply in many localities. Priority for intensive community-based services often goes to youth deemed to be at risk for out-of-home placement. As a practical matter, such risk is quite often demonstrated by prior hospitalization. Consequently, a more prominent function of inpatient and residential settings has become liaison with community-based care providers and schools to recommend and arrange implementation of appropriate postdischarge services from within this continuum of care. Several states and service regions have also implemented a centralization mechanism whereby a common application for services is submitted to the single point of entry (SPOA) reviewing body for appropriate assignment to community-based intensive treatment options. As it happens, though, there is little empirical basis to support these recommendations, or the prognostic judgments that are implicit in them.

A form of extended psychiatric triage has also emerged that may divert some admissions. Such services usually constitute an enhanced psychiatric emergency room service by providing a small number of "holding beds" for up to 72 hours, a mobile crisis team that can be called to a home, school, or other community setting by a parent, concerned citizen, police officer, etc. Such an enhanced emergency service usually has 24-hour socialwork coverage to work rapidly on community-based disposition whenever possible. Referred to as CPEPs in some localities (comprehensive psychiatric emergency program), their general objective is to treat in the emergency room if possible, and thus avoid inpatient hospitalization. Only rarely, however, do these settings have a separate section for children.

In hospital settings, daily rounds nowadays typically begin with the question, "Why does this child need to be in the hospital?" All hospitalizations covered by managed care plans are constantly monitored by the insurance companies' reviewers. Publicly funded care is also subject to retroactive denial of payments if inspection of the medical record is judged to lack sufficient justification for inpatient care. Although minimizing the time a child spends in a hospital is not a controversial goal, a widespread sentiment is that aggressive cost containment may have compromised care. For instance, payers often regard as inertia the observation of a child after withdrawing preadmission medications, which biases the system toward initiating new, possibly superfluous pharmacotherapy. This is another area deserving more systematic study.

OVERVIEW OF TYPES OF MILIEU SETTINGS AND THEIR PURPOSE IN A SYSTEM OF CARE

Inpatient Care

As noted earlier, acute care is now only deemed appropriate when less restrictive alternatives have been considered, have failed, or are not available. The most common reason for admission is behavior felt to place the child or others in danger. This may translate to suicidal ideation, intent, or attempt, or may reflect sufficient threat of aggression or actual aggression such that the caretaking system, school or home, is concerned and unable to handle the youth. It is difficult nowadays to get authorization from payers to admit for a purely diagnostic assessment. Indeed, many components of such evaluations, say, psychological testing, MRI, lab tests, and the like can generally be secured on an outpatient basis, and payers seldom find the putative value of inpatient observation a cogent rationale for admission.

Specialty acute inpatient care is a locked and therefore secure setting, which includes round-the-clock staffing, and the capacity to restrain or seclude an out-of-control patient. Despite the emphasis on the therapeutic value of the "structure of the unit," structure is a generic attribute of several other less restrictive settings, though it must be conceded that the locked setting confers a special level of environmental control.

The majority of short-term psychiatric treatment is provided in units located in freestanding psychiatric hospitals or in units located in general medical/surgical hospitals. Acute care was arbitrarily defined as being for 30 days or less. This was driven by the typical 30-day insurance policy rather than having any established relationship to diagnosis, progress, or prognosis. Nevertheless, this time frame certainly became embedded in the format of inpatient assessments and in the mindset driving disposition planning and implementation. The time frame, in turn, influenced many aspects of the inpatient therapeutic structure, such as how long it took to earn privileges, obtain an off-unit pass, etc. Beyond 30 days, applications for intermediate care (30–180 days) will be entertained, usually in the regional state facility.

Acute and intermediate care facilities generally serve children age 4 to 18 years. Very few programs serve a preschool population in an inpatient setting. The developmental disorders that in the past had occasioned the need for hospital care in this age group are now, thankfully, more successfully addressed by the universally available early intervention system and the significant growth of highly specialized education settings for very young children. It is customary to have separate inpatient settings for children up to age 12 or 13 and for adolescents up to age 18. Some inpatient units treat children and adolescents together, or those over the age of 16 may be admitted to adult settings, but these practices more often derive from necessity than philosophy.

Municipal and county facilities often have a public mandate to serve the local court system. Judges have the authority to mandate assessments in such units for defined timeframes (21 days is common). A complete assessment of the child's mental condition, including psychological testing, and a psychosocial assessment of the child's family, school, and community culminate in an advisory report to the court. In 2003, 2.2 million youth in the United States were arrested for delinquency or status offenses, of whom 1.8 million appeared in juvenile courts; 329,000 of these were detained in a residential setting for assessment. In addition, the census of youth in residential correctional facilities following adjudication was just under 100,000 (26). This population is considered to be massively underserved with respect to psychiatric illness, the prevalence of which is now known to be quite high (27). To the extent that mental health services variously exist within the juvenile justice system's residential programs, they constitute another version of a psychiatric inpatient provider system for incarcerated youth.

Inpatient units can be subspecialized for the care of unique psychiatrically impaired populations. Eating disorder services are one example which enable the more intensive medical management these youth require initially with the specialized psychiatric care that does most of the heavy lifting toward recovery adequate for the resumption of outpatient treatment. Special psychiatric units for the deaf, the blind, and for youth with cooccurring developmental disabilities also exist. Such facilities represent a type of nursing home care for the medically fragile who also have significant psychiatric problems, and whose families are unable to care for these children with the available community support services.

Partial Hospitalization and Day Treatment

Of the varieties of noninpatient programs, partial hospitalization is the most intensive. The clinical challenge for this level of care is the provision of short-term, crisis stabilization as an alternative to inpatient care or as a step down from inpatient care.

Partial hospital programming may be provided on an inpatient unit. Some refer to this as unit-based aftercare. It allows the patient to continue working with the same treatment team and the same peer group rather than forcing a change for a short period of time. Partial day hospital licenses require treatment to be no longer than 6 weeks, as well as daily chart documentation of progress, much like in an inpatient setting. However, most inpatient units have a high inpatient census and staffing is not necessarily easily expanded to cope with "day patients," so the model has obvious practical limitations.

More typically, partial hospital programs have their own staff, space, and school. Despite commonly being licensed for 6-week lengths of stay, managed care review generally constrains the actual duration of the patient's involvement to only days or a couple of weeks at most. Since the setting is generally open, and regulation does not allow restraint or seclusion but does permit therapeutic hold and use of a quiet room (no locked door), there are practical limitations on the degree of psychopathology for which these settings are suitable. Programmatically, the range of therapeutic services are similar to inpatient settings, and include individual, group, and family therapies, recreation and rehabilitation therapies, medical care, and psychopharmacology.

Day treatment, sometimes referred to as continuing day treatment, differs from partial hospitals in several ways. Length of stay is much longer, often driven by the school year's calendar. Children attending day treatment must usually be certified as being in need of that level of care by their local school district's committee on special education, since these authorities generally assume the cost of the program's educational component. The district is often intending that a child's stay in day treatment will last for at least a full school term or even for the entire academic year. Day treatment settings are as likely to be, fundamentally, schools with high psychiatric involvement as they are to be psychiatric settings as such. Even when a psychiatric facility houses a day treatment program, it is often partnered with a local education systems' special education division. The school service may therefore have some independence from the rest of the facility that the psychiatric staff should be aware of and respect to maintain good rapport with all those involved in the children's care.

Since most commercial payers generally cover only acute short-term care, it is Medicaid that more commonly covers the cost of day treatment, with eligibility based upon either the family's precarious finances or the child's own chronic disability. Some day treatment programs are funded entirely by units of state and local government and are therefore available regardless of means.

Partial and continuing day hospital programs occupy open settings, and these programs tend to be rather selective in whom they admit. Imminent danger to self or others, repeated need for restraint even by therapeutic holding, elopement risk, or bringing contraband to the program (especially drugs or alcohol) all preclude successful treatment in such settings. To date, limited treatment effectiveness research suggests that partial/day treatment is a cost-effective approach for some children in crisis in lieu of hospitalization, and/or as a step down for inpatients (28).

Residential Treatment

This title carries a connotation of a boarding school–like setting where the child lives, goes to school, and receives therapeutic services and all necessary medical care and psychiatric medicines in one location. Indeed, the prototype for residential treatment is the "cottage" model. This model, in turn, derived from the heritage of many of these facilities as turn-of-the-century orphanages or shelters for children of destitute families, especially in the eastern United States. These facilities were often founded by sectarian philanthropic groups to meet the needs of immigrants and had relocated from cramped urban quarters to home-like cottages, arranged spaciously as a campus to evoke a small neighborhood in more salubrious semirural (now suburban) settings. The explicit goal was to emulate family living, complete with live-in cottage parents, to the extent possible. Child guidance clinics were established at some of these facilities. The Child Welfare Act of 1915 provided widows with at least minimal support, and the orphanage population decreased significantly. Later in the twentieth century, support for foster care, adoption, and small group homes eclipsed large congregate care for the parentless. However, during the Great Depression, these same charitable entities partnered with the states and could draw down public funding to provide a wide array of services, which included care for emotionally troubled youth. The coming decades essentially completed the transformation of many of these facilities into therapeutic schools reliant on public funding serving children regardless of their faith or ethnicity.

Residential treatment facilities (RTFs) are typically licensed by state departments of mental health, and have the mission of caring for the severely psychiatrically impaired youth who do not need the constraints of an inpatient setting. By contrast, residential treatment centers (RTCs) generally come under the auspices of state departments of social service. The setting and range of services are similar, but the RTC population is generally less psychiatrically impaired and would probably be suitable for outpatient treatment were it not for adverse psychosocial circumstances that make community living inadequately supportive. Reasons may include absent or mentally ill family members or seriously damaged parent–child relationships. In some cases, an RTF may be collocated as a cottage within an RTC but with different staffing and capability for managing behavioral crises, including specialized staff training and a "quiet room."

One of the more controversial aspects of admission to RTCs has been the requirement in many states that parents relinquish custody of their children. Having parents make this wrenching decision seems intended to prevent parents fobbing off care of their children for economic reasons alone. Family advocates, however, perceive that the practice perpetuates flawed reasoning that blames the family for the child's illness, and that it discriminatorily inflicts pain on the families of mentally ill children.

Coordination of Care

Behavioral health entities, public and private, in certain parts of the country have tried to develop as many parts of the continuum of care as possible. This allows for internal control of transfer between the parts in as efficient a manner as possible. The ideal is the appropriate matching of patient need with the most appropriate level of care, with easy and seamless transfer to the next level of care as needed. Public single point of entry (SPOA) efforts have a similar goal.

However, institutional and clinical limitations impede the advancement of this ideal from noble rhetoric into practice. Individual facilities have been reluctant to abandon control over whom they will admit and when discharge is appropriate, as discussed in the next section. On the clinical side, mental health remains so riddled with huge areas of uncertainty and debate regarding diagnosis, treatment needs, and the efficacy of intervention, that discontinuity in treatment approach when changing providers is almost guaranteed. Pharmacotherapy, for example, is often modified as a function of setting to accommodate a new treatment team's predilections.

Another limitation in our clinical knowledge is a weak basis for determining level of service needs. It is easy to conclude that a child is not doing well and needs a more supportive or restrictive level of care, since severe symptomatology speaks for itself. However, clinicians have a much harder time trying to decide whether *success* in a setting better demonstrates a) that a youngster may now flourish in a "lower" level of care, or b) that the current setting is highly appropriate to his or her needs and should continue with it.

Thus, although administrative streamlining is necessary to the coordination of timely treatment that promotes a child's right to develop in normal, age-typical settings to the extent possible, it is alone probably not sufficient to bring about the seamless transitioning that many advocate.

REFERRAL AND ADMISSION

Admission Policies

Any healthcare service is duty bound to help as many people as possible. On the other hand, each setting has to have a realistic appraisal of its limitations, since no useful purpose is served by making commitments that diminish the service's overall quality of care or safety.

Acute inpatient services tend to be the least "selective," consistent with their mission to be accessible ports of last resort in a storm. Nevertheless, difficult situations still present themselves. For instance, many units cannot readily accommodate those with severe developmental disabilities experiencing acute behavioral disturbances, especially those lacking language, or at least need skillful 1 : 1 staffing and special milieu accommodations to serve them. These days, that level of care often means diverting available staff to the needs of the patient, rather than obtaining an addition to the staff complement for the child's stay. It is tempting to admit children with such severity as a temporizing measure and starting treatment with the necessary accommodations until a more appropriate care setting develops, but there is no guarantee that these alternatives will materialize or that a child will be well enough for discharge in the timeframe one hopes for.

Without the pressure to address acute crises, long-term inpatient, partial, day, and residential programs can be far more selective, and, as less secure settings, are obliged to be. Policies vary widely as a function of facilities, resources, expertise, and availability of alternatives in the region. Facilities weigh, to varying degrees, factors like histories of substance abuse, fire setting, sexual misconduct, running away and truancy, criminal involvement, developmental needs, medical needs, prospects for family involvement, and so forth to judge appropriateness. These are not always straightforward determinations and sometimes can cause facilities, their payers, and those making referrals to collide. In any event, admission policies should be based on soul-searching and strong programmatic and resource justifications. There has been increased concern about by the public agencies that fund care that facilities have been "cherry picking" children with less complex situations, and that some of these admission policies may discriminate against particular ethnic communities.

Emergency vs. Planned Hospital Admissions

Hospitals with psychiatric emergency rooms have constant capacity to assess all who present in psychiatric crisis. Hospitals with no mental health staff or programs usually transfer cases to those that do. The planned hospital admission is something of a contrivance today. Where a preauthorization assessment must be performed on the day of admission, the receiving unit may agree to hold a bed, with the expectation that the intended patient will be seen in the emergency room early in the day and authorization quickly obtained. This only works where all parties agree on the obvious and compelling need for hospitalization in the first place. Since Medicaid does not require preauthorizations, planning an admission days in advance is still feasible. This allows the referring person or agency to forward all relevant reports of previous assessments, laboratory findings, psychological testing, school reports, etc. to the receiving inpatient unit ahead of time. Conversation with unit staff on the part of referral sources may even produce a clearcut therapeutic or investigational agenda before the patient ever arrives. Transfer between hospitals or other institution, whether mandated by insurance or requested by parents, can also be planned in advance.

Entry to intermediate and long-term facilities is invariably planned, since an elaborate application screening and acceptance process is a required preliminary.

Referral Sources and Screening

Precise referral patterns are unique to particular facilities and their place in the local continuum of care. Parents generally prefer that their child be served as close to home as possible, so they can avail of visitation opportunities. All referring persons rely to a large degree on the reputation of the local, inpatient service. According to the business literature, it is well recognized that if a patient/family has a good experience, they will tell one or two people. However, if the experience is negative, eight to 10 people are likely to learn of it. Local schools are often the major source of referral to emergency departments, followed by families themselves. A portion of referrals comes from community agencies, especially those caring for foster children who are often overrepresented among psychiatrically hospitalized children.

Screening may involve a phone call by the referring source to the units' physician. Some hospitals have centralized intake systems where a socialwork assistant or higher level mental health professional obtains as much clinical information as possible to ensure that the child does indeed need inpatient care, that a legally appropriate parent or guardian is available to complete admission forms, that the family or personnel in place of family (foster parent, case worker) will be available to work with unit staff. Sometimes parents may want to tour the unit and meet with staff as they struggle with the decision to hospitalize a child. The evaluation also serves to ensure that no exclusion criteria apply. DSM-IV V-code diagnoses are generally not reimbursable. Some insurance plans will not cover hospitalization for a diagnosis of conduct disorder in the absence of a compelling acutely treatable cooccurring psychiatric condition. Sadly, it is not unusual that acute inpatient treatment is not covered for youth suffering from autism spectrum conditions.

Preauthorization

This refers to the process by which the patient's insurer, via a managed care intermediary, accepts or rejects the referral source's clinical information. This is intended to substantiate the need for inpatient care. Sometimes, rejection by a reviewing professional leads to an immediate doctor-to-doctor review of the circumstances. Because of the time-consuming nature of the authorization exercise, hospitals may employ resource management nurses or social workers, whose sole job is to interface with the managed care company.

Parents are often unaware of their mental health benefits until a crisis develops. Only in the emergency room is it suddenly determined that the insurance plan has a unique contract for the provision of psychiatric inpatient care with one particular facility that may be geographically remote from the patient's home, to the chagrin of already stressed parents.

A symptom picture that puts the child or others at imminent risk of harm, failure, or lack of available alternative services often tip the balance in favor of hospitalization. A multiaxial diagnosis and an initial intended treatment plan are typical parts of the preauthorization conversation. Approval for a hospital stay of one to a few days allows the admission to proceed. "Concurrent review" refers to subsequent conversations between the managed care company's reviewer and the resource management or physician staff about the child's progress and readiness for discharge.

Engaging and Supporting Families

Some units, when time permits, allow parents to come and view the unit and discuss the program with staff in advance of a child's admission. A small brochure generally provides useful information about visiting, phone calls, clothing and laundry considerations, how a child's education will be managed, and how medical problems will be addressed, as well as rules about forbidden items, such as lighters, matches, cigarettes, pocket knives, drugs, etc. The same or an additional document will describe the unit's points or levels system (usually a version of a token economy program) and how aggression to self and others may be dealt with. It is important that caregivers appreciate that the safety of all is paramount and that seclusion or restraint may be needed if someone is out of control or in imminent danger of losing control. The role of the members of the interdisciplinary team and whom to contact for different concerns must be made clear. Although the minor voluntary admission forms already signed by the parent or guardian permits the full panoply of needed psychiatric services, certain other levels of consent are now commonplace.

While units may administer any medication in an emergency circumstance, it is common to seek separate permission for the administration of standing psychotropics. Justifications differ on whether this permission must be via a special consent form or an oral discussion, but the discussion, including the indication for the medication and its risks and benefits, is documented in the patient record.

Every effort to join families as allies in helping the child to cope with whatever is believed to have led to hospitalization is essential to a good ongoing working relationship. The availability of chaplaincy services and interpreter services when needed can be a considerable consolation to parents. Units may run parent management training groups, general support groups, discharge preparation groups, disease-specific psychoeducation groups, and medication education groups, as well as traditional individual family therapy meetings. Timetables, schedule compatibility, and priorities for an individual family need to be established at the time of admission.

Realistic Expectations

Given the brevity of a hospital stay, caregivers and those making referrals need to be educated that the focus of treatment on acute units is acute stabilization of the presenting problems, rather than resolution of all difficulties a child may have. Where it is evident that a child will require a different type of school placement upon discharge, the child may not be able to remain on an inpatient unit while the school district deliberates the options according to its own time guidelines. Expectations for parental involvement in treatment, such as shadowing nursing staff in implementing a behavior modification plan, being available for family meetings, and participating in prescribed passes off the unit to test out newly acquired skills and indicating readiness for discharge all need to be spelled out.

Children in Surrogate/Foster Care

A foster parent has no legal standing and therefore a representative of the foster care agency, who in turn is acting as the agent of the state department of social services, must be available to sign admission papers. Even after admission, consent must be obtained again for the administration of standing psychotropic medications. Many placements in foster care are voluntary, that is, a court proceeding has not terminated a parent's rights, in which case the foster care agency must make reasonable efforts to obtain the parent's consent. This can be extremely difficult for hospital units with very ill, dyscontrolled children who, without appropriate consent, cannot get on with needed treatment. If a parent refuses consent, the agency may have to go to court to override the refusal.

It sometimes becomes clear, once the child is hospitalized, that the foster placement has irretrievably broken down. It is often difficult to secure a new foster home and to carry out the necessary courtship process between the child and the new foster parent on the time schedule of most inpatient units. Clarity of communication as to the limits of the stabilization role of the hospital's and the agencies' ongoing responsibilities to provide a suitable domicile for the child should be extensively documented, prior to admission if possible. The disordered and compromised attachments of these children are often reenacted in the inpatient setting, either with guarded, mistrustful, or unengaged behaviors. Other patterns include traumatic reenactments, or angry aggression meted out indiscriminately.

MULTIDISCIPLINARY ASSESSMENT

Diagnostic, Psychosocial/Developmental, Family and Academic Assessments

Beyond the rather generic principles of good clinical practice in psychiatric assessment, we should note some special aspects of evaluation in milieu settings. Barring the occasional true first-episode, usually adolescent, patient with de novo onset, children coming to inpatient or residential care these days tend to have extensive prior psychiatric histories because the conditions themselves are often chronic and with early onset. Nonetheless, it is important to elucidate whether the crisis at hand represents a *major departure* from prior level of disturbance or whether it is an intensification of the same ongoing difficulties. Indeed, a behaviorally dyscontrolled youngster may be no worse symptomatically relative to the past few years, but admission is indicated just because he or she is now much larger and so now exceeds the caregivers' capacity to provide containment. Abrupt changes, especially if linked to a current stressor, may dispose to a better postdischarge prognosis (29).

It is common to augment traditional history-taking with the use of rating scales, such as the Conners' Scales, the Child Behavior Checklist, or the Behavioral Assessment Scale for Children. Structured diagnostic interviews are no more common in inpatient than outpatient settings, which is to say they are not routine. Behavioral rating scales have parent-, teacher-, and often, self-report versions. We strongly recommend the acquisition of teacher input, which staff can readily obtain via fax, with appropriate parental consent. Severe dysfunction in the school setting has to be a factor in discharge planning. It is not uncommon for children to function significantly better in school than at home, whether by dint of structure, generally greater behavioral inhibition outside the home, or uniquely problematic interactions within the family. Obviously, the situational specificity of problems is a key aspect of evaluation.

Psychological testing was at one time nearly routine, but now is performed only as indicated. One tangible benefit in particular involves the elucidation of academic skill difficulties related to a hitherto unidentified learning disorder. Even if a child has been evaluated by the committee on special education of the child's home school district, major areas of dysfunction elude detection, such as problems with written expression, and the academic struggles that ensue greatly exacerbate the child's problems, or even lead to psychiatric manifestations that ultimately lead to admission. School failure is at times wrongly attributed to poor effort or emotional disturbance, when in fact neuropsychological deficits are the main culprit.

Beyond these aspects of psychiatric assessment, each discipline will probably do its own assessment. Hospital charts and RTC records are often chock full of separate initial evaluations by nursing, social work, rehabilitation, school, speech and language, and so on.

Prior Treatment History

Previous trials of medications should be inquired about with respect to target symptoms, compound used, optimum dose utilized, characterization of the medication trial, and patient response. Parents are not always able to provide the necessary detail, so consent to speak with previous prescribers should be sought.

Previous psychosocial treatments, including type (individual, group, family), duration, therapeutic targets, and response must similarly be ascertained.

The mental health of parents is particularly relevant to the wellbeing of the child. Parent past psychiatric history, substance use/abuse history, past and present treatment, and current mental functioning are highly relevant to parental capacity to care for a now ill child.

Prior placement, why it came about, duration, ability of the parent to stay involved with the child during the period of placement, the perspectives of child and parent regarding the placement, the status of reunification plans and or actual efforts—all provide a picture of the stability or its lack in the rearing environment. Such history also sheds light on discharge options.

Quality of Relationships with Family and Peers

Unfortunately, psychopathology among young people is often associated with quite corrosive relationships with their caregivers. By the time of inpatient admission, some families have come to see extrusion of the child as the solution to many of their problems. While this does not bode well, it is important to understand this level of antagonism at the front end. On the other hand, children whose caregivers acknowledge feeling quite stressed and worried by their child's problems seem less hostile, and there is some evidence that they experience better outcomes (29, 30). Siblings, too, may figure prominently in the histories of the presenting problems, as targets and/or provocateurs of problem behavior.

It is always appropriate to inquire about preferred activities, perceived strengths and talents, and with whom the child socializes, but these take on special significance in inpatient or residential settings. This information can serve practical purposes for treatment planning, as in the development of incentive plans, or by designating prosocial skills to encourage. Among young children, how many friends they have and keep is important; many of our patients can not report one out-of-school relationship and parents often relate that the child's behavior hampers development of friendships and deters the parents of their peers. Adolescents, on the other hand, usually identify with some peer group, and it is important to learn whether these youth are prone to troubles of their own, if they are invested in school, how much risk-taking behavior they engage in, etc. A lot of progress can be undone if a youngster gravitates back toward a problematic peer group, so alternative social venues that enable the child to gain status and recognition through some strength or talent are important aspects of discharge planning.

Nowadays, youngsters can link up in various electronic meeting places on the Internet. Sometimes this serves as a useful source of empathy and support that may be lacking in the nonvirtual world. On the other hand, patients can just as easily find reinforcement for nihilistic and self-destructive impulses, or just morbid self-absorption, which does not help in the struggle to manage psychiatric illness.

Observation in Setting

For all of the value of history taking, unit staff are in a unique position to assess how children tolerate the necessary separation from family, as well as how parents and children interact at visiting time, during on-ground passes, extent of phone contact, etc. The inpatient unit provides a readymade peer group that allows for some assessment of a given child's ability to share, take turns, play, and solve conflicts.

The unique capacity of staff across multiple domains of functioning, from getting up in the morning to going to bed at night, provides a rich tapestry upon which historical data and presenting symptoms are confirmed or refuted. Such observational data helps detangle purely "situational pathology" from inherent dysfunction in the child him/herself. Strengths and weakness observed, as well as the precise context and patterning of behavioral difficulties, form the basis for individualized behavioral therapeutic plans.

However, there is evidence for a "honeymoon" type of phenomenon, where the child looks nearly asymptomatic for a time and then begins to display more difficulties (31). Shorter lengths of stay may permit staff to observe only the period of suppressed behavioral difficulty.

Medical Consultations

When there are reasonable grounds to suspect that nonpsychiatric illnesses or conditions can cause or exacerbate the presenting problems, speedy consultation is paramount. To ascribe physical complaints to "somatization" may be an apt characterization at times, but the inpatient clinician should be especially alert to the psychiatric sequelae of disease. When a youngster with a history of anxiety and worry complains about joint pain or abdominal pain, he or she is no more immune to borreliosis, celiac disease or asthma than anyone else is. For better or worse, the medicolegal liability exposure for hospital services is exceptionally high, leading clinicians to err in the direction of caution in evaluating such possibilities. Occasionally, treatments for medical conditions can also be contributory, as with, for example, severely asthmatic children treated with high corticosteroid doses, and consultation from the appropriate specialist can identify such issues and manage the shift to alternative treatment.

Inpatient units colocated in general medical settings usually have no difficulty obtaining timely consultations. When consultants have to come from further afield or the patient needs to be transported to a medical facility for examination, logistical problems can interfere. It behooves such settings to establish policies that stipulate the acceptable window for accomplishing consultation that takes urgency into account, since that will be an important aspect of quality assurance auditing.

Laboratory Tests

Nearly all facilities have a panel of standard laboratory tests to obtain at admission, including complete blood counts (CBCs), routine blood chemistry, and tests of liver and thyroid function. Blood levels of measurable psychotropic medications as soon as possible upon presentation are essential, particularly when the behavior that occasions the admission is a departure from more typical functioning. High levels may raise the specter of behavioral toxicity, while unexpectedly low levels may suggest poor adherence that might restrain the impulse to jettison an agent for apparent lack of efficacy. Newly started medicines may also affect the bioavailability of other therapeutic drugs, and our understanding of potential metabolic interactions is incomplete. Pregnancy tests are often routine among female patients of child-bearing potential, regardless of the stated means of contraception, given the teratogenic potential of many current therapies.

Among adolescents, toxicological analysis of urine for substances of abuse is often a routine element of admission labs. While not infallible, they may help the youth to own up to clandestine drug use that can enable appropriate treatment.

Electroencephalography was at one time routine, but in more cost-conscious times its low yield in childhood psychiatric illness has largely shelved it. In rare instances it may be useful, such as with decline in language skills in a very young child that can conjure the possibility of PDD, but acquired epileptiform aphasia (Landau-Kleffner syndrome) may be part of the differential, even without obvious seizures. Likewise, brain imaging presently has no demonstrated diagnostic utility, and its use to aid in ruling out alternative etiology in psychosis (tumor, hemorrhage, lesion, etc.) is now less common and felt to be most indicated among children with acute onset, neurological symptoms, catatonia, or poor response to antipsychotics.

PROGRAMMING

Most of the therapeutic modalities that milieu settings incorporate receive detailed treatments elsewhere in this volume. Therefore, our discussion emphasizes special issues concerning their implementation on inpatient, day, and residential services.

General Principles

Special Factors in Milieu Settings

One of the risks of congregate care for youth with psychiatric disorders is that they may not bring out the best in each other, and instead may mutually reinforce self-defeating or antisocial conduct (32). Young children, for the most part, are still motivated more by adult approval and esteem than by that of their peers. By adolescence, though, this preference largely inverts, even in nonclinical groups, and those who challenge the adult-established order provide their peers with vicarious pleasure and may enjoy high status. Psychiatrically involved youngsters can rightly claim they have been allocated more than their fair share of misfortune, and it is well known that misery loves miserable company. However, little good comes when resentment leads to generalized rejection of available treatment and help. An important goal for any milieu setting is to create and sustain a "culture" that recognizes and values progress toward therapeutic goals, while dimming the allure of defeatism that often masquerades as rebellious grandstanding.

Another key milieu feature that requires vigilance concerns the treatment of more vulnerable patients, especially those with cognitive disabilities, odd behavior, or other stigmata, who are incapable of sticking up for themselves. Peer harassment of these individuals may well fall under old-fashioned meanness, but for some youth this inappropriate behavior may serve to counteract their anxieties about how much they may really have in common with such highly impaired individuals that they end up in the same setting.

Multidisciplinary Therapeutic Components

Most settings incorporate a fairly standard menu of therapeutic modalities, including individual, group, family, vocational, behavioral, milieu, rehabilitation/activities, and art therapies in addition to school, medications and specialized services for those with substance abuse or other cooccurring problems.

Specific disciplines often are associated with specific treatments. It is human nature to have personal views about the relative value of each of these from the perspective of one's specialty and training. Those with such prejudices usually have the social skills not to proclaim them outright, but there are more subtle ways in which one may give offense to the efforts of colleagues and thereby degrade the camaraderie on which the service depends. For instance, taking a patient out of another therapeutic activity for individual therapy is not only disruptive to the child, but implicitly devalues the work of a colleague. Ideally, there should be a consistent policy about when such interruptions are appropriate. When scheduling makes such conflict unavoidable, the other staff member should be alerted ahead of time. In staff meetings, everyone has an implicit theory about why a child is or is not getting better, and it is wise to recognize such perspectives. The child psychiatrist may correlate improvement with a medication change, for instance, while another therapist may emphasize a particular development in family therapy. Good leaders try to educate without being dismissive of other perspectives, and take into account reasonable attributions besides one's own.

Maintaining Social Development in an Atypical Environment

Treatment settings that segregate youth from usual community and home-living experiences for extended periods also pose a risk of institutionalization. Most facilities' programming therefore includes community trips and other off-campus activities. In fact, many RTCs provide greater opportunities for athletic and cultural enrichment (pools, gymnasia, art studios, music lessons) with skillful supervision than would otherwise be available to many youth in their homes. A careful balance has to be struck between appropriate supervision and allowing a youngster to develop age-typical skills, such as going to the store, traveling independently, and making choices about leisure time, purchases, etc. Often, excursions and other related activities are considered privileges that have to be earned, but a case can be made that at least some exposure should be contingent only on the current behavioral control to manage the outing successfully.

Inpatient

Psychiatric Care

Medications. The time pressures on acute inpatient care often do not allow adequate trials of medication that may have a long latency to determine response. On the other hand, the close observation these settings afford does permit faster titration than is typical in outpatient care. The combined effect is that many children admitted to inpatient care accrue several medications during their stay, layered in efforts to achieve stability as soon as possible and possibly at higher doses than necessary.

Another quandary for the hospital setting arises when children are relatively asymptomatic after admission, depriving the clinician of obvious target symptoms. This may be a short-term "honeymoon" phenomenon, but may nowadays encompass the whole authorized length of stay. In this case, there is a strong temptation to relate the child's difficulties to situational factors outside the hospital, and this is always appropriate to consider in therapy, but it does not diminish the significance of real psychopathology that warrants pharmacotherapy. In some instances, collaboration with the outpatient provider may lead to a decision to undertake a new treatment and monitor its tolerability so that the trial is well underway by the time the child returns for outpatient care.

Psychiatric inpatient units, particularly for children and adolescents, tend to be closed-staff units, where the attending psychiatrists are full-time hospital employees, in marked contrast to the rest of medicine, where community-based physicians have admitting privileges and continue to treat their patients while in hospital as the attendings of record. The rationale for a child's preadmission regimen is therefore often unclear to hospital attendings or house staff, or hospital clinicians may disagree with its appropriateness and even the outpatient prescribers' diagnoses as well. Inpatient clinicians may conclude that treatments they initiated are helping, but this is inevitably confounded with some degree of remission that the hospitalization itself may occasion (31). Trials often start with the anticipation that outpatient providers will continue monitoring or titration, but the aftercare provider often has only increasingly perfunctory discharge summaries to explain things, and even these are commonly not yet available by the time the patient is seen after discharge. One consequence is that when things do not go well right after discharge, the outpatient clinician changes treatment yet again according to his or her predilections. The potential impact of these organizational issues on quality of care seems like an important area warranting further study. But in the meantime, communication and collegiality with preadmission and postdischarge providers seem the best remedies.

Settings that operate in the context of longer lengths of stay can take a more methodical approach to disentangling the complex medication regimens of children admitted to these services. To do so, some means to quantify response in relation to treatment is highly advisable. Validated rating scales completed on a weekly basis, or even brief versions done daily, can be completed by nursing staff or others involved with the patient and scored for presentation alongside information about concurrent treatment. This approach may incur a large initial investment in computer programming and data management resources, as well as staff time to complete these items, but scannable forms can reduce the data entry burden. The investment, though, seems justified relative to the alternatives. Many of these patients experience only modest responses to treatment. Memory or plowing through weeks or months of medical record narratives alone are fallible sources for guidance on which of several attempted treatments and dosages yielded the most, if suboptimal, improvement.

Behavioral-Social Engineering to Achieve Individual Therapeutic Goals. As we discussed earlier, the high environmental control of an inpatient setting confers an almost unique ability to implement individualized behavior therapy plans. Since most often there is already a general unit-wide behavior therapy program whose implementation may be hard enough to maintain consistently, individualized plans should be used sparingly. Many individualized goals can be incorporated into unit-wide systems, as discussed later. Common individualized plans may involve exposure and response prevention for severe obsessive-compulsive disorder, a toileting plan for encopresis, special mealtime and postprandial supervision for those with eating disorders, habit reversal training or overcorrection for certain tics or stereotypies, adherence to diabetic or other medical regimens, desensitization for difficulties swallowing pills or tolerating phlebotomy, or inappropriate or harmful sexual behavior, to name a few. Youngsters with major developmental handicaps often need modifications to the more general system owing both to the idiosyncrasies of the problem behaviors and the need to make antecedent prompts and consequences available more quickly and more salient. Careful assessment following the principles of functional behavioral assessment (33) is imperative.

One of the major challenges in these plans is maintaining staff consistency, both between individuals and over time. Round-the-clock settings pose the added complication that each shift may tend to drift toward its own possibly idiosyncratic implementation when it has limited contact with the staff most involved in training and development. It is vital that those who coordinate the overall milieu program periodically spend time on, say, evening or night shifts, to acquaint themselves better with programmatic issues that these times of day entail, as well as guidance to staff on implementation.

Inpatient services can also utilize behavioral techniques to leverage changes in certain out-of-hospital difficulties. For instance, school refusal that has been refractory to outpatient treatment can be addressed by graduated exposure on passes, sometimes with the therapist in attendance to provide coaching and support. In some instances, hospital staff may bring the child unaccompanied by parents to dissociate somewhat school-related stimuli with separation anxiety when the latter seems to be the main problem.

Individual and Family Therapies. These modalities can profit from the therapist's ability to help the patient learn from daily experiences with the benefit of a more objective report of incidents that seemed to trigger the child's upsets than the child is likely to provide. This is particularly useful for cognitive approaches that can help the youngster reconsider incidents where a fairly benign event was construed as a major provocation.

Shorter stays have increased the prominence of family-oriented treatment, both to address the typical problems pertaining to relationships and parenting practices, and to plan ahead for discharge. Whereas acute units usually featured weekly sessions, and long-term settings rather less often, the frequency of these meetings may need to increase although the staffing complement is no greater.

Milieu Management

Policies and Staff Training. Nearly all regulatory and accrediting authorities mandate that inpatient services have a written procedures and policies manual. In addition, it is very useful to have a written description for parents that orients them to the unit and its procedures. A separate version for patients will usually depict, as appropriate to age, the rules for the unit.

Service-Wide Behavioral Programs. Milieu-based therapeutic programs based on behavior modification principles are nearly ubiquitous, and go by various names, such as level, point, token economy, or behavioral systems, and we mentioned some of their underlying principles earlier. These types of programs can serve at least three purposes. First, as a means of direct therapy they can be a rather efficient means of promoting target behaviors that are applicable to a large number of patients and that can readily incorporate some individualized behavioral goals as well.

Second, they can help provide the unit with structure, through establishment of basic for rules to aid in the management of the service. Therefore, not only may such programs benefit a child's own difficult behavior, they also offer a form of "governance" that includes consistency and fairness. Many patients, especially younger ones, need to better restrain retaliatory impulses following provocations by peers. This goal is easier when the child can count on other ways to address grievances, including consequences for the other child's misbehavior.

Third, these procedures have the potential to provide quantitative information on the nature and extent of patients' problems, their progress while in the hospital, and their response (or lack thereof) to different treatments. These data can supplement other types of clinical information, and at times they serve to correct overly broad and exaggerated reports based on global narratives, such as when one recent difficult day obscures the improvements evident on those that preceded it.

As with any good behavioral therapy program, the consistency of feedback is paramount, especially praise and recognition, which should be abundant but sincere. This would in many cases accompany assignment of points or tokens for achieving the positive behavioral goals of the activity or time of day, which is well defined. In addition, each patient has up to three or so individualized goals for which he or she obtains praise, encouragement, or corrections, as well as points earned. The actual privileges or rewards toward which points accrue can involve some that are earned daily (video game time) and some based on accumulation over several days (privilege level). The former enable the patient to begin each day with a new start and to benefit accordingly.

Overall "generic" programs of this sort may require further individualization or tailoring for the developmental or cognitive needs of patients. Modifications might include reducing exposure to triggers of upset or behavioral dyscontrol, having expectations more commensurate with current capabilities, prompts and consequences that are more tangible/visual/frequent and that are individually meaningful. Ideally, each milieu-based behavioral plan would, of course, be individualized and informed by thorough functional assessment of the problem behaviors that takes account of antecedents, consequences, and the context of these difficulties. On the other hand, it is extremely difficult to maintain consistency with a large number of staff attempting to implement even one plan, and many permutations may vitiate the whole endeavor further. With short lengths of stay, the effort is perhaps better directed toward helping families to develop behavioral support strategies most appropriate for their particular situations and working to promote generalization from hospital to community. Nonetheless, the overall point is that the rigidity of an exclusive one-size-fits-all approach and the infeasibility and possible inconsistencies in highly idiographic programming can each have detrimental extremes.

Education, Rehabilitation, and Life Skills Development

Different acute care units implement diverse arrangements for meeting the educational needs of patients. These can range from teachers coming to the unit for a few hours and giving assignments and instruction in a multipurpose area, to classrooms situated within the unit or elsewhere in the facility where children spend in essence a full school day. The more the hospital schooling arrangement resembles its community counterpart, though, the more reasonable the extrapolations one can make about a youngster's functioning in that critical setting. Teachers are these days only rarely employed by the facility itself, and more often for a public educational jurisdiction whose special education branch is responsible for the schooling of hospital inpatients. Despite administrative independence, coordination with clinical/hospital staff is typically smooth and collegiality high. One has to be mindful, though, of how programmatic, clinical, and administrative decisions affect school personnel, and vice-versa (such as budgetary constraints, personnel changes, placement determinations, and so forth, over which clinical staff do not generally have direct-line authority). Teachers provide an extremely valuable source of information about patients' functioning and clinical progress, and their participation in clinical meetings, and even in on-unit community meetings with patients, is worth any scheduling or other accommodation to enable it. Short-term units will often want to have some mechanism for supplying materials and assignments from the child's home school for teachers to work from so that the patient stays current; this is most significant for patients in the middle grades not in special education settings.

Other program components, for recreation and socialization, are typically led by staff aligned with the facility's rehabilitation, child life, activities therapy, or other similar department whose title varies by institution and custom. Personnel are often occupational therapists and from other related disciplines. In the best of situations, patients can have some choice about which of a few concurrent activities to participate in. This helps keep the group sizes more manageable, and enables more meaningful interaction. Off-unit and off-grounds trips can be important experiences and a corrective to institutionalizing effects of longer term services. Staff may consider involvement in these outings privileges to be earned, a point with some merit, but some exposure is a developmental necessity and might be considered for all but the most dysfunctional of patients who could not handle it.

Partial Hospitalization and Day Treatment

Psychiatric Care

Medications. In many respects, this is the ideal setting to optimize pharmacological treatment. It blends the observation and close monitoring that involvement in the program affords with the ecological validity of feedback from family and nonprogram social venues. Longer lengths of stay in day treatment in a noncrisis context also permit less frenzied efforts to evaluate and optimize medication treatment than acute inpatient stays allow.

Many patients in these settings will take at least part of their medications at home, and the youngster's behavior may often pose questions about adherence much more quickly and tangibly than in outpatient practice. Adherence problems may arise from principled ambivalence or opposition, on the part of the child or family, or from disorganization and forgetfulness. When the prospects for fixing the latter are faint, one can modify the regimen so that most or all of treatment is given in the program itself.

Behavioral-Social Engineering to Achieve Individual Therapeutic Goals. Many of the same principles of inpatient settings apply, but one also has the opportunity to emphasize functioning at home in the development, promotion, and monitoring of behavioral goals. Reports from home can be instrumental in this regard, and give parents some leverage in their efforts to promote behavioral change. Recognizing that many youth will have ongoing exposure to adverse conditions at home for which they need support in coping, it is also appropriate to cultivate skills in communicating and focus on prosocial adaptation to these problems. Self-expression and active participation in program components are the alternatives to withdrawal and preoccupation that these treatment settings can promote. Likewise, supportive and constructive words to peers are also behaviors that the milieu program can cultivate.

Education, Rehabilitation, and Life Skills Development

Time in academic activities will constitute the majority of the day for most programs. It is often reasonable for the overall clinical program to play a direct role in helping to address difficulties around the completion of homework and other assignments. For many patients, it may be useful to help youth become involved in activities, organization, jobs, volunteer work, sports, etc. outside of the program, and incentivize such participation accordingly.

Milieu Management

Many of the same principles of inpatient settings apply, but one also has the opportunity to emphasize functioning at home in the development, promotion and monitoring of behavioral goals. By the same token, the more open day program settings require even greater vigilance to issues around contraband and substance use on or off campus. The potential for off-campus harassment between peers is relatively uncommon, perhaps a result of the wider geographic range of patients' residences, but nonetheless rules and consequences to address it should be in place.

Residential Treatment

Much of the prior discussion of inpatient and day treatment settings has relevance to residential treatment centers. We will focus on a few areas of particular importance to child and adolescent psychiatrists' participation in the clinical team of these facilities.

First, settings differ in how the child psychiatrist is integrated into the treatment team. Most common is a consultative model, where the psychiatrist may care for a rather large number of patients and sits on many different treatment teams. In some instances, the psychiatrist is quite literally a consultant whom the facility engages part time and whose main professional obligations may be elsewhere. While not exactly at arm's length, this arrangement commonly does not enable the steady stream of *in situ* observation as hospital-based services and can resemble outpatient practice, but with a higher overall level of complexity. Seeing the patient individually and learning about his or her clinical status in staff meetings may be adequate in many situations. But just as outpatient practice usually entails seeing parents and children in one another's company, a lot may be learned by joining cottage meetings with staff and youngsters together. Ideally, such time will be incorporated into consultation agreements when appropriate.

Many youth in residential treatment do not necessarily have the severity of psychiatric illness that compels round-the-clock care. More moderate psychiatric problems otherwise manageable in community settings often come to require out-of-home treatment because of the absence or dysfunction of suitable caregivers. Common hardships that contribute to these situations include parental substance abuse, incarceration, and psychiatric and physical illness; the latter not infrequently involves diseases with bleak prognoses, and, at least until recently, parents with AIDS. Abuse and neglect are especially prevalent (34, 35). Extended family and foster care may have already proved unsuccessful for reasons not always attributable solely to the child's intrinsic psychopathology. Helping children to cope with these adversities in a supportive, consistent environment is pivotal. Components of a child's pharmacotherapy regimen may prove to be but temporizing measures that permit other interventions to gain traction and facilitate children's attainment of a sense of security, competence and control and optimism over one's destiny, rather than essential to the long-term treatment of a chronic mental illness (36).

Similarly, the extent and the quality of family involvement and visiting can be highly variable. One might anticipate waxing and waning of behavioral dysfunction, or at least of interest in academic and other pursuits, accordingly. Visiting times and holidays when children are apt to have overnight trips home can be especially difficult and lonely for those who lack consistent adults in their lives and special attention and programming at these times to compensate is commonplace and important. Relatedly, discharge planning is another potentially difficult issue, and ambivalence about leaving and uncertainty about what lies ahead may at times ignite a resurgence of mood and conduct difficulties.

That said, there are numerous specialized forms of residential treatment besides the more general case. Facilities devoted to treatment of substance abuse problems, eating disorders, and subdelinquent conduct problems, to name but a few, all entail specific variations on treatment philosophy, approach, and the extent of psychiatrists' involvement. Facilities operated or licensed by the juvenile corrections or rehabilitation authorities constitute yet another rather different category of setting that seek psychiatric input.

ADMINISTRATION

Team Building

It is not unusual among nontraining inpatient units that the unit chief/unit manager is not a psychiatrist. The rationale for this is often economic, allowing the psychiatrist to focus exclusively on the tasks that doctors must do. Regardless of discipline, the individual in charge of the unit must take the lead in galvanizing team members to work in a cohesive and coordinated way, all focused on that goal of stabilizing the patients' presenting problems, such that the transition to a lower level of care is effected as rapidly as possible.

Team members' efforts, competence, and rule adherence are susceptible to 1) external motivating factors and 2) internal factors that derive from one's personal identification to the organization, its mission, and internalization of its mores (37). High commitment to one's work role seems to derive more from the latter, and may have particular relevance for health-care workers (38). The leadership factors that cultivate such personal identification include demonstrated recognition of an individual's value to the organization, fairness in decisionmaking, providing autonomy that legitimates a favorable view of their competence, and an environment that supports morale to unify the group around a common mission (39, 40).

However, we noted early on that hospitals are complex organizations. Although the unit's leadership may direct the orchestra, many aspects of one's performance are determined by the leader of the relevant "section," or in this case the administrators of an employee's professional discipline (nursing, social work, rehab, psychology). So, when local interventions to address a performance problem are inadequate, the head of the discipline of the employee may become involved. The input of the personnel specialist of the institution's human resources department is often needed to ensure adherence to institutional and legal guidelines in these unpleasant situations.

Relevant formal administrative training may be obtained at the university levels through masters programs in business administration, public administration, or healthcare administration. The American Psychiatric Association conducts an examination in administrative psychiatry each year, coinciding with its annual meetings. While this certification process has not quite reached the same standing as subspecialty board qualifications, it is a useful mechanism to ensure reading across a broad range of administrative issues, such as organizational theory and function, management practices, finance, laws, and ethics.

Financial Issues and Clinicians

Utilization management refers to a set of techniques used by purchasers of healthcare benefits to manage costs by influencing patient care decisionmaking through case-by-case assessment of the appropriateness of care prior to and during its provision. Case review is mostly done by telephone. Prior review/authorization is usually required to enable payment for inpatient care. Typically a multiaxial DSM IV diagnosis must be provided, as well as past history of present or other relevant conditions. The goals of treatment, anticipated length of treatment, mechanisms used to measure patient's progress, services to be used to achieve treatment goals, risk assessment—including suicidality and homicidal potential, medication complications, initial discharge plan, current global assessment of functioning and current mental status, and other physiological/laboratory assessments if available—must also be communicated clearly and succinctly to the reviewer.

Concurrent review during hospitalization requires a recounting of the current treatment progression and that patient's response so far. The reason for the necessity for continued hospital treatment, the next step in treatment planning, as well as the steps taken to implement the past hospital care plan must all be clearly addressed (41).

Quality Assurance

Quality management may be said to have its origins in Deming's pioneering work in General Electric and in revolutionizing the quality of Japanese products after World War II. Their main concepts persist in the "plan, do, check, act" (PDCA) cycle commonly employed in hospitals to correct a problem. At the present time several national patient safety goals are promulgated by the Joint Commission on Accreditation of Hospital Organizations, such as forbidding the writing of certain prescription formats to reduce medication errors. Reducing medication errors is the goal for mandating that patients wear identification bracelets at all times, and that the nurse administering the medication always use two forms of identification (name and date of birth, name and photograph for younger children or those with severe language impairment) before giving medicine. Computerized order entry by the physician also lowers the risk of errors engendered by the well-known problem of doctors' illegible writing!

Projects to reduce the number of restraints and seclusions are commonplace in psychiatric units, and may involve constant retraining of staff in deescalation techniques, monitoring noneffective decisions, and making proactive use of prn medications as well as iteratively adjusting standing pharmacologic agents (42–45).

CONCLUSION

Designed for those burdened with more severe illness or psychosocial circumstances suboptimally equipped to meet their needs, milieu settings seem destined to be with us for some time. Developing community-based services that can provide equivalent levels of safety and treatment remains a worthy goal, but it is likely that the milieu settings considered in this chapter will still be a major conduit for access to these alternatives.

The structure and the form of milieu-based treatments in child and adolescent psychiatry have shown remarkable changes in recent decades. Psychiatry has, arguably, perhaps been more reactive to the social and economic pressures that gave rise to these changes than proactive in addressing the concerns that motivated them. One lesson is that complacency with comfortable procedures and institutions risks unpreparedness when demands come along either to update the model or to justify its continuance. Consequently, our field's newfound attunement to outcomes, to the quality of the science that underlies what we do, and the value for money our efforts yield are critical to the evolution of these settings. The coming years will show whether we have the rigor and vision to innovate and enhance still further the quality of the children's inpatient, residential and other hospital-based day treatments that constitute such a formidable responsibility for our discipline.

References

1. Murray DJ: *A History of Western Psychology*, Englewood-Cliffs, NJ, Prentice Hall, 1983.
2. Celsus AC: *De Medicina*. (Spencer WG, trans.) Cambridge, MA, Harvard University Press, 1935 (orig. c. 38AD).
3. *Metropolitan Life Insurance Co. v. Massachusetts*. 471 U.S. Sup Ct 724; 1985.
4. *Parham v. J.R.* 442 U.S. Sup Ct 584; 1979.
5. Wickizer TM, Lessler D: Do treatment restrictions imposed by utilization management increase the likelihood of readmission for psychiatric patients? *Med Care* 36:844–850, 1998.
6. Wickizer TM, Lessler D, Travis KM: Controlling inpatient psychiatric utilization through managed care. *Am J Psychiatry* 153:339–345, 1996.
7. Knitzer J: *Unclaimed Children: The Failure of Public Responsibility to Children and Adolescents in Need of Mental Health Services*. Washington, DC, Children's Defense Fund, 1982.
8. Stroul BA, Friedman RM: *A System of Care for Severely Emotionally Disturbed Children and Youth*. Washington, DC, CASSP Technical Assistance Center, Georgetown University Child Development Center, 1986.
9. Bickman L, Guthrie PR, Foster EM, et al.: *Evaluating Managed Mental Health Services: The Fort Bragg Experiment*. New York: Plenum; 1995.
10. Blader JC, Carlson GA: Trends in U.S. psychiatric inpatient admissions of children and adolescents. Paper presented at: 53rd Annual Meeting of the American Academy of Child and Adolescent Psychiatry, 2006, San Diego, CA.
11. Barker P: *The Residential Psychiatric Treatment of Children*. London: Crosby, Lockwood, & Staples; 1974
12. Hughes JM: *Reshaping the Psychoanalytic Domain: The Work of Melanie Klein, W.R.D. Fairbairn, and D.W. Winnicott*, Berkeley, CA; University of California Press, 1989.
13. Saxe E, Lyle J: The function of the psychiatric residential school. *Bull Menninger Clin* 4:163–171, 1940.
14. Winnicott DW: The theory of the parent–infant relationship. In: Buckley P (ed): *Essential Papers on Object Relations*. New York: New York University Press; 1986: pp. 233–253.
15. Azrin NH: A strategy for applied research: Learning based but outcome oriented. *Am Psychol* 32:140–149, 1977.
16. Lovaas OI, Schreibman L, Koegel RL: A behavior modification approach to the treatment of autistic children. *J Autism Child Schizophr* 4:111–129, 1974.

17. Bellack AS, Hersen M, Turner SM: Generalization effects of social skills training in chronic schizophrenics: An experimental analysis. *Behav Res Ther* 14:391–398, 1976.
18. Hersen M, Bellack AS: A multiple-baseline analysis of social-skills training in chronic schizophrenics. *J Appl Behav Analysis* 9:239–245, 1976.
19. Jones KW: *Taming the Troublesome Child: American Families, Child Guidance, and the Limits of Psychiatric Authority.* Cambridge, MA, Harvard University Press, 1999.
20. National Institute of Mental Health Survey and Reports Branch. *Use of Inpatient Psychiatric Services by Children and Youth under Age 18, United States, 1980* (Statistical note no. 175), Bethesda, MD; U.S. Department of Health and Human Services, April 1986.
21. Blader JC: Pharmacotherapy and postdischarge outcomes of child inpatients admitted for aggressive behavior. *J Clin Psychopharmacol* 26:419–425, 2006.
22. Martin A, Leslie D: Psychiatric inpatient, outpatient, and medication utilization and costs among privately insured youths, 1997–2000. *Am J Psychiatry* 160:757–764, 2003.
23. Connor DF, Ozbayrak KR, Kusiak KA, et al.: Combined pharmacotherapy in children and adolescents in a residential treatment center. *J Am Acad Child Adolesc Psychiatry* 36:248–254, 1997.
24. Chamberlain P: The Oregon Multidimensional Treatment Foster Care model: Features, outcomes, and progress in dissemination. *Cognitive and Behavioral Practice* 10:303–312, 2003.
25. Halliday-Boykins CA, Henggeler SW, Rowland MD, et al.: Heterogeneity in youth symptom trajectories following psychiatric crisis: Predictors and placement outcomes. *J Consult Clin Psychol* 72:993–1003, 2004.
26. Snyder HN, Sickmund M: *Juvenile Offenders and Victims: 2006 National Report.* Washington, DC, U.S. Department of Justice, Office of Juvenile Justice and Delinquency Prevention, 2006.
27. Teplin LA, Abram KM, McClelland GM, et al. Psychiatric disorders in youth in juvenile detention. *Arch Gen Psychiatry* 59:1133–1143, 2002.
28. Kiser LJ, Heston JD, Paavola M: Day treatment centers/partial hospitalization settings. In: Petti TA, Salguero C (eds): *Community Child and Adolescent Psychiatry: A Manual of Clinical Practice and Consultation.* Washington, DC, American Psychiatric Publishing, 2006: pp. 189–203.
29. Blader JC: Which family factors predict externalizing behavior among children discharged from inpatient psychiatric treatment? *J Child Psychol Psychiatry* 47:1133–1142, 2006.
30. Blader J: Symptom, family, and service predictors of children's psychiatric rehospitalization within one year of discharge. *J Am Acad Child Adolesc Psychiatry* 43:440–451, 2004.
31. Blader JC, Abikoff H, Foley C, et al.: Children's behavioral adaptation early in psychiatric hospitalization. *J Child Psychol Psychiatry* 35:709–721, 1994.
32. Dishion TJ, Dodge KA: Peer contagion in interventions for children and adolescents: Moving towards an understanding of the ecology and dynamics of change. *J Abnorm Child Psychol* 33:395–400, 2005.
33. O'Neill RE, Horner RH, Albin RW, et al.: *Functional Assessment and Program Development for Problem Behavior: A Practical Handbook*, 2nd ed. Pacific Grove, CA; Brooks/Cole Publishing, 1997.
34. Rosen M: Treating child welfare children in residential settings. *Child Youth Serv Rev* 21:657–676, 1999.
35. Kisiel CL, Lyons JS: Dissociation as a mediator of psychopathology among sexually abused children and adolescents. *Am J Psychiatry* 158:1034–1039, 2001.
36. Connor DF, McLaughlin TJ: A naturalistic study of medication reduction in a residential treatment setting. *J Child Adolesc Psychopharmacol* 15:302–310, 2005.
37. Kelman HC: Compliance, identification and internalization. *J Conflict Resolut* 2:51–60, 1958.
38. Franco LM, Bennett S, Kanfer R: Health sector reform and public sector health worker motivation: A conceptual framework. *Soc Sci Med* 54:1255–1266, 2002.
39. Tyler TR, Blader SL: Can businesses effectively regulate employee conduct? The antecedents of rule following in work settings. *Acad Manage J* 48:1143–1158, 2005.
40. Tyler TR, Blader SL: The group engagement model: Procedural justice, social identity, and cooperative behavior. *Pers Soc Psychol Rev* 7:349–361, 2003.
41. American Psychiatric Association Committee on Managed Care: *Utilization Management: A Handbook for Psychiatrists.* Washington, DC; American Psychiatric Publishing, 1992.
42. Donovan A, Plant R, Peller A, et al.: Two-year trends in the use of seclusion and restraint among psychiatrically hospitalized youths. *Psychiatr Serv* 54:987–993, 2003.
43. Richards D, Bee P, Loftus S, et al.: Specialist educational intervention for acute inpatient mental health nursing staff: Service user views and effects on nursing quality *J Adv Nurs* 51:634–644, 2005.
44. Measham TJ: The acute management of aggressive behaviour in hospitalized children and adolescents. *Can J Psychiatry* 32:199–203, 1995.
45. Greene RW, Ablon JS, Martin A: Use of collaborative problem solving to reduce seclusion and restraint in child and adolescent inpatient units. *Psychiatr Serv* 57:610–612, 2006.

CHAPTER 6.3.2 ■ INTENSIVE HOME-BASED FAMILY PRESERVATION APPROACHES, INCLUDING MULTISYSTEMIC THERAPY

MELISA D. ROWLAND, JOSEPH L. WOOLSTON, AND JEAN ADNOPOZ

The origins of intensive home-based family preservation treatments can be traced to services provided by our nation's first social workers in the early 1900s. Gleaning knowledge and experience from volunteers or "friendly visitors" of charitable organizations, these social workers helped impoverished families maintain custody of their children, primarily through the provision of concrete and pragmatic services. Home-based family visits were used to engage families and increase the accuracy of needs assessments. By focusing on the mobilization of help networks and emphasizing the coordination of services, these social workers laid the early foundations for today's home-based services (1).

While child welfare agencies experimented with home-based services, a similar trend was developing to serve families of delinquent youths. Juvenile courts were developed in both Chicago and Boston at the turn of the century to help manage the needs of delinquent children. While some of the court's services involved the suspension of parental rights and placement of children away from their homes, other services were community based and aimed to improve parental supervision. The early youth probation officers providing these services were charged with trying to help the parents maintain the youth in the home and community before recommending placement. Yet, despite the early focus on family preservation in both child welfare and juvenile justice, child protection (removal from the home) and incarceration strategies have dominated the field for most of the twentieth century. Furthermore, the psychoanalytic movement supported this process as it contributed substantially to an individually oriented treatment approach in social work practice and a shift away from recognizing the critically important roles of families and the social context in childhood problems (2).

It wasn't until the 1970s and '80s that the social and political climates, enhanced by new theoretical and treatment models, began to change in ways that supported the development of home-based family-centered treatments for youths with serious clinical problems and their families. Important political proponents of this development included the Department of Health and Human Services Children's Bureau's leadership and financial funding to support program development as well as research and resources for the expansion of family-based services. The Adoption Assistance and Child Welfare Act of 1980 (Public Law 96–272) required that states take reasonable efforts to prevent placement, hence further accelerating the growth of family-preservation programs. The Edna McConnel Clark Foundation became instrumental in promoting one model, the Homebuilders Program; and the Child Welfare League of America helped to establish prevention and reunification as necessary parts of the service continuum (3). These factors, among others, combined with a growing theoretical knowledge base that conceptualized human problems as contextually driven (4, 5) and amenable to intervention (6–8) laid the foundation for the growth of short-term, largely home-based family strengthening programs designed to support family capacity to care for their own children and to reduce the out-of-home placement of children (1).

DEFINITIONS

Unifying Themes

The term "intensive home-based family preservation" actually refers to a variety of treatment services and interventions provided in various formats, often with very different underlying treatment models and implementation strategies. Moreover, several different terms are used in the literature to denote these types of interventions, including family preservation services (the most common), intensive-in-home services, and home-based family therapy. Yet, despite the multiple terminologies, these interventions share a common theme and goal of trying to preserve the home and family. Indeed, several aspects of the underlying model of service delivery and corresponding ideologies generally serve to unify these programs and set them apart from other interventions.

STRUCTURE

The intensive home-based family preservation model of service delivery differs from traditional office-based interventions in several ways. Specifically: Services are provided in the home and community at times convenient for family members, treatment is time limited (1–5 months), therapists have low caseloads (two to six families) and make multiple visits weekly, and team members are available to families around the clock to respond to crises and treatment needs.

THEORETICAL UNDERPINNINGS

The vast majority of services provided within the intensive home-based family preservation model of service delivery base their intervention and implementation strategies on one or several compatible theoretical models of human behavior. These theories include social learning theory (6, 8); structural (9), strategic (5), or problem-focused (10) family therapy; crisis theory; and behavioral theories (11). As a group, intensive home-based family preservation services tend to offer present-focused, family-centered interventions designed to empower the youth's caregiver(s) to provide an appropriately nurturing and structured environment, thus reducing risk of placement.

DIFFERENCES: THREE MODELS

Within the broad category of intensive family preservation services, three relatively distinct practice models have been identified (3, 12).

Crisis Intervention Model

The *crisis intervention model*, exemplified by the Homebuilders approach, was the first family preservation model developed. Based on social learning principles, interventions in this model are very brief (4–6 weeks) and emphasize concrete services (food, clothing) and counseling that targets family communication, behavior management, and problemsolving skills (13).

Home-Based Model

Services provided under the rubric of the *home-based model* tend to be more clinically oriented than crisis models, are often provided by masters' level therapists, and are longer in duration (3–5 months). Interventions in this model frequently target problematic interactions among family members and between family members and the community (14). Clinical procedures are more complex than those in the crisis intervention model and involve a range of family, behavioral, and parent training intervention strategies. Multisystemic therapy (MST) (15) is an example of this type of treatment program.

Family Treatment Model

Although services provided under this model share similar theoretical underpinnings and treatment goals with the two home-based models mentioned, they differ in that concrete services are generally provided by case managers rather than therapists, and therapists generally provide clinical services in the outpatient office. Functional family therapy is an example of this type of intervention (10). Given this chapter's intended focus on the home-based treatment setting, the two types of intensive home-based family preservation that are primarily provided in home and community-based settings, the crisis intervention and home-based models are highlighted.

FAMILY PRESERVATION SERVICES IN CHILD WELFARE

Background

The first home-based family preservation services were provided in the early 1900s to families at risk of losing their children due to poverty and neglect. While these types of services fell by the wayside during the early part of the century, they reemerged in the 1970s, largely due to political concerns for youth in the child welfare system. In response to national unease about the rising numbers of children without permanent placement in foster care, the Adoption Assistance and Child Welfare Act of 1980 (Public Law 96–272) brought new focus and resources to home- and family-based intervention programs. Foundations (e.g., the Edna McConnel Clark Foundation's support of the Homebuilders model) played substantial roles in dissemination of these services (3). Yet, like most psychotherapeutic and psychosocial interventions, dissemination of home-based services preceded evidence of their effectiveness.

Research Findings

Early evaluations of intensive home-based family preservation programs consisted largely of descriptive information and quasiexperimental studies, primarily of the Homebuilders model. Homebuilders is a short-term (30–60 days) crisis intervention model variety of home-based treatment consisting mostly of concrete case management and behavioral interventions provided by bachelors' level child protection workers. While some of the early outcome data concerning these programs seemed promising, closer observation revealed substantial methodological problems in many of the evaluations (selection bias, nonequivalent control groups). As these methodological issues were addressed and more rigorous research was performed, the early positive findings did not hold. Two comprehensive reviews on the effectiveness of intensive home-based family preservation services for children at risk of out of home placement due to abuse or neglect (2, 16) indicate that crisis intervention types of intensive home-based family preservation services have had little impact in averting out-of-home placement. For example, in what is considered to be the most substantial, comprehensive, and methodologically sound evaluation of a family preservation project for child welfare youths to date; (17) researchers of a program in Illinois found that the 995 families that received the crisis intervention family preservation intervention fared no better than the 569 families that received regular services. No significant differences were found between the groups in terms of types and duration of out-of-home placement or subsequent child maltreatment. Three additional large studies (18–20) also considered to be methodologically sound and comprehensive, have found that crisis intervention family preservation services failed to produce statistically significant outcomes. Thus, despite widespread dissemination, crisis intervention family preservation services have not proven to be effective on closer evaluation.

Challenges

A number of factors have been proposed (21) by researchers and policymakers to explain the apparent lack of effectiveness for crisis intervention types of intensive home-based family preservation services for children in the child welfare system. Lindsey, Martin, and Doh (16) have outlined five explanations that summarize current thoughts in this regard. First, intensive home-based services in the child welfare sector have largely relied on casework intervention and, thus, might be founded on intervention models that do not have established effectiveness with youth and families experiencing significant difficulties (22, 23). Second, the intensive home-based family preservation treatment models employed in these studies might not have been flexible and comprehensive enough to meet the complex needs and problems often presented by the families. Third, the programs might not have been capable of addressing the severe psychosocial difficulties associated with the poverty experienced by many of the participating families. Fourth, the interventions might have been too brief as most problems presented by these families were chronic and enduring. And finally, it is notable that most studies did not actually succeed in targeting children truly at risk of placement (17). In summary, a general consensus is developing that suggests that children and families served by the child welfare system have needs that outstrip those provided by intensive home-based family preservation programs that employ the crisis intervention model.

Promising Directions

Rather than serving as a setback, this research provides helpful information that can be used to chart new courses for developing effective home-based interventions for youths in the child welfare system. Project 12-Ways (24) and multisystemic therapy (25) are two examples of intensive family and community-based interventions provided within the home-based model of service delivery that are promising for working with this population. Project 12-Ways is a systemically focused intervention, based on the eco-behavioral model, designed to work with families at risk of having their children placed due to abuse or neglect. The model defines intervention targets across the family's social ecology and implements interventions in the home and social contexts to address these behaviors. Program evaluations indicate that in the short term, families served by Project 12-Ways were less likely to be rereported for child maltreatment or have children removed than comparison families (26, 27). MST is also founded in ecological theory (4) and involves the implementation of empirically validated interventions to youth and family members with attention to the contexts within which they are embedded. An early randomized trial with maltreating families demonstrated that MST was more effective than parent training for improving family interactions (28). Importantly, a recently completed National Institute of Mental Health–funded randomized clinical trial compared MST with parent training plus standard mental health services (29) for adolescents at risk of placement due to physical abuse. Short-term results from this study suggest that MST holds promise for reducing youth out-of-home placement, and symptoms of depression as well as increasing youth perceptions of safety and parental use of nonphysical discipline (30).

MST, and the home-based service model within which it is delivered, differs from the intensive home-based family preservation programs that employ the crisis intervention model in several key ways that address the aforementioned challenges noted by Lindsey et al. (16). First, MST is well grounded conceptually and several randomized clinical trials support its effectiveness with juvenile delinquents and substance-abusing youths at risk of out-of-home placement (31). MST therapists are masters level and receive substantial supervision and ongoing training from doctoral-level clinicians who are trained in evidence-based practice. As adherence to the MST treatment model has been linked with improved youth and family outcomes (32–34), an ongoing quality assurance process (35) is used to support therapist fidelity to the treatment model. Thus, MST involves trained professionals implementing evidence-based practice in an environment that provides ongoing support and evaluation of outcomes.

Also addressing the challenges noted by Lindsey and colleagues (16), MST interventions can flex to meet the complex needs and problems often presented by families in the child welfare system. Interventions are based on the therapist and family's shared understanding of the drivers of the referral problems. Therapists are trained to be generalists who can assess and provide evidence-based interventions to individuals within and across the multiple systems that affect families (36, 37). For example, MST therapists working with families at risk of losing their children due to physical abuse must be able to provide interventions that address individual and family safety, abuse clarification, and psychopathology and substance abuse in the youths and their family members, as well as peer, school, and community difficulties that are contributing to the identified problems. A third concern expressed by Lindsey and colleagues (16) was that the severe psychosocial difficulties and poverty often found in child welfare populations adversely affects attempts to provide family preservation services. While it is certainly true that these factors often serve as barriers to intervention on MST teams, the model promotes therapists doing whatever it takes to help families achieve sustainable outcomes. Thus, MST therapists are encouraged to provide case management as well as treatment interventions when indicated. For example, therapists might help families secure better housing, apply for financial assistance, obtain transportation, enroll in vocational training or any number of interventions as long as they are considered key in promoting clinical goals. This broad view of clinical services is designed to help lessen the impact of poverty and other adverse social circumstances that often surround families who qualify for intensive home-based services.

A fourth limitation regarding the crisis intervention model of intensive home-based family preservation programs is that their short duration of intervention is not sufficient to address the chronic and enduring problems often found in families served by child welfare. To address this issue, MST teams serving child welfare populations have averaged 6 to 8 months of treatment, and research to better understand the length of treatment needed to adequately serve this population is currently underway (38). Finally, to deal with the issue that many youths in the early child welfare studies were not truly at risk of placement, studies of MST for this population have taken great care to involve youths who are already targeted for potential placement, as evidenced by the 29% placement rate for youths in the control condition of the aforementioned randomized MST trial with child welfare youths (29). Hence, MST as modified for physically abused youths in the child welfare system at risk of out-of-home placement serves as an example of one potentially effective home-based method of treating these families. Importantly, key features of MST address some of the critiques of the early family preservation treatment models.

HOME-BASED FAMILY PRESERVATION IN JUVENILE JUSTICE

Background

While innovative programs to separate juveniles from adults in the prison systems of Boston and Chicago at the turn of the last century set a promising tone for the potential of community-based services for delinquents, these rapidly devolved to current practices that largely consist of probation officers monitoring youths for compliance to court orders (2). This individualistic and often family-alienating focus prevailed throughout the 1900s, helping to create a multibillion-dollar juvenile prison industry that currently consists of more than 3,600 facilities estimated to house more than 110,000 juvenile offenders on any given day (39). Far from evidence based, current probationary and incarceration services are available nationwide. In contrast, it is estimated that fewer than 10% of families of youths on probation have access to evidence-based programs in their community, despite a growing national trend to make such services available (40, 41).

Family preservation services for delinquents first gained a foothold alongside similar services for youths in the child welfare programs in the 1970s and '80s. Given the prevalence of intensive home-based family preservation services utilizing the crisis intervention service delivery model at that time, this model also quickly became the most common type of home-based services provided for delinquents. Yet, unlike child welfare, a more intensive family preservation service, utilizing the home-based model of service delivery, emerged in the mid- to late 1980s. From the onset, this service, MST, was based on research findings in the field of child psychopathology and integrated intervention strategies that had emerging empirical support (15). MST has continued to expand its research base through almost 3 decades.

Research Findings

Initial research results of intensive home-based family preservation treatments for youths at risk of placement due to delinquency largely mirror those of similar services for youths in the child welfare system. That is, while initial reports were promising, more empirically sound evaluations showed that short-term crisis intervention models did not prevent out-of-home placement and rearrest for youths in the juvenile justice system (2). On the other hand, research concerning MST has demonstrated this model's substantial success in significantly reducing youth criminal behavior, incarceration, and out-of-home placement (31). Three randomized trials published during the 1990s and involving more than 400 families established the short- and long-term effectiveness of MST in reducing antisocial behavior, arrests, and incarcerations, as well as improvements in family functioning, and decreases in youth substance use (42–45). Moreover, a very long-term followup (46) of one of the projects (42) demonstrated that MST participants had 54% fewer arrests and spent 57% fewer days of confinement in adult detention facilities than their counterparts 14 years after entering the study.

Another important finding for MST involves its replication in community-based settings. MST has been transported into community-based settings as an intervention for juvenile delinquents since the mid-1990s. This has provided an opportunity for independent evaluations of the effectiveness of MST in treating adolescent antisocial behavior. Two of these replications have been published in peer-reviewed journals. The first evaluation was conducted in Norway and included four sites in a trial that randomized delinquent youths to MST or usual services. Results from this study revealed significant short- (6-month) and long-term (2-year) decreases in out-of-home placements and internalizing symptoms and externalizing symptoms for MST youths relative to their counterparts (47, 48). In the United States, Timmons-Mitchell and her colleagues (49) have also provided an independent replication of MST effectiveness with juvenile offenders in community settings. In this randomized study youths in the MST condition evidenced significantly fewer rearrests than their counterparts at 18-month followup. These results provide further support for the capacity of MST to achieve favorable outcomes when implemented in community practice settings.

To summarize, across several trials with violent and chronic juvenile offenders, MST produced 25% to 70% decreases in long-term rates of rearrest, and 47% to 64% decreases in long-term rates of days in out-of-home placements (31). A recent metaanalysis that included most of these studies (50) indicated that the average MST effect size for both arrests and days incarcerated was 55.

Overview of MST for Delinquents: Clinical Components

Originally developed as an alternative to incarceration for serious juvenile offenders, MST is an intensive home- and community-based intervention grounded in social ecological theories of behavior (15). As described previously, MST is delivered utilizing the home-based model of family preservation services. Hence, services are intensive, provided in the home and community to the entire family, and are available 24 hours a day, 7 days a week. Several key aspects of MST, however, differentiate this model from most family preservation services. Importantly, MST therapists are nested within an extensive quality assurance system designed to promote therapist capacity to provide effective interventions and facilitate treatment fidelity. As such, a typical MST team consists of four masters' level therapists, supervised by an experienced, 50% time, preferably doctoral level, mental health professional trained in MST supervision procedures. MST supervisors play an active, integral role in treatment, providing weekly group supervision, field-based assistance, and ongoing promotion of therapist skill development. MST supervisors are, in turn, supported by MST expert consultants. These doctoral level mental health professionals provide weekly team consultation as well as initial and quarterly booster trainings and ongoing assistance with implementation difficulties that can arise.

In terms of the specific work provided, MST therapists typically treat four to six families for 4–5 months, averaging approximately 60 hours of face-to-face contact per family during treatment. Initially, therapists engage with family members and others in the youth's ecology (teachers, peers, neighbors) to determine the drivers of the youth's referral behaviors across school, neighborhood, peer, and family systems. Once the therapist and caregivers have a shared understanding of the factors sustaining the problem behavior, evidence-based interventions are developed targeting these drivers. Therapists draw from a number of intervention techniques including behavioral, cognitive-behavioral, parent management, behavioral family systems, and pharmacological treatments. Interventions may be conducted with or target any number of individuals within and across these systems. For example, if an MST therapist determines that the most proximal driver of a particular youth's delinquent behavior is association with deviant peers and that poor parental monitoring and low youth engagement in school are drivers of this problem, then she would develop interventions based on this information. As such the therapist may work to help caregivers develop an appropriate monitoring plan with age-appropriate rewards and consequences, and be prepared to address barriers that arise in implementing that plan. Common barriers include youth behavioral outbursts, poor social support, parental skill deficits, or parental mental health problems. The therapist might help the parents learn to monitor peers more closely, interface with parents of peers, facilitate prosocial activities, and restrict access to deviant peers. Interventions involving the school might include helping the parent establish a cooperative relationship with the school, assistance in obtaining appropriate testing and placement, and facilitating a behavioral plan to reward appropriate school behavior and punish inappropriate behavior. In turn, should family or individual problems arise that impede therapeutic progress (marital discord or maternal depression) the therapist would endeavor to treat these problems as well with evidence-based interventions such as behavioral marital therapy, cognitive behavioral therapy, or psychiatric consultation for evidence-based pharmacotherapy to treat, for example, maternal depression. In summary, though short term, MST interventions are designed to bring intensive clinical focus and expertise to problems presented by antisocial youths and their families. An extensive quality assurance system built into this model helps to sustain clinical integrity and prevent program drift. Both the intensive focus of evidence-based clinical expertise and the careful monitoring of treatment fidelity are core features underlying MST's success in treating delinquents (35).

Promising Directions

While MST is the leading intensive home-based family preservation treatment for juvenile offenders that utilizes the home-based model of service delivery, two other intensive family preservation treatments that utilize the family treatment model have shown substantial promise in serving this population as well. Both multidimensional treatment foster care (51) (MTFC) and functional family therapy (10) (FFT) have data supporting their effectiveness in diminishing youth problem behavior and preserving community placement for youths with serious behavioral problems (52). While neither of these interventions is, technically speaking, a home-based family preservation program, both would fall under the category of family treatment model programs designed to treat youths at risk of placement due to delinquency.

Youths receiving MTFC are placed with highly trained foster parents as an alternative to residential placement. A treatment team consisting of the foster parents, a full-time case manager, individual and family therapists, and other resource staff provide intensive care over a 6- to 12-month period. MTFC interventions are based on social learning theory and strive to provide a) close supervision, b) fair and consistent limits, c) predictable consequences for rule breaking, d) a supportive relationship with a mentoring adult, and e) reduced exposure to delinquent peers while encouraging prosocial youth relationships. The ultimate goal of MTFC is to transition the youth to the family of origin by the end of treatment (53). One quasiexperimental investigation and two randomized controlled trials (54–56) have demonstrated the effectiveness of this model in decreasing youth delinquency and reducing out-of-home placement.

FFT consists of a behavioral family therapy targeting delinquent youths, their families, and aspects of the ecology that impact outcome. Treatment is provided by a therapist in the office and community, with most families averaging 12 sessions over 3 months. FFT relies on evidence-based interventions such as parent training and communication skill interventions to help families change the behaviors that are sustaining youth delinquency. One randomized controlled trial with juvenile status offenders and two quasiexperimental interventions with serious juvenile offenders have supported the efficacy of this intervention in improving family functioning and reducing delinquency (57).

Common Themes and Next Steps

Themes common to all three of these established treatment models (MST, MTFC, FFT) include a) a foundation in social-ecological and social learning theories, b) a problem-centered pragmatic approach, c) a strength-focused view of caregiver importance in treatment, and d) a quality assurance program designed to establish and help maintain therapist fidelity to the treatment model. These similarities, along with each program's unique way of applying evidence-based practice to empirically proven drivers of delinquency (poor family and school functioning, deviant peers), suggest a formula for success in treating delinquents (53). An important direction for future research focuses on determining the conditions needed to transport effectively these empirically tried interventions into the community to serve real-world populations without losing efficacy.

HOME-BASED FAMILY PRESERVATION IN MENTAL HEALTH

Background

Home- and community-based interventions for youths served by the mental health sector have their origins in the system of care (SOC) movement. This movement began with a seminal publication, entitled *Unclaimed Children* (58), which uncovered substantial inadequacies in our national mental health system's response to the problems encountered by children with serious emotional disturbance and their families. *Unclaimed Children* served as a rallying point for advocates, who ultimately helped to facilitate congressional funding of the Child and Adolescent Service System Program (CASSP), the Comprehensive Community Mental Health Services for Children and Their Families Program, and numerous other federal-, state-, and foundation-led initiatives to tackle mental service system inadequacies (59). These factors, combined with the forces of healthcare reform, rising psychiatric placement rates, and the realization that 50% of the nation's child mental health dollars were being spent on inpatient and residential treatments (60), served as catalysts to promote the development of alternative community-based services for youths with serious mental health problems.

Several important treatment trends or processes developed during this time. One was the dissemination of SOC initiatives into numerous communities. These initiatives were funded by foundation as well as federal dollars and were designed to provide a well organized and comprehensive spectrum of mental health and other necessary services to seriously emotionally disturbed youths and their families (61). As these initiatives emphasized the importance of providing a full spectrum of treatments that centered on caregiver empowerment and family involvement, they helped to promote the development of intensive home-based family preservation services. Another important trend was the introduction of the wraparound services concept. Wraparound is a process used to pull families, agencies, and service providers together to tailor or create services for children with significant needs. Composed of a multiagency team including the wraparound team leader and a family member, the goals of the team are to broker services and clinical treatment. While often confused with the family-based services that might be brokered by the team, wraparound is not, in and of itself, a home-based intervention (62).

Research

Research on the effectiveness of crisis family preservation services to prevent out-of-home placement by youths in the mental health sector has focused on the prevention of psychiatric hospitalization and residential placements. Given the high costs of such placements and lack of empirical data to support their effectiveness, it is surprising how little research has been done in this area. A handful of small studies, published between 1968 and 1982 (63–66), suggested that intensive family-based services had potential in reducing the rates of hospitalization for children and adolescents presenting with serious clinical problems. Likewise, researchers in New York City (67) demonstrated that psychiatric hospitalization can be avoided by providing intensive Homebuilders Crisis Intervention Services for youths not perceived by hospital staff as posing a danger to themselves or others. While these evaluations are informative, they do not directly address the question of the viability of intensive home-based family preservation services to address the clinical and safety needs of youths who qualify for emergent psychiatric hospitalization.

To address this issue, the National Institute on Mental Health (NIMH) funded a randomized clinical trial including 156 families to examine the capacity of home-based MST to serve as an alternative to the emergency psychiatric hospitalization of youths in psychiatric crisis (68, 69). In this study, youths who lived in the catchment area; were 10–17 years of age; had Medicaid or no funding; and were about to be admitted to a university-based hospital due to suicidal, homicidal, at-risk, or psychotic behaviors were randomized at the intake office of the hospital to receive either MST home-based services or psychiatric hospitalization with usual aftercare services. The clinical portion of this trial was conducted between 1995 and 1999, and the specific adaptations made to the MST model are highlighted in the Promising Directions section following. Initial post-treatment (4 months) outcomes were favorable, with youth who received MST demonstrating a 75% reduction in days hospitalized and a 50% reduction in days in other out-of-home placements compared to youths in the hospitalization condition (69). Youths in the MST condition also exhibited significant improvements in externalizing symptoms, family relations, school attendance and higher consumer satisfaction compared to the controls (68). At approximately 1 year posttreatment, MST was significantly more effective at decreasing rates of attempted suicide (70). On the other hand, youths in both treatment conditions generally improved to subclinical ranges on indices of individual psychopathology (youth internalizing and externalizing symptoms) by 12 to 16 months, with no significant differences in final outcome, although the groups reached improved symptoms with significantly different trajectories. Similarly, for functional outcomes such as school- and community-based placements, the gains initially found for MST at 4 months slowly dissipated. By 16 months postreferral, youths in both treatment conditions showed an overall deterioration in time spent living in the community and attending school (71).

These data are important, as they represent the first large well controlled trial of an intensive home-based service used as an alternative to emergency psychiatric hospitalization. The initial 4-month outcome studies (68, 69) provide solid evidence that an intensive well specified and well validated family- and home-based intervention can serve as a safe and clinically effective alternative to emergency psychiatric hospitalization. Importantly, the authors noted that considerable clinical resources were needed to stabilize safely and effectively psychiatric crisis situations; and hospitalization was still needed to ensure the safety of some MST youths, albeit in an altered form and on a less frequent basis. This suggests that psychiatric hospitalization has an important role to play in the continuum of services provided to youths with serious emotional disturbance, and services designed to avert or minimize hospitalization need to be well conceptualized, evidence based, and implemented with fidelity. Long-term functional outcomes for youths in this study were somewhat disappointing, as MST for delinquent youths has a track record for significantly reducing criminal behavior and out-of-home placement as long as 14 years posttreatment (46). Yet, these mental health findings are consistent with the broader literature concerning the longitudinal course for youths with serious emotional and psychiatric symptoms (72–74), which indicates that while measures of individual psychopathology tend to normalize over time, the youths continue to be at high risk for failure to meet critical developmental challenges. Thus, poor academic and job performance, criminal behavior, low financial achievement, high rates of early pregnancy, divorce, substance abuse, and mental health problems are potential outcomes for many of the youths represented in this study. The severity and chronic nature of problems found in this population have impacted the modifications to the MST mental health (MST-MH) model described below.

PROMISING DIRECTIONS

MST

The developers of MST for mental health populations or MST-MH have moved into community-based settings to test the effectiveness of this intervention. A study of MST-MH services in Hawaii of 31 youths randomized to MST or the integrated Hawaiian Continuum of Care yielded results at 6 months that are similar to those found in the hospitalization study: significantly reduced days in placement, externalizing symptoms, and risk-taking behavior. While followup data were not collected, this small study is promising and has provided a clinical venue for the developers to further hone the model adaptations (75). These adaptations are substantial and consist of both administrative and clinical additions (76, 77). Administratively, modifications include the integration of psychiatrists and psychiatric services into the team clinical structure, and the addition of a crisis caseworker to provide crisis intervention and case management assistance for MST therapists. Therapists are required to have a master's degree, and their time with the doctoral level team supervisor is increased both in the office and in the community. Therapist caseload is reduced from a maximum of four families (rather than five), and treatment is often extended from 4–6 to 6–8 months. Clinical modifications include additional training in crisis intervention; supplementary booster trainings and ongoing supervision in contingency management interventions for both youth and adult substance abuse; and additional training in assessment and evidence-based treatment of common psychiatric disorders in both youth and adults, such as attention-deficit hyperactivity disorder, mood, and thought disorders. These adaptations are provided within the context of basic MST; hence the core treatment principles and process for training, supervision, and quality assurance remain intact, but are supplemented by the adaptations.

Importantly, other promising home-based programs are being developed for youths with serious mental health problems. These programs are noteworthy, as each has specified treatment protocols and evaluations are being conducted in real-world settings to test the effectiveness of these interventions for youths with serious emotional problems and their families.

Intensive In-Home Child and Adolescent Psychiatric Service (IICAPS)

The Intensive In-Home Child and Adolescent Psychiatric Service (IICAPS) was developed in 1997 at the Yale Child Study Center as an intensive, psychiatric home-based intervention for children and adolescents with serious emotional and behavioral problems at risk of requiring institutional-based care or unable to be discharged from such care without intensive services (78). The IICAPS model is manualized and uses concepts and findings from developmental psychopathology to understand the multiple determinants that contribute to child and families presenting problems. Interventions are grounded in three broad sets of constructs: developmental psychopathology; psychology of motivation, action and problemsolving; and systems of care philosophy. Concepts from developmental psychopathology further the understanding of the child who is the focus of the IICAPS treatment.

Services are provided using the home-based model of service delivery with a master's-level clinician and bachelors' level mental health counselor providing services to the youth and family in the home and community for approximately 4–6 months. The services provided include assessment, evaluation, treatment, service coordination, and advocacy. Supervision and training are essential components of the IICAPS model. All individuals working in IICAPS complete 15 hours of training. A senior mental health clinician supervises the two-person clinical team weekly and a child and adolescent psychiatrist functions as medical director and coleader of regularly scheduled multidisciplinary rounds.

Fidelity to the IICAPS model (79) is measured by the degree of clinician adherence to the IICAPS tools and structures of treatment. Evidence supporting the continuous and simultaneous use of the engagement, assessment, treatment and quality assurance tools is required for programs to maintain their status as a recognized IICAPS site. IICAPS intervention outcomes are monitored with the help of a Web-based data collection system. This is used to collect both outcome and process measures for each site in the IICAPS network and can be used to evaluate the effectiveness of IICAPS in improving functioning and reducing the need for out-of-home placement. IICAPS services have been replicated in 14 sites within Connecticut, and steps are currently being taken both to develop measures of fidelity to the model and to evaluate its effectiveness.

While IICAPS appears to be a promising practice to maintain children at risk of hospitalization in their homes and communities safely, it has yet to be empirically evaluated. A pilot study with a comparison group is currently underway to begin assessment of the efficacy of IICAPS in impacting the serious mental health symptoms of youth at risk of psychiatric hospitalization and the parenting practices of their caregivers. This research represents an important step in helping to ensure that intensive home-based family preservation treatments maintain high standards to help ensure that the best possible care is provided to youths and families.

The Mental Health Services Program for Youth (MHSPY)

The Mental Health Services Program for Youth (MHSPY) is located in eastern Massachusetts and was established in 1998 to treat children and adolescents with severe and persistent mental health needs who failed usual service care and were at risk of placement. The theory of change underlying MHSPY is based on "continuity of intent theory" and grounded in CASSP principles (80, 81). MHSPY services are designed to provide a highly coordinated, individualized combination of mental health and pediatric care; substance abuse treatment; special education and social services to at-risk youth and their families. This treatment approach involves creation of a care planning team, made up of the family, a MHSPY care manager (a masters'-level clinician who chairs the team), and those providers or informal supports identified by the family as involved in their child's care. These additional provider team members may include: traditional therapists (psychologist or social worker), a child psychiatrist, family therapists (psychologist or social worker), and in-home "family skill builders."

The team engages with the family to define treatment goals and to determine how interventions will be delivered. These interventions may be implemented by the members of the clinical team, or brokered from other service providers. The classic intensive family preservation home-based model of service delivery is partially followed in that care managers carry a low caseload, provide services in the home and community, and are available around the clock. Two differences are that the timeframe is substantially longer (16 months) than the usual 3–6 months typically found in home-based programs, and services are implemented by a number of different providers, some of which are purchased by dollars under control of the case manager, which is more consistent with teams using the crisis intervention model or wraparound services concept.

A formal audit process exists to ensure quality and inform ongoing training and support of clinical staff, as well as evaluation of program implementation and outcomes. All purchased services are supervised and monitored for quality by the MHSPY care manager, who in turn receives weekly supervision and support from a clinical site supervisor (a senior clinician, usually a LICSW), as well as regular access to consultation from a child psychiatrist. All staff participate in monthly training and program development support. Outcome measures consist of data collected at baseline and every 6 months to assess functional outcomes, as well as level of care, service utilization and cost and care experience data. Aggregate analyses based on 6 years of multiwave, longitudinal data from the initial site, as well as replication results from a second site implemented in 2003, show that over 88% of days in the MHSPY program are spent at home and the majority of youths display clinical improvement, including a 45% reduction in risk to self and others. Hospitalization and other placement rates are lowered postenrollment by 55%, primary health maintenance visits are higher compared to similar Medicaid populations, while emergency room usage is lower. Importantly, the program has a 95% retention rate among previously "noncompliant" families. While these findings are encouraging, an important next step will involve further evaluation with a control group. The developers of the model are currently pursuing funds to assist with evaluations (81).

The programs highlighted in this section are important, as they represent emerging treatment approaches for trying to bring empirically validated intensive home-based family preservation services to youths with serious mental health problems and their families. While each of the programs still has substantial work to do toward reaching this goal, early findings are promising. Some of the challenges faced in developing, implementing, and evaluating empirically grounded home-based treatments are outlined below.

Challenges and Next Steps

Clinicians and researchers face a number of barriers in their attempts to validate and disseminate community and home-based interventions for youth presenting serious mental health problems and their families. Many of the challenges result from the unconventional nature and relatively novel approach represented by home-based services in the context of services and systems that have been parceled out and delivered with an individual focus for more than a century. These barriers include difficulties finding funding streams for relatively new and unconventional services, organizational and administrative adjustments needed to support home- rather than office-based therapists (cell phones, overtime, realistic safety training), and lack of prior training for therapists educated in traditional treatment models. Likewise, research of these interventions is difficult to conduct due to the complex nature of both the treatments and the real-world settings in which they are delivered and evaluated. For example, the first step is to develop and specify the treatment protocols. This involves the creation of a treatment manual, training program, and clinical process to facilitate clinical integrity to the model. Likewise, a measure of treatment fidelity must be established and validated. Once treatment is specified, the process of conducting research with heterogeneous samples of children and families presenting multiple problems in complex treatment, service and funding environments can be daunting in terms of methodological, clinical, and systems barriers.

CONCLUSION

Although home-based services for families of youths presenting serious clinical problems in the child maltreatment, juvenile justice, and mental health service systems have just recently become established, there are increasing signs that the use of these interventions will continue to grow. A confluence of factors currently exist that may help to promote the adoption of these interventions. Clinically, there is growing national interest in promoting evidence-based practice; which bodes well for empirically supported home-based interventions that offer alternatives to existing services (prison, foster care, and hospitalization) that have little demonstrated effectiveness. Financially, home-based interventions have the potential to produce substantive cost savings to service systems if they can be targeted at youths who are truly at imminent risk of placement. Ethically, home-based programs are consistent with the SOC movement and appeal to family-strengthening proponents on both sides of the political agenda. Yet it is important that empirically supported home-based services not fall into the same traps that ensnared their predecessors, that is, care must be taken to ensure the treatments provided are safe and effective. Families and youths with serious clinical problems have complex needs that are multiply determined and effective solutions require sophisticated, well implemented, evidence-based strategies. Critically, an infrastructure must exist that provides therapists and supervisors who are well trained and adequately paid, with strong organizational support; and funding streams must facilitate rather than hinder clinical progress. Most important, a quality assurance system must be in place to help ensure that the services provided continue to meet adequately and safely the growing and shifting needs of these complex clinical populations. As we enter the twenty-first century, with continued careful research, empirically supported home-based services may become a much-needed mainstream intervention.

References

1. Woodford MS: Home-based family therapy: Theory and process from "friendly visitors" to multisystemic therapy. *The Family Journal: Counseling and Therapy for Couples and Families* 7:265–269, 1999.
2. Fraser MW, Nelson, KE, Rivard, JC: Effectiveness of family preservation services. *Social Work Research* 21:138–153, 1998.
3. Nelson KE: Family-based services for families and children at risk of out-of-home placement. In: Barth R, Berrick JD, Gilbert N (eds): *Child Welfare Research Review* (vol 1). New York, Columbia University Press, 1994, pp. 83–108.
4. Bronfenbrenner U: *The Ecology of Human Development: Experiments by Design and Nature*. Cambridge, MA: Harvard University Press, 1979.
5. Haley J: *Problem Solving Therapy*. San Francisco: Jossey-Bass, 1976.
6. Bandura A: *Social Learning Theory*. Englewood Cliffs, NJ: Prentice Hall, 1977.
7. Nelson KE, Landsman, MJ: *Alternative Models of Family Preservation: Family-Based Services in Context*. Springfield, IL: Charles C Thomas Publisher, 1992.
8. Patterson GR, Reid, JB: Social interactional processes in the family: The study of the moment by moment family transactions in which human social development is embedded. *Journal of Applied Developmental Psychology* 5:237–262, 1984.
9. Minuchin S: *Families and Family Therapy*. Cambridge, MA: Harvard University Press, 1974.
10. Alexander JF, Parsons, BV: *Functional Family Therapy: Principles and Procedures*. Carmel, CA: Brooks/Cole, 1982.
11. Barth R: Theories guiding home-based intensive family preservation services. In: Whitaker J, Kinney J, Tracy E, Booths C, eds. *Improving Practice Technology for Work with High Risk Families: Lessons Learned from the*

"Homebuilders" Social Work Education Project. Seattle, WA: University of Washington, Center for Social Welfare Research, 6:91–113, 1988.
12. Nelson KE: Family based services for juvenile offenders. *Children and Youth Services Review* 12:193–212, 1990.
13. Kinney J, Haapala D, Booth C, Leavitt S: The homebuilders model. In: Whittaker JK, Kinney J, Tracey EM, Booth C (eds): *Reaching High-Risk Families: Intensive Family Preservation in Human Services*. New York, Aldine, 1990, pp. 31–64.
14. Lloyd JC, Bryce ME: *Placement Prevention and Family Reunification: A Handbook for the Family-centered Service Practitioner*. Iowa City, IA: University of Iowa, National Resource Center for Family Based Services, 1984.
15. Henggeler SW, Schoenwald SK, Borduin CM, Rowland MD, Cunningham PB: *Multisystemic Treatment of Antisocial Behavior in Children and Adolescents*. New York, Guilford Press, 1998.
16. Lindsey D, Martin S, Doh J: The failure of intensive casework services to reduce foster care placements: An examination of family preservation studies. *Children and Youth Services Review* 24:743–775, 2002.
17. Schuerman JR, Rzepnicki TL, Littell JH: *Putting Families First: An Experiment in Family Preservation*. Hawthorne, NY, Aldine De Gruyter, 1994.
18. Feldman L: *Evaluating the Impact of Family Preservation Services in New Jersey*. Trenton, NJ: Bureau of Research, Evaluation, and Quality Assurance, New Jersey Division of Youth and Family Services, 1990.
19. Meezan W, McCroskey J: Improving family functioning through family preservation services: Results of the Los Angeles experiment. *Family Preservation Journal* 1:9–29, 1996.
20. Yuan YT: *Evaluation of AB 1562 In-Home Care Demonstration Projects* (vols 1–2) Sacramento, CA, Walter R. MacDonald and Associates, 1990.
21. Swenson CC, Henggeler SW, Schoenwald SK: Family-based treatments. In: Hollin CR (ed): *The Essential Handbook of Offender Assessment and Treatment*. London, John Wiley & Sons Ltd., pp. 79–94, 2004.
22. Fischer J: Is casework effective: A review? *Soc Work* 18:5–20, 1973.
23. Sheldon B: Social work effectiveness experiments: Review and implications. *British Journal of Social Work* 16:223–242, 1986.
24. Lutzker JR, Frame JR, Rice JM: Project 12-Ways: An ecobehavioral approach to the treatment and prevention of child abuse and neglect. *Education and Treatment of Children* 5:141–155, 1982.
25. Swenson CC, Chaffin M: Beyond psychotherapy: Treating abused children by changing their social ecology. *Aggression and Violent Behavior* 11:120–137, 2006.
26. Lutzker JR, Rice JM: Using recidivism data to evaluate Project 12-Ways: An ecobehavioral approach to the treatment and prevention of child abuse and neglect. *Journal of Family Violence* 2:283–289, 1987.
27. Wesch D, Lutzker JR: A comprehensive 5-year evaluation of Project 12-Ways: An ecobehavioral program for treating and preventing child abuse and neglect. *Journal of Family Violence* 6:17–35, 1991.
28. Brunk M, Henggeler SW, Whelan JP: A comparison of multisystemic therapy and parent training in the brief treatment of child abuse and neglect. *J Consult Clin Psychol* 55:311–318, 1987.
29. Saldana L, Swenson CC, Ward D: The cost of treating youth and families traumatized by child physical abuse: Comparison of services outcomes for two evidence based practices and implications for dissemination. Toronto, Canada: 21st Annual Meeting—Transforming Lives Through Transforming Care. International Society for Traumatic Stress Studies, 2005.
30. Swenson CC: *Treatment for families experiencing child physical abuse*. Seattle, WA, Foster Care Assessment Program of the Children's Hospital, 2005.
31. Henggeler SW, Sheidow AJ, Lee T: Multisystemic treatment (MST) of serious clinical problems in youths and their families. In: Roberts AR, Springer DW (eds): *Forensic Social Work in Juvenile and Criminal Justice Settings: An Evidence-Based Handbook*, 3rd ed. Springfield, IL, Charles C Thomas, in press.
32. Henggeler SW, Melton GB, Brondino MJ, Scherer DG, Hanley JH: Multisystemic therapy with violent and chronic juvenile offenders and their families: The role of treatment fidelity in successful dissemination. *J Consult Clin Psychol* 65:821–833, 1997.
33. Huey SJ, Henggeler SW, Brondino MJ, Pickrel SG: Mechanisms of change in multisystemic therapy: Reducing delinquent behavior through therapist adherence and improved family and peer functioning. *J Consult Clin Psychol* 68:451–467, 2000.
34. Schoenwald SK, Sheidow AJ, Letourneau EJ: Toward effective quality assurance in evidence-based practice: links between expert consultation, therapist fidelity, and child outcomes. *Journal of Clinical Child and Adolescent Psychology* 33:94–104, 2004.
35. Henggeler SW, Schoenwald SK: The role of quality assurance in achieving outcomes in MST programs. *Journal of Juvenile Justice and Detention Services* 14:1–17, 1999.
36. Swenson CC, Saldana L, Joyner CD, Caldwell E, Henggeler SW, Rowland MD: *Multisystemic Therapy for Child Abuse and Neglect*. Charleston, SC, Family Services Research Center, Medical University of South Carolina, 2005.
37. Swenson CC, Saldana L, Joyner CD, Henggeler SW: Ecological treatment for parent to child violence. *Interventions for children exposed to violence*. New Brunswick, NJ, Johnson & Johnson, in press.
38. Schaeffer CM, Saldana L, Rowland MD, Henggeler SW, Swenson CC: New initiatives in improving youth and family outcomes by importing evidence-based practices. *Journal of Child and Adolescent Substance Abuse*, in press.
39. Sickmund M: *Juvenile Residential Facility Census: 2000, Selected Findings*. Washington, DC, Office of Juvenile Justice and Delinquency Prevention, 2002.
40. Elliott DS, Hamburg BA, Williams KR (eds): *Violence in American Schools: A New Perspective*. New York, Cambridge University Press, 1998.
41. Howel JC: *Preventing and Reducing Juvenile Delinquency: A Comprehensive Framework*. Thousand Oaks, CA: Sage Publications, 2003.
42. Borduin CM, Mann BJ, Cone LT, Henggeler SW, Fucci BR, Blaske DM, Williams RA: Multisystemic treatment of serious juvenile offenders: Long-term prevention of criminality and violence. *J Consult Clin Psychol* 63:569–578, 1995.
43. Henggeler SW, Melton GB, Brondino MJ, Scherer DG, Hanley JH: Multisystemic therapy with violent and chronic juvenile offenders and their families: The role of treatment fidelity in successful dissemination. *J Consult Clin Psychol* 65:821–833, 1997.
44. Henggeler SW, Melton GB, Smith LA: Family preservation using multisystemic therapy: An effective alternative to incarcerating serious juvenile offenders. *J Consult Clin Psychol* 60:953–961, 1992.
45. Henggeler SW, Melton GB, Smith LA, Schoenwald SK, Hanley JH: Family preservation using multisystemic treatment: Long-term follow-up to a clinical trial with serious juvenile offenders. *Journal of Child and Family Studies* 2:283–293, 1993.
46. Schaeffer CM, & Borduin CM: Long-term follow-up to a randomized clinical trial of multisystemic therapy with serious and violent juvenile offenders. *J Consult Clin Psychol* 73:445–453, 2005.
47. Ogden T, Halliday-Boykins CA: Multisystemic treatment of antisocial adolescents in Norway: Replication of clinical outcomes outside of the U.S. *Child and Adolescent Mental Health* 9:77–83, 2004.
48. Ogden T, Hagen KA: Multisystemic therapy of serious behaviour problems in youth: Sustainability of therapy effectiveness two years after intake. *Journal of Child and Adolescent Mental Health*, in press.
49. Timmons-Mitchell, J, Bender MB, Kishna MA Mitchell CC: An independent effectiveness trial of multisystemic therapy with juvenile justice youth. *Journal of Clinical Child and Adolescent Psychology* 35(2):227–236, 2006.
50. Curtis NM, Ronan KR, Borduin CM: Multisystemic treatment: A meta-analysis of outcome studies. *Journal of Family Psychology* 18:411–419, 2004.
51. Chamberlain P: *Treating Chronic Juvenile Offenders: Advances Made Through the Oregon Multidimensional Treatment Foster Care Model*. Washington, DC, American Psychological Association, 2003.
52. Elliott DS: *Blueprints for Violence Prevention, Series Ed*. Boulder, CO, University of Colorado, Center for the Study and Prevention of Violence, 1998.
53. Sheidow AJ, Henggeler SW: Community-based treatments. In: Heilbrun K, Sevin Goldstein NE, Redding R (eds): *Juvenile Delinquency*. New York, Oxford University Press, 1995, pp. 257–281.
54. Chamberlain, P: Comparative evaluation of specialized foster care for seriously delinquent youths: A first step. *Community Alternatives: International Journal of Family Care* 2:21–36, 1990.
55. Chamberlain P, Reid JB: Comparison of two community alternatives to incarceration for chronic juvenile offenders. *J Consult Clin Psychol* 66:624–633, 1998.
56. Leve LD, Chamberlain P, Reid JB: Intervention outcomes for girls referred from juvenile justice: Effects of delinquency. *J Consult Clin Psychol* 73:1181–1185, 2005.
57. Alexander J, Barton C, Gordon D, Grotpeter J, Hansson K, Harrison R, Mears S, Mihalic S, Parsons B, Pugh C, Schulman S, Waldron H, Sexton T: *Blueprints for Violence Prevention, Book Three: Functional Family Therapy*, Boulder, CO, Center for the Study and Prevention of Violence, 1998.
58. Knitzer J: *Unclaimed Children: The Failure of Public Responsibility to Children and Adolescents in Need of Mental Health Services*. Washington, DC: The Children's Defense Fund, 1982.
59. Kutash K, Duchnowski AJ, Friedman RM: The system of care 20 years later. In: Epstein M, Kutash K, Duchnowski A (eds): *Outcomes for Children and Youth with Emotional and Behavioral Disorders and Their Families: Programs and Evaluation Best Practices*. Austin, TX, Pro-Ed, Inc., 2005, pp. 3–22.
60. Burns BJ: Mental health service use by adolescents in the 1970s and 1980s. *J Am Acad Child Adolesc Psychiatry* 30:144–150, 1991.
61. Stroul BA, Friedman RM: *A System of Care for Severely Emotionally Disturbed Children and Youth*. Washington, DC, Georgetown University Development Center, 1986.
62. Burns BJ, Schoenwald SK, Burchard JD, Faw L, Santos AB: Multisystemic therapy and the wraparound process. *Journal of Child and Family Studies* 9:283–314, 2000.
63. Amini F, Zilberg NJ, Burke EL, Salasnek S: A controlled study of inpatient vs. outpatient treatment of delinquent drug abusing adolescents: One year results. *Compr Psychiatry* 23(5):436–444, 1982.
64. Flomenhaft K: Outcome of treatment for adolescents. *Adolescence* 9(33):57–66, 1974.

65. Langsley DG, Pittman FS, Machotka P, Flomenhaft K: Family crisis therapy: Results and implications. *Fam Process* 7(2):145–158, 1968.
66. Winsberg BG, Bailer I, Kupietz S, Botte E, Balka EB: Home vs. hospital care of children with behavior disorders: A controlled investigation. *Arch Gen Psychiatry* 37(4):413–418, 1980.
67. Evans ME, Boothroyd RA, Armstrong MI: Development and implementation of an experimental study of the effectiveness of intensive in-home crisis services for children and their families. *Journal of Emotional and Behavioral Disorders* 5(2):93–105, 1997.
68. Henggeler SW, Rowland MD, Randall J, Ward DM, Pickrel SG, Cunningham PB, Edwards JE, Miller SL, Zealberg JJ, Hand LD, Santos AB: Home-based multisystemic therapy as an alternative to the hospitalization of youths in psychiatric crisis: Clinical outcomes. *J Am Acad Child Adolesc Psychiatry* 38:1331–1339, 1999.
69. Schoenwald SK, Ward DM, Henggeler SW, Rowland MD: MST vs. hospitalization for crisis stabilization of youth: Placement outcomes 4 months post-referral. *Mental Health Services Research* 2:3–12, 2000.
70. Huey SJ, Henggeler SW, Rowland MD, Halliday-Boykins CA, Cunningham PB, Pickrel SG, Edwards J: Multisystemic therapy effects on attempted suicide by youths presenting psychiatric emergencies. *J Am Acad Child Adolesc Psychiatry* 43:183–190, 2004.
71. Henggeler SW, Rowland MD, Halliday-Boykins C, Sheidow AJ, Ward DM, Randall J, Pickrel SG, Cunningham PB, Edwards J: One-year follow-up of multisystemic therapy as an alternative to the hospitalization of youths in psychiatric crisis. *J Am Acad Child Adolesc Psychiatry* 42:543–551, 2003.
72. Bickman L, Lambert EW, Andrade AR, Penaloza RV: The Fort Bragg continuum of care for children and adolescents: Mental health outcomes over 5 years. *J Consult Clin Psychol* 68:710–716, 2000.
73. Bickman L, Noser K, Summerfelt WT: Long-term effects of a system of care on children and adolescents. *J Behav Health Serv Res* 26:185–202, 1999.
74. Manteuffel B, Stephens RL, Santiago R: Overview of the national evaluation of the comprehensive community mental health services for children and their families program and summary of current findings. *Child Services Social Policy and Research Practice* 5:3–20, 2002.
75. Rowland MD, Halliday-Boykins CA, Henggeler SW, Cunningham PB, Lee TG, Kruesi MJ, Shapiro S: A randomized trial of multisystemic therapy with Hawaii's Felix Class Youths. *Journal of Emotional and Behavioral Disorders* 13(1):13–23, 2005.
76. Henggeler SW, Schoenwald SK, Rowland MD, Cunningham PB: *Serious Emotional Disturbance in Children and Adolescents: Multisystemic Therapy*. New York, Guilford Press, 2002.
77. Rowland MD, Halliday-Boykins CA, Schoenwald SK: Multisystemic therapy with youth exhibiting significant psychiatric impairment. In: Epstein M, Kutash K, Duchnowski A (eds): *Outcomes for Children and Youth with Emotional and Behavioral Disorders and Their Families: Programs and Evaluation Best Practices*. Austin, TX, Pro-Ed, Inc., 2004.
78. Woolston J, Berkowitz S, Schaefer M, Adnopoz J: Intensive, integrated, in-home psychiatric services: The catalyst to enhancing outpatient intervention, the child psychiatrist in the community. In: Berkowitz S, Adnopoz J (eds): *Child and Adolescent Psychiatric Clinics of North America*. Philadelphia, W.B. Saunders Company, 1998, pp. 615–633.
79. Woolston JL, Adnopoz J, Berkowitz S: (in press) *IICAPS: A Home-Based Psychiatric Treatment Model for Children with Serious Emotional Disturbance*. New Haven, Yale University Press.
80. Emmons KM: Health behaviors in a social context. In: Berkman LF, Kawachi I (eds): *Social Epidemiology*. New York, Oxford University Press, 2000, pp. 242–266.
81. Grimes KE, MHSPY: A children's health initiative for maintaining at-risk youth in the community. *J Behav Health Serv Res*, in press.

CHAPTER 6.3.3 ■ COMMUNITY-BASED TREATMENT AND SERVICES

ANDRES J. PUMARIEGA AND NANCY C. WINTERS

HISTORY AND CHALLENGES IN CHILDREN'S COMMUNITY MENTAL HEALTH SERVICES

The early origins of mental health services for children in the United States emphasized a community and even a systems orientation. The context for the birth of these services was America in the 1890s, which, much as today, was undergoing rapid sociocultural changes due to immigration, industrialization, and urbanization. These social strains and their impact on children and families led to marked increases in juvenile crime and status offenses. Enlightened reformers saw the need for detaining young offenders separately from adults and adjudicating them in a separate court system (juvenile courts) that provided an opportunity for rehabilitation. The first community-based mental health services began in response to the perceived need for counseling juvenile offenders and their families. Thus, the new juvenile courts in Chicago and Boston established clinics that comprised the first child mental health services in the nation (1).

Their success led the Commonwealth Foundation to commission a study in the 1920s (and later start-up funding) that promoted the development of child guidance clinics throughout the nation, staffed with interdisciplinary teams of professionals who could serve children and their families. These clinics were first primarily staffed by social workers, but later attracted psychosocially oriented pediatricians, psychologists, and later psychoanalysts (as they emigrated from Europe) and psychiatrists (as the specialty grew and developed). These clinics later served as the bases of the first child psychiatry programs in the nation. They were removed from the specialty-oriented, hospital-based medical system evolving at tertiary medical centers. They provided low-cost services oriented to the needs of the child and the family, with treatment modalities evolving to include individual psychodynamic psychotherapy, family therapy, crisis intervention, and even day treatment programs. Many have survived to this day, and they even served as the model for the community mental health centers advocated in the 1960s community mental health legislation championed by the Kennedy administration, and later implemented throughout America in the 1960s (1).

The "medicalization" of psychiatry, starting in the 1970s and '80s, served to move child and adolescent psychiatric services toward a more hospital-based, tertiary care model. This left the child guidance clinics, and the community mental health centers that followed them, without significant child psychiatric input, adding to the relative neglect of the development of children's services. Many of the children previously served in these clinics were served in inpatient or residential facilities, or placed in foster care or juvenile detention facilities if they lacked third-party payment.

The modern era of community-based systems of care for children was ushered in by the publication of Jane Knitzer's (2) groundbreaking book, *Unclaimed Children*, which exposed the aforementioned consequences of neglecting the provision of community-based mental health services for children and their families. Her advocacy and that of others led to the development of the Child and Adolescent Service System Program (CASSP), which assisted all 50 states in the development of an infrastructure for publicly funded community-based services. The CASSP initiative was supported by the conceptual work of Stroul and Friedman (3), which coined the term "community-based system of care for seriously emotionally disturbed children and their families" and enunciated the principles behind such systems of care. Stroul and Friedman's work spurred the development of various innovative community-based treatment modalities, as well as a number of model demonstration programs in different parts of the United States that exemplify the use of these modalities within the context of an organized interagency system of care. In the early 1990s, the Robert Woods Johnson Foundation established eight pilot demonstration community systems of care programs in different parts of the country that demonstrated the viability of the system of care approach and demonstrated cost savings as well as less restrictive levels of care. Starting in 1994, the CASSP program was transformed into the Child and Adolescent Branch of the Center for Mental Health Services of the Substance Abuse and Mental Health Services Administration, which established the Comprehensive Community Mental Health Services for Children and Their Families Program. This program has funded over 80 community systems of care sites throughout the nation in widely diverse communities and American Indian communities, with over 75,000 children and families served by them, accompanied by a national evaluation. The Surgeon General's Report on Mental Health (4) also focused many of its recommendations in the area of children's mental health around the system of care model and its benefits for service system reform and community-based, individualized care.

INTERFACE OF CHILD MENTAL HEALTH SERVICES WITH OTHER CHILD-SERVING SYSTEMS

A number of health and human service agencies (schools, social welfare agencies, child protective agencies, juvenile justice, and public health) have experienced the increasing impact of psychosocial morbidity experienced by these children and youth. These agencies typically address pieces of the service system puzzle, with little to no coordination with other agencies often serving the same youth (5).

Juvenile Justice

In spite of the similarities in their populations, the juvenile justice and mental health systems have significant differences in their service orientations and philosophies. The juvenile justice system has faced a recent split in its orientation, between those who still promote the principles of rehabilitation advocated by its original founders, versus those who promote a more purely punitive and public safety approach. The latter viewpoint, with its push for longer sentences and even waivers into adult courts and prisons, gathered currency as the nation witnessed a major increase in juvenile crime in the 1980s (largely in poor inner city and rural areas), culminating in the widely publicized school shootings like that at Columbine, Colorado. This often clashes with the treatment and services orientation of the mental health system, though the latter suffers due to the lack of focus on behavioral containment and long-term followup. The service focus in the juvenile justice system shifted more toward detention/containment, either in juvenile detention facilities or in residential programs with some mental health programming and services (6).

The pressures to detain and incarcerate juveniles have led to overcrowded conditions and poor services in juvenile detention and incarceration facilities that violated several federal mandates. Chief among them is the Civil Rights of Institutionalized Persons Act (CRIPA), which mandates that states provide adequate health, mental heath, and human/social services to people detained on a long-term basis under state custody. However, other mandates, such as the Individuals with Disabilities Education Act, also apply to such youth. There have been well over 20 class action lawsuits involving juvenile justice systems all across the nation (7). Additionally, an increasing proportion of incarcerated youth are youth of color, with significant overrepresentation of underserved racial/ethnic minority groups as youth go deeper into the juvenile justice system. A mandate to reduce disproportionate minority confinement, requiring that states implement efforts to reduce such disparities, existed in federal law up until the late 1990s, but it was discontinued in spite of this serious continuing trend (6).

A number of studies have documented high rates of serious emotional disturbance among youth in the juvenile justice system, with estimates of approximately 50–70% (8, 9). Youth are referred to juvenile justice due to their propensity to display aggressive or disruptive behaviors, and after multiple disciplinary interventions in schools and out of home placements. They have similar histories as described for youth in child welfare, and were often previously served by that system. However, these youth typically have underutilized mental health services over their lifetime when compared to cohorts in other systems (10, 11). There is also disproportionate representation of minorities in the population of youth served by juvenile justice, especially of African Americans and Latinos. This is both due to the poverty and adversity faced by these youth, as well as the lack of culturally competent services in mental health and other agencies. The poor level of services within juvenile justice facilities also deprives them of adequate services, with racial bias further preventing access to services (12).

This trend toward the juvenile justice system becoming the "mental health system of last resort" for juveniles, as well as the public support for crime prevention, has led to increasing funding for services for juvenile offenders, including mental health services. They are leading either to the development of closer alliances between juvenile justice and mental health, or at times to the development of separate mental health services within the juvenile justice system. The latter trend may increase the access and control over these services for juvenile justice, but may result in unnecessary and costly duplication of services (6).

Areas of natural collaboration between these systems are in the prevention of entry into juvenile justice, particularly into detention/incarceration, and the treatment of youth with SED into the juvenile justice system. Multisystemic therapy (MST) has been tested extensively with youth at risk of detention and incarceration, and has resulted in significant reductions in out-of-home placement, externalizing criminal behaviors, rates of arrest and incarceration, and treatment costs (13). The significant reduction of incarceration by the CMHS system of care demonstration sites also supports the value of the system of care model in addressing the needs of this population of youth (14). The Surgeon General's report on youth violence (15) also reviews a number of effective preventive interventions for youth violence and delinquency.

Child Welfare

The original mission of the child welfare system was to provide custodial care for children and youth who were abandoned or abused by their families. This mission was initially met through the operation or support of orphanages in years past, and foster homes and group homes in later years. However, in recent years there has been greater recognition that children in the child welfare system have extremely high mental health needs, with prevalence rates estimated at about 50 percent, yet are significantly underserved with respect to mental health services (16). This is understandable considering the enormous stresses these children experience. Already traumatized by the abuse and neglect that led to removal from their parents' care, children placed in foster care are confronted with the additional traumas of the loss of their parents, multiple relocations, uncertainty about their future, and the difficult task of establishing positive attachments to new parent figures and foster siblings. In addition to having symptoms related to trauma and disrupted attachments, they are also at high risk for disruptive behaviors. They have greater difficulties in functioning at home, school, and in their communities, placing them at high risk for additional failed placements and need for residential treatment (16).

These needs led to the proliferation of residential treatment centers focused on the custodial and at times treatment needs of children in custody, particularly adolescents. Many of these facilities provide quality therapeutic and support services, but others in many states are largely unregulated in terms of the level or quality of service provision. Additionally, efforts to pursue effective permanency and transition plans back to the community are hampered by inadequate case management and community mental health services both for the youth and the family. These factors have led to a rapid increase in the number of children and youth cared for within such facilities for extended periods of time. Serious problems in the delivery of their care, such as indiscriminate polypharmacy, overuse of seclusion and restraints, and abuse at the hands of direct care staff, continue to hamper the system in spite of Knitzer's (2) original admonitions in the early 1980s.

The legal and social structures responsible for the care of children in state custody further complicate the situation for children in the child welfare system. The courts may make decisions supporting reunification that compromise the child's physical and/or emotional safety. Ninety percent of children in foster care are returned to their biological parents (17), and mental health services needed to support the reunification process are often inadequate. An additional challenge is the length of time children are spending in foster care without permanent plans for them being developed. There is the additional risk of further abuse in poorly monitored and overcrowded foster homes. Recent legislation such as the Adoption and Safe Families Act of 1997 attempts to shorten the time children spend in foster care (16).

When children are in foster care, there are unique challenges to establishing effective collaboration. There is first the challenge of forming a child–family team with multiple individuals who have varying levels of emotional commitment to and willingness to advocate for the child. These include the foster parent(s), child welfare worker, mental health professionals, court-appointed advocates (or attorney) for the child, possibly the biological parent(s), and/or extended family. The child- and family-centered system of care model works best when the child's parents are very invested. This may be difficult for foster parents, who are often caring for multiple high-need children and are not able to commit emotionally to a child who may live with them for a short period. Foster parents also suffer from inadequate training, support (including respite services and ongoing mental health consultation), and reimbursement for the care of children, particularly those who are seriously emotionally disturbed.

Another serious problem is the child welfare system being used by families in many states as a way to access intensive mental health services for children with inadequate insurance benefits. Intensive services (residential or day treatment), which may exceed $75,000 per year, are funded for children in state custody but are not covered by private insurance or Medicaid. In extreme cases, parents are forced to claim that they have neglected or abused their children. Parents lose control over the treatment their child receives while in state custody and, upon return home, their child may again have inadequate mental health coverage, compromising aftercare. These policies highlight the underlying problem of discriminatory policies toward childhood psychiatric illness.

These factors operate in the context of increasing numbers of children with complex mental health needs is soaring mental health costs, and are resulting in many federal class-action lawsuits. This is especially true for the Early Periodic Screening Detection and Treatment mandate for Medicaid. EPSDT mandates periodic health and mental health screening for covered children and medical necessity authorization of treatments and services to address abnormal findings, a benefit often omitted from managed Medicaid plans (7). Another arbitrary constraint within mental health systems that increase the risk of children being placed in foster care is the lack of needed parenting support services for individuals with mental illness, while states will fund the placement of their children in foster care. A different challenge is presented by the Welfare to Work law, which requires low-income parents to return to work to maintain some of their benefits. For some parents of at-risk children, this requirement makes it exceedingly difficult to spend the time needed to address the child's emotional or behavioral problems (16).

Children in foster care and those at risk for being placed in foster care are ideal candidates for the system of care approach, which can prevent out-of-home placement, support the strengths of the child and family, and use natural supports in the community. Wraparound programs, intensive case management programs, and therapeutic foster care are community-based interventions that have demonstrated effectiveness with this population of children and families (18). The American Academy of Child and Adolescent Psychiatry and the Child Welfare League of America (19) have developed specific screening, evaluation, and service standards to address the unique needs of children in the child welfare system. There is also a growing evidence base for psychosocial interventions for children with trauma-related disorders (20). Another positive trend is that of supporting foster care within a kinship network (extended family), allowing for relationships with family members to be sustained. More states are allowing families to retain custody of their children while they are in state-supported residential care (Oregon is one example); such changes to existing laws are usually accomplished only through significant advocacy by parent groups. (Also, see Chapters 5.15.1, 5.15.4, and 7.3.3)

Education

The educational system faces the impact of increased educational demands for average students due to the increased technological and informational demands on our society. In addition, the increasing needs of children with learning disorders and serious emotional disturbances are placing added burdens on schools. This occurs in the context of the underfunding of school districts due to downward pressures on property taxes (as exemplified by Proposition 13 in California) and other means of funding education. This lack of funding is especially felt in the area of special education services. Many school districts actively avoid the mandates of federal laws such as the Individualized Disability Education Act (IDEA) and Section 504 (which outlines services for mentally ill/emotionally disturbed children), often underidentifying children with covered disabilities and temporizing their needs informally through the services of regular classroom teachers so as to prevent added service commitments (21).

A recent salutary development in the area of interagency systems of care is the renewed interest in school-based services. These go beyond traditional school mental health consultation services and involve the colocation of health and mental health professionals within schools to provide a wide array of direct and indirect/preventive health and mental health services. School-based mental health services serve as an as ideal core service for a children's system of care, providing an excellent accessible portal of entry which is nonstigmatizing, and a naturalistic setting to observe behavior and integrate interventions into a child's environment. These services are often funded through blended Medicaid fee-for-service and managed care funding augmenting limited school funding. A number of models have been implemented in communities such as Baltimore, Maryland, rural South Carolina, the state of Hawaii, and Charlotte, North Carolina, with documented success in reducing adverse morbidity and increasing access to needed services (22–24). Innovative approaches through legislation to ensure interagency collaboration in IDEA-mandated services have been promoted in California through a law that mandates interagency collaboration in the development and implementation of individualized educational plans when these involve areas outside of educational services (25; Also, see Chapter 7.2).

Developmental Disabilities

Children and youth with developmental disabilities have significant mental health and social services needs. The prevalence of comorbidity of developmental disorders and behavioral/emotional disturbances are estimated to be quite high. In addition to mental health services, the service needs of children and youth with developmental disorders are often wideranging, including educational services, medical services (including general pediatric, neurological, and genetic), child welfare and social supports (with high rates of abuse and abandonment), and even juvenile justice services. The latter need is highlighted by the high prevalence of youth with Asperger's disorder found in juvenile justice populations (26). However, there is little recognition of these multiple service needs in the developmental disabilities service sector, much less adequate resources to meet them. Most state governments assign responsibility for serving children with developmental disabilities to the educational system under IDEA and ignore interagency collaborative approaches for their care. However, this system is overwhelmed in meeting its educational mission and dealing with more straightforward learning disabilities. The adult developmental disabilities sector is also moving rapidly to deinstitutionalize individuals currently in state training schools or facilities to community care, including the few youth in such programs. However, the behavioral support resources and staffing needed for successfully moving such individuals to community care are very limited, leaving them functioning at lower levels than their potential, and at risk of frequent utilization of psychiatric emergency services, hospitalization, and overmedication. This has led to many states experiencing class action lawsuits over the access and quality of care for its developmentally disabled citizens (26).

Primary Health Care

Primary care providers (including pediatricians, family physicians, some internists, and primary nurse practitioners) are the first line of mental health services for children in our nation, especially in rural and underserved areas. Studies (27) have demonstrated a high prevalence of mental health need among children and youth seen in primary care practices and settings. This role is even more critical in the Medicaid covered population, where the EPSDT benefit includes the requirement for annual screening, referral, and treatment for mental, emotional, and developmental disorders as well as physical illness. Potentially, the primary care system could be the most important (besides the educational system) in any effective effort to prevent the developmental morbidity of undetected and untreated mental illness in our children and youth (28).

In spite of these well known facts and mandates, very little has been or is being done to effectuate this role and function for the primary care sector. Primary care providers receive little to no training in child mental health and mental illness in their preservice or residency training. They are generally not provided (and not trained to use) the increasing number of evidence-based tools for effective screening and identification of youngsters with such needs. Access to specialist child mental health consultants and collaborators is hampered by problems with access and reimbursement. Additionally, the reimbursement mechanism for the direct delivery of entry-level mental health services by primary care practitioners is shrouded in mystery and bureaucracy, as if in an effort to reduce access to such services. The carve-out model primarily used for mental health benefits under managed Medicaid keeps "medical" and "mental health" sources of funding artificially separated (28).

There are some encouraging efforts toward enhancing and improving models of collaborative care between primary care and mental health providers, including child and adolescent psychiatrists. A few state Medicaid plans, particularly Vermont and Massachusetts, have adopted model or statewide programs to facilitate access to child mental health consultants by primary care practitioners. Some others have invested in training for primary care practitioners on EPSDT tools and referral procedures and support and consultative programs to enhance their function as mental health providers to high-risk populations. Other more formal models of collaborative care, using such technologies as telemedicine, are being evaluated and found to be effective in improving access to community-based care (28).

Current Crisis: Problems with Access and Overlap Across Populations

There continues to be increasing need for child mental health services in the United States. Recent studies suggest overall prevalence rates for childhood mental illness of 15 to 19%, with 3 to 8% for serious mental illness and emotional disturbance. However, less than one percent of children in the United States receive mental health treatment in hospital or residential settings, and another five percent in outpatient or community-based settings, with the majority of children in need receiving insufficient or no mental health services whatsoever (5). By contrast, the budgets dedicated to the financing of public mental health services for children have grown exponentially since the 1970s. For example, total Medicaid expenditures for mental health (largely applied to children) will grow to an estimated $14 billion by 2010, comprising a large portion of the total national mental health budget. A disproportionate level of these expenditures have been dedicated to inpatient and residential treatment, which are viewed with increasing skepticism given their high cost as well as limited documentation of outcome (4). In addition, the care of many children with mental illness and emotional disturbances is still shifted to the child welfare and juvenile justice systems, with many studies demonstrating a significant overlap between the children they serve and those served by mental health (7e).

COMMUNITY-BASED SYSTEMS OF CARE: AN INTEGRATIVE MODEL

In 1970 the report of the Joint Commission on the Mental Health of Children (29) documented serious problems in the quality of mental health care for children and adolescents with serious emotional and behavioral disturbances. The response, however, did not materialize until the study *Unclaimed Children* (2), published by the Children's Defense Fund, described disturbingly fragmented, uncoordinated care for this group of children, frequently separated from their families and communities and sent to institutions far from their homes. In 1984 the federal government responded by establishing the Child and Adolescent Service System Program (CASSP) under the auspices of the National Institutes of Mental Health (NIMH) to promote development of an integrated system of care for children and adolescents with serious emotional disturbance. CASSP provided seed money to states to expand mental health services to children and adolescents and established a set of core values and guiding principles for a system of care for children with serious emotional disturbances. CASSP principles comprise what became known as the system-of-care approach, defined as a comprehensive spectrum of mental health and other services and supports organized into a coordinated network to meet the diverse and changing needs of children and adolescents with severe emotional disorders and their families (3, 30).

The CASSP principles, now referred to as community systems of care principles, are based on a flexible and individualized approach to service delivery for the child and family within the context of his/her home and community as an alternative to treatment in out-of-home settings, while attending to family and systems issues that impact such care. These include access, utilization, child and family empowerment, financing, and clinical and cost effectiveness of mental health services provided to children and adolescents, as well as the functioning and effectiveness of systems of care for child mental health. Psychiatry, which was central in the traditional model, has only recently reengaged itself as a discipline in this new model. Psychiatrists face a major challenge in reaffirming their valued position in this model and integrating their developing clinical and scientific knowledge and skills base (3).

The CASSP initiative set forth the initial principles inherent in community-based systems of care. The key principles include: access to a comprehensive array of services, treatment individualized to the child's needs, treatment in the least restrictive environment possible, full utilization of family and community resources, full participation of families as partners in services planning and delivery, interagency coordination, the use of case management for services coordination, no ejection or rejection from services due to lack of "treatability" or "cooperation" with interventions, early identification and intervention, smooth transition of youth into the adult service system, effective advocacy efforts, and nondiscriminating, culturally sensitive services (3).

Another important principle inherent in this approach is that of the targeting of services to what are termed "seriously emotionally disturbed children." This designation includes the presence of an Axis I diagnosis under the diagnostic and statistical manual of the American Psychiatric Association (31), but places equal emphasis on the child's inability to function in at least one of his/her life domains (school, home, socially with peers). This reflects the difficulty in accurately diagnosing many children with serious functional problems, the bias against disruptive disorders (and failure to identify comorbid serious mental illness), and the lack of clarity and validity in clinical child diagnosis. Studies also suggest that the level of care received by children is only partially accounted by their clinical diagnosis, while level of function and psychosocial stressors are stronger predictors (32).

Implementation at the Clinical Level

The system-of-care model places the child and family at the center of the clinical process and as full partners at all levels of system planning (33, 34). Federal support and technical assistance to family advocacy organizations such as the Federation of Families for Children's Mental Health, National Association for the Mentally Ill, and others has facilitated expanded roles for family members in the mental health system and family empowerment through increased involvement in clinical and programmatic decisionmaking (4). The perspective of youth served in the mental health system is now being heard as family and consumer organizations are developing a cadre of youth advocates who can provide meaningful guidance to mental health professionals based on their own experience as recipients of services (35).

Family-driven care is a cornerstone of the system-of-care approach and has had a significant influence on national policy for both child and adult mental health (36, 37). The child and family drive the clinical planning process through determining the goals and desired outcomes of services, selecting the composition of the interagency planning team, evaluating the effectiveness of services, and having a meaningful role in all decisions, including those that impact funding of services. The interagency planning team has representatives from all the agencies involved with the child, and the team process facilitates interagency and interdisciplinary collaboration. The complementary contributions of various team members function synergistically in identifying system and community resources to promote better outcomes.

Some children and youth enter the system of care with discrete problems that can be addressed by a specific and/or time-limited service. For children with complex problems involved in multiple child-serving agencies, assessment and treatment planning should be accomplished through interdisciplinary clinical teams. The emphasis within these teams should be on the child and family's strengths, addressing specific clinical needs and supporting the child in his/her family and community environment. Mobilizing natural and normative resources (such as churches, community groups, recreational and extracurricular school-based activities) assures that the child is fully included in the life of the community and that developmental and clinical needs are served. This model emphasizes the need for a single case manager who will coordinate and manage these collaborative efforts. Interagency multidisciplinary teams invite full participation of consumer families and, when appropriate, the youth being served. Family advocates are involved coequally with professionals. Such teams function as treatment teams, coordinating multidimensional assessments, creating a crisis plan and a comprehensive care plan that embraces the clinical treatment plan. Such teams strive to bring professionals with very different goals and perspectives into a working relationship, defining the scope of each agency's work so as to assure that there is no duplication of efforts and no gaps in care. Funding constraints due to legally mandated categorical limits could leave some needs of a child unfulfilled. Many families can be well served by such interagency collaborative efforts, but often a parent or a youth surrounded by a team of professionals finds the experience intimidating and has trouble feeling that they are full participants in the planning process (38).

The wraparound process is a specific model of a child- and family-driven team planning process that has been empirically tested. Wraparound is a definable, integrated planning process that results in a unique set of community services and natural supports that are individualized for a child and family to achieve a set of positive outcomes. The wraparound process builds on the strengths of the child and family, is community-based using a balance of formal and informal supports, is outcome-driven, and provides unconditional care (39). Use of a strength-based orientation and discussion of needs rather than problems promotes more active engagement of families in service planning activities. Interventions designed to reinforce strengths of the child and family may include nontraditional therapies such as specific skills training or mentored work experiences that remediate or offset deficits. These interventions generally are not included in traditional categorical mental health funding and may require flexible funds that are not assigned to specific service types (40). For example, a youth at risk for substance abuse might receive funding for prosocial activities such as a health club membership or computer training. It has been noted that services are more likely to be effective if the wraparound process is informed by comprehensive clinical assessment addressing diagnostic and treatment issues and if the specific interventions are evidence based (41, 42).

Central to this process is the development of a child and family team (CFT). Such teams are composed primarily of nonprofessional members led by the consumer family, usually a parent. In cases of older youth as consumers, and with no parents available, the youth may serve as team leader. Empowering youth and families to assume a central role in outlining treatment goals and planning demands the involvement of specially trained individuals who can guide such families to develop a support network. Family advocates, partnering with professionals, provide the backbone of such a process. The goals for team development are to mobilize the natural support system for the family, including extended family, friends, neighbors, and natural helpers in communities. CFTs may include professionals to whom families have come to feel close, but the general rule is that teams should comprised no more than 50% professionals. Teams should employ professional advisors, including child and adolescent psychiatrists, who can offer advice on services, how best to access them, and on the various agencies in which the child is involved (35).

Such teams collaborate with professionals in agencies providing services. An empowered family accompanied by an advocate or a trusted professional care manager can more fully participate with a treatment team. The CFT creates an overall care plan, including a crisis plan. The clinical team then negotiates their role in the crisis and care plans. This negotiation further educates families about how their child's needs could be addressed through treatment, and enables professionals to learn about the realities faced by the family. In this model, the role of the case manager is supplanted by the CFT, which is responsible for maintaining and modifying the overall care plan, with the assistance of family advocates. The most complete evolution of a system of care that supports family-centered care involves agencies blending funds and undoing categorical constraints on the use of funds, with CFTs having control over the expenditure of such funds for services they deem needed and relevant. This radically alters the relationships of service providers to consumer families, enabling poor families to have control similar to middle or upper class families in their child's care and encouraging programs to develop new types of resources based on the common needs of families in that community (35).

A number of studies of wraparound in different communities with diverse populations of at-risk children and families have been described, generally reporting positive outcomes in terms of reduction of externalizing behavioral problems, level of function, reduction in out-of-home placement, improved family management skills and function, and increased consumer/family satisfaction (43–45). There have been recent efforts to operationalize wraparound as a *planning* model, as there has been some confusion about whether wraparound refers to the services themselves or the planning process. Recent studies on wraparound have incorporated measures such as the Wraparound Fidelity Index to ensure fidelity to the model (46).

Integration of services is fundamental to the community systems of care philosophy and approach. Service integration can be implemented in a variety of ways. The most fundamental is the interagency planning team, in which representatives from each agency involved with the child meet as a team to collaborate on the child and family's behalf and develop a single, integrated service plan. Integrated treatment models allowing mental health services to be provided in schools, juvenile justice, or child welfare settings have become quite prevalent. Another integration strategy is to colocate providers from different agencies in a single facility to enhance their collaboration and simplify the usually onerous task for families of accessing services from multiple agencies. Equally important in achieving service integration is the combining of funds from different agencies to form "blended" or "braided" funds to pay for services. This allows for the sharing of clinical and fiscal responsibility among agencies and decreases the likelihood of uncoordinated efforts driven by separate funding "silos" (47).

New Professional, Family, and Consumer Roles

Given the complexity of systems of care, the skills and roles that psychiatrists must display go far beyond clinical roles that are usually circumscribed and limited. These roles include serving as a front-line clinician, clinical consultant and collaborator to other professionals, collaborator with family advocates and consumers, clinical team leader, administrative leader in a delivery organization/system, quality assurance/improvement consultant, consultant to interagency teams, and outcome evaluator/researcher in systems of care. Child and adolescent psychiatrists, given their broad biopsychosocial and developmental perspectives, should be best able to integrate and coordinate community-based treatment delivered by multiple professionals with diverse skills. They have played critical roles in supporting some model blended-funding programs, and assuring that family-driven systems of care incorporate the most recent scientific advances in child and adolescent mental health. However, given the emphasis on tertiary care models of care in the training of most child and adolescent psychiatrists, they often have not developed many of the skills needed to serve as effective members, collaborators, and leaders of these new systems (48).

There is also a need for different professional roles for other disciplines and professionals. Social workers and other masters' level professionals assume a different type of care management role in addition to their therapy roles. These new functions involve collaborating and sharing roles with family advocates, and a new approach to partnering with consumer families. Psychologists are involved in the implementation of newer evidence-based practices, such as functional behavioral analysis and systematic measurement of behavior and strengths along with their psychodiagnostic and therapeutic roles. They may have new roles in program evaluation and quality assurance systems that involve working collaboratively with families in their design. Nurses are involved in a number of important roles, including greater involvement as psychiatric extenders (or, in some states, as primary psychiatric providers), as well as serving in liaison roles to pediatric and health systems. Community systems of care also have important roles for educators, formalizing their role as mental health coproviders involved in detection, triage, and behavioral interventions. Recreational and occupational therapists also have greater community involvement in schools and nonpsychiatric settings, rather than more traditional institutional settings. These roles require greater preprofessional training on development, psychopathology, and behavioral approaches (48).

The scope of family and consumer empowerment has been extended beyond the treatment setting to include their participation in a number of other roles within systems of care. These include providing case management and support services to other families, serving in quality assurance and consumer satisfaction assessment, participating in governance over system of care programs, and advocating for the maintenance and expansion of these programs. Organizations such as the Federation of Families for Children's Mental Health and other advocacy groups are helping to move the family and youth advocacy agenda (35).

Implementation at the Intervention Level

The President's New Freedom Commission goals and recommendations for a transformed mental health system included the dissemination of evidence-based practices as one of six major goals (36). This has provided the impetus for many states to legislate requirements around the use of evidence-based interventions. The system of care approach has provided a context for development of an evidence base for community-based interventions that provides alternatives to intensive treatment traditionally delivered in more restrictive settings, such as hospitals and residential treatment centers. These have been classified under the categories of community-based residential interventions (including therapeutic foster care and group homes), multimodal interventions (such as multisystemic therapy), service coordination and facilitation (including wraparound and intensive care management), and auxiliary and supportive services (including family education and support, mentoring, and respite services) (44). The evidence supporting these interventions will be described below, according to the schema proposed by Hoagwood et al. (49) for determining the level of evidence for mental health interventions, which includes efficacy, fidelity, and transportability, as well as Kazdin's (50) proposed levels of evidence: 1) not evaluated; 2) evaluated but unclear effects, no effects, or possible negative effects; 3) promising (some evidence); 4) well established (criteria by one system used for identifying evidence-based practice; and 5) better/best treatments (studies shown to be more effective than one or more other well established techniques).

The treatment foster care (TFC) model was developed by Chamberlain and colleagues at the Oregon Social Learning Center to address problematic behaviors in children with multiple mental disorders (51). It includes training of foster parents, in-home therapists and skills builders, and uses a specific model of behavior modification involving consistency, discipline and careful monitoring of behavior and consequences (44). Results of several studies indicate that TFC can reduce institutionalization, bring about more rapid improvement, and involves lower costs than other residential placements (51). In contrast to TFC, group homes involve creating a structured family environment for six to eight youths at a time, and the treatment model relies on the peer group milieu rather than parent–child interaction as the mediator of change. Group homes appear to be more common in the child welfare literature and have a less substantial literature than TFC (44). There have been questions about the potential for negative effects of grouping youth with similar problems together (52). Multisystemic therapy (MST) is regarded as among the most robust evidence-based interventions for youth (44). It combines home-based, wraparound, and cognitive-behavioral interventions that are individualized to the youth's ecological systemic context. Its developers have paid significant attention to manualizing MST and ensuring that it is applied with adequate fidelity in their research sites. It has been evaluated in eight randomized trials, including youth at risk of detention or incarceration and youth at risk of psychiatric or substance abuse hospitalization. It has shown significant results in reducing out-of-home placement, reducing externalizing behaviors, reducing rates of recidivism, and lowered costs of treatment (53, 54; Also,see Chapter 6.3.2).

Case management as an intervention has some overlap with wraparound, as both incorporate an assigned coordinator who participates in developing an individualized array of services and supports. Case management is a heterogeneous category that can refer to a variety of functions existing on a continuum from utilization management (or "gatekeeeping"), brokering or providing access to services, coordination of services, services monitoring and evaluation, advocacy, assessment, direct family support, and direct therapeutic service provision (38). Although definitions vary, the most consistent functions include service coordination and maintaining a coherent array of services and supports that meet the child and family's needs. Several types of studies on case management have been published. One study compared a full-time case manager with a primary therapist acting as case manager, finding that youth with the full-time case manager had better retention in services and a wider array of services, less restrictive services, and greater satisfaction, but not necessarily improved outcomes (55). In four randomized trials and a quasiexperimental study, case management has been compared to other interventions. The more intensive case management models (closer to direct service on the continuum) generally compare favorably with other interventions in reducing out-of-home placements and other functional outcomes, but the more common broker model shows primarily changes in service use as opposed to better individual outcomes (44). Additional work would be needed to define the model more systematically and determine what level of intensity is needed to produce favorable outcomes.

In the family support area, the most well examined intervention is mentoring. Mentoring programs have become fairly widespread. Dubois et al. (56) reviewed 55 mentoring programs, finding that better results were associated with greater number of best practices, which include having more explicit structure and monitoring of expectations, screening and training of mentors, parent involvement, and youth with more limited risk factors as opposed to serious mental health problems. Respite services involve providing temporary care to provide relief to caregivers of individuals with various disabilities. With the increased emphasis in systems of care on keeping children with serious disturbances at home, families have a greater need for relief to diminish caregiver burden. There has only been one quasiexperimental study on respite, which did show decreased caregiver strain and greater optimism, fewer out-of-home placements, and improvement of children's behavioral problems in the community (57). Although the rationale for respite in a system of care that is responsive to the needs of families and seeks to keep children at home is not disputed, more research is needed to demonstrate its effectiveness.

The recent Surgeon General reports on mental health (4) and on youth violence (15) point to research evidence supporting the effectiveness of a number of community-based interventions for children and youth, such as intensive case management, therapeutic foster care, partial hospitalization, and intensive in-home wraparound interventions. Other community-based interventions that show promise include school-based interventions, mentoring programs, family support and education programs, wilderness programs, crisis mobile outreach teams, time-limited hospitalization with coordinated community services, and family support services (41, 55, 58–60). Studies involving these modalities have demonstrated significantly better outcomes than traditional outpatient or residential services. These include reduced levels of externalizing and internalizing symptoms, improved family functioning, reduced utilization of more restrictive services, and improved cost-effectiveness.

One of the challenges facing community systems of care serving youth is the integration of evidence-based psychotherapeutic modalities, especially well tested, manualized interventions with demonstrated efficacy. Such interventions hold promise as broadly applicable interventions that could help address the considerable gap between mental health problems in children and the services needed to address these problems. However, there is still much work to be done in evaluating these interventions in real-world or community-based settings (61). Psychosocial interventions having the most empirical support include cognitive-behavioral therapy, interpersonal therapy, parent management training, parent–child interactive therapy (PCIT), and psychoeducational and cognitive-behavioral family interventions (60). Many newer systems of care demonstration programs are integrating such interventions into their programs, along with community-based interventions.

Pharmacotherapy in Systems of Care

Psychopharmacology has become increasingly prevalent in community settings as newer and more effective psychotropic agents have become available. These agents play an important role in the treatment of children with serious emotional and behavioral disturbance who have high rates of psychiatric comorbidity, psychosocial adversity, involvement with multiple agencies, and who are at highest risk for placement in restrictive settings (62, 63). Advances in pharmacotherapy have engendered increased expectations that medications can help stabilize and improve the functioning of this high-risk, high-need population. It is important for systems of care to integrate effectively and fully prescribing practitioners into interdisciplinary teams and integrate pharmacological therapies into children's wraparound plans (40). Effective use of pharmacotherapy includes systematic assessment of target symptoms, behaviors, function, and adverse effects by the whole team (including both synergistic and interfering side effects and issues such as optimal administration and dosing schedules). Ideally the team would also participate in the assessment of the efficacy of medications and interactions between pharmacotherapy and other treatment modalities and strength-based activities.

Effective pharmacotherapy requires that prescribing physicians have access to the inherent resources in a system of care, such as multiple informants to evaluate the child's symptom patterns and function in different contexts, and child and family education and support for treatment adherence. Lack of adequate contact of the children and families with the prescribing physician or medical practitioner often leads to children and families feeling uninformed, disempowered, and mistrustful of pharmacological therapies. Pharmacotherapy in systems of care should focus on functional improvement as well as on symptomatic relief. It should also include collaboration and psychiatric consultation around medication management with other prescribing medical professionals (64). Prescribing physicians in systems of care should promote use of evidence-based systematic assessment and symptom-rating tools and become actively involved in quality improvement around pharmacologic decisionmaking (40, 65). Attention to ethnic and cultural factors in diagnosis, metabolism of different agents, consent procedures, and attitudes towards medications are also important (66; Also, see Chapters 6.1.1 and 6.1.2).

Implementation at the Programmatic and Service Delivery Level

Following CASSP, several early demonstration projects were initiated to develop systems of care, including those in Ventura County in California (67) and Vermont (68) and the continuum of care established by the Department of Defense CHAMPUS program at Fort Bragg, North Carolina. From 1990 to 1995, the Robert Wood Johnson Mental Health Services Program for Youth funded eight national demonstration programs. More recently, the Center for Mental Health Services (CMHS) Comprehensive Community Mental Health Services Program for Children and Their Families has funded more than 80 demonstration projects in diverse communities throughout the nation to implement systems of care. The goals of these programs have been to implement CASSP values, reduce out-of-home placements, reduce service fragmentation, and promote earlier mental health intervention to reduce functional morbidity. The current phase of the grant program concerns culturally diverse populations and early childhood grants (47).

Service delivery features of the system-of-care model have been somewhat more difficult than specific interventions to operationalize and evaluate systematically, as until recently there have been no fidelity measures characterizing the essential features of a system of care (69). The Fort Bragg study was one of the few randomized designs of a system of care and showed that system coordination produced improved access to and satisfaction with services and also reduced restrictive forms of care (70). However, the fact that the system of care group showed clinical and functional outcomes similar to those of the traditional services group contributed to a shift towards more interest in the interventions themselves (71). More positive findings have been reported in other studies. A longitudinal study of the Vermont system of care concluded that the model was cost effective and resulted in reduced rates of out-of-home placement (72). Attkison et al. (67) reported reduced group home and foster care expenditures in three California counties using system-of-care approaches as compared with three counties that had more traditional services. Rosenblatt (73) reviewed results of 20 community-based system-of-care studies, concluding that there were improvements in most domains assessed, including clinical status, cost, and use of restrictive placements. The multisite national evaluation of the Comprehensive Mental Health Services Program for Children and Their Families has shown improved child and family functioning, increased stability of living situation, and reduced cost of care when cost offsets in education, juvenile justice, child welfare, and general health are considered (14, 74).

The system-of-care model appears to be beneficial in reducing use of residential and out-of-state placements and achieving improvements in functional behavior in youth with severe emotional and behavioral disorders who are served in multiple systems (4, 14). However, questions remain about the effectiveness of such systems in relation to more traditional systems, which specific outcomes are most meaningful to measure in evaluating the model, and what the active ingredients are that produce desired outcomes. Conducting research in complex systems of care is challenging because of the difficulty of identifying comparison groups and the near impossibility of using randomized assignment since the model has been embraced nationally and to offer less would be perceived as unethical (75). As a result the focus has shifted from measuring system-level outcomes to measuring clinical and functional outcomes of individual children (76).

A number of system-of-care demonstration programs that were originally grant funded have been successfully sustained. Two such programs with unique features are Wraparound Milwaukee in Milwaukee, Wisconsin, and The Village Project in Charleston, South Carolina. In existence since 1995, Wraparound Milwaukee was initially a CMHS funded system-of-care grant. It evolved into a sustainable publicly operated care management organization that focuses on providing a range of mental health, substance abuse, social, and other supportive services to children and adolescents who are identified by child welfare or juvenile justice as being at immediate risk of placement in a residential treatment center or psychiatric hospital based on emotional, behavioral, or mental health needs (45). Wraparound Milwaukee serves approximately 600 youth during a fiscal year using a child and family team process overseen by a care coordinator. Services are purchased from a blended pool from all the contracting agencies. Some of the unique features of Wraparound Milwaukee include the use of a mobile urgent treatment team that has dramatically reduced psychiatric hospital admissions, use of informal services and natural supports, and wraparound resource teams that provide specialized consultation for clinically complex youth (47).

The Village Project in inner city Charleston, South Carolina also began as a CMHS project, with an emphasis on serving a high-risk population of children and their families, many living in poverty and exposed to high levels of drug use and crime. The Village Project adopted an innovative strategy of colocating offices for each of the collaborating agencies in a large storefront shopping area in inner city Charleston. The Village Project provides community-based case management, clinical services, wraparound planning, and support services out of this site, as well as school-based programs, after-school programs, community mentoring programs, home-based intervention, and even specialty programs for young sexual offenders. Key elements that appear to be related to the program's success included a strong relationship between the directors of juvenile justice and mental health, the colocation of services in a single community facility improving ease of access, significant involvement of advocates and families as participants in the program, and support from state-level administrators (6).

CHALLENGES FOR COMMUNITY-BASED SYSTEMS OF CARE

Governmental Policy Imperatives

The Surgeon General's report on mental health in 1999 (4) was a watershed event in children's mental health, as it documented emerging evidence for a variety of psychopharmacologic, psychotherapeutic, and community-based interventions. It also provided support for reorganization of care according to CASSP principles. This was followed by the President's New Freedom Commission on Mental Health report (36), which was charged with conducting a comprehensive study of the U.S. mental health service delivery system and providing recommendations to the President for improving the system. The report documented pervasive fragmentation and disorganization and called for a fundamental transformation of the nation's approach to mental health care. The report presented six major goals and recommendations for a transformed mental health system: 1) Americans understand that mental health is essential to overall health; 2) mental health is consumer and family driven; 3) disparities in mental health care are eliminated; 4) early mental health screening, assessment, and referral are common practice; 5) excellent mental health care is delivered and research is accelerated; and 6) technology is used to access mental health care and information (77). This report contains elements consistent with the system-of-care model for children with serious emotional disturbance (consumer-driven care, emphasis on resilience and recovery rather than pathology, early intervention), but applies them to all of mental health care in the United States. The President's New Freedom Commission report has provided a strong impetus for states to develop comprehensive state mental health plans containing fundamental changes in adult and children's mental health. Such changes include wide implementation of initiatives toward consumer-driven care, treatment models promoting recovery and resilience, expanded prevention efforts and increased funding for early childhood mental health, and legislation of evidence-based practices.

Funding Challenges

As a result of the growth in mental health expenditures, the resources available to fund child mental health and human services are increasingly restricted. Medicaid, the public insurance program for the poor and disabled, funds a significant proportion of child mental health services in the United States, both through the coverage of AFDC recipients as well children with disabilities. Approximately 18% of children and adolescents 18 years of age and under are enrolled in the Medicaid program (including up to 25% of those under 3 years of age), with over 500,000 having severe emotional disturbances. However, the great majority of these children and youth are poor, underserved children of ethnic minority backgrounds. Children from these populations experience higher levels of stressors, such as poverty, discrimination, immigration, acculturation stress, and exposure to violence and trauma, and are likely to have higher levels of need for services. The cost of serving these populations of children and adolescents is in contrast to the high cost of the psychosocial morbidity they contend with, including lost productivity and the costs of welfare dependency and institutionalization (5).

These trends have increased pressures on public child mental health and social service agencies to demonstrate improved clinical and cost effectiveness, increasingly turning to managed care approaches to finance and organize mental health and social services. For example, over 60% of children who are Medicaid beneficiaries are under managed care plans, the largest beneficiary group in these programs. However, most managed care methods were developed with adult and private sector populations in mind, and are usually accompanied by the privatization of services. Managed care methodology is being implemented increasingly within Medicaid-funded children's mental health services with the aim of reducing utilization and costs, including such newer approaches as restrictive formularies, level of care criteria, and restrictive case rates. When applied to public child mental health services, these approaches have often resulted in fragmentation of care and the shifting of the burden of services and cost to the other child-serving agencies and systems, with the potential for significantly increased morbidity (78, 79). Such methodology also is being used to manage services funded by the child welfare system and juvenile justice systems, with significant potential impact on access to and quality of care.

A result of these pressures for cost containment has been an exponential growth of class action lawsuits over the past 15 years against state Medicaid, educational, child welfare, and juvenile justice agencies for failing to meet federal service mandates (7). However, rather than increase funding or make better use of resources, the response by the federal government has been to pursue legislation to undo many of the mandates associated with Medicaid, Title IX child welfare funding, and the Civil Rights for Instutionalized Persons Act (CRIPA), which are the bases of these lawsuits.

Mental Health Disparities and Needs of Culturally/Ethnically Diverse Populations

The United States is becoming increasingly culturally and ethnically diverse. More than 36% percent of all children and youth in the United States are from non-European racial and ethnic backgrounds, and this figure is expected to rise to more than 50% by the year 2030. Children and youth from non-European backgrounds and their families face many adversities, including language barriers, social discrimination, and socioeconomic and educational disparities. The Surgeon General's supplement on culture, race, ethnicity, and mental health (80) has highlighted the serious racial/ethnic disparities in child mental health and social services in our nation. For example, African American children remain in foster care for a longer period of time and have more foster care placements than European American children. Ethnically diverse children are overrepresented in child welfare and juvenile justice settings compared to nonminority youth, even when they have equal psychiatric morbidity.

Children and families from ethnically diverse cultures are distinctly different from those of European origins, with different beliefs, values, normative expectations for development and adaptive behaviors, parenting practices, relationship and family patterns, symptomatic expressions of distress, and explanations of mental illness (66). Consequently they have specific mental health needs with respect to treatment approaches, modalities, and support services. Studies support the presence of significant racial and ethnic disparities in a number of areas relating to children's mental health, including access to community-based services, accurate diagnostic assessment, access to evidence-based interventions, increasing rates of various forms of psychopathology in some populations, and significantly higher rates of out-of-home placements and institutionalization (particularly in child welfare and juvenile justice). In addition, there is evidence of subtle differences in the metabolism of psychopharmacological agents in diverse populations, related to both genetic and environmental (dietary) factors (66, 80).

There is an increasing consensus that mental health services should be provided within the cultural competence model This model indicates the need to identify and address the special mental health needs of diverse populations through both clinician-related factors (such as acquiring knowledge, skills, and attitudes that enable them to serve populations different from their own) and system factors (such as reviewing and changing policies and practices that present barriers to diverse populations, staff training around cultural competence, and the recruitment of diverse staff and clinicians for planning service pathways and delivering care). This model also calls for the use of natural strengths and resources in concert with professional services that are protective and support children and families in diverse communities and cultures dealing with emotional disturbance. It also includes the adoption of culturally specific therapeutic modalities (such as use of native healers or cultural mediators), mainstream modalities evaluated with diverse populations, and the appropriate use of language interpreters (66).

The cultural competence model has been operationalized in consensus health and mental health cultural competence standards, such as the Center for Mental Health Services standards (81). These standards address cultural adaptations and modifications in clinical processes (such as assessment, treatment planning, case management, and linguistic support) and system processes (such as staff training and development, access protocols, governance of service systems, quality assurance and improvement, and information management). There is beginning evidence that adopting such practices results in improved access to services and retention in treatment (81; Also, see Chapter 1.7.1).

Prevention and the Problems of the Very Young

One of the guiding principles of CASSP is to promote early identification for children with emotional disturbances, and therefore communities bear responsibility to assign some of their resources to prevention efforts (3). Examples of vulnerable populations include children experiencing violence, abuse, neglect, or other trauma, and children showing signs of depression or other mental health problems in the school or childcare setting. The integration of mental health services into schools, child welfare, and juvenile justice settings provides early intervention opportunities for children and youth with early symptoms of mental health disorders.

The early childhood population (generally ages 0–5, defined by their preschool-aged status) is a particularly vulnerable group of children for whom it has been shown that environmental risks can have significant long-term developmental impact, and that early intervention has the potential to be very beneficial over the long term (83). Until CMHS recently started funding of system-of-care projects for 0–6 year olds, the early childhood age group had not benefited from system of care reform (84). Since many agencies are involved with young children, the system-of-care model that promotes integrated planning and service strategies is extremely suitable for this age group. System of care integrated service strategies may include such activities as providing mental health consultation to Head Start, early intervention, primary care practitioners, community health nurses, and childcare workers; and providing mental health services to adults whose children are at risk of out-of-home placement. Examples of effective preventive approaches include nurse home visiting (85), referral to early intervention services, advocacy for stable placement, support for prenatal care, provision of substance abuse and mental health services and parenting supports to parents of infants at risk for abuse (86), and early mental health services for children at risk for psychiatric disturbance (87).

Barriers to these efforts persist, however, some of which are related to funding and eligibility for services. Mental health agencies may be unable to provide services to children who do not yet meet the full criteria for a mental health diagnosis, and addressing the parents' mental health or substance abuse issues may not be possible if they are uninsured. To address this issue, the state and local funding agencies need to adopt alternative eligibility criteria for services, have contractual agreements with other child-serving agencies that obviate the need for formal diagnosis, or allow the parent to be the recipient of services. For young children who are already showing some early symptoms of disorder, use of a more age-appropriate Diagnostic System for Zero to Three, Revised (DC:0–3R; 88) is more likely to identify conditions making them eligible for services. A crosswalk to ICD-9 diagnoses is needed for billing under the Medicaid system, however. States such as Maine, Florida, Washington, and California have developed crosswalks from DC:0–3 to ICD-9 diagnoses as part of their statewide early childhood plans. Another barrier is that there are few clinicians trained to diagnose and treat mental health conditions in very young children. States are beginning to invest resources in training to improve the skills of early childhood clinicians.

Challenges in Replication on a Larger Scale

The greatest challenge experienced by system-of-care demonstration programs is how to sustain the model after the grant period ends. Without external funding, the system often reverts to fragmentation and lack of coordination due to the separate funding and organizational structures of mental health, education, juvenile justice, child welfare, developmental disabilities, and substance abuse services. More recent system of care projects have benefited from lessons learned as to how to build in sustainability factors early in their projects. Some of the factors supporting sustainability include developing specific targeted outcomes agreed upon by all stakeholders from the outset, developing effective strategies for tracking and reporting those outcomes, and "social marketing," informing the wider community and legislature of successes of the project in socially meaningful terms (14, 89, 90).

An additional potentially daunting challenge is how to replicate a small demonstration project on a larger scale that addresses an entire population at a community or state level. It is generally not fiscally viable to apply all aspects of the model on a large scale. For example, regular meetings of interagency teams are costly in terms of personnel time, and may not be needed for children at lower levels of severity. Yet, the systems-level data are not robust enough to guide decision as to which elements of the model to select for the larger population. Thus, states have chosen different elements to implement on a larger scale, as will be described below.

Response to Challenges

The Robert Wood Johnson Foundation Mental Health Services Program for Youth (RWJ-MHSPY) and CMHS Comprehensive Community Mental Health Services Program for Children and Their Families ushered in a new level of activism in the United States by providing an unprecedented level of support for system reform in children's mental health. There has also been active support of these reform efforts by professional organizations such as the Academy of Child and Adolescent Psychiatry (AACAP), which in 1994 established a Work Group on Community-Based Systems of Care. The AACAP Work Group on Community-Based Systems of Care has developed policy guidelines on relevant topics, including structure of Medicaid managed care programs, training and roles of mental health professionals toward systems of care, outcomes in systems of care, and early childhood systems of care. It has developed tools for assessing service intensity need using a community-based paradigm, and systems-based practice educational materials (48, 91–94).

Systems of care reforms have also occurred at the state level. Incremental changes have occurred in many states through national trends, such as managed care Medicaid and the advent of Medicaid waivers that have allowed for innovations and more flexible use of treatment dollars (96). However, reforms associated with managed care Medicaid have not always been positive, as privatization of Medicaid has resulted in some instances in attenuation rather than expansion of appropriate community-based services (47). Some states have legislated very expansive systems reform. Notable examples include the states of Hawaii and New Mexico. Hawaii provides an integrated services model through providing mental health services in schools throughout the state. It has also implemented evidence-based interventions on a wide scale, developing its own classification system for levels of evidence for each treatment modality by diagnosis, and analysis of effective components of each treatment model (97). Hawaii also adopted statewide the Child and Adolescent Service Intensity Instrument (CASII) (94), a tool that provides a uniform procedure for assessment and planning intensity of service need using a community-based paradigm. In 2003, New Mexico legislated a comprehensive approach to planning, redesigning, financing, and oversight of services funded, provided, or managed by 15 state departments (98). The legislation established a purchasing collaborative that will procure a single statewide entity responsible for all behavioral health services and all mental health and substance abuse dollars. It is hoped that creation of a single integrated system will eliminate duplicative administrative structures and provide opportunities for agencies to maximize limited resources. The challenge for this sweeping innovation in New Mexico is for the new structure to provide a base to encourage more family- and consumer-driven and evidence-based services.

CONCLUSION

The Child and Adolescent Service System Program (CASSP) defined a system of care approach to providing mental health and related services to children and adolescents with serious emotional and behavioral disturbances. It has had a major influence on community systems of care through extensive federally funded projects, along with state and national initiatives that have embraced CASSP values. The system of care model emphasizes that care should be tailored to the individual needs and strengths of the child and family, culturally competent, coordinated and integrated, and provided in the most community-based and least restrictive setting that meets their needs. Families are included as full partners in the clinical process, and are involved in program development and evaluation. Services are coordinated and integrated into a comprehensive care plan. CASSP has fostered development of a number of evidence-based, community-based interventions that can represent meaningful alternatives to traditional institution-based care. Integrated system of care approaches to service delivery have produced favorable outcomes in reducing use of residential and out-of-state placements and achieving improvements in functional behavior in youth with severe emotional and behavioral disorders who are served in multiple systems. Family and consumer organizations, now strengthened by youth participation, have made substantial contributions to the reform of mental health care in this country.

References

1. Berlin I: Development of the subspecialty of child and adolescent psychiatry in the United States. In: J Weiner (ed): *Textbook of Child and Adolescent Psychiatry*, 2nd ed. Washington, DC, American Psychiatric Press, 1997, pp. 8–15.
2. Knitzer J: *Unclaimed Children: The Failure of Public Responsibility to Children and Adolescents in Need of Mental Health Services.* Children's Defense Fund, Washington, DC, 1982.
3. Stroul B, Friedman R: *A System of Care for Severely Emotionally Disturbed Children and Youth.* Georgetown University Child Development Center, CASSP Technical Assistance Center, Washington, DC, 1986.
4. U.S. Department of Health and Human Services: *Mental Health: A Report of the Surgeon General.* Center for Mental Health Services, Substance Abuse and Mental Health Services Administration, U.S. Department of Health and Human Services, Washington, DC, 1999.
5. Pumariega A, Nace D, England M, Diamond J, Mattson A, Fallon T, Hansen G, Lourie I, Marx L, Thurber D, Winters N, Graham M, Weigand D: Community-based systems approach to children's managed mental health services. *J Child Family Stud* 6:149, 1997.
6. Heffron W, Pumariega AJ, Fallon T Jr., Carter D: Youth in the juvenile justice system. In: Pumariega AJ and Winters NC (eds): *Handbook of Community-Based Systems of Care: The New Child and Adolescent Community Psychiatry.* New York, Jossey-Bass, 2003, pp. 224–249.

7. Vaughan T, Pumariega, A J, Klaehn R: Systems of care under legal mandates. In: Pumariega AJ, Winters NC (eds): *Handbook of Child and Adolescent Systems of Care: The New Community Psychiatry.* San Francisco: Jossey-Bass, 2003, pp. 414–431.
8. Atkins DL, Pumariega AJ, Montgomery L, Rogers K, Nybro C, Jeffers G, Sease F: Mental health and incarcerated youth. I: Prevalence and nature of psychopathology. *J Child Family Stud* 8:193, 1999.
9. Teplin L, Abram K, McClelland G, Dulcan M, Mericle A.: Psychiatric disorders in youth in juvenile detention. *Arch Gen Psychiatr* 59:1133–1143, 2002.
10. Pumariega AJ, Atkins DL, Rogers K, Montgomery L, Nybro C, Caesar R, Millus D: Mental health and incarcerated youth. II: Service utilization in incarcerated youth. *J Child Family Stud* 8:205, 1999.
11. Rogers K, Pumariega AJ, Atkins DL, & Cuffe, S: Factors associated with identification of mentally ill youth in the juvenile justice system. *Community Mental Health J* in press, 2006.
12. Rogers K, Powell E, Zima B, & Pumariega AJ: Who receives mental health services in the juvenile justice system. *J Child Family Stud* 10(4):485–494, 2001.
13. Borduin C: Multisystemic treatment of criminality and violence in adolescents. *J Am Acad Child Adol Psychiatr* 38:242–249, 1999.
14. Holden EW, Santiago, RL, Manteuffel, BA, Stephens R, Soler R, Liao Q, Branshears F, Zaro S, Brannan, A: Systems of care model demonstration projects: Innovation, evaluation, and sustainability. In: Pumariega AJ, Winters NC (eds): *Handbook of Child and Adolescent Systems of Care: The New Community Psychiatry.* San Francisco: Jossey-Bass, 2003, pp. 432–459.
15. U.S. Department of Health and Human Services: *Youth Violence: A Report of the Surgeon General.* Center for Mental Health Services, Substance Abuse and Mental Health Services Administration, U.S. Department of Health and Human Services, Washington, D.C. 2001a.
16. Marx K, Benoit M, Kamradt B: Foster children in the child welfare system. In: Pumariega AJ, Winters NC (eds): *Handbook of Child and Adolescent Systems of Care: The New Community Psychiatry.* San Francisco, Jossey-Bass, 2003, pp. 332–352.
17. Nordhaus BF, Solnit AJ: Foster placement. *Child Adol Psychiatr Clinics of North Am* 7:345–356, 1998.
18. Clark HB, Prange, ME, Lee B, Stewart ES, McDonald BB, Boyd LA: An individualized wraparound process for children in foster care with emotional/behavioral disturbances: Follow-up findings and implications from a controlled study. In: Epstein MH, Kutash K, Duchnowski AJ (eds): *Outcomes for children and youth with emotional and behavioral disorders and their families: Programs and evaluation best practices.* Austin, TX, Pro-Ed, 1998, pp. 686–707.
19. American Academy of Child & Adolescent Psychiatry and Child Welfare League of America (2002): *Joint Policy Statement on Mental Health Screening and Evaluation of Children in Foster Care.* Washington, DC, Author.
20. Pine DS, Cohen JA: Trauma in children and adolescents: Risk and treatment of psychiatric sequelae. *Biol Psychiatry* 51:519–531, 2002.
21. Porter G, Pearson G, Keenan S, Duval-Harvey, J: School-based mental health services: A necessity, not a luxury. In: Pumariega AJ, Winters NC (eds): *Handbook of Child and Adolescent Systems of Care: The New Community Psychiatry*, San Francisco, Jossey-Bass, 2003, pp. 250–275.
22. Flaherty L, Weist M, Warner B: School-based mental health services in the United States: History, current models, and needs. *Comm Ment Health J* 32:341–352, 1996.
23. Stone-Motes P, Melton G, Pumariega AJ, Simmons W: Ecologically oriented school-based mental health services: Implications for service system reform. *Psychol in the Schools* 36(5):391–402, 1999.
24. Casat C, Rigsby M, Sobelewski J, Gordon J: School-based mental health services (SBS): A pragmatic view of a program. *Psychol in the Schools* 36:403–414, 1999.
25. Schacht T, Hansen G: The evolving climate for school mental health services under the Individual with Disabilities Education Act. *Psychol in the Schools* 36:415–426, 1999.
26. O'Malley K: Youth with co-morbid disorders. In: Pumariega AJ, Winters NC (eds): *Handbook of Child and Adolescent Systems of Care: The New Community Psychiatry.* San Francisco, Jossey-Bass, 2003, pp. 276–315.
27. Asarnow JR, Jaycox LH, Duan N, LaBorde AP, Rea MM, Tang L, Anderson M, Murray P, Landon C, Tang B, Huizar DP, Wells KB: Depression and role impairment among adolescents in primary care clinics. *J Adolesc Health* 37:477–483, 2005.
28. Grimes K: Collaboration with primary care: Sharing risks, goals, and outcomes in an integrated system of care. In: Pumariega AJ, Winters NC (eds): *Handbook of Child and Adolescent Systems of Care: The New Community Psychiatry.* New York, Jossey-Bass, Chapter 14, pp. 316–331.
29. Joint Commission on the Mental Health of Children: *Crisis in child mental Health: Challenge for the 1970s.* New York, Harper and Row, 1970.
30. Lourie I: A history of community child mental health. In: Pumariega AJ and Winters NC (eds): *Handbook of Community-Based Systems of Care: The new Child and Adolescent Community Psychiatry* New York, Jossey-Bass, 2003.
31. American Psychiatric Association *Diagnostic and Statistical Manual for Mental Disorders*, 4th ed. (DSM-IV). Washington, DC, 1994.
32. Silver S, Duchnowski A, Kutash K, Friedman R, et al.: A comparison of children with serious emotional disturbance served in residential and school settings. *J Child Fam Stud* 1:43–59, 1992.
33. Friesen BJ, Koroloff NM: Family-centered services: Implications for mental health administration and research. *J Mental Health Admin* 14:13–25, 1990.
34. Osher T, de Fur E, Nava C, Spencer S, and Toth-Dennis, D: New roles for families in systems of care. In: *Systems of care: Promising Practices in Children's Mental Health*, 1998 series, (vol I). Washington, DC, Center for Effective Collaboration and Practice, American Institutes for Research.
35. Huffine C, Anderson D: Family advocacy development in systems of care. In: Pumariega AJ, Winters NC (eds): *Handbook of Child and Adolescent Systems of Care: The New Community Psychiatry.* San Francisco, Jossey-Bass, 2003, pp. 35–65.
36. U.S. Department of Health and Human Services: *New Freedom Commission on Mental Health: Achieving the promise: Transforming mental health care in America.* Rockville, MD: Department of Health and Human Services, 2003. Available at: www.mentalhealthcommission.gov/reports/finalreport/fullreport-02.htm.
37. Federation of Families for Children's Mental Health Web page: Family Leadership in Systems of Care. Retrieved in January 2006, www.ffcmh.org/systems_whatis.htm.
38. Winters NC, Terrell L: Case management: The linchpin of community-based systems of care. In: AJ Pumariega & NC Winters (Eds.) *Handbook of child and adolescent systems of care: The new community psychiatry,* San Francisco, Jossey-Bass, 2003, pp. 171–202.
39. VanDenBerg JE, Grealish EM: Individualized services and supports through the wraparound process: Philosophy and procedures. *J Child and Family Stud* 5:7–21, 1996.
40. American Academy of Child and Adolescent Psychiatry, Practice parameter on child and adolescent mental health care in community systems of care. *J Am Acad Child Adolesc Psychiatry* (in press).
41. Burns BJ, Hoagwood K: *Community Treatment for Youth: Evidence-Based Interventions for Severe Emotional and Behavioral Disorders.* Oxford University Press, New York, 2002.
42. Solnit AJ, Adnopoz J, Saxe L, Gardner J, Fallon T: Evaluating systems of care for children: Utility of the clinical case conference. *Am J Orthopsychiatry* 67:554–567, 1997.
43. Burchard JD, Bruns JD, Burchard SN: The wraparound approach. In: Burns BJ and Hoagwood K (eds): *Community Treatment for Youth: Evidence-Based Interventions for Severe Emotional and Behavioral Disorders.* New York, Oxford University Press, 2002.
44. Farmer EM, Dorsey S, Mustillo SA: Intensive home and community interventions. *Child Adolesc Psychiatr Clin N A* 13:857–884, 2004.
45. Kamradt B, Meyers MJ: Curbing violence in juvenile offenders with serious emotional and mental health needs: The effective utilization of wraparound approaches in an American urban setting. *Intl J Adolesc Med Health* 11:381–399, 1999.
46. Bruns EJ, Burchard JD, Suter JC, Leverentz-Bracy K, Force MM: Assessing fidelity to a community-based treatment for youth: The Wraparound Fidelity Index. *J Emotional Behav Disorders* 12:79–89, 2004.
47. Winters NC, Marx L, Pumariega AJ: Systems of care and managed care: Are they compatible? In: AJ Pumariega & NC Winters (Eds.) *Handbook of child and adolescent systems of care: The new community psychiatry.* San Francisco, Jossey-Bass, 2003, pp. 380–413.
48. American Academy of Child & Adolescent Psychiatry: *Guidelines for training towards community-based systems of care for children with serious emotional disturbances.* Washington, DC, Author, 1996.
49. Hoagwood K, Burns B, Kiser L, Ringeisen H, Schoenwald S: Evidence-based practice in child and adolescent mental health services. *Psychiat Svcs* 52:1179, 2001.
50. Kazdin A: Evidence-based treatments: Challenges and priorities for practice and research. *Child Adolesc Psychiatr Clin N Am* 13:923–940, 2004.
51. Chamberlain P: Treatment foster care. In: Burns BJ and Hoagwood K (Eds.) *Community Treatment for Youth: Evidence-Based Interventions for Severe Emotional and Behavioral Disorders.* New York, Oxford University Press, 2002.
52. Dishion T, McCord J, Poulin J: When interventions harm: Peer groups and problem behavior. *Am Psychol* 54:755–764, 1999.
53. Henggeler SW, Schoenwald SK, Rowland MD, Cunningham PB: *Multisystemic Treatment of Children and Adolescents with Serious Emotional Disturbance.* New York, Guilford Press, 2001.
54. Henggeler SW, Rowland MD, Halliday-Boykins C, Sheidow AJ, Ward DM, Randall J, Pickrel SB, Cunningham PB, Edwards J: One-year follow-up of multisystemic therapy as an alternative to the hospitalization of youths in crisis. *J Am Acad Child Adolesc Psychiatry* 42:543–551, 2003.
55. Burns B, Farmer E, Angold A, Costello E, Behar L: A randomized trial of case management for youths with serious emotional disturbance. *J Child Clin Psychol* 25:476, 1996.

56. Dubois DL, Holloway BE, Valentine JC, Cooper H: Effectiveness of mentoring programs for youth: A meta-analytic review. *Am J Community Psychol* 30:157–197, 2002.
57. Bruns EJ, Burchard JD: Impact of respite care services for families with children experiencing emotional and behavioral problems. *Children's Services: Social Policy, Research, and Practice* 3:29–61, 2000.
58. Kutash K, Rivera VR: Effectiveness of children's mental health services: A review of the literature. *Educ Treat Children* 18:443–477, 1995.
59. Grizenko N: Outcome of multimodal day treatment for children with severe behavior problems: A five year follow-up. *J Am Acad Child Adol Psychiatr* 36:989–997, 1997.
60. Rogers, K: Evidence-based community-based interventions. In: Pumariega AJ, Winters NC (eds): *Handbook of Child and Adolescent Systems of Care: The New Community Psychiatry.* San Francisco, Jossey-Bass, 2003, pp. 149–170.
61. Weisz JR: Lab-clinic differences and what we can do about them. I. The clinic-based treatment development model. *Clinical Child Psychol Newsletter* 15, 2000.
62. Costello EJ, Angold A, Burns BJ, Erkanli A, Stangl DK, Tweed DL: The Great Smoky Mountain Study of Youth: Functional impairment and serious emotional disturbance. *Arch Gen Psychiatry* 54:1137–1143, 1996.
63. Mattison RE, Morales J, Bauer MA: Adolescent schoolboys in SED classes: Implications for child psychiatry. *J Am Acad Child Adolesc Psychiatry* 32:1223–1228, 1993.
64. Pumariega AJ, Fallon T: Psychopharmacology in systems of care. In: Pumariega AJ, Winters NC (eds): *Handbook of Child and Adolescent Systems of Care: The New Community Psychiatry.* San Francisco, Jossey-Bass, 2003, pp. 120–148.
65. Zima BT, Hurlburt MS, Knapp P, Ladd H, Tang L, Duan N, Wallace P, Rosenblatt A, Landsverk J, Wells KB: Quality of publicly funded outpatient specialty mental health care for common childhood psychiatric disorders in California. *J Am Acad Child Adolesc Psychiatry* 44:130–144, 2005.
66. Pumariega A: Cultural competence systems of care for children's mental health. In: Pumariega AJ, Winters NC (eds): *Handbook of Child and Adolescent Systems of Care: The New Community Psychiatry.* San Francisco, Jossey-Bass, 2003, pp. 82–106.
67. Attkisson C, Rosenblatt AB, Dresser KL, Baize HR, Clausen JM, Lind SL: Effectiveness of the California system of care model for children and youth with severe emotional disorders. In: Nixon CT, Northrup CA (eds): *Evaluating Mental Health Services: How Do Programs for Children Work in the Real World?* Thousand Oaks, CA, Sage, 1997, pp. 146–208.
68. Bruns E, Burchard J, Yoe J: Evaluating the Vermont system of care: Outcomes associated with community-based wraparound services. *J Child Family Stud* 4:321, 1995.
69. Hernandez M, Gomez A, Lipien L, Greenbaum PE, Armstrong KH, Gonzalez, P: Use of the system-of-care practice review in the national evaluation: Evaluating the fidelity of practice to system-of-care principles. *J Emotional and Behavioral Disorders* 9:43–52, 2001.
70. Bickman L, Summerfelt WT, Noser K: Comparative outcomes of emotionally disturbed children and adolescents in a system of services and usual care. *Psychiatr Serv* 48:1543–1548, 1997.
71. Hoagwood K, Burns B, Kiser L, Ringeisen H, Schoenwald S: Evidence-based practice in child and adolescent mental health services. *Psychiat Svcs* 52:1179, 2001.
72. Santarcangelo S, Bruns EJ, Yoe JT: New directions: Evaluating Vermont's statewide model of individualized care. In: Epstein MH, Kutash K, Duchnowski AJ (eds): *Outcomes for Children and Youth with Behavioral and Emotional Disorders and Their Families: Programs and Evaluation best Practices.* Austin TX, Pro-Ed, 1998, pp. 55–80.
73. Rosenblatt A: Assessing the child and family outcomes of systems of care for youth with severe emotional and behavioral disturbance. In Epstein MH, Kutash K, and Duchnowski AJ (eds): *Outcomes for Children and Youth with Behavioral and Emotional Disorders and Their Families: Programs and Evaluation best Practices.* Austin, TX, Pro-Ed, 1998, pp. 55–80.
74. Foster EM, Connor T: Public cost of better mental health services for children and adolescents. *Psychiatr Serv* 56:50–55, 2005.
75. Duchnowski A, Kutash K, Friedman R: Community-based interventions in a system of care and outcomes framework. In: Burns BJ and Hoagwood K (eds): *Community Treatment for Youth: Evidence-Based Interventions for Severe Emotional and Behavioral Disorders,* 2002.
76. Stephens RL, Connor T, Nguyen H, Holden EW, Greenbaum P, Foster EM: The longitudinal comparison study of the national evaluation of the Comprehensive Community Mental Health Services for Children and Their Families Program. In: Epstein MH, Kutash K, Duchnowski AJ (eds): *Outcomes for Children and Youth with Emotional and Behavioral Disorders and Their Families: Programs and Evaluation Best Practices.* Austin: Texas, Pro-Ed, Inc., 2005.
77. Hogan MF: The President's New Freedom Commission: Recommendations to transform mental health care in America. *Psychiat Serv* 54:1467–1476, 2003.
78. Chang CF, Kiser LJ, Bailey JE, Martins M, Gibson WC, Schaberg KA, Mirvis DM, Applegate WB: Tennessee's failed managed care program for mental health and substance abuse services. *J Am Medical Association* 279:864–869, 1998.
79. Heflinger CA, Northrup DA: What happens when capitated behavioral health comes to town? The transition from the Fort Bragg demonstration to a capitated managed behavioral health contract. *J Behav Health Services and Research* 27:390–405, 2000.
80. U.S. Department of Health and Human Services: *Culture, Race, and Ethnicity: A Supplement to Mental Health: A report of the Surgeon General.* Center for Mental Health Services, Substance Abuse and Mental Health Services Administration, U.S. Department of Health and Human Services, Washington, DC, 2001b.
81. Four Racial Ethnic Panels. *Cultural Competence Standards for Managed Mental Health Services for Four Underserved/Underrepresented Racial/Ethnic Groups.* Rockville, MD, Center for Mental Health Services, Substance Abuse and Mental Health Administration, U.S. Department of Health and Human Services, 1999.
82. Pumariega AJ, Rogers, K, & Rothe, E: Culturally competent systems of care for children's mental health: Advances and challenges. *Comm Mental Health J* 41(5):539–556, 2005.
83. Shonkoff J, Phillips D: *From Neurons to Neighborhoods: The Science of Early Childhood Development. Committee on Integrating the Science of Early Childhood Development, Board on Children, Youth, and Families, Commission on Behavioral and Social Sciences and Education, National Research Council and Institute of Medicine.* Washington, DC, National Academy Press, 2000.
84. Knitzer J: Early childhood mental health services: A policy and systems development perspective. In: Shonkoff JP, Meisels SJ (eds): *Handbook of Early Childhood Intervention.* New York, Cambridge University Press, 1998.
85. Olds DL, Pettitt LM, Robinson J, Henderson, C Jr., Eckenrode J, Kitzman H, Cole B, Powers J: Reducing the risks for antisocial behavior with a program of prenatal and early childhood home visitation. *J Community Psychol* 26:65–83, 1998.
86. Zeanah CH, Larrieu JA, Heller SS, Valliere J, Hinshaw Fuselier S, Aoki Y, & Drilling M: Evaluation of a preventive intervention for maltreated infants and toddlers in foster care. *J Am Acad Child Adol Psychiat* 40:214–221, 2001.
87. Webster-Stratton C, Reid MJ, Hammond M: Treating children with early-onset conduct problems: Intervention outcomes for parent, child, and teacher training. *J Clin Child Adoles Psychol* 33:105–124, 2004.
88. ZERO TO THREE: *Diagnostic Classification of Mental Health and Developmental Disorders of Infancy and Early Childhood,* rev ed. Arlington, VA: ZERO TO THREE/National Center for Clinical Infant Programs, 2005.
89. Friesen BJ, Winters NC: The role of outcomes in systems of care: Quality improvement and program evaluation. In: Pumariega AJ and Winters NC (eds): *Handbook of Community-Based Systems of Care: The New Child and Adolescent Community Psychiatry.* New York, Jossey-Bass, 2003, pp. 459–486.
90. Woodbridge M, Furlong M, Casa JM, Sosna T: Santa Barbara's Multiagency Integrated System of Care. In: Hernandez M and Hodges (eds): *Developing Outcome Strategies in Children's Mental Health.* Baltimore: Paul H. Brookes Publishing, 2001.
91. American Academy of Child & Adolescent Psychiatry: *Best Principles for Managed Medicaid RFP's.* Washington, DC, Author, 1996.
92. American Academy of Child and Adolescent Psychiatry: *Best Principles for Measuring Outcomes in Managed Medicaid Mental Health Programs.* Washington, DC, Author, 1998.
93. Pumariega AJ, Winters NC, (eds): *Handbook of child and adolescent systems of care: The new community psychiatry.* San Francisco, Jossey-Bass, 2003.
94. American Academy of Child and Adolescent Psychiatry: *Child and Adolescent Service Intensity Instrument.* Washington, DC, Author, 2004.
95. American Academy of Child & Adolescent Psychiatry (Winters NC & Pumariega AJ, lead authors). Practice Parameters for Child Mental Health in Systems of Care. *Journal of the American Academy of Child and Adolescent Psychiatry,* 46(2):284–299.
96. Stroul BA, Pires SA, Armstrong MI: *Health Care Reform Tracking Project: Tracking State Health Care Reforms as They Affect Children and Adolescents with Behavioral Health Disorders and Their Families—2000 state survey.* Tampa, FL, Research and Training Center for Children's Mental Health, Department of Child and Family Studies, Division of State and Local Support, Louis de la Parte Florida Mental Health Institute, University of South Florida, 2001.
97. Daleiden EL, Chorpita BF: From data to wisdom: Quality improvement strategies supporting large-scale implementation of evidence-based services. *Child Adolesc Psychiatr Clin N Am* 14:329–349, 2005.
98. Hyde PS: A unique approach to designing a comprehensive behavioral health system in New Mexico. *Psychiat Serv* 55:983–985, 2004.

CHAPTER 6.4 ■ CHILD AND ADOLESCENT PSYCHIATRIC EMERGENCIES

LYNELLE E. THOMAS AND ROBERT A. KING

NATURE AND SCOPE

The emergency nature of a child or adolescent psychiatric problem is defined both by the severity and urgency of the potential threat to the child's and family's safety and wellbeing and by the community and clinical resources the family is able to access and use to address it. Thus some situations, such as intense aggressive or homicidal threats or outbursts, acute psychotic or anxiety states, serious suicide attempts, ingestions or intoxications, or acute toxic metabolic states, usually require immediate psychiatric attention in a setting that can muster the full range of immediate medical and psychiatric diagnostic and therapeutic interventions. Conversely, the presentation of many other more chronic or less urgent cases to the pediatric psychiatry emergency service (PES) reflects the absence of adequate mental health resources in the community or the family's relative inability to access or use clinical and social resources that could have prevented the crisis or permitted its management in a less acute outpatient setting. Although it is usually clear that these latter cases require prompt intervention, the perception that the case is an emergency and should be seen in a tertiary emergency service setting is more relative. For example, under what circumstances does an unhappy, neglected child's suicidal ruminations or threats indicate an imminent risk and need for crisis intervention? When does normative adolescent oppositionality or risk-taking evolve to illicit substance use, unprotected sexual activity, and other antisocial and high-risk behaviors, and at what point do these become so severe that emergency psychiatric intervention becomes urgently imperative?

The judgment that a given child's thoughts, feelings, or actions constitute a psychiatric emergency reflects some adult's perception that the child's condition is serious, urgent, or unmanageable in the current environment. As a corollary, a multiplicity of adults or agencies may potentially initiate the referral to a child psychiatric emergency service. These include parents, extended family members, teachers, police, mental health clinicians in the community, and child welfare workers (1). In addition, many facilities such as youth shelters, residential treatment centers, and juvenile detention use the hospital-based child psychiatric emergency service in the absence of adequate on-site emergency psychiatric capacities. During the academic year, middle and high schools are primary emergency department (ED) referral sources. Local and nationally publicized violence within school settings has sensitized communities and administrators to problematic behaviors. Many schools have, in turn, adopted a "zero tolerance policy" whereby youngsters must obtain "psychiatric clearance" before returning to school after having behaved in a way that was perceived as being threatening or dangerous to themselves or others (2).

Psychiatric emergencies were once considered uncommon in childhood. In recent years, however, the number of child and adolescent emergency patients has been on the rise. For example, between October 1, 1963 and July 31, 1964, the number of psychiatric consultations in the Yale–New Haven Hospital emergency department (ED) in New Haven, Connecticut, for children less than 15 years of age represented only 0.6% of the pediatric ED population (3). In contrast, the annual number of child psychiatry-related visits to the same ED was 2.5% of all pediatric visits in 1995 and 3.9% of those in 1999. Thus, by 1999, as a percentage of all ED cases, the proportion of child psychiatric emergency cases increased almost 60% over 1995 and more than five-fold compared with 1963 (4). In May 2006, psychiatry-related visits to the Yale–New Haven Hospital pediatric ED reached an all-time high of 6.6% of visits to the pediatric ED [unpublished data]. The magnitude of this clinical burden is apparent if this referral rate is extrapolated to the more than 31 million annual child and adolescent ED visits occurring nationally (5).

The root causes of these dramatic changes are unclear given the relative paucity of national data on child psychiatric ED use.

One contributing factor, the high prevalence of youth behaviors likely to result in an ED visit involving psychiatric evaluation or consultation, is amply documented by epidemiologic data. According to the national Youth Risk Behavior Survey (6), 16.9% of high school students have seriously considered suicide in the past 12 months, 13% made a suicide plan, 8.4% attempted suicide once or more, and 2.3% made a suicide attempt that resulted in an injury, poisoning, or overdose that had to be treated by a doctor or nurse. Furthermore, during the prior 12 months, 7.9% of students had been threatened or injured at least once with a weapon on school property; 3.6% of students had been in a physical fight in which they were injured and had to receive medical treatment; and 7.5% of students had ever been physically forced to have sexual intercourse when they did not want to.

In addition, dwindling funds and efforts at cost containment in mental health and community-based social service systems in many states have transformed hospital-based emergency services into a major provider of mental health services. Low Medicaid provider reimbursement rates and managed care–driven strictures have further eroded the availability of mental health resources in the community and have dramatically shortened lengths of hospital stay, thus denying many children and families adequate outpatient treatment in the community and effective inpatient treatment when that becomes necessary. Indeed, in many communities, the crisis in child PES parallels the overall crisis in ED care, as the ED becomes the primary care provider of last resort, particularly for Medicaid beneficiaries and the 45 million uninsured Americans (7).

This dearth of adequate child mental health facilities not only results in increased PES utilization, but also impacts the disposition of cases from the PES. The changing ecology of emergency psychiatric care for youth can be seen in recent trends in ED utilization and dispositions for self-injury. During the period 1997–2002, the annual rate of emergency visits for self-harm among young people aged 7 to 24 years of age was 225.3 per 100,000 (8). Approximately half of these visits (56.1%) resulted in an inpatient admission. Reflecting managed care restrictions, however, the length of stays of youngsters psychiatrically hospitalized after deliberate self-harm decreased significantly from 1990 to 2000, despite a dramatic increase in the severity of diagnoses (9, 10). (This trend of increased severity and decreased length of hospital stay for self-injury parallels that seen in overall admissions to child inpatient psychiatric services (11, 12)).

Because of a shortage of outpatient and inpatient child psychiatric services, a log jam or bottle neck crisis often prevails in hospital PES, where timely, appropriate dispositions cannot be found for many of the youngsters seen (2, 13). As a result, youngsters who cannot be discharged may end up being "boarded" on pediatric wards or in the ER itself pending the availability of an inpatient psychiatric bed. Additionally, the PES is burdened by frequent "bounceback" visits, as partially treated youngsters are discharged from inpatient services, but shortly return to the ED because they cannot be maintained at home by available outpatient resources.

Indeed, this log jam or gridlock too often prevails along the entire length of the child mental health care system, with a shortage of resources and pileup of untreated, undertreated, or inappropriately placed children at each level of care. Some children wait months for outpatient therapy and case management. Other youngsters ready for discharge from psychiatric hospitals cannot be discharged for lack of suitable subacute, residential, or community-based treatment resources. And, as always, when the predictable crises occur, the PES remains the access point of least resistance and resource of last resort.

With this background in mind, this chapter discusses the complexities of child and adolescent psychiatric emergencies and hospital-based assessment, and examines the problems confronting ED-based child and adolescent psychiatrists. We also discuss approaches to assessment, treatment, and disposition planning that are unique to this population, with a special focus on the uncooperative patient. (For the broader topics of the psychiatric evaluation of the child and the assessment of the suicidal child, see Chapter 4.2.2; Chapter 5.3.3; King et al. (14) For emergency psychiatric evaluation in the inpatient pediatric setting see King and Lewis (15).

HOSPITAL-BASED CHILD PSYCHIATRIC EMERGENCY EVALUATION

Adaptive Context of Child Psychiatric Emergencies

Child psychiatric emergencies presenting in the hospital setting are most often characterized by intense symptoms, perceived danger, and a sense of urgency complicated by the perception of imminent catastrophic outcome and frequent conflict among the parties involved. Despite this acuity, child psychiatric emergencies are usually the outcome of complex, ongoing processes rather than sudden, discrete events. Occasionally, a previously well functioning child with some underlying vulnerabilities may abruptly decompensate and display psychiatric symptoms in the presence of some critical or traumatic event or organic process. More often, however, the acute emotional or behavioral symptom that bring the youngster to the attention of the emergency service have been preceded by a longer history of emotional or behavioral difficulties. Thus, a key element of the emergency child psychiatric assessment is to answer the questions: "Who is concerned about the child?" and "Why now?"

A child's functioning and psychological wellbeing are highly dependent on the family, school, and community setting in which he or she lives and studies. Anything that adversely affects this system has the potential to precipitate a crisis. A child psychiatric emergency usually represents some perturbation or pathology in one or several of the elements in this delicately balanced ecosystem. Either an efflorescence of the child's psychopathology has overwhelmed the caretaking system and/or the caretaking system has, in some fashion, become less sufficient or less adequate. From this perspective, many child psychiatric emergencies can be conceptualized as a mismatch between needs and resources (16). The corresponding goal of child psychiatric emergency services evaluation is then to clarify the nature and the cause of the imbalance that has arisen and to identify the resources needed (safe environment, psychoeducation, psychopharmacotherapy, outpatient therapist, family support services) to restore equilibrium. Systematically clarifying the details of the precipitants to the crisis is thus paramount in determining the needed interventions and disposition.

Goals and Aims of the Hospital-Based Child Psychiatric Emergency Assessment

The primary goals of the child psychiatric emergency evaluation are, as expeditiously as possible:

1. To obtain each informant's account of the reason for referral
2. To develop a working alliance, if possible, with the patient and other involved parties around the assessment and disposition planning
3. To obtain a focused developmental history of the child's current difficulties and prior functioning against the backdrop of the child's family, current living situation, and any involved clinicians or agencies, with particular attention to the possible precipitants of the current crisis
4. To perform a mental status examination, with particular attention to evidence of suicidal or homicidal ideation, hallucinations, delusions, or thought disorder; evidence of confusion, disorientation, or other signs of delirium; and intense anxiety
5. To develop a differential diagnosis, including a formulation of what changing factors have precipitated the need for emergency evaluation at the present time
6. To arrive at a judgment regarding the degree of probable risk to the patient's safety or that of others
7. To identify interventions that will help to contain and ameliorate the patient's difficulties
8. To plan and implement a disposition
9. To collaborate effectively with other clinicians and care providers involved in the case, both within and beyond the hospital setting

General Considerations

The hospital ED is designed to contain and resolve urgent or life-threatening situations. The "triage model"—rapid determination of imminent dangerousness, containment, and referral—typifies the process of most hospital-based psychiatric emergency consultation and care. Some beleaguered psychiatric emergency services confine themselves to addressing only two questions: a) Is the child a danger to himself or others? b) Does the child need to be hospitalized or can he or she be discharged back home? Although these dispositional questions must remain at the forefront of the busy emergency clinician's mind, circumscribing the evaluation too narrowly to these areas both precludes an accurate understanding of the clinical situation and renders the ED visit of little ongoing value to the child, family, or treatment effort. Given that most crisis referrals arise out of multiple factors in the child's life, it is important that, no matter how expeditiously the evaluation is conducted, it provides the child, family, and clinicians with some useful perspective on how the crisis came about and how it fits into the overall trajectory of the child's life and clinical care.

The assessment and management of child psychiatric emergencies differ from the routine office evaluation in several important ways. The severity, dangerousness, or urgency of the symptoms usually requires rapid clinical decision-making and treatment implementation. Furthermore, the emergency assessment must often proceed under unpropitious circumstances constrained by time pressures, in the relative absence of trained support personnel or optimal physical arrangements, with unfamiliarity with the patient and family, the unavailability of key informants, and the lack of timely, appropriate alternatives for disposition.

Yet another constraint on emergency evaluations is the inconvenient hours at which they often occur—late at night or on weekends, when important informants, such as primary clinicians, teachers, or social welfare agency workers may be unavailable. The already difficult task of arranging an appropriate disposition at such hours is further complicated by the frequent unavailability of insurance reviewers needed for precertification, psychiatric hospital admissions staff members who can provide prompt information regarding bed availability, or outpatient clinicians who can undertake the responsibility of seeing the patient promptly for follow-up. The availability of sufficient social work, psychiatric nursing, or other professional staff members to assist in these information-gathering and coordinating tasks is essential to prevent burnout of clinicians faced with large volumes of child emergency evaluations.

Time constraints and the urgency of the situation do, of course, require that the clinician be active in eliciting the most relevant data in a time-efficient manner. Right from the onset of the interview process, the experienced emergency clinician begins to prioritize symptoms and to formulate and test tentative etiologic and diagnostic hypotheses that guide further questions. At the same time, the clinician also begins to ponder what interventions and dispositions these diagnostic hypotheses imply. Unlike less urgent settings, the emphasis is on clarifying the child's current symptoms and functioning, the factors in the child's living situation that have served to stabilize or exacerbate difficulties, and the resources and competencies available to the patient and the family.

Physical Setting

It is important to find a quiet evaluation area, where the clinician, adults, and child will not be frequently distracted by the sights and sounds of physically ill and upset children and their families. The area needs to be free enough of dangerous or delicate medical equipment or furnishings so the clinician need not be preoccupied with keeping the room and the patient safe. The spot needs to be secluded enough that the belligerent or uncooperative psychiatric patient will not disturb other families in the ED, yet near enough to other staff that reinforcements can be called on if needed for safety or calming or to prevent elopement.

Informants

The clinician's first task is to identify why this particular child has been brought to the ED at this particular time. The impetus for child psychiatric emergency referrals, with few exceptions, comes from adults in the child's life, rather than from the child. Obtaining a full and accurate diagnostic picture for any child psychiatric assessment requires gathering information from diverse sources, including the family, school staff, clinicians, and the child himself. In the emergency situation, however, the initial or primary informant may be an adult other than the primary caretaker, for example, police or corrections officers, school personnel, or representatives of various social service agencies. The wide array of potential referents and perspectives complicates the task of the evaluator, who must efficiently interview multiple informants and, like a detective, rapidly consolidate and reconcile sparse, often conflicting data.

From a practical standpoint, data are collected as they become available. At a minimum, the emergency assessment entails direct interviews with the child and all adults who accompany the child to the hospital setting, as well as any caretakers, clinicians, or caseworkers who are accessible by telephone. On a practical level, if the child is brought in by nonparental parties (friends, police, correctional officers, or child welfare workers) who may not want to remain in the ED for the evaluation, it is essential to speak with them directly and to obtain immediate contact information for those persons with direct knowledge of the precipitating crisis and the child's recent circumstances and responsibility for the child's care and disposition. Even when the child is not accompanied by a custodial parent or legal guardian, most states give the emergency clinicians the latitude to initiate emergency treatment of a child, including contacting of collateral informants, without parental consent. In such cases, it is always clinically desirable to contact and to involve the parents as soon as possible. Many states also permit adolescents to seek mental health services without a parent's involvement. These patients should also be encouraged to involve parents and other adult supports.

The presenting complaint and reasons for the referral are often described very differently, depending on the informant. These discrepancies, referred to in the research literature as *informant variance,* arise for a variety of reasons (17). Although these discrepancies complicate the diagnostician's task, when markedly differing accounts or divergences of perspective do occur, they provide potentially important clues to the nature of the child's crisis. At the very least, they point to troublesome lacks of continuity in the child's holding environment and a lack of shared consensus between the child and important adults.

Differences may stem from the different contexts in which the child is observed, the standard of judgment employed, and variations in the demands or stressors impinging on the child in each setting. This is particularly the case when children's symptoms are situation specific (occurring only at school, only at home, or only at one parent's house, but not the other's).

Informants may differ in their access to information concerning the child's feelings and behavior. Parents may be quick to report a behavior of the child that they find disturbing or annoying, especially externalizing behavior, but they may be less aware of internalizing problems (18) and may fail to recognize how discord within the family system (domestic violence, separation, divorce) may directly precipitate crisis symptoms within the child.

The child, in contrast, even if aware of and able to describe the problematic behavior verbally, may refrain from doing so out of defensiveness, shame, or fear of reproach. The interviewer must also be aware that vagueness and minimization of problems can sometimes indicate an attempt to maintain some secret within the family system, such as a parental mental illness, illegal activity, child or parental substance abuse, domestic violence, or physical or sexual abuse. In these cases, the evaluation can be extremely difficult, because the events surrounding the crisis may never be completely clarified.

Child Interview

In traditional office-based child psychiatric assessment, several hours and more than one interview with the child are usually desirable to place the child at ease with the interviewer and to obtain a full picture of the child. In contrast, the emergency assessment must be completed within the confines of a single interview. The emergency child interview and mental status examination must also reckon with the characteristic lability of children and their propensity to fall back to more immature or oppositional ways of coping, especially when they are confronted with the anxiety and distress associated with a hospital ED setting. Although it may not accurately reveal the child's optimal or characteristic level of functioning, this "snapshot" of the child in the ED often provides a valid picture of the child's vulnerability to regress under stress and how such regression may have led to the emergency referral.

Although every effort must be made to place the child at ease and to obtain his or her cooperation in understanding what has brought about the crisis, this is often difficult. The high levels of expressed emotion in the events leading up to ED referrals and the coercive processes required to bring the child to the ED often stimulate the child's oppositionality. As a result, the child in the ED is often sullen, mute, withdrawn, or antagonistic.

To the child who is aggrieved or sullenly refusing to talk, the clinician can validly invoke what has been termed the "constructive use of ignorance" by observing that, because they have never met before, the clinician really does not know what has led up to the ED visit and would genuinely like to hear the child's view of what has been happening.

Child Mental Status Examination

The mental status examination is of particular importance in the emergency evaluation (see Chapter 4.2.2) (19). In trying to understand the nature of the crisis and the interventions needed, the clinician will be especially attentive to evidence of psychosis, delirium, or other organic process, intoxication, dissociation, or extreme anxiety, depression, or elation. The presence of any of these factors is likely to render the patient more labile and vulnerable and points to the need for more intensive interventions and diagnostic studies. Hence, the clinician must be alert to and explicitly note the presence of the following:

- Disorientation, confusion, and fluctuating levels of consciousness
- Incoherence of thought or speech
- Evidence of hallucinations or delusions
- Impaired memory
- Slurred speech, ataxia, or apraxia

Assessment of safety additionally requires explicit attention to the following:

- The presence of suicidal or homicidal ideation
- Aggressive threats or ideation
- Impulsivity
- Proneness to regression or agitation during the interview
- Poor judgment and insight and limited intelligence
- Mood lability

Family Mental Status

The child's and parents' attitudes toward the examiner and toward each other during the interview provide valuable clues to whether the child and family can be effectively and safely worked with in an outpatient setting if the child is discharged home from the ED. Hence, the examiner will note carefully how the child and family interact, how the child relates to the examiner, and to what extent the child can own and reflect on the behaviors that have led to the ED visit.

To what extent can the child and parents, with the examiner's help, at least partially agree about the problems that must be addressed and achieve a working consensus about possible realistic (nonmagical) ways of working on them? In the absence of such a consensus, outpatient followup is not likely to be feasible or successful, as for example, when the child persists in denying any problem or when the child and parent remain locked in mutual recrimination. If the referral for emergency assessment comes from adults or agencies other than the parents (neighbors, police responding to a family disturbance, or school personnel concerned about a student's behavior), both child and family may portray the "problem" as the result of the school or neighbors' unreasonable expectations or the derelictions of others. This posture of defensive externalization also bodes ill for enlisting the child's and family's cooperation with any treatment recommendations. Conversely, families and children who, with admitted concern, recognize that certain problematic behavior patterns recur in their family may be more likely to have the commitment to make the transition from crisis intervention to ongoing outpatient treatment.

UNCOOPERATIVE OR AGGRESSIVE PATIENT

Special Considerations

We now consider special challenges posed by the uncooperative or aggressive patient. Oppositional and aggressive outbursts at school or at home are frequent precipitants of ED visits. Many such youngsters are brought to the ED by either police or emergency medical services, sometimes in physical restraints. In the ED, such children and adolescents often continue to be agitated, belligerent, and impulsive. Profanity, yelling, and verbal threats are unnerving and upsetting to the clinician, ED staff, and other families and children in the ED.

Aggressive or violently oppositional behavior is perhaps the most difficult management challenge facing the child psychiatry emergency clinician. The clinician must approach the potentially violent patient calmly but cautiously, with the twin goals of performing an assessment and simultaneously bolstering the child or adolescent's capacity to remain in behavioral control.

Establishing the Differential Diagnosis

The assessment of the aggressive, agitated patient begins with an evaluation of the possible causes. Aggressive behavior can occur in the context of a wide spectrum of psychiatric conditions. Thus, establishing a differential diagnosis is important in choosing short-term interventions and developing a disposition and longer term treatment plans.

The cause of oppositional, aggressive, and ultimately violent behavior in children and adolescents is usually multidetermined. It evolves from a transaction between the child's temperament and immediate environment, and both social and psychological factors and neurobiological processes influence it.

Poor impulse control is an important risk factor for aggressive outbursts. Impulsivity is a symptom common to several mental disorders of childhood and adolescence, most notably attention deficit disorders, hypomania, and conduct disorder. Children with cognitive deficits and developmental delays, such as mental retardation, autism, or other pervasive developmental disabilities, may have a limited repertoire of social coping skills and hence may react to stress and frustrations with aggressive behaviors.

Children reared in poorly structured, chaotic, or violence-prone families, and children who have been chronically or acutely traumatized may exhibit maladaptive, aggressive behaviors in response to stress or confrontation. Especially in adolescents, substance use is a common precipitant of disruptive, aggressive behavior by virtue of impairing judgment, increasing irritability, disinhibiting behavior, and exposing the youngster to potentially threatening situations. Underlying psychotic states, especially those characterized by mania, paranoia, or command auditory hallucinations, are also associated with agitated, aggressive behaviors.

It is also important to be alert for various organic conditions that can result in irritable, aggressive, or disorganized behavior (20). Toxic metabolic states, whether from ingestions, medication side effects, encephalopathies, or other medical illness, can produce delirium with disorganized and aggressive behavior. Neurologic conditions associated with irritability and aggressive behavioral outbursts include postconcussive states, frontal lobe lesions, and temporal lobe epilepsy. Hence, a careful medical history, including medications and substance use, is important (15). Finally, the overstimulating, chaotic, and confining nature of the ED itself can exacerbate anxiety, irritability, and aggressive impulses for many patients and families.

Specific Aspects of the Assessment

Data crucial for rendering an accurate portrayal of the context include a history of recent and past aggressive behavior, as well as psychiatric, family, and social information. A detailed history of the presenting violent episode is mandatory. This includes preceding and precipitating events, the details of the episode itself, and its aftermath. It is important to elicit the patient's own perspectives regarding the episode and to compare these with the perspectives of the other involved or witnessing parties. The social setting and behavior of the victim and the response of others in the environment should be clarified. The precipitant of such challenges is often a clash between the child and an adult authority figure over limit setting. The role of narcissistic injury, humiliation, intense anxiety, or challenges to the child's autonomy, self-concept, or inability of the youngster to escape from such challenges should be sought in the interview. It is important to assess and document the following in the child or adolescent (21):

1. The degree of premeditation and planning versus impulsiveness (22)
2. Ego syntonicity or dystonicity
3. Consistency with the patient's past behaviors or style (including chronic bullying)
4. Extraordinary or uncontrolled rage and use of weapons
5. The validity of perceived self-defense
6. Evidence of grossly impaired judgment or consciousness
7. Bizarre or delusional behavior or thought content
8. Risk of self-injury during the violent episode
9. The extent to which the child can remember the details of the episode (including his actions and their consequence), accept responsibility, or express remorse

Each of these variables has implications for diagnosis and disposition.

Management

Basic Tenets

In approaching the emergency assessment of the potentially violent patient, the first and overriding consideration should be that of safety: the safety of the patient, the safety of others, and the clinician's own safety. A patient must be under behavioral control before a thorough medical and psychiatric evaluation can be conducted. Safety can be maintained and harm averted in the following ways.

The clinician should always be polite and respectful to the patient and concerned parties. Maintaining a calm atmosphere and avoiding irritable and counteraggressive responses go a long way toward diffusing hostile interactions. The clinician should never be isolated with an aggressive patient without the ability to summon assistance. Placing oneself between the patient and the door permits exiting without obstruction, should the need arise. It is important to be attentive to one's own feelings of discomfort, anger, or threat, because these feelings provide important cues alerting the clinician to the potential for violence and the need to seek help.

Setting

The interview and waiting area should also be free of sharps, cords, or other potentially hazardous furnishings or medical equipment that are unfortunately ubiquitous to most emergency examination rooms. Interviews should be conducted in a space that will allow some degree of privacy and decreased stimulation. The interview area should, however, also allow some level of visual surveillance from the outside and ease of physical access should summoning staff assistance or security personnel become necessary. An easily identifiable alarm code should be used to alert other staff members to potential or actual violence. The space must also be adaptable to facilitate seclusion and restraint, if needed; restraints should be available nearby in areas where violence could occur.

Behavioral Interventions

Protocols for managing disruptive or aggressive pediatric patients should include algorithms for the progression of interventions, from least to most restrictive and invasive. Clarity of communication and firm limit-setting are essential and may be effective at de-escalating a potentially violent situation. Staff should supportively and firmly communicate to the patient and family what will and will not be tolerated in the ED, while at the same time offering a small range of acceptable alternatives.

When agitation is the result of organic causes and is accompanied by confusion and disorganization, particular attention is necessary to try to keep the patient carefully monitored and oriented. This can be accomplished by diminishing stimulation while maintaining adequate levels of lighting to avoid sensory ambiguity. It is often helpful to provide a staff companion or family member to remind the patient of where they are and to inform him or her of what is happening. Caution with sedation is needed, so as not to obscure fluctuations in level of consciousness.

"Chemical Restraint"

If these behavioral measures do not succeed, it is at this stage that the need for immediate medication should be assessed. The Centers for Medicare and Medicaid Services defines chemical restraint as "a drug used to control behavior or to restrict a patient's freedom of movement that is not standard treatment for the patient's medical or psychiatric condition" (23). There is no specific acute pharmacologic treatment for violent behavior per se. However, "nonspecific sedation" is frequently used in the management of acutely agitated patients, whatever the cause. The choice of agent is based on consideration of: 1) the severity of the target symptom; 2) the goals of the intervention; 3) the underlying diagnosis; 4) the patient's current other medications, allergies, medical problems, side effect profile, and if available, past history of medication response (24).

Antipsychotic and/or benzodiazepines are the most commonly used agents. Haloperidol and lorazepam are perhaps the most commonly used agents and are available in most pediatric EDs. Lorazepam is a nonspecific, sedative-hypnotic benzodiazepine that is readily absorbed after oral or intramuscular administration. It has a relatively short half-life (10 to 20 hours) and produces no active metabolites. In addition to sedation and anxiolytic properties, benzodiazepines have the advantage of reversibility with the benzodiazepine antagonist, flumazenil. Dosing in children ranges from 1 to 2 mg orally or intramuscularly every hour until sedation is achieved. Although useful at times, the benzodiazepines can also be associated with paradoxical disinhibition, particularly at lower doses, and in children and adolescents as compared to adults.

Haloperidol (Haldol) is a high-potency butyrophenone antipsychotic that has been has been shown to be more efficacious than lorazepam in controlling violent behavior in adult psychiatric patients (25). Haloperidol may be given in doses of 2 to 5 mg intramuscularly or orally. The dose may be repeated in 1 hour if necessary to achieve sedation. When compared with the lower potency antipsychotics (such as chlorpromazine), haloperidol causes less hypotension and less decrease of the seizure threshold, and it has fewer anticholinergic side effects. Despite these advantages, many clinicians prefer the more sedating low-potency agents, such as chlorpromazine (Thorazine), which is given at 0.25 to 0.50 mg/kg per dose orally or intramuscularly. This dose may be repeated in 1 hour if necessary to achieve sedation. Caution must be exercised when administering chlorpromazine intramuscularly, as it can easily lead to orthostatic hypotension and tachyarrhythmias when dosed too aggressively. As a general rule, IM doses should be half of oral equivalents (25 mg im corresponding to 50 mg po).

Some pediatric settings use the soporific antihistamine diphenhydramine (Benadryl) for sedating agitated, nonpsychotic pediatric psychiatric patients. It is readily available and is safely administered orally as well as intramuscularly. Caution is required, however, because both diphenhydramine and the benzodiazepines can idiosyncratically cause behavioral disinhibition or agitation in some children (particularly those with brain injury or mental retardation), thereby increasing behavioral dyscontrol. In addition, caution must be exercised not to compound anticholinergic/antihistamine "load." For example, the unintended or overzealous combination of chlorpromazine and diphenhydramine can easily lead to disinhibition, confusion, or frank delirium.

When choosing a pharmacologic approach to rapid tranquilization of children and adolescents, any concurrent medications and medical conditions must be taken into consideration to identify possible adverse drug interactions or contraindications. If there appears to be an underlying psychotic process, delirium, or agitation caused by substance abuse, a neuroleptic may be indicated. If an antipsychotic is used, the physician should also consider the prophylactic administration of diphenhydramine (Benadryl), 25 to 50 mg per dose, or benztropine (Cogentin) 1 to 2 mg, to prevent acute dystonic side effects, while taking into account any other anticholinergic drugs the patient is receiving. As with any other medication, ED staff should monitor the patient's vital signs and level of consciousness and should be alert to the possibility of side effects such as acute dystonic reactions (oculogyric crisis, torticollis).

There is less experience with the use of the newer atypical antipsychotics (olanzapine, quetiapine, risperidone, ziprasidone) for acute chemical restraint. These agents may also be helpful in the management of acute aggression, underlying psychosis or delirium, but their use in acute contexts is limited by several factors, including the lack of an injectable form for many of these agents (24).

If the indication for an antipsychotic is less clear (as is often the case in pediatric populations), the choice of sedating agent will depend more on the balance of the risk-to-benefit profiles of antipsychotic versus benzodiazepines, on the patient's history of previous treatment with a similar agent, and on physician and institutional experience, preferences, and practices.

The choice of route of administration also depends on the severity of the target symptoms and the cooperation of the youngster, as well as the available drug formulations. In general, intramuscular injection of a sedative has a faster onset of action than oral medication. Liquid oral preparations are preferable to tablets, because they cannot be as easily "cheeked" or sequestered. Some children and adolescents may calm down readily after accepting an oral medication. Perhaps this is the result of some anticipatory sedation and the sense of relief that the adults have taken action to control the situation. Offering the child the option of taking the medication orally, rather than by injection, is preferable if the situation permits. Not only is it less invasive, but also it enlists the child in the task of exerting control over his upset. Often, however, the threat of violence quickly escalates beyond the point at which a child or adolescent can ally and cooperate with these less restrictive and invasive measures. Such patients must often be physically restrained before they can be approached to offer or give sedative medication.

Physical Restraint

The Centers for Medicare and Medicaid Services and the Joint Commission on Accreditation of Healthcare Organizations mandate the standards and guidelines for hospital-based use of behavioral restraint and seclusion and subsequent monitoring. The Centers for Medicare and Medicaid Services standards specify that "restraint or seclusion should only be reserved for those situations when a patient's behavior becomes aggressive or violent, presenting an immediate danger to his/her safety or that of others" (23). Patients must be released from restraints when the goals of the treatment have been achieved, that is, when the patient and the patient's behavior are under control and no longer pose a threat to self or others or a further disruption to the therapeutic milieu.

Every accredited facility must have explicitly formulated restraint and seclusion policies and procedures particular to its institution. Staff members of all disciplines should be knowledgeable and trained in protocols for managing dangerous behavior. Elements of such a protocol should include the following:

1. *The indications for ordering and application of restraint. Example*: Restraints must be used only when less restrictive measure have been found to be ineffective in preventing risk of harm to self or others.
2. *Clarification of personnel and roles. Example*: The selected leader of the restraint determines the number of staff members required for a restraint and the need for hospital security staff and assigns each staff member to a specific task (e.g., restraining a particular limb, clearing a room).
3. *Guidelines for monitoring the restrained child. Example*: A staff person must be assigned to monitor the child continuously and to assess for restriction of airway, change in breathing pattern, decreased circulation, or increased body temperature.
4. *Guidelines for evaluation, reassessment, and removal of restraints. Example*: A physician or other licensed,

independent practitioner must see the patient and evaluate the need for restraint within 1 hour after the initiation of this intervention. Reassessment and contemporaneous documentation of the need for continuation of restraint must be done by a designated staff person every 2 hours for a child aged 9 to 17 years and every hour for a child less than 9 years old. Orders for continuation of restraint must be written by a physician or other licensed, independent practitioner. When a child shows behavioral control and can verbally contract for safety, he or she must be removed from restraints.

RISK ASSESSMENT AND DISPOSITION PLANNING

The assessment of risk is a difficult and anxiety-provoking task for the clinician, yet it is an inescapable part of the psychiatric emergency service assessment process. Child psychiatric and forensic psychiatric clinical researchers continue to search for clinical tools and algorithms that might permit richer, more accurate contextualized risk predictions of future violent outcome (22, 26, 27). Despite these efforts, there remains a paucity of empirically validated guidelines for acute risk assessment.

The history, interview of child and adult informants, and the mental status examination usually provide the emergency clinician with the data for a tentative formulation of diagnostic possibilities and the factors that have led to the current crisis and emergency referral. The crucial dispositive question facing the emergency clinician, however, is whether the child can now return to the current living situation with additional interventions and supports or whether some other more intensive, secure, or restrictive disposition must be found, such as admission to an inpatient psychiatric or pediatric ward or other therapeutic residential setting. This crucial decision hinges, in turn, largely on an estimation of the child's probable risk to self or others.

Some cases are clear cut. The child with a medically serious ingestion or other suicide attempt, active delirium or acute intoxication, or florid psychosis requires medical or psychiatric hospitalization. Similarly, a child who remains acutely aggressive or agitated despite crisis assessment and interventions in the ED also requires a secure placement.

In other cases, however, the assessment of risk and its implications are more complex. For example, a child's immediate suicidality or assaultiveness may subside during the course of the ED evaluation, but some youngsters remain prone to precipitous decompensations because of psychotic regression, ongoing substance abuse, or extreme reactivity to a chaotic or hostile living situation. When, as is often the case, it appears that these conditions are very likely to recur, hospitalization may be desirable, especially if outpatient treatment or intensive in-home services have already proved unfeasible or insufficient. Among the relative factors suggesting the need for more intensive intervention are a deteriorating course with recurrent crises; poor impulse control, judgment, and insight; escalating risky behaviors (dangerous driving, promiscuous or unsafe sexual activity, physical fights, substance use); or increasing self-mutilative behavior, such as self-cutting, even if not with suicidal intent.

Assessing the Context-Specific Aspects of the Crisis

Assessing the context-specific aspects of the crisis is particularly important in weighing risk in these more relative cases. For example, many children and adolescents can become violent or destructive in one setting, such as home or school, and yet show little or no dangerous propensities in other settings, such as in the hospital or outpatient clinic. Making a prediction based solely on the child's behavior in the ED, then, may have little predictive value as to subsequent behavior after discharge. By the same token, a child who initially presents as aggressive or threatening may not always require inpatient hospitalization if appropriate interventions can be made in the setting in which the crisis occurred (21). For example, most child and adolescent emergency visits for aggressive or suicidal threats or behaviors occur in the context of conflict with immediate caretakers. Effective crisis family intervention, psychoeducation, and short-term problem solving in the ED may result in temporary amelioration and resolution of the family crisis.

Although managed care has disingenuously perpetrated the myth that "medical necessity" is an unambiguously determined criterion and synonymous with imminent risk to self or others, the judgment of risk and clinical indications for hospitalization are not easily decided in many cases. Disposition is often "the art of the possible." Locating an inpatient bed and obtaining insurance authorization when needed are often difficult and time consuming. It is important, however, for the clinician not to confuse these pragmatic considerations with his or her own clinical judgment of what is optimal for a given child.

LEGAL CONSIDERATIONS

Mental health clinicians should be familiar with the state laws and institutional regulations that apply to the emergency psychiatric evaluation and treatment of minors, as well as those mandating reporting of physical or sexual abuse (28). The clinician should also know whom to contact in the hospital administration to obtain legal guidance when necessary.

In terms of the clinician's own legal vulnerability, one of the most important elements in decreasing legal exposure is scrupulous documentation of a thorough clinical assessment and good faith judgment in weighing the risks and benefits of one's actions for the patient. The duty to warn a clearly identified potential victim of a serious threat of imminent harm by a patient (e.g., divulging relevant findings about an adolescent's expressed intent to harm a another person) takes precedent over confidentiality (29). Needs for communication should be documented and handled openly, in adherence to state laws and institutional rules.

State statutes vary in their provisions and due process rights governing the certification, psychiatric hospital admission, and discharge of mentally disabled minors. In the state of Connecticut, for example, the statute regarding involuntary psychiatric hospitalization states that "if a physician determines that a child is in need of immediate hospitalization for evaluation or treatment of a mental disorder, the child may be hospitalized under an emergency or diagnostic certificate" (30). In many states, these statutes provide greater latitude in compelling the involuntary psychiatric inpatient treatment of minors than of adults. States vary as to the age under which parents may psychiatrically hospitalize a minor under a "voluntary" admission status, even without the minor's assent, as well as the age at which a minor may contest such a hospitalization or may be entitled to a court hearing.

SYSTEMS ISSUES

Optimizing the Emergency Department Setting for Emergency Child Psychiatric Services

Even in specialized pediatric hospitals, ED personnel often have little training or comfort in handling child behavioral health emergencies. Preoccupied with large numbers of seriously ill children, ED staff members may look on psychiatric patients as a nuisance, tangential to the ED's perceived "real" mission and diverting vital space, time, and personnel resources away from the "truly medically ill patients." This skeptical atmosphere often pervades the setting and results in implicit and explicit pressures for the mental health clinicians to be quick in their assessment and to discharge psychiatric emergency patients who may appear to the medical and nursing staff as disruptive, uncooperative, or unpleasant.

To counteract these potentially divisive staff tensions and resolve obstacles, ongoing collaborative efforts are needed at both the individual and system levels to communicate with ED staff and for the different services involved to communicate effectively regarding their goals and activities. Periodically scheduled meetings that bring together ED psychiatric and pediatric physicians, nursing, and social work leadership are important, because the large numbers of rotating staff involved (reflecting the nature of emergency work as occurring 24 hours a day, 7 days a week) make collaboration difficult.

The use of child psychiatric nurses to provide in-service training and consultation to ED nursing staff helps to bridge some of the interdisciplinary issues that arise in the ED. In addition, the availability of trained childcare workers with inpatient psychiatric experience who can assist with the management of child psychiatric patients in the ED decreases some of the demands on busy ED nursing staff.

Unless designed with mental health service needs in mind, the physical setting of many EDs is also suboptimal for conducting child psychiatric evaluations. One important focus of collaborative planning with ED staff is the identification or development of designated areas suitable for these purposes.

Coordination of Emergency Department Services with Outside Systems of Care

All too often, child psychiatric emergency visits contribute to a pattern of fragmented care by taking place in isolation from the child's ongoing treatment (if any) and with little or no assurance of adequate followup. To some extent, the lack of adequate communication is often the result of the late hour and the unavailability (even by telephone) of key informants and care providers (outpatient therapists, school personnel), as well as the constraints of busy ED clinicians who may have to deal with large numbers of patients with little time, sleep, or support staff.

Both in individual cases and on an institutional basis, however, it is essential to foster better communication. An attempt to contact referring or treating outpatient clinicians should always be made, and, even if not available, they should be notified (with the requisite consents) that their patient has been seen in the ED. Community clinicians and institutions (residential treatment centers, detention centers, shelters) should be encouraged to call before or at the time of sending a child to the ED, to provide necessary history, information, and disposition collaboration. To as great an extent as possible, it is also important to develop good institutional relationships with referring institutions and receiving acute psychiatric hospitals, including regular channels for communication about children sent from the ED for hospitalization.

When children are discharged home from the ED with recommendations for outpatient follow-up, definite arrangements (specifying time and therapist) should be made if possible before the child leaves the ED. There are a number of studies demonstrating that when the referring clinician contacts the accepting agency rather than simply suggesting that the patient or family do it, the rate of completed treatment can be increased significantly, even doubled (31). Obviously, this is easiest if the child and family will be returning to the ongoing care of a familiar clinician. Some child outpatient clinics reserve one or two appointment slots each day for urgent visits, to which patients seen in the ED the previous evening can be referred. If the child is not already in treatment, the likelihood of timely followup care is more uncertain. In the days following an emergency presentation, other priorities (such as family constraints, employment/financial stressors, lack of transportation) may loom larger than the original psychiatric crisis now abated by a brief ED-based crisis intervention. Some families seek out crisis-based care because they have difficulty sustaining the commitment of longer term outpatient therapies. Empirical studies of young suicide attempters seen in the ED and referred for outpatient therapy find that only about one-third ever keep even a single outpatient followup appointment (32–35).

In order to maximize the probability of successful followup referral, some programs have developed promising innovative interventions to build a preliminary alliance between the mental health care system and the family while still in the ED. For example, Spirito et al. successfully implemented an ED-based problem solving intervention that increased adolescent suicide attempters' overall adherence to outpatient treatment (36).

Beyond the practical constraints of individual and family factors, physical proximity, and actual availability of follow-up care, "cultural proximity and accessibility" or lack thereof is an often ignored but critical obstacle to behavioral health access. This is particularly true within cultural minority groups and other disadvantaged communities (2). For more information on cultural considerations in child and adolescent psychiatric emergency assessment and disposition planning see Pumariega and Rothe (37).

FUTURE DIRECTIONS

Restructuring the Mental Health Care System

In many cases, emergency clinicians struggle with the quandary that it appears unsafe to permit a given child to return home with only traditional clinic-based outpatient services in place. Yet hospitalization, even if available, seems unlikely to provide more than a brief respite, especially if only very short term and at a great geographic remove from home (hence precluding effective family work). Because of the frequent dearth of accessible inpatient psychiatric services for children seen in the ED, there has been an urgent need to develop alternative dispositions, as exemplified by the federally sponsored Comprehensive Community Mental Health Services for Children and Their Families Program initiative (10). Such alternative paradigms and programs focus on diverting child patients in crisis from inpatient hospital settings to a spectrum of well integrated wraparound community-based services that include intensive in-home services, multisystemic therapy (38), and/or day treatment facilities that emphasize existing family strengths, resources and problem solving (39) (see Chapter 6.3.2 on MST/IICAPS). The wider availability of such services has been shown to obviate the need for less urgent ED child psychiatry visits and ultimately to contain behavioral health care costs. Some models include mobile capacity and afford crisis evaluation and treatment with a focus on rapid stabilization and follow-along until access to the next level of care becomes available (40). Another innovative model is the "rapid response" approach of Greenfield et al. (41), which provided vigorous systematic clinical followup by a designated outpatient team for youngsters discharged from the pediatric ER following assessment for a suicidal event; compared to patients receiving standard care, the rapid response group at follow up had a significantly lower rate of hospitalization and suicidality and improved functioning.

Emergency Department-Based Interventions

The high emotions and crisis atmosphere generated by an ED PES visit presents a brief period of a few hours in which the youngster as well as the family may be, for the first time, ready to receive help and engage in change (42, 43). Recent studies demonstrate the potential benefits of structured emergency room interventions for specific psychiatric problems that seek to better leverage this window of opportunity by fostering structural change or shifts in patients' and families' perception of the events leading up to the ER visit (44, 45).

Rotheram-Borus et al. (43), for example, developed an ER-based intervention that helped families and youngsters reframe their understanding of the child's suicidal crisis. This brief intervention, targeted at a Hispanic population, consisted of the child and family viewing a soap opera–style video about a teen's suicide attempt, followed by participation in a family therapy session while still in the ER. Extensive training was also provided to staff in implementing the intervention. Follow up found that the intervention was effective, at modest cost, in improving adherence to outpatient therapy and reducing subsequent depression scores.

Comparing the impact of a specialized, structured motivational interview intervention with standard care in adolescents presenting to the ED with elevated blood alcohol level and history of problematic alcohol use, Spirito et al. (46) found the structured intervention resulted in significantly greater improvement in alcohol use outcomes (average number of drinking days per month and frequency of high-volume drinking).

CONCLUSION

Hospital-based PES continue to operate on the frontline of a child and adolescent behavioral health system in which service access remains delayed, limited, or unavailable. The high rates and shifting ecology of child psychiatric ED service use and limitations highlight largely understudied important questions regarding how child psychiatric services are actually used and how they might be more efficiently organized. If the hospital-based PES is to provide more than a Band-Aid or triage function for the increasing volume of seriously emotionally disturbed youth seen, it will be essential to develop more effective, rigorously evaluated acute interventions and means of linking the PES to more comprehensive systems of care.

References

1. Halamanaris PV, Anderson TR: Children and adolescents in the psychiatric emergency setting. *Psychiatr Clin North Am* 22:865–874, 1999.
2. Thomas LE: Trends and shifting ecologies: Part I. *Child & Adolescent Psychiatric Clinics of North America* 12(4):599–611, 2003.
3. Schowalter JE, Solnit AJ: Child psychiatry consultation in a general hospital emergency room. *J Am Acad Child Psychiatry* 5:534–551, 1966.
4. Santucci KA, Sather J, Baker MD: Psychiatry-related visits to the pediatric emergency department: A growing epidemic? (abstract). *Ambulatory Pediatric Association annual meeting*, Boston, MA, 2000.
5. American Academy of Pediatrics: Care of children in the emergency department. *Pediatrics* 107:777–781, 2001.
6. Centers for Disease Control and Prevention. Youth risk behavior surveillance, United States, 2005. *Morb Mortal Wkly Rep* 55(SS-5):1–108, 2006.
7. Institute of Medicine. Hospital-based emergency care: At the breaking point. *The Future of Emergency Care* (www.iom.edu/CMS/3809/16107/35007.aspx). Accessed July 21, 2006.
8. Olfson M, Gameroff MJ, Marcus SC, Greenberg T, Shaffer D: Emergency treatment of young people following deliberate self-harm. *Archives of General Psychiatry* 62(10):1122–1128, 2005.
9. Olfson M, Gameroff MJ, Marcus SC, et al.: National trends in hospitalization of youth with intentional self-inflicted injuries. *Am J Psychiatry* 162:1328–1335, 2005.
10. Harpaz-Rotem I. Commentary on Olfson M, Gameroff MJ, Marcus SC, et al.: [National trends in hospitalization of youth with intentional self-inflicted injuries. *Am J Psychiatry* 162:1328–1335, 2005.] *Evid. Based Ment. Health* 9:26–, 2006.
11. Harpaz-Rotem I, Leslie DL, Martin A, et al.: Changes in child and adolescent inpatient psychiatric admission diagnoses between 1995 and 2000. *Soc Psychiatry Psychiatr Epidemiol* 40:642–647, 2005.
12. Martin A, Leslie D. Psychiatric inpatient, outpatient, and medication utilization and costs among privately insured youths, 1997–2000. *American Journal of Psychiatry* 160(4):757–764, 2003.
13. Goldberg C: Children trapped by the gaps in treatment of mental illness. *The New York Times*, July 09, 2001.
14. King RA, Schwab-Stone M, Peterson B, Thies A: Psychiatric assessment of the infant, child, and adolescent. In: Kaplan HI, Kaplan VA (eds): *Comprehensive Textbook of Psychiatry* (vol II) 8 ed. Baltimore, Williams and Wilkins, 2005, pp. 3044–3075.
15. King RA, Lewis M: The difficult child. *Child Adolesc Psychiatr Clin North Am* 3:531–541, 1994.
16. Allen MH: Level one psychiatric emergency services: The tools of the crisis sector. *Psychiatr Clin North Am* 22:713–734, 1999.
17. American Academy of Child and Adolescent Psychiatry. Practice parameters for the psychiatric assessment of children and adolescents. *J Am Acad Child Adolesc Psychiatry* 34:1386–1402, 1995.
18. Velting DM, Shaffer D, Gould MS, Garfinkel R, Fisher P, Davies M: Parent–victim agreement in adolescent suicide research. *Journal of the American Academy of Child & Adolescent Psychiatry* 37:1161–1166, 1998.
19. Dryfoos JG: *Safe Passage: Making It Through Adolescence in a Risky Society*. Oxford, U.K., Oxford University Press, 1998.
20. Guerrero AP: General medical considerations in child and adolescent patients who present with psychiatric symptoms. *Child & Adolescent Psychiatric Clinics of North America* 12(4):613–628, 2003.
21. Reid WH. Clinical evaluation of the violent patient. *Psychiatric Clinics of North America* 11(4):527–537, 1988.
22. Skeem JL, Mulvey EP, Odgers C, et al.: What do clinicians expect? Comparing envisioned and reported violence for male and female patients. *Journal of Consulting & Clinical Psychology* 73(4):599–609, 2005.
23. Health Care Financing Administration: *Quality of Care Standards J, sect, Interpretive HCoPfPsR, Guidelines*. Washington DC, Health Care Financing Administration, 2000.
24. Heyneman EK. The aggressive child. *Child & Adolescent Psychiatric Clinics of North America* 12(4):667–677, 2003.
25. Citrome L, Volavka J: Violent patients in the emergency setting. *Psychiatr Clin North Am* 22:789–801, 1999.
26. Gillig PM: An adolescent crisis service in a rural area. *Psychiatric Services* 55(12), 2004.
27. Horwitz LM, Wang PS, Koocher GP, et al.: Detecting suicide risk in a pediatric emergency department: Development of a brief screening tool. *Pediatrics*. 107, 2001.
28. Fortunati FG, Jr., Zonana HV: Legal considerations in the child psychiatric emergency department. *Child & Adolescent Psychiatric Clinics of North America* 12(4):745–761, 2003.
29. Simon RI, Goetz S: Forensic issues in the psychiatric emergency department. *Psychiatr Clin North Am* 22:851–864, 1999.
30. State of Connecticut Social and Human Services, Department of Children and Families: *Commitment of Mentally Ill Children*, 1991.
31. Ellison JM, Wharff EA: More than a gateway: The role of emergency psychiatry service in the community mental health network. *Hosp Community Psychiatry* 36:180–185, 1985.
32. Rotheram-Borus MJ, Piacentini J, Van Rossem R, et al.: Treatment adherence among Latina female adolescent suicide attempters. *Suicide & Life-Threatening Behavior* 29:319–331, 1999.
33. Trautman PD, Stewart N, Morishima A: Are adolescent suicide attempters noncompliant with outpatient care? *J Am Acad Child Adolesc Psychiatry* 32:89–94, 1993.
34. Piacentini J, Rotheram-Borus MJ, Gillis JR, et al.: Demographic predictors of treatment attendance among adolescent suicide attempters. *Journal of Consulting & Clinical Psychology* 63(3):469–473, 1995.
35. Shaffer D: Demographic predictors of treatment attendance among adolescent suicide attempters. *J Consult Clin Psychol* 63:469–473, 1995.
36. Spirito A, Boergers J, Donaldson D, Bishop D, Lewander W: An intervention trial to improve adherence to community treatment by adolescents after a suicide attempt. *Journal of the American Academy of Child & Adolescent Psychiatry* 41:435–442, 2002.
37. Pumariega AJ, Winters NC: Trends and shifting ecologies: Part II. *Child & Adolescent Psychiatric Clinics of North America* 12(4):779–793, 2003.
38. Henggeler SW, Rowland MD, Halliday-Boykins C, et al.: One-year followup of multisystemic therapy as an alternative to the hospitalization of youths in psychiatric crisis. *J Am Acad Child Adolesc Psychiatry* 42:543–551, 2003.
39. American Psychiatric Association *Task force: A Vision for the Mental Health System* Washington, DC, April 3, 2003.

40. Edelsohn GA, Braitman LE, Rabinovich H, et al.: Predictors of urgency in a pediatric psychiatric emergency service. *J Am Acad Child Adolesc Psychiatry* 43:10:1197–1202, 2003.
41. Greenfield B, Larson C, Hechtman L, Rousseau C, Platt R: A rapid-response outpatient model for reducing hospitalization rates among suicidal adolescents. *Psychiatric Services* 53:1574–1579, 2002.
42. Feiguine RJ, Ross-Dolen MH, Havens J: The New York Presbyterian pediatric crisis service. *Psychiatric Quarterly* 17:139–152, 2000.
43. Rotheram-Borus MJ, Piacentini J, Cantwell C, Belin TR, Song J: The 18-month impact of an emergency room intervention for adolescent female suicide attempters. *Journal of Consulting & Clinical Psychology.* 68(6):1081–1093, 2000.
44. Glick R, Ghaemi S: The emergency treatment of depression complicated by psychosis or agitation. *J Clin Psych* 61:43–48, 2000.
45. May V: Attitudes to patients who present with suicidal behavior. *Emrg Nurse* 9:26–32, 2001.
46. Spirito A, Barnett NP, Colby SM, et al.: A randomized clinical trial of a brief motivational intervention for alcohol-positive adolescents treated in an emergency department. *Journal of Pediatrics* 145:396–402, 2004.

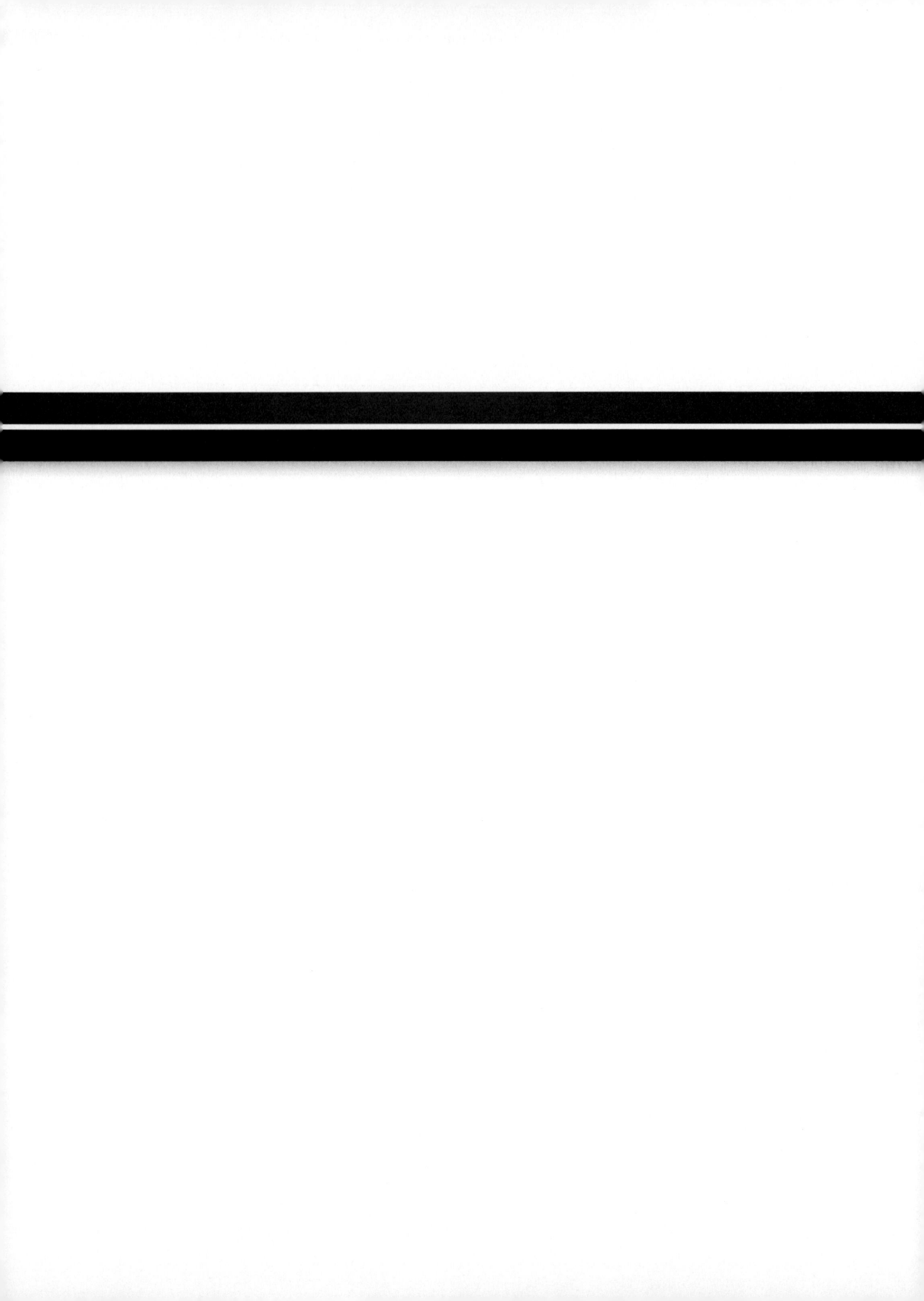

SECTION VII
INTERFACE AREAS OF CHILD AND ADOLESCENT PSYCHIATRY

7.1 ■ PEDIATRICS

CHAPTER 7.1.1 ■ THE CONSULTATION AND LIAISON PROCESSES TO PEDIATRICS

JONATHAN M. CAMPBELL AND LAURIE CARDONA

Children with medical disorders present with psychiatric and psychosocial concerns, frequently at rates that are much higher than expected when compared to the general population. For example, psychological disorders have been documented at rates 2–4 times higher in populations of children with chronic medical illness when compared to estimates within the general population (1). Although children with medical illness appear to be at greater risk for psychopathology, the presence of symptoms appears to vary somewhat according to medical illness (2). In addition to psychosocial needs expressed by children with medical illness, family members may also present with coping and adjustment difficulties resulting in requests for consultation. Parents of child survivors of cancer, for example, report posttraumatic stress symptoms associated with the distress of a life-threatening illness and its treatment, with roughly 14% of mothers and 10% of fathers meeting formal diagnostic criteria for posttraumatic stress disorder (3). The fairly common occurrence of child and family psychosocial needs within pediatric populations has resulted in the professional specialties of consultation-liaison (C/L) child psychiatry and pediatric psychology. Although consultation requests for C/L services may come from outpatient settings and the emergency department, the present chapter is focused on the consultation processes of C/L services to inpatient pediatric departments, arguably the most frequently used mechanism for C/L services.

DIFFERENCES IN THEORETICAL ORIENTATION, TRAINING, AND CULTURE BETWEEN CHILD PSYCHIATRY/PSYCHOLOGY AND PEDIATRICS

Prior to introducing models of consultation and describing the "nuts and bolts" of C/L consultation, it is useful to delineate and describe differences between pediatric and psychiatric/psychological orientations, training, and treatment cultures, which have been identified as challenges to effective C/L work (4). Despite each specialty area being concerned with child-based healthcare, there is surprisingly limited shared training experience for child psychiatry and pediatrics. The overlap is even less for training within pediatric psychology, which results in less appreciation for service provision within medical settings, such as care that occurs within inpatient hospital wards. Another important difference between pediatrics and child psychology/psychiatry is the conceptualization of a child's functioning and adjustment from a primarily biomedical as opposed to a biopsychosocial framework. Pediatric training and treatment typically occurs within a biomedical model whereby psychological and social factors are less emphasized in understanding a child's functioning. In contrast, child psychiatrists and pediatric psychologists often employ biopsychosocial conceptualizations to understand a child's functioning in which psychological and social contextual factors are emphasized.

Two practical differences between pediatrics and child psychiatry/psychology also impact consultation work: pace of work and work setting. The pace of work frequently differs between pediatric and psychiatric/psychological service settings, with a faster pace in pediatric settings when compared to child psychiatry and psychology. For example, C/L psychiatry consultations may take several hours to complete due to interviewing the child, family, and performing other assessments in response to the referral question. Psychotherapeutic interventions may take longer to initiate and realize benefits during the child's hospitalization. The treatment culture of the inpatient pediatric ward also stands in contrast to psychiatric and psychological approaches to intervention. Inpatient treatment settings involve multiple treatment members who operate under time constraints, thus leading to a reduced amount of confidentiality and privacy. In contrast, contact over time and privacy are two basic ingredients that are typically necessary for psychotherapeutic interventions to be implemented and effective.

BIOPSYCHOSOCIAL INFLUENCES ON PEDIATRIC ILLNESS

For child and adolescent psychiatrists and pediatric psychologists, C/L processes involve an array of intersecting domains of knowledge and diverse areas of competency. Content knowledge in the areas of typical child development, child psychopathology, psychological and psychiatric treatment, and consultation with multiple professional disciplines has been identified as prerequisite to effective C/L work (5). The domain of pediatric C/L service is fertile ground for collaboration between child and adolescent psychiatrists and pediatric psychologists; for the latter, a basic understanding of disease process and its medical management as well as general understanding of pediatric hospital practice are also necessary for effective consultation.

Research has documented the complex interplay between a child's biological functioning, psychological adjustment, social context, and development. An appreciation of each domain of the child's functioning is important in approaching C/L work with pediatric populations. Examples of the interplay between child-centered variables, family context, treatment providers, and psychological adjustment abound within the pediatric psychiatry and psychology literatures. To illustrate the complex relationships between these domains, several research findings from the pediatric psychology literature are reviewed briefly.

Biological Variables

Medical conditions vary in the degree of central nervous system involvement, both in terms of disease pathology and its medical management and treatment. For example, children with traumatic brain injury or brain malignancy, by definition, have direct involvement of the central nervous system. Other conditions are not directly linked to central nervous system impairment but result in increased risk of brain involvement; for instance, children with sickle cell disease are at significant risk of central nervous system involvement, with up to 17% suffering cerebrovascular accidents (6). Other pediatric illnesses appear to pose little risk of central nervous system involvement, such as chronic allergies or asthma (7).

Pediatric treatment regimens may also be associated with psychosocial difficulties, due to involvement of the central nervous system, procedural pain, and other untoward effects of treatment. For example, declines in overall cognitive functioning and other neurocognitive abilities, such as attention, concentration, fine motor skills, and memory are well documented untoward "late effects" of cranial irradiation. The use of intrathecal chemotherapy to prevent central nervous system involvement in the treatment of acute lymphoblastic leukemia has also been associated with neurocognitive declines in such areas as nonverbal reasoning and academic achievement (8). Acute painful medical procedures, such as lumbar puncture, are associated with greater psychological distress and acute behavioral disruption.

Psychological Variables

Children hospitalized for pediatric illness vary in terms of prior psychological functioning as well as coping and adjustment to a diagnosis of medical illness, repeated hospitalization, and painful medical procedures (e.g., lumbar punctures). A psychological variable frequently examined in this area consists of a child's cognitive appraisal and coping style, with children being variously categorized as information seeking/sensitizer or information avoiding/repressor. Research generally shows that children who use an information-seeking style of coping enjoy better outcomes when managing distress associated with medical procedures (9).

Social Variables

Family and caretaker variables are associated with children's adjustment in a variety of areas such as functional outcomes, distress during medical procedures, and treatment adherence. For example, greater psychological adjustment of caregivers is associated with more favorable outcomes for children sustaining a traumatic brain injury (10). Parent behavior during painful medical procedures, such as lumbar puncture, is associated with children's distress behavior, with parent apologizing for the procedure, explaining procedural events, and consoling correlated with greater child distress. Conversely, caregivers' use of distracting techniques, such as blowing noisemakers or watching videotapes during procedures, has been shown to result in less child distress and better adaptation (11). Within the type I diabetes literature, the presence (versus absence) of parents during adolescents' blood glucose testing has been associated with greater likelihood of *inappropriate* responding to episodes of hyperglycemia (12). Although participants were adolescents, findings suggest that additional educational intervention may be needed for parents to improve appropriate responding to hyperglycemia in management of type I diabetes.

Outside of the family context, there is growing recognition of the importance of peer relationships in affecting medical outcomes, such as the degree of support for treatment regimens. Researchers have begun to examine the influence of peer relationships in disease management and include peers in intervention programming. For example, peer involvement in an intervention for type I diabetes resulted in improved glycemic control (13). Specifically, the number of supportive peers involved in treatment was correlated with better controlled diabetes.

Developmental Perspectives

Children vary in their capacity to understand and cope with medical illness in terms of their cognitive development. Built upon Piaget's theory of cognitive development, Lewis (14) described characteristic changes in children's understanding of physical functioning and disease over time and recommended intervention be tailored to meet such perspectives. For example, as children develop from infancy to preschool age, they acquire greater knowledge and awareness of their bodies, as well as greater capacity to tend to bodily needs. Typically, preschoolers are able to name multiple body parts and verbalize concerns about bodily injury, such as "ouchies" or "boo-boos" (14). Cognitive development from preschool age to school age is associated with greater awareness and accuracy of the body in terms of its proportions, details, and internal structure. For example, preschool-aged children may view the body as a fluid-filled sac that will leak fluid if the skin is compromised. Later cognitive development results in greater understanding that separate organ systems exist within the body and that these organs can cause discomfort or pain, such as stomachaches.

Children's beliefs and knowledge about the causes of disease and illness also develop in concert with greater cognitive reasoning abilities. Therefore, the consultant's understanding of cognitive development may be used to guide patient education to increase understanding of the illness and improve adjustment (15). Children in the preoperational stage of development often fail to connect cause and effect between an event and illness. As children progress through concrete

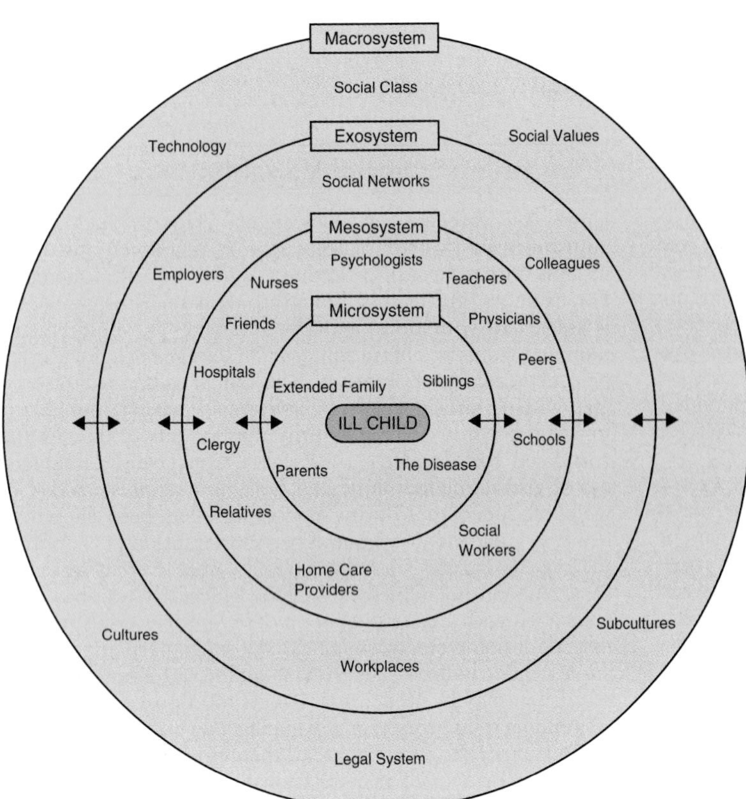

FIGURE 7.1.1.1. A social-ecological model of children with pediatric illness. (Reprinted from: Kazak AE, Segal-Andrews AM, and Johnson K. In: Roberts MC (ed): *Handbook of Pediatric Psychology*, 2nd ed. Guilford Press, 1995, p. 88, with permission.)

operational stages to formal operations, their capacity to link cause and effect increases. For example, children in early stages of concrete operations (6–8) may identify themselves as bringing about their own illness, punishment for misdeeds (14). Children in this stage may need education that dispels belief that they have brought about their own illness. As children progress to formal operations, reasoning about the causes of illness are characterized by abstract thought, with explanations about illness invoking internal organs, dysfunction, and biological mechanisms that may be compromised. Adolescents are equipped cognitively to understand illness, treatment procedures, and make planful decisions about contributing to the management of their illness. Greater cognitive sophistication in adolescence, however, is often accompanied by beliefs of invincibility, which may impede adherence to treatment.

INTRODUCTION OF TWO BIOPSYCHOSOCIAL MODELS

As briefly illustrated earlier in the chapter, the interplay between biological, psychological and social functioning is important in informing psychiatric assessment and treatment of children and adolescents. Although historically a child-focused endeavor, more recent conceptualizations of C/L service have begun to incorporate biopsychosocial notions in understanding child and adolescent functioning (16). As such, broader theories of pediatric illness have been proposed to account for connections between medical disorder, child variables, family functioning, and community-based contexts.

Social-Ecological Framework

An exemplar of the biopsychosocial approach to psychological adjustment within pediatric populations has been adapted from Bronfenbrenner's (17) social-ecological model of child development. Kazak's adaptation of Bronfenbrenner's model (18) provides a comprehensive organization of influences on child and adolescent adaptation to disease and illness (Figure 7.1.1.1). Akin to Bronfenbrenner's model, Kazak's adaptation to pediatric populations features basic theoretical tenets of a) *multiple layers of influence* (nested systems) and b) *bidirectionality of influence* on psychological functioning and adjustment. Factors influencing a child's functioning and adaptation are nested within systems that extend from intra-individual (e.g., cognitive functioning) to larger ecological influences (e.g., medical technology).

Orientation to Different Systems

As illustrated in Figure 7.1.1.1, systems of influence are nested within one another and represent diminishing causal influence on the patient's adaptation and functioning. The innermost circle is symbolic of the child with pediatric illness and intra-individual factors that impact the child's psychological adjustment and functioning. Examples of intra-individual variables include several of those introduced earlier, such as cognitive functioning and capacities for coping. The microsystem involves the patient's most immediate social relationships, including parents, siblings, and extended families, and, particularly relevant for pediatric consultation, disease-related influences. Microsystem influences are deemed the most proximal and salient causal influences on the child's adjustment. Mesosystem influences consist of more distal social and ecological influences on the patient's adaptation, exemplified by peers, school personnel, and an array of medical and mental health providers within the hospital setting and beyond. Exosystem influences consist of a variety of contexts that impact social relationships and functioning within the mesosystem. Finally, macrosystem influences are those that impact the entire system, such as cultural beliefs, social values, and, particularly relevant to pediatrics, medical technology.

The Disability-Stress-Coping Model of Adjustment

Another example of a biopsychosocial approach to working with pediatric populations is the disability-stress-coping model of adjustment to chronic illness (9). Similar to Kazak's model, the model represents a conceptual framework to organize and specify links between a range of biological, psychological, and social variables impacting psychosocial functioning. Built upon a risk-and-resilience framework, the model identifies biological, intrapersonal, and social-ecological variables that contribute to the child's psychosocial adjustment. Within the model, stress is identified as the primary source for elevating the risk of maladjustment to chronic disease. Various sources of stress are identified, such as functional disability associated with illness and psychosocial stressors. A range of psychosocial stressors are identified, such as life transitions (e.g., moving; new school placement) and hassles associated with disease management. Resilience factors are identified as *moderating* the link between stress and psychosocial adjustment. Factors are identified in the areas of stress processing (e.g., coping), within-person factors (e.g., competencies), and social-ecological variables (e.g., parental adjustment).

HISTORY OF CONSULTATION AND LIAISON TO PEDIATRICS

In the United States, the first consultation-liaison/psychosomatic medicine units were formally founded in the 1930s through the Rockefeller Foundation at Massachusetts General, Duke and Colorado. During the 1970s NIH began funding training grants to promote the growth of C/L psychiatry. By 2003, the field had formally adopted the name of psychosomatic medicine and gained approval as a subspecialty by the American Board of Medical Specialties (19). In parallel, in the 1960s the field of pediatric psychology began to formally emerge, through which psychologists also began to conduct a range of clinical and research activities in similar medical settings. In 2001, the Society of Pediatric Psychology was formally designated as Division 54 of the American Psychological Association (20).

RANGE OF SETTINGS AND ACTIVITIES

Pediatric psychologists and psychiatrists conduct clinical services, research activities, preventive educational programs, and public advocacy across diverse settings. Roberts (20) delineated five settings in which pediatric psychology services are most commonly provided: 1) Inpatient medical center units (C/L services for acute and chronic illnesses such as neonatal intensive care units, oncology units, respiratory care units); 2) outpatient medical clinics (emergency departments, primary care centers, pain clinic, craniofacial, genetics, neurology); 3) outpatient clinics providing care for children with psychiatric problems; 4) specialty facilities (physical rehabilitation centers, developmental disabilities centers, hospice); and 5) camps or groups (summer camps for children with diabetes, support groups for parents of chronically ill children).

There is an equally broad range of clinical service activities that are performed by pediatric psychiatrists and psychologists. Accordingly, psychiatric assessment of child, adolescent and family adjustment is a core service provided by mental health consultants. Depending on the setting and concerns presented by the medical team, psychiatric assessments can be quite focused in scope, or involve a comprehensive multisystem evaluation approach as described above. Structured interview methods, including the formal mental status exam, as well as standardized behavioral or psychological instruments are typically included in assessment procedures.

Psychiatric consultants are also familiar with a broad range of psychotherapeutic interventions to address presenting problems such as depression, anxiety, adherence difficulties, procedural pain, and chronic pain. Increasingly, there has been an emphasis in the field on the dissemination and implementation of evidence-based or empirically supported treatments (21). Such treatments typically target disease-specific problems such as acute and chronic pain, medication adherence, coping deficits, or family conflict. Finally, the psychiatric consultant is also required to have the most current knowledge of psychopharmacological interventions for the pediatric patient to address a broad range of psychiatric symptoms, including depression, anxiety, delirium, withdrawal, and behavioral agitation.

In addition to these patient-based clinical services, pediatric psychiatrists and psychologists develop expertise in activities such as: development of programs for promotion of health and prevention of health and psychological problems; education programs for pediatricians and family physicians regarding general child development issues; advocacy regarding child health and mental health at the public health and public policy level; and applied clinical research (20).

EMPIRICALLY SUPPORTED TREATMENTS WITH PEDIATRIC POPULATIONS

Professional organizations within the fields of medicine and psychology have identified numerous Empirically Supported Treatments (EST) that are effective for addressing a broad range of psychosocial difficulties experienced by children and adolescents (22). In 1998, the American Psychological Association's Division 12 approved a set of stringent criteria (the Chambless Criteria) by which interventions would be evaluated with regard to empirical support (23). Published research treatment protocols are ranked in three categories: well established, probably efficacious treatment, and promising intervention. For example, the criteria for a treatment to be considered well established are as follows: 1) at least two good between-group design experiments demonstrating efficacy in one or more of the following ways: superior to pill or psychological placebo or alternative treatment, or equivalent to an already established treatment in experiments with adequate statistical power (about 30 per group); or 2) a large series of single case design experiments ($n > 9$) demonstrating efficacy that have used good experimental design and compared the intervention to another treatment (e.g., pill, psychological placebo); 3) experiments must be conducted with treatment manuals; 4) characteristics of client samples must be clearly specified; and 5) effects must have been demonstrated by at least two different investigators or teams.

Treatments that are categorized as probably efficacious are those that 1) include two experiments showing the treatment is more effective than a wait list control group; or (2) one or more experiments meeting the well established treatments criteria, with the exception of the two investigators/teams criterion.

There have been numerous careful reviews of the pediatric literature examining EST across a variety of medical conditions. For example, Chen (24) completed a review of ESTs in sickle cell disease, McGrath (25) for constipation and encopresis, Powers (26) for pediatric pain, and Saelens (27) for pediatric obesity. The review conducted by Powers (26) concluded that cognitive behavioral therapy is a well established treatment for procedure-related pain in children and adolescents. Treatments include breathing exercises and other forms of relaxation and distraction, cognitive coping skills (e.g., teaching positive self-statement), mental imagery, filmed models, behavioral reinforcement with rehearsal, and directed coaching by parent or practitioner in which they prompt the child to engage in coping skills. Within the same special series journal review, Holden, Deichmann, and Levy (28) found that relaxation and self-hypnosis are well established and efficacious treatments for recurrent headache.

A more recent review conducted by Lemanek, Kamps, and Chung (29) regarding ESTs in regimen adherence for asthma, juvenile rheumatoid arthritis, and type 1 diabetes revealed that while no interventions were identified as well established, numerous cognitive-behavioral treatments met criteria for probably efficacious. Accordingly, within the area of asthma, interventions to address patient adherence, such as "organization strategies" that include increased supervision from a physician and tailoring the medication regimen, appear to fall within the category of probably efficacious. For type I diabetes, the reviewers found that operant learning procedures that focus on direct reinforcement interventions (token system, tangible rewards such as money, points exchanged for daily privileges, weekly bonuses) for increased adherence to regimen components such as blood glucose monitoring are considered probably efficacious.

The later reviews also reveal that much work is still needed to further our knowledge of the most effective treatments for children with medical and psychiatric problems. Powers (26) emphasized that "children, families, our medical colleagues, and insurance providers want helpful interventions that work over time and in a number of situations, that are cost-effective, and that can be learned and used by a number of health care providers." Thus, a future direction for the EST movement is the publication of well established and promising treatments as manuals so that there is greater dissemination and application of trials of empirically supported treatments in real-world contexts or clinical practices. Furthermore, in order for the field to advance, there must also be systematic research into how ESTs are best implemented across various population and setting types.

EMPIRICALLY SUPPORTED ASSESSMENTS WITH PEDIATRIC POPULATIONS

Analogous to the movement toward ESTs, there is growing interest in the identification and dissemination of empirically supported assessments (ESA) for use with pediatric populations. The Society of Pediatric Psychology (Division 54 of the American Psychological Association) has created a task force to review the empirical support for measures used with pediatric populations in the following areas: quality of life, family functioning, psychosocial functioning and psychopathology, social support and peer relations, adherence, pain, stress and coping, and cognitive functioning. Guidelines produced by the task force utilize a structure similar to the Chambless and Hollon criteria, with three outcomes identified. A well established assessment requires that the measure has been presented in at least two peer-reviewed articles by different investigators or investigatory teams along with sufficient detail documenting good reliability and validity. An approaching well established assessment is a measure that has been presented in at least two peer-reviewed articles, which might be by the same investigator or investigatory team with sufficient detail documenting moderate reliability and validity. Finally, a promising assessment is a measure that has been presented in at least one peer-reviewed article with sufficient detail documenting moderate reliability and validity. Results from the task force reviews will be published in future issues of the *Journal of Pediatric Psychology*.

FRAMEWORKS FOR CONSULTATION AND LIAISON PROCESSES

Numerous theoretical models and procedural frameworks have been described to capture the complex nature of the pediatric consultation process (Table 7.1.1.1). The models all share the common features of providing guidelines to psychiatric consultants for fostering professional relationships with healthcare providers and patients in order to improve patient care, and to promote the understanding of child and family adjustment to illness or hospitalization (30).

Resource Consultation

The models vary with regard to the degree of involvement the psychiatric consultant establishes and maintains with the medical team, patient, and family. The most time limited is the resource consultation model (31), also known as the independent functions model (32). Typically, the primary pediatrician or resident will contact the psychiatric consultant regarding a specific diagnostic question. For example, the team may request assessment of depressive symptoms and risk for suicide in a patient with a history of substance abuse, or request an assessment of possible ADHD symptoms in a child who has completed chemotherapy. In the resource consultation model, the consultant functions as a specialist who provides diagnostic clarification and suggests a set of recommendations to the medical team and family regarding possible intervention strategies for the identified problem area. Typically, once the specific question is addressed, the consultant does not provide followup monitoring or further evaluation. This approach is the most common type of consultation model among other medical professionals within a hospital setting. For example, a number of specialists (cardiology, pulmonology, and neurology) may provide evaluations and opinions regarding the medical management of a single patient, but ultimately the integration of the findings and comprehensive plan of care is carried out by the primary physician. One advantage of resource consultation is that it provides expert diagnostic information to the primary physician about a delineated problem area. The other principal advantage of this model for a psychiatric consultant is that it can serve as a powerful point of entry for the development of collaborative relationships with a variety of medical colleagues. Successful resource-type consultations often lead to the development of professional relationships that can result in more comprehensive models of pediatric consultation. The primary limitation of this model, as detailed by Drotar (33), is the limited communication and dialogue that exists among the professionals consulting on the care. Limited contact between professionals can result in an overly simplistic or narrow view of the patient's functioning or the types of psychiatric or psychosocial interventions available.

Process and Process/Educative Consultation

A second type of consultative model is the process-educative approach (31). Within this framework, the psychiatric consultant offers indirect psychological services to patients by means

TABLE 7.1.1.1

COMPARING AND CONTRASTING CONSULTATION MODELS TO PEDIATRICS

Model	Consultee	Nature	Methods	Duration
Resource consultation	Patient	Contact with patient and pediatrician	Telephone, face-to-face; "curbside" consultation	Limited; PRN
Process—educative consultation	Pediatrician	Contact with pediatrician	Educational	Ongoing relationship with pediatrician
Collaborative team	Patient and treatment team (e.g., pediatrician; nursing staff)	Contact with patient and healthcare providers	Interdisciplinary and multidisciplinary approach; "shared care giving"	Ongoing relationships with teams of healthcare providers
Family systems consultation	Patient, family and staff	Contact with patient, family and healthcare providers. Entire system is unit of consultation.	Joining with family; acknowledge strengths and competencies of family.	Time-limited
Multisystemic	Hospital and other systems	Contact with patient, family, healthcare providers, other systems (e.g., school settings)	Consultation with multiple care providers within and outside of the hospital setting	Proposed model; unknown

of advising and educating the medical staff about psychological or pharmacological management and treatment strategies. The consultant may not actually have contact with the patient directly, but instead the pediatrician presents the pertinent medical and psychosocial background and concerns to the consultant. The consultant may then, for example, provide education to the pediatrician regarding standardized assessment measures for diagnosis (e.g., ADHD) or suggest treatment protocols to address a specific psychosocial problem (medical adherence in chronically ill children). This type of educational consultation might take place in the context of phone calls or even formal seminars and lectures. For example, the C/L service of the Yale Child Study Center provides a lecture series to pediatric house staff and residents on topics ranging from psychological approaches to pain management in the chronically ill child to pediatric palliative care. As is evident, this level of collegial collaboration often emerges following prior successful collaborative efforts, such as those described above. One of the principal advantages of this type of educational consultation is that a potentially larger number of patients and families can be assisted by influencing a pediatrician's methods of assessment and intervention. The primary disadvantage of the process-educative approach is that the consultant is reliant on the pediatrician's observations and interpretation of the child and family's difficulties, which may be incomplete, or even flawed (30).

Collaborative Team Model

A third type of approach, the collaborative team model (32), is viewed by many as the ideal. Within this framework, the psychiatric consultant and the medical team are involved in "shared caregiving" (31) through which both professionals have equal responsibility, commitment, and decision-making in the care of the patient. The model therefore leads to intensive collaboration between the psychiatric consultant and all medical personnel involved with the child and family and may result in increased rates of referral due to visibility and interest shown by the consultant (1). Consequently, the consultant can develop interventions that address multiple levels of influence (34). The primary limitation of this model of care is that it requires a substantial commitment of time and resources.

Family, Systems, and Multisystemic Consultation

More recently, models of psychological intervention with medically ill children have emphasized the need for a broader systems perspective to guide consultation work. Specifically, clinical researchers such as Kazak (18) have developed models of consultation that address the context of social systems, including families, school, and hospital systems that influence a child's health outcomes. Within the family systems or social ecological frameworks, the psychiatric consultant evaluates the complex interactions between child–family, family–hospital, and family–community relationships that have direct and indirect impacts on child health outcomes. The family-systems framework emerged within the context of a growing body of literature that demonstrates that family interaction styles, disease management practices, family belief system, and communication patterns impact child health and psychological outcomes (35).

There is also a growing recognition that schools have an important role in child mental health outcomes, particularly for children with chronic illnesses. Involving educational systems during consultation work is important because many children with pediatric illness also present with educational concerns, such as comorbid learning and intellectual disabilities, attention-deficit hyperactivity disorder, and psychosocial adjustment problems related to school reentry. The confluence of medical, psychosocial, and educational needs in pediatric populations has resulted in the emergence of a subspecialty defined as pediatric school psychology. The proposed subspecialty is built on the notion that hospital-based psychiatric consultation/pediatric psychology and school psychology practice are inadequate to address the psychoeducational needs of children with medical illness. Proponents of the subspecialty argue that child psychiatrists and pediatric psychologists frequently lack prerequisite knowledge and experience to work effectively within school settings. For example, child psychiatrists and pediatric psychologists do not typically receive training in special education laws that pertain to children with medical illness. Similarly, child psychiatrists/psychologists often do not receive didactic training and supervised experience consulting with school professionals. Likewise, school psychologists typically do not receive didactic training relevant to the psychosocial and educational needs of children with medical illnesses or how to collaborate effectively with medical professionals.

The shortcomings of both child psychiatry/pediatric psychology and school psychology training traditions are problematic for several important reasons. First, children with severe medical illnesses are surviving due to advances in medical treatment. Second, special education laws exist to protect the rights of children with medical illnesses that interfere with educational progress. As such, federal legislation calls for children with medical illnesses and special education needs to be educated in public school settings that are least restrictive and educationally appropriate. Third, schools have become the de facto mental health service providers for children with psychosocial needs, not merely those children with medical illnesses. All told, the confluence of the three trends in public education results in public schools as important providers of psychiatric, psychosocial, and educational services to children with medical illnesses. As such, trends and needs of children with medical illness make strong arguments for increased collaborations between hospital-based practice and school settings (36).

DESCRIPTION OF CONSULTATION AND LIAISON REQUESTS IN INPATIENT SETTINGS

Due to the heterogeneity associated with inpatient hospital patient populations, psychiatric consultation requests within this treatment setting are characterized by a wide range of referral questions posed from varied hospital services (Table 7.1.1.2). Consultation requests may involve questions of differential diagnosis of psychiatric disorders, problems with managing patient behavior on the hospital ward, assistance with post-discharge treatment planning, and adherence with medical regimens, among others. Results from multiple reports indicate the most frequent reasons for psychiatric consultation are for coping/adjustment, noncompliance with treatment, depression, suicide attempt, pain management, psychosomatic problems, and anxiety (1, 37, 38). However, reasons for referral may also vary according to the expertise of the C/L service, such as a greater preponderance of neuropsychological and comprehensive psychological evaluation requests found for C/L services at the University of Florida (39). Research has also documented the multifaceted nature of consultations, with many requests involving more than one domain of psychosocial functioning. For example, in the Carter et al. study (37), 104 patient referrals yielded more than 240 specific concerns.

Referral rates to inpatient C/L services have been found to range widely, with 1–14% of inpatient hospitalization populations referred across a range of published studies (1). C/L consultation requests appear to be generated frequently from general pediatric and hematology/oncology services. For example, in a case-controlled prospective study of 104 referrals to an inpatient C/L service, Carter et al. (37), also found that 41% of referral requests were generated from hematology/oncology and general pediatrics, while Rodrigue et al. (39) found that over 70% of inpatient consult requests were from these two services. Within inpatient settings, other referrals were found to be generated from surgery/trauma, pulmonology, rehabilitation, and intensive care, among other departments.

Psychiatric referral has been shown to be associated with increased length of hospitalization, although it is not clear whether the increased length of stay results in greater likelihood of problem detection, if referral reflects a more complicated course of treatment due to psychiatric problems, or a combination of these factors (1). Despite the degree of psychopathology documented for children with medical illness and the relationship between psychopathology and hospital course, under referral for psychiatric consultation has been a consistent finding in the literature. Potential sources of under referral include resistance of family members to C/L psychiatry services or dissatisfaction of C/L services by physicians; however, nonidentification of psychosocial difficulty remains a significant problem in under referral.

TABLE 7.1.1.2

FREQUENT CONSULTATION REQUESTS ACROSS THREE PEDIATRIC SETTINGS

Setting	Presenting Concerns (%)	Primary Clinical Activities
Primary care	Heterogeneity of concerns: 1. Behavioral noncompliance (16.2) 2. Tantrums (12.8) 3. Aggression (8.1)	Assessment; parent guidance; psychotherapy.
Inpatient ward	Heterogeneity of concerns: 1. Adjustment problems (14.9) 2. Noncompliance (13.3) 3. Depression/Suicide (12.9) 4. Anxiety (6.6) 5. Pain management (6.6) 6. Parent coping (6.2)	Wide range of activities: Assessment; time-limited psychotherapy; staff consultation; psychopharmacological consultation; parent guidance.
Emergency department	1. Suicidal behaviors (47%) 2. Oppositional behavior (24%) 3. Threats of violence and/or aggression (17%)	Assessment, diagnosis, and disposition.

Note. Percentages reported are from Carter et al. (2003) and Drotar, Spirito, and Stancin's (2003) review.

CONSULTATION PROCEDURAL GUIDELINES

Several consultation protocols based on these theoretical models have been proposed (14, 40). C/L consultation protocols include procedural guidelines in the consultation process such as: 1) defining the referral questions; 2) review of records; 3) interview of primary caretakers; 4) assessment of the patient; 5) referral for additional tests or procedures; 6) assessment of interdisciplinary relationships between medical personnel; 7) collaboration with community agencies or schools; 8) diagnostic feedback and recommendations; 9) intervention phase; and 10) followup.

Referral Phase

Initially, the psychiatric consultant should speak directly to the primary physician, and other members of the medical team (primary nurse, residents, or pediatric social worker) to generate a list of concerns or diagnostic questions that are to be addressed during the consultation. It is critical for the consultant to listen for both implicit as well as the explicit messages from the physician (40). For example, the team may actually have more concerns about parental coping than they do about child psychological adjustment. During the referral phase, it is also important that the consultant take a thorough medical history and current treatment regimen from the referring physician. Finally, it is important that the consultant confirm that the parents and patient have been informed by the medical team about their concerns and that they have agreed to participate with the evaluation.

Record Review

Prior to meeting the family and patient, it is important for the consultant to review the medical chart, including prior medical records, for treatment information that may have been omitted by the referring physician. For example, for those patients who have multiple medical subspecialties involved in their care, it is important to review the treatments or consultations provided under their care. Additionally, oftentimes nurses document important observations regarding a child's mental status, mood states, and behavioral functioning that are important sources of data. As part of the record review, it is also critical that the consultant take note of all the medications prescribed to the patient, with particular emphasis on those medications that have psychoactive effects or withdrawal symptoms.

Interview with Primary Caretakers

It is usually most informative to begin the evaluation phase with a structured interview with the primary caretakers, which may include biological parents, foster or adoptive parents. Designated social service agency workers may also need to be contacted in the case of children who are in state custody. During this interview, the consultant should gather information regarding the patient's birth, developmental, social, and educational histories. Of particular importance is the history of past psychiatric treatments. Additionally, the consultant should inquire about the parents' social and psychiatric histories, the marital relationship, sibling relationships, extended family supports, economic and community resources available to the family. As highlighted earlier, difficulties within any of these areas have been identified as potential risk factors for children with serious medical conditions.

Child and Adolescent Assessment

A comprehensive mental status examination should be conducted with the child, as is permissible given the patient's age and developmental level of functioning. Play interviews and observations of the child's behavior during inpatient ward activities are also valuable sources of data. During the evaluation phase, formal diagnostic procedures such as self-report inventories for depression or anxiety may also be included. For those patients with altered states of consciousness, possible delirium, or other central nervous system dysfunction, repeated serial interviews are often critical in order to establish levels of baseline functioning and to explore possible etiological factors.

Referral for Other Tests or Procedures

Over the course of the evaluation, a range of differential diagnostic questions may arise that will lead the consultant to request additional tests or procedures from the medical team. For example, the consultant may suggest neuroimaging studies or an EEG for a patient with acute changes in mental status. Additionally, neuropsychological testing is often indicated in the context of further clarifying functional capacities for children with central nervous system insults.

Systems Assessment

The final two components during the assessment phase involve examining the relationships that exist amongst medical personnel, the child–family system, and relationships among medical personnel and community systems such as schools and social service agencies. The consultant may need to conduct systematic interviews and observations of all these various systems relationships in order to determine whether there are communication or collaboration difficulties contributing to the child's observed difficulties. Clinical researchers such as Kazak (41) suggest that a systems assessment is important because oftentimes family or family–staff interactional factors can play a central role in the child's problematic functioning.

Diagnostic Feedback Phase

Once the consultant has concluded all of the components of the assessment, the next step is to share the diagnostic formulation and set of recommendations with members of the medical team, parents, child, and other systems of care. Traditionally, consultation findings are summarized within the context of a report placed in the medical chart. It is of paramount importance, however, that the consultant communicate orally with the medical team and family regarding the findings and the recommendations for intervention. Direct discussion of the multiple factors that are contributing to the child's adjustment difficulties can then lead to candid discussions regarding the roles that each member of the medical team or family can assume in promoting improved child adaptation.

Interventions and Followup

Numerous evidence-based treatments have been developed to address child and family coping with acute and chronic illness. For example, there are highly effective cognitive-behavioral treatments such as progressive muscle relaxation and guided imagery training to address pain and anxiety during invasive medical procedures (42). Additionally, there are home-based, manualized, behavioral family systems therapy treatments targeting issues such as poor medical adherence and family conflict (18). Cognitive-behavioral methods are also useful in addressing more broadbased psychological problems such as anxiety and depression (21). Pharmacotherapy may also become an important component of a medically ill child's treatment regimen. For example, the psychiatric consultant may offer recommendations for medical management of symptoms such as behavioral agitation, delirium, depression, or anxiety. Additionally, a host of psychosocial interventions may be required. Accordingly, the family may require assistance in securing public assistance, special education services, or supportive marital therapy. Some interventions may be possible to introduce within the context of a hospitalization, but oftentimes the psychiatric consultant must provide the family and medical team with suggestions regarding other community-based mental health professionals that can begin to develop a psychological plan of care. If the child will return to the school setting, an important part of intervention should include guidance regarding the child's reentry to school.

BARRIERS (AND PROPOSED SOLUTIONS) TO EFFECTIVE CONSULTATION AND LIAISON SERVICES TO PEDIATRICS

Several barriers to effective C/L service to pediatrics have been identified in the literature, such as lack of availability of child psychiatry/psychology consultants, time constraints, and contrasts between illness-oriented versus biopsychosocial conceptualizations (14). Perhaps the most damaging barrier to effective C/L consultation to pediatrics is the difference between pace of work between clinical traditions. The typical length of psychiatric/psychological evaluation and consultation takes several hours, while the work pace within pediatric hospital settings moves much more quickly.

Flexible consultation and treatment approaches have been identified as mechanisms to increase satisfaction and subsequent use of consultation services. Other matters of practical importance involve accessibility of the psychiatric consultant, responsiveness to the consultation request, and minimal time to complete assessment and share findings (4). Consultation services are also enhanced with effective communication of assessment findings, treatment planning, and practical recommendations to both the referring pediatrician and the child and family. For both family and professional audiences, communication should be practical, action-oriented, and free of psychological jargon; for the pediatrician, written communication should be concise. The use of concise communication, particularly producing a concise chart note, may be most difficult for pediatric psychologists, who are less familiar with this method of professional communication.

Lewis (14) suggested that the consultant's presence during clinical rounds, departmental meetings, or other conferences may facilitate improved C/L service. Another useful guideline to reduce barriers to effective consultation involves defining role and functions of the consultant *prior* to the onset of service use. All told, an effective C/L consultant is one who is available and provides prompt and practical recommendations (14).

References

1. Shugart MA: Child psychiatry consultations to pediatric inpatients: A literature review. *General Hospital Psychiatry* 13:325–336, 1991.
2. Lavigne JV, Faier-Routman J: Psychological adjustment to pediatric physical disorders: A meta-analytic review. *Journal of Pediatric Psychology* 17:133–157, 1992.
3. Kazak A, Alderfer M, Rourke MT, et al.: Posttraumatic stress disorder (PTSD) and posttraumatic stress symptoms (PTSS) in families of adolescent childhood cancer survivors. *Journal of Pediatric Psychology* 29:211–219, 2004.
4. Kush SA, Campo JV: Consultation and liaison in the pediatric setting. In: Ammerman RT, Campo JV (eds): *Handbook of Pediatric Psychology and Psychiatry*. Needham Heights, MA, Allyn & Bacon, pp. 23–40, 1998.
5. Bronheim HE, Fulop G, Kunkel EJ, et al.: The Academy of Psychosomatic Medicine Practice Guidelines for Psychiatric Consultation in the General Medical Setting. *Psychosomatics* 39:S8–S30, 1998.
6. Bonner MJ, Gustafson KE, Schumacher E, et al.: The impact of sickle cell disease on cognitive functioning and learning. *School Psychology Review* 28:182–193, 1999.
7. Bender BG: Learning disorders associated with asthma and allergies. *School Psychology Review* 28:204–214, 1999.
8. Montour-Proulx I, Kuehn SM, Keene DL, et al.: Cognitive changes in children treated for acute lymphoblastic leukemia with chemotherapy only according to the Pediatric Oncology Group 9605 Protocol. *Journal of Child Neurology* 20:129–133, 2005.
9. Wallander JL, Thompson RJ, & Alriksson-Schmidt, A: Psychosocial adjustment of children with chronic physical conditions. In Roberts MC (ed): *Handbook of Pediatric Psychology* (pp. 141–158). New York, Guilford Press, 2003.
10. Ewing-Cobbs L, Bloom DR: Traumatic brain injury: Neuropsychological, psychiatric, and educational issues. In: Brown RT (ed): *Handbook of Pediatric Psychology in School Settings* Mahwah, NJ: Lawrence Erlbaum, 2004, pp. 313–331.
11. Blount RL, Piira T, Cohen LL: Management of pediatric pain and distress due to medical procedures. In Roberts MC (ed): *Handbook of pediatric psychology* (3rd ed. pp. 216–233). New York, Guilford Press, 2003.
12. Johnson SB, Perwien AR, Silverstein, JH: Response to hypo- and hyperglycemia in adolescents with Type I diabetes. *Journal of Pediatric Psychology* 25:171–178, 2000.
13. Pendley JS, Kasmen LJ, Miller DL, et al.: Peer and family support in children and adolescents with Type I diabetes. *Journal of Pediatric Psychology* 27:429–438, 2002.
14. Lewis M: The consultation process in child and adolescent psychiatric consultation-liaison in pediatrics. In Lewis M (ed): *Child and adolescent psychiatry: A comprehensive textbook* (3rd ed., pp. 1111–1115). Philadelphia, Lippincott, Williams & Wilkins, 2002.
15. LeBlanc LA, Goldsmith T, Patel DR: Behavioral aspects of chronic illness in children and adolescents. *Pediatric Clinics of North America* 50:859–878, 2003.
16. Knapp PK, Harris ES: Consultation-liaison in child psychiatry: A review of the past 10 years: Part I: Clinical findings. *Journal of the American Academy of Child and Adolescent Psychiatry* 37:17–25, 1998.
17. Bronfenbrenner, U. *The ecology of human development*. Cambridge, MA: Harvard University Press, 1979.
18. Kazak A, Rourke MT, Crump TA: Families and other systems in pediatric psychology. In Roberts MC (ed): *Handbook of pediatric psychology* (3rd ed., pp. 159–175). New York, Guilford Press, 2003.
19. Levenson JL: *Textbook of Psychosomatic Medicine* Washington, DC, American Psychiatric Publishing, 2005, p. xix.
20. Roberts MC, Mitchell MC, McNeal R. The evolving field of pediatric psychology: Critical issues and future challenges. In Roberts MC (ed): *Handbook of pediatric psychology* (3rd ed., pp. 3–18). New York, Guilford Press, 2003.
21. Chambless DL, Ollendick TH: Empirically supported psychological interventions: Controversies and evidence. *Annual Review of Psychology* 52:685–716, 2001.
22. Spirito A, Kazak AE: *Effective and Emerging Treatments in Pediatric Psychology*. New York, Oxford University Press, 2006.
23. Chambless DL, Hollon SD: Defining empirically supported therapies. *Journal of Consulting and Clinical Psychology* 66:7–18, 1998.
24. Chen E, Cole SW, Kato PM: A review of empirically supported psychosocial interventions for pain and adherence outcomes in sickle cell disease. *Journal of Pediatric Psychology* 29:197–209, 2004.
25. McGrath ML, Mellon MW, Murphy L: Empirically supported treatments in pediatric psychology: Constipation and encopresis. *Journal of Pediatric Psychology* 25:225–254, 2000.
26. Powers SW: Empirically supported treatments in pediatric psychology: Procedure related pain. *Journal of Pediatric Psychology* 24:131–145, 1999.
27. Saelens BE: Empirically supported treatments in pediatric psychology: Pediatric obesity. *Journal of Pediatric Psychology* 24:223–248, 1999.
28. Holden EW, Deichmann MM, & Levy JD: Empirically supported treatments in pediatric psychology: Recurrent pediatric headache. *Journal of Pediatric Psychology* 24, 91–109, 1999.
29. Lemanek KL, Kamps J, Chung NB: Empirically supported treatments in pediatric psychology: Regimen adherence. *Journal of Pediatric Psychology* 26, 279–282, 2001.
30. Hamlett KW, Stabler B: The developmental progress of pediatric psychology consultation. In: Roberts MC (ed): *Handbook of Pediatric Psychology*, 2nd ed. New York, Guilford Press, pp. 39–54, 1995.
31. Stabler B: Pediatric consultation-liaison. In: Routh DK (ed): *Handbook of pediatric psychology* (pp. 538–566). New York, Guilford, Press (1988).

32. Roberts MC. & Wright L: The role of the pediatric psychologist as consultant to pediatricians. In: Tuma J (ed): *Handbook for the practice of pediatric psychology* (pp. 251–289). New York, Wiley, 1982.
33. Drotar D: *Consulting with pediatricians: Psychological perspectives.* New York, Plenum, 2004.
34. Huszti HC, Walker CE: Critical issues in consultation and liaison. In: Sweet JJ, & Tovian SM (eds): *Handbook of clinical psychology in medical settings* (pp. 165–185). New York, Plenum Press, 1991.
35. Fiese BH: Introduction to the special issue: Time for family-based interventions in pediatric psychology. *Journal of Pediatric Psychology* 30, 629–630, 2005.
36. Brown RT (ed): *Handbook of Pediatric Psychology Applied to School Settings.* Mahwah, NJ, Lawrence Erlbaum, 2004.
37. Carter BD, Kronenberger WG, Baker J, et al.: Inpatient pediatric consultation-liaison: A case-controlled study. *Journal of Pediatric Psychology* 28:423–432, 2003.
38. Olson RA, Holden EW, Friedman A, et al.: Psychological consultation in a children's hospital: An evaluation of services. *Journal of Pediatric Psychology* 13, 479–492, 1988.
39. Rodrigue JR, Hoffman RG, Rayfield A, et al.: Evaluating pediatric psychology consultation services in a medical setting: An example. *Journal of Clinical Psychology in Medical Settings* 2:89–107, 1995.
40. Smith FA, Querques J, Levenson J, Stern TA: Psychiatric assessment and consultation. In: Levenson J (ed): *Textbook of psychosomatic medicine* (pp. 3–14). Washington, DC, American Psychiatric Publishing, 2005.
41. Kazak A, Simms S, & Rourke M: Family systems practice in pediatric psychology. *Journal of Pediatric Psychology* 27:133–143, 2002.
42. Cardona L. Behavioral approaches to pain and anxiety in the pediatric patient. *Child and Adolescent Psychiatric Clinics of North America* 3, 449–464, 1994.

CHAPTER 7.1.2 ■ INTEGRATING BEHAVIORAL SERVICES INTO PEDIATRIC CARE SETTINGS: PRINCIPLES AND MODELS

DAVID J. SCHONFELD AND JOHN V. CAMPO

SCOPE OF THE PROBLEM

Primary care is the label applied to community-based medical settings that offer first-contact personal health care that is comprehensive and longitudinal (1). Most American children make at least one primary care medical visit annually (2), and parents look to pediatric primary care providers (PCPs) as resources for addressing psychosocial problems (3). The public health relevance of pediatric mental health problems is increasingly being appreciated; it is estimated that between 15% to more than 25% of pediatric patients have a mental health (MH) problem or disorder (4, 5). The prevalence of MH problems of concern to pediatricians would be even greater if the MH needs of the parents of pediatric patients (e.g., maternal depression) were considered within the purview of pediatric PCPs (6). Due to the high prevalence of MH concerns in children and adolescents and the frequency of their contact with PCPs, it stands to reason that pediatricians and other PCPs are important resources for identification and early management of common MH problems and disorders.

Mental health disorders are among the most disabling of pediatric conditions, and are associated with interpersonal difficulties, poor school performance, and school absenteeism, with one-third of all school days missed by adolescents being MH related. It is therefore not surprising that psychosocial problems are the most common chronic conditions presenting during pediatric ambulatory health visits, with a broad range of severity and high rates of comorbidity, comparable to chronic conditions such as asthma and diabetes. Not only are MH disorders highly prevalent across the lifespan, but early onset is more the rule than the exception, with pediatric psychiatric disorder being powerfully predictive of adult disorder and impairment. As demonstrated by the National Comorbidity Study, the onset of approximately half of all MH disorders occurs at or before age 14, with approximately three of four MH disorders beginning by age 24 years (7).

DUALISM IN PEDIATRIC HEALTH CARE

Despite a growing awareness of the biopsychosocial model of health and an appreciation that physical and mental health are inextricably linked, our health care delivery system is split into parallel systems of care depending on whether a problem is conceptualized as physical (general medical conditions) or psychological (MH disorders). While it is true that most professionals, when pressed, will agree that health is a unitary construct that cannot be parsed into physical and mental components, our behavior, the organization of health care, the systems of healthcare reimbursement, and the behaviors of our patients suggest otherwise. Whether a disorder is conceptualized as physical or mental thus has profound implications for how and where the disorder is cared for, which professionals are expected to bear primary responsibility for care delivery, and how that care is reimbursed. Due to the persistent stigma associated with MH disorders, there are additional societal implications resulting from whether a disorder is considered to be a general medical condition or a MH disorder. In contrast to physical disease, MH disorders are often viewed by our society as being under the voluntary control of the affected individual, the consequence of individual weakness, inadequacy, or moral failing, and thus associated with stigma, shame, and embarrassment.

Physical symptoms are a common presentation of psychiatric disorder in general medical settings, with disorders conceptualized as mental (e.g., anxiety and depressive disorders) commonly presenting to PCPs and medical specialists with very real and disabling physical complaints and distress (functional abdominal pain and headaches) (8–10). Such patients tend to utilize more health services and can be quite costly to society (11). Potentially serious physical health consequences have also been associated with pediatric MH disorders, most notably increased risks of suicide, violence, and accidental injury, as well as overweight, early pregnancy and alcohol, drug, and tobacco abuse (12–15).

It is also well known that physical disease is a significant risk factor for the development of emotional and behavioral problems, with several studies documenting that chronic physical disorder is a risk factor for MH problems and disorders in both community-based and clinical samples across the lifespan (16–19). In part due to the success of modern medicine, chronic physical illness is a growing problem; approximately 1–3% of all youth suffer from significant functional impairment resulting from chronic physical illness (17). Physical diseases or injuries that affect the brain (e.g. epilepsy, cerebral palsy, head trauma) are especially potent risk factors for comorbid emotional, behavioral, and learning problems (19, 20). The presence of a MH disorder can also influence the course of physical disease, as demonstrated in juvenile diabetes, where comorbid depression has been identified as an independent risk factor for the development of diabetic retinopathy (21), repeat hospitalization (22), overall adaptation to the disease (e.g., adherence to treatment), and possibly metabolic control (23). From this, it should be evident that disorders considered to be mental can have profound physical health consequences and vice versa.

IMPLEMENTING BEST PRACTICES WITHIN PRIMARY CARE SETTINGS

Research has demonstrated the efficacy of a growing number of treatments for common pediatric MH disorders (24), but most affected youth do not receive any treatment (4). Of those who do receive services, many are not treated in accordance with available best practices, with considerable gaps existing between research-driven knowledge and routine clinical practices (25, 26). Interventions that have been proven efficacious for attention-deficit/hyperactivity disorder (ADHD) (25), anxiety disorders (27–29), and depressive disorders are generally not systematically or effectively applied on the population level, with routine care often falling short of best practices (30). Finding the means to translate advances in treatment efficacy into practical effectiveness strategies will thus be necessary to maximize public health benefits of new advances in therapeutics, and will likely require commitment, multidisciplinary collaboration, and systemic changes in the way that professionals in primary care and specialty MH care work together (31–33). One example of such an initiative to improve the quality of care for pediatric MH disorders in pediatric primary care settings is the effort by the American Academy of Pediatrics (AAP) to develop practice guidelines for the diagnosis and management of attention-deficit/hyperactivity disorder (34, 35).

THE EMERGENCE OF DEVELOPMENTAL-BEHAVIORAL PEDIATRICS (DBP)

The high prevalence of psychosocial problems in children within pediatric primary care settings was described by Haggerty in 1975 and termed the new morbidity. Due in part to the successes in preventive medicine (e.g., immunizations) and medical therapeutics (antibiotics), the nature of the pediatric needs of children and their families has changed, resulting in a growing emphasis on developmental and behavioral issues in pediatric care. Much of this alteration in practice pattern was also the result of a changing environment. Major changes in family, school, and neighborhood contexts over the past few decades resulted in an exacerbation and increase in developmental and behavioral problems along with a dramatic decrease in formal and informal social networks that might have in the past provided advice and guidance on their management.

The field of developmental-behavioral pediatrics (DBP) arose from the need to enhance the capacity of pediatricians to identify, manage, and when necessary, refer children with developmental and behavioral concerns and to implement effective prevention approaches. The goal was not to create a cadre of independent clinical subspecialists which might compete with child and adolescent psychiatrists, but to produce academic leaders and researchers that can enhance the training of general pediatricians so that they will be better prepared to address the developmental and behavioral needs of their own patients.

DBP focuses on the evaluation and management of common behavioral problems such as temper tantrums, attention-deficit disorders, or sleep problems, common developmental disabilities such as mental retardation, and physical complaints best addressed via a biobehavioral approach, such as recurrent abdominal pain. DBP aims to be eclectic and committed to multidisciplinary collaboration, with developmental-behavioral pediatricians striving to integrate a wide range of complementary theories derived from the medical, biological, behavioral, and social sciences, and drawing upon clinical skills and research approaches that are otherwise associated with a range of disparate disciplines. As a result, there is significant overlap between conditions appropriate for management by developmental-behavioral pediatricians and other disciplines, such as child and adolescent psychiatry, neurodevelopmental specialists, pediatric neurologists, and child psychologists.

As the field of DBP matured, it became desirable to have a recognized subspecialty so that there could be a core faculty within academic medical programs to organize the teaching of medical students, residents, fellows, and other allied health professionals, to conduct relevant research, and to assist in the delivery of clinical care. The Society for Developmental and Behavioral Pediatrics (initially called the Society for Behavioral Pediatrics) was formed in 1982; it is an international, interdisciplinary organization with approximately 750 members whose goal is to improve the health of infants, children, and adolescents by promoting research, teaching, and clinical practice in developmental-behavioral pediatrics (www.sdbp.org). SDBP has a well regarded professional journal, *Journal of Developmental and Behavioral Pediatrics* (www.jdbp.org), which is devoted entirely to the developmental and psychosocial aspects of pediatric health care and written for physicians, psychologists, and other clinicians and researchers.

In 1999, the field of developmental-behavioral pediatrics was approved as a subspecialty by the American Board of Medical Subspecialties and the first subboard of DBP within the American Board of Pediatrics was established to work with the Residency Review Committee to develop guidelines for subspecialty fellowship training and to develop an examination for certification of subspecialists in DBP. The first applications for accreditation of Fellowship Programs in DBP were accepted by the Accreditation Council for Graduate Medical Education in October 2002. Accredited fellowship programs in DBP accept trainees upon completion of an accredited pediatric residency program and are 3 years in duration. The fellowships comprise experiences in patient care to lead to the development of clinical proficiency, involvement in community or community-based activities, and development of skills in teaching, program development, research, and child advocacy. The first board certification examination in DBP was administered in November 2002, with the first certified subspecialists in the field in March 2003.

Both DBP and child and adolescent psychiatry are relatively young fields that share many commonalities. While DBP is firmly identified with traditional medicine by virtue of its subspecialty relationship to pediatrics, and child and adolescent psychiatry typically is considered to fall under the rubric of "mental health," DBP is increasingly integrating the insights offered by modern psychiatry and child and adolescent psychiatry is increasingly acknowledging its medical roots and connections to both pediatrics and psychiatry. The popularity of "triple board" training in pediatrics, psychiatry, and child and adolescent psychiatry, an alternative training pathway that also reflects a growing appreciation of the need to bridge the apparent gap between pediatric physical and mental health care, also validates the importance of active collaboration among the disciplines.

SHARING THE CHALLENGE

Although collaboration between pediatrics and psychiatry has been a topic of considerable interest and discussion for at least half a century, the hope of integrating MH services into pediatric general medical settings has yet to be realized. Parallel systems of care for physical and MH problems persist despite governmental recommendations to better integrate existing research-based knowledge into routine clinical practice (33), and existing models of reimbursement impair rather than facilitate meaningful collaboration. The scope and impact of pediatric emotional and behavioral problems nevertheless dictate that a response limited to the specialty MH sector is unlikely to prove successful in the short or long term, and is particularly unsuited to prevention efforts. Success in addressing the public health challenge presented by pediatric MH disorders will likely depend on multidisciplinary collaboration between child and adolescent psychiatrists, developmental-behavioral pediatricians, general pediatricians, family physicians, and affiliated MH professionals such as nurses, psychologists, and social workers, as well as efforts that span existing parallel systems of physical and MH care and reimbursement.

The public health importance of the primary care setting in the identification and management of common pediatric MH disorders is well recognized (3, 33, 36). PCPs manage the vast majority of recognized psychosocial problems (4) and prescribe the majority of psychoactive medications to American children and adolescents (32, 37). Psychosocial problems are increasingly becoming the major focus of primary pediatric care for school-age children, but surveys of pediatricians suggest that they are among the most time consuming and frustrating problems to deal with in routine practice. PCPs report inadequate training in the management of pediatric MH problems (4, 38), and low rates of PCP recognition of youth with MH disorders are the rule rather than the exception (3, 36, 38). Standardized assessment tools and/or diagnostic criteria are not in common use by PCPs in most clinical settings (39, 40).

While pediatricians do identify many MH concerns in their patients (in most cases, identifying far more children in need of treatment than are able to access child MH care), most children with MH needs still go unnoticed. It has been estimated that roughly 20% of children and adolescents have MH problems that are severe enough to warrant treatment (that have a diagnosable mental, emotional, or behavioral disorder), but of this group, less than 20–30% receive appropriate MH services in the United States (41) In one study, pediatricians' overall sensitivity for the identification of emotional/behavioral problems among preschool children 2–5 years of age was only 21%, while specificity was 93% (42). As a result, just over half (52%) of the children who had an emotional/behavioral problem, based on an independent assessment by two psychologists who performed an evaluation of children who had a positive initial screen, did not receive any counseling, medication, or MH referral from the pediatrician. Pediatricians' assessments tend to have far higher specificity than sensitivity. While they may miss most children with emotional or behavioral problems, they tend not to overdiagnose. Recognition is better in children or adolescents with more severe disturbance and in those with stressful family situations. However, it is likely that early detection, when problems are less severe and less recalcitrant to change, may respond better to less intensive interventions that could be provided in a primary care setting by the pediatrician.

Fortunately, studies have shown that the rate of identification of MH problems by pediatricians in the United States has increased dramatically over the past few decades. In one study, the rates of identification by pediatricians of any MH disorders, psychological symptoms, or social situations warranting clinical attention or intervention increased almost three-fold between 1979 and 1996, from 7–19% of all pediatric visits among 4- to 15-year-olds (43). Identification, though, represents only the first step in addressing MH needs in children. Pediatricians require additional skills if they are being expected to assist with management of some MH problems. Studies have shown that even when such problems are identified by pediatricians, most are handled through watchful waiting and/or primary care counseling alone; the vast majority of children identified with a MH or psychosocial problem never obtain services from a traditional MH provider, but instead continue to receive services from their primary care provider (38). Available research suggests that only one in four children with newly recognized psychosocial problems is referred for specialty MH services, with less than half of those referred ever seeing a MH specialist (4). Professional expectations as to the scope of practice are also relevant. While pediatricians have increasingly focused on the evaluation and treatment of common behavioral problems such as ADHD, which is often a major focus of DBP practice, there is considerably more variability in comfort and practice with regard to other problems such as depression and anxiety. For example, while pediatricians tend to consider themselves responsible for the recognition of pediatric depression, most do not consider the treatment of depression to be a core pediatric responsibility (44).

Barriers to accessing adequate MH services for youth presenting in primary care settings include stigma, insufficient access to specialty services, a shortage of child and adolescent psychiatrists and other MH professionals, imbalances in the geographic distribution of available MH professionals, prolonged delays in scheduling appointments, administrative practices that restrict access, and reimbursement problems (4, 33, 38). Even when credible referral is offered and available, family compliance with referral is quite low (4), with less than half of youth referred to specialty MH services ever receiving any treatment. In addition, PCP management of common disorders such as ADHD often fails to meet recommended standards for treatment intensity and followup (25), and PCPs are especially uneasy caring for disorders other than ADHD such as depression (44, 45). Professional expectations are clearly important and evolving. Uncomplicated ADHD is increasingly viewed as a disorder that is best managed in the primary care setting and by a pediatrician or family physician, whereas the management of pediatric depression is more commonly viewed as the purview of the MH specialist (44). Finally, while it is almost certainly true that professionals across disciplines are dedicated to improving services for youth with MH disorders, differences in training, classification systems, and reimbursement, as well as stigma and guild-related issues, can interfere with mutually respectful collaboration among professionals. There is often ambiguity with regard to role definition among MH professionals, and the role of PCPs in the management of MH disorders is even less clear (46, 47).

Despite the high prevalence of MH and behavioral concerns in children and the reality that most identification and treatment of these conditions falls to pediatricians and other PCPs, up until fairly recently there was limited training for most pediatricians in this area. In 1978, the Task Force on Pediatric Education of the American Academy of Pediatrics identified child development and chronic disabling conditions as areas of graduate pediatric education that were in need of enhancement. About that time (and subsequently), surveys completed by primary care pediatricians confirmed that they felt they were not adequately prepared to handle developmental and behavioral problems.

The Residency Review Committee governing pediatric training responded to these concerns by requiring, in 1997, that all accredited pediatric residency programs include at least a 1-month block rotation, as well as additional integrated training experiences, in developmental-behavioral pediatrics (DBP) which are directly supervised by faculty "with training in behavioral-developmental pediatrics." The vast majority of programs are now in compliance with this requirement, yet residency programs have found that providing quality training in DBP can be time consuming and difficult. The assessment and management of behavioral concerns are highly dependent on the context; there is rarely a simple and direct approach that will work in all situations. Teaching pediatric trainees about the management of behavioral problems therefore requires opportunities for clinical practice under direct supervision and quality faculty who are able to model clinical management, precept the trainee's clinical care, and engage the trainee in a discussion of alternative management approaches, all of which take considerable faculty time and resources. Given the limited number of highly qualified DBP faculty in the country and the low reimbursement rate by health insurers for their clinical services, this poses a significant challenge. In addition, many pediatric training programs provide only limited exposure to child and adolescent psychiatry, and sometimes no exposure whatsoever.

Behavioral or MH problems in children may result from parent–child, family, or simply parent problems. Assessment and treatment of the child, the identified patient, often requires assessment and intervention with the parents, yet unlike child and adolescent psychiatrists, pediatricians have very limited training or exposure to the care of adults, particularly adults with serious MH disorders. Despite these barriers, there appears to be a growing recognition among practicing pediatricians of the importance and value of continuing education in DBP and MH topics, which currently are highly prevalent among continuing medical education offerings geared to the practicing pediatrician.

Just as pediatricians may have insufficient training in the diagnosis and treatment of pediatric MH problems, child and adolescent psychiatrists typically have insufficient training on how to establish effective consultative or collaborative relationships with pediatricians and in developmental-behavioral pediatric issues. Child and adolescent psychiatrists often have not been exposed to, or lack sufficient experience with, anticipatory guidance and supportive management of common pediatric concerns and problems (e.g., management of common sleep problems and feeding difficulties), and neurodevelopmental issues have been relatively deemphasized as part of child and adolescent psychiatric training in many venues, at least until more recently. Likewise, developmental-behavioral pediatricians have focused considerably more than psychiatrists on neurodevelopmental issues and on the management of common pediatric problems, but have traditionally been less interested in the assessment and management of youth with serious psychopathology (e.g., bipolar disorder). Differences in training and experience likely have influenced relatively different orientations toward emotional and behavioral problems for child and adolescent psychiatrists and pediatricians, with the former tending to focus on the identification and treatment of MH disorders and the latter more oriented towards promoting overall child developmental health and wellness. One concrete illustration of these perceived differences in orientation was the development of the Diagnostic and Statistical Manual for Primary Care (DSM-PC) (48), which aims to help pediatricians identify and address the full spectrum of psychosocial situations or symptoms, ranging from developmental variations to problems to full disorders, that would benefit from intervention, even if the child's symptoms are not severe enough to meet the criteria for a specific MH disorder within the DSM used by child and adolescent psychiatrists. Furthermore, guild-related issues in these relatively young fields of child and adolescent psychiatry and DBP may not have provided sufficient time for the development of successful collaboration across respective clinical, educational, and research missions.

The traditional isolation and private office orientation of child and adolescent psychiatrists and other MH professionals may also have served to limit and restrict meaningful collaboration with pediatricians. Different expectations about standards of confidentiality in MH and general medical settings can also serve to constrain artificially the sharing of information between PCPs and MH specialists. Current healthcare practices also undermine efforts to promote collaboration between pediatricians and child and adolescent psychiatrists. Increasing use of behavioral health carve-outs may diminish the willingness and ability of MH providers to establish creative collaborative care models with PCPs. Managed behavioral healthcare organizations usually restrict their focus to specialty MH and substance abuse services and fail to address MH services that are provided in primary care or general pediatric settings. Innovative practices and prevention models that depend on screening, evaluation, and early treatment in primary care for MH needs may not be recognized or reimbursed by either the general managed care company or the managed behavioral healthcare organization, and obtaining reimbursement for MH services provided in a general medical setting may often seem akin to trying to fit a square peg in a round hole. The escalating productivity demands placed on pediatricians and other PCPs requiring increased throughput of patients, coupled with the historically inadequate reimbursement for MH services provided by pediatricians (and indeed most cognitive services), place enormous time pressure on pediatricians who attempt to deliver such services within their practice setting or to engage in substantive collaborative care with child and adolescent psychiatrists or other MH professionals.

PRIMARY CARE: A BRIDGE TO COLLABORATION

Despite the challenges outlined earlier, the advantages of targeting quality improvement efforts in the primary care setting to address MH needs are quite clear and include familiarity, proximity, and relative acceptability for youth with MH disorders and their families. PCPs remain an important resource for families to address pediatric psychosocial problems, and can deliver services in the context of an established relationship (3). There are many reasons why families might wish to rely on their pediatrician to assess and manage many behavioral and MH problems. Pediatricians are one of the most trusted sources of health information and services and have established relationships with children and their families that often start at the time of the birth of the child, or may even begin during a prenatal visit. The frequent well child checkups and sick visits, especially during the first few years of life, help to develop the relationship further; the frequent contact promotes both accessibility and convenience. For pediatricians who adopt a biopsychosocial orientation, it is especially clear that it is counterproductive, and indeed impossible, to try to separate the physical and MH care components of pediatric services. Coupled with the limited accessibility to MH providers in many communities and the stigma associated with mental illness, it is understandable why most MH and behavioral concerns present first to the child's pediatrician. A focus on primary care also acknowledges the reality that primary care is the de facto MH care system for most youths with recognized MH disorders (4) and that PCPs prescribe the vast majority of psychoactive medications to youth (32, 37). Delivering MH services in primary care powerfully communicates that physical and mental health are inseparable, and may aid in efforts to overcome stigma, improve communication between and among patients, families, and providers, and establish the foundation for meaningful educational and preventive interventions (38). Surveys of patients and families suggest that there is a preference to be seen in primary care for such problems rather than specialty care (1).

While it is recognized that high quality services for emotional and behavioral difficulties in primary care are generally multidisciplinary and collaborative (47), the evidence base necessary to make informed decisions about how to proceed in pediatric primary care is lacking. MH disorders such as ADHD, anxiety, and depression are most often chronic conditions that present with a broad range of severity, are commonly comorbid with other physical and MH disorders, and can exert their impact across the lifespan with a wide range of individual and family implications. Possible quality improvement strategies to address chronic MH problems in primary care settings include expanding the role of PCPs in managing common MH disorders, as well as the use of MH specialists as consultants to support the directed efforts of PCPs and/or to directly provide MH services within primary care (49). Adult depressive and anxiety disorders have been successfully managed in primary care using strategies that employ MH professionals as educators, consultants, supervisors, and/or direct service providers (50–52). Specialist participation in primary care beyond that of traditional off-site referrals can improve communication between PCPs and specialists, improve rates of referral completion, and enhance provider satisfaction (53). The collaborative office rounds model has been one attempt to support small case-oriented discussion groups that focus on MH needs of children presenting to primary care settings and are jointly led by pediatricians and child and adolescent psychiatrists (54). Available research nevertheless suggests that specialist involvement alone is less potent in improving care than are systemic changes in care system design (55–57).

The *chronic care model (CCM)* provides a framework to address the complexities associated with integrating MH services into general medical settings, and shifts the focus of care toward a longitudinal rather than an acute or cross-sectional perspective. Goals include ensuring that a mutually understood and agreed-upon care plan is in place, that patients and families have the skills and confidence necessary to manage the condition, that the most appropriate treatments are available for optimal illness control and the prevention of complications, and that accessible and continuous followup care is available (56, 58). There are six core elements of the CCM: 1) a *leadership* team composed of organizational partners, with leadership including specialists, generalists, and administrators with accountability for implementing the model; 2) *decision support* for direct care providers in general medical settings, which may include access to MH specialists and evidence-based guidelines to aid in the recognition and management of common MH disorders; 3) improvements in *delivery system design* to promote access to management guidelines and protocols. The use of a *care manager* responsible for coordinating care with PCPs and specialists has been promoted as an especially important element of delivery system design. The goal of a care manager is not to provide a nonphysician substitute for the PCP, but to complement and supplement the PCP's role by delivering services that the PCP does not have the skills or the time necessary to provide, such as formal psychiatric assessment, psychoeducation, and triage (56, 57), as well as to facilitate communication among families, PCPs, and supporting specialists (50, 57, 58). Ideally, the care manager mediates specialty input to the primary care setting (50, 55). The use of *patient care registries* to identify, manage, and track affected children can also modify the delivery system; 4) the use of *clinical information systems* to provide the technological underpinnings necessary to facilitate the roles of PCPs, care managers, and MH specialists; 5) *self-management support* for patients and families that includes materials and processes that promote understanding of common MH disorders and treatment options in order to facilitate patient activation and shared decisionmaking; and 6) access to *community resources* independent of healthcare providers to aid patients and families (57, 58).

A core value of the CCM is that optimal care is achieved when informed and motivated patients and families interact with a well prepared and proactive care team that is comprised of a multidisciplinary and diverse group of clinicians who communicate and participate regularly in the care of a defined group of patients (57, 58). As an adjunct, a "stepped care" approach emphasizes different levels of care depending on the type of specific disorder, its severity, complexity, and/or persistence in the face of intervention, and acknowledges the need for specialty MH care for selected or treatment refractory patients and families (50, 55). For example, a low severity disorder may initially be addressed through discussion of the disorder, basic psychoeducation for the patient and family, and watchful waiting, with higher levels of care being reserved for individuals suffering with the disorder at greater levels of severity and/or complexity. These higher levels of care might include initial management of the disorder in primary care by the PCP, followed by collaborative management in the primary care setting with the assistance of a care manager with specialty MH training, followed by referral for off-site specialty care. The CCM and stepped care approaches acknowledge that high quality illness management is multidisciplinary and collaborative, and a range of services and service delivery settings are indicated based on patient and family needs, since not all MH issues can be practically managed in the primary care setting (55–57, 59).

INTEGRATED MENTAL HEALTH SERVICES IN A RURAL PEDIATRIC PRACTICE

While there are many examples of a stepped collaborative care approach to the management of MH disorders in primary care for adults, few appear in the pediatric literature. We recently described a program within a large rural primary care practice in western Pennsylvania that relies on the relationship between PCPs and an on-site collaborative MH care team consisting of an advanced practice nurse (APN) with specialty MH training, a psychiatric social worker, and a child and adolescent psychiatrist (60). In this model, the PCP is the physician of record with responsibilities that include initial case identification, presumptive diagnosis, and ensuring the overall continuity of patient care. The APN serves as the primary liaison between the PCPs and psychiatrist (who is on-site infrequently), and functions as a bridge between primary and specialty care. The APN works closely with the PCP to complete an initial assessment and to triage each patient with an identified problem, with the goal of determining whether the child might benefit from services, and if so, where and how such services are best delivered. Treatment options include: 1) collaborative management with the PCP in primary care (generally appropriate for relatively straightforward, uncomplicated patients or those on a stable treatment regimen); 2) on-site MH comanagement by the PCP in collaboration with the primary care–based specialty MH team (such an approach might be appropriate for patients who failed earlier treatment by the PCP or patients of intermediate complexity or severity); and 3) off-site specialty MH referral (for patients with more complicated and/or severe disorders and psychosocial circumstances likely to render management within the primary care setting unsuccessful).

The APN provides patient and family education, ongoing case management and coordination, school liaison (e.g., requests and obtains teacher reports of patient behavior and performance), and treatment support services (psychopharmacology safety and outcome monitoring; brief psychotherapeutic support and intervention, including parent management training, simple behavior programs, and training in self-management strategies). The psychiatric social worker delivers brief psychotherapy for selected patients and families on site and the child and adolescent psychiatrist provides MH team leadership, supervision, education, psychiatric consultation for selected cases (diagnostic dilemmas, treatment failures), and will occasionally comanage cases requiring input from an experienced psychopharmacologist with the PCP. Approximately two-thirds of newly evaluated patients are triaged to routine services delivered by the PCP with APN support, 20% are managed on site by the PCP and MH team, and the remainder are referred to off-site specialty MH services. This rural program has been well received by PCPs, patients, and families, and patient and family compliance with initial assessment and triage visits has been quite high (91%) (60). This collaborative approach allows for MH services to be delivered and supported by blending both general medical and behavioral health funding streams, but other approaches may be even more feasible, such as those built around an APN capable of billing for the assessment and primary care based management of youth with emotional and behavioral problems via medical funding streams. A stumbling block for collaborative care approaches implemented outside a research setting arises from the practical difficulties of deriving fiscal support for specialist involvement in such models that does not involve directly billable, face-to-face time. Novel approaches such as telephone interventions (61), telephone care management for youth on psychoactive medications, and telemedicine may prove to be "nonstarters" in the real world unless innovations in systems of compensation for the delivery of behavioral health care services are permitted to parallel innovations in care delivery models. Nevertheless, while challenging from a fiscal perspective, collaborative models that flexibly incorporate pediatric MH specialists into primary care appear to be feasible and compatible with the workings of medical practice.

CONCLUSION

Health is a unitary construct that cannot be effectively parsed into physical and mental health, and thoughtful collaboration between child and adolescent psychiatrists, developmental-behavioral pediatricians, general pediatricians, and other professionals involved in pediatric care is critical to ensure the quality improvement efforts deserved by children everywhere. The familiarity, proximity, and acceptability of the primary care setting builds on established child and family relationships with PCPs. The PCP's attention to MH concerns communicates the powerful message that physical health and MH are inseparable. Equipping PCPs with the requisite knowledge and skills to identify, evaluate, and manage common developmental and behavioral concerns is a major goal of the field of developmental-behavioral pediatrics. The integration of MH services into primary care may aid in efforts to overcome previously identified barriers to intervention, such as cost and transportation problems, stigma and perceptions that treatment is not relevant, and strained relationships with MH service providers (62). Stepped collaborative care approaches that bridge primary and specialty care, as well as traditional medical care and behavioral health care, have the potential to facilitate patient and family access to MH services, improve adherence with initial MH contacts, decrease time between initial MH referral and active treatment, increase the quality of MH services in primary care, reduce stigma, efficiently integrate specialty MH professionals into primary care medical practice, and challenge false dichotomies between physical and MH care and reimbursement strategies. The ongoing operation and dissemination of such efforts will require attention to current funding mechanisms that segregate traditional medical and MH service delivery. Formal research addressing the effectiveness and design of collaborative care models for pediatric MH disorders is warranted.

References

1. Kelleher K: Prevention and intervention in primary care. In: Remschmidt, Belfer, Goodyer (eds): *Facilitating Pathways: Care, Treatment and Prevention in Child and Adolescent Mental Health*. 2004, Chapter 23.
2. Costello EJ, Burns BJ, Costello AJ, Edelbrock C, Dulcan M, Brent D: Service utilization and psychiatric diagnosis in pediatric primary care: The role of the gatekeeper. *Pediatrics* 82:435–441, 1988.
3. Horwitz SM, Leaf PJ, Leventhal JM, Forsyth B, Speechley KN: Identification and management of psychosocial and developmental problems in community-based, primary care pediatric practices. *Pediatrics* 89:480–485, 1992.
4. Rushton J, Bruckman D, Kelleher KJ: Primary care referral of children with psychosocial problems. *Arch Pediatr Adolesc Med* 156:592–598, 2002.
5. Frazer C, Emans SJ, Goodman E, Luoni M, Bravender T, Knight J: Teaching residents about development and behavior: Meeting the new challenge. *Arch Pediatr Adolesc Med* 153:1190–1194, 1999.
6. Olson AL, Kemper KJ, Kelleher KJ, Hammond CS, Zuckerman BS, Dietrich AJ: Primary care pediatricians' roles and perceived responsibilities in the identification and management of maternal depression. *Pediatrics* 110:1169–1176, 2002.
7. Kessler RC, Berglund P, Demler O, Jin R, Walters E: Lifetime prevalence and age of onset distributions of DSM-IV disorders in the National Comorbidity Survey Replication. *Archives General Psychiatry* 62:593–602, 2005.
8. Campo JV, Bridge J, Ehmann M, Altman S, Lucas A, Birmaher B, Di Lorenzo C, Iyengar S, Brent DA: Recurrent abdominal pain, anxiety, and depression in primary care. *Pediatrics* 113:817–824, 2004.
9. Egger HL, Costello EJ, Erkanli A, et al.: Somatic complaints and psychopathology in children and adolescents: Stomach aches, musculoskeletal pains and headaches. *J Am Child Adolesc Psychiatry* 38:852–860, 1999.
10. Liakopoulou-Kairis M, Alifieraki T, Protagora D, Korpa T, Kondyli K, Dimosthenous E, et al.: Recurrent abdominal pain and headache: Psychopathology, life event and family functioning. *Eur Child Adolesc Psychiatry* 11:115–122, 2002.
11. Campo JV, Comer D, Jansen-McWilliams L, Gardner W, Kelleher KJ: Recurrent pain, emotional distress, and health service use in childhood. *J Pediatrics* 141:76–83, 2002.
12. Bernstein G, Shaw K: Practice parameters for the assessment and treatment of children and adolescents with anxiety disorders. *J Am Acad Child Adolesc Psychiatry* 36(10 Suppl):S69–84, 1997.
13. Birmaher B, Ryan N, Williamson D, Brent D, Kaufman J, Dahl R, et al.: Childhood and adolescent depression: A review of the past 10 years. Part I. *J Am Acad Child Adolesc Psychiatry* 35(11):1427–1439, 1996.

14. Costello EJ, Angold A, Burns BJ, Erkanli A, Stangl DK, Tweed DL: The Great Smoky Mountains Study of Youth: Functional impairment and serious emotional disturbance. *Arch Gen Psychiatry* 53:1137–1143, 1996.
15. Lumeng JC, Gannon K, Cabral H, Frank DA, Zuckerman B: Association between clinically meaningful behavior problems and overweight in children. *Pediatrics* 112:1138–1145, 2003.
16. Dew MA: Psychiatric disorder in the context of physical illness. In: Dohrenwend BP (ed): *Adversity, Stress, and Psychopathology*, New York, Oxford University Press, pp. 177–218, 1998.
17. Gortmaker SL, Walker DK, Weitzman M, Sobol AM: Chronic conditions, socioeconomic risks, and behavioral problems in children and adolescents. *Pediatrics* 85:267–276, 1990.
18. Kovacs M, Goldston D, Obrosky DS, Bonar L: Psychiatric disorders in youths with IDDM: Rates and risk factors. *Diabetes Care* 20:36–44, 1997.
19. Rutter M, Tizard J, Whitmore K. *Education, health, and behavior*. London: Longman Group 1990.
20. Max JE, Koele SL, Smith WL, Sato Y, Lindgren SD, Robin DA, Arndt S: Psychiatric disorders in children and adolescents after severe traumatic brain injury: A controlled study. *J Am Acad Child Adolesc Psychiatry* 37:832–840, 1998.
21. Kovacs M, Mukerji P, Drash A, Iyengar S: Biomedical and psychiatric risk factors for retinopathy among children with IDDM. *Diabetes Care* 18:1592–1599, 1995.
22. Garrison MM, Katon WJ, Richardson LP: The impact of psychiatric comorbidities on readmissions for diabetes in youth. *Diabetes Care* 28:2150–2154, 2005.
23. Dantzer C, Swendsen J, Maurice-Tison S, Salamon R: Anxiety and depression in juvenile diabetes: A critical review. *Clin Psychol Rev* 23:787–800, 2003.
24. Weisz JR, Jensen PS: Efficacy and effectiveness of child and adolescent psychotherapy and pharmacotherapy. *Mental Health Serv Res* 1:125–157, 1999.
25. Jensen PS, Hinshaw SP, Swanson JM, Greenhill LL, Conners CK, Arnold LE et al.: Findings from the NIMH Multimodal Treatment Study of ADHD (MTA): Implications and applications for primary care providers. *J Dev Behav Pediatr* 22:60–73, 2001.
26. Olfson M, Gameroff MJ, Marcus SC, Waslick BD: Outpatient treatment of child and adolescent depression in the United States. *Arch Gen Psychiatry* 60:1236–1242, 2003.
27. Birmaher B, Axelson DA, Monk K, Kalas C, Clark DB, Ehmann M, et al.: Fluoxetine for the treatment of childhood anxiety disorders. *Journal of the American Academy of Child & Adolescent Psychiatry* 42(4):415–423, 2003.
28. Kendall P, Flannery-Schroeder E, Panichelli-Mindel S, Southam-Gerow M, Henin A, Warman M: Therapy for youths with anxiety disorders: A second randomized clinical trial. *Journal of Consulting and Clinical Psychology* 65:366–380, 1997.
29. Walkup J, Labellart M, Riddle M, Pine D, Greenhill L, Klein R: Fluvoxamine for the treatment for anxiety disorders in children and adolescents. *New England Journal of Medicine* 344:1279–1285, 2001.
30. Asarnow J, Jaycox LH, Duan N, LaBorde AP, Rea MM, Murray P et al.: Effectiveness of a quality improvement intervention for adolescent depression in primary care clinic: A randomized controlled trial. *JAMA* 293:311–319, 2005.
31. Institute of Medicine Committee on Quality of Health Care in America: *Crossing the Quality Chasm: A New Health System for the 21st Century*. Washington, DC, National Academy Press, 2001.
32. Ringeisen H, Oliver KA, Menvielle E: Recognition and treatment of mental disorders in children. *Pediatr Drugs* 4:697–703, 2002.
33. *U.S. Public Health Service Report of the Surgeon General's conference on children's mental health: A national action agenda*. Washington, DC: Department of Health and Human Services, 2000.
34. American Academy of Pediatrics, Committee on Quality Improvement: Diagnosis and evaluation of the child with attention-deficit/hyperactivity disorder. *Pediatrics* 105:1158–1170, 2000.
35. American Academy of Pediatrics, Committee on Quality Improvement: Clinical practice guidelines: Treatment of the school-aged child with attention-deficit/hyperactivity disorder. *Pediatrics* 108:1033–1044, 2001.
36. Costello EJ, Edelbrock C, Costello AJ, Dulcan MK, Burns BJ, Brent D: Psychopathology in pediatric primary care: The new hidden morbidity. *Pediatrics* 82:415–424, 1988.
37. Kelleher K, Hohmann AA, Larson DB: Prescription of psychotropics to children in office based practice. *Am J Dis Child* 143:855–859, 1989.
38. Kelleher KJ, Childs GE, Wasserman RC, McInerny TK, Nutting PA, Gardner WP: Insurance status and recognition of psychosocial problems: A report from PROS and ASPN. *Arch Pediatr Adolesc Med* 151:1109–1115, 1997.
39. Gardner W, Kelleher KJ, Pajer KA, Campo JV: Primary care clinicians' use of standardized tools to assess child psychosocial problems. *Ambulatory Pediatrics* 3(4):191–195, 2003.
40. Gardner W, Kelleher KJ, Pajer KA, Campo JV: Primary care clinicians' use of standardized psychiatric diagnoses. *Child: Care, Health, and Development* 30(5):401–412, 2004.
41. National Conference of State Legislatures Children's Policy Initiative: The Consortium on the School-Based Promotion of Social Competence, 2002.
42. Lavigne JV, Binns HJ, Christoffel KK, Rosenbaum D, et al.: Behavioral and emotional problems among preschool children in pediatric primary care: Prevalence and pediatricians' recognition. Pediatric Practice Research Group. *Pediatrics* 91:649–655, 1993.
43. Kelleher KJ, McInerny TK, Gardner WP, Childs GE, Wasserman RC: Increasing identification of psychosocial problems: 1979–1996. *Pediatrics* 105(6):1313–1321, 2000.
44. Olson AL, Kelleher KJ, Kemper KJ, Zuckerman BS, Hammond CS, Dietrich AJ: Primary care pediatricians' roles and perceived responsibilities in the identification and management of depression in children and adolescents. *Ambulatory Pediatrics* 2:91–98, 2001.
45. Rushton JL, Clark SJ, Freed GL: Pediatrician and family physician prescription of selective serotonin reuptake inhibitors. *Pediatrics* 105(6):E82, 2000.
46. Costello EJ, Pantino T: The new morbidity: Who should treat it? *J Dev Behav Pediatr* 8:288–291, 1987.
47. Pincus H: The future of behavioral health and primary care: Drowning in the mainstream or left on the bank? *Psychosomatics* 44:1–11, 2003.
48. Wolraich M, Felice M, Drotar D: *The Classification of Child and Adolescent Mental Diagnoses in Primary Care: Diagnostic and Statistical Manual for Primary Care (DSM-PC), Child and Adolescent Version*. Elk Grove Village, IL: American Academy of Pediatrics, 1996.
49. Bower P, Garralda E, Kramer T, et al.: The treatment of child and adolescent mental health problems in primary care: A systematic review. *Family Practice* 18:373–382, 2001.
50. Katon W, Von Korff M, Lin E, Simon G, Walker E, Unutzer J, et al.: Stepped collaborative care for primary care patients with persistent symptoms of depression: A randomized trial. *Arch Gen Psychiatry* 56:1109–1115, 1999.
51. Rollman BL, Belnap BH, Mazumdar S, Houck PR, et al.: A randomized trial to improve the quality of treatment for panic and generalized anxiety disorders in primary care. *Archives of General Psychiatry* 62(12):1332–1341, 2005.
52. Schulberg HC, Katon WJ, Simon GE, Rush AJ: Best clinical practice: Guidelines for managing major depression in primary medical care. *J Clin Psychiatry* 60:19–26, 1999.
53. Forrest CB, Glade GB, Baker AE, Bocian AB, Kang M, Starfield B: The pediatric primary-specialty care interface: How pediatricians refer children and adolescents to specialty care. *Arch Pediatr Adolesc Med* 153:705–714, 1999.
54. Fishman ME, Kessel W, Heppel DE, Brannon ME, Papai JJ, Bryn SD, Nora AH, Hutchins VL: Collaborative office rounds: Continuing education in the psychosocial/developmental aspects of child health. *Pediatrics* 99:e5, 1997.
55. Katon W, Von Korff M, Lin E, Simon G: Rethinking practitioner roles in chronic illness: The specialist, primary care physician, and the practice nurse. *Gen Hosp Psychiatry* 23:138–144, 2001.
56. Von Korff M, Gruman J, Schaefer J, Curry SJ, Wagner EH: Collaborative management of chronic illness. *Ann Inter Med* 127:1097–1102, 1997.
57. Wagner EH: The role of patient care teams in chronic disease management. *BMJ* 320:569–572, 2000.
58. Rothman AA, Wagner EH: Chronic illness management: What is the role of primary care? *Annals of Internal Medicine* 138:256–261, 2003.
59. Pincus HA, Hough L, Houtsinger JK, Rollman BL, Frank RG: Emerging models of depression care: Multi-level ("6P") strategies. *Int J Methods Psychiatr Res* 12:54–63, 2003.
60. Campo JV, Shafer S, Lucas A, Strohm J, Cassesse CG, Shaeffer D, Altman H: Managing pediatric mental disorders in primary care: A stepped collaborative care model. *Journal of the American Psychiatric Nurses Association* 11:1–7, 2005.
61. Borowsky IW, Mozayeny S, Stuenkel K, Ireland M: Effects of a primary care based intervention on violent behavior and injury in children. *Pediatrics* 114(4):e392–399, 2004.
62. Kazdin AE, Holland L, Crowley M: Family experiences of barriers to treatment and premature termination from child therapy. *J Consult Clin Psychol* 65:453–463, 1997.

7.1.3: MENTAL HEALTH ISSUES IN THE MEDICALLY ILL CHILD OR ADOLESCENT

CHAPTER 7.1.3.1 ■ CANCER

BRADLEY J. ZEBRACK

The American Cancer Society and the National Cancer Institute estimate that approximately 9,000–12,400 children and adolescents in the United States are diagnosed with cancer each year (1), which corresponds to roughly 1 in 6,500 young people under the age of 20 (2). Although childhood cancer is rare, it is the leading cause of death from disease among children age 1 to 14, resulting in an estimated 1,500 deaths in the United States in 2004 (3).

Prior to the 1970s and the advent and use of multimodal chemotherapy, children diagnosed with cancer had little hope of long-term survival. However, advances in treatment, including the large-scale coordination of treatment through clinical trials, have greatly increased the long-term life chances of these young people. Recent reports indicate that 78% of children diagnosed with various forms of cancer in the United States are expected to survive their disease and treatment, as compared to only 25% in the early 1970s (4). Today, 3 decades later, surviving childhood cancer is considered the norm rather than the exception.

Due to successes in treatment, much of the older literature on psychosocial outcomes for children with cancer is no longer appropriate to current and future cohorts of patients, survivors, and their family members. Psychosocial studies of children with cancer and their parents were initiated in the 1970s (studies of off-treatment survivors began in the early 1980s with Koocher & O'Malley's (5) groundbreaking work entitled *The Damocles Syndrome*), and occurred at a time when childhood cancer survivors were considered miracle children.

Contemporary trends in the psychosocial literature on childhood cancer encompass some or all of the following elements: 1) a developmental approach in which the issues experienced by children of various ages are treated in the context of their normative physical and psychosocial maturation; 2) a family systems approach emphasizing interactive impacts and responses in families and among family members; and 3) a stress-coping framework recently amended with a focus on posttraumatic effects. For people diagnosed with cancer it also is useful to examine their experiences in the context of "survivorship"—a continuum or trajectory initiated at diagnosis and extending through periods of treatment and then off-treatment survival or end–of–life (6, 7).

The research presented in this chapter reinforces the importance of examining the impact of cancer on children of different ages and developmental stages and within the context of family. The chapter also serves to orient the reader to the unique and sometimes subtle psychological, social, and behavioral effects of cancer on children and their families.

DEVELOPMENTAL CONTEXT

The boundaries used by theorists and researchers for classifying a "child" (as opposed to an adolescent or young adult) are varied. Some studies of pediatric cancer patients involve primarily elementary school–age children, while others combine younger school-age children with teenagers. Across this broad age range, the bulk of psychosocial research has been carried out with older school-age children. Very little work has been done with children under the age of 8 or 9 due in part to challenges related to literacy, human subjects' consent, and measurement.

From a developmental standpoint, younger school-age children are increasing their ability to think logically, understand cause and effect, and engage in formal reasoning (8). In addition, school-age children are acquiring a social and personal identity and are developing the ability to regulate themselves and their emotions (9). That said, the diagnosis and treatment of cancer will be interpreted and experienced differently by children of various ages and life stages. These differences are reflected in the literature presented in this chapter.

FAMILY SYSTEMS

The growth of "family systems theory" (10, 11) has emphasized how childhood illnesses, especially childhood cancer, may place psychological as well as physical strains on the family as a social system (12–14). In one of the first comprehensive studies of the family impact of childhood cancer, Chesler & Barbarin (15) suggested that childhood cancer is a "family disease" in that it "challenges the life course not only of the ill child but of the entire family."

General parenthood literature suggests that the centrality of one's role as a parent ranks quite high, higher even than that of marriage and employment, as a source of self-identity (16, 17). Parents worry about their children, about their physical and psychosocial wellbeing, and about their own ability/inability to protect them from fear, pain, temptation, or failure (18). For those parents whose children have experienced a medical trauma or serious life-threatening illness like cancer, these concerns and worries are likely to be intensified. Furthermore, when a brother or sister is diagnosed with cancer, siblings experience intrusive changes in family life. Siblings of pediatric cancer patients need to adapt to these changes and to the intrusive emotions such as fear, anger, isolation, jealousy, shame and guilt, which may be related to the illness of their sibling (19). They have to adjust to changes in family routines, to new ways of relating with their ill brother or sister, to increased responsibilities, and often to a decreased physical and emotional availability of their parents.

STRESS-COPING

While older notions of stress in cancer assume only negative or psychopathological outcomes are possible, recent research indicates that stress can be growth-producing as well as debilitating; thus, current investigations necessitate a broader conceptualization of stress and coping that allows for understanding reports of both positive and negative outcomes. Chesler and Barbarin's (15) stress-coping model is useful in organizing issues across five dimensions of stress and coping: intellectual, practical, interpersonal, emotional, and existential. The utility of this model comes from its organization of the cancer experience into observable categories of stress, coping responses and strategies, and sources of social support. It is applicable in that it identifies patient and survivor needs from perspectives incorporating quality of life, positive adaptation and family systems, thereby informing the development of interventions that address psychopathologic disease prevention as well as health promotion.

INTELLECTUAL ISSUES

Knowledge about Cancer, Treatment, and Life Threat

At the diagnostic stage, and immediately thereafter, children may experience stress in understanding the seriousness of the situation and in dealing with uncertainty. How do children become aware that they are in a serious situation, that they have a condition they ought to worry about? Sometimes parents or staff members tell them directly, but information may not be complete, may be delayed or not presented in a manner appropriate to the developmental stage of the child. Children and family members whose primary language is not English may struggle with simply understanding what hospital personnel are telling them, let alone the complexities and implications of impending medical procedures and treatment. Also, children will draw conclusions from the many cues consciously or unconsciously exhibited by parents, family members, friends and medical staff and by reading between the lines of what is said directly and what is whispered out of earshot. Many children note the rapidity and drama with which they are hospitalized; siblings are allowed to stay home from school in order to be at the hospital; grandparents travel long distances to come to the bedside; friends and relatives visit in large numbers; nurses and doctors visit often; and, almost everyone is extra attentive or looks scared or sad.

When a child is diagnosed with cancer, parents report feeling overwhelmed by the shock of the diagnosis, the stresses of uncertainty, and feelings of being trapped on an unpleasant emotional roller coaster (20). They report being faced with a strange and unfamiliar disease (21) and confronted with the challenges of understanding medical information, standard and alternative treatment options and possible complications, preparations for home care, and education about subsequent stages of illness and treatment (22). Part of the issue here is the diagnosis of a rare and potentially fatal disease that threatens the life of an innocent child, and that this occurs in a Western and affluent society where it is assumed that parents will die before their children. In addition, parents become introduced to a world of health utilization, governmental and community entitlements, hospital policies, health insurance regulations and limitations, and models of health care delivery (22). Even the language used by doctors and nurses can often be alien and strange to parents. The experience of hearing one's precious child referred to impersonally as "the host" or "the osteo in room 3" can be alienating. Parents also report feeling powerless in watching their child suffer and governed by the disease and its effects on everyday life and work (23).

Siblings of all ages struggle as well. Several studies indicate that siblings desire yet lack information about their brother or sister's cancer, the cause of it, and about the ill child's condition and prognosis (24, 25). They mention having to observe their brother or sister undergo painful procedures, and particularly at the end of life (24) (see Chapter 7.1.2.). They often feel left out of important family discussions with the healthcare team, and in some instances feeling left out of the information loop can result in siblings creating or imagining conditions that manifest fear (26).

PRACTICAL ISSUES

The Hospitalization Experience, Including Pain and Painful Procedures

Pediatric cancer treatment often involves multiple administrations of highly aversive medical procedures such as lumbar punctures, bone marrow aspirations, spinal taps and venipunctures over a prolonged period of time. Distress may be manifest by crying, screaming, requesting emotional support or physical contact, verbal resistance, verbal expression of fear, information seeking, and requesting delays in the administration of procedures or nonadherence with treatment (27). As treatment progresses, the seriousness of the situation may be brought home to the child by drastic medical procedures. Surgery, chemotherapy, radiation, repeated hospitalization, tests, and injections all debilitate the child physically and emotionally. In addition to pain, the illness and the side effects of treatment disrupt family life, school attendance, friendships and social activities.

As the amount of time spent in treatment increases, children inevitably experience the deaths of other children whom they have befriended. These deaths bring home very clearly the life-threatening nature of their own illness. The fragility of life becomes apparent when children realize that death could affect them as well (28). While we do not know how children deal with the imminence of approaching death, their clarity and straightforward approach in conversations represent a powerful coping strategy (15).

In adapting to the disease and its treatment, children with cancer also experience stress arising from relationships with staff members and medical personnel, and anxiety often is exacerbated when they are not allowed to be active participants in discussions of their illness. In the absence of adequate information, children may fantasize an even worse scenario, fearing the worst because they do not know what is wrong with them (29). Children also may experience anticipatory symptoms, including nausea and vomiting. Through repeated associations with chemotherapy and its aftereffects, certain environmental stimuli (e.g., smells and sights of the clinic) that are initially neutral come to elicit symptoms similar to those induced by chemotherapy (27). These impacts can influence siblings as well, in that brothers and sisters report having to "take care" of their ill brother or sister or parents, to take on extra tasks at home, and to be shuffled around to other family, friends, and neighbors, resulting in disruptions or limited involvement in social activities (24, 30).

Managing and balancing family home life and care for a child with cancer are the ultimate in challenge for parents. Many parents have indicated that uncertainty about their parent role and anticipating their child's distress during medical procedures are primary sources of stress, with uncertainty about the parenting role being associated with other measures of psychological distress (31). In addition, parents are confronted with decisionmaking and practicalities of informing their child's school officials about the child's illness, overseeing the process of actually facilitating the child's return to school, monitoring his/her health and needing to teach school personnel about unexpected health problems and signs to watch for (32). Parents also express concerns about their child's safety and of teasing by peers, and about academic progress and physical stamina (33) when returning to school. Concerns about the high financial costs of treatment and the need to devote much time to the sick child both at home and at the hospital are paramount (34) as another source of stress.

Adherence to Treatment

Nonadherence to prescribed treatments constitutes one of the most frequently encountered impediments to therapy administration in children with cancer, and these behaviors may take the form of refusing a procedure or treatment, failure to keep an appointment, or choosing alternative "unorthodox" treatment modalities (27). Recent discussions suggest that the rapport between medical staff, parents and children may be a key ingredient in overcoming resistance and promoting adherence to medical regimens. Thus, increased participation of children and adolescents in medical conversations and decisionmaking and treatment planning may help counter the possibility of nonadherence.

Cultural differences between patient, family, and medical staff also may interfere with treatment administration. Culture defines a family's response to an ill child and may explain behaviors such as nonadherence to prescribed therapies, parental preferences not to say the word "cancer" or not to discuss the issues with the child, degree and quality of parental involvement in patient care, and the family's relationship with healthcare staff (27, 35). Thus, physicians who wish to develop the most effective practical relationship with the child and family should carefully understand the cultural frame of the family.

School

While most patients are able to resume school activity in early outpatient phases of the treatment, complexities of treatment regimens, frequency of routine followup, disease status, neutropenia and infections can contribute to school difficulties (27). Hospitalizations result in missed school days and often necessitate assistance with schoolwork (obtaining assignments, learning materials, completing homework) (22). Many children's hospitals have inpatient schools where teachers help patients keep up with their schoolwork, often communicating with the child's teachers to obtain assignments.

How much school a child misses, and his or her level of achievement, will be factors in making plans for educational needs during treatment. Some children end up missing the academic year, others are able to keep up with peers, utilizing a tutor perhaps whenever not feeling well enough to attend school (36). Increased school absence, which can interfere with academic progress and peer socialization, is a common problem for children with cancer as they miss an average of 21–45 days of school per year (37, 38). Missing school is associated with reporting cancer-related stress and lower adjustment to cancer, and children with lower adjustment ratings also reported having fewer friends (39). On the other hand, other research shows that, within limits and with proper assistance, school attendance is not in and of itself a good predictor of academic performance and success.

Barriers to school reentry include changes in the child's appearance, cognitive abilities, emotional status, and physical activity, and misconceptions by peers and school personnel about cancer (40). Before returning to school, children have reported being most concerned about their ability to keep up with schoolwork and participate in extracurricular activities. They also expressed worry about their peers' reactions to changes in their physical appearance and the possibility that they may no longer fit in with friends as before (33).

Returning to school after an extended absence can be exciting but also anxiety provoking. Most children express concerns about returning to school after a long absence (36) or about keeping up in school both academically and physically (33). A study of children with cancer found perceived classmate social support to be the best predictor of adaptation in the child with cancer (41). Once having returned, these children's worries about academic performance and medical problems diminish, but concerns about keeping up with peers in extracurricular activities due to physical impairments persist.

Findings regarding childhood patients' experiences in school and social adaptation are mixed. Some investigators have examined social interactions between children with cancer returning to school and their healthy peers, and have reported that teachers and healthy peers perceived children with cancer as more socially isolated or withdrawn, low in leadership and social skills and disengaged from peers; yet, peer perceptions did not affect the child's popularity, their number of mutual friends, or their ratings of social competencies (42, 43). Some children returning to school have reported positive and rewarding friendships, whereas others recount negative experiences like "feeling invisible" and being bullied or "picked on." (44, 45) In contrast, others have reported generally adequate social adjustment for children with cancer as they return to school (46–48). In some cases the children describe themselves as more prosocial, teachers describe them as less aggressive, and peers perceive them as more sick, tired, and having missed school (49, 50).

Lahteenmaki and colleagues (45) report that as many as one-half of their sample of 43 childhood cancer patients were unsure whether their illness had been disclosed to classmates, and this concern reflects how peer reactions to the ill child and teachers' limited understanding of cancer may interfere with proper school reintegration. Peers may tease children with cancer because of their appearance or may avoid them for fear of contagion. Teachers may give the child "special" treatment, reinforcing the differences with peers, or may place excessive academic demands on a cognitively impaired child, or may reduce expectations or workload for patients who may be intellectually capable of completing assignments.

Cognitive Impairment

It is now generally accepted that central nervous system treatments for childhood cancer can result in significant cognitive impairment, most commonly in the areas of attention and concentration (51). Children who have received certain treatments, particularly to the central nervous system, are at risk for developing learning problems. Among areas frequently affected are attention, concentration, memory, handwriting, math, and organizing or sequencing of tasks (36). Children who have been irradiated and children diagnosed under 6 years of age are at greatest risk for difficulties in school functioning (52).

INTERPERSONAL ISSUES

Peer Relationships

Prolonged courses of cancer treatment often become an inevitable series of events (doctor visits, periods of nausea and illness, fatigue) in which children feel no respite or escape. Frequent disruptions, including hospitalizations or confinement to home often lead to periods of social isolation. Although most children with cancer experience a great deal of positive attention at first, some feel forgotten and eventually isolated from friends and peers as time goes by (15). This sense of isolation is particularly true for children with brain tumors who are perceived by peers as being sick and fatigued, are often absent from school, and identified less often than healthy peers as being a best friend (53).

Relationships outside the family, particularly with friends, often are a source of stress. Frustration and pain from social isolation and stigmatization by peers are experienced, as peers may have misconceptions and fears. Zeltzer et al. (54) have reported that youngsters with cancer report that the illness decreases their popularity with peers. This may be in part the result of chronic and repeated hospitalizations that decrease access to their peers; however, it may also relate to the stigma of cancer and to ill youngsters' experiences (or fears) of rejection. At the same time, research suggests that many school-age children with cancer report themselves feeling more mature than their peers, leading to the development of peer-type relationships with older youngsters (55, 56).

The introduction of cancer into the family can change family dynamics and roles dramatically. Often parents face a struggle to cope with their own emotional needs while also being attentive to the needs of the patient and other family members. Frequently this struggle leaves siblings receiving the least amount of time and attention, despite their growing concerns.

Studies indicate that siblings of children in treatment report feelings of anger, resentment, jealousy, frustration, and isolation from their family; of being overwhelmed by fear for their brother/sister's health; of fear of contagion of cancer; guilt for not being sick themselves; and of being treated differently by their parents (26, 57–64). They also report concerns about change in peer relationships in that peers would react to the illness in negative ways that affect their social lives (65). Other studies indicate that siblings experience feeling no control over a family situation in which they cannot influence the disease process, and frustrated that decisions about the illness and care are in the hands of doctors, nurses and other adults (parents) (57, 66). In cases involving death and bereavement, siblings often indicate that they feel unprepared (67). As a result, siblings may experience anxiety or guilt, or they may distance themselves or ignore the entire situation in response to feelings of being left out or isolated, or as a means of protecting themselves from the experience (68).

While changes in daily routines are accompanied by shifts in attention and being treated differently by their parents (61), siblings also have indicated that they felt positively about this treatment and that it was "only fair," given the circumstances. In turn, siblings may tend to treat their parents differently in that they perceive the need to protect their parents as well as the child with cancer by not making them worry (59, 69). Yet siblings still characterize these changes as a lack of communication or poor communication between themselves and their parents (59–61, 64, 70, 71). On the other hand, some siblings report, in retrospect, that despite these strains and tensions their family grew closer as a function of the ways in which they dealt with the illness together (30).

Effects on Child Rearing

Raising a child with cancer may alter a parent's ability to parent effectively (27). Overprotectiveness, difficulty with maintaining consistent discipline and expressing appropriate anger toward the child, and concerns about "spoiling" the child challenge parents throughout treatment and recovery (72). While data suggest that parents of children with cancer do not differ from community-matched parents of children without cancer with regard to basic orientation to childrearing (73), their ability to carry out the tasks of childrearing over the longterm certainly is impacted. Work by Zebrack and colleagues (74) has demonstrated that mothers of survivors of childhood cancer continue to worry about their children's medical and social futures, especially when they perceive that their children worry about these issues. The investigators' overall conclusion is that parental concerns and wellbeing and those of the child survivor have reciprocal influences on one another. Indeed, there is much agreement among researchers that family functioning and distress are integrally connected to the survivors' adjustment; that there exists a reciprocal nature of coping and adjustment among parents and children (31, 47, 75–78).

Effects on Marriage

Of particular concern to parents are the effects of childhood cancer on their marriage. With mothers and fathers assuming distinct and different roles in the face of childhood cancer, they also may exhibit different coping styles. The stress created by these differences, compounded by the disease-related stresses on personal and family time, finances, and family, can lead to marital strain for parents. Some studies show profound changes and marital discord in the parental dyad (79), while others show that marital relationships remain stable or actually improve over the course of the child's cancer (80). For some, the cancer experience compounds or exacerbates preexisting marital stresses (81).

EMOTIONAL ISSUES

Distress

As might be expected, children and their families experience and exhibit emotional and behavioral problems during the initial phases of diagnosis and treatment, with investigators reporting behavioral and emotional disturbances manifested in increased anxiety, depression, regression, and withdrawal among children in treatment for cancer. For instance, Cavusoglu (82) reports that rates of depression for both males and females aged 9 to 13 and at least 1 year after initial diagnosis were significantly higher than in a healthy age-matched control group and that rates also were significantly higher among patients in treatment than those off treatment and in remission. Some investigators have reported increased levels of distress associated with longer periods of active disease and treatment (83), and others have found that children with cancer ranked school reentry as a primary source of psychological pain, due in large part to their falling behind academically and the negative reaction of classmates. The authors conclude from their findings that younger children may be more adaptable to adverse situations than older children, or alternatively, that adjustment difficulties may not appear until much later after treatment and may manifest as posttraumatic stress symptoms.

In contrast, others report few emotional or behavioral problems in children with cancer and demonstrate normal psychosocial functioning during treatment administration (27). Several cross-sectional and comparative studies indicate that, for the most part, aggregate scores on measures of depression, distress, or anxiety for children and adolescents with cancer generally fall within the normal range or are no different from peers (48, 84, 85), and in some cases are reported at lower levels when compared to healthy controls (86, 87). Several prospective and long-term followup studies suggest that for many patients and survivors, emotional and behavioral problems are alleviated over time (88–91).

In addition to the research suggesting that for many school-age children emotional problems are either of short duration or not severe, recent work suggests that some children surviving cancer may be emotionally stronger than their healthy peers, and significantly more emotionally coherent and centered than they themselves were prior to their cancer treatment. New studies, consisting mostly of adolescents and young adults, suggest that some survivors of childhood cancer experience or manifest positive adaptation, or "posttraumatic growth." (92–95) In brief, these aging childhood cancer survivors attribute such growth and maturity to a sense of "seeking balance in my life," "not being afraid of emotions," and "having been through a crisis and come out whole." (96)

Parents also experience a wide range of emotional reactions to the diagnosis and ongoing treatment of their child. These feelings, common to children with cancer, include shock or confusion after receiving a diagnosis, disbelief/denial about the accuracy or extent of the disease, fear and anxiety, guilt, sadness or feelings of depression, and anger (97). They certainly experience greater levels of uncertainty and distress when compared to parents of children without cancer, as well as to parents of children who have survived cancer and are no longer in treatment (98, 99). How parents handle these emotions usually reflects variations in life situations, cultural norms, and their individual coping styles in responding to major distress.

In one of the earliest studies of parents of survivors of childhood cancer, Peck (100) suggested that parents continue to experience elevated levels of general anxiety, especially connected to uncertainty about the stability of the "cure" and the potential of the cancer returning. Other investigators report that some parents of childhood cancer patients and survivors are at elevated risk for psychosocial difficulties, including posttraumatic stress disorder (101–103), depression (104, 105), anxiety (5), and marital discord (106). In contrast, others report that most parents of survivors are mentally healthy and coping well, despite having ongoing concerns (85, 107–109). While distress becomes alleviated over time for parents of off-treatment survivors (110, 111), uncertainty and fears related to cancer can remain. There also is evidence to suggest that parent worries differ from those of their child, and that parents experience more distress and negative affect than survivors or siblings themselves (74, 112).

As for differences in mother and father coping, studies are mixed with regard to differences in affective/emotional responses and predictors of these responses. For instance, some investigators report that parents did not differ with regard to exhibiting symptoms of depression or anxiety or distress (98, 113), while others report significant differences (114). Other studies identify differences in affect and coping response (115, 116). For instance, Sloper (115) found that appraisal of the extent of strain posed by the illness and their own ability to deal with it, along with family cohesion, were most strongly predictive of stress for mothers. In contrast, employment problems and number of hospital admissions, along with family cohesion, were the most significant predictors of distress for fathers. Chesler and Parry (21) add that fathers can and do experience emotionally strong feelings with regard to feelings of terror, powerlessness, anticipatory loss, and guilt in spite of societal pressures to remain stoic and in control, and that many fathers did indeed find it difficult to express feelings of sadness, pain, weakness or vulnerability. Others indicate fathers as more likely than mothers to use more active problem-focused coping strategies or to accept that there was no known cause for the child's illness, whereas mothers relied more upon seeking social support or were more likely to feel some level of blame for their child's illness (98, 117).

Among siblings, significant internalizing problems, such as emotional and social withdrawal, anxiety, feelings of guilt, hopelessness, shame and sadness; or externalizing problems, such as anger, noncompliance or other acting-out behavior, have been reported (59, 68–70, 118–120). Anxiety, isolation, and loneliness have been reported as stress responses (59, 69, 121), along with feelings of unimportance, low self-esteem, and internalized hostility (59). Siblings also have been found to express fears, worries, and concerns that their brother or sister might not survive their illness (61), and they experience anxiety around a lack of communication within the family (59, 69). Notably, Havermans and Eiser (61) found that siblings in families that scored high on communication also were more likely to report worrying about death of their sibling than did siblings in families scoring low on communication.

Others report that siblings may have increased rates of emotional symptoms compared to the general population (112). For example, nearly half of a sample of adolescent siblings reported mild posttraumatic stress symptoms and 32% indicated moderate to severe levels (122). These siblings reported more posttraumatic stress symptoms than a reference group of nonaffected teens. Posttraumatic stress symptoms also were found associated with thoughts that the patient would die during treatment and finding the experience scary and difficult (122). In contrast, others have reported no substantial social-emotional problems in siblings of pediatric cancer patients (123–125), that a majority of siblings do not appear to have adjustment or behavioral problems (112, 126, 127), and that rates of distress are similar to those found in the general population (63, 125). In addition, resilience outcomes like those reported among survivors also have been reported in sibling studies, with siblings reporting benefits that include feeling more mature, adopting a different attitude toward life, becoming more caring toward others, and experiencing greater family closeness (61, 62).

Over time, impaired psychosocial functioning and quality of life improves for most siblings, although adolescent siblings experience more impaired emotional and social functioning when compared to younger school-age siblings (19). Also, with increasing age, sisters reported more physical problems, whereas brothers reported more behavioral and social problems. Ronen (128) suggests that gender socialization roles influence girls to talk more freely about anxieties and boys to hide them, thus resulting in observable differences in siblings' adjustment. Yet, negative attention-seeking and acting out may represent emotional reactions of siblings to the cancer experience (69).

EXISTENTIAL/SPIRITUAL ISSUES

Uncertainty

Mishel (129) defines uncertainty within the context of illness as the "inability to determine the meaning of illness-related events," which is brought about by "unpredictable and inconsistent symptom onset, continual questions about recurrence or exacerbation, and unknown future due to living with debilitating conditions." While many aspects of cancer and treatment in children remain uncertain (survival, effectiveness of treatment), children may not necessarily characterize themselves or their lives as uncertain. For example, in a study involving 9–12 year-old children with a variety of cancer diagnoses, Stewart (130) reports that these children quickly came to view their lives as routine and ordinary despite the unpredictable nature of the course of their illness. They described a process of getting used to cancer that allowed them to keep their focus on the ordinary nature of their everyday lives within the uncertain context of their illness, thus providing important insight into children's psychological adjustment to life-threatening illness. Although children with cancer live with symptoms of treatment on a daily basis, they also suggest that the symptoms are an integral part of overcoming cancer and do not expect complete symptom relief (131). While they suggest that one never gets used to symptoms and that symptoms contribute to discomfort and suffering, there also exists an attitude or belief among some children that they must exchange short-term pain for long-term gain, that they must feel a lot worse before they can feel better (131). This is all part of what Woodgate and Degner (132) theorize and call "keeping the spirit alive."

Over time, and with long-term remission and cure, many parents report positive aspects emerging from the cancer experience. Having once experienced the devastation and shock of diagnosis and the intensity and focus of treatment, many parents move to a new or renewed sense of valuing and living life to the fullest, improved quality of life, increased family closeness, and an ability to deal with other life stressors (133). Resilience after cancer does not occur in denial of a negative, life-threatening experience. Indeed, parents acknowledge that life goes on but cancer could come back, that life was difficult living through cancer, and that there is now a need to increase attention to their child's health (133).

COPING WITH CANCER

Normalizing the Experience

As a consequence of dealing simultaneously with normal social situations and with a unique medical situation, children with cancer sometimes feel they are living in two social worlds. One is a world of health, and children in remission and doing well spend most of their time in this world. The other is a world of medicine and illness, and even children doing well continually enter this world for checkups and treatments. There are different rules in these different worlds. At home and school, ill children try to be normal and to live according to the same rules as everyone else, trying to grow up and master the many challenges of everyday existence. In the hospital and medical center, they are special people—patients, struggling with life and death, seeing sickness and pain on every side. Here they relate to doctors and nurses, not solely to parents, teachers, and friends. Here, too, they often see friends die and may have to confront their own mortality.

Young people with cancer overwhelmingly report that their primary goal in relation to these two worlds is to resume a path through a normal life as soon as possible. At the root of this quest is a concern about being different or being treated differently than other young people (55). Most resist this, avoid an identity as a victim of cancer, and try to remain physically and socially active.

Normalizing School, Education, and Social Lives

As children with cancer undergo treatment, they also continue with their lives. For children between the ages of 6 and 18, school attendance is an important part of life, and a vital social and developmental activity. School represents the continuation of children's normal life as well as the primary source of social activity. Regular school attendance is vital to foster normal development and to prevent social regression and isolation from peers (134, 135). Positive school experiences can reduce children's maladaptive emotional responses to the disease and its treatments by helping them feel academically accomplished and socially accepted (27). For these reasons, children with cancer are encouraged to participate in school activities as fully as possible. Yet, parents may be reluctant to entrust to the school a child whose health is seen as fragile. Communication about the child's health condition with school personnel frequently becomes the responsibility of the parents, who are often still overwhelmed by the diagnosis and unsure of what information school personnel need (136).

Normalizing participation in school and social life involves participating in or avoiding social involvement and linking to friendships. Just as parents must decide what to tell their children at the point of diagnosis, young people with cancer must decide if, when, and how to share this information with their school-age peers. An even more delicate issue is what and how much to say about their illness to new acquaintances. Faced with the potential for varied reactions, young people with cancer may lose confidence because of their uncertainty about whether and how they will be accepted. When loss of opportunities for social interaction with peers is severe, it is experienced as a major deprivation that multiplies other stresses of the illness. When positive interaction with peers occurs, it helps ease the stress of coping with the illness and renews youngsters' adaptive capacities. Thus, participation in oncology camps, cancer survivor day picnics, and family retreats offer opportunities for life experiences that promote successful development of age-appropriate developmental tasks.

For students needing special attention/education, under some federal and state laws, states and local school districts must provide a free, appropriate elementary and secondary education in the least restrictive environment for all children with disabilities from ages 6 through 21. Students with cancer or a cancer history whose medical problems adversely affect their educational performance are considered to have a disability—to be "other health impaired," and as such entitled to receive needed special educational services (36). For children whose physical conditions place them at risk of further health problems, homebound education may be called for. Homebound instruction, while often indicated for patients at risk for exposures to infection in public, was recalled by 8 to 17-year-old off-treatment survivors as being academically inadequate and socially isolating (44).

Receiving detailed information about a child's disease and treatment plans will help school faculty and administrators better provide educational programming during and after treatment. Also, some treatment centers have special programs for school personnel to learn about cancer, while others have members of the treatment team visit the school on request. In other cases, parents become responsible for communicating directly with school personnel.

Communicating with Children about Cancer

There is a wide variety of opinion and practice regarding what and how much should be told to a school age child about their diagnosis, treatment, and prognosis. Some practitioners still endorse the practice popular decades ago, when children were deliberately told nothing or little about their condition. Others adopt a stance of sharing information if and when, and about what, the child asks for. And still others advocate relatively full sharing of information, hopefully in a realistically positive tone and with age-appropriate language and content. The Psychosocial Committee of the International Society of Pediatric Oncologists (SIOP) recommends full disclosure to the child, after or during a conference with the parents (137). Enabling honest and open family communication, receiving parental/family support, and utilizing psychological counseling (individual/group) all have been demonstrated to have positive associations with various psychosocial adjustment outcomes (15, 135, 138). Conversely, poor family communication and a lack of sharing/expressing emotion has been associated with worse coping (139).

Current research indicates that both the child's age and their preferences for information are associated with psychosocial outcomes. For example, in a study of 56 children with cancer, aged 8–16, two-thirds of the sample wanted to know everything about their disease; one-third wanted to know as little as possible; and those who received information were significantly less anxious and depressed than children who received less information (83). Ross (140) indicates that while most of a sample of 32 children aged 5–12 had at least a cursory understanding of why treatment was necessary, their preferences for information about cancer treatment varied widely: nine of the 32 children desired information regarding the specific details and timing of treatments, while five preferred no advance information at all. Several children indicated that a thorough understanding of certain medical procedures made the process even more painful. In contrast, Hockenberry-Eaton and colleagues (141) report that children's fears about medical procedures were allayed to some degree through a truthful understanding of what to expect, and that "knowing" about their cancer and its treatment made therapy easier to handle. These findings suggest the importance of open communication among parents, health care providers, and children when it comes to discussing cancer and its treatment, and that communication should also include an assessment of how much, if any, information a child prefers and can integrate. It also suggests that parents and staff members should encourage young patients to ask questions, and to provide them with the information from which intelligent questions can flow.

To aid in the communicative process, some clinics have developed visual aids, including a videotape of the diagnostic conference held with physicians, nurses, social workers, parents and child present. This tape can be taken home by the family and played and replayed at their leisure, thus aiding their understanding, their communication with one another, and their dissemination of accurate information to other family members, friends, and neighbors (142).

Coping Styles

Questioning, cheerfulness, denial, talkativeness, depression, humor, withdrawal, optimism, and low energy level all may be initial coping responses to therapy in children. These strategies tend to change and alternate over time as children pass through various stages of therapy and off-treatment survivorship (27). For example, investigators have identified differences in coping styles. For instance, 66 children with cancer in treatment, aged 6–15 years, endorsed greater use of avoidance as a coping strategy than did 414 healthy school-age children (143). In general, von Essen and colleagues (144) suggests that amusement, clinical competence, emotional support, family participation, honest communication and information, parent participation in decisionmaking, satisfaction of basic needs and normalizing social competence are the most important aspects of care, as they assure the child that he/she feels cared for. Emotional adjustment among children with cancer, ages 8–18, also was predicted by having positive expectations about the course of the illness (145). Others have demonstrated children's coping to be related to parent coping. For example, parent anxiety was found to be associated with a greater likelihood of children's coping difficulties (146).

As with psychological and emotional growth, some school age children surviving cancer exhibit signs of greater spiritual centeredness and a more coherent philosophy or outlook on life, although there exists little empirical research examining these outcomes in school-age children. Among patients ranging in age from 6.5 to 14.5 years, those of lower socioeconomic status were reported to use religious coping strategies significantly more often than others (147).

Childhood cancer is a potentially life-changing experience for parents. It often promotes change by challenging them to adopt new identities and/or coping styles, requiring new social role behaviors, and providing opportunity for new and different relationships with surrounding social environments and institutions, and constructing meaning from the illness (21, 117, 131, 148). Parents tend to use cognitive control and coping strategies that include being optimistic about the situation (predictive control), attributing power to medical caregivers (vicarious control); hoping for a miracle or wishful thinking (illusory control); and searching for information in order to better understand emotional reactions and to derive meaning from the situation (interpretative control) (149).

Although there exists a literature reporting parent outcomes with regard to coping and adjustment, Chesler and Parry (21) point out that mothers often are more willing to participate in studies and that many investigators have used maternal responses as a proxy for parental responses. In a study of fathers of childhood cancer survivors, Chesler and Parry demonstrate that fathers may in fact experience childhood cancer quite differently from their spouses, due largely to imposed gender identities and social role constructions in the United States. For example, fathers are often expected to control their emotions and remain stoic in the face of stress. In addition, the primary role assumed by fathers is that of breadwinner and provider. The authors also indicate that several fathers expressed frustration over the perceived differences in the ways fathers and mothers are treated by employers during childhood illness. Fathers believed that employers expected mothers to take leave from work when a child became ill and accommodated them for absences, whereas fathers were often expected to balance work and home life. Chesler and Parry concluded that to the extent that men subscribe to beliefs or enact behaviors and emotional styles congruent with social constructions of male gender identity, they may experience particular difficulties in handling the existential and emotional stresses of cancer.

Interventions that meet sibling needs for emotional and informational support are most important (57, 150) and may be met in several ways. Siblings report that accessing information is most helpful (67) and they identify mothers as being a primary source of information (61). They also express a desire to receive more in-depth information from the healthcare team (61). Indeed, sibling social competence has been reported to be associated with sibling self-report of possessing knowledge about their brother's or sister's cancer (151). Yet, while increasing sibling knowledge or understanding of cancer is important, Evans and colleagues (151) demonstrated that on its own, provision of information does not necessarily promote successful adjustment.

Houtzager et al. (66) suggest that the following coping strategies, delivered through a supportive group for siblings, may enhance adjustment: enhancing optimism about the situation, attributing power to medical caregivers, hoping for a miracle or wishful thinking, search for information in order to better understand emotional reactions and to derive meaning from the situation (66, 152). Others have suggested that reinforcing self-control as a coping skill (self-instruction, positive thinking, problemsolving methods, imagery exercises) may reduce anxiety and loneliness (153), and that enabling siblings to provide comfort to their sibling with cancer is an important emotional component of support (67). Many of these needs may be met by nursing and socialwork interventions (154, 155) or through support from family and friends (67). Specific books and Internet Websites aimed at siblings and appropriate for different developmental stages also could be valuable sources of information.

Current literature reinforces the importance of support groups for siblings and opportunities for peer involvement with other siblings, including special camps and family retreats, although data are scarce (71, 156, 157). Group programs may provide information about the illness, which can reduce fears (156). Meeting peers who also have a brother or sister with cancer is a unique opportunity for siblings to supply their need for recognition, communication, information and reality testing (66). One outgrowth of such activities is the advice some siblings of children with cancer have offered to other siblings: Be good so that you do not add to your family's burden; help take care of your ill brother or sister; and take care of yourself—talk to someone who cares about and can help you, like a relative, teacher, or friend (30).

SOCIAL SUPPORT

Many parents seek education and support to help them identify, express, and master the powerful feelings evoked by the difficult events of childhood cancer. Some need only validation of their feelings or that they are managing life adequately given the circumstances. Others need more intensive therapy or emotional support from trained mental health professionals. For many, parental hope is integral to helping parents cope with the illness experience, as is social and family communication (139). Receiving peer support from friends, from other parents of children with cancer and from community-based organizations composed of health professionals or laypersons is critically important (77, 158).

Chesler and Barbarin (159) note some of the difficulties experienced by parents of children with cancer in their effort to gain support from formerly close friends. On occasion, parents' own lack of skill or ability to ask for help, their own emotional overload, and their fear of stigma constrained their efforts to reach out for support. In reciprocal fashion, family friends often noted their desire to avoid intruding on parents' privacy, their fear or concern about their own emotional stability, and their lack of knowledge of what kind of help was useful, constrained their efforts to provide help. These strains sometimes resulted in old friends disappearing or distancing and others coming closer. Many parents of children with cancer reported finding new and helpful friends among the population of other parents of children with cancer. Whether through the medium of hospital waiting rooms and hallways or via the formation of support and self-help groups, many parents of children with cancer bonded with others in their same situation.

Locally organized parent groups exist in over 300 communities and medical sites across the United States. Some are large and formally organized, with bylaws, elected officers and nonprofit legal status, and others are small and informal gatherings. Some include members of the medical staff and others are exclusively parent led and attended. While not all (nor even a majority) of parents of children with cancer become active members of such groups, those who do report many benefits. The Candlelighters Childhood Cancer Foundation remains the preeminent national clearinghouse and resource for support groups for families of children with cancer (www.candlelighters.org).

Involvement in supportive social networks and having opportunities to express feelings and worries related to cancer may improve parents' adjustment to illness over the long term (160, 161). For example, some parents experience improvements in emotional functioning and adjustment from participating in professionally lead support groups or nonprofessional parent-lead self-help groups; supportive programs and interventions appear to offer important coping skills for parents of children in treatment. In one of few reported intervention studies, 19 families of childhood cancer survivors participated in a 1-day family group intervention combining the cognitive-behavioral and family therapy approaches. In this study by Kazak and colleagues (162), families reported positive outcomes, including reduction in posttraumatic stress and anxiety symptoms from pre- to postintervention time periods. Testing an 8-week educational program to increase problem-solving skills and reduce feelings of depression, distress, guilt, and anger, Sahler and colleagues (163) demonstrated positive changes for mothers participating in the program.

CONCLUSION

School-age children diagnosed with cancer enter a world of unfamiliar and threatening people and things, emotional confusion, physical discomfort, and pain. Diagnostic procedures are painful and scary, and the child often exists in the midst of a world of uncertainty—his own and his parents'. This uncertainly is escalated when parents and the medical staff fail to provide the child with information that is adequate, coherent, and tuned to an appropriate developmental level. Even with adequate information, young children often worry about their future, whether they will endure repeated hospitalizations and time away from home. Subsequent hospitalizations, of short or long duration, separate and often isolate the child from peers and schoolmates, as well as from the ordinary routines of family and neighborhood life. In addition, the long-term effects of the disease and treatments may compromise cognitive capacities and social or physical functioning (especially in the case of major surgery or radiation to critical organ systems).

Parents of children diagnosed with cancer typically experience shock and surprise. The stress of having a child diagnosed with a frightening and potentially fatal or disfiguring disease is escalated by the necessary entry into the culture of tertiary care medical facilities and their language, jargon, and status systems. Parents feel dependent upon the medical staff for the very survival of their child, and this forced dependency often disempowers parents, makes them feel unable to act positively in their child's behalf, and sometimes creates difficulty in parent–staff relationships. Parents' central role as a parent is to protect their children from harm, and a diagnosis of cancer in a child challenges the core definition of parentage.

Parents are often called upon to spend time in the hospital with the ill child, and for many the child's response to the illness raises concern about maintaining normal childrearing practices and discipline. In addition, parents are faced with balancing the competing needs of the ill child, family chores and relationships, and employment requirements. If employers are not responsive to these concerns, the family may face added financial stress. Maintaining normal and satisfying family routines and relationships often is difficult under these circumstances. Siblings often feel left out or overlooked, marital stress may occur (especially when mothers and fathers cope differently and with difficulty) and relationships with parents' parents and friends may also suffer.

When compared to early research on families of childhood cancer patients that focused on presumed psychopathological responses to coping with illness and death, current literature reflects a more complete account of the numerous components contributing to childhood cancer patients' and family members' feelings and responses, including the multitude of positive outcomes that may arise from their experience (57). Still to come are longitudinal studies that will offer a depth of insight into the extent to which patients, survivors, and family members describe, in their own words and on their own terms, their experiences living with, through, and beyond cancer.

References

1. Hewitt M, Weiner SL, Simone JV: *Childhood Cancer Survivorship: Improving Care and Quality of Life*. Washington, DC, National Academy Press, 2003.
2. Ries LAG, Eisner MP, Kosary CL, Hankey BF, Miller BA, Clegg L: *SEER Cancer Statistics Review, 1973–1999*. Bethesda, MD, National Cancer Institute, 2002.
3. Society AC: *Cancer Facts and Figures, 2004*. Atlanta: American Cancer Society, 2004.
4. Jemal A, Thomas A, Murray T, Thun M: Cancer statistics, 2002. *CA: A Cancer Journal for Clinicians* 52(1):23–47, 2002.
5. Koocher G, O'Malley J: *The Damocles Syndrome*. New York, McGraw Hill, 1981.
6. Mullan F: Seasons of survival: Reflections of a physician with cancer. *New England Journal of Medicine* 313:270–273, 1985.
7. Hassey Dow K: The enduring seasons in survival. *Oncology Nursing Forum* 17(4):511–516, 1990.
8. Giammona AJ, Malek DM: The psychological effect of childhood cancer on families. *Pediatric Clinics of North America* 49:1063–1081, 2002.
9. Cole M, Cole SR: *The Development of Children*, 4 ed. New York: Worth Publishers, 2001.
10. Rolland JS: *Families, Illness, and Disability: An Integrative Treatment Model*. New York: Basic Books, 1994.
11. Rosenblatt P: *Metaphors of Family Systems Theory* New York: Guilford Press, 1994.
12. Kazak A, Christiakis D: The intense stress of childhood cancer: A systems perspective. In: Pfeffer C (ed): *Severe Stress and Mental Disturbance in Children* Washington, D.C.: American Psychiatric Press, 1996.
13. Kazak AE, Simms S, Rourke MT: Family systems practice in pediatric psychology. *Journal of Pediatric Psychology* 27(2):133–143, 2002.
14. Ostroff J, Steinglass P: Psychosocial adaptation following treatment: A family systems perspective on childhood cancer survivorship. In: Baider L, Cooper CL, et al. (eds): *Cancer and the Family*. New York, John Wiley and Sons, 1996, pp. 129–147.
15. Chesler M, Barbarin O: *Childhood Cancer and the Family*. New York: Brunner/Mazel, 1987.
16. Rogers SJ, White LK: Satisfaction with parenting: The role of marital happiness, family structure and parents' gender. *Journal of Marriage and the Family* 60:293–308, 1998.
17. Thoits PA: Identity structures and psychosocial well-being: Gender and marital status comparisons. *Social Psychology Quarterly* 55:236–256, 1992.
18. McClelland J: Sending children to kindergarten: A phenomenological study of mothers' experiences. *Family Relations* 44:177–183, 1995.
19. Houtzager BA, Grootenhuis MA, Hoekstra-Weebers JE, Caron HN, Last BF: Psychosocial functioning in siblings of pediatric cancer patients one to six months after diagnosis. *European Journal of Cancer* 39(10):1423–1432, 2003.
20. McGrath PJ: Beginning treatment for childhood acute lymphoblastic leukemia: Insights from the parents' perspective. *Oncology Nursing Forum* 29(6):988–996, 2002.
21. Chesler M, Parry C: Gender roles and/or styles in crisis: An integrative analysis of the experiences of fathers of children with cancer. *Qualitative Health Research* 11(3):363–384, 2001.
22. Freeman K, O'Dell C, Meola C: Issues in families of children with brain tumors. *Oncology Nursing Forum* 27(5):843–848, 2000.
23. Enskar K, Carlsson M, Golsater M, Hamrin E, Kreuger A: Parental reports of changes and challenges that result from parenting a child with cancer. *Journal of Pediatric Oncology* 14(3):156–163, 1997.
24. Freeman A, O'Dell C, Meola C: Childhood brain tumors: Children's and siblings' concerns regarding the diagnosis and phase of illness. *Journal of Pediatric Oncology Nursing* 20(3):133–140, 2003.
25. Williams P, Hanson S, Karlin R, Ridder L, Liebergen A, Olson J: Outcomes of a nursing intervention for siblings of chronically ill children: A pilot study. *Journal of the Society of Pediatric Nurses* 2:127–137, 1997.
26. Wang RH, Martinson IM: Behavioral responses of healthy Chinese siblings to the stress of childhood cancer in the family: A longitudinal study. *Journal of Pediatric Nursing* 11(6):383–391, 1996.
27. Die-Trill M, Stuber ML: Psychological problems of curative cancer treatment. In: Holland JC (ed): *Psycho-Oncology*. New York, Oxford University Press, pp. 897–906, 1998.
28. Pendleton E: *Too Old to Cry ... Too Young to Die*. Nashville: Thomas Nelson, 1980.
29. Orr DP, Hoffmans MA, Bennetts G: Adolescents with cancer report their psychosocial needs. *Journal of Psychosocial Oncology* 2(2):47–59, 1984.
30. Chesler M, Allswede J, Barbarin O: Voices from the margin of the family: Siblings of children with cancer. *Journal of Psychosocial Oncology* 9(4):19–42, 1991.
31. LaMontagne LL, Wells N, Hepworth JT, Johnson BD, Manes R: Parent coping and child distress behaviors during invasive procedures for childhood cancer. *Journal of Pediatric Oncology Nursing* 16(1):3–12, 1999.
32. Kliebenstein MA, Broome ME: School re-entry for the child with chronic illness: Parent and school personnel perceptions. *Pediatric Nursing* 26(6):579–582, 2000.
33. McCarthy AM, Williams J, Plumer C: Evaluation of a school re-entry nursing intervention for children with cancer. *Journal of Pediatric Oncology* 15(3):143–152, 1998.
34. Rocha-Garcia A, Alvarez Del Rio A, Hernandez-Pena P, Martinez-Garcia Mdel C, Marin-Palomares T, Lazcano-Ponce E: The emotional response of families to children with leukemia at the lower socio-economic level in central Mexico: A preliminary report. *Psycho-oncology* 12(1):78–90, 2003.
35. Fadiman A: *The Spirit Catches You and You Fall Down: A Hmong Child, Her American Doctors, and the Collision of Two Cultures*. New York: Farrar, Straus and Giroux, 1997.
36. Brophy P, Kazak AE: Schooling. In: Johnson FL, O'Donnell EL (eds): *The Candlelighters Guide to Bone Marrow Transplants in Children*. Bethesda, MD, Candlelighters Childhood Cancer Foundation, pp. 68–73, 1994.
37. Brown RT, Madan-Swain A: Cognitive, neuropsychological, and academic sequelae in children with leukemia. *Journal of Learning Disabilities* 26:74–90, 1993.
38. List M, Ritter-Stier C, Lansky S: Enhancing the adjustment of long-term survivors: Early findings of a school intervention study. In: Green DM, D'Angio JJ (eds): *Late Effects of Treatment for Childhood Cancer*. New York: Wiley-Liss, Inc.; 1992.
39. Hockenberry M, Manteuffel B, Bottomley S: Development of two instruments examining stress and adjustment in children with cancer. *Journal of Pediatric Oncology Nursing* 14(3):178–185, 1997.
40. Peckham VC: Children with cancer in the classroom. *Teaching Exceptional Children* 26:26–32, 1993.
41. Varni JW, Katz ER, Colegrove Rea: Perceived social support and adjustment of children with newly diagnosed cancer. *Developmental and Behavioral Pediatrics* 15:20–26, 1994.
42. Noll RB, LeRoy S, Bukowski WM, Rogosch FA, Kulkarni R: Peer relationships and adjustment in children with cancer. *Journal of Pediatric Psychology* 16(3):307–326, 1991.
43. Noll R, Bukowski W, Davies W, Koontz K, Kulkarni R: Adjustment in the peer system of adolescents with cancer. *Journal of Pediatric Psychology* 18(3):351–364, 1993.
44. Bessell AG: Children surviving childhood cancer: Psychosocial adjustment, quality of life, and school experiences. *Exceptional Children* 67(3):345–359, 2001.
45. Lahteenmaki PM, Houostila J, Hinkka S, Salmi TT: Childhood cancer patients at school. *European Journal of Cancer* 38(9):1227–1240, 2002.
46. Kupst MJ: Coping with pediatric cancer: Theoretical and research perspectives. In: Bearison DJ, Mulhern RK (eds): *Pediatric Psycho-oncology: Psychological Perspectives on Children with Cancer*. New York, Oxford University Press, pp. 35–60, 1994.
47. Madan-Swain A, Brown RT, Sexson SB, Baldwin K, Pais R, Ragab A: Adolescent cancer survivors: Psychosocial and familial adjustment. *Psychosomatics* 35:1–7, 1994.
48. Spirito A, Stark L, Cobiella C, Drigan R, Androkites A, Hewett K: Social adjustment of children successfully treated for cancer. *Journal of Pediatric Psychology* 15(3):359–371, 1990.
49. Noll RB, Bukowski WM, Rogosch FA, LeRoy S, Kulharni R: Social interactions between children with cancer and their peers: Teacher ratings. *Journal of Pediatric Psychology* 15(1):43–56, 1990.
50. Reiter-Purtill J, Vannatta K, Gerhardt CA, Correll J, Noll RB: A controlled longitudinal study of the social functioning of children who completed treatment of cancer. *J Pediatr Hematol Oncol* 25(6):467–473, 2003.
51. Butler RW, Copeland D: Attentional processes and their remediation in children treated for cancer: A literature review and the development of a therapeutic approach. *Journal of the International Neuropsychological Society* 8(1):115–124, 2002.
52. Adamoli L, Deasy-Spinetta P, Corbetta A, et al.: School functioning for the child with leukemia in continuous first remission: Screening high-risk children. *Hematology and Oncology* 14:121–131, 1997.
53. Vannatta K, Gartstein MA, Short A, Noll RB: A controlled study of peer relationships of children surviving brain tumors: Teacher, peer, and self ratings. *Journal of Pediatric Psychology* 23(5):279–287, 1998.
54. Zeltzer LK, Kellerman J, Ellenberg L, Dash J, Rigler D: Psychologic effects of illness in adolescence: II. Impact of illness in adolescents—Crucial issues and coping styles. *Journal of Pediatrics* 97(1):132–138, 1980.
55. Chesler MA, Weigers M, Lawther T: How am I different? Perspectives for childhood cancer survivors on change and growth. In: Green DM, D'Angio G (eds): *Late Effects of Treatment for Childhood Cancer*. New York, John Wiley and Sons, 1992.

56. Weigers ME, Chesler MA, Zebrack BJ, Goldman S: Self-reported worries among long-term survivors of childhood cancer and their peers. *Journal of Psychosocial Oncology* 16(2):1–24, 1998.
57. Murray JS: Siblings of children with cancer: A review of the literature. *Journal of Pediatric Oncology Nursing* 16(1):25–34, 1999.
58. Williams P, Hanson S, Karlin R, et al.: Outcomes of a nursing intervention for siblings of chronically ill children: A pilot study. *Journal of the Society of Pediatric Nurses* 2:127–137, 1997.
59. Bendor SJ: Anxiety and isolation in siblings of pediatric cancer patients: The need for prevention. *Social Work Health Care* 14:17–35, 1990.
60. Martinson IM, Giliss C, Collaizzo Coughlin D, Freeman M, Bossert E: Impact of childhood cancer on healthy school-age siblings. *Cancer Nurs* 13(183–190), 1990.
61. Havermans T, Eiser C: Siblings of a child with cancer. *Child Care Health Dev* 20:309–322, 1994.
62. Sargent JR, Sahler OJ, Roghmann KJ, et al.: Sibling adaptation to childhood cancer collaborative study: Siblings' perceptions of the cancer experience. *Journal of Pediatric Psychology* 20(2):151–164, 1995.
63. Zeltzer LK, Dolgin M, Sahler O, et al.: Sibling adaptation to childhood cancer collaborative study: Health outcomes of siblings of children with cancer. *Medical and Pediatric Oncology* 27:98–107, 1996.
64. Houtzager BA, Grootenhuis MA, Last BF: Adjustments of siblings to childhood cancer: A literature review. *Support Care Cancer* 7:302–320, 1999.
65. Freeman K, O'Dell C, Meola C: Issues in families of children with brain tumors. *Oncol Nurs Forum* 27(5):843–848, 2000.
66. Houtzager BA, Grootenhuis MA, Last BF: Supportive groups for siblings of pediatric oncology patients: Impact on anxiety. *Psycho-Oncology* 10:315–324, 2001.
67. Freeman K, O'Dell C, Meola C: Childhood brain tumors: Children's and siblings' concerns regarding the diagnosis and phase of illness. *J Pediatr Oncol Nurs* 20(3):133–140, 2003.
68. Heffernan SM, Zanelli A: Behavior changes exhibited by siblings of pediatric oncology patients: A comparison between maternal and sibling descriptions. *Journal of Pediatric Oncology Nursing* 14(1):3–14, 1997.
69. Carpenter PJ, Sahler OJZ: Sibling perception and adaptation to childhood cancer: Conceptual and methodological considerations. In: Johnson JH, Johnson SB (eds): *Advances in Child Health Psychology*, Gainesville, University of Florida, 1991.
70. Breyer J, Kunin H, Kalish LA, Patenaude AF: The adjustment of siblings of pediatric cancer patients—A sibling and parent perspective. *Psycho-oncology* 2(201–208), 1993.
71. Heiney SP, Goon-Johnson K, Ettinger RS, Ettinger S: The effects of group therapy on siblings of pediatric oncology patients. *J Pediatr Oncol Nurs* 7:95–100, 1990.
72. Hillman KA: Comparing child-rearing practices in parents of children with cancer and parents of healthy children. *Journal of Pediatric Oncology Nurses* 14(2):53–67, 1997.
73. Davies WH, Noll RB, DeStefano L, Bukowski WM, Kulkarni R: Differences in the child-rearing practices of parents of children with cancer and controls: The perspectives of parents and professionals. *Journal of Pediatric Psychology* 16(3):295–306, 1991.
74. Zebrack B, Chesler M, Orbuch T, Parry C: Mothers of survivors of childhood cancer: Their worries and concerns. *Journal of Psychosocial Oncology* 20(2):1–26, 2002.
75. Manne SL, Lesanics D, Meyers P, Wollner N, Steinherz P, Redd W: Predictors of depressive symptomatology among parents of newly diagnosed children with cancer. *Journal of Pediatric Psychology* 20(4):491–510, 1995.
76. Kazak AE, Barakat LP: Brief report: Parenting stress and quality of life during treatment for childhood leukemia predicts child and parent adjustment after treatment ends. *Journal of Pediatric Psychology* 22(5):749–758, 1997.
77. Gilbar O: Parent caregiver adjustment to cancer of an adult child. *Journal of Psychosomatic Research* 52:295–302, 2002.
78. Barakat L, Kazak A, Meadows AT, Casey R, Meeske K, Stuber M: Families surviving childhood cancer: A comparison of post-traumatic stress symptoms with families of healthy children. *Journal of Pediatric Psychology* 22(6):843–859, 1997.
79. Dahlquist LM, Czyzewski DI, Copeland KG, Jones CL, Taub E, Vaughan JK: Parents of children newly diagnosed with cancer: Anxiety, coping, and marital distress. *Journal of Pediatric Psychology* 18(3):365–376, 1993.
80. Brown RT, Kaslow NJ, Hazzard AP, et al.: Psychiatric and family functioning in children with leukemia and their parents. *Journal of the American Academy of Child and Adolescent Psychiatry* 31(3):495–502, 1992.
81. Koocher GP: Psychosocial issues during the acute treatment of pediatric cancer. *Cancer* 58(2):468–472, 1986.
82. Cavusoglu H: Depression in children with cancer. *International Pediatric Nursing* 16(5):380–385, 2001.
83. Last B, Veldhuizen V: Information about diagnosis and prognosis related to anxiety and depression in children with cancer aged 8–16 years. *Eur J Cancer* 32A(2):290–294, 1996.
84. Noll RB, Gartstein MA, Vannatta K, Correll J, Bukowski WM, Davies H: Social, emotional, and behavioral functioning of children with cancer. *Pediatrics* 103(1):71–78, 1999.
85. Radcliffe J, Bennett D, Kazak AE, Foley B, Phillips PC: Adjustment in childhood brain tumor survival: Child, mother, and teacher report. *Journal of Pediatric Psychology* 21(4):529–539, 1996.
86. Worchel FF, Nolan BF, Wilson VL, Purser JS, Copeland DR, Pfefferbaum B: Assessment of depression in children with cancer. *Journal of Pediatric Psychology* 13:101–112, 1988.
87. Canning EH, Canning RD, Boyce WT: Depressive symptoms and adaptive style in children with cancer. *Journal of the American Academy of Child and Adolescent Psychiatry* 31:1120–1124, 1992.
88. Noll RB, MacLean WE, Whitt JK, Kaleita TA, Stehbens JA, Waskerwitz MJea: Behavioral adjustment and social functioning of long-term survivors of childhood leukemia: Parent and teacher reports. *Journal of Pediatric Psychology* 22(6):827–841, 1997.
89. Sawyer M, Antoniou G, Rice M, Baghurst P: Childhood Cancer: A 4-year prospective study of the psychological adjustment of children and parents. *Journal of Pediatric Hematology/Oncology* 22(3):214–220, 2000.
90. Sawyer M, Antoniou G, Toogood I, Rice M: Childhood cancer: A two-year prospective study of psychological adjustment of children and parents. *J Ac Child Adolesc Psychiatry* 36:1736–1743, 1997.
91. Kazak AE, Penati B, Boyer BA, Himelstein B, Brophy P, Waibel MKea: A randomized controlled prospective outcome study of a psychological and pharmacological intervention protocol for procedural distress in pediatric leukemia. *Journal of Pediatric Psychology* 21(5):615–631, 1996.
92. Arnholt U, Fritz G, Keener M: Self-concept in survivors of childhood and adolescent cancer. *Journal of Psychosocial Oncology* 11(1):1–16, 1993.
93. Elkin D, Phipps S, Mulhern R, Fairclough D: Psychological functioning of adolescent and young adult survivors of pediatric malignancy. *Medical and Pediatric Oncology* 29:582–588, 1997.
94. Gray RE, Doan BD, Schermer P, FitzGerald AV, P. BM, Jenkin Dea: Psychologic adaptation of survivors of childhood cancer. *Cancer* 70:2713–2721, 1992.
95. Zebrack BJ, Chesler MA: Quality of life in long-term survivors of childhood cancer. *Psycho-Oncology* 11(2):132–141, 2002.
96. Parry C: Embracing uncertainty: An exploration of the experiences of childhood cancer survivors. *Qualitative Health Research* 13(1):227–246, 2003.
97. Lauria MM: Common issues and challenges for families dealing with childhood cancer. In: Lauria MM, Clark EJ, Hermann JF, Stearns NM (eds): *Social Work in Oncology: Supporting Survivors, Families, and Caregivers*. Atlanta, American Cancer Society, 2001, pp. 117–142.
98. Hoekstra-Weebers JE, Jaspers JP, Kamps WA, Klip EC: Gender differences in psychological adaptation and coping in parents of pediatric cancer patients. *Psycho-oncology* 7(1):26–36, 1998.
99. Santacroce S: Uncertainty, anxiety, and symptoms of posttraumatic stress in parents of children recently diagnosed with cancer. *Journal of Pediatric Oncology* 19(3):104–111, 2002.
100. Peck B: Effects of childhood cancer on long-term survivors and their families. *British Medical Journal* 1:1327–1329, 1979.
101. Best M, Streisand R, Catania L, Kazak AE: Parental distress during pediatric leukemia and posttraumatic stress symptoms (PTSS) after treatment ends. *Journal of Pediatric Psychology* 26(5):299–307, 2001.
102. Manne Sl, Hamel KD, Gallelli K, Sorgen K, Redd WH: Posttraumatic stress disorder among mothers of pediatric cancer survivors: Diagnosis, comorbidity, and utility of the PTSD checklist as a screening instrument. *Journal of Pediatric Psychology* 23(6):357–366, 1998.
103. Pelcovitz D, Goldenberg B, Kaplan S, et al.: Posttraumatic stress disorder in mothers of pediatric cancer survivors. *Psychosomatics* 37:116–126, 1996.
104. Magni G, Messina C, DeLeo D: Psychosocial distress in parents of children with acute lymphoblastic leukemia. *Acta Psychiatrica Scandinavia* 68:297–300, 1983.
105. Speechley KN, Noh S: Surviving childhood cancer, social support, and parents' psychosocial adjustment. *Journal of Pediatric Psychology* 17:15–31, 1992.
106. Adams-Greenly M: Psychosocial staging of pediatric cancer patients and their families. *Cancer* 58:449–553, 1986.
107. Eiser C: Psychosocial effects of chronic disease. *Journal of Child Psychology and Psychiatry* 31:85–98, 1990.
108. Kupst M, Schulman J, Maurer H: Psychosocial aspects of pediatric leukemia—From diagnosis through the first six months of treatment. *Medical and Pediatric Oncology* 11:269–278, 1983.
109. Leventhal-Belfer L, Bakker A, Rossu C: Parents of childhood cancer survivors: A descriptive look at their concerns and needs. *Journal of Psychosocial Oncology* 11:19–41, 1993.
110. Steele RG, Long A, Reddy KA, Luhr M, Phipps S: Changes in maternal distress and child-rearing strategies across treatment for pediatric cancer. *Journal of Pediatric Psychology* 28(7):447–452, 2003.
111. Boman K, Lindahl A, Bjork O: Disease-related distress in parents of children with cancer at various stages after the time of diagnosis. *Acta Oncol* 42(2):137–146, 2003.
112. Taylor V, Fuggle P, Charman T: Well sibling psychological adjustment to chronic physical disorder in a sibling: How important is maternal awareness of their illness attitudes and perceptions? *Journal of Child Psychology and Psychiatry* 42(7):953–962, 2001.
113. Frank NC, Brown RT, Blount RL, Bunke V: Predictors of affective responses of mothers and fathers of children with cancer. *Psycho-oncology* 10:293–304, 2001.

114. Dahlquist LM, Czyzewski DI, Jones CL: Parents of children with cancer: A longitudinal study of emotional distress, coping style, and marital adjustment two and twenty months after diagnosis. *Journal of Pediatric Psychology* 21(4):541–554, 1996.
115. Sloper P: Predictors of distress in parents of children with cancer: A prospective study. *Journal of Pediatric Psychology* 25(2):79–91, 2000.
116. Goldbeck L: Parental coping with the diagnosis of childhood cancer: Gender effects, dissimilarity within couples, and quality of life. *Psycho-oncology* 10(4):325–335, 2001.
117. Eiser C, Havermans T, Eiser JR: Parents' attributions about childhood cancer: Implication for relationships with medical staff. *Child: Care, Health and Development* 21(1):31–42, 1995.
118. Barbarin OA, Sargent JR, Sahler OJZ, et al.: Sibling adaptation to childhood cancer collaborative study: Parental views of pre- and post-diagnosis adjustment of siblings of children with cancer. *Journal of Psychosocial Oncology* 13(3):1–20, 1995.
119. Sahler OJ, Roghmann KJ, Carpenter PJ, et al.: Sibling adaptation to childhood cancer collaborative study: Prevalence of sibling distress and definition of adaptation levels. *Journal of Developmental and Behavioral Pediatrics* 15(5):353–366, 1994.
120. Sloper P, While D: Risk factors in the adjustment of siblings of children with cancer. *Journal of Child Psychology, Psychiatry, and Allied Disciplines* 37:597–607, 1996.
121. Sahler OJZ, Roghmann KL, Mulhern RK, et al.: Sibling adaptation to childhood cancer collaborative study: The association of sibling adaptation with maternal well-being, physical health, and resource use. *Developmental and Behavioral Pediatrics* 18(4):233–243, 1997.
122. Alderfer MA, Labay LE, Kazak AE: Brief report: Does posttraumatic stress apply to siblings of childhood cancer survivors? *Journal of Pediatric Psychology* 28(4):281–286, 2003.
123. Dolgin MJ, Blumensohn R, Mulhern RK, et al.: Sibling adaptation to childhood cancer collaborative study: Cross-cultural aspects. *Journal of Psychosocial Oncology* 15:1–14, 1997.
124. Madan-Swain A, Sexson SB, Brown RT, Ragab A: Family adaptation and coping among siblings of cancer patients, their brothers and sisters, and non-clinical controls. *American Journal of Family Therapy* 21:60–70, 1993.
125. van Dongen-Melman J, Pruyn J, DeGroot A, Koot H, Hahlan K, Verhulst F: Late psychosocial consequences for parents of children who survived cancer. *Journal of Pediatric Psychology* 20:567–586, 1995.
126. Zebrack BJ, Zeltzer LK, Whitton J, et al.: Psychological outcomes in long-term survivors of childhood leukemia, Hodgkin's disease and non-Hodgkin's lymphoma: A report from the Childhood Cancer Survivor Study. *Pediatrics.* 110(1):42–52, 2002.
127. Zebrack B, Gurney JG, Oeffinger KC, et al.: Psychological outcomes in long-term survivors of childhood brain cancer: A report from the Childhood Cancer Survivor Study. *Journal of Clinical Oncology* 22(6):999–1006, 2004.
128. Ronen T: *Cognitive Developmental Therapy with Children.* Chichester, Wiley, 1997.
129. Mishel M: Uncertainty in chronic illness. *Annual Review of Nursing Research* 17:269–274, 1999.
130. Stewart JL: "Getting used to it": Children finding the ordinary and routine in the uncertain context of cancer. *Qual Health Res* 13(3):394–407, 2003.
131. Woodgate RL, Degner LF: Expectations and beliefs about children's cancer symptoms: Perspectives of children with cancer and their families. *Oncol Nurs Forum.* 30(3):479–491, 2003.
132. Woodgate RL, Degner LF: A substantive theory of keeping the spirit alive: The spirit within children with cancer and their families. *Journal of Pediatric Oncology Nursing.* 20(3):103–119, 2003.
133. Mellon S: Comparisons between cancer survivors and family members on meaning of the illness and family quality of life. *Oncol Nurs Forum* 29(7):1117–1125, 2002.
134. Deasy-Spinetta P: School issues and the child with cancer. *Cancer* 71(10):3261–3264, 1993.
135. Spinetta JJ: Behavioral and psychological research in childhood cancer. An overview. *Cancer* 50:1939–1943, 1982.
136. Larcombe I: Back to normality. *Nursing Times* 87:68–69, 1991.
137. Masera G, Chesler MA, Jankovic M, et al.: Guidelines for communication of the diagnosis. *Medical and Pediatric Oncology* 28(5):382–385, 1997.
138. Moore I, Glasser M, Ablin A: Late psychosocial consequences of childhood cancer. *Journal of Pediatric Nursing* 3(3):150–158, 1987.
139. Eapen V, Revesz T: Psychosocial correlates of pediatric cancer in the United Arab Emirates. *Support Care Cancer* 11:185–189, 2003.
140. Ross SA: Childhood leukemia: The child's view. *Journal of Psychosocial Oncology* 7(4):75–90, 1989.
141. Hockenberry-Eaton M, Minick P: Living with cancer: Children with extraordinary courage. *Oncology Nursing Forum* 21(6):1025–1031, 1994.
142. Eden T, Black I, Emery A: The use of taped parental interviews to improve communication with childhood cancer families. *Pediatric Hematology/Oncology* 10(2):157, 1992.
143. Phipps S, Fairclough D, Mulhern RK: Avoidant coping in children with cancer. *Journal of Pediatric Psychology* 20(2):217–232, 1995.
144. Von Essen L, Enskar K, Haglund K, Hedstrom M, Skolin I: Important aspects of care and assistance for children 0–7 years of age being treated for cancer. Parent and nurse perceptions. *Support Care Cancer* 10(8):601–612, 2002.
145. Grootenhuis MA, Last BF: Children with cancer with different survival perspectives: defensiveness, control strategies, and psychological adjustment. *Psycho-oncology* 10:305–314, 2001.
146. Frank NC, Blount RL, Brown RT: Attributions, coping, and adjustment in children with cancer. *Journal of Pediatric Psychology* 563–576, 1997.
147. Landolt MA, Vollrath M, Ribi K: Predictors of coping strategy selection in pediatric patients. *Acta Paediatrica* 91(9):954–960, 2002.
148. Clarke-Seffen L: Reconstructing reality: Family strategies for managing childhood cancer. *Journal of Pediatric Nursing* 12(5):278–287, 1997.
149. Grootenhuis MA, Last BF, De Graaf-Nijkerk JH, Van Der Wel M: Secondary control strategies used by parents of children with cancer. *Psycho-oncology* 5:91–102, 1996.
150. Walker C, Adams J, Curry D, et al.: A Delphi study of pediatric oncology nurses' facilitative behaviors. *Journal of Pediatric Oncology Nursing* 10:126–132, 1992.
151. Evans CA, Stevens M, Cushway D, Houghton J: Sibling response to childhood cancer: A new approach. *Child Care Health and Development* 18(229–244):229–244, 1992.
152. Last BF, Grootenhuis MA: Emotions, coping, and the need for support in families of children with cancer: A model for psychosocial care. *Patient Educ Couns* 33:169–179, 1998.
153. Hamama R, Ronen T, Feigin R: Self-control, anxiety, and loneliness in siblings of children with cancer. *Social Work in Health Care* 31(1):63–83, 2000.
154. Murray JS: Social support for school-age siblings of children with cancer: A comparison between parent and sibling perceptions. *Journal of Pediatric Oncology Nursing* 18:90–104, 2001.
155. Murray JS: A qualitative exploration of psychosocial support for siblings of children with cancer. *J Pediatr Nurs* Oct 17(5):327–337, 2002.
156. Carpenter PJ, Sahler OJZ, Davis MS: Use of a camp setting to provide medical information to siblings of pediatric cancer patients. *J Cancer Educ* 5:21–26, 1990.
157. Spinetta JJ, Jankovic M, Green D, et al.: Guidelines for assistance to siblings of children with cancer: Report of the SIOP working committee on psychosocial issues in pediatric oncology. *Med Pediatr Oncol* 33(395–398), 1999.
158. Chesler M, Chesney B: *Cancer and Self-Help.* Madison, WI, University of Wisconsin Press, 1995.
159. Chesler M, Barbarin O: Difficulties of providing help in a crisis: Relationships between parents of children with cancer and their friends. *Journal of Social Issues* 40(4):113–134, 1984.
160. Kazak A. B, L., Meeske K, Christakis D, Meadows A, Penati B, Stuber M: Posttraumatic stress, family functioning and social support in survivors of childhood leukemia and their mothers and fathers. *Journal of Consulting and Clinical Psychology* 65:120–129, 1997.
161. Manne S: Association of psychological vulnerability factors to post-traumatic stress symptomatology in mothers of pediatric cancer survivors. *Psycho-Oncology* 9:372–384, 2000.
162. Kazak AE, Simms S, Barakat L, et al.: Surviving cancer competently intervention program (SCCIP): A cognitive-behavioral and family therapy intervention for adolescent survivors of childhood cancer and their families. *Family Process* 38(2):175–191, 1999.
163. Sahler LJ, Varni JW, Fairclough DL, Butler RW, Noll RB, Dolgin MJ (eds): Problem-solving skills training for mothers of children with newly diagnosed cancer: A randomized trial. *J Dev Behav Pediatr* 23:77–86, 2002.

CHAPTER 7.1.3.2 ■ THE ROLE OF THE CHILD AND ADOLESCENT PSYCHIATRIST ON THE PEDIATRIC TRANSPLANT SERVICE

STEVEN C. SCHLOZMAN AND LAURA PRAGER

INTRODUCTION AND HISTORY

Any discussion of the psychiatric aspects of pediatric transplantation must begin with a brief history of the field of pediatric transplantation itself. Both solid organ and bone marrow transplant procedures have made remarkable progress over the last 30 to 40 years, with pediatric technological expertise keeping pace with the rapid development of new and better means of keeping transplant patients healthy and highly functional. In fact, if one examines the relatively high morbidity and mortality rate of all forms of transplantation 30 years ago compared to the state of the art today, it perhaps makes sense that interest in the psychosocial and psychiatric wellbeing of transplant patients is a relatively new and still understudied aspect of the field.

The first solid organ transplant procedures in children involved cardiac transplant attempts in infants during the late 1960s. These patients lived at most a few days, and although physicians and scientists tried valiantly to understand the limits of these potentially life-saving procedures, the results were plagued by infection, organ failure, and graft rejection. The introduction of cyclosporine as an immunosuppressing agent in 1980 marked perhaps the beginning of a fundamental change in the outcome of these procedures. Although powerful and increasingly specific antibiotic and physiologic medications were vastly improving outcomes, medications such as cyclosporine made possible the resistance to graft rejection that paved the way for a substantially more normal existence for transplant recipients. Patients lived longer, fared substantially better, and transplant services became gradually more interested in the psychosocial development of the younger patients whose lives had been saved, but permanently altered, inherent in the transplant itself and in the treatment of subsequent complications makes the medical training of the consultation-liason psychiatrist ideally suited for this service.

In a similar fashion, bone marrow transplantation began as a desperate attempt to prevent the development of otherwise fatal conditions, most commonly hematological malignancies. Since its somewhat rocky beginnings, great strides have been made in this difficult and unique procedure. While the first bone marrow transplant procedures took place in the late 1960s, unlike solid organ transplant procedures, bone marrow transplantation had its genesis in the pediatric population. In addition, perhaps because of the severe isolation that very young patients must endure during bone marrow transplantation, attention to the psychosocial needs of these patients received greater initial emphasis than did solid organ procedures on similar-age patients. However, for both solid organ and bone marrow transplant procedures, transplant services are increasingly recognizing the need for participation by, and integration with, pediatric mental health specialists. In addition to assisting transplant services with decisions regarding suitability and preparation of the patient and family for the imminent surgery, problems such as medication compliance, maintaining a normal developmental trajectory, the onset and treatment of emerging psychiatric disorders, and the management of psychological aspects of the still frequent medical crises all involve active participation of child mental health services. Furthermore, our experience suggests that the understanding of the medical challenges inherent in the procedure itself and in the treatment of subsequent complications make the physician training of the consultation-liaison child psychiatrist ideally suited for this service.

All of these developments gave rise to the somewhat new field of transplant psychiatry. Early consultants such as Owen Surman at Massachusetts General Hospital and Margaret Stuber at UCLA paved the way for greater acceptance of the psychiatric needs of solid organ and bone marrow transplant recipients. Interestingly, as with other significant, chronic, and severe medical conditions, there is some evidence that attention to the psychiatric concerns of transplant patients became more palatable to medical and surgical services as the overall capacity to keep these patients healthy continued to improve (1).

This chapter will summarize the psychiatric aspects of pediatric solid organ and bone marrow transplant patients. We will focus on the evaluation and preparation of patients and their families for the procedure itself, on the management of the patient and family during and immediately following the procedure, and on the long-term management of these patients as they move forward in their lives. In many ways, pediatric transplant psychiatry epitomizes the fundamental aspects of good consultation-liaison work. The principal challenge for the transplant psychiatrist is achieving balance in the dual role of helping the patient and family maintain a normal developmental trajectory while at the same time assisting the transplant team with the often charged and intense emotions that accompany working with these young patients.

PSYCHIATRIC SIMILARITIES AND DIFFERENCES BETWEEN SOLID ORGAN AND BONE MARROW TRANSPLANTATION PROCEDURES

Important Similarities

Patients who face either solid organ transplant or bone marrow transplant are gravely ill. Transplants are a viable option when other treatment modalities cannot prevent death or progressive, debilitating illness. Patients who require a new solid organ or organs, or patients who require bone marrow transplantation, are reckoning with the most basic of existential quandaries. If the patients are old enough, they will often be acutely aware of the risks to their life and wellbeing. They and their families are under enormous stress. Both patient populations must process the complex array of risks and benefits of multiple options and then make a decision about whether or not to proceed with a potentially life-threatening and most certainly life-changing treatment.

The risks of the surgery itself are difficult to contemplate, as is the meaning of the commitment to a lifetime of medications with both short- and long-term side effects. Both populations and their families will wonder about issues as immediate as whether academic and developmental progress will continue, and as distant as whether or not fertility will be at risk.

Immunosuppressive medications are still the mainstay of antigraft rejection treatment, and many patients experience neuropsychiatric side effects from those medications. Cyclosporine and tacrilomus, two major antirejection agents, as well as corticosteroids, have been associated with anxiety, depression, agitation, delirium, paranoia, potentially some cognitive changes, and worsening of preexisting psychiatric conditions. These effects will be discussed in detail below. The transplant psychiatrist must be aware of the potential for these side effects and monitor patients carefully.

Case Illustration 1: Side Effects of Immunosuppression

A 13-year-old boy with a history of autoimmune hepatitis and subsequent hepatic failure received a deceased donor liver transplant at age 12. Before his liver disease and surgery, he carried the psychiatric diagnoses of ADHD and an atypical mood disorder, and was treated with stimulant medications and atypical antipsychotics to prevent his often aggressive outbursts. Given the severity of his psychiatric disorder, his medication was continued throughout his perioperative course. However, after his transplant, he developed significant emotional lability that correlated with the addition of prednisone as a necessary part of his immunosuppressant regimen. This behavior was managed by increasing dosages of his atypical antipsychotic medications. As atypical agents are hepatically metabolized, increased monitoring of his liver function tests was necessary to ensure that the added psychotropics were not further compromising his graft.

In addition, in both populations of transplant recipients there is a high potential for drug–drug interactions. Many transplant recipients are on multiple agents, and these may affect each other with significant neuropsychiatric sequelae (refer to Chapter 6.1.1). The transplant psychiatrist may be the member of the team most likely to recognize these interactions given that vigilance regarding drug–drug interactions is a mainstay of psychopharmacology.

Case Illustration 2: Drug–Drug Interactions

An 18-year-old woman who underwent a deceased donor liver transplant for biliary atresia at age 2 presented to the pediatric transplant service for ongoing management of her transplant, as well as for care of her inflammatory bowel disease. Important psychiatric issues included diagnoses of depression and anxiety for which she was prescribed clonazepam and paroxetine. Her history was also significant for recreational marijuana use and a complex partial seizure disorder. Finally, she had persistent difficulties with medication compliance, often stopping her anti-rejection medications. After her arrest for possession at age 19, she abruptly stopped using marijuana, and almost immediately thereafter experienced another round of graft rejection for which she was admitted to the hospital with the assumption that she had stopped taking her medications. A low tacrolimus level made her insistence that she was indeed compliant all the more puzzling. The transplant service eventually concluded that the sudden withdrawal of marijuana likely increased gastric motility, such that she absorbed less immunosuppressing agents than before and thus was not able to maintain her graft without immediate treatment with steroids and a higher overall immunosuppressive regimen. Appropriate adjustments in immunosuppressant dosages adequately addressed the problem, and the patient was able to maintain her graft.

Apart from the psychiatric effects of the immunosuppressing agents themselves, recipients of transplant surgery often carry all of the incertainty and psychological distress that characterize the onset of a chronic medical condition. Indeed, there is mounting evidence that both bone marrow and solid organ recipients are at risk for posttraumatic syndromes and in some instances will meet full criteria for posttraumatic stress disorder. Mental health members of transplant services need to watch for these symptoms, both in patients and in their families. There is in fact some evidence that the extent to which parents feel traumatized correlates with the psychological and medical wellbeing of the pediatric transplant recipient (2, 3). These challenges, along with the normal adolescent drive toward independence and separation, contribute to the high rate of medication noncompliance that characterizes the most common cause of graft rejection in pediatric populations.

The issue of posttraumatic syndromes stemming from severe medical conditions and intense treatment regimens deserves special mention. As mentioned above, there is growing evidence that children who undergo frequent and often noxious treatments for chronic medical illness can develop subclinical traumatic reactions or the full syndrome of posttraumatic stress disorder (PTSD). A recent review by Stuber and colleagues (3) suggested that parental trauma was a strong predictor of patient traumatic reaction among medically ill pediatric cancer patients. Similarly, in pediatric transplant patients, new research stresses that the sense among families and patients of the seriousness of the illness, regardless of how physicians tended to view the severity of the condition, is a potent predictor of pathological stress reactions (2). As one might expect, sudden events, such as abrupt rupture of esophageal varicies in patients with portal hypertension, are associated with more traumatic responses than are insidious serious illnesses, such as slowly progressive cardiomyopathies. These data stress the need for clear, straightforward, developmentally and educationally tailored discussions with patients and families about the risks of the current condition. Assumptions that families will view their predicament exactly as the transplant team assesses the severity of the situation can lead to gross misunderstandings, the possibility of significant psychological stress for patients and caregivers, and potentially serious psychiatric syndromes such as PTSD or depression.

For all patients who undergo transplant procedures, there exists a difficult equilibrium in allowing their children to develop and grow as normally as possible, while remaining constantly vigilant and increasingly anxious about the possibility of graft rejection. Graft rejection is not always obvious, though in some instances it is preceded by a clearly worsening course. In other situations, however, possible graft rejection is discovered on routine laboratory tests, leading to an element of hypervigilance that both patient and parents can experience and that is neither helpful nor healthy. The transplant psychiatrist can be helpful in managing this particular form of anxiety. His or her unique understanding of transplant medicine may encourage a frank discussion by the patient and family about their heightened concerns.

Finally, given the natural epidemiology of childhood psychosocial and psychiatric difficulties, there will inevitably be some children and adolescents who will suffer psychological difficulties not directly related to their transplant, but whose transplant will complicate effective treatment. For these patients, though no clear guidelines exist, keeping in mind drug–drug interactions, the means by which medications are metabolized, and the possible neuropsychiatric side effects of immunosuppressants are all important considerations. In general, one should prescribe psychotropic agents in lower initial dosages and monitor closely both the mental status exam and laboratory values that might suggest adverse drug effects. In addition, one cannot underestimate the effectiveness of supportive, psychodynamic, and behavioral interventions for some patients. Undergoing and living with a transplant is trying at best, and for children and adolescents, the therapist can help them cope with shaping a developing identity, such that they do not necessarily assume a sickly sense of self.

Important Differences

In spite of the similarities noted above, there are differences to note as well. Patients who require solid organ transplant (heart, kidney, lung, liver) often see their disease as limited to that organ. Bone marrow transplantation is performed for patients who have an underlying systemic illness, i.e., cancer. As cancer itself carries particular emotional valence in our culture, patients receiving transplant procedures for malignancies may require extra attention given the associated stress that the diagnosis and all of its cultural signifiers can entail. Although some pediatric patients may receive solid organ transplantation for cancer, this is less common than for organ malformation or metabolic and autoimmune diseases. Additionally, the isolation associated with bone marrow transplantation is particularly harrowing for all patients, and attention to the developmental needs of these patients is crucial for their psychological and medical wellbeing.

Transplantation, is a final common pathway for a group of heterogeneous and not always related conditions. This poses a special challenge to the child psychiatrist working with the transplant team. To be effective, the child psychiatrist must have an understanding of the medical and surgical components of the underlying disease as well as an understanding of the risks and benefits of the transplant itself. He or she must then tailor any treatment to the temperament and preexisting psychological and developmental challenges facing the child and the family, keeping in mind the inherent limitations posed by both the disease and the treatment. As many patients are quite young, there is the added challenge of balancing the involvement of an extended family and multiple systems of care. The work is complex but immensely rewarding.

THE PRETRANSPLANTATION EVALUATION

The child and adolescent psychiatrist plays an important and complex role in the evaluation of the child who is approaching transplantation. Initially, the psychiatrist is responsible for conducting a thorough psychiatric evaluation of the patient and family. In addition, the psychiatrist must be familiar with the medical problems facing the patient, both before and after surgery, in order to educate the family about the risks and benefits or transplantation and to assess the family's ability to provide informed consent. The psychiatrist also acts as a liaison between the family and the transplant team. The family will need support, direction, and clarification of the transplant team's expectations and concerns. The team in turn will also need support, direction, and sometimes interpretation of the family's behavior. The psychiatrist may also serve to focus the team's attention on ethical conflicts that may arise, particularly those that involve directed living donation by a related or unrelated donor.

There are no universally accepted guidelines for the psychiatric evaluation of children who are potential candidates for organ transplantation. Some centers routinely offer an open-ended, face-to-face clinical interview with a mental health provider, some require formal psychological testing, and yet others rely on structured or semistructured interviews. Not all transplant teams have psychiatric consultants. In many centers, psychologists and/or social workers complete psychosocial assessments. There are differences among transplant centers as to what constitutes an acceptable candidate for transplant. Common exclusion criteria include active substance abuse, active psychotic symptoms, suicidal ideation with plan or intent, history of self-injurious behavior or suicide attempts.

As with a standard psychiatric evaluation, the order and style of the interview is dependent on the child's age and developmental stage. With a prepubertal child, it is appropriate, perhaps even necessary, first to meet with the parents in order to get a coherent, longitudinal history. With the adolescent, it is beneficial to interview the child alone before meeting the parents in order to reinforce the primacy of the adolescent's concerns and feelings. At some point, it is imperative to meet with the patient and the parents/caregivers together in order to be sure that all parties hear (and hopefully understand) the same information and that all are in agreement as to how to proceed.

The pretransplantation psychiatric evaluation should be primarily diagnostic but can also be educational and, sometimes, even therapeutic. In addition to the developmental, social, educational, family, and past psychiatric history, the evaluation should address the following aspects:

1. Screening of potential recipients for the presence of significant Axis I diagnoses such as mood, anxiety, or psychotic disorders, as well as potential learning disabilities or frank cognitive impairment
2. History of past or current drug or alcohol abuse, particularly in the adolescent patient
3. Assessment of child's relationship with caregivers
4. Determination of the child and family's motivation for transplant

Because young children do not always have a full understanding of either the gravity of their illness or of the ramifications of transplant, it is their parents and/or other caregivers/guardians who "consent" to the surgery and postoperative care. Nevertheless, a verbal child patient must be able to "assent" to the surgery and be willing to participate actively in the treatment process. Both parent and child must be able to work together toward the common goal of transplant. If parent or child is not fully engaged in the process, then it is difficult for the transplant team to know how best to proceed.

Case Illustration 3: Whose Transplant Is It, Anyway?

An 11-year-old girl with advanced cystic fibrosis (CF) and no past psychiatric history was brought by her mother for a living donor pretransplant psychiatric evaluation. She had already been placed on the waiting list for a deceased donor transplant at another center several years earlier and the family knew that she was close to the top of that list. However, despite reassurance by the transplant team at the original center, the mother was worried that her daughter would die before she received her deceased donor's lungs. She herself volunteered to be a living lobar lung donor and she aggressively pursued other potential donors until she found one. On initial interviews, the patient was cheerful and appeared to have a good understanding of why her mother and a local schoolteacher each wished to donate a lung lobe. In her final meeting with the transplant team pulmonologist, however, the patient curled into a ball on the couch, cried quietly, and refused to talk about the impending living donor transplant. Ultimately, the team decided that it was the patient's mother and not the patient who was the motivating force for living donor transplant. The child did not feel ready to have an elective transplant with her mother as a donor. The team again reassured the family that the child could wait for a deceased donor transplant.

5. Evaluation of the child and family's ability to comply with treatment recommendations of caregivers

Candidacy for transplant demands consistent attention to and compliance with the recommendations of the treatment team. Pre- and posttransplant patients must take many medications every day; often they are asked to endure time-consuming and uncomfortable procedures such as chest physical therapy for patients with bronchiectasis or CF. The patient's willingness to adhere to the pretransplant regimen is an important determinant of their readiness for transplant and the complicated posttransplant regimen that follows.

Case Illustration 4: Compliance

A high school girl with end-stage CF met with the child psychiatrist as part of a standard pretransplant evaluation. The patient asked her parents to be present for the entire interview. The young woman was strikingly thin. The transplant psychiatrist asked the patient if her CF doctor had ever suggested that she have a G-tube placed for nutritional supplementation. The patient burst into tears and stated that she could never tolerate a G-tube even though she had been told that she could not gain weight regardless of how many calories she consumed during meals. She acknowledged, also, that she had been instructed to start continuous oxygen but had been unable to do that either because she was too embarrassed to be seen in public with a nasal cannula. The psychiatrist tried to explore with the patient other ways that she might improve her ability to adhere to the recommendations of her doctors but ultimately had to deny her candidacy for transplant based on her history of noncompliance and her inability to adhere to the recommendations of her physicians.

6. Understanding of the social supports available to the family
7. Assessment of psychosocial stressors in the family, such as financial pressures or marital discord
8. Assessment of the patient and family's understanding of the risks and benefits inherent in transplantation
9. Determination of the ability of the patient and family to collaborate with the transplant team with the shared goal of improving the patient's quality of life

The question of past or ongoing substance abuse in adolescents facing transplant is particularly important and warrants further discussion. In adult liver transplantation programs, ongoing alcohol or addictive drug use is usually a contraindication to transplant (4). Most programs require demonstration of 6 months to 1 year sobriety. With lung transplantation programs, tobacco use is an absolute contraindication to transplant and, again, candidates must demonstrate that they have abstained from cigarettes for over 6 months. Adolescents are less likely than adults to have a longstanding problem with substance abuse but frequently they have tried recreational drugs or alcohol in social situations. Sometimes they drink heavily or smoke marijuana on the weekends with their friends. It can be challenging to help these young people understand that such behavior could jeopardize their eligibility for transplant and could, if it continues after transplant, precipitate failure of the allograft. Individual transplant programs are left to determine what degree of risk they are willing to tolerate.

Indeed, the issue of alcohol use among adolescent transplant recipients and candidates requires special attention. This is of course particularly important when discussing liver transplantation. Although there is ample evidence that many adolescents experiment with alcohol, the use of alcohol by liver transplant patients is potentially extremely dangerous. Because liver failure can be insidious and unpredictable, it is difficult to assess when and to what extent alcohol use is likely to contribute to liver dysfunction. For these reasons, most child psychiatric consultants to liver transplant services feel that they must explicitly convey to their patients the seriousness of alcohol use. However, lecturing to teenagers about the dangers of alcohol use is likely to be met with resistance and defensiveness. Normal adolescent drives toward independence, coupled with the adolescent's unique susceptibility to peer pressure, often lead to alcohol use even among patients who understand intellectually that their liver disease makes this behavior particularly dangerous and unhealthy. At the same time, most transplant services do not view occasional experimentation with alcohol as an absolute contraindication for future transplants in adolescent populations. We have found that frank, developmentally appropriate discussions with adolescent transplant patients about alcohol use are substantially more effective at quelling and preventing experimentation and use of alcohol. While alcohol use is not under any circumstances acceptable, especially in adolescents with liver disease, helping teens to grasp the limitations of their disease in as mature a matter as possible is the best way to ensure healthy behavior.

Adolescents with liver failure are not the only ones vulnerable to the effects of recreational drugs. Adolescents with other forms of end-organ failure are also prone to experimentation, use, and even abuse of alcohol and other drugs. Cigarette smoking is an absolute contraindication to lung transplant, but other drugs that suppress the respiratory drive also have the potential for lethality. As the time for transplant nears, it is often very difficult to know whether the adolescent with substance abuse issues has "reformed" and stopped using simply because he or she has become gravely ill or because he or she has passed through the experimentation phase and recognized the limitations of such behavior. Transplant teams usually hope that the latter is true, but that is not always the case.

Case Illustration 5: Substance Abuse

A recent high school graduate with CF was hospitalized in the setting of declining pulmonary function for a course of intravenous antibiotics and aggressive chest physical therapy. Her pulmonologist noted that her pulmonary function tests (PFTs) had declined precipitously since her last admission and were not improving with standard medical care. He asked the transplant team to evaluate her for candidacy. On psychiatric evaluation, the patient acknowledged that in the year prior to admission she had developed an addiction to OxyContin (oxycodone) and had actually been arrested for a drug-related crime 6 months earlier. She had been charged as a juvenile and placed on probation. She had been "clean" since then and had completed a mandatory drug treatment program. The transplant team was aware of her difficulty but felt that her drug use was probably adolescent "experimentation." All agreed that she would die without a transplant. She subsequently underwent living donor transplant approximately 9 months later and recovered well following the surgery. However, several months after her transplant she was rushed to the hospital in respiratory distress secondary to inadvertent narcotic overdose. She struggled with intermittent abuse for many months thereafter before finally agreeing to join a methadone maintenance program.

PERITRANSPLANT TREATMENT

For patients undergoing bone marrow or solid organ transplantation, the stress of the procedure and the resulting hospitalization can be particularly trying. In addition, in cases where deceased donor organs suddenly become available, families find themselves thrown into the hospital with little time to prepare. These aspects of transplantation require special attention by mental health clinicians, especially around the time of admission and during the ensuing hospital stay. However, as with the pretransplant evaluation, there are no clear guidelines to instruct the most appropriate intervention. Some centers employ an educational approach, requiring patients and families to undergo orientation to the hospital well before the transplant itself. Other centers focus attention on the patient and family directly after the transplant takes place. We have found that discussing these options with patients and families and allowing them to choose is the best approach. As we have stressed, intervention should focus on individual needs and temperamental differences.

Once the transplant takes place, it is imperative that the transplant psychiatrist be available to the patient, the family, and to the transplant team. Issues such as abrupt mental status changes, acute anxiety, poor medical outcomes, and treatment team stress all are often part of the transplant psychiatrists' responsibilities. These responsibilities are best met by frequent visits with all parties, developmentally appropriate explicit discussion of unfavorable outcomes with the team and with the patient and family, and vigilance for increasing stress and frustration surrounding the posttransplant course. To the extent that families can be made aware of the possibility of difficult postsurgical courses, they will be likely to cope more effectively with whatever outcomes transpire.

WORKING WITH THE TRANSPLANT TEAM

Transplant psychiatrists work with and are part of large multidisciplinary teams. In this setting the psychiatrist who evaluates the child or adolescent for transplant candidacy can sometimes come into conflict with the treatment team. Because many transplant patients endure lengthy hospital admissions, pediatricians (residents and staff), physical therapists, social workers and child-life specialists often form long-term and extremely close relationships with children and adolescents with end-stage organ failure. To these caregivers, referral for transplant evaluation represents an acknowledgement of the failure of current management and, at the same time, a plea for the only viable treatment option.

These children and adolescents may not meet criteria for candidacy for transplant for many reasons. Sometimes the patient is referred for transplant when they are too close to death and would not be able to tolerate the actual operation. Sometimes, the patient and family may be denied on psychosocial grounds. Regardless of the reason for denial of candidacy, the treatment team may be disappointed and angry with the transplant team. This is particularly difficult when the patient is denied because of a history of noncompliance with medical care in the outpatient setting and/or lack of social supports. Sometimes in these situations, caregivers promise that the patient will "do better" and appeal to the psychiatrist to reevaluate the situation. It is often helpful for the psychiatrist to meet with the treatment team to review the evaluation and to let all involved share their feelings.

Case Illustration 6: Conflict among Caregivers

A high school student with CF was hospitalized frequently on the pediatric service for treatment with antibiotics and chest physical therapy. The patient lived with her mother and her older sister. Her mother was an immigrant who worked long hours and was not home during the day. Her older sister was frequently out of the house as well. The patient spoke English but the mother did not. The patient had a very hard time complying with her outpatient regimen of multiple daily medications, breathing treatments, and chest physical therapy. She had had frequent hospitalizations over the years due to noncompliance with her outpatient self-care. The CF staff had tried many times to effect change in her social situation, without success. When asked why she was not able to take better care of herself, the patient said that she was too embarrassed to go to the nurse during school hours to take her midday medications and that at night she preferred to go out with friends. When the psychiatrist interviewed the patient regarding her interest in and suitability for transplant, the question of compliance took on more importance. The patient insisted that she wanted a transplant and that she would try harder to do all of what the treatment team asked of her. The patient's mother felt that her daughter's health was in God's hands and that she could not do anything more to help her. The transplant psychiatrist, after discussion with the treating pulmonologist, agreed to a trial period of 6 months during which the patient would be monitored carefully on the outpatient basis to assess compliance. Unfortunately, the patient was not able to follow a schedule at home for even a period of a few weeks and was soon readmitted to the hospital in respiratory distress. The transplant team ultimately denied her candidacy.

THE LIVING DONOR TRANSPLANT

As there are many more patients who need organ transplant than there are available organs, living organ donation has become much more widely accepted in the United States. Living donation is a viable option for kidney, lung, and liver transplants. Potential donors also undergo a comprehensive psychological evaluation as well as a medical workup in order to ensure full autonomy, informed consent, and the absence of coercion. In some centers, the child psychiatrist or mental health provider working with the transplant team plays a crucial role in the evaluation of potential living donors. In other centers, the psychiatric screening evaluation of living donors is cursory. Additionally, some centers stress the need for a psychiatrist other than the transplant psychiatrist to evaluate the donor candidate. In all instances, great emphasis is placed on the absence of coercion in these unique situations. Living donors may be biologically related to the recipient, emotionally connected but not biologically related, or unrelated and anonymous. Lung transplantation is unique in that two donors are necessary.

It is very common for a parent to volunteer to donate an organ or part of an organ to a child. In those cases, the issue of benefit to the donor, i.e., preservation of the life of a child, is incontrovertible. However, the psychiatrist must help the team to consider the wellbeing of other members of an immediate family if both a child and a parent have surgery simultaneously. The psychiatrist also has an obligation to the patient to ensure that the parents' motivation for transplantation is in the best interest of the child, both physically and emotionally.

Potential donors who are siblings also merit close attention during a screening evaluation. It can be very difficult for a sibling who is blood type identical to refuse to donate, particularly if one or both parents are ineligible. Even though a sibling might deny feeling family pressure, it undoubtedly exists. A lobectomy is a painful and potentially debilitating operation. Siblings who volunteer to be living lobar lung donors must anticipate a 4- or 5-day hospital stay followed by 6 to 8 weeks of recovery before they will be able to resume normal activities. Little work has been done on the followup of medical and psychological sequelae of living lung donors. A recent study suggests that many donors feel that they did the right thing, but feel undervalued and unrecognized by both the family and by the transplant team (5).

The screening evaluation of an unrelated but emotionally connected donor or of a donor who has no connection at all with the recipient can present other challenges. Families of transplant recipients often advertise for donors on the Internet or in local community settings. Donors often come with an incomplete understanding of the process and unrealistic expectations for the outcome. Sometimes donors expect payment; sometimes donors are actively struggling with psychiatric illness or substance abuse. Studies of kidney donors have shown that as many as 50% of donors who presented themselves as completely sure that they wanted to donate, expressed ambivalence about donation on self-report questionnaires (6). Again, it is left to the individual transplant center to determine who will make an appropriate, unrelated donor.

NEUROPSYCHIATRIC EFFECTS OF IMMUNOSUPPRESSING AGENTS

The risks of rejection and infection are constants in the life of a posttransplant child or adolescent. All transplant patients are maintained for the rest of their lives on immunosuppressive medications. These medications and their interactions with other agents can have significant neuropsychiatric side effects that can be difficult to distinguish from psychiatric illness and that can complicate any planned psychopharmacologic regimen. It is also important to remember that a child's pharmacodynamics and pharmacokinetics can be different. A child's hepatic metabolic rate is faster that that of an adult and, although pediatric kidney function is similar to that of an adult, children (specifically between the ages of 9 and 12 years) may have a higher glomerular filtration rate as well (see Chapter 6.1.1). Children tend to metabolize common psychotropic medications such as neuroleptics, anticonvulsants, antidepressants and benzodiazepines more rapidly. However, any psychotropic medication that inhibits the cytochrome P450 IIIA3/4 isoenzyme system can potentially increase the levels of immunosuppressive medication. Conversely, some agents, including the herbal antidepressant Saint John's wort can be associated with decreased immunosuppressant levels and subsequent graft rejection. Some of the most common neuropsychiatric profiles of immunosuppressant agents are summarized in Table 7.1.3.2.1.

Cyclosporine (Neoral, Sandimmune) is a polypeptide derived from a fungus and is the mainstay of immunosuppressive therapy. Common adverse effects include nephrotoxicity, hypertension, hypomagnesaemia, hyperkalemia, gastroparesis and hyperlipidemia. Neuropsychiatric effects are particularly problematic at high serum levels and include delirium, often accompanied by frank psychotic symptoms (auditory and visual hallucinations). These side effects often resolve spontaneously as serum levels decrease, but patients often have a clear memory of their hallucinations. Patients with central nervous system effects sometimes have periventricular white matter changes on MRI. Cyclosporine is metabolized in the liver by the P450 IIIA3/4 system; it is possible that the selective serotonin uptake inhibitors could increase its serum levels through inhibition of the cytochrome system, but this has not been convincingly demonstrated (7). Carbamazepine may decrease its levels through hepatic induction. Patients who undergo bone marrow transplants may be particularly vulnerable to the neuropsychiatric toxic effects of cyclosporine (8).

FK506 (Tacrolimus, Prograf) is a macrolide produced by bacteria, and is also used as a primary immunosuppressive, sometimes as a substitute for cyclosporine. The neuropsychiatric side effects are similar to those of cyclosporine, including delirium, seizures, and akinetic mutism. MRI scans may also reveal white matter changes in patients showing toxicity. Psychotropic medications such as the selective serotonin uptake inhibitors that inhibit the cytochrome P450IIIA3/4 system can cause increases in serum levels of FK506 and must be used with caution.

Mycophenolate mofetil (Cellcept) suppresses T and B cell lymphocyte proliferation and is used as rescue therapy for those patients who cannot tolerate cyclosporine or FK506. It can also sometimes be used as adjunctive immunosuppression with cyclosporine. Central nervous system side effects can include anxiety, depression and sedation.

TABLE 7.1.3.2.1

POTENTIAL PSYCHIATRIC SIDE EFFECTS OF IMMUNOSUPPRESSANT AGENTS

Immunosuppressant Agent	Description	Potential Psychiatric Side Effects	Laboratory Findings
Cyclosporin *Neoral; Sandimmune*	Polypeptide fungal product	Delirium, auditory hallucinations, visual hallucinations, other psychotic symptoms	Side effects more prominent at high serum values and tend to resolve as serum levels decrease, SSRI's may increase levels, carbamezapine may decrease levels, herbal agents such as Saint Johns' wort may decrease levels, question of increased sensitivity to neuropsychiatric side effects among bone marrow transplant recipients
Tacrolimus *Prograf*	Also called FK506 or 5FK; macrolide antibiotic	Delirium, auditory and visual hallucinations, other psychotic symptoms, seizures, akinetic mutism	Side effects more prominent at high serum values and tend to resolve as serum levels decrease, MRI may reveal white matter changes in toxic patients
Mycophenolate Mofetil *Cellcept*	Suppresses T and B cell proliferation as adjunct immunosuppressant or for patients who cannot tolerate cyclosporine or tacrolimus	Anxiety, depression, sedation	
Muromonab-CD3 *OKT3*	Given immediately postoperatively to prevent rejection, monoclonal antibody that suppresses CD3 T cell function	Aseptic meningitis, hallucinations during administrations	
Corticosteroids	Mainstay of most transplant regimens, usually started high and tapered over weeks to months, though many patients remain on small dose indefinitely	Increased appetite, anxiety, depression, hypomania, mania, paranoia	Often dose-related and resolve with lowered dose

OKT3 is a monoclonal antibody that is used in the immediate postoperative period to prevent rejection. It can cause aseptic meningitis. Patients can hallucinate during administration, but those symptoms usually abate fairly quickly.

Corticosteroids continue to be a mainstay of treatment for transplant patients. Very high doses in the immediate postoperative period are gradually tapered over several months. Most patients remain on a small daily dose of oral prednisone for the remainder of their lives. Their numerous side effects include weight gain, easy bruising, osteoporosis, hirsutism, affective lability, hypomania, or mania. Some patients can manifest psychotic symptoms at very high doses (9). The neuropsychiatric side effects are sometimes dose related and generally subside with gradual taper of medication. Sudden discontinuation of steroids can result in depression, irritability, or anxiety.

Case Illustration 7: Neuropsychiatric Side Effects of Immunosuppressant Treatment

A young woman with CF underwent bilateral living donor lung transplantation. After a rocky postoperative course, she stabilized and was transferred to the transplant floor. Although her overall condition continued to improve, the nurses often found her crying in her room and the psychiatrist was asked to assess her for a question of depression. On evaluation, the patient's mood was upbeat but she explained that she frequently burst into tears with the smallest stimulus. She felt that she was overreacting to "everything" but she could not help herself. She was embarrassed by how often she cried and puzzled because in between she did not feel sad. When asked about how things had gone for her in general, she reported that she had a vivid memory of her postoperative stay in the intensive care unit. She told the psychiatrist that she had had visions of people she knew coming and going although later her parents had told her that no one was there. She had a picture in her mind of her surgeon as a "prankster," dressed up in a costume. She remembered feeling incredibly fearful of him but also unable to help herself. The patient was relieved to learn that her affective lability was most likely secondary to her high-dose steroids and that her "hallucinations" were also a side effect of the cyclosporine treatment.

GRAFT VERSUS HOST DISEASE

Graft versus host disease (GVH) is a relatively rare occurrence in modern transplant medicine. The efficacy of current immunosuppressant agents, careful graft selection, and vigilance for early signs of complications all contribute to the relative decrease in this very serious complication of transplantation. However, clinicians need to be aware that GVH is still a possibility, especially with bone marrow transplantation, and that it can be associated with significant delirium and encephalopathy (10).

LONG TERM PSYCHIATRIC CARE OF THE PEDIATRIC TRANSPLANT PATIENT

Transplant patients are typically followed closely by the transplant team well after the transplant takes place. They frequently have medical and surgical complications, they sometimes require a second or even a third transplant, and they often suffer significant psychological distress as they attempt to grapple with the long-term implications of their disease. Throughout all of this, the transplant psychiatrist continues to play an important role. The meaning of the transplant will change as patients develop cognitively and emotionally. Issues of medication noncompliance are frequent, especially in adolescents, and constitute one of the most common causes of graft rejection. Additionally, as we mentioned above, psychiatric illnesses can occur either as a function of the transplant, or as unrelated conditions.

Management of all of these issues again calls for the careful reckoning of both psychiatric and nonpsychiatric phenomena. For example, a change in mental status may be secondary to a medication effect, a metabolic encephalopathy, a seizure disorder, a newly presenting psychiatric illness, or a combination of some or even all of these issues. Again, the medical expertise of the psychiatrist makes him or her ideally suited for these complicated issues.

CONCLUSION

As transplant procedures have become more successful, transplant teams have increasingly embraced the notion that the fundamental goal for young transplant patients is assuming the most normal life possible in spite of the obstacles that their diseases potentially pose. Transplant patients play on soccer teams, go on dates, graduate from school, and often want most of all to be thought of as an ordinary child or adolescent. Empathy for this desire, coupled with the simultaneous vigilance for the numerous problems outlined above, make the job of the pediatric transplant psychiatrist complicated, challenging, and undeniably rewarding.

References

1. Rauch PK, Jellinek MS: Paediatric consultation. In: Rutter M (ed): *Child and Adolescent Psychiatry*, 4th ed. Malden, MA, Blackwell, 2002, pp. 1051–1066.
2. Mintzer LL, Stuber ML, Seacord D, Castaneda M, Mesrkhani V, Glover D: Traumatic stress symptoms in adolescent organ transplant recipients. *Pediatrics* 115 (6):1640–1644, 2005.
3. Stuber ML, Kazack AE, Meeske K, et al.: Predictors of posttraumatic stress symptoms in childhood cancer survivors. *Pediatrics* 100:958–964; 1997.
4. Levinson JL, Olbrisch ME: Psychosocial screening and selections of candidates for organ transplantation. In Trepacz, DiMartini (eds): *The Transplant Patient*. Cambridge, U.K., Cambridge University Press, 2000, pp. 27–28.
5. Prager LM, Ginns LC, Wain JC, Roberts, DH: Medical and psychological follow-up of living lung donors *ISHLT*, 2006, in press.
6. Simmons RG, Klein SD, Simmons RL: (1977) *Gift of Life: The Social and Psychological Impact of Organ Transplantation*. A Wiley-Interscience: New York.
7. Markowitz JS, Gill HS, Hunt NM, Monroe RR Jr, DeVane CL: Lack of antidepressant-cyclosporine pharmacokinetic interactions. *Journal of Clinical Psychopharmacology* 18(1):91–93, 1998.
8. Atkinson K, Biggs J, Darveniza P, Boland J, Concannon A, Dodds A: Cyclosporine-associated central-nervous-system toxicity after allogeneic bone-marrow transplantation. *NEJM* 310(8):527, 1984.
9. Patton SB, Neutel CL: Corticosteroid-induced adverse psychiatric side effects: Incidence, diagnosis and management. *Drug Safety* 22:111–122, 2000.
10. Antonini G, Ceschin V, Morino S, Fiorelli M, Gragnani F, Mengarelli A, Iori AP, Arcese W: Early neurologic complications following allogeneic bone marrow transplant for leukemia: A prospective study. *Neurology* 50(5):1441–1445, 1998.

CHAPTER 7.1.3.3 ■ PSYCHOSOCIAL ASPECTS OF HIV/AIDS

ROBERT A. MURPHY, KAREN J. O'DONNELL, KATHRYN WHETTEN, AND JEAN ADNOPOZ

PSYCHOSOCIAL ASPECTS OF HIV INFECTION

The epidemic of human immunodeficiency virus (HIV) and acquired immunodeficiency syndrome (AIDS) represents a major world crisis affecting the health and psychological well being of tens of millions of persons, causing devastation among families, and threatening the social welfare of communities. With recent advances for early diagnosis, the prevention of mother-to-child transmission, and more effective drug treatments, there is an increasing gap in the impact of this disorder between wealthy and low resource countries of the world. In countries such as the United States, where newer, expensive drug therapies are available, there have been significant decreases in morbidity and mortality; countries with more limited resources are experiencing horrifying escalations in the spread and effects of infection with HIV/AIDS. The contrast is particularly true for children. In areas where treatments aimed at reducing perinatal transmission are readily available and affordable, there has been a dramatic decrease in the rate of perinatally infected children (1). In countries where resources are low, the treatment of pregnant women to prevent perinatal transmission has not yet become general practice. Combinations of antiretroviral (ART) drugs that have turned a deadly disease into a chronic one in wealthier countries are not generally available to poorer ones. However, throughout the world, the increasing focus is on children and adolescents, because 1) they are the age cohorts experiencing the highest rate of new infections, and 2) when effective treatments are available, children with HIV infection are living into adolescence and adulthood.

WORLD VIEW OF THE EPIDEMIC

According to estimates from the Joint United Nations Programme on HIV/AIDS (UNAIDS), by the end of 2005, approximately 40.3 million people, including between 2 and 2.6 million children, were living with HIV infection; 95% of these children live in low resource countries (2). In 2005 alone, 3 million adults and 600,000 children were newly infected with HIV. More than 500,000 children with HIV/AIDS die each year. Translated to a daily basis, 1,800 children under age 15 are newly infected and 1,400 die of AIDS-related illnesses. In excess of 15 million children have been orphaned due to HIV/AIDS, yet less than 10% of these children receive any form of assistance from their governments. As a result, children are deprived of parental, family, and other stable, loving relationships; medical care, education, nutrition, and sanitation; and the opportunity to prevent another generation from becoming infected. UNAIDS has set an ambitious goal of reducing mother-to-child transmission and improving pediatric treatment each by 80% by 2010, while dramatically reducing rates of HIV infection among youth and increasing levels of psychosocial support.

Sub-Saharan Africa continues to dominate the world HIV/AIDS epidemic in sheer numbers. Approximately 64% of all new infections and 85% of pediatric infections occur in the region (3). AIDS has dramatically heightened child mortality rates across the continent, while life expectancy has declined in many nations due to the disease. Although rates of infection are relatively lower in other parts of the world, the numbers remain significant and show a rapid increase in some areas. By the end of 2005, HIV infections were growing at their fastest rates in Eastern Europe and Central and East Asia, where spread of the epidemic is affected by patterns of migration and accompanying risk behaviors as people move to and from urban areas as economies and unemployment expand and contract. In Russia, the rapidly rising epidemic has been driven largely by injection drug use among young people of reproductive age. The HIV epidemic in Latin America is highly diverse, largely concentrated in urban areas, and typified by varied modes of transmission, including via heterosexual and homosexual contact and intravenous (IV) drug use. Rates of infection in some Caribbean islands are the highest of any area outside of sub-Saharan Africa. In Middle Eastern and North African nations, AIDS may go unrecognized and unaddressed due to cultural prohibitions regarding reproductive and sexual health (2). In general, the spread of the epidemic has been related to serious economic failure and concomitant increases in poverty and the disenfranchisement of young people, which lead to higher rates of IV drug use and greater reliance on prostitution as a means of livelihood (4).

EPIDEMIC IN THE UNITED STATES

In the United States, 1996 marked a major turning point in the epidemic, when the introduction of new therapies and combination therapy slowed the progression of HIV/AIDS for children and adults and led to an increase in the number of persons living with AIDS, accompanied by a dramatic decrease in HIV-related deaths. With the successful prevention of mother-to-child transmission in the United States as well as effective drug therapies for those who are infected, HIV/AIDS has come to affect disproportionately women and minorities who are adolescents and young adults. In 2003, women represented 27% of all those reported with HIV, compared with 7% of those reported with AIDS in the first 5 years of the epidemic (5). African-American and Hispanic youth have markedly higher rates of infection than their Caucasian peers, and adolescents with HIV/AIDS represent a fast-growing population, presenting new needs for their medical and psychological care compared to an earlier focus on infants and younger children (6).

Importantly, statistics on prevalence using the Centers for Disease Control and Prevention (CDC) surveillance case definition for AIDS fail to portray the true nature of the epidemic. With the advent of more effective therapies that delay or prevent the onset of AIDS-defining symptoms, many HIV-positive persons went unreported because they did not meet criteria for the AIDS diagnosis. Because of the delay between the time of infection and the development of symptoms, data on HIV infection and classifications of disease progression based on the CD4+ T lymphocyte count provide more pertinent and potentially useful information on the epidemiology of the disease among youth. It is significant that, unlike the declining rates of AIDS (7), the rate of spread of HIV infection remains fairly constant and has increased in some instances. For example, in the U.S. deep South, rates of HIV/AIDS have been consistently and dramatically increasing since 1997 (8). In this chapter, the term HIV/AIDS is used to refer to the continuum of infection, asymptomatic status, and symptomatic states increasing to life-threatening conditions.

CHILDREN AND HIV/AIDS

Changes in the incidence of AIDS have been even more dramatic among children than HIV among adults. For example, in 2003, only 59 children were reported to the CDC with perinatally acquired infection, a small fraction of the 8,749 children under age 13 diagnosed to date in the United States (9). The greatest contribution to this decline is the success of decreasing perinatal transmission from mother to child through treatment of HIV-infected pregnant women with antiretroviral treatment (ART) (1, 10). Before 1994, the rate of transmission of HIV infection from an infected mother to her child was approximately 25%; this rate has now fallen to less than 5% (9, 11). The effectiveness of antiretroviral drugs for the prevention of transmission is associated with the significantly reduced viral load for the pregnant woman (12), thereby reducing perinatal exposure for the newborn. Delivery by elective cesarean section has also been used as a method for preventing transmission (2, 13, 14); however, the success of ART may argue for its sole use as a prevention measure.

Some studies have demonstrated that shorter, less expensive courses of treatment with ART can be efficacious in decreasing transmission of infection from mother to child (15–18). For example, Lallemant et al. (10) demonstrated in Thailand that a single dose of nevarapine (NVP) reduced perinatal transmission to 2.8% relative to a placebo group (6.3%) and not significantly more than a group receiving NVP and zidovudine (ZDV). Nonetheless, without ART, mother-to-child transmission of HIV still occurs in approximately 35% of births in resource poor nations (2).

This picture is further complicated by the finding that HIV is transmitted by breast-feeding at rates three to four times higher than for formula-fed infants (19). Substituting infant formula for breast-feeding is an alternative in wealthy countries, but it is not the obvious answer for less wealthy ones due to the high rates of infant death from diarrheal disorders that are promoted through infected water. WHO/UNAIDS/UNICEF infant feeding guidelines stress the importance of sole breastfeeding for 6 months for women for whom HIV status is unknown or known to be negative (20). Even for women with known infection, breast feeding is recommended unless the preparation of infant formula is known to be safe and affordable, allowing a woman a choice about replacement feeding as well as counseling about risks and breast feeding techniques to prevent conditions that increase the risk of transmission, e.g., breast abscesses, nipple fissures, mastitis, as well as sores in the infant's mouth. In most poor countries, safe replacement feeding is simply not feasible and can be the cause of life threatening diarrhea and pneumonia as well as other infections. In other words, the risk of replacement feedings is seen as too high for otherwise healthy HIV uninfected infants (21, 22). There is a great need for programs that make replacement feedings safe and sustainable in high HIV/AIDS prevalence, low resource countries.

When and how the countries that have the highest rates of HIV/AIDS will be able to provide universal programs to prevent perinatal transmission remains to be seen. In wealthier nations, ART has effected dramatic improvements in HIV related mortality and morbidity, and in the past several years in less wealthy regions access to antiretroviral therapy is expanding. For example, at the end of 2003 approximately 400,000 people were receiving ART in less wealthy nations (low- and middle-income countries), but by mid-year 2005, approximately 1 million people were receiving ART in these countries (23). In sub-Saharan Africa, the region of the world with the largest burden of HIV cases, programs such as the Global Fund to Fight HIV, Malaria, and Tuberculosis and the President's Emergency Package for AIDS Relief (PEPFAR) have facilitated a three-fold increase in access to antiretroviral therapy over the past 12 months alone, and it is anticipated that these programs will continue to grow in the neediest countries. Continued implementation of such interventions requires access to affordable medications and a sound system for providing prenatal and perinatal care, as well as HIV testing and counseling (2). Even when women agree to be tested, many may not return for the results (24). Fears of stigmatization and, even worse, fear of abuse or being thrown out of their homes prevent women from being tested or returning for test results.

Orphans

Although a real opportunity exists to decrease the number of children infected with HIV, the number of infected adults of childbearing age continues to increase, resulting in a rapidly escalating number of children orphaned by the epidemic. With 15 million HIV orphans worldwide and many more children whose parents are incapacitated by illness, orphaned children are often looked after by family members, frequently by aging grandparents, or adolescent siblings, in institutional settings, or by other street children (2). However, as the infection rate in a community increases, there are fewer working adults; the result is a decrease in the resources available to care for orphaned children.

Few studies exist that describe the actual psychosocial symptoms of orphans in low resource countries, though it is increasingly recognized that many who have been orphaned by HIV/AIDS do not thrive. A study of orphans in Uganda found that those whose parents died of AIDS had higher depression scores than other orphans (25). The children showed signs of unresolved grief, and the study called for professional counseling interventions for orphans. Another study found that orphans were more likely to experience internalizing symptoms such as anxiety, a sense of failure, and suicidal thoughts when compared with non–orphan matched controls (26). Not addressing these issues results in children growing into adults who are not able to be as functional as others in their society and who are more likely to engage in high risk behavior, including sexual activity and criminality (27–29).

Adolescents and Youth

At least half of new HIV infections worldwide occur in adolescents and young adults, with higher rates among females and those of ethnic minority backgrounds (2, 30). Although mother-to-child transmission has become infrequent in the

United States, youth who were infected when rates of mother-to-child transmission were higher represent approximately one-fifth of HIV-infected persons (7, 31). The advent of ART, decreases in HIV prevention funding, and numbing to the fear of the disease are all reasons for a resurgence of unsafe sexual practices among youths and adults (32). Rates of infection with other sexually transmitted diseases (STDs) continue to be very high among youth and serve as indicators of their elevated risk of HIV infection. Of the 12 million cases of STDs that occur each year in the United States, one-fourth occur among teenagers, and two-thirds are acquired by 25 years of age (33). Drug use among adolescents can also increase the risk of HIV infection, not only through direct infection from injecting drug use but also through increased risk for unsafe sexual practices. Persons under the influence of alcohol or other drugs experience both decreased inhibitions and physical sensitivity, resulting in sexual practices that are more likely to result in damaged membranes and therefore transmission of HIV.

CLINICAL CHARACTERISTICS OF CHILDREN WITH HIV/AIDS

The clinical characteristics of HIV/AIDS in children are similar in many ways to those in adults, although there are several important differences. In addition to natural disease course differences, with more effective treatment regimens available since the mid-1990s, features of the disease have shifted from those illnesses secondary to a severely compromised immune system to those that represent damage to organ systems through multiple threats from long term infection.

Early signs of infection in untreated newborns and infants can include fever, persistent candidasis, poor weight gain, hepatomegaly and splenomegaly, lymphadenopathy, parotiditis, and diarrhea (6). Early treatment regimes, where early diagnosis and drug therapies are available, include ART (e.g., zidovudine) used to suppress viral replication and antibiotics (e.g., trimethoprim-sulfamethoxazole) used to prevent opportunist infections, such as *Pneumocystis carinii* pneumonia (PCP). Without this care, children may present early with life threatening illnesses such as PCP, lymphoid interstitial pneumonitis (LIP), bacterial infections, central nervous system disease, and other opportunistic infections. Liver and renal diseases are not uncommon; and malignancies, such as non-Hodgkin's lymphoma (NHL), can be associated with immune deficiency for children infected with HIV. Even with early identification and highly active antiretroviral treatment (HAART), many young children will show signs of their infection, predominately growth failure, fevers, and developmental delays. Fortunately, the emergence of newer treatment regimens has lessened the prevalence and severity of these symptoms.

PCP was formerly the leading cause of death in HIV-infected children; however, since the mid-1990s and the advent of HAART, PCP has become increasingly rare, especially in children for whom drug therapy results in CD4+ counts greater than 200 (34). Other bacterial infections that used to occur more frequently (e.g., sepsis, meningitis), also occur much less frequently for children with the advantage of early antiretroviral and antibiotic treatments. Of opportunistic infections, *Mycobacterium avium intracellulare* (MAI) complex disease and *Candida* esophagitis ("thrush") are the most prevalent among children, but, again, present rarely for children with preserved immune function. *Lymphoid interstitial pneumonia* (LIP) occurs only rarely in adults, and, now, with HAART, infrequently with children.

Other manifestations of HIV disease are varied, can affect all organ systems, and are seen more frequently now that children and adolescents are not dying from the early consequences of severe immune suppression (6, 35). These include the lymphoreticular system and hematologic abnormalities, gastrointestinal and hepatobiliary disease, cardiomyopathies, and renal disease. Growth stunting is still associated with HIV/AIDS in children; (7, 36) as HIV+ children approach adolescence, they struggle to adapt to their unusual appearance and their physical immaturity. Improvement in disease management has resulted in better weight gain, but not improved linear growth. Stunting is thought to be a side effect of some of the protease inhibitors (37).

Central Nervous System Disease

Neurological, neuropsychological, and developmental manifestations of HIV disease can be the earliest and most devastating markers of infection in children. In fact, neurodevelopmental dysfunction was one symptom of HIV infection that brought children to the attention of a medical community that still saw AIDS as an adult disease in the early 1980s (38). The virus was shown to cross the blood brain barrier readily and create both direct and indirect injury in the central nervous system (CNS). Early studies of CNS manifestations of HIV disease suggested that between 40% and 90% of infected children had some degree of neurologic involvement (39, 40). These studies, however, were generally conducted in cohorts of children with more advanced disease. Later prospective studies documented rates of serious neurodevelopmental signs in 8% to 13% in HIV-infected children and in 19% to 31% in children who met diagnostic criteria for AIDS (13, 41–43). Although early, aggressive, and well monitored treatment has dramatically reduced progressive HIV encephalopathy for children, there remain aspects of CNS effects that warrant attention by infectious disease specialists and also by mental health professionals monitoring the child's wellbeing.

Prior to the widespread use of HAART in the United States and other industrialized countries, three-fourths of children with HIV encephalopathy were diagnosed before the age of 36 months (42). HIV encephalopathy is a general term for HIV-associated CNS pathology resulting in structural damage (e.g., atrophy) and/or impaired function. This is predominately a clinical diagnosis, at times supported by neuroimaging and laboratory findings; and, in children, it usually refers to a progressive process. The definition of HIV encephalopathy adopted by the Pediatric AIDS Clinical Trials Group identifies three criteria: 1) impaired brain growth, 2) loss of or failure to achieve developmental milestones, and 3) clinically apparent neurological dysfunction. Impaired brain growth refers to acquired microcephaly and/or cerebral atrophy, or other findings from imaging studies. Decline in or failure to achieve developmental and cognitive milestones is evaluated by clinical observation, parental report, and serial neuropsychological testing. Clinical neurological difficulties often present as progressive motor dysfunction, most often symmetrical deterioration of previously attained functional motor skills, diffuse and symmetric loss of power or strength, diffuse and symmetric abnormalities of tone, and diffuse, symmetric, and pathologically increased deep tendon reflexes. HIV encephalopathy in the newborn and infant can also be manifested by significant changes in neurobehavioral status, including changes in range and regulation of arousal and attention, and decrements in alertness, responsivity, and attention. Improved neurodevelopmental status in these domains was one important marker of the effects of early, single drug ART for symptomatic children; and neurodevelopmental decline was seen as an indicator of the ineffectiveness of specific drug therapy (36).

Children with HIV/AIDS can also exhibit static neurodevelopmental deficits. They do not lose milestones; but as they grow older, deficits in neuromotor or cognitive development become more evident, and new skills are acquired at a slower rate than normal. It is often not clear whether these developmental difficulties are a direct or indirect effect of HIV infection, are unrelated to the disease, or are the result of a complex interaction of direct effects on the CNS, indirect toxicities of disease or drug treatment on the brain, or the various economic and psychosocial adversities faced by many children with HIV/AIDS.

Important for the medical or mental health practitioner, however, the devastating, early, and progressive manifestations of HIV activity in the brain are all but eliminated for children diagnosed early and treated successfully with HAART, that is, for whom viral activity in the brain is suppressed. The neurodevelopmental and behavioral risks for children with HIV disease in wealthier countries have changed dramatically but certainly have not been eliminated. To date there are few studies of the neurodevelopmental and psychological consequences of HIV and its treatments for the new cohort of children living with HIV/AIDS as a chronic disease. It is likely that the effects represent not only neurological injury to the CNS when viral suppression is not adequate but also the toxicities of drugs used to treat HIV/AIDS over a long period of time. In addition, the development and mental health of children living with HIV/AIDS will be affected by the economic and other psychosocial difficulties in their lives, e.g., the death of parents, changes in caregivers, the stigma of the disease.

Evaluation of Central Nervous System Abnormalities in HIV-Infected Children

An extensive history focusing on developmental milestones and a detailed neurologic examination are important in alerting the clinician to the possibility of the neurodevelopmental and learning effects of HIV/AIDS. A full neurodevelopmental assessment is warranted when there is any suggestion of developmental abnormalities or sign of neurologic disease. Neuropsychological testing can be useful in establishing an initial baseline, monitoring subsequent alterations in cognitive processing secondary to CNS involvement, and devising appropriate developmental or educational interventions.

In general, results of cerebrospinal fluid studies are normal in HIV encephalopathy, although there may be slightly elevated protein and a mild, predominantly lymphocytic pleocytosis. Abnormalities in imaging studies associated with HIV encephalopathy are nonspecific and include enlargement of the ventricles, cortical atrophy, attenuation of periventricular white matter, and cerebral calcifications (44). The calcifications, when they occur, are usually symmetrical and are located in the basal ganglia and periventricular frontal white matter, or occasionally in the cerebellar regions. Computed tomography scanning is most helpful in demonstrating cerebral calcifications, whereas magnetic resonance imaging is better at detecting the abnormalities in white matter. Abnormalities can be seen on neuroimaging studies, even in the absence of other signs of encephalopathy; however, repeated assessments are usually helpful in assessing progression of disease and failure of treatment in an individual patient.

Treatment of HIV Infection

Formerly, the approach to treating HIV/AIDS in children was to reserve the use of antiretroviral medications for patients who already had fairly advanced disease, as evidenced by a decline in CD4+ T lymphocyte cells or the development of symptoms of their disease. However, once it was understood that the period that preceded clinical signs of disease was not a period of latency, but, in fact, a period characterized by continuous replication of the virus and destruction of the immune system, newer recommendations for treatment were developed (45, 46). In addition, the current treatment of HIV infection in adults and children has progressed from the use of a single antiretroviral drug designed to thwart the entry of the virus into the blood stream, to multiple drugs that, taken at the same time, attack the virus and its replication at different points in its pathophysiological process. The advent of a new class of drugs in the 1990s, the protease inhibitors, resulted in dramatic improvements in HIV-associated mortality and morbidity by preventing viral replication. It is now recommended that treatment decisions, such as when to start and when to change a treatment regime, be made from measures of the extent of viral replication and CD4+ T lymphocyte count. The extent of viral replication, commonly referred to as the *viral load*, is quantified by measuring the HIV ribonucleic acid (RNA) by polymerase chain reaction amplification.

The present treatment approach, referred to as highly active antiretroviral treatment (HAART), includes starting treatment early and achieving maximal suppression of viral replication using a combination of at least three different antiretroviral medications, including nucleoside reverse transcriptase inhibitors, nonnucleoside reverse transcriptase inhibitors, protease inhibitors, and fusion inhibitors. Fortunately, these combination drug protocols have successfully reduced viral load to undetectable levels and preserved immune functioning in as many as one-half of the children who adhered to the protocol (47, 48). Of course, these successes have been documented in wealthy countries in which these expensive treatments are feasible, but not in low resource countries where HIV/AIDS in children is most prevalent.

Unfortunately, there is a potential for the virus to develop resistance to antiretroviral medications, particularly if someone has already been treated with a single medication before starting triple therapy and if adherence is inconsistent. In such cases, once there is a rebound in the viral load, the virus is likely to be resistant to all three medications, and all three will need to be changed. In addition, within the different classes of medications is a tendency for cross-resistance to develop: If the virus is resistant to one medication in a class, it may also be resistant to others within the same class. Thus, even in this era of multiple medications from which to choose, the choices become limited once viral resistance has developed, and chronic medication nonadherence should be considered in selection of pharmacotherapy strategies. Despite this limitation, some evidence indicates that although patients may have a rebound in viral load measurements on triple therapy, they continue to do better and have a slower progression of disease than would otherwise be expected (49). As with other manifestations of HIV disease in children, advances in management are almost certainly having an effect on decreasing the prevalence and severity of CNS disease among children. Such a decrease in CNS manifestations of HIV disease has been well documented in adults, has been observed in children, but awaits further study in children and adolescents (50).

All of the antiretroviral medications have adverse effects, some of which may be mitigated by the use of other medications, including psychotropic medications. The finding that antiretroviral medications, particularly the protease inhibitors, can cause significant derangements in metabolic processes resulting in abnormal lipid profiles and glucose levels, and alterations in body composition, are among the most important adverse effects (51). This latter, referred to as the *lipodystrophy syndrome,* may be very distressing to patients because of the changes in physical appearance. There is wasting and disappearance of fat from the face and limbs but an increase in fat in the abdominal region and over the lower part of posterior neck.

A major challenge posed by the advances in therapy of HIV disease has been the need to ensure that patients consistently are able to take all of their medicines. Inconsistent adherence can provide the window for resistant viral strains to replicate and dominate, increasing viral load, this time with a virus that is not affected by the current treatment. One study reported a linear association between self-reported adherence and level of HIV viral suppression. Patients taking fewer than 80% of their prescribed doses of antiretroviral medications had a significant increase in viral load measurements compared with those who took more of their medications. As noted above, successes of HAART have been documented for those children with good adherence (6). Despite this serious risk, adherence is not simple or easy for children and families. Treatment regimens often call for a large number of medications, taken at regular intervals each day. Some of the medications are available only as large capsules that are difficult to swallow; others have a particularly bad taste. Important interventions for the care of children with HIV/AIDS include support and strategies for children and families in taking medications on time and more easily.

CHILD DEVELOPMENT AND HIV/AIDS

Findings of an expectable developmental progression in children's understanding of HIV and AIDS should inform pediatric prevention and intervention efforts, because they highlight the importance of practices that are tailored to children's psychological and cognitive capacities. As with their overall cognitive development and capacity for logical reasoning, children's understanding of HIV/AIDS follows a predictable sequence. Preschool and early school-age children explain HIV/AIDS in terms of contiguous events. At this age, children may begin to recognize that symptoms are the result of an underlying illness, but they are likely unable to explain its viral origin. With development, the causation of HIV/AIDS can be described as a sequential process related to actions and events, including sexual behavior, blood exposure, or drug use. Typically, these explanations may provide older school-age children with a factually accurate account of how HIV/AIDS may be contracted. The final stage of understanding is based on the expanded capacity for abstract reasoning that accompanies adolescence. Youth become able to describe the origins of HIV/AIDS in terms of its underlying disease (52, 53). The child's understanding of his or her own death and that of family members follows a similar progression.

For parents of infants, preoccupation with the medical and psychological demands of coping with HIV disease may deplete families of the energy and psychological resources available to attend to normative aspects of early childhood development. For example, parents of an infant with HIV/AIDS may be overcome with anxiety and remorse at having transmitted the virus to their child, as well as the distress and possible depression related to their own disease. The parents may then be less responsive to the infant's cues related to basic needs involving nurturance, warmth, or sustenance that form the basis for attentive and reciprocal interactions. In one study, the motor development and adaptive behavior of children with HIV/AIDS decreased with changes in caregivers, something not uncommon when a child's mother is sick or dying (54).

As young children develop the capacity for imaginative or pretense play that allows them to mediate between internal states and actions, children may enact repeated scenarios related to illness or loss, even though the same child may never be able to verbalize these concerns. Although children may gradually be able to understand basic facts about HIV illness and death, their ideas will likely remain concrete and specific to their life experiences. Metaphors about death may engender greater confusion, because young children are unable to abstract the basic concept that death represents a final cessation of life. At this stage of development, children may feel threatened and upset by conflicts stemming from experiencing their own loving and competitive feelings toward their parents, to which already emotionally fragile parents may be unable to respond effectively. With their egocentric orientation, young children may assume that their actions play a causal role in a parent's illness, resulting in feelings of guilt and responsibility.

For school-aged children, independence and engagement with peers and a broader social world may be experienced by the child as a rejection of the caregiver, and some children may find themselves unable to negotiate this natural developmental step. Children who have been unable to resolve conflicting feelings concerning medically compromised parents may remain tied to their caregivers in a manner that precludes their developmentally appropriate ventures into the world of peers and school, that is, fear of loss of the parent could result in undue separation distress. Mastery of basic logical principles allows a child to infer cause-and-effect relationships regarding HIV/AIDS, and language serves a regulatory as well as a communicative function.

CHILDREN AFFECTED BY HIV/AIDS

The numbers of children affected by parents or caregivers with HIV/AIDS continues to rise in poverty stricken areas of the world, including poor areas of the United States, (8) with substantial rates of HIV infection among young, minority women, 50% of whom are estimated to bear children (29, 55). Unfortunately, family members as well as professionals may fail to recognize the unique concerns and obstacles that threaten the development of HIV-affected children. As witnesses to repeated periods of acute, incapacitating parental illness, these children anticipate the death of one or both parents and worry about who will take care of them when their parents are no longer available. They may be left to contend with feelings of sorrow, anger, guilt, and confusion in isolation as other family members turn their attention to the infected adult or struggle with their own histories of loss (56–58). Many children in HIV-affected families face additional burdens related to parental instability and incarceration, family and residential instability, exposure to violence, caregiver substance abuse, and social isolation (59–61).

In an effort to redress the paucity of data on the functioning of HIV-affected children, Forehand et al. developed a multidisciplinary, longitudinal study of HIV-infected mothers and their affected children (55). Researchers followed an urban sample of 105 6- to 11-year-old HIV-affected African-American children and a matched comparison group of 150 mothers and children where HIV was absent. After controlling for the severity of AIDS symptoms, 3-year results indicated higher levels of internalizing and externalizing psychiatric symptoms among the HIV-infected mothers and their affected children, as well as greater impairments in children's social competence. Children who had been orphaned due to parental death from HIV/AIDS demonstrated higher levels of clinically significant internalizing and externalizing symptoms prior to their parent's death and at 2 year followup relative to HIV affected children whose parent remained living and to those of uninfected parents (62). At three assessment points (prior to death, 6 months postdeath, and 2 years postdeath), between 52% and 73% of children demonstrated clinically significant symptoms. Another study suggested that HIV-affected children had increased rates of anxiety and depressive disorders (63), with symptoms most acute during early disease stages (64).

The unpredictable course of HIV/AIDS, marked by multiple episodes of relapse and recovery and a chronic course of illness, limits parents' ability to provide consistent and stable care and perpetuates a sense of anxiety and dread among their children (65, 66). Ironically, many parents may neglect their own health as they focus on the pressing needs of their children, and children's longer term needs for permanency and security may be sacrificed by their parent's unwitting neglect of their own important health issues. Affected children often are unable to express their expectable feelings of anger and guilt because of an unrecognized fear that they may become overwhelmed by their distress or may hasten the death of their loved one (65). Adolescents affected by parental HIV infection and AIDS are particularly vulnerable. Adolescents residing with a parent diagnosed with AIDS consistently report high levels of parent–child conflict, academic failure, peer relationship problems, and criminal behavior, with estimates that 25% to 73% present with clinically significant difficulties (66). As Zayas and Romano (67) noted, "Perhaps no group of children in modern time has been more battered by the combination of social and familial decay and a devastating illness, coupled with the normal storms of adolescence."

Adolescents and Risk Behaviors

HIV infection has become an increasing problem among adolescents, particularly those who engage in high levels of risk-taking behaviors (68). In the United States, 2,050 new cases of AIDS were reported among 13 to 24 year olds in 2003 for a cumulative total of 38,490 adolescents and young adults who have had HIV/AIDS (9). Because existing prevention and intervention programs have resulted in significant decreases in prenatal and perinatal HIV infection, the majority of the new cases may involve persons who contracted HIV during adolescence (69). As in the general population, HIV infection among adolescents affects young women and youth of African-American and Latino descent disproportionately relative to their representation in the general population (70).

Although most adolescents strive to loosen the ties of childhood dependency by substituting intimate and romantic relationships with peers (71), those who must contend with personal or familial HIV may be compromised in these behaviors, which subserve adolescent individuation and the formation of an independent sense of self. The expectable rule transgressions and rebellions against parental strictures become fraught with danger, real and imagined, about the potential consequences of their emerging sexuality and the strength of their angry or defiant feelings. Peers exert a strong influence on adolescents' attitudes toward the practice of safer sex, and peer attitudes that favor or discourage condom use are strong predictors of their actual use (72). Nonetheless, initial sexual encounters among teens are rarely planned, and this spontaneity decreases the likelihood of the use of birth control or engagement in sexual practices aimed at reducing the chances of HIV transmission (72, 73).

Among affected youth for whom childhood has not been a normative process, the tasks of adolescence become even more challenging (68). These adolescents appear at greater risk of poor health outcomes, as well as maladaptive behaviors leading to truancy, high risk sexual behavior, criminal activity, substance abuse, and psychiatric disturbances (72). This cohort of adolescents often does not seek needed medical treatment, thus increasing their own risk of contracting both STDs and other strands of HIV. Moreover, youth who are truant or who withdraw from school prematurely miss receiving information promoting healthy behaviors and preventing STDs (74). Adolescents within the criminal justice system, who present with high reported rates of infectious diseases, including HIV/AIDS, and limited histories of primary prevention and healthcare are thought to be among those at highest risk for becoming infected (75).

PSYCHOPATHOLOGY AND HIV DISEASE

Depression has been consistently associated with less self-care, including the practice of unprotected sexual intercourse. HIV-positive individuals who engage in high-risk sexual behavior appear more pessimistic and hopeless about their future and possess fewer strategies for coping with stress. As a result, they appear less likely to disclose their serostatus to potential sex partners or to initiate discussion of safer sex practices. Efforts at primary prevention may be confounded by this compromised sense of self-worth, and a pessimistic outlook may interfere with the ability to apply HIV knowledge to actual behaviors. High-risk sexual behavior or drug abuse may also be symptomatic of a depressive disorder, in which the behavior represents a self-destructive act or an attempt to minimize experience and awareness of affective disturbance, a finding that has received empirical support from studies of adult samples (11, 72, 76, 77).

Children with attention deficit hyperactivity disorder or conduct disorder are more likely to engage in impulsive actions that increase their risk of HIV infection (78–80). In addition, children with HIV/AIDS (including those with perinatal infection) exhibit a high prevalence of ADHD-related symptoms, suggesting that the relationship between HIV infection and difficulties with attention and hyperactivity is a factor in transmission as well as a manifestation of the effects of the disease on the CNS and behavior after infection (81).

Adolescents diagnosed with psychiatric disorders, particularly externalizing disorders, may engage in a range of behaviors that potentiates their risk for HIV/AIDS (72, 80). Compared with nonpsychiatrically disordered peers, adolescents with comorbid psychiatric disorders engage in more frequent substance abuse, including IV drug abuse, unprotected sexual intercourse, and sexual activity with partners of unknown risk history. Even among runaway and homeless adolescents, who are much more likely than most adolescents to engage in high risk sexual activity and IV drug use, those with a diagnosis of conduct disorder are still more likely to have engaged in an exchange of sexual activity in return for money or drugs and to have unprotected sex with multiple partners (72). A diagnosis of conduct disorder increases the likelihood of IV drug more than two-fold (OR, 2.3), and the likelihood of exchanging sex for drugs or money almost three-fold (OR, 2.8). Adolescents who know someone infected with HIV are also at greater risk of drug injection (OR, 1.4) or sexual exchange (OR, 1.3). Other disorders associated with impulsivity or sexual preoccupation, such as bipolar, borderline personality, or impulse control disorders, may also interfere with the use of safer sexual practices. Whether the psychopathology arises from separate causes or is the result of the associated stress of HIV infection, comorbid psychiatric disorders further compromise the functioning and quality of life for youth infected with HIV (77, 82).

To date, there are insufficient studies for a full understanding of the neurological and behavioral health consequences of HIV/AIDS in children. There is reason, however, to believe that these children present at higher risk for various psychiatric conditions than their noninfected peers. For example, children with HIV/AIDS are known to be at increased risk for psychiatric hospitalization (83, 84), and the primary reasons for admission involve depression and behavioral difficulties (e.g., oppositional defiant disorder and ADHD). Results from the Women and Infants Transmission Study (WITS) indicated higher rates of behavioral problems among young children with HIV/AIDS, but when socioeconomic factors were analyzed, it seemed that HIV/AIDS and psychiatric disorders were linked to the psychosocial adversity in the child's life as opposed to the disease itself. This is consistent with a study by Lester et al., (85) who found that child emotional distress was related to major life events and parental anxiety even more than knowledge of HIV status.

Children with chronic illnesses, in general, are found to be at higher risk for psychiatric problems, including depression, anxiety, and feelings of isolation (84, 86–88). However, children with HIV/AIDS have additional factors in the complexity of their illness and treatment, as well as in the adverse psychosocial circumstances and poverty in which many live. Children who know about their HIV status live in fear of their disease (the worry that every cold or flu symptom is a potential sign of pending deterioration and death), and they live in fear of the loss of caregivers and other family members with HIV/AIDS. As a result, the psychiatric status, needs, and concerns of the child and adolescent with HIV infection is an essential part of their care, even with the advancements in HAART (89–91). Indeed, higher rates of mental health disorders would have multiple effects on: high risk sexual behavior (resulting in not only risk to another but also the risks of contracting resistant viral strains); less optimal compliance with drug treatment; lower school attendance, learning, and adaptive behavior with peers; and limited achievement of an adulthood with the personal competences of self-care. It must be considered also that these affective and behavioral associations with HIV/AIDS in children and adolescents may predict more severe conditions as the child grows up, including severe affective disorders and suicide risk.

Cognitive deficits may place youth at heightened risk of contracting HIV. Those diagnosed with mental retardation or borderline intellectual functioning may lack important skills related to judgment and logical decisionmaking that would allow them to conduct accurate appraisals of the risks associated with a range of behaviors, including those related to sexual activity and substance use. They may lack accurate information about prevention and routes of HIV transmission, which may lead to erroneous conclusions about HIV. Their judgments may mirror those of younger children, who may overgeneralize their risk to common and innocuous situations, such as touching and sharing household items.

Despite the decrease in severe progressive HIV encephalopathy for those with access to HAART, there is increasing awareness that neurodevelopmental and psychiatric effects of the disease are still present and are likely multiply determined. Behavioral health problems can contribute to risk behavior that results in HIV infection. HIV/AIDS can also be accompanied by behavioral health problems that are the results of multiple factors, including direct and indirect injury to the CNS, the toxic effects of extended use of specific ART and other drugs, as well as the multiple emotional and socioeconomic factors associated with living with HIV/AIDS.

Sexual Abuse and HIV Transmission

In some instances, HIV infection has been found to be a sequela of sexual abuse, with estimates of its extent ranging from 0.2% to 14.6% of HIV-positive samples (92, 93). Factors that put children at greater risk of HIV disease, such as substance abuse, social and economic marginalization, and dysfunctional lifestyles, are the same factors that put them at greater risk of sexual abuse. Some evidence indicates that the experience of sexual abuse in childhood may result in increased sexual risk taking and drug use in adolescence and adulthood, thus increasing a person's lifetime risk of HIV infection (94–96). Recommendations for HIV testing of children who are being evaluated for sexual abuse vary from testing all children undergoing evaluation to testing only those for whom information suggests an increased risk of exposure to HIV due to the specific nature of the sexual assault. Risk of transmission of HIV should be a particular consideration if a child is evaluated immediately after an incident of sexual abuse, because of the possibility of providing prophylactic antiretroviral medications to prevent transmission. Such postexposure prophylaxis has been shown to be beneficial in needle sticks and other types of occupational accidents (97), and it is now being used with children and adults who have been raped, sexually assaulted, or have put themselves at risk of sexual transmission (98).

STIGMA AND SECRECY

The guilt, shame, and anxiety of living with a family member whose illness may not be discussed or even revealed represents a notable challenge to the development of HIV-affected youth (99, 100). Although children may know of a parent's illness, they may not be provided with opportunities for identifying the illness and discussing its ramifications in order to organize their ideas, fears, and feelings (101). Should death occur in the absence of disclosure about the illness, children may be unable to metabolize their complex reactions and may be left to struggle with their poorly understood and painful memories and feelings. Ironically, even though many parents are reluctant to inform their children of their own HIV infection, some children become caregivers to sick parents and younger siblings without ever being able to name the illness that has debilitated their family members. In the presence of social disapprobation, many parents elect to keep their diagnosis secret from family, friends, and society as a whole. Self-imposed secrecy and reactions to social stigma may preclude families from procuring necessary treatment, seeking assistance with permanency planning for affected children, and obtaining needed forms of social support.

DISCLOSURE OF AN HIV/AIDS DIAGNOSIS

Despite emerging findings for the benefits of disclosure, many parents are unable to reveal an HIV diagnosis to an infected child. Disclosure forces parents to confront their personal responsibility and to acknowledge the negatively sanctioned behaviors related to substance abuse or sexual activity (102, 103). Unable to tolerate their own guilt, remorse, and psychological pain, parents may withdraw and may deny an illness that is evident to their children and loved ones (104). Other parents struggle with their knowledge of HIV but equate disclosure with harming their children and instead attempt to protect them from this painful knowledge, to preserve the mystique of childhood innocence. Lipson (103) suggested that this conscious fear that children cannot understand the ramifications of HIV masks a deeper fear that children will indeed grasp its fatal implications.

The issues of disclosure and permanency planning become still more important with the evolution of HIV/AIDS from an acute, fatal illness to a chronic condition that nevertheless portends a shortened life span (101). Studies have indicated that upwards of 75% of HIV-positive parents inform children of an HIV/AIDS diagnosis (105). Older children are more likely to be told of a personal or parental diagnosis, and infected parents tended to disclose more information as they became more symptomatic (106, 107).

From one perspective, disclosure may be viewed as occurring over the course of several stages (56, 58, 108, 109). At the outset, Tasker (109) identified a *secrecy phase* during which parents struggle with their own acceptance of the illness and their wish to deny its implications. Their unwillingness to reveal health status, their own or that of the infected child, may be influenced by the negative associations among HIV and AIDS, promiscuous sexual activity, and the use of illicit substances. Children whose parents are unable to move beyond this phase are left to cope with reactions to their overwhelming sense of loss, guilt, and abandonment in secrecy and isolation. Progressing toward an *exploratory phase*, parents demonstrate ambivalence about disclosing the diagnosis, although the need to guard against revelation diminishes over time. Parents engage in tentative attempts to name the disease through the use of euphemisms or report secondary illnesses associated with HIV/AIDS. Parents may enter a *readiness phase* in which they rehearse possible disclosure scenarios, either explicitly or in fantasy, with a trusted friend or professional helping to guide them through the process. Practicing the form, timing, and content of disclosure provides opportunities for parents to consider the possible reactions of their children and to identify strategies to assist their coping responses. The final, *disclosure phase*, occurs when children are told of an HIV/AIDS diagnosis. Disclosure provides the words to name a condition that is pervasive in its effects but has not been discussed openly. It allows menacing secrets to be replaced by knowledge, and it shifts the developmental tasks toward coping with a painful reality.

Although the American Academy of Pediatrics has recommended that HIV-infected children be informed of their diagnosis (110), there are few protocols to guide the clinician and family through the ambivalence and regret preceding the actual disclosure. Parents who disclose a diagnosis to their children report less personal depression, accompanied by observed improvements in children's behavior problems, self-competence, and receipt of social support (111, 112). Although disclosure of other life-threatening illnesses, such as cancer, appears to alleviate anxiety directly (113), the social stigma and isolation associated with HIV infection may cause some children to experience periods of heightened distress. Symptoms may abate as children are afforded continued opportunities for discussion and expression. Once additional stressors are accounted for, disclosure of an HIV diagnosis does not appear to result in further decrements in children's emotional or social functioning. Instead, disclosure may alleviate the burden of unspoken fears and may become a basis for further integration of painful knowledge and a foundation for permanency planning efforts.

With burgeoning rates of HIV infection among adolescents, disclosure will increasingly become a decision that will be made by youth as well as their adult caregivers (111). For example, a comparison of mother–child dyads in which the child had a positive HIV status found that children who had disclosed their diagnosis to similarly aged friends reported no decrements in their behavior or self-concept. Importantly, children who disclosed their status to their peers experienced a statistically significant increase in their immune response (CD4 percent) relative to their nondisclosing, HIV-positive peers, a difference that was apparent regardless of age or medication regimen (114).

PERMANENCY PLANNING

For many families, disclosure of HIV can be seen as preparation for the task of permanency planning for children who will be orphaned by the disease. Permanency planning attempts to sustain continuity in the face of illness and loss by increasing stability and psychological security for children as they experience parental death. Efforts involve assisting parents to identify a familiar and accepted surrogate caregiver willing to accept the legal responsibility of guardianship and able to offer children affective support, reassurance, and understanding during periods of acute illness and following death (30, 58, 115).

The interrelationship between disclosure and permanency planning was demonstrated in a study of 151 HIV-infected parents and their 171 adolescent children (105). Almost three-fourths of the teens in the study had been told of their parent's HIV diagnosis, and most were aware of plans for their future custody. Virtually all parents who made a permanency plan consulted the potential guardian, and almost all plans were agreed to by the chosen guardian. Legal custody arrangements were rare, however, occurring in less than one-fourth of cases, a statistic attesting to the difficulty parents experience in taking the final step toward the release of their custodial interest in their children. The high rates of permanency planning attempts are encouraging, because they indicate that many parents are able to address their children's needs in a planned and thoughtful manner. However, the relative lack of legally sanctioned custody arrangements raises concern. Without legal intervention, it is quite possible that the plan developed by the parent may be jeopardized by the trauma, stress, anger, frustration, and disorganization that frequently follow parental death.

The process of developing a workable plan that names adults who will serve as parental replacements and calls into view a future for children in which parents will not participate is long and painful. Many parents assume that a relative or older sibling will take custody of younger children, yet they may be unaware that without specific planning these assumptions can easily go awry. Although efforts can be made to identify a potential guardian earlier in the disease process, most frequently this work does not begin in earnest until the terminal stages of the disease. Many states now provide legal remedies designed to ease the strain on parents of making custodial decisions and to allow for a more flexible approach to guardianship. It is now possible for children to be cared for by a temporary or standby guardian who is responsible only when parents are too ill to fulfill their familial obligations. Guardianship reverts to parents as their acute symptoms remit and they are able to resume responsibility.

The caregivers selected by parents most frequently are members of the extended family who represent the most realistic option for supporting the psychological and physical development of affected children and providing continuity in the midst of loss (108). Although strenuous attempts may be made to place children who lose a parent to HIV/AIDS in the care of relatives or others known to them through their family's social networks, siblings remain together in fewer than 50% of these cases (116, 117). The separation from other siblings can be experienced as a replication of the loss of the parent, a situation that could be avoided with careful planning and a commitment to maintaining the integrity of sibling groups.

PREVENTIVE INTERVENTIONS

Efforts to address "life skills," which range from educational and vocational preparation to reduction in specific risk behaviors, appear promising and may be delivered across a range of settings, including schools, homes, and other contexts in which youth are present (2, 118, 119). Prevention curricula based on a psychoeducational and problem-solving approach to sexual and other risk behaviors have demonstrated a range of positive outcomes in school and community settings, including increased condom use during sexual intercourse, decreased high-risk (unprotected) sexual behavior, decreased sexual activity with multiple partners, increased age at time of first intercourse, and increased discussion of sexual practices between parents and children (120–123). Across studies, increased condom use represents the most consistent positive finding, while delayed age of first intercourse the least consistent, albeit positive, finding. HIV prevention program effectiveness has been consistently linked to a skills-based focus on reducing sexual risk behaviors, increased duration and number of sessions, and reliance on trained facilitators (119). The extent to which primary preventive approaches may generalize to high risk, psychiatrically impaired, or juvenile delinquent cohorts outside these mainstream settings remains untested (52, 124, 125), yet those at greatest risk of contracting HIV or AIDS tend to be these same adolescents whose isolation from traditional health and mental health treatment systems complicates their receptivity to primary and secondary prevention efforts.

EVIDENCE BASED MENTAL HEALTH INTERVENTIONS

Children who are infected and affected by HIV/AIDS present with a range of psychiatric disorders that warrant treatment. An increasingly strong empirical basis has emerged in support of disorder- and population-specific psychotherapeutic and pharmacologic interventions. Primarily cognitive-behavioral in orientation, efficacious models are available that target depression, attention deficit hyperactivity disorder, disruptive behavior disorders, and anxiety disorders, including posttraumatic stress disorder (126, 127). Recent efforts have addressed the transportability of efficacious interventions from research to community settings, emphasizing an effectiveness paradigm that integrates issues of treatment fidelity and clinical competence with those related to sustaining practice changes over time.

Rotheram-Borus and her colleagues (128–130) have compiled 6-year outcome data from a randomized controlled trial of a cognitive-behaviorally oriented coping intervention for HIV-affected adolescents. This 24-session intervention included modules related to a) cognitive and emotional coping with an HIV diagnosis, b) skills acquisition related to emotional distress, risk behaviors, and permanency planning, and c) postbereavement adjustment and transition to a new caregiver. At 2 years following CBT-based counseling, the adolescents experienced declines in symptoms of psychological distress, including depression, anxiety, and conduct problems. After 4 years, unwanted pregnancies were fewer in the treatment condition, as were stressful family events. By 6 years, problem and conduct behaviors increased in both conditions, albeit at a lesser rate in the treatment condition. Differences in symptomatology were no longer apparent at 6 years posttreatment; however, those who had received treatment were more likely to be employed or enrolled in school, to have better problem-solving skills, and to have positive future expectations. They were less likely to receive public welfare benefits.

Children infected with and affected by HIV/AIDS may be especially vulnerable to symptoms of posttraumatic stress disorder (PTSD) with its hallmark symptoms of persistent reexperiencing and recollection of traumatic events, avoidance of traumatic reminders, and physiological hyperarousal (131, 132). Studies in the United States have identified traumatic stress in children whose parents are terminally ill (133), and a host of adjustment difficulties in children with HIV+ parents (134). A U.S.-based study found that traumatic stress for orphans included their exposure to the "fact" of the impending death of their parent as well as their exposure to other family members who are experiencing fear and anxiety about the impending death (133). For many children it is likely that HIV/AIDS represents only one of many traumatic events that may include multiple caregiver and family losses; responsibility for a dying parent; residential, educational, and economic instability; abuse and adversity in the context of new living situations; and exposure to community and family violence (135, 136). As with other types of trauma, the adjustment of children to the sequelae of HIV/AIDS remains heavily influenced by premorbid functioning and the stability of subsequent caregiving relationships (137, 138).

The loss of a loved one, particularly a parent or other primary caregiver, under circumstances that are experienced as unexpected, shocking, or terrifying, may give rise to a constellation of symptoms and reactions described as childhood traumatic grief (CTG) (139, 140). For many HIV-affected youth, the death of a parent has been preceded by multiple disruptions of attachments because of the instability and relapses attributable to the progression of HIV/AIDS. The child may become preoccupied with the death and manifest pronounced behavioral and emotional symptoms that interfere with normative bereavement and effective coping with loss. The acuity of distress can preclude the child from processing cognitive and emotional reactions to the loss and result in an inability to recall even positive memories of the deceased. In addition to grief-specific symptoms, the child may exhibit symptoms of PTSD, depression, or disruptive behavior that further impair functioning.

Children whose PTSD is overlaid with the experience of traumatic grief and loss are unable to grieve normally and arrive at a conception of their loss as a painful, regrettable aspect of their life history. Instead, the death itself is continually reexperienced via intrusive thoughts, feelings, or images, or is warded off to the detriment of psychological and social functioning (140, 141). A child may experience both PTSD and CTG in terms of a significant impairment in their capacity to reminisce and cope with the loss of a loved one. Alternatively, a child may experience PTSD in the absence of impaired reminiscence of the deceased, or may be unable to complete a normative and expectable grieving process without meeting diagnostic criteria for PTSD. In contrast, uncomplicated bereavement, although a source of distress, represents a normative process that neither interferes with a child's capacity to sustain positive memories of the deceased nor impinges excessively on psychosocial functioning.

Rotheram-Borus et al. (134) compared bereaved adolescents following parental death due to HIV/AIDS to nonbereaved peers. Prior to death, the yet-to-be bereaved adolescents experienced higher levels of distress, adverse life experiences, and contact with the criminal justice system. In the acute aftermath of parental death, they experienced higher levels of depressive symptoms and passive problem-solving approaches relative to nonbereaved peers. At 1 year following parental death, the acute symptoms had dissipated, yet the same adolescents continued to engage in high risk sexual behaviors at a rate well beyond that of their peers.

Although not specific to situations involving HIV/AIDS, several researchers have integrated cognitive behavioral strategies for treating PTSD and CTG with a range of clinical settings and patient populations. In one approach, Layne et al. provided a group intervention in U.S. and Bosnian school settings following, respectively, exposure to a school shooting and wartime violence. Relative to controls, those who received the active treatment were 2, 1.5, and 4 times more likely to experience respective improvements in PTSD, depression, and grief (142–144).

Cohen, Mannarino, and Deblinger (145, 146) have adapted their well supported CBT intervention for sexually abused children experiencing posttraumatic stress to circumstances of traumatic grief (140, 141, 145). In a 16-week model, which has been delivered in individual and group settings to children who have experienced traumatic deaths due to illness and violence, children receive eight sessions of CBT focused on posttraumatic stress followed by an additional eight directed toward symptoms of CTG. Results indicate that children experienced significant decreases in symptoms of PTSD and traumatic grief, accompanied by improvements in adaptive functioning. Consistent with the sequencing of PTSD and grief focused sessions, PTSD symptomatology improved earlier during the course of treatment, followed by alleviation of traumatic grief symptoms.

In each of the models, early intervention sessions focused on trauma-related symptoms, and later sessions targeted specific symptoms of CTG. Sessions were focused on the traumatic experience itself, reminders of trauma and loss, stress and adversity, bereavement, and developmental impact. Through psychoeducation about loss and trauma, enhancement of coping skills, development of a narrative about the trauma or loss, and group process–oriented activities, children experienced reductions in posttraumatic stress, grief, and depressive symptoms. Those who experienced the greatest symptom relief also improved to the greatest extent in psychosocial functioning. Although primarily child focused in nature, both models involve remaining parents and caregivers in learning effective management of symptoms and behavior, and supporting children during the course of their treatment.

COMMUNITY BASED MENTAL HEALTH INTERVENTIONS

In contrast to the diagnosis based perspective, research on community interventions has taken a broader perspective that incorporates system of care tenets and recognizes the complex comorbidities among child psychiatric patients. Traditional modalities of office and clinic based care may be ill suited to families struggling with HIV/AIDS, who must contend with multiple medical appointments and complex treatment regimens within a sometimes disorganized and overstressed family environment (147, 148). In light of obstacles to traditional service use, home and community based approaches to the mental health care of children and families offer promising alternatives that may increase treatment engagement, service utilization, and clinical outcome (56, 58, 149). Clinical services, including their duration, intensity, and location, should be distinguished by their comprehensive and flexible nature, and designed to care for children in biological, extended, and foster care families. Specific intervention components may be directed toward medical compliance, family and psychiatric stabilization, and permanency planning. Modalities may include home and community based psychological assessment, psychotherapy, psychiatric consultation and medication management, clinically informed case management, support groups, family stabilization, 24-hour emergency consultation, formal collaboration with pediatric AIDS providers, and consultation with a range of social service systems. In addition to approaches designed specifically for families and children contending with HIV/AIDS, other home based interventions may be utilized, based on consideration of presenting problems or risk factors (149), including home visitation for high risk infants and young children (150), multisystemic therapy for delinquent and psychiatrically disturbed youth (151), and community based posttraumatic stress interventions (152).

CONCLUSIONS

With advances in medical treatments, particularly HAART, HIV/AIDS has been transformed from an acute illness with a vastly foreshortened life span to a condition with many characteristics of a serious chronic illness. These hard-won gains have improved the quality of life for many infected persons, yet for others throughout the world, HIV infection continues to proliferate at truly epidemic proportions. Within the United States, perinatally acquired HIV has diminished from approximately 25% to less than 5% of births to HIV-infected women. Like the virus itself, the demographics of HIV/AIDS have mutated and evolved. Most new HIV infections appear among adolescents and young adults, with women of childbearing age and minority communities experiencing a disproportionate share of new diagnoses. Although fewer American infants and children are newly infected, increasing numbers are affected by the illness of parents, caregiving adults, and family members. These youth are themselves at increased risk of becoming infected because of their own risk-taking behaviors.

A coordinated national and international effort towards the prevention of new HIV infections and the provision of appropriate care to those who are already infected is required. The availability of effective treatment for HIV/AIDS does not, at present, portend a cure. Given the myriad psychosocial stressors encountered by HIV-infected and affected children and youth, comprehensive and effective medical and mental health services remain crucial. Mental health providers should draw upon the large array of evidence based treatment models for those conditions that are prevalent among infected and affected children, including depression, posttraumatic stress, and externalizing behaviors. Access to care must be extended to children, adolescents, and families who have traditionally existed at the margins of the health care delivery system. To be maximally effective, psychiatric treatment must address children's wellbeing through a comprehensive strategy that addresses the medical and mental health needs of individual children, supports family functioning, addresses permanency planning for infected and affected youth, and coordinates care among psychiatric, medical, and social service providers, offers the most likely pathway to the stability, safety, and wellbeing that is essential for each child's growth and development.

References

1. Conner EM, Sperling RS, Gelber R, et al.: Reduction of maternal–infant transmission of human immunodeficiency virus type 1 with zidovudine treatment. Pediatric AIDS clinical trials group protocol 076 study group. *New England Journal of Medicine* 331:1173–1180, 1994.
2. Joint United Nations Programme on HIV/AIDS: *A Call to Action: Children, the Missing Face of AIDS*. New York, United Nations Children's Fund, 2005.
3. Newell ML, Brahmbhatt H, Ghys PD: Child mortality and HIV infection in Africa: A review. *AIDS* 18(2):S27–S34, 2004.
4. Dehne KL, Pokrovskiy V, Kobyschcha Y, Schwartlander B: Update on the epidemics of HIV and other sexually transmitted infections in the newly independent states of the former Soviet Union. *AIDS* 14(3):S75–S84, 2000.
5. Centers for Disease Control and Prevention. HIV/AIDS surveillance report, 2003. Accessed November 4, 2005.
6. Brady MT: Pediatric human immunodeficiency virus-1 infection (review). *Advances in Pediatrics* 52:163–193, 2005.
7. Centers for Disease Control and Prevention: *Young People at Risk: HIV/AIDS among America's Youth*. Washington, DC, 1999.
8. Reif SS, Lowe K, Whetten K: HIV and AIDS in the Deep South. *American Journal of Public Health* 26(6):970–973, 2006.
9. Centers for Disease Control and Prevention. *HIV/AIDS Surveillance Report: HIV Infection and AIDS in the United States*. Atlanta: U.S. Department of Health and Human Services, Centers for Disease Control and Prevention; 2003.
10. Lallemant M, Jourdain G, Le Couer S, et al.: Single dose perinatal nevirapine plus standard zidovudine to prevent mother-to-child transmission of HIV-I in Thailand. *New England Journal of Medicine* 351(3):217–228, 2004.
11. Cooper ER, Charurat M, Burns DN, Blattner W, Hoff R: Trends in antiretroviral therapy and mother–infant transmission of HIV. The woman and infants transmission study group. *Journal of Acquired Immune Deficiency Syndrome* 24:45–47, 2000.
12. Edwards SG, Larbalestier N, Hay P, et al.: Experience of nevirapine use in a London cohort of HIV-infected pregnant women. *HIV Medicine* 2(2):89–91, 2001.
13. European Mode of Delivery Collaboration. Elective caesarean section versus vaginal delivery in prevention of vertical transmission: A randomized clinical trial. *Lancet* 353:1035–1039, 1999.
14. International Perinatal HIV Group. The mode of delivery and the risk of vertical transmission of human immunodeficiency virus type I. *New England Journal of Medicine* 340:977–987, 1999.
15. De Cock KM, Fowler MG, Mercier E, et al.: Prevention of mother-to-child HIV transmission in resource-poor countries. *Journal of the American Medical Association* 283:1175–1182, 2000.
16. Rouet F, Elenga N, Msellati P, et al.: Primary HIV-1 infection in African children infected through breastfeeding. *AIDS* 16:2303–2309, 2002.

17. Saba J. The results of the PETRA intervention trial to prevent perinatal transmission in sub-Saharan Africa. Paper presented at: Sixth Conference on Retroviruses and Opportunistic Infections, 1999, Chicago.
18. Shaffer NH, McConnell M, Bolu O, et al.: Prevention of mother-to-child HIV transmission internationally. *Emerging Infectious Diseases* 10:2027–2028, 2004.
19. Magoni M, Bassani L, Okong P, et al.: Mode of infant feeding and HIV infection in children in a program for prevention of mother-to-child transmission in Uganda. *AIDS* 19:433–437, 2005.
20. United Nations Children's Fund: *HIV and Infant Feeding*. New York, United Nations Children's Fund HIV/AIDS Unit, 2002.
21. Kuhn L, Stein Z: Infant survival, HIV infection and feeding alternatives in less-developed countries. *American Journal of Public Health* 87:926–931, 1997.
22. Ross JS, Labbok MH: Modeling the effects of different infant feeding strategies on infant survival and mother-to-child transmission of HIV. *American Journal of Public Health* 94:1174–1180, 2004.
23. Joint United Nations Programme on HIV/AIDS, World Health Organization. Progress on global access to HIV antiretroviral therapy: An update on "3×5": UNAIDS/WHO; 2005.
24. Cartoux M, Meda N, Van de Perre P, Newell ML, de Vincenzi I, Dabis F: Acceptability of voluntary HIV testing by pregnant women in developing countries: An international survey. Ghent international working group on mother-to-child transmission of HIV. *AIDS* 12(18):2489–2493, 1998.
25. Sengendo J, Nambi J: The psychological effects of orphanhood: A study of orphans in Rakai district. *Health Transition Review* 7(Suppl):105–124, 1997.
26. Makame V, Ani C, Grantham-McGregor S: Psychological well-being of orphans in Dar El Salaam, Tanzania. *Acta Paediatrica* 91(4):459–465, 2002.
27. Bachanas PJ, Morris MK, Lewis-Gess JK, et al.: Psychological adjustment, substance use, HIV knowledge, and risky sexual behavior in at-risk minority females: Developmental differences during adolescence. *Journal of Pediatric Psychology* 27(4):373–384, 2002.
28. Bor R, du Plessis PH: The impact of HIV/AIDS on families: An overview of recent research. *Families, Systems, and Health* 15:413–427, 1997.
29. Pilowsky DJ, Wissow L, Hutton NH: Children affected by HIV: Clinical experience and research findings. *Psychiatric Clinics of North America* 9:451–464, 2000.
30. Joint United Nations Programme on HIV/AIDS: *Children on the Brink 2002: A Joint Report on Orphan Estimates and Program Strategies*. Washington, DC, U.S. Agency for International Development, 2002.
31. Centers for Disease Control and Prevention: *Enhanced Perinatal Surveillance—United States, 1999–2001*. Atlanta, U.S. Department of Health and Human Services, Centers for Disease Control and Prevention, 2004.
32. Joint United Nations Programme on HIV/AIDS: *Report on the Global HIV/AIDS Epidemic: June 2000*. Geneva, United Nations, 2000.
33. Chabon B, Futterman D: Adolescents and HIV. *AIDS Clinical Care* 11:9–15, 1999.
34. Morris A, Lundgren JD, Masur H, et al.: Current epidemiology of pneumocystic pneumonia. *Emerging Infectious Diseases* 10:1713–1720, 2004.
35. Forsyth BWCH: The AIDS epidemic: Past and future. *Psychiatric Clinics of North America* 9:267–278, 2000.
36. McKinney REJ, Johnson GM, Stanley K, et al.: A randomized study of combined zidovudine-lamivudine versus didanosine monotherapy in children with symptomatic therapy-naïve HIV-1 infection. The pediatric AIDS clinical trials group protocol 300 study team. *Journal of Pediatrics* 133:500–508, 1998.
37. Miller TL, Mawn BE, Orav EJ, et al.: The effect of protease inhibitor therapy on growth and body composition in human immunodeficiency virus type 1–infected children. *Pediatrics* 107:E77, 2001.
38. Oleske J, Minnefor A, Cooper RJ, et al.: Immune deficiency syndrome in children. *Journal of the American Medical Association* 249:2345–2349, 1983.
39. Belman AL: Acquired immune deficiency syndrome and the child's central nervous system. *Pediatric Clinics of North America* 39:691–714, 1992.
40. Epstein LG, Sherer LR, Oleske JM: Neurological manifestations of human immunodeficiency virus infection in children. *Pediatrics* 78:678–687, 1986.
41. Blanche S, Rouzioux C, Moscato LM, et al.: A prospective study of infants born to women seropositive for human immunodeficiency virus type 1. *New England Journal of Medicine* 320:1643–1648, 1989.
42. Lobato LM, Caldwell B, Ng P, Oxtoby MJ: The pediatric spectrum of disease clinical consortium: Encephalopathy in children with perinatally acquired human immunodeficiency virus infection. *Journal of Pediatrics* 126:710–715, 1995.
43. Msellati P, Lepage P, Hitimana D, Van Goethem C, Van de Perre P, Dabis F: Neurodevelopment testing of children born to human in immunodeficiency virus type 1 seropositive and seronegative mothers: A prospective cohort study in Kigali, Rwanda. *Pediatrics* 92:843–848, 1993.
44. Exhenry C, Nadal D: Vertical human immunodeficiency virus-1 infection: Involvement of the central nervous system and treatment. *European Journal of Pediatrics* 155:839–850, 1996.
45. Perelson AS, Neumann A, Markowitz M: HIV-1 dynamics in vivo: Virion clearance rate, infected cell life span, and viral generation time. *Science* 271:1582–1586, 1996.
46. Saag MS, Holodny M, Kuritzkes DR: HIV viral load markers in clinical practice. *National Medicine* 2:625–629, 1996.
47. Krogstad P, Wiznia A, Luzuriaga K, et al.: Treatment of human immunodeficiency virus-1 infected infants and children with the protease inhibitor nelfinavir mesylate. *Clinical Infectious Diseases* 28:1109–1118, 1999.
48. Soh CH, Oleske JM, Brady MT, et al.: Long-term effects of protease-inhibitor-based combination of CD4 T-cell recovery in HIV-1 infected children and adolescents. *Lancet* 362:1522–1528, 2003.
49. Kauffman D, Pantaleo G, Sudre P: CD4-cell count in HIV-1-infected individuals remaining viremic with highly active antiretroviral therapy (HAART). *Lancet*:723–724, 1998.
50. Mascke M, Kastrup O, Esser S: Incidence and prevalence of neurological disorders associated with HIV since the introduction of highly active antiretroviral therapy (HAART). *Journal of Neurology, Neurosurgery, and Psychiatry* 69:376–380, 2000.
51. Carr A, Samaras K: Diagnosis, prediction and natural course of HIV-1 protease-inhibitor-associated lipodystophy, hyperlipidemia, and diabetes mellitus: A cohort study. *Lancet* 353:2093–2099, 1999.
52. Schonfeld DJ: Teaching young children about HIV and AIDS. *Child and Adolescent Psychiatric Clinics of North America* 9:375–387, 2001.
53. Walsh ME, Bibace RH: Children's conceptions of AIDS: A developmental analysis. *Journal of Pediatric Psychology* 16:273–285, 1991.
54. Holditch-Davis H, Miles M, Burchinal M, O'Donnell K, McKinney R, Lim W: Parental caregiving and development caregiving of infants of mothers with HIV. *Nursing Research*. 50:5–14, 2001.
55. Family Health Project Research Group H: The family health project: A multidisciplinary longitudinal investigation of children whose mothers are HIV infected. *Clinical Psychology Review* 18:839–856, 1998.
56. Gossart-Walker S, Murphy RA: Children and HIV: A model of home-based mental health treatment. In: Lightburn A, Sessions P (eds): *Handbook of Community-Based Clinical Practice*. New York, Oxford University Press, 2006, pp. 285–301.
57. Ickovics JR, Druley JA, Morrill AC, Grigorenko E, Rodin JH: "A grief observed": The experience of HIV-related illness and death among women in a clinic-based sample in New Haven, Connecticut. *Journal of Consulting and Clinical Psychology* 66:958–966, 1998.
58. Murphy RA. Life care planning for the child with HIV/AIDS. In: Riddick-Grisham S (ed): *Pediatric life care Planning and case Management*. Boca Raton, FL, CRC Press, 2004, pp. 609–625.
59. Gewirtz A, Gossart-Walker SH: Home-based treatment for children and families affected by HIV/AIDS: Dealing with stigma, secrecy, disclosure, and loss. *Psychiatric Clinics of North America* 9:313–330, 2000.
60. Maman S, Campbell J, Sweat MD, Gielen ACH: The intersections of HIV and violence: Directions for future research and interventions. *Social Science and Medicine*. 50:459–478, 2000.
61. Wright W, Draimin BH: Providing clinical opportunities for youths affected by HIV. *Psychiatric Clinics of North America* 9:347–358, 2000.
62. Pelton J, Forehand R: Orphans of the AIDS epidemic: An examination of clinical level problems of children. *Journal of the American Academy of Child and Adolescent Psychiatry* 44:585–591, 2005.
63. Lee MB, Lester P, Rotheram-Borus MJ: The relationship between adjustment of mothers with HIV and their adolescent daughters. *Clinical Child Psychology & Psychiatry* 7(1):71–84, 2002.
64. Dorsey S, Forehand R, Armistead L, Morse E, Morse P, Stock M: Mother knows best? Mother and child report of behavioral difficulties of children of HIV-infected mothers. *Journal of Psychopathology and Behavior Assessment* 21:191–206, 1999.
65. Gossart-Walker S, Moss NEH: Groups: An effective strategy for intervention. *Psychiatric Clinics of North America* 9:331–346, 2000.
66. Rotheram-Borus MJ, Robin L, Reid HM, Draimin BHH: Parent–adolescent conflict and stress when parents are living with AIDS. *Family Process* 37:83–94, 1998.
67. Zayas LH, Romano K: Adolescents and parental death from AIDS. In: Dane BO, Levine C (eds): *AIDS and the New Orphans*. Westport, CT, Auburn House, 1994.
68. Donenberg GR, Pao M: Youth and HIV/AIDS: Psychiatry's role in a changing epidemic. *Journal of the American Academy of Child and Adolescent Psychiatry* 44:728–747, 2005.
69. Ruland CD, Finger W, Williamson N, et al.: *Adolescents: Orphaned and vulnerable in the time of HIV/AIDS*. Arlington, VA, Family Health International, 2005.
70. Anderson MM, Morris REH: HIV and adolescents. *Pediatric Annals*. 22:436–446, 1993.
71. Blos P. *On Adolescence*. New York, Free Press, 1962.
72. Brown LK, Danovsky MB, Lourie KJ, DiClemente RJ, Ponton LEH: Adolescents with psychiatric disorders and the risk of HIV. *Journal of the American Academy of Child and Adolescent Psychiatry* 36:1609–1617, 1997.
73. Hein K, Dell R, Futterman D, Rotheram-Borus MJ, Shaffer NH: Comparison of HIV+ and HIV− adolescents: Risk factors and psychosocial determinants. *Pediatrics* 95:96–104, 1995.
74. Slonim-Nevo V, Auslander WF, Ozawa MN: Education options and AIDS-related behaviors among troubled adolescents. *Journal of Pediatric Psychology* 20:41–60, 1995.
75. Hammett TM, Gaiter JL, Crawford C: Reaching seriously at-risk populations: Health interventions in criminal justice settings. *Health Education and Behavior* 25:99–120, 1998.

76. Kalichman SCH: HIV transmission risk behaviors of men and women living with HIV-AIDS: Prevalence, predictors, and emerging clinical interventions. *Clinical Psychology: Science and Practice* 7:32–47, 2000.
77. Sherbourne CD, Hays RD, Fleishman JA, et al.: Impact of psychiatric conditions on health-related quality of life in persons with HIV infection. *American Journal of Psychiatry* 157:248–254, 2000.
78. Booth RE, Zhang Y, Kwiatkowski CFH: The challenge of changing drug and sex risk behaviors of runaway and homeless adolescents. *Child Abuse & Neglect* 23:1295–1306, 1999.
79. Booth RE, Zhang YH: Conduct disorder and HIV risk behaviors among runaway and homeless adolescents. *Drug and Alcohol Dependence* 48:69–76, 1997.
80. Donenberg GR, Emerson E, Bryant FB, Wilson H, Weber-Shifrin E: Understanding AIDS-risk behavior among adolescents in psychiatric care: Links to psychopathology and peer relationships. *Journal of the American Academy of Child & Adolescent Psychiatry* 40:642–653, 2001.
81. Brown LK, Lescano CM, Lourie KJ: Children and adolescents with HIV infection. *Psychiatric Annals* 31(1):63–68, 2001.
82. Cooper ML, Wood PK, Orcutt HK, Albino A: Personality and predisposition to engage in risk or problem behaviors during adolescence. *Journal of Personality and Social Psychology* 84:390–410, 2003.
83. Gaughan DM, Hugher MD, Oleske JM, Malee K, Gore CA: Psychiatric hospitalization among children and youths with human immunodeficiency virus infection. *Pediatrics* 113:e544–e551, 2004.
84. Hein K, Dell R, Futterman D, Rotheram-Bonus MJ, Shaffer N: Comparison of HIV+ and HIV− adolescents: Risk factors and psychosocial determinants. *Pediatrics* 95:96–104, 2000.
85. Lester P, Chesney M, Cooke M, et al.: Diagnostic disclosure to HIV-infected children: How parents decide when and what to tell. *Clinical Child Psychology & Psychiatry* 7(1):85–99, 2002.
86. Mellins CA, Smith R, O'Driscoll P, et al.: NIH/NIAID/NICHD/NIDA-sponsored women and infant transmission study group: High rates of behavioral problems in perinatally HIV-infected children are not linked to HIV disease. *Pediatrics* 111:384–393, 2003.
87. Reiter-Purtill J, A. GC, Vannatta K, Passo MH, Noll RB: A controlled longitudinal study of the social functioning of children with juvenile rheumatoid arthritis. *Journal of Pediatric Psychology* 28:17–28, 2003.
88. Weiland SK, Pless IB, Roghmann KJ: Chronic illness and mental health problems in pediatric practice: Results from a survey of primary care providers. *Pediatrics.* 89:445–449, 1992.
89. Colebunders R, Verdonck K: Reply to Gonzalez and Everall: Lest we forget: Neuropsychiatry and the new generation of anti-HIV drugs. *AIDS* 13:869, 1991.
90. DeLuca A, Ciancio BC, Larussa D, et al.: Correlates of independent HIV-1 replication in the CNS and of its control by antiretrovirals. *Neurology* 59:342–347, 2002.
91. Leserman J: The effects of depression, stressful life events, social support, and coping on the progression of HIV infection. *Current Psychiatry Reports* 2:495–502, 2000.
92. Gutman LT, Herman-Giddens ME, McKinney RE: Pediatric acquired immunodeficiency syndrome: Barriers to recognizing the role of child sexual abuse. *American Journal of the Disabled Child* 147:775–780, 1993.
93. Lindegren ML, Hanson IC, Hammett TA, Beil J, Fleming PL, Ward JW: Sexual abuse of children: Intersection with the HIV epidemic. *Pediatrics* 102:E46, 1998.
94. Allers CT, Benjack KL, White J, Rousey JT: HIV vulnerability and the adult survivor of childhood sexual abuse. *Child Abuse & Neglect* 17:291–298, 1993.
95. Gellert GA, Berkowitz CD, Durfee MJ: Testing the sexually abused child for HIV: Reducing uncertainty in clinical decisionmaking. *Journal of Child Sexual Abuse* 2:83–93, 1992.
96. Johnsen LW, Harlow LL: Childhood sexual abuse linked with adult substance use, victimization, and AIDS risk. *AIDS Education & Prevention* 8:44–57, 1996.
97. Henderson DK: Postexposure chemoprophylaxis for occupational exposures to the human immunodeficiency virus. *Journal of the American Medical Association* 281:931–936, 1999.
98. Centers for Disease Control and Prevention. Sexually transmitted diseases treatment guidelines. *Morbidity and Mortality Weekly Report* 51:1–80, 2002.
99. Hamra M, Karuri K, Orrs M, D'Agostino A: The relationship between expressed HIV/AIDS-related stigma and beliefs and knowledge about care and support of people living with AIDS in families caring for HIV-infected children in Kenya. *AIDS Care* 17:911–922, 2005.
100. Nagler SF, Adnopoz J, Forsyth BWCH: Uncertainty, stigma, and secrecy: Psychological aspects of AIDS for children and adolescents. In: Geballe S, Gruendel J, Andiman W (eds): *Forgotten Children of the AIDS Epidemic.* New Haven, Yale University Press, 71–82, 1995.
101. Murphy RA: Disclosure: The challenges and benefits for children affected by HIV. *The Source* 10:23–25, 30, 2000.
102. Lipson MH: Disclosure of diagnosis to children with human immunodeficiency virus or acquired immunodeficiency syndrome. *Developmental and Behavioral Pediatrics* 15:S61–S65, 1994.
103. Lipson MH: What do you say to a child with AIDS? *Hastings Center Report* 23:6–12, 1993.
104. Faithfull JH: HIV-positive and AIDS-infected women: Challenges and difficulties of mothering. *American Journal of Orthopsychiatry* 67:144–151, 1997.
105. Rotheram-Borus MJ, Draimin BH, Reid HM, Murphy DAH: The impact of illness disclosure and custody plans on adolescents whose parents live with AIDS. *AIDS* 11:1159–1164, 1997.
106. Armistead L, Tannenbaum L, Forehand R, Morse E, Morse PH: Disclosing HIV status: Are mothers telling their children? *Journal of Pediatric Psychology* 26:11–20, 2001.
107. Ledlie SWH: Diagnosis disclosure by family caregivers to children who have perinatally acquired HIV disease: When the time comes. *Nursing Research* 48:141–149, 1999.
108. Adnopoz JH: Relative caregiving: An option for permanency. *Psychiatric Clinics of North America* 9:359–374, 2000.
109. Tasker MH: *How can I tell you? Secrecy and Disclosure with Children when a Family Member has AIDS.* Bethesda, MD, Institute for Family-Centered Care, 1995.
110. American Academy of Pediatrics: Disclosure of illness status to children and adolescents with HIV infection. *Pediatrics* 103:164–166, 1999.
111. Battles HB, Wiener LS: From adolescence through young adulthood: Psychosocial adjustment associated with long-term survival of HIV. *Journal of Adolescent Health* 30(3):161–168, 2002.
112. Wiener LS, Battles HB, Heilman NEH: Factors associated with parents' decision to disclose their HIV diagnosis to their children. *Child Welfare* 77:115–135, 1998.
113. Reeve J, Kline WHH: Pediatric/adolescent AIDS: From disclosure to dialogue in psychotherapy. *Psychotherapy* 32:180–183, 1995.
114. Sherman BF, Bonanno GA, Wiener L, Battles HBH: When children tell their friends they have AIDS: Possible consequences for psychological well-being and disease progression. *Psychosomatic Medicine* 62:238–247, 2000.
115. Ryder RW, Munkolenkole K, Nkusu M, Batter V: AIDS orphans in Kinshasa, Zaire: Incidence and socioeconomic consequences. *AIDS* 8:673–679, 1994.
116. Draimin BH: A second family? Custody and placement decisions. In: Geballe S, Gruendel J, Andiman W (eds): *Forgotten Children of the AIDS Epidemic.* New Haven: Yale University Press; pp. 125–139, 1995.
117. Draimin BH, Gamble I, Shire A, Hudis JH: Improving permanency planning in families with HIV disease. *Child Welfare* 77:180–194, 1998.
118. Magnani R, MacIntyre K, Karim AM, Brown L, Hutchinson P: The impact of life skills education on adolescent sexual risk behaviors in KwaZulu-Natal, South Africa. *Journal of Adolescent Health* 36:289–304, 2005.
119. Robin L, Dittus P, Whitaker D, et al.: Behavioral interventions to reduce incidence of HIV, STD, and pregnancy among adolescents: A decade in review. *Journal of Adolescent Health* 34:3–26, 2004.
120. Jemmott JB, Jemmott LS, Fong GTH: Reductions in HIV risk-associated sexual behaviors among black male adolescents: Effects of an AIDS prevention intervention. *American Journal of Public Health* 82:372–377, 1992.
121. Lefkowitz ES, Sigman M, Au TKH: Helping mothers discuss sexuality and AIDS with adolescents. *Child Development* 71:1383–1394, 2000.
122. Main DS, Iverson DC, McGloin J, et al.: Preventing HIV infection among adolescents: Evaluation of a school-based education program. *Preventive Medicine* 23:409–417, 1994.
123. St. Lawrence JS, Brasfield TL, Jefferson KW, Alleyne E, O'Bannon RE, Shirley AH: Cognitive-behavioral intervention to reduce African-American adolescents' risk for HIV infection. *Journal of Consulting and Clinical Psychology* 63:221–227, 1995.
124. McKay MM, Chasse KT, Paikoff R, et al.: Family-level impact of the CHAMP family program: A community collaborative effort to support urban families and reduce youth HIV risk exposure. *Family Process* 43:79–93, 2004.
125. Schoeberlein DR, Woolston JL, Brett JH: School-based HIV prevention: A promising model. *Psychiatric Clinics of North America* 9:389–406, 2000.
126. Burns BJ: Children and evidence-based practice. *Psychiatric Clinics of North America* 26:955–970, 2003.
127. McClellan JM, Werry JS: Evidence-based treatments in child and adolescent psychiatry: An inventory. *Journal of the American Academy of Child & Adolescent Psychiatry* 42:1388–1400, 2003.
128. Rotheram-Borus MJ, Lee M, Leonard N, et al.: Four-year behavioral outcomes of an intervention for parents living with HIV and their adolescent children. *AIDS* 17:1217–1225, 2003.
129. Rotheram-Borus MJ, Lee M, Lin YY, Lester P: Six-year intervention outcomes for adolescent children of parents with the human immunodeficiency virus. *Archives of Pediatric and Adolescent Medicine* 158:742–748, 2004.
130. Rotheram-Borus MJ, Lee MB, Gwadz M, Draimin B: An intervention for parents with AIDS and their adolescent children. *American Journal of Public Health* 91(8):1294–1302, 2001.
131. American Psychiatric Association: *Diagnostic and Statistical Manual of Mental Disorders*, 4th ed. Washington, DC, American Psychiatric Association, 1994.
132. Pynoos RS, Steinberg AM, Piacentini JC: A developmental psychopathology model of childhood traumatic stress and intersection with anxiety disorders. *Biological Psychiatry* 46:1542–1554, 1999.
133. Saldinger AKP, Cain AC: Meeting the needs of parentally bereaved children: A framework for child-centered parenting. *Psychiatry* 67:331–352, 2004.

134. Rotheram-Borus MJ, Weiss R, Alber S, Lester P: Adolescent adjustment before and after HIV-related parental death. *Journal of Consulting and Clinical Psychology* 73:221–228, 2005.
135. Atwine B, Cantor-Graae E, Bajunirwe F: Psychological distress among AIDS orphans in rural Uganda. *Social Science & Medicine* 61:555–564, 2005.
136. Foster G, Makufa C, Drew R, Mashumba S, Kambeu S: Perceptions of children and community members concerning the circumstances of orphans in rural Zimbabwe. *AIDS Care* 9:391–405, 1997.
137. Pine DS, Cohen JA: Trauma in children and adolescents: Risk and treatment of psychiatric sequelae. *Biological Psychiatry* 51:519–531, 2002.
138. Forehand R, Pelton J, Chance M, et al.: Orphans of the AIDS epidemic in the United States: Transition-related characteristics and psychosocial adjustment at 6 months after mother's death. *AIDS Care* 11:715–722, 1999.
139. Cohen JA, Mannarino AP, Greenberg T, Padlo S, Shipley C: Childhood traumatic grief: Concepts and controversies. *Trauma, Violence, & Abuse* 3:307–327, 2002.
140. Cohen JA, Mannarino AR, Knudsen K: Treating childhood traumatic grief: A pilot study. *Journal of the American Academy of Child and Adolescent Psychiatry* 43:1225–1233, 2004.
141. Cohen JA, Berliner L, Mannarino AP: Treating traumatized children: A research review and synthesis. *Trauma, Violence, & Abuse* 1:29–46, 2000.
142. Layne CM, Davies R, Burlingame GM, Saltzman WR, Thomas N, Pynoos RS: *Technical Report: Evaluation of the UNICEF School-Based Psychosocial Program for War-Exposed Adolescents as Implemented During the 2000–2001 School Year*. Provo, UT, Brigham Young University, 2002.
143. Layne CM, Pynoos RS, Saltzman WS, et al.: Trauma/grief focused group psychotherapy: School-based post-war intervention with traumatized Bosnian adolescents. *Group Dynamics Theory, Research and Practice* 5:277–290, 2001.
144. Saltzman WR, Pynoos RS, Layne CM, Steinberg AM, Aisenberg E: Trauma/grief-focused intervention for adolescents exposed to community violence: Results of a school-based screening and group treatment protocol. *Group Dynamics Theory, Research and Practice* 5:291–303, 2001.
145. Cohen JA, Deblinger E, Mannarino AP, Steer RA: A multisite, randomized controlled trial for children with sexual abuse–related PTSD symptoms. *Journal of the American Academy of Child & Adolescent Psychiatry* 43:393–402, 2004.
146. Hensler D, Wilson C, Sadler BL: *Closing the Quality Chasm in Child Abuse Treatment: Identifying and Disseminating Best Practices. The Findings of the Kauffman Best Practices Project to Help Children Heal from Child Abuse*. Kansas City, MO, Ewing Marion Kauffman Foundation, 2004.
147. Murphy RA, Forsyth BWC, Adnopoz J: Neurobiological and psychosocial sequelae of HIV disease in children and adolescents. In: Lewis M (ed): *Comprehensive Textbook of Child and Adolescent Psychiatry*. Baltimore, Williams & Wilkins, 2002.
148. O'Hare BAM, Venables J, Naluberg JF, Makakeeto M, Kibirige M, Sothall DP: Home-based care for orphaned children infected with HIV/AIDS in Uganda. *AIDS Care* 17:443–450, 2005.
149. Adnopoz J. Working with high-risk children and families in their own homes: An integrative approach to the treatment of vulnerable children. In: Lightburn A, Sessions P (eds): *Handbook of Community-Based Clinical Practice*. New York: Oxford University Press, 2006, pp. 364–378.
150. Eckenrode J, Zielinski D, Smith E, et al.: Child maltreatment and the early onset of problem behaviors: Can a program of nurse home visitation break the link? *Development and Psychopathology* 13:873–890, 2001.
151. Curtis NM, Ronan KR, Borduin CM: Multisystemic treatment: A meta-analysis of outcome studies. *Journal of Family Psychology* 18(411–419), 2004.
152. Saxe GN, Ellis BH, Fogler J, Hansen S, Sorkin B: Comprehensive care for traumatized children. *Psychiatric Annals* 35:443–448, 2005.

CHAPTER 7.1.3.4 ■ EPILEPSY

GUATAMI RAO, YANN B. PONCIN, AND JOSEPH GONZÁLEZ-HEYDRICH

Epilepsy, or recurrent seizures, is one of the more prevalent chronic disorders affecting children. Studies have consistently found that children and adolescents with epilepsy are at greater risk for psychiatric illness when compared to children with other chronic illnesses. Psychiatric disorders are often undiagnosed and poorly managed in these children, despite parent perceptions that the emotional problems are among the more burdensome parts of the illness (1, 2). The arrows of directionality go the other way as well: Children with ADHD and adults with major depressive disorder (MDD) are at increased risk for developing epilepsy (3, 4). Moreover, some psychiatric medications can worsen seizures, while certain anticonvulsants are useful as treatments for psychiatric disorders. Thus, the study of the pathophysiology of epilepsy may shed light on that of the psychiatric disorders with which it is associated, and vice versa. Child psychiatrists have important contributions to make to the recognition, treatment, and research into the psychiatric repercussions of epilepsy in children. This chapter will provide an overview of epilepsy, its epidemiology, management, and prognosis. Finally, it will also focus on psychiatric disorders associated with epilepsy and offer guiding principles for psychopharmacologic management.

DEFINITIONS

A seizure results from a disturbance in the brain's electrical system in the form of an abnormal, hypersynchronous firing of cortical neurons. Its manifestations may be behavioral or sensory and these may be obvious or subtle. An individual seizure may have a variety of causes, such as fever in a young child, hypoxia, or infection. Recurrent seizures in the absence of provoking stimuli, such as active infection or fever, are known as epilepsy (5). Nonepileptic seizures, under which psychogenic seizures are classified, may appear similar to epileptic seizures but are not caused by electrical disruptions in the brain. The time leading up to a seizure, the seizure itself, and the time immediately after a seizure are respectively referred to as the preictal, ictal and postictal periods. The time in between seizures is called the interictal period. While seizures are the defining and most dramatic manifestation of epilepsy, they are episodic, whereas the brain dysfunction underlying them continues during the interictal periods, as can the associated psychosocial impact. Thus seizures themselves are rarely what is most impairing for children with epilepsy (Table 7.1.3.4.1).

TABLE 7.1.3.4.1

COMMON CAUSES OF SEIZURES

High fever*
■ Systemic infection
■ Hyperthermia
Congenital disorders*
■ Cerebral palsy
■ Tuberous sclerosis
■ Phenylketonuria
CNS infections
■ Meningitis
■ Encephalitis
Structural damage
■ Head trauma*
■ Intracranial bleed
■ Neoplasm
Metabolic derangements
■ Hypoglycemia
■ Electrolyte disturbance
Anoxia
■ Hanging
■ Carbon monoxide poisoning
■ Cardiac disorders
Substances
■ Lead toxicity
■ Medications
■ Cocaine
Inflammatory disorders
■ Multiple sclerosis
■ Lupus
*Most common in children.

EPIDEMIOLOGY

Each year, approximately 150,000 children and adolescents in the United States will have a seizure of some type (6). The vast majority are children under the age of 5 who experience a febrile seizure. Each year, recurrent unprovoked seizures, or epilepsy, will develop in up to 7 in 10,000 children under the age of 15 (7), or in approximately 42,000 children. Across developed countries the annual incidence is similar (8, 9). In U.S. surveys, the incidence of epilepsy is greatest among the very young and the elderly and is generally higher in males, after the age of 5 (10). Whether the incidence of epilepsy is higher in African Americans or populations with lower socioeconomic status, as reported by some (11, 12), is contradicted by others (13, 14). In any given year 1 in 200 children under 15 will have epilepsy (7), or about 300,000 children. Across age groups, in two-thirds of patients the etiology is unknown (10). Populations at special risk for epilepsy are those with a single unprovoked seizure, autism (15), mental retardation, cerebral palsy (16), and children of parents with epilepsy (17).

PROGNOSIS

Approximately 70% of people with epilepsy will go into remission, defined as five or more seizure-free years, whether on or off medication (18). Prognosis will vary according to age and seizure type, with a better prognosis for childhood onset epilepsy without neurological or developmental disabilities. Only 35% of those with mental retardation, cerebral palsy, or other neurological condition will enter remission (19). A decade's longitudinal followup study found that more than one-third of patients with childhood onset epilepsy with more than 5 years of remission who then stopped their medications relapsed within the next 5 years (20). Approximately 10% of child patients newly diagnosed with epilepsy will go on to have intractable epilepsy (21). The course and prognosis for the most common psychiatric comorbidities of epilepsy have not been well studied. However, it is clear that for many patients these continue long after seizures have stopped.

INTERTWINING OF EPILEPSY AND PSYCHIATRY: PAST AND PRESENT

The first recorded description of epilepsy dates to Babylonian clay tablets from 2000 BC (22). Hippocrates also wrote about epilepsy in 400 BC. He described it as having a natural cause, like other medical conditions, rather than being a divine curse as previously thought. He noted the association with depression and wrote that *"melancholics ordinarily become epileptics, and epileptics melancholics: what determines the preference is the direction the malady takes; if it bears upon the body, epilepsy, if upon the intelligence, melancholy."* (23). In the middle ages, some held the view that seizures were characteristic of witches or that witches caused epilepsy (24). Mid-nineteenth century England considered epilepsy a form of insanity (25). In the late nineteenth century, with the advent of neurology as a specialty and the successful use of bromide to treat epileptic patients, epilepsy became increasingly viewed as a brain disorder, and its social stigma attenuated. However, into the twenty-first century, some segments of the public continue to have highly negative perceptions of epilepsy (26).

Although epilepsy in modern medicine is not viewed as a simple causal explanation for severe psychiatric illness, the overlap between epilepsy and psychiatry is extensive and has been increasingly recognized. Seizures can produce alterations in consciousness that can mimic psychiatric symptoms in the ictal and periictal periods, such as commonly occurs, for example, when the seizure starts in the temporal lobes (27). There is also a high prevalence of psychiatric comorbidity in the interictal period. Clearly, the presence of epilepsy has neuropsychiatric and psychological associations, if not sequelae. These problems can be conceptualized along two domains: 1) The brain dysfunction causing seizures, the seizures themselves, and adverse effects of antiepileptic drugs, and their potential contribution to psychiatric pathology, through common physiologic mechanisms, and 2) the psychosocial and psychological consequences of epilepsy or its treatment, irrespective of any biological overlap.

Regardless of etiology, the psychiatric considerations include the child's concerns about self-image and self-esteem, which can be related to the seizure disorder itself or side effects of drug treatment; intrapsychic issues related to temperament and coping skills; psychosocial issues, such as withdrawal and social isolation in contrast to affiliation; the cognitive impact of seizures or their treatment, including decrements in IQ or other neuropsychologic changes; the impact of the disorder or its treatment on daily living (28); and the developmental impact of any or all of these on the individual child in maintaining his or her developmental trajectory.

Learning to live with this chronic, at times severe, disorder while remaining psychiatrically healthy can be a challenge for some children. Child psychiatrists can play an active role in recognizing and treating these psychiatric repercussions or in helping to educate others to do so. With the aim of better helping children who have epilepsy and comorbid psychiatric disorders, it is useful to have a familiarity with the fundamental diagnostic, classification, and treatment considerations in epilepsy. This is reviewed in the following sections, before turning back to psychiatric aspects in more detail.

DIAGNOSIS AND EVALUATION

Most evaluations begin, naturally, with the clinical suspicion that a child is having some form of seizure activity. These can range from the dramatic, such as outright tonic-clonic activity, to the subtle, such as brief staring spells. Other common presentations include unusual sensations, repetitive movements, automatic behaviors, or altered consciousness. Most seizures are brief, lasting from a few seconds to several minutes. Afterward, depending on the type of seizure, a person may have a headache, confusion, muscle soreness, fatigue, odd sensations, or feel nothing at all. Like all diagnostic evaluations, one begins with a detailed clinical history, which is the single most important exam in making a diagnosis, as frequently, diagnostic testing, including EEG—which may not capture definitive interictal clues of seizure activity—will not yield any findings. Since the patient himself may have a poor recollection of the event, collateral information is essential. Generally, one wants to know at minimum the time and speed of onset; the presence of abnormal movements; whether bladder control was maintained; whether the patient bit his lips or tongue; how long the episode lasted; and how long it took for the patient to recover after the episode. The patient can be asked directly how he felt after the event and whether or not he had any premonitions of the event; these can include aural, visual, tactile, or olfactory sensations, among others. The clinical history and exam will help determine the additional workup needed. This usually includes an encephalogram (EEG). Unless the exam is suggestive of obvious triggering pathology, such as a high fever in an infant or a headache, vomiting, and focal neurological findings in a teenager, which would suggest the need for other diagnostic testing first, the single most useful tool in evaluating unprovoked seizures is the EEG.

THE ELECTROENCEPHALOGRAM (EEG): BASIC TERMINOLOGY

In the late nineteenth and early twentieth century, the EEG was an experimental tool applied to the scalp of animals to examine electrical currents in the brain. In 1929 German psychiatrist Hans Berger published a report on his experiments using it to record the fluctuating electrical potentials of the human cortex (29). Soon, the EEG became the prime tool in diagnosing seizures and it remains decades later, now along with neuroimaging, a key instrument in diagnosing epilepsy.

To understand epilepsy and its various syndromes, one must also be familiar with the basic terminology used to describe EEG tracings. EEGs are traditionally acquired using the 10–20 international electrode placement system, in which electrodes are placed in a bipolar fashion from the nasion, where the frontal and nasal bones join, to the inion, the prominent point of the occipital bone.

The EEG starts with the technician asking the patient to close her eyes, or in the case of children, placing a hand over the child's eyes. This is done to bring out the alpha rhythm, which is the predominant rhythm of the brain during wakefulness.

TABLE 7.1.3.4.2

TYPICAL FREQUENCIES AND AMPLITUDES OF SYNCHRONIZED BRAINWAVES

Rhythm	Typical Frequencies (Hz)	Typical Amplitude (uV)
Alpha	8–13	20–200
Beta	13–30	5–10
Delta	1–5	20–200
Theta	4–8	10

Opening the eyes will usually attenuate the rhythm, and other waveforms, such as theta and beta, will appear. While drowsy, more theta and delta waveforms appear in the brain, slowly progressing to more attenuation and the onset of stage 1 sleep. During the acquisition of the EEG, certain maneuvers are attempted to provoke seizures, including hyperventilation and photic stimulation. The response of the brain to these maneuvers helps the observer to determine if the patient is within the normal range, or may be encephalopathic. For example, an encephalopathic child will have prolonged delta after hyperventilation, and may have a slower than normal background at baseline. A patient with absence epilepsy can have an otherwise normal background, but with the onset of hyperventilation, a 3 Hz spike and wave morphology appears along with behavioral arrest. The EEG is also useful because certain epilepsy syndromes have typical and at times diagnostic EEG patterns.

Several elemental EEG waveforms are presented in Table 7.1.3.4.2. In most children, an alpha rhythm with an 8 Hz frequency is reached by age 3 years.

EPILEPSY: CLASSIFICATION

A seizure's manifestations depend on where it starts and where it spreads. Recalling that the definition of epilepsy is recurrent seizures that occur spontaneously in the absence of provoking stimuli, an isolated seizure is not considered to be epilepsy. An epilepsy syndrome is defined by a distinguishing pattern of signs, symptoms, and history. These include the seizure type, whether it starts at an identifiable place or focus in the brain (a focal, partial or localization-related seizure), or whether it does not (a generalized seizure or one with bi-hemispheric involvement from the start). Partial seizures are further classified according to whether they cause alterations in consciousness (complex partial) or consciousness remains intact (simple partial seizure), and whether they progress to generalized tonic-clonic seizures (with secondary generalization) or not. Seizures are called unclassified or undetermined if there is insufficient information on whether they have a focal onset or if they occur in the neonatal period. The definition of an epilepsy syndrome also commonly includes the age of onset, history, including family history, physical exam, EEG findings during and between seizures, etiology, imaging findings, and prognosis. An idiopathic epilepsy syndrome is one in which there is only epilepsy with no underlying structural brain lesions or other neurologic signs or symptoms. These are usually presumed to be genetic and are usually age dependent. An epilepsy syndrome is considered "symptomatic" if there is an identifiable structural cause such as a tumor or infarct. An epilepsy syndrome is considered "cryptogenic" if it is presumed that there is an underlying structural cause even though it is undiscoverable at this time, for example if a child has moderate mental retardation plus epilepsy but normal neuroimaging studies. A benign epilepsy syndrome is one characterized by epileptic seizures that are easily treated, or require no treatment, and remits without sequelae.

In 1989, the International League Against Epilepsy (ILAE) met to determine a classification scheme for epilepsy syndromes. The currently approved ILAE classification divides epilepsies into focal- or localization-related syndromes versus generalized ones, and according to etiology. There is also a newer classification system that is under development to further classify seizures according to ictal semiology, seizure type, and syndromes. The complete ILAE classification of epilepsy syndromes is presented in Table 7.1.3.4.3.

TABLE 7.1.3.4.3

INTERNATIONAL LEAGUE AGAINST EPILEPSY CLASSIFICATION, 1989

Localization-related epilepsy and syndromes

1. Idiopathic
   a. Benign childhood epilepsy with centrotemporal spikes
   b. Childhood epilepsy with occipital paroxysms
   c. Primary reading epilepsy
2. Symptomatic
   a. Chronic progressive epilepsia partialis continua of childhood
   b. Reflex seizures, startle seizures
   c. Temporal lobe epilepsies
   d. Frontal lobe epilepsies
   e. Parietal lobe epilepsies
   f. Occipital lobe epilepsies
3. Cryptogenic

Generalized epilepsies and syndromes

1. Idiopathic
   a. Benign neonatal familial convulsions
   b. Benign neonatal convulsions
   c. Benign myoclonic epilepsy in infancy
   d. Childhood absence epilepsy
   e. Juvenile absence epilepsy
   f. Juvenile myoclonic epilepsy
   g. Epilepsy with grand mal seizures on awakening
2. Cryptogenic or symptomatic
   a. West syndrome
   b. Lennox-Gastaut syndrome
   c. Epilepsy with myoclonic-astatic seizures
   d. Epilepsy with myoclonic absences

Symptomatic

1. Nonspecific etiology
   a. Early myoclonic encephalopathy
   b. Early infantile epileptic encephalopathy with suppression burst

Undetermined epilepsies and syndromes

1. With both generalized and focal features.
   a. Neonatal seizures
   b. Severe myoclonic epilepsy in infancy
   c. Epilepsy with continuous spike waves during slow wave sleep
   d. Acquired epileptic aphasia (Landau-Kleffner)
2. Without generalized or focal features

Special syndromes

1. Febrile seizures
2. Isolated seizures or status epilepticus
3. Seizures precipitated by metabolic or toxic event

TABLE 7.1.3.4.4

RELATIVE FREQUENCY OF EPILEPSY SYNDROMES IN A COMMUNITY SAMPLE OF CHILDREN AGED 0 TO 15 YEARS (N = 613)

Epilepsy Syndrome	Relative Frequency (%)
Localization-related	58.6
Symptomatic	31.8
Cryptogenic	16.8
Idiopathic	10
Generalized	29
Primary generalized	20.6
Cryptogenic/symptomatic	7
Other syndromes	12.4

(Adapted from Berg AT, Shinnar S, Levy SR, Testa FM: Newly diagnosed epilepsy in children: Presentation at diagnosis. *Epilepsia* 40 (4):445–452, 1999.)

Common causes of seizures in the first year of life are perinatal complications, febrile seizures, infections, metabolic problems, and ischemic events. In adolescents and young adults, common causes are trauma, congenital abnormalities, tumors, and central nervous system infections. A concern germane to psychiatrists is differentiating paroxysmal nonepileptic events and nonepileptic seizures from true epilepsy. Complicating matters, patients with nonepileptic seizures may also have concomitant epileptic seizures. Video EEG monitoring is the ideal modality to differentiate these events.

In the first year of life, generalized seizures are the most common type. The incidence then declines and remains constant throughout childhood and adulthood. Thereafter, partial seizures are the most common type in childhood (30), and the incidence is constant until after age 65 years, when a precipitous increase occurs attributable to cerebrovascular disease. Absence (or *petit mal*) seizures, considered in the differential diagnosis of ADHD, rarely occur in the first year, peak from the ages of 5 to 10 years, and then decline, being quite rare by the age of 30. The incidence of various epilepsy syndromes in newly diagnosed children is described in Table 7.1.3.4.4, while clinical features and treatment of the various epilepsy syndromes commonly found in children is described in Table 7.1.3.4.5.

BEHAVIORS THAT MIMIC EPILEPSY

Children often have behaviors that are paroxysmal and may be mistaken for seizures. In most cases, these events are easily defined and there is no treatment needed. There are some instances, however, when the only way to differentiate these events from true seizures is to use video EEG to confirm an EEG correlate. To ascertain a true seizure, determining the duration of the event, observing the presence of a postictal state, and obtaining a history to uncover any provocative stressors are all useful.

Behavioral events that may appear epileptiform were examined by Kotagal and colleagues in a retrospective study looking at 134 children and adolescents admitted to their pediatric epilepsy unit. They found that in children less than 5 years the common diagnoses were parasomnias and sleep jerks. In the older age group, nonepileptic seizures were common (31).

Behaviors that can raise the concern for epilepsy but are not epileptiform in etiology are outlined in Table 7.1.3.4.6.

TABLE 7.1.3.4.5

EPILEPSY SYNDROMES COMMONLY SEEN IN CHILDHOOD (INFANCY SYNDROMES AND ATYPICAL ABSENCE NOT INCLUDED IN THIS TABLE)

Epilepsy Type, Localization, Related Epilepsy	Clinical Features	Treatment
Rolandic epilepsy	Mouth twitching, drooling, nocturnal predisposition	If indicated, carbamazepine or lamotrigine
Temporal lobe epilepsy	Gastric aura, automatisms, tonic posturing	Carbamazepine, lamotrigine, oxcarbazepine
Frontal lobe epilepsy	Hypermotor activity (bicycling, etc.) with change in behavior	Phenytoin, carbamazepine, lamotrigine; zonisamide also helpful
Parietal/occipital lobe epilepsy	Somatosensory/visual phenomena	Carbamazepine, lamotrigine
Generalized idiopathic epilepsy syndromes	Features	Treatment
JME	Brief myoclonic jerks, at times repetitive; can secondarily generalize if untreated	Divalproex, lamotrigine, levetiracetam
Childhood absence	Staring and brief multiple episodes of behavioral arrest	Divalproex, lamotrigine, ethosuximide
Juvenile absence	Myoclonic jerks and staring spells with older age of onset	Divalproex, ethosuximide, lamotrigine, levetiracetam, topiramate
Epilepsy with generalized tonic-clonic seizures	Generalized tonic-clonic seizures that can occur upon awakening or at any time of day with no partial onset	Lamotrigine or divalproex; levetiracetam, topiramate also helpful

TABLE 7.1.3.4.6

BEHAVIORS THAT CAN BE MISTAKEN FOR SEIZURE ACTIVITY

Behavior of Psychiatric or Undefined Origin	Clinical Manifestations
Nonepileptic seizure	May appear very much like a true seizure, but there is no epileptiform activity on EEG. Duration greater than 10 minutes, the lack of a postictal state, and motor movements incongruent with seizure activity are clues.
Breath-holding	Crying followed by cessation of breathing. Within seconds, cyanosis occurs, followed by loss of consciousness and falling. Quick return to consciousness. No neurological damage. Triggered by fear, frustration, or minor injury.
Staring	May need to rule out epilepsy, depending on clinical presentation.
Cyclic vomiting	Repeated, spontaneous vomiting lasting days, followed by asymptomatic periods. May have an EEG correlate.
Stereotyped movements	Tics or other stereotypes
Violent attacks	Violence associated with epilepsy is nondirected thrashing. If violence is organized this does not suggest epilepsy.
Shuddering	Shakes and shudders. No loss of consciousness. Lasts seconds.
Jitteriness	Jittering movements in infants. Stopped by holding down the arms.
Head drops	Can be mistaken for infantile spasms, but no EEG correlate.
Behavior associated with defined syndromes	
Syncope	
1. Sandifer. Seen in children with gastroesophageal reflux 2. Chiari malformations 3. Cardiac conditions	1. Intermittent contractions of the neck with flexion and syncope. 2. Syncope from increased intracranial pressure. Torticollis, ataxia, opisthotonus, nystagmus. 3. Lightheadedness, palpitations, pallor. May need EEG with EKG strip running to clarify etiology.
Cataplexy (e.g., of narcolepsy)	Atonia; partial or full loss of tone
Paroxysmal movement disorders (e.g., channelopathies, dysfunction of ion channels)	Hard to differentiate at times, but no loss of consciousness.
Episodic Ataxia Type I and II	Brief attacks of cerebellar ataxia. Type 2 also involves eye movement difficulties.
Paroxysmal kinesigenic dyskinesia	Choreathetosis or dystonia lasting seconds to minutes. Triggered by, e.g., getting up from chair or out of car.
Paroxysmal exercise-induced dyskinesia	Dystonia occurs 10–15 minutes after starting exercise.
Benign paroxysmal upgaze of childhood	Spells, lasting hours or days, of intermittent upgaze deviation associated with ataxia; language delay is often present.
Benign paroxysmal torticollis	Starts in infancy with attacks of torticollis lasting minutes or hours.

NONEPILEPTIC SEIZURES IN CHILDREN

Nonepileptic seizures (NES) can be classified as physiologic or psychogenic. Physiologic NES are events that resemble seizures but are not caused by epileptiform discharges; these include, for example, syncopal episodes or hypoglycemia. Psychogenic NES refer to behaviors that may resemble seizure activity, but which also are not epileptiform, and are rooted in a psychological etiology. In DSM IV TR, if they are volitional, NES might be classified as factitious disorder with predominantly psychological signs and symptoms or as malingering if secondary gain is a motive. If the NES are not volitional, conversion disorder with seizures or convulsions is the appropriate diagnosis. NES are well documented in adult populations, and approximately 5 to 20% of patients with epilepsy also have nonepileptic seizures. Nonepileptic seizures occur in children, but can be more difficult to delineate from true epilepsy as they are not as common. Moreover, children diagnosed with paroxysmal nonepileptic seizures (PNES) also often carry a diagnosis of EEG-confirmed epilepsy. For example, one study of children with intractable seizures found that one-fifth had nonepileptic seizures, and three-quarters of these children also had documented epileptic seizures (32). Kotagal and colleagues found that 15% of all patients monitored on their pediatric epilepsy unit had PNES; of these, close to half also had epilepsy (31).

The presence of nonepileptiform seizures in children is attributable to a variety of precipitants, most of which have some identifiable psychological or psychosocial component. In adults they are frequently attributed to dissociative phenomena (33), posttraumatic stress disorder (34), and mood disorders. In one study designed to study the psychiatric features of children with nonepileptic seizures, severe environmental stress and major mood disorders were the most common findings (35). The most common environmental stressor involved the family, including parental divorce, parental discord, or the death of a close family member. Sexual abuse was the second most common environmental stressor, occurring in 32% of children. Separation anxiety with school refusal was found in 24% of the children. In their study, Bhatia and Sapra found that school phobias and fear of examinations were the most common precipitating factors (36). Some investigators have found that a family history of epilepsy is commonly found in children with nonepileptic seizures (37).

What does PNES look like? Many patients mimic their own seizures (38). Lancman and colleagues found unresponsiveness with generalized violent and uncoordinated movements or generalized trembling to be the most common manifestations (37). Others have found that tremors, intermittent stiffening, out of phase hand movements, and kicking and thrashing of the legs are most common, especially among adolescents; younger children often present less dramatically with staring or closing of the eyes and no responsiveness (39).

Diagnosing nonepileptic seizures can be difficult. If a typical nonepileptic event is captured on video without an EEG correlate, there is a greater likelihood that the event is nonepileptic. However, frontal lobe seizures occasionally present without an EEG correlate. Hence, clinical observation is crucial. Generally, an event that has a duration of more than 10 minutes, that does not have a postictal state, and in which the movements are neuroanatomically incongruent with a seizure, is unlikely to be epileptic. Early psychiatric intervention is warranted to address these behaviors and prevent them from becoming more entrenched (40).

MENTAL RETARDATION AND EPILEPSY

Epilepsy is a common comorbidity in children with mental retardation, with a direct correlation between the severity of intellectual compromise and the severity of chronic epilepsy. The prevalence of mental retardation is about 1% of the general population (41), but epilepsy is found in approximately 20–40% of children with mental retardation, depending on its severity (42). In addition, about 40% of children with epilepsy have mental retardation. The age at which epilepsy presents is related to the etiology of the mental retardation.

In children with mental retardation, it can be difficult to differentiate seizures from behavior, as this population has more frequent repetitive and stereotyped behaviors than the general population. Several types of nonepileptic events are associated with mental retardation and include self-stimulation, hyperventilation, Sandifer syndrome, spasticity, clonus, dystonic posturing, and choreoathetosis (43). A study by Donat and Wright examined the most common types of behavior in a sample of 31 girls with mental retardation. They found 23% had behavioral staring, 40% had abnormal eye movements, and 42% had tonic posturing (44). As a result, a misdiagnosis of seizures can occur.

Several studies have investigated the age at which seizures present in mental retardation. One study of 98 children found that the average age of the first seizure was 1.3 years, with an earlier onset in children with severe mental retardation and a later onset for patients with mild mental retardation (1). Another study of 151 children with mental retardation, found that 69% had epilepsy by age 3 years without difference between severe and mild mental retardation for onset before or after age 3. Partial seizures predominated, with 72% of the children having these and 28% having generalized seizures. In this population, as in most studies, a prenatal cause for the epilepsy was found in more than 40% (45). When severe epilepsies occur in infancy, they profoundly impact neuropsychological development (46). They are also usually quite difficult to control with AEDs, with many patients undergoing multiple AED trials before seizure control is improved.

Several epilepsy syndromes can result in significant mental retardation, including infantile spasms, Lennox-Gastaut, and the epileptic encephalopathies.

Infantile spasms, or West syndrome, is classified as either cryptogenic or symptomatic, and based on seizure semiology. This syndrome can be catastrophic. There is a better prognosis associated with the cryptogenic type (47). Cryptogenic infantile spasms are not associated with findings on neuroimaging, whereas patients with symptomatic infantile spasms will have an MRI lesion, such as cortical dysplasia, hemimegalencephaly, arterio-venus malformation (AVM), stroke, or other lesion. Patients present as neonates, or in the first month or two of life, with extensor or flexor spasms or a combination of both. They typically have multiple seizures daily, at times causing profound lethargy. Early diagnosis and treatment is crucial, and carries a more favorable long-term prognosis.

Lennox-Gastaut syndrome is commonly known as a mixture of seizure types, including tonic, atonic, myoclonic, and atypical absence seizures. Patients are usually intellectually compromised. The majority of children have onset between 3 to 5 years. Most cases have an underlying brain abnormality and are therefore classified as symptomatic. The intracranial pathologies linked to Lennox-Gastaut include focal cortical dysplasias, diffuse subcortical laminar heterotopias, and, rarely, Sturge-Weber syndrome. Seizures occur multiple times daily, especially during sleep. At times, one seizure type predominates over others. In general, tonic seizures are the most common, and can be mild. They may, however, lead to falls. Children may require a helmet. Atypical absence seizures are the second most common type of spell in Lennox-Gastaut, and are associated with some loss of muscle tone, or jerks. Myoclonic jerks are less common. Approximately 50–75% of Lennox-Gastaut patients will go into nonconvulsive status epilepticus.

The intellectual disability in Lennox-Gastaut is severe in most cases, but on occasion, further decline may be halted by controlling the seizures, since the seizures themselves seem to play a role in the cognitive deterioration. Successful treatment with complete seizure control is rare.

Epileptic encephalopathy is a condition in which the epileptiform abnormalities are thought to contribute to progressive cerebral deterioration, which impacts cognition and functioning. It can be associated with nearly continuous spike and wave discharges, leading to an alteration in consciousness.

Landau-Kleffner syndrome (LKS), also called acquired epileptiform aphasia, involves progressive neuropsychological impairment linked to the appearance of rhythmic EEG activity. Landau and Kleffner first described the correlation between language loss, in previously normally developing children, and paroxysmal EEG discharges in the speech centers (48). LKS is characterized by acquired aphasia and EEG findings that show bilateral, independent temporal spikes that are activated by early sleep. Secondary symptoms include behavioral and psychomotor disturbances. Males are more affected than females, with a 2:1 ratio. Children present between the ages of 3 and 9. Word deafness is a first sign; the child does not respond to commands from parents, or if a phone or doorbell rings, the child is confused and is unable to perform the appropriate action, although previously he or she was able to. Children are invariably referred for audiograms, which are normal. This initial symptom can develop into complete unresponsiveness and impaired communication. The child speaks in a brief, telegraphic manner, and communication may be limited to gestures. In an older child, reading and writing skills can be lost. LKS can also be mistaken for autism. Several important differences are present. Children with autism have language regression before the age of 3, whereas most children in LKS have regression between the ages of 5 and 7 (49). Children with LKS also retain their social skills and do not generally have stereotyped behaviors.

ANTIEPILEPTIC DRUGS (AEDS): GENERAL CONSIDERATIONS

Patients are rarely started on an AED after a single seizure. Rather, an AED is started if the seizure recurs or if there are compelling risk factors for recurrence. Choice of AED depends on evidence of efficacy for that seizure type, adverse effect profile, interactions with other medications, and cost. Treatment is started with a single AED. If that AED is not effective, a second AED is chosen. A drug with a different mechanism of action and lack of drug–drug interaction with the first AED is preferred. The first AED is maintained until the second AED is at a therapeutic dose. Then if seizures are controlled, an attempt to taper off the first one is made. Monotherapy is preferred but some patients will require more than one AED to control their seizures. Use of multiple AEDs simultaneously is associated with more adverse effects.

Neuropsychiatric Effects of Antiepileptic Drugs (AEDs)

AEDs are of particular interest to psychiatry for three reasons: 1) Many have cognitive and behavioral adverse effects (AEs); 2) many have desirable psychotropic effects such as mood stabilization and anxiolysis; and 3) both these sets of effects could provide clues into the pathophysiology of psychiatric disorders.

There have been a number of studies that have investigated the cognitive and behavioral side effects of antiepileptic drugs over the last 30 years. However, there are fewer studies examining the specific side effects of these drugs in children. As a group, AEDs are thought to affect attention, vigilance, and psychomotor speed (50). Attempts to study these effects have been hampered by the difficulties of designing studies in a population with neurological and developmental heterogeneity. Lack of consensus on how to test for these potential AED effects limits the power to detect effects, to generalize from findings, and to compare across studies. The field continues to struggle to develop consistent study designs, testing paradigms, and ways of controlling for confounding variables (51, 52). The effect of AEDs on cognition is difficult to disentangle from the effects of seizures and changes in seizure frequency and severity. Importantly, many of the studies on new AEDs are funded by their manufactures to satisfy FDA requirements for approval. In these studies, efficacy in attenuating seizures is the primary outcome. Measurement of any effects on cognition or behavior has received much less scientific attention in these trials. Adequate studies are also lacking that relate potential cognitive and behavioral side effects of AEDs to schooling and social adjustment (66). The impact of AEDs on the developing brain is unclear. While decreasing seizures is expected to have a beneficial effect, some studies have raised concerns. For example, in one study of the developing rat brain, AEDs have been found to lead to neurodegeneration (53).

Several representative studies examine the effects of AEDs as a group on cognition. Williams and coworkers (1998) administered neuropsychological testing to 32 children with newly diagnosed epilepsy, prior to and after initiation of medication monotherapy. They compared this group to a chronic condition comparator group of diabetic children. They found no significant difference between groups on measures of attention, immediate memory, delayed memory, complex motor speed, or behavior problems (54). Likewise Mandelbaum and Burack also followed children prospectively and found no cognitive declines directly attributable to treatment with AEDs (55). The relatively small sample size in both of these studies, however, limits their power to detect anything but large effects. In another study looking at subjective impressions, children and parents differed in their reports of cognitive side effects. Children reported no change in symptoms before and after AED discontinuation, whereas parents found their children to be more alert and active off the AEDs (56).

Despite the lack of conclusive data, it is helpful to examine what is known about the cognitive and behavioral effects of some individual AEDs. A more complete listing of AEDs can be found in Table 7.1.3.4.7. Some of the new AEDs seem to produce fewer adverse effects than the older ones but this is not consistent across all types of adverse effects.

Phenobarbital is used to treat partial seizures and generalized seizures except absence. It can have significant adverse effects on cognition, mood, and behavior. It can also cause hyperactivity, irritability, and depression. Studies have raised the concern that phenobarbital is associated with decreases in IQ, whereas others have not supported this finding (57, 58). Cognitive deficits may be reversible with treatment discontinuation but deficits may persist over several years (59). This raises the concern that there exist cumulative impairments that are not completely reversible with extended periods of treatment with some AEDs.

Carbamazepine is one of the more commonly used medications in pediatric epilepsy. It is used to treat partial seizures and generalized tonic-clonic seizures, and to treat mania. It is converted to an active metabolite, carbamazepine epoxide, which also has some associated toxicity. Carbamazepine

TABLE 7.1.3.4.7

COMMON ANTIEPILEPTIC DRUGS (AEDS) AND THEIR MECHANISMS OF ACTION

Drug	Site of Action	Clearance	Indications
Carbamazepine	Blocks Na^+ channel	>95% hepatic	Partial seizures
Ethosuximide	Blocks Ca^{2+} channels	80% hepatic 20% renal	Childhood absence
Felbamate	Blocks NMDA receptor, modulates Na^+ channel conductance	50% hepatic 50% renal	Lennox-Gastaut; focal seizures
Gabapentin	Modulates Ca^{2+} channel	100% renal	Partial seizures, as add on
Lamotrigine	Blocks Na^+ channels, attenuates Ca^{2+} channels	85% hepatic	Lennox-Gastaut, partial seizures
Levetiraceteam	Under Investigation	Body water, needs to be renally dosed	Partial seizures, complex partial status
Oxcarbazepine	Blocks Na^+ channels, increases K^+ channel conductance, attenuates Ca^{2+} channels	45% renal 45% hepatic	Partial and generalized seizures
Phenobarbital	Increases GABAa receptor activity, decreases glutamate excitability, decreases Na^+, K^+, and Ca^{2+} conductance	75% hepatic 25% renal	Partial and generalized seizures.
Phenytoin	Blocks Na^+ channels, some Ca^{2+} and Cl^- action	>90% hepatic	Partial and generalized; frontal lobe seizures
Topiramate	Blocks Na^+ channels, modulates GABAa, NMDA, and AMPA	30–50% hepatic 50–70% renal	Partial and generalized seizures
Valproate	May affect GABA glutaminergic activity, decreases Ca^{2+} and K^+ conductance thresholds	>95% hepatic	Childhood absence, JME, idiopathic generalized, and add on for partial
Zonisamide	Inhibits glutamate excitation, blocks NA^+, K^+, Ca^{2+} channels	>90% hepatic	Idiopathic generalized and partial.

induces its own metabolism as well as that of several psychotropic agents. It can cause sedation, mild psychomotor slowing, and decreased attention and memory, even within the therapeutic range (60). Studies have demonstrated decreased performances on the continuous performance test (CPT) (61). However, other studies have found that this initial slowing improves after one month of treatment (62).

Valproic acid (commonly administered as divalproex) is used for the treatment of absence, generalized tonic-clonic, partial, and myoclonic seizures, infantile spasms, and migraines. It is also used for mania and aggression. It is highly protein bound and can displace other drugs that are protein bound, like phenytoin. It can inhibit the metabolism of phenobarbital. These effects can lead to toxicity. It has a range of potential somatic adverse effects. Additionally, in therapeutic ranges it has been shown to cause impaired decisionmaking and attention. In children these effects can be more pronounced. Despite its efficacy against mania, it has also been known to cause aggression, irritability, and hyperactivity in some children in a dose-dependent fashion. In other children however, it is quite effective in many epilepsy syndromes, and by monitoring AED levels, its side effects can be minimized.

Phenytoin is active against partial seizures and generalized seizures, except absence. It is known to cause a decrease in mental speed and concentration, even at therapeutic ranges in adults (63). In children, there is less literature, but a dose-related slowing in mentation has been observed. It can also cause gingival hyperplasia, hirsutism, and coarsening of facial features.

Benzodiazepines, such as clonazepam and clobazam (not approved for use in the United States), are used to treat a range of seizures, including myoclonic, akinetic, and absence seizures, as well as Lennox-Gastaut. They can cause profound sedation and impairment. For example, clonazepam has been shown to cause decreased attention, irritability, hyperactivity, and disinhibition (64). Tolerance can develop after 1 to 6 months. These adverse effects are offset by the excellent efficacy of benzodiazepines in pediatric epilepsy syndromes.

While there is data investigating the cognitive effects of the newer AEDs, more research is needed on this topic. *Lamotrigine* treats partial and generalized seizures and is used in bipolar disorder. Its metabolism is inhibited by valproic acid and stimulated by enzyme-inducing AEDs such as carbamazepine. Lamotrigine has been associated with a high risk of Stevens-Johnson syndrome, but the risk of this serious complication is decreased if lamotrigine is titrated upwards slowly and not coadministered with valproic acid. If a rash occurs, the patient should be evaluated right away and serious consideration given to discontinuing the lamotrigine. Sedation is not usually a problem, even on initial titration. It causes little or no cognitive impairment, and as yet has no detectable effect on attention, psychomotor speed, or memory (60). In addition, some authors suggest it may even improve alertness (65).

Levetiracetam has activity against partial and myoclonic seizures. It has been associated with reports of irritability and aggression, especially in children with mental retardation, and baseline behavioral problems. In an open label study in patients with autism, it was found to have a favorable effect on attention, hyperactivity, and mood instability (66).

Oxcarbazepine is structurally similar to carbamazepine and is used for many of the same seizure types. It is not, however, converted to the toxic, epoxide metabolite of carbamazepine and causes less induction of enzymes that metabolize other medications. There has been interest in its use for bipolar disorder but its efficacy, especially in pediatric bipolar disorder, has been recently cast into doubt (67, 68). It has been associated with only mild cognitive impairment.

Topiramate is useful in the treatment of partial and generalized seizures. It is the one newer AED for which there are significant concerns that it adversely affects cognition (69). Specifically, it has been found that it causes declines in word fluency and attention, and poorer attention after one month's treatment in young adults (70). Compared to pediatric clinical practice, higher doses and faster titration schedules are used in adult studies. Some suggest that the titration schedule may influence the degree of cognitive adverse effects. For example, in one such study patients were randomized to the addition of topiramate or valproic acid to already existing carbamazepine monotherapy (71). A slow titration schedule was used. Psychometric testing was done after 8 weeks. There was little difference in cognitive effects between the two drugs. Still, it is advisable to monitor an individual patient's response to topiramate and to monitor school performance. Psychiatric side effects such as depression, paranoia, and acute confusional psychosis have also been reported with topiramate. It can be associated with weight loss. An initial interest in the use of topiramate for bipolar disorder has not been substantiated in controlled trials.

Zonisamide is used to treat partial seizures. There is little sedation associated with this drug. Some patients lose weight because of decreased appetite. A study examining cognition in patients with refractory partial epilepsy before and during zonisamide treatment showed that high plasma concentrations of zonisamide were linearly associated with deficits in verbal acquisition, but did not affect psychomotor abilities (72). Another study looked at patients on zonisamide or carbamazepine with phenytoin. There were lower verbal IQ and performance IQ scores in patients on zonisamide compared to carbamazepine (73). Here, too, the effect increased with dose.

Gabapentin is used for partial seizures. It has also been shown to have some efficacy against anxiety and chronic pain. It has essentially no drug–drug interactions. It is not useful for the treatment of mania. It can cause behavioral disinhibition, especially in children with preexisting behavioral problems or mental retardation.

Tiagabine is a specific gamma-aminobutyric acid (GABA) reuptake inhibitor that is used to treat partial seizures. It is not recommended for anxiety, bipolar disorder, or any psychiatric use at this time because of a high rate of neurological adverse effects, including de novo seizures, emotional lability, and dizziness.

PSYCHIATRIC DISORDERS IN CHILDREN WITH EPILEPSY

General Considerations

Children with epilepsy have high levels of psychiatric comorbidity. The Isle of Wright study by Rutter and colleagues (74) found that children with idiopathic seizures showed a 29% rate of psychiatric disorders. In contrast, the rate for psychiatric disorders was 7% for children in the general population and 12% for those with other physical problems outside the CNS. More recently, in a population survey of more than 10,000 children aged 5 to 15 in the United Kingdom, Davies and colleagues found similar rates adjusting symptoms to DSM-IV. Psychiatric disorders were 37% in children with epilepsy, 9% in controls, and 11% in the chronic condition comparator, diabetes (75). Rodenburg and coworkers conducted a series of metaanalyses, involving 46 studies and 2,434 subjects to examine the types and severity of psychopathology in children with epilepsy. They found a medium to large effect size of psychopathology for children with epilepsy compared to healthy controls. The researches noted a smaller effect size for psychopathology when comparing children with epilepsy to those with chronic illnesses, leading them to conclude that some, but not all, of the psychopathology in epilepsy is attributable to a "generic feature" of chronic illness (76). Considering gender, some have found that chronically ill females tend to fare less well emotionally than chronically ill males, and have more suicidal thinking (77). As for treatment, it seems to be underutilized in this population (78). In order to improve recognition and treatment of psychiatric dysfunction in children with epilepsy, it is useful to consider the specific psychiatric disorders associated with epilepsy.

Autism and Epilepsy

The link between autism and epilepsy was first noted by Leo Kanner. The incidence of epilepsy in autism has been estimated to range from 5% to over 30%, with a bimodal distribution in age of onset. The first peak is before 5 years and the other after 10 years. There does not appear to be a gender difference (79). Any seizure type can be associated with autism.

The different subtypes of autism spectrum disorders have different rates of epilepsy. In classic autism, epilepsy has been found to develop in a third of children, with risk linked to intracranial pathology (79). Childhood disintegrative disorder carries a risk of 70% for the development of epilepsy. In Rett disorder, over 90% of patients have epilepsy (80).

A specific EEG pattern that correlates with autism has not been found. About 10% of children with autism have a paroxysmal EEG pattern, such as that found in Landau Kleffner syndrome or with electrical status epilepticus in sleep. EEGs are not routinely requested for patients with autism. A retrospective study by Gabis and colleagues examined the EEG findings in 56 children with pervasive developmental disorders to examine the value of obtaining an EEG in this patient population. They found that only two children without clinical seizures, or a history of language regression, as in LKS, had an epileptiform EEG (81). In general, a patient who has autism and displays paroxysmal stereotyped behaviors raises the suspicion of epilepsy. In addition to EEG, home or school videos are helpful to clarify the event. If regression is present, then an EEG should be obtained. A higher index of suspicion is warranted in those patients with autism who are lower functioning or severely impaired, as seizure disorders are more common in those with lower IQ (82).

Depression and Anxiety

As in adults, depression and anxiety are commonly found in children with epilepsy. Caplan and colleagues interviewed 100 children with epilepsy and found that 33% had a depressive or anxiety disorder. Those with mood and anxiety disorders had lower IQ scores (83). Only 33% of those with identified disorders had received prior mental health treatment, surprising given their involvement in the health care system as a result of their epilepsy. Other studies have found depressive symptoms to be the most common psychiatric symptom in children with epilepsy (84).

A variety of factors have been proposed and studied to explain depression in epilepsy, yielding contradictory results. The epilepsy factors include age of onset, duration of epilepsy, seizure type, and seizure severity. Iatrogenic factors include treatment with AEDs and surgery. Psychosocial factors include stigma, discrimination, sense of control, attributional style, and social supports. Ultimately the likely explanation is multifactorial (85). The etiology of anxiety is less well explored. Some have considered the role of limbic structures, which include the amygdale and hippocampus, as an area of pathogenesis for anxiety (86).

Suicide

In adults, rates of suicide or self harm in those with epilepsy are thought to be five times that of the general population, with the highest risk for those with temporal lobe epilepsy (87). Robertson reviewed studies that examined causes of death in epilepsy and found that the rate of death by suicide was 10 times that of the general population (85). The data in children also suggest high rates of suicidal thinking or behavior. A chart review of pediatric suicide attempters with epilepsy found a rate 15 times that of the general population (88). In the Caplan study cited above, 20% of the subjects reported suicidal thinking, compared to 9% of controls. Of those with suicidal thinking 37% had plans. Those with disruptive behaviors comorbid with depression and anxiety were 12 times more likely to have suicidal thinking. Duration of illness also corresponded to suicidal thinking.

Psychosis

Psychosis and its relationship to epilepsy has generated a robust literature. Since the mid-nineteenth century, there have been generally two lines of thinking regarding psychosis. In one, epilepsy and active psychosis are thought to be incompatible. ECT for the treatment of psychosis emerged in part from this perspective. The other line of thought views epilepsy as coexisting with or facilitating psychoses (86). The concept of forced normalization and alternative psychoses introduced by Landolt illustrates a reciprocal coexistence (89); patients whose EEGs were abnormal but which normalized with treatment were observed to develop psychopathology. Slater and Beard described schizophrenia-like psychoses related to duration of epilepsy and amount of brain damage; this association was especially strong in temporal lobe epilepsy (90). The concept of kindling as an etiologic theory for epilepsy may also help explain the emergence of psychotic phenomena (91).

Psychotic symptoms have been considered according to their temporal relationship with seizure activity; that is, whether they are preictal, ictal, postictal or interictal. The psychiatrist is most likely to be concerned with inter-ictal presentations of psychosis, although the hospital-based consultant may be called in during any of the other states. Occasionally, the hospital-based psychiatric consultant may be the first to evaluate a psychotic presentation, before the epilepsy history is revealed through chart records, by a late-arriving family member, or by the patient himself after he recuperates.

There are no epidemiologic studies examining the comorbidity of psychosis and epilepsy in children. Adult studies have methodological limitations but provide some information. Mendez and colleagues retrospectively compared outpatients in a neurology clinic who had epilepsy or migraine headaches. They found that 9% of the patients with epilepsy had interictal schizophrenia symptoms, versus 1% of the patients with migraine (92). Shaw and colleagues found that 3% of patients with temporal lobectomy for intractable seizures developed schizophrenia-like psychoses (93).

In addition to methodological issues, studies and descriptions of psychotic states in epilepsy patients have been plagued by matters of semantics in describing both psychotic symptoms and epilepsy. Parnas and Korsgaard observed in 1982 that the descriptions of psychosis seldom fit the Bleulerian definition of schizophrenia and advised against the use of the term schizophrenia-like to describe psychoses in epilepsy (94). With this concern in mind, Kanemoto and colleagues set out to reexamine the matter of interictal psychoses using DSM-IV criteria definitions of psychotic disorders in conjunction with the International League Against Epilepsy Classification criteria. In a retrospective review of all outpatient records from 1984 to 1999 at their regional epilepsy center, they found 132 patients to have interictal psychoses, or 4.5% of all patients. The researches excluded ictal or postictal psychotic phenomena. Schizophrenia was found in 1.9% of the total sample. Temporal lobe epilepsy made up the vast majority of seizure types with psychosis, accounting for 56% of cases. The patients with schizophrenia were more likely to have had early onset psychosis (< 20 years old) and to have lower IQ. One significant limitation of the study is its retrospective design (95).

An epidemiological question mark remains for both adults and children regarding epilepsy and psychosis. The sum of the data suggests that perhaps interictal psychotic states are more commonly seen than would be expected in the general population and that temporal lobe epilepsy seems to be the predominant type accountable for this.

ADHD and Disruptive Behavior Disorders

Symptoms of ADHD in epilepsy syndromes tend to be ones of inattention rather than hyperactivity-impulsivity. Some suggest that ADHD and epilepsy share common risk factors and that both may share common neuropsychological impairments, especially the inattentive type (96). Others have also observed that a number of children with uncomplicated ADHD and without epilepsy have epileptiform discharges (97).

Several studies have examined the prevalence of ADHD in epilepsy populations. In one, a history of ADHD was 2.5 times more common in children newly diagnosed with epilepsy compared to controls (98). Several other studies have looked at the prevalence of ADHD in pediatric epilepsy. Dunn and coworkers found that 25% to 37% of children and adolescents scored in the clinical range on the attention scale of the Child Behavior Checklist (CBCL); using a symptom inventory which gives symptom profiles according to DSM-IV, they found 24% of children had ADHD with predominantly inattentive type and 11.4% with combined type (99). In the U.K. population study by Davies, the rate of DSM-IV ADHD in complicated epilepsy was 12% and in uncomplicated epilepsy, 0%, suggesting degree of illness may account for ADHD symptoms (75).

The data for other disruptive disorders is generally embedded in data on ADHD. Caplan and colleagues found ADHD, oppositional defiant disorder or conduct disorder in 25% of patients with complex partial epilepsy or generalized primary seizures (100). Ott and coworkers found disruptive behavior disorders in up to 23% of those with complex partial epilepsy or primary generalized seizures (2).

Neuropsychological Functioning and Education

The literature generally suggests that epilepsy negatively impacts cognitive functioning. Although findings are variable, this is related to specific epilepsy syndromes, age of onset, duration, seizure frequency, and number of AEDs.

Williams and colleagues found that children with epilepsy had a full scale IQ in the low average to average range (101). O'Leary and colleagues also found that children with epilepsy had lower IQs. They administered the WISC-III to 32 child patients with epilepsy, without comorbid conditions and IQ greater than 70, and to matched controls and found a mean difference of one standard deviation on the full scale IQ, 107 versus 92 (102). Hoie and colleagues studied nonverbal intelligence in 198 children with epilepsy using Raven matrices. Severe nonverbal performance problems were found in 43% of children with epilepsy, compared to 3% of controls (103). These studies reflect group trends and do not reflect how an individual child will perform; for example Smith and colleagues also found IQs in the low to average range, but individual scores ranged from the < 1% to > 99% (104).

Regarding IQ stability, Bourgeois and colleagues prospectively followed children yearly over 4 years, administering their first psychological evaluation within 2 weeks of initial diagnosis. They found that overall IQ did not decrease, but that in a subset of subjects, IQ scores persistently showed a decrease of 10 points or more. This was related to a higher incidence of drug levels in the toxic range, difficulty controlling seizure activity, and an earlier age of seizure onset (105). Rodin and colleagues readministered the WISC to children with epilepsy 5 years after initial testing and found that WISC IQ estimates decreased slightly over time; they suggested that decreased mental growth rather than loss of function was responsible (106).

Regarding education and achievement, Farwell and colleagues studied 118 children with epilepsy and found they had repeated a grade or been placed in special education at twice the normal rate. In this study, years of seizure activity correlated with lower intelligence (107). Aldenkamp and colleagues examined several factors related to achievement and concluded that epilepsy type is the main factor underlying educational achievement. They speculated that since epilepsy type is correlated with intelligence, this may be the primary cognitive factor underlying educational underachievement (108). Regarding achievement, it seems that that only those children with high severity epilepsy have lower school administered achievement scores compared to national norms, but not those children with inactive or low severity epilepsy (109). Whether epilepsy itself or, more generally, the presence of a chronic condition, affects achievement has also been studied; those with epilepsy generally do less well (110).

Learning Disorders

Difficulties in reading, writing, and mathematics may be found in one-third of children with epilepsy (111). One study examining children with epilepsy found that academic problems were highest in math, followed by spelling, reading, and comprehension. Children also did less well than expected for age and IQ level (112). Seizure onset in the language-dominant hemisphere is thought to affect reading comprehension, written language and calculation abilities, more so than seizure onset in the nondominant hemisphere (113).

Family

Rodenburg and colleagues in a literature review found that compared to control children, families with a child with epilepsy had a lower quality of parent–child relationship, more depression in mothers, and had problems with family functioning (114). Family factors seem to be stronger predictors of psychopathology than epilepsy-related factors (115).

Quality of Life

Adolescents' perceptions of epilepsy can be highly negative. Cheung and Wirrell interviewed healthy controls and children with chronic conditions. When asked about the physical and social impact of eight chronic diseases (epilepsy, leukemia, HIV infection, Down syndrome, migraine, asthma, diabetes, and arthritis), epilepsy was viewed as having a worse physical impact than all illnesses except Down syndrome. The perceptions included the view that epilepsy commonly causes mental handicap and commonly leads to self-injury and death or injury in others. In addition, healthy controls viewed individuals with epilepsy as less honest, popular, fun, and less adept at sports than healthy teens (116).

Children with epilepsy often have a poorer self-concept than do those with other chronic conditions (117–119). Older adolescents perceive a greater negative impact on life and general health and have more negative attitudes about epilepsy. Those with severe seizures and female patients seem have the greatest difficulty (120). Each AED also has its own side effect profile which may impact self esteem, such as weight gain. Mitchell argued, however, that family, socioeconomic, and cultural factors are the primary determinants of social, academic and other problems in epilepsy and that medications, seizures, or cognition play a minor role (121).

Driving restrictions may impact adolescents with epilepsy. Restrictions on driving after a seizure are mandated by law and vary from state to state, usually lasting 3 to 12 months after an index seizure. If no new seizures occur during the restricted time, driving privileges are reinstituted (122).

Examining outcome, Jalava and colleagues followed a cohort of childhood onset epilepsy into adulthood with a mean followup of 35 years. They found that those with epilepsy and no other neurological problems did less well than controls in education, employability, marriage rate, and—depending on seizure activity and polypharmacy—satisfaction with present life (123).

PSYCHOPHARMACOLOGICAL TREATMENT OF CHILDREN WITH EPILEPSY AND COMORBID PSYCHIATRIC DISORDERS

Psychopharmacological treatment in children with epilepsy should always be embedded in a full biopsychosocial approach to the child's problems. Different domains of dysfunction should be conceptualized and each given treatments specific to that domain. Thus, academic and social skills deficits may require remediation. School failure may require modification of the educational plan. Relationship problems benefit from psychotherapy, as will low self-esteem and coping difficulties. Family and individual misconceptions should be countered with psychoeducation. The primary symptoms of the patient's DSM-IV Axis I disorder may, depending on the disorder, benefit from psychotherapy or psychopharmacology, or both.

When the time comes to choose a psychopharmacological agent, four considerations should be borne in mind: efficacy, seizure threshold, interactions, and adverse effects. Considering efficacy first, for nearly all the psychiatric disorders comorbid with epilepsy, specific randomized controlled trials in children with epilepsy plus that disorder have not been done. Thus clinicians will need to use as a guide the efficacy data from children without seizures, but more circumspectly. Similarly, while many psychotropics have been assumed to lower the threshold for having a seizure, randomized controlled data, with the exception of methylphenidate, does not exist for the risk of exacerbating seizures. For most psychotropics, practitioners must rely on the FDA trial data for that agent, comparing the rate of new-onset seizures in patients receiving active medication versus those receiving placebo, even though patients with epilepsy are excluded from almost all these trials. Other ways to estimate the risk include considering the rate of seizures when the psychotropic has been taken in an overdose and examining the literature for uncontrolled case reports and case series.

Drug–drug interactions between psychotropics and AEDs can be pharmacodynamic (e.g., additive sedation) or pharmacokinetic (e.g., decreased antipsychotic plasma level when the patient is taking carbamazepine). These interactions must

TABLE 7.1.3.4.8

RECOMMENDATIONS FOR COMMONLY USED PSYCHOTROPICS IN THE CHILD WITH A SEIZURE DISORDER

Medication or Class	Recommendations (Low Seizure Risk ≠ Absent Risk)	Key Drug–Drug Interactions with AEDs
First generation antipsychotics	■ Use not advised for chlorpromazine and loxapine ■ Use others judiciously ■ Haloperidol has among lowest risk	Carbamazepine, phenobarbital, phenytoin, and perhaps oxcarbazepine may reduce levels through cytochrome P450 3A4 induction.
Second generation antipsychotics	■ Use not advised for clozapine ■ Seizure risk low for others	Risperidone, quetiapine, aripiprazole, and ziprasidone may be reduced by above AEDs through 3A4.
SSRIs/SNRIs	■ Seizure risk low ■ Venlafaxine may have increased risk over others	Fluoxetine and fluvoxamine may increase carbamazepine levels through 3A4 inhibition.
Trazodone	Seizure risk low	Substrate of 3A4; above AEDs may reduce
Alpha agonists	Seizure risk low	No known drug interactions with AEDs
Bupropion	Use not advised	Phenytoin and phenobarbital may reduce levels through 2B6 induction.
Atomoxetine	Seizure risk unclear. Use judiciously	No known drug interactions with AEDs
Lithium	Use judiciously. Considered proconvulsant	Neurotoxicity with carbamazepine and phenytoin
Stimulants	FDA contraindicates when comorbid seizures are present, but data suggest can be used judiciously	No known drug interactions with AEDs
TCAs/tetracyclic antidepressants	■ Use not advised for clomipramine, amoxapine, and loxapine ■ Use others judiciously	Valproate may increase and carbamazepine may decrease TCA levels.
Benzodiazepines	Anticonvulsant, but proconvulsant if suddenly discontinued	Alprazolam, diazepam midazolam, and triazolam are substrates of 3A4.

be considered when adding or removing an AED or a psychotropic. It is useful to anticipate that the rate of adverse effects from a psychotropic might be higher in patients with epilepsy than in patients without it. This will result in a frank discussion of risks with the family and "starting low and going slow" with the psychotropic. Table 7.1.3.4.8 summarizes recommendations for the more commonly prescribed psychotropics when epilepsy is comorbid.

Just as we would not have a patient's seizures go untreated, we and our colleagues in neurology should not overlook the psychiatric and psychological comorbidities commonly present in children with epilepsy, and ensure that these do not go undiagnosed and untreated.

References

1. Steffenburg S, Gillberg C, Steffenburg U: Psychiatric disorders in children and adolescents with mental retardation and active epilepsy. *Arch Neurol* 53(9):904–912, 1996.
2. Ott D, Caplan R, Guthrie D, Siddarth P, Komo S, Shields WD, et al.: Measures of psychopathology in children with complex partial seizures and primary generalized epilepsy with absence. *J Am Acad Child Adolesc Psychiatry* 40(8):907–914, 2001.
3. Hesdorffer DC, Ludvigsson P, Olafsson E, Gudmundsson G, Kjartansson O, Hauser WA: ADHD as a risk factor for incident unprovoked seizures and epilepsy in children. *Arch Gen Psychiatry* 61(7):731–736, 2004.
4. Kanner AM: Depression in epilepsy: Prevalence, clinical semiology, pathogenic mechanisms, and treatment. *Biol Psychiatry* 54(3):388–398, 2003.
5. Szabo CA: Patient page. Risk of fetal death and malformation related to seizure medications. *Neurology* 67(3):E6–7, 2006.
6. Hauser WA: The prevalence and incidence of convulsive disorders in children. *Epilepsia* 35(suppl 2):S1–6, 1994.
7. Cowan LD: The epidemiology of the epilepsies in children. *Ment Retard Dev Disabil Res Rev* 8(3):171–181, 2002.
8. Kurtz Z, Tookey P, Ross E: Epilepsy in young people: 23 year follow up of the British national child development study. *BMJ* 316(7128):339–342, 1998.
9. Oka E, Ohtsuka Y, Yoshinaga H, Murakami N, Kobayashi K, Ogino T: Prevalence of childhood epilepsy and distribution of epileptic syndromes: A population-based survey in Okayama, Japan. *Epilepsia* 47(3):626–630, 2006.
10. Hauser WA, Annegers JF, Rocca WA: Descriptive epidemiology of epilepsy: Contributions of population-based studies from Rochester, Minnesota. *Mayo Clin Proc* 71(6):576–586, 1996.
11. Shamansky SL, Glaser GH: Socioeconomic characteristics of childhood seizure disorders in the New Haven area: An epidemiologic study. *Epilepsia* 20(5):457–474, 1979.
12. Heaney DC, MacDonald BK, Everitt A, Stevenson S, Leonardi GS, Wilkinson P, et al.: Socioeconomic variation in incidence of epilepsy: Prospective community based study in south east England. *BMJ* 325(7371):1013–1016, 2002.
13. Annegers JF, Dubinsky S, Coan SP, Newmark ME, Roht L: The incidence of epilepsy and unprovoked seizures in multiethnic, urban health maintenance organizations. *Epilepsia* 40(4):502–506, 1999.
14. Reading R, Haynes R, Beach R: Deprivation and incidence of epilepsy in children. *Seizure* 15(3):190–193, 2006.
15. Tuchman R, Rapin I: Epilepsy in autism. *Lancet Neurol* 1(6):352–358, 2002.
16. Hauser WA, Annegers JF, Kurland LT: Incidence of epilepsy and unprovoked seizures in Rochester, Minnesota: 1935–1984. *Epilepsia* 34(3):453–468, 1993.
17. Ottman R, Annegers JF, Hauser WA, Kurland LT: Higher risk of seizures in offspring of mothers than of fathers with epilepsy. *Am J Hum Genet* 43(3):257–264, 1988.
18. Annegers JF, Hauser WA, Elveback LR: Remission of seizures and relapse in patients with epilepsy. *Epilepsia* 20(6):729–737, 1979.
19. Epilepsy Foundation. Epilepsy and seizure statistics. Available at: http://www.epilepsyfoundation.org/answerplace/statistics.cfm. Accessed August 15, 2006.
20. Sillanpaa M, Schmidt D: Prognosis of seizure recurrence after stopping antiepileptic drugs in seizure-free patients: A long-term population-based study of childhood-onset epilepsy. *Epilepsy Behav* 8(4):713–719, 2006.
21. Berg AT, Shinnar S, Levy SR, Testa FM, Smith-Rapaport S, Beckerman B: Early development of intractable epilepsy in children: A prospective study. *Neurology* 56(11):1445–1452, 2001.
22. World Health Organization. Epilepsy: Historical overview. February 2001. Available at: http://www.who.int/mediacentre/factsheets/fs168/en/. Accessed August 16, 2006.
23. Lewis A: Melancholia: A historical review. *J Ment Sci* 80:1–42, 1934.

24. Masia SL, Devinsky O: Epilepsy and behavior: A brief history. *Epilepsy Behav* 1(1):27–36, 2000.
25. Roberts A: The 1844 Report of The Metropolitan Commissioners in Lunacy. Available at: http://www.mdx.ac.uk/WWW/STUDY/4_09.htm#4.9.2. Accessed August 16, 2006.
26. Spatt J, Bauer G, Baumgartner C, Feucht M, Graf M, Mamoli B, et al.: Predictors for negative attitudes toward subjects with epilepsy: A representative survey in the general public in Austria. *Epilepsia* 46(5):736–742, 2005.
27. Mace CJ: Epilepsy and schizophrenia. *Br J Psychiatry* 163:439–445, 1993.
28. Lossius MI, Clench-Aas J, Roy BV, Mowinckel P, Gjerstad L: Psychiatric symptoms in adolescents with epilepsy in junior high school in Norway: A population survey. *Epilepsy Behav* Aug 4, 2006.
29. Haas LF: Hans Berger (1873–1941), Richard Caton (1842–1926), and electroencephalography. *J Neurol Neurosurg Psychiatry* 74(1):9, 2003.
30. Berg AT, Shinnar S, Levy SR, Testa FM: Newly diagnosed epilepsy in children: Presentation at diagnosis. *Epilepsia* 40(4):445–452, 1999.
31. Kotagal P, Costa M, Wyllie E, Wolgamuth B: Paroxysmal nonepileptic events in children and adolescents. *Pediatrics* 110(4):e46, 2002.
32. Holmes GL, Sackellares JC, McKiernan J, Ragland M, Dreifuss FE: Evaluation of childhood pseudoseizures using EEG telemetry and video tape monitoring. *J Pediatr* 97(4):554–558, 1980.
33. Bowman ES: Why conversion seizures should be classified as a dissociative disorder. *Psychiatr Clin North Am* 29(1):185–211, x, 2006.
34. Mondon K, de Toffol B, Praline J, Receveur C, Gaillard P, El Hage W, et al.: Psychiatric comorbidity in patients with pseudoseizures: Retrospective study conducted in a video-EEG center. *Rev Neurol (Paris)* 161(11):1061–1069, 2005.
35. Wyllie E, Glazer JP, Benbadis S, Kotagal P, Wolgamuth B: Psychiatric features of children and adolescents with pseudoseizures. *Arch Pediatr Adolesc Med* 153(3):244–248, 1999.
36. Bhatia MS, Sapra S: Pseudoseizures in children: A profile of 50 cases. *Clin Pediatr (Phila)* 44(7):617–621, 2005.
37. Lancman ME, Asconape JJ, Graves S, Gibson PA: Psychogenic seizures in children: Long-term analysis of 43 cases. *J Child Neurol* 9(4):404–407, 1994.
38. Vincentiis S, Valente KD, Thome-Souza S, Kuczinsky E, Fiore LA, Negrao N: Risk factors for psychogenic nonepileptic seizures in children and adolescents with epilepsy. *Epilepsy Behav* 8(1):294–298, 2006.
39. Kramer U, Carmant L, Riviello JJ, Stauffer A, Helmers SL, Mikati MA, et al.: Psychogenic seizures: Video telemetry observations in 27 patients. *Pediatr Neurol* 12(1):39–41, 1995.
40. Brunquell P, Mc Keever M, Russman BS: Differentiation of epileptic from nonepileptic head drops in children. *Epilepsia* 31(4):401–405, 1990.
41. McLaren J, Bryson SE: Review of recent epidemiological studies of mental retardation: Prevalence, associated disorders, and etiology. *Am J Ment Retard* 92(3):243–254, 1987.
42. Bowley C, Kerr M: Epilepsy and intellectual disability. *J Intellect Disabil Res* 44(Pt 5):529–543, 2000.
43. Paolicchi JM: The spectrum of nonepileptic events in children. *Epilepsia* 43(suppl 3):60–64, 2002.
44. Donat JF, Wright FS: Episodic symptoms mistaken for seizures in the neurologically impaired child. *Neurology* 40(1):156–157, 1990.
45. Airaksinen EM, Matilainen R, Mononen T, Mustonen K, Partanen J, Jokela V, et al.: A population-based study on epilepsy in mentally retarded children. *Epilepsia* 41(9):1214–1220, 2000.
46. Shields WD: Catastrophic epilepsy in childhood. *Epilepsia* 41(suppl 2):S2-6, 2000.
47. Riikonen R: Long-term outcome of West syndrome: A study of adults with a history of infantile spasms. *Epilepsia* 37(4):367–372, 1996.
48. Landau WM, Kleffner FR: Syndrome of acquired aphasia with convulsive disorder in children. 1957. *Neurology* 51(5):1241, 8 pages following 1241, 1998.
49. Tuchman RF, Rapin I: Regression in pervasive developmental disorders: Seizures and epileptiform electroencephalogram correlates. *Pediatrics* 99(4):560–566, 1997.
50. Meador KJ: Cognitive outcomes and predictive factors in epilepsy. *Neurology* 58(8 suppl 5):S21-6, 2002.
51. Kwan P, Brodie MJ: Neuropsychological effects of epilepsy and antiepileptic drugs. *Lancet* 357(9251):216–222, 2001.
52. Loring DW, Meador KJ: Cognitive side effects of antiepileptic drugs in children. *Neurology* 62(6):872–877, 2004.
53. Bittigau P, Sifringer M, Ikonomidou C: Antiepileptic drugs and apoptosis in the developing brain. *Ann N Y Acad Sci* 993:103–114; discussion 123-124, 2003.
54. Williams J, Bates S, Griebel ML, Lange B, Mancias P, Pihoker CM, et al. Does short-term antiepileptic drug treatment in children result in cognitive or behavioral changes? *Epilepsia* 39(10):1064–1069, 1998.
55. Mandelbaum DE, Burack GD: The effect of seizure type and medication on cognitive and behavioral functioning in children with idiopathic epilepsy. *Dev Med Child Neurol* 39(11):731–735, 1997.
56. Aldenkamp AP, Alpherts WC, Sandstedt P, Blennow G, Elmqvist D, Heijbel J, et al.: Antiepileptic drug-related cognitive complaints in seizure-free children with epilepsy before and after drug discontinuation. *Epilepsia* 39(10):1070–1074, 1998.
57. Farwell JR, Lee YJ, Hirtz DG, Sulzbacher SI, Ellenberg JH, Nelson KB: Phenobarbital for febrile seizures: Effects on intelligence and on seizure recurrence. *N Engl J Med* 322(6):364–369, 1990.
58. Camfield CS, Chaplin S, Doyle AB, Shapiro SH, Cummings C, Camfield PR: Side effects of phenobarbital in toddlers: Behavioral and cognitive aspects. *J Pediatr* 95(3):361–365, 1979.
59. Sulzbacher S, Farwell JR, Temkin N, Lu AS, Hirtz DG: Late cognitive effects of early treatment with phenobarbital. *Clin Pediatr (Phila)* 38(7):387–394, 1999.
60. Meador KJ: The cognitive effects of antiepileptic medication. In: Wyllie E, Gupta A, Lachhwani DK (eds): *The Treatment of Epilepsy: Principles and Practice*, 4th ed. Philadelphia, Lippincott Williams and Wilkins, pp. 33–62, 2006.
61. Mandelbaum DE, Burack GE, Bhise V: Effects of anticonvulsant therapy on cognition and attention in children with new-onset, idiopathic epilepsy: Prospective study. Abstract E-07. *Ann Neurology* 2003;56.
62. Larkin JG, McKee PJ, Brodie MJ: Rapid tolerance to acute psychomotor impairment with carbamazepine in epileptic patients. *Br J Clin Pharmacol* 33(1):111–114, 1992.
63. Gillham RA, Williams N, Wiedmann KD, Butler E, Larkin JG, Brodie MJ: Cognitive function in adult epileptic patients established on anticonvulsant monotherapy. *Epilepsy Res* 7(3):219–225, 1990.
64. Bensch J, Blennow G, Ferngren H, Gamstorp I, Herrlin KM, Kubista J, et al.: A double-blind study of clonazepam in the treatment of therapy-resistant epilepsy in children. *Dev Med Child Neurol* 19(3):335–342, 1977.
65. Franz DN, Tudor C, Leonard J, Egelhoff JC, Byars A, Valerius K, et al.: Lamotrigine therapy of epilepsy in tuberous sclerosis. *Epilepsia* 42(7):935–940, 2001.
66. Rugino TA, Samsock TC: Levetiracetam in autistic children: An open-label study. *J Dev Behav Pediatr* 23(4):225–230, 2002.
67. MacMillan CM, Korndorfer SR, Rao S, Fleisher CA, Mezzacappa E, Gonzalez-Heydrich J: A comparison of divalproex and oxcarbazepine in aggressive youth with bipolar disorder. *J Psychiatr Pract* 12(4):214–222, 2006.
68. Wagner KD, Kowatch RA, Emslie GJ, Findling RL, Wilens TE, McCague K, et al.: A double-blind, randomized, placebo-controlled trial of oxcarbazepine in the treatment of bipolar disorder in children and adolescents. *Am J Psychiatry* 163(7):1179–1186, 2006.
69. Salinsky MC, Storzbach D, Spencer DC, Oken BS, Landry T, Dodrill CB: Effects of topiramate and gabapentin on cognitive abilities in healthy volunteers. *Neurology* 64(5):792–798, 2005.
70. Martin R, Kuzniecky R, Ho S, Hetherington H, Pan J, Sinclair K, et al.: Cognitive effects of topiramate, gabapentin, and lamotrigine in healthy young adults. *Neurology* 52(2):321–327, 1999.
71. Aldenkamp AP, Baker G, Mulder OG, Chadwick D, Cooper P, Doelman J, et al.: A multicenter, randomized clinical study to evaluate the effect on cognitive function of topiramate compared with valproate as add-on therapy to carbamazepine in patients with partial-onset seizures. *Epilepsia* 41(9):1167–1178, 2000.
72. Berent S, Sackellares JC, Giordani B, Wagner JG, Donofrio PD, Abou-Khalil B: Zonisamide (CI-912) and cognition: Results from preliminary study. *Epilepsia* 28(1):61–67, 1987.
73. Wilensky AJ, Friel PN, Ojemann LM, Dodrill CB, McCormick KB, Levy RH: Zonisamide in epilepsy: A pilot study. *Epilepsia* 26(3):212–220, 1985.
74. Rutter M, Graham P, Yule W: A neuropsychiatric study in childhood. *Clinics in Developmental Medicine, No. 35/36*. Philadelphia, J.B. Lippincott Co., 1970.
75. Davies S, Heyman I, Goodman R: A population survey of mental health problems in children with epilepsy. *Dev Med Child Neurol* 45(5):292–295 2003.
76. Rodenburg R, Stams GJ, Meijer AM, Aldenkamp AP, Dekovic M: Psychopathology in children with epilepsy: A meta-analysis. *J Pediatr Psychol* 30(6):453–468, 2005.
77. Suris JC, Parera N, Puig C: Chronic illness and emotional distress in adolescence. *J Adolesc Health* 19(2):153–156, 1996.
78. Ott D, Siddarth P, Gurbani S, Koh S, Tournay A, Shields WD, et al.: Behavioral disorders in pediatric epilepsy: Unmet psychiatric need. *Epilepsia* 44(4):591–597, 2003.
79. Tuchman RF, Rapin I, Shinnar S: Autistic and dysphasic children: II. Epilepsy. *Pediatrics* 88(6):1219–1225, 1991.
80. Steffenburg U, Hagberg G, Hagberg B: Epilepsy in a representative series of Rett syndrome. *Acta Paediatr* 90(1):34–39, 2001.
81. Gabis L, Pomeroy J, Andriola MR: Autism and epilepsy: Cause, consequence, comorbidity, or coincidence? *Epilepsy Behav* 7(4):652–656, 2005.
82. Volkmar FR, Nelson DS: Seizure disorders in autism. *J Am Acad Child Adolesc Psychiatry* 29(1):127–129, 1990.
83. Caplan R, Siddarth P, Gurbani S, Hanson R, Sankar R, Shields WD: Depression and anxiety disorders in pediatric epilepsy. *Epilepsia* 46(5):720–730, 2005.
84. Ettinger AB, Weisbrot DM, Nolan EE, Gadow KD, Vitale SA, Andriola MR, et al.: Symptoms of depression and anxiety in pediatric epilepsy patients. *Epilepsia* 39(6):595–599, 1998.
85. Lambert MV, Robertson MM: Depression in epilepsy: Etiology, phenomenology, and treatment. *Epilepsia* 40(suppl 10):S21-47, 1999.

86. Torta R, Keller R: Behavioral, psychotic, and anxiety disorders in epilepsy: Etiology, clinical features, and therapeutic implications. *Epilepsia* 40(suppl 10):S2–20, 1999.
87. Harris EC, Barraclough B: Suicide as an outcome for mental disorders: A meta-analysis. *Br J Psychiatry* 170:205–228, 1997.
88. Brent DA: Overrepresentation of epileptics in a consecutive series of suicide attempters seen at a children's hospital, 1978–1983. *J Am Acad Child Psychiatry* 25(2):242–246, 1986.
89. Krishnamoorthy ES, Trimble MR, Sander JW, Kanner AM: Forced normalization at the interface between epilepsy and psychiatry. *Epilepsy Behav* 3(4):303–308, 2002.
90. Slater E, Beard AW, Glithero E: The schizophrenia like psychoses of epilepsy. *Br J Psychiatry* 109:95–150, 1963.
91. Krishnamoorthy ES, Trimble MR: Forced normalization: Clinical and therapeutic relevance. *Epilepsia* 40(Suppl 10):S57–64, 1999.
92. Mendez MF, Grau R, Doss RC, Taylor JL: Schizophrenia in epilepsy: Seizure and psychosis variables. *Neurology* 43(6):1073–1077, 1993.
93. Shaw P, Mellers J, Henderson M, Polkey C, David AS, Toone BK: Schizophrenia-like psychosis arising de novo following a temporal lobectomy: Timing and risk factors. *J Neurol Neurosurg Psychiatry* 75(7):1003–1008, 2004.
94. Parnas J, Korsgaard S: Epilepsy and psychosis. *Acta Psychiatr Scand* 66(2):89–99, 1982.
95. Kanemoto K, Tsuji T, Kawasaki J: Reexamination of interictal psychoses based on DSM IV psychosis classification and international epilepsy classification. *Epilepsia* 42(1):98–103, 2001.
96. Noeker M, Haverkamp F: Neuropsychological deficiencies as a mediator between CNS dysfunction and inattentive behaviour in childhood epilepsy. *Dev Med Child Neurol* 45(10):717–718, 2003.
97. Hemmer SA, Pasternak JF, Zecker SG, Trommer BL: Stimulant therapy and seizure risk in children with ADHD. *Pediatr Neurol* 24(2):99–102, 2001.
98. Hesdorffer DC, Ludvigsson P, Olafsson E, Gudmundsson G, Kjartansson O, Hauser WA: ADHD as a risk factor for incident unprovoked seizures and epilepsy in children. *Arch Gen Psychiatry* 61(7):731–736, 2004.
99. Dunn DW, Austin JK, Harezlak J, Ambrosius WT: ADHD and epilepsy in childhood. *Dev Med Child Neurol* 45(1):50–54, 2003.
100. Caplan R, Arbelle S, Magharious W, Guthrie D, Komo S, Shields WD, et al.: Psychopathology in pediatric complex partial and primary generalized epilepsy. *Dev Med Child Neurol* 40(12):805–811, 1998.
101. Williams J, Griebel ML, Dykman RA: Neuropsychological patterns in pediatric epilepsy. *Seizure* 7(3):223–228, 1998.
102. O'Leary SD, Burns TG, Borden KA: Performance of children with epilepsy and normal age-matched controls on the WISC-III. *Child Neuropsychol* 12(3):173–180, 2006.
103. Hoie B, Mykletun A, Sommerfelt K, Bjornaes H, Skeidsvoll H, Waaler PE: Seizure-related factors and non-verbal intelligence in children with epilepsy: A population-based study from Western Norway. *Seizure* 14(4):223–231, 2005.
104. Smith ML, Elliott IM, Lach L: Cognitive skills in children with intractable epilepsy: Comparison of surgical and nonsurgical candidates. *Epilepsia* 43(6):631–637, 2002.
105. Bourgeois BF, Prensky AL, Palkes HS, Talent BK, Busch SG: Intelligence in epilepsy: A prospective study in children. *Ann Neurol* 14(4):438–444, 1983.
106. Rodin EA, Schmaltz S, Twitty G: Intellectual functions of patients with childhood-onset epilepsy. *Dev Med Child Neurol* 28(1):25–33, 1986.
107. Farwell JR, Dodrill CB, Batzel LW: Neuropsychological abilities of children with epilepsy. *Epilepsia* 26(5):395–400, 1985.
108. Aldenkamp AP, Weber B, Overweg-Plandsoen WC, Reijs R, van Mil S: Educational underachievement in children with epilepsy: A model to predict the effects of epilepsy on educational achievement. *J Child Neurol* 20(3):175–180, 2005.
109. Austin JK, Huberty TJ, Huster GA, Dunn DW: Does academic achievement in children with epilepsy change over time? *Dev Med Child Neurol* 41(7):473–479, 1999.
110. Austin JK, Huberty TJ, Huster GA, Dunn DW: Academic achievement in children with epilepsy or asthma. *Dev Med Child Neurol* 40(4):248–255, 1998.
111. Aldenkamp AP, Alpherts WC, Dekker MJ, Overweg J: Neuropsychological aspects of learning disabilities in epilepsy. *Epilepsia* 31(Suppl 4):S9–20, 1990.
112. Seidenberg M, Beck N, Geisser M, Giordani B, Sackellares JC, Berent S, et al.: Academic achievement of children with epilepsy. *Epilepsia* 27(6):753–759, 1986.
113. Butterbaugh G, Olejniczak P, Roques B, Costa R, Rose M, Fisch B, et al.: Lateralization of temporal lobe epilepsy and learning disabilities, as defined by disability-related civil rights law. *Epilepsia* 45(8):963–970, 2004.
114. Rodenburg R, Meijer AM, Dekovic M, Aldenkamp AP: Family factors and psychopathology in children with epilepsy: a literature review. *Epilepsy Behav* 6(4):488–503, 2005.
115. Rodenburg R, Marie Meijer A, Dekovic M, Aldenkamp AP: Family predictors of psychopathology in children with epilepsy. *Epilepsia* 47(3):601–614, 2006.
116. Cheung C, Wirrell E: Adolescents' perception of epilepsy compared with other chronic diseases: "Through a teenager's eyes". *J Child Neurol* 21(3):214–222, 2006.
117. Austin JK: Comparison of child adaptation to epilepsy and asthma. *J Child Adolesc Psychiatr Ment Health Nurs* 2(4):139–144, 1989.
118. Austin JK, Huster GA, Dunn DW, Risinger MW: Adolescents with active or inactive epilepsy or asthma: A comparison of quality of life. *Epilepsia* 37(12):1228–1238, 1996.
119. Hoare P, Mann H: Self-esteem and behavioural adjustment in children with epilepsy and children with diabetes. *J Psychosom Res* 38(8):859–869, 1994.
120. Devinsky O, Westbrook L, Cramer J, Glassman M, Perrine K, Camfield C: Risk factors for poor health-related quality of life in adolescents with epilepsy. *Epilepsia* 40(12):1715–1720, 1999.
121. Mitchell WG: Social outcome of childhood epilepsy: Associations and mechanisms. *Semin Pediatr Neurol* 1(2):136–143, 1994.
122. Richards KC: Patient page. The risk of fatal car crashes in people with epilepsy. *Neurology* 63(6):E12–3, 2004.
123. Jalava M, Sillanpaa M, Camfield C, Camfield P: Social adjustment and competence 35 years after onset of childhood epilepsy: A prospective controlled study. *Epilepsia* 38(6):708–715, 1997.

CHAPTER 7.1.4 ■ LIFE-LIMITING ILLNESS, PALLIATIVE CARE, AND BEREAVEMENT

JOHN P. GLAZER AND DAVID J. SCHONFELD

PEDIATRIC PALLIATIVE MEDICINE

Some 500,000 children suffer from life-limiting illness and 50,000 die annually in the United States (1). This reflects two parallel trends: 1) the shift from acutely life-threatening infectious disease to chronically life-limiting noninfectious disease in pediatrics and 2) the expanding recognition of the need for, and capacity to identify and intervene with functionally impairing and distressing pain, depression, and anxiety, and the challenges to communication typical of these children and their families. Originating as "respite for weary travelers" in ancient times, the modern hospice movement began in the twentieth century with Dame Cicely Saunders' groundbreaking efforts at St. Christopher's Hospice, London, on behalf of adults dying of cancer, coming to the United States in the 1970s, proliferating rapidly, and only recently extended to children (1).

The term palliative care does not appear in the indexes of the first two editions of this text. It appears in the third edition in passing reference in chapters on pain and cancer. But pediatric palliative medicine has come of age in the new millennium and is the lens through which issues not only of death and dying but the more inclusive and accurate concept of *life-limiting illness* is now seen. This chapter addresses the principles and practice, from a psychiatric perspective, of pediatric palliative medicine by reviewing in a biopsychosocial fashion the major elements of diagnosis and treatment of children with life-limiting illness and their families. The term "life-limiting" deserves emphasis: Himelstein and colleagues (1) state that "palliative care is appropriate for children with a wide range of conditions, even when cure remains a distinct possibility." This broad view of palliative care, the notion that "palliative care is not all about death" (2) is recognized by the American Academy of Pediatrics practice guidelines: "the components of palliative care are offered at diagnosis and continued throughout the course of illness, whether the outcome ends in cure or death" (3). This crucial distinction recognizes both the unpredictability of medical prognostics and the role of hope, "the weight of a feather on the side of optimism" (4): the denial of hope differs from realistic appraisal and acceptance of life threat. While hospice and palliative medicine grew out of care for individuals with cancer, the scope is now much broader. Pediatric life-limiting illness is of course seen in a broad range of diagnostic categories, from cancer to chronic renal disease, cystic fibrosis, neurological disorders, mitochondrial disorders, sickle cell disease, and others. Pediatric palliative care services have recently been extended to the perinatal setting (5).

Himelstein et al. (1) have proposed the following "essentials" of pediatric palliative care (Figure 7.1.4.1): physical concerns such as pain assessment and management; 2) psychosocial concerns, including child and family fears, communication and coping styles; 3) spiritual concerns; 4) advanced care planning, including identification of decisionmakers, illness trajectory, care goals, and end of life care; 5) practical concerns regarding location of care and familiarity with the child and family's community and school environment; and finally, 6) bereavement care for families if the child dies. Communication with and among child patient and family members, and relationships between pain and psychiatric symptom expression, are central to the focus and expertise of the child psychiatrist in a medical setting, as is the grounding of care longitudinally. As such, child and adolescent psychiatry and pediatric palliative medicine are natural partners in the management of children with life-limiting illness as reviewed below.

SCOPE

This chapter addresses psychiatric aspects of pediatric life-limiting illness through review of cognitive-developmental acquisition of the concepts of death, assessment, and management of psychiatric symptoms, and management of pain in the life-limited child, as well as parental loss, the psychosocial needs of caregivers, and approaches to systems of care. "Palliative care" and "bereavement" are meant as inclusive terms: As children with life-limiting illness live longer, with advances in chemotherapy, transplant technology (see Chapters 7.1.3.1 and 7.1.3.2), radiation oncology and other modalities, old distinctions blur. To palliate is to "relieve pain and distress" without cure (6); as already noted, this definition is expanded to include children with life-limiting illness who survive and those who do not. Similarly, bereavement is "a deprivation causing grief and desolation, especially the death or loss of a loved one" (6). In addition to the 50,000 children and adolescents who will face their own deaths each year in the United States, another 4% of children will lose a parent before age 15 years (7). Professionals responsible for the care of children must address the psychosocial needs of children and families in all of these settings. Speaking to the experience of children and families with life-limiting illness more than 20 years ago, Solnit wrote that "the adults and the children don't know whether to prepare for life or for death" (4). The principles discussed here address the universal experience of separation and loss by children, whether they, their parents, or their siblings have life-limiting illness from which they may recover or die.

CHILDREN'S CONCEPTS OF DEATH

Children experience life-limiting illness in themselves or others through the prism of psychological, physical, and social development. Health professionals must therefore approach such children and their families with expertise in child and adolescent development and family systems (1). Central to this approach is an appreciation of the developmental acquisition of the concepts of death (8). The stages in children's understanding of the concepts of death have been well studied (9–13). Four major concepts related to death have been noted consistently: irreversibility, finality (also termed nonfunctionality), causality, and inevitability (also termed universality). Acquisition over time of a mature understanding of each of these concepts inevitably shapes a child's response to life-limiting illness in herself or loved ones. Speece and Brent (12) concluded that most studies found the age of acquisition of the three concepts they reviewed (irreversibility, nonfunctionality, and universality) to occur between 5 and 7 years; earlier studies citing an older age of acquisition typically were noted to have significant methodological flaws.

Since infants have been shown to respond to maternal depression with altered feeding patterns and failure to thrive, it is not surprising that they can similarly respond to the affective tone within the household after the serious illness or death of a family member (14). In this way, infants and toddlers are capable of reacting to someone else's death, even if they "understand" little of what has occurred. But once infants have developed object permanence, they are capable of appreciating the permanence of loss. It is therefore probably no coincidence that infants and toddlers engage universally in the game of peek-a-boo (or hide and seek) which has been suggested may be an attempt for children to understand and cope with separation and loss. Indeed, the translation for "peek-a-boo" from Old English is literally "alive-or-dead" (15, 16).

Infants, toddlers, and young children generally equate death with disappearance or separation. However, when faced with traumatic events, such as the death of a parent or other family member, some children 2–3 years of age or even younger have been able to demonstrate a beginning understanding of some of the concepts of death. In general, the role of personal exposure to the death of others has been controversial; although several studies have shown that such personal experience may promote the acquisition of the concepts of death (17, 18), other studies have failed to support this conclusion (19, 20). Cross cultural comparisons (21–23) have illustrated both cultural variations and important cross cultural consistencies, suggesting that although the underlying developmental framework is likely to be robust across cultures, sociocultural variables may have a significant impact on the rate of acquisition of individual concepts. In addition, developmentally based and conceptually focused education have been demonstrated to have a positive impact on children's rate of acquisition of these concepts (24).

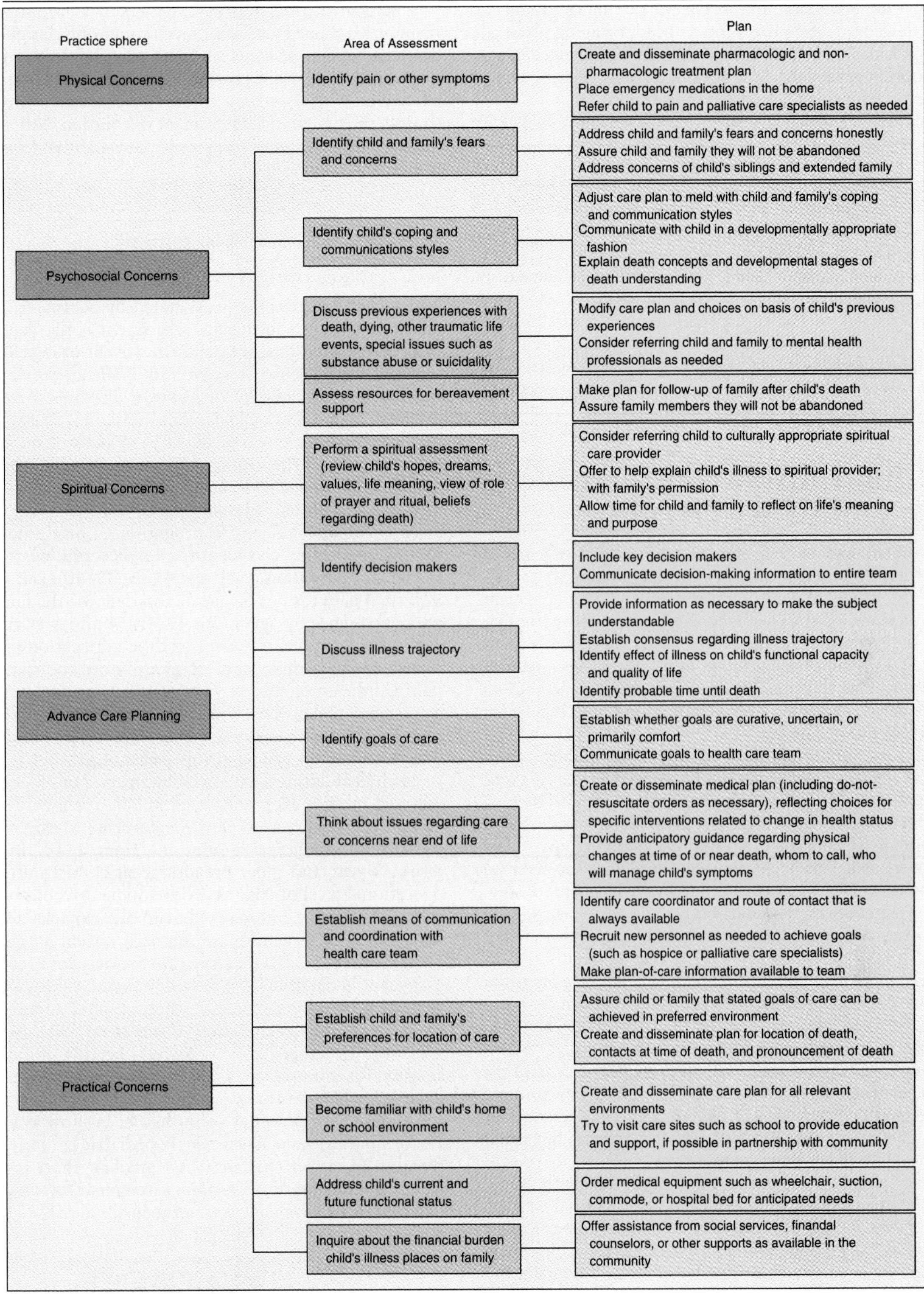

FIGURE 7.1.4.1. Essential elements in the approach to pediatric palliative care. (From Himelstein BP, Hilden JM, Boldt AM, Weissman D: Pediatric palliative care. *N Engl J Med* 22;350(17):1752–1762, 2004, with permission.)

From preschool age to early childhood, children continue to clarify their concepts of death but are still confused at times, remaining prone to misconceptions and literal misinterpretations. Children in this age group with a life-limiting illness have been shown to have a marked awareness of the seriousness of their illness, even if never told that their illness is fatal, and often develop a conceptual understanding of death more typical of an older child (25, 26).

During adolescence, reactions to life-limiting illness are influenced both by emerging formal operational cognitive capacities for abstract thought and by intense developmental striving for physical, sexual, social, psychological, and intellectual independence and mastery. Life-limiting illness turns this developmental process on its head, bringing physical immobility and dependence rather than independence, isolation from peers rather than the forging of new relationships, and may stop educational progress in its tracks.

Intervention

Study and recognition of the developmental acquisition of concepts of life-limiting illness and mortality by children and adolescents has led to effective tools for and approaches to intervention. The pediatric and child psychiatric literature increasingly reflect development of sophisticated, evidence guided approaches to the care of children with life-limiting illness and their families. These include the advent of multidisciplinary pediatric palliative care teams that strive to become involved early in illness trajectory (27), and specialized approaches to psychotherapy (28), among others.

PAIN AND SYMPTOM MANAGEMENT

Pain assessment and management is at the heart of care of children with life-limiting illness. The International Association for the Study of Pain defines pain as "an unpleasant sensory and emotional experience associated with actual or potential tissue damage or described in terms of such damage (29)". This definition has much utility for psychiatrists in its recognition that emotional factors are inherent and that its magnitude varies according to factors not limited to the extent of measurable tissue damage.

The historic undertreatment of pain in children and its adverse medical and emotional consequences is well documented (30). Eland's pioneering work in the 1970s (31) found in a chart review that of 25 children undergoing major surgery (traumatic amputation, nephrectomy, cleft palate repair) at a major children's hospital, 13 received no postoperative analgesia at any point in their hospital stay. Among the 12 children who did receive analgesic drugs, only 24 total doses were given, compared to 372 opioid and 299 nonopioid analgesic doses given to a comparison series of 18 adult postoperative patients. Reflecting prevailing attitudes toward the experience and management of pediatric pain, Swafford and Allen reported that just 26 of 180 children (14%) admitted to a pediatric intensive care unit over a 4 month period "required" opioid analgesia, stating "pediatric patients seldom need medication for the relief of pain. They tolerate discomfort well. The child will say he does not feel well or that he is uncomfortable, that he wants his parents but often he will not relate the unhappiness to pain" (32).

Pediatric pain management has improved with time, particularly after Anand and colleagues' influential studies in the 1980s showing that preterm infants undergoing surgery with minimal anesthesia exhibited marked, physiologically documented stress responses, with adverse effects on morbidity and mortality (33). However, adequate pain management in children with life-limiting illness continues to be a major challenge, best documented in children with cancer. Wolfe et al. (34) interviewed parents of 103 children dying of cancer at a major pediatric oncology center between 1990 and 1997 a mean of 3.1 years after the child's death, regarding symptoms and suffering experienced in the last month of life. Of the 103 children, parents reported that 80% were treated for pain in the last month of life but only 30% were treated "successfully." Noting that palliative care is now an expected standard, the authors caution that it is unclear whether the care of children with cancer meets that standard, concluding that "89 percent of the children experienced substantial suffering from at least one symptom, most commonly fatigue, pain, or dyspnea," treatment was "seldom successful, even in the case of symptoms that are typically considered to be amenable to treatment" (34) .Pain may mimic "psychiatric" symptoms (35); thus, in the psychiatric assessment of children with life-limiting illness, cancer or otherwise, pain assessment and management is a critical component.

Assessment

Pain assessment in children with life-limiting illness has recently been reviewed (36). As noted by Schechter (37), while developmentally appropriate assessment is the "cornerstone" of pediatric pain management, the advent of developmentally sensitive instruments is recent and challenges remain, including the limited capacity of younger children to report pain directly. McCulloch and Collins (36) include the following major factors in clinical pediatric pain assessment: 1) developmental stage, 2) intelligence, 3) personality, 4) temperament, 5) previous pain experience, 6) expectation and acceptance of pain, 7) child and parent coping strategies, anxieties, and cultural background, and 8) prognosis. Clinical studies suggest that most children can identify presence and location of pain by age 2, pain intensity by age 4 (36, 38–40), can participate in formal pain ratings by age 5, and describe the quality of the pain experience by age 8 (36, 41–43). Gaffney et al. (44) conceptualize pain measurement as "the application of a specific metric to some dimension of pain," note the challenge that pain is inherently subjective, and point out two fundamental assessment dimensions: 1) the sensory dimension of intensity, and 2) the affective dimension of level of distress. Any pain measure must specify what it is measuring.

In clinical settings, pain in children age 8 or older is typically assessed using a 10-point visual analog scale with "no pain" at one end and "most pain imaginable" at the other, with or without numerical gradations from 1–10. In Piagetian terms, 8 year and older preadolescent children at a concrete operational level of cognitive development would be expected to have a simple, internalized symbolic capacity to rate pain severity, thus the utility of numeric visual measures (36). Several well validated measures appropriate for preoperational 3–8 year old children have been developed, using cartoon faces at graded pain intensity (45), photographed faces ("Oucher" scale (46)) and poker chips ("pieces of pain (47)"). Pain measures developed for relatively healthy children (after surgery, for example) may be invalid when applied to seriously ill children (48). Fortunately, a measure specifically applicable to children with cancer as young as age 2 is now available (50). Performing *any* pain assessment in pediatric palliative medicine remains an unmet challenge: A Canadian chart review study found documentation of pain assessment in only 5 of 77 children (6%) who had died in the hospital (51).

TREATMENT

Pharmacologic

The cornerstone of addressing pain pharmacotherapy in adults is the analgesic ladder of the World Health Organization (52) shown in Figure 7.1.4.2, and is applicable to children (52, 53).

The WHO analgesic ladder grades pain severity and matches an analgesic category to each level: Acetaminophen or another NSAID for mild pain, the "mild" opiate codeine for mild to moderate pain with or without an adjuvant, and the potent opiates morphine or fentanyl with or without adjuvants

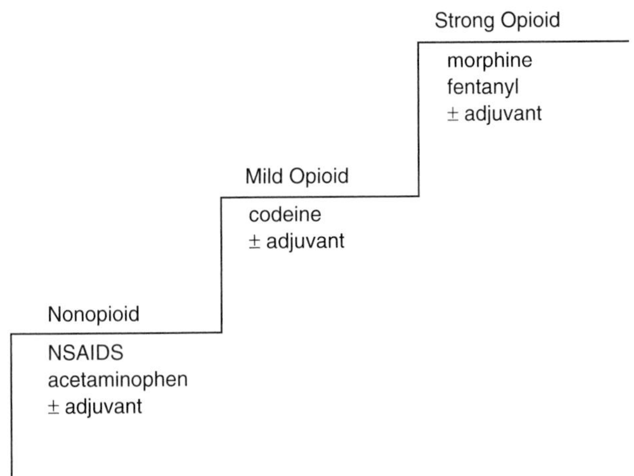

FIGURE 7.1.4.2. The analgesic ladder. (Adapted from World Health Organization Ladder: *Cancer Pain Relief and Palliative Care*, Technical Report Series 804. Geneva, World Health Organization, 1990.)

for moderate to severe pain. Caveats include avoidance of acetylsalicylic acid (aspirin) due to antiplatelet effects, agonist/antagonist opioids because of their ceiling effect, and the opioid meperidine (Demerol) because of toxic metabolite accumulation with extended use (54).

There are now many published studies of pediatric analgesic pharmacotherapy, but interpretation must be cautious because of the heterogeneity of populations studied, the small numbers of children at a given age (neonates to adolescents), illness severity, and etiological category (nociceptive or neuropathic) and the needed ethical constraints on clinical trials involving life-limited children (55). Drug pharmacokinetics and pharmacodynamics are age dependent (55) and analgesic response by drug category varies by mechanism. Thus, pain assessment and management must distinguish nociceptive (from tissue damage with an intact nervous system) and neuropathic (from damage to nervous tissue) pain, as well as being age specific (55).

Acetaminophen is the accepted standard bottom rung of the analgesic ladder, followed for moderate pain by nonsteroidals (NSAIDS) such as Ketorolac, now widely used in pediatric patients with safety and efficacy demonstrated by the oral and intravenous routes. Both acetaminophen and NSAIDS have opioid-sparing effects and are appropriate adjuvants in treating severe pain, with morphine or fentanyl at the upper rung of the analgesic ladder, both for additional analgesia and to reduce opioid side effects by allowing lower doses. Acetaminophen may be administered rectally in palliative care situations if the oral route is unavailable, provided dose and pharmacokinetic guidelines are observed (56). Monitoring for NSAID gastrointestinal, renal and hematologic toxicity is mandatory. Evidence supporting safety and efficacy of selective COX-2 inhibitors in children is not available and their use is not recommended.

Opioids are the mainstay of analgesic pharmacotherapy for severe pain in pediatric palliative care. Underutilization of opioids in pediatric pain management is common, and clinical studies establish the rarity of opioid dependence in appropriately treated medically ill children (57). Codeine, metabolized by the liver to an active morphine metabolite, is typically chosen for moderate pain, and morphine remains the opioid of choice for severe pain. Morphine is the only opioid for which safety, efficacy, pharmacokinetics, pharmacodynamics, and safety have been well studied in children (36). Morphine elimination half life with parenteral administration is about 2 hours in children, and much longer, 6–8 hours, in neonates (58). Oxycodone and hydromorphone are potential alternatives to morphine; these may be chosen when morphine side effects are limiting or analgesia inadequate (36, 59–61). The synthetic opioid Fentanyl has particular utility in palliative care settings in its transdermal form when oral or intravenous routes are distressing or otherwise limited. An important limitation of transdermal Fentanyl is that neither rapid dose adjustment nor effect offset are possible or predictable due to its absorption characteristics (62).

70 percent of adults with cancer pain achieve adequate analgesia with opioids (63) but special circumstances, particularly neuropathic pain, may require adjuvant pharmacotherapy. Adult trials demonstrating efficacy of tricyclic antidepressants and anticonvulsants for the treatment of neuropathic pain are the only systematic data available. Anecdotally, tricyclics such as imipramine and amitriptyline, and the anticonvulsants gabapentin and pregabalin have been used to treat pediatric pain but with no evidence base. Tricyclics lack antidepressant effects in children. If they are used for pain management, standard electrocardiographic and plasma level monitoring are mandatory. Psychostimulants have been reported to reduce somnolence in children with cancer (64) and to have an opiate-sparing effect in adults (65). Clinical wisdom suggests pairing adequate analgesia with alertness through the addition of psychostimulants to opioids in terminally ill children is desirable but systematic clinical trials have not been reported.

Psychological and Behavioral

"Health professionals cannot choose to avoid using psychology to treat pain." McGrath and coworkers' (66) formulation provides a useful working model of the role of an array of psychological interventions for pediatric pain management. The evidence base is limited but growing, and as McGrath (66) notes, "informal psychological interventions accompany every medical intervention ... our choice is whether to use psychology in a conscious, constructive fashion or to leave the psychological aspect of our interventions to chance." The task of pain management for seriously ill children is to have command of empirically supported psychological and behavioral treatments, integrate them with pharmacologic treatment, and understand the "myths (66)" that needlessly limit them, especially that the need for psychological intervention implies psychopathology.

Empirical support for psychological/behavioral pediatric pain management modalities is strongest for medical procedures and for headache (66).

Most fundamentally, controlled clinical trials demonstrate that the presence of parents with their children undergoing painful medical procedures reduces the child's distress (67).

Progressive muscle relaxation, first described by Jacobson (68), in which serial muscle groups are first tensed then relaxed, has demonstrated efficacy in treating pediatric medical procedure pain (69). Patients and parents typically like learning it, and it has no adverse effects, though muscle groups that have been the focus of tissue damage and pain should be avoided. Innovative clinical trials in adults show that training partners in such skills as muscle relaxation has both analgesic efficacy for the patient and enhances a sense of self-efficacy in the partner. Clinical experience suggests similar effects in pediatric pain management where the "partner" is a parent (70).

Jay, Elliott, and Katz (71), using a controlled repeated-measures counterbalanced design, studied a package of cognitive behavioral (CB) interventions including guided imagery, distraction, and deep breathing in 56 children with leukemia between ages 3½ and 13 years undergoing bone marrow aspiration. Compared to the control condition of 30 minute preprocedure cartoon watching, children in the CB group exhibited significantly less behavioral distress, self-reported pain, and lower heart rate during the procedure. Kuttner (72) reviews the evidence for hypnosis in treating pediatric pain and suggests benefit in children as young as age 3 years (73).

Appropriate use of empirically validated pediatric pain management techniques both pharmacologic and psychologic requires that they be embedded within "good clinical pain practice (66)", including the principles that pain is inherently subjective and the child's report of it should be taken at face value, that pediatric pain should be measured and monitored over time, that sick children should be told, in developmentally appropriate terms, what is going to happen to them, and that parents should accompany their children undergoing medical procedures. Finally, one would expect that family functioning and relationship quality would have mediating effects on pain control, as suggested by a recent study of pain management in adolescents (74).

Skilled and timely assessment and management of pain are necessary but often insufficient in the care of the child with life-limiting illness. Dyspnea, somnolence, nausea, vomiting and sialorrhea, among other symptoms, must also be addressed to assure the best possible quality of life even at the end of life. Two such measures are opiates to relieve dyspnea, and psychostimulants for opiate augmentation and promotion of alertness while maintaining analgesia (1).

ROLE OF THE CHILD PSYCHIATRIST

The evidence base guiding psychiatric intervention for children with life-limiting illness is limited but growing. The child psychiatrist should be guided both by wisdom accrued from years of informed clinical observation and practice and through an emerging understanding of developmental neurobiology, mediated by clinical judgment.

Psychiatric and psychological outcome studies most applicable to palliative care are those addressing the epidemiology of psychological and functional outcome of childhood cancer. Taken together, these studies consistently indicate a favorable psychosocial outcome for most children, with a small subset at risk for psychopathology (75–77). Koocher and O'Malley (75), for example, found 17% of 117 childhood cancer survivors had moderate or severe psychological sequellae. More recent studies have focused specifically on posttraumatic stress disorder as an outcome of life-limiting pediatric illness (78), a useful conceptual model. Finally, the limitations of categorical psychiatric diagnosis in pediatric psychiatry have been noted (79).

Pharmacotherapy

Pharmacotherapy for children and adolescents with life-limiting illness is an urgent priority where evidence is limited and attention and evidence growing. The topic has recently been reviewed (80). In one of the first clinical trials of pediatric pharmacotherapy in a medically ill population, Gothelf and colleagues (81) reported their experience with SSRI treatment of depression and anxiety in children with cancer. In this 8 week open label trial, fifteen 7–20 year olds with cancer were treated for major depression or an anxiety disorder with fluvoxamine 25 mg, increasing by 25 mg every 2–3 days until reaching a predetermined dose of 100 mg/day. All subjects were assessed with the Schedule for Affective Disorders and Schizophrenia (K-SADS) and screened for depression and anxiety with the Child or Beck Depression Inventory and the Screen for Child Anxiety Related Emotional Disorders (SCARED), respectively. For depression, 14 of 15 subjects showed a significant decrease in Child Depression Inventory—Revised scores from baseline to weeks 4 and 8 ($p<0.001$). Seven of 14 patients with major depressive disorder and 4 of 5 patients with anxiety disorders were judged by predetermined criteria to have achieved remission by week 8. Most subjects were in the early phases of cancer treatment yet 9 were judged to have survival probability of $\leq$ 30%, suggesting applicability to a palliative care population (81).

Psychological Care of Life-Limited Children

Very young children with a terminal illness are mostly preoccupied with the discomfort of the illness, whether acute or chronic, and the separation and withdrawal that occur when hospitalization is necessary. Somewhat older children, although also troubled by pain and separation, interpret their illness according to their level of cognitive and emotional development. Thus, school-age children may interpret the illness as an act of "immanent justice" for the guilt they feel about some real or imagined misdeed. Many children show regressive behavior in the face of serious illness, hospitalization, and its treatment. Excessive regressive behavior is uncomfortable for children as well as for those caring for them, and should be gently but firmly managed by the parents and hospital staff. Adolescents may deny psychological symptoms but exhibit outbursts of anger, anxiety, and sadness unpredictably. On the other hand, some children are astoundingly courageous and steadfast in the face of serious illness or death.

It is important to inform children with honesty about their health status, even though parents and healthcare providers may initially voice discomfort when children question or acknowledge an awareness of the seriousness of their condition. Children in turn perceive this discomfort in adults and may join parents and other caring adults in a mutual pretense that they are unaware of the seriousness of their condition, often in an attempt to provide support to their parents. Parents need to understand that children may fear the process of dying as much as death itself. Without the ability to communicate their concerns, children are left alone to deal with their worries and are deprived of possible supports and assistance with coping.

When informing children about their serious or life-threatening condition, it is best to do so in the form of a conversation over time, initially being sure to convey that they have a serious illness. The amount of detail provided depends in part on the developmental level of the child and his typical coping style; unnecessary details and graphic information are best avoided. It is important to avoid false reassurances, while maintaining a sense of hope. Children should be treated more as children living with a life-limiting illness than children dying of one—to the extent possible, it is important to optimize the quality of their remaining time, minimizing pain and discomfort, supporting their ability to sleep and eat, and allowing them to maintain valued routines with family, friends, school, and the community as much as possible.

Especially for young children who have a limited sense of time, focus initially on immediate and short term concerns; remembering that "dying soon" may be interpreted quite differently based on the child's perception of time. Given children's magical thinking and egocentrism, it is important to reassure children whenever possible of their lack of personal responsibility. Throughout the process of discussing their illness and its treatment, it is useful for adults to ask children to explain back what they have been told, in this manner, misconceptions and misinterpretations can often be identified and corrected.

Children who are terminally ill may at other times ask directly if they are going to die. Before answering the question, it is important to explore the likely motivation for such a question. If the underlying concern relates to a fear of pain or discomfort, then the child should be invited to communicate any pain or discomfort and be reassured that all measures will be taken to keep the child physically comfortable. If the underlying fear relates to abandonment, the child can be reassured that a family member will remain with the child throughout the hospitalization or time in hospice.

Patients—adults and children alike—feel threatened by the passivity imposed on them by illness. Every effort must be made to give children a feeling of active participation in treatment. Children should be informed at each stage what is being done, why it is being done, and what to expect. Children vary in their capacity to deal with the inevitability of their impending death or with a diagnosis that implies it (82). In some cases, older children and adolescents possess the cognitive and emotional maturity to render them competent to take part in even the most difficult decisions in their medical care, including the decision to forego life-sustaining treatment for terminal illness (83).

BEREAVEMENT

Loss of a Child

Potential Risk Factors

Rando (84) identifies several characteristics of the loss or the mourner that increase the risk of a complicated mourning process for adults. Several factors relate to the nature of the death: sudden, unexpected death, especially when traumatic, violent, mutilating, or random; death resulting from an overly lengthy illness; death of a child; and death the mourner perceives as preventable. If the premorbid relationship with the deceased was marked by anger, ambivalence, or excessive dependence or the mourner has unaccommodated losses or stressors or mental illness, then there is also an increased risk of a complicated mourning process. In addition, complicated mourning is increased if the grief is "disenfranchised" such that the mourner does not perceive adequate social support for grieving because of invalidation of the loss (e.g., early pregnancy losses which are often not met with much overt social support) or the relationship (death of an ex-spouse).

Anticipatory grieving allows parents and others to experience graduated feelings of grief, while being reassured by the child's continued presence when such feelings become overwhelming. In this manner, anticipatory grieving may allow some of the "work" of grieving to be completed prior to the child's death. Unfortunately, family members (and hospital staff) often engage in anticipatory grieving at a different pace. At times, a parent (or often a hospital staff member) may prematurely disengage from a child who is dying and be seen by others, including the child who is dying, as abandoning the child. Often, unacceptable thoughts arise. For example, parents may find themselves wishing that the child would finally die and relieve everyone of the emotional and financial burden and suffering. Such a wish may horrify a parent and lead to the immediate mobilization of certain defense mechanisms. A common defense mechanism is that of reaction formation whereby the parent becomes extra protective in caring for the dying child. The parent also may feel guilty and express his or her guilt (and anxiety) by asking repetitive questions that require tactful answers. As a chronically ill child nears death, the parents may be filled with remorse and may experience a resurgence of love. Rarely, a denial that death is imminent may remain in force. After the death of a chronically ill child, parents may feel a mixture of relief and guilt, perhaps with feelings of remorse being uppermost.

While it is critical to involve parents in decisionmaking regarding their child's treatment, the healthcare team should not use this as an excuse to avoid assuming the difficult responsibility of formulating treatment recommendations. In particular, when further treatment is futile and when the child is being maintained on life support, the healthcare team should convey to the family that the child has died and invite input from the family members about whether they would like to be present when life support is removed and their preferences on timing, without leading them to believe they are being asked whether they believe treatment is likely be effective or whether or not they "wish to allow (their child) to die."

Funeral Attendance

Parents should be provided information about the potential benefits for grieving children of attending funerals and participating in other observances and offered advice on how to provide support to children in these settings. Based on clinical experience, it has been shown to be helpful to advise family members to appoint someone, preferably who is not directly impacted by the death, that understands children's developmental needs and that the child knows and trusts to explain in simple terms what should be expected during the funeral or other ritual, to invite the child to participate to the level that he or she is comfortable, and to accompany the child throughout the event(s). This adult can then monitor the child's reactions and allow the child to leave the ceremony whenever desired. Children often can use the funeral rite in the same way adults do, especially if they have adults in attendance who can help them understand their feelings and describe what is taking place. Children who do not wish to attend the funeral should not be made to feel guilty. Rather, arrangements should be made for them to be in the company of an understanding adult during the time of the funeral. Older children should be encouraged to participate in the rites and rituals with the adults because these practices usually help them to deal with the reality of death and to access comfort and support from family members and friends. If older children choose not to attend the funeral, the reason for the choice should be explored, but if they continue to feel that they do not want to attend, this wish should be respected. Children should not be forced or coerced to participate directly in any portion of the ceremony that they find distressing, such as throwing dirt on the casket or kissing or touching the body of the deceased (85).

Advance Planning

As noted, comprehensive care of children with life-limiting illness is not limited to dying children. Whether the ultimate outcome is cure, chronic illness, or death, early intervention by the palliative medicine team is crucial: "Until we define the palliative medicine clientele as *all* children who have a life-limiting condition, even while they are receiving the most aggressive curative therapy possible, we will remain in the untenable position we are in: Palliative medicine teams are allowed in the door for children only when children are very close to death, far too late for the team to forge relationships (27)." Moreover, legal and ethical tensions and uncertainties often complicate end of life decisionmaking and take time to be resolved. Psychiatrists and ethicists may recognize the appropriateness of a competent adolescent to decline aggressive treatment, for example, but state laws may forbid it (1). Himelstein outlines four components to advance planning: 1) identification of the decisionmakers; 2) clarification of patient and parents' understanding of the illness and prognosis; 3) establishment of care goals: curative, uncertain, or comfort care; and 4) joint decisionmaking regarding use or nonuse of life-sustaining medical interventions such as mechanical ventilation, intravenous hydration or phase I chemotherapy. Clearly, decisions of this breadth and depth take *time*. Ideally, palliative care teams become involved early as partners of the primary team: "Palliative care teams work alongside of, not instead of, the primary team. Rather than taking over, they complement that team's efforts. They ease some of the burden of caring for and communicating with the family when complex medical and psychosocial decisions must be made (27)."

Special Situations

Parents and Siblings

Parents' response to the death of a child has been addressed in several studies (86). In a study of 21,062 Danish parents with a child who died, mortality from "natural" (cancer, cardiovascular, digestive) and "unnatural" (motor vehicle accidents and suicide) causes was statistically significantly higher 10–18 years after childhood death than in control parents who had not lost a child (87). "Bereavement" is classified in DSM-IV-TR as a "condition that may be the focus of clinical attention," not a psychiatric disorder per se, though clinical resemblance to major depressive disorder is common. Purported differences in symptom expression and impairment in "normal" and "complicated" grief may not be robust (88). Siblings also require clinical attention (89, 90). Active outreach to siblings is important prior and subsequent to a child's death. In particular, the impact on older children and adolescents of sibling death is often underappreciated. Parents who are themselves mourning and feeling overwhelmed may be reluctant to appreciate the suffering of the siblings and may in fact turn to them for their own support. It is vital for the medical team, whether hospital, hospice or outpatient based, to provide systematic, clinically sophisticated support and intervention either from a member of the palliative care team or through referrals to community-based psychological, pediatric, school-based (22, 92, 94) and if appropriate, religious resources. Critical to this process is the palliative care team's active followup contact with the family after the child's death.

Child's Loss of a Parent

Four percent of children will experience the death of a parent before their fifteenth birthday (7). Since adults as well as children with life-limiting illness are living longer, needed attention is being paid to the psychosocial needs of these children. After a review of the literature on bereavement in childhood, the Institute of Medicine (91) summarized the factors that are associated with an increased risk of psychological morbidity for children after the death of a parent or sibling:

1. Loss in a child younger than 5 years of age, or during early adolescence
2. Loss of a mother for girls younger than 11 years of age, and loss of a father for adolescent boys
3. Premorbid psychological difficulties in the child or lack of prior knowledge about death
4. When the relationship with the deceased had been conflicted or when the parent remarries and there is a poor relationship between the child and the stepparent
5. When the surviving parent is psychologically vulnerable and excessively dependent on the child, or the environment is unstable and inconsistent
6. When there is a lack of adequate family or community supports, or when the surviving parent is unable to access available supports
7. When the death was unanticipated or the result of suicide or homicide

Swick and Rauch (95) have described their innovative program Parenting at a Challenging Time (PACT), which provides consultation and intervention to adults with cancer who have young children (≤ 18), using a parent guidance model. "Clinicians can help the parents of these children facilitate their children's best possible adjustment by emphasizing the principles of facilitating communication, minimizing disruption, preserving family time, and attending to their legacy. Clinicians place their children's behaviors within the context of their developmental stage and help the parents find language and an approach that feels comfortable to them (95)."

Providers

Hospital staff members also experience anxiety in the presence of a dying child or a grieving parent, and they tend at times to deal with that anxiety by withdrawal and a conspiracy of silence. These reactions may impair their ability to give the dying child and his or her family the best care possible.

The death of a patient is one of the most stressful personal and professional experiences faced by healthcare providers. Clinicians need to understand their personal feelings about death in order to be effective in providing support to children who have experienced the death of a loved one, or who are faced with their own impending death. Often this will involve on the part of the physician some introspection about prior personal losses. But perhaps most important, healthcare providers should remain conscious of the impact that helping children who are dying or grieving has on both their professional and personal lives, and they should seek and establish means of meeting their own personal needs regarding bereavement.

Jellinek (96), Frader (97), and others have addressed the special challenges to physicians and allied professionals in the care of seriously ill children, particularly physicians in training. Biological and psychological patient outcomes, from glucose homeostasis to pain control, are strongly associated with the quality of provider–patient communication. Models for training physicians and allied professionals in patient-centered communication exist, have been evaluated, and are effective (98). Operationalizing provider communications training is challenging, but possible, and is now required in residency training programs by ACGME mandate. The new Cleveland Clinic Lerner College of Medicine has a structured curriculum with defined standards of professionalism and communication in which all medical students must demonstrate competency (99).

SUMMARY: PALLIATIVE CARE, RELATIONSHIPS AND MEDICAL EDUCATION

Bowlby's marriage of ethology, neuroscience, and psychoanalysis gave child psychiatry a language for understanding and investigating attachment, separation, and loss (100). This biological substrate, mediating and mediated by experience, is brought sharply into focus by life-limiting illness. Loss is universal, but the loss of a child—jarring, unexpected, and unnatural—is as severe a stress as the child or the child's parents can experience. Fortunately, clinical studies demonstrate that gravely ill children and their parents may both endure and even grow under the right circumstances at least some of the time. Hinds et al. (101) evaluated 10–20 year olds with advanced cancer within 7 days of one of three decisions: 1) whether to enroll in a phase I clinical trial; 2) whether to support a do not resuscitate order; or 3) whether to limit care to comfort measures and forgo life sustaining treatment. Both children and adolescents in the study understood they were making end-of-life decisions, and strikingly, expressed altruistic motives—the wish to help others unknown to them—in their decisionmaking, for example, participation in a phase I trial knowing it would not be lifesaving for them but could be for others. Similarly, Mack et al. (102) found in an interview study of parents whose children died of cancer that parent ratings of the quality of the child's care was directly proportional to the quality of physician communication. Parent-reported attributes of "quality communication" by physicians included providing clear information about what to expect at the end of life, conveying bad news sensitively, and including the child patient in discussion when appropriate.

Pediatric palliative medicine is an established, growing multidisciplinary subspecialty. Child and adolescent psychiatrists and psychologists as well as developmental-behavioral pediatricians and allied professionals are uniquely qualified to play key roles on palliative care teams with their special expertise in addressing issues of attachment, separation, and loss universally experienced. Historically, there has been little attention in medical school curricula to training students in the competencies necessary to provide quality communication and caregiving to life-limited children and their families; as noted, medical educators are recognizing and remediating this. Solomon and coworkers have pioneered pediatric palliative medicine curricula through the Initiative for Palliative Care (103). Such efforts must be encouraged, expanded, and their impact on the quality of medical education and clinical care systematically evaluated.

Acknowledgments

The authors wish to acknowledge Melvin Lewis, MB, BS, FRCPsych, DCH for his important contributions to earlier editions of this chapter.

References

1. Himelstein BP, Hilden JM, Morstad Boldt A, Weissman D: Pediatric palliative care. *New England Journal of Medicine* 350:1752–1762, 2004.
2. Hilden JM: Personal communication, 2006.
3. Palliative care for children. *Pediatrics* 106:351–358, 2000.
4. Solnit AJ: Changing perspectives: Preparing for life or death. In: Schowalter JE, Patterson PR, Tallmer M, Kutscher AH, Gullo SV, Perets D (eds): *The Child and Death*. New York, Columbia University Press, 1983.
5. Carter BS, Hubble C, Weise KL: Palliative medicine in neonatal and pediatric intensive care. In: *Child and Adolescent Psychiatric Clinics of North America*. Edited by Glazer J, Hilden J, Yaldoo-Poltorak D, Martin A. Philadelphia, PA, Elsevier Saunders, 2006, pp. 759–777.
6. *Stedman's Medical Dictionary*. Baltimore, Williams & Wilkins, 1966.
7. Rauch PK, Muriel AC: *Raising an Emotionally Healthy Child When a Parent Is Sick*. Chicago: McGraw-Hill; 2005.
8. Schonfeld D: Talking with children about death. *J Pediatr Health Care* 7:269–274, 1993.
9. Hostler S: The development of the child's concept of death, in *The Child and Death*. Edited by Sahler O. St. Louis, Mosby, 1978, pp. 1–25.
10. Kastenbaum R: The child's understanding of death: How does it develop? in *Explaining Death to Children*. Edited by Grollman E. Boston, Beacon, 1967, pp. 89–108.
11. Smilansky S: *On Death: Helping Children Understand and Cope*. New York, Peter Lang, 1987.
12. Speece M, Brent S: Children's understanding of death: A review of three components of a death concept. *Child Dev* 55:1671–1686, 1984.
13. Wass H: Concepts of death: A developmental perspective. In: Wass H, Corr C (eds): *Childhood and Death*. Washington, DC, Hemisphere, 1984, pp. 3–24.
14. Lansky S, Stephenson L, Weller E, Cairns G, Cairns N: Failure to thrive during infancy in siblings of pediatric cancer patients. *American Journal of Pediatric Hematology/Oncology* 4:361–366, 1982.
15. Betz C, Poster E: Children's concepts of death: Implications for pediatric practice. *Nursing Clinics of North America* 19:341–349, 1984.
16. Maurer A: Maturation of concepts of death. *British Journal of Medical Psychology* 39:35–41, 1966.
17. Kane B: Children's concepts of death. *J Gen Psychol* 134:141–153, 1979.
18. Reilly T, Hasazi J, Bond L: Children's conceptions of death and personal mortality. *J Pediatr Psychol* 8:21–31, 1983.
19. Jenkins R, Cavanaugh J: Examining the relationship between the development of the concept of death and overall cognitive development. *Omega* 16:193–199, 1986.
20. Townley K, Thornburg K: Maturation of the concept of death in elementary school children. *Educ Res Q* 5:17–24, 1980.
21. Florian V, Kravetz S: Children's concepts of death: A cross-cultural comparison among Muslims, Druze, Christians, and Jews in Israel. *J Cross Cult Psychol* 16:174–189, 1985.
22. Schonfeld D, Smilansky S: A cross-cultural comparison of Israeli and American children's death concepts. *Death Stud* 13:593–604, 1989.
23. Wass H, Guenther Z, Towry B: United States and Brazilian children's concepts of death. *Death Educ* 3:41–55, 1979.
24. Schonfeld D, Kappelman M: The impact of school-based education on the young child's understanding of death. *J Dev Behav Pediatr* 11:247–252, 1990.
25. Clunies-Ross C, Landsdown R: Concepts of death, illness, and isolation found in children with leukemia. *Child Care Health Dev* 14:373–386, 1988.
26. Spinetta J: The dying child's awareness of death: A review. *Psychol Bull* 81:256–260, 1974.
27. Glazer, JP, John P, Hilden, MD, Joanne M, Yaldoo-Poltorak PD, Dunya: Pediatric palliative medicine. In: Glazer JP, Hilden JM, Yaldoo-Poltorak D, Martin A (eds): *Child and Adolescent Psychiatric Clinics of North America*. Philadelphia, Elsevier, 2006, pp. xvii–xx.
28. Brown MR, Sourkes B: Psychotherapy in pediatric palliative care. In: *Child and Adolescent Psychiatry Clinics of North America*. Edited by Glazer JP, Hilden JM, Yaldoo-Poltorak D, Martin A. Philadelphia, PA, Elsevier Saunders, 2006, pp. 585–596.
29. Merskey H, Albe-Fessard D, Bonica J, et al.: Pain terms: A list with definitions and notes on usage. *Pain* 1979; 6:249.
30. Schechter NL, Berde CB, Yaster M: Pain in infants, children, and adolescents an overview. In: *Pain in Infants, Children and Adolescents*. Edited by Schechter NL, Berde CB, Yaster M. Philadelphia, PA, Lippincott Williams & Wilkins, 2003, pp. 3–18.
31. Eland J: The experience of pain in children, in *Pain: A Source Book for Nurses and Other Health Professionals*. Edited by Jacox A. Boston, Little Brown, 1977.
32. Swafford L, Allen D: Relief in pediatric patients. *Med Clin North Am* 52:131–136, 1968.
33. Anand KJ, Hansen DD, Hickey PR: Hormonal metabolic stress response in neonates undergoing cardiac surgery. *Anesthesiology* 73:661–670, 1990.
34. Wolfe J, Grier HE, Klar N, Levin SB, Ellenbogen M, Salem-Schatz S, Emanuel EJ, Weeks JC: Symptoms and suffering at the end of life in children with cancer. *New England Journal of Medicine* 342:326–333, 2000.
35. Heiligenstein E, Jacobson P: Differentiating depression in medically ill children and adolescents. *J Am Acad Child Adolesc Psychiatry* 27:716, 1988.
36. McCulloch R, Collins JJ: Pain in children who have life-limiting conditions. In: Glazer JP, Hilden JM, Yaldoo-Poltorak D, Martin A (eds): *Child and Adolescent Psychiatric Clinics of North America*. Philadelphia, Elsevier Saunders, 2006, pp. 657–682.
37. Schechter NL: The development of pain perception and principles of pain control. In: *Child and Adolescent Psychiatry: A Comprehensive Textbook*. Lewis M (ed): Philadelphia, PA, Lippincott Williams & Wilkins, 2002, p. 408.
38. Champion G, Goodenough B, von Baeyer C, et al.: Measurement of pain by self-report. In: *Measurement of Pain in Infants and Children*. Edited by Finley G, McGrath P. Seattle, Washington, IASP Press, 1998, pp. 5–20.
39. Hicks C, von Baeyer C, Spafford P, et al.: The faces pain scale revised: Toward a common metric in pediatric pain measurement. *Pain* 93:173–183, 2001.
40. Hunter M, McDowell L, Hennessy R, et al.: An evaluation of the faces pain scale with young children. *J Pain Symptom Manage* 20:122–129, 2000.
41. McGrath PA, Gillespie JM: Pain assessment in children and adolescents. In: *Handbook of Pain Assessment*. Edited by Turk DC, Melzick R. Guilford Press, 2001, pp. 97–118.
42. Shih A, von Baeyer C: Preschool children's seriation of pain faces and happy faces in the affective facial scale. *Psychol Rep* 74:659–665, 1994.
43. St-Laurent-Gagnon T, Bernard-Bonnin A, Villeneuve E: Pain evaluation in preschool children and their parents. *Acta Paediatr* 88:422–427, 1999.
44. Gaffney A, McGrath PJ, Dick B: Measuring pain in children: Developmental and instrument issues. In: *Pain in Infants, Children, and Adolescents*. Edited by Schechter NL, Berde CB, Yaster M. Philadelphia, PA, Lippincott Williams & Wilkins, 2003, 129.
45. Bieri D, Reeve R, Champion G, et al.: The faces pain scale for the self-assessment of the severity of pain experienced by children: Development, initial validation, and preliminary investigation for ratio scale properties. *Pain* 41:139–150, 1990.
46. Beyer J, Wells N: The assessment of pain in children. *Pediatr Clin North Am* 36:837–854, 1989.

47. Hester N, Foster R, Kristensen K: Measurement of pain in children: Generalizability and validity of the pain ladder and the poker-chip tool. *Pediatric Pain* 15:79–84, 1990.
48. Biersdorff K: Incidence of significantly altered pain experience among individuals with developmental disabilities. *Am J Ment Retard* 98:619–631, 1994.
49. Collins J, Devine T, Dick G, et al.: The measurement of symptoms in young children with cancer: The validation of the memorial symptom assessment scale in children aged 7–12. *J Pain Symptom Manage* 23:10–16, 1994.
50. Gauvain-Piquard A, Rodary C, Rezvani A, et al.: The development of the DEGR(R): A scale to assess pain in young children with cancer. *Eur J Pain* 3(2):165–176, 1999.
51. McCallum D, Byrne P, Bruera E: How children die in hospital. *J Pain Symptom Manage* 20:417–423, 2000.
52. World Health Organization Ladder. *Cancer Pain Relief and Palliative Care*. Technical report series 804. Geneva, World Health Organization, 1990.
53. World Health Organization. *Cancer pain relief and palliative care in children*. Geneva: World Health Organization 1998.
54. Goldman A, Frager G, Pomietto M: Pain and palliative care. In: *Pain in Infants, Children, and Adolescents*. Edited by Schechter NL, Berde CB, Yaster M. Philadelphia, PA, Lippincott Williams & Wilkins, 2003, pp. 539–562.
55. McCulloch R, Collins JJ: Pain in children who have life-limiting conditions. In: *Child and Adolescent Psychiatry Clinics of North America*. Edited by Glazer JP, Hilden JM, Yaldoo-Poltorak D, Martin A. Philadelphia, PA, Elsevier Saunders, 2006, p. 665.
56. McCulloch R, Collins JJ: Pain in children who have life-limiting conditions. In: *Child and Adolescent Psychiatry Clinics of North America*. Edited by Glazer JP, Hilden JM, Yaldoo-Poltorak D, Martin A. Philadelphia, PA, Elsevier Saunders, 2006, p. 655–656.
57. Berde CB, Ablin AR, Glazer J, et al.: American Academy of Pediatrics: Report of the sub-committee on disease-related pain in childhood cancer. *Pediatrics* 86:818–825, 1990.
58. Bhat R, bu-Harb M, Chari G, et al.: Morphine metabolism in acutely ill preterm newborn infants. *J Pediatr* 120(5):795–799, 1992.
59. Bruera EB: Randomized, double-blind, cross-over trial comparing safety and efficacy of oral controled-release oxycodone with controlled-release morphine in patients with cancer pain. *J Clin Oncol* 16(10):3222–3229, 1998.
60. Lawlor P, Turner K, Hanson J, et al.: Dose ratio between morphine and hydromorphone in patients with cancer pain: a retrospective study. *Pain* 72(1–2):79–85, 1997.
61. Moriarty M, McDonald CJ, Miller AJ: A randomized crossover comparison of controlled release hydromorphone tablets with controlled release morphine tablets in patients with cancer pain. *Journal of Clinical Research* 2:1–8, 1999.
62. Collins JJ, Dunkel IJ, Gupta SK, et al.: Transdermal fentanyl in children with cancer pain: Feasibility, tolerability, and pharmacokinetic correlates. *J Pediatr* 134(3):319–323, 1999.
63. Wiffen P, Collins S, McQuay H, et al.: Anticonvulsant drugs for acute and chronic pain. Cochrane Database Syst Rev 20:CD001133, 2005.
64. Yee J, Berde C: Dextroamphetamine or methylphenidate as adjuvants to opioid analgesia for adolescents with cancer. *J Pain Symptom Manage* 9:122–125, 1994.
65. Forrest WH Jr., Brown BW Jr., Brown CR, et al.: Dextroamphetamine with morphine for the treatment of postoperative pain. *N Engl J Med* 296:712–715, 1977.
66. McGrath PJ, Dick B, Unruh AM: Psychologic and behavioral treatment of pain in children and adolescents. In: Schechter NL, Berde CB, Yaster M (eds): *Pain in Infants, Children, and Adolescents*. Philadelphia, Lippincott Williams & Wilkins, 2003, pp. 303–316.
67. Bauchner H, Vinci R, Bak S, et al.: Parents and procedures: A randomized controlled trial. *Pediatrics* 1996; 98:861–867.
68. Jacobson E: You Must Relax. New York, McGraw-Hill, 1957.
69. Powers S: Empirically supported treatments in pediatric psychology: Procedure-related pain. *J Pediatr Psychol* 24:131–145, 1999.
70. Yaldoo-Poltorak D, Benore E: Cognitive-behavioral interventions for physical symptom management in pediatric palliative medicine. In: *Child and Adolescent Psychiatric Clinics of North America*. Edited by Glazer J, Hilden J, Yaldoo-Poltorak D, Martin A. Philadelphia, PA, Elsevier Saunders, 2006, pp 683–691.
71. Jay S, Elliot C, Katz E, Siegal S: Cognitive-behavioral and pharmacologic interventions for children's distress during painful medical procedures. *J Consult Clin Psychol* 55:861–865, 1987.
72. Kuttner L, Solomon R: Hypnotherapy and imagery for managing children's pain. In: *Pain in Infants, Children, and Adolescents*. Edited by Philadelphia, PA, Lippincott Williams & Wilkins, 2003, pp. 317–328.
73. Felt B, Mollen E, Diaz S, et al.: Behavioral interventions reduce infant distress at immunization. *Arch Pediatr Adolesc Med* 154:719–724, 2000.
74. Elliott E, Connell H: *Family cognitive behavioral pain management for adolescents: A process model to guide decisions and interventions*. Poster session presented at the International Symposium on Paediatric Pain, London, 2000.
75. Koocher G, O'Malley J: *The Damocles Syndrome*. New York, McGraw-Hill, 1981.
76. Wasserman A, Thompson E, Wilimas I, et al.: The psychological status of survivors of childhood/adolescent Hodgkin's disease. *Am J Dis Child* 1987; 141:626.
77. Fritz G, William J, Amylan M: After treatment ends: Psychosocial sequelae in pediatric cancer survivors. *Am J Orthopsychiatry* 1988;58:552.
78. Stuber ML, Shemesh E: Post-traumatic stress response to life-threatening illnesses in children and their parents. In: Glazer J, Hilden J, Yaldoo-Poltorak D (eds): *Child and Adolescent Psychiatric Clinics of North America*. Philadelphia, Elsevier Saunders, 2006, pp. 597–609.
79. Glazer JP, Ivan TM: Psychiatric aspects of cancer in childhood and adolescence, In: *Child and Adolescent Psychiatry: A Comprehensive Textbook*. Edited by Lewis M. Baltimore, MD, Williams & Wilkins, 1996, pp. 956–968.
80. Stoddard FJ, Usher CT, Abrams AN: Psychopharmacology in pediatric critical care, in *Child and Adolescent Psychiatric Clinics of North America*. Edited by Glazer JP, Hilden JM, Yaldoo Poltorak D. Philadelphia, PA, Elsevier Saunders, 2006, pp. 611–655.
81. Gothelf D, Rubinstein M, Shemesh E, et al.: Pilot study: Fluvoxamine treatment for depression and anxiety in children and adolescents with cancer. *J Am Acad Child Adolesc Psychiatry* 44:1258–1262, 2005.
82. Greenham D, Lohmann R: Children facing death: Recurring patterns of adaptation. *Health Social Work* 7:89–94, 1982.
83. Leikin S: A proposal concerning decisions to forgo life-sustaining treatment for young people. *J Pediatr* 115:17–22, 1989.
84. Rando T: *Treatment of Complicated Mourning*. Champaign, IL, Research Press, 1993.
85. Lewis M, Lewis DO, Schonfeld DJ: Dying and death in childhood and adolescence, in *Child and Adolescent Psychiatry: A Comprehensive Textbook*. Edited by Lewis M. Baltimore MD, Williams & Wilkins, 1991, pp. 1057.
86. Dyrgroven, A: Parental reactions to the loss of an infant child: a review. *Scand J Psychol* 31:266–280, 1990.
87. Li J, Precht D, Mortensen P, Olsen J: Mortality in parents after death of a child in Denmark: A nationwide follow-up study. *Lancet* 361:363–367, 2003.
88. Ginzburg K, Geron Y, Solomon Z: Patterns of complicated grief among bereaved parents. *Omega J Death Dying* 45:119–132, 2002.
89. Davies B: *Shadows in the Sun: The Experiences of Sibling Bereavement in Childhood*. Philadelphia, Brunner/Mazel, 1999.
90. Christ G, Bonanno G, Malkinson R, Rubin S: Bereavement experiences after the death of a child. In: *When Children Die: Improving Palliative and End-of-Life Care for Children and their Families*. Edited by Field M, Behrman R. Washington, DC, National Academies Press, 2003, pp. 553–579.
91. Osterweis M, Solomon F, Green M (eds): Bereavement: Reactions, Consequences, and Care. Washington, DC, National Academy Press, 1984.
92. Newgass S, Schonfeld D: School crisis intervention, crisis prevention, and crisis response. In: Roberts A (ed): *Crisis Intervention Handbook: Assessment, Treatment and Research*, 3rd ed. New York, Oxford University Press, 2005, pp. 499–518.
93. Schonfeld D, Smilansky S: A cross-cultural comparison of Israeli and American children's death concepts. *Death Stud* 13:593–604, 1989.
94. Schonfeld D, Lichtenstein R, Kline M, Speese-Linehan D: *How to Respond to and Prepare For a Crisis*, 2nd ed. Alexandria, VA, Association for Supervision and Curriculum Development, 2002.
95. Swick SD, Rauch PK: Children facing the death of a parent: The experiences of a parent guidance program at the Massachusetts General Hospital Cancer Center. In: *Child and Adolescent Psychiatric Clinics of North America*. Edited by Philadelphia, PA, Elsevier Saunders, 2006, pp. 779–794.
96. Jellinek MS, Todres ID, Catlin EA, et al.: Pediatric intensive care training: Confronting the dark side. *Critical Care Medicine* 21:775–779, 1993.
97. Frader, JE, Joel E: Difficulties in providing intensive care. *Pediatrics* 64:10–16, 1979.
98. Stewart M: Effective physician-patient communication and health outcomes: A review. *Can Med Assoc J* 152:1423–1433, 1996.
99. Fishleder A: Cleveland Clinic Lerner College of Medicine, personal communication, 2006.
100. Bowlby J: The making and breaking of affectional bonds. I. Aetiology and psychopathology in the light of attachment theory: An expanded version of the fiftieth Maudsley lecture, delivered before the Royal College of Psychiatrists. *Br J Psychiatry* 130:201–210, 1977.
101. Hinds P, Drew D, Oakes L, et al.: End-of-life care preferences of pediatric patients with cancer. *J Clin Oncol* 23:9146–9154, 2005.
102. Mack J, Hilden J, Watterson J, et al.: Parent and physician perspectives on quality of care at the end of life in children with cancer. *J Clin Oncol* 23:9155–9161, 2005.
103. Solomon MZ, Browning D: Pediatric palliative care: Relationships matter and so does pain control. *J Clin Oncol* 23:9055–9057, 2005.

CHAPTER 7.2 ■ SCHOOLS

JEFF Q. BOSTIC, BRADLEY STEIN, AND MARY SCHWAB-STONE

Schools are among the most valuable sites for child psychiatrists to promote mental health. Almost all children attend schools, where many of their unique needs can be addressed daily by committed professional school staff. Symptoms of psychopathology usually manifest across home and school settings, yet the range of interventions is often much wider in schools where classrooms, school staff, and instructional/behavioral approaches to the child can be configured to optimize the fit between child and school.

As psychiatric hospitalization continues to give way to treatment efforts in more naturalistic settings, schools have become primary venues for management of mental health by child psychiatrists. At one end of the spectrum, the *school psychiatrist* provides *direct* treatment to students or staff. This direct treatment usually occurs on site at the school and may include face-to-face evaluations of students or staff, individual or group therapy, or medication management. This allows teachers and staff to access the child psychiatrist for specific mental health issues, and allows the child psychiatrist to factor in the school's resources and philosophy in devising interventions. At the other end of the spectrum, the *school consultant* advises school staff, providing *indirect* services to students by assisting school personnel. The consultant may meet with administrators concerned about how best to respond to the death of a teacher, or to provide recommendations to help teachers work with students who have depression, attention deficit hyperactivity disorder, autism, or other special needs. Child psychiatrists often blend these roles, sometimes treating and advocating for a patient, and sometimes consulting to various school staff around complex problems (1).

Child psychiatrists will continue to become essential partners in schooling children, not just those children identified with psychopathology, but all children. The mental health consultant is often able to benefit many more children than would be possible through providing direct service on site at a school. Eight million children and youth are estimated to need mental health services in schools, yet less than one-fourth currently receive appropriate services (2, 3). Proactive efforts to prevent and impede psychopathology will continue to supplant treatment only after full blown psychiatric disorders or crises are evidenced. Child psychiatrists will continue to provide input on specific emotional disabilities, and increasingly promote mental health for all students, providing input on programs and principles found effective for everything from combating depression to decreasing bullying, and by working directly with educators to adapt effective treatments to diverse school environments (4).

EMERGENCE OF SCHOOL MENTAL HEALTH SERVICES

Mental health entwined with schools over the last half of the twentieth century following four significant social moments. First, after hundreds of thousands of refugee students were displaced at the end of World War II, Gerald Caplan used school-based interventions to assist teachers working with these students. Second, the civil rights movement in the 1960s brought about federal education rights legislation. No longer could schools require students with disabilities to fit into their existing programs. Systematic identification of students with emotional and behavioral disabilities began, accompanied by a need for clinical advice about assessing and treating these students in the least restrictive school settings. Third, increased social change in the late 1960s and wider recognition of problem behaviors among students, such as substance abuse, unprotected sexual intercourse, and more recently, bullying and school violence, caused schools to turn to mental health clinicians for advice. Fourth, the decrease in the 1990s in psychiatric hospitalizations and residential placements, coupled with the lack of access to mental health care among those most in need, resulted in proliferation of school-based mental health treatment, and delivery of psychiatric services within schools (5). Most recently the No Child Left Behind legislation has required intervention earlier for those students not progressing as expected. These events, and some important lessons learned from them, are provided in Table 7.2.1.

MODELS OF CONSULTATION

Multiple models of psychiatric consultation to schools have emerged, including the mental health model, the behavioral model, and the organizational model (6). These models are summarized in Table 7.2.2, as well as differences in their approach to the same problems. Regardless of the specific model, the child psychiatrist role appears broadening as collaborator, expert consultant, and partner in prevention, early intervention, and service delivery efforts (7).

Mental Health Consultation (MHC)

Mental health consultation (MHC) (8) stresses that the consultant's goals are both to be helpful with the problem at hand and also to provide the consultee new knowledge and skills to handle similar problems in the future. This type of consultation is frequently indirect, as the consultant may hear about a troublesome student from a parent or staff, and make recommendations to these staff, sometimes without ever seeing the student. The consultant is usually paid by the school, and the consultee is free to follow (or not) the consultant's recommendations.

Behavioral Consultation

Behavioral consultants attempt to change the behavior of teachers and students by focusing on: a) problem identification, b) problem analysis, c) plan implementation, and d) problem evaluation. During the *problem identification* stage, the consultant and teacher identify a specific problem to address.

TABLE 7.2.1

MAJOR EVENTS IN PSYCHIATRIC CONSULTATION TO SCHOOLS

Social Event	Mental Health Impacts on Schools	Child Psychiatry Response	Lessons Learned
Aftermath of WWII	Displaced orphan students required emotional support to contend with school	Mental health providers worked with educators to manage displaced students	Life events require mindful planning to promote mental health and resiliency in children
Civil rights movement	Equality for all, including those with disabilities, required schools to accept and respond to diverse students	Child psychiatrists identified psychiatric disorders that schools considered as possible educational disabilities	1. Psychiatric disorders did not necessarily "fit" educational disability categories 2. No consensual or empirical school interventions for identified disorders/disabilities existed
Social change and problem Behaviors	Problematic behaviors spilled into the classroom and interfered with schooling	Child psychiatrists provided input on lifestyle variables influencing quality of life	1. Little empirical evidence supported child psychiatry recommendations 2. Efforts to identify the prevalence of substance abuse and other problem behaviors helped illuminate mental health issues
Decrease in psychiatric hospitaliza-tion	Students managed in nonschool environments returned to schools to receive an education appropriate for them, given complex needs	Child psychiatrists focused on discharge planning to provide outpatient treatment, including in school settings	Psychiatrists and educators partnered, by necessity, to address mental health issues impacting children in daily environments

TABLE 7.2.2

CONTEMPORARY MODELS OF SCHOOL CONSULTATION

	Consultation Model		
Aspect of the Consultation	Mental Health Consultation	Behavioral Consultation	Organizational Consultation
Initial focus	Consultee's understanding of problem	Problematic behaviors exhibited by students/staff	How school contributes to problem
How information is obtained from consultee	Listen to staff's description of problem	Direct observation in classroom, counting frequency, length of specified behaviors	Review of school philosophy, curriculum, instructional philosophy, administrative procedures for problem class or group
Objective	Help consultee arrive at and implement new strategy/techniques	Help consultee measure problem behaviors, alter and shape student responses leading to problem behaviors	Help consultee refine organizational configuration and goals to diminish circumstances
Evaluation of model	Do students/staff identify and address specific issues? Do staff feel empowered/able to enact a solution?	Do specific problem behaviors diminish in frequency/intensity? What does "data collection" reveal?	Does this specific problem illuminate larger problems in policy impacting multiple students? Does the proposed solution benefit everyone?
Example case (17 year-old student who does not attend regularly the year after becoming a teen parent)	Consultee thinks back to when student attended, aware that family changes occurred, guides student to teen parent support services while adjusts schedule at school for student to attend later in day	Consultee keeps track of days/times missed, addresses directly with student, and they construct plan for student to be there on time by having others care for child on certain days; they measure success of plan, and revise as needed	Consultee identifies well intended but misattuned policies for attendance for current school population, and provide alternative schedule for students with children, course credit that can be completed at home, and course credit shifted to allow parenting study/work to count toward graduation

Usually, a "problem" occurs when the student's observed behavior is not what is desired and expected by the teacher or other school personnel. When a discrepancy exists between current and desired behavior, the consultant and teacher establish goals for the resolution of the problem, formulating the problem in behavioral terms. During *problem analysis,* the consultant and the school staff generate hypotheses about factors that influence the behavior and design a plan to solve the problem. During *plan implementation,* the consultant and school staff enact the plan and also collect data to measure how the problem behavior changes following implementation. During *program evaluation,* the consultant and school staff examine whether the goals have been attained, if new problems have arisen, and how the plan should be continued, modified, or phased out (9–11).

Behavioral consultation has advanced through the *collaborative problemsolving* model described by Greene and Ablon (12). This behavioral approach diverges from preexisting behavioral models by suggesting that students often lack a repertoire of other behaviors to employ when in complex situations, and so revert, almost inflexibly, to primitive or aggressive behaviors in such circumstances. Problem behaviors require adults (teachers or parents) to respond to the "message" attempted by the student's behavior, rather than efforts to stop the behavior immediately or to ignore or tolerate it. Rather than conventional reinforcement when desirable behaviors spontaneously emerge, or punishment when misbehaviors occur, desirable behaviors have to be identified, agreed upon by the student and teacher, and practiced so that they become familiar parts of the student's repertoire.

Organizational Consultation

Organizational consultation focuses on schools as systems and seeks to facilitate improvement in school functioning through the application of behavioral science concepts and the involvement of usually multiple system members (e.g., administrators and teachers) in the process of organizational change. Difficulties may emerge because of mismatches between the students and requirements of the educational system. Systemic problems such as communication breakdowns and ambiguity about responsibilities can cause anxiety and frustration among school staff, and impact student progress and behavior. Individual student problems may illuminate school system factors that contribute to the problem, and should be modified. For example, in one inner city charter school, a large number of students failed to graduate. During consultation it emerged that most students could not complete a swimming requirement, necessitating adjustment to this well intended, but misattuned, requirement. Models addressing low-achieving schools, such as the Comer School Development Program, precipitated school restructuring and change in school culture and climate, positively impacting student self-esteem, motivation, and achievement (13).

THE ROLES OF SCHOOL STAFF WITHIN SCHOOL CONSULTATION

Most commonly, child psychiatrists interact with schools to coordinate treatment for their patients. Establishing an effective partnering relationship with school staff usually most benefits patients, particularly if the school sees the child differently or resists making accommodations for this student. Child psychiatrists often need to be aware of the staff options at a patient's school so that helpful school staff can be accessed and empowered to address the patient's needs.

Roles of School Personnel

As the demands on schools have intensified, staff roles have changed, such that consultants must have realistic expectations about who can perform specific interventions with students as recommendations are provided. The consultee may be anyone within the school hierarchy, and the consultant must address these needs while being mindful of how the consultation will impact everyone else within the system. The consultant must also consider who is in a position to implement recommendations when providing consultation.

Teachers remain the front-line staff most involved with students. Elementary teachers usually have approximately 25 students for 6 hours each day. By middle school, teachers usually teach in a specific content area, providing instruction to approximately 150 different students each day. *Special education teachers* are credentialed to provide alternative instruction to smaller groups of students with learning disabilities, including dyslexia, nonverbal learning disorders, or emotional disorders that interfere with learning. For students to receive instruction from special education teachers, they must have an individualized education plan (IEP). *Aides* often do not possess a 4-year college degree or teacher certification, but may work under a classroom teacher, or work with a specific student who has different teachers.

School psychologists either are employed by the school or have a contract with the school to test and help construct individualized educational plans (IEPs) for students to address their specific learning difficulties. They may also provide individual and group therapy to students. *Guidance counselors* sometimes provide psychotherapy to students, although their primary role is to assist students in college or vocational planning and class selection. *School adjustment counselors and/or social workers* have been added to school staffs in many locations, where their primary role is to provide psychosocial treatments to students, and sometimes their families.

School nurses address acute health care needs of students, and administer medications to students; however, school nurses sometimes travel between several schools each day so that complex or frequent medication regimens become difficult.

Occupational therapists work with students individually or in small groups to help students with basic activities of daily living, and alternative strategies for students who have sensory integration issues to help them learn to cope with various stimuli. *Speech-language therapists* meet with students who have communication and social skills difficulties individually and in small groups.

School administrators liaison between the school and the community. *Principals* manage all services (from teaching to custodial) within their school building, and report to the superintendent. The *superintendent* guides educational activities among all the schools within a school district, and reports to an elected *school board* in public schools, or an appointed board in private, parochial, or charter schools.

ESTABLISHING A RELATIONSHIP WITH A SCHOOL

Schools today face great demands to impart knowledge, to prepare students vocationally, to socialize children to interact with others effectively, and to protect their health and safety. These varied, often competing agendas impact every intervention proposed by the child psychiatrist, regardless of the child psychiatrist's role "identified" by the school. Moreover, public, private, parochial, and charter schools not only vary widely in their priorities, but also in their system hierarchy and their accountability to the community. Familiarity with each individual school, its priorities, and its staff is a prerequisite to any meaningful consultation.

Evaluating a School

When the child psychiatrist has the opportunity to visit a school, a framework for evaluating the school can help discern the fit between that school and a particular student, as well as better match interventions to the culture of that school. Table 7.2.3 provides a sample approach child psychiatrists can use when entering a school. Awareness of the general reaction the consultant has to the school and its staff helps clarify the likely fit between a school and an identified student. Depending on the needs of the student, the child psychiatrist may employ relevant questions from Appendix A.

THE SCHOOL CONSULTATION PROCESS

The goal of school consultation is to build alliances and to share information that helps the school staff recognize and resolve problems. This process can be broken down into three tasks: 1) *allying with consultees;* 2) *aligning consultee objectives;* and 3) *mobilizing consultees to follow through with interventions* (14). Allying with consultees requires the consultant to empathize with consultees and to decrease their possible resistance. In aligning consultees, the consultant reframes people's comments, behaviors, or positions to establish unifying goals attractive to all participants. Mobilizing consultees to act requires the consultant to invest the participants in solving the problem and to empower consultees with the skills to be successful with the intervention. Consulting techniques helpful in accomplishing these tasks are described in Appendix B.

SPECIAL EDUCATION

Child psychiatrists often identify psychiatric disorders that require changes within the school setting for patients to benefit. The child psychiatrist is expected to identify specific disabilities (disorders) that impact a child's performance in the classroom, and to clarify changes, such as additional time for test-taking for students with ADHD, or deviations from certain readings for patients with mood disorders or writing activities in patients with nonverbal learning disorder. Child psychiatrists may recommend services, such as social pragmatics instruction in patients with Asperger syndrome, and may comment on educational settings, although child psychiatrists should not recommend specific placements for their patients. Based on services needed, the child's educational team is obligated to identify the most appropriate site for service delivery. Many options now exist for schools to educate students with psychiatric disorders, so the child psychiatrist must have some familiarity with the special education process, and the legal parameters surrounding educational planning for these students (15).

Special education refers to specialized instruction for students who cannot benefit from traditional classroom instruction. Eventually, all students will be appreciated as unique learners, as every child, wherever on the disability spectrum, deserves specialized instruction to optimize potential. Schools continue to become more sophisticated in addressing the needs of all their students, currently propelled by legal efforts to support education of each child in the United States. Legal protections have evolved beyond the equal protection clause of the 14th Amendment to the U.S. Constitution to provide every student with an appropriate education. Any child who is not progressing appropriately in school is entitled to an evaluation to determine if a disability is present, whether this disability interferes with school performance, *and* whether specialized teaching is needed. Anyone, including the student, the student's family, school staff, or a clinician (such as a child psychiatrist) can request an evaluation for a student. This eligibility process is summarized in Appendix C and Table 7.2.4.

The American with Disabilities Act and Section 504 of the Rehabilitation Act of 1973

The *Americans with Disabilities Act* (ADA) prohibits the denial of educational services, programs, or activities to students with disabilities, and prohibits discrimination against all such students once enrolled. If parents suspect their child has a disability, they may request an evaluation to determine if a disability is present and interferes with educational progress. This is usually provided in writing to the school's principal. A child with a suspected disability is usually referred to a child study team at the school to provide accommodations. Theoretically, *accommodations* refer to classroom changes that help the student meet requirements, without "lowering" academic standards.

Schools may generate an accommodation plan for such a student called a *504 Plan*. These plans derive from *Section 504 of the Rehabilitation Act* (1973), which ensures that all disabled children receive a "free and appropriate public education" (FAPE) in the "least restrictive environment" (LRE). Both the ADA and Section 504 are managed by the Office for Civil Rights; the focus of both is to ensure that all students have an equal opportunity to benefit from the educational opportunities available to students in a given school. ADA is broader since Section 504 only pertains to school districts that receive federal funding. Section 504 services apply to any person who has a "physical or mental impairment which substantially limits a major life activity" so schools often attempt a 504 plan for students with disabilities minimally impacting educational progress. Students qualifying for a 504 plan may receive special *accommodations* to help them meet educational requirements, usually within regular school classrooms.

The Individual with Disabilities Education Act (IDEA)

For students with more severe psychiatric disorders, additional safeguards have been provided by Public Law 94–142 (1975), revised as the *Individual with Disabilities Education Act* (IDEA), and most recently reauthorized in 2004 (technically as the Individual with Disabilities *Improvement* Act). IDEA extended a free appropriate public education to students with disabilities, mandating specialized instruction and related services if necessary to meet these students' unique needs. The IDEA defines "children with disabilities" to mean children with autism; deaf–blindness; deafness; emotional disturbance; hearing impairment; mental retardation; multiple disabilities; orthopedic impairment; other health impairment (ADHD historically has been included in this category); specific learning disability; speech or language impairment; traumatic brain injury; and visual impairment, including blindness. IDEA defines "emotionally disturbed" (previously called "serious emotional disturbance") as a condition having one or more of the following over a long period of time, to a marked degree, and which adversely affect educational performance: An inability to learn that cannot be explained by intellectual, sensory, or health factors; an inability to build or maintain satisfactory interpersonal relationships with peers

TABLE 7.2.3

FRAMEWORK FOR EVALUATING A SCHOOL

School Component	What to Observe	Potential Questions for Staff
School building	Safety/security: Does the building appear safe? Is the building comfortable (temperature, chairs beyond desks, lighting, noisy)? Does the building prize students (student art on the walls, recognition of student achievements, evidence of parent–teacher alliance)? Is this a place a child would want to be in?	How does one enter/exit the building? Where do students go if they are having a hard time? Where are students' classwork or projects kept or displayed? What happens after school is over? Do students stay in the building before or after school?
Classrooms	What do classrooms look like? How big is the room? How many students are in this room, and how many adults? How many learning areas are there, and are they separated so children can be in a quiet place within the classroom? How stimulating (visual, auditory, tactile) is this classroom, and do the students appear over/understimulated?	What's the average number of students in each classroom? How are teachers encouraged to set up their classroom? If a student is having a hard time in the classroom, where does he/she go? How did you (teacher) decide what to put up in your classroom?
School atmosphere	How is a stranger greeted? Does the school seem organized for students or for staff? Do most students appear engaged with instruction (students within classrooms, alert, attentive, answering/asking questions)? How do students and staff interact (smiling, directives, calm, tense)? Do children thrive here?	Whom should I meet when I enter the building? How do students move between classes/to lunch/recess? What do students do when they've finished classroom assignments? What do staff expect from students here? What do staff most worry about here regarding students?
School staff Administrators	Are administrators present/accessible? What kind of tone/impression does the administrator convey? Do staff appear comfortable around the administrator? Who does this administrator best serve (students, teachers, parents, other administrators)? What led to this administrator being selected for this building (student needs, up/down move for this administrator)?	What kind of interactions does the administrator have with students (discipline, earned reward time, common interests discussed in halls/lunch)? What is the administrator's priority in this building? What do staff seek from the administrator (support, camaraderie, ideas, discipline, avoidance)?
Teachers	Do teachers want to be in this school (eager to be with students or staff)? Do teachers stay in this building? How do teachers engage students (time to work, demonstrate content, model enthusiasm, surprise students)? How often do teachers alter the instructional approach (every 10 minutes, something different [lecture, student reading, class discussion], or employ different modalities [visual, auditory, tactile] employed during instruction?	How many teachers left this building last year? Average over the last several (5) years? What is the student : teacher ratio? What's the average length of time teachers have been in this district/building? How many teachers here have advanced (masters, doctoral) degrees? What kind of teachers do best in this school (independent, orderly, collaborative, creative)?
Special staff	Are other school staff present? How do teachers and other school staff interact (take student out, coteach, friendly/tense)? How do teachers describe other staff (particularly contributions of special educators)?	What kind of special educational staff work here? How often are they in this building (always, weekly)? What kind of other teachers are in the classroom (parent aides, "paraprofessional" aides)? Do they work with particular students, with everyone in the classroom. . . ?
Support staff	Are support staff friendly? Do they appear open about discussing the school and students? Do support staff work well with other staff?	What kind of support staff are in this building? How long have most of them been here? How are support staff paired with other staff?

TABLE 7.2.4

SCHOOL SERVICE PLANS FOR STUDENTS WITH PSYCHIATRIC DISORDERS

Type of School Service Plan	District Service Plan	504 Plan	Individualized Educational Plan (IEP)
Purpose	To respond quickly to mild changes in the student's life that impact learning; focus is on mild and/or brief circumstances that may impact learning	To ensure that all students have equal opportunity to learn, even if they have a disability; focus is student's opportunities as compared to other students in that school	To remediate symptoms of a student's disability; student's unique needs are the focus
Criteria to receive this plan	Student has a symptom or disorder that impacts learning	Student has an impairment that limits a major life activity, but may not require specialized instruction	Student has a disability which interferes with educational progress, and which requires specialized instruction
Who develops this plan	Teacher and administrator, usually with parental input	Teacher, administrator (often the school's designated 504 coordinator, school counselor and usually parent, student (if appropriate)	Educational team, including staff certified in special education; may include evaluations by school psychologist, social worker; parent may bring friends, advocates, own evaluators to be part of team
What is usually provided	Changes within classroom to enable student to perform better	Changes within classroom or school building to enable student to complete curriculum expectations	Changes within classroom setting(s) to provide student different instruction, and may substantially alter what is required of student
Example of what is provided	Student is allowed to sit closer to teacher during instruction; student is met by familiar staff to decrease anxiety	Student is allowed more time to complete tests; Student may be provided device to hear better	Student may leave regular language arts class and receive specialized reading program; student may be exempted from course requirements
Which staff deliver services	Usually regular education staff	Usually regular education staff	Staff with specialized training (special education teachers, speech therapists, occupational therapists)
Where the student receives services	Regular classroom	Regular classroom with regular peers "to the maximum extent appropriate"	Wide ranging, from regular education classrooms (inclusion) to pullout for special education classrooms, to offsite day school programs, to 24 hr/day residential schools
Review of the plan	As needed	Plan reviewed at least every year	At least every year plan is reviewed, and every 3 years the student is retested to see if still qualifies
Disciplinary actions	Usually not applicable	If "manifestation hearing" indicates student's impairment or disability caused misbehavior, then student cannot be suspended/expelled; school is not required to provide free, appropriate education for suspended or expelled students	If "manifestation hearing" indicates student's disability caused misbehavior, then student cannot be suspended/expelled; if student is suspended or expelled, school must still provide free, appropriate education
Appeal recourses	None provided	School may alter 504 plan immediately should circumstances indicate need; "notice" may be provided verbally; family may appeal to the Office for Civil Rights if perceive school is discriminating against child because of a disability	School must provide "prior written notice" before changes in educational plan or placement are made; family may appeal decisions or plan to local, then state, departments of education

and teachers; inappropriate types of mood or behavior under normal circumstances; a general mood of unhappiness or depression; or a tendency to develop physical symptoms or fears associated with personal or school problems.

In addition to having a diagnosed disability, to qualify for services under IDEA, the child must require *specialized instruction* (instruction from a special education teacher) because he or she is *not* making effective progress in school (which includes social and interpersonal progress–not just academic progress). If any of the above conditions are *not* met, the child is *not* eligible for IDEA services, but may be eligible for a 504 plan or for other services.

The evaluation for IDEA eligibility is more comprehensive than for a 504 plan. A multidisciplinary team of school-based professionals may conduct a comprehensive individual analysis of *all* suspected areas of disability. Usual components include assessment of the student's: 1) cognitive abilities; 2) communication abilities; 3) academic performance; 4) social/emotional status; 5) medical history/health status; 6) vision/hearing screening; and 7) motor abilities. Additional components (specialized evaluations) may be added as deemed necessary, such as intelligence testing, speech/language testing, achievement testing, neuropsychological testing physical examination, occupation/physical therapy evaluations, and psychiatric assessment (4). If the parent feels the evaluation is inaccurate, an independent evaluation may be requested, although the school is *not* "bound" to follow recommendations from an outside evaluator (including the patient's child psychiatrist).

The IDEA provides for educational services to include disabled children under the age of 6, and when necessary, up to the student's twenty-second birthday. IDEA ensures that all disabled children receive an *individualized education plan (IEP)* with parental input and consent, and includes due-process guarantees if parents disagree with this IEP or with the student's placement in an alternative setting or school. The IDEA prevented "troublesome" children from being refused admittance or from being ejected from a school because the school contended that it did not offer an appropriate program; instead the school *must* provide a free, appropriate education in the least restrictive setting. IDEA goes beyond Section 504 by allowing *modifications* so that the student does not, depending on that student's disability, have to meet the same academic requirements as students in regular education. For example, just as a wheelchair-bound student would not be required to meet physical education requirements applicable to students without a disability, students with a psychiatric disability might not be required to contend with upsetting curriculum content (PTSD), or complete the same amount of problems (ADHD), or participate in certain class requirements such as speaking in front of the class (social anxiety disorder). The multidisciplinary team devises the IEP; components of an IEP are provided in Table 7.2.5.

The authority of school officials has increased with subsequent amendments to the IDEA. At this time, administrators may immediately remove and place a student into an alternative setting if the student brings a weapon to school or to a school function, or if the student sells, uses, or attempts to buy drugs at school or at a school function. The alternative placement is decided by an emergency IEP team meeting. The amendments also include a provision for dealing with other conduct considered to be dangerous. School officials can suspend a child for up to 10 days (total within a school year) and in the interim ask for an expedited administrative hearing at which an order changing placement can be obtained on a showing by "substantial evidence that maintaining the current placement of the child is substantially likely to result in injury to the child or to others." This process can be repeated during a formal dispute by parents over the change of placement or of the appropriateness of the alternative placement.

Important protections for students have also emerged with amendments to the IDEA. For students with disruptive behaviors, the school may be required to conduct a *manifestation determination review* to determine if a student's misbehaviors are a result of a disability. For example, a child with Tourette's might not be able to sit still, or quietly, because of tics, or a student with bipolar disorder might not be deemed capable of speaking softly or remaining seated. The educational team must determine whether the student understood that his or her behavior was inappropriate, whether the student could control the behavior, and whether the IEP and placement had been appropriate. If it is determined that the misconduct was not a manifestation of the child's disability, the school may apply the same disciplinary sanctions to that child as apply to children without disabilities. If the conduct is found to be a manifestation of the disability, the school is obligated to continue programming, embodied in an IEP, in the alternative setting. Children subject to discipline, but who have not been evaluated for and/or identified as eligible for special education, but who are suspected of having qualifying disabilities are entitled to the same protections as children already found eligible.

The IDEA provides extensive procedural protections to parents of children with disabilities, including "the right to participate in the development of the IEP, the right to independent evaluations, the right to inspect educational records" and "the opportunity to present complaints with respect to any matter relating to the identification, evaluation, or educational placement of the child, or the provision of a free appropriate public education to such child." Such a proceeding, referred to as a *due process* hearing, requires a neutral adjudicator, a right to counsel at the parent's expense, and the right to present evidence and cross-examine witnesses. If dissatisfied, either party has a right to judicial review in the appropriate state or federal court.

EDUCATIONAL INTERVENTIONS FOR STUDENTS WITH SELECTED PSYCHIATRIC DISORDERS

Psychiatrists may be asked for specific classroom and school environment modifications by the school, the legal system, and/or the parents. The sample interventions in Table 7.2.6, derived from www.schoolpsychiatry.org, may be appropriate for particular students having various psychiatric disorders, depending on the needs of the child and the resources of the school. Such interventions should always be paired with the individual needs of each student rather than categorically applied to every student with that disorder, so interventions addressing several comorbid conditions are often required. Interventions may be adapted to a student's district service plan, 504 plan, or to an (IEP) as modifications/accommodations, or informally implemented in regular classroom settings. The success or failure of these interventions often helps clarify whether a child can remain in the current school environment or requires a different educational setting. While students are entitled to an education in the least restrictive environment, this parameter may necessitate a student receive instruction in a regular classroom, receive some instruction outside the regular classroom, receive all instruction in a self-contained special education classroom, go to a program at another site, or attend an off-site 24 hour/day residential school. Accordingly, the psychiatrist's report should clarify diagnoses ("rule-out" diagnoses are not helpful to schools), appropriate accommodations for symptoms that impair school progress, recommendations for services (e.g., social pragmatics training through speech therapy), and program recommendations (staff trained to work with students with autism spectrum disorders).

TABLE 7.2.5

COMPONENTS OF AN INDIVIDUALIZED EDUCATIONAL PLAN (IEP)

Component	Example	Comments
Usual Components		
Present level of functioning	"Although in the 5th grade, [student] is currently reading at 3rd grade level."	Both strengths and weaknesses should be described, with current functioning identified for each area of need requiring a goal
Educational goals	"In normal classroom discussions, [student] will repeat back accurately instructions for a task, 4/5 times daily."	Goals should include: 1) circumstances or setting; 2) observable behavior; and 3) performance measure, as well as staff person responsible for implementing
Educational accommodations and modifications	"[Student] will be allowed to take tests verbally or untimed."	Intervention necessary to allow student to access curriculum, or how curriculum will be modified
Special education and related services	"[Student] will receive specialized reading instruction 60 minutes/day for 4 days/week in the learning center."	Clarification of staff with special expertise to assist student and how that will occur (teaching, consult to teacher, group instruction)
Placement and participation specifications	"[Student] will receive reading, math, and social group instruction in a pullout resource classroom."	Least restrictive environment for student to receive services
Transition services planning	"[Student] will work at ______ 2 days/wk starting April 1st."	For all students by age 16, although may start at age 14
Transfer of rights planning	"[Student] is aware of right to participate."	Student informed, allowed to participate by age 16, and parental rights transfer when reaches age 18
Additional Components/ Related Services		
Adapted physical education	"[Student] will be allowed to ride bicycle for PE requirement in place of group PE."	Changes in physical education requirements based on disability
Behavioral intervention plan	"[Student] will access [staff] and follow deescalation steps when irritated."	A *Functional Assessment of Behavior* usually includes 1) antecedents to the negative behaviors, 2) specific negative behavior, and 3) consequences (benefits) of this behavior so that interventions can occur at any of these three points
Counseling services	"[Student] will receive 30 minutes of individual counseling per week."	Counseling is usually to help student function better at school; counseling may include parents or family training
Extended school year services	"[Student] will receive tutoring 2 hrs/day for 4 wks in summer."	Extended year services are required to "prevent regression" rather than to increase new skills throughout the year
Occupational therapy	"[Student] will receive keyboarding training."	Often includes additional training in activities of daily living; may also include special cushions, devices, or techniques to address sensory-motor symptoms
Physical therapy	"[Student] will practice writing with special paper and pencil."	Includes development of gross and fine motor skills
School health services	"[Student] will have blood pressure checked weekly."	Medication administration, vital sign or other check (blood glucose), or nutritional services may occur
Speech/language therapy	"[Student] will receive speech therapy with another student 30 minutes/wk to develop conversation skills"	Includes social-pragmatic training as well as training for dysarticulation
Transportation services	"[Student] will ride a van with an assistant."	May include special vehicles or configurations based on student's needs

TABLE 7.2.6

CLASSROOM INTERVENTIONS FOR SPECIFIC PSYCHIATRIC SYMPTOMS

Target Symptoms	Interventions	Examples
	To be Implemented by Teacher/School Staff	To be Adapted According to Student's Age, Interests, Capabilities
Anxiety		
Worry	Forewarn the student of transitions, and have "tasks" for the student to focus on during transitions.	If the student is worried about a school trip, provide tasks that distract from anxiety, such as checking attendance, or holding the door at the site.
	Devise a desensitization approach agreeable to the student.	If the student fears speaking in front of the class, allow the student to: have the speech read by a peer; read the speech into a recorder outside class; do the speech with a peer reading some part.
	Help the student examine other perspectives.	The student says "I can't go to the school dance because everyone will notice that I'm nervous." Ask the student: "How would your best friend/someone you admire handle a situation like this? What does your friend think you should do?"
	Provide the student with competing responses to negative thoughts or behaviors.	The student says "I'm afraid I'll start crying in class." Ask the student: "If you start to feel sad, what can you do before you start to cry? Can you distract yourself by doodling?"
Emotionality	Provide specific steps the student can take to relax, or provide a relaxation ritual.	Take three deep breaths; tense fingers or toes for five seconds, then relax.
	Provide alternative foci to distract the student from somatic symptoms.	Provide the student a phrase to think of or an activity (doing three problems then standing up, 10 problems then walking to the fountain).
Separation Difficulty	Provide desirable activity/responsibility for the student upon entering school.	Before school begins, allow the student to feed fish, clean boards, play with peers, or discuss music/sports with another student who shares interests.
	Provide times during the school day for the student to convey brief (30 second) messages to his/her family.	Have a brief script/message the student can phone to a parent ("Hi Mom, made it through Science—now we're going to make penguins in art class. I love you."); prepare the parent not to overreact to tearful messages.
	Have a parent send notes to the student to read as a reward for staying at school for increasing intervals.	Have a parent place a brief note to the student in his/her lunchbox that the student can read at lunchtime ("Dear [name], I know you're at lunch now—enjoy the cupcake. Have a great afternoon, and when I pick you up today we'll get to play soccer. Love, Dad").
Social Fears	Allow the student to observe several other students before attempting a task.	If the student resists speaking in class, allow the student to observe others, focusing on how they start, how long they speak, where they look, and how they stop.
	Have the student rehearse social skills in a smaller or more relaxed setting.	In a small group facilitated by a counselor, have students review and role-play how to make and keep friends. Give students homework to practice skills in other settings (classroom, playground, home play date, etc.).
Obsessive Thoughts	Establish acceptable teacher comments to "unstick" the student when he/she is obsessing.	With the student and parents, identify useful statements to break an obsessive cycle ("Move to your seat on 3—1, 2, 3." "Now think about your coach—what would he/she say to your "rut," "stuck moments"?).
	Allow the student to dictate or tape record if he/she cannot touch the pencil or paper.	Teacher or voice dictation software can "transcribe" the student's ideas to avoid touching/erasing the paper.

(continued)

TABLE 7.2.6

(CONTINUED)

Target Symptoms	Interventions	Examples
	To be Implemented by Teacher/School Staff	To be Adapted According to Student's Age, Interests, Capabilities
Compulsions	Allow the student to alter the work sequence.	If the student gets stuck doing problems in a certain way, allow the student to start with even numbers, or start from the end and work backwards to #1.
	Have the student identify and substitute less disruptive compulsive behaviors.	Allow the student to touch underneath the desk, flex fingers, or do versions of compulsions that are not disruptive to others.
Mood Symptoms		
Sad Mood	Check in with the student to quantify his/her mood status each day.	Allow the student to complete a mood scale (10 = very happy to 1 = very sad) at first check-in time each morning.
	Help the student identify "all the evidence" surrounding his/her negative perceptions of self or events.	Examine specific events that led to the student's conclusion that "I'm no good." "What happened that led to this conclusion? Did anything happen that disputes your conclusion? What else happened in your other classes that day?"
	Help the student identify automatic negative thoughts.	The student says "I'm no fun. No one wants to be around/play with me." Ask the student: "What happened that made you think this?" or "what evidence leads you to reach this conclusion?"
	Acknowledge the student's feelings (rather than dispute/argue with feelings).	"It's sad when . . . ," "discouraging," "frustrating" rather than "it's not so bad," or "aw, come on, things will be better soon."
Irritable Mood	Model appropriate responses to replace irritable responses.	Provide an alternative, appropriate comment: "I know you have something important to say, and I want to hear it, but I can't hear your point when you use sarcasm. It sounds like your point (without sarcasm) is ______." Could you please say your point again without relying on sarcasm?"
	Allow the student to take him/herself out of a situation (self-timeout) when irritability is starting to disrupt others.	Provide specific steps for the student to remove him/herself from situations ("I [student)] feel myself getting frustrated, so I am going to leave this kickball game and swing on the swings for five minutes. After I watch others, and think I understand what I'm supposed to do, I'll try kickball again.")
	Provide opportunities for the student to "fix" problems or inappropriate classroom behaviors.	Allow the student a chance to "redo" with an appropriate comment or behavior; if the student tears up paper, allow him/her to tape it together.
Manic Mood	Allow the student to complete schoolwork or tests in a less stimulating environment.	Identify a calm, comfortable area (with limited distractions, noise, and sensory stimuli) where the student can complete work/tests.
	Allow the student alternative modes of expression if he/she cannot verbalize in a useful way or is speaking too rapidly.	Provide the student with an opportunity to write, dictate, or draw ideas.
	Allow the student to have homebound instruction during manic periods.	Determine the conditions that warrant homebound instruction (for example, the student is sleeping during the school day while awake at night; the student's fears or delusions are causing conflicts in the classroom). Home instruction may need to be provided by specialized (therapeutically trained) staff.

TABLE 7.2.6

(CONTINUED)

Target Symptoms	Interventions	Examples
	To be Implemented by Teacher/School Staff	To be Adapted According to Student's Age, Interests, Capabilities
Appetite Changes	Encourage the student to use snacks and/or physical activity to enhance functioning. Change food reinforcers to nonedibles.	Provide snack breaks when the student finishes tasks. Encourage the student to be physically active at appropriate times by taking attendance to the office, standing and moving books, etc. Instead of chips or candy, reinforce the student with stickers, computer time, or points to earn a lunch date with a preferred peer (if increased appetite/weight).
Fatigue; Energy Loss	Augment classroom instruction with recordings of instruction.	Tape-record or videotape lectures and provide recordings to the student.
	Identify study partners who can support and assist with assignments.	Allow a peer to study with the student and to assist in academic assignments.
	Introduce physical activity throughout the day.	Provide the student physical responsibilities (taking attendance to the office, emptying trash, putting up class materials) throughout the day to encourage physical activity.
	Grade the student based on work completed or attempted (rather than work assigned).	Grade items completed (for example, even numbers only), and do not count the items the student does not get to (odd items).
Suicidal or Self-Harm Thoughts	Identify appropriate methods for expressing feelings of hopelessness or self-destruction.	Encourage the student to draw pictures, write songs or poems, or use sculpting to depict feelings of sadness, anger, or despair.
	Establish a hierarchy of people for the student and staff to contact if the student has suicidal thoughts.	Specify multiple staff and treatment providers, and the order or circumstances for contacting them, when the student is feeling or appearing unsafe.
Psychosis Symptoms **Hallucinations** **Delusions**	Identify and avoid the student's exposure to known distressing stimuli.	Clarify with the student or family the items, places, or topics that trigger delusional thinking and find alternatives, particularly when the student is stressed or currently experiencing psychosis symptoms.
	Allow the student alternative schoolwork or activities to avoid provoking delusions.	If the student cannot proceed with a task, provide an alternative, "grounding" task which requires little creativity, such as reading, moving items, or doing rote tasks.
	Devise steps to employ when the student is delusional or hallucinating.	Employ a series of steps to deescalate the student when he/she is becoming more delusional (first: change topic, second: change activity, third: change setting, fourth: change staff).
Attention-Deficit/ Hyper Activity Symptoms **Inattention**	Define classroom expectations in positive terms.	"Please sit down, get our your pencils and paper, and let's look at the board to find our first task."
	Give the student duplicate materials.	Keep a set of classroom materials in the student's desk and another set at home in case essential items are forgotten.
	Affix materials to the student's desk.	Keep regularly needed materials such as pencils attached to the student's desk where they cannot be misplaced.
	Provide organizational devices in the classroom.	Use colored folders to distinguish math vs. reading vs. social studies work; use a clipboard to hold papers or current activities.
	Keep a sample model of a correctly formatted paper for the student to refer to.	Keep formatted (even laminated) paper showing where name, date, etc., should appear on the student's assignments.
	Have the student repeat directions back to the teacher.	After giving directions, have the student repeat back the sequence.

(continued)

TABLE 7.2.6

(CONTINUED)

Target Symptoms	Interventions	Examples
	To be Implemented by Teacher/School Staff	To be Adapted According to Student's Age, Interests, Capabilities
	Provide check-in points during lessons.	"Raise your hand when you finish the first three problems, and we'll come by to check them."
	Provide untimed or extended time for tests or assignments.	Allow the student to work at his/her own pace, even "rest," so he/she can demonstrate all that he/she has learned.
	Diminish external distractions.	Minimize noise in the classroom by using headphones, tennis balls on chair legs, or rugs.
	Use a daily progress book or email between school and parents.	Send a small book or email between school and home to keep parents and teacher aware of the student's daily progress, and of any events that might influence the student's attention.
Hyperactivity	Clarify volume and movement expectations of the student before unstructured activities. Specify acceptable personal space.	"As we go through the hall, we'll only use our whispering voices if we have to speak, then in the lunchroom we'll remember to use our 'inside' voices." Clarify space boundaries with visuals such as "each person has the space of four tiles." Put tape on the floor to demonstrate that others stand outside this distance.
Impulsivity	Establish a waiting routine.	Develop with the student a multi-step plan for waiting, such as "count to five then raise your hand and look the teacher in the eyes."
	When behavior is inappropriate, first remind the student what he/she is expected to do, then reinforce efforts closer to classroom expectations.	During misbehavior, clarify what you want the student to do rather than describing the misbehavior ("next time you turn in a paper, make sure your name is at the top" instead of "don't turn in a paper without your name at the top").
Autism Spectrum Symptoms **Communication Difficulties**	Create situations to motivate language use.	Structure situations so that language becomes helpful (choose the flavor of ice cream from a list).
	Allow the student time to process information and respond.	Provide sufficient time for the student to understand direction and to respond (wait 10 seconds for student response).
	Ensure that the teacher is positioned strategically to engage the student's attention.	Align at the student's eye level. Touch the student's desk or chair while quietly saying something like, "Look at the ———(checklist or material) and listen. I need you to know..." Pause to give the student time to shift attention.
	Provide choice boards for the student to communicate preferred activities.	Show the student different options for tasks (picture of a book [for reading], food [for snack], counting cubes [for math]).
	Develop visual cues to reduce sensory overload.	Devise visual cues such as hand signals or use of pictures to diminish reliance on verbal and physical prompts.
	Use scaffolding techniques to promote spontaneous language.	Add "parts" (sentence starters, transition statements to connect ideas) to facilitate conversation with the student.
Difficulties with Social Interaction	Pair the student with a "typical" peer/buddy to help carry out social interactions in structured settings. Divide social skills into successive steps and teach the steps incrementally.	Team the student with a "typical" peer during a structured recess kickball game to show the student how to kick, run, and catch. Break down social encounters and teach multiple ways to accomplish each part (you can introduce yourself by saying your name, by asking what the other person is doing, by showing the other person an interesting object, by just saying "hi," or by having a friend who already knows someone introduce that person).

TABLE 7.2.6

(CONTINUED)

Target Symptoms	Interventions	Examples
	To be Implemented by Teacher/School Staff	To be Adapted According to Student's Age, Interests, Capabilities
	Provide explicit teaching about how to start conversations, respond to comments, and end conversations.	Describe specific phrases and behaviors to create conversations ("stand this far from a person, look at their eyes, say 'hi,' ask if they want to play four square with you," "say 'maybe another time' if they say 'no.')
Restrictive Routines/Interests	Provide alternative tasks, particularly when the student is sensory overloaded.	Allow the student several choices within his/her daily tasks. The student can choose the order of tasks, or when/where to take a break.
	Specify the student's routine for asking questions or describing topics when the student seeks or presents information.	Explain that the procedure for asking questions is to limit him/herself to two questions, then allow others to ask ("You can ask the two most important questions to begin work.")
Sensory Issues Includes extreme over-sensitivity or under-responsiveness to sound, light, or other sources of stimulation	To control sensory inputs, allow the student to be first or last in line or to leave class early.	Allow the student to change classes 5 minutes before the other students, or have him/her hold the door open for other students and then join the end of the line as the "caboose."
	Teach students who use distracting vocalizations or other self-stimulating behaviors to employ other intrusive vocalizations or behaviors.	Practice humming loudly and softly and have the student role-play appropriate times to hum loudly and appropriate times to hum softly.

From these recommendations the student's educational team can identify a specific placement to address the student's unique needs.

MENTAL HEALTH SERVICES IN SCHOOLS

Approximately 20% of students aged 6–17 years currently suffer from significantly impairing psychopathology (Chapter 2.2.1). Less than one-fifth of these students receive any treatment for these disorders. Minority groups and the uninsured are less likely to receive mental health services. One-quarter of public schools have no counselors, and over half do not have a social worker, yet schools are being asked to deal with more of the mental health needs of their students (16). In addition, reports of increased bullying and school shootings accent the importance of recognizing and responding to the psychic pain of students.

School psychiatry has expanded to address school violence, sexual harassment, bullying, substance abuse, discrimination, and discipline. New school arenas include the after-school setting, with increased rates of crime, drug use, and sexual behaviors during the afternoon hours when many youth are without adult supervision. Psychiatrists and other mental health professionals continue to refine child psychiatry's role in schools, incorporating business and educational principles in effecting change and improving system functioning. Modern school consultation focuses more on early identification and intervention at the individual and system levels to help attain short-term educational and behavioral goals and to prevent later long-term negative outcomes.

School-Based Mental Health Services

School-based mental health (SBMH) centers provide direct mental health services to students in about 1,500 (10% of) American schools. Prominent in New Mexico, Hawaii, Maryland, and Ohio, as well as Los Angeles, Dallas, Baltimore, and Memphis, SBMH has continued to proliferate and address the needs of students, particularly when they might otherwise not have access to mental health services. The Dallas Public Schools Family and Children's Centers (DPS-FCC) established a modern school-based health center in the United States in 1969, with mental health accounting for almost 50% of visits there. Students who have utilized the health centers have demonstrated better attendance, fewer discipline referrals, and achieved higher standardized test scores (7). The Baltimore School-Based Health Centers provides similar mental health care currently in over 40 school-based health centers. These sites provide direct service that allow students ready access to mental health services, and appear particularly important in school districts with a high percentage of uninsured and minority students. On-site school mental health services provide greater access to youth and their families, with less stigma and the opportunity for early intervention (17, 18).

Expanded SBMH incorporates the important elements of 1) school-family-community agency partnerships; 2) a full continuum of mental health education, promotion, assessment, prevention and intervention, and treatment; and 3) services for all youth in both general and special educational programs (19). Expanding on existing programs and personnel already present through collaborative relationships that establish seamless linkages between schools and agencies has become a favored strategy within SBMH (20).

Intervention and Prevention Programs

There are many prevention and early intervention models targeting both high-risk and all children in schools. Successful school models integrate the school, family, and community in coordinating services. Common elements in successful intervention and prevention programs include: youth being connected to a trusted adult, access and coordination of appropriate programs and services with ongoing evaluation, program continuity with school support, and emphasis on early identification and intervention. Psychiatrists can help schools identify and implement appropriate programs depending on the needs and resources of the school system. Kratchowill and colleagues (11) have identified useful Websites where clinicians can monitor programs as these programs evolve and as independent evaluations occur (Appendix D).

Universal prevention programs address the school system as a whole, and aim to improve the overall educational

TABLE 7.2.7

UNIVERSAL SCHOOL PROGRAMS PROMOTING MENTAL HEALTH

Name	Objective	Key Features	Outcome
Comer School Development Process (New Haven) Elementary school	To create a safe and supportive school environment through indirect service and system consultation	No-fault atmosphere, collaboration of all levels of school staff, health professionals, parents and community leaders, and consensus decisionmaking	Quasiexperimental and randomized control trials: increase in long-term academic achievement, better self-concept, improved class and school environment
PATHS (Promoting Alternative Thinking Skills) (24)	To promote skills that decrease violence and delinquency	~100 classroom lessons addressing emotional literacy, self-control, social competence, positive peer relations and interpersonal problemsolving skills	Emotional competence improved and aggression decreased; administrator support and teacher adherence important variables (25)
CAPSLE (Creating a Peaceful School Learning Environment)	To decrease violence, including bystander effects	Psychodynamic consultation about school system to alter patterns contributing to bullying/aggression: positive classroom climate campaign, teacher behavioral management, physical education promoting relaxing and self-defense, peer/adult mentorship	Decreased disciplinary referrals, school exclusions, increased student perceptions of safety (26) Improved student achievement scores in students attending CAPSLE schools ≥2 years (27)
Bullying Prevention Project (28)	To decrease aggression, violence, bullying	Zero tolerance of bullying, school staff, student and parent training for early identification and recognition of bullying, increased supervision of high risk areas, noncoercive school discipline, conflict resolution skills	Decreased bullying and antisocial behavior, increased social climate and positive attitude in classroom and school
FRIENDS Program (School-Based Cognitive Behavioral Treatment to Decrease Anxiety) (29)	To decrease stress, anxiety, and to promote self esteem, resilience, and positive relationships	10 classroom sessions providing CBT techniques to manage stress, anxiety	Controlled trials: Reduced anxiety symptoms, increased self-esteem (30)
School-Based Cognitive-Behavioral Treatment for Depression	To decrease negative thoughts and depression symptoms	Group sessions teaching relationship of cognitions, emotions, and behaviors, then student practice recognizing and replacing: social competence training	Inconsistent results; some decrease or stabilization in depression symptoms (31)
Signs of Suicide (SOS)	To reduce suicidal behaviors among youth	Youth view video to recognize signs of suicide in self and others, then respond by "ACT" (acknowledging, caring, and telling others)	Significantly lower rates of suicide attempts; greater knowledge about suicidality and more adaptive attitudes about depression (32)
Life Skills Training	To reduce substance use among youth	In class curriculum: 15 sessions first year, yearly booster sessions for self-management skills (decisionmaking and problemsolving), social skills	Decreased alcohol, marijuana, and tobacco use (33)
DARE (Drug Abuse Resistance Education)	To reduce substance use among youth	10 session curriculum with police officers teaching skills to resist influences to use drugs; "Plus" adds peer/parent sessions, reinforcing postcards mailed to families, extracurricular activities and neighborhood action teams	DARE: mild decreases in tobacco use (34) DARE PLUS: decreased substance use and violence among boys (35)
Gatehouse Project	To increase emotional wellbeing and decrease risky behaviors (e.g., substance use) among youth	10 week curriculum for 14-year-olds to address conflicting emotional responses and practice strategies for dealing with these	3–5% less substance use than nontreated peers (36)

TABLE 7.2.8

SCHOOL-BASED PROGRAMS FOR SPECIFIC MENTAL HEALTH ISSUES

Target Group	Program Name	Grade Level	Program Length	Skills/Components	Outcome Measurements
Social anxiety	SASS (Skills for Academic and Social Success)	9–11	14 sessions	Realistic thinking (1); social skills (5); exposure (5); relapse prevention (1); two unstructured sessions	Controlled trial: treated students less likely to meet social phobia criteria (37)
PTSD	CBITS (Cognitive Behavioral Intervention for Traumatized Students) (38)	6–8	10 sessions	CBT education, relaxation, imaginal exposure to stress/trauma; practice combating negative thoughts and using social problemsolving	Controlled trial: decreases in PTSD, depression, and psychosocial dysfunction symptoms (38)
Depression	IPT (Interpersonal Therapy)	6–12	12 sessions	Interpersonal skills; implemented with economically disadvantaged Latino girls	Controlled trial: decreased depression, improved functioning
Inattentive, disruptive behaviors (77% students had ADHD)	YESS (Youth Experiencing Success in Schools)	K–6	Biweekly parenting sessions; teacher inservice (6 hrs) and biweekly consultation throughout school year; clinician meetings with students	Parent training in behavioral management, "daily report card," monitoring of student's performance, procedures and rewards reevaluated	Controlled trial: Teacher and parent reported improvements in attention, grades, peer relationships (39)

climate and learning environment while inculcating skills useful to all students (Table 7.2.7). *Specific (selected) intervention/prevention* models are for students experiencing significant difficulty and are usually reserved for students who "screen" positive for significant impairment, rather than being administered to all students. Sample selected intervention programs are described in Table 7.2.8.

Video Consultation

Video technology has improved alternatives available to schools seeking psychiatric input, particularly those in remote areas with limited access to mental health services. Some of these programs provide indirect service to schools through consultation with school staff provided by a psychiatrist or psychologist around mental health issues impacting students (21). Video consultation can provide individual student evaluations, indirect consultation to teachers and school staff, and opportunities to demonstrate interventions for students whose psychiatric issues impair learning (22). Such technological advances increase options for collaboration with schools, although new problems such as billing, confidentiality parameters, providing consultation or treatment across states, receptiveness by staff and students, and potential losses of important observations by not being "in the room" must be anticipated when employing this modality (23).

APPENDIX 1

SCHOOL CONSULTATION FRAMEWORK

The psychiatric school consultant should consider how *micro problems can lead to macro solutions,* that is, how individual student problems can be addressed to improve circumstances for all subsequent students and staff. Five components should be considered in every consultation:

1. Who is the actual **consultee,** and what are the *confidentiality* parameters?
2. What is the Consultation **question,** and what is the consultee seeking and wishing will happen?
3. How is the larger **system** experiencing this problem?
4. What **legal or ethical factors** should be considered?
5. How does the consultant understand this problem **biopsychosocially?**

The Consultee and Confidentiality Parameters

The consultant must establish procedures to clarify who is appropriate to contact or to evaluate. When requested to meet with students, the consultant must obtain parental permission before interviewing any student. If parents refuse for the consultant to evaluate their child, the consultant may still observe the student unobtrusively, and consult to staff about their questions on how best to work with this student. Clarification of confidentiality should occur, sometimes recurrently, with staff, students, and parents. Anyone meeting with the consultant should understand how information is shared and whether written clinical information is placed in the student or personnel records.

Clarification of the Consultation Question and Needs/Wishes of the Consultee

Consultants help others define the problem and envision solutions. While consultees may ask for interventions to assist a student, sometimes they actually wish the consultant would address administrators, or recommend the student be removed from this consultee's classroom. Consultants must read between the lines to clarify both the consultee's overt request as well as underlying desires. The success of every consultation depends on the consultant understanding the consultee's concerns and wishes, such that both agree on the problem and on realistic goals for any intervention.

The System Reaction to the Problem

The problem will affect various school staff members differently, and each may have different goals for this consultation. Consultants should clarify who requested a consultation, who knows about the consultation, who has consented to the consultation, and who should be informed about the findings for this consultation. The more that differing goals can be aligned, the higher the probability that participants will invest in a proposed solution.

Legal and Ethical Factors

Special educational laws may provide the student different opportunities, yet families or schools may not see the applicability of such laws in a particular case. Similarly, the case may be confounded by ethical dilemmas, particularly in cases of suspected abuse. If abuse is suspected, the consultant may help staff articulate concerns to the appropriate agency, or assist parents and the school in addressing circumstances or staff perceived as abusive. In acutely dangerous situations such as suicidality or homicidality, the consultant can help consultees facilitate emergency treatment or how to warn others who may be at risk. Potential legal and ethical ramifications should be considered for every proposed intervention.

Biopsychosocial Understanding of the Problem

Child psychiatrists consider people's biologic vulnerabilities to psychopathology, their past experiences, and current family, peer, school, or other social stressors in explaining dysfunctional behaviors. These different influences may provide multiple intervention targets for a particular problem and should take into consideration existing services in the school and community. A student may need interventions biologically, psychologically, and socially, such as a referral for a medication evaluation, a behavioral plan at school and home, and connection to social groups such as sports teams, choir or band, or summer camps.

APPENDIX 2

SCHOOL CONSULTING TECHNIQUES

Ally

1. *Validate consultees' perceptions before proposing any solutions.* Validating perceptions cultivates consultee trust that the consultant understands their predicament. If in doubt, ask questions or pose solutions as questions ("What would likely happen if we...?").
2. *Bind anxiety.* Everything the consultant does either increases or decreases anxiety within the system. The more people who share the problem, the less anxious each individual will be. While consultants may not know the answer to various problems, thinking through how they would find an answer can diminish the consultee's anxiety.
3. *Create respect for everyone involved.* Minimizing splitting of staff, students, and parents decreases the probability that individuals will oppose an intervention. The consultant can attempt to separate personalities from the problem by focusing on terms used, by identifying the common goals between parties, and by identifying the circumstances each party uniquely faces.

Align

4. *Find the good intent gone awry.* When students or staff act inappropriately, the consultant can back up to the good intention that motivated the person's (mis)behavior so that self-esteem, and thus willingness to attempt different behaviors, is maximized. For example, if a teacher "yells" at students, the consultant can backtrack to the diligent efforts by the teacher to get the student's attention and to feel responsible that the student learns the material. Then the consultant is positioned to examine alternatives (visually signal the child, use a very soft voice), which will seem less critical of the teacher's yelling.
5. *Help others to see the child (or staff member) differently.* Maladaptive behaviors may be used to solve problems when no other solution is available (e.g., talking in class may be the only way a student "knows" to slow down instruction or to obtain positive attention from others since the student cannot garner positive attention by doing the academic task).
6. *Connect others.* To benefit the staff or student, by utilizing existing services in the school and community.
7. *Appeal to shared values by giving people options they cannot argue with.* Explore and identify appropriate desires of students and staff so that interventions can be provided to realize those appropriate goals. For example, identifying that a student seeks to attend college, or hold a particular job, provides a "frame" for posed interventions ("You've indicated you want to attend/work at _____, and they require you to show up on time, so we have to practice going to sleep at 10 PM so that you can be ready the next morning.").

Mobilize

8. *At every opportunity, expand the consultee's skills.* Whenever possible, the consultant attempts to assist the consultee in selecting and implementing skills helpful for that situation. The consultant aspires to provide the consultee facility with multiple skills that the consultee can use subsequently independently.
9. *Use the consultee's own words to frame interventions.* Framing interventions with terms used by the consultee, by staff, and by students, increases each person feeling heard, and improves the probability of each investing in proposed solutions.
10. *Identify one step up from the current situation.* Consultees may need help seeing the steps in a sequence toward appropriate behavior (e.g. cursing may be "a step up" from physically assaulting others). Even small positive changes generate momentum to achieve greater changes.
11. *Move toward anticipating problems rather than reacting to them.* Efforts to help consultees see how problems arise, and how they might be prevented in the future, can empower consultees to find and face problems early. More importantly, initial reactions may not represent optimal solutions, but instead create additional conflicts or problems.

APPENDIX 3

DETERMINING SPECIAL EDUCATION ELIGIBILITY

1. Does the child have *one or more of the following types of disability* (documented by medical evaluation/diagnosis, educational/psychological testing.)?
   - Autism
   - Developmental delay
   - Intellectual disability
   - Sensory-hearing, vision, deafness, blindness
   - Neurological
   - Emotional
   - Communication
   - Specific learning
   - Other health
2. If one or more of these disabilities is present, is the child *making effective progress in school?* If the student is being *reevaluated* to determine if a disability is still impacting the child, would the child continue to make progress in school without the currently provided special education services?
3. Is the lack of progress a *result of the child's disability?*
4. *Does the child* require specially designed instruction in order to make effective progress in school *or does the child require related services in order to access the general curriculum?*

APPENDIX 4

WEB SITES

Sites for:

Social-emotional competence	www.casel.org
Violence prevention	www.colorado.edu/cspv/blueprints
Substance abuse prevention	www.modelprograms.samhsa.gov
	www.drugstrategies.org/pubs.html
	www.surgeongeneral.gov/library/youthviolence/report.html
	www.nida.nig.gov/prevention/prevopen.html
HIV/AIDS prevention	www.cec.gov/hiv/projects/repo/compend.html

Sites for School Consultation

http://www.schoolpsychiatry.org: Mental health information for school staff, parents, and clinicians; interventions for psychiatric disorders and symptoms; rating scales to assess disorders and monitor treatments

http://smhp.psych.ucla.edu: Clearinghouse for important mental health, school, and education materials

http://csmha.umaryland.edu: Up-to-date information about school-based health centers

http://www.ldonline.org: Information on classroom changes for students with learning disabilities, including ADHD

http://www.ideapartnership.org: Up-to-date information on changes in the IDEA parameters

http://www.wrightslaw.com: Information about legal aspects of education, including IDEA 504 plans

References

1. Bostic JQ, Bagnell A: Psychiatric school consultation: An organizing framework and empowering techniques. *Child Adolesc Psychiatr Clin N Am* 10(1):1–12, 2001.
2. Kestenbaum CJ: How shall we treat the children in the 21st century? *J Am Acad Child Adolesc Psychiatry* 39(1):1–10, 2000.
3. Rappaport N: Emerging models. *Child Adolesc Psychiatr Clin N Am* 10(1):13–24, 2001.
4. Walter HJ, Berkovitz IH: Practice parameter for psychiatric consultation to schools. *J Am Acad Child Adolesc Psychiatry* 44(10):1068–1083, 2005.
5. Weist MD, Lever NA, Stephan SH: The future of expanded school mental health. *J Sch Health* 74(6):191, 2004.
6. Erchul WP, Martens BK: *School Consultation: Conceptual and Empirical Bases of Practice*. New York, Plenum, 1997.
7. Jennings J, Pearson G, Harris M: Implementing and maintaining school-based mental health services in a large, urban school district. *J Sch Health* 70(5):201–205, 2000.
8. Caplan G: Types of mental health consultation. *Am J Orthopsychiatry*. 33(4):470–481, 1963.
9. Putnam RF, Handler MW, Rey J, McCarty J: The development of behaviorally based public school consultation services. *Behav Modif* 29(3):521–538, 2005.
10. Kratochwill TR: Applied behavior analysis and school psychology. *J Appl Behav Anal* 27(1):3–5, 1994.
11. Kratochwill TR, Albers CA, Shernoff ES. School-based interventions. *Child Adolesc Psychiatr Clin N Am* 13(4):885–903, vi–vii, 2004.
12. Greene RW, Ablon JS: *Treating Explosive Kids: The Collaborative Problem-Solving Approach*. New York, Guilford Press, 2006.
13. Comer JP, Woodruff DW: Mental health in schools. *Child Adolesc Psychiatr Clin N Am* 7(3):499–513, viii, 1998.
14. Bostic JQ, Rauch PK: The 3 R's of school consultation. *J Am Acad Child Adolesc Psychiatry* 38(3):339–341, 1999.
15. Mattison RE: School consultation: A review of research on issues unique to the school environment. *J Am Acad Child Adolesc Psychiatry* 39(4):402–413, 2000.
16. Waddell C, McEwan K, Shepherd CA, Offord DR, Hua JM: A public health strategy to improve the mental health of Canadian children. *Can J Psychiatry* 50(4):226–233, 2005.
17. Bruns EJ, Walrath C, Glass-Siegel M, Weist MD: School-based mental health services in Baltimore: Association with school climate and special education referrals. *Behav Modif* 28(4):491–512, 2004.
18. Walrath CM, Bruns EJ, Anderson KL, Glass-Siegal M, Weist MD: Understanding expanded school mental health services in Baltimore City. *Behav Modif* 28(4):472–490, 2004.
19. Paternite CE: School-based mental health programs and services: Overview and introduction to the special issue. *J Abnorm Child Psychol* 33(6):657–663, 2005.
20. Health PsNFCoM: *Achieving the Promise: Transforming Mental Health Care in America*. SMA pub. no. 03-3832. Rockville, MD, 2003.
21. Harper RA, Santos CW: Teaching school consultation through video conferencing. Paper presented at: 29th Annual Meeting of the American Association of Directors of Psychiatric Residency Training, San Juan, Puerto Rico, 2000.
22. Young TL, Ireson C: Effectiveness of school-based telehealth care in urban and rural elementary schools. *Pediatrics* 112(5):1088–1094, 2003.
23. Whitten P, Kingsley C, Cook D, Swirczynski D, Doolittle G: School-based telehealth: An empirical analysis of teacher, nurse, and administrator perceptions. *J Sch Health* 71(5):173–179, 2001.
24. Greenberg MT, Kusche CA: *Blueprints for Violence Prevention: The PATHS Project*. Boulder, CO, Institute of Behavioral Science, Regents of the University of Colorado, 1998, p. 10.
25. Kam CM, Greenberg MT, Walls CT: Examining the role of implementation quality in school-based prevention using the PATHS curriculum. Promoting Alternative THinking Skills Curriculum. *Prev Sci* 4(1):55–63, 2003.
26. Twemlow SW, Fonagy P, Sacco FC, Gies ML, Evans R, Ewbank R: Creating a peaceful school learning environment: A controlled study of an elementary school intervention to reduce violence. *Am J Psychiatry* 158(5):808–810, 2001.
27. Fonagy P, Twemlow SW, Vernberg E, Sacco FC, Little TD. Creating a peaceful school learning environment: the impact of an antibullying program on educational attainment in elementary schools. *Med Sci Monit* 11(7):CR317–325, 2005.
28. Olweus D. Bullying at school. Basic facts and an effective intervention programme. *Promot Educ* 1(4):27–31, 48, 1994.
29. Shortt AL, Barrett PM, Fox TL: Evaluating the FRIENDS program: A cognitive-behavioral group treatment for anxious children and their parents. *J Clin Child Psychol* 30(4):525–535, 2001.
30. Stallard P, Simpson N, Anderson S, Carter T, Osborn C, Bush S: An evaluation of the FRIENDS programme: A cognitive behaviour therapy intervention to promote emotional resilience. *Arch Dis Child* 90(10):1016–1019, 2005.
31. Possel P, Horn AB, Groen G, Hautzinger M: School-based prevention of depressive symptoms in adolescents: A 6-month follow-up. *J Am Acad Child Adolesc Psychiatry* 43(8):1003–1010, 2004.
32. Aseltine RH, Jr, DeMartino R: An outcome evaluation of the SOS Suicide Prevention Program. *Am J Public Health* 94(3):446–451, 2004.
33. Botvin GJ, Griffin KW: Life skills training as a primary prevention approach for adolescent drug abuse and other problem behaviors. *Int J Emerg Ment Health* 4(1):41–47, 2002.
34. Ennett ST, Tobler NS, Ringwalt CL, Flewelling RL: How effective is drug abuse resistance education? A meta-analysis of Project DARE outcome evaluations. *Am J Public Health* 84(9):1394–1401, 1994.
35. Perry CL, Komro KA, Veblen-Mortenson S, et al.: A randomized controlled trial of the middle and junior high school D.A.R.E. and D.A.R.E. Plus programs. *Arch Pediatr Adolesc Med* 157(2):178–184, 2003.
36. Bond L, Patton G, Glover S, et al.: The Gatehouse Project: Can a multilevel school intervention affect emotional wellbeing and health risk behaviours? *J Epidemiol Community Health* 58(12):997–1003, 2004.
37. Masia-Warner C, Klein RG, Dent HC, et al.: School-based intervention for adolescents with social anxiety disorder: Results of a controlled study. *J Abnorm Child Psychol* 33(6):707–722, 2005.
38. Stein BD, Jaycox LH, Kataoka SH, et al.: A mental health intervention for schoolchildren exposed to violence: A randomized controlled trial. *JAMA* 290(5):603–611, 2003.
39. Owens JS, Richerson L, Beilstein EA, Crane A, Murphy CE, Vancouver JB: School-based mental health programming for children with inattentive and disruptive behavior problems: First-year treatment outcome. *J Atten Disord* 9(1):261–274, 2005.

7.3 ■ THE LAW

CHAPTER 7.3.1 ■ THE CHILD AND ADOLESCENT PSYCHIATRIST IN COURT

SARGHI SHARMA AND CHRISTOPHER R. THOMAS

This chapter is intended to serve as a guide for the child and adolescent psychiatrist who will need to work within the legal system; to help clarify and demystify the complex legal realm and hopefully empower child and adolescent psychiatrists when they interface this system (Table 7.3.1.1). Whether or not a child and adolescent psychiatrist has any interest in forensic work, there may come a time when he or she will have to deal with the legal system. There are many scenarios in which child and adolescent psychiatrists and the legal system may interact, involving not only those offering forensic testimony, but clinical practitioners with no intent for legal involvement. The chapter begins with a brief overview followed by sections that clarify the two distinct roles that a child and adolescent psychiatrist may serve within the judicial process. Many of the dilemmas encountered will not have a clear-cut answer and since factors within any legal situation are complex and often jurisdiction specific, it is more important for the child and adolescent psychiatrist to understand the general guiding principles and be able to apply them appropriately.

OVERVIEW

The court structure in the United States has both state and federal systems. The state and federal courts consist of general trial courts that can have appellate review. That means that at times a case can be decided by a lower court, but a party in the case can later appeal the decision or proceedings to a higher court. General courts in both systems handle criminal and civil cases. Civil cases encompass a wide variety of legal actions ranging from personal injury claims to breach of contracts, while criminal courts involve cases brought by the government against a defendant for allegedly committing illegal acts. Psychiatrists are increasingly being called upon to testify in cases involving children and adolescents for varying purposes in all types of legal proceedings.

The state legal systems also provide a series of specialized courts for matters that are better handled in a court of limited jurisdiction. Juvenile court is the type of specialized civil court that is most familiar to many child and adolescent psychiatrists. The creation of a juvenile court in 1909 focused on the rehabilitation of delinquents rather than their punishment and thus was meant to be different from adult criminal courts. The criminalization of juvenile justice over the past decades has resulted in what were previously adult forensic psychiatric evaluations, such as competency examinations, being requested in juvenile court.

The extent to which a child and adolescent psychiatrist needs to be familiar with the court system will depend upon their practice. Those who are involved in forensic work need to and will be held accountable to have an understanding of the various court systems and different procedures to a much greater extent than the child and adolescent psychiatrist whose only involvement with the court is when subpoenaed as a fact witness.

Many psychiatrists are understandably apprehensive of any contact with the court. Unfamiliarity with the processes and procedures of the judicial system is a major factor in these misgivings and anxieties. Most information child and adolescent psychiatrists have about the judicial system is based on fictional depictions from books, television, and movies, or from news reports about high profile cases. Imagine the distorted view others have of child and adolescent psychiatry based on the same sources and it is easy to see how unfamiliarity exists on both sides of psychiatry and the law. It is not only the difficulty of dealing with unfamiliar rules, but also very different approaches to evaluating information and making decisions from those used in medicine. While child and adolescent psychiatrists frequently must address conflict in the clinical care of patients, the methods of reaching resolution focus on reducing confrontation through amicable mediation or reconciliation. In contrast, the judicial system relies primarily on an adversarial approach, where opposing parties are allowed the opportunity to present their strongest arguments supporting their position and attacking the other so that a judge or jury may decide between the two. The aggression of cross-examination can be very intimidating and feel more like a personal attack rather than a dispute of ideas. Medical professionals are often baffled by judicial rulings that go against their opinions or recommendations when they fail to see that the court must consider and balance a wider range of viewpoints or evidence. Previous experience with litigious families and rising general concern about medical malpractice also add to misgivings about any contact with the courts for child and adolescent psychiatrists. As in any consultation setting, knowledge and practice can correct most uncertainties and improve the ability of the child and adolescent psychiatrist working with courts and attorneys.

TREATMENT OR FACT WITNESS

Process of Involvement

Subpoena

At times child and adolescent psychiatrists becomes aware of their role in a legal situation by way of a subpoena. A subpoena is a legal document that, in most cases, will result in being compelled to either appear at a specified proceeding, produce specified documents, or both. In most cases being served with a subpoena does not mean that the child and adolescent psychiatrist has done something wrong. Generally, it simply means that the recipient possesses information that is relevant to a legal dispute involving other parties. If the child and adolescent psychiatrist works for an organization, be it state or private, they should contact their legal department and inform them of the subpoena as soon as possible. If a recipient is in private

TABLE 7.3.1.1

DEFINITIONS OF LEGAL TERMS

Confidentiality:
Secrecy; the state of having the dissemination of certain information restricted.
Cross-examination:
The questioning of a witness at a trial of hearing by the party opposed to the party who called the witness to testify. The purpose of cross-examination is to discredit a witness before the fact-finder in any of several ways, as by bringing out contradictions and improbabilities in earlier testimony, by suggesting doubts to the witness, and by trapping the witness into admissions that weaken the testimony. The cross-examiner is allowed to ask leading questions, but is traditionally limited to matters covered on direct examination and to credibility issues.
Defendant:
A person sued in a civil proceeding or accused in a criminal proceeding.
Deposition:
A witness's out-of-court testimony that is reduced to writing (usually by a court reporter) for later use in court for discovery purposes.
Direct examination:
The first questioning of a witness in a trial or other proceedings, conducted by the party who called the witness to testify.
Expert witness:
A witness qualified by knowledge, skill, experience, training, or education to provide a scientific, technical, or other specialized opinion about the evidence or a fact issue.
Fact witness:
A witness who may testify only to information that is based on firsthand knowledge.
Guardian ad litem:
A caretaker, usually a lawyer, appointed by the court to appear in a lawsuit on behalf of an incompetent or minor party.
Plaintiff:
The party who brings a civil suit in a court of law.
Preponderance of evidence:
The greater weight of the evidence; superior evidentiary weight that, though not sufficient to free the mind wholly from all reasonable doubt, is still sufficient to incline a fair and impartial mind to one side of the issue rather than the other. It is also referred to as preponderance of proof or balance of probability.
Privilege:
A special legal right, exemption, or immunity granted to a person or class of persons; an exception to a duty.
Reasonable doubt:
The doubt that prevents one from being firmly convinced of a defendant's guilt, or the belief that there is a real possibility that a defendant is not guilty.
Redirect examination:
A second examination, after cross-examination, the scope ordinarily being limited to matters covered during cross-examination.
Subpoena:
A writ commanding a person to appear before a court or other tribunal, subject to a penalty for failing to comply.
Subpoena duces tecum:
A subpoena ordering the witness to appear and to bring specified documents or records.
Voir dire:
A preliminary examination to determine the qualifications of a prospective witness or evidence.

practice, s/he may want to discuss the subpoena with an attorney as it may have later implications related to another type of legal claim. The attorney named on the subpoena does not need to be contacted, but may be called to clarify the reason for the issuance of the request. While the child and adolescent psychiatrist may ask the attorney questions about the pending legal case, it is important to remember that attorneys, including those who work for the state or other government agencies, can lack an understanding of privacy laws that direct clinical practice disclosure of information regarding protected health information. It is possible for the child and adolescent psychiatrist to violate the Health Insurance Portability and Accountability Act (HIPAA) Privacy Rule under these circumstances, as subpoenas do not necessarily provide the authority to release confidential personal health information.

When it is time for the child and adolescent psychiatrist to provide the information requested in the subpoena, he or she needs to ensure that the patient or the individual who controls the privilege, as in the case of a minor child, has consented to the information's release, there has been a judicial determination that the privilege does not apply or has been waived by some conduct of the patient's, such as making their mental health a part of the legal claim. If there has been no waiver by the patient or when it is uncertain who has the ability to consent, such as in the course of custody disputes or with divorced parents, the child and adolescent psychiatrist should contact the issuing attorney to notify him or her that they will not be able to provide any information about the patient without authorization by the patient, the valid representative, or a court order. If the child and adolescent psychiatrist is not provided with any of the above, then he or she must still appear at the court proceeding or deposition and provide information about himself, but when asked information regarding the patient the psychiatrist would respond that the information is confidential and privileged and follow the direction of the judge if in court (1).

There are occasions when the underlying legal dispute may involve, or have the potential to involve, professional liability claims that could expose the practitioner to legal liabilities and would involve different HIPAA regulations that are not covered in this chapter and for which the reader is referred to Chapter 7.3.4 on medical malpractice.

As mentioned above, the subpoena could also require the production of all the relevant medical records. Child and adolescent psychiatrists that work for an institution or do contract work are not responsible for maintaining the information and will not be the custodian of record for the medical records. They would thus not have any documents that are responsive to a subpoena. For clinicians in private practice however, arrangements for the entire medical record that is responsive to the subpoena must be made available.

The child and adolescent psychiatrist may be asked by the family of their patients or the patients themselves to provide legal testimony regarding psychiatric treatment rendered. This may at times be appropriate to agree to as it may offer more flexibility regarding appearance versus a subpoena. However, when the testimony requested is regarding an expert opinion and not a rendition of treatment facts, the requesting party should be informed of the impropriety of the request and that this type of service is best handled by a nontreating psychiatrist. Further information regarding the role of forensic testimony by child and adolescent psychiatrists is detailed in the following section. The child and adolescent psychiatrist should avoid serving as both treating clinician and forensic expert for any given individual.

General Court Procedures

For the child and adolescent psychiatrist who has never been to court before, it is strongly recommended to visit the courthouse prior to testifying. Knowing where to park, where the courtroom in located, where to sit, and the general layout of the courtroom can be helpful to alleviate anxiety and increase the overall comfort level. Juvenile, or family, courts are generally not open to the public and only the parties involved in the current case are allowed attendance without prior permission.

The child and adolescent psychiatrist should dress appropriately for court, with either a suit or blazer for both men and women. If bringing files into court they should be contained properly and organized for ease. Avoid unnecessary items to avoid delay with security clearance. Cell phones and pagers are not allowed to be on during court, so other arrangements for coverage will be required. When the physician arrives at court it is important to let the attorneys be aware of the arrival and any time constraints. Although the psychiatrist will be given a specific time for testimony there is often a significant wait time which is why is it wise to keep the day clear of clinical duties. Many people will bring reading materials to court, but watching the legal process is an interesting way to spend the time as well.

In general, the layout of the courtroom will have a judge presiding on an elevated podium, referred to as a bench, with the court personnel below and to the side of the bench. The attorneys, as there may be several, will be seated at tables facing toward the judge. There will also be a court officer present. If it is an open court, there may be many other people not involved in the case in attendance in the gallery. Depending upon the type of case and the state, a jury may be seated for testimony. When the child and adolescent psychiatrist is called to testify, he or she is sworn in by the officer of the court and then allowed to sit in the witness box which is usually to the side of the judge. The psychiatrist will be asked to state name and business address. It may be helpful to bring a business card to give to the court reporter for difficult spellings, although many courtrooms now do not have court reporters, but audio record proceedings. Either way, the testimony will be put into the official court record. The psychiatrist will be asked to state his or her credentials, training and experience in a process known as *voir dire*.

The psychiatrist may not bill the patient or an insurance company for time spent for testimony or any aspect of the subpoena. In general there will be no reimbursement for the time spent in court as a fact witness.

Testimony

There may be many lawyers involved in the case and all of them will have an opportunity to question the psychiatrist. There will be initial questioning by the side that has asked the fact witness to testify, usually the patient's attorney, which is called direct testimony, after which they will be asked further questions related to the topic of the earlier testimony or submitted records by an opposing attorney, referred to as cross-examination. The first attorney then is able to ask the physician further questions if they choose to "redirect", after which the other attorney has the right again to ask questions. The types of questions and the goals of the questioning will vary depending upon the case and the attorney's relationship to it. When the witness is finished with his testimony, the judge will excuse him and the psychiatrist will now be free to leave the courtroom. There may be times when the psychiatrist may have to return to court the next day or on a later date. The court will try to work within the physician's schedule, so a prudent physician may wish to bring an appointment book to expedite the process of rescheduling.

When testifying in court, it is important to speak clearly and loudly and allow time to think about a question before supplying an answer. Since the testimony is being recorded or transcribed, all the responses must be verbal. It is important to remain calm and professional regardless of the actions of the attorneys or others involved in the case. The fact witness should give only factual information and not speculate or give an opinion in their answer. The simplest and best advice for testifying in court seems to often be the hardest to follow: Answer the question asked and do not offer further information. There will be times when a question can not be answered as posed and the psychiatrist should feel free to say so to the attorney or presiding judge. This may be the case when the fact witness is asked to give a yes or no only answer to misleading questions, which at times the psychiatrist would be able to clarify if given the opportunity. The psychiatrist does not have to be able to answer each question asked. He or she should feel comfortable saying that aspect was not evaluated or s/he simply does not know the answer to the question. The psychiatrist should expect to understand the question and be comfortable in asking for it to be repeated or rephrased. If a question of a fact is asked, the witness has the option, which should be exercised liberally, of checking it against the medical records before responding. The law requires that the fact witness testify according to the best memory or with the aid of written records. This allows the psychiatrist to indicate either uncertainty regarding the answers or no recollection regarding the specific question. Sometimes, attorneys and judges may ask questions regarding the psychiatrist's opinion as an expert. It is very important to not cross the boundary as a clinician testifying as a fact witness and become instead an expert witness, as this can compromise treatment. If this occurs, the psychiatrist can politely raise the issue and express to the judge the problem of providing expert opinion and serving as therapist. Sometimes, questions for expert opinion can be deflected by the fact witness clinician by stating that the question was never addressed or evaluated as part of the routine care of the patient.

Attorneys can raise several types of objections during the course of testimony. The specific legal meaning of each type of objection is beyond the scope of this chapter. The psychiatrist only needs to know that when an objection is made that they should either not answer the question or stop speaking if in the middle of a reply. The judge will then make a ruling on the objection and then the psychiatrist will be informed if they should answer the question or the attorney will move on to another line of inquiry.

The physician may be asked if his answer is of "medical certainty," which can be a confusing and misleading term to physicians unfamiliar with the legal system. Most competent physicians are able to acknowledge that there is always the possibility of an incorrect diagnosis, treatment, report, or laboratory result regardless of how unlikely the chances. This may serve the psychiatrist well in a clinical setting and enable them to constantly question and reexamine the diagnosis or treatment plan. However, in a court of law the answer to questions of "reasonable medical certainty" will usually be "yes" if the physician has reached a conclusion or diagnosis and started an appropriate treatment plan. The common legal interpretation of "reasonable medical certainty" is that the physician has sufficient information to be assured that the answer is "more likely than not accurate" (2).

There are some tactics that lawyers may use in their questioning that can be unsettling to the physician who is new to the court process.

1. An attorney will "summarize" the testimony that the physician gave earlier, in direct testimony for example, and then ask the physician if that is correct or use it as an introduction to a question. The physician should be aware of this approach and realize that more often than not the testimony has been altered intentionally in some way. When this occurs the physician can state that the statement is not entirely correct or have the court record read back.
2. The physician should be aware of any question starting with "Would you agree that . . . ?" This is because there is often a second question after the seemingly innocuous question the physician probably would not agree with and oftentimes the question is intentionally worded to be misleading. This can be done to have the physician answer the question in a way he or she would not have if phrased otherwise. At the same time, the physician does not need to constantly look for traps and try to outmaneuver the lawyer, but instead stick to the basic principles of testifying as a fact witness.
3. Another type of question that may be difficult for physicians to answer in court is: "Is that everything?" It is more likely than not that the physician has forgotten some information and should thus leave the availability of going back to topics at a later time by responding: "That is everything that I recall at this time."

The witness may have to answer questions about previous violations or legal actions in the course of their testimony. There may be occasions when a witness may feel harassed by an attorney, but it is not helpful for the child and adolescent psychiatrist to attempt to argue or show their anger while on the stand. Ultimately, if the witness either needs to take a break or feels ill, they can indicate this to the presiding judge. The judge may either decide to take a short break or adjourn the testimony until another day.

Depositions

Depositions are that part of litigation called discovery and they serve several purposes. They result in both sides showing their hand; they also give attorneys a chance to observe a witness, which may shape legal strategy. Should the case go to trial, a deposition provides a record of answers given by the child and adolescent psychiatrist that, if contradicted in subsequent court testimony, could raise the question of credibility of the practitioner. Deciding to have personal legal counsel present for deposition or testimony depends on the circumstances, but most situations present little or no exposure to the child and adolescent psychiatrist. However, there may be valid reasons why an attorney would prepare and/or accompany a child and adolescent psychiatrist. If the case is volatile or may have further legal implications, it would be prudent to discuss with personal counsel.

If required to by the subpoena and with valid authorization the psychiatrist may be required to bring the entire clinical file which may be taken at that time, but will be returned later. The psychiatrist can also request to be deposed versus making a courtroom appearance, as a deposition will in general provide more convenience in location and scheduling. The psychiatrist will be sworn in and usually both attorneys will be present along with a court reporter. A deposition usually occurs outside of the courtroom, often at a lawyer's office. One lawyer may object to another lawyer's questions, but the psychiatrist will still be asked to answer. At a later time the lawyers may argue in front of a judge and the testimony may be stricken. The psychiatrist should be treated respectfully and allowed to have appropriate breaks. A copy of the deposition transcript may be requested for review.

Case Illustration: Subpoena for Custody Case

Dr. Jones has worked with a family for approximately one year. The 6-year-old daughter, Anna, has been treated for an anxiety disorder while Dr. Jones also has worked with the parents for some behavioral problems. Mrs. Smith was the parent that usually brought Anna to her appointments and Mr. Smith came for the initial evaluation and for two other sessions. The parents during this period have had a breakdown in their marriage and the mother has told Dr. Jones about numerous family problems that are affecting Anna that were discussed in the course of treatment. Dr. Jones has not seen the family for several months and then receives a phone call from Mrs. Smith stating that the parents have decided to divorce, and she asks Dr. Jones to write a letter to the court in support of her having full custody of Anna. She feels that Dr. Jones knows the problems in the family well and would be the best person to explain to the court why she would be the better primary parent for their daughter. Dr. Jones tries to explain that he does not feel comfortable complying with the request and feels that it would be unethical of him to do so. The mother then asks Dr. Jones if she can bring Anna in for a custody evaluation to allow Dr. Jones to feel comfortable writing the letter. Dr. Jones explains that it would be inappropriate for him to change roles from treating psychiatrist to forensic evaluator. Shortly thereafter, Dr. Jones is issued a subpoena duces tenem from Mrs. Smith's lawyer, as he feels Dr. Jones' testimony will be helpful to her case. There is also a release of information included from both parents that will allow Dr. Jones to discuss protected health information. Dr. Jones blocks his entire clinic day, gathers his case materials, and is in court on the scheduled date and time. During direct examination, the mother's attorney asks him if he thinks the father is emotionally capable of taking care of Anna alone if the parents divorce, and what custody arrangement would be in the child's "best interests" in terms of visitations. Dr. Jones is later asked regarding the child's specific medical treatment rendered and what the long-term prognosis and plan would be for the patient. Dr. Jones has a release to discuss any specifics of the evaluation and treatment of Anna and is required to answer those questions to the best of his ability. However, regarding the earlier questions about the father's capability to raise Anna alone or what type of custody arrangement should be undertaken, Dr. Jones did not evaluate those aspects and thus does not have an opinion on those topics relating to Anna, and informs the court of this through his answers.

COURT-ORDERED EVALUATIONS OR EXPERT WITNESS

Child and adolescent psychiatrists may also contribute to judicial cases as expert witnesses. An expert witness is recognized by the court as being able to offer valuable information based on training and experience. Courts have long recognized that the information provided by individuals with special learning or knowledge can assist in deciding certain cases, such as child custody. A survey of judges and attorneys found that mental health issues were involved in one-third of juvenile cases (3). Unlike the fact witness, the expert witness can provide opinions that the court will treat as evidence in guiding its decision. Expert witnesses are permitted to testify about conclusions or opinions they have reached based on their professional skills and analysis, as well as provide information about their area of expertise. Serving as an authority for the court is a very different role for child and adolescent psychiatrists from involvement with the legal system on behalf of patients. It is critical for anyone serving as an expert witness to know the procedural, legal and ethical differences in undertaking evaluations and providing reports for the court from clinical practice with patients and families.

Expert testimony is used in both civil and criminal litigation, two very different judicial settings. It is helpful for any expert appearing in either court to know the differences in the types of cases that are heard and the procedures used in them. Child and adolescent psychiatrists may be called to serve as expert witnesses in civil or family court for custody evaluations, termination of parental rights, or liability claim cases where no one has been charged with a crime. They may also be called to serve as expert witnesses in juvenile or adult criminal court for cases where a minor has been charged with an offense. While juvenile court differs in many aspects from adult criminal court, many of the processes and procedures are the same and the differences have decreased over time. In some states, juvenile courts are referred to as family courts, which can be confusing. Typically in civil or family courts, a plaintiff brings a claim against a defendant for the court to decide. The burden of proof is on the plaintiff and standard is for a preponderance of the evidence. In juvenile or adult criminal court, the district attorney brings charges against a minor. The district attorney must meet a much higher standard of proof, beyond a reasonable doubt. In both civil and criminal litigation, the cases may be decided by a judge or by a jury.

Serving as an expert witness ethically requires the avoidance of any potential conflict of interest. A child and adolescent psychiatrist should not provide both therapy and expert testimony for anyone. The impartiality and objective position of the expert witness is undermined by having a therapeutic relationship with a plaintiff or defendant. Likewise, the ability to provide treatment is compromised by also offering expert testimony for any patient. Other potential conflicts of interests for expert witnesses include any outside relationships with any of the parties that create an interest in the outcome of a case, such as serving on the speaker's panel for a drug company involved in a lawsuit.

It is also important to be familiar with the laws and rules concerning expert medical testimony, as these may differ from state to state. Some states require licensure within that state in order to conduct an evaluation and testify (4). Some states require specific training or certification in order to perform certain types of forensic exams, such as competency evaluations.

Process of Involvement

Child and adolescent psychiatrists are usually contacted directly by the court or by an attorney involved with a case to request expert testimony. The request might also come from a guardian ad litem appointed to represent a minor involved in court litigation or from child protective services pursuing an investigation of a child and family. Sometimes attorneys may have their clients make the initial call seeking expert testimony. This can be confusing, as it may appear that the client is seeking clinical evaluation and care as a patient, rather than services from an expert witness. It is best if the initial contact is with the court or the attorneys requesting expert testimony in order to clarify not only the role but also the specific questions to be addressed in any evaluation, as well as details like scheduled trial date. The involvement of an expert witness in a legal case can be required and ordered by a judge, such as a juvenile disposition hearing, or it can be the choice of an attorney in preparing a case, such as a liability claim with emotional injuries for posttraumatic stress disorder. When it is ordered by a judge, it is usually as a court-appointed impartial expert. In this situation the opposing parties before the court accept that there will be only one expert viewpoint providing testimony, rather than having their own separate or "dueling" experts present.

The first and most important step is to determine the question or questions that prompted the court or attorneys to seek expert testimony, just as in providing any mental health consultation. Sometimes the expectations on what child and adolescent psychiatry can answer or provide are unrealistic, and at other times a request is made for vague or unclear reasons. It is best to clarify the specific request for expert testimony from the start, in order to direct the evaluation and avoid unnecessary complications and confusion later on. This also helps to ascertain the level and extent of expertise required by the case and determines if the child and adolescent psychiatrist is qualified to comment as an expert. Being qualified as an expert for the court does not require that the child and adolescent psychiatrist be recognized as a national authority on the specific area in question, such as post traumatic stress disorder in a liability claim, but that his or her background include sufficient experience to render a professional opinion. Outlining the specific question or questions for the potential expert will also provide information necessary to judge the relative merits of the case and if the psychiatrist is interested in undertaking the time and effort required to address the issues fully. Finally, along with the details of the parties involved, determining the questions for the expert permits the opportunity to uncover any potential conflicts of interests that might undermine or compromise an objective opinion.

It is also important to determine when and if any court dates have been set. Quite often, expert testimony is the last thing that is arranged as a case develops or a court hearing is scheduled. The psychiatrist must be very clear about the amount of time that will be needed to prepare any evaluation for the court and delays can be expected in arranging appointments or receiving requested documents. Usually, allowances can be made for the requested evaluations in civil cases and attorneys can request a continuance, but juvenile and criminal courts do not have as much flexibility in their schedules. The child and adolescent psychiatrist should not feel pressured into undertaking cases when adequate time is not permitted to complete a thorough evaluation.

Contract and Payment

Following a decision to take on a forensic evaluation, it is best to have a letter of agreement or service contract outlining the type of evaluation to be performed, rates for fees and related expenses, and how payment will be received. Fees for forensic evaluation will vary from area to area but are typically higher than routine clinical psychiatric services because the nature of the work is more exacting and requires of a certain level of expertise. The rates are usually set by the hour rather than a flat fee, since it is impossible to predict how much time any forensic evaluation might take. Charges are for all services, including direct clinical interview of involved parties, review of records, discussion with attorneys, preparation of report and time spent in deposition or court. There may also be other incurred expenses for travel with certain cases. It is unethical for experts to seek contingent reimbursement based on a percentage of any potential settlement in a civil case. This creates a vested interest in the outcome of the court's decision, undermining the objective position of the expert and compromising the integrity of any opinion expressed. Mental health insurance will not cover the expenses for forensic evaluation. Billing should be directed to those requesting the service, although some attorneys in civil cases may request that it go to the client. Sometimes court appointments for an impartial expert will also define who and what portion of the evaluation will be paid by parents involved in a custody hearing. With any court-ordered forensic evaluation, it is important to request a copy of the order. Quite often, the attorney will request a copy of the child and adolescent psychiatrist's curriculum vitae to be entered in support of the court's determination of expert status. It is important to have an updated curriculum vitae readily handy for court appearance and offer it even when it is not requested in advance.

Evaluation

Forensic evaluations are more complicated than routine clinical evaluations. It is not sufficient to determine if a mental disorder is present or not, but often whether it was present at a specific point in time and what relation it has to the question before the court. For example, the child and adolescent psychiatrist appearing as an expert must be able to say not only that a child has attention deficit hyperactivity disorder, but also how it might have contributed to his specific behaviors that resulted in charges. For custody evaluations, it is insufficient just to identify the child's developmental needs; there must also be an assessment of both parents' abilities to meet those needs. Questions in a child abuse evaluation must be carefully fashioned to avoid leading the child and suggesting answers. Information must be collected in a fashion that will provide the basis for opinions within reasonable medical certainty.

Offering a psychiatric opinion on anyone requires a thorough evaluation of that individual by the child and adolescent psychiatrist. Interviews should be preceded by obtaining informed consent in which the purpose of the evaluation is made clear, especially that it will serve in preparing a report and who will see it. It is important to remember that those interviewed will probably be influenced in answering any questions by how they desire to see the case decided. Juvenile delinquents may minimize or conceal certain aspects of their life. Parents in custody disputes will want to present themselves favorably. The child and adolescent psychiatrist will want to take this into account and try to obtain the most complete picture by obtaining information from other sources, especially those that are more objective. For example, school records of behavior can be helpful in cases claiming psychiatric trauma, where it is critical to determine exactly when symptoms first appeared in relation to the incident in question. Sometimes evaluations will require interviewing participants opposing each other in court who may not want to cooperate with an interview, such as parents involved in a custody dispute. In those cases, the child and adolescent psychiatrist should inform them that an opinion must be made with or without their participation and that it is in their interest to tell their side of the case.

It is very important to have access to and review all materials relating to the questions presented by the evaluation. The child and adolescent psychiatrist conducting the exam may need the assistance of the court or attorneys as well as consent of parents in obtaining copies of previous evaluations, school reports, psychological testing and medical records. Courts or attorneys requesting expert opinion can also be instrumental in arranging clinical interviews with all those necessary to the evaluation. Sometimes, additional consultations or testing may be indicated as part of a forensic evaluation. The recommendation for any referrals should be made to the court or attorney that arranged the initial evaluation.

Report

A written report is usually prepared and submitted prior to any testimony. It is useful to discuss the findings with the retaining attorney or judge prior to composing the report in order to be sure that all questions have been covered. The child and adolescent psychiatrist must not let such conversation influence his or her conclusions unless new facts are presented that had not been previously known. The report should clearly state the psychiatric opinion regarding the legal questions that have been asked and summarize the data on which that opinion is based. It should indicate that all information has been considered, both for and against, and that alternative conclusions have been ruled out. The format is similar to other psychiatric consultative evaluations, but must be more detailed. It should document all sources of information, list all those examined, with both the date and length of interviews, and all records reviewed. The text should be clear and understandable to lay readers, avoiding psychiatric jargon. Pejorative language should not be used. It is important to remember that the opposing side will review any report in detail, and unwise language will be brought up in court. Information included in the body of the report should indicate the source, such as "the child described" or "the mother alleged." It is useful to include direct quotations from those interviewed to illustrate specific points. The conclusion should offer a clear formulation from a psychiatric perspective and provide specific responses to all the legal issues raised by the request for expert opinion. If treatment is indicated, an appropriate plan should be outlined; for liability cases, it should include the estimated length and costs of all necessary interventions. A well prepared report sometimes results in reaching a settlement outside of court.

Testimony

The court procedures and advice presented in the section on treatment or fact witness apply to expert testimony as well. Attorneys retaining expert witnesses will most likely want to go over the material that will be presented in court and the questions likely to come up. Depositions are frequently used by attorneys to determine what type of evidence may be presented by an expert witness. Depositions are exactly like courtroom testimony and follow the same procedures in the sequence of examination. Attorneys will object to some questions, but unlike the court, the witness will answer the question and the judge will decide later if the objection will be sustained or overruled. Experts will receive a transcript of the deposition for authentication, and quite frequently it will need correction for medical terms. If followed by later courtroom testimony, statements made in the deposition may be used to challenge the consistency of expert opinion by answers that the expert has made in court.

The process of establishing qualifications may be more detailed if the child and adolescent psychiatrist is appearing for one side of the case and especially if opposing experts might testify. The opposing attorney may try to undermine the value of any subsequent opinion offered by indicating during establishment of qualifications that the child and adolescent psychiatrist is inexperienced, particularly in the areas in question, less worthy than the opposing side's expert, or is just an opinion for sale. The volume of forensic work done by the child and adolescent psychiatrist might be raised not only to challenge experience but also to demonstrate if that is the primary work activity and that the expert is merely a "hired gun."

The process and the advice for handling of direct, cross-, redirect and recross-examination in expert testimony are essentially the same as with fact witnesses. In addition to the qualifications of expertise, the testimony of a child and adolescent psychiatrist is expected to meet the general acceptance rule or *Frye* test, named after the case of *Frye v. United States* (5). This standard holds that a medical test, procedure, or disorder has been generally accepted in the scientific community. For example, describing a person as suffering from a particular syndrome is unlikely to be considered unless it is included in the *Diagnostic and Statistical Manual* of the American Psychiatric Association. A new standard for scientific opinion in federal cases was set by the U.S. Supreme Court's ruling in *Daubert v. Merrill Dow Pharmaceuticals, Inc.* (6). Unlike the *Frye* standard, *Daubert* states that the judge is the one to determine if the offered evidence is scientifically valid and that it will assist the court in understanding or determining facts relevant to the case. In addition, this assessment by the judge of expert opinion must be made prior to its being presented in court before a jury. Sometimes opposing attorneys will object to expert testimony as "hearsay," as evidence based on the statements or experience of those other than the expert witness. Such evidence is permitted for expert witnesses, as the use of others' statements and experience gathered as part of clinical evaluation is a recognized practice in formulating psychiatric opinions. Opposing attorneys may also ask if the child and adolescent psychiatrist accepts or recognizes another professional as an expert in the field or a particular study, paper, or book as authoritative. This is usually in order to present information that may conflict, or appear to contradict, the evidence presented by the expert witness. It is important to maintain objectivity throughout testimony and avoid the appearance of personal bias. The expert is not a patient advocate in such situations, but presents psychiatric opinion and the data on which it is based.

Specialized Forensic Evaluation

The role and use of psychiatric expert testimony has increased over time and just as the body of knowledge has grown, so have the types of litigation it is used for in court. The specialized topics of child abuse and child custody are handled in separate chapters in this volume. Juvenile justice and tort litigation represent the oldest and newest areas respectively of psychiatric expert opinion.

It is understandable that child and adolescent psychiatry be called on to evaluate the problems and needs of youthful offenders in disposition hearings. Child and adolescent psychiatry plays a crucial role not only in understanding antisocial behavior but also assessing the frequent comorbid and contributing psychiatric disorders of delinquents (7). Beyond the assessment of juvenile delinquents and recommendations for treatment and rehabilitation, child and adolescent psychiatrists are called upon to perform a variety of other assessments for juvenile court. All states permit transfer or waiver of delinquency cases from juvenile to adult criminal court, usually for serious or violent offenses, and many require that a psychological evaluation be performed prior to doing this. The case of *Kent v. United States* (8) established due process and the standards for juvenile transfer. A transfer evaluation usually requires the child and adolescent psychiatrist to assess the amenability to intervention and developmental maturity of the youthful offender. Evaluation for competency to stand trial is especially relevant for adolescents, as research has shown that few below age 15 meet the adult standard (9).

Previously, the only liability cases involving child and adolescent psychiatric expert testimony were claims of malpractice or negligent care. Courts were reluctant to consider any claims for allegations of psychological trauma. The growing scientific understanding of posttraumatic stress disorder and public awareness have resulted in courts considering claims related to psychological trauma (10). Claims for compensation require not only that the child be suffering from posttraumatic stress disorder, but that the incident in question be a major contributing cause for the symptoms.

Case Illustration: Disposition Hearing for Juvenile Case

Dr. Smith is contacted by the local juvenile court with a request to conduct a transfer evaluation of Jim, a 16-year-old boy currently held in juvenile detention following his arrest for armed robbery. A court hearing has been scheduled, but the district attorney and judge agree to reschedule in order to allow time for the completion of the forensic evaluation. Dr. Smith agrees, and arrangements are made for billing the court. A copy of the court order, arrest reports, probation record, and psychological testing are sent to Dr. Smith. He contacts the juvenile detention center and arranges times to interview both Jim and his mother, his legal guardian.

Dr. Smith reviews the records and learns that Jim was on probation for possession of a controlled substance (marijuana) when he was arrested for allegedly robbing a pizza delivery boy at gunpoint. No one was injured and apparently the gun was not loaded. He has one other recorded arrest for shoplifting (beer at a convenience store) when he was 13. Psychological testing reveals no current psychiatric complaints other than symptoms associated with his drug use. In addition, it notes that he would be considered competent to stand trial as an adult, although the psychologist expresses the opinion that Jim's needs would be better met by the juvenile court system.

On interview with Jim, Dr. Smith explains that she is preparing a report for the court as it considers sending his case for trial in adult criminal court. Jim understands and agrees to the interview. Jim describes feeling sad since his incarceration but does not have sufficient symptoms for a diagnosis of major depression. He admits to using alcohol and marijuana on almost a daily basis, having begun drinking at age 11 and smoking at age 12. He has drunk until he passed out, but denies blackouts or other symptoms associated with alcohol use. He has had hallucinations associated with marijuana use. He has experimented with cocaine by snorting it on two occasions and has tried Ecstasy several times but denies using or trying any other drugs. He also does not think that the marijuana that he uses is laced with other drugs but is not sure. He admits to arrests listed in his criminal record and to having stolen some money from his mother in order to pay for marijuana but denies other antisocial behavior, including physical fights, firesetting, vandalism, cruelty to animals, rape, and involvement with a gang. He states that he had been using both alcohol and marijuana with friends at the time that the pizza delivery boy arrived. He also remembers taking his friend's gun and threatening the delivery boy as a joke, although now he thinks what he did was stupid. His probation officer had made plans to refer him for drug treatment, but that had not taken place at the time of the incident. He also was noncompliant with his probation visits, since he did not want to be found in violation with a positive drug screen. He was a student in ninth grade at the time of his arrest, having been held back for failing due to truancy and poor academic performance. He expresses a desire to get his GED and enter a trade school.

His mother also understands the purpose of the interview and agrees to answer Dr. Smith's questions. She reports that she and Jim's father were never married and that they amicably separated when Jim was 3 years old. His father has stayed involved with Jim, taking him every other weekend. She admits that both she and Jim's father have problems with drinking. She currently works evenings cleaning offices and says that it has been hard to supervise Jim. She corroborates Jim's description of his behavior and previous troubles with the law.

Dr. Smith considers that while Jim is mature, his offense was serious and previous probation has not contained his behavior, he does not have a pattern of violent offense and that there has never been a serious effort made to deal with the drug use that is central to his antisocial behavior. She calls the district attorney to learn why the request for a transfer hearing was made. The district attorney points out the history of arrests, the appearance of threatening and potentially violent behavior and that Jim will soon be 17 and beyond the scope of juvenile probation. Dr. Smith asks if the court has the option of deferred or concurrent sentencing, where Jim would be sent for drug treatment by court order and his progress reviewed at age 17, when he would either be released or sentenced as an adult. The district attorney said that was possible but did not know of treatment facilities that would take Jim. Dr. Smith then prepares a report for the court outlining her findings and opinion that Jim should not be transferred because there was no prior rehabilitation for his drug use and the lack of previous violent offenses. She recommends a facility that would accept Jim for drug treatment on court order. The court and district attorney accept Dr. Smith's report and recommendation at the hearing and she does not have to testify.

CONCLUSION

There have been numerous changes in the judicial and legal system in recent years that affect the role of the child and adolescent psychiatrist in court (11). It is critical for any professional to keep abreast of these changes, even if forensic child psychiatry is not a part of their clinical practice. Practitioners may not choose to perform custody evaluations, but new laws and judicial decisions regarding custody will affect the children and families they care for. Understanding the judicial process improves the chances of being a more effective advocate for mental health, either as a fact or expert witness.

References

1. Macbeth J: Legal issues in the treatment of minors. In: Schetsky and Benedek (ed,): *Principles and Practice of Child and Adolescent Psychiatry*, American Psychiatric Publishing, Inc., 2005.
2. Harney D: *Medical Malpractice*. Mitchie Company, 1993.
3. Mossman D, Kapp J: Courtroom whores—or why do attorneys call us? Findings from a survey on attorneys' use of mental health experts. *J Am Acad Psychiatry Law* 26:27–36, 1998.
4. Simon R, Shuman D: Conducting forensic examinations on the road: Are you practicing your profession without a license? *J Am Acad Psychiatry Law*, 27:75–82, 1999.
5. *Frye v. United States*, 293 F. 1013–1014 D.C. Cir., 1923.
6. *Daubert v. Merrill Dow Pharmaceuticals, Inc.*, 113 S Ct 2786, 1993.
7. Thomas C, Penn J: Juvenile justice mental health services. *Child Adolesc Psychiatr Clin N Am*, 11:731–748, 2002.
8. *Kent v. United States* 383 U.S. 541, 566–567, 1966.
9. Grisso T, Steinberg L, Woolard J, et al.: Juveniles' competence to stand trial: A comparison of adolescents' and adults' capacities as trial defendants. *Law Hum Behav*. 27:333–363, 2003.
10. Schetky DH, Guyer MJ: Civil litigation and the child psychiatrist. *J Am Acad Child Adolesc Psychiatry* 29:963–968, 1990.
11. Ash P, Derdeyn AP: Forensic child and adolescent psychiatry: A review of the past 10 years. *J Am Acad Child Adolesc Psychiatry* 36:1493–1502, 1997.

CHAPTER 7.3.2 ■ DIVORCE AND CHILD CUSTODY

ANLEE D. KUO AND JOHN B. SIKORSKI

INTRODUCTION

The evolution of current American attitudes and concepts of family, marriage, divorce, and childrearing responsibilities has been highly influenced by technological innovations, and by changing legal concepts, economic conditions, and governmental policies (1). These factors include the development and availability of birth control and family planning options in the 1960s and the women's and children's rights movements in the 1960s and '70s (2–4).

During these decades, the U.S. Supreme Court affirmed constitutional rights to privacy regarding the sexual behaviors of adults (5, 6). The past 3 decades have also seen large changes in the labor market and increase in educational and employment options for women. There have also been various governmental tax policies (marriage penalties) and transfer payments (social welfare and dependency support) that impact individual decisions about marriage, cohabitation, and childrearing arrangements (7–9).

These same sociocultural changes impelled the divorce reform pressures in the 1960s, resulting in the divorce reform state statutes in the 1970s, enabling no fault divorce, community property rights, and variable child custody arrangements. Recent demographic trends indicate that approximately one-half of marriages in the United States end in divorce, with increasing numbers of children living with an unmarried or single parent. Approximately one-third of American children will experience significant family instability and grow up living with only one parent, especially if they are poor and minority children (7).

These sociocultural changes and legal reforms in turn have generated a demand for competent psychiatric evaluators who are knowledgeable about the complex clinical, legal, and ethical considerations involved with child custody work, and who are capable of integrating and translating the multidimensional aspects of this evaluation into a comprehensive and useful format for the courts.

THE IMPACT OF DIVORCE ON CHILDREN

While some parents may think or hope that their conflicting or untoward behavior may have little impact on the child, our clinical experience with these children reveals the heartfelt sensitivity and anguish that the child may feel. For example, one 5-year-old boy when discussing with the child custody evaluator his experience in his family, apprehensively stated, "My parents are having a tug of war and I am the rope." An 8-year-old girl, after overhearing part of her mother's angry telephone exchange with her father, anxiously asked her mother, "Do you hate the part of me that is Daddy?"

The psychological sequelae on children of divorce are dependent on many risk and protective factors, but a large body of research over the past 30 years confirms that divorce increases the overall risk for adjustment problems in children and adolescents (10–14). Overall, the data indicate the psychological risk to be at approximately two times greater for children of divorce families as compared to children from intact families (12, 15). More specifically, about 10% of children in married families had serious psychological and social problems compared to 20–25% of children from divorced families (12, 13, 16).

Several important longitudinal studies have investigated the short- and long-term effects of divorce on children (13, 17). According to these studies, the initial period of separation is immensely stressful for the majority of children and adolescents, partially due to the fact that most children are uninformed by their parents about the separation or divorce (13). Thus, a large number of children are unprepared for their parents' separation and react with an acute, intense sense of shock, disbelief, distress, sorrow, anxiety, and anger (13, 15). Developmental factors dictate how children and adolescents manifest their distress at the time of marital rupture (12, 15, 18, 19). Preschool children can experience regression, intensified anxiety, fears and neediness, sleep disturbances, and increased aggression. Middle school–aged children may experience anxiety, loneliness, and a sense of powerlessness. They may also struggle with feelings of responsibility for the divorce, conflicts of loyalty between the parents, and have fantasies of reconciliation. Their school performance and peer relationships may also be negatively affected. Adolescents may experience acute depression, intense anger, and anxiety about their own future relationships. They may also withdraw socially and accelerate their separation and individuation process from the family. In general, this acute response diminishes or disappears over a period of 1 to 2 years (13). Interestingly, the initial responses of children do not necessarily predict the longer term consequences for psychosocial adjustment (15).

Regarding the longer term consequences, children of divorce are significantly more likely to have externalizing problems such as conduct disorder and antisocial behaviors, relationship problems with peers, parents and authority figures, academic problems, and internalizing symptoms such as depression, anxiety, and low self–esteem (16). Other potentially long-term negative effects of divorce include a significant decline in the economic stability of their family and the loss of important relationships with close friends and extended family members, including nonresident parents, who are typically the fathers. As young adults, these children are at risk for weaker marital relationships, earlier pregnancies and lower socioeconomic attainment (16).

The psychological impact of the divorce on any individual child is dependent on a number of risk and protective factors. High levels of interparental conflict—whether in the conflict of the marriage or in high conflict divorce situations—appear to have an especially negative influence on the psychological adjustment of children (20). Protective factors include a good relationship with at least one parent or caregiver, parental warmth, and the support of siblings and peers (13, 16). The effect of the parent and child's gender on postdivorce adjustment is another increasingly important area of study. The data on this subject is unclear, with some studies indicating boys are more vulnerable than girls in both short-term and long-term consequences (15, 21). In mother-custody families, boys may have improved adjustment with regular paternal contact, provided the father is reasonably healthy (21). Overall, interparental conflict, the psychological health of the parents, and the quality of the parent–child relationships appear to be among the most important predictors of a child's adjustment to divorce (16, 22).

Despite the increased risk of psychopathology in children of divorce, it is important to recognize that the majority of controlled research findings demonstrate that no significant difference exists between children from divorced and married families (13, 18). More specifically, about 75 to 80% of children and adolescents who come from a divorced family do not suffer major psychological problems (13). In other words, the majority of children demonstrate resiliency rather than dysfunction as an outcome of divorce.

LEGAL CONCEPTS

Changing values and perceptions of women and children's rights in the 1970s (2) have largely driven the evolution of current concepts of divorce. Historically, the father had inherent custody of the children since they were considered to be his "chattels" or property and women had few legal rights (18, 23, 24). From the mid-nineteenth century through the later part of the twentieth century, the courts emphasized the importance of the mother–infant bond and adopted the "tender years doctrine," with custody presumptively going to the mother (23). During the 1970s, the courts also relied on the concept of the "psychological parent," with the presumption that the mother fulfilled this role (15). The current social and legal trend has moved away from assuming single parent custody and increasingly recognized the importance of the father's role in parenting (25). Currently, the legal doctrine of the "best interests of the child" is the guiding principle in deciding child placement and custody disputes (26). The model legislation of the Uniform Marriage and Divorce Act (the "Act") approved by the American Bar Association in 1974 (27) further established the language and definition regarding the "best interests" criteria. According to the relevant section (section 402), the court shall consider the wishes of the parents and the child; the interactions of the child with those who may significantly affect his or her best interests; the child's adjustment to his or her home, school and community; and the mental and physical health of all individuals involved (26, 27).

The majority of states have adapted their statutes from the concept of and language in this Act (26). For example, in California, the court makes a determination in the "best interests of the child," considering "among any other factors it finds relevant," "the health, safety, and welfare of the child," "allegations of abuse and neglect" and "the habitual and continued illegal use of controlled substances or the continual abuse of alcohol (28)." California Family Code Section 3040 further delineates the "best interest of the child" definition: "The court shall consider, among other factors, which parent is more likely to allow the child frequent and continued contact with the non-custodial parent ... and shall not prefer a parent as custodian because of the parent's sex." California Family Code Section 3042 also states, in part, "If a child is of sufficient age and capacity to reason so as to form an intelligent preference as to custody, the court shall consider and give weight to the wishes of the child in making an order and granting or modifying custody (29)." Despite the general acceptance of the "best interests" principle (30, 31) the concept remains ambiguous, leaving judges wide discretion to interpret it in a variety of ways. As a result of this vagueness, the courts have increasingly relied on the expertise of mental health professionals to assist in the determination of the "best interests" concept (23).

Another important legal concept in child custody work involves the two usual outcomes of a custody dispute, namely joint or sole custody (31). In joint legal custody, both parents have legal decisionmaking powers regarding their child's welfare. In sole legal custody, one parent has the legal authorization to make major decisions for the child. In joint physical custody, the child resides for periods of time in each parent's home. The schedule regarding the time spent in each household and transitions between residences varies on a case-by-case basis. In sole physical custody, the child resides with one parent all the time. Current literature reflects a lack of consensus on the best custody arrangement for children (21).

GENERAL CONSIDERATIONS IN THE EVALUATION PROCESS

Competence as a forensic specialist in child custody work involves a well trained clinician with sufficient skills in evaluation, diagnosis, and treatment of mental health problems (18, 23, 32). Other important skills include knowledge of child development, an understanding of family dynamics, and familiarity with family law and the legal process of divorce and custody in the relevant jurisdiction. In many states, clinicians must remain current in their knowledge of child custody issues by participating in relevant court approved continuing education requirements. For example, court appointed child custody evaluators must document that they have obtained appropriate training as specified by the Judicial Council of California (33).

To further promote and maintain standards of care in this exceedingly complicated area of forensic work, guidelines for evaluating child custody disputes have been published by practitioners and other mental health and legal associations. Professional organizations have taken the lead in developing guidelines and practice parameters. The AACAP has published Practice Parameters for Child Custody Evaluations (23); other guidelines have been published by the American Psychological Association (34), the American Association of Family and Conciliation Courts (35), the American Psychiatric Association (36), the Judicial Council of California (37) and other mental health professionals (19, 32, 38).

Prior to beginning the evaluation, the expert should familiarize himself with the common ethical issues and pitfalls frequently encountered in child custody work (19). Wearing "two hats," therapist and forensic evaluator, is a common mistake and inappropriate in the setting of a custody evaluation (31, 39). As a therapist, the clinician acts as an advocate for the child and attempts to establish a therapeutic alliance with him/her for the purpose of treatment. As a forensic evaluator, the clinician is acting as a neutral expert who assesses the child and then provides objective information and informed opinions to the attorney or court. Before starting the evaluation, the clinician should be clear about his role and convey this information to all parties involved. The evaluator should also avoid situations that might bias the evaluation or suggest a conflict of interest such as prior involvement with either of the parties in the case (23, 39). Finally, the expert should be careful about conducting unilateral evaluations with only one parent–child interaction assessed. This type of one-sided participation inherently leads to biased assessments (40).

The psychiatric evaluation process itself has several phases. The initial phase essentially involves acceptance of the referral, clarification of the questions to be answered and determination of the fee schedule (40). In order to avoid a biased assessment, the referrals should come from both attorneys and the judge. Experts should talk to the attorneys in a conference regarding clarification of the questions to be answered. Evaluation and court time fees should be determined up front and full or partial retainers requested prior to starting the evaluation process (23).

The next phase of the evaluation consists of the clinical interview and collection of data from a variety of sources. Prior to beginning the interview process, the expert may explain to the parents that information provided in the evaluation is not a confidential or privileged communication; the information can be disclosed in the written evaluation and to the attorneys and judges during the court process (18). The expert should obtain written waivers regarding this issue. Interviews typically include an interview with each parent individually, the child alone, and the child with each parent (18, 23, 32). Some evaluators prefer to make home visits to put the information they are gathering in a larger context. In the interview with parents, the expert may obtain the history of the marriage and separation and each parent's psychosocial history, work schedule, financial stability, social support network, parent capacities and understanding of the child's needs, plan for meeting these needs, disciplinary style, daily routine with the child, and relevant cultural and religious beliefs (23, 32).

Psychological testing may be used when the mental health of a parent is an issue (19, 32). However, the testing results should only be used adjunctively and not relied on as the sole support of an opinion (18, 32).

In the interview with the child, the expert should use a nonthreatening, comforting, friendly style of interaction and developmentally appropriate language while assessing for level of attachment and evidence of indoctrination by the parents (23). The interview with child and parent is used to assess the child's way of relating to each parent and vice versa (32, 40). More specifically, the expert may assess attachment to and degree of comfort with each parent and look for signs of anxiety in the child. The expert may also look at the home environment to get a sense of the child's daily life and the parent's attunement to the developmental needs of the child. Other important sources of collateral information include therapists, teachers, healthcare providers, alternate caregivers, extended family members and friends, as well as records from or interviews with schools, therapists, mental health experts and pediatricians.

The written report is a comprehensive description of all the information gathered that supports the final conclusion and recommendation (23, 32). The first part of the report essentially states the referral source, the basic question to be addressed and all the sources of information for the report. The second part describes the information obtained from the clinical interviews and collateral sources. The third part includes the results of any relevant psychological testing such as the MMPI or medical data. The final section of the writeup consists of a conclusion and recommendations. The AACAP lists factors that should be considered when the expert determines the final recommendations: the arrangement that offers the most continuity for the child; the child's preference; the quality of attachment between the child and each parent; the parent's attunement to the child's developmental needs and ability to meet these needs; the impact of gender in the parent–child relationship; and the level of conflict between the parents (23). No studies have adequately supported the idea that one gender fares better with the mother or father, but parents should be sensitive to the gender role model needs of the child (23). After the report is completed and delivered to the court or the parties specified by the court, the expert may need to participate in a chamber's conference or a deposition or be required to testify directly in a court hearing. In general, 4–5% of cases end up with a need for expert testimony (18). However, the expert should be aware that the actual trial may not take place for another year after the evaluation and she may need to update the evaluation at that time (23).

The role and use of child custody evaluations in family law proceedings has generated considerable controversy based on empirical, due process, and ethical considerations.

The Association of Family and Conciliation Courts recently devoted a symposium issue on child custody evaluations (41).

Clinicians and court personnel engaged in the complicated process of custody evaluations, struggling to ascertain the "best interests of the child," may be guided by the commentary of the California Supreme Court's perception (42) that:

> The essence of parenting ... lies in the ethical, emotional and intellectual guidance the parent gives to the child throughout his formative years, and often beyond. The source of this guidance is the adult's own experience of life; its motive power is parental love and concern for the child's wellbeing; and its teachings deal with such fundamental matters as the child's feelings about himself, his relationships with others, his system of values, his standards of conduct and his goals and priorities in life.

SPECIAL CONSIDERATIONS

Current societal forces have generated special issues in child custody evaluations and created a new set of challenges for the forensic expert. The special issues involve topics such as rights of stepparents and grandparents, infant placement and custody, homosexual parenting, parental kidnapping, parental alienation, allegations of sexual abuse, parental relocation, and the impact of reproductive technologies. As these complex issues become more prevalent in custody cases, courts have grown to rely more heavily on the expertise of the child and adolescent psychiatrist for guidance (41).

One of the special issues encountered with increasing frequency involves society's changing perception and definition of the concept of "family" which has evolved into a more complicated structure than the traditional form of previous generations. The current family structure can include biological parents, stepparents, adoptive parents, biological and step-grandparents, stepsiblings, biological siblings, adoptive siblings and, with the new reproductive technologies, surrogate mothers, donor fathers, or birth others (43). These extended family members are increasingly seeking visitation rights or custody of children. Custody law surrounding this issue is evolving and varies from state to state. However, some general trends exist.

With respect to stepparents, the courts generally favor a presumption of the natural parents obtaining custody. However, this presumption can be overcome by "clear and convincing evidence" that the best interests of the child require placement with a nonbiological parent (44). All states have enacted some form of grandparent visitation legislation, but they vary in degree of permissiveness. In the case of *Troxel v. Granville*, the U.S. Supreme Court placed limitations on the grandparent's visiting rights and concluded that the broad language of a Washington State visitation statute allowing "any person" to petition for visitation rights "at any time" unconstitutionally infringed on the parents' "fundamental right" under the 14th Amendment to raise their family free from governmental interference (45). Through future case law, the courts will continue to ascertain the meaning of the "best interest of the child" through a determination of the boundary between parental autonomy and custody rights of extended family members (46).

Infant custody and visitation litigation is on the rise due to fathers more frequently seeking custody of their children and weakening of the presumption for sole maternal custody (the "tender years" presumption) over the past 2 decades (8, 47). Historically, the court's focus was to preserve the mother–infant attachment. However, current research indicates that most infants form meaningful attachments to both parents at about 6 or 7 months of age (9, 19). Thus, the trend now in evaluations is on identification of the child's attachment figures prior to the divorce and the preservation of these relationships postdivorce. For example, most states have laws that emphasize "frequent and continuing contact" between children and their primary caretakers to minimize separation anxiety and maintain continuity in attachments (48). For children under 2 or 3 years of age, "frequent and continuing contact" involves multiple contacts each week (2 to 3 days) with both parents (49). In further support of this trend, current research indicates that infants and toddlers readily adapt to consistent transitions between various environments such as alternative care facilities (19, 49). These studies indicate that the prior emphasis on one-household stability has apparently been overrated. Consistency of schedule appears to be a more important factor in a child's adapting to multiple transitions rather than maintenance of one household (19).

The topic of infant overnights is evolving and a heated ongoing topic of debate within family law (49–52). In support of overnights for infants, ample evidence indicates children significantly benefit from maintaining close relationships with both parents (48, 49). No evidence exists to support the theory that overnights are harmful to infants (48, 49, 52). On the contrary, research with daycares, preschools, communal based sleeping arrangements and other alternative care facilities indicate toddlers and infants can readily adapt their sleeping schedules to different environments. Although the current research data is useful in determining custody arrangements for infants, the forensic expert should always take into account the individual differences in temperament among infants and toddlers with respect to coping with change. Also, frequent and continuing contact between parents may not be preferable if one parent is abusive, neglectful, or has serious mental health issues (19).

The topic of gay and lesbian parenting has been particularly complex and challenging. Arising out of historical prejudices and stereotypes, the current literature on homosexual parenting indicates no significant differences in parenting abilities or in the psychological health or sexual orientation of the child (21, 40). Some state legislatures and state courts have taken varied approaches to aspects of this issue, and it behooves the evaluator to obtain the relevant and current legal authorities in their jurisdiction (53). Rather than focus on issues of sexual stereotyping, the forensic evaluator in these cases should assess the child's needs, the parent's ability to meet these needs and the quality of the parent–child relationship without being influenced by sexual stereotypes (18, 44).

Parental kidnapping, the abduction or withholding of a child by one parent, is a potentially serious and tragic outcome of some child custody disputes (18). An underground network has even developed to assist parents who are fleeing from what is perceived as an unjust legal system (44). Some risk factors have been identified with parental abduction such as narcisstic/sociopathic personality traits, child abuse allegations, and low socioeconomic and ethnic minority status (54). Schetky and Haller (55) have described the trauma experienced by children in these situations and the legal aspects of these kidnappings (55). These children often suffer emotional traumas from their parent's irrational behavior and develop mistrust of their parents and feelings of a lack of safety and protection from the law. Forensic experts confronted with this issue should familiarize themselves with relevant state laws, federal laws (the Uniform Child Custody Jurisdiction and Enforcement Act and the Parental Kidnapping Prevention Act) and international agreements (the 1988 International Child Abduction Remedies Act and the 1980 Hague Convention on the Civil Aspects of International Child Abduction) that have been established to deal with this problem and provide some procedures and sanctions to address it (56, 57).

The phenomenon of parental alienation has generated considerable discussion and debate since Dr. Richard Gardner originally coined the term "parental alienation syndrome" in the 1980s. Scholars have debated over whether such a syndrome exists, and use of the term has engendered considerable criticism and controversy (19, 23, 58, 59). Kelly and Johnston (58) have developed a new formulation of this phenomenon focusing on the alienated child rather than on the parent's alienating behavior (58). According to their new formulation, an alienated child is "one who expresses, freely and persistently, unreasonable negative feelings and beliefs toward a parent that are significantly disproportionate to the child's actual experience with that parent." They also list factors contributing to a child's alienation of one parent such as the aligned parent's negative beliefs reinforcing the child's beliefs, the parent's enmeshment or overidentification with the child, the personality and response of the rejected parent, high conflict in the divorce leading the child to choose a side, alignment of professionals, family, friends and siblings contributing to the child's feelings and the child's age, temperament, vulnerability and cognitive capacity. The children in these situations often suffer symptoms typical of high conflict divorces such as anxiety, splitting, insecurity, distortion, difficulties in relationships, anger and low frustration tolerance, and psychosomatic symptoms (19). Assessment of these cases is complicated and potentially fraught with problems due to *oversimplification*, inaccurate assumptions and inadequate training or knowledge about the complex dynamics involved in these cases (60). Stahl (19) has indicated that the evaluator's primary task is to understand the emotional dynamics of the family, the impact of the alienation on the family, the overall functioning of the child, the history of the family relationships and the level of parental conflict in the divorce. Due to the complexity of these cases, experts should be familiar with the current literature regarding the evaluation and assessment of these children both from a legal and psychological standpoint (19, 60, 61).

Allegations of child sexual abuse are unfortunately a common occurrence in high conflict child custody disputes. Assessing the validity of such allegations is a complicated process involving consideration of the various potential causes for such allegations, careful interviewing techniques, and an understanding of normal child development regarding sexual behavior, memory, and suggestibility (18, 19). Bernet (32) has described a variety of possibilities in considering the differential diagnosis of an allegation including parental misinterpretation, parental delusions, parental indoctrination, interview suggestion, fantasy, miscommunication, lying, group contagion and perpetrator substitution (32). The controversies surrounding this issue have led to a proliferation of literature on the appropriate way to assess children and minimize bias and distortion (32, 62–64).

In general, the current literature suggests that interviewers utilize open ended questions and avoid leading questions, repetitive questioning and manipulation of the emotional tone to direct the interviewee (65, 66). The controversies have also led to a large amount of research on the topic of children's memory and suggestibility (23, 64, 65, 67–70). Regardless of the validity of the allegation, the allegation itself indicates emotional risk for the child (23, 63). Thus, the evaluator's responsibility extends beyond a mere determination of the validity of the allegation and should include a thorough understanding of the family and individual dynamics surrounding the accusation.

Accusations of psychiatric illness are another unfortunate special circumstance arising in child custody disputes with one parent attempting to demonstrate the mental unfitness of the other parent. In these cases, AACAP urges evaluators to focus on the assessment of "parenting" and the impact of the psychiatric illness on the parent–child relationship (23). The mere existence of such a mental disorder in and of itself is not the critical issue in these custody cases.

The issue of parental relocation is a growing topic of concern in the child custody field due to increasing demands for mobility by both parents. Most jurisdictions recognize a presumptive right of the custodial parent to be able to move (71, 72). However, a determination of whether the parent may relocate with the child and the ultimate custodial arrangement in such cases is based on consideration of all the relevant facts and circumstances specific to each individual case (40, 72, 73), with a focus on an outcome that is in the "best interest of the child."

For the child custody evaluator, these cases are among the most complicated and emotionally difficult assessments to conduct due to the inherent physical limits on arriving at a middle ground or compromise with one parent attempting to move to a different location. In addition, there is a dearth of literature and research on move-away evaluations. Thus, experts and the courts have been grappling with this issue and continue to do so through the evolving case law on the subject. Based on the information rising out of these cases, the courts generally consider several factors when confronted with move-away cases: the children's relationship with both parents, the age of the children, the developmental needs of the children, the distance of the move, the children's preference (if the age is appropriate), the parents' ability to cooperate effectively, the current custodial arrangement, and the reasons for the move (72, 74, 75).

Three landmark cases regarding this issue that were decided by the California Supreme Court are *In re Marriage of Burgess* (72), *In re Marriage of LaMusga* (74) and *In re Marriage of Nicole F. Brown and Anthony Yana* (76). In the case of *In re Marriage of Burgess*, the court determined that a custodial parent seeking to relocate with the children is not required to establish the necessity of the move. However, the court can restrain such a removal if the move would prejudice the rights or welfare of the child. In the case of *In re Marriage of LaMusga*, the court determined that the noncustodial parent bears the initial burden of showing that the proposed relocation of the children would cause detriment to the children, requiring a reevaluation of the children's custody. If the parent makes such an initial showing of detriment, then the court must determine whether a change in custody is in the best interest of the children. The case of *In re Marriage of Nicole F. Brown and Anthony Yana* (76) makes clear that the noncustodial parent is not entitled to a full evidentiary hearing on the move-away until he has made a showing of detriment to the child. Since this is clearly an evolving area of child custody work, experts confronted with move-away cases should review the current case law and legislation in the relevant state to guide them in this regard.

In the past few decades, there has been an increased focus on the issue of domestic violence in the context of divorce (77–79) Its increasing importance is reflected in the fact that most state legislation currently includes domestic violence as one factor for courts to consider in determining the "best interest of the child" in custody cases. Many states such as California have a rebuttable presumption against sole or joint custody for a perpetrator of violence (80). A comprehensive assessment in these cases includes evaluation of a broad range of issues such as the veracity of the allegations, an understanding of the extent and form of violence, the impact of the violence on the children, the level of danger or risk to all the parties involved, the parenting ability of both parents, and the developmental needs of the children (19). Recommendations can include dynamic therapy, psychiatric medications, anger management or batterer's programs, parenting skills classes, substance abuse treatment, or attendance at a divorce workshop (79). Supervised or limited visitation or supervised transfers may also need to be implemented. Experts involved with this type of evaluation should stay current with the trends in the relevant state legislature. Some states also require the evaluator to attend training in domestic violence in order to participate in court ordered assessments (81).

The technological developments in reproductive endocrinology and in vitro fertilization (IVF) during the past 25 years have brought desired childbearing to individuals and couples who could not, in prior generations, have experienced the joys and challenges of biological parenthood.

The first IVF birth in the United States occurred in 1982. There are now over 400 fertility clinics and over 45,000 babies born in the United States in 2002 with the assistance of some reproductive technology. The processes and terminology of donor insemination, egg (ovum) donation, surrogacy, gestational care, and embryo adoption have developed in this burgeoning enterprise (43). It remains to be seen what differential developmental variations, family and social cultural adaptations, and psychosocial outcomes may develop with these children and families.

In this arena, new psychological, ethical, and legal issues are pressed to keep up with the developing technology and service demands. In 2004, the Ethics Committee of the American Society for Reproductive Medicine reported that "The Ethics Committee finds that disclosure to the child of the facts of donor conception and, if available, characteristics of the donor may serve the best interests of the offspring (82)."

A recent case involving parental rights was brought to the California Supreme Court. This matter involved a same sex couple, one of whom provided the ovum, and the other became the gestational mother, with assisted reproductive technology from an anonymous sperm donor. The couple reared the twin children as partners until they separated when the children were 5 years old. The California Supreme court ruled that the prenatal waiver of the egg-donating parent was invalid because she was a biological parent, and the couple "intended" to raise the children together. The California Supreme Court ruled that there were equal parental rights and obligations to these same sex parents, adding that "we perceive no reason why both parents of a child cannot be women (83)."

DISPUTE RESOLUTIONS

The concepts of alternative dispute resolution in divorce and child care matters has developed in the past two decades, in part because of the persistent ill effects and undesirable consequences of hostile and costly adversarial court proceedings (84).

Even after the divorce decree, property settlement, and custody and visitation, or co-parenting, orders are filed, parents continue to be parents, with relational bonds, overlapping histories, and moral responsibilities to their children. It is therefore in the best interests of the children, families, and society that the disruptive scars and dark shadows of divorce related conflict be minimized.

To meet this challenge, alternative dispute resolution techniques and divorce education programs have been developed within the court systems, as well as by community agencies and the private sector. These alternative resolution techniques seek to minimize the adversarial and polarizing tendencies inherent in civil litigation. They also seek to provide a more internal locus of control and responsibility in each parent. These programs also seek to provide a larger scope of educational information and experience to the parents, to facilitate more informed judgments and dispute resolution.

Over the past 2 decades, several states have provided legislation to encourage or mandate court-provided or private mediation services prior to court trial scheduling. California enacted mandatory mediation in 1981, and has developed specific definitions, procedures, and training requirements for court-authorized mediators (85). In general, parents utilizing mediation services report a higher level of coparenting communication and cooperativeness than parents utilizing adversarial litigation (40, 89).

During the past decade, a new form of alternative dispute resolution has developed, known as collaborative law (86, 87). The collaborative law process binds the two parties and their respective attorneys to engage in good faith, problemsolving negotiations, defining the legitimate needs of each party and coming to a binding agreement that is then turned into a marital settlement agreement order.

This model is purported to provide incentives to cooperation and disincentives to escalating conflicts. However, either party can withdraw from the process and not forfeit their rights to take the case to court for more traditional and costly litigation (86). Child psychiatrists and other mental health experts may be consulted by the parties to inject information or opinions into this process.

Another procedure for minimizing parental conflict and facilitating decisionmaking, short of a formal court hearing, has been legislation to allow the family court to appoint a special master with limited and specific recommendations and decisionmaking authority, but always subject to the appeal and review of the court. State laws and jurisdictions vary in this partial delegation of this judicial authority, within specific parameters subject to review of the court of jurisdiction to persons with specific credentials and experience relative to the matter of the case (88).

The past 2 decades have seen the development of a variety of psychoeducational and preventive intervention programs in the public sector, court systems, and in private and community based settings. These programs have focused on the impact of family conflict and disruptions, and the negative adversarial process effects on children's postdivorce adaptation. They have also focused on parent's ability to more competently parent, communicate and reestablish domestic nurturance and stability (89).

Some curriculum-based parent or parent-child educational programs have begun to show evidence of improvements in parental satisfaction, reconstituted family communication, and reduction in post divorce adjustment symptoms (90, 91).

One such innovative community based program, *Kids Turn*, in San Francisco, utilizes curriculum-based educational workshops of 1½ hours each for 6 consecutive weeks, with concurrent parallel parent workshops and workshops for their children according to the children's developmental status (91). In addition to these court recommended but voluntary programs, *Kids Turn* has developed curriculum based educational programs for parents of infants and toddlers, workshops for stepparents, and workshops for adolescent parents and men, focusing on nonviolent family skills and nurturing parenting. Some of these workshops are translated and conducted in Spanish and Cantonese, to be more accessible to ethnically and culturally diverse communities (92).

FUTURE DIRECTIONS

In the last half of the twentieth century, we have seen how technological innovation and sociocultural changes have impacted family structure and functioning, and have driven changes in clinical practice and the law.

Child and adolescent psychiatrists and other mental health professional will continue to be called upon to develop the knowledge base, utilize evidence based practices, consult with distressed children and families, and provide relevant expertise to policymakers, community agencies, and the courts, in the evolving complexities of divorce and custody in the twenty-first century.

References

1. Mc Lanahan, et al.: Marriage and child wellbeing; Introducing the issue. *Future of Children* 15(2):3–12, 2005.
2. Nock S: Marriage as a public issue. *Future of Children* 15(2):12–32, 2005.
3. Kay HH: From the second sex and the joint venture: An overview of women's rights and family law in the United States during the 20th century. *California Law Review* 88(6):2019–2093, 2000.
4. Rodham, H: The rights of children. *Harvard Education Review* 1973; 43:487–514
5. *Griswold v. Connecticut*, 381 U.S. 479 (1965)
6. *Roe v. Wade*, 410 U.S. 113 (1973)
7. Cerlin, AJ: American marriage in the early 21st century. *The Future of Children* 15(2):33–57, 2005.
8. Thomas A, Sawhill, I: For love and money? The impact of family structure on family income. *The Future of Children* 15(2):58–76, 2005.
9. Carasso, A, Steuerle, CE: The hefty penalty on marriage facing many households with children. *The Future of Children* 15(2):157–175, 2005.
10. Wallerstein JS, Kelly JB: *Surviving the Breakup*. New York, Basic Books, 1980.
11. Kalter, N: Long term effects of divorce on children: A developmental vulnerability model. *Amer. J. Orthopsychiat* 57(4):587–600 1987.
12. Hetherington, ME, Kelly, J: *For Better or For Worse*. New York, W.W. Norton Company, Inc., 2002.
13. Kelly, JB, Emery, R: Children's adjustment following divorce: Risk and resilience perspectives. *Family Relations* 52:352–262, 2003.
14. Amato PR: The consequences of divorce for adults and children. *Journal of Marriage and Family* 62:1269–1287, 2000.
15. Wallerstein JS, Corbin S: The child and the vicissitudes of divorce. In: *Child and Adolescent Psychiatry: A Comprehensive Textbook*, 3rd ed. Philadelphia, Lippincott, Williams and Wilkins, 2002, pp. 1275–1285.
16. Kelly JB: Children's adjustment in conflicted marriage and divorce: A decade review of research. *Journal of American Academy of Child and Adolescent Psychiatry* 39(8):963–973, 2000.
17. Wallerstein JS, Lewis JM, Blakeslee S: *The Unexpected Legacy of Divorce*. New York, Hyperion, 2000.
18. Billick SB, Ciric SJ: Role of the psychiatric evaluator in child custody disputes. In: *Principles and Practice of Forensic Psychiatry*, 2nd ed. London, 2003, pp. 331–347.
19. Stahl P: *Complex Issues in Child Custody Evaluations*, Thousand Oaks, CA, Sage Publications, Inc., 1999.
20. Roseby V, Johnston JR: Children of Armageddon: Common developmental threats in high conflict divorcing families. *Child and Adolescent Psychiatry Clinics of North America* 7(2):295–309, 1998.
21. Binder R: American Psychiatric Association Resource Document on Controversies in Child Custody: Gay and Lesbian Parenting, Transracial Adoptions, Joint Versus Sole Custody and Custody Gender Issues. *Journal of the American Academy of Psychiatry and the Law* 26(2):267–276, 1998.
22. Ash P, Derdeyn A: Forensic child and adolescent psychiatry: A review of the past ten years. *Journal of American Academy of Child and Adolescent Psychiatry* 36: pp. 1493–1501, 1997.
23. American Academy of Child and Adolescent Psychiatry: Practice parameters for child custody evaluations. *Journal of the American Academy of Child and Adolescent Psychiatry* 36:57S–67S, 1997.
24. Schetky D: History of child and adolescent forensic psychiatry. In: *Principles and Practice of Child and Adolescent Forensic Psychiatry*. Washington, DC, American Psychiatric Publishing, Inc., 2002, pp. 3–14.
25. Lamb ME: The development of infant–father attachments. In: *The Role of the Father in Child Development*, 3rd ed. New York, Wiley, 1997.
26. Nurcombe B, Partlett DF: *Child Mental Health and the Law*, New York, Free Press, 1994.
27. Group for the Advancement of Psychiatry: *Divorce, Child Custody and the Family*. New York, Mental Health Materials, 1980.
28. California Family Code, Section 3011.
29. *In re Marriage of Rosson*, 178 Cal. App. 3d 1094, 224 Cal. Rptr. 250 (Mar 1986).
30. Goldstein J, Freud A, Solnit AJ, et al.: *In the Best Interest of the Child*. New York, Free Press, 1996.
31. Skolnick A: Solomon's Children: The New Biologism, Psychological Parenthood, Attachment Theory, and the Best Interests Standard. In *All Our Families*. New York, Oxford University Press, 1998.
32. Bernet W: The Child and Adolescent Psychiatrist and the Law. In: *Handbook of Child and Adolescent Psychiatry*, New York, Wiley, 1998, pp. 438–468.
33. Judicial Council of California: Education, Experience and Training Standards for Court Appointed Child Custody Investigators and Evaluators. California Rules of Court, Rule 5.225, 2004.
34. American Psychological Association: Guidelines for child custody evaluations in divorce proceedings. *Am Psychol* 49:677–680, 1994.
35. American Association of Family and Conciliation Courts: *Model standards of practice for child custody evaluations*. Madison, WI, American Association of Family and Conciliation Courts, 1994.
36. American Psychiatric Association Task Force on Clinical Assessment in Child Custody Disputes: *Child Custody Consultation*. Washington, DC, American Psychiatric Association, 1988.
37. Judicial Council of California: Court-Ordered Child Custody Evaluations. California Rules of Court, Rule 5.220, 2004.
38. Herman S: Child custody evaluations and the need for standards of care and peer review. *Journal of the Center for Children and the Courts* 1:139–150, 1999.
39. Schetky D: Forensic ethics. In: *The Principles and Practice of Child and Adolescent Psychiatry*. Washington, DC, American Psychiatric Publishing, 2002, pp. 15–20.
40. Herman SP: Child custody evaluations. In: *Principles and Practice of Child and Adolescent Forensic Psychiatry*. Washington, DC, American Psychiatric Publishing, Inc., 2002, pp. 69–78.
41. *Family Court Review* 43(2):187–282, 2005.
42. *In re Marriage of Carney*, 24 Cal. 3d. 725 (1979).
43. Ehrensaft D: *Mommies, Daddies, Donors, Surrogates*. New York, Guilford Press, 2005.
44. Herman S: Special issues in child custody evaluations. *J Am Acad Child Adolesc Psychiatry* 29:969–974, 1990.
45. *Troxel v. Granville*, 530 U.S. 57 (2000).
46. Scott CL: Troxel, et vir, *Petitioners v. Granville*: Grandparents' rights or parental autonomy? *J Am Acad Psychiatry Law* 28:465–468, 2000.
47. Horner TM, Guyer MJ: Infant placement and custody. In: *Handbook of Infant Mental health*. New York, Guilford, 1993, pp. 462–479.
48. Warshak R: Blanket restrictions. *Family and Conciliation Courts Review* 38(4):422–445, 2000.
49. Kelly J, Lamb ME: Using child development research to make appropriate custody and access decisions for young children. *Family and Conciliation Courts Review* 38(3):297–311, 2000.
50. Pruett M, Ebling R, Insabella G: Critical aspects of parenting plans for young children. *Family Court Review* 42(1):39–59, 2004.
51. Solomon J: Another look at the developmental research: Commentary on Kelly and Lamb's "Using Child Development Research to Make Appropriate Custody and Access Decision." *Family Court Review* 39(4):355–365, 2001.
52. Gould J, Stahl P: Never paint by the numbers. *Family Court Review* 39(4):372–6, 2001.
53. Serra R: Sexual orientation and Michigan law. *Michigan Bar Journal* September 76(9):948–54, 1997.
54. Johnston JR, Girdner LK, Sagatun-Edwards I: Developing profiles of risk for parental abduction of children from a comparison of families victimized by abduction with families litigating custody. *Behavioral Sciences and the Law* 17:305–322, 1999.
55. Schetky DH, Haller L: Parental kidnapping. *J Am Acad ChildPsychiatry* 22:279–285, 1983.
56. Weiner MH: International child abduction and the escape from domestic violence. *Fordham Law Review* 69(2):593–706, 2000.
57. Morganroth Fred: The Hague Convention: Understanding and handling abduction and retention cases. *Michigan Bar Journal* 78(1):28–35, 1999.
58. Kelly JB, Johnston JR: The alienated child: A reformulation of parental alienation syndrome. *Family Court Review* 39(3):249–266, 2001.
59. Williams, Justice R: James, Should judges close the gate on PAS and PA? *Family and Conciliation Courts Review* 39(3):267–281, 2001.
60. Lee SM, Olesen NW: Assessing for alienation in child custody and access evaluations. *Family Court Review* 39(3):282–298, 2001.
61. Sullivan M, Kelly JB: Legal and psychological management of cases with an alienated child. *Family Court Review* 39(3):299–315, 2001.
62. American Academy of Child and Adolescent Psychiatry: Practice parameters for the forensic evaluation of children and adolescents who may have been physically or sexually abused. *J Am Acad Child Adolesc Psychiatry* 36:423–442, 1997.
63. Schuman T: Allegations of sexual abuse. In *complex issues in child custody evaluations*. Thousand Oaks, CA, SAGE Publications, Inc, 1999, pp. 43–68.
64. Poole DA, Lindsay DS: Interviewing preschoolers: Effects of nonsuggestive techniques, parental coaching and leading questions on reports of nonexperienced events. *J Exp Child Psychol* 60:129–154, 1995.
65. Bruck M, Ceci SJ: Reliability and suggestibility of children's statements: From science to practice. In: *Principles and Practice of Child and Adolescent Forensic Psychiatry*. Washington, DC, American Psychiatric Publishing, Inc., 2002, pp. 137–149.
66. Quinn KM: Interviewing children for suspected sexual abuse. In: *Principles and Practice of Child and Adolescent Psychiatry*. Washington, DC, American Psychiatric Publishing, Inc. 2002, pp. 149–159.
67. Clark BK: Developmental aspects of memory in children. In *Principles and Practice of Child and Adolescent Forensic Psychiatry*. Washington, DC, American Psychiatric Publishing, Inc., 2002, pp. 129–137.
68. Loftus E: Creating false memories. *Sci Am* 277(3):70–75, 1997.
69. Loftus E, Pickerell J: The formation of false memories. *Psychiatric Ann* 25:720–725, 1995.
70. Poole MK, Lindsay DS: Children's eyewitness reports after exposure to misinformation from parents. *J. Exp. Psychol Appl* 7:27–50, 2001.
71. California Family Code, Section 7501.
72. *In re Marriage of Burgess* (1996) 13 Cal. 4th 25.
73. *Tropea v. Tropea* (1996), 87 NY 2d 727.
74. *In re Marriage of LaMusga* (2004) 32 Cal. 4th 1072, 12 C.R.3d 576, 88 P3d 81.
75. *In re Marriage of Nicole F.: Brown and Anthony Yana* (2006), S131030, Ct. App 2/6 B170252, San Luis Obispo County, Super. Ct. No. DR 21998.
76. *Gordon v. Goertz* (1996) 195 N.R. 321.

77. Lieberman AF, Van Horn P: Attachment, trauma and domestic violence. *Child and Adolescent Psychiatric Clinics of North America* 7(2):423–443, 1998.
78. Johnston J, Roseby V: Domestic violence and parent–child relationships in families disputing custody. In *The Name of the Child*. New York: Free Press, 1997:25–45
79. Dickstein LI: Domestic abuse as a risk factor for children and youth. In: *Principles and Practice of Child and Adolescent Forensic Psychiatry*. Washington, DC, American Psychiatric Publishing, Inc., 2002, pp. 205–212.
80. California Family Code, Section 3044.
81. Judicial Council of California, California Rule of Court, Rule 5.215, 2004.
82. Ethics Committee of the American Society for Reproductive Medicine: Informing offspring of their conception by gamete donation. *Fertility and Sterility* 81(3):527–531, 2004.
83. *K.M. vs. E.G.* (S125643) 37 Cal. 4th 130, 33 Cal. Rptr.3d 61 (2005).
84. Sullivan L: Alternative dispute resolution offers what the bench cannot. *Michigan Bar Journal* 85(2):16–18, 2006.
85. Judicial Council of California, California Rule of Court, Rule 5.210: Court-Connected Child Custody Mediation, 2004
86. Tesler P: *Collaborative Law: Achieving Effective Resolution in Divorce without Litigation*. Washington, DC, American Bar Association, 2001.
87. Fletcher CA, et al.: Collaborative practice: Divorce without litigation. *Michigan Bar Journal* 85(2):25–27, 206.
88. California Code of Civil Procedure, Section 638 and California Family Code No. 3160.
89. Kelly JB: Psychological and legal interventions for parents and children in custody and access disputes: Current research and practice. *Virginia Journal of Social Policy and the Law* 10(1):129–163, 2002.
90. Wolchik SA, et al.: Six year follow-up of preventive interventions for children of divorce: A randomized controlled trial. *JAMA* 288(15):1874–1881, 2002.
91. Hannibal ME: *Good Parenting through Your Divorce*. New York, Marlow and Co., 2002.
92. *Kid's Turn*. www.kidsturn.org (email: Kidsturn@earthlink.net)

CHAPTER 7.3.3 ■ ADOPTION

RACHEL MARGARET ANN BROWN

Adoption refers to a formal action in which an adult assumes primary legal and other parental responsibilities for another, usually a minor. Although this formal action has the potential for enormous psychological significance for all the participants involved in the process, many of them never encounter child and adolescent psychiatrists. As our professional pathways intersect the lives of people involved in the adoption process at different places (but almost always at times when there are problems), we see only the fragmented parts of a complex and multifaceted picture. This chapter is directed at providing a cohesive overview of adoption.

HISTORICAL ASPECTS OF ADOPTION

Adoption is an ancient practice, although not a universal one, since some Islamic interpretations of the Koran ban adoption, while supporting other means of looking after orphaned or abandoned children. It was codified more than 4,000 years ago by the Babylonians, and is described in the Bible, for example, in the adoption of Moses by the daughter of Pharaoh. The ancient Romans practiced both the adoption of children and that of adults, in order to provide a suitable heir for the family. Similar practices, with similar motivation, are described in China, in ancient Egypt, Greece, and, until fairly recently, in the Polynesian societies of Tahiti, and Hawaii. Originally, adoption was designed to benefit the adopter, by providing them with a successor, someone to carry out rituals after their death, someone to work on their behalf and support them, or someone to cement a critical power alliance.

Informal adoption has been part of American society since before the institutionalization of the world's first adoption statute by the Commonwealth of Massachusetts in 1851. The formalization of adoption developed in the context of the "boarding out" in foster care of babies from almshouses, the system of apprenticing and indenturing impoverished children, and the practice of sending homeless children from the Northeast by orphan trains to work in farming communities in the Midwest. In the first part of the twentieth century, most adoptions in the United States were still informal, without confidentiality for any of the parties, sometimes driven by financial motives on the part of the mother, and frequently accompanied by the stigma of illegitimacy and fear of the inheritance of defective genes. Throughout the twentieth century, the states, and later the federal government, have steadily formalized the practice of adoption even where it continues to be independently organized by physicians, lawyers, and the families involved. Significant social change has also affected the numbers and context in which adoption takes place. The adoption of infants was a particularly common practice in the 20 years prior to 1970. Many unmarried mothers chose (or were pressured to choose) adoption over single parenthood, and many healthy infants (mostly white) were placed, often in great secrecy because of the stigma associated with illegitimacy, with unrelated, childless, adoptive parents. The number of nonrelative adoptions increased from about 33,800 in 1951 to 89,200 in 1970.

In the 1970s, a number of social forces impacted on the numbers of children available for adoption, and their age and status. The widespread use of birth control, the availability of abortion, and the acceptance of single parenthood had a significant impact on the availability of infants, especially white infants, for adoption by unrelated couples. The number of unrelated adoptions declined from 89,200 in 1970 to 47,700 in 1977. The adoption of a healthy infant is now an often-expensive undertaking, out of the reach of many middle class couples.

In parallel with these social changes affecting the availability of babies for adoption, two other groups of children became increasingly recognized as suitable for adoptive placements. First, in the mid-1970s, there was a new recognition of the numbers of children living, often in significant instability and for many years, in temporary foster care family placements because of neglect and abuse in their families of origin. In the 1980s, there was a move toward planning for permanency, and an acceptance that children, even older children previously seen as "unadoptable," might benefit from adoptive placement. The Adoption Assistance and Child Welfare Act of 1980 was designed to prevent children in foster care from languishing in temporary situations, and to facilitate adoptions for children who could not be reunified with biological families. After conclusions from policy and social science that adoption was more stable than long-term foster care, Congress passed the Adoption and Safe Families Act (ASFA) in 1997. This legislation requires planning for permanence for children in foster care within a year of removal, and termination of parental rights for children who have been in foster care 15 out of the last 22 months. The Adoption Promotion Act (2003) gave enhanced incentives for adoption of older children. As a result of these shifts in policy and legislation, over the last 15 years increasing numbers of children from the foster care system have been placed for adoption. The numbers rose nationwide from approximately 25,000 in 1995 to around 50,000 in each of the last 5 years. The focus for these children has shifted from adoption for the psychological or financial benefit of adults to adoption for the psychological benefit of the child. More recently, increasing numbers of children have been adopted from foster care by relatives into so-called "kinship" placements.

The second largest group of children affected by changes in adoption practices has been children adopted from overseas. These so-called "international" adoptees arrived in the United States and in European homes initially in the aftermath of World War II, and then after the wars in Korea and Vietnam. Korean adoptees began arriving in the United States and Europe in 1955; originally, many of these children were the offspring of non-Korean military fathers and Korean mothers, but international adoption from Korea has continued, though in lesser numbers, ever since. More than 150,000 Korean children have been adopted by U.S. parents. As time has passed, American parents have continued to adopt children from other countries, including China, Russia, India, Romania, Guatemala, and Colombia. Since 1989, for example, more than 20,000 Chinese children, mostly baby girls, have been adopted by American parents (2) and more than 17,000 have arrived from Guatemala (3). In the United States and other countries—Sweden, Denmark and the UK—similar practices have resulted in a phenomenon known as "visible" adoption: that is, because of the child's and parents' physical appearance, it is obvious that the child is adopted.

As a result of these developments in social policy and legislation, clinicians are likely to encounter the adoption triad of adopted child, biological parent(s), and adoptive families, affected by adoption in notably different ways. First, there are children relinquished by their biological parents, and adopted through private, often church-affiliated, agencies, or independently through attorneys, clergy, or physicians. Statistics on such adoptions are not routinely collected (4); however, the most recent figures from the mid-'90s suggest numbers approaching 50,000 a year, a significant decline from the peak of the 1950s and '60s. Most children adopted by this route are adopted as babies and young infants, either directly from hospital or after short periods in relatively good quality foster homes. Many biological parents, especially mothers, retain some contact with these children, either directly with the adoptive families, or indirectly through the placing agency, through "open" adoption. The adoptive families of many privately adopted U.S.-born and international adoptees are, because of the expense of private adoption, relatively socioeconomically advantaged. Second, the practice of international adoption means that many young children, most between the ages of 3 months and 3 years, arrive in the United States from overseas, often after spending time in orphanages or foster homes, where their care may have been less than optimal and about which reliable information may be missing. Most of these children have scant access to information or contact with their biological parents, and some have little experience with the culture and language of their country of origin. Third, about 50,000 children a year are adopted, either by unrelated families who may also have been their foster parents, or by relatives, from the publicly funded child welfare system. More than half of these children are adopted after the age of 6, many of them in adolescence, and they are likely to be from racial or ethnic minorities. Most have been in temporary custody for more than 4 years, and have suffered significant trauma and neglect. Their adoptive families may be more likely to be older, single parents, and financially less well off.

Adoption has a long history and has affected many millions of children and adults. Most estimates range from 2.5% to 3.5% of the population, and the most recent U.S. data (for 2001) suggest that between 120,000 and 130,000 children are adopted each year (4). It is a practice that is likely to continue, driven by the needs of orphaned, abandoned, and neglected children worldwide, and by the profound desire of adults to parent and nurture children of their own. Even though the majority of adoptions result in well adjusted, well loved children and contented families, child and adolescent psychiatrists will continue to see all three members of the adoption triad—birth parents, adoptive parents, and especially adopted children—in their clinical practices. Attempts to answer some of the questions that arise from the natural experiments of adoption will continue to give rise to fascinating and productive research.

NORMAL DEVELOPMENT IN ADOPTIVE FAMILIES

Most adopted children and families appear to fare well, and, in the context of a relatively unusual family composition, follow a normal developmental track, albeit with some characteristic differences and challenges not faced by children raised by their biological parents. Some authors have suggested that adoption in itself is always a loss or an injury to a child's self-esteem—it is unlikely that we have the evidence to prove that this is indeed always the case, and we run the risk, in taking this view, of assuming that the merely different is in fact pathological. Most clinicians, and most adoptive professionals and families, today support the practice of telling children early about their origins and the circumstances of adoption. Perhaps the increasing numbers of domestic and international transracial adoptions has had the effect of lessening the secrecy and stigma that used to surround it. Giving children information early, even before they are ready to wholly comprehend the information (5), leads to a process of understanding governed by the external facts, the child's internal cognitive and emotional development, and the family's ability to talk comfortably about the issues.

At some point, however, adopted children become more curious about their origins and relationship with the parents, real or fantasy, who gave birth to them, and cared for them prior to their adoption. As their toddlers and preschool children become aware of the realities of pregnancy and child birth, adoptive parents will face questions about the adopted child's origins and early life, and will need to find ways to answer them honestly and openly. Just as young children whose parents divorce are likely to see themselves as responsible for the divorce, because of their behavior or attitude, so adoptive preadolescent children may assume that they were given for adoption because they were in some way damaged or defective, or unwanted because they were a boy, not a girl, or vice versa. As in other families referred for clinical intervention, it is not uncommon to find that the children have not shared such feelings or thoughts, sometimes because of a wish to protect their parents' perceived vulnerabilities. Although systematic research has not demonstrated it, it is also not uncommon, or surprising, to find adoptive children anxious about being removed from their adoptive families.

Adolescence appears to be a particularly sensitive time for many adoptive families, and possibly a significant stressor for adopted children, for a number of reasons, some inherent to the normal developmental process of adolescence, and some unique to the adoptive situation. The process of developing and focusing self-identity is clearly impacted by the reality of adoption; adopted adolescents may have little actual information about their biological roots and families, and may find their adopted parents are uncomfortable and guarded about their child's curiosity. The wish of the adopted adolescent or young adult to search for their biological family, and meet their first parents, almost universally welcomed by those biological parents, is, sadly, for some adoptive parents exquisitely painful and may be experienced as rejection, even when the adolescent does not have that intent. In some families, this issue becomes focused on the idealization of the biological parent, and used as a weapon in a war of control around the adolescent's emerging independence.

The challenges of normal parenting are focused in somewhat different ways for adoptive parents, even when the adoption takes place in infancy. Adoptive parents face relating to children who may not resemble them physically or psychologically, may be placed with them abruptly, and with little preparation, or with whom the legal course of adoption may delay the development of confidence in a future with the child. Moreover, many adoptive couples have already faced the considerable and often prolonged trauma and grief of infertility and its treatment. Research and clinical experience supports the view that unresolved grief over the loss of the potential for a natural child may interfere with the emotional availability of new adoptive parents. As their children grow, adoptive parents face questions and doubts, from themselves, the child and from others, about their role and abilities in comparison to "real" parents. Some extended families may perceive, and at times voice, rejection of the adopted child in comparison to "real" children. Even where such overtly pathological attitudes are not apparent, there are some clinical situations in which parents clearly experience difficulties in attaching to, owning, and accepting their adopted child, especially (6) that child's expression of instinctuality—soiling, sexual curiosity, aggression, and eating. It has been suggested (7) that such difficulties result in strong prohibitions and negative expectations, and may even contribute to the referral of adopted children to clinical settings.

IS ADOPTION PATHOGENIC?

Even before the recent upsurge in the adoption of children from the welfare system, it was fairly clear that adopted children were overrepresented in clinical populations. Some of the literature supporting this finding dates from a time when most adopted children were placed in their adoptive families as infants. Studies from the 1960s, cited by Durdeyn (7) in a previous edition of this text (8–13), establish that adopted children were overrepresented in outpatient settings, and tended to be referred for externalizing behaviors.

More recent studies of inpatient settings (14–16) support the conclusion that adopted children are more commonly referred and admitted, with rates as high as 21% of inpatient adolescents in one study (15), though generally falling around 10% of admissions. Warren's (16) study showed that the referrals among adopted children were for generally lesser problems. Some evidence (17) suggests that differences seen between adopted, foster, and nonadopted children in behavioral problems and rates of referral were the result of a small group of influential cases, rather than a reflection of the group as a whole.

Adoption alone brings relatively low risks (18–20). Among these are slightly higher rates of externalizing symptoms in adolescence, of self-reported offending and substance abuse (18), higher scores on items reflecting unhappy, anxious behavior and problems with peer relationships (21), and the suggestion of an increased risk for suicide during adolescence (22). Studies of school and court populations support the finding that problems in psychological and social adjustment are more common in adopted children than in the general population.

Although these studies appear to demonstrate that adoption for a minority of children appears to be a risk factor for psychopathology, it only seems so when adopted children are compared to the general population. When compared to children returned to their families of origin, or to those raised in long-term foster care, adoption is, in fact, clearly beneficial. For most adopted children, the practice has an overwhelmingly positive outcome, and most adopted children are happy and well adjusted.

The natural experiment of adoption has played an important role in the exploration of the etiology of mental illness, particularly schizophrenia, demonstrating the biological underpinnings of the disorder (23–26). Studies of adopted children at high risk for schizophrenic illnesses demonstrate that these children exhibit subtle developmental delays, cognitive problems, and poor interpersonal relationships. More recent studies have also examined the contribution of environment, including family environment, to the manifestation of the schizophrenic illness, and support the notion of gene–environment interactions. Using a Finnish sample of children adopted by unrelated parents, Tienari et al. (24) showed that disordered adoptive rearing assessed in the adoptive families predicts schizophrenia-spectrum disorders at 21-year followup. The finding was only apparent, however, in adoptees at high genetic risk for schizophrenia, and suggests that adoptees at high genetic risk may be more sensitive to adverse environmental effects in an adoptive rearing environment than are adoptees at low genetic risk. The presumed genotype appears to be "sensitive" not only to dysfunction in the family environment but to protective environmental factors.

Studies like this suggest that adoptive rearing in a quality home environment may be of particular value for those at higher genetic risk. As the possibility that children at high genetic risk for schizophrenia (and other mental illnesses) may be identified in early childhood becomes more realistic, it is possible that adoptive parents, and the psychiatrists working with them, will have new challenges and possibilities in prevention. They, and we, as their psychiatrists, also face the challenge of counseling the children of such high-risk adoptees as they move into the age of risk for onset of schizophrenic disorders.

INTERNATIONAL ADOPTION

Just as the practice of domestic adoption for children of parents with mental illness has shed new light on the etiology of schizophrenia, so has the practice of international adoption brought new insights into the importance of early childhood experiences (1), even when those are relatively brief, as well as an awareness of the relevance of transracial adoption and immigration in the context of already prejudiced and racist societies. Internationally adopted children grown to adult life have begun to tell their own moving and fascinating stories, describing their vague memories of early childhood, their sense of loss and disconnection from their countries of origin, and the tremendous care and attachment they experienced in their adoptive families.

Studies of children recently adopted from overseas show that growth and developmental delays are frequent (2, 3), particularly where the child is raised in an orphanage rather than in a foster family setting. Three-quarters of the Chinese-born adoptees evaluated in a New England adoption clinic (2) had significant developmental delays, with gross motor delays being the most common. Medical problems were also common, some being minor and easily correctable (anemia, elevated lead levels, hepatitis antibodies, parasites, and positive TB skin tests). Others, though less common, were more serious and included hearing loss, syphilis, orthopedic problems and congenital anomalies. Many internationally adopted children are also inadequately vaccinated (27). Similar findings (3) come from a cohort of children adopted to the United States from Guatemala, though the problems are not as severe as those in the Chinese children. Adopted children were diagnosed with neurological problems, including hypo- and hypertonia, clonus, mental retardation and developmental disorders, and with emotional problems, the latter including depression, posttraumatic stress and eating disorders. They were also commonly seen to exhibit self-comforting behaviors, such as rocking and banging. This study again demonstrates the significant growth and cognitive advantages experienced by children in foster placements rather than orphanages, prior to adoption. Children who were younger at placement also did better, with those younger than 2 being less likely to be developmentally delayed.

After the resolution of initial medical problems most internationally adopted young children appear to adapt well to their new environment (28), and progress satisfactorily during early school age. It has, however, been of concern to clinicians in a variety of different countries that internationally adopted children appear more commonly in clinical settings than might be expected (29). Although not all studies are in agreement, most suggest that a larger minority than would be expected do experience significant mental health problems in childhood, adolescence, and early adult life. Dutch studies (30–32) show elevated rates of behavioral problems, anxiety, and depression, especially in the home setting, and especially for boys, with adjustment problems increasing into adolescence, even among those adopted as infants. Evidence from the Swedish national registers for those born in 1970–1979, comparing inter country adoptees to the general population found that the adoptees were more than three times more likely to die from suicide, attempt suicide, or be admitted to a psychiatric hospital, and more than five times more likely to use drugs, twice as likely to use alcohol, and somewhat more likely to commit a crime (33, 34). Some evidence supports the view that the problems are not that of the whole sample, but rather a result of small group of significant outliers. Cederblad's (28) study found that preadoption conditions, rather than age at placement, increased the risk of later maladaptation, and that the rate of children with poor attachments increased if the child had been in an orphanage or foster home for a longer time. Similar findings emerge from other studies (22, 25, 35–38). It is possible that the minority at risk is the group of children that suffered more significant early childhood neglect or abuse; it is, however, also possible that the small group are those who were biologically more sensitive to such experiences (30). Whatever the cause, and even though this is a group at significant risk, the vast majority of internationally adopted children (92% of the girls, and 82% of the boys) had no indication of mental health disorders, or maladjustment.

Cederblad et al. (28) also found that a substantial number of their subjects had been teased or felt ill at ease because of foreign looks, and two-thirds had been regarded as foreigners. Indicators that the young person was struggling with identity were related to level of symptom load and self-esteem, though most subjects coped well with their "special outsider" status. The issue of transracial adoption has been a sensitive and emotive topic, not only as regards international adoption, but as it pertains to the adoption of (mostly) black children by (mostly) white families in the United States. In a comprehensive review of the issue, Rushton and Minnis (39) acknowledge the highly contentious nature of this subject, and its political and social context. Most empirical research has been done on black infants in white adoptive families in the United States, but other transracial placements include Australasian peoples and gypsies in central Europe. Rushton and Minnis conclude that the available evidence suggests that such placements have satisfactory outcomes in over 70% of placements, comparing favorably with other samples.

Overall, studies of internationally adopted children demonstrate that most fare well, and that it is the minority who experience mental health problems. A number of factors may play a part in increasing the risk. Those factors include being male, being placed with a single parent, or in an adoptive white collar family, older age at placement, and placement in an orphanage rather than a foster home prior to adoption. It is also important to remember that adoptive parents may be, to some degree, supercompetent, and that children who fare well in adoptive families may be at genetically higher risk than the general population, but environmentally somewhat protected. These studies also bring forth the subtle, and sometimes not so subtle, challenge of growing up with a distinct and different appearance, in a culture that may not welcome difference, or may even be overtly racist and discriminatory.

Many internationally adopted children come to the United States, and other Western countries, with the assistance of long established international adoption agencies that have worked extensively in the social welfare systems of the countries of origin of the adoptive children, and cooperate with them in providing enhanced orphanage or foster care environments. In contrast, the children adopted into largely middle class American and European families after the fall of the Ceaucescu regime in Romania had experienced extraordinarily deprived orphanage conditions. Their story (40, 41) illustrates both the impact of early emotional and social deprivation on child development, as well as the degree of recovery possible in an enhanced family environment. For this group of children, exposed to extreme early global deprivation, duration of emotional deprivation predicted cognitive outcomes at the time of adoption, as well as recovery in the adoptive family. In these studies, the age of "late" adoption was 24–42 months—in earlier studies, children placed under the age of 5 are mostly classified as "early" placements; this shift acknowledges the growing understanding in the adoption field of the importance of experiences in the first years of life. Children exposed to longer periods of deprivation were more delayed; those placed at an older age appeared to recover less completely; and, even for those placed at younger ages, the most extensive recovery took place in the first two years after placement. Studies of these children as they move into adolescence suggest that a minority, at least, continue to experience particular ongoing problems in social relationships. Some of the behaviors typical of such children when referred for clinical evaluation are described in Stein et al. (42). They include inappropriate social behaviors, attachment problems, odd and bizarre behaviors, language delays, defiance, noncompliance, and anger.

CHILDREN FROM THE WELFARE SYSTEM

For many years, social policy dictated that although babies and young infants could be adopted, children removed from their families by the welfare system or placed by their families after infancy were considered unsuitable for adoption. Social policy shifted significantly, however, in the seventies, as the numbers of children in foster care (and the public expense of their care) grew, and evidence emerged that even older children adopted after adverse care experiences did well after adoption, many better than those who went home to their biological families (20, 21, 43, 44). It is clear, however, that children adopted older, especially after adverse childcare experiences, have more psychosocial difficulties than those adopted as babies. Howe (45) looked at a group of more than 200 adopted children, now young adults, and interviewed their parents. The subjects were baby adoptions, children adopted older who had good care as babies, and children adopted older who had poor care as babies. The latter group was the only one with higher rates of adolescent problems; however, no problem behaviors were reported in more than one-fourth of the group. Behavior problems include peer relationship difficulties and the lower likelihood of having a special friend (43, 46). The findings from more recent studies, including those of the Romanian orphans, as well as research on the infancy attachment process, suggest that for infants the timing of placement for permanency (which in most cases means adoption) is a matter of some urgency and that the infant's development (or maldevelopment) proceeds at a pace that is unlikely to be congruent with the timelines of juvenile courts. Although the evaluation of potentially abusive families, and the associated legal processes, can be quite lengthy, it is possible (47) and, from a child developmental point of view clearly advisable, for these processes to continue while the child is given the potential for permanence through so-called "concurrent planning."

It is unlikely that child and adolescent psychiatrists will have extensive involvement with those children adopted from the welfare system who are doing well. However, many clinicians work with the children and families of those who are doing poorly. As a result, clinicians are likely to see adoptive families struggling with children with extreme behavioral and emotional difficulties, especially in relationships within and outside the family, and, at times, be involved in the heartbreaking situations with adoptive families where the placement is disrupted (family breakdown prior to the finalization of the adoption) or dissolved (family breakdown after the adoption is finalized). Breakdown rates of older adoptions are 10–50% (48).

CONCLUSION

Adoption touches many lives. Many adults joyfully become parents through adoption, and would be insulted by the suggestion that this is in any way a lesser means of becoming parents. Many babies and children of all ages find permanent families through adoption; for most of them, adoption has a positive outcome, contributes to positive psychological adjustment, and is clearly protective; for a minority, adoption may contribute to, or be associated with, emotional and behavioral problems, and psychiatric disorders. Children at particular risk include those adopted later in life, after early adverse experiences, as well as those at particular genetic risk. It is also important not to neglect, or ignore, the biological parents and families of children relinquished or removed and placed for adoption. They too may be our patients. Clinicians working with adopted children and their families should be aware of the complexity and variability of the circumstances in which adoption takes place, as well as the meaning of the process for all the individuals involved.

References

1. Tizard B: Intercountry adoption: A review of the evidence. *J Child Psychol Psychiatry* 32:743–756, 1991.
2. Hendrie NW: Health of children adopted from China. *Pediatrics* 105:6:e76, 2000.
3. Miller L, Comfort K, and Tirella L: Health of children adopted from Guatemala: Comparison of orphanage and foster care. *Pediatrics* 115:e710–e717, 2005.
4. National Adoption Information Clearinghouse: How Many Children Were Adopted Between 2000 and 2001? Accessed through www.childwelfare.gov/adoption/index.cfm, June 26, 2006.
5. Brodzinsky DM, Singer LM, Braff AM: Children's understanding of adoption. *Child Dev* 55:869–878, 1984.
6. Brinich PM: Some potential effects of adoption on self and object representations. *Psychoanal Study Child* 35:107–133, 1980.
7. Derdeyn A. Adoption. In: Lewis M (ed): *Child and Adolescent Psychiatry: A Comprehensive Textbook*, 1996.
8. Silberstein RM, Mandell W: Adopted children brought to child psychiatric clinics. *Arch Gen Psychiatry* 158:451–456, 1963.
9. Humphrey M, Ounsted C: Adoptive families referred for psychiatric advice. I: The children. *Br J Psychiatry* 109:599–608, 1963.
10. Menlove FL: Aggressive symptoms in emotionally disturbed adopted children. *Child Dev* 36:519–532, 1965.
11. Offord DR, Aponte JF, Cross LA: Presenting symptomatology of adopted children. *Arch Gen Psychiatry* 20:110–116, 1969.
12. Schechter MD, Carlson P, Simmons J, Work H: Emotional problems in the adoptee. *Arch Gen Psychiatry* 10:37–46, 1964.
13. Simon NM, Senturia AG: Adoption and psychiatric illness. *Am J Psychiatry* 122:858–867, 1966.
14. Kotsopoulos S, Cote A, Joseph L, et al.: Psychiatric disorders in adopted children: A controlled study. *Am J Orthopsychiatry* 58:608–612, 1988.
15. Senior N, Himadi E: Emotionally disturbed, adopted, inpatient adolescents. *Child Psychiatry Hum Dev* 15:189–197, 1963.
16. Warren, SB: Lower threshold for referral for psychiatric treatment for adopted adolescents. *J Am Acad Child Adolesc Psychiatry* 31:512–517, 1992.
17. Brand AE, Brinich PM: Behavior problems and mental health contacts in adopted, foster and nonadopted children. *J Child Psychol Psychiatry* 40(8):1221–1229, 1999.
18. Fergusson DM, Lynskey M, Horwood LJ: The adolescent outcomes of adoption: A 16 year longitudinal study. *J Child Psychol Psychiatry* 36:597–615, 1995.
19. Hersov L: The seventh Jack Tizard memorial lecture: Aspects of adoption. *J Child Psychol Psychiatry* 31:493–510, 1990.
20. Fratter J, Rowe J, Sapsford D, Thoburn J: *Permanent Family Placement: A Decade of Experience*, London, BAAF, 1991.
21. Maughan B, Pickles A: Adopted and illegitimate children grown up. In: L Robins and M Rutter (eds): Straight and devious pathways from childhood to adulthood. New York, Cambridge University Press, 1990.
22. Slap G, Goodman E, Huan B: Adoption as a risk factor for attempted suicide during adolescence. *Pediatrics* 108:E30, 2001.
23. Kety SS, Wender PH, Jacobsen B, et al.: Mental illness in the biological and adoptive relatives of schizophrenic adoptees: Replication of the Copenhagen Study in the rest of Denmark. *Arch Gen Psychiatry* 51:442–445, 1994.
24. Tienari P, Wynne LC, Sorri A, et al.: Genotype-environment interaction in schizophrenia-spectrum disorder: Long-term follow-up study of Finnish adoptees. *Br J Psychiatry* 184:216–222, 2004.
25. Howe OD, McDonald C, Cannon M, Arseneault L, Boydell J, Murray RM: Pathways to schizophrenia: The impact of environmental factors. *Int J Neuropsychopharmacol* 7 Suppl 1:S7–S13, 2004.
26. Wahlberg K-E, Wynne LC, Oja H, et al.: Gene-environment interaction in vulnerability to schizophrenia: Findings from the Finnish adoptive family study of schizophrenia. *Am. J Psychiatry* 154:355–362, 1997.
27. Hostetter MK: Infectious diseases in internationally adopted children: The past five years. *Pediatr Infect Dis J* 17:517–518, 1998.
28. Cederblad M, Hook B, Irhammar M, Mercke AM: Mental health in international adoptees as teenagers and young adults: An epidemiological study. *J Child Psychol Psychiatry* 40:1239–1248, 1999.
29. Kim WJ: International adoption: A case review of Korean children. *Child Psychiatry Hum Dev* 25:141–154, 1995.
30. Stams GJ, Juffer F, Rispens J, Hoksberger RAC: The development and adjustment of 7 year old children adopted in infancy. *J Child Psychol Psychiatry* 41:1025–1037, 2000.
31. Verhulst FC, Althaus M, Versluis-den Bieman HJ: Problem behavior in international adoptees. I: An epidemiological study. *J Am Acad Child Adolesc Psychiatry* 19:94–103, 1990.
32. Verhulst FC, Versluis-den Bieman HJ: Developmental course of problem behaviors in adolescent adoptees. *J Am Acad Child Adolesc Psychiatry* 34:151–159, 1995.
33. Hjern A, Lindblad F, Vinnerljung B: Suicide, psychiatric illness, and social maladjustment in intercountry adoptees in Sweden: A cohort study. *Lancet* 10, 360:443–447, 2002.
34. Von Borczyskowski A, Hjern A, Lindblad F, Vinnerljung B: Suicidal behavior in national and international adult adoptees: A Swedish cohort study. *Soc Psychiatry Psychiatr Epidemiol* 41:95–102, 2006.
35. Fisher L, Ames EW, Chisholm K, Savoie L: Problems reported by parents of Romanian orphans adopted to British Columbia. *Int J Behav Development* 20:67–82, 1997.
36. Hoksbergen RAC: Turmoil for adoptees during their adolescence? *Int J Behavioral Dev* 20:33–46, 1997.
37. Juffer F, Rosenboom LG: Infant-mother attachment of internationally adopted children in the Netherlands. *Inter J Behav Dev* 20:93–107, 1997.

38. Moracovitch S, Goldberg S, Gold A, et al.: Determinants of behavioral problems in Romanian children adopted in Ontario. *Inter J Behav Dev* 20:17–30, 1997.
39. Rushton A, Minnis H. Annotation: Transracial family placements. *J Child Psychol Psychiatry* 38:147–159, 1997.
40. Rutter M, Andersen-Wood L, Becket C, et al.: Developmental catch-up, and deficit, following adoption after severe global early privation. *J Child Psychol Psychiatry* 39:465–476, 1998.
41. O'Connor TG, Rutter M, Beckett C, Keaveney L, Kreppner JM, and the English and Romanian Adoptees Study Team: The effects of global severe privation on cognitive competence: Extension and longitudinal follow-up. *Child Dev* 71:376–390, 2000.
42. Stein M: International adoption: A four-year-old child with unusual behaviors adopted at six months of age. *Dev Behav Pediatrics* 24:63–69, 2003.
43. Hodges J, Tizard B: Social and family relationships of ex-institutional adolescents. *J Child Psychol Psychiatry* 30:77–97, 1989.
44. Seglow J, Pringle MK, Wedge P: *Growing Up Adopted* Windsor, U.K.; NFER, 1972.
45. Howe D: Parent reported problems in 211 adopted children: Some risk and protective factors. *J Child Psychol Psychiatry* 38:401–411, 1997.
46. Rushton A, Treseder J, Quinton. D: An eight year prospective study of older boys placed in permanent substitute families: A research note. *J Child Psychol Psychiatry* 36:687–696, 1995.
47. Zeanah CH, Larrieu JA, Heller SS, et al.: Evaluation of a preventive intervention for maltreated infants and toddlers in foster care. *J Am Acad Child Adolesc Psychiatry* 40:214–221, 2001.
48. Borland M, O'Hara G, Triseliotis J: Placement outcomes for children with special needs. *Adoption and Fostering* 15:18–28, 1991.

CHAPTER 7.3.4 ■ MALPRACTICE AND PROFESSIONAL LIABILITY

PETER ASH AND BARRY NURCOMBE

Malpractice litigation and other forms of formal legal investigation of medical care, such as state medical licensing board investigations, are society's means of holding physicians to appropriate standards and compensating patients who have been negligently harmed. There are problems with utilizing litigation to achieve these goals: It is an inefficient way of compensating patients, since many who have been harmed do not sue (1), many who have suffered damage and do sue were not harmed by negligence, and the costs of litigation, both financially and emotionally, are very high. Physicians who have been sued describe the process as extremely painful emotionally, even when they prevail (2). Practicing defensive medicine is common (3), though probably less of an issue in child psychiatry than in more technological medical specialties, and some psychiatrists may avoid taking on the most difficult patients. Physicians understandably hate being sued. Malpractice premiums have increased markedly over the past 30 years, triggering calls for legislative tort reform. Over half the states now have limits on noneconomic damages (pain and suffering) (4). More systematic reforms of the system have been called for, such as moving to a no-fault system adjudicated administratively, along the lines of the worker's compensation system, but such proposals currently have very limited political support.

Compared to many medical specialties, child and adolescent psychiatry is not high risk. Even when sued, child and adolescent psychiatrists prevail most of the time. While accurate national data are difficult to come by because insurance companies keep much of their loss experience as proprietary information, analysis of the psychiatry dataset of the Physician Insurers Association of America from 1985 to 2000 for child and adolescent patients indicated that only about 14% of claims resulted in a payment, and the average payment was less than the average payment in adult psychiatric malpractice cases (5). These positive outcomes are reflected in the practice of some insurers of giving discounted premiums to child and adolescent psychiatrists.

Malpractice litigation is not the only arena in which physicians have professional liability: Medical licensing boards investigate complaints, as do ethics committees of professional associations. While such investigations do not directly result in monetary damage payments, in medical licensing investigations the ability of the clinician to practice may be at stake, and findings of fault may later be admitted as evidence in a malpractice case.

THE LAW OF MALPRACTICE

The term malpractice refers to an act or omission by a professional in the course of his or her professional duty that causes or aggravates an injury to a patient or client and is the consequence of a failure to exercise a reasonable degree of prudence, diligence, knowledge, or skill. To substantiate malpractice, the plaintiff must establish the following four points, known as the 4 Ds, by a preponderance of the evidence:

1. The clinician had a *Duty of reasonable care* to the patient.
2. There was a *Dereliction of that duty*, when judged by the standard of the average, prudent practitioner.
3. The patient sustained *Damage, a compensable injury or harm.*
4. The damage was a *Direct result* of the clinician's failure to exercise a reasonable standard of care.

Duty of Care: The Doctor–Patient Relationship

The clinician owes a duty of reasonable care toward a patient when a professional relationship exists between them. This relationship is formed when a clinician explicitly or implicitly agrees to provide care to a patient. The clinician thus enters into a contract that binds him or her to provide a reasonable level of care in return for a valuable consideration (the fee). Unless the clinician has unwisely promised a cure, he or she is not bound to provide more than a reasonable level of care.

The doctor–patient relationship cannot be imposed on a competent patient, nor can a doctor be forced to care for a patient, except in special situations, such as an emergency room. Controversial situations arise when it is argued that a relationship has been implied by the physician's actions or words. For example, the discussion of a patient's condition by telephone before transfer to a different hospital has been held to imply a contractual relationship (6). Payment is not necessary; even free advice can create a professional relationship. The clinician should be careful about giving casual advice at cocktail parties and the like, lest it be construed that a contractual relationship has been formed.

Conversely, a physician cannot be forced to treat patients who are unable to pay for services or to use a treatment that he or she is not competent to implement. The physician also has a legal (though perhaps not an ethical) right to refuse to give aid in an emergency. Good Samaritan laws have been enacted to protect from liability those physicians who do render emergency aid, unless they have been grossly negligent (e.g., abandoning a live patient who is still hemorrhaging).

When working with minor patients, it is important to be clear with the family who the patient is. In some types of family work, the "family" is defined as the patient, and the clinician may thereby establish a doctor–patient relationship with each member of the family. When the minor is the identified patient, the physician is not taking on responsibility for treating the parents, and communications from the parent about the child are placed in the child patient's record. However, when advice is given to a parent in a separate parent session (e.g., "Your child would be better off if the two of you divorced"), the physician is likely to be held responsible for the foreseeable consequences of that advice.

The Internet allows doctors to communicate with patients in new ways. E-mail communications between a patient who is or will be seen in the office clearly fall within an established doctor–patient relationship. Responding to a nonpatient's email with therapeutic advice may establish a doctor–patient relationship, much as if a similar communication was conducted over the telephone (7). Simply responding to a prospective patient's email with a referral to someone in their geographic area does not establish a doctor–patient relationship. While the law is still evolving in this area, the trend is that the medicine is practiced in the state where the patient resides, not where the physician practices (8), so physicians who conduct email treatment with a patient who resides in a state where the clinician does not have a license may be practicing without a license. Prudent risk management dictates that professional email communications with nonpatients that might be construed as therapeutic contain a clear disclaimer that the email does not constitute professional advice and refer the patient to their physician for such advice. Similarly, general information about mental health conditions which a physician may post on his or her website should likewise contain a disclaimer. Professional risk management organizations have developed guidelines for practitioner websites (9, 10).

As psychiatric practice has become more focused on psychopharmacology, collaborative treatment relationships in which the psychiatrist handles medications while another mental health professional conducts psychotherapy have become more common. These relationships often leave ambiguous which clinician is responsible for what. Simon (11) recommends that these understandings be made explicit through written agreement or that the physician write the collaborating mental health provider a letter detailing such issues as what the physician's role will be, who is providing emergency coverage, and the expectations of communication between the collaborating providers.

After the termination of the contract, the physician owes no further obligation to the patient other than that of confidentiality. Physicians who terminate contracts unilaterally and without reasonable cause are at risk of actions for *abandonment*. The physician must give the patient due notice of termination and must ensure that necessary arrangements are made for alternative care. If the patient resists termination, failure to refer to another physician may be construed as negligence. Some risk managers advise that patients be notified at the outset that noncompliance with treatment is deemed a termination of treatment.

Vicarious Liability

In accordance with the doctrine of *respondeat superior* (let the master answer), a physician is legally responsible for the negligent actions of employees or supervisees. Thus, a psychiatrist may be held liable for the negligent or outrageous actions of his secretary and office staff or house officers whom he or she supervises. In malpractice cases involving inpatients, the hospital is often a defendant because of its vicarious liability for the actions of nurses, ward staff, and house officers.

Supervising and Consulting Relationships

Supervisors who provide care, supervise the care of residents, or are the attending physician of record face malpractice exposure for the care they direct, and may be held liable for care they supervise, either as vicariously liable for the actions of a house officer, or as directly liable for inadequate supervision. Consider a suit filed subsequent to an adolescent's suicide after the adolescent was brought to an emergency room and examined by a resident who discharged the patient after discussion with the chief resident but without telephoning the attending child psychiatrist. Assuming the overall care was found negligent, courts may apportion blame differently, depending on local interpretations of whether residents are held to the standard of specialists and the nature of the contract of the on-call attending (who has been found vicariously liable in some cases even when not contacted). If the attending had been called, then the apportioning problem is still complex. At this time there exists no clear standard as to what constitutes reasonable supervision (12).

When the physician is asked by another clinician to see a patient, the consulting physician's liability for malpractice is governed by whether a doctor–patient relationship was created. If the consulting physician provides consultation to the treating doctor, but does not write orders or otherwise direct the treatment, then ordinarily no doctor–patient relationship is formed, and the consultant's duty is only to the consultee doctor. However, if the consulting physician writes orders or otherwise directs care, then the court will usually find that a doctor–patient relationship was created.

Clinicians may examine people on behalf of a third party, such as a school or insurer, to whom they owe a contractual duty. However, if the examination causes the examinee harm, for example, by failure to detect suicidality or the possibility of child abuse, the liability risk is ambiguous. Some courts have held that the clinician's duty is to the employer; others have held that, if the person being examined reasonably relied on the examination for diagnosis, a duty may be owed. The physician is advised to inform the examinee that the purpose of the examination is not therapeutic. In court-ordered evaluations, courts typically find that the evaluator is immune as an agent of the court (13).

Fiduciary Relationship

The clinician's obligations toward the patient go beyond the duty to provide reasonable care. The relationship between psychiatrist and patient is analogous to that between guardian and ward. The patient has a right to expect the physician to show good faith, that is, to act in the patient's best interest.

This, the physician's *fiduciary duty*, is especially onerous in psychiatry, because emotionally disturbed people share their most private experiences with their mental health clinicians and are thus very vulnerable. Improper sexual contact, invasion of privacy, breach of confidentiality, outrageous manipulation of the patient's emotions, and the exploitation of patients for financial gain are all examples of *double agentry* and *breaches of fiduciary trust.* These *intentional torts* are discussed later in this chapter.

Dereliction of Duty: Breach of the Standard of Care

In accordance with the contract inherent in the doctor–patient relationship, the physician is bound to provide a reasonable level of care. In other words, the physician contracts to provide reasonable, prudent, diligent, knowledgeable, and skillful medical care. Unless the clinician has unwisely promised a cure, the contract does not call for exceptional care, only a level of expertise equivalent to that exercised under similar circumstances by the average practitioner in the same field of medicine. *The clinician is not liable for an error of judgment unless the error represented a substandard level of care.* If the clinician exercised reasonable judgment, the clinician is not responsible simply because the patient suffers a bad outcome. If clinicians differ as to how a particular issue should be addressed, it is enough to show that there is a respectable minority who endorse the approach that was taken. The considerable variation among clinicians in methods of treatment has made standards difficult to establish, particularly in regard to psychotherapy, where there are many different approaches. The standard is tighter with regard to precautions against suicide or violence or the monitoring of medication.

The standard of care traditionally required that the clinician be judged by the professional standard in the locality. However, the emergence of national standards has caused the courts to move in this direction, with allowance for the paucity of resources in some areas. Since the statute of limitations typically does not begin to toll until a child reaches the age of majority, cases involving children may be filed many years after the alleged malpractice took place. The standard of care is linked to the standard of professional practice at the time of the alleged breach of duty. If a clinician practices medicine in a specialty area for which he or she is not trained, the clinician is likely to be held to the standard applying to that specialty.

Breach of the Duty of Care

Malpractice suits are founded in the legal theories of intentional and negligent torts. An *intentional tort* involves deliberate intent on the part of the wrongdoer or wrongful conduct that the wrongdoer ought to have known was unacceptable (in which case it is known as a *quasi-intentional tort*). Examples of intentional torts are assault, battery, false imprisonment, fraudulent commitment, defamation, invasion of privacy, sexual exploitation, and the intentional infliction of emotional distress. Expert testimony is not required to substantiate an intentional tort, and malpractice insurance may not cover it. A *negligent tort* involves an unintentional error that reflects a failure by the clinician to exercise a reasonable standard of medical care. Expert testimony is required for proof of negligence.

In determining whether treatment fell below the standard of care, the courts may look to a variety of sources (14), and inquire whether the treatment:

1. Violates a statute (such as the child abuse reporting law or HIPAA regulations)
2. Violates a licensing board regulation or other regulatory agency holdings (such as FDA guidelines)
3. Violates an ethical principle of the profession (such as confidentiality)
4. Violates case law (such as the *Tarasoff* duty to protect)
5. Violates the professional consensus of the community

Professional consensus is the least clear of these elements, and the one about which expert opinion at trial most often differs. When there is no disagreement about what treatment the defendant doctor actually provided, the difficult question is whether that course was reasonable in the specific case at issue. When professional organizations began developing published practice parameters or practice guidelines, clinicians were concerned that such guidelines would create liability by setting the standard of practice. In response to this concern, published guidelines typically contain disclaimers stating the guidelines do not define a standard of practice. Guidelines have often proved useful to defendant doctors by indicating that a range of approaches are acceptable. In day-to-day work, in considering a course of action, a clinician should ask himself, "What would my peers think of this?" and "What would I think if a colleague told me he was going to do this?" If the answer is to be one of concern, then the physician should consider the approach carefully and document the rationale fully.

Damage, Harm, or Injury

Harm may be physical or psychological. Physical harm or damage resulting from negligence includes, for example, side effects of medication such as tardive dyskinesia, physical injury incurred when a patient is improperly restrained, or homicide or suicide. Psychological damages may be of two types: general pain and suffering, and damages to the patient's mental health. Expert testimony is not needed to establish pain and suffering: The jury can draw its own conclusion as to how much suffering it thinks a normal person would suffer given a particular harm. Psychiatric evidence may be utilized to inform the jury about the impact of an injury on the plaintiff's capacity to enjoy life. Mental health damages typically require expert testimony, as, for example, when a plaintiff alleges that her major depressive disorder has been aggravated by traumatic treatment. Injury to a parent or child may give rise to an action for loss of consortium, that is, loss of the care, comfort, and society of a spouse, parent, or child.

Proximate Cause

The plaintiff must substantiate that the defendant's wrongful act or omission directly caused or aggravated the patient's injury. In other words, it must be proven that, but for the wrongful conduct, the damage would not have occurred or would not have been aggravated or that a direct, uninterrupted link or foreseeable chain of events exists between the wrongful conduct and the injury or its aggravation. The legal concept of *cause* is analogous to the psychiatric concept of *precipitation* or *aggravation*.

Some states have comparative or contributory negligence rules that instruct juries to consider whether the plaintiff's negligence, such as failing to inform the clinician of a worsening condition, or failing to cooperate with treatment, contributed to the bad outcome, and reduce damages accordingly. Because a child or adolescent patient's responsibility is generally held to be lower than that of an adult, comparative negligence issues are uncommon in child or adolescent malpractice cases.

Restitutive Payment

If the defendant is found liable, the judge or jury may award damages. Damages are designed to be *compensatory,* that is, to recompense the victim for medical expenses, pain, suffering, loss of enjoyment of life, impairment of capacity, and future loss of earnings and to restore the plaintiff to his or her original position, so far as money is able to do so. If the defendant's behavior has been egregiously outrageous, malicious, or wanton, *punitive* damages may be imposed over and above compensatory damages, but are rare in malpractice cases. By federal law, all payments whether as a result of settlement talks or by trial verdict, are reported to the National Practitioner Data Bank (15).

Managed Care

Although managed care has had considerable impact on clinical practice, it has had rather little impact on malpractice litigation. From the law's perspective, the clinician is responsible for prescribing needed treatment, and managed care deals only with payment of fees. In *Wickline v. State of California* (1986) (16), the court affirmed the physician's duty to prescribe care, and suggested that the physician had a duty to appeal adverse decisions made by managed care reviewers. In clinical practice, clinicians routinely take into account the ability of the patient to pay in making treatment recommendations.

A number of states have attempted to pass laws holding managed care entities liable for denying authorization or payment for needed care. However, most managed care contracts are employee benefits, and are covered under the federal Employee Retirement Income Responsibility Act (ERISA). Congress originally passed ERISA to regulate pensions, but it has been interpreted to cover employee health care benefits as well. ERISA has two major prongs that limit the liability of managed care companies: First, it preempts any state law with which it conflicts, and second, it limits the damage for error to the amount of the benefit denied (the cost of treatment). Thus, state laws which assign liability to managed care are voided, and the most the patient can recover for improperly denied care is the cost of the care. The courts have recognized that this leaves patients with little redress (17), but reform, so called "patient rights" legislation, requires congressional action.

In malpractice litigation, managed care issues rarely surface: Physicians are reluctant to argue that their care, which resulted in a bad outcome, was limited by financial considerations, and plaintiffs are reluctant to assert that they happily would have paid for expensive care out of pocket if only the doctor had recommended it.

COURSE OF A TYPICAL CASE

If a clinician's patient suffers a serious adverse treatment-related event, the clinician should report the matter to his or her insurer and follow their risk management advice. With minor patients, the parents control access to information, so no formal release is necessary to discuss with them what occurred, unlike in cases involving adults. A number of states have passed legislation which prohibits apologies or expressions of sympathy or regret from later being admitted as evidence of physician negligence. Peer-review activities, such as morbidity and mortality conferences, are not discoverable to prove liability. The clinician then enters an uneasy waiting period to see if suit is filed. For minor patients, the statute of limitations (the period during which suit can be filed) does not begin to run until the child becomes an adult, so the wait can be quite long. Attorneys for plaintiffs in malpractice actions typically work on a contingency fee basis in which they initially bear the costs of litigation. Attorneys therefore screen cases carefully before making a judgment that spending the time and money to pursue the case is likely to be profitable. If the physician is served with notice of being sued, the malpractice insurance carrier should immediately be notified.

After suit is filed, the discovery phase begins, which will involve both sides retaining experts and taking depositions, including the deposition of the defendant doctor. Settlement talks also occur in this period. Whether the malpractice insurer can settle without the agreement of the defendant doctor depends on the terms of the insurance contract. If the case does not settle, it progresses to trial. Halleck (18), an experienced forensic psychiatrist who had himself testified in numerous malpractice actions, has described how emotionally wrenching even he found being a defendant. If money is paid to the plaintiff, either as a product of settlement negotiations or a court verdict, the amount and doctor's name are reported to the National Practitioner Data Bank, and the information is available to credentialing bodies, licensing boards, insurers, and managed care entities. This publicity has reduced doctors' willingness to settle a case for "nuisance value."

CIRCUMSTANCES IN WHICH MALPRACTICE IS MOST LIKELY TO OCCUR

While in many ways child and adolescent malpractice cases are similar to adult malpractice cases, only involving younger patients, they differ from adult cases in a number of respects. First, minors are less responsible for their acts, which tends to shift responsibility to the clinician and the parents. Second, minors typically cannot consent to treatment, which introduces a third party decisionmaker, usually the parents, into the case. Third, parents are often involved as quasipatients because they receive advice from the clinician. And finally, juries are sympathetic to injured children. While an allegation of malpractice can involve any aspect of practice, the vast majority of cases fall into one of the several areas shown in Table 7.3.4.1 and described here.

Issues Pertaining to Dangerousness

From a malpractice perspective, the central questions are first, whether the danger was reasonably foreseeable, and second, if it was, whether the clinician took adequate steps to protect the patient and potential victims. Foreseeability focuses on the adequacy of the assessment of risk, and protection focuses on the interventions employed once significant risk is found. While there is general acceptance that psychiatrists lack the ability to accurately predict violence, there is increasing agreement on the standards for assessing the risk of violence.

Suicide

Suicide of a young person is a tragedy. Assessment and treatment of suicidal children and adolescents are covered in detail in Chapter 5.4.3. Assessment of suicidal intent is more difficult in adolescents than it is in adults because the rate of suicidal ideation is so high in middle to late adolescents. In 2003, the Youth Risk Behavior Surveillance study found that 16.9% of high school students had seriously considered suicide in the previous 12 months, 16.5% had made plans, 8.5% had attempted suicide, and 2.9% had made an attempt that required medical attention (19). When these rates are compared to the completed suicide rate of approximately .007%, it is clear that the ratio of suicidal ideation to completed suicide is very high (over 2000:1). Assuming that an adequate assessment was conducted, documentation of the assessment is key. The oft-seen suicide assessment note of "SI–"

TABLE 7.3.4.1

COMMON ISSUES IN MALPRACTICE LITIGATION

Area of Practice	Example Plaintiff Allegation
Dangerousness	
Suicide	Weak suicide assessment documentation: "SI–"
Homicide	No violence risk assessment in chart
Failure to protect from danger	Inpatient sexually assaulted by another inpatient
Failure to protect third parties	Dangerous patient escapes from hospital and family not notified
Protecting and releasing information	Confidential information released without authorization
Treatment	
Failure to obtain informed consent	Possible side effects not discussed
Psychotherapy	Implanted memories of sexual abuse
Sex with patient	Therapist had sex with patient
Medication	Girl with bipolar disorder treated with sodium divalproex for 8 months gives birth to baby with birth defects and there is no documentation of pregnancy status when medication is started
Ending treatment	
Negligent discharge	Patient discharged while still suicidal
Abandonment	Therapist terminated treatment without referral when patient failed to pay bill

(suicidal ideation negative) does not offer much protection to a defendant psychiatrist because it fails to document the components of the suicide assessment, such as what history was obtained about prior attempts, family history, plan, etc. Where some suicide risk is present, assessment entails weighing risk factors and protective factors. Good documentation of risk and protective factors, and of the physician's reasoning about intervention, is the best protection in the event of an adverse outcome. On an inpatient unit, the psychiatrist should also document his or her review of the assessments of others, such as nurses and house officers. Timely, clear, legible, pertinent, thorough, dated, timed, and signed records are the key to communication and the best proof that the hospital and staff have exercised reasonable care. In *Abille v. United States* (20), after a psychiatrist transferred a patient from a suicidal status to a less dangerous status, the patient committed suicide. The finding of negligence against the defendant hinged on the psychiatrist's failure to keep detailed records that explained his decision to transfer the patient, even though it was conceded that, under the circumstances, the decision may have been reasonable. Finally, it is important to keep in mind that suicide assessment is a process, and for depressed or suicidal youth, repeated assessments need to be documented.

If a physician determines that the patient is at significant risk for suicide, then he or she has a duty to institute reasonable precautions. If the clinician decides not to hospitalize the patient, it is important to document the protective factors and interventions that were employed. For youthful patients, this often involves utilizing the family to monitor the patient's condition, provide some protection, and alert the clinician if the situation deteriorates. The child or adolescent's risk for suicide should be discussed with the parents. If the patient is in the hospital, it is important to document the physician's review of observations of other care providers and to document the reasons when levels of supervision are reduced.

What if the patient refuses to cooperate with the admitting psychiatrist, who consequently does not elicit and diagnose an imminent suicide risk? In *Skar v. City of Lincoln, Nebraska* (21), a recalcitrant patient injured himself in a suicide attempt. The court found for the defendant and held that the patient had a duty to cooperate with his physician as far as he was able. However, it is essential in such a case that the psychiatrist record the questions put to the patient and the patient's responses or failure to respond. Also, with minor patients who can not legally consent to treatment, courts are likely to apportion less responsibility to the patient.

Failure to Protect or Control a Violent or Sexually Aggressive Patient

Clinicians and hospitals assume a duty of care toward patients with a potential for violence. The psychiatrist must carefully assess the potential for danger and must ensure that the hospital staff takes adequate precautions to protect a violent patient from harming others. Past medical records should be scrutinized concerning violence potential, and referring agents and parents should be questioned. In accordance with the imminence of the risk, housing in a secure unit, confinement to a room, close observation, a search of clothing and personal effects, and removal of all dangerous objects (belts, mirrors), may be required. If the patient is medicated, staff members should check that medication is actually swallowed. It is essential that the degree and nature of risk be communicated to all staff who care for the patient.

The prevalence of sexual abuse and its relationship to psychiatric disorder mean that many minors admitted to psychiatric hospitals are at risk of precocious sexual activity and unwanted pregnancy. Suicide and sexual activity involving latency-aged inpatients have been reported to be the most common types of malpractice action brought against child psychiatry training programs (22). These cases may involve two patients cared for by different doctors, and raise complicated confidentiality problems (can the plaintiff-victim get access to the medical file of the perpetrator?). The central issues are the foresight involving the risk of the activity occurring, and the adequacy of nursing monitoring of patient interaction. Known perpetrators should be closely observed and housed in single rooms, if necessary. However, the closeness of the possible observation decreases if the therapeutic environment is less restrictive, for example, in a residential treatment center.

Negligent Release or Discharge of a Suicidal or Violent Patient

A patient may harm himself or herself or others while on pass in the grounds of the hospital, on leave with relatives or friends, after discharge, or after absconding from a hospital. Was the tragedy foreseeable by a reasonably prudent psychiatrist? This is the question that the courts seek to answer. In doing so, they are aware that the safety of the public must be balanced against the need to rehabilitate patients, that reasonable, calculated risks must often be taken, and that *bona fide* errors of clinical judgment are unavoidable (23).

Increasing pressure by managed-care organizations, Medicaid agencies, and insurers has raised the specter of premature discharge against medical advice forced by withdrawal of funding. The clinician should be aware that legal responsibility for any harm that consequently befalls the patient or community will be placed on his or her shoulders. The risk may be so great that the hospital should bear the cost of continued hospitalization.

Wrongful Injury, Assault, and Battery

A patient injured by staff members who use excessive force to subdue him or her may have a claim against the hospital for battery or wrongful injury. Wrongful injury may also be claimed when one patient is harmed by another whom the staff could not control; however, the plaintiff would have to establish that the hospital was derelict in its duty to control the violent patient.

Seclusion and restraint present serious liability risks. They may be legitimate management techniques when the risk of harm is imminent and there are no alternatives; but they should not be used to compensate for understaffing. Physical control should be time limited, and the patient should be examined by a physician if the maximum permissible time (e.g., 1 hour) requires extension. Seclusion and restraint should never be ordered "as needed." Quality assurance tracking is required to ensure that the use of physical controls does not become excessive.

If the person causing the harm is a hospital employee, the hospital may be liable, particularly if it were known that the employee had a propensity for violence or sexual misbehavior (24). The hospital may also be liable for the misbehavior of physicians, agency nurses, or others who work in a hospital but who are not employed by it. State institutions may claim *sovereign immunity,* which precludes litigants from suing governmental institutions; however, most jurisdictions have greatly limited or abolished this doctrine.

Failure to Protect Endangered Third Parties

Prior to the first *Tarasoff* decision (25) in 1974, clinicians had duties to their patients, but not to third parties. So, if a patient harmed a third party, the patient might have grounds to sue the clinician for failing to treat or restrain him, but the victim could not successfully sue the clinician. This was in line with general negligence principles which hold that in most situations, one does not have a duty to protect third parties. Thus, if a man sees someone drowning in a river, he has no legal duty to help (although he may have a moral duty). In the clinical situation, it was also thought that the patient's confidentiality prevented notifying a potential victim of threats, and that psychiatrists' inability to accurately predict violence limited their ability to intervene.

The first time the California Supreme Court heard the *Tarasoff* case, it found that clinicians did have a duty to potential victims, and that duty overrode the need for confidentiality, holding "The protective privilege ends where the public peril begins" (*Tarasoff I* at 561). The Court also decided that the duty could be discharged by warning the potential victim, which became known as the "duty to warn."

Concerned by the serious implications for patient confidentiality of this judgment, the American Psychiatric Association pressed the appellate court to reopen the case. In an unusual move, the court did so, and in *Tarasoff II* (26), the issue of failure to warn was debated. The court decided that there was a *duty to protect* rather than a duty to warn: *If there is a serious danger of violence, the clinician must take reasonable care to protect the foreseeable victim.* The court failed to define what constituted "reasonable care" and how dangerous the patient must be before precautions should be taken.

Following *Tarasoff*, courts and legislatures in other jurisdictions have wrestled with these issues. The key dimensions that need to be decided are:

1. Is there a duty to protect?
2. If there is a duty, who needs to be protected? Only identifiable victims? The general public?
3. What triggers the duty? Is a specific threat required, or only a clinical judgment of risk?
4. How can the duty be discharged? A warning? Calling the police?

Jurisdictions have answered these questions differently, with about half the states finding a duty, a minority holding there is no duty, and some leaving the question unresolved. The trend has been toward legislation specifying what the duty is and how clinicians can fulfill it to avoid liability (27). Clearly, clinicians need to be aware of the law in their own jurisdiction.

Despite the attention paid to *Tarasoff* issues, clinical cases involving a need to breach confidentiality are uncommon with adolescent patients, because in the vast majority of cases where an adolescent is judged an imminent risk to others, the adolescent is hospitalized and kept in the hospital until he no longer poses serious risk. Further, in working clinically with dangerous minors, parents control consent to release information, and they will often consent to involving victims (as in family treatment), so problems of breaching confidentiality without consent may often be sidestepped. *Tarasoff* situations most commonly arise in two situations: first, when the patient is not available for intervention, as when a therapist hears about a threat over the telephone or the patient escapes from the hospital, and second, in situations of contingent threats ("I think I'll pass, but if that teacher gives me an 'F,' I'll shoot her").

What, then, should a clinician do if a patient threatens violence and the situation can not be managed clinically? First, undertake and document a violence risk–resource analysis. If the risk is serious, take precautions to protect endangered parties, and with minors, discuss the situation with the parents. Second, if the patient is already hospitalized, take precautions against elopement, consider limiting visitation and leave, and do not discharge the patient unless you are convinced that the risk of violence has diminished. Ask for a consultation if you are in doubt. Third, if a potentially violent hospitalized patient elopes or fails to return from leave, seek consultation from a colleague and from the hospital's attorney and inform the parents. If the risk of harm is significant, inform the local police and the police department of the area where the patient lives, by telephone and certified letter. If certain people (family, friends, or acquaintances) could be in danger, warn them by telephone, through the police, and by certified letter. Fourth, if you warn a third party by telephone or letter, take care to divulge only as much as necessary to let them know they are at risk. Fifth, involve the patient in the warning process. The patient may agree to having a warning given. If you have control of the patient, let the patient be present when you telephone the police and the third party, allow him or her to read the contents of the letters sent to the endangered third party and the police, and encourage the patient to discuss his or her reactions to these interventions. Knowing the potential victim has been warned may bolster the patient's own self-control.

If the situation is unclear in the home state, the clinician would be well advised to act as though the broadest interpretation of the doctrine applies. However, as Simon (28) points out, one should not allow concern about *Tarasoff* liability to interfere with sound clinical practice. Instead, the clinician should make reasonable efforts to control potentially violent patients before breaching confidentiality; and if warnings are required, they should be incorporated into treatment whenever possible.

Failure to Report Child Abuse or Neglect

All states have mandatory reporting laws requiring mental health clinicians to report a reasonable suspicion of child abuse or neglect, and failure to do so is malpractice (29). The statutes immunize a clinician making a good faith report, so a report to protective services that is later deemed unfounded is not a basis for malpractice. However, other interventions taken by the clinician based on a conclusion of abuse may be actionable. In *Montoya v. Bebensee* (30), a clinician advised a mother to withhold visitation from a father who was suspected of abuse. The father sued, and the court held that the report to protective services was immune from suit, even if made negligently, but the advice to the mother fell outside the reporting statute and could be grounds for suit, a holding Guyer (31) characterized as "you can sound an alarm, but you can't form a posse." Litigation over recovered memories has addressed similar issues, and is discussed further below.

Protecting and Releasing Information

The Hippocratic oath includes a precept regarding confidentiality: "What I may see or hear in the course of the treatment or even outside of the treatment in regard to the life of men, which on no account one must spread abroad, I will keep to myself, holding such things shameful to be spoken about." Confidentiality has always been seen as especially central in psychiatry. The issue is complex in child and adolescent psychiatry because the clinician needs to weigh the child's need for privacy against the parents' right to know by virtue of their legally controlling the release of information until the child patient becomes an adult. In many jurisdictions, the extent to which an adolescent can enforce a privacy right against the parents' control of the record is legally murky. It is clear that parents have a right to know if the adolescent is involved in a dangerous clinical situation. Many states have allowed minors some control over the record, generally in parallel to the degree that minors in that jurisdiction can consent to treatment. Aside from the legal precedents, children and adolescents value confidentiality in psychotherapy as necessary for feeling comfortable to share sensitive material. While clinicians are advised to be aware of the rules in their jurisdiction, from a clinical perspective, it is important at the outset of treatment to discuss with patients and their parents what information will be shared with parents and under what conditions.

Confidentiality and Privilege

Confidentiality precludes the physician from divulging private matters revealed by the patient in the context of the doctor–patient relationship. *Privilege* is the patient's right to bar the physician from disclosing confidential matters in a court of law. Testimonial privilege derives from statutes in some states, and from court holdings in other states. In *Jaffee v. Redmond* (32), the U.S. Supreme Court held that there was a mental health privilege in federal court. Physicians should consult their local statutes to understand the extent of this privilege and its exceptions. Confusion may occur when a clinician receives a *subpoena* to appear in court (with or without records). A subpoena merely requires the clinician to appear in court. It does not compel him or her to testify about confidential matters unless the patient has specifically authorized the clinician to do so, or has waived privilege, or unless the clinician is ordered to do so by the judge. Although states vary somewhat in the exceptions allowed to the rule of privilege, the following are the most usual:

1. *Waiver by patient.* The clinician should seek specific written authorization from the patient before disclosing confidential material in court or to other parties (e.g., other mental health agencies).
2. *The patient-litigant exception.* If a patient offers his or her mental health as evidence in litigation, he or she generally waives privilege concerning the specific issue in evidence. Similarly, if the patient pleads insanity as a criminal defense, the psychiatric examination conducted to evaluate that matter is not privileged (33).
3. *Evaluation for a reason other than psychiatric treatment.* For example, the psychiatric evaluation of a disputant in a child custody case is not privileged if the evaluation was conducted as part of the case. A similar exclusion applies to evaluations for the purpose of civil commitment.
4. *Duty to protect endangered third parties.* The *Tarasoff* exclusion discussed above applies when the community is endangered.
5. Other limited exceptions authorized by law, such as mandatory reporting of child abuse and civil commitment proceedings.

HIPAA

The Health Insurance Portability and Accountability Act of 1996 (HIPAA) authorized the U.S. Department of Health and Human Services to establish regulations regarding the privacy of medical records, which they did in what is known as the Privacy Rule (34) which went into effect in 2003. The Privacy Rule establishes a federal floor for the protection of protected health information (PHI). If state law provides for a higher level of protection of privacy, state law controls. "Covered entities," which includes practitioners who have transmitted PHI electronically, are covered by the Privacy Rule. The Privacy Rule is complex, and a complete summary will not be attempted here. The Office for Civil Rights in the Department of Health and Human Services provides considerable information on its website regarding the details of the Privacy Rule and federal "guidances" giving their interpretations of the Privacy Rule (35), and many professional organizations provide information and recommendations to their members. Despite this assistance, there are as yet some situations where it is unclear what is required of practitioners: There are still few court cases interpreting the Privacy Rule, and how each state's laws may preempt the Privacy Rule is often confusing. Violations of HIPAA and the Privacy Rule can be investigated and prosecuted.

HIPAA has implications for psychiatric practice. First, clinicians covered by the Privacy Rule are required to give patients (or parents) a *Notice of Privacy Practices* at the patient's first appointment. The notice must spell out how clinicians assure privacy and under what conditions and to whom protected health information can be released without obtaining consent. Second, HIPAA gives patients the right to see their records, with very limited exceptions. Third, the Privacy Rule restricts third party payer requests for information to the "minimum necessary" information. Previously, insurance companies, relying on the patient's release signed as a condition of obtaining coverage, could, and often did, ask for a copy of the entire chart. The American Psychiatric Association (36) has taken a formal position on what constitutes the minimum necessary information necessary for payment which includes identifying information, diagnosis, treatment plan, and dates of treatment, but excludes much of the detailed material often found in progress notes. Fourth, the Privacy Rule creates a new category of medical record which it terms psychotherapy notes. Psychotherapy notes, as defined in the Privacy Rule, are notes that are part of the medical record, and so are different from process notes, which the clinician typically holds apart from the medical record and can destroy whenever he or she wishes (except to avoid a subpoena!). However, psychotherapy notes are kept separately from the regular medical record, and can only be released with the consent of the patient, giving such notes substantially greater protection than the regular medical record. Clinicians are permitted, but not required, to maintain psychotherapy notes. Psychotherapy notes are the only special category of notes in the Privacy Rule: Advocates for AIDS patients and substance abuse patients were unsuccessful in getting special protection for their records. Keeping a second set of records is somewhat cumbersome, and many clinicians do not keep psychotherapy notes, but rather choose not to document highly sensitive fantasy material.

HIPAA has drawn attention to the electronic transmission of information, of which one common form is emailing patients. The potential problems with email are that it can be intercepted and may inadvertently be delivered to the wrong person. For emails that involve sensitive information, it is best to use Web-based email that is encrypted. For email that simply has to do with arranging appointment times, encryption is probably not necessary.

Improper Release of Information from Medical Records

The unauthorized disclosure of confidential information from a patient's record could be actionable on the ground of breach of confidentiality and also may constitute a HIPAA violation. Medical records should be kept in a locked place in the ward or medical records department to bar access to unauthorized people. The patient or legal guardian must give written consent for the transfer of information to legitimate professionals or agencies (other involved clinicians, attorneys, hospitals, schools, social welfare departments, and insurance companies).

If a subpoena is served without the written consent of the patient or guardian, the clinician has three alternatives: to seek the patient's consent; to have a motion filed by an attorney to quash the subpoena; or to refuse to testify unless ordered by the judge to do so. If the clinician persists in refusing to testify despite the judge's instruction to do so, he or she may be held in contempt of court (37).

Defamation

Defamation involves communication by one party about a second party to a third party that damages the reputation of the second party. Defamation is most likely to occur in child psychiatry when carelessly written medical records are released to third parties. For example, the patient may have been described in the record as a "psychopath" or "malingerer," labels that could be extremely damaging in the hands of later employers or creditors. Clinicians who gossip about patients over coffee or in elevators put themselves at risk of liability on the grounds of defamation or breach of confidentiality.

Defenses against defamation include *substantial truth* and *conditional privilege.* Conditional privilege allows communication when both parties have a duty and an interest to receive and report such matters. For example, when one doctor refers a patient to another, conditional privilege in most jurisdictions allows the two doctors to discuss the patient's condition. (However, a prudent outpatient practice is to have the referring doctor have the patient sign a release.) No such privilege applies to those who have no such duty and interest. Testimony given in court or provided to the court in documents such as medical reports or medical records attract *absolute privilege* insofar as they refer to the broadly defined matter at issue. *Malice*, if proven, destroys conditional privilege. Malice is substantiated by the author's evident self-interest, excessive distribution of the defamatory material, reckless disregard of the truth, or the vituperative style of the documents involved in the case.

Improper Treatment

Failure to Obtain Informed Consent

The doctrine of informed consent is founded on the constitutional right of the individual to control what is done to his or her own body (38). A patient cannot give informed consent unless he or she has a) *sufficient information* on which to base a decision, b) *mental competency* to make a rational decision, and c) freedom to exercise *voluntary choice.* All states require informed consent, and psychiatrists are also ethically bound to obtain it.

The physician must therefore disclose sufficient information to enable the patient, or the patient's legal representative, to weigh all material pros and cons. How much is that? The earlier "professional" standard (39, 40) referred to *what a reasonable medical practitioner would disclose* under similar circumstances. Following two 1972 cases, *Canterbury v. Spence* (41) and *Cobbs v. Grant* (42), some jurisdictions may have adopted the "patient" standard, that is, *as much information as a reasonable patient would require* to make a rational decision under similar circumstances. *Canterbury* and other cases suggest that the physician should discuss the following matters with the patient:

1. The nature of the condition that requires treatment
2. The nature, purpose, and benefits of the proposed treatment, and the probability that it will succeed
3. The risks and consequences of the proposed treatment
4. Alternatives to the proposed treatment (including no treatment) and their attendant risks and consequences
5. The prognosis with and without the proposed treatment

The courts have held that *not all risks need be disclosed—only the material ones.* Unfortunately, there are no clear guidelines concerning what is "material," except to suggest that, even if the likelihood be slight, the more serious the risk, the greater the probability that it should be discussed. *A risk is material when a reasonable person would be likely to attach significance to the risk or cluster of risks.* Risk is linked not only to the procedure but also to the physician and his or her competence to perform the procedure (e.g., if the physician has alcoholism or suffers from human immunodeficiency virus infection). The plaintiff must prove that nondisclosure of material risk caused the injury of which he or she complains. Some courts require that the plaintiff prove that a reasonable person would have refused the procedure had the risks been disclosed.

Therapeutic privilege countervails the clinician's duty to disclose. The physician is obliged to protect a vulnerable patient from the emotional trauma that could be sustained if upsetting risks were prematurely revealed. However, therapeutic privilege should never be invoked merely because the clinician fears that, if apprised of the facts, the patient would reject a desirable treatment. If the clinician proposes to limit disclosure on the ground of therapeutic privilege, clear documentation and expert consultation are required concerning the patient's exceptional sensitivity.

Consent is not required for emergency treatment in which the harm from failure to treat is imminent and outweighs the potential danger of the treatment. However, if possible, a relative's consent should be obtained.

For most children and adolescents, informed consent of a parent or guardian is necessary for psychiatric treatment. In treating a child whose parents are divorced, the clinician should be sure that the parent requesting treatment is legally empowered to give consent. It is generally prudent to keep a copy of the legal custody order in the chart. On a clinical basis, it is generally best to obtain the consent and participation of both divorced parents. Problems can arise if both divorced parents have the power to consent, and one consents but the other refuses. In that case, the clinician should have the requesting parent obtain court authorization for the decision to pursue treatment.

In some cases, minors can consent to treatment on their own behalf. Competence is extended to emancipated minors. When should an unemancipated minor be regarded as sufficiently mature to participate in health care decisions? It depends on the jurisdiction and the condition being treated. All states allow minors to seek treatment for venereal disease. Most allow treatment for substance abuse. Landmark federal decisions (43, 44) extended to "mature minors" the right to make health decisions concerning contraception and abortion, and required the availability of a judicial bypass procedure for minors who are not mature, but they left unclear what a mature minor was. Many states have "mature minor" rules which allow "mature" youth to seek treatment on their own. In some jurisdictions, "mature minor" is undefined, while in others it is defined by statute. Some states allow adolescents to seek outpatient psychiatric care. The present situation is very confused, and the practitioner should ascertain the law on the matter in his or her own state. The minor's ability to consent, however, does not generally require the parents to pay for treatment, so youth obtaining psychiatric treatment on their own remains fairly rare. Although it may not be legally required, the desirability of promoting a treatment alliance suggests that it is judicious to promote the understanding and cooperation of all minors mature enough to comprehend. For patients more than 13 years of age, it is prudent to obtain formal assent.

The third element of informed consent, *voluntariness,* is easily compromised. True voluntary consent requires that the patient be free of coercion. However, even a mature minor can be susceptible to threat, cajolement, bribery, or false inducement by parents, physicians, or hospital staff. The inmates of correctional institutions and psychiatric hospitals are particularly vulnerable to therapeutic coercion.

Problems with Admission

A physician who causes a patient to be admitted to a psychiatric hospital without proper evaluation may be sued for *negligent diagnosis* or *false imprisonment.* A falsely imprisoned plaintiff may recover damages for *loss of dignity* and *emotional distress.* Ignorance of the mental health statutes is no defense; failure to comply with statutory requirements could be actionable. For example, in *Johnson v. Greer* (45), a patient recovered damages after being forcibly detained in hospital for several days beyond the 24 hours permitted on an emergency warrant. Malice, spite, ulterior motive, bad faith, or fraud during involuntary hospitalization could also result in damages for false imprisonment or *malicious prosecution* (46). Parents or guardians may admit unemancipated minors against their will, and healthcare providers should be able to rely on parental consent (46, 47). However, the psychiatric justification for admission should be carefully documented.

Negligent Diagnosis

The physician must distinguish organic disease from functional disorders and, within the latter, must differentiate the major psychoses from each other and from other Axis I and II conditions. The physician who admits patients to a psychiatric hospital must be alert for signs that could indicate a toxic condition. In *Hirschberg v. State* (48), for example, a patient who had taken an overdose of salicylates died after having been hospitalized without adequate physical examination, special investigations, or proper precautions. The hospital was found liable.

The physician who fails to diagnose the patient accurately (e.g., by missing psychosis when it is present or by confusing bipolar disorder with schizophrenia) may found treatment on a false premise and thus may be open to a liability suit. However, there have been few actions on these grounds. Lawyers have been reluctant to pursue such cases in view of the reputedly widely varying expert opinion concerning the most appropriate treatment for different psychiatric conditions. As child psychiatry becomes more empirically based, it is likely that such actions will increase in frequency.

Psychotherapy

There are so many schools of psychotherapy that failure to use a particular type of therapy or not conducting psychotherapy very skillfully seldom gives rise to a successful malpractice action for several reasons. There is a lack of consensus in the field as to appropriate methods. It is difficult to prove harm as a result of negligent psychotherapy, because mental injury is hard to substantiate when the plaintiff was already emotionally disturbed before the alleged negligence. In the 1990s, however, suits involving allegations that recovered memories of abuse were "implanted" by therapists became frequent, and some led to large jury verdicts or settlements (49). In the highly publicized *Ramona* case (50), the father of a patient was allowed to sue on his own behalf for damages allegedly flowing from memories implanted in his daughter because the court found that he was a "direct victim" of the psychotherapy. The "direct victim" theory gives rise to many problems, such as who may sue and what the nature of the victim-plaintiff's relationship to the therapist must be (51), and is particularly an issue in child psychiatry because of the therapist's involvement with parents. The direct victim test has not been adopted in many states other than California. In a variant of this genre, the patient sues the therapist for failing to recognize that dissociative identity disorder is confabulatory or for accepting uncritically the patient's recovered memories of abuse.

Sexual Exploitation and the Tort of Outrage

Expert testimony is not required to substantiate the impropriety of sexually molesting a patient. As an intentional tort, *res ipsa loquitur* ("the thing speaks for itself"), and the burden of proof shifts to the defendant. In *Roy v. Hartogs* (52), the court held that public policy protected patients from such malicious abuses of authority, power, and fiduciary trust. The perpetrator faces criminal sanctions for rape, aggravated assault, or child abuse, as well as civil actions for malpractice or battery (unconsented touching). Most malpractice policies will cover the cost of a defense if the clinician denies the sexual contact occurred, but exclude payment for damages for a sexual relationship with a patient. Liability for improper sexual relations may extend beyond the patient to others involved, such as the spouses of patients so harmed. Residual transference has persuaded courts that cessation of treatment does not open the door to a sexual relationship. Indeed, *negligent management of the transference* is often adopted as the theory behind the action for damages.

The tort of *outrage* refers to the intentional infliction of severe emotional distress on a patient, as a result of reckless and intolerable behavior. For example, in *Abraham v. Zaslow* (53), damages were awarded to a woman who had sustained bruising and renal failure after exposure to "rage-reduction therapy," an intrusive intervention involving several hours of physical restraint, poking, tickling, and verbal insult. Patients have a right to expect that clinicians will adhere to established methods of treatment. If exceptional methods are proposed, full informed consent is required, supportive consultation from a colleague would be advisable, and adequate reference to the scientific literature should be made.

Medication

The points in the medication of a patient at which negligence is most likely to occur are as follows:

1. The diagnosis of the psychiatric disorder
2. The adoption of an appropriate rationale for drug therapy
3. The choice of a particular drug to treat the patient's psychiatric disorder

4. Inquiry concerning a past history of excessive therapeutic response, severe side effects, or allergic reaction to the drug in question or to related drugs
5. The search for coexistent medical conditions that would contraindicate the medication in question or would indicate the need for caution in its use
6. Obtaining informed consent
7. The administration of an appropriate dose of the drug in question, by an approved route
8. The prescription of drugs in combination, or the addition of a drug or drugs to an existing medication regimen
9. The choice of a drug not approved by the U.S. Food and Drug Administration or the use of a drug in a way, or for a purpose, that deviates from that recommended in the package insert or *Physician's Desk Reference* (PDR)
10. Monitoring the therapeutic effect and side effects of the medication
11. Ceasing the medication after a therapeutic effect has been achieved or maintaining long-term medication at the lowest effective dosage

Decision to Medicate

In *Osheroff v. Chestnut Lodge* et al. (54), suit was brought against a private hospital for negligent failure to disclose all treatment alternatives. The plaintiff, who suffered from mixed affective and personality disorder, had been treated for several months with individual psychotherapy. After transfer to a different hospital, he responded to antidepressant medication within a few weeks. Several eminent psychiatrists testified for the plaintiff that antidepressant medication was the treatment of choice, and the plaintiff had had insufficient opportunity to consider it as a treatment alternative. The suit was settled out of court in favor of the plaintiff. Such cases are less common with children because medications are more controversial in this age group.

Inappropriate Rationale for Treatment

Psychotropic drugs are sometimes prescribed to control inmates in correctional or mental retardation institutions. These situations warrant close scrutiny; the physician may have been induced to medicate the patient by the urgings of harassed staff, rather than by the medical needs of the patient, a practice that has been specifically criticized in at least one class action suit (55) and one malpractice case (56).

Choice of An Inappropriate or Unapproved Drug or Route of Administration

This kind of error occurs when the physician orders a drug that is inadequate to treat the patient's disorder (a benzodiazepine for major depressive disorder) or when the physician prescribes a drug for which there are less risky alternatives (a neuroleptic for anxiety disorder). A different problem arises when the clinician prescribes a drug not approved by the Food and Drug Administration. Undoubtedly, the risk of malpractice is greater if approved guidelines have not been followed. However, because of the great expense of generating data to persuade the FDA to approve an indication for a drug's use in children, more than 70% of all PDR entries either have no dosing information for children or have explicit statements that safety and efficacy in children has not been determined (57). Courts generally find that the PDR does not set the standard of practice, and expert testimony is necessary to determine whether a particular use is an accepted treatment. Usage that is more experimental or investigational requires providing considerably more information about benefits, risks, and alternatives to obtain informed consent.

An intravenous or intramuscular route of administration carries an increased risk of excessive or adverse response. This is particularly likely if the patient is predisposed to side effects as a result of hepatic, renal, cardiac, or brain dysfunction. The clinician should be cautious if such conditions are detected. Parenteral administration should generally be reserved for emergencies or long-term depot treatment.

Failure to Obtain a Medication History

The patient's past medication history should be ascertained by interview, by review of medical records, and by telephone contact, if required, with other clinicians. The physician may be held liable for excessive side affects, allergic reactions, idiosyncratic responses, or drug interactions, if these had been foreseeable.

Failure to Detect Contraindicative Conditions

The physician may fail to check for conditions or disorders that would render the patient vulnerable to severe side effects. For example, preexisting hypothyroidism may be overlooked when lithium is prescribed. Different classes of psychotropic drug require different assessments prior to prescribing. If a contraindicative condition is uncovered but the medication is still considered potentially justified, a risk-to-benefit analysis should be documented, expert consultation should be obtained, and specific informed consent should be recorded. Hospitals should mandate, as policy, standard diagnostic workups for all psychotropic drugs. Since a very high proportion of adolescent pregnancies are unplanned and psychotropic drugs cross the placenta, when prescribing medication to an adolescent girl, the clinician should document pregnancy status and use of contraception.

Forcible Administration

The involuntary commitment of a patient to a psychiatric hospital does not permit involuntary medication, except in narrowly defined circumstances, generally having to do with the safety of the patient or others. Forcible medication can place the practitioner at risk of an action for the intentional tort of battery. The legal doctrine most pertinent to this issue, *the right to refuse treatment*, has been most clearly articulated in two convoluted cases, *Rennie v. Klein* (1981) (58) and *Rogers v. Commissioner of Mental Health* (59). In *Rennie*, a New Jersey case, it was determined that the mentally ill had a sufficient liberty interest to require due process before treatment was forcibly administered, but due process was satisfied by an in-hospital review. In considering this case, the U.S. Supreme Court deferred to the professionalization standard articulated in *Youngberg v. Romeo* (1982) (60), in effect declining to uphold a constitutional right to refuse treatment. In *Rogers*, the Massachusetts Supreme Court held that involuntarily committed patients should be presumed competent to refuse treatment except in emergencies. An "emergency" was defined as a situation fraught with the need to prevent violence or associated with the likelihood that the patient's health would significantly deteriorate without treatment. In nonemergency situations, forcible treatment may be administered only after a judicial hearing in which the court approves a "substituted judgment" treatment plan. "Substituted judgment" requires the court to determine what the patient would have decided if he or she were competent.

The failure of the U.S. Supreme Court to clarify this matter means that each state must make its own determination of the boundaries of the right to refuse treatment. The legal situation with regard to children is unclear. The right to refuse treatment apparently extends to the legal guardians of minors, to emancipated minors, and to those minors otherwise empowered to consent. What of the mature minor? Arguably, except in emergencies, the clinician should seek the consent of both mature minor and parent before starting treatment. If the mature minor refuses treatment, and the treatment is regarded vital, a judicial determination of competence should be requested.

Failure to Monitor Treatment

The case of *Clites v. State of Iowa* (1982) illustrates negligent failure to monitor psychotropic medication, in addition to other errors. The plaintiff, a mentally retarded patient, was admitted to a state residential facility at the age of 11 years. Between the ages of 17 and 22 years, he was treated with various psychotropic drug combinations, until tardive dyskinesia was noticed. The appellate court held that the hospital had failed to document behavior sufficiently aggressive or self-abusive to warrant neuroleptic treatment, that the medication appeared to be designed primarily for the staff's convenience, that the practice of prescribing polypharmacy was substandard, that the treatment had not been monitored adequately by a physician, that "drug holidays" should have been employed, that the staff had been too slow in recognizing the patient's dyskinesia, and that informed consent had not been sought from the patient's parents. Damages of more than $750,000 were affirmed.

Adequate monitoring of drug effects requires baseline and regular mental status examinations, physical examinations, vital signs, and laboratory testing, in accordance with the pharmacology of the drug and its potential side effects. "Drug holidays" should be considered if long-term medication is required. Physicians run a serious risk if they write "as-needed" orders for potent drugs, if they telephone prescriptions into a pharmacy without examining their patients, or if they provide multiple repeat refills without proper monitoring. In 2004, the FDA began issuing guidelines for SSRI use (61) regarding the frequency of monitoring patients for suicidal ideation. The FDA guidelines exceed what many clinicians think is appropriate. However, in the event of a child or adolescent suicide shortly after beginning an SSRI, a defendant psychiatrist would likely have a difficult time persuading a jury that such monitoring was not necessary. Recent actions by national regulatory agencies in the U.S., U.K., and Canada suggest that psychotropic medications are being exposed to increased regulatory scrutiny.

Abandonment

Psychiatrists are most at risk of liability when they terminate the treatment of patients without adequate safeguards, when they are unavailable and either no covering physician is provided or the covering physician has not been given sufficient information, or when adequate steps are not taken to protect endangered third parties.

The physician has the duty to provide continued care, as long as needed, until the doctor–patient relationship is terminated. This relationship may be severed by mutual consent or by the patient. However, unilateral termination of care by the clinician, if abrupt or premature, may put him or her at risk of breach of contract should harm (e.g., suicide) befall the patient. Failure to provide a telephone number for a disturbed patient to call, failure to provide adequate substitute care during absences, or failure to convey adequate precautionary information to substitute physicians may all be construed as abandonment if the patient is found to have suffered harm as a consequence.

When is the therapist warranted in unilaterally terminating the relationship? Lack of cooperation or threatening behavior may justify termination; failure to pay the bill does not (62). If the clinician does decide to terminate the relationship, the following safeguards are required (28):

1. The reason for the termination should be discussed with the patient. The clinician should give at least 1 month's notice of termination, to allow the patient to locate another therapist.
2. The patient should be provided with the names and telephone numbers of alternative therapists or agencies.
3. The clinician should mail to the patient a certified letter (return receipt requested) reflecting this discussion and containing the reasons for termination. The letter should also convey the names and telephone numbers of alternative clinicians or agencies.

These problems are most likely to occur in highly ambivalent adolescent patients with personality disorder whose suicide risk is aggravated by loss, separation, or rejection.

SUPERVISING, TEACHING, RESEARCH, AND PUBLICATION

The torts of *invasion of privacy, breach of confidentiality,* and *defamation* are the liability risks most commonly incurred by teachers, researchers, and writers.

These torts stem from the ethical, contractual, and (in some jurisdictions) statutory obligation of the clinician not to disclose private information that should be kept within the doctor–patient relationship. In invasion of privacy, the plaintiff alleges that details from his or her private life have been publicized. This may occur, for example, if a clinician publishes an article in which the identity of the subject is insufficiently disguised. It has been held that a patient undergoing psychotherapy cannot give proper informed consent to the publication of a book concerning the treatment (63).

A patient has the right to bar nonessential onlookers when he or she is being examined or treated or when his or her case is discussed. The teacher should seek informed consent before exposing patients to case conferences or discussing cases for teaching purposes. The use of videotapes for teaching necessitates written informed consent, the continuation of which should be requested on a yearly basis.

Research with children poses complex ethical issues over and above issues with adults because of children's vulnerability and lack of legal competence. Federal law includes special protections for children involved in federally sponsored research (64). These include the requirement that, in addition to the parent's consent, the child's assent is required for participation for research that is not expected to benefit the child (assuming the child can give assent). The Privacy Rule authorized by HIPAA carries further requirements for protecting the privacy of actual or prospective research subjects. Institutional review boards (IRB) in universities and most organizations have adopted these principles for all research they review, even if technically the research would not be governed by federal rules. Any practitioner involved in research would be well advised to meet these standards. If research procedures are later questioned, especially if an adverse event befalls a research subject, documentation of approval by an IRB is a crucial component in demonstrating the research was undertaken thoughtfully and with due regard to the wellbeing of the research subjects.

COMPLAINTS TO OTHER REGULATORY BODIES

Malpractice cases are not the only arena in which child and adolescent's care is scrutinized. Complaints may be made to state licensing boards, professional ethics committees, and, for HIPAA violations, to the Office of Civil Rights of DHHS.

Unlike in a malpractice case, harm to the patient does not need to be proved for a complaint to be found justified: all that is needed is proof of unethical or incompetent behavior or violation of a regulation. For example, if a clinician is found to have practiced while intoxicated, he can be sanctioned even if his actual care has not been shown to be poor. Furthermore, the range of professional work that can be scrutinized is wider, because a doctor–patient relationship is not necessary for a complaint to go forward. For example, child psychiatrists who conduct child custody evaluations on court order are generally immune from malpractice suits, both because such evaluations, like most forensic evaluations, do not create a doctor–patient relationship, and because the evaluator is an agent of the court and so usually has the immunity of other court personnel. However, disgruntled parents are free to pursue complaints to ethics committees and state licensing boards, and such grievances are not uncommon.

From the perspective of the investigated doctor, complaints to these agencies trigger a process that is similar in many ways to being sued. Sometimes, particularly with ethics committee investigations, the psychiatrist may feel that the whole matter can be disposed of informally by discussion with members of the committee and submitting records for review. Unless the clinician is extremely confident or very familiar with the proceedings, however, he or she is well advised to obtain an attorney before proceeding, rather than run the risk of making admissions that may later prove damaging, or in agreeing to waive due process protections in order to "wrap this up in a hurry." Many malpractice insurance policies cover the cost of attorney representation in licensing board investigations. While money is not at stake directly (although results of these investigations are often admissible in later malpractice actions), the psychiatrist's license to practice medicine may be threatened, and one should proceed cautiously.

RISK MANAGEMENT IN CHILD PSYCHIATRY

Clinical practice is fraught with error, and error can have serious consequences. Confronted by the catalogue of litigation in this chapter, even the insouciant may quail. However, defensive psychiatry is no answer, because overly timid treatment can also put the clinician at risk of negligent malpractice. What, then, is the best way to avoid litigation? General risk management principles that apply to adult psychiatry, such as the importance of clear communication with patients and parent and good documentation by the clinician apply to work with children and adolescents as well. Some special considerations that apply to child and adolescent psychiatry are shown in Table 7.3.4.2. The best precaution is to practice careful medicine while fully apprising the patient and family of the diagnosis, the treatment plan, and the progress of therapy. Many malpractice suits arise from a neglect of this simple principle. Hospitals provide many opportunities for failed communication, particularly when the attending physician delegates to other members of the team the responsibility for keeping parents informed of their children's progress. A good therapeutic alliance is the key to good medicine and the avoidance of lawsuits. Used for this purpose, informed consent can be transformed from an empty legalism into the foundation of a true collaboration.

Documentation

The clinician should keep a good record of the rationale for treatment. Progress notes should be timely, regular, dated, and signed. Gutheil, in his classic 1980 article on paranoia and progress notes (65), recommends imagining a plaintiff attorney looking over your shoulder while writing progress notes. Issues that potentially may come in court, such as those described above, should be documented fully. If you disagree with the diagnosis, investigation, or treatment plan in the record, respectfully note that you disagree and insert your amended diagnosis and plan. If you merely sign off on a trainee's notes, you could be concurring with erroneous observations, diagnosis, or treatment. One of the most common errors is to raise a diagnostic question but not follow through by investigating it or, having ordered investigation, to lose sight of the results.

Note any discrepancies between the nurses', the therapist's, and the physician's progress notes. If there is such a

TABLE 7.3.4.2

RISK MANAGEMENT PRINCIPLES

General Principle	Special Consideration in Child and Adolescent Work	Example of Potential Problem
Open communication	Clear understanding of minor's confidentiality and exceptions	Parents have right to see chart Parents need to be told of dangerous situations
Clarity of role definition	Whether the child or the whole family is the patient	In family work, there may be a doctor–patient relationship with each person in the family
Need to obtain informed consent	Assent from minor is useful; consent from parents is usually required	In nontraditional family or postdivorce situations, need to be sure which parent(s) have authority to consent
Appropriate medication use	Much use is off label	Insufficient explanation of possible side effects
Compliance and cooperation with treatment	May be reduced by immaturity or minor's lack of agreement	Child's being less legally responsible may shift more responsibility for safety to clinician
Documentation of treatment	Documentation of communications with collateral sources (parents, school) is important	Failure to document telling parents that their son had some suicidal symptoms
Careful risk assessment	Risk factors less researched and less predictive than with adults Ratio of suicidal ideation to completed suicide is much higher than with adults	Unforeseen impulsive suicide

discrepancy, try to account for it. Do not allow a nursing progress note concerning suicide risk to go unremarked.

If you detect an error in your notes, do not erase it. Draw a line through the error, write "error," and date and sign your correction in the margin. Do not criticize or argue with other professionals or agencies in your notes, and avoid gratuitous or extravagant commentary ("This child has had an appalling home life"). Do not record psychodynamic speculations in the clinical record; those unconscious incestuous strivings may come back to haunt you. You may consider keeping your psychotherapy *process notes* separate from the official record of therapy *progress notes.*

Dangerousness Assessment

A risk–resource analysis should be conducted whenever a patient presents a risk of violence to self or others. Such an assessment is most likely to be required in the following circumstances: when the risk of violence is raised during outpatient evaluation or treatment; when a potentially violent patient presents for admission to hospital; when the leave or discharge from hospital of a potentially violent patient is being considered; or when such a patient elopes. Areas of assessment when considering violence towards others commonly cited in the literature are shown in Table 7.3.4.3.

Predatory violence, that is, violence that is planned, is more difficult to assess because the youth has a clear motive to conceal his thinking. In the wake of highly publicized school shootings, many schools have developed so called "zero tolerance" policies for direct or implied threats of school violence that may be triggered when a child or adolescent makes a threat, brings a weapon to school, or writes a story that includes violence toward peers. In such situations, schools frequently require a psychological evaluation before allowing a child to return. The clinician should be aware that a single individual assessment alone is of very limited value in these situations, and only tentative conclusions about dangerousness should be drawn. More accurate evaluations require corroborative interviews, especially with friends of the evaluated youth, to assess whether the youth is on a path of escalating interest and planning of hurting others. In such interviews, one is looking not only for direct threats and violent ideation, but for "leakage," a spilling over of preoccupation with violence, such as might be found in diaries, being fascinated with weapons, following prospective victims, drawing plans of the school, etc. (66, 67).

TABLE 7.3.4.3

AREAS FOR ASSESSMENT OF RISK OF VIOLENCE TO OTHERS

Past history of violent threats or actions
Nature of Threat
Direct threat
Has potential victim been bullied or provoked patient?
Plan for harming the victim
Access to lethal weapons?
Leakage of preoccupation with violence in journals, Web surfing, and writings
Taking steps toward action, such as following or stalking victim, obtaining a weapon, rehearsing an attack
Threat communicated to others, especially peers
Past History
History of being abused
History of alcohol or drug abuse
Demographic Factors
Late adolescent
Male
Disadvantaged ethnic groups with a cultural tradition of masculine defensiveness
Psychological Factors
Copes with anxiety or hostility by externalizing or projecting it in the form of impulsive, explosive actions, suspicious vigilance, or frank persecutory delusions
Command hallucinations that instruct the patient to take violent action or that threaten violence to the patient or his or her family
Inner controls against violent actions subjectively or objectively reduced
Strong inner urge to be violent
Social environment
Family psychopathology in the form of rejection, neglect, physical or sexual abuse, or family violence
Parental mental or physical health impaired
Intelligence below average
Impairment of the sensorium
Alcohol or substance abuse
Repeatedly victimized or scapegoated at school
Therapeutic Alliance
Has the patient lost or terminated a therapeutic relationship?
Is he or she competent and motivated to enter into one?
Protective factors
Younger, female, white, religious, middle-class
No access to lethal means
If there has been a threat of violence, a threat without plan or identified victim
Secure family without major psychopathology
Positive relationship with a therapist

Treatment

Before a particular treatment is commenced, be careful to check that the patient harbors no conditions and is taking no drugs that would contraindicate it, and inquire about previous allergic or idiosyncratic reactions to drugs. For drugs with known teratogenic effects in early pregnancy, such as sodium divalproex, the rationale for use in girls should be carefully documented, even for a girl who states she is not planning to become pregnant. Avoid polypharmacy. Monitor the progress of medication regularly. In patients taking long-term medication, "drug holidays" should be considered. Unless there are good reasons for departing from them, follow recommended guidelines for dosage and administration. Avoid prescribing medication "as needed" and automatic refills, and be careful of telephone requests for repeat prescriptions. If the suicide risk is serious, only small amounts of a potentially lethal drug should be prescribed. Hospitals should check that potentially suicidal patients are not cheating, concealing, and hoarding medication.

When a patient is admitted to the hospital, the degree of risk of suicide or violence should be assessed, and each degree of risk should be linked to a set of nursing precautions that are automatically activated when the clinician indicates the degree of risk. Every attempt should be made to obtain past records and to scan them for risk factors.

If you are unavailable in case of emergency during treatment, the name of a fully informed substitute physician should be provided to the patient. Do not terminate treatment unilaterally without preparing the patient, giving adequate notice, and providing him or her with the names of other clinicians or agencies that could help.

In outpatient practice, the duty to protect is precipitated when the patient makes a specific threat to harm a specified victim. When possible, incorporate the protection in therapy. Psychotherapy, hospitalization, and medication may be both more protective and more therapeutic than warning the foreseeable victim or alerting the police.

Be vigilant to avoid unauthorized disclosure of confidential information to external agencies, do not gossip about patients, and do not publish articles about patients without adequately disguising their identity. Obtain the parents' consent before releasing reports to external agencies. Blanket consent forms, obtained during the rush of admission, may not hold water legally.

Identified High Risk Situations

There are often clinical situations which the physician recognizes to carry a higher risk of an adverse outcome, such as when a chronically suicidal adolescent is to be discharged from the hospital, or standard medications have been tried and failed, and a less tested medication with the potential for serious side effects is being considered. A number of strategies can lessen the liability risk in managing such situations. First, document in more than usual detail the pros and cons of the intervention being considered. Second, be especially attentive to informed consent issues, discuss such issues fully with the parent or guardian, document the discussion, and, if medications are involved, have a parent sign a written consent form. Third, when in doubt, shout (68)! Get a second opinion and have it documented. In case of a malpractice suit, the test will be what a reasonable clinician would have done under the circumstances. A consulting clinician's contemporaneous second opinion will likely carry greater weight than the opinion of a hired expert who wasn't there peering through the retrospect-oscope with full knowledge of the subsequent events.

CONCLUSION

When Bellamy (69) examined appellate psychiatric malpractice cases in the 15 years after World War II, he could identify 18 cases, none of which involved child or adolescent patients. The situation is not so rosy today, but defendant doctors still win most cases. The law has no wish to penalize physicians for honest errors. Its purpose is to protect patients from being harmed by reckless, careless, or incompetent clinical practice, and if they have been so harmed, to compensate them for injury. In most successful suits for negligent malpractice, the errors are glaring. Attention to the safeguards described in this chapter will protect clinicians from litigation while allowing them to practice nondefensive psychiatry.

References

1. Studdert DM, Mello MM, Brennan TA: Medical malpractice. *N Engl J Med* 350:283–292, 2004.
2. Charles SC, Wilbert JR, Kennedy EC: Physicians' self-reports of reactions to malpractice litigation. *Am J Psychiatry* 141:563–565, 1984.
3. Studdert DM, Mello MM, Sage WM, et al.: Defensive medicine among high-risk specialist physicians in a volatile malpractice environment. *JAMA* 293:2609–2617, 2005.
4. National Conference of State Legislatures. Table of state medical malpractice tort laws. 2005; available at: http://www.ncsl.org/standcomm/sclaw/medmaltorttable205.htm. Accessed December 14, 2005.
5. Ash P.: Malpractice in child and adolescent psychiatry. *Child Adolesc Psychiatr Clin N Am* 11:869–886, 2002.
6. *O'Neill v. Montefiore Hosp.*, 11 AD2d 132; 202 NYS2d 436 (NY App 1960).
7. Recupero PR.: E-mail and the psychiatrist-patient relationship. *J Am Acad Psychiatry Law* 33:465–475, 2005.
8. Reed J: Cybermedicine: Defying and redefining patient standards of care. *Indiana Law Review* 37:845–877, 2004.
9. American Medical Association. H-120.949 Guidance for Physicians on Internet Prescribing. 2005; available at: http://www.amaassn.org/apps/pf_new/pf_online?f_n=browse&doc=policyfiles/HnE/H-120.949.htm. Accessed Jan. 19, 2006.
10. eRisk Working Group for Healthcare. eRisk Guidelines. 2002; available at: http://www.medem.com/phy/phy_eriskguidelines.cfm. Accessed Jan. 24, 2006.
11. Simon RI: *Assessing and Managing Suicide Risk: Guidelines for Clinically Based Risk Management*. Washington, DC, American Psychiatric Press, Inc., 2004.
12. Kachalia A, Studdert DM: Professional liability issues in graduate medical education. *JAMA* 292:1051–1056, 2004.
13. *LaLonde v. Eissner*, 405 Mass 207, 539 NE2d 538 (Mass Sup Jud Ct 1989).
14. Caudill OB. Standard of care analysis (on panel: Risk Management Concerns for Child Psychiatry, Eric Marine, chair). Paper presented at: American Academy of Child and Adolescent Psychiatry 52nd Annual Meeting; Oct. 20, 2005; Toronto, ON.
15. Health Care Quality Improvement Act of 1986, 42 USC § 11101 et seq Title IV (1986).
16. *Wickline v. State*, 239 Cal Rptr 810, 819 (Cal 1986).
17. *Pegram v. Herdrich*, 530 US 211 (2000).
18. Halleck SL. Malpractice in psychiatry. *Psychiatr Clin North Am.* 1983;6:567–583.
19. Grunbaum JA, Kann L, Kinchen S, et al.: Youth risk behavior surveillance—United States, 2003. *MMWR* 53:1–96, 2004.
20. *Abille v. United States*, 482 F Supp 703 (ND Cal 1980).
21. *Skar v. City of Lincoln, Nebraska*, 599 F2d 253 (8th Cir 1979).
22. Wagner KD, Pollard R, Wagner RF, Jr.: Malpractice litigation against child and adolescent psychiatry residency programs, 1981–1991. *J Am Acad Child Adolesc Psychiatry* 32:462–465, 1993.
23. *Higgins v. State*, 24 AD2d 147, 265 NYS2d 254 (NY 1965).
24. *Samuels v. Southern Baptist Hospital*, 594 So2d 571 (La App 1992).
25. *Tarasoff v. Regents of the University of California* (Tarasoff I), 529 P 2d 553, 118 Cal Rptr 129 (Cal 1974).
26. *Tarasoff v. Regents of the University of California* (Tarasoff II), 551 P 2d 334, 131 Cal Rptr 14 (Cal 1976).
27. Kachigian C, Felthous AR: Court responses to Tarasoff statutes. *J Am Acad Psychiatry Law* 32:263–273, 2004.
28. Simon RI: *Clinical Psychiatry and the Law*. Washington, DC, American Psychiatric Press, Inc., 1987.
29. *Landeros v. Flood*, 131 Cal Rptr 69, 555 P2d 389 (Cal 1976).
30. *Montoya v. Bebensee*, 761 P2d 285 (Colo App 1988).
31. Guyer MJ: Child psychiatry and legal liability: Implications of recent case law. *J Am Acad Child Adolesc Psychiatry* 29:958–962, 1990.
32. *Jaffee v. Redmond*, 518 US 1 (1996).
33. *Bremer v. State*, 18 MdApp 291, 307 A2d 503 (Md App 1973).
34. Standards for Privacy of Individually Identifiable Health Information (the Privacy Rule), 45 CFR Parts 160 and 164 (adopted April, 2001).
35. Office of Civil Rights (DHHS). Medical Privacy—National Standards to Protect the Privacy of Personal Health Information. 2006; available at: http://www.hhs.gov/ocr/hipaa/privacy.html. Accessed Jan. 2, 2006.
36. American Psychiatric Association: Minimum Necessary Guidelines for Third-Party Payers for Psychiatric Treatment: Position Statement (APA Document Reference No. 200211). 2002; available at: http://www.psych.org/edu/other_res/lib_archives/archives/200211.pdf. Accessed Dec. 1, 2005.
37. *In re Lifschutz*, 2 Cal3d 415, 467 P2d 557 (Cal 1970).
38. *Schloendorff v. New York Hospital*, 211 NY 125, 105 NE 92 (NY 1914).
39. *Aiken v. Clary*, 396 SW2d 668 (Mo 1965).
40. *Natanson v. Kline*, 350 P2d 1093 (Kan 1960).
41. *Canterbury v. Spence*, 464 F2d 772 (DC Cir 1972).
42. *Cobbs v. Grant*, 8 Cal3d 229, 502 P2d 1 (Cal 1972).
43. *Planned Parenthood of Central Missouri v. Danforth*, 428 US 52 (1976).
44. *Bellotti v. Baird*, 428 US 132 (1976).
45. *Johnson v. Greer*, 477 F2d 101 (5th Cir 1973).
46. *Pendleton v. Burkhalter*, 432 SW2d 724 (Tex. Civ App 1968).
47. *Parham v. J.R. and J.L.*, 442 US 584 (1979).
48. *Hirschberg v. State*, 91 Misc2d 590, 398 NYS 2d 470 (NY 1977).
49. Partlett DF, Nurcombe B: Recovered memories of child sexual abuse and liability: Society, science, and the law in a comparative setting. *Psychology, Public Policy, and Law* 4:1253–1306, 1998.
50. *Ramona v. Ramona*, (judgment on jury verdict), No. 61898 (Napa [Cal] Cty Super Ct 1994).
51. Appelbaum PS, Zoltek-Jick R.: Psychotherapists' duties to third parties: Ramona and beyond. *Am J Psychiatry* 153:457–465, 1996.
52. *Roy v. Hartogs*, 81 Misc2d 350, 366 NYS2d 297 (1975), *affd*, 85 Misc 2d 891, 381 NYS 2d 587 (1976).
53. *Abraham v. Zaslow*, No 245862 (Santa Clara Cty Sup Ct 1970).
54. *Osheroff v. Chestnut Lodge* et al., Maryland Health Claims Arbitration (1987).
55. *Nelson v. Heyne*, 355 FSupp 451 (ND Ind. 1972), *affd*, 491 F 2d 352 (7th Cir), *cert denied*, 417 US 976 (1974).
56. *Clites v. State*, 322 NW 2d 917 (Iowa Ct App 1982).
57. Blumer JL: Off-label uses of drugs in children. *Pediatrics* 104:598–602, 1999.
58. *Rennie v. Klein*, 720 F 2d 266, 653 F2d (3rd Cir 1983), *vacated* 458 U.S. 1119 (1982).

59. *Rogers v. Commissioner of Mental Health*, 458 NE2d 308 (Mass 1983), began as *Rogers v. Okin*, 478 F Supp 1342 (D Mass 1979), *affd in part, revd in part*, 634 F 2d 650 (1st Cir 1980), *vacated subnom.* and was later reviewed by the U.S. Supreme Court as *Mills v. Rogers*, 457 US 291 (1982).
60. *Youngberg v. Romeo*, 457 US 307 (1982).
61. Food and Drug Administration. Class Suicidality Labeling Language for Antidepressants. 2005; available at: http://www.fda.gov/cder/drug/antidepressants/PI_template.pdf. Accessed March 5, 2005.
62. Smith JT: *Medical Malpractice: Psychiatric Care.* Colorado Springs, CO, New York, Shepard's/McGraw Hill, McGraw Hill, 1986.
63. *Doe v. Roe & Poe*, 400 NYS2d 668 (1977).
64. Protection of Human Subjects: Additional Protections for Children, 45 Code of Federal Regulations [CFR], Subtitle A, Part 46, Subpart D, 10-1-99 Edition.
65. Gutheil TG: Paranoia and progress notes: A guide to forensically informed psychiatric recordkeeping. *Hospital & Community Psychiatry* 31:479–482, 1980.
66. Borum R, Fein R, Vossekuil B, Berglund J: Threat assessment: Defining an approach for evaluating risk of targeted violence. *Behav Sci Law* 17:323–337, 1999.
67. Federal Bureau of Investigation [FBI]. *The School Shooter: A Threat Assessment Perspective.* Washington, DC, U.S. Dept. of Justice, 2000.
68. Rappeport JR.: Malpractice prevention. Paper presented at: Spring Grove State Hospital Center; May, 1984; Catonsville, MD.
69. Bellamy WA: Malpractice risks confronting the psychiatrist: A nationwide fifteen year study of appellate court cases, 1946 to 1961. *Am J Psychiatry* 118:769–780, 1962.

POSTSCRIPT ■ LOOKING BACK, DREAMING FORWARD: REFLECTIONS ON THE HISTORY OF CHILD PSYCHIATRY

LEON EISENBERG

Anyone willing to write a chapter entitled Looking Back, Dreaming Forward must hesitate on recalling Yogi Berra's quip, "The future ain't what it used to be." However cloudy my vision forward, what I see when I look back (it's 60 years since my graduation) may be instructive for younger readers (by now almost everyone is younger than I am). What I see when I remember the child psychiatry of the 1950s is both ignorance (for which we cannot be blamed) and arrogance (for which we can). As Bertolt Brecht has Galileo say in his play:

> One of the chief causes of poverty in science is imaginary wealth. The purpose of science is not to open the door to an infinitude of wisdom, but to set some limits on the infinitude of error (1).

When I was trained by Leo Kanner, there was no subspecialty certification, and hence no ABPN-approved residencies. In the 1950s, most departments of psychiatry were heavily psychoanalytic in orientation; departments of psychology were behavioristic; the word *neuroscience* had yet to be coined. When I say I was trained by Kanner, I mean that quite literally. I acknowledge that I did gain a great deal of practical knowledge from the one social worker (Barbara Ashenden) and the one psychologist (Charlotte Waskowitz) on the staff, but neither was academic in orientation. When I joined the full-time staff of the Children's Psychiatric Service after completing my training, I effectively doubled the number of psychiatrists.

Leo Kanner was a polymath. If there is such a thing as *eidetic* imagery, he had it. He could picture in his mind the page on which he had read a poem in high school. He recalled the names of teachers who had attended his evening adult education classes at Hopkins when he saw them on the city streets. They were astonished to be remembered by name (and often he added the names of their seatmates) 5 or 10 years after a one-semester course (and I was equally astonished as I looked on!). A graduate of the Sophien-Gymnasium in Berlin who had earned his M.D. from the University of Berlin with a thesis on electrocardiography, he knew classical Greek and Latin (and frequently quoted Homer and Virgil). As a child he had learned Polish, Hebrew, and German, went on to learn English, and had familiarized himself with other languages as well. He was vain enough to display his erudition with multilingual puns that kept a monolingual American (with only remnants of high school Latin and German) hopping trying to figure them out.

His principal mode of teaching was extending to me the privilege of sitting in on his consultations with patients and families. The "price" for the privilege was taking notes and writing up the case report for the formal record (once he had come to trust the fidelity of my accounts). And it was an extraordinary privilege. He was polite and gentle but his questions were penetrating. He listened intently. He was unfailingly courteous, even to the most arrogant and dismissive parents. He charmed children and adolescents alike. His secret psychiatric technique (no longer permissible) was smoking a cigar. He blew lingering smoke rings (in those days, no one knew of the risks of second-hand smoke; those who objected to smoking did so on aesthetic grounds). The children were invariably fascinated. While he saw the parents, the clinic psychologist did a Binet or a WISC on the youngster and provided a brief and usually quite insightful report on her findings before he met the parents again. He wrapped up the 2- to 3-hour sessions with a sagacious review of what he had learned, with what he thought might be helpful to child and family, and with appropriate referrals (his was primarily a consulting practice). Then, he and I would have another 30 minutes together. I was free to pose any questions I wanted. I was encouraged to challenge his conclusions. I often did but usually came around to his position when he mustered the grounds for it.

During the other 4½ days of the week, I saw and treated clinic patients referred from pediatrics and, with the other fellows and occasional rotating pediatric residents, participated in a weekly case conference chaired by Dr. Kanner with the social worker and psychologist in attendance. There was no journal club, no regular supervision. It was catch as catch can with colleagues.

Kanner had come to America in 1924 amid the economic chaos in Berlin for a job in the State Hospital in Yankton, South Dakota (German inflation was on an exponential curve). In this unlikely setting, he found a way to do research and to publish several papers, one of which (on the rarity of general paresis among Native Americans) attracted the attention of Kraepelin, who visited Yankton to meet Kanner. In 1928, he applied for and received a Commonwealth Foundation Fellowship from Adolf Meyer, then the doyen of American psychiatry, at the Henry Phipps Clinic of the Johns Hopkins Hospital. At the completion of the 2-year fellowship, Meyer and Edwards A. Park, the Professor of Pediatrics, chose Leo Kanner to inaugurate a new clinic in pediatrics, charged with "investigating the rank and file of patients in the pediatric clinic for the form(ul)ation of psychiatric problems, the mastery of which should be made accessible to the pediatrician to serve him as the psychopathological principles in dealing with children."

The clinic was initiated in 1930 with support from the Rockefeller Foundation. His office was a small pediatric examining room with a sink and a table. Five years later, based on his intensive study of the world literature and his clinical experience, Kanner wrote the first English-language textbook on child psychiatry (2). Its first edition paid homage to Meyer's psychobiological terminology, but by the second (3), the Meyerian neologisms were abandoned. Kanner's most outstanding and lasting contribution was the identification of the syndrome he called "autistic disturbances of affective contact" (4). On the basis of 11 patients who had been brought to him because of their unusual psychopathology, he formulated the characteristics of a syndrome still identified by these very features. In Michael Rutter's words (5): "Kanner's paper was a model of clarity in its combination of systematic, thorough, and objective observation with deep clinical understanding and appreciation of the personal problems faced by each child, and his family:... Nearly all the basic points made in the original paper have been amply confirmed by other writers."

Kanner had concluded his 1943 article with the statement: "Here we seem to have a pure culture example of an inborn autistic disturbance of affective contact." That conclusion, at a time when child psychiatric disorders were uniformly attributed to psychogenic causes, left him out on a limb and probably delayed widespread acceptance of the syndrome as a clinical entity. His syndrome remains unique.

MENTAL RETARDATION

The very terms in the official classification for the mentally retarded offend today's sensibilities. The terms ran from feebleminded to moron to imbecile to idiot. Down syndrome was still known as Mongolian idiocy, a label reflecting Langdon-Down's belief that it was an atavistic throwback to a more primitive "Mongolian race" (6). We did know that risk increased with the mother's age, but trisomy 21 was not identified until the late 1950s (7, 8). That is hardly surprising, given that the correct human chromosome number was not established until 1948! Whatever the terminology and whatever the ignorance about pathophysiology, what remains distressing is that most child guidance clinics of the '50s and '60s screened out retarded children as if retardation excluded treatable psychiatric disorders. A recent study of an epidemiological cohort of almost 600 children with intellectual disability has provided documentation of the substantial and persistent level of psychopathology and the need for effective interventions (9).

Few things epitomize Kanner's personal commitment to the rights of all children more than his concern for the "feebleminded" at a time when most psychiatrists assiduously excluded them from their clinics and offices. The Superintendent of the Maryland State Training School for the Retarded, knowing of Kanner's concern for such patients, appealed to Leo Kanner for help in controlling an appalling problem. Female patients were being removed from the training school by court orders and were being exploited in the community for cheap domestic labor. The superintendent was at his wits' end; he simply didn't know what to do. With the assistance of Miss Mabel F. Kraus, a social worker, Kanner (10) did a followup study on 166 patients who had been released from the school via habeas corpus writs secured by lawyers over the previous two decades. Three-quarters of these releases had been obtained by enterprising attorneys who, for a fee, secured what were essentially indentured domestic servants for affluent Baltimore households; others had been claimed by relatives who suddenly appeared to manipulate estates that had been left them; a few were demanded by parents who, after years of neglect, asserted their "natural rights."

Kanner was able to follow 102, of whom only 13 were making even a modestly satisfactory adjustment in the community at the time of the study; 11 had died of illness and neglect before they reached 30; 17 had tuberculosis, syphilis, or gonorrhea; 29 were prostitutes; 8 had been committed to mental hospitals; and 6 were in prison. In total, these released patients had given birth to 165 offspring, 18 of whom had died from neglect, 30 of whom had been committed to orphanages, and 108 of whom tested at a "feebleminded level" when examined. The customary sequence had been a period of domestic servitude, followed by peremptory release when the young women proved to be inadequate as maids, and then a mournful hegira through the whorehouses and flophouses of the Baltimore slums. Few now remember Kanner's paper in the *American Journal of Psychiatry*, but in 1938, the study had a dramatic impact. The release of the information produced a double row of inch-high headlines across the front page of the April 8th edition of the *Baltimore Sun* and provided the impetus to end an evil practice that had arisen from the collusion of attorneys and judges against the valiant but unsuccessful opposition of the superintendent of the Training School. It is a study worth remembering (10). Clinical precision joined with social conscience in a clinical project with immediate benefit for the lives of a despised minority.

In 1942, amid the war against the Nazis, Foster Kennedy, a well known neurologist, published a paper in the *American Journal of Psychiatry* entitled: "The problem of social control of the congenital defective: Education, sterilization, euthanasia" (11). In it, he proposed that defective children with no future or hope of a worthwhile life "should be relieved of the agony of living," language remarkably similar to the Nazi policy to *end life unworthy of life*. In a vigorous response to Kennedy, Kanner (12) wrote: "Let us try to recall one single instance in the history of mankind when a feeble-minded individual or group of individuals was responsible for the retardation or persecution of humaneness and sciences. They who caused Galileo to be jailed were not feeble-minded. They who instituted the Inquisition were not mental defectives. The great man-made catastrophes resulting in wholesale slaughter and destruction were not started by idiots, imbeciles, morons, or borderlines. The one man, Schicklgruber, whose IQ is probably not below normal, has in a few years brought infinitely more disaster and suffering to this world than have all of the innumerable mental defectives of all countries and all generations combined."

Kanner's revulsion against euthanasia for the severely retarded was not universal; in the same issue of the *Journal* an unsigned editorial argued that the role of psychiatrists should be to persuade parents to agree to release their defective children from "the burden of living" (13). Euthanasia never became official policy, but sterilization was widespread in U.S. institutions for the mentally retarded.

EARLY RESEARCH ON THE HERITABILITY OF EARLY INFANTILE AUTISM

When Leo Kanner (4) first identified infantile autism as a diagnostic entity, he concluded that his patients had:

> ... come into the world with an innate inability to form the usual, biologically provided affective contact with people, just as other children come into the world with innate physical or intellectual handicaps.... [W]e seem to have pure culture examples of inborn autistic disturbances of affective contact (p. 250).

Kanner believed that his emphasis on an "inborn" disturbance delayed the acceptance of early infantile autism as a clinical entity. Recognition of the impact of severe maternal deprivation on child development had brought psychogenesis to the fore (14–16). Psychiatry was dominated by Don Jackson's "schizophrenogenic mother" and Gregory Bateson's "double-bind" (17). When Kanner coined the term "refrigerator mother," the diagnosis of autism became more fashionable; it suggested that a "refrigerator mother" produced a "frozen child" (something he later regretted). Kanner was aware of the frequency of obsessional and schizoid traits among the parents and even suggested that the parents might be "successfully autistic adults." Indeed, in my paper on the fathers of autistic children I suggested that the severe obsessional traits and relative social isolation some displayed might represent a *forme fruste* of the complete entity (18). Thirty years later, Sula Wolff and her colleagues (19) compared the parents of autistic patients with the parents of other child psychiatric patients and confirmed Kanner's observations on the predominance of schizoid and socially gauche characteristics. But neither he nor I seriously pursued the genetic hypothesis. At Kanner's invitation, I reviewed the charts of his first 100 patients and found 131 siblings, of whom 3 were autistic (20). I did not have a clue about the significance of what I had found. All I knew of genetics was Mendelian; it was clear that Mendelian laws were not operative in autism. Autism, I concluded, was not inherited because it was not Mendelian. No one called attention to my error.

In the 1950s, there were no published data on the prevalence of autism; but assuredly we knew it was rare. It was not until 10 years later that modern child psychiatric epidemiology began with the Isle of Wight study by Rutter and his colleagues (21, 22). In a total population of 2,200 children, they found only one autistic child, a prevalence similar to the estimate of 4 to 5 per 10,000 published in the same year by Lotter (23). But I didn't understand what finding three autistic children among 131 sibs implied. The rate I observed among siblings was two orders of magnitude greater than expected and established a genetic risk. Not until the mid-1970s did Folstein and Rutter (24) provide unequivocal proof of inheritance by comparing the identical and fraternal cotwins of autistic probands in a total population sample. I call attention to my failure to understand the data I analyzed to remind readers that the prevalent concepts, ideas, and methods of any given era act as blinders to all but the very gifted.

"ADHD" IN THE 1950s

When my professional career began, what is now known as ADHD had not yet been recognized as a diagnostic entity. Symptoms of overactivity and inattentiveness existed, of course, but were allocated to such categories as "behavioral disorder," "minimal brain damage," "minimal brain dysfunction," or "post-encephalitic syndrome" (even though an episode of encephalitis had never been documented). The patients were not of much interest to most child guidance clinics because of the supposition of "organicity." The one symptomatic treatment that seemed to be as effective was dextroamphetamine. It was not in wide use and had never been put to an exacting test. Indeed, when the Psychopharmacology Service Center of the NIMH convened a conference in 1958 on Child Research in Psychopharmacology (25), "there was essentially no research on drugs in children" (26). Randomized controlled trials were being introduced into psychiatry in the late 1950s. Our research group at Hopkins received the first NIMH grant for RCTs on tranquilizers and stimulants for treating hyperkinesis in children (27). Tranquilizers proved to be worse than placebos (28), but stimulants were clearly effective (29), a finding that has been repeatedly confirmed.

What was entirely unexpected was the explosion in the use of these agents in subsequent decades for a condition that had been regarded as uncommon, so uncommon that the first edition of the APA *Diagnostic and Statistical Manual* (DSM I), published in 1952, had no such categories as hyperactivity or attention deficit disorder. In 1967, I participated in a World Health Organization Symposium on Diagnosis and Classification in Child Psychiatry (30). Mike Rutter and I had to argue vigorously for the inclusion of hyperkinesis as a syndrome. The other participants were highly skeptical of the diagnosis hyperkinesis. Most U.K. psychiatrists allocated it to the category "behavior disorder." We won the day, and hyperkinetic reaction of childhood appeared in DSM II in 1968; however, it was not until DSM III (1980) that attention deficit/hyperactivity disorder (ADHD) entered the official lexicon.

It is, of course, not possible to find data on rates before a given disease has entered the official nomenclature. The Centers for Disease Control (31) estimate ADHD population prevalence based on parental reports from the National Survey of Children's Health in 2003 at about 4.4 million American children aged 4–17 years of age. More than 50% of those children (2.5 million) were reported currently to be taking medication for the disorder. The survey reports a remarkably wide difference in the percentage of children with ADHD between Colorado (~ 5.1%) and Alabama (~ 11.2%), with an overall U.S. average of about 7.8%. Can these disparities possibly be valid? Are there localized "epidemics" of ADHD or is it that there are epidemics of diagnosis? Do the variations reflect differences in the availability of specialists, in fashions in diagnosis, and in their administrative consequences in particular communities?

It is useful to recall, in this connection, Judy Rapoport's studies in the late 1970s. At the time, dextroamphetamine was labeled pharmacologically as a stimulant. Because hyperkinetic children responded to the stimulant by slowing down as if it were a sedative, their response was termed paradoxical. When Judy (alone of all of us with the courage to do the study!) put the matter to empirical test by giving dextroamphetamine to normal children (including several of her own), they slowed down just as the patients did (32). The "paradox" was age-related, not "disease"-related. That lesson continues to elude most child psychiatrists. A "therapeutic" response to the drug is taken as "confirmation" of a diagnosis. Are we converting a dimensional spectrum that covers the entire population arbitrarily into a diagnostic category? Have we become carpenters with hammers who see all problems as nails?

WHAT ESTABLISHED AND WHAT ERODED PSYCHOANALYTIC HEGEMONY?

When I completed my training in psychiatry, a half-century ago, psychoanalysis was in and genetics was out. Fifty years later, genetics is in and psychoanalysis is out. What happened? Did the change result from scientific progress? Science had a good deal to do with the blossoming of genetics, but economics proved decisive for practice.

How had an untestable theory and a treatment without proof of effectiveness come to be so dominant a half-century ago? Three characteristics of medicine (*all* of medicine, including psychiatry) in the 1950s help to explain it: treatment recommendations were based on "clinical experience" rather than exacting trials; there were few therapeutic alternatives in psychiatry and no equally comprehensive theory; and, most important of all, psychoanalysis taught psychiatrists to listen to their patients.

As to the first, treatment decisions in all of medicine as well as in psychiatry rested largely upon expert opinion (33). The first randomized clinical trial in medicine (on streptomycin for tuberculosis) was not published until 1948 (34).

As to the second, other than ECT, there were no reliably effective treatments for psychotic patients. Psychiatric patients were being warehoused in state mental hospitals in ever-growing numbers. So desperate was the state of affairs that more than 20,000 frontal lobotomies were performed in the United States in the 20 years following its introduction in 1936! What led to the abandonment of lobotomy was not the moral sensitivity of science, but rather the appearance of the dramatically effective psychotropic drugs that replaced it (35).

No other psychological theory provided as comprehensive an account of the origins of psychopathology. The brain sciences of the era were entirely irrelevant to clinical practice. Diagnosis was unreliable and made little difference for treatment. Psychoanalysis seemed to "explain" the bizarre symptoms patients exhibited. Its very complexity and counter-intuitiveness enhanced its allure. It connected the symptoms of mental illness to the psychopathology of everyday life.

As to the third, many patients improved when we listened to them and offered what other specialists derided as "talk therapy." Proof that talk therapies do work had to wait another 30 years. Psychiatry as a profession remained remarkably indifferent to the absence of empirical justification. Warnings that lack of data would threaten our credibility (and likelihood of being reimbursed for our services!) were simply ignored. In the late '60s I wrote (36):

> What is remarkable is how little effect these studies [of psychotherapy outcomes] with their scots verdict of "not proven" have had on professional practice. Surely ... they should have led to ... studies to define the indications for, the best methods of, and the limitations to, psychotherapy rather than what can only be compared to a religious conviction in possessing an exclusive road to salvation.

At the 1962 APA Conference on Psychiatric Training (37), I spoke from the floor at the final plenary session. During the preceding 4 days, there had been general agreement on the importance of further training in newly arising or rediscovered disciplines (psychopharmacology, sociology, anthropology); at the same time, the acknowledged shortage of psychiatrists and the financial burden precluded lengthening residency training. I made the obvious point that something had to go. No one had indicated what should be cut back to make room for the new, even though more sausage could not be squeezed into the same casing. Accordingly, I volunteered a modest proposal: namely, that the time devoted to psychoanalytic theory and practice be sharply reduced. I questioned psychoanalysis as a "science" because its propositions were formulated in such a way that they could not be disconfirmed. A didactic analysis for psychiatric house officers, I added, limited their geographic mobility, necessitated moonlighting to secure supplementary income, prepared them for practice patterns limited to middle- and upper class patients, turned them away from research because they had been fed readymade "answers," and isolated them from public service (38).

I had never before, nor have I ever since, had such an electrifying effect on a professional audience. I was barely able to get out of the way of a veritable stampede of eminent department chairmen who lined up behind the floor microphones to challenge my facts, my conclusions, my credentials, and my lineage! (I say "chair*men*" advisedly; there was not a single chair*woman*.) My modest proposal disappeared with the merest trace: a footnote on page 8 of the Conference Report (37). However, by the 1976 APA Conference on training (39), the influence of psychoanalysis had ebbed markedly, not because of my or other theoretical challenges, but because of the rising tide of psychopharmacology.

REFLECTIONS ON MY CRITIQUE OF PSYCHOANALYSIS

Do I still believe what I said then? My scientific critique is unchanged. The "research" method of psychoanalysis follows none of the accepted scientific principles of prediction, design, control, and quantification. Freud's ideas had been revolutionary in their time, but "the history of science... is replete with instances in which an initially liberating conceptualization, once institutionalized, becomes a barrier to progress" (40).

What I failed to acknowledge was the powerful and lasting contribution psychoanalysis had made to psychiatry by teaching trainees to listen to patients and to try to understand their distress, rather than merely to classify them with a diagnostic algorithm, or snow them with drugs, or lock them away, or release them to homelessness. Basing care on what is unique to the individual patient is central to clinical competence, whether in medicine or surgery or psychiatry. Psychoanalysis made a dynamic psychological approach central to general psychiatry. It emphasized the importance of memory, its vulnerability to distortion, and its centrality to each person's life narrative, the way we explain ourselves to ourselves and to others. Because those narratives can be self-defeating, therapy must be designed to help patients to reconstruct their autobiographies in ways that permit growth. Those principles remain as important in caring for patients today as they were then, but the paymasters of the healthcare marketplace are making time less and less available to patients (41). The economic barriers that hinder psychiatrists in providing psychotherapy have impoverished clinical psychiatry.

Psychoanalysis itself continues to do well in private institutes and conclaves, but it is largely missing from the academic scene in psychiatry, where it was once dominant (42). There has been, however, a sea change in psychotherapy research. Whereas there were no psychotherapies of proven efficacy 50 years ago (36), randomized controlled clinical trials have shown that a number of nonanalytic psychotherapies do work for particular disorders (43). Does the new evidence explain the recession of psychoanalysis? Not at all! Despite proof of efficacy, the provision of any brand of psychotherapy is diminishing. HMOs and insurance companies simply won't pay for more than a soupçon. Psychiatrists now make DSM-IV diagnoses and prescribe drugs. Money is shaping practice (44).

I hope I have persuaded readers of the importance of skepticism toward received wisdom. Psychoanalysis circa 1950 was no more the royal road to salvation than the human genome project is 60 years later. The challenge is the integration of concepts of mind and brain: Can we invent paradigms that will give new meanings to an old term, "psychogenetic?" For that, we will need to provide an education for our successors that will bridge disciplines among the brain, behavioral, and clinical sciences (45). We would do well to heed the admonition of Sir Aubrey Lewis (46), late head of Maudsley Hospital in London:

> The philosophers thought it proper to put not one but two mottoes on the Temple at Delphi: one, the better remembered, was "Know Thyself": but the second, equally imperative, enjoined "Nothing in Excess." It might be worth inscribing that over the Temple of Psychiatry.

DREAMING AHEAD

What are my credentials as a futurologist? I offer a prediction I made 20 years ago (44), which readers can check against the two decades that have followed to make an informed decision about the believability of my dreams.

A PARABLE FOR OUR TIME

I invented a virtual experiment as a metaphor for a clear and impending danger: the threat that reliance on technology would replace concern for the patient and the patient's story (44). The starting point for the studies in our Laboratory of Mental Science was the neurobiological breakthrough by René Descartes, identifying the pineal glad as the seat of the soul (47).

> The part of the body in which the soul exercises its functions immediately is in nowise the heart, nor the whole of the brain, but merely the most inward of all its parts, to wit, a certain very small gland which is situated in the middle of its substance and so suspended above the duct whereby the animal spirits in its anterior cavities have communication with those in its posterior, that the slightest movements which take place in it may alter very greatly the course of these spirits; and reciprocally that the smallest changes which occur in the course of the spirits may do much to change the movements of this gland ... The whole action of the soul consists of this, that solely because it desires something, it causes the little gland with which it is closely united to move in the way requisite to produce the effect which relates to this desire.

Accordingly, our research team grew pineal cells in tissue culture and eluted a unique protein from the supernatant. Against this pineal-specific protein, we prepared a monoclonal antibody made radioactive by incubating the hybridoma cells with oxygen-labeled acetate. Administered parenterally, the tracer molecule, modified to permeate the blood-brain barrier in the region of the pineal body, binds to the gland tightly and specifically. As the positrons emitted by O collide with electrons in the adjacent tissues, the gamma rays produced by particle annihilation are detected and converted by appropriate instrumentation into a visual image. A major step forward occurred when our engineers succeeded in constructing a luminescent screen on which moment-to-moment changes could be displayed. Thus, displacements in the pineal (accompanied, as Descartes had predicted, by ventricular currents) could be correlated with fluctuations in the state of the soul.

That must suffice for an account of the science of the matter. Now consider its economics. The instrument, destined to be patented as *PinealPet®*, can be guaranteed to increase the earning capacity of American psychiatrists handsomely, when they work in a fee-for-service system. Because its immediate imaging properties make it ideal for office use, psychiatrists rather than radiologists can bill for it, and thus attain economic parity with other technology-based disciplines. Because it will no longer be necessary to inquire of the patient about the state of his or her soul, a notoriously time-consuming, uncertain, and altogether messy procedure, time savings will be prodigious; productivity will increase; cost-effectiveness will please both supply side and free market economics. For myself, I intended to ask no profit (other than the Nobel Prize money).

Furthermore, the therapeutic potential of this technological advance will not have escaped notice. It should prove possible, in principle, by a kind of psychochiropractic, to correct the subluxations of the pineal which result in existential *angst*. By means of the piezoelectric effect, the therapist should be able to manipulate the pineal body with pulses of current under direct visual control to align it in such fashion as to produce harmony in the soul.

Yet, at the very point that the device was ready to be marketed, I was afflicted by an acute crisis of conscience, in all probability resulting from *mal de mer* of the pineal. I melted the instrument down; I shredded blueprints and protocols before they could be copied by sinister commercial interests. In the nick of time, I had realized the consequences of my thought experiment. Once at hand, PinealPet, like the endoscope, the stent, and the cardiac catheter before it, would have come to dominate clinical practice through its potential for increasing earnings *and* its capacity to generate nominally objective data. A technology invested with the authority of science is irresistible to patient and doctor alike in reifying disease.

How good was that prediction? Psychochiropractics, of course, have not quite arrived (though brain stimulation techniques are multiplying). There has been an enormous increase in technological capabilities for brain imaging. For an understanding of the brain-mind interface, that bodes only good. For practice, it carries the risk of premature application, as PinealPet did. What the thought experiment left out—until I at the very last moment "melted the instrument down and shredded the blueprints"—is *agency*; that is, the responsibility of physicians committed to patient care to resist and even roll back the tide of reductionism.

Until recently, financial subsidies from industry and uncontrolled access for pharmaceutical sales representatives have been "embedded" in departments of academic medicine much as journalists were with military units in the invasion of Iraq. The ubiquity of drug company–sponsored meals, lectures, and visits from PSRs during medical residency training represented a very considerable investment by the industry. Reflecting a conviction that this investment pays off, big Pharma has been spending two to three times as much on marketing and administration as it does on research and development (48, 49). However, in the past 10 years, leading teaching hospitals have ended "pizza lunches" for house staff and have limited the access of drug detail representatives to faculty and house staff. Academic psychiatry is beginning to assert the primacy of evidence-based medicine and alerting physicians to the risks of seduction by gifts and blandishments.

In a second major step forward, the American Board of Psychiatry and Neurology now requires that residents demonstrate familiarity with and competence in a set of evidence-based psychotherapies, in addition to competence in psychopharmacology. The impact of this requirement depends on progress in developing reliable measures of competence and making these measures a key to accreditation. Once again, it will be up to all of us to assure the achievement of that goal.

A third major deficit in academic psychiatry—the decades-long decline in the number of psychiatrist-investigators—is being addressed in a serious and credible way. In 2003, the Institute of Medicine issued a scholarly document *Research Training in Psychiatry Residency: Strategies for Reform* (50). Among its many excellent recommendations (51) was a proposal that a public–private consortium be created to carry the program forward. With support from NIMH and leading psychiatric societies, precisely such a consortium was created: the National Psychiatry Training Council. In 2005, it completed its work with a report, *Educating a New Generation of Psychiatrist Investigators* (52). Its recommendations include a call for the Residency Review Committee to give greater flexibility to program directors in designing the order of training (so that child and adolescent training within the first 2 years counts toward subspecialty training, for example) and to permit the creation of research tracks by shortening mandated requirements. No less important, it emphasizes that "research literacy" be made the goal for all residents. To reinforce that proposal, the ABPN examination must include questions to demonstrate literacy in assessing methodology and outcome of research protocols. It calls for a "national academy" of senior research mentors to be available on an ad hoc basis to all trainees.

These recommendations have been presented at a number of professional psychiatric meetings; several model child psychiatry research training fellowships have come into being, the most notable being the Albert J. Solnit Integrated Child and Adult Research Residency Pathway at the Yale Child Study Center (53). Once again, how far this effort to recruit a new generation of child psychiatry investigators will proceed will depend upon the support it receives from the old (faculty) as well as the young (students in training). Our fate is in ourselves, not in our stars.

THE FUTURE OF PATIENT CARE: ECONOMICS AND ETHICS

Nothing has shaken my conviction that the superiority of patient-centered, psychologically sensitive, integrative medicine will become ever more evident. Patients as well as physicians will serve as its advocates and assure its ascendancy. In his surrealistic short story, *A Country Doctor*, written early in the last century, Franz Kafka wrote: "To write prescriptions is easy; to come to an understanding with people is difficult." The first part of the aphorism no longer rings quite true; choosing the right prescription for the individual patient at the appropriate moment is a real challenge in an era when we have powerful medications (with powerful side effects) at our command. However, it remains true that coming to an understanding with people is even more difficult and demands more time than writing a script. Time is the essence of good medical care. It is time that is at threat.

I conclude with a passage from Plato's *The Laws*, written about 350 BC (54). An Athenian "Stranger" addresses Cleinias, a Cretan, and Megillus, a Spartan. The Athenian Stranger (in effect, Plato himself) has this to say about "slave" and "free" physicians in Greek society:

> Slaves . . . are almost always treated by other slaves who either rush about on flying visits or wait to be consulted in their surgeries. This kind of doctor never gives any account of the particular illness of the individual slave, or is prepared to listen to one; he simply prescribes what he thinks best in the light of experience, as if he had precise knowledge, and with the self-confidence of a dictator. Then he dashes off on his way to the next slave-patient, and so takes off his master's shoulders some of the work of attending the sick.
>
> The visits of the free doctor, by contrast, are mostly concerned with treating the illnesses of free men; *his* method is to construct an empirical case history by consulting the invalid and his friends; in this way he himself learns something from the sick and at the same time he gives the individual patient all the instruction he can. He gives no prescription until he has somehow gained the invalid's consent; then, coaxing him into continued cooperation, he tries to complete his restoration to health.
>
> The Stranger asks: "Which of the two methods do you think makes a doctor a better healer. . .?"

The reader of this textbook will have no difficulty in choosing the preferred option. In return for what that reader has learned, he and she have incurred an obligation: to fight to preserve that option. Commitment to assuring children access to the best professional care is the precondition for child psychiatry to flourish.

References

1. Brecht B (1943): *Life of Galileo*, trans. Willett J. In: Willett J, Manheim R (eds): *Bertolt Brecht: Plays, Poetry and Prose. The Collected Plays* vol. 5, p 1. Methuen, London, 1980.
2. Kanner L: *Child Psychiatry*. Springfield, IL, Charles C Thomas, 1935.
3. Kanner L: *Child Psychiatry*, 2nd ed. Springfield, IL, Charles C Thomas, 1948.
4. Kanner L: Autistic disturbances of affective contact. *Nervous Child* 2:217–250, 1943.
5. Rutter M: Foreword to *Childhood Psychosis* by Kanner L. Washington, DC, Winston and Sons, 1973, p. viii.
6. Down JLH: Observation on an ethnic classification of idiots. *London Hospital Clinical Lecture Reports* 3:259, 1866.
7. LeJeune J, Gauthier M, Turpin R: Les chromosomes humaines en culture de tissus. *Compte du Rendu Academy of Science* 248:602, 1958.
8. Jacobs PA, Baikie AG, Court Brown. WM, Strong JA: The somatic chromosomes in Mongolism. *The Lancet* 1:710–711, 1959.
9. Einfeld SL, Piccinin AM, Mackinnon A, et al.: Psychopathology in young people with intellectual disability. *Journal of the American Medical Association* 296:1981–1989, 2006.
10. Kanner L: Habeas corpus releases of feebleminded persons and their consequences. *American Journal of Psychiatry* 94:1013–1033, 1938.
11. Foster Kennedy R: The problem of social control of the congenital defective: Education, sterilization, euthanasia. *American Journal of Psychiatry* 99:13–16, 1942.
12. Kanner L: Exoneration of the feebleminded. *American Journal of Psychiatry* 99:17–22, 1942.
13. Editorial: Euthanasia. *Journal of Psychiatry* 99:141–143, 1942.
14. Goldfarb W: Effects of psychological privation in infancy and subsequent stimulation. *American Journal of Psychiatry* 102:18–33, 1945.
15. Spitz RA: Hospitalism: An inquiry into the genesis of psychiatric conditions in early childhood. *Psychoanalytic Study of the Child* 1:53–74, 1945.
16. Bowlby J: *Material Care and Mental Health*. Geneva, WHO Monograph Series, no. 2, 1951.
17. Bateson G, Jackson DD, Haley J, Weakland JH: Toward a theory of schizophrenia. *Behavioral Science* 1:251–264, 1956.
18. Eisenberg L: The fathers of autistic children. *American Journal of Orthopsychiatry* 27:715–714, 1957.
19. Wolff S, Narayan S, Moyes B: Personality characteristics of parents of autistic children: A controlled study *Journal of Child Psychology and Psychiatry* 29:143–154, 1988.
20. Kanner L, Eisenberg L: Follow-up studies in infantile autism. In: Hoch PH, Zubin J (eds): *Psychopathology of Childhood*, New York, Grune & Stratton, 1957, pp. 227–239.
21. Rutter M, Graham P: Psychiatric disorder in ten and eleven year old children. *Proceedings of the Royal Society of Medicine* 59:382–387, 1966.
22. Rutter M, Tizard EJ, Whitmore K: *Education Health and Behavior*. London: Longman, 1970.
23. Lotter V: Epidemiology of autistic conditions in young children: Part I. Prevalence. *Social Psychiatry* 1:124–137, 1966.
24. Folstein S, Rutter M: Infantile autism: A genetic study of 21 twin pairs. *Journal of Child Psychology and Psychiatry* 18:297–321, 1977.
25. Fisher S (Ed.): *Child Research in Psycho-Pharmacology*. Springfield IL: Charles C Thomas Publisher, 1959.
26. Cole J: Introduction. In: Conners CK (ed) In: *Clinical Use of Stimulant Drugs in Children: Proceedings of a symposium held at Key Biscayne, Florida*, March 5–8, 1972. New York, American Elsevier Publishing Co., Inc., pp. xi–xii, 1974,.
27. Lipman RS: NIMH—Pre-support of research in minimal brain dysfunction in children. In: Conners CK (ed) *In Clinical Use of Stimulant Drugs in Children: Proceedings of a symposium held at Key Biscayne, Florida*, March 5–8, 1972. New York: American Elsevier Publishing Co., Inc., pp. 202–206, 1974.
28. Cytryn L, Gilbert A, Eisenberg L: The effectiveness of tranquilizing drugs plus supportive psychotherapy in treating behavior disorders of children. *American Journal of Orthopsychiatry* 30:113–129, 1960.
29. Eisenberg L, Lachman R, Molling P, Lockner A, Mizelle J, Conners K: A psychopharmacologic study in a training school for delinquent boys. *American Journal Orthopsychiatry* 33:431–447, 1963.
30. Rutter M, Lebovici S, Eisenberg L, et al.: A triaxial classification of mental disorders in childhood. *Journal of Child Psychology and Psychiatry* 10:41–61, 1969.
31. Centers for Disease Control and Prevention: Prevalence of diagnosis and medication treatment for attention/deficit/hyperactivity disorder: United States 2003. *Morbidity and Mortality Weekly Reports* 54:842–847, 2005.
32. Rapoport JL, Buchsbaum MS, Zahn TP, et al.: Dextroamphetamine: Cognitive and behavioral effects in normal prepubertal boys. *Science* 199:560–563, 1978.
33. Doll R: Development of controlled trials in preventive and therapeutic medicine. *Journal of BioSocial Science* 23:365–378, 1991.
34. Medical Research Council: Streptomycin treatment of tuberculous meningitis. *Lancet* 1:582–596, 1948.
35. Pressman JD: *Last Resort: Psychosurgery and the Limits of Medicine*. New York, Cambridge University Press, 1998.

36. Eisenberg L: Child psychiatry: The past quarter century. *American Journal of Orthopsychiatry* 39:389–401, 1969.
37. Barton WE, Malamud W (eds): *Training the Psychiatrist to Meet Changing Needs* Washington, DC: American Psychiatric Association; p.8 1963.
38. Eisenberg L: If not now, when? *American Journal of Orthopsychiatry* 32:781–793, 1962a.
39. Rosenfeld AH (ed): *Psychiatric Education: Prologue to the 1980s.* Washington, DC, American Psychiatric Association 1976.
40. Eisenberg L: Discussion. In: Hoch PH, Zubin J (eds): *The Future of Psychiatry*, New York, Grune & Stratton, 1962b pp. 251–255.
41. Eisenberg L: Whatever happened to the faculty on the way to the Agora? *Archives of Internal Medicine* 159:2251–2256, 1999.
42. Eisenberg L: The "ecology" of psychiatry and neurology. In: Hagar M. (ed) *The Convergence of Neuroscience, Behavioral Science, Neurology, and Psychiatry*. New York; Josiah Macy Jr. Foundation, 2005.
43. Kazdin AE: Developing a research agenda for child and adolescent psychotherapy. *Archives of General Psychiatry* 57:829–835, 2000.
44. Eisenberg L: Mindlessness and brainlessness in psychiatry. *British Journal of Psychiatry* 148:497–508, 1986.
45. Pellmar T, Eisenberg L (eds): *Bridging Disciplines in the Brain, Behavioral and Clinical Sciences*. Washington, DC: National Academy Press, 2000.
46. Lewis A: Ebb and flow in social psychiatry. *Yale Journal of Biology and Medicine* 35:62–83, 1962.
47. Descartes R: The passion of the soul. In *Philosophical Works (vol. I)*, trans. Haldane ES and Ross GRT, New York: Dover, 1649.
48. Angell M: *The Truth About the Drug Companies: How They Deceive Us and What to Do About It*. New York: Random House, 2004.
49. Avorn J: *Powerful Medicines: The Benefits, Risks, and Costs of Prescription Drugs*. Knopf, 2004.
50. Abrams MT, Patchan KM, Boat TF: *Research Training in Psychiatry Residency: Strategies for Reform*. Washington, DC: National Academies Press, 2003.
51. Eisenberg L: Review of Abrams MT, Patchan KM, Boat TF: *Research Training in Psychiatric Residency: Strategies for Reform*. Washington, DC: National Academies Press. *American Journal of Psychiatry* 161:1930–1931, 2004.
52. *National Psychiatry Training Council: Educating a New Generation of Psychiatrist Investigators*, (unpublished manuscript), Washington, DC, 2005.
53. Martin A, Block M, Pruett K, et al.: From too little too late to early and often: Child psychiatry education during medical school (and before and after). *Child & Adolescent Psychiatric Clinics of North America*, doi:10.1016/j.chc.2006.07.005.
54. *Plato (350 BC) The Laws*. Trans Saunders TJ, London, Penguin Classics, 1970, pp. 181–182.

INDEX